CLINICAL NATUROPATHIC MEDICINE

SECOND EDITION

Leah Hechtman

PhD (Cand), MSciMed (RHHG), BHSc, ND

Director, The Natural Health and Fertility Centre
Natural Health and Fertility Pty Ltd

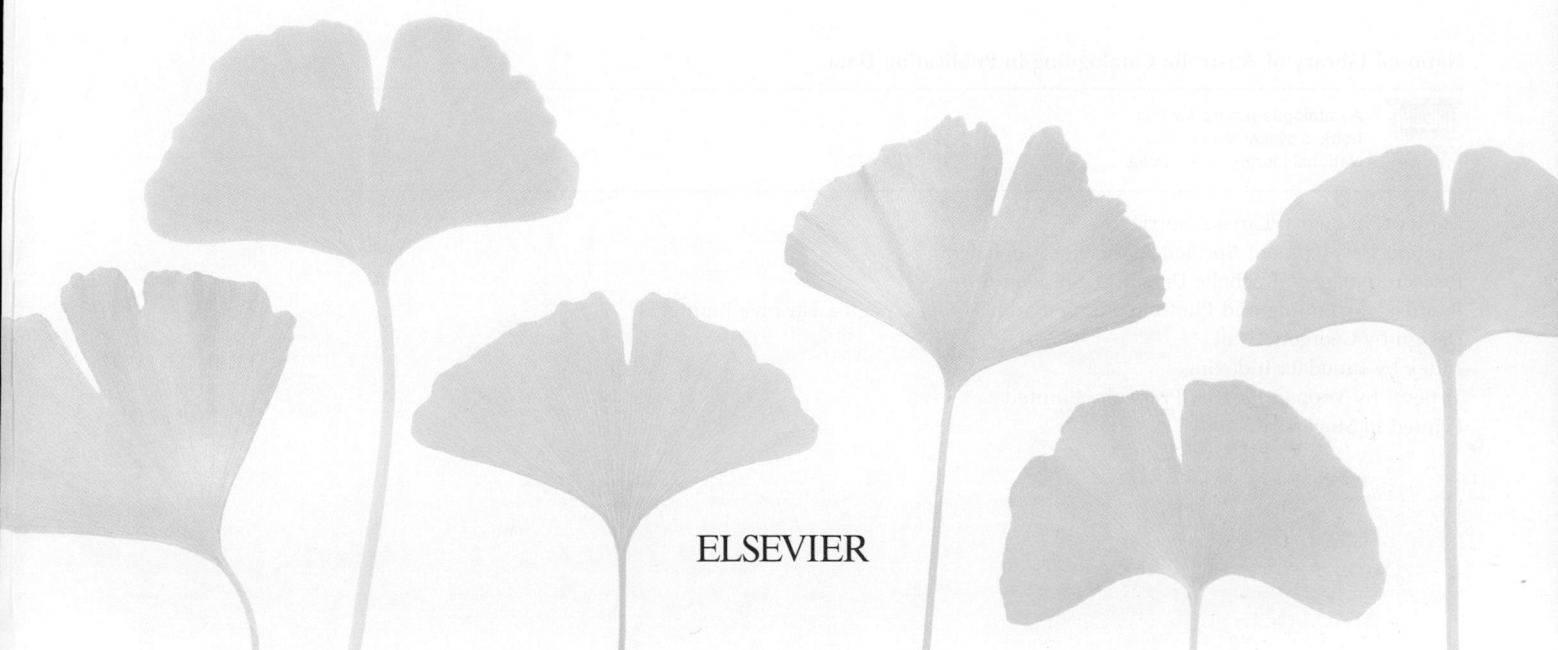

ELSEVIER

ELSEVIER

Elsevier Australia. ACN 001 002 357
(a division of Reed International Books Australia Pty Ltd)
Tower 1, 475 Victoria Avenue, Chatswood, NSW 2067

1st edition 2012; Reprinted 2014 (twice), 2016, 2021, 2022

ISBN: 978-0-7295-4242-5

National Library of Australia Cataloguing-in-Publication Data

NATIONAL LIBRARY OF AUSTRALIA

A catalogue record for this book is available from the National Library of Australia

Content Strategist: Larissa Norrie
Content Development Specialist: Vanessa Ridehalgh
Project Managers: Rochelle Deighton, Shravan Kumar
Permissions Editing and Photo Research: Sarah Thomas, Regina Lavanya Remigius
Design by Georgette Hall
Index by Innodata Indexing
Typeset by Toppan Best-set Premedia Limited
Printed in Singapore

CLINICAL NATUROPATHIC MEDICINE

Foreword

One of the greatest problems limiting the reemergence of naturopathic medicine has been the lack of modern textbooks, especially those based on science. When I was a student back in the early 1970s, the most current textbook in the US had been published the year I was born!

For almost a century, the mantra of conventional medicine and its apologists had been that naturopathic medicine is not only not scientific but misguided, giving patients 'false hope' at best and delaying needed medical intervention at worst. I still remember a debate I had with an MD while I was working as a research associate at a medical school before I decided to enter naturopathic school. I had become a vegetarian and noticed many changes in my body and health. I asked one of my fellow researchers what these changes meant and was told, 'These are errors in your observations; diet does not affect you'! This may sound unbelievable today, but remember this was the doctrine of conventional medicine until recently. The problem for me in the debate, however, was that as a pre-professional I was not aware of research to refute him, only my personal experience. Shortly thereafter, I learned from the woman who married my roommate from college that her juvenile rheumatoid arthritis had been cured. This was quite a surprise to me as I was happily working with MDs and PhDs to find a cure for this incurable disease. When I asked how this happened, her response was that she had seen a naturopathic doctor. 'What is that?' I wondered. I had the opportunity to meet him and ask what he did for my friend. His answer: 'I taught her how to eat properly and detoxified her liver.' This was quite intriguing and a totally different way of thinking about health and disease. I then asked the ND the same question I had asked the MD. He took Guyton's *Medical Physiology* — then a standard textbook for medical schools — off his bookshelf and showed me what was happening to my body as I changed my diet. I was very impressed that the naturopath knew physiology better than the MDs/PhDs I was working with in medical research. I then asked him if I could spend a few days with him watching him see patients. After seeing 'incurable' after 'incurable' patient get better with his expert care, I was convinced that there was something special here. Clearly diet and natural therapies — though discounted by conventional medicine — were indeed effective. But when I asked him for research supporting his therapies or modern books on naturopathic medicine to read, he had nothing to offer.

Happily, this problem is now being substantively addressed.

The first modern textbook of naturopathic medicine was co-authored in 1985 by Michael Murray, ND and me, the *Textbook of Natural Medicine* — breaking an almost four-decade hiatus. Now in its 5th edition, the *Textbook*'s major contribution was beginning the documentation of the research support for natural medicine. The 2200-page text cites over 12 000 references to the peer-reviewed scientific literature documenting the efficacy of natural therapies. Another important contribution was that we brought together for the first time multiple naturopaths as the experts for a scholarly publication. And finally, we developed and documented protocols for the use of natural therapies to promote health, prevent disease and even reverse a wide range of diseases. Unfortunately, it had for far too long been the lone standard for the profession. Finally, this changed with the emergence of Hechtman's excellent *Clinical Naturopathic Medicine*. The first edition provided great detailed guidance on how to practise natural medicine. This second edition provides a welcome update and advancement in depth and breadth.

The major contribution of *Clinical Naturopathic Medicine* that differentiates it from *Textbook of Natural Medicine* is that it is unabashedly focused entirely on the practice of naturopathic medicine. Hechtman and her colleagues expertly look at the historic origins of naturopathic concepts and therapies then integrate these with scientific research to provide a strong foundation for modern clinical naturopathy. While there is plenty of science, I especially appreciate how the authors carefully considered traditional naturopathic approaches and therapies in the context of modern science to provide students and practitioners with guidance on how to think about and treat patients. This is a key strength of *Clinical Naturopathic Medicine*: practical guidance and how to think about patients.

As appropriate, almost every chapter covers not only what to do, but also how to do it and how to optimise for the uniqueness of each patient. Nutrient dosages, herbal combinations, potential adverse interactions with conventional drugs, laboratory tests and clinical criteria identifying patient characteristics that require modification of the intervention, etc. are all covered. Truly, a remarkable compilation of how to practise naturopathic medicine conscientiously, effectively and safely.

Another very interesting aspect of *Clinical Naturopathic Medicine* is that it is systems, rather than disease, oriented. This means that most of the content is oriented towards physiological systems and what goes wrong rather than the disease the person has and how to treat it. While there is plenty of guidance on how to treat diseases, there is far more attention to understanding the function of the system, why it goes wrong and what to do about it.

Included also is some very sophisticated guidance on understanding the adverse effects of the drugs used by conventional medicine for each disease and how to mitigate their effects without impairing their efficacy. This later guidance is extremely important as few realise the prevalence of adverse drug reactions. Research has shown that 25% of patients suffer an adverse event as a result of medical care.[1] Worse, in the US adverse reactions to **properly prescribed** drugs is the fourth leading cause of death.[2] And for the elderly (over age 60!), the numbers are alarming: one in ten hospital admissions are due to adverse drug reactions.[3] Fortunately, many of these adverse events can be prevented by the expert use of natural therapies — as fully described in *Clinical Naturopathic Medicine*. We clearly need conventional medicine: it has many almost miraculous successes which benefit all. However, it is an incomplete system and is very well balanced by naturopathic medicine. We need to stop using the term 'alternative' and instead focus on 'collaborative' medicine. For the benefit of our patients, we need to integrate the best of natural and conventional medicine.

I am extremely impressed with this work and wish it had been available when I was a student. Conscientious clinicians will use the great resource every day. Congratulations Leah Hechtman, ND and her skilled colleagues. This outstanding textbook will have a profound impact on improving the clinical quality and efficacy of our profession.

Joseph Pizzorno ND
Editor-in-Chief, *Integrative Medicine, a Clinician's Journal*
Founder, Bastyr University
Commissioner, U.S. White House Commission on Complementary and Alternative Medicine Policy
Licensed naturopathic physician with prescriptive rights, State of Washington since 1975

[1] Gandhi TK, Weingart SN, Borus J, et al. Adverse drug events in ambulatory care. New Engl J Med 2003;348:1556–64.
[2] Lazaraou J, Pomeranz BH, Corey PN. Incidence of drug reactions in hospitalized patients: a meta-analysis of prospective studies. JAMA 1998;279:1200–5.
[3] Oscanoa TJ, Lizaraso F, Carvajal A. Hospital admissions due to adverse drug reactions in the elderly. A meta-analysis. Eur J Clin Pharmacol 2017;73(6):759–70.

Contents

CHAPTER APPENDICES

Preface

As we release the second edition of this text, it is a perfect opportunity to reflect on the growth and change in naturopathy since the first edition.

The practice of naturopathy worldwide has continued to achieve greater recognition and acceptance in the wider medical communities. Improved research pathways, educational opportunities and greater evidence for our practice mean the profession continues to evolve positively. This in turn ensures that people are receiving the help they need. As naturopaths, we continue to strive for more, to push the limits, to stretch the boundaries. We continue to help people in need with a form of medicine that supports the body's innate ability to heal itself.

The intention to help others is undoubtedly the primary driver in our profession as evidenced by our standards of patient care. Naturopathic clinicians strive to find the cause of a patient's complaint. We seek to empower people through education and we choose to support them in their health concerns with the gentlest, yet most effective treatments available. We know what we do works. We are simply supporting the development of our time-tested treatments with research and modern medical practices.

We need to continue to take on more responsibility for the welfare of our patients as we strive for healthcare excellence. We need to validate and translate our practice into the language of modern medicine to enable greater access to more individuals who dearly need our care.

We need to share our knowledge and historical wisdom; formulate and share our strategies and work together to push forward. If we truly want to be at the table of modern healthcare, we cannot hide away and shield our methods. As naturopaths, we offer a unique perspective of healthcare and provide significant support and relief for patients. Our treatments encourage self-responsibility and involvement in the healing process.

The structure of this text was crucial to the design of the project. It was important that the content is easily accessible, logical and articulate. The textbook has been divided into three parts: Part 1 — Principles of naturopathic medicine — providing an overview to our main treatment approaches; Part 2 — Naturopathic treatments — giving a specific overview of the two main treatments, nutrition and herbal medicine; and Part 3 — Body systems — detailing each system of the body and relevant major conditions. There are also appendices relevant for the student and the clinician, both in the book and online at Expert Consult. This text is accompanied by a second volume of advanced principles, topics and conditions.

Each component of this book has been arranged in a systematic manner: each chapter pertains to a specific system of the body or unique topic; and each condition is organised according to pedagogy that ensures the content is comprehensively and systematically covered. Within each condition, the reader can view the content in overview for quick access or as a detailed discussion that may provoke critical thought, reflection and consideration. The traditional approach to the topic has been incorporated and integrated into the carefully researched content that follows. Each reference was included not solely because it supported a statement, but because it ensured that the content delivered was sound and accurate. At the conclusion of each condition, the reader is provided with a comprehensive case study. This ensures that each contributor's unique clinical perspective enriches the content and translates the theory into realistic clinical practice.

At the heart of naturopathy, we must lean on our elders whose traditional system demonstrated that the essence of our treatment relies on the relationship between the patient and the clinician. Evidence-based medicine forms a component of our system of knowledge. It provides us with a lens to explain the efficacy of our treatment but can never replace the healing relationship. The relationship between clinician and patient continues to be the greatest teacher for growth and understanding and ultimately the platform for change and healing.

Leah Hechtman
July 2018

About the author

Leah Hechtman is an experienced and respected clinician who specialises in fertility, pregnancy and reproductive health for men and women. She is the Director of The Natural Health and Fertility Centre in Sydney, Australia.

She has completed extensive advanced training and is a university lecturer, keynote speaker, author, contributor to various professional texts and journals, and educator to her peers.

Leah is currently completing her PhD through the University of New South Wales, Faculty of Medicine, School of Women's and Children's Health, Sydney, Australia.

She holds memberships and fellowship status with numerous groups and organisations in naturopathy and the wider medical and fertility communities.

Leah leads by example, remembering to live life to the fullest and believes that ill health is merely a stepping stone to help you reclaim your true state of being.

Acknowledgments

As we conclude working on the second edition, I reflect on the journey myself and my co-contributors have taken. We have had our share of loss, birth, personal challenge and prosperity. Sadly, two of the contributors from the first edition have passed away — Dr Tini Gruner and David Kirk. Two individuals whose passion for our profession was clearly evident. Their contributions remain in the text and have been respectfully updated. They both contributed to our profession significantly and are greatly missed.

It has been an honour and a privilege to work again with some of the first edition's contributors and to meet and work with some wonderful new individuals. I am deeply humbled and inspired by what has been possible and what we have collectively achieved. A book of this magnitude is near impossible without the support, dedication and commitment of everyone involved in the project.

In the order of their contribution, my appreciation to Dr Kate Broderick, Dr Sue Evans, Rachel Arthur, Annalies Corse, Michael Colenso, Liesl Blott, Gabrielle Covino, Lisa Costa Bir, Justin Sinclair, Jane Frawley, Emily Bradley, Susan Hunter, Dr Ses Salmond, Dr Janet Schloss, Kathy Harris, Dr Karen Bridgman, Annmarie Cannone, Dr Bradley McEwen, Dr Matthew Leach, Teresa Mitchell-Paterson, Daniel Robson, Ian Breakspear, Cheryl le Roux, Dr Erica McIntyre and Dr Kate Worsfold.

A special note of gratitude goes to Liesl Blott for her contribution of both Chapter 6 and each of the interaction tables within each system. Additionally, much gratitude to Lisa Costa Bir for Chapter 8 and her expertise provided for the dietary plans within each condition.

I have learnt much from working with you all. Your dedication to the project and commitment to sharing your knowledge and improving the education standards of our profession have been inspiring. Additionally, my deepest gratitude to Dr Joseph Pizzorno. Joe, it is again a privilege to include your foreword and have you involved once more.

My sincere appreciation goes to the team at Elsevier. The second edition certainly took longer than anyone planned. As we ploughed through the project the integrity of those involved was highly evident and I am most appreciative of their respective kindness, commitment and dedication to producing the best possible text. Much gratitude to Larissa Norrie, Vanessa Ridehalgh, Rochelle Deighton and others.

Thank you to Cheryl le Roux for your dedication and commitment to the project as my research assistant. You provided much support to get through what was needed and your skill and knowledge are highly evident. I know I will see much success for you in the future.

To my colleagues at UNSW — my supervisors, study collaborators and clinicians, and fellow researchers — you have provided me with growth, opportunity and challenge. You have helped me to expand and develop as a researcher and this has supported me to develop in ways I am truly grateful for.

To my fellow clinicians and colleagues, past lecturers, teachers and mentors — you each hold a place in my development, have provided me with inspiration and guidance and have helped me become the person and clinician that I am today. Thank you.

To all herbalists and naturopaths — both past and present — we share this journey together. The more we collaborate and support each other, the more we can achieve collectively and contribute to the greater good for all.

Special thanks to my family and friends. Your love, patience and understanding have given me much support to achieve and contribute to the betterment of others.

Finally, my gratitude to each patient I have ever worked with or will work with. It is the unanswerable and the mysterious that propels me as I yearn to understand and discover the answers. Each patient is my greatest teacher. Each story, each journey, each experience my master class. Each person reminds me to respect the innate healing ability of the body, the wisdom and gifts from nature, and the tenderness and humility of the human spirit.

Contributors

Rachel Arthur
BHSc, BNat(Hons), NA

Liesl Blott
PGradDip(MM), BPharm, BHSc(Herbal Med), AdvDip(Nat), Cert IV Assessment & Workplace Training
Adjunct Senior Lecturer, School of Pharmacy and Biomedical Sciences, Curtin University, Perth, Western Australia, Australia

Emily Bradley
MNutrMed, BHlthSc(Nat)
Lecturer and Clinic Supervisor, Laureate International Universities (Southern School of Natural Therapies) and Endeavour College of Natural Health, Melbourne, Victoria, Australia
Naturopath, Private Practitioner, St Kilda, Victoria, Australia

Ian Breakspear
MHerbMed, ND, DBM, CertPhyto
Fellow, Naturopaths and Herbalists Association of Australia
Member, Boundary Bend Olives Expert Scientific Steering Committee, Australia
Senior Lecturer, Endeavour College of Natural Health, Sydney, New South Wales, Australia
Private Practitioner, King Street Clinic, Sydney, New South Wales, Australia

Karen Bridgman
PhD, MSc(Hons), MAppSci, MEd(Higher Ed)
Director, Starflower Pty Ltd and Starflower Herbals, Warriewood, New South Wales, Australia
Clinical Practice, Fayworth Health Centre at Australian Biologics Testing Services, Sydney, New South Wales, Australia

Kate Broderick
BSc, JD, DNM, DipAcu
Lecturer, Naturopathic Medicine, Endeavour College of Natural Health, Adelaide, South Australia, Australia
Anam Chara Natural Health, Adelaide, South Australia, Australia

Annmarie Cannone
MHumNut, GradDip(Nat), BAppSci(Nat Stud)
Contract Academic, Endeavour College of Natural Health, Sydney, New South Wales, Australia
Clinical Nutritionist/Naturopath, Owner at Empowered Health and Wellbeing, Mortlake, New South Wales, Australia

Michael Colenso
GCert eLearning, AdvDipHltSc(Nat), DipHltSc (HM)
Examiner, Naturopaths and Herbalists Association of Australia
Director, All Good Medicine, Brisbane, Queensland, Australia

Annalies Corse
BMedSc, BHSc
Senior Lecturer, Health and Medical Sciences, Laureate Universities, Sydney, New South Wales, Australia
Naturopathic Practitioner, Private Clinical Practice, Sydney, New South Wales, Australia
Academic Writer, Postgrad Lecturer, Presenter, Medical and Health Sciences, New South Wales, Australia

Lisa Costa Bir
BAppSc(Nat), GradDip(Nat), MWomens Health (currently completing), MATMS
Lecturer and Supervisor, Nutrition and Naturopathy, Endeavour College of Natural Health, Sydney, New South Wales, Australia

Gabrielle Covino
BHealthSc (Naturopathy), MHumNutr
Lecturer and Clinical Supervisor, Southern School of Natural Therapies (Think Education), Victoria, Australia
Committee Member (Melbourne Branch), Nutrition Society of Australia
Private Practitioner, Melbourne, Victoria, Australia

Sue Evans
PhD
Senior Lecturer in Complementary Medicines, School of Medicine, University of Tasmania, Tasmania, Australia

Jane Frawley
PhD
Lecturer Public Health, Faculty of Health, University of Technology Sydney, Sydney, New South Wales, Australia

Kathy Harris
MHSc, BEd, ND, FNHAA, MATMS
Lecturer, Endeavour College of Natural Health, Sydney, New South Wales, Australia
Private Practitioner, Wholistic Medical Centre, Surry Hills, New South Wales, Australia

Susan Hunter
BA, BHSc, ND
Director, Healthful Clinic
Private Practitioner, Melbourne, Victoria, Australia

Matthew J. Leach
BN(Hons), ND, DipClinNutr, PhD
Senior Research Fellow, Department of Rural Health, University of South Australia, Adelaide, South Australia, Australia

Cheryl le Roux
BHSc(NutMed), BSc
Writer, Researcher, Nutritional Medicine, Clear Nutrition, Sydney, New South Wales, Australia

Bradley McEwen
PhD, MHSc (HumNutr), BHSc, ND(Adv), DBM, DNutr, DSM
Practitioner, Educator, Researcher, National Centre for Naturopathic Medicine
Practitioner and Student Mentor, Optimum Mentoring

Erica McIntyre
BHSc, BSocSc(Psych)(Hons), PhD (Psych)
Postdoctoral Research Fellow, Australian Research Centre in Complementary and Integrative Medicine (ARCCIM), Faculty of Health, University of Technology Sydney, Sydney, New South Wales, Australia

Teresa Mitchell-Paterson
Adv Dip(Nat), BHSc(CompMed), MHSc(HumNut)
Senior Lecturer, Nutritional Medicine, Torrens University, Sydney, New South Wales, Australia

Daniel Robson
BNat
Private Practitioner, Goulds Natural Medicine, Hobart, Tasmania, Australia

Ses Salmond
PhD, BA, ND, DBM, DHOM, DRM, DNUT
Naturopath, Clinical Services, Leichhardt Women's Community Health Centre, Sydney, New South Wales, Australia
Naturopath, Clinical Services, Liverpool Women's Health Centre, Sydney, New South Wales, Australia
Director, Arkana Therapy Centre, Sydney, New South Wales, Australia

Janet Schloss
PhD, PostGradCert(Nut), AdvDipHS, BARM, DipNut, DipHM
Clinical Trial Coordinator, Office of Research, Endeavour College of Natural Health, Fortitude Valley, Queensland, Australia

Justin Sinclair
MHerbMed, BHSc(Nat)
Research Fellow, NICM Health Research Institute, Western Sydney University, New South Wales, Australia
Principal Consultant, Traditional Medicine Consultancy, Miranda, New South Wales, Australia
Contract Academic, Naturopathic and Bioscience Departments, Endeavour College of Natural Health, Sydney, New South Wales, Australia

Kate Worsfold
MClinPsych, BPsych(Hons), PostGradDip(Nut), AdvDip(NutMed)
Director, Compass Health Group
Private Practitioner, Gold Coast, Queensland, Australia

Reviewers

Madelaine Bishop
Adv Dip(Nat), BHlthSc (Comp Med), GradCert (ClinEd Teaching), Cert IV TAE
Practitioner, Lecturer in Nutritional Medicine and Clinical Supervisor, Paramount College of Natural Medicine, Perth, Western Australia, Australia

Robyn Carruthers
MHSc, BEd, AdvDipHerbMed, AdvDipNat
Deputy Director: Clinical & Research, South Pacific College of Natural Medicine, Auckland, New Zealand

Ruth Fellowes
MPH, BHSc, AdvDipNutrMed, AdvDipWHM, DipNutr
Practitioner, Educator, WEA Newcastle Academy of Complementary Health, Newcastle, New South Wales, Australia

Jeffery Flatt
ND (CCNM), BNatTher (SCU), PhD (candidate)
Discipline Lead for Complementary Health, Lecturer in Complementary Health, School of Health, University of New England, Armidale, New South Wales, Australia

Nicole Quaife
BHSc, MHealthProm
Naturopath, Education and Training, Australasian College of Nutrition and Environmental Medicine (ACNEM), Melbourne, Victoria, Australia

PART 1

Principles of naturopathic medicine

1

Naturopathic philosophy

Kate Broderick

INTRODUCTION

Naturopathic medicine is categorised as a 'whole medical system'. Whole medical systems are 'complete systems of theory and practice that have evolved independently over time in different cultures and apart from conventional medicine or Western medicine.'[1] Perhaps the greatest part of this categorisation is attributable to the comprehensive and seamless philosophical basis of naturopathic medicine and the closely aligned clinical theory and practice that flow from that philosophy. The foundation of naturopathic philosophy and clinical theory as the basis of practice can be compared to that of Eastern whole medical systems such as traditional Chinese medicine or Ayurveda, as well as to other Western whole medical systems such as homeopathy, though certainly naturopathic medicine is the youngest of these systems.

The evolution of naturopathic medicine since its establishment as a profession just over 100 years ago has run parallel in time to the evolution of modern conventional medicine, and this has resulted in influences that have shaped and galvanised both the naturopathic professional body and the practice of naturopathic medicine. It has been more heavily influenced by modern technological medical advances than by the older whole medical systems, while it has also been challenged to define its philosophy and clinical theory clearly and comprehensively in order to strengthen its identity and its approach to disease and healing.

Origins of naturopathic medicine

The history of naturopathic medicine can be traced back to ancient roots in Greco-Roman medicine, but a full exposition of the ancient period is beyond the scope of this text. This chapter will limit itself to a concise overview of the more immediate history of the profession, from the mid-1800s hydrotherapy and nature cure movements in Europe to the first two decades of professional formation in 20th century America. This will provide a basis for understanding the roots of modern naturopathic philosophy and clinical theory.

EUROPEAN HYDROTHERAPY AND NATURE CURE

While there are a number of key players in the development of the European hydrotherapy and nature cure movements, the two most influential figures were Vincenz Priessnitz (1799–1851) and Father Sebastian Kneipp (1821–97). Their pioneering work in hydrotherapy was the subject of provincial rivalry and unrelenting professional jealousy from the medical community yet it laid the foundation for the development of a new system of medicine following on their traditions.

Born into a peasant family in Austrian Silesia, Priessnitz received no official medical training. He began treating injuries from local farmyard accidents with cold-water applications, wet bandages and compresses. From these early beginnings Priessnitz experienced overwhelming clinical success as he developed his art of water cure, with Chopin and Napoleon III among those who sought his clinical expertise.[2] His fame soon spread far beyond the confines of Austria and patients from Britain, France, Italy, Turkey, America and Germany soon sought his guidance.[3]

Like Priessnitz, Father Kneipp came from humble beginnings in Bavaria, Germany. Too poor to afford medical help, he cured himself of tuberculosis with cold-water therapy; nightly dips in the icy waters of the Danube were the key to his success.[2] After attending a seminary and becoming a priest, he began to successfully treat the people of his parish using his water cure and herbal medicines. Word of his successful water cure spread, and one of his patients, Benedict Lust, would go on to take Kneipp's water cure across the Atlantic to America, providing the foundation for the creation of a new system of medicine.[2,4] But the formation of this new system would draw from other roots already in America.

THOMSONIANISM, PHYSIOMEDICALISM AND THE ECLECTICS

Samuel Thomson (1769–1843) developed a method of healing that was predominantly based on the use of Native American herbal remedies and sweat baths. His approach was labelled heroic but was considered less harmful than the orthodox medicines being used at the time, which included the use of bleeding, mercury and arsenic. Thomson's simple healing system was based on the concepts of heat and cold; heat was considered life supporting and cold was considered life threatening. Substances that stimulated heat in the body, such as diaphoretics, were considered therapeutic, while substances that introduced cold into the body, such as mercury, aconite and opium, were avoided.[5]

Thomson had a strong belief in an individual's ability and right to self-treat and firmly believed that the practice of healing should remain with lay people. Underpinning his adamant belief that his system of healing should only be practised by householders was his strong aversion to medical education. He sold franchises to his healing method, which he called 'friendly botanic societies', until the time of his death in 1843.[6]

The physiomedicalist movement was initiated by one of Thomson's assistants in reaction to Thomson's rejection of educational progression. In 1835, Thomson enlisted the support of Alva Curtis, a young and popular practitioner from Ohio who claimed to have lost only one out of 200 patients. Curtis used the position bestowed upon him by Thomson to gather support for his own system of healing and led a breakaway movement in 1838 with the establishment of his *Independent Thomsonian Botanic Society*.[7] In contrast to Thomson's aversion to furthering medical knowledge, Curtis established medical schools to teach and develop his system of healing, which was largely based on the use of herbal medicine.

The physiomedicalist movement also initiated the use of an energetic diagnostic system. Patients in deficient states were regarded as 'asthenic', and those in excess states were regarded as 'sthenic'. Diagnostic procedures such as tongue analysis and pulse diagnosis were also employed so that the most appropriate herbal remedies could be selected.

After initial work by Curtis and Cook, the physiomedicalist movement was further refined by Thurston in 1900 as a:

> *... medical philosophy founded on the Theorem of a vital force or energy, inherent in living matter of tissue-units, whose aggregate expression in health and disease is the functional activities of the organism and whose inherent tendency is integrative and constructive; resistive, eliminative, and reconstructive to inimical invasion, or disease-causations.*[8]

The detailed and comprehensive work of Thurston provided the physiomedicalist movement with a philosophical basis. In his 400-page document, Thurston provided a rational outline of the failure of 'regular' medicine and went on to set out the theorems of physiomedicalism, the principles of the physiomedicalist movement, and a comprehensive manifesto on medical education, medical terminology, body systems, pathology, disease states, symptoms, diagnosis, food, immunity and the role of the physician.

Wooster Beach (1794–1868) established the 'reformed botanic movement', which drew on the professionalism of medicine and the heritage of indigenous herbal medicine and European and American healing traditions.[9] As the numbers of practitioners and the popularity of this new movement increased, Beach's influence diminished, and the practice of this system of healing came to be known as the 'Eclectic' movement, with Beach widely considered to be the founder of Eclectic medicine.[10] This movement allowed practitioners to incorporate treatment modalities of other healing systems into their repertoire. Free to experiment with a range of healing modalities, the numbers of Eclectic practitioners soared. At its peak, Eclecticism claimed over 20000 practitioners in the United States; these numbers presented serious competition for the practice of orthodox medicine.[11]

Formation of a profession

Naturopathy was formalised as a system of medicine in the United States under the stewardship of Benedict Lust in the early 20th century. As mentioned, Lust was a disciple of Father Kneipp and he formally introduced the practice of Kneipp's hydrotherapy to the United States, opening the Kneipp Water Cure Institute in New York in 1896 at the age of 27.[12] Lust is considered to be the father of naturopathy. Trained in osteopathy and chiropractic, he opened the first health food shop in America and founded massage and chiropractic schools in New York. He also obtained degrees in homeopathy and in Eclectic medicine in 1913 and 1914.[13] Lust purchased the rights to the term 'naturopathy' from Dr John Scheel in 1902.[14,15]

The formation of naturopathy as a profession and a system of medicine was based on European and American nature cure and similar systems described earlier in this section. Lust's overarching perspective was that if something was natural and it worked, then it could be considered part of naturopathy. Lust was a tireless and avid advocate of naturopathy, speaking and writing prolifically to both medical audiences and the lay public. His dedication and that of other early pioneers of naturopathy, as well as the popularity of naturopathy as compared to the orthodox medicine of the early 20th century, resulted in a rapid rise in the profession for the next 40 years.

Perhaps the most comprehensive and well-known text demonstrating the early philosophical foundations of naturopathy is *Nature Cure*, by Dr Henry Lindlahr, first published in 1913.[16] Lindlahr was also a former patient and disciple of Father Kneipp, and was a major figure in the early American naturopathic landscape. *Nature Cure* perhaps went beyond any other contemporary writings to set out a cohesive and comprehensive philosophy and theory for naturopathy, though Lindlahr did not use that term, and this work is still used as a seminal text in the study of modern naturopathic philosophy and clinical theory.

But, despite the prolific writing of these early naturopathic pioneers, the profession went forward for more than half a century without any clear and concise statement of professional identity and without a philosophical or theoretical approach to practice that was documented and widely agreed to by the members of the profession. Political and cultural forces, as well as advancements in conventional medicine, negatively affected the ability of the profession to remain cohesive and the profession in America became almost non-existent by mid-century. A resurgence in the profession that can be correlated to the rise of the counter-culture in the late 1960s and the 1970s, and the political and legal battles that ensued from that resurgence, provided a galvanising force for organising and regulating the profession. From that came the coalescing of the body of modern naturopathic philosophy and clinical theory that is the subject of the remainder of this chapter.

DEFINING NATUROPATHIC MEDICINE

> *Naturopathic medicine is a distinct method of primary health care — an art, science, philosophy and practice of diagnosis, treatment, and prevention of illness. Naturopath[s] seek to restore and maintain optimum health in their patients by emphasizing nature's inherent self-healing process, the vis medicatrix naturae. This is accomplished through education and the rational use of natural therapeutics.*[17]

The development of naturopathic medicine in America and the political forces it has defended itself against have resulted in America leading the charge to define the profession and its philosophies and clinical approach, with the above definition being a core part of early efforts. However, the philosophy and clinical theory of naturopathic medicine have migrated worldwide with the profession itself and have been adapted to align with different regulatory, educational, political and economic structures wherever it is practised. The philosophy and clinical theory presented in this chapter represent an adaptation that is suitable to the Australian landscape.

An Australian definition of naturopathy was developed in 2000 by the Naturopathy and Nutrition Forum, a working group of naturopathic practitioners and educators at a retreat coordinated by Southern Cross University. This definition, as follows, was subsequently adopted within the Naturopathy National Training Package of 2002:[18]

> *Naturopathy is a distinct method of healing, underpinned by a philosophical perspective which recognises that all living forms possess a self-regulatory, inherent ability for self-healing. This inherent ability, or Vital Force, operates in an intelligent, orderly fashion. Naturopathic approaches to health care are aimed at supporting and enhancing the body's own ability to heal itself.*
>
> *Expressions of health and disease are considered reflections of the dynamic interchange between the physical, mental, social, environmental and spiritual landscape of the individual.*
>
> *Naturopathy is both an art and a science, drawing upon several lines of evidence, which range from qualitative, quantitative, cultural and traditional.*
>
> *Naturopathic practice integrates a number of modalities, principally nutrition, herbal medicine and tactile therapy. These modalities are applied on the basis of specific principles, and within the context of a healing environment which endeavours to empower the individual, motivate and educate them in order to restore, maintain and optimise wellbeing.*

The comprehensiveness of the Australian definition of naturopathy as compared to the more brief US definition, above, is reflective of both the differences in the regulatory and educational frameworks of the two countries and the aims of the two definitions. It also reflects the fact that the brief US definition is part of a larger document that includes a longer definition, in addition to the six principles of naturopathic medicine, each of which is discussed in the next section. The key commonality of the two definitions is the concept of the healing power of nature, which is one of the primary distinguishing philosophical underpinnings of naturopathic medicine.

Concepts of health and disease

The preamble to the Constitution of the World Health Organization as adopted by the International Health Conference in 1946 defines 'health' as 'a state of complete physical, mental and social well-being and not merely the absence of disease or infirmity.'[19] This definition has not been amended since. In taking a holistic view of health and wellbeing, it is in complete alignment with the naturopathic approach to disease and healing.

Whereas the conventional model of diagnosis and treatment of disease approaches disease as a discrete entity that can be identified and eliminated through application of drugs or surgery, the naturopathic model approaches disease from a baseline presumption of health as the natural state of being. Naturopathic treatment seeks to restore health by removing the causes of disease or illness.[20] A concise summary of the naturopathic model for restoration of health is shown in Fig. 1.1. This model gives us a preview of the principles of naturopathic medicine and the other important frameworks of naturopathic clinical theory detailed below.

1. Universe is ordered, intelligent, wise and benign
2. Health is a constant and natural state of being
3. Ill health is an adaptive response to disturbance in organism
4. Removal of disturbing factors will result in potential return of normal health
5. Intervention should involve least force necessary to stimulate self-healing mechanisms

FIGURE 1.1 Naturopathic model for restoration of health

Zeff J, Snider P. Course syllabus: NM5131, Naturopathic clinical theory. Seattle: Bastyr University; 1997–2005. Used with permission of Jared Zeff.

Relevance of philosophy and clinical theory to naturopathic practice

The existence of a unified philosophy and clinical theory to underpin naturopathic practice is not only vitally important to the definition of the profession for regulatory bodies and the general public, but also critical to guide both the education of future naturopaths and the foundational approach of the practice of naturopathic medicine. As with any healing system, the view of a practising naturopath regarding what naturopathic medicine is will guide and shape what they do in the consulting room, how they justify what they do, and what they expect the outcomes to be. It is the lens through which all patients can be viewed to guide diagnosis and treatment or preventive care. Naturopathic philosophy and clinical theory serve as guideposts for the collective of a highly eclectic profession — they are the glue that holds the profession together — as well as serving to distinguish naturopathic medicine from other systems of natural therapeutics.

And importantly, a cohesive philosophy and clinical theory creates a foundation for thinking deeply about what we do and why we do it. It guards against the loss of individualisation of patient care and the movement of naturopathic medicine towards short cuts, protocols, loss of connection to our traditions, and the replacement of meaningful restoration of health with long-term reliance on symptom-based interventions.

PRINCIPLES OF NATUROPATHIC MEDICINE

There are six commonly recognised principles of naturopathic medicine, which provide the philosophical underpinnings out of which grow naturopathic clinical theory and practice. These six principles are the foundations for how naturopaths approach patient care. They are summarised in Fig. 1.2.

1. *Vis Medicatrix Naturae:* The Healing Power of Nature
2. *Primum Non Nocere:* First Do No Harm
3. *Tolle Totum:* Treat the Whole Person
4. *Tolle Causam:* Treat the Cause
5. *Docere:* Naturopath as Teacher
6. *Preventare:* Prevention

FIGURE 1.2 Six principles of naturopathic medicine

Vis Medicatrix Naturae (The Healing Power of Nature)

> *The healing power of nature is the inherent self-organizing and healing process of living systems which establishes, maintains and restores health. Naturopathic medicine recognizes this healing process to be ordered and intelligent. It is the naturopath[/s] role to support, facilitate and augment this process by identifying and removing obstacles to health and recovery, and by supporting the creation of a healthy internal and external environment.*[17]

This principle is the key commonality between the US and Australian definitions of naturopathic medicine and naturopathy (see above), though the Australian definition uses the term 'vital force' to name this principle. It is the first principle of naturopathic medicine because it defines the major distinguishing philosophy of the naturopathic approach to healing, as compared to conventional or other medicines. As the cornerstone of naturopathic practice, it highlights the nature of the organism to operate according to an intelligent and ordered process and it also underscores the naturopath's reliance on this intelligence to bring the organism back to health when the correct internal and external environments are provided.

The recognition of a 'life force' that is distinguished from the known laws of nature or the material sciences is common to the whole medical systems. These systems all carry a presumption that some form of energetic force provides the catalyst for life and for the capacity of the human organism to heal. The concept is described in ancient healing systems of both the East and West, some of which are still in practice today: Hippocrates named this force the *physis*, Galen named it the *pneuma*, Paracelsus dubbed it 'the inner alchemist' or *archeus*, in Ayurveda and yoga it is *prana*, and in Chinese medicine it is *qi/chi*. Across all of these systems of thought the concept of the vital force is defined somewhat differently. For example, in Chinese medicine, in the concept of *qi*, there is no distinction between matter and energy — both are comprised of *qi*.[21] However, the core concept of this force being what enlivens the organism and guides it back to health from illness is shared across the systems.

As with these historical systems, the concept of the vital force was established as a core philosophy in naturopathic medicine at a time when the material sciences were much less advanced than they are at present. Thus, much of what might have been considered vitalistic in historical naturopathic practice can now be explained in materialistic/mechanistic terms, via the laws of chemistry and physics. And it is possible that at some time in the future, with the growing understanding of quantum physics, all aspects of what we refer to as the *Vis Medicatrix Naturae* will be explained in mechanistic terms. Certainly, in the fields of nutritional research and pharmacognosy (the study of medicinal drugs of natural origin, i.e. from plants or other natural sources), much of what a naturopath does can already be explained via modern scientific mechanisms of action. However, that does not negate the fact that, absent a full scientific exposition of the nature of the energetics and consciousness of human and other organisms, the concepts of *qi*, *prana* or vital force and the knowledge of how to support or encourage their movement via traditional therapeutics have great utility in the establishment and maintenance of human health.

The principle of the *Vis Medicatrix Naturae* aims to guide the naturopath to work with, rather than against, nature. As an important part of this aim, the naturopath's view of the symptoms of illness is framed in the context of the body's own innate natural healing mechanisms:

> *Rather than viewing the ill patient as suffering from a 'disease,' the naturopath views the ill person as functioning within a process of disturbance and recovery in the context of nature and natural systems ... Disease is the process whereby the intelligent body reacts to disturbing elements. It employs such processes as inflammation and fever to help restore its health.*[20]

Thus, the *Vis Medicatrix Naturae* is a 'self-organising and healing process', and disease is seen as something caused by disturbance of that process and the body's attempt to recover from that disturbance. Symptoms of acute disease, such as fever and acute inflammation, are seen as tools that the body uses to bring itself back to health — they are self-healing processes that express the *Vis Medicatrix Naturae* and enable the possibility of a complete cure. Suppressing those processes poses an obstacle to cure. Of course, in some instances, it can be necessary to suppress severe symptoms. This is discussed further in the section on the therapeutic order below.

There is a common variant in the discussion of the *Vis Medicatrix Naturae* that should be addressed: the *Vis Medicatrix Naturae* is often equated to 'vitality', which is somewhat of a sidestep from the principle. Certainly, the level of a person's vitality is something in which a naturopath is keenly interested. The level of vitality tells us what type of response a person may or may not mount to a treatment intervention and what level of intervention is best called for in a given case; that is, lower force vs higher force, among other things. However, the level of a person's vitality is not the same as the *Vis Medicatrix Naturae*. The *Vis Medicatrix Naturae* is the intelligence and order in natural processes, the tendency towards balance and health, whereas vitality can be considered as the power behind or within this intelligence. Perhaps the easiest way to distinguish these concepts is by analogy. If the *Vis Medicatrix Naturae* is very simplistically equated to the blueprint for an engine, then vitality can be equated to the fuel for the engine. The blueprint is always there, the level of the fuel can be higher or lower.[22]

Primum Non Nocere (First Do No Harm)

> *Naturopath[s] follow three precepts to avoid harming the patient:*
>
> *Naturopath[s] utilize methods and medicinal substances that minimize the risk of harmful effects, and apply the least possible force or intervention necessary to diagnose illness and restore health.*
>
> *Whenever possible the suppression of symptoms is avoided as suppression generally interferes with the healing process.*
>
> *Naturopath[s] respect and work with the Vis Medicatrix Naturae in diagnosis, treatment and counseling, for if this self-healing process is not respected the patient may be harmed.*[17]

This principle is familiar from its roots in Hippocratic medicine, and on the surface has commonality to the Hippocratic oath still taken by medical doctors in the contemporary world. Hippocrates said, 'As to diseases, make a habit of two things: to help, or at least to do no harm.'[23]

This first precept or principle provides the clearest connection between the principles of naturopathic medicine and the therapeutic order, discussed below. This first precept has two important components: using therapies that minimise risk of harmful effects and applying the least force necessary to diagnose and affect a cure. The first component shows a contrast to conventional medicine, where negative side effects of medications tend to be accepted as the norm and both surgeries and medicines can put the patient at substantial risk. Of course, in any system of medicine, there is a balancing of the risk of not treating against the risk of providing the available treatment.

However, in naturopathic medicine, the therapies used are generally much lower force interventions than those in conventional medicine. In both diagnostics and treatment, 'lower force' generally refers to procedures and examinations that are least invasive to the patient's body and expose the patient to the least amount of risk. With regard to treatment, it also refers to using more gentle therapies, those with a more subtle action, whenever possible, and using more aggressive therapies only when absolutely necessary to avoid risk.

The second precept points to the naturopath's avoidance of suppressing symptoms of disease, as to do so will interfere with the healing process. Symptoms, particularly those characterised by inflammation or discharge, are seen as expressions of the body's attempt to heal, and barring any harm from allowing them to run their course, suppression of symptoms is generally avoided. Suppression can be defined as anything that prevents the development, action or expression of a symptom, inhibiting or stopping a normal healing process from occurring. The concept of a normal healing process is discussed in the section on the process of healing below.

Palliation of symptoms is sometimes necessary when a disease process has risen to the level of being dangerous to the patient or when the patient is in a great deal of pain or discomfort. Palliation can be defined as making a disease or its symptoms less severe or unpleasant without removing the cause. It can be done in a way that is suppressive or in a way that is not suppressive, although both possibilities are not always available in every case. As an example, the palliation of a fever higher than 40°C can be achieved in a suppressive way by bringing the body temperature down to normal or close to normal with a non-steroidal anti-inflammatory drug, or it can be achieved in a non-suppressive way by gently lowering the core temperature using hydrotherapy to a level that is no longer dangerous but which allows the fever to still do its important work in the healing process. The different forms of palliation generally present the decision of whether or not to suppress — if there is a possibility for cure, for return to normal health, the second principle urges us to avoid suppression to the greatest extent possible while ensuring patient safety.

The third precept ties in with the foundational first principle and calls for choosing therapies that rely upon the *Vis Medicatrix Naturae* for healing. In general, the more aggressive a therapy is, the more it is supplanting or potentially counteracting the intelligence of the *Vis Medicatrix Naturae*, and in cases where no harm will result from using only lower force interventions to support the body's natural healing processes, this precept urges that approach. This minimises to the greatest extent possible the potential of harm, because the naturopath is then working with the body's own innate healing capacity instead of trying to force healing by substituting a stronger intervention and their own judgment about what is right for the patient. The *Vis Medicatrix Naturae* knows what is right to bring the patient to health. In this, the importance of teaching the patient about the healing process is clear so that both the naturopath and the patient understand the diagnostic and treatment approach and respect the body's innate capacities.

It is often said that the corollary to the principle First Do No Harm is First Do Nothing. This acknowledges that it is not what the naturopath does that returns a person to health, but when the vitality is strong enough and the causes of illness are not overpowering the system, the *Vis Medicatrix Naturae* will return the patient to health without intervention.

Tolle Totum (Treat the Whole Person)

> *Health and disease result from a complex of physical, mental, emotional, genetic, environmental, social, and other factors. Since total health also includes spiritual health, naturopath[s] encourage individuals to pursue their personal spiritual development. Naturopathic medicine recognizes the harmonious functioning of all aspects of the individual as being essential to health. The multi-factorial nature of health and disease requires a personalized and comprehensive approach to diagnosis and treatment. Naturopath[s] treat the whole person taking all of these factors into account.*[17]

Treat the whole person is the third of the six principles of naturopathic medicine. This principle sets out a bio-psycho-social-spiritual approach to assessing and treating patients. Naturopaths take into account not just the physical body, but also the patient's state of mind and mental functioning, their emotional state and emotional intelligence, the exposures that their particular environment presents, the nature of their family and social relationships, and their connection with their spirituality. This holistic approach recognises that the various aspects of a person are intimately interconnected such that no part can be understood without reference to the whole, and the whole is greater than the sum of the parts. It is also an approach that puts the patient at the centre, rather than the disease.

In contrast to holism, a reductionist approach will tend to look at the minute parts of a system and extrapolate or attribute behaviours of that system to its isolated parts, essentially analysing the complex human organism in terms of its fundamental constituents — for example, biochemical pathways, cellular mechanisms or organ functions — and treating that analysis as sufficient explanation of the whole. This can be seen very clearly in the therapies of conventional medicine.

However, just because naturopathic medicine is a holistic pursuit, one cannot deny that it also has its reductionist components. Particularly as the realms of functional medicine and naturopathic nutrition increasingly overlap, and pharmacognosy continues to elucidate the specific biochemical and pharmacological actions of many herb constituents, naturopathic medicine is showing a tendency to gravitate more towards a reductionist approach. The third principle of naturopathic medicine might serve as a caution against moving too far in that direction. This is not to say that reductionist information about the workings of the minute aspects of the human organism does not have value — of course it does. But naturopathic philosophy and clinical theory urge that this information be seen within the wider scheme of things, rather than being considered as the 'truth' that ends the conversation. Any amount of understanding that we have from the material sciences must be considered in light of the organism as a whole, as well as the limits of the human intellect to process the full complexity of the human organism.

Naturopaths examine many facets of a person when considering what may be causing and what may remedy illness in an individual — each person's experience of illness is different — and a truly individualised view of the patient is necessary to a holistic approach. Taking an individualised view of both the patient and their experience of illness is necessarily a patient-centred approach. In 'Towards a global definition of patient centred care',[24] Stewart defines patient-centred care as that which:

> *(a) explores the patients' main reason for the visit, concerns, and need for information; (b) seeks an integrated understanding of the patients' world — that is, their whole person, emotional needs, and life issues; (c) finds common ground on what the problem is and mutually agrees on management; (d) enhances prevention and health promotion; and (e) enhances the continuing relationship between the patient and the doctor.*

Despite the source of this definition being a conventional medical journal, it is an apt description of the patient-centred naturopathic approach.

Tolle Causam (Treat the Cause)

> *Illness does not occur without cause. Causes may originate in many areas. Underlying causes of illness and disease must be identified and removed before complete recovery can occur. Symptoms can be expressions of the body's attempt to defend itself, to adapt and recover, to heal itself, or may be results of the causes of disease. The Naturopath seeks to treat the causes of disease, rather than to merely eliminate or suppress symptoms.*[17]

The fourth of the six principles of naturopathic medicine, Treat the Cause, flows naturally from the preceding principle, because treating the whole person necessarily implies treating the primary causes of illness, and *Tolle Totum* indicates where to look for the causes: the physical, the mental, the emotional and the spiritual.

Lindlahr's unity of disease as outlined in *Nature Cure* states that there are three primary causes of disease: lowered vitality, abnormal composition of blood and lymph, and accumulation of morbid matter and poisons in the system.[16] Of course, the era in which this book was published explains its dated language, and we would describe these causes somewhat differently today. Lindlahr's three primary causes of disease point to the conditions of the body that are setting up an environment for illness to take hold. If disease were a plant, then the condition of the body is the soil in which the plant of illness may grow. A person can give illness a fertile soil in which to take root or can deny it that fertile soil through appropriate habits that follow natural laws. A modern naturopath would refer to this foundational condition of the body as the 'terrain' for disease. Contrast this to a pathogen, which is like the seed being planted in that terrain.

To describe briefly each of Lindlahr's three primary causes, the concept of vitality has been discussed above as related to the principle of the *Vis Medicatrix Naturae*, as the 'fuel that runs the engine'. Lowered vitality is a state of depletion that occurs as the body, mind, emotions and spirit are denied the conditions needed to maintain their healthy function, or it can occur constitutionally. In naturopathic philosophy and clinical theory, anything that negatively affects the state of the vitality is termed a 'disturbing factor', and the longer that disturbing factor persists, the more depleted the vitality becomes.

'Abnormal composition of blood and lymph' relates primarily to the proper access of the body to necessary nutrients. If a person doesn't ingest, digest or absorb well the essential proteins, fats, carbohydrates, vitamins, minerals, and other micronutrients, or they don't breathe properly to maintain the appropriate levels of the various blood gases, then they do not have what they need in their blood and lymph to nourish their cells. 'Accumulation of morbid matter and poisons' in the system relates to the build-up of toxins over time, whether from endogenous or exogenous sources. If the cells and tissues, and perhaps especially the organs of elimination and extracellular fluids, are burdened with a large toxic load, then cellular function is disturbed or compromised, and organ systems begin to experience dysfunction.

As an aside, Lindlahr goes deeper than these three primary causes and states that they are, themselves, caused by a greater underlying common cause: 'transgression of natural laws in thinking, breathing, eating, dressing, working, resting, as well as in moral, sexual and social conduct.'[16] Again, this comports with the language of his time, but these ideas are reflected in modern language in the section below on the determinants of health. From his three primary causes, it appears as if Lindlahr places all causes of illness in the physical body. However, his list of 'transgressions of natural law' demonstrates that he also considered mental and emotional influences and elsewhere in *Nature Cure* he lists 'mental afflictions' as a secondary cause of illness. Finally, it is worth noting that Lindlahr's three primary causes of disease are closely interrelated, because not only do they all spring from the same deeper causes in lifestyle, but also once one has begun, it is more likely that the others will follow.

Returning to the concept of the terrain as the internal environment of an organism that provides the setting for either health or disease, as well as determining an individual's tendencies or susceptibilities to illness, we must consider the endogenous production of toxins in the body and the condition of toxaemia. Toxaemia is the production of high levels of metabolic waste created by maldigestion — the dysbiotic bacterial metabolism of poorly digested food in the intestines. These toxins enter the blood, irritate tissues systemically, interfere with organ function and become the basis for chronic illness, inflammatory processes, autoimmune processes and other dysfunctions.[25]

Endogenous toxicity sourced in gastrointestinal dysfunction and inflammation is one framework from which to look at all three of Lindlahr's primary causes of disease. Though this is a long-standing traditional naturopathic theory, it is clear from recent research that the absence of beneficial bacteria in the colon and/or the presence or overgrowth of non-beneficial bacteria or other organisms, in either the small intestine or the colon, are correlated to various diseases, particularly those involving dysregulation of the immune system. From a more traditional perspective, we can surmise that the action of dysbiotic flora on various foods during digestion, as well as the failure of proper digestion in the absence of necessary beneficial bacteria, forms toxic by-products, which then increase the total toxic load on the body's systems of elimination and which can overwhelm these systems, producing symptoms of illness. Chronic gastrointestinal dysfunction and inflammation will reduce digestive and absorptive capacities for essential nutrients and ultimately devitalise the entire system via chronic impacts on lymphatic and nervous tissues associated with the gastrointestinal tract (GIT). It is this line of thought that supports the traditional naturopathic approach of seeking the cause of illness in the digestive system and treating the cause accordingly.

Of course, it is important to note that even the normal metabolic processes produce a regular baseline load of endogenous toxins that must be eliminated from the body. This is what our eliminative organs are designed to do. When they are overwhelmed by a heavy load of toxins from other sources, or when the body's organs of elimination are not functioning optimally, even the accumulation of our normal metabolic wastes can create the symptoms of illness. Finally, we are exposed in the modern world to a plethora of exogenous toxins throughout our daily lives, all of which contribute to the body's total toxic load and affect the capacity of the eliminatory organs to maintain a balanced internal environment. We can draw from this an understanding of the naturopathic approach to placing a primary treatment emphasis on detoxification, depuration and elimination in order to address the accumulation of toxins as a cause of disease.

Docere (Doctor as Teacher)

> *The original meaning of the word 'doctor' is teacher. A principal objective of Naturopathic medicine is to educate the patient and emphasize self-responsibility for health. Naturopath[s] recognize and employ the therapeutic potential of the [practitioner]-patient relationship.*[17]

This is the fifth of the six principles, and despite its brevity, there are several very important concepts within it. Educating the patient is just one component; it is well understood that naturopaths teach their patients about how their bodies function, the nature of disease and healing, and the importance of health-supporting behaviours. Second is the idea of emphasising self-responsibility. If a naturopath is teaching their patient how to support their own health and also emphasising self-responsibility, then they are not acting in a paternalistic way; that is, the naturopath is not directing the patient nor acting as an authority above them. Instead, they are working in partnership with the patient, serving as a guide and allowing them to access and use the information to empower their own behaviour.

The third important component of this principle is the recognition and employment of the therapeutic potential of the practitioner–patient relationship. This underscores the idea that the cultivation of a meaningful therapeutic relationship with patients is a type of teaching or guiding in itself, and it has value in the healing process of the patient. In order to work with patients in this way, a naturopath must get to know them well, within the context of a long-term, continuing therapeutic relationship, and develop trust so that they will share their full range of experiences and challenges to allow the constructing of a picture of who they are as a whole person. The naturopath provides a safe, non-judgmental space for the patient to be the whole of who they are. This can call for significant time and patience on the part of both the naturopath and the patient.

The ability to be a therapeutic presence for patients can be one of the most valuable skills that a naturopath can apply in the treatment room. Therapeutic presence can be defined as 'bringing one's whole self into the encounter with clients, by being completely in the moment on multiple levels: physically, emotionally, cognitively, and spiritually.'[26] This includes being unconditionally present with the patient, deeply listening from a place of discernment and non-judgment, and an ability to take on a witness perspective on both self and other. Attention is given to both verbal and non-verbal communication, and the cultivation of self-awareness of attitudes, words and judgments, as well as emotional intelligence on the part of the naturopath, is a foundational practice.

The emphasis placed on self-responsibility in this principle points to the benefits of an egalitarian relationship between practitioner and patient in naturopathy. In Western culture, the conventional healthcare system has historically tended to create more of an active–passive or guidance–cooperative relationship between doctor and patient, with the doctor assuming a more authoritarian role sitting hierarchically above the patient. Within this healthcare culture, it can sometimes be a challenge for a naturopath to facilitate the creation of a more egalitarian relationship with a patient. However, it is quite often the case that patients seeking care from a naturopath are looking for a space where their concerns will be fully heard and where they are a full partner in their own health decisions, making those decisions based upon an understanding of their body and their condition and the treatment options and potential outcomes available. It is this type of empowerment that the naturopath seeks to create.

The act or action of 'teaching' may be accomplished by a naturopath in any number of ways and in a wide array of settings. Providing information or sharing specific knowledge with a patient one-on-one can help them understand some aspect of themselves (body, mind, emotions, spirit) better, and that understanding then becomes a framework around why certain recommended treatments or behaviour changes can be useful. This can be most powerful when the naturopath can identify where the largest gaps are in a person's knowledge about health. But this type of informational support results in action or behaviour change in the patient only when the underlying reason for a detrimental behaviour is a lack of understanding or information. For example, providing information to a smoker regarding the negative health impacts of smoking is unlikely to motivate them to change that behaviour, because most smokers are already very aware of the increased incidence of some diseases that result from smoking.

Beyond providing informational support to patients, or even providing that support via community lectures or writing, naturopaths often support and teach patients by assisting them in their own process of self-evaluation, helping them to see where their own blind spots are, or misalignments between their beliefs and actions. This also generally will include emotional support via counselling and assisting patients to understand how various mental and emotional patterns can be connected to problems with physical health. The connection between early childhood trauma and various types of chronic illness that are often present in patients who seek care from a naturopath, such as autoimmune disease, is an important consideration and the 'safe space' afforded in a naturopathic consultation can often provide a place for past traumas to rise to the surface to be healed. Thus, it is crucial for a naturopath to have a good referral network of practitioners who are more highly trained in working with mental and emotional conditions to work with in partnership in complex cases.

Preventare (Prevention)

> *Naturopathic colleges emphasize the study of health as well as disease. The prevention of disease and the attainment of optimal health in patients are primary objectives of naturopathic medicine. In practice, these objectives are accomplished through education and the*

promotion of healthy ways of living. Naturopath[s] assess risk factors, heredity and susceptibility to disease, and make appropriate interventions in partnership with their patients to prevent illness. Naturopathic medicine asserts that one cannot be healthy in an unhealthy environment and is committed to the creation of a world in which humanity may thrive.[17]

This is the sixth and final principle of naturopathic medicine. It is important to note in introducing this principle that, whether a naturopath is aiming to assist a patient in healing from disease, or preventing potential future disease, the therapeutic approach still follows the same strategies. All six of the principles apply in a preventive context as well as in the context of illness, and the clinical theory as discussed in the following sections likewise applies to both contexts.

There are many different types of preventive care, and naturopathic medicine approaches these from all levels. Primary prevention can be defined as actions taken to prevent a state of illness from ever occurring. In naturopathic medicine, primary prevention might include diet and lifestyle modification; instruction on health supportive daily habits; smoking, drug or alcohol abuse cessation; weight loss; or counselling that assists a patient in resolving mental or emotional patterns that might eventually lead to either physical or mental illness. Primary prevention also commonly falls into the public health arena, with measures such as infectious disease reporting, sanitation and food safety regulations.

Secondary prevention can be defined as early detection of sub-clinical disease; that is, disease that is not yet showing outward signs and symptoms. In large part, this type of prevention falls into the realm of conventional medicine. Examples of secondary prevention are PAP smears, mammograms, scheduled screening blood tests and bowel cancer screening. A naturopath can still play a vital role in ensuring appropriate secondary prevention for patients. Naturopaths, in working holistically, will tend to gather significantly more information from patients and to see patients more frequently than their GP, and thus, naturopaths are uniquely situated to identify any concerns that might signify a need for further investigation to detect early development of diseases. Referral to the GP is the responsibility of a naturopath in such instances. Naturopaths also play a role in directly addressing early risk factors for more severe disease, such as high blood pressure, chronic inflammation or blood sugar dysregulation.

Lastly, there is tertiary prevention, which can be defined as actions taken to reduce the negative effects of disease or treatments or minimise reduced function from established disease. For patients with severe chronic or terminal illnesses, this can be an important role of the naturopath, to assist in support of a higher quality of life, a subjective sense of greater wellbeing, palliating of side effects of high force medications, or assisting healing from surgery. In conventional healthcare, tertiary prevention falls primarily into the realm of palliative care, though heroic conventional treatments quite often prevent a disease or injury from having more profound impacts on structures or functions of the body.

At the beginning of this section on prevention, the point was made that all the other five principles also apply in a preventive care context. Now, coming full circle, we will close this discussion of the six principles of naturopathic medicine by noting that the opposite is also true: the concept of prevention is also built into all the other five principles. A naturopath's support of the *Vis Medicatrix Naturae* is naturally preventive, as it assists in maintaining a high level of vitality, which supports health generally. A naturopath's recommendation of the least invasive treatment methods under the principle of First Do No Harm will focus on foundational health behaviours first, which are naturally preventive as well as being curative. Recommendations aimed at the cause of an illness will help to prevent recurrence by making the patient aware of the causes of disease and how to avoid them. Treating the whole person will serve to give the naturopath a view over all parts of a person, even those that are not at present dysfunctional, allowing treatment recommendations that support the wellness of the whole both curatively and preventively. And finally, it would be hard to conceptualise a naturopath as teacher separate from the concept of prevention, as naturopaths empower and motivate their patients to a state of wellness through these two concepts hand-in-hand.

People are beginning to realize that it is cheaper and more advantageous to prevent disease, rather than to cure it.

Dr Henry Lindlahr, **Nature Cure**[16]

NATUROPATHIC CLINICAL THEORY: CONCEPTUAL FRAMEWORKS

While the six principles discussed in the preceding section provide the main philosophical foundation that guides the naturopathic approach, clinical practice requires further conceptual frameworks that guide how a naturopath views disease and healing processes, how a naturopath approaches development of a treatment strategy for each patient, and what the specific components are of a holistic view of health. These frameworks are discussed below.

The process of disease and healing

The naturopathic view of the process of healing,[20] as conceptualised and defined by Dr Jared Zeff, is represented in Fig. 1.3.

Beginning at the top of this schematic, the naturopathic perspective of the process by which acute illness ('reaction') occurs is shown as: a person begins in a state of normal health, then disturbing factors are introduced which cause a disturbance of function, then the disturbance of function causes a reaction — an acute illness. Disturbing factors are discussed further in the

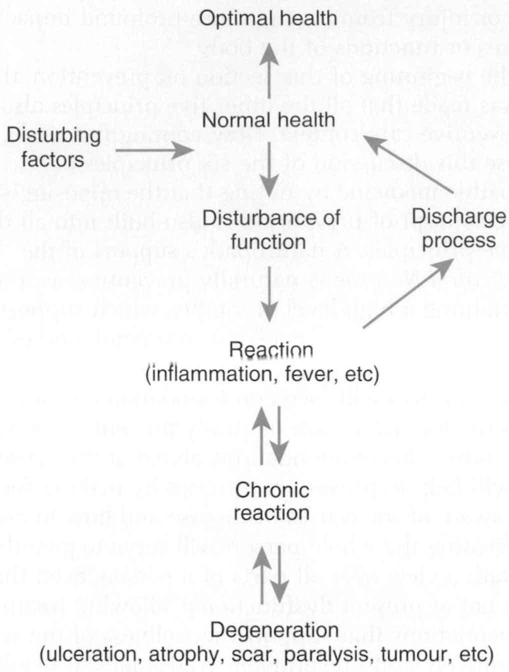

FIGURE 1.3 The process of healing

Zeff JL, Snider P, Myers SP et al. A hierarchy of healing: the therapeutic order. In Pizzorno JE, Murray MT, editors. Textbook of natural medicine. 4th edn. St Louis: Elsevier; 2013.

section below on the therapeutic order. However, a few examples to consider would be inappropriate diet, overworking/stress or excessive alcohol or caffeine intake. These speak to the concept of setting up the 'terrain' for illness, discussed earlier in this chapter.

Setting aside for now the possibility of more severe or damaging acute illnesses or injuries, when the acute reaction is not suppressed and the process is allowed to run its course, the disturbing factors are removed. Then the person has a high enough level of vitality and the acute reaction guided by the *Vis Medicatrix Naturae* will result in the body going through a discharge process, which returns the body to normal health. This is represented in the schematic by the arrows moving upwards to the right from the reaction stage back towards the top and normal health. Note that a person does not travel in reverse from the reaction stage to normal health without going through the discharge process. A discharge can come in many forms, from those that we are familiar with in acute illness such as a runny nose, coughing, sneezing, vomiting or diarrhoea, to those that might be less easily recognised as a discharge, such as sweating, skin rashes, odours, crying or other emotional outbursts.

This will obviously not be an appropriate approach for all acute conditions. Acute conditions are generally those that are self-resolving within a relatively short period, and they have an inflammatory component. But this is a broad spectrum of illness or injury, from the common cold, minor skin infection or low-grade gastrointestinal virus to severe bleeding or life-threatening illnesses such as appendicitis, severe asthma or meningitis. The self-resolving nature of an acute illness must be recognised as either return to health in a relatively short time, or potentially death if appropriate intervention is not applied. One of the tasks of the naturopath is to make a judgment in the case of acute illness as to whether a higher force intervention is needed to preserve life or prevent major damage to the organism and to refer appropriately and in a timely manner. But in the event of an acute illness that can safely be left to run its course, supported by advice to remove any disturbing factors and to rest to conserve the vitality, this will allow the reaction to proceed through all of the stages of inflammation to the discharge process and result in a return to health.

We return to the process of healing schematic in Fig. 1.3. Consider what occurs when there is suppression of the acute reaction: the continuation of disturbing factors, which creates a cumulative burden on the body and/or a lowered state of vitality that prevents a sufficient discharge process, will drive the human organism into a state of chronic reaction.[20] In contrast to an acute reaction, which is generally brief and self-resolving, a chronic disease/reaction is of longer duration and, by its nature, generally does not self-resolve as long as the factors that led to the chronic reaction remain in place. If the chronic reaction is of a great enough severity or long enough duration, it can then result in a degenerative state, including structural changes to the body that may ultimately be irreversible.

A chronic reaction, or disease state, is viewed as reversible within this framework, with the approach being to remove the disturbing factors that are placing a continuing burden on the body, stimulate the *Vis Medicatrix Naturae* to support self-healing, and avoid suppression of any resultant discharge process, within the bounds of safety for the patient in that process. More specific discussion of how this is done in the context of patient treatment can be found in the section on the therapeutic order, below. This general approach supports the patient in moving from the chronic reaction state back to a state of acute reaction, from which the discharge process can proceed, resulting in return to health. However, depending on the patient and their condition, multiple iterations of this process can be necessary to fully regain normal health, with each iteration of discharge moving the patient closer to that state.

The process whereby a patient moves from a chronic reaction and devitalised state to an acute reaction and discharge is often referred to as a 'healing crisis', though the term 'healing reaction' is more apt. According to Lindlahr, '[a] healing crisis is an acute reaction, resulting from the ascendancy of Nature's healing forces over disease conditions.'[16] The primary thing to note with regard to a true healing reaction is that it is an expression of the action of the *Vis Medicatrix Naturae* in the body's attempt to return itself to normal health. In that sense, it is the same as a discharge process in any acute illness. A healing reaction is usually short-lived and self-limiting and generally, while the patient may feel acutely worse in some symptoms, they will have an overall sense of feeling more well.

When a patient experiences an increase in symptoms during treatment, it is the task of the naturopath to discern whether it is a healing reaction or an actual increase of symptoms due to a worsening underlying condition. An examination of the pattern of the acute reaction within the overall history of the patient's case will often elucidate the difference. And naturopaths are assisted by Hering's rules of cure in this differentiating process. Hering's rules state that healing, that is resolution of symptoms and/or pathology, will generally occur from the top of the body downwards, from the deeper, more vital organs to the more superficial or less vital organs, from the centre to the periphery (i.e. core to extremities), and from the most recent to the oldest, with reference to the original occurrence of a symptom or pathology.[27] An examination of the patient's symptoms during an acute reaction often reveals these patterns, indicating a movement towards return to health and, if these patterns are not seen in the patient's symptom picture, it can indicate that the healing process is not moving in the right direction or the disease state is actually moving deeper.

In the process of the healing reaction, the symptoms of the reaction, as an expression of the *Vis Medicatrix Naturae,* must not be suppressed except in cases where it is necessary for the safety of the patient, and in that event, as minimal a level of suppression as possible. A suppression during the process of a healing reaction will stop the healing process and reverse it, driving the chronic reaction back to a deeper state.

The therapeutic order

The therapeutic order is a natural hierarchy of therapeutic intervention, based on or dictated by observations of the nature of the healing process, from ancient times through the present.[20]

The therapeutic order, presented in Fig. 1.4, represents the framework within which a naturopath works to develop specific treatment recommendations for individual patients. It is deeply interwoven with the six principles and with the process of healing. The therapeutic order 'operationalises' the general philosophy that crosses all six principles to use the lowest force interventions possible to both support the natural work of the *Vis Medicatrix Naturae* and avoid harm to the patient. This first addresses the cause(s) of illness, and does so in a holistic manner with regard to all aspects of the body, mind and spirit of the patient, allowing the patient to learn through the therapeutic process how to heal and maintain their own health.

The therapeutic order itself can be viewed through different lenses. It can be very helpful when first learning to work with this framework to view each level discretely — to compartmentalise the types of interventions or therapies that can fall at each level and to view the levels in a step-wise manner to maximise understanding of the underlying philosophy. However, an experienced practitioner mind can view the framework through a more complex lens, with an understanding that each level of the order will tend to be iterative of the level(s) above it, and that compartmentalisation of certain treatments at a given level can be an over-simplification. For example, if a practitioner prescribes a herb to support liver function in a patient with an overload of toxins or signs of liver compromise, one view of this is to put that therapy at level 3 of the therapeutic order, as tonifying a weakened system. However, it can also be argued that a well-functioning liver is essential to vitality, and so strengthening it is perhaps also falling at level 2, as stimulating the *Vis Medicatrix Naturae* (an argument that is even more compelling if the energetic aspects of the herbs are taking into consideration). For the purposes of this chapter, we will adopt the more compartmentalised view in order to establish firmly an understanding of the general tenor of each level of the order.

1. Establish the conditions for health
   - *Identify and remove disturbing factors*
   - *Institute a more healthful regimen*
2. Stimulate the healing power of nature (*Vis Medicatrix Naturae*); the self-healing processes
3. Address weakened or damaged systems or organs
4. Correct structural integrity
5. Address pathology: use specific natural substances, modalities or interventions
6. Address pathology: use specific pharmacological or synthetic substances
7. Suppress or surgically remove pathology

FIGURE 1.4 The therapeutic order: hierarchy of healing

Zeff JL, Snider P, Myers SP et al. A hierarchy of healing: the therapeutic order. In Pizzorno JE, Murray MT, editors. Textbook of natural medicine. 4th edn. St Louis: Elsevier; 2013.

LEVEL 1: ESTABLISH THE CONDITIONS FOR HEALTH

The therapeutic order starts with the lowest force interventions that naturopaths can recommend — those that are at the heart of a person's daily lifestyle, diet and habits. The first level of the order establishes this as a two-pronged approach: to identify and remove disturbing factors and to institute a more healthful regimen. This level provides a direct connection to the process of healing, where we see that disturbing factors are the causative force that pushes the organism into a state of reaction. We have discussed the removal of those disturbing factors as a vital component of the healing process — this is treating the cause. Another term that can be used to describe disturbing factors is 'obstacles to cure'. The terms are relatively synonymous, but the difference in description can provide insight to a naturopath who is working to discern the patient's needs at this level of the therapeutic order. A disturbing factor might be readily identifiable as an active force in a person's life, whereas an obstacle to cure might look more like a blockage. In practice, these often turn out to be the same things — the things causing illness are the same things that are getting in the way of a return to health.

If the first prong is viewed as 'non-healthful things to be removed', then the second prong, instituting a more healthful regimen, can be viewed as 'healthful things to be added' to a patient's way of life. Again, at this first level, the naturopath is focused on the lowest force interventions, which generally will consist of behavioural or dietary changes on the part of the patient. The guidance for the many different areas of life and habit that might be addressed in a holistic manner at this level is provided by the determinants of health, which are discussed in the final section below.

Even though this first level of the order contains the lowest force interventions, it is important to note that, depending upon the patient's overall condition, state of vitality or toxicity, and specific pathological conditions, the safety of the patient must always be taken into consideration with any treatment recommendation in order to avoid harm. For example, advising a patient with pronounced kidney dysfunction to change their water intake, or advising a patient with insulin-controlled diabetes mellitus to alter their dietary patterns, must be done cautiously and with close attention to the potential negative outcomes of these recommendations, which would be safe in other types of patients.

LEVEL 2: STIMULATE THE *VIS MEDICATRIX NATURAE*

When using the lowest force interventions at the first level of the therapeutic order, the naturopath is partnering with the patient to give the *Vis Medicatrix Naturae* what it needs to bring the person back to normal health and to remove things that are getting in the way of it doing its job. But in that first level we are relying on the patient's vitality in its current state to drive the process of healing. Some patients can be helped at the first level alone, but many patients, especially those with chronic illnesses, have a lowered vitality and need additional intervention.

At the second level of the therapeutic order, the naturopath is providing a slightly higher level of intervention, while still relying on the patient's innate healing capacity. This acknowledges that the patient's current state of vitality may need support or stimulation in order for the first-level interventions to return the patient to health. At the second level, the *Vis Medicatrix Naturae* is stimulated in order to increase the effectiveness or strength of the patient's innate healing processes.

There are several ways that this can be accomplished, and the particular intervention chosen for an individual patient will depend on the condition of the patient, their level of vitality and their choices as to what to pursue. Perhaps the simplest ways to stimulate the *Vis Medicatrix Naturae* are by exposure to the natural elements: fresh air, sunshine, time spent in nature, honouring of the rhythms of nature in daily life, and the therapeutic use of water are some examples. With hydrotherapy being one of the core therapeutic modalities of traditional naturopathy, the modern body of knowledge on the therapeutic use of water is vast, can be applied in a highly individualised way and is perhaps underappreciated in modern naturopathic practice.

Other methods for increasing vitality and stimulating the *Vis Medicatrix Naturae* are modalities that we might call 'energetic' in nature, such as breath work or gentle body movement, ingestibles such as homeopathy or flower essences, and acupuncture or other related therapies that move or unblock the flow of energy. The latter of these are considered to be stimulations that are more specific because they tend to be administered according to the particular presentation of the patient. However, their effects nonetheless result in a stimulation of the vital force.

LEVEL 3: ADDRESS WEAKENED SYSTEMS

If interventions or treatments applied at the first two levels of the therapeutic order are insufficient to start the patient on the path towards healing and support them in continuing to move in that direction, then naturopaths move on to the third level, the next higher level of force in treatment. This is often the case in longer-standing chronic reactions or in cases of more severely lowered vitality, in which organs can be compromised, blocked or congested from long-term stresses. Naturopaths select treatments at this level based upon the particular systems in each patient that are showing signs of decreased or compromised function. Naturopaths often tend to gravitate to looking first at the digestive and detoxification systems, as these systems are considered the foundation of health as discussed earlier in this chapter. However, beyond this, the nervous, endocrine, cardiovascular, respiratory, genitourinary, musculoskeletal and integumentary systems must be considered, as well as placing some focus on systems within systems, such as the menses within the endocrine system.

This level will tend to include natural therapies that are ingestible and are providing specific support to an organ or a system. Many, but not all, clinical nutrients (referring to nutraceuticals rather than nutrition via food) and herbal medicines used nutritively or to stimulate or support particular biochemical pathways or cellular systems fall at this level. It is also at this level where there begins to be cross-over between naturopathic medicine and functional medicine, with specific testing being conducted to look at biomarkers of system or organ function prior to prescribing treatments aimed to stimulate or support specific biochemical or physiological processes. This implies a reduced deference to the *Vis Medicatrix Naturae* — it is a movement into the realm of being slightly more forceful, of isolating and encouraging certain functions in the body rather than allowing the body to return to balance on its own design. However, when systems or organs have been overloaded or compromised for some time, this level of treatment has great utility, and it is still working *with* constructive natural processes rather than *against* pathological processes, as will be seen in the fifth level, below.

LEVEL 4: CORRECT STRUCTURAL INTEGRITY

Structure and function are closely intertwined. If a structure is compromised, for example blood flow or nerve conduction is impeded to an organ, then the function of that organ will be changed — weakened, irritated/inflamed, stagnated. Sometimes a structural change precedes a functional change, as in an injury that causes some skeletal misalignment or scar tissue formation, and sometimes functional change can precede structural problems, as in chronic inflammation that causes muscles to place asymmetrical stresses on the skeleton, nerves and blood vessels.

Naturopathic manual therapies can be used to address some structural issues. If a functional change caused the structural problem, then the underlying functional problem must also be addressed at the preceding levels of the therapeutic order, or the structural therapy will likely have only short-lived effect. If a structural problem was created by a forceful trauma to the body or postural habits, then the treatment may be more straightforward. Along with manual therapy by the naturopath, often chiropractic, osteopathy, specialised forms of massage, exercise prescriptions, or physiotherapy can be great adjunctive therapies when addressing structural integrity. Naturopathy has a long history of being intertwined with chiropractic and osteopathy, and many early naturopaths were also trained in these medical systems.

LEVEL 5: ADDRESS PATHOLOGY WITH NATURAL INTERVENTIONS

In the first four levels of the therapeutic order, the specific nature of the pathology is not directly considered in relation to the Western pathological diagnosis — the naming of the disease in those terms — except as it is relevant to ensuring the safety of the patient and avoidance of harm. Instead, the person as a whole has been considered, as well as their lifestyle and environment, along with identifying what organ systems or structures might be under-functioning or compromised. At the fifth level of the therapeutic order, the naturopath turns to look directly at the identified pathology and pathophysiology. Most patients will improve and move towards the direction of healing when the first three to four levels of the therapeutic order are applied. But in some cases, it is necessary to move to a higher level of force in our interventions.

At the fifth level, the naturopath is using natural interventions from the same point of view as a medical doctor uses synthetic pharmacological agents. Hence, this level of the therapeutic order is often referred to as 'green allopathy'. At this level, the natural intervention is being used to directly address —that is, counteract — the pathogenesis or the signs and symptomatology of the disease. For example, in a case of type 2 diabetes mellitus, herbs or nutrients used to target lowering elevated blood sugar or increasing insulin sensitivity of cells directly, or in a case of an inflammatory disease, herbs or nutrients used with a directly anti-inflammatory action. As the second of these examples indicates, treatments at this level can be suppressive, and this is one of the key reasons why this level is considered to contain higher force interventions. But in addition this level is where the naturopath turns from working with the organism to working against the disease, taking the naturopath a step away from the foundational philosophies.

LEVELS 6 AND 7: CONSIDER PHARMACOLOGICAL DRUGS AND SURGERY

The inclusion of these levels within the therapeutic order is critical in order to acknowledge both the full range of treatments that are available in any given case and the ultimate necessity of these high force interventions in some cases. Because these two levels of therapeutics are beyond the scope of a naturopath's practice in Australia and most of the world, they will not be discussed in any detail here. However, again, it is incumbent upon a naturopath to use their training and experience to assess risk correctly for all patients and to make appropriate referrals to the GP, specialist or emergency department when these levels of treatment are indicated. Conversely, use of suppressive therapies when it is not necessary will pose an obstacle to the process of healing and can ultimately prevent a cure.

The determinants of health

In considering disturbing factors in the process of healing, or what constitutes 'establishing the conditions for health' at the first level of the therapeutic order, the naturopath is guided by a final framework, the determinants of health. Within this framework, there are three major categories: inborn traits, disturbances and lifestyle factors.[15,20]

Inborn traits include a person's genetic make-up; maternal diet, lifestyle, emotional state, general health and toxic exposures; and the individual's constitution.[15,20] Historically, naturopaths and other practitioners alike might have considered that most of these would be beyond the reach of any type of therapy to influence after birth. However, the growing field of epigenetics and the concept of neuroplasticity are demonstrating that our environment, stressors, emotional state and many other factors will influence which of our genes are being expressed at any given time and how our nervous system might adapt to overcome innate traits. It is possible that changes in lifestyle, diet, energetics, emotions and psychological and mental patterning can influence the impact that genes or other inborn traits have on who a person ultimately becomes. Likewise, with a person's constitution, it will always be what it is — it does not change — but the particular expression and robustness of our constitution can be influenced with constitutional remedies/therapies and positive lifestyle choices.

The second major category is disturbances, or disturbing factors, which connects directly to the process of healing and the first level of the therapeutic order. Disturbances can be events that have happened in the past that have left a longer-term lack of wellness in the body, such as past illnesses (particularly chronic or recurrent ones), injuries, medical interventions, traumas or toxic exposures. They can also be current disturbances which

Spiritual life	Digestion, toxaemia
Fresh air	Rest
Exposure to nature	Sleep
Clean water	Exercise
Natural light	Socioeconomic factors
Loving and being loved	Culture and community
Diet, nutrition	Meaningful work
Unadulterated food	

FIGURE 1.5 Determinants of health: behavioural, environmental and other life factors

Zeff J, Snider P. Course syllabus: NM5131. Naturopathic clinical theory. Seattle: Bastyr University; 1997–2005. Used with permission of Jared Zeff.

consist of any aspect of the person's current life that is pushing the body, mind, emotions or spirit towards reaction or towards maintaining a state of chronic reaction.[15,20] As with the first category, there may be factors here that are beyond treatment; for example, if a patient has had an organ removed. In development of treatment recommendations, the naturopath and patient work in partnership to identify these past and present disturbances, remove them where possible from present life conditions, and work retrospectively on any lingering effects from past disturbances that were not fully resolved, which can be on the physical, mental, emotional or spiritual levels. On this last point, it is important to look at whether and how past illnesses or symptoms may have been suppressed for a view into what may arise to be healed as the treatment process continues.

The third major category covers lifestyle factors across a holistic array of considerations that include socioeconomic, relational, environmental and other factors outside the realm of the individual patient.[15,20] Fig. 1.5 features a list of some of these determinants of health, though it is not exhaustive. The principle of treat the whole person is perhaps seen most in operation in this list of factors that contribute to human health, and the second prong of level 1 of the therapeutic order is represented here. Instituting a more healthful regimen, viewed holistically, will seek to address what can be addressed across all these factors, while acknowledging that the naturopath, and indeed the patient, can often have only minimal, if any, influence in some of these areas.

REFERENCES

[1] US National Center for Complementary and Alternative Medicine. Whole medical systems: an overview; 2012.

[2] Kirchfield F, Boyle W. Nature doctors: pioneers in naturopathic medicine. East Palestine, OH: Buckeye Naturopathic Press; 1994.

[3] Scoutetten H. Hydrotherapy in Germany. Graefenberg and Priessnitz. Lancet 1843;40(1029):274–6.

[4] Boyle W, Saine A. Lectures in naturopathic hydrotherapy. Sandy, OR: Eclectic Medical Publications; 1988.

[5] Winston D, Dattner AM. American system of medicine. Clin Dermatol 1999;17:53–6.

[6] Willard TL. Textbook of modern herbology. 2nd ed. Calgary: Wild Rose College of Natural Healing; 1993.

[7] Griggs B. Green pharmacy: a history of herbal medicine. London: Robert Hale; 1983.

[8] Thurston JM. The philosophy of physiomedicalism: its theorem, corollary, and laws of application for the cure of disease. Richmond, IN: Nicholson Printing; 1901.

[9] Haller JS. Medical protestants, the Eclectics in American medicine, 1825–1939. Carbondale, IL: Southern Illinois University Press; 1994.

[10] Wood M. Vitalism — the history of herbalism, homeopathy and flower essences. Berkeley: North Atlantic Books; 1992.

[11] Ody P. The Herb Society's complete medicinal herbal. London: Dorling Kindersley; 1993.

[12] Czeranko S. Past pearls: the trials of Benedict Lust. Naturopathic doctor news and review; 2010. Available from: http://ndnr.com/education-web-articles/past-pearls-the-trials-of-benedict-lust/.

[13] Cody GW, Hascall H. The history of naturopathic medicine: the emergence and evolution of an American school of healing. In: Pizzorno JE, Murray MT, editors. Textbook of natural medicine. 4th ed. St Louis: Elsevier; 2013.

[14] Micozzi MS. Historical aspects of complementary medicine. Clin Dermatol 1998;16:651–8.

[15] Pizzorno JE, Snider P. Naturopathic medicine. In: Micozzi MS, editor. Fundamentals of complementary and integrative medicine. 3rd ed. St Louis: Elsevier; 2006.

[16] Lindlahr H. Nature cure. 20th ed. Holicong, PA: Wildside Press; 1922.

[17] Select Committee on the Definition of Naturopathic Medicine, Snider P, Zeff J, co-chairs. Definition of naturopathic medicine: AANP position paper. Rippling River, OR; 1989.

[18] Australian National Training Authority. Qualifications framework health training package; 2002. Available from: www.ntis.gov.au/~ntis2/pdf_files/hlt02rul.pdf.

[19] World Health Organization. Constitution of the World Health Organization; 2006. Available from: www.who.int/governance/eb/who_constitution_en.pdf.

[20] Zeff JL, Snider P, Myers SP, et al. A hierarchy of healing: the therapeutic order. In: Pizzorno JE, Murray MT, editors. Textbook of natural medicine. 4th ed. St Louis: Elsevier; 2013.

[21] Kaptchuk T. The web that has no weaver: understanding Chinese medicine. New York: Rosetta Books; 2010.

[22] Selected excerpts from dialogs with various naturopathic elders. Foundations Project. The heart of naturopathic medicine. Unified Energetics 2007;3:8–17. Available from: www.foundationsproject.com/documents/articles/FoundationsInteview.pdf.

[23] Grammaticos PC, Diamantis A. Useful known and unknown views of the father of modern medicine, Hippocrates and his teacher Democritus. Hell J Nucl Med 2008;11(1):2–4.

[24] Stewart M. Towards a global definition of patient centred care. BMJ 2001;322(7284):444–5.

[25] Zeff JL. The process of healing: a unifying theory of naturopathic medicine. J Naturopathic Med 1997;7(1):122–5.

[26] Geller SM, Greenberg LS, Watson JC. Therapist and client perceptions of therapeutic presence: the development of a measure. Psychother Res 2010;20(5):599–610.

[27] Saine A. Hering's law: law, rule or dogma? Second Annual Session of the Homeopathic Academy of Naturopathic Physicians; 1988. Available from: www.homeopathy.ca/articles_det12.shtml.

Principles of herbal medicine

2

Sue Evans

BRIEF HISTORY OF WESTERN HERBAL MEDICINE

The use of plants as medicines predates humans on the planet, as birds and animals have been observed to use plants in ways that benefit their health and treat disease.[1,2] With regard to our own species, there is evidence that medicinal plants, including those used today, have been highly valued since prehistoric times.[3,4]

Given their widespread and continuous use, medicinal plants have been called 'the birthright of mankind'. They belong in the kitchen as much as in the clinic or laboratory, as they continue to play a role with household medicine providing immediate care for minor ills. Older generations, including those who do not see themselves as knowledgeable about the use of medicinal plants, may use plant-based remedies for dealing with day-to-day health problems, such as ginger root for nausea or a spicy hot lemon drink for colds.[5]

In addition, medicinal plants continue to be used across the world as a stand-alone therapy or as part of naturopathic treatment.

Hippocratic writings and humoral medicine

Early documentation of Western herbal medicine (WHM) is found in the 60 treatises that comprise the Hippocratic Corpus. These are the works of the followers of the Greek healer Hippocrates of Cos, and were written over a period of about 700 years between the fifth (or early fourth) century BCE and the second century CE. They contain references to 380 plant species and their uses in 3100 different conditions.[6] Many of the plants documented in these works are well known today. They include garlic and fennel, oregano and elder, pomegranate and chaste tree, among others.

The origins of humoral medicine, central to Western medical thought until the Age of Enlightenment (18th century), are also found in these writings. Humoral medicine is based on the idea that the four elements — earth, water, fire and air — are the basis of all existence and are expressed in four humours — melancholic, phlegmatic, choleric and sanguine — each of which is related to a particular season and has its own qualities (see Table 2.1).

In this system, individual personality traits were understood to be related to specific humours (see Box 2.1 for an early description of these traits), and disease was seen as largely due to an imbalance of the humours. Consequently, the actions of medicinal plants were understood as assisting in rebalancing the humours. This is also the origin of plants being described as heating, cooling, moistening and drying.

Middle Ages and the spice trade

Throughout the Middle Ages medicinal plants were fundamental to medical care, both among the social and medical elites, and within the monasteries and nunneries which provided primary healthcare to their communities. Medieval herbals document the detail of plant use.[7] At this time some medicinal plants were cultivated and traded locally, and others were imported.[8] The most valuable of the imported plants were the spices.

Spice plants have been traded for medicinal, culinary and ritual uses since biblical times, their Asian origins shrouded in mystery for centuries. When ingested, they promote a sense of warmth. This was a particularly important quality in the cold winters of northern Europe and these plants were understood in humoral terms to counter the problems of the phlegmatic (damp) humour. Spices were traded over vast distances overland via long supply chains. They changed hands (and increased in price) many times between, for example, the islands of Banda and Run, now part of Indonesia (source of nutmeg and clove), Sri Lanka (source of cinnamon) and India (source of black pepper).

The long supply chains of these valuable commodities were controlled by Muslim traders. The high level of distrust between Christians and Muslims in the Middle Ages motivated European leaders to find ways to disrupt the Muslim domination of this lucrative market. This was one of the factors behind the instigation in the 15th to 17th centuries of maritime journeys which became known as the voyages of exploration. Individuals including Vasco da Gama, Christopher Columbus and Ferdinand Magellan led these expeditions. Of particular interest in the context of the history of Western herbal medicine is that these journeys not only were seeking alternative supply routes for spices, but their brief was also to seek out other medicinal plants that might be useful in Europe.[9–11]

TABLE 2.1 Humoral theory and related phenomena

Humour	Sanguine	Choleric	Melancholic	Phlegmatic
Substance	Blood	Yellow bile	Black bile	Phlegm
Quality	Hot and moist	Hot and dry	Cold and dry	Cold and moist
Season	Spring	Summer	Autumn	Winter
Element	Air	Fire	Earth	Water

Source: Trickey Enterprises (Victoria) Pty Ltd. The humoral theory, p. 8. Women, hormones and the menstrual cycle. 3rd ed. Melbourne.

BOX 2.1 The Regimen Sanitatis Salernitanum (a Salernitan regimen of health)

Poem by unknown author of 12th or 13th century.

Fat and jolly of nature are those of sanguine humor.
They always want to hear rumors,
Venus and Bacchus delight them, as well as good food and laughter;
They are joyful and desirous of speaking kind words.
These people are skillful for all subjects and quite apt;
For whatever cause, anger cannot lightly rouse them. They are
Generous, loving, joyful, merry, of ruddy complexion,
Singing, solidly lean, rather daring, and friendly.
Next is the choleric humor, which is known to be impulsive:
This kind of man desires to surpass all others.
On the one hand he learns easily, he eats much and grows quickly;
One the other hand, he is magnanimous, generous, a great enthusiast.
He is hairy, deceitful, irritable, lavish, bold,
Astute, slender, of dry nature, and of yellowish complexion.
There remains the sad substance of the black melancholic temperament,
Which makes men wicked, gloomy, and taciturn.
These men are given to studies, and little sleep.
They work persistently toward a goal; they are insecure.
They are envious, sad, avaricious, tight-fisted,
Capable of deceit, timid, and of muddy complexion.

(Note: The phlegmatic temperament is not mentioned in this poem.)

Matterer JL. A boke of gode cookery — regimen sanitatis salernitanum. 2001. Available from: www.godecookery.com/regimen/regimn14.htm

These expeditions led to widespread European colonisation of the Americas, and parts of Asia, Africa and Oceania. The 'New World' of the Americas provided a pharmacopoeia of medicinal plants new to the Europeans. Information about these discoveries was widely disseminated; for example, in 1577 an English translation of a Spanish herbal, Monardes' *Joyfull News from the Newe World*, became available.[12,13]

Culpeper

The trade in imported medicinal plants — and the prices they commanded — drew criticism from some herbalists who were sceptical of the need for new and expensive commodities. Throughout the writings of that most enduring of English herbal figures, Nicholas Culpeper (1616–54),[14] such criticism is evident. Abandoning his medical studies at Cambridge, Culpeper became apprenticed to an apothecary and fought for Cromwell in the English Civil War. He was committed to empowering his patients by sharing knowledge about local (English) medicinal plants. From his practice in central London he dismissed the use of new imported plants, arguing that they were being promoted in order to 'line the pockets' of the medical elites. In his view, local plants were not only easily available and cheap, but they were more than adequate to address local health problems. In his opinion 'a Man may preserve his Body in Health, or cure himself when sick, with such things only as grow in England, they being most fit for English constitutions'.[15] He had a colourful, productive and relatively short life, and although he died at the age of 38, his herbals have remained popular through the centuries.

The classification system that he popularised, ascribing qualities or 'degrees' of heating, cooling, moistening or drying, was based on humoral medicine and is described in Table 2.2. Although these concepts are no longer used to describe disease, some aspects remain useful in a modern understanding of herbal medicine. For example, spices are still considered hot, bitters and sedatives cooling, mucilages moistening and astringents drying.[15]

Western herbal medicine in the colonies

Colonisation led to an exchange of medicinal plants between Europe and its colonies. In the case of North America this process was clearly two-way. European

TABLE 2.2 Temperaments of herbal medicines

Hot	Examples of actions	Dry	Examples of actions
1st degree	To enhance sweating	1st degree	To strengthen
2nd degree	To open pores; clear obstructions	2nd degree	To bind
3rd degree	To inflame, cause fevers	3rd degree	To stop fluxes
4th degree	To cause inflammation, blisters (externally)	4th degree	To dry up radical moisture
Cold	**Examples of actions**	**Moist**	**Examples of actions**
1st degree	To cool	1st degree	To ease coughs
2nd degree	To abate fevers; refresh the spirits	2nd degree	To loosen the belly
3rd degree	To suppress perspiration	3rd degree	To make whole body watery and phlegmatic
4th degree	To stupefy the senses and ease pain	4th degree	Not possible

Source: Culpeper N. Culpeper's complete herbal. Ware, Herts: Wordsworth; 1653/1995.

medicinal plants were brought to the New World with the English colonists and cultivated by them in their 'dooryard gardens' of food and medicine. Indigenous medicinal plants were incorporated into this herbal tradition, albeit after some initial reluctance. This cross-fertilisation between European and native American medicinal plants provided the basis for the 19th century botanic medicine movements.[16]

A similar transfer of medicinal plant knowledge between Indigenous and non-Indigenous peoples in Australia is not evident. There are records of European medicinal plants being among the plants transported from England to Australia with the First Fleet and subsequent supply ships. In addition, a medicinal plant garden was established in the Rocks area of Sydney to 'provide the needs of Sydney General Hospital' within weeks of the arrival of the first Europeans. Some early medical practitioners showed an interest in local medicinal plants, and collected information about their use.[17] However, this interest did not result in the widespread use of indigenous plants as medicines, and very few Australian native plants will be found in the dispensaries of Australian practitioners today.

Rather the North American experience and use of plants indigenous to that continent is reflected in the development of the botanical medicine movements of the 18th and 19th centuries. It is this knowledge which was exported throughout the English-speaking world and consequently these plants are well represented in the dispensaries of contemporary practitioners of WHM.[18]

Thomsonianism

The early botanic medicine movement originated with the work of Samuel Thomson, who bridged the domestic and professional uses of herbal medicine, and promoted the use of local (North American) plants over imported ones.

Thomson developed a system of medicine based on herbal formulations to treat common health problems. He patented this system in 1813 and developed a highly successful business selling a year's worth of medical supplies to a family for $20. He also established a network of 'chapters' or support groups, where individuals could share the practical application of his ideas and medicines. In the pioneering society that was the US of the time, this approach to healthcare proved to be enormously successful in a situation where 'regular' medical treatment was not well regarded or trusted, and was often unavailable or unaffordable.

Thomson's system of medicine had clear links with humoral medicine, and could be followed by anyone, regardless of their level of education. His rationale for healing was based on stimulating the individual's vital force. He promoted a very simple idea that illness was largely to do with an excess of 'cold' which could be countered through the application of heat. This was achieved by the use of steam baths and the ingestion of 'heating' plants, especially cayenne. He also used emetics in order to 'cleanse' the body before treatment.

In the years following, these simple ideas were developed further by the physiomedicalists and Eclectics. Figures such as Alva Curtis and Wooster Beach in the US and Albert Coffin in the UK were influential in herbal medicine both politically and philosophically during the 19th century. They were among the leaders of a large group of herbal practitioners who provided medical care in the US and UK. These practitioners documented their work, including many case histories, in books and professional journals. This work remains a rich resource of clinical data available to herbal historians and scholars on the use of medicinal plant preparations in the treatment of a wide range of conditions, many of them serious and acute.

One of the continuing ideas expressed in these works is the importance of treating the vital force which regulates the body. Obstruction of the vital force was thought to cause cellular, organ or system dysfunction. Symptoms of disease were explained as expressions of the body's attempts to resolve problems facing the vital force. The greatest obstruction to it was the accumulation of metabolic wastes associated with poor elimination. The emphasis of treatment was on assisting the body to rid itself of this 'toxic encumbrance', primarily through promoting diaphoresis (sweating), emesis and enemas ('purging and puking'). While the techniques may have changed, the emphasis on organ dysfunction and on toxicity as a potential contributing factor in disease can be seen in contemporary herbal practice (see Ch 1).

The botanic medicine movements of the 19th century flourished in what has been described as a period of 'free trade in physic', or 'medical sectarianism' where herbalists, homeopaths and 'regular' ('allopathic') practitioners and others practised freely. However, from the 1850s this freedom of practice began to be challenged, as allopathic practitioners and their supporters began to introduce legislation to advantage them over those who practised herbal medicine and homeopathy.[16,18–21]

These attempts to professionalise medicine took place over half a century and were eventually highly successful. They resulted in the medical profession developing 'one of the most privileged, autonomous positions in the marketplace in the contemporary Anglo-American context'.[20] As a consequence of this privilege, other approaches to medicine, including herbal medicine, became marginalised. Interestingly, it was in this climate that the new discipline, naturopathy, was developed at the dawn of the 20th century.

This marginalisation was challenged in the 1960s and 1970s with the development of the counter-culture. The re-emergence of herbal medicine at this time was and continues to be consumer-led and has occurred despite the initial opposition of both the state and the medical profession.[20,22] Commercial interests have been quick to recognise the opportunities this new field offered, as the burgeoning markets in over-the-counter remedies attest.

MODERN PRACTICE

Modern Australian herbal medicine, similar to its European and North American counterparts, is largely founded on the Anglo-Thomsonian model as described above and the philosophies of Hippocrates and his successors. Humoral theory, doctrine of signatures, planetary influences and vital force are all aspects of herbal medicine that have influenced its past practices and the ways in which practitioners have traditionally understood the activity of these plants.

However, in recent decades WHM has become more and more firmly rooted in biomedical disease concepts that are based on scientific principles and research. These principles can be seen when reading influential books by authors such as Simon Mills, Kerry Bone, Rudolf Fritz Weiss, and others.

Many traditional concepts are not accepted by, and may be incompatible with, contemporary scientific understandings. At the same time, public popularity of herbal medicine arises from a perception that herbalists offer 'something different'.[23] Consequently, WHM is in a philosophical dilemma. On the one hand, we are indebted to our ancestral herbal forefathers for our distinctive approach which is being demanded by the public. On the other hand, we try to fit our knowledge and practice into the prevailing scientific worldview.

The way out of the dilemma has been to adopt a biopsychosocial system which is based on current scientific knowledge and rationale, while also considering holistic aspects including the social, environmental, spiritual, psychological, cultural and economic aspects of a person.

The following principles are founded on the action-based method and principles advocated by a number of key figures within WHM.

CURRENT WESTERN HERBAL MEDICINE — PHILOSOPHICAL PRINCIPLES

Western herbal medicine is based on the concept that a normal human body is free of disease and capable of resisting disease and maintaining homeostasis.

In the physiomedical tradition the following three principles are fundamental and are still in place today:

1 A belief in a vital force that underlies all living organisms. It is this force that unifies all living organisms and is responsible for restoration and preservation of health.
2 A holistic philosophical framework that believes in treating individuals within the wider framework of their emotional, social, economic, spiritual and cultural aspects.
3 The principle of 'do no harm' — specifically the use of non-toxic medicines.

Individualised and holistic treatment

These naturopathic approaches are based on a belief that every person is unique; thus diagnosis and treatment of ailments is always individualised. No-one is ever in perfect health and each person has their own individual limitations on their potential for good health. Or, to put it another way, each person has areas of weakness that require support to enable them (or, more particularly, their organs) to function optimally within their limits. The task of the herbalist is to assess and enable each person's potential. Diagnosis is based on assessment of the individual's vitality and their level of toxic encumbrance.

This model for understanding health and disease has similarities with other traditional health systems which also classify people into constitutional types and which understand disease states as springing from excesses or deficiencies of substances considered elemental within these traditions. Traditional Chinese medicine, for example, includes concepts such as *qi* (vitality), *yin* and *yang*, and five elements of wood, fire, earth, metal and water. The Indian Ayurvedic tradition describes *prana* (energy), and three constitutional types of *kapha* (water and earth), *pitta* (fire and water) and *vata* (air). Causes and classification of diseases, qualities of different foods and herbal medicines, and broader cosmology are all explained by complex interactions of these elements, influences and forces. Diagnosis and holistic treatments are individualised within these frameworks.

Individualisation of diagnosis and holistic treatment are also central to contemporary approaches to Western herbal medicine. Treating people, rather than diseases, and assessing the cause of health problems in a way that incorporates the whole picture of a person, are key aspects of the naturopathic paradigm. It is useful to have classificatory models, such as theories of the elements, to understand temperaments of both people and herbs. Such frameworks enable practitioners to distinguish between possible treatments, and promote accurate and appropriate prescribing of herbal medicines.

Contemporary Western herbalism still aims primarily to stimulate vitality. This is achieved through addressing four key aspects essential to healthy functioning: enhancing digestion and assimilation of nutrients, encouraging elimination of metabolic wastes, ensuring adequate circulation (of blood to provide nutrients to all cells, and lymph to carry away wastes), and enervating nerve supply. Addressing these fundamental physiological functions enhances vitality by providing an environment that maximises the body's innate healing capacity. Treatment regimens are individualised, holistic and natural (herbs, foods, fasting, rest, sweating, massage, exercise) and without side effects. Ideally, attention is focused on correcting functional disturbances before they cause more structural change and deteriorate into chronic problems.

TRADITION AND SCIENCE

The enduring nature of herbal practice demonstrates its ability to adapt to change. Any tradition needs to maintain contemporary relevance in order to survive. Herbals from different historical periods demonstrate how herbalists reflect contemporary understandings of health and disease in their descriptions of the medicinal actions of the herbs. The concepts they use in their descriptions demonstrate these understandings. Box 2.2 details the challenges of the transmission of traditional knowledge.

A challenge for maintaining contemporary relevance is to decide which aspects of a tradition are central to the tradition and should be retained, and which aspects should be reinterpreted or discarded.

These challenges face the 21st century practitioners of WHM. The way that Western societies understand the world around them is firmly based in the scientific method. Therefore an adaptation required of contemporary herbalists is to reassess and reinterpret traditional understandings in light of current science.

BOX 2.2 Herbals

A herbal is a book which describes the uses of individual medicinal plants. Herbals document the uses of herbs in particular eras. 'Reading the old herbals' has been the major source of transmission of herbal knowledge in WHM and they are a major source of what is generally understood by herbalists to be 'traditional knowledge'. Herbals are often associated with a particular person, for example *Culpeper's Complete Herbal* by Nicholas Culpeper.

However, herbals are informed by practical use and they need to be read in their own specific historical context. They contain a lot of assumed knowledge. Some of this is knowledge which was general knowledge at that time — for example, Culpeper does not include a description of barberry (*Berberis vulgaris*) in his herbal because *'This shrub is so well known by every boy or girl that has attained to the age of seven years, that it needs no description'*. While this knowledge may have been common in 17th century London, few children or adults among his current readers have such knowledge.

This means that the interpretation of herbals from specific historical periods requires specialist understanding — ideally from those who have not only an understanding of the period in question, but also a detailed understanding of the ways that herbalists use plants. The historian Anne Van Ardsdall suggests that we think about herbals as abbreviated texts, or notes for practitioners that must be read with the understanding that they are built upon years of apprenticeship. As she says:

> *The texts make sense because an unwritten text can be assumed to lie between each line of written text: that unwritten text is the voice of the teacher and the memory of the apprentice healer, neither of which we can hear.*
>
> Van Arsdall 2014

Another historian, John Riddle, gives an example of the mistakes and omissions that can occur when researchers depend only on the written record, without an understanding of the assumed knowledge of the underpinning practice. In his research on the historical use of contraceptives, he found many references to the use of the seeds of Queen Anne's lace (*Daucus carota*) for this purpose in some cultures. However, it was only after many years of historical research, and after a conversation with a herbalist, that he learned that the seeds should be crushed, This brings home the limitations of the written record. For if the seeds were swallowed whole,

> *they go through the alimentary canal without absorption, or, in other words, 'they go right through you' ... Nothing in the historical sources specified this critical piece of information. Experienced herbalists may know instinctively to crush the seeds. It makes me all the more aware that medical writings themselves were not sufficient to explain the continuous use of natural products over many centuries. By and large the information about these drugs has been transmitted orally.*

Culpeper N. Culpeper's complete herbal. Ware, Herts: Wordsworth; 1653/1995; Riddle J. Eve's herbs: a history of contraception and abortion in the West. Cambridge, Mass: Harvard University Press; 1997; Van Arsdall A. Evaluating the content of medieval herbals. In Francia S, Stobart A, editors. Critical approaches to the history of Western herbal medicine. London: Bloomsbury; 2014.

The published research on herbs and their therapeutic actions, particularly regarding their pharmacological constituents, is ever increasing and often, but not always, empirical knowledge of herbal actions has been validated by scientific research. This is consistent with the well-cited finding that 74% of plant-derived compounds used in pharmaceuticals were used for similar uses by traditional healers.[24]

New actions and uses of herbal medicines have also been discovered. And further, while there has always been cross-cultural exchange of herbal medicines, scientific investigation of herbs from other cultural traditions has increased knowledge and accessibility of these herbs in the Western herbal tradition. The body of knowledge about herbal medicines continues to expand for the Western herbalist.

Scientific research into herbal medicines has evolved alongside a worldwide movement towards a stronger evidence base for health practices, linking research findings with clinical application (see, for example, Box 2.3 on evidence for the usefulness of St John's wort). Evidence-based medicine is increasingly valued by both practitioners and consumers and it is perceived to legitimise health practices.

BOX 2.3 Tradition and science — St John's wort

St John's wort is named for its red sap which in old Christian beliefs was connected with the blood and wounds of Jesus. It is a very good wound healer, especially as an infused oil applied topically to injuries and strains. It has affinity for the nerves and traditional uses include nerve injuries and nervous complaints, from physical conditions such as neuralgic pain (e.g. sciatica or shingles) to chronic nervous conditions such as restlessness, irritability, anxiety, depression and nervous debility.

Scientific research in the last decade has confirmed the usefulness of St John's wort for treating depression. Numerous clinical trials have found St John's wort as effective as SSRI drugs for the treatment of mild to moderate depression, but with fewer side effects. Mechanisms of action have been clarified as inhibition of synaptic reuptake of several neurotransmitters. The constituent largely responsible for these actions is hyperforin, although other constituents also support this activity. Scientific research has also discovered new actions and uses for St John's wort. For example, hyperforin and other constituents such as hypericin and pseudohypericin have demonstrated antiretroviral and antibacterial actions, and hypericin also has anticancer effects. St John's wort has demonstrated activity against herpes infection and has potential to reduce nicotine withdrawal and to contribute to the treatment of some cancers.

Combining traditional and scientific knowledge expands our knowledge base about actions and uses for St John's wort as well as confirming its efficacy and safety for traditional uses.

Braun L, Cohen M. Herbs and natural supplements: an evidence-based guide. 2nd edn. Sydney: Churchill Livingstone Elsevier; 2007.

Evidence-based approaches already have a strong foothold in the fields of pharmacy and medicine and are increasingly being applied to Western herbal medicines. There are a number of levels of evidence. In vitro studies explore pharmacological activity, usually of single active constituents, and help to scientifically explain mechanisms of action. In vitro studies can also give cause for speculation on new uses for herbal medicines. In vivo animal studies examine the practical application of herbs or their constituents and give some indication of their efficacy and dosage. Human clinical trials provide the most relevant information regarding application of herbal medicines, and randomised controlled studies are considered to provide the highest quality of evidence.

Evidence-based medicine does have some limitations. First, it is very expensive and time-consuming to conduct clinical trials. Scientific investigations of drugs and herbs tend to proceed only if there are foreseeable profits to be made. Patenting herbal medicines can be difficult as many herbs grow as weeds and grow in many parts of the world, so pharmaceutical companies are often not motivated to invest money in researching herbal medicines. Meanwhile herbal medicine manufacturers may not have the necessary infrastructure or resources to conduct their own research. Second, testing herbal medicines as they are used in clinical practice is not straightforward. Scientific investigation of drugs tends to focus on the mechanism of action of specific molecules or constituents. This may have limited clinical applicability in practice as herbs are usually prescribed in their whole form, in combination with other herbs, and alongside other treatments such as dietary changes or nutritional supplementation. Third, scientific research offers a particular type of information that may be applicable across populations but does not necessarily account for a herb's usefulness in individual cases. And last, the prioritising of scientific evidence means that those herbal medicines that do not have an evidence base are rejected as ineffective, rather than simply being viewed as unsubstantiated by clinical research.[25]

In summary, while evidence-based research usefully adds to the existing knowledge about herbal medicine, this kind of information should not necessarily be valued over and above traditional empirical knowledge. In the abovementioned example of St John's wort, it is valuable to have proven the efficacy and safety of St John's wort for treating depression through clinical investigation. However, depression is not the only nervous disorder for which St John's wort has traditionally been prescribed. By valuing scientific research over empirical evidence, other traditional uses for St John's wort, for example as a nerve tonic in the treatment of nervous debility, risk becoming undervalued and eventually lost. Emphasising evidence-based medicine changes the knowledge base completely and is causing shifts in the way herbal medicine is both taught and practised.[26]

Scientific exploration and an evidence base are important but they are not the only valid sources of knowledge about herbs. Accessing historical, empirical knowledge as well as scientific information provides a rich array of material about herbal medicine. Familiarity with both empirical and scientific understanding of herbal medicines, using the vitalist approach, and focusing on the unique presentation of each individual, are all essential aspects of modern Western herbalism.

HERBAL ACTIONS AND CONSTITUENTS

Traditionally herbs have been classed according to their actions on the body and this has been a large component of empirical knowledge about herbal medicines. The ways in which herbalists have understood and described these actions has varied in different historical eras, depending on larger cultural influences of the times. For example, in Galen's time cosmological influences included both natural and supernatural forces and, among other uses, some herbal medicines offered protection against evil spirits. In Culpeper's era imbalances of humours were thought to cause diseases and astrological influences conferred particular activity on herbs. By the time of the physiomedicalists and the Eclectics herbs were classified according to effect on an organ or on tissue. And by the 20th century, the branch of pharmacology dealing with natural medicines and their constituents, pharmacognosy, had evolved as a scientific discipline.

Herbalists use whole extracts of herbs rather than isolated single constituents, not only because they believe that this provides most benefit and protects against unwanted side effects, but also because this is the basis of the way that they understand the action of the herbs which are their tools of trade.

Herbs contain hundreds of chemical constituents, some more pharmacologically active than others, and the development of the study of pharmacognosy has once again changed our understanding of how herbs work. The therapeutic actions of herbal medicines are due to one, or more usually some, of these active principals. Constituents can be classified by their chemical structure, and each class of compound has recognisable therapeutic actions. As plants contain many different kinds of compounds, they usually have multiple actions. This may include protective actions (for example, one constituent may be toxic, another protective) or synergistic actions (constituents that enhance the activity of other constituents). What follows is merely a brief description of some of the major constituent classes of herbal medicines and some examples of herbal medicines containing these compounds.[27,28]

Carbohydrates

Carbohydrates form a large class of compounds which includes the gums and mucilages (examples include *Linum* spp., *Plantago psyllium* and *Ulmus fulva*) that are strongly hydrophilic (absorb moisture) and thus make useful bulking laxatives. Pectin is another carbohydrate found in many fruits and is used medicinally to absorb toxins and encourage elimination through the bowels. The gums, mucilages and pectin are cleansing and soothing to mucous membranes. The branched long-chain polysaccharides are very important compounds in herbal medicine as their main action is immune-modulating. Herbs containing these constituents include *Eleuthrococcus senticosus*, *Astragalus membranaceus*, *Echinacea* spp., *Chlorella*, and shiitake and reishi mushrooms.

Glycosides

Glycosides are sugar ethers composed of a sugar (usually glucose) component, the glycone, and a non-sugar component, the aglycone. This is a large and diverse class of constituents with a variety of therapeutic roles in herbal remedies, including:

- Anthraquinone glycosides have an osmotic effect in the large intestine causing a laxative action. Examples include *Aloe vera, Rhamnus purshiana* and *Cassia senna.*
- Saponin glycosides (discussed further under sterols) have a bitter, acrid taste and are often irritating to mucous membranes.
- Cyanogenic glycosides, used as flavouring agents, nervines and anti-carcinogens. Laetrile and amygdalin, found in apricot kernels, are examples of cyanogenic glycosides; however, they are too toxic to be used as medicine. Prunasin (found in *Prunus serotina* and *Prunus amygdalus*), which converts to hydrocyanic acid, can be extremely poisonous but in small quantities is an excellent expectorant.
- Isothiocyanate glycosides, found in the seeds of many cruciferous plants. These cause local vasodilation and can be used therapeutically as counter-irritants to loosen phlegm in bronchial or sinus areas. Examples include mustard (*Brassica nigra*), horseradish (*Armoracia rusticana*) and nasturtium (*Tropaeolum majus*).
- Cardiac glycosides which have powerful effects on the heart, increasing the force of systolic contractions. Traditionally herbs containing these constituents (such as *Convallaria majalis, Digitalis purpurea, Urginea scilla*) were used to treat congestive heart failure, but as these herbs have a very low therapeutic index they are considered unsafe and are no longer available to naturopaths to use therapeutically.
- Iridoid glycosides which are monoterpenoids and give herbs their bitter principle. Bitters stimulate digestive secretions from stomach, pancreas and liver. Bitter herbs include *Gentiana lutea, Andrographis paniculata* and *Artemisia absinthium.*

Flavonoids

Flavonoids are plant pigments that give flowers, fruits and berries their colour. Examples such as quercetin, rutin and bioflavonoids (e.g. hesperidin) are found in citrus fruit, rosehips and green peppers and act to strengthen and tone capillaries. Other types of flavonoids include flavones, flavonols, isoflavones and flavins, which are anti-inflammatory, anti-allergic, antiviral and antioxidant (e.g. *Silybum marianum, Crataegus oxycantha, Ginkgo biloba* and *Scutellaria baicalensis*).

Phenols

Phenols are one of the largest group of chemical components in plants and have a variety of physiological effects. The simple phenols include salicylates and salicins (such as found in *Filipendula ulmaria* and *Salix alba*) which convert to salicylic acid in the body and have analgesic, antipyretic (reducing fever) and anti-inflammatory effects:

- Phenylpropanoids, which may also be glycosides, include cynarin (found in *Cynara scolymus*) which is hepatoprotective and hypocholesterolaemic, and curcumin (found in *Curcuma longa*), also hepatoprotective as well as anti-inflammatory and hypotensive.
- Lignans are common phenolic compounds found in grains (for example linseed or flaxseed) and pulses (especially soybean). They have phyto-oestrogenic (phytosterolic) properties and can also be antioxidant and anti-carcinogenic. Herbal examples include *Schisandra chinensis* and *Silybum marianum*.
- Coumarins commonly have mild anticoagulant, antimicrobial or antispasmodic effects. Herbal examples include *Aesculus hippocastanum*, *Angelica archangelica* and *Medicago sativa*.
- Quinones can have significant antioxidant, antimicrobial and antifungal effects (for example *Drosera rotundifolia*, *Juglans cinerera*, *Tabebuia avellanedae*), a subset, the anthraquinones, have laxative effects (for example *Rumex crispus* and *Rhamnus purshiana*).
- Tannins are also polyphenolic compounds, discussed below.

Tannins

Tannins form a very large and complex group of substances made from phenolic acid and found in isolated parts of plants such as unripe fruit, bark, leaves or stems. Tannins have an astringent action and are used for treating diarrhoea and topically for skin abrasions. Examples include *Agrimonia eupatoria*, *Geranium maculatum* and *Hamamelis virginiana*.

Oils

This class of compounds includes volatile (essential) oils and fixed oils (lipids). Essential oils are the component that gives plants their scent and they have been used therapeutically for thousands of years. They have a complex chemistry but are mainly terpenes and terpenoids (see below). They are very potent and not usually used internally as isolated compounds. The ketone volatile oils, for example, can be neurotoxic internally. However, in whole herbs the volatile components are generally safe and have a great variety of effects, from antiseptic to expectorant to spasmolytic. Some examples of herbs with reasonably high levels of volatile oils include *Apium graveolens*, *Mentha x piperita* and *Rosmarinus officinalis*.

The fixed oils are completely different chemical compounds and include the essential fatty acids, which are an essential component of cell membranes and regulate inflammation and cholesterol. Plant sources of essential fatty acids include borage (*Borago officinalis*) and evening primrose (*Oenothera biennis*).

Resins

Resins are a more concentrated form of volatile oil, exerting antimicrobial, astringent and anti-inflammatory properties. Herbal examples include *Boswellia serrulata*, *Calendula officinalis* and *Commiphora molmol*.

Terpenes

These compounds are commonly found in medicinal herbs, with varying effects depending on their level of chemical complexity. The monoterpenes are the major class of chemical compounds found in essential oils (e.g. *Eucalyptus* spp. and *Pinus* spp.) and the iridoid glycosides. The diterpenes are the most bitter of all terpenoid compounds (e.g. in *Marrubium vulgare*) and are commonly in Lamiaceae family herbs (e.g. *Salvia officinalis*) and can have pronounced activity (e.g. vasodilatory, hypotensive, bronchodilatory effects of *Coleus forskohlii*, and antimitotic activity of *Taxus baccata*). The sesquiterpenes are found in the essential oil component of plants and are, for example, responsible for the blue colour of chamazulene essential oil in *Chamomilla recutita*. Sesquiterpene lactones are bitter and are characteristic of Asteraceae family plants (e.g. *Achillea millefolium*, *Arnica montana* and *Artemisia* spp.), where they are known to commonly cause contact dermatitis.

Sterols and saponins

Phytosterols are tetracyclic triterpenoids and include the saponin glycosides which are characterised by producing a lather in water. Phytosterols contain precursors to cortisone (steroidal sapogenins) and are found in *Aesculus hippocastanum*, *Bupleurum falcatum*, *Dioscorea villosa*, *Glycyrrhiza glabra* and *Withania somnifera*.

Alkaloids

Alkaloids are nitrogen-containing compounds and form one of the most diverse and complex group of chemicals found in plants. Alkaloids are usually highly active pharmacologically as they can cross the blood–brain barrier and depress or stimulate the central nervous system and interact with neurotransmitter receptors.[29] Many alkaloid-containing herbs cause adverse reactions or are toxic, thus many are on the poisons schedule and are not available for use by herbalists. Examples of alkaloids include caffeine, nicotine, morphine and cocaine. The different types of alkaloids include:

- Xanthine alkaloids are mild stimulants and can temporarily raise blood pressure; examples include caffeine and theobromine, found in tea, coffee and chocolate.
- Pyrrolizidine alkaloids are toxic in large doses; examples include nicotine (in tobacco, *Nicotiana tabacum*) and senecionine in comfrey (*Symphytum officinalis*).
- Tropane alkaloids activate the central nervous system and paralyse the peripheral nervous system, and have been used ritually to alter states of consciousness. Hyoscyamine, hyoscine and scopolamine are all tropane alkaloids that are found in deadly nightshade (*Atropa*

belladonna), thornapple (*Datura stramonium*) and henbane (*Hyocyamus niger*). These herbs have a history of medicinal use for their anticholinergic and antispasmodic actions. However, they are toxic even in low doses and their effects are cumulative as the alkaloids are not well excreted.[27] As herbs containing these alkaloids can cause respiratory and circulatory failure (and death) they are not available for use by herbalists today.

- Indole alkaloids, including vincristine and vinblastine (from the herb *Catharanthus roseus*), have been isolated for use as chemotherapeutic agents in the treatment of leukaemia and Hodgkin's lymphoma. However, they have major side effects and can only be prescribed by medical practitioners.[30] Another herb scheduled due to its powerful effects, notably on the central nervous system, is *Rauwolfia serpentina*, as its alkaloid reserpine has toxic side effects.
- Phenylalkylamine alkaloids include ephedrine, found in *Ephedra sinica*, which acts as a central nervous system stimulant.
- Quinoline alkaloids include quinine (from *Cinchona* spp.), used to treat malaria. Isoquinoline alkaloids exert sedative and analgesic properties and are found in *Corydalis cava* and *Eschscholzia californica*; more potent examples are morphine and codeine (both found in the opium poppy, *Papaver somniferum*). Other examples of isoquinoline alkaloids include berberine and hydrastine, which are strongly antimicrobial and found in *Berberis* spp. and *Hydrastis canadensis*.

Herbal medicines are prescribed according to their known effects or actions. These effects may be understood through empirical knowledge or through evidence provided by the study of pharmacognosy (Box 2.4). Both sources of knowledge have validity and relevance to the modern practice of WHM. There are complex interactions and synergy between the multiple constituents of each herbal medicine and supposition of activity based on chemical analysis needs to be balanced with demonstrated clinical usefulness.

BOX 2.4 Different approaches — traditional and scientific

An example of different approaches to the application of herbal medicines is *Echinacea* spp.: its historical use by native Americans for the treatment of snakebites; and its properties as a stimulating alterative lymphatic blood cleanser by physiomedicalists. It is specifically used to treat acute toxic conditions and as part of the naturopathic approach to the treatment of chronic infective conditions.

Modern science supports this knowledge but from a different perspective. Research demonstrates that different chemical constituents of *Echinacea* stimulate immune activity in humans in various ways: nonspecific cellular immunity, macrophage, leucocyte and natural-killer cell activation, antiviral, antifungal and anti-inflammatory actions. Science thus supports the use of *Echinacea* in the treatment of both acute and chronic infections.

Bartram T. Encyclopedia of herbal medicine. Christchurch, Dorset: Grace Publishers; 1995; Braun L, Cohen M. Herbs and natural supplements: an evidence-based guide. 2nd edn. Sydney: Churchill Livingstone Elsevier; 2007.

SAFETY AND INTERACTIONS

Empirical knowledge of plants and their actions forms the basis of herbal medicine. This includes knowledge of herbal indications, contraindications, dosage and safety issues and is based on generations of clinical experience and observation in both oral and written forms. However, herbs are now being used in new forms and concentrations which require reassessment of traditional understandings. In the last few decades in particular there has also been much scientific investigation of efficacy and safety of many herbal medicines. With the increasing popularity of herbal medicine use in Australia, it is particularly important to understand and clarify issues around the safety of herbal medicines and the interactions between herbs and drugs (Box 2.5).

Interactions between herbal medicines and drugs will become increasingly important to assess as stronger and more refined herbal medicines are produced. There are a number of sources of information regarding the safety of herbal medicines;[25,29] however, many popular herbs have not been scientifically studied. No evidence of safety does not mean that herbs are unsafe, but rather that no scientific investigation has confirmed safety.

BOX 2.5 A case of herbal medicine safety

The importance of investigating the safety of herbal medicines can be demonstrated in the case of black cohosh (*Cimicifuga racemosa*). Black cohosh is used extensively for the treatment of menopausal symptoms and its efficacy for this purpose has been well established in multiple clinical trials. However, there have been reports of serious adverse events and concerns about its use in pregnancy and in women with breast cancer. Recent systematic analyses have demonstrated, however, that black cohosh is generally safe to use. As a precautionary measure, it is recommended that black cohosh be avoided in the first trimester of pregnancy (which empirical information sources also suggest). Preliminary investigation of the mechanism of action of black cohosh also leads to speculation that black cohosh may have a beneficial interaction with anticancer treatments such as tamoxifen, and thus women on these medications may require lower doses.

It has been important to explore and understand the mechanisms of action of black cohosh and to rigorously test its safety for women in vulnerable and complex situations. A positive outcome has been the discovery that in fact this herb may enhance the action of anticancer treatments in women with breast cancer.

Braun L, Cohen M. Herbs and natural supplements: an evidence-based guide. 2nd edn. Sydney: Churchill Livingstone Elsevier; 2007.

Safety in pregnancy

The issue of the safety of herbal medicines is particularly fraught when it comes to treating women during pregnancy or lactation. Concerns for the viability of the pregnancy and the health of the fetus need to be foremost in the herbalist's mind. Avoiding herbs that may be toxic to mother or child, teratogenic substances (that may cause fetal abnormalities) or herbs that stimulate the uterus (and may cause miscarriage) is essential. Proving safety of herbal medicines for pregnant or lactating women is a vexed proposition, as it is for all medicines, as it is unethical to conduct research on this population. Empirical evidence suggests that only a small number of herbs are contraindicated in pregnancy and during lactation, but there has been very little scientific research supporting (or negating) this knowledge. There is speculation about the safety of many — some would say any — herbs in pregnancy, usually based on understandings of individual pharmacological constituents of herbs and their bioactivity. This has led to much conflicting advice in the literature. Common practice in this situation is to rely on data from empirical sources of evidence and animal studies.

There is a general consensus that it is best to avoid or minimise the use of internal herbal treatments in the first trimester of pregnancy, as this is the time of greatest embryonic development. This includes using caution when treating women who are trying to conceive. Exceptions to this rule are treating health issues particular to this period of time, such as threatened miscarriage or nausea ('morning sickness').

It is generally agreed that all toxic herbs (e.g. *Phytolacca decandra*) should be avoided throughout pregnancy and lactation. This stipulation also includes concentrated essential oil extracts (taken internally) and large doses of laxative herbs, especially those containing anthraquinone glycosides.

Some herbs that are contraindicated in pregnancy, such as uterine stimulants, may be usefully employed in the last 6 weeks of pregnancy to prepare for labour. A full discussion can be found in Chapter 18.

Historical note

The use of herbal medicine during pregnancy was discussed by John Scudder in 1898:

> *The state of the uterine system too must not be overlooked, for the periods of menstruation, pregnancy and lactation are attended with peculiarities in relation to the action of medicines. Thus the employment of aloëtic and drastic purgatives must be suspended during the catamenia and period of pregnancy; agents likewise which exert any powerful influence upon the system should not be administered at these times. Agents which are absorbed and communicate injurious properties to the blood, should be avoided during pregnancy and lactation; so too should all cathartic or other medicines which communicate their properties to the milk of the mother, while she is nursing.*[31]

Potential interactions

Through scientific endeavour knowledge of interactions, both herb–herb and herb–drug, has steadily evolved over the last few decades. Interactions can be either positive (beneficial) or negative (adverse) and may be mild, moderate or severe. An example of a negative herb–herb interaction is combining tannins with alkaloids as the tannins form complexes and precipitates and inhibit absorption. Other herb–herb interactions may be beneficial, such as saponins enhancing lipid solubility. Traditional herbal prescribing using a combination of herbs in a formula relies on positive herb–herb interactions as a way of enhancing particular herbal actions within a formula.

Herb–drug interactions can similarly be either mild or severe, positive or negative. In-depth knowledge of pharmacokinetics and pharmacodynamics allows for better understanding of the potential for interactions; however, much is still speculative as there have not been enough clinical studies conducted to confirm outcomes of many herb–drug combination therapies. Those drugs with a narrow therapeutic index, such as digoxin and warfarin, warrant special attention when it comes to their potential to interact with herbs or other drugs, as small changes to any aspect of their pharmacokinetic properties can have serious consequences.

PRINCIPLES OF HERBAL TREATMENT

The contemporary Western herbalist considers the historical principles of herbal treatment and the naturopathic approach combined with the best modern science has to offer. A good grounding in the naturopathic paradigm, empirical knowledge and the latest scientific research, a thorough understanding of herbal actions and herbal pharmacognosy and up-to-date expertise on issues of interactions and herbal safety, are all essential components of knowledge for professional herbalists today.

FORMULATING A HERBAL PRESCRIPTION

Herbal treatment usually involves a multifaceted approach and a combination of different herbs in a coordinated prescription or formula. While in some situations it may be appropriate to use 'simples', that is prescription of only one herb usually given in drop doses (see below), more commonly illnesses and their causes are complex and a more sophisticated approach is required. This takes some thought and planning and, of course, sound knowledge of herbal materia medica.

The following is a systematic approach to arrive at an individual prescription:

- Patient presents with condition(s)
- Practitioner takes a case history, physical examination, laboratory investigations and (if applicable) traditional evaluation (e.g. iris diagnosis, pulse diagnosis)

- All the gained information is condensed into a diagnosis (or provisional diagnosis if there is not enough information to come up with a definitive diagnosis)
- Practitioner considers probable underlying causes
- Practitioner decides on a final diagnosis and treatment approach
- Other medical and non-medical treatments as well as current pharmacological treatments are considered
- Holistic aspects including social, cultural, environmental, economic and spiritual are considered
- Final treatment and management plan is developed.

Case taking and diagnosis

To attain the desired outcome of recovery from illness, correct diagnosis in the first instance is essential. Once the patient's history has been attained, a therapeutic strategy can be devised with clear aims. Individualising aetiology complicates the process of diagnosis because establishing the underlying causes of illness is often not straightforward. Where in conventional medicine diagnostics are increasingly technical, relying on laboratory tests or the use of sophisticated equipment, naturopathic diagnosis relies heavily on detailed case taking. However, the medical diagnosis does not need to be as precise (and often cannot be) as is the case in orthodox practice. We are often dealing with functional disorders rather than pathologies. This is not to say that we cannot manage a patient's pathology; it merely emphasises the fact that many of our clients fall into the medical 'too hard basket'. For example, the patient has consulted a medical doctor for a range of symptoms, has undertaken several pathological investigations which have returned negative, and therefore, according to the current medical viewpoint, because there is no pathology the patient is well. However, the patient is clearly unwell and suffers several debilitating functional problems such as nausea in the morning, low appetite, aching lower back and extreme fatigue. Obviously the patient's metabolism is not functioning as it should; however, it has not yet progressed to a pathological state. The range of tests has demonstrated this and so a medical system that relies almost exclusively on medical tests would view this patient as well and thus belonging in the medical 'too hard basket'. However, as holistic practitioners we recognise dysfunction and prescribe remedies to correct dysfunction; and good case taking will usually provide enough information to indicate how this person ended up with their symptoms.

Case taking

When taking a case, questions about each body system are asked to determine other health issues that may be impacting on the initial concern or that need to be considered overall. This is consistent with the paradigm of holistic practice. Questions on sleep, mood, energy levels and ability to recover from illness help the herbalist to assess the patient's vitality. Personal and family medical histories are useful indicators to potential areas of weakness (for example, a family history of hypertension might lead the herbalist to pay particular attention to function of the heart, kidneys and nervous system). Details of diet and other lifestyle factors such as exercise and stressors provide information on nutritional deficiencies or excesses and other adverse influences on health. Physical examinations are another source of information and an opportunity to both assess and reassure the patient through touch. Iridology provides insight into a patient's constitution and areas of weakness, tension or 'toxicity'.

Diagnosis

Diagnosis for the modern herbalist should contain elements of both medical and naturopathic frameworks. This means that the herbalist needs to have knowledge of pathology and also of naturopathic philosophy. Take endometriosis as an example. This is a medical diagnosis, confirmed on laparoscopy (a surgical procedure), and is usually treated surgically and/or hormonally. The herbalist, however, would view this as a condition of pelvic congestion and differentiate between the need to cleanse, relax or tonify the pelvic region according to other signs and symptoms in the individual patient. An understanding of the physiological and pathological mechanisms is essential, especially given the implications for fertility. But herbalists also need to recognise what is unique about what they have to offer for the treatment and prevention of this disorder. Understanding the medical framework is important, especially in order to effectively communicate with other medical personnel; however, herbalists need to frame diagnosis and focus treatment within the naturopathic paradigm. Working alongside other health professionals, such as doctors, is often of great benefit for patients.

Therapeutic strategy

The therapeutic strategy of the Western herbal medicine practitioner focuses on the concept that the human body, when in a state of optimal health, has the ability to resist disease and heal itself of common ailments, and maintain homoeostasis. The concept of enhancing or compensating physiological functions within the patient is essential to ensuring a holistic therapeutic strategy enabling both short- and long-term patient health outcomes to be addressed. It is important that the more traditional approach of enhancement is used simultaneously with the more allopathic strategy of compensation.

ENHANCING STRATEGIES

By enhancing normal physiological processes, individuals have the greatest opportunity to prevent and fight disease and maintain good health, as evidenced in the metaphor about attending to the soil to nourish the seed, so that it grows into a strong plant and is more resistant to disease. Similarly the concept of enhancing a patient's own bodily functions can ensure that their inherent healing ability can be enhanced. This concept draws on the traditional idea of 'vitality' or the innate energy of a person, and seeks to enhance this through physiological means. This may involve correcting underlying disharmony within the patient, by balancing areas of over- or under-stimulation. Of particular importance in this strategy is the use of tonifying, adaptogenic and trophorestorative herbs. One of the prime differences between conventional and naturopathic medicine is that the former looks for common causes of a given illness in different people (e.g. a pathogen), while the latter looks for unique causes in different individuals (e.g. the cause of the immune system's inability to fight off infection). Where medicine focuses its attempts on killing the pathogen (e.g. with antibiotics), naturopathy focuses on enhancing the individual's innate ability to fight the infection (e.g. boosting vitality). It is vital that the modern Western herbal medicine practitioner continues to focus on using enhancing strategies when composing a treatment plan.

COMPENSATION STRATEGIES

The use of herbs in a direct compensatory function can ensure that the symptomatic complaints of a patient are promptly addressed, while the aforementioned enhancing strategies work on the underlying cause(s). A wide range of bodily functions can be directly enhanced by the use of herbal medicines. Herbal subgroups commonly starting with 'anti' are a good example of this, such as anti-inflammatory, antibacterial, antiviral or anti-allergic.[32] These herbs assist the patient by doing the job for them. Herbs that act directly on hormonal cascades or organ function without also tonifying or restoring them also fall into this category (e.g. sedative herbs).

CASE STUDY

John, aged 40, presented with symptoms of a mild head cold, complicated by swollen and painful glands in the neck and throat area. He complained that he developed these symptoms every few weeks. Case taking revealed that 12 months previously John had glandular fever and had only taken a couple of days off before 'soldiering on' back to work full-time. He admitted to feeling tired and run down since then.

Clearly John's recurring acute symptoms stemmed from his unresolved glandular fever, and his lymphatic (glandular) and immune systems were compromised. The herbalist gave priority to the treatment of John's immediate symptoms (compensation strategies) and encouraged him to take time off work 'as if he had the glandular fever now', to allow for a more complete recovery. A herbal formula and dietary advice were dispensed.

In the longer term the herbalist made plans to cleanse and strengthen John's lymphatic system and to build up his vitality (enhancement strategies). In this way John would be better able to fight off any infections and eventually prevent them from recurring at all.

Treatment aims and strategy

Devising a therapeutic strategy is at the heart of treatment of any illness. The strategy needs to be clearly and consciously designed and appropriate to both the management of the illness and the circumstances of the patient.

There are a number of steps along the way, each involving skills and knowledge. Of fundamental importance to the herbalist is a thorough understanding of pathophysiology, naturopathic philosophy, herbal materia medica and sources of good nutrition. Some knowledge of other related fields is also helpful, such as botany, iridology, nutritional medicine and mineral therapies. These are all building blocks of knowledge necessary for the contemporary professional herbalist. Other skills help to make a well-rounded practitioner: an understanding of human psychology, reasonable counselling skills, a calm disposition and a clear mind will all help the practitioner to focus and the patient to feel heard. This fosters a positive therapeutic relationship, which is essential to deep healing.

Notwithstanding the importance of seeking and treating underlying causes of illness, it is also imperative that patients get symptomatic relief from any pain or discomfort. Determining priorities of treatment should occur early on in the consultation and acute problems need to be given first priority. Acute illnesses are usually expressed as sudden onset of marked symptoms, often accompanied by fever, and often short-lived. Giving priority to the treatment of acute illnesses is important for a number of reasons. First, because they are usually uncomfortable and demanding of immediate attention. Second, acute problems can also indicate 'fault lines' or areas of weakness that need to be strengthened to prevent more serious problems in the long term. Third, good resolution of acute illnesses is very important to prevent problems being driven deeper into the body where over time they may become more chronic. And finally, it is important to focus on acute treatment and not address chronic conditions in the acute state.

Historical note

The following paragraph was written by the Eclectic physician Eli Jones in 1911 and is highly relevant to the modern practitioner:

> *An old gentleman had a sick child and called a doctor, who examined the child about as described above and then began to prepare the medicine. The father asked, 'What ailed the child?' The doctor replied, 'Oh, it's a little cold and some fever.' The old gentleman said, 'Doctor, I will pay you for the visit but you need not leave any medicine.' The second doctor came and examined the child in about the same manner and his diagnosis was as indefinite as the other. He was not allowed to leave any medicine for the child. The third doctor came; he examined the child and then began to prepare the medicine. The father said, 'What ails the child, doctor?' 'Why it's measles, any fool ought to know that,' was the doctor's answer. 'All right, doctor, you may prescribe for the child.' The old gentleman was sensible. No doctor should be allowed to give a dose of medicine unless he can give an intelligent reason why he gives it, what he gives it for, and what he expects it to do.*

Once causes of illness have been established, the next step is to decide what treatments are needed to rectify the situation. This step can be usefully compartmentalised into short- and long-term treatment aims. In the short term priority should be given to relief of symptoms and the processes of cleansing, tonifying, stimulating or relaxing should begin. In the longer term lifestyle factors such as diet, exercise and stress management are particularly needed to address imbalances. Once the herbal practitioner has clarified what needs to be achieved in the short term, appropriate herbal actions can be determined immediately.

Approaches to treatment using herbal medicines are either traditional or scientific. The traditional approach focuses on herbal actions and the scientific approach focuses on active constituents. Many herbalists use a combination of both understandings of herbal medicines in their treatment of patients.

CASE STUDY

Using the case study above we can use different approaches to herbal treatment. The herbalist planned to cleanse and strengthen John's lymphatic system and to build up his vitality. Using a traditional interpretation, the following herbal actions could be considered appropriate: lymphatic alterative, immune stimulant, antiviral/antimicrobial, trophorestorative, tonic. The scientific approach, focusing on active constituents, may look to use herbs containing long-chain polysaccharides to stimulate aspects of the immune system, flavonoids for their antiviral and anti-inflammatory properties, resins for their anti-inflammatory, astringent and antimicrobial properties and phytosterols for their tonic properties.

HERBAL ACTIONS

Choosing herbal actions can be based either on traditional understandings of herbal materia medica, or on knowledge of active constituents of herbs and the physiological effects they have. What is most important is to match desired herbal actions to treatment aims. Using the case study cited above, the herbalist's aim in the short term was to treat John 'as if he had the glandular fever now'. This would entail initiating treatment of an acute viral illness. Diaphoretic teas or therapeutic baths could be used to stimulate perspiration and promote proper resolution of fever. As this is a debilitating state, bedrest would be essential. Enhancing immune function through prescription of antiviral, immune-stimulating and lymphatic cleansing herbs would also be appropriate actions at this initial stage of treatment. This approach of cleansing, resting and supporting the body's natural defence mechanisms allows for more complete recuperation from the acute phase of the illness. As glandular fever can have long-term consequences, follow-up treatment, especially the use of herbal tonics, is essential. A 'clean' diet and plenty of bedrest are also important components of long-term treatment. Alternating acute treatment strategies whenever acute symptoms return, followed by some weeks of restorative herbal tonics between bouts of infection, will ensure complete resolution of the glandular fever symptoms and the underlying viral overload. This protocol will ensure that vitality is gradually restored and the patient will become more robust and energetic, and more able to fight off infection.

CONSTRUCTING A HERBAL FORMULA

Before constructing a herbal formula there are a number of steps, of which making a naturopathic diagnosis is by far the most difficult. To diagnose accurately relies on knowledge of the patient, knowledge of pathophysiology, and comprehensive understanding of naturopathic principles. Thorough case taking is essential, including past health history, assessment of nutritional status and levels of stress. This information enables assessment of the patient's vitality and an understanding of why this person has this problem at this time. A solid grounding in both medical and naturopathic paradigms allows for an understanding of the patient's illness from different perspectives. What a doctor calls endometriosis, a herbalist might diagnose as pelvic congestion; what a doctor calls anxiety, a herbalist might diagnose as nervous debility.

Assessment of vitality also helps to determine the appropriate force or depth of treatment: the more vital the patient the more robust they are, and the deeper the treatment can be. For patients with poor vitality, time must be given to nourishing and restoring them, to enable them to withstand more aggressive treatment of underlying problems.

Having clarity about the cause(s) of illness in this person at this time enables the herbalist to clarify what needs doing now and over time. From this a treatment plan can be devised.

CASE STUDY

Maria had a history of severe constipation. Medical investigation had led to a diagnosis of irritable bowel syndrome. Maria was advised to try over-the-counter laxatives; however, these caused painful abdominal cramping. So Maria sought the help of a herbalist. The herbalist took a thorough case history and diagnosed Maria with pelvic congestion caused by inappropriate diet and nervous tension. For symptomatic relief she prescribed a herbal formula containing antispasmodic and carminative herbs, bitters and nervine relaxants. She made some dietary modifications emphasising high-fibre foods, and showed Maria some relaxation techniques as a way of helping to manage stress.

Devising a herbal formula requires clarity of purpose and sound knowledge of materia medica and herbal pharmacognosy. It is important that the herbal prescriptions reflect the treatment aims. Aside from these considerations, herbal formulas may vary between practitioners according to their preference and the availability of herbs.

One example of a herbal formula for Maria could be a combination of:

- Chamomile (*Chamomilla recutita*)
- Wild yam (*Dioscorea villosa*)
- Fennel (*Foeniculum vulgare*)
- Liquorice (*Glycyrrhiza glabra*)
- Cascara (*Rhamnus purshiana*)
- Gentian (*Gentiana lutea*).

Easing spasm and tension in the lower digestive tract is achieved through the antispasmodic action of chamomile and wild yam, the carminative action of chamomile and fennel, the gently warming action of fennel, the demulcent action of liquorice and the relaxing nervine action of chamomile. Gentle stimulation of the bowels is achieved through the action of the bitter cholagogues gentian, wild yam, cascara and chamomile, and through the mild purgative effects of liquorice and cascara. Generalised soothing and relaxation are achieved through the use of liquorice with its adaptogenic properties, as well as the nervine action of chamomile. Liquorice and fennel improve the overall taste of the familiar and are a counterbalance to the extreme bitterness of gentian.

The process of devising a treatment strategy that would lead to construction of a herbal formula can be summarised into a number of steps:

- Decide upon a naturopathic diagnosis
- Assess vitality
- Clarify treatment aims, both short and longer term
- Construct a treatment strategy, including medicines, dietary and lifestyle advice
- Clarify what herbal actions will achieve these aims
- Select the most appropriate herbs
- Choose appropriate amounts of each herb in the formula
- Decide on appropriate dosage of the overall formula.

Amounts of each herbal medicine in the formula will vary according to the emphasis of action. For example, in Maria's case, if the tension is considered to be the main contributing factor to the constipation, herbs with relaxing and antispasmodic actions will dominate the mixture. If it is more an issue of underactivity of digestive processes, then bitter action will predominate. Overall dosage will depend on individual requirements, and is discussed in a later section on dosage.

While individualisation of diagnosis and treatment is the mainstay of naturopathy, there are situations where treatment can be generalised. This is particularly true of acute conditions such as common viral illnesses. In these instances a more generic herbal formula can be dispensed to the majority of patients.

The process of constructing a herbal formulation

In order to design a herbal treatment formula the following points must be considered.

HERB SELECTION

The type of herb selected will depend on a number of factors:

1. Treatment principles selected and the type of person presenting. For example, the patient's constitution.
2. Treatment method required, i.e. will the herbal medicine be prescribed to tonify, regulate, eliminate or other?
3. Type of condition treated. Each type of condition will require varying approaches. For example, chronic conditions typically require mild herbal medicines for long-term use whereas acute treatment typically requires medium to strong herbal medicines in medium to high doses.
4. Consideration of existing presentation. Presence of injuries, infection, fever, etc. will also require symptomatic treatment.
5. Patient's constitution. Those with strong constitutions can benefit from stimulating herbal medicines, whereas those with weak constitutions require combinations of restorative medicines when prescribing eliminative regimens.
6. Intensity of effect desired/outcome. Always remember that different herbal medicines produce varied effects. The quality of the herbal medicine must be considered as well as the dose prescribed.
7. Season, climate and environment. The season will determine the type of prescription. In summer, cooler herbal medicines are encouraged due to the natural increase in body temperature. Conversely during winter, warmer herbal medicines are prescribed to stimulate the body and warm the patient.
8. Availability of herb. Clinic stock and local availability of particular herbs will determine the final selection of a herb.

DURATION OF TREATMENT

In general the duration of treatment will be determined by the following factors.

Nature of the botanical

The strength of the chosen herb/s will determine how long this particular herb or the formula containing this herb can be used:

Mild herbs (e.g. marshmallow)	Long-term — more than 3 months
Medium herbs (e.g. echinacea)	Medium term — between 1 and 3 months
Strong herbs (e.g. *Lactuca virosa*)	Short term — less than 1 month

Principle of the treatment

Depends if the treatment is aimed at:

Constitutional and preventive treatment	Long-term
Rebalancing the disharmony	Short to long-term
Symptom relief	Short term

Nature of the condition treated

Treatment length will be determined whether the condition in general is:

Acute–subacute	Usually short-term treatment with relative high doses in short succession — up to every ½ hour
Chronic–degenerative	Usually long-term treatment with relative low doses dispensed possibly only 1–2 times per day
Local	Usually short to medium term. Dosages medium to high depending on the particulars of the condition. Often uses topical application
Systemic	Usually medium to long-term. Dosages low to high depending on the condition. Usually internal
Of endogenous or exogenous cause	Short to long-term depending on cause and presentation. Dosages low to high depending on the severity of the symptoms and condition
Internal	Medium to long-term. Medium to low doses
External	Short to medium-term. Medium to high doses
Deficient nature	Medium to long-term. Medium to low doses
Excess nature	Short to medium-term. Medium to high doses
Cold	Medium to long-term. Medium to low doses
Hot nature	Short to medium-term. Medium to high doses

Individual constitution

Some constitutions are more sensitive than others consequently they will require different duration of treatment:

Strong constitution	Short- to long-term treatment. Medium to high dose
Weak constitution	Medium- to long-term treatment. Medium to low doses

PREPARATION OF HERBAL MEDICINES

Quality of herbal medicines

The quality of a herbal medicine can be affected by all stages of production, from the raw material through to all processes of manufacture of the end-product medicine. Sourcing of medicinal plants is particularly complex because the chemical composition of the plant will vary due to such factors as climate (temperature, rainfall, hours of sunlight) and soil quality as well as processes of harvesting, drying and storage of plant material. In addition, each step in the manufacturing process can affect the quality of the end product.[33]

Sourcing of herbal medicines

The sourcing of medicinal plants is a complex issue as these plants are sourced from around the world. Supply chains are long, and in most cases it is not possible for herbalists to understand the provenance of the plants they use. This is particularly the case in Australia, where almost all plants are grown overseas. Most species are wild harvested. In Europe, of the 1500 plant species traded in and native to Europe, only 120–130 are under cultivation.[34] In India, most of the estimated 177 000 tonnes of medicinal plants used domestically each year are collected in the wild.[35]

Plant populations are under threat, with 15 000 of the estimated 50–80 000 plant species used medicinally worldwide being threatened with extinction.[36]

Three factors contributing to the threats can be identified. First, overharvesting is common, largely due to increased demand, which means all medicinal plant populations are under pressure. This is largely due to an increase in the use of herbal medicines in developed countries and the increased use of concentrated extracts as opposed to simple preparations of medicinal plants.[37]

Second, changes in land use, through the clearing of land for agricultural use and the demands of increased urbanisation, or through natural or human-made disasters including civil unrest, can destroy the habitat of medicinal plants.

Third, climate change requires the plants to adapt. For example, as increases in temperatures occur, plants requiring cool or cold temperatures move further from the equator and/or to higher ground in order to survive.

IS INCREASED CULTIVATION THE ANSWER?

Cultivation is appropriate for some plants, particularly those for which large amounts are required, such as chamomile and peppermint. Cultivation can also provide manufacturers with control over the growing and harvesting of the raw materials used in their products. However, not all plants are easily cultivated: many require a particular ecosystem in order to survive. In addition, there are social and cultural reasons why wild-grown medicinals are important.

In an era where both practitioners and patients are increasingly interested in the provenance of coffee, food and clothes, and the demand for sustainable, fair trade and organic products is ever-increasing, both herbal practitioners and their patients would like more information about the provenance of the medicinal plants they use.[38,39]

Stringent plant identification techniques are essential to ensure the correct species is being used and that there is no adulteration of medicines with mistaken plant product. Plant identification is most accurately achieved through a laboratory-based technique of thin layer chromatography, which can also be used to test for the presence of marker compounds. Marker compounds are constituents that can indicate medicinal activity and can be used as a measure of quality. Quality of raw herbal matter should also be assessed through sight, smell and touch. Plant material should be of a good colour, smell fresh (not mouldy or musty), and be well dried but not powdery.

In Australia, the manufacture of herbal medicines is legislated under the Good Manufacturing Practice (GMP) code for quality assurance. This includes controls on processes of screening for contaminants, hygiene of the manufacturing environment, testing and identification of plant material, documentation of manufacturing processes, labelling and post-production quality control. Two exceptions to the GMP code are products made by practitioners for individual supply to patients, and home manufacturing of medicines for personal use. For home manufacture, naturally it is sensible to be mindful of the need for accurate plant identification, and appropriate hygienic measures. Labelling end products is imperative, as is the keeping of accurate and complete records of manufacture. The GMP code is in place to ensure minimal microbial contamination and to safeguard against substitution of the correct plant product for another that may be ineffective or unsafe. In general, Australia has excellent quality control and standards of manufacture, although unfortunately this is not true of all countries, even industrialised ones.

Quality of raw materials and proper manufacturing techniques determine the efficacy of herbal medicines. The higher the quality of the starting material and the better the manufacturing processes, the more effective the herbal medicine.

Historical note

The following extract is taken from John Scudder's 1898 book *The American Eclectic Materia Medica and Therapeutics*:

> *That the physician may be certain as to the quality of these remedies when he makes his purchases, it is well that he should prepare some of them himself. Office pharmacy is profitable in this way if in no other. It may be very simple. You gather the agent in the season when its virtues are greatest, pound it up in a mortar, if you have one, on a board with a hatchet or hammer if you have no mortar, put it in a glass or glazed vessel that can be tightly stoppered, cover it with twice its weight of alcohol (76 to 98 per cent, as the crude article contains resinous substances), and let it stand fourteen days. It is now ready for use. Pour off the tincture, express all you can get out of the drug, and if you want a very nice article, filter through paper. Your Pharmacist turns up his nose at the crude process, but it won't turn up when he is shown the product and has it compared with the 'fluid extracts' on his shelves. It is a sound and reliable remedy, and will give success in practice.*[40]

Standardisation

The standardisation of herbal medicines is a vexed issue. Theoretically standardisation ensures consistency of strength of a medicine. It tests that levels of certain chemical components, marker compounds, are consistent to ensure uniformity between batches of medicine. From the scientific perspective standardised extracts of herbs are useful in research where reproducibility and predictability are important concerns.[25] However, for the practising herbalist there are a number of concerns with this process. Herbs are chemically complex and there may not be agreement about which are the main active constituents to use as marker compounds. In fact there are often multiple active constituents that may work synergistically, so the presence of one constituent in a standardised amount may not be a useful indicator of overall activity. In herbal medicine the saying that the 'whole is greater than the sum of its parts' is generally true. A further concern about standardisation is that herbs may be manipulated to ensure high levels of marker compounds at the expense of other constituents. Given that this may impact on synergistic actions, this kind of manipulation may affect both safety and efficacy of the herbal medicine. Another concern is that extreme forms of standardisation processes involve isolation of particular constituents, in much the same manner as drugs are formulated. The problem with this is one of philosophy as much as practice: in this form the herb is more akin to a drug and is, like drugs, more likely to cause side effects and other adverse events.

Types of herbal preparation

In addition to those factors influencing quality of herbs and variations of standardisation processes, another variable that affects potency of herbal medicines is the different forms of herbal preparations (Table 2.3). Herbs can be used medicinally in a number of forms. What form is administered depends on the condition being treated, availability and convenience, as noted by John Scudder in his 1898 text when he states: 'the most convenient and agreeable form of exhibiting [the herbal medicine], whether it should be given alone, or combined with other ingredients, and how far these are likely to impede, modify, or facilitate its operation [should be taken into account when prescribing]'.

POSOLOGY — HERBAL MEDICINE DOSAGE

Posology, the study of dosage, is a highly controversial area of herbal medicine. In part this arises from the variation in quality, form and type of preparation, but there are also different philosophical approaches to treatment which determine dosage protocols. There are multiple traditions and sources of information, including the pharmacopoeias, other herbal traditions and clinical trials.

Historical perspective

In the late 19th century the Eclectic physician John Scudder[40] wrote in his book *Specific Medication and*

TABLE 2.3 Different herbal preparations

Preparation	Process	Advantages	Disadvantages
Topical preparations Poultices Compresses Creams Ointments Liniments Suppositories Pessaries Infused oils	Water- or oil-based or both	Useful to treat local wounds or inflammation	Messy Oil-based preparations only dissolve lipid-soluble constituents and easily become rancid
Dry preparations Powders	Powdered dried herbs (barks, seeds or roots)	Easily incorporated into food or drinks	Can be difficult to swallow May have an unpleasant taste Have a short shelf life
Dry preparations Tablets Capsules	Compressed powdered dried herbs or spray-dried concentrated liquid extracts	Convenient Bypass unpleasant tastes Can be enteric-coated, useful to avoid irritating the stomach or to avoid alcohol	Excipients added for binding, lubricating, colouring, flavouring and coating Generally low dose Not as well absorbed as liquid forms Lack flexibility for individual prescribing
Liquid preparations (water extracts) Infusions Decoctions	Dried herbs steeped in boiling water (leaves, flowers) or simmered (roots, bark)	Avoids alcohol Hot preparations encourage diaphoresis Increase fluid intake, useful for treating urinary tract problems Pleasant taste	Water a poor solvent, limits extraction of some constituents (e.g. resins) Do not preserve well Need to be prepared daily — inconvenient
Liquid preparations (glycerine extracts) Syrups Oxymels Glycetracts	Syrups and oxymels are a combination of liquid preparations (fluid extracts, juices, decoctions) with sugar or honey Glycetracts use glycerine as solvent	Sweet taste Emollient and demulcent — soothe mucous membranes Avoids alcohol Sugar preserves the medicine for many months	Not as potent as alcohol extracts
Liquid preparations (alcohol extracts) Tinctures Fluid extracts	Water and alcohol combined as solvents Tinctures 1 : 3 (weight:volume) or weaker Fluid extracts most concentrated, usually 1 : 1 or 1 : 2 but can be made up to 8 : 1 concentrations	Most concentrated preparation, so require the smallest dose Alcohol preserves the extract, allowing for a long shelf life Readily absorbed Easy to make into individualised prescriptions	Generally taste unpleasant

Source: Adams J, Tan E. Herbal manufacturing: how to make medicines from plants. Melbourne: Adams & Tan, 1999, p. 15. With permission of Melbourne Polytechnic.

Specific Medicines, that 'As a rule, the dose of medicine should be the smallest quantity that will produce the desired result'. His philosophy was to use minimal medicinal dosing of singular herbs (made largely from fresh herb tinctures) that matched the patient's symptom picture as evident in yet another of his rules: 'it is best to employ remedies singly, or in simple combination of remedies acting in the same way'. In this he differed from his contemporary John Uri Lloyd, who used drop doses of more concentrated herbal liquids, maintaining that the doses used by Scudder were not potent enough. The issue of dosage has been a highly contentious one throughout the long history of herbal medicine practice, and continues to be so to this day.

Modern perspective

Provided that the practitioner has been appropriately trained in one form of dosing with consideration given to philosophical and practical approaches (namely vitalistic or pharmacological), the results for their patient are likely to be positive, as the practitioner will be acutely aware of what is in the best interests of the health of the patient. The merits of each philosophy should be emphasised, rather than deciding that one or the other is more correct. Fittingly, Eli Jones commented in his book *Definite Medication* in 1911:

> *In our grand and noble profession we have no place for a narrow-minded man, a bigoted man. A physician who*

cannot see anything good outside of his own particular school of medicine is a small-minded man and will find his level as such men always do.

Both approaches acknowledge an innate energetic quality of the herbs involved, and that a unique synergy can come from either a well-chosen single herb or a combination of herbs, providing patients with many health benefits. Indeed, at the centre of each philosophy is the understanding that each patient is an individual and requires a unique formulation and dosage. This was described aptly in Scudder's 1898 text when he stated that 'in prescribing a medicine, it is necessary to consider the age, sex, temperament, habits and idiosyncrasy of the patient, before the dose can be properly apportioned'.[31]

VITALISTIC APPROACH

Simples

Some herbalists prefer to treat using 'simples' (the use of one herb at a time). This approach which, as previously mentioned, largely stems from the philosophies of the Eclectic physicians Scudder and Lloyd, has some similarities with homoeopathy in that herbs are matched to the patient's symptom picture, and only very small doses, from 10 to 50 drops daily, are prescribed. In this approach the 'energetics' of the herb is felt to be as influential as any physical action they have on the patient's biochemistry. This approach is practised by some, but not the majority, of Western herbalists.

Polypharmacy

Another kind of approach is polypharmacy where multiple herbs, perhaps 8–15 different herbal medicines, are combined together into a formulation. This system is used popularly in Ayurvedic medicine and traditional Chinese medicine, where herbs are formulated into prescriptions based on a particular framework. Within the Western herbal tradition, some herbalists follow a similar approach when they find that particular herbs work together synergistically, but caution needs to be taken so that this does not end up as a 'shotgun' approach that indicates an inability to properly diagnose or clarify priorities of treatment. Using many herbs in a formula also means only small amounts of each herb can be included and this may lead to less effective treatment.

PHARMACOLOGICAL APPROACH

The most popular guidelines for dosage are based on pharmacopoeias like the British Herbal Pharmacopoeia (BHP) and the German Commission E monographs. Dosage recommendations in the BHP come from combining recorded historical accounts with average doses used by UK herbalists surveyed in the 1980s and from information gathered in earlier texts such as the British Pharmacopoeia and the British Pharmaceutical Codex. There are some problems and inconsistencies in this method but it is still a very useful guide. The Commission E, established by the German Health Department, also in the 1980s, comprised a committee of industry and academic experts who reviewed clinical research and combined this information with traditional knowledge.[32] The resultant herbal monographs were then compiled, released for public comment and reviewed again. Thus the German Commission E monographs are considered to be of exceptional quality and of great use to the modern practitioner.

The dose of each herb in the pharmacological approach is usually expressed as a range of either daily or weekly amounts. For example, dosage of chamomile (*Chamomilla recutita*) can be calculated at:

- 2–8 g dried herb (taken as an infusion) three times daily
- 1–4 mL of a 1 : 1 fluid extract three times daily, or
- 20–40 mL fluid extract per week.

There is a broad dosage range listed for most herbs as they have a wide therapeutic index, and thus a wide margin for safety (and efficacy), when compared with pharmaceutical drugs. However, care should be taken for herbs that have a low safety margin (e.g. *Phytolacca decandra*), ensuring that the patient is given small, incremental doses in order to avoid side effects from occurring. Further discussion regarding dosage for different subgroups of the population (such as children) can be found later in this chapter.

The pharmacological approach often employs a relatively small number of herbs in a formula (4–6 herbs), although the daily dose for the whole formula can be quite high, for example between 4 and 10 mL two to four times per day (a total of 8–40 mL/day). When comparing the modern dosages of herbal medicines to the traditional dosages of their Indian and Chinese counterparts, the ranges in general are strikingly similar (and tend to be in the higher dosage range).[32]

MANUFACTURERS' DOSAGE RECOMMENDATIONS

Herbal medicine manufacturers label each liquid extract with a suggested dosage range and this can be used as a guideline; however, there is merit in checking multiple sources, including the pharmacopeias mentioned above, for dosage recommendations. The herbalist can then construct a herbal formulation which includes a number of herbs within the recommended dosage range. The way in which an extract is produced can greatly impact on the dosage range, and for this reason the manufacturer dosage guidelines are useful. Extracts that are produced from reconstituting more concentrated extracts produce vastly different end results to those that are made from more traditional methods such as reserved percolation.[32] Theoretically a 1 : 5 extract has more than five times the activity than a 1 : 1 extract, and this should be taken into account by the practitioner.

CONSIDERATIONS FOR LIQUID FORMULATIONS

There are many ways to think about constructing a herbal formula, and the goal is always to ensure that the practitioner maintains the fundamental therapeutic objectives when choosing the herbs to include in a particular herbal mix. The following is one example of a framework that can be used to achieve this end.

Type of desired herbal action

When considering which herbs within a formula should have a higher dose, it is important to consider the actions that the practitioner desires:

1 *Prime mover herbs* are given dosage emphasis within the formula, and are those that are most highly indicated. These herbs can often be included to treat the patient's symptomatic complaints, such as sedatives to improve sleep.
2 *Adjuvant herbs* are those that are indicated, but are included more for their supportive or tonifying actions, that work over a longer time frame. These herbs are often enhancement herbs, such as adaptogens, that help aid the stress response over a longer time frame. Further subgroups of adjuvant herbs are described below:
   a *Helper herbs* help the prime mover work. They are not always necessary; however, for example, you may want to include *Marrubium vulgare* in a cough formula to help loosen mucus.
   b *Assistant herbs* are those that are included for secondary health problems. For example, if you include *Matracaria recutita* in a digestive formula it will strengthen the digestive system and improve sleep.
   c *Moderator herbs* reduce any overtly strong effect in the prescription. These are not always necessary. An example may be where you include a warm herb such as ginger to a mixture to reduce the mixture's cooling effects.
   d *Messenger herbs* are included only if necessary and ensure that the energy of the prescription goes to the organ most affected. For example, you may want to combine goldenseal and elecampane to direct both herbal medicines to reduce mucus from the lungs (both would work on the lungs; however, the combination would enhance the effect).
   e *Harmonising herbs* can be included to harmonise and integrate a prescription. A good example is liquorice; it is not always necessary nor is there always room in the bottle, however, it is advantageous if possible.

Synergy

Synergy is a concept used to describe the philosophy that the overall result of the combined formula is greater than the effects of its individual constituents.[32] This concept (difficult to quantify and qualify) is widely accepted as fact by many herbalists, although it should be questioned, especially since there is considerable traditional evidence for using singular rather than combined herbs. Some early trials are being conducted that support the concept of synergy, but not all combinations of herbal medicines should be considered 'synergistic' simply because they are in the same bottle. Overlapping actions of different herbs within a formula need to be taken into account when devising a prescription and dosage, in order to ensure that the desired actions are enhanced and the undesired minimised. The synergy of herbal medicines should not be underestimated as they can provide profound results, given the right circumstances, although future research needs to be conducted.

Nature of the herb

The nature of the herb in question needs to be considered, for example in the case of bitters, only small amounts are needed to stimulate digestive secretions, so lower doses are preferred.

Quality

The quality of the raw material (see above) affects the final dosage required. As already discussed, this factor is difficult to control. Even if all manufacturing and processing techniques remain the same, individual batches of herbs from different raw materials can deliver vastly different end products. Therefore manufacturing companies often standardise levels of certain constituents, in an attempt to ensure a higher degree of consistency.

Preparation form

The form of preparation, as mentioned previously, can significantly affect the dosage range. This is due to the nature of the active components and the method of extraction that ensures their best mode of delivery to the patient. For example, a larger amount of fresh ginger is required in a herbal infusion (tea) as compared with an alcoholic extract (tincture).

Individual response

Variations to dose depend on individual circumstances such as sex, weight, organ function, absorption and metabolism, timing (e.g. before or after food), current medication, tolerance and route of administration.[33]

Dosage methods for modern herbal prescriptions

The following comments relate to the dosage of alcoholic extracts, which in Australia are most commonly prepared from dried plants as 1:1s and 1:2s. Some herbalists prefer 1:5s and/or to use extracts prepared from fresh plant material.

AMOUNT PER WEEK METHOD (Table 2.4)

The amount per week method is the most common method of determining dosage and dispensing quantities. It is calculated by the fact that a daily dose can be converted into a weekly dose for convenience of dispensing. The therapeutic dosage of herbs is listed in this form (i.e. mL/week). Dispensing dosages are then based on the fact that 105 mL can fit into a 100 mL bottle or 210 mL can often fit into a 200 mL bottle, allowing for a dosage of 5 mL t.d.s. or 7.5 mL b.i.d. or a single daily dose of 15 mL to be prescribed. Thus if a herb dose of 2–3 mL three times daily (t.d.s.) is required, this is converted into the weekly dose of 42–63 mL (rounded to 40–65 mL). So if this herb was a prime mover a dose of 55–65 mL would be included in the 100 mL bottle, leaving 35–45 mL for 'adjuvant' herbs to be included. This would

TABLE 2.4 Example — Amount per week method

Herbal medicine	Ratio	Dosage range (per week)	Dosage per week	Dosage for 2 weeks
Chamomilla recutita	1:2	20–40 mL	40 mL	80 mL
Glycyrrhiza glabra	1:1	10–30 mL	30 mL	60 mL
Gentiana lutea	1:1	5–15 mL	10 mL	20 mL
Rosmarinus officinalis	1:2	15–30 mL	20 mL	40 mL
Dosage: 5 mL t.d.s.				
TOTAL			100 mL	200 mL

TABLE 2.5 Amount per dose method 1

Herbal medicine	Ratio	Dosage range (per week)	Quantity per dose	Dosage per week
Chamomilla recutita	1:2	0.95–1.9 mL	1.51 mL	31.51 mL
Glycyrrhiza glabra	1:1	0.75–1.42 mL	1.41 mL	29.41 mL
Gentiana lutea	1:1	0.23–0.71 mL	0.51 mL	10.51 mL
Rosmarinus officinalis	1:1	0.71–1.42 mL	1.36 mL	28.61 mL
TOTAL			5 mL t.d.s.	105 mL

then be dispensed at a dose of 5 mL t.d.s., or 7.5 mL b.i.d. If the practitioner wanted to see the patient in 2 weeks, the amount of prime mover herb would be multiplied by 2. (See Table 2.4.)

AMOUNT PER DOSE METHOD 1 (Table 2.5)

The amount per dose, for each herb, is calculated by dividing the weekly range by the number of doses per week (i.e. a prescription of 5 mL t.d.s. over 1 week = approximately 21 doses). This can give the practitioner a higher degree of accuracy when determining how much of each herb the patient is consuming in each dose. To make up the final formula the amount of each herb per dose is scaled to the total required for the bottle, as shown in Table 2.5.

This technique is of particular use when prescribing herbs that have a high level of toxicity, or potency (e.g. *Phytolacca decandra*) or if you wish to prescribe herbs at a dose other than at 5 mL t.d.s. or 7.5 mL b.i.d. (See Table 2.5.)

AMOUNT PER DOSE METHOD 2 (Tables 2.6 and 2.7)

An alternative method of amount per dose method is as follows.

Dosage formula

$$\frac{\text{total amount}}{\text{total minimum amount}} = X$$

$$X \times \text{each minimum dose} = \text{mL}$$

EXAMPLE

Herbal formula including the following herbs:

TABLE 2.6 Amount per dose method 2 (sample formula)

	Daily dosage range	
Herbal medicine	Minimum	Maximum
Rehmannia glutinosa	4.3 mL	8.6 mL
Iris versicolor	2.9 mL	5.7 mL
Cynara scolymus	2.9 mL	7.9 mL
Calendula officinalis	1.4 mL	4.3 mL
Thymus vulgaris	2.1 mL	5.7 mL
TOTAL	13.6 mL	32.2 mL

As we have 5 herbs in this formula, we can determine how many millilitres are required for each herb at the minimum therapeutic dose.

For example:

$$\frac{\text{total mL}}{\text{total minimum dose of all herbs in formula}} = \text{n}$$

In a 200 mL bottle (that can fit 220 mL) we divide the total mL by the total minimum dose of all herbs in formula, that is:

$$\frac{220}{13.6} = 16.18\,(\text{n})$$

We then take n (16.18) and multiply it by the minimum quantity of each herb (as listed in Table 2.6) to

TABLE 2.7 Amount per dose method 2 (calculation of formula)

Herbal medicine	Minimum	Calculated qty	Qty required
Rehmannia glutinosa	4.3 mL	69.57 mL	70 mL
Iris versicolor	2.9 mL	46.92 mL	45 mL
Cynara scolymus	2.9 mL	46.92 mL	45 mL
Calendula officinalis	1.4 mL	22.65 mL	25 mL
Thymus vulgaris	2.1 mL	33.98 mL	35 mL
TOTAL	13.6 mL	220.04 mL	220 mL

Qty, quantity.

determine the total quantity of each herb required for a therapeutic effect.

This can be best summarised as shown in Table 2.7.

OUTCOME

Therefore, the dosage calculation is between 13.6 and 32.2 mL/day (calculated minimum and maximum dosage range of all herbal medicines), and the realistic recommendation for your patient will depend on the speed of action required, the patient's condition and temperament.

Dosage could be 15 mL/day (5 mL t.d.s.) or could increase to 30 mL/day (10 mL t.d.s.) or anything in between.

Treating children

Deciding on the dosage required for each patient is basically an art that improves with time. Each child has a different temperament, a different constitution and a different metabolic rate. Once the practitioner has connected with the patient they will begin to determine what 'type' they are. Each person will respond to the same herbal medicines differently. Some people have very strong affinities and aversions to certain medicines and some people are very sensitive to dose fluctuations. As a general rule, always start with a low dose and be selective with the herbal medicines. If presented with an 'allergenic' child, be realistic and start them on one drop of the medicine, preferably in the clinic, and watch their reaction. It is unlikely that they will have any reaction; however, it will give great insight into their connection and response to the medicine so that their therapeutic dosage can be recommended confidently and accurately.

In pre-pubescent children it is usual to avoid very stimulating or heating herbs, all toxic herbs, and hormonally active herbs. The bitter taste of many herbal medicines and the alcohol content of fluid extracts can be off-putting for children, although if they have taken this type of medicine since infancy they will not flinch. Disguising the medicine's flavour with syrups, cordials or fruit juice helps with compliance — and medicinal syrups can be used to enhance the overall medicinal activity too. Children are usually given small, frequent doses as they generally metabolise very quickly.

Generally speaking, all herbal medicines are fine to give to children in theory, provided they are given at the correct dosage. Understandably some herbal medicines resonate more strongly with children than others. Both of these points should be taken into account when preparing formulations. Teenage children can be given adult doses unless they are particularly small for their age.

THERAPEUTIC DOSAGE

For a herbal medicine to work it must be given at a therapeutic dosage; that is, the amount required to produce a therapeutic result. Higher amounts of the plant are appropriate when your aim is to give more of the plant material; lower amounts of the plant are appropriate when your aim is to give a more energetic level of the plant. In fact, both therapeutic ranges work best for different types of patients.

It is essential to recognise that some children will be incredibly sensitive to the energy of the plants and will have wonderful reactions to the teas, while others may require stronger therapeutic dosages.

SAFE DOSAGE

The safe dosage of a herbal medicine is the amount of the herb that can be administered safely. The recommended dosages in the example below are safe therapeutic amounts (for an adult). It is imperative that you adhere to the recommended dosages. Please note that dosages are calculated for adult long-term use. Short term (acute conditions), the dosage *may* be increased above the maximum (though never for *Tylophora indica* or *Phytolacca decandra*); however, do not exceed the dosage drastically. This is especially important in smaller children and babies. It is best to be safe and adhere to recommendations and use the therapeutic freedom when treating older children and adults.

RECOMMENDED DOSAGE

When working with children you will notice that small dosages are very successful. Children have a wonderful ability to respond very quickly to herbal medicines. Therapeutic recommendations of herbal medicines are general guidelines. Always start at the lower end of the therapeutic margin and if the dosage is not sufficient, it may be increased *gradually* towards the upper limit. The art of giving herbal medicine is finding the correct amount for the person (child) you are treating.

There may be times when it is appropriate to give a higher dosage:

- When the patient does not respond to small dosages
- In acute conditions, when there is no time to waste and you feel it is essential to get things moving.

In these instances it is imperative to use your discretion and monitor your patient closely.

CHILD DOSAGE

Calculating the dosage for children can be easily achieved by using some simple formulas. Please note that these methods are only approximates as metabolic changes can interfere.

Ausberger's rule — based on weight

In kilograms: (1.5 × weight in kg) + 10

EXAMPLES

Child weighs 20 kg: (1.5 × 20) + 10 = 40, so they should receive 40% adult dose.

Child weighs 10 kg then they should receive 25% of adult dose.

Clark's rule — based on weight in kilograms

Weight in kg/67 kg × adult dose = child's dose

Young's rule — based on age

$$\frac{\text{Age in years}}{\text{Age} + 12} \times \text{adult dose} = \text{child's dose}$$

Fried's rule — best for infants (1–2 years)

$$\frac{\text{Age in months}}{150} \times \text{adult dose} = \text{child's dose}$$

EXAMPLE

A child presents in clinic requiring the following herbal formula:

Althaea officinalis 30 mL
Angelica archangelica 15 mL
Inula helenium 30 mL
Tilia spp. 30 mL
TOTAL: 105 mL
Adult dose: 5 mL t.d.s.

For example:

Using the calculation in the example we have provided for Ausberger's rule listed above:

Child weighs 20 kg then they should receive: (1.5 × 20) + 10 = 40% adult dose

Therefore this child requires 40% of adult dosage of 5 mL t.d.s. Therefore the child requires (5 mL × 40%) = 2 mL t.d.s.

> **Historical note**
>
> **John M. Scudder**
>
> *I recall the old practice in diseases of children as being especially unpleasant; and the little fellows were unpleasantly prejudiced against the doctor. It was almost as good as a whipping to threaten a child with the doctor or with medicine. Now the physician is the child's favourite (the small dose physician), and it is a pleasure to see them gather around one when he visits the house. It is also a pleasure to treat the little ones. The remedies are nice and clean, tasteless, and their effects are pleasant and certain. I should be willing to rest my claim to kindly consideration when I finish my work, upon the little I have done to make the practice of medicine pleasant for children.*[41]

Constitution/temperament

Constitution is defined as the whole of an individual's inherited and acquired characteristics.

Generally speaking, people with a strong constitution tend not to have as many illnesses, and when they do, they seem to recover quite quickly. These are the types of people that usually grow up abusing their health because they can get away with it without any ill consequences. They also tend to be less receptive to someone with a weaker constitution, thus showing little consideration for their needs. Please note that someone with a very good constitution can only burn their candle for so long.

Those with a weaker constitution have a greater amount of inherent weaknesses in their body. They need to take extra care of their body — more than someone with an inherited strong constitution needs to take — to stay well. They are more sensitive to foods, environment and stress and tend to take longer to recover from illnesses that occur more frequently in them than in someone with a strong constitution.

Constitution is based on two complementary factors:

1 Genotype, and
2 Phenotype.

GENOTYPE = HEREDITARY FACTORS

Genotype is defined as the person's entire genetic inheritance, including those characteristics that result from the interaction carried by the recessive genes but not expressed in the phenotype. This does not automatically result in all of these genes being expressed.

PHENOTYPE = ENVIRONMENTAL INFLUENCES

Phenotype is defined as 'the entire physical, biochemical, and physiological makeup of an individual as determined both genetically and environmentally, as opposed to genotype'.[42]

The phenotype of any given characteristic arises from two levels of interaction:

- The interaction of the proteins synthesised from the specific genes that affect the characteristic
- The ongoing interaction between the genotype and the environment (gene–environment interaction).

The genotype inheritance may be modified within limits by the phenotype — such as nutrition, climate, home and social life.

The evaluation of a constitution assesses the ability of an individual to withstand diseases and the pathways of weakness which would precipitate disease.

Those patients with a 'strong' constitution require and can withstand high dosing, in contrast to patients with a 'weaker' constitution who require and respond to much lower dosage levels.

Treating the elderly, frail or debilitated

Elderly, frail or debilitated patients also need to be given smaller doses than the average adult dose. Kidney and

Historical note

Temperament: It is doubtless true that temperament exercises a great and important influence over the action of medicines; yet temperaments are so poorly described, and the facts so ill defined in regard to their therapeutic relations that we are almost tempted to pass the subject by, as one that can only be learned by long practice. The sanguine temperament does not bear stimulants well, and is very readily affected by quinine and morphia, as is also the encephalic; while persons of a lymphatic temperament will generally require increased quantities of all remedies to produce a certain effect. We might consider the bilious temperament as the medium between the two named, the sanguine and the encephalic being more and the lymphatic less sensitive to the action of remedies.[31]

liver function naturally decline in those over the age of 60, even in healthy individuals. Consequently the ability of the elderly to metabolise and excrete drugs and herbs occurs at a slower rate than in younger adults, and there is a risk of overdosing. Frailty and debility also indicate the need for lower dosage due to suboptimal organ function and/or hypersensitivity of the nervous system. For all elderly, frail or debilitated patients, calculating dose according to weight of the individual, as per Clark's rule (see above), is a reasonable approach.

Treating overweight or underweight patients

It is also useful to apply Clark's rule to vary doses from the standard when treating noticeably overweight or underweight individuals. For a 90 kg patient, dose could be calculated as 90/60 = 1½ (or 1.5) times the standard adult dose; for example, 1.5 × 5 mL = approximately 7.5 mL three times daily.

Treating hyperallergenic patients

Individuals who suffer from allergies or who have a history of sensitivity to other medications are more likely to react hypersensitively to herbal medicines too. When treating these patients it is prudent to start with very low doses (for example, 10–20 drops per dose in normal weight adults) and instruct patients to gradually increase dosage amounts. They are likely to respond well to lower doses of herbal medicines than might normally be given and so, by keeping to the principle of prescribing the minimum effective dose, may only need substantially smaller doses than the standard measure of 5 mL three times daily. Including a herb to enhance liver function in the herbal prescription would also be most appropriate for these patients.

Acute illness

In acute conditions symptoms are usually extreme and changeable. It is necessary to keep pace with the symptoms with frequent dosing and changes of herbal prescription as required. For instance a common cold, caused by a rhinovirus, often starts with sore throat and fever. Within 24 hours the throat starts to ease but the sinuses and nose fill with phlegm. Initially the phlegm may be clear but it may change to cream or yellow, or even green, indicating secondary bacterial infection. Ears or lungs may become congested with mucus. In each of these phases of the infection the herbal actions required will change: diaphoretics, demulcents and alternatives initially, then later anticatarrhals and astringents, with antiseptic expectorants needed later still. Diaphoresis is best achieved with hot infusions taken frequently. Dosage of other liquid extracts would also be given frequently, for example 3 mL five times daily.

CASE STUDY

Michael brought his 4-year-old son, Oliver, to see the herbalist. Oliver had a history of recurrent ear infections, usually preceded by a head cold, with fever, runny nose and sore throat. The doctor suggested Oliver have grommets implanted to drain fluid from behind his eardrum, but Michael wanted to explore other treatment options first. Oliver had a sore throat now, and his ears were starting to hurt.

The herbalist discussed Oliver's diet in detail and made some suggestions for modification. She prepared a dried herb mixture of diaphoretic, decongestant and anticatarrhal herbs for Michael to take home and make into an infusion for Oliver. She suggested he drink 3 small cups daily with ½ teaspoon of honey. She also prescribed a mixture of fluid extracts containing alterative, antiviral and expectorant herbs, based in a marshmallow syrup, 25 drops to be taken four times daily. She asked Michael to call her the next week to let her know how Oliver was progressing.

REFERENCES

[1] Gwinner H. Male European starlings use odorous herbs as nest material to attract females and benefit nestlings. In: East LM, Dehnhard DM, editors. Chemical signals in vertebrates 12. New York: Springer; 2013.

[2] Huffman M. 2003. Animal self-medication and ethno-medicine: exploration and exploitation of the medicinal properties of plants. Proc Nutr Soc 2003;62:371–81.

[3] Lietava J. Medicinal plants in a middle paleolithic grave Shanidar IV? J Ethnopharmacol 1991;35:263–6.

[4] Martkoplishvili I, Kvavadze E. Some popular medicinal plants and diseases of the upper palaeolithic in Western Georgia. J Ethnopharmacol 2015;166:42–52.

[5] Hatfield G. Memory, wisdom and healing: the history of domestic plant medicine. Stroud: Sutton Publishing; 1999.

[6] Touwaide A, Appetiti E. 2014. Food and medicines in the Mediterranean tradition. A systematic analysis of the earliest extant body of textual evidence. J Ethnopharmacol 2015;167:11–29.

[7] Van Arsdall A. Evaluating the content of medieval herbals. In: Francia S, Stobart A, editors. Critical approaches to the history of Western herbal medicine. London: Bloomsbury; 2014.

[8] Francia S. The use of trade accounts to uncover the importance of cumin as a medicinal plant in medieval England. In: Francia S, Stobart A, editors. Critical approaches to the history of Western herbal medicine. London: Bloomsbury; 2014.

[9] Corn C. The scents of Eden: a narrative of the spice trade. New York: Kodansha International; 1998.
[10] Dalby A. Dangerous tastes, the story of spices. London: The British Museum Press; 2000.
[11] Schivelbusch WT. Tastes of paradise: a social history of spices, stimulants and intoxicants. New York: Random House; 1993.
[12] Aguirre Marco CP. Nationalism and science: Amerindian contribution, Spanish tradition and the "new" American plants in the rise of the United States medical botany. Revista de Fitoterapia 2005;5:103–7.
[13] Monardes N. Joyfull nevves out of the newe founde worlde. London, in Poules Churche-yarde: Willyam Norton; 1577.
[14] Tobyn G. Culpeper's medicine: a practice of western holistic medicine. Shaftesbury, Dorset: Element Books; 1997.
[15] Culpeper N. Culpeper's complete herbal. Ware, Herts: Wordsworth; 1653/1995.
[16] Berman M, Flannery M. America's botanico-medical movements: vox populi. New York: Pharmaceutical Products Press; 2001.
[17] Evans S. Joseph Banks and the continuing influence of European colonisation on Australian herbal practice. Australian Journal of Medical Herbalism 2009;21:3–5.
[18] Griggs B. New green pharmacy. London: Vermillion; 1997.
[19] Martyr P. Paradise of quacks: an alternative history of medicine in Australia. Sydney: Macleay Press; 2002.
[20] Saks M. Orthodox and alternative medicine. politics, professionalization and health care. London: Continuum; 2003.
[21] Willis E. Medical dominance. Sydney: Allen and Unwin; 1989.
[22] Coulter I, Willis E. Explaining the growth of complementary and alternative medicine. Health Sociology Review 2007;16:214–25.
[23] Avila C, Evans S, Morgan A. Herbal wisdom: memory and migration. Coolabah 2011;5:15–33.
[24] Farnsworth NR. Screening plants for new medicines. In: Wilson EO, editor. Biodiversity. Washington DC: National Academy Press; 1988.
[25] Braun L, Cohen M. Herbs and natural supplements: an evidence-based guide. 2nd ed. Sydney: Churchill Livingstone Elsevier; 2007.
[26] Evans S. Changing the knowledge base of Western herbal medicine. Soc Sci Med 2008;67:2098–106.
[27] Evans W. Trease and Evans pharmacognosy. London: Elsevier; 2009.
[28] Bruneton J. Pharmacognosy, phytochemistry, medicinal plants. Paris: Lavoisier; 2008.
[29] Mills S, Bone K. The essential guide to herbal safety. St Louis, Missouri: Elsevier Churchill Livingstone; 2005.
[30] Weiss R. Herbal medicine. Beaconsfield. UK: Beaconsfield Publishers; 1988.
[31] Scudder J. American eclectic materia medica and therapeutics. Cincinnati: Scudder Brothers; 1898.
[32] Bone K, Mills E. Principles and practice of phytotherapy. Edinburgh: Churchill Livingstone Elsevier; 2013.
[33] Adams J, Tan E. Herbal manufacturing: how to make medicines from plants. Melbourne: North Melbourne Institute of TAFE; 2012.
[34] Hamilton AC. Medicinal plants, conservation and livelihoods. Biodiversity and Conservation 2004;13:1477–517.
[35] Booker A, Johnston D, Heinrich M. The welfare effects of trade in phytomedicines: a multi-disciplinary analysis of turmeric production. World Dev 2016;77:221–30.
[36] Robertson E. Medicinal plants at risk. Tuscon: Centre for Biological Diversity; 2008.
[37] Jagtenberg T, Evans S. Global herbal medicine: a critique. Journal of Alternative and Complementary Medicine 2003;9:321–9.
[38] Engels G, Brinkmann J. Chamomile. American Botanical Council Herbalgram 2015;108:8–17.
[39] Evans S, Avila C. Partners in practice: practitioners' perceptions of herbal medicine manufacturers revealed through dispensary decisions. Australian Journal of Herbal Medicine 2016;28:41–7.
[40] Scudder J. Specific medications and specific medicines. Cincinnati: Scuddder Brothers; 1870.
[41] Eclectic Medical Journal; 1877.
[42] Dorland WAN. Dorland's illustrated medical dictionary with CD. Cincinnati: Saunders; 2007.

Principles of nutritional medicine

3

Rachel Arthur

NATUROPATHIC NUTRITION

The international naturopathic literature is unanimous that[1–3] 'nutrition forms the basis of complementary medical practice'.[1] However, this modality, unlike herbal medicine, is not the domain of naturopaths alone, and there are many other health professionals, such as dietitians, nutritionists and integrative medical practitioners, practising nutritional medicine. Differences exist, however, in both the underpinning knowledge and the application of this modality by naturopaths when compared with other professionals. Some would argue that these differences are of such significance as to constitute a distinct modality, hence the term 'naturopathic nutrition'.

The delineation is the result of underpinning naturopathic philosophy which is distinct from medical philosophy, in its promotion of six central tenets:[3]

- The Healing Power of Nature *Vis Medicatrix Naturae*
- First Do No Harm *Primum Non Nocere*
- Treat the Whole Person *Tolle Totum*
- Find the Cause *Tolle Causum*
- Naturopath as Teacher *Docere*
- Prevention *Preventare*

Preventive medicine

While these tenets appear to emphasise vitalism over a mechanistic approach, naturopathy and naturopathic nutrition are a combination of both and, arguably, in the current context move increasingly towards a mechanistic model, with its growing reliance on evidence-based medicine (EBM). However, naturopathic nutrition evolved from 'nature cure', in which dietary correction and therapy constituted the only nutritional intervention. Modern practice of naturopathic nutrition spans the whole spectrum, from more traditional practitioners who restrict their prescriptions to whole foods, to others who employ nutrients, sometimes at supraphysiological doses: for example B_3 for cholesterol lowering; and in highly modified forms, for example liposomal vitamin C; and nutraceuticals, for example DIM, to intentionally manipulate biochemical processes.[3]

Bio-individuality

In its application, naturopathic nutrition upholds as the ideal a diet based on whole, natural foods, particularly one that emphasises quality, fresh, seasonal and organic produce and demonstrates reduced dependence on animal foods.[1,2,4] Equally important, however, is the concept that all individuals have a unique interaction with their nutritional environment and therefore the 'ideal naturopathic diet' may take many different forms within this basic framework in order to meet the diverse needs of patients.

This core principle has attracted the name 'bio-individuality',[1] which is derived from the term 'biochemical individuality' coined by the nutritional biochemist Roger Williams in the 1970s, to articulate the wide inter-individual variability in levels of enzyme activity.[2] Naturopathic adoption of this concept has also led to a broadening of its meaning in order to encompass all the influences that make an individual truly individual, and in the context of nutrition, alter their requirements for nutrients.[5] These influences include:

- Genetics; for example, individuals with the methylenetetrahydrofolate reductase (MTHFR) polymorphism have greater folate requirements than other individuals[6]
- Age; for example, vitamin D synthesis, activity and tissue sensitivity decline with age[7]
- Gender; for example, women typically absorb a greater proportion of the mineral manganese than men, as a result of lower ferritin levels and therefore increased expression of intestinal divalent metal transporter-1 (DMT-1)[8]
- Environmental exposures — heavy metals, toxins; for example, excessive lead exposure can increase an individual's requirements for calcium to prevent toxicity of this heavy metal[9]
- Drug consumption — both prescription and recreational; for example, excessive consumption of alcohol will deplete a large number of nutrients leading to increased requirements[10]
- Pathology; for example, patients with poorly controlled diabetes mellitus type 1 or 2 demonstrate increased urinary losses of chromium compared with individuals not suffering the condition[10]
- Emotional response;[5] for example, increased cortisol release secondary to a stress response is associated with increased losses of vitamin C and decreased adrenal concentration of this nutrient.[11]

Although most practitioners of nutrition may recognise that not everyone who eats salt, for example, will develop high blood pressure, the naturopath's adoption of the concept of bio-individuality forces them to formally consider the physiological idiosyncrasies of each patient.[1] This becomes a lens through which the practitioner can view the adequacy or appropriateness of each individual's diet and, accordingly, assists the naturopath to reassess the merits of nutrient reference values (NRV), such as recommended daily intake (RDI), with respect to the individual patient.

A natural evolution for naturopathic nutrition it would seem then, with regard to the central tenet of bio-individuality, is the much publicised promise of personalised medicine, made possible by the sequencing of the human genome and increased accessibility to genetic testing, which opens the door to an understanding of nutrigenetics and nutrigenomics in our treatment of the individual.[12,13] Although arguments both for and against this approach being incorporated into naturopathic nutrition have been made, it is important to know that while some genetic testing has become highly accessible, the research required to support the depth of understanding necessary for comprehensive and accurate interpretation and application of this remains in the future. (See Nutrigenetics, nutrigenomics, epigenetics and the promise of personalised medicine below.)

THE FUNCTIONAL PRACTITIONER

The traditional orthodox approach to the nutritional medicine prescription is characterised by correction of deficiencies and avoidance of problematic foods.[1] Even while acknowledging patient bio-individuality, a practitioner can continue to practise in this stopgap fashion. Increasingly synonymous with modern naturopathy and naturopathic nutrition, however, is the emerging concept of the functional approach and the functional practitioner:[5] 'The concept of biochemical individuality is central to every aspect of the practice of functional medicine, from clinical assessment and diagnosis to the broad spectrum of treatment modalities'.[5]

The functional approach differentiates itself from the traditional orthodox one primarily by seeking to identify the alteration in function that underpins the presenting problem.[1] Consistent with this is the naturopath's endeavour to bring together seemingly disparate pieces of information and synthesise them into an integrative picture of the whole patient's health and wellbeing, a process referred to as pattern recognition.[5] With respect to nutrition, in which there already exists substantial dynamic interconnectedness between nutrients (agonistic, antagonistic, conditional) and between nutrients in any given specific physiological or pathological context — for example, iodine, selenium and mercury in thyroid conditions — being alert to patterns and using illness as information about the underpinning aberrant biochemistry appears to make sense. The functional practitioner also demonstrates increased attentiveness to the possibility of marginal and subclinical deficiency states and evidence of suboptimal functioning in any part of the body, even in the absence of confirmed pathology (see Clinical picture assessment below).

NATUROPATHIC NUTRITIONAL ASSESSMENT

There is an absence of information in the scientific literature detailing the methods of nutritional assessment employed by naturopaths, their frequency of use, or the weight attributed by practitioners to their results, for example as a diagnostic algorithm. Two previous Australian studies, however, have surveyed naturopaths regarding their general diagnostic methods.[14,15] In addition to orthodox techniques such as vital signs and pathology results, practitioners in both studies reported frequent use of iris, face, tongue and nail diagnosis. Recently another Australian naturopathic survey investigated the assessment methods used in relation to zinc.[16] While these results relate specifically to this mineral and therefore may not be generalisable to other nutritional contexts, they currently provide the only information about how naturopaths assess patients' nutrition.

The results of this study confirm widespread use of both clinical picture assessment and qualitative dietary analysis, considered the cornerstones of traditional naturopathic diagnosis. In particular there was a statistically significant positive relationship between practitioners' use of the two methods, revealing two subgroups: (a) practitioners who exclusively use traditional diagnostic methods, and (b) practitioners who have largely abandoned the use of traditional diagnostic methods. The bulk of surveyed practitioners, however, fell somewhere in between, using a combination of these traditional skills and additional functional or pathological testing.

Clinical picture assessment

Clinical picture assessment (CPA) is the observation and recording of the patient's collective signs and symptoms, a proportion of which may be caused by the inadequate supply of a given nutrient(s), for example koilonychia, or spoon-shaped fingernails, as evident in iron deficiency anaemia. CPA forms the basis of both orthodox and naturopathic nutritional diagnosis[1,17] and when used by clinicians familiar with each nutrient's deficiency picture, provides an important, first-line, non-invasive nutritional assessment technique.

Naturopathic CPA differs from dietetic practice in that a larger range of signs and symptoms may be considered indicative of suboptimal nutrition, including sometimes the specific consideration of nail, tongue and pulse characteristics.[14,15] The principal reason for this is the increased attention awarded by naturopaths to the potential for marginal as well as overt deficiency states. Similarly, there is recognition of functional in addition to pathological impairment.[1] For example, a patient may report experiencing episodes of discomfort in the epigastric region following the consumption of certain foods, such as steak and chicken. In light of negative results for *Helicobacter pylori* and endoscopic investigations, the condition may be declared idiopathic and the dietitian may be at a loss to provide either an explanation or a solution. On the other hand the naturopath may note that the patient's fingernails are particularly fragile and brittle and that their mucous membranes, while not having a pallor indicative of anaemia, are not as red as expected with optimal iron status. When this is combined with the apparent impaired digestion of concentrated proteins, an underlying pattern of hypochlorhydria and secondary suboptimal mineral status may be deduced. In this way the naturopath, while continuing to observe and use orthodox nutritional diagnoses where appropriate, is also a specialist in pattern recognition,[5] bringing individual pieces of information together to form an understanding of the whole.

CPA, however, possesses a range of limitations and weaknesses which make it unsuitable as a stand-alone nutritional assessment method. These include:

- The time taken to manifest characteristic features of long latency deficiency diseases associated with some nutrients, e.g. calcium
- Non-specificity as a result of the overlapping signs and symptoms between multiple nutrient deficiency pictures;[18] for example, angular stomatitis is seen in both iron and riboflavin deficiency
- The potential for deficiency signs and symptoms to remain past the point of repletion with a given nutrient; for example, goitre and iodine deficiency
- Being a non-quantitative method.

Dietary analysis methods

A variety of formal and informal data collection techniques may be used by naturopaths to elicit patients' dietary habits, including 24-hour food recalls, prospective food diaries and food frequency questionnaires. Following this, the nutritional adequacy of the diet is determined using a method that can be essentially categorised as either qualitative or quantitative.

Qualitative dietary analysis (QUALD), while being the traditional method, remains the most dominant practice. It is based on practitioners' knowledge of food nutrient distribution, such that when a patient provides information about food types and quantities, any significant excesses and deficiencies can be recognised.[15] In addition to this, a qualitative analysis offers the advantage of taking into consideration additional key influences such as food processing, cooking methods and nutrient interactions (for example, ≥ 300 mg calcium from dairy reduces iron absorption from other foods by 70%)[10] to determine the true overall nutritive value of the diet.

Other perceived merits of QUALD include the fact that a comprehensive understanding of the individual's dietary habits forms a central part of the naturopathic management and corresponding individualised treatment of the patient. An addition to this is, ideally, that the patient should at the same time be re-educated regarding optimal dietary choices. QUALD, however, also possesses limitations, including the fact that, in the absence of a formalised process, it is unlikely that a practitioner's knowledge of nutrient distribution will be absolute or that they will demonstrate the same degree of familiarity for all individual nutrients, from the macro through to the most ultra-trace. Consequently, the potential for assessor blind spots arises.

In comparison, quantitative dietary analysis (QUAND) methods use a software database for nutrient distribution information rather than relying on the practitioner's own memory. Practitioners using QUAND enter dietary information into a database, which calculates the average daily intake with respect to energy and a select number of nutrients. The results, in comparison to general indications of deficiencies and excesses flagged by QUALD, identify, for each nutrient, whether intake meets, falls below or exceeds the corresponding dietary reference intake (DRI) and by how much. Other advantages of QUAND include the consistency and congruency inherent in computerised analysis; for example, ensuring the comparison of 'apples to apples' when reviewing a patient's dietary changes over time. The depth of analysis provided in some areas also offers an advantage, such as macronutrient contributions to total kilojoule intake and distribution of dietary fatty acids; however, due to a lack of food distribution information, a significant disadvantage is the omission of many trace minerals from these analyses.

In addition to the labour-intensive nature of data entry, which may deter practitioners from employing these methods,[16] QUAND has a number of established limitations.[18] The primary issue rests with the presumption that nutrient composition is both static and generic. The database nutrient values for an orange, derived from a calculated average of a particular sample determined at one time, are applied to all oranges regardless of farming method, time of harvest, region cultivated, period in storage, etc. Critiques of QUAND acknowledge that this is a necessary though problematic artefact,[19] as variables such as these can have a profound influence on the nutrient composition of both primary and secondary foods.[20] Processed foods such as orange juice demonstrate even greater variability (between batches and brands) for additional reasons relating to manufacturing and packaging differences.[21] Another issue presents itself with those database values which have been borrowed from overseas food tables.[19] Particularly in relation to mineral content, these values have shown themselves to be non-transferable from one country to another due to differences in both soil chemistry and agricultural practices.[22,23]

Regardless of whether QUALD or QUAND is used, the naturopath typically applies an additional level of analysis that accounts for the bio-individuality of the patient. In particular the adequacy of the diet would need to be considered in light of digestive efficacy, potential drug–nutrient interactions and environmental exposures. An example of this additional level of analysis is presented in Table 3.1.

Specific nutritional testing

In some instances, the naturopathic practitioner may opt to use additional testing to determine patient nutriture, for example to confirm the preliminary CPA and QUALD findings, monitor changes during supplementation or

TABLE 3.1 Additional levels of analysis performed as part of naturopathic nutrition

Source of influence	Example	Increased nutrient requirements	Decreased nutrient requirements
Genetics	Hereditary haemochromatosis	Chromium and other divalent metals	Iron
Digestive function and efficiency	Fat malabsorption	All fat-soluble vitamins and essential fatty acids	
Lifestyle	High exercise frequency and intensity	Magnesium, vitamin C, chromium, potassium	
Nutrient interactions	Frequent consumption of cola soft drink	All alkaline minerals, e.g. calcium, magnesium, potassium	
Drug–nutrient interactions	Proton pump inhibitor	Impaired solubilisation and digestion of range of nutrients including iron, zinc, calcium, magnesium, copper, chromium, folate, B_{12}, protein	
Environmental and occupational exposure	Lead	Increased calcium and iron will help to minimise lead uptake	

Source: Lukaski HC. Chromium as a supplement. Annu Rev Nutr 1999; 19:279–302; Martí N, Mena P, Cánovas JA et al. Vitamin C and the role of citrus juices as functional food. Nat Prod Commun 2009;4(5):677–700; Moore BJ, Rolls BJ, Mennella JA et al. Soda isn't only low in calcium. J Bone Miner Res 2004;19(5):872; [reply]; Padayatty S, Doppman JL, Chang R et al. Human adrenal glands secrete vitamin C in response to adrenocorticotrophic hormone. Am J Clin Nutr 2007;86(1):145–9; Rolfs A, Hediger MA. Metal ion transporters in mammals: structure, function and pathological implications. J Physiol 1999;518(1):1–12.

assess for toxicity. A number of tests are available for most nutrients including static measures using different biological samples (e.g. hair, blood, saliva) or dynamic indices (e.g. red blood cell transketolase activity as a measure of thiamine nutriture), each with a different level of scientific validation.[24]

The seemingly small proportion of naturopaths currently referring patients for either static or dynamic biological nutritional testing[16] may be the result of a variety of practical and philosophical issues including cost, limited knowledge/education regarding testing options, the invasive nature of some procedures and concerns regarding their validity.[16] Knowledge of nutritional testing options and the adoption of some biological testing, however, appear to be increasing among naturopaths. This is consistent with the emerging recognition that diagnostic techniques, which are essentially reductive, can be an important part of the holistic management of patients.[5]

There is increasing interest among the naturopathic profession in nutritional tests that fall into a third category, functional testing, with some overlap between the three groups.[5] The premise of the functional test is that it facilitates the practitioner's understanding of how the patient's function has been impacted by pathology or suboptimal nutrition. Rather than focusing on diagnoses that compartmentalise diseases into known entities, these tests, while recognising such categories, principally investigate any underlying patterns and processes.[5]

In relation to nutrition, the results generated, rather than comparing how much nutrient 'X' was found in the patient's blood compared with 1000 other patients' blood samples, simply compare the patient to their optimal or unimpeded self. Loading urine tests, for example oral or IV administration of magnesium followed by 24-hour urine collection to determine the rate of retention, are a good illustration of this concept. The results of a magnesium loading test may indicate that the patient has retained a large proportion of the administered mineral; these values are not used as a point of comparison with other individuals' test responses, however, but simply reflect that regardless of level of intake this patient continues to exhibit a functional magnesium deficiency and, in so doing, may help to elucidate the patient's unique requirements for this nutrient.[25] In many instances a combination of both static/dynamic and functional tests can help to paint a more comprehensive picture of the individual's nutriture. Table 3.2 provides a comparison between orthodox and functional assessments of several nutrients.

A small number of these functional tests may be performed within the clinic, for example urinary indican testing and live blood analysis, while others may be performed independent of mainstream laboratories including hair mineral analysis, gastrointestinal (GI) profiles and urinary organic acids. Some functional tests originally familiar only to naturopaths and integrative medical practitioners have attracted the attention of mainstream medicine and are increasingly employed by orthodox practitioners, for example reverse T_3. From the naturopath's perspective, the attractiveness of being able to perform such tests without having to send the patient back to the doctor and in some instances without significant out-of-pocket expense to the patients, should not be underestimated. There are questions, however, regarding the validity of some of these assessments[16] and more research is urgently required to validate them.

TABLE 3.2 Comparison between static/dynamic and functional assessments for several nutrients

Nutrient	Static/dynamic assessment	Comment	Functional assessment	Comment
Magnesium	Serum	Serum magnesium concentrations demonstrate poor sensitivity and specificity due to the small percentage of this nutrient in the extracellular environment and the tight homeostatic control of these levels	Magnesium retention test: IV magnesium loading followed by 24-hr urinary magnesium analysis	Renal magnesium excretion decreases in a deficiency; therefore, those individuals who retain > 20–25% of magnesium are considered to have suboptimal magnesium body levels. The test protocol, however, is currently non-standardised and therefore limits its reproducibility
Chromium	Plasma	Although a plasma level of 0.5 ng/mL is typical this is not believed to be indicative of individual status due to a lack of equilibrium with tissue levels	Pre- and post-supplementation assessment of blood lipids and blood glucose levels	Relative chromium status is retrospectively determined through the observation of changes in parameters affected by chromium nutriture. Chromium supplementation in deficient patients may produce a significant reduction in both blood glucose and lipid levels
Iodine	Random urine test or spot urine test	Although internationally the most established iodine assessment method, this test reflects only short-term dietary intake of iodine and is confounded by several variables, e.g. diurnal variation, hydration	Full thyroid function test: TSH, T_3, T_4 and thyroid antibodies	Although not a substitute for urinary iodine (UI), thyroid assessment constitutes an important illustration of the impact that iodine status (both deficiency and excess) is having on its key endocrine action
Mercury	Blood	This test reflects current levels of mercury exposure and can be used as a monitoring technique in this capacity	DMPS chelation followed by urinary mercury analysis	Heavy metals tend to bioaccumulate, partly due to impaired excretion. Provocation testing such as this reflects not only current exposure levels but also total body content

Source: McKelvey W, Gwynn RC, Jeffery N et al. A biomonitoring study of lead, cadmium, and mercury in the blood of New York City adults. Environ Health Perspect 2007;115(10):1435–41; Padayatty S, Doppman JL, Chang R et al. Human adrenal glands secrete vitamin C in response to adrenocorticotrophic hormone. Am J Clin Nutr 2007;86(1):145–9; Ristic-Medic D, Piskackova Z, Hooper L et al. Methods of assessment of iodine status in humans: a systematic review. Am J Clin Nutr 2009;89(6):S2052–69; Vamnes JS, Eide R, Isrenn R et al. Blood mercury following DMPS administration to subjects with and without dental amalgam. Sci Total Environ 2003;308(1–3):63–71; Wilcken D, Dudman NP, Tyrrell PA et al. Folic acid lowers elevated plasma homocysteine in chronic renal insufficiency: possible implications for prevention of vascular disease. Metabolism 1988;37(7):697–701.

NUTRIGENETICS, NUTRIGENOMICS, EPIGENETICS AND THE PROMISE OF PERSONALISED MEDICINE

Thanks to the sequencing of the human genome and increased accessibility to genetic testing, there is intense interest in exploring gene–nutrition interactions including nutrigenetics (how genes modify nutritional requirements and the individual's response to diet), nutrigenomics (how genes are affected by the individual's diet) and epigenetics (how gene expression is affected by diet and nutrient intake). These technological and research developments are being hailed as the road to 'personalised nutrition' and have been embraced by some practitioners of naturopathic nutrition — as a natural extension of the practice of bio-individuality — and by more orthodox nutritional researchers alike.[12] There are also substantial direct-to-consumer (DTC) testing options available, which add the potential for a consumer-driven change in our practice model and assessment approach.[13]

While the future of gene–nutrition research may hold the promise of ultimately matching the individual's nutriome with their genome to provide optimal genetic and physiological health, our current level of knowledge falls overwhelmingly short.[26] In particular, at this time in the clinical context we are limited to the identification of specific single nucleotide polymorphisms (SNPs), deletions and insertions for a limited number of specific genes that suggest a nutrient interaction. We are not yet able to look at the interaction between these SNPs, their impact on metabolomics or thoroughly ascertain the efficacy of altered nutrition on a range of outcomes in individuals with these.[26]

On a positive note, mainstream nutrition and nutritional science is embracing the naturopathic concept of bio-individuality at last.

NATUROPATHIC NUTRITIONAL TREATMENT

Consistent with the tenets of both bio-individuality and the functional approach, each of the naturopath's nutritional prescriptions, even for the same pathology, is individualised, taking into account the unique contributions to each patient's state of imbalance. The starting point for improved nutrition is the diet, either in terms of modifications to patients' existing habitual eating patterns or with the application of a short-term dietary therapy such as detoxification or an elimination and challenge period as a diagnostic tool for food allergy or intolerance. Unique to the naturopath's nutritional prescription may be the incorporation of some functional foods[20] such as flaxseed oil, broccoli sprouts, seaweeds, spirulina and LSA (linseed/flaxseed, sunflower seed and almond mix).

The implementation of nutritional supplements ideally is considered only when dietary changes, as a vehicle for improved nutriture, have been maximised[2,18] or when the effective dose required cannot feasibly be achieved through food, for example pharmacological actions. There are many clinical scenarios, however, meeting such criteria and therefore necessitating the use of supplements, such as poor-quality food, compromised nutrient absorption, and presence of anti-nutrients in the diet and lifestyle. In fact, a large American study concluded that routine supplementation of a multivitamin across all individuals aged > 65 years would have significant positive economic consequences due specifically to the subsequently improved immune function and reduced risk of cardiovascular disease.[27]

Nutritional supplementation

The variety of nutritional supplements recommended by naturopaths is broad, extending beyond the essential micronutrients to the ultra-trace minerals, individual amino acids, various fatty acid preparations, meal replacements, isolated vegetable constituents, plant-based antioxidants, etc. Traditionally the majority of these supplements were in the form of low-dose combinations, with formulations aimed at treatment of specific imbalances or conditions, for example vitamins A, C and E with zinc for immune boosting. While many products such as these continue to be prescribed by naturopaths (although nutrient doses generally appear to be increasing), recently there has been an influx of higher dose single nutrient products into the market. The latter offers practitioners the opportunity to use some nutrients in 'pharmacological doses', evoking a response distinct from simple nutrient repletion, and supports the tenets of individualistic prescribing.

In addition to this there has also been a shift towards incorporating nutrients wherever possible in forms more comparable with their presentation in food; for example, mixed tocopherols and carotenoids, rather than single isolated isomers and constituents. The rationale behind this pertains to both increased breadth and magnitude of nutrient actions, as well as possibly improved safety.[20,28]

Another burgeoning area of nutritional supplementation, consistent with the evolution of the functional practitioner, is the inclusion of nutrients in their active forms such as methyltetrahydrafolate (MTHF), 5-hydroxytryptophan (5-HTP) and pyridoxal-5-phosphate (P5P). Active nutrients or intermediates are believed to better address patients' bio-individuality in cases where there is evidence of biochemical or metabolic pathway impairment, for example nutrient activation. They also help fulfil the primary treatment goal of the functional practitioner: optimising patient physiology. For example, a patient may demonstrate features of a vitamin B_6 deficiency regardless of high levels of intake. Taken together with the results of functional nutritional testing, a tentative diagnosis of an impaired ability to convert this vitamin into its main active form pyridoxal phosphate (PLP) may be reached. In this instance, the most individualised and effective approach may be the administration of the pre-phosphorylated form.

In spite of the increasing range of novel oral treatment options, in specific scenarios naturopathic practitioners may recommend parenteral administration (e.g. IM or IV). These situations, however, are likely to be in the minority of cases and with specific justification, for example IM B_{12} injections in patients with evidence of B_{12} malabsorption.[10]

Naturopathic nutrition research

Research pertaining to the effects of single nutrient interventions becomes more prolific with each year that passes. For example, while folate's role in homocysteine lowering and reduced cardiovascular risk made its debut almost 30 years ago,[29] at the time of writing 86 articles are cited by PubMed as having been published in the last 12 months on this topic alone. The reason for this burgeoning interest in nutritional research appears multifactorial but it is surely spurred on in part by the push for both more preventive focused approaches to health and the desire to reduce dependence on pharmaceutical interventions, which typically have a higher associated risk of adverse outcomes. It is important also to remember that for many nutrients, the elucidation of their essentiality has occurred only relatively recently, for example zinc in 1961,[30] and accordingly our understanding of these nutrients in human physiology remains in its infancy, with much still to discover.

Nutritional research may take the form of randomised controlled trials (RCTs) of single or small nutrient combinations; for example, selenium and vitamin E, for the prevention or treatment of a condition within a specific patient population, such as the prevention of prostate cancer in healthy men.[31] The nutrient or nutrient combination may be investigated as a stand-alone therapy or as an adjuvant to pharmaceuticals to improve response rates and treatment efficacy and/or to reduce side effects.[32] Similarly specific dietary interventions may be investigated for the prevention or treatment of select conditions.[33]

One particular research growth area is nutrigenomics, investigating the effects of nutrients on genomic stability, which adds weight to both the concept of bio-individuality and the profound influence nutrition ultimately has on disease expression.[20] However, does any of this constitute naturopathic nutritional research? Many would argue that it does not because naturopathic nutrition by definition is about the individualistic prescription, a construct that is the antithesis of current RCT methodology, which seeks to control as many variables as possible.[34] Many argue that effective research into naturopathic nutrition necessitates the inception of a new scientific paradigm and research methodology that can accommodate for individualisation of treatment, combination therapies and non-specific healing effects, in particular. One flagged model is whole practice research, whereby the selected participants, for example patients with the same orthodox diagnosis, are treated by one of a cluster of highly trained practitioners using an individualised approach and prescriptions, such that the practitioner becomes the 'black box'. Advocates of a new practitioner-centred model of naturopathic research argue that this will ultimately produce evidence that more accurately reflects practice realities.[35]

The future of naturopathic nutrition

The current positive momentum of naturopathic nutrition suggests a bright future, in which mainstream medicine has a renewed interest in individualised nutrition as a key preventive strategy against increasing morbidity and mortality in developed countries. The principle of bio-individuality, at the core of naturopathic nutrition, continues to receive scientific validation from both our growing understanding of nutrigenomics and the consistent failings of 'one size fits all' nutritional intervention studies, for example selenium supplementation to reduce cancer incidence.[36,37] As part of this future, particularly in light of the potential for broader adoption of naturopathic nutrition by other health professionals, ongoing vigilance to bio-individuality and the development of diagnoses from both a functional and a pathological perspective are imperative. To lose these fundamental principles in the rush to jump aboard the nutritional bandwagon will simply constitute a misappropriation of our knowledge and will fail to improve health outcomes for patients; for example, homocysteine lowering with high-dose folate and B_{12} fails to improve survival in cardiovascular patients.[38] Hand in hand with this, we urgently need a new research methodology that can accurately reflect and assess holistic naturopathic nutritional medicine and therefore direct new treatments and forms of intervention, and an audience of receptive practitioners who remain committed to discovering and practising best medicine.

REFERENCES

[1] Bridgman K. Nutrition. In: Robson T, editor. An introduction to complementary medicine. Crows Nest, New South Wales: Allen and Unwin; 2005. p. 245–62.
[2] Murray M, Pizzorno J. Nutritional medicine. In: Pizzorno J, Murray M, editors. Textbook of natural medicine. St Louis: Churchill Livingstone Elsevier; 2006. p. 461–73.
[3] Bradley R. Philosophy of naturopathic medicine. In: Pizzorno J, Murray M, editors. Textbook of natural medicine. St Louis: Churchill Livingstone Elsevier; 2006. p. 79–87.
[4] Haas A. Staying healthy with nutrition. Berkeley: Celestial Arts; 1992. p. 222.
[5] Levin B, Bland J, Schmidt M. Functional medicine in natural medicine. In: Pizzorno J, Murray M, editors. Textbook of natural medicine. St Louis: Churchill Livingstone Elsevier; 2006. p. 13–26.
[6] Solis C, Veenema K, Ivanov AA, et al. Folate intake at RDA levels is inadequate for Mexican American men with the methylenetetrahydrofolate reductase 677TT genotype. J Nutr 2008;138(1):67–72.
[7] Food and Agriculture Organization/World Health Organization. Report of a joint FAO/WHO expert consultation. Bangkok, Thailand, Rome: FAO/WHO; 2002.
[8] Higdon J. An evidence-based approach to vitamins and minerals. New York: Thieme; 2006.
[9] Chuang H, Tsai SY, Chao KY, et al. The influence of milk intake on the lead toxicity to the sensory nervous system in lead workers. Neurotoxicology 2004;25(6):941–9.
[10] Gropper S, Smith J, Groff J. Advanced nutrition and human metabolism. 5th ed. Belmont: Wadsworth Thomson Learning; 2009.
[11] Padayatty S, Doppman JL, Chang R, et al. Human adrenal glands secrete vitamin C in response to adrenocorticotrophic hormone. Am J Clin Nutr 2007;86(1):145–9.
[12] Kohlmeier M, De Caterina R, Ferguson LR, et al. Guide and position of the international society of nutrigenetics/nutrigenomics of personalized nutrition: Part 2 — Ethics, challenges and endeavors of precision nutrition. J Nutrigenet Nutrigenomics 2016;9(1):28–46.
[13] Fallaize R, Macready AL, Butler LT, et al. An insight into the public acceptance of nutrigenomic based personalized nutrition. Nutr Res Rev 2013;26(1):39–48.
[14] Grace S, Vemulpad S, Beirman R. Training in and use of diagnostic techniques among CAM practitioners: an Australian study. J Altern Complement Med 2006;12(7):695–700.
[15] Bensoussan A, Myers SP, Wu SM, et al. Naturopathic and western herbal medicine practice in Australia — a workforce survey. Complement Ther Med 2004;12(1):17–27.
[16] Arthur R, et al. Zinc assessment in Australian naturopathic practice: its influences, methodology and perceived validity. Unpublished research 2008.
[17] Walsh C, et al. Zinc: health effects and research priorities for the 1990s. Environ Health Perspect 1994;102(Suppl. 2):5–46.
[18] Holman P. Assessment of nutritional status. In: Jamison J, editor. Clinical guide to nutrition and dietary supplements in disease management. Sydney: Churchill Livingstone; 2003.
[19] Food Standards Australia New Zealand. NUTTAB 2006. Available from: www.foodstandards.gov.au/monitoringandsurveillance/nuttab2006/.
[20] Braun L, Cohen M. Herbs and natural supplements: an evidence-based guide. 3rd ed. Marrickville: Elsevier; 2010.
[21] Martí N, Mena P, Cánovas JA, et al. Vitamin C and the role of citrus juices as functional food. Nat Prod Commun 2009;4(5):677–700.
[22] Ashton J, Barclay AW, Louie M, et al. The chromium content of some Australian foods. Food Australia 2003;55(5):201–4.
[23] Thorn J, Robertson J, Buss DH, et al. Trace nutrients. Selenium in British food. Br J Nutr 1978;39(2):391–6.
[24] Gibson R. Principles of nutritional assessment. New York: Oxford University Press; 1990.
[25] Arnaud MJ. Update on the assessment of magnesium status. Br J Nutr 2008;99(Suppl. 3):S24–36.
[26] Fenech M, El-Sohemy A, Cahill L, et al. Nutrigenetics and nutrigenomics: viewpoints on the current status and applications in nutrition research and practice. J Nutrigenet Nutrigenomics 2011;4:69–89.

[27] DaVanzo J. A study of the cost effects of multivitamins in selected populations. Report of the Lewin Group to Wyeth Consumer Healthcare 2003.
[28] Higdon J. An evidence-based approach to vitamins and minerals. New York: Thieme; 2003.
[29] Wilcken D, Dudman NP, Tyrrell PA, et al. Folic acid lowers elevated plasma homocysteine in chronic renal insufficiency: possible implications for prevention of vascular disease. Metabolism 1988;37(7):697–701.
[30] King J, Cousins R. Zinc. In: Shils M, Shike M, Ross AC, editors. Modern nutrition in health and disease. Baltimore: Lippincott Williams & Wilkins; 2006. p. 271–85.
[31] Dunn B, Ryan A, Ford L. Selenium and vitamin E cancer prevention trial: a nutrient approach to prostate cancer prevention. Recent Results Cancer Res 2009;181:183–93.
[32] Sarris J, Schoendorfer N, Kavanagh D. Major depressive disorder and nutritional medicine: a review of monotherapies and adjuvant treatments. Nutr Rev 2009;67(3):125–31.
[33] Barnard N, Cohen J, Jenkins DJA, et al. A low-fat vegan diet and a conventional diabetes diet in the treatment of type 2 diabetes: a randomized, controlled, 74-wk clinical trial. Am J Clin Nutr 2009;89(5):S1588–96.
[34] Calabrese C. Research in natural medicine. In: Pizzorno J, Murray M, editors. Textbook of natural medicine. St Louis: Churchill Livingstone; 2006. p. 117–26.
[35] Adams J, Wardle J. Engaging practitioners in research. J Complement Med 2009;8(5):5.
[36] Hatfield DL, Gladyshev VN. The outcome of Selenium and Vitamin E Cancer Prevention Trial (SELECT) reveals the need for better understanding of selenium biology. Mol Interv 2009;9(1):18–21.
[37] Schrauzer GN. RE: lessons from the Selenium and Vitamin E Cancer Prevention Trial (SELECT). Crit Rev Biotechnol 2009;29(2):81.
[38] Marcus J, Sarnak MJ, Menon V. Homocysteine lowering and cardiovascular disease risk: lost in translation. Can J Cardiol 2007;23(9):707–10.

4

Diagnostics

Annalies Corse

INTRODUCTION

The clinical practice landscape of naturopathy is shifting significantly. While naturopathic practitioners continue to uphold our founding philosophy to address the true causes of human illness with herbal medicine, nutrition, homoeopathy, manual therapies and more traditional forms of physical examination, we are met with the inevitable need to be more scientific, clinically experienced and evidence based. This is especially the case in the area of clinical diagnostics and pathology testing. We could argue these changes were firmly assimilated into naturopathic education and practice many decades ago. However, the requirement to improve and maintain a thorough understanding of orthodox medical diagnostics most certainly exists.

In orthodox medicine, disease causation and characteristics are encompassed within the specialisation of pathology. Pathology supports every facet of medicine, from initial laboratory diagnosis and the observance of patterns and trends in chronic disease, through to monitoring therapeutic medications and innovative medical research. Pathology has evolved over centuries in the laboratory, producing testing methods that cover potential disease development, the presence of disease, the cause or severity of disease and both the positive and negative effects of treatment. From preconception to postmortem, it has been said, 'Medicine IS pathology'.[1]

Interpretation of laboratory and diagnostic medical reports can be challenging for the naturopathic practitioner. For medical professionals, pathology is considered a pillar of medical practice, used and interpreted by most doctors on an hourly basis. Despite the inclusion of medical laboratory reports and their interpretation in naturopathic curricula, there are many possible reasons why practitioners may not feel confident or may avoid interpreting these reports. Traditionally, pathology testing was not part of naturopathy; symptomatology, history taking and physical examination were and remain the cornerstones of holistic health. The inclusion of pathology testing in our clinical decision making may at times be met with resistance in our profession. Naturopathic practitioners may avoid requesting, querying or discussing pathology tests with medical staff, in the belief that their requests may be dismissed. Universities and colleges delivering naturopathy degrees and courses do introduce diagnostics as a subject but, as with all clinically based areas of practice, real life clinical experience with patients fortifies knowledge and instills confidence. Unless a new graduate displays initiative in continuing their education regarding diagnostics, it is an area of practice that may unfortunately be underutilised.

Pathology testing is a reality for all patients in the care of doctors. Naturopaths will continually be expected to have an understanding of routine and some specialist pathology. Additionally, a sound understanding of pathology testing by a naturopath can facilitate the detection of illness, especially if a patient is encouraged to seek previously unwanted medical advice.

Advances in pathology have developed extensively in the past two decades. It is difficult to extrapolate what pathology will involve in 20 years' time, particularly in the areas of genomics, data processing and personalised medicine.[2] Currently, nine areas of sub-specialisation exist within the broader context of pathology. These comprise anatomical pathology, chemical pathology, clinical pathology, forensic pathology, general pathology, genetic pathology, haematology, immunopathology and microbiology.[1] Pathology tests are an integral part of clinical decisions and patient care, with more than 70% of all medical diagnoses requiring their use.[3] The need for naturopaths to be abreast of these new techniques has never been so great; almost all of our patients will continue to have extensive pathology reporting. These reports and results can provide essential clinical data to inform our own holistic assessments and prescriptions.

Interpretation of pathology tests is at times quite simple, as some tests are reported as either a positive or a negative result (species identification of microorganisms is one of many examples). However, many test results are quantitative and reported as numerical values. This is where result interpretation requires comparison with a reference range. Reference ranges are sometimes determined by testing a particular parameter in a 'normal, healthy' patient population. If these results show a Gaussian or bell-shaped curve, the central 95% is set as the normal range.[4] It is important to always use reference ranges supplied by the laboratory that performed the test, as some laboratories set their own reference ranges for certain tests.

For naturopathic practitioners, quantitative results interpreted as normal/abnormal do not comply with the holistic model of healthcare. Many patients with results considered 'normal' by standard reference ranges still experience symptoms and display signs of significant clinical disease. These patients may be considered as having sub-clinical or functional problems as opposed to extensive clinical pathology. Both integrative medicine and naturopathy have suggested the emergence of the 'optimal range'. Optimal ranges still sit within normal reference ranges but are much more narrow. Arguments supporting the concept of the optimal range specify that pathology results can be used to practise preventive medicine. Those critical of the optimal range concept contend that the establishment of such ranges is difficult to achieve with studies, and relies more on lengthy clinical experience.

Pathology relies on the analysis of tissues (hair, blood, organ sections), cells (free cells within body fluids or tissues) and body fluids (semen, saliva, urine, cerebrospinal fluid, mucous membrane secretions, serous fluids) and faeces. Blood is the most commonly sampled tissue for pathology testing.[5] Despite being relatively non-invasive to sample, blood perfuses the entire body; virtually all organs and systems can be monitored via the cellular and non-cellular components of blood. Blood is involved in transportation of nutrients, hormones and metabolic wastes, chemical regulation of pH and protection via immunity and blood coagulation. In certain situations, blood is an inappropriate medium for clinical accuracy, hence the sampling of hair, urine, faeces, etc. In this chapter we discuss the reasons for selecting specific body tissues for each test in relation to human physiology.

All forms of diagnostic pathology services incur great financial costs. For routine and some specialist pathology services, cost to patients is minimised via Medicare. Functional pathology is not scheduled under Medicare, with costs directly incurred by the patient. Ethical issues arise if a financial benefit exists for the practitioner (e.g. using testing equipment for which additional fees are charged). This also occurs when clinicians routinely test patients at a cost of many hundreds of dollars before imparting advice and treatment. Ethically, each health and medical practitioner must evaluate whether the results of any clinical investigations will change the patient's treatment plan or prescription. If the answer is no, practitioners must justify their clinical reasoning for requesting investigations, particularly when a cost to the patient exists. The same level of evaluation is expected of medical practitioners when requesting clinical investigations via Medicare.

Thorough clinical interpretation of a patient's pathology results requires an understanding of units of measurement used for reporting. Systeme International (SI) units, or the international system of units, are a set of units for scientific and commercial work. These were established in 1960 by the International Bureau of Weights and Measures.[6] SI units allow the measurement and reporting of values in a uniform manner throughout the world. Clinical laboratories worldwide have adopted many SI units, though some countries continue to use non-SI units.[6] Table 4.1 presents the seven SI base units and Table 4.2 presents SI-derived units used by the vast majority of laboratories throughout the world.

TABLE 4.1 SI base units

Quantity	Name	Symbol
Length	metre	m
Mass	kilogram	kg
Time	second	s
Electric current	ampere	A
Thermodynamic temperature	kelvin	K
Luminous intensity	candela	cd
Amount of substance	mole	mol

Pincus M, Abraham N. Interpreting laboratory results. In McPherson R, Pincus M, editors. Henry's clinical diagnosis and management by laboratory methods. 23rd edn. St Louis: Elsevier; 2017, pp. 84–101.

TABLE 4.2 SI-derived units

Quantity	Name	Symbol
Area	square metre	m^2
Volume	cubic metre litre	m^3 L
Concentration		
Mass	kilogram/litre	kg/L
Substance	mole/litre	mol/L
Molality	mole/kilogram	mol/kg
Density	kilogram/litre	kg/L
Mass fraction	kilogram/kilogram	kg/kg
Mole fraction	mole/mole	mol/mol
Number concentration	number/litre	L-1
Clearance	litre/second	L/s

Pincus M, Abraham N. Interpreting laboratory results. In McPherson R, Pincus M, editors. Henry's clinical diagnosis and management by laboratory methods. 23rd edn. St Louis: Elsevier; 2017, pp. 84–101.

HAEMATOLOGY

Haematology is the subspecialisation of pathology concerning the study of blood and bone marrow, particularly the cellular components and coagulation properties of blood. The formation of blood cells is known as haematopoiesis and occurs in the red bone marrow. Haematopoiesis is an active process that replenishes red blood cells (RBCs or erythrocytes), white blood cells (WBCs or leucocytes) and platelets (thrombocytes). All blood cells arise from a pluripotent stem cell and differentiate under the influence of specific growth factors.[6]

Full blood count (FBC)

TOTAL RED CELL COUNT (RCC)

Mature RBCs form from erythroid progenitor cells (erythroblasts or normoblasts). Immature RBCs are

TABLE 4.3 Reference range (RCC)

Age	RCC range ($\times 10^{12}$/L)
Infant (cord blood)	4–6
3 months	3.2–4.8
12 months	3.6–5.2
3–6 years	4.1–5.5
10–12 years	4.0–5.4
Adult female	3.8–5.8
Adult male	4.5–6.5

Osei-Bimpong A, Burthem J. Supplementary techniques including blood parasite diagnosis. In Bain B, editor. Dacie and Lewis practical haematology. 11th edn. Elsevier Churchill Livingstone; 2012, pp. 101–21.

nucleated and accumulate haemoglobin as they mature. During maturation, the nucleus becomes highly condensed and is extruded; this first, non-nucleated RBC is known as a reticulocyte.[6]

Terminology

Erythrocytosis: increased total RCC, usually reported as polycythaemia.
Erythropenia: decreased total RCC, usually reported as anaemia.

Clinical significance

The total RCC varies at different stages of life, and between genders. It must be interpreted based on these differences. Abnormalities must be interpreted in context with RBC indices, blood films, haemoglobin (Hb) and haematocrit (Hct) levels and possibly iron studies, folate and B_{12} levels. Importantly, reference ranges may vary between laboratories; always note the reference range supplied with the report. Refer to Table 4.3 for reference ranges.

TOTAL WHITE CELL COUNT (WCC)

WBCs are further divided into granulocytes (neutrophils, eosinophils and basophils) and agranulocytes (monocytes and lymphocytes). The total WCC represents all five populations, though thorough and meaningful interpretation of WBCs requires viewing the white cell differential. The WCC detects all nucleated cells in blood samples; the count is corrected if nucleated RBCs are present.

Terminology

Leucocytosis: increased total WCC.
Leucopenia: decreased total WCC.

Clinical significance

WBCs are involved in many diverse pathological processes, including infection, inflammatory conditions, immunological disorders, bone marrow failure and haematological and other malignancies. Interpretation depends entirely on other tests including the WBC differential, blood and bone marrow films, immunological tests or investigations for malignancy. Again, reference ranges may vary between laboratories; always note the reference range supplied with the report. Refer to Table 4.4 for reference ranges.

TABLE 4.4 Reference range (WCC)

Age	WCC range ($\times 10^{9}$/L)
Neonate	6.0–22.0
12 months	6.0–18.0
4–7 years	5.0–15.0
8–12 years	4.5–13.5
Adult	4.0–11.0

Naushad H. Leucocyte count. eMedicine Drugs and Diseases, 2016. Available from: http://emedicine.medscape.com/article/2054452-overview

TABLE 4.5 Reference range: reticulocyte count

Age	Reference range
Term infant, cord blood	2–6%
Children	0.2–2.0%
Adults	0.5–1.5%

Reproduced with permission from the Royal College of Pathologists of Australasia (RCPA). RCPA manual of use and interpretation of pathology tests. 7th ed. Sydney: RCPA, 2015. https://www.rcpa.edu.au/Library/Practising-Pathology/RCPA-Manual/Home.

RETICULOCYTE COUNT

Reticulocytes are immature RBCs. After reticulocytes form in bone marrow, they are released into the general circulation and usually require three days to fully mature.[6]

Terminology

Reticulocytosis: increased reticulocyte count.

Clinical significance

Reticulocytosis indicates increased erythropoiesis in bone marrow. Reasons can include anaemia and erythropoietin (EPO) therapy in renal disease. Reticulocytosis may be naturally occurring in those living/training at altitude, or induced by EPO abuse in elite endurance sport. A low reticulocyte count often indicates anaemia in conjunction with either bone marrow failure or nutritional deficiency of iron, folate or B_{12}. Findings must be interpreted in conjunction with the entire FBC, blood or bone marrow films and possibly iron, folate, B_{12} levels, and genetic studies for inherited anaemias (e.g. G6PD and thalassaemia studies).[7] Reference ranges vary in different laboratories depending on the instrumentation method used; the ranges in Table 4.5 are a general guide based on microscopy.

HAEMATOCRIT (HcT)

The Hct level or packed cell volume represents the proportion of RBCs in relation to whole blood and is

TABLE 4.6 Reference range: Hct levels

Age	Reference range
Adult male	40.7–50.3%
Adult female	36.1–44.3%
Newborn	45–61%
Infant	32–42%

Reproduced with permission from the Royal College of Pathologists of Australasia (RCPA). RCPA manual of use and interpretation of pathology tests. 7th ed. Sydney: RCPA, 2015. https://www.rcpa.edu.au/Library/Practising-Pathology/RCPA-Manual/Home.

expressed as a ratio or percentage.[8] It is one of very few tests where gross examination via the naked eye provides information often as valuable as automated results.

Clinical significance

Decreased Hct levels indicate a low concentration of RBCs and therefore anaemia. Hct must be interpreted with Hb levels, the RCC, red cell indices and blood films to elicit the precise cause of the anaemia (e.g. dietary deficiency of haematinic nutrients, blood loss or intravascular destruction of RBCs).[9] High Hct levels can indicate dehydration, as blood plasma levels can be reduced with poor hydration, making the RCC artificially elevated. If dehydration is not a factor, the increased Hct is indicative of polycythaemia, and a cause for this must be found on further testing. Some conditions associated with polycythaemia include haemochromatosis, multiple myeloma and polycythaemia rubra vera.[9] Refer to Table 4.6 for reference ranges.

PLATELET COUNT

Platelets are derived from progenitor cells known as megakaryocytes. These large cells fragment to produce up to 3000 platelets per megakaryocyte.[6] Platelets are involved in clot formation and inflammation.

Terminology

Thrombocytosis: increased platelet count.
Thrombocytopenia: decreased platelet count.

Clinical significance

Thrombocytopenia must be confirmed via a repeat sample or blood/bone marrow films, as low platelet counts are often induced artificially due to clotted blood samples. Thrombocytopenia may occur as a result of chronic infection (especially infectious mononucleosis, malaria or HIV) or hypersplenism. Medications and drugs can reduce platelet counts (e.g. thiazide diuretics, gold salts, heparin, some antibiotics and alcohol abuse). As platelets are involved in the acute phase of inflammation, thrombocytosis can indicate chronic inflammation, neoplasia and infection. Thrombocytosis is also common post splenectomy.[7] Abnormal platelet counts must be viewed in conjunction with the entire FBC and blood/bone marrow films. Reference ranges depend on the automated method used by the laboratory, but the reference range (thrombocyte count) 150–400 × 10^9/L[7] may be used as a guide.

HAEMOGLOBIN (Hb)

Hb is synthesised endogenously and is specifically adapted for the transport of gases such as oxygen and carbon dioxide to and from the lungs. The protein component is comprised of four globin chains (two alpha chains and two beta chains). Each globin chain contains an iron-rich pigment known as haeme. The chemical structure of haeme is based on porphyrin rings.

Clinical significance

The clinical term 'anaemia' is often used to describe a low Hb concentration, low RCC or low Hct. However, anaemia is an exceedingly common complication of many diseases. Hb testing is preferred over the RCC and Hct for this situation.[8] Hb alone cannot determine the exact cause of anaemia. Additionally, Hb levels can be elevated in hypoxic conditions of high altitude living (>1000 metres above sea level) and smoking.[10] Laboratories can differ greatly with reference ranges due to instrumentation; Table 4.7, adapted from the World Health Organization, is a guide for reference ranges.

RBC INDICES

The various RBC indices represent the size, content and Hb concentration of erythrocytes.[8] They are a method of determining morphological characteristics of erythrocytes via automated methods as opposed to blood film

TABLE 4.7 Reference range: Hb (g/L)

Age	Non-anaemia	Mild anaemia	Moderate anaemia	Severe anaemia
0.5–5 yrs	110 or higher	100–109	70–99	<70
5–11 yrs	115 or higher	110–114	80–109	<80
12–14 yrs	120 or higher	110–119	80–109	<80
> 15 yrs (females: non-pregnant)	120 or higher	110–119	80–109	<80
> 15 yrs (females: pregnant)	110 or higher	100–109	70–99	<70
> 15 yrs (males)	130 or higher	110–129	80–109	<80

Reprinted from World Health Organization (WHO). Haemoglobin concentrations for the diagnosis of anaemia and assessment of severity [Internet]. Vitamin and Mineral Nutrition Information System. WHO, 2016 [cited 20 July 2016]. Available from: http://www.who.int/vmnis/indicators/haemoglobin.pdf.

examination via microscopy. RBC indices are incredibly useful for characterising anaemias.

MEAN CELL VOLUME (MCV)

MCV is the average volume of RBCs. It is calculated by dividing the Hct by the RCC. The reference ranges in Table 4.8 are a guide only, as ranges may depend on the laboratory.

MEAN CELL HAEMOGLOBIN (MCH)

MCH is the weight of Hb in the average RBC. It is calculated by dividing the Hb concentration by the RCC. Variation also occurs in reference ranges. Refer to Table 4.9 for reference ranges.

MEAN CELL HAEMOGLOBIN CONCENTRATION (MCHC)

MCHC is the average concentration of Hb in a given volume of packed RBCs. It is calculated by dividing the Hb concentration by the Hct. Again due to laboratory instrumentation, ranges vary considerably. Refer to Table 4.10 for reference ranges.

TABLE 4.8 Reference range: MCV

Age	MCV (fL)
Term infant (cord blood) mean	106
3 months	95
12 months	70–86
3–6 yrs	73–89
10–12 yrs	77–91
Adult	80–100

Reproduced with permission from the Royal College of Pathologists of Australasia (RCPA). RCPA manual of use and interpretation of pathology tests. 7th ed. Sydney: RCPA, 2015. https://www.rcpa.edu.au/Library/Practising-Pathology/RCPA-Manual/Home.

TABLE 4.9 Reference range: MCH

Age	MCH (pg)
<3 months	24–34
<12 months	23–31
3–12 yrs	24–30
Adult	27–32

Reproduced with permission from the Royal College of Pathologists of Australasia (RCPA). RCPA manual of use and interpretation of pathology tests. 7th ed. Sydney: RCPA, 2015. https://www.rcpa.edu.au/Library/Practising-Pathology/RCPA-Manual/Home.

TABLE 4.10 Reference range: MCHC

Age	MCHC (g/L)
Adults and children	300–350

Reproduced with permission from the Royal College of Pathologists of Australasia (RCPA). RCPA manual of use and interpretation of pathology tests. 7th ed. Sydney: RCPA, 2015. https://www.rcpa.edu.au/Library/Practising-Pathology/RCPA-Manual/Home.

RED CELL DISTRIBUTION WIDTH (RDW)

The RDW is used to help with classification of anaemia, in conjunction with the MCV, MCH and MCHC. It helps to quantify the degree of variation in RBC size and volume.[11] Reference ranges are entirely dependent on the method used, therefore always use the reference range supplied by the laboratory.

Terminology

Microcytosis: RBCs with low volume and small size.
Macrocytosis: RBCs with high volume.
Anisocytosis: RBCs display significant variation in size and volume (may be a mix of macrocytosis, microcytosis and normocytosis; the key word here is variation).

Clinical significance

Microcytic anaemia often shows a decreased MCV. Microcytosis is found in iron deficiency anaemia, thalassemias, lead (Pb) toxicity and some patients with anaemia of chronic disease.[11] In macrocytic anaemia, the MCV is elevated, MCH is low and MCHC is usually normal or decreased. Macrocytosis is found in many types of anaemia including megaloblastic, aplastic, dyserythropoeitic and sideroblastic anaemias. Liver disease, alcohol excess, myxoedema and hypoxic conditions of the lungs can also lead to macrocytosis.[11] Abnormalities of the RBC indices will always be followed with a blood film and results must be interpreted in conjunction with this report.

WBC DIFFERENTIAL

Neutrophils

Neutrophils are the most abundant leucocytes in adult blood. Neutrophils identify, phagocytise and destroy foreign particulate matter and microbes. Neutrophils are easily recognised on microscopy by their multilobed nucleus and cytoplasmic granules. These granules, enzymes and other proteins are required to digest and kill phagocytised microbes.[6]

TERMINOLOGY

Neutrophilia: increased neutrophil count.
Neutropenia: decreased neutrophil count.
Agranulocytosis: severe neutropenia.

CLINICAL SIGNIFICANCE

Neutrophilia represents an above-normal-for-age concentration of neutrophils in peripheral blood. Causes of neutrophilia range from short-lived acute infections through to chronic and life-limiting disease. Six areas of pathophysiology can lead to neutrophilia:

1. Acute inflammation
2. Acute infection (e.g. often bacterial; some viral, fungal and parasitic infections)
3. Tissue necrosis (e.g. burns, tissue trauma and myocardial infarction)
4. Physiological alteration (e.g. pregnancy, smoking, intense exercise and the stress response)

5 Neoplasia (e.g. carcinomas, sarcomas and myeloproliferative disorders)
6 Metabolic alterations (e.g. corticosteroid use, uraemia, ketoacidosis).[12]

The degree of neutrophilia is host dependent; children display greater degrees of neutrophilia, while those who are iron, folate or B_{12} deficient can have an impaired neutrophilic response.[12]

Neutropenia can be inherited (e.g. Fanconi's anaemia, though there are many other examples), autoimmune (e.g. rheumatoid arthritis), toxin/drug associated (e.g. alcohol, chemotherapy agents, radiation, some antibiotics, thiazides, anthithyroids, anticonvulsants to name a few), haematological (e.g. bone marrow failure, megaloblastic anaemia) or as the result of any overwhelming infection.[12]

Lymphocytes

The lymphocyte count on a WBC differential represents all the diverse sub-populations of T- and B-lymphocytes found in peripheral blood. B-lymphocytes secrete immunoglobulins (antibodies) against a specific antigen (humoral immunity) while T-lymphocytes are the cells of the cell-mediated response.[13]

TERMINOLOGY

Lymphocytosis: increased lymphocyte count.

CLINICAL SIGNIFICANCE

Lymphocytosis is uncommon in bacterial infection and often increases during viral infection (non-viral infections include pertussis, tuberculosis, toxoplasmosis and rickettsial infection). Chronic ulcerative colitis and Crohn's disease can display a lymphocytosis. It may be a feature of autoimmune diseases (e.g. Graves' disease and Sjögren's syndrome). Acute lymphocytic leukaemia (ALL), chronic lymphocytic leukaemia (CLL) and lymphoma can all induce lymphocytosis.[12]

Monocytes

TERMINOLOGY

Monocytosis: increased monocyte count.
Monocytopenia: decreased monocyte count.

CLINICAL SIGNIFICANCE

Monocytosis is a common finding in specific infections such as tuberculosis, subacute bacterial endocarditis, and protozoal and rickettsial infection. It can be observed in haematological malignancies (leukaemias, lymphomas, multiple myelomas). Many chronic inflammatory disorders show monocytosis (e.g. chronic ulcerative colitis, coeliac disease and autoimmune vascular conditions). Monocytosis can occur during recovery from both acute infection and neutropenia. Monocytopenia is uncommon, but can be observed in the initial hours after prednisone therapy.[12]

Eosinophils

Being granulocytes, eosinophils release their cache of toxic granules in order to damage an invading microbe or erroneous cell. Eosinophils are also immunoregulatory and pro-inflammatory; they can enhance the process of inflammation.[12]

TERMINOLOGY

Eosinophilia: increased eosinophil count.

CLINICAL SIGNIFICANCE

Eosinophilia is a hallmark of the allergic response in all clinical manifestations (including asthma, allergic rhinitis, eczema, urticaria). Parasitic infections can induce eosinophilia, particularly with helminths (worms). Some forms of haematological malignancy show eosinophilia (e.g. Hodgkin's lymphoma, chronic myeloid leukaemia [CML] and T-cell lymphomas). In the gut, eosinophilia is seen in eosinophilic oesophagitis. Pulmonary eosinophilic syndromes affect the respiratory syndrome.[12]

Basophils

TERMINOLOGY

Basophilia: increased basophil count.

CLINICAL SIGNIFICANCE

Basophilia is most common in allergic responses and hypersensitivity reactions (food, drugs and antigenic proteins). It is sometimes seen in CML and during varicella infection. Some patients with hypothyroidism may show basophilia.[12] Reference ranges may differ between laboratories.

Refer to Table 4.11 for reference ranges for the WBC differential.

TABLE 4.11 Reference range: WBC differential

Age	Cell count × 10^9/L				
	Neutrophils	Lymphocytes	Monocytes	Eosinophils	Basophils
Neonate	4.5–12.0	2.2–7.0	0.2–1.6	<2.0	<0.1
1–3 yrs	1.5–7.0	2.2–5.5	0.1–1.5	0.2–0.5	<0.1
4–7 yrs	1.6–9.0	2.0–5.0	0.06–1.0	0.1–1.4	<0.2
8–12 yrs	1.4–7.5	1.4–3.8	0.06–0.8	0.04–0.75	<0.2
Adult	2.0–7.5	1.5–4.0	0.2–0.8	0.04–0.4	<0.1

Reproduced with permission from the Royal College of Pathologists of Australasia (RCPA). RCPA manual of use and interpretation of pathology tests. 7th ed. Sydney: RCPA, 2015. https://www.rcpa.edu.au/Library/Practising-Pathology/RCPA-Manual/Home.

APPT TEST

The APTT test is requested with a PT or INR when a coagulopathy (bleeding disorder) is suspected. Again, it measures the time taken for blood to clot.

Clinical significance

The APTT provides an assessment of the intrinsic and common coagulation pathways and assesses clotting factors VIII, IX, XI and XII. It is used to monitor intravenous (IV) heparin therapy.[11] APTT reference ranges differ between laboratories, so the reference range of 25–35 seconds is a guide only.[11]

INR TEST

The INR test applies a correction factor to the prothrombin ratio in order to standardise result reporting for warfarin therapy across laboratories.

Clinical significance

The INR is indicated in the monitoring of oral anticoagulant therapy, such as warfarin. It is also used in broader testing of anticoagulation. Reference ranges can vary and can be set to reflect expected ranges for warfarin and non-warfarin patients.

Other specialised tests for the assessment of bleeding and coagulation include:

- D-dimer (indicated to confirm or rule out inappropriate thrombus formation)
- Fibrinogen (to further assess possible bleeding disorders)
- Coagulation factors (to determine whether one specific clotting factor is decreased/normal/ increased).[14]

ERYTHROCYTE SEDIMENTATION RATE (ESR)

The ESR is a surrogate marker of inflammation. Its use dates back almost a century and, despite the nonspecific nature of the results, the ESR remains the most frequently employed laboratory measure of inflammation.[15] The nonspecificity of the ESR arises from the fact that inflammation is a pathological process in many syndromes and diseases; the ESR cannot reveal or diagnose the source or cause of inflammation. Additionally, the ESR can be influenced by many conditions other than inflammation; for example, pregnancy, obesity and anaemia.[16]

The ESR is measured via recording the rate of RCB sedimentation in 1 hour. In the non-inflammatory state, RBCs generally resist sedimentation and rouleaux formation (stacking) due to the net negative charge of RBCs.[15] In the pro-inflammatory state excess fibrinogen, immunoglobulins and other pro-inflammatory proteins coat RBCs, thereby increasing both their density and rate of sedimentation. A highly elevated ESR (>100 mm/hr) can be related to metastatic cancer, polymyalgia rheumatica, chronic infection and hyperfibrogenaemia.[17] See C-reactive protein for further discussion of inflammatory markers. Refer to Table 4.12 for reference ranges.

TABLE 4.12 Reference range: ESR

Age	Female (mm/hr)	Male (mm/hr)
Newborn	0–2	0–2
Newborn to puberty	3–13	3–13
Adult <50 yrs	<20	<15
Adult >50 yrs	<30	<20
Pregnancy	<100	n/a

Kellner C. Erythrocyte sedimentation rate. Medscape Drugs and Diseases, 2016. Available from: http://emedicine.medscape.com/article/2085201-overview#a2

PERIPHERAL BLOOD FILMS AND MORPHOLOGY STUDIES

Despite the evolution of haematology towards the automation of many tests, the peripheral blood film retains its crucial interpretive role in laboratory medicine, and is unlikely to be replaced. It involves the use of staining techniques to visually appraise and analyse peripheral blood with light microscopy. It is performed by senior medical scientists and pathologists.

In addition to routine peripheral blood films, bone marrow aspirates can be examined microscopically. Bone marrow aspirates are used in the diagnosis of haematological malignancies (the various leukaemias and lymphomas). The following lists describe some common morphological findings from routine examination of peripheral blood.

ERYTHROCYTE MORPHOLOGY

Hypochromasia: shows increased central pallor of RBCs. Very common in iron deficiency and thalassaemia and other microcytic conditions such as lead toxicity and anaemia of chronic disease. Refer to Fig. 4.1 to see a healthy mature RBC and to Fig. 4.2 for RBC hypochromasia.

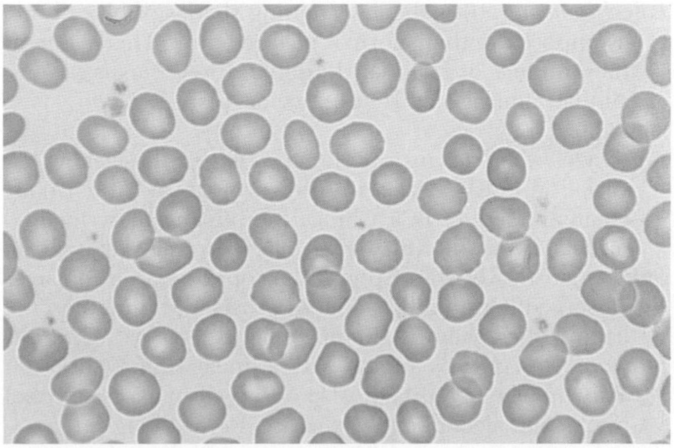

FIGURE 4.1 Mature RBCs in peripheral blood

Rozenberg G. Microscopic haematology. 3rd edn. Chatswood NSW: Elsevier; 2011.

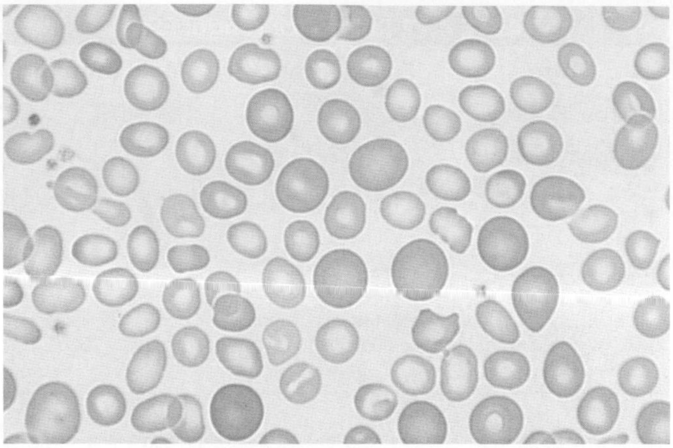

FIGURE 4.2 RBC hypochromasia

Rozenberg G. Microscopic haematology. 3rd edn. Chatswood NSW: Elsevier; 2011.

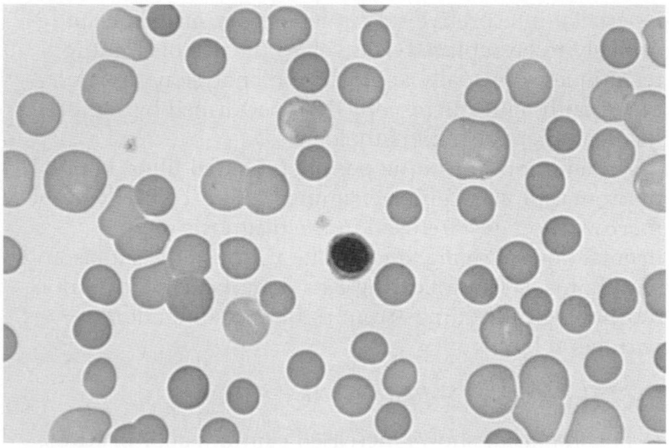

FIGURE 4.3 Autoimmune haemolytic anaemia (warm antibody): peripheral blood film showing spherocytes, reticulocytes (polychromasia) and a nucleated red cell

Rozenberg G. Microscopic haematology. 3rd edn. Chatswood NSW: Elsevier; 2011.

Polychromasia: RBCs display staining shades of blue-grey as opposed to their normal pale red-pink. This is due to the presence of residual ribosomal RNA, thus is a similar clinical picture to reticulocytosis. Refer to Fig. 4.3.

Anisocytosis, microcytosis and *macrocytosis:* these show variation in RBC size with little uniformity. Abnormally small and large RBCs. Clinical significance described previously in the RBC indices. Refer to Fig. 4.4.

Spherocytosis: RBCs are spherical as opposed to biconcave. Observed in hereditary spherocytosis and immune haemolytic anaemias. Refer to Fig. 4.5.

Stomatocytosis: RBCs appear with a linear stoma (slit). This may be hereditary. Also observed in excess alcohol intake and alcoholic liver disease. Refer to Fig. 4.6.

Acanthocytosis: spherical RBCs have multiple surface spicules. Commonly seen in liver disease, postsplenectomy and in anorexia nervosa and starvation. Refer to Fig. 4.7.

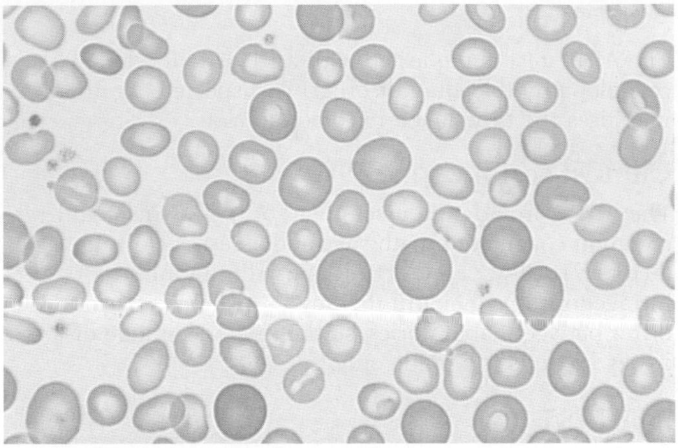

FIGURE 4.4 RBC anisocytosis and dimorphic blood picture with microcytic and normocytic RBCs

Rozenberg G. Microscopic haematology. 3rd edn. Chatswood NSW: Elsevier; 2011.

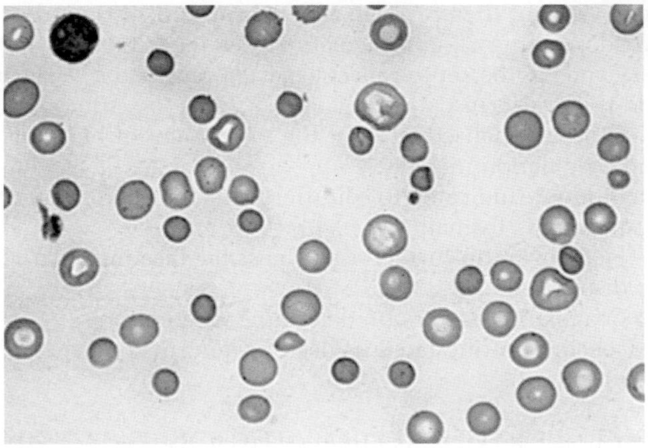

FIGURE 4.5 RBC spherocytosis. Dense staining RBCs devoid of central pallor

Engorn B, Flerlage J, editors. The Harriet Lane handbook. 20th edn. Saunders; 2015.

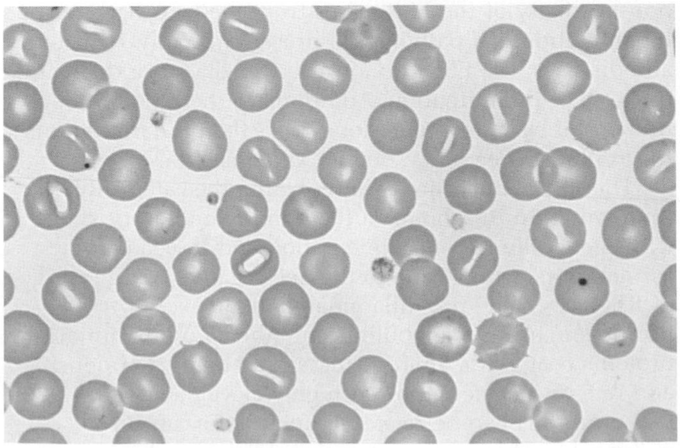

FIGURE 4.6 RBC stomatocytosis

Rozenberg G. Microscopic haematology. 3rd edn. Chatswood NSW: Elsevier; 2011.

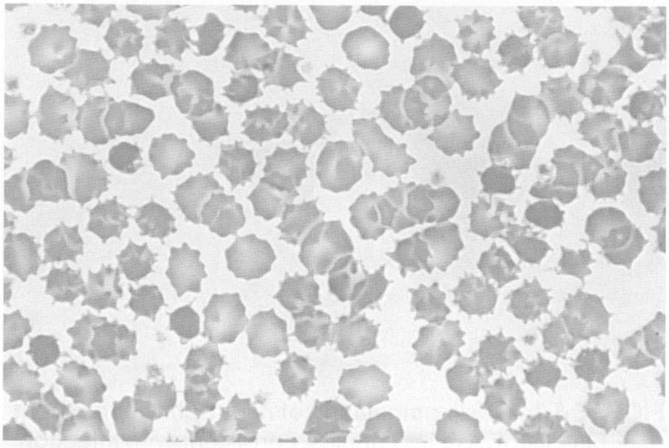

FIGURE 4.7 RBC acanthocytosis

Rozenberg G. Microscopic haematology. 3rd edn. Chatswood NSW: Elsevier; 2011.

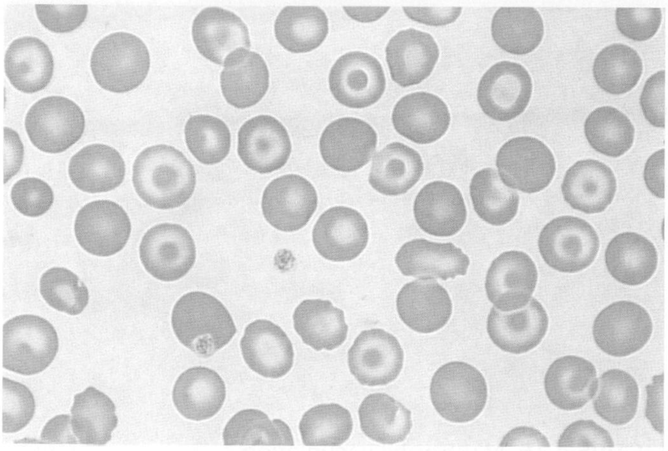

FIGURE 4.8 RBC target cells

Rozenberg G. Microscopic haematology. 3rd edn. Chatswood NSW: Elsevier; 2011.

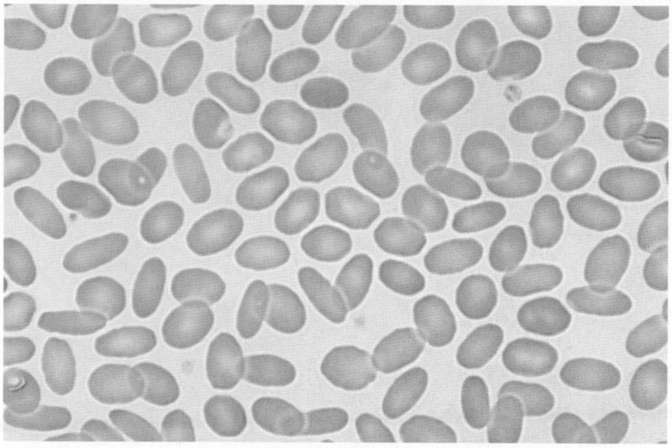

FIGURE 4.9 RBC elliptocytosis as observed in hereditary elliptocytosis

Rozenberg G. Microscopic haematology. 3rd edn. Chatswood NSW: Elsevier; 2011.

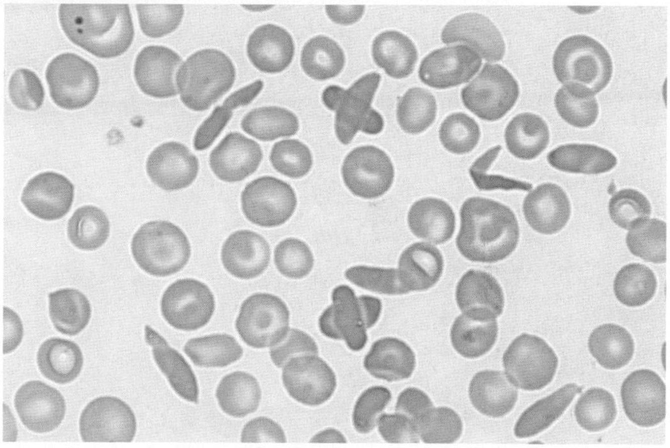

FIGURE 4.10 RBC sickle cells

Rozenberg G. Microscopic haematology. 3rd edn. Chatswood NSW: Elsevier; 2011.

Target cells: RBCs show areas of increased central staining. Noted in severe iron deficiency, obstructive liver disease, thalassaemia and postsplenectomy. Refer to Fig. 4.8.

Elliptocytosis: shows elliptically shaped RBCs with loss of biconcave shape. May be hereditary, but also noted in megaloblastic anaemia, iron deficiency and thalassaemia. Refer to Fig. 4.9.

Sickle cells: sickle-shaped RBCs. Can be hereditary (sickle cell anaemia) or observed postsplenectomy. Refer to Fig. 4.10.

Schistocytosis: fragmented RBCs are found commonly in haemolytic anaemia. Refer to Fig. 4.11.

RBC inclusions: these include Howell-Jolly bodies (various anaemias and postsplenectomy) and basophilic stippling (various anaemias, liver disease and postsplenectomy). Malaria parasites (*Plasmodium falciparum)* are easily observed in RBCs on peripheral blood films. Refer to Fig. 4.12.[18]

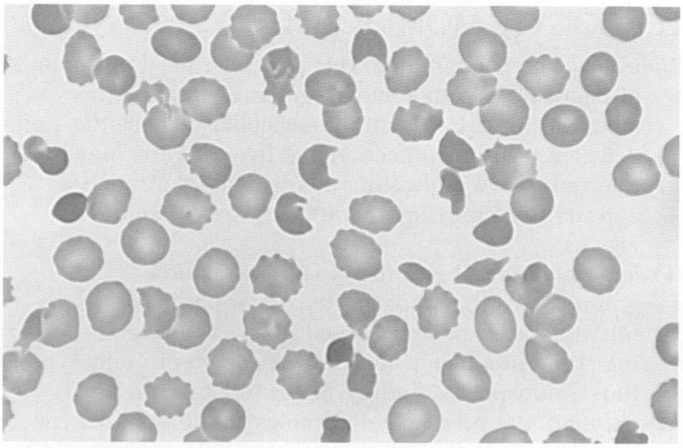

FIGURE 4.11 RBC schistocytosis cells

Rozenberg G. Microscopic haematology. 3rd edn. Chatswood NSW: Elsevier; 2011.

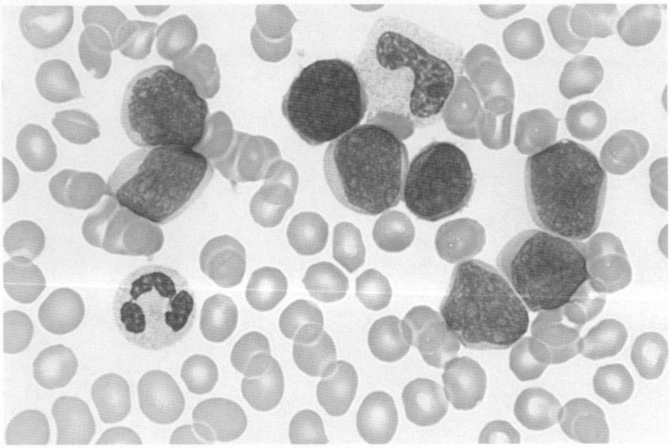

FIGURE 4.12 Lymphoblastic leukaemia/lymphoma. Peripheral blood infiltrated with blast cells

Rozenberg G. Microscopic haematology. 3rd edn. Chatswood NSW: Elsevier; 2011.

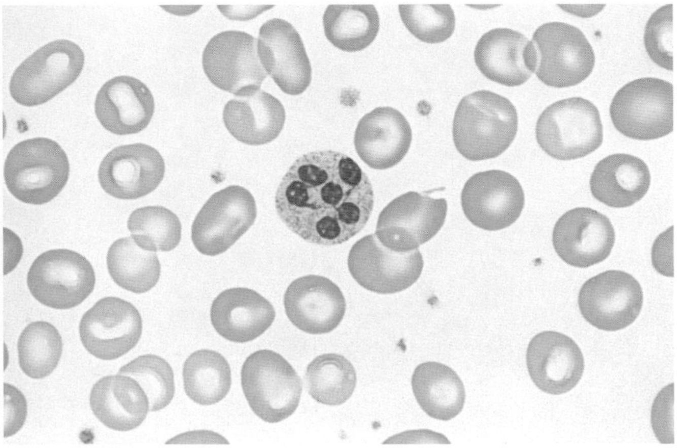

FIGURE 4.13 Hypersegmented neutrophils

Rozenberg G. Microscopic haematology. 3rd edn. Chatswood NSW: Elsevier; 2011.

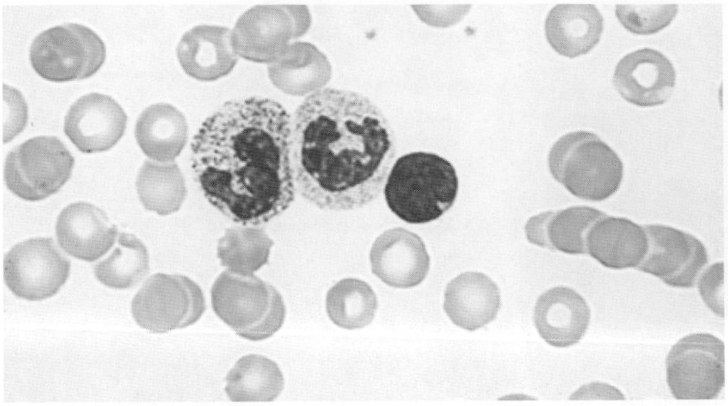

FIGURE 4.14 Toxic granulation of neutrophils. Prominent dark blue cytoplasmic granules, consistent with infection and other toxic states

Engorn B, Flerlage J, editors. The Harriet Lane handbook. 20th edn. Saunders; 2015.

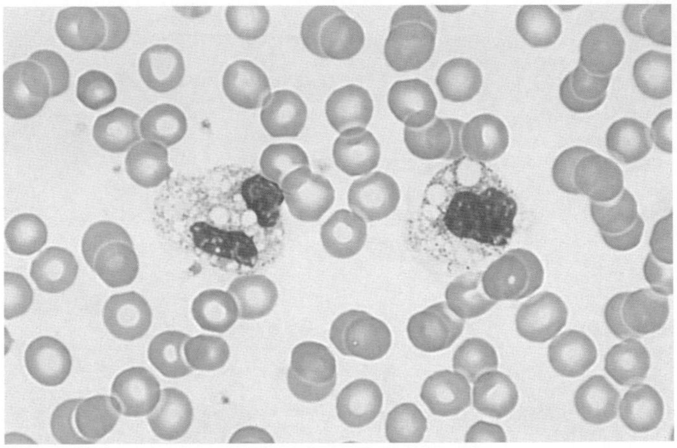

FIGURE 4.15 Neutrophil vacuolation

Rozenberg G. Microscopic haematology. 3rd edn. Chatswood NSW: Elsevier; 2011.

LEUCOCYTE MORPHOLOGY

Hypersegmented neutrophils: this is an increased percentage of neutrophils with a hypersegmented nucleus (five lobes or more). Common in megaloblastic anaemia, iron deficiency, chronic infection and liver disease. May be referred to as a 'right shift' (neutrophil maturation appears to be moving forwards in excess). Refer to Fig. 4.13.

Toxic granulation: this is increased granulation of all granulocytes that appears more basophilic on microscopy. May be observed in severe bacterial infection, pregnancy and tissue damage of many types, thus a nonspecific finding. Refer to Fig. 4.14.

Vacuolation: the presence of vacuoles in the granulocytic cytoplasm usually indicates infection. Vacuolation is a physiological response to many forms of cellular damage and is seen as a protective response. Refer to Fig. 4.15.

Dohle bodies: are pale-blue staining cytoplasmic inclusions. Observed in pregnancy, infection, inflammation, severe burns, tuberculosis and postchemotherapy.

Auer rods: are small, pale-blue staining rod-shaped cytoplasmic inclusions in myeloblasts and promyelocytes which are immature cells of myelocytic series. They are seen in some myelodysplastic syndromes and acute myeloblastic leukaemia (AML).

Left shift: is the presence of immature/precursor granulocytes. It may be due to pregnancy, infections or bone metastases by malignancies. In pregnancy and infection it may represent an immune system under duress, as granulocytes are required in peripheral blood and are released from bone marrow early. Refer to Fig. 4.16.

Atypical lymphocytes: are enlarged lymphocytes with a large cytoplasm, at times abnormally granulated. They are common in viral infections (particularly Epstein-Barr virus [EBV], cytomegalovirus [CMV], hepatitis A and measles) and may be observed postimmunisation. Refer to Fig. 4.17.[18]

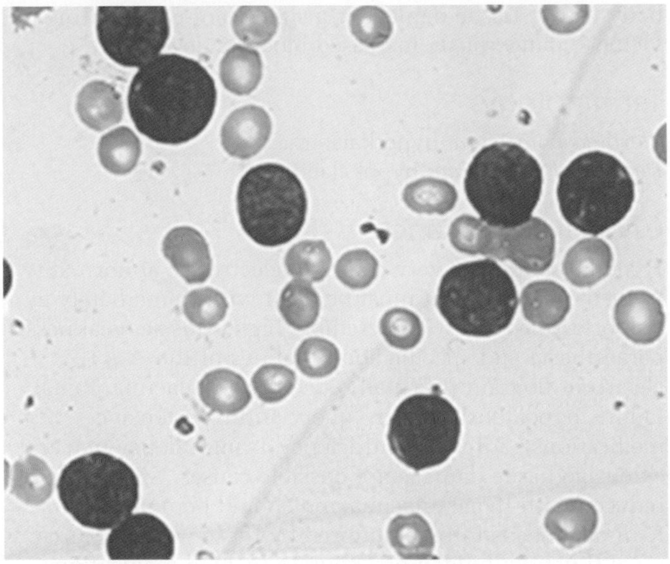

FIGURE 4.16 Leucocytic left shift. Leucocyte blasts with increased nucleus-to-cytoplasmic ratio

Engorn B, Flerlage J, editors. The Harriet Lane handbook. 20th edn. Saunders; 2015.

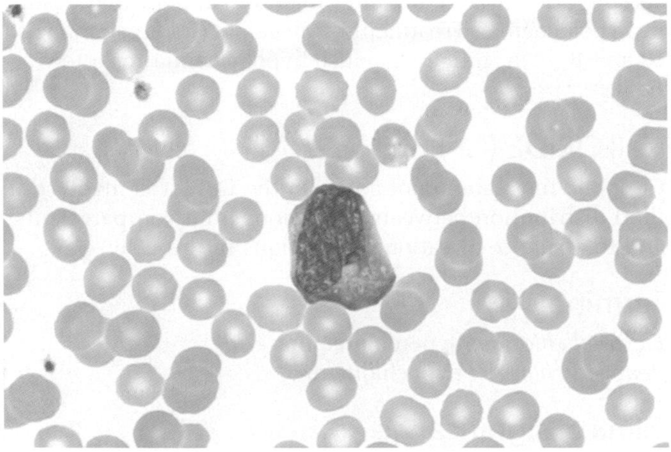

FIGURE 4.17 Reactive lymphocyte with irregular nucleus and basophilic cytoplasm

Rozenberg G. Microscopic haematology. 3rd edn. Chatswood NSW: Elsevier; 2011.

THALASSAEMIA TESTING

Thalassaemia comprises a group of inherited genetic blood disorders. Gene mutations in thalassaemia affect the normal production of haemoglobin, leading to mild-to-severe forms of anaemia. Haematology laboratories can specifically test for and classify the various types of thalassaemia. This group of conditions is an excellent example of the synergistic interpretation of many haematology tests for both diagnosis and planning treatment. From the FBC the RCC, Hb concentrations and RBC indices are often all low. On peripheral blood smear, RBCs are most often noted as microcytic, hypochromic, nucleated and target cells.[14] In conjunction with iron studies, these simple yet elegant tests lead the pathologist and clinician to order tests that identify the exact form of thalassaemia, such as Hb electrophoresis, and DNA analysis for the specific mutations involved.[14]

Coagulation profile

Coagulation profiles or panels are requested to assess the risk of bleeding. Coagulation profiles include the activated partial thromboplastin time (APTT) and the prothrombin time (PT). The FBC is often included, to quantify the platelet count. Other specialised tests can be added, including fibrinogen levels, the thrombin time (TT) and D-dimer levels.[11] The panels are often used for the preoperative assessment of patients with specific clinical indications (e.g. liver disease and positive bleeding history). They may be used as screening tests for the investigation of inherited clotting factor deficiencies, but are not diagnostic in this respect.

Special attention is required when assessing coagulation profiles of female patients. Factor VIII and von Willebrand's factor (VWF) both increase due to the effect of oestrogen. Both can display increased activity during high oestrogen phases of the menstrual cycle, pregnancy and any form of oestrogen therapy.[11]

The PT measures the time taken for blood to clot. It measures the extrinsic pathway (tissue factor pathway) of blood coagulation and assesses clotting factors I, II, V, VII and X.[11]

CLINICAL SIGNIFICANCE

Elevated PT can be due to liver disease, vitamin K deficiency, warfarin therapy or disseminated intravascular coagulation (DIC). When used in monitoring warfarin therapy, the PT is reported as the International Normalised Ratio (INR). PT reference ranges differ between laboratories so the reference range of 12–13 seconds is a guide only.[11]

BIOCHEMISTRY

Clinical biochemistry is the subspecialty of pathology concerning the biochemical aspects of disease and health. In practice, testing focuses on the analysis of blood serum (the non-cellular, fluid portion of blood where clotting factors have been removed) and urine. Other fluids used for specialised biochemical tests include CSF (cerebrospinal fluid) and fluid aspirates from joints or gastric sources. Biochemistry assesses the function of almost all internal organs and systems; every field of medicine uses certain biochemical profiles. It is a significant pathology service used in general practice as well as emergency and highly specialised areas of medicine.

The biochemistry profile is the most frequently requested testing panel in biochemistry. This panel includes electrolytes, urea and creatinine (EUCs), and liver function tests. Additionally, testing panels may be requested to assess the function of a specific internal organ. Reference ranges in clinical biochemistry are becoming far more standardised for international interpretation of results. This is evidenced by the adoption of the 'harmonisation' concept by many countries, including Australia.[19] The harmonisation concept highlights the difference in reference ranges for different ages and, in some cases, gender.

Electrolytes, urea and creatinine (EUCs)

EUCs are part of the standard biochemistry profile, but may also be requested as a separate testing panel. Electrolytes tested include sodium (Na^+), potassium (K^+), chloride (Cl^-) and bicarbonate (HCO_3^-) ions. Body water (H_2O) and electrolytes are in constant flux via eating, drinking, sweating and urination, yet we must maintain their steady state.[20] Maintaining our extracellular fluid (ECF) volume is essential for survival; blood circulation, O_2 and nutrient delivery to tissues with consequent removal of metabolic wastes all rely on the healthy maintenance of the ECF volume.[20] EUCs are also essential for monitoring renal function, cardiac function and IV fluid replacement.

SODIUM (Na^+)

Na^+ is the most abundant extracellular cation. Serum Na^+ concentration reflects our state of hydration; body Na^+ content and osmotic (water) shifts between blood and other fluid compartments. One-quarter of our sodium is unavailable for fluid exchange and is incorporated into other tissues such as bone and hair. Na^+ input is highly variable due to diet; output via urine is regulated by the hormones aldosterone (renal origin: increases renal Na^+ reabsorption) and atrial natriuretic peptide (ANP) (cardiac origin: increases renal Na^+ excretion).[20]

Terminology

Elevated sodium: hypernatraemia
Decreased sodium: hyponatraemia.

Clinical significance

Hypernatraemia may be caused by IV isotonic saline therapy and excess mineralocorticoid (aldosterone). Hyponatraemia may be observed in fluid retention (cardiac and renal disease), deficiency of mineralocorticoid, excess H_2O intake, gastrointestinal loss (vomiting/diarrhoea), renal loss and excessive sweating. It is occasionally seen in diuretic therapy. Severe hyperlipidaemia or hyperproteinaemia can cause 'pseudohyponatraemia'.[11]

POTASSIUM (K^+)

K^+ is the most abundant intracellular cation and has a significant role in maintaining cellular resting membrane potential. Electrically excitable tissues (nerve and all forms of muscle tissue) are incredibly sensitive to changes in blood K^+ concentration, which is maintained within a very narrow range. Dietary K^+ intake is highly variable and renal excretion should mirror intake.[20] K^+ excretion is determined by the glomerular filtration rate (GFR) and blood K^+ concentration. 98% of total body K^+ is within body tissue. Tissue damage is a significant contributing factor to dangerously increased blood K^+ levels.[20]

Terminology

Elevated potassium: hyperkalaemia.
Decreased potassium: hypokalaemia.

Clinical significance

Hyperkalaemia is a very common electrolyte abnormality in medical practice; it must be dealt with immediately as risk of cardiac arrest is incredibly high. Muscle weakness, paraesthesia and specific abnormalities of the electrocardiogram (ECG) all reflect hyperkalaemia. Renal failure, hypoaldosteronism (query antihypertensive medications), adrenal insufficiency, insulin deficiency and extensive tissue damage are possible causes. GFR will be reduced with hyperkalaemia and should be noted. Dietary K^+ intake needs to be monitored by those with impaired renal function; hidden oral sources include medications and supplements administered as K^+ salts. Hypokalaemia mostly results from increased loss (gut), reduced intake (rare, but possible in severe hypocaloric diets) or redistribution of K^+ into cells.[20] Again, muscle weakness and specific changes on ECG can be noted. Insulin therapy can initiate hypokalaemia. Re-feeding of a high carbohydrate (CHO) diet after malnourishment may result in hypokalaemia. Treatment of megaloblastic anaemia with B_9 and B_{12} can initially produce hypokalaemia for a few days.[20]

CHLORIDE (Cl^-)

Cl^- is the most abundant anion in the ECF. It is involved in fluid distribution between the various fluid compartments and the balance of cations and anions in the ECF.

Terminology

Elevated chloride: hyperchloraemia.
Reduced chloride: hypochloraemia.

Clinical significance

Hyperchloraemia may be observed in dehydration, metabolic acidosis, prolonged vomiting/diarrhoea and excessive IV saline therapy. Hypernatraemia and hyperchloraemia are often noted together. Hypochloraemia may be seen in over-hydration. Hyponatraemia is also associated with hypochloraemia.[11]

BICARBONATE

The human body produces a number of endogenous buffers to stabilise abrupt changes in hydrogen ion (H^+) concentration. Buffers are solutions of a weak acid or base, plus their salt. In the ECF, the bicarbonate anion (HCO_3^-) is the most significant. HCO_3^- can bond with H^+ to form carbonic acid (H_2CO_3), which then dissociates into H_2O and CO_2.

Terminology

Not specific, but the test is also known as the total bicarbonate and total carbon dioxide.

TABLE 4.13 Reference range: major blood electrolytes		
Electrolyte	Age	Range (mmol/L)
Na⁺	<1 week	132–147
	1 week to <18 yrs	133–144
	>18 yrs	135–145
K⁺	<1 week	3.8–6.5
	1 week to <26 weeks	4.2–6.7
	26 weeks to <2 yrs	3.9–5.6
	2 yrs to <18yrs	3.6–5.3
	>18 yrs	3.5–5.2
Cl⁻	<1 week	98–155
	1 week to <18 yrs	97–110
	>18 yrs	95–110
HCO₃⁻	<1 week	15–28
	1 week to <2 yrs	16–29
	2 yrs to <10 yrs	17–30
	10 yrs to 18 yrs	20–32
	>18 yrs	22–32

NPS MedicineWise. Erythrocyte sedimentation rate [Internet]. 2016. Available from: www.nps.org.au (accessed 17 June 2016)

TABLE 4.14 Reference range: anion gap	
	All ages
With K+	8–16 mmol/L
Without K+	4–13 mmol/L

NPS MedicineWise. Erythrocyte sedimentation rate [Internet]. 2016. Available from: www.nps.org.au (accessed 17 June 2016)

TABLE 4.15 Reference range: urea	
Age	Urea (mmol/L)
Neonate	1.0–4.0
Adult	3.0–8.0

Reproduced with permission from the Royal College of Pathologists of Australasia (RCPA). RCPA manual of use and interpretation of pathology tests. 7th ed. Sydney: RCPA, 2015. https://www.rcpa.edu.au/Library/Practising-Pathology/RCPA-Manual/Home.

Clinical significance

Mostly used in the assessment of acid–base disorders (respiratory and metabolic acidosis or alkalosis). HCO_3^- is increased in metabolic alkalosis (vomiting, excess ingestion of sodium bicarbonate, K⁺ depletion from diuretic therapy) and compensated respiratory acidosis.[20] It is decreased in metabolic acidosis (renal disease, diabetic ketoacidosis, lactic acidosis, chronic diarrhoea).[11] While blood HCO_3^- levels are essential for the diagnosis of acid–base disorders, they must be interpreted in conjunction with the other blood gases (O_2, CO_2) (see blood gases).

Refer to Table 4.13 for reference ranges for the major blood electrolytes.

ANION GAP

The anion gap value is reported with EUCs. It is a calculation based on the difference between measured cations (Na⁺ and K⁺) and anions (Cl⁻ and HCO_3^-) in serum, but can also be determined from urinary electrolyte measurements. In health, the measured serum cations should be higher than the measured anions. The resulting anion gap should be positive.[20]

Clinical significance

An elevated anion gap indicates the presence of excess, unmeasured non-chloride anions (commonly lactate, ketone bodies, phosphate and sulfate). An increased anion gap usually occurs in metabolic acidosis and renal failure.[11] Some laboratories do not include K⁺ ions in their calculations. Refer to Table 4.14 for reference ranges.

UREA

Urea is the predominant waste product of nitrogenous compounds in the body. It is used as a measure of renal dysfunction. Serum urea concentration is dependent upon renal function, but also the amount of urea produced by the body. Urea production is heavily influenced by dietary protein intake. Urea forms via the urea cycle in the liver and kidneys, and is then excreted from the body via the renal glomerulus. There is a substantial capacity for renal reabsorption of urea.[21]

Terminology

Elevated urea: hyperuraemia.
Decreased urea: hypouraemia.

Clinical significance

Hyperuraemia can reflect reduced glomerular filtration from renal or non-renal causes, for example hypercatabolic states (e.g. diabetic ketoacidosis, severe fever and infection, thyrotoxicosis).[11] Hypouraemia may be noted in pregnancy, fluid retention, reduced protein intake and severe liver disease.[11] Refer to Table 4.15 for reference ranges.

CREATININE

Creatinine is produced in muscle tissue from creatine and creatine phosphate. It is used as a marker of renal GFR, and in the assessment of renal function.[21] The rate of endogenous creatinine production is fairly constant, but there is considerable individual variation due to dietary meat intake (a significant source of creatine).

Clinical significance

Increased blood creatinine levels occur in conditions that reduce the GFR. Causes include hypovolaemia, hypotension, renal disease and renal obstruction. Low blood creatinine may be noted in any state of muscle wasting (e.g. malnutrition, disordered eating, the elderly, rapid weight loss).[11] Reference ranges vary considerably and are dependent on age. Refer to Table 4.16 for reference ranges.

TABLE 4.16 Reference range: creatinine

Age	Range (umol/L)
<1 week	22–93
1 week–<4 weeks	17–50
4 weeks–<2 yrs	11–36
2 yrs–<6 yrs	20–44
6 yrs–<12 yrs	27–58
Female	
12 yrs–<15 yrs	35–74
15 yrs–<19 yrs	38–82
19 yrs–<60 yrs	45–90
Male	
12 yrs–<15 yrs	35–83
15 yrs–<19 yrs	50–100
19 yrs–<60 yrs	60–110

NPS MedicineWise. Erythrocyte sedimentation rate [Internet]. 2016. Available from: www.nps.org.au (accessed 17 June 2016)

TABLE 4.17 Reference range: calcium

	Age	Range (mmol/L)
Calcium	<1 week	1.85–2.80
	1 week–<26 weeks	2.20–2.80
	26 weeks–<2 yrs	2.20–2.70
	2 yrs–<18 yrs	2.20–2.65
	>18 yrs	2.10–2.60
Calcium corrected for albumin	>18 yrs	2.10–2.60
Ionised calcium		1.16–1.30

NPS MedicineWise. Erythrocyte sedimentation rate [Internet]. 2016. Available from: www.nps.org.au (accessed 17 June 2016)

GLOMERULAR FILTRATION RATE (GFR)

The GFR is a calculation based on a patient's age, gender and blood creatinine results. Assessment of the GFR is the main indicator test for kidney function. A reduced GFR is generally assessed at frequent points over many months and can indicate chronic kidney disease. Rapid reductions in GFR can indicate acute renal failure.

A GFR result of >90 mL/min/1.73 m^2 is considered normal. A GFR of 60–89 mL/min/1.73 m^2 is only mildly reduced. A reading in this range constitutes renal pathology only if serum creatinine is elevated or other signs of renal damage are clinically evident. GFR generally declines with age. Additionally, GFR is less accurate with extremes of body composition, including emaciation, obesity, paraplegia and elevated muscle mass.[11] It is not a suitable renal assessment in pregnancy.[11]

- 30–59 mL/min/1.73 m^2—GFR moderately reduced.
- 15–29 mL/min/1.73 m^2—GFR severely reduced.
- <15 mL/min/1.73 m^2—end-stage kidney damage.[11]

CALCIUM (Ca OR Ca^{2+})

Calcium is the most abundant cation in the body, with approximately 99% of body Ca stored as hydroxyapatite in skeletal tissue. Only 1% is found distributed between the ECF and soft tissues.[23] Ca exists as three forms:

(1) Free (ionised) Ca (this is the physiologically active form, accounting for 50% of blood Ca)
(2) Complexed Ca (bound with bicarbonate, lactate, phosphate and citrate anions to form Ca salts), accounting for 10% of blood Ca
(3) Blood plasma protein bound Ca (the remaining 40% of blood Ca).[26]

Ca is involved in mineralisation of skeletal tissue, blood coagulation, nerve-impulse transmission, some blood buffer systems and normal muscle tone/excitability and is essential for nucleic acid synthesis. It plays a critical role in cell membrane function.[25]

Blood Ca levels are maintained within a very narrow range, sometimes to the detriment of skeletal health. EFC Ca adjustments are achieved via the actions of parathyroid hormone (PTH), calcitonin and 1, 25-dihydroxyvitamin D_3.[25]

Terminology

Elevated blood calcium: hypercalcaemia.
Reduced blood calcium: hypocalcaemia.

Clinical significance

Hypercalcaemia produces marked clinical features and may be caused by hyperparathyroidism, many malignancies, bone metastases, states of high bone turnover (e.g. prolonged immobilisation, hyperthyroidism) and certain vitamin toxicities (e.g. vitamin D and vitamin A).[11] In all cases, blood Ca should not be interpreted in isolation; phosphate, creatinine, urea, ALP, FBC and blood PTH are all useful. Hypocalcaemia is only clinically significant if the ionised Ca level is reduced. It may be caused by hypoparathyroidism, vitamin D deficiency, osteomalacia, hypomagnesaemia and hypoalbuminaemia.[11] Refer to Table 4.17 for reference ranges.

MAGNESIUM (Mg OR Mg^{2+})

Magnesium is the fourth most prevalent cation in the body: 50–60% of the body's Mg is in skeletal tissue, with 40–50% dispersed among soft tissues. Only 1% is present in the ECF.[26] Over half of this ECF Mg is in the ionised/free state, 30% is associated with plasma proteins and 15% exists in salt form with anions such as phosphate and citrate.[25]

More than 300 enzymes require Mg^{2+} as a cofactor. Every reaction in the body that requires adenosine triphosphate (ATP) requires Mg. The transcription/translation of DNA, translation of mRNA, nerve conduction, maintenance of resting membrane potential, K^+ homeostasis and Ca channel activity all rely on Mg.[25]

Terminology

Elevated blood magnesium: hypermagnesaemia.
Reduced blood magnesium: hypomagnesaemia.

TABLE 4.18 Reference range: magnesium

Age	Range (mmol/L)
<1 week	0.60–1.00
1 week–<18 yrs	0.65–1.10
>18 yrs	0.70–1.10

Klemm K, Klein M. Biochemical markers of bone metabolism. In McPherson R, Pincus M, editors. Henry's clinical diagnosis and management by laboratory methods. 23rd edn. St Louis: Elsevier; 2017, pp. 188–204.

Clinical significance

Unexplained cardiac arrhythmias and neuromuscular disorders may be investigated with suspicion of hypomagnesaemia. Clinical features of hypocalcaemia, but with normal blood Ca, should have blood Mg measured to check for hypomagnesaemia.[11] Decreased levels suggest either reduced intake, or loss via the renal or gastrointestinal systems. Hypermagnesaemia is generally due to renal failure.[11] Normal blood Mg levels do not exclude underlying deficiency.[25] Refer to Table 4.18 for reference ranges.

PHOSPHATE (PO_4^-)

Some 80–85% of the phosphate content of the body resides in skeletal tissue (as hydroxyapatite and calcium phosphate), with approximately 15% present in the ECF as the inorganic phosphate compound (PO_4^-). Phosphate not in the ECF is complexed into biomolecules such as the nucleic acids, phospholipids and ATP.[25] It is an essential structural component of skeletal tissue, the nucleic acids, phospholipids, phosphoproteins, ATP and the high-energy cofactor nicotinamide adenine dinucleotide phosphate (NADPH). It is an essential compound for highly metabolically active tissue. It is lowered by PTH and increased by growth hormone and vitamin D.[25]

Clinical significance

Elevated phosphate levels are observed in response to low PTH levels (e.g. hypoparathyroidism, hypercalcaemia of malignancy). Elevated blood phosphate may also be noted in renal failure. Decreased phosphate may be found in hyperparathyroidism, hypercalcaemia of malignancy and the long-term use of magnesium- and aluminium-based antacids.[11] Refer to Table 4.19 for reference ranges.

TABLE 4.19 Reference range: phosphate

Age	Range (mmol/L)
< 1 week	1.25–2.85
1 week–< 4 weeks	1.50–2.75
4 weeks–< 26 weeks	1.45–2.50
26 weeks–< 1 yr	1.30–2.30
1 yr–< 4 yrs	1.10–2.20
4 yrs–< 15 yrs	0.90–2.00
15 yrs–< 18 yrs	0.80–1.85
18 yrs–< 20 yrs	0.75–1.65
> 20 yrs	0.75–1.50

NPS MedicineWise. Erythrocyte sedimentation rate [Internet]. 2016. Available from: www.nps.org.au (accessed 17 June 2016)

Liver function tests (LFTs)

Liver function tests (LFTs) are part of a full biochemical profile. They are very useful in the assessment and longer-term management of patients with hepatic disorders. The term 'liver function test' is actually less preferred than the term 'liver biochemical test (LBT)'. This is largely because some analytes measured in this panel are ubiquitous in many organs; they do not measure a known function of the liver.[22]

A major argument against the validity of LFTs is they do not measure the functional capacity of the liver. However, it is worth remembering the liver performs thousands of biochemical reactions—gluconeogenesis, clotting factor biosynthesis, cholesterol biosynthesis, protein biosynthesis and xenobiotic detoxification, to name a few. No one testing panel could measure all this. The usefulness of LFTs comes from the ability to identify liver disease and distinguish which type is present, determine the severity of hepatic disease and monitor its progression or response to therapy. In this sense, they are a useful testing panel for both medical and naturopathic treatments.

BILIRUBIN

Bilirubin is generated by the body as a breakdown product of haeme (from senescent RBCs, prematurely destroyed erythroid bone marrow and haemoproteins such as myoglobin and cytochromes).[22] Bilirubin formation begins predominantly in the spleen before being completed in the liver. Unconjugated bilirubin (i.e. not bound to protein, lipid soluble and non-water soluble) enters hepatocytes to become conjugated (lipid insoluble, water soluble), which is more readily excreted by the body via bile. Interestingly, hepatic conjugation of bilirubin requires a number of important proteins, including the glutathione S-transferase superfamily.[22]

Terminology

Direct bilirubin: conjugated bilirubin.
Indirect bilirubin: unconjugated bilirubin.
Total bilirubin levels: represent both fractions together.
Hyperbilirubinaemia: elevated serum bilirubin.

Clinical significance

Hyperbilirubinaemia must be assessed by determining which fraction (conjugated versus unconjugated) is responsible for the elevation. Elevated total and conjugated bilirubin is seen in hepatocellular and biliary disease.[11] Elevated unconjugated bilirubin (i.e. elevated total bilirubin with normal direct bilirubin) reflects a rate of bilirubin production in excess of conjugation. Haemolysis, megaloblastic anaemia and Gilbert's syndrome are common causes.[11] Neonatal jaundice represents the

TABLE 4.20 Reference range: bilirubin

Bilirubin	Range (umol/L)
Total	<20
Direct	<7

Reproduced with permission from the Royal College of Pathologists of Australasia (RCPA). RCPA manual of use and interpretation of pathology tests. 7th ed. Sydney: RCPA, 2015. https://www.rcpa.edu.au/Library/Practising-Pathology/RCPA-Manual/Home.

accumulation of unconjugated bilirubin.[23] Refer to Table 4.20 for reference ranges.

AMINOTRANSFERASES

Aminotranferases include alanine aminotransferase (ALT) and aspartate aminotransferase (AST). They are sometimes referred to as transaminases. AST is found (from highest to lowest concentration) in both the cytoplasm and mitochondria of hepatic cells, cardiac muscle, skeletal muscle, kidneys, brain, pancreatic and lung tissue. It is also found in leucocytes and erythrocytes.[22] AST catalyses the biochemical interconversions between aspartate, a-ketoglutarate, oxaloacetate and glutamate. ALT is cytoplasmic and present in many tissues, though the greatest concentration by far is in hepatic tissue. Therefore, ALT is a more specific indicator of liver pathology over AST.[22] ALT catalyses two steps of the alanine cycle (for removal of nitrogen and glucose recycling). These enzymes serve no function in blood plasma; their presence in serum or plasma is indicative of cellular and tissue injury.

Clinical significance

Elevated levels are observed in all forms of liver pathology and may be nonspecific when viewed in isolation. Symptomatology, clinical history and physical examination help to determine the diagnosis. Mild elevations with ALT > AST may indicate chronic viral hepatitis, haemochromatosis, medication use and toxin damage, coeliac disease, hyperthyroidism, steatosis or Wilson's disease. Mild elevations with AST > ALT may indicate ethanol-related liver injury, hypothyroidism, myopathy and strenuous exercise. Severe, acute elevations with ALT > AST may indicate acute bile duct obstruction, acute viral hepatitis, medications and toxins, Wilson's disease. Severe, acute elevations with AST > ALT may indicate ethanol-related liver injury and medication or toxin damage, acute rhabdomyolysis.[22]

When recognising ethanol-related liver disease, a ratio of AST to ALT of more than 2 is often seen. A ratio of 3 is highly suggestive of alcoholic liver disease. Hepatic ALT synthesis requires pyridoxal 5′-phosphate (B_6), which is deficient in these patients.[22] Laboratories may supply their own reference ranges, and the ranges in Table 4.21 are a guide.

TABLE 4.21 Reference ranges: LFT enzymes

Enzyme	Neonate (U/L)	Adult (U/L)
ALT	<50	<35
AST	<80	<40
GGT		<30 (F) <50 (M)
LDH		120–250

NPS MedicineWise. Erythrocyte sedimentation rate [Internet]. 2016. Available from: www.nps.org.au (accessed 17 June 2016)

ALKALINE PHOSPHATASE (ALP)

The ALP enzyme is responsible for removing phosphate groups (dephosphorylation) from base nucleotides, nucleosides, phosphate-containing proteins and alkaloids. Substantial amounts of ALP are found in liver and skeletal tissue, but also in the small intestine, kidneys and placenta.[20] There are many isoenzyme forms of ALP that are tissue specific; these can be separated and detected by electrophoresis. Generally, elevations of other LFTs will indicate that the source of a raised ALP is hepatic.

TABLE 4.22 Reference ranges: ALP

Age	Range (U/L)
<1 week	80–380
1 week– <4 weeks	120–550
4 weeks–<26 weeks	120–650
26 weeks–<2 yrs	120–450
2 yrs–<6 yrs	120–370
6 yrs–<10 yrs	120–440
Female	
10 yrs–<13 yrs	100–460
13 yrs–<14 yrs	70–330
14 yrs–<15 yrs	50–280
15 yrs–<16 yrs	45–170
16 yrs–<22 yrs	35–140
22 yrs and over	30–110
Male	
10 yrs–<14 yrs	130–530
14 yrs–<15 yrs	105–480
15 yrs–<17 yrs	80–380
17 yrs–<19 yrs	50–220
19 yrs–<22 yrs	45–150
22 yrs and over	30–110

NPS MedicineWise. Erythrocyte sedimentation rate [Internet]. 2016. Available from: www.nps.org.au (accessed 17 June 2016)

Clinical significance

ALP is elevated in cholestasis and infiltrative diseases of the liver (e.g. space-occupying tumours).[20] It is also elevated in bone diseases with high osteoblast activity. Transient elevations are seen throughout infancy and childhood; hence the requirement for comprehensive reference ranges reflective of age.[11] Refer to Table 4.22 for reference ranges.

GAMMA GLUTAMYLTRANSFERASE (GGT)

The enzyme GGT plays a role in the gamma glutamyl cycle, which is involved in the synthesis and degradation of glutathione, plus xenobiotic detoxification.[24] It is found in many tissues besides liver tissue, including the bile duct, gallbladder, pancreas, seminal vesicles and spleen.[22]

Clinical significance

GGT is elevated in cholestatic liver disease. Levels may also be increased in diabetes and non-alcoholic fatty liver disease (NAFLD). Some causes of NAFLD include enzyme induction from medications and chronic alcohol ingestion. Elevations in GGT have been observed in pancreatitis and prostatitis. Acute hepatocellular damage from acute viral hepatitis and paracetamol hepatotoxity often show a normal GGT in the early course of disease.[11] Refer to Table 4.21 for reference ranges.

LACTATE DEHYDROGENASE (LDH)

The enzyme LDH has a copious tissue distribution throughout the body and is a very nonspecific indicator of disease. LDH catalyses the reversible conversion of lactate to pyruvate.

Clinical significance

Elevated levels can be seen in many liver diseases, but in any pathology that involves tissue damage. Some examples include myocardial infarction (MI), skeletal muscle disease/damage, some malignancies, haemolytic anaemia and hepatic metastases of cancers.[11] Refer to Table 4.21 for reference ranges.

TOTAL PROTEIN

Also known as total plasma protein, this test is representative of total albumin and immunoglobulin levels (the only serum proteins in high enough quantities contributing to this measurement). It is mainly used with the albumin level to calculate globulin levels. Refer to Table 4.23 for a summary of protein reference ranges.

Clinical significance

Useful in the diagnosis of malnutrition and protein-losing states, as well as the diagnosis and monitoring of both hyper- and hypogammaglobulinaemias.[11] Postural influences induce inaccuracies of results, with recumbent position collections falsely lowering results. Venous stasis and dehydration can show falsely elevated results. Refer to Table 4.24 for reference ranges.

ALBUMIN

Albumin is the most prolific protein in normal blood plasma and is usually representative of two-thirds of total protein. Albumin is synthesised in the liver and can be negatively affected by liver disease/dysfunction, malnutrition, malabsorption and protein loss via gastrointestinal or renal disease. Low albumin leads to impaired intravascular oncotic pressure, which manifests clinically as peripheral oedema.[26] Albumin is also important for the transportation of amino acids, thyroxin, bilirubin, free fatty acids, oestrogen, cortisol, haeme, Ca and Mg.[26] Albumin can become glycosylated as a consequence of hyperglycaemia (see fructosamine test)

TABLE 4.23 Reference range: proteins

	Age	Range (g/L)
Total protein	Neonate <2 yrs >18 yrs	40–75 50–75 60–80
Albumin	All	32–45
Globulin	Neonate >18 yrs	12–36 25–35

Reproduced with permission from the Royal College of Pathologists of Australasia (RCPA). RCPA manual of use and interpretation of pathology tests. 7th ed. Sydney: RCPA, 2015. https://www.rcpa.edu.au/Library/Practising-Pathology/RCPA-Manual/Home.

TABLE 4.24 Reference range: total protein

Age	Reference range (g/L)
Neonate	40–75
Infant <2 yrs	50–75
18 yrs and over	60–80

Reproduced with permission from the Royal College of Pathologists of Australasia (RCPA). RCPA manual of use and interpretation of pathology tests. 7th ed. Sydney: RCPA, 2015. https://www.rcpa.edu.au/Library/Practising-Pathology/RCPA-Manual/Home.

Terminology

Elevated blood albumin: hyperalbuminaemia.
Decreased blood albumin: hypoalbuminaemia.

Clinical significance

Albumin levels are tested in the assessment of hydration, nutritional status, protein-losing disorders (nephrotic syndrome) and liver disease. Hypoalbuminaemia may be noted in chronic liver disease, malnutrition, overhydration and burns. It may also be observed during the acute phase response.[11] Blood collection in the erect position rather than supine can increase the albumin level. Hyperalbuminaemia may be observed in dehydration.[11] Albumin levels are critical in the interpretation of Ca and Mg levels (both ions are bound to albumin; a decrease in albumin may be responsible for their reduced levels).

GLOBULINS

Terminology

Elevated levels: hypergammaglobulinaemia.
Reduced levels: hypogammaglobulinaemia

Clinical significance

Elevated gammaglobulins are observed in response to chronic inflammation, infection, autoimmune disease and liver disease. Reduced levels are seen in protein-losing enteropathies, B lymphocyte (humoral) immunodeficiency and sometimes in nephrotic syndrome.[11]

AMYLASE

Amylase is a digestive enzyme secreted by salivary glands and the pancreas. Amylase is able to hydrolyse the glycosidic bonds of polysaccharides (e.g. starches and glycogen) to yield free glucose.

Terminology

Elevated level: hyperamylasaemia

Clinical significance

Very high blood amylase levels are seen in acute pancreatitis, but elevations are not diagnostic. Elevated blood amylase is also observed in severe cases of duodenal ulcer (perforated) and upper small intestinal obstruction. Pelvic infection, mumps and diabetic ketoacidosis can all lead to hyperamylasaemia.[11] Age-specific reference ranges vary between laboratories; the reference range 20–100 U/L is a guide.[11]

LIPASE

Lipase is a digestive enzyme also secreted by the salivary gland and the pancreas. Lipase breaks down triglycerides into free fatty acids and glycerol.

Clinical significance

Elevated blood lipase levels indicate pancreatitis, which is often observed before increases in blood amylase levels. Additionally, blood lipase is not elevated by salivary gland disease, thus lipase provides a better indication of pancreatic cell damage.[11] Age-specific reference ranges vary between laboratories; the reference range <61 U/L is a guide.[11]

Iron studies

IRON (Fe)

Iron is an essential nutrient mineral for most living organisms; Fe is incorporated into haemoglobin and myoglobin for oxygen transportation and is an essential component of the electron transfer chain in mitochondria. Serum iron levels show significant diurnal variation; morning levels can be 30% higher than at other times of day.[27] Serum iron levels fall rapidly during both acute and chronic infection. Iron deficiency may or may not be accompanied by anaemia, thus results from the FBC should be considered in conjunction with iron profiles. Iron deficiency without anaemia is still a depleting problem, leading to impaired cognition, and physical and intellectual underperformance in both children and adults.[28] The interpretation of iron studies may be difficult at times, due to the shared relationship of iron metabolism and inflammation.[27]

Clinical significance

Serum iron values are of little significance when viewed in isolation. This test should be interpreted in conjunction with the full iron profile. It is used in the detection of iron deficiency anaemia; however, elevated serum iron is a common clinical manifestation. Serum iron may be elevated by some medications and supplements (e.g. oestrogens, Fe supplementation), alcohol and medical conditions such as haemochromatosis and hepatitis.[28] In the absence of an iron-deficient diet, potential blood loss should be investigated. Reference ranges are 4.5–27 umol/L (child) and 9–27 umol/L (adult).[11]

FERRITIN

Ferritin is an intracellular Fe storage protein, with the capacity to store up to 4000 Fe atoms. Serum ferritin levels correlate well with the amount of stored tissue iron.[27]

Clinical significance

Ferritin levels are both age and gender dependent. Reduced serum ferritin levels are indicative of iron deficiency. Elevated levels are observed during inflammation, infection, liver disease or malignancy, due to the acute phase response. Soluble transferrin receptor levels may be useful in these situations.[28] Ferritin levels are increased in cases of iron overload (e.g. haemochromatosis, haemosiderosis and iron supplementation). Higher ferritin levels are seen with increasing body mass index (BMI).[27] Note: reference ranges for postmenopausal women tend to reflect adult male reference ranges. Refer to Table 4.25 for reference ranges.

TRANSFERRIN

Apotransferrin (synthesised in liver tissue) is the circulating transporter protein for iron and refers to the protein without any bound iron. Transferrin refers to apotransferrin that has bound with one to two atoms of iron.[27] Transferrin binds with the transferrin receptor on cells, resulting in the uptake of iron and its subsequent usage or storage.

Clinical significance

Elevated transferrin levels may be observed in iron deficiency or high oestrogen states such as pregnancy and

TABLE 4.25 Reference range: ferritin

Population	Range (micrograms/L)
Adult female	15–200
Pregnant female	<30 (low Fe status) <15 (depleted Fe stores)
Adult male	30–300
Children	20–200

Royal College of Pathologists of Australasia (RCPA). Education online. RCPA, 2016. Available from: https://www.rcpa.edu.au/Education; Women and Newborn Health Service, King Edward Memorial Hospital. Complications in pregnancy. Clinical Guidelines. Government of Western Australia, 2013. Available from: www.kemh.health.wa.gov.au/development/manuals/O&G_guidelines/sectionb/2/b2.23.pdf

oestrogen therapy.[27] Reduced transferrin levels may reflect iron loading or poor synthetic functions of the liver as seen in liver disease.[27] The reference ranges are 2.0–3.5 g/L for children and 2.0–3.2 g/L for adults.[27]

TOTAL IRON BINDING CAPACITY (TIBC)

TIBC measures the maximum amount of iron that may be carried by transferrin. Some laboratories may measure TIBC as an alternative to a direct measurement of transferrin.

Clinical significance

A calculation known as the transferrin saturation is the ratio between serum iron and the TIBC.

SOLUBLE TRANSFERRIN RECEPTOR (sTfR)

sTfR for transferrin is membrane bound. Blood levels become elevated during an increased demand for iron. Reference ranges vary considerably based on age, gender, pregnancy and laboratory method used.

Clinical significance

Iron deficiency, megaloblastic anaemia, increased erythropoiesis and haemolysis can all lead to elevated sTfR levels. This measurement is not used routinely in the general detection or assessment of anaemia, though it is very useful in distinguishing iron deficiency anaemia from the anaemia of chronic disease. In the acute phase response of infection/inflammation, blood levels of iron and transferrin both fall, while ferritin levels increase.[11] Thus, these three parameters become unreliable indicators of iron deficiency until the acute phase passes. sTfR may be added on at this time for measurement, or a repeat test of iron studies at a later date may be requested. It is a useful parameter when investigating anaemia in a patient with a preexisting inflammatory state. The reference ranges are 2.2–5.0 mg/L (males) and 1.9–4.4 mg/L (females).[28]

Refer to Table 4.26 for a clinical interpretation of the full iron studies testing panel.

C-reactive protein (CRP)

CRP is synthesised in the liver and is present only in very small amounts in blood. It is one of the proteins synthesised in the acute phase response of inflammation.[29] The role of CRP as an acute phase reactant is to bind with phospholipids, invading microorganisms and some proteins. CRP is generally considered a marker of bacterial infection when levels are greatly elevated. More specifically, CRP is considered as a marker of general inflammation. It is often preferred over the ESR in this respect, as CRP rises and falls more rapidly than the ESR in response to inflammation.

CLINICAL SIGNIFICANCE

CRP is useful in monitoring disease activity of chronic inflammatory disorders. Infective, neoplastic and septic disorders can also be monitored via CRP. High sensitivity (hs) CRP assays are used to determine risk of coronary artery disease.[11] The reference range (CRP) target is <5 mg/L.[11] Reference range (hs-CRP) low risk is <1.0 mg/L and average risk is 1.0–3.0 mg/L.[11]

Tumour markers

Tumour markers are not screening tests for malignancies, nor do the results diagnose or rule out malignant disease. Additionally, some tumour markers are elevated due to a range of malignancies.[11] Pre- and post-treatment tumour marker levels are often compared to determine the efficacy of cancer therapies. Decreased levels may indicate that only small amounts of tumour remain, or destruction of the tumour.[11] Refer to Table 4.27 for reference ranges of some commonly tested tumour markers.

Cardiac enzymes and markers

Cardiac enzymes and markers are protein-based structures released into the bloodstream during damage to cardiac muscle tissue. Along with the electrocardiogram (ECG), these markers help to diagnose acute coronary syndromes (ACS) and myocardial infarction (MI). There is one very clinically important cardiac enzyme, cardiac troponin (cTn), which is derived only from cardiac muscle.[30]

Troponin is actually a complex of three protein subunits found in striated muscle tissue: tropomyosin-binding troponin (TnT), the inhibitory subunit (TnI) and the Ca-binding subunit (TnC). Each protein has a specific role. TnI has a cardiac-specific form (cTnI) and cardiac TnT (cTnT) specificity approaches

TABLE 4.26 Overall interpretation of iron studies

	Iron	TIBC	Transferrin saturation	Ferritin	sTfR
Fe deficiency	Decreased	Increased	Decreased	Decreased	Increased
Fe deficiency + acute phase response	Decreased	Normal or decreased	Normal or decreased	'Normal' <100 ug/L	Increased
Acute phase response	Decreased	Decreased	Decreased	Increased	Normal
Fe overload	Increased	Normal or decreased	Increased	Increased	Decreased

Reproduced with permission from the Royal College of Pathologists of Australasia (RCPA). RCPA manual of use and interpretation of pathology tests. 7th ed. Sydney: RCPA, 2015. https://www.rcpa.edu.au/Library/Practising-Pathology/RCPA-Manual/Home.

TABLE 4.27 Tumour marker physiology and reference ranges

Marker	Physiological role	Conditions	Reference range
Alpha fetoprotein (AFP)	In health, AFP is produced by the fetal yolk sac and liver	Used in the assessment and monitoring of liver carcinoma and germ cell tumours (ovarian and testicular). AFP is also used in pregnancy for assessing risk of neural tube defects and trisomy 21 (low AFP). May be seen in liver regeneration of non-malignant disease	<16 ng/L (non-pregnant, adult). Varies with gestational age in pregnancy
Beta-human chorionic gonadotrophin (beta-HCG)	Produced by an embryo after implantation as part of normal pregnancy	Use in non-malignant disease: diagnosis of pregnancy, ectopic pregnancy and threatened abortion. hCG-producing tumours include uterine carcinoma, germ cell tumours and hydatidiform mole	<5 mIU/L (non-pregnant). Varies with gestational age in pregnancy
Cancer antigen 15.3 (CA 15.3)	Cancer antigen	Breast malignancy	<30 U/mL
Cancer antigen (19.9) 19.9	Cancer antigen	GIT malignancy, particularly pancreatic	<37 U/mL
Cancer antigen 125 (CA 125)	Cancer antigen	Ovarian carcinoma, peritoneal disease of any cause	<35 U/mL
Carcinoembryonic antigen (CEA)	Produced in gastrointestinal tissue during normal fetal development	Often used to monitor colorectal or breast adenocarcinoma. Elevations also possible in lung, liver and pancreatic carcinoma. Inflammatory bowel disease and smoking may increase levels	<2.5 ng/L; <5 ng/L (smokers)
NSE	Functions in mature neurons in glycolytic pathways	Used to monitor neural crest tumours, including small cell lung carcinoma	<12 ng/L
Prostate-specific antigen (PSA)	In health, PSA is believed to be involved in the liquefaction of semen	Used in the assessment of prostatic carcinoma, benign prostatic hypertrophy (BPH) and prostatitis. PSA results that do not correlate with physical exam and symptomatology are generally repeated	≤4 ng/mL was considered normal, but this is being replaced by the practice that the higher the PSA, the more likely further investigations are required

Sharma S. Tumour markers in clinical practice: general principles and guidelines. Indian Journal of Medical and Paediatric Oncology 2009; 30(1):1–8.

almost 100%.[30] cTnI and cTnT are released slowly from damaged cardiac muscle, for 1 to 2 weeks post-MI. These levels decline slowly after cardiac injury.[30]

CLINICAL SIGNIFICANCE

CTnT and CTnI are almost absent in normal blood serum. It is important to note that cardiac troponin levels can rise in other pathologies such as pericarditis, myocarditis, pulmonary embolism, sepsis, renal failure and other critical illnesses.[30] Even intense physical exercise such as endurance events can induce minor elevations in cTn. Cardiac markers play a secondary role to clinical presentation, the ECG and history taking with regard to any case of ACS. Cardiac markers become important once patients are stable, particularly if ECG results are negative. As cardiac markers rise slowly, testing at presentation is not useful; some protocols suggest testing at 0 and 2 hours, others at 0–3–6 or 0–4–8 hours. Ultimately, all protocols look for gradual elevation in troponin levels. Point-of-care testing at the bedside is available in emergency departments for troponin testing. Troponin testing is also utilised for determining infarct size and prognosis if tested approximately 72–96 hours after an MI event.[30]

Other parameters measuring potential risk and progression of cardiac disease include lipids and the lipid fractions, homocysteine, CRP and B-type natriuretic peptide (BNP). Clotting studies for potential embolism may be relevant for some patients. Reference range thresholds for troponin testing are extremely method dependent; the significant issue here is collecting blood samples according to the time intervals specified by the method used.

Carbohydrate metabolism

Laboratory assessment of metabolic syndromes and all forms of diabetes (type 1, type 2, gestational diabetes and diabetes insipidus) is increasingly common in clinical biochemistry, medicine and naturopathy. The assessment of metabolic syndromes, insulin resistance and diabetes involves an analysis of both carbohydrate metabolism and lipid metabolism. The testing of energy substrates, specific hormones and end products is important in these assessments. Consequently, testing panels for carbohydrate and lipid metabolism have developed extensively in the past decade or so.

Glucose: The blood glucose level (BGL) is the most important parameter for testing fuel metabolism, and must be assessed in accordance with a patient's feed-fast cycle.

Blood glucose is best assessed after an 8 to 12 hour fast.[31] A random blood plasma glucose level is measured irrespective of meal times. A random BGL is not diagnostic of diabetes, but can be useful in assessing hypoglycaemia and severe hyperglycaemia.

TERMINOLOGY

Elevated BGL: hyperglycaemia.
Decreased BGL: hypoglycaemia.
Normal BGL: normoglycaemia.

CLINICAL SIGNIFICANCE

Hyperglycaemia is indicative of prediabetic conditions such as impaired fasting glucose (IFG) and impaired glucose tolerance (IGT). Fasting hyperglycaemia constitutes a higher risk of microvascular events.[31] Hyperglycaemia on fasting BGL must be confirmed with further testing via an oral glucose tolerance test.

Oral glucose tolerance test (OGTT)

The OGTT series of blood measurements assesses the physiological response to a standardised oral CHO load (75 g of glucose in 300 mL of H_2O) after approximately 10 hours of fasting.[31] Due to the effects of physiological stress on CHO metabolism, the OGTT cannot be performed during or after acute illness or exercise. Blood is then sampled at specific time intervals.

CLINICAL SIGNIFICANCE

In normoglycaemia, the BGL should reach a maximum concentration at approximately 60 minutes; and it should return to a near fasting level at approximately 120 minutes. Diabetes is diagnosed if the BGL is >11.1 mmol/L at the 120-minute mark. IGT is diagnosed if the BGL is between 6.1 and 7.8 mmol/L in the post-load sample.[31] Refer to Table 4.28 for reference ranges.

TABLE 4.28 Reference range: plasma glucose

Condition	Diagnostic criteria (mmol/L)
Normal fasting plasma glucose	<6.1
Impaired fasting glucose	≥6.1 but <7.0
Impaired glucose tolerance	OGTT 2-hr glucose: ≥7.8 but <11.1
Diabetes mellitus	
Criterion 1	Random BGL 11.1 or higher
Criterion 2	Fasting BGL 7.0 or higher
Criterion 3	OGTT 2-hr glucose: 11.1 or higher
Criterion 4	HbA_{1c} >48 mmol/L

Shaikh N, Borrell J, Evron J, Leeflang M. Procalcitonin, C-reactive protein, and erythrocyte sedimentation rate for the diagnosis of acute pyelonephritis in children. Cochrane Database Syst Rev, 2015: 1:CD009185.

Glycated haemoglobin (HbA_{1c})

Specific proteins are susceptible to the process of glycation, an irreversible process in which proteins become bound to glucose derivatives. Haemoglobin in erythrocytes can become glycated over a period of time, particularly in cases of sustained hyperglycaemia. Glycated haemoglobin is known as HbA_{1c} and remains with erythrocytes for their entire life span. The HbA_{1c} level represents the average plasma glucose concentration throughout the 8–12 weeks prior to its measurement.[31]

CLINICAL SIGNIFICANCE

A raised HbA_{1c} level of >48 mmol/L is not necessarily diagnostic of diabetes. OGTT must be performed to confirm a diagnosis. Additionally, some physiological states may reduce the HbA_{1c} level in diabetic patients with poor control and hyperglycaemia. These include increased erythropoiesis (e.g. EPO therapy, chronic liver disease, iron, B_{12} or folate therapy), erythrocyte destruction (e.g. haemolytic anaemia, rheumatoid arthritis, some medications) and reduced glycation (aspirin, vitamin C and vitamin E therapy).[32] The HbA_{1c} is used to monitor the long-term control of diabetes, to set targets for dietary and drug therapies. Most diabetic associations recommend an HbA_{1c} of <53 mmol/L. Refer to Tables 4.29 and 4.30 for reference ranges for type 1 and type 2 diabetes mellitus respectively.

TABLE 4.29 Reference range: type 1 diabetes HbA_{1c}

Type 1 diabetes	HbA_{1c} target (mmol/L)
General target	≤53
Children and adolescents	≤58
Pregnant or planning pregnancy	≤53
Recurrent and severe hypoglycaemia	≤64
Hypoglycaemia unawareness	≤64

Jones G, Barker G, Goodall I et al. Change of HbA_{1c} reporting to the new SI units. MJA 2011; 195(1):45–46.

TABLE 4.30 Reference range: type 2 diabetes HbA_{1c}

Type 2 diabetes	HbA_{1c} target (mmol/L)
General target	≤53
Children and adolescents	≤53
Pregnant or planning pregnancy	≤42
Diabetes and clinical cardiovascular disease	≤53
Recurrent and severe hypoglycaemia	≤64
Hypoglycaemia unawareness	≤64
Lifestyle modification + metformin	≤42
Antidiabetic agents (other than metformin and insulin)	≤48
Patients on insulin therapy	≤53

Jones G, Barker G, Goodall I et al. Change of HbA_{1c} reporting to the new SI units. MJA 2011; 195(1):45–46.

Ketones

Ketone synthesis occurs in the liver, via the oxidation of free fatty acids. In the normoglycaemic fed state, insulin rises and lipolysis is inhibited. These conditions favour triglyceride synthesis, thus reducing fatty acid oxidation (breakdown for energy) and ketone body formation. During a fasting/non-fed state, insulin levels decline and glucagon increases, favouring fatty acid oxidation and ketogenesis.[33] The main ketones are acetoacetate, hydroxybutyrate and acetone, though hydroxybutyrate is the only one used in diagnostic testing. Ketone measurement is indicated for investigating the causes and progression of metabolic acidosis and hypoglycaemia.

CLINICAL SIGNIFICANCE

Increased hydroxybutyrate levels are indicative of ketosis (induced by diabetes mellitus, fasting and possibly alcoholism). Low levels may accompany hypoglycaemia, thus indicating a non-ketotic cause such as hyperinsulinism.[11] Reference range: < 1.2 mmol/L.[11]

Insulin

CLINICAL SIGNIFICANCE

Elevated levels are observed in insulin therapy and type 2 diabetes. If insulin/glucose ratio is measured, elevations are associated with beta cell hyperplasia an insulinomas.[11] Plasma glucose levels must be interpreted with insulin results, looking for elevations in both. Reference ranges: <5 mU/L (during hypoglycaemia); 4–10 mU/L (post 8-hour fast with a normal plasma glucose).[11]

Fructosamine

Like HbA_{1c}, fructosamines are end products produced via glycation reactions. Fructosamines form when a monosaccharide (fructose or glucose) attaches to a primary amine. Fructosamine levels are occasionally used in diabetes management, and generally reflect the BGL over the past 2–3 weeks.[14]

CLINICAL SIGNIFICANCE

In practice, HbA_{1c} levels are preferred for the long-term management of diabetes. Fructosamine levels can be useful when evaluating a patient's response to diet or medication after a few weeks, as opposed to waiting a few months. Fructosamine levels may be preferred over HbA_{1c} levels in clinical situations where HBA_{1c} levels are falsely reduced (e.g. pregnancy, haemolytic anaemia or blood loss).[14] Elevated fructosamine levels indicate hyperglycaemia over the previous 2–3 weeks. Reduced fructosamine may be falsely low in clinical states of low protein (view total protein and albumin levels). Again, vitamin C therapy can lead to reduced fructosamine levels.[14] Reference ranges depend on the individual laboratory. Reference range: 200–290 umol/L.[11]

Homeostasis model assessment (HOMA)

Various methodologies are used for both the assessment and the diagnosis of insulin resistance, with an overall clinical picture obtained from fasting BGL, glucose tolerance, serum insulin and HbA_{1c} results. Insulin resistance assessment can also be determined via Homeostasis Model Assessment (HOMA). HOMA testing has been used extensively for the assessment of insulin resistance in NAFLD clinical studies.[34]

HOMA is an estimation of steady state beta cell function and insulin sensitivity. HOMA measurements correspond well with non-steady state assessments of beta cell function and insulin resistance such as hyperinsulinaemic and hyperglycaemic clamp models (considered gold standard) and oral and IV glucose tolerance testing.[35] HOMA testing is a calculation based on fasting plasma glucose and insulin levels. It provides values for %B, %S and an insulin resistance (IR) index.[35] The equations from which HOMA results are derived, provide calculations as to the degree and extent of any insulin resistance currently active in a patient.[35] When using HOMA calculation software, special attention needs to be paid regarding the units of measure used for substituted results.

By comparing the relationship between insulin and glucose in the basal state, the balance between hepatic glucose output and insulin secretion is estimated. Patient results are compared to response curves.[36] Some studies argue that HOMA testing is not superior to fasting insulin levels, while others suggest a use for the collection of longitudinal results in patients with abnormal glucose tolerance.[36]

Lipid profile

Laboratory assessment of lipids and their transport proteins links closely with the assessment of carbohydrate metabolism. Like disorders of CHO metabolism, altered lipid profiles outside of normal physiological ranges are linked with metabolic syndromes and increased risk of cardiovascular disease. As with CHO testing, lipid profiles should be assessed on fasting samples, as the feed–fast cycle alters the results.

Cholesterol (chol), free fatty acids (FFAs) and triglycerides (trigs) require protein transporters for their passage throughout the body. These include:

- High-density lipoproteins (HDL): protein rich
- Low-density lipoproteins (LDL): cholesterol rich
- Intermediate-density lipoproteins (IDL): cholesterol and triglyceride rich
- Very low-density lipoproteins (VLDL): liver synthesised triglyceride rich
- Chylomicrons: dietary triglyceride rich.[37]

CHOLESTEROL

This steroid is synthesised in the liver and is essential for correct cellular anatomy and physiology. Cholesterol is a precursor substrate for the formation of all steroid hormones, the calciferols (vitamin D group), co-enzyme Q10 and bile acids. Blood cholesterol (chol) levels are maintained via hepatic synthesis (approximately 1 g/day) and intake of dietary cholesterol.[37]

Cellular uptake of cholesterol occurs via the ECF, as cholesterol is delivered to the tissues via LDL. LDL receptors on cell membranes mediate this uptake. Expression of the LDL receptor gene is regulated by intracellular chol concentration.[37] HDL particles transport cholesterol from peripheral tissues back to the liver for potential excretion.

TRIGLYCERIDES

While FFAs are the predominant metabolic fuel (in addition to glucose), they are often not present in free form in blood plasma.[37] FFAs are packaged into triglycerides (3 fatty acids bonded to a glycerol molecule). Trigs are either supplied by the diet or generated in the liver and adipose tissue via lipogenesis. Trigs are transported to cells for use as energy via beta-oxidation of fatty acids, or stored in adipose tissue.

Terminology

Hypercholesterolaemia: elevated blood cholesterol.
Hyperlipidaemia: elevation of certain lipoproteins.
Dyslipidaemia: defective lipoprotein metabolism.

Clinical significance

Measurement of total cholesterol appears to be becoming less clinically relevant, though high elevations do prompt clinicians to initiate further testing. Testing the individual cholesterol carrying lipoprotein ratios is more informative. It is worth remembering that trig levels represent not only dietary triglyceride content but also liver-generated triglycerides from CHO consumption. Assessments should not be made during an acute illness (this is associated with lower cholesterol levels). Dyslipidaemias represent a vast array of pathologies: genetic (familial hypercholesterolaemia, hypertryglyceridaemia) and a host of secondary causes (diabetes, hypothyroidism, glucocorticoid therapy, Cushing's syndrome, obesity, cholestasis and pancreatitis are some common examples).[11] Refer to Table 4.31 for reference ranges.

APOLIPOPROTEINS

These proteins include apolipoprotein A-I (apo A-I), apolipoprotein B (apo B), lipoprotein (a) and apolipoprotein E (apo E). They provide the protein components for lipoproteins and have other metabolic roles. There are at least 10 known apolipoproteins. For simplicity, apo A-I is found predominantly in HDL, whereas apo B is associated with LDL.[37]

Clinical significance

Apo A-I and apo B are sometimes measured as an alternative to HDL and LDL. Reduced apo A-I and elevated apo B are both associated with increased risk of vascular pathology. They may offer a better prediction of atherosclerotic risk.[11] Apo B tested with LDL is used to investigate hyperapobetalipoproteinaemia, which is indicative of increased atherosclerotic risk. Lipoprotein (a) is tested in early-onset coronary or cerebral arterial disease, particularly in the case of a strong family history. Apo E genotyping is performed when investigating inherited forms of hyperlipidaemia.[11] Refer to Table 4.32 for reference ranges.

HOMOCYSTEINE

The amino acid homocysteine is an intermediate molecule in the biosynthesis and regulation of methionine (a sulfur-containing amino acid).[37] Both inherited (genetic) and acquired defects of this biochemical pathway can result in elevated levels of homocysteine and an increased risk of thrombosis. Acquired causes are usually related to insufficient dietary supply of folate, vitamin B_6 and vitamin B_{12}.[37]

Terminology

Hyperhomocysteinaemia: elevated blood homocysteine.

Clinical significance

Mild hyperhomocysteinaemia is a known risk factor for atherosclerosis, vascular disease and thrombus formation. A number of inherited defects (including MTHFR genetic polymorphisms) lead to elevated homocysteine levels. Low levels of folic acid, vitamin B_6 or vitamin B_{12} are linked with elevated homocysteine levels.[11] Reference range: 5–15 umol/L.[11] Target range (established vascular disease): <-10 umol/L (fasting).[11]

IMMUNOLOGY

Allergy testing

Allergic conditions involve IgE mediated hypersensitivity reactions involving the skin (urticarial, dermatitis),

TABLE 4.31 Reference range: lipid profile

Analyte	Reference range (mmol/L)
Total chol	Target <4.0
HDL (female)	1.0–2.2 (therapeutic target >1.0)
HDL (male)	0.9–2.0 (therapeutic target >1.0)
LDL	2.0–3.4 (therapeutic target <2.5)
Trigs	<1.7

Reproduced with permission from the Royal College of Pathologists of Australasia (RCPA). RCPA manual of use and interpretation of pathology tests. 7th ed. Sydney: RCPA, 2015. https://www.rcpa.edu.au/Library/Practising-Pathology/RCPA-Manual/Home.

TABLE 4.32 Reference range: apolipoproteins

Lipoprotein	Range (g/L)
Apo A-I	1.0–1.8
Apo B	<0.9
Lipoprotein (a)	<0.2
Apo E	Method dependent

Reproduced with permission from the Royal College of Pathologists of Australasia (RCPA). RCPA manual of use and interpretation of pathology tests. 7th ed. Sydney: RCPA, 2015. https://www.rcpa.edu.au/Library/Practising-Pathology/RCPA-Manual/Home.

respiratory system (allergic rhinitis and asthma), gastrointestinal tract and systemic anaphylaxis. IgE testing investigates true allergic reactions and is not used for the assessment of food intolerance (see functional pathology for food intolerance testing).

TOTAL IMMUNOGLOBULIN E (IgE)

IgE is one of the five human immunoglobulin isotypes (immunoglobulins A, D, G and M make up the remaining four isotypes). Of these 5 isotypes, IgE is present in the lowest amounts in human serum, but IgE concentration is also very age dependent. Half of this amount is present in the extravascular space (outside the vasculature).[38] IgE present in the intravascular pool has a very short half-life of 1–5 days.[38]

Clinical significance

Serum IgE tends to increase steadily in healthy children up to approximately 10–15 years of age. IgE decline usually commences in the 20s, with this gradual decline ceasing around 80 years of age.[38] All patients' serum IgE levels must be compared to age-stratified, non-atopic references ranges, not to a general 'all-ages' reference range. Atopic infants and children have an earlier and much steeper rise in IgE in early life than non-atopic juveniles.[38] Elevated IgE is highly likely in atopic conditions such as allergic rhinitis (hay fever), extrinsic (allergic) asthma and atopic dermatitis (eczema). Severely raised IgE levels are commonly observed in parasitic infections. Asthmatic patients with normal or low IgE are unlikely to have an allergic mechanism in their pathogenesis, thus a diagnosis of intrinsic (non-allergic) asthma is more likely.

Total serum IgE is nonspecific and cannot identify reactions to specific allergens. Total IgE has been largely superseded by allergen-specific IgE. Total IgE is still used in clinical screening for allergy, as well as for investigating the extent of allergic-based reactions. Refer to Table 4.33 for reference ranges.

TABLE 4.33 Reference range: IgE

Age	Range (IU/mL)
6–12 months	2–34
1–2 yrs	2–97
3 yrs	2–199
4–6 yrs	2–307
7–8 yrs	2–403
9–12 yrs	2–696
13–15 yrs	2–629
16–17 yrs	2–537
18 yrs and over	2–214

Martins T, Bandhauer M, Bunker A et al. New childhood and adult reference intervals for total IgE. Journal of Allergy and Clinical Immunology. 2014; 133(2) 589–591.

SCRATCH TESTING

Scratch testing is a form of in vivo provocation testing. A three-stage reaction involving capillary restriction, erythematous flare and circular wheal formation indicates a positive response to an allergen.[38] These liquid allergens are introduced just under the epidermis, via a very shallow needle puncture. Some laboratories may administer the test via intradermal injection. Bleeding from puncture sites can induce false positive results. Reactions are usually maximal at 15–20 minutes post allergen exposure, though late-phase reactions can be noted within 24 hours post test. Results are measured via a visual grading of wheal and flare reactions, often with the use of millimetre callipers. Most grading systems grade from 0 to 5+. Scratch testing commonly tests airborne allergens (e.g. moulds, dust mites, animal epidermals, pollens, insect venoms) and some common food allergens. Any positive result indicates true allergy to specific allergens.

ALLERGEN-SPECIFIC IgE

Allergen-specific IgE antibodies (if present) are located on basophils, mast cells and serum. The development of the radioallergosorbent test (RAST) has allowed for the detection of allergen-specific IgE. This test is preferred over skin testing when patients have taken antihistamines, beta-receptor stimulants or high-dose steroids (all reduce the provocation reaction required for skin testing).[38] It may also be a better-tolerated form of allergy testing in children and elderly patients. It is preferable in many instances to test potential IgE food allergies via RAST, as food reagents for skin testing can be labile or extremely variable.[38] The RAST generally offers more food-based allergens for analysis.

AUTOIMMUNITY MARKERS

Autoimmunity and autoimmune disease are two distinct pathologies, though they are commonly mistaken as being the same type of disease. Autoimmunity is the classic reaction involving aberrant immunity to self.[39] Autoimmunity is prevented via our immune system building tolerance to self-structures and only directing an immune response towards non-self antigens such as pathogenic microorganisms, or antigens located on malignant cells. Autoimmunity is a much more broad term than autoimmune disease.[39] Autoimmunity involves the production of *autoantibodies* directed against self-antigens. This type of humoral autoimmunity is rather common in the general population.[39] Only a small portion of people with autoantibodies will go on to develop an actual autoimmune disease.

Autoimmune diseases are usually classified as either organ-specific or non-organ specific. In some autoimmune diseases, the organ specificity involves targets at subcellular level, for example proteins or receptors as targets (type 1 diabetes being a classic example). Other examples of organ-specific autoimmune diseases include Graves' disease, Hashimoto's thyroiditis, atrophic thyroiditis, autoimmune Addison's disease, coeliac disease, pernicious anaemia, multiple sclerosis, myasthenia gravis, autoimmune alopecia, autoimmune vitiligo and discoid lupus.[11] Non-organ specific autoimmune disease may also be referred to as systemic autoimmune disease. These diseases often involve joints, connective tissue and blood vessels. Some examples include systemic lupus erythematosus (SLE), scleroderma, rheumatoid arthritis, reactive arthritis and Sjögren's syndrome.[39]

Clinical significance

The detection of autoantibodies via laboratory testing is simply indicative of a state of autoimmunity; positive autoantibody results do not indicate or diagnose autoimmune diseases. Clinical history, physical examination, results of tissue biopsies (if relevant) and imaging studies are all used collectively by doctors to decide whether autoimmunity is elevated to autoimmune disease. Interpretation of results within the full clinical context is paramount. Refer to Table 4.34 for a summary of commonly tested autoantibodies with clinical interpretation.

COELIAC SEROLOGY

Dietary gluten (from wheat, barley, rye and oats) exists in two forms: polymeric (glutenin) and monomeric (gliadin) gluten.[40] Large gluten peptides traverse the gut epithelial lining and bind with specific antigen presenting cells (APCs) located in gut lymphoid tissue. When gluten peptides are presented to T-lymphocytes via APCs, these now 'activated' T-lymphocytes produce pro-inflammatory cytokines and induce the maturation of B-lymphocytes to plasma cells (antibody producing cells).[40] The specific antibodies produced either act against gluten (the anti-gliadin antibodies) or are autoantibodies (anti-tissue transglutaminase antibodies). Tissue transglutaminase is produced endogenously for the deamination of gliadin peptides.[40]

A diagnosis of coeliac disease in never based on antibody levels alone, but on an assortment of clinical findings. Anti-tissue transglutaminase levels (IgA TTG) are usually the first test requested (high specificity and sensitivity for coeliac disease). Other antibody testing includes serum IgA levels for anti-gliadin antibodies and endomysial proteins.[11] False negative results do occur if the patient is tested while on a gluten-free diet. As most antibodies tested here are of the IgA class, IgA deficiency can also lead to false negative results. Genetic testing may be necessary and may have been requested based on the patient's clinical and family history (see genetic testing). In most instances, results are reported as either positive or negative for the individual antibodies tested. This may differ between laboratories, which will supply their own ranges depending on the methodology used.

Clinical significance

Gluten sensitivity without coeliac disease is another common clinical presentation, for which antibody testing is

TABLE 4.34 Summary of autoantibody tissue targets and potential autoimmune diseases

Auto-antibody	Tissue target	Possible autoimmune disease
Anti-nuclear antibodies (ANA) Note: at least a dozen subtypes known.	Usually nuclear structures such as DNA, RNA, histones and specific nucleoproteins	Found in many diseases including SLE, connective tissue diseases and Sjögren's syndrome
Adrenal cytoplasmic autoantibodies (ACA)	Adrenal cell membrane	Addison's disease
Antitransglutaminase antibodies (anti-tTG)	Transglutaminase	Coeliac disease
Rheumatoid factor	IgG	Rheumatoid arthritis
Anti-thrombin antibodies	Thrombin	SLE
Anti-thyrotrophin receptor antibodies (TRAb)	TSH receptor	Graves' disease
Anti-thyroglobulin antibodies (TgAb)	Thyroglobulin	Hashimoto's thyroiditis
Thyroid peroxidase autoantibodies (TPOAb)	Thyroid peroxidase	Graves' disease and Hashimoto's thyroiditis
Parietal cell autoantibodies (PCA)	Gastric parietal cell	Pernicious anaemia
Intrinsic factor antibodies (IFAb)	Intrinsic factor (gastric parietal cells)	Pernicious anaemia
Extractable nuclear antigens (ENA)	Specific components of nuclear components	Like the ANA, found in many including SLE, connective tissue diseases, Sjögren's syndrome, scleroderma
Anti-cardiolipin antibody (ACL)	Cardiolipin is a lipid component of the inner mitochondrial membrane	SLE, connective tissue diseases, many non-autoimmune conditions including certain infections and thrombotic events. Positive results should be confirmed with re-testing after 2–3 months

Hughes T. Basic guide to autoimmune testing: part 1 ANA, ENA and dsDNA antibodies [Internet]. Clinpath Pathology, 2016 [cited 29 June 2016]. Available from: http://clinipathpathology.com.au/media/85920/autoimmune%20testing.pdf; Royal College of Pathologists of Australasia (RCPA). Education online [Internet]. RCPA, 2016 [cited 19 August 2016]. Available from: https://www.rcpa.edu.au/Education.

often negative. Gluten allergy may be observed as a specific IgE gluten response (which would be determined on IgE specificity testing) but is not related to true coeliac disease.[40] Anti-tissue transglutaminase may also be elevated in patients with inflammatory bowel disease, arthritis and type 1 diabetes mellitus. Anti-gliadin antibodies are sometimes observed in inflammatory arthritis, peripheral neuropathy and infertility (including miscarriage).[40]

If coeliac disease is diagnosed, or other gluten pathologies are confirmed, other pathology tests for possible malabsorption should be viewed, for example FBC and iron profiles for anaemias, vitamins D and B_{12} and red cell folate levels, total protein, albumin and globulin levels. ESR and CRP may indicate levels of inflammation, but are not essential to view. Faecal fat analyses may be performed to investigate the extent of malabsorption.

Reference range: results for transglutaminase, gliadin and endomysial antibodies are usually reported as qualitative results (positive/negative); some methodologies use reference ranges, thus check ranges supplied by the laboratory.

SEROLOGY

A host of antibodies are present in blood serum and are indicative of adaptive immune responses facilitated via B lymphocyte humoral immunity. Our individual antibody inventory is a reflection of our lifetime exposure to microbes and immunisations, plus our genetic heritage, potential autoantigens and age.[41] Clinical laboratory diagnostics can identify such antibodies and they can also be quantified to indicate the precise level present in serum.

Serology is the specialisation of medical science concerning the study of antibodies in blood serum. Serology has developed over the decades to also include the study of antibodies in other secretions such as saliva, and to investigate other proteins in sera and saliva that do not function as antibodies.

Serology and the ability to detect antibody and/or antigen in clinical specimens allow laboratories to offer powerful clinical tools. Serology not only detects, identifies and quantifies antigens, but also measures a patient's antibody response to infection.[42] Virology is technically a sub-specialty of microbiology. However, viruses are not able to be cultured in the same way as other microorganisms using traditional nutrient media; viruses require a living host or tissue in order to survive, grow and replicate. For this reason, clinical diagnosis of viral infection occurs via antibody–antigen interactions, capitalising on serological methods for this purpose. Some serological methods used in the detection of viruses include immunofluorescence, enzyme-linked immunosorbent assay (ELISA), western blot analysis and complement fixation.

Clinical significance

In many cases, serology can determine whether a current viral infection is acute or chronic. Serology can differentiate between a primary infection and a re-infection.[42] Detection of virus-specific immunoglobulin M (IgM) antibodies generally indicates a recent primary infection (these antibodies are usually present for the initial 2–3 weeks of a primary infection). Testing during the convalescent phase may reveal seroconversion; a fourfold increase of the specific antibody titre compared to serum tested in the acute phase.[42]

Some viruses are not detected via serological methods, and may require tissue culture or detection of their DNA/RNA for diagnosis. Examples of viral nucleic acid detection methods include the polymerase chain reaction (PCR). See the microbiology section for further explanation. Refer to Table 4.35 for viruses commonly tested via serological methods, with a corresponding clinical interpretation.

Viral hepatitis screening

Worldwide, viral causes of hepatitis are estimated to affect as many as 400 million individuals, making these infections a significant public health concern.[43] As such, serological testing for the five major viral hepatitis subtypes is an important clinical service performed by pathology laboratories. Hepatitis serology also represents some of the most thorough testing seen in serology. Results are usually reported as positive or negative for each analyte tested. If a titre is quantified, it is usually based on a reference range set by the laboratory, thus reference ranges may vary.

Many viral hepatitis infections present clinically in the same way as other systemic viral infections with fever, malaise, fatigue, myalgia, anorexia, arthralgia, headaches and possibly pharyngitis, coryza and cough.[43] In addition to hepatitis serology, LFTs, FBC and albumin/globulin levels may show abnormal results and are useful in assessing the extent of pathology. Viral hepatitis subtyping serology is necessary to determine the exact viral subtype present, which then determines treatment, prognosis and potential for infectivity of others. Refer to Table 4.36 for a summary of viral hepatitis subtypes and their clinical interpretation.

STOOL ANALYSIS

Stool analysis refers to a broad spectrum of testing parameters in the assessment of digestion, GIT inflammation and GIT bleeding. Stool analysis is also a cornerstone test in microbiology for the identification of microorganisms and the diagnosis of infection.

Gross microscopic examination

Some microbes, their larvae or eggs are identified via microscopy.

Stool culture

Stool culture assists in determining the aetiology of bacterial diarrhoea, and can identify the bacterium responsible. Most cases of acute diarrhoea are infectious, and determining the causative microbe is necessary for correct treatment. A variety of culture mediums are required, with incubation periods of 24–48 hours required for sufficient growth of potential pathogens to occur. Examples of microorganisms detected by stool culture include *Campylobacter* spp., *Salmonella* spp., *Shigella* spp., *Vibrio* spp., *Aeromonas* spp., *Clostridium* spp. and

TABLE 4.35 Selected viruses and their diagnostic interpretation

Virus	Serological analyte	Positive result interpretation	Other tests for evaluation
Adenovirus	Adenovirus antibody	Useful to determine the cause of atypical pneumonia. Generally only used in cases of serious disease. May be useful in determining cause of severe chronic infection	Also note FBC report, WCC, blood film and LFTs for abnormalities
Arbovirus	Arbovirus IgM antibody (these are arthropod based-infections)	Arbovirus family includes causative viruses for Ross River, dengue, Barmah Forest, West Nile and yellow fever, and Murray Valley, Japanese and tick-borne encephalitis. Current or recent infection. Exception is Ross River virus, where specific IgM may be elevated for several years	Useful for investigating infections in returned travellers. Also consider blood films for malarial parasites if fitting with clinical presentation. PCR of CSF may be used in cased of encephalopathy
	Arbovirus IgG antibody	Generally indicates past infections	As above
Epstein-Barr virus (EBV)	Viral capsid antigen (VCA) IgM	Acute infection. Detected during clinical presentation, usually present for 4 weeks	Also note FBC report, WCC, blood film and LFTs for abnormalities
	Viral capsid antigen IgG	Persist for life and are occasionally noted during acute infection. Usually indicative of recent infection	Also note FBC report, WCC, blood film and LFTs for abnormalities
	Epstein-Barr nuclear antigen (EBNA) antibodies	Develop 2–3 months post initial infection; lifelong persistence and indicative of past infection	Also note FBC report, WCC, blood film and LFTs for abnormalities
Human immunodeficiency virus (HIV)	HIV-1 and HIV-2 antibodies	HIV-1 common worldwide, HIV-2 more confined to Africa. In terminal disease, HIV antibodies may be negative	Positive result must be confirmed via immunoblot testing on a separate sample. HIV-1 RNA and HIV p24 antigen can be used in diagnosis, but are better determinants of response to therapy and monitoring disease progression
Herpes simplex viruse	HSV 1 and HSV 2	Limited use for diagnosis of oral or genital herpes. Seroconversion of negative to positive, or a four-fold rise in antibody titres between acute and convalescent samples	Viral culture, CSF serology, serology of vesicle fluid and PCR are often used for diagnosis over serum antibody testing
Measles virus	IgM	May be negative during rash; can remain positive for 4–6 weeks. Generally only tested in non-immunised populations, particularly children	Severe infection may lead to encephalitis, thus organ function tests like LFTs, EUCs and inflammatory markers help with full clinical investigation
	IgG	Consistent with previous infection or immunisation	As above

Royal College of Pathologists of Australasia (RCPA). Education online. RCPA, 2016. Available from: www.rcpa.edu.au/Education

Escherichia spp. Some parasites and protozoa are also detected via stool culture.[44]

Stool PCR

A variety of faecal bacterial pathogens are detected via faecal PCR, though stool cultures are still necessary for the detection of parasites and protozoa. PCR is considered a superior testing methodology regarding sensitivity and rapid testing times. One limitation is that stool PCR is based on a single stool sample, whereas stool culture follows the 3-day collection protocol, and potentially captures sufficient quantities of shed microorganisms, which are notorious for evading detection via low sample numbers. *Blastocystis* spp. and *Dientamoeba fragilis*, *Giardia lamblia*, *Entamoeba histolytica* and *Cryptosporidium* spp. (in addition to bacterial infections) can be determined via stool PCR.[45]

TOXOPLASMA

While toxoplasmosis is essentially a parasitic infection and may be considered as part of the study of microbiology, laboratory diagnosis of this infection relies on the detection of toxoplasma antibodies in serum, thus the test is classified as part of serology. The aetiological

TABLE 4.36 Hepatitis viral subtypes and their diagnostic interpretation

Viral subtype	Analyte tested	Result interpretation
Hepatitis A (HAV)	IgM anti-HAV IgG anti-HAV	Recent infection Previous infection or immunisation
Hepatitis B (HBV)	Anti-HBV surface antigen (Anti-HBs) HBV surface antigen (HBsAg) Anti-HBV core antigen (Anti-HBc) IgM Anti-HBV core antigen (Anti-HBc) IgG HBV e antigen Anti-HBe	Positive result can be used to confirm immunity Acute HBV infection or carrier status. Both imply infectivity Recent infection Past infection or carrier status. Full significance depends on HBsAg result and anti-HBs result If present in HBsAg positive patients: greater infectivity and increased risk of chronic liver diseases Lesser risk of infectivity and better prognosis
Hepatitis C (HCV)	HCV RNA	Used to detect HCV as a possible cause of acute hepatitis, cirrhosis and hepatocellular carcinoma; monitoring of HCV treatment, testing blood and tissues of donor patients and post needle-stick injury
Hepatitis D (HDV)	Anti-HDV	Rising titres = acute infection; continual high titres = chronic infection. HDV infection only occurs in patients with HBV infection
Hepatitis E (HEV)	Anti-HEV	Antibodies develop early in HEV infection. Often tested when clinical picture is consistent with hepatitis, but other hepatitis serology is negative

Royal College of Pathologists of Australasia (RCPA). Education online. RCPA, 2016. Available from: www.rcpa.edu.au/Education

agent is *Toxoplasma gondii*. This parasite is omnipresent in the environment and shows an ability to infect most mammals. Immunocompromised individuals, pregnant women and neonates are most at risk of this infection.[46]

Clinical significance

A four-fold increase in IgG titres when comparing acute and convalescent samples (at least 2 weeks apart) is considered a positive diagnosis for toxoplasmosis.[11] The clinical term 'toxoplasmosis' is only used in cases where clinical signs/symptoms of the disease are present, while 'toxoplasma infection' describes an asymptomatic patient with a positive serology result.[46] Reference range: IgG titre <16. IgM ≥ 16: infection within the past 12 months.[11]

ABO BLOOD GROUPING AND CROSS-MATCHING

ABO blood typing is a serological test, as the method uses the detection of antibody in blood serum. The ABO red cell antigen system was first discovered in the early 1900s.[47] This system forms the basis of compatibility testing of blood products from donors to recipients. Doctors often request a 'group and hold' for patients likely to require blood transfusions. Such clinical situations include trauma patients, surgical patients, obstetric patients and some cancer patients. The group and hold determines the ABO blood group, rhesus (Rh) factor status and an antibody screen for any non-ABO, non-Rh antibodies.[47] A group and hold expedites the process of obtaining cross-matched blood should the situation arise.

For ABO grouping, a patient's RBCs are tested/mixed with two reagent sera; the first reagent contains anti-A antibodies, the second contains anti-B antibodies (the body forms antibodies against the A and/or B red cell antigens it lacks).[47] Refer to Table 4.37 for a summary of the ABO antigen combinations, with their corresponding ABO blood types.

TABLE 4.37 ABO blood types and their associated antigens

Blood type	A antigen	B antigen	Rhesus factor
A positive	Present	Absent	Present
B positive	Absent	Present	Present
AB positive	Present	Present	Present
O positive	Absent	Absent	Present
A negative	Present	Absent	Absent
B negative	Absent	Present	Absent
AB negative	Present	Present	Absent
O negative	Absent	Absent	Absent

Clinical significance

O negative patients are deemed as 'universal donors'. O negative blood contains no Rh factor and no antigens for A or B; it can be transfused to patients of all blood types. AB positive patients are deemed as 'universal recipients'. Their blood contains A, B and Rh antigens and will not produce antibodies against any donor blood type received.

RED CELL ANTIBODY SCREENING

This screening method looks for unexpected antibodies in patients' serum.[47] These antibodies develop from previous exposure to rare and foreign red cell antigens via a pregnancy or transfusion of blood products. Less than 2% of the general population will be positive for any of these red cell antigens.[47] Any positive result here dictates further compatibility testing with donor blood before a patient transfusion can proceed. Hundreds of rare red cell antigens exist, but some more commonly known antigens include Duffy, Kell, Kidd and Lewis antigens.

MICROBIOLOGY

Microbiology encompasses the study of viruses, bacteria, fungi (yeasts and moulds) and parasites. The microbiology laboratory is a true amalgamation of old and new, with techniques used for hundreds of years remaining as important as new genomic methodologies for diagnosing the causative agent of infections. Additionally, serological studies are also used to confirm and rule out infections as the cause of many clinical presentations. Highly specific nutrient media, the Gram stain and traditional microscopy all help to identify the causative agents of infections, from common mild infections through to rare and life-threatening microbial diseases. A select few are expanded upon in this chapter.

Terminology

Cocci: round.
Diplococci: cocci occurring in pairs.
Bacilli: rod-shaped.
Coccobacilli: rounded rod-shaped.
Spirochete: spiral-shaped.
Aerobic: with oxygen.
Anaerobic: without oxygen.

For the past three decades, molecular biological techniques such as the polymerase chain reaction (PCR) have pushed the specialisation of microbiology towards the study of genetics. PCR is a nucleic acid amplification (NAA) technique, in which microorganisms with fastidious growth requirements and poor growth response in traditional culture mediums may be detected. PCR is also useful when very small numbers of microbes are present, yet infection is clinically apparent. Some pathogens are intracellular, making culture and isolation techniques unreliable for diagnostic purposes. PCR is routinely used for the detection of some bacterial species including *Mycoplasma* spp., *Haemophilis* spp., *Ureaplasmas*, *Chlamydia* spp. and *Borrelia* spp. PCR is especially useful when traditional culturing techniques are negative, or when specimens are not traditionally related to microbiology, such as tumour tissue.

HELICOBACTER

Of the various species of *Helicobacter*, *H. pylori* is the most significant regarding infection in humans. The *Helicobacter* genus preferentially colonises the stomach and the intestinal tract.[48] Humans are the primary reservoir and faecal–oral transmission is a significant issue. This infection shows a worldwide distribution with many individuals having an asymptomatic carrier status. *H. pylori* is an important cause of gastritis (acute and chronic), peptic ulceration, gastric adenocarcinomas and lymphomas.[48]

Specific biochemical characteristics of *H. pylori* are capitalised upon for diagnostics; the high production of urease is the basis of the urea breath test. Patients receive radiolabelled ^{13}C or ^{14}C urea (oral dosing). CO_2 from exhaled breath samples is analysed 15 minutes pre and 30 minutes post dosing. Rapid hydrolysis of urea (high CO_2 levels) indicates the presence of urea-cleaving microbes and their enzyme (urease) in the stomach.[11]

- Microscopy: curved Gram-negative bacilli, highly motile, multiple flagella. Classically spiral-shaped if viewed in fresh culture
- O_2 requirement: aerobic
- Differentiate from: *Campylobacter*
- Clinical specimens required: method dependent; blood, tissue, faeces, exhaled breath
- Use of NAA: not applicable. Non-invasive testing includes stool and serology testing (antigen detection), culture/susceptibility testing and the urea breath test. Invasive detection methods include endoscopy (with biopsy) and histological sampling
- Other *Helicobacter* species: *H. heilmanni*, *H. fennelliae* and *H. cinaedi*.[48]

BLASTOCYSTIS

The *Blastocysis* genus represents some of the most common protozoa to infect the gastrointestinal tract of humans. The most clinically important species to human health is *B. hominis*. This protozoan has been classified as vegetable matter, yeast and a fungus, though current scientific knowledge has established it as a protozoan parasite with at least ten recognised subtypes.[49] Transmission appears to occur via zoonotic and human-to-human contact. At least six different forms of this parasite have been identified via electron microscopy: cyst, amoeboid, granular, avacuolar, vacuolar and multivacuolar forms. Vacuolar cells are the most distinctive.[49]

B. hominis infection remains controversial for several reasons:

1. Various transmission routes
2. Varying pathogenicity of subtypes
3. Doubts surrounding infectious stage of life cycle
4. The possibility that *B. hominis* is a commensal organism in humans
5. No serological antibody response occurs, ruling out serological confirmation of infections.

Despite this, infection is more likely in patients with high exposure to pets, farm animals, contaminated water and a recent travel history to developing countries. Diarrhoea, vomiting, abdominal cramping, weight loss and IBS are all clinical manifestations of *B. hominis* infection.

- Microscopy: vacuolar form is very distinct; however, their numbers can be reduced in clinical specimens
- O_2 requirement: anaerobic, though possible mitochondrial structures are evident on microscopy
- Differentiate from: *Giardia*, *Campylobacter*, rotavirus. Other self-limiting GIT infections include norovirus, enterovirus and adenovirus

- Clinical specimens required: faecal sample for microscopy. Highly trained laboratory staff may identify the less obvious cyst form. Organism may be noted on biopsy
- Use of NAA: not applicable.[49]

BORDETELLA

B. pertussis is the bacterial species responsible for pertussis (whooping cough). Despite the introduction of a pertussis vaccine in 1949, the infection remains endemic worldwide, with approximately 16 million infections and 200 000 deaths each year (primary population is non-vaccinated children).[50]

- Microscopy: Gram-negative coccobacilli
- O_2 requirement: strictly aerobic
- Differentiate from: *Legionella, H. influenzae, C. pneumoniae, Mycobacterium* and viral respiratory pathogens
- Clinical specimens required: blood, nasopharyngeal swab
- Use of NAA: yes
- Other *Bordetella* species: *B. parapertussis, B. bronchiseptica* and *B. holmesii.*[50]

BORRELIAE

Two human diseases are associated with the *Borreliae* genus: relapsing fever (*B. recurrentis* and several different *Borrelia* species) and Lyme borreliosis (*B. burgdorferi*).[51] The arthropod vector of transmission is the *Ixodes* tick (several species). *Ixodes* reservoirs include small mammals (e.g. mice) and some birds.[52] Specialised structural features enhance this bacterium's adaptation to aquatic sediments, biofilms and mucosal surfaces.[53] Lyme borreliosis is the most common vector-borne infection in the United States, and is a significant public health issue in Europe and Asia.[53]

Testing should be initiated for any patient with recent travel to or residence in Lyme endemic areas, particularly when the characteristic erythema migrans skin lesion is noted.[53] Lymphopenia may be present with an FBC, and abnormal LFTs (ALT and AST) are possible. (Haematogenous spread to distant organ sites is a possibility, including joints, the nervous system and cardiac tissue.)[53] The existence of Lyme borelliosis via native Australian vectors and animal reservoirs remains controversial, though testing is available in Australia.

- Microscopy: motile spirochaetes (helical rods). Not visualised on Gram stain due to small size; live bacteria may be visible on darkfield or phase contrast microscopy
- O_2 requirement: microaerobic
- Clinical specimens required: blood, skin lesion biopsy. Synovial fluid and CSF may be used for investigation of late neurological Lyme disease
- Differentiate from: *Plasmodium* infection, SLE, CFS, arthritic diseases (systemic symptomatology), contact dermatitis, urticaria, pityriases rosea or spider bite (cutaneous lesion)
- Use of NAA: yes, though only available via specialist laboratories. Serological testing is useful, but antibodies are notoriously slow to develop, and immune complexes can also affect the results
- Other *Borrelia* species: *B. duttoni, B. hermsii, B. parkeri, B. afzeli, B. garinii* and *B. turnicata.*[52]

CAMPYLOBACTER

Campylobacter spp. infections cause acute gastrointestinal illness associated with considerable abdominal pain and diarrhoea. *C. jejuni* is most common in humans. It is considered one of the most common bacterial infections of humans worldwide.[54] This infection may be responsible for systemic disease in compromised patients. It shares considerable morphological similarities with *Helicobacter.*

- Microscopy: curved Gram-negative bacilli. Highly motile
- O_2 requirement: microaerophilic
- Differentiate from: *Helicobacter*
- Clinical specimens required: faeces or blood for culture
- Use of NAA: not available
- Other *Campylobacter* species: *C. coli, C. lari, C. fetus, C. hyointestinalis* and *C. upsaliensis.*[54]

CANDIDA

The genus *Candida* represents fungi with the potential to cause superficial, subcutaneous and systemic infections. *Candida* fungi reproduce via budding, and because of this growth pattern are classified as yeasts. *Candida* is not particularly pathogenic; it is considered opportunistic as it generally only causes disease in compromised hosts.[55] *Candida* is also classified as commensal yeast; it naturally resides in humans as part of the normal microbiota, only flourishing when the biochemical environment of the host changes condition to favour *Candida* growth. The most clinically relevant species is *Candida albicans.* The yeast is generally non-infectious, but it may be sexually transmitted. Infection is also due to a patient's own endogenous reservoir.[55]

- Microscopy: Gram-positive unicellular yeast with budding
- O_2 requirement: anaerobic
- Differentiate from: other (bacterial) STIs and other skin/nail fungi such as *Trichophyton* spp. and *Malassezia* spp.
- Clinical specimens required: urogenital and oropharyngeal swabs
- Use of NAA: PCR available. Antibody detection may be required. Antigen detection via ELISA is common
- Other *Candida* species: *C. krusei, C. parapsilosis, C. tropicalis, C. guilliermondii* and *C. glabrata.*[55]

ROTAVIRUS

Worldwide, Group A rotaviruses are the most significant cause of acute gastroenteritis in infants and young children.[56] A range of clinical outcomes is observed with rotavirus infection, from asymptomatic illness to severe, life-threatening gastroenteritis (infants in particular).[56] The oral rotavirus vaccine is part of childhood immunisation schedules.

- Microscopy: characteristic wheel-shaped viral particles
- O_2 requirement: anaerobic

TABLE 4.38 *Chlamydia* spp. infections and their associated conditions

Organism	Conditions
C. trachomatis	Ocular trachoma, adult and neonatal conjunctivitis and infant pneumonia, urogenital STI. Associated with maternal transfer in neonates
C. pneumoniae	Respiratory infections including severe pneumonia, inflammatory atherosclerotic plaques
C. psittaci	Respiratory infections including severe bronchopneumonia. Associated with avian zoonotic infection

Geisler W. Diseases caused by *Chlamydiae*. In Goldman L, Schafer A, editors. Goldman-Cecil medicine. 25th edn. Philadelphia: Elsevier Saunders; 2016, pp. 2007–13.

- Differentiate from: other viral, parasitic or bacterial causes of gastroenteritis
- Clinical specimens required: faecal sample
- Use of NAA: not common. Detection of viral antigen via ELISA is very reliable.[56]

CHLAMYDIA

Three species of *Chlamydia* are relevant to human infections: *C. trachomatis, C. pneumoniae* and *C. psittaci. C. trachomatis* infection is one of the most common STIs worldwide.[57] *Chlamydia* spp. are obligate intracellular parasites and display a unique developmental cycle: the infectious form (elementary bodies) are metabolically inactive, while the non-infectious form (reticulate bodies) are metabolically active.[57] Refer to Table 4.38 for a summary of the three most common *Chlamydia* species in humans, with their associated clinical states.

Chlamydial infections are a notifiable infection in Australia. Correct laboratory testing and diagnosis are essential and often involve more than simple swabs and microscopy.

- Microscopy: Gram-negative bacilli. Strict intracellular parasite. Elementary body morphology is important to distinguish between the different *Chlamydia* species
- O_2 requirement: aerobic
- Clinical specimens required: blood, eye swab, urogenital swab, pharyngeal swab, sputum
- Differentiate from: other microbial causes of pneumonia, ocular infection and STIs
- Use of NAA: yes. PCR available and very sensitive for all species.[57]

NEISSERIA

The two most clinically important infections related to the *Neisseria* genus are caused by *N. gonorrhoeae* (causative agent of gonorrhoea) and *N. meningitidis* (causative agent of bacterial meningitis). Despite the use of effective antibiotic therapy for *N. gonorrhoeae,* it remains one of the most common STIs.[58] The identification of *N. gonorrhoeae* from any specimen is always clinically significant. *N. meningitidis* does colonise the nasopharyngeal mucosa of healthy people not causing disease, though it is responsible for community-acquired meningitis and bronchopneumonia and can lead to overwhelming or fatal sepsis.[58]

- Microscopy: Gram-negative cocci (as diplococci). Gram-negative diplococci may be identified within neutrophils
- O_2 requirement: obligate aerobe
- Clinical specimens required: *N. gonorrhoea:* pharyngeal, rectal or urogenital swab. *N. meningitidis:* cerebrospinal fluid, blood, urine, sputum (CSF)
- Use of NAA: yes
- Other *Neisseria* species: *N. sicca* and *N. mucosa* (oropharyngeal commensals).[58]

CLOSTRIDIUM

The *Clostridium* genus is a large group of spore-forming bacteria.[59] The most clinically significant species in this group include: *C. difficile* (antibiotic use), *C. tetani* (tetanus) and *C. botulinum* (botulism). *C. difficile* produces spores that have become highly resistant to antibiotics and hospital decontamination efforts. Overgrowth of *C. difficile* in the gut of some patients with antibiotic exposure is considered an endogenous infection.[59]

- Microscopy: Gram-positive bacilli
- O_2 requirement: anaerobic
- Clinical specimens required: *C. difficile:* faeces. *C. tetani:* blood, though clinical history and presentation are more reliable than cultures. *C. botulinum:* blood, faeces, wound swab
- Use of NAA: not common
- Other *Clostridia* species: *C. perfringens* and *C. speticum.*[59]

GIARDIA

Giardiasis is an intestinal parasitic infection caused by the water-borne protozoan, *Giardia lamblia.* Diarrhoea and malabsorption are common complications. *Giardia* infections may result in IBS, CFS and food allergies after the infection has resolved.[60] The parasite is transmitted via contaminated water and has two distinct phases to its life cycle: the trophozoite (proliferative phase) and the cyst (infectious phase).[60]

- Microscopy: characteristic kite-shaped trophozoite; other specific features include two nucleated sucking pads and four flagella[61]
- O_2 requirement: anaerobic
- Differentiate from: other infective and non-infective forms of diarrhoea
- Clinical specimens required: faecal sample for microscopy
- Use of NAA: not common.[60]

LEGIONELLA

The most common and clinically relevant bacterium in this group is *L. pneumophila,* the causative agent of Legionnaires' disease. This respiratory illness ranges from a mild pneumonia-like illness to a rapidly progressive fatal pneumonia.[62] This infection is a significant concern for any patient who is already debilitated or immunocompromised. Outbreaks occur in communities exposed to contaminated water from cooling towers (e.g. hotels, hospitals), as the natural habitat of this bacterium is water.[62]

- Microscopy: Gram-negative bacilli
- O_2 requirement: aerobic
- Clinical specimens required: sputum, bronchial aspirates or washings, blood
- Differentiate from: *M. pneumoniae*, *C. pneumoniae*, *B. pertussis* and viral respiratory pathogens
- Use of NAA: yes. Additionally, antibody detection via fluorescent staining is very useful
- Other *Legionella* species: a total of 18 *Legionella* species have been associated with human disease.[62]

PLASMODIUM

The *Plasmodium* genus represents parasitic protozoa that invade and infect erythrocytes to cause malaria.[63] Parasites are transmitted to the bloodstream via bites from the malaria vector, the female *Anopheles* mosquito. In medical practice, patients with febrile illness are recommended for malaria evaluation if they have travelled to endemic countries (which include Mexico; Central and South America; Africa; India; Middle, Central and Southeast Asia; Oceania; and Papua New Guinea). Severe infection is a medical emergency.[64] The defining characteristic of malaria is the visual identification of malaria parasites on peripheral blood films: *P. falciparum, P. vivax, P. ovale* and *P. malariae*. Malaria is a concerning public health issue worldwide, particularly within developing countries.[64]

With any case of suspected malaria, several laboratory evaluations are required: (1) FBC (anaemia possible, thrombocytopenia seen in severe disease), (2) biochemistry: EUCs and LFTs (renal failure, hypoglycaemia and metabolic acidosis are indicative of poor prognosis), (3) peripheral blood films (thin and thick) for microscopy (thick films are more sensitive). The percentage parasitaemia is then calculated.[63] Species identification is determined via morphological studies.

- Microscopy: parasites show eosinophilic nucleus and basophilic cytoplasm
- O_2 requirement: both, depending on stage of life cycle
- Clinical specimens required: blood
- Differentiate from: other infectious diseases accompanied by fever, rigor and malaise including *B. burgdorferi* (Lyme disease), *S. typhi* (typhoid fever), influenza viruses, dengue fever virus, *M. tuberculosis* (TB), viral and bacterial meningitis and viral hepatitis
- Use of NAA: yes, though only available through research facilities. ELISA testing available.[63]

STAPHYLOCOCCI

The most clinically important human pathogen in this genus is *S. aureus*. This bacterium causes a myriad of infections, from wound and skin infections through to mastitis, septicaemia and endocarditis.[65] It is a commonly isolated bacterium from healthy people, particularly from the skin and nasal passages. Infection is generally due to lowered host resistance at the site of infection. Methicillin-resistant *S. aureus* (MRSA) is increasingly present in hospitals and the wider community.[65]

- Microscopy: Gram-positive cocci arranged in 'grape-bunch' clusters
- O_2 requirement: facultative anaerobe
- Clinical specimens required: pus, sputum, faeces, urine or blood depending on site of infection
- Differentiate from: dependent upon site of infection; possible number of similar microbes is extensive due to widespread nature of *S. aureus* infections
- Use of NAA: yes
- Other *Staphylococci* species: *S. epidermidis*, *S. saprophyticus*.[65]

STREPTOCOCCI

The *Streptococcus* genus is a large group covering many diverse infections in humans. Many classification systems exist for the various species within this group, but for practical reasons they are either known as beta-haemolytic or alpha/gamma haemolytic streptococci.[66] Refer to Table 4.39 for a summary of the most common *Streptococcus* organisms affecting humans, with their associated clinical states.

- Microscopy: Gram-positive cocci arranged in chains, diplococci (*S. pneumonia*)
- O_2 requirement: facultative anaerobes
- Clinical specimens required: swabs of the affected and relevant mucosal or cutaneous surface, blood
- Differentiate from: dependent upon the organ system affected; for example: *Enterococcus*, *M. pneumoniae*, *C. pneumoniae*, *B. pertussis* and viral respiratory pathogens; for urogenital infections: *N. gonorrhoea*, *C. trachomatis*, *E. coli*, *Candida*, *G. vaginalis* and *Trichomonis* (parasitic)
- Use of NAA: available for some species. Also Group A antigen test, culture/sensitivity testing.[66]

TABLE 4.39 Selected *Streptococcus* species and associated clinical conditions

Species	Diseases
S. pyogenes (group A *Streptococcus*)	Pharyngitis, skin and soft-tissue infections, bacteraemia, rheumatic fever, acute glomerulonephritis
S. agalactiae (group B *Streptococcus*)	Neonatal disease, endometritis, wound infections, urinary tract infections, bacteraemia, pneumonia, skin and soft-tissue infections
S. pneumoniae	Subacute endocarditis, sepsis in neutropenic patients, pneumonia, meningitis
S. mutans	Dental caries, bacteraemia
S. anginosus	Abscesses in brain, oropharynx or peritoneal cavity

Kilian M. *Streptococcus* and *Enterococcus*. In Greenwood D, editor. Medical microbiology. 18th edn. Elsevier Churchill Livingstone; 2012, pp. 183–98.

In both orthodox medical and naturopathic clinical practice, special attention is afforded for all communicable diseases defined as notifiable infections. The Communicable Disease Network Australia (CDNA) and the National Notifiable Diseases Surveillance System (NNDSS) establish which infections must be reported.[67] More than 50 communicable infections belong to this register; it is important for all health professionals to be familiar with the infections included on this list. While some are rarely encountered in clinical practice, others are common, including varicella, all STIs and influenza.[67] In Australia, laboratories and primary healthcare providers are legally obliged to report all cases of notifiable infections to the Department of Health in their state.[67]

ENDOCRINOLOGY

Please note, the following endocrinology discussion with reference ranges is based on serum analyses, unless otherwise specified (e.g. urine). Salivary hormone testing is discussed specifically in Naturopathic assessments.

CORTISOL

Two physiological triggers cause the adrenal cortex to secrete cortisol: (1) the circadian secretion of adrenocorticoid hormone (ACTH) from the anterior pituitary gland and (2) physiological stress.[68] Cortisol secretion is part of a much larger hypothalamic–pituitary–adrenal (HPA) axis involving several feedback loops. Pituitary ACTH release is under the control of the hypothalamic corticotrophin-releasing hormone (CRH).

The circadian pattern of ACTH release reveals a surge in secretion between 4 am and 8 am with declining levels throughout the day. In normal sleep–wake cycles, the lowest levels of secretion are seen just after midnight. Ultradian rhythms for ACTH are responsible for 10–18 secretory bursts in a 24-hour period. Physiological stress sources include surgical trauma, pyrogenic infections, hypoglycaemia, significant haemorrhage and prolonged psychological stress.[68]

In primary adrenal pathologies, the adrenal glands cannot respond to ACTH due to damage or disease (low cortisol/high ACTH). In diseases affecting pituitary function, ACTH does not form or is not released and cortisol levels are low. Damage to the hypothalamus is also associated with low ACTH and low cortisol. Testing with exogenous ACTH (Synacthen) is useful in pinpointing the source of the adrenal pathology. This test is called the Synacthen stimulation test (SST) and examines the ability of the adrenal gland to respond to a stimulus.

A possible source of adrenal pathology is primary adrenal cortex insufficiency or adrenal suppression/atrophy due to glucocorticoid-based pharmacotherapy.

The CRH stimulation test is used when hypothalamic dysfunction is suspected. The results may be interpreted as follows:

- Hypothalamic dysfunction: elevated ACTH after CRH dose (sampled at 30 min or 1 hr, depending on protocol)
- Pituitary dysfunction: no significant ACTH response (sampled at 30 min or 1 hr)
- Adrenal dysfunction: elevated ACTH at 30 min and a further rise at 1 hr with little or no rise in cortisol.[68]

Dexamethasone suppression testing involves administration of oral dexamethasone (synthetic glucocorticoid) under a number of different protocols; as a single dose or for 2 days at low dose, followed by 2 days at high dose. Blood collections commence prior to dosing for a total of 7 days (morning peak is captured by sampling at 9 am). Additionally, 24-hour urine collections are used for cortisol measurement and are usually collected corresponding to baseline, low and high dose time points.

Clinical significance

- Dexamethasone suppression test (long): the inability to suppress ACTH is associated with pituitary Cushing's syndrome. No suppression of cortisol at the 8 mg dose is associated with adrenal neoplasms[11]
- Elevated ACTH levels are associated with both corticosteroid deficiency (adrenal insufficiency) and corticosteroid excess (through pituitary oversecretion)
- Reduced ACTH can be seen in corticosteroid excess (due to adrenal tumours) and corticosteroid deficiency (due to pituitary deficiency)
- Urinary cortisol levels are sometimes used and only significant when a full 24-hour urine collection is provided for analysis. Increased cortisol excretion is associated with adrenal hyperfunction.[11]

Reference ranges are:

DST: suppression is defined as a reduction in blood cortisol to <50% of the basal value[11]

SST: a baseline (pre-Synacthen), post-Synacthen or an increment of >200 nmol/L at 30 minutes all indicate a normal response to Synacthen and excludes adrenal atrophy. A normal result does not ensure an adequate adrenal response to severe stress[11]

ACTH: <10 pmol/L (time of day dependant; ideal sample timing is 8 am to 9 am)[11]

Random cortisol: 200–650 nmol/L (morning peak). Trough level should be ≤50% of the morning peak (sample at 8 pm). Higher peak and trough levels are observed in stressed patients and during oral contraceptive therapy[11]

Urinary cortisol: 100–300 nmol/24 hr.[11]

ALDOSTERONE

Aldosterone is one of several hormones based on the steroid ring structure. It is believed its evolutionary emergence was for the need to conserve both the electrolyte sodium and water.[69] The most well-known actions of aldosterone include stimulation of sodium retention in the distal nephron, distal colon and the salivary glands. Sodium retention increases plasma volume via water retention and is one defence mechanism against low plasma volume and low blood pressure. Aldosterone also functions in the cardiovascular system, the inflammatory response and the central nervous system.[70]

Aldosterone is a key hormone in the renin–angiotensin–aldosterone system (RAAS). When serum Na is low (with its consequent low water/low blood volume effects), renal renin secretion is stimulated. Renin release stimulates angiotensinogen secretion, resulting in angiotensin I release. Angiotensin-converting enzyme (ACE) converts angiotensin I to angiotensin II (primarily in the pulmonary vasculature). Angiotensin II has several actions in defending against drops in blood volume and blood pressure, one of which is stimulating the adrenal cortex to release aldosterone.[69]

Terminology

Hyperaldosteronism: elevated blood aldosterone levels.

Clinical significance

Hyperaldosteronism is also known as Conn's syndrome. The clinical presentation often involves hypertension and muscle weakness. Hypokalaemia may also be present. There are various causes of hyperaldosteronism, including adrenal hyperplasia, adrenal aldosterone-secreting tumours and renal disease. Determining the precise cause warrants further diagnostic testing, including serum and urine electrolyte levels and specialised testing measuring the patient's physiological response to pharmacological agents such as dexamethasone and captopril.[11] Screening is suggested for hypertension unresponsive to medications/interventions, or hypertension/cerebrovascular accidents in patients <20 years of age.[70]

A measurement of the aldosterone/renin ratio is of more diagnostic value than individual aldosterone levels.[11] An elevated aldosterone/renin ratio indicates excessive mineralocorticoid, or primary hyperaldosteronism. If aldosterone and renin are both elevated to a similar extent, secondary hyperaldosteronism is suspected (source of pathology is renal).[11] Patients are advised not to restrict salt intake and remain in an upright position for approximately 2 hours pre test (both actions increase the test sensitivity). Unfortunately, various antihypertensive medications affect the results, which must be interpreted in consultation with a pathologist.[69]

The recommended angiotensin/renin ratio (ARR) is the ratio of plasma aldosterone (ng/L) to plasma renin activity (ng/mL/h): 20–40. ARR of 35 or higher is highly indicative of primary hyperaldosteronism (PAA). Some clinicians require serum aldosterone levels of >15 ng/dL for a PAA diagnosis.[70]

CATECHOLAMINES

The catecholamines include adrenaline (epinephrine), noradrenaline (norepinephrine) and dopamine. Dopamine is synthesised in the brain from tyrosine. Dopamine is also the precursor substrate for both adrenaline (epinephrine) and noradrenaline (norepinephrine), both of which are synthesised in the adrenal medulla. It is well known that the catecholamines are imperative to the function of the autonomic nervous system.

Clinical significance

Elevated blood catecholamines are suggestive of catecholamine-secreting tumours, such as phaeochromocytoma (adrenaline [epinephrine] or noradrenaline [norepinephrine]) or neuroblastoma (dopamine). Urinary catecholamines are measured more often in these suspected cases (urinary excretion is increased in phaeochromocytoma.[11] Further testing may be indicated in cases of clinical uncertainty, where a suspected tumour cannot be identified via diagnostic imaging. This test is known as the clonidine suppression test.

Some laboratories may test the breakdown metabolites of catecholamines in urine; these metabolites include metanephrine, normetanephrine, homovanillic acid and vanillylmandelic acid (all are elevated in cases of aforementioned tumours). Stress, certain recreational drugs and other stimulants such as nicotine and caffeine heavily influence blood testing of catecholamines, thus false positive results can occur.[11] The blood test may be useful for investigating the cause of persistent hypertension. A certain amount of patient preparation is required prior to testing, to reduce the possibility of false positive results. Serial measurements are also recommended. Refer to Tables 4.40 and 4.41 for reference ranges for serum and urine catecholamines respectively.

THYROID FUNCTION TESTS (TFTs)

For normal thyroid function, a healthy and intact hypothalamic–pituitary–thyroid (HPT) axis and a steady source of dietary iodine are required. The hypothalamus produces thyrotrophin-releasing hormone, which then triggers the anterior pituitary gland to release thyroid-stimulating hormone (TSH), also known as thyrotrophin.[71] TSH stimulates production and release of thyroid hormones by the thyroid gland. Negative feedback from thyroid hormones on the hypothalamus/pituitary gland keeps TSH within a narrow normal range.

TABLE 4.40 Reference range: catecholamines (blood)

Catecholamine	Reference range (nmol/L)
Adrenaline (epinephrine)	<0.3
Noradrenaline (norepinephrine)	<2.5
Dopamine	<0.5

Reproduced with permission from the Royal College of Pathologists of Australasia (RCPA). RCPA manual of use and interpretation of pathology tests. 7th ed. Sydney: RCPA, 2015. https://www.rcpa.edu.au/Library/Practising-Pathology/RCPA-Manual/Home.

TABLE 4.41 Reference range: catecholamines (urine)

Catecholamine	Reference range (nmol/24 h)
Adrenaline (epinephrine)	<80
Noradrenaline (norepinephrine)	<780
Dopamine	<3500

Reproduced with permission from the Royal College of Pathologists of Australasia (RCPA). RCPA manual of use and interpretation of pathology tests. 7th ed. Sydney: RCPA, 2015. https://www.rcpa.edu.au/Library/Practising-Pathology/RCPA-Manual/Home.

Via the action of TSH, iodine enters thyroid follicular cells as inorganic iodide and is incorporated into two hormones: thyroxin (T4) and 3,5,3'- triiodothyronine (T3) via several biochemical steps, some of which involve the amino acid tyrosine. All circulating T4 is produced by the thyroid, while only 20% of T3 is made in the thyroid (the majority is synthesised by the liver).[71] Most circulating T3 and T4 are bound to plasma proteins, including thyroxin-binding globulin, transthyretin and albumin.[72] A small percentage of T3 and T4 are free and represent biologically active hormones.

Another testing parameter is reverse T3 (rT3). Upon hepatic conversion of T4 to T3, a small portion of rT3 (the inactive form of T3) is produced. During prolonged physiological stress (psychological and physical), it is believed more rT3 than T3 is synthesised to conserve energy metabolism in T3-dependent peripheral tissues. rT3 does not deliver O_2 molecules to peripheral tissues for cellular respiration and ATP production with the same efficiency as active T3.[14] This is one proposed mechanism of non-thyroidal illness (sick euthyroid syndrome).

Conventional endocrine pathology testing does not usually involve rT3 testing for hypothyroidism. However, integrative pathology considers rT3 to be a valuable parameter in the assessment of a hypothyroid state. rT3 elevations can be observed in cases of chronic illness and stress, where it binds to T3 receptors, blocks T3 physiology and has hypothyroid effects. This rT3 can be seen in conjunction with normal TSH/T4/free T4 levels.[73]

Terminology

Hyperthyroidism: elevated thyroid function.
Hypothyroidism: reduced thyroid function.
Euthyroidism: normal thyroid function.

Clinical significance

Many clinical circumstances make the interpretation of TFTs challenging. Hyperthyroidism classically shows low TSH with high T3/T4, while hypothyroidism involves elevated TSH, with normal or low T3/T4. In most cases, further testing is usually required to determine the cause or source of thyroid dysfunction. This requires additional testing beyond simple TFTs to include a free T4 (FT4) level to measure the unbound (bioavailable) T4 fraction. A host of thyroid antibodies can be tested, though this may require referral to an endocrinologist. The testing of TSH only (without fT4) is a limitation imposed by laboratories, not clinicians. Laboratories will automatically add the fT4 test if TSH is abnormal.

Longitudinal testing can prove valuable for determining baseline levels of HPT axis homeostasis for individual patients, in the non-diseased state. The average fT3, fT4 and TSH are determined and any deviation from the average is considered clinically significant. Tables 4.42 and 4.43 help to summarise the many result patterns seen when investigating thyroid diseases via laboratory tests.

Special clinical considerations are required when interpreting TgAb levels in cases of Hashimoto's hypothyroidism. While many pathology resources indicate the presence of elevated TgAbs, the clinical reality reflects a different situation entirely, where TgAb levels are often not elevated. Pathophysiological reasons for such clinical variety can include the natural ebb and flow of an

TABLE 4.43 Characterisation of thyroid conditions based on thyroid antibody testing

Condition	aTPO	TgAb	TRAb
Primary hypothyroidism	N	N	N
Congenital hypothyroidism	N	N	N
Hashimoto's hypothyroidism	High	High or N	N
Graves' disease	High or N	High or N	High
Neonatal Graves' disease	High or N	High or N	High
TSH deficiency (central hypothyroidism)	N	N	N
Non-thyroidal illness	N	N	N

Abbreviations: TgAb: antithyroglobulin Abs; aTPO: anti-thyroid peroxidase Abs; TRAb: thyroid receptor Abs
McAuley D. Common laboratory values. Global RPh, The clinician's ultimate reference, 2016. Available from: www.globalrph.com/labs_t.htm

TABLE 4.42 Classification of thyroid conditions based on TFTs

Condition	TSH	FT_3	FT_4	rT_3
Primary hypothyroidism	High	Low or N	Low	Low
Congenital hypothyroidism	High	Low	Low	Low
Hashimoto's hypothyroidism	High	Low or N	Low or N	Low
Hypothyroidism (other)	N	N	N	High
Graves' disease	Low	High	High	High or N
Neonatal Graves' disease	Low	High	High	High or N
TSH deficiency (central hypothyroidism)	Low or N	Low	Low	Low
Non-thyroidal illness	Variable	Low	Variable	High

McAuley D. Common laboratory values. Global RPh, The clinician's ultimate reference, 2016. Available from: www.globalrph.com/labs_t.htm

individual's immune response (TgAb levels often change when tested frequently) and dietary intake at the time of testing (e.g. pro-inflammatory foods can precipitate a pro-inflammatory immune response). Negative antibody TgAb results can also result in Hashimoto's patients with low immune competence.

While TPO elevations are definitive results in Hashimoto's hypothyroidism, caution is required to not always expect elevated TgAbs, and rely on the full spectrum of physical examination, clinical history/presentation and pathology tests before clinical decisions are made. This will assist to avoid overlooking such cases in clinical practice. Hashimoto's thyroiditis has an insidious onset, and many patients do not present at the time of overt disease.[71]

Subclinical hypothyroidism is a medical term for patients with elevated TSH, but a normal T3/T4/fT4 (when low levels are usually expected). Additionally, there are many non-thyroidal illnesses that can cause both increased and decreased TSH. This is observed as low TSH in the acute phase of illness, normal to high TSH during healing of the illness, and normal TSH upon resolution of the illness. Another concern is that many pharmaceuticals can supress TSH secretion, including opioids, glucagon, glucocorticoids and dopamine.[74]

It is well known in clinical endocrinology that a TSH-centred testing strategy has limitations when evaluating thyroid disease. This approach assumes the hypothalamic-pituitary axis is stable and intact. It is well known that prolonged stress, illness and altered sleep–wake cycles can affect the correct functionality of this axis.[14] It does not take into account the patient's recent dynamic clinical state regarding illness or medications. It is often more useful to look at the TSH result and note any results at the extreme ends of the normal range, especially for patients with minor symptoms of thyroid dysfunction. Looking at TSH trends over time is very useful, particularly if a patient is continually approaching the high-end of normal, or the low-end of normal.

With TSH deficiency (central hypothyroidism) there is a loss of physiological secretion of TSH, where the pulsatile secretion of TSH and the total amount in 24 hours is diminished. This results in normal or low TSH results, despite a clinical (signs/symptoms) or biochemical hypothyroid state (low fT3 and fT4). In this case, the pituitary gland is not responsive to the hypothyroid state. This clinical situation is only common in patients with a history of cranial irradiation and neurosurgery (especially in childhood).[72,74] Refer to Table 4.44 for reference ranges for the full thyroid testing panel.

TABLE 4.44 Reference ranges: full thyroid testing panel

Hormone	Normal range
TSH	0.4–4.0 mIU/L (Note: some biochemistry institutes recommend an upper limit of 2.5 mIU/L, which may or may not be adopted by conventional laboratories. Subclinical hypothyroidism: 4.0–10 mIU/L.) (Other thyroid parameters are often normal. Antibody screening may be beneficial, as is longitudinal serial TSH monitoring.)
Free T3	4.0–8.0 pmol/L
Free T4	10–25 pmol/L
rT3	10–24 ng/dL

American Association for Clinical Chemistry (AACC). Thalassaemia laboratory tests. AACC, 2016. Available from: https://labtestsonline.org/understanding/conditions/thalassemia/start/2; Australian Prescriber. Managing subclinical hypothyroidism. NPS Medicinewise. Available from: www.nps.org.au/australian-prescriber/articles/managing-subclinical-hypothyroidism; Mayo Medical Laboratories. T3 (triiodothyronine), reverse, serum. Mayo Clinic. Available from: www.mayomedicallaboratories.com/test-catalog/Clinical+and+Interpretive/9405

fT_3:fT_4 RATIO

This ratio represents the level of free T3 to free T4. With T3 representing active thyroid hormone, the normal ratio in euthyroid, healthy individuals is expected to be constant. Approximately 20% of T3 synthesis occurs in thyroid tissue, with the remaining 80% occurring via the extra-thyroidal conversion of T4 to T3 via deiodination.[75] This ratio may reflect the extent of extrathyroidal T4 to T3 conversion.[75] Decreased ratios have been noted in post-thyroidectomy patients treated with levothyroxine and patients with metabolic syndrome. The establishment of reliable reference ranges remains the subject of clinical research.[75]

fT_3:rT_3 ratio

This ratio examines the extent to which active T3 is synthesised in comparison to inactive rT3. A lower ratio here indicates excess production of rT3 when compared to fT3. Such results have been noted in kilojoule restriction, fasting, post-surgery and some cardiovascular events such as stroke.[76]

ANTIDIURETIC HORMONE (ADH)

ADH may also be referred to as vasopressin. ADH is a peptide hormone that shares a highly similar amino acid structure to another peptide hormone, oxytocin. Both are released by the posterior pituitary gland. ADH is responsible for maintaining the normal osmolarity (solute to solvent ratio) of body fluids and normal blood volume. Renal tissue is the main target for ADH action, increasing water permeability from the renal lumen to the renal interstitial tissue.[70] This helps to decrease urine flow and volume (known as antidiuresis).

Clinical significance

ADH is stimulated by increased ECF osmolality and decreases in blood volume or blood pressure.[77] Several drugs can increase ADH secretion, including opiates, nicotine and barbiturates to name a few.[70] Alcohol suppresses the secretion of ADH. Increased levels are noted in many cancers, diabetes insipidus (renal origin), pneumonia and syndrome of inappropriate ADH secretion (SIADH).[77] Decreased levels may be observed in nephrotic syndrome, enuresis and diabetes insipidus (pituitary origin).[77] ADH levels are interpreted in conjunction with

TABLE 4.45 Reference ranges: serum osmolarity and ADH

Serum osmolarity (mOSm/L)	ADH level (pmol/L)
270–280	< 1.4
280–285	< 2.3
285–290	0.9–4.6
290–295	1.9–6.5
295–300	3.7–11.1

Royal College of Pathologists of Australasia (RCPA). Education online. RCPA, 2016. Available from: www.rcpa.edu.au/Education; White B, Porterfield S. Hypothalamus-pituitary complex. In White B, editor. Endocrine and reproductive physiology. 4th edn. Philadelphia: Elsevier Mosby; 2013, pp. 99–128.

blood plasma osmolality levels. Refer to Table 4.45 for reference ranges.

GROWTH HORMONE (GH)

Human GH is actually a group of hormones, primarily secreted by somatotrophs of the anterior lobe of the pituitary gland.[77] The functions of growth hormone include metabolic effects, tissue growth and cellular differentiation.[78] GH enhances the cellular uptake of amino acids, protein synthesis, catabolism of fatty acids and hepatic secretion of insulin-like growth factor 1 (IGF-1). GH also inhibits tissue utilisation of glucose, thus increasing BGL.[78] Severe deficiencies in GH lead to decreased height, while excess GH secretion leads to acromegaly and its consequent decrease in normal life span. GH levels are stimulated by exercise and remain elevated immediately after exercise.[79] GH is also stimulated by stress, starvation and acute hypoglycaemia.[77]

A distinct diurnal rhythm exists for GH secretion, with peak secretion occurring in the early hours of the morning. Alterations occur due to changes in sleep–wake patterns (e.g. night and shift workers), as opposed to following light–dark patterns.[79] Secretion of GH is pulsatile, thus testing of GH in isolation is of little clinical value. Abnormal GH secretion is one of several hormones implicated in dwarfism and gigantism. In adults, GH deficiency is linked to changes in body composition, hypoglycaemia, sarcopenia, muscle weakness and early exhaustion.[79]

Clinical significance

Testing GH in isolation is of limited diagnostic value. Dynamic testing of GH is needed for diagnostics. Additional testing of IGF-1 assists in screening for acromegaly and gigantism.[11] IGF-1 varies with age, nutritional status and gender. It generally is not tested during times of malnutrition, with severe illness or during puberty.

Diagnosis of GH deficiency requires a *growth hormone stimulation test*. The testing protocol involves fasting, then a period of moderate exercise, followed by testing of both GH and BGLs. BGL must decrease to <2.2 mmol/L. The *growth hormone suppression test* investigates the possibility of excessive GH secretion and is the definitive test for acromegaly or pituitary gigantism.[11] After an initial blood sample, the patient ingests a 75 g glucose load. Blood is then sampled every 30 minutes for 3 hours.

Reference ranges are:

- GH stimulation test: a GH result of ≥20 mU/L (10 ug/L) shows normal stimulation and excludes GH deficiency
- GH suppression test: a GH result of <1 mU/L shows adequate suppression and excludes excessive GH secretion
- IGF-1: 30–50 nmol/L (adults).[11]

β-hCG

Human chorionic gonadotropin (hCG) is produced by the placenta during pregnancy, but is also produced by some germ cell and other tumours.[80] hCG is a glycoprotein hormone and contains two subunits, the alpha and the beta subunit. Testing of the beta subunit is essential, as the alpha subunit shares structural similarities with FSH, LH and TSH, thus false positives may occur.

Clinical significance

Serial testing of β-hCG is used to monitor the health of a pregnancy and to determine gestational age. It is also used to monitor health after surgery or chemotherapy for germ-cell tumours.[80] For pregnancy testing, it is important for females to recall the dates of their last menstrual cycle to obtain a more meaningful clinical interpretation. A positive pregnancy test can be detected 6–10 days post ovulation.

Both qualitative (positive/negative) and quantitative (numerical values) testing for β-hCG is available. Qualitative testing involves urine testing; however, any positive urine testing must be confirmed with a positive serum β-hCG. In addition to some forms of cancer, elevated levels are noted in ectopic pregnancy, though levels here are often lower than usual for the suspected gestational age. β-hCG levels are often measured after miscarriage, post dilation and curettage (D&C) procedures and after medical termination of pregnancy to ensure the absence of products of conception.

The reference range is: negative result = <2 ug/L or <5 IU/L.[11]

Due to the significant variation in hCG levels between individual females week by week of pregnancy, reference ranges are very wide and used only as a guide. β-hCG is not routinely monitored in normal pregnancy, only in cases such as threatened miscarriage, suspicion of twins or triplets, or for women who conceive with assisted fertility techniques.

CALCITONIN

Parafollicular cells (also known as C cells) located within the thyroid gland are the site of calcitonin production (a peptide hormone). The function of calcitonin is to decrease plasma calcium concentration.[81] This occurs in two ways. First, osteoclasts are inhibited from resorbing bone, thus encouraging the deposition of Ca in bone. Second, calcitonin reduces the formation of new osteoclasts.[81]

TABLE 4.46 Reference range: calcitonin

Population	Normal range (ng/L)
Adult females	<5
Adult males	<12
0–6 months	<40
6 months–3 years	<15

Paediatric reference ranges are similar to adults in children over 3 years of age. Reproduced with permission from the Royal College of Pathologists of Australasia (RCPA). RCPA manual of use and interpretation of pathology tests. 7th ed. Sydney: RCPA, 2015. https://www.rcpa.edu.au/Library/Practising-Pathology/RCPA-Manual/Home.

Neoplastic activity of C cells results in medullary thyroid carcinoma, the most aggressive from of thyroid cancer.[82]

Clinical significance

As an inhibitor of bone resorption, calcitonin prevents bone loss during stresses on Ca conservation, such as pregnancy, lactation and times of increased growth.[82] Blood calcitonin levels may be important when investigating the various causes of both hyper- and hypocalcaemia, along with vitamin D and serum PTH levels. Elevated blood calcitonin is considered a significant tumour marker for medullary thyroid carcinoma (MTC). It is also used to detect residual thyroid tissue and metastasis post MTC surgery.[82] Elevations in calcitonin may be observed in non-cancerous pathologies, such as benign C cell hyperplasia (an autoimmune thyroid disease), and some renal pathologies.[82] Refer to Table 4.46 for reference ranges.

DEHYDROEPIANDROSTERONE SULFATE (DHEAS)

DHEAS is the sulfated form of DHEA, an adrenal steroid hormone. Like all steroid hormones, DHEA is derived from cholesterol. Diagnostic tests measure the DHEAS form, as this is much easier to detect in serum. In the adrenal cortex, DHEA is the precursor substrate for androstenedone, which is ultimately converted to testosterone and oestrogens (in both males and females).[83] Adrenal androgens appear to have a minor physiological role in males, as their secondary sexual characteristics are maintained by testosterone produced in the testes.[84]

Clinical significance

Elevated DHEAS is indicative of an adrenal source of androgens. This is typical of congenital adrenal hyperplasia or adrenal tumours. Testing DHEAS is useful when investigating infertility, hirsutism and virilisation in female patients.[11] DHEAS is measured in females to investigate polycystic ovary syndrome (PCOS) and amenorrhoea. It is useful when investigating precocious puberty in both young girls and boys. Decreased levels are seen in adrenal insufficiency (primary and secondary), chronic fatigue syndrome and poorly controlled diabetes mellitus.[83]

Reference ranges are 3.4–14.4 umol/L (adult male) and 1.6–8.9 umol/L (adult female, premenopausal). (Paediatric ranges are not clearly established due to significant variability.)[83]

Note: DHEAS levels increase significantly in children 6–8 years of age, and DHEAS peaks at approximately 20–30 years. During the ageing process, DHEAS levels reduce significantly.[83]

FOLLICLE-STIMULATING HORMONE (FSH)

FSH is a glycoprotein hormone secreted by gonadotrophic cells of the anterior pituitary gland.[84] Its primary role is the stimulation of ovarian follicles in females, and the regulation of spermatogenesis in males. FSH secretion is regulated by hypothalamic gonadotrophin-releasing hormone (GnRH). FSH levels are negligible in both boys and girls until the onset of puberty. FSH helps to establish menarche in females as well as regular monthly menstrual cycles. In males, FSH stimulates Sertoli cells for the conversion of immature spermatids to mature sperm cells.[84]

Clinical significance

FSH is used in the investigation of gonadal hypofunction, onset of the menopause, delayed menarche, infertility and suspected pituitary tumours. Elevated FSH is due to pituitary secretion from a lack of negative feedback from gonadal androgens/oestrogens (causes here include primary gonadal hypofunction and the postmenopausal state).[11] Pituitary tumours involving gonadotrophic hormones may also cause elevations. Decreased FSH is likely due to pituitary or hypothalamic disease.[11] When investigating ovarian reserves for female infertility patients, anti-mullarian hormone (AMH) measurements are more reliable.

LUTEINISING HORMONE (LH)

LH is the second gonadotrophic hormone secreted by the anterior pituitary gland. This hormone is responsible for causing ovulation and development of the ovarian corpus luteum. In females, LH stimulates the synthesis of oestrogen by the ovary and progesterone by the corpus luteum.[84] LH secretion is also regulated by GnRH. Again, LH levels are negligible before the onset of puberty in both sexes. In females, ovarian follicles stimulated by FSH will not proceed to ovulation. Approximately 48 hours prior to ovulation, LH secretion surges, increasing 6 to 10-fold.[84] In males, LH stimulates testosterone secretion by Leydig cells in the testes.

Clinical significance

Single LH results are misleading, due to the marked pulsatile nature of LH secretion. It is essential to know the stage of the menstrual cycle when interpreting results, though this proves difficult with amenorrhoea. Testing must be performed at the time of suspected mid-cycle LH peak to investigate whether this peak is actually occurring. LH testing is used extensively when investigating most menstrual cycle disorders (e.g. oligomenorrhoea, amenorrhoea), for infertility testing and to identify the presence/absence of ovulation.

Elevated LH levels are seen in primary gonadal failure (again, there is a lack of negative feedback on the pituitary from gonadal androgens/oestrogens). Elevations may also

TABLE 4.47 Reference ranges: FSH and LH

Population	LH	FSH
Adult female	2–15 U/L	1.0–1.8 U/L
Female (postmenopausal)	15–100 U/L	>18 U/L
Adult male	2–10 U/L	1.0–5.0 U/L (age related)

Reproduced with permission from the Royal College of Pathologists of Australasia (RCPA). RCPA manual of use and interpretation of pathology tests. 7th ed. Sydney: RCPA, 2015. https://www.rcpa.edu.au/Library/Practising-Pathology/RCPA-Manual/Home.

TABLE 4.48 Reference ranges: oestradiol

Phase	Reference range (pmol/L)
Early follicular	100–200
Preovulatory	500–1700
Luteal	500–900
Postmenopausal	70–200

Reproduced with permission from the Royal College of Pathologists of Australasia (RCPA). RCPA manual of use and interpretation of pathology tests. 7th ed. Sydney: RCPA, 2015. https://www.rcpa.edu.au/Library/Practising-Pathology/RCPA-Manual/Home.

be due to LH secreting pituitary tumours.[11] Decreased LH levels are associated with hypothalamic or pituitary failure. Refer to Table 4.47 for reference ranges for both FSA and LH.

OESTRADIOL (E_2)

E_2 is a steroid hormone with marked physiological importance in females and minor functions in males. In addition to its reproductive functions, oestrogen is important for non-reproductive tissues such as bone, liver, cardiovascular organs, integument, CNS and adipose tissue. Approximately 60% of serum oestrogen is transported via sex-hormone-binding globulin (SHBG), 20% via albumin and 20% in free (bioavailable) form.[85] Oestrogen is primarily synthesised in the ovaries; however, some peripheral tissues such as breast tissues do convert androgens to oestrogens (aromatisation) to yield elevated local oestrogen levels.

Oestrogen secretion increases throughout the follicular phase of the menstrual cycle and has numerous functions on the oviducts, mucus secretion and muscle tone in reproductive structures to help facilitate fertilisation.[85]

Clinical significance

Elevated oestrogen is seen in PCOS. High levels are used to confirm precocious puberty in young females. E2 is tested extensively during assisted fertility treatments, particularly when monitoring ovulation induction. It is important to take the timing of blood sampling into account, as the range for E2 changes throughout the menstrual cycle. Decreased levels are often noted in delayed onset of puberty or after menopause. Refer to Table 4.48 for reference ranges.

TABLE 4.49 Reference range: progesterone

Phase	Reference range (nmol/L)
Follicular	2.0–4.5
Luteal	7.0–70

Reproduced with permission from the Royal College of Pathologists of Australasia (RCPA). RCPA manual of use and interpretation of pathology tests. 7th ed. Sydney: RCPA, 2015. https://www.rcpa.edu.au/Library/Practising-Pathology/RCPA-Manual/Home.

PROGESTERONE

Progesterone is a steroid-based sex hormone important in both male and female reproduction. In females, progesterone is primarily produced by the corpus luteum, which forms only after successful ovulation. In males and females, progesterone is the intermediate substrate for producing testosterone, oestrogen and corticosteroid hormones.

Clinical significance

Progesterone levels should steadily increase in the latter half of the menstrual cycle (luteal phase). This steady rise in progesterone indicates that ovulation has taken place (due to the presence of the corpus luteum). Absence of increased luteal progesterone indicates an anovulatory cycle or inadequacy of corpus luteum function.[11] Testing is often performed on day 28 of the menstrual cycle, to capture the luteal phase rise in progesterone. For women undergoing assisted fertility treatments, progesterone levels are often monitored after the confirmation of early pregnancy. Rising progesterone levels in this situation indicate progression of the pregnancy. Refer to Table 4.49 for reference ranges.

TESTOSTERONE

The steroid hormone testosterone is the main androgen in males, responsible for male secondary sexual characteristics. While typically a 'male' hormone, testosterone is present in small amounts in females and is often tested in female reproductive disorders. Approximately two-thirds of testosterone circulates bound to SHBG, with a small amount bound to albumin. Less than 4% circulates as free testosterone.[86]

Clinical significance

Testosterone is used when investigating the cause of virilisation, hirsutism or possibly infertility in females (all conditions may show testosterone elevations). In males, testosterone levels are elevated in juvenile males with precocious puberty, and reduced in males with testicular failure.[11] Results are sometimes interpreted in conjunction with the free androgen index (FAI) or SHBG result. In most cases, a laboratory will measure the total testosterone level. Free testosterone levels can be added if total levels appear abnormal. Refer to Table 4.50 for reference ranges.

PROLACTIN

Prolactin is an anterior pituitary hormone with a polypeptide-based structure. Normally, secretion is very low, due to inhibition via dopamine. Prolactin secretion

TABLE 4.50 Reference range: total testosterone

Population	Reference range (nmol/L)
Males	6.7–28.9
Females	<2.1

Monash University. Testosterone and androgens in women. Women's Health Program, Monash University, 2010. Available from: http://med.monash.edu.au/sphpm/womenshealth/info-4-health-practitioners/index.html

does follow a circadian rhythm, with pulsatile secretions influenced by stimuli such as stress, pregnancy and exercise.[84] High prolactin in pregnancy and breastfeeding stimulates lactation in breast tissue. It also acts on the hypothalamus via negative feedback to inhibit GnRH secretion. This in turn reduces FSH.

Terminology

Hyperprolactinaemia: elevated serum prolactin levels.
Hypoprolactinaemia: reduced serum prolactin levels.

Clinical significance

Elevated prolactin levels are seen in prolactinomas of the pituitary gland and in some hypothalamic disorders associated with amenorrhoea and galactorrhoea.[11] Elevated levels are a normal finding during pregnancy and lactation. Certain pharmaceutical medications cause elevations in prolactin, including oestrogen therapy, metoclopramide and phenothiazine.[11]

Reference ranges are <750 mU/L (females) and 150–500 mU/L (males).[11]

SEX HORMONE-BINDING GLOBULIN: (SHBG)

Significant amounts of steroid hormones require assistance for transportation in blood plasma (steroids are lipophilic and hydrophobic, while blood plasma is an aqueous environment). As noted in previous sections, these transport proteins are synthesised in hepatic tissue. SHBG is a glycoprotein with binding specificity for androgens and oestrogens, and is important in both male and female reproductive endocrinology. Some SHBG is produced in extra-hepatic tissues, including the brain, uterine, testicular and placental tissues.[84] Any steroid hormone bound to SHBG is not free or is unavailable for binding with receptors. Free hormone is biologically active and can enter cells to initiate receptor activation.

Clinical significance

The amount of SHBG influences the bioavailability of androgens and oestrogens. Elevated SHBG is caused by oestrogenic states, such as pregnancy and oestrogen therapy. Reduced levels are observed in conditions of androgen excess. Refer to Table 4.51 for reference ranges.

TABLE 4.51 Reference range: SHBG

Population	Reference range (nmol/L)
Male (adult)	20–60
Male (pubertal)	16–100
Female (adult and pre-menopause)	40–120
Female (adult and post-menopause)	28–112
Female (pubertal)	36–125
Infants (1–2 yrs)	60–252
Males and females (pre-pubertal, 2–8 yrs)	72–220

Royal College of Pathologists of Australasia (RCPA). Education online. RCPA, 2016. Available from: www.rcpa.edu.au/Education; Wilson G, Sheikh-Ali M. Endocrinology. In Rakel R, Rakel D, editors. Textbook of family medicine. 9th edn. Philadelphia; Elsevier Saunders; 2016, pp. 817–66.

FREE ANDROGEN INDEX (FAI)

The FAI value represents the ratio of androgen (total testosterone) to SHBG, thus determining the bioavailability of free testosterone. It is more clinically relevant than total testosterone testing, as it shows the portion of bioavailable (free and unbound) androgen.

Clinical significance

A high FAI is often observed in hirsutism and virilisation in females. Precocious puberty in young males requires FAI testing to look for elevations, while decreased levels are often associated with testicular failure in males.[11] The FAI may be unreliable if SHBG levels are low.[84]

Reference ranges are highly dependent on the methodology used by laboratories, and are also adjusted for age, gender and Tanner stage development (pubertal staging).[11]

PARATHYROID HORMONE (PTH) AND PTH-RELATED PEPTIDE (PTHrP)

Both PTH and PTHrP are calcitropic hormones. PTH is secreted by the parathyroid glands, while PTHrP is produced by a variety of fetal and adult tissues. PTHrP is multifunctional, while PTH is one of the principle regulators of blood calcium concentration.[84] Both the synthesis and the secretion of PTH are stimulated by hypocalcaemia, and are conversely inhibited by hypercalcaemia.[84]

Hyperparathyroidism can be a primary pathology, or a secondary result of other abnormalities. In primary hyperparathyroidism, there is an over-proliferation of PTH secreting cells in one or more of the four parathyroid glands.[87] The excess in PTH leads to hypercalcaemia. Secondary hyperparathyroidism results from compensation of the parathyroid gland, where PTH is secreted in excess in response to vitamin D deficiency (vitamin D is required for maintaining blood Ca levels) and chronic kidney disease (inefficient renal reabsorption of Ca).[88]

Terminology

Hyperparathyroidism: PTH level is either increased, or high end of the normal range when hypercalcaemia is also present.
Hypoparathyroidism: PTH levels are decreased.

TABLE 4.52 Common anatomical locations for cytological sampling and testing

Tissue or cavity of origin	Specimens	Conditions
Cervical/vaginal	Brushings	Cervical intraepithelial neoplasia (CIN. Grades I, II and III). Malignancies, infections
Respiratory tract and mediastinum	Sputum, FNA, bronchial washings and brushings	Malignant, inflammatory and infective conditions
Urinary bladder	Urine and bladder washings	Bladder cancer, urothelial malignancy. Investigation of chronic haematuria
Pleural, pericardial and peritoneal fluids	Transudate or exudate fluids from pathological effusions	Malignancies, congestive heart failure, cirrhosis, pneumonia, lupus, trauma. Common site for metastases
Peritoneal fluids	Ovarian or fallopian tube washings	Gynaecological malignancies, pancreatic and gastric malignancies
Cerebrospinal fluid (CSF)	Mostly obtained via lumbar puncture	Malignancy
Gastrointestinal tract	FNA and brushings	Malignancy, Barrett's oesophagitis, infection
Breast	Nipple discharge and FNA	Malignancy, non-malignant cysts
Thyroid	FNA	Thyroid nodules (determining malignancy or non-malignancy)
Salivary gland	FNA	Infection, malignancy
Lymph nodes	FNA	Infection, malignancy (including sentinel nodes for non-lymphatic tumours)
Liver	FNA and brushings	Malignancy, monitoring rejection in liver transplantation
Pancreas and biliary tree	FNA and brushings	Malignancy, inflammatory conditions, cystic conditions
Kidney and adrenal gland	FNA	Wilms' tumour in children, malignancy, cystic conditions, infection
Ovary	FNA	Benign ovarian cysts, malignancy, abscess

Fletcher C. Introduction. In Fletcher C, editor. Diagnostic histopathology of tumours. 4th edn. Philadelphia: Elsevier Saunders; 2013, pp. 1–5.

Clinical significance

Serum PTH is an essential test for determining the cause of either hypocalcaemia or hypercalcaemia.

If hypercalcaemia is associated with malignancy, PTH levels are usually low. PTHrP can be tested here, if malignancy is suspected but cannot be detected via other tests.[11] In this sense, PTHrP is considered a tumour marker, and elevated levels in patients with hypercalcaemia are highly suggestive of malignancy. PTHrP testing is used to monitor progression in some cancers.[88]

A recommended PTH range of 1.0–7.0 pmol/L is a general guide; some laboratories may supply reference ranges based on their testing methodology. PTHrP normal range is <5 pmol/L (also method dependent).[11]

Cytopathology and histopathology

Cytopathology is described as the medical discipline 'devoted to the diagnosis of cellular tissue obtained by minimally invasive methods'.[89] Such methods include tissue scrapings, brushings and aspirations. Cytopathology is primarily performed via microscopy, thus the skill, interpretation and accuracy of cytopathologists is imperative with regard to the clinical implications for all patients undergoing such tests. Clinical decisions about medication prescription, surgery (both major and minor), treatment planning, diagnosis, prognosis and staging of many malignancies all rely on accurate cytological interpretation.

The most well-known of all cytological tests is the Papanicolaou (Pap) test; this is largely due to its success in contributing to the worldwide decline in cervical cancer mortality (developed nations).[90]

The array of clinical terminologies, specific cellular identifications and descriptions used by cytopathologists in their reporting is immense. Very simply, terms such as 'invasive', 'atypical', 'suspicious' and 'normal' feature heavily in cytological reporting. Refer to Table 4.52 for a summary of cytopathological samples, with corresponding significance of any clinical abnormalities.

Histopathology is the medical specialisation dealing with the study of diseased tissues. Like cytology, histopathology is centred on the skill of microscopy to help identify, diagnose or stage disease. Unlike cytopathology, histological examination involves viewing entire tissue cross-sections, from the cells of the apical surface to the anatomy of the basement membrane (cytopathology examines free cells and exfoliated tissue fragments).[90]

In the majority of cases, tissue samples for histopathological examination will be obtained via a tissue biopsy or tissue sample obtained during surgery. In some cases, whole organs removed in a surgical procedure (e.g. uterus, tonsils) will undergo a gross macroscopic examination by a histopathologist. Some common biopsy techniques include:

- Cone biopsy (cervix)
- Soft-tissue biopsy (e.g. breast, testes)
- Punch biopsy (skin, moles).

Tissue sections are then frozen and cut to prepare extremely thin tissue sections for fixing and staining on glass slides for examination. Interpretation involves the findings and medical opinions of a specialist histopathologist. Many malignancies are diagnosed via histopathology. Surgical removal of cancer involves histopathology, looking for the clearance of surgical margins or whether malignant tissue remains postsurgery.[90]

In reality, cancer diagnoses are determined by histopathologists, not surgeons, oncologists or other clinicians. The histopathology report often stages the grade of malignancy and outlines what progression the malignancy make take. Clinical treatment decisions in oncology are often based entirely on histopathology reports.[90] Interpretation is complex, organ specific and as such, reporting reflects the vast array of tissue descriptions of the unique organs of the human body.

Terminology used in cytopathology and histopathology reporting is extensive and instilled with medical language. In the past, non-standardised reporting strategies have complicated reports, though many professional pathology bodies worldwide are working towards standardised reporting systems. Most reporting is highly organ specific, as organs and tissues have their own unique macroscopic and microscopic appearance. A brief list (non-organ specific) of terminology includes the following:

- Adenocarcinoma: malignant tumour cells originating from glandular tissue
- Anaplasia: loss of differentiation and loss of normal growth orientation of cells; a hallmark of potential malignancy
- Benign: non-malignant growth
- Chromatin:
- CIS: carcinoma in situ. Neoplastic growth where tumour cells remain confined to epithelium; no evidence of invasion of the basement membrane. Invasive growth potential is usually still high
- Dysplasia: abnormally developing cells; abnormal size, morphology and organisation of mature cells
- Hyperplasia/hypoplasia: increased/decreased numbers of normal cells, in normal arrangement
- In situ: in its original anatomical location
- Karyolysis: swelling of the nucleus, with loss of chromatin
- Metaplasia: change in mature cells to an abnormal form for that tissue
- Neoplasia: new and abnormal growth; may be benign or malignant.[91]

CLINICAL GENETICS

Genomic diseases and disorders represent some of the most commonly encountered conditions in many areas of health and medicine. The astonishing progress observed in the areas of the Human Genome Project, gene therapies, cytogenetic testing and molecular genetics testing have provided medical science with a means for chromosomal, sub-chromosomal, single gene and even genome-wide analysis. Many diseases of unknown cause can now be attributed to specific errors within the genome.

Genetic abnormalities arise from abnormal chromosome segregation, extra chromosome replication, chromosomal translocation, nucleotide deletions and duplications, and genomic imprinting.[92] The specialty of genetics encompasses many areas of subspecialisation; however, only two generally deal with and perform laboratory diagnostics of genetic disorders: cytogenetics (microscopic analysis of chromosomes examining their structure and numbers) and molecular genetics (the study of the structure and function of genes at the molecular level—molecular genetics techniques include fluorescence in situ hybridisation [FISH] and comparative genomic hybridisation [CGH] studies).[93] There are hundreds of specific genetic abnormalities that can now be identified through genetic testing. The vast majority of genetic testing is performed by specialist medical scientists, pathologists and geneticists from laboratories dedicated to genetics.

Reporting of genetic diseases usually involves qualitative analysis, where specific genetic mutations are reported as detected/not detected. Other reports involve a descriptive and thorough appraisal of chromosomal abnormalities. It is impossible to list the interpretive terminology for all genetic diseases here, but some commonly encountered clinical genetics terminology includes:

- Aneuploidy: chromosomes are missing or extra chromosomes are present
- Autosome: any chromosome that is not a sex chromosome (i.e. chromosomes 1 to 22 in humans)
- Carrier testing: genetic testing of a patient at risk of familial genetic disease, to determine whether they carry the faulty gene in question
- Chromosome: thread-like structures found in the nucleus of all cells (except erythrocytes). Location of genetic material (DNA) anchored to proteins. Humans have 23 pairs of chromosomes; one chromosome from each pair is inherited from each parent. There are 22 pairs of autosomes, and 1 pair of sex chromosomes (XX for females and XY for males)
- Congenital: refers to presence at birth; not always an inherited trait
- Deletion: loss of genetic material; may be large and visible as missing areas of chromosomes on the karyotype, or may be very small and requiring gene analysis
- Diploid: the number of chromosomes in human cells, existing as pairs
- Dominant: a genetic condition or disease where only one copy of the two gene alleles is mutated, yet the patient displays all signs/symptoms of the condition in question
- Duplication: extra chromosomal material present in two or more copies and may be visible on the karyotype

- Genotype: the specific genes present in an individual
- Haploid: the number of chromosomes in gametes (ova and sperm). There is only one copy of each chromosome in gametes. The human haploid number is 23
- Heterozygous: in relation to genetic disease, heterozygous means the inheritance of one normal and one abnormal copy of a gene. Many carriers of genetic diseases are heterozygous for the mutation in question
- Homozygous: in relation to genetic disease, homozygous means the inheritance of two abnormal copies of a gene
- Insertion: the addition of chromosomal material in an abnormal chromosome location. This results in abnormal transcription and translation
- Inversion: two breaks within a chromosome, with a chromosomal segment inverting direction. This may lead to abnormal transcription and translation
- Karyotype: the description of a patient's chromosomes after photography and analysis via microscopy
- Locus: the position on a chromosome or segment of a gene
- Monosomy: only one copy of a chromosome pair is present
- Mosaicism: some cells display abnormal genetics for a particular trait, while other cells have normal genetics. This determines the level of severity of the associated condition, with many genetic diseases existing as a spectrum of signs/symptoms
- Oncogene: a gene with the potential to cause cancer, if triggered by epigenetic factors
- Phenotype: the anatomical, physiological or biochemical features of a living organism, based upon their genes or environment
- Polymorphisms: changed chromosomal structures. They occur naturally in the population
- Predictive testing: used for patients with a family history of particular genetic diseases, but who do not currently have signs/symptoms, e.g. familial breast cancers
- Recessive: a genetic condition or disease where both copies of gene alleles are mutated, one each inherited from the mother and the father. The patient displays all signs/symptoms of the condition in question
- Single-nucleotide polymorphisms: changes in a single nucleotide within a gene. MTHFR gene differences are an example
- Somatic mutation: a mutation in any cells of the body apart from sex cells (ova and sperm), thus they cannot be passed on to offspring
- Translocation: when a section on one chromosome detaches and attaches to another. Genetic material may be lost, gained or remain the same after a translocation
- Trisomy: the presence of three copies of a specific chromosome, instead of two. The resulting karyotype shows 47 chromosomes, not the normal number of 46
- X-linked gene: any gene normally found on the X chromosome.[92]

Some examples of genetic testing include newborn screening, cancer genetic testing and prenatal testing. Some genetic conditions commonly tested for include Tay Sachs diseases, Down syndrome (trisomy 21), Patau's syndrome, (trisomy 13), Edwards' syndrome (trisomy 18) Klinefelter's syndrome, Turner's syndrome, cystic fibrosis and phenylketonuria.

Clinical genetic testing is incredibly vast, therefore categories exist according to their purpose. This helps clinicians understand their use and interpret their results with greater accuracy:

- Diagnostic: diagnostic testing can both diagnose and rule out specific genetic diseases in an individual. It is used only when physical/clinical signs and symptoms of a certain disease are present. Clinical examples include fragile X testing in young males with severe developmental delays. More than 1000 genetic tests are available for the more common autosomal dominant, autosomal recessive and X-linked disorders.
- Predictive/pre-symptomatic: this is useful to detect genetic mutations associated with serious diseases that may not have yet manifested clinically. They are of great use when a patient's family member is known to have a specific genetic condition; in many cases, the mutation can be identified well before a disease process has initiated. Examples include hereditary haemochromatosis and Huntington's disease. This form of testing may help with treatment initiation, life or reproductive planning.
- Predisposition testing: informs clinicians and patients of the potential risk associated with specific genetic-based illnesses. Many cancers are associated with this form of genetic testing. A positive result implies increased surveillance, but does not guarantee the disease in question will ever occur. Similarly, a negative result is not completely negligible.
- Carrier: this involves families and individuals for which a known genetic mutation or disease is present. Clinical examples include Tay-Sachs disease, cystic fibrosis and thalassaemia.
- Prenatal: this is used during a pregnancy for which certain genetic diseases may be suspected. For example, amniocentesis and chorionic villus sampling can be used in the detection of cystic fibrosis and sickle cell anaemia.
- Pre-implantation: pre-implantation testing of embryos conceived via IVF and ICSI can detect serious genetic conditions such as Huntington's disease, cystic fibrosis, thalassaemia and muscular dystrophy. This is a heavily regulated process in most countries, reserved for families with known serious or terminal genetic conditions.
- Newborn: performed after an infant's birth, newborn screening is able to identify serious genetic conditions early in life. Many of these conditions can be well managed and increase infant survival rate if detected and treated early. Examples include cystic fibrosis, phenylketonuria, galactosaemia and many genetic metabolic conditions.
- Pharmacogenomic: genetic testing of a patient's biological response to pharmacological agents will increase in this new era of personalised medicine. Pharmacogenomic testing of a patient's unique

physiological and biochemical response to medicines can help formulate drug choice, dosing regimens and drug selection.
- Research based: not used in the immediate clinical setting, however genetic research adds to the growing knowledge of the human genome and its contribution to ill health and disease.
- Forensic: forensic analysis of genetic material is most often used in legal proceedings or to establish biological relationships between individuals. It does not serve a clinical use in living individuals.[94,95]

TOXICOLOGY

Much of healthcare, medicine and naturopathy are devoted to the study of the natural components of normal and abnormal body functions. Conversely, the specialty of toxicology focuses on exogenous substances, and how they may adversely affect human health. Many chemical compounds introduced into the body significantly impact upon our physiology and biochemistry; these effects can be beneficial (in the case of therapeutic medications) or harmful (e.g. heavy metals, drugs of abuse, environmental contaminants).

As the science of toxicology has grown, naturally it has required subdivision. There are four key areas of toxicology: (1) detection of drugs of abuse, (2) therapeutic drug monitoring, (3) exposure testing for environmental toxins and (4) detection of DNA markers explicit for damage by specific environmental compounds.[96] The majority of toxicological testing is performed on blood and urine. Some methods require faecal or hair samples.

Drugs of abuse

Testing drugs of abuse is less a general practice or naturopathic matter; this is more a feature of emergency medicine, employment screening and forensic medicine.[97] As a summary, the drugs of abuse frequently tested include opiates, tranquillisers, barbiturates, cocaine, amphetamines and hallucinogens (e.g. cannabinoids, tryptamines and piperazines).[97] In general, laboratory reports will show findings as 'detected' or 'not detected'.

Medications

A host of therapeutic medications require very close monitoring in patients. Many medications do have toxic side effects and must not reach toxic levels in order to remain therapeutic. In addition, poor patient compliance is a significant issue in all areas of health; sub-therapeutic levels of medications require medical intervention.[97] The following classes of medications require regular monitoring via laboratory testing (the vast majority are conducted via blood testing):
- Anti-asthmatics (theophylline)
- Anticonvulsants
- Antidepressants
- Anti-inflammatories and analgesics
- Antipsychotics
- Cardiotrophics
- Chemotherapeutic agents
- Immunosuppressives
- Lithium.[97]

Generally, results of individual drugs are quantified, with results reported as a numerical value. These results are then compared to a desired therapeutic range for the drug in question.

Heavy metals

One area of toxicology involving urine sampling is heavy metal testing. The desired specimen for testing is a 24-hour plain urine (a collection of all urine produced in a continual 24-hour period). Most screening tests for heavy metals will investigate aluminium, arsenic, cadmium, cobalt, lead and mercury levels. When looking to determine the chronicity of heavy metal exposures, other tissues will be sampled for testing (including hair and nails).[96]

VITAMIN AND TRACE ELEMENTS

Routine pathology testing of vitamin and trace element levels is common for specific micronutrients, namely vitamins D, B_9 and B_{12} and the mineral iron. As previously discussed, other minerals are assessed via blood as electrolytes (Na, K, Ca, Mg). Despite the lack of routine testing of vitamins, laboratory methods have been developed to analyse blood levels of all the water and lipid-soluble vitamins. Testing of all vitamins is not common for a number of reasons:
- Many deficiencies are easily recognised via thorough physical examination/clinical history taking, negating the need for blood testing
- Some methodologies serve as surrogate markers of vitamin activity only
- Testing of vitamins may only be indicated for very specific clinical concerns.[96]

Clinical significance

With any nutrient deficiency diagnosed via pathology testing (vitamin or mineral) it is important to remember that poor dietary intake is not the sole reason for deficiencies. Poor dietary intake, malabsorption, increased excretion and increased physiological requirements all require careful consideration. Refer to Tables 4.53 and 4.54 for reference ranges and clinical significance of micronutrient vitamins and trace elements, respectively.

The assessment of trace elements requires accessing tissue, as most trace elements are readily stored within various body tissues. No single body tissue or fluid reigns supreme in the assessment of gross or trace elements. The assessment of each element must be based on its own unique physiology, storage, route of absorption and excretion. Both limitations and merits exist for all commonly tested tissues, including hair, urine, whole blood, serum, plasma and cellular blood components.[98] Plasma or serum levels of elements can fluctuate due to changes in transport proteins, the response to stress and changes in blood volume.[96] Hair is useful for routine screening of some elements.[98]

TABLE 4.53 Reference ranges: water and lipid-soluble vitamins

Vitamin	Specimen and test name	Reference range	Other possible tests/ clinical significance
Retinoids	Serum (retinol)	0.7–2.8 umol/L	Liver retinol stores Most serum tests are insensitive Used when investigating fat malabsorption syndromes
Carotenoids	Serum (carotenoids)	Supplied by laboratory	Testing indicates recent intake only
Tocopherols	Serum (tocopherol)/lipid ratio)	Child: 7–35 umol/L Adult: 11–46 umol/L	Hyperlipidaemia may disguise underlying deficiency Used in paediatric testing of haemolysis and fat malabsorption
Calciferols	Serum (25-OH vitamin D)	50–200 nmol/L 30–49 nmol/L (mild deficiency) 12.5–29 nmol/L (moderate deficiency) <12.5 nmol/L (severe deficiency)	Used in the investigation of rickets, osteomalacia, osteoporosis and fat malabsorption syndrome
Phyloquinones	Plasma (PT, APTT, INR). Surrogate markers of vitamin K activity	See coagulation studies (haematology)	Used in the investigation of fat malabsorption syndromes, haemorrhagic disease of the newborn
Thiamine	Erythrocytes (transketolase activity)	A ratio expressed with/without TPP	24 h thiamine (urine) reflects recent intake, not stores May be used in suspected alcoholic or nutritional cardiomyopathy/neuropathy
Riboflavin	Erythrocytes (glutathione reductase activity)	A ratio expressed with/without FAD	24 h riboflavin (urine) reflects recent intake, not stores
Niacin	Erythrocytes (NAD/NADP ratio)	<1 (deficiency)	Pyridine/nicotinamide ratio
Pantothenic acid	Whole blood	<100 ug/L (inadequate intake)	24 h pantothenic acid (urine)
Pyridoxines	Serum (P-5-P)	>30 nmol/L (adequate) >0.8 nmol/L (acceptable) <0.5 nmol/L (inadequate)	Aminotransferase levels (RBCs) Pyridoxic and xanthenuric acid and tryptophan load tests (urine)
Folate/folic acid	Erythrocytes (RBC folate level)	<368 nmol/L (depleted) <322 nmol/L (deficient) <227 nmol/L (anaemia) 7–45 nmol/L (serum)	Formiminoglutamic acid (urine) Histidine load test (urine) Used for suspected megaloblastic anaemia, haemolytic anaemia and pregnancy nutritional screening
Cobalamin	Serum	120–680 pmol/L (though varies depending on methodology)	Methylmalonic acid (urine) B_{12} assays generally measure total B_{12} (not bioavailable B_{12}) Used for suspected megaloblastic anaemia
Ascorbates	Serum (ascorbic acid)	<11.4 umol/L (deficient)	WBC ascorbic acid (reflects tissue stores) 24 h ascorbic acid (urine) reflects recent intake

FAD: flavin adenine dinucleotide; NAD: nicotinamide adenine dinucleotide; TPP: thiamin pgyrophosphate

Royal College of Pathologists of Australasia (RCPA). Education online. RCPA, 2016. Available from: www.rcpa.edu.au/Education; Salwen M. Vitamins and trace elements. In McPherson R, Pincus M, editors. Henry's clinical diagnosis and management by laboratory methods. 23rd edn. Philadelphia: Elsevier Saunders; 2017, pp. 416–27.

TABLE 4.54 Selected trace element transport and tissue storage

Trace element	Primary function	Transport protein	Tissue markers
Boron	Steroid metabolism; osteoporosis prevention	NaBC1	Serum, urine, hair
Chromium	Insulin receptor binding factor	Transferrin	RBCs, urine, hair
Copper	Erythrocyte superoxide dismutase cofactor	Ceruloplasmin, albumin and transcuperin	RBCs, serum ceruloplasmin
Iodine	Thyroid hormone synthesis	Thyroxin-binding protein, transthyretin	Urine
Iron	Porphyrin structure and function (haeme, cytochromes). Enzyme cofactor and erythrocyte production	Transferrin	Serum ferritin
Manganese	Enzyme cofactor; occasional cofactor substituent for Zn and Mg	n/a	RBCs
Molybdenum	Sulfur metabolism and catabolism of purine nucleotides	a-1- macroglobulin (RBC protein)	Hair
Selenium	Cofactor for glutathione peroxidase and thyroxin oxidase	Selenoprotein P	Serum, whole blood, hair
Zinc	Enzyme cofactor, DNA structural role (zinc fingers)	Albumin and a-2- macroglobulin (RBC protein)	RBCs, hair, plasma

Fitzgerald K, Nelson-Dooley C, Lord R. Nutrient and toxic elements. In Lord R, Bralley J, editors. Laboratory evaluations for integrative and functional medicine. 2nd edn. Duluth, Georgia: Metametrix Institute; 2008, pp. 68–151; Royal College of Pathologists of Australasia (RCPA). Education online. RCPA, 2016. Available from: www.rcpa.edu.au/Education; Salwen M. Vitamins and trace elements. In McPherson R, Pincus M, editors. Henry's clinical diagnosis and management by laboratory methods. 23rd edn. Philadelphia: Elsevier Saunders; 2017, pp. 416–27.

NATUROPATHIC ASSESSMENTS

Since the ancient inception of naturopathy as a healing modality, a multitude of naturopathic physical examination techniques have been refined and used. Many of these physical assessments are exactly the same as those performed by doctors, including sphygmomanometry for blood pressure measurements, basic measurement of body temperature, measurement of heart rate at various pulse points, measurement of the respiratory rate and auscultation of internal organs such as the heart, lungs and gut. The electrocardiogram (ECG) for measuring cardiac function, spirometry for respiratory function and Holter monitors for blood pressure measurements offer a more detailed analysis of any problems identified on a basic physical exam.

Physical examination is a cornerstone of both naturopathy and modern medicine and should still be performed by naturopaths on new patients and regarded as clinically relevant with ongoing patients. Physical examination can detect many minor and major health problems, thus bringing them to the attention of your patients and their medical team.

Some physical examination techniques are no longer used in modern medicine (or used less) as they are too time-consuming or have been replaced by other modern investigative tests. This does not negate the wealth of information to be gleaned from naturopathic assessments, particularly when viewing the results under a nutritional, holistic and constitutional lens.

Oral exam and tongue diagnosis

The inability to effectively masticate affects every aspect of health. It enables the ability to efficiently digest, assimilate and absorb essential macro- and micronutrients. An oral exam involves not only questions around oral health, but also a brief examination of the gums, teeth, lips, palate, buccal mucosa and of course tongue.[99] While a detailed oral exam is the specialist area of dentists and some doctors, naturopathic practitioners may find the first signs of nutritional deficiencies and systemic poor health via an oral exam, which can alert the patient and their dentist/doctor to investigate further. The oral exam often relates to systemic inflammation, toxicity, heavy metal concerns or dietary and nutritional imbalances. Infections, autoimmune disease and signs of oxidative stress all present in the oral cavity.[99] Temperomandibular joint (TMJ) dysfunction can be assessed and referred to a dentist, physiotherapist or osteopath if necessary for a thorough examination.

Other features to look for are an unbalanced bite (may affect cognitive function),[100] amalgam fillings, root canals and angular stomatitis/chelitis (B complex vitamin deficiencies). Observe the presence of the lips at rest (abnormalities include possible nerve palsy or potential mouth breathing).[99] Cracked and fissured lips can indicate multiple micronutrient deficiencies and food intolerances.[96] Enlarged tonsils can indicate infection, poor antioxidant status, Th1/Th2 imbalance, allergies, food intolerances and breathing disorders, which will often require a referral.[100]

THE TONGUE

The tongue should look pink and moist, with no furrows or ulceration. The ventral surface should be smooth. Coffee, green tea and dairy-based foods can all alter the colour of the tongue if consumed just prior to the examination. Question if the patient has brushed their tongue prior to examination, as this may affect the observance of any tongue coatings. Look for deviation of the tongue on protrusion or fasiculations, both of which may indicate nerve damage. Look for glossitis (smooth, swollen and 'beefy' red), which can indicate iron, folate or B_{12} deficiency. Low oestrogen states in postmenopausal women may cause 'menopausal glossitis'.[101]

On the lateral borders, a scalloped tongue can indicate bruxism (chronic jaw clenching) and dehydration.[98] Geographic tongue with uneven papilla distribution or areas of 'bald spots' often corresponds with gluten sensitivity.[102] 'Hairy tongue' (leukoplakia) of the lateral borders usually indicates severe infections, particularly EBV and some fungal infections.[102] A coated tongue usually indicates general poor digestion and dehydration (particularly if the coating disappears from morning to evening with the general consumption of daily fluids).

Transverse furrows of the tongue are known as fissured tongue, which is believed to be inherited and can lead to halitosis and infection from trapped food particles.[102] Ulcers should be examined for size, number and colour. Poor-healing, aphthous ulcers are often seen in systemic inflammatory conditions such as Crohn's disease, ulcerative colitis, HSV and reactive arthritis.[100] Non-healing ulcers must be referred for medical examination for oral cancer; question the patient's use of tobacco and alcohol (including mouthwash).

In traditional Chinese medicine (TCM) the tongue is related to many energetic meridians and physiological pathways. This is a special area not traditionally taught in Western naturopathic modalities, but may be used by some practitioners with further education.

THE GUMS

Gums are important to examine, as periodontal disease often corresponds with cardiovascular disease. The gums should be pink, well perfused with colour and not pale. Erythematous (red and spongy) gums indicate active inflammation. The presence of bleeding or exudate is significant; bleeding can be due to periodontitis and gingivitis, but from a nutritional standpoint, gum health is at risk with macronutrient deficiencies of protein and micronutrient deficiencies of folate and antioxidants such as vitamin C and coenzyme Q10. The minerals calcium, iron and zinc are all critical to the structural integrity of the gums.[103]

THE MUCOSA

An examination of the buccal mucosa involves observing the inside tissue of the lips and cheeks, looking for any signs of lesions for referral. Question salivation, as xerostomia (severe dry mouth and poor salivation) can be induced by certain medications and possibly gluten sensitivity. There are now strong links between gluten intolerance and Sjögren's disease and poor hydration is an obvious factor.[100] Candidiasis of the oropharynx is noted during the mucosal exam and is due to immunocompromise, diabetes and chronic antibiotic therapy.[103]

THE TEETH

Ask whether the patient has all their teeth. If teeth are missing, asking why gives a very useful indication of their medical and health history.[103] Look at the general condition of the teeth. Look for the presence of dental caries. Query the presence of metals (especially dissimilar metals) and any dental restorations that are present. Any problems here may require referral for holistic dental intervention and treatment.

Nail and skin diagnosis

NAIL PLATE

The nail plate is a keratin-rich structure. Keratin is high in sulfur-containing amino acids and the essential elements zinc (Zn), selenium (Se), magnesium (Mg), iron (Fe) and copper (Cu). The main inference with nail diagnosis is that any deficiency in sulfur-rich amino acids or the aforementioned elements will present in the nail plate. Additionally, toxic accumulation of certain elements can be observed in the nail plate; these include Mees' lines (arsenic toxicity), whitening (Se toxicity) and the Fe overload of haemochromatosis.[104] The following anatomical landmarks are examined during the nail assessment.

NAIL BED

The nail bed is a vascular-rich area. Colour changes are known as chromonychia:

- Brown, vertical lines: may be seen in melanoma, vitamin B_{12} deficiency, vitamin D deficiency and Addison's disease. Pallor of the nail bed may indicate Fe deficiency anaemia. Cyanosis corresponds with poor tissue oxygenation. Refer to Figs 4.18 and 4.19.
- Leukonychia (white spots): several types exist. Mees' lines (transverse white lines on the nail plate) are observed in arsenic toxicity. Leukonychia striata (from hypoalbuminaemia) are white transverse lines present in the nail bed. Blanching the nail bed differentiates these two nail features; leukonychia striata lines disappear upon blanching. Leukonychia are classically caused by nail trauma. Check if the white spots are only on one nail, or only on the dominant hand. If so, trauma should be suspected first. If the white spots continue to the other hand or to the toenails, trauma is a less likely cause. Refer to Fig. 4.20.
- Splinter haemorrhages: classically observed in sub-acute bacterial endocarditis, but very common in vitamin C deficiency. Also common due to nail trauma. Check if the splinter haemorrhages are only on one nail, or only on the dominant hand. If so, trauma should be

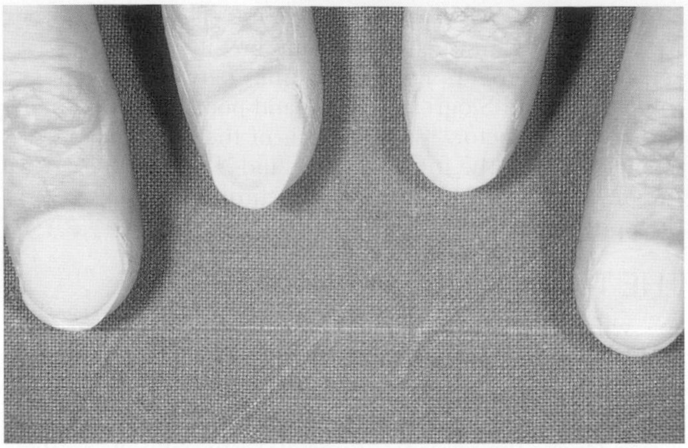

FIGURE 4.18 Pallor of nail bed

Hoffbrand A, Pettit J, Vyas P. Colour atlas of clinical hematology. 4th edn. Elsevier; 2010.

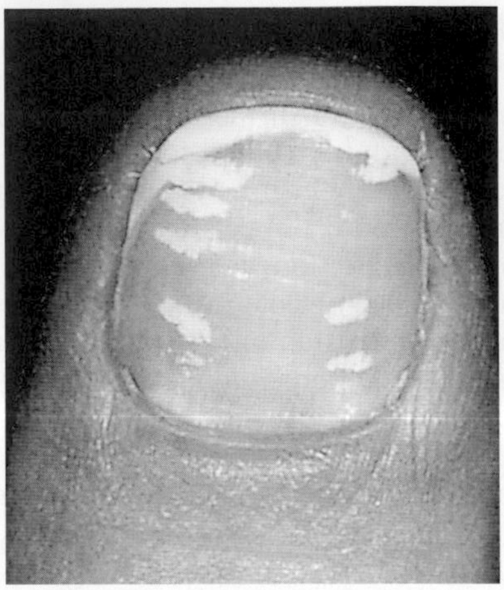

FIGURE 4.20 Leukonychia

Habif T. Clinical dermatology. 6th edn. Elsevier; 2016.

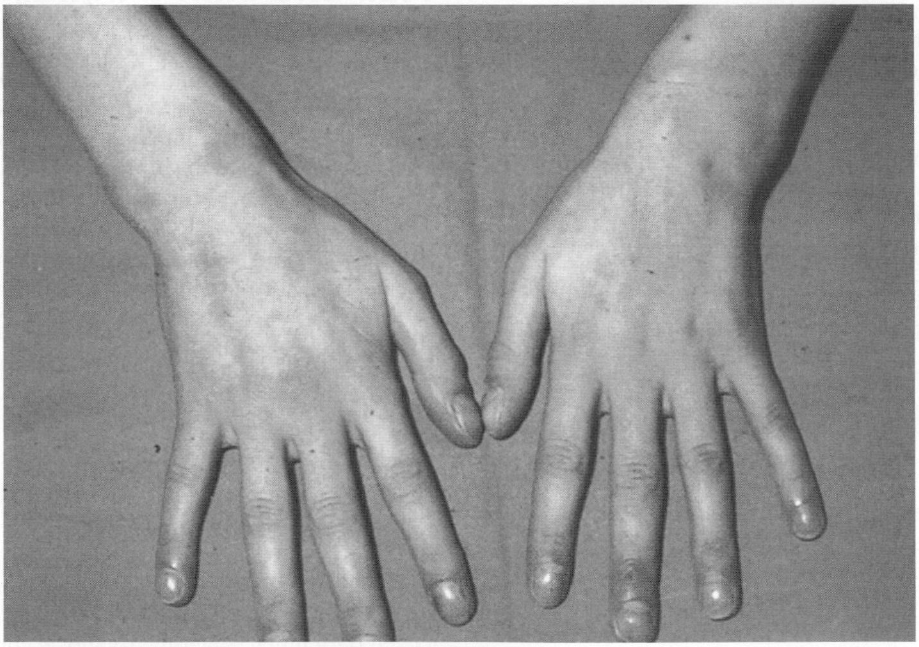

FIGURE 4.19 Cyanosis of nail bed

Goljan E. Rapid review pathology. 4th edn. Saunders; 2014.

suspected first. If the haemorrhages continue to the other hand or to the toenails, trauma is a less likely cause. Refer to Fig. 4.21.

- Capillary refill test: simple test of circulation. The nail plate is depressed until blanching is seen in the nail bed. Pink colouration should ideally return in 1 to 2 seconds. Repeat the test on the nail of the big toe.[104]

NAIL TEXTURE

Look for trachyonychia (atopic dermatitis, psoriasis and psoriatic arthritis). Trachyonychia includes pitting, thickening and flaking of the nails. Protein, mineral and B vitamin deficiencies are also related to the various forms of trachyonychia.[105] Refer to Fig. 4.22.

LUNULA

The lunula is the proximal area of the nail plate, supporting its growth. Blue-coloured hues in the lunula may indicate either Cu, silver (Ag) or mercury (Hg) toxicity. Absence of the lunula may indicate protein deficiency.[106]

NAIL GROWTH

Fingernails are renewed in adults every 6 months (though nail growth is slower in the elderly or in severe chronic

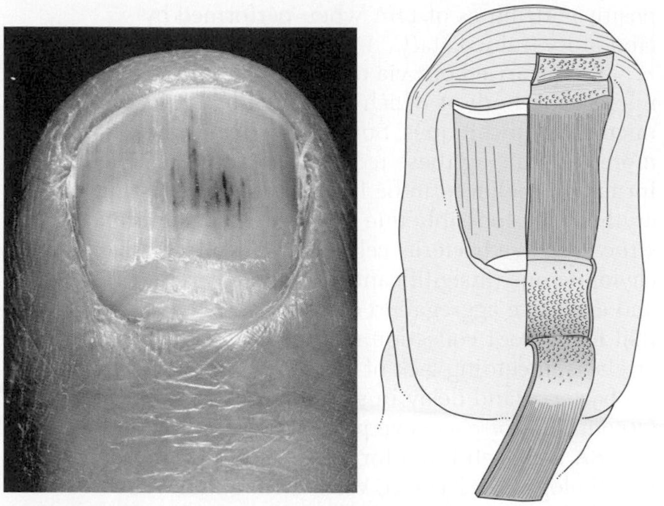

FIGURE 4.21 Splinter haemorrhage
Habif T. Clinical dermatology. 6th edn. Elsevier; 2016.

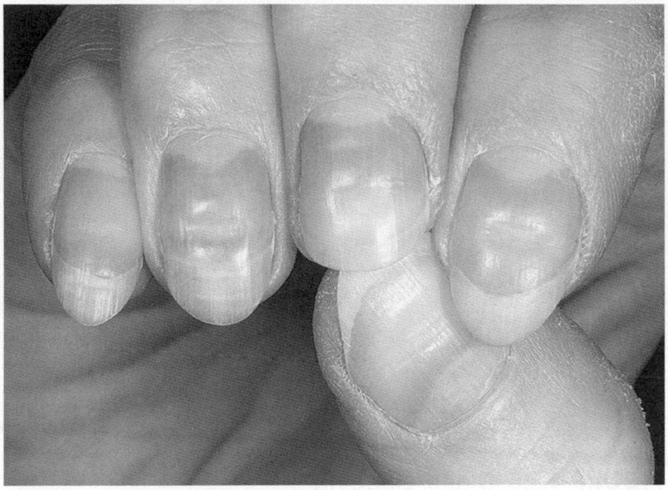

FIGURE 4.23 Beau's lines
Habif T. Clinical dermatology. 6th edn. Elsevier; 2016.

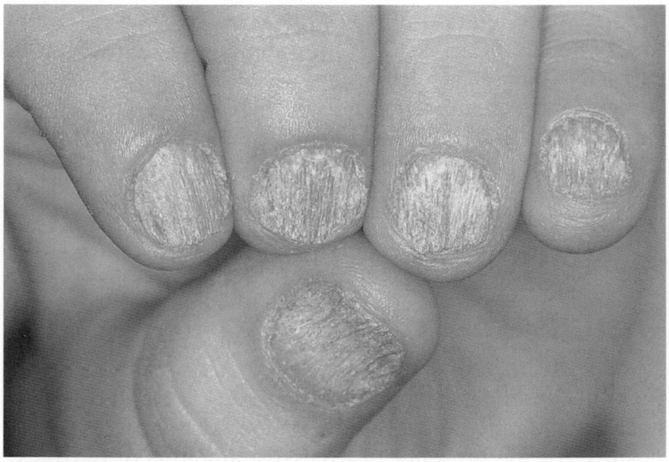

FIGURE 4.22 Trachyonychia
Chu DH, Rubin AI. Diagnosis and management of nail disorders in children. Pediatr Clin N Am, 61(2), pp 293–308, Copyright © 2014 Elsevier Inc.

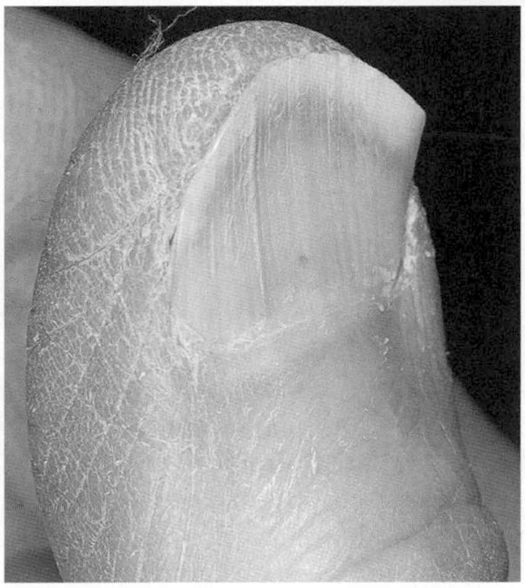

FIGURE 4.24 Koilonychia
Habif T. Clinical dermatology. 6th edn. Elsevier; 2016.

illness). Fingernail and toenail growth is much faster in children. Brittle and soft nails are often due to biotin and Mg deficiency or general malnutrition. Beau's lines are transverse canals/furrows. They are markers of acute illness, with the degree of the furrow corresponding to the severity of illness. Diarrhoeal illnesses often manifest with a Beau's line in nails. The timing of the illness can be inferred via the location of these lines in nails.[105] Refer to Fig. 4.23.

PARONYCHIUM

The paronychium is the lateral and proximal tissue border of the nail plate. The presence of inflammation or infection should be traced back to a source, if possible. Inflammation is often seen in arthritic conditions, while infection may be due to a host of sources including nail treatments.[106] Shape changes are relatively common in nutrient deficiencies, with koilonychia the most common (Fe deficiency, Zn deficiency, plus sulfur, protein, vitamin B and vitamin C deficiency). Koilonychia may be associated with diabetes, solvent exposure, SLE and Raynaud's disease. Clubbing is an enlarged distal area of fingers. Most common causes are pulmonary and cardiovascular disease. Shamroth's window test is used for the assessment of potential clubbing.[106] Findings should always be correlated with other medical physical examinations, laboratory diagnostics, medical imaging and clinical presentation/ history.[106] Refer to Figs 4.24 and 4.25.

The skin

The importance of a general skin examination should never be underestimated. This examination starts the moment you first see your patient, whether you have formally begun the examination, or not. Texture, colour

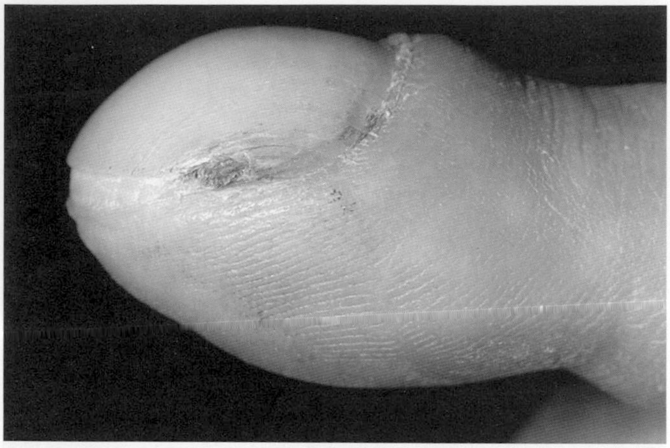

FIGURE 4.25 Digital clubbing

Habif T. Clinical dermatology. 6th edn. Elsevier; 2016.

and hydration levels are all important. Aside from the face and hands, the scalp, orbits, ears, neck, shoulders and arms can all be examined with relative ease.

Common skin complaints include follicular hyperkeratosis (related to vitamin A assimilation), acne (location is important, but dysbiosis, hormonal imbalance, infection and toxicity are all possible causes), acanthosis nigricans (insulin resistance), hair loss or abnormal hair growth (many underlying reasons), poor healing of lesions (global nutrient concerns), petechiae and easy bruising (vitamin C or vitamin K deficiency). Dry skin is indicative of vitamin A, zinc and omega 3 deficiencies.[106] Any skin issues should lead you to question absorption and assimilation of nutrients, or the presence of an increased physiological demand for these nutrients in your patient. Always keep in mind that low nutrient levels may not be a straightforward dietary deficiency.

Live blood analysis (LBA)

Live blood analysis is the microscopic examination of a capillary blood sample, viewed immediately after specimen collection. In contrast to a routine peripheral blood film (non-living cells, stained and preserved/fixed to a glass slide), LBA views blood cells that remain viable for a minimal period after sampling, approximately 20–30 minutes. Routine blood films are prepared from venous blood samples. Some proponents of LBA state capillary blood provides a more accurate reflection of blood components at the tissue level compared to venous blood, though no evidence currently exists to support this.

LBA is offered as a functional pathology test via various names and methods. There is no standardisation for the reporting of results and currently, no minimum scientific qualification for those who offer LBA testing. Most LBA testing is performed by the same practitioner making the supplement/medicine prescription, as opposed to an independent laboratory. These aspects diminish the positive attributes of LBA when performed by laboratory-trained staff.

LBA is carried out via darkfield and phase contrast microscopy, both of which are scientifically valid microscopy techniques. Some components are viewed more easily using these techniques, including spicule formation (believed to be fibrin strands), 'ghosting' of erythrocytes (possibly due to weak RBC membrane structure), live bacteria, cell-wall deficient organisms, chylomicrons (insignificant if the patient is not fasting) and excessive aggregation of platelets. It must be noted that many poor collection methods can lead to blood artefacts, including lack of aseptic sampling (accounting for bacteria) and delay in sampling blood from the finger (accounting for excessive platelet aggregation and fibrin).

LBA is a useful tool for haematology screening, as RBC morphology, WBC count, WBC differential, WBC morphology and neutrophil motility can all be assessed. WBC motility is one parameter that cannot be measured via routine blood films, making LBA a useful assessment of phagocytic function in neutrophils. RBC morphology problems tend to be over-estimated with LBA, as a significant population of RBCs may not be assessed. Even for trained pathologists, RBC morphology is the most subjective part of blood film analysis.[8] Proficiency in recognising true abnormal morphology comes with extensive haematology training, lengthy experience and the ability to interpret results in an appropriate clinical context.

FUNCTIONAL PATHOLOGY

Urinary pyrrole testing

Reliable pathology testing for pyroluria is available in Australia and overseas. The methodology is based on urine analysis and determines whether the patient's urine tests positive for the presence of excessive amounts of pyrroles and determines (quantifies) the actual level present in the urine. Pathology testing is essential for both adults and children with pyroluria, and correct diagnosis is essential to rule out other possible conditions that can often present in the same way. Most methodologies measure hydroxyhaemopyrrolin-2-one (HPL).[107] HPL production with subsequent urinary excretion occurs as a result of normal haemoglobin synthesis. Nutrient deficiencies, toxic exposure, intestinal dysbiosis, stress and genetic predispositions are all linked with elevated urinary HPL levels.

Clinical significance

Increased urinary HPL levels are linked to a range of cognitive, affective and neurobehavioural disorders.[107] Quantitative results are useful in this context, as response to treatment can be ascertained in conjunction with determining pyroluria status. Screening is useful for patients with Down syndrome, autism, epilepsy, ADHD, depression or anxiety, as some of these individuals respond well to nutritional interventions specific for pyroluria.[108] Refer to Table 4.55 for reference ranges.

TABLE 4.55 Reference range: urinary HPL	
Condition	**HPL reference range (ug/dL)**
Negative for pyroluria	<10
Borderline pyroluria	10–20
Positive for pyroluria	>20

McGinnis W, Audhya T, Walsh W et al. Discerning the mauve factor, Part 2. Alternative Therapies in Health and Medicine 2008; 14(3):56–62.

Salivary hormones

The aqueous environment of urine and saliva is advantageous for pathology testing for several reasons: it is relatively non-invasive, unbound fractions of hormones are measured (the need for transport proteins is redundant in saliva and urine) and these fluids are under less physiological homeostatic control than blood plasma. Saliva and urine are common specimens for testing hormones, especially glucocorticoids, sex steroids, DHEA and thyroxin.[109]

- Clinical significance: results for hormones with circadian (glucocorticoids) or ultradian (oestrogen, progesterone) secretion patterns are interpreted as for blood samples. It is also important to note that significant oral or even systemic immune illness can affect salivary flow rate, leading to concentration/dilution effects. Specimens need to be obtained when patients are free of infection.[109]
- Defined reference levels are not well established, due to the niche use of saliva testing, mainly for psychiatry, sports medicine, clinical endocrinology and stress physiology. Broad standardisation may occur in the future, as saliva is a widely acceptable sample from a medical research perspective.

Functional liver detoxification profile (FLDP)

As explained with respect to routine LFTs, the liver performs thousands of biochemical reactions, including gluconeogenesis, clotting factor biosynthesis, cholesterol biosynthesis, protein biosynthesis and xenobiotic detoxification. No testing panel can reflect the capacity of all hepatic functions. The FLDP differs from routine LFTs in that it specifically evaluates the detoxification capacity of the liver, by challenging both phase I and phase II enzymatic pathways:

- Phase I (CYP 450): hydrolysis, reduction and oxidation reactions. Challenged by low-dose caffeine
- Phase II (conjugation reactions): glutathione and amino acid conjugation, glucoronidation, sulfation, acetylation and methylation. Challenged by low-dose aspirin and paracetamol.[107]

Ultimately, detoxification of both endotoxic and exotoxic chemicals produces waste metabolites made water-soluble for excretion, thus they can be accessed and detected in saliva and urine samples. The FDLP measures both the conversion of the challenge chemicals, plus their removal from the body.[107]

Clinical significance

Phase I (elevated activity) indicates increased free radical synthesis. Phase I (reduced activity) indicates diminished enzyme activity. Phase II (reduced activity) indicates broad-range clinical issues, especially multiple chemical sensitivities.

Varying situations of normal physiology can affect the result. Oestrogen flux, progesterone flux, BMI and insulin production can all affect the results.[107] Clinicians should not rely on this one test in isolation, but with the full spectrum of diagnostics, especially thorough case history taking.

Complete digestive stool analysis (CDSA)

Functional pathology laboratories conduct CDSA testing. Panels will differ slightly depending on the laboratory, though many offer a tiered approach to testing to suit the clinical situation:

- Level 1: macroscopic and microscopic analysis (and parasite visualisation). Basic cultures for beneficial, dysbiotic, pathogenic bacteria and yeasts. Some laboratories offer antimicrobial sensitivity testing in the panels
- Level 2: level 1; additional digestion, absorption and metabolic markers
- Level 3: level 2; additional markers of inflammation and possibly GIT tumour markers
- Level 4: level 3; additional parasitology via serological techniques.[107]

Macroscopic and microscopic examination of faeces is an important clinical tool. Stool consistency (liquid through to formed), adult parasites, cyst form parasites, parasitic oocytes, spores, erythrocytes, frank blood, mucus, leucocytes and undigested food particles or plant fibres may be present. Plant cells, pollen grains, fungal spores and plant fibres may all resemble some helminths, protozoans, parasites and their eggs; hence an experienced microbiologist or scientist should conduct this phase of testing.[110]

Reference ranges: reporting strategies differ between laboratories. Generally, microorganism growth is expressed as being at, above or below an expected norm. Macroscopic and microscopic descriptions are qualitative to describe both normal and pathological features of the faecal specimen. Serological antigen/antibody results may be qualitative (positive versus negative) or quantitative depending on the methodology employed.

COMPREHENSIVE PARASITOLOGY

In addition to faecal parasite identification, most functional pathology laboratories offer faecal parasitology panels that include bacterial and yeast profiling (including pathogenic, beneficial and dysbiotic flora). Generally, parasitology testing requires a 3-day faecal specimen collection. Some laboratories also offer antimicrobial susceptibility testing to both synthetic and natural pharmacological agents.

Clinical significance

These investigations are useful for chronic gastrointestinal issues (IBD, IBS, malabsorption), autoimmune diseases, chronic fatigue syndromes, chronic inflammatory conditions and food/chemical intolerances. Thorough clinical/lifestyle history taking will help to confirm whether this testing is necessary. Recent travel, food intake, socioeconomic history and transfusion history are all important.[60,61] Results can be affected by antibiotic and other antimicrobial therapies, thus specimen collection during or close to recent therapy should be avoided.

Commonly tested microbial species include *Cryptosporidium* spp., *Giardia* spp., *trichomes, Candida* spp., *E. coli, Streptococci, Bifidobacteria* spp., *Lactobacilli* spp., plus various intestinal anaerobes or specifically requested parasitic cultures. Parasite serology, PCR or specialised cultures may be required.[60,61]

Reference ranges vary according to the laboratory; however, reports often indicate results as either above/below an ideal range, or qualify results as positive/negative.

ALTERED INTESTINAL PERMEABILITY

Addressing this anatomical and physiological concern is a bastion of naturopathic practice. While increased intestinal permeability is a normal and much needed feature of neonatal and infant anatomy and physiology, its presence or reoccurrence is a problematic clinical manifestation of many chronic health conditions. As such, diagnostic testing measuring the level of intestinal permeability is used in conjunction with a comprehensive case history analysis.

This methodology involves the administration of non-metabolised saccharides such as lactulose (a synthetic saccharide normally used as an osmotic laxative) or mannitol (a sugar alcohol).[111] After administration, these challenge substances are recovered and measured in urine samples. Patients generally provide a first morning urine specimen after an 8-hour fast. An oral liquid challenge substance is ingested, with urine samples collected for another 6 hours.[111] Both sensitivity and specificity of this test increase greatly when two challenge substances are administered.[111]

Clinical significance

Many situations can disrupt the normal membrane composition of the gastrointestinal mucosa, including acute and chronic disease, pharmacological agents, disease treatments, some phytochemicals and dietary habits. This test gives information regarding the integrity of the small intestine only, and not the large intestine.

Reference ranges are:

- 20–30% recovery of mannitol; <1% recovery of lactulose = normal.
- Unchanged/no decrease in mannitol; >1% recovery of lactulose (an increased L/M ratio) = impaired small intestinal permeability.[111]

Hair tissue mineral analysis (HTMA)

The analysis of hair tissue is common in a number of highly specific areas of medicine. These include toxicology studies for detecting drugs of abuse and heavy metal exposure, and HTMA for nutrient mineral levels. Methodologies such as high-performance liquid chromatography (HPLC) and mass spectronomy (MS) analyse hair tissue for trace amounts of these substances. Both are common techniques used in analytical chemistry.

Blood plasma analysis does not necessarily reflect current levels of most minerals (as a result of homeostatic mechanisms maintaining the very narrow plasma mineral ranges). Urine reflects the amount of mineral eliminated from the body, not necessarily storage. Hair is a significantly mineralised tissue, thus the concentration of elements is considered higher here than for blood or urine.[112]

Before considering HTMA for a patient, they must be a suitable candidate for analysis. Hair colours, hair dyes, perming/chemical straightening solutions and use of anti-dandruff shampoo all render hair inappropriate for analysis. Mineralisation of water sources can also influence HTMA results.[113] Hair must be sampled from growth immediately adjacent to the scalp (usually within a 1–2 cm margin). Any hair collected past this length will not provide results for recent heavy metal levels/mineral levels.

Hair analysis techniques are not standardised, with laboratories generally using different analytical methods. For this reason, reference range guidelines are difficult to provide, and rely entirely on using ranges provided by the testing facility. Some laboratories also place greater relevance on mineral ratios, as opposed to individual mineral levels. HTMA is a legitimate and valuable screening tool for toxic metal exposure (including arsenic, cadmium, lead, mercury and selenium), though HTMA is not considered a diagnostic tool.[113] As HTMA is a form of toxicological analysis, eliminating the source of toxin exposure is the first priority of treatment.

Urinary iodine

Iodine deficiency can present in patients of all ages and demographics inducing goitre, hypothyroidism and some neurological deficits. Natural dietary goitrogens can be problematic for people who are already iodine deficient. Blood levels of iodine do not reflect iodine status, thus testing the amount of iodine excretion via urine can determine recent intake of iodine. The excretion rate does fluctuate throughout the day, thus repeated monitoring may be necessary for some individuals.[114]

Clinical significance

Urinary iodine excretion should be evaluated in conjunction with serum TSH, thyroid hormones, TG levels and approximation of thyroid size. Thyroid function tests may show elevated TSH, low fT4 and elevated T3 when iodine deficiency is present. Urinary iodine levels are accepted by the WHO as a good marker of dietary intake of iodine.[114] This test is useful for determining the degree

TABLE 4.56 Reference ranges: urinary iodine

Population	Median urinary iodine (ug/L)	Iodine intake	Iodine status
Children (6 yrs and over)	<20 20–49 50–99 100–199 200–299 ≥300	Insufficient Insufficient Insufficient Adequate Above requirements Excessive	Severe deficiency Moderate deficiency Mild deficiency Adequate levels Slight risk of excess levels of iodine Risk: iodine-induced hyperthyroidism
Pregnant women	<150 150–249 250–499 ≥500	Insufficient Adequate Above requirements Excessive	Iodine deficient Adequate levels Slight risk of excess levels of iodine Risk: iodine-induced hyperthyroidism
Lactating women and infants (<2 yrs)	<100 ≥100	Insufficient Adequate	Iodine deficient Adequate levels

Reprinted from World Health Organization (WHO). Urinary iodine concentrations for determining iodine status deficiency in populations [Internet]. Vitamin and Mineral Nutrition Information System. WHO, 2016 [cited 12 August 2016]. Available from: http://apps.who.int/iris/bitstream/10665/85972/1/WHO_NMH_NHD_EPG_13.1_eng.pdf.

of iodine deficiency and monitoring a patient's response to iodine replacement therapy.[115] A urinary iodine level does not provide explicit information about the function of the thyroid gland.[115]

Calculation of urinary iodine: when conducting urinary spot iodine analysis, health practitioners must ascertain whether the reported result is corrected for creatinine. This often involves direct liaison with any laboratory used for urinary iodine levels in the first instance. If the laboratory does not correct for creatinine, and the patient's creatinine result has been measured, a simple correction calculation can be applied: *urinary iodine (ug/L) ÷ creatinine (mmol/L) × 8.85 = corrected urinary iodine.*

Refer to Table 4.56 for reference ranges.

WHO defines the three populations in Table 4.56 as most 'at risk' for the adverse clinical consequences of iodine deficiency. The reference ranges for adult males and non-pregnant females are:

- Median urinary iodine >100 ug/L: no iodine deficiency.
- Median urinary iodine 50–99 ug/L: mild iodine deficiency.
- Median urinary iodine 20–49 ug/L: moderate iodine deficiency.
- Median urinary iodine <20 ug/L: severe iodine deficiency.[116]

REFERENCES

[1] Royal College of Pathologists of Australasia (RCPA). What is pathology? RCPA, 2016. Available from: www.rcpa.edu.au/About/What-is-Pathology.

[2] Gu J, Taylor C, Phil D. Practicing pathology in the era of big data and personalised medicine. App Immunohistochem Mol Morphol 2014;22(1):1–9.

[3] RCPA. Pathology. The facts. RCPA, 2016. Available from: www.rcpa.edu.au/getattachment/7a64de30-cf76-45f8-ac85-868f864e86b4/Path-Fcts-Booklt.aspx.

[4] Ozarda Y. Reference intervals: current status, recent developments and future considerations. Biochemica Medica 2016;26(1):5–11.

[5] Australian Government Department of Health. Pathology under Medicare. Australian Government Department of Health, 2016 Available from: www.health.gov.au/internet/main/publishing.nsf/Content/health-pathology-aboutus-index.htm.

[6] Walker S. Laboratory reference ranges. In: Walker B, editor. Davidson's principles and practice of medicine. 22nd ed. Elsevier Churchill Livingstone; 2014. p. 1307–12.

[7] Osei-Bimpong A, Burthem J. Supplementary techniques including blood parasite diagnosis. In: Bain B, editor. Dacie and Lewis practical haematology. 11th ed. Elsevier Churchill Livingstone; 2012. p. 101–21.

[8] Vajpayee N, Graham S, Bem S. Basic examination of blood and bone marrow. In: McPherson R, Pincus M, editors. Henry's clinical diagnosis and management by laboratory methods. 23rd ed. Philadelphia: Elsevier Saunders; 2017. p. 510–39.

[9] Gersten T Haematocrit. Medline Plus. US National Library of Medicine, 2016. Available from: www.nlm.nih.gov/medlineplus/ency/article/003646.htm.

[10] World Health Organization (WHO). Haemoglobin concentrations for the diagnosis of anaemia and assessment of severity. Vitamin and Mineral Nutrition Information System. WHO, 2016. Available from: www.who.int/vmnis/indicators/haemoglobin.pdf.

[11] RCPA. Education online. RCPA, 2016. Available from: www.rcpa.edu.au/Education.

[12] Huchison R, Schexneider K. Leucocytic disorders. In: McPherson R, Pincus M, editors. Henry's clinical diagnosis and management by laboratory methods. 23rd ed. Philadelphia: Elsevier Saunders; 2017. p. 606–58.

[13] Howard M, Hamilton P. Lymphocytes. In: Howard M, editor. Haematology: an illustrated colour text. 4th ed. Elsevier Churchill Livingston; 2013. p. 8–9.

[14] American Association for Clinical Chemistry (AACC). Thalassaemia laboratory tests. AACC, 2016. Available from: https://labtestsonline.org/understanding/conditions/thalassemia/start/2.

[15] Saxena A, Cronstein B. Acute phase reactants and the concept of inflammation. In: Firestein G, editor. Kelley's textbook of rheumatology. 9th ed. Philadelphia: Elsevier Saunders; 2013. p. 818–29.

[16] Australian Association for Clinical Biochemistry (AACB). Table 6: Reference intervals for harmonised chemical pathology. AACB Committee for Common Reference Intervals and AACB Paediatric Biochemistry Special Interest Group, 2014. Available from: www.rcpa.edu.au/getattachment/5feedb34-6ca0-401b-8851-740b82508081/Table-6-Reference-intervals-harmonised-chemical.aspx.

[17] Kellner C. Erythrocyte sedimentation rate. Medscape 2016. Available from: http://emedicine.medscape.com/article/2085201-overview#a2.

[18] Ford J. Red blood cell morphology. Int J Lab Hematol 2013;35(3): 351–7.

[19] AACB. Reference intervals for harmonised chemical pathology. AACB Committee for Common Reference Intervals and AACB Paediatric Biochemistry Special Interest Group, 2014. Available from: www.rcpa.edu.au/getattachment/5feedb34-6ca0-401b-8851-740b82508081/Table-6-Reference-intervals-harmonised-chemical.aspx.

[20] Gaw A, Murphy M, Srivastava R, et al. Water and sodium balance. In: Gaw A, editor. Clinical biochemistry: an illustrated colour text. 5th ed. Elsevier Churchill Livingstone; 2013. p. 14–15.

[21] Oh M, Briefel G. Evaluation of renal function, water, electrolytes and acid–base balance. In: McPherson R, Pincus M, editors. Henry's clinical diagnosis and management by laboratory methods. 23rd ed. Philadelphia: Elsevier Saunders; 2017. p. 162–87.

[22] Pratt D. Liver chemistry and function tests. In: Feldman M, editor Sleisenger and Fordtran's gastrointestinal and liver disease. 10th ed. Philadelphia: Elsevier Saunders; 2016. p. 1243–53.

[23] Hansen T. Neonatal jaundice: background, pathophysiology, aetiology. Medscape 2016. Available from: http://emedicine.medscape.com/article/974786-overview.

[24] Valdavino-Flores CH, Gonsebatt M. The role of amino acid transporters in GSH synthesis in the blood–brain barrier and central nervous system. Neurochem Int 2012;61(3):405–15.

[25] Klemm K, Klein M. Biochemical markers of bone metabolism. In: McPherson R, Pincus M, editors. Henry's clinical diagnosis and management by laboratory methods. 23rd ed. Philadelphia: Elsevier Saunders; 2017. p. 188–204.

[26] McPherson R. Specific proteins. In: McPherson R, Pincus M, editors. Henry's clinical diagnosis and management by laboratory methods. 23rd ed. Philadelphia: Elsevier Saunders; 2017. p. 253–66.

[27] Lam Q. Interpreting serum ferritin. Common sense pathology. RCPA. October 2013.

[28] RCPA. Iron studies standardised reporting protocol. 1st edn. RCPA 2013. Available from: www.rcpa.edu.au/Library/Practising-Pathology/NCRPQF/Docs/Iron-Studies-Standardised-Reporting-Protocol.

[29] Shaikh N, Borrell J, Evron J, et al. Procalcitonin, C-reactive protein, and erythrocyte sedimentation rate for the diagnosis of acute pyelonephritis in children. Cochrane Database Syst Rev 2015;(1):CD009185.

[30] Bock J. Cardiac injury, atherosclerosis, and thrombotic disease. In: McPherson R, Pincus M, editors. Henry's clinical diagnosis and management by laboratory methods. 23rd ed. Philadelphia: Elsevier Saunders; 2017. p. 244–52.

[31] d'Emden M, Shaw J, Jones G, et al. Guidance concerning the use of glycated haemoglobin (HbA1c) for the diagnosis of diabetes mellitus. MJA 2015;203(2).

[32] Jones G, Barker G, Goodall I, et al. Change of HbA_{1c} reporting to the new SI units. MJA 2011;195(1):45–6.

[33] DeFronzo A, Ferrannini E. Regulation of intermediary metabolism during fasting and feeding. In: Jameson L, editor. Endocrinology: adult and paediatric. 7th ed. Philadelphia: Elsevier; 2016. p. 598–626.

[34] Farias de Azevedo Salgado A, de Carvalho L, Oliviera C, et al. Insulin resistance index (HOMA-IR) in the differentiation of patients with non-alcoholic fatty liver disease and healthy individuals. Arch Gastroenterol 2010;47(2):165–9.

[35] Diabetes Trials Unit. HOMA calculator. University of Oxford; 2016. Available from: www.dtu.ox.ac.uk/homacalculator/.

[36] Wallace T, Levy J, Matthews D. Use and abuse of HOMA modelling. Diabetes Care 2004;27(6):1487–95.

[37] Mitsios J, Rand J. Laboratory approach to thrombotic risk. In: McPherson R, Pincus M, editors. Henry's clinical diagnosis and management by laboratory methods. 23rd ed. Philadelphia: Elsevier Saunders; 2017. p. 834–41.

[38] Hamilton R. Assessment of human allergic diseases. In: Rich R, editor. Clinical immunology. 4th ed. Elsevier Saunders; 2013. p. 1192–201.

[39] Winter W, Harris N, Merkel K, et al. Organ-specific autoimmune diseases. In: McPherson R, Pincus M, editors. Henry's clinical diagnosis and management by laboratory methods. 23rd ed. Philadelphia: Elsevier Saunders; 2017. p. 1032–56.

[40] Mannon P. Immunologic diseases of the gastrointestinal tract. In: Rich R, editor. Clinical immunology. 4th ed. Philadelphia: Elsevier; 2013. p. 896–909.

[41] Wine Y, Horton A, Ippolito G, et al. Serology in the 21st century: the molecular level analysis of the serum antibody repertoire. Curr Opin Immunol 2015;35:89–97.

[42] Murray P, Rosenthal K, Pfaller M. Laboratory diagnosis of viral disease. In: Murray P, Rosenthal K, Pfaller M, editors. Medical microbiology. 8th ed. Philadelphia: Elsevier Saunders; 2016. p. 392–9.

[43] Deinstag J, Delemos A. Viral hepatitis. In: Bennett J, editor. Mandell, Douglass and Bennett's principles and practice of infectious diseases. 8th ed. Philadelphia: Elsevier Saunders; 2015. p. 1439–68.

[44] Hewison C, Heath C, Ingram P. Stool culture. Aust Fam Physician. Reprod Health 2012;41(10):775–9.

[45] RCPA. Faecal pathogen testing by PCR and the detection of *Dientamoeba fragilis* and *Blastocystis* species, Guideline, RCPA. 2015. Available from: www.rcpa.edu.au/getattachment/cec7ecb1-632d-4102-8087-117a471c7c31/Faecal-pathogen-testing-by-PCR.aspx.

[46] Montoya J. Toxoplasmosis. In: Goldman L, Schafer A, editors. Goldman-Cecil medicine. 25th ed. Philadelphia: Elsevier; 2016. p. 2125–33.

[47] Emery M. Blood and blood components. In: Marx J, editor. Rosen's emergency medicine. 8th ed. Philadelphia: Elsevier; 2014. p. 75–80.

[48] Cover T, Blaser M. *Helicobacter pylori* and other gastric *Helicobacter* species. In: Bennett J, Dolin R, Blaser M, editors. Mandell, Douglas, and Bennett's principles and practice of infectious diseases. 8th ed. St Louis: Elsevier Saunders; 2015. p. 2494–502.

[49] Hotez P. *Blastocystis hominis* and *Blastocystis spp* infection. In: Cherry J, editor. Feigin and Cherry's textbook of paediatric infectious diseases. 7th ed. Philadelphia: Elsevier Saunders; 2014. p. 2875–6.

[50] Long S. Pertussis (*Bordetella pertussis* and *Bordetella parapertussis*). In: Kliegman R, editor. Nelson textbook of paediatrics. 20th ed. Philadelphia: Elsevier; 2016. p. 1377–82.

[51] Cockayne A. *Treponema* and *Borrelia*. In: Greenwood D, editor. Medical microbiology. 18th ed. Elsevier Churchill Livingstone; 2012. p. 365–74.

[52] Wormser G. Lyme disease. In: Goldman L, editor. Goldman-Cecil medicine. 25th ed. Philadelphia: Elsevier Saunders; 2016. p. 2021–7.

[53] Todar K *Borrelia burgdorferi* and Lyme disease. Todar's online textbook of bacteriology, 2016. Available from: http://textbookofbacteriology.net/kt_toc.html.

[54] Allos B, Iovine N, Blaser M. *Campylobacter jejuni* and related species. In: Bennett J, editor. Mandell, Douglas and Bennett's principles and practice of infectious diseases. 8th ed. St Louis: Elsevier; 2015. p. 2485–93.

[55] Warnock D. Fungi. In: Greenwood D, editor. Medical microbiology. 18th ed. Elsevier Churchill Livingstone; 2012. p. 616–41.

[56] Cunliffe N, Nakagomi O. Reoviruses. In: Greenwood D, editor. Medical microbiology. 18th ed. Elsevier Churchill Livingstone; 2012. p. 559–65.

[57] Geisler W. Diseases caused by *Chlamydiae*. In: Goldman L, Schafer A, editors. Goldman-Cecil medicine. 25th ed. Philadelphia: Elsevier Saunders; 2016. p. 2007–13.

[58] Murray P, Rosenthal K, Pfaller M. *Neisseria* and related genera. In: Murray P, Rosenthal K, Pfaller M, editors. Medical microbiology. 8th ed. Philadelphia: Elsevier; 2016. p. 234–42.

[59] Onderdonk A, Garrett W. Gas gangrene and other *Clostridium*-associated diseases. In: Bennett J, Dolan R, Blaser M, editors. Principles and practice of infectious diseases. 8th ed. Philadelphia: Elsevier Saunders; 2015. p. 2768–72.

[60] Einarsson E, Ma'ayeh S, Svard S. An update on *Giardia* and giardiasis. Curr Opin Microbiol 2016;34:47–52.

[61] Greenwood D. Protozoa. In: Greenwood D, editor. Medical microbiology. 18th ed. Elsevier Churchill Livingstone; 2012. p. 642–54.

[62] Hood J, Edwards G. *Legionella*: Legionnaires' disease; Pontiac fever. In: Greenwood D, editor. Medical microbiology. 18th ed. Elsevier Churchill Livingstone; 2012. p. 339–42.

[63] Bannister L, Sherman I. Plasmodium. In: Encyclopaedia of life sciences. John Wiley and Sons; 2009. Available from: http://onlinelibrary.wiley.com/doi/10.1002/9780470015902.a0001970.pub2/full.

[64] Schleyer A, Sisson S, Baustian G, et al. First Consult. Malaria. Elsevier; 2013.

[65] Rupp M, Fey P. *Staphylococcus epidermis* and other coagulase-negative *Stapylococci*. In: Bennett J, Dolin R, Blaser M, editors. Principles and practice of infectious diseases. Philadelphia: Elsevier Saunders; 2015. p. 2272–82.

[66] Kilian M. *Streptococcus* and *Enterococcus*. In: Greenwood D, editor. Medical microbiology. 18th ed. Elsevier Churchill Livingstone; 2012. p. 183–98.

[67] Australian Government Department of Health. Australian National Notifiable Diseases and Case Definitions. Australian Government, 2017. Available from: www.health.gov.au/casedefinitions.

[68] Guber H, Farag A. Evaluation of endocrine function. In: McPherson R, Pincus M, editors. Henry's clinical diagnosis and management by laboratory methods. 23rd ed. St Louis: Elsevier; 2017. p. 362–99.

[69] Fuller P, Young M. Aldosterone secretion and action. In: Jameson L, editor. Endocrinology: adult and paediatric. 7th ed. Philadelphia: Elsevier Saunders; 2016. p. 1756–62.

[70] Chrousos G, Sertedaki A, Magdalini Kyritsi E Hyperaldosteronaemia Workup. eMedicine Drugs and Diseases, 2016. Available from: http://emedicine.medscape.com/article/920713-workup?pa=sSPExbSmRXCJLcMG6x1TB5QotebmzDvooc5A1lxEHy9tQoq D9S35SkZ8mza4Q2K2VrJxKJt4DRD8mxYr6kYfOw%3D%3D.

[71] Esposito T, Lobaccaro J, Esposito M, et al. Effects of low carbohydrate diet therapy in overweight subjects with autoimmune thyroiditis: possible synergism with ChREBP. Drug Des Dev Ther 2016;10:2939–46.

[72] Rivkees S. Thyroid disorders in childhood and adolescence. In: Sperling M, editor. Paediatric endocrinology. 4th ed. Philadelphia: Elsevier Saunders; 2014. p. 444–70.

[73] van den Beld A, Visser T, Feelders R, et al. Thyroid hormone concentrations, disease, physical function, and mortality in elderly men. J Clin Endo Metab 2005;90(12):6403–9.

[74] McAuley D. Common laboratory values. Global RPh, The clinician's ultimate reference, 2016. Available from: www.globalrph.com/labs_t.htm.

[75] Oto Y, Muroya K, Hanakawa J, et al. The ratio of serum triiodothyronine to free thyroxine in children: a retrospective database survey of healthy short individuals and patients with severe thyroid hypoplasia or central hypothyroidism. Thyroid Res 2015;8:10.

[76] Douyon L, Schteingart D. Effect of obesity and starvation on thyroid hormone, growth hormone and cortisol secretion. Endocrinol Metab Clin North Am 2002;31(1):173–89.

[77] White B, Porterfield S. Hypothalamus-pituitary complex. In: White B, editor. Endocrine and reproductive physiology. 4th ed. Philadelphia: Elsevier Mosby; 2013. p. 99–128.

[78] Kopchick J, List E, Frohman L. Growth hormone. In: Jameson L, editor. Endocrinology: adult and paediatric. 7th ed. Philadelphia: Elsevier Saunders; 2016. p. 325–58.

[79] Safran M, Zachazewski J, Stone D. Growth hormone. In: Safran M, Zachazewski J, Stone D, editors. Instructions for sports medicine patients. 2nd ed. Philadelphia: Elsevier Saunders; 2012. p. 438.

[80] Chernecky C, Berger B. Human chorionic gonadotrophin. In: Chernecky C, Berger B, editors. Laboratory tests and diagnostic procedures. 6th ed. St Louis: Elsevier Saunders; 2013. p. 602–67.

[81] Hall J. Parathyroid hormone, calcitonin, calcium and phosphate metabolism, vitamin D, bone and teeth. In: Hall J, editor. Guyton and Hall textbook of medical physiology. 13th ed. Philadelphia: Elsevier; 2016. p. 1001–19.

[82] Findlay D, Sexton P, Martin J. Calcitonin. In: Jameson L, editor. Endocrinology: adult and paediatric. 7th ed. Philadelphia: Elsevier Saunders; 2016. p. 1004–17.

[83] Auchus R, Miller W. The principles, enzymes and pathways of human steroidogenesis. In: Jameson L, editor. Endocrinology: adult and paediatric. 7th ed. Philadelphia: Elsevier Saunders; 2016. p. 1695–716.

[84] Wilson G, Sheikh-Ali M. Endocrinology. In: Rakel R, Rakel D, editors. Textbook of family medicine. 9th ed. Philadelphia: Elsevier Saunders; 2016. p. 817–66.

[85] Mayo Clinic. Oestradiol free, serum (includes oestradiol and SHBG). Mayo Medical Laboratories. Mayo Foundation for Medical Education and Research; 2016. Available from: www.mayomedicallaboratories.com/test-catalog/print.php?unit_code=91215.

[86] Monash University. Testosterone and androgens in women. Women's Health Program, Monash University, 2010. Available from: http://med.monash.edu.au/sphpm/womenshealth/info-4-health-practitioners/index.html.

[87] Gardella T, Juppner H, Brown E, et al. Parathyroid hormone and the parathyroid hormone receptor type 1 in the regulation of calcium and phosphate homeostasis and bone metabolism. In: Jameson L, editor. Endocrinology: adult and paediatric. 7th ed. Philadelphia: Elsevier Saunders; 2016. p. 969–90.

[88] Levi R, Pearson R, Toth D, et al. First Consult. Hyperparathyroidism. Elsevier; 2010.

[89] Cibas E. Pleural, pericardial and peritoneal fluids. In: Cibas E, Ducatman B, editors. Cytology. Diagnostic principles and clinical correlates. 4th ed. St Louis: Elsevier Saunders; 2014. p. 127–53.

[90] Fletcher C. Introduction. In: Fletcher C, editor. Diagnostic histopathology of tumours. 4th ed. Philadelphia: Elsevier Saunders; 2013. p. 1–5.

[91] Western University. Glossary of medical terms. Schulich School of Medicine and Dentistry, 2016. Available from: www.schulich.uwo.ca/pathol/about_us/resources/glossary_of_medical_terms.html.

[92] Nussbaum R, McInnes R, Huntington W. Principles of clinical cytogenetics and genome analysis. In: Nussbaum R, editor. Thompson and Thompson genetics in medicine. 8th ed. Philadelphia: Elsevier Saunders; 2016. p. 57–74.

[93] Bacino C, Lee B. Cytogenetics. In: Kliegman R, editor. Nelson textbook of paediatrics. 20th ed. Philadelphia: Elsevier; 2016. p. 604–27.

[94] McPherson E. Genetic diagnosis and testing in clinical practice. Clin Med Res 2006;4(2):123–9.

[95] Wieacker P, Steinhard J. The prenatal diagnosis of genetic diseases. Dtsch Arztebl Int 2010;107(48):857–62.

[96] Salwen M. Vitamins and trace elements. In: McPherson R, Pincus M, editors. Henry's clinical diagnosis and management by laboratory methods. 23rd ed. Philadelphia: Elsevier Saunders; 2017. p. 416–27.

[97] Pincus M, Bluth M, Abraham N. Toxicology and therapeutic drug monitoring. In: McPherson R, Pincus M, editors. Henry's clinical diagnosis and management by laboratory methods. 23rd ed. Philadelphia: Elsevier Saunders; 2017. p. 324–61.

[98] Fitzgerald K, Nelson-Dooley C, Lord R. Nutrient and toxic elements. In: Lord R, Bralley J, editors. Laboratory evaluations for integrative and functional medicine. 2nd ed. Duluth, Georgia: Metametrix Institute; 2008. p. 68–151.

[99] Escott-Stump S. Orofacial conditions: dental difficulties and oral disorders. In: Escott-Stump S, editor. Nutrition and diagnosis-related care. 7th ed. Baltimore: Lippincott Williams & Wilkins; 2012. p. 96–102.

[100] Woo V. Nutrition and inflammation. In: Touger-Decker R, Mobley C, Epstein J, editors. Nutrition and oral medicine. 2nd ed. Newark: Humana Press; 2014. p. 129–52.

[101] Sheetal A, Hiremath V, Patil A, et al. Malnutrition and its oral outcome: a review. J Clin Diag Res 2013;7(1):178–80.

[102] Migliario M, Rimondini L. Oral and non-oral diseases and conditions associated with bad breath. Minerva Stomatol 2000;60(3):105–15.

[103] Stone P. Functional nutrition evaluation: eight-step mouth exam. Federal Way (WA): Institute for Functional Medicine; 2014.

[104] Cashman M, Sloan S. Nutrition and nail disease. Clin Dermatol 2010;28(4):420–5.

[105] Baran R, Dawber R, Haneke E, et al. Modification of nail surface. In: Baran R, editor. A text atlas of nail disorders — diagnosis and treatment. London: Martin Dunitz; 2002. p. 17–48, 49–66, 139–153.

[106] Heimburger D. Clinical manifestations of nutrient deficiencies and toxicities. In: Ross A, Caballero B, Cousins R, et al, editors. Modern nutrition in health and disease. 11th ed. Philadelphia: Lippincott Williams & Wilkins; 2013. p. 757–70.

[107] Schoendorfer N, Roytas D. Naturopathic diagnostic techniques. In: Sarris J, editor. Clinical naturopathy. 2nd ed. Chatswood NSW: Elsevier Churchill Livingstone; 2014. p. 19–52.

[108] McGinnis W, Audhya T, Walsh W, et al. Discerning the mauve factor, Part 2. Altern Ther Health Med 2008;14(3):56–62.

[109] Groschl M. Current status of salivary hormone analysis. Clin Chem 2008;54(11):1759–69.
[110] Winters R. Macroscopic mimics of helminths in stool specimen examination. Lab Med 2008;39(2):114–18.
[111] Humphreys C. Intestinal permeability assessment. In: Pizzorno J, editor. Textbook of natural medicine. 4th ed. St Louis: Elsevier; 2013. p. 169–78.
[112] Szynkowska M, Marcinek M, Pawlaczyk A, et al. Human hair analysis in relation to similar environmental and occupational exposure. Environ Toxicol Pharmacol 2015;40(2):402–8.
[113] Austin S, Soloway N. Hair mineral analysis. In: Pizzorno J, Murray M, editors. Textbook of natural medicine. 4th ed. St Louis: Elsevier Churchill Livingstone; 2013. p. 150–6.
[114] Medeiros-Neto G, Rubio I. Iodine-deficiency disorders. In: Jameson L, editor. Endocrinology: adult and paediatric. 7th ed. Philadelphia: Elsevier Saunders; 2016. p. 1584–600.
[115] WHO. Urinary iodine concentrations for determining iodine status deficiency in populations. Vitamin and Mineral Nutrition Information System. WHO, 2016. Available from: http://apps.who.int/iris/bitstream/10665/85972/1/WHO_NMH_NHD_EPG_13.1_eng.pdf.
[116] Lee S, Ananthakrishnan S, Pearce E, et al. Iodine deficiency workup. Drugs and diseases. endocrinology. Medscape, WebMD. 2017. Available from: http://emedicine.medscape.com/article/122714-workup#c7.

5

Case taking and treatment

Michael Colenso

PRINCIPLES INTO PRACTICE

Core to the education and professional performance of naturopathy is the ability to effectively document the clinical experience, serving immediate practical considerations related to the individual practitioner and broader aspects relevant to the continuous improvement of the profession. There are a range of professional and logistical considerations in relation to patient records, case taking and documentation of treatments. More broadly, clinical case taking is integral to the personal and professional development of the practitioner, providing scaffolding for patient engagement and a framework for case investigations and for directing further learning. Individual cases may be reviewed in collaboration with colleagues or be developed as case studies to serve in additional research or education activities that benefit the naturopathic profession.

For naturopathy students, the commencement of clinic practicum represents an exciting period of implementing learning (propositional knowledge) into practice (forming process knowledge). The documentation of patient records, case taking and treatment proposals facilitates the ability to assimilate foundation knowledge with individual perspectives and research undertakings. It assists critical thinking and enables problem solving in real-world scenarios under clinical supervision. Continuing through the career of the practitioner, case documents serve to inform their reflective practice, enabling collaboration with peers and mentors in ongoing engagements and contributing to the refinement of personal and professional values of the individual professional. Fig. 5.1 represents this progression of professional epistemology for health practitioners.

The importance of case taking and treatment plans endures for all practitioners, irrespective of their experience, as documentation is essential to meet with legislative obligations, association membership requirements and matters of professional indemnity. At a fundamental level, ensuring consistent quality of naturopathic care in the community requires a coherent operating framework for practitioners, with adherence to defined professional standards and regulatory requirements.

Effective case taking and documented treatment delivery are central to achieving both compliance and best practice, commencing with the coordination of initial patient engagement and the efficient collation of personal details. Initial naturopathic consultations are standardly 60–90 minutes, with an extensive patient history being recorded. Follow-up and subsequent consultations may vary in duration from 30 to 45 minutes, depending on diagnostic reports and evolving patient cases. With experience and increasing competence, practitioners may progress with shorter and less structured consultations. Known as the novice–expert shift this advancement represents a departure from predetermined protocols, with increasing adaptation and independence in the consultations of proficient and expert practitioners.[1]

All consultations involve effective communication and accurate information gathering, progressing to then detail the clinical decision making, treatment planning and recommendations of the practitioner. With a range of assessment and therapeutic approaches that can be adapted for the individual patient, there is additional variance in how practitioners may consult and provide naturopathic treatment. There is no universal approach or set of templates for naturopathic case taking, with practitioners often developing their own clinic documents including patient intake forms, and initial and follow-up consultation forms. Structured forms with logical question formats and systematic checklists can be useful in guiding lines of inquiry during consultation. These forms and other clinical assessment documents are particularly valuable in supporting the development of skills and confidence in naturopathic students and emerging practitioners.

The practices and methods detailed in this chapter are not to be construed as prescriptive, nor should they be interpreted in any way that may contravene relevant regulations or governance as related to naturopathic practice in specific regions. This considered, there are benefits in working towards a consistent case-taking methodology that contributes to professional cohesion with both domestic and international colleagues, while preserving the unique holistic approaches of individual practitioners.

It is advisable to consider this chapter in parallel with collated governance documents currently relevant to your region. The information supplied here is not to be decontextualised or to supersede professional guidelines or legislation relevant to your place and time of clinical

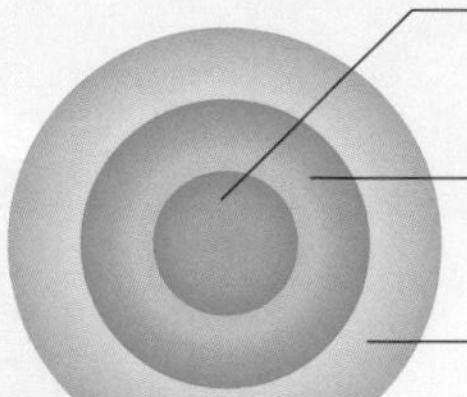
Propositional knowledge
Knowing what needs to be done
Can be taught and learned
Process knowledge
Knowing how to proceed
Gained tacitly by experience
Personal and professional values
The practitioner as an individual
Developed through reflection and analysis

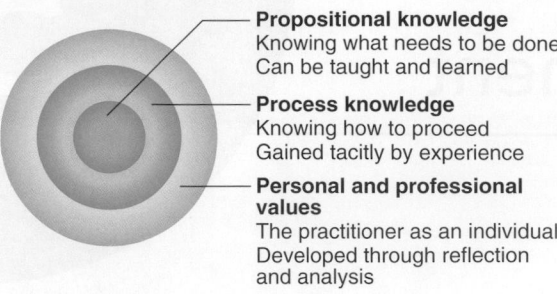

FIGURE 5.1 Personal and professional development of a practitioner

Adapted from Walker B. Davidson's principles and practice of medicine. 22nd edn. Edinburgh: Churchill Livingstone; 2014.

practice. With this considered, you may also find value in reviewing the professional code of conduct from various associations or bodies both in your region and abroad.

CLINIC RECORDS

The standards of records and the ability to report on specifics are consistently established for naturopathy professionals by the relevant bodies internationally. The nature of naturopathic consultation and treatment generates a high volume of information related to individual patients. Their confidence that this information will be recorded accurately and stored securely is paramount to their trust in a practitioner. This is an aspect that many patients will be conscious of and how you are perceived to operate in this regard will impact on both their choice of you as a practitioner and the information that they may choose to disclose with you.

Privacy ethics are not only clearly required by professional associations; health record privacy is specifically both legislated for and stringently regulated in most countries. Significant to all, the Universal Declaration of Human Rights refers to privacy and protection by law in Article 12.[2] Considerations of the right to privacy in the digital age have been advanced by the Office of the United Nations High Commissioner for Human Rights (OHCHR) and are enshrined in the current and emerging privacy legislations of individual nations and states.[3] It is your responsibility as a health professional to ensure that patient records and privacy are managed effectively with compliance by yourself and all relevant staff with access in your clinic.

Obligations relevant to privacy commence from your initial engagement with individuals. This may precede any formal patient arrangement or consent to treatment. Information acquired via your website or email are examples of this. Having a published privacy policy on the clinic website is recommended as it addresses legal considerations while presenting your business as professional and conscious of the concerns of the individual. Similarly, having an email signature that details aspects related to privacy and intended recipients (either specifically in the email or via a link to the privacy policy on your website) serves to protect the interests of all parties.

Recently implemented Australian Privacy Principles (APPs) commence with aspects of personal information and highlight the importance of an organisational privacy policy that informs the open and transparent management of personal information.[4] The primary purpose of the APPs may be for entities larger than your clinic, but they do provide a clear and easily accessible set of guidelines that may assist you in developing your privacy policy. There are likely to be specific health information handling guidelines relevant to your region that are supplied to support establishing business operations, similar to the business resources published with the APPs.[5]

Records management

Records management may have an impact on the manner practitioners choose to implement business systems and distribute information to patients. Increasingly, practitioners are implementing clinic software solutions that handle patient bookings and clinic logistics. These may extend to management of all email communications and provide the ability to enter all consultation information directly into the system. This may not suit the communication style of many practitioners, such as those taking notes during consultations on paper-based forms or less formal and unstructured notepads. Similarly, prescriptions, treatment advice, and other information are frequently provided in paper-based form to patients — all of which need to somehow be recorded within a patient record.

Most clinics currently operate with some form of digital information (which may be limited to emails) in conjunction with paper-based documents. This necessitates the storage of dual records management and some means to link all aspects of patient information as a complete record.

Whether a clinic is entirely or partially paper-based, the scanning and digital archiving of documents is often undertaken in order to back-up paper documents and reduce long-term storage. When and how digitisation occurs is relevant, as it may impact on business efficiency in relation to how practitioners prepare for upcoming consultations, how cases are reviewed and any later date access requirements.

Regardless of the business systems in place, the benefit of multiple and secure back-ups cannot be overemphasised. Compliance and indemnity requirements for record keeping can persist for decades after consultations, even for deceased patients. It is important to be aware of the duration required for clinic record keeping in the region of your practice. This may be legislated nationally and can vary between states. This responsibility endures after a practitioner has closed a clinic or retired from practice. It is in both practitioner and business interests to maintain records securely for as long as necessary.

There is also the need to satisfy a patient's right to information. Clinic record requests from patients must be complied with and in a timely manner; standardly the clinic record is to be supplied to the patient at no cost within 30 days. The record must include all information collected and recorded relevant to the individual, which includes email exchanges and any notes made by the practitioner during consultations.

Many practitioners may record notes in shorthand or with abbreviations. While it may not be necessary to explain these to patients, they may require explanation at a later date in litigation or other compliance situations. It may seem obvious, but ensure that you can later understand your own notes and remain aware that the information could be made public. Some practitioners may make audio or other recordings of consultations with patients for later reference. It is not only ethical to ensure that patients are aware of this practice, but also in many circumstances it is a legal requirement to ensure disclosure prior to the event. Storage of recordings is largely onerous. The practice often involves deletion of the media or files within a short timeframe.

Patient records may be adapted to share with other parties for a number of purposes, such as peer collaboration, mentoring, case study publication or research purposes. It is important that the patient's privacy is protected at all times, requiring de-identification of the individual. This includes any photographs shared, particularly in today's society as social media platforms have facial recognition in place.

CONSULTATION CASE TAKING

Traditionally patient engagement may commence with a telephone enquiry, consultation booking and the completion of a patient intake form that may be completed at the clinic reception prior to an initial consultation. The information supplied on arrival and on completion of the intake form serves to formalise the therapeutic arrangement and document the initial legal premise of ethical practice, part of the process of ensuring the informed consent of the patient. Valid consent is a crucial undertaking to be established for safe and ethical practice and requires that:

- the person is adequately informed as to the nature of the therapeutic engagement
- the person has the capacity to make treatment decisions (or has an appropriate parent, guardian or caretaker as legal signatory for the treatment to occur as relevant)
- the consent covers the specific practitioner performing the act
- the consent covers the therapeutic act to be performed.[6]

New technologies are enabling variations to these traditional processes, with websites and social media emerging as the forward-facing aspect of a clinic — supporting the ability to inform patients about services, and extending to receiving enquiries and managing bookings. Online booking systems may be contained within the website functionality or be integrated with clinic software. Patient intake forms can be also sent, completed and returned by email in advance of the consultation. It is relevant to consider these approaches as a means to facilitate and record informed consent early in the engagement. They may also serve to assist in more complicated consent situations, such as when engaging with consulting for children, patients with an intellectual disability or older patients who are cognitively impaired.

Clinic records, be they paper-based, digital or a combination, should include specific personal details of the patient such as full name, address, contact details and an emergency contact/next-of-kin. Practitioner details should also be clearly stated on records including invoices and receipts, detailing their full name, contact details, professional association or registration membership number, and business and taxation numbers. The date and location of sessions should be accurately recorded for each consultation with patients, along with details of treatment provided, prescription written and advice given.

The ergonomics of providing online clinic information and patient intake forms being received in advance of sessions may free up more time for meaningful engagement, rather than by rote progressing through consultation forms. Informing new patients of the consultation process, fees and possible treatments in advance supports their self-determined decision making. Intake forms received in advance can assist practitioners to be prepared for initial consultations. This may be of particular benefit to new practitioners, providing the opportunity to review information and prepare for consultations related to a presentation or current medication not previously encountered.

Purposes of case taking

In discussing clinic records management and privacy we have introduced the logistical aspects that underpin a core purpose of case taking, serving as a record of the consultation. Before any health professional can attend to the needs of others it is essential that their ability to perform safely and effectively is ensured. Central to the importance of clinical case taking is protecting yourself as a practitioner, providing a clear and accurate record of your engagement with patients, with detailed information acquired during all consultations and documented in case-taking notes.

Irrespective of level of education, any additional health qualifications attained, actual competence or experience in clinical practice, without a record of effective case taking, for any and every consultation, a practitioner is in a precarious and indefensible position. In Australia, for example, for any possible court actions related to professional negligence, or malpractice, a defendant must demonstrate that they have met the required standard of care. It must be substantiated that the defendant practitioner has acted in a consistent manner as accepted by peer professional opinion.[7] Without appropriate case notes they would be at high risk of liability for the offence and also risk loss of coverage under the terms of any existing professional indemnity insurance policy.

More positively, effective case taking is aligned with the widely known health idiom and the naturopathic principle of *First Do No Harm* (*Primum Non Nocere*.) Patient intake forms highlight preexisting conditions or medications and the information gathered through the consultation may identify potential items of concern. It is possible that a health issue beyond the scope of practice of the practitioner is identified, indicating a need for the patient to be referred to other medical services. Confirmation of a patient's current medications, achieved through case-taking enquiry, may identify any potential herb–drug interactions and inform appropriate prescribing that ensures that no harm comes to the patient from recommended treatment.

The purpose of detailed case taking holds particular relevance in the holistic healthcare model of naturopathy and alignment with the naturopathic principles of *Treat the Whole Person* (*Tolle Totum*) and *Treat the Cause* (*Tolle Causam*). With initial consultations, standardly of an hour duration at least, the practitioner collates and documents a high volume of information about the whole person in order to identify cause and establish treatment goals. The initial naturopathic consultations can be considered as a hybrid approach encompassing standard physical examination, nutritional assessment and psychology consultation methods. In addition to the volume of data collated, efforts to understand and respect the patient holistically as an individual with unique circumstances, beliefs and values is core to traditional naturopathic practice.[7]

The process of individualisation in naturopathy involves the assessment of both the morphology of a patient and their constitution, as may be revealed by family history investigation or diagnostic tools.[8] Concepts of naturopathic constitution can be understood in terms of familial predispositions or iridology grading. Traditional medicine systems, such as Ayurvedic or traditional Chinese medicine, may also be incorporated as part of a practitioner's approach in charting a constitutional picture of the individual to inform diagnosis and treatment. The approach of naturopathy is valued by both consumers and emerging health professionals.[9,10] Accordingly, health service managers are choosing to incorporate complementary practitioners within mainstream integrative healthcare services.[11]

Documentation from case taking supports referencing requirements at a later date, such as when called on by patients to communicate with other health professionals or make referrals. Case taking of multiple consultations enables efficient assessment of the treatments provided, as practitioners undertake reflective practice, mentoring and professional development activities. Reviewing cases in parallel with emerging evidence substantiating therapeutic agents is part of the increasing practice of evidenced-based medicine (EBM) in naturopathy. Reservations related to applying EBM to naturopathy are being overcome as implementation is found effective in education programs.[12–14] Practitioners use traditional knowledge in guiding their EBM research undertakings and to implement biomedical science knowledge in their understanding of traditional practices.[15]

Consultation variations

Initial consultations are of longer duration than subsequent consultations, involve thorough patient history investigation and are focused on the primary presenting complaint. Questioning and case taking will vary accordingly to the patient themselves, with considerations of their age (infant, child or adult) and presenting condition (acute, chronic, simple, multiple or complex). It is important for practitioners to be conscious of time, ensuring that adequate time is reserved for the coordination of prescription and treatment information to be transferred. With multiple and complex presenting conditions, the initial consult may need to be narrowed to the identified primary presentation.

The second consultation is then dependent on the extent of the initial consultation and whether additional presenting complaints are to be further investigated at this time. The second and other follow-up consultations are primarily focused on checking the patient's symptoms, reviewing the results of any diagnostics that may have been undertaken and comparing information against previous records to gauge the effectiveness of treatments. The end section of consultation notes may include a final 'To follow-up' section that details symptoms to review and is a reminder of other items to investigate. The structure of consultation forms, consistency of note taking, recording of treatment provided and follow-up notes assist in reviewing cases prior to each engagement.

Although it may not be possible to address all aspects of interest within a single consultation, it is important to ensure that each session has a sense of closure — especially if patients are in a distressed emotional state. With broad variations between patients and consultations it becomes relevant for practitioners to develop a sense of timing and rhythm for their engagements. This extends beyond individual consultations and more broadly across the treatment and multiple sessions with patients. Case notes are a cohesive resource for clinical practice and may also serve to facilitate reconnection, conversation and rapport with patients.

COMMUNICATION

Naturopathy demonstrates a patient-centred care approach, involving a 'whole-person' consultation exploring the individual's history, needs, values and environment while promoting active patient participation via shared decision making and lifestyle education.[16] Patient-centred care, practitioner empathy and patient empowerment are aspects sought by those seeking complementary medicine services and consistently experienced by patients of naturopathy.[17,18] Communication with patients is central to the success of the naturopathic model and its practitioners.

Practitioner communications should be articulate, accessible, emotionally balanced and professionally focused. In considering communication basics this extends to non-verbal aspects of a clinic, such as ensuring an appropriate environment and personal presentation.[19] Both the reception counter and consultation room are to provide privacy and ensure that communications, including phone calls, are not overheard. Initial engagements must include clear communication regarding clinical services provided, with particular regard to any

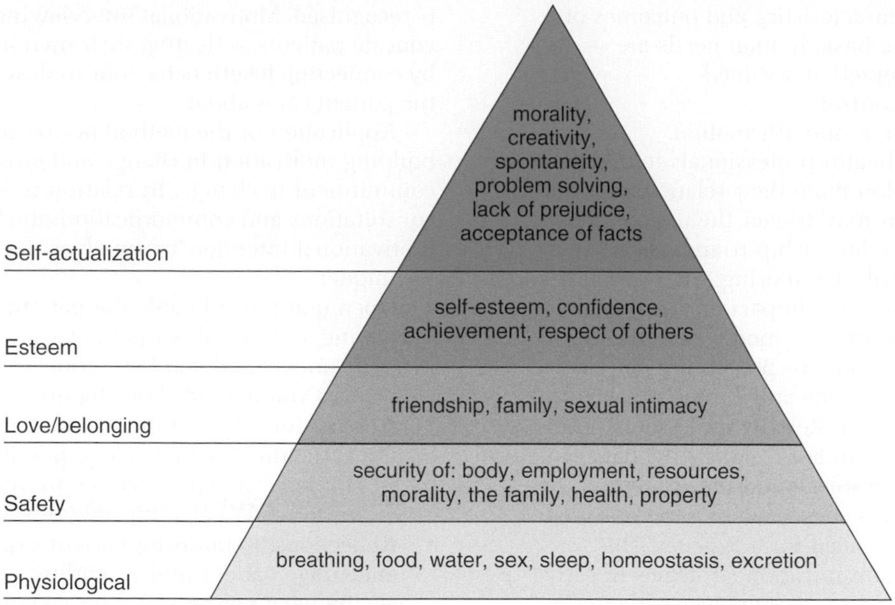

FIGURE 5.2 Maslow's hierarchy of needs

Saul McLeod/CC BY SA 4.0, https://commons.wikimedia.org/wiki/Category:Maslow%27s_hierarchy_of_needs#/media/File:Maslow%27s_Hierarchy_of_Needs_Pyramid.png

physical examination to take place and announcement of each and every physical contact to occur during sessions.

There should be no disruptions to consultations; patients should feel that the practitioner is attentively focused for the duration of all engagements. Practitioners should encourage a free-flowing exchange, avoiding scripted sessions and over-direction, and ensuring that information is received from patients who are not simply being passive in responding to questions. Open questioning is used where possible as it encourages patients to present information in their own words and can lead to additional information being revealed through their responses.

Active listening is a key aspect to effective consultations and increases the likelihood that the patient knows you are listening to them. It involves:

- Paying attention: face the patient, maintain eye contact, and avoid distractions and fidgeting
- Listening demonstratively: have an open posture, and use nodding and encouragers such as 'Yes' and 'Go on'
- Providing feedback: seek clarification, summarise and redirect with further questions
- Responding appropriately: avoid interruptions, use a relaxed and calm tone of voice, and provide open and honest responses
- Deferring judgment: avoid assumptions, be empathetic and allow time for full responses.[20]

There can be challenges in maintaining appropriate eye contact during consultation sessions and balancing the recording of case notes. Reflective paraphrasing can be used in exchanges to validate the patient's responses and provide the opportunity to pause the dialogue and record notes.

Consultation tools

There are a range of psychology models and counselling methods that may be implemented to support patient engagement and relationship development. Understanding a patient's purpose for engaging with naturopathic treatment and their expressed desires or expected outcomes can be relevant for directing communications both through consultation and in effectively providing relevant recommendations. Developing an appreciation for where a patient is situated in relation to their needs can be facilitated with application of, for example, Maslow's hierarchy (see Fig. 5.2).

Maslow's model can be useful in aiding considerations of an initial consultation and is most useful in longer term treatment planning. Knowing in advance that a patient is presenting with the primary condition of abdominal pain and constant diarrhoea simply shows that the consultation should first focus on the basic physiological needs that must be addressed. This approach may assist practitioners in preparing various lines of questioning with screening tools and coordinating for certain diagnostic procedures; it does not serve to differentiate actions at the physiological level.[21] Maslow's hierarchy provides a useful construct for evolving treatment plans with patients over a series of consultations, where basic physiological issues may be resolved and underlying personal aspects then addressed.

The process of exploring such models can elucidate and highlight one of the most critical practitioner resources, self-awareness. Knowing yourself and your own personality aspects enables nuanced engagement with others. All individuals have human relationship needs that can unconsciously create typical patterns of relating with others, affecting the characteristics and outcomes of relationships. The three basic human needs are:

1 The need to be accepted and valued
2 The need to be in control
3 The need for affection and affirmation.

It is important for health professionals to understand which of these needs dominate their relationships and be aware of situations that may trigger the unconscious need.[22] The Karpman relationship triangle is another model that can be useful in exploring self-awareness and personal tendencies that may impact on interpersonal communications. The Karpman model explores the connection between personal responsibility and power in conflict or human interactions and is built on the three primary roles of Persecutor, Rescuer and Victim. The dynamic can be effective in appreciating the default nature of people (including therapists) and the related expectations that patients may have in a therapeutic relationship, such as the need for a Rescuer. This potentially informs communication strategies in early engagement and progression to empower patients.

Jungian types, various psychometrics, homeopathy and iridology constitutions are all models which practitioners may implement in their own unique practice of naturopathy, informing personality interpretations and communication strategies. Irrespective of models used, it is important to recognise how they may be perceived by individual patients if introduced to them. It is important to ensure that communications with patients are appropriately aligned with their values and worldview.

Similarly with prescribed treatment regimens, discernment is advised in making recommendations for individual patients. A particular diet, nutritional protocol or lifestyle regimen that may work for yourself and others you have treated will not be suitable for every patient encountered. Narrow and rigid treatment approaches may lead to non-compliance with recommendations or for ongoing health issues following treatments. At the extreme, the inflexibility of a practitioner can be paternalistic, where patients may feel 'victims' to lack of progress and a 'naturopath knows best' treatment dynamic can unfold. A practitioner's duty of care is to provide a treatment appropriately suited to the patient, not to make the patient fit the practitioner's treatment or philosophical approach.[6]

Motivational interviewing is a counselling method that is well suited to naturopathic consultations, aligned with principles of respecting the individual and educating in the process of supporting health improvement. The method originated in the treatment of alcoholism and addictions in the 1980s, drawing on the phrase 'ready, willing and able.' It outlines three components of motivation:

- Readiness: whether change is an immediate priority
- Willingness: importance of the change as identified by the patient
- Ability: patient confidence in their ability to change.[23]

Aligned with respect for the individual in naturopathic practice, motivational interviewing honours the patient's autonomy and acknowledges the right and freedom not to change. Similarly it is a collaborative approach, where the individual's knowledge of self and ability to change, or heal, is recognised. Motivational interviewing also seeks to educate patients, activating their own motivation to change by connecting health behaviour to desired outcomes that the patient cares about.

Application of the method occurs in two phases — building motivation to change and strengthening commitment to change. In relation to initial naturopathy consultations and communication, the first phase of motivational interviewing involves the OARS counselling technique:

- Open questions: Enable the patient to do most of the talking, to learn about patient values.
  - 'I understand you have concerns about drinking. Can you tell me about them?'
- Affirmations: Compliments or statements of understanding. Acknowledge possibilities.
  - 'I appreciate your courage to discuss drinking habits with me. We can improve this.'
- Reflections: Rephrasing patient expressions to encourage patient understanding.
  - 'By what you've said, you recognise the impact drinking is having on your health.'
- Summaries: Ensure mutual understanding, highlight discrepancies between status and goals.
  - 'If it's okay with you, please let me check that I understand what we've been discussing. You are concerned about your drinking on most days and you are noticing that it has been impacting on your health and family life. Your partner and a close friend have also shared concerns about your daily habit. You've tried drinking less and have been finding it difficult to stop when you start. Does this sound right?'

The method generally involves one open question and a couple of reflections that follow the patient's response, assisting in the process of building rapport and establishing a therapeutic relationship.[24]

CLINICAL DECISION MAKING

Clinical decision models in healthcare have been emerging over recent decades, and many (such as the SOAP notes model: Subjective data, Objective data, Assessment and Plan see below) originated as documentation methodologies. The Ballard-Reisch Participative Model is one of the earliest specific decision-making models, designed for doctors in 1990 in efforts to provide a structured approach to patient-centred care.[25] The Nutrition Care Model was first adopted by the American Dietetic Association in 2003 for registered dietitian nutritionists and dietetic technicians.[26] These various frameworks have been taught in naturopathic curricula for several decades and continue to hold relevance in contemporary education and practice.

The role of naturopaths as primary healthcare providers varies significantly in different international jurisdictions, with the ability to make diagnoses and prescribe therapeutic procedures varying accordingly with professional scope of practice. Broadly, naturopaths assess patients over a range of health aspects, employing a unique body of knowledge that evaluates not only in relation to pathological aetiologies but also in terms of normal physiological function and subclinical functional disturbances.[27] Employing a diverse array of assessment and treatment modalities in an individualised approach to patients adds to the difficulty of defining a single practice model and decision-making framework.

SOAP

Before advancing to explore a naturopathic decision-making framework, there is value in first appreciating conventional medical frameworks. These may be presented to naturopaths by patients in consultation or may be encountered in multidisciplinary integrative practices by some practitioners. SOAP notes were developed as a problem-oriented medical record in the 1960s and continue to be used widely in healthcare today as admission notes, medical histories and other documents of a patient's chart.

Subjective data

Subjective data comprise the patient's statement as to the purpose for the consultation, outlining the presenting or chief complaint, and describing the condition in narrative form. Enquiry will seek to outline a history of the present illness with clarifiers to detail the state of experienced symptoms in the patient's own words. SAMPLE is a mnemonic for a key method used to remember key areas of enquiry, and is detailed in Box 5.1. SAMPLE case history may be taken in conjunction with vital signs, a review of physiological systems and aligned questioning.

In efforts to detail symptoms and elucidate aetiology, the nature of the pain being experienced is investigated by questioning to define and clarify aspects. The OLD CHARTS mnemonic, in Box 5.2, is one of several used to clarify the presenting complaint and pain sensation (SOCRATES, LOCQSMAT and OPQRST are others). Additional screening tools may be implemented in conjunction and can assist in tracking signs over time and progression via treatments.

When gauging the severity of pain various scaling tools may be used, such as the visual Wong-Baker Faces Pain Rating Scale, which may overcome communication barriers such as language and age — it is particularly useful for young children.

Other screening tools may be used to help define current signs and symptoms; some also being supplied to the patient to assist in logging and journalling efforts. The Bristol Stool Scale (also known as the Meyers Scale in the UK) is an example; it defines seven stool types as a clinical communication aid.

Objective data

The objective component of SOAP involves measures from the observations of the practitioner and results from diagnostics, pathology and other testing. Some anthropometric data, such height and weight, and other information from medication lists, medical records and diagnostic test results may be collected in advance of the initial consultation or at the time. During consultations a statement of vital signs and findings from physical examination can be produced.

Assessment

A summary of the patient's condition(s), including differential diagnosis assessment and confirmed aetiologies, may be detailed by the health professional in SOAP notes. Where a definitive diagnosis has not been made, multiple possible diagnoses may be detailed.

Plan

The plan can extend from organising diagnostic testing and referrals through to treatment, with procedures or exercises to be performed, medicines prescribed and patient education included. Where multiple health problems are assessed, the plan is ideally prioritised and may well specify actions, each according to consideration of the severity of and urgency for diagnosis and treatment.

BOX 5.1 SAMPLE history: History of Present Illness (HPI) questioning in medical assessment

S Symptoms and signs of presenting complaint, be that an injury or illness. Additional mnemonics are used to assist in clarifying the pain being experienced (see Box 5.2)
A Adverse reactions or known allergies to any medications, foods or other triggers
M Medications that are being taken currently or have been previously taken
P Past medical history detailing diagnosed conditions, injuries, surgeries and the like
L Last oral intake, where food/drink was consumed. Last menstruation may also be detailed
E Environment or Events known to relate to the injury or illness, covering family and social history.

Adapted from SAMPLE history, https://en.wikipedia.org/wiki/SAMPLE_history. CC BY SA 3.0.

BOX 5.2 OLD CHARTS: Symptom or nature or pain clarification questioning

O Onset: When and how did it start? Was it sudden or gradual? Progressive or regressive?
L Location: Where is it? Where does it hurt most?
D Duration: When did/does it occur? Does the pain follow any patterns?
CH Character: What is the pain like? Can you describe it for me? An ache? Stabbing?
A Alleviating/Aggravating factors: Does anything change the pain?
R Radiation: Does the pain radiate anywhere? Where does it move or extend from?
T Temporal pattern: Is it every morning? All day? What time during the night?
S Severity. How bad is the pain? On a scale from 0 as no pain up to 10 as worst possible pain?

Adapted from SOAP note, https://en.wikipedia.org/wiki/SOAP_note. CC BY SA 3.0.

Decision-making framework for naturopathy

As the philosophies and practices of healthcare systems are continuously evolving it can be difficult to stipulate a robust and all-encompassing framework for any specific modality. This is certainly the case for naturopathy. Phytotherapy and the herbalist approach to patient care have a long history and recent texts focusing on this core modality are of benefit in harmonising various schools of patient engagement in relation to herbal medicine practices.[28] Naturopathic practices are diverse across regions and among individual practitioners. It is helpful to reflect on broader complementary and alternative medicine (CAM) consultation processes and case studies.[29]

DeFCAM

A distinct decision-making framework for complementary and alternative medicine (DeFCAM) was published in 2010 and serves well in application here for naturopathy. The framework builds on existing medical models (such as SOAP and the Participative Decision-making Model) and is contextualised specifically for CAM and integrative healthcare practitioners. DeFCAM aligns with several overarching concepts that influence CAM decision making:

- Evidence-based medicine and critical analysis
- Modality or profession-specific principles and philosophies
- Practitioner knowledge, skills and scope of practice
- Patient income, culture, values and education.

There are six stages of the DeFCAM framework, presented linearly here as RADPAR (Rapport, Assessment, Diagnosis, Planning, Application, Review), although they are to be considered as existing in a unidirectional and dynamic model of intersecting phases. The framework was initially drafted in relation to the naturopathic process in 2008 and continues to hold close alignment with naturopathy concepts outlined previously in this text.[25]

RAPPORT

Establishing rapport with patients is considered the most important phase in the model, with consideration of initial dedication to building trust and ongoing development through the therapeutic relationship. Key aspects of communication skills and counselling techniques relevant to naturopathy and building rapport have been presented throughout this chapter.

ASSESSMENT

The assessment phase involves the acquisition, validation and organisation of patient information. This encompasses both subjective and objective data as highlighted in the SOAP model and demonstrated as relevant in naturopathy via implementation of patient intake and consultation documentation, open questioning, active listening methods and reflective paraphrasing methods. DeFCAM also details Maslow's hierarchy as a model that is supportive of the consultation assessment approach for CAM practitioners, as expanded in Box 5.3.

> **BOX 5.3 Application of Maslow's hierarchy model within naturopathic assessment framework**
>
> **Physiological:** Evaluation of physiological function via physical assessment, health history and diagnostics such as pathology, imaging and iridology. May be ordered by practitioner or acquired via patient records and/or correspondence with other healthcare professionals
>
> **Safety-security:** Assessment of the patient's environment, socioeconomic considerations such as occupation, finances, residence and domestic arrangements
>
> **Love and belonging:** Identification of significant others in the patient's life; includes partners, family, friends, social network and community. Considers cultural identity, religious and spiritual needs
>
> **Self-esteem:** Assessment of the patient's self-respect level and perceived self-image, demonstrated independence, self-control and life competence, expressed dignity and perception of body image
>
> **Self-actualisation:** Enquiry to appreciate the patient's happiness and fulfilment in life, expanding to gauge their perceived level of self-determination. Identify next aspirational and/or spiritual needs.
>
> Adapted from Leach M. The naturopathic process: a framework for naturopathic practice. J Aust Trad Med Soc 2008;14(1):7–10.

The assessment process in DeFCAM extends beyond the limitations of a body systems overview, reaching beyond physical examination and health history to incorporate the relevant diagnostics used in CAM modalities to identify underlying causes of presenting conditions. In naturopathy this relates to clinical picture assessment (CPA) and qualitative and quantitative (QUALD/QUAND) dietary analysis methods introduced in Chapter 7.

Likewise the principles of Western herbal medicine previously detailed are encompassed here, involving the holistic assessment of the patient, their vitality, constitution, family history, environmental and personal health, and lifestyle. In naturopathy disease is considered broadly as a process rather than a single pathophysiological entity. The naturopathic model sees disease as any disturbance to normal function and assesses determinants of health.[30] How all this information is organised, recorded and managed is a consideration within DeFCAM.

DIAGNOSIS

The logical clustering of patient assessment data is the third phase of the DeFCAM framework, which is known as diagnostic reasoning. Although the formulation of 'medical' diagnoses is beyond the scope of practice for naturopaths in some countries such as Australia, there is a precedent of other health professions (nursing and dietetics) developing diagnostic lists that mitigate associated concerns. Traditional naturopathic diagnosis encompasses review of physical states involving detailed inspection of skin, hair, nails, eyes and the tongue. Symptomatic presentations, such as the colour and form of mucus and exudates, are also incorporated as part of the naturopathic diagnostic methodology.

In recent years there has been improved accessibility and affordability of pathology services for naturopaths and their patients, contributing to increased implementation in contemporary practice. Services used may include functional pathology testing (such as full liver function testing), metabolic and hormone profiling, heavy metal and organic toxicology screening, comprehensive diagnostic stool analysis (CDSA) and single-nucleotide polymorphism (SNP) profiling. These reductive diagnostic tools may be implemented for differential diagnosis, to identify subclinical functional disturbances and underlying familial influences as part of a holistic approach to individual patient care. Differential diagnostic flowcharts provide a visual means to support decision making, such as in Fig. 5.3.[31]

Traditional naturopathic diagnosis can be appreciated as a bottom-up inductive reasoning approach where specific data can be interpreted to inform generalisations (such as the development of a constitution picture of an individual.) In contrast, modern bioscience diagnostics are aligned with a top-down deductive reasoning approach where generalisations are narrowed in a process of forming specific conclusions. In exploring the diagnosis phase of DeFCAM, Leach provides examples of various decision-making models and distilled comparisons in relation to alignment with inductive or deductive reasoning approaches.

With the diverse factors that influence unique CAM modality practices considered, no single model provides an all-encompassing suitability for CAM, significantly relevant to naturopathy as a broad modality in itself. Versatile adoption of multiple models is proposed as relevant, providing flexibility for diverse practices between individual practitioners and agility to suit the increasing inductive reasoning of experienced clinicians. Experienced practitioners may be selective in the implementation of specific diagnostic tools and agile in the adoption of a particular clinical decision-making approach for a patient and the complexity of the presenting condition.

This progression of decision-making competency can be appreciated in relation to theories of expertise development in nursing and in parallel with the

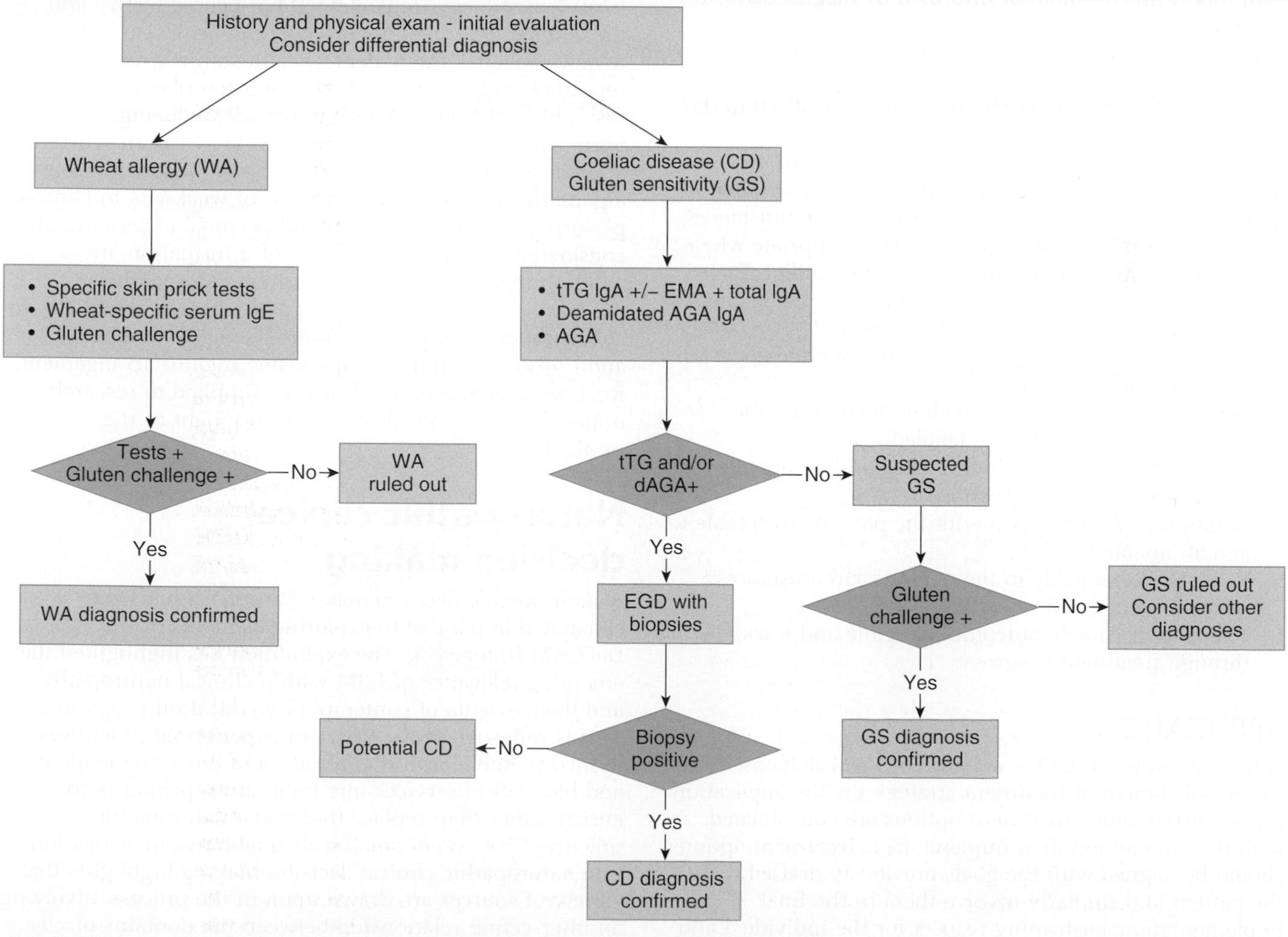

FIGURE 5.3 Flowchart for the differential diagnosis of gluten-related disorders

EMA: anti-endomysial antibodies; AGA: anti-gliadin antibodies; EGD: esophagogastroduodenoscopy Adapted from Sapone A, Bai J, Ciacci C et al. Spectrum of gluten-related disorders: consensus on new nomenclature and classification. BMC Med 2012; 10:13. © Sapone et al; licensee BioMed Central Ltd 2012.

novice–expert shift introduced earlier.[32] The ability to depart from deductive frameworks and extend into inductive approaches is proportionate with increased clinical experience; expert practitioners can confidently make accurate decisions drawing from observed cues thus mitigating the delays and expenses related to excessive reliance on clinical tests.[33]

PLANNING

The DeFCAM planning phase involves the development of goals for the identification and prioritisation of strategies to address the needs of the patient. Strategies may be focused on the prevention, reduction or resolution of health issues or on facilitation of the improvement of function or wellbeing for the patient. Coordination of required referrals identified through consultation may take precedence to the implementation of any treatment plans. The scheduling of diagnostics and interpretation of results may also be a precursor for broader treatment planning, via facilitation of differential diagnosis or provision of deeper insights to presenting conditions. Initial treatment may be focused on ameliorating presenting symptoms, with follow-up consultation informed by diagnostic results that enable more narrow clinical determinations and inform planning for the effective deployment of targeted therapeutics.

The goals of treatment should be individualised to the patient, with various options clearly presented and explained so that they are aware and involved in the process. This may be particularly relevant in providing treatments that are suited to their personal circumstances, such as ensuring recommendations are appropriate when considering value and affordability for the patient. Each goal should be aligned to one problem and provide one outcome, with clear and accessible direction.

Establishing SMART goals is a recommended approach, where treatment goals are:

- **S**pecific: Significant to the patient, focused on the problem of the goal being detailed
- **M**easurable: Meaningful with value and potentially motivational with progression
- **A**chievable: Agreed upon with the patient, acceptable to and attainable by them
- **R**ealistic: Reasonable to the patient's circumstances, results-oriented and rewarding
- **T**ime-based: Timely outcomes, tangible and trackable through treatment progress.

APPLICATION

Following on from the formulation of CAM diagnoses and the establishment of treatment strategies is the application phase during which treatment options are consolidated with the patient and then implemented. Treatment options should be aligned with the goals previously drafted with the patient and similarly involve them in the final implementation, enshrining respect for the individual and contributing to improved compliance with treatments.

There are broad approaches to treatment in CAM modalities and it is not possible to establish a single methodology of applying treatments. This extends to naturopathy itself, as a modality with diverse means of delivery and extensive treatment options possible. Naturopathic interventions should be based on the most robust evidence available, substantiating clinical decisions and the safety and efficacy of treatments used. Such an EBM approach uses external clinical evidence to inform, but never to replace, individual practitioner expertise.[34]

Effective implementation of EBM in healthcare curricula is demonstrated to both improve practitioner confidence and contribute to high-quality healthcare.[35,36] Both experienced naturopathy practitioners and emerging graduates of EBM-inclusive naturopathy curricula desire information sources that contain traditional and scientific information, with randomised trials increasingly rated as essential by recent graduates.[37] Evidence-based practice is highly valued by contemporary practitioners and is highlighted in representations to substantiate the validity of naturopathy in the advocacy efforts of professional associations.[38]

REVIEW

The review phase of DeFCAM assesses whether the treatment strategy implemented has been effective and the defined treatment goals have been achieved. The review evaluates the patient's health status, with a focus on resolution of the primary presenting complaint and the restoration of homeostasis and overall wellbeing. Systematic reflective practice serves to evolve the current approaches and methods of the practitioner, identifying any ineffective treatments or areas of weakness in clinical performance. Patient records and personal experience are considered as important sources of information, in addition to scientific publications, by naturopathy practitioners.[37] Review may be undertaken individually, in collaboration with peers, or more formally via a clinic audit procedure under a supervising mentor arrangement. Reviews may also be published or supplied to research undertakings to contribute to advancement of the profession.

Naturopathic clinical decision making

A naturopathic decision-making approach has been elucidated in parallel to exploring elements of the DeFCAM framework. The exploration has highlighted the emerging relevance of EBM within clinical naturopathy and the curricula of contemporary education programs. This is reflective of the desire of experienced practitioners to incorporate a critical application of emerging evidence and biomedical services into their clinic, primarily to enrich rather than replace traditional naturopathic practices.[39] A recent small-scale qualitative investigation into naturopathic clinical decision making highlights that a variety of sources are drawn upon in the process, involving an intersecting relationship between the domains of conventional information sources, clinical experience and practitioner intuition.[40] This is represented in Fig. 5.4.

The significance of intuition in clinical decision making can be appreciated via the dual-process theory of

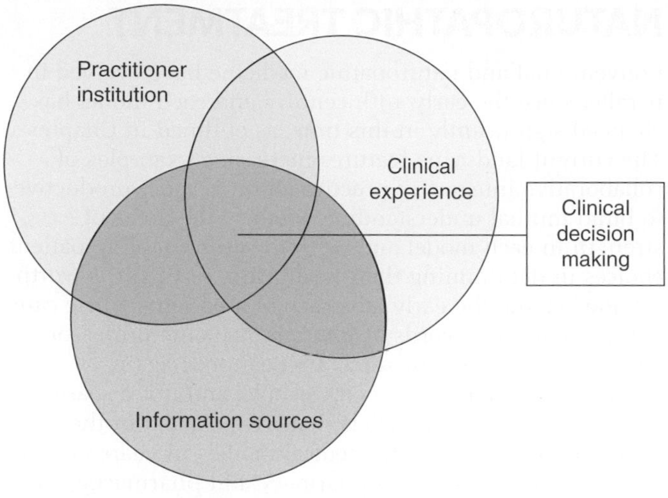

FIGURE 5.4 Relationship of input sources to naturopathic clinical decision making

Adapted from Steel A, Adams J. Approaches to clinical decision-making: a qualitative study of naturopaths. Comp Thera Clin Prac 2011;17(2):81–4.

cognition, where reasoning is understood to occur through both an intuitive, experiential, automatic and affective system (System One) and an analytical, deliberative and logical processing system (System Two). In dual-process theory System One is akin to 'subconscious' decision making, typically deployed when short cuts and heuristic techniques are used to make decisions with minimal effort, which can increase cognitive efficiency.[41] System Two is used for more complex circumstances and for decisions that require significant contemplation, but with repeated exposure and experience the thinker may switch to System One processing for these types of situations.

Traditional medical decision making involves models in which a single system of thought is implemented (such as expected-utility theory and prospect theory.) Hybrid dual system models involving integrated System One and System Two processes have been developed and applied to the medical field, linked to the threshold concept of decision making. System One may be approximate and prone to increased margins of error, yet it is adaptive and minimises time to action and in doing so may be more effective in the final analysis. In clinical decision making it can be considered a means to circumvent 'paralysis by analysis'.[42]

This adaptability is not only critically useful in triage, emergency medicine and paramedic decision making, its relevance also permeates through all medical fields and it is particularly apt in application to the intersecting naturopathic decision-making theorem — encompassing the elements of critical analysis of information sources, merged with evolving clinical experience and intuitive practices of naturopathic practitioners. Intuition, linked to the individual's expertise and its essential role in making clinical judgments, has been appreciated for several decades in the nursing profession as a result of Benner's 'novice to expert' theory of clinical expertise published in the early 1980s.[43] The model details aspects relevant to the education of naturopathic practitioners, recognising that novice practitioners rely more heavily on analytical resources and principles in guiding their decision making and implementation of treatment strategies. It is a sensible approach in formative clinic training and early practice, as clinical experience is acquired and intuition developed.

The value of intuition in the medical practice of general practitioners, hospital physicians and surgical doctors is increasingly recognised in emerging clinical efficacy research, extending to embrace emotion and neuroscience data in appreciating the 'gut feelings' experienced in complex and uncertain diagnostic circumstances.[44] Emerging cognitive research further substantiates this understanding of clinical decision making, via fuzzy-trace theory where gist-based intuition is recognised as being used by experienced practitioners in medicine and public health.[45]

As we considered the value of consultation forms and clinical assessment resources useful in supporting student and emerging practitioners, similarly a methodical analytic approach and utilisation of structured diagnostic and treatment protocols can be considered valuable in facilitating the formative clinical experience of practitioners. In ongoing professional development and efforts to embrace mindful practice it is advised that, as clinicians undertake reflective practice, there is ongoing audit of how intuition and potential cognitive biases may be evident in their evolving clinical decision-making processes.[46]

DETERMINANTS OF HEALTH

It is relevant to revisit naturopathic philosophy in efforts to further contextualise the unique decision-making approach of the modality. Naturopathic clinical theory recognises the innate ability of the body to seek balance to optimise health and wellness. As illness can be understood as a process of disturbance to health, naturopathic practitioners seek to identify areas of abnormal function and the origins of disturbances. Naturopathic medicine requires practitioners to understand what determines health in a broad and holistic assessment of the individual; these determinants may be either health promoting or health disturbing in nature.[30]

Determinants of health may originate from genetic inheritances or be a result of congenital expressions or intrauterine influences on the preborn. Determinants may be a result of physical and emotional exposure, stresses and trauma. They may be influenced by environment, including air, water and food quality, and exposure to toxins via these or the homes in which we live. They may involve modifiable behavioural factors such as poor hygiene, unsafe sexual practices, a sedentary lifestyle, poor dietary habits, alcohol consumption, drug usage and/or substance abuse.

Socioeconomic aspects may influence various behavioural factors and broader sociocultural aspects have an impact on psychoemotional and spiritual components. Disruptions in these areas create increased stress on both individuals and families, with associated consequences to each entity and even on communities more broadly.

BOX 5.4 FORSEE: Socioeconomic questioning in naturopathic assessment

F Family environment, encompasses living arrangements, family dynamics and responsibilities
O Occupation and employment status, insight into daily pattern, responsibilities, stress and finances
R Religion and cultural background, informing aspects of worldview, philosophy and aspirations
S Social support, informs elements of personal network, distance and accessibility to support
E Education, level of education attained. Field of study may provide additional insight into outlook
E Environment (work and residence), extending to school or childcare details in paediatric cases.

Adapted from Leach M. Clinical decision making in complementary and alternative medicine. Churchill Livingstone: Sydney; 2010.

BOX 5.5 DISEASE: Lifestyle history questioning in naturopathic assessment

D Diet and fluid intake, extending to QUALD and QUAND dietary analysis methods
I Illicit drug use, may extend to include self-medication with pharmaceuticals
S Smoking status, both current status and prior history of habitual tobacco smoking
E Exercise frequency and duration, to include history of current training regimen/pattern
A Alcohol use, frequency and volume. Types of drinking habits, past and present
S Sleep quality and duration. Can extend to assessment of energy and/or stress levels
E Entertainment or recreation choices; extends to outdoor activities and connection with nature.

Adapted from Leach M. Clinical decision making in complementary and alternative medicine. Churchill Livingstone: Sydney; 2010.

Naturopathic consultation (especially the initial consultation) involves thorough investigation of both socioeconomic and lifestyle aspects of an individual's current circumstances and personal history. Additional mnemonics to guide assessment in these domains are detailed in Boxes 5.4 and 5.5. Lines of questioning in these areas are crucial to the holistic approach and unique decision-making model of naturopathy.

These efforts to delve deeply into the underlying socioeconomic, lifestyle and spiritual aspects of an individual patient's life are a core foundation that defines clinical naturopathic practice. The efforts to understand a person holistically are appreciated by patients and are primary to building rapport, acknowledged as the most important phase in the DeFCAM model. The quality time spent listening to patients is demonstrated to not only strengthen the therapeutic relationship, but also contribute to improved patient health outcomes.[10]

NATUROPATHIC TREATMENT

Conventional and naturopathic medicine have evolved in parallel since the early 19th century and each model has changed significantly in this time, as outlined in Chapter 1. The current landscape features increasing examples of collaborative integrative practice and it is most productive to build mutual understanding, identify the areas of strength in each model and work towards enabling patient choices in determining their healthcare. In this it is worth acknowledging the early advocacy of a patient-centric care approach and the words of internal medicine professor Hermann Nothnagel in 1882: 'I repeat once again, medicine is about treating sick people, and not diseases.'[47] This is one of many parallels that have existed in the evolution of the disparate medical models in years past, as is the entwined history of pharmacy and pharmacognosy that extends over many centuries.[48]

Homeostatic principles that appreciated the body's ability to maintain itself in a normal state of health and advocacy of the practitioner's role in facilitating the self-healing of patients were consistent principles in emerging naturopathic practice. Disease was appreciated as resulting from disturbances in normal function and inflammatory processes were recognised as acute reactions of the body in mitigating causative elements. Henry Lindlahr is considered a founder of scientific naturopathy. In addition to implementing a therapeutic regimen that aligned with the six principles, he was an early pioneer in the implementation of vitamin and mineral preparations in practice. Lindlahr is recognised for advancing a holistic physiological model for disease — rather than a simple reduction, where invasion of a pathogen created presentation; for example, symptoms were recognised as a physiological response and evidence of the body fighting against causal factors.

In Lindlahr's *Nature Cure: Philosophy and Practice Based on the Unity of Disease and Cure*, published in 1913, a cohesive naturopathic treatment model was developed in relation to an understanding of progression from acute expressions through to chronic disease states.[49] Five stages of inflammation were identified:

- Incubation: Period between exposure to an infectious disease and subsequent development
- Aggravation: Phase during which natural responses to pathogenic agents and toxins commences, accompanied by an increase of fever and inflammation processes
- Destruction: As healing occurs there are morbid changes such as the destruction of phagocytes, pathogenic microbes, tissues and blood vessels. The disintegration of tissues occurs with the accumulation of exudates, with pus formation leading to the development of conditions such as abscesses, boils and open sores. If supported by treatment that builds blood, increases vitality and promotes elimination then infection may be overcome and toxins eliminated. A worsening of symptoms in this stage is considered as a healing crisis
- Abatement: A gradual lowering of temperature and the other symptoms of inflammation, with the absorption and elimination of exudates and toxins

- Reconstruction: As affected areas have been cleared of accumulations and obstructions, with abatement running its course, the work rebuilding the injured tissue and organs commences. As reconstruction is the last stage of the inflammatory process, it can be considered the most important. Restoring damage and normal function in the injured areas resolves the effect of acute disease in the individual.

In contrast to orthodox medicine, naturopathic treatment allows inflammatory processes to run their normal course through the stages of Destruction, Absorption and Reconstruction, unless the individual is so debilitated or the condition is so severe (e.g. meningitis or appendicitis) that this cannot safely be achieved.[50] In this process Lindlahr documented that intestinal membranes and glandular structures would be rebuilt. However, with suppressive treatment (such as quinine, mercury, purging salts or opiates used in pharmacological treatments at that time) sloughed membranes and absorbent vessels are not reconstructed. He suggested that via suppression the individual experiences symptom resolution and may think they are cured, but reconstruction in the affected area has not occurred and the intestinal tract remains in an atrophied condition — resulting in poor absorption, malnutrition and ongoing disorders.

Lindlahr extended appreciation of the inflammatory model to the perspective that continued suppression of self-healing efforts in acute diseases leads to the creation of chronic conditions, which can never be resolved by ongoing suppressive treatments. Naturopathic treatment, over 100 years ago and today, requires effort to address fundamental disturbances of health in the individual and acknowledges that symptomatic treatment by itself only contributes to ongoing health complications. A contemporary example is symptomatic treatment of asthma with steroidal anti-inflammatory and antihistamine drugs, effectively opening the airways yet weakening the individual with prolonged use. The overuse of corticosteroid anti-inflammatories can contribute to the individual becoming immunocompromised, further reducing respiratory defences while creating additional chronic side effects such as osteoporosis.[31]

The naturopathic treatment model identifies chronic disease as a continuation and accumulation of health disturbance factors. Healing is achieved by reducing disturbances to health and stimulating and supporting the self-healing processes of individuals. In progressing the health of individuals with chronic conditions they can return to an acute state, where reactive symptoms may arise before the achievement of normal full health. Without addressing underlying disturbances, further deteriorations are projected in the naturopathic health process model. The naturopathic process of healing that informs treatment planning is demonstrated in Fig. 5.5.

The naturopathic healing process developed over a hundred years ago is robust and increasingly relevant today. Biomedicine has transformed the impact of injuries and diseases that were largely fatal in the past, improving outcomes and extending life spans. The predominant health morbidities of the developed world today are non-communicable chronic diseases, recently accounting

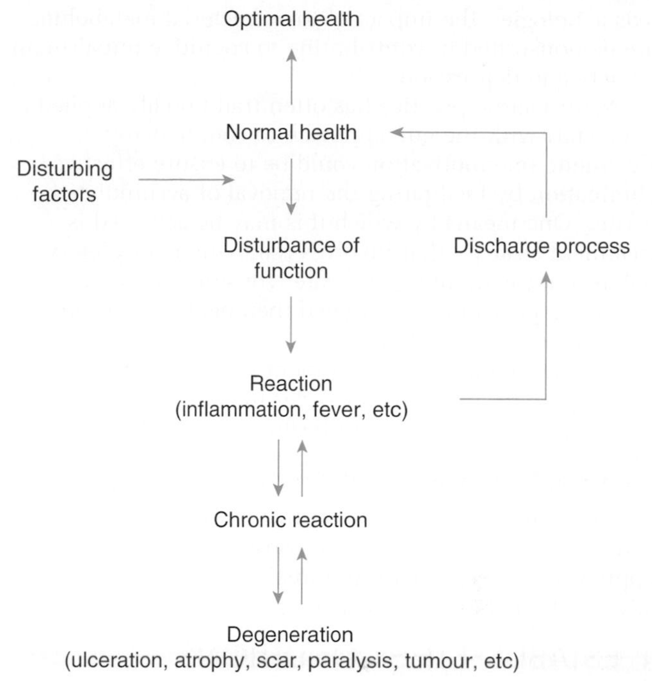

FIGURE 5.5 The process of healing in naturopathic medicine

Adapted from Zeff J, Snider P, Myers S, et al. A hierarchy of healing: the therapeutic order — a unifying theory of naturopathic medicine. In Pizzorno J, Murray M. Textbook of natural medicine. 4th edn. St Louis: Churchill Livingstone; 2013.

for 85% of the total burden of disease in Australia for example.[51] These include obesity, cardiovascular disease, type 2 diabetes, Alzheimer's disease and depression.

The bulk of chronic diseases are recognised to be preventable, with lifestyle factors responsible, which is the primary focus of the naturopathic treatment approach. There is also an increasing realisation that inflammation is intimately linked with the advancement of most diseases.[52] This is concordant with the naturopathic healing process perspective and inflammation is demonstrated to be responsive to therapeutic approaches used by naturopaths, such as low-reactive diets, probiotics and phytotherapeutics.

Naturopathic therapeutic order

More than 2000 years ago Hippocrates stated that 'All disease begins in the gut' and the traditional naturopathy perspectives developed in recent centuries have embraced this approach to treatments. The approach is increasingly validated by volumes of evidence from recent research identifying that many chronic metabolic diseases have their origins in the gut. The integrity of the gut lining and the health of microbiota are demonstrated to be involved in contributing to immune-mediated diseases, the inflammatory cascade and chronic diseases such as obesity.[53] Dysbiosis can result in the production of bacterial endotoxins that leak through the gut and contribute to metabolic syndrome once in the circulation, contributing to systemic inflammation and insulin resistance.[54–56] In consideration of microbiome–gut–brain axis aetiologies, the impact of toxic bacterial metabolites are demonstrated in contributing to cognitive impairment, anxiety and depression.[57–59]

Naturopathic practice has often traditionally applied a 'First start with the gut' approach to commencing treatment; one motivation could be to ensure effective elimination by facilitating the removal of accumulated wastes. One means by which this may be achieved is a treatment strategy that involves removing poor dietary habits, increasing fibre and water consumption and deploying probiotics or targeted therapeutics to improve gastrointestinal conditions.

Broader naturopathic treatment planning involves the deployment of a therapeutic order in alignment with the six principles and process of healing previously outlined. The order (outlined below) is specific but not necessarily fixed, being adapted to each patient's current presentation and need for safe and effective treatment strategies that address acute and chronic care considerations. The approach is to begin with minimal intervention and advance to higher levels as necessary.[10]

1. ESTABLISH THE CONDITIONS FOR HEALTH

The importance of determinants of health and the result of challenges to them have been highlighted as core to naturopathic decision making. Disturbing factors are to be identified and removed in consideration of their impact, as guided by the naturopathic principle *Treat the Cause* (*Tolle Causam.*)

In the broader application of treatment the role of naturopathy can be considered in alignment with the principles *Doctor as Teacher* (*Docere*) and *Prevention* (*Preventare*), where the practitioner can promote a healthier regimen with patients and educate them in this. The may involve aspects such as informing about healthier food choices, revising alcohol and/drug consumption, stress management, promoting physical activity and connection with natural environments — *Treat the Whole Person* (*Tolle Totum.*)

2. STIMULATE SELF-HEALING

This order involves the implementation of the *Healing Power of Nature (Vis Medicatrix Naturae),* with consideration of *First Do No Harm* (*Primum Non Nocere.*) This can be understood in relation to the implementation of enhancing strategy via the use of nutraceuticals to stimulate digestive and/or metabolic functions or immunostimulant herbal therapeutics to mitigate infectious conditions. This could be considered as 'trigger-point phytotherapy', implemented in coordination with the first order and 'long-term repair' considerations as practitioners consider immediate needs and develop a treatment plan suited to the patient.[8]

3. SUPPORT WEAKENED OR DAMAGED SYSTEMS

Chronic disease development in the traditional naturopathic process of healing was understood in terms of diminishing vital organ functions, akin to the general adaptation syndrome concept developed by endocrinologist Hans Searle in the late 1930s. The impact of prolonged stress is recognised in relation to dysfunctional physiology or endocrine systems; for example, reduced adrenal function and disruption of the hypothalamic–pituitary–adrenal axis, in which case trophorestorative phytotherapeutics (such as *Glycyrrhiza glabra*) could be considered as part of therapeutic planning at this level of order. Similarly, a damaged and weakened gastrointestinal system could be supported by slippery elm (*Ulmus rubra*), which could act to both alleviate inflammatory symptoms while also supporting the repair of mucous membranes in the gut.

4. CORRECT STRUCTURAL INTEGRITY

Structural problems in the body may be considered in naturopathic treatment in relation to prescribing exercise activities and/or physical therapies such as remedial soft-tissue massage. An example of implementing structural integrity into treatment could include recommending certain stretching methods or remedial mid-back treatments to address misalignment (T1–T12) issues often associated with underlying stress on digestive organs and diminished function.[30] Where the techniques are beyond the training and scope of practice of individual naturopaths, referral to physical therapists such as chiropractors, osteopaths or musculoskeletal therapists is coordinated.

5. ADDRESS PATHOLOGY USING SPECIFIC NATURAL SUBSTANCES

Patients have often experienced benefit from therapeutic interventions via the first four orders of the treatment hierarchy. Chronic conditions and limited progression towards health from previous interventions may be considered in parallel to incoming pathology results that inform differential diagnosis. Breaking a case down in this manner and implementing a pathology-specific treatment in naturopathic treatment is not generally preferred; however, the contemporary practice of the modality has increased accessibility to diagnostic tools, and modern therapeutics are demonstrated to achieve consistent high-quality results in addressing specific pathophysiologies.

This could involve the use of a specific phytotherapeutic demonstrated to be effective against a particular pathogen, such as using the antibiotic efficacy of peppermint oil (*Mentha x piperita*) in addressing intestinal dysbiosis involving *Escherichia coli*.[60] This approach is sometimes referred to as 'green allopathy', where a natural antimicrobial is substituted for a pharmaceutical equivalent in a targeted effort to resolve a pathology on behalf of the host. This can extend to the implementation of other compensatory strategies to address presenting symptomatic complaints; for example, the use of anti-inflammatory phytotherapeutics (such as *Curcuma longa*) in initial treatment. In alleviating symptoms it is important to recognise that, without deployment in a holistic manner involving the initial steps of the naturopathic therapeutic order, results are likely to be transitory.[50]

6. ADDRESS PATHOLOGY USING PHARMACEUTICAL OR SYNTHETIC SUBSTANCES

Misperceptions of contemporary naturopathy endure, including the notion that naturopaths are opposed to any and all pharmaceutical and/or surgical interventions. The naturopathic therapeutic order recognises that such approaches are necessary in circumstances to preserve life and limb. In the case of naturopathic physicians, the ability to prescribe pharmaceuticals may be within scope of practice (as relevant in accordance with their training and statutory regulation). The choice to take such a path is in accordance with the therapeutic order and is implemented as relevant to safely protect patient health and influence recovery.[30]

Similarly where naturopaths are not trained to prescribe pharmaceuticals, treatment of patients involves respectful recognition of currently prescribed medical treatments and prohibits recommendations to circumvent or modify. Accordingly, naturopaths refer to relevant medical services at all times when and where required by presenting patient circumstances. In advancing patient-centric care naturopaths standardly seek to work in an integrative medical model with general practitioners, medical specialists and allied health professionals, involving interprofessional communication and collaborations wherever possible.

7. EMPLOY SURGICAL CORRECTION AND 'HIGHER FORCE' THERAPIES

Employing surgical intervention and other therapies such as chemo- and/or radiotherapy is recognised as the last line of the therapeutic order, in both naturopathic and conventional medicine. As with the previous step in the order, naturopathic physicians in some jurisdictions may perform minor surgical procedures as do general practitioners. More broadly, naturopaths are not directly involved in the decision making and deployment of surgery or 'higher force' therapies, but act to support the medical treatments being undertaken by patients. Contemporary naturopathy is widely recognised to be a useful complementary therapy in support of pre- and postoperative surgical recovery and in integrative oncology treatments. It is crucial to establish interprofessional communication in collaborative patient healthcare for such complicated circumstances, ensuring that the timing and deployment of therapeutics are effective and patients are informed of potential interactions.

Deploying naturopathic treatment

Just as initial engagement and consultations are guided by individual clinic practices, systems and patient record documentation, so too is the deployment of naturopathic treatment strategies and individual prescriptions supplied following consultations. The layout of clinic spaces may inform how prescriptions are organised. A dispensary separate from the consulting room can give the practitioner time and space to review and verify various therapeutics, checking for possible contraindications, drug interactions and optimal doses in the process. Other practitioners may dispense from the consultation room itself, with the process as part of their consultation method.

Initial and follow-up consultation forms may feature a prescription section at the end of the document, possibly broken down to include various sections such as lifestyle and/or exercise recommendations, diet plans, nutrient supplements and/or phytotherapeutic prescriptions detailing doses and consumption advice. Alternatively, recommendations and prescriptions may be provided with use of carbon-copy pads that are used to supply the patient with a copy simultaneously. Regardless of paperwork, clinic software or other dispensing systems used, it is crucial that all prescription information from each consultation is recorded and can be effectively aligned with patient records.

All treatment information supplied to patients must be legible and in accessible language that avoids jargon. The process of providing and explaining treatments to patients again necessitates effective communication skills, ensuring that the individual patient (or their guardian) is clear on the appropriate dosage and implementation of therapeutics. All information supplied should include clinic and practitioner details, specifying contact information and clear guidance in relation to ceasing treatment and/or contacting the practitioner as required. Increasingly, clinic software and practitioner websites may provide an effective means to distribute information, which can be customised for individual patients, tracked via their records and support the practitioner's intellectual property.

Planning long-term treatment strategies and the aligned supply of information at appropriate conjectures is an important element of deploying naturopathic treatment. In providing information to patients be conscious of their ability and enthusiasm to engage so as to ensure that they are not overloaded. Similarly it is not necessary to overload patients with the full specifications of your treatment strategy; be mindful of the SMART principles in providing information for current recommendations and the broader approach. Practitioners may track a patient's various conditions and symptoms on software or a spreadsheet, supporting the tracking of treatments over consultations and ensuring that secondary issues are not forgotten by practitioners over time.

INTRODUCTION TO CASE STUDIES

Throughout this text as various body systems and lifecycle stages are reviewed, associated pathologies and naturopathic approaches are detailed. For each there is a brief case study provided that highlights an example of patient presentation, with relevant diagnostics and naturopathic treatments outlined. In addition to the Overview and Treatment Protocol sections consistently presented in that text, the following case study will include additional rationale elements that serve to illustrate the principles introduced in this chapter.

The case is aligned to the first four conditions of the text, those being:

- Food allergy and hypersensitivity
- Irritable bowel syndrome
- Ulcerative colitis
- Crohn's disease.

These conditions may have a similar initial presentation. The purpose here is to focus on the initial and follow-up consultation processes, considering differential diagnosis and treatment planning. Later case studies will be scaffolded by the preceding introduction to the system and will not require the contextualisation and detailed narrative that is provided for the following introduction case.

CASE STUDY

OVERVIEW

A patient booking is received via email and the initial consultation is booked for the following week. The patient is currently working overseas in South-East Asia and is not able to supply further details via the patient intake form that is standardly supplied and returned by new patients to your clinic.

The information available at present is as follows:

Steven is 37 years old and has been experiencing lower abdominal pain on and off for the past few months. It commenced with a bout of bloody diarrhoea, which has persisted with alternating periods of diarrhoea and constipation since. He has been treated initially with a course of antibiotics and continues with a prescription of Imodium to address episodes of diarrhoea. He has consistently been taking pain medication, tablets with ibuprofen plus codeine, to manage severe episodes of pain. Steven is returning home for a few weeks before returning to work overseas. He is concerned by weight loss and the impact that diarrhoea is having on his work performance.

PRE-CONSULTATION CONSIDERATIONS

Although there may not be the opportunity to have the initial consultation informed by a complete patient intake form, there is a significant volume of detail that can be used to inform preparation for the initial consultation. There are a number of insights that may already assist in narrowing considerations of the possible pathologies involved, in turn informing lines of enquiry that a practitioner could prepare for. In consideration of the patient returning overseas in a few weeks, efforts could be made to ensure relevant diagnostic and treatment resources are available for the initial consultation with Steven — whom you are already aware is work and performance focused.

For example, consideration of South-East Asian travel and the initial condition could indicate a novel microbial infection — this could inform preparation to ensure kit is

CASE STUDY CONTINUED

available to expedite pathology for a comprehensive diagnostic stool analysis. Practitioners may also ensure the dispensary is currently stocked with a specific probiotic product and/or antimicrobial phytotherapeutic. Some may also consider investigating contact with a travel specialist medical clinic in the area in case coordination of referral and/or collaboration is required — this would be of particular importance if it is revealed through consultation that Steven is experiencing ongoing blood in stools.

The experience of the practitioner may impact on their preliminary considerations and efforts to prepare for this initial consultation. A novice practitioner may choose to undertake further reading in relation to South-East Asian gastrointestinal infections and prepare with various diagnostic tools in advance. Fig. 5.6 outlines some thinking that could occur prior to the first consultation in this case, guiding enquiry and planning for the session (with shorthand abbreviated notes and prompts.)

INITIAL CONSULTATION

Your initial consultation is 90 minutes; you commence your session with Steven by enquiring about his current work project and time spent in South-East Asia, opening dialogue and rapport. Steven explains that he is a civil engineer who is project managing the development of a new industrial precinct in northern Indonesia. He has consulted for similar projects previously, yet this is his first time as lead for such a large project. He travelled to the region 3 months ago and has been working primarily in Indonesia since, with trips to Malaysia and Thailand also during the period.

He is enjoying the challenge, but is finding adapting to company catering and local food difficult as he is a fussy eater. Steven expressed frustration at the ongoing health issues he is experiencing and the lack of results achieved through the medical treatment he has so far received from the company doctor on site overseas. His work has organised for him to see a travel specialist GP, who he is booked to see in the coming days. His wife had also encouraged him to see a naturopath. He adds that this is his first engagement with a CAM practitioner. He is cautious with regard to the possible costs related with naturopathic consultations and treatment; you are able to explain your processes with him and highlight his involvement in all decision making prior to organisation of diagnostics or prescriptions.

Much can be revealed as the patient expresses themselves in this opening dialogue, both through explicit information and less formal inferences. Steven has revealed himself to be a logically minded and results-focused professional, and this will have an impact on his communication preferences and expectations from treatment. In building trust and rapport the initial tactic of the consultation would best involve a directed line of questioning and physical examination, as opposed to opening with acknowledgement of the emotional considerations related to stress and separation from family. It is a presumption but it could be considered that a person like Steven may be more likely to open up in relation to emotional factors at the end of a consultation, following logical enquiry, diagnostics and discussion related to his upcoming specialist GP appointment (about whom you are well-informed, following your initial

CASE STUDY CONTINUED

preparations and review of local travel health medical services available).

Subjective enquiry

A practitioner's questioning regarding Steven's history of the presenting illness could follow the SAMPLE line of enquiry and involve OLD CHARTS pain clarification questioning. The symptoms of diarrhoea and pain do not feature significantly prior to the past 3 months, Steven stated in his own words that he is a particularly fussy eater and that he had occasionally experienced upset digestion when he lost employment several years ago. The initial bout of diarrhoea was experienced with mild fever 2 weeks after working in Indonesia, was especially watery and lasted for several days with some blood in stools encountered at the end. He was treated at the time with a full course of antibiotics (ciprofloxacin) and the antidiarrhoeal Imodium, which appeared to resolve the initial disturbance within several days. No watery diarrhoea, rectal bleeding or blood in stools has been encountered since.

The onset of the condition did not follow a particular meal and was not associated with colleagues becoming ill. Steven had been eating primarily from the company-provided catering, which is largely akin to a basic Western diet that he is accustomed to. On further questioning it was confirmed that he had been exclusively drinking bottled water, black espresso coffee, no tea and consuming 1 or 2 beers most evenings. On further questioning there was one night before the illness where he did visit a bar and had a cocktail. (He was not sure of the source of the ice used.)

The pain commenced suddenly with the first bout of diarrhoea and reappeared again 1–2 weeks after all other symptoms had subsided. He had taken Imodium at the time of the initial bout and recommenced this when pain and mild diarrhoea recommenced (noting that he had been somewhat

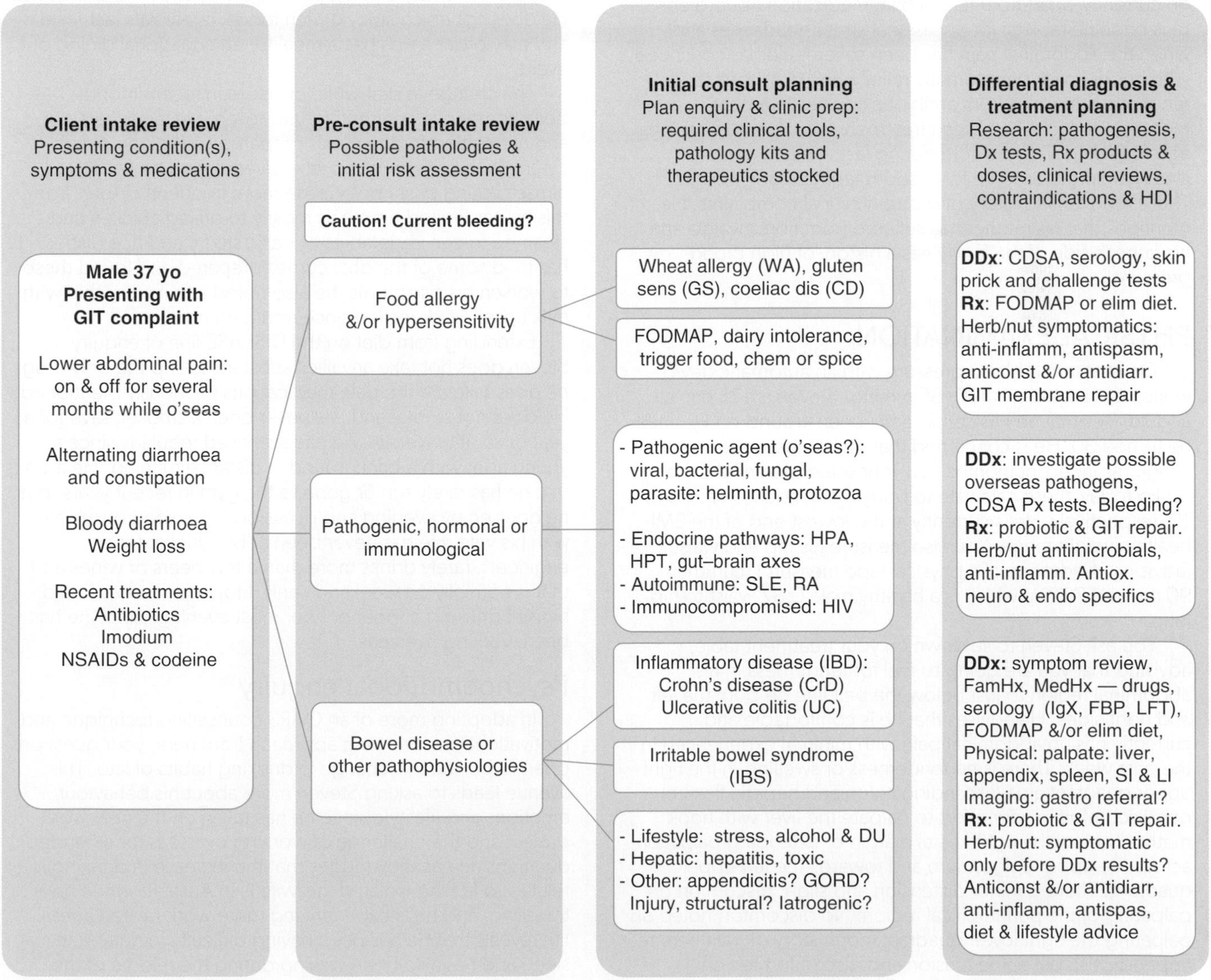

FIGURE 5.6 Case study: patient intake and possible pre-consultation considerations

CASE STUDY CONTINUED

constipated during this period). After a couple of days of the second bout Steven visited the onsite GP and a second round of ciprofloxacin was prescribed, again relieving all symptoms within several days. Electrolyte solutions were provided during treatment of the initial and secondary bouts also.

Ongoing episodes involving pain are generally occurring once or twice a month and last for several days; no trigger foods or events have been distinctly noticed. The onset of pain is generally sudden. It is a severe cramping (colic) pain that starts centrally in the lower abdomen and sometimes then focuses in the left lower abdomen. It is not experienced every day or week and is noted to occur when stool patterns change, when stools loosen before diarrhoea bouts reoccur. Increased abdominal bloating and flatus are noticed during bouts. Defecating relieves the pain somewhat. He last ate breakfast several hours ago and passed motions the evening of the day before yesterday.

Steven has no known allergies to medications or foods that he is aware of. He has no other medications that he is on currently, apart from taking pain medication (ibuprofen plus codeine tablets) for occasional stress headaches and when the abdominal pain has been severe. He has continued with Imodium for symptomatic relief when diarrhoea bouts recommence. Apart from antibiotic courses in recent months, the last time of such treatment was about 12 months ago following a severe cold during last winter. No major illness or surgeries, save for wisdom teeth surgery at age 21. There is no family history of gastrointestinal complaints. He mentions that his mother has suffered from fibromyalgia and his father's side of the family has a history of high blood pressure.

PHYSICAL EXAMINATION

On measuring blood pressure with an automatic device while he is seated it is 130/85 mmHg. Steven is 175 cm tall and advises that he has consistently been around 65 kg since he turned 30. He is concerned that he has lost several kilograms in recent months. On your scales he weighs in at 62 kg today, these calculate to body mass indexes of 21 and 19, respectively. He is currently at the lowest end of the BMI healthy weight range. You also measure his hip and waist (advising in advance of a physical tape measure), currently 90 cm and 78 cm, which is a healthy male 0.87 waist-to-hip ratio.

You ask Steven to lie down on your treatment table, advising that you are going to feel for tenderness in his abdominal region to just below the belt line on both the left and right sides. He advises that he is comfortable and currently has no abdominal pain with minimal experienced in the past week. There is no tenderness or swelling in the right upper quadrant area (ascending colon and hepatic flexure), nor discomfort in your effort to palpate the liver with hook method below the right costal margin or extending palpation across the upper epigastrium and towards the left upper quadrant. There is minor distension and slight discomfort on palpating of the periumbilical region. No discomfort noted on palpating the right lower quadrant (nor history of pain here re: appendicitis), but some tension and discomfort felt on palpation of the left lumbar region extending down to the left iliac region.

CASE STUDY CONTINUED

Dietary investigation

It's about 30 minutes into your consultation and you both return to seating around your desk as you commence the dietary investigation. In brief Steven provides insight into his normal daily intake; he prefaces again by highlighting he is a 'fussy' or non-adventurous eater with a 'meat and three veg' family background. He has never been a big breakfast eater, tending towards juice and coffee normally in his adult life. He will often have a banana, muesli bar or a yoghurt around morning tea time, followed by another coffee. He has up to 3 or 4 espresso coffees each day; he consciously drinks up to 2 litres of water during the day.

Steven does not eat a lot of bread. His lunch is normally a salad with chicken or left-overs from the previous evening meal. He does continue with red meat, mash and steamed vegetables as a staple dinner meal, varying with grilled chicken with vegetables or fish and garden salad. Steven is active in the kitchen and alternates cooking meals with his wife, who he appreciates is more adventurous and often prepares Asian-style meals such as stir fry with noodles or rice. He does not enjoy spicy or rich foods, rarely eats fast food and may order a rich pasta meal for an occasional dining out event.

The change in diet while overseas in recent months has been somewhat confronting for Steven. He rarely eats out and has settled for the meals prepared by the company's caterers. This has involved little diversity and he has found himself eating pasta bolognese more frequently. Apart from this he has limited his meals mostly to grilled chicken and steamed frozen vegetables or basic stir fry and rice dishes. He has tried some of the dhal curries prepared and found these to worsen his symptoms; he also noted a fruit smoothie with milk upset his digestion since returning home.

Extending from diet on the DISEASE line of enquiry, Steven does not take any illicit substances and the only drugs he does take are the pain medications previously mentioned. He does not smoke and has never been a smoker, save for a year or so at university. He has exercised regularly since a young age, with a background in distance running. He admits that he has rarely run or gone to the gym in recent years, but he does enjoy evening and occasional weekend bushwalks with his wife. He has never been a 'big drinker for an engineer', rarely drinks more than a few beers or wines and that is normally on weekends only. However, he has found himself drinking a 'beer or two' most evenings since he has been working overseas.

Psychoemotional enquiry

In adopting more of an OARS counselling technique and motivational interviewing approach from here, your questions open to pursue this change in drinking habits of late. This avenue leads to asking Steven more about his behaviour, emotions and lifestyle since he has taken on the new work project and the challenge of working overseas for extended durations. He acknowledges that the increase in drinking is related to feeling isolated (his wife is in Australia when he is travelling) and he is experiencing more work-related stress. He reveals that he has been having difficulty in getting to sleep and has also been waking during the middle of the night, leaving him fatigued and depressed at the end of most days.

CASE STUDY CONTINUED

With affirmation that you appreciate the difficulty in discussing these challenges, Steven continues to open up and reveals that he has been increasingly anxious during the day at work and especially since his health has been inconsistent. You are able to extend with a couple of additional questions related to broader family circumstances, relationship status and finance concerns. In reflecting and summarising back to Steven there is agreement that these factors are weighing on his mind daily, compounded by work pressures and being distant from his network of friends. In the process you are able to provide assurances, highlighting that this is an important aspect of the holistic approach of naturopathy in providing treatment and supporting his return to good health.

Diagnostic considerations

Entering into the final 30 minutes of the initial consultation you have been able to consolidate a clearer picture of the presenting condition, influencing factors and the underlying circumstances of the patient. This all serves to inform differential diagnosis considerations from here, being able to draft a therapeutic strategy that encompasses options for initial pathology testing and treatments. The flowchart for differential diagnosis of gluten-related disorders presented earlier in Fig. 5.3 is one diagnostic avenue that could prove helpful in narrowing focus for immediate actions: wheat allergy, gluten sensitivity or coeliac disease could be the pathophysiology of this case. This is relevant given the dietary changes and increased pasta consumption during the period of illness.

The subjective information acquired early in the consultation does tend to indicate that an infectious agent may have first triggered the gastrointestinal issues and catalysed ongoing symptomatic presentations. The periodic nature of the bouts of diarrhoea, aligning with the timing and clarified experience of the pain do align with the Rome III criteria as detailed later in the diagnosis of irritable bowel syndrome (IBS). In combination with other presenting factors such as stress and indications of alteration to gut flora, IBS leads as the most likely pathophysiology at play ahead of inflammatory bowel diseases (IBD) such as ulcerative colitis and Crohn's disease. Initial pathology testing and treatments are best focused towards IBS as opposed to food sensitivities alone or IBD.

In explaining your initial interpretation and various pathology options to Steven it is possible to consider ways in which ergonomic and more affordable solutions may be possible in collaboration with his planned engagement with the travel specialist medical services. For instance, you are aware that blood pathology and stool analysis are likely avenues to be pursued by a specialist GP. It may be possible to have these diagnostics performed via this medical service, which is to be reimbursed by Steven's company and/or under public health fee scheduling.

This is not likely a consideration for naturopathic physicians who provide primary healthcare medical services as part of their training and status, but it may be an integrative approach considered by naturopaths in other regions where coordination of pathology tests may be at additional expense to patients. In approaching this as an option it would be relevant to detail that you are interested in conducting various blood tests (such as full blood count, iron studies, vitamin B_{12} status, liver function, C-reactive protein and gliadin antibodies) as well as a comprehensive diagnostic stool analysis with parasitology (CDSA/Px1 or Px3), relevant in consideration of water-borne parasitic infections (such as *Entamoeba histolytica*, *Giardia lamblia* and *Schistosoma japonicum*) which are prevalent in undeveloped regions of Indonesia.[61–63]

In this effort, you can explain to Steven that pathology costs may be mitigated and that you welcome a collaborative integrative treatment approach that is centred on his health outcomes. This serves to respect his initial concerns expressed in relation to naturopathic treatment costs, acknowledge the financial pressures impacting on health raised during the consultation and continue to build trust and rapport. You can explain to Steven that you can order these tests now if preferred, he can leave with the order form and CDSA kit and choose to organise following his GP consult or the tests may be ordered by the GP with results to be forwarded to yourself when available (which can be supported by a referral letter to the GP, detailing your pathology test considerations).

The affordable option of a blood spot gluten sensitivity test can be presented as a diagnostic that can be undertaken in this session, being useful in expediting insight into the status of some gliadin antibodies in advance of the broader serology results from a blood test. It is most likely that practitioners would recommend an elimination or low FODMAP diet in this initial consultation as both a differential diagnosis process and effort to reduce inflammation in the initial dietary treatment of the presenting condition. Naturopathic diagnostics including iridology and other observations of hair, skin, nail, eyes and tongue may also be performed at this stage.

TREATMENT PROTOCOL

The implementation of an elimination and/or low FODMAP diet at this stage is valuable in helping to reduce factors contributing to the condition and serving to identify possible allergens or sensitivities in the first weeks of treatment in this case. The elimination would include recommendations to avoid lactose and fructose, as these short-chain carbohydrates may have poor absorption and contribute to diarrhoea via osmotic effect. (Recollect the fruit smoothie that Steven mentioned upset his system when consumed recently.) Legumes, beans, onion and wheat also present short-chain carbohydrates that may be fermenting due to dysbiosis and in turn create intestinal gas and pain.

Removing these potential irritants is a first therapeutic order intervention in establishing the conditions for health. Advising reduced use of non-steroidal anti-inflammatory drugs and codeine could also serve to mitigate NSAID gastrointestinal irritation and opioid-induced constipation. Other dietary modifications to implement at this stage would include the elimination of alcohol and coffee, substituting with alternatives such as lemon, lime and bitters in the place of beer, and peppermint and chamomile teas in the place of coffee. All these substitute options also serve to stimulate digestion and/or ameliorate gastrointestinal symptoms being encountered and are a second order intervention in stimulating self-healing.

CASE STUDY CONTINUED

Other therapeutic functional foods may be included in the low inflammatory diet, such as carrots and small amounts of sweet potato that are high in beta-carotene and serve to repair intestinal walls. Oats (steel-cut or rolled) are another food that may provide multiple benefits; although containing a small amount of fructose, the bran provides soluble fibre to mitigate constipation and mucilage to soothe and heal intestinal linings. Oats are high in iron to replenish lost stores following blood loss and infection, with fatty acids, lecithin, phosphorous and vitamin B_{12} all nourishing the nervous system. Oats (*Avena sativa*) are also useful for IBS as the compound avenine acts as a phytotherapeutic nervous sedative, this nervine action of oats is useful in alleviating anxiety and depression. Encouraging the use of oats in Steven's diet is of additional benefit as *Avena sativa* has been demonstrated to be effective in lowering arterial hypertension, addressing his slightly high blood pressure at present and ongoing predisposition in familial history.

HERBAL MEDICINE

Slippery elm (*Ulmus rubra*) is another phytotherapeutic that is especially high in mucilage and can be considered to work at the third therapeutic order level, supporting transition through the weakened digestive system, removing toxins and simultaneously repairing damaged intestinal walls. The mucilage of *Ulmus rubra* is so high that it must be considered in safe prescribing due to the potential for herb–drug interaction, with its absorbent capacity reducing the efficacy of other ingested medicines. *Ulmus rubra* can be prescribed at 1 tablespoon/day during periods of constipation or reduced to 1 teaspoon/day during bouts of diarrhoea. It is best taken mixed in water or orange juice (low FODMAP permissible) and is advised to be taken at least 2 hours away from ingesting other medications (pharmaceutical, herbal or nutritional), first thing in the morning may be optimal.

An antidiarrhoeal herbal formula could be tailored for Steven, for use pre-emptively in advance and during episodic bouts (in trial as a substitute for Imodium as currently used). The formula would contain spasmolytic, carminative, nervine and astringent liquid extract (LE) herbs (the extraction ratios of LE are displayed in the formulas): 5 mL to be taken 3 times a day: mid-morning, pre-lunch and pre-dinner.

Viburnum opulus	1:2 LE 20 mL
Matricaria chamomilla	1:2 LE 30 mL
Humulus lupus	1:2 LE 25 mL
Agrimonia eupatoria	1:2 LE 20 mL
Zingiber officinalis	1:2 LE 5 mL

Peppermint (*Mentha x piperita*) oil has been demonstrated to be of direct benefit for IBS, in fifth level therapeutic order intervention addressing microbial infection as a phytotherapeutic antibiotic.[60] In addition to this direct effect peppermint oil also performs symptomatic relief via its phytotherapeutic actions as a spasmolytic, carminative and chologogue. Peppermint oil could be deployed in capsules prepared with other antimicrobial essential oils such as the selective antimicrobial caraway (*Carum carvi*) seed oil, which is recognised not to impact beneficial bacteria.[64]

CASE STUDY CONTINUED

Myrrh (*Commiphora molmol*) is an additional phytotherapeutic that could be added to the antimicrobial capsules, demonstrated effective as a powerful broad-spectrum antimicrobial, effective against methicillin resistant *Staphylococcus aureus* (MRSA), enterocolitis and a range of parasitic infections such as schistosomiasis.[65,66] Various naturopathic antimicrobial products exist in the market; such formulations are frequently deployed in a 'Weed and Seed' approach that features phased alternating deployment with probiotic supplements in an effort to eliminate undesired bacteria and replenish the microbiome with beneficial bacteria in therapeutic doses.

NUTRITIONAL MEDICINE

The restoration of beneficial microflora is the initial focus of nutritional supplementation efforts, coordinated with the restorative dietary approaches previously detailed. Probiotic formulas may be deployed by themselves or in combination with prebiotic nutritional support that may include lactulose, galacto-oligosaccharides (GOS) and fructo-oligosaccharides (FOS). Multi-strain probiotics are shown to be specifically effective in the treatment of IBS, in addition to their generally restorative function suitable in the treatment of broader gastrointestinal conditions.[67,68]

Initial probiotic prescribing requires caution as they may result in digestive upset, gas and/or bloating with pain in some individuals. The phased deployment with phytotherapeutic antimicrobials may be structured so that the 'weeding' occurs on weekends and 'seeding' is deployed during the week only. The treatment following the initial consultation may be deployed with a request for Steven to maintain a daily journal, recording any symptomatic events in conjunction with a food diary that could be supported by pain and/or stool measurement charts. There are various applications that may facilitate these efforts; their use would be appropriate for a patient with the capabilities and focus such as Steven has. The treatment information you supply provides clear direction and details the planning for the restrictive diet to be undertaken for the fortnight ahead, followed by efforts to gradually reintroduce foods in the following weeks.

Second consultation

The first follow-up consultation is booked for 2 weeks' time, with an hour reserved for the next session. Diagnostic results may be received prior to the next consult and the opportunity to review in advance can again inform diagnostic and treatment planning for the next session. An email is received from Steven within the first week: he did experience a minor flare-up of diarrhoea and pain for 1 day — which was resolved without use of Imodium in this instance. He also advised that full blood pathology and CDSA with parasitology tests were organised in his consultation with the GP.

You receive the results of both your blood spot gluten sensitivity test and the bloodwork from the GP a few days in advance of your next consultation with Steven. The sensitivity test did not present any antibody (IgA or IgG) markers for either gluten or gliadin. The other results indicated normal white blood cell counts and liver function test results, and the blood panel did not have any other indications save for low in

CASE STUDY CONTINUED

normal range results for ferritin (the order did not include total iron binding capacity [TIBC], vitamin B_{12} or gliadin antibody testing). The CDSA/Px3 results are not expected to be returned for at least another week.

Your follow-up consultation with Steven is focused on reviewing the journal documentation he has supplied and discussing his response to the prescribed diet and initial treatments. Save for the minor episode encountered for a day in the first week there have been no significant pain or bouts of diarrhoea in the past fortnight. Some discomfort with gas and bloating was experienced at various times through the period, recognised to occur at times of switching between the antimicrobial and probiotic phases. Steven found the limited diet to be challenging, but was compliant for most of the time.

TREATMENT PROTOCOL

The focus for the next fortnight is to continue with intestinal repair, increasing the dose of probiotics to be now consumed daily. The reintroduction of excluded foods is discussed, highlighting the potential for symptoms to flare up in the challenge phase of the process. It is advised that one food group be introduced for a day with results to be recorded in the journal, followed by a day without challenge. A food plan is drafted, detailing where dairy is to be introduced one day with a banana smoothie for breakfast and then cheese in the afternoon if no issues are experienced. A day break and then a test of honey with oats for breakfast the next day, introduction of a FODMAP limited fruit on another, garlic and onion in a stir fry on another day, and toast and pasta later in the fortnight.

In discussing challenge testing with Steven you present the option of lactulose/mannitol breath test diagnostics to be organised in the fortnight ahead, as a means to test intestinal permeability. He advises that this was part of the planning recommended by the GP, who awaits the results of the CDSA before their confirmation of any possible prescription or coordination of additional diagnostics, which could include a colonoscopy examination. Steven is eager to organise as much as possible before returning overseas in a few weeks, yet he is cautious in extending treatment strategies in advance of further insights arising from pathology results.

You advise that it is possible to continue with the current naturopathic treatment strategy, working to restore gastrointestinal tract integrity, improving microbiome culture and digestive function. You advise that you are able to continue support in the months ahead, with the ability to engage in teleconsulting and dispatch of therapeutics overseas. It is ideal that you have undertaken the initial consultations in person, being able to perform physical examination, make direct observations and build a solid rapport in the process. This is another example of how traditional naturopathy principles robustly endure in contemporary clinical practice, which is increasingly sophisticated and conscious in the adoption of new technologies to support holistic healthcare services.

Herbal medicine

The initial antidiarrhoeal formula is repeated and supplied to again be taken daily in the fortnight ahead, with the option to gradually reduce from three doses to as-needed. Recipes for the introduction of turmeric (*Curcuma longa*) into the daily regimen are provided, with a high bioavailability curcumin capsule recommended to be taken once daily for anti-inflammatory benefit and mitigation of visceral hypersensitivity.[69,70]

Nutritional medicine

You supply a ferric iron formula and sublingual B_{12} tablets at this consultation also, with explanation of their benefits in consideration of recent poor absorption and other indicators you have observed. Probiotic dose is to be increased, discontinuing with antimicrobial 'weeding' at the current moment (pending further insights from CDSA/Px3 results.) Additional dietary advice and recipes are supplied, with additional prebiotic food and yoghurt product advice also provided. This is supplied in parallel with extending recommendations for establishing daily routines for physical activity and stress management exercises.

This narrated case has ideally provided insights into the implementation of communication and case-taking techniques as critically deployed in strategic diagnostics and treatment planning. There are clearly still several unknowns in relation to the exact pathophysiologies involved with this case. It has, however, been possible to advance a reasoned naturopathic treatment strategy in the interim. The decision-making framework presented provides a measure of consistency in the deployment of naturopathy principles within the contemporary clinic environment of the modern profession. The approach facilitates the ability for practitioners to be agile in their own clinical practices, supporting the capability to design and deploy customised treatments that are well informed and suited to the unique circumstances of each person in their care.

REFERENCES

[1] Walker B. Davidson's principles and practice of medicine. 22nd ed. Edinburgh: Churchill Livingstone; 2014.

[2] The United Nations. Universal Declaration of Human Rights. 1948.

[3] United Nations Office of High Commissioner for Human Rights. The right to privacy in the Digital Age. New York: OHCHR; 2014. Available from: www.ohchr.org/EN/Issues/DigitalAge/Pages/DigitalAgeIndex.aspx.

[4] Office of the Australian Information Commissioner. Privacy fact sheet 17: Australian privacy principles. Canberra: OAIC; 2014. Available from: www.oaic.gov.au/individuals/privacy-fact-sheets/general/privacy-fact-sheet-17-australian-privacy-principles.

[5] Office of the Australian Information Commissioner. Business resource. Handling health information under the Privacy Act: a general overview for health service providers. Canberra: OAIC; 2014. Available from: www.oaic.gov.au/engage-with-us/consultations/health-privacy-guidance/business-resource-handling-health-information-under-the-privacy-act-a-general-overview-for-health-service-providers.

[6] Zetler J, Bonello R. Essentials of law, ethics and professional issues for CAM. Sydney: Churchill Livingstone; 2012.

[7] Lord D. Person-centred care and naturopathy: patient beliefs and values. Aust J Herb Med 2015;27(4):132–4.

[8] Bone K, Mills S. Principles and practices of phytotherapy. 2nd ed. Sydney: Churchill Livingstone; 2013.

[9] Stock-Schröer B, Huber R, Joos S, et al. Are students of health professions in Germany interested in naturopathy and complementary medicine? Europ J Int Med 2015;7:51.

[10] Fleming S, Gutknecht N. Naturopathy and the primary care practice. Prim Care 2010;37(1):119–36.
[11] Singer J, Adams J. Integrating complementary and alternative medicine into mainstream healthcare services: the perspectives of health service managers. BMC Complement Altern Med 2014;14:167.
[12] Jagtenberg T, Evans S, Grant A, et al. Evidence-based medicine and naturopathy. J Altern Complement Med 2006;12(3):323–8.
[13] Connelly E, Elmer P, Morris C, et al. The Vanguard Faculty program: research training for complementary and alternative medicine faculty. J Altern Complement Med 2010;16(10):1117–23.
[14] Zwickey H, Schiffke H, Fleishman S, et al. Teaching evidence-based medicine at complementary and alternative medicine institutions: strategies, competencies, and evaluation. J Altern Complement Med 2014;20(12):925–31.
[15] Steel A, Adams J. The interface between tradition and science: Naturopaths' perspectives of modern practice. J Altern Complement Med 2011;17(10):967–72.
[16] Morgan S, Yoder L. A concept analysis of person-centered care. J Holist Nurs 2012;30:6–15.
[17] Franzel B, Schwiegershausen M, Heusser P, et al. Individualised medicine from the perspectives of patients using complementary therapies: A meta-ethnography approach. BMC Complement Altern Med 2013;13:124.
[18] Foley H, Steel A. Patient perceptions of clinical care in complementary medicine: a systematic review of the consultation experience. Patient Educ Couns 2017;100(2):212–23.
[19] Geldard D, Geldard K. Basic personal counselling: A training manual for counsellors. 7th ed. Sydney: Pearson; 2012.
[20] University of Adelaide. Active listening learning guide. [PDF online]. Adelaide: UA; 2014. Available from: www.adelaide.edu.au/writingcentre/learning_guides/learningGuide_activeListening.pdf.
[21] Leach M. The naturopathic process: a framework for naturopathic practice. J Aust Trad Med Soc 2008;14(1):7–10.
[22] O'Toole G. Communication: core interpersonal skills for health professionals. 3rd ed. Sydney: Elsevier; 2009.
[23] Miller R, Rollnick S. Motivational interviewing: preparing people for change. 2nd ed. New York: Guilford Press; 2002.
[24] Hall K, Gibbie T, Lubman S. Motivational interviewing techniques: facilitating behaviour change in the general practice setting. Aust Fam Physician 2012;41(9):660–7.
[25] Leach M. Clinical decision making in complementary and alternative medicine. Sydney: Churchill Livingstone; 2010.
[26] Academy of Nutrition and Dietetics. NCP101: What is the nutrition care model? Chicago: AND; 2016. Available from: www.eatrightpro.org/resources/practice/nutrition-care-process/ncp-101.
[27] Bettenburg R, Milliman B, Oberg E, et al. Naturopathic physicians and primary care. In: Goldstein M, Weeks J, editors. Meeting the nation's primary care needs. Washington: Academic Consortium for Complementary and Alternative Health Care (ACCAHC); 2013. Available from: www.naturalmedicinejournal.com/sites/default/files/ACCAHC.pdf.
[28] Conway P. The consultation in phytotherapy: the herbal medicine practitioner's approach to the patient. London: Churchill Livingston; 2011.
[29] Galvin K, Bishop M. Case studies for complementary therapists: a collaborative approach. Sydney: Churchill Livingstone; 2011.
[30] Zeff J, Snider P, Myers S, et al. A hierarchy of healing: the therapeutic order — a unifying theory of naturopathic medicine. In: Pizzorno J, Murray M, editors. Textbook of natural medicine. 4th ed. St Louis: Churchill Livingstone; 2013.
[31] Sapone A, Bai J, Ciacci C, et al. Spectrum of gluten-related disorders: consensus on new nomenclature and classification. BMC Med 2012;10:13.
[32] Benner P. From novice to expert. Amer J Nurs 1982;82(3):402–7.
[33] Crespo K, Torres J, Recio M. Reasoning process characteristics in the diagnostic skills of beginner, competent and expert dentists. J Dent Educ 2004;68(12):1235–44.
[34] Sackett D, Rosenberg W, Gray J, et al. Evidence based medicine: what it is and what it isn't. Br Med J 1996;312:71.
[35] Hecht L, Buhse S, Meyer G. Effectiveness of training in evidence-based medicine skills for healthcare professionals: a systematic review. BMC Med Educ 2016;16:103.
[36] Young T, Rohwer A, Volmink J, et al. What are the effects of teaching evidence-based health care (EBHC)? Overview of systematic reviews. PLoS ONE 2014;9(1):e86706.
[37] Braun L, Spitzer O, Tiralongo E, et al. Naturopaths and Western herbalists' attitudes to evidence, regulation, information sources and knowledge about popular complementary medicines. Complement Thera Med 2012;21(1):58–64.
[38] National Herbalists Association of Australia (NHAA). Submission to review of the Australian Government rebate on private health insurance for natural therapies. Sydney: NHAA; 2013. Available from: www.nhaa.org.au/docs/Submissions/NHAA_Private_Health_Insurance_Submission__29_01_2013_.pdf.
[39] Wardle J, Adams J, Lui C-W, et al. Current challenges and future directions for naturopathic medicine in Australia: a qualitative examination of perceptions and experiences from grassroots practice. BMC Complement Altern Med 2013;13:15.
[40] Steel A, Adams J. Approaches to clinical decision-making: a qualitative study of naturopaths. Complement Thera Clin Pract 2011;17(2):81–4.
[41] Evans J. Dual processing accounts of reasoning, judgment and social cognition. Annu Rev Psychol 2008;59:255–78.
[42] Jensen J. Paramedic clinical decision making. Nova Scotia; 2010. Available from: www.australianparamedicalcollege.com.au/learning-material/adv-dip-healthcare/paramedic-clinical-decision-making.pdf.
[43] Benner P. From novice to expert, excellence and power in clinical nursing practice. Menlo Park CA: Addison-Wesley; 1984.
[44] Stolper E, Van de Wiel M, Van Royen P, et al. Gut feelings as a third track in general practitioners' diagnostic reasoning. J Gen Intern Med 2011;26(2):197–203.
[45] Corbin J, Reyna V, Weldon R, et al. How reasoning, judgment, and decision making are colored by gist-based intuition: a fuzzy-trace theory approach. J Appl Res Mem Cogn 2015;4(4):344–55.
[46] Croskerry P. From mindless to mindful practice: cognitive bias and clinical decision making. N Engl J Med 2013;368:2445–8.
[47] Reach G. Simplistic and complex thought in medicine: The rationale for a person-centered care model as a medical revolution. Patient Prefer Adherence 2016;10:449–57.
[48] Heinrich M, Barnes J, Gibbons S, et al. Fundamentals of pharmacognosy and phytotherapy. 2nd ed. London: Churchill Livingstone; 2012.
[49] Lindlahr H. Nature cure: philosophy and practice based on the unity of disease and cure. Miami: Hardpress Publishing; 1913.
[50] Zeff J. Nature cure and the process of healing. Vancouver; 2001. Available from: http://salmoncreekclinic.com/articles-by-dr-zeff/clinical-theory/nature-cure-and-the-process-of-healing.
[51] Australian Institute of Health and Welfare. Leading types of ill health. Canberra: AIHW; 2014. Available from: www.aihw.gov.au/australias-health/2014/ill-health.
[52] Hunter P. The inflammation theory of disease. EMBO Rep 2012;13(11):968–70.
[53] Vajro P, Paolella G, Fasano A. Microbiota and gut-liver axis: a mini-review on their influences on obesity and obesity related liver disease. J Pediatr Gastroenterol Nutr 2013;56(5):461–8.
[54] Jialal I, Rajamani U. Endotoxemia of metabolic syndrome: a pivotal mediator of meta-inflammation. Metab Syndr Relat Disord 2014;12(9):454–6.
[55] Escobedo G, López-Ortiz E, Torres-Castro I. Gut microbiota as a key player in triggering obesity, systemic inflammation and insulin resistance. Rev Invest Clin 2014;66(5):450–9.
[56] He C, Shan Y, Song W. Targeting gut microbiota as a possible therapy for diabetes. Nutr Res 2015;35(5):361–7.
[57] Zhang S, Jiao T, Chen Y, et al. Methylglyoxal induces systemic symptoms of irritable bowel syndrome. PLoS ONE 2014; 9(8):e105307.
[58] Foster J, McVey-Neufeld K. Gut-brain axis: how the microbiome influences anxiety and depression. Trends Neurosci 2013; 36(5):305–12.
[59] Dash S, Clarke G, Berk M, et al. The gut microbiome and diet in psychiatry: Focus on depression. Curr Opin Psychiatry 2015; 28(1):1–6.
[60] Thompson A, Meah D, Ahmed N, et al. Comparison of the antibacterial activity of essential oils and extracts of medicinal and

culinary herbs to investigate potential new treatments for irritable bowel syndrome. BMC Complement Altern Med 2013;13:338.
[61] Lim Y, Vythilingam I. Parasites and their vectors: a special focus on Southeast Asia. Vienna: Springer; 2014.
[62] Dib H, Lu S, Wen S. Prevalence of *Giardia lamblia* with or without diarrhea in South East, South East Asia and the Far East. Parasitol Res 2008;103(2):39–51.
[63] World Health Organization. Schistosomiasis fact sheet. Geneva: WHO; 2016. Available from: www.who.int/mediacentre/factsheets/fs115/en.
[64] Hawrelak J, Cattley T, Myers S. Essential oils in the treatment of intestinal dysbiosis: a preliminary in vitro study. Altern Med Rev 2009;14(4):380–4.
[65] Abdallah E, Khalid A, Ibrahim N. Antibacterial activity of oleo-gum resins of *Commiphora molmol* and *Boswellia papyrifera* against methicillin resistant *Staphylococcus aureus* (MRSA). Sc Res Ess 2009;4(4):351–6.
[66] Tonkal A, Morsy T. An update review on *Commiphora molmol* and related species. J Egypt Soc Parasitol 2008;38:763–96.
[67] Yoon J, Sohn W, Lee O, et al. Effect of multispecies probiotics on irritable bowel syndrome: a randomized, double-blind, placebo-controlled trial. J Gastroenterol Hepatol 2014;29(1):52–9.
[68] Didari T, Mozaffari S, Nikfar S, et al. Effectiveness of probiotics in irritable bowel syndrome: updated systematic review with meta-analysis. World J Gastroenterol 2015;21(10):3072–84.
[69] Dulbecco P, Savarino V. Therapeutic potential of curcumin in digestive diseases. World J Gastroenterol 2013;19(48):9256–70.
[70] Farzaei M, Bahramsoltani R, Abdollahi M, et al. The role of visceral hypersensitivity in irritable bowel syndrome: pharmacological targets and novel treatments. J Neurogastroenterol Motil 2016;22(4):558–74.

6 Interactions

Liesl Blott

WHAT IS A HERB/NUTRIENT–DRUG INTERACTION?

A drug–drug interaction occurs when the pharmacological effect of, or response to, one drug is altered in some way by the concurrent use of another drug.[1,2] This pharmacological principle can be extended to include interactions between drugs and herbal or nutritional medicines. Thus, the use of pharmaceutical medicines in combination with complementary medicines has the potential to alter the usual effect of, or response to, the drug, the herb, the nutrient, or a combination of these agents, with many of these interactions being regarded as clinically significant.[3–11]

Given that there is a meaningful and growing trend towards the use of integrative treatment approaches that incorporate both pharmaceutical and complementary medicines, health practitioners are encouraged to exercise caution and professional discretion so as to reduce the risks of unwanted interactions and negative outcomes.[4,6–12]

POTENTIAL OUTCOMES OF INTERACTIONS

The most important concerns with regards to interactions are that they may result in decreased drug effectiveness or increased drug toxicity.[1,3] The term 'interaction' therefore often has negative connotations; however, interactions may also be beneficial and may lead to an improved therapeutic response or to a decreased risk of adverse effects, or help to reduce the risk of drug-induced nutrient depletions.[2,4]

The key outcomes of herb/nutrient–drug interactions can be summarised as follows:[1,4,6]

1. Interactions may potentially increase the risk of drug toxicity due to increased absorption or decreased metabolism of drugs or other agents
2. Interactions may potentially reduce drug efficacy and therapeutic benefits due to decreased absorption or increased metabolism of drugs or other agents
3. Interactions may lead to an increased likelihood or greater severity of adverse effects due to similar adverse effect profiles
4. Interactions may lead to enhanced therapeutic benefits or disease outcomes due to additive or synergistic effects
5. Interactions may lead to reduced therapeutic effects due to antagonistic pharmacological actions
6. Use of certain medications may lead to depletions of or increased demand for certain nutrients.

CLASSIFICATION OF DRUG INTERACTIONS

Drug interactions are usually broadly classified as either pharmacodynamic or pharmacokinetic, based on the underlying pharmacological mechanisms governing the interaction.[5] Drug–disease interactions may also occur, although less commonly.[2–4]

Pharmacodynamic herb/nutrient–drug interactions refer to interactions where the intrinsic action of the herbal or nutritional medicine either antagonises or enhances the activity of the pharmaceutical medicine.[4,6,8]

Pharmacokinetic herb/nutrient–drug interactions refer to interactions where the combination of herbal or nutritional medicine with a pharmaceutical medicine leads to a change in the absorption, metabolism, distribution or excretion of one or more of these compounds. This usually results in either reduced or increased pharmacological activity of the drug, and may increase the risk of adverse effects or toxicity.[6,7,12]

Drug–disease interactions are those in which an existing disease or health condition can lead to unintended drug effects. Certain diseases can alter drug pharmacodynamic and pharmacokinetic parameters. This process may lead to a greater risk of toxicity, reduced therapeutic outcomes or physiological changes or it may exacerbate other existing conditions and disease states.[3]

PHARMACODYNAMIC HERB/NUTRIENT–DRUG INTERACTIONS

Pharmacodynamic herb/nutrient–drug interactions occur when the herbal or nutritional substance modifies the pharmacological effect of a drug, without changing the plasma concentration of the drug, resulting in an additive, synergistic or antagonistic outcome.[3,4,8] This type of interaction occurs when the two interacting agents affect a common target, such as the same organ systems, receptor sites, hormones, neurotransmitters or enzymes.[2,5] Pharmacodynamic interactions include those relating to agonist or antagonistic effects between two different substances that act on the same receptor site or which both have an effect on the release of the same hormones, enzymes or neurotransmitters.[13]

In theory, pharmacodynamic interactions may be fairly predictable, based on knowledge of the mechanisms of action of both substances; however, the magnitude and clinical relevance of the effect are often unknown.[2,4,8] Factors such as the individual's age, state of health and personal characteristics, the nature of the drug, the indication for use, the dose and the form of dose administration will also lead to wide and unpredictable variations between individuals.[3–6]

Health practitioners often intentionally combine two or more substances with a similar effect for an additive or synergistic effect to improve outcomes. Doctors may, for example, prescribe a combination of two antihypertensive drugs with different mechanisms of action to improve response. Likewise, herbalists frequently combine several herbal medicines with similar, synergistic actions to improve therapeutic benefits. In much the same way, complementary medicines may be used in combination with pharmacological drugs to enhance patient management; for example, in the combination of fish oils with an anti-inflammatory agent in a patient with rheumatoid arthritis.[2–4] Drugs and herbs or nutrients with similar actions or characteristics can therefore produce an exaggerated response, which may be beneficial.

However, these additive or synergistic interactions also have the potential to be detrimental, since they may result in an associated increased risk of adverse effects or toxicity. An example is the use of herbal medicines with antiplatelet properties in combination with anticoagulant drugs such as warfarin, leading to an increased risk of bleeding and bruising. Another example is the use of drugs and herbal medicines both of which have sedative properties, potentially leading to excessive drowsiness when used concurrently.[3,4,8]

Pharmacodynamic interactions may also be antagonistic in nature. This occurs when the different therapeutic agents have opposing effects and concurrent use may compromise drug efficacy, leading to a diminished therapeutic benefit. The clinical significance of such interactions often relates to the characteristics of the drug itself, as well as the severity of the condition being treated. An example of this type of interaction is the use of immunostimulant herbs such as *Andrographis paniculata* or *Echinacea* spp. in a patient taking immunosuppressant drugs to prevent organ transplant rejection. Although data about specific interactions between immunosuppressive drugs and immunostimulating herbs are limited, and largely theoretical, caution is strongly advised because the consequences of such an interaction are serious, with an increased risk of treatment failure.[6,9] Another example of an antagonistic interaction is the use of the herbal medicine *Vitex agnus-castus* — which has agonist effects on dopamine D_2 receptors — in combination with a dopamine antagonist drug (e.g. domperidone), thereby theoretically reducing drug effect. Conversely, *Vitex agnus-castus* may theoretically potentiate the effects of dopamine agonist drugs (e.g. bromocriptine).[1,14]

It should be noted that pharmacodynamic interactions may also occur between certain drugs and food substances that either oppose or potentiate the drug's pharmacological action. An example is a sudden increased intake of vitamin K-containing foods, such as kale, cabbage, Brussels sprouts and broccoli in a patient who is taking warfarin. Warfarin exerts its anticoagulant action by inhibiting the synthesis of vitamin K-dependent clotting factors. Therefore, a significant increased intake of dietary vitamin K has the potential to oppose the anticoagulant action of warfarin and reduce drug effectiveness.[3]

In summary, pharmacodynamic interactions can result in additive, synergistic or opposing effects and have the potential to be either beneficial or detrimental. Although these types of interactions may be predicted in theory, the clinical significance of pharmacodynamic interactions between drugs and herbs, nutrients or foods is often largely unknown. Many interactions are theoretical and speculative and are based on an understanding of the actions of the various agents, rather than on controlled clinical studies.[8]

Caution is advised with combined use of herbs and nutrients with drugs where there is a known risk of a pharmacodynamic interaction, especially where the severity of the interaction — such as treatment failure or risk of toxicity — is of significant clinical concern.

PHARMACOKINETIC HERB/ NUTRIENT–DRUG INTERACTIONS

Pharmacokinetic herb/nutrient–drug interactions occur when the combination of a drug with a herbal medicine, nutrient or nutritional supplement results in an alteration in drug absorption, distribution, metabolism or excretion. The change relates to the *duration* or magnitude of the drug effect, rather than the *type* of effect.[2,7,10–12] Most of the current evidence of clinically relevant pharmacokinetic interactions between drugs and herbal medicines appears to relate to changes in the rate and extent of drug metabolism due to alterations in the activity of the CYP450 enzyme system. Interactions due to changes in the activity of the drug transporter P-glycoprotein (P-gp) are also emerging as an important consideration.[4,7,10]

Absorption

Drug absorption interactions involve changes to either the extent or the rate of absorption. These interactions apply mainly to orally administered substances, with absorption being influenced by a number of factors including gastric pH, rate of gastric emptying and the physiochemical interplay between different agents taken at the same time.[2]

Drugs that alter gastric pH may reduce absorption of several compounds, including minerals such as iron and calcium. Proton pump inhibitors (PPIs), for example, are prescribed for the treatment of stomach ulcers, heartburn and gastric reflux because they decrease gastric acidity.

This effect can, however, affect solubility and absorption of several drugs or other substances.[2,3,12]

Drugs that reduce gastric motility, such as hyoscine, may delay gastric emptying time, which in turn can affect the rate but not the extent of absorption of several other drugs, herbs or nutrients. Similarly, drugs that shorten gastric emptying time, such as metoclopramide, may cause substances to reach the duodenum quicker, allowing for an increased rate of absorption.[2,3,12]

Absorption may also be influenced by the activity of intrinsic drug transporters. A notable example is P-glycoprotein (P-gp), a protein that acts as an efflux pump to expel drugs out of cells, thus reducing the potential pharmacological action. Some herbal medicines, especially St John's wort, have been shown to induce P-gp, resulting in clinically significant reductions in the efficacy of some drugs. Conversely, some substances such as grapefruit juice, rosemary and quercetin may inhibit P-gp activity, thereby theoretically increasing the cellular concentration of some drugs. The clinical significance of most interactions relating to the expression of P-gp is still under investigation. Until more information becomes available, caution is advised with use of any herbal medicines or nutritional compounds identified as having an effect on P-gp activity.[4,15]

Physiochemical interactions refer to interactions in which there is an intrinsic incompatibility between two or more substances, leading to a physical or chemical change when used in combination. This can affect both the extent and rate of absorption of one or more of the medicines or substances. Examples of this include the co-administration of minerals such as calcium, magnesium or iron with tetracycline or quinolone antibiotics. The combination may lead to the formation of an insoluble complex between the drug and the mineral and consequent decreased absorption of both agents.[4,12] Herbal medicines with a high tannin content also have the potential to bind to minerals, and may form precipitates with some other compounds such as alkaloids, glycosides, proteins and polysaccharides. Physiochemical interactions can usually be minimised by dosage separation.[4]

Theoretical concerns have also been raised that highly mucilaginous herbs such as slippery elm and marshmallow may form a physical barrier that impairs drug absorption. The clinical significance of this is, however, unclear.[4]

Distribution

Following absorption from the gastrointestinal tract, drugs circulate in the bloodstream mainly reversibly and bound to plasma proteins such as albumin or α-1-acid glycoprotein. A portion of the drug will be unbound, and this is the part that is pharmacologically active and able to bind to the target receptor sites. Competition for bind sites is common and a drug or substance can therefore cause displacement of another drug or substance from the plasma proteins. Theoretically, this displacement can trigger a higher concentration of free drug and result in an exaggerated effect and increased risk of toxicity. Clinically significant interactions due to drug displacement are considered rare, as the higher concentration of free drug leads to a subsequent increase in drug elimination and steady state balance is reinstated.[2,3,5]

Metabolism

Most medicines are metabolised primarily by the liver, and the extent and rate of this metabolism directly affects the pharmacological effect. Clinically important interactions can occur if one or more substances that alter drug metabolism are used concurrently.[15]

Liver metabolism occurs via a two step process known as Phase I and Phase II. During Phase I various compounds including drugs, herbal medicines, nutrients, alcohol, chemicals, pollutants, microbes and byproducts of normal physiological processes enter the liver via the blood. They are then transformed from active compounds into inactive, yet chemically reactive, intermediary metabolites by the cytochrome P450 (CYP450) enzymes. In Phase II, these intermediary compounds are then further transformed into water-soluble forms that can be eliminated in the urine or faeces.[2,3,5]

Some pharmaceutical and complementary medicines can affect the activity of the metabolising CYP450 enzymes, and this action is responsible for many of the reported drug–drug, drug–herb or drug–food/nutrient interactions. Substances that inhibit CYP enzyme activity may lead to decreased drug metabolism, which can result in an increased drug effect and risk of toxicity. Conversely, substances that induce CYP enzyme activity may increase the rate of metabolism, which can result in a faster rate of drug clearance, with a risk of diminished effect or treatment failure.[2,3] The majority of metabolism-related drug interactions, are due to six CYP450 enzymes, namely CYP1A2, CYP2C9, CYP2C19, CYP2D6, CYP2E1 and CYP3A4. Of these, CYP3A4 has been identified as being responsible for the metabolism of 40–45% of drugs, while 20–30% are metabolised by CYP2D6 and about 10% by CYP2C9, with the other enzymes being responsible for the rest.[3] From this it can be understood that drugs or natural medicines that affect the activity of CYP3A4 and CYP2D6 in particular have the greatest potential for metabolism-related interactions.[4,13]

St John's wort is the most highly studied of the herbal medicines in terms of interactions. It is well established that this herbal medicine can significantly induce CYP450 enzyme activity, especially CYP3A4, and to a lesser extent CYP2C19, an effect that is mainly due to the constituent hyperforin.[4] There is a substantial risk of clinically relevant interactions between St John's wort and multiple different drugs, given that up to 45% of drugs are metabolised by CYP3A4. Caution is strongly advised with the use of St John's wort in combination with many drugs, the most common outcome being an increased rate of metabolism due to enzyme induction, resulting in diminished drug activity and a risk of treatment failure. Several other herbal medicines also affect CYP450 enzyme activity, including *Ginkgo biloba, Allium sativum, Camellia sinensis, Glycyrrhiza glabra, Zingiber officinale, Piper nigrum, Rosmarinus officinalis, Curcuma longa, Panax ginseng, Hydrastis canadensis* and *Schisandra chinensis.*[4,15] It should be noted that the magnitude of enzyme

TABLE 6.1 Examples of medicines metabolised by different cytochrome P450 enzymes

Cytochrome P450	Percentage of pharmaceutical drugs metabolism by enzyme	Examples of substrates (drugs metabolised by the enzyme)
CYP1A2	Approximately 5%	Amitriptyline, caffeine, diazepam, imipramine, naproxen, estradiol, olanzapine, ondansetron, paracetamol, propranolol, tamoxifen, theophylline, terbinafine, verapamil, warfarin
CYP2C9	Approximately 10%	Amitriptyline, carvedilol, celecoxib, diclofenac, fluoxetine, fluvastatin, glibenclamide, glipizide, ibuprofen, imipramine, indometacin, irbesartan, losartan, montelukast, naproxen, phenytoin, rosiglitazone, rosuvastatin, tamoxifen, terbinafine, warfarin
CYP2C19	Approximately 10%	Amitriptyline, citalopram, cyclophosphamide, diazepam, escitalopram, esomeprazole, lansoprazole, moclobemide, nelfinavir, omeprazole, pantoprazole, phenytoin, propranolol, topiramate, warfarin
CYP2D6	Approximately 20–30%	Amitriptyline, carvedilol, citalopram, clozapine, codeine, dextromethorphan, donepezil, fluoxetine, haloperidol, labetalol, methadone, metoclopramide, metoprolol, oxycodone, paroxetine, pethidine, promethazine, risperidone, tamoxifen, tramadol, venlafaxine
CYP2E1	Approximately 5%	Ethanol, halothane, paracetamol, theophylline
CYP3A4	Approximately 40–45%	Alprazolam, amiodarone, amlodipine, atazanavir, atorvastatin, bromocriptine, budesonide, carbamazepine, citalopram, clarithromycin, clindamycin, cocaine, cyclophosphamide, ciclosporin, dexamethasone, dextromethorphan, diazepam, diltiazem, doxorubicin, ethinylestradiol, hydrocortisone, ifosfamide, imatinib, indinavir, itraconazole, lapatinib, lopinavir, methadone, midazolam, nifedipine, ondansetron, paclitaxel, ritonavir, saquinavir, sertraline, sildenafil, simvastatin, sirolimus, sodium valproate, tacrolimus, tamoxifen, tramadol, vinblastine, vincristine, voriconazole, zolpidem

This table is not exhaustive and is intended to provide examples of medicine substrates only.

induction or inhibition by these herbal medicines is variable and may not always lead to clinically significant interactions. Caution is, however, generally recommended with co-administration with drugs that act as CYP enzyme substrates, especially if outcomes are uncertain.[4,11,15]

Table 6.1 provides a summary of examples of medicines (i.e. substrates) that are metabolised by the different cytochrome P450 enzymes. Risk of an interaction exists when complementary medicines that either inhibit or induce the CYP450 enzymes are used in combination with these medicines.[3,13]

Excretion

The main organs of excretion are the kidneys and the bowels, although some excretion also occurs through the lungs, sweat, saliva and breastmilk.[4] Factors that alter renal function in some way will interfere with the normal urinary excretion of drugs and their metabolites. This in turn influences herb/nutrient–drug interactions, particularly with regard to substances that change urinary pH. For example, high doses of vitamin C can acidify the urine, which potentially decreases the excretion of acidic drugs such as aspirin. The opposite may occur with ingestion of substances such as bicarbonate that significantly alkalinise the urine.[3,4] Competition occurs between some drugs for the same active renal transport systems, which may lead to clinically significant interactions.[2,3] This type of interaction has not been noted to any great extent between drugs and herbs or nutrients.

FACTORS INFLUENCING DRUG INTERACTIONS

The outcomes of drug interactions can be highly variable between different individuals. A number of factors may influence the likelihood, magnitude and clinical significance of an interaction. These factors should be taken into consideration when assessing the risks and benefits associated with concurrent use of pharmaceutical and complementary medicines in an individual.[2-4,6,16]

1. **Drug characteristics:** Specific drug characteristics impact on the risk and severity of interactions. Drug interactions of greatest concern are those with drugs with a narrow therapeutic index. With these drugs, even minor changes in drug concentration at the target site can result in major changes in response. Notable examples are warfarin, digoxin and lithium. In addition, drugs that significantly induce or inhibit CYP450 enzymes are more likely to interact with other agents.
2. **Duration, frequency and dose:** The duration of therapy, dose used, frequency and route of administration all influence the likelihood and

potential severity of an interaction. This applies to drugs as well as herbal or nutritional medicines.

3 **Multiple therapies:** Individuals who are taking multiple drugs may be more vulnerable to herb/nutrient–drug interactions. The term 'polypharmacy' is generally used to describe simultaneous use of five or more medicines, including prescription drugs, over-the-counter drugs and complementary medicines. While the use of multiple therapies may be beneficial and appropriate, great caution needs to be applied to prevent unwanted interactions and adverse effects.

4 **Disease:** Preexisting disease states may predispose an individual to interactions, especially those that cause impaired liver or renal function. The liver is the primary site for drug metabolism and the kidneys are the primary site for urinary excretion. Compromised liver or renal function may result in increased drug serum concentrations, placing the individual at increased risk of drug interactions and toxicity. The nature of the disease is another important consideration, especially where compromised treatment may have life-threatening consequences such as in patients with cancer or HIV, or in those who have undergone organ transplant.

5 **Age:** Elderly people are at greatest risk of interactions due to age-related physiological changes which affect their ability to absorb, metabolise and eliminate drugs and natural medicines.

6 **Heredity factors:** Genetic variability can affect the individual's ability to metabolise certain drugs. People who lack the gene to form the enzyme CYP2D6 are, for example, at a greater risk of toxicity when taking drugs or herbal medicines that are metabolised by this particular liver enzyme. Genetic polymorphisms can also lead to idiosyncratic reactions which can be difficult to predict.

7 **Environment:** Chronic exposure to chemicals and pesticides can increase the activity of liver enzymes. This may increase the rate of drug metabolism and potentially decrease drug effects.

8 **Diet and nutrition:** Nutritional status and dietary intake of essential nutrients can affect the risk and severity of drug–nutrient interactions. Certain medications can lead to nutrient depletions, some of which are of major concern. Those with poor dietary intake or with other dietary or lifestyle factors that compromise nutritional status will be at a greater risk of the depletions becoming clinically relevant. Sudden changes in dietary intake of certain foods can also affect the safety and efficacy of some drugs.

9 **Alcohol:** Alcohol affects the liver's ability to metabolise drugs, herbs and nutrients. The effect is variable, depending on whether intake is acute or chronic. Alcohol intake may also contribute to several nutrient depletions.

10 **Smoking:** Smoking may increase the rate of liver metabolism of some drugs.

11 **Poor communication:** Patient non-disclosure to their medical doctors about the complementary medicines being taken has been identified as a factor that can increase the risk of interactions.

COMPLEXITY OF HERB/NUTRIENT–DRUG INTERACTIONS

The evidence for herb/nutrient–drug interactions is often based on data which are derived from laboratory or animal studies or anecdotal case reports, or which are theoretical in nature, based on known pharmacological activity. However, there is often a poor correlation between these and clinical effects.[4] A lack of sufficient well-designed, controlled clinical studies investigating herb–drug or nutrient–drug interactions has been identified.[4] Furthermore, a systematic review reported that many of the studies that have been conducted to date have been of poor methodological quality, yielding conflicting and unreliable results.[12]

In addition, unlike pharmaceutical compounds, herbal medicines are a complex mixture of chemical constituents and bioactive substances. For many herbal medicines, only some of the bioactive compounds have been identified and characterised. It is not always clear to what extent the various constituents contribute to herbal actions and interactions. Other factors contributing to the complexity of herb–drug interactions are a result of the variability in plant constituents. Variability depends on the part of the plant used, the climate, the growing and harvesting conditions, the storage and extraction methods and whether or not herbal medicines are standardised during the manufacturing process. Similarly, wide variations can occur between nutritional supplements and their potential for interactions, depending on the source and specific compound or salt used (as this influences bioavailability), as well as the extraction, manufacturing processes and storage methods used. This complex range of factors adds to the challenge of predicting the likelihood, severity and nature of many herb–drug and nutrient–drug interactions.[2-4,6,7,9,10,12]

The validity of existing evidence on herb/nutrient–drug interactions is therefore often uncertain, clinical relevance is often unclear and prevalence is often unknown and possibly underreported.

THE HERB/NUTRIENT–DRUG INTERACTION TABLES IN THIS TEXT

Tables detailing potential herb–drug and nutrient–drug interactions are included at the back of the book.

The tables have been formulated to include information on interactions between herbal medicines, nutrients/nutritional supplements and drugs. The tables include a summary of the potential outcome, a graded recommendation and a comments section that explains the nature of each interaction in more detail. The recommendations are broadly divided into four categories, namely Avoid, Caution, Monitor/Observe and Beneficial. Factors that were taken into account when determining these interaction categories included currently available evidence and safety data, potential severity and clinical consequences, the likelihood of an interaction, whether the interaction is based on clinical studies or extrapolated from case studies or laboratory or animal studies, as well as commonly applied integrative prescribing principles. New safety data and evidence are, however, constantly emerging and best practice regarding some of these interactions may change with time.

The tables do not include information on possible contraindications, for example use in pregnancy, nor do they include herb–herb, herb–nutrient or nutrient–nutrient interactions.

Practitioners are encouraged to use the interactions tables as a guide, but to apply professional judgment on the appropriateness of use of a combination of herb–drug or nutrient–drug for each patient. It is imperative that health practitioners remain vigilant when prescribing herbal or nutritional medicines for patients already taking pharmaceutical medicines and that practitioners investigate whether there are any known safety concerns or interactions. Health practitioners of all disciplines are encouraged to make use of the available resources to allow for informed decisions, so as to optimise patient wellbeing without compromising patient safety. When recommending complementary medicines in combination with pharmaceutical medicines both anticipated benefits and potential risks should be taken into consideration.

REFERENCES

[1] Australian Medicines Handbook 2017 (online). Adelaide: Australian Medicines Handbook Pty Ltd; 2017 July. Available from: https://amhonline.amh.net.au/.

[2] Bryant B, Knights K. Pharmacology for health professionals. 4th ed. Sydney: Elsevier; 2014.

[3] Arcangelo VP, Peterson AM. Pharmacotherapeutics for advanced practice: a practical approach. 4th ed. Lippincott, Williams & Wilkins; 2016.

[4] Braun L, Cohen M. Herbs and natural supplements. An evidence-based guide, vol. 1. 4th ed. Sydney: Elsevier; 2015.

[5] Rang HP, Dale MM, Ritter JM, et al. Rang and Dale's pharmacology. 8th ed. Churchill Livingston Elsevier; 2015.

[6] Kotsirilos V, Vitetta L, Sali A. A guide to evidence-based integrative and complementary medicines. Churchill Livingston Elsevier; 2011.

[7] Oga EF, Sekine S, Shitara Y, et al. Pharmacokinetic herb–drug interactions: insight into mechanisms and consequences. [Review] Eur J Drug Metab Pharmacokinet 2016;41(2):93–108.

[8] Choi JG, Eom SM, Kim J, et al. Comprehensive review of recent studies on herb–drug interaction: a focus on pharmacodynamic interaction. Review] J Altern Complement Med 2016;22(4):262–79.

[9] Posadzki P, Watson L, Ernst E. Herb–drug interactions: an overview of systematic reviews. Review] Br J Clin Pharmacol 2013;75(3):603–18.

[10] Gurley BJ. Pharmacokinetic herb–drug interactions (part 1): origins, mechanisms, and the impact of botanical dietary supplements. Review] Planta Medica 2012;78(13):1478–89.

[11] Gurley BJ, Fifer EK, Gardner Z. Pharmacokinetic herb–drug interactions (part 2): drug interactions involving popular botanical dietary supplements and their clinical relevance. Review] Planta Med 2012;78(13):1490–514.

[12] Chen XW, Sneed KB, Pan SY, et al. Herb–drug interactions and mechanistic and clinical considerations. Review] Curr Drug Metab 2012;13(5):640–51.

[13] Australian Pharmaceutical Formulary and Handbook. 23rd ed. Pharmaceutical Society of Australia; 2015.

[14] Natural Medicines Professional Comprehensive Database. 2017. Available from: http://naturaldatabase.therapeuticresearch.com.

[15] Cho HJ, Yoon IS. Pharmacokinetic interactions of herbs with cytochrome P450 and P-glycoprotein. Evid Based Complement Alternat Med 2015;2015:736431.

[16] Hilmer SN. The dilemma of polypharmacy. Aust Prescr 2008;31:2–3.

PART 2

Naturopathic treatments

7

Nutritional medicine (supplementation)

Gabrielle Covino

INTRODUCTION TO NUTRITIONAL MEDICINE

In modern naturopathic clinical practice the use of nutritional supplementation has attained an increased level of acceptance, and plays an increasingly important role in the design and implementation of patient treatment protocols. The nutritional armamentarium that practitioners have to draw upon is quite considerable and specific nutrients are often available in many forms. In recent times, to conform to the rigorous requirements of evidence-based medicine, it has become necessary that this practice attain greater sophistication and specificity.

At the most basic level broad-spectrum multivitamin and mineral supplements are prescribed to provide a 'tune-up' of micronutrient metabolism.[1] In many cases this can be achieved using a broad spectrum of nutrients contained in a single formula. In general these kinds of formulations provide nutrients in concentrations that equate with the dietary reference ranges established by various regulatory bodies throughout the world.

In many instances, however, the nutrient dose would be in the higher reference range and equate more with the 'tolerable upper limit' (when and where this can be defined). In these concentrations, 'nutritional benefits appear to outweigh the theoretical risk of toxic effects at normal or modestly elevated physiological intake levels'.[2]

In some instances nutrients are used in what many practitioners consider to be a 'therapeutic range'. Also referred to as 'pharmacological dosing', this approach moves beyond the deficiency/repletion model of nutrition. Often this would mean prescribing a nutrient in a specific form or dose, in the absence of a pronounced deficiency of that nutrient. Using higher doses during the acute phase of an illness (vitamin C and zinc are examples of this) is representative of this approach. While it remains controversial, this approach is now finding increasing support in the medical literature.

In this chapter the essential vitamins, minerals and trace elements are evaluated and assessed, with a detailed section assigned to each nutrient. The biochemical function and the basic physiological requirements for each nutrient are presented, in conjunction with the pharmacological or therapeutic dose ranges and the accompanying clinical applications.

Wherever possible, the clinical applications and dose ranges are supported by evidence from peer-reviewed journals. Provided there are sufficient reliable data, the various commercial supplemental forms of nutrients are evaluated. Additionally, important nutrient interactions with prescription medications are included.

Of course the lure of scientifically endorsed nutritional supplements should not draw our attention away from the primary importance of a healthy diet. By and large a healthy diet is one that emphasises high-quality, fresh, natural produce; foods that are micronutrient dense, ethically produced and not 'pharmed', modified or adulterated with pesticides or hazardous chemicals. This chapter covers nutrient deficiencies and how they relate to diet, and how they can be addressed in both the diet and with supplementation. See Appendix 3 available online at Expert Consult for a full dosage discussion of each nutrient, including pharmacological dosing.

Dietary reference intakes

The quantitative recommendations for nutrient intakes used as reference values or standards for planning and evaluating the nutrient intakes of healthy people are collectively referred to as the 'dietary reference intakes' or 'dietary intake standards'. These include the estimated average requirement (EAR) and three other reference values: the recommended dietary allowance (RDA), the adequate intake (AI) and the tolerable upper level (TUL). These designated terms (and their relative intake levels) vary slightly from country to country. In this chapter the figures and estimates used for the dietary reference intakes are those provided by regulatory organisations, primarily in Australia and New Zealand.[3] Occasionally these figures will be compared with the intake levels given by other organisations worldwide, depending on the context and the nutrient under discussion.

In this text the terms RDA and RDI (recommended dietary intake) are considered as interchangeable. The RDI/RDA is the amount of a nutrient required to meet the needs of 97–98% of the population, and is the level of intake that would generally maintain tissue pools and prevent deficiency. Generally these intake levels are calibrated based on body weight, ethnicity, life stage and

TABLE 7.1 Dietary reference ranges (Australia and New Zealand)

Range	Description
EAR — estimated average requirement	The EAR is the median usual intake estimated to meet the requirement of half the healthy individuals in a life stage/gender group
RDI — recommended dietary intake	The RDI is the average daily dietary intake level sufficient to meet the nutrient requirements of nearly all healthy individuals (97–98%) in a life stage/gender group
AI — adequate intake	Where an EAR (and therefore an RDI) for the nutrient cannot be determined because of limited or inconsistent data, an AI is determined. The AI can be used as a goal for individual intake but is based on experimentally derived intake levels or approximations of observed mean nutrient intakes by a group of apparently healthy people maintaining a defined nutritional state
UIL (or TUL) — upper intake limit (or tolerable upper limit)	Highest level of continuing daily nutrient intake likely to pose no adverse health effects in almost all individuals

Source: Nutrient Reference Values for Australia and New Zealand including Recommended Dietary Intakes. Commonwealth Department of Health and Ageing, Australia Ministry of Health, New Zealand National Health and Medical Research Council; 2004.

gender, and adjusted to accommodate periods of increased nutrient requirement or demand, such as during menstruation, pregnancy and lactation, or during recovery from major illness (Table 7.1).

BEYOND THE BASIC REQUIREMENTS

Dietary reference intakes, while useful as a general guide for the various life phases and population groups, do little to address the needs of the individual. They are based primarily on the prevention of deficiency, rather than the prevention of chronic disease and the promotion of optimal health.

While they can be very useful in assessing the upper limits and safety thresholds for specific nutrients, dietary reference intakes such as the RDI were never designed to cover the optimal daily intake requirements of individuals. 'The precise amount of a nutrient that will be adequate for any given individual is therefore unknown. It can be stated only in terms of probabilities.'[4]

There is now a growing consensus that the biochemical threshold for deficiency has been set too low and needs to be re-evaluated.[5] The current RDIs can serve as a useful general guide, especially with respect to nutrients that can cause toxicity, even at relatively low intakes. However, the recommended intake levels are often less than acceptable to many practitioners of nutritional medicine, who seek not only to prevent and treat deficiencies, but also to go that one step further, using nutrients to enhance wellbeing and extend life.

This does not simply mean increasing our life span, as longevity per se is an inadequate marker of quality of life. But increasing quality of life can certainly make increased longevity more a meaningful objective rather than a purely statistical one. It is often observed that in the developed world we are living longer but getting sicker. It is a primary aim of naturopathic nutritional medicine to change this trend. Certainly much has already been achieved — with regard not only to increasing our essential daily nutrient intakes, both qualitatively and quantitatively, but also to encouraging individuals to improve their health potential. The application of therapeutic nutrient regimens not only improves quality of life but may also decrease the likelihood of inherited genetic diseases.[6]

It is not enough that we remain within the average range, and maintain average health. Certainly this would appear to be the aim of the regulatory bodies that have established the dietary reference ranges that are currently in place. In this case the average, as far as our health is concerned, would most probably equate with fulfilling our basic needs for subsistence and survival. Yet this average is certainly well below what many of us aspire to when we talk of gaining and attaining 'health'.

Seeking to establish the optimal needs of the individual is to fulfil the unique set of requirements presented by that individual. We are all 'subtly and beautifully different',[1] with our own idiosyncrasies, unique traits and metabolic strengths and weaknesses. We are also uniquely susceptible. While this susceptibility blueprint may seem indelible and our metabolic fate predestined, through nutritional means (diet and supplements) there is still much that can be done to change the seemingly inevitable course of events that determine the quality and extent of human life.

It is now recognised that higher doses of vitamins, minerals and trace elements are often necessary to accommodate our individual needs, our unique 'biochemical individuality'. As Roger Williams (who originally devised the term) has observed, 'individuality in nutritional needs is the basis for the genetotrophic approach and for the belief that nutrition applied with due concern for individual genetic variations, which may be large, offers the solution to many baffling health problems.'[6]

The World Health Organization now acknowledges that:

> *we have gone beyond the era of requirements to prevent deficiency and excess to the present goal of preserving micronutrient-related functions. The next step in this evolution will surely be the incorporation of the knowledge and necessary tools to assess genetic diversity in the redefinition of nutritional requirements for optimal health throughout the life course.*[7]

This idea certainly resonates with the nutritional objectives of naturopathic clinical medicine, as it does with other emerging fields in nutritional science, such as 'nutrigenomics', which seeks to 'expand comprehension of how nutrients affect the human body and to personalise nutrition, making possible individualised nutritional recommendations'.

Therapeutic dose

When working outside the deficiency/repletion model, it is possible to prescribe nutrients within what is considered to be the 'therapeutic range'. This is also known as 'pharmacological dosing' or 'supranutritional dosing'. Nutrients prescribed within this range would have benefits without the risk of toxic effects.

Vitamins, minerals and other compounds may be prescribed in higher doses during the acute phase of illness to stimulate the body's endogenous defences (such as when prescribing high-dose vitamin C or zinc). When the illness or condition being treated is resolved, the nutrient is then withdrawn or the dose scaled down considerably. This would avoid the possibility of habituation or 'conditioned deficiency', which may result in a relative lack of responsiveness to the nutrient in doses required for adequacy.[8]

VITAMINS

Vitamins are organic compounds that are needed in the diet in small amounts in order to prevent specific deficiency diseases and to support a state of optimal health. The term 'organic' means that a substance contains carbon, and often hydrogen — this means that all the macronutrients are also organic.

As vitamins are organic substances they can be both created and destroyed. Human bodies are unable to manufacture most vitamins, but some plants, animals and bacteria can. Thus vitamins that cannot be synthesised in the body, or cannot be synthesised in adequate amounts to prevent deficiency, must therefore be present in our food intake. Vitamins generally need to be handled with care during processes such as cooking and storage. Some vitamins are less stable than others; the water-soluble vitamins B_1, B_2 and C are particularly vulnerable.

The term 'vitamine' was coined by Dr Casimir Funk in 1911 after he isolated what was then thought to be 'anti-beriberi factor' (vitamin B_1) from rice polishings. The term was derived from 'vital amine', reflecting both the structural and functional properties of the compound, as it was regarded as being 'vital' (from the Latin *vita* meaning 'life') and an 'amine' (a nitrogen-containing compound). It is now known that not all vitamins contain nitrogen and, as a result, these vital compounds are simply called vitamins, a name that still reflects their life-giving importance.

The diseases associated with vitamin deficiencies have been described from at least 2000 BC, but it was not until the beginning of the 20th century that the idea of vitamin-deficiency diseases was accepted. Prior to this time, the traditional view was that these diseases were caused by toxic agents in the body rather than by something that was missing from the diet.

The vitamins were discovered between 1911 (vitamin B_1) and 1940 (vitamin B_{12}) and were named according to an alphabetical system (A, B, C, D and E) devised by two American scientists, McCollum and Davis, in 1915.

Functions of vitamins

- Vitamins cannot be broken down to provide energy, but they do assist in the reactions that release energy from carbohydrates, proteins and fats.
- Vitamins regulate metabolism and form parts of coenzymes that are involved in chemical reactions in the body.
- Many of the vitamins act as antioxidants.
- Vitamins prevent deficiency diseases, such as scurvy, beriberi and rickets, and also protect against some diseases such as cancer, heart disease and neural tube defects.

Salient aspects

Vitamin supplements do not offer the many benefits and advantages that come from consuming vitamin-rich foods. Although for the most part in this chapter nutrients are discussed individually, it should be remembered that vitamins are not found in isolation in nature. In many instances it has been shown that, while consuming foods that are high in a particular vitamin may have beneficial effects, laboratory studies have failed to show similar effects from supplementation; a good example of this is vitamin C intake and reduced rates of cancers.

Remember that there is much more to food than just carbohydrates, proteins, fats, vitamins and minerals. Also present is a vast array of phytochemicals, the actions of many of which we are only just starting to understand. We also need to be aware of the combinations of vitamins (and other nutrients) as they are found in foods. Different vitamins and minerals are needed for the absorption, transport and use of other vitamins and minerals. For example, vitamin C is better absorbed and remains active in the body longer if taken with flavonoids.

Remember also that everyone is an individual. We all have different requirements and may respond differently to supplements or dietary changes. It is therefore necessary to be aware of these differences when gathering information and when making therapeutic recommendations. Supplementation should not replace a good diet. In an ideal world we would attain adequate nutrition from the food that we eat. However, in reality this is not always the case, and is not always practical. Often when recommending the use of a particular supplement we are also making changes to the diet to ensure that the individual continues to receive adequate intakes of nutrients once supplementation is ceased. It is also important to be able to distinguish between a vitamin deficiency caused by a dietary lack of a nutrient, and a state of deficiency that is in fact due to poor absorption or utilisation of a nutrient. The assimilation and use of nutrients may be affected by such factors as poor gastrointestinal health or function, the use of drugs, stress, hormone imbalances, illness and other lifestyle factors. It is useful to consider increased need, reduced intake and absorption/assimilation capacity when we think of

TABLE 7.2 Comparison of the characteristics of water-soluble and fat-soluble vitamins

	Water-soluble vitamins	Fat-soluble vitamins
Name	Vitamins B_1, B_2, B_3, B_5, B_6, B_9, B_{12}, biotin (B_7) and C	Vitamins A, D, E and K
Food sources	Grains, legumes, fruits, vegetables, meats, dairy products	Fats, animal and plant oils, liver, egg yolk, leafy green vegetables
Stability	Easily destroyed or removed from foods by incorrect cooking	Usually not as unstable as water-soluble vitamins
Absorption	Directly into the bloodstream	First into the lymph and then enter the blood
Storage	Minimal storage in the body (except for B_{12} which may be stored primarily in the liver for 3–5 years)	Significant storage in the body, mainly in the liver and fatty tissue
Excretion	Excess is readily excreted, mainly via the kidneys	Usually not readily excreted. Excretion mainly via the liver in bile
Transport	Can travel freely in blood and lymph	Many require protein carriers for transport around the body
Requirement	Must be in the diet daily	Not essential in the diet every day
Chemistry	Contain carbon, hydrogen, oxygen and other elements (e.g. nitrogen, sulfur, cobalt)	Contain carbon, hydrogen and oxygen only
Toxicity risk	Toxicity is generally unlikely, unless supplementation is given at extremely high doses	Excess is stored rather than excreted, so toxicity may be a problem
Deficiency risk	Deficiency symptoms may develop rapidly	Deficiency symptoms develop slowly

nutritional requirements and the potential for supplementation.

Classification of vitamins

Vitamins are placed into one of two general groups according to whether they are *fat soluble* or *water soluble.* It should be noted that the compounds in each group vary considerably in terms of their structure and function, but because of their solubility they have some general characteristics in common. The use of solubility as a means of classification is practical and provides general information about how that vitamin is handled by the body.

Knowing the solubility characteristics of a vitamin gives an indication of the types of foods that the vitamin will be found in and the best ways of handling these foods, and also provides information on the way the body will absorb, transport, distribute, store and excrete the vitamin.

In total there are 13 vitamins: four are fat soluble and the remaining nine are water soluble. Table 7.2 outlines the major differences and similarities between the fat-soluble and water-soluble vitamins.

Water-soluble vitamins

The water-soluble vitamins are the various B complex vitamins, including inositol and choline, and vitamin C.

The B complex vitamins are thiamine (B_1), riboflavin (B_2), niacin (B_3), pantothenic acid (B_5), pyridoxine (B_6), folate (B_9), cyanocobalamin (B_{12}) and biotin (B_7). Each has a very specific role in the body, but when viewed as a group it is seen that many of them have similar functions, including:

- An involvement with carbohydrate, protein and lipid metabolism and the conversion of these substances into energy
- Acting as coenzymes in many chemical reactions (i.e. they are necessary for these reactions to take place)
- Required for digestive system function (e.g. hydrochloric acid production and gut motility)
- Required for red blood cell production and iron metabolism
- Required for immune system function
- Required for the manufacture of hormones and neurotransmitters
- Required for the metabolism of other vitamins.

As a general rule, the following foods are good sources of the B group vitamins: wholegrains, legumes, eggs, organ meats (liver and kidneys), meats, yeast extracts, nuts and seeds. In addition, folic acid is found in the highest amounts in vegetables (particularly leafy green vegetables) and a range of fruits, while vitamin B_{12} is found exclusively in animal foods (although some plant foods, such as breakfast cereals, are fortified with this vitamin).

VITAMIN B_1 (THIAMINE)

Forms of nutrient

Thiamine exists in four forms in the human body: thiamine monophosphate (TMP), diphosphate (TDP), triphosphate and unphosphorylated thiamine. Vitamin B_1 functions in the body as part of the coenzyme thiamine pyrophosphate (TPP) (previously known as cocarboxylase). The conversion of thiamine to TPP is dependent on an enzyme and the presence of magnesium. This reaction is inhibited by alcohol. 80% of thiamine in the body is in the form of TPP.

Distribution and storage

A continuous supply of vitamin B_1 is required to prevent deficiency. Body turnover is rapid, and storage is minimal. There is 30 mg of thiamine in the average adult, with approximately 50% of this being in muscle tissue. The highest concentrations are in the heart, liver, kidneys and brain.

Absorption

Vitamin B_1 is well absorbed in the small intestine (jejunum, ileum). Factors that increase absorption are small frequent doses and vitamin C. Factors that decrease absorption are alcohol, thiaminase, sulfite preservatives, digestive diseases, high intake of tea and coffee, and folate or protein deficiency.

Excretion

Vitamin B_1 is typically excreted in urine. Factors that increase excretion are an intake greater than requirements, consumption of diuretics or alcohol, or any factor that increases the urine flow rate.

Interactions (medication, nutrient, dietary)

Antibiotics may reduce the bacterial biosynthesis of thiamine by disrupting the gastrointestinal microbiota or gut flora. Prescription diuretics can also reduce thiamine levels, and levels should be monitored in people on long-term therapy, as thiamine deficiency can worsen heart conditions in this group. Chemotherapeutic drugs such as fluorouracil may increase the breakdown of thiamine or interfere with its activation. Metformin may reduce the activity of thiamine and could lead to lactic acidosis. Similarly, anticonvulsant medication (e.g. phenytoin) has been shown to lower thiamine levels. Horsetail (*Equisetum arvense*) contains a thiaminase-like compound that can destroy thiamine in the stomach and (theoretically at least) lead to symptomatic thiamine deficiency. It is probably best to avoid using this herb in people at risk of thiamine deficiency.[6]

Function

Thiamine combines with adenosine triphosphate (ATP) to form thiamine diphosphate, a coenzyme in several enzymes involved in carbohydrate metabolism. These enzymes include pyruvate dehydrogenase, transketolase and α-ketoglutarate, and the branched-chain α-keto acid dehydrogenase complex involved in amino acid catabolism. Thiamine is also involved in the biosynthesis of the neurotransmitters acetylcholine and γ-aminobutyric acid (GABA).

Therapeutic applications

- All forms of beriberi and its associated symptoms
- Some digestive disturbances
- Nerve disorders, depression, fatigue, low morale, irritability, anxiety
- Alcoholism
- Insect-bite protection
- Alzheimer's disease.

Deficiency signs

- *Subclinical deficiency:* anxiety, irritability, fatigue, headaches, anorexia, easy exhaustion, gastrointestinal tract disturbances (constipation, discomfort), muscle fatigue and pain, confusion.
- *Severe deficiency:* beriberi in infants (aged 2–3 months) — more common if mother deficient; acute attacks result in death within hours; loud piercing crying (can be hoarse, soundless); cyanosis; dyspnoea; vomiting; tachycardia; cardiomegaly; nystagmus; convulsions; improves rapidly with thiamine administration. Adults — wet beriberi (affects primarily the cardiovascular system); cerebral beriberi (Wernicke–Korsakoff syndrome) in chronic alcoholics.

Biochemical testing

- Serum thiamine
- Urinary thiamine
- Red blood cell transketolase activity
- Red blood cell thiamine pyrophosphate (TPP)
- α-keto acids in urine.

Supplemental forms

Thiamine hydrochloride (thiamine HCl) consists of 89% thiamine and 11% hydrochloric acid (HCl) and is the most common form of vitamin B_1 used in supplements. Other forms include thiamine nitrate and benfotiamine — a synthetic thiamine monophosphate derivative.[9,10]

Toxicity

There is no evidence of toxic effects from oral administration, even with high doses, as the kidneys can clear excessive amounts.

Dosage requirements

The RDI is 1.3 mg/day for adult males and 1.1 mg/day for women. During pregnancy and lactation 1.4 mg/day is recommended. The safe upper limit for thiamine in Australia has not been established.[11]

The therapeutic range is quite wide and depends on the condition being treated. Doses as high as 4000 mg have been used to treat Leigh's disease, and a dose of 300 mg/day has been used to treat severe deficiencies (100 mg 3 times a day). A dose of 50 mg/day may be helpful for alcoholics without encephalopathy. A dose of 5–15 mg/day has been used in patients on a refined grain diet.[12]

Food sources

Beef, pork, chicken, fish, liver, wheatgerm, wholegrain cereals and unprocessed wheat, rice, peas, beans and peanuts, milk and milk products, green leafy vegetables, nuts and seeds. Brewer's yeast and yeast-extract spreads are also good sources.[13]

Dietary intake and the need for supplementation

Factors that affect thiamine status include a diet high in carbohydrates; excess alcohol intake; excess consumption of tea, coffee or raw fish; malabsorption syndromes; long-term intravenous feeding; dialysis; hypermetabolism; and increased requirement states.

Wholegrains are potentially good sources of thiamine, but much of the thiamine is lost when the grain is milled.[13] For example, the thiamine content of one cup of cooked brown rice is 0.14 mg but that of cooked white rice is only 0.01 mg, and the thiamine content of wholewheat flour is 0.50 mg compared with 0.10 mg in white flour.[14] In Australia there is mandatory thiamine-enriched baking flour.[11] As a result an overreliance on refined cereals and a low intake of animal foods rich in B vitamins could result in subclinical thiamine deficiency.

Stored thiamine is depleted within 2 weeks of a thiamine-deficient diet, with the clinical manifestation of deficiency appearing at about 3 months.[15]

Raw fish and shellfish contain enzymes (thiaminases) that destroy thiamine, and a too frequent consumption of raw fish can result in thiamine deficiency.[14] People who drink alcohol excessively have greater requirements for thiamine (10–100 mg/day). The caffeic acid and polyphenolic compounds present in tea and coffee (tannins) can also antagonise thiamine, although moderate tea and coffee consumption is unlikely to disrupt thiamine absorption to any appreciable degree.

There is also evidence suggesting that thiamine is used less efficiently as we age, and that supplementation should be considered at different life stages. The need for additional thiamine increases during severe diarrhoea, fever, stress and surgery. A well-formulated multivitamin formula with thiamine in levels above the average daily requirement should ensure sufficiency and prevent deficiency in these situations.

In a study published in the *Journal of the American Dietetic Association,* which reviewed 64 gluten-free foods for vitamin content, it was shown that many of these products contained inferior amounts of thiamine, riboflavin and niacin when compared with wheat products. The study concluded that people with coeliac disease may run the risk of deficiency of these nutrients and should be routinely assessed for deficiency, and that pregnant and nursing women with coeliac disease should be provided with recommendations to help increase their intake of these vitamins.[13]

VITAMIN B_2 (RIBOFLAVIN)

Forms of nutrient

In body tissues, riboflavin is present mainly in the coenzyme form as flavin adenine dinucleotide (FAD) or flavin mononucleotide (FMN).

Distribution and storage

Conversion of riboflavin to its coenzyme forms mainly takes place in the small intestine, liver, heart and kidneys, but occurs to a limited degree in most tissues.

Absorption

The maximum amount of riboflavin that can be absorbed from a single dose is 27 mg in an adult; therefore higher doses should be administered as a divided dose.[15] It is possible that the absorption of riboflavin supplements is increased when taken with food because bile salts facilitate intestinal uptake of riboflavin.[8]

Excretion

Riboflavin is excreted in the urine, mainly as metabolites. Levels of riboflavin exceeding 27 mg are excreted. Riboflavin is a yellow-green naturally fluorescent compound, and this is the reason for the yellow colour of urine often observed by those taking supplements.

Interactions (medication, nutrient, dietary)

Interactions occur with diuretics, flurouracil, pyrithiamine, nitrites, sulfites, insulin, levothyroxine, tannic acid and caffeic acid.[16] Tricyclic antidepressants, antipsychotic medication (e.g. chlorpromazine), antimalarial medication (quinacrine) and certain chemotherapy agents (doxorubicin) inhibit the incorporation of riboflavin into FAD and FMN.[17] Some studies have shown that probenecid reduces renal tubular secretion and total urinary excretion of both supplemental and dietary riboflavin, although the clinical significance of this interaction is unknown. Anticholinergic drugs may decrease riboflavin absorption.

Function

Riboflavin is a constituent of two coenzymes: riboflavin-5-phosphate and FAD. The riboflavin coenzymes are essential parts of oxidative enzyme systems involved in electron transport. Riboflavin plays an essential role in nutrient metabolism and antioxidant protection.[18] Riboflavin supports the activity of antioxidants, such as glutathione peroxidase, and is involved in the production of adrenaline by the adrenal glands. Clinically, riboflavin promotes normal growth and assists in the synthesis of steroids, red blood cells and glycogen. Riboflavin helps to maintain the integrity of the mucous membranes, skin, eyes and nervous system. It is thought that riboflavin also aids the body in absorbing iron, as it is common for anaemia to accompany a deficiency of riboflavin.

Riboflavin also plays an important conversion role in the body: vitamin B_6 to its active form pyridoxal phosphate, tryptophan to niacin and methylentetrahydrofolate (MTHF) to methylTHF by the MTHFR enzyme.[19]

Therapeutic applications

- Ariboflavinosis (riboflavin deficiency)
- Migraine
- Ocular cataract
- Skin conditions — acne, dermatitis, eczema, ulcers
- Stress (with other B vitamins)
- Faulty vitamin B_6 and B_9 metabolism
- Anaemia and sickle cell anaemia
- Leg cramps.

Deficiency signs

Angular stomatitis (cracking at the corners of the lips), cheilosis, glossitis (inflammation of the tongue), lethargy, depression, generalised weakness in the limbs, oedema of the pharyngeal and oral mucous membranes, seborrhoeic dermatitis, scrotal dermatitis or dermatitis affecting the labia majora and nasolabial folds, photosensitivity, burning and itching of the eyes, corneal vascularisation, leucopenia and thrombocytopenia.

Biochemical testing

- Serum or urine riboflavin
- Erythrocyte glutathione reductase activity coefficient (EGRAC).[17,20]

Supplemental forms

The most common forms of riboflavin used in nutritional supplements are riboflavin 5′-monophosphate and riboflavin sodium phosphate.

Toxicity

Vitamin B_2 is generally considered non-toxic at the doses recommended for clinical use. High doses can result in flavinuria, the fluorescent yellow colouration of the urine, although this does not result in adverse events. Apart from rare documented cases of allergic reactions to riboflavin, toxicity in humans is unknown.

Dosage requirements

The RDI for riboflavin in Australia is 1.33 mg/day for men (increased to 1.6 mg/day >70 years) and 1.1 mg/day for women (increased to 1.3 mg/day >70 years. The RDI during pregnancy is 1.4 mg/day and lactation is 1.6 mg/day.[19] For preventing migraine headaches, a dose of 400 mg/day has been used, although the benefits can take up to 3 months to be fully realised.[21]

For preventing cataracts, a daily dietary intake of approximately 2.6 mg of riboflavin has been used.[22] A combination of riboflavin 3 mg plus niacin 40 mg/day has also been used.[22]

Food sources

Eggs, lean meat, organ meats, yeast extracts, green leafy vegetables and milk are important sources of riboflavin in Western diets.[23]

Dietary intake and the need for supplementation

Riboflavin status is adversely altered by infection.[24] Requirements may increase to some extent as a result of heavy exercise or dieting, and lowered riboflavin status has been observed in the presence of anorexia nervosa. Some cancers, congenital heart disease and alcoholism result in a greater risk of riboflavin deficiency.[25] A deficiency of riboflavin may result in a secondary deficiency in vitamin-B_6-dependent pathways. Some studies have shown reduced levels of enzymes (consistent with riboflavin deficiency) in women taking oral contraceptives, although this is probably only relevant in women with marginal riboflavin deficiency.[26] People taking tricyclic antidepressants will need to take supplemental riboflavin, in the form of a multivitamin containing adequate levels of B complex vitamins. Riboflavin is synthesised by the gut flora of the large bowel but very little of it is absorbed.[27] Riboflavin requirements are also increased during pregnancy and lactation and supplementation may be necessary.

VITAMIN B_3 (NIACIN, NIACINAMIDE)

Niacin has a wide variety of dietary sources and can also be synthesised from dietary tryptophan. Intake of niacin from the diet is based on niacin equivalents: 60 mg tryptophan = 1 mg niacin — (60 : 1).[28]

Forms of nutrient

The main forms of niacin are niacinamide and nicotinic acid. Nicotinamide adenine dinucleotide (NAD) and nicotinamide adenine dinucleotide phosphate (NADP) are the active coenzyme forms.

Distribution and storage

Niacin is found in high concentration in the liver, muscles, kidneys and heart. On entering the cell, niacin is converted into its coenzyme forms (NAD and NADP). Most NAD is found attached to enzymes; however, some may remain unattached. 'Free NAD' is referred to as 'storage NAD', and it has a high rate of turnover (clinical signs of pellagra have developed within 50–60 days).

Absorption

In low concentrations, niacin is rapidly absorbed in the proximal small intestine via facilitated diffusion, and at high concentrations it is absorbed via passive diffusion.

Excretion

Niacin is metabolised in the liver and excreted renally through the urine.[28] Any excess is methylated in the liver and excreted in the urine. Some may be excreted to the gastrointestinal tract and will then be excreted or reabsorbed.

Interactions (medication, nutrient, dietary)

Niacin (the nicotinic acid form) at pharmacological doses may affect glucose control and increase fasting blood glucose levels.[16] It may increase uric acid production in those prone to gout. It can also lead to mild-to-quite-severe episodes of flushing, tingling and itching.

- Oral contraceptive pill: this may reduce vitamin B_3 levels.
- Allopurinol: large doses of niacin can reduce urinary excretion of uric acid, potentially resulting in hyperuricaemia.[29]
- Isoniazid, rifampicin and other antitubercular agents may lead to drug-induced niacin depletion.[30]
- Mercaptopurine and azathioprine can induce niacin deficiency, and vitamin co-administration can reverse this.
- Tetracycline antibiotics: if taking niacin, ensure the supplement and antibiotic are administered at least 4 hours apart.
- Phenothiazines: there is a synergistic (beneficial) effect of concomitant niacin supplementation.
- Tricyclic antidepressants: co-administration of niacin and L-tryptophan has a potential synergistic (beneficial) effect.
- Cholesterol-lowering agents (e.g. ursodeoxycholic acid): this combination appears to be incompatible.

- Aspirin, paracetamol and non-steroidal anti-inflammatory drugs (NSAIDs): concomitant use may increase bleeding risk.
- HMG co-A reductase inhibitors (statins): beneficial interaction when administered concurrently.[31]

Function

Niacin and niacinamide have a very wide range of metabolic function and activity. Niacin and niacinamide are precursors of the enzymes NAD and NADP, which are essential for oxidation–reduction reactions, ATP synthesis and ADP–ribose reactions. The main function of NAD is the liberation of energy from dietary fuels, while NADP is mainly involved in fatty acid biosynthesis.

Therapeutic applications

The nicotinic acid form of vitamin B_3 is used in pharmacological doses (≥500 mg) for blood-lipid modification, but caution should be exercised as adverse events can occur in susceptible individuals at these high doses (e.g. flushing, hypotension, headaches). These adverse effects are not experienced with the niacinamide form.[28] For mild vitamin B_3 deficiency, niacin or niacinamide 50–100 mg/day is used. For pellagra in adults, the WHO recommends niacinamide (to avoid the flushing caused by niacin) at 300 mg/day in divided doses.[32] Doses of 2000–3000 mg of niacin in combination with simvastatin have been shown to increase high-density lipoproteins and decrease the frequency of cardiovascular events.[33] Supplementation of niacin has been used in psychiatric medicine to treat schizophrenia and recent scientific advances support the use of nutrient supplementation such as niacin.[34]

Reducing the 'niacin flush'

According to the leading orthomolecular physician Abram Hoffer, to reduce side effects such as flushing and itching it may be necessary to begin with a smaller dose. It may be necessary to start with 25 mg, taken after a meal with 1 g of vitamin C (vitamin C counteracts histamine released into the blood). As the flush moderates, the dose is gradually increased by 25 mg/week. Hoffer also recommends taking an aspirin before taking niacin, to decrease the side effects, and to have a high water intake.[35]

Deficiency signs

- *Mild deficiency*: indigestion, canker sores, unrelenting fatigue, vomiting, depression.
- *Severe deficiency*: pellagra — niacin deficiency presents with skin, mucous membrane, central nervous system and gastrointestinal symptoms. These are characterised as the 'four Ds': dermatitis, diarrhoea, dementia and death. The skin appears cracked, thick and scaly, with a darkly pigmented rash, which is made worse by sun exposure. The tongue and mouth become inflamed, with a burning sensation and a bright, beefy-red appearance. As the condition progresses dementia becomes a feature, with accompanying headaches, irritability and, followed by mental confusion, hallucinations, amnesia and severe depression.

Biochemical testing

- *N*-methylnicotinamide in urine
- 2-Pyridone (urine)
- Lactate and pyruvate in urine.

Supplemental forms

Niacinamide (also known as nicotinamide) is the main form of vitamin B_3 present in dietary sources and nutritional supplements. Vitamin B_3 is also available in the nicotinic acid form, which can be used to meet the daily requirements for this nutrient; it is also used in pharmacological doses but is treated as a prescription medicine at these ranges and can cause adverse effects. The inositol hexanicotinate (slow-release) form of vitamin B_3 can be used in higher doses without these side effects but is ineffective in modifying blood-lipid profiles.

Toxicity

Niacin from food does not cause adverse effects; however, there are many side effects associated with toxic doses of B_3 including hyperuricaemia, flush, hypotension, GI upset, hypothyroidism, hepatotoxicity and headache. Nausea, vomiting, elevated liver enzymes and jaundice have been associated with intakes of 3 g/day for longer than 3 months. Rare cases of liver toxicity have been reported in doses higher than 3.5 g/day.[36] Nicotinamide does not generally cause flushing and is mostly better tolerated than niacin; however, there have been observed signs of liver toxicity at doses of 3000 mg/day.[37]

Dosage requirements

The Australian RDI for niacin is 16 mg/day for adult males and 14 mg/day for women. This is increased to 17 mg/day during lactation and 18 mg/day during pregnancy. The upper level of intake of niacin (as nicotinic acid) is 35 mg/day for men and women (including in pregnancy and lactation). The upper level of intake of niacin (as nicotinamide) is 900 mg for men and women. An upper level of nicotinamide intake during pregnancy and lactation cannot be established — recommendations are that intake should be sourced from food only during these periods.[38]

Food sources

Meat, fish, poultry, wholegrain breads and bread products, fortified cereals, legumes, nuts and molasses. Brewer's yeast and yeast-extract spreads are also rich sources.

Dietary intake and the need for supplementation

Niacin adequacy in the diet is dependent on intake of tryptophan. It has been estimated that 60 mg of tryptophan is converted to 1 mg of niacin, although this varies from individual to individual. In a study conducted among Japanese women in 2004 it was shown that 67 mg of tryptophan was required to produce 1 mg of niacin.[39] The need for niacin is greater during pregnancy, and supplementation may be warranted. However, pregnancy greatly enhances the conversion of tryptophan to niacin. Therefore, if protein requirements are maintained during pregnancy, supplementation may not be necessary. If dietary protein levels and quality are high, it is possible for tryptophan alone to provide the daily requirement of niacin equivalents.[27]

Reduced kilojoule intake can lead to lowered tryptophan levels, and niacin deficiency is seen in those suffering from malnutrition, in the homeless and in anorexia nervosa.[40] For those who try to lose weight by consuming fewer kilojoules, blood tryptophan levels can be lowered substantially.[39] Niacin is lost when foods are cooked and these losses are particularly high for vegetables and rice. Perhaps ironically, heating can increase the niacin content of coffee. Espresso coffee can contain up to 24.1 mg of niacin per 100 g (niacin is released from trigonelline in coffee beans by the roasting process).[27]

VITAMIN B_5 (PANTOTHENIC ACID)

Forms of nutrient

The active form of pantothenic acid is coenzyme A (CoA).

Distribution and storage

Serum contains free pantothenic acid, while it is present in erythrocytes as coenzyme A.

Absorption

Approximately 50% of pantothenic acid is absorbed in the jejunum.

Excretion

Pantothenic acid is excreted in the urine.

Interactions (medication, nutrient, dietary)

Theoretically, antibiotics may interfere with pantothenic acid synthesised by the intestinal microflora, although it is not known if this is a significant source of the vitamin. Alcohol consumption can deplete this nutrient.

Function

Pantothenic acid is the precursor of CoA, which is essential for 4% of known enzymatic reactions. CoA is involved in over 100 different reactions in the intermediary metabolism.[41] CoA is required in the metabolism of carbohydrates, proteins and lipids. CoA is required in: acetylation reactions in glucogenesis; the release of energy from carbohydrates; and the biosynthesis and degradation of fatty acids, cholesterol, steroid hormones, porphyrins, acetylcholine and other compounds. Bacteria synthesise CoA from aspartate, α-ketovalerate, cysteine and ATP.

Therapeutic applications

The therapeutic dose is 50–100 mg/day; the safe upper limit has been reported as 550 mg/day.[41] Doses of 200 mg/day (in animals) have been trialled to enhance wound healing.[42]

Deficiency signs

- Sensation of 'burning' in the feet; fatigue.
- An induced deficiency in humans resulted in muscle weakness, malaise, vomiting, abdominal distress, cardiovascular symptoms and burning cramps.[43]

Biochemical testing

Pantothenic acid deficiency or insufficiency is difficult to establish conclusively, although urinary α-keto acids and pyruvate can provide a clue.

Supplemental forms

Calcium pantothenate is the most stable form commonly used in nutritional supplements.[44] It is composed of 91.5% pantothenic acid and 7.5% calcium. Pantothine — a pantothenic acid derivative — is available in Japan and the US as a cholesterol-lowering agent.[45]

Toxicity

Pantothenic acid is not known to be toxic in humans. When administered in doses of 10–20 g the only dated evidence of toxicity is occasional episodes of diarrhoea.[46]

Dosage requirements

Australian and New Zealand RDI for vitamin B_5 is 6 mg/day for men and 4 mg/day for women. The RDI in pregnancy is 5 mg/day and lactation is 6 mg/day.[47] In the US 10 mg/day is recommended for adults (both male and female).

Food sources

Chicken, beef, potatoes, oats, cereals, tomato products, liver, kidney, egg yolk, broccoli, avocados, sweet potatoes, wholegrains, milk and leafy green vegetables. Royal jelly contains significant amounts of pantothenic acid.[48]

Dietary intake and the need for supplementation

Due to the ubiquitous nature of pantothenic acid (*panto* is the Greek for 'everywhere'), deficiency of this nutrient is not a concern in clinical practice — it is essential to all forms of life and is present (to a degree) in all foods.[43] The amounts found in a well-formulated multivitamin and mineral supplement should provide adequate insurance against deficiency.

Oestrogen- and progestin-containing oral contraceptives may increase the requirement for pantothenic acid.[46]

VITAMIN B_6 (PYRIDOXINE)

Forms of nutrient

Vitamin B_6 is made up of a group of six related compounds: pyridoxal, pyridoxine, pyridoxamine and their 5′-phosphates. Pyridoxal is a form of vitamin B_6 obtained via the diet from animal food sources. Pyridoxine is the primary form of B_6 used in clinical treatment.[49] The liver very efficiently and rapidly converts pyridoxine to the pyridoxal form. The active form is pyridoxal 5-phosphate (PLP).

Distribution and storage

Pyridoxine and pyridoxal are transported to the liver, where they are oxidised to their active forms (pyridoxine and PLP) and distributed to tissue. A significant amount of PLP is found in muscle tissue (bound to phosphorylase) and in the liver.

Absorption

Pyridoxine and its related compounds are absorbed by simple diffusion in the upper small intestine. A more acidic environment increases absorption.

Excretion

Pyridoxine is rapidly and efficiently excreted in the urine.

Interactions (medication, nutrient, dietary)

- Drugs such as penicillamine, isoniazid and hydralazine: can lead to the depletion of vitamin B_6.[17]
- Antibiotic administration (due to disruption to the intestinal microbiota): can lead to reduced vitamin B_6. Broad-spectrum antibiotics used to treat tuberculosis (cycloserine) increase urinary excretion of pyridoxine.[50]
- Oral contraceptive pill: increases vitamin B_6 requirements.[16]
- Alcohol: increases requirements.
- Antiepileptic medicine (valproic acid, carbamazepine and phenytoin) reduces plasma PLP and can result in hyperhomocysteinaemia.[51]
- Phenobarbital (phenobarbitone): those taking this drug should avoid high doses of pyridoxine (data suggest that pyridoxine 200 mg/day can reduce plasma levels of phenobarbital [phenobarbitone]).[6]
- Theophylline: when used long-term this drug may induce a pyridoxine deficiency; supplementation may be required.[50]

Function

As a coenzyme vitamin B_6 is involved in a wide variety of metabolic reactions. These include: the transanimation of amino acids; the conversion of tryptophan to niacin; the synthesis of γ-aminobutyric acid (GABA) in the central nervous system; the metabolism of serotonin, noradrenaline and dopamine; the metabolism of polyunsaturated fatty acids and phospholipids; and the synthesis of the haem component of haemoglobin. It is also involved in protein, carbohydrate and lipid metabolism.[6,49] The presence of B_6 (and B_9 and B_{12}) is essential in homocysteine metabolism — the deficiency of any of these nutrients results in hyperhomocysteinaemia.[52] PLP is a coenzyme in a diverse range of biochemical reactions — more than 140 enzymes are PLP dependent.[49]

Therapeutic applications

For the treatment of deficiency states a dose of 5–25 mg/day is given.[16] Large US population studies found significantly more users or oral contraceptives (compared to women who have never used an OCP) had low plasma PLP levels.[53] For vitamin B_6 deficiency in women taking oral contraceptives the dose is 25–30 mg/day. For symptoms associated with premenstrual syndrome (PMS), controlled trials suggest a dose up to 100 mg/day may be of value.[54] Doses of 30–40 mg/day have been used for the treatment of hyperemesis gravidarum (nausea and vomiting) in pregnancy. Higher doses (25 mg every 8 hours for 3 days) used in studies suggest B_6 may be beneficial in reducing nausea.[55] Doses of 100–200 mg/day have been recommended for carpal tunnel syndrome.[56] For lowering elevated homocysteine, an effective daily regimen includes 50 mg pyridoxine in combination with vitamin B_{12} 1000 micrograms with 0.8 mg (800 micrograms) folic acid.[57]

Deficiency signs

Vitamin B_6 deficiency affects the metabolism of fatty acids, and can thus lead to skin lesions, seborrhoeic dermatitis, impaired immune function, depressive illness, feelings of confusion, irritability, tongue inflammation, skin ulceration at the corners of the mouth, and sores or ulcers of the mouth. Deficiency can also lead to decreased haemoglobin synthesis and microcytic anaemia. Hyperhomocysteinaemia as a result of B_6 deficiency is associated with cardiovascular disease (CVD), neurodegenerative disorders and complications in pregnancy.[52]

Biochemical testing

- Xanthurenate in urine
- Kynurenate in urine (organic acids produced from tryptophan)
- Homocysteine in plasma: >15 nmol/mL
- Homocysteine in urinare: >25 micrograms/mg creatine
- EGOT index — red blood cell count: >1.5 million cells/μL
- Plasma PLP (the most common measure of vitamin B_6 status): >30 nmol/L.

Supplemental forms

Pyridoxine hydrochloride is the most common supplemental form of vitamin B_6: 1 mg of pyridoxine hydrochloride typically yields 0.8227 mg of pyridoxine.

Toxicity

There are no reported adverse effects from high intakes of B_6 from food sources.[58] High doses (100–200 mg/day) may lead to toxicity when taken long-term — doses of 1000 mg have been associated with neuropathy.[49]

Dosage requirements

In Australia the RDI is 1.3 mg/day for male adults (19–30) and 1.7 mg/day for men >51 years. The RDI for women aged 19–50 is 1.3 mg/day and >51 years is 1.5 mg/day. The RDI is 1.9 mg/day in pregnancy and 2 mg/day in lactation. The upper level of intake for both men and women (including pregnancy and lactation) is 50 mg.[57,59]

Food sources

Wholegrain cereals, meat, organ meats, poultry, legumes, bananas and eggs. Yeast-extract spreads (Vegemite,

Marmite) are a rich source for supplementation during pregnancy or labour for improved maternal and neonatal outcomes.[60]

Dietary intake and the need for supplementation

As the levels of vitamin B_6 in basic foods can be reduced significantly by processing, preservation and refining, marginal deficiencies of this nutrient are probably more widespread than is currently recognised. Vitamin B_6 is present in a wide range of foods of both plant and animal origin, although it is highly unstable when subjected to heat, radiation and chemical oxidants.[61] Heavy alcohol use (and the metabolic byproduct acetaldehyde) has been shown to deplete vitamin B_6.[62] Long periods of unresolved stress may also lead to the depletion of vitamin B_6. Where lowering homocysteine levels is an important risk-reduction strategy, the administration of supplemental vitamin B_6 in combination with vitamin B_{12} and folic acid should prove an effective nutritional intervention. Reducing the dietary intake of methionine has also been suggested to be a relevant dietary consideration in this case.[61]

During pregnancy the requirement for vitamin B_6 is increased, especially in the third trimester, and supplementation is an important clinical consideration during this time.[60] Vitamin B_6 at doses up to 75–100 mg/day appears to be an effective measure for the treatment of hyperemesis gravidarum (morning sickness).[63] Requirements are also increased during lactation.

The intestinal flora synthesise relatively large amounts of B_6, although just how much is absorbed is open to speculation.[64] Theoretically, the administration of probiotics should lead to an improved biosynthesis of pyridoxine.

Taking vitamin B_6 at night should be avoided as it may evoke vivid dreams and cause sleep disruption.[16]

VITAMIN B_9 (FOLATE)

Forms of nutrient

The generic term 'folate' refers to a group of structurally related compounds, which are derivatives of the parent compound pteroylmonoglutamate (PGA) and exert the biological activity of folic acid. Folate occurs naturally in different forms, including 5-methyltetrahydrofolate (5-MTHF), 5-formyltetrahydrofolate (5-formyl-THF), 5,10-methyltetrahydrofolate and 5,10-methylene tetrahydrofolate. PGA is the principal intracellular form of folate in human tissue, and 5-MTHF is the principal form in plasma.

Distribution and storage

After absorption, folic acid enters the circulation and is delivered to a wide variety of tissues. The liver is the main storage site for folate, and accounts for 50% of total body stores. A considerable amount of folate is also recycled enterohepatically and reabsorbed.[65]

Absorption

Ingested folate is first hydrolysed by pancreatic folate conjugase and mucosal conjugase, and is then transported across the proximal small intestine (jejunum) via active transport and diffusion. A small percentage is passively absorbed, as is the case with vitamin B_{12}.

Excretion

Some folate is eliminated through the bile, although the kidneys are the predominant route of excretion.

Interactions (medication, nutrient, dietary)

- Sulfasalazine, cimetidine and antacids impede folate absorption.
- Aminopterin, methotrexate, pyrimethamine, trimethoprim and triamterene are all folate antagonists.
- Anti-epileptic medications (phenytoin, valproate, carbamazepine) and cholestyramine increase the requirement for folate.
- Proton pump inhibitors, anticonvulsants, antituberculosis drugs, alcohol and oral contraceptives lead to lowered serum and tissue levels of folate.[65]

Folic acid supplementation can mask neurological complications in people with vitamin B_{12} deficiency. Use of pancreatic enzymes might impair absorption of folic acid. It is suggested that folic acid supplementation is given at different times from enzyme supplementation if both are being used therapeutically.[66] It has been proposed that folic acid supplementation may interfere with zinc absorption, although there is little current evidence to support this.[67]

Function

Folate coenzymes within the cell are involved in one-carbon transfer reactions, including those involved in phases of amino acid metabolism, nucleotide biosynthesis (purine and thymidine), repair and synthesis of DNA and the remethylation of homocysteine to methionine. Methionine is used for protein synthesis or conversion to S-adenosylmethionine (the body's primary methyl donor).[68]

Therapeutic applications

- *Moderate deficiency:* doses of 250–1000 micrograms have been recommended
- *Severe deficiency:* in severe deficiency states such as megoblastic anaemia higher dose — 5 mg/day — can correct the anaemia. (Note: this can potentially delay diagnosis of B_{12} deficiency which, if left untreated, can cause permanent cognitive decline and nerve damage).[68]

400 micrograms/day is recommended for the prevention of neural tube defects. In women with a history of complications associated with neural tube defects 5 mg/day prior to conception and continuing throughout the first trimester is recommended.[69]

To improve cognitive function in the elderly a daily regimen of 800 micrograms folic acid, 500 micrograms vitamin B_{12} and 20 mg vitamin B_6 has shown benefits. These benefits were particularly observed in patients with higher baseline homocysteine, suggesting an important role in lowering homocysteine to prevent cognitive decline and dementia.[70]

To lower homocysteine levels, an effective daily regimen includes 0.8 mg (800 micrograms) folic acid in combination with 1000 micrograms vitamin B_{12} and 50 mg pyridoxine.[57] Folic acid supplementation (alone) at 0.5–5 mg/day has also been shown to lower plasma homocysteine concentrations on average by 25%.[71]

To improve response to antidepressants doses of 200–500 micrograms have been used. To reduce the toxicity of methotrexate used to treat rheumatoid arthritis and psoriasis doses of 1–5 mg have been used.[65] While the timing of taking folic acid in relation to methotrexate still lacks consensus, most trials avoid administration of folic acid on the same day as methotrexate.[72]

Deficiency signs

Macrocytic anaemia, megaloblastic anaemia (severe deficiency), hyperhomocysteinaemia, peripheral neuropathy, neurological symptoms,[67] mental confusion, depression, insomnia, nausea, fatigue, headaches, anorexia, glossitis, gastrointestinal disturbances, irritability, diarrhoea, frequent infections, paranoid behaviour.[31]

Biochemical testing

The following marker levels indicate deficiency:

- Serum folate: <3 ng/mL (the first sign of suboptimal intake and reflects recent dietary intake)[73]
- Erythrocyte folate: <140 ng/mL (a decrease in RBC folate follows serum folate reductions — erythrocyte folate reflects tissue stores and folate status over 120 days)[73]
- Homocysteine in plasma: >15 nmol/mL (follows serum folate and RBC folate. Note: this is a useful functional indicator of folate status; however, elevated concentrations of homocysteine can be seen in other situations e.g. B_6, B_{12})[73]
- Homocysteine in urine: >25 micrograms/mg creatinine[74]
- Leucocyte folate: <500 ng/mL.

Supplemental forms

Oral folates are generally available in two supplemental forms: folic acid (or pteroylmonoglutamic acid) and folinic acid. Folic acid is stable and inexpensive and is the common form used in dietary supplementation and food fortification.[68] Some researchers claim that folinic acid may be the optimal form of supplemental folate. It bypasses the deconjugation and reduction steps required for standard folic acid and is more metabolically active — it is capable of boosting levels of folic acid in circumstances where regular folic acid has little effect.[65] Folate found in food is in the form of pteroylpolyglutamate. Folinic acid is available as a supplement in the form of calcium folinate.

Toxicity

Supplemental folic acid is generally considered non-toxic, even at high doses. At nutritional doses it is quite safe.

Dosage requirements

The recommended daily intake of folic acid is 400 micrograms/day for adult men and women. The dose should be increased to 600 micrograms/day during pregnancy and to 500 micrograms/day during lactation.[75] To avoid masking vitamin B_{12} deficiency, the upper level of intake for men and women (including pregnancy and lactation) is 1000 micrograms/day.[76]

Food sources

Leafy green vegetables, dark-green vegetables (broccoli and Brussels sprouts), fruits, brewer's yeast, beans, legumes, liver and kidney contain high amounts of folate. Australian millers are required (by law) to add folic acid to wheat flour for the purposes of making bread (plain, sweet, rolls, bagels, English muffins, focaccia and both commercial and domestic flour mixes).[77]

Dietary intake and the need for supplementation

Folate in food is less bioavailable (~50%) than synthetic folic acid, which is 100% bioavailable ingested on an empty stomach.[68] Before folate in food can be absorbed it must first be enzymatically deconjugated in the small intestine to the monoglutamate form. After absorption it is then reduced to the tetrahydrofolate form before entering the methylation cycle. Folate repletion would therefore be more effective using a supplement, although dietary sources should be increased to provide long-term sufficiency.

The cooking and processing of foods readily destroys folate. A diet that is high in animal proteins and low in fresh vegetables and leafy greens is likely to contribute to folate deficiency, although some animal foods such as liver contain high levels of folate. It has been suggested by one researcher that the low incidence of cardiovascular disease among the French may be due to their high intake of artisan foods made from organ meats (pâté, terrines, foie gras), which are excellent and palatable sources of folate.

Folic acid deficiency is common in the elderly. In the elderly, folate supplementation should be accompanied by vitamin B_{12} in case there is masking of a B_{12} deficiency, which exacerbates neurological symptoms.[78]

The biological requirement for folate and the risk of deficiency is highest during the anabolic phases of the life span including pregnancy, the development of the fetus and lactation, and supplementation is warranted during these periods of high demand.[68]

Individuals who are homozygous for the genetic variation that causes MTHF reductase deficiency (C667T polymorphism) may have an increased requirement for folate.

There is an association with suboptimal folate intake and the development of some cancers, including breast, prostate and colorectal cancer thought to be related to folate's role in DNA synthesis, stability and repair.[79]

The administration of folic acid, vitamins B_6 and B_{12} and betaine remains a useful nutritional strategy for lowering homocysteine levels in people at risk of the complications of cardiovascular disease.[80]

VITAMIN B_{12} (COBALAMIN)

Forms of nutrient

Methylcobalamin and 5-deoxyadenosylcobalamin.

Distribution and storage

Vitamin B_{12} is actively transported into the blood via protein binding to transcobalamin II. The major storage sites for vitamin B_{12} are the liver, the kidneys and the adrenal glands. It is distributed throughout the body tissues, where it is converted to its active coenzymes methylcobalamin and 5-deoxyadenosylcobalamin. The extensive capacity for the liver to store B_{12} means it may be 5–10 years between deficiency and onset of clinic symptoms.[81]

Absorption

Gastric acid initially liberates B_{12} from animal proteins. Following this, the absorption of cobalamin is highly dependent on the presence of intrinsic factor, a protein that is secreted by the parietal cells of the stomach. Bound to intrinsic factor, vitamin B_{12} is transferred across the gastrointestinal mucosa to the ileum, where it is absorbed.[82] When the secretion of intrinsic factor is impaired, as little as 1% of vitamin B_{12} is absorbed. Inflammatory disorders affecting the terminal ileum, such as Crohn's disease and coeliac disease, may also decrease absorption.

Excretion

Vitamin B_{12} is primarily excreted through the urine; however, approximately 0.6–6 micrograms/day is excreted via the bile and almost all is reabsorbed in the ileum.

Interactions (medication, nutrient, dietary)

- Steroid drugs, such as prednisone, have been reported to increase the absorption of vitamin B_{12} in patients with pernicious anaemia.
- Excessive alcohol consumption and some drugs may decrease absorption of B_{12}.
- Administration of chloramphenicol may lead to antagonism of the haematopoietic response to vitamin B_{12}.
- Prolonged metformin use may increase the risk of B_{12} deficiency.[83]
- Phenobarbital (phenobarbitone) and phenytoin may lead to markedly elevated serum B_{12} levels, which may be responsible for the neuropsychiatric side effects of these drugs.
- The oral contraceptive pill lowers concentrations of B_{12}, as do gastric acid inhibitors, proton pump inhibitors and H_2 receptor antagonists.
- Folic acid deficiency can bring about a deficiency of B_{12}. Large doses of vitamin C may diminish the effectiveness of B_{12} and should be administered separately.

Function

Vitamin B_{12} is a name used to describe a group of compounds known collectively as 'cobalamins'. Vitamin B_{12} serves as a cofactor for three enzymatic processes: homocysteine to methionine, methylmalonic acid to succinyl CoA and 5-methyltetrahydofolate to tetrahydrofolate (needed for red blood cell production and DNA synthesis).[84]

Therapeutic applications

For pernicious anaemia, cyanocobalamin doses of 1000–2000 micrograms/day for life.[85] For mild malabsorption, 500–1000 micrograms/day (or every other day) for 1 week then weekly for 4–8 weeks.[85] For lowering elevated homocysteine, an effective daily regimen includes vitamin B_{12} 1000 micrograms in combination with 0.8 mg (800 micrograms) folic acid and 50 mg pyridoxine.[57]

Deficiency signs

Confusion and memory loss (key presenting features in the elderly). Depression, irritability, fatigue, feelings of agitation, psychosis, poor blood clotting and a tendency to bruise easily, pernicious anaemia (the most common cause of severe B_{12} deficiency), macrocytic anaemia, infertility, hyperhomocysteinaemia, progressive peripheral neuropathy, impaired coordination, unsteady gait, paraesthesia, loss of appetite, nausea, glossitis, irregularities of the tongue and mouth, achlorhydria, dermatitis and skin sensitivity.[85]

Biochemical testing

- Serum vitamin B_{12}: <150 pmol/mL.(sub-clinical deficiency 150–220 pmol/L)[86]
- Methylmalonic acid in blood: >0.4 mol/mL
- Homocysteine in urine: >25 micrograms/mg creatinine
- Homocysteine in plasma: >9.8 nmol/mL.

Supplemental forms

Cyanocobalamin is the form of vitamin B_{12} most commonly found in vitamin B_{12} supplements. It is also available as adenosylcobalamin, hydroxocobalamin and methylcobalamin. Vitamin B_{12} is available in sublingual, nasal and oral preparations, and can also be administered intramuscularly.

Toxicity

No toxicity for vitamin B_{12} has been recorded, even at high oral doses (>10 mg/day).

Dosage requirements

The absolute minimum requirement for vitamin B_{12} for the maintenance of haematological status and basic serum vitamin B_{12} values is 2.4 micrograms/day — this is reflected in the Australian RDI for men and women. The RDI is increased during pregnancy (2.6 micrograms/day) and lactation (2.8 micrograms/day).[87] In the elderly, daily supplementation with 10–25 micrograms/day has been recommended. Vegans will benefit from 2–3 micrograms/day (minimum).

Food sources

Fortified cereals, cheese, milk, lamb's liver, beef, kidney, sardines, poultry, fish, shellfish and eggs. About 25% of B_{12} is consumed from animal sources and 30–50% from milk and dairy products.[87] Vitamin B_{12} is also present in trace amounts in some plant-based sources such as edible algae, mushrooms, fermented soya foods such as tempeh.

Dietary intake and the need for supplementation

Absorption of vitamin B_{12} is reduced with increasing age (10–30% of older people malabsorb food-bound vitamin B_{12}). As people age they become susceptible to deficiencies in key nutrients. Vitamin B_{12} deficiency can occur in up to 20% of the older population. Because many of the symptoms of vitamin B_{12} deficiency can be very similar to the litany of complaints attributable to 'getting old', such as fatigue, lassitude, malaise, vertigo and cognitive impairment, B_{12} deficiency should be considered in any differential diagnosis of the older population. Despondency and depression are almost always a feature of this deficiency as well.

Causes of the deficiency include, most frequently, food-cobalamin malabsorption syndrome (>60% of all cases), pernicious anaemia (15–20% of all cases), insufficient dietary intake and malabsorption. Hypochlorhydria or low stomach gastric acid production can also lead to B_{12} deficiency. In older people there is a greater incidence of hypochlorhydria.[88] Vegans and vegetarians (including exclusively breastfed children of vegetarian mothers) are at greater risk of becoming vitamin B_{12} deficient.[82]

Despite the fact that it is possible to obtain vitamin B_{12} from some non-animal sources (e.g. tempeh, nori seaweed) the trace amounts found in these foods are unlikely to prevent deficiency. It is highly advisable for people whose diet excludes all animal proteins (vegans and strict vegetarians) to take a supplement that fulfils the basic requirements for this nutrient. Unlike folate, cobalamin is resistant to destruction by cooking. To improve the absorption of vitamin B_{12}, even when the diet contains rich sources of this nutrient, it would still seem clinically relevant to ensure that the gastrointestinal environment is balanced and functioning correctly. In hypochlorhydria (lowered stomach hydrochloric acid (HCl)), neither the separation from protein nor the binding to intrinsic factor can take place, significantly decreasing the bioavailability of vitamin B_{12}.[89] In some instances supplementation with betaine hydrochloride to increase gastric pH may be necessary.

Vitamin B_{12} (as cyanocobalamin or methylcobalamin) has been shown to be an effective, cost-effective and safe method of treating and preventing vitamin B_{12} deficiency. Administered orally or sublingually, it is a highly effective therapy and a less invasive alternative to receiving an intramuscular injection.[82] Research suggests high-dose oral supplementation is as effective as intramuscular vitamin B_{12}, except potentially in those with poor absorption due to pernicious anaemia.[90] Even when intrinsic factor is not present a percentage of cobalamin is passively diffused and absorbed. People aged 50 years and over are less likely to absorb vitamin B_{12} from food, and a daily oral or sublingual supplement would help prevent deficiency.

BIOTIN (B_7)

Forms of nutrient

The active form of biotin (or vitamin H) is biocytin.

Distribution and storage

Biotin is distributed in whole blood and serum. The liver is an important storage site.

Absorption

Studies in animals have shown that biotin is absorbed from the upper portion of the small intestine, probably via active transport. It is also absorbed in the distal colon in humans. Once absorbed by the mucosal cells of the digestive system it is bound to protein and cannot diffuse back into the lumen of the gastrointestinal tract. Biotin can be produced by gut bacteria but limited absorption is shown from this route.

Avidin and biotin

Avidin, the glycoprotein from raw egg white, binds to biotin in the gut to form an insoluble complex that cannot be absorbed. Once heated, avidin is denatured, becomes inactive and no longer affects biotin absorption.

Excretion

Biotin is excreted via the urine and faeces.

Interactions (medication, nutrient, dietary)

- Some anticonvulsant drugs and alcohol may inhibit intestinal carrier-mediated transport of biotin and renal absorption.
- Steroid hormones and some anticonvulsant drugs may accelerate the catabolism of biotin in the tissues.
- Antibacterial sulfa drugs and other antibiotic therapy may decrease bacterial synthesis of biotin; however, the degree of bacterial synthesis of biotin still remains to be fully elucidated.[50]
- Biotin taken together with either alpha lipoic acid or vitamin B_5 (panthothenic acid) can reduce the body's absorption of both nutrients.

Function

Biotin is a coenzyme in synthesis of fat, glycogen and amino acids. It acts as an essential cofactor for the acetyl-CoA, propionyl-CoA, β-methylcrotonyl-CoA and pyruvate carboxylase enzymes, which are important in the synthesis of fatty acids, the catabolism of branched-chain amino acids and the gluconeogenic pathway. Biotin may also have a role in the regulation of gene expression arising from its interaction with nuclear histone proteins.

Therapeutic applications

To date there is very scant information regarding the amount of dietary biotin required to promote optimal health or prevent chronic disease. Oral biotin supplementation has been well tolerated in doses up to 200 mg/day in people with hereditary disorders of biotin metabolism. In people without disorders of biotin metabolism, doses of up to 5 mg/day for 2 years were not associated with adverse effects. Supplemental biotin alone (9 mg) and in combination with chromium picolinate has proved effective in the maintenance of glycaemic control and reduction in plasma triglycerides.[91] High-dose biotin (100–330 mg/day) may positively impact disability in progressive multiple sclerosis due to its role in activating acetyl-CoA carboxylase (a rate-limiting enzyme in myelin synthesis).[92]

Deficiency signs

Dietary biotin deficiency is rare. Early signs of biotin deficiency may include changes in skin quality and integrity, such as depigmentation, scaly dermatitis, abnormal hair loss (alopecia), conjunctivitis, central nervous system abnormalities and impaired immunity.

Biochemical testing

- Urinary α-hydroxyisovalerate.
- Plasma biotin is not a sensitive marker for deficiency.

Supplemental forms

Occurs as D-biotin, also known as vitamin H. Biotin contains not less than 97.5% and not more than the equivalent of 100.5% of 5-[(3a*S*, 4*S*, 6a*R*)-2-oxohexahydrothieno[3,4-D]imidazol-4-yl] pentanoic acid.

Toxicity

There is no known toxicity for biotin.

Dosage requirements

There is no RDI for biotin. The AI is 30 micrograms/day for males and 25 micrograms/day for females. Requirements increase during pregnancy (30 micrograms/day) and lactation (35 micrograms/day).[93] In Europe the recommended daily intake is 40 micrograms/day.[94] In deficiency states 100–600 micrograms/day has been well tolerated.[95]

Food sources

Egg yolk, liver and yeast are rich sources of biotin.

Dietary intake and the need for supplementation

Those who avoid rich food sources of biotin, such as eggs, liver, some cheeses and yeast, should consider taking a supplement that contains B complex vitamins including biotin. Biotin requirements may increase during pregnancy. Recent studies also suggest that individuals who consume a ketogenic diet have an increased biotin requirement.[96]

INOSITOL

Forms of nutrient

The free form of inositol in humans is myo-inositol (1,2,3,5/4,6-cyclohexitol), the structure of which closely resembles glucose. It appears in combined forms as esters, phosphates and as a component of phospholipids (phosphatidylinositol).

Distribution and storage

Myo-inositol is widely distributed and is found in virtually all human cells. The highest concentrations are found in the kidneys and the brain. Lesser amounts are found in muscle tissue, red blood cells, body fluids, and in the liver and pancreas.

Absorption

Dietary inositol is converted in the intestine through the endogenous microflora, although the major supply pathway of inositol monophosphate is via a receptor-mediated salvage system and from glucose-6-phosphate.[31]

Excretion

The kidney is the main site for excretion (urinary). Understandably, high intake of caffeine and diabetes will increase excretion.

Interactions (medication, nutrient, dietary)

Carbamazepine reduces inositol levels in the brain by inhibiting enzymatic synthesis of inositol. Valproic acid and pharmacological lithium carbonate also reduce inositol levels in the brain, probably by a similar mechanism.

Function

The primary function of inositol is in cell membrane structure and integrity. It is an essential component of cell membrane phospholipids. Inositol is linked to serotonin, noradrenaline and cholinergic receptors, as a constituent of the intracellular phosphatidyl second messenger system. It works closely with choline. Recent data also suggest that inositol functions as a mediator in the insulin signalling pathway.[97]

Therapeutic applications

Clinical trials have been conducted using inositol to treat central nervous system disorders such as Alzheimer's disease, eating disorders, panic disorder, depression and obsessive–compulsive disorder. Supplementation between 12 g and 18 g has proven effective in treating panic disorders.[98] Supplementation of inositol has shown promising results on maternal metabolic profiles in pregnancy and as a potential treatment for non-insulin-resistance with PCOS.[99,100]

Deficiency signs

Decreased growth, alopecia (hair loss), dermatitis and weight loss have been seen in animal studies, although there is no reliable consensus on the signs and symptoms of inositol deficiency in humans.

Biochemical testing

At present there are no clinical evaluations available for inositol status.

Supplemental forms

An alternative name for inositol is hexahydroxy-cyclohexane. Inositol hexaphosphate (InsP6; IP6) is a form of inositol present in some foods (e.g. grains, soya beans). It is available in supplement form. Myo-inositol (also known as mesoinositol; *cis*-1,2,3,5-*trans*-4,6-inositol) is the nutritionally active form and the most prevalent natural isomer of inositol. It is the most commonly available supplemental form of inositol.

Toxicity

There is no known toxicity of inositol, even at quite high levels (3 g), although it may have a laxative effect.

Dosage requirements

No RDI or RDA for inositol has been established. The estimated daily average intake (US) ranges from 300 mg/day to 1000 mg/day.

Food sources

Wholegrains, citrus fruits, brewer's yeast and molasses are rich sources of inositol.

Dietary intake and the need for supplementation

Levels of inositol supplied in a supplement containing the B group vitamins should be adequate to ensure adequacy of intake. As a precautionary measure against deficiency inositol is included in infant formulas.

CHOLINE

Forms of nutrient

Choline has three methyl groups that are available for transfer to homocysteine or tetrahydrofolate. Although choline can be synthesised in human tissue by methylation of glycine, there are many conditions that limit the rate of synthesis, making it a conditionally essential nutrient. It is dependent on glycine, folic acid, vitamin B_{12} and methyl donor compounds.

Distribution and storage

Choline accumulates in all tissues but is concentrated in fatty tissues such as the liver, kidneys, breast tissue, placenta and brain.

Absorption

Absorption of choline occurs in the small intestine by passive diffusion and it is transported by chylomicrons to the liver. Absorption is best when given as lecithin (phosphatidyl choline).

Excretion

Excretion is via the hepatobiliary route with eventual elimination via faeces.

Interactions (medication, nutrient, dietary)

Methotrexate has been shown to decrease choline levels, and administration of choline has been shown to decrease liver damage caused by the drug.[101]

Function

Choline is essential for: cell membrane structure and signalling; as a methyl donor via betaine (it is involved in the regulation of homocysteine concentration in the blood); as a neurotransmitter (acetylcholine); as a precursor to phospholipids (phosphatidylcholine and sphingomyelin); and in the metabolism and transport of cholesterol and lipids.

Therapeutic applications

- Liver conditions, including alcohol related liver damage, non-alcoholic fatty liver disease (NAFLD), gallstones and hepatitis[102]
- Improves methylation in people with impaired MTHFR (C677T) function
- Pregnancy
- Heart disease, including hypercholesterolaemia and hypertension
- Disorders of the central nervous system, including dementia, Alzheimer's disease and senile dementia, panic disorder.

Deficiency signs

Deficiency results in fatty liver changes (NAFLD) and abnormalities in liver function.[103] The primary marker of deficient choline is liver damage identified by elevated alanine aminotransferase (ALT).

Biochemical testing

Phosphocholine in the liver (highly correlated with dietary choline).[104]

Supplemental forms

Choline chloride or choline bitartrate, and lecithin (commercial lecithins contain between 20% and 90% phosphatidylcholine). Phosphatidylcholine provides choline (4.2 g phosphatidylcholine = 550 mg of choline).[45]

Toxicity

Excessive consumption (10 000–16 000 mg/day) has been associated with reduced appetite (anorexia), nausea, vomiting, gastrointestinal distress, and fishy body odour.[105]

Dosage requirements

There is no established RDI. AI in men is 550 mg/day, women 425 mg/day, pregnancy 550 mg/day, lactation 550 mg/day. The upper level of intake is 3500 mg/day.[104] Between 300 mg and 1100 mg improves methylation in those with impaired MTHFR function.[106]

Food sources

Soya and egg are the sources with the highest choline content (2200 mg choline per 100 g). Also found in milk, liver and peanuts.

Dietary intake and the need for supplementation

Diets high in lecithin have been shown to double plasma choline concentrations. The requirements for choline are influenced by other methyl group donors. Strict vegetarians (no milk or eggs) are at risk of inadequate choline intake.

VITAMIN C

Forms of nutrient

Vitamin C is a name used to describe a range of compounds that exhibit the biological activity of ascorbic acid. Naturally occurring vitamin C appears in both the reduced form (L-ascorbic acid) and its oxidised form (L-dehydroascorbic acid).

Distribution and storage

Ascorbate and dehydroascorbate circulate in the bloodstream both in free solution and bound to albumin. After it enters the circulation, vitamin C is taken up and concentrated in a wide range of tissues. There is no specific storage site for vitamin C, although it does concentrate in the adrenal glands, with other glandular tissues, such as the thymus and pituitary, also exhibiting relatively high concentrations. White blood cells have a marked ability to concentrate ascorbate.[107] Skeletal muscle is also highly responsive to vitamin C intake and has exhibited a greater relative uptake than leucocytes.[108]

Absorption

Vitamin C is absorbed in the middle region of the small intestine (jejunum) and to some degree in the mouth, stomach and proximal small intestine, through active transport mechanisms and passive diffusion. Plasma concentrations of oral doses of vitamin C increase significantly at doses between 30 mg and 100 mg/day with approximately 70–90% absorption up to 180 mg/day,[109] with some research suggesting doses up to 200 mg at a time have a 100% absorption efficiency.[110] Absorption of doses above 1 g/day falls to less than 50%.[109]

Excretion

Vitamin C is excreted primarily through the urine. The kidneys regulate vitamin C levels by conserving energy stores when intake is low and excreting excess when intake is high. Any excess is excreted within 2–3 hours and most is excreted in urine as ascorbic acid or its metabolites. Even with very low intakes of vitamin C 5–10% is in the form of oxalic acid, but excretion in this form is limited when intake is high.

Factors that increase the breakdown or excretion are:

- psychological, chemical, emotional or physiological stress
- alcohol, smoking, antibiotics, cortisone, aspirin and heavy metals
- fever, viral illnesses.

Interactions (medication, nutrient, dietary)

- Patients with renal failure who take aluminium-containing compounds such as phosphate binders should avoid high dose supplemental vitamin C.
- Warfarin: vitamin C doses of 5–10 g/day can reduce warfarin absorption. Individuals on anticoagulants should limit their vitamin C intake to 1 g/day and have their prothrombin time monitored by the clinician following their anticoagulant therapy.
- People on sodium-restricted diets may be advised to avoid megadoses of sodium ascorbate.[111]

Function

The functions of vitamin C are primarily due to its ability to undergo reversible oxidation and reduction. This characteristic allows vitamin C to act as a cofactor for reactions that require a metal ion (such as Fe^{2+} or Cu^{1+}) and to serve as a protective antioxidant.

Vitamin C (ascorbic acid, ascorbate) is involved in a wide range of metabolic processes, including oxidation–reduction reactions and cellular respiration, carbohydrate metabolism, synthesis of lipids and proteins, conversion of cholesterol to bile acids and conversion of folic acid to folinic acid. Vitamin C increases the bioavailability of iron from food by promoting intestinal absorption of non-haem iron.[112] An important biochemical function of vitamin C is to act as a reducing agent and as a cofactor for metalloenzymes, copper-containing hydroxylases and the 2-oxoglutarate-linked, iron-containing hydroxylases.

Vitamin C is a potent reducing agent; it reduces hydrogen peroxide and also acts as a free-radical-quenching antioxidant. It is also important for regeneration of other antioxidants, α-tocopherol and glutathione.[107] Vitamin C acts to reduce the tocopheroxyl radical formed by oxidation of the vitamin in cell membranes and plasma lipoproteins. It also reacts with nitrite to form NO, NO_2 and N_2, preventing the formation of carcinogenic *N*-nitrosamines.[107]

Vitamin C is required for the synthesis of collagen, an important structural component of blood vessels, tendons, ligaments and bone. Vitamin C also plays an important role in the synthesis of the neurotransmitter, noradrenaline.

Therapeutic applications

The therapeutic applications of vitamin C are summarised in Appendix 3 available online at Expert Consult.

- Lowers blood cholesterol concentration and improves blood lipid profile.[113]
- Reduces the severity of allergic reactions.[114]

Deficiency signs

- *Severe deficiency*: appears definitively as scurvy, although this condition is rare in the developed world.
- *Subclinical deficiency*: is quite common and has various clinical manifestations. These may include: fatigue; psychomotor decline; listlessness, anorexia, irritability and failure to thrive (in infants); increased susceptibility to colds and infections; poor collagen synthesis; degenerative changes in capillaries, bone and connective tissue; bleeding gums; easy bruising; poor wound healing; dry skin; arthralgia, aching bones, joints and muscles; personality changes.

Biochemical testing

- Ascorbate in serum (reflects recent dietary intake).
- Ascorbate in leucocytes (reflects tissue stores).
- Ascorbate in urine after a 500 mg oral load.

Supplemental forms

Mineral ascorbates are the preferred form used in the majority of dietary supplements, and all appear to be equally well absorbed. They are also less acidic than non-buffered vitamin C supplements, and are less irritating to the gastrointestinal tract than pure ascorbic acid. Sodium ascorbate and calcium ascorbate are the most common supplemental forms, although a number of other mineral ascorbates are available. Sodium ascorbate generally supplies 111 mg of sodium per 1000 mg of ascorbic acid, and calcium ascorbate provides 90–110 mg of calcium per 1000 mg of ascorbic acid. Natural and synthetic L-ascorbic acid are chemically identical, and there appears to be very little difference in their biological activity.[115]

Toxicity

Vitamin C is non-toxic, even at extremely high doses. Common issues associated with high-dose intake include nausea, diarrhoea and abdominal cramping as a result of the osmotic effect of unabsorbed vitamin C.[109]

Dosage requirements

The dietary reference ranges of vitamin C for various life stages are given in Appendix 3 available online at Expert Consult.

The RDI for men and women is 45 mg/day, increasing to 60 mg/day in pregnancy and 80 mg/day during breastfeeding.[116] The upper tolerable limit (while not established) is conservatively recommended at 1000 mg/day. US recommendations (RDA) are higher — men (90 mg/day), women (75 mg/day), pregnancy (85 mg/day), breastfeeding (120 mg/day) and a set RDA for smokers of 125 mg/day for men and 110 g/day for women.[117]

Note: International RDI/RDAs for vitamin C are set to prevent vitamin C deficiency (scurvy) and vary widely. Some countries (e.g. France) are looking beyond the prevention of deficiency to the broader benefits of vitamin C in disease prevention, and are adjusting their RDAs accordingly. This approach is echoed by some in the wider scientific community who believe clinical data from scientific studies strongly suggest that vitamin C intake above the RDA can contribute to the prevention of chronic disease (e.g. CVD and certain cancers).[118]

Food sources

Capsicum, kiwi fruit, papaya, blackcurrants, oranges, strawberries, grapefruit, melon, sweet potato, spinach, redcurrants, pineapple, Brussels sprouts, mangoes, satsumas, tangerines, turnips, gooseberries, broccoli, swedes, spring onions, artichokes, potatoes, avocados, leeks, lemons, okra, peas, raspberries, tomatoes, blackberries, bananas, cauliflower, broad beans, cabbage, nectarines, parsnips, rhubarb, etc.[119]

Dietary intake and the need for supplementation

In developed countries it would certainly seem that overt vitamin C deficiency (scurvy) has been consigned to history as a nutritional relic of less enlightened times. Nevertheless, 'hypovitaminosis C' lingers as a clinical reality in the contemporary world — particularly in at-risk populations.[120] This is despite the urgings of government health authorities, who have repeatedly conveyed the message of the importance of a regular daily intake of fresh fruit and vegetables. And given that a relatively small amount (<100 mg/day) of vitamin C is required to maintain total storage pools in those without a deficiency, this advice would seem sound. However, when fresh fruit and vegetables are not a regular part of the diet there is a strong rationale for supplementation. The amount of vitamin C present in well-formulated multivitamin and mineral supplements would certainly meet the requirements for the prevention of overt deficiency, and would account for shortfalls in the diet, although higher doses are often warranted during times of acute stress and during illness. The vitamin C requirement of smokers is twice that of non-smokers. Bioavailability is also reduced in stress, viral illnesses, fever, heavy metal toxicity, antibiotic use and painkillers.[114] While it has been demonstrated that plasma and circulating cells are saturated at 300 mg/day, with urinary elimination of higher doses,[109] empirical evidence suggests that the effective dose range and tolerability of vitamin C are relative to individual requirements, and that oral doses of more than 1 g/day are often effective for clinical conditions.

Fat-soluble vitamins

VITAMIN A (RETINOL, RETINAL AND RETINOIC ACID)

Retinol activity equivalents

Vitamin A activity is expressed in microgram retinol equivalents (RE):

- 1 microgram RE = 1 microgram retinol
  = 6 micrograms β-carotene
  = 12 micrograms α-carotene and other provitamin A carotenoids
- 1 IU retinol = 0.3 micrograms RE.[121]

Forms of nutrient

Vitamin A is a general term used to describe a group of compounds that demonstrate the biological activity of retinol. The term 'retinoids' applies to the compounds retinol (an alcohol) and retinal (an aldehyde), which appear in animal products and are classified as 'preformed vitamin A'. Another class of compounds related to vitamin A are the 'provitamin A carotenoids', which are found in plant foods. These compounds (α-carotene, β-carotene, lutein, zeaxanthin, lycopene, etc.) can be metabolised to retinol in humans. These compounds also have antioxidant activity and other roles independent of retinol.

The retinoids are the three forms of vitamin A that are active in the human body. They are:

Retinol:
- alcohol form
  - major storage and transport form of vitamin A
  - involved in reproduction.

Retinal:
- aldehyde form
  - important for vision
  - intermediate in the conversion of retinol and retinoic acid.

Retinoic acid:
- acid form
  - acts like a hormone
  - involved in regulating growth and embryonic development.

Distribution and storage

More than 90% of vitamin A present in the body is found in the liver, although some is present in all tissues. The supply of vitamin A in the liver is enough to last for several months. About 80–90% is stored in the stellate cells, and 10–20% is stored in the hepatocytes. It is also concentrated in the retina, kidneys, lungs, adrenal glands and intraperitoneal fat.

Absorption

Vitamin A is absorbed in the duodenum and jejunum. Absorption is enhanced by gastric secretions, bile salts, pancreatic and intestinal lipase, as well as protein and dietary fat — if there is approximately 10 g or more of fat in a meal, the absorption of dietary preformed vitamin A is 70–90%.[122]

Excretion

Retinol is mainly excreted through the urine, although some is lost (as inactive metabolites) through the breath and faeces. When intake is excessive, biliary excretion increases: 10% is unabsorbed and appears in faeces, 20% is excreted in faeces after secretion into the gastrointestinal tract in bile, 17% is excreted in urine, 3% is exhaled as carbon dioxide and the remaining 50% is stored, primarily in the liver.

Interactions (medication, nutrient, dietary)

- Zinc is a component of retinol-binding protein (RBP). It is also required for the enzymatic converstion of retinol to retinal (required for rhodopsin synthesis involved in dark adaptation).[123]
- Drugs such as ketoconazole, which inhibit cytochrome P450, can significantly increase the half-life of retinoic acid.
- Vitamin A may potentiate the development of intracranial hypertension when taken in combination with tetracycline-type antibiotics, and thus this combination should be avoided.
- Anticoagulant medication, when combined with long-term or high-dose vitamin A, may increase the risk of bleeding.
- Orlistat reduces vitamin A levels.
- Competitive inhibition of alcohol dehydrogenase may lead to decreased synthesis of retinoic acid, resulting in functional vitamin A deficiency, which has been postulated to be involved in fetal alcohol syndrome.
- In people who take antacids, concomitant supplementation with vitamin A interacts in a beneficial (supportive) way, and has been shown to help heal gastric ulcers.
- Anthelmintic drugs (for worm infestation): vitamin A supplementation is a beneficial or supportive interaction, as vitamin A is depleted by helminth infection and low vitamin A status increases the likelihood of infestation.
- Cytotoxic chemotherapeutic drugs: an additive (synergistic) effect of vitamin A enhancing the antitumour effect of these agents has been noted.
- Cholesterol-lowering medication (bile acid sequestrants) reduce the absorption of fat-soluble vitamins, and vitamin A supplementation can avoid nutrient depletion and adverse effects.
- Oral colchicine may lead to vitamin A depletion.
- In people taking corticosteroids vitamin A can prevent or reduce adverse drug events.
- Avoid concurrent vitamin supplementation in conjunction with pharmaceutical retinoid prescriptions (e.g. Roaccutane) and topical high-strength retinols used for acne and anti-ageing treatments.

Function

Vitamin A (retinol) is an essential nutrient for the normal functioning of the visual system; for growth and development and the maintenance of normal cellular differentiation; and for maintenance of epithelial cellular integrity, immune system function, red blood cell production and reproduction.[124] These dietary needs for vitamin A are normally provided for as preformed retinol (mainly as retinyl ester) and provitamin A carotenoids.

Therapeutic applications

- To correct an overt vitamin A deficiency (hypovitaminosis A) without corneal changes: 10 000–15 000 IU/day for 1–2 weeks. Short-term doses of 10 000–50 000 IU have been used to correct deficiency.
- To reduce secondary infection in children with measles doses of 200 000 IU over 2 consecutive days are effective in reducing mortality from measles in children under 2 years old.[125]
- Complications in pregnancy: a dose of 23 300 IU/week of retinol acetate has been used to reduce maternal anaemia and night blindness; however, doses >10 000 IU in pregnancy are contraindicated. These studies are primarily related to developing countries where vitamin A deficiency is common.[126]
- Vitamin A and β-carotene intake may also be inversely associated with risk of developing cataracts.[127]

Deficiency signs

Blindness, poor tooth and bone formation, visual impairment, poor adaptation to darkness (nyctalopia), dry skin, dry hair, poor fingernail quality, pruritus, reduced synthesis of steroid hormones, diminished immune function, keratomalacia, xerophthalmia, corneal degeneration, Bitot's spots and follicular hyperkeratosis (phrynoderma) secondary to blockage of hair follicles with plugs of keratin.[128]

Biochemical testing

- Retinol in serum.
- Beta carotene in serum.

Levels <1.05 mmol/L are indicative of a deficiency state.

Supplemental forms

Vitamin A is generally used in the form of esters such as acetate, propionate and palmitate. Retinyl palmitate (also known as vitamin A palmitate) is the usual form of vitamin A stored in the liver. This is the principal form of vitamin A used in supplements. Unlike the alcohol esters (retinol), retinyl palmitate is a highly stable form of supplemental vitamin A.

Toxicity

Acute toxicity following doses of 15 mg (50000 IU) produces nausea, vomiting, headache, increased cerebrospinal fluid pressure, dizziness, blurred vision and muscular miscoordination. Acute toxicity poses less of a problem than chronic toxicity; for example, daily intakes of >25000 IU for more than 6 years or >100 000 IU for more than 6 months are considered toxic. Toxicity from a single dose is more common in children than in adults. Children and the elderly are particularly sensitive to vitamin A toxicity.[129] As the main storage site for retinol, the liver is the primary target for retinol toxicity.

Dosage requirements

In Australia and New Zealand the RDI is 900 micrograms/day for adult men and 700 micrograms/day for women. This is increased to 800 micrograms/day during pregnancy and 1100 micrograms/day during lactation. The upper intake limit in Australia and New Zealand has been set at 3000 micrograms/day for adult men and women (the same during pregnancy and lactation).[121] Note: children's dosages vary depending on where they are in the life span and their gender. Therefore, it is best to calculate using Clark's rule for each patient.

Food sources

Preformed vitamin A is found almost exclusively in animal products, such as human breast milk, glandular meats, liver and fish-liver oils (a very rich source), egg yolk, whole milk and other dairy products. Provitamin A carotenoids are found in dark-green, leafy vegetables, yellow-orange vegetables, and in yellow and orange non-citrus fruits.

Dietary intake and the need for supplementation

In the 99%-fat-free world we currently live in it is highly probable that the intake of fat-soluble vitamins has decreased. It is expected that, if people reduce their fat intake to comply with the current recommendations of 10–29% of energy in the diet, the intake of fat-soluble vitamins may be reduced to very low levels.[130]

The majority of dietary retinol (in the esterified form) is found in animal-derived foods such as eggs, whole milk, butter, meat and oily ocean fish. Freshwater fish also contain retinol but it is less biologically active. Animal liver is probably the richest source of this nutrient. Provided that these foods are included in the diet on a regular basis, there should be no need for supplementation, but if the avoidance of fat results in the avoidance of rich sources of vitamin A, and if the diet is also low in fresh fruit and vegetables, supplemental vitamin A may be required.

Plant foods provide a rich source of vitamin A, as carotenes, which are then converted to vitamin A in the body. Carotenoid pigments are present in grains, dietary oils, leafy greens, yellow-orange vegetables, carrots and fruit. If fresh fruit and vegetables remain a central and important part of the daily diet, they should provide enough vitamin A, although the bioconversion of carotenes to active vitamin A may be compromised if digestive function is impaired.

Vitamin A deficiency can occur in malabsorption syndromes such as coeliac disease. Lifestyle patterns that contribute to poor vitamin A status include the regular consumption of tobacco, which increases the demand for vitamin A and may result in the depletion of tissue reserves, as does a reliance on commercial snack foods, fast foods and sucrose, which replace fresh fruit and vegetables in the diet. If these dietary patterns prevail, taking a daily supplement that contains adequate levels of retinol would help prevent deficiency and maintain tissue levels of vitamin A. As preformed retinol has less antioxidant activity than β-carotene, it is important to maintain an intake of both preformed vitamin A and carotenes in the diet to help quench singlet oxygen radicals and maintain a healthy immune system.[88]

As alcohol accelerates the breakdown of vitamin A and interferes with the conversion of carotenoids to retinol, people with a history of heavy alcohol use run the risk of deficiency. Supplementation may be necessary, although caution is advised, and under no circumstances should supplements and alcohol be taken concomitantly.

VITAMIN D_3 (CHOLECALCIFEROL) AND VITAMIN D_2 (ERGOCALCIFEROL)

Vitamin D_3 quantities are expressed as follows:

- 1 microgram of cholecalciferol (vitamin D) = 40 IU of vitamin D_3
- 0.025 microgram of cholecalciferol (vitamin D) = 1 IU of vitamin D_3.

Forms of nutrient

In humans, vitamin D_3 (cholecalciferol) is manufactured from 7-dehydroxycholesterol in the skin (Box 7.1). The action of ultraviolet (UV) light on the skin, followed by thermal isomerisation, produces cholecalciferol. Cholecalciferol is bound to carrier protein in the blood and hydroxylated in the liver to form 25-hydroxycholecalciferol,

BOX 7.1 Sunlight: the naturopathic view

Our perception of the sun as a life-giving force has changed. In fact the sun is now viewed as something of an environmental enemy. Environmental changes, such as the thinning of the ozone layer, have magnified our fears. Nevertheless, we have evolved to make use of the complete solar spectrum for the regulation of various body functions. The use of solar radiation in medicine, now called phototherapy, began with the early research conducted by the Nobel Prize winning physician Niels Ryberg Finsen. Finsen successfully treated lupus vulgaris and tuberculosis with ultraviolet radiation. The early pioneering naturopaths (sometimes referred to as 'sun doctors') also regarded regular sun exposure as a necessary requirement for robust good health.

Source: Margherita T, Cantorna YZ, Froicu M et al. Vitamin D status, 1,25-dihydroxyvitamin D_3, and the immune system. Am J Clin Nutr 2004; 80(Suppl):1717S–1720S.

and then is again hydroxylated in the kidneys to form the active form, 1,25-dihydroxycholecalciferol (calcitriol).

The nutrient also appears as vitamin D_2 (ergocalciferol), which is produced by UV irradiation of the fungal steroid ergosterol. Vitamin D_2 is the form present in foods such as mushrooms.

Distribution and storage

After vitamin D_3 is produced in the skin it is picked up by the plasma transport protein vitamin-D-binding protein (DBP) and delivered to the liver, where it is converted to 25-hydroxyvitamin D_3. The next target organ is the kidney, which produces the steroid hormones 1α,25-dihydroxyvitamin D_3 (calcitriol) and 24(*R*),25-dihydroxyvitamin D. These hormones are then delivered to other target tissues.[131] Vitamin D reserves are stored in body fat for use in periods without sun exposure.

Absorption

Dietary vitamin D is absorbed from the small intestine, in the presence of bile, and is then transported into the circulation via the lymph in chylomicrons.

Excretion

Excretion is via the hepatobiliary route, being excreted in bile and faeces.

Interactions (medication, nutrient, dietary)

Lipid-lowering drugs, glucocorticoids, calcium-channel blockers, topical antifungal agents (e.g. ketoconazole), anticonvulsants, antituberculosis medications, anti-rejection medications and HAART (AIDS treatment).[132,133]

Function

The key function of vitamin D is to maintain serum calcium and phosphorus levels within the normal range, in order to sustain a wide variety of metabolic and physiological functions as well as optimising bone health and normal neuromuscular function.[134]

Adequate vitamin D is required to upregulate calcium absorption during times of increased demand, such as during growth periods and pregnancy, and when dietary calcium intake is low. Vitamin D also appears to have other roles within the body, such as enhancing immune function, and deficient levels may play a role in autoimmune disease physiology.

Therapeutic applications

It has been suggested that doses as high as 50 000 IU of vitamin D_2 administered once a week for 8 weeks will correct a vitamin D deficiency.[135] An oral intake of 4000 IU/day has been used without adverse effects.[136] In the absence of adequate sun exposure, 1500–2000 IU/day of cholecalciferol is necessary to raise the blood level of 25-hydroxyvitamin D_3 (25OHD) above 75 nmol/L.[135]

Deficiency signs

Rickets, osteomalacia, osteoporosis, increased fracture risk, muscle weakness and pain, osteoporosis, psoriasis, pregnancy and breastfeeding (infants exclusively breastfed beyond 6 months), to protect against cancers, especially breast and colon cancer, seasonal affective disorder (SAD), chronic kidney disease and autoimmune diseases.

Biochemical testing

- Serum 25OHD is the marker for vitamin D status: a blood level of 50 nmol/L (20 ng/mL) is considered the minimum necessary to meet the body's needs; levels below this are considered as a deficiency. Levels of 21–29 ng/mL (52–72 nmol/L) are considered 'insufficient' with a goal that both children and adults are at a level of >30 ng/mL (75 nmol/L).[133]
- Assessment may be conducted in conjunction with parathyroid hormone (PTH) tests, as PTH levels are elevated when the blood concentration of 25OHD is lowered.

Supplemental forms

While 'vitamin D' refers to a range of related fat-soluble sterols, cholecalciferol (vitamin D_3) is widely recognised as the most appropriate supplemental form and displays greater bioavailability than ergocalciferol (vitamin D_2).

Toxicity

Toxicity from dietary vitamin D or sun exposure is practically impossible; however, toxicity can be caused by excess oral intake through supplementation.[137] Hypervitaminosis D induces hypercalcaemia, which has been observed as a result of daily doses of >50 000 IU of vitamin D. However toxicity is unlikely in healthy people where intake levels are <10 000 IU/day.[133,137]

Dosage requirements

1. 1 microgram cholecalciferol is equal to 0.2 microgram 25OHD. Vitamin D is also sometimes expressed in international units where 1 IU equals 0.025 microgram cholecalciferol or 0.005 microgram 25OHD.

2 RDI 5–15 micrograms/day (200 IU–600 IU) with a UL of 80 micrograms/day (3200 IU).

Australian recommendations for adequate daily intake of vitamin D are: birth to 50 years of age, 200 IU (5 micrograms); adults, 51–70 years old, 400 IU (10 micrograms); adults > 70 years old, 600 IU (15 micrograms).[138] The upper safe level of intake for adults is 80 micrograms/day and for infants is 25 micrograms/day.[138]

Data from supplementation studies and expert consensus indicate that, without adequate sun exposure, a vitamin D intake of at least 800–1000 IU/day is required by both children and adults.[133]

Food sources

Very few foods contain significant amounts of vitamin D. Rich sources are fish, especially high-fat fish such as salmon, herring and mackerel. Other important sources include meat, milk and eggs. Mushrooms provide a reasonable vegetarian source.

Dietary intake and the need for supplementation

Obtaining enough vitamin D from dietary sources can be difficult. Oily fish, including salmon, mackerel and herring, and cod liver oil are some of the best sources of this nutrient (as vitamin D_3). Vitamin D is also available from vegetable sources (as vitamin D_2), although it is not as well absorbed as the vitamin D_3 found in animal foods.[139] Cholecalciferol (vitamin D_3) is converted to 25OHD up to five times faster than is vitamin D_2. Furthermore, meat products also contain some 25OHD, which displays greater activity than vitamin D_3.[131] Nevertheless, for those avoiding animal products, probably the richest source of food-bound vitamin D (as D_2) occurs in mushrooms. Sun-dried mushrooms typically provide 400–500 IU of vitamin D per serving (1 cup = 156 g).

Many everyday foods are fortified with vitamin D. These include milk, orange juice, cereals and some breads. Some yoghurts and cheeses are now fortified with vitamin D, although other dairy products are not. Most European countries forbid the fortification of milk with vitamin D, but permit the fortification of margarine and some cereals.

Adequate intake of vitamin D is unlikely to be achieved through dietary means, particularly in the groups at greatest risk of deficiency, although vitamin D-fortified foods may assist in maintaining vitamin D status in the general population.[140] Fortification is unlikely to be effective in sectors of the population that avoid dairy foods and processed foods in general, and if regular sun exposure is unattainable, supplementation should be considered. People who are at risk of vitamin D deficiency, such as dark-skinned and veiled women (particularly in pregnancy), their infants, and older people living in residential care, should consider taking supplemental cholecalciferol. In people with malabsorption conditions such as irritable bowel syndrome (Crohn's disease and ulcerative colitis), vitamin D supplementation is recommended to maintain bone mineral density and to normalise circulating vitamin D concentrations.[141]

In general, the exposure to sunlight of the hands, face and arms for 5–15 minutes/day, 2–3 times a week should provide adequate amounts of vitamin D_3. The concentration of previtamin D in the skin reaches equilibrium in white skin within 20 minutes of exposure to UV light, although it can take 3–6 times longer for pigmented skin to reach equilibrium. Despite this, dark skin pigmentation does not affect the amount of vitamin D that can be produced by sun exposure. Conversely, ageing lowers the amount of 7-dehydrocholesterol in the skin and lowers the capacity for vitamin D production.[142]

VITAMIN E (α-, β-, γ- AND δ-TOCOPHEROLS)

Equivalent doses of tocopherols

TABLE 7.3 Conversion table for the tocopherols

Form	Alternative name	mg α-tocopherol equivalence
d-α-tocopherol	RRR-α-tocopherol	1
d-α-tocopherol acetate	RRR-α-tocopherol acetate	0.91
d-α-tocopherol acid succinate	RRR-α-tocopherol acid succinate	0.81
dl-α-tocopherol	all-rac-α-tocopherol	0.74
dl-α-tocopherol acetate	all-rac-α-tocopherol	0.67
d-β-tocopherol	RRR-β-tocopherol	0.25–0.40
d-?-tocopherol	RRR-?-tocopherol	0.10
α-tocotrienol		0.25–0.30

Source: Vitamin E|Nutrient Reference Values [Internet]. Nrv.gov.au. 2014 [cited 2 August 2016]. Available from: https://www.nrv.gov.au/nutrients/vitamin-e (c) © Commonwealth of Australia (Department of Health) 2015-2017. CC BY 4.0

Forms of nutrient

Vitamin E is a generic term used to describe any of a group of chemically related compounds that exhibit the activity of α-tocopherol. α-tocopherol is the form of vitamin E found in animal tissues and plasma. However, naturally occurring vitamin E is a complex chemical entity, comprising eight distinct isoforms: α-, β-, γ- and δ-tocopherol, and the tocotrienol (α, β, γ and δ) subfamily.

THE FOUR TOCOPHEROLS: α, β, γ AND δ

This family of four tocopherols are molecules consisting of a complex ring structure and a long saturated chain. The members vary according to the number and position of methyl groups on the benzene ring, and each has a different degree of biological activity. The most abundant and most biologically active of the tocopherols is the naturally occurring D-isomer of α-tocopherol.

THE FOUR TOCOTRIENOLS: α, β, γ AND δ

This family of four tocotrienols are molecules that have a similar basic structure to the tocopherols but with unsaturated side chains. They have less vitamin E activity than the tocopherols.

SYNTHESISED AND NATURALLY OCCURRING VITAMIN E

α-tocopherol is naturally found in foods as the D-isomer (D-α-tocopherol or RRR- α-tocopherol). This is thought to be the most biologically active form. Synthesised forms produce a mixture of D- and L-isomers. The L-isomers are not as active as the D-isomers. The synthetic form D,L-α-tocopherol is cheaper but not as active. Therefore it is essential to assess supplements accurately to ensure that they contain naturally occurring D-α-tocopherol.

Distribution and storage

Vitamin E is distributed to all tissues, although it accumulates and is stored to a greater extent in adipose tissue. It is also stored for a brief time in the liver.

Absorption

Vitamin E absorption takes place in the presence of bile. It is incorporated into tissue and transported between membranes through the action of α-tocopherol transfer protein, a lipophilic binding protein.

Excretion

Vitamin E is metabolised in the liver and excreted via the urine.

Interactions (medication, nutrient, dietary)

Medications that reduce the absorption of dietary fats will also impede vitamin E absorption. These include cholestyramine, colestipol, isoniazid, orlistat and sucralfate.

Vitamin E may inhibit the activity of chlorpromazine and chloroquine.

Those on antiplatelet drugs such as clopidogrel and dipyridamole, and non-steroidal anti-inflammatory drugs (aspirin, ibuprofen, etc.) may be at increased risk of bleeding when taking vitamin E supplements. High-dose vitamin E (>300 mg/day) may also have a potentiating effect on warfarin and close medication supervision is advised, particularly in those who are vitamin K deficient. Consumption of vitamin E at these doses may also lead to interactions with tamoxifen and ciclosporin.[143]

Function

Vitamin E is recognised to be the most important lipid-soluble antioxidant in the body. The antioxidant capacity of vitamin E comes from its superior ability to interrupt free radical chain reactions.[144] The major role of vitamin E is to protect polyunsaturated fatty acids (PUFAs). In this regard, vitamin E is thought to have basic functional importance in the maintenance of membrane integrity in virtually all cells of the body. Other processes involving vitamin E include the modulation of cellular signalling, enzymatic activity and the modification of gene transcription and expression.[145]

Therapeutic applications

- Deficiency due to fat malabsorption syndromes (e.g. chronic cholestasis, cystic fibrosis, chronic steatorrhoea, coeliac disease)
- Anaemia in haemodialysis
- Age-related macular degeneration and cataracts
- Alzheimer's dementia
- Cerebral infarction prevention
- Diabetic neuropathy
- Dysmenorrhoea
- Hyperlipidaemia
- Tardive dyskinesia
- Rheumatoid arthritis
- Osteoarthritis
- Cardiovascular disease risk prevention
- Nitrate tolerance
- Premenstrual syndrome
- Intermittent claudication
- Improving male fertility
- Menopausal symptoms
- Improving immunity in the elderly
- General antioxidant effects
- Prostate cancer prevention
- Sunburn prevention.

Deficiency signs

Severe deficiency in humans is considered to be rare and would usually only occur with concurrent fat malabsorption conditions, in premature infants and in certain rare genetic disorders. Premature infants are at risk of deficiency as they are born with limited vitamin E stores, have inefficient absorption and quickly use up any stores due to their rapid growth. Cigarette smoking increases the utilisation of α-tocopherol resulting in smokers having an increased risk of deficiency compared with non-smokers.[146] Marginal subclinical deficiency may be relatively common, with studies demonstrating an increased risk of heart disease, cancer, diabetes and stroke in those with low levels.

DEFICIENCY SIGNS AND SYMPTOMS

- *First sign.* Erythrocyte haemolysis (red blood cell destruction) when blood levels fall below a critical level. If left untreated this may result in haemolytic anaemia.
- *Progressive symptoms.* Neuromuscular dysfunction and muscle atrophy. This involves the spinal cord and retina, and results in loss of coordination and reflexes, and impaired vision and speech. All these symptoms are rapidly corrected with supplementation if the cause is a deficiency of vitamin E.
- *Animal studies.* Animal studies indicate reproductive symptoms in animals, such as infertility, resorption of a fetus and abortion. However, these have not been found in human studies.
- *Increased risk of certain conditions.* Individuals with inadequate intakes of vitamin E have a greater risk of developing heart disease, cancers (gastrointestinal tract, breast, cervix, lung) and diabetes. Intermittent claudication and fibrocystic breast disease, while not

caused directly by deficiency states, are known to occur more often in those with low levels of vitamin E.
- *General signs and symptoms.* Lethargy, apathy, reduced concentration, lowered immune response.

Biochemical testing

A plasma level of vitamin E (α-tocopherol) of <12 μmol/L is associated with anaemia, increased infections, poor pregnancy outcomes and stunted growth. In normal, healthy adults, plasma concentrations average between 20 and 30 μmol/L.[147]

Supplemental forms

D-α-tocopherol is the form most often used in supplements and is known as 'natural vitamin E'. It has the highest bioavailability of the forms of vitamin E. It is also the most studied form because it is retained within the body, and vitamin E deficiency is corrected with this form. However, in nature, eight substances have been found to have vitamin E activity: α-, β-, γ- and δ-tocopherol and α-, β-, γ- and δ-tocotrienol. Many supplements now contain a mixture of vitamin E isomers. Current clinical research suggests that the tocotrienols may be more effective than α-tocopherol in some clinical conditions, and may possess more potent antioxidant activity.[148] α-tocopherol esters such as α-tocopherol succinate and acetate are more stable than the non-esterified forms, displaying greater resistance to oxidation during storage. These esters are also water soluble.

SUMMARY OF α-TOCOPHEROL OPTIONS

- *Natural vitamin E.* This is derived from vegetable oils. All forms are D-isomers. It is available in the following forms: D-α-tocopherol (an oil), D-α-tocopheryl acetate (an oil) and D-α-tocopheryl succinate (a solid).
- *Synthetic vitamin E.* This is derived from purified petroleum oil. All forms are DL-isomers. It is available in the following forms: DL-α-tocopherol (an oil), DL-α-tocopheryl acetate (an oil) and DL-α-tocopheryl succinate (a solid).

Toxicity

Although rare, toxicity and adverse events from ingesting high doses of supplemental vitamin E for extended periods have been reported. Toxic levels produce a variety of symptoms, such as nausea, fatigue, headache, disturbed vision, haemorrhage, flatulence, diarrhoea, gastrointestinal distress and muscle weakness.[31]

Dosage requirements

In Australia and New Zealand an adequate intake (AI) of 10 mg/day is recommended for adult men and 7 mg/day for women.[149] In the US, the RDA for vitamin E in both men and women is 15 mg/day and is based on the use of α-tocopherols as they are the only form maintained in plasma.[150] The Australian upper limit (UL) has been established as 300 mg for both men and women. In the US, the UL is 1000 mg/day (1100 IU of synthetic tocopherol or 1500 IU of natural tocopherol).

Note: Indiscriminate supplementation with vitamin E should be cautioned in the general population given recent reports that may demonstrate an association with increased all-cause mortality and supplementation in doses >400 IU/day.[151,152]

Food sources

Vitamin E is found mainly in cold-extracted vegetable oils, wheatgerm oil being a particularly rich source, as are tree nuts, peanuts and avocados. Some vitamin E is also found in the fats of meat, poultry and fish. Egg yolk contains some vitamin E, as does animal milk and butter. It is also available in dark-green leafy vegetables such as spinach and kale, and in some vegetables such as sweet potato and asparagus. Both palm oil and rice bran oil are rich sources of the tocotrienols. Tocotrienols are also found in wholegrains such as barley and oats.

Dietary intake and the need for supplementation

While vitamin E deficiency leading to neurological symptoms is rare in humans, vitamin E insufficiency states are likely to occur, especially when the dietary intake of vitamin E is less than optimal. The efficient uptake and distribution of vitamin E can also be impaired in certain disease states, such as short bowel syndrome and other lipid and hepatic malabsorption states.[153] These conditions can be prevented, and in some instances be reversed, by supplementation with vitamin E.[145] Replete vitamin E status is highly important during pregnancy and lactation, and supplementation is likely to be warranted, particularly if dietary intake of vitamin E is low.

VITAMIN K (PHYTOMENADIONE)

Forms of nutrient

Vitamin K is not a single compound but a group of fat-soluble compounds derived from 2-methyl-1,4-naphthoquinone. Vitamin K is a general term used to describe a group of chemically related compounds that exhibit the activity of phytomenadione. This family of compounds includes:
- *Phylloquinone or vitamin K_1.* This originates from green leafy plants and green vegetables and is the main dietary source of vitamin K. It is fat soluble
- *Menaquinones or vitamin K_2.* This is produced by gut bacteria in the jejunum, ileum and colon. It is found in fermented foods, and is fat soluble
- *Menadione or vitamin K_3.* This is a synthetic, water-soluble form of the vitamin. It is no longer used in humans due to toxicity concerns.

Distribution and storage

Vitamin K_2 is transported via plasma lipoproteins, and concentrates mainly in the liver, although it does occur in other tissues, such as bone and blood vessels. Only small amounts of vitamin K are stored in body tissues and a regular supply through the diet is required.

Absorption

The vitamin K_2 series is synthesised by various Gram-positive bacteria present in the jejunum and ileum.

Excretion

About 60–70% of ingested phytomenadione is metabolised by the liver, and excreted in the urine and bile within a few days. Excretion of other forms of vitamin K may be by similar routes.

Interactions (medication, nutrient, dietary)

The effects of vitamin K_1 are also antagonised by excessive oral intakes of vitamin A. Vitamin K_1 significantly interacts with coumarin anticoagulants (warfarin) by inhibiting the production of vitamin K-dependent clotting factors.[154] The effect of 2-methyl-1,4-naphthoquinone (vitamin K_3) is antagonised by dactinomycin D. Individuals on anticoagulant therapy should monitor their vitamin K intake.

Antibiotics can reduce vitamin K status by destroying vitamin K-producing bacteria in the gut.

Function

Vitamin K catalyses the carboxylation of a number of protein factors involved in blood clotting, including prothrombin, forming the calcium binding sites on glutamyl side chains in the protein. Once carboxylated, the glutamates are referred to as γ-carboxyglutamic acid (GLA). GLA proteins may be involved in reabsorption of calcium by the kidney tubules and solubilisation of calcium salts in the urine. Vitamin K-dependent proteins are involved in coagulation, preservation of bone mineral density (osteocalcin is a vitamin K-dependent protein which may stabilise hydroxyapatite), protection against vascular calcification, cell signalling and brain lipid metabolism.[155,156] In all cases, vitamin K exerts its effects by being involved in a chemical reaction that alters a protein so that it can interact with calcium.

Therapeutic applications

Doses of 45 mg/day of MK-4 (menatetrenone, synthetic form of vitamin K) for 6 months have been used in clinical trials in postmenopausal women to reduce bone fracture risk.[157] Newborn babies are routinely given vitamin K to prevent bleeding due to vitamin K deficiency (babies have very low levels of vitamin K when born as the gut is still sterile).

Deficiency signs

Tendency to bruise easily, presence of blood in the stool, poor clotting/prolonged bleeding, impaired bone remodelling, impaired bone mineralisation and soft-tissue calcification.

Biochemical testing

The following levels are indicative of deficiency:

- Phylloquinone[158]
- Circulating uncarboxylated osteocalcin (ucOC) and desphospho-uncarboxylated matrix Gla-protein (dp-ucMGP) — markers of bone and vasculature vitamin K status[159]
- Uncarboxylated prothrombin (PIVK-II).[160]

Supplemental forms

Phylloquinone or phytomenadione (synthetic K1)[161] or menaquinone (MK) (vitamin K_2) is commonly used in nutritional supplements. Menatetranone (MK-4) (synthetic vitamin K) is also available.[157]

Toxicity

No tolerable upper limit has been established for vitamin K, although in its naturally occurring form (vitamin K_1) it is generally thought to be non-toxic. In its synthetic form, menadione (vitamin K_3), it can be toxic at high doses, especially in those who display vulnerability, such as infants.

Dosage requirements

In Australia and New Zealand no RDI has been established, although an adequate intake of 70 micrograms/day for adult males and 60 micrograms/day for adult females has been suggested.[158] The US adequate intake for vitamin K is 120 micrograms/day for adult males and 90 micrograms/day for females (this dose is constant throughout pregnancy and lactation).[162]

Experimental data indicate that these levels are well above the level needed to maintain a normal prothrombin time.[163]

Food sources

Dietary vitamin K_1 is available mainly in leafy green vegetables, whereas the menaquinones (vitamin K_2) are produced by bacteria and are mostly found in fermented foods such as cheese, curd and the Japanese food natto (fermented soya beans).[164]

Dietary intake and the need for supplementation

Vitamin K (phylloquinone) is available from dietary sources, such as mushrooms and dark-green leafy vegetables, but it must be converted in the body to vitamin K_2 (menaquinone) before it can be utilised. Vitamin K can also be produced endogenously by the intestinal microflora. Despite this, when the diet contains few viable food sources of vitamin K, deficiency can still occur relatively quickly, as vitamin K, unlike other fat-soluble vitamins, is not stored in the body. Due to these variables in the way vitamin K is absorbed and converted, it has been suggested that daily supplementation is likely to be of benefit to most people.[165]

US recommendations for daily intake of vitamin K (all forms) is 100–120 micrograms/day, but this value is based on the hepatic vitamin K requirement for the synthesis of blood clotting factor and not for other target tissues, such as bone.[3] Clinical studies in the US have suggested that the recommended intake of vitamin K is probably too low, and that 'usual dietary practices' are unlikely to provide enough of this nutrient for the maintenance of healthy bone mass. Supplements provide greater vitamin K bioavailability than food, and a comparable intake from the diet would require consumption of 2000–5000 micrograms/day of vitamin K. Current evidence would indicate that vitamin K is most effective for osteoporosis prevention when it is co-administered with minerals (calcium, magnesium, zinc) and vitamin D. Vitamin K_1 tends to accumulate in the liver, whereas vitamin K_2 is far more abundant in other tissues, including the pancreas, bone and vessel walls.[166] High-risk groups for vitamin K deficiency include people with chronic gastrointestinal disorders such as coeliac disease, Crohn's disease, ulcerative colitis and irritable bowel syndrome.[167] Other population demographics at risk include newborn children, cystic fibrosis patients, individuals with cholestatic liver diseases (bile duct obstruction, cirrhosis) or pancreatitis and the institutionalised elderly.[155]

COENZYME Q10

Forms of nutrient

The form of coenzyme Q10 (CoQ10) found in humans consists of a polyisoprene chain containing 10 isoprene units (five carbon atoms each).[168] Over 90% of CoQ10 in human serum and biological tissue exists as reduced ubiquinol-10 ($CoQ10H_2$). It also exists in other oxidative states: as a radical semiquinone intermediate ($CoQH_2$) and as the fully oxidised ubiquinone form (CoQ).

Distribution and storage

CoQ10 is found in virtually all cell membranes, particularly those of the mitochondria, and in lipoproteins. In its quinol form, the amount of CoQ10 in various membranes and in the blood ranges from 30% to 90%, depending on the metabolic state of the cell.[168] CoQ10 is concentrated in tissues with high-energy requirements, such as the heart and skeletal muscle. It also concentrates in the brain, liver, kidneys, adrenals, pancreas and spleen, as well as in the fibroblasts and epidermis of skin.[169] In adults the total body pool is estimated to be approximately 0.5–1.5 g.[170]

Absorption

Endogenous synthesis of CoQ from tyrosine (or phenylalanine) and mevalonate occurs in all cells. The current understanding is that, when endogenous biosynthesis is unimpaired, cell membrane CoQ10 reaches saturation level.[168] The intestinal absorption of CoQ10 is limited and slow (due to its hydrophobicity and high molecular weight) and varies depending on metabolic function, oxidative stress and the body's requirements during the ageing process.[170] CoQ10 is fat soluble and is best absorbed alongside fats in a meal.[171]

Excretion

CoQ is excreted through the urine and faeces.

Interactions (medication, nutrient, dietary)

As cholesterol-lowering drugs inhibit the HMG-CoA reductase enzyme, which is required for synthesis of cholesterol as well as CoQ10, the result can be decreased serum CoQ10.[172] The beta blockers propranolol and metoprolol, and phenothiazines and tricyclic antidepressants have been shown to inhibit CoQ10-dependent enzymes. In people on warfarin therapy high doses of CoQ10 should be used with caution due to the vitamin K-like properties of CoQ10.[173]

Function

CoQ10 is a crucial component of the oxidative phosphorylation process in mitochondria (electron transport) and of the conversion of energy from carbohydrates and fatty acids into ATP to drive cellular machinery and synthesis.[168] CoQ10 also functions as an intercellular antioxidant, and is essential for the health of all tissues and organs, particularly the heart. It has a sparing effect on vitamin E, preventing damage to lipid membranes and plasma lipids.[8]

Therapeutic applications

A typical therapeutic dose of CoQ10 for most conditions has been set at 60–200 mg/day (in divided doses). Two studies on breast cancer used 390 mg/day and research examining the use of CoQ10 in Parkinson's disease and other neurological conditions found doses up to 1200 mg/day to be safe and effective.[174] A daily dose of CoQ10 of up to 900 mg orally has been used in the treatment of congestive heart failure[175] and 100 mg t.d.s. has been used successfully in the treatment of coronary artery disease.[176] Optimal doses in heart disease appear to be 50–300 mg/day.[173] In migraine prophylaxis, 300 mg of CoQ10 (100 mg t.d.s.) has been used in adults;[177] childhood studies suggest a dose of 1–3 mg/kg/day.[178] In the treatment of essential hypertension, 225 mg/day has been trialled, and this dose was found to significantly improve systolic and diastolic blood pressure and reduce the need for medication.[179,180] The administration of CoQ10 may play a positive role in treatment of male infertility, increasing sperm volume and motility.[180] Doses of 300 mg have been used successfully to improve subjective fatigue sensation and physical performance during exercise[181] and in the treatment of fibromyalgia.[182] CoQ10 may also be beneficial in diabetes, by improving blood pressure and long-term glycaemic control.[183]

Deficiency signs

At present there are no clearly defined signs of deficiency of CoQ10. Heart function irregularities and functional impairments in skeletal muscle could well have an association with lowered CoQ10 levels and altered endogenous biosynthesis. Other general symptoms may include fatigue, irritability and reduced immunity. CoQ10 deficiency is seen in a variety of clinical conditions including heart disease, diabetes, Parkinson's disease, Huntington's disease and myopathy.[173]

Biochemical testing

The following are tests for deficiency:

- CoQ10 in serum: a low value signals tissue depletion
- Hydroxymethylglutarate (HMG) in urine: high or low levels indicate blockage to the biosynthetic metabolic pathway

- Lactate, succinate, fumarate, malate in urine: high levels indicate a potential mitochondrial functional insufficiency.[74]

Supplemental forms

In its reduced form as the hydroquinone (ubiquinol) CoQ10 is a potent lipophilic antioxidant and functions to protect the intra- and extracellular components from free radical damage. Apart from the fact that an efficient mechanism is in place to convert orally administered CoQ10 as ubiquinone to ubiquinol, there is evidence that the reduced form displays superior bioavailability.[184] CoQ10 is available as a powder in hard-shell capsules, and as an oil suspension in both hard-shell and soft-gel delivery mediums. Water-soluble formulations are also being investigated.[185] A synthetic analogue of CoQ10, idebenone (2,3-dimethoxy-5-methyl-6-(10-hydroxydecyl)-1,4-benzoquinone), has also been developed.[172]

CoQ10 combined with oil is a common form of CoQ10 supplementation, with soft gelatin capsules containing soy bean oil suspension of CoQ10 displaying the highest bioavailability (compared to polyscorbate or lecithin additives).[184] Research also shows that solubilised forms may be better absorbed (3–6 times higher compared to powder).[184] In the official pharmacopoeias (British and US), CoQ10 is also called ubidecarenone. High-grade CoQ10 formulations use the *trans*-isomer, which has an affinity for the interior of cell membranes.[168] Cheaper formulations that use the *cis*-isomer are best avoided.

Toxicity

There is no known toxicity for CoQ10, and it appears to be safe even at relatively high doses (600–3000 mg), although mild gastrointestinal symptoms such as nausea and stomach upsets have been experienced at these doses. Safety and tolerability of pharmacological doses of 30–300 mg/day have been confirmed.[173]

Dosage requirements

The reference range for plasma CoQ10 in healthy adults is 0.4–1.91 micrograms/mol/L.

Food sources

Meat, poultry and fish. Vegetables and fruit are relatively low in this compound.

Dietary intake and the need for supplementation

Levels of CoQ10 present in the diet (typically 3–5 mg/day) are probably not sufficient to increase serum levels significantly, which would require at least 100 mg/day.[169] A good deal of the CoQ10 requirement is met from its manufacture within the body (mainly within the liver). In healthy people CoQ10 requirements are usually met through the synthesis of tyrosine, phenylalanine and mevalonate. However, coenzyme levels are lowered when metabolic efficiency is compromised by disease processes, oxidative stress, inflammation and ageing.[186] The endogenous biosynthesis of the quinone nucleus of CoQ from tyrosine is dependent on adequate amounts of vitamin B_6.

Biotin, folic acid and vitamins B_2, B_3, B_5, B_6 and B_{12} are all involved in the endogenous synthesis of CoQ10. Vitamin C is also important in this regard, as is lipoic acid, which helps to regenerate CoQ10 in the body. It may take up to 8 weeks before the clinical effects of CoQ10 supplementation are noticed. Because of the action of secreted bile acids CoQ10 bioavailability is greatest when ingested with meals.[184]

MINERALS

Of the more than 100 elements in nature, just four (carbon, hydrogen, oxygen and nitrogen) make up 96% of the weight of the human body. The remaining 4% is made up of minerals. Minerals are naturally occurring elements found in nature as mineral salts. These mineral salts make up rock formations that, as they are eroded over time, form the basis of soil.

All the food that we eat relies on the minerals in soil or water for its own mineral content. If the soils in a particular area are depleted the crops grown in those soils will also lack minerals, as will the animals that feed there. The mineral concentrations of soils can vary considerably according to geographic location. Modern fertilisers do not replace all the minerals that were once found in soils. Different countries will have different mineral imbalances in their soils, which will lead to varying signs and symptoms of mineral deficiency in their populations.

Modern agriculture can be considered to be a recipe for mineral deficiencies, which is worsened by the losses caused by processing and manufacturing methods. Consider also that the pollutants and chemicals associated with modern farming techniques have changed the mineral content and ratios of both water and soils.

Minerals are *inorganic,* meaning that they do not contain carbon — in fact minerals are individual elements. Being inorganic minerals cannot be destroyed or changed. Iron for example will always be iron; it may reversibly combine with other elements but it cannot be changed into anything else or be destroyed by factors such as heat, air and light (compare this with vitamins, which are organic and easily destroyed).

Unlike vitamins, minerals cannot be synthesised by the body, and therefore they must come through the diet. Note also that, as minerals are inorganic, they cannot be produced by plants, animals or microorganisms.

Mineral classification

Minerals can be broadly categorised into the following groups:

- *The major elements.* These elements are present in and required in the largest amounts by the body. The major elements include calcium, magnesium, potassium, sodium, phosphorus and chlorine.
- *Trace elements.* These elements are present in and required in smaller amounts in the body. Trace

elements include iron, zinc, copper, manganese, iodine, selenium, molybdenum, chromium, boron, cobalt and silicon.
- *Elements of uncertain human requirement.* Some elements are thought to possibly be essential, or to have some role in the body, while others are known to have no biological function at all. Minerals for which essentiality has been suggested include fluorine, nickel, lithium, vanadium, strontium, germanium and rubidium.
- *Toxic elements.* The toxic elements are often collectively known as the 'heavy metals'. These minerals build up in the body over a period of time and interfere with physiological function. They include aluminium, arsenic, lead, cadmium and mercury. All minerals are toxic in large enough amounts; however, the heavy metals are toxic in very small amounts.
- *Elements of potential toxicity.* Some elements are considered to be potentially toxic, and avoidance of these is encouraged. Like the toxic elements, they build up in the body over a period of time and interfere with physiological functions. They include thallium, uranium, tin, antimony and titanium.

Biological functions of minerals

The minerals have several general functions, including roles that are both *structural* and *functional*. Again this is different to the vitamins, which do not form part of body structures.

The general functions of minerals include the following. They:
- act as cofactors to enzymes, allowing enzymes to function
- do not supply energy, but may be involved in activating enzymes necessary for energy production
- form part of the structures of the body, such as bone, connective tissue and proteins
- form part of the physiologically important substances; for example, iron is part of the structure of haemoglobin
- form part of some hormones; for example, iodine is a part of thyroid hormone
- are essential for proper tissue fluid balance (homoeostasis), osmotic pressure and electrical conductivity across the cell membrane
- regulate fluid distribution and blood volume
- regulate the function of muscle and nervous tissue
- maintain and regulate the pH of body fluids
- are essential constituents of glandular secretions; for example, chlorine is part of the hydrochloric acid secretions in the stomach.

Mineral relationships

- This is covered under 'Deficiency and toxicity'.
- The relationship of minerals to one another is critical. Too much of one mineral can push another mineral out of the body, resulting in deficiency symptoms.
- Often these interactions are complex and poorly understood.

Mineral imbalances

There are many factors that may lead to mineral imbalance, including:
- Farming and agricultural methods: these may deplete the soil of certain minerals, resulting in deficiencies of those minerals in crops.
- Fertilisers: these may exclude some essential minerals and add high amounts of others. This ultimately affects the mineral balance in the crops being grown, as well as in the animals fed these crops
- Refining and processing methods: these may remove nutrients, some of which may be added back to the food (fortification).
- Toxic metals: minerals such as lead, copper, mercury and aluminium may enter the food chain.
- Digestion: if digestive function or structure is poor, absorption will be impaired.
- Dietary sources: some minerals, such as sodium, are often added to foods in excessive amounts as preservatives or flavour enhancers.

Deficiency and toxicity

Every mineral has an optimal range of intake. Intake below this range causes deficiency, while intake above this range causes toxicity. Either way, the body's optimal state of functioning is impaired. Often, the symptoms of mineral deficiency are similar to those of mineral toxicity. The 'healthy' range of a mineral will vary from person to person, but general guidelines are given for everyone.

CAUSES OF MINERAL DEFICIENCY

- Decreased food intake or intake of food that is low in minerals.
- Modern farming techniques.
- Kidney disease, metabolic disorders or alcoholism.
- Malabsorption.
- Consumption of coffee, tea, alcohol or certain preservatives.
- The use of some prescription or non-prescription medications.

CAUSES OF MINERAL TOXICITY

- The addition of individual minerals to the diet in excessive amounts; for example, phosphorus in carbonated beverages or sodium chloride in table salt.
- Toxic metals via technology or the environment; for example, copper pipes used in water supply.
- High ingestion of supplements, either deliberate or accidental.
- Hereditary diseases that affect an individual's mineral metabolism; for example, Wilson's disease is a genetic disorder of poor copper metabolism which presents as an inability to excrete this mineral.

Major elements

CALCIUM (CA)

Forms of nutrient

Calcium occurs in many forms, each of which has a different solubility in water (Table 7.4). Hydroxyapatite, a

TABLE 7.4 Characteristics of various forms of calcium

Form of calcium	Percentage of elemental calcium	Percentage solubility in water
Calcium ascorbate	10.27	na
Calcium acetate	25.34	40
Calcium aspartate	12–20	na
Calcium biglycinate	21.30	na
Calcium oxolate	31.29	0.00067
Calcium carbonate	40.04	0.0014–0.0056
Calcium citrate	24.12	0.096
Calcium citrate malate	23.70	1.1
Calcium lactate	18.37	9
Calcium gluconate	9.31	40
Microcrystalline hydroxyapatite	na	0.08
Calcium fumarate	26.00	1.22
Calcium glycinate	21.30	na
Tricalcium phosphate	39.00	0.97
Calcium lysinate	12.06	na
Dicalcium phosphate	29.46	0.02
Calcium chloride	36.11	74

Source: Straub DA. Calcium supplementation in clinical practice: a review of forms, doses, and indications. Nutr Clin Pract 2007; 22:286–296.

crystalline compound comprising calcium carbonate and calcium phosphate, is the form of calcium found primarily in the teeth and bones.

Distribution and storage

The majority of calcium (99%) is stored in the teeth and bones. The remaining 1% is stored in the cells of the soft tissues, the bloodstream and in extracellular fluid.[187]

Absorption

Calcium is absorbed in the duodenum, jejunum and ileum through a saturable active transport system that involves vitamin D and parathyroid hormone activity. Some calcium is also passively absorbed. Calcium absorption is greatest when the intake of calcium is low and the demand is high. Absorption is highest when taken in doses <500 mg.[187] Calcium absorption decreases with age, lowered stomach acidity, lowered oestrogen levels, alcohol, coffee, salt, phosphorous, smoking and high levels of dietary fibre.[188] If vitamin D deficiency is present, very little available calcium is absorbed.

Excretion

Main excretion pathways: 50–70% of ingested calcium is unabsorbed and remains in the gastrointestinal tract to be lost in the faeces. The calcium that is absorbed is excreted by the kidneys. Normally, 90% of calcium is filtered from the blood in the kidneys and is reabsorbed, while the remaining 10% is excreted in the urine.

Minor excretion pathways: some calcium is lost in sweat, although this represents a minimal loss except during very heavy sweating. There are also small losses in bile and pancreatic secretions.

Factors that increase excretion: these include high intakes of salt, protein (especially meat), phosphorus, processed foods, refined sugar, caffeine, alcohol or cigarettes; high calcitonin, cortisol, glucocorticoids and stress hormones; low exercise; ageing; and excessive intakes of lysine.

Interactions (medication, nutrient, dietary)

Sodium chloride, when taken in high amounts, can increase urinary calcium loss — for every 2.5 g of sodium chloride excreted by the kidneys, 2.6 mg of calcium is drawn into the urine.[189] A high intake of phosphoric acid (e.g. from carbonated soft drinks, meat) may increase the renal elimination of calcium. A high caffeine intake can also increase renal calcium excretion. Drugs where interactions with calcium are possible include cardiac glycosides (digoxin), calcium-channel blockers, quinolone and tetracycline antibiotics, thiazide diuretics, corticosteroids, H2 blockers and proton pump inhibitors.[190]

It has been suggested that calcium can decrease the absorption of other divalent cations such as magnesium, and that supplements of these should be taken separately (2 hours apart). This is an important consideration if a person has low magnesium stores (high intakes of calcium can exacerbate low magnesium status and vice versa), but calcium does not have a clinically significant effect on magnesium balance in individuals whose magnesium stores are adequate.[191]

Function

Calcium is a macro mineral essential for the optimal functioning of virtually every cell in the body. Over 99% of total body calcium is found in the teeth and bones (to support their structure and function). However, only the remaining 1% of total body calcium — found in the blood, extracellular fluid and the soft tissues — is needed to support critical metabolic functioning.[192] Various physiological functions requiring calcium include muscle contraction, neurotransmission, signal transduction, enzyme secretion, vascular function, blood coagulation and glandular secretion.

Therapeutic applications

For osteoporosis risk reduction 1000 mg/day of calcium is recommended, together with key accessory nutrients such as vitamin D (400 IU), zinc, copper, manganese and silica.[193] In premenstrual syndrome 1000–1200 mg/day is recommended.[194] During pregnancy where there is a history or risk of pre-eclampsia the calcium dose is 2000 mg/day. To help ameliorate gastric hyperacidity 500–1500 mg/day as required.[16] In Asian populations and those with low calcium intake, an increase of 300 mg/day of calcium is associated with a 18–22% decrease in stroke risk.[195] Calcium requirements also increase with amenorrhoea (anorexia and/or exercise induced), individuals with cow's milk allergy or lactose intolerance and vegans.[196,197]

Deficiency signs

- *Children*: long-term deficiency may result in growth impairment and poor tooth development.
- *Adults*: osteoporosis, osteomalacia, bone deformities, bone pain and increased fracture rates, muscle spasms, nausea and vomiting (advanced deficiency), dry skin and nails, hair loss, convulsions, anxiety, insomnia, depression.

Biochemical testing

- Serum calcium (Note: does not indicate levels of bone calcium)
- Urinary calcium
- Assessment of adequacy: hair and urine calcium, markers of bone resorption, serum 25-hydroxy vitamin D, parathyroid hormone (PTH).

Supplemental forms

There are numerous supplemental forms of calcium available. These include calcium citrate, calcium orotate and calcium citrate malate; hydroxyapatite (bovine) is also available as a supplement.

Calcium carbonate is the most common form, and is the one used in the majority of clinical trials. It yields the highest amount of elemental calcium (see Table 7.4), although its absorption and distribution are inferior to other forms.[187,198] Its absorption is dependent on stomach acid so is best taken with food. Calcium citrate is equally absorbed with or without food and is useful for patients with absorption disorders, inflammatory bowel disease or achlorhydria (particularly those treated with H2 blockers and proton pump inhibitors).[187,192]

Toxicity

As levels in the body are tightly regulated, toxicity is rare. Ingestion of extremely high amounts (2–5 g for extended periods) can result in acute toxicity, although toxicity is more likely to result from pathology.

Dosage requirements

In Australia and New Zealand the RDI for adult men and women is 1000 mg/day and 1000 mg/day during pregnancy and lactation. The RDI increases for men >70 years to 1300 mg/day and women >51 years to 1300 mg/day. The upper limit intake/tolerable upper limit for calcium has been calculated at 2500 mg/day for both men and women.[199]

Food sources

Dairy products, leafy greens such as mustard greens, lamb's quarters, etc. Chinese broccoli, bok choy, fish with edible bones such as tinned salmon and sardines, tahini and molasses. Pulses, cereals, nuts and seeds, dried fruit, and green vegetables contain reasonable amounts of calcium. 'Hard' water in some areas of the country may provide significant amounts. Mineral water can also be a valuable dietary source of calcium.[200]

Dietary intake and the need for supplementation

Dairy products are an excellent source of dietary calcium, as well as other important nutrients such as protein, phosphorus, potassium, magnesium and zinc. For people accustomed to obtaining their calcium in this way, and for whom dairy products (with the possible exception of plain milk) are well tolerated and enjoyed on a daily basis, their consumption should not be discouraged. In clinical naturopathic medicine this is a controversial subject, and a 'no-dairy' policy has often been seen as a hallmark of the profession. Yet, despite the fact that milk and milk-based products are problematic for some, it would seem ill advised to insist on the a priori exclusion of this food group in the belief that this will bring benefits to all. In fact the exclusion of dairy products has the potential to increase the risk of calcium deficiency. However, dairy products should never be seen as the sole source of calcium in the diet. Fermented milk products, such as yoghurt, kefir and cultured butter, offer viable alternatives and may be better tolerated and assimilated. As butterfat helps in the absorption of calcium it is probably a good idea to avoid non-fat milk, especially in children. In infants and young children, goat's milk and goat's milk formulas, which more closely resemble human milk in their nutrient profile, are also an option.[201]

In people whose traditional diets contain very little or no dairy foods, it would seem inadvisable to insist that they suddenly increase their calcium intake by loading up on dairy. Calcium requirements vary quite markedly, and no two individuals handle calcium in the same way. There may also be genetic and ethnic differences in calcium requirements and the ways in which the body uses calcium. Calcium is absorbed more effectively in people of Asian and African descent, and less so by Caucasians. There are also those people who choose to avoid milk and dairy products for ethical or health reasons. In addition, dairy foods simply 'disagree' with some people. In other instances dairy foods may trigger an immune response, manifesting as allergy or food intolerance.

To achieve an adequate intake of dietary calcium in this situation would mean emphasising plant and other non-dairy sources. Plant foods are an excellent source of calcium, provided they are selected and prepared correctly. To achieve adequate absorption of calcium from plant foods it is important to avoid exposure to high levels of phytates and oxalates, which can impede calcium absorption. Foods rich in oxalic acid include spinach, rhubarb and legumes, and phytic acid occurs at high levels in seeds, wholegrains, nuts and legumes. Fermentation, soaking and sprouting of these foods is one way to make the calcium more absorbable. Leafy greens with low oxalate content, such as bok choy and Chinese broccoli, are also a good way of increasing calcium intake from vegetables. Plant foods may not have the calcium content of dairy foods, but do contain significant amounts of other alkaline minerals, such as potassium and magnesium, which confer additional benefits on bone health by reducing the acid load of the diet.[201]

Absorption of calcium from supplements is greatest when taken with food. Doses of 500 mg or less are more efficiently absorbed, as the active transport system for calcium in the intestine is easily saturated.[202] Calcium supplements are best taken in a divided dose in order to increase absorption.

ANIMAL PROTEIN CONSUMPTION AND RENAL ACID LOAD

The avoidance of animal protein in the belief that it will contribute to renal calcium loss, systemic acidity and the leeching of calcium from bone is only a relevant consideration if intake is excessive. In fact it has been shown that adequate protein intake is more likely to have a positive effect on bone mineral density as a high protein intake increases calcium absorption.[203]

An adequate supply of protein is essential for maintaining bone density (bone is approximately 50% protein), and low-protein diets may in fact have a negative effect on bone development.[204] It is more likely that a high intake of sucrose and other acid-forming components of the diet, such as refined flour products, are more likely to increase systemic acidity and incidental calcium loss than are meat and other protein sources. A balanced strategy would be to maintain an adequate protein intake while increasing the intake of fresh vegetables and fruit, which would help to ensure that a balanced calcium/phosphorus ratio is maintained. In addition to being excellent calcium sources, fruits, vegetables and leafy greens also provide key micronutrients such as magnesium, potassium, boron, and vitamins C, A and K.

MAGNESIUM (MG)

Forms of nutrient

Magnesium plays a key role in more than 300 enzymes, primarily as the Mg–ATP complex in energy-dependent activities. It is the fourth most plentiful cation in the body and is the dominant intracellular cation. Magnesium is found in the body both in its free state and bound to protein.

Overall, the level of free magnesium is very low because it is highly reactive.

Distribution and storage

In the human body the majority of magnesium (>60%) is found in bone. Muscle tissue contains 25% of total body magnesium, while extracellular magnesium accounts for only 1%. Some magnesium is found in plasma, and half of this is ionised and actively involved in physiological reactions, bound to proteins or complexed with anions. Magnesium is associated with various intracellular structures, such as the nucleus and intracellular organelles, and free magnesium accounts for 1–5% of total cellular magnesium. Intracellular free magnesium is maintained at a relatively constant level, even if the extracellular level varies.

Absorption

Dietary magnesium is absorbed in the intestinal tract, primarily in the distal small intestine (jejunum and ileum), in the presence of bile, as well as gastric and pancreatic juice. In healthy adults, 30–50% of dietary magnesium is absorbed. Absorption is essentially a passive intercellular process across the electrochemical gradient. However, active transport does occur, usually when the dietary magnesium intake is extremely low.[205]

Excretion

A process of filtration/resorption in the kidneys regulates the magnesium balance in the body. Urinary magnesium excretion increases when the magnesium intake is in excess, whereas the kidney conserves magnesium when there is magnesium deprivation.

Interactions (medication, nutrient, dietary)

- Potassium-sparing diuretics may potentiate the physiological effects of magnesium.
- Antiarrhythmic drugs, tetracycline and fluoroquinolone antibiotics should be administered 2 hours apart from magnesium supplementation.
- Loop diuretics and thiazide diuretics can cause magnesium wasting.
- Calcium channel blockers may enhance the hypotensive effect.
- Loop diuretics, foscarnet, azathioprine, aminoglycosides, amphotericin B, cisplatin, beta blockers, corticosteroids, aluminium laxatives, antacids that cause hypophosphataemia, prednisone.

Long-term use of proton-pump inhibitors (3+ months) increases risk of hypomagnesaemia.[206]

Function

Magnesium, the fourth most abundant intracellular cation, has been identified as a cofactor in over 300 enzymatic reactions.[207] It is required for protein synthesis, for both anaerobic and aerobic energy generation, and for glycolysis, either indirectly as a part of the magnesium–ATP complex, or directly as an enzyme activator. Magnesium plays a multifunctional role in cell metabolism (particularly at the level of key phosphorylations), and has a critical role in cell division. It has been suggested that magnesium is necessary for the maintenance of an adequate supply of nucleotides for the synthesis of RNA and DNA. Magnesium regulates the movement of potassium in myocardial cells and is also known to act as a calcium channel blocker. Magnesium is needed to create the powerful antioxidant, glutathione. It is also important in the regulation of blood glucose. Magnesium is an important element in the metabolism and/or action of vitamin D, and is essential for the synthesis and secretion of parathyroid hormone (PTH). Magnesium (with calcium) is also involved in the formation of hard tooth enamel, which is resistant to decay.[208]

Therapeutic applications

In the treatment of hypertension, 600–1000 mg/day has been used — normal serum magnesium is associated with a 30% lower risk of CVD and 22% lower risk of ischaemic heart disease (IHD).[209,210] For migraine headache (particularly with aura and in the prevention of premenstrual migraine), 400–600 mg/day of the oxide form is effective.[211,212] In patients without aura, 600 mg/day for 3 months is associated with reduced migraine severity.[213] For osteoporosis, 150–750 mg/day has been used, both alone and in combination with calcium or other supplements.[214] For premenstrual syndrome 200–300 mg/day has been used.[215] For pregnancy-related leg cramps 240 mg in the morning and 440 mg in the evening has been used.[216,217] There is a significant inverse relationship between magnesium intake and risk of type 2 diabetes — 300–400 mg/day reduces fasting blood glucose and improves insulin sensitivity.[218,219] In alcoholism, 30–60% of patients have hypomagnesaemia.[212] For attention deficit hyperactivity disorder (ADHD) 6 mg/kg/day for 6 months has been used in children aged 7–12 years.[220] For multiple sclerosis, 1 g/day as magnesium glycerophosphate for about a month then increased to 1.5 g has been used.[221]

Deficiency signs

Hypocalcaemia, hypokalaemia (due to an inhibition of Na^+,K^+-ATPase activity),[205] prediabetes, insulin resistance, neuromuscular abnormalities, including positive Chvostek and Trousseau signs, muscular fasciculations, tremor, tetany, nausea and vomiting.[222] Deficiency is associated with inflammatory bowel disease, renal disorders, chronic alcoholism, ageing and is seen with muscle tightness and pain as a result of accumulating lactic acid.[207]

Biochemical testing

Currently there is no sensitive and specific biomarker for magnesium status.[191] Red blood cell, whole blood, plasma, serum, urine are some tests currently used. The tight regulation of blood magnesium concentration means a 'normal' range is often maintained — even in the presence of low dietary magnesium intake and increased magnesium excretion. Therefore a chronically low magnesium intake and/or a high calcium (dietary) to magnesium ratio would likely present with normal serum magnesium concentration, alongside potentially low tissue magnesium concentrations and reduced bone magnesium content.[191]

Supplemental forms

There are many forms available for supplementation, including magnesium lactate, magnesium malate, magnesium orotate, magnesium citrate, magnesium aspartate, magnesium diglycinate, magnesium fumarate, magnesium gluconate, magnesium amino acid chelate, magnesium phosphate, magnesium taurinate, magnesium carbonate, magnesium acetate, magnesium hydroxide, magnesium oxide and magnesium sulfate (Table 7.5). Bioavailability of magnesium supplements is dependent on their water solubility — organic magnesium salts have a higher solubility than inorganic salts. Recent data suggest that magnesium citrate is the most appropriate form for therapeutic and supplementation purposes.[223]

Toxicity

Magnesium has a strong safety profile and toxicity is rare, although it can occur in individuals with impaired renal function or during massive intravenous administration of magnesium. The most frequent side effect is diarrhoea and abdominal cramping. Lowering the dose or decreasing the frequency of supplementation usually mitigates this.[211]

TABLE 7.5 Comparison of magnesium supplement forms

Form	Bioavailability	Uses	Elemental magnesium (per 100 mg)
Magnesium amino acid chelate	Good	Treating and preventing hypomagnesaemia	20 mg
Magnesium aspartate	Very good	Treating and preventing hypomagnesaemia	6.75 mg
Magnesium carbonate	Poor	Antacid	40 mg
Magnesium chloride	Well absorbed	In solution for treating and preventing hypomagnesaemia	11.8 mg
Magnesium citrate	Excellent (25–30%)	Treating and preventing hypomagnesaemia	16.2 mg
Magnesium citrate malate	Very good	Food fortification; treating and preventing hypomagnesaemia	15 mg
Magnesium diglycinate	Reasonable	Treating and preventing hypomagnesaemia	na
Magnesium fumarate	Very good	Treating and preventing hypomagnesaemia	na
Magnesium gluconate	Excellent	Treating and preventing hypomagnesaemia	5.3 mg
Magnesium lactate	Very good	Treating and preventing hypomagnesaemia	Approx. 12 mg
Magnesium orotate	Excellent	Heart and cardiovascular health	6.9 mg
Magnesium sulfate	Poor absorption orally	Laxative, parenteral infusions	9.7 mg
Magnesium taurinate	Crosses blood–brain barrier	Depression[221]	25 mg
Magnesium oxide	Low bioavailability (4–5%)		

Dosage requirements

The RDI for magnesium in Australia and New Zealand is 400 mg/day for adult men and 320 mg/day for women (increased to 350–360 mg/day during pregnancy and 310–320 mg/day during lactation). The upper level intake is 350 mg/day.[224]

Food sources

Magnesium is ubiquitous in foods, but the content varies substantially. Leafy vegetables, as well as grains and nuts, generally have a greater magnesium content than do meats and dairy products. The magnesium content of water is variable, depending on the region of its source and the manner of storage. 'Hard' water has a higher concentration of magnesium salts and contains approximately 120 mg/L. Magnesium from water is usually better absorbed than magnesium from foods.

Dietary intake and the need for supplementation

As Johnson[225] so aptly described the situation: 'in an age of sky-rocketing medical costs due to astronomical investments in high-tech gadgets that allow us to look inside the body in a myriad of ever more complicated ways, and in miracle drugs that can achieve amazing feats, it seems incredible that a deficiency of one of the cheapest nutrients may be at the roots of a colossal tree of pathologies that inflict untold pain and monetary losses worldwide'.

A varied diet rich in fresh vital foods, grown in healthy soil, should provide adequate magnesium and ensure magnesium sufficiency, yet many factors can affect the magnesium economy in the body, making supplementation of this mineral a key clinical consideration. When supplementing magnesium to correct a magnesium deficiency or insufficiency state, it is important to provide correct accessory nutrients. Magnesium requires selenium, PTH and vitamins B_6 and D for its absorption. Pyridoxine is only converted into its coenzyme form in the presence of magnesium. Simply supplementing magnesium without taking into account the variables that affect its absorption and elimination may result in less than spectacular clinical outcomes. Some forms of magnesium (oxide, sulfate) can result in a cathartic reaction (laxative effect) when used at therapeutic doses. Clinical studies support the superior bioavailability of magnesium citrate, magnesium diglycinate, magnesium orotate, magnesium chloride, magnesium lactate and magnesium aspartate.[225] Organic magnesium salts such as gluconate, lactate and aspartate are better absorbed than non-organic forms.

Magnesium, like calcium, is regulated by PTH, and people who are magnesium deficient can run the risk of being calcium deficient as well. Some forms of magnesium are now being identified as having specific clinical applications. Magnesium orotate, for example, has benefits for the heart. As a cellular fixative of magnesium, orotic acid has antiarrhythmic, vasodilatory and cardioprotective effects.

POTASSIUM (K)

Forms of nutrient

Potassium is the principal cation in intracellular fluid.

Distribution and storage

Approximately 98% of the body content of potassium is held in the intracellular fluid.

Absorption

Absorption occurs rapidly through the whole length of the small intestine via passive diffusion along its concentration gradient (as long as the concentration in the contents of the gastrointestinal tract (GIT) is higher than that in the blood). Potassium is absorbed extremely well, with 85–90% of potassium salts and dietary potassium being absorbed in the small intestine. It is secreted into the GIT as part of bile and pancreatic juices, and is reabsorbed.

Excretion

Of the total dietary potassium 80% is excreted in the urine with 90% reabsorbed along the kidney tubule. Approximately 15% is excreted in faeces and 5% in sweat.[226] Body levels are controlled by renal excretion. There are minimum daily losses of approximately 7% of circulating blood levels, even at low potassium levels, and therefore daily replacement is essential.

Interactions (medication, nutrient, dietary)

ACE inhibitors, angiotensin receptor blockers, NSAIDs, anticoagulants, digoxin and potassium-sparing diuretics can increase the risk of hyperkalaemia.[227] Drugs such as aminoglycosides, β2-agonists, loop and thiazide diuretics, glucocorticoids, bronchodilators, mineralocorticoids, penicillins and tetracyclines can all lead to potassium loss and electrolyte imbalance.[228]

Function

Potassium is the major cation of intracellular fluid, and maintains the water balance within cells. A high intracellular concentration of potassium is maintained by the Na^+/K^+-ATPase pump. The movement of potassium out of cells, and sodium into cells, changes the electrical potential during the depolarisation and repolarisation of nerves and muscles. Potassium plays an essential role in many physiological processes, including nerve impulse transmission; cardiac, smooth and skeletal muscle contraction; gastric secretion; renal function; tissue synthesis; and carbohydrate synthesis. In conjunction with bicarbonate, phosphate, sodium, calcium and magnesium, potassium preserves the acid–alkali balance of the body.

Therapeutic applications

An oral dose of 2000–4000 mg/day has been suggested for the correction of mild deficiency or to help correct blood pressure.[229]

A dose of 500 mg/day has been used successfully for the treatment of congestive heart failure or cardiomyopathy.[230]

Deficiency signs

Muscle weakness, fatigue, mental confusion, listlessness, irritability, apprehension, nerve conduction irregularities, impeded or absent reflexes, hypotension, muscle cramping and spasms, anorexia, abdominal bloating, nausea, constipation, polydypsia, polyuria. Deficiency (hypokalaemia) is most commonly related to prolonged vomiting, the use of diuretics, alcoholism, laxative overuse, congestive heart failure, some forms of kidney disease and metabolic disturbances.[231]

Biochemical testing

- Serum potassium
- Urinary potassium (24-hour)
- Erythrocyte potassium.

Supplemental forms

Many forms of supplemental potassium are available, including potassium acetate, potassium ascorbate, potassium bicarbonate, potassium chloride, potassium citrate, potassium gluconate, potassium glycerophosphate, potassium orotate, potassium phosphate and potassium sulfate. Potassium gluconate and potassium citrate are the most common supplemental forms.

Toxicity

In moderate to high doses potassium salts (taken orally) have been shown to cause nausea, vomiting, abdominal discomfort, diarrhoea and ulcers.[232] Toxicity symptoms may also include tingling of the hands and feet and muscular weakness. Potassium chloride can cause gastric irritation, especially when taken on an empty stomach. Dietary potassium is not associated with adverse events or toxicity.[233]

Dosage requirements

The RDI in Australia and New Zealand is 3800 mg/day for men and 2800 mg/day for women. The RDI for lactation is 3200 mg/day.[232]

Food sources

Fruit is generally a rich source of potassium, dried fruit particularly so. Other rich sources include vegetables, nuts, parsley, blackstrap molasses, kelp and tea.

Dietary intake and the need for supplementation

Diets rich in potassium favourably affect the acid–base balance in the body, as the foods are rich in bicarbonate and can thus counteract diet-induced acidity. Potassium intake from the diet is often lower than required for optimum health and peak metabolic function. Ideally, dietary potassium intake should be twice that of sodium.

As a supplement, potassium citrate appears to be the superior form, and has benefits due to its citrate content as well as its potassium content. Citrate is useful for reducing the formation of kidney stones, and has a similar effect to oranges and grapefruit (citrate mostly complexes with potassium in orange and grapefruit juices). Potassium citrate can have a protective effect against bone loss by inhibiting bone resorption.

SODIUM (NA)

Forms of nutrient

Sodium is the major electrolyte present in the extracellular fluid.

1 mmol sodium = 23 mg sodium

1 g sodium chloride salt contains 390 mg (17 mmol) of sodium.[234]

Distribution and storage

Approximately 95% of the total sodium content of the body is found in extracellular fluid. It is also found in the kidney, gut, and salivary and sweat glands. Sodium is also found in bone.

Absorption

Sodium absorption is rapid and efficient. It occurs primarily by passive diffusion (some absorbed by active transport). Approximately 98% is absorbed even with excessive intakes.

Dietary intake often provides more than the body requires. Due to rapid and efficient absorption there is a very real risk that these high intakes may result in adverse effects.

Excretion

Sodium is excreted through the urine via the kidneys. Some sodium is lost in the sweat when exercising in hot weather.

Interactions (medication, nutrient, dietary)

There is evidence that excess sodium can have adverse effects on calcium, leading to increased bone loss. Increased sodium excretion leads to increased urinary calcium elimination, which may be due to the competition between sodium and calcium for reabsorption in the kidney. It may also be due to the effect of sodium on parathyroid hormone (PTH) secretion.

Function

All body fluids contain sodium, and it is required for many biochemical processes, including water-balance regulation, fluid distribution on either side of the cell walls, muscle contraction and expansion, nerve stimulation and acid–alkaline balance. Sodium is a cation needed to maintain extracellular volume and serum osmolality. Approximately 95% of the total sodium content of the body is found in extracellular fluid, being maintained outside of the cell via the Na^+/K^+-ATPase pump. Sodium is also important for maintaining the membrane potential of cells and for active transport of molecules across cell membranes. Sodium is vital in the proper functioning of the adrenal glands.

Therapeutic applications

Sodium is sometimes used therapeutically in extreme cases, for example to treat heat stroke and leg cramps.

Exercise, particularly in a warm environment, and diarrhoeal illness are two situations that will increase the requirement for salt to substantially greater levels.

Deficiency signs

Sodium depletion is mainly caused by enteric, renal or adrenal disease, and sodium retention is caused by renal disease (healthy kidneys are well able to excrete excess dietary salt). The most common cause of sodium loss is acute diarrhoea.

Low sodium levels may also cause (these symptoms can also be due to dehydration): blurred vision, oedema, decreased fluid volume, hypotension, nausea and vomiting, dizziness, poor memory and impaired concentration.

Biochemical testing

Sodium blood tests are used to detect hyponatraemia and hypernatraemia as part of an electrolyte panel or basic metabolic panel. Urinary sodium can also be measured in sodium-sensitive individuals with hypertension who need to lower their sodium intake.

Supplemental forms

Sodium is ubiquitous in the diet and is rarely supplemented. As tissue salts, sodium chloride, sodium phosphate and sodium sulfate are commonly used therapeutically in very dilute concentrations (6×).

Toxicity

Provided the kidneys are healthy and functioning efficiently, sodium toxicity from the diet is highly unlikely. High intakes of salt correlate with an increased incidence of hypertension in both adults and children.[235]

Dosage requirements

There are no established dosage requirements for sodium. The human body requires approximately 0.5 g/day of sodium for the maintenance of fluid homeostasis and cell function. The average intake range in Australia and New Zealand has been set at 460–920 mg/day (20–40 mmol) for adults (including pregnancy and lactation). The upper level of intake recommendation is 2300 mg/day (110 mmol).[234] Importantly, international consensus on recommendation is divided with the recommended intake of salt varying considerably between countries. The British health authorities advise a maximum of 6 g/day, but in Germany a maximum of 10 g/day is recommended. In contrast, Sweden recommends a maximum of 2 g/day, and Poland recommends a minimum of 1.4 g/day.

Food sources

The majority of foods contain at least some sodium, as sodium chloride (known as salt). Reasonable amounts are found in seafood, beef and poultry. Some sodium is present in vegetables, including celery, beets, carrots and artichokes. It is present in high amounts in processed and cured meats, brine-soaked foods such as pickles, olives and sauerkraut, salted and smoked fish, caviar and most cheeses, particularly processed cheeses

Dietary intake and the need for supplementation

It is estimated that Australians (including children) have a mean salt (sodium chloride) intake of 5.5 g/day, which delivers about 2000 mg/day (110 mmol) of sodium. About 80% of salt intake comes from processed foods and 20% from discretionary use (table salt/cooking).[236] Current intakes of sodium well and truly meet the relatively low requirements of the body and mitigate the need for supplementation.

Nevertheless, sodium is an essential element for human physiological and metabolic function, and should be present in the diet to a limited degree. Prudent use of unrefined ocean salt is probably the best way to obtain this element. Unrefined ocean salt has only 31% sodium by volume and contains other minerals such as calcium and magnesium, as well as a wide range of other elements in trace amounts. Some of these, such as iodine, are present in amounts too low to meet adequacy. However, ocean salt does contain a range of trace elements which are probably toxic in higher amounts, but in a very low dose (i.e. at hormetic exposure) may have additional benefits across the life span.

According to the Weston Price Foundation, another way to supply sodium in the diet is by consuming mineral-rich broths made with animal bones. These broths contain not only sodium, but also other key macrominerals in a bioavailable 'ionised electrolyte solution'. Increasing the amount of potassium in the diet should also help to ameliorate the hypertensive effects of sodium.

PHOSPHORUS (P)

Forms of nutrient

Phosphate salts or organophosphate molecules. The majority of dietary phosphorus is in the form of free phosphate.

Distribution and storage

Most phosphorus is concentrated in the bones, with some found in the teeth. Phosphorus is also found to an appreciable degree in red blood cells.

Absorption

About 70% of phosphorus is absorbed from the intestines, although absorption is dependent to some extent on the levels of calcium and vitamin D and the activity of parathyroid hormone (PTH), which regulates phosphorus and calcium metabolism.

Excretion

Phosphate is reabsorbed in the kidneys and eventually excreted in the urine. Small amounts are lost in bile, which regulates body levels of phosphorus. Estimated losses are approximately 1400 mg/day (540 mg in faeces and 860 mg in urine).

Interactions (medication, nutrient, dietary)

Unsaturated fatty acids, iron and aluminium can interfere with phosphorus absorption. The calcium/phosphorus ratio of dairy milk is lower than that of human breast milk, which may contribute to hypocalcaemia in formula-fed infants. Phosphoric acid (found in soft drinks) can bind with calcium in the intestines and prevent calcium absorption.[237] Excessive use of antacids can deplete phosphorus.[8]

Function

Second to calcium, phosphorus is the most abundant mineral in the human body. Phosphorus (as phosphate) accounts for more than half of the mineral mass of bone. It is critical for bone mineralisation, cell signalling and energy storage in the form of ATP.[238] The phosphate ion is essential for the metabolism of carbohydrate, lipids and protein, and functions as a coenzyme in multiple enzyme systems.

Therapeutic applications

1 Oxaluric renal stone disease and some cases of uric acid stone disease. Prevention of stone formation in patients with renal polycystic disease. Prevention of stone relapse after ESWL (extracorporeal shock wave lithotripsy) or lithotomy
2 Distal renal tubular acidosis complicated by hypercalciuria, mainly in children
3 Renal hypercalciuria and hyperoxaluria
4 Prevention of renal complications at the time of glaucoma treatment with acetazolamide
5 Potassium supplementation during treatment of hypertension.[239]

Deficiency signs

A syndrome resulting from the prolonged and excessive use of antacids, leading to acute phosphorus depletion, is characterised by weakness, anorexia, malaise and bone pain.

Biochemical testing

Blood and urine values are used to diagnose parathyroid, bone and calcium disorders, kidney conditions and vitamin D imbalances.

Supplemental forms

Sodium phosphate is widely used in supplements. Other forms include calcium phosphate, iron phosphate and potassium phosphate.

Toxicity

Toxicity is extremely rare, given that the kidneys are capable of excreting large volumes of phosphorus on a daily basis, and usually arises in chronic renal disease. This can result in neuroexcitability, tetany and convulsions.[8]

Dosage requirements

The RDI for adults is 1000 mg/day (including in pregnancy and lactation). The upper level (UL) of intake is 4000 mg/day for adults and during lactation. The UL decreases to 3500 mg/day during pregnancy and 3000 mg/day in adults >-70 years.[240]

Food sources

The primary dietary sources of phosphorous are animal and plant proteins. Inorganic phosphorous is found in food preservatives and in soft drinks as phosphoric acid.[241] Phosphorus is abundant in milk, poultry, fish and meat. Cheese and eggs also contain substantial amounts, while seeds and nuts contain reasonable levels of phosphorus. It is also found in wholegrains, brewer's yeast and wheatgerm.

Dietary intake and the need for supplementation

Phosphorus is usually abundant in the diet and there is rarely a need for supplementation. High dietary and serum phosphorous may promote cardiovascular calcification; however, it appears the calcium/phosphorus ratio is more relevant than absolute phosphorus intake. High phosphorus intake can be mitigated by increasing calcium intake.[242]

CHLORINE (CL)/CHLORIDE (CL)

Forms of nutrient

Chloride is the major anion (negatively charged ion) in the human body.

Distribution and storage

Low concentrations (extracellular) of chloride are found in bone and in connective tissue. Intracellular chloride is found in the highest concentration in the erythrocytes, and to a lesser degree in the gastric mucosa, gonads and skin.[8] Chloride is a component of stomach hydrochloric acid (HCl).

Absorption

Chloride absorption is rapid and easy in the small intestine via passive diffusion (less so in the large intestine). Chloride ions follow the cations that are actively transported, such as sodium ions. Much of the chloride secreted into the gastrointestinal tract as part of gastric juices (including HCl) is reabsorbed.

Excretion

Chloride is normally lost in the urine, sweat and stomach secretions. Excessive loss can occur from heavy sweating, vomiting, and adrenal gland and kidney disease.

Interactions (medication, nutrient, dietary)

Adverse physiological events such as sweating, vomiting or diarrhoea can deplete chloride levels. Chloride levels can also be affected by surgical procedures and during acute illness.

Function

Chloride accompanies sodium and water and helps generate the osmotic pressure of body fluids. Chloride is a key constituent of stomach HCl. Chloride helps to maintain the body's acid–base balance.

Therapeutic applications

Note: Chloride is typically prescribed with other electrolytes.

- Electrolyte losses — prolonged vomiting, diarrhoea, excessive sweating, dehydration.
- Metabolic alkalosis.

- Cushing's disease (excess excretion of potassium and chloride).
- Hypochlorhydria.
- Poor wound healing and clot formation after an injury.
- Potassium deficiency.

Deficiency signs

Heat exhaustion, muscle cramps, hair loss, nausea.

Biochemical testing

The normal serum range for chloride is 9–106 mmol/L.

Supplemental forms

Chloride is usually abundant in the diet and is rarely supplemented. Chloride is a component of potassium chloride, calcium chloride and chromium chloride.

Toxicity

Associated symptoms and high levels are typically attributed to the sodium and potassium ions due to consumption of high levels of table salt (NaCl) or potassium chloride (KCl).

It is thought that chloride may play a role in the increased incidence of high blood pressure and other conditions associated with high intakes of table salt. This is supported by the fact that blood pressure elevation occurs more strongly and consistently when sodium and chloride are consumed together than it does if either mineral is taken on its own.

Dosage requirements

The AI of chloride for adults is 2.3 g/day (including pregnancy and lactation). AI in adults >71 years is 1.8 mg/day.[243]

Food sources

The main dietary source of chloride is through table salt or sea salt. It is also present in vegetables, sea vegetables (e.g. wakame, kelp, dulse), olives, rye, lettuce, tomatoes and celery.

Dietary intake and the need for supplementation

Chloride is usually abundant in the diet and supplementation is not really of clinical significance.

Trace elements

IRON (FE)

Forms of nutrient

Iron appears commonly in aqueous oxidation states as ferrous (Fe^{2+}) iron and ferric (Fe^{3+}) iron. In the body it is important that iron is chemically bound in order to facilitate appropriate physiological function, transport and storage and to minimise the presence of free ionic iron, which can lead to harmful oxidation reactions.

Distribution and storage

After absorption, iron is transported by ferritin to specific sites for use. Approximately two-thirds of the body's iron is concentrated in haemoglobin (erythroid precursors and mature erythrocytes), a percentage of which is recycled to form new red blood cells.[244,245] Iron is stored in the liver, spleen and bone marrow. Lactoferrin (present in neutrophils, plasma and human breast milk), which is structurally similar to transferrin, is also involved in iron transport.[246]

Absorption

Iron is absorbed as ferrous iron. The absorption of both haem and non-haem iron occurs primarily in the upper portion of the duodenum. Haem iron from animal sources is absorbed more efficiently than non-haem iron from plant-based sources, although when iron stores are low, non-haem iron is absorbed almost as efficiently as haem iron.[245] Non-haem iron is more efficiently absorbed in the presence of vitamin C, which facilitates the conversion of ferric iron to ferrous iron.[247]

Excretion

The body's iron economy is typically under tight physiological control, although some iron is lost daily via the faeces, from exfoliated mucosal cells, bile, exuded red blood cells, and small amounts in desquamated skin cells and sweat. A minimal amount is excreted in the urine.[245]

During menstruation, adolescent girls and premenopausal women excrete considerable amounts of iron, although these losses vary considerably between individuals, in the range 14–50 mg.

Interactions (medication, nutrient, dietary)

- Antacids, cholestyramine, cimetidine, H_2-receptor antagonists, haloperidol and omeprazole have the potential to interfere with iron absorption.
- Bisphosphonates, such as alendronate, etidronate, risedronate (Actonel) and tiludronate, should be separated by at least 2 hours from iron, as iron can decrease the absorption of bisphosphonates by forming insoluble complexes.
- Iron may reduce the absorption of levodopa, and so it is advisable to separate the doses.
- Supplemental iron can reduce the effect of some medications (ACE inhibitors and some antibiotics) and should be administered 2 hours apart from one another.[16]
- Iron can decrease the absorption and efficacy of levothyroxine by forming insoluble complexes in the gastrointestinal tract. Doses should be separated by 2 hours.
- Concomitant use of iron can decrease absorption of methyldopa, resulting in increases in blood pressure. Doses should be separated by at least 2 hours.
- Oral iron supplements can markedly reduce absorption of mycophenolate mofetil. Iron should be taken 4–6 hours before or 2 hours after mycophenolate mofetil.
- Oral iron supplements can reduce absorption of penicillamine by 30–70%, most probably due to chelate formation. Take penicillamine at least 2 hours before or after iron-containing supplements.
- Iron decreases the absorption of quinolone antibiotics due to the formation of insoluble complexes. These

antibiotics should be taken at least 2 hours before or 2 hours after iron-containing supplements.

- Concomitant use of iron can decrease the absorption of tetracycline antibiotics by 50–90%. Tetracyclines should be taken at least 2 hours before or after iron-containing supplements.

Black tea (can reduce iron absorption by up to 90%) and coffee (tannic acid) can reduce absorption of both dietary and supplemental iron and should not be consumed at the same time.[248]

Function

The majority of functional iron in the body is present in haem proteins, such as the haemoglobin of red blood cells and the myoglobin of muscle cells — where it is required for oxygen and carbon dioxide transport. Iron is also found in cytochromes, which are involved in oxygen transport or mitochondrial electron transfer. Many other enzymes also contain or rely on iron for their biological function (e.g. catalase, xanthine oxidase, glutathione peroxidase), and iron is found in the functional groups of most enzymes in the Krebs cycle.[246] Many of the key biological functions of iron rely on its high redox potential, enabling rapid conversion between the Fe^{2+} and Fe^{3+} forms. The redox potential of iron is also potentially harmful and can lead to oxidative damage to cell components such as fatty acids, proteins and nucleic acids. Fortunately, within the body iron is usually bound to carrier proteins and/or molecules with antioxidant properties, which minimise the capacity of the free ion to cause oxidative stress. Iron is also an essential cofactor in the synthesis of neurotransmitters such as dopamine, noradrenaline (norepinephrine) and serotonin.

Therapeutic applications

For iron deficiency anaemia in adults, 100–200 mg elemental iron can be given daily or in 2 or 3 divided doses.[249] For children with iron deficiency anaemia, the dose is 2 mg/kg/day (0–5 years) or 30 mg/day (5–12 years).[250] During menstruation, doses of 60 mg/day (of elemental iron) have been suggested.[251] Australian recommendations suggest it is reasonable to continue iron supplementation and replenish stores for 3–6 months in adults and 2–3 months in children.[252]

Deficiency signs

Initially, iron deficiency leads to depletion of ferritin (tissue iron stores) and clinical symptoms are minimal.[246] Impaired immune function, impaired physical and cognitive performance; adverse pregnancy outcomes; angular stomatitis; glossitis; oesophageal webs; gastritis; koilonychia, thin and brittle fingernails, 'spoon nails'; pica; pagophagia (the compulsive consumption of ice or iced drinks); cold intolerance; pale skin, conjunctiva and nail beds; breathlessness on exertion; fainting; vertigo; headache; tachycardia.[253] Restless leg syndrome has also been associated with iron deficiency anaemia.[254] Iron deficiency anaemia is frequently associated with chronic kidney disease, inflammatory bowel disease, cancer and chronic heart failure. Women of child-bearing age, pregnant women, adolescent girls and children aged 0–5 are most at risk of iron deficiency anaemia.[253]

Biochemical testing

Biochemical tests for iron status include serum iron, haemoglobin, mean cell volume, haematocrit, serum transferrin, transferrin saturation, serum ferritin, total iron-binding capacity, transferring receptor, erythrocyte protoporphyrin, and the zinc protoporphyrin haem ratio test. Serum ferritin is the most specific test that correlates with total body iron stores.[253]

When assessing supplementation from testing, the formula 1 mmol iron = 55.8 mg iron is used.

Supplemental forms

Most supplemental iron is in the ferrous form, in which the elemental iron is bound to a carrier molecule. These include ferrous aspartate, ferrous carbonate, ferrous chloride, ferrous citrate, ferrous fumarate, ferrous gluconate, ferrous oxide, ferrous succinate and ferrous sulfate (see Table 7.6). The ferrous salts (fumarate, sulfate and gluconate) are better absorbed than ferric iron.[246] Of the supplemental forms available, ferrous fumarate yields the most elemental iron. Intravenous iron infusions may be offered in anaemia.

TABLE 7.6 Comparison of iron supplements

Form	Absorption/ Tolerability	% of elemental iron
Ferrous lactate	Well tolerated and absorbed	19
Ferrous sulfate (heptahydrate)	Gastrointestinal side effects in higher doses (>40 mg)	20–22
Ferrous sulfate (monohydrate)	Gastrointestinal side effects in higher doses (>40 mg)	33
Ferrous fumarate	Well tolerated and absorbed	33
Ferrous succinate	Well tolerated and absorbed	35
Ferrous carbonate	Well tolerated and absorbed	24
Ferrous gluconate	Well tolerated and absorbed	12
Ferrous citrate	Well tolerated and absorbed	24
Ferrous amino acid chelate, including: ferrous *bis*-glycine chelate (FeBC), ferric *tris*-glycine chelate, ferric glycinate and ferrous *bis*-glycinate hydrochloride	Well tolerated and absorbed	Varies depending on type

Toxicity

Symptoms of iron toxicity include vomiting, diarrhoea, organ dysfunction (cardiovascular, neurological, renal, hepatic and haematological) and even death. Toxicity most commonly manifests in people with genetic disorders associated with iron metabolism (haemochromatosis, sickle cell disease and thalassaemia). Iron toxicity can occur in small children who have inadvertently swallowed iron tablets, the severity of symptoms being dependent on the amount ingested. Excess iron intake impairs the absorption of other minerals. The tolerable upper intake level for iron has been set at 45 mg/day, and levels higher than this may produce the first symptoms of toxicity (gastrointestinal distress, constipation, nausea and vomiting).

Dosage requirements

In Australia and New Zealand the RDI for iron is: infants 7–12 months, 11 mg/day; adult males, 8.0 mg/day; and women under 50 years old, 18 mg/day. In women 51–70 years the RDA is reduced to 5.0 mg/day. During pregnancy the RDI is increased to 27 mg/day, and reduced to 9 mg/day during lactation. The upper intake limit for iron has been set at 45 mg/day.[255]

Food sources

Iron in the diet is present in two forms: haem (ferrous iron) and non-haem (ferric iron). Approximately 40% of iron in meat, fish and poultry is haem iron and the rest is non-haem iron. Haem iron is well absorbed (25%). Non-haem iron is poorly absorbed (2–20%), and is present in plant-based foods and iron enriched/iron fortified foods. Non-haem iron absorption is inhibited by phytates, tannins, calcium, soybean proteins and polyphenols.[246]

Main food sources of iron are eggs, fish, liver, meat and green leafy vegetables.

Dietary intake and the need for supplementation

For marginal iron deficiency emphasis on iron-rich foods in the diet should be the first consideration. As the haem iron found in animal foods is better absorbed than that from plant-based sources, adequate meat intake is important for the maintenance of healthy iron status. Avoidance of red meat increases the risk of iron and zinc deficiencies.[256] Younger women in particular are more likely to avoid red meat. Men are less likely to be deficient than women, although vegans and vegetarian men also run the risk of low iron status. Menstruating women are more likely to run the risk of iron deficiency, and if repletion of iron through dietary means is unattainable supplementation should be considered. For individuals who choose to avoid meat for religious or ethical reasons, well-absorbed plant sources of dietary iron should be emphasised. The traditional naturopathic approach was to include concentrated iron sources such as kelp, brewer's yeast and blackstrap molasses in the diet, although these foods are not to everyone's taste, in which case iron supplementation may be necessary. There are many forms of ferrous iron available as supplements, all of which display a similar degree of bioavailability.

The amount of iron absorbed decreases with increasing dose. For this reason, it is recommended that iron supplements be taken in two or three doses equally spaced across the course of the day. Iron supplements can cause nausea and constipation in some instances, and are best taken with food to avoid these effects. These effects are more pronounced when ferrous sulfate is used, although this is probably dose dependent. Substitution with an alternative form of ferrous iron may help to overcome the unwanted effects. There is some evidence that lactoferrin (from whey protein) enhances iron metabolism.[257]

Iron deficiency also impairs both vitamin A and iodine metabolism, and this should be considered when evaluating the clinical picture. Maintaining iron levels during pregnancy is crucial. Demands for iron are increased during pregnancy, and most of this is needed during the last two trimesters.[258] In the latter part of pregnancy, it is difficult to meet daily iron requirements through food intake alone, even from the most optimal diet, and supplementation should be instigated.[247] In pregnant and lactating women a riboflavin deficiency can reduce the effectiveness of iron supplements. Riboflavin and iron deficiencies often coexist when animal product intake is low.[259]

Vitamin C improves bioavailability of dietary iron; however, it can increase the frequency of side effects associated with oral iron supplementation including nausea, diarrhoea and constipation. Recent meta-analyses have found side effects occur in 30–70% of patients.[260]

ZINC (ZN)

Forms of nutrient

In the human body zinc is present as a positively charged ion. In contrast to other trace elements, such as iron and copper, zinc has a single redox state, which means that it poses no threat of oxidative damage to cells.[261]

Distribution and storage

After absorption zinc passes through the liver and then to the general circulation. Zinc is distributed throughout the body, and circulates bound to albumin and α_2-macroglobulin, with approximately 3% being complexed with amino acids. A large percentage (about half) of zinc is contained in skeletal muscle, and bone (30%). The pancreatic B-cells contain some of the highest concentrations of zinc in the body.[262] The liver also represents a labile pool for zinc, containing about 5%.[263] There is, however, no storage form of zinc in the body as a consequence of a highly effective homeostatic mechanism.[264]

Absorption

Zinc absorption takes place via saturable and non-saturable processes, with the highest rates of absorption taking place in the jejunum. The gastrointestinal environment influences the efficiency of zinc absorption; for example, zinc binds to protein hence the amount of dietary protein contributes to the efficiency of zinc absorption.[265]

Excretion

- The faeces is the major route of excretion for zinc, with a minor amount lost in the urine. Renal excretion varies, depending on intake levels, and the kidneys are involved in the maintenance of zinc homeostasis. Zinc is also lost through sloughed skin cells, sweat, hair, menstrual blood and semen.

Interactions (medication, nutrient, dietary)

- Zinc and copper are mutually antagonistic, each interfering with the gastrointestinal uptake of the other, thus potentially leading to an imbalance. To avoid potentiating a copper deficiency, high-dose zinc should not be used long term. When zinc is supplemented, copper intake should be proportionate.
- Some research suggests zinc and iron can negatively interact — transferrin (the main iron transporter) can also bind zinc and zinc can block the iron storage capacity of ferritin.[266] Supplemental iron can also decrease zinc absorption.
- Quinilone and tetracycline antibiotics interact with zinc in the GI tract inhibiting absorption of both zinc and the antibiotic — take antibiotics either 2 hours before zinc or 4–6 hours after.[267]
- Long-term use of thiazide and loop diuretics can increase urinary zinc excretion and zinc levels should be monitored carefully in people using these medications.
- Non-steroidal anti-inflammatory drugs (NSAIDs) interact with zinc and doses should be separated by 2 hours.
- Captopril and enalapril can also lead to the renal loss of zinc and levels should be monitored.
- Absorption of penicillamine (a drug used to treat rheumatoid arthritis) is reduced with zinc supplementation — take zinc either 2 hours before or after taking penicillamine.
- Amiloride can lead to zinc retention, and concomitant zinc supplementation is inadvisable in people using this drug.[16]

Function

Zinc is essential for growth and development and functions in the structure of proteins. It has a critical involvement in the proliferation, differentiation, cell signalling and apoptosis of cells. Zinc plays a crucial role in the pathways involved in inflammation and it is involved in up to 300 different enzymes. Functions that require zinc include immunity, carbohydrate and protein metabolism, DNA metabolism and repair, reproduction, vision, taste, bone health and cognition/behaviour. Zinc is also essential for neurogenesis, synaptogenesis, neuronal growth and neurotransmission. Zinc is required for cell division and differentiation, and is an essential nutrient for normal embryogenesis.[261]

Therapeutic applications

To address an established zinc deficiency, 25–50 mg/day elemental zinc is recommended. Clinical studies suggest that effective acute prescribing for the common cold is best achieved by taking higher doses of zinc as lozenges containing 13–14 mg elemental zinc (as acetate or gluconate).[268] Results are beneficial when taking supplements within 24 hours of onset and can reduce both the severity and duration of a cold.[269] Supplementation with 25 mg/day has been used to augment antidepressant therapy.[270] In Wilson's disease, 50 mg zinc (as acetate) taken 3 times daily has been shown to be effective. In the treatment of type 2 diabetes, 30 mg has been shown to be effective, without inducing a copper deficiency.

Deficiency signs

Impaired growth, impaired immune function, impaired reproductive function, acrodermatitis enteropathica (severe), deficits in taste and smell, lesions of the skin, mouth and nose, delayed sexual maturation and impotence, behavioural changes, irritability and impaired cognitive function, birth defects, spontaneous abortion, dermatitis and alopecia. Deficiency can be a consequence of low dietary intake, compromised absorption, increased excretion and an increase in need (e.g. growth and development and pregnancy).[261]

Biochemical testing

- Plasma, urine and hair are reliable markers of zinc status.[271]
- Functional markers: delta 6-desaturase activity linolenic acid:gamma linolenic acid (LA:GLA) and zinc metallothionen.[74]

Supplemental forms

Many forms of zinc are available, including zinc acetate, zinc ascorbate, zinc aspartate, zinc citrate, zinc gluconate, zinc methionine, zinc orotate, zinc picolinate and zinc sulfate. Zinc oxide is used in topical preparations. Zinc sulfate is commonly used in liquid zinc preparations. Zinc gluconate is commonly used in solid-dose preparations, such as tablets and lozenges.

Toxicity

Zinc toxicity from dietary sources is unlikely, but it can occur when excessive amounts of zinc are ingested as supplements. Symptoms of toxicity include nausea, vomiting, metallic taste, abdominal cramps, diarrhoea and headaches. Long-term excessive intake of zinc can also induce a copper deficiency, and may lead to suppressed immune function and reduced levels of high-density lipoprotein cholesterol.

Dosage requirements

In Australia and New Zealand the RDI for zinc is 14 mg/day for men and 8 mg/day for women, increasing to 11 mg/day in pregnancy and 12 mg/day in lactation. The upper level of intake for adults is 40 mg/day.[272]

Food sources

Sources include oysters (contain more zinc per serve than any other source), red meat, pulses, chicken, fish, nuts, seeds and ginger.

Dietary intake and the need for supplementation

To date, no single reliable marker for individual zinc status has been established. Serum zinc is inadequate, as the effects of zinc deficiency on specific functions are often present before plasma zinc levels are decreased. As is the case with magnesium, zinc is stored intracellularly and only a small percentage is found in the plasma.

Zinc supplementation is clinically relevant in treating skin conditions such as acne and acrodermatitis enteropathica. In combination with other primary antioxidants zinc may also be beneficial in slowing the progression of age-related macular degeneration. Recent studies have found a strong relationship between zinc and type 2 diabetes, with decreases in pancreatic zinc found in diabetic patients.[262]

Supplementation should also be considered in attention deficit and attention deficit hyperactivity disorders. The use of zinc pharmacologically during the acute phase of infection remains clinically relevant, despite some inconsistent results from clinical trials. Generally zinc supplementation reduces the duration and severity and symptoms of the common cold, even though an overt zinc deficiency may not be present. Loss of taste (hypogeusia) can be corrected in some people with zinc deficiency. In cases of male infertility, zinc assessment and supplementation should be given priority in the implementation of a nutritional treatment protocol. Low zinc status has been associated with reduced serum testosterone levels, reduced seminal volume and reduced sperm mobility, which should improve with the tissue repletion of zinc. A large systematic review also found zinc supplementation in pregnancy lowers the risk of preterm birth.[273] Therapeutic supplementation of zinc is also beneficial in treating Wilson's disease (genetic disorder of copper metabolism).

As is the case with iron, menstruating women who avoid red meat and other animal foods should carefully monitor their zinc status. Men also run the risk of zinc deficiency, particularly if they adopt a diet that relies on white poultry and fish as the main sources of protein.[263]

Zinc from plant-based sources is difficult to absorb, particularly zinc from foods that have high phytate levels, such as wholegrains and seeds. Absorption of zinc from animal proteins is greater than from a diet rich in plant proteins and the requirement for dietary zinc for vegetarians may be up to 50% greater.[274] Organic acids, such as citric, lactic, acetic, butyric and formic acids, produced during fermentation enhance zinc absorption from wholegrains, possibly by forming soluble ligands with zinc or by preventing the formation of the insoluble zinc–phytate complex.[275] To obtain adequate trace elements such as zinc from grains, it is therefore advisable that they be fermented or sprouted. Children adapt less well to a vegetarian diet, making them more vulnerable to suboptimal zinc status.[276]

COPPER (CU)

Forms of nutrient

Copper occurs in multiple valence states, with Cu^+ (cuprous) and Cu^{2+}(cupric) being the most common biologically active forms.[277]

Distribution and storage

Bound to albumin or histidine, copper is transported to the liver, where it is bound to ceruloplasmin, for release into the bloodstream and transport to tissues. Approximately 2 mg/day is directly absorbed across the gastrointestinal tract and then incorporated in blood, serum, liver, brain, muscle and kidneys. The liver is the primary storage organ for copper, followed by muscle and bone.[277]

Absorption

Depending on the bioavailability of dietary sources, 20–70% of ingested copper is absorbed, primarily in the duodenum, where it diffuses across the intestinal mucosa via the divalent metal transporter DMT1. Copper is absorbed to a lesser extent in the stomach.

Excretion

Of the total amount of copper absorbed only about 15% is actually transported to the tissues, the remaining 85% being excreted. The majority of copper is excreted in the bile, with a small percentage being in the urine.

Interactions (medication, nutrient, dietary)

- High levels of zinc as supplements (>50 mg/day for extended periods) can result in copper deficiency.[278]
- Penicillamine significantly increases urinary excretion of copper. Doses should be separated by at least 2 hours and patients taking this medication should be monitored for copper deficiency.[278]
- Patients receiving haemodialysis seem to be at risk of copper deficiency, and copper supplementation may be needed in these patients.
- As iron and copper use the same transport system, the excessive intake of either element can cause deficiency in the other. A high copper intake can also reduce zinc absorption.
- Excessive used of antacids interferes with copper absorption.

Function

Copper is an essential micronutrient in the function of several enzymes, including cytochrome c oxidase, amino acid oxidase and monoamine oxidase. As a cofactor of the antioxidant enzymes copper–zinc superoxide dismutase and ceruloplasmin, copper plays a crucial role in antioxidant defence. Copper is required for infant growth, host defence mechanisms, bone strength, red and white cell maturation, iron transport, cholesterol and glucose metabolism, myocardial contractility and brain development.

Therapeutic applications

For copper deficiency, cupric sulfate in doses of up to 0.1 mg/kg/day have been used. For osteoporosis, 2.5 mg/day copper combined with zinc 15 mg, manganese 5 mg and calcium 1000 mg has been used.[230] However recent research is conflicting in the therapeutic role of copper in the treatment of osteoporosis.[279]

Deficiency signs

Dietary copper deficiency is uncommon. Deficiency signs include: anaemia (that is unresponsive to iron therapy), neutropenia, leucopenia, osteoporosis, osteoporosis in children, arthritis, glucose intolerance, altered immunity.

Biochemical testing

Serum, platelet, leucocyte and urinary copper can be used; however, there is no definitive copper status biomarker. Other tests include ceruloplasmin concentration, erythrocyte superoxide dismutase activity, cytochrome c oxidase activity. Serum copper appears to be the most useful biomarker.[280] However serum copper reflects serum ceruloplasmin and is not a sensitive indicator of nutritional copper status.[281]

Supplemental forms

Copper citrate, copper gluconate, copper sulfate, copper chloride, copper amino acid chelates, cupric oxide and cupric sulfate are forms commonly used in supplements; however, cupric oxide is a less bioavailable form of copper.[282]

Toxicity

Copper toxicity leads to gastrointestinal effects such as abdominal pain, cramps, nausea, diarrhoea and vomiting. Recent research has shown no adverse effects in taking up to 8 mg/day for 6 months except in conditions where excess copper intake poses a risk (e.g. Wilson's disease).[283]

Dosage requirements

In Australia and New Zealand the adequate intake level has been set at 1.7 mg/day for adult men and 1.2 mg/day for adult women increasing to 1.3 mg/day in pregnancy and 1.5 mg/day in lactation. The safe upper limit is 10 mg for both men and women.[284]

Food sources

Legumes, mushrooms, nuts, seeds, kidney, cocoa, shellfish, egg yolk, blackstrap molasses and brewer's yeast. Beef liver and oysters are the best sources of copper.[285]

Dietary intake and the need for supplementation

As beef liver is the best and most easily assimilated source of copper, the consumption of traditional foods such as pâtés and terrines is a good dietary vehicle for providing adequate copper in the diet. A well-formulated multivitamin and mineral formula should provide enough copper to maintain sufficiency.

Infants receiving a diet that is predominantly or exclusively based on bovine milk run the risk of developing a copper deficiency. Cow's milk has substantially less copper than human breast milk and is also less bioavailable.[277] Elevated plasma copper has also been linked to high homocysteine levels.[286]

MANGANESE (MN)

Forms of nutrient

Manganese is a group VII transition metal that exists in a number of oxidation states. In biological systems the most prevalent are Mn^{2+} and Mn^{3+}. Manganese citrate is the main form concentrated in the blood.

Manganese is a cofactor for enzymes involved in the metabolism of amino acids, lipids and carbohydrates. Manganese-dependent enzyme families include oxidoreductases, transferases, hydrolases, lysases, isomerases and ligases. These enzymes include arginase, glutamine synthase and mitochondrial superoxide dismutase (SOD2 or MnSOD).

Distribution and storage

When manganese enters the portal blood from the gastrointestinal tract it may remain in its free state or be taken up by α2-macroglobulin, which is subsequently taken up by the liver. A small amount enters the systemic circulation, where it may undergo oxidisation to Mn^{3+} bound to transferrin. Uptake by the liver occurs through a unidirectional, saturable process similar to passive mediated transport.[287]

The manganese concentration is highest in tissues rich in mitochondria. Bone, liver, pancreas and kidney also have high concentrations, and manganese is also found in the hair and in pigmented structures, such as the retina, dark skin and melanin.[287]

Absorption

Absorption of manganese occurs throughout the small intestine through the divalent metal transporter. In adults absorption has been reported to be in the range 2–15%.

Excretion

Levels are regulated by excretion. Most manganese is secreted via bile, which may be reabsorbed. If bile flow is obstructed, manganese is found in intestinal or pancreatic juices and small amounts may be lost in urine or sweat.

Interactions (medication, nutrient, dietary)

Manganese and iron compete for absorption sites. Fibre, phytate, calcium, phosphorus and magnesium may also interfere with manganese absorption. It has been suggested that ethanol may enhance manganese toxicity. Manganese can also decrease the effectiveness of antibiotics.

Function

Manganese is a component of a number of enzymes and activates a range of others. Manganese metalloenzymes include manganese superoxide dismutase, arginase, phosphoenolpyruvate decarboxylase and glutamine synthetase (where it converts glutamate to glutamine in the glial cells). Glycosyl transferases are specifically activated by manganese. It is an essential element in the formation of bone, and is also involved in carbohydrate, cholesterol and amino acid metabolism.

Therapeutic applications

There are no established therapeutic applications.

Deficiency signs

Impaired growth; skeletal abnormalities; impaired reproductive performance; ataxia; defects in lipid and carbohydrate metabolism; poor bone development/ thickened limbs, curvature of the spine, and swollen and enlarged joints; insulin resistance.

Biochemical testing

While no direct biomarker for the assessment of manganese status has been established, erythrocyte (red blood cell) manganese may be a useful indicator of manganese status. Currently, most measures of manganese concentrations are highly variable. Hair analysis is valid for measuring manganese toxicity but not deficiency.

Supplemental forms

TABLE 7.7 Supplemental forms of manganese

Form (no bioavailability data available)	Elemental level
Manganese ascorbate	13%
Manganese aspartate	17%
Manganese amino acid chelate	10%
Manganese chloride	27.7%
Manganese citrate	30%
Manganese gluconate	11.0–12.2%
Manganese orotate	31.5%
Manganese picolinate	20%
Manganese sulfate	31.8–37.2%

Toxicity

Manganese toxicity in humans is primarily a concern for those exposed to high airborne concentrations in the workplace where it is a known neurotoxin. Environmental exposure is a serious concern, and toxicosis can result in a permanent and crippling neurological disorder of the extrapyramidal system, similar to Parkinson's disease. In its milder form, toxicity is expressed by hyperirritability, violent acts, hallucinations, disturbances of libido and incoordination. Contamination of water supplies may also cause manganese toxicity, but exposure to trace amounts through diet and supplements should not be a cause for concern.

Dosage requirements

The Australian adequate intake level has been set at 5.5 mg/day for men and 5 mg/day for women (including pregnancy and lactation).

Food sources

Nuts (especially pecans), seeds, wholegrains, butterfat and leafy vegetables. Alfalfa tea is a particularly rich source of manganese.[288]

Dietary intake and the need for supplementation

A diet containing a range of foods, organically grown in manganese-rich soil, should provide enough of this nutrient to meet an individual's daily requirements. Non-phytate sources are probably a better option, as high phytate levels can hinder manganese absorption, although, as with other trace elements such as zinc, fermentation, soaking and sprouting of wholegrains can overcome this problem and make these nutrients more absorbable. Additional amounts of manganese in supplements would not be of concern, as manganese is safe and well tolerated, even at tolerable upper intake levels.

Vegetarians consuming large quantities of soya products may be susceptible to manganese deficiency due to the high phytate levels of soya. Conversely, vegetarians who are iron deficient may have elevated manganese levels.[74]

IODINE (I)

Forms of nutrient

After ingestion, dietary iodine is converted to iodide ions (I^-). Iodine refers to the atom and the molecule I_2, which in its gaseous form is toxic. Iodide refers to the ion I^-, which is often found bound to other minerals in food.

Distribution and storage

Once they enter the circulation, iodide ions are distributed throughout the extracellular fluid. Iodine is bound to a significant degree in plasma. In the human body the thyroid gland contains the highest concentration of iodine. The average healthy human adult contains 20–50 mg of iodine: 70–80% of this is converted in the thyroid gland, and almost all of this is in the form of thyroglobulin (the storage form of thyroid hormone). Iodine is found to a lesser extent in the salivary glands, breast, choroid plexus and gastric mucosa.[289] Only 1 mg is found in blood (as thyroid hormones).

Absorption

Absorption occurs very rapidly through the stomach and small intestine. Any dietary iodine is largely converted to iodide in the intestine. Iodine is also absorbed rapidly and efficiently through the skin.

Excretion

90–97% of iodine (175 micrograms/day) is excreted via the kidneys, and 3–10% (20 micrograms/day) via the bile (reabsorbed) and faeces. Small amounts are lost via sweat, saliva and gastric juices (6 micrograms/day). Total excretion is approximately 200 micrograms/day.

Interactions (medication, nutrient, dietary)

- ACE inhibitors: there is a moderate risk that using these drugs with potassium iodide increases the risk of hyperkalaemia, so caution is warranted.
- The antiarrhythmic amiodarone contains 37.3% iodine.
- Plasma iodide levels may be increased with iodine supplements, and thyroid function should be monitored.
- The angiotensin receptor blockers losartan, valsartan, irbesartan, candesartan, telmisartan and eprosartan increase the risk of hyperkalaemia and caution should be exercised if these are used in combination with iodine supplements.
- Anti-thyroid drugs: co-administration with iodine is contraindicated.
- Lithium: when lithium is used pharmacologically, iodine may have an additive or synergistic hypothyroid effect.
- Potassium-sparing diuretics: co-administration with potassium iodide increases the risk of hyperkalaemia. Potassium-sparing diuretics include spironolactone, triamterene and amiloride.[6]
- Deficiencies in selenium, iron, zinc and vitamin A can exacerbate the effects of iodine deficiency.[290]

DIETARY GOITROGENS

Some foods contain goitrogenic substances that prevent the utilisation of iodine. These compounds are primarily isothiocyanates, which are similar in action and structure to propylthiouracil (a thionamide drug used to treat hyperthyroidism). They are found in cruciferous vegetables (cabbage, broccoli, cauliflower, Brussels sprouts, cassava root, soya beans, peanuts, pine nuts and millet).[291] In order to achieve clinical results (i.e. in hyperthyroid patients), large amounts of these foods must be consumed in their raw state, and iodine intake must be restricted. The highest levels of isothiocyanates are found in raw soya milk (0.46–2.5 mg/dL). Isoflavones in soya beans (genestein and daidzein) have been found to inhibit thyroid synthesis.[45] In the *Brassica* family, swedes, cabbage and turnips usually contain the highest levels. However, the quantity varies considerably according to climate and soil factors. Cooking deactivates (breaks down) dietary goitrogens.

Function

Iodine is an essential micronutrient and is present in the human body in low concentrations, almost exclusively in the thyroid gland. Iodine is an essential component of the thyroid hormones, levothyroxine (T4) and triiodothyronine (T3), with iodine comprising 65% and 59% of their weights, respectively. These hormones are involved in the maintenance of metabolic rate, cell metabolism and integrity of connective tissue. Thyroid hormones are necessary for the development of the brain and nervous system in the developing fetus and infant.

Therapeutic applications

The optimal level of iodine intake to prevent thyroid disease lies within a relatively narrow range — optimal status for adults is 150–250 micrograms.[292] During pregnancy and lactation, the WHO recommends 250 micrograms/day.[293] High-dose supplementation with 1500–6000 micrograms/day (with no adverse effects) has been used successfully to treat breast pain, tenderness and nodularity in women with fibrocystic breast disease.[294]

Deficiency signs

The most critical time for iodine status is in early life.[295] Iodine-deficiency disorders include:

- *Fetus*: abortion; stillbirth; congenital anomalies; neurological cretinism (mental deficiency, deaf mutism, spastic diplegia, squint); hypothyroid cretinism: mental deficiency, dwarfism, hypothyroidism
- *Neonate*: psychomotor defects, increased perinatal mortality, neonatal hypothyroidism
- *Children and adolescents*: retarded mental and physical development, impaired hearing, increased infant mortality[293]
- *Adults*: goitre and its complications, iodine-induced hyperthyroidism
- *All ages*: goitre (may also occur with high iodine levels); hypothyroidism, including impaired mental function
- *Breast disorders*: iodine deficiency may play a role in fibrocystic breast disease — the presence of iodine may modulate the effects of oestrogen on breast tissue
- *Vegetarians and vegans who do not consume seaweed*: rates of deficiency as high as 25–80% (respectively) have been reported.[296]

Note: even a mild deficiency during pregnancy is associated with reduced educational outcomes in children — including significant reductions in spelling, grammar and literacy.[297]

Biochemical testing

Urinary iodine (UI):

- <20 micrograms/L — severe iodine deficiency
- 20–49 micrograms/L — moderate deficiency
- 50–99 micrograms/L — mild iodine deficiency
- 100–199 micrograms/L — acceptable levels
- 200–299 micrograms/L — excessive
- ≥300 micrograms/L — excessive levels (risk of hypothyroidism, autoimmune thyroid disease).[298]

Supplemental forms

Potassium iodide (KI), potassium iodate (KIO_3) and sodium iodide (NaI) are the forms commonly used in supplements and food fortification. Kelp is often used as a source of iodine in nutritional supplements.

Toxicity

Intakes of up to 10 times the levels considered adequate should not lead to adverse events in people with a healthy functioning thyroid.

Excessive intake of iodine can cause metallic taste, soreness in teeth and gums, burning in mouth and throat, increased salivation, coryza, sneezing, eye irritation and eyelid swelling, headache, cough, pulmonary oedema, swelling of the parotid and submaxillary glands, inflammation of the pharynx, larynx and tonsils, acneform skin lesions, gastric upset, diarrhoea, anorexia and depression. Prolonged use of iodides can cause thyroid gland hyperplasia, thyroid adenoma, goitre and severe hypothyroidism.[291]

Dosage requirements

In Australia and New Zealand the RDI for adult men and women is 150 micrograms/day. This is increased to 220 micrograms/day during pregnancy and 270 micrograms/day during lactation. The upper level of intake (UL) is 1100 micrograms/day (caution needs to be exercised in those with thyroid cancer, autoimmune thyroid disease or a significant history of deficiency as they may adversely respond to levels below the UL or the levels considered safe for the general public.[299]

Food sources

Sources include saltwater fish, iodised salt, kelp and other sea vegetables, butter, pineapple, artichokes, asparagus and dark-green vegetables.

Dietary intake and the need for supplementation

Iodine deficiency remains a serious public health problem worldwide. In 2003, WHO estimated that 54 countries were still affected by iodine deficiency as a public health problem, and nearly 2 billion people have inadequate iodine nutrition. Pregnant/lactating women and young infants are the most vulnerable to the consequences of the deficiency, and close attention to iodine status in these individuals remains a priority in clinical practice. Iodine assessment is paramount in women before conception and pregnancy, and should be part of a balanced periconception nutritional protocol. In people with low iodine status, based on relevant diagnostic markers (urinary testing and circulating thyroid-stimulating hormone (TSH) and T4 levels), a combination of dietary/supplemental measures should be undertaken to ensure that iodine nutriture is established and maintained. Proper iodine utilisation requires sufficient levels of pro-vitamin A. A selenium deficiency will also have a negative impact on iodine status.

To meet the daily requirements for iodine sufficiency and adequacy (in individuals not using iodised salt as a regular component of the diet), a supplement that contains iodide or iodate would be an effective way of supplying this vital nutrient. In addition to the consumption of iodine-rich marine foods 2–3 times a week (approximately 300 micrograms), a supplement containing 250 micrograms of elemental iodine has been recommended during pregnancy and lactation. Substances and pollutants with antithyroid effects (including some natural polyphenolics) should also be avoided during this period.[300]

Note: Unrefined ocean salt (Celtic sea salt), despite having a wide range of minerals and trace elements not present in table salt, has iodine levels too low to meet the recommended daily intake levels for iodine adequacy and the prevention of iodine spectrum disorders.[301]

SELENIUM (SE)

Forms of nutrient

Selenium exists in different oxidation states, which allows it to form to several organic compounds, including selenomethione (the major form in food), selenocysteine, dimethyl selenide, trimethyl selenium, iodothyronine deiodinase (a component of glutathione peroxidase) and selenoprotein P.24. Selenocysteine is the predominant seleno-compound present in the seleno-proteins of body tissues. Inorganic forms are selenite and selenite.[302]

Distribution and storage

The thyroid glands contains the largest amount of selenium in human tissue. The skeletal muscles contain significant body selenium, with relatively high concentrations in the kidneys, testes and liver. Selenium is also found in immune cells, erythrocytes and platelets.[303]

Absorption

Selenium is absorbed throughout the small intestine via both active and passive transport. Organic selenium (selenomethionine) is actively transported via the same mechanism as used by methionine. The selenate form is also actively transported, via a mechanism common to sulfate, while selenocysteine and selenite are both passively absorbed.[304] Organic forms (selenomethionine and selenium-rich yeasts) are better absorbed than inorganic forms (sodium selenite). All selenium from food is organic and is bound to the amino acids cysteine, cystine and methionine. 80% of the selenium derived from food is absorbed and is actively transported across the brush border of the intestine. 60% of the inorganic forms of selenium is absorbed, although this amount is greatly improved if the inorganic forms are taken with food, especially protein foods.

Excretion

Selenium excretion is regulated via the kidneys. However, small amounts are excreted via sweat and in the breath. Excretion through the breath is as the garlicky smelling dimethylselenide; unabsorbed selenium is excreted in the faeces.

Interactions (medication, nutrient, dietary)

- Anticoagulant and antiplatelet drugs: combining selenium with these drugs may increase the risk of bleeding.
- Barbiturates: selenium can inhibit the hepatic metabolism of barbiturates and may prolong the sedative effects of barbiturates.
- HMG-CoA reductase inhibitors (statins): theoretically, selenium could reduce the effectiveness of these drugs.
- Cisplatin (a chemotherapeutic agent) can reduce selenium levels.

Function

Selenium is an essential micronutrient that exerts its biological functions through more than 25 seleno-proteins. Families of seleno-proteins include the glutathione peroxidases, the iodothyronine deiodinases and the thioredoxin reductases. Selenium plays a role in the antioxidant enzyme glutathione peroxidase, which protects cell membranes from damage caused by the peroxidation of lipids (including thyroid cells). Selenium is used for thyroid hormone synthesis and metabolism and for thyroid gland functioning.[305] As an essential component of the enzyme iodothyronine deiodinase, which converts levothyroxine (T4) to triiodothyronine (T3), selenium plays a major role in the synthesis and metabolism of thyroid hormones. Selenium also plays a role in immune defence, liver function, fertility and reproductive function in both males and females, visual health, and chemoprevention. Selenium also reduces the toxicity of heavy metals.[304]

Therapeutic applications

Many studies have suggested there is an inverse association between the risk of some cancers and selenium status; however, definitive therapeutic recommendations for selenium require more research.[306] Current data suggest there is a negative relationship between selenium status and type 2 diabetes: while the use of supplements is unlikely to increase the risk of type 2 diabetes in otherwise healthy individuals, supplementation should be avoided in those with high selenium status and at increased risk of the development of type 2 diabetes.[307]

Any supplementation of selenium should always be considered in relation to the u-shaped effects of selenium — it shows major benefits in selenium-deficient individuals yet poses health risks in those with excess selenium.[305]

Deficiency signs

Severe deficiency appears in regions where the selenium content of soil is extremely low (China) and leads to Keshan's disease or Kashin–Beck disease. Keshan's disease is characterised by cardiomyopathy, and mainly affects young children and women of childbearing age. Kashin–Beck disease leads to structural deformities of bone. Selenium deficiency is also associated with male infertility.[308]

Subclinical selenium deficiency can play a part in the development of clinical conditions such as cardiovascular disease, altered immune function, male infertility, inflammatory disorders, autoimmune thyroid disease and viral infection.

Other signs and symptoms of deficiency include haemolytic anaemia, muscle pain and tenderness, reproductive failure, increased risk of spontaneous abortion, neural tube defects, placental retention and worsening of autoimmune conditions.

Biochemical testing

Plasma, erythrocyte, urine, hair and nails. An elevated T4 and a lowered T3 serum level is a functional marker of deficiency (due to depressed iodothyronine deiodinase activity). Whole-blood selenium is a good indicator of long-term selenium status. Glutathione peroxidase is probably a better indicator of total body pool selenium (approximately 14 mg). The urinary seleno-metabolites monomethylselenium and methylseleno-*N*-acetyl-D-galactosamine may also be useful markers.[302]

Supplemental forms

The organic form of selenium, selenomethionine, is commonly used in both liquid and solid preparations. Organic selenomethionine is the safest and most effective form of selenium to use as a supplement (90% absorption). Supplements can also contain selenium-rich yeasts (grown in a high-selenium medium).[309] Sodium selenite (50% absorption) has specific clinical applications when used in pharmacological doses (200–400 micrograms), although it should be used with caution and glutathione peroxidise levels should be monitored to prevent toxicity.[310]

Toxicity

High blood levels of selenium can lead to selenium toxicity (selenosis), which can manifest symptomatically as severe gastrointestinal distress, changes to (and loss of) hair and nails, mottled teeth, garlic breath odour, fatigue, numbness and tingling and a suspected role in ischaemic heart disease, cardiomyopathy, renal disease and some neurological diseases.[311,312]

Dosage requirements

The RDI in Australia and New Zealand is 70 micrograms/day for adult men and 60 micrograms/day for women. This is increased to 65 micrograms/day during pregnancy and 75 micrograms/day during lactation. The upper level of intake is 400 micrograms/day for those aged ≥14 years.[313]

Food sources

Brazil nuts, butter, garlic, broccoli, onions and grains grown in selenium-rich soil. Meat, chicken, fish and eggs also contain relatively high levels of selenium.

Dietary intake and the need for supplementation

The selenium content of plants varies considerably depending on the selenium concentration of the soil in which they are grown, which varies regionally. This can mean that the levels of selenium in foods manufactured from these plants are inadequate. The same can be said of animal foods, and the selenium content of animal foods reflects the selenium content and availability in the diet consumed by the animal.

While severe selenium deficiency diseases do occur, they tend to be isolated and rare. However, marginal selenium deficiencies do occur, even in areas where selenium concentrations in the soil appear to be adequate. Selenium supplements can be beneficial for people living in regions with very low environmental levels of this element.[304] A low intake of selenium-rich foods in the diet may lead to marginal deficiency, as can nutrient antagonists such as alcohol and tobacco, resulting in increased losses or reduced hepatic storage of selenium.[314]

As selenium is well absorbed (70–95%) from dietary sources,[304] emphasising selenium-rich foods is probably the best way to treat a subclinical or marginal selenium deficiency. The best dietary source of selenium is Brazil nuts (provided they are from Brazil). The selenium in Brazil nuts is both highly concentrated and highly bioavailable. Consuming as little as two Brazil nuts a day provides the equivalent of 100 micrograms selenium, with other studies suggesting that only one nut daily is enough to recover from deficiency.[315,316] Other important selenium-containing foods include broccoli, Brussels sprouts, cabbage, cauliflower, collards, kohlrabi, mustards and kale, which display additional chemoprotective benefits over and above their selenium content.

People from low socioeconomic backgrounds, the elderly, pregnant and lactating women, and infants are also at risk of low selenium status. Low selenium status during pregnancy has been associated with adverse pregnancy outcomes such as miscarriages, neural tube defects, premature birth and low birth weight.[317]

MOLYBDENUM (MO)

Forms of nutrient

Molybdenum is a metal that exists in three valence states: Mo^{4+}, Mo^{5+} and Mo^{6+}. As a cofactor it appears in enzymes, particularly xanthine oxidase, sulfite oxidase and aldehyde oxidase.

Distribution and storage

After absorption some molybdenum is deposited in the liver, muscle and bone, and a proportion in the adrenal glands and gastrointestinal tract. Molybdenum stored in the liver, muscle and bone is considered 'slow turnover' compared with that which is stored in the adrenal glands and gastrointestinal tract (fast turnover), the latter being mobilised more quickly to meet physiological requirements.

Absorption

Of the ingested molybdenum 25–80% is absorbed in the stomach and small intestine (upper jejunum). Molybdenum absorption is passive and not saturable, and may be decreased by high copper intake (due to mineral competition).

Excretion

The body levels of molybdenum are regulated by excretion rather than absorption. Once absorbed, the metal is mainly excreted via urine; however, considerable amounts are excreted in bile as molybdate.

Interactions (medication, nutrient, dietary)

High molybdenum intake (dietary or supplemental) may interfere with copper absorption, just as a high copper intake may interfere with molybdenum absorption.[318]

Caution: Care should be taken when supplementing molybdenum in those with gout. High doses (10–15 mg/day) have been associated with elevated levels of uric acid, leading to a condition closely resembling gout. This is probably due to molybdenum complexing with copper in the kidneys, making it unavailable to aid in uric acid elimination.

Function

The basis of the importance of molybdenum is in its role in metalloenzymes. In humans, molybdenum is a cofactor for three important enzymes: xanthine oxidase/dehydrogenase, sulfite oxidase and aldehyde oxidase.

Therapeutic applications

To date no therapeutic range for molybdenum has been adequately assessed. Doses of 50 micrograms to 6.0 mg have been suggested.[319] A dose of 120 mg/day (as tetrathiomolybdate) has been recommended in the treatment of Wilson's disease.[320]

Deficiency signs

Frank deficiency is extremely rare and no deficiency has been observed in otherwise healthy humans.[319,321]

Biochemical testing

- Molybdenum intake: Plasma molybdenum concentration (reflects longer term intake) and 24-hour urinary excretion (relates to recent intake and is a suitable biomarker for short-term intake). There is no useful biomarker for molybdenum status.[321]
- Hair: direct assessment of molybdenum status.

Supplemental forms

Supplemental molybdenum is available in several forms: sodium molybdate, ammonium molybdate, molybdenum picolinate, molybdenum citrate and molybdenum aspartate. All forms of supplemental molybdenum seem to be well absorbed.

Toxicity

Through the diet and water supply molybdenum toxicity is rare, which is probably due to the fact that clearance through the kidneys is quite rapid. One study has shown that doses of up to 1500 micrograms/day for 24 days do not result in elevated blood or urinary levels of molybdenum.[322] However, toxicity has been observed in animals, such as cattle grazing in pastures in high-molybdenum areas. A high incidence of gout has been observed in regions with a high molybdenum content of soil and high dietary intakes.[322]

Dosage requirements

In Australia and New Zealand the RDI has been set at 45 micrograms/day for adult men and women, increasing to 50 micrograms/day during pregnancy and lactation. The upper level of intake is 2000 micrograms/day.[323] In Europe, the adequate intake is 65 micrograms/day for adults.[321]

Food sources

Plant foods growing above ground, such as legumes, leafy vegetables and cauliflower, contain relatively high concentrations of molybdenum compared with food from tubers or animals. The highest levels of molybdenum appear in legumes such as lentils and beans, with peas being the richest source, followed by nuts and grains. Plants grown in alkaline or neutral soils with high molybdenum concentrations can be expected to have the highest molybdenum levels. Most drinking water has low levels of molybdenum.

Dietary intake and the need for supplementation

Like many of the trace elements, molybdenum is difficult to obtain through the diet, particularly if foods are grown in soils that are low in this element. Therefore, a broad-spectrum micronutrient supplement that contains adequate levels of molybdenum is a good way to ensure regular exposure. Molybdenum has been reported to be beneficial to various groups of individuals, including those with sulfite sensitivity and asthmatics with an elevated urinary sulfite/sulfate ratio.

CHROMIUM (CR)

Forms of nutrient

Chromium exists in multiple valence states (from Cr^{2+} to Cr^{6+}). After ingestion, dietary chromium (as the divalent (chromous) ion) is rapidly oxidised and reduced by gastric acid to form Cr^{3+} (the trivalent chromic form), which is able to bind to ligands to form molecular coordination complexes.

Distribution and storage

Chromium is transported bound to albumin and transferrin and rapidly stored in tissue. Tissues with the highest chromium concentration are the kidneys, followed by the spleen, liver, lungs, heart and skeletal muscle.

Absorption

Chromium absorption is inversely related to dietary intake, and is under a basal control mechanism, which ensures that a minimum level of absorbed chromium is maintained. Absorption of chromium is in the range 0.5–2%, depending on intake.[324]

Excretion

Most excess chromium is excreted in the urine, and as much as 3050 micrograms/day may be excreted. Small amounts are lost in the hair, perspiration and bile and unabsorbed chromium is excreted via the faeces.

Interactions (medication, nutrient, dietary)

- Chromium interacts with iron by affecting its binding to transferrin, and theoretically it should impair iron metabolism and storage, although this interaction has been disputed.
- Chromium supplementation may reduce the requirement for hypoglycaemic agents (by as much as 50% in some clinical studies), and the dosage of these medications should be closely monitored.
- Patients taking statin drugs for lipid modification also need to monitor their dose requirements if using pharmacological doses of chromium.
- Corticosteroids can lead to significant renal excretion of chromium.

Function

Trivalent chromium has been shown to have functions in carbohydrate, lipid, protein and corticosteroid metabolism. A role for chromium has been proposed as a component of the chromium-loaded oligopeptide chromodulin (holochromodulin), which may function in the amplification system for insulin signalling.[318] It plays an essential role in normal glucose function and lipid metabolism.[325]

Therapeutic applications

Recent evidence suggests that low chromium status correlates with an increased relative risk of coronary heart disease and diabetes.[324]

Doses of 200–1000 micrograms/day have been used in clinical studies to improve glucose and lipid control in patients with type 2 diabetes.[326]] However, doses closer to 400–660 micrograms/day have been shown to be highly effective.[325,327] In people with type 2 diabetes, chromium picolinate supplementation has been shown to reduce mean HbA1c levels from >9% to <7%, and improved glycaemic control meant that their antidiabetic medication was reduced by 50%. There is also evidence of the beneficial effects of chromium picolinate supplementation in women with gestational diabetes.[328]

Chromium supplementation, in the form of chromium picolinate, has been shown to be safe and effective for use in conditions such as prediabetes, diabetes, dyslipidaemia, depression, metabolic syndrome and other clinical conditions associated with insulin resistance.[329]

Deficiency signs

Impaired glucose tolerance, elevated circulating insulin, glycosuria, fasting hyperglycaemia, impaired growth, hypoglycaemia, elevated serum cholesterol and triglycerides, nerve disorders, neurological disorders, ocular eye pressure, decreased insulin binding, decreased insulin receptor number, decreased lean body mass, elevated body fat, gestational diabetes, atypical depression.[330]

Biochemical testing

At present there is no single reliable test for chromium status. Chromium status is challenging to determine as blood, urine and hair levels are not necessarily a reflection on stores.[331]

Supplemental forms

Chromium picolinate, chromium nicotinate and chromium chloride are the most widely studied forms.

Toxicity

Trivalent chromium, the form of chromium found in foods and nutrient supplements, is one of the least toxic nutrients as chromium is poorly absorbed and rapidly excreted.[332]

Dosage requirements

No RDI for chromium has been established. In Australia and New Zealand an adequate intake of 35 micrograms for men and 25 micrograms for adult women has been recommended. During pregnancy the RDI is increased to 30 micrograms/day and 45 micrograms/day during lactation.

Food sources

Broccoli, legumes, spices, beef, fish, hard wheat, hazelnuts, mussels, oysters, raw sugar, butter and egg yolk.

Dietary intake and the need for supplementation

Even well-balanced diets can contain suboptimal levels of chromium, and the intestinal absorption of trivalent chromium is low (0.5–2.0%).[333] To increase absorption and improve tissue pools of chromium, supplementation is often warranted, and this should also address subclinical deficiency states. A high intake of simple sugars increases chromium loss.[334] A high level of exercise can also increase chromium excretion.[335]

For therapeutic use, chromium picolinate is probably the best form to use as a supplement. Chromium supplementation in the form of chromium picolinate has been shown to be safe and effective for use in conditions such as prediabetes, diabetes, dyslipidaemia, depression, metabolic syndrome and other clinical conditions associated with insulin resistance.[329]

At present there is no reliable marker available for the assessment of chromium deficiency. Serum is currently the only method employed, and this is probably inadequate. Thus a great deal is left to the judgment of the clinician when it comes to identifying individual requirements for this nutrient. The best assessment may be the response of glucose and insulin to chromium supplements. In those whose impaired glucose and insulin function is related to a suboptimal intake of chromium, supplementation will be beneficial.

It has been noted by researchers that people with diabetes or glucose intolerance may not respond to supplementation as readily as non-diabetics and may require higher doses to achieve significant clinical effects. Doses of 400–600 micrograms/day or more may be required.[324]

BORON (B)

Forms of nutrient

Boron is found in the body as boric acid in $B(OH)_3$ and the tetrahydroxyborate ion $B(OH)_4^-$.

Distribution and storage

After absorption, boron tends to concentrate in the bone, nails, dental enamel (teeth), spleen, parathyroid gland and, to a lesser extent, the blood.

Absorption

Approximately 90% of dietary boron is absorbed in the intestines and metabolised to form $B(OH)_3$.

Excretion

Boron is excreted primarily through the urine, although some is excreted through the faeces, sweat and breath.[336]

Interactions (medication, nutrient, dietary)

As boron may increase serum oestrogen levels, women on oestrogen therapy should exercise caution if taking boron concomitantly.[74]

Function

Boron is a non-metallic trace element. It is found abundantly in nature as compounds formed in combination with sodium and oxygen. Boron has yet to be recognised as an essential nutrient for humans, although data from several animal and human studies suggest that it may play a role in cell membrane function, mineral and hormone metabolism, and enzyme reactions.[337] Research also suggests that boron is needed, or is beneficial, for embryogenesis, bone growth and maintenance, and immune function. It also plays a role in the metabolism of calcium and magnesium, energy substrates such as triacylglycerols and glucose, nitrogen-containing substances such as amino acids and proteins, reactive oxygen species, and hormones such as insulin, oestrogen, calcitonin and vitamin D.[338]

Therapeutic applications

The common supplemental dose of boron lies in the range 3–9 mg/day. A dose of 6–9 mg/day has been used to alleviate the symptoms of arthritis, and 10 mg/day has been used to increase steroid hormone production (testosterone) in males. Doses of 0.25–3.25 mg/day have been reported to increase plasma 17β-oestradiol in women by more than 50%. Boric acid powder 600 mg/day intravaginally for 2 weeks has been used to treat vulvovaginitis.[339]

Deficiency signs

Animal data have shown that boron deficiency impairs calcium metabolism, brain function and energy metabolism. As boron affects the composition, structure and strength of bone, deficiency symptoms are similar to those seen in osteoporosis; that is, decreased absorption coupled with increased excretion of calcium and magnesium.

Biochemical testing

No definitive biochemical test for boron deficiency has been established. Possible markers: serum, urine, hair (use with care as many shampoos and hygiene products contain boron).

Supplemental forms

Boric acid is the mineral acid form of boron. Boric acid contains 36% elemental boron. Other forms of supplemental chelated boron include boron aspartate, boron citrate, boron glycinate, boron orotate, boron picolinate, calcium borate, calcium borogluconate and sodium tetraborate decahydrate.

Toxicity

Boron has limited toxicity when administered orally, but toxicity results from acute ingestion of large doses, with symptoms of anorexia, indigestion, dermatitis and alopecia

Dosage requirements

The WHO states an acceptable range of intake as 1–13 mg/day for adults. A TUL for adults has been set at 20 mg/day.

Food sources

Foods rich in boron include avocado, ground cinnamon, peanuts, pecans, grapes, raisins and wine. Pulses, nuts and avocados contain 1.0–4.5 mg boron/100 g, while fruits and vegetables provide 0.1–0.6 mg boron/100 g.[340] Boron is well absorbed from dietary beverages, including prune and grape juice, wine, coffee and milk. Depending on the geographical region, boron can also be available in the water supply.

Dietary intake and the need for supplementation

As for many trace elements, it is the boron level in soil that determines the intake by a population in any given area and the incidence of disease related to a deficiency or inadequate intake of this element. As the naturopath and boron researcher Rex Newnham has noted, in places where there is a greater than usual amount of boron in the soil there is much less arthritis. He also makes the observation that some of the benefits of health spas — where people bathed to restore their health and ease their aches and pains — may have been due to the high boron content of the water. He mentions Ngawha in New Zealand, where spa pools containing 300 ppm of boron have served as a popular curative place for arthritics.[340] Commercial crops grown with fertiliser tend to have lower levels of boron, as superphosphate inhibits the uptake of trace minerals such as boron. People who rely on convenience foods and fast foods are also less likely to have an adequate intake of boron, as this trace element tends to be concentrated in fruit and vegetables. In those unwilling to improve their intake of fresh fruit and vegetables, a boron supplement of 3 mg/day is recommended.

As boron appears to improve the mineral economy (retention) in the body, it is advisable to include boron in nutrient supplement protocols for the treatment and prevention of osteoporosis. In menopausal women who have difficulty absorbing calcium, boron supplementation may be of considerable benefit, due to the fact that it increases 17β-oestradiol levels and influences the metabolism of vitamin D, and other steroid hormones. Boron should also be considered in supplementation protocols for the treatment and prevention of rheumatoid arthritis.

COBALT (CO)

Forms of nutrient

Cobalt is a trace element that is essential for normal growth and life span but only as part of the vitamin B_{12} molecule — hence the name 'cobalamin'. One atom of cobalt is found at the centre of the porphyrin-like corrin ring structure of vitamin B_{12}. Inorganic cobalt salts are toxic.

Distribution and storage

Cobalt is found within the body as a functional part of the vitamin B_{12} molecule. In total there is less than 1 mg in the average adult body, and it is found in the bone, muscle, liver and kidneys.

Absorption

Cobalt is absorbed as part of the vitamin B_{12} molecule. Optimal absorption requires intrinsic factor, calcium, hydrochloric acid, pancreatic secretions and levothyroxine.

Humans and animals are unable to incorporate cobalt into vitamin B_{12} and therefore it must be ingested as the preformed vitamin.

Iron status and the chemical form of cobalt can cause discrepancies in dietary absorption rates.

Excretion

Ingested cobalt is largely excreted in the urine. Gastrointestinal absorption varies in the range 5–45%.

Interactions (medication, nutrient, dietary)

All interactions are as for vitamin B_{12} (see earlier in this chapter).

Function

The role of cobalt is as part of the vitamin B_{12} molecule. Many of the functions of vitamin B_{12} in the body are due to the cobalt portion of the molecule, and include red blood cell production, DNA synthesis, and maintenance of the nervous system and nervous system function.

Therapeutic applications

These are as for vitamin B_{12} (see earlier in this chapter).

Deficiency signs

Deficiency is essentially a vitamin B_{12} deficiency. Therefore, symptoms include pernicious anaemia and potentially fatal macrocytic anaemia, abnormalities in cell formation, central nervous system disorders and neural degeneration.

Biochemical testing

No definitive biochemical test for cobalt deficiency has been established. Assessment of vitamin B_{12} parameters is also advisable.

Supplemental forms

Cobalt is only useful as part of vitamin B_{12}. Supplementation with cobalt will *not* treat the symptoms of a vitamin B_{12} deficiency.

Toxicity

Toxicity occurs within the range of 25–30 mg/day or above; however, there are very limited clinical data on cobalt.

Dosage requirements

These are unknown. The average daily intake in Australia is 34 micrograms/day.[341]

Food sources

Meat, potatoes, internal organs (offal), nuts and yeast extract.

SILICON (SI)

Forms of nutrient

Silicon as $Si(OH)_4$ appears abundantly in the soil, in minerals and in human tissues. Orthosilicic acid is the form predominantly absorbed by humans.[342]

Distribution and storage

In humans the highest concentrations of silicon are located in the connective tissues such as the aorta, trachea, tendon, bone and skin, and to a lesser degree in the liver, heart and muscle. Significant amounts are also found in the epidermis and hair.

Absorption

Little is known about silicon absorption, but it is not protein-bound in the bloodstream.[342] Absorption appears to mainly occur in the small intestine, although some may be absorbed in the lungs in the form of silicic acid from the dust of stone, sand, flint or glass blowing. It is believed that parathyroid hormone (PTH) affects silica as it has a role in calcium and phosphorus metabolism (PTH may increase the absorption of silica as well as of calcium and phosphorus).

Excretion

Silicon is eliminated primarily through the kidneys (urinary excretion).

Interactions (medication, nutrient, dietary)

Silicon can impede the uptake of aluminium (beneficial) and is involved in the metabolism of calcium and other bone minerals such as phosphorus and magnesium.

Function

Silicon is involved in a number of biochemical reactions leading to the synthesis of glycoproteins and polysaccharides in the extracellular matrix of connective tissue. Silicon is an important cross-linking agent in connective tissue and, in conjunction with calcium, is an important element for maintaining skeletal integrity. Silicon is involved in the biochemistry of subcellular enzyme structures, and is the main component of osteoblasts.

Therapeutic applications

None clinically established.

Deficiency signs

Poor hair, nail and skin quality; skeletal abnormalities and poorly formed joints; reduced contents of cartilage and collagen, and disruption of mineral balance in the femur and vertebrae.[342]

Biochemical testing

Not applicable.

Supplemental forms

There are several water-soluble forms of silica which are referred to collectively as silicic acid. Orthosilicic acid is the form predominantly absorbed by humans.[342] The form present in food is silicon dioxide and is used in over-the-counter supplements.

Toxicity

To date no clear evidence of adverse health risks of dietary silicon has been found. A 'no observed adverse effects level' (NOAEL) of 50000 ppm (mg/L) for dietary silica has been suggested.[342] The safe upper limit is 700 mg/day. Toxicity is associated with environmental inhaled particles.[343]

Dosage requirements

There are no established dosage requirements, although a daily intake of 10–25 mg/day on the basis of the 24-hour urinary excretion of silicon has been suggested.[344]

Food sources

Silicon is abundant in plant foods, vegetables and wholegrains. Lettuce, cucumber, avocado, strawberries, onions, dandelion and other dark leafy greens are good sources. Beer is also a good source of silicon that is highly bioavailable.[187] Large amounts of silicon are also present in the hulls of wheat bran, barley, oats, rice bran and mussels. Plant pectin is a particularly rich source, as are potatoes.[188] Other traditional sources include the herbal medicine *Equisetum arvense* (horsetail). Drinking water (albeit dependent on geography) appears to be the most bioavailable source in the diet as fluid ingestion appears to account for >20% of total dietary silica.[343]

Dietary intake and the need for supplementation

The best way to obtain adequate silicon is through the diet. Silicon is more bioavailable in beverages than in solid foods. This is because beverages contain orthosilicic acid, which is absorbed more efficiently than silicon dioxide. Diets that are predominantly high in animal fat and protein but low in plant foods, particularly wholegrain cereals, are generally low in silicon. While it is not considered an essential trace element, silicon has long been recognised in naturopathic clinical medicine as a key nutritive factor in the structural system, and silicon is often included in calcium supplements as an important accessory nutrient for the maintenance of bone mineral density and healthy connective tissue. Silicon levels decrease with age, and close attention should be given to silicon in the diet or as supplement when the clinical picture includes presenting conditions such as poor hair, nail and skin quality. Psoriasis and acne may also respond favourably to improvements in silicon status, either through supplementation or increased dietary intake.

ESSENTIAL FATTY ACIDS

Forms of nutrient

The essential fatty acids are divided into two classes: n-6 and n-3, also known as ω-3 and ω-6. They are called essential fatty acids as they cannot be manufactured by the body (de novo synthesis) and must be derived from the diet. The n-6 fatty acids occur in the form of linoleic acid (LA), and the n-3 fatty acids as α-linolenic acid (ALA). Both forms are metabolised to longer chain fatty acids. ALA is metabolised to arachidonic acid (AA), a fatty acid which is essential for the synthesis of hormones, leucotrienes, prostaglandins and thromboxanes. ALA is converted to eicosapentaenoic acid (EPA) and docosahexaenoic acid (DHA). The majority of fatty acids are found in the esterified form in lipoproteins, although some free fatty acids are present in plasma and bound to albumin.

Distribution and storage

After they have been hydrolysed and absorbed, fatty acids are distributed through the body, via the lymph (on chylomicrons) and bloodstream, to the liver, the principal site of fat metabolism. Fatty acids are typically deposited in cell membranes, particularly those of platelets, erythrocytes, neutrophils, monocytes and liver cells. Fatty acids are also fundamental building blocks for the synthesis of the majority of lipids, including phospholipids, sphingolipids and cholesterol esters.[190]

Absorption

After ingestion fatty acids are dispersed into small particles by the action of the bile, and then hydrolysed by digestive enzymes and absorbed through the intestinal mucosa. A variety of enzymes are involved in this process, depending on the chain length of the fatty acid. Before entry into the mitochondria, medium- and long-chain fatty acids must first be esterified to coenzyme A.[345]

Excretion

Excretion is by the hepatobiliary route via the bile and faeces.

Interactions (medication, nutrient, dietary)

Some authors suggest that high doses of fish oils should be used with caution in people taking anticoagulant medication, although there is research refuting this.[346] It is advisable that people with bleeding disorders use caution when taking fish oil supplements. Despite this (justified) caution, there is research to suggest that EPA/DHA supplementation is effective as an anti-coagulant in patients with stable coronary artery disease on low-dose aspirin.[347] There are potentially beneficial interactions (added effect) between non-steroidal anti-inflammatory drugs (NSAIDs) and statins (pravastatin). As fish oils (EPA content) can lower blood pressure, there is the possibility of an added effect in people currently using antihypertensive medication.[230] Gamma linolenic acid (GLA) supplements should be used in cancer patients only after careful evaluation of fatty acid status, as high levels of n-6 fatty acids can enhance the formation and growth of tumours.[346] Men with prostate cancer and those at increased prostate cancer risk should avoid flax seed and ALA supplements.[348]

Deficiencies of biotin, vitamin E, protein, zinc, vitamin B_{12} and B_6 all interfere with the action of Δ^6-desaturase.[349] There is also evidence that copper deficiency may disturb the balance of fatty acids.[350]

Function

The biological functions of the essential fatty acids include: the stimulation of growth and reproduction; the health and growth of skin and hair; wound healing; reducing plasma cholesterol levels; reducing platelet aggregation; as a precursor of all main eicosanoids (e.g. prostaglandins, leucotrienes, lipoxins); regulation of gene function; neural development; balancing ω-6-eicosanoid production; cardiac function; involvement in ion transport; apoptosis; and regulation of gene function. They are an essential component of the phospholipids that serve as structural units of cell membranes, mitochondria and nuclei, and play a major and vital role in the properties of most membranes, improving cell membrane fluidity.[351] Polyunsaturated fatty acids are made up of long-chain hydrocarbons containing two or more double bonds and a carboxyl group.

Therapeutic applications

Studies have indicated that the anti-inflammatory dose of fish oil is 2.7 g or more daily, and that higher doses are also safe and effective.[352] In moderate hypertension fish oils 4 g/day have been recommended. To reduce elevated triglyceride levels 1–4.6 g/day have been recommended. A meta-analyse found supplementation with between 1 g and 4.5 g/day of ω-3 fatty acids reduces the risk of cardiovascular disease by improving endothelial function.[353] Doses of 1–7 g/day with an average dose of 3.5 g/day (or 50 mg/kg of bodyweight) of n-3 PUFAs have been used successfully in RA patients to reduce swollen joints, morning stiffness, pain and the need for NSAIDs.[354] Doses of 3.8 g/day and 3.6 g/day of DHA and EPA from fish oils have been used to increase immunity.[355] For depression, EPA 1 g twice a day has been used. In schizophrenia 1–4 g of EPA has been used, and in borderline personality disorder EPA 1 g/day as ethyleicosapentaenoic acid has been used.[356] Improved brain function, executive function, grey matter volume and vascular markers have been found in older adults taking 2200 mg/day of ω-3 fatty acids.[357]

Deficiency signs

Scaly dermatitis, alopecia, eczema, cracked heels, dry hair, dandruff, brittle nails, thrombocytopenia, growth retardation. In children, learning disorders, attention deficits. Deficiency occurs in malabsorptive disorders (e.g. cystic fibrosis), in chronic liver disease and in anorexia nervosa and other conditions of severe malnutrition.[358]

Biochemical testing

Red blood cell and fasting plasma. The omega-3 index — blood cell EPA/DHA levels that are expressed as a percentage of the total fatty acids — is used as a risk marker and risk factor for cardiovascular disease and major depressive disorder.[359] For CV risk: <4 = high risk, 4–8 = intermediate risk, >8 = low risk.[360,361] Routine use of this test is currently limited clinically as population clinical reference values have not been established.[362]

Supplemental forms

Essential fatty acid supplements are commonly derived from either seed oils or marine oils. Various seed oils (across the spectrum from almond to walnut) provide a rich source of α-linolenic and α-linoleic fatty acids. Hemp and flax contain the highest ratio of linoleic acid for supplementation (3 : 1), and proponents of hemp seed oil believe this source to have the optimum ratio. Supplements that provide ω-3 fatty acids, EPA and DHA are best sourced from oils derived from deep-sea, cold-water fish. Salmon, both wild and farmed, provides the highest DHA content, followed by herring and anchovy.

Supplemental fish oils are available primarily as soft gel capsules and as liquids. The liquids vary in palatability, although they can be disguised in drinks and juices when used to supplement the diets of children, who generally have a low tolerance to fish products. Oils derived from fish livers (halibut and cod) are not a reliable source of essential fatty acids and are generally used for their vitamin A and D content.

Toxicity

Nutrient supplements containing nutritive oils from animal and plant-based sources have an excellent safety profile at the recommended doses.

Dosage requirements

TABLE 7.8 Australian adequate intakes of essential fatty acids

	Linoleic acid	α-linolenic acid	Total n-3 fatty acids
Men	13 g/day	1.3 g/day	160 mg/day
Women	8 g/day	0.8 g/day	90 mg/day
Pregnancy	10 g/day	1 g/day	115 mg/day
Lactation	12 g/day	1.2 g/day	145 mg/day

WHO recommends 0.250–2 g/day of EPA/DHA.
Source: Fats: Total fat & fatty acids.|Nutrient Reference Values [Internet]. Nrv.gov.au. 2014 [cited 5 September 2016]. Available from: https://www.nrv.gov.au/nutrients/fats-total-fat-fatty-acids © Commonwealth of Australia (Department of Health) 2015-2017. CC BY 4.0

Food sources

ALA is found primarily in vegetable oils. Flax, canola and soya are just a few of the seed oils rich in this fatty acid. Edible nuts such as walnuts also contain significant amounts, and ALA is also found in meat and dairy products, and to a lesser extent in leafy green vegetables.[363]

The most concentrated sources of EPA and DHA are deep-sea, cold-water fish such as salmon, mackerel, halibut and herring. The EPA/DHA ratio varies depending on the species of fish (e.g. one serve of cod provides 0.2–0.3 g of n-3 fatty acids whereas a serve of salmon or mackerel provides 1.5–3 g of n-3 fatty acids).[364] Egg yolk can also be a rich source of DHA, as long as the chicken's diet contains or is enriched with linolenic acid (from flax meal, fish meal or insects).

Dietary intake and the need for supplementation

Compared with the diets of a generation ago, modern diets contain significantly fewer ω-3 fatty acids.[365] Modern farming methods have the effect of increasing the amount of ω-6 and oleic acid in vegetables, fruits, fish, eggs, grains and legumes, while decreasing the amount of valuable ω-3.[366] Commercial animal feeds are also rich in n-6 fatty acids, which has resulted in the production of meat that is rich in n-6 yet poor in n-3 fatty acids.[367] To ensure an adequate balance of fatty acids in the diet, it is best if sources of ω-3 fatty acids are incorporated in meals on a daily basis. It has been suggested that a 4 : 1 ratio of ω-6/ω-3 fatty acids may be optimal[365] — current intakes are within the range of 10 : 1–20 : 1.[368] Vegans and vegetarians who choose to avoid fish and fish products are also likely to be deficient in ω-3 fatty acids, especially DHA. While vegetable sources of ALA (e.g. flax seed oil) can be converted to EPA and DHA, this process is heavily reliant on enzymes such as δ^6-desaturase. The activity of this enzyme is impaired when the diet is high in ω-6 fatty acids. δ^6-desaturase activity decreases with age, and the ability to convert ALA to EPA and DHA is also limited in premature infants, hypertensive individuals and some diabetics.[367] Increasing the intake of ω-3 fatty acids has been shown to reduce asthma symptoms and severity. Boys with attention deficit hyperactivity disorder have been shown to have a deficiency of essential fatty acids. Gender differences appear to exist in relation to conversion of ALA to DHA which may be related to oestrogen and which results in a better conversion efficiency in young women compared to men.[369]

Fatty acid status and the individual requirements for supplementation vary enormously, and this is largely dependent on intake, assimilation, absorption and degradation.[370] Both deficiencies and excesses of fatty acids do occur, and both can be problematic, as an excess of one can create a deficiency of another.

In ω-6 deficiencies the routine supplementation with ω-3 fatty acids can lead to competition for desaturase enzymes and the worsening of clinical conditions. In such cases it has been suggested that supplementation with a good source of ω-6, such as evening primrose oil, will be effective.[370]

While an excess of ω-3 fatty acids is more probable than an excess of ω-6, excesses of ω-3 do occur and are clinically relevant. An intake of DHA that is too high can disturb membrane permeability and the activity of some enzymes, and without adequate antioxidants can cause the accumulation of lipid peroxides. (It is always a good idea to supplement vitamin E when EPA and DHA are used.)

A good way to reduce the amount of n-6 fatty acids in the diet is to substitute with monounsaturated oils (e.g. olive oil, avocado). Olive oil also helps to increase the incorporation of n-3 fatty acids into tissues.[367] It is important to note that the body uses essential fatty acids most efficiently when the diet contains an adequate ratio of saturated fat.[366] ALA is, despite its bad reputation, an essential fat and should be a natural part of the diet, either from animal sources or from good-quality plant-based sources such as organic coconut oil.

In specific clinical conditions where high doses of fish oils are required to achieve an anti-inflammatory effect (e.g. in rheumatoid arthritis), supplementation would be preferable to simply increasing the amount of fish in the diet, which would be impractical for many people and probably would not produce a significant clinical effect. Supplementation with fish oils is recommended during the third trimester of pregnancy. An adequate dietary intake of n-3 fatty acids, particularly DHA, is necessary for the growth of the brain of the fetus at this time. Deficiencies can result in visual and cognitive impairment and disturbances in mental function in infants.[371]

This also has implications in later life, for improved cognitive function in adults, and meeting fatty acid requirements in early life may prevent the development of cerebrovascular disease and dementia.[372] Dietary precursors such as LA and ALA are not a reliable way to increase DHA during pregnancy, and it is necessary to supplement the mother's diet with preformed long-chain polyunsaturated fatty acids, as found in deep-sea fish and the supplements derived from them. Sacrifice of maternal DHA to the developing fetal nervous system has been identified as a factor in postpartum depression.

FLAX SEED AS A SOURCE OF EPA AND DHA

Ingested ALA (from flax seed oil, etc.) is converted to EPA or DHA. However, the conversion is not very efficient, and would not be sufficient to provide these nutrients during times of increased requirement. EPA and DHA from fish oils are more rapidly incorporated into plasma and membrane lipids, and produce more rapid effects than ALA from plant-based sources. Fish oil supplements are far superior in the provision of EPA — DHA particularly — during this important developmental period.

THE MERCURY QUESTION

Fish oil supplements made in a facility that complies with the stringent requirements of Good Manufacturing Practice (GMP) will have very low levels of mercury and other contaminants such as lead. In Australia, for example, manufacturers must subject their oils to tests to show that they contain no more than NMT 1 ppm of mercury and NMT 10 ppm of lead. These are acceptable levels, which conform to international requirements, such as those in the *British Pharmacopeia* (BP) and *United States Pharmacopeia* (USP). Both are well regarded as official authorities for setting public standards for prescription and over-the-counter medicines and other healthcare products.

THE FISHY AFTERTASTE

Some people state that fish oil supplements 'repeat' on them, and eructation and an unpleasant aftertaste of fish can occur in susceptible people. The best way to avoid this is to take the supplement just before a full meal. This allows the oil to be incorporated in the food contents of the stomach and carried to the small intestine.[352] The oil is also more likely to be partially emulsified by the action of bile, particularly if there are other fats present in the meal. These problems are less likely to occur when the fish oil supplement is taken in capsule form rather than as a liquid, although it has been noted that some patients with persistent oesophageal reflux may not be able to take fish oil at all.[352]

VEGETABLE OILS: A NATUROPATHIC PERSPECTIVE

Food products such as margarine made from vegetable oils are often touted as good sources of essential fatty acids, yet there is increasing concern about these products. The vegetable oils used to manufacture them are subjected to hydrogenation, which essentially saturates the fatty acid chains, so that they remain solid at room temperature. This is convenient from a storage and shelf-life perspective, but not from a nutritional perspective, as these industrial processes lead to the generation of *trans* fats, which are hazardous to human health.

There are numerous papers in the medical literature which show that the *trans* fats generated by hydrogenation of vegetable oils are harmful.[373–377] *Trans* fats calcify cells and cause inflammation of the arteries, which are known risk factors in heart disease. In the journal *Atherosclerosis* it was concluded that '*Trans* fat should be banned from the food supply'.[378]

Modern vegetable oils also go through caustic refining, bleaching and degumming processes during which they are subjected to high temperatures or chemicals of questionable safety. They are also deodorised. Canola oil, which contains high levels of ω-3 fatty acids, becomes rancid and foul smelling when subjected to oxygen and high temperatures,[378] and the deodorisation process removes a large portion of the ω-3 fatty acids by turning them into *trans* fatty acids. In the naturopathic context these products are anything but 'natural' (in any sense of the word). In fact, in the case of hydrogenated margarines, they are really 'imitation foods' and are best avoided.

REFERENCES

[1] Ames BN, Elson-Schwab I, Silver EA. High-dose vitamin therapy stimulates variant enzymes with decreased coenzyme binding affinity (increased K(m)): relevance to genetic disease and polymorphisms. Am J Clin Nutr 2002;75(4):616–58.

[2] Eastmond DA, Macgregor JT, Slesinski RS. Trivalent chromium: assessing the genotoxic risk of an essential trace element and widely used human and animal nutritional supplement. Crit Rev Toxicol 2008;38(3):173–90.
[3] Nutrient Reference Values for Australia and New Zealand including Recommended Dietary Intakes. Commonwealth Department of Health and Ageing, Australia Ministry of Health, New Zealand National Health and Medical Research Council; 2004. Available from: www.nrv.gov.au.
[4] Dwyer T. Dietary requirements of adults. Marrickville, NSW: Elsevier; 2003.
[5] Dainty JR, Bullock NR, Hart DJ, et al. Quantification of the bioavailability of riboflavin from foods by use of stable-isotope labels and kinetic modeling. Am J Clin Nutr 2007;85(6): 1557–64.
[6] Shils ME, Shike M, Ross AC, et al. Modern nutrition in health and disease. 10th ed. Baltimore, MD: Lippincott Williams & Wilkins; 2005. p. 2146.
[7] World Health Organization. Vitamin and mineral requirements in human nutrition: report of a joint FAO/WHO expert consultation, Bangkok, Thailand, 21–30 September 1998. Available from: http://apps.who.int/iris/bitstream/handle/10665/42716/9241546123.pdf?sequence=1&isAllowed=y.
[8] Cleland LG, James MJ. The role of fats in the lifecycle stages. Adulthood — prevention: rheumatoid arthritis. Med J Aust 2002;176(Suppl.):S119–20.
[9] Thiamin (vitamin B_1). Hendler S, Rorvik D, editors. In: PDR for nutritional supplements. 2nd ed. Montavale: Physicians' Desk Reference Inc.; 2009. p. 609–15.
[10] Fraser D, Diep L, Hovden I, et al. The effects of long-term oral benfotiamine supplementation on peripheral nerve function and inflammatory markers in patients with type 1 diabetes: a 24-month, double-blind, randomized, placebo-controlled trial. Diabetes Care 2012;35(5):1095–7.
[11] Thiamin. Nutrient Reference Values for Australia and New Zealand including Recommended Dietary Intakes. Commonwealth Department of Health and Ageing, Australia Ministry of Health, New Zealand National Health and Medical Research Council; 2004 Available from: www.nrv.gov.au/nutrients/thiamin.
[12] Sriram K, Manzanares W, Joseph K. Thiamine in nutrition therapy. Nutr Clin Pract 2012;27(1):41–50.
[13] DiNicolantonio J, Niazi A, Lavie C, et al. Thiamine supplementation for the treatment of heart failure: a review of the literature. Congest Heart Fail 2013;19(4):214–22.
[14] Rahmani N, Muller HG. The fate of thiamin and riboflavin during the preparation of couscous. Food Chem 1996;55:23–7.
[15] Wooley J. Characteristics of thiamin and its relevance to the management of heart failure. Nutr Clin Pract 2008;23(5):487–93.
[16] Bates CJ, Benjamin C. Niacin. Encyclopedia of human nutrition. Oxford: Elsevier; 1998. p. 253–9.
[17] Powers H. Current knowledge concerning optimum nutritional status of riboflavin, niacin and pyridoxine. Proc Nutr Soc 1999;58(02):435–40.
[18] Pompella A, Visvikis A, Paolicchi A, et al. The changing faces of glutathione, a cellular protagonist. Biochem Pharmacol 2003;66(8):1499–503.
[19] Riboflavin. Nutrient Reference Values for Australia and New Zealand including Recommended Dietary Intakes. Commonwealth Department of Health and Ageing, Australia Ministry of Health, New Zealand National Health and Medical Research Council; 2004 Available from: www.nrv.gov.au/nutrients/riboflavin
[20] Graham J. Erythrocyte riboflavin for the detection of riboflavin deficiency in pregnant Nepali women. Clin Chem 2005;51(11):2162–5.
[21] Boehnke C, Reuter U, Flach U, et al. High-dose riboflavin treatment is efficacious in migraine prophylaxis: an open study in a tertiary care centre. Eur J Neurol 2004;11(7):475–7.
[22] Cumming RG, Mitchell P, Smith W. Diet and cataract: the Blue Mountains Eye Study. Ophthalmology 2000;107:450–6.
[23] Ashoori M, Saedisomeolia A. Riboflavin (vitamin B_2) and oxidative stress: a review. Br J Nutr 2014;111(11):1985–91.
[24] Sperduto RD, Hu TS, Milton RC, et al. The Linxian cataract studies. Two nutrition intervention trials. Arch Ophthalmol 1993;111:1246–53.
[25] Siassi F, Ghadirian P. Riboflavin deficiency and esophageal cancer: a case control-household study in the Caspian Littoral of Iran. Cancer Detect Prev 2005;29(5):464–9.
[26] Scrimshaw NS, SanGiovanni JP. Synergism of nutrition, infection, and immunity: an overview. Am J Clin Nutr 1997;66:464S–77S.
[27] Magnúsdóttir S, Ravcheev D, de Crécy-Lagard V, et al. Systematic genome assessment of B-vitamin biosynthesis suggests co-operation among gut microbes. Front Genet 2015;6:148.
[28] Rennie G, Chen A, Dhillon H, et al. Nicotinamide and neurocognitive function. Nutr Neurosci 2015;18(5):193–200.
[29] Bates CJ, Benjamin C. Niacin. Encyclopedia of human nutrition. Oxford: Elsevier; 1998. p. 253–9.
[30] Bilgili S, Karadag A, Calka O, et al. Isoniazid-induced pellagra. Cutan Ocul Toxicol 2011;30(4):317–19.
[31] Jusko WJ, Levy G. Effect of probenecid on riboflavin absorption and excretion in man. J Pharm Sci 1967;56:1145–9.
[32] World Health Organization (WHO). United Nations High Commission for Refugees. Pellagra and its prevention and control in major emergencies. 2000. Available at http://www.who.int/nutrition/publications/emergencies/WHO_NHD_00.10/en/.
[33] Brown B, Zhao-Q X, Chait A, et al. Simvastatin and niacin, antioxidant vitamins, or the combination for the prevention of coronary disease. N Engl J Med 2001;345(22):1583–92.
[34] Messamore E. Niacin subsensitivity is associated with functional impairment in schizophrenia. Schizophr Res 2012;137(1–3): 180–4.
[35] Hoffer A. Negative and positive side-effects of vitamin B_3. J Orthomol Med 2003;18:146–60.
[36] Knip M, Douek IF, Moore WP, et al. Safety of high-dose nicotinamide: a review. Diabetologia 2000;43:1337–45.
[37] Hendler S, Rorvik D, editors. PDR for nutritional supplements. Montvale, NJ: Medical Economics Co.; 2001.
[38] Niacin. Nutrient Reference Values for Australia and New Zealand including Recommended Dietary Intakes. Commonwealth Department of Health and Ageing, Australia Ministry of Health, New Zealand National Health and Medical Research Council; 2004. Available from: www.nrv.gov.au/nutrients/niacin.
[39] Fukuwatari T, Ohta M, Kimtjra N, et al. Conversion ratio of tryptophan to niacin in Japanese women fed a purified diet conforming to the Japanese Dietary Reference Intakes. J Nutr Sci Vitaminol (Tokyo) 2004;50:385–91.
[40] Jagielska G, Tomaszewicz-Libudzic C, Brzozowska A. Pellagra: a rare complication of anorexia nervosa. Eur Child Adolesc Psychiatry 2007;16(7):417–20.
[41] Expert Group on Vitamins and Minerals. Safe upper levels for vitamins and minerals. 2003. Available from: www.food.gov.uk/multimedia/pdfs/vitmin2003.pdf.
[42] Leonardi R, Zhang Y-M, Rock CO, et al. Coenzyme A: back in action. Prog Lipid Res 2005;44:125–53.
[43] Lanska D. The discovery of niacin, biotin, and pantothenic acid. Ann Nutr Metab 2012;61(3):246–53.
[44] Kelly G. Pantothenic acid. Altern Med Rev 2011;16(3):263–74.
[45] Hendler S, Rorvik D. PDR for nutritional supplements. 2nd ed. Montvale: Thomson Reuters; 2008.
[46] Flodin N. Pharmacology of micronutrients. New York: Alan R. Liss, Inc; 1988.
[47] Pantothenic acid. Nutrient Reference Values for Australia and New Zealand including Recommended Dietary Intakes. Commonwealth Department of Health and Ageing, Australia Ministry of Health, New Zealand National Health and Medical Research Council; 2004 Available from: www.nrv.gov.au/nutrients/pantothenic-acid.
[48] Vaxman F, Chalkiadakis G, Olender S, et al. Improvement in the healing of colonic anastomoses by vitamin B5 and C supplements. Experimental study in the rabbit. Ann Chir 1990;44:512–20.
[49] Ahmad I, Mirza T, Qadeer K, et al. Vitamin B6: deficiency diseases and methods of analysis. Pak J Pharm Sci 2013;26(5):1057–69.
[50] Natural Medicines Comprehensive Database. Vitamin B6. 2011.
[51] Apeland T, Frøyland E, Kristensen O, et al. Drug-induced perturbation of the aminothiol redox-status in patients with epilepsy: Improvement by B-vitamins. Epil Res 2008;82(1):1–6.
[52] Lippi G, Plebani M. Hyperhomocysteinemia in health and disease: where we are now, and where do we go from here? Clin Chem Lab Med 2012;50(12):2075–80.

[53] Morris M, Picciano M, Jacques P, et al. Plasma pyridoxal 5′-phosphate in the US population: the National Health and Nutrition Examination Survey, 2003–2004. Am J Clin Nutr 2008;87(5):1446–54.
[54] Whelan A, Jurgens T, Naylor H. Herbs, vitamins and minerals in the treatment of premenstrual syndrome: a systematic review. Can J Clin Pharmacol 2009;16(3):e407–29.
[55] Magee L, Mazzotta P, Koren G. Evidence-based view of safety and effectiveness of pharmacologic therapy for nausea and vomiting of pregnancy (NVP). Am J Obstet Gynecol 2002;186(5): S256–61.
[56] Gerritsen AA, de Krom MC, Struijs MA, et al. Conservative treatment options for carpal tunnel syndrome: a systematic review of randomised controlled trials. J Neurol 2002;249:272–80.
[57] Varga E. Homocysteine and MTHFR mutations: relation to thrombosis and coronary artery disease. Circulation 2005;111(19):e289–93.
[58] Institute of Medicine. Food and Nutrition Board. Dietary Reference Intakes: thiamin, riboflavin, niacin, vitamin B6, folate, vitamin B12, pantothenic acid, biotin, and choline. Washington DC: National Academy Press; 1998.
[59] Vitamin B6. Nutrient Reference Values for Australia and New Zealand including Recommended Dietary Intakes. Commonwealth Department of Health and Ageing, Australia Ministry of Health, New Zealand National Health and Medical Research Council; 2004 Available fromwww.nrv.gov.au/nutrients/vitamin-b6.
[60] Salam RA, Zuberi NF, Bhutta ZA. Pyridoxine (vitamin B6) supplementation during pregnancy or labour for maternal and neonatal outcomes (Review). Cochrane Database Syst Rev 2015;(6):CD000179.
[61] Kronenburg AF, Fugh-Berman A. Complementary and alternative medicine (CAM) in reproductive-age women: a review of randomised controlled trials. Reprod Toxicol 2003;17:137–52.
[62] Clayton P. B6-responsive disorders: a model of vitamin dependency. J Inherit Metab Dis 2006;29(2–3):317–26.
[63] Matok I, Clark S, Caritis S, et al. Studying the antiemetic effect of vitamin B6 for morning sickness: pyridoxine and pyridoxal are prodrugs. J Clin Pharmacol 2014;54(12):1429–33.
[64] Vech RL, Lumeng L, Li TK. Vitamin B_6 metabolism in chronic alcohol abuse. The effect of ethanol oxidation on hepatic pyridoxal 5′-phosphate metabolism. J Clin Invest 1975;55:1026–32.
[65] McPartlin J, Benjamin C. Folic acid. Encyclopedia of human nutrition. Oxford: Elsevier; 2005. p. 257–64.
[66] Gregory S, Kelly ND. Folates: supplemental forms and therapeutic applications. Altern Med Rev 1998;3:208–20.
[67] Butterworth CE Jr, Tamura T. Folic acid safety and toxicity: a brief review. Am J Clin Nutr 1989;50:353–8.
[68] Chan Y-M, Bailey R, O'Connor D. Folate. Adv Nutr 2013;4(1): 123–5.
[69] Talaulikar V, Arulkumaran S. Folic acid in obstetric practice: a review. Obstet Gynecol Surv 2011;66(4):240–7.
[70] Smith A, Smith S, de Jager C, et al. Homocysteine-lowering by B vitamins slows the rate of accelerated brain atrophy in mild cognitive impairment: a randomized controlled trial. PLoS ONE 2010;5(9):e12244.
[71] Liu Y, Tian T, Zhang H, et al. The effect of homocysteine-lowering therapy with folic acid on flow-mediated vasodilation in patients with coronary artery disease: a meta-analysis of randomized controlled trials. Atherosclerosis 2014;235(1):31–5.
[72] Whittle S. Folate supplementation and methotrexate treatment in rheumatoid arthritis: a review. Rheumatology 2003;43(3):267–71.
[73] Bailey LB, editor. Folate in health and disease. 2nd ed. Baca Raton: CRC Press; 2010.
[74] Clarke R. Lowering blood homocysteine with folic acid-based supplements: meta-analysis of randomised trials. Indian Heart J 2000;52:S59–64.
[75] Folate. Nutrient Reference Values for Australia and New Zealand including Recommended Dietary Intakes. Commonwealth Department of Health and Ageing, Australia Ministry of Health, New Zealand National Health and Medical Research Council; 2004 Available from: www.nrv.gov.au/nutrients/folate.
[76] Lohner S, Fekete K, Berti C, et al. Effect of folate supplementation on folate status and health outcomes in infants, children and adolescents: a systematic review. Int J Food Sci Nutr 2012;63(8):1014–20.
[77] Food Standards Australia New Zealand. Folic acid fortification. 2016. Available from: www.foodstandards.gov.au/consumer/nutrition/folicmandatory/Pages/default.aspx.
[78] Laird E, McNulty H, Ward M, et al. Low vitamin B12 and elevated folate status in older adults: a risk factor for cognitive impairment? Proc Nutr Soc 2015;74:OCE4.
[79] Kim Y. Folic acid supplementation and cancer risk: point. Cancer Epidemiol Biomarkers Prev 2008;17(9):2220–5.
[80] McCully KS. Homocysteine, vitamin deficiency and prevention of arteriosclerosis. Integrative Med 1998;1:3–9.
[81] Carmel R. Current concepts in cobalamin deficiency. Annu Rev Med 2000;51:357–75.
[82] Langan R. Zawistoski K. Update on vitamin B12 deficiency. Am Fam Physician 2015;83(12):1425–30.
[83] de Jager J, Kooy A, Lehert P, et al. Long-term treatment with metformin in patients with type 2 diabetes and risk of vitamin B-12 deficiency: randomised placebo controlled trial. Br Med J 2010;340:c2181.
[84] Evatt M, Mersereau P, Bobo J, et al. Why vitamin B12 deficiency should be on your radar screen. Centers for Disease Control and Prevention. 2010.
[85] Stabler S. Vitamin B12 deficiency. N Engl J Med 2013;368(2):149–60.
[86] Allen L. How common is vitamin B-12 deficiency? Am J Clin Nutr 2009;89(2):693S–6S.
[87] Vitamin B12. Nutrient Reference Values for Australia and New Zealand including Recommended Dietary Intakes. Commonwealth Department of Health and Ageing, Australia Ministry of Health, New Zealand National Health and Medical Research Council; 2004. Available from: www.nrv.gov.au/nutrients/vitamin-b12.
[88] Zeisel SH. Is there a metabolic basis for dietary supplementation? Am J Clin Nutr 2000;507S–11S.
[89] Takenaka S, Sugiyama S, Ebara S, et al. Feeding dried purple laver (nori) to vitamin B_{12}-deficient rats significantly improves vitamin B_{12} status. Br J Nutr 2001;85:699–703.
[90] Devalia V, Hamilton M, Molloy A. Guidelines for the diagnosis and treatment of cobalamin and folate disorders. Br J Haematol 2014;166(4):496–513.
[91] Geohas J, Daly A, Juturu V, et al. Chromium picolinate and biotin combination reduces atherogenic index of plasma in patients with type 2 diabetes mellitus: a placebo-controlled, double-blinded, randomized clinical trial. Am J Med Sci 2007;333(3):145–53.
[92] Sedel F, Papeix C, Bellanger A, et al. High doses of biotin in chronic progressive multiple sclerosis: a pilot study. Mult Scler Relat Disord 2015;4(2):159–69.
[93] Biotin. Nutrient Reference Values for Australia and New Zealand including Recommended Dietary Intakes. Commonwealth Department of Health and Ageing, Australia Ministry of Health, New Zealand National Health and Medical Research Council; 2004. Available from: www.nrv.gov.au/nutrients/biotin.
[94] European Food Safety Authority. Scientific opinion on dietary reference values for biotin. 2016. Available from: www.efsa.europa.eu/en/efsajournal/pub/3580.
[95] Tourbah A, Edan G, Clanet M, et al. Effect of MD1003 (high doses of biotin) in progressive multiple sclerosis: results of a pivotal phase II randomised double-blind placebo-controlled study. Paper presented at: American Association of Neurological Sciences (AANS) Annual Scientific Meeting 2015; Washington DC. Available from www.neurology.org/content/84/14_Supplement/PL2.002.
[96] Yuasa M, Matsui T, Ando S, et al. Consumption of a low-carbohydrate and high-fat diet (the ketogenic diet) exaggerates biotin deficiency in mice. Nutrition 2013;29(10):1266–70.
[97] Bañuls C, Rovira-Llopis S, Falcón R, et al. Chronic consumption of an inositol-enriched carob extract improves postprandial glycaemia and insulin sensitivity in healthy subjects: a randomized controlled trial. Clin Nutr 2016;35(3):600–7.
[98] Palatnik A, Frolov K, Fux M, et al. Double-blind, controlled, crossover trial of inositol versus fluvoxamine for the treatment of panic disorder. J Clin Psychopharmacol 2001;21(3):335–9.
[99] Bevilacqua A, Bizzarri M. Physiological role and clinical utility of inositols in polycystic ovary syndrome. Best Pract Res Clin Obstet Gynaecol 2016;37:129–39.
[100] Ferrari F, Facchinetti F, Ontiveros A, et al. The effect of combined inositol supplementation on maternal metabolic profile in

pregnancies complicated by metabolic syndrome and obesity. Am J Obstet Gynecol 2016;215(4):503, e1–8.
[101] Hardwick R, Clarke J, Lake A, et al. Increased susceptibility to methotrexate-induced toxicity in nonalcoholic steatohepatitis. Toxicol Sci 2014;142(1):45–55.
[102] Yu D, Shu X, Xiang Y, et al. Higher dietary choline intake is associated with lower risk of nonalcoholic fatty liver in normal-weight Chinese women. J Nutr 2014;144(12):2034–40.
[103] Zeisel S. Choline. In: Ross A, Caballero B, Cousins R, et al, editors. Modern nutrition in health and disease. 11th ed. Lippincott Williams & Wilkins; 2014. p. 416–26.
[104] Choline. Nutrient Reference Values for Australia and New Zealand including Recommended Dietary Intakes. Commonwealth Department of Health and Ageing, Australia Ministry of Health, New Zealand National Health and Medical Research Council; 2004 Available from: www.nrv.gov.au/nutrients/choline.
[105] Busby M, Fischer L, Da Costa K, et al. Choline- and betaine-defined diets for use in clinical research and for the management of trimethylaminuria. J Am Diet Assoc 2004;104(12):1836–45.
[106] Yan J, Wang W, Gregory J, et al. MTHFR C677T genotype influences the isotopic enrichment of one-carbon metabolites in folate-compromised men consuming d9-choline. Am J Clin Nutr 2010;93(2):348–55.
[107] Pigdon J. Vitamin C fact sheet. Corvallis, OR: Linus Pauling Institute, Oregon State University.
[108] Carr A, Bozonet S, Pullar J, et al. Human skeletal muscle ascorbate is highly responsive to changes in vitamin C intake and plasma concentrations. Am J Clin Nutr 2013;97(4):800–7.
[109] Jacob R, Sotoudeh G. Vitamin C function and status in chronic disease. Nutr Clin Care 2002;5(2):66–74.
[110] Levine M, Wang Y, Padayatty S, et al. A new recommended dietary allowance of vitamin C for healthy young women. Proc Natl Acad Sci U S A 2001;98(17):9842–6.
[111] Bender DA, Benjamin C. Ascorbic acid. Physiology, dietary sources and requirements. Encyclopedia of Human Nutrition. Oxford: Elsevier; 2005. p. 169–76.
[112] Trinidad T, Kurilich A, Mallillin A, et al. Iron absorption from NaFeEDTA-fortified oat beverages with or without added vitamin C. Int J Food Sci Nutr 2013;65(1):124–8.
[113] Ashor A, Siervo M, van der Velde F, et al. Systematic review and meta-analysis of randomised controlled trials testing the effects of vitamin C supplementation on blood lipids. Clin Nutr 2016;35(3):626–37.
[114] Chambial S, Dwivedi S, Shukla K, et al. Vitamin C in disease prevention and cure: an overview. Indian J Clin Biochem 2013;28(4):314–28.
[115] Linus Pauling Institute. Supplemental forms. Oregon State University.; 2016. Available from: http://lpi.oregonstate.edu/mic/vitamins/vitamin-C/supplemental-forms.
[116] Vitamin C. Nutrient Reference Values for Australia and New Zealand including Recommended Dietary Intakes. Commonwealth Department of Health and Ageing, Australia Ministry of Health, New Zealand National Health and Medical Research Council; 2004 Available from: www.nrv.gov.au/nutrients/vitamin-c.
[117] Office of Dietary Supplements. Vitamin C. 2016. Available from: https://ods.od.nih.gov/factsheets/VitaminC-HealthProfessional/.
[118] Frei B, Birlouez-Aragon I, Lykkesfeldt J. Authors' perspective: what is the optimum intake of vitamin C in humans? Crit Rev Food Sci Nutr 2012;52(9):815–29.
[119] USDA National Nutrient Database for Standard Reference. 2016. Available from: www.ars.usda.gov/ba/bhnrc/ndl.
[120] Bender AE, Benjamin C. Fruits and vegetables. Encyclopedia of human nutrition. Oxford: Elsevier; 1998. p. 356–60.
[121] Vitamin A. Nutrient Reference Values for Australia and New Zealand including Recommended Dietary Intakes. Commonwealth Department of Health and Ageing, Australia Ministry of Health, New Zealand National Health and Medical Research Council; 2004. Available from: https://www.nrv.gov.au/nutrients/vitamin-a.
[122] Ross C, Tan L. Vitamin A deficiencies and excess. In: Kliegman R, Stanton B, St. Geme J, editors. Nelson textbook of pediatrics. 20th ed. Philadelphia: Elsevier; 2016. p. 317–21.
[123] Linus Pauling Institute. Zinc. 2017. Oregon State University. Available from: http://lpi.oregonstate.edu/mic/minerals/zinc.
[124] Akhtar S, Ahmed A, Randhawa M, et al. Prevalence of vitamin A deficiency in South Asia: causes, outcomes, and possible remedies (Review). J Health Popul Nutr 2014;31(4):413–23.
[125] Huiming Y, Chaomin W, Meng M. Cochrane review: vitamin A for treating measles in children. Evidence-Based Child Health 2006;1(3):743–66.
[126] McCauley M, van den Broek N, Dou L, et al. Vitamin A supplementation during pregnancy for maternal and newborn outcomes. Cochrane Database Syst Rev 2015;(10):CD008666.
[127] Wang A, Han J, Jiang Y, et al. Association of vitamin A and β-carotene with risk for age-related cataract: a meta-analysis. Nutrition 2014;30(10):1113–21.
[128] Mayo-Wilson E, Imdad A, Herzer K, et al. Vitamin A supplements for preventing mortality, illness, and blindness in children aged under 5: systematic review and meta-analysis. BMJ 2011;343(1):d5094.
[129] Penniston K, Tanumihardjo S. The acute and chronic toxic effects of vitamin A. Am J Clin Nutr 2006;83:191–201.
[130] Jellin J, Gregory P. Pharmacist's letter/prescriber's letter. Natural Medicines Comprehensive Database. 2010. Available from: www.naturaldatabase.com.
[131] Norman AW. Sunlight, season, skin pigmentation, vitamin D, and 25-hydroxyvitamin D: integral components of the vitamin D endocrine system. Am J Clin Nutr 1998;67:1108–10.
[132] Salonen RM, Nyyssonen K, Kaikkonen J, et al. Six-year effect of combined vitamin C and E supplementation on atherosclerotic progression: the Antioxidant Supplementation in Atherosclerosis Prevention (ASAP) Study. Circulation 2003;107:947–53.
[133] Holick M. Vitamin D deficiency. N Engl J Med 2007;357:266–81.
[134] Bischoff-Ferrari H, Dietrich T, Orav E. Higher 25-hydroxyvitamin D concentrations are associated with better lower-extremity function in both active and inactive persons aged > or =60 y. Am J Clin Nutr 2004;80:752–8.
[135] Holick M, Binkley N, Bischoff-Ferrari H, et al. Evaluation, treatment, and prevention of vitamin D deficiency: an Endocrine Society Clinical Practice Guideline. J Clin Endocrinol Metab 2011;96(7):1911–30.
[136] Holick MF. The vitamin D epidemic and its health consequences. J Nutr 2005;135:2739S–48S.
[137] Vieth R. Vitamin D supplementation, 25-hydroxyvitamin D concentrations, and safety. Am J Clin Nutr 1999;69:842–56.
[138] Vitamin D. Nutrient Reference Values for Australia and New Zealand including Recommended Dietary Intakes. Commonwealth Department of Health and Ageing, Australia Ministry of Health, New Zealand National Health and Medical Research Council; 2004. Available from: www.nrv.gov.au/nutrients/vitamin-d.
[139] Wagner CL, Greer FR. Prevention of rickets and vitamin D deficiency in infants, children, adolescents. Pediatrics 2008;122(5):1142–452.
[140] Nowson C, Ebeling P, Mason R, et al. Vitamin D and health in adults in Australia and New Zealand: a position statement. Med J Aust 2012;197(10):553–4.
[141] Armas LAG, Hollis BW, Heaney RP. Vitamin D_2 is much less effective than vitamin D_3 in humans. J Clin Endocrinol Metab 2004;89:5387–91.
[142] Nowson CA, Margerison C. Vitamin D intake and vitamin D status of Australians. Med J Aust 2002;177:149–52.
[143] Podszun M, Frank J. Vitamin E drug interactions: molecular basis and clinical relevance. Nutr Res Rev 2014;27(02):215–31.
[144] Holden R, Ki V, Morton A, et al. Fat-soluble vitamins in advanced CKD/ESKD: a review. Sem Dial 2012;25(3):334–43.
[145] Møller KI, Kongshoj B, Philipsen PA, et al. How Finsen's light cured lupus vulgaris. Photodermatol Photoimmunol Photomed 2005;3:115–17.
[146] Leonard S, Bruno R, Ramakrishnan R, et al. Cigarette smoking increases human vitamin E requirements as estimated by plasma deuterium-labeled CEHC. Ann N Y Acad Sci 2004;1031(1):357–60.
[147] Traber M. Vitamin E inadequacy in humans: causes and consequences. Adv Nutr 2014;5(5):503–14.
[148] Zingg J-M. Molecular and cellular activities of vitamin E analogues. Mini Rev Med Chem 2007;7:545–60.
[149] Vitamin E. Nutrient Reference Values for Australia and New Zealand including Recommended Dietary Intakes. Commonwealth Department of Health and Ageing, Australia Ministry of Health,

New Zealand National Health and Medical Research Council; 2004. Available from: www.nrv.gov.au/nutrients/vitamin-e.
[150] Food and Nutrition Board, Institute of Medicine. Vitamin E. Dietary reference intakes for vitamin C, vitamin E, selenium, and carotenoids. Washington, DC: National Academy Press; 2000. p. 186–283.
[151] Miller E. Meta-analysis: high-dosage vitamin E supplementation may increase all-cause mortality. Ann Intern Med 2005;142(1):37.
[152] Holden R, Ki V, Morton A, et al. Fat-soluble vitamins in advanced CKD/ESKD: a review. Sem Dial 2012;25(3):334–43.
[153] European Commission. Health and Consumer Protection. Opinion of the scientific community on food on tolerable upper level intake of vitamin E. 2016. Available from: http://ec.europa.eu/food/fs/sc/scf/out195_en.pdf.
[154] Kabagambe E, Beasley T, Limdi N. Vitamin K intake, body mass index and warfarin maintenance dose. Cardiology 2013;126(4):214–18.
[155] Nowak J, Grzybowska-Chlebowczyk U, Landowski P, et al. Prevalence and correlates of vitamin K deficiency in children with inflammatory bowel disease. Sci Rep 2014;4:4768.
[156] Shiraki M, Tsugawa N, Okano T. Recent advances in vitamin K-dependent Gla-containing proteins and vitamin K nutrition. Osteopor Sarcopen 2015;1(1):22–38.
[157] Shiraki M, Itabashi A. Short-term menatetrenone therapy increases gamma-carboxylation of osteocalcin with a moderate increase of bone turnover in postmenopausal osteoporosis: a randomized prospective study. J Bone Miner Metab 2009;27(3):333–40.
[158] Vitamin K. Nutrient Reference Values for Australia and New Zealand including Recommended Dietary Intakes. Commonwealth Department of Health and Ageing, Australia Ministry of Health, New Zealand National Health and Medical Research Council; 2004. Available from: www.nrv.gov.au/nutrients/vitamin-k.
[159] Theuwissen E, Magdeleyns E, Braam L, et al. Vitamin K status in healthy volunteers. Food Funct 2014;5(2):229–34.
[160] Westenfeld R, Krueger T, Schlieper G, et al. Effect of vitamin K2 supplementation on functional vitamin K deficiency in hemodialysis patients: a randomized trial. Am J Kidney Dis 2012;59(2):186–95.
[161] National Institutes of Health. Dietary supplement label database. 2014. Available from: https://ods.od.nih.gov/Research/Dietary_Supplement_Label_Database.aspx.
[162] Food and Nutrition Board, Institute of Medicine. Vitamin K. Dietary reference intakes for vitamin A, vitamin K, arsenic, boron, chromium, copper, iodine, iron, manganese, molybdenum, nickel, silicon, vanadium, and zinc. Washington, DC: National Academy Press; 2001. p. 162–96.
[163] Pizzorno L, Pizzorno J. Vitamin K, beyond coagulation to uses in bone, vascular and anti-cancer metabolism. IMCJ 2008;7(2):24–30.
[164] Cranenburg E, Schurgers L, Vermeer C. Vitamin K: The coagulation vitamin that became omnipotent. Thromb Haemost 2007;98:120–5.
[165] Ziaei S, Faghihzadeh S, Sohrabvand F, et al. A randomised placebo-controlled trial to determine the effect of vitamin E in the treatment of primary dysmenorrhoea. BJOG 2001;108:1181–3.
[166] Knapen MH, Schurgers LJ, Vermeer C. Vitamin K_2 supplementation improves hip bone geometry and bone strength indices in postmenopausal women. Osteoporos Int 2007;18:963–72.
[167] O'Connor E, Grealy G, McCarthy J, et al. Effect of phylloquinone (vitamin K1) supplementation for 12 months on the indices of vitamin K status and bone health in adult patients with Crohn's disease. Br J Nutr 2014;112(07):1163–74.
[168] Crane FL. Biochemical functions of coenzyme Q10. J Am Coll Nutr 2001;20:591–8.
[169] Thomson CD, Chisholm A, McLachlan SK, et al. Brazil nuts: an effective way to improve selenium status. Am J Clin Nutr 2008;87:379–84.
[170] Yamamoto Y, Yamashita S. Plasma ratio of ubiquinol and ubiquinone as a marker of oxidative stress. Mol Aspects Med 1997;18(Suppl.):S79–84.
[171] Linus Pauling Institute. Coenzyme Q10. Oregon State University. 2016. Available from: http://lpi.oregonstate.edu/mic/dietary-factors/coenzyme-Q10.
[172] Bargossi AM, Grossi G, Fiorella PL, et al. Exogenous CoQ10 supplementation prevents plasma ubiquinone reduction induced by HMG-CoA reductase inhibitors. Mol Aspects Med 1994;15 (Suppl.):s187–93.
[173] Gao L, Mao Q, Cao J, et al. Effects of coenzyme Q10 on vascular endothelial function in humans: A meta-analysis of randomized controlled trials. Atherosclerosis 2012;221(2):311–16.
[174] Beal M. Therapeutic approaches to mitochondrial dysfunction in Parkinson's disease. Parkinsonism Relat Disord 2009;15: S189–94.
[175] Langsjoen P, Langsjoen A. Supplemental ubiquinol in patients with advanced congestive heart failure. Biofactors 2008;32(1–4):119–28.
[176] Tiano L, Belardinelli R, Carnevali P, et al. Effect of coenzyme Q10 administration on endothelial function and extracellular superoxide dismutase in patients with ischaemic heart disease: a double-blind, randomized controlled study. Eur Heart J 2007;28(18):2249–55.
[177] Baggio E, Gandini R, Plancher AC, et al. Italian multicenter study on the safety and efficacy of coenzyme Q10 as adjunctive therapy in heart failure. CoQ10 Drug Surveillance Investigators. Mol Aspects Med 1994;15(Suppl.):s287–94.
[178] Gofshteyn J, Stephenson D. Diagnosis and management of childhood headache. Curr Prob Pediatr Adolesc Health Care 2016;46(2):36–51.
[179] Sandor PS, Di Clemente L, Coppola G, et al. Efficacy of coenzyme Q10 in migraine prophylaxis: a randomized controlled trial. Neurology 2005;64:713–15.
[180] Langsjoen P, Langsjoen P, Willis R, et al. Treatment of essential hypertension with coenzyme Q10. Mol Aspects Med 1994; 15(Suppl.):S265–72.
[181] Balercia G, Buldreghini E, Vignini A, et al. Coenzyme Q10 treatment in infertile men with idiopathic asthenozoospermia: a placebo-controlled, double-blind randomized trial. Fertil Steril 2009;91:1785–92.
[182] Cordero M, Santos-García R, Bermejo-Jover D, et al. Coenzyme Q10 in salivary cells correlate with blood cells in fibromyalgia: improvement in clinical and biochemical parameter after oral treatment. Clin Biochem 2012;45(6):509–11.
[183] Mizuno K, Tanaka M, Nozaki S, et al. Antifatigue effects of coenzyme Q10 during physical fatigue. Nutrition 2008;24:293–9.
[184] Jankowski J, Korzeniowska K, Cieślewicz A, et al. Coenzyme Q10 — a new player in the treatment of heart failure? Pharmacol Rep 2016;68(5):1015–19.
[185] Evans M, Baisley J, Barss S, et al. A randomized, double-blind trial on the bioavailability of two CoQ10 formulations. J Funct Food 2009;1:65–73.
[186] Alehagen U, Johansson P, Björnstedt M, et al. Cardiovascular mortality and N-terminal-proBNP reduced after combined selenium and coenzyme Q10 supplementation: A 5-year prospective randomized double-blind placebo-controlled trial among elderly Swedish citizens. Int J Cardiol 2013;167(5):1860–6.
[187] Straub DA. Calcium supplementation in clinical practice: a review of forms, doses, and indications. Nutr Clin Pract 2007;22:286–96.
[188] Ramsubeik K, Keuler N, Davis L, et al. Factors associated with calcium absorption in postmenopausal women: a post hoc analysis of dual-isotope studies. J Acad Nutr Diet 2014;114(5):761–7.
[189] Weaver CM. Calcium. In: Erdman J, Macdonald I, Zeisel S, editors. Present knowledge in nutrition. 10th ed. John Wiley & Sons, Inc; 2012.
[190] Wright M, Proctor D, Insogna K, et al. Proton pump-inhibiting drugs, calcium homeostasis, and bone health. Nutr Rev 2008;66(2):103–8.
[191] Rosanoff A, Dai Q, Shapses S. Essential nutrient interactions: does low or suboptimal magnesium status interact with vitamin D and/or calcium status. Adv Nutr 2016;7(1):25–43.
[192] Committee to Review Dietary Reference Intakes for Vitamin D and Calcium, Food and Nutrition Board, Institute of Medicine. Dietary reference intakes for calcium and vitamin D. Washington, DC: National Academy Press; 2010.
[193] Prentice R, Pettinger M, Jackson R, et al. Health risks and benefits from calcium and vitamin D supplementation: Women's Health Initiative clinical trial and cohort study. Osteoporos Int 2012;24(2):567–80.
[194] Whelan A, Jurgens T, Naylor H. Herbs, vitamins and minerals in the treatment of premenstrual syndrome: a systematic review. Can J Clin Pharmacol 2009;16(3):e407–29.
[195] Larsson S, Orsini N, Wolk A. Dietary calcium intake and risk of stroke: a dose-response meta-analysis. Am J Clin Nutr 2013;97(5):951–7.

[196] Jankowski C. Calcium and Vitamin D supplementation decreases incidence of stress fractures in female Navy recruits. Yearb Sports Med 2009;2009:17–19.
[197] Appleby P, Roddam A, Allen N, et al. Comparative fracture risk in vegetarians and nonvegetarians in EPIC-Oxford. Eur J Clin Nutr 2007;61(12):1400–6.
[198] Reinwald S, Weaver CM, Kester JJ. The health benefits of calcium citrate malate: a review of the supporting science. Adv Food Nutr Res 2008;54:219–346.
[199] Calcium. Nutrient Reference Values for Australia and New Zealand including Recommended Dietary Intakes. Commonwealth Department of Health and Ageing, Australia Ministry of Health, New Zealand National Health and Medical Research Council; 2004. Available from: https://www.nrv.gov.au/nutrients/calcium.
[200] Patrick L. Comparative absorption of calcium sources and calcium citrate malate for the prevention of osteoporosis. Altern Med Rev 1999;4:74–85.
[201] Rutherfurd SM, Moughan PJ, Lowry D, et al. Amino acid composition determined using multiple hydrolysis times for three goat milk formulations. Int J Food Sci Nutr 2008;59:679–90.
[202] Goldberg G. Nutrition and bone. Women Health Med 2006;3: 157–9.
[203] Kerstetter J, O'Brien K, Caseria D, et al. The impact of dietary protein on calcium absorption and kinetic measures of bone turnover in women. J Clin Endocrinol Metab 2005;90(1):26–31.
[204] Heaney RP. Constructive interactions among nutrients and bone — active pharmacologic agents with principal emphasis on calcium, phosphorus, vitamin D and protein. J Am Coll Nutr 2001;20:403S–9S, 417S–20S. (discussion).
[205] Enig MG Mineral primer. Weston A. Price Foundation; 2008. Available from: http://www.westonaprice.org/abcs-of-nutrition/166-mineral-primer.html.
[206] Wilhelm S, Rjater R, Kale-Pradhan P. Perils and pitfalls of long-term effects of proton pump inhibitors. Expert Rev Clin Pharmacol 2013;6(4):443–51.
[207] Benson J. Magnesium. Altern Med Rev 2015;23:58–9.
[208] Elson M, Haas MD. Staying healthy with nutrition. The complete guide to diet and nutritional medicine. Berkeley, CA: Celestial Arts; 1992.
[209] Del Gobbo L, Imamura F, Wu J, et al. Circulating and dietary magnesium and risk of cardiovascular disease: a systematic review and meta-analysis of prospective studies. Am J Clin Nutr 2013;98(1):160–73.
[210] Sanjuliani AF, de Abreu Fagundes VG, Francischetti EA. Effects of magnesium on blood pressure and intracellular ion levels of Brazilian hypertensive patients. Int J Cardiol 1996;56:177–83.
[211] Tepper D. Magnesium. Headache 2013;53:1533–4.
[212] Campbell A. Magnesium: not to be overlooked. Altern Ther Health Med 2013;19(3):8–9.
[213] Köseoglu E, Talaslıoglu A, Gönül AS, et al. The effects of magnesium prophylaxis in migraine without aura. Magnes Res 2008;21(2):101–8.
[214] Stendig-Lindbergl G, Tepper R, Leichter I. Trabecular bone density in a two year controlled trial of peroral magnesium in osteoporosis. Magnes Res 1993;6(2):155–63.
[215] Quaranta S, Buscaglia M, Meroni M, et al. Pilot study of the efficacy and safety of a modified-release magnesium 250 mg tablet (Sincromag) for the treatment of premenstrual syndrome. Clin Drug Investig 2007;27(1):51–8.
[216] Dahle LO, Berg G, Hammar M, et al. The effect of oral magnesium substitution on pregnancy-induced leg cramps. Am J Obstet Gynecol 1995;173:175–80.
[217] Young GL, Jewell D. Interventions for leg cramps in pregnancy. Cochrane Database Syst Rev 2002;CD000121.
[218] Dong J, Xun P, He K, et al. Magnesium intake and risk of type 2 diabetes: meta-analysis of prospective cohort studies. Diabetes Care 2011;34(9):2116–22.
[219] Mooren F, Krüger K, Völker K, et al. Oral magnesium supplementation reduces insulin resistance in non-diabetic subjects - a double-blind, placebo-controlled, randomized trial. Diabetes Obes Metab 2011;13(3):281–4.
[220] Starobrat-Hermelin B, Kozielec T. The effects of magnesium physiological supplementation on hyperactivity in children with attention deficit hyperactivity disorder (ADHD). Positive response to magnesium oral loading test. Magnes Res 1997;10:149–56.
[221] Firoz M, Graber M. Bioavailability of US commercial magnesium preparations. Magnes Res 2001;14:257–62.
[222] Rude R, Shils M. Magnesium. In: Shils M, Shike M, Ross A, et al, editors. Modern nutrition in health and disease. 10th ed. Baltimore: Lippincott Williams & Wilkins; 2006. p. 223–47.
[223] Rylander. Bioavailability of magnesium salts – a review. J Pharm Nutr Sci 2014;4:57–9.
[224] Magnesium. Nutrient Reference Values for Australia and New Zealand including Recommended Dietary Intakes. Commonwealth Department of Health and Ageing, Australia Ministry of Health, New Zealand National Health and Medical Research Council; 2004. Available from: https://www.nrv.gov.au/nutrients/magnesium.
[225] Johnson S. The multifaceted and widespread pathology of magnesium deficiency. Med Hypotheses 2001;56:163–70.
[226] Daly K, Farrington E. Hypokalemia and hyperkalemia in infants and children: pathophysiology and treatment. J Pediatr Health Care 2013;27(6):486–96.
[227] Mandal A. Hypokalemia and hyperkalemia. Med Clin North Am 1997;81(3):611–39.
[228] Gennari F. Hypokalemia. N Engl J Med 1998;339(7):451–8.
[229] Whelton P. Effects of oral potassium on blood pressure. JAMA 1997;277(20):1624.
[230] Braun L, Cohen M. Herbs and natural supplements: an evidence-based guide. Sydney: Elsevier Mosby; 2005.
[231] Sheng H-W. Sodium, chloride and potassium. In: Stipanuk M, editor. Biochemical and physiological aspects of human nutrition. Philadelphia: WB Saunders; 2000. p. 686–710.
[232] Potassium. Nutrient Reference Values for Australia and New Zealand including Recommended Dietary Intakes. Commonwealth Department of Health and Ageing, Australia Ministry of Health, New Zealand National Health and Medical Research Council; 2004. Available from: www.nrv.gov.au/nutrients/potassium.
[233] Food and Nutrition Board, Institute of Medicine. Potassium. Dietary reference intakes for water, potassium, sodium, chloride and sulfate. Washington DC: National Academies Press; 2005. p. 186–268.
[234] Sodium. Nutrient Reference Values for Australia and New Zealand including Recommended Dietary Intakes. Commonwealth Department of Health and Ageing, Australia Ministry of Health, New Zealand National Health and Medical Research Council; 2004. Available from: www.nrv.gov.au/nutrients/sodium.
[235] He F, MacGregor G. Reducing population salt intake worldwide: from evidence to implementation. Prog Cardiovasc Dis 2010;52(5):363–82.
[236] Food Standards Australia New Zealand. How much sodium do Australians eat? 2015. Available from: www.foodstandards.gov.au/consumer/nutrition/salthowmuch/pages/howmuchsaltareweeating/howmuchsaltandsodium4551.aspx.
[237] Tucker K. Osteoporosis prevention and nutrition. Curr Osteoporos Rep 2009;7(4):111–17.
[238] Nicoll R. Cardiovascular calcification and bone: a comparison of the effects of dietary and serum calcium, phosphorous, magnesium and vitamin D. Int Cardiovasc Forum J 2015;1(5):209.
[239] Zmonarski SC, Klinger M, Puziewicz-Zmonarska A, et al. Therapeutic use of potassium citrate. Przegl Lek 2001;58(2):82–6.
[240] Phosphorus. Nutrient Reference Values for Australia and New Zealand including Recommended Dietary Intakes. Commonwealth Department of Health and Ageing, Australia Ministry of Health, New Zealand National Health and Medical Research Council; 2004. Available from: www.nrv.gov.au/nutrients/phosphorus.
[241] Kremsdorf R, Hoofnagle A, Kratz M, et al. Effects of a High-protein diet on regulation of phosphorus homeostasis. J Clin Endocrinol Metab 2013;98(3):1207–13.
[242] Palacios C. The role of nutrients in bone health, from A to Z. Crit Rev Food Sci Nutr 2006;46(8):621–8.
[243] MedlinePlus Medical Encyclopedia. Chloride in diet. 2014. Available from: https://medlineplus.gov/ency/article/002417.htm.
[244] Newnham R. Discovering the cure for arthritis. Nutr Health 2004;17:281–4.
[245] Ganz T, Nemeth E. Regulation of iron acquisition and iron distribution in mammals. Biochim Biophys Acta 2006;1763: 690–9.
[246] McDermid J, Lonnerdal B. Iron. Adv Nutr 2012;3(4):532–3.
[247] Hunt JR, Benjamin C. Iron. Encyclopedia of human nutrition. Oxford: Elsevier; 2005. p. 82–9.

[248] Hurrell R, Reddy M, Cook J. Inhibition of non-haem iron absorption in man by polyphenolic-containing beverages. Br J Nutr 1999;81:289–95.
[249] Beutler E. Disorders of iron metabolism. In: Lichtman MA, Williams WJ, Beutler E, et al, editors. Williams hematology. 7th ed. New York: McGraw-Hill Medical; 2006. p. 511–53.
[250] WHO. Guideline: intermittent iron supplementation for preschool and school-age children. Geneva: WHO; 2011.
[251] Fernández-Gaxiola A, De-Regil L. Intermittent iron supplementation for reducing anaemia and its associated impairments in menstruating women. Cochrane Database Syst Rev 2011;(12):CD009218.
[252] Grant C, Wall C, Brewster D, et al. Policy statement on iron deficiency in pre-school-aged children. J Paediatr Child Health 2007;43(7–8):513–21.
[253] Lopez A, Cacoub P, Macdougall I, et al. Iron deficiency anaemia. Lancet 2016;387(10021):907–16.
[254] Allen R, Auerbach S, Bahrain H, et al. The prevalence and impact of restless legs syndrome on patients with iron deficiency anemia. Am J Hematol 2013;88(4):261–4.
[255] Iron. Nutrient Reference Values for Australia and New Zealand including Recommended Dietary Intakes. Commonwealth Department of Health and Ageing, Australia Ministry of Health, New Zealand National Health and Medical Research Council; 2004. Available from: https://www.nrv.gov.au/nutrients/iron.
[256] Institute of Medicine FNB. Dietary reference intakes for vitamin A, vitamin K, arsenic, boron, chromium, copper, iodine, iron, manganese, molybdenum, nickel, silicon, vanadium and zinc. Washington, DC: National Academy Press; 2001.
[257] Yokoi K, Alcock NW, Sandstead HH. Iron and zinc nutriture of premenopausal women: associations of diet with serum ferritin and plasma zinc disappearance and of serum ferritin with plasma zinc and plasma zinc disappearance. J Lab Clin Med 1994;124:852–61.
[258] Paesano R, Pietropaoli M, Gessani S, et al. The influence of lactoferrin, orally administered, on systemic iron homeostasis in pregnant women suffering of iron deficiency and iron deficiency anaemia. Biochimie 2009;91:44–51.
[259] Allen LH, Graham JM, Sabel JE. Pregnancy, dietary guidelines and safe supplement use. Oxford: Elsevier; 2005.
[260] Cancelo-Hidalgo M, Castelo-Branco C, Palacios S, et al. Tolerability of different oral iron supplements: a systematic review. Curr Med Res Opin 2013;29(4):291–303.
[261] Huang L, Drake V, Ho E. Zinc. Adv Nutr 2015;6(2):224–8.
[262] Chimienti F. Zinc, pancreatic islet cell function and diabetes: new insights into an old story. Nutr Res Rev 2013;26(01):1–11.
[263] Freake HC, Benjamin C. Zinc. Physiology. Encyclopedia of human nutrition. Oxford: Elsevier; 2005. p. 447–54.
[264] King J, Shames D, Lowe N. Effect of acute zinc depletion on zinc homeostasis and plasma zinc kinetics in men. Am J Clin Nutr 2001;74:116–24.
[265] Zinc. Nutrient Reference Values for Australia and New Zealand including Recommended Dietary Intakes. Commonwealth Department of Health and Ageing, Australia Ministry of Health, New Zealand National Health and Medical Research Council; 2004. Available from: https://www.nrv.gov.au/nutrients/zinc.
[266] Olivares M, Pizarro F, Ruz M, et al. Acute inhibition of iron bioavailability by zinc: studies in humans. Biometals 2012;25(4):657–64.
[267] Hooper P. Zinc lowers high-density lipoprotein-cholesterol levels. JAMA 1980;244(17):1960.
[268] Prasad A, Beck F, Bao B, et al. Duration and severity of symptoms and levels of plasma interleukin-1 receptor antagonist, soluble tumor necrosis factor receptor, and adhesion molecules in patients with common cold treated with zinc acetate. J Infect Dis 2008;197(6):795–802.
[269] Singh M, Das R. Zinc for the common cold. Cochrane Database Syst Rev 2011;(2).
[270] Maret W, Sandstead HH. Zinc requirements and the risks and benefits of zinc supplementation. J Trace Elem Med Biol 2006;20:3–18.
[271] Lowe N, Fekete K, Decsi T. Methods of assessment of zinc status in humans: a systematic review. Am J Clin Nutr 2009;89(6):2040S–51S.
[272] Zinc. Nutrient Reference Values for Australia and New Zealand including Recommended Dietary Intakes. Commonwealth Department of Health and Ageing, Australia Ministry of Health, New Zealand National Health and Medical Research Council; 2004. Available from: https://www.nrv.gov.au/nutrients/zinc.
[273] Gebraselassie S, Gashe F. A systematic review of effect of prenatal zinc supplementation on birthweight: meta-analysis of 17 randomized controlled trials. J Health Popul Nutr 2011;29(2):134–40.
[274] Institute of Medicine, Food and Nutrition Board. dietary reference intakes for vitamin a, vitamin k, arsenic, boron, chromium, copper, iodine, iron, manganese, molybdenum, nickel, silicon, vanadium, and zinc. Washington, DC. National Academy Press, 2001.
[275] Levenson CW. Zinc: the new antidepressant? Nutr Rev 2006;64:39–42.
[276] Gibson RS, Yeudall F, Drost N, et al. Dietary interventions to prevent zinc deficiency. Am J Clin Nutr 1998;68:484S–7S.
[277] Gibson RS. Content and bioavailability of trace elements in vegetarian diets. Am J Clin Nutr 1994;59:1223S–32S.
[278] Turnlund JR. Copper. In: Shils ME, Shike M, Ross AC, et al, editors. Modern nutrition in health and disease. 10th ed. Philadelphia: Lippincott Williams & Wilkins; 2006. p. 286–99.
[279] Linus Pauling Institute. Copper. 2014 Available from: http://lpi.oregonstate.edu/mic/minerals/copper.
[280] Harvey L, Ashton K, Hooper L, et al. Methods of assessment of copper status in humans: a systematic review. Am J Clin Nutr 2009;89(6):2009S–24S.
[281] Bertinato J. Zouzoulas A. Considerations in the development of biomarkers of copper status. J AOAC Int 2009;92(5):1541–50.
[282] Baker D. Cupric oxide should not be used as a copper supplement for either animals or humans. J Nutr 1999;129:2278–9.
[283] Rojas-Sobarzo L, Olivares M, Brito A, et al. Copper supplementation at 8 mg neither affects circulating lipids nor liver function in apparently healthy Chilean men. Biol Trace Elem Res 2013;156(1–3):1–4.
[284] Copper. Nutrient Reference Values for Australia and New Zealand including Recommended Dietary Intakes. Commonwealth Department of Health and Ageing, Australia Ministry of Health, New Zealand National Health and Medical Research Council; 2004. Available from: https://www.nrv.gov.au/nutrients/copper.
[285] Weber T, Solioz M. Evaluation of chocolate as a source of dietary copper. Eur Food Res Technol 2014;238(6):1063–6.
[286] Celik C, Bastu E, Abali R, et al. The relationship between copper, homocysteine and early vascular disease in lean women with polycystic ovary syndrome. Gynecol Endocrinol 2013;29(5):488–91.
[287] Arthur R The dynamic balance. How to assess and correct mineral deficiencies in clinical practice. Workshop. Unpublished. 2008.
[288] Sánchez-Castillo CP, James WPT, Benjamin C. Sodium. Salt intake and health. Encyclopedia of human nutrition. Oxford: Elsevier; 2005. p. 154–67.
[289] Cavalieri RR. Iodine. In: Goodhart RS, Shils ME, editors. Modern nutrition in health and disease. 6th ed. New York: Lea & Febiger; 1980. [Ch 9].
[290] Hess S. The impact of common micronutrient deficiencies on iodine and thyroid metabolism: the evidence from human studies. Best Pract Res Clin Endocrinol Metab 2010;24(1):117–32.
[291] Zimmermann MB. Iodine and iodine deficiency disorders. In: Erdman JWJ, Macdonald IA, Zeisel SH, editors. Present knowledge in nutrition. 10th ed. John Wiley & Sons; 2012. p. 554–67.
[292] Zimmerman M. Iodine deficiency. Endocrinol Rev 2009;30:376–408.
[293] WHO, UNICEF, International Council for the Control of Iodine Deficiency Disorders. Assessment of iodine deficiency disorders and monitoring their elimination. 3rd ed. Geneva: WHO; 2007.
[294] Kessler J. The effect of supraphysiologic levels of iodine on patients with cyclic mastalgia. Breast J 2004;10(4):328–36.
[295] Błażewicz A, Makarewicz A, Korona-Glowniak I, et al. Iodine in autism spectrum disorders. J Trace Elem Med Biol 2016;34:32–7.
[296] Krajčovičová-Kudláčková M, Bučková K, Klime I, et al. Iodine deficiency in vegetarians and vegans. Ann Nutr Metab 2003;47(5):183–5.
[297] Hynes K, Otahal P, Hay I, et al. Mild iodine deficiency during pregnancy is associated with reduced educational outcomes in the offspring: 9-year follow-up of the gestational iodine cohort. J Clin Endocrinol Metab 2013;98(5):1954–62.

[298] WHO. Urinary iodine concentrations for determining iodine status deficiency in populations. Vitamin and Mineral Nutrition Information System. Geneva: World Health Organization; 2013. Available from: http://www.who.int/vmnis/en/.
[299] Iodine. Nutrient Reference Values for Australia and New Zealand including Recommended Dietary Intakes. Commonwealth Department of Health and Ageing, Australia Ministry of Health, New Zealand National Health and Medical Research Council; 2004. Available from: www.nrv.gov.au/nutrients/iodine.
[300] Hetzel BS, Benjamin C. Iodine. Deficiency disorders. Encyclopedia of human nutrition. Oxford: Elsevier; 2005. p. 74–82.
[301] Berbel P, Obregon MJ, Bernal J, et al. Iodine supplementation during pregnancy: a public health challenge. Trends Endocrinol Metab 2007;18:338–43.
[302] Lajin B, Kuehnelt D, Jensen K, et al. Investigating the intra-individual variability in the human metabolic profile of urinary selenium. J Trace Elem Med Biol 2016;37:31–6.
[303] Nacamulli D, Mian C, Petricca D, et al. influence of physiological dietary selenium supplementation on the natural course of autoimmune thyroiditis. Clin Endocrinol (Oxf) 2010;73(4):535–9.
[304] Navarro-Alarcon M, Cabrera-Vique C. Selenium in food and the human body: a review. Sci Total Environ 2008;400:115–41.
[305] Duntas L, Benvenga S. Selenium: an element for life. Endocrine 2014;48(3):756–75.
[306] Dennert G, Zwahlen M, Brinkman M, et al. Selenium for preventing cancer. Cochrane Database Syst Rev 2011;(5): CD005195.
[307] Steinbrenner H. Interference of selenium and selenoproteins with the insulin-regulated carbohydrate and lipid metabolism. Free Radic Biol Med 2013;65:1538–47.
[308] Sunde RA. Selenium. In: Ross AC, Caballero B, Cousins RJ, et al, editors. Modern nutrition in health and disease. 11th ed. Philadelphia: Lippincott Williams & Wilkins; 2012. p. 225–37.
[309] Institute of Medicine, Food and Nutrition Board. Dietary reference intakes: vitamin C, vitamin E, selenium, and carotenoids. Washington, DC: National Academy Press; 2000.
[310] Benton D, Cook R. The impact of selenium supplementation on mood. Biol Psychiatry 1991;29:1092–8.
[311] Vinceti M, Bonvicini F, Rothman K, et al. The relation between amyotrophic lateral sclerosis and inorganic selenium in drinking water: a population-based case-control study. Environ Health 2010;9(1):77.
[312] Jäger T, Drexler H, Göen T. Human metabolism and renal excretion of selenium compounds after oral ingestion of sodium selenate dependent on trimethylselenium ion (TMSe) status. Arch Toxicol 2014;90(1):149–58.
[313] Selenium. Nutrient Reference Values for Australia and New Zealand including Recommended Dietary Intakes. Commonwealth Department of Health and Ageing, Australia Ministry of Health, New Zealand National Health and Medical Research Council; 2004. Available from: www.nrv.gov.au/nutrients/selenium.
[314] Stewart MS, Spallholz JE, Neldner KH, et al. Selenium compounds have disparate abilities to impose oxidative stress and induce apoptosis. Free Radic Biol Med 1999;26:42–8.
[315] Martens I, Cardoso B, Hare D, et al. Selenium status in preschool children receiving a Brazil nut–enriched diet. Nutrition 2015;31(11–12):1339–43.
[316] Snook JT. Effect of ethanol use and other lifestyle variables on measures of selenium status. Alcohol 1991;8:13–16.
[317] Mariath A, Bergamaschi D, Rondó P, et al. The possible role of selenium status in adverse pregnancy outcomes. Br J Nutr 2011;105(10):1418–28.
[318] Anderson RA, Benjamin C. Chromium. Encyclopedia of human nutrition. Oxford: Elsevier; 2005. p. 396–401.
[319] Molybdenum. Monograph. Altern Med Rev 2006;11:156–61.
[320] Anderson RA, Polansky MM, Bryden NA, et al. Effect of exercise (running) on serum glucose, insulin, glucagon, and chromium excretion. Diabetes 1982;31:212–16.
[321] EFSA NDA Panel (EFSA Panel on Dietetic Products, Nutrition and Allergies). Scientific opinion on dietary reference values for molybdenum. EFSA J 2013;11(8):3333–5.
[322] Falcão DA, Isaac L. Clinical aspects and molecular basis of primary deficiencies of complement component C3 and its regulatory proteins factor I and factor H. Scand J Immunol 2006;63:155–68.
[323] Molybdenum. Nutrient Reference Values for Australia and New Zealand including Recommended Dietary Intakes. Commonwealth Department of Health and Ageing, Australia Ministry of Health, New Zealand National Health and Medical Research Council; 2004. Available from: www.nrv.gov.au/nutrients/molybdenum.
[324] Vincent JB. Elucidating a biological role for chromium at a molecular level. Acc Chem Res 2000;33:503–10.
[325] Paiva A, Lima J, Medeiros A, et al. Beneficial effects of oral chromium picolinate supplementation on glycemic control in patients with type 2 diabetes: a randomized clinical study. J Trace Elem Med Biol 2015;32:66–72.
[326] Abdollahi M, Farshchi A, Nikfar S, et al. Effect of chromium on glucose and lipid profiles in patients with type 2 diabetes; a meta-analysis review of randomized trials. J Pharm Pharm Sci 2013;16(1):99.
[327] Anderson R. Chromium and insulin resistance. Nutr Res Rev 2003;16(02):267.
[328] Jovanovic L, Gutierrez M, Peterson CM. Chromium supplementation for women with gestational diabetes. J Trace Elem Exp Med 1999;12:91–7.
[329] Jovanovic-Peterson L, Peterson CM. Vitamin and mineral deficiencies which may predispose to glucose intolerance of pregnancy. J Am Coll Nutr 1996;15:14–20.
[330] Anderson RA, Polansky MM, Bryden NA, et al. Supplemental-chromium effects on glucose, insulin, glucagon, and urinary chromium losses in subjects consuming controlled low-chromium diets. Am J Clin Nutr 1991;54:909–16.
[331] Gibson RS. Principles of nutritional assessment. 2nd ed. New York: Oxford University Press; 2005.
[332] Nielsen FH. Manganese, molybdenum, boron, chromium, and other trace elements. In: Erdman JJ, Macdonald I, Zelssel S, editors. Present knowledge of nutrition. John Wiley & Sons; 2012.
[333] Langard S, Costa M, Gunnar FN, et al. Chromium. Handbook on the toxicology of metals. Burlington, CA. Academic Press; 2007. p. 487–510.
[334] Anderson RA, Bryden NA, Polansky MM. Dietary chromium intake. Freely chosen diets, institutional diet, and individual foods. Biol Trace Elem Res 1992;32:117–21.
[335] Anderson RA. Recent advances in the clinical and biochemical effects of chromium deficiency. Prog Clin Biol Res 1993;380:221–34.
[336] Devirian T, Volpe S. The physiological effects of dietary boron. Crit Rev Food Sci Nutr 2003;43(2):219–31.
[337] Blaurock-Busch E, Griffin V. Mineral and trace element analysis, laboratory and clinical application. Boulder, CO: TMI/MTM Inc; 1996.
[338] Penland JG. Dietary boron, brain function, and cognitive performance. Environ Health Perspect 1994;102(Suppl. 7):65–72.
[339] Forrest H, Nielsen P. The emergence of boron as nutritionally important throughout the life cycle. Nutrition 2000;16(7–8): 512–14.
[340] Monograph. Boron. Altern Med Rev 2004;9:434–7.
[341] Hokin B, Adams M, Ashton J, et al. Comparison of the dietary cobalt intake in three different Australian diets. Asia Pac J Clin Nutr 2004;13(3):289–91.
[342] Martin KR. The chemistry of silica and its potential health benefits. J Nutr Health Aging 2007;11:94–7.
[343] Jugdaohsingh J. Silicon and bone health. J Nutr Health Aging 2007;11(2):99–110.
[344] Han M, Schiavone-Gatto P, Compher C, et al. Minerals and trace elements. Clin Nutr. 4th ed. Philadelphia: WB Saunders; 2005. p. 140–54.
[345] Lichtenstein A, Jones P. Present knowledge in nutrition. 10th ed. ILSI Wiley-Blackwell; 2012.
[346] Cleland L, James M, Proudman S. Fish oil: what the prescriber needs to know. Arthritis Res Ther 2006;8:202.
[347] Lev E, Solodky A, Harel N. Treatment of aspirin-resistant patients with omega-3 fatty acids versus aspirin dose escalation. J Vasc Surg 2010;52(2):520.
[348] Lord R, Bralley J. Laboratory evaluations for integrative and functional medicine: fatty acids. Duluth, GA: Metametrix Institute; 2008.
[349] Basch EM, Ulbricht CE, editors. Natural standard herb & supplement handbook. The clinical bottom line. St Louis, MO: Mosby Elsevier; 2005.

[350] Horrobin DF. The regulation of prostaglandin biosynthesis by the manipulation of essential fatty acid metabolism. Rev Pure Appl Pharmacol Sci 1983;4:339–83.
[351] Patterson E, Wall R, Fitzgerald G, et al. Health implications of high dietary omega-6 polyunsaturated fatty acids. J Nutr Metab 2012;2012:1–16.
[352] Watkins PA, Benjamin C. Fatty acids. Metabolism. Encyclopedia of human nutrition. Oxford: Elsevier; 2005. p. 186–98.
[353] Wang Q, Liang X, Wang L, et al. Effect of omega-3 fatty acids supplementation on endothelial function: a meta-analysis of randomized controlled trials. Atherosclerosis 2012;221(2):536–43.
[354] Calder P. Session 3: Joint Nutrition Society and Irish Nutrition and Dietetic Institute Symposium on 'Nutrition and autoimmune disease' PUFA, inflammatory processes and rheumatoid arthritis. Proc Nutr Soc 2008;67(04):409.
[355] Kapoor R, Huang YS. Gamma linolenic acid: an anti-inflammatory omega-6 fatty acid. Curr Pharm Biotechnol 2006;7:531–4.
[356] Irving CB, Mumby-Croft R, Joy LA. Polyunsaturated fatty acid supplementation for schizophrenia. Cochrane Database Syst Rev 2006;(3):CD001257.
[357] Witte A, Kerti L, Hermannstadter H, et al. Long-chain omega-3 fatty acids improve brain function and structure in older adults. Cereb Cortex 2013;24(11):3059–68.
[358] Forbes D, Parsons H. Essential fatty acids: food for mind and body. Acta Paediatr 2012;101(8):808–10.
[359] Baghai T, Varallo-Bedarida G, Born C, et al. Major depressive disorder is associated with cardiovascular risk factors and low omega-3 index. J Clin Psychiatry 2010;72(09):1242–7.
[360] Block R, Harris W, Reid K, et al. EPA and DHA in blood cell membranes from acute coronary syndrome patients and controls. Atherosclerosis 2008;197(2):821–8.
[361] Harris W. The omega-3 index: from biomarker to risk marker to risk factor. Curr Atheroscler Rep 2009;11(6):411–17.
[362] Harris W, Pottala J, Varvel S, et al. Erythrocyte omega-3 fatty acids increase and linoleic acid decreases with age: Observations from 160,000 patients. Prostaglandins Leukot Essent Fatty Acids 2013;88(4):257–63.
[363] Akter K, Gallo D, Martin S, et al. A review of the possible role of the essential fatty acids and fish oils in the aetiology, prevention or pharmacotherapy of schizophrenia. J Clin Pharm Ther 2011;37(2):132–9.
[364] Calder P. Omega-3 polyunsaturated fatty acids and inflammatory processes: nutrition or pharmacology? Br J Clin Pharmacol 2013;75(3):645–62.
[365] Anderson B, Ma D. Are all n-3 polyunsaturated fatty acids created equal? Lipids Health Dis 2009;8(1):33.
[366] Meyer BJ, Mann NJ, Lewis JL, et al. Dietary intakes and food sources of omega-6 and omega-3 polyunsaturated fatty acids. Lipids 2003;38:391–8.
[367] Enig MG Know your fats. Weston A. Price Foundation; 2008. Available from: http://www.westonaprice.org/know-your-fats.html.
[368] Molendi-Coste O, Legry V, Leclercq I. Why and how meet n-3 PUFA dietary recommendations? Gastroenterol Res Pract 2011;2011:1–11.
[369] Burdge G. α-Linolenic acid metabolism in men and women: nutritional and biological implications. Curr Opin Clin Nutr Metab Care 2004;7(2):137–44.
[370] Stevens LJ, Zentall SS, Deck JL, et al. Essential fatty acid metabolism in boys with attention-deficit hyperactivity disorder. Am J Clin Nutr 1995;62:761–8.
[371] Swanson D, Block R, Mousa S. Omega-3 fatty acids EPA and DHA: health benefits throughout life. Adv Nutr 2012;3(1):1–7.
[372] Lord RS, Bralley JA. Laboratory evaluations for integrative and functional medicine: fatty acids. Duluth, GA: Metametrix Institute; 2008.
[373] Dansinger M. Ban trans fats in 2007. Medgenmed 2006;8:58.
[374] Caramia G. Omega-3: from cod-liver oil to nutrigenomics. Minerva Pediatr 2008;60:443–55.
[375] Gerberding JL. Safer fats for healthier hearts: the case for eliminating dietary artificial trans fat intake. Ann Intern Med 2009;151:137–8.
[376] Bu SY, Mashek DG. Trans fats: foods, facts, and biology. Minn Med 2008;91:41–4.
[377] Destaillats F, Moulin J, Bezelgues JB. Letter to the editor: healthy alternatives to trans fats. Nutr Metab (Lond) 2007;4:10.
[378] Kummerow FA. The negative effects of hydrogenated trans fats and what to do about them. Atherosclerosis 2009;205(2):458–65.

8

Nutritional medicine (dietary)

Lisa Costa Bir

FOOD AS MEDICINE

INTRODUCTION

The concept of food as medicine, for both prophylactic and therapeutic purposes, can be traced back to the Hippocratic Corpus of Ancient Greece[1] where the idea of food as medicine and its importance is discussed. The idea that food can be used medicinally has always formed an integral part of naturopathic treatment philosophy. Early texts describe the importance of individuals understanding the curative powers of food, with Hippocrates stating 'He who does not know food — how can he cure the disease of man?[2] as well as perhaps his most mentioned quote 'Let food be thy medicine, and medicine be thy food', a direct reference to the understanding and benefits of nutritional therapy, both for prevention and cure of disease.

The naturopathic holistic approach to nutritional therapy is centred on consumption of whole, natural and minimally processed foods, with the understanding that they protect against disease, while more heavily refined and processed foods, depleted of nutrients, may promote disease. Naturopaths seek to impart the wisdom that food provides a medium to influence the vital force, enabling the body's inherent ability to heal itself when the correct tools, for example healthy diet, are provided.

The use of food as medicine is highly sophisticated, with components in food displaying the ability to target receptor sites in the body, exerting physiological benefits to reduce the risk of chronic diseases such as cardiovascular disease (CVD) and osteoporosis. Diet-based nutritional therapy using wholefoods provides not only energy, essential nutrients and phytochemicals but also safe and effective preventive interventions that can be used to complement allopathic recommendations. A reduction in side effects as well as improved treatment outcomes for the patient may be seen when combining medicinal foods with conventional therapy. This can be seen with the use of pantry staples such as ginger root and honey, both of which have been shown to reduce the side effects associated with cancer,[3,4] thus improving quality of life for the patient.

Other benefits of using food as medicine include the relatively low cost, easy availability, fewer side effects and lack of resistance to synthetic antibiotics. There is also the immediate benefit to the patient: empowerment by being an active participant in their own healing through cooking and food selection while the naturopath works as a facilitator to educate and empower them not only about what to eat but also about other factors including behaviours around food. Contemporary research examining nutrition interventions highlights the importance of education, with studies showing that food education increases knowledge of nutrition leading to positive and long-lasting changes in nutrition-related behaviour.[5]

Though dietary guidelines that detail ideal recommended daily intakes, kilojoule intakes and proportions exist, chronic disease rates are higher than ever in the West,[6] perhaps due to the current reductionist approach to nutrition. While this reductionist approach has both pros and cons, the naturopathic focus on nutrition encompasses both reductionist and holistic perspectives, integrating empirical and scientific evidence. Using the Western reductionist framework, holistic nutritional therapy examines cause and effect but interweaves a holistic approach influenced by integrating philosophies from traditional Eastern medicine (such as Ayurveda and traditional Chinese medicine) which consider the whole person, including spiritual and physical needs. This allows a move away from the ideas that food is something that merely supplies energy and that food can be reduced to its macronutrient component, for example a 'carb' or 'protein'. Food provides all these things and more. The naturopath seeks to understand the social and cultural factors influencing dietary choices and behaviours while acknowledging that the act of eating is an opportunity for enjoyment and nourishment. Clearly, the practitioner must ensure the diet meets psychological as well as physical needs. Building upon this idea, we can see that the naturopathic nutritionist does more than educate the patient on macronutrient composition; they provide counselling around food and lifestyle habits such as food selection and diversity and examine factors such as constitution, behaviour, seasonality, affordability, availability and environment as influences affecting the patient and their diet.

In contemporary times, interest in Hippocrates' philosophy that diet is a source of medicine has been renewed. This is highlighted by the example of fermented foods. Fermented foods were traditionally a well-established part of the human diet for thousands of years but use and knowledge of them had declined considerably until recently. An appreciation for fermented foods has once again grown, in part due to researchers gaining an understanding of their underlying microbial functionality and ability to reduce disease. As a result, many fermented foods such as sauerkraut, kefir and kim chi that were once resigned to grandma's kitchen are now available in the mainstream environment and may be recommended as part of a patient's treatment protocol.

The importance of how a wholefood diet is vital to health is highlighted by epidemiological and clinical studies that examine the role of dietary and disease prevention. Studies on specific dietary patterns such as a plant-based diet can be associated with reduced rates of cardiovascular disease,[7] while numerous studies justify the protective role of diets rich in fruits and vegetables in disease prevention. A 2016 study showed that low fruit and vegetable consumption was inversely related to all-cause mortality in a large Australian cohort,[8] a sobering fact since diet is a modifiable risk factor for many diseases.

Sustainability

Truly holistic nutrition considers more than what we consume, understanding the importance of the interaction between ourselves and our environment. The naturopathic nutritionist also seeks to impart respect for the environment itself, considering the environment in which the food is grown, animal welfare and food miles. In keeping with these principles seasonal produce that is pesticide free and not genetically modified is advocated in an attempt to reduce exposure to harmful substances and promote environmental sustainability. And the importance of food processing methods in relation to health cannot be forgotten. Brazil provides an example of the growing interest in this area since it has recently included recommendations on food processing in its dietary guidelines, suggesting a growing understanding of the importance of not just nutritional composition on overall health and wellbeing but also of food preparation methods.[9]

Supplements versus wholefoods

While supplements are often required, the naturopathic practitioner understands that food-based treatment should form first-line options, as supplements cannot replace the foundations of a healthy diet. Although therapeutic amounts of certain nutrients may not be obtainable through diet alone and may at times be required in supplement form, a large body of scientific evidence suggests that the intake of foods in their whole state is more beneficial than supplements in isolation because of the synergistic effects of other active components within the wholefood. The combined effect of these phytochemicals and nutrients is deemed to be far more beneficial than the effect of any isolated compound. This is seen with the example of tomatoes: current research suggests that tomato-based foods used as a first-line approach to cardiovascular health are superior to supplementation with lycopene, the active constituent found within tomatoes.[10] Similarly in mice, kiwifruit in wholefood form was shown to be a better delivery vehicle for restoring depleted vitamin C tissue levels than supplemental vitamin C.[11] Clearly, as eloquently noted by Rodrigo et al (2014),[12] nature provides synergy amongst substances, something that scientists cannot always concoct in a pill.

The resurgence in interest in the concept of food as medicine has led to more research being conducted to confirm the beneficial effects of the traditional use of many foods. Below is a summary of current research using food as medicine.

AVOCADO (*PERSEA AMERICANA*)

Native to Mexico, the avocado is a single seed berry that differs from most of the other commonly consumed fruits in the West in that it is low in sugar and high in fat, in particular monounsaturated fats (MUFAs). Avocados contain optimal quantities of fibre, both soluble (30%) and insoluble (70%),[13] as well as folate and fat-soluble antioxidants such as carotenoids and vitamin E. The high fat content of avocados allows for greater absorption of some other lipophilic phytochemicals within the avocado as well as from other foods consumed with the avocado.

Adding 150 g of avocado (approximately one avocado or 24 g of avocado oil) to a salad has been shown to improve absorption of carotenoids by 5–15 times.[14] Alpha carotene, beta-carotene and lutein absorption were all enhanced compared to intake of an avocado-free salad. Similarly, consuming avocado in combination with tomato salsa has been shown to increase lycopene and beta-carotene levels in humans compared to when salsa is consumed alone.[15]

Applying this clinically, the naturopath could use food as medicine principles by recommending avocado be combined with a tomato-based salsa to a patient wanting to reduce the risk of prostate cancer. Combining avocado with salsa would increase absorption of lycopene, reducing cancer risk, since dietary lycopene has been shown to decrease prostate cancer risk.[16] Food as medicine principles could also be used for a patient with macular degeneration. Adding avocado to their lunchtime salad or sandwich would increase absorption of lutein; lutein has been shown to reduce macular degeneration.

Avocados for transitional feeding

Avocados are an excellent first food for infant transitional feeding because of their wide array of nutrients (see Table 8.1). In particular, they are a rich source of oleic acid, a monounsaturated fatty acid found abundantly in breast milk.[17] The high fat content of avocados makes them an ideal food, since high fats are required for adequate brain development as well as for energy to support rapid growth. Additionally, the high fibre content of avocado has been hypothesised to be useful for the infant gut as a possible prebiotic source for the developing microbiota.[18]

Avocado and satiety

Because of their high fat content, avocados may mistakenly be avoided, particularly when it comes to weight loss.

TABLE 8.1 One half (68 g) of a Hass avocado contains

Nutrients	Quantity
Fibre	4.6 g
Sugar	0.2 g
Potassium	345 mg
Sodium	5.5 mg
Magnesium	19.5 mg
Vitamin A	43 micrograms
Vitamin C	6 mg
Vitamin E	1.3 mg
Vitamin K	14 micrograms
Folate	60 micrograms
Choline	10 mg
Lutein/zeaxanthin	185 micrograms
Phytosterols	75 mg

Adapted from Dreher ML, Davenport AJ. Hass avocado composition and potential health effects. Crit Rev Food Sci Nutr 2013; 53(7):738–750.

Conversely, research suggests that avocados appear to have similar effects on weight control as low fat fruits and vegetables, possibly in part due to their combination of high fibre, high fat and water content (the fresh pulp equates to 72% of water). A randomised controlled single-blind study observed that the addition of an avocado at lunch increased satiety and decreased desire to eat compared with the alternative control meal.[19] It is known that high fat meals take longer to digest and this in combination with fibre may help to keep blood sugar levels stable for longer, thus reducing the desire to eat.

RED BEETROOT (*BETA VULGARIS RUBRA*)

Beetroot has been used since Roman times as a medicinal food. It is an exceptional source of many nutrients and phytochemicals including ascorbic acid, carotenoids, phenolic acids, flavonoids as well as highly antioxidant and anti-inflammatory constituents known as betalains, which are responsible for the bright colour of beetroot.[20] Modern science reveals beetroot as a rich source of inorganic nitrate, the reduction of which provides a natural means of generating nitric oxide (NO) availability in the body. This has led to beetroot being studied for its therapeutic efficacy in conditions characterised by diminished NO bioavailability.

Hypertension

A 2013 systematic review and meta-analysis observed that consumption of beetroot juice was associated with a reduction in hypertension.[21] Duration of the interventions with beetroot juice ranged from 2 hours to 15 days with participants consuming approximately 140 to 500 mL/day. The daily amount of nitrate in the beetroot juice consumed varied between 5.1 and 45 mmol/dose (321–2790 mg). Greater changes were noted in systolic blood pressure (BP) (−4.5 mmHg) than diastolic BP (−1.1 mmHg). A more recent systematic review and meta-analysis also observed an improvement in vascular and endothelial function following consumption of beetroot juice.[22] Duration of treatment with beetroot juice was between 1.5 hours and 28 days. Of note, most of the studies were undertaken in young, healthy men, thus further studies need to be undertaken in hypertensive individuals and/or older adults, particularly as research suggests that vascular responsiveness to inorganic nitrate may be modified by mechanisms of vascular ageing, limiting the ability to convert inorganic nitrate into NO.[23]

The results from the latter studies provide positive connotations for guidelines in improving patient outcomes. A systolic BP reduction of at least 5 mmHg has been suggested to decrease the risk of mortality due to stroke by 14% and mortality from cardiovascular diseases by 9%.[24] Thus including a daily beetroot juice in the diet of patients at risk of CVD would appear prudent and a way in which to use food as medicine.

Exercise performance

Beetroot juice has been shown to improve exercise performance in healthy individuals in a systematic review and meta-analysis.[25] Consumption of beetroot juice has been shown to reduce time to exhaustion significantly. Performance for time trials and graded exercise tests improved though these outcomes were not statistically significant; however, as noted by the researchers, despite not reaching statistical significance, any positive effect on time trial or graded exercise performance may be useful to an elite sports person wishing to gain a competitive edge. Nitrates in beetroot appear to increase exercise capacity, reduce oxygen cost of exercise, enhance exercise tolerance and performance and improve muscle contractibility.[26] Acute consumption of beetroot juice (150–250 mL) following exercise has also been shown to reduce muscle soreness induced by eccentric exercise, suggesting beetroot may also function as an anti-inflammatory.[27]

BITTER MELON (*MOMORDICA CHARANTIA*)

Bitter gourd/melon (also known as karela) is a vegetable with a distinctly bitter taste belonging to the Cucurbitaceae family. It contains a range of constituents including charantin, vicine and polypeptide-p that have been identified as having antidiabetic effects, while the non-toxic alkaloid momordicine provides a bitter flavour.

Diabetes

A number of animal studies have documented the antidiabetic and hypoglycaemic effects of *Momordica charantia* with multiple mechanisms reported for its antidiabetic potential including the ability to:

- Transport glucose into the cells
- Repair damaged β-cells and increase secretion and sensitivity of insulin in the pancreas
- Increase glucose uptake in adipocytes and skeletal muscle

- Inhibit the absorption of glucose by inhibiting glucosidase
- Suppress the activity of disaccharidases in the intestine.[28]

A Cochrane Review found insufficient evidence to recommend *Momordica charantia* for type 2 diabetes mellitus;[29] however, this nutritive vegetable is the most popular food used for management of diabetes by people from India, China and Malaysia.[30] A small preliminary trial investigating bitter gourd in supplement form observed a decrease in the risk of metabolic syndrome at the end of 3 months.[31] Bitter gourd is found in many fruit and vegetable shops in Australia as well as in Asian grocers. When used traditionally in the diet, bitter gourd is cooked in a curry or the fruits may be dehydrated or pickled. Blanching or soaking in salt water before cooking will reduce the bitter taste.[32]

BLUEBERRIES (*VACCINIUM* SPP.)

Blueberries are a rich source of antioxidants, in particular polyphenols known as anthocyanins. These are found mostly concentrated in the outer layer of the fruit and are responsible for the bright pigments seen in berries.[33]

Cognitive function

Anthocyanins exert significant anti-inflammatory and antioxidant potential, visible in the brain. This has important consequences, particularly as the brain is vulnerable to oxidative stress and inflammation, both of which have been shown to influence age-related decline. Following ingestion, rat studies reveal the presence of anthocyanins in areas of the brain involved with learning and memory retention such as the neocortex and the hippocampus; the presence of anthocyanins in the brain correlates with improved cognition.[34] As well as their antioxidant and anti-inflammatory effects, blueberries have been shown to have other neuroprotective actions in the brain including the ability to enhance neuronal signalling, buffer excess calcium, improve neurogenesis and increase extracellular signal-regulated kinase activation and insulin-like growth factor-1, the latter two of which are associated with increased spatial memory.[35]

Dietary intake of berries in animal studies is associated with less cognitive decline and thus blueberries have also been studied therapeutically for reducing dementia and Alzheimer's disease-related symptomatology in humans. Over 3 months consumption of 6–9 mL/kg of wild blueberry juice for 12 weeks in nine elderly participants with early memory decline was shown to improve memory function, in particular paired associate learning and word list recall.[36] An additional positive outcome was an improvement in mood; inflammation is known to play a role in depression, thus an anti-inflammatory mechanism is one way in which blueberry consumption may have reduced depressive symptoms. A more recent study examined 6 weeks of daily consumption of 2 cups of frozen blueberries on functional mobility in older adults.[37] Improvements were seen in a number of measures such as usual gait speed and number of step errors during single-task adaptive gait, leading to the hypothesis that blueberry supplementation may provide an effective countermeasure to age-related decline in functional mobility. These positive results suggest that many dysfunctions associated with ageing could be partially ameliorated by supplementing the diet with blueberries.

BROCCOLI SPROUTS

Young broccoli sprouts contain a range of beneficial constituents including vitamin C, carotenoids, flavonoids as well as several glucosinolates including glucobrassicin and glucoraphanin.[38] Broccoli sprouts contain higher levels of glucosinolates and display higher upregulation of phase II enzyme activity compared to adult cruciferous vegetables,[39] making them a highly functional food.

Sulforaphane is an isothiocyanate and hydrolysis product of glucoraphanin via the enzyme myrosinase. In healthy adults, absorption of sulforaphane has been shown to be sevenfold higher than when consuming the equivalent amount of broccoli sprout powders due to the fact that the powders often do not contain active myrosinase, which is required for the formation of sulforaphane.[40]

Immunity and detoxification

Broccoli sprouts have been shown to reduce viral replication and inflammation in the nasal fluid of smokers inoculated with influenza[41] as well as to enhance bodily antiviral defence responses in non-smoking healthy volunteers.[42] A beverage containing broccoli sprouts was also shown to enhance detoxification of some airborne pollutants in a randomised clinical trial conducted in China,[43] while a recent study showed the ability of sulforaphane to suppress the nasal inflammatory response when exposed to diesel exhaust particles.[44] The dose of sulforaphane used in the latter study was equivalent to consumption of 100–200 g of broccoli, highlighting the potential preventive and therapeutic potential of broccoli or broccoli sprouts for reducing the impact of particulate pollution on allergic disease and asthma.

CHIA SEEDS (*SALVIA HISPANICA*)

Chia seeds are native to Central and South America, however they are now cultivated in other areas of the world including Australia. Chia seed is made up of fats (30–33%), carbohydrates (26–41%) and protein (15–25%) as well as high quantities of fibre and antioxidants.[45] Chia seed contains optimal levels of the essential fatty acid (EFA), alpha-linolenic acid (ALA; 18:3*n*-3). ALA can be metabolically converted to long-chain *n*-3 polyunsaturated fatty acids (PUFAs) including eicosapentaenoic acid (EPA) and docosahexaenoic acid (DHA); however, enzymatic conversion of ALA to EPA and particularly DHA has been suggested to be inefficient.[46]

Anti-inflammatory

In spite of its long history of traditional use as a medicinal food, and its popularity today, there have been relatively few trials conducted in humans assessing the health benefits of chia seeds. A 7-week trial in ten postmenopausal women observed an increase in polyunsaturated fatty acid content particularly in eicosapentaenoic acid (EPA) following supplementation with 25 g milled chia daily,[47] however no increases were seen in DHA levels.

Pregnant women who received 16 mL chia oil daily from the third trimester of pregnancy until the first 6 months of nursing were shown to have significantly increased milk content of ALA during the 6 months of nursing, as well as an increase in DHA, though the latter was only apparent during the first 3 months of nursing.[48] It has been proposed that consuming ALA-rich foods in high amounts may result in transformation to DHA in women who are low in DHA. This study has positive implications for individuals who choose not to consume fish and may be missing out on DHA, as well as for their infants, for whom DHA is essential for adequate brain development.

CINNAMON (*CINNAMOMUM* SPP.)

Cinnamon is a sweet woody bark of which there are more than 200 species. True or Ceylon cinnamon (*Cinnamomum verum*) (formerly *C. zeylanicum*) and Chinese cassia cinnamon (*Cinnamomum cassia*) are the most commonly used. Cinnamon is available in whole quill form (cinnamon sticks) or as a ground powder. Cinnamon contains a range of constituents which have been shown to increase insulin receptors and their substrates, promote insulin release, enhance insulin sensitivity, and increase insulin disposal and GLUT4 receptors, facilitating glucose entry into cells.[49]

Cinnamon has been demonstrated to be effective for its glycaemic effects in healthy and diabetic patients. A systematic review and meta-analysis involving six randomised controlled studies observed a significant decrease in mean HbA1c levels in people with type 2 diabetes;[50] however, in a meta-analysis of ten randomised controlled studies released slightly later, cinnamon intake of between 120 mg/d and 6 g/d for 4 to 18 weeks was shown to reduce levels of fasting plasma glucose, though no significant effects were observed with haemoglobin A1c levels.

Consumption of cinnamon tea in healthy individuals has been shown to slightly decrease postprandial blood glucose levels,[51] suggesting improved glycaemic control. The study used cinnamon sticks (*Cinnamomum burmannii* bark) soaked in water for 24 hours, which were then heated for 1 hour, cooled and filtered; this method could be easily replicated by patients. Six grams of cinnamon added to a rice pudding was shown to moderate postprandial glucose response in normal weight and obese adults,[52] suggesting the usefulness of adding cinnamon to high GI meals in an attempt to help regulate blood sugar.

DATES (*PHOENIX DACTYLIFERA*)

Dates have been used as a medicinal food for more than 6000 years and more than 2000 different varieties exist.[53] Dates are rich in carbohydrates (total sugars, 44–88%) as well as fibre (6.4–11.5%).[54]

Dates for improved labour and delivery

In the first study of its kind, consumption of dates in the final month of pregnancy has been shown to improve labour and delivery outcomes.[55] Women in their last month of pregnancy were instructed to consume six dates per day (totalling 60–67 g of fruit) until the onset of their labour pains, whereas the placebo group were asked to abstain from consuming dates for the period of the study. Date consumers experienced greater cervical dilation than their non-date-consuming counterparts, as well as a significantly higher rate of intact membranes (83% versus 60%).

Consumption of dates also resulted in a significant reduction in induction compared to non-date consumers, with lower use of prostin and oxytocin (28% versus 47%); higher rates of spontaneous labour were also recorded (96% versus 79%) for date consumers. The mean time for first stage of labour was also significantly lower for date consumers (510 minutes versus 906 minutes), a statistic that would convince most pregnant women to increase their consumption of date fruits.

FISH

Consumption of fish provides a range of nutrients, in particular n-3 long-chain PUFA (polyunsaturated fatty acid) (n-3 LC-PUFA), mainly EPA and DHA which are associated with a range of health benefits throughout the life span.

Cognition

A meta-analysis of 21 studies observed that dietary fish consumption at least once per week was associated with lower risk of cognitive dysfunction, in particular Alzheimer's disease and dementia.[56] Dietary consumption of baked or grilled fish at least once a week has been found to improve structural brain integrity in cognitively normal older adults.[57] Fish consumption was positively associated with larger grey matter volumes in the hippocampus, precuneus, posterior cingulate and orbitofrontal cortex. Interestingly, these results were found to be independent of omega-3 fatty acids, suggesting that other constituents within the fish may also be important.

Safety

While numerous health benefits have been associated with fish consumption, concerns have also been raised because of the presence of environmental pollutants such as heavy metals, polycyclic aromatic hydrocarbons, polychlorinated biphenyls (PCBs), polybrominated diphenyl ethers, dioxins, furans and chlorinated pesticides contained in seafood. While many still question whether we really still call fish a medicinal food, at this point the benefits of consuming it appear to outweigh the negatives.

FLAXSEED (*LINUM USITATISSIMUM*)

Flaxseed is a red-brown nutty seed that provides a rich dietary source of α-linolenic acid, phyto-oestrogenic lignans, as well as dietary fibre. Ground (milled) flaxseed added to the diet provides substantially more bioavailable α-linolenic acid and lignan metabolites than whole flaxseed, suggesting it is preferable for patients to consume ground flaxseed to obtain best possible therapeutic benefits.

Hormone regulation

Flaxseeds are used for their hormone-regulating actions. Enterolactone and enterodiol are lignans found in flaxseed that have been hypothesised to assist in preventing proliferation of tumours by inhibiting activation of nuclear factor kappa B (NFκB) and vascular endothelial growth factor (VEGF). A systematic review and meta-analysis examining efficacy of flaxseed on hot flushes, vaginal atrophy and oestrogen-dependent cancers in menopausal women found consumption of flaxseed assisted to reduce hot flush frequency and intensity, including night sweats. However, though clinically significant, the results were not statistically significant.[58]

In males with prostate cancer waiting to undergo radical prostatectomy, flaxseed consumption has been shown to reduce proliferation rates pre-surgery.[59] The men were assigned to either their usual (control) diet, flaxseed (30 g/d) low-fat diet, or flaxseed and low-fat diet for 30 days. Proliferation rates were significantly lower among men assigned to the flaxseed arms. However, no differences between apoptotic rate, median change in prostate-specific antigen (PSA) or median change in IGF-I were noted. Azrad et al[60] also noted a reduction in tumour proliferation in males with localised prostate cancer consuming 30 g of flaxseed for 30 days prior to surgery. However, once again, the results while clinically significant were not statistically significant.

Hypertension

A systematic review and meta-analysis of 11 studies involving 1004 participants observed that consumption of 30–50 g of flaxseed per day resulted in a small but significant reduction in blood pressure. It is important to note that even a reduction of 2 mmHg in systolic blood pressure is associated with a lower stroke mortality of 10%.[61] While the majority of studies were all conducted in normotensive or pre-hypertensive populations, it is hypothesised that the same results would be applicable to hypertensive individuals.

GARLIC (*ALLIUM SATIVUM*)

Botanically *Allium sativum* is a member of the Lillaceae family. Its use as a medicinal food for both prevention and management of disease is seen worldwide in many cultures. Garlic contains a range of vitamins and minerals; however, the therapeutic properties of garlic have been largely described as being due to the presence of organosulfur compounds (OSCs). Allicin (diallyl thiosulfinate) is the main sulfur compound responsible for the flavour of garlic and is also thought to be responsible for many of the biological functions of garlic. When garlic is chopped or crushed, the enzyme allinase is activated and produces allicin from alliin. Allicin is converted into other OSCs, including ajoene which is largely responsible for the potent antiviral activity of garlic.

Garlic displays many mechanisms of action including demonstrated anticoagulant, antioxidant, anticarcinogenic, anti-inflammatory, antimutagenic, antifungal, antiviral, antibiotic, anthelmintic, hypolipideamic, antihypertensive, enhanced detoxification, hepatoprotective and immunomodulatory activity. In spite of its many actions, there is unfortunately a lack of high-quality studies detailing the benefits of garlic as a medicinal food, with much of the positive research undertaken on garlic supplements. Despite the lack of evidence-based research on garlic in its food form, the benefits observed with garlic supplements along with traditional recommendations provide a good rationale for fresh garlic to be recommended in the diet.

TABLE 8.2 Dosage for various forms of ginger equivalent to 1000 mg standardised ginger

1 tsp (5 g) of freshly grated ginger rhizome
2 mL of ginger liquid extract
2 tsp (10 mL) of ginger syrup
4 cups (237 mL) of pre-packed ginger tea
2 mL of ginger liquid extract
4 cups of fresh ginger tea (prepared by infusing ½ tsp of freshly grated ginger root in hot water for 5–10 minutes)
1 cup of ginger ale (made with real ginger)
2 pieces of crystallised ginger, each 25 mm square, 6 mm thick

Adapted from Ding M, Leach M, Bradley H. The effectiveness and safety of ginger for pregnancy-induced nausea and vomiting: a systematic review. Women Birth Mar 2013; 26(1):e26–e30. doi: 10.1016/j.wombi.2012.08.001. Epub 201

GINGER (*ZINGIBER OFFICINALE*)

The use of ginger as a medicinal food can be traced back thousands of years where it featured dominantly in both Ayurvedic and traditional Chinese medicine. Ginger contains pungent constituents including gingerols, shogaols, zingerone and paradol which have been shown to exert a number of effects including gastrointestinal, antioxidant, analgesic and anti-inflammatory. As a medicinal food it may appear in numerous forms, including fresh, dried, pickled, preserved, crystallised, candied, powdered, ground or liquid form as a tea or ginger syrup or beer. (See Table 8.2.)

Dysmenorrhoea

A meta-analysis involving six trials suggested that ginger may be effective in reducing dysmenorrhoea in women.[62] While there are many methodological issues associated with the studies, ginger was found to be more effective than a placebo at reducing the severity of crampy, colicky pain and was found to be just as good as NSAIDs. The daily dose of powdered ginger ranged from 750 mg to 2000 mg, with the most common duration and timing of ginger treatment being in the first 3 days of menstruation, though one study started dietary supplementation of ginger 2 days before menstruation began. Increased production of prostaglandins derived from cyclooxygenase-2 (COX-2) and other inflammatory mediators is associated with excessive contractions of the uterus which result in pain and cramping; it is thought that the ability of ginger to inhibit COX-2 and other inflammatory mediators is in part responsible for the beneficial effects seen in reducing dysmenorrhoea.

Chronic pain

As well as its anti-inflammatory properties, a systematic review suggests ginger also displays analgesic properties that make it a useful tool for pain management.[63] Use of ginger was found to reduce delayed muscle onset soreness as well as reduce pain associated with osteoarthritis. A further meta-analysis also observed less disability in participants with osteoarthritis using ginger.[64]

Nausea and vomiting associated with pregnancy and chemotherapy

Ginger displays antiemetic properties whereby it increases tone and motility in the gut due to anticholinenergic and anti-serotonergic actions. A systematic review and meta-analysis of ginger extracts for nausea and vomiting associated with pregnancy observed a reduction in severity of nausea but did not notice a change in vomiting episodes.[65] The majority of studies suggest a daily dosage of <1500 mg for nausea relief. Adverse effects with use of ginger are mild and infrequent.

Chemotherapy-induced nausea and vomiting (CINV) is a common symptom experienced by patients receiving cancer treatment. A recent study undertaken on breast cancer participants observed that oral ginger taken for the first 3 days of the chemotherapy cycle reduced nausea severity and the number of vomiting episodes compared to the control.[66] However, a systematic review of seven studies found mixed results for ginger as an anti-CINV treatment in patients receiving chemotherapy, with three demonstrating a positive effect, two in favour but with caveats, and two showing no significant benefits.[67]

GREEN TEA (*CAMELLIA SINENSIS*)

Camellia sinensis has been consumed as a medicinal tea in Asia for thousands of years. It contains a range of antioxidant phenolics including epigallocatechin-3-gallate (EGCG) which appears to have an antioxidant activity about 25–100 times more potent than that of vitamins C and E.[68] In vitro studies reveal that green tea polyphenols exert a number of anticancer effects including acting as antioxidants and blocking histone deacetylases (HDAC) which are found in large amounts in cancer cells.

Green tea and the prostate

In an exploratory, open label, phase II trial of 113 men diagnosed with prostate cancer, randomised to consume six cups daily of brewed green tea, black tea or water (control) prior to radical prostatectomy (RP), researchers observed bioavailable tea polyphenols in prostate tissue samples from 32 of 34 men and evidence of a profound systemic antioxidant effect in those consuming green tea but not in the other groups.[69] Using tissue analysis following radical prostatectomy as an end point, green tea consumption resulted in a reduction of the prostate cancer tumour marker NFkB. A small but statistically significant decrease in serum prostate-specific antigen (PSA) levels was also seen in the green tea consumers only. Green tea shows benefit over black tea as a means to assist in reducing oxidative stress in the prostate region. Low-caffeine varieties may be preferable for the naturopathic patient due to the high quantity required.

HONEY

Honey has been used since ancient times for the treatment of several diseases both internally as well as topically.

Radiation-induced oral mucositis

Topical application of honey has been shown to protect from the effects of radiation-induced oral mucositis formation, a complication of radiation therapy for head and neck cancers. Oral mucositis manifests as inflammation of the mucous membranes of the mouth, with ulceration, pain, and difficulty swallowing, eating and drinking, as well as a reduction in quality of life. Destruction of the mucous membranes often results in bacterial and fungal infections which may cause further complications.

Honey has wound healing, antimicrobial and anti-inflammatory properties that favourably influence the positive therapeutic effects seen in reducing complications of radiation-induced oral mucositis. A meta-analysis of nine studies involving 476 participants observed lower incidence and severity of oral mucositis as well as later onset in participants consuming honey compared with the control groups.[70] Incidence of weight loss was also significantly less in the honey group, important since weight loss is a predictor of poorer outcomes.[71]

The addition of turmeric, also known for its anti-inflammatory and antimicrobial properties, to the honey mixture has been shown to be helpful.[72] Participants undergoing radiotherapy applying honey and turmeric powder 5 minutes before and after each treatment also observed favourable results. The most common protocol used for the majority of studies in terms of honey administration was 20 mL of pure honey applied topically 3 times per day (before, immediately after and several hours after therapy) throughout the course of radiation therapy. A number of studies used Manuka honey and other honeys including thyme honey and Dabur honey were also used.

KIWIFRUIT (*ACTINIDIA DELICIOSA*)

Kiwifruit are berries of the woody vine *Actinidia*. They are rich in nutrients, particularly vitamin C, potassium and vitamin E as well as fibre and carotenoids such as beta-carotene, lutein and zeaxanthin.[73] Kiwifruit come in a number of varieties, the most common being *Actinidia deliciosa* (Hayward kiwis — green kiwifruit) as well as *Actinidia chinensis* (the gold variety).

Cardiovascular health

In men with high cholesterol levels consumption of two green kiwifruits per day in combination with a healthy diet has been shown to improve high-density lipoprotein (HDL) cholesterol and decrease total cholesterol compared to consuming a healthy diet alone.[74] Consuming two green kiwifruits per day was also shown to reduce cholesterol as well as improve markers of inflammation in hypercholesterolaemic male patients with moderate inflammation (observed via elevated levels of C-reactive protein, CRP).[75] A cross-sectional study observed that consuming at least one kiwifruit per week was associated with lower plasma concentrations of fibrinogen and a favourable lipid profile in the context of consuming a normal diet.[76] Elevated fibrinogen levels are associated with an increased risk of adverse cardiovascular events.

Constipation

Consumption of two Hayward green kiwifruits per day for 4 weeks in patients with irritable bowel syndrome with constipation has been shown to increase defecation frequency and decrease colon transit time, resulting in improved bowel function.[77] This study confirms older studies that showed kiwifruit reduced constipation and decreased laxative use.[78] While the dietary fibre is one mechanism of action related to its laxative action, kiwifruit also contains a proteolytic enzyme of thiol proteases, known as actinidin, which facilitates laxation via stimulating receptors in the colon, increasing motility.

MUSHROOMS

Mushrooms are fungi that have enjoyed a long history of use as a food. The ancient Greeks are said to have used them for strength in battle, while the Romans believed they were the 'Food of the Gods.[79]

Cancer protection

A meta-analysis of observational studies has suggested that dietary consumption of mushrooms is associated with a reduced risk of breast cancer.[80] Polysaccharides, in particular beta-glucans, within mushrooms exert immune-modulating actions by enhancing innate and cell-mediated immune responses as well as displaying anti-tumour actions.

Additionally, *Agaricus bisporus* (white button mushrooms) have been shown to protect against breast cancer in vitro due to their ability to suppress the aromatase enzyme.[81] Other edible mushrooms such as *Lentinus edodes* (shiitake) are associated with health benefits and have a long history of use; however, there is a paucity of research available investigating their dietary use.

Source of vitamin D

White button mushrooms are typically grown in the dark and thus contain negligible amounts of vitamin D but mushrooms that have been exposed to the sun or UV radiation have been found to be an excellent source of vitamin D. Mushrooms contain ergoserol, a sterol which can be converted to vitamin D under the presence of UV irradiation.[82] A randomised placebo controlled study in adults with 25(OH)D levels below 20 ng/mL observed that serum 25(OH)D levels increased significantly when consuming vitamin D-enriched mushrooms and that consuming vitamin D from UV-irradiated mushrooms was equally as effective at raising 25(OH)D levels as ingesting the same amount of vitamin D as a supplement.[83]

NUTS

Nuts are nutrient dense and provide high-quality fats, protein, fibre, minerals, tocopherols, phytosterols and other phenolic compounds.[84] Their consumption can be traced back as far as 7000 BC. Consumption of nuts in countries with a Mediterranean-style diet has been estimated to be twice that of those with an American diet.[85]

Cardiovascular disease

A number of studies have investigated the association between nut consumption and risk of coronary artery disease (CAD). In a number of meta-analyses high consumption of nuts appears to decrease the risk of CAD.[86,87] Risk of CAD was found to decrease by 5–10% for every increase in the serving of nuts per week. A protective effect for CAD was found when more than two servings of nuts were consumed per week. A further systematic review and meta-analysis also observed that consumption was associated with lower total cholesterol, low-density lipoprotein (LDL) cholesterol, triglycerides and ApoB (the latter of which was seen more strongly in diabetic populations than healthy groups); the major determinant of cholesterol lowering appeared to be related to the nut dose rather than nut type.[88] In spite of the large number of studies undertaken examining the health benefits of nuts, as well as the positive results obtained, a Cochrane Review determined there to be a lack of evidence for the effects of nut consumption on CVD clinical events in primary prevention.[89]

Glycaemic control

A number of reviews have also observed a positive relationship between nut consumption and better glycaemic control.[90] A systematic review of twelve trials found that diets containing a median dose of 56 g/d of nuts significantly lowered HbA1c and fasting glucose levels compared with control diets.[91]

Prebiotic

Nuts are rich in fibre as well as other components suggesting that they could be a useful prebiotic to modify the gut microbiota. Healthy participants consuming a daily dose of roasted almonds (56 g) and almond skins (10 g) for 6 weeks experienced a significant increase in faecal *Bifidobacterium* spp. and *Lactobacillus* spp. while the growth of pathogenic *Clostridium perfringens* was significantly repressed.[92] Interestingly, consumption of pistachio nuts has been shown to have a greater effect on gut microbiota composition than almond consumption.[93] Participants consuming pistachios experienced an increase in the number of potentially beneficial butyrate-producing bacteria compared to those consuming almonds, suggesting that pistachios may be a superior choice for people wanting to transform the composition of their microbiota.

OATS (*AVENA SATIVA*)

Oats have been farmed for more than 2000 years, though one of the earliest references to their use comes from Pliny who described use of oat porridges by Germanic tribes in

TABLE 8.3 Oats can be classified according to their degree of processing

Groats	Hulled oats from which the hard unpalatable outer hull is removed from the whole oat grain, keeping the outer bran layer intact.
Steel-cut oats/pinhead oats	Made by passing groats through steel cutters which chop each one into three or four pieces. Very nutritious as they contain the whole grain including the oat bran.
Rolled oats	Prepared by steaming groats and flattening them with a roller.
Instant oats	Made in a similar way to rolled oats, except they are steamed for a longer period and rolled more thinly.

Singh R, De S, Belkheir A. *Avena sativa* (oat), a potential neutraceutical and therapeutic agent: an overview. Crit Rev Food Sci Nutr 2013; 53(2):126–144. doi: 10.1080/10408398.2010.526725. Reprinted by permission of the publisher (Taylor & Francis Ltd, http://www.tandfonline.com).

the 1st century (CE) in his *Encyclopedia Naturalis Historia*. Oats are regarded both as a food and medicine. They are high in soluble fibre (10.3/100 g)[94] including β-glucan, a polysaccharide with many of the health benefits associated with oat consumption. (See Table 8.3.)

Cholesterol

Oat consumption is believed to lower cholesterol with a meta-analysis involving 28 randomised clinical trials observing that adding ≥3 g oat beta glucans daily to the diet reduces LDL and total cholesterol by 0.25 mmol/L and 0.30 mmol/L, respectively, though no change was seen with regards to HDL cholesterol or triglycerides.[95] The analysis did not find that duration of oat consumption (range between 2–12 weeks) influenced the results. Oats appear to owe their cholesterol-lowering action in part to their beta-glucan content. Beta-glucans form a viscous mass in the small intestine, preventing reabsorption of bile salts and limiting intestinal absorption of dietary cholesterol, resulting in lower cholesterol levels.[96]

Glycaemic control

A number of studies have reported beneficial effects of oat consumption on people with poor glycaemic control. A systematic review and meta-analysis investigating oat intake in patients with type 2 diabetes found that consumption of oats reduced concentrations of glycosylated haemoglobin A1c, fasting blood glucose, total cholesterol and low-density lipoprotein cholesterol.[97] Consumption of oats significantly reduced the acute postprandial glucose and insulin responses compared with the control meal. β-glucan increases the viscosity of food, delaying gastric emptying and lengthening gut transit time, which slows absorption of carbohydrates, resulting in better glucose control for diabetic patients. An intake of 3 g or more per day of β-glucan is thought to be beneficial.

OLIVES (*OLEA EUROPAEA*)

The traditional Mediterranean diet is rich in olives, and their presence in the diet has been proposed to influence the positive health outcomes observed in this population group. Olives are a rich source of monounsaturated fats as well as antioxidants and the bitter-tasting phenolic glycoside oleuropein,[98] which has been identified as possessing a number of different beneficial properties including anti-inflammatory and antimicrobial activity.

Digestive

As olives mature, oleuropein content is reduced as a result enzymatic and chemical changes. Though their content is reduced compared to immature olives, green olives have been identified as still having noteworthy content of oleuropein, suggesting that from a naturopathic perspective they could be used as an aperitif or digestive to stimulate digestive juices prior or following a meal.[99] Black olives signify the presence of anthocyanin and levels of oleuropein are very low, in some cases zero, thus it is unlikely they exert any bitter action.

Anti-inflammatory

As well as their use for healthy digestive function, olives appear to possess powerful anti-inflammatory activity and may be a useful way of using food as medicine in the diet to protect from free radical damage. A clinical study in 25 healthy adults, albeit underpowered, observed that consumption of 12 green olives per day for 30 days resulted in a decrease in interleukin-6 and malondialdehyde, signifying a reduction in both inflammation and oxidative stress.[100] This is the first study of its kind and further studies are required to confirm these promising anti-inflammatory effects attributed to olives.

POMEGRANATE (*PUNICA GRANATUM*)

Pomegranates have been used as a medicinal food for centuries. They display potent anti-inflammatory properties, inhibiting arachidonic acid eicosanoid pathways as well antioxidant properties. Unbeknownst to many, pomegranate displays higher antioxidant activity than red wine or green tea, both of which are renowned for their ability to fight oxidative stress.[101] The main antioxidants in pomegranate juice are polyphenols including ellagitannins and anthocyanins.

Prostate cancer

Pomegranate juice has been shown to inhibit the growth of prostate cancer cells in vivo and in vitro where it has been shown to prevent angiogenesis and metastasis. In human clinical studies consumption of 236 mL pomegranate juice daily has been shown to result in a 12% decrease in cell proliferation and a 17% increase in apoptosis, as well as significant reductions in oxidative state in men with rising PSA after surgery or chemotherapy.[102] Mean PSA doubling time significantly increased with treatment from a mean of 15 months at baseline to 54 months post-treatment, with no patients developing metastases during the trial, leading the authors to suggest the potential of pomegranate juice for reduction of prostate cancer risk. It should be noted, however, that this study had no control group so it is difficult to interpret the findings and further studies are required.

PRUNES (*PRUNUS DOMESTICA*)

Prunes are dried plums. They are produced industrially by drying plums at 85–90°C for 18 hours.[103] Prunes contain high levels of phenols including flavonoids and anthocyanins.

Constipation

Traditionally prunes have been used for the management of constipation; modern research confirms this use, with a systematic review of four studies observing prune consumption to be more efficacious than psyllium, another commonly recommended nutritional for constipation.[104] The review found that in constipated subjects, 3 weeks supplementation with 100 g/d of prunes resulted in an improvement in both stool frequency and consistency, citing prunes to be an effective dietary tool for relief from constipation. Prunes contain 6 g of fibre/100 g and this fibre content may be one mechanism by which they exert their action. However, prunes also contain sorbitol and phenolic compounds which are poorly absorbed by the small intestine, creating an osmotic effect and increasing laxation.

It should be noted that there is a risk of aggravating symptoms of bloating and abdominal discomfort in patients with irritable bowel syndrome that is constipation predominant, as sorbitol can be rapidly fermented by colonic bacteria, causing luminal distension.[105] Additionally, since sorbitol is not FODMAPS friendly, prunes may also cause discomfort in this population group.

Bone health

A 2016 systematic review[106] observed that prunes may be a worthy addition to the diet for those wanting to reduce osteoporosis and osteopenia risk. In vitro and animal studies observed that prunes may reverse and prevent bone loss even at relatively low intakes.[107] Polyphenols within prunes appear to impede osteoclastogenesis, reducing osteoclast activity by downregulating activated T-cells, cytoplasmic 1 (NFATc1) and inflammatory mediators.[108]

Daily consumption of prunes in combination with calcium and vitamin D by postmenopausal women was shown to result in a decrease in serum levels used to measure bone turnover including bone-specific alkaline phosphatase and tartrate-resistant acid phosphatase-5b.[109] The women experienced increases in bone mineral density in the ulna and spine that was not seen in the placebo group consuming dried apple. A more recent study also observed similar benefits. Daily consumption of 50 g of dried plums (equivalent to 5–6 dried plums) for 6 months was shown to be as effective as 100 g of dried plums in preventing bone loss in older, osteopenic postmenopausal women, compared to the placebo group.[110] This is hypothesised to be due to the ability of dried plums to prevent bone resorption.

SOY (*GLYCINE MAX*)

Soy foods are rich in phytoestrogens including isoflavones such genistein, daidzein and glycitein. Isoflavone constituents within soy foods exhibit both oestrogen-dependent and independent properties that potentially inhibit the development of a number of hormone-related cancers such as breast cancer. Isoflavones mimic naturally occurring oestrogen, binding to oestrogen receptors and manifesting weak oestrogenic effects where required. Alternatively, isoflavones may also perform as naturally occurring selective oestrogen receptor modulators (SORMs) where, depending upon the tissue, they may exert oestrogen antagonistic effects, agonist effects or no effects at all.[111]

The notion that soy-containing foods may be a useful addition to the diet came to the attention of researchers who noted that in Japan, where soy consumption was high, the yearly rate of breast cancer was low at approximately 33 cases per 100 000 women.[112] Conversely, they noted that in Western European countries and the US, where dietary soy intake was low, breast cancer incidence was more than double, ranging from 80 to 100 per 100 000 women. The phyto-oestrogenic action of soy foods has led to it being studied for its role in a range of conditions including breast cancer, prostate cancer, perimenopause and osteoporosis.

Breast cancer

Epidemiological studies show positive results with reduced risk of breast cancer for population groups consuming high quantities of naturally derived soy products (tofu, soybeans, miso). However, as noted by Zhong,[113] these positive results seem to be seen primarily in Asian countries, not their Western counterparts, where frequently little or no effect is observed. This variation in results has been hypothesised to be due to a number of factors discussed in the following section.

Are all soy foods created equal?

The answer to this question is 'No'. The quality of soy products consumed in the West is vastly different to that of Asian countries. The majority of soy products in the West come from second-line soy products that are heavily processed (e.g. soy yoghurt, soybean oils, mock meats such as soy bacon and baked goods to which soy has been added) whereas in Asian countries people tend to consume wholefood soy that still retains its fibre and fatty acids (e.g. edamame, natto, tempeh, miso, tofu) in combination with a largely plant-based diet that is low in saturated fat. The quantity of isoflavones found in second-line soy foods has been said to be low and may not be enough to confer any real health benefits.[114] From a naturopathic perspective, these foods are also highly processed and often contain high quantities of preservatives and additives, making them less than ideal as a medicinal food source.

In addition, the quantity of soy foods consumed by the two populations is vastly different: in Asia people consume an average of between 25 and 50 mg of isoflavone per day[115] but soy isoflavone intake in the Western diet is considerably less, with estimates of approximately 0.8 to 0.15 mg per day. Also, Asian populations are exposed to soy products over a long period of time, generally their whole lifetime, whereas Westerners are typically not. Researchers have suggested that early exposure is important[116] as well as the long-term cumulative effect of soy isoflavones, rather than acute or short-term ingestion.

Last but by no means least, our microflora appear to influence the therapeutic effects associated with soy foods. Equol is an isoflavone that is a bacterially derived metabolite of daidzein. Only 30% of the Western population carries colonic bacteria that convert daidzein to equol, compared to 60% of Asian populations, suggesting that equol producers are likely to get more profound effects from soy foods than non-equol producers, who convert daidzein to a less oestrogenic metabolite, *O*-desmethylangolensin.[117] Equol has been shown to have stronger oestrogenic activity than daidzein; however, it also exhibits anti-oestrogenic activity where required, suggesting it functions as a SORM, increasing oestrogen where it is low, or decreasing it where it is high.

Did you know?

- Battered tempeh, deep-fried for 30 minutes, loses almost 45% of the total isoflavones found in raw tempeh, highlighting the fact that cooking methods influence the therapeutic effect an individual receives when consuming soy foods.
- The isoflavone concentration of some processed soy proteins may be only 20% of that found in traditional soy foods.

Murphy PA, Song T, Buseman G et al. Isoflavones in retail and institutional soy foods. J Agric Food Chem 1999; 47:2697–704; Zaheer K, Akhtar MH. An updated review of dietary isoflavones: nutrition, processing, bioavailability and impacts on human health. Crit Rev Food Sci Nutr 2017 Apr 13; 57(6):1280–93.

Osteoporosis

Soy foods have been shown to preserve bone mineral density, and their high intake in the traditional Asian diet has been suggested to be one reason why Asian populations experience a lower incidence of osteoporosis, despite their low consumption of dairy products. Soy isoflavones stimulate osteoablast activity through activation of oestrogen receptors. Additionally, while some animal proteins have been associated with increased urinary calcium excretion, soy protein has not.[118] Dietary inclusion of whole soy foods containing approximately 60 mg/d of isoflavones has been shown to improve bone health, in particular increasing serum osteocalcin, a marker of bone formation, in postmenopausal women.[119] It also reduces bone turnover during early menopause,[120] in part due to a reduction in urinary deoxypyridinoline, a marker of bone reabsorption. Reductions in several key clinical risk factors for CVD such as LDL cholesterol have also been observed.

Soy for climacteric complaints

Dietary soy has been shown to help reduce a number of complaints attributed to perimenopause. In a recent open-label, controlled, crossover clinical trial involving perimenopausal women regular consumption of ViveSoy®, a soy milk drink containing 50 mg of isoflavones and 15 g of protein, was found to reduce climacteric symptoms by 20.4% as well as urogenital complaints by 21.3%. Participants also reported improved health-related quality of life by 18.1%.[121]

Safety

Many studies of soy supplements have produced negative results with some even showing that it may increase risk of cancer. It is important to note that many studies on supplements use isolated constituents and these work very differently to wholefoods. Thus while research may not support the use of soy isoflavone in supplement form, dietary use, provided it is with wholefoods, appears to be safe consumed long term to obtain benefits.

A systematic review involving seven prospective cohort studies investigating the relationship between dietary soy intake and risk of a primary breast cancer diagnosis observed no significant association between dietary soy intake and primary breast cancer.[122] A meta-analysis of five cohort studies investigating women for 4–7 years post first breast cancer diagnosis observed that higher intake of soy was associated with decreased recurrence and mortality in oestrogen receptor negative women as well as decreased mortality, but not less recurrence in women who were oestrogen receptor positive.[123]

TOMATOES (*SOLANUM LYCOPERSICUM*)

Tomatoes belong to the nightshade family and are a rich source of nutrients including vitamin C (when consumed raw) as well as carotenoids, such as lycopene, alpha-carotene, beta-carotene and lutein. Dietary use of tomatoes includes their fresh wholefood form; surprisingly however, the bulk of tomato consumption comes from processed forms such as canned and sun-dried tomatoes, ketchup, tomato pastes, juices, purees, soups and sauces.

A large body of evidence has focused on lycopene, a carotenoid within tomatoes, that has been identified as an antioxidant agent with potential anticancer properties including inhibition of the cancer cell cycle, interference with growth factors that stimulate cancer cell proliferation such as insulin-like growth factor 1 (IGF-1), induction of phase two enzymes involved in detoxification of harmful metabolites as well as regulation of transcription.[124] Despite the primary focus on lycopene, it is important for the naturopathic practitioner to remember the therapeutic potential of recommending the wholefood rather than being reductionist and focusing on one constituent. This is illustrated by rat studies that demonstrated consumption of whole tomato was more effective than isolated lycopene for the prevention and development of progression of prostate cancer, leading the authors to hypothesise that the tomato must contain other compounds as well as lycopene that modify risk of prostate cancer.[125]

Reduction of prostate cancer risk

Consumption of tomato products and estimated lycopene intake have been linked to reduced risk of prostate cancer. Decreased risk of prostate cancer was observed in an epidemiological study conducted over 23 years involving 46 719 men, whereby increasing tomato sauce intake to at least two serves per week was associated with a decreased risk of prostate cancer overall.[126] A meta-analysis of twenty-six studies that included 17 517 cases of prostate cancer reported from 563 299 participants observed an inverse association between lycopene consumption and risk of prostate cancer.[127] The authors suggested that lycopene consumption decreased incidence of prostate cancer by 3% for every 10 micrograms/dL rise in circulating lycopene levels, though interestingly no greater risk reduction was observed with intake above 85 micrograms/dL.

A 3-week nutritional intervention with tomato products alone (containing at least 30 mg of lycopene) or in combination with selenium, grape juice, soy isoflavones, tea and omega-3 fatty acids was found to lower PSA in patients with non-metastatic prostate cancer compared to those with low dietary intakes.[128] Median PSA-values were found to decrease by 1% in patients with the highest increases in plasma lycopene, selenium and omega-3 fatty acids, compared to an 8.5% increase in the patients with the lowest intake of lycopene, selenium and omega-3 fatty acids.

Tomato juice for sperm health

Daily consumption of tomato juice may help to promote male fertility in individuals with poor sperm motility. Lycopene is found in high quantities in the male testis and because of its free radical scavenging capabilities may be useful as an antioxidant for spermatozoa which are highly susceptible to oxidative stress, which may contribute to male infertility. In a small study involving 54 participants, males who had been diagnosed with infertility and poor sperm concentration and/or poor sperm motility were separated into three groups: a tomato juice group, an antioxidant supplement group and a control group.[129] Those in the tomato juice group were asked to consume one can of tomato juice for 3 months containing approximately 30 mg of lycopene, 38 mg of vitamin C and 3 mg of vitamin E. At the end of the 12 weeks, researchers observed that the tomato juice group experienced a significant increase in seminal plasma lycopene levels compared to the other groups. While there was no change in sperm concentration, the tomato juice group experienced a significant increase in sperm motility at week 6 as well as a decrease in semen WBCs. Interestingly, the improvement seen in sperm motility was not observed at the 12th week in the tomato group; the authors hypothesised that may be due to individual variations in sperm motility as well as other factors such as abstinence. This early study suggests that daily consumption of tomato juice containing lycopene offers an exciting and palatable food as medicine option for males with impaired sperm motility; however, further research is required to understand why the effects may be short term.

Preparation information

- Carotenoids within tomato products are lipophilic thus use of olive oil or coconut oil in the cooking process would greatly increase the absorption of lycopene and other carotenoids.
- Lycopene concentration is increased from cooked rather than raw foods. However, conversely, vitamin C content diminishes with cooked compared to raw, thus a mix of cooked and raw tomato products is suggested.

VINEGAR

Vinegar has been used medicinally for thousands of years. Hippocrates is said to have used it as a topical for wound healing due to its antimicrobial effects. Modern medicine has also discovered a range of health benefits associated with ingestion.[130] Acetic acid is the main constituent found in vinegar and is responsible for its strong smell. Acetic acid is a short-chain fatty acid which has been shown to improve glycaemic control, reducing type 2 diabetes risk. Its mechanism of action is likely to be multifaceted involving a complex interplay between facilitating insulin secretion, upregulating flow-mediated vasodilation, decreasing hepatic glucose production plus much more. (See Fig. 8.1.)

PCOS

Impaired insulin sensitivity is involved in the aetiology of polycystic ovary syndrome (PCOS), thus the use of vinegar, known for its antiglycaemic effects, would be a useful addition to the diet. Consumption of 15 g of apple cider vinegar (approximately 1 tbsp) in seven patients with PCOS seeking non-pharmacological treatment resulted in improvements in hormone parameters.[131] Intake of the vinegar resulted in a decrease in insulin resistance in six patients, as well as a decrease of the LH/FSH ratio in five of seven patients. Ovulatory menstruation was observed within 40 days in four of seven patients.

Antidiabetic and cholesterol lowering effects

The majority of studies undertaken suggest the effects of vinegar for glycaemic control appear to be more efficacious in normal glucose-tolerant individuals than in either those with type 2 diabetes or those with impaired glucose tolerance (see Fig. 8.1). However recent studies have found that consumption of vinegar prior to a meal reduces postprandial hyperinsulinaemia and hypertriglyceridaemia in individuals with impaired glucose tolerance[132] and type 2 diabetes.[133]

YOGHURT

Yoghurt is an ancient fermented milk product. Its use can be traced back to 100 BC to the Greeks;[134] however, it was in the early 20th century that the health benefits of yoghurt became widely recognised, leading to it being sold in pharmacies as a medicinal food. Dietary ingestion of yoghurt provides a range of nutrients including calcium as

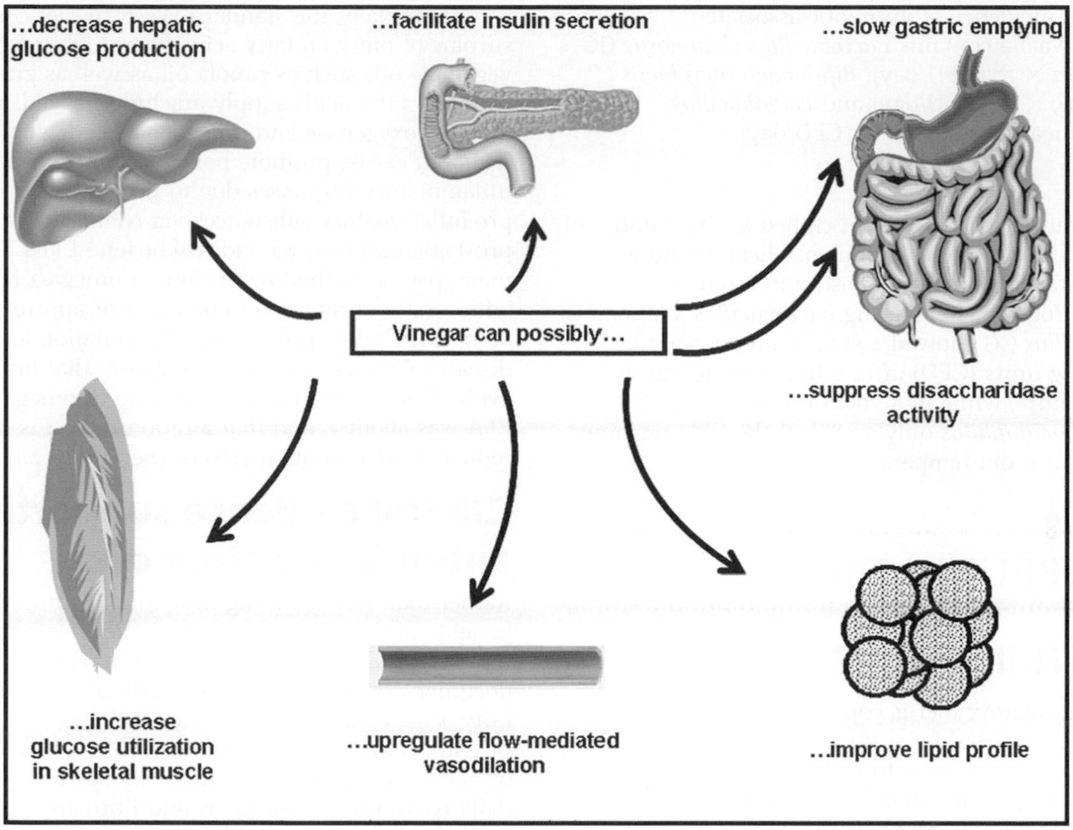

FIGURE 8.1 Possible proposed mechanisms of action for vinegar.

Petsiou E, Mitrou P, Raptis S, et al. Effect and mechanisms of action of vinegar on glucose metabolism, lipid profile, and body weight. Nutr Rev Oct 2014; 72(10) 651–61. By permission of Oxford University Press.

well as viable bacterial strains (*Streptococcus thermophilus* and *Lactobacillus bulgaricus*). Other beneficial bacterial strains such as *Lactobacillus acidophilus* and *Bifidobacterium bifidus* are often added for therapeutic benefit.

Yoghurt for bacterial vaginosis

Bacterial vaginosis is the most common lower genital tract infection in women of reproductive age[135] and is characterised by increased vaginal pH as well as loss of lactobacilli with facultative bacterial dominance.[136] Yoghurt provides a source of lactobacilli that are able to survive digestive processing to colonise the vagina via migration from the anus. However, it has been noted that lactobacilli from yoghurt shows less ability to adhere to vaginal epithelial cells compared to naturally occurring lactobacillus strains in the vagina.[137] This suggests that for optimal therapeutic benefit, it may be useful to use both oral yoghurt ingestion and topical yoghurt to gain best results.

Oral consumption of a probiotic-rich yoghurt (100 g twice per day) has been shown to be just as effective as standard antibiotic therapy at reducing the incidence of bacterial vaginosis in pregnant women.[138] The women consumed yoghurt for 1 week and experienced a decrease in vaginal pH with 80% of women experiencing symptomatic cure. Other studies also highlight the efficacy for topical application of yoghurt into the vagina for management of bacterial vaginosis. Yoghurt may be syringed into the vagina[139] but as application is associated with soiling underclothes with yoghurt, patients may prefer to soak tampons in yoghurt and then insert overnight for adequate colonisation to occur.

Yoghurt for candidiasis

Vulvovaginal candidiasis is characterised by vulvovaginal inflammation due to various *Candida* species. A small pilot study observed lower fungal colonisation rates in both HIV-infected women and non-HIV-infected women consuming probiotic-rich yoghurt compared to no intervention.[140] Topical yoghurt has also been shown to be useful in the management of vulvovaginal candidiasis, particularly when combined with honey.[141] Participants experienced a reduction in symptoms such as itching, discharge and redness. Topical application can be followed using the same instructions above for bacterial vaginosis.

Yoghurt for prevention of antibiotic-associated diarrhoea

Diarrhoea due to antibiotic therapy is a common complication but dietary probiotic yoghurt may help. Consumption of 100 g of the probiotic yoghurt known as Vaalia, a commonly available brand in supermarkets, twice a day in children aged between 1 and 12 years who were prescribed antibiotics (for the same duration as their treatment) reduced gastrointestinal disturbance; in particular, the incidence of antibiotic-associated diarrhoea.[142] Vaalia contains *Lactobacillus rhamnosus* GG (mean dose 5.2 × 109 CFU/day), *Bifidobacterium lactis* (mean dose 5.9 × 109 CFU/day) and *Lactobacillus acidophilus* (mean dose 8.3 × 109 CFU/day).

Storage

Probiotic yoghurts should be kept chilled as the number of living bacteria in probiotic yoghurt has been found to decrease substantially under exposure to room temperature. Yoghurts containing *Lactobacillus johnsonii* and *Lactobacillus* GG showed a significant decrease in colony-forming units (CFU) after 6 hours of storage at room temperature, while in a yoghurt containing *Lactobacillus acidophilus* only 53.8% of the CFU remained after 6 hours at room temperature.[143]

THERAPEUTIC DIETS

THE ANTI-INFLAMMATORY DIET

The anti-inflammatory diet is commonly prescribed for conditions characterised by systemic, chronic inflammation. Its premise is to manipulate the diet to include food components that decrease inflammatory processes, while decreasing foods that are pro-inflammatory. An anti-inflammatory diet is largely plant based and thus rich in antioxidant and anti-inflammatory phytochemicals. Research reveals that a predominantly animal-sourced diet may increase inflammation levels, while a plant-dominant dietary pattern may reduce inflammation.[144,145]

Movement towards a diet that is anti-inflammatory is associated with a decrease in levels of C-reactive protein, a marker of inflammation,[146] as well as a reduced incidence of many chronic conditions including rhinosinusitis,[147] diabetes,[148] heart disease[149] and autoimmune diseases such as rheumatoid arthritis and inflammatory bowel disease. Many key dietary patterns exhibit anti-inflammatory properties including the Mediterranean diet and the traditional Okinawan diet. However, from a naturopathic perspective these diets still feature gluten and alcohol, both of which are inflammatory, and thus an anti-inflammatory diet omitting these may be required, depending on the needs of the individual patient.

Rationale for prescription

Research shows that the standard Western diet is highly inflammatory with consumption linked to increased rates of inflammatory diseases including irritable bowel disease, diabetes and non-alcoholic fatty liver disease,[150] as well as increased risk of the anti-inflammatory diseases mentioned above. This style of diet is characterised by consumption of energy-dense, processed foods high in saturated fat and sugar[151] which are promoters of inflammation. The diet contains little in the way of beneficial items such as fruits and vegetables, known detractors of inflammation.

Additionally, the standard Western diet contains a surplus of omega-6 fatty acids from highly refined vegetable oils such as canola oil as well as grain-fed meats. Omega-6 fatty acids supply arachidonic acid, a substrate for cyclooxygenase and lipoxygenase enzyme pathways which in excess promote both local and systemic inflammatory responses due to the release of pro-inflammatory substances via NF-kB activation such as prostaglandin (PG) E2 and leukotriene LTB4.The diet of many people in the West is low in omega-3 fatty acids with a ratio of omega-6 to omega-3 of approximately 15/1 to 16.7/1,[152] thus promoting inflammation and chronic diseases. Empirical evidence suggests that human beings evolved on a diet in which the ratio of omega-6 to omega-3 EFA was about 1, and that a ratio under 4 is best for reducing inflammation effects. (See Fig. 8.2.)

Clinical evidence supporting an anti-inflammatory diet

Rather than just featuring individual components, the benefits of the anti-inflammatory diet relate to it being followed as a specific dietary pattern. Foods with documented anti-inflammatory efficacy include omega-3 fatty acids from nuts and seeds, fish and avocado, ample brightly coloured fruits and vegetables as well as a variety of herbs and spices. All of these should be included on a daily basis. Fermented foods and fibre are also imperative to ensure modulation of the gut microbiota to reduce short-chain fatty acid secretion by dysbiotic microflora and resultant inflammation.

INCLUSIONS IN AN ANTI-INFLAMMATORY DIET

Oily fish

Consumption of salmon has been shown to reduce the severity of mild ulcerative colitis, a bowel condition characterised by inflammation. In a small pilot study involving twelve subjects, participants consumed 200 g of Atlantic salmon three times per week in combination with their conventional medicine for 8 weeks.[153] A reduction in simple clinical colitis activity index (SCCAI), a marker examining general wellbeing, day- and night-time stool frequency, urgency of defecation, amount of blood in the stool and extra-intestinal complications was observed. Inflammatory markers such as C-reactive protein were also reduced, though these were not statistically significant.

Despite the lack of statistical significance with regards to inflammation, any reduction in inflammation is clinically significant for the patient and this, combined with the decrease in SSCAI score, suggests the addition of salmon or any other oily fish to the diet combined with other anti-inflammatory foods (see Fig. 8.2) would be beneficial for any patient wanting to reduce inflammation. Other fish rich in omega-3 fatty acids include mackerel, tuna, mullet, bluefish, anchovies, sardines, herring and trout. Omega-3 fatty acids decrease the arachidonic acid content of cell membranes, leading to the synthesis of eicosanoids with weaker inflammatory properties than those manufactured from omega-6 fatty acids.

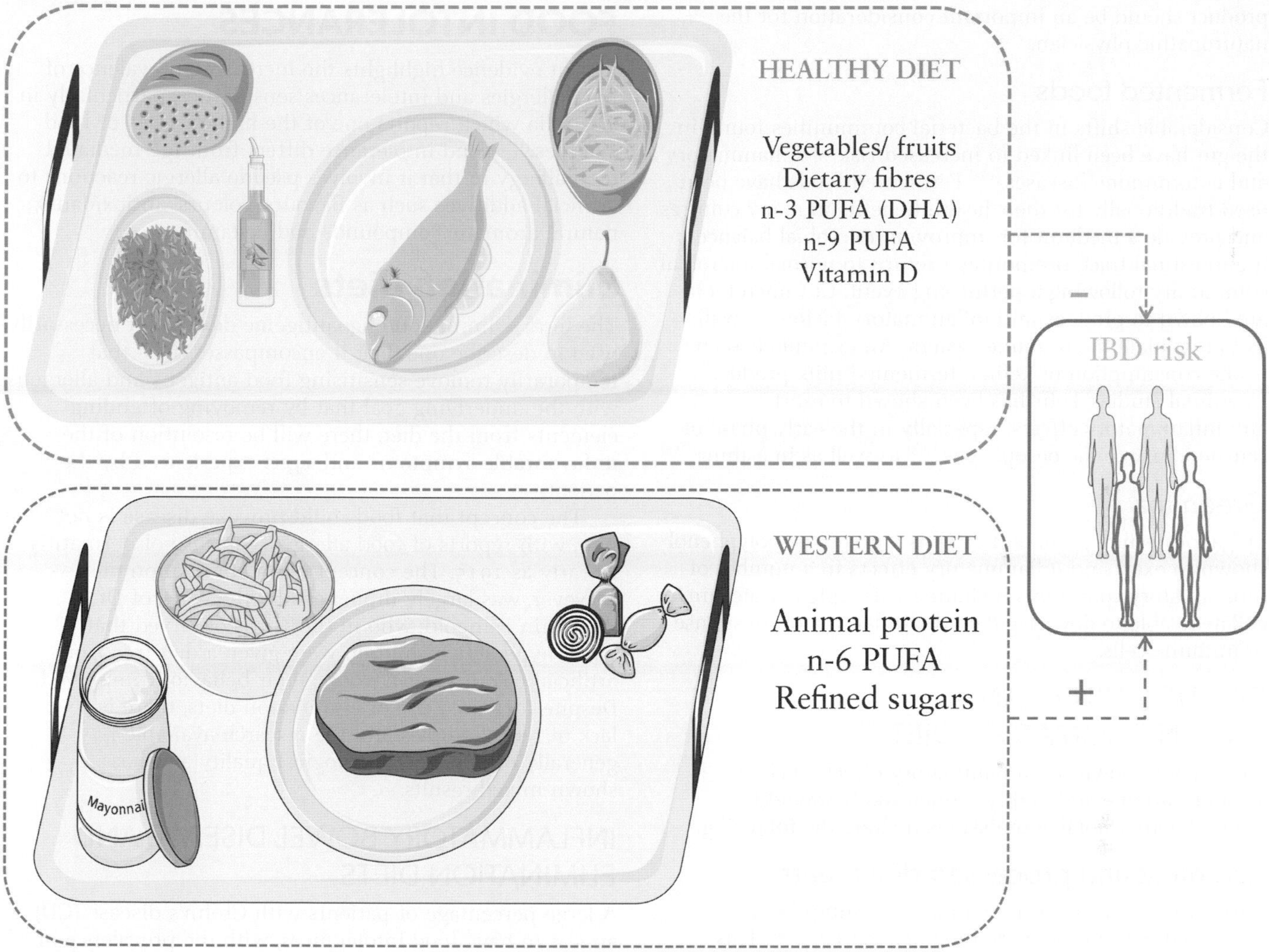

FIGURE 8.2 Influence of dietary choices on inflammatory bowel disease.

Marion-Letellier R, Savoye G, Ghosh S. IBD: in food we trust. J Crohns Colitis 2016 Nov; 10(11):1351–61. By permission of Oxford University Press.

Herbs and spices

Substantial anti-inflammatory effects can potentially be produced by a diet rich in spices.[154]

Ginger inhibits cyclooxygenase-1 and cyclooxygenase-2 as well as 5-lipoxygenase (5-LOX) and genes that encode for inflammatory cytokines and chemokines.[155] Consumption has been shown to decrease markers of inflammation such as CRP and PGE_2.[156] Curcumin, the active ingredient in the Indian spice turmeric, has been found to suppress the TNF-α-induced activation of NFκB and COX-2 expression.[157]

Fruits and vegetables

As outlined previously in this chapter, fruits and vegetables contain phytochemicals and antioxidants that are instrumental in reducing inflammation. Higher consumption of fruits and vegetables is associated with lower levels of C-reactive protein compared to lower consumption.[158,159] A variety of seasonal fruits and vegetables are suggested with a good mix of both raw and cooked fruits and vegetables, since many phytochemicals and antioxidants are altered with heat and processing. The addition of juicing can provide a large quantity of anti-inflammatory constituents delivered in a concentrated form.

Cocoa

Cocoa is rich in flavonols such as epicatechin and catechin, which have been proposed to reduce inflammation via modulating signalling pathways involved in inflammation. A number of studies of in vitro and animal studies have unequivocally demonstrated that cocoa flavonols reduce pro-inflammatory cytokines and inhibit inflammatory mediators such as NFκB, COX-2 and iNO. However, a 2016 review observed lack of long-term effect in healthy participants, though participants with diabetes and impaired glucose control experienced more pronounced benefits.[160] An Italian cohort study revealed that consumption of small quantities of dark chocolate (approx. 20 g) was associated with low concentrations of CRP.[161] Flavonol content among cocoa and chocolate products is variable: milk chocolate, dark chocolate and natural cocoa powder contain 3 mg/g, 14 mg/g and 40 mg/g of flavonols, respectively.[162] Thus recommendations on choice of cocoa product should be an important consideration for the naturopathic physician.

Fermented foods

Considerable shifts in the bacterial communities found in the gut have been linked to increased risk of inflammatory and autoimmune diseases.[163] Fermented foods have been used traditionally for their health benefits in many cultures and provide a medium for improving microbial balance in the intestinal tract, promoting a return to normal microbial community following a perturbing event. Gut microbiota are known to produce anti-inflammatory factors as well as to modulate the immune system. An example is seen in the consumption of kefir, a fermented milk product. In animal studies, kefir has been shown to exert anti-inflammatory effects, especially in the early phase of caustic injury to the oesophagus,[164] as well as in asthma.[165]

Green tea

Epigallocatechin-3-gallate [EGCG] is a green tea polyphenol shown to exert anti-inflammatory effects in a number of inflammatory conditions including IBD. Epigallocatechin-3-gallate is able to downregulate the inflammatory response in immune cells.

EXCLUSIONS ON AN ANTI-INFLAMMATORY DIET

Foods with known pro-inflammatory effects such as alcohol, caffeine and highly refined foods should be omitted. Other notable omissions include the following.

Red meat and processed deli meats

Current research suggests red meat consumption is associated with higher inflammatory markers.[166] This appears particularly true for processed meats such as bacon, salami and ham. Grass-fed beef is lower in overall fat and higher in carotenoids and omega-3 fatty acids and would thus appear to be a superior choice over grain-fed beef.[167] Other studies have suggested that the cut of meat may influence the inflammatory response, with Hodgson et al[168] finding that lean cuts of meat were less inflammatory.

Trans fats

Results from the Nurses' Health Study suggest that consumption of trans fats is associated with a pro-inflammatory effect. Participants consuming the most trans fats had higher levels of inflammatory markers such as CRP, IL-6, and TNF-α receptors in comparison to those consuming the least.[169]

Gluten

Gluten consumption has been shown to increase intestinal permeability, in part due to its effect on zonulin, a protein required for modulation of intracellular tight junctions; these effects are seen even in individuals without coeliac disease. Intestinal permeability is linked to a range of inflammatory disorders. A gluten-free diet in participants with autoimmune disease without coeliac serology has been shown to be useful, particularly with disease remittance.

FOOD INTOLERANCES

Recent evidence highlights the increasing prevalence of food allergies and intolerances/sensitivities, particularly in Australia which reports one of the highest rates of food allergies.[170] Food intolerance differs from IgE-mediated food allergy in that it involves pseudo allergic reactions to artificial additives such as flavours, colours, antioxidants, natural aromatic compounds and histamine.

Elimination diets

The term 'elimination/oligoantigenic diet' is not necessarily used to describe one diet; it encompasses diets that temporarily remove sensitising food antigens and allergens with the underlying goal that by removing offending elements from the diet, there will be resolution of the unfavourable symptoms and signs experienced by the patient.

The concept that food could provoke disease is not new, with reports of food allergy as a cause of dermatitis as early as 1915. The concept of an elimination diet, however, was largely influenced by the work of Dr Benjamin Feingold, who in the 1970s observed that when hyperactive children were given a diet free from artificial colours and flavours, their behaviour improved. Despite increased use of elimination diets, there is a lack of recent studies and the research available is generally of poor methodological quality and has shown mixed results.

INFLAMMATORY BOWEL DISEASE AND ELIMINATION DIETS

A large percentage of patients with Crohn's disease (CD) appear to have food intolerances, with the prevalence of immunoglobulins (IgGs) against various foods, especially vegetables, grains and nuts, shown to be significantly higher in CD patients compared to healthy controls.[171] A review of nine clinical trials examining the use of an elimination diet in patients with CD observed mixed results, with six showing positive results and three showing no significant benefit.

Food sensitivities in CD patients appear to be individualised, leading researchers to suggest that CD patients would benefit from a tailored elimination diet that could be individually modified for their own specific symptoms and responses. From a naturopathic perspective this could be done via IgG testing, with a number of trials successfully using this approach by targeting sensitivities that elicited a high IgG response in blood serum and removing these foods from the diet. In animal studies,[172] intestinal inflammation via CD4(+) T-cell hyperactivation was induced by food antigens associated with high serum IgG levels; however, this was ameliorated by removing the offending food antigens — the premise behind an exclusion diet. Rajendran and Kumar[173] conducted one of the studies that used IgG testing. They tested reactions to 14 specific food antigens, and removed each patient's four most reactive foods from their diet for 4 weeks. Disease activity was reduced, as were the number of bowel movements per day (on average four to two) and pain.

EXAMPLE OF AN ANTI-INFLAMMATORY DIET

BREAKFAST	
Turmeric scrambled eggs (season with pepper) with gluten-free toast and avocado	Turmeric in the eggs/golden milk functions as an anti-inflammatory agent. Curcumin, one of the active constituents within turmeric, inhibits TNF-α-induced activation of NFκB and COX-2, reducing inflammation. Piperine in black pepper increases absorption of curcumin. Additionally, since curcumin is lipohilic, absorption is further enhanced in the presence of the lipid-rich avocado. Fruits such as avocado contain a range of anti-inflammatory and antioxidant constituents shown to reduce response to inflammation.
SNACK	
Chia seed pudding with seasonal fruits Green tea	Chia seeds have been shown to increase EPA which exerts an anti-inflammatory action. Green tea contains polyphenols which have been shown to reduce the release of pro-inflammatory mediators in people at risk of chronic inflammation.
LUNCH	
Steamed salmon with ginger and shallots + 2 tbsp sauerkraut Mixed greens + rice	Omega-3 fatty acids found in salmon play an important role in moderating propensity for arachidonic acid cascade overreactions when n-6 mediators dominate. Use of fermented foods helps to reduce dysbiosis, a known contributor to inflammation. Low-grade inflammation of the intestine results in metabolic dysfunction, in which dysbiosis of the gut microbiota is involved.
DINNER	
Vegetable and lentil curry	Plant-based meals are shown to be anti-inflammatory compared with a standard Western diet. It makes ample use of antioxidant-rich spices; diets rich in spices have been attributed to low rates of inflammatory diseases.
SUPPER	
'Golden milk' latte (non-dairy)	As above for recommendations for curcumin.

Benefits seen in other studies also included better quality of life, symptom reduction and increased remission rates, leading researchers to state that there is sufficient evidence to try an elimination diet as the first line of treatment for people with mild or moderate CD.[174,175]

Though not strictly classified as an inflammatory bowel disease, trials in participants with irritable bowel syndrome have also found some improvements with dietary avoidance guided by IgG4 reactivity.[176,177] Thus practitioners may wish to recommend IgG testing in IBS patients who are not responding to herbal medicines and other naturopathic interventions.

BEHAVIOURAL IMPROVEMENT AND ELIMINATION DIET OF ADDITIVES

A number of reviews detail the efficacy of elimination diets for behavioural improvements in children, with two of the most recently conducted meta-analyses and systematic reviews revealing that in children with ADHD, restriction of sugar and sweeteners and elimination of colours and preservatives improves behavioural and attention performance.[178–181]

The behavioural effects of additives are not limited to children with ADHD. In 2007, in a community-based, double-blind, placebo-controlled food challenge, McCann et al[182] observed that dietary combinations of certain artificial colours together with the preservative sodium benzoate increased hyperactivity in 3-year-old and 8–9-year-old children in the general population, compared to their usual diet.

However more recently Lok et al (2013)[183] conducted a randomised controlled study that showed lack of effect of artificial colours and a preservative (sodium benzoate) on the behaviour of Chinese children aged 8–9 years old. This may in part be due to genetic differences existing between population groups since gene polymorphisms have been shown to influence the way in which the individual reacts or not to additives in the diet. Stevenson et al (2010)[184] showed that adverse effects of food additives on ADHD symptoms were moderated by histamine degradation gene polymorphisms in children, in part explaining the mixed results seen in studies conducted thus far.

ATOPIC DERMATITIS AND ELIMINATION DIETS

Exclusion diets are common in patients with atopic dermatitis (AD) however there is a lack of high-quality research to substantiate their use. A 2008 Cochrane Review found little evidence to support the use of exclusion diets (in particular egg and milk), suggesting this may be because the participants were not allergic to the food substances in the first place.[185] From a naturopathic perspective it would be interesting to see if the results would be more positive if other common allergens such as gluten were removed from the diet, in combination with milk and dairy. The Cochrane Review did find there may be some benefit in using an egg-free diet in infants with suspected egg allergy who have positive specific IgE to eggs. The Review cites one study which found 51% of the children involved had a significant improvement in body surface area without atopic dermatitis with the exclusion diet compared to normal diet at the end of 6 weeks.

Supporting the use of an exclusion diet, Johnston et al (2004)[186] investigating dietary manipulation by parents of children with atopic dermatitis found that 39% of families reported subjective improvement of symptoms when using an elimination diet. Of the participants who completed their questionnaire, 75% had tried some form of dietary exclusion; the most common foods omitted were dairy products (48%), eggs (27%) and cow's milk (25%).

ASTHMA AND ELIMINATION DIETS

A 2015 case report discusses the benefits of implementing an exclusion diet that eliminates reactive foods as measured by ELISA for management of asthma symptoms.[187] Both patients discussed in the cases demonstrated a reduction in symptoms of asthma (such as less shortness of breath and wheezing), as well as a reduced need for medication while following an IgG antibody-guided elimination diet.

Time frame: how soon should patients see results?

Improvement in symptoms was seen in 4 weeks by 98.4% of participants following an elimination diet for non-IgE-mediated gastrointestinal food allergies.

Lozinsky AC, Meyer R, De Koker C et al. Time to symptom improvement using elimination diets in non-IgE-mediated gastrointestinal food allergies. Pediatr Allergy Immunol 2015 Aug; 26(5):403–438.

Histamine

Histamine is an amine and the product of decarboxylation of the amino acid and L-histidine. Intolerance to histamine is estimated to affect 1% of the population, though this number may be underestimated as many patients go undiagnosed due to the wide array of signs and symptoms experienced.[188]

Histamine intolerance may arise as the result of excessive consumption of a histamine-containing food in combination with an inability to break down histamine in the intestines. Dysfunction in the enzymes that break down histamine such as monoamine oxidase (MAO), diamine oxidase (DAO) and histamine-N-methyltransferase (HNMT) are implicated in the pathogenesis of histamine intolerance.[189] Dysfunctions in these enzymes may be due to genetic variations, with several single-neucleotide polymorphisms observed in the DAO enzyme, though acquired causes such as inflammatory bowel disease due to altered enterocytes causing decreased production of DAO[190] may also influence intolerance to histamine.

Histamine intolerance manifests as a non-IgE mediated hypersensitivity reaction but may cause similar signs to an allergic reaction, with common complaints related to gastrointestinal disturbances such as diffuse abdominal pain, colic, flatulence and intermittent diarrhoea, as well as other symptoms such as urticaria and pruritus, headaches, sneezing, rhinorrhoea and congestion of the nose, arrhythmias and flushing.[191–193] Diagnosis of histamine intolerance may include a thorough patient history and elimination of histamine-rich foods followed by oral histamine provocation.[194]

DIETARY RECOMMENDATIONS

Bacteria and yeasts have the ability to manufacture vasoactive amines such as histamine as they ferment, thus contamination by microbes often increases histamine content in food, particularly the longer a food is stored. Taking this into consideration, food should be consumed when as fresh as possible to prevent microbial contamination. Food that is more than a few day's old may aggravate the condition. Foods containing large quantities of histamine should also be avoided. These include aged and fermented cheeses, yoghurt, processed meats such as salami, alcoholic beverages such as red wine, fermented foods such as sauerkraut and soy foods, fish that has been frozen, smoked or tinned, as well as certain fruits and vegetables containing higher quantities of histamine including oranges, tomatoes, avocados, spinach and eggplant.

An additional consideration is to remove foods that liberate histamine release such as citrus fruits and tea (see Table 8.4). An upper limit of 100 mg histamine/kg in foods has been suggested; however, this quantity may still be too high for some. Alongside dietary modifications, the modern naturopath also works to support healthy gut function, understanding that excess histamine can promote inflammation in the gut so increasing intestinal permeability,[195] as well as supporting methylation because low methylation is associated with inadequate breakdown of histamine. A low histamine diet has been shown to have a therapeutic benefit by reducing atopic dermatitis[196] as well as gastrointestinal complaints.[197]

Low histamine and salicylate diet meal planner

ADULT OPTION

BREAKFAST	
Omelette made with low-amine vegetables such as peeled white potato, chives and grated zucchini. Season with sea salt Serve with pan-fried Brussels sprouts and broccoli Quicker option: rolled oats with maple syrup and pear	Eggs are a quality source of protein. Teamed with carbohydrate-containing potato they will provide sustained energy throughout the day. Peeled white potato, zucchini and chives are low-amine vegetables. Broccoli and Brussels sprouts contain sulforaphane which helps to support healthy methylation. Methylation may be impaired in those with histamine intolerance. Breakfast cereals containing cocoa, nuts, fruit and honey need to be avoided due to their histamine content. They can be replaced with rolled oats and maple syrup which are low-amine and salicylate options.
SNACK	
Raw cashews Pear, vanilla and oat muffin	Raw cashews are low in salicylates and amines Pears are a low-histamine fruit. They can be used to make muffins using low-histamine flours such as buckwheat, rice and GF wheat as well as rolled oats. Vanilla and maple syrup are low-histamine and salicylate options.
LUNCH	
Quinoa and wild rice salad with shredded carrot, red cabbage and poached chicken	Rice and quinoa are both low-histamine sources of starchy carbohydrates for energy and fibre. Low-histamine salad vegetables such as carrots, cucumber, parsley and spring onion can be added for flavour. Team with chicken with no skin but make sure the chicken or other low-amine meat such as lamb, beef or veal is not prepared too long in advance to prevent histamine build-up. Use fresh herbs such as parsley and chives as well as a pinch of sea salt for flavour, as olive oil and vinegar contain high quantities of amines.
SNACK	
Sparkling water Rice/goats/soy/cow's milk hot chocolate made using carob and flavoured with maple syrup	Milk options listed are low histamine. Chocolate is high in histamine therefore should be replaced with carob and maple syrup which are both low in amines and salicylates. Tea and coffee contain moderate levels of histamine and thus should be avoided.
DINNER	
Fish tacos Ceviche kingfish with lime. Serve in iceberg lettuce cups Serve with sweet potato wedges	Tinned fish and oily fish are considered to be high histamine sources, but white fish is considered to be relatively low. Team with low-histamine vegetables such as iceberg lettuce and sweet potato.

Salicylates

Like histamine intolerance, intolerance to salicylates involves a nonspecific antigen-induced pseudo-allergic hypersensitivity reaction that results from consumption of items containing salicylic acid.[198] Signs and symptoms include but are not limited to urticaria, angio-oedema, migraine, irritable bowel syndrome (IBS), asthma and eczema.[199] A low-salicylate diet is recommended for those exhibiting sensitivity to salicylates, naturally occurring chemicals found in a number of foods (see Table 8.5).

Salicylic acid is found in plants and functions naturally to protect the plant from stressors. It should thus come as no surprise that common dietary sources are found in plant foods. A systematic review examining common sources of dietary salicylates in the Scottish population observed alcoholic beverages to be the most prominent source (22%), followed by herbs and spices (17%), fruits (16%), non-alcoholic beverages including fruit juices (13%), tomato-based sauces (12%) and vegetables (9%).[200]

Dietary salicylates have been linked to a number of adverse health issues including urticaria, angio-oedema,[201] asthma and gut disturbances such as diarrhoea and colitis.[202] Consumption of high doses of supplemental fish oil have been reported to control salicylate intolerance,[203] thus it could be hypothesised that frequent consumption of oily fish in the diet may also confer similar benefits. A low-salicylate diet has been shown to help manage aspirin-induced respiratory disease;[204] however, a review of the available current literature reveals that more well-controlled studies detailing successful implementation of a low-salicylate diet are required to elucidate its usefulness and practicality in clinical practice.

TABLE 8.4 Common high-histamine foods

Order	Items	Content (mg/kg)
1	Sausage	3572
2	Tuna	2927
3	Mackerel	2467
4	Pork	2067
5	Mackerel pike	1391
6	Spinach	1358
7	Green tea	878
8	Peeled orange	743
9	Peanut	635
10	Orange	632
11	Tomato	557
12	Cheese	533
13	Banana	495
14	Orange juice	462
15	Tangerine	429
16	Grape	315
17	Red wine	287
18	Coffee	282
19	Strawberry	257
20	Cocoa	177
21	Chocolate	162
22	White wine	162
23	Pineapple	158
24	Egg	136
25	Beer	118
26	Milk	38
27	Pickle	23
28	Distilled liquor	16

Choi JH, Park CW, Lee CH. A study of histamine content in food in Korea. Korean J Dermatol 2007;45:768–771. Reproduced with permission.

TABLE 8.5 Salicylate content of common wholefoods

Food item	Salicylates (mg/kg)	Food item	Salicylates (mg/kg)
Fruits		Vegetables	
Banana	0.34	Asparagus	1.29
Blackberries	0.81	Broccoli	0.0
Blueberries	0.57	Cabbage green	0.0
Galia melon	0.62	Carrots	0.16
Grapefruit	0.44	Cauliflower	0.01
Green apple	0.55	Celery	0.04
Kiwifruit	0.31	Cucumber	0.02
Lime	0.0	Eggplant	0.0
Mango	0.03	Green bean	0.07
Nectarine	3.29	Green capsicum	0.01
Orange	0.11	Lettuce (iceberg)	0.05
Peach	0.12	Mushroom (button)	0.13
Pear	0.23	Onion (white)	0.80
Plum	0.01	Potato	0.02
Raspberry	0.09	Red capsicum	0.09
Red grape	0.02	Snow peas	0.20
Strawberry	0.61	Swede	0.07
White grape	0.02	Tomato	0.13
Yellow melon	0.11	Yellow capsicum	0.09
		Zucchini	0.0
Juices		Spices	
Apple	0.83	Black cumin	25.05
Cranberry	0.99	Cumin	29.76
Grapefruit	0.10	Chat masala	5.74
Orange	0.68	Cinnamon	0.78
Pineapple	4.06	Garam masala	12.85
Tomato	1.32	Paprika	28.25
		Turmeric	20.88

Wood A, Baxter G, Thies F et al. A systematic review of salicylates in foods: estimated daily intake of a Scottish population. Mol Nutr Food Res 2011 May; 55 Suppl 1:S7–S14.

Final thoughts

Of note, exclusion diets need to be as varied as possible to reduce risk of nutritional deficiencies as well as preventing negative long-term effects on the patient's relationship and behaviour with food, particularly in children.[205] Because elimination diets can be restrictive and complicated, practitioners should ensure they support the patient with adequate resources. Depending on the patient's needs this may include a personalised menu adapted to individual patient taste and nutritional needs.

Elimination diets are associated with nutritional deficiencies including vitamin D, zinc and calcium, thus the patient must be managed appropriately with supplementation where required.[206] Lastly, it should be noted that in most cases an elimination diet should not be followed forever, a point that needs to be discussed with the patient. The ultimate goal of the practitioner should be to improve overall function of the body, in particular gut and immune health so that a wide range of foods can be consumed once again without negative reactions.

VEGETARIAN DIET

The number of people choosing to follow a vegetarian eating pattern is increasing. The last national nutrition survey in Australia[207] suggested that approximately 2–3% of people identified with being vegetarian; however, with the growing interest in plant-based diets it is likely this number has increased considerably. The health benefits associated with a plant-based diet, as well as ethical, ecological and economic concerns, are some of the reasons cited for following this dietary style.[208]

The main defining feature of a vegetarian diet is the absence of animal products but there are many variations on a vegetarian diet, with some advocates consuming the flesh of chicken and fish while others omitt all animal protein but eggs (see Table 8.6).

Benefits

A 2014 study examining the nutritional quality of a range of diets observed vegetarian diets to be mostly better in terms of nutrient quality than the typical omnivorous diet.[209] As with most dietary styles, if it is well balanced and managed well, a vegetarian dietary pattern can be compatible with a healthy lifestyle and optimal nutritional status. Studies examining the health benefits in populations following a vegetarian diet show that followers exhibit:

- Lower blood concentrations of total cholesterol, low-density lipoprotein cholesterol, high-density lipoprotein cholesterol and non-high-density lipoprotein cholesterol[210]
- Less visceral fat and greater improvements in insulin resistance and oxidative stress markers than those following conventional diets[211]
- Reduced body weight[212]
- Protection against coronary heart disease[213]
- Diverse gut microbiota due to the high fibre and variation in the diet
- Reduced blood pressure.[214]

These beneficial effects are likely due to high consumption of unrefined vegetable products, such as wholegrains, legumes, nuts, fruits and vegetables which are rich in disease-protecting phytochemicals.

Nutritional considerations for the practitioner

In spite of the health benefits associated with a vegetarian diet, problems arise where it is not planned appropriately and leads to nutritional deficiencies. In particular, adequate intake of protein, vitamin B_{12},[215] omega-3 fatty acids, iron, zinc[216] and calcium all need to be considered by the naturopathic practitioner in the planning of a nutritionally adequate vegetarian diet, as these are commonly deficient.

IRON

The naturopathic practitioner must determine the cause of iron deficiency and manage it appropriately. Iron deficiency in vegetarians may occur as a result of:

TABLE 8.6 Classification of different styles of vegetarianism

Pesco-vegetarians	Omit all animal products other than fish
Lacto-ovo vegetarians	Omit all animal products but include eggs and dairy products
Lacto-vegetarians	Omit all animal products but dairy products
Ovo-vegetarians	Omit all animal products but eggs
Vegans	Omit all animal products including honey

- Inadequate dietary intake
- Poor absorption due to higher content of absorption inhibitors such as phytates found in plant-based foods or a coexisting disease impeding absorption such as hypothyroid or inflammatory bowel disease (iron is absorbed in the small intestine)
- Blood loss, for example menorrhagia.

It has been suggested that vegetarians have 80% higher iron requirements than non-vegetarians. This is based on the belief that only 10% of iron is absorbed from a vegetarian diet, compared to 18% in a mixed diet containing meat.[217] It is debatable how relevant this is since an adaptive mechanism occurs in those with lower stores of iron allowing them to first absorb more iron and second excrete less faecal ferritin than those with higher stores.[218] Additionally, vegetarian diets are typically rich in vitamin C, which is known to enhance absorption of iron up to six-fold because it aids the conversion of Fe^{3+} (ferric) to Fe^{2+} (ferrous) iron, the best absorbed form of iron.[219]

Iron intakes in vegetarians and omnivores in industrialised countries have been shown to be similar, and a review published in the *Medical Journal of Australia* suggested that vegetarians who eat a balanced diet are at no greater risk of iron deficiency anaemia than non-vegetarians.[220] Interestingly, before the age of 11, children who are vegetarian may even have higher levels of iron than their omnivore counterparts,[221] though despite similar intakes, vegetarians often have lower serum ferritin concentrations than omnivores. The majority of dietary iron in Australian diets comes from cereal-based foods that have been fortified,[222] not from meat, even in non-vegetarians. The naturopathic practitioner seeking to encourage their patient to adopt more of a wholefood diet may need to take this into consideration, particularly if the patient is avoiding iron-fortified cereals.

Iron and brain function in infants and small children

Parents bringing their children up as vegetarian should be aware of the importance of adequate iron in their child's diet as well as the consequences of iron deficiency anaemia (IDA) on their child's brain function and development. Lack of iron results in poor brain myelination and impaired monoamine metabolism, particularly with regards to dopamine.[223] Deficiency, even mild, causes long-term effects on behaviour and cognition that can persist despite iron replacement therapy. Iron deficiency anaemia in infancy is associated with slower reaction times and poorer inhibitory control in 10-year-olds, even after long-term iron therapy.[224] IDA has been shown to cause permanent changes in the nuclei of the basal ganglia leading to deficits in spatial intelligence and IQ in small children.[225] In spite of the permanent damage afflicted, a systematic review involving 14 studies did observe a modest positive effect with supplementation of iron in anaemic infants and children on cognitive outcomes following intake of at least 2 months' duration.

> While most naturopaths focus on vitamin C as an enhancer of iron, it is important to note that other nutrients including vitamin A and β-carotene can also enhance non-haem iron absorption in a vegetarian diet.
>
> Refrain from drinking tea with meals. The higher the polyphenol content of the tea, the less absorption of iron that takes place. In tea made from 3 g of tea leaves concentrated at 396 mg/275 mL/serve polyphenols decreased iron absorption by 91%, while the same tea diluted to 99 mg/275 mL/serve polyphenols decreased iron absorption by 82%.
>
> Hurrell RF, Reddy M, Cook JD. Inhibition of non-haem iron absorption in man by polyphenolic-containing beverages. Br J Nutr 1999; 81:289–95.

Vitamin B_{12}

Vitamin B_{12} is required for the manufacture of nucleic acids and erythrocytes and in the maintenance of myelin. Individuals following vegetarian diets may be at risk of developing vitamin B_{12} deficiency due to the fact that it is found primarily in animal products. Dairy, eggs and fish contain very small amounts of vitamin B_{12} thus, depending on how restrictive the vegetarian diet is, vitamin B_{12} may need to be supplemented. Pregnant and lactating women as well as infants may be particularly vulnerable to B_{12} deficiency due to additional demands. A systematic review observed that 45% of vegetarian infants may be deficient in vitamin B_{12}.[226] Given the importance of vitamin B_{12} in the body, adequate nutritional planning if following a vegetarian diet is imperative, particular as many of the neurological manifestations of vitamin B_{12} deficiency are irreversible.

Zinc

Zinc has roles in cellular metabolic processes, reproduction, immunity, neurology, and growth and development, hence its deficiency in the body can be wide ranging. Meat, fish and poultry are the main contributors of zinc in the adult non-vegetarian diet;[227] however, vegetarians are able to obtain zinc from other sources including pulses, legumes, nuts and seeds. A systematic review observed zinc intake as well as zinc levels to be lower in vegetarians compared to omnivores,[228] while another systematic review and meta-analysis observed zinc intakes and serum zinc concentrations of pregnant vegetarian women were significantly lower compared with pregnant non-vegetarian women. Interestingly, in the latter study, both groups (omnivore and vegetarians) were not meeting the recommended dietary allowance (RDA) for zinc.[229] A higher percentage of Australian vegetarian children (13.3%) consume zinc supplements, compared with non-vegetarian children (8.6%).[230] This may be warranted given the high percentage of people deficient, combined with the importance of zinc in the body, particularly for growth and development.

Omega-3 fatty acids

Intakes of eicosapentaenoic acid (EPA) and docosahexaenoic acid (DHA) are low in vegetarians who do not consume fish, since EPA and DHA are primarily obtained from consuming fish. Consumption of chia seeds, walnuts and flaxseeds may be helpful as a source of α-linolenic acid (ALA), though efficiency of conversion of ALA to EPA and DHA is dependent on a number of factors. Consumption of omega-3 enriched eggs (6 per week) in lacto-ovo-vegetarians has been shown to increase DHA.[231] Chickens may be fed flaxseed, soy or algal marine sources which results in the production of n-3 fatty acid enriched eggs.

BONE MINERAL DENSITY AND VEGETARIANISM

Vegetarian diets often have lower amounts of calcium, vitamin D, vitamin B_{12}, protein and n-3 (ω-3) fatty acids. As a result of the lower amount of these nutrients some have hypothesised that vegetarians may be at increased risk of osteoporosis due to the importance of these nutrients for bone health.

A 2009 meta-analysis suggested lower bone density in those following a vegetarian diet;[232] however, it should be noted that most of the studies reviewed examined a vegan diet, rather than a vegetarian diet, thus the accuracy in concluding that a vegetarian diet is associated with decreased bone mineral density (BMD) is disputed. Other studies conducted show that while vegetarians consume lower quantities of calcium than omnivores, that quantity is not vastly different. Perhaps this is why much of the research conducted solely on vegetarian diets suggests no link with decreased bone mineral density.[233]

A recent cross-sectional study observed that vegetarian diets were not detrimental to bone health in young adults, in part due to the fact that healthy vegetarian diets often had higher intakes of protective anti-inflammatory and antioxidant nutrients that alkalised the body, protecting against loss of bone mineral density.[234] Low acid load is associated with lower bone resorption and as a result higher bone mineral density. This lower acid load comes from a diet that is rich in fruits and vegetables, particularly those that are potassium rich, since potassium has a sparing effect on calcium being leached from the bones.[235]

Other bone protective effects associated with a vegetarian diet include a higher intake of phytoestrogen foods such as soy and lignans which also exert bone protective effects. Tempeh, a commonly consumed fermented food, offers one of the highest food sources of vitamin K_2, which is required for bone formation through osteocalcin formation.

In order to ensure an adequate intake of essential nutrients, the planning of a vegetarian diet requires emphasis on the use of wholegrains, legumes, nuts and seeds.

VEGETARIAN MEAL PLANNER

BREAKFAST	
Green smoothie 1 mango, ½ bunch of parsley, kale, 1 scoop natural protein powder, water	Parsley is a rich source of iron. By combining it with vitamin C found in the fruit, the bioavailability of the iron is increased.
LUNCH	
Bibimbap-style bowl: serve steamed rice with marinated tofu, shiitake mushrooms, carrots, wilted spinach, shredded red cabbage and spring onions. Add a fried egg on top and a sprinkle of chilli	Tofu and eggs are both excellent sources of protein for vegetarians. A large quantity of wholefoods that are plant based and high in fibre help to promote the diverse microbiota seen in vegetarians.
DINNER	
Stir fry of marinated tempeh with Asian-style vegetables with rice noodles made in cast iron skillet	Tempeh provides a highly nutritious source of protein. Cooking with cast iron kitchenware in conjunction with increasing dietary iron and vitamin C rich foods has been shown to help increase ferritin stores.
SNACKS	
Boiled eggs Trail mix made from walnuts, pepitas and two dates Nori sheets Fresh seasonal fruit	Eggs provide an excellent source of protein. Pumpkin seeds provide zinc which may be low in vegetarians. Nori is a plant-based source of vitamin B_{12} which may be low in vegetarians.

GLUTEN-FREE DIET

A gluten-free diet (GFD) has become increasingly popular and is the most commonly adopted special diet worldwide. Controversially, a GFD is followed not only by those with recognised allergy to gluten, but also by those without a gluten-related disorder. The percentage of individuals adopting a GFD for non-medical reasons, including as a lifestyle choice, reportedly surpasses those with a permanent gluten-related disorder. A 2015 survey conducted in the USA involving 1500 people found that 26% of individuals stated they followed it because it was 'a healthy option', while 19% stated it was 'better for my digestion'.[236] Interestingly, 'I have gluten sensitivity' was the least-cited reason for implementation of a gluten-free diet.

In an Australian cross-sectional population survey of over 1000 adults approximately 10.6% had chosen to avoid wheat, with nearly half of those being gluten free, despite less than 1% of them actually being diagnosed with coeliac disease.[237] In contrast to the American survey where the majority of individuals followed a GFD for health reasons, the Australian study found the majority of individuals followed a GFD to assist with reducing unfavourable gut symptoms such as bloating and abdominal pain.

It is estimated that the average Westerner consumes approximately 10–20 g of gluten per day in their diet,[238] most of which is consumed in foods that would not appear to the average consumer to contain gluten. A survey of gluten-containing products in Australian supermarkets found the presence of gluten in nearly 2000 different food items, including vinegars and ice-creams. Gluten was also found in over 100 non-foods including pain relievers and vitamins.[239] This highlights the importance of the naturopathic practitioner to educate the patient who is trying to avoid gluten to be aware of all possible sources of gluten exposure.

What is gluten?

Gluten is a protein composed of gliadin and glutenins. Glutenins do not appear to be a causative factor in the signs and symptoms associated with coeliac disease. However, research has implicated gliadin in the pathogenesis of coeliac disease with a large percentage of individuals producing antigliadin antibodies in response to exposure to gluten. Four fractions of gliadin have been described, including α, β, γ and ω subunits; the α-gliadin subunit has been found to have the most profound deleterious effects, while β, γ and ω exhibit milder toxicity.

Following ingestion of gluten, glutamine and proline-rich gluten-composing gliadin proteins are partially hydrolysed by proteases in the small intestine of the gastrointestinal tract. As a result of only partial hydrolysis, relatively large residual proline and glutamine-rich peptides can remain intact in the intestinal lumen, resulting in the production of gluten peptides, which may be toxic or immunogenic.[240]

Gluten-related disorders are characterised by the adverse reactions exerted following ingestion of gluten-containing products. They can be classified into three different disorders: coeliac disease, wheat allergy and non-coeliac gluten sensitivity (NGCS).

COELIAC DISEASE

Coeliac disease is an autoimmune disease characterised by the production of serum antibodies against tissue transglutaminase-2 (TG2) following ingestion of gluten in genetically predisposed individuals carrying the HLA-DQ2 and/or HLA DQ8 genotypes. This immunological T-cell mediated reaction results in subsequent inflammation and atrophy of the villi, decreasing absorption of many nutrients, as well as the presence of increased intraepithelial lymphocytes and intestinal permeability.

Management of gluten intolerance and/or sensitivity requires exclusion of wheat and other gluten-containing foods such as rye and barley from the diet. The only treatment is a life-long gluten-free diet, which is effective and well tolerated by the majority of patients. Individuals with coeliac disease report significantly improved health-related quality of life when adhering to a gluten-free diet[241] and respond promptly with resolution of clinical symptoms through histological changes in the gut. As a result of the autoimmune reaction against intestine tissue, transglutaminase may take a longer time to resolve. In children with coeliac disease, implementation of a GFD for just 2 months has been shown to rapidly decrease coeliac disease antibody concentrations by 50%.[242]

WHEAT ALLERGY

Wheat allergy involves cross-linking of IgE by repeat sequences in gluten peptides and non-gluten proteins, resulting in the release of immune mediators such as histamine from degranulated mast cells and basophils.[243] It is characterised by activation of T-cells in the intestinal mucosa against gluten.[244] Though peptides different from those in coeliac disease may be involved, a gluten-free diet is considered to be the gold standard for those suffering from wheat allergy, and needs to be implemented as consciously as for those with coeliac disease.

NON-COELIAC GLUTEN SENSITIVITY

The concept that only individuals with coeliac disease and wheat allergy will respond to a GFD has become disproven in recent years with the surfacing of evidence supporting NCGS, the term given to a reaction following consumption of gluten that does not appear to involve allergic or autoimmune mechanisms and is not coeliac disease or wheat allergy. Little is known about the prevalence of NCGS due to the fact that many individuals self-diagnose. Diagnosis of NCGS is typically undertaken by excluding gluten via an elimination diet then rechallenging to observe for the presence of intestinal or extra-intestinal symptoms such as foggy mind, chronic fatigue, joint and muscular pain and anaemia.

It should be noted that while gluten is the protein often attributed to a wide array of symptoms, other candidates for signs and symptoms produced following ingestion of gluten-containing products include non-gluten wheat proteins such as amylase-trypsin inhibitors or wheatgerm agglutinin, and exorphins released during the digestion of gluten, as well as fructans. These other dietary components should be investigated as well.[245]

Gluten proteins

Wheat: Gliadin and glutenin
Barley: Harden
Rye: Secalin
Oats: Avenin

Saturni L, Ferretti G, Bacchetti T. The gluten-free diet: safety and nutritional quality. Nutrients 2010; 2:16–34.

Implementing a gluten-free diet

A number of studies exist detailing the therapeutic benefits of a GFD for conditions including autism, irritable bowel syndrome, autoimmune disorders and depression. Organisation and emotional support for individuals implementing a GFD are associated with higher adherence to a gluten-free diet.[246] Thus the naturopathic practitioner's role is to support the patient with education on how to implement a healthy gluten-free diet as well as strategies to follow it, making sure it is not only gluten-free but nutritionally sound. Frequent evaluation in the first 6 months is required to ensure compliance and to provide advice on factors such as interpreting labels correctly, availability and access of gluten-free foods, trouble-shooting dilemmas faced when eating out, travelling and socialising, as well as navigating the organoleptic properties of gluten-free food. Additionally, the naturopathic nutritionist will need to provide advice on how to repair the gut mucosa to improve nutrient absorption. Individuals with coeliac disease have a higher risk of osteoporosis and a 40% increased risk of bone fractures.[247] Anaemia is also a common nutritional deficiency as a result of impaired absorption, so care should be taken by the naturopathic practitioner to address risk factors and correct nutritional deficiencies.

HOW MUCH GLUTEN CAN BE TOLERATED?

Contrary to popular opinion, gluten-free products are not totally devoid of gluten. The definition for what constitutes 'gluten-free' in Australia is set by Food Standards Australia and New Zealand (FSANZ) which allows a limit of 3 ppm of gluten in gluten-free products. It is suggested that approximately 10–100 mg of gluten may be tolerated by individuals with coeliac disease.[248]

NUTRITIONAL CONSIDERATIONS

Many individuals assume that GF alternatives are healthier than their gluten-containing counterparts; however, like any dietary style, a gluten-free diet that is not planned properly may be low in a number of nutrients.

Refined, energy-dense foods

There is a plethora of processed/packaged GF products available (e.g. cereal bars, biscuits and potato crisps) which many individuals may mistakenly consume excessively on the understanding that they are healthy, simply because they are gluten-free. Higher content of both saturated and hydrogenated fatty acids and an increase in the glycaemic index and glycaemic load of the meal have been noted in some individuals following a gluten-free diet.[249] However, an analysis of Australian GF products showed that they were not significantly different in their nutritional quality compared with their gluten-containing counterparts.[250] Individuals following a GFD should be counselled on wholefood GF versus refined GF products.

Fibre

Research has shown that individuals adhering to a gluten-free diet may consume less fibre than those not avoiding gluten.[251] This may be due to patients' individual preferences, avoidance of grain foods high in fibre and the fact that many packaged gluten-free products are highly refined and devoid of or low in fibre. A 7-day prospective study investigating food intake in 55 patients adhering to a GFD for more than 2 years and compared to 50 newly-diagnosed age- and sex-matched patients studied prospectively over 12 months on GFD found that fibre intake was inadequate in the majority of participants when intake was compared with Australian Nutritional Recommendations and Australian population data.[252] Adequate fibre may be obtained on a GFD that is planned appropriately with abundant fruits, vegetables and GF grains, pseudo-grains and legumes.

Micronutrients

Micronutrient intake may be inadequate in those following a gluten-free diet. More than 10% of both newly-diagnosed women and women experienced in gluten-free eating had inadequate thiamin, folate, vitamin A, magnesium, calcium and iron intakes, while in men, more than 10% had inadequate thiamin, folate, magnesium, calcium and zinc intakes, in part due to habitual poor dietary choices.[253] Similar results were seen in a small Swedish study undertaken on 30 children. Researchers observed that children on GFD appear to follow the same trends as healthy children on a normal diet, with high intakes of saturated fat and sucrose and low intakes of dietary fibre, vitamin D and magnesium compared to recommendations. Vitamin D, riboflavin, niacin, thiamine, magnesium and selenium were lower in children with coeliac disease than in healthy children. However, children with coeliac disease did have high iron and calcium levels.[254]

Fish, meat, fruit and vegetables are sources of minerals in the diet and their presence in the diet can help to counterbalance possible micronutrient deficiencies associated with a GFD. Individuals following a GFD are advised to consume these foods in their diet, with particular emphasis on all fruits and vegetables because they are low in energy and rich in nutrients.[255]

Quinoa and flaxseed are recommended to improve the amount of omega-3 fatty acids in gluten-free diets while meals based on amaranth, quinoa and buckwheat will have higher levels of protein, fat, fibre and minerals than those based on rice and corn, and are thus good alternative ingredients for gluten-free diets.[256]

There are numerous cereals, grains, seeds, legumes and nuts that may replace gluten:

- Amaranth
- Arrowroot
- Buckwheat
- Corn
- Legumes
- Millet
- Nuts
- Potato
- Quinoa
- Rice
- Sorghum
- Tapioca
- Soy
- Teff.

AVOID (DUE TO GLUTEN CONTENT)

- Wheat, e.g. durum, semolina
- Kamut
- Barley
- Rye.

CAN OATS BE CONSUMED ON A GLUTEN-FREE DIET?

Oats contain a prolamin fraction, called avenin, which is similar to gliadins, secalins and hordeins.[257] Oats that have been uncontaminated by gluten-containing cereals (i.e. gluten-free oats) can be safely consumed by most individuals with coeliac disease.[258] This is because oat avenins are structurally different and represent a smaller percentage of protein than is found in wheat. It should be noted, however, that many individuals with coeliac disease may find it difficult to digest oats.

Gluten-free diet and type 1 diabetes

In adolescents with type 1 diabetes and coeliac disease, adherence to a GFD has been shown to increase quality of life and result in better glycaemic control compared to those with poor adherence.[259] A gluten-free diet in participants with autoimmune disease without coeliac serology has also been shown to be useful, particularly with disease remittance. Fifteen children aged 2–15 years, newly diagnosed with type-1 diabetes administered a gluten-free diet for 1 year, displayed improved HbA1c as well as a three times higher prevalence of partial remission 1 year after diagnosis, signifying better metabolic control after 1 year. A 2012 report details the case of a 6-year-old boy, newly diagnosed type 1 diabetes, who was started on a gluten-free diet and who remained without the need for exogenous insulin after 20 months. At the initiation of gluten-free diet, HbA1c was 7.8% and was stabilised at 5.8%–6.0% without insulin therapy with a GFD. At 16 months after diagnosis fasting blood glucose was 4.1 mmol/L and after 20 months he was still without daily insulin therapy.

Svensson J, Sildorf SM, Pipper CB et al. Potential beneficial effects of a gluten-free diet in newly diagnosed children with type 1 diabetes: a pilot study. Springerplus 2016 Jul 7; 5(1):994; Sildorf SM, Fredheim S, Svensson J et al. Remission without insulin therapy on gluten-free diet in a 6-year-old boy with type 1 diabetes mellitus. BMJ Case Rep 2012 Jun 21; 2012. pii: bcr0220125878.

GLUTEN-FREE DIET PLANNER

BREAKFAST	
Slow-cooked spiced lamb with sauerkraut, salad and natural yoghurt, serve with quinoa	Leftovers can be advocated for those following a GFD as eating out can pose problems due to contamination with gluten. Slow-cooked lamb provides a source of vitamin B_{12} and iron (both of which are commonly deficient in coeliac disease) that is easily digestible. If tolerated, natural live yoghurt and sauerkraut can be consumed to improve the gut microflora which may help to reverse gluten-induced dysbiosis. Quinoa is GF.
SNACKS	
Tapioca pudding with seasonal fruit, flaxseeds and pumpkin seeds	Tapioca is gluten-free and lends itself well to desserts. Adequate fruit intake is emphasised to increase vitamin content in the diet and reduce oxidative damage associated with inflammation. Zinc deficiency is common in coeliac disease, thus pumpkin seeds which are rich in zinc provide an ideal snack.
LUNCH	
Salmon sashimi rice bowl: 200 g salmon sashimi served on top of ½ cup steamed rice. Serve with 1 slice of nori, pickled carrots and cucumber, ¼ avocado, sprinkle of sesame seeds and 1 tsp tamari	Patients should be counselled that gluten-free can be quick, wholefood oriented and still tasty. A fishmonger can provide sashimi-grade salmon/trout/kingfish. Serve with rice, which is a cost-efficient, easily available gluten-free alternative. Tamari is a by-product of miso and is a gluten-free alternative to soy sauce which contains wheat. Nori provides a source of minerals.
DINNER	
Vietnamese rice flour and turmeric pancake served with shredded chicken (or tofu for vegan alternative), bean sprouts, mint, Thai basil and shredded carrot	Rice flour can be mixed with coconut milk and turmeric to make a savoury pancake that is gluten-free. Ample vegetables are included to boost fibre, antioxidants and vitamins.

VEGAN DIET

A vegan diet is one that excludes all animal-derived substances including meat, fish, eggs, dairy-based products such as butter, cheese and yoghurt, as well as honey. As noted by the American Dietetic Association, a vegan diet, if planned adequately, may be healthy and may be used to help treat and protect against a range of diseases.

Vegan diets have gained traction among the general population in the last few years, with the proportion of individuals choosing to follow a vegan diet increasing. Reasons for choosing to adopt a vegan diet are varied. 'Health' is one of the top reasons cited (with 47% of individuals stating this), followed by animal welfare (27%).[260] The reason an individual follows a vegan diet may offer a clue as to how nutritious their diet is. Individuals adopting a vegan diet for health reasons have been shown to have diets with higher nutritional value and also appear to engage in other healthier lifestyle behaviours such as regular exercise, compared to those following a vegan diet for ethical reasons.[261] However, while total nutritional value has been shown to be lower in the diets of those following a vegan diet for ethical reasons, soy consumption and vitamin supplementation has been shown to be higher, highlighting the differences in vegan diets that are a result of the individual's belief system.

It is now far easier for vegans to compose an adequate vegan diet than it was 10 years ago. The market is more versatile, with increased availability of vegan foods which have been supplemented with key nutrients that may otherwise be commonly deficient in the vegan diet. However, adequate planning by the naturopathic practitioner may still be required to ensure the patient's optimal health and prevention of nutritional deficiencies.

The vegan microbiome

Differences have been observed in the gut microbiota of vegans compared to their omnivore counterparts. Because the diets of vegans are higher in carbohydrates and fibre than that of omnivores, vegans' stool samples have been shown to have significantly reduced pH, which influences bacterial preference.[262,263] Lower pH has been shown to correlate with reduced counts of *E. coli* and *Enterobacteriacea* species as they are not tolerant of the more acidic environment. Conversely, a greater abundance of protective species such as *F. prausnitzii* have been seen in vegans, in part due to low pH.[264] In this way, the naturopath may be able to manipulate the microbiota by suggesting a vegan diet if a patient's comprehensive digestive stool analysis (CDSA) has shown an overgrowth of *E. coli*. Statistically significant differences in bacterial composition but no difference in measures of diversity were observed in Northeastern US urban-dwelling vegan and omnivorous citizens.[265] This highlights the fact that diet can contribute to the quantity and associated bacterial community shifts in faecal microbiota composition; however, diversity is more challenging. Interestingly, 40% of vegans have been found to be equol producers.[266]

Nutritional considerations

Vegan diets are higher in fibre and contain optimal fat profiles compared to their omnivorous counterparts.[267]

A well-planned vegan diet may be also be higher in magnesium, folate, and vitamins C and E and is therefore useful for increasing quantities of protective nutrients and phytochemicals and for reducing the intake components of the diet implicated in several chronic diseases. This is largely the result of increased consumption of plant foods, in particular fruit and vegetables, compared to their omnivorous counterparts.

A vegan diet, if not planned correctly, may be devoid of fundamental nutrients such as protein, omega-3 fatty acids, vitamin B_{12}, iron, calcium and zinc due to omission of nutrients found primarily within animal products. A Finnish study observed decreased dietary intake of vitamins B_{12} and D in vegans compared to non-vegetarians as well as lower concentrations of iodine and selenium. However, vegan individuals displayed better fatty acid profiles as well as much higher concentrations of antioxidants such as genistein and daidzein, the latter of which are commonly found in soy products.[268] Similarly, a Danish study[269] noted that vegan participants had better dietary macronutrient composition than the average Nordic population. However, micronutrient content was insufficient, with selenium, iodine and vitamin D all below the recommended levels. It should be noted that nutritional deficiencies are not unique to a vegan diet. A small Swiss study examining macronutrients and macronutrients among omnivores, vegans and vegetarians noted different deficiencies existed depending on the style of diet; 58% of omnivores were found to be deficient in folate while 47% of vegans were deficient in zinc. Interestingly, contrary to popular opinion, iron deficiency was comparable among all three groups.[270]

VITAMIN B_{12}

As with a vegetarian diet, vitamin B_{12} is a known high-risk nutrient for vegans, because it is available almost exclusively from animal products. Individuals following a vegan diet need to take a supplement or consume adequate quantities of fortified foods to meet vitamin B_{12} requirements. Small, frequent doses of vitamin B_{12} appear to be better absorbed than larger, less frequent doses.[271] Individuals following a vegan diet should also have their vitamin B_{12} status assessed regularly to identify a potential problem and rectify it, particularly as many vegans take B_{12} supplements irregularly or refuse to use them, deeming them to be synthetic. Vitamin B_{12} is required for synthesis of DNA and for maintaining the health of the myelin sheath, thus deficiency can result in demyelinisation of peripheral nerves, the spinal cord, cranial nerves and the brain, leading to damage of the nerves and neuropsychiatric abnormalities such as dementia, loss of memory, psychosis and generalised weakness. Vegans may need to consume a vitamin B_{12} supplement, particularly if they are not regularly consuming vitamin B_{12} fortified foods.

Food sources of vitamin B_{12}

TEMPEH

Tempeh is a fermented soy product that is a source of vitamin B_{12}. Tempeh contains very small quantities of vitamin B_{12} (0.7–8.0 micrograms/100 g). Bacterial contamination during tempeh production may contribute to the vitamin B_{12} content of tempeh.

NORI

Nori is a great source of vitamin B_{12}.[272] Consumption of approximately 4 g of dried purple laver (about 2 sheets of nori) supplies about 2.4 micrograms of vitamin B_{12} per day.[273] In Japan, nori is often served for breakfast; however, in the West this may be unpalatable for many patients. A large amount of nori can be consumed in the form of nori chips, or by using nori sheets as wraps for homemade sushi. Nori can also be torn and scattered through Japanese-inspired salads, rice or soups. In a nutritional analysis of six vegan children aged between 7 and 14 years who for 4–10 years consumed a vegan macrobiotic diet made up primarily of brown rice, sea vegetables such as kombu and hijiki as well as sheets of dried nori seasoned with sesame oil, shoyu and miso, researchers found that none of the children were deficient in vitamin B_{12}. The researchers suggested that the consumption of nori, hijiki and kombu may help to prevent vitamin B_{12} deficiency in vegans.[274]

MUSHROOMS

Contrary to popular opinion, mushrooms are not an optimal source of vitamin B_{12} with many varieties containing zero or trace levels.[275] Shiitake mushrooms have been found to contain vitamin B_{12}; however, the quantity needed to be consumed to meet RDIs of vitamin B_{12} would not be possible on a daily basis.

Protein

Vegan diets may not meet RDI targets for protein if not planned correctly.[276] Supplemental protein in the form of a low-allergen protein shake is an option if nutrient requirements are not being met but may not be needed for most patients who can carefully construct their diet, paying attention to the higher-protein plant foods such as tofu, tempeh, quinoa, black beans and chickpeas. There is no need to consciously combine different protein foods as long as a variety of these foods are consumed, as the body will maintain a pool of amino acids that can be used to

TABLE 8.7 Proteins at a glance

Brand	Food	Serving size	Protein
Annalisa	Brown lentils (canned)	120 g	8.2 g
Annalisa	Chickpeas (canned)	120 g	7.4 g
Absolute Organic	Black beans (canned)	200 g	17.8 g
Absolute Organic	Red kidney beans (canned)	200 g	8.8 g
Soyco	Tofu — Malaysian	100 g	16 g

complement protein from the diet. The protein quality in foods can be assessed by the protein digestibility-corrected amino acid score (PDCAAS).[277] This score assesses the quality of protein according to amino acid requirements as well as ability to digest the food. Most animal proteins and soy protein have a PDCAAS score close to or equal to 1.0 (the maximum score); however, scores for other plant proteins are generally lower. (See also Table 8.7.)

Omega-3 fatty acids

Optimal sources of the omega-3 fatty acid linolenic acid should be emphasised to enhance synthesis of the long-chain fatty acid docosahexanoic acid. Vegans have much lower plasma concentrations of omega-3 fatty acids when compared to individuals who eat fish. The plant-based n–3 fatty acid α-linolenic acid (ALA; 18:3n–3) can be converted into EPA and DHA; however, as discussed in the section on vegetarianism, this is at a fairly low efficiency. Seven intervention studies published in the last 10 years suggest ALA from nut and seed oils is not converted to DHA at all.[278] However, vegan individuals do respond well to a relatively low dose of a vegetarian omega-3 supplement made from micro-algae oil which has been shown to significantly increase blood erythrocyte and plasma DHA algae.[279] The oil from brown algae (kelp) is a source of DHA and could also be promoted as a dietary addition.

Calcium

Plant foods that are rich in calcium such as green leafy vegetables, tofu and tahini should be consumed to ensure adequate intake of calcium and co-factors such as magnesium. Soy milk fortified with calcium carbonate has been shown to be absorbed similarly to calcium in cow's milk.

Zinc and iron

There are virtually no studies assessing zinc and iron status in vegans; however, as both minerals are associated with meat intake in the Western diet, it can be hypothesised that both minerals may be lacking in some vegan diets. Plant foods contain an abundance of zinc though as with a vegetarian diet phytate content may impact absorption. Processing methods such as soaking, heating and sprouting may help to reduce the phytate-limiting effects on zinc bioavailability.

Research

Because a vegan diet tends to be lower in protein, and protein and its amino acids are essential for healthy mood, it has been postulated that a vegan diet may negatively impact mood. But contrary to this, a small study showed that vegan individuals were less likely to be stressed and experienced less anxiety than their omnivore counterparts.[280] The researchers hypothesised that a vegan diet may promote mood benefits because it is high in plant-based foods which are anti-inflammatory, and which thus negate inflammation in the brain, which is implicated in the pathogenesis of depression.

A large systematic review and meta-analysis comprised of 98 cross-sectional studies and 10 cohort prospective studies involving a total population of more than 130 000 vegetarians and 15 000 vegans observed that the risk of many chronic diseases could be reduced by following a plant-based diet.[281] Vegetarian and vegan participants showed significantly lower BMI, lipid variables and fasting glucose (all risk factors for chronic disease), compared with non-vegetarians and non-vegans. Following a vegan diet was also associated with a significant decrease in total cancer mortality. This is likely to be in part due to the fact that a well-rounded vegan plant-based diet provides ample fruit, vegetables, soybeans, legumes and nuts, all of which are known to be chemo protective as well as highly anti-inflammatory. In fact, following a vegan diet that is rich in anti-inflammatory wholefoods has been shown to decrease systemic inflammation in the presence of obesity, as measured by circulating CRP.[282]

VEGAN DIETS IN PREGNANCY

Diet in pregnancy affects not only the mother, but also her baby. Dietary deficiencies may affect the long-term health of the child, hence the interest in examining vegan diets in pregnancy. The most recent systematic narrative review available highlights that the evidence on vegan–vegetarian diets in pregnancy is scant and suggests more randomised studies are required to allow for distinguishing the effects of diet from confounding factors.[283] From the research available at this time it appears that a well-planned (and the emphasis is on well- planned!) vegan diet in a healthy pregnant woman does not appear to be associated with worse outcomes than are seen in omnivores. Close attention should be paid, however, to vitamin and trace element requirements, particularly vitamin B_{12}, iron, vitamin D and calcium: deficiencies in these are prevalent in the vegan diet and requirements are increased during pregnancy.

Breastfed infants born to vitamin B_{12}-deficient mothers have a high risk of vitamin B_{12} deficiency. A number of case reports exist of infantile vitamin B_{12} deficiency encountered in the offspring of strict vegan and vegetarian mothers.[284] Low serum levels of B_{12} have been linked to negative impacts in cognitive, motor and growth outcomes, thus care should be taken to ensure women following a vegan diet are meeting vitamin B_{12} requirements and that supplementation is continued into lactation.[285]

VEGAN MEAL PLANNER

BREAKFAST	
Tempeh, potato and kale hash	Nutrient considerations for an individual following a vegan diet are specifically focused on key nutrients such as protein and calcium which may otherwise be obtained from animal products. Tempeh is a fermented soy product that is vegan and is a rich source of absorbable protein as well as calcium and isoflavones. Kale is a nutrient-dense green that exhibits excellent absorbability for its calcium content. This could be made as a dinner and then consumed for breakfast the next day.
SNACKS	
Chilli-flavoured nori chips Chia pudding Fresh seasonal fruit with 30 g almonds	Nori is rich in iodine and may be a possible source of vitamin B_{12} for vegans. Chia seeds are a source of fatty acids and fibre. Almonds are a plant-based source of calcium.
LUNCH	
Vegan falafel bowl Falafels (chickpea base) served with salad containing hummus and quinoa tabouli	Plant sources of protein include chickpeas, found in the hummus and falafels, as well as quinoa. Quinoa contains all 8 essential amino acids and when combined with chickpeas would provide a complete source of protein.
DINNER	
Mexican dinner Black beans with Mexican-style rice. Serve with corn tortilla, guacamole, corn on the cob and fresh tomatoes	Black beans contain an optimal source of protein. By combining them with corn and rice, the PDCAAS content of the meal is further enhanced. Patients can be counselled on nutrient-dense vegan meals based on wholefoods so that they do not have to rely on processed vegan foods such as faux meats.

DAIRY-FREE DIET

Dairy products feature dominantly in the Western diet; however, emergence of the ability to digest lactose is a relatively recent event in human history, occurring 7500 to 10000 years ago. Inability to digest dairy products, in particular the cow's milk protein casein and the carbohydrate lactose, requires implementation of a dairy-free diet for amelioration of symptoms. Removal of dairy products from the diet has been shown to improve a range of conditions including constipation in children[286] as well as to reduce the risk of prostate cancer.[287]

Lactose

Lactose is a disaccharide made up of galactose bound to glucose. Absorption of lactose in the intestines is dependent upon hydrolysis to its component monosaccharides by the brush-border enzyme lactase.[288]

Deficiency of lactase has been described in three different conditions:[289]

- Congenital absence of the lactase enzyme — rare disease of the newborn associated with a locus (2q21)
- Primary late-onset lactose deficiency — autosomic recessive condition characterised by a gradual reduction in lactase activity, usually non-existent before ages 5–6 years
- Secondary lactose deficiency — typically occurs following gastrointestinal infection by viruses and parasites, coeliac disease or IBD, precipitating damage to the villi where lactase is produced, leading to partial atrophy. Reversible upon repair of the gut.

From week 8 of gestation, lactase activity can be detected at the mucosal surface in the human intestine and continues to increase, peaking by birth.[290] Lactose concentration in mother's milk is considerably higher (7.2 mg/100 mL) compared to cow's milk which contains 4.7 mg/100 mL.[291] Most children, with the exception of those who suffer from congenital absence of the intestinal enzyme lactase, are able to digest lactose from breast milk. As children wean, lactase activity decreases and the genes that encode lactase expression are down-regulated and switched off as a result of normal maturation, with concurrent loss of the brush border enzyme lactose in the intestines. In those without the lactase enzyme, unabsorbed lactose molecules osmotically attract fluid into the lumen of the colon, increasing fluidity of the contents in the intestines. In addition, bacteria in the colon ferments the undigested lactose into short-chain fatty acids such as methane and CO_2. This results in symptoms such as gas and urgency commonly associated with lactose intolerance.[292]

LACTOSE INTOLERANCE

Lactose intolerance related to primary or secondary lactase deficiency is characterised by:[293]

- Abdominal pain
- Abdominal distension
- Cramping
- Borborygmi
- Flatus
- Diarrhoea induced by lactose in dairy products
- Vomiting (in severe cases).

While inability to digest cow's milk is often viewed as an intolerance or defect of the body, the inability to digest lactose is actually a natural state of being for the majority of the world's population who are not able to digest it post weaning; in fact, it is estimated that by age 7 years and beyond only 35% of the human population can actually digest lactose.[294] Certain ethnic groups display the ability to tolerate lactose better than others, with this appearing to be attributed to race and gene pool. Descendants from Northern European populations and their offspring in America and Australia, which traditionally practised cattle domestication, have a high frequency of 'lactose persistence trait' with up to 90% showing lactose persistence. Conversely, this trait is low in Asian populations where lactose persistence is estimated to be only about 1%.[295]

Effect of raw milk on lactose intolerance

In recent times, consumption of unpasteurised raw milk has increased in popularity. It has been hypothesised that because raw milk is not pasteurised, the retention of microflora that occurs due to the milk not being heated may aid digestion of lactose, reducing malabsorption, in a similar manner that occurs for yoghurt. Unfortunately, a small randomised controlled pilot study found this hypothesis was not supported; in fact, there appeared to be higher lactose malabsorption for raw vs pasteurised milk on day 1, though by day 2 results were comparable between the two different types of milk.[296]

Management

- Management of lactose intolerance requires implementation of a lactose-free diet; however, some studies suggest that up to 7 g of lactose may be tolerated before symptoms arise.[297]
- Altered forms of dairy food ingestion may be helpful. Consumption of live yoghurts and fermented dairy products such as kefir are often tolerated by those with lactose intolerance as the lactose is fermented by the probiotic strains within the yoghurt/fermented dairy.
- Lactose-free cheese and milks have the lactase enzyme added to them to aid digestion of lactose, while other individuals may wish to supplement with an enzyme supplement containing lactase before consuming a lactose-containing meal.

Casein

Intolerance to dairy is usually attributed to lactose though intolerance to casein, a protein found in dairy products, is becoming more recognised.

DIFFERENT TYPES OF CASEIN

Beta-casein proteins make up approximately one-third of the total protein of cow's milk and can be found in two genetic variants: A1 and A2. Either or both of these genetic variants may be expressed in cow's milk, depending on the individual cow's genetic makeup. In recent years, increasing evidence has pointed to the fact that A1 beta-casein, a protein produced by a large percentage of European-origin cattle — but not purebred Asian or African cattle — is associated with cow's milk intolerance. Animal studies show that when digestive enzymes within the gut meet with A1 beta-casein proteins it results in the release of the peptide beta-casomorphin-7 (BCM-7), which activates μ-opioid receptors found throughout the gastrointestinal tract, increasing T-helper 2 pathways[298] and gut transit time[299] and creating inflammation. BCM-7 is released from consumption of not only milk but also cheese and yoghurt. Notably, A2 beta-casein also causes release of BCM-7, however this appears to be in much smaller quantities.

Research

A small double-blind, randomised 8-week cross-over study was conducted at Curtin University in Western Australia to evaluate the differences in gastrointestinal effects in adults consuming milk containing A1 versus A2 beta-casein. The researchers observed that consumption of A1 beta-casein milk led to significantly higher stool consistency values (Bristol Stool Scale) and more abdominal pain and gut inflammation compared with consumption of A2 beta-casein milk.[300]

Similar results were seen in a double-blind, randomised, 2×2 crossover trial involving 45 Chinese participants. Consumption of milk containing a mix of both A1 and A2 beta-casein types was associated with higher gastrointestinal inflammation, significantly greater postdigestive symptoms, longer gastrointestinal transit times and lower levels of short-chain fatty acids compared to consumption of milk containing only A2 beta-casein.[301] Interestingly, as well as the aforementioned gastrointestinal complaints, participants also exhibited decreased cognitive processing speed and accuracy, suggesting that casein, like gluten, appears to impact cognitive function. Larger trials are required to confirm these findings.

DAIRY-FREE MEAL PLANNER

BREAKFAST	
Coconut yoghurt served with seasonal fruit and seeds Cinnamon chai almond milk	Coconut yoghurt is made with coconut milk and is dairy free. Most brands contain live cultures; however they are higher in fat and lower in carbohydrates and protein than their dairy-based counterparts. Nut-based milks can be used in place of dairy milks. Homemade almond milk is preferable because it is higher in calcium and other nutrients compared to conventionally bought almond milk which may be flavoured with almond essence.
LUNCH	
Pesto chicken pizza with mixed leaf salad dressed with balsamic	Pizza can be made using a vegan cheese, or by using dairy-free pesto as a replacement for cheese. Vinegars can be used as substitutes for creamy dairy-based salad dressings.
DINNER	
Dairy-free lasagne Serve with green vegetables	White sauces typically contain cheese and butter but these can easily be replaced by non-dairy-containing ingredients such as silken tofu, pureed white beans or pureed cauliflower, all of which contain the right consistency and texture to use in place of dairy products. The addition of green vegetables provides a non-dairy source of calcium.
SNACKS	
Fruit smoothie Fruit-based gelato	Water, rice and nut milks are useful dairy alternatives. Smoothies can be made using frozen banana as a base to obtain a thick, creamy texture in place of milk. Fruit-based gelatos can be used as an alternative to ice-cream and frozen yoghurts, provided they are free from dairy.

REFERENCES

[1] Chilton SN, Burton JP, Reid G. Inclusion of fermented foods in food guides around the world. Nutrients 2015;7(1):390–404.

[2] Clarke JO, Mullin GE. A review of complementary and alternative approaches to immunomodulation. Nutr Clin Pract 2008;23(1):49–62.

[3] Marx W, Kiss N, Isenring L. Is ginger beneficial for nausea and vomiting? An update of the literature. Curr Opin Support Palliat Care 2015;9(2):189–95.

[4] Jayalekshmi JL, Lakshmi R, Mukerji A. Honey on oral mucositis: a randomized controlled trial. Gulf J Oncolog 2016;1(20):30–7.

[5] Rustad C, Smith C. Nutrition knowledge and associated behavior changes in a holistic, short-term nutrition education intervention with low-income women. J Nutr Educ Behav 2013;45(6):490–8.

[6] Fardet A, Rock E. Toward a new philosophy of preventive nutrition: from a reductionist to a holistic paradigm to improve nutritional recommendations. Adv Nutr 2014;5(4):430–46.

[7] Jacobs DR Jr, Tapsell LC. What an anticardiovascular diet should be in 2015. Curr Opin Lipidol 2015;26(4):270–5.

[8] Nguyen B, Bauman A, Gale J, et al. Fruit and vegetable consumption and all-cause mortality: evidence from a large Australian cohort study. Int J Behav Nutr Phys Act 2016;13:9.

[9] Ministry of Health Brazil. Dietary guidelines for the Brazilian population; 2014. 2nd edn. Available online: http://www.fao.org/nutrition/education/food-dietary-guidelines/regions/brazil/en/.

[10] Burton-Freeman B, Sesso HD. Whole food versus supplement: comparing the clinical evidence of tomato intake and lycopene supplementation on cardiovascular risk factors. Adv Nutr 2014;5(5):457–85.

[11] Vissers MCM, Bozonet SM, Pearson JF, et al. Dietary ascorbate intake affects steady state tissue concentrations in vitamin C-deficient mice: tissue deficiency after suboptimal intake and superior bio- availability from a food source (kiwifruit). Am J Clin Nutr 2011;93(2):292–301.

[12] Rodrigo R, Libuy M, Feliu F, et al. Polyphenols in disease: from diet to supplements. Curr Pharm Biotechnol 2014;15(4):304–17.

[13] Dreher ML, Davenport AJ. Hass avocado composition and potential health effects. Crit Rev Food Sci Nutr 2013;53(7):738–50.

[14] Unlu NZ, Bohn T, Clinton SK, et al. Carotenoid absorption from salad and salsa by humans is enhanced by the addition of avocado or avocado oil. J Nutr 2005;135(3):431–6.

[15] Unlu NZ, Bohn T, Clinton SK, et al. Carotenoid absorption from salad and salsa by humans is enhanced by the addition of avocado or avocado oil. J Nutr 2005;135(3):431–6.

[16] Chen P, Zhang W, Wang X, et al. Lycopene and risk of prostate cancer: a systematic review and meta-analysis. Medicine (Baltimore) 2015;94(33):e1260.

[17] Comerford KB, Ayoob KT, Murray RD, et al. The role of avocados in complementary and transitional feeding. Nutrients 2016;8(5).

[18] Comerford KB, Ayoob KT, Murray RD, et al. The role of avocados in complementary and transitional feeding. Nutrients 2016;8(5).

[19] Wien M, Haddad E, Oda K, et al. A randomized 3 × 3 crossover study to evaluate the effect of Hass avocado intake on post-ingestive satiety, glucose and insulin levels, and subsequent energy intake in overweight adults. Nutr J 2013;12:155.

[20] Clifford T, Howatson G, West DJ, et al. The potential benefits of red beetroot supplementation in health and disease. Nutrients 2015;7(4):2801–22.

[21] Siervo M, Lara J, Ogbonmwan I, et al. Inorganic nitrate and beetroot juice supplementation reduces blood pressure in adults: a systematic review and meta-analysis. J Nutr 2013;143(6):818–26.

[22] Lara J, Ashor AW, Oggioni C, et al. Effects of inorganic nitrate and beetroot supplementation on endothelial function: a systematic review and meta-analysis. Eur J Nutr 2016;55(2):451–9.

[23] Siervo M, Lara J, Jajja J, et al. Ageing modifies the effects of beetroot juice supplementation on 24-hour blood pressure variability: an individual participant meta-analysis. Nitric Oxide 2015;47:97–105.

[24] Siervo M, Lara J, Ogbonmwan I, et al. Inorganic nitrate and beetroot juice supplementation reduces blood pressure in adults: a systematic review and meta-analysis. J Nutr 2013;143(6):818–26.

[25] Hoon MW, Johnson NA, Chapman PG, et al. The effect of nitrate supplementation on exercise performance in healthy individuals: a systematic review and meta-analysis. Int J Sport Nutr Exerc Metab 2013;23(5):522–32.

[26] Jones AM. Dietary nitrate supplementation and exercise performance. Sports Med 2014;44(Suppl. 1):S35–45.

[27] Clifford T, Bell O, West DJ, et al. The effects of beetroot juice supplementation on indices of muscle damage following eccentric exercise. Eur J Appl Physiol 2016;116(2):353–62.

[28] Chaturvedi P. Antidiabetic potentials of *Momordica charantia*: multiple mechanisms behind the effects. J Med Food 2012;15(2):101–7.

[29] Ooi CP, Yassin Z, Hamid TA. *Momordica charantia* for type 2 diabetes mellitus. Cochrane Database Syst Rev 2012;(8):CD007845.

[30] Ching SM, Zakaria ZA, Paimin F, et al. Complementary alternative medicine use among patients with type 2 diabetes mellitus in the primary care setting: a cross-sectional study in Malaysia. BMC Complement Altern Med 2013;13:148.

[31] Tsai C, Chen E, Tsay H-S. Wild bitter gourd improves metabolic syndrome: a preliminary dietary supplementation trial. Nutr J 2012;11(1):4.

[32] Krawinkel M, Keding GB. Bitter gourd (*Momordica charantia*): a dietary approach to hyperglycemia. Nutr Rev 2006;64(7):331–7.

[33] Michalska A, Łysiak G. Bioactive compounds of blueberries: post-harvest factors influencing the nutritional value of products. Int J Mol Sci 2015;16(8):18642–63. doi:10.3390/ijms160818642.

[34] Andres-Lacueva C, Shukitt-Hale B, Galli RL, et al. Anthocyanins in aged blueberry-fed rats are found centrally and may enhance memory. Nutr Neurosci 2005;8:111–20.

[35] Shukitt-Hale B, Bielinski DF, Lau FC, et al. The beneficial effects of berries on cognition, motor behaviour and neuronal function in ageing. Br J Nutr 2015;114(10):1542–9.

[36] Krikorian R, Shidler M, Nash T, et al. Blueberry supplementation improves memory in older adults. J Agric Food Chem 2010;58(7):3996–4000.

[37] Schrager MA, Hilton J, Gould R, et al. Effects of blueberry supplementation on measures of functional mobility in older adults. Appl Physiol Nutr Metab 2015;40(6):543–9.

[38] Bahadoran Z, Mirmiran P, Azizi F. Potential efficacy of broccoli sprouts as a unique supplement for management of type 2 diabetes and its complications. J Med Food 2013;16(5):375–82.

[39] Natella F, Maldini M, Nardini M, et al. Improvement of the nutraceutical quality of broccoli sprouts by elicitation. Food Chem 2016;201:101–9.

[40] Atwell LL, Hsu A, Wong CP, et al. Absorption and chemopreventive targets of sulforaphane in humans following consumption of broccoli sprouts or a myrosinase-treated broccoli sprout extract. Mol Nutr Food Res 2015;59(3):424–33.

[41] Noah TL, Zhang H, Zhou H, et al. Effect of broccoli sprouts on nasal response to live attenuated influenza virus in smokers: a randomized, double-blind study. PLoS ONE 2014;9(6):e98671.

[42] Müller L, Meyer M, Bauer RN, et al. Effect of broccoli sprouts and live attenuated influenza virus on peripheral blood natural killer cells: a randomized, double-blind study. PLoS ONE 2016;11(1):e0147742.

[43] Egner PA, Chen JG, Zarth AT, et al. Rapid and sustainable detoxication of airborne pollutants by broccoli sprout beverage: results of a randomized clinical trial in China. Cancer Prev Res (Phila) 2014;7:813–23.

[44] Heber D, Li Z, Garcia-Lloret M, et al. Sulforaphane-rich broccoli sprout extract attenuates nasal allergic response to diesel exhaust particles. Food Funct 2014;5(1):35–41.

[45] Mohd Ali N, Yeap SK, Ho WY, et al. The promising future of chia, *Salvia hispanica*. J Biomed Biotechnol 2012;2012:171956.

[46] Nieman DC, Gillitt ND, Meaney MP, et al. No positive influence of ingesting chia seed oil on human running performance. Nutrients 2015;7(5):3666–76.

[47] Jin F, Nieman DC, Sha W, et al. Supplementation of milled chia seeds increases plasma ALA and EPA in postmenopausal women. Plant Foods Hum Nutr 2010;67:105–10.

[48] Valenzuela R, Bascuñán KA, Chamorro R, et al. Modification of docosahexaenoic acid composition of milk from nursing women who received alpha linolenic acid from chia oil during gestation and nursing. Nutrients 2015;7(8):6405–24.

[49] Medagama AB. The glycaemic outcomes of cinnamon, a review of the experimental evidence and clinical trials. Nutr J 2015; 14:108.

[50] Akilen R, Devendra D, Robinson N. Cinnamon in glycaemic control: systematic review and meta-analysis. Clin Nutr 2012;31(5):609–15.

[51] Bernardo MA, et al. Effect of cinnamon tea on postprandial glucose concentration. J Diabetes Res 2015;2015:913651.

[52] Magistrelli A, Chezem JC. Effect of ground cinnamon on postprandial blood glucose concentration in normal-weight and obese adults. J Acad Nutr Diet 2012;112(11):1806–9.

[53] Alkaabi JM, Al-Dabbagh B, Ahmad S, et al. Glycemic indices of five varieties of dates in healthy and diabetic subjects. Nutr J 2011;10:59.

[54] Habib HM, Ibrahim WH. Nutritional quality of 18 date fruit varieties. Int J Food Sci Nutr 2011;62(5):544–51.

[55] Al-Kuran O, Al-Mehaisen L, Bawadi H, et al. The effect of late pregnancy consumption of date fruit on labour and delivery. J Obstet Gynaecol 2011;31(1):29–31.

[56] Zhang Y, Chen J, Qiu J, et al. Intakes of fish and polyunsaturated fatty acids and mild-to-severe cognitive impairment risks: a dose-response meta-analysis of 21 cohort studies. Am J Clin Nutr 2016;103(2):330–40.

[57] Raji CA, Erickson KI, Lopez OL, et al. Regular fish consumption and age-related brain gray matter loss. Am J Prev Med 2014;47(4):444–51.

[58] Ghazanfarpour M, Sadeghi R, Latifnejad Roudsari R, et al. Effects of flaxseed and *Hypericum perforatum* on hot flash, vaginal atrophy and estrogen-dependent cancers in menopausal women: a systematic review and meta-analysis. Avicenna J Phytomed 2016;6(3):273–83.

[59] Demark-Wahnefried W, Polascik TJ, George SL, et al. Flaxseed supplementation (not dietary fat restriction) reduces prostate cancer proliferation rates in men presurgery. Cancer Epidem Biomark 2008;17(12):3577–87.

[60] Azrad M, Vollmer RT, Madden J, et al. Flaxseed-derived enterolactone is inversely associated with tumor cell proliferation in men with localized prostate cancer. J Med Food 2013;16(4):357–60.

[61] Lewington S, Clarke R, Qizilbash N, et al. Age-specific relevance of usual blood pressure to vascular mortality: a meta-analysis of individual data for one million adults in 61 prospective studies. Lancet 2002;360:1903–13.

[62] Chen CX, Barrett B, Kwekkeboom KL. Efficacy of oral ginger (*Zingiber officinale*) for dysmenorrhea: a systematic review and meta-analysis. Evid Based Complement Alternat Med 2016;2016:6295737.

[63] Lakhan SE, Ford CT, Tepper D. Zingiberaceae extracts for pain: a systematic review and meta-analysis. Nutr J 2015;14:50.

[64] Bartels EM, Folmer VM, Bliddal H, et al. Efficacy and safety of ginger in osteoarthritis patients: a meta-analysis of randomized placebo-controlled trials. Osteoarthritis Cartilage 2015;23(1):13–21.

[65] Viljoen E, Visser J, Koen N, et al. A systematic review and meta-analysis of the effect and safety of ginger in the treatment of pregnancy-associated nausea and vomiting. Nutr J 2014;13:20.

[66] Arslan M, Ozdemir L. Oral intake of ginger for chemotherapy-induced nausea and vomiting among women with breast cancer. Clin J Oncol Nurs 2015;19(5):E92–7.

[67] Marx WM, Teleni L, McCarthy AL, et al. Ginger (*Zingiber officinale*) and chemotherapy-induced nausea and vomiting: a systematic literature review. Nutr Rev 2013;71(4):245–54.

[68] Cao Y, Cao R, Bråkenhielm E. Antiangiogenic mechanisms of diet-derived polyphenols. J Nutr Biochem 2002;13(7):380–90.

[69] Henning SM, Wang P, Said JW, et al. Randomized clinical trial of brewed green and black tea in men with prostate cancer prior to prostatectomy. Prostate 2015;75(5):550–9.

[70] Cho HK, Jeong YM, Lee HS, et al. Effects of honey on oral mucositis in patients with head and neck cancer: a meta-analysis. Laryngoscope 2015;125(9):2085–92.

[71] Balakrishnan VS. Low BMI linked to worse colorectal cancer outcomes. Lancet Oncol 2015;16(16):e593.

[72] Francis M, Williams S. Effectiveness of Indian turmeric powder with honey as complementary therapy on oral mucositis: a nursing

perspective among cancer patients in Mysore. Nurs J India 2014;105(6):258–60.
[73] Stonehouse W, Gammon CS, Beck KL, et al. Kiwifruit: our daily prescription for health. Can J Physiol Pharmacol 2013;91(6):442–7.
[74] Gammon CS, Kruger R, Minihane AM, et al. Kiwifruit consumption favourably affects plasma lipids in a randomised controlled trial in hypercholesterolaemic men. Br J Nutr 2013;109(12):2208–18.
[75] Gammon CS, Kruger R, Conlon CA, et al. Inflammatory status modulates plasma lipid and inflammatory marker responses to kiwifruit consumption in hypercholesterolaemic men. Nutr Metab Cardiovasc Dis 2014;24(1):91–9.
[76] Recio-Rodriguez JI, Gomez-Marcos MA, Patino-Alonso MC, et al. Effects of kiwi consumption on plasma lipids, fibrinogen and insulin resistance in the context of a normal diet. Nutr J 2015;14:97.
[77] Chang CC, Lin YT, Lu YT, et al. Kiwifruit improves bowel function in patients with irritable bowel syndrome with constipation. Asia Pac J Clin Nutr 2010;19(4):451–7.
[78] Chan AO, Leung G, Tong T, et al. Increasing dietary fiber intake in terms of kiwifruit improves constipation in Chinese patients. World J Gastroenterol 2007;13(35):4771–5.
[79] Valverde ME, Hernández-Pérez T, Paredes-López O. Edible mushrooms: improving human health and promoting quality life. Int J Microbiol 2015;2015:376387.
[80] Li J, Zou L, Chen W, et al. Dietary mushroom intake may reduce the risk of breast cancer: evidence from a meta-analysis of observational studies. PLoS ONE 2014;9(4):e93437.
[81] Chen S, Oh SR, Phung S, et al. Anti-aromatase activity of phytochemicals in white button mushrooms (*Agaricus bisporus*). Cancer Res 2006;66(24):12026–34.
[82] Urbain P, Singler F, Ihorst G, et al. Bioavailability of vitamin D_2 from UV-B-irradiated button mushrooms in healthy adults deficient in serum 25-hydroxyvitamin D: a randomized controlled trial. Eur J Clin Nutr 2011;65(8):965–71.
[83] Urbain P, Singler F, Ihorst G, et al. Bioavailability of vitamin D_2 from UV-B-irradiated button mushrooms in healthy adults deficient in serum 25-hydroxyvitamin D: a randomized controlled trial. Eur J Clin Nutr 2011;65(8):965–71.
[84] Brufau G, Boatella J, Rafecas M. Nuts, source of energy and macronutrients. Br J Nutr 2006;96:S24–8.
[85] Martin N, Germanò R, Hartley L, et al. Nut consumption for the primary prevention of cardiovascular disease. Cochrane Database Syst Rev 2015;(9):CD011583.
[86] Ma L, Wang F, Guo W, et al. Nut consumption and the risk of coronary artery disease: a dose-response meta-analysis of 13 prospective studies. Thromb Res 2014;134(4):790–4.
[87] Zhou D, Yu H, He F, et al. Nut consumption in relation to cardiovascular disease risk and type 2 diabetes: a systematic review and meta-analysis of prospective studies. Am J Clin Nutr 2014;100:270–7.
[88] Del Gobbo LC, Falk MC, Feldman R, et al. Effects of tree nuts on blood lipids, apolipoproteins, and blood pressure: systematic review, meta-analysis, and dose-response of 61 controlled intervention trials. Am J Clin Nutr 2015;102(6):1347–56.
[89] Martin N, Germanò R, Hartley L, et al. Nut consumption for the primary prevention of cardiovascular disease. Cochrane Database Syst Rev 2015;(9):CD011583.
[90] Blanco Mejia S, Kendall CW, Viguiliouk E, et al. Effect of tree nuts on metabolic syndrome criteria: a systematic review and meta-analysis of randomised controlled trials. BMJ Open 2014;4(7):e004660.
[91] Viguiliouk E, Kendall CW, Blanco Mejia S, et al. Effect of tree nuts on glycemic control in diabetes: a systematic review and meta-analysis of randomized controlled dietary trials. PLoS ONE 2014;9(7):e103376.
[92] Liu Z, Lin X, Huang G, et al. Prebiotic effects of almonds and almond skins on intestinal microbiota in healthy adult humans. Anaerobe 2014;26:1–6.
[93] Ukhanova M, Wang X, Baer DJ, et al. Effects of almond and pistachio consumption on gut microbiota composition in a randomised cross-over human feeding study. Br J Nutr 2014;111(12):2146–52.
[94] Singh R, De S, Belkheir A. *Avena sativa* (oat), a potential neutraceutical and therapeutic agent: an overview. Crit Rev Food Sci Nutr 2013;53(2):126–44.
[95] Whitehead A, Beck EJ, Tosh S, et al. Cholesterol-lowering effects of oat β-glucan: a meta-analysis of randomized controlled trials. Am J Clin Nutr 2014;100(6):1413–21.
[96] Nwachukwu ID, Devassy JG, Aluko RE, et al. Cholesterol-lowering properties of oat β-glucan and the promotion of cardiovascular health: did Health Canada make the right call? Appl Physiol Nutr Metab 2015;40(6):535–42.
[97] Hou Q, Li Y, Li L, et al. The metabolic effects of oats intake in patients with type 2 diabetes: a systematic review and meta-analysis. Nutrients 2015;7(12):10369–87.
[98] Ramírez E, Brenes M, García P, et al. Oleuropein hydrolysis in natural green olives: importance of the endogenous enzymes. Food Chem 2016;206:204–9.
[99] Charoenprasert S, Mitchell A. Factors influencing phenolic compounds in table olives (*Olea europaea*). J Agric Food Chem 2012;60(29):7081–95.
[100] Accardi G, Aiello A, Gargano V, et al. Nutraceutical effects of table green olives: a pilot study with *Nocellara del Belice* olives. Immun Ageing 2016;13:11.
[101] Wang L, Martins-Green M. Pomegranate and its components as alternative treatment for prostate cancer. Int J Mol Sci 2014;15(9):14949–66.
[102] Pantuck AJ, Leppert JT, Zomorodian N, et al. Phase II study of pomegranate juice for men with rising prostate-specific antigen following surgery or radiation for prostate cancer. Clin Cancer Res 2006;12(13):4018–26.
[103] Igwe EO, Charlton KE. A systematic review on the health effects of plums (*Prunus domestica* and *Prunus salicina*). Phytother Res 2016;30(5):701–31.
[104] Lever E, Cole J, Scott SM, et al. Systematic review: the effect of prunes on gastrointestinal function. Aliment Pharmacol Ther 2014;40(7):750–8.
[105] Halmos EP, Gibson PR. Dried plums, constipation and the irritable bowel syndrome. Aliment Pharmacol Ther 2011;34(3):396–7, author reply 397–398.
[106] Igwe EO, Charlton KE. A systematic review on the health effects of plums (*Prunus domestica* and *Prunus salicina*). Phytother Res 2016;30(5):701–31.
[107] Hooshmand S, Arjmandi BH. Viewpoint: dried plum, an emerging functional food that may effectively improve bone health. Ageing Res Rev 2009;8(2):122–7.
[108] Igwe EO, Charlton KE. A systematic review on the health effects of plums (*Prunus domestica* and *Prunus salicina*). Phytother Res 2016;30(5):701–31.
[109] Hooshmand S, Chai SC, Saadat RL, et al. Comparative effects of dried plum and dried apple on bone in postmenopausal women. Br J Nutr 2011;106(6):923–30.
[110] Hooshmand S, Kern M, Metti D, et al. The effect of two doses of dried plum on bone density and bone biomarkers in osteopenic postmenopausal women: a randomized, controlled trial. Osteoporos Int 2016;27(7):2271–9.
[111] Messina M. Impact of soy foods on the development of breast cancer and the prognosis of breast cancer patients. Forsch Komplementmed 2016;23(2):75–80.
[112] Jemal A, Bray F, Center MM, et al. Global cancer statistics. CA Cancer J Clin 2011;61(2):69–90.
[113] Zhong C. Soy food intake and breast cancer risk: a meta-analysis. Wei Sheng Yan Jiu 2012;41:670–6.
[114] Zaheer K, Akhtar MH. An updated review of dietary isoflavones: nutrition, processing, bioavailability and impacts on human health. Crit Rev Food Sci Nutr 2017;57(6):1280–93.
[115] Wu AH, Yu MC, Tseng CC, et al. Epidemiology of soy exposures and breast cancer risk. Br J Cancer 2008;98(1):9–14.
[116] Messina M. Impact of soy foods on the development of breast cancer and the prognosis of breast cancer patients. Forsch Komplementmed 2016;23(2):75–80.
[117] Rafii F. The role of colonic bacteria in the metabolism of the natural isoflavone daidzin to equol. Metabolites 2015;5(1):56–73.
[118] Bawa S. The significance of soy protein and soy bioactive compounds in the prophylaxis and treatment of osteoporosis. J Osteoporos 2010;2010:891058.
[119] Scheiber MD, Liu JH, Subbiah MT, et al. Dietary inclusion of whole soy foods results in significant reductions in clinical risk factors for osteoporosis and cardiovascular disease in normal postmenopausal women. Menopause 2001;8(5):384–92.

[120] Sathyapalan T, Aye M, Rigby AS, et al. Soy reduces bone turnover markers in women during early menopause: a randomized controlled trial. J Bone Miner Res 2017;32(1):157–64.
[121] Tranche S, Brotons C, Pascual de la Pisa D, et al. Impact of a soy drink on climacteric symptoms: an open-label, crossover, randomized clinical trial. Gynecol Endocrinol 2016;32(6):477–82.
[122] Chen M, Rao Y, Zheng Y, et al. Association between soy isoflavone intake and breast cancer risk for pre- and post-menopausal women: a meta-analysis of epidemiological studies. PLoS ONE 2014;9:e89288.
[123] Chi F, Wu R, Zeng YC, et al. Post-diagnosis soy food intake and breast cancer survival: a meta-analysis of cohort studies. Asian Pac J Cancer Prev 2013;14:2407–12.
[124] Holzapfel NP, Holzapfel BM, Champ S, et al. The potential role of lycopene for the prevention and therapy of prostate cancer: from molecular mechanisms to clinical evidence. Int J Mol Sci 2013;14(7):14620–46.
[125] Boileau TW, Liao Z, Kim S, et al. Prostate carcinogenesis in N-methyl-N-nitrosourea (NMU)-testosterone-treated rats fed tomato powder, lycopene, or energy-restricted diets. J Natl Cancer Inst 2003;95:1578–86.
[126] Graff RE, Pettersson A, Lis RT, et al. Dietary lycopene intake and risk of prostate cancer defined by ERG protein expression. Am J Clin Nutr 2016r;103(3):851–60.
[127] Chen P, Zhang W, Wang X, et al. Lycopene and risk of prostate cancer: a systematic review and meta-analysis. Medicine (Baltimore) 2015;94(33):e1260.
[128] Paur I, Lilleby W, Bøhn SK, et al. Tomato-based randomized controlled trial in prostate cancer patients: effect on PSA. Clin Nutr 2017;36(3):672–9.
[129] Yamamoto Y, Aizawa K, Mieno M, et al. The effects of tomato juice on male infertility. Asia Pac J Clin Nutr 2017;26(1):65–71.
[130] Budak NH, Aykin E, Seydim AC, et al. Functional properties of vinegar. J Food Sci 2014;79(5):R757–64.
[131] Wu D, Kimura F, Takashima A, et al. Intake of vinegar beverage is associated with restoration of ovulatory function in women with polycystic ovary syndrome. Tohoku J Exp Med 2013;230(1):17–23.
[132] Mitrou P, Petsiou E, Papakonstantinou E, et al. The role of acetic acid on glucose uptake and blood flow rates in the skeletal muscle in humans with impaired glucose tolerance. Eur J Clin Nutr 2015;69(6):734–9.
[133] Mitrou P, Petsiou E, Papakonstantinou E, et al. Vinegar consumption increases insulin-stimulated glucose uptake by the forearm muscle in humans with type 2 diabetes. J Diabetes Res 2015;2015:175204.
[134] Fisberg M, Machado R. History of yogurt and current patterns of consumption. Nutr Rev 2015;73(Suppl. 1):4–7.
[135] Chapman DK, Bartlett J, Powell J, et al. Bacterial vaginosis screening and treatment in pregnant women. J Midwifery Womens Health 2016.
[136] Nasioudis D, Linhares IM, Ledger WJ, et al. Bacterial vaginosis: a critical analysis of current knowledge. BJOG 2017;124(1):61–9.
[137] Van Kessel K, Assefi N, Marrazzo J, et al. Common complementary and alternative therapies for yeast vaginitis and bacterial vaginosis: a systematic review. Obstet Gynecol Surv 2003;58(5):351–8.
[138] Hantoushzadeh S, Golshahi F, Javadian P, et al. Comparative efficacy of probiotic yoghurt and clindamycin in treatment of bacterial vaginosis in pregnant women: a randomized clinical trial. J Matern Fetal Neonatal Med 2012;25(7):1021–4.
[139] Tasdemir M, Tasdemir I, Tasdemir S, et al. Alternative treatment for bacterial vaginosis in pregnant patients; restoration of vaginal acidity and flora. Arch AIDS Res 1996;10(4):239–41.
[140] Hu H, Merenstein DJ, Wang C, et al. Impact of eating probiotic yogurt on colonization by *Candida* species of the oral and vaginal mucosa in HIV-infected and HIV-uninfected women. Mycopathologia 2013;176(3–4):175–81.
[141] Abdelmonem AM, Rasheed SM, Mohamed AS. Bee-honey and yogurt: a novel mixture for treating patients with vulvovaginal candidiasis during pregnancy. Arch Gynecol Obstet 2012;286(1):109–14.
[142] Fox MJ, Ahuja KD, Robertson IK, et al. Can probiotic yogurt prevent diarrhoea in children on antibiotics? A double-blind, randomised, placebo-controlled study. BMJ Open 2015;5(1):e006474.
[143] Scharl M, Geisel S, Vavricka SR, et al. Dying in yoghurt: the number of living bacteria in probiotic yoghurt decreases under exposure to room temperature. Digestion 2011;83(1–2):13–17.
[144] Cao Y, Wittert G, Taylor AW, et al. Nutrient patterns and chronic inflammation in a cohort of community dwelling middle-aged men. Clin Nutr 2017;36(4):1040–7.
[145] Barbaresko J, Koch M, Schulze MB. Dietary pattern analysis and biomarkers of low-grade inflammation: a systematic literature review. Nutr Rev 2013;71:511–27.
[146] Cavicchia PP, Steck S, Hurley TG, et al. A new dietary inflammatory index predicts interval changes in serum high-sensitivity C-reactive protein. J Nutr 2009;139:2365–72.
[147] Nayan S, Maby A, Endam LM, et al. Dietary modifications for refractory chronic rhinosinusitis? Manipulating diet for the modulation of inflammation. Am J Rhinol Allergy 2015;29(6):e170–4.
[148] McGeoghegan L, Muirhead CR, Almoosawi S. Association between an anti-inflammatory and anti-oxidant dietary pattern and diabetes in British adults: results from the national diet and nutrition survey rolling programme years 1–4. Int J Food Sci Nutr 2015;67(5):553–61.
[149] Saita E, Kondo K, Momiyama Y. Anti-inflammatory diet for atherosclerosis and coronary artery disease: antioxidant foods. Clin Med Insights Cardiol 2015;8(Suppl. 3):61–5.
[150] Huang EY, Devkota S, Moscoso D, et al. The role of diet in triggering human inflammatory disorders in the modern age. Microbes Infect 2013;15(12):765–74.
[151] Thorburn AN, Macia L, Mackay CR. Diet, metabolites, and "western-lifestyle" inflammatory diseases. Immunity 2014;40(6):833–42.
[152] Simopoulos AP. Evolutionary aspects of diet, the omega-6/omega-3 ratio and genetic variation: nutritional implications for chronic diseases. Biomed Pharmacother 2006;60(9):502–7.
[153] Grimstad T, Berge RK, Bohov P, et al. Salmon diet in patients with active ulcerative colitis reduced the simple clinical colitis activity index and increased the anti-inflammatory fatty acid index — a pilot study. Scand J Clin Lab Invest 2011;71(1):68–73.
[154] Gardener SL, Rainey-Smith SR, Martins RN. Diet and inflammation in Alzheimer's disease and related chronic diseases: a review. J Alzheimers Dis 2015;50(2):301–34.
[155] Grzanna R, Lindmark L, Frondoza CG. Ginger — an herbal medicinal product with broad anti-inflammatory actions. J Med Food 2005;8(2):125–32.
[156] Arablou T, Aryaeian N, Valizadeh M, et al. The effect of ginger consumption on glycemic status, lipid profile and some inflammatory markers in patients with type 2 diabetes mellitus. Int J Food Sci Nutr 2014;65(4):515–20.
[157] Prasad S, Gupta SC, Tyagi AK, et al. Curcumin, a component of golden spice: from bedside to bench and back. Biotechnol Adv 2014;32(6):1053–64.
[158] Esmaillzadeh A, Kimiagar M, Mehrabi Y, et al. Fruit and vegetable intakes, C-reactive protein, and the metabolic syndrome. Am J Clin Nutr 2006;84(6):1489–97.
[159] Lee Y, Kang D, Lee SA. Effect of dietary patterns on serum C-reactive protein level. Nutr Metab Cardiovasc Dis 2014;24(9):1004–11.
[160] Ellinger S, Stehle P. Impact of cocoa consumption on inflammation processes — a critical review of randomized controlled trials. Nutrients 2016;8(6):321.
[161] di Giuseppe R, Di Castelnuovo A, Centritto F, et al. Regular consumption of dark chocolate is associated with low serum concentrations of C-reactive protein in a healthy Italian population. J Nutr 2008;138:1939–45.
[162] Gu L, House SE, Wu X, et al. Procyanidin and catechin contents and antioxidant capacity of cocoa and chocolate products. J Agric Food Chem 2006;54:4057–61.
[163] Coit P, Sawalha AH. The human microbiome in rheumatic autoimmune diseases: a comprehensive review. Clin Immunol 2016;170:70–9.
[164] Yasar M, Taskar AK, Kaya B, et al. The early anti-inflammatory effect of kefir in experimental corrosive esophagitis. Ann Ital Chir 2013;84(6):681–5.
[165] Lee MY, Ahn KS, Kwon OK, et al. Anti-inflammatory and anti-allergic effects of kefir in a mouse asthma model. Immunobiology 2007;212(8):647–54.

[166] Ley SH, Sun Q, Willett WC, et al. Associations between red meat intake and biomarkers of inflammation and glucose metabolism in women. Am J Clin Nutr 2014;99(2):352–60.
[167] Daley CA, Abbott A, Doyle PS, et al. A review of fatty acid profiles and antioxidant content in grass-fed and grain-fed beef. Nutr J 2010;9:10.
[168] Hodgson JM, Ward NC, Burke V, et al. Increased lean red meat intake does not elevate markers of oxidative stress and inflammation in humans. J Nutr 2007;137(2):363–7.
[169] Mozaffarian D, Pischon T, Hankinson SE, et al. Dietary intake of trans fatty acids and systemic inflammation in women. Am J Clin Nutr 2004;79:606–12.
[170] Allen KJ, Koplin JJ. Why does Australia appear to have the highest rates of food allergy? Pediatr Clin North Am 2015;62(6):1441–51.
[171] Kawaguchi T, Mori M, Saito K, et al. Food antigen-induced immune responses in Crohn's disease patients and experimental colitis mice. J Gastroenterol 2015;50(4):394–405.
[172] Kawaguchi T, Mori M, Saito K, et al. Food antigen-induced immune responses in Crohn's disease patients and experimental colitis mice. J Gastroenterol 2015;50(4):394–405.
[173] Rajendran N, Kumar D. Food-specific IgG4-guided exclusion diets improve symptoms in Crohn's disease: a pilot study. Colorectal Dis 2011;13:1009–13.
[174] Gunasekeera V, Mendall MA, Chan D, et al. Treatment of Crohn's disease with an IgG4-guided exclusion diet: a randomized controlled trial. Dig Dis Sci 2016;61(4):1148–457.
[175] Brown AC, Roy M. Does evidence exist to include dietary therapy in the treatment of Crohn's disease? Expert Rev Gastroenterol Hepatol 2010;4(2):191–215.
[176] Kalliomäki MA. Food allergy and irritable bowel syndrome. Curr Opin Gastroenterol 2005;21(6):708–11.
[177] Mansueto P, D'Alcamo A, Seidita A, et al. Food allergy in irritable bowel syndrome: the case of non-celiac wheat sensitivity. World J Gastroenterol 2015;21(23):7089–109.
[178] Heilskov Rytter MJ, Andersen LB, Houmann T, et al. Diet in the treatment of ADHD in children — a systematic review of the literature. Nord J Psychiatry 2015;69(1):1–18.
[179] Nigg JT, Lewis K, Edinger T, et al. Meta-analysis of attention-deficit/hyperactivity disorder or attention-deficit/hyperactivity disorder symptoms, restriction diet, and synthetic food color additives. J Am Acad Child Adolesc Psychiatry 2012;51(1):86–97.e8.
[180] Heilskov Rytter MJ, Andersen LB, Houmann T, et al. Diet in the treatment of ADHD in children — a systematic review of the literature. Nord J Psychiatry 2015;69(1):1–18.
[181] Nigg JT, Lewis K, Edinger T, et al. Meta-analysis of attention-deficit/hyperactivity disorder or attention-deficit/hyperactivity disorder symptoms, restriction diet, and synthetic food color additives. J Am Acad Child Adolesc Psychiatry 2012;51(1):86–97.e8.
[182] McCann D, Barrett A, Cooper A, et al. Food additives and hyperactive behaviour in 3-year-old and 8/9-year-old children in the community: a randomised, double-blinded, placebo-controlled trial. Lancet 2007;370:1560–7.
[183] Lok KY, Chan RS, Lee VW, et al. Food additives and behavior in 8- to 9-year-old children in Hong Kong: a randomized, double-blind, placebo-controlled trial. J Dev Behav Pediatr 2013;34(9):642–50.
[184] Stevenson J, Sonuga-Barke E, McCann D, et al. The role of histamine degradation gene polymorphisms in moderating the effects of food additives on children's ADHD symptoms. Am J Psychiatry 2010;167(9):1108–15.
[185] Bath-Hextall F, Delamere FM, Williams HC. Dietary exclusions for established atopic eczema. Cochrane Database Syst Rev 2008;(1):CD005203.
[186] Johnston GA, Bilbao RM, Graham-Brown RA. The use of dietary manipulation by parents of children with atopic dermatitis. Br J Dermatol 2004;150(6):1186–9.
[187] Virdee K, Musset J, Baral M, et al. Food-specific IgG antibody–guided elimination diets followed by resolution of asthma symptoms and reduction in pharmacological interventions in two patients: a case report. Glob Adv Health Med 2015;4(1):62–6.
[188] Maintz L, Novak N. Histamine and histamine intolerance. Am J Clin Nutr 2007;85(5):1185–96.
[189] Manzotti G, Breda D, Di Gioacchino M, et al. Serum diamine oxidase activity in patients with histamine intolerance. Int J Immunopathol Pharmacol 2016;29(1):105–11.
[190] Maintz L, Novak N. Histamine and histamine intolerance. Am J Clin Nutr 2007;85(5):1185–96.
[191] Wantke F, Götz M, Jarisch R. Histamine-free diet: treatment of choice for histamine-induced food intolerance and supporting treatment for chronic headaches. Clin Exp Allergy 1993;23(12):982–5.
[192] Siebenhaar F, Melde A, Magerl M, et al. Histamine intolerance in patients with chronic spontaneous urticarial. J Eur Acad Dermatol Venereol 2016;30(10):1774–7.
[193] Rosell-Camps A, Zibetti S, Perez-Esteban G, et al. Histamine intolerance as a cause of chronic digestive complaints in pediatric patients. Rev Esp Enferm Dig 2013;105:201–7.
[194] Siebenhaar F, Melde A, Magerl M, et al. Histamine intolerance in patients with chronic spontaneous urticaria. J Eur Acad Dermatol Venereol 2016;30(10):1774–7.
[195] Bischoff SC, Barbara G, Buurman W, et al. Intestinal permeability — a new target for disease prevention and therapy. BMC Gastroenterol 2014;14:189.
[196] Chung BY, Cho SI, Ahn IS, et al. Treatment of atopic dermatitis with a low-histamine diet. Ann Dermatol 2011;23(Suppl. 1):S91–5.
[197] Rosell-Camps A, Zibetti S, Pérez-Esteban G, et al. Histamine intolerance as a cause of chronic digestive complaints in pediatric patients. Rev Esp Enferm Dig 2013;105(4):201–6.
[198] Raithel M, Baenkler HW, Naegel A, et al. Significance of salicylate intolerance in diseases of the lower gastrointestinal tract. J Physiol Pharmacol 2005;56(Suppl. 5):89–102.
[199] Swain AR. The role of natural salicylates in food. PhD thesis. Allergy Unit, Royal Prince Alfred Hospital, Sydney. Available from: www.slhd.nsw.gov.au/rpa/allergy/resources/foodintol/development.html.
[200] Wood A, Baxter G, Thies F, et al. A systematic review of salicylates in foods: estimated daily intake of a Scottish population. Mol Nutr Food Res 2011;55(Suppl. 1):S7–14.
[201] Fernando SL, Clarke LR. Salicylate intolerance: a masquerader of multiple adverse drug reactions. BMJ Case Rep 2009;pii.
[202] Raithel M, Baenkler HW, Naegel A, et al. Significance of salicylate intolerance in diseases of the lower gastrointestinal tract. J Physiol Pharmacol 2005;56(Suppl. 5):89–102.
[203] Healy E, Newell L, Howarth P, et al. Control of salicylate intolerance with fish oils. Br J Dermatol 2008;159(6):1368–9.
[204] Sommer DD, Rotenberg BW, Sowerby LJ, et al. A novel treatment adjunct for aspirin exacerbated respiratory disease: the low-salicylate diet: a multicenter randomized control crossover trial. Int Forum Allergy Rhinol 2016;6(4):385–91.
[205] Maslin K, Grundey J, Glasby G, et al. Cows' milk exclusion diet during infancy: is there a long-term effect on children's eating behaviour and food preferences? Pediatr Allergy Immunol 2016;27(2):141–6.
[206] Meyer R, De Koker C, Dziubak R, et al. A practical approach to vitamin and mineral supplementation in food allergic children. Clin Transl Allergy 2015;5:11.
[207] McLennan W, Podger A. National Nutrition Survey: selected highlights; 1995. Australia, 1995. ABS cat. no. 4802.0. Canberra; Australian Bureau of Statistics.
[208] Gibson RS, Heath AL, Szymlek-Gay EA. Is iron and zinc nutrition a concern for vegetarian infants and young children in industrialized countries? Am J Clin Nutr 2014;100(Suppl. 1):459S–68S.
[209] Clarys P. Comparison of nutritional quality of the vegan, vegetarian, semi-vegetarian, pesco-vegetarian and omnivorous diet. Nutrients 2014;6(3):1318–32.
[210] Wang F, Zheng J, Yang B, et al. Effects of vegetarian diets on blood lipids: a systematic review and meta-analysis of randomized controlled trials. J Am Heart Assoc 2015;4(10):e002408.
[211] Kahleova H, Pelikanova T. Vegetarian diets in the prevention and treatment of type 2 diabetes. J Am Coll Nutr 2015;34(5):448–58.
[212] Barnard ND, Levin SM, Yokoyama Y. A systematic review and meta-analysis of changes in body weight in clinical trials of vegetarian diets. J Acad Nutr Diet 2015;115(6):954–69.
[213] Navarro JA, de Gouveia LA, Rocha-Penha L, et al. Reduced levels of potential circulating biomarkers of cardiovascular diseases in apparently healthy vegetarian men. Clin Chim Acta 2016;461:110–13.
[214] Yokoyama Y, Nishimura K, Barnard ND, et al. Vegetarian diets and blood pressure: a meta-analysis. JAMA Intern Med 2014;174(4):577–87.

[215] Pawlak R, Lester SE, Babatunde T. The prevalence of cobalamin deficiency among vegetarians assessed by serum vitamin B_{12}: a review of literature. Eur J Clin Nutr 2014;68(5):541–8.

[216] Foster M, Herulah UN, Prasad A, et al. Zinc status of vegetarians during pregnancy: a systematic review of observational studies and meta-analysis of zinc intake. Nutrients 2015;7(6):4512–25.

[217] Reid MA, Marsh KA, Zeuschner CL, et al. Meeting the nutrient reference values on a vegetarian diet. Med J Aust 2013;199(Suppl. 4):S33–40.

[218] Reid MA, Marsh KA, Zeuschner CL, et al. Meeting the nutrient reference values on a vegetarian diet. Med J Aust 2013;199(Suppl. 4):S33–40.

[219] Saunders AV, Craig WJ, Baines SK, et al. Iron and vegetarian diets. Med J Aust 2013;199(Suppl. 4):S11–16.

[220] Saunders AV, Craig WJ, Baines SK, et al. Iron and vegetarian diets. Med J Aust 2013;199(Suppl. 4):S11–16.

[221] Gibson RS, Heath AL, Szymlek-Gay EA. Is iron and zinc nutrition a concern for vegetarian infants and young children in industrialized countries? Am J Clin Nutr 2014;100(Suppl. 1):459S–68S.

[222] Reid MA, Marsh KA, Zeuschner CL, et al. Meeting the nutrient reference values on a vegetarian diet. Med J Aust 2013;199(Suppl. 4):S33–40.

[223] Lozoff B. Early iron deficiency has brain and behavior effects consistent with dopaminergic dysfunction. J Nutr 2011;141(4):740S–746S.

[224] Algarín C, Nelson CA, Peirano P, et al. Iron-deficiency anemia in infancy and poorer cognitive inhibitory control at age 10 years. Dev Med Child Neurol 2013;55(5):453–8.

[225] Carpenter KL, Li W, Wei H, et al. Magnetic susceptibility of brain iron is associated with childhood spatial IQ. Neuroimage 2016;132:167–74.

[226] Pawlak R, Lester SE, Babatunde T. The prevalence of cobalamin deficiency among vegetarians assessed by serum vitamin B_12: a review of the literature. Eur J Clin Nutr 2014;68(5):541–8.

[227] Foster M, Samman S. Vegetarian diets across the lifecycle: impact on zinc intake and status. Adv Food Nutr Res 2015;74:93–131.

[228] Foster M, Chu A, Petocz P, et al. Effect of vegetarian diets on zinc status: a systematic review and meta-analysis of studies in humans. J Sci Food Agric 2013;93:2362–71.

[229] Foster M, Herulah UN, Prasad A, et al. Zinc status of vegetarians during pregnancy: a systematic review of observational studies and meta-analysis of zinc intake nutrients. Nutrients 2015;7(6):4512–25.

[230] Rangan A, Jones A, Samman S. Zinc supplement use and contribution to zinc intake in Australian children. Public Health Nutr 2015;18(4):589–95.

[231] Burns-Whitmore B, Haddad E, Sabaté J, et al. Effects of supplementing n-3 fatty acid enriched eggs and walnuts on cardiovascular disease risk markers in healthy free-living lacto-ovo-vegetarians: a randomized, crossover, free-living intervention study. Nutr J 2014;13:29.

[232] Ho-Pham LT, Nguyen ND, Nguyen TV. Effect of vegetarian diets on bone mineral density: a Bayesian meta-analysis. Am J Clin Nutr 2009;90:943–50.

[233] Lanham-New SA. Is "vegetarianism" a serious risk factor for osteoporotic fracture? Am J Clin Nutr 2009;90:910–11.

[234] Knurick JR, Johnston CS, Wherry SJ, et al. Comparison of correlates of bone mineral density in individuals adhering to lacto-ovo, vegan, or omnivore diets: a cross-sectional investigation. Nutrients 2015;7(5):3416–26.

[235] Burckhardt P. The role of low acid load in vegetarian diet on bone health: a narrative review. Swiss Med Wkly 2016;146:w14277.

[236] Reilly NR. The gluten-free diet: recognizing fact, fiction, and fad. J Pediatr 2016;175:206–10.

[237] Golley S, Corsini N, Topping D, et al. Motivations for avoiding wheat consumption in Australia: results from a population survey. Public Health Nutr 2015;18:490–9.

[238] Bascuñán KA, Vespa MC, Araya M. Celiac disease: understanding the gluten-free diet. Eur J Nutr 2017;56(2):449–59.

[239] Atchison J, Head L, Gates A. Wheat as food, wheat as industrial substance; comparative geographies of transformation and mobility. Geoforum 2010;41(2):236–46.

[240] Balakireva AV, Zamyatnin AA. Properties of gluten intolerance: gluten structure, evolution, pathogenicity and detoxification capabilities. Nutrients 2016;8(10):pii: E644.

[241] Burger JP, de Brouwer B, IntHout J, et al. Systematic review with meta-analysis: dietary adherence influences normalization of health-related quality of life in coeliac disease. Clin Nutr 2016;36(2):399–406.

[242] Lund F, Hermansen MN, Pedersen MF, et al. Decrease by 50% of plasma IgA tissue transglutaminase antibody concentrations within 2 months after start of gluten-free diet in children with celiac disease used as a confirming diagnostic test. Scand J Clin Lab Invest 2016;76(2):128–32.

[243] Fassano A, Sapano A, Zevallos V, et al. Nonceliac gluten sensitivity. Gastroenterology 2015;148:1195–204.

[244] Fassano A, Sapano A, Zevallos V, et al. Nonceliac gluten sensitivity. Gastroenterology 2015;148:1195–204.

[245] Gibson PR, Muir JG, Newnham ED, et al. Other dietary confounders: FODMAPS. Dig Dis 2015;33(2):269–76.

[246] White LE, Bannerman E, Gillett PM. Coeliac disease and the gluten-free diet: a review of the burdens; factors associated with adherence and impact on health-related quality of life, with specific focus on adolescence. J Hum Nutr Diet 2016;29(5):593–606.

[247] Pantaleoni S, Luchino M, Adriani A, et al. Bone mineral density at diagnosis of celiac disease and after 1 year of gluten-free diet. Scientific World Journal 2014;2014:173082.

[248] Balakireva AV, Zamyatnin AA. Properties of gluten intolerance: gluten structure, evolution, pathogenicity and detoxification capabilities. Nutrients 2016;8(10):pii: E644.

[249] Vici G, Belli L, Biondi M, et al. Gluten-free diet and nutrient deficiencies: a review. Clin Nutr 2016;35(6):1236–41.

[250] Wu JH, Neal B, Trevena H, et al. Are gluten-free foods healthier than non-gluten-free foods? An evaluation of supermarket products in Australia. Br J Nutr 2015;114:448–54.

[251] Vici G, Belli L, Biondi M, et al. Gluten-free diet and nutrient deficiencies: a review. Clin Nutr 2016;35(6):1236–41.

[252] Shepherd SJ, Gibson PR. Nutritional inadequacies of the gluten-free diet in both recently-diagnosed and long-term patients with coeliac disease. J Hum Nutr Diet 2013;26(4):349–58.

[253] Shepherd S, Gibson P. Nutritional inadequacies of the gluten-free diet in both recently-diagnosed and long-term patients with coeliac disease. J Hum Nutr Diet 2013;26(4):349–58.

[254] Ohlund K, Olsson C, Hernell O, et al. Dietary shortcomings in children on a gluten-free diet. J Hum Nutr Diet 2010;23(3):294–300.

[255] Penagini F, Dilillo D, Meneghin F, et al. Gluten-free diet in children: an approach to a nutritionally adequate and balanced diet. Nutrients 2013;5(11):4553–65.

[256] Alvarez-Jubete L, Arendt EK, Gallagher E. Nutritive value and chemical composition of pseudocereals as gluten-free ingredients. Int J Food Sci Nutr 2009;60(Suppl. 4):240–57.

[257] La Vieille S, Pulido OM, Abbott M, et al. Celiac disease and gluten-free oats: a Canadian position based on a literature review. Can J Gastroenterol Hepatol 2016;2016:1870305.

[258] La Vieille S, Pulido OM, Abbott M, et al. Celiac disease and gluten-free oats: a Canadian position based on a literature review. Can J Gastroenterol Hepatol 2016;2016:1870305.

[259] Pham-Short A, Donaghue KC, Ambler G, et al. Quality of life in type 1 diabetes and celiac disease: role of the gluten-free diet. J Pediatr 2016;179:131–8, e1.

[260] Dyett PA, Sabaté J, Haddad E, et al. Vegan lifestyle behaviors: an exploration of congruence with health-related beliefs and assessed health indices. Appetite 2013;67:119–24.

[261] Radnitz C, Beezhold B, DiMatteo J. Investigation of lifestyle choices of individuals following a vegan diet for health and ethical reasons. Appetite 2015;90:31–6.

[262] Glick-Bauer M, Yeh MC. The health advantage of a vegan diet: exploring the gut microbiota connection. Nutrients 2014;6(11):4822–38.

[263] Zimmer J, Lange B, Frick JS, et al. A vegan or vegetarian diet substantially alters the human colonic faecal microbiota. Eur J Clin Nutr 2012;66(1):53–60.

[264] Miquel S, Martín R, Rossi O, et al. *Faecalibacterium prausnitzii* and human intestinal health. Curr Opin Microbiol 2013;16:255–61.

[265] Wu GD, et al. Comparative metabolomics in vegans and omnivores reveal constraints on diet-dependent gut microbiota metabolite production. Gut 2016;65(1):63–72.

[266] Patman G. Gut microbiota: the difference diet makes to metabolites and microbiota. Nat Rev Gastroenterol Hepatol 2015;12(2):63.

[267] Clarys P, Deliens T, Huybrechts I, et al. Comparison of nutritional quality of the vegan, vegetarian, semi-vegetarian, pesco-vegetarian and omnivorous diet. Nutrients 2014;6(3):1318–32.
[268] Elorinne AL, Alfthan G, Erlund I, et al. Food and nutrient intake and nutritional status of Finnish vegans and non-vegetarians. PLoS ONE 2016;11(2):e0148235.
[269] Kristensen NB, Madsen ML, Hansen TH, et al. Intake of macro- and micronutrients in Danish vegans. Nutr J 2015;14:115.
[270] Schüpbach R, Wegmüller R, Berguerand C, et al. Micronutrient status and intake in omnivores, vegetarians and vegans in Switzerland. Eur J Nutr 2017;56(1):283–93.
[271] Zeuschner CL, Hokin BD, Marsh KA, et al. Vitamin B_{12} and vegetarian diets. Med J Aust 2013;199(Suppl. 4):S27–32.
[272] Watanabe F, Takenaka S, Katsura H, et al. Dried green and purple lavers (nori) contain substantial amounts of biologically active vitamin $B_{(12)}$ but less of dietary iodine relative to other edible seaweeds. J Agric Food Chem 1999;47(6):2341–3.
[273] Watanabe F, Yabuta Y, Bito T, et al. Vitamin B_{12}-containing plant food sources for vegetarians. Nutrients 2014;6(5):1861–73.
[274] Suziki H. Serum vitamin B_{12} levels in young vegans who eat brown rice. J Nutr Sci Vitaminol 1995;41:587–94.
[275] Watanabe F, Yabuta Y, Bito T, et al. Vitamin B_{12}-containing plant food sources for vegetarians. Nutrients 2014;6(5):1861–73.
[276] Kristensen NB, Madsen ML, Hansen TH, et al. Intake of macro- and micronutrients in Danish vegans. Nutr J 2015;14:115.
[277] Marsh KA, Munn EA, Baines SK. Protein and vegetarian diets. Med J Aust 2013;199(Suppl. 4):S7–10.
[278] Lane K, Derbyshire E, Li W, et al. Bioavailability and potential uses of vegetarian sources of omega-3 fatty acids: a review of the literature. Crit Rev Food Sci Nutr 2014;54(5):572–9.
[279] Sarter B, Kelsey KS, Schwartz TA, et al. Blood docosahexaenoic acid and eicosapentaenoic acid in vegans: associations with age and gender and effects of an algal-derived omega-3 fatty acid supplement. Clin Nutr 2015;34(2):212–18.
[280] Beezhold B, Radnitz C, Rinne A, et al. Vegans report less stress and anxiety than omnivores. Nutr Neurosci 2015;18(7):289–96.
[281] Dinu M, Abbate R, Gensini GF, et al. Vegetarian, vegan diets and multiple health outcomes: a systematic review with meta-analysis of observational studies. Crit Rev Food Sci Nutr 2017;57(17):3640–9.
[282] Sutliffe JT, Wilson LD, de Heer HD, et al. C-reactive protein response to a vegan lifestyle intervention. Complement Ther Med 2015;23(1):32–7.
[283] Piccoli GB, Clari R, Vigotti FN, et al. Vegan vegetarian diets in pregnancy: danger or panacea? A systematic narrative review. BJOG 2015;122(5):623–33.
[284] Guez S, Chiarelli G, Menni F, et al. Severe vitamin B_{12} deficiency in an exclusively breastfed 5-month-old Italian infant born to a mother receiving multivitamin supplementation during pregnancy. BMC Pediatr 2012;12:85.
[285] Pepper MR, Black MM. B_{12} in fetal development. Semin Cell Dev Biol 2011;22(6):619–23.
[286] Crowley ET, Williams LT, Roberts TK, et al. Does milk cause constipation? A crossover dietary trial. Nutrients 2013;5(1):253–66.
[287] Aune D, Navarro Rosenblatt DA, Chan DS, et al. Dairy products, calcium, and prostate cancer risk: a systematic review and meta-analysis of cohort studies. Am J Clin Nutr 2015;101(1):87–117.
[288] Deng Y, Misselwitz B, Dai N, et al. Lactose intolerance in adults: biological mechanism and dietary management. Nutrients 2015;7(9):8020–35.
[289] Vandenplas Y. Lactose intolerance. Asia Pac J Clin Nutr 2015;24(Suppl. 1):S9–13.
[290] Deng Y, Misselwitz B, Dai N, et al. Lactose intolerance in adults: biological mechanism and dietary management. Nutrients 2015;7(9):8020–35.
[291] Vandenplas Y. Lactose intolerance. Asia Pac J Clin Nutr 2015;24(Suppl. 1):S9–13.
[292] Di Rienzo T, D'Angelo G, D'Aversa F, et al. Lactose intolerance: from diagnosis to correct management. Eur Rev Med Pharmacol Sci 2013;17(Suppl. 2):18–25.
[293] Misselwitz B, Pohl D, Frühauf H, et al. Lactose malabsorption and intolerance: pathogenesis, diagnosis and treatment. United European Gastroenterol J 2013;1(3):151–9.
[294] Lukito W, Malik SG, Surono IS, et al. From 'lactose intolerance' to 'lactose nutrition'. Asia Pac J Clin Nutr 2015;24(Suppl. 1):S1–8.
[295] Deng Y, Misselwitz B, Dai N, et al. Lactose intolerance in adults: biological mechanism and dietary management. Nutrients 2015;7(9):8020–35.
[296] Mummah S, Oelrich B, Hope J, et al. Effect of raw milk on lactose intolerance: a randomized controlled pilot study. Ann Fam Med 2014;12(2):134–41.
[297] Vandenplas Y. Lactose intolerance. Asia Pac J Clin Nutr 2015;24(Suppl. 1):S9–13.
[298] Ul Haq MR, Kapila R, Sharma R, et al. Comparative evaluation of cow β-casein variants (A1/A2) consumption on Th2-mediated inflammatory response in mouse gut. Eur J Nutr 2014;53(4):1039–49.
[299] Pal S, Woodford K, Kukuljan S, et al. Milk intolerance, beta-casein and lactose. Nutrients 2015;7(9):7285–97.
[300] Ho S, Woodford K, Kukuljan S, et al. Comparative effects of A1 versus A2 beta-casein on gastrointestinal measures: a blinded randomised cross-over pilot study. Eur J Clin Nutr 2014;68(9):994–1000.
[301] Jianqin S, Leiming X, Lu X, et al. Effects of milk containing only A2 beta casein versus milk containing both A1 and A2 beta casein proteins on gastrointestinal physiology, symptoms of discomfort, and cognitive behavior of people with self-reported intolerance to traditional cows' milk. Nutr J 2016;15:35.

9

Herbal medicine

Justin Sinclair, Leah Hechtman

If you would understand anything, observe its beginning and its development.
Aristotle (384–322 BCE)

INTRODUCTION

This chapter explores the evolution of the herbal classes of the Western herbal materia medica, from both a traditional and modern standpoint. A brief history of the development of this approach to classification is discussed, followed by current lists of the herbal classes categorised by organ systems.

HERBAL MEDICINE CLASSIFICATION

Origins

The use, development and progression of the knowledge of medicinal plants are intrinsically interconnected with human evolution. Herbal knowledge began with our early Palaeolithic hominid ancestors,[1,2] and has slowly unfolded over the millennia to become more encompassing and systematic, thus shaping and moulding the great palette of properties that modern-day herbalists employ. This evolving knowledge base was built on the foundations of observation, experience and experimentation, and represents what is now called 'traditional knowledge'. It led to the establishment of sciences such as botany, pharmacology, medicine and toxicology, and also to the classification of our materia medica into therapeutic classes based on pharmacological action. This chapter discusses the different traditional and modern systems of herbal classes, and explores the history behind their developmental evolution.

Western herbal medicine has a rich and varied history. It is largely believed that our modern herbal paradigm evolved mainly from the Mediterranean world from the Greeks and Romans; however, other ancient cultures, such as Mesopotamia, Egypt and the Arabic world, also contributed heavily to form a collective knowledge base that has expanded over the centuries. The medical paradigms of these cultures were strongly linked with shamanic, religious and ritualistic practices, and it was not until the 5th century BCE that disease was seen not as an affliction passed on to humans by the gods, but as a natural occurrence due to internal, inherent, constitutional or environmental disturbances within the organism.

The collation and organisation of the medicinal properties of plants have been uniquely and ubiquitously established throughout all cultural paradigms. It therefore appears logical to hypothesise that this organisation is based on the current medical model employed within the culture at the time. Consequently, it is paramount to look at the historical progression of these various cultures to investigate how they have contributed to our modern herbal paradigm.

While archaeologists have shown evidence that early humans had knowledge of various plants, the oldest written evidence originates from Mesopotamia (modern-day Iraq). The people of ancient Mesopotamia, namely the Sumerians (ca. 5400 BCE) and Akkadians (ca. 2270–2083 BCE) were the first to write on the topic of health and disease, as did the Egyptians. Medical writing from this time was based largely on prescriptions listing potential ailments, with an ingredient list and preparation instructions for the remedy,[3,4] along with the requisite prayers and sacred ritual that were also deemed equally important. While the people of Mesopotamia were the first to write on the topic of herbal remedies, it was the Egyptians who infused this knowledge into their own culture and expanded on it greatly.

The Smith Papyrus was written in the 17th century and incorporated over 700 specific medicines of plant, animal and mineral origin, along with surgical procedures and formulations for various illnesses.[5] Likewise, the Ebers Papyrus (1600 BCE) describes many herbal formulations and guidelines for herbal compounding and is four times the length of the Smith Papyrus. An unfortunate circumstance surrounding many of these texts is that the actual plants and ingredients were not elaborated on, and in many cases the correct botanical description of the plants used in the prescriptions of this time was not accurate. Furthermore, the information being presented was classified by the ailment being treated (i.e. by indication), and at that time there was no discussion of herbal medications based on action or class.

Over 1000 kilometres away the Greeks similarly started collating vast amounts of knowledge on the subject of medicine and the natural world. Of particular note were the Hippocratic physicians who, like Hippocrates of Kos (ca. 460–370 BCE), sought to demystify the causes of disease and separated them from supernatural causes. The body of work attributed to Hippocrates is known as the *Corpus Hippocraticum*. It was actually written from the 5th century BCE to the 2nd century BCE, and is a collection of 62 treatises on several medical topics, mentioning over 250 different plant species. Interestingly, there is no classification of herbs; the only parameter is the presenting disease of the patient (i.e. the indication), and not the specific pharmacological actions of the herbs themselves.

Further great contributions to herbal medicine occurred over the next 400 years. Theophrastus (371–287 BCE), a pupil of the eminent Aristotle (384–322 BCE), took over the *Peripatos* and continued his investigation into the natural world. A prolific writer, Theophrastus authored the *Historia Plantarum* (*History of Plants*) and *De Causis Plantarum* (*On the Causes of Plants*), which is why many scholars consider him to be the Father of Botany. These two works represent the first systematic analysis of the botanical world.

The *Historia Plantarum* was devoted to the classification of plants based on morphological characteristics. Conversely, *De Causis Plantarum* highlighted topics such as plant growth, soil preparation and techniques for sowing crops. Not having the medical training of a physician, but instead an interest in natural sciences and biology, Theophrastus failed to propose a classification of medical plants based on their action, although his contribution to botany should not be forgotten.

Gaius Plinius Secundus (23/24–79 CE), a Roman encyclopaedist and writer, relied heavily on the writings of Theophrastus in his monumental *Naturalis Historia* (*Natural History*). This work, completed around 77 CE, comprises topics such as anthropology, geography, arts, age-specific technology, zoology, metallurgy and botany (including the medicinal uses of plants), but still lacks a classification of plants according to their therapeutic action.

It was not until Pedanius Dioscorides (1st century CE) that the first true classification of herbal medicines into therapeutic classes occurred. Born in Anazarba in Cilicia (Asia Minor), Dioscorides was a Greek with a keen interest in pharmacotherapy. Dioscorides is supposed to have travelled all over the Mediterranean and Asia Minor, cataloguing and documenting all the plant life he came across and, most importantly, he obtained local knowledge about their medicinal virtues. He produced the five-book magnum opus known simply as *De Materia Medica*, which is the foundation upon which subsequent traditions have been constructed. Beautifully illustrated with hand-painted renditions of the herbal medicines used (it is not known if these drawings date back to Dioscorides or not), this work classifies medicines on the basis of their pharmacological action. This book was to remain an important source for physicians well into the 16th century, being used by Arabic, Greek, Roman and European physicians for almost 1500 years.

From works such as *De Materia Medica*, the interest in herbal pharmacotherapy ignited, with many texts adding to the knowledge already available in the early Middle Ages. Galen (129–200 CE) was a prolific author who wrote many treatises on pharmacotherapy and therapeutics, although many of his works are now lost. Of particular interest is the contribution that physicians of the Arabic world made to the advancement of herbal classes by adding to the knowledge base established by Dioscorides and Galen. Of note is Abu Ali Sina (980–1037 CE), better known as Avicenna, who wrote the *Canon of Medicine* in 1025 CE, which provided a discussion on pharmacology and evidence-based medicine and documented over 700 different medications. Other Arabic contemporaries of Avicenna, such as Abu al-Qasim, Al-Razi,[6] Maimonides and Hunayn ibn-Ishaq,[6] wrote compendiums that were essentially pharmaceutical encyclopaedias, which would form the basis for the birth of the pharmacopoeia during the early stages of the European Renaissance.

During the early centuries of the Common Era, not only did the birth of herbal classes come to fruition, but also one of the great philosophies quite specific to herbal medicines is thought to have originated, although supportive evidence for this is lacking. The Doctrine of Signatures was a belief that the gods gave clues to the keen observer as to the potential indications and therapeutic actions for which plants may be used. The taste, shape, colour or scent of plants led humans to potential drugs with healing virtues. While the origin of this system seems to be lost in remote history, it was particularly favoured by the enigmatic Paracelsus (1493–1541 CE).

Some examples of the Doctrine include:

- Colour: *Taraxacum officinale* (Dandelion) was used for liver conditions because of its yellow flowers (yellow being associated with bile),[7,8] the same of which could be said for other herbs such as *Chelidonium majus* (greater celandine) and *Gentiana lutea* (yellow gentian).
- Shape: the shape of leaves or other morphological characteristics. For example, the heart-shaped fruit of *Capsella bursa pastoris* (Shepherd's purse) look like a uterus, and thus the herb has been used for female reproductive complaints, especially conditions such as menorrhagia and dysmenorrhoea. Similarly, William Coles thought that the fruit of the walnut (*Juglans regia*) looked like the brain and would assist in any such ailment of this organ.[9] Lastly, Paracelsus commented on the shape of the leaves of *Hepatica acutiloba*, suggesting that they resemble the liver, and they were therefore indicated for hepatic afflictions.

The Doctrine of Signatures was developed further and formalised by the writing of a 17th century shoemaker Jakob Böehme (1575–1624 CE), who wrote about it in his work *Signatura Rerum* (*The Signature of All Things*). He is said to have had a mystical experience in which God revealed the relationships between man and all things. This concept was passed on to later authors such as Nicholas Culpeper (1616–1654 CE), but was soon lost to the imagination of the many seeking the rationalism and clarity that came with the scientific revolution.

THE ADVENT OF SCIENCE

With the Renaissance came a fascination with natural philosophy, and it is widely accepted that it was from this period that the scientific revolution sprang forth. Rationalism and reductionism became the model by which science progressed, projecting from it a confidence that shook the very foundations on which medicine, and indeed how we viewed the world, had stood for millennia. As the medical paradigm underwent a transmutation, so too did the practice and influence of herbal medicine, as we better understood the afflictions of the body and their causes.

In our thirst for knowledge, we started to categorise the world and the machinations of what had previously been mysterious and seen as a work of God. Publications such as *De Revolutionibus Orbium Coelestium* (*On the Revolutions of the Heavenly Spheres*) by Copernicus, *De Humani Corporis Fabrica* (*On the Structure of the Human Body*) by Andreas Vesalius, *Dialogue Concerning the Two Chief World Systems* by Galileo Galilei, *The Sceptical Chymist* by Robert Boyle, *Meditations of First Philosophy* by Rene Descartes and *Philosophiae Naturalis Principia Mathematica* by Sir Isaac Newton became the new cornerstones for the birth of the sciences as we now know them. Evidence and substantiation became all important, and soon displaced Aristotelian elemental theory and the concept of humoral medicine.

Soon it was not plants themselves but rather the chemicals within them that became the focus of scientific investigation. While herbals, such as those by Gerard and Culpeper, gained popularity with commoners, medicine, and with it pharmacotherapy, had evolved and changed astronomically. Over the next 200 years the dominance of plants in the materia medica of orthodox medicine slowly waned, and instead the reductionist view began to prevail; that is, that the active constituents of plants were the true 'essence' behind their medicinal virtues.

THE CONJUNCTION

The observation of the evolution of herbal medicine, regardless of epoch, suggests that it is continuing to improve and advance. Modern science, although still in its adolescence when compared with the ancient traditions from which it sprang, has much to offer. A veritable explosion of technology has led to the development of sophisticated experimental procedures and machinery which allows the observer to analyse the specific chemistry and active-constituent profiles of plants, and thus to define their action and individual concentrations. High-performance liquid chromatography, mass spectrometry and high-throughput screening represent the modern-day 'Doctrine of Signatures', with peaks and troughs in a graph identifying what a herbal medicine may potentially be used for, and therefore guiding researchers to a myriad of as yet unfound actions and novel medical discoveries.

With over 255 000 flowering plants currently known, and an estimated 5000 of these having been studied for their medicinal virtue, the mind boggles at the as yet unrealised potential for plant-based pharmacotherapy. In truth, it could be argued that such statistics suggest that the knowledge base of our materia medica may only now, after 60 000 years, be entering an embryonic stage of evolution, and it is science that will fertilise and enrich it to grow to new heights. Metaphorically, if the evolution of herbal classes is viewed as a tree, science has allowed new branches and shoots to sprout forth in a far-reaching canopy that continues to grow. However, we must be careful to remember that it is the roots, the foundational support, that allows such growth to occur.

The modern herbalist is confronted with a quandary: to rely on the traditional knowledge obtained over millennia of usage, or to repudiate such wisdom and bow to the authority of, and acceptance now afforded by, modern science? Fortunately the two standpoints are not mutually exclusive, but rather complement each other, and the erudite herbal practitioner should equally value both systems of evidence. In fact, scientific empiricism is commonly validating the ancient use and actions of plant-based medicines, and in many cases is adding to our previous knowledge, for the betterment of all. It is the authors' heartfelt belief that it will only be through the conjunction of ancient wisdom and scientific techniques that herbal medicine will continue to evolve and prosper.

By understanding the origins and development of the herbal classes over the ages, we can undoubtedly observe that they have evolved in harmony with the knowledge base that was popular during a particular time. Many of the terms developed by the authors of the traditional texts are still used today by modern herbalists. Such terms as 'tonics', 'analgesics', 'aromatics', 'purgatives', 'astringents', 'digestives', 'carminatives', 'cathartics', 'purgatives', 'emetics' and 'bitters' all come from the ancient past, and still find a rightful pride of place in our modern herbal monographs and pharmacopoeias, even if some of the actions are now considered somewhat heroic. Modern science, with its plethora of analytical and experimental techniques, now adds to this list a wealth of information that shows how remarkably complex the secondary metabolites of plants really are. For example, the antiarrhythmic, aldose-reductase inhibiting and thyroid-suppressing actions of some plants are now well known and accepted, and direct the clinician to using such plants in more effective ways.

The following descriptions include both modern and ancient herbal actions, classified according to body system for ease of information retrieval. In addition to the herbal action, the descriptions include a definition, known indications, cautions and contraindications for the specific herbal class, the application of the medicine (duration of treatment and dispensing advice) and a list of herbs known to have the particular action.

GASTROINTESTINAL SYSTEM

Antacids

DEFINITION

Antacids are herbal medicines that counteract or neutralise the acidity in the gastrointestinal tract, most specifically the stomach. The main herbal antacid is meadowsweet (*Filipendula ulmaria*), also known as meadwort or queen of the meadow.

TRADITION

Meadowsweet has an incredible ability to regulate hydrochloric acid (HCl) secretions in a simple and effective manner. It is important to ensure that the patient is not consuming pharmaceutical antacids (especially those containing aluminium) as these can interfere with its effectiveness. Meadowsweet encourages normal digestive function, while pharmaceutical antacids suppress symptoms and impede normal digestive function. Most patients will develop further digestive problems from the use of pharmaceutical antacids. It is axiomatic that the suppression of a symptom will almost always cause detrimental effects in other areas.

INDICATIONS

- Gastro-oesophageal reflux disease (GORD) as an (adjunct)
- Hyperchlorhydria
- Acid reflux.

CONTRAINDICATIONS

- Hypochlorhydria
- Achlorhydria
- Concurrent administration with pharmaceutical antacids (e.g. Mylanta).

APPLICATION

- Best taken before meal
- Caution concurrent use with aspirin
- Medium- to long-term application is advisable for extended benefits.

HERBAL MEDICINES

- *Filipendula ulmaria* (meadowsweet).

Anthelmintics

DEFINITION

Anthelmintic herbal medicines assist in killing or expelling intestinal worms or parasites. They are generally very bitter, and patient compliance may be a challenge. Most of the major herbal manufacturers have developed high-quality herbal tablets that are very effective. It is important for the herbalist to taste some of these herbal medicines before making up a formula for a patient. Flavouring agents such as liquorice or fennel are very useful, but due to their high sugar content may be contraindicated in some cases of infestation, blood sugar control, fructosaemia and dental caries.

TRADITION

The term 'anthelmintic' derives from the Greek *anti,* meaning 'against', and *helmins,* a term denoting a 'worm', generally of parasitic origin. This class of herbal medicine is one of the oldest in our long tradition, with many remedies being used in Egyptian and Roman times when parasitic infections were highly prevalent. In many developing nations with poor sanitation and hygiene, parasitic worms are still responsible for the poor health of millions.

INDICATIONS

- Known worm infestation (round worm, pin worm, etc.).

CONTRAINDICATIONS

- Serious worm infestation causing intestinal obstruction.

APPLICATION

- Best taken before meals
- Short- to medium-term application is advisable for extended benefits.

HERBAL MEDICINES

- *Allium sativum* (garlic)
- *Artemisia absinthium*/*A. annua* (wormwood)
- *Citrus* spp.
- *Handroanthus impetiginosus* (pau d'arco)
- *Juglans nigra* (black walnut) hulls
- *Tanacetum vulgare* (tansy)
- *Thymus vulgaris* (thyme).

Antiemetics

DEFINITION

Antiemetic herbal medicines reduce nausea and may relieve or prevent vomiting. Nausea can be challenging to treat due to its many potential causes (e.g. hyperemesis gravidarum, medication side effects, gastritis, food poisoning). However, the antiemetic herbs are fast acting and are usually required in small, frequent doses. If all else fails, a warm ginger (*Zingiber officinale*) tea with a little honey can usually settle a temperamental stomach.

TRADITION

The term 'antiemetic' derives from the Greek *anti,* meaning 'against', and *emesis* meaning 'to vomit'.[10] This herbal class was described in ancient literature as preventing nausea and emesis. Many plants from this category also belong to the carminative class, which relies on essential oils to exert a calming and antispasmodic effect to the gastrointestinal tract.

INDICATIONS

- Nausea and emesis
- Hyperemesis gravidarum (morning sickness)
- Mild food poisoning/mild gastritis.

CONTRAINDICATIONS

- None known for this class
- Specific to the individual herbal medicines within the class.

APPLICATION

- Best taken before meals
- Short- to medium-term application is advisable for extended benefits.

HERBAL MEDICINES

- *Ballota nigra* (black horehound)
- *Berberis aquifolium* (Oregon mountain grape)
- *Chionanthus virginica* (fringe tree)
- *Cinnamomum zeylanicum/C. verum* (Ceylon cinnamon)
- *Mentha x piperita* (peppermint)
- *Zingiber officinale* (ginger).

Carminatives

DEFINITION

Carminative herbal medicines relieve flatulence, usually by relaxing the intestinal sphincter muscles. Most of the medicines are culinary herbs and have been used for this benefit for a long time. Many herbs in this class belong to the Lamaiaceae and Apiaceae families, which are known to contain essential oils.

TRADITION

The term 'carminative' is uniquely medical in origin, and suggests a remedy that is able to expel wind. However, Hensleigh Wedgwood suggests in *A Dictionary of English Etymology* (1859–1865) that 'the theory was that they dilute and relax the gross humours from whence the wind arises, combing them out like knots in wool'.[10] Interestingly, these herbs and their known essential oil constituents also contribute to an antispasmodic action, which is why they are so effective in alleviating wind and griping conditions.

INDICATIONS

- Colic, especially in infants
- Griping and excessive flatulence
- Gastrointestinal upset from overindulgence
- Irritable bowel syndrome
- Mild epigastric pain.

CONTRAINDICATIONS

- Specific to the individual herbal medicines within the class.

APPLICATION

- Can be taken during or after meals, or as required (prn)
- Short- to medium-term application is advisable for extended benefits.

HERBAL MEDICINES

- *Anethum graveolens* (dill)
- *Capsicum* spp. (chilli)
- *Carum carvi* (caraway)
- *Cinnamomum zeylanicum/C. verum* (Ceylon cinnamon)
- *Foeniculum vulgare* (fennel)
- *Lavandula angustifolia* (English lavender)
- *Matricaria chamomilla* (German chamomile)
- *Melissa officinalis* (lemon balm)
- *Mentha x piperita* (peppermint)
- *Pimpinella anisum* (aniseed)
- *Valeriana officinalis* (valerian)
- *Zingiber officinale* (ginger).

Demulcents

DEFINITION

Demulcent herbal medicines soothe inflamed surfaces such as the skin and mucous membranes. A perfect example is slippery elm bark powder, which is mixed with warm/hot water to form a paste, and cool water added before drinking. This preparation has a mucilaginous quality, and it coats the mucous membranes as it passes through the gastrointestinal tract. The coating protects, soothes and heals all the way from the mouth to the anus.

TRADITION

The term 'demulcent' derives from the Latin *mulcere* meaning 'to soothe'.[10] Demulcents have been used medicinally for millennia, both internally and externally, for their healing and soothing properties. They often contain mucopolysaccharides, and many of the herbs belonging to this class contain mucilage (e.g. the members of the Malvaceae family [marshmallow], and the hardy succulent aloe). As a class, demulcent herbs are part of our traditional knowledge base, and their therapeutic activity is typically due to mucilage as the active constituent.

INDICATIONS

- Inflammation of the gastrointestinal tract (peptic ulceration, inflammatory bowel disease)
- Ulceration (topically)
- Burns, scalds and rashes (topically).

CONTRAINDICATIONS

- Specific to the individual herbal medicines within the class
- Herbs rich in mucilage may reduce the absorption of other medicines.

APPLICATION

- Best taken before meals
- Medium- to long-term application is advisable for extended benefits.

HERBAL MEDICINES

- *Aloe vera* (aloe)
- *Althea officinalis* (marshmallow) (root is more mucilaginous)
- *Glycyrrhiza glabra* (liquorice)
- *Trigonella foenum-graecum* (fenugreek)
- *Ulmus rubra* (slippery elm).

Gastrointestinal anti-inflammatories

DEFINITION

Anti-inflammatory herbal medicines reduce inflammation. The herbal medicines selected for inclusion in this class are specific to the gastrointestinal tract.

TRADITION

The term 'inflammation' is derived from the Latin *inflammare,* meaning 'to set on fire'. The term has been associated with redness and inflammation of the body since the early 16th century.[10] Herbal lore suggests that our ancient ancestors used herbal medicine effectively and efficaciously for all manner of inflammatory disorders, from simple burns and scalds of the skin, to gastrointestinal disorders such as mucus colitis.

INDICATIONS

- Medically diagnosed irritable bowel syndrome
- Inflammatory bowel disease (Crohn's disease, ulcerative colitis)
- Mild food poisoning, mild gastritis
- Peptic or duodenal ulceration.

CONTRAINDICATIONS

- Specific to the individual herbal medicines within the class.

APPLICATION

- Best taken before meals
- Short- to medium-term application is advisable for extended benefits.

HERBAL MEDICINES

- *Andrographis paniculata* (andrographis)
- *Bosewellia serrata* (boswellia/Indian frankincense)
- *Calendula officinalis* (calendula)
- *Curcuma longa* (turmeric)
- *Dioscorea villosa* (wild yam)
- *Filipendula ulmaria* (meadowsweet)
- *Glycyrrhiza glabra* (liquorice)
- *Matracaria chamomilla* (German chamomile)
- *Picrorhiza kurroa* (picrorhiza)
- *Rehmannia glutinosa* (rehmannia)
- *Scutellaria baicalensis* (baikal skullcap)
- *Smilax officinalis* (sarsparilla) and *S.ornata* (brown sarsaparilla).

Gastrointestinal astringents

DEFINITION

Astringent herbal medicines cause the contraction of mucous membranes and exposed tissues. This is often due to the tannin content that binds to proteins on the exposed surface.

TRADITION

Astringent herbal medicines, those which coat the surface of and protect tissues, are not exclusively beneficial for external use. Conditions such as leaky gut syndrome may also benefit from this class of medicines.

INDICATIONS

- Leaky gut syndrome
- Ulcerative colitis
- Gastric ulcer
- Diarrhoea.

CONTRAINDICATIONS

- Constipation.

APPLICATION

- Best taken before meals
- Short- to medium-term application is advisable for extended benefits.

HERBAL MEDICINES

- *Agrimonia eupatoria* (agrimony)
- *Ballota nigra* (black horehound)
- *Cnicus benedictus* (blessed thistle)
- *Commiphora myrrha* (myrrh)
- *Filipendula ulmaria* (meadowsweet)
- *Geranium maculatum* (geranium/cranesbill).
- *Hamamelis virginiana* (witch hazel)
- *Hydrastis canadensis* (goldenseal)
- *Leptandra virginica* (black root)
- *Myrica cerifera* (bayberry)
- *Quercus robur* (English oak).

Gastrointestinal spasmolytics

DEFINITION

Also known as 'antispasmodics', spasmolytic herbal medicines reduce cramping. Many of the digestive antispasmodics, much akin to the carminative and antiemetic classes, contain essential oils as primary active constituents.

TRADITION

The term 'antispasmodic' is derived from the Greek *anti,* meaning 'against', and *spasmodes,* meaning 'of the nature of a spasm'.[10] The term 'spasm' is also derived from the Greek for 'convulsion' or 'to contract violently'.[10] Interestingly, antispasmodics do not apply only to the gastrointestinal system, but also have the ability to reduce spasm in the visceral smooth muscle, bronchial tubes, bile and urinary ducts, and blood vessels,[11] making this class useful in a multitude of conditions.

INDICATIONS

- Colicky pain
- Excessive flatulence
- Dysmenorrhoea, menstrual cramping and discomfort
- Irritable bowel syndrome.

CONTRAINDICATIONS

- Specific to the individual herbal medicines within the class.

APPLICATION

- Best taken before meals
- Short- to medium-term application is advisable for extended benefits.

HERBAL MEDICINES

- *Ballota nigra* (black horehound)
- *Carum carvi* (caraway)

- *Cinnamomum zeylanicum/C. verum* (Ceylon cinnamon)
- *Dioscorea villosa* (wild yam)
- *Foeniculum vulgare* (fennel)
- *Fumaria officinalis* (fumitory)
- *Lavandula angustifolia* (English lavender)
- *Leptandra virginica* (black root)
- *Matricaria chamomilla* (German chamomile)
- *Mentha x piperita* (peppermint)
- *Valeriana officinalis* (valerian)
- *Viburnum opulus* (cramp bark)
- *Vibernum prunifolium* (black haw).

Laxatives

DEFINITION

Laxative herbal medicines promote the evacuation of the bowels. It is important to not overuse these herbal medicines as dependence can ensue. Retraining the bowel and fostering healthy bowel habits are recommended, as are improvements of diet and lifestyle. Adequate water intake is essential.

TRADITION

The term 'laxative' comes from the Latin *laxus,* meaning 'loose' or 'lax', and has been used in the context as a form of medicine since the late 14th century.[10] Laxatives comprise a traditional herbal class which have also been called purgatives in more recent times. Anthroquinone glycosides are one of the main active constituents present in this class. These chemicals give rise to a direct laxative action, although the mucilage of the bulk demulcents is not to be discounted in this respect, especially when a softer stool is desired.

INDICATIONS

- Constipation
- Detoxification
- Softening of the stool to ease passing.

CONTRAINDICATIONS

- Specific to the individual herbal medicines within the class
- Caution should be exercised in patients with inflammatory bowel disease.

APPLICATION

- Short-term application is advisable.

HERBAL MEDICINES

- *Aloe vera* (aloe)
- *Berberis vulgaris* (barberry)
- *Fumaria officinalis* (fumitory)
- *Glycyrrhiza glabra* (liquorice)
- *Handroanthus impetiginosus* (pau d'arco)
- *Juglans nigra* (black walnut)
- *Leptandra virginica* (black root)
- *Rhamnus purshiana* (cascara)
- *Rheum palmatum* (Turkey rhubarb)
- *Rumex crispus* (yellow dock)
- *Senna alexandrina* (senna)
- *Taraxacum officinale radix* (dandelion root).

Anthraquinone-containing laxatives

- *Aloe vera* (aloe)
- *Handroanthus impetiginosus* (pau d'arco)
- *Juglans cinerea* (butternut)
- *Rhamnus purshiana* (cascara)
- *Rheum palmatum* (Turkey rhubarb)
- *Rumex crispus* (yellow dock)
- *Senna alexandrina* (senna).

Mucous membrane trophorestoratives

DEFINITION

Also known as 'mucous membrane tonics', mucous membrane trophorestorative herbal medicines normalise and help restore the function, secretion and morphology of the mucous membrane. Specifically, these herbal medicines have an affinity for healing the lining of the gastrointestinal tract and improving its integrity and function. They are specifically indicated for gastric hyperpermeability or for individuals suffering from food intolerances and digestive disturbances.

TRADITION

While the herbs in this category have traditionally been used for complaints of the gastrointestinal tract, the fact that this class of agents is specific to the mucous membranes suggests it is a more recent and modern definition. The term 'trophorestorative' is a recent one. However, when the definition of the term is compared with that of 'tonic' there does not seem to be a great deal of difference, as both restore tone and function to a specific organ or tissue. It seems that the term 'trophorestorative' is just a modern name for what is simply a tonic herbal class.

INDICATIONS

- Leaky gut syndrome
- Malabsorption disorders
- Irritation and inflammation of the mucous membranes (ulcers, etc.).

CONTRAINDICATIONS

- Specific to the individual herbal medicines within the class.

APPLICATION

- Best taken before meals.
- Medium- to long-term application is advisable for extended benefits.

HERBAL MEDICINES

- *Hydrastis canadensis* (goldenseal)
- *Plantago lanceolata* (English plantain/ribwort).

HEPATOBILIARY SYSTEM

Bitters

DEFINITION

Also known as 'bitter tonics', 'digestive stimulants' and 'aromatic digestives', bitter herbs stimulate the digestive system via the vagus nerve and local gut effects. Their purpose is to help improve the function of the digestive system. A practical example of a bitter is the popular lemon, lime and bitters drink (i.e. Angostura bitters) which is typically drunk before or during a meal, the aim of which is to assist in the proper digestion of the meal.

TRADITION

The term 'bitters' belongs to ancient history, and has been used therapeutically for centuries. It seems to originate from the Old English *biter*, meaning 'bite', which changed in meaning to 'acrid tasting' over time.[10] Bitters are akin to a tonic for an underfunctioning gastrointestinal system, promoting not only more lively secretions, but also better assimilation and absorption.

INDICATIONS

- Dyspepsia and poor digestive function
- Nausea
- Hypochlorhydria
- Decreased bile flow

CONTRAINDICATIONS

- Hyperchlorhydria
- Stomach ulcers
- Gastritis/gastroenteritis.

APPLICATION

- Best taken before meals
- Medium- to long-term application is advisable for extended benefits.

HERBAL MEDICINES

- *Agrimonia eupatoria* (agrimony)
- *Andrographis paniculata* (andrographis)
- *Angelica archangelica* (angelica)
- *Artemisia absinthium*/*A. annua* (wormwood)
- *Berberis aquifolium* (Oregon mountain grape)
- *Bupleurum falcatum* (bupleurum)
- *Centaurium erythraea* (centaury)
- *Chelone glabra* (balmony)
- *Chionanthus virginica* (fringe tree)
- *Cnicus benedictus* (blessed thistle)
- *Cynara cardunculus* var. *scolymus* (globe artichoke)
- *Gentiana lutea* (gentian)
- *Hydrastis canadensis* (goldenseal)
- *Picrorhiza kurroa* (picrorhiza)
- *Stachys officinalis* (wood betony).

Cholagogues

DEFINITION

Cholagogue herbal medicines increase the flow and release of stored bile from the gallbladder by stimulating gallbladder contraction. A simple way of remembering the difference between a choleretic and a cholagogue is that cholagogue contains a 'g', and 'g' is for 'gallbladder'. Many of the herbal medicines in this class also exhibit other actions that affect the entire hepatobiliary system.

TRADITION

This class of herbal medicines belongs to traditional lore. The term 'cholagogue' is derived from the Greek *chole*, meaning 'bile', and *agein*, meaning 'to lead forth'.[12]

INDICATIONS

- Poor digestion, especially of lipids
- Steatorrhoea
- Prophylaxis of cholelithiasis.

CONTRAINDICATIONS

- Caution should be exercised in patients with known cholelithiasis (gallstones) as this may cause blockage and/or pain
- Specific to the individual herbal medicines within the class.

APPLICATION

- Best taken before meals
- Medium- to long-term application is advisable for extended benefits.

HERBAL MEDICINES

- *Agrimonia eupatoria* (agrimony)
- *Andrographis paniculata* (andrographis)
- *Artemisia absinthium*/*A. annua* (wormwood)
- *Artemisia vulgaris* (mugwort)
- *Berberis aquifolium* (Oregon mountain grape)
- *Calendula officinalis* (calendula)
- *Chelidonium majus* (greater celandine)
- *Chionanthus virginicus* (fringe tree)
- *Curcuma longa* (turmeric)
- *Cynara cardunculus* var. *scolymus* (globe artichoke)
- *Fumaria officinalis* (fumitory)
- *Gentiana lutea* (gentian)
- *Hydrastis canadensis* (goldenseal)
- *Iris versicolor* (blue flag)
- *Juglans cinerea* (butternut)
- *Leptandra virginica* (black root)
- *Peumus boldus* (boldo)
- *Picrorhiza kurroa* (picrorhiza)
- *Silybum marianum* (St Mary's thistle)
- *Taraxacum officinale* radix (dandelion root)
- *Verbena officinalis* (vervain).

Choleretics

DEFINITION

Choleretic herbal medicines increase the production and flow of bile from the liver specifically. Most of the herbal medicines in this class also exhibit other actions that affect the entire hepatobiliary system.

TRADITION

Like cholagogues, choleretics belong to the traditional knowledge base. The term 'choleretic' is derived from the Greek *chole,* meaning 'bile', and *hairesis,* meaning 'removal'.[10]

INDICATIONS

- Poor digestion
- Liver insufficiency.

CONTRAINDICATIONS

- Specific to the individual herbal medicines within the class
- Caution should be exercised in patients with known cholelithiasis (gallstones) as this may cause blockage and/or pain. Equally, caution should be exercised in patients with known acute or chronic liver disease.

APPLICATION

- Best taken before meals
- Medium- to long-term application is advisable for extended benefits.

HERBAL MEDICINES

- *Andrographis paniculata* (andrographis)
- *Artemisia absinthium/A. annua* (wormwood)
- *Berberis vulgaris* (barberry)
- *Calendula officinalis* (calendula)
- *Chelidonium majus* (greater celandine)
- *Curcuma longa* (turmeric)
- *Cynara cardunculus* var. *scolymus* (globe artichoke)
- *Hydrastis canadensis* (goldenseal)
- *Mentha x piperita* (peppermint)
- *Picrorhiza kurroa* (picrorhiza)
- *Silybum marianum* (St Mary's thistle).

Hepatics

DEFINITION

Otherwise known as 'hepatotonics' or 'hepatic tonics', hepatic herbal medicines improve the tone, vigour and function of the liver. They are similar to hepatoprotectives and hepatotrophorestoratives in that many of these medicines will exhibit multiple effects on the liver and hepatobiliary system.

TRADITION

The term 'hepatic' is derived from the Greek *hepatos,* meaning 'liver'. This class of herbal medicine is of ancient origin. Texts such as *De Materia Medica* discuss a multitude of herbs specific for the liver which we have now scientifically identified as possessing hepatic activity.

INDICATIONS

- Poor liver function or digestion (dyspepsia)
- Liver-specific conditions (hepatitis, etc.)
- Alcoholic liver damage such as fatty liver and cirrhosis
- Detoxification of the liver.

CONTRAINDICATIONS

- Specific to the individual herbal medicines within the class.

APPLICATION

- Best taken before meals
- Medium- to long-term application is advisable for extended benefits.

HERBAL MEDICINES

- *Andrographis paniculata* (andrographis)
- *Berberis aquifolium* (Oregon mountain grape)
- *Berberis vulgaris* (barberry)
- *Bupleurum falcatum* (bupleurum)
- *Cynara cardunculus* var. *scolymus* (globe artichoke)
- *Panax ginseng* (Korean ginseng)
- *Peumus boldus* (boldo)
- *Phyllanthus amarus* (phyllanthus)
- *Picrorhiza kurroa* (picrorhiza)
- *Salvia miltiorrhiza* (dan shen)
- *Schisandra chinensis* (schisandra)
- *Silybum marianum* (St Mary's thistle)
- *Taraxacum officinale radix* (dandelion root).

Hepatoprotectives

DEFINITION

Hepatoprotective herbal medicines protect hepatocytes (the main liver cells) against damage. Similar to the cholagogue and choleretic herbal medicines, many of the hepatoprotective agents exhibit multiple effects on the liver and hepatobiliary system.

TRADITION

Even though many of the herbs specific to this category are also known hepatics, it seems that this class is of more modern origin. As knowledge of anatomy, physiology and phytochemistry evolves, we are learning more about the therapeutic applications of these herbs. One extraordinary example is *Silybum marianum.* Scientific studies show that this herb has the ability to increase hepatocyte regeneration as well as to augment these cells against toxins. Silybin and silymarin have been shown to have hepatoprotective activity, both in vitro and in vivo, against all manner of liver toxins, from *Amanita phalloides* or *A. virosa* poisoning to chemical and heavy-metal toxicity.[13]

INDICATIONS

- Poor liver function and digestion (dyspepsia)
- Liver-specific conditions (hepatitis, etc.)
- *Amanita* fungus poisoning
- Heavy-metal toxicity

- Alcoholic liver damage (e.g. fatty liver and cirrhosis)
- Chemical exposure.

CONTRAINDICATIONS

- Specific to the individual herbal medicines within the class.

APPLICATION

- Best taken before meals
- Medium- to long-term application is advisable for extended benefits.

HERBAL MEDICINES

- *Andrographis paniculata* (andrographis)
- *Angelica polymorpha* (dong quai)
- *Bupleurum falcatum* (bupleurum)
- *Camellia sinensis* (green tea)
- *Curcuma longa* (turmeric)
- *Cynara cardunculus* var. *scolymus* (globe artichoke)
- *Panax ginseng* (Korean ginseng)
- *Phyllanthus amarus* (phyllanthus)
- *Picrorhiza kurroa* (picrorhiza)
- *Salvia miltiorrhiza* (dan shen)
- *Schisandra chinensis* (schisandra)
- *Silybum marianum* (St Mary's thistle).

Hepatotrophorestoratives

DEFINITION

Hepatotrophorestorative herbal medicines restore the integrity of liver tissue. They are similar to hepatotonics and hepatoprotectives in that many will exhibit multiple effects on the liver and hepatobiliary system.

TRADITION

Worthy of note is a mythological reference to the liver's regenerative powers. In Greek mythology, Prometheus was punished by Zeus (for stealing fire and giving it to mankind) by being tied to a rock and having an eagle peck out and eat his liver during the day as a form of torture. During the night, the liver would regrow and regenerate, and the entire process could begin once more. Whether or not the ancient Greeks knew of the liver's regenerative powers is uncertain.

INDICATIONS

- Liver-specific conditions (hepatitis, etc.)
- *Amanita* fungus poisoning
- Heavy-metal toxicity
- Alcoholic liver damage (e.g. fatty liver and cirrhosis)
- Chemical exposure.

CONTRAINDICATIONS

- Specific to the individual herbal medicines within the class.

APPLICATION

- Best taken before meals
- Medium- to long-term application is advisable for extended benefits.

HERBAL MEDICINES

- *Bupleurum falcatum* (bupleurum)
- *Cynara cardunculus* var. *scolymus* (globe artichoke)
- *Salvia miltiorrhiza* (dan shen)
- *Silybum marianum* (St Mary's thistle).

IMMUNE SYSTEM

Anti-allergics

DEFINITION

Anti-allergic herbal medicines temper an overactive immune response, often by stabilising or inhibiting the degranulation of mast cells. Anti-allergics are indicated for allergic skin disorders such as eczema, and also for respiratory conditions such as asthma and seasonal pollinosis.

TRADITION

The immune system is one of the most complex physiological systems in the human body. The term 'allergy' was first coined by the Austrian paediatrician von Pirquet in 1906, who took it from the Greek *al*, meaning 'beyond' and *ergon*, meaning 'activity'.[10] Considering that our understanding of allergies has matured and grown so much in the last two to three decades, this class of agents should be considered of more modern origin.

INDICATIONS

- Skin conditions of an allergic nature (eczema, etc.)
- Hay fever/seasonal pollinosis
- Asthma (mild to moderate cases).

CONTRAINDICATIONS

- Specific to the individual herbal medicines within the class.

APPLICATION

- Best taken with meals
- Medium- to long-term application is advisable for extended benefits.

HERBAL MEDICINES

- *Albizia lebbeck* (albizia)
- *Ephedra sinica* (ma huang)
- *Ganoderma lucidum* (reishi)
- *Hemidesmus indicus* (hemidesmus)
- *Matricaria chamomilla* (German chamomile)
- *Picrorhiza kurroa* (picrorhiza)
- *Scutellaria baicalensis* (baikal skullcap)
- *Tanacetum parthenium* (feverfew)
- *Tylophora indica* (tylophora)
- *Urtica dioica folia* (nettle leaf).

Antibacterials

DEFINITION

Antibacterial herbal medicines elicit a specific immune response to bacterial agents, or have a direct antibacterial activity upon certain species of bacteria. More modern terminology has been introduced to be more specific, 'bacteriostatic' meaning a substance that can reduce or inhibit the growth of bacteria, and 'bactericidal' meaning a substance that kills the bacterium in its entirety.[13]

TRADITION

The term 'bacterial' is derived from the Greek *baketerion,* meaning 'small staff', or *baktron,* meaning 'stick or rod', based on the fact that when viewed under a microscope the first bacteria identified were rod shaped.[10] The term was first used in the mid-19th century and so belongs to our more recent traditional knowledge.

INDICATIONS

- Suspected bacterial infection (topically and systemically).

CONTRAINDICATIONS

- Serious bacterial infections, such as bacterial meningitis, are medical emergencies and require acute medical intervention
- Specific to the individual herbal medicines within the class.

APPLICATION

- Best taken with meals
- Medium- to long-term application is advisable for extended benefits.

HERBAL MEDICINES

- *Allium sativum* (garlic)
- *Berberis vulgaris* (barberry)
- *Calendula officinalis* (calendula)
- *Commiphora myrrha* (myrrh)
- *Echinacea* spp. (echinacea)
- *Hydrastis canadensis* (goldenseal)
- *Salvia officinalis* (sage)
- *Scutellaria baicalensis* (baikal skullcap)
- *Thymus vulgaris* (thyme).

Antibiotics

DEFINITION

Antibiotic herbal medicines eradicate or inhibit the growth of bacteria, in many cases without the mass destruction of microflora within the bowel. Antibiotics are one of the broader group of antimicrobial compounds, which are used to treat infections caused by microorganisms, including fungi and protozoa.

TRADITION

The term 'antibiotic' is derived from the Greek *anti,* meaning 'against', and *biotikos,* meaning 'fit for life'. The term was first coined by Selman Waksman in the early 1940s.[10] Antibiotics are similar to antimicrobials in that they kill or inhibit the growth of microorganisms, although modern science has revealed that pharmaceutical antibiotics generally have no effect against viruses or fungal agents, with better drugs having been developed specifically for infections with these organisms.

INDICATIONS

- Mild to moderate infections of bacterial, viral or fungal origin.

CONTRAINDICATIONS

- None known for this class
- Specific to the individual herbal medicines within the class.

APPLICATION

- Best taken before meals
- Short- to medium-term application is advisable for extended benefits
- Best to support the bowel flora with active cultures during and after treatment.

HERBAL MEDICINES

- *Allium sativum* (garlic)
- *Andrographis panniculata* (andrographis)
- *Artemisia* spp. (wormwood)
- *Berberis vulgaris* (barberry)
- *Calendula officinalis* (calendula)
- *Cnicus benedictus* (blessed thistle)
- *Cinnamomum zelyanicum/C. verum* (Ceylon cinnamon)
- *Echinacea* spp. (echinacea)
- *Handroanthus impetiginosus* (pau d'arco)
- *Hydrastis canadensis* (goldenseal)
- *Juglans nigra* (black walnut)
- *Lavandula angustifolia* (English lavender)
- *Salvia miltiorrhiza* (dan shen)
- *Thymus vulgaris* (thyme).

Antifungals

DEFINITION

Antifungal herbal medicines elicit a specific immune response to, or act directly on, fungi of various genuses and species. Fungi include not only the more well-known mushrooms, but also moulds and yeasts. Perhaps surprisingly, eukaryotic fungi are more closely related phylogenetically to animals than to plants,[14] and this may be the reason why they can be quite difficult to treat. Examples of fungal pathogens include *Candida albicans, Aspergillus* spp., *Cryptococcus neoformans, Histoplasma* spp. and *Pneumocystis jiroveci.*

TRADITION

The term 'antifungal' is derived from the Greek *anti,* meaning 'against', and Latin *fungus,* which could have been derived from the Greek *sphongos,* meaning 'sponge'.[10]

INDICATIONS

- Suspected fungal infection (topical or systemic), such as tinea pedis (athlete's foot)
- *Candida albicans* infection (candidiasis).

CONTRAINDICATIONS

- Specific to the individual herbal medicines within the class.

APPLICATION

- Best taken with meals
- Medium- to long-term application is advisable for extended benefits.

HERBAL MEDICINES

- *Allium sativum* (garlic)
- *Azadirachta indica* (neem leaf)
- *Handroanthus impetiginosus* (pau d'arco)
- *Thuja occidentalis* (thuja)
- *Thymus vulgaris* (thyme).

Topical antifungals

- *Calendula officinalis* (calendula)
- *Melaleuca alternifolia* (tea tree oil).

Antimicrobials

DEFINITION

Antimicrobial herbal medicines elicit a general immune response to any microbial agent (viruses, bacteria, fungi). These remedies are often prescribed together with immune-enhancing herbs and other indicated remedies. It is beneficial to know exactly which microbe is to be eradicated in order to specify further the desired action (e.g. antiviral, antifungal, antibacterial).

TRADITION

The term 'microbial' was coined in the late 19th century from the Greek *mikros*, meaning 'small', and *bios*, meaning 'life'[10] as a general term for bacteria, viruses and fungi. This class of agents is of relatively modern origin, although many of the great minds throughout history, such as Avicenna, Marcus Varro and Susruta, hinted at the existence of microbes long before they were discovered by science in the late 17th century.

INDICATIONS

- All manner of mild to moderate viral, bacterial or fungal infections (topical and systemic).

CONTRAINDICATIONS

- Specific to the individual herbal medicines within the class.

APPLICATION

- Best taken with meals
- Medium- to long-term application is advisable for extended benefits.

HERBAL MEDICINES

- *Achillea millefolium* (yarrow)
- *Agathosma betulina* (buchu)
- *Allium sativum* (garlic)
- *Arctostaphylos uva-ursi* (bearberry)
- *Armoracia rusticana* (horseradish)
- *Azadirachta indica* (neem leaf)
- *Baptisia tinctoria* (wild indigo)
- *Berberis aquifolium* (Oregon mountain grape)
- *Berberis vulgaris* (barberry)
- *Calendula officinalis* (calendula)
- *Camellia sinensis* (green tea)
- *Citrus* spp. (citrus seed extract)
- *Commiphora myrrha* (myrrh)
- *Echinacea* spp. (echinacea)
- *Euphorbia hirta* (euphorbia)
- *Foeniculum vulgare* (fennel)
- *Handroanthus impetiginosus* (pau d'arco)
- *Hydrastis canadensis* (goldenseal)
- *Hypericum perforatum* (St John's wort)
- *Hyssopus officinalis* (hyssop)
- *Inula helenium* (elecampane)
- *Juniperus communis* (juniper)
- *Matricaria chamomilla* (German chamomile)
- *Melissa officinalis* (lemon balm)
- Propolis (resinous production of bees)
- *Salvia miltiorrhiza* (dan shen)
- *Salvia officinalis* (sage)
- *Scutellaria baicalensis* (baikal skullcap)
- *Thuja occidentalis* (thuja)
- *Thymus vulgaris* (thyme).

Antipyretics

DEFINITION

Also known as 'febrifuges', antipyretic herbal medicines reduce or prevent fever. They are not to be confused with antihydrotic herbal medicines, which reduce sweating. Antihydrotics are indicated in instances such as hot flushes during the menopause, while antipyretics are used to reduce fever often of infectious origin.

It is important to reflect on Thomsonian medicine, which encouraged fever as the body's natural way of eliminating toxins and eradicating infection. This process is still encouraged in herbal medicine, although there are instances where fever needs to be reduced, such as in children or in chronic or dire situations.

Interestingly, many of the medicines within this class exhibit multiple actions, and some show immune-stimulating effects.

TRADITION

The term 'antipyretic' is derived from the Greek *anti*, meaning 'against', and *pyretos*, meaning 'fever'.[10] In ancient times fever was seen as a normal occurrence as a response to disease within the body, and was encouraged and nurtured rather than suppressed (using diaphoretic herbs). Only in acute and dangerous fevers would temperature be reduced.

HERBAL MEDICINES

- *Achillea millefolium* (yarrow)
- *Alchemilla vulgaris* (lady's mantle)
- *Andrographis panniculata* (andrographis)
- *Azadirachta indica* (neem leaf)

- *Baptisia tinctoria* (wild indigo)
- *Melissa officinalis* (lemon balm)
- *Rehmannia glutinosa* (rehmannia)
- *Salix alba* (white willow)
- *Scutellaria baicalensis* (baikal skullcap).

Antivirals

DEFINITION

Antiviral herbal medicines help to eradicate viral organisms.

TRADITION

First described in the 18th century, the term is derived from the Latin *virus*, meaning 'poisonous' or 'noxious'.[10] The use of specific antiviral herbal substances is largely a modern application, as our knowledge of the phytochemistry of plants expands and highlights those herbs that have antiviral activity or that can elicit an immune response such that the body can respond to a viral infection.

INDICATIONS

- Suspected mild to moderate viral infections.

CONTRAINDICATIONS

- Specific to the individual herbal medicines within the class.

APPLICATION

- Best taken with meals
- Medium- to long-term application is advisable for extended benefits.

HERBAL MEDICINES

- *Azadirachta indica* (neem leaf)
- *Hypericum perforatum* (St John's wort)
- *Melissa officinalis* (lemon balm)
- *Thuja occidentalis* (thuja).

Diaphoretics

DEFINITION

Also known as 'sudorifics', diaphoretic herbal medicines promote sweating during a fever. It is this action that enables the medicines to control a fever. Note that diaphoretics should not be confused with antipyretics, which reduce a fever (see above).

TRADITION

The term 'diaphoresis' is defined in *Webster's Dictionary* as 'to throw off by perspiration', which reflects the fact that this class of medicines is used to raise the body temperature in order to assist in fighting infections of viral or bacterial origin. Diaphoretics have been employed across all known cultural paradigms of herbal medicine, and found particular importance in Native American herbal medicine, which heavily influenced the Thomsonian system, which itself later evolved into what we know today as naturopathy and Western herbal medicine.

INDICATIONS

- Suspected mild to moderate viral infections (systemic).

CONTRAINDICATIONS

- Specific to the individual herbal medicines within the class.

APPLICATION

- Best taken with meals
- Short-term application is advisable.

HERBAL MEDICINES

- *Achillea millefolium* (yarrow)
- *Asclepias tuberosa* (pleurisy root)
- *Bryonia dioica* (red bryony)
- *Bupleurum falcatum* (bupleurum)
- *Capsicum* spp. (cayenne, chilli)
- *Eupatorium perfoliatum* (boneset)
- *Hemidesmus indicus* (hemidesmus)
- *Hyssopus officinalis* (hyssop)
- *Inula helenium* (elecampane)
- *Matricaria chamomilla* (German chamomile)
- *Melissa officinalis* (lemon balm)
- *Mentha x piperita* (peppermint)
- *Nepeta cataria* (catmint)
- *Sambucus nigra* (elderflower)
- *Solidago virgaurea* (goldenrod)
- *Tilia cordata* (lime or linden flowers)
- *Zanthoxylum clava-herculis* (prickly ash)
- *Zingiber officinale* (ginger).

Immune enhancers

DEFINITION

Also called 'immune stimulants', immune enhancer herbal medicines stimulate one or more aspects of the immune system. They enhance immune function and/or stimulate an immune response when required.

Some of the herbal medicines in this class have been described above and these should be reviewed in the context of their immunostimulant action.

TRADITION

While our ancient ancestors used many of the herbs within this class to treat infections, it seems that they did so because of their observations of the therapeutic effects of the herbs rather than because of knowledge that the herbs directly stimulate what we now know as the immune system. The first mention of the concept of immunity was not made until relatively recent times, but the concept was discussed by Thucydides in ca. 430 BCE regarding the Plague of Athens. He observed that the strong who survived the plague were able to tend to the sick and dying without fear of contracting the disease a second time.[15]

INDICATIONS

- Infections of bacterial, viral or fungal origin.

CONTRAINDICATIONS

- Specific to the individual herbal medicines within the class
- Caution should be exercised in patients receiving immunosuppressive therapy (e.g. patients taking medication to suppress organ rejection).

APPLICATION

- Best taken with meals
- Medium- to long-term application is advisable for lasting benefit.

HERBAL MEDICINES

- *Allium sativum* (garlic)
- *Aloe vera* (aloe)
- *Andrographis panniculata* (andrographis)
- *Angelica polymorpha* (dong quai)
- *Arctostaphylos uva-ursi* (bearberry)
- *Astragalus membranaceus* (astragalus)
- *Azadirachta indica* (neem leaf)
- *Baptisia tinctoria* (wild indigo)
- *Codonopsis pilosula* (codonopsis)
- *Echinacea* spp. radix (echinacea root)
- *Eleutherococcus senticosus* (Siberian ginseng)
- *Handroanthus impetiginosus* (pau d'arco)
- *Hydrastis canadensis* (goldenseal)
- *Paeonia lactiflora* (white peony)
- *Panax ginseng* (Korean ginseng)
- *Phytolacca decandra* (poke root)
- *Picrorrhiza kurroa* (picrorhiza)
- Propolis (resinous production of bees)
- *Rehmannia glutinosa* (rehmannia)
- *Thuja occidentalis* (thuja)
- *Uncaria tomentosa* (cat's claw).

Immune modulators

DEFINITION

Immune-modulator herbal medicines modulate and balance the activity of the immune system.

TRADITION

Members of this herbal class have only been recently found, via scientific investigations, especially in vitro and in vivo studies, to exert an immunomodulatory activity. Much like tonics (or, the lesser used term, amphoterics), immune-modulator herbal medicines restore balance to an under or overfunctioning immune system, thus making their use effective in people susceptible to recurrent infections and the elderly. Many of the herbs within this class are adaptogens, which may account in part for this normalising effect. Dammarane saponins, glycosides, alkylamides and polysaccharides are important active constituents of this class of herbal medicines.

INDICATIONS

- Recurrent infectious disease from weakened immune function
- Age-related reduction in function of the immune system.

CONTRAINDICATIONS

- Specific to the individual herbal medicines within the class
- Caution should be exercised in patients receiving immunosuppressive therapy (e.g. those taking medication to suppress organ rejection).

APPLICATION

- Best taken with meals
- Medium- to long-term application is advisable for lasting benefit.

HERBAL MEDICINES

- *Cordyceps sinensis* (cordyceps)
- *Echinacea* spp. *radix* (echinacea root)
- *Eleutherococcus senticosus* (Siberian ginseng)
- *Ganoderma lucidum* (reishi)
- *Grifola frondosa* (maitake)
- *Lentinula edodes* (shitake)
- *Panax ginseng* (Korean ginseng)
- *Withania somnifera* (withania, ashwagandha).

Immune suppressants

DEFINITION

In contrast to immune enhancers, immune suppressant herbal medicines reduce or dampen the immune response. Also known as 'immune depressants', they are indicated in instances where the immune system is overactive. Traditionally they are used in cases of autoimmune conditions or hyperimmune situations. The most commonly used and known immunosuppressant is the herb *Hemidesmus indicus*.

TRADITION

Like the immune enhancers and immune modulators, the class immune suppressants has only been identified in relatively recent times, owing to the English nomenclature. During the last 60 years, drugs such as cortisone, azathioprine and ciclosporin have been shown to have pronounced immunosuppressant activity, and these have given rise to the possibility of organ transplantation and the treatment of serious autoimmune disorders. Herbs within this class, while not as therapeutically effective for more serious conditions, have a place in the management of conditions such as hay fever and asthma.

INDICATIONS

- Overactivity of the immune system.

CONTRAINDICATIONS

- Specific to the individual herbal medicines within the class
- Caution should be exercised in patients who have a weakened immune system, the elderly and other susceptible patients.

APPLICATION

- Best taken with meals
- Medium- to long-term application is advisable for lasting benefit.

HERBAL MEDICINES

- *Albizia lebbeck* (albizia)
- *Hemidesmus indicus* (hemidesmus)
- *Tylophora indica* (tylophora).

Lymphatics

DEFINITION

Lymphatic herbal medicines improve the flow of lymphatic fluid or increase lymphatic drainage (detoxification).

TRADITION

The lymphatic system was first discussed by the physician Rufus of Ephesus, and later by Herophilus and Galen.[16] The term 'lymphatic' is derived from the Latin *lympha,* meaning 'clear water', which relates to the clear nature of lymphatic fluid.[10]

Herbs within this class are typically used to assist in the cleansing and detoxification of the body, and have a specific role with regard to the glands and nodes.[11] While not specifically classified as a lymphatic at the time, herbs within this class have been used for centuries to achieve such an action. In 1653 Culpeper wrote about the virtue of cleavers, alluding to its use in lymphatic conditions: 'It helps all sorts of hard swellings or kernels in the throat ... to cleanse the blood and keep the body in health'. Writings such as this illustrate how, in certain cases and classes, the herbal knowledge that we still value today does not necessarily come from scientific testing, but from observation and experimentation over hundreds of years and generations of patients. To know that not much has changed in our use and knowledge of this herbal class since the day of Culpeper should not only drive us to understand better the pharmacology and mechanisms by which this class of medicines works, but also enable us to realise the great wisdom and insight our herbal forebears possessed and passed down to us.

INDICATIONS

- Lymphatic congestion or stagnation
- Detoxification.

CONTRAINDICATIONS

- Specific to the individual herbal medicines within the class
- Caution should be exercised in patients with lymphoma (cancer of the lymphatic system).

APPLICATION

- Best taken with meals
- Medium- to long-term application is advisable for lasting benefit.

HERBAL MEDICINES

- *Baptisia tinctoria* (wild indigo)
- *Calendula officinalis* (calendula)
- *Echinacea* spp. (echinacea)
- *Galium aparine* (cleavers)
- *Iris versicolor* (blue flag)
- *Phytolacca decandra* (poke root).

RESPIRATORY SYSTEM

Anti-asthmatics

DEFINITION

Anti-asthmatic herbal medicines ameliorate the symptoms of mild to moderate asthma.

TRADITION

The term 'asthma' is derived from the Greek *asthma,* meaning 'panting' or 'to breathe hard'.[10] The condition has appeared in many ancient texts, from the *Huang Ti Nei Ching* of ancient China,[17] to the Ebers Papyrus of ancient Egypt,[18] and therefore asthma should be considered an ancient disease. Historically, *Ephedra sinensis* and *Tussilago farfara* were used to manage asthmatic patients, but these herbs are now scheduled by the Therapeutic Goods Administration (TGA) due to certain constituents (i.e. alkaloids) they contain, and can no longer be used by herbal medicine practitioners in Australia. Many of the herbs that remain in this category are anti-allergic, anti-inflammatory or immune suppressants.

INDICATIONS

- Asthma (atopic asthma, etc.)
- Bronchial asthma
- Breathlessness or wheezing.

CONTRAINDICATIONS

- Specific to the individual herbal medicines within the class
- Severe cases of asthma need to be managed with pharmaceutical medication. However, complementary and herbal medicines can still work effectively as adjunct therapy.

APPLICATION

- Best taken with meals
- Medium- to long-term application is advisable.

HERBAL MEDICINES

- *Albizia lebbeck* (albizia)
- *Angelica polymorpha* (dong quai)
- *Ephedra sinica* (ma huang)
- *Hemidesmus indicus* (hemidesmus)
- *Ganoderma lucidum* (reishi)
- *Tanacetum parthenium* (feverfew)
- *Tylophora indica* (tylophora).

Anti-catarrhals

DEFINITION

Anti-catarrhal herbal medicines reduce the formation of mucus. The resolution of catarrh will aid in relieving the discomfort that characterises many upper and lower respiratory tract conditions.

TRADITION

The term 'anti-catarrhal' is derived from the Greek *anti*, meaning 'against', and *katarrhous*, which literally translates as 'a flowing down'.[10] The term was developed in the late 14th century, and thus this is a traditional class of herbal medicines dating back to our ancient knowledge base.

INDICATIONS

- Catarrhal conditions, especially upper respiratory tract infections progressing to lower respiratory tract infections and/or catarrh.

CONTRAINDICATIONS

- Specific to the individual herbal medicines within the class.

APPLICATION

- Best taken with meals
- Short- to medium-term application is advisable.

HERBAL MEDICINES

- *Allium sativum* (garlic)
- *Armoracia rusticana* (horseradish)
- *Berberis aristata* (Indian barberry)
- *Euphrasia officinalis* (eyebright)
- *Glechoma hederacea* (ground ivy)
- *Hydrastis canadensis* (goldenseal)
- *Hyssopus officinalis* (hyssop)
- *Nepeta cataria* (catmint)
- *Pimpinella anisum* (aniseed)
- *Polygala tenuifolia* (polygala)
- *Polygonum bistorta* (bistort)
- *Salvia officinalis* (sage)
- *Sambucus nigra* (elderflower)
- *Solidago virgaurea* (goldenrod).

Antitussives

DEFINITION

Antitussive herbal medicines reduce coughing. Most antitussive herbs work by depressing the cough reflex, often due to the presence of cyanogenic glycosides or saponins. This depression is most useful for cases of nervous or dry cough, especially in children.

TRADITION

The term 'antitussive' is derived from the Greek *anti*, meaning 'against', and the Latin *tussis*, meaning 'cough'.[10] In ancient times antitussive herbal medications contained opiates, but these are considered too risky in modern practice.

INDICATIONS

- Non-productive cough
- Severe or persistent cough that is stubborn to expectorant usage
- Nervous cough
- Cough due to external irritation or obstruction (neoplasia, tumour, reflux).

CONTRAINDICATIONS

- Specific to the individual herbal medicines within the class
- Use only when specifically indicated and only for the short term
- Contraindicated in congestive pulmonary conditions/ productive cough due to potential suppression of mucus elimination leading to complications.

APPLICATION

- Best taken before meals
- Long-term therapy is not advised.

HERBAL MEDICINES

- *Althaea officinalis radix* and *folia* (marshmallow root and leaf)
- *Glycyrrhiza glabra* (liquorice)
- *Hedera helix* (English ivy)
- *Humulus lupulus* (hops)
- *Inula helenium* (elecampane)
- *Prunus serotina* (wild cherry bark)
- *Thymus vulgaris* (thyme)
- *Tussilago farfara* (coltsfoot).

Bronchodilators

DEFINITION

Bronchodilator herbal medicines dilate the bronchioles to assist with breathing. They are especially beneficial in asthmatic conditions.

TRADITION

The term 'bronchodilator' is derived from the Greek *bronchos*, meaning 'windpipe' or 'throat', and the Latin *dilatare*, meaning 'to make wider' or 'to enlarge'.[10] While it is certain that herbs were employed for this action in ancient times, this class is of more recent origins and became accepted as our knowledge of the pulmonary tree and its physiology become better known in the last century.

INDICATIONS

- Asthma and related complaints
- Breathlessness
- Wheeze.

CONTRAINDICATIONS

- None known.

APPLICATION

- Take at any time for immediate effect
- Long-term therapy is safe with gentler options, but the underlying cause must always be treated.

HERBAL MEDICINES

- *Coleus forskolii* (coleus)
- *Euphorbia hirta* (euphorbia)
- *Jusicia adhatoda* (adhatoda).

Decongestants

DEFINITION

Decongestant herbal medicines remove congestion of the mucous membranes, especially those within the upper respiratory tract.

TRADITION

The term 'congestion' is derived from the Latin *congestus* and *congerere*, meaning 'to bring together' or 'to pile up'.[10] Decongestants are infinitely valuable in conditions such as sinus congestion, seasonal pollinosis and blocked noses due to infections.

INDICATIONS

- Asthma and related complaints
- Sinusitis and sinus congestion.

CONTRAINDICATIONS

- Specific to the individual herbal medicines within the class.

APPLICATION

- Take at any time for immediate effect
- Long-term therapy is safe with gentler options, but the underlying cause must always be treated.

HERBAL MEDICINES

- *Armoracia rusticana* (horseradish)
- *Capsicum* spp. (cayenne, chilli)
- *Hydrastis canadensis* (goldenseal).

Expectorants

There are various classes of expectorants:

- Stimulating
- Warming
- Relaxing
- Amphoteric/general.

Each of these is outlined in an individual section below.

TRADITION

The term 'expectorant' comes from the Latin *expectoratus* (*ex* meaning 'to expel' and *pectus* meaning 'breast'), which literally translates as 'making a clean breast/chest'.[10] The term seems to have come into use in the late 17th century.

Stimulating expectorants

DEFINITION

Otherwise known as 'reflex expectorants', stimulating expectorant herbal medicines provoke increased mucociliary activity by reflex stimulation of the upper digestive wall. Historically, an emetic was shown to also stimulate expectoration. There are many historical examples such as ipecacuanha, *Lobelia*, squills, *Primula*, *Bellis*, *Saponaria* and *Polygala*. A high saponin content is a feature of this class.

INDICATIONS

- Cough linked with bronchial congestion
- Bronchitis
- Emphysema.

CONTRAINDICATIONS

- Dry and irritable conditions of the lungs
- Asthma
- Young children
- Can irritate dyspeptic conditions of the gastrointestinal tract.

APPLICATION

- Best taken before food as a hot infusion/decoction.

HERBAL MEDICINES

- *Angelica archangelica* (angelica)
- *Asclepias tuberosa* (pleurisy root)
- *Grindelia camporum* (grindelia)
- *Inula helenium* (elecampane)
- *Polygala tenuifolia* (polygala)
- *Viola odorata* (sweet violet).

Warming expectorants

DEFINITION

Warming expectorants are typically composed of herbs of a culinary nature. Many spices are used for their ability to counteract cold and damp conditions. Note that most of these remedies are rich in essential oils.

Due to the warming nature of these remedies, they are particularly indicated in conditions characterised by cold and damp (i.e. conditions in which the patient feels cold and the lungs are very congested [damp]).

INDICATIONS

- Productive cough associated with cold
- Bronchitis
- Emphysema
- Profuse catarrhal conditions
- Aromatic digestives
- Congestive chronic infections and inflammatory conditions.

Traditional applications

Warming expectorants were seen to also act on digestive/assimilation functions:

- Abdominal distension
- Loss of appetite
- Loose stools.

CONTRAINDICATIONS

- Gastro-oesophageal reflux.

APPLICATION

- Best taken immediately before food as a hot infusion/decoction.

HERBAL MEDICINES

- *Allium sativum* (garlic)
- *Cinnamomum zeylanicum*/*C. verum* (Ceylon cinnamon)
- *Foeniculum vulgare* (fennel)
- *Pimpinella anisum* (aniseed)
- *Zingiber officinale* (ginger).

Relaxing expectorants

DEFINITION

Relaxing expectorant herbal medicines promote the expulsion of excessive mucus by relaxing spasm to promote natural expectoration. Most of the herbal medicines in this category exhibit spasmolytic actions concurrently with demulcent properties.

INDICATIONS

- Debility and weariness from repeated coughing
- Spasmodic coughing, bronchitis, pneumonia causing inflammation and irritation to the respiratory tract.

CONTRAINDICATIONS

- Specific to the individual herbal medicines within the class.

APPLICATION

- Best taken before or with food as a warm infusion/concoction.

HERBAL MEDICINES

- *Drosera rotundifolia* (sundew)
- *Euphorbia hirta* (euphorbia)
- *Glycyrrhiza glabra* (liquorice)
- *Hedera helix* (English ivy)
- *Marrubium vulgare* (white horehound)
- *Pimpinella anisum* (aniseed)
- *Thymus vulgaris* (thyme)
- *Tussilago farfara* (coltsfoot).

Amphoteric/general expectorants

DEFINITION

Many respiratory conditions are characterised by abnormal mucus (catarrh), which can narrow airways. Often the mucus is thick and difficult to expectorate, as it 'saturates' and flattens the cilia, thereby interfering with normal expulsion.

Amphoteric or general expectorants are those that balance expectoration. They are especially indicated when debility from repeated coughing and expectoration have exhausted the patient. As an amphoteric they bring balance and regulation to the system and general wellbeing.

INDICATIONS

- Debility and weariness from repeated coughing
- Spasmodic coughing, bronchitis, pneumonia causing inflammation and irritation of the respiratory tract.

CONTRAINDICATIONS

- Specific to the individual herbal medicines within the class.

APPLICATION

- Best taken before or with food as a warm infusion/concoction.

HERBAL MEDICINES

- *Hedera helix* (English ivy)
- *Plantago lanceolata* (ribwort)
- *Trifolium pratense* (red clover)
- *Verbascum thapsus* (mullein)
- *Viola tricolor* (heartsease)
- *Zingiber officinale* (ginger).

Respiratory anti-inflammatories

DEFINITION

Herbal medicines having this action have an anti-inflammatory effect on the respiratory tract, and are especially beneficial in instances of acute pain in inflammation and irritation of the respiratory system. The following herbal medicines all exhibit a dual action on the respiratory tract and so will undoubtedly be a major component of a respiratory formula.

TRADITION

Herbs in this category cross over into many other classes of respiratory herbal medicines. Diseases of the respiratory tract commonly involve inflammation (e.g. asthma, bronchitis, pleurisy and laryngitis), and therefore this class of herbal medicines is often employed for respiratory conditions.

INDICATIONS

- Any respiratory condition with associated inflammation (asthma, bronchitis, etc.).

CONTRAINDICATIONS

- Specific to the individual herbal medicines within the class.

APPLICATION

- Best taken with meals
- Short- to medium-term application is advisable.

HERBAL MEDICINES

- *Asclepias tuberosa* (pleurisy root)
- *Glycyrrhiza glabra* (liquorice)
- *Plantago lanceolata* (ribwort)
- *Solidago virgaurea* (goldenrod)
- *Thymus vulgaris* (thyme).

Respiratory antiseptics

DEFINITION

Antiseptics are akin to the antimicrobials in that they inhibit the growth of or destroy microorganisms. They are therefore useful for respiratory tract infections.

TRADITION

Even though our knowledge about microbiology was attained only relatively recently, herbs in this class have been employed traditionally for all manner of respiratory complaints. Many herbs rely on the antiseptic activity of the essential oils that they contain.

INDICATIONS

- Respiratory tract infections
- Damp infective conditions.

CONTRAINDICATIONS

- Specific to the individual herbal medicines within the class.

APPLICATION

- Best taken with meals
- Short- to medium-term application is advisable. Long-term application should be avoided.

HERBAL MEDICINES

- *Asclepius tuberosa* (pleurisy root)
- *Echinacea* spp. (echinacea)
- *Inula helenium* (elecampane)
- *Picrorrhiza kurroa* (picrorhiza)
- *Salvia officinalis* (sage)
- *Solidago virgaurea* (goldenrod)
- *Thymus vulgaris* (thyme).

Respiratory demulcents

DEFINITION

Demulcent herbal medicines soothe inflamed surfaces such as the skin or mucous membranes. They are indicated for dry mucous membranes, and will soothe and restore normal mucus production by reflex demulcency. They should be used with caution in cases of overproduction of mucus. Respiratory tract demulcents are indicated for hot, dry, irritated and tickly coughs.

Demulcents are cool and moist energetically and, using the system of opposites, are indicated for conditions characterised by heat and dryness. These herbal medicines contain mucilage and have a soothing and anti-inflammatory action on the lower respiratory tract. They appear to have an opposite effect to stimulating expectorants; that is, they exert a reflex demulcent action on the pharynx and upper gastrointestinal tract rather than a stimulating and expectorant one.

INDICATIONS

- Cough in children
- Dry, irritable, non-productive and tickly coughing
- Asthmatic wheezing and tightness.

CONTRAINDICATIONS

- Wet, damp chest problems. However, they are also useful if there is an irritable component
- Profuse catarrhal or congestive conditions of the mucosa.

APPLICATION

- Best taken before meals
- A cold, aqueous infusion is best
- Long-term therapy is well tolerated.

HERBAL MEDICINES

- *Althaea officinalis folia* and *radix* (marshmallow leaf and root)
- *Asparagus racemosus* (shatavari)
- *Drosera rotundiflora* (sundew)
- *Glycyrrhiza glabra* (liquorice)
- *Plantago lanceolata* (ribwort)
- *Plantago major* (plantain)
- *Polygonum bistorta* (bistort)
- *Trigonella foenum-graecum* (fenugreek)
- *Tussilago farfara* (coltsfoot)
- *Ulmus rubra* (slippery elm)
- *Verbascum thapsus* (mullein).

Respiratory tonics

DEFINITION

Respiratory tonic herbal medicines are general tonics for the lungs and respiratory system.

TRADITION

Not surprisingly, tonics for the lungs date back to early times, with references to herbs such as cinnamon being used for 'watery lungs' attributed to Pedanius Disocorides in his section on aromatics in *De Materia Medica*. As a herbal class, they can be used in any lung deficiency to assist in restoring tone and function, albeit that they will do little for serious structural (e.g. tumours, obstructions) problems.

INDICATIONS

- Any instance where a lung tonic is required.

CONTRAINDICATIONS

- Specific to the individual herbal medicines within the class.

APPLICATION

- Best taken before meals
- Due to the required tonic action, medium- to long-term application is best.

HERBAL MEDICINES

- *Inula helenium* (elecampane)
- *Verbascum thapsus* (mullein).

Respiratory spasmolytics

DEFINITION

Otherwise known as 'antispasmodics for the respiratory system', respiratory spasmolytics relax the bronchioles.

TRADITION

As this is a modern class, extrapolation from bronchodilator herbal medicines can be considered.

INDICATIONS

- Tight chest, breathlessness
- Non-productive cough
- Wheezing
- Other asthmatic symptoms.

Traditional usage

- Europe — Solanaceae family (nightshades):
  - Atropine-related antiparasympathetic constituents enabled them to be prominent anti-asthmatics
  - Potent neuroactive properties
  - *Datura* spp., *Atropa belladonna, Solanum* spp. (strictly scheduled herbal medicines)
- Asia — *Ephedra sinica* (ma huang):
  - Sympathomimetic action
  - Culinary herbal medicines traditionally used as relaxants
  - Hyssop, thyme, horehound, grindelia.

CONTRAINDICATIONS

- Solanaceae family: glaucoma, urinary obstruction, paralytic ileus, intestinal atony and obstruction
- *Ephedra*: appetite disorders, glaucoma, concurrent monoamine oxidase inhibitor (MAOI) usage.

APPLICATION

- Take at any time for immediate effect
- Long-term therapy is safe with gentler options (never with Solanaceae family or *Ephedra*), but the underlying cause should always be treated.

HERBAL MEDICINES

- *Angelica archangelica* (angelica)
- *Asclepias tuberosa* (pleurisy root)
- *Coleus forskolii* (coleus)
- *Drosera rotundifolia* (sundew)
- *Euphorbia hirta* (euphorbia)
- *Glycyrrhiza glabra* (liquorice)
- *Grindelia camporum* (grindelia)
- *Hyssopus officinalis* (hyssop)
- *Inula helenium* (elecampane)
- *Justicia adhatoda* (adhatoda)
- *Marrubium vulgare* (white horehound)
- *Prunus serotina* (wild cherry bark)
- *Thymus vulgaris* (thyme).

Cough sedatives

DEFINITION

Sedatives typically reduce activity, particularly in the nervous system, and decrease nervous tension. The herbal medicines listed below reduce spasm and induce sleep. Both are antitussive in action, and have a spasmolytic action on the respiratory tract in conjunction with their sedative action.

TRADITION

The term 'sedative' derives from the Latin *sedatives,* meaning 'to calm' or 'to allay'.[10] The origin of the term is attributed to the late 18th century.

INDICATIONS

- Sleeplessness associated with long-term coughing
- Non-productive, tickly cough preventing sleep
- Severe or persistent cough stubborn to expectorant usage and thereby preventing sleep
- Nervous cough preventing sleep
- Cough due to external irritation or obstruction (neoplasia, tumour) preventing sleep.

CONTRAINDICATIONS

- Use only when specifically indicated and only for the short term.

APPLICATION

- Best taken before meals
- Long-term therapy is not advised.

HERBAL MEDICINES

- *Humulus lupulus* (hops)
- *Prunus serotina* (wild cherry bark).

MUSCULOSKELETAL SYSTEM

Anti-inflammatories

DEFINITION

Anti-inflammatory herbal medicines reduce inflammation. The herbal medicines listed below are specifically for the treatment of musculoskeletal inflammatory diseases. They may either be directly anti-inflammatory or act via some other mechanism, and have an important and very specific activity in chronic joint inflammation.

INDICATIONS

- Muscle cramps, pain and inflammation (lumbago, etc.)
- Osteoarthritis.

CONTRAINDICATIONS

- Specific to the individual herbal medicines within the class
- Caution should be exercised in patients with lymphoma (cancer of the lymphatic system).

APPLICATION

- Best taken with meals
- Medium- to long-term application is advisable for lasting benefit.

HERBAL MEDICINES

Antirheumatic agents

- *Actaea racemosa* (black cohosh)
- *Apium graveolens* (celery)
- *Boswellia serrata* (Indian frankincense)
- *Capsicum* spp. (cayenne, chilli)
- *Curcuma longa* (turmeric)
- *Guaiacum officinale* (guaiacum)
- *Harpagophytum procumbens* (Devil's claw)
- *Menyanthes trifoliata* (bogbean)
- *Salix alba* (white willow bark)

- *Smilax officinalis* (sarsaparilla) and *S. ornata* (brown sarsaparilla)
- *Zanthoxyylum clava-herculis* (prickly ash)
- *Zingiber officinale* (ginger).

Salicylate anti-inflammatories

- *Betula pendula* (silver birch)
- *Filipendula ulmaria* (meadowsweet)
- *Gaultheria procumbens* (wintergreen) — volatile oil, topical use only
- *Iris versicolor* (blue flag)
- *Populus tremuloides* (American poplar)
- *Salix alba* (white willow bark).

Steroidal anti-inflammatories

- *Bupleurum falcatum* (bupleurum)
- *Dioscorea villosa* (wild yam)
- *Glycyrrhiza glabra* (liquorice)
- *Rehmannia glutinosa* (rehmannia).

Anti-inflammatories of unknown mode of action

- *Apium graveolens* (celery)
- *Centella asiatica* (gotu kola)
- *Guaiacum officinale* (guaiacum)
- *Menyanthes trifoliata* (bogbean).

Musculoskeletal spasmolytics

DEFINITION

Musculoskeletal spasmolytic herbal medicines reduce or relieve smooth-muscle spasm (involuntary contractions). The herbal medicines given below have specific antispasmodic effects on the musculoskeletal system.

TRADITION

Spasmolytics, better known as 'herbs with an antispasmodic action', have many applications in human health. They are particularly useful in female reproductive health. This class of herbal medicines is of traditional origin.

INDICATIONS

- Muscle spasms
- Menstrual pain/cramping (dysmenorrhoea).

CONTRAINDICATIONS

- Specific to the individual herbal medicines within the class
- Pregnancy.

APPLICATION

- Best taken with meals
- Short-term application is advisable until pain relief is achieved.

HERBAL MEDICINES

Spasmolytic

- *Actaea racemosa* (black cohosh)
- *Dioscorea villosa* (wild yam)
- *Glycyrrhiza glabra* (liquorice)
- *Lavandula angustifolia* (English lavender) — volatile oil
- *Matricaria chamomilla* (German chamomile)
- *Piper methysticum* (kava)
- Rubefacients
- *Valeriana officinalis*/*V. edulis* (valerian)
- *Viburnum opulus* (cramp bark)
- *Viburnum prunifolium* (black haw).

Spasmolytic and sedative

- *Actaea racemosa* (black cohosh)
- *Dioscorea villosa* (wild yam)
- *Eschscholzia californica* (Californian poppy)
- *Lavandula angustifolia* (English lavender) — volatile oil
- *Matricaria chamomilla* (German chamomile)
- *Piper methysticum* (kava)
- *Piscidia piscipula* (Jamaican dogwood)
- *Scutellaria lateriflora* (skullcap)
- *Valeriana officinalis*/*V. edulis* (valerian)
- *Viburnum opulus* (cramp bark)
- *Viburnum prunifolium* (black haw).

DERMATOLOGICAL SYSTEM

Astringents

DEFINITION

Astringent herbal medicines cause the contraction of mucous membranes and exposed tissues. This is often due to the presence of tannins, which precipitate proteins on the exposed surface. When used in wound management, or to staunch bleeding, astringent herbs are called 'haemostatics' or 'styptics'.

TRADITION

Astringent herbs have been used in wound management for millennia. The term 'astringent' derives from the Latin *astringere*, meaning 'to bind fast', 'tighten', 'contract' or 'draw tight'.[10] It is this same action which has been used for centuries to tan hides and produce leather. The main phytochemical constituents responsible for this action are tannins, both hydrolysable and condensed.

INDICATIONS

- Minor skin abrasions, lacerations and wounds.

CONTRAINDICATIONS

- Specific to the individual herbal medicines within the class
- Tannins have the ability to bind to various substances and cause them to precipitate out of solution. Of note is the tendency for tannins to bind to alkaloids, a problem many a herbalist has encountered in the dispensary.

APPLICATION

- Topically, as a cream or salve for wound management
- Short- to medium-term application is needed for lasting benefit.

HERBAL MEDICINES

- *Achillea millefolium* (yarrow)
- *Agrimonia eupatoria* (agrimony)
- *Ballota nigra* (black horehound) — mild
- *Cnicus benedictus* (blessed thistle)
- *Commiphora myrrha* (myrrh)
- *Filipendula ulmaria* (meadowsweet)
- *Hamamelis virginiana* (witch hazel)
- *Hydrastis canadensis* (goldenseal)
- *Leptandra virginica* (black root)
- *Myrica cerifera* (bayberry)
- *Quercus robur* (English oak)
- *Phytolacca decandra* (poke root).

Depuratives

DEFINITION

Also known as 'alteratives' or 'blood purifiers', depurative herbal medicines improve detoxification of the body (by improving digestion, and the function of the liver/gallbladder, kidney/bladder and/or the immune system). They aid in the elimination of and reduce the accumulation of metabolic waste products within the body. They are largely used to treat chronic skin conditions and musculoskeletal disorders.

TRADITION

Just as our understanding of the exact mechanism of action of depurative herbal medicines is poor, so too is the etymology of the terms 'alterative' and 'depurative'. However, these terms are used uniquely in herbal and naturopathic medicine. On this basis it can be concluded that this class belongs to our traditional knowledge base. This class is still very popular for treating stagnant and chronic skin conditions and conditions of toxicity.

INDICATIONS

- Chronic skin conditions (eczema, psoriasis, etc.)
- Musculoskeletal disorders (osteoarthritis, etc.).

CONTRAINDICATIONS

- Specific to the individual herbal medicines within the class.

APPLICATION

- Best taken with meals
- Medium- to long-term application is advisable for lasting benefit.

HERBAL MEDICINES

- *Arctium lappa* (burdock)
- *Berberis aquifolium* (Oregon mountain grape)
- *Hemidesmus indicus* (hemidesmus)
- *Iris versicolor* (blue flag)
- *Rumex crispus* (yellow dock)
- *Schisandra chinensis* (schisandra)
- *Scrophularia nodosa* (figwort)
- *Silybum marianum* (St Mary's thistle)
- *Smilax officinalis* (sarsaparilla) and *S.ornata* (brown sarsaparilla)
- *Taraxacum officinale radix* (dandelion root)
- *Trifolium pratense* (red clover)
- *Urtica dioica folia* (nettle leaf)
- *Viola tricolor* (heartsease).

Emollients

DEFINITION

Herbal medicines that express emollient activity are used to soothe the surface of the skin to alleviate discomfort, and are also softening, protective and healing in nature. Some authors, such as Mills,[11] have suggested that this term is interchangeable with that of 'demulcent', whereas other authors suggest that emollient herbal medicines are for topical application only, and demulcents are for internal use on mucous membranes.[13] The term 'vulnerary' is also sometimes used synonymously with emollient.

TRADITION

The use of herbs in this way comes from our traditional knowledge base, and such herbs were most likely some of the earliest medicines used by our Palaeolithic ancestors. The term 'emollient' is French and is derived from the Latin *emollientum*, meaning 'to soften'.[10] Typically it is mucilage that allows this therapeutic class to exert its physiological effect.

INDICATIONS

- Minor burns, scalds and abrasions
- Inflammatory skin conditions
- Dry skin.

CONTRAINDICATIONS

- Specific to the individual herbal medicines within the class
- Caution should be exercised when treating blistered skin from burns. Use only on unbroken skin to reduce the risk of secondary infection.

APPLICATION

- Topically as a cream to maximise absorption into the skin. Ointments are less effective
- Short-term application is required for lasting benefit.

HERBAL MEDICINES

- *Althaea officinalis* (marshmallow)
- *Stellaria media* (chickweed).

Vulneraries

DEFINITION

Vulnerary herbal medicines promote the healing of wounds. They are similar to and work synergistically with anti-ulcer, astringent and demulcent herbal medicines.

TRADITION

The term 'vulnerary' derives from the Latin *vulnerarius*, from the nominative singular term *vulnus*, meaning 'wound'. The term was first coined in the last decade of the 16th century.[19] The use of herbs in wound management precedes the written word, so vulneraries are a strong traditional representative of our herbal lore.

INDICATIONS

- Minor burns, scalds and abrasions
- Inflammatory skin conditions
- Dry skin.

CONTRAINDICATIONS

- Specific to the individual herbal medicines within the class
- Caution should be exercised when treating blistered skin from burns. Use only on unbroken skin to reduce the risk of secondary infection.

APPLICATION

- Short- to medium-term application is needed for lasting benefit.

HERBAL MEDICINES

- *Aloe vera* (aloe) gel
- *Althaea officinalis folia* and *radix* (marshmallow leaf and root)
- *Arnica montana* (arnica)
- *Astragalus membranaceus* (astragalus)
- *Calendula officinalis* (calendula)
- *Centella asiatica* (gotu kola)
- *Echinacea* spp. (echinacea)
- *Geranium maculatum* (cranesbill)
- *Glechoma hederacea* (ground ivy)
- *Hypericum perforatum* (St John's wort)
- *Lamium album* (white dead nettle)
- *Matricaria chamomilla* (German chamomile)
- *Mitchella repens* (squaw vine)
- *Plantago lanceolata* (ribwort)
- Propolis (resinous production of bees)
- *Stellaria media* (chickweed)
- *Symphytum officinale* (comfrey)
- *Uncaria tomentosa* (cat's claw)
- *Verbascum thapsus* (mullein).

Topical vulneraries

- *Calendula officinalis* (calendula)
- *Commiphora myrrha* (myrrh)
- *Echinacea* spp. (echinacea)
- *Handroanthus impetiginosus* (pau d'arco)
- *Hydrastis canadensis* (goldenseal)
- *Hypericum perforatum* (St John's wort)
- *Melissa officinalis* (lemon balm)
- Propolis (resinous production of bees)
- *Stellaria media* (chickweed)
- *Symphytum officinale* (comfrey)
- *Thymus vulgaris* (thyme)
- *Ulmus rubra* (slippery elm)
- *Urtica dioica folia* (nettle leaf).

URINARY SYSTEM

Diuretics

DEFINITION

Diuretic herbal medicines increase urinary output and/or the excretion of metabolic waste products.

TRADITION

The term 'diuretic' is derived from the ancient Greek *diouretikos*, meaning 'prompting urine'. The term has been used in medical circles since the late 15th century.[10] Traditionally, herbs from this class have been employed to treat such conditions as urinary tract infections and dropsy, and to assist in detoxifying the body. Dioscorides mentions the term diuretic over 28 times in Book One (Aromatics) alone of his *De Materia Medica*, and suggests plants such as juniper, kupeiros (cypress), kinamomon (*Cinnamomum zeylanicum*) and krokos (*Crocus sativus*) possess this therapeutic activity.[20] Other ancient scholars and clinicians, such as Pliny the Elder, Hildegard von Bingen, Pietro Mattioli, Leonard Fuchs and William Withering (who discovered digitalis), also took an interest in plants that have this action.[21]

INDICATIONS

- Dysuria and oliguria linked to urinary tract infection or stones
- As an adjunct to cardioactive glycoside medication for heart failure
- Ascites
- Nocturnal enuresis
- Functional disturbances of micturition
- Urinary stones
- Haematuria
- Arthritis and other musculoskeletal disorders
- Integumentary disorders
- Premenstrual syndrome.

CONTRAINDICATIONS

- Renal failure or serious renal disorders
- Specific to the individual herbal medicines within the class
- Caution should be exercised in patients already taking loop or thiazide diuretics, as electrolyte imbalance and increased diuresis may occur
- Diabetes.

APPLICATION

- Best taken in high doses with meals
- Phased treatments or long-term therapy are acceptable applications.

HERBAL MEDICINES

- *Aphanes arvensis* (parsley piert)
- *Apium gravelolens* (celery seed)
- *Asparagus racemosa* (shatavari)
- *Astragalus membranaceus* (astragalus)
- *Betula pendula* (silver birch)

- *Camellia sinensis* (green tea)
- *Cynara cardunculis* var. *scolymus* (globe artichoke)
- *Daucus carota* (wild carrot)
- *Elymus repens* (couch grass)
- *Equisetum arvense* (horsetail)
- *Eupatorium purpureum* (gravel root)
- *Galium aparine* (cleavers, clivers)
- *Guaiacum officinale* (guaiacum)
- *Hydrangea aborescens* (hydrangea)
- *Iris versicolor* (blue flag)
- *Juniperus communis* (juniper)
- *Parietaria judaica* (pellitory of the wall)
- *Petroselinum crispum* (parsley)
- *Plantago major* (plantain)
- *Smilax officinalis* (sarsaparilla) and *S.ornata* (brown sarsaparilla)
- *Solidago virgaurea* (goldenrod)
- *Taraxacum officinale folia* and *radix* (dandelion leaf and root)
- *Tilia cordata* (lime tree)
- *Urtica dioica folia* and *radix* (nettle leaf and root)
- *Zanthoxyylum clava-herculis* (prickly ash)
- *Zea mays* (corn silk).

Diuretic — anti-gout

- *Apium graveolens* (celery seed)
- *Juniperus communis* (juniper)
- *Taraxacum officinale folia* (dandelion leaf)
- *Urtica dioicafolia* and *radix* (nettle leaf and root).

Urinary tract antiseptics

DEFINITION

Urinary tract antiseptic herbal medicines inhibit the growth of or destroy microorganisms in the urinary tract.

TRADITION

Reports of disorders of the genitourinary system date back to the Hippocratic and pre-Hellenistic Egyptian eras, and these disorders have been treated successfully with certain key herbs for over 2000 years. While modern science argues that the ancients were unaware that foreign bacteria and other microorganisms are responsible for these disorders (although there is evidence to suggest that scholars such as Varro [116–27 BCE] and other earlier physicians described microorganisms in their writings such as *De Re Rustica*), the herbs that they used, most likely on the basis of experimentation and observation over hundreds of years, have now been found to have antimicrobial and antiseptic actions. That said, this specific herbal class can be considered to be of a relatively recent origin, but is heavily influenced by the clinical experimentation and herbal knowledge of our forebears.

INDICATIONS

- Mild urinary tract infection
- Urinary stones
- Prostatitis
- Interstitial cystitis.

CONTRAINDICATIONS

- Specific to the individual herbal medicines within the class
- Renal failure or kidney impairment
- Pregnancy.

APPLICATION

- Best taken before or with meals.
- Long-term treatment is not advisable.

HERBAL MEDICINES

- *Agathosma betulina* (buchu)
- *Arctostaphylos uva-ursi* (bearberry)
- *Berberis vulgaris* (barberry)
- *Capsella bursa-pastoris* (shepherd's purse)
- *Echinacea* spp. (echinacea)
- *Filipendula ulmaria* (meadowsweet) — mild
- *Glycyrrhiza glabra* (liquorice)
- *Hydrastis canadensis* (goldenseal)
- *Juniperus communis* (juniper)
- *Piper methysticum* (kava)
- *Thymus vulgaris* (thyme)
- *Vaccinium macrocarpon* (cranberry)
- *Zea mays* (corn silk).

Urinary tract anti-inflammatories

DEFINITION

Urinary tract anti-inflammatory herbal medicines reduce inflammation in the urinary tract by acting locally, and may also exert a demulcent activity.

TRADITION

Many of the herbs within this class are also very well established urinary demulcents, and thus are effective in managing minor to moderate urinary tract inflammation. Much akin to the urinary antiseptics, they are members of a class which has been founded on the recently acquired understanding of the phytochemical constituents of the plants. The history of use of this herbal class dates back at least as far as Dioscorides, as he mentions the use of such herbs as *Prunus amygdalus, Cassia acutifolia,* amarakinon (*Cotula foetida*) and phoenix elate (*Borassus flabellifer*) for various inflammations of the kidneys and urinary tract.[20]

INDICATIONS

- Any mild to moderate infection, inflammation or irritation of the urinary tract
- Prostatitis or urinary stricture
- Cystitis, urethritis
- Kidney or bladder stones.

CONTRAINDICATIONS

- Renal failure or serious kidney disease
- Pregnancy.

APPLICATION

- Best taken before or with meals.

HERBAL MEDICINES

- *Althaea officinalis folia* and *radix* (marshmallow leaf and root).
- *Betula pendula* (silver birch)
- *Crateva nurvala* (crataeva)
- *Elymus repens* (couch grass)
- *Glycyrrhiza glabra* (liquorice)
- *Plantago lanceolata* (ribwort)
- *Solidago virgurea* (goldenrod)
- *Zea mays* (corn silk).

Urinary tract anti-lithics

DEFINITION

Urinary tract anti-lithic herbal medicines reduce the formation of calculi (stones) in the urinary tract.

TRADITION

The term 'anti-lithic' is derived from the Greek *anti*, meaning 'against', and *lithos*, meaning 'stone'.[10] The knowledge of urinary stones dates back millennia, and they are mentioned specifically in the Hippocratic Oath. Whether or not the herbs listed below are effective treatments for this condition is uncertain, as there is very little clinical evidence to suggest they are. In acute presentations of renal colic due to ureter blockage or obstruction it is highly unlikely that a patient would seek the help of a herbalist or naturopath; rather, they would go to the accident and emergency department for opiate analgesia. However, herbal medicine is excellent in preventing recurrence of such conditions. In addition to herbal medicines, the diet should be modified and water intake increased.

INDICATIONS

- Kidney and bladder stones.

CONTRAINDICATIONS

- Renal failure or kidney disease
- Specific to the individual herbal medicines within the class
- Pregnancy.

APPLICATION

- Best taken before or with meals
- Medium- to long-term treatment is advisable.

HERBAL MEDICINES

- *Alchemilla vulgaris* (lady's mantle)
- *Althaea officinalis folia* and *radix* (marshmallow leaf and root)
- *Crateva nurvala* (crataeva)
- *Equisetum arvense* (horsetail)
- *Eupatorium purpureum* (gravel root)
- *Hydrangea aborescens* (hydrangea)
- *Tylophora indica* (tylophora)
- *Zea mays* (corn silk).

Urinary tract astringents

DEFINITION

Urinary tract astringent herbal medicines cause constriction or contraction of mucous membranes and exposed tissues, usually by precipitating proteins, which create a barrier on the exposed surface of the membrane.

TRADITION

Astringent herbal medicines date back to ancient times. In his magnum opus, *De Materia Medica*, Dioscorides praises the use of astringent herbal medicines, such as amomon (*Elletaria cardamommum*) and juniper berries,[20] in all manner of inflammatory conditions.

INDICATIONS

- Haematuria — requires further medical investigation and is potentially serious
- Urethral stricture.

CONTRAINDICATIONS

- Renal failure or kidney disease
- Specific to the individual herbal medicines within the class
- Pregnancy

APPLICATION

- Best taken before or with meals
- Medium-term treatment is advisable; however, the cause of bleeding must first be investigated to ensure that it is not more serious (cancer, etc.).

HERBAL MEDICINES

- *Achillea millefolium* (yarrow)
- *Agrimonia eupatoria* (agrimony)
- *Alchemilla vulgaris* (lady's mantle)
- *Arctostaphylos uva- ursi* (bearberry)
- *Capsella bursa-pastoris* (shepherd's purse)
- *Equisetum arvense* (horsetail)
- *Plantago major* (plantain)
- *Rehmannia glutinosa* (rehmannia)
- *Rubus idaeus* (raspberry)
- *Urtica dioica folia* and *radix* (nettle leaf and root)
- *Vitis vinifera* (grape seed).

Urinary tract demulcents

DEFINITION

Urinary tract demulcent herbal medicines have a soothing effect on the mucous membranes of the urinary tract.

TRADITION

These herbs are used to exert a soothing action on the urinary system, typically the lower urinary tract. They combine well with urinary antiseptics and anti-inflammatory herbs used in urinary tract infections.

INDICATIONS

- Urinary infection
- Urinary stones

- Prostatitis
- Interstitial cystitis.

CONTRAINDICATIONS

- Renal failure and serious kidney disease
- Specific to the individual herbal medicines within the class.

APPLICATION

- Best taken with meals, typically at high doses. Excellent as infusions
- Phased treatment or long-term therapy are acceptable applications.

HERBAL MEDICINES

- *Alchemilla vulgaris* (lady's mantle)
- *Althea officinalis folia* and *radix* (marshmallow leaf and root)
- *Elymus repens* (couch grass)
- *Zea mays* (corn silk).

Renal tonics/protectives

DEFINITION

Renal tonic/protective herbal medicines improve the tone and function of the kidneys.

TRADITION

The term 'renal' is derived from the Latin *renalis*, roughly meaning 'belonging to the kidneys'.[10] Renal tonics are not of recent origin, having been used by those knowledgeable in wortcunning for centuries. Interestingly, however, the herbs in this class are not of a traditional Western herbal origin (i.e. Mediterranean/European or American) but come from Ayurvedic and traditional Chinese medical paradigms which modern Western herbalists have incorporated in their own materia medica.

INDICATIONS

- Any condition affecting the renal system.

CONTRAINDICATIONS

- Specific to the individual herbal medicines within the class
- Kidney function requires careful consideration before prescription of herbal medicines within this class.

APPLICATION

- Best taken with meals
- Long-term application is advisable for lasting benefit, provided the specific herbal medicine used is considered suitable for use as long-term treatment.

HERBAL MEDICINES

- *Astragalus membranaceus* (astragalus)
- *Bupleurum falcatum* (bupleurum)
- *Rehmannia glutinosa* (rehmannia)
- *Schisandra chinensis* (schisandra).

FEMALE REPRODUCTIVE SYSTEM

Emmenagogues (uterine stimulants)

DEFINITION

Emmenagogue herbal medicines increase the amplitude of uterine contractions and therefore affect the expulsive activity of the uterus.

TRADITION

Traditionally these herbal medicines were also prescribed as an abortifacient (i.e. a substance that induces abortion). This practice is illegal, frequently unsuccessful, dangerous and potentially lethal, and therefore is no part of naturopathic practice.

INDICATIONS

- Any condition with excessive bleeding associated with poor uterine tone
- For the expulsive activity of an emmenogogue to aid in the removal of retained tissue, and to assist in the healing and regenerative potential of the uterine lining
- After a termination of pregnancy to eliminate tissue remnants that may later cause a pelvic infection
- Heavy menstrual flow caused by a lack of tone (often by repeated pregnancies).

CONTRAINDICATIONS

- Generally should only be prescribed by qualified and experienced herbalists because of the nature of these herbal prescriptions.

APPLICATION

- Best taken with meals
- Long-term application is advisable for lasting benefit, provided the specific herbal medicine used is considered suitable for use as long-term treatment.

HERBAL MEDICINES

- *Artemisia vulgaris* (mugwort)
- *Caulophyllum thalictroides* (blue cohosh)
- *Mentha pulegium* (pennyroyal)
- *Ruta graveolens* (rue)
- *Salvia officinalis* (sage)
- *Tanacetum parthenium* (feverfew).

Female tonics

DEFINITION

Female tonic herbal medicines tonify and restore the organs and functions of the female reproductive system.

TRADITION

Herbs used for female sexual health belong to the traditional knowledge base, and are deeply rooted in not only Western herbal lore but also Ayurvedic and Chinese medicine.

INDICATIONS

- Low libido
- Reduced reproductive function and health (generally)
- Poor ovulation
- Menstrual cycle irregularities
- Infertility.

CONTRAINDICATIONS

- Specific to the individual herbal medicines within the class.

APPLICATION

- Best taken with meals
- Medium- to long-term application is advisable for lasting benefit.

HERBAL MEDICINES

- *Angelica polymorpha* (dong quai)
- *Asparagus racemosa* (shatavari)
- *Chamaelirium luteum* (false unicorn root).

Galactagogues

DEFINITION

Galactagogue herbal medicines encourage the production, quality and release of breast milk. The importance of breastfeeding human infants and the need for clinicians to help patients with delayed or insufficient milk production are both well established.

TRADITION

Herbs have a long history of use in all cultures to stimulate milk production both in women and in dairy animals. Application was as simple as drinking fennel seeds boiled in barley water, providing relief for both mothers and their children.

INDICATIONS

- Poor breast milk production
- Infant colic
- Mastitis.

CONTRAINDICATIONS

- Specific to the individual herbal medicines within the class.

APPLICATION

- Best taken with meals
- Medium- to long-term application is advisable for lasting benefit.

HERBAL MEDICINES

- *Anethum graveolens* (dill)
- *Asparagus racemosa* (shatavari)
- *Foeniculum vulgare* (fennel)
- *Galega officinalis* (goat's rue)
- *Medicago sativa* (alfalfa)
- *Pimpinella anisum* (aniseed)
- *Rubus idaeus* (raspberry leaf)
- *Trigonella foenum graecum* (fenugreek)
- *Urtica dioica folia* (nettle leaf)
- *Vitex agnus-castus* (chaste tree).

Antigalactagogues

- *Salvia officinalis* (sage).

Uterine astringents (haemostatics)

DEFINITION

Uterine astringent herbal medicines have a vasoconstrictive action on the endometrial circulation and thus reduce or stop blood loss associated with menstruation. These herbal medicines typically contain tannins, which act as astringents specifically on the proteins within bleeding tissues.

TRADITION

Uterine astringents were prescribed in instances of excessive bleeding or threatened blood loss. Their application is extensive and they were often also prescribed for the treatment of leucorrhoea.

INDICATIONS

- Any female reproductive condition that causes menorrhagia or metrorrhagia (e.g. fibroids, growths, premenopausal bleeds).

CONTRAINDICATIONS

- Due to the nature of these herbal medicines, constipation and other drying side effects can occur. Furthermore, long-term administration may affect the uptake of nutrients. Close monitoring of the patient is advisable
- Specific to the individual herbal medicines within the class.

APPLICATION

- Best taken with meals
- Short-term application is advisable for acute benefits; however, specific consideration of presentation is advised.

HERBAL MEDICINES

- *Achillea millefolium* (yarrow)
- *Alchemilla vulgaris* (lady's mantle)
- *Capsella bursa-pastoris* (shepherd's purse)
- *Hydrastis canadensis* (goldenseal)
- *Lamium album* (white deadnettle)
- *Panax notoginseng* (tienchi ginseng)
- *Trillium erectum* (beth root).

Uterine spasmolytics

DEFINITION

Uterine spasmolytic herbal medicines slow the rate and decrease the amplitude of uterine contractions, thus affecting the number of contractions in the uterine muscle per unit of time. They also have an effect on peristaltic activity in the bowel, and are frequently used to alleviate organ pain caused by excessive muscle contraction and/or associated ischaemia.

TRADITION

The term 'antispasmolytic' is derived from the Greek *anti*, meaning 'against', and *spasmodes*, meaning 'of the nature of a spasm'.[10] 'Spasm' itself is translated from the Greek for 'a convulsion' or 'to contract violently'.[10] Uterine spasmolytics have a strong history of use in female reproductive health and treatment, dating far back into herbal folklore. Their application is wide and consistent with modern application and clinical outcomes.

INDICATIONS

- Any condition that requires symptomatic relief of spasm and excessive uterine activity
- Prevention of early labour or miscarriage when this is associated with uterine overactivity.

CONTRAINDICATIONS

- Specific to the individual herbal medicines within the class.

APPLICATION

- Best taken with meals
- Long-term application is advisable for lasting benefit, provided the specific herbal medicine used is considered suitable for use as long-term treatment.

HERBAL MEDICINES

- *Dioscorea villosa* (wild yam)
- *Ligusticum wallichii* (Szechuan lovage)
- *Viburnum opulus* (cramp bark)
- *Viburnum prunifolium* (black haw).

Uterine tonics

DEFINITION

Uterine tonic herbal medicines improve the lining of the uterine muscle, regulate the activity of the uterus, increase the tone of the muscle and improve the overall strength of the uterus. They are said to normalise and assist with normal uterine functions.

TRADITION

Rubus idaeus is one of the oldest prescriptions and has been prescribed as a traditional *partus preparator* and general uterine tonic prior to pregnancy for centuries. As a tonic class, these herbal medicines have a strong traditional basis and proven clinical efficacy.

INDICATIONS

- Any condition associated with uterine pain
- For all complaints associated with abnormal bleeding patterns
- Conditions associated with prolapse, malposition or enlargement of the uterus
- As partus preparators
- Any condition that requires an improvement in the microenvironment of the uterus and endometrium (e.g. threatened miscarriage, preconception preparation, infertility).

CONTRAINDICATIONS

- Specific to the individual herbal medicines within the class.

APPLICATION

- Best taken with meals
- Long-term application is advisable for lasting benefit, provided the specific herbal medicine used is considered suitable for use as long-term treatment.

HERBAL MEDICINES

- *Alchemilla vulgaris* (lady's mantle)
- *Aletris farinosa* (true unicorn root)
- *Angelica polymorpha* (dong quai)
- *Caulophyllum thalictroides* (blue cohosh)
- *Chamaelirium luteum* (false unicorn root)
- *Mitchella repens* (squaw vine)
- *Rubus idaeus* (raspberry leaf).

Phyto-oestrogenics

DEFINITION

Phyto-oestrogens, or plant-based oestrogens, have the ability to occupy oestrogen receptors, but elicit a weaker physiological response than the endogenous, or indeed synthetic, hormones. Dietary oestrogens and isoflavones contain a phenolic ring, which is a prerequisite for binding to oestrogen receptors. Dietary oestrogens are about 100–1000 times less potent than human oestrogens (estradiol or estriol). Herbs that exhibit this activity typically contain isoflavones[22] or, in some cases, lignins. Herbs that contain isoflavones typically belong to the Fabaceae family and can be used in oestrogen deficiency.

INDICATIONS

- Decreased oestrogen production (e.g. menopause).

CONTRAINDICATIONS

- Known oestrogen excess. Some practitioners recommend dietary soy for its oestrogen-modulating activity via competitive inhibition
- Specific to the individual herbal medicines within the class.

APPLICATION

- Best taken with meals
- Medium- to long-term application is advisable for lasting benefit.

HERBAL MEDICINES

- *Trifolium pratense* (red clover).

Specific hormone modulators

DEFINITION

Hormone-modulating herbal medicines have the ability to modulate and balance various hormones, including progesterone, oestrogen, follicle-stimulating hormone (FSH), luteinising hormone (LH) and prolactin.

The following herbal classes and the herbal medicines within these classes are highly specialised. Due to their modern classification, they have no traditional categorisation.

TRADITION

Our understanding of hormones can only be considered as recent, as the term 'hormone' was first coined by Ernest Starling in 1905 at University College London.[23] His experimental work caused an explosion of interest in what we now call 'endocrinology', and paved the way for the elucidation of oestrogen, progesterone and testosterone in 1929 by Butenandt, Reichstein and Doisy, who received the Nobel Prize for their contribution to science and medicine.[23] In the 1950s further important advances in endocrinology were made, with the identification of LH, adrenocorticotropic hormone, FSH and prolactin.[23] These discoveries paved the way for our interpretation of how various phytochemicals modify the behaviour of these hormones.

INDICATIONS

- Hormone imbalance specific to the therapeutic application required.

CONTRAINDICATIONS

- Specific to the individual herbal medicines within the class.

APPLICATION

- Best taken with meals
- Medium- to long-term application is advisable for lasting benefit.

HERBAL MEDICINES

Follicular phase modulators

- *Chamaelirium luteum* (false unicorn root)
- *Paeonia lactiflora* (white peony)
- *Tribulus terrestris* (tribulus).

FSH inhibitors

- *Lycopus virginicus* (bugleweed).

FSH stimulants

- *Actaea racemosa* (black cohosh)
- *Tribulus terrestris* (tribulus).

Hormone balancers

- *Angelica polymorpha* (dong quai)
- *Chamaelirium luteum* (false unicorn root)
- *Actaea racemosa* (black cohosh)
- *Paeonia lactiflora* (white peony)
- *Serenoa repens* (saw palmetto).

Hypothalamic–pituitary ovarian modulators

- *Actaea racemosa* (black cohosh)
- *Chamaelirium luteum* (false unicorn root)
- *Glycyrrhiza glabra* (liquorice)
- *Paeonia lactiflora* (white peony)
- *Trillium erectum* (beth root)
- *Vitex agnus-castus* (chaste tree).

LH inhibitors

- *Actaea racemosa* (black cohosh)
- *Humulus lupulus* (hops)
- *Lycopus virginicus* (hugleweed).

LH stimulants

- *Vitex agnus-castus* (chaste tree).

Luteal phase modulators

- *Paeonia lactiflora* (white peony)
- *Vitex agnus-castus* (chaste tree).

Menstrual cycle regulators

- *Chamaelirium luteum* (false unicorn root)
- *Paeonia lactiflora* (white peony)
- *Vitex agnus-castus* (chaste tree).

Oestrogen modulators

- *Actaea racemosa* (black cohosh)
- *Alchemilla vulgaris* (lady's mantle)
- *Asparagus racemosa* (shatavari)
- *Chamaelirium luteum* (false unicorn root)
- *Dioscorea villosa* (wild yam)
- *Foeniculum vulgare* (fennel)
- *Glycyrrhiza glabra* (liquorice)
- *Hypericum perforatum* (St John's wort)
- *Paeonia lactiflora* (white peony)
- *Panax ginseng* (Korean ginseng)
- *Smilax officinalis* (sarsaparilla) and *S.ornata* (brown sarsaparilla)
- *Trigonella foenum-graecum* (fenugreek)
- *Trillium erectum* (beth root)
- *Vitex agnus-castus* (chaste tree).

Oestrogen stimulators

- *Alchemilla vulgaris* (lady's mantle)
- *Aletris farinosa* (true unicorn root)
- *Angelica polymorpha* (dong quai)
- *Asparagus racemosa* (shatavari)
- *Chamaelirium luteum* (false unicorn root)
- *Cimicafuga racemosa* (black cohosh)
- *Dioscorea villosa* (wild yam)
- *Foeniculum vulgare* (fennel)
- *Glycyrrhiza glabra* (liquorice)
- *Paeonia lactiflora* (white peony)
- *Panax ginseng* (Korean ginseng)
- *Salvia officinalis* (sage)
- *Serenoa repens* (saw palmetto)
- *Verbena officinalis* (vervain).

Ovarian tonics

- *Caulophyllum thalictroides* (blue cohosh)
- *Chamaelirium luteum* (false unicorn root)
- *Hydrastis canadensis* (goldenseal)
- *Vitex agnus-castus* (chaste tree).

Ovulation stimulators

- *Tribulus terrestris* (tribulus)
- *Vitex agnus-castus* (chaste tree).

Progesterone stimulators

- *Alchemilla vulgaris* (lady's mantle)
- *Caulophyllum thalictroides* (blue cohosh)
- *Vitex agnus-castus* (chaste tree).

Prolactin inhibitors

- *Glycyrrhiza glabra* (liquorice)
- *Paeonia lactiflora* (white peony)
- *Vitex agnus-castus* (chaste tree).

Prolactin stimulants

- *Humulus lupulus* (hops).

Testosterone/androgen inhibitors

- *Glycyrrhiza glabra* (liquorice)
- *Paeonia lactiflora* (white peony)
- *Serenoa repens* (saw palmetto)
- *Vitex agnus-castus* (chaste tree).

Testosterone stimulants

- *Avena sativa* seed (oat seed)
- *Centella asiatica* (gotu kola)
- *Ginkgo biloba* (ginkgo)
- *Panax ginseng* (Korean ginseng)
- *Smilax officinalis* (sarsaparilla) and *S.ornata* (brown sarsaparilla)
- *Turnera diffusa* (damiana).

MALE REPRODUCTIVE SYSTEM

Male tonics

DEFINITION

Male tonics are herbal medicines that tonify and restore the organs and functions of the male reproductive system.

TRADITION

Herbs used for male sexual health belong to the traditional knowledge base, and are deeply rooted in not only Western herbal lore but also Ayurvedic and Chinese medicine.

INDICATIONS

- Impotence
- Erectile dysfunction
- Benign prostatic hyperplasia.

CONTRAINDICATIONS

- Specific to the individual herbal medicines within the class.

APPLICATION

- Best taken with meals
- Medium- to long-term application is advisable for lasting benefit.

HERBAL MEDICINES

- *Panax ginseng* (Korean ginseng)
- *Serenoa repens* (saw palmetto)
- *Smilax officinalis* (sarsaparilla) and *S.ornata* (brown sarsaparilla)
- *Tribulus terrestris* (tribulus)
- *Turnera diffusa* (damiana).

Antiprostatics/antihyperprostatics

DEFINITION

Antiprostatic herbal medicines tonify and restore the prostate gland and functions of the male reproductive system.

TRADITION

This is a modern classification of herbal medicines, and a solid traditional definition is limited. The following herbal medicines have been used for a significant period of time, and their strong reputation highlights the importance of their prescription.

INDICATIONS

- Benign prostatic hyperplasia and associated symptoms
- Incontinence
- Prostatitis.

CONTRAINDICATIONS

- Specific to the individual herbal medicines within the class.

APPLICATION

- Best taken with meals
- Medium- to long-term application is advisable for lasting benefit.

HERBAL MEDICINES

- *Cucurbita pepo* (pumpkin seeds)
- *Epilobium parviflorum* (willow herb)
- *Pygeum americanum* (pygeum)
- *Serenoa repens* (saw palmetto)
- *Urtica dioica/radix* (nettle root).

Specific hormone modulators

DEFINITION

Specific hormone-modulating herbal medicines have the ability to modulate and balance various hormones, including progesterone, oestrogen, FSH, LH and prolactin.

The following herbal classes and the herbal medicines within these classes are highly specialised. Due to their modern classification, they have no traditional categorisation.

TRADITION

Our understanding of hormones can only be considered as recent, as the term 'hormone' was first coined by Ernest Starling in 1905 at University College London.[23] His experimental work caused an explosion of interest in what we now call 'endocrinology', and paved the way for the elucidation of oestrogen, progesterone and testosterone in 1929 by Butenandt, Reichstein and Doisy, who received the Nobel Prize for their contribution to science and medicine.[23] In the 1950s further important advances in endocrinology were made, with the identification of LH, adrenocorticotropic hormone, FSH and prolactin.[23] These discoveries paved the way for our interpretation of how various phytochemicals modify the behaviour of these hormones.

INDICATIONS

- Specific hormone imbalance (treated with appropriate specific therapeutic application).

CONTRAINDICATIONS

- Specific to the individual herbal medicines within the class.

APPLICATION

- Best taken with meals
- Medium- to long-term application is advisable for lasting benefit.

HERBAL MEDICINES

Anaphrodisiacs

- *Vitex agnus-castus* (chaste tree).

FSH inhibitors

- *Lycopus virginicus* (bugleweed).

FSH stimulants

- *Tribulus terrestris* (tribulus).

LH inhibitors

- *Humulus lupulus* (hops)
- *Lycopus virginicus* (bugleweed).

LH stimulators

- *Vitex agnus-castus* (chaste tree).

Prolactin inhibitors

- *Glycyrrhiza glabra* (liquorice)
- *Panax ginseng* (Korean ginseng)
- *Serenoa repens* (saw palmetto)
- *Vitex agnus-castus* (chaste tree).

Testosterone stimulators

- *Avena sativa* seed (oat seed)
- *Centella asiatica* (gotu kola)
- *Ginkgo biloba* (ginkgo)
- *Panax ginseng* (Korean ginseng)
- *Smilax officinalis* (sarsaparilla) and *S.ornata* (brown sarsaparilla)
- *Turnera diffusa* (damiana).

CARDIOVASCULAR AND HAEMATOLOGICAL SYSTEM

Antiarrhythmics

DEFINITION

Antiarrhythmic herbal medicines normalise or stabilise the heart rhythm. The term 'antiarrhythmic' is derived from the Greek *anti,* meaning 'opposed' or 'against', *a,* meaning 'not', and *rhythmos,* meaning 'rhythm'. Arrhythmia is defined as an irregularity or loss of rhythm associated with the heartbeat. In many cases this can include fibrillation, extrasystole and tachycardia,[11] some of which can be life-threatening.

TRADITION

Herbs in this class, such as *Crataegus monogyna, Corydalis ambigua* and *Angelica polymorpha,* have been shown in animal studies to have the pharmacological ability to prolong the refractory period and to correct experimentally induced atrial fibrillation.[24,25] More clinical studies are required to confirm the efficacy and safety of these herbs. It is due to the growing knowledge base of pharmacology and physiology that this action has been identified, and this classification is therefore a modern development.

While the antiarrhythmic activity of various herbal medicines has only come to light in the last 30 years, all these herbs have a strong historical association with the cardiovascular system. The herbs within this class have a diverse phytochemistry, active constituents of note including oligomeric procyanthocyanidins flavonoids, dammarane saponins and alkaloids.[26]

INDICATIONS

- Known cardiac arrhythmias.

CONTRAINDICATIONS

- Caution should be exercised in patients already taking antiarrhythmic or cardiac glycoside (e.g. Lanoxin) medications
- Caution should be exercised in patients taking medication for high blood pressure, as many herbs within this class may have an additive hypotensive effect
- Caution should be exercised in patients taking anticoagulant medication, as a potential additive effect may occur (herb specific).

APPLICATION

- Best taken with meals
- Medium to long-term application is advisable.

HERBAL MEDICINES

- *Angelica polymorpha* (dong quai)
- *Corydalis ambigua* (corydalis)
- *Crataegus* spp. (hawthorn leaves and berries)
- *Panax notoginseng* (tienchi ginseng)

- *Salvia miltiorrhiza* (dan shen)
- *Withania somnifera* (withania, ashwagandha).

Antioxidants

DEFINITION

Antioxidant herbal medicines protect against oxidation and free radical damage. The term 'antioxidant' is derived from the Greek *anti,* meaning 'against', and the English *oxidant,* meaning 'a substance that can cause oxidation or is oxidising in action'.

TRADITION

Commonly, practitioners forget about the antioxidant effects of herbal medicines and instead place significant importance on dietary supplements such as vitamins A, C and E and bioflavonoids. An example of a herbal medicine that has powerful antioxidant activity is grape seed extract, which has been shown in both animal and in vitro studies to have a greater free-radical scavenging activity than vitamins C and E and β-carotene.[27] The most important constituents in this respect are the oligomeric proanthocyanidin complexes (OPCs) and flavonoids.

The use of antioxidants in phytotherapy is a relatively modern concept that is a direct result of the emergence of the 'free radical' theory in health and disease, which was first proposed by Professor Denham Harman in the 1950s. There is little doubt about the significance of the proposal that oxidative processes are intimately linked with many chronic modern-day diseases, including cardiovascular disease. The antioxidant defence system of the body is coming under increasing stress due to factors such as poor diet (i.e. one that is low in fruits and vegetables), environmental influences (e.g. pollution), inflammation and nervous system stress, to name just a few. The term 'oxidative stress' is used to describe a situation in which the body's antioxidant defences are overwhelmed by oxidative processes. The ideal herbal antioxidant is one that is effective in both a lipid and an aqueous environment.

Herbs in this class are typically rich in flavonoids, OPCs, flavonol glycosides, stilbenes (e.g. resveratrol) and polyphenols.

INDICATIONS

- Patients with known history of a cardiovascular disease, disorder or condition
- Patients with family history of a cardiovascular disease, disorder or condition who wish to be proactive about their health (preventive approach)
- As a general tonic or as part of a regular detoxification program.

CONTRAINDICATIONS

- Caution should be exercised in patients taking anticoagulants (e.g. warfarin), as certain herbs in this class may have an additive effect.

APPLICATION

- Best taken with meals
- Medium- to long-term application is advisable.

HERBAL MEDICINES

- *Allium sativum* (garlic)
- *Andrographis paniculata* (andrographis)
- *Astragalus membranaceus* (astragalus)
- *Camellia sinensis* (green tea)
- *Crataegus* spp. (English hawthorn leaves and berries)
- *Curcuma longa* (turmeric)
- *Ginkgo biloba* (ginkgo)
- *Larrea tridentate* (chaparral)
- *Lycopersicon esculentum* (tomato)
- *Olea europaea* (olive leaves)
- *Polygonum cuspidatum* (Japanese knotweed)
- *Rosmarinus officinalis* (rosemary)
- *Salvia officinalis* (sage)
- *Schisandra chinensis* (schisandra)
- *Scutellaria baicalensis* (baikal skullcap)
- *Silybum marianum* (St Mary's thistle)
- *Thymus vulgaris* (thyme)
- *Uncaria tomentosa* (cat's claw)
- *Vaccinium myrtillus* (bilberry)
- *Vitis vinifera* (grape seed extract).

Anti-tachyarrhythmics

DEFINITION

Anti-tachyarrhythmic herbal medicines prevent and/or alleviate palpitations and reduce the heart rate (i.e. have a negatively chronotropic activity). The term 'anti-tachyarrhythmic' is derived from the Greek *anti,* meaning 'against', *tachy,* meaning 'speed', and *rhythmos,* meaning 'rhythmic'.[10]

TRADITION

Herbs in this class have a range of pharmacological activities, including sedative and anxiolytic actions. While the terminology used for this class is modern, the herbs have been used to manage cardiac disorders for centuries. For example, motherwort was noted as being effective for cardiac weakness and nervousness by Gerard in the late 16th century,[28] and was listed in *King's American Dispensatory* (1905) for nervous conditions, hysteria and neuralgia.[29]

The main active constituents of the anti-tachyarrhythmic class include volatile oils (mainly linalol and linalyl acetate), dammarane saponins,[13] flavonoids and alkaloids (leonurine and stachydrine).[30]

INDICATIONS

- Known cardiac palpitations or uncomplicated tachycardia
- Cardiac symptoms associated with neurosis
- Conditions characterised by nervousness, restlessness and anxiety
- Catecholamine-induced tachycardic episodes (i.e. panic disorders), in combination with other herbal classes (nervine tonics, sedatives, anxiolytics, adaptogens, etc.).

CONTRAINDICATIONS

- Caution should be exercised in patients already taking antiarrhythmic medications or those that can induce a negative chronotropic state
- Caution should be exercised in patients taking medication for high blood pressure, as certain herbs within this class may have an additive hypotensive effect
- Caution should be exercised in cases with hypothyroidism (motherwort specifically)
- Caution should be used when prescribing to pregnant or lactating women (herb-specific contraindication).

APPLICATION

- Best taken with meals
- Medium- to long-term application is advisable.

HERBAL MEDICINES

- *Lavandula angustifolia* (English lavender)
- *Leonurus cardiaca* (motherwort)
- *Lycopus virginica* (bugleweed)
- *Salvia miltiorrhiza* (dan shen)
- *Terminalia arjuna* (terminalia)
- *Withania somnifera* (withania, ashwagandha)
- *Zizyphus jujube* (zizyphus).

Blood tonics

DEFINITION

Blood tonic herbal medicines improve the quality of the blood. They tonify, build and strengthen the blood quality, and synergistically act as a nutritive and whole-body tonic.

TRADITION

Blood tonics have been used for centuries and within many different herbal paradigms. The traditional 'spring tonic' is an excellent example of herbs being employed to wake the body from its winter stasis and reinvigorate the organs and blood. Many of the herbs in this class also contain good amounts of iron, which modern science has confirmed is vital for healthy haemoglobin formation.

INDICATIONS

- Chronic skin conditions (e.g. eczema), when combined with alteratives
- Systemic infections, in conjunction with orthodox medication in moderate to severe cases
- Convalescence after illness, or as part of a regular healthy lifestyle.
- Mild anaemia.

CONTRAINDICATIONS

- None known.

APPLICATION

- Best taken with meals
- Medium- to long-term application is advisable.

HERBAL MEDICINES

- *Angelica polymorpha* (dong quai)
- *Codonopsis pilosula* (codonopsis)
- *Rehmannia glutinosa* (rehmannia)
- *Withania somnifera* (withania, ashwagandha).

Cardiac tonics

DEFINITION

Cardiac tonic herbal medicines increase the force of contraction of the heart (i.e. are positively inotropic), and restore tone and vigour to the heart muscle (i.e. myocardium). The term 'tonic' is derived from the Greek *tonikos*, meaning 'stretching', which evolved by the 18th century to have the meaning of 'having the property of restoring to health'.[10]

TRADITION

Tonics, by definition, work by restoring tone and proper function to a particular body system. Simon Mills describes them as being 'nourishing, supportive and restorative'.[11] Due to the type of action they have, they may need to be taken for a relatively long time for a therapeutic effect to be achieved. However, the effect is relatively long lasting. Cardiac tonics have the ability to improve the tone, strength, vigour and function of the myocardium.

Tonics, regardless of the body system at which they are aimed, comprise one of the most ancient classes in herbal lore. Modern day herbalists rely heavily on tonic classes, which are often used to treat organ-specific chronic disorders and disease states, in many cases as adjunct treatment to primary orthodox medications.

INDICATIONS

- Patients with mild symptoms of heart failure (Stage I or II of the New York Heart Association Guidelines)
- Hypotensive patients
- Age-related cardiac and/or vascular decline.

CONTRAINDICATIONS

- Caution should be exercised in patients with hypertension and those taking medication for high blood pressure
- Caution should be exercised in patients taking cardiac glycosides (digoxin).

APPLICATION

- Best taken with meals
- Medium- to long-term application is advisable.

HERBAL MEDICINES

- *Albizia lebbeck* (albizia)
- *Angelica polymorpha* (dong quai)
- *Astragalus membranaceus* (astragalus)
- *Coleus forskholii* (coleus)
- *Crataegus* spp. (English hawthorn leaves and berries)
- *Leonurus cardiaca* (motherwort)
- *Olea europaea* (olive leaves)

- *Panax ginseng* (Korean ginseng)
- *Panax notoginseng* (tienchi ginseng).

Cardioprotectives

DEFINITION

Cardioprotective herbal medicines protect the myocardium and decrease the risk of heart damage due to toxins or ischaemia.

TRADITION

The concept of the cardioprotective class is of recent origin. The herbs within this class do not show a single pharmacological activity, but rather a combination of many different cardiac-specific actions work synergistically to protect the myocardium. Actions of note in this class include antiplatelet, hypotensive, antiarrhythmic, antioxidant, antiatherogenic and cardiac tonic, which all work together to provide the cardioprotective activity of this class.

Scientific studies have confirmed that herbs within this class have the ability to reduce a range of cardiac events, including, but not limited to, myocardial ischaemia, reperfusion injury, hypertension, paroxysmal atrial fibrillation and heart failure (mild cases only).

INDICATIONS

- Patients with a known history of a cardiovascular disease, disorder or condition
- Patients with a family history of a cardiovascular disease, disorder or condition (preventive treatment).

CONTRAINDICATIONS

- Caution should be exercised in patients with hypertension and those taking medication for high blood pressure (herb-specific contraindication). Some of the herbs listed below may have an additive effect, although the likelihood of this is low.

APPLICATION

- Best taken with meals
- Medium- to long-term application is advisable.

HERBAL MEDICINES

- *Andrographis paniculata* (andrographis)
- *Corydalis ambigua* (corydalis)
- *Crataegus* spp. (English hawthorn leaves and berries)
- *Inula racemosa* (inula)
- *Panax ginseng* (Korean ginseng)
- *Panax notoginseng* (tienchi ginseng)
- *Rosmarinus officinalis* (rosemary)
- *Salvia miltiorrhiza* (dan shen).

Circulatory stimulants

DEFINITION

Circulatory stimulant herbal medicines improve the peripheral circulation and blood flow through body tissues. The term 'circulatory stimulation' is derived from the Latin *circulationem,* meaning 'to form a circle', and *stimulare,* meaning 'to goad' or 'to urge into action'.[10] The term 'circulation' is attributed to William Harvey (1578–1657 CE), who is said to be the first Western physician to correctly elucidate the pumping mechanism of the heart and its importance in the systemic and peripheral blood flow.

TRADITION

Circulatory stimulants belong to the traditional knowledge base. In ancient times heat was always intrinsically linked with life and, conversely, conditions of cold were related to death and loss of function. Herbal medicines that can increase blood flow, and in so doing increase the circulation of oxygen-rich blood to areas that require it, while also bringing nutriment and immune cells to defend against infection, and removing toxins and cell debris, are of great value in conditions of deficiency. Herbs in this class are those traditionally considered energetically to be hot or pungent. Active constituents such as glucosinolates, volatile oils, capsaicinoids and alkaloids are typically responsible for this action.

INDICATIONS

- Fever management
- Lowered vitality
- Conditions of poor circulation.

CONTRAINDICATIONS

- Caution should be exercised in patients with inflammatory disorders of the gastrointestinal tract (e.g. ulceration), as pungent herbs may cause irritation and pain.

APPLICATION

- Best taken with meals
- Short- to medium-term application is advisable.

HERBAL MEDICINES

- *Angelica polymorpha* (dong quai)
- *Armoracia rusticana* (horseradish)
- *Brassica alba/B. nigra* (mustard)
- *Capsicum* spp. (cayenne, chilli)
- *Cinnamomum zeylanicum/C. verum* (Ceylon cinnamon)
- *Ginkgo biloba* (ginkgo)
- *Juniperus communis* (juniper berry)
- *Myrica cerifera* (bayberry)
- *Panax ginseng* (Korean ginseng)
- *Rosmarinus officinalis* (rosemary)
- *Urtica dioica* (nettle)
- *Zanthoxylum clava-herculis* (prickly ash)
- *Zingiber officinale* (ginger).

Warming circulatory stimulants

- *Armoracia rusticana* (horseradish)
- *Capsicum* spp. (cayenne, chilli)
- *Cinnamomum zeylanicum/C. verum* (Ceylon cinnamon)
- *Panax ginseng* (Korean ginseng)
- *Zanthoxylum clava-herculis* (prickly ash)
- *Zingiber officinale* (ginger).

Fibrinolytics

DEFINITION

Fibrinolytic herbal medicines prevent and reduce the development of insoluble fibrin clots. The term 'fibrinolytic' is derived from the English word *fibrin*, and the Greek word *lysis*, meaning 'loosening' or 'dissolving'.[10] In modern medicine, fibrinolytic drugs are commonly called 'clot busters', and are also known as 'thrombolytics'.

TRADITION

The use of the fibrinolytic class is relatively recent. With a greater understanding of conditions such as acute myocardial infarction and ischaemic stroke through the theory of 'reperfusion',[31] this class of herbs has become invaluable in modern orthodox medicine. Considering the seriousness and acute nature of the conditions that require fibrinolytics, clinicians must apply common sense to patient management from a herbal or naturopathic perspective.

INDICATIONS

- Patients with a family history of cardiovascular and/or cerebrovascular thrombus development
- Conditions such as deep vein thrombosis (DVT).

CONTRAINDICATIONS

- Caution should be exercised in patients currently taking orthodox fibrinolytic medications, as there is the potential for an additive effect
- Caution should be exercised in patients with haemorrhagic conditions.

APPLICATION

- Best taken with meals
- Short- to medium-term application is advisable.

HERBAL MEDICINES

- *Allium sativum* (garlic)
- *Capsicum* spp. (cayenne, chilli)
- *Centella asiatica* (gotu kola)
- *Salvia miltiorrhiza* (dan shen).

Hypertensives

DEFINITION

Hypertensive herbal medicines increase both systolic and diastolic blood pressure. The term 'hypertensive' is derived from the Greek *hyper,* meaning 'over, beyond or above measure', and the Latin *tensionem,* meaning 'stretching'.[10] This is an interesting definition when you consider the physiological effect that increased blood pressure has on the vessel walls.

TRADITION

As a herbal class the hypertensives are seldom used as part of patient management except in patients with low blood pressure (e.g. orthostatic hypotension). More often a hypertensive action is an adverse reaction or interaction, or a side effect of the use of a specific herb. Herbs that are known to have a hypertensive activity should be avoided in patients with hypertension.

INDICATIONS

- Patients with known hypotension.

CONTRAINDICATIONS

- Caution should be exercised in patients with hypertension and those taking medications for high blood pressure.

APPLICATION

- Best taken with meals
- Medium-term application is advisable.

HERBAL MEDICINES

- *Coffea arabica* (coffee)
- *Cytisus scoparius* (broom)
- *Glycyrrhiza glabra* (liquorice)
- *Hydrastis canadensis* (goldenseal).

Hypocholesterolaemics

DEFINITION

Hypocholesterolaemic herbal medicines reduce cholesterol levels within the blood. The term 'hypocholesterolaemic' is derived from the Greek *hypo,* meaning 'under' or 'low', the English word *cholesterol* (descriptive of the specific substance involved) and the Greek *haima,* meaning 'blood'.[10]

TRADITION

The use of hypocholesterolaemics as a herbal class is a recent development. While cholesterol was first isolated and its molecular composition determined in the early 20th century, research into the effect of cholesterol on the cardiovascular system and its negative implications for human health has been done only in the last 30 years. Cholesterol, and more specifically the ratio of low-density lipoprotein (LDL) to high-density lipoprotein (HDL), has serious ramifications for the health of the cardiovascular and circulatory systems, and it is now understood that high cholesterol levels have contributed heavily to the increased mortality from cardiovascular disease in Western societies.

Other classes of herbal medicines that combine well with hypocholesterolaemics are antioxidants, bitter digestives, choleretics and cholagogues. The active constituents thought to be most relevant in this class include caffeoylquininc acids, flavonoids, polyphenols and amino acids.

INDICATIONS

- Confirmed hypercholesterolaemia or hyperlipidaemia
- Familial hyperlipidaemia.

CONTRAINDICATIONS

- Caution should be exercised in patients taking hypocholesterolaemic medication, as theoretically the use of herbal medicine may have an additive effect (potentially beneficial interaction).

APPLICATION

- Best taken with meals
- Medium- to long-term application is advisable.

HERBAL MEDICINES

- *Albizia lebbeck* (albizia)
- *Allium sativum* (garlic)
- *Avena sativa* (oats)
- *Camellia sinensis* (green tea)
- *Curcuma longa* (turmeric)
- *Cynara cardunculus* var. *scolymus* (globe artichoke)
- *Gymnema sylvestre* (gymnema)
- *Olea europaea* (olive leaves)
- *Panax notoginseng* (tienchi ginseng)
- *Plantago ovata* (psyllium)
- *Polygonum multiflorum* (polygonum)
- *Trigonella foenum-graecum* (fenugreek).

Other

- Mucilaginous herbal medicines: *Ulmus* spp. (slippery elm); *Plantago psyllium* (ipshagula)
- Dietary soluble and insoluble fibre.

Hypolipidaemics

DEFINITION

Hypolipidaemic herbal medicines reduce the concentration of blood lipids. The term 'hypolipidaemic' is derived from the Greek *hypo*, meaning 'under' or 'low', *lipos*, meaning 'fat' or 'grease', and *haima*, meaning 'blood'.[10] Hypolipidaemics are broader in their scope of action than hypocholesterolaemics (the effect of which is limited to activity on cholesterol and triglycerides), having an effect on phospholipids (chylomicrons, very-low-density lipoproteins [VLDLs], intermediate-density lipoproteins [IDLs], LDLs and HDLs[32]) and cholesterol esters.

TRADITION

Like the hypocholesterolaemic class, the hypolipidaemics are a modern development that have a broad scope and clinical application. Research has shown that herbs such as turmeric have in vivo hypolipidaemic activity, which has been attributed to the curcumin component of the herb[33] and has far-reaching implications for improving outcomes in patients with chronic cardiovascular disease.

INDICATIONS

- Patients with elevated triglycerides, LDL/HDL ratio and cholesterol
- Familial hyperlipidaemia and hypercholesterolaemia.

CONTRAINDICATIONS

- Caution should be exercised in patients taking hypocholesterolaemic medication, as theoretically the use of herbal medicine may have an additive effect (potentially beneficial interaction).

APPLICATION

- Best taken with meals
- Medium- to long-term application is advisable.

HERBAL MEDICINES

- *Curcuma longa* (turmeric)
- *Cynara cardunculus* var. *scolymus* (globe artichoke)
- *Polygonum multiflorum* (polygonum)
- *Terminalia arjuna* (terminalia)
- *Trigonella foenum-graecum* (fenugreek).

Hypotensives

DEFINITION

Hypotensive herbal medicines decrease both systolic and diastolic blood pressure. The term 'hypotensive' is derived from the Greek *hypo*, meaning 'under' or 'low', and the Latin *tensionem*, meaning 'stretching'.[10] They usually work well in combination with other herbal medicine classes (i.e. nervine tonics, anxiolytics, adaptogenics, etc., as needed), especially in cases of catecholamine-induced hypertension. They combine well with peripheral vasodilators.

TRADITION

Herbal medicines have been used to reduce blood pressure for hundreds of years, although it was only in the last century that it was understood how complex this mechanism is and the hypertensives were established as a specific class. The action of these herbs arises typically from specific phytochemicals, such as OPCs, iridoid glycosides and flavonoids. Seldom does a herb in this class exert a single action; many herbs in this class work on many facets of the cardiovascular system simultaneously (i.e. cardiac tonic, antiplatelet and cardioprotective, etc.).

INDICATIONS

- Patients with known pre- or mild hypertension such as seen in Stage 1 (both primary and secondary hypertension).

CONTRAINDICATIONS

- Caution should be exercised in patients with hypotension and those taking medication for low blood pressure.

APPLICATION

- Best taken with meals
- Medium- to long-term application is advisable.

HERBAL MEDICINES

- *Achillea millefolium* (yarrow)
- *Allium sativum* (garlic)
- *Astragalus membranaceus* (astragalus)
- *Coleus forskholii* (coleus)
- *Crataegus* spp. (English hawthorn leaves and berries)
- *Harpagophytum procumbens* (Devil's claw)
- *Inula racemosa* (inula)
- *Leonurus cardiaca* (motherwort)
- *Olea europaea* (olive leaves)
- *Salvia miltiorrhiza* (dan shen)
- *Scutellaria baicalensis* (baikal skullcap)

- *Valeriana officinalis* (valerian)
- *Viburnum opulus* (cramp bark)
- *Vinca minor* (lesser periwinkle)
- *Viscum album* (mistletoe)
- *Withania somnifera* (withania, ashwagandha)
- *Zizyphus jujube* (zizyphus).

Peripheral vasodilators

DEFINITION

Peripheral vasodilatory herbal medicines dilate (widen) the peripheral blood vessels and thereby improve circulation to peripheral tissues and assist in reducing blood pressure. The term 'peripheral vasodilator', although recent, is derived from the Greek *peripheria*, meaning 'circumference' or 'outer surface', from the Latin *vaso*, meaning 'vessel', and the Latin *dilatare*, meaning 'to make wider' or 'to enlarge'.[10]

TRADITION

This is a modern class born from our expanding knowledge of anatomy and physiology. However, many of the herbs listed below have been used for centuries for cardiovascular health, although the clinicians did not fully understand the physiological or pharmacological action being elicited.

INDICATIONS

- Mild to moderate hypertension (prehypertension and Stage 1 hypertension)
- Patients with poor peripheral circulation (cold hands and feet)
- Potential for use in Raynaud's phenomenon.

CONTRAINDICATIONS

- Caution should be exercised in patients with hypotension and those taking medication for low blood pressure, as this herbal class may have an additive effect.

APPLICATION

- Best taken with meals
- Medium- to long-term application is advisable.

HERBAL MEDICINES

- *Achillea millefolium* (yarrow)
- *Crataegus* spp. (English hawthorn leaves and berries)
- *Ginkgo biloba* (ginkgo)
- *Tilia cordata* (lime or linden flowers)
- *Viburnum opulus* (cramp bark)
- *Viscum album* (mistletoe).

Platelet aggregation inhibitors (antiplatelets)

DEFINITION

Antiplatelet herbal medicines reduce platelet aggregation and hence prolong bleeding time and prevent thrombus formation. The term 'antiplatelet' is derived from the Greek *anti*, meaning 'against', and the English *plate + let*, used to describe the plate-like structure of many blood cells.

TRADITION

Antiplatelet action is a modern classification for herbs that are of particular use in primary prevention (i.e. prophylaxis) of thrombotic cerebrovascular or cardiovascular diseases. Clinical trial evidence to support herbal use is still unavailable.

INDICATIONS

- History of deep vein thrombosis
- History of veno-occlusive disease (peripheral vascular disease).

CONTRAINDICATIONS

- Caution should be exercised in patients taking prescription antiplatelet medication, as an additive effect may occur
- Herbs with known antiplatelet activity should be discontinued for a minimum of at least 2 weeks prior to undergoing surgery. Individual hospitals and surgeons may have different requirements, which are to be respected.

APPLICATION

- Best taken with meals
- Medium- to long-term application is advisable.

HERBAL MEDICINES

- *Allium sativum* (garlic)
- *Andrographis paniculata* (andrographis)
- *Angelica polymorpha* (dong quai)
- *Coleus forskholii* (coleus)
- *Commiphora myrrha* (myrrh)
- *Crataegus* spp. (English hawthorn leaves and berries)
- *Curcuma longa* (turmeric)
- *Ginkgo biloba* (ginkgo)
- *Salix alba* (white willow bark)
- *Salvia miltiorrhiza* (dan shen)
- *Vaccinium myrtillus* (bilberry)
- *Vitis vinifera* (grape seed extract)
- *Zingiber officinale* (ginger).

Tissue perfusion enhancers

DEFINITION

Herbs that act as tissue perfusion enhancers are those that enhance the flow of nutrients, via improvements in blood rheology, to specific target tissues.

TRADITION

Ginkgo biloba, the sole member of this herbal class, has been used for centuries as a tonic for the memory and for whole body. Modern research suggests that extracts of this herb have the ability to positively affect blood rheology, and therefore to increase blood flow and nutrient delivery to poorly perfused tissues. This is especially true of the microvasculature, such as the capillaries, which is the site of most nutrient delivery and waste disposal.[11]

INDICATIONS

- Elderly patients, with potential for use in dementia
- Poor cognitive function and memory
- Tinnitus.

CONTRAINDICATIONS

- While recent reports have suggested that ginkgo has the potential to increase bleeding in people taking anticoagulant medication, more recent studies have shown that this is unlikely. That said, it is still wise to monitor patients closely.

APPLICATION

- Best taken with meals
- Medium- to long-term application is advisable.

HERBAL MEDICINES

- *Ginkgo biloba* (ginkgo).

Vasoprotectives

DEFINITION

Vasoprotective herbal medicines protect the integrity of the blood vessels, and by so doing support their normal function.

TRADITION

It is only with the advent of modern phytochemical analysis and the understanding of the biological activity of the active constituents that the full potential of the vasoprotective action of these herbs for improving health has been recognised. Certain herbs that have this ability also have venotonic activity. Constituents such as OPCs,[28] flavonoids and flavonol glycosides[34] are considered important contributors to the actions of this class.

INDICATIONS

- Varicose veins, spider veins or other vessel disorders.

CONTRAINDICATIONS

- None known for the class, but specific contraindications may exist for the individual herbs mentioned below.

APPLICATION

- Best taken with meals
- Medium- to long-term application is advisable.

HERBAL MEDICINES

- *Ginkgo biloba* (ginkgo)
- *Vaccinium myrtillus* (bilberry)
- *Vitis vinifera* (grape seed extract).

Venotonics

DEFINITION

Venotonic herbal medicines maintain the structure and integrity of veins and improve venous return. As a tonic herbal medicine, they improve the tone, vigour and function of the venous system.

TRADITION

The tonic nature of this class suggests that it is of a traditional origin. Like the venoprotective class, venotonics rely on OPCs and flavonoids for their action, but also on triterpene saponins,[27] such as aescin, and steroidal saponins, such as ruscogenin.[28] Herbs in this class are used as supportive therapy for discomforts of chronic venous insufficiency, including symptoms of pain, heaviness, itching and swelling.[28]

INDICATIONS

- Patients with poor venous return
- Patients with varicose veins, spider veins or other vessel disorders.

CONTRAINDICATIONS

- None known for the class, but specific contraindications may exist for the individual herbs mentioned below.

APPLICATION

- Best taken with meals
- Medium- to long-term application is advisable.

HERBAL MEDICINES

- *Aesculus hippocastanum* (horse chestnut)
- *Dioscorea villosa* (wild yam)
- *Ginkgo biloba* (ginkgo)
- *Ruscus aculeatus* (butcher's broom)
- *Vitis vinifera* (grape seed extract).

Specific cardiovascular herbal medicines

DEFINITION

The following herbal medicines and classes are highly specialised classifications. They have no traditional definition as a group, but each of them can be found in other traditional classes for this system.

INDICATIONS

- Poor cardiovascular health, the specific herbal medicine used depending on the specific presentation.

CONTRAINDICATIONS

- Specific to the individual herbal medicines within the class.

APPLICATION

- Best taken with meals
- Medium- to long-term application is advisable for lasting benefit.

HERBAL MEDICINES

Anti-ischaemics

- *Crataegus* spp. (English hawthorn leaves and berries)
- *Inula racemosa* (inula)

- *Salvia miltiorrhiza* (dan shen)
- *Terminalia arjuna* (terminalia).

Beta blockers

- *Inula racemosa* (inula). (Note: this herb has an action similar to that of pharmaceutical beta blockers)

Cardiac vascular tonifiers

- *Achillea millefolium* (yarrow)
- *Aesculus hippocastanum* (horse chestnut)
- *Ginkgo biloba* (ginkgo)
- *Ruscus aculeatus* (butcher's broom)
- *Vaccinium myrtillus* (bilberry)
- *Vitis vinifera* (grape seed extract).

Cardiovascular-specific diuretics

- *Olea europaea* (olive leaves)
- *Taraxacum officinale folia* (dandelion leaf).

Cerebrovascular stimulants

- *Ginkgo biloba* (ginkgo)
- *Rosmarinus officinalis* (rosemary)
- *Vinca minor* (lesser periwinkle).

Coronary vascular antispasmodics

- *Coleus forskholii* (coleus)
- *Justica adhatoda* (adhatoda)
- *Viburnum opulus* (cramp bark).

Coronary vasodilators

- *Corydalis ambigua* (corydalis)
- *Crataegus* spp. (English hawthorn leaves)
- *Viburnum opulus* (cramp bark).

Myocardial oxygen utilisation improvers

- *Crataegus* spp. (English hawthorn leaves and berries).

Negative chronotropics

- *Crataegus* spp. (English hawthorn leaves and berries)
- *Valeriana officinalis* (valerian)
- *Verbena officinalis* (vervain)
- *Withania somnifera* (withania, ashwagandha).

Positive chronotropics

- *Coffea arabica* (coffee) — and other coffee species
- *Crataegus* spp. (English hawthorn leaves and berries)
- *Ephedra sinica* (ephedra)
- *Panax ginseng* (Korean ginseng)
- *Paullinia cupana* (guarana)
- *Theobroma cacao* (cocoa).

Positive inotropics

- *Astragalus membranaceus* (astragalus)
- *Crataegus* spp. (English hawthorn leaves and berries)
- *Cytisus scoparius* (broom)
- *Eleutherococcus senticosus* (Siberian ginseng)
- *Panax ginseng* (Korean ginseng)
- *Theobroma cacao* (cocoa).

ENDOCRINE SYSTEM

Adaptogens

DEFINITION

Adaptogen herbal medicines increase the body's resistance to physical, environmental, emotional or biological stressors, and restore normal physiological function to the body. They are also known as a 'whole-body tonics'.

TRADITION

The term 'adaptogen' is of recent origin, and is attributed to Hans Selye (1907–1982) and his research into the general adaptation syndrome in the late 1940s. His research outlined the way in which organisms respond to stress, and highlighted the detrimental impact stress can have on the human organism, especially if exposure is prolonged. Many of the adaptogenic herbal medicines contain saponins in their profile of active constituents.

INDICATIONS

- Poor health due to excessive stress (anxiety, etc.)
- Intensive exercise
- Convalescence
- Adrenal exhaustion (in combination with adrenal tonics).

CONTRAINDICATIONS

- Specific to the individual herbal medicines within the class.

APPLICATION

- Best taken with meals
- Medium- to long-term application is advisable for lasting benefit.

HERBAL MEDICINES

- *Andrographis paniculata* (andrographis)
- *Asparagus racemosus* (shatavari)
- *Astragalus membranaceus* (astragalus)
- *Atractylodes macrocephala* (atractylodes)
- *Bacopa monnieri* (bacopa)
- *Codonopsis pilosula* (codonopsis)
- *Cordyceps sinensis* (cordyceps)
- *Eleutherococcus senticosus* (Siberian ginseng)
- *Ganoderma lucidum* (reishi)
- *Glycyrrhiza glabra* (liquorice)
- *Grifola frondosa* (maitake)
- *Lentinula edodes* (shitake)
- *Panax ginseng* (Korean ginseng)
- *Panax notoginseng* (tienchi ginseng)
- *Panax quinquefolium* (American ginseng)
- *Rehmannia somnifera* (rehmannia)
- *Rhodiola rosea* (rhodiola)
- *Schisandra chinensis* (schisandra)
- *Withania somnifera* (withania, ashwagandha).

Adrenal restoratives

DEFINITION

Adrenal restorative herbal medicines restore the functioning of the adrenal glands by rebuilding and rebalancing function.

TRADITION

The adrenal glands are so named as they are located relative to the kidneys. The term 'adrenal' is derived from the Latin *ad*, meaning 'near', and *renes*, meaning 'kidney'.

In traditional Chinese medicine, physicians relied on herbal medicines such as liquorice to restore tone and function to the kidneys and adrenal glands. Herbal medicines were chosen to nourish them after or during periods of high stress.

INDICATIONS

- Adrenal fatigue/exhaustion
- Extreme states of stress, or prolonged period of stress.

CONTRAINDICATIONS

- Specific to the individual herbal medicines within the class
- Avoid in instances of headache and epilepsy
- Avoid excessive caffeine use concomitantly.

APPLICATION

- Best taken with meals
- Medium- to long-term application is advisable.

HERBAL MEDICINES

- *Glycyrrhiza glabra* (liquorice)
- *Rehmannia somnifera* (rehmannia).

Aldose reductase inhibitors

DEFINITION

These herbal medicines inhibit aldose reductase, an enzyme involved in the production of harmful sugar metabolites in diabetes.

TRADITION

Aldose reductase is an enzyme involved primarily in carbohydrate metabolism, and is responsible for the conversion of glucose to substances such as sorbitol. While this description of the action is modern, the condition known as diabetes has been treated for centuries. For example, in traditional Chinese medicine, diabetes was known as wasting and thirsting disease, and was mentioned in the magnum opus *Huang Ti Nei Ching*, which was in existence during the Han dynasty. Diabetes has been mentioned in the Ebers Papyrus (1600 BCE) of Ancient Egypt, in which it is outlined how to 'eliminate urine which is too plentiful'.[35]

INDICATIONS

- Diabetes mellitus (type 1 and type 2).

CONTRAINDICATIONS

- Specific to the individual herbal medicines within the class.

APPLICATION

- Best taken with meals
- Short-term application is advisable for specific requirements.

HERBAL MEDICINES

- *Glycyrrhiza glabra* (liquorice)
- *Scutellaria baicalensis* (baikal skullcap).

Anti-obesity agents

DEFINITION

Anti-obesity herbal medicines stimulate weight loss.

TRADITION

It is unlikely that this herbal class has been used, or indeed has been required, prior to the last century. With massive changes in personal dietary intake, food accessibility, the use of hormones in food and the overrefining of foodstuffs in developing nations, this class of herbal medicines has come to pass as a result of our modern lifestyle. Obesity is not a problem in developing nations, but is a scourge of affluent societies. Herbs in this class work, in conjunction with healthy dietary habits and an exercise regimen, by increasing the rate of the metabolism.

INDICATIONS

- Obesity and weight gain.

CONTRAINDICATIONS

- Specific to the individual herbal medicines within the class.

APPLICATION

- Best taken with meals
- Medium-term application is advisable.

HERBAL MEDICINES

- *Coffea arabica* (coffee)
- *Cola nitida* (cola)
- *Coleus forskohlii* (coleus)
- *Fucus vesiculosus* (bladderwrack)
- *Panax notoginseng* (tienchi ginseng)
- *Paullinia cupana* (guarana)
- *Theobroma cacao* (cocoa).

Appetite-inhibiting agents

DEFINITION

Appetite-inhibiting herbal medicines interfere with the sense of satiety, hunger and cravings for certain foods (especially simple or refined carbohydrates).

TRADITION

The word 'appetite' is derived from the Latin *appetere*, meaning 'to long for' or 'to desire', and it was only in the 14th century that the term 'appetite' came to mean a craving for food.[10]

INDICATIONS

- Diabetes mellitus
- Obesity, weight gain.

CONTRAINDICATIONS

- Specific to the individual herbal medicines within the class.

APPLICATION

- Best taken before meals
- Duration specific to the individual.

HERBAL MEDICINES

- *Gymnema sylvestre* (gymnema).

Hypoglycaemics/antidiabetics

DEFINITION

Hypoglycaemic herbal medicines regulate and balance blood sugar levels. The term 'hypoglycaemic' is derived from the Greek *hypo*, meaning 'under' or 'low', *glycos*, meaning 'sugar', and *aemia*, meaning 'blood'. Patients with diabetes can experience low blood sugar levels, which can present with sweating, tremulousness, hunger, palpitations, confusion, stupor and even coma.[36]

TRADITION

Insulin was first isolated in the 1920s by Nicolae Paulesco.[37] Banting and MacLeod went on to research and produce the first insulin for the treatment of diabetes, and received the Nobel Prize in 1923. Herbs in this class have been shown experimentally and clinically to have an antidiabetic/hypoglycaemic action by reducing the intestinal absorption of glucose,[38] stimulating insulin secretion,[39] and increasing the amount of pancreatic β-cells and islets of Langerhans.[40]

INDICATIONS

- Diabetes mellitus
- Insulin resistance
- Obesity.

CONTRAINDICATIONS

- Specific to the individual herbal medicines within the class
- Caution should be exercised when using herbs that can lower blood sugar levels (BSLs)
- Caution should be exercised when treating patients taking insulin, as an additive effect, potentially causing hypoglycaemia, is possible.

APPLICATION

- Best taken before or during meals
- Short- to medium-term application is advisable initially
- Close patient monitoring is required.

HERBAL MEDICINES

- *Galega officinalis* (goat's rue)
- *Gymnema sylvestre* (gymnema)
- *Olea europaea* (olive leaves)
- *Panax ginseng* (Korean ginseng)
- *Phyllanthus amarus* (phyllanthus)
- *Stevia rebaudiana* (stevia)
- *Trigonella foenum graecum* (fenugreek).

Pancreatic trophorestoratives

DEFINITION

Trophorestorative herbal medicines restore the function and morphology of the pancreas (endocrine functions).

TRADITION

Although conditions such as diabetes were treated centuries ago, there is little evidence to suggest that the practitioners at that time had made the link identifying these conditions as being due to a disorder of the pancreas. The pancreas was first described by the little known Greek physician and anatomist Herophilus (335–280 BCE),[41] but it is only in recent times that the islets of Langerhans and the inner workings and biochemistry of this complex organ have been identified and elucidated.

The leaves of *Gymnema sylvestre* have been shown to assist in regenerating the islets of Langerhans in vivo,[42] but more research is required to understand this mechanism more clearly.

INDICATIONS

- Any condition that affects the endocrine function of the pancreas
- Diabetes mellitus
- Syndrome X/insulin resistance
- Obesity.

CONTRAINDICATIONS

- None known.

APPLICATION

- Long-term application is advisable for lasting benefit.

HERBAL MEDICINES

- *Gymnema sylvestre* (gymnema).

Thyroid stimulants

DEFINITION

Thyroid stimulant herbal medicines restore the function and morphology of the thyroid gland, stimulate this gland's secretion of thyroid hormones and increase their metabolism.

TRADITION

The thyroid gland was first described by Thomas Wharton in 1656, but thyroid disorders were treated in the Medicinal School of Salerno in ca. 1180 CE. The author and surgeon Rogerius Salernitanus, who wrote *Post Mundi Fabricam*, described several surgical cures and pharmacotherapy which would prove efficacious by modern standards.[43] It would therefore seem that this is a traditional herbal class, even though modern science has contributed greatly to our current understanding of thyroid disorders and their treatment.

INDICATIONS

- Hypothyroidism
- Subclinical hypothyroidism
- Obesity
- Weight gain.

CONTRAINDICATIONS

- Hyperthyroidism.

APPLICATION

- Best taken with meals
- Medium- to long-term application is advisable for lasting benefit.

HERBAL MEDICINES

- *Bacopa monniera* (bacopa)
- *Coleus forskohlii* (coleus)
- *Fucus vesiculosus* (bladderwrack)
- *Salvia miltiorrhiza* (dan shen)
- *Withania somnifera* (withania, ashwagandha).

Thyroid suppressants

DEFINITION

Thyroid suppressant herbal medicines reduce the secretion of thyroid hormones, restore metabolism, and alleviate the associated signs and symptoms of thyroid excess.

TRADITION

Serious presentations of hyperthyroidism, such as Grave's disease, were first characterised and described in the late 19th century. Herbs that can suppress thyroid function by reducing the secretion of thyroid hormones have an important place in our current material medica, although caution and common sense should be exercised when prescribing them. Herbs within this class, especially bugleweed, have been shown in vivo to reduce T3, T4 and TSH levels.[13]

INDICATIONS

- Hyperthyroidism.

CONTRAINDICATIONS

- Hypothyroidism
- Pregnancy and lactation.

APPLICATION

- Best taken with meals
- Medium- to long-term application is advisable for lasting benefit.

HERBAL MEDICINES

- *Leonurus cardiaca* (motherwort)
- *Lycopus virginicus* (bugleweed).

NEUROLOGICAL SYSTEM

Analgesics

DEFINITION

Otherwise known as anodynes, analgesic herbal medicines are those that relieve pain.

The term 'analgesic' is derived from the Greek *an*, meaning 'without', and *algia*, meaning 'pain'. This class incorporates whole herbs and active constituents that have the ability to reduce and ameliorate pain. Analgesics generally work on either the peripheral or the central nervous system and via multifarious pathways.

TRADITION

The analgesic class of medicines is probably one of the oldest known to humankind. Pain has plagued people throughout history, and therefore its amelioration has been of top priority. This is an area in which orthodox pharmaceuticals have been quite successful, but herbal analgesics also work effectively, although they generally take longer to take effect.

INDICATIONS

- Mild to moderate pain of any cause.

CONTRAINDICATIONS

- Potential potentiation of orthodox pain medications
- Allergies (especially to salicylates such as in *Salix alba*)
- Serious, acute pain may require pharmaceutical medication or medical intervention.

APPLICATION

- Best taken with meals
- Medium- to long-term application is advisable for lasting benefit.

HERBAL MEDICINES

- *Anemone pulsatilla* (pasque flower)
- *Cannabis* spp. (cannabis)
- *Capsicum* spp. (cayenne, chilli)
- *Corydalis ambigua* (corydalis)
- *Eschscholtzia californica* (Californian poppy)
- *Gaultheria procumbens* (wintergreen) — topical use of volatile oil
- *Gelsemium sempervirens* (gelsemium)
- *Harpagophytum procumbens* (Devil's claw)
- *Hypericum perforatum* (St John's wort)
- *Matricaria chamomilla* (German chamomile)
- *Piper methysticum* (kava)
- *Piscidia piscipula* (Jamaican dogwood)

- *Salix alba* (white willow bark)
- *Scutellaria lateriflora* (skullcap).

Anti-epileptics

DEFINITION

Anti-epileptic herbal medicines prevent seizures, typically by improving nervous system communication with the brain. These herbal medicines act as supportive adjuncts to other treatments. They should not be relied on as the sole treatment.

TRADITION

While the disease known as epilepsy has been documented for millennia, with it affecting people such as Julius Caesar, our understanding of the disease, and therefore the birth of this herbal class, is of more recent origins.

INDICATIONS

- Tonic–clonic seizures
- Absence seizures
- Epilepsy.

CONTRAINDICATIONS

- Specific to the individual herbal medicines within the class
- Potential interaction with pharmaceutical anti-epileptic/antiseizure medication.

APPLICATION

- Best taken with meals
- Short- to medium-term application is advisable.

HERBAL MEDICINES

- *Bacopa monnieri* (bacopa)
- *Cannabis* spp. (cannabis) particularly high CBD extracts
- *Paeonia lactiflora* (white peony)
- *Piper methysticum* (kava)
- *Polygala tenuifolia* (polygala)
- *Scutellaria lateriflora* (skullcap)
- *Valeriana officinalis* (valerian)
- *Viscum album* (mistletoe)
- *Zizyphus jujube* (zizyphus).

Anti-headache/anti-migraine agents

DEFINITION

These are herbal medicines that prevent headaches and/or migraines.

TRADITION

Headache, also called 'cephalalgia', is a relatively common condition that can be caused by benign effects such as dehydration, or by serious medical emergencies such as haemorrhagic stroke or aneurysm. Migraine is defined as a severe and sustained headache that is most often accompanied by concomitant emesis, nausea and photophobia. It is not surprising, therefore, that many herbs in this class are also strong analgesics.

INDICATIONS

- Tension/cluster headaches
- Migraine prophylaxis.

CONTRAINDICATIONS

- Specific to the individual herbal medicines within the class.

APPLICATION

- Best taken with meals
- Short- to medium-term application is advisable.

HERBAL MEDICINES

- *Curcuma longa* (turmeric)
- *Lavandula angustifolia* (English lavender)
- *Mentha x piperita* (peppermint)
- *Piscidia piscipula* (Jamaican dogwood)
- *Rosmarinus officinalis* (rosemary)
- *Stachys officinalis* (wood betony)
- *Tanacetum parthenium* (feverfew)
- *Verbena officinalis* (vervain)
- *Vitis vinifera* (grape seed extract).

Cerebral circulatory stimulants

DEFINITION

These herbal medicines improve circulation to the brain.

TRADITION

With a paucity of ancient material to substantiate this action, and a plethora of scientific studies validating the circulatory activity of herbs such as *Ginkgo biloba*, it would appear that this is a relatively recent class of herbal medicines.

INDICATIONS

- Difficulty with memory
- Cognitive impairment.

CONTRAINDICATIONS

- Specific to the individual herbal medicines within the class.

APPLICATION

- Best taken with meals
- Short- to medium-term application is advisable.

HERBAL MEDICINES

- *Centella asiatica* (gotu kola)
- *Ginkgo biloba* (ginkgo)
- *Vinca minor* (lesser periwinkle).

Cognitive enhancers

DEFINITION

These herbal medicines positively affect cognition and memory.

TRADITION

Like the cerebral circulatory stimulants, cognitive enhancers, also known as 'nootropics', are of recent discovery. That said, authors such as Culpeper discussed the ability of herbs such as rosemary to address conditions of the brain and so, while the term is of recent origin, the herbs within this class belong to the realm of ancient history.

INDICATIONS

- Difficulty with memory
- Cognitive impairment.

CONTRAINDICATIONS

- Specific to the individual herbal medicines within the class.

APPLICATION

- Best taken with meals
- Short- to medium-term application is advisable.

HERBAL MEDICINES

- *Bacopa monnieri* (bacopa)
- *Coffea arabica* (coffee)
- *Cola nitida* (cola)
- *Ginkgo biloba* (ginkgo)
- *Paeonia lactiflora* (white peony)
- *Paullinia cupana* (guarana)
- *Rosmarinus officinalis* (rosemary)
- *Theobroma cacao* (cocoa)
- *Vinca minor* (lesser periwinkle).

Hypnotics/sedatives

DEFINITION

Hypnotic herbal medicines induce sleep and concomitant relaxation.

TRADITION

The term 'hypnotic' is derived from the Greek *hypnotikos*, meaning 'inclined to sleep' or 'putting to sleep'.[10] Also known as 'soporifics', hypnotic herbs are described in the ancient literature, and were even used to sedate patients prior to surgery. Pedanius Dioscorides, Galen and Gaius Plinius Secundus highly praised herbs such as the opium poppy (*Papaver somniferum*), *Mandragora officinarum* and *Hyoscyamus niger* for their hypnotic qualities.[44] However, modern knowledge and practice recognise the potential fatal consequences of using such herbs in crude doses. The herbs within this class work effectively to reduce insomnia and calm restlessness, and do so without the risks of the herbs used by our forebears.

INDICATIONS

- Insomnia (both falling and staying asleep)
- Restlessness and anxiety associated with poor sleep habits.

CONTRAINDICATIONS

- Specific to the individual herbal medicines within the class
- Potential interaction with pharmaceutical hypnotic medication.

APPLICATION

- Best taken with meals
- Short- to medium-term application is advisable.

HERBAL MEDICINES

- *Corydalis ambigua* (corydalis)
- *Eschscholzia californica* (Californian poppy)
- *Humulus lupulus* (hops)
- *Lactuca virosa* (wild lettuce)
- *Lavandula angustifolia* (English lavender)
- *Passiflora incarnata* (passion flower)
- *Piper methysticum* (kava)
- *Piscidia piscipula* (Jamaican dogwood)
- *Valeriana officinalis* (valerian)
- *Zizyphus jujube* (zizyphus).

Mild hypnotics

- *Matricaria chamomilla* (German chamomile).

Nervine relaxants

DEFINITION

These herbal medicines have a sedative effect on the nervous system and decrease nervous tension. Some of the following herbal medicines may also alleviate pain and spasm.

TRADITION

Interestingly, the term 'relaxant' has a close tie etymologically with 'laxative'. Both terms are derived from the Latin *laxus*, meaning 'to loosen' or 'to become less tense'.[10]

INDICATIONS

- Insomnia (both falling and staying asleep)
- Restlessness and anxiety.

CONTRAINDICATIONS

- Specific to the individual herbal medicines within the class
- Potential interaction with pharmaceutical hypnotic/relaxant medication.

APPLICATION

- Best taken with meals
- Short- to medium-term application is advisable.

HERBAL MEDICINES

- *Actaea racemosa* (black cohosh)
- *Anemone pulsatilla* (pulsatilla)
- *Apium graveolens* (celery)
- *Avena sativa* green (green oat)
- *Corydalis ambigua* (corydalis)
- *Eschscholzia californica* (Californian poppy)
- *Humulus lupulus* (hops)
- *Hyssopus officinalis* (hyssop)

- *Lavandula angustifolia* (English lavender)
- *Leonurus cardiaca* (motherwort)
- *Matricaria chamomilla* (German chamomile)
- *Melissa officinalis* (lemon balm)
- *Passiflora incarnata* (passion flower)
- *Piper methysticum* (kava)
- *Piscidia piscipula* (Jamaican dogwood)
- *Scutellaria lateriflora* (skullcap)
- *Tilia cordata* (lime flowers)
- *Valeriana officinalis* (valerian)
- *Verbena officinalis* (verbena)
- *Viburnum opulus* (cramp bark)
- *Viscum album* (mistletoe)
- *Withania somnifera* (withania, ashwagandha)
- *Zizyphus jujube* (zizyphus).

Nervine tonics

DEFINITION

These herbal medicines restore tone to the nervous system. This class is of particular importance in dealing with nervous exhaustion, anxiety and restlessness.

TRADITION

Remedies that restore tone to frayed nerves have been listed in pharmacopoeias and materia medica for centuries, and thus belong to the traditional knowledge base. These herbs gently restore tone and vigour to the nervous system, although some, such as rosemary, can have a more stimulating effect.

INDICATIONS

- Anxiety and restlessness
- Nervous exhaustion
- Poor sleep habits.

CONTRAINDICATIONS

- Specific to the individual herbal medicines within the class.

APPLICATION

- Best taken with meals
- Medium- to long-term application is advisable.

HERBAL MEDICINES

- *Avena sativa* green (green oats)
- *Avena sativa* seed (oat seed)
- *Bacopa monnieri* (bacopa)
- *Centella asiatica* (gotu kola)
- *Dioscorea villosa* (wild yam)
- *Hypericum perforatum* (St John's wort)
- *Lavandula angustifolia* (English lavender)
- *Matricaria chamomilla* (German chamomile)
- *Passiflora incarnata* (passion flower)
- *Piper methysticum* (kava)
- *Piscidia piscipula* (Jamaican dogwood)
- *Rosmarinus officinalis* (rosemary)
- *Schisandra chinensis* (schisandra)
- *Scutellaria baicalensis* (baikal skullcap)
- *Scutellaria lateriflora* (skullcap)
- *Stachys officinalis* (wood betony)
- *Turnera diffusa* (damiana)
- *Valeriana officinalis* (valerian)
- *Verbena officinalis* (vervain).

Specific trophorestoratives

- *Avena sativa* green (green oats)
- *Avena sativa* seed (oat seed)
- *Bacopa monnieri* (bacopa)
- *Hypericum perforatum* (St John's wort).

Nervine stimulants

DEFINITION

These herbal medicines stimulate the nervous system and increase energy levels.

TRADITION

While it is only relatively recently that the mechanism of action of this class of herbs has been fully identified and understood, the herbs themselves have been used for thousands of years to give people that wanted 'pick-me-up'. Short-term use (a couple of days) is usually all that is required. From a phytochemical point of view, alkaloids (methylxanthines) and essential oils are the active ingredients in these herbs.

INDICATIONS

- Fatigue, excessive tiredness
- Short-term use during periods of physical stress.

CONTRAINDICATIONS

- Specific to the individual herbal medicines within the class
- Avoid excessive caffeine use concomitantly.

APPLICATION

- Best taken with meals
- Short- to medium-term application is advisable.

HERBAL MEDICINES

- *Camellia sinensis* (green tea)
- *Coffea arabica* (coffee) — and other coffee species
- *Cola nitida* (cola)
- *Eleutherococcus senticosus* (Siberian ginseng)
- *Ephedra sinica* (ephedra)
- *Occimum basilicum* (sweet basil)
- *Panax ginseng* (Korean ginseng)
- *Paullinia cupana* (guarana)
- *Rosmarinus officinalis* (rosemary)
- *Theobroma cacao* (cocoa).

Mild nervine stimulants

- *Avena sativa* seed (oat seed)
- *Nicotiana* spp. (tobacco).

Other

- Thujone-containing plants (use with caution in high dose or excessive use)
- Camphor-containing plants or their extracts.

PSYCHOLOGICAL SYSTEM

Antidepressants

DEFINITION

These herbal medicines assist in alleviating depression.

TRADITION

Only in the last two decades has mental health begun to get the attention it deserves from a research point of view, and it still has some way to go. But is depression a disease of the modern ages, or was it experienced in the distant past? Perhaps unsurprisingly, 'depression' is simply a modern name for a rather old condition. Melancholy has been the subject of many authors throughout history, from Keats to Wordsworth, and from Plath to Shakespeare. The term 'melancholy' is derived from the Greek *melancholia*, meaning literally 'black' (*melanin*) and 'bile' (*khole*).[10] Students of our herbal past will remember that excess black bile, from an ancient physiological perspective, was attributed to sadness, sullenness, gloom and irritability[10] — what we now know as depression. This latter term comes from the Latin *depressionem*, meaning 'to press down' or 'to depress'. The term only came to mean dejection or depression of the spirit in the late 17th century.[10]

INDICATIONS

- Mild to moderate depression
- Anxiety and restlessness (generalised anxiety disorder, panic attacks, etc.).

CONTRAINDICATIONS

- Specific to the individual herbal medicines within the class
- Caution should be exercised in patients taking pharmaceutical medications (selective serotonin reuptake inhibitors [SSRIs], etc.)
- Patients with severe depression should be referred to the appropriate medical personnel.

APPLICATION

- Best taken with meals
- Medium- to long-term application is advisable
- Remember that certain herbs can take up to 4–6 weeks before the full therapeutic effect is experienced.

HERBAL MEDICINES

- *Avena sativa* green (green oats)
- *Avena sativa* seed (oat seed)
- *Cola nitida* (cola nut)
- *Hypericum perforatum* (St John's wort)
- *Lavandula angustifolia* (English lavender)
- *Melissa officinalis* (lemon balm)
- *Rosmarinus officinalis* (rosemary)
- *Turnera diffusa* (damiana).

Mild antidepressants

- *Nepeta cataria* (catmint)
- *Schisandra chinensis* (schisandra)
- *Verbena officinalis* (vervain).

Anxiolytics

DEFINITION

Anxiolytic herbal medicines reduce anxiety.

TRADITION

Another term used for this class of herbs is 'thymoleptics'. This term is of recent origin, and is used in both orthodox and complementary medicine. The term 'anxiolytic' is derived from the Latin *anxius*, meaning 'solicitous, uneasy and troubled in the mind'.[10]

INDICATIONS

- Anxiety and restlessness (generalised anxiety disorder, panic attacks, etc.).

CONTRAINDICATIONS

- Specific to the individual herbal medicines within the class.

APPLICATION

- Best taken with meals
- Medium to long-term application is advisable.

HERBAL MEDICINES

- *Eschscholzia californica* (Californian poppy)
- *Humulus lupulus* (hops)
- *Hypericum perforatum* (St John's wort)
- *Lavandula angustifolia* (English lavender)
- *Matricaria chamomilla* (German chamomile)
- *Passiflora incarnata* (passion flower)
- *Piper methysticum* (kava)
- *Valeriana officinalis* (valerian)
- *Withania somnifera* (withania, ashwagandha)
- *Zizyphus jujube* (zizyphus).

Dopaminergic agonists

DEFINITION

Dopaminergic agonist herbal medicines bind to and activate dopamine receptors. They affect the neurotransmitter dopamine or the components of the nervous system that use dopamine. (Dopamine is produced in the synthesis of all catecholamine neurotransmitters, and its production is the rate-limiting step for this synthesis.)

HERBAL MEDICINES

- *Vitex agnus castus* (chaste tree).

Serotonergic agonists

DEFINITION

Serotonergic agonist herbal medicines bind to and activate serotonin receptors. They affect the neurotransmitter serotonin or the components of the nervous system that use serotonin.

HERBAL MEDICINES

- *Ganoderma lucidum* (reishi)
- *Grifola frondosa* (maitake)

- *Hypericum perforatum* (St John's wort)
- *Lentinula edodes* (shitake).

Thymoleptics

DEFINITION

Otherwise known as 'euphorics' or 'mood elevators', thymoleptics are herbal medicines that elevate mood. This term is also used in orthodox medicine for a pharmaceutical medication that 'favourably modifies mood in serious affective disorders such as depression and mania'[45] and includes medications such as tricyclic antidepressants, monoamine oxidase inhibitors (MAOIs) and lithium compounds.[45]

TRADITION

The term 'thymoleptic' is of recent origin, and is used in both orthodox and complementary medicine.

INDICATIONS

- Mild to moderate depression (affective mood disorders)
- Anxiety and restlessness (generalised anxiety disorder, panic attacks, etc.).

CONTRAINDICATIONS

- Specific to the individual herbal medicines within the class
- Severe cases of depression should be referred to the appropriate medical personnel.

APPLICATION

- Best taken with meals
- Medium- to long-term application is advisable
- Remember that certain herbs can take up to 4–6 weeks before the full therapeutic effect is experienced.

HERBAL MEDICINES

- *Avena sativa* green (green oats)
- *Avena sativa* seed (oat seed)
- *Coffea arabica* (coffee) — and other coffee species
- *Cola nitida* (cola nut)
- *Crocus sativus* (saffron)
- *Eleutherococcus senticosus* (Siberian ginseng)
- *Ephedra sinica* (ephedra)
- *Lavandula angustifolia* (English lavender)
- *Melissa officinalis* (lemon balm)
- *Panax ginseng* (Korean ginseng)
- *Paullinia cupana* (guarana)
- *Schisandra chinensis* (schisandra)
- *Scutellaria lateriflora* (skullcap)
- *Theobroma cacao* (cocoa)
- *Turnera diffusa* (damiana).

REFERENCES

[1] Leroi-Gourhan A. The flowers found with Shanidar IV: a Neanderthal burial in Iraq. Science 1975;190:562–4.
[2] Lietava J. Medicinal plants in a middle paleolithic grave: Shanidar IV. J Ethnopharmacol 1992;35:263–6.
[3] Estes JW. The medical skills of Ancient Egypt. Canton: Science History Publications; 1989.
[4] Buenz EJ, Schnepple DJ, Bauer BA, et al. Techniques: bioprospecting historical herbal texts by hunting for new leads in old tomes. Trends Pharmacol Sci 2004;25(9):494–8.
[5] Di Stefano V. Holism and complementary medicine. Crows Nest, NSW: Allen and Unwin; 2006.
[6] Mills S, Bone K. Principles and practice of phytotherapy. London: Churchill Livingstone; 2000.
[7] Faber K. Dandelion — *Taraxacum officinale* Weber. Pharmazie 1958;13:423–36.
[8] Schutz K, Carle R, Schieber A. *Taraxacum* — a review on its phytochemical and pharmacological profile. J Ethnopharmacol 2006;107(3):313–23.
[9] Pearce JMS. The doctrine of signatures. Eur Neurol 2008;60:51–2.
[10] Harper D. Online etymology dictionary. 2001. Available from: www.etymonline.com.
[11] Mills S. The complete guide to modern herbalism. London: Harper Collins; 1989.
[12] Thomas CL, editor. Choleresis. In: Taber's cyclopedic medical dictionary. Philadelphia: F.A. Davis; 1993.
[13] Bone K. A clinical guide to blending liquid herbs: herbal formulations for the individual patient. St Louis, MO: Churchill Livingstone; 2003.
[14] Baldauf SL, Palmer JD. Animals and fungi are each other's closest relatives: congruent evidence from multiple proteins. Proc Natl Acad Sci USA 1993;90(24):11558–62.
[15] Retief FP, Cilliers L. The epidemic of Athens, 430–426 BC. S Afr Med J 1998;88(1):50–3.
[16] Ambrose C. Immunology's first priority dispute: an account of the 17th-century Rudbeck–Bartholin feud. Cell Immunol 2006;242(1):1–8.
[17] Saavedra-Delgado AM, Cohen SG. Huang-Ti, the Yellow Emperor and the Nei Ching: antiquity's earliest reference to asthma. Allergy Proc 1992;12(3):197–8.
[18] Cohen SG. Asthma in antiquity: the Ebers Papyrus. Allergy Proc 1992;13(3):147–54.
[19] Vulnerary. In Merriam–Webster online dictionary. Available from: www.merriam-webster.com.
[20] Gunther RT. The Greek herbal of Dioscorides. New York: Hafner; 1933.
[21] Kinne-Saffran E, Kinne RK. Herbal diuretics revealed: from 'wise women' to William Withering. Am J Nephrol 2002;22(2–3):112–18.
[22] Pengelly A. The constituents of medicinal plants: an introduction to the chemistry and therapeutics of herbal medicine. Crows Nest, NSW: Allen and Unwin; 1996.
[23] Tata JR. One hundred years of hormones. EMBO Rep 2005;6(6):490–6.
[24] Chang HM, But PP. Pharmacology and applications of Chinese materia medica, vol. 2. Singapore: World Scientific; 1987.
[25] Thompson EB, Aynillian GH, Gora P, et al. Preliminary study of potential antiarrhythmic effects of *Crataegus monogyna*. J Pharm Sci 1974;63(12):1936–7.
[26] Bone K. Clinical applications of Ayurvedic and Chinese herbs: monographs for the Western herbal practitioner. Warwick, Queensland: Phytotherapy Press; 1996.
[27] Braun L, Cohen M. Herbs and natural supplements: an evidence-based guide. 2nd ed. Marrickville, NSW: Elsevier; 2007.
[28] Blumenthal M. Herbal medicine: expanded Commission E monographs. Austin, TX: American Botanical Council; 2000.
[29] Felter HW, Lloyd JU. King's American dispensatory. 18th ed. Portland, OR: Eclectic Medical Publications; 1905. Reprinted 1983.
[30] Bradley PR, editor. British herbal compendium: a handbook of scientific information on widely used plant drugs, vol. 1. Exeter: British Herbal Medicine Association; 1992.
[31] Rickles F. Throbolytic (fibrinolytic) drugs and progress in treating cardiovascular disease. FASEB J 2005;19:671.
[32] Hyperlipidaemia. New York: American Heart Association; 2009.
[33] European Scientific Cooperative on Phytotherapy. *Curcumae longae* rhizoma. Monographs. Stuttgart: Thieme; 2003.
[34] Blumenthal M. The ABC clinical guide to herbs. Austin, TX: American Botanical Council; 2003.
[35] Sanders LJ. From Thebes to Toronto and the 21st century: an incredible journey. Diabetes Spectrum 2002;15(1):56–60.
[36] Beers MH, Berkow R. The Merck manual of diagnosis and therapy. 17th ed. Whitehouse Station, NY: Merck Research Laboratories; 1999.

[37] Murray I. Paulescso and the isolation of insulin. J History Med Allied Sci 1971;26(2):150–7.
[38] Shimizu K, Ozeki M, Iino A, et al. Structure–activity relationships of triterpene derivatives extracted from *Gymnema inodorum* leaves on glucose absorption. Jpn J Pharmacol 2001;86(2):223–9.
[39] Persaud SJ, Al-Majed H, Raman A, et al. *Gymnema sylvestre* stimulates insulin release in vitro by increased membrane permeability. J Endocrinol 1999;163(2):207–12.
[40] Prakash AO, Mather S, Mather R. Effect of feeding *Gymnema sylvestre* leaves on blood glucose in beryllium nitrate treated rats. J Ethnopharmacol 1986;18(2):143–6.
[41] von Staden H. Herophilus: the art of medicine in early Alexandria. Cambridge: Cambridge University Press; 1989.
[42] Shanmugasundaram KR, Rojendran VM. Possible regeneration of the islets of Langerhans in streptozotocin — diabetic rats given *Gymnema sylvestre* leaf extracts. J Ethnopharmacol 1990;30(3):265–79.
[43] Bifulco M, Cavalio P. Thyroidology in the medieval medical school of Salerno. Thyroid 2007;17(1):39–40.
[44] Ramoutsaki IA, Askitopoulou H, Konsolaki E. Pain relief and sedation in Roman Byzantine texts: *Mandragora officinarum, Hyoscyamos niger* and *Atropa belladonna.* Int Cong Ser: History Anaesth 2002;1242:43–50.
[45] Thymoleptic. Dorland's pocket medical dictionary. Philadelphia, PA: WB Saunders; 1995. p. 817.

PART 3

Body systems

The gastrointestinal system

10

Jane Frawley, Emily Bradley, Susan Hunter

SECTION A

OVERVIEW OF THE GASTROINTESTINAL SYSTEM

The gastrointestinal tract encompasses the mouth, oesophagus, stomach, small intestine and large intestine. Accessory organs include the pancreas, liver and gallbladder (see Ch 11). The overall primary function of the gastrointestinal tract is to break down food into its basic macro and micro nutrients and to further absorb and assimilate these. Below is an overview of the process of digestion, focusing on the main organs. See Fig. 10.1 for an overview of the gastrointestinal system.

CEPHALIC PHASE

The thought, sight and smell of food triggers appetite, oral secretions and gastric secretions via the vagal nerve. This is a key part of the digestive process that initiates secretions in the mouth and stomach, enabling the upper digestive tract to prepare for the arrival of food.

THE ORAL CAVITY AND OESOPHAGUS

Mastication is the act of chewing that initiates the breakdown of the food into smaller particles, increasing its surface area and mixing it with saliva. Saliva is produced and emptied into the oral cavity by various glands including the sublingual, submandibular and parotid glands. Each day healthy people produce about 1.5 L of saliva which contains many substances such as minerals, enzymes and antibacterial substances. Lingual lipase and salivary amylase are two of the main enzymes in saliva. Lingual lipase initiates the first stages of fat digestion and salivary amylase initiates carbohydrate digestion. Protein digestion is also commenced in the oral cavity by mechanical mastication. The oesophagus propels the bolus of food down through the oesophageal sphincter and into the stomach.

STOMACH

The stomach can be divided into three major sections: the fundus (most proximal), corpus (also called the body) and antrum. The wall of the stomach consists of three layers, namely the mucosal, muscularis and serosal (outermost layer). The innermost layer, the mucosa, contains primarily parietal cells (responsible for secreting hydrochloric acid), chief cells (responsible for secreting pepsinogen) and mucus-secreting cells. Approximately 1–3 L of gastric fluid containing hydrochloric acid (0.1 mol/L), digestive enzymes and certain binding products is secreted in a day. When the bolus of food has been propelled through the oesophagus and reaches the stomach it is then mixed with gastric juice to facilitate further breakdown. The pH of hydrogen chloride (HCl) is approximately 1–1.5 and this maintains a largely sterile environment.

Primary functions of the stomach include unfolding tertiary and secondary proteins, converting pepsinogen to pepsin, solubilising certain nutrients (calcium, B_{12}) and the reduction of non-haem iron to its bioavailable ferrous state. Water, iodine, copper, fluoride and molybdenum are all absorbed from the stomach.

SMALL INTESTINE

The small intestine is a long tubular organ that is approximately 500–600 cm in length. The three major sections of the small intestine are called the duodenum (most proximal and approximately 30 cm long), jejunum (approximately 200 cm long) and ileum (most distal and approximately 300 cm long). By far the greatest amount of digestion occurs in the small intestine, predominantly in the duodenum and the upper jejunum. A series of finger-like projections called villi are present on the mucous membrane of the small intestine, largely increasing surface area and therefore absorption. The most common cell types in the small intestine include the enterocytes (95%), goblet cells, enteroendocrine cells and Paneth cells.

Carbohydrate digestion is completed here by the release of enzymes produced in the pancreas, namely pancreatic amylase, maltase, lactase, sucrase and isomaltase. Protein digestion is facilitated by the release of trypsin, chymotrypsin, carboxypeptidases, elastase, aminopeptidases and dipeptidases, and fat digestion is completed by bile released from the gallbladder, pancreatic lipase, phospholipase and cholesterol esterase.

Many substances are absorbed from the small intestine including vitamins A, B, C, D, E and K, calcium, phosphorus, magnesium, iron, copper, selenium, zinc, chromium, manganese, molybdenum, lipids, amino acids and monosaccharides.

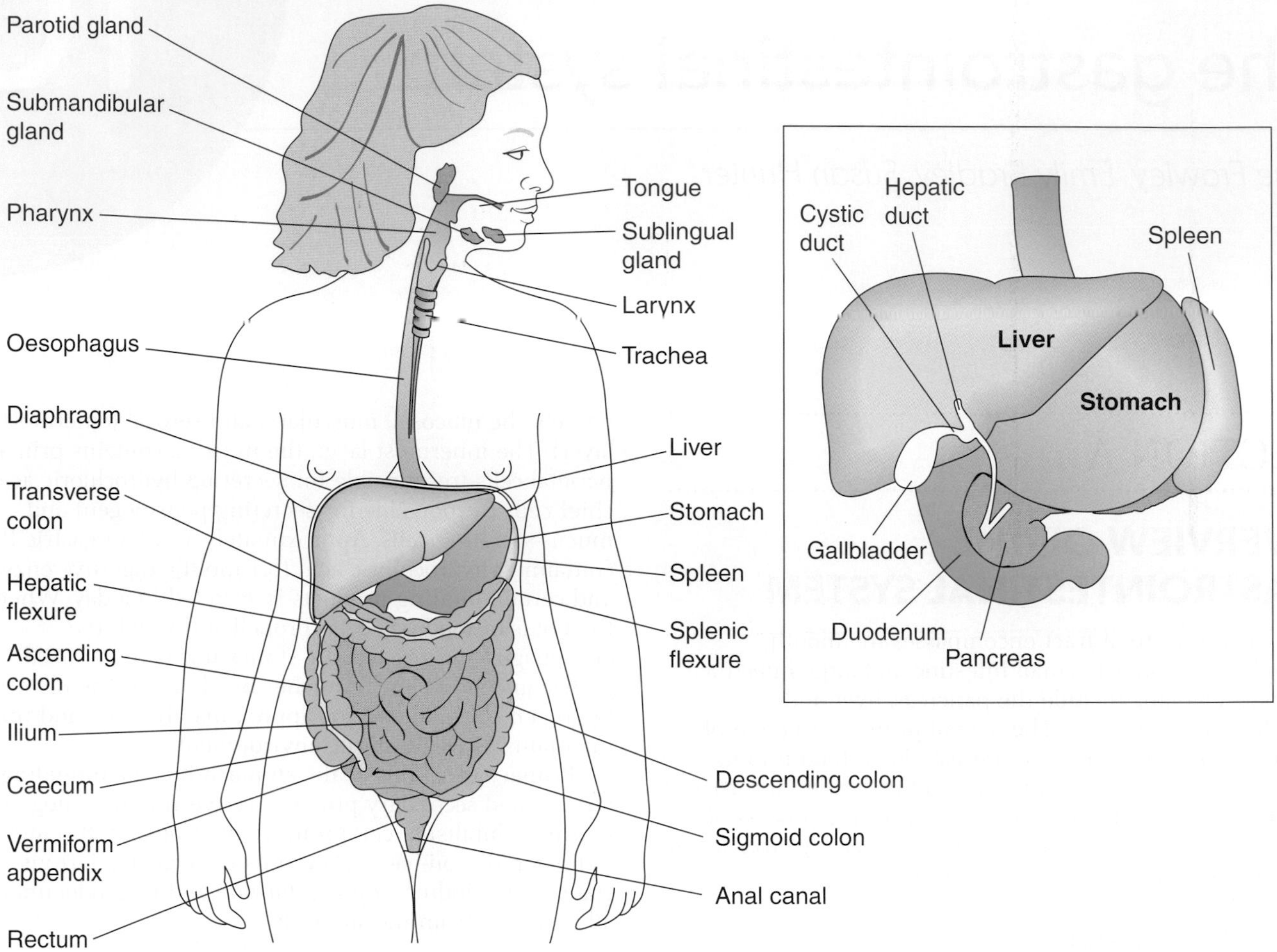

FIGURE 10.1 Anatomical diagram of the gastrointestinal system.

LARGE INTESTINE

The large intestine consists of four sections: the caecum, colon, rectum and anus. It is on average about 120–150 cm long. The mucosa of the colon is much smoother than that of the small intestine and does not contain crypts, folds or villi. Mucin-producing goblet cells are much more abundant, facilitating the movement of faeces through the large intestine. A normal colonic transit time from ingestion to defecation is considered to be less than 72 hours.[1]

Bacteria in the large bowel ferment and break down any remaining carbohydrates, producing short chain fatty acids (SCFAs), hydrogen, carbon dioxide and methane. Any remaining proteins are converted to amino acids and bilirubin is broken down to form stercobilin. Vitamin K and some B vitamins are also produced via this fermentation process. Some substances are absorbed from the large intestine including water, vitamin K, biotin, sodium, potassium and chloride.

ROLE OF THE NATUROPATH

Traditional interpretation

The gastrointestinal tract (GIT) is integral to the function of every other organ and organ system of the body. It is responsible for the digestion, absorption and assimilation of nutrients without which the body would cease to function. Traditionally it was considered that poor or sluggish digestion led to poor vitality and diminished health. Poor digestion is believed to exert a wide range of effects on other systems of the body and to contribute to conditions such as skin disorders (acne, psoriasis and dermatitis), allergies (asthma, hay fever and sinusitis), nervous system complaints (depression and insomnia due to poor amino acid and cofactor absorption and assimilation) and endocrine disorders (thyroid disease and diabetes) among others. A healthy gastrointestinal tract is therefore viewed as one of the most important factors needed to obtain and maintain optimal health and vitality.

Modern interpretation

Healthy digestion begins in the mouth and ends in the colon, thus if problems arise in the upper digestive tract they are likely to have a follow-on effect in the lower digestive system. For example, if the pH of the stomach is too high, food transit and breakdown in the stomach may be compromised and slowed. This may lead to symptoms such as acid reflux or dyspepsia as food tends to stay in the stomach for an extended period of time and is not broken down efficiently and moved on. The bolus of food entering the proximal end of the small intestine may not have a low enough pH to trigger the series of events needed, such as enzymatic release, leading to further compromised digestion. If the food is not sufficiently broken down macro and micro nutrient absorption is compromised. A higher pH than optimal may also provide an environment where bacteria survive or translocate from the distal bowel. Symptoms of these conditions in the small intestine include bloating, pain, flatulence, diarrhoea and constipation. If foods are not properly broken down by the time they reach the large bowel excessive fermentation can result, causing further pain and bloating. Increased intestinal permeability, food sensitivities, malabsorption and nutrient deficiencies can result, having wide implications for other bodily systems.

When consulting a patient with a chronic health problem a naturopath will always ask about digestion to ensure that this is not part of the complex picture. If symptoms indicate that digestion is involved this is often where treatment will commence.

Specific nutritional objectives

POTENTIAL DEFICIENCIES AND REQUIREMENTS

As all nutrients are absorbed from the gastrointestinal tract, a deficiency of any nutrient is theoretically possible. Certain disease states also increase the likelihood of nutrient deficiencies; for example, iron deficiency anaemia in Crohn's disease of the terminal ileum. Deficiencies can also occur due to low dietary intake as a result of poor dietary practices, food intolerances or anorexia due to psychiatric disease, certain medications or chronic illness. The following are some common deficiencies that occur in the gastrointestinal tract.

Magnesium

Magnesium depletion may be due to chronic diarrhoea. In patients where diarrhoea is a common symptom, magnesium status should be clinically evaluated. Conditions such as food intolerance, irritable bowel syndrome (IBS) and inflammatory bowel disease (IBD) all have the propensity to cause excessive losses.

Iron

Iron deficiency anaemia may occur as a result of the reduced intake of meat or as a consequence of chronic disease. Some people with poor digestive function believe that they cannot adequately digest meat protein and subsequently remove it from their diet. This is often a problem that can be fixed by improving digestive function. Certain diseases of the gastrointestinal tract also inhibit absorption and/or cause excessive losses due to bleeding; supplementation is always required in such cases.

Zinc

Zinc deficiencies can occur as a result of reduced or absent meat intake. Zinc is required for the production of many enzymes in the gastrointestinal tract as well as hydrochloric acid. Deficiencies can also lead to poor healing of mucous membranes and hyperpermeability of the wall of the small intestine. Zinc also contributes to the healthy function of the immune system which is integral to the healthy function of the gastrointestinal tract.

Vitamin B_{12}

Vitamin B_{12} is abundant in meat and is therefore also commonly low in vegetarians, vegans and those who consume very limited amounts of meat. Vitamin B_{12} is primarily absorbed from the terminal ileum, also a common site for Crohn's disease activity. In any of these cases supplementation is crucial to obtain healthy levels.

Essential fatty acids

Unfortunately the Western diet contains abundant amounts of omega-6 (n-6) fatty acids and considerably fewer omega-3 (n-3) fatty acids. An imbalance of these essential fatty acids is common where vegetable oils are over-consumed and fish is under-consumed. The current guidelines for seafood consumption recommend eating fish (low mercury, sustainable) 3–4 times a week and this should always be advised. Supplementation is often warranted to both re-establish balance and work therapeutically to decrease inflammation.

Fibre

Low-fibre diets are a characteristic feature of conditions such as diverticulitis, constipation and bowel cancer in the West. Poor-quality grains are often consumed which are highly refined and processed. The addition to the diet of high-fibre foods such as vegetables, fruit, nuts and seeds, and wholegrains should always be encouraged and supplementation is necessary in many conditions of the gastrointestinal tract.

Protein

Low-protein diets are common among patients with chronic disease, the elderly, vegetarians and vegans. The breakdown products of protein, amino acids, are required for many varied digestive functions in the gastrointestinal tract such as carbohydrate digestion (production of salivary amylase, pancreatic amylase, maltase, lactase, sucrase and isomaltase), protein digestion (production of hydrochloric acid, pepsin, trypsin, chymotrypsin, carboxypeptidases, elastase, aminopeptidases and dipeptidases), fat digestion (production of lingual lipase, bile and pancreatic lipase) and pancreatic function (manufacture of the digestive enzymes gastrin, cholecystokinin and secretin). In some conditions of the gastrointestinal tract supplementation is necessary.

Dietary influences and objectives

Poor dietary practices will impact widely on the health of the whole body as well as having a direct impact on the function of the gastrointestinal tract. A diet high in sugar, salt, trans or saturated fat and processed foods not only limits the amount of healthy food consumed, it directly impacts on stomach function and bowel health. Accessory organs such as the pancreas, gallbladder and liver are also adversely affected.

Furthermore poor diets increase the risk of developing further nutritional deficiencies such as iron, magnesium, zinc, protein and essential fatty acids. As all nutrients are absorbed from the gastrointestinal tract, poor dietary practices and certain malabsorption syndromes have the ability to cause long-term deficiencies of any vitamin, mineral, amino acid or essential fatty acid. This further impacts on the manufacture of enzymes and other gastric secretions needed for healthy gastrointestinal function.

A healthy diet should contain abundant amounts of fresh produce. Fruits, vegetables, lean red meat, chicken and turkey, fish, wholegrains, legumes and nuts and seeds should all be incorporated. Unfortunately there are many conditions, such as coeliac disease and lactose intolerance, where certain dietary components need to be avoided. If this is the case, special diets need to be devised, taking into consideration alternative foods to minimise the chance of developing nutrient deficiencies; for example, calcium deficiency in lactose intolerance.

People should also be encouraged to drink adequate amounts of pure water and to eat consciously. This entails eating slowly and chewing food adequately. Food should never be eaten in a hurry or 'on the run'. Food should also be as fresh as possible, be in season and of good quality.

Specific herbal medicine classes for the gastrointestinal system

ANTHELMINTIC

An anthelmintic substance kills intestinal worms. Herbal medicines in this class include *Andrographis paniculata, Artemisia annua, Artemisia vulgaris* and *Tanacetum parthenium.*

ANTIBACTERIAL

An antibacterial substance kills bacteria. In the gastrointestinal system bacterial infection can be found anywhere from the mouth to the large bowel. Herbal medicines in this class that are relevant to the gastrointestinal tract include: *Allium sativum, Andrographis paniculata, Azadirachta indica, Berberis vulgaris, Commiphora mol mol, Hydrastis canadensis, Salvia officinalis* and *Thymus vulgaris.*

ANTIDIARRHOEAL

An antidiarrhoeal substance eases diarrhoea. Herbal medicines in this class that are relevant to the gastrointestinal tract include *Achillea millefolium, Agrimonia eupatoria, Geranium maculatum, Hamamelis virginiana* and *Quercus robur.*

ANTIEMETIC

An antiemetic substance relieves nausea and vomiting. Examples include *Balota nigra, Berberis vulgaris, Cynara scolymus, Mentha x piperita* and *Zingiber officinalis.*

ANTI-INFLAMMATORY

An anti-inflammatory substance reduces inflammation. This may be by a variety of mechanisms including the reduction of certain inflammatory mediators. Inflammation may be either localised in the gastrointestinal tract or systemic. Herbal medicines in this class that are relevant to the gastrointestinal tract include: *Achillea millefolium, Aloe vera, Bupleurum falcatum, Calendula officinalis, Chamomilla recutita, Curcuma longa, Filipendula ulmaria, Glycyrrhiza glabra, Hydrastis canadensis, Salix alba, Scutellaria baicalensis, Vaccinium myrtillus* and *Zingiber officinalis.*

ANTIOXIDANT

An antioxidant substance either reduces or protects against oxidative damage. Oxidation and the generation of free radicals may happen either locally in the gastrointestinal tract or systemically. Herbal medicines in this class include: *Andrographis paniculata, Astragalus membranous, Camellia sinensis, Curcuma longa, Ginkgo biloba, Rosmarinus officinalis, Salvia officinalis, Schisandra chinensis, Scutellaria baicalensis, Silybum marianum* and *Vaccinium myrtillus.*

ANTIPARASITIC

An antiparasitic is a substance that kills parasites. Herbal medicine examples include *Artemisia annua, Artemisia absinthium* and *Tabebuia avellanedae.*

ANTISPASMODIC

An antispasmodic is a substance that reduces spasm. In the gastrointestinal tract spasm can occur in the stomach, small intestine or large intestine. Herbal medicines in this class that are relevant to the gastrointestinal tract include: *Achillea millefolium, Chamomilla recutita, Dioscorea villosa, Foeniculum vulgare, Melissa officinalis, Mentha x piperita, Rosmarinus officinalis, Valeriana officinalis, Viburnum opulus* and *Zingiber officinale.*

ASTRINGENT

An astringent is a substance that astringes tissues and mucous membranes in the gastrointestinal tract, often by precipitating proteins. Herbal medicines in this class include *Achillea millefolium, Agrimonia eupatoria, Cinnamomum zeylanicum, Commiphora mol mol, Filipendula ulmaria, Geranium maculatum, Hamamelis virginiana, Salvia officinalis* and *Viburnum opulus.*

BITTERS

Bitters work by stimulating the bitter taste receptors on the tongue. This in turn directly stimulates the secretion of saliva, HCl and gastrin in the stomach. Bitters also stimulate increased production of bile by the liver and increase the production of pancreatic enzymes. Bitters may be indicated for anorexia, sluggish dyspepsia, food allergies or intolerances, gallbladder disease and liver disease.

Some common bitter herbs are: *Andrographis paniculata, Artemisia absinthium, Artemisia annua, Berberis vulgaris, Calendula officinale, Chelidonium majus, Cynara scolymus, Erythrea centaurium, Gentiana lutea, Humulus lupulus, Hydrastis canadensis* and *Taraxacum officinale.*

CARMINATIVE

A carminative is a substance that relaxes sphincters in the gastrointestinal tract, therefore easing flatulence. Examples of carminative herbs include: *Anethum graveolens, Chamomilla recutita, Cinnamomum zeylanicum, Curcuma longa, Foeniculum vulgare, Melissa officinalis, Mentha x piperita, Rosmarinus officinalis* and *Zingiber officinalis.*

DEMULCENT

A demulcent is a substance that soothes irritated tissue. In the gastrointestinal tract these substances are useful for irritation that occurs in the oesophagus, stomach or intestines. Demulcents are also sometimes used to ease constipation. Herbal medicines in this class that are relevant to the gastrointestinal tract include: *Althea officinalis, Glycyrrhiza glabra, Plantago major* and *Ulmus rubra.*

LAXATIVES

A laxative is a substance that reduces transit time by causing defecation. Laxatives may be bulking agents such as *Linum* spp. or *Plantago psyllium* or stimulating substances such as *Cassia* spp., *Rhamnus purshiana,* rhubarb spp. and *Rumex crispus.*

INVESTIGATIONS

ALLOPATHIC INVESTIGATIONS

Helicobacter pylori breath test

This urea breath test is used to determine the presence of *Helicobacter pylori* (*H. pylori*) in the stomach. A small amount of 13C or 14C (radioactive) isotope-labelled urea is given orally and a breath sample is collected 20 to 30 minutes later. *H. pylori* produces vast amounts of urease which hydrolyses the labelled 13C or 14C to produce ammonia and carbon dioxide. A test is considered positive when labelled 13C is detected in the breath sample.[2] A positive result indicates the presence of *H. pylori.*

Stool analysis

Stool samples are used to determine the presence of a parasite or bacteria in the bowel. A routine culture can identify *Campylobacter, Salmonella* and *Shigella* while tests for *Yersinia,* enterohaemolytic *Escherichia coli* and parasites, ova and cysts need to be specially ordered.[3] A positive result indicates the presence of a bacteria or parasitic infestation; however, positive diagnoses from stool culture are poor (1.5–5.6%).[3] A stool sample may also be used to identify the presence of blood, white blood cells or red blood cells.

Gastroscopy/colonoscopy

A gastroscopy (also called an upper endoscopy) is a procedure used to examine the upper gastrointestinal tract, mainly the oesophagus, stomach and duodenum. The patient is anaesthetised under general anaesthetic while a gastroenterologist uses an endoscope to gently navigate through the upper gastrointestinal tract. This test may be suggested if Barrett's oesophagus, peptic ulcer, duodenal ulcer, Crohn's disease, coeliac disease, oesophageal or stomach cancer is suspected. Biopsies are also frequently taken.

A colonoscopy is a similar procedure using a colonoscope, inserted into the anus to examine the large bowel. This test may be suggested if bowel cancer, polyps, diverticular pockets or inflammatory bowel disease are suspected. Interpretation of these tests is straightforward and usually detailed on the gastroenterologist's report.

Serum tests

Blood tests may also be useful for diagnostic purposes. Tests such as erythrocyte sedimentation rate (ERS) and C-reactive protein (CRP) may be indicative of inflammation; however, not necessarily in the digestive tract. They may be useful to indicate active disease in inflammatory bowel disease. Certain nutrient values may also be helpful, such as iron and B_{12}. If these are low in the absence of other factors such as bleeding or poor nutrition, disorders that commonly present with malabsorption may be present such as Crohn's disease or coeliac disease. Antiendomysial IgA and tissue transglutaminase IgA (often called a coeliac panel) is another common screening that may be performed if coeliac disease is suspected. It should be noted that this test needs to be performed with the presence of gluten in the diet or a false negative may result.

NATUROPATHIC FUNCTIONAL ASSESSMENTS

Functional stool analysis

A functional stool analysis may be crucial to understanding the function of the gastrointestinal tract. These are comprehensive stool tests designed to identify pathogenic and commensal microbiota along with exogenous bacteria and parasites. They also investigate markers of digestion and maldigestion together with certain markers of disease activity such as blood, pus, mucus, white blood cells and lactoferrin.

Correct interpretation of these tests is imperative. Digestive markers such as the presence of meat fibres and vegetable fibres may indicate poor HCl production or decreased enzymatic breakdown. Depressed elastase 1 may indicate compromised pancreatic function, and high triglycerides, long chain fatty acids, total fat and cholesterol in the stool may indicate fat malabsorption or high dietary fat intake.

SCFAs are produced via the fermentation of fibre by gut microbes. High levels of SCFAs may indicate carbohydrate malabsorption, low HCl levels or bacterial overgrowth of the small intestine. Low levels may indicate a fibre-deficient diet or reduced levels of bowel flora. Healthy populations of anaerobic bacteria such as *Lactobacillus* spp. and *Bifidobacter* spp. are integral to colonic health. Low levels indicate dysbiosis, increasing the likelihood of developing larger populations of opportunistic bacteria or acquiring pathogenic organisms. Pathogenic bacteria (e.g. *Clostridium difficile, Campylobacter* spp., *Klebsiella* spp., *Salmonella* spp., *Shigella, Pseudomonas*), yeasts (e.g. *Candida* spp., *Rhodotorula* spp.) and parasites (e.g. *Blastocystis* spp., *Cryptosporidium* spp., *Clonorchis sinensis, Dientamoeba fragilis, Entamoeba histolytica, Giardia lamblia*) can all be diagnosed using these tests.

IgG food allergy testing

IgG radioallergosorbent test (RAST) measures IgG4 antibodies for specific antigens using the ELISA technique. It is very sensitive and useful for the identification of food sensitivities. It tests blood IgG4 reactions to 90 or so different foods. The results of this test should be interpreted with caution. Food sensitivities are graded from 1+ to 4+. Many 1+ and 2+ foods can be kept in the diet if rotated regularly with other less allergenic foods. If these foods produce symptoms, however, they should be avoided for a period of time. Foods that elicit a 3+ or 4+ result should be avoided until the underlying causes have been established and rectified.

Breath tests for carbohydrate malabsorption

These tests are useful for the identification of lactose and fructose malabsorption. Breath tests use either hydrogen or methane to check for malabsorption. Patients drink the test medium (lactose or fructose) and the amount of hydrogen/methane excreted in the breath over the next few hours is recorded. If lactose/fructose malabsorption exists the carbohydrate is not absorbed and it travels to the large bowel where it is degraded by colonic flora, producing large amounts of hydrogen/methane that are then partially absorbed into the bloodstream and excreted via the lungs. There should always be a baseline test done first using lactulose to ensure that the patient produces hydrogen (up to 28% do not produce hydrogen and methane should be used).[4] A positive test results from breath hydrogen readings above 20 ppm within the 3–4 hour test period for lactose and fructose.[5]

A lactulose breath test may also be helpful to diagnose small intestinal bacterial overgrowth. A positive test result indicates high breath levels (>10 ppm) of hydrogen (produced by bacteria in the small intestine and excreted in the breath) after 15 minutes and before 1.5 hours after ingestion.[5]

Intestinal permeability

This test may be useful to identify the presence of intestinal permeability. It involves drinking two substances, lactulose and mannitol, and examining their ratio when recovered in the urine. Increased urinary excretion of lactulose indicates intestinal permeability as the sugar molecule is generally too large (>150 daltons) to be absorbed between the mucosal cells of a healthy digestive system. If high levels result, the junctions between the cells are larger and the mucosa can be said to be permeable. Low levels of urinary mannitol (under 9%) indicate malabsorption.[6] The lactulose/mannitol ratio should be below 0.035 in a healthy gut.[6]

Allopathic treatment

ACID SUPPRESSIVE MEDICATION

Over-the-counter antacids and H_2 receptor antagonists (H_2RAs) are commonly used for the relief of reflux. Antacids are very popular as they quickly relieve heartburn. H_2RAs have a longer duration of action and appear to work better if taken before an event likely to cause reflux (i.e. a large meal).[7]

Proton pump inhibitors (PPIs) are the mainstay of both acute and chronic reflux treatment. Their main advantage over the H_2RAs is that they are able to increase gastric pH for 15 to 21 hours as compared with 8 hours for H_2RAs.[7] They are part of the triple or quadruple therapy used for *H. pylori* eradication.

TRIPLE THERAPY

All cases of peptic ulcer disease associated with *H. pylori* are treated with a combination of antibacterial treatments and proton pump inhibitors.[2] Triple therapy is the first line of treatment (any proton pump inhibitor with clarithromycin, amoxycillin or metronidazole) for 1 week and, if treatment fails, quadruple therapy or an alternative triple therapy will be offered.[2]

LAXATIVES

Bulk laxatives such as psyllium, wheat bran, oat bran and linseeds are often recommended as an initial treatment. These laxatives work by attracting water to bulk the stool and increase stool weight: however, poor fluid intake may result in further constipation. Laxatives such as lactulose, mannitol and polyethylene glycol are osmotic laxatives.[3] They are non-absorbable and work by keeping water in the bowel. Stool-softening agents may also be used. They are used to lubricate the stool to assist defecation. Examples include paraffin oil and dioctyl sodium.[3] Neuromuscular agents such as tegaserod, a serotonin type 4 receptor antagonist, may also be used to stimulate peristalsis and fluid secretion.[2]

ANTIDIARRHOEALS

Antidiarrhoeal drugs may be used to reduce diarrhoea. Examples are loperamide or diphenoxylate and atropine. These drugs are used largely for symptomatic relief and may be used in inflammatory bowel disease, irritable bowel syndrome or acute diarrhoea.

ANTIBIOTICS

Antibiotics are used to attenuate a bacterial or parasitic infection. Examples include norfloxacin, ciprofloxacin, doxycycline and rifaximin.[3] These medications are often necessary to eradicate infection; side effects may include diarrhoea and abdominal discomfort for some.

ANTI-INFLAMMATORY MEDICATION

Anti-inflammatory drugs such as the 5-aminosalicylates sulfasalazine and mesalazine may be used in inflammatory bowel conditions such as Crohn's disease and ulcerative colitis. These are salicylate-based drugs that work by reducing inflammation either locally or systemically.

SECTION B

ADVERSE FOOD REACTIONS, FOOD ALLERGY AND HYPERSENSITIVITY

Epidemiology

The prevalence of reported adverse reactions to food varies around the world, with Europe, Sweden and Australia estimating that about 19% of their populations have an adverse reaction to one or more foods.[8] The reported prevalence in some countries, for example Spain, is lower at 4%.[8] The prevalence of food allergy in the developed world is increasing, with levels estimated to be between 5 and 10%.[9] Further, it has been reported that in developed countries, 3–8% of children and 1–3% of adults suffer from true food allergy.[10] Reactions to food can be divided into toxic and non-toxic reactions. Toxic reactions involve food toxins that may be naturally present in food or a consequence of food processing, contaminants or additives. In the contemporary world these reactions are rare, thanks to diet variety and food processing standards. They are dose-dependent reactions and have the same effect on everybody. Non-toxic food reactions can be further divided into immune and non-immune mediated reactions. Reactions that involve immune activation are mediated by immunoglobulins, especially immunoglobulin E (IgE) but also possibly IgG, IgA and IgM. Non-immune mediated food hypersensitivity reactions are often termed 'food intolerances' and include fructose and lactose intolerance. There is also another general category, called 'undefined', about which little is known. The group includes idiosyncratic and psychosomatic food reactions. The following section focuses on food allergies and food intolerances.

Differentiating between food allergy and hypersensitivity

FOOD ALLERGY

Most food allergies are IgE mediated. IgE is associated with receptors on mast cells, fixed cells in the mucosa and skin and basophils in the blood.[11] Conjugation of IgE with an allergen leads to cell granulation and the subsequent release of mediators (primarily histamine) and the synthesis of new mediators namely prostaglandins (PGs), leukotrienes and cytokines. This causes an immediate reaction which results in vasodilation, exudation, smooth muscle contraction and mucus secretion (largely due to histamine). There is also a late phase response 4–6 hours after the initial reaction,[11] due to chemotactic mediators released at the same time as the immediate reaction, which involves inflammatory cells (neutrophils and eosinophils). This reaction usually lasts a few days.

A food allergy reaction is usually to the protein component of the food. Common culprits include milk, egg, nuts, soy, sesame, fish and shellfish. Food allergy commonly causes gastrointestinal, respiratory, dermatological and cardiovascular symptoms, and sometimes results in anaphylaxis. Symptoms include urticaria, angio-oedema, atopic eczema, dermatitis syndrome, asthma, gastrointestinal anaphylaxis (nausea, pain, cramping, vomiting and diarrhoea), proctocolitis, enteropathy, enterocolitis and Heiner's syndrome, a pulmonary disease usually seen in children as a reaction to milk.[11] Oral allergy syndrome may also occur; it has four clear stages as follows:

1 Oral mucosal symptoms only
2 Oral mucosal and gastrointestinal symptoms
3 Oral mucosal and systemic symptoms (e.g. urticaria, asthma)
4 Oral mucosal and life-threatening problems (glottis oedema, anaphylactic shock).[11]

TABLE 10.1 Common reactions to foods

Reaction	Most common foods
Urticaria/angio-oedema	Common culprits are milk, egg, peanut, food additives, mustard and cod
Atopic eczema dermatitis syndrome	Common in children, common culprits are milk, egg, wheat and soy

Ortolani C, Pastorello EA. Food allergies and food intolerances. Best Pract Res Clin Gastroenterol 2006; 20:467–483.

Although any severe food allergy may culminate in anaphylaxis, reactions to fish, shellfish and peanuts are most likely to do so.[12] Some foods produce common reactions; for example urticaria is commonly a result of milk, egg, peanut, food additives, mustard and/or cod while eczema and dermatitis may be due to milk, egg, wheat and soy.[11] See Table 10.1.

Infants are often more likely to develop tolerance than older children or adults. Those allergic to milk, eggs, wheat or soy may develop tolerance by 3–5 years. However, children allergic to fish, shellfish, peanuts or nuts rarely lose their hypersensitivity. A small percentage of children tolerate peanuts by 5 years but if not, tolerance is unlikely to develop.

Other less well-defined food allergies may also occur, these may be IgG, IgM or IgA mediated. These may be due to a defective mucosal barrier.

Aetiology

GASTROINTESTINAL MUCOSAL HYPERPERMEABILITY

The gastrointestinal tract has three main functions: to act as a barrier and defend against microbial invasion, to determine tolerance or ignorance to dietary agents and to digest and assimilate nutrients. This mucosal barrier consists of epithelial cells held together by tight junctions. Various cellular and chemical factors also help to ensnare pathogens or render them harmless, including extremes of pH, mucus, bile salts, brush border enzymes, together with innate and adaptive immune responses.[13] Many factors including pathogens, vitamin D deficiency, alcohol, anti-inflammatory drugs, the microbiome and stress appear to increase intestinal permeability.[10,14] If this intestinal barrier is compromised, proteins, pathogens and antigens may pass through the intestinal wall.

GENETICS

It appears that genetic predisposition is a strong determining factor in allergic disease. There is an 11–13% risk of developing allergies if there is no parental history, a 40% risk if the patient has one allergic parent, and 80% if both parents are allergic.[9] Twin studies show that environmental factors are important in the development of atopic disease.

MATERNAL CONSUMPTION AND EARLY CONSUMPTION OF ALLERGENIC FOODS

Consumption of allergenic foods by the mother during gestation and/or lactation was once thought to predispose children to food allergy;[12] however, this is now being questioned. Additionally, the optimal time for introducing highly allergenic foods to prevent development of food allergies is not yet known. While previous studies suggested early exposure increased risk, recently the notion that prolonged avoidance may actually increase risk is being investigated. Delaying induction of oral tolerance to the allergenic food may result in sensitisation initially occurring through exposure via the skin.[14]

COELIAC DISEASE

Coeliac disease (CD) is a chronic gluten-sensitive immune-mediated enteropathy in genetically predisposed individuals carrying the HLA class II haplotype DQ2 or DQ8. The prevalence of CD is 1% in the USA and Europe, up to 5.6% in parts of Africa.[15] Some studies suggest prevalence has increased in the last few decades.[16] The highest prevalence is in the first-degree relatives of an individual with CD and only 10–15% of those with CD are diagnosed.[16] CD is also associated with a range of complex, chronic conditions including IgA deficiency, Down syndrome, myaglias, liver function abnormalities, autoimmune thyroiditis, type I diabetes, inflammatory bowel disease, Sjögren's syndrome and Addison's disease.[15–17]

Diagnosis

Serological tests that measure the autoantibodies produced in response to gluten ingestion are used to both diagnose and monitor CD. Anti-tissue transglutaminase antibodies IgA-ELISA test (tTG-IgA) and endomysial antibodies (EMA-IgA) are commonly used as they have high sensitivity and specificity. Deamidated gliadin peptide antibodies (DGP-IgG) is also used, and is currently the most accurate test for CD in young children.[17] Test kits, which use a blood spot from the fingertip using anti-tTG, also appear to be accurate[17] and may be a useful clinical method of investigation.

Small intestinal endoscopy and biopsy are regarded as the gold standard diagnostic test. Histological changes including increased intraepithelial lymphocytes, crypt hyperplasia and villous atrophy are rated using the Marsh Scale from 0 (preinfiltrative) to 3c (total atrophy). It should be noted however that mild changes are not unique to CD.

Gluten needs to be consumed for the serology and small intestinal biopsy to be accurate, or there is a high risk of a false negative result.[17] Recommendations for the amount and duration of gluten exposure required vary, though daily consumption for 6 weeks is usually recommended. If a patient has been on a gluten-free diet (GFD), HLA typing for the genetic alleles is used to rule out CD. However further testing is necessary for confirmation if susceptibility is indicated. The accurate diagnosis of CD is important to differentiate the condition from wheat allergy and non-coeliac gluten sensitivity (NCGS), which respond to a gluten-free diet, but have different associated complications and risks.

Aetiology

Genetics confer susceptibility in CD. Human leucocyte antigen class II genes (HLA)-DQ2 (located on chromosome 6p21) are found in 95% of cases, with HLA-DQ8 identified in a minority of cases.[18] Recently, additional genes involved in the pathogenesis of CD have been identified, including COELIAC337 and COELIAC438, at positions 2q33 and 19p13.1. While genetic susceptibility is necessary for this condition, not everyone with these genes will develop CD.[15] Consumption of gluten, present in wheat (gliadin), rye (secalin) and barley (horedin), is the trigger; however, other environmental factors are frequently involved such as the gut microbiota, feeding patterns, and the amount and timing of gluten exposure.[16]

The glutamine and proline-rich fraction in gluten, called gliadins in wheat, secalin in rye and horedin in barley, is poorly digested in humans. Some of the gliadin peptides may cross the intestinal barrier and subsequently the glutamine residues are deamidated, increasing binding to the HLADQ2 or DQ8 molecules, triggering an abnormal immune and inflammatory response. The intestinal mucosa is subsequently damaged with flattening of the villi, infiltration of lymphocytes in the epithelium, and increased density and depth of the crypts.[16]

There is significant variation in expression and severity of the signs symptoms of CD;[17] however, clinical presentation tends to have a predominantly gastrointestinal picture (classical) in young children, while a greater prevalence of extraintestinal symptoms (atypical) is present in older CD patients.[16] Classical symptoms relate to the digestive system and include diarrhoea (or constipation), steatorrhoea, abdominal pain, failure to thrive, and weight loss due to malabsorption. Atypical symptoms include few or no intestinal symptoms, and extraintestinal conditions such as osteopenia/osteoporosis, peripheral neuropathy, infertility, coeliac hepatitis, oral apthous ulcers, dermatitis herpetiformis, depression, anaemia and other mineral/vitamin deficiencies (iron, vitamin D, calcium, folate, vitamin B_{12}, vitamin B_6, vitamin K and zinc) are more common. Sometimes 'silent' CD is diagnosed upon screening with no apparent symptoms.

FOOD HYPERSENSITIVITY/INTOLERANCE

Food hypersensitivity or tolerance reactions to foods may be explained by the following quote: 'Hypersensitivity causes objectively reproducible symptoms or signs, initiated by exposure to a defined stimulus at a dose tolerated by normal subjects.'[19]

The reaction has to be reproducible, be the result of a particular substance and in a dose that most people could tolerate. The final point on dose is important as large amounts of certain foods or food components would cause symptoms in most people. Fructose is a great example of this as a 25 g dose will cause symptoms in up to 50% of the general population.[4]

Food intolerances differ in that they are much more insidious and may cause delayed symptoms. Food intolerances can be enzymatic, pharmacological or idiosyncratic in nature and are generally thought to be

TABLE 10.2 Sources and examples of FODMAPs

FODMAP	High FODMAP	Low FODMAP alternative
Monosaccharides	Fructose (in excess of glucose) Fruits: apples, pears, watermelon, mango, cherries, boysenberries and fruit juice from high-fructose foods Vegetables: asparagus, broad beans, sugar snap peas Sweeteners: high-fructose corn syrup, honey	Fruits: banana, grapes, honeydew melon, kiwifruit, lemon, lime, mandarin, orange, passionfruit, paw paw and most berries (except boysenberries and blackberries) Sweeteners: maple syrup, golden syrup
Disaccharides	Lactose Dairy products: cow's/goat's milk, yoghurt	Dairy products: lactose-free, almond or rice-based milk, yoghurt and ice-cream, hard cheese, feta, cottage cheese
Oligosaccharides (fructans/FOS, GOS)	*FOS* Grains: wheat-, rye-, and barley-based products Vegetables: onion, garlic, artichokes, leeks, beetroot, savoy cabbage, peas Fruits: watermelon, peaches, persimmon, prunes, nectarines, most dried fruit Nuts: pistachios *GOS* Legumes: red kidney beans, lima beans, mung beans, black beans, baked beans, soya beans, lentils, chickpeas	Fruits: banana, most berries (except boysenberries and blackberries), grapes, lemon, lime, mandarin, orange, kiwifruit, pineapple, passionfruit, rhubarb Vegetables: capsicum, bok choy, green beans, parsnip, silverbeet, cucumber, carrots, celery, eggplant, lettuce, potatoes, yams, tomatoes, zucchini Grains: wheat-free grains/flour, gluten-free bread or cereal products, quinoa
Polyols (sorbitol, mannitol, maltitol, xylitol, isomalt)	*Sorbitol* Fruits: apples, pears, avocado, apricots, blackberries, nectarines, peaches, plums, prunes, watermelon *Mannitol* Vegetables: sweet potato, mushrooms, cauliflower, snow peas	Sweeteners: maple syrup, sugar (sucrose) Fruits: banana, grape, honeydew melon, kiwifruit, lemon, mandarin, orange, passionfruit, paw paw

Adapted from Gibson PR, Shepherd SJ. Food choice as a key management strategy for functional gastrointestinal symptoms. Am J Gastroenterol 2012 May; 107(5):657–666; quiz 667; Nanayakkara WS, Skidmore PM, O'Brien L et al. 2016. Efficacy of the low FODMAP diet for treating irritable bowel syndrome: the evidence to date. Clin Exp Gastroenterol 2016; 9:131–142.

non-immune activated.[11,12] Incidence appears to be on the rise, which is possibly due to a reduction in food quality, the addition of preservatives and food additives, early weaning and early introduction of solids to infants, insecticides, pesticides and food processing practices.

FODMAPs

FODMAPs stands for fermentable oligosaccharides, disaccharides, monosaccharides and polyols. These are poorly absorbed carbohydrates, which either in isolation or in combination often cause gastrointestinal symptoms such as bloating, flatulence, discomfort, nausea and abdominal cramps in susceptible individuals. In very large amounts, FODMAPs often cause symptoms in healthy people.[20] As humans lack the enzymes to digest fructans, fructo-oligosaccharides, galacto-oligosaccharides and polyols, these carbohydrates are incompletely absorbed in the small intestine, exacerbating digestive symptoms. Several mechanisms contribute to symptom development. These undigested carbohydrates increase osmotic load and subsequently intestinal water content, often causing diarrhoea. Small intestinal and colonic transit time is also accelerated, and the carbohydrate fractions are rapidly fermented by gastrointestinal microbiota and degraded by colonic flora into SCFAs, and gases (H_2, CH_4 and CO_2). FODMAPs restriction may be beneficial in those with functional gastrointestinal symptoms in conditions such as irritable bowel syndrome, non-coeliac gluten sensitivity and possibly inflammatory bowel disease.[21]

While some people require restriction of all FODMAPs groups to alleviate digestive symptoms, fructose and lactose are only malabsorbed by some. See Table 10.2 for sources and examples.

One of the clinical challenges in implementing a low FODMAPs diet is the limited information regarding the FODMAPs composition of a particular food, as well as variation of the content.[20]

Aetiology

LACTOSE INTOLERANCE

Food intolerance can be caused by an enzyme deficiency, for example lactose intolerance is the direct result of the body not producing enough lactase to break down the lactose in milk. Lactose is the most common food intolerance caused by an enzyme deficiency. Lactose is a disaccharide that is metabolised by β-galactosidase (lactase is a sub-class) to glucose and galactose. Lactose intolerance is characterised by bloating, borborygmi, flatulence, pain and diarrhoea. As with all malabsorbed FODMAPs, two effects occur when the undigested lactose reaches the colon: firstly, it increases the osmotic load and subsequently intestinal water content; and secondly it is fermented by colonic bacteria into SCFAs and gases (H_2, CH_4, and CO_2) causing pain and discomfort. Lactose maldigestion affects up to 20% of Caucasians.[22,23]

Incidence in some ethnic groups is up to 60% (Africa, Asia, Baltic states, Mediterranean).[22] The prevalence of lactose intolerance in IBS is between 17% and 86%, but a study reported a 17–24% incidence.[24] Studies have shown that self-reported lactose intolerance is frequently inaccurate.

Lactase deficiency can be secondary to conditions in the small intestine causing mucosal damage or reduced expression of lactase such as in gastroenteritis, small intestinal bacterial overgrowth, inflammatory bowel disease, irritable bowel syndrome or coeliac disease. In these cases, lactase production can recover when the underlying issue is addressed. The activity of lactase declines with age (called lactase non-persistence); however, the extent of this varies with ethnicity and genetics, with a number of alleles and polymorphisms involved. Lactase persistence occurs in approximately 25% of the population,[25] and is highest in northern European populations (more than 90% in Scandinavia), and lowest in Asia and Africa — believed to have evolved in response to both cultural changes such as the domestication of mammals for their milk, and genetics.[26] The severity of symptoms depends on how much lactase is being produced by the small intestine, as well as factors such as the dose of lactose consumed, the presence of other nutrients, gastrointestinal motility, the composition of the intestinal microflora, and visceral sensitivity of the gut.[27] Studies indicate that most people can tolerate doses of up to 12 g of lactose (up to 15–18 g if consumed with other nutrients).[28] This suggests low dairy intake may be required, but complete exclusion is not necessary for most.

FRUCTOSE INTOLERANCE

Fructose malabsorption occurs when the amount of ingested fructose exceeds the level that can be metabolised and absorbed by the small intestine. Fructose is a 6-carbon monosaccharide. It is ingested as a monosaccharide, as the disaccharide sucrose (glucose + fructose), or as fructan polymers such as oligosaccharides and polysaccharides. If the degree of polymerisation (DP) is <10, they are usually referred to as fructo-oligosaccharides and if the DP is ≥10 they are usually called inulins. Another form of dietary fructose is the galacto-oligosaccharides (fructose + glucose + galactose), usually present as raffinose. As fructose is frequently present in foods that contain other poorly absorbed carbohydrates (FODMAPs), symptoms in susceptible individuals may be due to fructose alone or a combined effect. The human digestive tract has a limited and variable ability to absorb fructose, which occurs via several routes.[29] GLUT 5 is a fructose transporter that is responsible for moving the sugar across the brush border; it has a low capacity but is present along the whole length of the small intestine.[4] GLUT 2 is a low-affinity transporter that will carry glucose, fructose and galactose and is found on the basolateral membrane.[4] When glucose is present in the small intestine GLUT 2 is shunted into the brush border to facilitate diffusion. Higher luminal concentrations of glucose are taken up by the cells via an active process, which in turn activates a system that can more efficiently take up all hexoses including fructose.[4] This also inadvertently facilitates the diffusion of fructose. This becomes very important when designing a diet for fructose intolerance as foods with equal or higher amounts of glucose as compared with the amount of fructose present are usually tolerated. Recent research has identified GLUT 8 and 12 may also play a role in fructose absorption.[30]

Symptoms of fructose malabsorption include abdominal bloating and pain, altered intestinal motility and flatulence.[29] It is associated with gastro-oesophageal reflux, small intestinal bacterial overgrowth (SIBO) and depression.[4]

Fructose intolerance may be a primary or secondary condition. Hereditary fructose intolerance is a rare autosomal recessive disorder that is due to a deficiency of the liver enzyme fructose-1,6-bisphosphate aldolase.[31] It is a particularly dangerous condition where fructose 1-phosphate accumulates in liver cells and competitively inhibits phosphorylase. This results in vomiting, failure to thrive, hypoglycaemia and liver failure with jaundice and bleeding in children.[31] Secondary fructose intolerance is quite different. In this case the incomplete fructose absorption is due to abnormalities in the expression of GLUT 5.[4] Research suggests that it affects 30% of the population,[32] and is more common in those with compromised gut function as a result of Crohn's disease, coeliac disease, IBS or gastroenteritis. Diabetes, metformin and a high glycaemic index (GI) diet all increase the uptake of fructose via insertion of GLUT 5 into the brush border.[4] Co-ingestion of amino acids and corticosteroids also increases uptake, however the mechanism is unknown.[4] A low GI diet, stress and TNF-α (tumour necrosis factor alpha) reduce uptake.[4]

Mutual considerations

DIFFERENTIAL DIAGNOSIS

The primary differential diagnoses for food allergies and hypersensitivities include post-infectious malabsorption due to villus atrophy, bile salt deconjugation and secondary disaccharidase deficiency, enterotoxigenic bacteria (*Vibrio cholera, Escherichia coli, Clostridium difficile*), cystic fibrosis, inflammatory bowel disease, neuroblastoma, short bowel syndrome, Hirschsprung's disease and ileal stenosis.[1]

INVESTIGATIONS

Skin prick test

This test is widely available and commonly used. It is best used for the identification of environmental and food allergens. The results appear to be variable and it is not sensitive enough to identify food intolerances. Cross reactivity and false positives are possible, leading to incorrect results.[11] The test can also be inconvenient.

Specific naturopathic investigations

IgE RADIOALLERGOSORBENT TEST (RAST)

This test uses enzyme-linked immunosorbent assay (ELISA) to measure IgE in the blood, for each allergen. It is convenient and appears to be accurate for airborne allergens. It detects IgE only and is quite expensive. The test can give false negative (more common) and false positive results.

IgG RAST

This test measures IgG4 antibodies for specific antigens using the ELISA technique. It is very sensitive and useful for the identification of food intolerances. It tests blood IgG4 reactions to 90 or so different foods. Various studies have found positive results.[33–36]

FOOD AVOIDANCE AND CHALLENGE

These diets are useful for the identification of food intolerances, but are unsafe for some allergies. See 'Elimination diet' below.

BREATH TESTS

These tests are useful for the identification of lactose and fructose malabsorption. Breath tests use either hydrogen or methane to check for malabsorption. Patients drink the test medium (lactose or fructose) and the amount of hydrogen/methane excreted in the breath over the next few hours is recorded. If lactose/fructose malabsorption exists the carbohydrate is not absorbed and it travels to the large bowel where it is degraded by colonic flora, producing large amounts of hydrogen/methane that are then partially absorbed into the blood-stream and excreted via the lungs. There should always be a baseline test done first using lactulose to ensure that the patient produces hydrogen (up to 28% do not produce hydrogen and methane should be used).[4]

LACTULOSE/MANNITOL TEST

May be useful for the identification of intestinal permeability. This test involves drinking the two substances, lactulose and mannitol. Increased lactulose indicates intestinal permeability as the sugar is only partially absorbed between the mucosal cells in a healthy gut. If high levels result, the junctions between the cells are larger and the mucosa can be said to be permeable. High levels of mannitol indicate malabsorption.

Therapeutic considerations

CLINICAL DECISION MAKING AND RATIONALE

Common allopathic treatments are as follows:[12]

- Adrenaline given if IgE mediated allergy is suspected. Antihistamines and sodium cromoglycate may also be given
- Strict dietary avoidance depending on severity of symptoms
- Hyposensitisation may be offered to reduce sensitivity.

Naturopathic perspective

The therapeutic approach is to ensure that inflammatory triggers are strictly avoided concurrent with repair and restoration of the impaired digestive system. This enables repletion of nutrient status and subsequent improvement in overall health and wellbeing.

Therapeutic application

NUTRITIONAL MEDICINE (DIETARY)

Dietary therapeutic objectives

Dietary therapeutic objectives include reducing the severity and frequency of symptoms and improving quality of life. Foods that precipitate attacks should be identified and avoided.

Specific dietary treatments

PREVENTIVE PROGRAM

- Breastfeeding (at least 4 months)
- Hydrolysed infant formula may be useful
- The optimal timing of the introduction of allergic foods is unknown. While previous studies have found delayed exposure until 1–3 years of age is beneficial, more recent studies are beginning to suggest that tolerance may even be increased with early introduction[37]
- Introduction of solids at 4–6 months (potentially including allergenic foods, though not as early weaning foods)
- Control exposure to dust, pets, tobacco, smoke and other irritants
- Probiotics taken during pregnancy and lactation have had mixed results in preventing allergy development[10]
- A varied diet during infancy, however, may protect against food sensitisation and the development of food allergy in childhood[9]
- Probiotics taken during pregnancy and then given postnatally to the infant may prevent food hypersensitivity in young children, especially if there was a caesarean delivery.[38]

AVOID TRIGGER FOODS

Treatment for IgE mediated food allergy usually involves strict avoidance and the person may need to carry adrenaline (epinephrine). It is not safe to use an elimination/food challenge diet for these patients and reactions can be life-threatening. IgG mediated food allergies may require herbal medicine treatment, while underlying problems are addressed.

Gluten needs to be avoided for life in those with CD and 70% of patients report an improvement in symptoms within two weeks of starting a gluten-free diet.[39] Significant patient education is needed to assist patients avoid gluten-containing grains (wheat, rye and barley), as well as products made from these grains. Gluten or gluten-containing ingredients are also used as ingredients in food processing, and thus sources can be 'hidden'.[39] See Box 10.1 for common sources of hidden gluten. As manufacturers sometimes change ingredients and thus products may no longer be gluten free, patients should also be encouraged to join a Coeliac Society to ensure they are working from an up-to-date list of 'safe' options. The definition of gluten-free also varies around the world, so imported products may contain larger amounts of gluten than those locally produced. While oats do not contain gluten, products are often contaminated by gluten-containing grains.[17] Though

BOX 10.1 Common sources of hidden gluten

Baked beans	Oatmeal contaminated with gluten
Blue cheese	Paté
Brown rice syrup	Playdough
Chutneys and pickles	Potato crisps/chips
Communion wafers	Salad dressings
Curry powder	Sausages and beef burgers
Farina	Seitan (wheat gluten)
Gravy powder and browning	Self-basting turkeys
Hard sweets	Shredded suet
Hydrolysed vegetable protein	Some chocolates and drinking chocolate
Imitation crab meat	Some lipsticks
Instant coffee	Some medicines containing starch or wheat derivatives
Liquorice	Some pharmaceutical products
Luncheon meat	Some toothpastes
Malt vinegar	Soups
Matzo flour/meal	Soy sauce and other sauces
Meat and fish pastes	Supplements
Mustards	White pepper

Nasr I, Leffler DA, Ciclitira PJ. Management of celiac disease. Gastroentest Endosc Clin N Am 2012; 22(4):695–704.

certified gluten-free oats are tolerated by most, 5–10% may be experience a reaction.[40]

There are many commercial gluten-free products available, however while 'safe', the nutritional value of these needs to be evaluated as they are often high in other undesirable ingredients.[41] Naturally gluten-free foods should be the basis of a gluten-free diet. If desired, alternative grains (and pseudograins) to consider include amaranth, buckwheat, millet, rice, quinoa, sorghum, teff and wild rice. Small intestinal damage can lead to secondary food intolerances such as lactose or FODMAPs, which should be evaluated in the newly diagnosed, and in patients with persistent symptoms despite a gluten-free diet.[17]

Monitoring of adherence to a gluten-free diet is recommended, especially if symptoms are persisting, as accidental exposure is the most common cause.[39] As little as 50 mg of gluten (a few crumbs of bread) may induce enteropathy in some individuals.[17] Retesting of anti-tTg-IgA antibodies is recommended to monitor response (and compliance) to a gluten-free diet.[40]

ELIMINATION AND ROTATION DIET

Some patients prefer to undertake an elimination and rotation diet, rather than use testing. This may be due to a variety of reasons such as cost or previous inconclusive results. A thorough rotation diet usually consists of two stages, the elimination stage, followed by dietary rotation.

Elimination diet

- Exclusion diet for 21–28 days
- Another 2 weeks may be necessary if symptoms are still present. Alternatively, the patient may need to reduce more foods
- Initially common for patients to complain of fatigue, headaches and food cravings; however these symptoms usually disappear after 3–5 days
- See Table 10.3 for an example of an elimination diet.

Note that many people with wheat intolerance appear to be able to cope with other gluten-containing grains — challenge separately. Also dairy foods can be problematic due to either their carbohydrate (lactose) or protein (casein) content. All dairy products contain casein whereas some dairy products contain negligible amounts of lactose so separate challenges are also recommended.

In cases with suggestive intestinal symptoms present but where breath testing has not been done, a low FODMAP diet is implemented. This is usually recommended for 4–6 weeks, followed by reintroduction of each group or type – fructose, lactose, sorbitol, mannitol, and finally fructans and galacto-oligosaccharides to determine the triggers and tolerance for a particular patient. However, if testing indicates that fructose and lactose are not malabsorbed, these groups can be included in the diet to minimise restriction.

Elimination diet — food challenge[41]

- Step 1: Follow elimination diet for 2–3 weeks.
- Step 2: Choose a food (usually the most inconvenient to eliminate, in case it can be returned to the diet) and serve 3 times during the day.
- Step 3: Record any symptoms. If a reaction is recorded for a single serving of the food on the challenge day, further challenges on that day are not necessary.
- Step 4: Return to elimination diet and continue to record any symptoms for 2 days.
- Step 5: If the challenged food was not problematic then it can be returned to the diet.
- Step 6: Start again at step 2 for all remaining foods.

Identification is only the first stage. Many factors may be responsible for food intolerances and until these are recognised and corrected the patient is at risk of becoming intolerant to more and more foods. Problems that may contribute to the development of food intolerances include intestinal hyperpermeability, dysbiosis and inflammation. Reintroduction of as many foods as possible is important.

TABLE 10.3 Example elimination diets

Food group	Include	Avoid
Dairy	Use rice milk as a substitute	Milk, butter, cream, ice-cream, yoghurt, cheese, custard
Cereals	Rice, millet and quinoa. This includes brown and white rice, rolled rice, rice noodles, rice cakes, rice flour, millet flour and puffed millet. Avoid rice crackers as they commonly contain artificial flavourings and MSG	Wheat, rye, buckwheat, oats, corn, barley and spelt. This includes bread, pasta, cakes, biscuits, breakfast cereals, noodles, soy sauce, gravy, most sauces
Soy	Use rice milk as a substitute for soymilk	Soybeans, soymilk, tofu, tempeh, miso, soy sauce, tamari, shoyu, soy yoghurt, many gluten-free products
Eggs		All eggs, egg-containing products
Vegetables	Avocado, asparagus, alfalfa, artichoke, beans, bok choy, broccoli, Brussels sprouts, cabbage, carrots, capsicum, cauliflower, cucumber, eggplant, fennel, garlic, ginger, lettuce, leeks, mushrooms, onion, parsley, peas, potato, pumpkin, radish, rocket, salad greens, silver beet, spinach, sprouts, squash, sweet potato, water cress, zucchini	Tomatoes, corn
Fruit	Apples, apricots, bananas, blackberries, blueberries, cherries, dates, figs, grapes, honeydew melon, kiwifruit, lychees, mango, nectarine, papaya, passionfruit, peaches, pears, plums, raspberries, rockmelon, star fruit, strawberries, watermelon	Oranges, lemons, limes, mandarins and grapefruit Tomatoes and all tomato products Canned and dried fruits
Nuts and seeds		Almonds, Brazil nuts, hazelnuts, macadamias, peanuts, pine nuts and walnuts Pepitas, sesame seeds, poppy seeds, sunflower seeds, linseeds
Meats	Beef, chicken, duck, kangaroo, lamb, pork, quail, turkey, veal	All processed meats, including sausages, salami, ham, stuffed and crumbed meats
Seafood		All seafood including fish, prawns, calamari, squid, lobster, crab, eel
Fats and oils	Olive oil	Butter, any other vegetable oils including canola, sunflower, flaxseed (linseed), safflower, sesame, almond, coconut, walnut
Beverages	Water (fresh and filtered), diluted fruit juice (no tomato or citrus juices), vegetables juices, soda water, mineral water, herbal teas	Beer, wine, spirits, coffee, black tea, green tea, chai tea, hot chocolate, soft drinks and cordial. Any juice containing citrus or tomato
Confectionery and sweeteners	Honey, fructose (small amounts), molasses, stevia, small amounts of sugar	All confectionery including chocolate and lollies. All artificial flavourings, sweeteners, colourings
Condiments	All herbs and spices, salt and pepper, apple cider vinegar, balsamic vinegar (if no preservatives), rice vinegar	All sauces, commercial marinades, salad dressings, lemon juice, lime juice, pesto, many dips, red wine vinegar, white wine vinegar, mayonnaise, soy sauce, tamari

Daley J. Managing a rotation diet. J Comp Med 2008; 7:26–30. Reproduced with permission of Australian Pharmaceutical Publishing Company Pty Ltd.

Rotation diet

Foods that have provoked symptoms in the elimination and challenge phase are avoided and the remaining foods are rotated in a 4-day cycle. Foods from the same family may be eaten every second day and the same food can be eaten once every 4 days.

The following foods are an exception and can be eaten at any time as they are the only members of their families: fish (as long as the variety is different), turkey, olive oil, olives, avocado, mushrooms, sesame seeds, Brazil nuts, flaxseeds, pine nuts, macadamia nuts, chestnuts, sweet potato, Jerusalem artichoke, banana, kiwifruit, papaya, guava, mango, pomegranate, pineapple and agar. See Table 10.4 for a sample rotation diet.[42]

LOW FODMAP AND FRUCTOSE MALABSORPTION DIET

Not all FODMAPs will be symptom triggers for all patients;[43] fructans and galacto-oligosaccharides are always malabsorbed and fermented by intestinal microflora.

A low-fructose diet restricts the amount of fructose consumed, particularly the free fructose (the amount in excess of glucose).[29] This diet is usually followed for 2–6 weeks to allow symptom reduction, followed by a

TABLE 10.4 Sample rotation diet

Food	Day 1	Day 2	Day 3	Day 4
Red meat	Lamb	Beef, veal	Rabbit, kangaroo	Pork
Chicken and fowl	Turkey, chicken flesh and eggs	Turkey, quail	Turkey	Turkey, duck
Seafood	Fish — salmon Mussels	Fish — bass Crab, lobster, octopus (calamari, squid)	Fish — trevally Oysters, scallops and abalone	Fish — e.g. barramundi Prawns
Dairy (or dairy alternative)	Sheep's milk yoghurt and cheese Soy milk, cheese, yoghurt	Cow's milk, yoghurt, cheese	Buffalo cheese	Goat's milk, yoghurt, cheese
Legumes	Kidney, soy (tofu), lima beans		Pinto, chickpeas, black beans, black-eyed, split peas	
Nuts and seeds	Soy, walnuts, sesame seeds, pine nuts, macadamia nuts, Brazil nuts	Almonds, sunflower seeds, sesame seeds, pine nuts, Brazil nuts	Peanuts, pecans, pumpkin seeds, sesame seeds, pine nuts, macadamia nuts, Brazil nuts	Cashew, pistachio, sesame seeds, pine nuts, macadamia nuts, Brazil nuts
Oils and fats	Soy oil, walnut oil, avocado oil, linseed oil, olive oil	Butter, ghee, avocado oil, linseed oil, olive oil	Avocado oil, linseed oil, olive oil	Safflower oil, avocado oil, linseed oil, olive oil
Grains and flours	Soy, buckwheat, quinoa, arrowroot, guar gum	Rice, millet, rye, potato	Amaranth, chickpea, kudzu root	Barley, oats, wheat, corn, tapioca, agar
Sweeteners	Honey, raisins	Dates, molasses, rice syrup	Figs, currants	Coconut, malt, sago, maple syrup
Vegetables	Beetroot, broccoli, cabbage, cucumber, garlic, green beans, kale, onion, rocket, squash, white radish	Avocado, carrots, capsicum, mushrooms, parsley, potato	Bok choy, horseradish, olives, red radish, rocket	Avocado, capsicum, celery, eggplant, iceberg lettuce, Jerusalem artichoke, parsnip, sweet potato, tomato
Fruits	Apple, boysenberry, blackberry, grapes, melons, papaya, rhubarb, strawberries	Apricot, cranberry, guava, kiwi fruit, lemon, orange, plum, prune	Melons, pear, pineapple, raspberry, quince	Cherries, blueberries, grapefruit, kiwifruit, limes, mango, nectarine, peach, tangerine

Adapted from a table by Dr SJ Rockwell in Pizzorno J, Murray M. The textbook of natural medicine. 3rd edn. Elsevier; 2006.

reintroduction phase when fructose-containing foods are increased slowly, one at a time, to determine individual tolerance. The aim is to determine the least restrictive diet that avoids symptoms. However, other poorly absorbed carbohydrates such as the polyols and oligos may also contribute to fructose malabsorption and symptoms, and may therefore need to be restricted.[43]

The glucose/fructose ratio is important when designing a low-fructose diet. If the amount of glucose is higher than that of fructose GLUT 2 will assist in absorption, reducing the amount of free fructose exposed to colonocytes. While glucose enhances the absorption of fructose it does not enhance the absorption of fructans, galactans and polyols.

Limit foods that contain fructose in higher or equal amounts to glucose or a large fructose load:[44–46]

- Fruits — apple, cantaloupe, grapes, guava, mango, nashi pear, quince, watermelon, fruit juice concentrates, fruit juices, dried fruits, pomegranate, persimmon, lychee
- Sweeteners — honey, molasses, high-fructose syrup, agave
- Sauces — chutney, barbecue sauce, tomato sauce, plum sauce, relish, tomato sauce
- Other — fortified wines, soft drinks with high-fructose syrup
- Vegetables (>100 mg/100 g food) — asparagus, beetroot, butter beans, cabbage, capsicum, carrot, eggplant, fennel, lettuce (cos), sweet potato, tomato.

FRUCTAN (CHAINS OF FRUCTOSE UNITS) CONTAINING FOODS

Vegetables such as artichokes, asparagus, garlic, green beans, leek, onions, spring onion and shallots, rye and wheat (many breakfast cereals, bread, biscuits, crackers, cakes, pies, pastas, pizzas and some noodles) should be avoided. Inulin and fructo-oligosaccharides should also be avoided. These commonly occur in health food products and prebiotic formulas.

Long-term food restriction from following a low-fructose or FODMAP diet may have undesirable effects including reduced intake of nutrients and alteration to the gastrointestinal microbiome.[26]

TABLE 10.5 Lactose content of common dairy foods

Food	Lactose (grams)
Butter 1 tbs	0.1
Hard cheese 100 g	0.1
Cream 1 tbs	1.0
Cottage cheese 100 g	1.9
Ricotta 100 g	2.0
Ice-cream 2 scoops	6.0
Goat's milk 1 cup	9.0
Yoghurt 200 g	9–10
Cow's milk 1 cup	12–14

LACTOSE MALABSORPTION DIET

If lactose malabsorption and not casein allergy is present only dairy foods high in lactose should be avoided. Studies indicate that single doses of up to 12 g of lactose are tolerated by most people with lactose intolerance, and up to 15–18 g if combined with other nutrients.[28] This suggests low dairy intake is advisable and complete exclusion is not necessary. See Table 10.5 for lactose content of common dairy foods. Aside from the impact on calcium status (which could be maintained from alternative sources), regular intake of lactose may lead to colonic adaptation. Studies of probiotics have resulted in mixed results; effects may be dependent on the specific strains. Lactase replacement may increase tolerance to lactose foods.[26] As lactose intolerance may occur as part of a bigger picture of FODMAP intolerance and other digestive conditions, further strategies addressing these may also be required.

NUTRITIONAL MEDICINE (SUPPLEMENTAL)

Nutritional medicine therapeutic objectives

Dietary therapeutic objectives include reducing the severity and frequency of symptoms, improving intestinal permeability if necessary, optimising digestion and improving quality of life. It should also be noted that if intake of food is reduced due to food intolerance or allergy (e.g. dairy foods) care should be taken to ensure dietary adequacy, and supplementation may be necessary. Correction of multiple nutritional deficiencies is often needed in newly diagnosed CD patients, and follow-up monitoring is recommended as studies have highlighted numerous nutritional deficiencies in those following a gluten-free diet.[47]

Repair gut hyperpermeability

While there is little clinical evidence to support the use of nutritional supplementation to repair intestinal hyperpermeability, the following nutrients are often used.

GLUTAMINE

Glutamine has been shown to decrease intestinal permeability in animal models.[48,49] Two randomised clinical trials have demonstrated promising results.[50,51] The more recent trial, in 48 burns patients, found that adding supplemental glutamine (0.5 g/kg) to enteral feeding for 14 days lessened intestinal permeability.[50]

ZINC

Zinc sulfate (110 mg 3 times a day, for 8 weeks) has been shown to decrease intestinal hyperpermeability in Crohn's disease patients in remission.[52] Zinc supplementation for intestinal permeability in food intolerance/allergy patients has not been studied to date. The dose in this study is extremely high and should be used only for short periods of time.

Increase dietary fibre

Dietary fibre (non-digestible carbohydrate) influences digestive function, provides bulk for the stool and acts as a substrate for colonic bacterial fermentation. Insoluble fibres include lignans, cellulose and some hemicelluloses, while viscous or soluble fibres include pectin, gums, beta-glucans and some hemicelluloses.

Probiotics

Lactobacillus spp., *Bifidobacter* spp., etc. Probiotics promote microflora homoeostasis, therefore improving the mucosal immune and barrier functions.[53] Various clinical trials have demonstrated the ability of probiotics to decrease permeability.[54–56] Specific strains that appear to be beneficial for the intestinal barrier are *E. coli* Nissle 1917, *L. salivarius* strains UCC118 and CCUG38008, *L. rhamnosus* GG, *Lactobacillus casei* strain DN-114 001, and *L. casei* strain Shirota.[57] These will also prevent bacterial translocation.

Other factors — more recent nutritional and dietary components have been identified which influence the intestinal barrier through a range of different mechanisms including vitamin D, the polyphenols epigallocatechin-3-gallate (EGCG), genistein and curcumin, and the flavonoids quercetin, myricetin, and kaempferol; however, clinical evidence is lacking.[58]

Optimise digestion

PANCREATIC/DIGESTIVE ENZYMES

Digestive enzymes given with food will aid digestion and given between meals will reduce inflammation. Patients with CD may have reduced exocrine pancreatic ability[59] and therefore benefit from supplementation.

BETAINE HYDROCHLORIDE

Betaine hydrochloride may be necessary to decrease the pH of the stomach and aid digestion.

Dosage requirements

- Glutamine: 1000 mg/day
- Zinc: 20 mg/day
- Probiotics multistrain formula: 25–50 × 109 organisms per day.

HERBAL MEDICINE

Herbal medicine therapeutic objectives

General therapeutic objectives include reducing symptoms and reducing the allergenic response. Many food sensitivities have an underlying cause such as dysbiosis, gut hyperpermeability, inflammation or poor digestion. In order to get lasting results, these elements must be addressed. Food intolerances such as secondary lactose and secondary fructose malabsorption syndromes nearly always have an underlying cause.

Herbal medicine classes

ANTI-INFLAMMATORY HERBAL MEDICINES

An anti-inflammatory herbal medicine decreases inflammation. Relevant examples here include *Curcuma longa, Boswellia serrata, Filipendula ulmaria, Salix alba, Urtica dioica* and *Aloe vera.*

BITTER HERBAL MEDICINES

Bitters stimulate the bitter taste receptors on the tongue, directly stimulating the secretion of saliva, hydrochloride and gastrin in the stomach. Bitters also stimulate increased production of bile by the liver, and increase the production of pancreatic enzymes. Notable examples that are relevant here include *Gentiana lutea, Taraxacum officinale (radix)* and *Hydrastis canadensis.*

ANTIMICROBIAL HERBAL MEDICINES

Substances that kill micro-organisms. Examples include *Hydrastis canadensis, Berberis vulgaris* and *Allium sativum.*

CHOLERETICS

Choleretics increase the production of bile by the liver. Examples include *Berberis vulgaris, Taraxacum officinale (radix), Cynara scolymus, Silybum marianum, Curcuma longa* and *Hydrastis canadensis.*

CHOLOGOGUES

Chologogues stimulate the release of bile from the gallbladder. Examples include *Gentiana lutea, Berberis vulgaris, Cynara scolymus, Rumex crispus* and *Iris versicolor.*

VULNERARY HERBAL MEDICINES

If indicated, this class of medicines decreases healing time. Examples include *Calendula officinalis, Achillea millifolium* and *Hydrastis canadensis.*

Specific herbal medicines

ALBIZIA LEBBECK (ALBIZIA)

Albizia is anti-inflammatory, anti-allergenic and antioxidant. The constituents and mechanisms of albizia are poorly understood. Albizia contains saponins (albiziasaponins A, B and C), epicatechin and procyanidins.[60] It has been shown to stabilise mast cell degranulation in vitro and in vivo.[61,62] Antioxidant activity has also been demonstrated in vivo.[63] Albizia may be useful to dampen down acute systemic reactions to food, especially those involving histamine such as urticaria. More severe reactions require medical attention. No clinical trials have been conducted.

Albizia may reduce male fertility. Reductions in sperm concentration, motility and testicular weight have been shown in vivo.[64,65] It is largely thought to be safe; however, it is probably best not to use with men wanting to procreate at around the same time.

Dose of the liquid extract (1 : 2) is 4–8 mL/day.

SCUTELLARIA BAICALENSIS (BAIKAL SKULLCAP)

Baikal skullcap contains baicalin, baicalein and wogonin and is anti-inflammatory, anti-allergenic and antioxidant.[60] Baicalein has been shown to decrease IL-6, IL-8 and MCP-1 inflammatory cytokines through inhibition of NF-κB activation in human mast cells.[66] Baicalein was also shown to inhibit inflammation through inhibition of COX-2 gene expression in vitro.[67]

Baicalein (and quercetin and luteolin) inhibits the release of histamine, leukotrienes and prostaglandin D2, from IgE-stimulated mast cells in a dose-dependent manner.[68] These compounds also inhibited IgE-mediated TNF-α and IL-6 production from bone-marrow derived mast cells.[69] In an animal study, baikal skullcap reduced the severity of food-induced allergy symptoms by regulating the immune response of T-helper cells, and the release of related inflammatory cytokines.[70] Baikal skullcap also has antioxidant and hepatoprotective effects. Baikal skullcap may be useful to dampen down acute but mild food reactions or to help prevent the systemic effects of food hypersensitivity. More severe reactions require medical attention.

Baikal skullcap may inhibit some P450 enzymes (CYP1A2, CYP2E1). However, no clinical reports have been made.[60] An increased risk of bleeding is theoretically possible with coadministration of warfarin and other anticoagulants.[60] There is conflicting data on safety in pregnancy — avoid.

Dose of the liquid extract (1 : 2) 4–8 mL/day, but in many cases the higher end of the range is necessary.

TYLOPHORA INDICA/ASTHMATICA (TYLOPHORA)

Tylophorine and its analogues are phenanthroindolizidine alkaloids.[70] Tylophora has antioxidant activity and has been shown to scavenge nitric oxide in vitro.[71] It also has antiasthmatic, antiproliferative, anti-inflammatory and antianaphylactic properties.[72,73] Tylophora inhibits contact sensitivity and delayed hypersensitivity in vivo.[72] Tylophora suppresses IL-2 production at the higher end of dose range and enhances IL-2 at low dose.[72]

Various older clinical trials show benefits in asthma.[74]

Dose: (1 : 5) 1–2 mL/day for the first 10–14 days of the month.[75]

Use short term and intermittently; not considered safe in pregnancy or lactation.[75] Tylophora may be useful to dampen down acute but mild food reactions. More severe reactions require medical attention.

URTICA DIOICA/URENS (NETTLE LEAF)

Nettle leaf is a traditional treatment for inflammation and allergy. The leaf extract IDS 30 was shown to reduce NF-κB leading to reductions in both COX and LOX reactions in vitro.[76] The extract may also reduce TNF-α.[77] An old double-blind, randomised study showed an improvement of allergic rhinitis symptoms in 69 patients taking a freeze-dried nettle preparation after 1 week.[78]

Dose of the liquid extract (1:2) is 2–6 mL/day.

Other useful herbal medicines

Although these herbal medicines have not been studied under clinical trial conditions, carminatives such as *Chamomilla recutita* (chamomile), *Zingiber officinale* (ginger), *Foeniculum vulgare* (fennel) and *Melissa officinalis* (lemon balm) are useful to decrease abdominal distension and flatulence. Bitter herbs such as *Gentiana lutea* (gentian) and *Taraxacum officinale* (dandelion root) may be useful to stimulate digestion.

Lifestyle recommendations

Lifestyle recommendations include:

- Avoid environmental allergens, if sensitive, such as excessive dust, tobacco smoke and pet hair
- Control stress levels by engaging in an activity that the patient enjoys such as exercise, tai chi, yoga or meditation
- Ensure adequate sleep and nutrition for healthy immune system function
- Use non-toxic household cleaning products
- Use natural body products and make-up.

CASE STUDY

FOOD INTOLERANCES

A 33-year-old women presents with a history of gastrointestinal symptoms including severe bloating, constipation (3–4 stools a week — type 1 on the Bristol Stool Chart) and haemorrhoids; fatigue, anxiety, and insomnia (both onset and maintenance). She had eliminated foods high in FODMAPs 18 months earlier which she found helped to reduce the bloating, though it exacerbated immediately again if she 'slipped up'. Blood tests conducted by her doctor revealed iron deficiency anaemia. Two courses of iron supplementation (Ferrogradumet) had been prescribed which had improved her mood and energy, though worsened her digestive discomfort considerably. A senna-based laxative taken at night had been used to address this. Despite mild improvement, she was frustrated with her symptoms and was aware of becoming increasingly stressed about what she could eat. Her diet was as follows:

Breakfast: porridge, with ½ cup of Zymil (lactose-free milk), LSA and strawberries. A cup of coffee (with milk)

Morning tea: A cup of coffee (with milk) and a banana low-FODMAP muffin

Lunch: Chicken and salad with dressing (varies type but always commercial brands) or sandwich (spelt bread)

Afternoon tea: A cup of coffee (with milk) and sweet treat (dark chocolate or lollies)

Dinner: Vegetables and rice or soba noodles with chicken/beef 2 days and fish/tofu 2 days a week. Omelette and salad 1–2 days a week. Eats out — often Asian restaurants 1–2 days a week.

CASE STUDY CONTINUED

TREATMENT PROTOCOL

The ongoing presence of symptoms despite the previous treatment suggests additional factors may be an issue. While the anaemia may be due to low iron take and increased losses from haemorrohoids, other causes need to be explored. The digestive symptoms indicate that factors inhibiting absorption may also be contributing (e.g. reduced digestive secretions, SIBO and damaged intestinal lining). A referral for coeliac serology was provided as this was a key differential diagnosis. As the patient was on a low gluten diet (due to wheat and rye being excluded on the FODMAP diet), genetic testing was also conducted. As follow-up testing for the anaemia had not yet been performed, this was also recommended to determine if repletion had occurred (less likely if coeliac disease is present, and within 2 months of treatment) and if not, to assist in determining the degree and duration of treatment required. Changes to the diet were minimal initially, pending the test results and to avoid adding to the patient's anxiety about what to eat. Recommendations included maintain adequate hydration (to avoid exacerbating fatigue and constipation), slightly increase fibre (5 g) by adding crushed flaxseeds as a source of both fibre and anti-inflammatory omega-3, and reduce caffeine by switching to green tea (to limit any exacerbation of abdominal discomfort and insomnia). Focus was placed on her eating habits such as eating slowly and chewing well, to increase vagal activation and trigger increased digestion. Lifestyle strategies were discussed to assist with sleep hygiene, and meditation and handouts were provided.

NUTRITIONAL MEDICINE

Supplementation with B-complex, magnesium and zinc was commenced to assist with energy production, mood and iron absorption/utilisation. Zinc was also recommended to support intestinal epithelial lining integrity and the production of digestive secretions.

HERBAL MEDICINE

Iberogast was started to reduced digestive distension and regulate motility. 20 drops diluted in water was prescribed — to be sipped slowly before each meal.

FOLLOW-UP

Coeliac testing was positive and full blood and iron tests confirmed that she was still anaemic. The patient decided not to confirm coeliac disease with an endoscopy.

TREATMENT RECOMMENDATIONS

Education about coeliac disease and the gluten-free diet — handouts were provided on a naturally gluten-free diet and a referral to join Coeliac Australia for up-to-date information about products which are 'safe'.

Continued avoidance of FODMAP foods (while epithelial repair is occurring) to reduce malabsorption symptoms. Support to increase the variety of foods which could be eaten was suggested (Monash FODMAPs app and associated cookbooks). Reintroduction of each FODMAP group would commence once digestive symptoms had reduced.

Repair of epithelial lining — vitamin A (2500 IU), vitamin D (4000 IU), EPA/DHA (3 g) and glutamine (3 g) were started.

CASE STUDY CONTINUED

These were chosen to increase recovery of the microvilli, and also to assist in replenishing deficiencies. Serum vitamin D testing was recommended to assist in determining adequate protocol needed for replenishment.

Iron supplementation was recommenced using 30 mg elemental bisglycinate, along with vitamin C. This was prescribed away from the zinc supplementation and with dinner (so absorption would be increased by the presence of animal protein and vitamin C, and side effects such as constipation and bloating would be minimised).

Treatment protocol was adjusted over the next 6 months, and follow-up testing of iron status and coeliac serology ordered to review progress. Diet re-evaluation was regularly performed to ensure nutritional levels were adequate. Pre- and probiotics were also introduced to support immune and digestive health.

IRRITABLE BOWEL SYNDROME

Epidemiology

IBS is thought to affect about 11.2% of the world's population, though this varies according to country and diagnostic criteria used. The prevalence is higher in women and in those under 50 years.[79]

Classification

Irritable bowel syndrome is a functional bowel disorder characterised by abdominal cramping and altered bowel motions.

Stool consistency is assessed using the Bristol Stool Form Scale which rates stool by appearance from 1 (hard and lumpy) to 7 (liquid) (without the use of antidiarrhoeals or laxatives).

Other signs and symptoms may include urgency, incomplete evacuation, abdominal distension and the passage of mucus. If blood is seen in the stool the patient must be immediately referred to a general practitioner for investigation.

Approximately one-third of IBS patients also suffer from dyspepsia.[80] Patients may also complain of a variety of other symptoms such as bloating, increased flatulence, nausea, fatigue and back pain.

Irritable bowel is commonly diagnosed using the Rome IV criteria, which always presume the absence of a structural or biochemical explanation for the symptoms. The criteria are based on the presence of recurrent abdominal pain or discomfort for at least 3 months' duration, with symptoms on at least 1 day a week including at least two of the Rome IV symptoms listed in Box 10.2.

Irritable bowel syndrome is a frustrating condition and no two cases ever appear to be the same. It is primarily a functional disorder, which means that it is due to the way the gastrointestinal tract functions rather than a result of pathology that is often easier to measure. This is a common source of frustration for patients as it often means there is no effective treatment available.

BOX 10.2 Comparing Rome III (2006) and IV (2016) criteria for diagnosing IBS

Rome III criteria

- Relieved with defecation
- Onset associated with a change in frequency of stool
- Onset associated with a change in form (appearance) of stool
- Subtyping by predominant stool pattern:
  - IBS-C — hard or lumpy stools ≥25% and loose or watery stools ≤25% of bowel movements
  - IBS-D — loose or watery stools ≥25% and hard or lumpy stools ≤25% of bowel movements
  - IBS-M — hard or lumpy stools ≥25% and loose or watery stools ≤25% of bowel movements
  - IBS-U — insufficient abnormality of stool consistency to meet criteria for IBS with constipation, diarrhoea, or mixed
- Stool consistency is assessed using the Bristol Stool Form Scale which rates stool by appearance from 1 (hard and lumpy) to 7 (liquid) (without the use of antidiarrhoeals or laxatives).

Other signs and symptoms may include urgency, incomplete evacuation, abdominal distension and the passage of mucus. If blood is ever seen in the stool patient must be immediately referred to a general practitioner for investigation.

Rome IV

Recurrent abdominal pain, on average, at least 1 day/week in the last 3 months, associated with two or more of the following criteria:

- Related to defecation
- Associated with a change in frequency of stool
- Associated with a change in form (appearance) of stool
- Criteria fulfilled for the last 3 months with symptom onset at least 6 months before diagnosis.

Rome IV now also identifies subtypes differently. Subtypes are based on how frequently a person experiences very loose or very hard stools.

Lacy BE, Mearin F, Chang L. Bowel disorders. Gastroenterology 2016; 150:1393–1407; Rome III Diagnostic Criteria for Functional Gastrointestinal Disorders: www.romecriteria.org/assets/pdf/19_RomeIII_apA_885-898.pdf

Aetiology

The pathophysiology of IBS appears to be multifactorial and intricate, often differing from person to person. Recent theories include dysregulation of the gut–brain axis, altered serotonin signalling, visceral hypersensitivity, infection, alterations to gut flora and food hypersensitivity.

GUT–BRAIN AXIS

The brain communicates with the digestive system via the parasympathetic, sympathetic and enteric nervous systems. The parasympathetic nervous system controls digestion and relaxation. It conserves energy, slows heart rate, increases digestion and relaxes sphincter muscles in the digestive tract. The sympathetic nervous system functions in opposition to this. It is responsible for the 'fight or flight' response and stimulates blood flow to major muscles, dilates the pupils, increases sweating, accelerates the heart rate, widens the bronchial passages and decreases gut motility. In a sense, it downregulates functions that are not seen as essential for immediate survival and increases those that are. Patients with IBS are commonly found to have an increase in sympathetic nervous system function and a decrease in parasympathetic function.[81] Both the sympathetic and parasympathetic nervous systems control gut function via their influence on the enteric nervous system. The enteric nervous system is sometimes called 'the second brain' as it is an extensive nervous system in the gut that controls its function. This may explain what has always been suspected: that stress has a huge effect on gastrointestinal function. In IBS, stress often leads to over-stimulation of the sympathetic nervous system, which interferes with the way food is digested, leading to pain, discomfort and altered bowel motility.

ALTERED SEROTONIN SIGNALLING

About 95% of the body's serotonin is located in the digestive tract.[82] Serotonin stimulates the enteric nervous system to initiate secretion and peristalsis.[83,84] Research has shown that too much serotonin in the gut causes diarrhoea and too little causes constipation.[84,85] Alterations in serotonin signalling in the GIT may be due to a variety of factors, including changes in the number of enterochromaffin (EC) cells, serotonin levels, tryptophan hydroxylase message levels and the expression of the serotonin-selective reuptake transporter (SERT).[86] Activation of the 5-HT 3 receptor increases motility, secretion and sensation, whereas activation of the 5-HT 4 receptor has various excitatory and inhibitory effects including increasing motility and secretion and decreasing visceral hypersensitivity.[82] Serotonin-selective reuptake transporter polymorphisms, reduced SERT mRNA and inflammation are all thought to cause SERT downregulation.[85,86] Interestingly, reduced levels of tryptophan hydroxylase were found in the mucosa of IBS patients.[81]

VISCERAL HYPERSENSITIVITY

Patients with IBS have increased awareness of gastrointestinal function (oesophagus, stomach, duodenum, ileum and rectum) and pain.[81,82] This is also possibly worse for stress and psychological factors.[81] In vivo data have shown that reduced levels of serotonin may increase visceral hypersensitivity.[87]

INFECTION

It is theorised that gastrointestinal infection may increase the risk of developing IBS due to the disruption of commensal flora and mucosal inflammation and damage.[88] Risk factors for developing post-infectious IBS include more toxigenic organisms, female gender, longer duration of illness, depression and possibly the presence of a fever.[88-90] A cohort study of Canadian participants with gastroenteritis found that 3.7% went on to develop post-infectious IBS.[89] Other studies have found the rate of post-infectious IBS to be in the realm of 4–31%.[88] In around 15% of these cases, IBS symptoms have been found to persist for at least 8 years.[91]

ALTERATIONS TO GUT FLORA

Gut flora is commonly altered in irritable bowel syndrome. Antibiotics, non-steroidal anti-inflammatory drugs (NSAIDs), the contraceptive pill, physical and psychological stress and a poor diet all damage good gut bacteria. Alterations in gut flora may lead to overgrowth of potentially pathogenic bacteria such as *Clostridium difficile*, decreased production of SCFAs and increased susceptibility to ingested pathogens.[92] More recent culture-independent molecular techniques have demonstrated qualitative and quantitative changes in mucosal and faecal microbiota in IBS patients. Abnormal microbiota may activate innate immune responses leading to increased intestinal hyperpermeability, activated nociceptive sensory pathways and further dysregulation of the enteric nervous system.[93]

Almost 50% of patients with diagnosed IBS have SIBO.[94,95] Proton pump inhibitors, antihistamines (H_2 antagonists), GIT surgery, immune deficiency and malnutrition are all possible causes although much more research into aetiological factors is needed. In a clinical trial, IBS patients with SIBO and restless leg syndrome had >80% improvement after treatment with the antibiotic rifaximin for the bacterial overgrowth together with zinc and probiotics.[96] SIBO has also been found to be associated with depression, diverticulitis, interstitial cystitis, acromegaly, cystic fibrosis and fibromyalgia.[97-101]

FOOD HYPERSENSITIVITY/INTOLERANCE

Many patients with IBS complain that ingestion of certain foods precedes their symptoms. While some food intolerances are caused by the absence of the enzyme needed to break them down (i.e. primary lactose intolerance), others appear to be due to other defective carrier mechanisms (i.e. fructose intolerance and FODMAPs). Inflammation of the mucosa may also impede enzyme release from the brush border as commonly happens in lactose intolerance that is secondary to gastroenteritis. This then causes further irritation and an ever-increasing number of intolerances. The relationship between food hypersensitivity and IBS appears to be a 'chicken and egg' scenario. Having food to which the person is intolerant within their diet causes further inflammation, luminal distension and pain, damaging the gut wall and leading to further inflammation and mucosal hyperpermeability. See also the section on adverse reactions, food allergy and hypersensitivity in this chapter.

Investigations

Haematological and biochemical investigations

Commonly include full blood examination, erythrocyte sedimentation rate, C-reactive protein, liver function test, iron studies, vitamin B_{12} and coeliac serology.

IgG radioallergosorbent test (RAST)

This test measures IgG4 antibodies for specific antigens using the ELISA technique. It is very sensitive and useful for the identification of food intolerances. It tests blood IgG4 reactions to 90 or so different foods. Various studies have found positive results in symptoms when allergens are isolated and removed from the diet.[33–36]

Colonoscopy

A colonoscopy may be offered to rule out other disorders such as inflammatory bowel disease or diverticulitis, or in those with 'alarm' symptoms (such as rectal bleeding, weight loss anaemia or a family history of bowel cancer, IBD or coeliac disease), but it is not routinely performed on those with typical IBS symptoms.

SPECIFIC NATUROPATHIC INVESTIGATIONS

Food avoidance and challenge

These diets are useful for the identification of food intolerances, but are unsafe for some allergies.

Breath tests

These tests are useful for the identification of lactose and fructose malabsorption.

Lactulose/mannitol test

Useful for the identification of intestinal permeability.

Complete digestive stool analysis/ GI effects profile

These are comprehensive stool tests designed to identify microbiota including anaerobes. They also investigate markers of digestion and certain biochemical parameters.

Therapeutic considerations

The treatment protocol for IBS is often multifactorial and long-term success often relies on identifying the cause or causes. Comprehensive clinical evaluations together with functional and standard pathology tests are required to determine the cause or at least factors that are contributing to the symptoms.

Where necessary, it is important to improve transit time, improve peristalsis, decrease mucosal permeability, correct dysbiosis, address neurotransmitter function, improve stomach function, decrease nausea, decrease flatulence, decrease abdominal distension, manage stress and identify and treat food intolerances or allergies.

Therapeutic application

NUTRITIONAL MEDICINE (DIETARY)

Many patients with IBS complain that certain foods aggravate their symptoms. For some these foods are obvious and for others they are vague and appear to change. Correct identification of food allergens is crucial. See also the section on adverse reactions, food allergy and hypersensitivity earlier in this chapter.

DIETARY THERAPEUTIC OBJECTIVES

Symptom control is the main motivation for suggesting dietary change. Many patients with IBS have already tried to restrict certain foods in the hope that they will discover the cause of their illness only to discover that they appear to react to more and more foods. Diets should be changed cautiously to avoid the development of macro- and micro-nutrient deficiencies.

SPECIFIC DIETARY TREATMENTS

Short chain carbohydrates/FODMAPs

Many patients with IBS find the avoidance of certain short chain carbohydrates such as FODMAPs, lactose and fructose helps with symptom control. This is often due to poor absorption and a subsequent osmotic effect. When the undigested saccharide reaches the colonic flora it is quickly metabolised to produce hydrogen and carbon dioxide. These gases are produced too quickly for the body to metabolise or pass them and abdominal distension and pain often result. In recent years, evidence of the benefits of a low-FODMAP diet in IBS has accumulated with positive results from several RCTs,[45,102–106] case-control studies, and observational studies.[107–113] While not all IBS patients will respond to a low-FODMAP diet, in these studies up to 86% reported a reduction in gastrointestinal symptoms. A study investigated the effects of dietary restriction in 62 patients with IBS and fructose malabsorption (diagnosed by breath hydrogen testing).[107] Compliance was reasonable with 77% of patients adhering to the diet always or frequently. A reduction in abdominal symptoms was noted in 74% of patients, being much more significant for those who followed the dietary guidelines (85% vs. 36%). For a full description and a list of foods to avoid see the section on adverse reactions, food allergy and intolerance earlier in this chapter.

Avoid trigger foods

Patients often recall particular foods that worsen their symptoms. Some common examples include alcohol, coffee, excessively fatty food, sugar, brassica vegetables, legumes, beans, onions and white bread. A food diary might be useful to help identify these trigger foods and, after identification, it may be easier to decipher what is wrong. For example, if legumes, beans, onions and wheat appear to be problematic the patient may have excessive gaseous production from the fermentation of short chain carbohydrates.

Gluten may be a trigger food in some patients and increase intestinal hyperpermeability, especially those positive HLA-DQ2/8.[114] However, in others it may be the short chain carbohydrate component that causes symptoms. In a recent double-blind crossover study conducted on 37 IBS patients with noncoeliac gluten sensitivity, gastrointestinal symptoms improved on the low-FODMAP diet, but no specific effects were found on a low-gluten diet.[115]

Identification of food allergies by IgG4 testing and the subsequent removal of trigger foods may be very useful if food allergies are suspected.

Fibre and prebiotics

Increasing fibre-rich foods in the diet will have a positive effect on IBS-C by improving transit time and therefore decreasing the associated symptoms that occur with constipation. This can be achieved by increasing wholegrains, vegetables, fruits and legumes in the diet.

Increasing dietary fibre will also stimulate the production of SCFAs.

Ensure adequate hydration

Adequate water intake is essential for healthy bowel motility. Unfortunately many patients drink inadequate amounts of water: a simple change can have a large therapeutic benefit — aim for 2.5 L/day. This recommendation may need to be modified according to weight, weather and exercise patterns.

OTHER DIETARY CONSIDERATIONS

- Avoid any foods that produce symptoms.
- Ensure adequate protein intake. Many people with IBS narrow their diet and self-restrict certain foods in the belief that it reduces symptoms. Meat is commonly eliminated and therefore protein intake is often reduced. Difficulty digesting meat is frequently an indication of insufficient digestion, which can be corrected with herbal medicines and nutritional supplements. Protein is essential for many aspects of a healthy digestive tract such as adequate production of HCl, digestive enzymes and neurotransmitters and providing amino acids for phase II liver detoxification.
- The consumption of fish should be encouraged. Fish is an easily digestible source of protein and essential fatty acids.
- Ensure adequate fluid intake to correct dehydration in diarrhoea predominant IBS or improve constipation in IBS-C.
- A healthy intake of fresh fruit and vegetables is essential for a steady supply of fibre, enzymes and nutrients. Vegetables should be lightly cooked, but not raw.
- Seeds such as flaxseeds (ground), and wholegrains should also be consumed for their abundant fibre content. Some of these may need to be restricted, however, for a period of time if SIBO, parasites or short chain carbohydrate intolerance are present.
- Diets usually need to be individually determined to avoid trigger foods and control symptoms.

NUTRITIONAL MEDICINE (SUPPLEMENTAL)

Nutritional medicine therapeutic objectives

The primary aims of nutritional medicine are to decrease inflammation and correct dysbiosis. The patient should also be thoroughly checked for any nutritional deficiencies due to food aversion, food avoidance, poor breakdown and assimilation, malabsorption, diarrhoea and anorexia. Any deficiencies need to be corrected.

SPECIFIC NUTRIENTS REQUIRED

Probiotics

Many people with IBS experience symptomatic improvement with the use of probiotics. Several meta-analyses have evaluated the use of probiotics for IBS.[116,117] Overall the use of probiotics was positively associated with less abdominal pain and a general improvement in symptoms. Some particular probiotics that have demonstrated positive results include VSL#3 (*Lactobacillus casei, L. plantarum, L. acidophilus* and *L. delbrueckii* subspp. *bulgaricus, Bifidobacterium longum, B. breve* and *B. infantis*, and *Streptococcus salivarius* subspp. *thermophilus*),[118,119] *B. infantis*,[120] *L. plantarum* 299v[121] and *L. plantarum*.[122,123]

Probiotics may be useful to improve transit time if dysbiosis is present. A double-blind, placebo-controlled, randomised study was conducted to investigate the effects of a probiotic beverage containing *Lactobacillus casei* Shirota in 70 patients with chronic constipation.[124] Patients were randomised to receive either 65 mL a day of the probiotic drink or placebo for 4 weeks. Consumption of the probiotic-containing beverage led to significant improvements in stool consistency in 89% of the probiotic group as compared with 56% in the placebo group.

Fibre

If dietary fibre intake is low, supplementation may be necessary. Supplementing with a mix of insoluble and soluble fibres may be best. Insoluble fibres include cellulose, hemicelluloses and lignin, which are responsible for creating the structure of plant cell walls and include wheat bran and rice bran. Soluble fibres include pectins, gums and mucilage and are found mainly in plant cells. Examples include psyllium, oat bran and flaxseeds.

A systemic review found that there was level B evidence to recommend psyllium for the treatment of constipation.[125] and a recent systematic review and meta-analysis of 14 RCTs found while supplementation with soluble fibre was beneficial in IBS patients, bran was not.[126] Any additional fibre supplementation must be started slowly and increased gradually with increasing water intake.

Dosage requirements

Probiotics: The strength of probiotic formulas varies between different strains; it is always best to follow the manufacturer's instructions.

HERBAL MEDICINE

Herbal medicine therapeutic objectives

Herbal medicine intervention aims to decrease pain, decrease abdominal distension, decrease flatulence, improve peristalsis, improve transit time and reduce any stress or anxiety that may be present.

Herbal medicine classes

ANTIDIARRHOEAL HERBAL MEDICINES

Antidiarrhoeals are used to decrease the volume and consistency of the stool. Examples include tannin-containing herbs such as *Hamamelus virginiana, Agrimonia eupatoria, Quercus robur, Geramium maculatum, Ulmus rubra, Camellia sinensis.*

SPASMOLYTIC HERBAL MEDICINES

Spasmolytics reduce spasm in the gastrointestinal tract. Examples include *Chamomilla recutita, Viburnum opulus, Mentha x piperita, Dioscorea villosa.*

CHOLERETIC HERBAL MEDICINES

Choleretics are used to increase the production of bile by the liver. Examples include *Silybum marianum, Chionanthus virginicus, Schisandra chinensis, Cynara scolymus.*

GIT ANTIMICROBIAL HERBAL MEDICINES

GIT antimicrobials are used to kill any microorganisms present. Examples include *Hydrastis canadensis,* propolis, *Commiphora molmol,* citrus seed extract.

LAXATIVE HERBAL MEDICINES

A laxative is indicated here to shorten transit time and increase defecation. Examples include *Rumex crispus, Juglans cinerea, Taraxacum officinale (radix), Aloe vera, Plantago ovata, Linum usitatissimum, Ulmus rubra, Rhamnus purshiana, Rheum palmatum.*

CARMINATIVE HERBAL MEDICINES

A carminative is used to relax the sphincters in the gastrointestinal tract and therefore ease flatulence. Examples include *Matracaria recutita, Zingiber officinale, Foeniculum vulgare, Mentha x piperita.*

SEDATIVE AND NERVINE HERBAL MEDICINES

Sedatives and nervines may be useful if stress or anxiety is also present. Examples include *Valeriana officinalis, Matracaria recutita, Humulus lupulus, Rosemarinus officinalis, Melissa officinalis, Verbena officinalis, Lavendula officinalis, Passiflora incarnata, Piper methysticum, Scutellaria lateriflora.*

Specific herbal medicines

Some herbal medicines that are particularly valuable include the following.

MENTHA X PIPERITA (PEPPERMINT)

Peppermint is used mainly as a whole plant extract, either as a tea, tincture or fluid extract. It is antispasmodic, antiemetic, antimicrobial, chologogue, carminative and bitter. Peppermint oil is possibly acceptable for short-term use or as needed. However, long-term safety has not been established. Peppermint oil contains around 50% menthol, which is thought to be largely responsible for the plant's spasmolytic activity. However, peppermint oil also contains small amounts of the ketones menthone (19%) and pulegone (0.1–2%), which have well-defined toxic properties. The longest trial of peppermint oil (0.2–0.4 mL/day) was for 6 months and the results were insignificant.[127] A recent 4-week RCT involving 72 IBS-D and IBS-M patients investigated the use of enteric peppermint oil, found a 40 % reduction in the total IBS symptom score from baseline (particularly abdominal discomfort, bloating, pain at evacuation and urgency).[128] Some improvements were noted by participants within 24 hours of commencing treatment.

Peppermint may be useful in the long term but if this is the case whole plant extract or tea would be safer and perhaps more beneficial because of other compounds such as flavonoids, tannins and bitter principle.

Dose: Leaf liquid extract (1 : 2): 1.5–4.5 mL/day.

Essential oil (diluted) 0.2–0.4 mL 3 times a day.

CYNARA SCOLYMUS (GLOBE ARTICHOKE)

Preliminary evidence suggests that globe artichoke extract might reduce the symptoms of IBS. In a post marketing surveillance study aimed to evaluate the efficacy of cynara in dyspepsia, a sub-group of 279 IBS patients were isolated and followed-up to see if cynara could also help IBS.[129] Artichoke leaf extract reduced abdominal pain, cramping, bloating, flatulence and constipation associated with IBS after 6 weeks of treatment. At the end of the study 96% of participants rated cynara as better than any previous treatment they had tried for IBS.

Cynara has also produced good results for the treatment of dyspepsia.[130,131] This is clinically relevant as up to one-third of all IBS patients suffer with concomitant dyspepsia.[80]

Dose: (1 : 2): 3–8 mL/day.

CHAMOMILLA RECUTITA (CHAMOMILE)

Many constituents of chamomile have been found to be anti-inflammatory including the flavonoids apigenin, apigetrin, rutin and quercetin. Chamomile is also antispasmodic, choleretic and antioxidant.[60] Chamomile may also be very useful for IBS associated with anxiety as it is sedative and appears to decrease stress.[132]

Dose: (1 : 2): 3–6 mL/day.

CURCUMA LONGA (TURMERIC)

Turmeric is anti-inflammatory, antioxidant, antimicrobial and hepatoprotective. A partially blinded, randomised, pilot study of 207 individuals with IBS (Rome II criteria) investigated the effects of one (72 mg) or two (144 mg) tablets of a standardised turmeric extract for 8 weeks.[133] Turmeric reduced the prevalence of IBS by 41% and 57% respectively. Approximately two-thirds of all participants reported symptom improvement and improved bowel habit. No major side effects were noted.

Dose: Liquid extract (1 : 1): 5–15 mL/day.

Powdered turmeric 1.5–3 g/day.

HYPERICUM PERFORATUM (ST JOHN'S WORT)

St John's wort is widely used for mood disorders including anxiety and depression, and may be beneficial in IBS to support stress tolerance and serotonin levels. In an animal model of IBS, St John's wort was found to have positive effects on intestinal inflammation and oxidative stress, and inhibit small intestine and colonic transit.[134] Women with IBS treated with St John's wort extract for 8 weeks were found to have less autonomic nervous system reactivity to stress, as well as significantly improved gastrointestinal symptoms.[135] However, a 12-week RCT did not find improvement in the overall bowel symptom score in the treatment group compared to placebo.[136]

Dose of St John's wort (1 : 2): 15–40 mL/week.

Example herbal formula

A formula for IBS would depend on the sub-classification and perceived causes.

CONSTIPATION

If constipation is the dominant symptom, the initial formula would most likely contain laxatives, carminatives and whatever else is deemed important. For example a formula for IBS-C with primary symptoms of constipation, flatulence, abdominal distension and pain may contain laxatives, bitters, choleretics and carminatives.

Rumex crispus 1:2 30 mL
Cynara scolymus 1:2 30 mL
Mentha x piperita 1:2 20 mL
Matracaria recutita 1:2 20 mL

Dose: 5 mL 3 times a day, 15–20 minutes before food.

If the constipation was more severe then use of a stronger anthraquinone-containing herb may be needed, for example *Rhamnus purshiana* (cascara), *Rheum palmatum* (turkey rhubarb) or senna. Additional carminatives may also be necessary.

DIARRHOEA

If diarrhoea predominates with spasm and pain the formula would contain primarily spasmolytics, carminatives and astringents.

Dioscorea vilosa 1:2 20 mL
Matracaria recutita 1:2 20 mL
Agrimonia eupatoria 1:2 20 mL
Viburnum opulus 1:2 15 mL
Zingiber officinale 1:2 5 mL

Dose: 5 mL 3 or 4 times a day.

OTHER

Slippery elm would also be useful for IBS-C or IBS-D. If using for IBS-C the dose needs to be larger so that the polysaccharides predominate; that is, 1 tablespoon/day. However, if dosing for IBS-D 1 teaspoon/day or 1 teaspoon 2 x/day is enough as the tannins will predominate.

LIFESTYLE RECOMMENDATIONS

Exercise

Exercise has been shown to improve the symptoms of IBS.[137,138] Exercise also helps to decrease stress which has a positive effect on IBS symptoms.

Psychosocial factors

A study comparing 347 IBS cases with 1041 age and sex matched controls from the general population found independent associations between IBS and work stress, anxiety, sleeping disturbances and a family history of IBS.[139] Stress is a well-known exacerbating factor in IBS, it may preempt symptoms or increase their severity.[140,141] Patients for whom stress is a contributing factor should be encouraged to undertake activities that reduce stress, for example tai chi, yoga, meditation and/or exercise. It is also important to identify patients who would benefit from counselling and refer them to the appropriate person.

CASE STUDY

OVERVIEW

A 39-year old man presented with a 4-year-old history of digestive problems, recently diagnosed as IBS-D. He related

CASE STUDY CONTINUED

the onset to the time he started looking after his mother who had colon cancer. The symptoms exacerbated with her passing, as did his hypervigilance on monitoring his daily bowel motions. He rated his anxiety as very high, due to both his health and work demands. Current symptoms include increased frequency of bowel motions 4–5 days of the week (usually 3 in morning within 3 hours of rising), increased sense of urgency, loose stools (Bristol Stool type 5 and 6), bloating after all meals, and noticeable undigested food in his stool. Previously, a colonoscopy and stool test had been performed. He had been prescribed an antidepressant by his GP, though he was reluctant to take it. He had not identified any specific foods which exacerbated things, though noted that alcohol and coffee were both triggers. A typical day's diet is as follows:

Breakfast: Natural muesli and low-fat milk
Morning tea: Apple, dry biscuits and hummus
Lunch: Sandwich with cheese and tomato
Dinner: Easy to prepare 'quick' meals — meat and vegetables with pasta or rice.

TREATMENT PROTOCOL

While he had already been diagnosed with IBS, a referral was made to identify if any other conditions were contributing to his symptoms. Blood testing for coeliac disease and breath testing for fructose and lactose intolerance and SIBO. Previous test results were also requested to review whether thyroid abnormalities had been excluded. A referral was also made to the GP to discuss a mental health care plan and referral to a psychologist to address both his grief and anxiety.

Initial prescription

Schisandra chinensis 1:2 25 mL
Mentha x piperita 1:2 30 mL
Hypericum perforatum 1:2 25 mL
Lavandula angustifolia 1:2 15 ml
Zingiber officinale 1:2 5 mL

Dose 5 mL 3 times daily diluted into 50 mL water.

This formula was focused on reducing his anxiety and stress, reducing visceral hypersensitivity and discomfort and reducing intestinal spasm.

His diet contained potential digestive triggers including gluten and FODMAPs, as well as numerous nutrient imbalances. As the recommended testing requires gluten intake for accuracy, the initial changes were to his eating habits (eating slowly and chewing thoroughly), switching the fruit to a low FODMAP option, and inclusion of additional protein sources (fish, eggs, ground seeds and nuts) and switching to low FODMAP vegetables. Lifestyle strategies including increasing exercise (preferably outside for added benefits for stress and vitamin D levels) and deep breathing meditation were also recommended to assist the gut–brain axis.

Pre- and probiotics, and digestive enzymes were not given prior to testing.

FOLLOW-UP

Test results revealed fructose and lactose intolerance were present, and the diet was adjusted to reflect this. Emphasis was placed on foods which could be eaten to maximise his nutritional intake. Recommendation was also made to trial

CASE STUDY CONTINUED

reintroduction after 8 weeks both to avoid nutritional restrictions and further disturbance to the microflora balance.

A probiotic of *L. plantarum* 299v was also introduced to reduce intestinal epithelial inflammation. Supplementation with magnesium, B-complex and glutamine was also commenced to support his anxiety and the adverse effects this had on his digestive function.

SMALL INTESTINAL BACTERIAL OVERGROWTH

Epidemiology

The overall prevalence of SIBO is unknown and appears to vary among patient groups. Prevalence rates of SIBO may also be higher in older adults, affecting up to 50% of persons over the age of 75.[142] A meta-analysis found that 56% of IBS sufferers have SIBO.[143] Prevalence levels of SIBO in coeliac disease have been reported to vary widely from 9–55% with up to 59% occurrence in adults with diverticulitis.[144,145] SIBO has also been detected in up to 60% of people with gastroparesis, 30–40% of patients with chronic pancreatitis and 56% of patients with cystic fibrosis.[146–148] A high prevalence of SIBO in patients with immunodeficiency has also been identified.[149]

Classification

SIBO is a heterogeneous syndrome characterised by an increase in the number and/or alteration in the type of bacteria in the small bowel.[150] In SIBO the bacterial population in the small intestine exceeds 10^5–10^6 organisms CFU m/L.[149]

Two types of SIBO have been identified using quantitative aerobic and anaerobic bacteria culture.[151] The first type is generally due to a defective gastric barrier and characterised by Gram-positive bacteria from the upper respiratory tract and oral cavity.[151] The second is the coliform type of SIBO and is usually due to failure of intestinal clearance or small bowel anatomical alterations[151] (see Table 10.6).

TABLE 10.6 Aerobic and anaerobic bacteria

Bacteria	Gram-positive flora	Coliform flora
Aerobic bacteria	*Streptococcus* *Staphylococcus* *Enterococcus* *Micrococcus* *Lactobacillus* *Corynebacterium*	*Escherichia coli* *Klebsiella* *Proteus* *Acinetobacter* *Enterobacter* *Neisseria* *Citrobacter*
Anaerobic bacteria	*Fusobacterium* *Peptostreptococcus*	*Bacteroides* *Clostridium*

Adapted from Bohm M, Siwiec RM, Wo JM. Diagnosis and management of small intestinal bacterial overgrowth. Nutr Clin Pract 2013; 28(3):289–299.

Identification of the type of SIBO is currently not available for clinicians with the current methods used for detection and to date it is only SIBO associated with bacteria that colonise the large bowel that is linked to gastrointestinal signs and symptoms.[149]

SIGNS AND SYMPTOMS

Signs and symptoms of SIBO may include frequent belching, intestinal bloating, flatulence, abdominal distension, abdominal pain, steatorrhoea and diarrhoea.[151] In some cases, malabsorption of nutrients may occur leading to secondary signs and symptoms including weight loss, malnutrition, muscle mass loss, peripheral oedema and osteoporosis.[150]

DIFFERENTIAL DIAGNOSIS

Differential diagnosis may include irritable bowel syndrome, parasite infection, large bowel bacterial overgrowth, infectious diarrhoea, yeast overgrowth, endometriosis, IBD (Crohn's disease and ulcerative colitis), coeliac disease, non-coeliac gluten sensitivity, small intestine obstruction, hypochlorydria, pancreatic enzyme insufficiency, fructose malabsorption, lactose intolerance, food allergies and/or intolerances and *Helicobacter pylori* infection.

Aetiology and pathogenesis

The development of SIBO may be multifactorial and can be due to disorders of the body's antibacterial protective mechanisms such as achlorydria, pancreatic exocrine insufficiency and immunodeficiency syndromes. Patients with inflammatory bowel disease, small bowel diverticula, pancreatitis, steatorrhoea and narcotic use are also at increased risk of having SIBO.[152]

Coeliac disease could also be a risk factor for developing SIBO. In a small study, 12 coeliac disease sufferers who did not improve on a gluten-free diet were found to have SIBO which was continuing to cause their symptoms.[153]

GASTRIC ACID BARRIER

Conditions associated with inhibition of gastric acid production such as pernicious anaemia, *Helicobacter pylori* infection, malnutrition and ageing increase the risk of development of SIBO.[154] Long-term use of proton pump inhibitors also causes reduced hydrochloric acid production and is associated with increased risk of developing SIBO.[155] One study with 450 participants found SIBO was detected in 50% of participants who used PPIs long term (>36 months).[156]

IMPAIRED INTESTINAL CLEARANCE

Disturbance of the body's digestive self-cleaning mechanism is associated with SIBO onset. Intestinal motility occurs with the action of phase III of the migrating motor complex, causing contraction and relaxation of the small bowel during the fasting state, in order to clear the lumen.[154] Individuals with dysmotility are at greater risk of developing SIBO. In a 2013 study with 150 people 63% of participants with diminished amplitude of antral/intestinal phasic activity and impaired antroduodenal coordination were found to have SIBO.[155]

There are quite a number of conditions that can interfere with normal gut motility. Motility disorders such as scleroderma, autonomic neuropathy in diabetes mellitus, post-radiation enteropathy and small intestinal pseudo-obstruction are all associated with SIBO.[150] Anatomical abnormalities such as small intestinal obstruction, diverticula, fistulae, surgical blind loop and previous ileocecal resections all interfere with intestinal motor activity.[150]

IMMUNITY

Increased numbers of duodenal and jejunal immunoglobulin A immunocytes have been detected in patients with SIBO.[149] Despite immune activation being present no damage to microvilli along the brush border of the small intestine is seen in SIBO.

MALABSORPTION

Malabsorption of carbohydrates, proteins, fats and vitamins is commonly seen in SIBO. Overgrowth of colonic bacteria in the small intestine is associated with carbohydrate malabsorption. Carbohydrate malabsorption in SIBO is thought to be due to reduced disaccharidase function, increased intraluminal carbohydrate degradation by bacteria and damage done to enterocytes that leads to the loss of absorptive surface along the brush border.[149,154]

Bacterial breakdown of carbohydrates in the small intestine causes fermentation to occur leading to increased intestinal gas production.[154] Increased gas and SCFA production results in pain, bloating and a change in stool pattern. Increased methane production also causes constipation in many patients. In many patients, SIBO is associated with increased incidence of fructose and lactose malabsorption.[157]

Bacterial proteases are thought to cause inactivation of pancreatic digestive enzymes and the intraluminal deamination of proteins, therefore causing reduced protein absorption resulting in loss of muscle mass and hypoalbuminaemia which causes peripheral oedema in some SIBO patients.[154] Steatorrhoea in SIBO is caused by bacterial deconjugation of bile acids resulting in deficiency of intraluminal bile acids.[158] Deconjugated bile acids are less effective at solubilising fats which may lead to decreased absorption of fat-soluble vitamins, that is vitamins A, E, D and K.[154] Vitamin B_{12} deficiency may also occur with reduced absorption of free and intrinsic factor bound vitamin B_{12} that is captured and used by bacteria and can result in megaloblastic anaemia and neurological disorders.[154] Iron deficiency may also be present in SIBO although the exact mechanism is not known. It is thought to be due to injury to gastric mucosa caused by bacterial toxin, SCFAs and/or unconjugated bile acids.[149]

ENDOTOXIN PRODUCTION

Bacteria overgrowing in the small intestine may produce excessive amounts of ammonia, D-lactate, indoles, amines and endogenous bacterial peptidoglycans that stimulate production of pro-inflammatory cytokines.[150]

Investigations

The diagnosis of SIBO is controversial with significant disagreement in the literature.[159] There are two tests that can be used: jejunal aspirate culture and breath testing.

JEJUNAL ASPIRATE CULTURE

There is no gold standard test for diagnosing of SIBO. The use of jejunal aspirate culture where there is the presence of coliform bacteria isolated from the proximal jejunum with >10(5) colony forming units/mL is one method.[160] This is an invasive, time consuming and impractical test that is rarely used in clinical practice.

BREATH TESTS

The lactulose breath test is commonly used to diagnose SIBO in clinical practice. It assesses the oro-caecum transit time and measures the amount of exhaled hydrogen and methane after the ingestion of 10 g of lactulose liquid.[161] Bacteria in the bowel produce hydrogen and methane gas on fermentation of carbohydrates that are not absorbed in the small intestine and remain undigested and move through to the large intestine. Most of the gas produced is transported in the blood to the lungs where it is exchanged into the airways of the lungs and breathed out. The breath test measures the parts per million (ppm) of these gases exhaled every 20 minutes for up to 2 hours.[162] A positive SIBO diagnosis is reached when there is a rise of over 20 parts per million of hydrogen in a 20-minute period within 90 minutes of testing. However research has questioned the validity of these studies by demonstrating that an abnormal rise in hydrogen as a result of the lactulose breath test is often a result of alterations to oro-caecal transit time in patients with IBS.[163]

The glucose breath test is used to more specifically measure proximal ileum bacterial overgrowth and is considered a more accurate test for diagnosing SIBO than the lactulose breath test.[159] Patients ingest 50 g of glucose and a hydrogen peak of >12 ppm is considered a positive result.[154]

There is no diagnostic test currently available to clinicians that can accurately determine the strains of bacteria that are overgrowing.[149] The fructose breath test can be useful to do if fructose malabsorption is a suspected comorbidity.

HAEMATOLOGICAL AND BIOCHEMICAL INVESTIGATIONS

Useful testing to investigate other possible causes of signs and symptoms, malnutrition and inflammation includes full blood examination, biochemistry, C-reactive protein, coeliac serology and genotyping, total IgE, total vitamin B_{12}, serum folate, iron studies, plasma zinc and vitamin D.

Specific naturopathic investigations

STOOL TESTING

Comprehensive stool analysis/GI effects profile is useful to identify microbiota in the large bowel as well as other stool testing that looks at digestive markers such as pancreatic elastase, faecal fats, faecal reducing sugars and parasite testing; for example, faecal PCR and MCS.

Therapeutic considerations

NATUROPATHIC PERSPECTIVE

The treatment of SIBO is multifactorial. The eradication of the bacterial overgrowth is just one part of SIBO treatment. In order to achieve long-term successful SIBO eradication it is important to identify and remove the causative factors. Where necessary it is important to correct achlorydria, poor pancreatic exocrine sufficiency and dysmotility. The use of prokinetic agents should be considered for patients with gastroparesis or intestinal dysmotility; however, the efficacy of these agents is not yet proven.[149] It is important to address bloating, flatulence, abdominal pain and changeable bowel habits; identify and treat any food allergies and/or intolerances that may be present, and correct nutritional deficiencies and comorbidities that arise.

ALLOPATHIC TREATMENT

Commonly used antibiotics to treat SIBO include ciprofloxacin, metronidazole, neomycin, norfloxacin and doxycycline.[149] Rifaximin is a non-systemic antibiotic that is used to restore gut microbiota imbalance.[164]

NUTRITIONAL MEDICINE (DIETARY)

Many SIBO patients report that symptoms begin each day once they begin eating. Identifying and removing trigger foods and high allergen foods are important to relieve gastrointestinal symptoms.

Dietary therapeutic objectives

The primary aim of treatment is to control symptoms while eradicating the bacterial overgrowth and correcting any dysmotility problems that are present. The objective is to improve gastric emptying to reduce bacterial fermentation of the ingested food.

Specific dietary treatments

No dietary changes have been clinically proven to improve SIBO, however a number of dietary changes have been postulated to help symptoms and are frequently recommended in clinical practice.

FODMAP-friendly diet

A low-FODMAP diet is often used to manage signs and symptoms of SIBO. The use of a low-FODMAP diet during this time may be useful for reduction in carbohydrate fermentation.

Avoidance of snacking

Eating three main meals a day and avoiding snacking to not disrupt migrating myoelectric complex activity may help relieve symptoms.

Low grain diet

The restriction of wholegrains during the bacterial eradication stage may help reduce further carbohydrate fermentation. Soaking grains overnight before cooking may help improve the digestion of wholegrains in SIBO patients.

Elemental diet

Some SIBO patients have used an elemental diet for 2 to 3 weeks to reduce hydrogen or methane production and eradicate bacterial overgrowth. A proprietary formula such as Vivonex or a diet formula that patients can make themselves is used. A combination of amino acid powder, medium chain triglyceride oil or coconut oil, honey, vitamins, minerals and sea salt is made up and consumed.

The specific carbohydrate (SCD) diet

The specific carbohydrate (SCD) diet is also used in some cases. The SCD diet is based on avoiding starches, oligosaccharides and disaccharides. It is thought that primarily eating protein and fats 'starves' the overgrowing bacteria. There is no evidence to support this diet being helpful in the treatment of SIBO.

Avoidance of trigger foods

Patients often tell their practitioner the foods and beverages that trigger their symptoms. Common examples include coffee, brassica family vegetables, legumes, gluten-containing grains and onions. Continue to avoid foods that trigger symptoms for the patient.

Other dietary considerations

- Ensure adequate fluid intake to correct dehydration in diarrhoea and to improve bowel motions in patients experiencing constipation.
- Aim for seven to eight serves of vegetables per day to provide prebiotic fibre sources of beneficial bacteria.
- Eating a diet high in polyphenol-rich foods increases beneficial bacteria counts during eradication. Examples include green tea, grapes, cocoa powder, berries, flaxseed meal and dark chocolate.
- Encourage increased consumption of fish to increase intake of essential fatty acids and protein.
- Adequate protein intake is needed for production of HCl, digestive enzymes, neurotransmitters and to support phase II liver detoxification.

NUTRITIONAL MEDICINE THERAPEUTIC OBJECTIVES

The aim of treatment is to reduce bacterial overgrowth in the small intestine, correct dysbiosis, reduce inflammation and address any nutritional deficiencies.

Nutritional medicine (supplemental)

SPECIFIC NUTRIENTS REQUIRED

Probiotics

Probiotics may be useful in improving migrating myoelectric complex function, healing leaky gut, reducing visceral hypersensitivity, decreasing inflammation and enhancing IgA production. They may also exhibit a selective antibacterial action.

The use of some probiotic strains can reduce intensity and severity of GI signs and symptoms as well as gas production in the small intestine. *Lactobacillus casei* (CRL 431) and *Lactobacillus acidophilus* (CRL 430) help reduce the number of bowel motions and production of hydrogen on glucose breath test (GBT) after 21 days of treatment.[165] Other strains that have been found to be beneficial in the treatment of SIBO include *Lactobacilli casei, Lactobacilli plantarum, Streptococcus faecalis, Bifidobacterium brevis* and *Bacillus clausii.*[166]

Bifidobacterium lactis HN019 may be of use to improve stool frequency and consistency in SIBO patients with constipation.[167]

The use of *Bifidobacterium bifidum, Bifidobacterium lactis, Bifidobacterium longum, Lactobacillus acidophilus, Lactobacillus rhamnosus* and *Streptococcus thermophilus* in patients with SIBO and chronic liver disease significantly improved clinical symptoms and eradicated SIBO.[168]

Lactobacillus rhamnosus GG has been found to be useful in reducing visceral hypersensitivity in SIBO.[169]

The use of *Saccharomyces ceravaseae var boulardii* (Biocodex strain) may also be beneficial with a reduction in GI symptoms and hydrogen concentrations seen in paediatric patients with SIBO.[170]

Dosage requirements

Probiotics: The strength of probiotic formulas varies between different strains; it is always best to follow the manufacturer's instructions.

PREBIOTICS

The use of prebiotics in SIBO is controversial as they theoretically would worsen symptoms by creating more gas production; however, there is research to suggest they play a beneficial role in treatment.

The use of partially hydrolysed guar gum (PHGG) was found to improve resolution of SIBO when given with rifaximin. It has a role to play in relieving symptoms in patients with SIBO. PHGG is anti-inflammatory, increases intestinal motility, decreases methane production and increases concentration of *Bifidobacteria* and butyrate producing bacteria counts.[171,172]

The use of lactulose at 10 g twice a day in SIBO patients was found to eradicate GI signs and symptoms and a significant reduction in bacteria concentration in the small intestine in 3 days.[173]

The use of galacto-oligosaccharide (GOS) powder reduced methane gas production in animal studies and may play a role in reducing gas production in SIBO.[174]

Note: PHGG and GOS will tend to be better tolerated in the treatment of SIBO and lactulose is not to be used in patients with fructose malabsorption.

Dosage requirements

PHGG dosage: 5 g per day

Lactulose dosage: Begin lactulose at ¼ teaspoon daily and increase slowly to 10 mL per day. Some patients may experience bloating and flatulence and will find they cannot tolerate the full dose. In those cases remain on the daily dose that the patient is comfortable taking.

GOS dosage: 5 g once a day

OTHER

The use of digestive enzymes and betaine hydrochloride may be useful in restoring upper digestive function in patients who have poor pancreatic digestive enzymes and suspected low gastric acid production.

Nutrients that are found to be in low levels due to SIBO will require supplementation. These may include iron, vitamin B_{12}, zinc and vitamin D.

Fish oil and glutamine assist in repair of the gastrointestinal tract by reducing inflammation of the gastrointestinal tract and providing fuel for enterocytes.

HERBAL MEDICINE

Herbal medicine therapeutic objectives

Herbal medicine intervention aims to eradicate bacterial overgrowth in the small intestine, decrease pain, decrease abdominal distension, decrease flatulence and improve peristalsis and transit time.

Herbal medicine classes

GIT ANTIMICROBIAL HERBS

Antimicrobial herbal medicines assist in the eradication of pathogenic bacteria. Examples include *Hydrastis canadensis, Punica granatum, Allium sativum*, propolis and *Camellia sinensis*. Herbal essential oils such as *Syzygium aromaticum, Thymus officinalis* and *Cinnamomum zeylanicum* are all effective antimicrobial agents that may help with the eradication of SIBO.[175]

Bitter herbal medicines

Herbs that are bitter to taste may assist in increasing vagal stimulation of hydrochloric acid (HCl) for patients with gastroparesis or insufficient gastric acid production. Examples include *Andrographis paniculata, Gentiana lutea* and *Taraxacum officinalis (radix)*.

Antidiarrhoeal herbal medicines

Antidiarrhoeal herbs decrease the volume and consistency of the stool. Examples include tannin-containing herbs such as *Hamamelus virginiana, Agrimonia eupatoria, Geranium maculatum, Ulmus rubra* and *Camellia sinensis*.

Laxative herbal medicines

Herbs that shorten transit time and increase defecation may be useful in SIBO patients with constipation. Examples include *Rumex crispus, Juglans cinerea, Taraxacum officinale (radix), Aloe vera, Plantago ovata, Linum usitatissimum, Ulmus rubra, Rhamnus purshiana* and *Rheum palmatum*.

Carminative herbal medicines

Herbs with a carminative action are used to relax the sphincters in the gastrointestinal tract and reduce flatulence. Examples include *Matracaria recutita, Zingiber officinale, Foeniculum vulgare* and *Mentha x piperita*.

Specific herbal medicines

A recent study of 396 patients who tested positive for SIBO found that 17 out of 37 patients who received herbal antimicrobial therapy for 4 weeks had a negative lactulose

TABLE 10.7 Herbal medicines to treat SIBO

FC Cidal	Dysbiocide	Candibactin-AR	Candibactin-BR
Proprietary blend 500 mg: 1 capsule contained:	Proprietary blend 950 mg per 2 capsules contained:	1 capsule contained:	2 capsules contained:
Tinospora cordifolia (stem), *Equisetum arvense* (stem), pau d'arco (inner bark), *Thymus vulgaris* (aerial part), *Artemisia dracunculus* (leaf), *Sida cordifolia* (aerial part), *Olea europaea* (leaf)	Dill seed, *Stemona sessilifolia* powder and extract, *Artemisia absinthium* shoots and leaves extract, *Pulsatilla chinensis* rhizome powder and extract, *Brucea javanica* powder and extract, *Picrasma excelsa* bark extract, *Acacia catechu* stem extract, *Hedyotis diffusa* powder and extract, yarrow leaf and flower extract (*Achillea millefolium*)	Red thyme oil (*Thymus vulgaris*, providing 30–50% thymol) 0.2 mL, oregano oil (*Origanum vulgare*, providing 55%–75% carvacrol) 0.1 mL, sage leaf 5.5 : 1 extract (*Salvia officinalis*) 75 mg, lemon balm leaf 5 : 1 extract (*Melissa officinalis*) 50 mg	Coptis root and rhizome extract (*Coptis chinensis*, containing berberine) 30 mg, Indian barberry root extract (*Berberis aristata*, containing berberine) 70 mg, berberine sulfate 400 mg. Proprietary 4 : 1 Extract 300 mg: Coptis root and rhizome (*Coptis chinensis*), Chinese skullcap root (*Scutellaria baicalensis*), philodendron bark (*Phellodendron chinense*), ginger rhizome (*Zingiber officinale*), Chinese liquorice root (*Glycyrrhiza uralensis*), Chinese rhubarb root and rhizome (*Rheum officinale*)

Chedid V, Dhalla S, Clarke JO et al. Herbal therapy is equivalent to rifaximin for the treatment of small intestinal bacterial overgrowth. Glob Adv Health Med 2014; 3(3):16–24.

breath test compared to 23 of 63 patients who were given rifaximin (200 mg 3 times a day) for eradication.[176]

The herbal antimicrobial combinations used were: dysbiocide and FC Cidal or Candibactin-AR and Candibactin-BR (see Table 10.7).

MENTHA X PIPERITA (ESSENTIAL OIL)

A case report about the use of *Mentha x piperita* essential oil to treat SIBO found it effective in reducing IBS signs and symptoms, and a reduction in hydrogen production on lactulose breath testing after treatment was noted.[177]

Example herbal formula

Herbal formula for the eradication of SIBO:
Punica granatum 1 : 5 LE 40 mL
Syzygium aromaticum 1 : 2 LE 20 mL
Propolis 1 : 2 LE 20 mL
Mentha x piperita 1 : 2 LE 20 mL
7.5 mL twice a day after food

LIFESTYLE RECOMMENDATIONS

Talk to general practitioner about weaning and removing pharmaceutical medications that may be contributing to SIBO; for example, proton pump inhibitors and narcotic medications.

Engaging in regular exercise should be encouraged.

PARASITES

Epidemiology

Prevalence rates for parasite infections vary within various communities and from country to country. Developing countries have a higher incidence of parasite infections than developed countries. Variation in detection is also determined by different diagnostic approaches.

Blastocystis hominis and *Giardia lamblia* are commonly isolated parasites with prevalence rates for *Blastocystis* ranging from 0.5% to 62%; worldwide incidence of *Giardia* is thought to be 20–60%.[178,179] Higher prevalence of *Blastocystis* in patients with irritable bowel syndrome (IBS) has also been found.[180,181]

Cryptosporidium infection rates are 6.1% in developed countries and between 1.4% and 41% in developing countries.[182] Incidence of *Campylobacter jejuni* infection has been found to in 5–6 people per 100 000 in an American hospital setting with the number of reported cases increasing.[183] It is thought that 6.3% to 29.8% of people with intestinal parasitosis have *Dientamoeba fragilis*.[184]

Classification

SIGNS AND SYMPTOMS

Common signs and symptoms seen in patients with parasite infection include nausea, vomiting, frequent belching, lack of appetite, flatulence, abdominal pain, diarrhoea and fatigue. Less commonly seen signs and symptoms in *Blastocystis* infection include fever, faecal leucocytes, rectal bleeding, hepatomegaly, splenomegaly, skin rashes and joint pain. Some people who test positive for parasites may be asymptomatic.

DIFFERENTIAL DIAGNOSIS

Viral gastroenteritis, irritable bowel syndrome, large bowel bacterial overgrowth, small intestinal bacterial overgrowth, yeast overgrowth, endometriosis, Crohn's disease, ulcerative colitis, coeliac disease, non-coeliac gluten sensitivity, diverticulitis, colitis, acute appendicitis, hypochlorydria, pancreatic enzyme insufficiency, fructose malabsorption, lactose intolerance, food allergies and/or intolerances and *Helicobacter pylori* infection.

Aetiology and pathogenesis

Parasite infestation typically occurs when a person drinks contaminated water or eats contaminated food, or it can happen via direct faecal–oral contact. Ingesting unpasteurised milk, contaminated water or undercooked poultry and pork products is a common cause of infection. Infection can also be passed on from animals including dogs, cats, rats, possums, kangaroos, wombats, cattle, chickens, birds and pigs.[183,185,186]

Travelling in developing countries, working with young children and animals, having concurrent gastrointestinal infection and lowered immunity are predisposing factors for contracting a parasite infection.

Giardia lamblia inhabits the small intestine and can cause malnutrition as it covers the surface of the brush border and scavenges nutrients in the intestinal lumen if left untreated. Giardiasis occurs with ingestion of the cysts; once the cysts reach the small intestine they excyst. *Giardia* are very hardy and are able to tolerate extreme pH and temperatures.[179]

Blastocystis hominis is characterised as an atypical stramenopile with numerous subtypes identified. There is some controversy surrounding pathogenicity and it is possible that certain subtypes are pathogenic while others are not.

After ingestion, *Cryptosporidium* oocysts travel through the gut lumen to the small intestine, where they release sporozoites that adhere to and invade the epithelial cells of the gastrointestinal tract.[187]

Parasites such as *Dientamoeba fragilis, Entamoeba histolytica* and *Blastocystis hominis* are found in the large intestine and infection results in tissue damage. In chronic infections tissue damage is often due to an immune response to the parasite, changes in cytokine profiles or toxic protozoal products and mechanical damage caused in the gut.[188]

Nitric oxide can inhibit the growth of many pathogenic microorganisms and macrophages and enterocytes produce and release nitric oxide in the intestinal lumen.[179] Activation of immune cells in response to parasite infections occurs and is often detected with elevated eosinophil levels on white cell count.

Low diversity of the gut microbiota may predispose individuals to parasite infections. The microbiota plays a protective role in the production of the antimicrobial compounds and metabolic byproducts that inhibit the growth of pathogens, provide specific competition for receptor sites on the intestinal mucosa, compete for nutritional substrates and enhance host immune responses.[189]

Investigations

Polymerase chain reaction (PCR) and microscopy stool testing in combination form the most accurate way to detect parasites. The PCR method is available with general pathology laboratories and accurately detects DNA for the following parasites:

Blastocystis hominis
Dientamoeba species
Giardia lamblia
Cryptosporidium species
Entamoeba histolytica.

It is important to note that the shedding of some parasites may be cyclical and may not be picked up on one sample so multiple samples may be needed if infection is suspected.[178]

Comprehensive stool analysis/GI effects profile is also useful to identify the role the microbiota in the large bowel is playing in gut function and to look at digestive and inflammatory markers such as pancreatic elastase, faecal fats, faecal calprotectin and faecal sIgA.

HAEMATOLOGICAL AND BIOCHEMICAL INVESTIGATIONS

Testing to investigate other possible causes of signs and symptoms, malnutrition and inflammation includes white cell count, full blood examination, biochemistry, ESR, C-reactive protein, coeliac serology and genotyping, total IgE, total vitamin B_{12}, serum folate, iron studies, plasma zinc and vitamin D.

Therapeutic considerations

ALLOPATHIC TREATMENT

Commonly used antibiotics to treat parasites include metronidazole, erythromycin, doxycycline, fluoroquinilone, nitazoxanide, iodoquinol, paromomycin and tetracycline.[183,190,191]

NATUROPATHIC PERSPECTIVE

The main aim of complementary medicine is to restore function of the gastrointestinal tract following a parasite infection that is causing gastric signs and symptoms and in any malnourishment. Eradication of parasites, reducing signs and symptoms, supporting restoration of the gut microbiota, reducing inflammation, healing the gut mucus layer and supporting immunity are important. Addressing any nutritional deficiencies detected is also an important treatment consideration.

Nutritional medicine (dietary)

DIETARY THERAPEUTIC OBJECTIVES

The aim with diet is to eat a diet that reduces digestive signs and symptoms and to include foods that will assist in eradicating the parasites, correcting imbalance of gut flora and healing the gastrointestinal tract after eradication.

Specific dietary treatments

HIGH-FIBRE DIET

A diet high in fibre including foods such as oat bran, ground flaxseeds, psyllium husks and slippery elm is useful in increasing mucus production in the colon to protect against continued infection and to reduce colonic pH to create a less than ideal environment for parasites to inhabit.

LOW LACTOSE AND SUGAR DIET

Avoidance of high-lactose dairy products such as milk, soft white cheeses and yoghurt during infection is important to avoid secondary lactose intolerance developing.[192] Avoiding foods and drinks high in simple sugars such as confectionery, sweeteners, fruit juices and soft drinks is useful as these sugars can feed *Giardia*.[179]

LOW-FAT DIET

Individuals with *Giardia* will benefit from a low-fat diet: avoid the use of oils and full-fat dairy products. This may reduce nausea, steatorrhoea and diarrhoea. Reduced release of bile acids into the gut lumen reduces *Giardia* growth.[179]

AVOIDANCE OF TRIGGER FOODS

Patients are often aware of foods and beverages that trigger their digestive symptoms. Common examples include coffee, *Brassica* genus vegetables, legumes, gluten-containing grains and onions. Continue to avoid trigger foods until gut healing is complete then look at slow reintroduction of these foods when appropriate.

Some individuals with chronic parasite infection can experience weight loss so it is important to ensure they are eating adequate protein and fats.

Blueberries (*Vaccinium myrtillus*)

Eating blueberries and drinking polyphenol-rich blueberry drink (Bouvrage) (at the equivalent of 40 g blueberries per day) reduces *Giardia duodenalis* and *Cryptosporidium parvum*.[193]

Wheatgerm

One small study found that eating 1 tsp of wheatgerm three times a day may assist in eradication of *Giardia* when given with metronidazole treatment.[194] The wheatgerm agglutinin binds to *Giardia* cysts and trophocytes, preventing excystation, replication and growth of the parasite.

OTHER DIETARY CONSIDERATIONS

- Use oral rehydration therapy to avoid dehydration.
- Avoid caffeine and alcohol to prevent further dehydration during infection.
- Focus on eating well-cooked vegetables to aid digestion and provide prebiotic fibre sources to beneficial bacteria.

NUTRITIONAL MEDICINE THERAPEUTIC OBJECTIVES

The aim of treatment is to eradicate parasites, reduce gastric signs and symptoms, correct dysbiosis, reduce inflammation and address any nutritional deficiencies.

NUTRITIONAL MEDICINE (SUPPLEMENTAL)

Probiotics

Probiotics are useful in the treatment of parasites as they compete with pathogens for adhesion sites and nutrients, improve intestinal barrier function and modulate mucus secretion. They also improve immune modulation by interacting with dendritic cells that cause differentiation of T-cells into Th1, Th2 or Treg lymphocytes, leading to different cytokine induction and/or through humoral immune response via IgA-producing cells and their secretory IgA.[187]

Strains of probiotics that have been found to be useful in the treatment of some parasites in animal and human studies are listed in Table 10.8.

SACCHAROMYCES BOULARDII

Saccharomyces boulardii is useful in reducing the severity and shortening the duration of diarrhoea in acute parasite infection.[195]

TABLE 10.8 Probiotic strains that may be useful for the treatment of parasitic infection

	Blastocystis	*Giardia*	*Cryptosporidium*
L. reuteri strains 4000 and 4020			•*
L. acidophilus NCFM			•
L. rhamnosus GG	•	•	•
L. casei shirota			•
VSL#3			•
Saccharomyces boulardii	•	•	
L. johnsonii La1		•	
L. plantarum 299V		•	
L. acidophilus LA5	•	•	
B. lactis BB12	•		

*Signifies strain is effective

Besirbellioglu BA, Ulcay A, Can M et al. *Saccharomyces boulardii* and infection due to *Giardia lamblia*. Scan J Infect Dis 2006; 38(6–7):479–481; Dinleyici EC, Eren M, Dogan N et al. Clinical efficacy of *Saccharomyces boulardii* or metronidazole in symptomatic children with *Blastocystis hominis* infection. Parasitol Res 2011; 108(3):541–545; Hawrelak J. Giardiasis: pathophysiology and management. Alt Med Rev 2003; 8(2):129–143; Travers MA, Florent I, Kohl L et al. Probiotics for the control of parasites: an overview. J Parasitol Res 2011; Art 610769, 11 pp.

Dosage requirements

Probiotics: The strength of probiotic formulas varies between different strains; it is always best to follow the manufacturer's instructions.
Saccharomyces boulardii: 250 mg 2 to 4 times a day.

OTHER

Nutrients that are found to be low due to parasite infection will require supplementation. These are commonly iron, vitamin B_{12}, zinc and/or vitamin D.

Fish oil, zinc and glutamine assist in repair of the gastrointestinal tract by reducing inflammation of the gastrointestinal tract during and post infection.

HERBAL MEDICINE

Herbal medicine therapeutic objectives

Herbal medicine intervention aims to eradicate parasites, decrease pain, decrease abdominal distension, decrease flatulence and improve peristalsis and transit time.

Herbal medicine classes

GIT ANTIPARASITIC HERBS

Antimicrobial herbal medicines assist in the eradication of parasites. Examples include *Hydrastis canadensis, Punica granatum, Allium sativum, Brucea javanica, Coptis chinensis* and propolis.[196,197] Herbal essential oils such as *Syzygium aromaticum, Origanum vulgare* and *Cinnamomum zeylanicum* are all effective antimicrobial agents that may help with the eradication of parasites.

ANTIDIARRHOEAL HERBAL MEDICINES

Antidiarrhoeal medicines help decrease the volume and consistency of the stool. Examples include tannin-containing herbs such as *Hamamelus virginiana, Agrimonia eupatoria, Geranium maculatum, Ulmus rubra* and *Camellia sinensis.*

MUCOPROTECTIVE HERBAL MEDICINES

Herbs that heal damaged gastric mucosa include *Ulmus rubra, Aloe vera, Althea officinalis* and *Glycyrrhiza glabra.*

ANTI-INFLAMMATORY HERBAL MEDICINES

Herbs that reduce inflammation in the small or large intestine include *Curcuma longa, Boswellia serrata, Filipendula ulmaria, Urtica dioica* and *Aloe vera.*

VULNERARY HERBAL MEDICINES

Herbs that heal the gastric mucosa include *Calendula officinalis, Achillea millefolium* and *Hydrastis canadensis.*

CARMINATIVE HERBAL MEDICINES

Herbs with a carminative action help relax the sphincters in the gastrointestinal tract and reduce any flatulence. Examples include *Matracaria recutita, Zingiber officinale, Foeniculum vulgare* and *Mentha x piperita.*

SPECIFIC HERBAL MEDICINES

Allium sativum

The allicin in garlic has been found to be effective for the removal of parasites, particularly *Giardia.*[198,199] Garlic has been found to be more effective than metronidazole in eradicating *Blastocystis.*[200]

Nigella sativa

Nigella sativa extract has been found in one in vitro study to be more effective in eradicating *Blastocystis* than metronidazole treatment.[201]

EXAMPLE HERBAL FORMULA

Herbal formula for the eradication of parasitic infection:
Punica granatum (rind) 1 : 5 LE 40 mL
Syzygium aromaticum 1 : 2 LE 20 mL
Propolis 1 : 2 LE 20 mL
Allium sativum 1 : 2 LE 20 mL
5 mL 3 times a day after food.

LIFESTYLE RECOMMENDATIONS

To avoid infection or re-infection:

- Ensure food eaten is well cooked and avoid eating uncooked or rare meat if eating out and unsure of the quality of the food
- Store cooked and uncooked food correctly
- Wash hands thoroughly with soap and warm water after handling animals, nappies, going to the toilet and before preparing food
- If using drinking water from a tank ensure a filter is installed to remove organisms that are less than 1 micron in size
- When travelling in developing countries drink only clean bottled water.

ULCERATIVE COLITIS

Epidemiology

The incidence and prevalence of ulcerative colitis (UC) is increasing, including in areas where it has previously been at low levels such as Asia and the developing world. The annual incidence of UC in Europe is 24.3 per 100 000 people, while in North America it is 19.2, and it is 6.3 in Asia and the Middle East.[202]

Classification

Unlike Crohn's disease, which can affect various parts of the gastrointestinal tract, UC is restricted to the rectum and colon. The disease usually follows a pattern of remissions and exacerbations and the severity can range from mild to severe. Ulcerative colitis usually requires lifetime management and patients frequently benefit from support services and counselling.

UC is always found in the large colon and can be either isolated to the rectum (proctitis), found in the rectum and descending colon (left-sided UC), extend to involve the descending colon and the transverse colon (extensive UC) or involve the whole colon (total UC).[101] Disease activity may be described as acute severe (usually in patients with extensive or total disease), moderately active (usually left-sided) or active proctitis.[203]

SIGNS AND SYMPTOMS

Signs and symptoms may include urgency, diarrhoea, rectal bleeding, rectal mucus, weight loss, anorexia, fever,

TABLE 10.9 Differentiation of Crohn's disease from ulcerative colitis

Variable	Crohn's disease	Ulcerative colitis
Mucosal lesions	Aphthous ulcers are common in early disease; late disease is notable for stellate, 'rake,' 'bear claw,' linear or serpiginous ulcers; cobblestoning	Micro-ulcers are more common than larger ulcers Pseudopolyps are more common
Distribution	Often discontinuous and asymmetrical with skipped segments and normal intervening mucosa, especially in early disease	Continuous, symmetrical and diffuse, with granularity or ulceration found throughout the involved segments of colon; periappendiceal inflammation (caecal patch) is common even when the caecum is not involved
Rectum	Completely, or relatively, spared	Typically involves the rectum with proximal involvement to a variable extent
Ileum	Often involved (75% of cases of Crohn's disease)	Not involved, except as 'backwash' ileitis in ulcerative pancolitis
Depth of inflammation	Submucosal, mucosal and transmural	Mucosal; not transmural except in fulminant disease
Serosal findings	Marked erythema and creeping fat (the latter is virtually pathognomonic)	Absent, except in severe colitis or toxic megacolon
Complications	Perianal findings are often prominent, including large anal skin tags and deep fissures; perianal fistulas are often complex	Perianal findings are not prominent (any fissures or fistulas are uncomplicated)
Strictures	Often present	Rarely present; suggestive of adenocarcinoma
Fistulas	Perianal, enterocutaneous, rectovaginal, enterovesicular and other fistulas may be present	Not present, except rarely for rectovaginal fistula
Granulomas	Present in 15–60% of patients (higher frequency in surgical specimens than in mucosal pinch biopsies)	Generally not present (micrgranulomas may be associated with ruptured crypt abscesses)
Other histological features	Crypt abscesses may be present Hallmark is focally enhanced inflammation, often on a background of normal mucosa	Crypt abscesses and ulcers are the defining lesions Ulceration on a background of inflamed mucosa
Serology	pANCA positive in 20–25%; ASCA positive in 41–76%	pANCA positive in 60–65%; ASCA positive in 5%

From Sands BE. From symptom to diagnosis: clinical distinctions among various forms of intestinal inflammation. Gastroenterology 2004; 126:1518.

abdominal pain, nausea and vomiting. Proctitis (disease activity in the rectum only) may present with constipation. Of these, urgency, diarrhoea and bleeding are by far the most common with the presence of fever, anorexia and weight loss indicating the risk of life-threatening complications such as toxic megacolon, perforation or haemorrhage.[3] See Table 10.9 for differentiation between ulcerative colitis and Crohn's disease symptoms and features.

DIFFERENTIAL DIAGNOSIS

Differential diagnosis may include Crohn's disease, infectious diarrhoea (*Campylobacter*, *Salmonella*, *Shigella*, *Clostridium difficile*, *Entamoeba histolytica*), other infections (cytomegalovirus, schistosomiasis, *Chlamydia*, *Herpes simplex*), carcinoma or ischaemic colitis.[3]

Aetiology and pathogenesis

GENETIC PREDISPOSITION

Family history is an important risk factor for the development of UC with 10–20% of those affected reporting a family member with the same condition.[1] The association is highest among first-degree relatives and stronger again in relatives of patients with early onset disease.[1] Certain ethnic groups have an increased risk also, for example a first-degree relative of a Jewish patient has a 4.5% chance of developing the condition compared with 1.6% for a non-Jewish patient.[204]

Susceptibility genes for UC appear to be located on chromosomes 2, 3, 6, 7 and 12 with the IBD2 locus on chromosome 12 having the strongest linkage.[1] The mutations in the NOD2/CARD15 gene on chromosome 16[205] are strongly related to Crohn's disease but not to UC. Other loci are common to Crohn's disease and UC such as IL23R, IL12B, HLA, NKX2–3 and MST1.[206] There is a plethora of research currently being conducted to isolate particular genes that both render an individual susceptible and augment the course of the disease. Several genetic polymorphisms appear to be associated with risk, including those related to vitamin D receptor, interleukin, and interleukin receptor gene.[207]

IMMUNE DYSREGULATION

The initiating factors for UC are largely unknown although immune dysregulation appears to be at the heart of the condition. This altered immune function results in mucosal inflammation with the infiltration of macrophages and lymphocytes. These cells then up-regulate nuclear transcription factors culminating in the local release of inflammatory mediators and cytokines leading to tissue damage.[203]

The most common autoantibody in UC is the perinuclear antineutrophil cytoplasmic antibody (pANCA), which is found in the serum of most patients.[1] The antigen to which this autoantibody is directed and the pathogenic nature of pANCA are currently unknown.[1]

DYSBIOSIS

Intestinal microflora may be a very significant factor in the development of UC. Interestingly, a study has found early and repeated antibiotic use is associated with increased risk of developing IBD,[208] potentially due to alterations of the microbiome. A study found disordered intestinal bacteria in 96 patients with IBD (73 UC and 23 Crohn's disease) compared with the non-UC control group.[209] The researchers found that the *Bacteroides fragilis* group was significantly decreased in the faeces of patients with IBD. *Bacteroides vulgatus* was also decreased in IBD patients and furthermore it was identified as the principal microflora present in healthy controls. Interestingly, propionic and butyric acids were significantly decreased in the faeces of IBD patients. The presence of *Bacteroides* (especially *B. vulgatus*) has been found to aggravate UC in animal models.[210] Other studies on the microflora in IBD patients have found conflicting results,[211] and more research needs to be conducted. Furthermore there have also been studies to suggest that the *Lactobacillus* species may be reduced in active UC.[1,212] One small study of 57 IBD patients found that 30% of UC patients had a significant reduction in diversity of mucosal flora.[213] This was mainly due to the loss of normal anaerobic bacteria such as *Bacteroides* species, *Eubacterium* species, and *Lactobacillus* species.

DEFICIENT MUCIN

Mucin is an important substance that helps to protect and repair the lining of the gastrointestinal tract. It is often found to be deficient in patients with UC and this is thought to be due in part to the immune system manufacturing antibodies that actively destroy it.[214,215] Reduced levels of mucin may lead to abnormal mucosal permeability rendering the mucosa more susceptible to contact from bacteria and other luminal contents. Cyclosporin also appears to reduce mucin.[216] Non-steroidal anti-inflammatory medication use may increase relapses in UC, potentially through reduced mucosal prostanoid synthesis.[217]

SEROTONIN ALTERATION

Molecular changes in serotonergic signalling in the gastrointestinal tract in UC may lead to alterations in motility, secretion and sensation.[85] Coates et al. found that mucosal serotonin, tryptophan hydroxylase 1 messenger RNA, serotonin transporter messenger RNA, and serotonin transporter immunoreactivity were all significantly reduced in UC.[85,87]

REDUCED APOPTOSIS

Mucosal T-cells appear to be resistant to apoptosis in UC.[205] It appears that these T-cells may be protected by interleukin 6 (IL-6), the transcription of which is regulated by nuclear factor kappa B (NF-κB).[218] Reactive oxygen species (ROS) stimulate tumour necrosis factor alpha (TNF-α), which leads to the transcription of NF-κB which in turn regulates the transcription of many inflammatory cytokines, including IL-6.[218,219]

OTHER ENVIRONMENTAL FACTORS

A number of large studies have investigated the effects of diet, smoking and infection on ulcerative colitis and the results to date appear to be inconclusive.[220–225] It is generally acknowledged, however, that smoking and an appendectomy are protective against the development of the disorder.[224,226] A high long-term intake of omega-3[227] and vegetable consumption[228] appear to be associated with a reduced risk of developing UC, while high intake of trans fats,[227] omega-6 fatty acids and meat intake[228] increases it. The use of the oral contraceptive pill has also been identified as a possible risk factor in developing IBD and increasing relapses (though this association was strongest in Crohn's disease).[229,230]

Investigations

Haematological and biochemical investigations commonly include full blood examination (particularly for haemoglobin, white cell count, electrolytes, creatinine and albumin), erythrocyte sedimentation rate, C-reactive protein, liver function test, iron studies, vitamin B_{12}, vitamin D and folate.[2] The MTHFR polymorphism may also be useful to identify altered folate metabolism, especially in those on folate — depleting medications such as sulfasalazine.

Other investigations include stool culture and examination, sigmoidoscopy/colonoscopy and radiography.[2] These investigations will identify and assess any histological changes.

Bone densitometry should be performed at 1–2 year intervals for those who have received corticosteroids at high doses or for long durations.

SPECIFIC NATUROPATHIC INVESTIGATIONS

Food avoidance and challenge

These diets are useful for the identification of food intolerances, but are unsafe for allergies. (See earlier in this chapter on adverse reactions, food allergy and hypersensitivity, specifically breath tests.) These tests are useful for the identification of lactose and fructose malabsorption. Breath tests use either hydrogen or methane to check for malabsorption. Patients drink the test medium (lactose or fructose) and the amount of hydrogen/methane excreted in the breath over the next few hours is recorded. If lactose/fructose malabsorption exists the carbohydrate is not absorbed and it travels to the large bowel where it is degraded by colonic flora, producing large amounts of hydrogen/methane that are then partially absorbed into the bloodstream and excreted via the lungs. There should always be a baseline test done first using lactulose to ensure that the patient produces hydrogen (up to 28% do not and methane should be used).[4]

Lactulose/mannitol test

Useful for the identification of intestinal permeability. This test involves drinking the two substances, lactulose and mannitol. Increased lactulose indicates intestinal permeability as the sugar is only partially absorbed between the mucosal cells in a healthy gut. If high levels result, the junctions between the cells are larger and the mucosa can be said to be permeable. High levels of mannitol indicate malabsorption.

Complete digestive stool analysis/ GI effects profile

These are comprehensive stool tests designed to identify pathogenic and commensal microbiota along with exogenous bacteria and parasites. They also investigate markers of digestion and maldigestion and certain markers of disease activity such as blood, pus, mucus, white blood cells and lactoferrin (GI effects profile only).

Therapeutic considerations

ALLOPATHIC TREATMENT

- Sulfasalazine, coated mesalazine or olsalazine may be prescribed.
- Corticosteroids (commonly prednisolone) may be required if the inflammation is more severe or if more of the bowel is involved.
- Antidiarrhoeal drugs, for example loperamide or diphenoxylate and atropine, may be helpful.
- Immune suppressants such as azathioprine or 6-mercaptopurine are also often used to induce and/or maintain remission.
- The anti-TNF antibody drug infliximab is approved for use in ulcerative colitis.[231]
- Surgery may also be an option for drug-refractory patients.

Therapeutic application

NATUROPATHIC PERSPECTIVE

One of the main aims of complementary medicine is to keep patients in remission for as long as possible. For some people this is achievable using complementary medicines only, while others need a more combined approach and benefit from using complementary medicines alongside standard medications. This may enable the patient to use lower doses of conventional medications less frequently, thus reducing unwanted side effects. Avoidance of surgical intervention is also a key aim. Treatment therefore aims to reduce inflammation, heal the ulcerated mucosa, protect the bowel mucosa, correct any dysbiosis, modulate immune system function, reduce diarrhoea, reduce bleeding and mucus secretion and reduce pain. Treatment also aims to address any consequences of the disease such as nutrient deficiencies and any unwanted side effects of medication.

NUTRITIONAL MEDICINE (DIETARY)

Dietary therapeutic objectives

While certain diets don't cause ulcerative colitis, dietary interventions can be useful to improve symptom control, reduce inflammation, alter the microbiota and mucosal integrity, correct nutritional deficiencies, prevent anaemia, prevent osteoporosis and improve general health. Weight loss is common in ulcerative colitis and may be due to anorexia, malabsorption, diarrhoea, vomiting, increased nutrient requirements due to inflammation and certain medications,[232] therefore adherence to good dietary practices is crucial.

Specific dietary treatments

FIBRE AND PREBIOTICS

IBD commonly reduces SCFAs, especially acetate, propionate, and butyrate production in the colon. Increasing fibre in the diet increases levels of these SCFAs, possibly negating the effects of compromised colonocyte energy supply due to intestinal inflammation.[233] A placebo-controlled trial found that psyllium (*Plantago ovate*) relieved gastrointestinal symptoms in UC patients in remission. Psyllium was associated with significant improvement in symptoms (69%) compared with placebo (24%).[234] A later open label, multicentre, randomised clinical trial examined the efficacy and safety of psyllium seeds (10 g b.i.d.) as compared with mesalazine (500 mg t.d.s.) for maintaining remission in 105 patients with UC.[235] After 1 year rates of continued remission were the same in all groups (mesalazine, psyllium), suggesting psyllium may be as effective as mesalazine for maintaining remission in UC. Additionally, a significant increase in faecal butyrate was observed with psyllium seed use.

A pilot study aimed to determine whether UC patients could increase faecal butyrate levels by dietary means.[236] Twenty-two patients added oat bran (60 g, corresponding to 20 g dietary fibre) to their daily food intake for 3 months. Faecal butyrate concentration increased by 36% after 1 month. Further long-term studies are needed to study the benefits of oat bran in UC, although these preliminary results are encouraging.

Three trials have demonstrated the efficacy of germinated barley foodstuff (GBF) in the treatment of UC.[237–239] GBF acts as a prebiotic, increasing luminal butyrate production. It consists of high amounts of fibre and glutamine-rich protein. In one of these investigations, a placebo controlled trial administered GBF (20 g/day) as an adjunct to conventional treatment to 57 UC patients in remission.[237] Significantly better Crohn's disease activity index (CDAI) values were seen in the GBF group compared with control. Additionally steroid tapering without exacerbation was more successful in the GBF group. An open label study evaluated the effects of GBF in active UC.[238] Twenty-one patients with mild to moderate UC received GBF (20–30 g/day for 24 weeks) as an adjunct to conventional treatments. A significant decrease in CDAI was observed after 24 weeks compared with control. The amounts of visible blood passed and nocturnal diarrhoea were particularly improved. The barley extract was well tolerated and no side effects were observed. This open label study is promising. However, larger double blind studies are required to confirm these results. An animal study has demonstrated that GBS reduced NF-κB and IL-6 by increasing butyrate in the lumen.[240]

ANTIOXIDANTS

Oxidative stress is common in inflammatory disorders as neutrophils, macrophages and inflammatory cells produce large amounts of reactive oxygen species (ROS).[241] Excessive oxidative stress has been linked to worsening inflammation and colorectal cancer.[241–243] A study of 167 patients with IBD found that levels of beta-carotene and vitamin C were significantly lower as compared with the aged matched, healthy control group.[244] Other studies have also demonstrated a reduced antioxidant capacity in UC.[245,246] While there have been no clinical trials conducted to examine the effects of dietary antioxidants in IBD it stands to reason that increased amounts of these substances could be extremely beneficial. Vitamins A, C, E, zinc, selenium are all crucial antioxidants that are bioavailable from fruits and vegetables.

ESSENTIAL FATTY ACIDS

While most research on the benefits of fish products has focused on fish oil supplementation it is still extremely advisable for IBD patients to include fish at least 4 times a week in their diet. The omega-3 fatty acids from fish reduce inflammation in IBD.

SHORT CHAIN CARBOHYDRATES

Many patients with UC find the avoidance of certain short chain carbohydrates such as lactose and fructose helps with symptom control. This is often due to poor absorption and a subsequent osmotic effect. A pilot study found that restriction of short chain carbohydrates in the diet greatly improved symptom control for patients with IBD (n = 72).[247] For a more thorough discussion of short chain carbohydrates see earlier in this chapter on adverse reactions, food allergy and hypersensitivity.

Other dietary considerations

In many cases dietary recommendations depend upon the patient's personal disease history and symptoms. Some general considerations might include:

- Avoid any foods that produce symptoms or increase risk factors, such as alcohol.[248]
- During an acute attack many patients need to eat a very simple and easily digestible diet. Foods such as soft-cooked vegetables, fish and chicken are recommended. Some patients prefer an elemental diet. This involves using a product that contains all essential nutrients in a pre-digested form. This allows the bowel to rest and is associated with attaining remission in many cases.[249] Unfortunately, the diet is often found to be unpalatable and the hyperosmolality may cause diarrhoea. The reoccurrence of symptoms is common once the diet is stopped.
- Ensure adequate protein intake. Many people with IBD narrow their diet and self-restrict certain foods in the belief that it reduces symptoms. Meat may be eliminated and therefore protein intake is reduced. Prospective studies have suggested an increased risk of development and relapse with high intake of animal meat, possibly due to the inflammatory components such as arachidonic acid.[250] Protein is essential for many aspects of a healthy gastrointestinal tract such as adequate production of HCl, digestive enzymes and neurotransmitters and providing amino acids for phase II liver detoxification.
- The consumption of fish should be encouraged. Fish is an easily digestible source of protein and essential fatty acids, which are anti-inflammatory.
- Ensure adequate fluid intake to correct dehydration for loose bowel motions or diarrhoea.
- A healthy intake of fresh fruit and vegetables is essential for a steady supply of fibre, enzymes and nutrients. Vegetables should be cooked and not eaten raw.
- Wholegrains should also be consumed if tolerated. Many patients, however, can only tolerate 'white' products.
- Diets need to be individually designed in order to counteract nutritional deficiencies as much as possible.

NUTRITIONAL MEDICINE (SUPPLEMENTAL)

Nutritional medicine therapeutic objectives

Nutritional medicine is used for very similar reasons and is an extension to dietary therapy. A study aimed at comparing the nutritional status of patients recently diagnosed with UC against age- and sex-matched controls found significant deficiencies in the serum concentrations of beta-carotene, magnesium, selenium and zinc.[251] Weight and body mass index were also significantly lower in UC patients and protein, calcium, phosphorus, and riboflavin intake were lower. While food intake is a common problem in chronic disease, patients with UC often require greater amounts of macro and micro nutrients due to the disease process and supplementation is crucial to obtain optimal levels.

Nutritional supplementation aims to improve symptom control, reduce inflammation, correct nutritional deficiencies, prevent anaemia, prevent osteoporosis and improve general health.

Specific nutrients required

FISH OILS

A higher intake of omega-3 fatty acids (especially DHA) may reduce the risk of developing UC,[252] and a diet with a higher omega-3 to omega-6 ratio has been found to be associated with reduced disease relapse.[253] In a study examining colonic mucosa biopsies in UC patients, the degree of inflammation was positively associated with levels of arachidonic, docosapentaenoic and docosahexaenoic acid and negatively associated with levels of linoleic, α-linolenic and eicosapentaenoic acids.[254] This suggests manipulation of dietary fats may influence mucosal inflammation.

Two Cochrane reviews found there was no evidence to support the use of fish oil for the maintenance of remission in UC.[255,256] Three small randomised controlled trials were included in the systematic review (total number of participants = 138) and overall results showed a similar relapse rate to the control group.

Another Cochrane review found mixed outcomes in trials designed to determine whether fish oil can induce remission in UC.[257] Six studies were included in the review: one found that fish oil induced remission while the others showed positive secondary effects such as improved sigmoidoscopic scores compared with placebo, a corticosteroid sparing effect and improvements in disease activity. Adverse events were reported as very low.

PROBIOTICS

There is evidence that shows that probiotics are important in both the treatment and long-term management of ulcerative colitis and pouchitis.[258–261] They appear to work in several ways by competitively excluding microbial pathogens, modulating immune function and enhancing gastric mucosal function.[262] Strains of bacteria that have been found to be effective include *Bifidobacterium longum*,[260] *Lactobacillus* GG[261] and *Escherichia coli* Nissle 1917.[263] Interestingly the probiotic *E. coli* Nissle 1917 has been shown to be as effective as mesalazine for maintaining remission in a 12-month double blind controlled trial.[263]

VSL#3 (Orphan Australia) is another probiotic that has been found to be effective in both UC and Crohn's disease. It contains four strains of lactobacilli (*Lactobacillus casei, L. plantarum, L. acidophilus* and *L. delbrueckii* subspp. *bulgaricus*), three strains of bifidobacteria (*Bifidobacterium longum, B. breve* and *B. infantis*), and *Streptococcus salivarius* subspp. *thermophilus*.

Randomised double blind studies have found that VSL#3 increases the diversity of intestinal microflora in patients in remission[264] and effectively maintains antibiotic-induced remission in recurrent pouchitis.[265] An open label study found that VSL#3 induced remission in 77% of medication-refractory UC patients after 6 weeks.[266] VSL#3 has also been found to induce remission in children with mild to moderate UC.[267] In vivo studies have shown that VSL#3 decreases mucosal inflammation and increases luminal mucin content by 60%.[268,269]

IRON

Iron levels need to be closely monitored owing to bleeding, anaemia of chronic disease and possible reduced intake. Anaemia in IBD is associated with worsening health, poorer quality of life and increased hospitalisations.[270] Increasing iron-rich foods such as lean meats is often helpful, but if levels are low a supplement is necessary. Iron should also be taken with certain other nutrients such as vitamin C, vitamins A, B_1, B_6, B_{12} and folate as these act as cofactors and facilitate not only intestinal absorption but also cellular uptake. It should also be noted that supplementary iron could bind with sulfasalazine, reducing the absorption of both, so taking these two separately is always advised.

CALCIUM

Rates of osteopenia and osteoporosis in patients with IBD are 40–50% and 15% respectively, with very little difference between UC and Crohn's disease.[271] Risk factors for osteoporosis in IBD include use of corticosteroids, malnutrition due to anorexia and malabsorption, smoking, lack of physical exercise, hormonal and genetic factors.[232,271] Patients who have undergone ileal pouch-anal anastomosis have a higher risk of developing osteoporosis.[272]

The British Society of Gastroenterology published guidelines in 2000 for the prevention and treatment of osteoporosis in IBD.[273] The guidelines recommend a calcium intake of 1500 mg/day. The guidelines were updated in 2007 to recommend 1000 mg/day and 1200–1500 mg/day for postmenopausal women and men respectively, due to studies showing a slight improvement in bone mineral density with doses of 500–2000 mg/day.[274]

VITAMIN D

A small study found that 55% of patients with UC had deficient vitamin D levels.[275] Vitamin D (1,25(OH)2D) enhances calcium and phosphate absorption from the intestine in order to improve bone mineralisation. Vitamin D also plays a role in bone formation, maintaining the epithelial barrier, modulating the immune system and inflammation.[276,277] Supplementation with vitamin D will also help with the absorption of calcium. There is very limited research evaluating the correct dose of vitamin D in IBD. However, a dose of 1000 IU/day is commonly recommended based on extrapolation from fracture prevention studies in osteoporosis. Due to the complex issues of IBD, including malnutrition, long-term medication, immune system involvement, and genetic variation in response to supplementation, extrapolation from these studies is problematic and it is very likely that much higher doses of vitamin D are in fact needed. Dose and duration of vitamin D supplementation should be adjusted in accordance with blood test results where possible. Randomised controlled trials are urgently necessary.

FOLATE

Hyperhomocysteinaemia is common in patients with UC, due to low levels of folate and B_{12}.[278] Plasma total homocysteine levels have also been found to be high in children with IBD most likely due to low folate levels.[279] Folate levels are often reduced in UC as a result of the disease process, poor intake, and certain medications. Supplemental folic acid may also assist in reducing the risk of IBD patients developing colorectal cancer.[280]

GLUTATHIONE

Glutathione is an important intracellular antioxidant that is biosynthesised from L-cysteine, L-glutaminic acid and glycine. Glutathione levels have been found to be low in UC, possibly due to low plasma cysteine levels.[281] Animal studies have demonstrated that N-acetylcysteine (NAC), a glutathione precursor, attenuates disease progression.[282,283]

GLUTAMINE

Glutamine is a major source of nutrition for enterocytes.[284] Small studies have suggested that glutamine may be beneficial in treating postoperative patients with pouchitis.[284]

ZINC

A study found that 15.2% of IBD patients tested were found to have low levels of serum zinc,[285] supporting other studies that have also demonstrated lower zinc levels in UC.[251,286] Zinc is a necessary cofactor for many proteins and the antioxidant compound Cu/Zn-superoxide dismutase. Low mucosal levels of zinc, vitamin A and folic acid may predispose the mucosa to injury.[287]

MAGNESIUM

Magnesium depletion is common in patients with UC owing to chronic diarrhoea and possibly also poor dietary intake. Magnesium deficiency in IBD can cause complications such as muscle cramps, tetany, fatigue, depression, bone pain, cardiac abnormalities, urolithiasis, impaired healing and colonic motility disorders.[288]

GERMINATED BARLEY FOODSTUFF

A pilot study on 46 patients with UC using GBF supplementation (30 g a day in 3 doses) for 8 weeks in addition to their medication, found a significant decrease in mean serum CRP levels and frequency of abdominal pain and cramping compared to the control group.[289]

Dosage requirements

- Fish oils: 2–6 g total fish oil/day
- Probiotics: VSL#3 1–3 sachets/day
- Iron: A daily dose for iron depends on many factors. If iron levels are very low and supplementation is well tolerated then a higher elemental dose is given (around 100 mg). If a maintenance dose is needed or if gastrointestinal symptoms are noted a lower elemental dose of 15–20 mg b.i.d. or t.d.s. may be used
- Calcium: 1500 mg/day
- Vitamin D: 1000–5000 IU/day
- Folate: 1 mg/day
- Glutathione: 300 mg/day
- Glutamine: 7 g 3 times daily
- Zinc: 30–50 mg/day
- Magnesium: 400 mg/day (in divided doses) is necessary to replenish levels.

HERBAL MEDICINES

Herbal medicine therapeutic objectives

Herbal medicines are employed to reduce inflammation, heal and protect the bowel mucosa, improve transit time, reduce blood and mucus loss, decrease pain and reduce any stress or anxiety that may be present.

Herbal medicine classes

ANTI-INFLAMMATORY HERBAL MEDICINES

Anti-inflammatory herbs to decrease inflammation. Examples include *Curcuma longa, Boswellia serrata, Filipendula ulmaria, Salix alba, Urtica dioica, Aloe vera.*

MUCOPROTECTIVE HERBAL MEDICINES

Mucoprotective herbs to protect the mucous membranes of the intestine. Examples include *Ulmus rubra, Aloe vera* and *Glycyrrhiza glabra.*

IMMUNE-MODULATING HERBAL MEDICINES

Immune-modulating herbs to modulate immune system function. Examples include *Echinacea purpurea/angustifolia, Astragalus membranous, Hemidesmis indicus, Tylophora asthmatica, Andrographis paniculata.*

ANTIOXIDANT HERBAL MEDICINES

Antioxidant herbs to reduce oxidation. They are crucial for immune function as free radical production leads to the stimulation of TNF-α. Herbs such as *Silybum marianum, Curcuma longa* and *Vaccinium myrtillus* may be important therapeutic considerations in ulcerative colitis to decrease excessive free radical production

HAEMOSTATIC AND ASTRINGENT HERBAL MEDICINES

Haemostatic and astringent herbs. Herbs such as *Geranium maculatum, Agrimonia eupatoria* and *Quercus robur* may be useful in mild disease to reduce blood and diarrhoea.

Specific herbal medicines

Some herbal medicines that are particularity valuable include the following.

CURCUMA LONGA (CURCUMIN)

A randomised, multicentre, double blind, placebo controlled clinical trial found that curcumin in combination with standard medication was more successful in maintaining remission than medication alone.[290] Patients were given either curcumin and sulfasalazine or mesalazine, or placebo and sulfasalazine or mesalazine. At the end of the study period 4.65% of patients receiving curcumin had relapsed compared with 20.51% for placebo. A pilot study found that curcumin improved ulcerative proctitis in all five patients and led to subsequent reductions in medication for four patients.[291] Extensive research over the last two decades has shown that curcumin exhibits powerful anti-inflammatory properties by acting on NF-κB, cyclooxygenase 2 (COX-2) and 5 lipoxygenase (5 LOX), TNF, IL-1,IL-6 and inducible nitric oxide synthase pathways, as well as influencing neutrophil chemotaxis.[292,293] Both turmeric and curcumin have been shown to be very safe.[294]

ALOE VERA

Forty-four UC patients were randomised to receive oral *Aloe vera* gel (2:1 ratio, 100 mL b.i.d.) or placebo for 4 weeks.[295] Clinical remission was achieved in 30% of participants, while 37% said their condition improved. The simple clinical colitis activity index (SCCAI) and histological scores also improved significantly during treatment compared with placebo. The extract was well tolerated.

ANDROGRAPHIS PANICULATA (ANDROGRAPHIS)

Andrographis paniculata has immune and anti-inflammatory actions, which may make it beneficial in the treatment of UC. It has been found to inhibit TNF-α, IL-1s, and NF-κB in vitro. In a large randomised, double-blind, placebo-controlled trial involving 224 adults with mild-to-moderate UC, 1800 mg of *Andrographis paniculata* extract (HMPL-004) improved clinical symptoms; however, there was no difference in the remission rates after 8 weeks.[296]

SILYBUM MARIANUM (MILK THISTLE)

An RCT in 80 patients with inactive ulcerative colitis examined the effect of a daily dose of 140 mg silymarin, the active constituent in *Silybum marianum*, for 6 months in addition to their medication. Compared to the placebo group, those on the silymarin had significantly improved haemoglobin levels, erythrocyte sedimentation rate and disease activity.[297]

LIFESTYLE RECOMMENDATIONS

Stress

It is advisable to control stress levels as much as possible. A study reported that 41.8% of IBD patients experienced anxiety. Interestingly, there was a positive correlation between the level of anxiety and disease knowledge.[298] Stress and anxiety appear to exacerbate symptoms for many patients with IBD. A study found that exercise, stress management training, behavioural techniques, self-care strategies and a Mediterranean diet significantly improved the quality of life for 30 patients with UC.[299] More recently, a study on mindfulness-based stress reduction in the prevention of flare-up in patients with inactive ulcerative colitis found no difference from the controls in the rate of flare-ups or severity, however sub-analysis based on their stress levels (perceived and measured by urinary cortisol) identified there was a positive effect on those with the highest stress levels.[300] This highlights the potential importance of stress management in reducing the risk of triggering a flare-up.

Other

- Ensure regular exercise.
- Encourage the patient to give up smoking if necessary. Smoking controls the symptoms of UC for many patients; however, it should be discouraged.

CASE STUDY

OVERVIEW

James, aged 42, was diagnosed with ulcerative colitis 4 years ago shortly after he quit smoking. He had not had a flare-up of digestive symptoms for 2 years. For the last 6 weeks he began having urgent, loose stools each morning and over those weeks he had now found himself moving his bowels 4 to 5 times a day. He reported there was now blood and mucus in the stool and he was experiencing lower abdominal pain after eating. James had also begun to lose weight and had very little appetite. He ate a grain- and dairy-free diet.

TREATMENT PROTOCOL

James was referred for further investigations to look into the likelihood of parasitic or pathogenic bacterial infection in the small or large bowel. He was also tested for faecal

CASE STUDY CONTINUED

calprotectin, white cell count, CRP, ESR, total vitamin B_{12} and iron studies.

James was provided with the following dietary advice:

- Reduce intake of omega-6 oils, i.e. sunflower, corn and safflower oil
- Cut out red meat and chicken until the flare-up subsides
- Increase intake of oily fish only and eat some vegetarian protein sources like legumes, quinoa and soy
- Increase omega-3 foods, preferably by eating fresh oily fish, chia seeds and fresh ground flaxseeds daily
- Aim to increase intake of walnuts and hemp seeds
- Focus on eating fruits and vegetables of varying colours, i.e. a rainbow diet
- Drink green tea daily
- Drink diluted fresh vegetable juices to increase antioxidants and add wheatgrass juice.

The initial prescription was:

HERBAL MEDICINE

Curcumin extract tablets 4000 mg/day in divided doses
Slippery elm powder 1 tsp mixed with water into a slurry, 3 times a day after meals

HERBAL FORMULA

Chamomilla recutita 30
Punica granatum (rind) 40
Agrimonia eupatoria 30
5 mL 4 times a day

NUTRITIONAL MEDICINE

Fish oil EPA/DHA equivalent 1800 mg EPA and 1200 mg DHA per day
VSL#3 probiotic 1 sachet per day with food
Oral rehydration powder: 1 serve a day in water to stop dehydration

CROHN'S DISEASE

Epidemiology

The incidence and prevalence of Crohn's disease is increasing, in both children and adults, suggesting environmental factors play a major role.[202] This is highlighted by the increase seen in migrants transitioning from developing to developed world countries.

Classification

Crohn's disease is a chronic inflammatory disease of the gastric mucosa that commonly affects the terminal ileum and colon, but can affect any part of the digestive tract from the mouth to the anus.[301] When disease activity is confined to the colon only, the term Crohn's colitis is often used.[1] The disease usually follows a pattern of remissions and exacerbations and the severity can range from mild to severe.

SIGNS AND SYMPTOMS

Symptoms often include pain, diarrhoea, rectal bleeding, fatigue, weight loss, constipation, fever, perianal fissures and loss of appetite. Fistulas and abscess are also common manifestations of the disease. Perianal fistulas are estimated to occur in 15% to 35% of patients.[1] Extraintestinal signs include musculoskeletal, ocular, mucocutaneous, hepatobiliary, genitourinary and vascular manifestations.[1] Crohn's disease is chronic and debilitating; patients frequently benefit from support services and counselling. See Table 10.9 for differentiation between Crohn's disease and ulcerative colitis symptoms and features.

DIFFERENTIAL DIAGNOSIS

Differential diagnoses may include ulcerative colitis, appendicitis, appendiceal abscess, neoplasm (caecal or ileal adenocarcinoma, lymphoma, metastatic cancer, carcinoid tumour), infection (including *Salmonella, Yersinia enterocolitica, Yersinia pseudotuberculosis, Mycobacterium tuberculosis*, cytomegalovirus), vascular disorders and gynaecological disorders.[1]

Aetiology and pathogenesis

The aetiology and pathophysiology of Crohn's disease is complex and as yet not fully understood. Data suggest that it may be due to a defective innate immune response as a result of genetic and environmental factors.[302–304]

THE INNATE IMMUNE SYSTEM AND THE NOD$_2$/CARD$_{15}$ GENE

Research in the past has focused much more on the adaptive immune system. However, some data have identified defects in the innate immune system as being more problematic.[305] The innate immune system responds immediately to pathogens that enter the gastrointestinal tract by activating local cells such as macrophages and natural killer cells.[305] Genome-wide scanning has identified that the NOD2/CARD15 gene on chromosome 16 is associated with Crohn's disease.[305,306] Patients carrying the NOD2 gene appear to have an increased innate immune response to commensal organisms as demonstrated by various mucosal and serum antibodies such as the anti-*Saccharomyces cerevisiae* antibodies.[307,308] In vivo research has demonstrated that defects in the NOD2 gene lead to increased stimulation of the innate immune system via activation of nuclear factor kappa B (NF-κB), interleukin-1beta (IL-1β) and interleukin-8 (IL-8), which are key inducers of inflammation in Crohn's disease.[309,310] The highest quantities of CARD15 mRNA are found in the paneth cells of the small intestine.[311] Paneth cells synthesise and release antibacterial proteins such as defensin, which are commonly depleted in Crohn's disease.[311]

OTHER IDENTIFIED GENES

The NOD2/CARD15 gene was the first discovered in 2001 and remains the most thoroughly researched. However, later examinations have identified other genes that may also be involved.[311] Defects have been found on the DRD2 gene, which codifies for the D2 dopamine receptor, but the significance of this is as yet unknown.[224,312] Although genetics appear to play a large part in the development of Crohn's disease it is generally accepted that certain environmental factors also need to be present.[311]

ENVIRONMENTAL FACTORS

Environmental factors are also thought to impair innate immune system function. Changes in microbiota composition and biodiversity, bacteria such as *Mycobacterium paratuberculosis*, and smoking have all been positively correlated with Crohn's disease.[224,313–315] Breastfeeding appears to decrease the risk of Crohn's disease while infantile diarrhoea and smoking appear to increase it.[316] Permeability of the intestinal wall may also be increased due to genetics, medication, allergy, infection or inflammation and this can lead to further digestive and immune problems.[317–319] Obesity has also been identified as a possible risk factor.[320,321]

DEFECTIVE INNATE IMMUNE RESPONSES

Crohn's disease is associated with overactivity of T-helper 1 (Th1) immune responses, which are characterised by the expression of IL-2, interferon-gamma (IFN-γ), IL-12 and tumour necrosis factor alpha (TNF-α).[305] TNF-α leads to multiple inflammatory effects within the mucosa of the small intestine. It induces the transcription factor NF-κB, which stimulates the release of many cytokines, cell-cycle proteins and enzymes that damage the bowel wall in Crohn's disease.[322] Advances in treatment have focused on suppressing TNF and therefore NF-κB.[323,324] In summary, the luminal barrier is compromised owing to NOD2/CARD15 defects, repeated injury or exogenous agents. This causes chronic inflammation further leading to defective immune responses to commensal bacteria (food antigens may also contribute). This causes the differentiation of type 1 T-helper cells (Th1) leading to the production of macrophages IL-12, IL-18, IL-1, IL-6, TNF (IL-12 and IL-18 in turn further increase macrophage production). All of this leads to an increase in TNF and therefore NF-κB which induces the expression of over 200 genes, further compromising barrier function.

STRESS

While the role of stress on Crohn's disease is not fully understood, it is believed to potentially influence both its development and its exacerbations.[325–327] This is thought to be due to its ability to increase intestinal permeability, alter immune function and increase inflammation.

DIET

While the role of diet in the development of Crohn's disease is not yet fully understood, a prospective study has found an association between long-term high-fibre intake, especially from fruit, and reduced risk.[328]

Investigations

Haematological and biochemical investigations commonly include a full blood examination (particularly for haemoglobin, white cell count, electrolytes, creatinine and albumin), erythrocyte sedimentation rate, C-reactive protein, iron studies, vitamin B_{12}, folate and antibodies (p-ANCA).[2] Vitamin D levels should also be checked.

Other investigations include stool culture and examination, sigmoidoscopy/colonoscopy and radiography.[2] These investigations will identify and assess any histological changes.

Bone densitometry should be performed at 1–2 year intervals for those who have received corticosteroids at high doses or for long durations.

SPECIFIC NATUROPATHIC INVESTIGATIONS

Food avoidance and challenge

These diets are useful for the identification of food intolerances, but are unsafe for allergies. (See earlier in the chapter on adverse reactions, food allergy and hypersensitivity, specifically breath tests.) These tests are useful for the identification of lactose and fructose malabsorption. Breath tests use either hydrogen or methane to check for malabsorption. Patients drink the test medium (lactose or fructose) and the amount of hydrogen/methane excreted in the breath over the next few hours is recorded. If lactose/fructose malabsorption exists the carbohydrate is not absorbed and it travels to the large bowel where it is degraded by colonic flora, producing large amounts of hydrogen/methane that are then partially absorbed into the bloodstream and excreted via the lungs. There should always be a baseline test done first using lactulose to ensure that the patient produces hydrogen (up to 28% do not and methane should be used).[4]

Lactulose/mannitol test

Useful for the identification of intestinal permeability. This test involves drinking the two substances, lactulose and mannitol. Increased lactulose indicates intestinal permeability as the sugar is only partially absorbed between the mucosal cells in a healthy gut. If high levels result, the junctions between the cells are larger and the mucosa can be said to be permeable. High levels of mannitol indicate malabsorption.

Complete digestive stool analysis/ GI effects profile

These are comprehensive stool tests designed to identify microbiota including anaerobes. They also investigate markers of digestion and certain biochemical parameters.

Therapeutic considerations

ALLOPATHIC TREATMENT

Primary classes of pharmaceutical drugs employed in the treatment of Crohn's disease include:[2]

- Antibiotics if infection is suspected
- Anti-inflammatories such as the 5-aminosalicylates sulfasalazine, mesalazine
- Corticosteroids; prednisolone is commonly used
- Immunomodulators such as azathioprine and 6-mercaptopurine
- Biological substances such as infliximab. Infliximab is a TNF-α antibody that is given as an infusion.

Surgery is undertaken in many cases.

Therapeutic application

NUTRITIONAL MEDICINE (DIETARY)

Dietary therapeutic objectives

While certain diets do not cause Crohn's disease, dietary interventions can be useful to improve symptom control, reduce inflammation, correct nutritional deficiencies, prevent anaemia, prevent osteoporosis and improve general health. Nutrient status may be reduced due to disease activity, malabsorption, anorexia or certain medications. Weight loss is estimated to occur in 65% to 75% of patients with Crohn's disease, therefore a healthy, well-balanced diet is essential.[232]

Specific dietary treatments

FIBRE AND PREBIOTICS

Various studies have found that IBD patients commonly have low luminal levels of SCFAs, primarily butyrate, acetate and propionate.[233] Fermentation of carbohydrates and dietary fibre produces these SCFAs in the large bowel. Most human trials investigating the effects of fibre in IBD have been done in ulcerative colitis. However, it is still reasonable to consider the use of fibre in Crohn's disease. In vitro and in vivo studies in IBD models have shown that fibre increases SCFA production in the colonic lumen, decreases inflammation and leads to the regeneration of colonic tissue.[233] Prebiotics also alter the intestinal microflora balance and can reduce dysbiosis. In an RCT, 67 patients with inactive and mild to moderately active Crohn's disease were given either oligofructose-enriched inulin or placebo 10 g twice daily for 4 weeks. Compared to the placebo, the treatment group had a significant increase in the number of *Bifidobacterium longum* and a decrease in *Ruminococcus gnavus*, along with improvement in disease activity in those with active disease.[329] As oligofructose and insulin are both FODMAPs, these may further increase intestinal symptoms such as visceral hypersensitivity. It is important for practitioners to carefully monitor patient response and increase the dose slowly.

Patients with extensive disease activity in the small bowel, however, may benefit from a low-fibre diet.

ESSENTIAL FATTY ACIDS

While most research on the benefits of fish products has focused on fish oil supplementation it is still extremely advisable for patients with Crohn's disease to include fish at least 4 times a week in their diet. The omega-3 fatty acids from fish reduce inflammation in Crohn's disease.

SHORT CHAIN CARBOHYDRATES

Many patients with Crohn's disease find the avoidance of certain short chain carbohydrates such as lactose and fructose helps with symptom control. This is often due to poor absorption and a subsequent osmotic effect. A pilot study found that restriction of short chain carbohydrates in the diet greatly improved symptom control for patients with IBD (n = 72).[247] For a more thorough discussion of short chain carbohydrates see earlier in the chapter on adverse reactions, food allergy and hypersensitivity.

Other dietary considerations

In many cases dietary recommendations depend upon the patient's personal disease history and symptoms. Some general considerations might include:

- Avoid any foods that produce symptoms.
- Diets need to be individually designed in order to counteract nutritional deficiencies such as B_{12}, iron and magnesium as much as possible.
- During an acute attack many patients need to eat a very simple and easily digestible diet. Foods such as soft-cooked vegetables, fish and chicken are recommended. Some patients prefer an elemental diet. This involves using a product that contains all essential nutrients in a pre-digested form. This allows the bowel to rest and is associated with attaining remission in many cases.[249] Unfortunately, the diet is often found to be unpalatable and the hyperosmolality may cause diarrhoea. The reoccurrence of symptoms is common once the diet is stopped.
- Ensure adequate protein intake. Many people with IBD narrow their diet and self-restrict certain foods in the belief that it reduces symptoms. Meat may be eliminated and therefore protein intake is reduced. Alternative protein sources should be recommended, along with support to promote digestion. Protein is essential for adequate production of HCl, digestive enzymes and neurotransmitters, nutrients for phase II liver detoxification and many other key components of a healthy gastrointestinal system.
- The consumption of fish should be encouraged. Fish is an easily digestible source of protein and essential fatty acids that are anti-inflammatory.
- Ensure adequate fluid intake to correct dehydration for loose bowel motions or diarrhoea.
- A healthy intake of fresh fruit and vegetables is essential for a steady supply of fibre, enzymes and nutrients. Vegetables should be cooked and not eaten raw.
- Wholegrains should also be consumed if tolerated. Many patients however can only tolerate 'white' products.
- Avoid additives. Experimental studies have indicated that some additives such as maltodextrin and emulsifying agents or thickeners such as carboxymethyl cellulose, carrageenan and xanthan gum, may have negative effects on the intestinal barrier, potentially due to decreasing the viscosity of mucosal mucus and increasing inflammation.[330]

FODMAP DIET

While there is limited research on a low-FODMAP diet in the management of IBD, a retrospective study on 72 adults (52 with Crohn's disease and 20 with ulcerative colitis) found it reduced digestive symptoms such as abdominal pain, bloating, flatulence and diarrhoea.[331]

SPECIAL CARBOHYDRATE DIET

Recently, a small amount of research has suggested possible benefits from a special carbohydrate diet (SCD). A retrospective study in 26 children with IBD found that an SCD increased remission and reduced disease activity.[332] Another small study in unmedicated children found similar results.[333] Positive results were also reported in a case series on adults with IBD.[334]

The diet focuses on monosaccharides (glucose, galactose and fructose) that are believed to be well absorbed, while restricting disaccharides due to an inability to digest and absorb them. This malabsorption is thought to increase bacterial and yeast overgrowth, inflammation and mucosal damage.[330] The diet focuses on fruits and vegetables containing a high ratio of amylose to amylopectin, nuts, nut-derived flours, dry-curd cottage cheese, homemade yoghurts (fermented for 24 hrs), meats, eggs, butters and oils, but excludes sucrose, maltose, isomaltose, lactose, grain-derived flours and all true and pseudograins, potatoes, okra, corn, liquid milk, soy, cheeses containing high amounts of lactose, as well as most food additives and preservatives.

NUTRITIONAL MEDICINE (SUPPLEMENTAL)

Nutritional medicine therapeutic objectives

Due to inflammation of the small intestine, a Crohn's sufferer will often have reduced absorption of essential nutrients, which further exacerbates their ill health. Common deficiencies include iron, zinc, calcium, folate and vitamin B_{12},[335] but levels of most nutrients are often altered. Nutrient deficiencies can lead to fatigue, muscle aches, further digestive problems, anaemia, osteoporosis, anxiety and depression.

Nutritional therapeutic objectives therefore aim to address these deficiencies and nutritional medicine is used as an extension to dietary therapy.

Specific nutrients required

OMEGA-3 FATTY ACIDS

Fish oils have been shown to reduce many inflammatory mediators involved in Crohn's disease.[336,337] A prospective study involving 229 702 participants found an inverse relationship between the intake of DHA and the development of Crohn's disease.[338] A recent Cochrane review found that while omega-3 fatty acids are safe, only a small benefit was found in preventing relapse after 1 year. However analysis of the two largest and highest quality studies found no benefit in using omega-3 fatty acids over placebo.[339] This was an update of an earlier review.[255,256,340] Six randomised, placebo-controlled trials of fish oil or other n-3 supplement for maintenance of remission in Crohn's disease were included. The trials involved 1039 participants who were in remission at the time of recruitment and who used the intervention for at least 6 months. Adult doses ranged from 1.8–3.3 g/day of EPA and from 0.8–1.8 g/day of DHA. By far the largest trial (EPIC-1) used a supplement containing 2.2 g of EPA and 0.8 g of DHA (n = 363).[341] The trials included were methodologically rigorous (especially the EPIC-1 and EPIC-2). However, the doses may have been inadequate.

PROBIOTICS

A Cochrane review of the use of probiotics to maintain remission in Crohn's disease found there was no evidence to support this practice.[342] The authors conclude, however, that they could locate only very small trials that lacked the statistical power needed to show differences should they exist. Larger trials are required to determine if probiotics are beneficial in Crohn's disease. Another more recent meta-analysis of eight studies also found that probiotics did not prevent clinical or histological relapse.[343]

There is some early evidence from a small trial that *Saccharomyces boulardii* might improve intestinal permeability in patients with Crohn's disease.[55] However, a prospective study involving 165 Crohn's patients in remission, found 1 g of *S. boulardii* for 52 weeks did not have a significant effect on the time to relapse, disease activity or inflammatory markers compared to controls.[344]

IRON

Approximately 60–80% of patients with Crohn's disease suffer from anaemia.[232] Iron is primarily absorbed from the terminal ileum which is a common area for active Crohn's disease. Deficiency may also be secondary to blood loss. Ferritin in combination with haemoglobin, transferrin, TIBC (total iron binding capacity), iron saturation and mean cell volume (MCV) will give the best indication of iron status. Care needs to be taken to differentiate iron deficiency anaemia from anaemia of chronic disease, which is also common in IBD.[345] As ferritin is an acute phase protein, erythrocyte sedimentation rate and C-reactive protein levels need to be taken into consideration. From time to time patients may need an iron infusion, especially those with severe iron deficiency anaemia.

Iron appears to binds to sulfasalazine, reducing the absorption of both. Separate doses by 2 hours and give away from other divalent cations such as calcium, phosphorus and zinc.

VITAMIN B_{12}

Vitamin B_{12} is also largely absorbed from the terminal ileum and it is estimated that 48% of Crohn's disease patients have a deficiency in the vitamin.[232] Injections are often given and sublingual B_{12} works well. There is a large reference range for B_{12}; however levels above 400 micrograms are optimal.

FOLIC ACID

Certain medications such as methotrexate (a folate antagonist drug) reduce folate levels. About 22% of Crohn's disease patients are folate deficient.[346]

ZINC

A study found that 15.2% of IBD patients tested were found to have low levels of serum zinc.[285] Zinc is important for healthy immune function, digestion, absorption, wound healing and epithelial barrier integrity. Zinc is a necessary cofactor for many proteins and the antioxidant compound Cu/Zn-superoxide dismutase. Low mucosal levels of zinc, vitamin A and folic acid may predispose the mucosa to injury.[287]

CALCIUM

Calcium depletion occurs in approximately 13% of Crohn's disease patients.[232] However, rates of osteopenia and osteoporosis in patients with IBD are 40–50% and 15% respectively, with very little difference between UC and Crohn's disease.[271] Poor bone density is a consequence of corticosteroid medication, malnutrition due to anorexia and malabsorption, smoking, lack of physical exercise, hormonal and genetic factors.[232,271] Caution should be taken with patients in whom calcium-containing kidney stones have developed (also a side effect of corticosteroids). Use only calcium citrate in this situation.

The British Society of Gastroenterology published a guideline in 2000 for the prevention and treatment of osteoporosis in IBD.[273] The guideline recommends a calcium intake of 1500 mg/day. The guideline was updated in 2007 to recommend 1000 mg/day and 1200–1500 mg/day for postmenopausal women and men due to studies showing a slight improvement in bone mineral density with doses of 500–1200 mg/day.[274] Supplementation of 500–100 mg calcium combined with 800 IU of vitamin D/day in osteopenic patients with Crohn's disease resulted in a small improvement in bone mineral density.[347] Dose away from zinc and magnesium.

VITAMIN D

Vitamin D is essential for calcium absorption and approximately 75% of patients are deficient.[232]] Low vitamin D levels have been associated with increased risk of Crohn's disease and disease activity.[276] Vitamin D (1,25(OH)2D) enhances calcium and phosphate absorption from the intestine in order to improve bone mineralisation. Vitamin D plays a role in bone formation, the intestinal barrier and also affects immune system function.[277,348] Supplementation with vitamin D will also help with the absorption of calcium. Correction of a vitamin D deficiency in Crohn's disease patients is associated with a reduced risk of surgery[348] and lower disease activity.[349] There is very limited research evaluating the correct dose of vitamin D in IBD. However, a dose of 1000 IU/day is commonly recommended based on extrapolation from fracture prevention studies in osteoporosis. More recently, a small study found the majority of Crohn's disease patients with mild to moderate disease activity required vitamin D at a dose of 5000 IU/day for 24 weeks to increase serum levels from 16±10 ng/mL to 45±19 ng/mL.[349] Further exploration of recommended doses for IBD patients is warranted. Due to the complex issues of IBD, including malnutrition, long-term medication and immune system involvement, extrapolation from these studies is problematic and it is very likely that much higher doses of vitamin D may be needed.

MAGNESIUM

Magnesium depletion is thought to occur in 14–32% of patients with Crohn's disease.[121] This is most likely due to chronic diarrhoea, terminal ileum disease and bowel resections. Magnesium deficiency in IBD can cause complications such as muscle cramps, tetany, fatigue, depression, bone pain, cardiac abnormalities, urolithiasis, impaired healing and colonic motility disorders.[170] Doses of 400 mg/day (in divided doses) are necessary to replete levels. High levels of supplemental zinc (142 mg/d) may reduce the absorption of magnesium, separate doses by 2 hours.

VITAMIN A

Many people with Crohn's disease have difficulty converting beta-carotene (and other pre-formed retinols) to the active retinol and retinal, as this requires riboflavin, niacin (B_3), zinc and iron. Half the daily intake of vitamin A is commonly from vegetables and therefore pre-formed retinols, often rendering supplementation necessary.

Dosage requirements

- Omega-3 fatty acids: It is expected that doses of 6 g/day are required to ameliorate inflammation in Crohn's disease
- Probiotics: Therapeutic effects vary between strains; consult manufacturer's instructions
- Iron: A daily dose for iron depends on many factors. If iron levels are very low and supplementation is well tolerated then a higher elemental dose is given (around 100 mg). If a maintenance dose is needed or if gastrointestinal symptoms are noted a lower elemental dose of 15–20 mg b.i.d. or t.d.s. may be used
- Vitamin B_{12}: Dose depends on vitamin B_{12} status. Consider doses of 500–2000 micrograms/day if levels are low and monitor
- Folic acid: If patients are taking methotrexate then folate supplementation is paramount. Dose: 500 micrograms/day. Note: Methotrexate works by antagonising folate, so folate supplement must only be undertaken in cooperation with the methotrexate prescriber. Incorrect supplementation may cause failure of the methotrexate therapy
- Zinc: 25–50 mg of elemental zinc a day in deficiency states. Supplement away from antibiotics, folate, iron and NSAIDs
- Calcium: 1000–1500 mg/day
- Vitamin D: 1000–5000 IU/day and monitor
- Vitamin A: 10 000 IU/day.

HERBAL MEDICINE

Herbal medicine therapeutic objectives

The use of herbal medicine aims to decrease pain, decrease abdominal distension, decrease flatulence, improve peristalsis, improve transit time and reduce any stress or anxiety that may be present.

Herbal medicine classes

ANTI-INFLAMMATORY HERBAL MEDICINES

Anti-inflammatory herbs to decrease inflammation. Examples include *Curcuma longa, Boswellia serrata, Filipendula ulmaria, Salix alba, Urtica dioica, Aloe vera.*

MUCOPROTECTIVE HERBAL MEDICINES

Mucoprotective herbs to protect the mucous membranes of the intestine. Examples include *Ulmus rubra, Aloe vera* and *Glycyrrhiza glabra.*

IMMUNE MODULATING HERBAL MEDICINES

Immune modulating herbs to modulate immune system function. Examples include *Echinacea purpurea/angustifolia, Astragalus membranous, Hemidesmis indicus, Tylophora asthmatica, Andrographis paniculata.*

ANTIOXIDANT HERBAL MEDICINES

Antioxidant herbs to reduce oxidation. They are crucial for immune function as free radical production leads to the stimulation of TNF-α. Herbs such as *Silybum marianum, Curcuma longa* and *Vaccinium myrtillus* may be important therapeutic considerations in ulcerative colitis to decrease excessive free radical production.

HAEMOSTATIC AND ASTRINGENT HERBAL MEDICINES

Herbs such as *Geranium maculatum, Agrimonia eupatoria* and *Quercus robur* may be useful in mild disease to reduce blood and diarrhoea.

Specific herbal medicines

CURCUMA LONGA (CURCUMIN)

Curcumin inhibits NF-κB, lipoxygenase (LOX), cyclooxygenase 2 (COX 2), phospholipase, thromboxane, nitric oxide (NO), inducible nitric oxide synthase (iNOS), collagenase, monocyte chemoattractant protein-1 (MCP-1), interferon-inducible protein, IFN-γ, TNF, IL- 1, 6 and 12, elastase and hyaluronidase.[322,350,351] NF-κB is involved in the production of various cytokines and chemokines that induce inflammation in Crohn's disease.[352] Curcumin appears to suppress the activation of NF-κB by inhibiting the I-kappa B kinase complex (IKK).[353–355] Curcumin has also been shown to both inhibit and improve experimentally induced colitis by reducing NF-κB, NO, iNOS and COX 2 in many in vivo studies.[352,356–362]

In a pilot trial, 5 patients with Crohn's disease received 360 mg of curcumin 3 times a day for 1 month, followed by 4 times a day for another 2 months.[291] The Crohn's disease activity index (CDAI), C-reactive protein (CRP) and erythrocyte sedimentation rate (ESR) all fell significantly in 4 out of 5 patients. Five patients with UC were also enrolled and received 550 mg of curcumin twice a day for 1 month, then 3 times a day for another month. Overall stool quality was greatly improved and frequency was significantly reduced. Two patients were able to eliminate their concomitant medications altogether, while another two patients were able to reduce them.

Curcumin has been found to be non-toxic in animal and human trials even at doses of up to 8000 mg/day for 3 months.[350] A common therapeutic dose of curcumin is 400–600 mg, 3 times a day, which is equivalent to 60 g of fresh turmeric root or 15 g of the powder.[322]

ARTEMISIA ABSINTHIUM (WORMWOOD)

A double blind, randomised controlled trial investigating the effects of *Artemisia absinthium* (wormwood) in Crohn's disease found that wormwood may have a steroid sparing effect.[363] Forty patients currently receiving a stable daily dose of 40 mg or less of prednisone for at least 3 weeks were randomised into two groups to receive either 150 mg a day of wormwood or placebo for 10 weeks while steroids were tapered off, The patients were observed for 20 weeks. After 8 weeks of treatment 65% of patients in the wormwood group experienced an almost complete remission compared with none in the placebo group. This remission persisted until the end of week 20. Only 10% of

patients in the wormwood group needed to start steroid therapy again compared with 80% in the placebo group. This was supported by a later 6-week study, where patients receiving wormwood (3 doses 750 mg/day of dried powder) in addition to their medication were more likely to achieve clinical remission and reduced levels of TNF-α compared to the placebo group.[364]
Dose: (1 : 5) 0.7–3.0 mL/day.
Note: Wormwood should not be used long term.

BOSWELLIA SERRATA (BOSWELLIA)

Boswellic acids appear to inhibit 5-lipoxygenase and possibly also various interleukins and TNF-α.[365] A double blind clinical trial randomised 102 patients with active Crohn's disease to receive either boswellia extract H15 (1200 mg) or mesalazine (1.5 mg) 3 times a day for 8 weeks.[366] The boswellia extract was proven to be as effective as mesalazine in reducing the CDAI. The authors concluded that boswellia is superior to mesalazine in terms of the risk-benefit ratio. However, in a double-blind, placebo-controlled, randomised, parallel study, *Boswellia serrata* extract (Boswelan, PS0201B0, 2400 mg capsules 3 times daily) was not more effective in maintaining remission or reducing disease activity compared to placebo after 52 weeks.[367]

Dose: 1200 mg–2000 mg of gum resin 3 times a day.

LIFESTYLE RECOMMENDATIONS

Stress

Stress is often a contributing factor in Crohn's disease as it affects both the systemic immune system and the local immune status of the intestine. Stress appears to play a role in exacerbating and accentuating the intestinal inflammation in IBD through brain–gut interactions.[368] A 5-year study of stable IBD patients investigated the influence of stress on rates of exacerbation. Those patients with prolonged stressful life events were found to have a 90% recurrence rate compared with only 40% recurrence in low stress patients.[368]

Other

- Ensure regular exercise
- Encourage the patient to give up smoking if necessary. Smoking is a risk factor for the development of Crohn's disease.

CASE STUDY

CROHN'S DISEASE CASE STUDY

Anita – a 24-year-old women – presented with Crohn's disease. Her ongoing symptoms included chronic diarrhoea, abdominal pain, flatulence and a reduced appetite. Anita had tested positive for fructose malabsorption 2 years ago and mentioned that nuts and seeds were not very well tolerated and would trigger her digestive symptoms. She had visited her gastroenterologist recently and he had prescribed budenoside, reducing her signs and symptoms, but she still

CASE STUDY CONTINUED

felt unwell. Anita was a smoker, continued to drink coffee and her diet was erratic with episodes of eating refined sugar and wheat products causing the diarrhoea and abdominal pain to worsen.

TREATMENT PROTOCOL

Anita was advised to follow the low-FODMAP diet closely, cease smoking and avoid caffeine. She was also advised to adopt a semi-vegetarian diet, trial ½ cup of bone broth to help with mucosal healing and to include small amounts of fermented food such as sauerkraut and kefir to help balance large bowel microbiota.

Anita was prescribed the following:

HERBAL MEDICINE

A herbal tablet formula containing:
Boswellia serrata 840 mg/day
Zingiber officinale 180 mg/day
Apium graveolens 500 mg/day
Curcuma longa 210 mg/day
This was to be taken in divided doses after meals
Curcumin extract tablets 4000 mg/day in divided doses
Slippery elm powder 1 tsp mixed with water into a slurry 3 times a day to be taken away from budenoside.

NUTRITIONAL MEDICINE

Fish oil EPA/DHA equivalent 1800 mg EPA and 1200 mg DHA per day
Saccharomyces boulardii 250 mg 4 times a day
L-glutamine powder 5 g 4 times a day for gastric mucosal healing
Oral rehydration powder — 1 serve a day in water to stop dehydration.

DIVERTICULAR DISEASE

Diverticulosis is one of the most common gastrointestinal tract disorders in the Western world, occurring in 60% of those over the age of 60.[369] While it is traditionally thought of as a Western disease, increased prevalence has been reported in some developing countries.[370]

Classification

Diverticular disease encompasses diverticulosis and diverticulitis. Diverticulosis is due to herniation of the bowel wall in the large colon leading to the formation of sacs. The condition is usually asymptomatic, but diverticular bleeding or haemorrhage may occur in some patients and is responsible for about 30% of cases of rectal bleeding.[371] Diverticulitis occurs when the diverticular become infected due to impacted faeces, resulting in inflammation and perforation of the colonic diverticulum. This occurs in 10% to 25% of patients with diverticulosis and is by far the most common complication.[371] Repeated inflammation may cause the lumen to narrow, leading to obstruction.

SIGNS AND SYMPTOMS

Many patients with diverticular disease are asymptomatic. If diverticulitis develops patients may have symptoms including abdominal pain, excessive flatulence, bleeding, bowel obstruction, nausea, anorexia, abscess, fistulas and perforation.[371]

DIFFERENTIAL DIAGNOSIS

The primary differential diagnoses for diverticulitis are appendicitis and IBS. Others include inflammatory bowel disease, infectious colitis, peptic ulcer disease, colorectal carcinoma and gynaecological conditions such as pelvic inflammatory disease or ovarian rupture.[1]

Aetiology and pathogenesis

DIET

Diverticulitis is a relatively new condition. It was not written about before World War I and, as noted above, is primarily a disease of the Western world.[372] Because of this there is much speculation that it may be due to changing diets. A Western diet that is low in fibre and high in saturated fat is often associated with diverticular disease. A vegetarian diet and having more than 25 g fibre daily are, respectively, associated with a 31% and a 41% lower risk of being hospitalised with diverticular disease.[373] Not all studies found a correlation with fibre intake,[374] though this may be influenced by the lack of patients with a high fibre intake (above 25 g). Fibre may not only influence colonic transit time and stool bulk, but also play an important part in the microbiome health.

Age

The incidence of diverticular disease increases with age. Less than 10% of cases occur in those aged under 40 years compared with 50–60% in patients aged 80 years or older.[1]

Constipation and colonic motility

Longer transit times and lower volume stools may predispose to diverticular pockets. This leads to an increase in intraluminal pressure that may cause herniation of the bowel wall.[375] Bulkier stools are associated with less colonic contraction and lower wall pressures.[1] However this theory has been challenged with the prevalence of constipation among diverticular disease patients not varying substantially from the population.[376] More recent theories regarding the changed colonic motility in diverticular disease include alterations in connective tissue strength of the intestinal wall, neural and musculature function within the enteric nervous system, which may result in symptoms such as abdominal pain and visceral hypersensitivity.[377,378]

OBESITY

Obesity increases the risk of diverticulitis and diverticular bleeding. A cohort study found that an increased BMI, waist circumference and waist-to-hip ratio significantly increased the risk of developing diverticular disease. The researchers found that a BMI of >30 led to a relative risk of 1.78 for diverticulosis and 3.19 for diverticular bleeding.[379] Diverticular disease in younger patients (<40 years) is positively correlated with male gender and obesity.[380]

OTHER FACTORS

Changes to the microbiome composition in diverticular disease have not yet been researched; however, preliminary data suggest a greater diversity in the phylum Proteobacteria.[381] Genetics may also play a role in the susceptibility and development of diverticular disease in up to 40% of cases.[382]

Investigations

A full blood test may be useful especially to see the white cell counts and any markers of anaemia. A further iron studies test may be necessary if results indicate low iron status or if bleeding is suspected. Erythrocyte sedimentation rate and C-reactive protein may be useful to ascertain the degree of inflammation. Increased levels indicate inflammation. An iron studies test is done to evaluate iron levels. Ferritin levels should be included in this testing. However, high ferritin is often more of an indication of inflammation than of adequate iron status as ferritin is an acute phase protein. Always evaluate ferritin in light of all other iron parameters.

A barium enema, ultrasound, CT scan and colonoscopy can assess the presence of diverticular pockets.[1]

Therapeutic considerations

ALLOPATHIC TREATMENT

- Antibiotics are usually given if diverticulitis develops[383]
- Anti-inflammatories such as mesalazine[384]
- Surgery may be recommended for severe recurrent or complicated diverticulitis[383]
- Increased fibre intake may be recommended to prevent diverticulitis.

Therapeutic application

NUTRITIONAL MEDICINE (DIETARY)

Dietary therapeutic objectives

Specific dietary treatments are used primarily to prevent infection. Once the pockets are formed, the most important therapeutic objective is to improve motility.

Specific dietary treatments

DIETARY INCLUSIONS

Fibre

Fibre will increase the bulk of the stool, reduce transit time and decrease luminal pressure. A dose of 20–30 g of fibre a day is needed.[371] This can be achieved by increasing wholegrains, vegetables, fruits and legumes in the diet. This is by far the most important dietary intervention.

Ensure adequate hydration

Adequate water intake is essential for healthy bowel motility. Unfortunately many patients drink inadequate amounts of water yet this simple change can have a large therapeutic benefit. Aim for 2.5 L/day. This recommendation may need to be modified owing to weight, weather and exercise patterns.

Foods to avoid

A review found that a diet high in fat and red meat is associated with diverticular disease.[385] The same review found that a high-fibre diet is associated with a reduced risk. More studies on diverticulitis and diets high in fat and red meat consumption are warranted in order to understand the connection. It is also comprehensible that because high fat and meat diets contain insufficient amounts of fibre this could be a primary reason for the association.

OTHER DIETARY CONSIDERATIONS

- Foods high in fibre should be encouraged in the diet. Fruit, vegetables, wholegrains, legumes and beans can all be added to the diet to increase fibre content. This also encourages a combination of soluble and insoluble fibres.
- If the patient is overweight, weight-loss guidelines should be given.
- Adequate water intake to reduce constipation should also be recommended if required.

NUTRITIONAL MEDICINE (SUPPLEMENTAL)

Nutritional medicine therapeutic objectives

Nutritional treatment largely aims to prevent an acute attack of diverticulitis by reducing risk factors such as constipation. Anti-inflammatory nutrients may also be used at the time of an acute attack.

Specific nutrients required

FIBRE

If dietary fibre intake is low for any reason, supplementation may be necessary. Supplementing with a mix of insoluble and soluble fibres may be best. Insoluble fibres include cellulose, hemicelluloses and lignin, which are responsible for creating the structure of plant cell walls and include wheat bran and rice bran. Soluble fibres include pectins, gums and mucilage and are found mainly in plant cells. Examples include psyllium, oat bran and flaxseeds.

There is level B evidence to recommend psyllium for the treatment of constipation.[125] Any additional fibre supplementation must be started slowly and increased gradually with increasing water intake. While a mixture of both insoluble and soluble fibres is desirable it is probably insoluble fibre that has the most therapeutic benefit in constipation.[385]

PROBIOTICS

Probiotics may be useful to improve transit time if dysbiosis is present. A double blind, placebo-controlled, randomised study was conducted to investigate the effects of a probiotic beverage containing *Lactobacillus casei* Shirota in 70 patients with chronic constipation.[124] Patients were randomised to receive either 65 mL a day of the probiotic drink or placebo for 4 weeks. Consumption of the probiotic-containing beverage led to significant improvements in stool consistency in 89% of the probiotic group compared with 56% in the placebo group. Probiotics have several additional beneficial actions in the treatment of diverticular disease including altering the gut microbial balance leading to inhibition of bacterial overgrowth, reducing the metabolism of pathogens, and anti-inflammatory effects.[386] There have been numerous studies investigating the effectiveness of probiotics in the reduction of symptoms and episodes of acute diverticulitis. While results are promising, Lahner et al's recent systematic review concluded that there was still insufficient high-quality evidence to draw conclusions. The heterogeneity in probiotic strains used, the dosage, the combination with other drugs as well as the different outcome measures make conclusions more difficult. [386] Several open-label studies[387–389] and one double-blind, placebo-controlled trial,[378] using a variety of different probiotic strains, have found positive results in treating symptomatic uncomplicated diverticular disease, reducing symptoms and episodes of diverticulosis and maintaining remission. Strains that may be useful include *L. casei* subspp. DG, VSL#3 (composed of *L. casei, L. plantarum, L. acidophilus, L. delbrueckii* subspp. *Bulgaricus, B. longum, B. breve, B. infantis, Streptococcus salivarius* subspp. *thermophilus), Escherichia coli* Nissle 1917 and *Proteus vulgaris.*

ANTI-INFLAMMATORY NUTRIENTS

Anti-inflammatory nutrients such as coenzyme Q10, vitamin C, selenium, quercetin and bromelain may be useful in addition to antibiotics to decrease inflammation during an acute episode of diverticulitis. There is currently no research to support the use of these supplements in diverticular disease. However, traditionally they are used to reduce inflammation, improve immune system function and enhance healing.

Dosage requirement

- Probiotics: Multistrain product 25–50 × 10^9 organisms/day

HERBAL MEDICINE

Herbal medicine therapeutic objectives

Herbal medicine may be used to prevent an attack of diverticulitis or perhaps as an early stage intervention in mild cases.

Herbal medicine classes

BITTER HERBAL MEDICINES

To stimulate digestion, increase the release of bile and reduce transit time. Examples include *Berberis vulgaris, Gentiana lutea, Taraxacum officinale* and *Hydrastis canadensis.*

ANTIBACTERIAL HERBAL MEDICINES

To kill any pathogenic bacteria present. Examples include *Berberis vulgaris, Baptisia tinctoria, Myrica cerifera, Allium sativum, Commiphora molmol, Andrographis paniculata* and *Hydrastis canadensis.*

IMMUNE STIMULATING HERBAL MEDICINES

To improve immune system surveillance and function. Examples include *Echinacea* spp., *Thuja occidentalis* and *Phytolacca decandra.*

ANTI-INFLAMMATORY HERBAL MEDICINES

These include *Curcuma longa, Salix alba* and *Filipendula ulmaria* to decrease inflammation.

Specific herbal medicines

There are no clinical trials evaluating the effects of herbal medicine for diverticular disease. Below is a brief outline of some specific herbal medicines which, because of their actions, may be useful for the treatment of diverticulitis.

HYDRASTIS CANADENSIS (GOLDENSEAL)

While there is no research for the use of goldenseal in diverticular disease the herb boasts broad range antibacterial activity.[390] Goldenseal could therefore be useful for the treatment of active diverticulitis.

ECHINACEA PURPUREA/ANGUSTIFOLIA

Echinacea has a strong traditional use for the treatment of infection.[391] It is well known for its ability to stimulate immune function and also has anti-inflammatory and antioxidant properties. Echinacea could be useful for the treatment of active diverticulitis.

ALLIUM SATIVUM (GARLIC)

Garlic is antibacterial, antioxidant, anti-inflammatory and immune enhancing. It may consequently be useful in the treatment of active disease.

Dose: fresh garlic 2–5 g/day; make sure it is bruised or crushed. Tablets are often also used.

Dosage requirements

- *Hydrastis canadensis* (goldenseal): Tincture (1 : 3) 2.0–4.5 mL/day.[74]
- *Echinacea purpurea/angustifolia:* liquid extract (1 : 2) 10–20 mL/day if acute infection is present.

LIFESTYLE RECOMMENDATIONS

Exercise

Lack of physical activity affects transit time and can lead to constipation, a major risk factor for diverticular disease.[392,393] One study found that intense exercise (jogging and running) was much more significantly correlated with a decreased risk of developing symptomatic diverticular disease.[392]

Water intake

Patients should be encouraged to drink adequate water as dehydration commonly leads to constipation.

CASE STUDY

OVERVIEW

A 64-year-old woman presented with recurrent episodes of lower abdominal cramp-like pain. This had escalated in the

CASE STUDY CONTINUED

previous day, and she now also felt generally unwell. Her temperature was mildly elevated. She had also become prone to constipation, skipping 3 to 4 days without a bowel motion. She had a past history of IBS-mixed, and though this was largely resolved, she continued to avoid garlic and onion as these still caused significant bloating.

The increased intensity of pain, temperature and feeling unwell suggested pathology and was immediately referred for investigations and blood tests. Diverticulitis was diagnosed and she was admitted to hospital for intravenous antibiotics.

In a follow-up consultation 6 weeks later, she reported that despite initial improvement, she was still struggling with discomfort. She had been prescribed two courses of oral broad-spectrum antibiotics, which reduced symptoms but only short term. She had also found that she felt worse when she tried to eat a high-fibre diet and had subsequently reduced her food intake to one to two small meals a day. She had also added an over-the-counter laxative to reduce the risk of constipation.

Since retiring 4 years ago, her exercise levels had decreased significantly and she was eating out often when catching up with friends.

TREATMENT PROTOCOL

The initial treatment aimed to reduce the inflammation, muscle spasm, infection and intestinal luminal pressure and promote motility. Due to the recent reduction in food intake, supporting nutritional status was also important.

A herbal prescription was given as follows:

Rumex crispus 1 : 2 30 mL
Hydrastis canadensis 1 : 3 20 mL
Matricaria chamomilla 1 : 2 20 mL
Andrographis paniculate 1: 2 30 mL
5 mL 3 times daily

NUTRITIONAL MEDICINE PROTOCOL

Vitamin C 1 g was prescribed to assist the immune defences and reduce inflammation.

Zinc equivalent to 30 mg and vitamin A 2500 IU daily to support the epithelial lining and immune system.

It was recommended that fluid intake was increased to 2.5 L/day to maintain adequate systemic and luminal hydration. Foods were slowly increased, initially focusing on soups and smoothies, which could be consumed in small portions. Fibre intake was slowly increased using fruits, vegetables, nuts and seeds (especially crushed flaxseeds) and wholegrains. As she had lost a considerable amount of muscle, protein was increased (high-quality sources including fish and initially a supplement) along with beneficial fats to reduce inflammation, and maintain kilojoule requirements.

Exercise, with regular yoga and walking, was recommended to improve bowel tone and peristalsis. Areas addressed as she improved included pre- and probiotic foods to support the microbiome health and probiotic supplements to assist in reducing antibiotic-induced side effects.

GASTRO-OESOPHAGEAL REFLUX DISORDER

Epidemiology

Gastro-oesophageal reflux disease (GORD), informally known as heartburn, refers to the repeated exposure of the oesophagus to gastric contents leading to symptoms or histological changes. The highest prevalence levels of at least weekly symptoms are reported in Western countries such as the US (9.8%). Intermediate rates have been found in Europe and the Middle East (15.2% and 14.4% respectively), with East Asia reporting lower rates of prevalence (5.2%).[394] Worldwide incidence appears to be on the rise owing to obesity, increased longevity and the increased use of certain medications that affect oesophageal function.[395]

Classification

SIGNS AND SYMPTOMS

Symptoms include the sensation of burning in the oesophageal region, feeling of chest pain, chronic cough, chronic hoarseness, teeth erosion, water brash and, less frequently, angina-like pain, belching and queasiness. Sometimes the condition is asymptomatic. Dysphagia with weight loss, anaemia or bleeding needs to be referred in order to exclude strictures or oesophageal adenocarcinoma.[3]

COMPLICATIONS

The severity of GORD varies from non-erosive disease to erosive disease and in severe cases may develop into Barrett's oesophagus. Non-erosive disease is by far the most common presentation with one-third of patients having erosive disease.[3] Barrett's oesophagus is a primary risk factor for the development for oesophageal adenocarcinoma.[7] Patients without visible damage to the oesophagus have been referred to as having endoscopy negative reflux disease (ENRD).[396]

GORD is associated with reflux cough syndrome, reflux laryngitis syndrome, reflux asthma syndrome and reflux dental erosion syndrome.[7] Interestingly, other proposed associations include pharyngitis, sinusitis, idiopathic pulmonary fibrosis and recurrent otitis media.[7] The severity of oesophageal injury is established by undergoing an endoscopy.

DIFFERENTIAL DIAGNOSIS

Differential diagnoses that should be considered include gastritis, peptic ulcer disease, functional dyspepsia, Barrett's oesophagus, adenocarcinoma of the oesophagus, angina and myocardial infarct.

Aetiology and pathogenesis

LOWER OESOPHAGEAL SPHINCTER FUNCTION

Gastro-oesophageal reflux disease is most commonly caused by poor tone of the lower oesophageal sphincter allowing the reflux of gastric acid secretions into the oesophagus. The lower oesophageal sphincter is a segment of smooth muscle at the distal end of the oesophagus that acts as a physical barrier preventing the refluxing of gastric contents into the oesophagus.[397] This sphincter opens in response to peristalsis to allow food and liquids into the stomach. However, in gastro-oesophageal reflux disease, the sphincter opens at other times (commonly after meals) to allow the reflux of acidic gastric content. Some patients suffer from a permanent lack of sphincter tone.[397] Other factors that may contribute to reflux include reduced oesphageal peristalsis and the subsequent clearance of gastric contents, delayed gastric emptying and distension.

Symptoms are particularly bad when the patient is lying down and the chronic reflux may lead to severe oesophagitis or Barrett's oesophagus.

OBESITY

Obesity is associated with a statistically significant increase in the risk of developing gastro-oesophageal reflux disease.[398–400] It is also positively associated with an increase in adenocarcinoma.[401–403] A study found that the increased risk of adenocarcinoma appears to be independent of other associated risk factors such as smoking.[403] Patients with a BMI over 35 who also suffered from gastro-oesophageal reflux had a significantly higher risk of developing cancer than people with obesity but no reflux or those with reflux but no obesity. Insulin resistance, which is often increased in obesity, has also been found to be associated with GORD.[228]

AGE

A retrospective study of 1307 patients found that oesophageal exposure to acid increased proportionally with age. However, the severity of reflux symptoms appeared to decrease.[404] This was due to an age-related decrease in abdominal lower oesophageal sphincter length and oesophageal motility. Dysmotility exacerbated reflux in the supine position.

MEDICATIONS

Some medications that relax the lower oesophageal sphincter may increase the exposure of the oesophagus to gastric contents. In a Swedish study, five classes of medication were identified that all had well-documented evidence of relaxation effects on the sphincter. They were the nitroglycerins, anticholinergics, β-adrenergic agonists, xanthines, and the benzodiazepines. These classes of medications appear to also increase the risk of oesophageal adenocarcinoma.[405]

STRESS

Many patients report that stress worsens their reflux symptoms. A study of 56 patients with reflux found that acute auditory stress exacerbated heartburn symptoms by enhancing the perceptual response to intra-oesophageal acid exposure.[406] Stress does not appear to alter oesophageal motility.[407]

HYPOCHLORHYDRIA

The traditional naturopathic understanding of reflux is that low stomach acid is commonly to blame. This may be due to a variety of reasons including certain medications, ageing, stress and parasympathetic nervous system dysfunction. It is hypothesised that food is inadequately broken down and stays in the stomach for longer periods of time, leading to the refluxing of gastric contents into the oesophagus. Hypochlorhydria may also contribute to the overgrowth of *Helicobacter pylori* and small intestinal bacterial overgrowth due to the higher pH.

DIET

Patients commonly list foods that appear to increase their symptoms. For many patients this includes fatty foods, chocolate, coffee, alcohol, spicy foods and 'acidic' foods such as oranges and soft drinks. Large carbohydrate-based meals (pasta and bread) may also be problematic. Caffeine and alcohol are thought to reduce oesophageal sphincter pressure, while the acidic foods are thought to add to the acidity in the stomach.

Investigations

Diagnostic tests for gastro-oesophageal reflux disease include barium oesophagram, endoscopy, oesophageal mucosal biopsy and an empirical trial of proton pump inhibitors (PPIs).[7] A hydrogen breath test may also be recommended if peptic ulceration needs to be ruled out.

Therapeutic considerations

ALLOPATHIC TREATMENT

- Individuals with mild or transient reflux often use over-the-counter antacids and H_2 receptor antagonists (H_2RAs). Antacids are very popular as they quickly relieve heartburn. H_2RAs have a longer duration of action and appear to work better if taken before an event likely to cause reflux (e.g. a large meal).[7]
- Proton pump inhibitors (PPIs) are the mainstay of both acute and chronic reflux treatment. Their main advantage over the H_2RAs is that they are able to increase gastric pH for 15 to 21 hours as compared with 8 hours for H_2RAs.[7]
- Surgery may be offered in some cases.[7,397]

Therapeutic application

NUTRITIONAL MEDICINE (DIETARY)

Dietary therapeutic objectives

General therapeutic objectives include improving symptoms, reducing the risk of erosive disease and/or cancer and improving quality of life. Foods that precipitate attacks should be identified and reduced and weight reduction is important if necessary.

SPECIFIC DIETARY TREATMENTS

Avoid trigger foods

Even though patients commonly list foods such as chocolate, coffee, fatty meals and alcohol as reflux precipitators, research does not support the removal of these from the diet.[408] Many patients, however, describe symptom relief by avoiding these dietary factors.

Weight loss

Weight loss should be recommended for individuals who are overweight or obese.[409] Therefore a weight-loss diet should be prescribed for these patients. Regular consultations to ascertain progress and provide support are crucial. Dietary intervention studies evaluating weight loss as a therapeutic strategy need to be carried out in patients with GORD concomitant with obesity.

Apple cider vinegar

Apple cider vinegar may be useful to gently lower the pH of the stomach. Patients can start by adding a teaspoon of apple cider vinegar to a glass of water before meals. This dose can be increased to a tablespoon if needed.

Protein

If sphincter tone is problematic, amino acids may help to strengthen the connective tissue. A diet rich in protein is therefore recommended to ensure healthy collagen production.

OTHER DIETARY CONSIDERATIONS

- Increase protein in diet up to 0.8–1.2 g/kg to ensure healthy collagen production.
- Increase fresh fruit and vegetables to ensure adequate antioxidant, vitamin and mineral intake. Low intake of fruits and vegetables in the diet is positively associated with GORD, Barrett's oesophagus and oesophageal cancer.[410]
- Use only wholegrain carbohydrates, this will increase fibre and increase satiety. An increase in dietary fibre has been associated with lower rates of GORD.[411,412]
- Avoid any trigger foods that cause an episode of reflux or increase the severity such as high-fat foods.[413]
- Cut down or restrict coffee and alcohol as these beverages may increase the frequency and severity of reflux; however research is conflicting.[412,414] These beverages are best avoided in patients who report increasing incidence or severity with consumption. Alcohol may increase mucosal inflammation, impair oesphageal motility and the clearance of gastric contents, and increase the risk for Barrett's oesophagus and oesophageal cancer.[415]

NUTRITIONAL MEDICINE (SUPPLEMENTAL)

Nutritional medicine therapeutic objectives

General therapeutic objectives include improving symptoms, reducing the risk of erosive disease and/or cancer and improving quality of life. If acid suppression medication has been used for a long time, assess nutritional status of nutrients such as calcium, magnesium, vitamin B_{12} and iron levels[416] and treat accordingly.

Specific nutrients required

BETAINE HYDROCHLORIDE

If low stomach acid is the cause of the reflux symptoms, betaine hydrochloride may be useful. This may help to improve digestion and move food more efficiently through the stomach. Betaine hydrochloride should only be taken with protein-containing meals and the dose should be built up slowly.

OTHER NUTRIENTS

Although there is no research to support their use in GORD, zinc and vitamins B_1, B_3 and B_6 could be useful to increase hydrochloric production and improve digestion. Antioxidants such as quercetin, flavonoids, vitamin E,[417,418] lycopene,[419] and rutin[420] may also assist in reducing oesphageal inflammation and damage.

Dosage requirement

- Betaine hydrochloride: 400–800 mg/meal.

HERBAL MEDICINE

Herbal medicine therapeutic objectives

General therapeutic objectives include improving symptoms, reducing the risk of erosive disease and/or cancer and improving quality of life. Herbal medicine treatment aims to reduce the reflux of gastric contents, improve stomach function, reduce pain, soothe mucous membranes and heal the oesophageal mucosa. Support for stress tolerance may also be indicated.

Herbal medicine classes

ANTI-INFLAMMATORY HERBAL MEDICINES

To reduce inflammation in the stomach or duodenum. Examples include *Curcuma longa, Boswellia serrata, Filipendula ulmaria, Salix alba, Urtica dioica, Aloe vera.*

MUCOPROTECTIVE HERBAL MEDICINES

To protect the gastric mucosa from damage. Examples include *Ulmus rubra, Aloe vera, Althea officinalis* and *Glycyrrhiza glabra.*

DEMULCENT HERBAL MEDICINES

To soothe the lining of the stomach and duodenum. Examples include *Ulmus rubra, Althea officinalis* and *Glycyrrhiza glabra.*

MUCOUS MEMBRANE TONIC HERBAL MEDICINES

To strengthen the mucosa. Examples include *Hydrastis canadensis* and *Plantago major.*

VULNERARY HERBAL MEDICINES

These are used to heal the gastric mucosa. Examples include *Calendula officinalis, Achillea millefolium* and *Hydrastis canadensis.*

Specific herbal medicines

GLYCYRRHIZA GLABRA (LIQUORICE)

Liquorice has a mucoprotective effect as it increases mucus secretions from the gastric mucosa, enhancing cell proliferation and healing time.[60] Liquorice is also anti-inflammatory and anti-ulcer.[421,422] Glycerrhitinic acid and glycyrrhizic acid appear to be responsible for the anti-inflammatory effects of liquorice.[421,423]

Adverse effects of liquorice are very rare with short term use; however, longer periods of use may cause hypertension, hypokalaemia, hypercortisolism and pseudohyperaldosteronism associated with sodium retention, potassium loss and suppression of the renin-angiotensin-aldosterone system. High doses (110–900 g) of liquorice have been associated with visual disturbance in 5 patients.[60] If longer term use is warranted deglycyrrhizinised liquorice may be useful.

ALTHEA OFFICINALIS (MARSHMALLOW)

Marshmallow is known to contain between 5 and 10% polysaccharides making it both demulcent and vulnerary.[75] It provides a soothing and protective barrier on the mucous membrane of the oesophagus and stomach, which is why marshmallow has enjoyed a long history of use in reflux and gastritis. No clinical trials have investigated the effects of marshmallow in gastro-oesophageal reflux disease. Marshmallow appears to be safe and well tolerated.

Dose: (1 : 5) 3–6 mL/day.

ULMUS RUBRA (SLIPPERY ELM)

No research has been done to investigate the effects of slippery elm in reflux; however, the bark contains a very high percentage of polysaccharides, which are thought to be responsible for the demulcent, soothing and healing effects.

Slippery elm also contains tannins, which quite possibly also contribute to the healing/vulnerary action of slippery elm.

Slippery elm has traditionally been used to soothe irritated and inflamed tissues internally and externally. Slippery elm appears to be safe and well tolerated.

Dose: 1 teaspoon (5 g = 1 metric teaspoon) 3 times a day before meals.

CHAMOMILLA RECUTITA (CHAMOMILE)

Many constituents of chamomile have been found to be anti-inflammatory including the flavonoids apigenin, apigetrin, rutin and quercetin. Chamomile may also have anti-ulcer properties as the constituent bisabolol has been shown to inhibit gastric ulcers in vivo.[60] Chamomile has a long history of use as a sedative. It could therefore be quite useful in gastritis and reflux that is associated with stress or anxiety.

Adverse reactions are rare but may include allergic reactions (common among the Asteraceae family).[424] German chamomile, which is the type of chamomile generally used in Western herbal medicine, is thought to be less allergic than Roman chamomile.

Dose: (1 : 2) 3–6 mL/day.

LIFESTYLE RECOMMENDATIONS

Stop smoking

Being a current smoker is positively associated with GORD.[425]

Changes to sleep arrangement

Raise the foot of the bed by 15–20 cm. This appears to decrease the episodes of night reflux due to postural change.[408,426]

Lie on the left side while sleeping as much as possible as this position appears to alleviate reflux.[408]

Lose weight

Obesity is associated with an increase in GORD, both symptomatically and on histological examination.[398,408,427]

Dietary intake

Eat evening meal 2–3 hours before retiring as going to bed with a full stomach will increase the likelihood of reflux.[428]

Do not overeat as this will cause the stomach to distend, increasing symptoms.[428]

EAT SLOWLY

Increase saliva production, which is often reduced in GORD sufferers, by chewing food thoroughly to help increase oesophageal clearance of gastric contents.

Exercise

Regular exercise appears to be protective against GORD.[412,429]

ADEQUATE HYDRATION

Drink adequate water over the course of the day. Water consumption should reach 2–2.5 L for an adult. Always refrain, however, from drinking large amounts of water with meals.

CASE STUDY

OVERVIEW

Sally, aged 57 years, presented with excessive belching, a burning sensation in the chest and throat approximately 20 minutes after eating and being quick to feel full after eating, despite trying to eat slowly. She had a chronic cough, halitosis and her dentist had observed erosion of enamel on her teeth at a recent dental visit. Her upper digestive symptoms were worse in the afternoon and evening and after eating meals.

The current upper gastric issues had begun after a very stressful time personally. Sally was eating large amounts of bread and drinking five to six coffees a day. She had been trying to manage the symptoms with Mylanta®.

She was becoming anxious and worried about what she could eat that would not trigger her symptoms. A review of her diet showed she was still consuming gluten-free white bread each morning and at lunch, fried foods for the evening meal and coffee twice a day.

TREATMENT PROTOCOL

Treatment began with the removal of trigger foods and drinks. Sally replaced coffee with chamomile (*Chamomilla recutita*) tea.

CASE STUDY CONTINUED

Sally was referred for further investigations to rule out the possibility of *Helicobacter pylori* infection and she had her pancreatic elastase, faecal fats and faecal reducing sugars tested to further investigate her upper gastric function.

The following initial prescription was given to provide some symptom relief until all investigations were completed:

Althea officinale 30 mL
Chamomilla recutita 30 mL
Melissa officinalis 20 mL
Glycyrrhiza glabra 20 mL

Dose: 5 mL diluted 4 times a day before eating.

Slippery elm (*Ulmus rubra*) powder 1 teaspoon mixed with warm water into a slurry taken after each meal.

PEPTIC ULCER DISEASE

Classification

Peptic ulcer disease is the ulceration of the mucous membrane of the stomach or duodenum. The term peptic ulcer is used to describe ulcerations of the stomach while duodenal ulcers denote ulcers found just out of the stomach in the duodenum. Peptic ulcer disease was seen as a chronic incurable disease characterised by stomach pain and discomfort until it was discovered that *Helicobacter pylori* (*H. pylori*) and non-steroidal anti-inflammatory drugs (NSAIDs) were largely to blame. Over 90% of duodenal ulcer patients and 80% of peptic ulcer patients have this infection.[3]

SIGNS AND SYMPTOMS

The most common symptom of peptic ulceration is pain, which is often described as gnawing or burning. The pain may occur 1 to 3 hours after eating or when the stomach is completely empty. Other symptoms may include nausea, vomiting, anorexia and weight loss. The main complication of peptic ulcer disease is perforation and bleeding. It appears that bleeding occurs more commonly in patients using NSAIDs, regardless of *H. pylori* status.[430,431]

DIFFERENTIAL DIAGNOSIS

The primary differential diagnoses for peptic ulcer disease are gastritis, gastric metaplasia, pancreatitis, pancreatic cancer, dyspepsia, sliding hernia and Barrett's oesophagitis.

Investigations

- Radiography is still occasionally used but endoscopy is by far the most common diagnostic test used today.[1]
- 13C urea or 14C urea breath test for *H. pylori*. A small amount of 13C or 14C (radioactive) isotope-labelled urea is given orally and a breath sample is collected 20–30 minutes later. *H. pylori* produces vast amounts of urease which hydrolyses the labelled 13C or 14C to produce ammonia and carbon dioxide. A test is considered positive when labelled 13C is detected in the breath sample.[2] A positive result indicates the presence of *H. pylori*.

- Stool antigen test may be useful to diagnose active disease.[2]
- A histology and culture may be performed if an endoscopy has been undertaken.[2]

Aetiology and pathogenesis

Numerous factors are involved in the pathogenesis of peptic ulcer disease. Gastric secretions, refluxed bile, increased oxidative stress and inflammatory eicosanoids, reduced gastric mucus barrier and mucosal blood flow result in defective mucosal barrier function and subsequent injury.[432]

HELICOBACTER PYLORI

H. pylori is significantly associated with stomach and duodenal ulcers. Early reports suggested that the prevalence in peptic ulcer disease was 100%, more recent reports appear to suggest it is more likely 80% in gastric ulceration and 90% in duodenal ulcers.[3]

NON-STEROIDAL ANTI-INFLAMMATORY DRUGS (NSAIDs)

Aspirin and other NSAIDs are popular medications commonly used for the relief of pain and inflammation; however, the most common side effect is gastric ulceration which is induced by damage to the mucosa suppressing the cyclo-oxygenase pathway, inhibiting prostaglandins, neutrophil infiltration and oxidative stress, along with delaying gastric healing.[432] NSAID use is positively correlated with perforation and bleeding and there appears to be an additive risk if the patient is also infected with *H. pylori*.[431]

Additional risk factors for ulcer development among patients using NSAIDs include previous peptic ulcer disease, prior NSAID-induced gastric inflammation, advancing age, concomitant use of glucocorticoids, anticoagulants and alcohol.[1]

STRESS

Before the realisation that *H. pylori* and NSAIDs were responsible for most cases of gastric ulceration it was thought that stress played a major role. Although many studies have attempted to evaluate this they are largely flawed as most did not control for the presence of NSAID use or *H. pylori*. The incidence of *H. pylori* negative disease is between 5% and 20% and it is thought that perhaps stress may be a causative factor here.[433] Acute physiological stress results in increased gastric acid secretion, decreased blood flow to the mucosa, decreased production of the protective mucin and mucosal ulceration.[434] The effects of emotional stress on the gastric mucosa are not as well defined, although many patients hypothesise a correlation.

Therapeutic considerations

ALLOPATHIC TREATMENT

All cases of peptic ulcer disease associated with *H. pylori* are treated with a combination of antibacterial treatments and proton pump inhibitors.[2] Triple therapy is the first line of treatment (any proton pump inhibitor with clarithromycin, and amoxicillin or metronidazole) for 1 week and if treatment fails quadruple therapy or an alternative triple therapy will be offered.[2] Surgery may be offered in rare cases.

Therapeutic application

NUTRITIONAL MEDICINE (DIETARY)

Dietary therapeutic objectives

Good dietary practices are important. A diet rich in good quality protein, complex carbohydrate, fruit and vegetables will enhance general and immune system health and improve healing times. It is wise to avoid alcohol consumption if at risk of developing peptic ulcer disease.

SPECIFIC DIETARY TREATMENTS

- Increase protein in diet up to 0.8–1.2 g/kg to ensure healthy collagen production.
- Increase fresh fruit and vegetables to ensure adequate phytochemical, vitamin and mineral intake.
- Restrict substances that aggravate the gastric lining such as alcohol and smoking.
- Increase high antioxidant containing foods and beverages such as blueberries, garlic, chillies, turmeric and green tea.

NUTRITIONAL MEDICINE (SUPPLEMENTAL)

Nutritional medicine therapeutic objectives

Nutritional medicine treatment goals include improving healing time and improving immune system function.

Specific nutrients required

VITAMIN C

Vitamin C has traditionally been used to facilitate healing in any part of the body. A randomised, controlled trial involving 171 *H. pylori*-infected participants found that the addition of 500 mg of ascorbic acid twice daily to the triple therapy regimen decreased the amount of clarithromycin that patients needed to take. The high elimination efficacy for clarithromycin-susceptible *H. pylori* infection was maintained.[435]

The addition of ascorbic acid to the NSAID acetylsalicylic acid, was found to protect the gastric mucosa against ulceration in 10 healthy patients.[436] An older double blind, randomised, crossover study demonstrated that doses of 1 g, twice daily, of ascorbic acid had a protective effect against aspirin-induced duodenal injury.[437] More recently however, the addition of vitamin C (500 mg/day) for 30 days to triple and quadruple therapy, did not significantly improve *Helicobacter pylori* eradication rates.[438]

ESSENTIAL FATTY ACIDS

In vitro and in vivo evidence suggests that polyunsaturated fatty acids (PUFAs) inhibit the growth of *H. pylori* and may heal gastric ulcers.[439–442] In animal studies omega-3 has been demonstrated to reduce gastric epithelium injury induced by NSAIDs, alcohol and stress.[443] Potential benefits of omega-3 include reduction of mucosal damage via the suppression of inflammatory leukotrienes, counteracting apoptosis induced from oxidative stress and acid secretion, while increasing protective factors such as mucus secretion, antioxidant enzymes activity.[443] Clinical trial evidence is needed.

PROBIOTICS

Probiotics may be useful to assist with *H. pylori* eradication and to help re-inoculate the gastrointestinal tract after conventional treatment. In vivo data have shown that *L. rhamnosus* GG enhances gastric ulcer healing.[444]

A previous review of the efficacy of probiotics in the treatment of peptic ulceration found that seven out of nine human studies showed a decrease in the symptoms and population of *H. pylori.* The use of probiotics with standard treatment improved eradication rates (81% vs 71%) and antibiotic associated side effects (23% with probiotics vs 46% with combination therapy alone).[445] *Lactobacillus casei* and *Lactobacillus johnsonii* La1 appear to be the most researched strains.

A randomised controlled trial investigated the effects of *Clostridium butyricum* when used in addition to standard *H. pylori* eradication therapy on changes to the intestinal microbiota. Nineteen patients with gastroduodenal ulcer were randomly assigned to one of three groups: group A (standard treatment only), group B (standard treatment and *C. butyricum*) and group C (standard treatment plus double doses of *C. butyricum*). Diarrhoea and loose stools were reported as 43% in group A, 14% in group B and 0% in group C. Levels of obligate anaerobes in group C were significantly higher than in group A ($P < 0.05$) and *C. difficile* toxin A was detected in both group A and group B but not in group C, indicating that the probiotics may have prevented the growth of this potentially pathogenic microbe.[446] More recently a meta-analysis of 19 RCTs evaluated six multistrain probiotic mixtures as an adjunct to *H. pylori* eradication therapy. Eradication rates were increased to over 90% with mixtures of *L. acidophilus/B. animalis, L. helveticus/ L. rhamnosus,* and *L. acidophilus/B. longum/Enterococcus faecalis.* The majority of studies used doses of >1010 cfu/day for 3–5 weeks.[447] A meta-analysis of 25 RCTs of one of six single probiotic strains as an adjunct to standard therapy was conducted by the same group as above. The most commonly tested strain studied was *Saccharomyces boulardii (S. boulardii)* CNCM I-745 (39% of RCT treatment arms). This was the only strain to significantly increase *H. pylori* eradication rates, and also reduce adverse side effects associated with standard treatment.[447]

Other nutrients

Other nutrients such as zinc, glutamine and vitamin A may also be appropriate. It is generally thought that these substances help to heal the gastric mucosa. However, there is currently little research base to support this. Several studies have recently found lower serum zinc levels to be associated with greater risk of gastric mucosal damage.[448,449] Animal studies have also found zinc has a protective effect of alcohol induced gastric ulcers.[450,451]

Dosage requirements

- Vitamin C: 1 g 2 or 3 times a day
- Essential fatty acids: 3 g/day
- Probiotics: Doses depend on product used. Follow manufacturer's instructions.

HERBAL MEDICINE

Herbal medicine therapeutic objectives

Herbal medicine treatment aims to support and quicken healing of the gastric mucosa. Triple antibiotic therapy works well in a very short period of time and is therefore the most common treatment choice for most patients. Herbs with demonstrated anti-*H. pylori* activity may be used alongside conventional treatment to potentially improve the outcome. It would be interesting to see a clinical trial investigate the effects of triple antigen treatment with and without additional herbal medicines to see whether outcome measures such as *H. pylori* eradication and healing times are improved.

Herbal medicine classes

ANTI-INFLAMMATORY HERBAL MEDICINES

To reduce inflammation in the stomach or duodenum. Examples include *Curcuma longa, Boswellia serrata, Filipendula ulmaria, Salix alba, Urtica dioica, Aloe vera.*

MUCOPROTECTIVE HERBAL MEDICINES

To protect the gastric mucosa from damage. Examples include *Ulmus rubra, Aloe vera, Althea officinalis* and *Glycyrrhiza glabra.*

DEMULCENT HERBAL MEDICINES

To soothe the lining of the stomach and duodenum. Examples include *Ulmus rubra, Althea officinalis* and *Glycyrrhiza glabra.*

MUCOUS MEMBRANE TONIC HERBAL MEDICINES

To strengthen the mucosa. Examples include *Hydrastis canadensis* and *Plantago major.*

VULNERARY HERBAL MEDICINES

These are used to heal the gastric mucosa. Examples include *Calendula officinalis, Achillea millefolium* and *Hydrastis canadensis.*

Specific herbal medicines

CURCUMA LONGA (TURMERIC)

Turmeric has been shown to have a strong antibacterial effect against *H. pylori* in vitro.[452] A more recent in vivo study has demonstrated the antibacterial effects of the primary constituent, curcumin, against *H. pylori.*[453] However, a study involving 36 patients with *H. pylori*-induced gastritis found that those receiving the curcumin were less likely to have eradicated the infection compared to those treated with triple therapy (78.9% vs 5.9%).[454]

A phase II clinical trial investigated the effects of turmeric on the healing time of gastric ulcers in 25 patients.[455] Two capsules containing 300 mg of turmeric were given 5 times a day (total of 5 g/day) for between 4 and 12 weeks. After 4 weeks 48% of participants were ulcer free, after 8 weeks 72% were ulcer free and after 12 weeks 76% were ulcer free. Turmeric and curcumin appear to be safe and generally well tolerated.

Dose: 10–15 mL of a 1 : 1 liquid extract a day or 5 g of the powder. If using a curcumin-only product, 200 mg, 2 or 3 times a day is advisable.

GLYCYRRHIZA GLABRA (LIQUORICE)

Liquorice has a mucoprotective effect as it increases mucus secretions from the gastric mucosa, enhancing cell proliferation and healing time.[60] Liquorice is also anti-inflammatory and anti-ulcer.[421,422] Glycerrhitinic acid and glycyrrhizic acid appear to be responsible for the anti-inflammatory effects of liquorice.[421,423] In a recent RCT involving 120 patients with peptic ulcer disease or non-ulcer dyspepsia, liquorice (D-Reglis (380 mg b.i.d.) (in addition to triple therapy) was found to be effective in increasing the eradication of *H. pylori* compared to the control group (83.3% and 62.5%).[456]

BRASSICA OLERACEA (CABBAGE)

Drinking the juice from white cabbage leaves is a very traditional treatment for peptic ulcers. Two small clinical trials were performed in 1949 and 1956; however, no follow-up investigation has ever been conducted.[457,458] The trials on the whole were positive, showing that 100 mL a day of cabbage juice in divided doses effectively healed ulcers in 7–22 days.

ALOE VERA

Aloe vera is anti-inflammatory and both protective and healing to the gastric mucosa. Two in vivo studies demonstrated the healing effects of aloe in experimental models.[459,460] Both studies showed a reduction in TNF-α, while Eamlamnam et al also demonstrated improved gastric ulcer healing.[459]

Dose: (1 : 2) 1–3 mL 3 times per day.

CHAMOMILLA RECUTITA (CHAMOMILE)

Many constituents of chamomile have been found to be anti-inflammatory, including the flavonoids apigenin, apigetrin, rutin and quercetin. Chamomile may also have anti-ulcer properties as the constituent bisabolol has been shown to inhibit gastric ulcers in vivo.[60,461] Chamomile has a long history of use as a sedative. It could therefore be quite useful in peptic ulcer disease that is associated with stress or anxiety.

Dose: 1–3 mL of the 1 : 2 liquid extract 3 times a day.

LIFESTYLE RECOMMENDATIONS

The following lifestyle recommendations may help to reduce the incidence and symptoms of peptic ulcer disease:

- Reduce alcohol consumption as this directly irritates the stomach lining
- Stop smoking as this is positively linked to gastric ulcers and gastric cancer
- Reduce stress: e.g. meditation, yoga, tai chi, exercise may be useful to reduce daily stress levels
- Eliminate NSAIDs as they directly contribute to gastric ulceration
- Avoid coffee and caffeine
- Avoid foods that irritate the stomach.

CASE STUDY

OVERVIEW

A 39-year-old male presented with a history of gastric pain that started when he began his own business as a carpenter 5 years ago. He had mostly 'just put up with it', taking over-the-counter antacid medication when needed. However, following a big birthday celebration the pain was exacerbated, prompting him to seek investigations. On endoscopy a gastric ulcer was diagnosed, though he was negative for *H. pylori*. The pain had reduced with esomeprazole (Nexium) 20 mg/day, and he was motivated to prioritise his health, stop the medication as soon as possible, and prevent a recurrence. Other key aspects identified were a BMI of 35, a long history of smoking (since he was a teenager) and regular binge drinking. As he was working long hours, most meals were purchased (takeaway) or pre-made.

TREATMENT PROTOCOL

The initial focus of treatment was to support the healing of the gastric mucosa, reduce inflammation and to address the underlying causes.

A herbal prescription was given to sooth the lining, support the gastric circulation and production of mucus and improve his stress resilience.

Calendula officinalis 1 : 2 20 mL
Glycyrrhiza glabra 1 : 1 high-grade 25 mL
Matricaria chamomilla 1 : 2 30 mL
Withania somnifera 2 : 1 25 mL

Dose: 8 mL twice daily

Zinc carnosine was given 1 tablet twice daily to support the gastric mucosa, and omega-3 EPA/DHA (equivalent to 2 g) for reducing inflammation and nervous system support.

Lifestyle strategies to reduce stress levels and prompt blood flow to the digestive system were important in this case. Initially this consisted of deep breathing exercises, short meditations, and counselling to assist him to identify ways to cope with the challenges he faced with his business, and reduce binge drinking. His diet and eating habits were likely to be contributing to the development of the ulcer due to the poor nutrient content, the presence of components which trigger inflammation, and overall excessive portion sizes consumed. Initial strategies to address this included education on foods to include — fruit, vegetables, good quality protein and healthy fats. A handout was provided to assist in making healthier choices (including takeaway options) to increase antioxidants, reduce inflammation and provide nutrients needed for healing.

Follow-up recommendations also included strategies to support digestion and the proper breakdown of food, the health of the microflora balance, integrity of the gastric/intestinal epithelial lining, and improvement in body composition.

REFERENCES

[1] Feldman M, Friedman L, Brandt L. Sleisenger and Fortran's gastrointestinal and liver disease: pathophysiology, diagnosis and management. 8th ed. Philadelphia: Saunders; 2006.

[2] Talley N, Martin C. Clinical gastroenterology: a practical problem-based approach. 2nd ed. Sydney: Elsevier; 2006.
[3] Talley N, Segal I, Weltman M. Gastroenterology and hepatology: a clinical handbook. Sydney: Elsevier; 2008.
[4] Gibson PR, Newnham E, Barrett JS, et al. Review article: fructose malabsorption and the bigger picture. Aliment Pharmacol Ther 2007;25:349–63.
[5] Sydney-Smith M. Breath tests. J Comp Med 2008;7:35–40.
[6] Allen R. Gut permeability and intestinal dysbiosis. J Comp Med 2005;4:35–40.
[7] Richter JE. Gastro-oesophageal reflux disease. Best Pract Res Clin Gastroenterol 2007;21:609–31.
[8] Burney P, Summers C, Chinn S, et al. Prevalence and distribution of sensitization to foods in the European Community Respiratory Health Survey: a EuroPrevall analysis. Allergy 2010;65(9):1182–8.
[9] Savage J, Johns CB. Food allergy: epidemiology and natural history. Immunol Allergy Clin North Am 2015;35(1):45–59.
[10] Valenta R, Hochwallner H, Linhart B, et al. Food allergies: the basics. Gastroenterology 2015;148(6):1120–31.
[11] Ortolani C, Pastorello EA. Food allergies and food intolerances. Best Pract Res Clin Gastroenterol 2006;20:467–83.
[12] Samartín S, Marcos A, Chandra RK. Food hypersensitivity. Nutr Res 2001;21:473–97.
[13] Sampson HA. Update on food allergy. J Allergy Clin Immunol 2004;113:805–19, quiz 820.
[14] Sicherer SH, Sampson HA. Food allergy: epidemiology, pathogenesis, diagnosis, and treatment. J Allergy Clin Immunol 2014;133(2):291–307.
[15] Mocan O, Dumitraşcu DL. The broad spectrum of celiac disease and gluten sensitive enteropathy. Clujul Med 2016;89(3):335.
[16] Guandalini S, Assini A. Celiac disease — a review. JAMA Pediatr 2014;168:3.
[17] Kelly CP, Bai JC, et al. Advances in diagnosis and management of celiac disease. Gastroenterology 2015;148(6):1175–86.
[18] Sapone A, Bai JC, Ciacci C, et al. Spectrum of gluten-related disorders: consensus on new nomenclature and classification. BMC Med 2012;10(1):1.
[19] Berstad A, Arslan G, Lind R, et al. Food hypersensitivity — immunologic (peripheral) or cognitive (central) sensitisation? Psychoneuroendocrinology 2005;30:983–9.
[20] Gibson PR, Shepherd SJ. Food choice as a key management strategy for functional gastrointestinal symptoms. Am J Gastroenterol 2012;107(5):657–66, quiz 667.
[21] Nanayakkara WS, Skidmore PM, O'Brien L, et al. Efficacy of the low FODMAP diet for treating irritable bowel syndrome: the evidence to date. Clin Exp Gastroenterol 2016;9: 131–42.
[22] Savaiano D, Hertzler S, Jackson KA, et al. Nutrient considerations in lactose intolerance. Nutrition in the prevention and treatment of disease. San Diego: Academic Press; 2001.
[23] Suarez FL, Savaiano D, Arbisi P, et al. Tolerance to the daily ingestion of two cups of milk by individuals claiming lactose intolerance. Am J Clin Nutr 1997;65:1502–6.
[24] Pimentel M, Kong Y, Park S. Breath testing to evaluate lactose intolerance in irritable bowel syndrome correlates with lactulose testing and may not reflect true lactose malabsorption. Am J Gastroenterol 2003;98:2700–4.
[25] Petruláková M, Valík L. Food allergy and intolerance. Acta Chimica Slovaca 2015;8(1):44–51.
[26] Deng Y, Misselwitz B, Dai N, et al. Lactose intolerance in adults: biological mechanism and dietary management. Nutrients 2015;7(9):8020–35.
[27] Misselwitz B, Pohl D, Frühauf H, et al. Lactose malabsorption and intolerance: pathogenesis, diagnosis and treatment. United European Gastroenterol J 2013;1(3):151–9.
[28] Shaukat A, Levitt MD, Taylor BC, et al. Systematic review: effective management strategies for lactose intolerance. Ann Intern Med 2010;152(12):797–803.
[29] Fedewa A, Rao SS. Dietary fructose intolerance, fructan intolerance and FODMAPs. Curr Gastroenterol Rep 2014;16(1):1–8.
[30] Putkonen L, Yao CK, Gibson PR. Fructose malabsorption syndrome. Curr Opin Clin Nutr Metab Care 2013;16(4):473–7.
[31] Wong D. Hereditary fructose intolerance. Mol Genet Metab 2005;85:165–7.
[32] Gibson PR, Shepherd SJ. Personal view: food for thought — western lifestyle and susceptibility to Crohn's disease. The FODMAP hypothesis. Aliment Pharmacol Ther 2005;21:1399–409.
[33] Atkinson W, Sheldon TA, Shaath N, et al. Food elimination based on IgG antibodies in irritable bowel syndrome: a randomised controlled trial. Gut 2004;53:1459–64.
[34] Zar S, Benson MJ, Kumar D. Food-specific serum IgG4 and IgE titers to common food antigens in irritable bowel syndrome. Am J Gastroenterol 2005;100:1550–7.
[35] Zar S, Kumar D, Benson MJ. Food hypersensitivity and irritable bowel syndrome. Aliment Pharmacol Ther 2001;15:439–49.
[36] Zar S, Mincher L, Benson MJ, et al. Food-specific IgG4 antibody-guided exclusion diet improves symptoms and rectal compliance in irritable bowel syndrome. Scand J Gastroenterol 2005;40:800–7.
[37] du Toit G, Tsakok T, Lack S, et al. Prevention of food allergy. J Allergy Clin Immunol 2016;137(4):998–1010.
[38] Zhang GQ, Hu HJ, Liu CY, et al. Probiotics for prevention of atopy and food hypersensitivity in early childhood: a PRISMA-compliant systematic review and meta-analysis of randomized controlled trials. Medicine (Baltimore) 2016;95(8):e2562.
[39] Bai JC, Fried M, Corazza GR, et al. World Gastroenterology Organisation global guidelines on celiac disease. J Clin Gastroenterol 2013;47(2):121–6.
[40] Nasr I, Leffler DA, Ciclitira PJ. Management of celiac disease. Gastrointest Endosc Clin N Am 2012;22(4):695–704.
[41] Daley J. Managing a rotation diet. J Comp Med 2008;7: 26–30.
[42] Pizzorno J, Murray M. The textbook of natural medicine. 3rd ed. St Louis: Churchill Livingstone; 2006.
[43] Barrett JS, Gibson PR. Fermentable oligosaccharides, disaccharides, monosaccharides and polyols (FODMAPs) and nonallergic food intolerance: FODMAPs or food chemicals? Therap Adv Gastroenterol 2012;5(4):261–8.
[44] Latulippe ME, Skoog SM. Fructose malabsorption and intolerance: effects of fructose with and without simultaneous glucose ingestion. Crit Rev Food Sci Nutr 2011;51(7):583–92.
[45] Shepherd SJ, Parker FC, Muir JG, et al. Dietary triggers of abdominal symptoms in patients with irritable bowel syndrome: randomized placebo-controlled evidence. Clin Gastroenterol Hepatol 2008;6(7):765–71.
[46] Food Standards Australia and New Zealand (FSANZ). NUTTAB 2010 online searchable database. 2010. Available from: www.foodstandards.gov.au/science/monitoringnutrients/nutrientables/nuttab/Pages/default.aspx.
[47] Theethira TG, Dennis M, Leffler DA. Nutritional consequences of celiac disease and the gluten-free diet. Expert Rev Gastroenterol Hepatol 2014;8(2):123–9.
[48] Basivireddy J, Jacob M, Balasubramanian KA. Oral glutamine attenuates indomethacin-induced small intestinal damage. Clin Sci 2004;107:281–9.
[49] Salman B, Oguz M, Akmansu M, et al. Effect of timing of glutamine-enriched enteral nutrition on intestinal damage caused by irradiation. Adv Ther 2007;24:648–61.
[50] Peng X, Yan H, You Z, et al. Effects of enteral supplementation with glutamine granules on intestinal mucosal barrier function in severe burned patients. Burns 2004;30:135–9.
[51] Zhou YP, Jiang ZM, Sun YH, et al. The effect of supplemental enteral glutamine on plasma levels, gut function, and outcome in severe burns: a randomized, double-blind, controlled clinical trial. JPEN J Parenter Enteral Nutr 2003;27:241–5.
[52] Sturniolo GC, Di Leo V, Ferronato A, et al. Zinc supplementation tightens 'leaky gut' in Crohn's disease. Inflamm Bowel Dis 2001;7:94–8.
[53] Miraglia Del Giudice M, De Luca MG. The role of probiotics in the clinical management of food allergy and atopic dermatitis. J Clin Gastroenterol 2004;38:S84–5.
[54] Alberda C, Gramlich L, Meddings J, et al. Effects of probiotic therapy in critically ill patients: a randomized, double-blind, placebo-controlled trial. Am J Clin Nutr 2007;85:816–23.
[55] Garcia Vilela E, De Lourdes De Abreu Ferrari M, Oswaldo Da Gama Torres H, et al. Influence of *Saccharomyces boulardii* on the intestinal permeability of patients with Crohn's disease in remission. Scand J Gastroenterol 2008;43:842–8.

[56] Rosenfeldt V, Benfeldt E, Valerius NH, et al. Effect of probiotics on gastrointestinal symptoms and small intestinal permeability in children with atopic dermatitis. J Pediatr 2004;145:612–16.
[57] Bischoff SC, Barbara G, Buurman W, et al. Intestinal permeability — a new target for disease prevention and therapy. BMC Gastroenterol 2014;14(1):1.
[58] De Santis S, Cavalcanti E, Mastronardi M, et al. Nutritional keys for intestinal barrier modulation. Front Immunol 2015;6:612.
[59] Leeds JS, Hopper AD, Hurlstone DP, et al. Is exocrine pancreatic insufficiency in adult coeliac disease a cause of persisting symptoms? Aliment Pharmacol Ther 2007;25(3):265–71.
[60] Braun L, Cohen M. Herbs and natural supplements: an evidence-based guide. 3rd ed. Sydney: Elsevier; 2010.
[61] Johri RK, Zutshi U, Kameshwaran L, et al. Effect of quercetin and *Albizzia* saponins on rat mast cell. Indian J Physiol Pharmacol 1985;29:43–6.
[62] Tripathi RM, Sen PC, Das PK. Studies on the mechanism of action of *Albizzia lebbeck*, an Indian indigenous drug used in the treatment of atopic allergy. J Ethnopharmacol 1979;1:385–96.
[63] Resmi CR, Venukumar MR, Latha MS. Antioxidant activity of *Albizzia lebbeck* (Linn.) Benth in alloxan diabetic rats. Indian J Physiol Pharmacol 2006;50:297–302.
[64] Gupta RS, Chaudhary R, Yadav RK, et al. Effect of saponins of *Albizzia lebbeck* (L.) benth bark on the reproductive system of male albino rats. J Ethnopharmacol 2005;96:31–6.
[65] Gupta RS, Kachhawa JB, Chaudhary R. Antispermatogenic, antiandrogenic activities of *Albizia lebbeck* (L.) benth bark extract in male albino rats. Phytomedicine 2006;13:277–83.
[66] Hsieh CJ, Hall K, Ha T, et al. Baicalein inhibits IL-1beta- and TNF-alpha-induced inflammatory cytokine production from human mast cells via regulation of the NF-kappaB pathway. Clin Mol Allergy 2007;5:5.
[67] Woo KJ, Lim JH, Suh SI, et al. Differential inhibitory effects of baicalein and baicalin on LPS-induced cyclooxygenase-2 expression through inhibition of C/EBPbeta DNA-binding activity. Immunobiology 2006;211:359–68.
[68] Kimata M, Shichijo M, Miura T, et al. Effects of luteolin, quercetin and baicalein on immunoglobulin E-mediated mediator release from human cultured mast cells. Clin Exp Allergy 2000;30:501–8.
[69] Kimata M, Inagaki N, Nagai H. Effects of luteolin and other flavonoids on IgE-mediated allergic reactions. Planta Med 2000;66:25–9.
[70] Goun E, Cunningham G, Chu D, et al. Antibacterial and antifungal activity of Indonesian ethnomedical plants. Fitoterapia 2003;74:592–6.
[71] Jagetia GC, Baliga MS. The evaluation of nitric oxide scavenging activity of certain Indian medicinal plants in vitro: a preliminary study. J Med Food 2004;7:343–8.
[72] Ganguly T, Badheka LP, Sainis KB. Immunomodulatory effect of *Tylophora indica* on Con A induced lymphoproliferation. Phytomedicine 2001;8:431–7.
[73] Ganguly T, Khar A. Induction of apoptosis in a human erythroleukemic cell line K562 by tylophora alkaloids involves release of cytochrome c and activation of caspase 3. Phytomedicine 2002;9:288–95.
[74] Bone K. A clinical guide to blending liquid herbs. St Louis: Elsevier; 2003.
[75] Mills S, Bone K. The essential guide to herbal safety. St Louis: Elsevier; 2005.
[76] Broer J, Behnke B. Immunosuppressant effect of IDS 30, a stinging nettle leaf extract, on myeloid dendritic cells in vitro. J Rheumatol 2002;29:659–66.
[77] Konrad A, Mahler M, Arni S, et al. Ameliorative effect of IDS 30, a stinging nettle leaf extract, on chronic colitis. Int J Colorectal Dis 2005;20:9–17.
[78] Mittman P. Randomized, double-blind study of freeze-dried *Urtica dioica* in the treatment of allergic rhinitis. Planta Med 1990;56:44–7.
[79] Lovell RM, Ford AC. Global prevalence of and risk factors for irritable bowel syndrome: a meta-analysis. Clin Gastroenterol Hepatol 2012;10(7):712–21.
[80] Spiller R. Clinical update: irritable bowel syndrome. Lancet 2007;369:1586–8.
[81] Ohman L, Simren M. New insights into the pathogenesis and pathophysiology of irritable bowel syndrome. Dig Liver Dis 2007;39:201–15.
[82] Gilkin RJ Jr. The spectrum of irritable bowel syndrome: a clinical review. Clin Ther 2005;27:1696–709.
[83] Garvin B, Wiley JW. The role of serotonin in irritable bowel syndrome: implications for management. Curr Gastroenterol Rep 2008;10:363–8.
[84] Spiller R. Recent advances in understanding the role of serotonin in gastrointestinal motility in functional bowel disorders: alterations in 5-HT signalling and metabolism in human disease. Neurogastroenterol Motil 2007;19(Suppl. 2):25–31.
[85] Coates MD, Mahoney CR, Linden DR, et al. Molecular defects in mucosal serotonin content and decreased serotonin reuptake transporter in ulcerative colitis and irritable bowel syndrome. Gastroenterology 2004;126:1657–64.
[86] Mawe GM, Coates MD, Moses PL. Review article: intestinal serotonin signalling in irritable bowel syndrome. Aliment Pharmacol Ther 2006;23:1067–76.
[87] Coates MD, Johnson AC, Greenwood-Van Meerveld B, et al. Effects of serotonin transporter inhibition on gastrointestinal motility and colonic sensitivity in the mouse. Neurogastroenterol Motil 2006;18:464–71.
[88] Spiller RC. Role of infection in irritable bowel syndrome. J Gastroenterol 2007;42(Suppl. 17):41–7.
[89] Borgaonkar MR, Ford DC, Marshall JK, et al. The incidence of irritable bowel syndrome among community subjects with previous acute enteric infection. Dig Dis Sci 2006;51:1026–32.
[90] Rhodes DY, Wallace M. Post-infectious irritable bowel syndrome. Curr Gastroenterol Rep 2006;8:327–32.
[91] Marshall JK, Thabane M, Garg AX, et al. and Walkerton Health Study Investigators. Eight year prognosis of postinfectious irritable bowel syndrome following waterborne bacterial dysentery. Gut 2010;59(5):605–11.
[92] Hawrelak JA, Myers SP. The causes of intestinal dysbiosis: a review. Altern Med Rev 2004;9:180–97.
[93] Simrén M, Barbara G, Flint HJ, et al. Intestinal microbiota in functional bowel disorders: a Rome foundation report. Gut 2013;62(1):159–76.
[94] Esposito I, de Leone A, Di Gregorio G, et al. Breath test for differential diagnosis between small intestinal bacterial overgrowth and irritable bowel disease: an observation on non-absorbable antibiotics. World J Gastroenterol 2007;13(45):6016–21.
[95] Majewski M, McCallum RW. Results of small intestinal bacterial overgrowth testing in irritable bowel syndrome patients: clinical profiles and effects of antibiotic trial. Adv Med Sci 2007;52:139–42.
[96] Weinstock LB, Klutke CG, Lin HC. Small intestinal bacterial overgrowth in patients with interstitial cystitis and gastrointestinal symptoms. Dig Dis Sci 2008;53(5):1246–51.
[97] Lin HC. Small intestinal bacterial overgrowth: a framework for understanding irritable bowel syndrome. JAMA 2004;292(7):852–8.
[98] Pimentel M, Wallace D, Hallegua D, et al. A link between irritable bowel syndrome and fibromyalgia may be related to findings on lactulose breath testing. Ann Rheum Dis 2004;63(4):450–2.
[99] Resmini E, Parodi A, Savarino V, et al. Evidence of prolonged orocecal transit time and small intestinal bacterial overgrowth in acromegalic patients. J Clin Endocrinol Metab 2007;92(6):2119–24.
[100] Tursi A, Brandimarte G, Giorgetti GM, et al. Assessment of small intestinal bacterial overgrowth in uncomplicated acute diverticulitis of the colon. World J Gastroenterol 2005;11(18):2773–6.
[101] Weinstock LB, Fern SE, Duntley SP. Restless legs syndrome in patients with irritable bowel syndrome: response to small intestinal bacterial overgrowth therapy. Dig Dis Sci 2008;53(5):1252–6.
[102] Ong DK, Mitchell SB, Barrett JS, et al. Manipulation of dietary short chain carbohydrates alters the pattern of gas production and genesis of symptoms in irritable bowel syndrome. J Gastroenterol Hepatol 2010;25(8):1366–73.
[103] Staudacher HM, Lomer MC, Anderson JL, et al. Fermentable carbohydrate restriction reduces luminal bifidobacteria and gastrointestinal symptoms in patients with irritable bowel syndrome. J Nutr 2012;142(8):1510–18.
[104] Halmos EP, Power VA, Shepherd SJ, et al. A diet low in FODMAPs reduces symptoms of irritable bowel syndrome. Gastroenterology 2014;146(1):67–75.
[105] Pedersen N, Andersen NN, Végh Z, et al. Ehealth: low FODMAP diet vs *Lactobacillus rhamnosus* GG in irritable bowel syndrome. World J Gastroenterol 2014;20(43):16215–26.
[106] Böhn L, Störsrud S, Liljebo T, et al. Diet low in FODMAPs reduces symptoms of irritable bowel syndrome as well as traditional

dietary advice: a randomized controlled trial. Gastroenterology 2015;149(6):1399–407.
[107] Shepherd SJ, Gibson PR. Fructose malabsorption and symptoms of irritable bowel syndrome: guidelines for effective dietary management. J Am Diet Assoc 2006;106:1631–9.
[108] Staudacher HM, Whelan K, Irving PM, et al. Comparison of symptom response following advice for a diet low in fermentable carbohydrates (FODMAPs) versus standard dietary advice in patients with irritable bowel syndrome. J Hum Nutr Diet 2011;24(5):487–95.
[109] Ostgaard H, Hausken T, Gundersen D, et al. Diet and effects of diet management on quality of life and symptoms in patients with irritable bowel syndrome. Mol Med Rep 2012;5(6):1382–90.
[110] Mazzawi T, Hausken T, Gundersen D, et al. Effects of dietary guidance on the symptoms, quality of life and habitual dietary intake of patients with irritable bowel syndrome. Mol Med Rep 2013;8(3):845–52.
[111] Roest RD, Dobbs BR, Chapman BA, et al. The low FODMAP diet improves gastrointestinal symptoms in patients with irritable bowel syndrome: a prospective study. Int J Clin Pract 2013;67(9):895–903.
[112] Wilder-Smith CH, Materna A, Wermelinger C, et al. Fructose and lactose intolerance and malabsorption testing: the relationship with symptoms in functional gastrointestinal disorders. Aliment Pharmacol Ther 2013;37(11):1074–83.
[113] Pedersen N, Vegh Z, Burisch J, et al. Ehealth monitoring in irritable bowel syndrome patients treated with low fermentable oligo-, di-, mono-saccharides and polyols diet. World J Gastroenterol 2014a;20(21):6680–4.
[114] Vazquez–Roque MI, Camilleri M, Smyrk T, et al. A controlled trial of gluten-free diet in patients with irritable bowel syndrome-diarrhea: effects on bowel frequency and intestinal function. Gastroenterology 2013;144(5):903–11.
[115] Biesiekierski JR, Peters SL, Newnham ED, et al. No effects of gluten in patients with self-reported non-celiac gluten sensitivity after dietary reduction of fermentable, poorly absorbed, short-chain carbohydrates. Gastroenterology 2013;145(2):320–8.
[116] McFarland LV, Dublin S. Meta-analysis of probiotics for the treatment of irritable bowel syndrome. World J Gastroenterol 2008;14:2650–61.
[117] Didari T, Mozaffari S, Nikfar S, et al. Effectiveness of probiotics in irritable bowel syndrome: updated systematic review with meta-analysis. World J Gastroenterol 2015;21(10):3072–84.
[118] Kim HJ, Camilleri M, McKinzie S, et al. A randomized controlled trial of a probiotic, VSL#3, on gut transit and symptoms in diarrhoea-predominant irritable bowel syndrome. Aliment Pharmacol Ther 2003;17:895–904.
[119] Kim HJ, Vazquez Roque MI, Camilleri M, et al. A randomized controlled trial of a probiotic combination VSL#3 and placebo in irritable bowel syndrome with bloating. Neurogastroenterol Motil 2005;17:687–96.
[120] Whorwell PJ, Altringer L, Morel J, et al. Efficacy of an encapsulated probiotic *Bifidobacterium infantis* 35624 in women with irritable bowel syndrome. Am J Gastroenterol 2006;101:1581–90.
[121] Ducrotté P, Sawant P, Jayanthi V. Clinical trial: *Lactobacillus plantarum*299v (DSM 9843) improves symptoms of irritable bowel syndrome. World J Gastroenterol 2012;18(30):4012–18.
[122] Niedzielin K, Kordecki H, Birkenfeld B. A controlled, double-blind, randomized study on the efficacy of *Lactobacillus plantarum* 299V in patients with irritable bowel syndrome. Eur J Gastroenterol Hepatol 2001;13:1143–7.
[123] Nobaek S, Johansson ML, Molin G, et al. Alteration of intestinal microflora is associated with reduction in abdominal bloating and pain in patients with irritable bowel syndrome. Am J Gastroenterol 2000;95:1231–8.
[124] Koebnick C, Wagner I, Leitzmann P, et al. Probiotic beverage containing *Lactobacillus casei* Shirota improves gastrointestinal symptoms in patients with chronic constipation. Can J Gastroenterol 2003;17:655–9.
[125] Ramkumar D, Rao SS. Efficacy and safety of traditional medical therapies for chronic constipation: systematic review. Am J Gastroenterol 2005;100:936–71.
[126] Moayyedi P, Quigley EM, Lacy BE, et al. The effect of fiber supplementation on irritable bowel syndrome: a systematic review and meta-analysis. Am J Gastroenterol 2014;109(9):1367–74.
[127] Pittler MH, Ernst E. Peppermint oil for irritable bowel syndrome: a critical review and meta-analysis. Am J Gastroenterol 1998;93:1131–5.
[128] Cash BD, Epstein MS, Shah SM. A novel delivery system of peppermint oil is an effective therapy for irritable bowel syndrome symptoms. Dig Dis Sci 2016;61(2):560–71.
[129] Walker AF, Middleton RW, Petrowicz O. Artichoke leaf extract reduces symptoms of irritable bowel syndrome in a post-marketing surveillance study. Phytother Res 2001;15:58–61.
[130] Marakis G, Walker AF, Middleton RW, et al. Artichoke leaf extract reduces mild dyspepsia in an open study. Phytomedicine 2002;9:694–9.
[131] Holtmann G, Adam B, Haag S, et al. Efficacy of artichoke leaf extract in the treatment of patients with functional dyspepsia: a six-week placebo-controlled, double-blind, multicentre trial. Aliment Pharmacol Ther 2003;18:1099–105.
[132] Yamada K, Miura T, Mimaki Y, et al. Effect of inhalation of chamomile oil vapour on plasma ACTH level in ovariectomized-rat under restriction stress. Biol Pharm Bull 1996;19:1244–6.
[133] Bundy R, Walker AF, Middleton RW, et al. Turmeric extract may improve irritable bowel syndrome symptomatology in otherwise healthy adults: a pilot study. J Altern Complement Med 2004;10:1015–18.
[134] Mozaffari S, Esmaily H, Rahimi R, et al. Effects of *Hypericum perforatum* extract on rat irritable bowel syndrome. Pharmacogn Mag 2011;7(27):213.
[135] Wan H, Chen Y. Effects of antidepressive treatment of Saint John's wort extract related to autonomic nervous function in women with irritable bowel syndrome. Int J Psychiatry Med 2010;40(1):45–56.
[136] Saito YA, Rey E, Almazar-Elder AE, et al. A randomized, double-blind, placebo-controlled trial of St John's wort for treating irritable bowel syndrome. Am J Gastroenterol 2010;105(1):170–7.
[137] Kim YJ, Ban DJ. Prevalence of irritable bowel syndrome, influence of lifestyle factors and bowel habits in Korean college students. Int J Nurs Stud 2005;42:247–54.
[138] Levy RL, Linde JA, Feld KA, et al. The association of gastrointestinal symptoms with weight, diet, and exercise in weight-loss program participants. Clin Gastroenterol Hepatol 2005;3:992–6.
[139] Faresjo A, Grodzinsky E, Johansson S, et al. Psychosocial factors at work and in every day life are associated with irritable bowel syndrome. Eur J Epidemiol 2007;22:473–80.
[140] Hertig VL, Cain KC, Jarrett ME, et al. Daily stress and gastrointestinal symptoms in women with irritable bowel syndrome. Nurs Res 2007;56:399–406.
[141] Murray CD, Flynn J, Ratcliffe L, et al. Effect of acute physical and psychological stress on gut autonomic innervation in irritable bowel syndrome. Gastroenterology 2004;127:1695–703.
[142] Gabrielli M, D'angelo G, Di Rienzo T, et al. Diagnosis of small intestinal bacterial overgrowth in the clinical practice. Eur Rev Med Pharmacol Sci 2013;17(Suppl. 2):30–5.
[143] Ford AC, Spiegel BM, Talley NJ, et al. Small intestinal bacterial overgrowth in irritable bowel syndrome: systematic review and meta-analysis. Clin Gastroenterol Hepatol 2009;7(12):1279–86.
[144] Tursi A, Brandimarte G, Giorgetti G. High prevalence of small intestinal bacterial overgrowth in celiac patients with persistence of gastrointestinal symptoms after gluten withdrawal. Am J Gastroenterol 2003;98(4):839–43.
[145] Tursi A, Brandimarte G, Elisei W, et al. Assessment of small intestinal bacterial overgrowth in uncomplicated acute diverticulitis of the colon. World J Gastroenterol 2005;11(18):2773–6.
[146] Trespi E, Ferrieri A. Intestinal bacterial overgrowth during chronic pancreatitis. Curr Med Res Opin 1999;15(1):47–52.
[147] Fridge JL, Conrad C, Gerson L, et al. Risk factors for small bowel bacterial overgrowth in cystic fibrosis. J Pediatr Gastroenterol Nutr 2007;44(2):212–18.
[148] George NS, Sankineni A, Parkman HP. Small intestinal bacterial overgrowth in gastroparesis. Dig Dis Sci 2014;59(3):645–52.
[149] Grace E, Shaw C, Whelan K, et al. Review article: small intestinal bacterial overgrowth — prevalence, clinical features, current and developing diagnostic tests, and treatment. Aliment Pharmacol Ther 2013;38(7):674–88.
[150] Bures J, Cyrany J, Kohoutova D, et al. Small intestinal bacterial overgrowth syndrome. World J Gastroenterol 2010;16(24): 2978–90.

[151] Bohm M, Siwiec RM, Wo JM. Diagnosis and management of small intestinal bacterial overgrowth. Nutr Clin Pract 2013;28(3):289–99.
[152] Chuoung RS, Ruff KC, Malhorta A, et al. Clinical predictors of small intestinal bacterial overgrowth by duodenal aspirate culture. Aliment Pharmacol Ther 2011;9:1059–67.
[153] Ghoshal UC, Ghoshal U, Misra A, et al. Partially responsive celiac disease resulting from small intestinal bacterial overgrowth and lactose intolerance. BMC Gastroenterol 2004;4(1):1.
[154] Parodi A, Dulbecco P, Savarino E, et al. Positive glucose breath testing is more prevalent in patients with IBS-like symptoms compared with controls of similar age and gender distribution. J Clin Gastroenterol 2009;43(10):962–6.
[155] Jacobs C, Coss Adame E, Attaluri A, et al. Dysmotility and proton pump inhibitor use are independent risk factors for small intestinal bacterial and/or fungal overgrowth. Aliment Pharmacol Ther 2013;37(11):1103–11.
[156] Lombardo L, Foti M, Ruggia O, et al. Increased incidence of small intestinal bacterial overgrowth during proton pump inhibitor therapy. Clin Gastroenterol Hepatol 2010;8(6):504–8.
[157] Nucera G, Gabrielli M, Lupascu A, et al. Abnormal breath tests to lactose, fructose and sorbitol in irritable bowel syndrome may be explained by small intestinal bacterial overgrowth. Aliment Pharmacol Ther 2005;21(11):1391–5.
[158] Dukowicz AC, Lacy BE, Levine GM. Small intestinal bacterial overgrowth: a comprehensive review. Gastroenterol Hepatol 2007;3(2):112.
[159] Rana SV, Sharma S, Kaur J, et al. Comparison of lactulose and glucose breath test for diagnosis of small intestinal bacterial overgrowth in patients with irritable bowel syndrome. Digestion 2012;85(3):243–7.
[160] Khoshini R, Dai SC, Lezcano S, et al. A systematic review of diagnostic tests for small intestinal bacterial overgrowth. Dig Dis Sci 2008;53(6):1443–54.
[161] Huang H, Chen L, Zhang B, et al. Clinical value of radionuclide small intestine transit time measurement combined with lactulose hydrogen breath test for the diagnosis of bacterial overgrowth in irritable bowel syndrome. Hell J Nucl Med 2016;19(2):124–9.
[162] Rana SV, Malik A. Hydrogen breath tests in gastrointestinal diseases. Indian J Clin Biochem 2014;29(4):398–405.
[163] Yu D, Cheeseman F, Vanner S. Combined oro-caecal scintigraphy and lactulose hydrogen breath testing demonstrate that breath testing detects oro-caecal transit, not small intestinal bacterial overgrowth in patients with IBS. Gut 2011;60(3):334–40.
[164] Ojetti V, Lauritano EC, Barbaro F, et al. Rifaximin pharmacology and clinical applications. Expert Opin Drug Metab Toxicol 2009;6:675–82.
[165] Gaon D, Garmendia C, Murrielo NO, et al. Effect of *Lactobacillus* strains (*L. casei, L. acidophilus* strains CERELA) on bacterial overgrowth-related chronic diarrhea. Medicina (B Aires) 2002;62(2):159–63.
[166] Soifer LO, Peralta D, Dima G, et al. [Comparative clinical efficacy of a probiotic vs. an antibiotic in the treatment of patients with intestinal bacterial overgrowth and chronic abdominal functional distension: a pilot study]. Acta Gastroenterol Latinoam 2010;40(4):323–7.
[167] Zhao Y, Yu YB. Intestinal microbiota and chronic constipation. Springerplus 2016;5(1):1130.
[168] Kwak DS, Jun DW, Seo JG, et al. Short-term probiotic therapy alleviates small intestinal bacterial overgrowth, but does not improve intestinal permeability in chronic liver disease. Eur J Gastroenterol Hepatol 2014;26(12):1353–9.
[169] Dai C, Zheng CQ, Jiang M, et al. Probiotics and irritable bowel syndrome. World J Gastroenterol 2013;19(36):5973–80.
[170] Goulet O, Joly F. Intestinal microbiota in short bowel syndrome. Gastroenterol Clin Biol 2010;34:S37–43.
[171] Furnari M, Parodi A, Gemignani L, et al. Clinical trial: the combination of rifaximin with partially hydrolysed guar gum is more effective than rifaximin alone in eradicating small intestinal bacterial overgrowth. Aliment Pharmacol Ther 2010;32(8):1000–6.
[172] Ohashi Y, Sumitani K, Tokunaga M, et al. Consumption of partially hydrolysed guar gum stimulates Bifidobacteria and butyrate-producing bacteria in the human large intestine. Benef Microbes 2015;6(4):451–5.
[173] Kurtovic J, Segal I, Riordan SM, et al. Culture-proven small intestinal bacterial overgrowth as a cause of irritable bowel syndrome: response to lactulose but not broad spectrum antibiotics. J Gastroenterol 2005;40(7):767–8.
[174] Mwenya B, Santoso B, Sar C, et al. Effects of including β1–4 galacto-oligosaccharides, lactic acid bacteria or yeast culture on methanogenesis as well as energy and nitrogen metabolism in sheep. Anim Feed Sci Technol 2004;115(3):313–26.
[175] Bhatta R, Baruah L, Saravanan M, et al. Effect of medicinal and aromatic plants on rumen fermentation, protozoa population and methanogenesis in vitro. J Anim Physiol Anim Nutr (Berl) 2013;97(3):446–56.
[176] Chedid V, Dhalla S, Clarke JO, et al. Herbal therapy is equivalent to rifaximin for the treatment of small intestinal bacterial overgrowth. Glob Adv Health Med 2014;3(3):16–24.
[177] Logan AC, Beaulne TM. The treatment of small intestinal bacterial overgrowth with enteric coated peppermint oil. a case report. (Peppermint oil). Altern Med Rev 2002;7(5):410–17.
[178] Clark CG, van der Giezen M, Alfellani MA, et al. Recent developments in *Blastocystis* research. Adv Parasitol 2013;82:1–32.
[179] Hawrelak J. Giardiasis: pathophysiology and management. (Giardiasis). Altern Med Rev 2003;8(2):129–43.
[180] Ramirez-Miranda ME, Hernandez-Castellanos R, Lopez-Escamilla E, et al. Parasites in Mexican patients with irritable bowel syndrome: a case-control study. Parasit Vectors 2010;3(3):96.
[181] Surangsrirat S, Thamrongwittawatpong L, Piyaniran W, et al. Assessment of the association between *Blastocystis* infection and irritable bowel syndrome. J Med Assoc Thai 2010;93(Suppl. 6):S119–24.
[182] Chen XM, Keithly JS, Paya CV, et al. Cryptosporidiosis. N Engl J Med 2002;346(22):1723–31.
[183] Blaser MJ. Epidemiologic and clinical features of *Campylobacter jejuni* infections. J Infect Dis 1997;176(Suppl. 2):S103–5.
[184] Barratt JL, Harkness J, Marriott D, et al. A review of *Dientamoeba fragilis* carriage in humans: several reasons why this organism should be considered in the diagnosis of gastrointestinal illness. Gut Microbes 2011;2(1):3–12.
[185] Noël C, Dufernez F, Gerbod D, et al. Molecular phylogenies of *Blastocystis* isolates from different hosts: implications for genetic diversity, identification of species, and zoonosis. J Clin Microbiol 2005;43(1):348–55.
[186] Parkar U, Traub RJ, Kumar S, et al. Direct characterization of *Blastocystis* from faeces by PCR and evidence of zoonotic potential. Parasitology 2007;134(03):359–67.
[187] Travers MA, Florent I, Kohl L, et al. Probiotics for the control of parasites: an overview. J Parasitol Res 2011;2011:610769.
[188] Levinson W, Jawetz E. Medical microbiology and immunology: examination and board review. Appleton & Lange; 1996.
[189] Pérez PF, Minnaard J, Rouvet M, et al. Inhibition of *Giardia intestinalis* by extracellular factors from Lactobacilli: an in vitro study. Appl Environ Microbiol 2011;67(11):5037–42.
[190] Smith HV, Corcoran GD. New drugs and treatment for cryptosporidiosis. Curr Opin Infect Dis 2004;17(6):557–64.
[191] Johnson EH, Windsor JJ, Clark CG. Emerging from obscurity: biological, clinical, and diagnostic aspects of *Dientamoeba fragilis*. Clin Microbiol Rev 2004;17(3):553–70.
[192] Swagerty DL, Walling AD, Klein RM. Lactose intolerance. Am Fam Physician 2002;65(9):1845–60.
[193] Anthony JP, Fyfe L, Stewart D, et al. The effect of blueberry extracts on *Giardia duodenalis* viability and spontaneous excystation of *Cryptosporidium parvum* oocysts, in vitro. Methods 2007;42(4):339–48.
[194] Grant J, Mahanty S, Khadir A, et al. Wheat germ supplement reduces cyst and trophozoite passage in people with giardiasis. Am J Trop Med Hyg 2001;65(6):705–10.
[195] Dinleyici EC, Eren M, Ozen M, et al. Effectiveness and safety of *Saccharomyces boulardii* for acute infectious diarrhea. Expert Opin Biol Ther 2012;12(4):395–410.
[196] Qiao JY, Li LJ, Zhang R, et al. Antiprotozoal effects of oregano oil and *Brucea javanica* on *Blastocystis hominis* in vitro. Journal of Pathogen Biology 2008;6:012.
[197] Zhang X, Qiao JY, Zhang R, et al. In vitro antiprotozoal effects of *Brucea javanica, Coptis chinensis, Radix pulsatillae* and Arecae on *Blastocystis hominis.* J Trop Med 2007;11:004.
[198] Ankri S, Mirelman D. Antimicrobial properties of allicin from garlic. Microbes Infect 1999;1(2):125–9.

[199] Anthony JP, Fyfe L, Smith H. Plant active components — a resource for antiparasitic agents? Trends Parasitol 2005;21(10):462–8.
[200] Yakoob J, Abbas Z, Beg MA, et al. In vitro sensitivity of *Blastocystis hominis* to garlic, ginger, white cumin, and black pepper used in diet. Parasitol Res 2011;109(2):379–85.
[201] El Wakil SS. Evaluation of the in vitro effect of *Nigella sativa* aqueous extract on *Blastocystis hominis* isolates. J Egypt Soc Parasitol 2007;37(3):801–13.
[202] Molodecky NA, Soon S, Rabi DM, et al. Increasing incidence and prevalence of the inflammatory bowel diseases with time, based on systematic review. Gastroenterology 2012;142(1):46–54.
[203] Langmead L, Rampton DS. Review article: complementary and alternative therapies for inflammatory bowel disease. Aliment Pharmacol Ther 2006;23:341–9.
[204] Yang H, McElree C, Roth MP, et al. Familial empirical risks for inflammatory bowel disease: differences between Jews and non-Jews. Gut 1993;34:517–24.
[205] Thompson-Chagoyán OC, Maldonado J, Gil A. Aetiology of inflammatory bowel disease (IBD): role of intestinal microbiota and gut-associated lymphoid tissue immune response. Clin Nutr 2005;24:339–52.
[206] Fisher SA, Tremelling M, Anderson CA, et al. Genetic determinants of ulcerative colitis include the ECM1 locus and five loci implicated in Crohn's disease. Nat Genet 2008;40:710–12.
[207] Cioffi M, Rosa AD, Serao R, et al. Laboratory markers in ulcerative colitis: current insights and future advances. World J Gastrointest Pathophysiol 2015;6(1):13–22.
[208] Kronman MP, Zaoutis TE, Haynes K, et al. Antibiotic exposure and IBD development among children: a population-based cohort study. Pediatrics 2012;130(4):e794–803.
[209] Takaishi H, Matsuki T, Nakazawa A, et al. Imbalance in intestinal microflora constitution could be involved in the pathogenesis of inflammatory bowel disease. Int J Med Microbiol 2008;298:463–72.
[210] Kishi D, Takahashi I, Kai Y, et al. Alteration of V beta usage and cytokine production of CD4+ TCR beta homodimer T cells by elimination of *Bacteroides vulgatus* prevents colitis in TCR alpha-chain-deficient mice. J Immunol 2000;165:5891–9.
[211] Sartor R. Microbial influences in inflammatory bowel diseases. Gastroenterology 2008;134:577–94.
[212] Bullock NR, Booth JC, Gibson GR. Comparative composition of bacteria in the human intestinal microflora during remission and active ulcerative colitis. Curr Issues Intest Microbiol 2004;5:59–64.
[213] Ott SJ, Musfeldt M, Wenderoth DF, et al. Reduction in diversity of the colonic mucosa associated bacterial microflora in patients with active inflammatory bowel disease. Gut 2004;53:685–93.
[214] Hayashi T, Ishida T, Motoya S, et al. Mucins and immune reactions to mucins in ulcerative colitis. Digestion 2001;63(Suppl. 1):28–31.
[215] Takaishi H, Ohara S, Hotta K, et al. Circulating autoantibodies against purified colonic mucin in ulcerative colitis. J Gastroenterol 2000;35:20–7.
[216] Phillips TE, McHugh J, Moore CP. Cyclosporine has a direct effect on the differentiation of a mucin-secreting cell line. J Cell Physiol 2000;184:400–8.
[217] Feagins LA, Cryer BL. Do non-steroidal anti-inflammatory drugs cause exacerbations of inflammatory bowel disease? Dig Dis Sci 2010;55(2):226–32.
[218] Mitsuyama K, Sata M, Rose-John S. Interleukin-6 trans-signaling in inflammatory bowel disease. Cytokine Growth Factor Rev 2006;17:451–61.
[219] Kaplan M, Mutlu EA, Benson M, et al. Use of herbal preparations in the treatment of oxidant-mediated inflammatory disorders. Complement Ther Med 2007;15:207–16.
[220] Delco F, Sonnenberg A. Birth-cohort phenomenon in the time trends of mortality from ulcerative colitis. Am J Epidemiol 1999;150:359–66.
[221] Delco F, Sonnenberg A. Exposure to risk factors for ulcerative colitis occurs during an early period of life. Am J Gastroenterol 1999;94:679–84.
[222] Halfvarson J, Jess T, Magnuson A, et al. Environmental factors in inflammatory bowel disease: a co-twin control study of a Swedish-Danish twin population. Inflamm Bowel Dis 2006;12:925–33.
[223] Mahid SS, Minor KS, Soto RE, et al. Smoking and inflammatory bowel disease: a meta-analysis. Mayo Clin Proc 2006;81:1462–71.
[224] Timmer A. Environmental influences on inflammatory bowel disease manifestations. Lessons from epidemiology. Dig Dis Sci 2003;21:91–104.
[225] Chan SS, Luben R, van Schaik F, et al. Carbohydrate intake in the etiology of Crohn's disease and ulcerative colitis. Inflamm Bowel Dis 2014;20(11):2013–21.
[226] Higuchi LM, Khalili H, Chan AT, et al. A prospective study of cigarette smoking and the risk of inflammatory bowel disease in women. Am J Gastroenterol 2012;107(9):1399–406.
[227] Ananthakrishnan AN, Khalili H, Konijeti GG, et al. Long-term intake of dietary fat and risk of ulcerative colitis and Crohn's disease. Gut 2014;63(5):776–84.
[228] Hou JK, Abraham B, El-Serag H. Dietary intake and risk of developing inflammatory bowel disease: a systematic review of the literature. Am J Gastroenterol 2011;106(4):563–73.
[229] Khalili H, Higuchi LM, Ananthakrishnan AN, et al. Oral contraceptives, reproductive factors and risk of inflammatory bowel disease. Gut 2013;62:1153–9.
[230] Cornish JA, Tan E, Simillis C, et al. The risk of oral contraceptives in the etiology of inflammatory bowel disease: a meta-analysis. Am J Gastroenterol 2008;103(9):2394–400.
[231] Hare NC, Arnott ID, Satsangi J. Therapeutic options in acute severe ulcerative colitis. Expert Rev Gastroenterol Hepatol 2008;2:357–70.
[232] O'Sullivan M, O'Morain C. Nutrition in inflammatory bowel disease. Best Pract Res Clin Gastroenterol 2006;20:561–73.
[233] Galvez J, Rodriguez-Cabezas ME, Zarzuelo A. Effects of dietary fiber on inflammatory bowel disease. Mol Nutr Food Res 2005;49:601–8.
[234] Hallert C, Kaldma M, Petersson BG. Ispaghula husk may relieve gastrointestinal symptoms in ulcerative colitis in remission. Scand J Gastroenterol 1991;26:747–50.
[235] Fernandez-Banares F, Hinojosa J, Sanchez-Lombrana JL, et al. Randomized clinical trial of Plantago ovata seeds (dietary fiber) as compared with mesalamine in maintaining remission in ulcerative colitis. Spanish Group for the Study of Crohn's Disease and Ulcerative Colitis (GETECCU). Am J Gastroenterol 1999;94: 427–33.
[236] Hallert C, Bjorck I, Nyman M, et al. Increasing fecal butyrate in ulcerative colitis patients by diet: controlled pilot study. Inflamm Bowel Dis 2003;9:116–21.
[237] Hanai H, Kanauchi O, Mitsuyama K, et al. Germinated barley foodstuff prolongs remission in patients with ulcerative colitis. Int J Mol Med 2004;13:643–7.
[238] Kanauchi O, Mitsuyama K, Homma T, et al. Treatment of ulcerative colitis patients by long-term administration of germinated barley foodstuff: multi-center open trial. Int J Mol Med 2003;12:701–4.
[239] Kanauchi O, Suga T, Tochihara M, et al. Treatment of ulcerative colitis by feeding with germinated barley foodstuff: first report of a multicenter open control trial. J Gastroenterol 2002;37(Suppl. 14):67–72.
[240] Kanauchi O, Serizawa I, Araki Y, et al. Germinated barley foodstuff, a prebiotic product, ameliorates inflammation of colitis through modulation of the enteric environment. J Gastroenterol 2003;38:134–41.
[241] Roessner A, Kuester D, Malfertheiner P, et al. Oxidative stress in ulcerative colitis-associated carcinogenesis. Pathol Res Pract 2008;204:511–24.
[242] Dincer Y, Erzin Y, Himmetoglu S, et al. Oxidative DNA damage and antioxidant activity in patients with inflammatory bowel disease. Dig Dis Sci 2007;52:1636–41.
[243] Rezaie A, Parker RD, Abdollahi M. Oxidative stress and pathogenesis of inflammatory bowel disease: an epiphenomenon or the cause? Dig Dis Sci 2007;52:2015–21.
[244] Hengstermann S, Valentini L, Schaper L, et al. Altered status of antioxidant vitamins and fatty acids in patients with inactive inflammatory bowel disease. Clin Nutr 2008;27:571–8.
[245] Koutroubakis IE, Malliaraki N, Dimoulios PD, et al. Decreased total and corrected antioxidant capacity in patients with inflammatory bowel disease. Dig Dis Sci 2004;49:1433–7.
[246] Kruidenier L, Kuiper I, Van Duijn W, et al. Imbalanced secondary mucosal antioxidant response in inflammatory bowel disease. J Pathol 2003;201:17–27.
[247] Croagh C, Shepherd SJ, Berryman M, et al. Pilot study on the effect of reducing dietary FODMAP intake on bowel function in patients without a colon. Inflamm Bowel Dis 2007;13:1522–8.

[248] Swanson GR, Tieu V, Shaikh M, et al. Is moderate red wine consumption safe in inactive inflammatory bowel disease? Digestion 2011;84(3):238–44.

[249] Ferguson LR, Shelling AN, Browning BL, et al. Genes, diet and inflammatory bowel disease. Mutat Res 2007;622:70–83.

[250] Andersen V, Olsen A, Carbonnel F, et al. Diet and risk of inflammatory bowel disease. Dig Liver Dis 2012;44(3):185–94.

[251] Geerling BJ, Badart-Smook A, Stockbrugger RW, et al. Comprehensive nutritional status in recently diagnosed patients with inflammatory bowel disease compared with population controls. Eur J Clin Nutr 2000;54:514–21.

[252] John S, Luben R, Shrestha SS, et al. Dietary n-3 polyunsaturated fatty acids and the aetiology of ulcerative colitis: a UK prospective cohort study. Eur J Gastroenterol Hepatol 2010;22(5):602–6.

[253] Uchiyama K, Nakamura M, Odahara S, et al. N-3 polyunsaturated fatty acid diet therapy for patients with inflammatory bowel disease. Inflamm Bowel Dis 2010;16(10):1696–707.

[254] Pearl DS, Masoodi M, Eiden M, et al. Altered colonic mucosal availability of n-3 and n-6 polyunsaturated fatty acids in ulcerative colitis and the relationship to disease activity. J Crohns Colitis 2014;8(1):70–9.

[255] Turner D, Steinhart AH, Griffiths AM. Omega-3 fatty acids (fish oil) for maintenance of remission in ulcerative colitis. Cochrane Database Syst Rev 2007;(3):CD006443.

[256] Turner D, Zlotkin SH, Shah PS, et al. Omega-3 fatty acids (fish oil) for maintenance of remission in Crohn's disease. Cochrane Database Syst Rev 2007;(2):CD006320.

[257] De Ley M, De Vos R, Hommes DW, et al. Fish oil for induction of remission in ulcerative colitis. Cochrane Database Syst Rev 2007;(4):CD005986.

[258] Gassull MA. Review article: the intestinal lumen as a therapeutic target in inflammatory bowel disease. Aliment Pharmacol Ther 2006;24(Suppl. 3):90–5.

[259] Haskey N, Dahl WJ. Symbiotic therapy: a promising new adjunctive therapy for ulcerative colitis. Nutr Rev 2006;64:132–8.

[260] Macfarlane S, Furrie E, Kennedy A, et al. Mucosal bacteria in ulcerative colitis. Br J Nutr 2005;93(Suppl. 1):S67–72.

[261] Zocco MA, Dal Verme LZ, Cremonini F, et al. Efficacy of Lactobacillus GG in maintaining remission of ulcerative colitis. Aliment Pharmacol Ther 2006;23:1567–74.

[262] Rioux KP, Fedorak RN. Probiotics in the treatment of inflammatory bowel disease. J Clin Gastroenterol 2006;40:260–3.

[263] Kruis W, Fric P, Pokrotnieks J, et al. Maintaining remission of ulcerative colitis with the probiotic *Escherichia coli* Nissle 1917 is as effective as with standard mesalazine. Gut 2004;53:1617–23.

[264] Kuhbacher T, Ott SJ, Helwig U, et al. Bacterial and fungal microbiota in relation to probiotic therapy (VSL#3) in pouchitis. Gut 2006;55:833–41.

[265] Mimura T, Rizzello F, Helwig U, et al. Once daily high dose probiotic therapy (VSL#3) for maintaining remission in recurrent or refractory pouchitis. Gut 2004;53:108–14.

[266] Bibiloni R, Fedorak RN, Tannock GW, et al. VSL#3 probiotic-mixture induces remission in patients with active ulcerative colitis. Am J Gastroenterol 2005;100:1539–46.

[267] Huynh HQ, Debruyn J, Guan L, et al. Probiotic preparation VSL#3 induces remission in children with mild to moderate acute ulcerative colitis: a pilot study. Inflamm Bowel Dis 2009;15(5):760–8.

[268] Caballero-Franco C, Keller K, De Simone C, et al. The VSL#3 probiotic formula induces mucin gene expression and secretion in colonic epithelial cells. Am J Physiol Gastrointest Liver Physiol 2007;292:G315–22.

[269] Soo I, Madsen KL, Tejpar Q, et al. VSL#3 probiotic upregulates intestinal mucosal alkaline sphingomyelinase and reduces inflammation. Can J Gastroenterol 2008;22:237–42.

[270] Giannini S, Martes C. Anemia in inflammatory bowel disease. Minerva Gastroenterol Dietol 2006;52:275–91.

[271] Bernstein CN. Osteoporosis in patients with inflammatory bowel disease. Clin Gastroenterol Hepatol 2006;4:152–6.

[272] Kuisma J, Luukkonen P, Jarvinen H, et al. Risk of osteopenia after proctocolectomy and ileal pouch-anal anastomosis for ulcerative colitis. Scand J Gastroenterol 2002;37:171–6.

[273] Scott EM, Gaywood I, Scott BB. Guidelines for osteoporosis in coeliac disease and inflammatory bowel disease. Gut 2000;46:I1.

[274] Lewis N, Scott BB. Guidelines for osteoporosis in coeliac disease and inflammatory bowel disease. Br Soc Gastroenterol 2007. Available from: www.bsg.org.uk/pdf_word_docs/ost_coe_ibd.pdf.

[275] Sinnott BP, Licata AA. Assessment of bone and mineral metabolism in inflammatory bowel disease: case series and review. Endocr Pract 2006;12:622–9.

[276] Mouli VP, Ananthakrishnan AN. Review article: vitamin D and inflammatory bowel diseases. Aliment Pharmacol Ther 2014;39(2):125–36.

[277] Feldman D, Malloy PJ, Krishnan AV, et al. Vitamin D: biology, action, and clinical implications. Osteoporosis. 3rd ed. San Diego: Academic Press; 2008.

[278] Zezos P, Papaioannou G, Nikolaidis N, et al. Hyperhomocysteinemia in ulcerative colitis is related to folate levels. World J Gastroenterol 2005;11:6038–42.

[279] Nakano E, Taylor CJ, Chada L, et al. Hyperhomocystinemia in children with inflammatory bowel disease. J Pediatr Gastroenterol Nutr 2003;37:586–90.

[280] Burr NE, Hull MA, Subramanian V. Folic acid supplementation may reduce colorectal cancer risk in patients with inflammatory bowel disease: a systematic review and meta-analysis. J Clin Gastroenterol 2017;51(3):247–53.

[281] Sido B, Hack V, Hochlehnert A, et al. Impairment of intestinal glutathione synthesis in patients with inflammatory bowel disease. Gut 1998;42:485–92.

[282] Ardite E, Sans M, Panes J, et al. Replenishment of glutathione levels improves mucosal function in experimental acute colitis. Lab Invest 2000;80:735–44.

[283] You Y, Fu JJ, Meng J, et al. Effect of N-acetylcysteine on the murine model of colitis induced by dextran sodium sulfate through up-regulating PON1 activity. Dig Dis Sci 2009;54(8):1643–50.

[284] Karp SM, Koch TR. Micronutrient supplements in inflammatory bowel disease. Dis Mon 2006;52:211–20.

[285] Vagianos K, Bector S, McConnell J, et al. Nutrition assessment of patients with inflammatory bowel disease. JPEN J Parenter Enteral Nutr 2007;31:311–19.

[286] Lih-Brody L, Powell SR, Collier KP, et al. Increased oxidative stress and decreased antioxidant defenses in mucosa of inflammatory bowel disease. Dig Dis Sci 1996;41:2078–86.

[287] Davidson G, Kritas S, Butler R. Stressed mucosa. Nestle Nutr Workshop Ser Pediatr Program 2007;59:133–42, discussion 143–6.

[288] Galland L. Magnesium and inflammatory bowel disease. Magnesium 1988;7:78–83.

[289] Faghfoori Z, Shakerhosseini R, Navai L, et al. Effects of an oral supplementation of germinated barley foodstuff on serum CRP level and clinical signs in patients with ulcerative colitis. Health Promot Perspect 2014;4(1):116.

[290] Hanai H, Iida T, Takeuchi K, et al. Curcumin maintenance therapy for ulcerative colitis: randomized, multicenter, double-blind, placebo-controlled trial. Clin Gastroenterol Hepatol 2006;4:1502–6.

[291] Holt PR, Katz S, Kirshoff R. Curcumin therapy in inflammatory bowel disease: a pilot study. Dig Dis Sci 2005;50:2191–3.

[292] Aggarwal BB, Sung B. Pharmacological basis for the role of curcumin in chronic diseases: an age-old spice with modern targets. Trends Pharmacol Sci 2009;30(2):85–94.

[293] Ali T, Shakir F, Morton J. Curcumin and inflammatory bowel disease: biological mechanisms and clinical implication. Digestion 2012;85(4):249–55.

[294] Aggarwal BB, Harikumar KB. Potential therapeutic effects of curcumin, the anti-inflammatory agent, against neurodegenerative, cardiovascular, pulmonary, metabolic, autoimmune and neoplastic diseases. Int J Biochem Cell Biol 2009;41(1):40–59.

[295] Langmead L, Feakins RM, Goldthorpe S, et al. Randomized, double-blind, placebo-controlled trial of oral aloe vera gel for active ulcerative colitis. Aliment Pharmacol Ther 2004;19:739–47.

[296] Sandborn WJ, Targan SR, Byers VS, et al. *Andrographis paniculata* extract (HMPL-004) for active ulcerative colitis. Am J Gastroenterol 2013;108(1):90–8.

[297] Rastegarpanah M, Malekzadeh R, Vahedi H, et al. A randomized, double blinded, placebo-controlled clinical trial of silymarin in ulcerative colitis. Chin J Integr Med 2015;21(12):902–6.

[298] Selinger CP, Lal S, Eaden J, et al. Better disease specific patient knowledge is associated with greater anxiety in inflammatory bowel disease. J Crohns Colitis 2013;7(6):e214–18.

[299] Elsenbruch S, Langhorst J, Popkirowa K, et al. Effects of mind-body therapy on quality of life and neuroendocrine and cellular immune functions in patients with ulcerative colitis. Psychother Psychosom 2005;74:277–87.
[300] Jedel S, Hoffman A, Merriman P, et al. A randomized controlled trial of mindfulness-based stress reduction to prevent flare-up in patients with inactive ulcerative colitis. Digestion 2014;89(2):142–55.
[301] Head K, Jurenka JS. Inflammatory bowel disease. Part II: Crohn's disease — pathophysiology and conventional and alternative treatment options. Altern Med Rev 2004;9:360–401.
[302] Abraham C, Cho JH. Functional consequences of NOD2 (CARD15) mutations. Inflamm Bowel Dis 2006;12:641–50.
[303] Abreu MT, Sparrow MP. Translational research in inflammatory bowel disease. Mt Sinai J Med 2006;73:1067–73.
[304] Yamamoto-Furusho JK, Korzenik JR. Crohn's disease: innate immunodeficiency? World J Gastroenterol 2006;12:6751–5.
[305] Sands BE. Inflammatory bowel disease: past, present, and future. J Gastroenterol 2007;42:16–25.
[306] Rogler G. Update in inflammatory bowel disease pathogenesis. Curr Opin Gastroenterol 2004;20:311–17.
[307] Wen Z, Fiocchi C. Inflammatory bowel disease: autoimmune or immune-mediated pathogenesis? Clin Dev Immunol 2004;11:195–204.
[308] Young Y, Abreu MT. Advances in the pathogenesis of inflammatory bowel disease. Curr Gastroenterol Rep 2006;8:470–7.
[309] Maeda S, Hsu LC, Liu H, et al. Nod2 mutation in Crohn's disease potentiates NF-kappaB activity and IL-1beta processing. Science 2005;307:734–8.
[310] Strober W, Fuss I, Mannon P. The fundamental basis of inflammatory bowel disease. J Clin Invest 2007;117:514–21.
[311] Gaya DR, Russell RK, Nimmo ER, et al. New genes in inflammatory bowel disease: lessons for complex diseases? Lancet 2006;367:1271–84.
[312] Magro F, Cunha E, Araujo F, et al. Dopamine D2 receptor polymorphisms in inflammatory bowel disease and the refractory response to treatment. Dig Dis Sci 2006;51:2039–44.
[313] Behr MA, Schurr E. Mycobacteria in Crohn's disease: a persistent hypothesis. Inflamm Bowel Dis 2006;12:1000–4.
[314] Kostic AD, Xavier RJ, Gevers D. The microbiome in inflammatory bowel disease: current status and the future ahead. Gastroenterology 2014;146(6):1489–99.
[315] De Diego C, Alcantara M, Valle J, et al. Influence of smoking habits and CARD15 mutations on the onset of Crohn's disease. Scand J Gastroenterol 2006;41:1209–11.
[316] Silbermintz A, Markowitz J. Inflammatory bowel diseases. Pediatr Ann 2006;35:268–74.
[317] Demeo MT, Mutlu EA, Keshavarzian A, et al. Intestinal permeation and gastrointestinal disease. J Clin Gastroenterol 2002;34:385–96.
[318] D'Inca R, Annese V, Di Leo V, et al. Increased intestinal permeability and NOD2 variants in familial and sporadic Crohn's disease. Aliment Pharmacol Ther 2006;23:1455–61.
[319] Kraus TA, Cheifetz A, Toy L, et al. Evidence for a genetic defect in oral tolerance induction in inflammatory bowel disease. Inflamm Bowel Dis 2006;12:82–8, discussion 81.
[320] Khalili H, Ananthakrishnan AN, Konijeti GG, et al. Measures of obesity and risk of Crohn's disease and ulcerative colitis. Inflamm Bowel Dis 2015;21(2):361.
[321] Suibhne TN, Raftery TC, McMahon O, et al. High prevalence of overweight and obesity in adults with Crohn's disease: associations with disease and lifestyle factors. J Crohns Colitis 2013;7(7):e241–8.
[322] Bengmark S. Curcumin, an atoxic antioxidant and natural NFkappaB, cyclooxygenase-2, lipooxygenase, and inducible nitric oxide synthase inhibitor: a shield against acute and chronic diseases. JPEN J Parenter Enteral Nutr 2006;30:45–51.
[323] Ghosh S. Anti-TNF therapy in Crohn's disease. Novartis Found Symp 2004;263:193–205, discussion 205–18.
[324] Korzenik JR. Crohn's disease: future anti-tumor necrosis factor therapies beyond infliximab. Gastroenterol Clin North Am 2004;33:285–301, ix.
[325] Ananthakrishnan AN, Khalili H, Pan A, et al. Association between depressive symptoms and incidence of Crohn's disease and ulcerative colitis: results from the nurses' health study. Clin Gastroenterol Hepatol 2013;11(1):57–62.
[326] Lerebours E, Gower-Rousseau C, Merle V, et al. Stressful life events as a risk factor for inflammatory bowel disease onset: a population-based case–control study. Am J Gastroenterol 2007;102(1):122–31.
[327] Bernstein CN, Singh S, Graff LA, et al. A prospective population-based study of triggers of symptomatic flares in IBD. Am J Gastroenterol 2010;105(9):1994–2002.
[328] Ananthakrishnan AN, Khalili H, Konijeti GG, et al. Long-term intake of dietary fat and risk of ulcerative colitis and Crohn's disease. Gut 2014a;63(5):776–84.
[329] Joossens M, De Preter V, Ballet V, et al. Effect of oligofructose-enriched inulin (OF-IN) on bacterial composition and disease activity of patients with Crohn's disease: results from a double-blinded randomised controlled trial. Gut 2012;61:958.
[330] Ruemmele FM. Role of diet in inflammatory bowel disease. Ann Nutr Metab 2016;68(Suppl. 1):33–41.
[331] Gearry RB, Irving PM, Barrett JS, et al. Reduction of dietary poorly absorbed short-chain carbohydrates (FODMAPs) improves abdominal symptoms in patients with inflammatory bowel disease-a pilot study. J Crohns Colitis 2009;3(1):8–14.
[332] Obih C, Wahbeh G, Lee D, et al. Specific carbohydrate diet for pediatric inflammatory bowel disease in clinical practice within an academic IBD center. Nutrition 2016;32(4):418–25.
[333] Suskind DL, Wahbeh G, Gregory N, et al. Nutritional therapy in pediatric Crohn's disease: the specific carbohydrate diet. J Pediatr Gastroenterol Nutr 2014;58(1):87–91.
[334] Kakodkar S, Farooqui AJ, Mikolaitis SL, et al. The specific carbohydrate diet for inflammatory bowel disease: a case series. J Acad Nutr Diet 2015;115(8):1226–32.
[335] Goh J, O'Morain CA. Review article: nutrition and adult inflammatory bowel disease. Aliment Pharmacol Ther 2003;17:307–20.
[336] Miura S, Tsuzuki Y, Hokari R, et al. Modulation of intestinal immune system by dietary fat intake: relevance to Crohn's disease. J Gastroenterol Hepatol 1998;13:1183–90.
[337] Trebble TM, Stroud MA, Wootton SA, et al. High-dose fish oil and antioxidants in Crohn's disease and the response of bone turnover: a randomised controlled trial. Br J Nutr 2005;94:253–61.
[338] Chan SSM, Luben R, Olsen A, et al. Association between high dietary intake of the n− 3 polyunsaturated fatty acid docosahexaenoic acid and reduced risk of Crohn's disease. Aliment Pharmacol Ther 2014a;39(8):834–42.
[339] Lev-Tzion R, Griffiths AM, Ledder O. Omega 3 fatty acids (fish oil) for maintenance of remission in Crohn's disease. Cochrane Database Syst Rev 2014;(2):CD006320.
[340] Turner D, Zlotkin SH, Shah PS, et al. Omega-3 fatty acids (fish oil) for maintenance of remission in Crohn's disease. Cochrane Database Syst Rev 2009;(1):CD006320.
[341] Feagan BG, Sandborn WJ, Mittmann U, et al. Omega-3 free fatty acids for the maintenance of remission in Crohn's disease: the EPIC randomized controlled trials. JAMA 2008;299:1690–7.
[342] Rolfe VE, Fortun PJ, Hawkey CJ, et al. Probiotics for maintenance of remission in Crohn's disease. Cochrane Database Syst Rev 2006;(4):CD004826.
[343] Rahimi R, Nikfar S, Rahimi F, et al. A meta-analysis on the efficacy of probiotics for maintenance of remission and prevention of clinical and endoscopic relapse in Crohn's disease. Dig Dis Sci 2008;53:2524–31.
[344] Bourreille A, Cadiot G, Le Dreau G, et al. *Saccharomyces boulardii* does not prevent relapse of Crohn's disease. Clin Gastroenterol Hepatol 2013;11(8):982–7.
[345] Stein J, Dignass AU. Management of iron deficiency anemia in inflammatory bowel disease: a practical approach. Ann Gastroenterol 2013;26(2):104.
[346] Bermejo F, Algaba A, Guerra I, et al. Should we monitor vitamin B12 and folate levels in Crohn's disease patients? Scand J Gastroenterol 2013;48(11):1272–7.
[347] Bakker SF, Dik VK, Witte BI, et al. Increase in bone mineral density in strictly treated Crohn's disease patients with concomitant calcium and vitamin D supplementation. J Crohns Colitis 2013;7(5):377–84.
[348] Ananthakrishnan AN, Cagan A, Gainer VS, et al. Normalization of plasma 25-hydroxy vitamin D is associated with reduced risk of surgery in Crohn's disease. Inflamm Bowel Dis 2013a;19(9):1921.

[349] Yang L, Weaver V, Smith JP, et al. Therapeutic effect of vitamin D supplementation in a pilot study of Crohn's patients. Clin Transl Gastroenterol 2013;4(4):e33.
[350] Chainani-Wu N. Safety and anti-inflammatory activity of curcumin: a component of turmeric (*Curcuma longa*). J Altern Complement Med 2003;9:161–8.
[351] Shishodia S, Sethi G, Aggarwal BB. Curcumin: getting back to the roots. Ann N Y Acad Sci 2005;1056:206–17.
[352] Salh B, Assi K, Templeman V, et al. Curcumin attenuates DNB-induced murine colitis. Am J Physiol Gastrointest Liver Physiol 2003;285:G235–43.
[353] Aggarwal S, Ichikawa H, Takada Y, et al. Curcumin (diferuloylmethane) down-regulates expression of cell proliferation and antiapoptotic and metastatic gene products through suppression of IkappaBalpha kinase and Akt activation. Mol Pharmacol 2006;69:195–206.
[354] Jobin C, Bradham CA, Russo MP, et al. Curcumin blocks cytokine-mediated NF-kappa B activation and proinflammatory gene expression by inhibiting inhibitory factor I-kappa B kinase activity. J Immunol 1999;163:3474–83.
[355] Shishodia S, Potdar P, Gairola CG, et al. Curcumin (diferuloylmethane) down-regulates cigarette smoke-induced NF-kappaB activation through inhibition of IkappaBalpha kinase in human lung epithelial cells: correlation with suppression of COX-2, MMP-9 and cyclin D1. Carcinogenesis 2003;24:1269–79.
[356] Camacho-Barquero L, Villegas I, Sanchez-Calvo JM, et al. Curcumin, a *Curcuma longa* constituent, acts on MAPK p38 pathway modulating COX-2 and iNOS expression in chronic experimental colitis. Int Immunopharmacol 2007;7:333–42.
[357] Jian YT, Mai GF, Wang JD, et al. Preventive and therapeutic effects of NF-kappaB inhibitor curcumin in rats colitis induced by trinitrobenzene sulfonic acid. World J Gastroenterol 2005;11:1747–52.
[358] Jiang H, Deng CS, Zhang M, et al. Curcumin-attenuated trinitrobenzene sulphonic acid induces chronic colitis by inhibiting expression of cyclooxygenase-2. World J Gastroenterol 2006;12:3848–53.
[359] Sugimoto K, Hanai H, Tozawa K, et al. Curcumin prevents and ameliorates trinitrobenzene sulfonic acid-induced colitis in mice. Gastroenterology 2002;123:1912–22.
[360] Ukil A, Maity S, Karmakar S, et al. Curcumin, the major component of food flavour turmeric, reduces mucosal injury in trinitrobenzene sulphonic acid-induced colitis. Br J Pharmacol 2003;139:209–18.
[361] Zhang M, Deng C, Zheng J, et al. Curcumin inhibits trinitrobenzene sulphonic acid-induced colitis in rats by activation of peroxisome proliferator-activated receptor gamma. Int Immunopharmacol 2006;6:1233–42.
[362] Zhang M, Deng CS, Zheng JJ, et al. Curcumin regulated shift from Th1 to Th2 in trinitrobenzene sulphonic acid-induced chronic colitis. Acta Pharmacol Sin 2006;27:1071–7.
[363] Omer B, Krebs S, Omer H, et al. Steroid-sparing effect of wormwood (*Artemisia absinthium*) in Crohn's disease: a double-blind placebo-controlled study. Phytomedicine 2007;14:87–95.
[364] Krebs S, Omer TN, Omer B. Wormwood (*Artemisia absinthium*) suppresses tumour necrosis factor alpha and accelerates healing in patients with Crohn's disease — a controlled clinical trial. Phytomedicine 2010;17(5):305–9.
[365] Ammon HP. Boswellic acids in chronic inflammatory diseases. Planta Med 2006;72:1100–16.
[366] Gerhardt H, Seifert F, Buvari P, et al. [Therapy of active Crohn disease with *Boswellia serrata* extract H 15]. Z Gastroenterol 2001;39:11–17.
[367] Holtmeier W, Zeuzem S, Preibeta J, et al. Randomized, placebo-controlled, double-blind trial of Boswellia serrata in maintaining remission of Crohn's disease: good safety profile but lack of efficacy. Inflamm Bowel Dis 2011;17(2):573–82.
[368] Hollander D. Inflammatory bowel diseases and brain-gut axis. J Physiol Pharmacol 2003;54(Suppl. 4):183–90.
[369] Ünlü C, Daniels L, Vrouenraets BC, et al. A systematic review of high-fibre dietary therapy in diverticular disease. Int J Colorectal Dis 2012;27(4):419–27.
[370] Fong SS, Tan EY, Foo A, et al. The changing trend of diverticular disease in a developing nation. Colorectal Dis 2011;13(3):312–16.
[371] Place RJ, Simmang CL. Diverticular disease. Best Pract Res Clin Gastroenterol 2002;16:135–48.
[372] Lorimer JW, Doumit G. Comorbidity is a major determinant of severity in acute diverticulitis. Am J Surg 2007;193:681–5.
[373] Crowe FL, Appleby PN, Allen NE, et al. Diet and risk of diverticular disease in Oxford cohort of European Prospective Investigation into Cancer and Nutrition (EPIC): prospective study of British vegetarians and non-vegetarians. BMJ 2011;343:d4131.
[374] Peery AF, Sandler RS, Ahnen DJ, et al. Constipation and a low-fiber diet are not associated with diverticulosis. Clin Gastroenterol Hepatol 2013;11(12):1622–7.
[375] Talley NJ, Lasch KL, Baum CL. A gap in our understanding: chronic constipation and its comorbid conditions. Clin Gastroenterol Hepatol 2009;7:9–19.
[376] Burgell RE, Muir JG, Gibson PR. Pathogenesis of colonic diverticulosis: repainting the picture. Clin Gastroenterol Hepatol 2013;11(12):1628–30.
[377] Böttner M, Wedel T. Abnormalities of neuromuscular anatomy in diverticular disease. Dig Dis 2012;30(1):19–23.
[378] Tursi A, Brandimarte G, Elisei W, et al. Assessment of small intestinal bacterial overgrowth in uncomplicated acute diverticulitis of the colon. World J Gastroenterol 2005;11(18):2773–6.
[379] Strate LL, Liu YL, Aldoori WH, et al. Obesity increases the risks of diverticulitis and diverticular bleeding. Gastroenterology 2009;136:115–122.e1.
[380] Cole CD, Wolfson AB. Case series: diverticulitis in the young. J Emerg Med 2007;33:363–6.
[381] Daniels L, Budding AE, de Korte N, et al. Fecal microbiome analysis as a diagnostic test for diverticulitis. Eur J Clin Microbiol Infect Dis 2014;33(11):1927–36.
[382] Granlund J, Svensson T, Olén O, et al. The genetic influence on diverticular disease — a twin study. Aliment Pharmacol Ther 2012;35(9):1103–7.
[383] Steel M. Colonic diverticular disease. Aust Fam Physician 2004;33:983–6.
[384] Petruzziello L, Iacopini F, Bulajic M, et al. Review article: uncomplicated diverticular disease of the colon. Aliment Pharmacol Ther 2006;23:1379–91.
[385] Aldoori W, Ryan-Harshman M. Preventing diverticular disease. Review of recent evidence on high-fibre diets. Can Fam Physician 2002;48:1632–7.
[386] Lahner E, Bellisario C, Hassan C, et al. Probiotics in the treatment of diverticular disease. A systematic review. J Gastrointestin Liver Dis 2016;25(1):79–86.
[387] Annibale B, Maconi G, Lahner E, et al. Efficacy of *Lactobacillus paracasei* sub. paracasei F19 on abdominal symptoms in patients with symptomatic uncomplicated diverticular disease: a pilot study. Minerva Gastroenterol Dietol 2011;57(1):13–22.
[388] Lahner E, Esposito G, Zullo A, et al. High-fibre diet and *Lactobacillus paracasei* B21060 in symptomatic uncomplicated diverticular disease. World J Gastroenterol 2012;18(41):5918.
[389] Tursi A, Brandimarte G, Giorgetti GM, et al. Mesalazine and/or *Lactobacillus casei* in preventing recurrence of symptomatic uncomplicated diverticular disease of the colon: a prospective, randomized, open-label study. J Clin Gastroenterol 2006;40(4):312–16.
[390] Scazzocchio F, Cometa MF, Tomassini L, et al. Antibacterial activity of Hydrastis canadensis extract and its major isolated alkaloids. Planta Med 2001;67:561–4.
[391] Tierra M. Echinacea: an effective alternative to antibiotics. J Herb Pharmacother 2007;7:79–89.
[392] Aldoori WH, Giovannucci EL, Rimm EB, et al. Prospective study of physical activity and the risk of symptomatic diverticular disease in men. Gut 1995;36:276–82.
[393] Simren M. Physical activity and the gastrointestinal tract. Eur J Gastroenterol Hepatol 2002;14:1053–6.
[394] Rubenstein JH, Chen JW. Epidemiology of gastroesophageal reflux disease. Gastroenterol Clin North Am 2014;43(1):1–14.
[395] Pandolfino JE, Kwiatek MA, Kahrilas PJ. The pathophysiologic basis for epidemiologic trends in gastroesophageal reflux disease. Gastroenterol Clin North Am 2008;37:827–43.

[396] van Pinxteren B, Numans ME, Bonis PA, et al. Short-term treatment with proton pump inhibitors, H2-receptor antagonists and prokinetics for gastro-oesophageal reflux disease-like symptoms and endoscopy negative reflux disease. Cochrane Database Syst Rev 2006;(3):CD002095.
[397] Moayyedi P, Talley NJ. Gastro-oesophageal reflux disease. Lancet 2006;367:2086–100.
[398] Anand G, Katz PO. Gastroesophageal reflux disease and obesity. Rev Gastroenterol Disord 2008;8:233–9.
[399] Ebrahimi-Mameghani M, Saghafi-Asl M, Arefhosseini S, et al. Is there any association between overweight, obesity and symptoms of reflux disease? Pak J Biol Sci 2008;11:443–7.
[400] Friedenberg FK, Xanthopoulos M, Foster GD, et al. The association between gastroesophageal reflux disease and obesity. Am J Gastroenterol 2008;103:2111–22.
[401] Hampel H, Abraham NS, El-Serag HB. Meta-analysis: obesity and the risk for gastroesophageal reflux disease and its complications. Ann Intern Med 2005;143:199–211.
[402] Veugelers PJ, Porter GA, Guernsey DL, et al. Obesity and lifestyle risk factors for gastroesophageal reflux disease, Barrett esophagus and esophageal adenocarcinoma. Dis Esophagus 2006;19:321–8.
[403] Whiteman DC, Sadeghi S, Pandeya N, et al. Combined effects of obesity, acid reflux and smoking on the risk of adenocarcinomas of the oesophagus. Gut 2008;57:173–80.
[404] Lee J, Anggiansah A, Anggiansah R, et al. Effects of age on the gastroesophageal junction, esophageal motility, and reflux disease. Clin Gastroenterol Hepatol 2007;5:1392–8.
[405] Lagergren J, Bergstrom R, Adami HO, et al. Association between medications that relax the lower esophageal sphincter and risk for esophageal adenocarcinoma. Ann Intern Med 2000;133:165–75.
[406] Fass R, Naliboff BD, Fass SS, et al. The effect of auditory stress on perception of intraesophageal acid in patients with gastroesophageal reflux disease. Gastroenterology 2008;134:696–705.
[407] Johnston BT, McFarland RJ, Collins JS, et al. Effect of acute stress on oesophageal motility in patients with gastro-oesophageal reflux disease. Gut 1996;38:492–7.
[408] Kaltenbach T, Crockett S, Gerson LB. Are lifestyle measures effective in patients with gastroesophageal reflux disease? An evidence-based approach. Arch Intern Med 2006;166:965–71.
[409] Kahrilas PJ, Shaheen NJ, Vaezi MF, et al. American Gastroenterological Association Medical Position Statement on the management of gastroesophageal reflux disease. Gastroenterology 2008;135:1383–91, 1391 e1–e5.
[410] Kubo A, Levin TR, Block G, et al. Dietary antioxidants, fruits, and vegetables and the risk of Barrett's esophagus. Am J Gastroenterol 2008;103:1614–23, quiz 1624.
[411] El-Serag HB, Satia JA, Rabeneck L. Dietary intake and the risk of gastro-oesophageal reflux disease: a cross sectional study in volunteers. Gut 2005;54:11–17.
[412] Nilsson M, Johnsen R, Ye W, et al. Lifestyle related risk factors in the aetiology of gastro-oesophageal reflux. Gut 2004;53:1730–5.
[413] Fox M, Barr C, Nolan S, et al. The effects of dietary fat and calorie density on esophageal acid exposure and reflux symptoms. Clin Gastroenterol Hepatol 2007;5:439–44.
[414] Anderson LA, Cantwell MM, Watson RG, et al. The association between alcohol and reflux esophagitis, Barrett's esophagus, and esophageal adenocarcinoma. Gastroenterology 2009;136: 799–805.
[415] Grad S, Abenavoli L, Dumitrascu DL. The effect of alcohol on gastrointestinal motility. Rev Recent Clin Trials 2016;11(3):191–5.
[416] Fashner J, Gitu AC. Common gastrointestinal symptoms: risks of long-term proton pump inhibitor therapy. FP Essent 2013;413:29–39.
[417] Rao CV, Vijayakumar M. Effect of quercetin, flavonoids and α-tocopherol, an antioxidant vitamin on experimental reflux oesophagitis in rats. Eur J Pharmacol 2008;589(1):233–8.
[418] Lukić M, egec A, egec I, et al. The impact of the vitamins A, C and E in the prevention of gastroesophageal reflux disease, Barrett's oesophagus and oesophageal adenocarcinoma. Coll Antropol 2012;36(3):867–72.
[419] Giri AK, Rawat JK, Singh M, et al. Effect of lycopene against gastroesophageal reflux disease in experimental animals. BMC Complement Altern Med 2015;15(1):1.
[420] Kumar S, Singh M, Rawat JK, et al. Effect of rutin against gastric esophageal reflux in experimental animals. Toxicol Mech Methods 2014;24(9):666–71.
[421] Aly AM, AL-Alousi L, Salem HA. Liquorice: a possible anti-inflammatory and anti-ulcer drug. AAPS PharmSciTech 2005;6:E74–82.
[422] Asl MN, Hosseinzadeh H. Review of pharmacological effects of Glycyrrhiza sp. and its bioactive compounds. Phytother Res 2008;22:709–24.
[423] Baltina LA. Chemical modification of glycyrrhizic acid as a route to new bioactive compounds for medicine. Curr Med Chem 2003;10:155–71.
[424] McKay DL, Blumberg JB. A review of the bioactivity and potential health benefits of chamomile tea (*Matracaria recutita* L.). Phytother Res 2006;20:519–30.
[425] Eslick GD, Talley NJ. Gastroesophageal reflux disease (GERD): risk factors, and impact on quality of life-a population-based study. J Clin Gastroenterol 2009;43:111–17.
[426] Gerson LB, Fass R. A systematic review of the definitions, prevalence, and response to treatment of nocturnal gastroesophageal reflux disease. Clin Gastroenterol Hepatol 2009;7:372–8, quiz 367.
[427] Festi D, Scaioli E, Baldi F, et al. Body weight, lifestyle, dietary habits and gastroesophageal reflux disease. World J Gastroenterol 2009;15:1690–701.
[428] Nowak M, Buttner P, Harrison S, et al. Effectiveness of lifestyle measures in the treatment of gastroesophageal reflux disease: a case series. Ther Clin Risk Manag 2006;2:329–34.
[429] Nocon M, Labenz J, Willich SN. Lifestyle factors and symptoms of gastro-oesophageal reflux — a population-based study. Aliment Pharmacol Ther 2006;23:169–74.
[430] Gisbert JP, Legido J, García-Sanz I, et al. *Helicobacter pylori* and perforated peptic ulcer. Prevalence of the infection and role of non-steroidal anti-inflammatory drugs. Dig Liver Dis 2004;36:116–20.
[431] Papatheodoridis GV, Sougioultzis S, Archimandritis AJ. Effects of *Helicobacter pylori* and nonsteroidal anti-inflammatory drugs on peptic ulcer disease: a systematic review. Clin Gastroenterol Hepatol 2006;4:130–42.
[432] Farzaei MH, Abdollahi M, Rahimi R. Role of dietary polyphenols in the management of peptic ulcer. World J Gastroenterol 2015;21(21):6499–517.
[433] Choung RS, Talley NJ. Epidemiology and clinical presentation of stress-related peptic damage and chronic peptic ulcer. Curr Mol Med 2008;8:253–7.
[434] Jones MP. The role of psychosocial factors in peptic ulcer disease: beyond *Helicobacter pylori* and NSAIDs. J Psychosom Res 2006;60:407–12.
[435] Chuang CH, Sheu BS, Kao AW, et al. Adjuvant effect of vitamin C on omeprazole-amoxicillin-clarithromycin triple therapy for *Helicobacter pylori* eradication. Hepatogastroenterology 2007;54:320–4.
[436] Konturek PC, Kania J, Gessner U, et al. Effect of vitamin C-releasing acetylsalicylic acid on gastric mucosal damage before and after *Helicobacter pylori* eradication therapy. Eur J Pharmacol 2004;506:169–77.
[437] McAlindon ME, Muller AF, Filipowicz B, et al. Effect of allopurinol, sulphasalazine, and vitamin C on aspirin induced gastroduodenal injury in human volunteers. Gut 1996;38: 518–24.
[438] Demirci H, Uygun İlikhan S, Öztürk K, et al. Influence of vitamin C and E supplementation on the eradication rates of triple and quadruple eradication regimens for *Helicobacter pylori* infection. Turk J Gastroenterol 2015;26:456–60.
[439] Manjari V, Das UN. Oxidant stress, anti-oxidants, nitric oxide and essential fatty acids in peptic ulcer disease. Prostaglandins Leukot Essent Fatty Acids 1998;59:401–6.
[440] Manjari V, Das UN. Effect of polyunsaturated fatty acids on dexamethasone-induced gastric mucosal damage. Prostaglandins Leukot Essent Fatty Acids 2000;62:85–96.
[441] Thompson L, Cockayne A, Spiller RC. Inhibitory effect of polyunsaturated fatty acids on the growth of *Helicobacter pylori*: a possible explanation of the effect of diet on peptic ulceration. Gut 1994;35:1557–61.

[442] Correia M, Michel V, Matos AA, et al. Docosahexaenoic acid inhibits *Helicobacter pylori* growth in vitro and mice gastric mucosa colonization. PLoS ONE 2012;7(4):e35072.

[443] Ianiro GI, Franceschi FR, Bibbo S, et al. Omega-3 fatty acids: a novel resort against gastrointestinal injury. Eur Rev Med Pharmacol Sci 2014;18(20):3086–90.

[444] Lam EK, Yu L, Wong HP, et al. Probiotic *Lactobacillus rhamnosus* GG enhances gastric ulcer healing in rats. Eur J Pharmacol 2007;565:171–9.

[445] Lesbros-Pantoflickova D, Corthesy-Theulaz I, Blum AL. *Helicobacter pylori* and probiotics. J Nutr 2007;137:812S–818S.

[446] Imase K, Takahashi M, Tanaka A, et al. Efficacy of *Clostridium butyricum* preparation concomitantly with *Helicobacter pylori* eradication therapy in relation to changes in the intestinal microbiota. Microbiol Immunol 2008;52:156–61.

[447] McFarland LV, Huang Y, Wang L, et al. Systematic review and meta-analysis: multi-strain probiotics as adjunct therapy for *Helicobacter pylori* eradication and prevention of adverse events. United European Gastroenterol J 2016;4(4):546–61.

[448] Abdelkader NA, Abdelhakam SM, Hamed AM, et al. Peptic ulcer disease and *Helicobacter Pylori* infection: Does serum zinc level play a role? Int J Curr Microbiol App Sci 2016;5(5): 227–34.

[449] Zhang WH, Wu XJ, Niu JX, et al. Serum zinc status and *Helicobacter pylori* infection in gastric disease patients. Asian Pac J Cancer Prev 2012;13(10):5043–6.

[450] Ineu RP, Oliveira CS, Oliveira VA, et al. Antioxidant effect of zinc chloride against ethanol-induced gastrointestinal lesions in rats. Food Chem Toxicol 2013;58:522–9.

[451] Salama SM, Gwaram NS, AlRashdi AS, et al. A zinc morpholine complex prevents HCl/ethanol-induced gastric ulcers in a rat model. Sci Rep 2016;6:29646.

[452] O'Mahony R, Al-Khtheeri H, Weerasekera D, et al. Bactericidal and anti-adhesive properties of culinary and medicinal plants against *Helicobacter pylori.* World J Gastroenterol 2005;11:7499–507.

[453] De R, Kundu P, Swarnakar S, et al. Antimicrobial activity of curcumin against Indian *Helicobacter pylori* and also during mice infection. Antimicrob Agents Chemother 2009;53(4):1592–7.

[454] Koosirirat C, Linpisarn S, Changsom D, et al. Investigation of the anti-inflammatory effect of *Curcuma longa* in *Helicobacter pylori*-infected patients. Int Immunopharmacol 2010;10(7):815–18.

[455] Prucksunand C, Indrasukhsri B, Leethochawalit M, et al. Phase II clinical trial on effect of the long turmeric (*Curcuma longa* Linn) on healing of peptic ulcer. Southeast Asian J Trop Med Public Health 2001;32:208–15.

[456] Hajiaghamohammadi AA, Zargar A, Oveisi S, et al. To evaluate of the effect of adding licorice to the standard treatment regimen of *Helicobacter pylori.* Braz J Infect Dis 2016;20(6):534–8.

[457] Cheney G. Rapid healing of peptic ulcers in patients receiving fresh cabbage juice. Calif Med 1949;70:10–15.

[458] Cheney G, Waxler SH, Miller IJ. Vitamin U therapy of peptic ulcer; experience at San Quentin Prison. Calif Med 1956;84:39–42.

[459] Eamlamnam K, Patumraj S, Visedopas N, et al. Effects of *Aloe vera* and sucralfate on gastric microcirculatory changes, cytokine levels and gastric ulcer healing in rats. World J Gastroenterol 2006;12:2034–9.

[460] Prabjone R, Thong-Ngam D, Wisedopas N, et al. Anti-inflammatory effects of *Aloe vera* on leucocyte-endothelium interaction in the gastric microcirculation of *Helicobacter pylori*-infected rats. Clin Hemorheol Microcirc 2006;35:359–66.

[461] El Souda SSED, Ahmed KM, Grace MH, et al. Flavonoids and gastroprotective effect of *Matricaria chamomilla* against indomethacin-induced ulcer in rats. J Herbs Spices Med Plants 2015;21(2):111–17.

11

The hepatobiliary system

Ses Salmond

SECTION A

OVERVIEW OF THE HEPATOBILIARY SYSTEM

The average adult liver weighs approximately 1.5 kg and is the second largest organ in the body after the skin. The liver is shielded by the rib cage and sits in the upper right abdominal cavity. From the front, two lobes of the organ are visible; the right lobe is much larger than the left. Closer inspection of the two anterior lobes of the liver reveal a connective fibre, referred to as the falciform ligament. The falciform ligament is actually an extension of the visceral peritoneum which houses the liver and separates and protects it from other organs in the abdominal cavity. A posterior view of the organ reveals the presence of the caudate and the quadrate lobes.

The liver is the metabolic powerhouse of the body; it requires a dedicated vascular and arterial blood supply. The portal vein brings deoxygenated blood that is nutrient rich from the spleen, stomach, pancreas and intestines. The hepatic artery supplies the liver with oxygenated blood from the aorta. The entry point of the portal vein, hepatic artery and common bile duct at the base of the liver is referred to as the porta hepatis. Inside the liver, both the portal vein and the hepatic artery branch into an intricate network of blood vessels which supply hepatocytes with blood and nutrients and facilitate metabolic functions. About 1.5 L of blood circulates through the liver every minute then exits the organ via the hepatic veins before entering the inferior vena cava for reoxygenation by the heart.

The larger lobes of the liver are made up of smaller lobules; these lobules are regarded as the liver's functional units and contain hepatocytes (see Fig. 11.1). The cellular structure of the liver is complex and highly specified. The liver has no capillaries and instead, blood moves through the organ via sinusoids that house the Kupffer cells which are responsible for phagocytosis.

The liver is the primary site for bile production and secretion to the gallbladder for storage. Newly formed bile is transported from the liver via the bile ducts and moves into the left and right hepatic ducts. The left and right ducts merge and bile then exits the liver through the common hepatic duct. This duct then joins the cystic duct of the gallbladder forming the common bile duct, which allows for the transport of bile to the gallbladder for storage.

The gallbladder is a small pear-shaped sac between 7 and 10 cm long and is tucked neatly behind the liver. The primary function of the gallbladder is the storage and release of bile into the duodenum. The presence of lipids in the duodenum stimulates the secretion of cholecystokinin; this causes the contraction of the gallbladder and the release of bile into the duodenum which emulsifies the lipids. Acid chyme in the duodenum increases the release of bicarbonate into the bile from the liver to reduce the pH of the contents of the duodenum.

The liver is involved in hundreds of metabolic processes, with much of its work centring on the metabolism of carbohydrates, proteins, lipids, vitamins and minerals (see Table 11.1). Processes of bile synthesis and detoxification are also major responsibilities. The liver is without question the most important organ of metabolism in the human body. The health and vitality of an individual are to a very large extent determined by the health and vitality of the liver. The maintenance of a well-functioning liver is pivotal when treating holistically. From a naturopathic perspective, there are several cardinal signs of liver dysfunction. The presence of dark circles under the eyes, halitosis and a yellow tongue immediately suggest liver insufficiency and these signs can be detected by simple observation. Investigation into the digestive functions and emotional health of a patient can also quickly reveal other symptoms of liver disharmony. The presence of fatigue, nausea, fat intolerance, anger, constipation and skin problems beg for urgent attention to be paid to hepatobiliary function.

Other signs of liver sluggishness are less obvious and not as widely recognised but are, however, of no lesser importance. Problematic digestion, flatulence and bloating, and headaches are also implicated in poor liver function. Naturopathy also recognises food and drug allergies and intolerances, premenstrual syndrome and morning sickness as clinical signs of liver dysfunction. Signs that indicate more sinister pathology include the presence of spider naevi, palmar erythema, right upper quadrant pain or discomfort, fluid retention, oedema and ascites.

The breakdown of both endogenous and exogenous substances by an optimally functioning liver is crucial for the maintenance of health and the treatment of disease

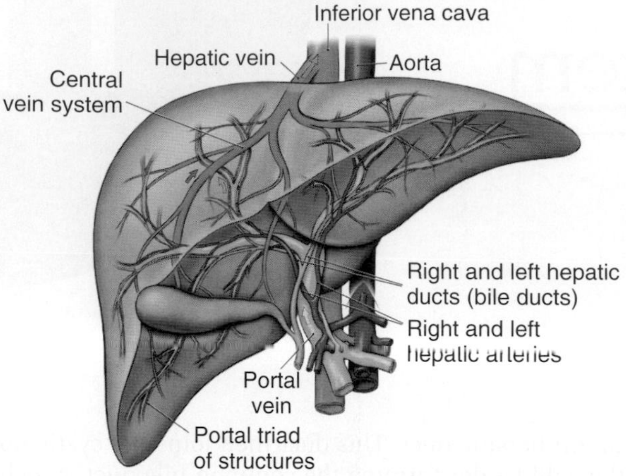

FIGURE 11.1 Anatomical diagram showing the two lobes of the liver, the central vein, portal vein and hepatic artery.
Source: Miller: Miller's anesthesia, 7th ed. Churchill Livingstone Elsevier, 2009.

states. Premenstrual syndrome can be linked to the improper breakdown of oestrogens by the liver. Likewise, exogenous chemicals found in foods or drugs or from environmental sources contribute heavily to the toxic load on the liver and ultimately to suboptimal performance. Conditions traditionally associated with liver disharmony and the mechanism of liver involvement are described in Table 11.2.

ROLE OF THE NATUROPATH

The role of the naturopath in the naturopathic treatment of the hepatobiliary system blends knowledge from early naturopathic pioneers and draws on current evidence. The modern naturopath has many more treatment options than traditional practitioners; however, the core of the treatment approach remains the same. A naturopath delivers treatments that combine the primary goal of supporting the body's own innate ability to heal (vitality, life force, vis medicatrix naturae) with a naturopathic therapeutic order. This means that symptomatic relief can be given while

TABLE 11.1 The role of the liver — the great mediator of human health

Substance	Creation	Destruction/Transformation	Storage
Carbohydrates	Carbohydrate metabolism: gluconeogenesis, glycogenesis	Carbohydrate metabolism: glycogenolysis and conversion of fructose and galactose to glucose Conversion of glucose to glycogen and triglycerides if intake exceeds requirements	Storage of glucose as glycogen
Lipids	Lipid metabolism: production of triglycerides, phospholipids, lipoproteins, cholesterol via lipogenesis	Lipid metabolism: lipolysis and transformation of fatty acids to acetyl-coA via β-oxidation	
Proteins	Protein metabolism: production of clotting factors (fibrinogen, prothrombin, albumin, globulins, transferrins and lipoproteins) Synthesis of non-essential amino acids and transport mechanisms for vitamin A, Fe, Zn, Cu	Protein metabolism: proteolysis, conversion of ammonia to urea, transamination and deamination of amino acids	
Vitamins and minerals		Conversion of carotene to vitamin A, folate to 5-methyl tetrahydrofolic acid, vitamin D to 25-hydroxycholecalciferol	Storage of fat-soluble vitamins (A, D) and storage of vitamins and minerals (B_{12}, Zn, Fe, Cu, Mg)
Bile	Bile salt synthesis	Destruction of red blood cells to form bilirubin	Secretion of bile, no storage function (gallbladder)
Hormones/ drugs		Destruction/detoxification of synthetic and natural drugs, alcohol, hormones and steroids: aldosterone, glucocorticoids, testosterone, progesterone and oestrogen, thyroid hormones	
Old material		Phagocytosis of red blood cells, white blood cells, bacterium by Kupffer cells	

TABLE 11.2 Conditions traditionally associated with liver disharmony

Disease	Mechanism of liver involvement
Skin conditions: acne, boils, eczema, psoriasis	One of the liver's main tasks is blood filtration; if this is compromised, the direction of cure allows for skin manifestations of hepatic and systemic toxicity
Premenstrual syndrome	PMS-A involves a relative excess of oestrogen and a relative deficiency of progesterone with a possible relation to poor liver clearance of oestrogens
Immune dysfunction	The liver has one of the largest populations of macrophages which are key components of the innate immune system. Kupffer cells are involved in phagocytosis, antigen processing and presentation and are intimately involved in the body's response to infections and toxins
Constipation	Bowel and digestive function are intimately linked to liver function. Liver dysfunction results in suboptimal formation and secretion of bile, resulting in impaired digestion. Longer bowel transit times also increase toxic burden on the liver
Arthritis	Primary diseases of the liver with joint involvement: primary biliary cirrhosis, hepatitis, haemochromatosis, Wilson's disease. Primary diseases of the joints with liver involvement: RA, Sjögren's syndrome, SLE, sclerosis
Autoimmune disorders	Disorders of immune regulation can direct immune cells against the liver and cause liver injury; the small intrahepatic bile ducts are the target of destruction by lymphocytes in autoimmune destructive cholangiopathy
Hepatitis	A destructive T-cell response is directed at liver cells in autoimmune hepatitis. In chronic hepatitis C, persistent Th1 stimulation results in gradual accumulation of liver injury induced by cytotoxic T lymphocytes, natural killer cells and macrophages
Chronic fatigue syndrome	A sluggish liver leads to increased toxic load in the body; blood has less oxygen-carrying capacity and increased strain on the liver has impacts on its metabolic functions including energy production and storage, neurotransmitter production and hormone production. Chronic liver disease is also associated with fatigue
Migraines	Liver involvement in several proposed causes of migraines: food allergy and intolerance, hormonal influences. General liver dysfunction and associated constipation may also result in bilious headaches

PMS-A: PMS anxiety; RA: rheumatoid arthritis; SLE: systemic lupus erythematosus; Th1: T helper 1.

Diehl AM. Nonalcoholic fatty liver disease abnormalities in macrophage function and cytokines. Am J Physiol Gastrointes Liver Physiol 2002; 282(1):G1–G5; Farrell GC. Hepatitis C, other liver disorders and liver health. A practical guide. Sydney: Maclennan and Petty; 2002; Mills PR, Sturrock RD. Occasional survey: clinical associations between arthritis and liver. Ann Rheum Dis 1982; 41(3):295–307; Trickey R. Women, hormones and the menstrual cycle. Rev edn. Sydney: Allen & Unwin; 1998; Tsutsui H, Nakanishi K, Matsui K et al. IFN-gamma-inducing factor up-regulates Fas ligand-mediated cytotoxic activity of murine natural killer cell clones. J Immunol 1996; 157(9):3967–3973.

gently addressing the underlying causes and supporting the patient's overall vitality.

A therapeutic order or treatment approach for gallstones would thus incorporate symptomatic treatment, removal of the cause of the condition and stimulation of the body's innate healing ability or the healing power of nature. Weakened body systems are tonified and restored to health so that metabolic function is improved, the immune system is strengthened, the body is detoxified and the life force is stimulated. This approach sees the prescription of herbal and nutritional supplements in therapeutic doses. The regulation of diet and lifestyle is also a primary intervention regardless of the presenting pathology.

Liver detoxification

The human body is exposed to an everyday onslaught of toxins, from toxic household cleaning chemicals, cosmetics and pesticides, to the air we breathe and the water we drink, to toxic deposits in food and ubiquitous plastics to the overuse of recreational and non-recreational drugs.

The liver plays a crucial role in detoxifying these molecules, many of which are fat-soluble and, if not removed by the liver, can be stored in the body's fat reserves for long periods of time.

The two major types of reactions involved in the detoxification and metabolism of metabolites in the liver are classified as Phase I and Phase II reactions.[1] Phase I detoxification reactions involve processes of oxidation (loss of electrons), reduction (gain of electrons) and hydrolysis (splitting a double bond or functional group and adding a hydroxyl group and a hydrogen). The Phase I process introduces or exposes functional groups to increase molecular hydrophilia. Phase I also involves cytochrome P450 enzymes. After Phase I processing, the metabolites are highly reactive and Phase II activity is required as a matter of urgency to prevent tissue damage by accumulated highly reactive compounds.

Phase II detoxification involves the process of conjugation via glucuronidation, amino acid conjugation, acetylation, sulfation, methylation and glutathionation. Both conjugants and enzymes are required for this activity that sees water-soluble side groups added to increase water solubility. Finally, during the process known as Phase III, the conjugated compound is removed from the liver via transporters on sinusoidal and canalicular membranes. This biotransformation can lead to the elimination of some metabolites and the activation of others.[2]

TABLE 11.3 The major detoxification mechanisms of the liver

Detoxification method	Substances detoxified
Filtering of the blood by Kupffer cells	Bacteria and bacterial products, immune complexes
Bile secretion	Cholesterol, haemoglobin breakdown products, extra calcium
Phase I detoxification	Prescription drugs (amphetamines, digoxin, phenobarbital), over-the-counter drugs (paracetamol, ibuprofen), caffeine, histamine, hormones, benzopyrene, aniline, CCL_4 (carbon tetrachloride), insecticides, arachidonic acid, tobacco
Phase II detoxification (glutathione conjugation)	Paracetamol, organophosphates, pesticides, alcohol, toxic metals, tetracycline, penicillin, alcohol
Amino acid conjugation	Benzoate, aspirin
Methylation	Dopamine, adrenaline (epinephrine), histamine, thiouracil
Sulfation	Oestrogen, aniline dyes, warfarin, paracetamol, methyldopa, steroid hormones, catecholamines, phenols, tamoxifen, apomorphine, ethinylestradiol
Acetylation	Sulfonamides, mescaline
Glucuronidation	Paracetamol, morphine, diazepam, digoxin, oestrogens, NSAIDs, paracetamol

Kauffman FC. Sulfonation in pharmacology and toxicology. Drug Metab Rev 2004; 36(3&4):823–843.

Therefore altering liver metabolism can increase the toxic side products of Phase I, increase the activation and concentration of some therapeutic drugs or decrease the therapeutic concentrations by increasing their elimination. Thus it is essential that detoxification processes in the liver are understood and treated with particular consideration (Table 11.3).

The cytochrome P450 (CYP) enzymes remove accumulated material from the body and are concentrated in the endoplasmic reticulum of the liver cells. The CYP enzymes are responsible for the majority of the oxidation of xenobiotic chemicals including drugs, pesticides and carcinogens as well as the metabolism of endobiotics such as steroids, fat-soluble vitamins and eicosanoids.[3] There are 57 known active P450 genes in the human genome and 58 pseudogenomes; those of families 1–3 are the enzymes involved in xenobiotic metabolism.[4] The following isoenzymes, expressed in the human liver, are primarily responsible for the metabolism of xenobiotics: CYP1A2, CYP2C9, CYP2C19, CYP2D6 and CYP3A4.[5] Tricyclic antidepressants and antipsychotics are metabolised by CYP2D6, while selective serotonin reuptake inhibitors and proton pump inhibitors are metabolised by CYP2C19.[4] Amitifadine, a triple reuptake inhibitor, is a moderate inhibitor of CYP2D6, CYP3A4, CYP2C9 and CYP2C19, and a potent inhibitor of CYP2B6.[6]

Bile acids and drugs activate the pregnane X receptor (PXR) to induce CYP3A4, which is the predominant cytochrome P450 enzyme expressed in the liver and intestine. CYP3A4 is critical in detoxifying bile acids and drugs and protects against cholestasis.[7] CYP3A4 makes up 30% of the total P450 content in the liver and metabolises nifedipine, ciclosporin, erythromycin, midazolam and alprazolam.[6]

Inducers of CYP3A4 can increase the clearance of other drugs, causing a reduced therapeutic effect. *Hypericum perforatum* can reduce the serum concentrations of indinavir and ciclosporin among others.[8,9] In addition, inducers may increase the activation of pro-drugs, resulting in an alteration in their efficacy and pharmacokinetics and also increase the bioactivation of drugs that contribute to hepatoxicity via reactive intermediates. On the other hand, inhibitors of CYP3A4 may increase the bioavailability of drugs. Grapefruit juice can increase the serum concentrations of calcium channel antagonists, an antihypertensive drug, and also statins.[10] Grapefruit juice is of concern for those drugs with a low therapeutic index.

Smoking increases caffeine metabolism as cigarettes induce CYP1A2, the isoenzyme that metabolises caffeine.[11] Smokers therefore require three to four times more caffeine doses compared with non-smokers to obtain comparable plasma caffeine levels and this may explain why caffeine intake is usually higher in smokers.[12] Required nutrients, activation and inhibition of liver detoxification are listed in Table 11.4.

Hepatobiliary nutritional objectives (dietary)

See Table 11.1 for an overview of the functions of the liver. Any form of liver disease will compromise the liver's ability to function. This will affect the metabolism of proteins, carbohydrates and fats; the transformation of amino acids, toxins and pharmaceutical drugs; the storage of fat-soluble vitamins such as vitamins A, D, E and K; the regulation of blood sugar via the storage and release of sugar via glycogen; the activation of substances such as vitamin D and pharmaceuticals. Also certain dietary and lifestyle factors will compromise the liver's ability to function either by creating deficiencies or by increasing the workload on the liver and accelerating disease. Nutritional and lifestyle recommendations that are the same for all types of liver disease are covered here with specific requirements mentioned in the relevant section.

The key objectives are weight management and digestive health through a high antioxidant and anti-inflammatory diet; adopting a wholefood diet with a wide variety of plant-based foods.

PROTEIN

The liver synthesises 80% of the blood proteins from amino acids in the diet. The liver is also able to convert

TABLE 11.4 Required nutrients, activation and inhibition of liver detoxification

Phase and conjugation	Required nutrients	Induced by	Inhibited by
Phase I	B_2, B_3, B_6, B_9, B_{12}, BCAA (branch-chain amino acid), glutathione, flavonoids and phospholipids	Tobacco (CYP1A2), omeprazole, ethanol *Hypericum perforatum* (hyperforin) *Anethum graveolens* *Camellia sinensis* *Carum carvi* Resveratrol *Schisandra chinensis* *Silybum marianum* *Zingiber officinale* (CYP1A2, CYP3A4) High-protein diet	Grapefruit juice (CYP3A4), quinidine, erythromycin, fluvoxamine *Vitis vinifera* (CYP2E1)
Phase II		*Allium sativum* *Curcuma longa* *Cymbopogon citratus (citral)* Resveratrol *Rosmarinus officinalis* *Salvia officinalis* *Schisandra chinensis* Cruciferous vegetables *Taraxacum officinale*	Deficiencies in Se, Zn, B_2, B_5, B_6, B_9, glutathione, vitamin C Low-protein diet NSAIDs Molybdenum Aspirin
Glutathione		Glutathione and B_6	
Amino acid		Cysteine and glycine	
Methylation		Methionine and SAM-e (S-adenosyl methionine)	
Sulfation		Glycine, cysteine, methionine, molybdenum	
Acetylation		N-acetylcysteine and B_5	
Glucuronidation		Taurine and glucuronic acid	
Phases I and II		Brassica family Oranges N-acetylcysteine Alpha lipoic acid *Camellia sinensis* *Curcuma longa* Resveratrol *Schisandra chinensis*	

Bagchi D, Ray SD, Bagchi M et al. Mechanistic pathways of antioxidant cytoprotection by a novel IH636 grape seed proanthocyanidin extract. Indian J Exp B 2002; 40(6):717–726; Brandin H, Viitanen E, Myrberg O et al. Effects of herbal medicinal products and food supplements on induction of CYP1A2, CYP3A4 and MDR1 in the human colon carcinoma cell line LS180. Phytotherapy Research 2007; 21(3):239–244; Liska D, Lyon M, Jones DS. Detoxification and biotransformational imbalances. Explore 2006; 2(2):122–140; Maliakal PP, Wanwimolruk S. Effect of herbal teas on hepatic drug metabolizing enzymes in rats. J Pharm Pharmacol 2001; 53(10):1323–1329; Murray KF, Messner DJ, Kowdleyz KV. Mechanisms of hepatocyte detoxification physiology of the gastrointestinal tract. In Johnson LR, Barrett KE, eds. Physiology of the gastrointestinal tract. 4th edn. Edinburgh: Academic Press; 2006, pp. 1483–1504; Nakamura Y, Miyamoto M, Murakami A et al. A Phase II detoxification enzyme inducer from lemon grass: identification of citral and involvement of electrophilic reaction in enzyme induction. Biochem Biophys Res Commun 2003; 302:593–600; Nho CW, Jeffery E. The synergistic upregulation of phase II detoxification enzymes by glucosinolate breakdown products in cruciferous vegetables. Tox App Pharmacol 2001; 174:146–152.

amino acids in the diet to other non-essential amino acids needed by the body.[13] When liver function is compromised, protein manufacture decreases and can lead to protein calorie malnutrition (PCM). Inflammation in the liver further compromises the production of important proteins.[13]

Protein calorie malnutrition is associated with an increased risk of morbidity and mortality in patients with cirrhosis and occurs in 50%–90% of these patients.[13] The protein albumin is important for maintaining oncotic pressure. Reduced oncotic pressure reduces the ability to hold water within the bloodstream and water leaks into the surrounding tissues. During liver disease, pressure in the liver increases, forcing water from the blood vessels into the abdominal cavity, a condition known as ascites. Protein is also important for the immune system (antibodies such as IgG), wound healing (collagen, elastin), transport structures (haemoglobin), peptide-based hormones (insulin, thyroxine), biochemical functions catalysed by enzymes (pepsin, collagenase), clotting factors, muscle, hair and nails. Ascites can hide malnutrition, giving the patient the appearance of being overweight;

further examination should show wasted arm and leg muscles and poor hair and nails and possibly excessive bruising due to lack of clotting factors.[14] Previously, protein intake was restricted in the liver patient due to the effects of ammonia on the development of hepatic encephalopathy (HE).[13,15]

Liver disease is often accompanied by anorexia, leading to reduced intake of protein and other foods. If kilojoules are sufficiently restricted this will lead to proteins being catabolised in the liver for energy. A reduced ability to manufacture bile leads to poor fat absorption and a further reduction in available kilojoules.

The storage of sugars as glycogen in the liver acts as a buffer for blood glucose levels, preventing an excess of sugar after meals and releasing sugar slowly as needed later. Changes to liver metabolism mean that glycogen is no longer efficiently stored and released by the liver. In PCM this leads to the catabolism of proteins from muscle and fat for energy and poor blood sugar regulation. An overnight fast in the cirrhotic patient is similar to that of a 72-hour fast in the healthy individual.[14] Cirrhotic patients are also prone to hypermetabolism, increasing the need for energy intake.

Higher than usual intakes of branched chain amino acids as well as vegetable proteins have shown benefits in patients with cirrhosis, but more research is needed on both topics. Sodium restrictions are necessary to prevent ascites development, but very strict limitations, which may lead to PCM, should be avoided.[13]

Blood tests showing albumin (20-day half-life) and prealbumin (2-day half-life) can be used to monitor liver status but these and many of the other hepatic proteins such as transferrin are negative acute-phase proteins, which means their levels decrease in response to infection/inflammation, injury or trauma.[16]

Patients with cirrhosis should consume 100–170 kJ per kg of body weight per day with 1.0–1.5 g/kg protein per day to prevent muscle catabolism. This should preferably be taken as four small meals a day with a late evening snack of protein and some carbohydrate to help balance blood sugars and prevent muscle wasting and cramps.[13] If hepatic encephalopathy (HE) occurs, temporarily restrict protein to 0.6–0.8 g/kg/day until the cause of the HE is determined and eliminated.[13] Studies have shown a benefit in using plant-based protein as it is lower in ammonia, reducing the risk of HE and is higher in fibre which improves digestive function.[13]

In cases of ascites, sodium intake should be limited but not to the extent that food becomes unpalatable and anorexia worsens.[13]

At the opposite scale liver disease is also associated with metabolic syndrome and excess nutrition in which case protein has the benefit of increasing satiety.

FIBRE

Fibre-like protein is important in all aspects of liver disease. Fibre increase satiety and helps regulate blood sugar, so is important in the metabolic picture in non-alcoholic fatty liver disease (NAFLD). Fibre absorbs bile and removes it from the body and improves intestinal transit time which is important for healthy digestive function. Many types of fibre also act as prebiotics supporting a healthy gut microbiome. Use caution with fibre in cachexic patients who are nutrient deficient as fibre can increase their satiety to the detriment of other nutrient intake. Fibre also reduces the formation of gallstones, especially during rapid weight loss.[17]

FATS

Biliary disease affects the body's ability to process fats so the intake of fats should be reviewed. In general avoid all trans fats, allow moderate amount of saturated fats, preferably from grass-fed animals, and game and fish. Increase the amount of essential fatty acids to reduce inflammation by including fish, nuts and seeds such as walnuts and flaxseed.[18] Fats in the diet are important to stimulate bile flow and prevent gallstones but excessive fat can lead to gallbladder attacks.[17]

ANTIOXIDANTS

Inflammation due to oxidative stress is a major factor in the pathogenesis of chronic liver disease in the hepatobiliary system leading to fibrosis and further loss of function. Reduced hepatobiliary function can also increase the reactive oxygen species (ROS) load on the body due to an accumulation of unprocessed toxins. Therefore a diet full of varied antioxidant-rich food is vital.

In hepatitis C virus infection, oxidative mediated pathways are involved in the progression of persistent infection to fibrosis, cirrhosis and carcinogenesis. In cholecystitis, damage to tissues releases ROS causing lipid peroxidation of membranes and inflammation.[19] ROS are also responsible for the release of inflammatory cytokines that further exacerbate the inflammatory process. Thus dietary antioxidants are crucial in the management of hepatobiliary conditions. Fruits and vegetables rich in vitamins E and C, selenium, carotenoids and anthocyanins are recommended for their powerful antioxidant activity and overall nutrient content. However, fruit consumption should remain at two pieces per day to avoid excessive sugar intake.

Oxygen radical absorbance capacity (ORAC) measurements indicate that garlic, curly cabbage and Brussels sprouts are the strongest source of vegetable antioxidants.[20]

Flavonoids occur naturally in the diet and can be found in tea, wine, fruit and vegetables. Quercetin is a flavone and can be found in onions, apples, broccoli and berries and exhibits significant anti-inflammatory and antioxidant activity.[21] The flavanone group exists in most citrus fruits. Hesperidin is a flavanone glycoside abundantly found in citrus fruits, cumin and peppermint[22] and has anti-inflammatory, analgesic, antibacterial, antifungal, antiviral, antioxidant and free radical scavenger activity.[23]

Catechins are found in tea and wine and anthocyanidins are found in berries, grapes, tea and wine. Research suggests that the flavonoids have anti-inflammatory, anti-allergic, antiviral, antioxidant and anti-carcinogenic activities.[24] Anthocyanins are responsible for the blue and purple colour pigmentation in fruits and vegetables and demonstrate both antioxidant and anti-inflammatory activity.[25] Research has shown that they may work to prime[26] the cell and enhance the ability to withstand stress.

Resveratrol decreased NAFLD severity in animal models through TNF-α inhibition; activation of AMPK; skeletal muscle SIRT1 and SIRT4 expression; increasing mitochondria; increasing hepatic uncoupling protein 2 expression; decreasing hepatic LDL receptor and SR-BI mRNA and protein expressions; and reducing nuclear factor kappaB (NF-kappaB) activity.[27]

Vitamin E is an important fat-soluble antioxidant which helps prevent the oxidation of lipids and reduces oxidative stress. The high oxidative stress associated with liver disease increases the need for vitamin E.[18] Many foods containing vitamin E are also high in cholesterol except for green and yellow vegetables; therefore it is important to incorporate green and yellow vegetables in the diet. Vegetables also tend to be lacking in patients with NAFLD.[28]

PROBIOTICS

The intestinal epithelial cells prevent the translocation of bacterial products to the portal circulation. When this barrier is damaged the liver cells are exposed to bacterial products such as lipopolysaccharide (LPS) and toxins. These products can trigger an immune response, oxidative stress, inflammation, fibrosis and promote insulin resistance, obesity and metabolic syndrome.[29–32]

A study investigating the correlation between intestinal permeability in patients with NAFLD and disease progression concluded that the severity of steatosis in NAFLD in humans is correlated with increased gut permeability due to small intestinal bacterial overgrowth (SIBO), causing disruption of intercellular tight junctions in the intestine.[33]

Evidence suggests that diet and lifestyle factors which are known to exacerbate NAFLD may do this by changing the gut microbiota.[30,31] Poor diet affects gut motility and that affects the microbiota and intestinal permeability which further degrades gut motility. A high-fat diet increases inflammatory microbiota and causes an increase in bile acids, which disrupts intestinal permeability.[30] A high-fructose diet increases bacteria that can extract energy from complex polysaccharides, resulting in an increase of free fatty acids and energy reaching the liver with consequent hepatic lipogenesis and gluconeogenesis.[30] In NAFLD the microbiota convert choline into methylamines; this reduced availability of choline, reduces the export of VLDL from the liver and increases fat accumulation and ROS.[30] Changes in bile acid metabolism increase bacteriostasis in the gut, which adversely affects the liver when combined with intestinal permeability.[30,32]

The use of probiotics has improved the pathology of NAFLD: in animal models and to some extent in human models, probiotics led to decreases in liver fat and serum ALT and lipid levels, and improvements in inflammation, liver fibrosis, oxidative stress and insulin resistance.[18,30,32]

Changes to diet within a few days lead to a change in microbiota; however, if the diet reverts so do the microbiota. Therefore changes to diet need to be sustainable, containing plenty of plant food and fermented foods.

Naturopathic wholefood diet and lifestyle

The above dietary principles can be achieved through the implementation of a naturopathic wholefood diet that includes plenty of plant-based foods, both fresh and dried legumes, seasonally varied fresh and local fruit and vegetables, organic if possible. This will ensure high-fibre, vitamin, mineral and antioxidant content. Include good fats such as fish, olive oil, avocado, walnuts and flaxseed. Include good-quality protein such as grass-fed beef, lamb, game, wild fish and eggs. Include vegetarian-based forms of protein with nuts, seeds, tempeh, legumes and gluten-free grains such as buckwheat and quinoa.

Exercise is a vital addition to a sensible wholefood diet. The exercise regimen should be based on the capabilities and time constraints of the patient, starting slowly and sustainably to incorporate activity into their lives. Make it fun and social with activities such as salsa, tennis and walking and advocate weight training and cardiovascular exercise. Include activities in the sunlight and fresh air.

Fasting and rapid weight loss

Fasting and weight loss are contraindicated in hepatobiliary disease as rapid weight loss and cycles of weight gain and weight loss are indicated in the aetiology of gallstones. Fasting is contraindicated in the treatment of NAFLD as it creates massive adipose lipolysis[34] and the free fatty acids are then able to flood the liver, worsening the condition, owing to the rapid transfer of fatty acids and enhanced production of TNF-α.[35] Furthermore, prolonged fasting has also been found to impair the free radical scavenging ability of liver cells[36] thus, according to the 'second hit' or more recently the multi-hit theory, oxidation exacerbates liver damage. In the worst case scenario, morbidly obese patients who undergo drastic weight loss have experienced fatal hepatic failure.[37]

SUGAR

There are strong links between metabolic syndrome and hepatobiliary disease therefore sugar must be reduced as much as possible in the diet. Compromised liver function reduces the liver's ability to store excess sugar in the liver as glycogen. Therefore meals should consist of a balance of protein, fats, fibre and complex carbohydrates to control the rate at which sugar is released.

Suggestions for reducing high sugar intake in diets include:

- Reduce sugar cravings by stabilising blood sugars through consumption of small regular meals
- Ensure adequate intake of protein and fibre to assist with blood sugar regulation
- Do not add sugar to food, and have a moderate intake of honey
- Ensure ingredients for healthy snacks are available
- Increase intake of fresh fruit and vegetables and of wholegrains if low.

Hepatobiliary nutritional objectives (nutrients)

Potential nutritional deficiencies that should be considered in all hepatobiliary disease are listed in Table 11.5. Poor diet, malabsorption and diminished reserves combined with hepatobiliary dysfunction mean that deficiencies are probable. The hepatobiliary disease itself often increases the need for some nutrients. This is definitely true of vitamins such as vitamin E to combat oxidative stress.[38] Fat soluble vitamin deficiencies are common manifestations of malnutrition and a retrospective study reported that the majority of liver disease patients being considered for liver transplantation presented with vitamin A and D deficiencies.[38]

Zinc, magnesium and selenium deficiencies are common in many types of chronic liver disease whereas manganese, copper and iron can be in excess and lead to complications that exacerbate neurological symptoms, cirrhosis and biliary obstruction.[38]

Hepatobiliary herbal medicine classes

There is an extensive array of herbal medicines available for the treatment of liver conditions and without a proper understanding of the traditional use of the herb and of current supportive evidence from the literature, the selection of the most condition-specific and appropriate medicines is a complex task. With experience and an inquiring mind, the herbal practitioner is able to develop an understanding that balances hard evidence, traditional knowledge and intuitive understanding.

The classes of herbal medicines that need to be considered in the treatment of any liver condition must include choleretics, cholagogues, hepatoprotectives and hepatotrophorestoratives. Choleretics are herbal medicines with the ability to increase bile production in the liver and optimise the flow of bile to the gallbladder; they are indicated in almost any disorder involving the hepatobiliary system. Cholagogues are herbal medicines that improve the flow of bile from the gallbladder by enhancing either gentle or strong contractions of the gallbladder wall. Bear in mind that treatment designed to restore and optimise health should focus on gentle support of the hepatobiliary organs. Overstimulation of the liver or gallbladder in chronic or severely suppressed cases will result in a healing crisis and patient compliance naturally wanes. Of course herbal therapy that is heroic is absolutely contraindicated in cases of acute inflammation, gallstones or end-stage liver disease.

Hepatotrophorestoratives protect and restore liver function and are important in the treatment of liver conditions. Hepatotrophorestoratives protect the liver from directly ingested toxins, such as alcohol and reactive metabolites, secondary to metabolism. *Silybum marianum* does this by upregulating glutathione, the liver's endogenous antioxidant. In vitro studies have confirmed the antiviral action of silymarin.[39–42] Two main hypotheses explored to explain the antiviral effect are: (1) improved cellular response and (2) inhibition of viral function. One in vitro study showed that silibinin inhibits HCV (hepatitis C virus) genotype 1b and 2a strain JFH1 replication in cell culture system by inhibiting polymerase activity.[39]

Hepatoprotective herbs are anti-inflammatory antioxidants and antifibrotics and are crucial to limit the damage from reactive oxygen species (ROS) and prevent the pathogenesis of inflammation due to fibrosis, cirrhosis and eventual carcinoma.

As cachexia is a key feature of any end-stage liver disease, the adaptogens and herbal nutritives will help rebuild the stressed body and reduce fatigue. Carminatives and bitter digestive herbs will work to restore appetite and reduce the flatulence, nausea and griping associated with liver dysfunction. Depending on the severity of the liver pathology, these herbs can be taken as extracts or as herbal teas. Nervines can be prescribed as gentle healing teas to tone and restore function to the nervous system, whether stress, anxiety, insomnia or depression predominates.

Depending on the cause of the hepatobiliary dysfunction and the resilience and attitude of the patient, several other classes of herbal medicine can be employed to restore health. In metabolic syndrome, blood sugar and cholesterol regulators can also be employed. In hepatitis antivirals and immune-stimulating herbs can be employed to reduce viral load and replication, and immune stimulants support any specific antiviral activity.

Please see Table 11.6 for a comprehensive discussion.

INVESTIGATIONS

Allopathic investigations

LIVER FUNCTION TEST (LFT)

The liver is comprised of three systems: the hepatocyte, involved with metabolic reactions, protein synthesis, and degradation and metabolism of xenobiotics (e.g. drugs); the biliary system, concerned with the metabolism of bilirubin and bile salts; and the reticuloendothelial system, involved with the immune system and the production of haem and globin metabolites (e.g. bilirubin).[43]

Laboratory tests can either be employed to measure physiological function (bilirubin, prealbumin and albumin), measure injury to the liver (ALT, AST, ALP and GGT) or measure reactions to liver injury (globulins and tissue antibodies). Liver tests are used to determine the presence of liver disease, assist with diagnosis and monitor the course of disease progression.[44] Alanine aminotransferase (ALT) and aspartate aminotransferase (AST) are common indicators of cell injury, as any damage to liver cell membranes results in the release of aminotransferases into the circulation. Aminotransferases are regarded as the most sensitive but nonspecific markers of liver cell damage. ALT is more specific as it is present in the liver while AST is present in other body tissues. Both enzymes (ALT and AST) require pyridoxal phosphate (B_6) as a co-factor. Thus an alcoholic who is deficient in B_6 may have lower ALT or AST serum levels. The introduction of a multivitamin containing B_6 and B_{12} will yield a more accurate level of ALT and AST in alcoholic patients.[43]

TABLE 11.5 Potential nutritional deficiencies			
Deficiency	**Reason**	**Daily requirement**	**Foods containing**
Vitamin A	Bile disorders interfere with fat-soluble vitamin absorption. Vitamin A deficiency linked to hepatic fibrosis and cirrhosis	2500 IU	Vitamin A: butter, cheese, eggs and meat Carotenoids: papaya, carrots, mango, spinach, pumpkin, broccoli, tomatoes, apricots, rock melon
Vitamin D	Bile disorders interfere with fat-soluble vitamin absorption	400 IU	Butter, oily fish, cheese, eggs
Vitamin E	Bile disorders interfere with fat-soluble vitamin absorption. Reduced vitamin E linked to increased oxidative damage and degree of fibrosis	500 IU	Wheatgerm, almonds, sunflower seeds, walnuts, cashews, avocado, brown rice, olive oil, oily fish, green vegetables
Vitamin K	Reduced liver function interferes with vitamin K synthesis	150–500 micrograms	Cauliflower, Brussels sprouts, kale, tomatoes, spinach, green beans, broccoli
Protein	Protein calorie malnutrition is common in cirrhosis; marked by reduced serum albumin and skeletal muscle volume	Complicated cirrhosis: 1–1.2 g/protein/kg per day Uncomplicated cirrhosis: 0.8–1 g/protein/kg/day	Legumes, lean cuts of meat, fish, chicken (organic), cheese, milk, eggs, bread, nuts and seeds, tofu, tempeh
Branched chain amino acids	Branched chain amino acid deficiencies noted in chronic liver disease	Leucine Isoleucine Valine	Eggs, poultry, meat and milk have significant BCAA content
Selenium	Low selenium levels directly associated with chronic liver pathologies. Needed for activity of glutathione peroxidase	150–400 micrograms	Brazil nuts, wholegrains, molasses, cashews, onion, garlic, broccoli
SAM-e	Deficiency impairs crucial functions of liver and increased susceptibility to damage. Most important methyl donor	600–1200 mg per day	Not found in food but produced from ATP and methionine
Zinc	Zinc deficiency is thought to complicate many liver diseases. Serum and hepatic zinc reduced in chronic HBV and HCV. Deficiencies linked to impaired activity of superoxide dismutase (CuZnSOD)	25–40 mg	Sesame seeds, pumpkin seeds, sunflower seeds, walnuts, almonds, homemade muesli, dhal, oysters, meat, fish, chicken, eggs, wholegrains
Magnesium	Deficiencies identified in pathogenesis of NAFLD, non-alcoholic steatohepatitis (NASH) and insulin resistance. Look for leg cramps in cirrhosis and supplement as a matter of course	250 mg–350 mg per day	Wholegrains, green leafy vegetables, legumes, almonds, cashews, pecans and Brazil nuts, soybeans and soy products, molasses
L-carnitine	Deficiency impairs beta oxidation which shifts hepatic fatty acid synthesis to VLDL and encourages hepatic triglyceride synthesis	1000 mg	Lamb, beef, poultry, fish, eggs with small amounts in mushrooms
Methyl factors (B_9, B_{12})	Reduced B_9, B_{12} methyl factors linked to increased insulin resistance, poor synthesis of methionine from homocysteine and SAM-e	B_9: 500 micrograms Methylcobalamin, active form of B_{12} is preferred over cyanocobalamin 50–200 micrograms	B_9: organ meats, green leafy vegetables and Brussels sprouts B_{12}: meat, fish, eggs, cheese, milk and oysters

TABLE 11.6 Herbal classes and application

Class	Key herbs within class
Gentle liver detoxifiers	*Juglans cinerea, Peumus boldo, Phyllanthus amarus, Rumex crispus, Silybum marianum, Taraxacum officinale, Verbena officinalis*
Moderate liver detoxifiers	*Andrographis paniculata, Bupluerum falcatum, Chionanthus virginicus, Cynara scolymus, Hypericum perforatum, Leptandra virginica, Schisandra chinensis, Silybum marianum*
Mighty liver detoxifiers	*Berberis vulgaris, Chelidonium majus, Curcuma longa, Iris versicolor, Peumus boldo, Picrorhiza kurroa, Silybum marianum*
Phase I detoxifiers	*Anethum graveolens, Carum carvi, Hypericum perforatum, Schisandra chinensis, Silybum marianum, Taraxacum officinale*
Phase II detoxifiers	*Allium sativum, Camellia sinensis, Curcuma longa, Cymbopogon citratus (citral), Rosmarinus officinalis, Salvia officinalis, Schisandra chinensis, Taraxacum officinale*
Phase I and II detoxifiers	*Curcuma longa, Rosmarinus officinalis, Schisandra chinensis, Silybum marianum*
Hepatoprotectives	*Andrographis paniculata, Angelica sinensis, Bupleurum falcatum, Curcuma longa, Cynara scolymus, Panax ginseng, Phyllanthus amarus, Picrorhiza kurroa, Salvia miltiorrhiza, Schisandra chinensis, Silybum marianum, Smilax ornata, Taraxacum officinale*
Hepatotrophorestoratives	*Cynara scolymus, Silybum marianum*
Cholagogues	*Chelidonium majus, Chionanthus virginicus, Curcuma longa, Cynara scolymus, Dioscorea* spp., *Matricaria recutita, Picrorhiza kurroa, Rumex crispus, Silybum marianum, Taraxacum officinale folia/radix*
Choleretics	*Andrographis paniculata, Berberis vulgaris, Calendula officinalis, Chelidonium majus, Curcuma longa, Cynara scolymus, Mentha x piperita, Silybum marianum, Zingiber officinale*
Bitters	*Achillea millefolium, Andrographis paniculata, Centaurium erythraea, Cynara scolymus, Gentiana lutea, Humulus lupulus, Hydrastis canadensis, Matricaria recutita, Scutellaria baicalensis*
Blood sugar improvers	*Codonopsis pilosula, Foeniculum vulgare, Galega officinalis, Glycyrrhiza glabra, Gymnena silvestre, Morus and Nigra alba, Phyllanthus amarus, Silybum marianum*
Carminatives	*Achillea millefolium, Angelica archangelica, Foeniculum vulgare, Lavendula angustifolia, Matricaria recutita, Melissa officinalis, Mentha x piperita, Rosmarinus officinalis, Zingiber officinale*
Nervines	*Avena sativa (green and seed), Centella asiatica, Hypericum perforatum, Melissa officinalis, Passiflora incarnata, Scutellaria lateriflora, Turnera diffusa, Verbena officinalis*
Adaptogens/tonics	*Andrographis paniculata, Astragalus membranaceus, Avena sativa, Centella asiatica, Codonopsis pilosula, Eleutherococcus senticosus, Ganoderma lucidum, Panax ginseng, Rehmannia glutinosa, Rhodiola rosea, Schisandra chinensis, Withania somnifera*
Hepatic anti-inflammatories	*Andrographis paniculata, Bupleurum falcatum, Curcuma longa, Glycyrrhiza glabra, Menyanthes trifoliata, Picrorhiza kurroa, Scutellaria baicalensis, Silybum marianum*
Alternatives	*Arctium lappa, Berberis vulgaris, Centella asiatica, Galium aparine, Iris versicolor, Juglans cinerea, Rumex crispus, Smilax ornata, Trifolium pratense, Urtica dioica folia/radix, Viola tricolor*
Anticholesterolaemics and hypocholesterolaemics	*Commiphora mol mol, Cynara scolymus, Curcuma longa, Silybum marianum, Trigonella foenum graecum*
Antifibrotics and fibrinolytics	*Astragalus membranaceus, Centella asiatica, Ginkgo biloba, Salvia miltiorrhiza, Scutellaria baicalensis, Urtica dioica*
Interferon production stimulators	*Astragalus membranaceus, Echinacea angustifolia, Eleutherococcus senticosus, Ganoderma lucidum, Hydrastis canadensis, Panax ginseng, Vitis vinifera*
Antioxidants	*Andrographis paniculata, Astragalus membranaceus, Bupleurum falcatum, Camellia sinensis, Curcuma longa, Rosmarinus officinalis, Schisandra chinensis, Silybum marianum, Vitis vinifera*
Hepatic antivirals	*Andrographis paniculata, Bupleurum falcatum, Hypericum perforatum, Phyllanthus amarus, Picrorhiza kurroa, Scutellaria baicalensis*
Immune stimulants	*Andrographis paniculata, Astragalus membranaceus, Baptisia tinctoria, Codonopsis pilosula, Echinacea* spp., *Eleutherococcus senticosus, Panax ginseng, Tabebuia avellanedae*

Bartram T. Bartram's encyclopedia of herbal medicine. London: Robinson Publishing; 1998; Choi EH, Lee N, Kim HJ et al. *Schisandra fructus* extract ameliorates doxorubicin-induced cardiomycytes: altered gene expression for detoxification enzymes. Genes Nutr 2008; 2:337–345; Salmond S. The mighty liver and beyond. Phytomedicine Seminar Series. Phytomedicine 2002; Thomsen M. Phytotherapy desk reference. 2nd edn. Dee Why (NSW): Institut For Phytoterapi; 2001.

Alkaline phosphatase (ALP) and gamma-glutamyl transferase (GGT) are regarded as cholestatic enzymes. They show minimal activity in normal hepatic tissue and are used to detect impaired bile flow. ALP is present in several body tissues but is often associated with the liver, bone, intestine and placenta.[45] If ALP is less than three times the normal value, biliary obstruction is less likely. However, if levels are greater than three times the normal value, biliary obstruction must be ruled out immediately.[46]

GGT is derived predominantly from the liver and as its activity closely matches the activity of ALP, it is often used to determine the source of raised ALP. If GGT is increased then the ALP source is often from the liver. However, if GGT is normal then bone is regarded as the ALP source. GGT is found in both hepatocytes and biliary epithelia cells and is more specific for diagnosis of hepatobiliary conditions as it is not found in other body tissues.[47]

The primary role of GGT is the extracellular catabolism of glutathione, the major thiol antioxidant, which protects cells against oxidants produced during normal metabolism, and is also involved in cellular defence.[48] GGT is often elevated in alcoholics, in some obese people and in the presence of high concentrations of therapeutic drugs such as acetaminophen.[43] In addition, circulating serum GGT has been linked to non-alcoholic fatty liver disease, vascular and nonvascular diseases and mortality outcomes.[48] For example, raised GGT alongside albuminuria may predict the development of hypertension.[43]

The ratios of elevated aminotransferases assist in the diagnosis of liver disorders. For example, an AST-to-ALT ratio higher than 4 is characteristic of Wilson disease, ratios between 2 and 4 are typical of alcoholic liver disease, and a ratio below 1 suggests nonalcoholic steatohepatitis (without cirrhosis). When elevations of AST and ALT are mild, ratios above 2 are consistent with alcoholic liver disease or cirrhosis of any aetiology.[49]Normal serum values for aminotransferases differ widely among laboratories, but the general consensus is moving towards values equal to or below 30 U/L for men and 19 U/L for women.[49]

As prealbumin and albumin are synthesised in the liver, decreased serum levels reflect liver disease and protein loss, malnutrition and generalised catabolic states. Decreased serum albumin usually indicates the presence of chronic disease due to its 21-day half-life.[44,47] Prealbumin has a half-life of 2 days and therefore is a more immediate indicator of liver status than albumin. Reduced serum prealbumin and albumin levels are good indicators of both disease progression and severity.

Increased bilirubin levels indicate levels of cell necrosis and cholestasis. Bilirubin can be classified as either direct (conjugated bilirubin) or indirect (unconjugated bilirubin). High levels of conjugated bilirubin indicate the presence of blockages in bile ducts. The compromised excretion of bile results in increased serum bilirubin. High levels of unconjugated bilirubin suggest bleeding disorders, resulting in the availability of haem supplies that exceed the liver's ability to conjugate bilirubin or diseased tissue with compromised ability to conjugate bilirubin.[50]

Prothrombin time (PT) relies on clotting factors I, II, V, VII and X which are all synthesised in the liver. Factors II, VII and X require vitamin K: thus, if liver damage is present and vitamin K synthesis is reduced, prothrombin times may be increased due to lack of clotting factors. Both albumin and prothrombin time are regarded as insensitive indicators of hepatic injury but are better indicators of disease severity.[51]

Transition from the immune–active phase of disease to the inactive carrier state in HBV treatment revolves around HBV DNA suppression, marked by the loss of serum hepatitis B e antigen (HBeAg) and the development of anti-HBe antibodies (HBeAg seroconversion). ALT should also be normal. These markers should be tested every 3 to 6 months; a flare-up of any of these markers could indicate a viral breakthrough and the patient should be referred to their GP or referred to a hepatology outpatient clinic at hospital for urgent treatment review.

Interpretation of investigations and mechanism of result is listed in Table 11.7.

Other investigations

Patients with liver disease can present with considerable alterations in blood profiles. Abnormalities in platelet number and function are common in patients who have liver disease, thus full blood counts are recommended to monitor haemolysis. Thrombocytopenia is also a feature of advanced stage liver disease and is associated with increased platelet sequestration in the spleen due to portal hypertension. Thrombocytopenia also may be a consequence of decreased thrombopoietin synthesis in the liver.[52]

There are two types of hepatobiliary autoimmune condition: primary biliary cirrhosis (PCB) and autoimmune hepatitis. Both conditions have similar signs and symptoms to other liver diseases and elevated liver enzymes; however, they also have detectable antibodies. For autoimmune hepatitis, test for antinuclear antibodies (ANAs), smooth-muscle antibodies (SMAs), liver-kidney microsomal type 1 (LKM-1) or anti–liver cytosol 1 (anti-LC1) antibodies. For PCB test for antimitochondrial antibodies.

The gold standard for the evaluation of liver disease is the liver biopsy which estimates the stage of liver disease by assessing the pattern and the degree of fibrosis. Tissue samples can be obtained through percutaneous, peritoneoscopic or open surgical evaluation. The size of the tissue sample obtained can be a limitation. Obtaining tissue samples from multiple areas of the liver is more beneficial but the procedure carries greater risk and is a less attractive option for patients.[53]

The Child score was first proposed in 1964. This test relied on bilirubin and albumin scores and assessed the presence of ascites, encephalopathy and nutritional status in order to classify and rate hepatic function. The Child–Pugh score was proposed a decade later and nutritional status was replaced by prothrombin time. This score is used to both determine mortality for surgical procedures and monitor the progression of disease.[54] The model for end-stage liver disease (MELD) was introduced to evaluate patients awaiting liver transplantation. The calculation of

TABLE 11.7 Interpretation of investigations and mechanism of result

Liver function test	Interpretation	Mechanism
↑ increased ALT	Any liver injury or liver necrosis	ALT is located in the cytosol of hepatocytes thus serum levels rise with liver cell injury
↑ increased GGT	Cholestatic liver disease Primary biliary cirrhosis Primary sclerosing cholangitis Liver cancer	GGT is found in both hepatocytes and biliary epithelial cells
AST>ALT	Cirrhosis Liver cancer Alcoholic liver disease (2 : 1)	Higher ratio of AST to ALT used as a diagnostic tool for identifying cirrhosis
↑ increased GGT, normal ALT, ↑ ALP	Cholestasis Liver cancer	Increased GGT and ALP means there is a hepatic source to the liver injury
↑ increased globulins	Cirrhosis Autoimmune liver disease	Failure of damaged liver to degrade immunoglobulins Increased globulin production Multiple reasons
↑ increased bilirubin	Poor liver function Acute liver injury Gilbert's syndrome Inherited syndromes Cirrhosis Haemolysis	Damaged hepatocytes cannot excrete bilirubin
↑ increased conjugated bilirubin	Gallstones Bile duct blockage (tumour, gallstone) Liver cancer Drug-induced cholestasis	Blockages in bile ducts result in compromised excretion of bile and blood levels rise
↑ increased unconjugated bilirubin	Hepatitis Cirrhosis Gilbert's syndrome Haemolytic or pernicious anaemia Criggler Najjar	Severe red blood cell destruction results in large amounts of haem needing catabolism. Levels exceed the liver's ability to conjugate. Diseased liver fails to conjugate bilirubin in cases of hepatitis or cirrhosis
↓ reduced albumin	Poor liver function Poor prognosis Liver failure	Albumin is synthesised in hepatocytes thus compromised liver function will decrease synthesis
Full blood count	**Interpretation**	**Mechanism**
↓ reduced platelets	Cirrhosis Liver failure	Increased destruction of platelets within spleen, reduced platelet production in bone marrow
Coagulation studies	**Interpretation**	**Mechanism**
Prolongation of prothrombin time	Cirrhosis	Clotting factors synthesised in the liver
Tumour marker	Interpretation	Mechanism
Alphafetoprotein (AFP)	Liver cancer	AFP levels increase in presence of hepatocellular carcinoma in 40–60% of cases

the MELD score is based on serum bilirubin, serum creatinine and prothrombin time.[55]

FibroMeters are specific blood tests for liver fibrosis. The two diagnostic targets of this test are the stage of fibrosis and the extent of fibrosis in chronic viral hepatitis, alcoholic liver disease and non-alcoholic fatty liver disease (NAFLD). FibroMeters have high diagnostic accuracy and are the only tests employed to ascertain and classify fibrosis and cirrhosis in HCV patients.[56]

Transient elastography (FibroScan) is a noninvasive ultrasound that uses shear wave velocity to measure liver stiffness (elasticity) in kilopascals (kPa)[57] for the assessment of hepatic fibrosis in patients with chronic liver disease.[58] The median value of the ten valid measurements is considered representative of liver elasticity (range 2.5–75 kPa)[59] FibroScan is now regarded as a reliable surrogate marker for grading the severity of liver fibrosis in patients with chronic liver disease (CLD), determining prognosis in patients with chronic hepatitis B (CHB) or chronic hepatitis C (CHC) and monitoring antiviral treatment outcome. It is useful in identifying HCV-related cirrhosis, but has a failure rate of 5%, primarily in obese patients, and has diminished accuracy in the earlier stages of fibrosis.[60]

In hepatitis B virus (HBV) infection, values less than 5–6 kPa indicate absent or minimal liver fibrosis, whereas the reported cut-off values for predicting cirrhosis in patients with chronic hepatitis B ranged from 9.4 to 12.9 kPa, with values greater than 12–14 kPa highly suggestive of cirrhosis.[61] In hepatitis C virus (HCV) infection the FibroScan cut-off values for the diagnosis of fibrosis F≥1, F≥2, F≥3 and F=4 are 5.3 kPa, 7.4 kPa, 9.1 kPa and 13.2 kPa respectively. This study verified these data with corresponding liver biopsy specimens.[62]

A 2014 meta-analysis suggested that FibroScan is excellent in diagnosing (fibrosis stage 3) F≥3 (85% sensitivity, 82% specificity) and cirrhosis (F=4) (92% sensitivity, 92% specificity), and it has a moderate accuracy for (fibrosis stage 2) F≥2 in NAFLD patients.[57]

Naturopathic investigations

FUNCTIONAL LIVER DETOXIFICATION PROFILE (FLDP)

The functional liver detoxification profile (FLDP) tests the Phase I and Phase II detoxification pathways of the liver by using low-dose caffeine, paracetamol and aspirin challenges. This test can be ordered by naturopaths and is available through private pathology laboratories in Australia. Caffeine is primarily absorbed by the intestine and is metabolised in the liver by Phase I cytochrome P450 enzyme 1A2. Paracetamol is metabolised through three of the Phase II pathways: glutathione conjugation, sulfation and glucoronidation. Aspirin is metabolised through glycine conjugation and glucoronidation. Caffeine, aspirin and paracetamol need to be eliminated from the diet 24 hours before the test.[63]

The FLDP employs both saliva and urine specimens which are collected at specific times by the patient. The samples are then sent to the laboratory where they are tested for the presence of metabolites. The ability of the liver to engage in Phase I and Phase II detoxification pathways is evident due to the absence or presence of metabolites from the ingestion of the three challenge substances.

Clinicians are provided with a comprehensive report where errors in a patient's detoxification pathways are identified. Although a skilled clinician should be able to determine poor liver detoxification ability and employ a treatment protocol to correct the detoxification problems, this test may be of value where patient compliance is low, where treatment has failed to produce the desired results and in cases where the patient requires evidence of functional derangement before embarking on a naturopathic treatment protocol.

HAIR TISSUE MINERAL ANALYSIS (HTMA)

The hair tissue mineral analysis (HTMA) test measures the levels and ratios of minerals and heavy metals in hair. However, this test is particularly useful for the diagnosis of heavy metal toxicity. This test is particularly useful in identifying chronic exposure to arsenic, lead, mercury and aluminium. There is debate about the usefulness of this test for the diagnosis of any diseases other than toxicity from heavy metal exposure. However, laboratories do offer hair mineral tests as a method of assessing nutrient status and deficiencies.

The discerning practitioner is advised to engage in comprehensive case taking and a thorough dietary analysis so that deficiencies can be elicited through personal communication, understanding and interpretation of a patient's dietary habits rather than solely relying on a laboratory test. Notwithstanding, the HTMA test is a valid tool for the assessment of suspected toxicity where a patient presents with headaches, nausea, fatigue, irritability, depression, anxiety and insomnia, and where other potential aetiological leads have been ruled out.

Allopathic treatment

OVERVIEW OF MEDICATIONS AND MODE OF ACTION

Hepatitis B

The current available treatments for chronic hepatitis B virus (HBV) infection include pegylated interferon alpha-2a (PEG-IFN-2A) or any of the five approved nucleos(t)ide analogues (NUC): lamivudine (LMV), entecavir (ETV), adefovir dipivoxil (ADV) and tenofovir disoproxil fumarate (TDF).[64–66]

The mechanism of action of PEG-IFN centres on the drug's ability to cause degradation of viral messenger RNA and inhibit protein synthesis. The nucleoside and nucleotide analogues act as competitive inhibitors of HBV reverse transcriptase and once incorporated into the DNA strand provoke chain termination.[65]

A small proportion of treatment-naive HBV mono-infected patients are treated with pegylated interferon.[65]

Lamivudine is often associated with the development of drug resistance, with resistance to LMV occurring in 20–23% of patients after 1 year and in 70–80% of patients after 5 years of treatment.[67,68] Entecavir (ETV) and tenofovir (TDF) are recommended as the first-line treatment for viral suppression with a low risk of antiviral resistance.[66] The drug-resistant mutations usually affect the reverse transcriptase domain of the HBV polymerase protein.[65]

Hepatitis C

Since 2013/2014 direct-acting antivirals (DAAs) have become the gold standard of treatment for chronic hepatitis C viral infection, leading to sustained viral response (SVR) in 91% of CHC patients in 12 weeks.[69] Treatment response depends on HCV genotype, the presence or otherwise of cirrhosis and whether the patient is treatment naïve or treatment experienced.[69] The SVR rates for each HCV genotype overall are as follows: genotype 1 (92.8% SVR), genotype 2 (82.6% SVR), genotype 3 (74.8% SVR) and genotype 4 (89.6% SVR).[69]

The new DAA drugs have different modes of action, therefore they are usually given in combination as double or triple therapy to ensure rapid eradication of the virus and to prevent the creation of drug-resistant strains.[70]

There are four classes of DAAs defined by their mode of action and therapeutic target:

- Nonstructural (NS3/4A) protease inhibitors inhibit NS3/4A serine protease, an enzyme involved in post-translational processing and replication of HCV. Examples are telaprevir, boceprevir, simeprevir, faldaprevir, dasabuvir.
- Nonstructural (NS5A) inhibitors include daclatasvir, ledipasvir, ombitasvir. The mode of action of these inhibitors is the redistribution of NS5A from the endoplasmic reticulum to lipid droplets which inhibits viral replication.[71]
- Nonstructural (NS5B) RNA-dependent RNA polymerase inhibitors are incorporated into the nascent RNA chain, causing premature chain termination. An example of a nucleoside polymerase inhibitor is sofosbuvir (SOF).
- Non-nucleoside polymerase inhibitors (NNPIs) make the enzyme ineffective, e.g. dasabuvir in combination with ombitasvir/paritaprevir/ritonavir.[70]

Overall the adverse events associated with DAAs are mild: nausea, fatigue and anaemia. Sofosbuvir is contraindicated in patients with severe renal impairment (it is metabolised through the kidneys)[72] and three case reports of severe pulmonary arterial hypertension have been associated with sofosbuvir-based therapy.[73]

However, the sustained viral clearance rates (SVR) in genotype 3 (GT3) HCV infection are low and even lower in cirrhotics.[74] Current treatment guidelines for hepatitis C GT3 patients recommend sofosbuvir plus pegylated interferon/ribavirin or sofosbuvir plus ribavirin or sofosbuvir plus daclatasvir.[75] A clinical trial of differing treatment regimens in genotype 3 HCV infection is as follows: ledipasvir (LDV), sofosbuvir (SOF) and ribavirin administered for 12 weeks had a 82.6% SVR, whereas sofosbuvir with pegylated interferon and ribavirin for 12 weeks achieved a SVR of 88.9% compared to sofosobuvir plus ribavirin for 24 weeks which only achieved a 76.1% SVR.[69]

Hepatitis D

Pegylated interferon is the only approved drug known to be active against hepatitis D virus (HDV).[76]

Hepatitis E

Ribavirin is the treatment of choice for patients chronically infected with hepatitis E virus (HEV), achieving a 85% sustained virological response (SVR) rate.[77]

PEG-interferon and ribavirin

Pegylated interferon is currently used in HBV and HDV infection and ribavirin is largely used in chronic hepatitis C genotype 3 infection in conjunction with the new direct-acting antivirals.

There is a range of side effects associated with PEG-IFN and ribavirin treatment. Influenza symptoms are the most commonly reported side effect, and the incidence of fatigue and headache, pyrexia and myalgia is high. Side effects including depression, insomnia, irritability and gastrointestinal symptoms including diarrhoea, nausea and anorexia are also frequently reported. Neutropenia and thrombocytopenia are commonly reported and dose reduction is required. Haemolytic anaemia is the most common side effect of ribavirin.[78,79] Additionally, ribavirin is teratogenic. Literature suggests that a 9 months wash-out period after ribavirin use rather than the current recommendation of 6 months may be prudent.

Ursodeoxycholic acid (UDCA)

The use of ursodeoxycholic acid (UDCA) in the treatment of hepatobiliary problems originated in China. Current medical practice is to use a synthesised preparation of UDCA. This preparation was synthesised by Japanese scientists as early as 1955.[80]

UDCA can alter the profile of the bile acid pool, and has choleretic, immunomodulatory and cytoprotective actions. It has been suggested that UDCA displaces the hepatotoxic bile acid pool by favourably expanding the hydrophilic bile acid pool and thus exhibits competitive displacement of toxic bile acids. Chenodeoxycholic acid (CDCA) was traditionally used to dissolve gallstones. However, UDCA largely replaced the use of CDCA in the 1980s because of safety issues. UDCA is used in the treatment of gallstones as an alternative to cholecystectomy because of its ability to solubilise cholesterol from the surface of the gallstone. The recommended dose of UDCA for gallstones is 8–10 mg/kg per day and a dissolution rate of 30% to 60% has been reported.[81]

A meta-analysis of randomised controlled trials reported that during weight loss UDCA and/or higher dietary fat content appeared to prevent formation of gallstones.[82]

SECTION B

CHOLELITHIASIS

Epidemiology

Cholelithiasis refers to the presence of gallstones in the gallbladder. Epidemiological studies suggest that between 10% and 15% of white adults in developed countries will develop gallstones.[83] Within this group females are diagnosed between two and three times more often than males of the same age.[84,85] Native American populations rank as the highest risk group for gallstone disease[86,87] and Pima Indian women over 30 years demonstrate 70% prevalence. Gallstone prevalence is, however, low in Asia and Africa.[88] Twin studies have further established a genetic component to stone formation; a Swedish study involving 43 141 twins born between 1900 and 1958 demonstrated that heritability and environmental factors influence gallstone disease.[89]

Independent determinants for gallstone formation are age, female sex, body mass index (BMI), high cholesterol and gallbladder polyps.[90]

AGE AND GENDER

Increases in age are associated with increased biliary cholesterol secretion and decreased biliary salt secretion.[91] Increases in age have been linked to a decline in cholesterol 7-α-hydroxylase activity;[92] this leads to increased biliary cholesterol secretion thus promoting an optimal environment for gallstone development. Gallstones are more prevalent in the female population because of the presence of endogenous oestrogens. Increased oestrogens especially during pregnancy have been linked to increased hepatic cholesterol uptake and synthesis, gallbladder hypomotility and decreased cholesterol 7-α-hydroxylase activity.[85,93]

Classification

Gallstones can be classified as cholesterol stones or pigment stones. Approximately 37–86% of gallstones are cholesterol-rich stones, 2–27% are pigment stones and 4–16% are mixed.[94] Black pigment stones are formed from bile precipitation, consist primarily of calcium bilirubinate and are present in haemolytic disorders, while brown pigment stones are linked to bacterial and helminthic infections in the biliary tree.[93,95] Cholecystectomies performed in Western countries reveal that cholesterol gallstones account for 80–90% of cases and cholesterol stones are the most common type of gallstones. Cholesterol gallstones are smooth in shape, can vary in size and are primarily composed of cholesterol crystals (70%), glycoproteins, bile pigments and calcium salts.[96]

Aetiology

OBESITY

The presence of metabolic syndrome is associated with an increased risk of gallstone disease.[97]

High-kilojoule diets, and diets high in refined carbohydrates and triglycerides and low in HDL cholesterol are linked to gallbladder disease.[98] Obesity is linked to gallstone formation as obese people demonstrate increased biliary secretion of cholesterol from the liver due to an increase in 3-hydroxy-3-methyl-glutaryl-CoA (HMG-CoA) reductase activity.[96] Women with a body mass index (BMI) greater than 32 are six times more likely to develop gallstones than women with a BMI less than 22.[99]

A cross-sectional study found waist-to-hip ratio, waist-to-height ratio, body mass index and visceral adipose tissue thickness were all associated with gallstone disease in women. The waist-to-hip ratio alone reflected gallstone disease in men.[100]

The first stages of rapid weight loss are also implicated in gallstone formation and a prolonged fat-restricted diet is thought to exacerbate gallbladder stasis.[85,96] Weight cycling is a process involving rapid loss of weight, followed quickly by regaining of that weight, and this process is strongly associated with gallstone formation.[101]

ENDOCRINE DISORDERS

Insulin resistance, chronic hyperglycaemia and disorders of lipid metabolism are also involved[102] thus implicating a metabolic syndrome symptom picture.[97] Diabetes mellitus may increase the risk of stone formation due to associated gallbladder dysfunction, dysfunctional cholesterol metabolism and altered glucose metabolism.[103]

GENETICS

Genetic factors account for 25–30% of total gallstone risk. This risk percentage is higher in Hispanic populations (45–65%). Gene polymorphisms in enterohepatic transporters, mucin gene expression and Gilbert's syndrome variants have a role in gallstone formation.[83]

DRUG THERAPY

Drugs that alter cholesterol metabolism include statins (HMG-CoA reductase inhibitors), fibrates and ceftriaxone, an antibiotic.[85,96] Ceftriaxone is contraindicated in gallbladder disease. Despite fibrates' ability to lower triglycerides, they have been implicated in cholelithiasis formation[98] by enhancing cholesterol secretion and impairing bile acid synthesis.[104,105] The presence of exogenous oestrogen from the use of tamoxifen as adjuvant hormonal therapy in breast cancer treatment has also been linked to gallstone formation.[106]

INTESTINAL TRANSIT TIME

Slow intestinal transit time has been linked to gallstone formation due to increased colonic absorption of deoxycholate, a byproduct of bile acid metabolism by gut bacteria. Deoxycholate promotes hepatic cholesterol secretion and stone crystallisation.[107]

HELICOBACTER SPECIES

A Chilean study[108] identified an association between bile-resistant *Helicobacter* species and gallbladder disease. However, no causative role for the infective organism was noted. A 2005 animal study[109] demonstrated that infection with *Helicobacter* species potentiated and accelerated the formation of cholesterol stones in mice fed a lithogenic diet. A 2007 meta-analysis[110] identified a slightly higher risk of gallstone formation or benign liver disease in the presence of *Helicobacter* infection; however, the authors were clear to identify problems with sample heterogeneity and methodology variations across the meta-analysis. An epidemiological study of 10 000 patients found a positive association between the presence of *Helicobacter* infection and gallstones.[111]

Pathogenesis

The pathogenesis of gallstones involves a process in which chemical components of bile precipitate in the gallbladder and occasionally in the bile duct.[93] Cholesterol stone formation is primarily associated with the hepatic hypersecretion of cholesterol and hyposecretion of bile acids and phosphatidylcholine (lecithin).[98,112] Cholesterol stones form if bile contains more cholesterol than bile salts and phospholipids can dissolve, resulting in the formation of microscopic cholesterol-rich vesicles and then macroscopic gallstones.

Development of gallstones has also been linked to hypomotility of the gallbladder and excess biliary mucin secretion.[87]

Gallbladder mucins are essential to offer protection against the detergent effect of high concentration of bile acids.[113] It has been demonstrated that mucin gene polymorphisms may influence susceptibility to gallstone disease.[113] In patients presenting with hypertriglyceridaemia, decreased sensitivity to cholecystokinin (CCK) is thought to impair gallbladder motility and thus increase the risk of gallstones.[112] Hypomotility and mucin hypersecretion[114] are linked back to hepatic cholesterol hypersecretion, thus revealing a self-perpetuating cycle of lithogenesis.

SIGNS AND SYMPTOMS

Gallstones are asymptomatic in 60–80% of cases; it is estimated that only 10–20% of asymptomatic patients will develop symptoms.[115] Gallstones lodged in the gallbladder can manifest clinically with the presence of biliary pain. The most common clinical manifestation of gallstones is the presence of episodic biliary pain which presents in the upper right abdominal or epigastric areas and can radiate to the right subscapular area, midback or right shoulder. Patients with biliary pain may complain they cannot get comfortable; milder cases can present with a feeling of bloatedness and pressure. In more serious presentations, patients complain of pain which is stabbing, cramping or like the pressure of a heavy weight. Episodes of biliary pain generally last between 30 minutes and a few hours and episodes may occur daily or once every few months. Nausea may present, but vomiting and fevers are uncommon.[116]

COMPLICATIONS

Pain that lasts longer than 12 hours may be an indicator of acute cholecystitis. Acute cholecystitis is attributed to gallstone impaction in the cystic duct and manifests with fever and upper abdominal pain with marked tenderness and guarding in the right upper quadrant. Murphy's sign is a key indicator of acute cholecystitis and is noted on inspiration, where the patient will demonstrate marked tenderness to palpation. This sharp abdominal pain can be attributed to elevated pressure within the gallbladder due to the obstruction of either the neck of the gallbladder or the cystic duct.[85] Acute cholecystitis is a serious complication of gallstones and urgent medical attention should be sought to avoid the serious complications of gallbladder perforation or fistulas.

DIFFERENTIAL DIAGNOSIS

Upper right abdominal pain may also present in conditions such as irritable bowel syndrome (IBS), peptic ulcer disease, pancreatitis, gastro-oesophageal reflux disease, angina pectoris, appendicitis, bowel obstruction, liver disease, oesophagitis and epigastric pain from myocardial infarction.[115,116] Elements of diagnostic confusion may exist as biliary pain is only a suggestive symptom of gallstone disease. The naturopathic clinician should direct questioning to elicit the nature or sensation of pain, its location, frequency, duration and onset, intensity and radiation, cessation, factors which aggravate or alleviate pain, and concomitant symptoms. Sound clinical judgment is necessary and the first line of action should be to refer the patient to a general practitioner for confirmatory diagnostic testing.

NATUROPATHIC DIAGNOSIS

Iridology

The gallbladder region can be located in the right iris and is positioned at 8 o'clock between the liver and the duodenal areas; all three regions are positioned on a straight radius extending from the pupil to the sclera border. The realm of iridology does not extend to the ability of being able to identify gallstones, as any markings in the iris refer to the tissues of the gallbladder rather than the gallbladder contents. Jensen[117] suggests that gallstones could be suspected if sluggishness and toxicity are located in the gallbladder area and most occurrences of gallbladder dysfunction will show closed lesions in the shape of a small football in the gallbladder area. Hall[118] makes a special reference to the gallbladder as the organ of resentment and suggests that some gallstone formation may be the internalising of anger, which can lead to dysregulation of homeostasis.

Nail analysis

Although there are no specific fingernail signs for the presence of gallstones, the patient's nails should be carefully analysed for indications of jaundice. If the nails are yellow, liver dysfunction is usually indicated. However, yellow nails may also be due to hypervitaminosis A, or fungal infections. The general quality of the fingernails needs to be assessed and any suspicions of protein deficiency or inadequate intake of vitamins and minerals should be addressed in the patient's nutritional analysis.

Tongue analysis

The liver and gallbladder regions are represented on each side of the tongue. Two thick yellow strips down each side of the tongue indicate heat in the hepatobiliary region. The left side of the tongue is traditionally associated with the liver and the right side with the gallbladder. In traditional Chinese medicine, the liver is regarded as the blood storer so if the sides of the tongue are pale, blood deficiency is indicated. Conditions involving heat in the hepatobiliary region will produce a red tongue with a yellow coating.[119]

Investigations

Liver function blood tests can show elevated bilirubin and alkaline phosphatase which may indicate a possible obstruction in the extrahepatic ducts (choledocholithiasis). If a stone migrates and obstructs the pancreatic duct, amylase and lipase levels may be elevated.[85,96] However, liver function tests may not indicate abnormalities even if biliary pain is present and there is severe pathology.

If gallbladder stones are suspected, a medical practitioner will order a transabdominal/endoscopic ultrasound which is regarded as the most accurate and sensitive diagnostic tool. Ultrasonography can detect the size of the gallbladder, common bile and hepatic ducts as well as the presence of wall thickening and pericholecystic fluid which is indicative of acute cholecystitis.[96] Cholecystography was the standard method for assessing the gallbladder but has now been replaced by ultrasonography as the diagnostic tool of choice.[120]

In cases of choledocholithiasis, the preferred diagnostic tool is endoscopic retrograde cholangiography (ERCP) as transabdominal ultrasound is less sensitive for the visualisation of stones in ducts and ERCP has the added benefit of being able to extract stones endoscopically.[87,121] When there are elevated serum amylase and lipase ERCP is used to rule out choledocholithiasis or gallstone pancreatitis before a cholecystectomy is performed. Abdominal CT (computed tomography), x-ray and MRI (magnetic resonance imaging) can also be used in diagnosis.

Hepatobiliary scintigraphy (HIDA) scans are used to rule out acute cholecystitis as this can detect obstruction of the cystic duct via an intravenously injected nuclear isotope.[85]

SPECIFIC NATUROPATHIC INVESTIGATIONS

There are no specific laboratory investigations available to naturopaths to assist in determining gallbladder function. During case history taking, investigations into bowel function and stool appearance could reveal fatty floating stools — steatorrhoea. Steatorrhoea could suggest excess bile, excess fat in the diet or the use of low-kilojoule fat substitutes such as olestra. Alternatively, very pale stools or clay-coloured stools could indicate reduced bile and bilirubin. Bilirubin gives stool its brown colour from the breakdown of red blood cells. Referred scapula pain can also be an indication of inflammation of the gallbladder and possibly stones.

A functional liver detoxification profile (FLDP) will highlight problems with liver function and may be of use if the patient presents with general biliousness and digestive concerns. A tongue analysis and a complete assessment of digestive function and associated digestive symptoms will greatly assist the clinician in determining a treatment approach. At all times, referral to a general practitioner for diagnosis is essential if gallstones are suspected.

Therapeutic considerations

CLINICAL DECISION MAKING AND RATIONALE

Suspected gallstones

If gallstones are suspected by the naturopath, best clinical practice suggests the patient should be referred to a general practitioner for appropriate diagnostic testing. Once gallstones or biliary obstruction have been ruled out, the naturopath is best advised to ensure optimal gallbladder, liver and gastrointestinal function in the treatment protocol.

Prevention of gallstones is better than an attempt to cure, thus a treatment plan that addresses risk factors and promotes optimal health will assist in procuring the client's health, especially in rapid weight loss.

Established gallstones

Informed clinical reasoning plays a vital role in the treatment of gallstones. If presented with a case of diagnosed gallstones, it is imperative that the naturopath is aware of the severity of the case and the treatment recommendations made by the client's general practitioner. If a client presents with gallstones and does not provide details of the size and number of stones, along with recommendations by a medical practitioner, it would be negligent to proceed to treat this patient. Any treatment designed to stimulate gallbladder contraction risks the lodgement of the stone in the neck of the gallbladder or the cystic duct.

Surgery

If surgery is not recommended by a general practitioner or gallbladder surgeon, the treatment approach attempts to manage symptoms, increase the bile solubility of cholesterol and effectively manage diet and lifestyle factors known to aggravate the condition. Early intervention in the pathophysiological development of gallstones may in fact reduce the risk and severity of complications arising from stone formation. If surgery is recommended, then a supportive naturopathic treatment plan that addresses presurgical preparation and postsurgical recovery is most appropriate.

Therapeutic application

HISTORICAL PERSPECTIVE

Before it was destroyed by German bombing in World War II, the Museum of the Royal College of Surgeons Collection housed an Egyptian mummy priestess (circa 1500 BC) complete with thirty gallstones. Gallstones were found in Catherine the Great of Russia after her death.

The biliary pain experienced by Sir Walter Scott as he wrote *The Bride of Lammermoor* was apparently so intense that his shirt was reportedly burned from constant applications of hot fomentations.[122,123]

NATUROPATHIC PERSPECTIVE

Gallstones are most effectively treated with a long-term approach — thus treatment should be regarded as management — rather than cure. Any short-term, quick fix attempts will not address the chronic nature of the problem and, as previously mentioned, can risk the patient's wellbeing. Heavy-handed treatments designed to instantly dissolve or flush gallstones are dangerous. The treatment should be based on diet and lifestyle advice and supporting bile formation and gallbladder function and motility.

The treatment of cholelithiasis requires the following considerations:

1. Assess the case presentation and obtain a diagnosis if not provided
2. Identify possible contraindications for treatment
3. Promote optimal bile formation in the liver
4. Promote effective gallbladder motility and function
5. Support gallstone dissolution

6 Support optimal digestive and GIT function
7 Support normal bile and cholesterol reabsorption in the small intestine
8 Support the body's carbohydrate and lipid metabolism pathways
9 Address dietary concerns and encourage intake of fresh fruit and vegetables, fibre and water
10 Address factors that hinder or obstruct the healing process.

NUTRITIONAL MEDICINE (DIETARY)

Dietary therapeutic objectives

See 'Hepatobiliary nutritional objectives (dietary)' for an overview.

1 Increase consumption of bitter herbs (dandelion greens, rocket, gentian) and raw foods to encourage bile production and release
2 Reduce or remove intake of refined carbohydrates, processed foods and takeaways (high in fat and sugar)
3 Reduce fatty and over-rich foods in the diet that can over-stimulate the gallbladder to produce bile and lead to an acute attack
4 Support lipid metabolism by reducing saturated and trans fatty acids and increasing essential fatty acid intake. Also monitor dietary cholesterol intake; make adjustments where appropriate, but do not blame lithogenesis on dietary cholesterol intake
5 Encourage fibre intake (soluble and insoluble fibre) to reduce risk of stone formation
6 Ensure adequate protein for weight management
7 Support optimal digestive and GIT function with wise food choices
8 Improve vitality and general wellbeing.

Specific dietary treatments

DIETARY INCLUSIONS

Fibre

Substantial evidence suggests that diets high in fibre may reduce the incidence of gallstones and several epidemiological studies substantiate this claim.[98,99] Moran and colleagues[124] demonstrated a beneficial link between psyllium fibre supplementation and gallstone formation in a study of obese patients on kilojoule restriction. Insoluble dietary fibre in the form of wheat bran has been noted for its ability to reduce the deoxycholic acid content and cholesterol saturation index of bile.[125]

Oat bran

A randomised controlled trial with a crossover design found that daily ingestion of 84 g of oat bran for 6 weeks significantly reduced serum cholesterol by 13% and LDL cholesterol by 17% ($P \leq 0.05$).[126,127]

Food allergy/sensitivity

A 1968 study made an interesting link between food allergy and stone formation. When the participants in this study were placed on an elimination diet, gallbladder symptoms ceased. Eggs, pork, onion, milk, coffee, fowl, oranges, corn, beans, nuts, apples and tomatoes were found to initiate gallbladder symptoms when introduced. The principal researcher in this study theorised that allergic reactions to these foods caused the bile ducts to swell, leading to stone formation through impaired bile flow, poor gallbladder motility and compromised function.[128]

Fruit and vegetables and vitamin C intake

A 2006[129] study reported that diets high in green leafy vegetables, citrus fruits, fruits and vegetables high in vitamin C and cruciferous vegetables were inversely associated with the risk of cholecystectomy. Recent studies have demonstrated an inverse relationship between ascorbic acid intake and gallstone formation in women because of the association between cholesterol 7α-hydroxylase activity and ascorbic acid concentrations in the liver.[130]

Fatty acids

Animal studies have shown promising results with monounsaturated fatty acid supplementation and reduced gallstone formation. However, studies on humans have shown less conclusive results with some studies showing a protective effect and some studies demonstrating no significant difference in gallstone formation after supplementation.[99] A double-blind, placebo controlled study[131] showed a beneficial effect of polyunsaturated fatty acid supplementation in obese women during weight loss. During this study, obese women on kilojoule restriction had decreased nucleation time and increased cholesterol saturation compared with women who were supplemented with polyunsaturated fatty acids.

DIETARY EXCLUSIONS

Fat

A 2005 study[132] observed that high intakes of trans fatty acids were associated with a higher risk of gallstone disease in men. In particular, the study isolated a positive relationship between intake of trans-oleic acid (a trans-isomer in partially hydrogenated vegetable oils) and gallstone disease. A drastic reduction and preferably total exclusion of all trans fats is desirable in this instance, not only to reduce the associated risk with gallstone formation, cardiovascular disease and cancer but also to optimise overall health. Any dietary modification should be recommended and supervised by the naturopath to avoid rapid weight loss and to reduce the effects of weight cycling on the pathogenesis of gallstones.

Suggestions for reducing saturated and trans fat intake include:

- Reduce trans fat intake by excluding margarine, commercially fried foods, baked goods
- Reduce saturated fat intake by choosing lean cuts of organic grass-fed meats, and game meats such as kangaroo
- Replace red meat intake with consumption of oily cold-water fish (salmon, tuna, mackerel, sardines, herrings, kippers)
- Reduce consumption of hard cheeses which are high in total fat and saturated fat

- Avoid cooking with saturated fats; do not deep fry anything
- Increase intake of omega-3 polyunsaturated fatty acids including wheatgerm, linseed and walnuts.

Refined sugar

Research indicates that the consumption of 40 g of sugar per day doubles the risk of symptomatic gallstone formation[98] and several studies have also found a direct correlation between refined sugar intake and gallstone formation. Misciagna et al[133] reported that a high intake of refined sugars led to gallstone development due to increased synthesis of cholesterol in the liver secondary to increased secretion of insulin. Mathur et al[134] reported that high dietary carbohydrate consumption altered biliary motility, enhanced crystal formation and mass, and decreased gallbladder volume in mice.

OTHER DIETARY CONSIDERATIONS

Kilojoule intake and meals

Excessive kilojoule intake is believed to be linked to gallstone formation due to the association with obesity.[98] A naturopathic treatment protocol should address excessive kilojoule intake. Conversely, low kilojoule intake of less than 3600 kJ per day as part of rapid weight loss can increase the risk of gallstones. A comprehensive dietary approach to the treatment of gallstones should include recommendations to eat small, frequent meals as this reduces the risk of gallstones by encouraging more frequent gallbladder contraction and emptying.[135]

Dietary cholesterol

The effects on dietary cholesterol intake and the pathogenesis of gallstones are unclear as reported in the literature. A study that investigated the effects of egg yolk supplementation in healthy males with normal lipid profiles demonstrated an increase in mean biliary cholesterol saturation, with four participants developing lithogenic bile and three developing cholesterol crystals.[136] Conversely, researchers found no increase in biliary cholesterol saturation with the administration of a high-cholesterol diet when healthy female college students were supplemented with egg yolk.[137]

Until 1985, the effect of dietary cholesterol in biliary cholesterol saturation had not in fact been studied in population cohorts with gallstones. Lee et al[138] conducted a study with both healthy subjects and subjects with gallstones and found an increase in biliary cholesterol saturation for short periods of time with the modest addition of dietary cholesterol in the form of egg yolk.

As most cholesterol is endogenously synthesised, dietary cholesterol may only have a limited role in stone formation. Best clinical practice would see the naturopathic clinician assess a patient's case thoroughly and attempt to build a picture based on the information gathered so that understanding of the patient's susceptibility to gallstones can be determined and modifications implemented. In this case, conflicting evidence in the literature should not cloud the application of common sense and informed clinical judgment, reasoning and decision making.

Protein and iron

Protein deficiency in the diet has been linked to increased susceptibility to bile acid induced cholestasis.[139] Iron deficiency has also been linked to cholesterol gallstone formation in both animal and human studies.[140,141] Researchers in one study[140] collected serum and bile samples from women at the time of cholecystectomy and concluded that elevated transferrin levels and iron deficiency without anaemia were prevalent.

Beneficial folk remedies

The benefits of dandelion root beverage in supporting optimal gallbladder function cannot be underestimated. Dorothy Hall regards dandelion root beverage as 'one of the best things that ever happened to a doubtful liver'.[142] Likewise, the bitter dark-green leaves of the dandelion or chicory plants can be either added to fresh carrot juices or tossed through garden salads to stimulate bile production and gallbladder contraction. Artichoke leaves can be cooked with garlic and lemon and eaten with bitter green salads. Foods that are viewed as traditional tonics for the gallbladder include pears, parsnips, seaweed, lemons, limes and turmeric.[143] The consumption of small quantities of grated radish regularly for any gallbladder or liver disorders is also recommended.

NUTRITIONAL MEDICINE (SUPPLEMENTAL)

See 'Hepatobiliary nutritional objectives (nutrients)'.

Nutritional medicine therapeutic objectives

- Potential nutritional deficiencies that should be considered in all hepatobiliary disease are listed in Table 11.5
- Promote optimal gallbladder motility and hepatobiliary function
- Assist with bile formation through the use of lipotrophic factors.

Specific nutrients required

VITAMIN C

Vitamin C is needed for the metabolism of cholesterol to bile acids and its use has been suggested in gallstone incidence.[130,144] Vitamin C supplementation in women has a demonstrated protective effect against gallstone formation.[98]

GLYCINE/BETAINE (TRIMETHYLGLYCINE) AND TAURINE

Necessary for the binding of Ca^{2+} to bile salts (with taurine) which reduced tendency of Ca^{2+} to precipitate as insoluble salts and develop into gallstones.[145] Bile acids are synthesised in the liver from cholesterol and conjugated with glycine or taurine.[146] Dosage at 500 mg/day on an empty stomach.

SAMPLE DAILY DIET

BREAKFAST	
Bircher muesli pot with soaked oats, grated apple, chia seeds, cinnamon, almond milk and live yoghurt	Oats and seasonal fruit in the bircher muesli provide a source of fibre; an inverse association between dietary fibre intake and prevalence of gallstones exists.[147] Yoghurt provides a source of beneficial live bacteria to assist in reducing dysbiosis. Dysbiosis is prevalent in individuals with gallstones. Elevated bacteria levels within the biliary tract have led to the hypothesis that dysbiosis may be a possible contributor to the presence of gallstones.[148]
LUNCH	
Baked globe artichokes with garlic, lemon, parsley and breadcrumbs. Serve with quinoa, haloumi and bitter greens such as radicchio and rocket	Globe artichoke stimulates bile secretion and may exert an anticholestatic action.[149] The addition of lemon and other bitter greens such as radicchio and rocket further gently stimulates secretion of bile.
DINNER	
Dhal containing ample onion, garlic, fenugreek and turmeric. Serve with rice and salad	Dietary garlic and onion display antilithogenic activity by decreasing hypersecretion of cholesterol into bile and increasing the bile acid output, reducing formation of lithogenic bile in animal studies.[150] Consumption of garlic and onion may also help with regression of reformed gallstones.[151] Fenugreek displays antilithogenic activity and reduces accumulation of fat in the liver and inflammation of the gallbladder membrane as well as enhancing regression of gallstones.
SNACK	
Smoothie made with fresh fruits rich in vitamin C and lecithin	Lecithin promotes dissolution of gallstones by increasing biliary phospholipid concentrations. Vitamin C is required for conversion of cholesterol to bile acids and may help to prevent gallstone formation by promoting the conversion of cholesterol to bile salts, thereby decreasing the lithogenicity of bile.

METHIONINE

Supplementation with methionine can prevent cholestasis by maintaining membrane integrity and function.[139]

LECITHIN

Research in 1975 examined the role of lecithin in gallstone dissolution. In one study researchers used a combination of 2250 mg of lecithin and 750 mg of cholic acid daily over a 6-month period to dissolve gallstones with success.[152,153] A study 1 year later in 1976 reported similar results with 1200 mg of lecithin a day successfully dissolving existing gallstones.[154] There have been few human studies on the efficacy of lecithin supplementation on gallstone reduction since this original research was conducted.

VITAMINS A, D, E AND K: THE FAT-SOLUBLE VITAMINS

The presence of bile salts is necessary for absorption of the fat-soluble vitamins[144,155] so interference with bile metabolism may warrant vitamin supplementation.[155]

Dosage requirement

- Vitamin C: 3–4 g per day in 500 mg divided doses
- Betaine (trimethylglycine): 500–1000 mg per day
- Taurine: 500 mg to 3 g daily in divided doses
- Methionine: 200–400 mg b.i.d. or t.d.s.
- Lecithin: 1200 mg
- Vitamin A: 2500 IU daily (do not exceed in pregnancy)
- Vitamin D: 400 IU daily
- Vitamin E: 300 IU daily
- Vitamin K: 2.5–5 mg weekly up to 5 mg daily.

HERBAL MEDICINE

Herbal medicine therapeutic objectives

- Reduce pain and inflammation
- Improve gallbladder function and motility
- Promote optimal formation, storage and release of bile

- Promote gentle gallbladder contraction where safe
- Promote dissolution of gallstones
- Improve sluggish bowel function
- Improve digestion and reduce digestive disturbance
- Improve vitality and wellbeing.

Herbal medicine classes

The role of herbal medicine in the treatment of gallstones is not solely limited to the treatment of lithiasis. Herbal remedies are indicated in gallstone prevention and reoccurrence, the symptomatic treatment of gallstones as well as both pre- and postoperative care where gallstone removal is necessary.

Cholagogue herbal medicines are agents that promote the release of stored bile from the gallbladder. This herbal class is specifically indicated where there is evidence of bile insufficiency, biliary tract dysfunction, gallbladder congestion or sluggishness and where symptoms of indigestion prevail. Because of the ability of this class of herbal medicines to stimulate gallbladder contraction, cholagogues are contraindicated in cases of acute cholelithiasis and bile duct obstruction. Cholagogues are best indicated in the prevention of gallstones, where small gallstones of a limited number have been detected and in situations where sluggish gallbladder motility has resulted in discomfort and gastrointestinal upset. In cases where gallstones have been successfully dissolved or passed, cholagogues may be beneficial in preventing the reoccurrence of such stones and in cases where surgical intervention has been necessary, cholagogues may be used to counteract postoperative dyskinesia.

Other classes of herbal medicines offer much in the treatment of gallstones. The anti-inflammatory herbal medicine *Matricaria recutita* (chamomile) is especially suited to digestive inflammation. Carminative herbs are high in volatile oils and target the mucosal lining of the gastrointestinal system, reducing symptoms of flatulence through a combined anti-inflammatory and spasmolytic action. Carminative herbs are indicated where gallstones produce symptoms of abdominal discomfort, flatulence, pain and griping.

Specific herbal medicines

TARAXACUM OFFICINALE (DANDELION ROOT)

Weiss[156] regards dandelion as the key herb for gallstones and with its additional tonic and nutritional properties, it allows the latent stage of gallstone disease to be reached more easily and quickly. Dandelion's affinity for gallstones is also acknowledged by Mills[157] who suggests dandelion improves the function of both the liver and kidneys by diluting bile and urine, thus reducing the potential for stone and crystal formation. This is reinforced by Bartram[158] who reports that dandelion is used in gallbladder inflammation and to prevent the tendency to form gallstones and also assists the elimination of plasma cholesterol. This herb stimulates the flow of bile and is contraindicated in the presence of a blocked bile duct.

Only limited scientific data are available to verify the empirical use of dandelion and no human or clinical studies thus far have been conducted on the efficacy of the herb in treating the conditions it is reputed to be effective for. The choleretic activity of *Taraxacum officinale* is limited to traditional knowledge and a 1959 study conducted by Bohm[159] that looked at bile secretion in rats after an intraduodenal injection of a leaf extract. A more recent animal study[160] concluded that *Taraxacum officinale* has anti-angiogenic, anti-inflammatory and antinociceptive activity through its ability to inhibit nitric oxide production and COX-2 expression.

CYNARA SCOLYMUS (GLOBE ARTICHOKE)

There are no studies on the efficacy of *Cynara scolymus* on gallstones directly. However, some studies do report favourable findings on bile composition, choleresis and cholesterol lowering activity. The choleretic effect of a single dose of dried artichoke extract significantly increased bile secretion after administration in one study.[161] In another study[162] the effect of artichoke extract on functional gallbladder disorders was investigated. Researchers reported decreases in nausea, stomach pains and loss of appetite and 80% of participants reported their symptoms had improved. A 2008 study reported a statistically favourable decrease in total cholesterol levels after administration of artichoke leaf extract over a 12-week period.[163]

CURCUMA LONGA (TURMERIC)

A 1991[164] rat study looked at the effect of curcumin, capsaicin, ginger, mustard, black pepper and cumin on cholesterol and bile acid metabolism. This study demonstrated significant elevation of hepatic cholesterol-7 α-hydroxylase (the rate-limiting enzyme of bile acid biosynthesis). The authors suggested that the spices turmeric, red pepper, ginger and mustard can stimulate the conversion of cholesterol to bile acids, an important pathway of elimination of cholesterol from the body. Research by Rasyid and Lelo[165] demonstrated that 20 mg of curcumin was capable of inducing gallbladder contraction by up to 29% with an observation time of 2 hours. Rasyid et al[166] then demonstrated that the administration of 40 mg of curcumin produced a 50% contraction of the gallbladders of a cohort of healthy volunteers.

DIOSCOREA VILLOSA (WILD YAM)

The saponins in *Dioscorea villosa* have been studied for their ability to lower cholesterol since the 1940s.[167] It has been suggested that saponins bind to and increase the faecal excretion of cholesterol salts, and can thus lower cholesterol.[168] Diosgenin, a saponin, is reported to be very similar to cholesterol in structure and it interferes with the esterification of cholesterol in the liver[169] leading to increased cholesterol excretion through the bile and overall cholesterol reduction.

PEUMUS BOLDO (BOLDO)

Boldo grows in Central Chile and the leaves are used for inflammation of the gallbladder, gallstones and biliary colic and liver disease.[170] Boldo is particularly useful for alleviating the pain of cholelithiasis. Boldo leaves are rich in the alkaloid boldine which is responsible for the antioxidant,[171] hepatoprotective, anti-inflammatory,[172] cholagogic and choleretic actions of the plant. In addition, Boldo has immuno- and neuromodulator actions. It reduces lipid peroxidation and enzymatic leakage of LDH and ALT.[171–173]

LIFESTYLE RECOMMENDATIONS

As obesity and a sedentary lifestyle have been implicated in the pathogenesis of gallstones, exercise is a priority in the treatment and management of this condition. Studies have demonstrated that exercise prevents gallstone formation in women.[174] It is important to highlight the importance of sensible weight reduction as both rapid weight loss and weight cycling have been implicated in stone formation. The role of the naturopath is to suggest an exercise regimen that is attainable, rewarding and empowers the patient in the management of their health. If the patient is overweight, it is essential that the naturopath is cognisant of injuries that can be sustained from high-impact exercise. Low-impact activities are suggested so that exercise can be used as a long-term and comprehensive approach to weight management and gallstone prevention.

CASE STUDY

OVERVIEW

A 58-year-old woman presented with a diagnosis of cholelithiasis with symptoms of episodic epigastric pain, epigastric tenderness and biliary colic. She has two children aged 28 and 25 and a history of oral contraceptive (OCP) use and uterine fibroids. Menopause was at 50.

She is a fussy eater with a history of cyclical fad diets (lemon detox, Atkins, cabbage diet) and has a very sweet tooth and an aversion to bitter foods, all fats and vegetables. She experiences slow intestinal transit with constipation and haemorrhoids and frequent headaches, possibly due to dehydration.

CLINICAL EXAMINATION

Weight: 72 kg, Height:165 cm, BMI: 26
Waist circumference: 82 cm

LABORATORY INVESTIGATIONS

ALT 150	U/L (5–30)
AST 200	U/L (10–35)
ALP 168	U/L (20–35)
GGT 140	U/L (5–35)

Abdominal ultrasound and abdominal CT shows cholelithiasis — two calculi 1.6 cm and 1.8 cm in diameter, with mobile biliary sludge. Common bile duct measures 0.5 cm in diameter which is within normal range. There was no evidence of intrahepatic or extrahepatic bile duct obstruction.

Patient has a history of oestrogen dominance (OCP, uterine fibroids, pregnancy, overweight), slow intestinal transit, high carbohydrate consumption aggravated by cyclical

CASE STUDY CONTINUED

dieting. These are all factors associated with cholelithiasis and are largely dependent on lifestyle factors, therefore patient education is key.

TREATMENT PROTOCOL

FIRST APPOINTMENT

The strong history of weight cycling played a significant role in the aetiology of the gallstones, so it is **crucial** that dietary and lifestyle advice is included alongside the herbal treatment. Address issues around cyclical fad dieting.

There was no evidence from the investigation of obstruction, therefore there were no contraindications and herbal treatment could be employed safely.

SPECIFIC MEDICINES

Chromium, 250 micrograms daily

HERBAL MEDICINE

Cynara scolymus is without doubt the key herb for the treatment of gallstones owing to its hypocholesterolaemic, anti-inflammatory and antioxidant activity. *Equisetum arvensis* is historically noted to prevent the precipitation of mineral oxalates from biliary sludge into cholelithiasis.

Crataegus oxyacantha is renowned for dissolving cholesterol[175] and this herb has been used in traditional Chinese medicine for food stagnation and is a powerful antioxidant due to the oligomeric procyandins.

Dioscorea villosa is a hypocholesterolaemic, antioxidant, anti-inflammatory and spasmolytic cholagogue. Maude Grieve recommends it for biliary colic and one of its common names is, aptly, colic root.

Schisandra chinensis is an inducer of Phase II liver detoxification, and an adaptogen, antioxidant and hepatoprotective. *Schisandra chinensis* is also known as supporting emotional and physical resilience.

Taraxacum officinale is a cholagogue, hepatoprotective, anti-inflammatory and diuretic. It is recommended as the key herb for gallstone disease by Weiss and has traditionally been noted for its affinity in the treatment of gallstones.

Herbal formula

Cynara scolymus 1 : 2	20 mL
Schisandra chinensis 1 : 2	30 mL
Taraxacum officinale radix 1 : 2	20 mL
Equisetum arvensis 1 : 2	15 mL
Crataegus oxyacantha (blend) 1 : 2	15 mL
Dioscorea villosa 1 : 2	10 mL
Total	110 mL

Dose: 7 mL twice daily before meals

NUTRITIONAL MEDICINE

As sedentary lifestyle is implicated in the aetiology of gallstones, exercise is crucial. Plan a weekly exercise schedule to help with gradual and sustainable weight loss.

Reduce sugar and refined carbohydrates

Re-educate the patient on the benefits of introducing good oils so long-term weight management can be achieved. Include rice bran oil in cooking, olive oil and nut oils in salads.

CASE STUDY CONTINUED

Include avocados, linseeds, walnuts, grilled salmon (good oils) and small oily fish.

Include fibre and protein for satiety and to reduce constipation. Fibre also absorbs bile in the GIT and removes it from the body, lowering cholesterol.

Increase fluid intake to reduce headaches and constipation. Try mint, fennel and liquorice teas.

Try to expand the palate away from predominantly sweet foods. Include lemon zest and berries (high in vitamin C) on yoghurt. Use herbs and spices such as turmeric (anti-inflammatory), cinnamon, cumin, fennel, dill and coriander to increase antioxidant herbs, stimulate taste and digestion and create a healthy appetite. Also include bitter foods.

SECOND APPOINTMENT (1 MONTH LATER)

On second presentation, there was considerable improvement in the patient's presenting signs and symptoms as there was no biliary discomfort or epigastric pain, so the initial herbal formula was repeated.

She had introduced olive oil in cooking, ate a healthy low-sugar breakfast daily and had reduced chocolate to one square a day after dinner and was enjoying 70% dark chocolate instead of family-size packets of M&Ms.

ADDITIONAL TREATMENT

Herbal medicine

Silybum marianum standardised to contain 140 mg silybin, twice daily.

Nutritional medicine

Lecithin, 1200 mg b.i.d. to assist cholesterol elimination.

FOLLOW-UP APPOINTMENT

Results of second ultrasound taken 6 months after initial presentation showed no presence of gallstones. All liver enzymes were within normal range.

Additional information

The gallbladder cleanse

The standard 2-day gallbladder cleanse has been practised in both traditional and modern naturopathy and Ayurveda. The cleanse involves consuming an Epsom salt and water solution followed by an olive oil and grapefruit juice solution, then repeating the Epsom salt solution again. Watery stools are expected on the morning of day 2 of the cleanse and cholesterol gallstones are reported to appear in this bowel movement. Reports of people passing 40 to 100 stones at one time are not uncommon. However, in most cases these stones are in fact not cholesterol gallstones.

The formation of such stones could be explained through a process of saponification involving the magnesium sulfate, olive oil and grapefruit juice. Weiss[156] indicates a similar theory when he reports on the traditional use of turpentine oil in the gallbladder cleanse and suggests the spherical objects are soaps formed from oil combining with bile in the intestines. The risk of undertaking the gallbladder cleanse in cases where stones detected in the gallbladder are larger than the opening of the neck of the gallbladder (2 cm) is risky. Large amounts of olive oil could overstimulate the gallbladder, leading to the expulsion of stones and gallstone impaction and resultant cholecystitis, cholangitis or pancreatitis. The gallbladder cleanse is unsafe and not recommended in current naturopathic practice.

What is cholesterol?

Cholesterol forms part of the structure of every cell membrane and is a precursor to bile acids and steroid hormones. The liver is the main site for cholesterol synthesis and lipoprotein metabolism. Hepatocytes (liver cells) produce the most cholesterol, but all cells in the body are capable of synthesising cholesterol. Cholesterol exists in two forms in the liver: cholesterol esters (storage form) or free cholesterol. Cholesterol catabolism is a more limited process where the liver and steroidogenic cells convert cholesterol to bile acids and steroid hormones. Limited locations for this catabolic process necessitate the transport of cholesterol from body tissues and organs to the liver. Cholesterol homeostasis is regulated by pathways that either increase or reduce hepatic cholesterol.[176]

Cholesterol is transported in the blood by two main types of plasma proteins: low-density lipoprotein (LDL) and high-density lipoprotein (HDL) (see Table 11.8).

Low-density lipoproteins (LDLs) transport cholesterol from the liver and encourage the deposition of cholesterol in the peripheral cells. High-density lipoproteins (HDLs) are responsible for the release of cholesterol from cells and transport cholesterol back to the liver for catabolism. A method of cholesterol transportation is needed in the body as somatic cells cannot degrade cholesterol to bile acids — this process must take place in the liver. In other words, the HDLs (good cholesterol) take cholesterol out of the tissues and ferry it to the liver, which converts it to bile salts. Eighty per cent of the cholesterol in the body is converted into cholic acid in the liver (conjugated with other substances to form bile salts).[177]

HDL is responsible for mediating the removal of cellular cholesterol via two independent pathways. Diffusion-mediated cellular cholesterol release involves the removal of cell cholesterol that has been trapped by lipoproteins. This process is mediated by the process of cholesterol acyl esterification on high density lipoproteins. Apolipoprotein mediated removal of cellular cholesterol is the second pathway for the removal of cholesterol from cells. This process involves the generation of new HDL particles via the removal of cholesterol and phospholipids and the process is mediated by ATP-binding cassette transporter (ABCA1).[178,179] The very low-density lipoproteins (VLDLs) are formed in the liver and transport triglycerides and carbohydrates to peripheral tissues.

TABLE 11.8 The principal lipoproteins
The plasma lipids include these components, free fatty acids from adipose tissue, which circulate bound to albumin and chylomicron remnants

		Composition percentage (%)					
	Size (nm)	Protein	Free cholesterol	Cholesteryl esters	Triglyceride	Phospholipid	Origin
Chylomicrons	75–1000	2	2	3	90	3	Intestine
Chylomicron remnants	30–80	–	–	–	–	–	Capillaries
Very low-density lipoproteins (VLDL)	30–80	8	4	16	55	17	Liver and Intestine
Intermediate-density lipoproteins (IDL)	25–40	10	5	25	40	20	VLDL
Low-density lipoproteins (LDL)	20	20	7	46	6	21	IDL
High-density lipoproteins (HDL)	7.5–10	50	4	16	5	25	Liver and intestine

CHOLECYSTITIS

Epidemiology

Cholecystitis refers to the acute or chronic inflammation of the gallbladder and this condition can either present as calculous or acalculous (without gallstones) cholecystitis. Acute calculous cholecystitis develops in only 1–3% of people who have symptomatic gallstones.[180] Acute calculous cholecystitis is estimated to be three times more common in women than men, matching the incidence and prevalence of cholelithiasis.[181]

Aetiology: acute cholecystitis

Approximately 95% of acute cholecystitis cases are associated with blockage of the cystic duct by gallstones followed by distension and subsequent chemical or bacterial inflammation.[182] Five to ten per cent are acalculous (without gallstones), attributable to infection, tumours, pregnancy or complications of terminal illness.[183,184]

INFECTION

Rarely gallbladder inflammation can be triggered by blockage of the cystic duct by gastrointestinal parasites or tumours.[185]

Acute acalculous cholecystitis may occur in cases of acute Epstein-Barr virus (EBV) infection, especially in patients with cholestatic hepatitis.[186,187]

PREGNANCY AND ORAL CONTRACEPTION

Symptomatic gallstones occur in about 0.1–0.2% of pregnancies[188] and biliary tract problems are the second most common surgical problem that presents with pregnancy. Increased oestrogen levels during pregnancy or from oral contraception increase the risk of gallstone and biliary sludge formation.[189,190]

CRITICAL ILLNESS

Acalculous cholecystitis occurs in only 1–5% of cases, usually in terminally ill patients as a result of cachexia, fever, dehydration and lack of oral feeding as a stimulus for bile production.[180,185,191]

Aetiology: chronic cholecystitis

Chronic cholecystitis is a longstanding inflammatory condition involving low-grade inflammation of the gallbladder and repeated mild attacks of acute cholecystitis. The aetiology of chronic cholecystitis is associated with gallstone formation.[192] However, this condition presents clinically with symptoms much milder than those seen in acute cholecystitis.

INFECTION

Helicobacter pylori infection has also been implicated in the aetiology of chronic cholecystitis,[193] with one study[194] showing specific histological evidence such as necrosis, degeneration and infiltration of inflammatory mediators found in tissues colonised by the *H. pylori* bacteria. Evidence of *H. pylori* infection in cases of chronic cholecystitis has also been linked in the literature to the pathogenesis of hepatobiliary tract cancer.[195]

IMPAIRED ACTIVITY OF MUSCULATURE

Chronic acalculous cholecystitis is characterised by recurrent episodes of biliary pain in cases where there is no radiographic evidence of gallstones.[196]

Pathogenesis: acute cholecystitis

Acute cholecystitis results from the partial or complete blockage of the cystic duct by cholelithiasis (gallstones) or blockage of the neck of the gallbladder (Hartmann's pouch) by biliary sludge (see Fig. 11.2). These blockages result in an increase in intraluminal pressure within the gallbladder

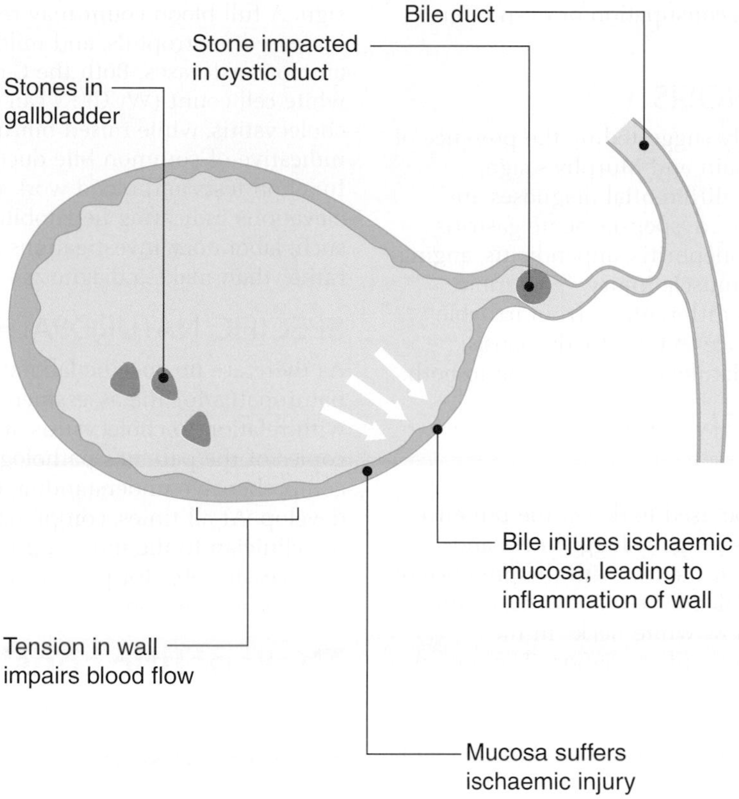
Bile duct
Stone impacted in cystic duct
Stones in gallbladder
Bile injures ischaemic mucosa, leading to inflammation of wall
Tension in wall impairs blood flow
Mucosa suffers ischaemic injury

FIGURE 11.2 Pathogenesis of acute cholecystitis.

and the oedematous thickening and distension of the gallbladder wall.

Prostaglandins play a significant role in the pathophysiology of cholecystitis; reduced anti-inflammatory mediators and increased inflammatory mediators result in inflammation and significant mucosal trauma. The inflammatory changes and damage to the mucosa of the gallbladder caused by prostaglandins initiate the release of mucosal phospholipases that hydrolyse bile lecithin into lysolecithins. Lysolecithins further exacerbate mucosal inflammation by damaging the protective glycoprotein mucosal epithelial layer of the gallbladder wall.[197] Infection is not believed to be an initiating factor involved in the aetiology of acute cholecystitis. However, secondary bacterial infection with *Escherichia coli*, *Klebsiella* or *Streptococcus faecalis* may present in approximately 20% of cases.[108]

Pathogenesis: chronic cholecystitis

Long-term histological changes in chronic cholecystitis due to chronic inflammation include epithelial metaplasia, hyperplasia, muscular thickening and adipose deposition. The serosal surface of the gallbladder may also thicken and significant fibrosis of the gallbladder mucosa is common. This thickening impairs proper organ function by preventing the contraction and expansion of the gallbladder. In cases of severe and longstanding pathology, dystrophic calcification of the gallbladder wall may occur, resulting in porcelain gallbladder. Approximately 20% of porcelain gallbladders harbour carcinomas.[198]

Overview

SIGNS AND SYMPTOMS

Patients with acute cholecystitis present clinically with severe midline abdominal pain that is rapid in onset. The cardinal sign required for the diagnosis of acute cholecystitis is constant pain that radiates to the right upper quadrant, right scapular and shoulder region. On palpation, the patient will demonstrate tenderness and guarding and deep breathing may exacerbate this pain (Murphy's sign). Anorexia, nausea, vomiting and fever are evident and mild jaundice may be evident if bile flow is significantly impaired.[182,185]

Nausea is the most common complaint in a patient with chronic gallbladder disease and is specifically associated with intolerance to fatty foods. In severe cases of chronic cholecystitis, the smell or sight of fatty foods may be enough to stimulate a response. Flatulent dyspepsia also presents clinically and patients most often complain of belching, heartburn, bloating, fullness and flatulence. Again, the consumption of fatty meals is a trigger for these complaints. Often, the signs and symptoms of chronic cholecystitis can be nonspecific and vague and the absence of clinical signs such as right upper quadrant pain or a palpable mass may result in delayed diagnosis or the confusion of organic symptoms with those of irritable bowel syndrome, constipation or even reflux oesophagitis.

DIFFERENTIAL DIAGNOSIS

Acute cholecystitis is strongly suggested by the presence of both right upper quadrant pain and Murphy's sign, possibly with fever. Possible differential diagnoses are gallbladder attack, cholangitis, dyspepsia, acute gastritis, peptic ulcer, IBS, acute pyelonephritis, appendicitis, angina, heart attack and intercostal muscle injury.[199] Chronic cholecystitis may be hard to differentiate from irritable bowel syndrome as intolerance to fatty foods, nausea, indigestion, dyspepsia and flatulence are common to both.

NATUROPATHIC DIAGNOSIS

Iridology

Although iridology cannot be used to detect the presence of gallstones, tissue weakness, organ sluggishness and toxicity are commonly seen in the iris with the presence of crypts or lacunae in the gallbladder region. Longstanding chronic cholecystitis may show white flecks in the hepatobiliary region indicating inflammation. The presence of jaundice in the sclera is, however, more suggestive of severe hepatobiliary dysfunction. An orange-brown central heterochromia is indicative of gallbladder dysfunction and may indicate liver and gastrointestinal dysfunction. According to Sharan, cholecystitis may appear as an inflammatory white or yellow-white cloud in the gall bladder area.[199]

Tongue analysis

In cholecystitis cases, the tongue may present with a creamy white or thick yellow and greasy coating.

Urine and stools

A biliary obstruction can cause white (acholic) stools because of the lack of bilirubin due to the suppression of bile and dark urine (bilirubinuria).

Investigations

Ultrasound is the investigation of choice where acute cholecystitis is suspected.[200] Ultrasound findings show fluid build-up around the gallbladder, gallbladder distension and an oedematous gallbladder wall with thickening and gallstones. If the cystic duct is obstructed, biliary scintigraphy is the most accurate diagnostic tool and is considered the gold standard if the diagnosis of cholecystitis is still unclear after ultrasonography is performed.[201] Ultrasonography is a useful tool before laparoscopic cholecystectomy and can be used to ascertain potential surgical complications. Magnetic resonance imaging (MRI) and computed tomography can be used as adjunct tools for the diagnosis of acute cholecystitis; however, this approach is less frequently used owing to expense and time factors.[202]

There are no laboratory tests available that can reliably diagnose acute cholecystitis.[203] Clinical judgment will prompt a diagnosis based on imaging results and an assessment of right upper quadrant pain and Murphy's sign. A full blood count may reveal leucocytosis with increased neutrophils, and mild elevation of aminotransferases. Both the C-reactive protein (CRP) and white cell count (WCC)[204] can be associated with acute cholecystitis, while raised bilirubin > 5 mg/dL can be indicative of common bile duct obstruction.[176] Liver function tests and blood work may only show mild elevations indicating hepatobiliary dysfunction and, as such, laboratory investigations should be used to support rather than make a diagnosis.

SPECIFIC NATUROPATHIC INVESTIGATIONS

As there are no specific laboratory tests available to naturopaths for the assessment of gallbladder function with relation to cholecystitis, it is advisable to obtain copies of the patient's pathology results so that a comprehensive understanding of the patient's health can develop. At all times, comprehensive case taking will direct the clinician to the most appropriate treatment plan and the need to refer for proper diagnosis if the patient does not present with one.

Therapeutic considerations

CLINICAL DECISION MAKING AND RATIONALE

The primary therapeutic consideration for acute cholecystitis is the acknowledgement that this condition may be a medical emergency. In extreme cases, if left untreated acute cholecystitis can result in either gangrene, necrosis of the gallbladder wall or rupture of the gallbladder wall with resultant peritonitis. Given the severity of implications of untreated acute cholecystitis it is crucial that the naturopathic clinician engages in a comprehensive case-taking process so that informed decisions can be made. If presented with a case of acute cholecystitis, it is essential that the clinician remains cognisant of the scope of naturopathy and practices within the limits of their qualifications and expertise. In this instance, direct referral to a general practitioner (or to hospital if gallbladder rupture is suspected) is considered best clinical practice.

Therapeutic application

The naturopathic approach to the treatment of cholecystitis involves recognising the strengths and limitations of naturopathic practice. Treatment relies heavily on the use of anti-inflammatory herbal medicines and long-term case management involves the use of herbal medicines and nutritional supplements that protect and restore function to the dysfunctional gallbladder. The naturopath must be aware of the signs and symptoms that characterise an acute attack of cholecystitis and refer immediately to a hospital for assessment. Assess patient dietary, lifestyle, medical and family history. This will give the clinician important understanding into their case presentation.

If cholecystectomy has been recommended to the patient, a pre- and postsurgical treatment plan is beneficial.

HISTORICAL PERSPECTIVE

The death of Alexander the Great at the age of 34 has been attributed to acute obstructive cholecystitis. Evidence suggests that on the 13th day of June in the 13th year of his rule he died from peritonitis secondary to acute cholecystitis. Historians have suggested that the fatal biliary tract disease was fuelled by excess consumption of alcohol and overeating at a banquet that Alexander threw for his leading officers in Babylon.[122]

NATUROPATHIC PERSPECTIVE

Do not treat acute cholecystitis, refer immediately.

Chronic cholecystitis

The treatment of chronic cholecystitis requires the following considerations:

- Assess the case presentation, consider differentials and obtain a diagnosis if one has not been provided
- Identify any possible contraindications for treatment
- Reduction in inflammation will provide symptomatic relief by reducing pain; it will also reduce histological damage and help return function by reducing swelling and therefore stasis. Begin hepatic and biliary trophorestoratives to assist organ function
- If safe to do so, gently stimulate gallbladder motility with choleretics (e.g. *Cynara scolymus*) and cholagogues (*Taraxacum officinale*) so stagnation can be reduced and gallbladder function restored
- Support optimal digestive and GIT function (*Gentiana lutea*) — prolonged intestinal transit time can increase stone formation. Encourage fibre and dietary bitters
- Address potential for bacterial infection as stone formation and cholecystitis have been linked to bacterial infection such as *H. pylori*; antimicrobials are the key herbal agents to employ
- Address any factors that hinder or obstruct the healing process
- Address obesity due to the link with gallstones but avoid rapid weight loss as this can enhance stone formation.

Post cholecystectomy support

The removal of the gallbladder or just the stones within the gallbladder can be by laparoscopic surgery (key hole) or laparotomy (open surgery).

Gallbladder surgery does not address the possible causative factors like gastrointestinal dysfunction, gallbladder dysmotility or free fatty acid dysregulation so it is still crucial to address these issues.

Removal of the gallbladder means that bile is still produced but not stored, therefore meals containing high quantities of fat should be avoided except for small amounts of essential fatty acids which will reduce inflammation.

Stimulate the digestive system before meals with bitters (*Gentiana lutea*), cholagogues (*Taraxacum officinale*), choleretics (*Curcuma longa*) and carminatives (*Matricaria recutita*) to maximise bile and pancreatic enzymes and digestive function.

Injuries to the bile duct during routine laparoscopic cholecystectomies may result in mild or moderate symptoms like abdominal tenderness, pain and distension, nausea and vomiting.[205] Gentle anti-inflammatory herbal medicines like *Glycyrrhiza glabra* and *Matricaria recutita* can serve to dampen any inflammatory response and mucous membrane trophorestoratives (*Hydrastis canadensis*) help repair damaged tissue postsurgery.

Postsurgery, to reduce bruising and trauma apply topically an arnica-based homoeopathic cream. To improve healing combine a vitamin E cream with *Calendula officinalis* and *Centella asiatica.*

A homoeopathic treatment plan will assist the healing process. Without doubt, arnica is the first choice and other remedies can be used depending on how the wound is healing.

NUTRITIONAL MEDICINE (DIETARY)

The role of dietary treatment in chronic cholecystitis is undeniably linked with any dietary guidelines designed to address gallstone formation and liver function. The dietary therapeutic guidelines for gallstone formation are presented below and additional suggestions for the inflammation associated with cholecystitis have been detailed.

Dietary therapeutic objectives

See 'Hepatobiliary nutritional objectives (dietary)' for an overview.

- Gently stimulate gallbladder motility and reduce gallbladder stagnancy through wise food choices (fresh fruits and vegetables, wholegrains, poultry and fish)
- Support optimal digestive and GIT function, increase consumption of bitters (dandelion greens, rocket, kale) and raw foods to encourage bile production and release
- Support lipid metabolism by reducing saturated and trans fatty acids and increase essential fatty acid intake
- Monitor dietary cholesterol intake; make adjustments where appropriate
- Reduce or remove intake of refined carbohydrates, processed foods and takeaways (high in fat and sugar)
- Encourage fibre intake (soluble and insoluble fibre) to reduce risk of stone formation.

Additionally, specific dietary suggestions for inflammation include:

- Increase intake of dietary anti-inflammatories by including pineapple (bromelain) and paw paw (papain)
- Increase intake of dietary antioxidants by including an array of berries and cherries
- Soothe inflamed mucous membranes by increasing the intake of demulcent foods like oats and slippery elm.

Specific dietary treatments

In addition to the hepatobiliary nutritional objectives (dietary) and the dietary suggestions recommended for the treatment of gallstones, the following recommendations will help with the management of chronic cholecystitis. A focus on anti-inflammatory and antioxidant rich foods will temper an inflamed gallbladder and lessen the severity and duration of mild cholecystic attacks noted in the progression of this condition.

DIETARY INCLUSIONS

Bromelain and papain

Both the stem and the fruit of *Ananas comosus* (pineapple) contain a variety of proteolytic enzymes known as bromelains. Bromelain enzymes are a digestive aid and an anti-inflammatory agent,[206,207] making fresh pineapple consumption beneficial in cases of chronic cholecystitis. Papain is an enzyme found in paw paw and it has demonstrated anti-inflammatory activity and may also assist with digestion to reduce symptoms of nausea, dyspepsia and indigestion.

DIETARY EXCLUSIONS

Saturated and trans fats

A reduction in both saturated and trans fat intake will reduce the potential for gallstone formation and reduce any inflammation associated with chronic cholecystitis as the consumption of saturated and trans fats has been directly linked to gallstone formation. The intake of trans fats, particularly in women, is also positively correlated with systemic inflammation.[208]

Refined sugar

Sugar intake needs to be reduced significantly owing to the increased risk of gallstone formation. Research has shown that diets high in refined sugars promote abnormal bile composition, altered gut microflora, hyperinsulinaemia and gallstone formation. Sugar intake has also been directly linked to inflammatory processes in the body;[209–211] thus a reduction or complete removal of refined sugar from the diet will reduce the risk of gallstone formation and reduce inflammation associated with chronic cholecystitis. *Foeniculum vulgare* (fennel) seed tea can reduce the taste/need for sugar with an initial dose of up to three cups per day until the management of symptoms, then two cups per day as a maintenance dose.

NUTRITIONAL MEDICINE (SUPPLEMENTAL)

See 'Hepatobiliary nutritional objectives (nutrients)' and Table 11.5.

Nutritional medicine therapeutic objectives

- Potential nutritional deficiencies that should be considered in all hepatobiliary disease are listed in Table 11.5. Address nutrient deficiencies or requirements
- Promote optimal gallbladder motility and function
- Support bile production and release with the use of lipotrophic factors
- Prevent and reduce inflammation during mild acute attacks of cholecystitis.

Specific nutrients required

Because of the associated aetiology the symptomatic treatment and long-term management of chronic cholecystitis needs to incorporate many of the nutritional supplements that are prescribed for gallstones.

SAMPLE DAILY DIET

BREAKFAST	
Papaya fruit boat: papaya cut open and filled with chopped banana and pineapple core, lecithin and live yoghurt	Lecithin may help to break down microlithiasis found in biliary sludge. Papaya and pineapple both contain enzymes that assist in reduction of inflammation. Vitamin C fruits are preferred as vitamin C accelerates the conversion of cholesterol to bile salts.
LUNCH	
Salmon with bitter green salad dressed with lemon juice and garlic	Salmon contains omega-3 fatty acids to reduce inflammation and reduce cholesterol saturation found in biliary sludge, while dark-green bitter leafy vegetables encourage the release of bile and gallbladder motility.
DINNER	
Legume curry made with garlic, onion, fenugreek and ginger served with green salad and rice	Consumption of a vegetarian diet is associated with less incidence of gallbladder disease.[212] Spices such as garlic, onion and fenugreek decrease hypersecretion of cholesterol into bile, reducing lithogenic bile in animal studies[213] and reducing accumulation of fat in the liver and inflammation of the gallbladder membrane.
SNACKS	
Dandelion tea Fresh fruit	Dandelion tea may help to support bile production and optimal gallbladder motility. Antioxidant and anti-inflammatory.

Essential fatty acids

Generally a low-fat diet is recommended in gallbladder disease to prevent gallbladder attacks caused by overstimulation of the gallbladder. However essential fatty acids are indicated in cholecystitis to assist in the prevention of gallstones and to reduce chronic inflammation. Fish oils are useful in reducing the inflammatory response by competing with inflammatory arachidonic acid (AA) in the cyclooxygenase and lipoxygenase pathways.[214]

Quercetin

Quercetin modulates the inflammatory response via inhibiting the NF-κB pathway[215] and inhibits cytokines, phospholipase A2, cyclooxygenase and lipoxygenase, thus reducing the concentrations of prostanoids and leukotrienes.[216] It is also reported to be antifibrotic[217] and antibacterial[218] and as such may be beneficial in the chronic cholecystitis picture.

Rutin

Rutin is a flavonol glycoside comprised of quercetin and rutinose and its anti-inflammatory action in the gastrointestinal system is due to its ability to deliver quercetin to the intestine for the mediation of TNF-α-induced NF-κB activation.[219] Rutin has free radical scavenging ability, can inhibit lipid peroxidation and may inhibit the oxidation of vitamin C.[220]

Hesperidin

Hesperidin is a citrus flavonoid with antioxidant activity that inhibits reactive oxygen species activity.[221]

Dosage requirement

- Essential fatty acids: 3–6 g per day of eicosapentaenoic acid (EPA) and docosahexaenoic acid (DHA)
- Quercetin: 1500 mg/day
- Rutin: 1200 mg/day
- Hesperidin: 1000 mg/day.

HERBAL MEDICINE

Herbal medicine therapeutic objectives

- Improve gallbladder function and motility
- Promote the optimal formation, storage and release of bile
- Promote gentle gallbladder contraction where safe to do so
- Promote the dissolution of gallstones if indicated
- Reduce inflammation and colic during mild acute attacks
- Improve bowel function
- Improve digestive function and reduce digestive disturbance
- Address sleeping difficulty, anxiety or associated stress.

Specific herbal medicine classes

Herbal medicine has a substantial role in the treatment and management of chronic cholecystitis and therapeutic effects can be achieved by targeting both symptoms and aetiological influences. The liver, gallbladder and gastrointestinal system can be treated with a range of hepatobiliary herbs that have a wide scope of therapeutic activity.

Cholagogue herbal medicines promote the release of stored bile from the gallbladder and can be used in cases where there is bile insufficiency, gallstone formation and evidence of poor digestion. Strong cholagogues are contraindicated in cases of chronic cholecystitis — the gentle approach is necessary here as this is a chronic condition and requires a gentle, long-term approach. Hepatics will support the function of the liver and the production of bile; many hepatics also have secondary anti-inflammatory and antioxidant activities and thus initiate substantial therapeutic effect when prescribed synergistically.

Anti-inflammatory and antispasmodic herbal medicines are essential in the long-term management of cholecystitis as they can reduce the length and severity of mild acute attacks and ease much of the gastrointestinal discomfort associated with the condition. Nervines may be indicated if the patient presents with anxiety, stress or sleep disturbances and antimicrobials should be considered if any pathogenic activity is reported.

Specific herbal medicines

DIOSCOREA VILLOSA (WILD YAM)

Dioscorea villosa has a significant choleretic activity owing to increased bile flow produced by the constituent diosgenin. It is reported to have a hypocholesterolaemic activity by reducing cholesterol absorption and increasing cholesterol secretion.[222] Diosgenin has been found to increase bile flow as well as the biliary output of cholesterol and glutathione.[223] *Dioscorea villosa* also has strong antioxidant activity[224] due to the presence of catechins, chlorogenic acids, proanthocyanadins and anthocyanadins.[225] This antioxidant activity of diosgenin reduces the cholestatic effects of oestrogen in rats.[226] Combined hypocholesterolaemic and antioxidant activity contribute significantly to this herb's therapeutic activity in the treatment of chronic cholecystitis. Dioscorea has traditionally been called colic root due to its marked anti-inflammatory and antispasmodic actions. Grieve suggests this herb provides the quickest and most effective relief for bilious colic.[227]

CYNARA SCOLYMUS (GLOBE ARTICHOKE)

Cynara has a broad therapeutic scope in the treatment of both gallstones and the dyspeptic picture associated with chronic cholecystitis. The choleretic, cholagogue, hepatoprotective and hypocholesterolaemic activities of *Cynara scolymus* have been noted in the literature[228,229] and as such this herb is regarded highly for its role in the treatment of gallstones. Cases of chronic cholecystitis often present with nausea, dyspepsia and biliousness and *Cynara scolymus* is well indicated in the treatment and management of such symptoms. Cynara has been noted for its ability to reduce symptoms in cases of functional dyspepsia[230,231] and the inulin present in *Cynara scolymus* contributes to this herb's beneficial activities in the gastrointestinal and immune systems by functioning as a prebiotic.[232] Inulin has been found to assist gastrointestinal and immune function, reduce cholesterol and serum lipids and reduce the inflammation of inflammatory bowel disease (IBD).[233]

MATRICARIA RECUTITA (CHAMOMILE)

Matricaria recutita is a key herb in the treatment and management of chronic cholecystitis and associated digestive disorders. The herb has a long history of therapeutic use with Asclepius, Galen and Hippocrates referring to its healing powers[234] and it has been traditionally regarded as the 'Plant's Physician' due to its ability to contribute to the health of the garden.[227] The presence of alpha-bisabolol content in chamomile oil is credited for providing the majority of antibacterial, antifungal and anti-inflammatory actions and further anti-inflammatory and antispasmodic actions are associated with the presence of chamazulene, apigenin and alpha-bisabolol.[234]

Matricaria recutita is a component of the well-researched formulation STW 5. STW 5 is a combination of traditionally used herbal medicines including *Iberis amara, Mentha x piperita, Matricaria recutita, Glycyrrhiza glabra, Angelica archangelica, Carum carvi, Melissa officinalis* and *Chelidonium majus.*[235] Efficacy of the STW 5 formulation has been demonstrated in numerous trials and its antispasmodic, anti-inflammatory and tonic effects have been noted extensively in the literature.[236–238] One study suggested that some of the most pronounced effects from this formulation come from the angelica root and chamomile flower components;[236] however, the therapeutic activity of the formulation is thought to be due to synergistic activity of the included herbal medicines and the high quality of the materials used.

VALERIANA OFFICINALIS (VALERIAN)

Valeriana officinalis has been traditionally regarded as a powerful nervine, carminative and antispasmodic.[227] It has a long use in Western European herbalism as a sedative due to its ability to inhibit the breakdown of gamma-amino butyric acid and has been used in traditional Chinese medicine for menstrual pain.[239] Although it is commonly regarded as an effective sedative, valepotriates in this herb exhibit spasmolytic activity in the gastrointestinal system.[240] Valerian is best administered in tincture or extract form to elicit the above effects. Valerian will provide most benefit in cases marked by gastrointestinal discomfort or constipation. For insomnia, valerian is prescribed as a herbal tea to promote sleep.

CHIONANTHUS VIRGINICUS (FRINGE TREE)

Chionanthus virginicus has been traditionally used for the treatment of bilious fevers, liver complaints and typhoid.[227] This herb is known for its mild laxative and cholagogue actions and has been cited as a specific for the treatment of gallstones and gallbladder inflammation.[241] Fringe tree is indicated in gallbladder inflammation/gallstones particularly when highly coloured urine, clay-coloured stools and right-sided pain are present.[158] There is a lack of evidence-based research to support its clinical use but this herb should be considered in cases marked by both gallbladder inflammation and constipation. This is an endangered herb.

CURCUMA LONGA (TURMERIC)

Turmeric has long been used in Asian and Ayurvedic herbal medicine as a bitter digestive, choleretic and anti-inflammatory agent. Initial reports on the biological activity of curcumin in 1937 suggested improvements in patients with chronic cholecystitis, owing to improved bile flow and gallbladder motility.[242] More recent research shows it may be beneficial for use in chronic cholecystitis owing to its ability to reduce flatulent dyspepsia.[243] *Curcuma longa* also demonstrates marked anti-inflammatory activity via the inhibition of arachidonic acid pathways and antioxidant activity.[244] This herb has been found to be effective in both acute and chronic inflammation[245] and is thus a key herb in the treatment of chronic cholecystitis.

SCUTELLARIA BAICALENSIS (BAIKAL SKULLCAP)

Histamine has been detected in the gallbladder epithelium of rodents[246] and it has been theorised that allergic responses mediated by mast cells in the gallbladder mucosa may be present in cases of cholecystitis.[247] Baikal skullcap is the herbal medicine of choice in these circumstances as it has demonstrated anti-allergic, anti-inflammatory and antioxidant activity.[248]

LIFESTYLE RECOMMENDATIONS

It is imperative that weight loss is addressed in cases of cholecystitis because of the link between obesity, gallstones and associated gallbladder inflammation. Weight loss can be achieved through the implementation of a daily exercise regimen. Alcohol and smoking should be avoided at all costs and naturopathic support to quit smoking should be offered to patients.

CASE STUDY

OVERVIEW

A 45-year-old man presented with a history of gastrointestinal discomfort. The patient reported constant flatulence, dyspepsia, intolerance to fatty food, constipation, abdominal distension and bloating, nausea and reflux. He reported he had been experiencing these symptoms for the past 5 years following an acute gallbladder attack.

He revealed that no further acute episodes had been experienced. However, a low-grade pain was evident. He was reluctant to see a naturopath but was encouraged to make an appointment by his wife to try to avoid starting cholesterol medication.

Dietary investigation revealed significant intake of takeaway food and alcohol. The patient reported daily consumption of takeaway pasta and curries for lunch and dinner and intake of up to one bottle of red wine per evening. The patient was drinking 5 cups of strong coffee a day. The patient reported headaches, high stress at work and constant deadlines with no time to exercise.

CLINICAL EXAMINATION

Weight: 110 kg, Height: 182 cm, BMI: 33
Waist circumference: 148 cm

LABORATORY INVESTIGATIONS

ALT 78 U/L	(5–30)
AST 65 U/L	(10–35)

CASE STUDY CONTINUED

ALP 180 U/L	(20–35)
GGT 100 U/L	(5–35)
Cholesterol 7 mmol/L	(3.9–5.5)
Triglycerides 2 mmol/L	(0.5–1.7)
HDL chol. 1.3 mmol/L	(0.9–2.1)
LDL chol. 3.8 mmol/L	(1.7–3.5)

Abdominal ultrasound showed cholecystitis — with mobile biliary sludge and gallbladder wall thickening, a consequence of long-term inflammation. There was no evidence of intrahepatic or extrahepatic bile duct obstruction.

The presence of *H. pylori* was not detected by the urea breath test.

TREATMENT PROTOCOL

INITIAL APPOINTMENT

The patient was reluctant to change and sceptical about non-allopathic treatment. Therefore it was decided to provide digestive symptom relief first. Hopefully then the patient would be open to change and well enough to implement sustainable change. Discussed need for immediate medical attention should the patient suffer another gallbladder attack involving radiating pain to the shoulder and back.

HERBAL MEDICINE

Silybum marianum — hepatotrophorestorative and protective against the patient's alcohol consumption. This herb was employed to reduce lipid peroxidation and for its antioxidant, anti-inflammatory, antifibrotic and hypocholesterolaemic properties

Scutellaria baicalensis — antioxidant, anti-inflammatory, antifibrotic. Has a history of use and efficacy within traditional Chinese medicine for chronic cholecystitis

Centella asiatica was used to reduce fibrosis and promote healing of gallbladder wall from chronic inflammation

Gentiana lutea for dyspepsia, flatulence and abdominal bloating

Curcuma longa for flatulent dyspepsia, nausea; antioxidant, anti-inflammatory

Matricaria recutita included for its anti-inflammatory and carminative properties

Cynara scolymus — cholagogue, choleretic, antioxidant, hypocholesterolaemic, to help with fatty food intolerance and constipation

Peumus boldo was used to manage the pain of chronic cholecystitis

Taraxacum officinale (root) to improve gallbladder motility, improve bile production and release, and improve digestion and constipation; also anti-inflammatory and reduces nausea.

Herbal formula

Silybum marianum (glycetract) 1 : 2	30 mL
Cynara scolymus 1 : 2	15 mL
Centella asiatica 1 : 2	15 mL
Scutellaria baicalensis 1 : 2	30 mL
Peumus boldo 1 : 2	10 mL
	100 mL

Dose: 9 mL twice daily before meals

CASE STUDY CONTINUED

Nutritional medicine

Curcuma longa: equivalent curcuminoids 161.5 mg twice daily

Multivitamin: with vitamin B complex

Fish oil EPA/DHA: 1000 mg twice daily

High-potency, multistrain probiotic containing *Lactobacillus* and *Bifidobacterium* strains.

Hydration

Patient was prepared to try to drink a litre of sparkling water a day to help with headaches, constipation and energy levels.

SECOND APPOINTMENT (4 WEEKS LATER)

The patient reported a significant improvement in his abdominal discomfort but only slight improvement in constipation. Reducing alcohol intake was discussed with a target of 50% alcohol reduction and 2 alcohol-free days a week.

Herbal formula and nutritional medicine prescription were repeated.

ADDITIONAL HERBAL MEDICINE

Digestive bitters (*Gentiana lutea* and *Zingiber officinale*): 4 drops in water 20 minutes before meals

HYDRATION, TEA AND COFFEE

Patient was managing to drink half a litre of sparkling water a day and was willing to try to increase.

Chamomile and mint tea after every meal for flatulence, stress and hydration.

Replace three cups of coffee with dandelion coffee (with honey for compliance).

THIRD APPOINTMENT (4 WEEKS LATER)

The patient was very happy with the improvement in digestive discomfort and constipation and his compliance in terms of alcohol reduction and water consumption. He was motivated to discuss dietary changes and exercise due to a total weight loss of 10 kg over 3 months. He also reported a reduction in headaches and stress levels.

LONG-TERM MANAGEMENT

Multivitamin: with vitamin B complex

Fish oil EPA/DHA: 1000 mg twice daily

Digestive bitters (*Gentiana lutea* and *Zingiber officinale*): 4 drops in water 20 minutes before meals

Switched herbal formula to a *Silybum marianum* tablet and a complex antioxidant to improve long-term compliance

Maintain hydration with herbal teas, reduced coffee and reduced alcohol

Exercise — plan an enjoyable and sustainable exercise program of at least 45 minutes five times a week and increase incidental exercise; reduce instances of being seated for long periods of time.

CASE STUDY CONTINUED

Diet — low carbohydrate; add plant protein, high fibre, healthy fats (omega-3), high antioxidant foods. Limit takeaway meals to just lunchtime and replace chips, pasta, bread and rice-based dishes at food courts for kebabs with salad, Japanese teriyaki salmon and miso soup, vegetable curry without rice. Dinner should be lean protein and green vegetables. Patient will visit GP to repeat blood tests and see if cholesterol levels are within normal range and liver enzymes have reduced.

NON-ALCOHOLIC FATTY LIVER DISEASE

Epidemiology

Non-alcoholic fatty liver disease (NAFLD) is the most common chronic liver disease in Western countries[249] and is associated with higher levels of overall and liver-related morbidity and mortality.[250] NAFLD is slightly more prevalent in male populations with a 1.1 : 1 male-to-female ratio and a 1.8 : 1 male-to-female ratio in Caucasian populations.

Non-alcoholic fatty liver disease (NAFLD) is a major health problem in Western countries, affecting 30% of the adult population.[18] It affects 60–80% of patients with diabetes mellitus and/or obesity,[18,251] and in the morbidly obese ranges from 75% to 92%.[251] Approximately 3–5% of the US population is estimated to have non-alcoholic steatohepatitis (NASH), which is the progressive form of NAFLD.[251]

Alarmingly the prevalence of NAFLD in children and adolescents is increasing, and has been reported to be about 10%.[18] Moreover, non-alcoholic steatohepatitis (NASH) has been diagnosed in 3% of children and adolescents.[18]

Progression to cirrhosis occurs in about 20–25% of adults with NASH within 10 years, with hepatocellular carcinoma occurring in 8.6% of cirrhotic NASH patients within 12 years or in 11.3% within 5 years.[18]

A diagnosis of non-alcoholic fatty liver disease (NAFLD) requires confirmation of hepatic steatosis with the additional exclusion of excessive intake of alcohol.[252] If fatty liver or macrovesicular steatosis exists in isolation, the condition is referred to as NAFLD and progression to cirrhosis is limited.[253] However, the diagnosis of non-alcoholic steatohepatitis (NASH) is made when steatosis exists with necro-inflammatory infiltration, hepatic injury and fibrosis; it can lead to cirrhosis, liver failure and hepatocellular carcinoma (HCC).[254,255]

Aetiology

INSULIN RESISTANCE AND METABOLIC SYNDROME

NAFLD is regarded as the hepatic manifestation of metabolic syndrome[253,254] and metabolic syndrome is noted as a strong predictor of NAFLD and progressive fibrosis.[256]

People with NAFLD display high levels of insulin resistance. Hepatic insulin resistance results in the failure to store sugar through glycogen synthesis and also a failure to suppress the release of sugar through gluconeogenesis.[257] Insulin resistance in adipose tissue is due to high lipolytic rates and an increase in circulating free fatty acids.[258] Visceral adipose tissue releases large amounts of hormones, inflammatory cytokines and free fatty acids into the portal vein,[259] which results in direct injury to the liver.

CARDIOVASCULAR DISEASE

NAFLD has been identified as a risk factor for diabetes and cardiovascular disease,[249] independent of already known risk factors such as metabolic syndrome and insulin resistance. Cardiovascular implications of NAFLD involve an increased risk of coronary heart disease and stroke with the accumulation of abdominal fat deemed the key indicator that drives both fatty liver and carotid artery disease.[260] There is little research available to prove that reducing liver fat will reduce levels of cardiovascular mortality despite the understanding that NAFLD is not only a marker for but also an early mediator of atherosclerosis.[261,262]

HIGH FRUCTOSE CONSUMPTION

High fructose consumption from corn syrup in the form of soft drinks has been linked with metabolic syndrome.[263] High fructose consumption is regarded as a contributing factor in NAFLD as fructose is lipogenic and stimulates triglyceride synthesis.[264] One case-controlled study[265] exists to suggest that fructose may be involved in the pathogenesis of NAFLD. This study examined the dietary history and analysis of serum and liver tissue in patients with NAFLD where cirrhosis was absent. Results of this study suggest that the hepatic metabolism of fructose favours de novo lipogenesis and ATP depletion causing hepatic ischaemia.

HEPATITIS C INFECTION

Over 55% of people infected with the hepatitis C virus (HCV) display evidence of hepatic steatosis[266] and NASH is reported in 4–10% of cases. Recent research details a link between insulin resistance and chronic hepatitis C (CHC), with estimates suggesting that 30–70% of hepatitis C patients demonstrate some level of insulin resistance.[267] HCV genotype 3a directly induces fatty liver deposition, namely viral steatosis.[268–270] The mechanism of hepatitis C-induced hepatic steatosis is not yet fully understood but it has been suggested that the HCV genotype 3a may interfere with triglyceride secretion.[271] Severity of steatosis has been linked significantly with the HCV RNA viral load; with steatosis resolution noted after HCV antiviral treatment.[272] The development of steatosis has not been linked to either autoimmune hepatitis or hepatitis B infection.[273]

ENDOCRINE DYSFUNCTION

The literature has reported links between insulin resistance and NAFLD for years. However, research has led to an expansion of the clinical associations of NAFLD to include hypopituitarism and hypothalamic dysfunction.[274] Hypothalamic and pituitary dysfunction can result in a similar presentation to the picture of insulin resistance. Patients with pituitary or hypothalamic disease are at risk of developing NAFLD via excessive weight gain, dyslipidaemia, impaired glucose tolerance and growth hormone deficiencies.[275] Augmenting the association between NAFLD and metabolic syndrome is an association between NAFLD and polycystic ovarian syndrome (PCOS). A prevalence of up to 42% has been reported[276] in the literature and advances to fibrotic liver disease[277] have been noted.

PETROCHEMICAL EXPOSURE

Exposure to petrochemicals has also been linked to the pathogenesis of NAFLD. A Bulgarian study[278] identified elevated liver enzymes, dyslipidaemia, decreased serum glutathione and evidence of hepatomegaly after 666 workers were studied a petrochemical plant. The impact of occupational exposure to petrochemicals was examined in a Brazilian study[279] which identified that the chance of developing liver changes was 3.56 times greater following such exposure than in the reference population, regardless of the presence of obesity, alcohol consumption, smoking or lack of exercise. Exposure to petrochemicals may also be involved in the presence of a more aggressive form of NAFLD with the absence of the metabolic syndrome.[253]

DYSBIOSIS

Recent evidence now links dysbiosis in both T2DM and NAFLD.[280] Dysbiosis increases intestinal permeability and is associated with a shift in the metabolic function of the gut microbiota.[31,281] Increased intestinal permeability increases hepatic exposure to bacterial products such as lipopolysaccharides, endotoxins and alcohols. Lipopolysaccharides, cell-wall components of Gram-negative bacteria, are delivered to the liver via the portal vein and promote the following cascade of events: oxidative stress, insulin resistance, hepatic inflammation and fibrosis.[30,31,282] Changes to the microbiome can also cause dysmotility, gut inflammation and other immunological changes in the gut that might contribute to liver injury.[31]

The gut microbiota profile can be associated with obesity, NAFLD and NASH, and in some cases may predict disease progression.[281,282] Specific bacteria such as *Bacteroides* are independently associated with NASH and *Ruminococcus* with significant fibrosis.[281]

Therefore the manipulation of gut microbiota by probiotics and prebiotics may be useful in the treatment and prevention of NAFLD due to high-fat-diet-induced obesity and insulin resistance.[281,282]

Pathogenesis

There is a two-hit theory of pathogenesis and more recently a multi-hit theory; the two theories overlapping on many aspects. We describe the multi-hit theory here. The multi-hit theory starts with an excess of triglycerides, insulin resistance and gut dysbiosis leading to increased oxidative stress and inflammation causing endoplasmic reticulum stress and mitochondrial dysfunction.[283] Progression from NAFLD to NASH is determined by a complex interplay of genetics and environmental factors.[283]

WHAT FACTORS LEAD TO THE ACCUMULATION OF FAT IN THE LIVER?

Triglycerides are the most predominant lipid that accumulates in the liver; hepatic steatosis occurs when the inflow and synthesis of fat exceed the export and catabolism of fat.[284]

There are several mechanisms that contribute to the excess presence of fatty acids in the liver. The plasma nonesterified fatty acid (NEFA) pool contributes most of the free fatty acids that move to the liver in NAFLD via the increased delivery of fatty acids to the liver from peripheral adipose tissue. An excess dietary intake of fatty acids can also contribute to the excess delivery of free fatty acids in the liver via the plasma NEFA pool. Free fatty acid accumulation in the liver can be a result of increased synthesis of fatty acids within the liver itself via a process of de novo lipogenesis. Free fatty acids can also accumulate if hepatic lipogenesis is inhibited or if the transport of fatty acids LDLs out of the liver in the form of low density lipoproteins is impaired.[249,285]

Both hepatic and peripheral insulin resistance and obesity are factors associated with an increase in circulating free fatty acids.[286,287] Free fatty acids interfere with insulin signalling in striated muscle and adipocytes by limiting the uptake of glucose. Excess glucose is then available for the conversion of more free fatty acids in the liver. A vicious cycle of insulin resistance that increases free circulating fatty acids, and interferes with insulin signalling, results in further fatty acid dysregulation.[271]

Oxidative damage involves the peroxidation of lipids accumulated in hepatocytes via induction of hepatic CYP2E1 and CYP3A4[288] and mitochondrial dysfunction leading to the development of reactive oxygen species (ROS).[289] This ROS oxidation results in a progression of NAFLD to NASH. Research suggests that the factors that increase hepatic oxidative damage also promote inflammatory cytokine production and insulin resistance. The enzyme I kappa kinase beta (IkKb) promotes the activation of NF-kB and also causes insulin resistance (see Fig. 11.3).[290] NF-kB also initiates inflammatory cytokine production and promotes the release of TNF-α. TNF-α production further potentiates insulin resistance and NAFLD.[291]

SIGNS AND SYMPTOMS

Non-alcoholic fatty liver disease usually occurs in the fourth to fifth decade of life[292] and although usually asymptomatic, fatigue and/or right upper quadrant abdominal discomfort with weight issues are often noted. Health problems associated with NAFLD due to obesity include arthritis, nonspecific body aches and pains, sleep disturbances and dyspnoea and this may lead to a lower quality of life and depression.

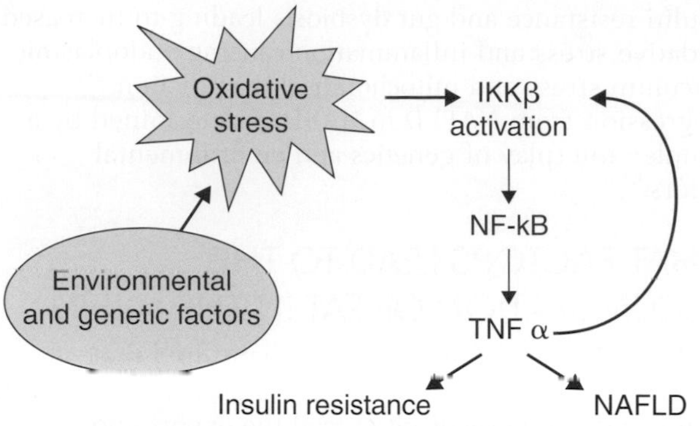

FIGURE 11.3 Relationship of IKKβ, insulin resistance and NAFLD.

Source: Solga SF, Diehl AM. Non-alcoholic fatty liver disease: lumen–liver interactions and possible role for probiotics. J Hepatol 2003;38:681–687.

DIFFERENTIAL DIAGNOSIS

Non-alcoholic fatty liver disease may present with upper right quadrant abdominal pain or discomfort and this may be easily confused with irritable bowel syndrome or gallbladder disease. A diagnosis of primary NAFLD can generally be made through rigorous case history taking and liver function tests and confirmed by ultrasound or FibroScan. A possible differential diagnosis is secondary NAFLD. Causes of secondary NAFLD include the presence of inborn errors of metabolism as evident in Wilson's disease, Andersen's disease, Mauriac syndrome and systemic carnitine deficiency. Nutritional disorders also contribute to secondary NAFLD via severe starvation or severe weight cycling, total parenteral nutrition or protein malnutrition. HIV infection and hepatitis C (genotype 3) infection as well as inflammatory bowel disease, acute fatty liver of pregnancy and environmental hepatotoxin exposure also contribute to secondary NAFLD.[259]

NATUROPATHIC DIAGNOSIS

Nail analysis

Nail analysis is more relevant in alcohol-induced diseases of the liver, where the nails can be very white. However, naturopathic clinicians are advised to check for ridges across the nails which indicate a severe disruption to systemic nutrition.

Tongue analysis

In cases of NAFLD, the tongue will be pale and corpulent with a greasy white or yellow coating.[293]

Investigations

NAFLD is often diagnosed in asymptomatic patients after raised aminotransferases are detected through routine screening or abnormal hepatic ultrasonography is detected during investigations for gallstones.[294] A precise diagnosis of NAFLD requires a liver biopsy. However, there is often reluctance to proceed with a biopsy.[295]

Where advanced disease is not present, blood tests are usually normal, with approximately 80% of the population with hepatic steatosis having aminotransferases within the normal range.[296] Often laboratory studies show only mild elevations in transaminases with alkaline phosphatase (ALP) and gamma glutamyl transpeptidase (GGT) between 1.5 and 3 times the normal level.

Alanine aminotransferase (ALT) levels can be either normal or only mildly elevated and they rarely exceed three times the normal level in this condition. The ALT to AST ratio is greater than 1 unless the disease process is advanced or the patient is a heavy drinker. Alkaline phosphatase is occasionally elevated but is usually less than twice the upper limit of normal. Serum ferritin is often raised in NAFLD patients and has also been associated with advanced fibrosis.[297] Autoantibodies associated with autoimmune hepatitis are often present in low titres in patients with NAFLD.[297] Other investigations related to metabolic syndrome that may lead to a diagnosis of NAFLD include tests for fasting serum glucose and insulin. A fasting blood glucose test (FBG) is indicated and if the results are ≥ 5.6 mmol/L, a 75 g oral glucose tolerance test (in the absence of type 2 diabetes) may be necessary. Cholesterol and triglyceride levels should be included along with a full blood count.

Imaging techniques that are currently used include ultrasound, FibroScan, CT and MRI and if more than one-third of the liver is affected, these techniques can reliably detect steatosis. These imaging techniques cannot be used for the reliable detection of NASH or fibrosis.[298] The FibroTest is a predictive score of liver fibrosis that involves the use of a mathematical algorithm and selective noninvasive markers. This test combines age, gender, bilirubin, gamma glutamyltransferase, apolipoprotein A1, haptoglobin and α2-macroglobulin results in an effort to determine the staging of fibrosis.[295]

SPECIFIC NATUROPATHIC INVESTIGATIONS

In the absence of specific laboratory tests available to naturopaths in the management of NAFLD, clinicians are advised to obtain copies of the patient's blood tests and any other investigations so that case progression can be managed and the most effective interventions prescribed. Because of the link between NAFLD and metabolic syndrome, body mass index (BMI) measurements are encouraged.

Therapeutic considerations

CLINICAL DECISION MAKING AND RATIONALE

In the first instance, if a patient presents in clinic with signs or symptoms that lead you to suspect NAFLD, referral to a general practitioner for diagnosis is needed. Care must be taken not to automatically assume that the patient is suffering from irritable bowel syndrome if gastrointestinal discomfort is apparent. Pay specific attention to any right upper quadrant pain or fatigue reported by the patient. Ascertaining the patient's dietary history is imperative so that alcohol consumption can be ruled out as a determinant of fatty liver disease.

Non-alcoholic fatty liver disease is an emerging health issue of high importance[299] and a clear link between obesity and NAFLD exists. With 70% of people in the

United States classed as overweight and 38% obese,[294] cause for concern is understandable.

The primary intervention is patient education on diet and lifestyle around obesity, metabolic syndrome, insulin resistance and cardiovascular disease — while understanding that there may be an underlying psychological component to their condition.

With training in symptomatology and diagnosis and pathophysiology, the naturopath has the skill set to understand the underlying aetiologies of this condition. Training in herbal medicine and nutritional supplementation allows for the design and application of prescriptive treatments so that metabolic function is optimised. Naturopaths are also in the best position to offer dietary and lifestyle suggestions so that risk factors and causes of NAFLD can be addressed long term.

Treatment begs for a grassroots approach — simplicity is the key here. Provide patients with simple and effective guidelines for weight management, exercise and optimal metabolic performance. Simplicity will assist with the dissemination of information to patients, and importantly, will allow patients to modify the dietary and lifestyle patterns of their children so that change is generational. The naturopathic approach to the treatment of NAFLD involves recognising the condition as a symptom of metabolic disharmony compounded by poor diet and lifestyle choices. Thus, naturopathic treatment involves recognising underlying conditions related to the aetiology of NAFLD and treating them, while improving liver function and fatty acid oxidation in the process.

Therapeutic application

HISTORICAL PERSPECTIVE

Non-alcoholic fatty liver disease was first reported in the literature in 1958 when Westwater and Fainer[300] recognised it in a cohort of obese patients. Non-alcoholic fatty disease was officially recognised in the literature in 1979 by Adler and Schaffer[301] and the term 'non-alcoholic steatohepatitis' was introduced in 1980 when Ludwig et al[302] identified similar histopathological findings in obese patients and patients with alcoholic liver disease.

NATUROPATHIC PERSPECTIVE

Naturopathic treatment should focus on stable and long-term weight loss without rapid loss or weight cycling. As insulin resistance can be a significant barrier to weight loss and may exacerbate symptoms of fatigue, strategies for reducing insulin resistance need to be incorporated.

Overall, treatment should be thorough and the patient should be guided towards eventual autonomous management of their dietary and lifestyle habits so that further hepatic inflammation and associated necrosis can be avoided.

The treatment of NAFLD requires the following considerations:

- Assess the case presentation and obtain a diagnosis if not provided
- Identify possible contraindications for treatment
- Patient education is critical. Provide dietary and lifestyle advice that is accessible to both adults and children
- Encourage weight loss through dietary and lifestyle changes — encourage the intake of fresh fruit and vegetables, fibre and adequate water
- Avoid rapid weight loss or weight cycling; encourage a healthy attitude to long-term weight loss, rather than short-term results
- Address insulin resistance
- Reduce oxidative stress
- Address any dysbiosis
- Support optimal digestive and GIT function
- Improve overall liver function and support fatty acid oxidation in hepatocytes
- Assess and address chemical toxicity in the liver (petrochemicals, fertilisers, pesticides, alcohol or heavy metals)
- Address any factors that hinder or obstruct the healing process.

NUTRITIONAL MEDICINE (DIETARY)

The role of dietary modification in the treatment of NAFLD is of paramount importance. This attitude is accepted by mainstream medical practitioners with conventional therapeutic guidelines suggesting dietary modification as the first line of treatment for NAFLD in place of drug therapy.[303] Diet and exercise improve both liver biochemistry and hepatic steatosis.[304]

The impact of obesity on the prevalence of NAFLD is clear, thus weight reduction is the principal goal of dietary modification. The benefits of the holistic and comprehensive approach of naturopathic dietary treatment are extensive and relevant in the treatment of NAFLD.

The following factors should be considered before weight management is attempted:

- Assessment of the patient's relationship to food so that underlying causes of obesity can be addressed
- Nutritional counselling will provide long-term benefits for the patient and family members
- Assessment of cultural barriers that may impede optimal nutrient intake and lead to overconsumption of the wrong type of foods
- Planning meals in advance to assist with weight loss and with the long-term management of weight
- Education on required daily kilojoule intake and portion sizes.

Dietary therapeutic objectives

See 'Hepatobiliary nutritional objectives (dietary)' for an overview.

- Reduce abdominal visceral fat in the first instance
- Reduce the influence of metabolic syndrome and insulin resistance by supporting metabolic process and blood sugar regulation
- Eliminate consumption of refined carbohydrates, processed foods and takeaway food (high in fat, salt and sugar)
- Encourage the consumption of a naturopathic wholefood diet (this should be detailed in patient handouts with meal planning and recipe ideas)

- Support lipid metabolism by reducing intake of saturated and trans fats and increasing consumption of essential fatty acids
- Support optimal digestive and hepatic function with foods that stimulate optimal organ function and performance such as bitter and fermented foods, prebiotics, fibre and probiotics.

Specific dietary treatments

DIETARY INCLUSIONS

Dietary antioxidants

Research indicates that mitochondrial dysfunction resulting from uncontrolled oxidative stress and the over-expression of TNF-α may contribute significantly to NAFLD progression,[305] stressing the need for antioxidant therapy. As the health benefits associated with fruits and vegetables are not due to specific phytochemicals in isolation, but from a mixture of compounds,[306] a distinct role for food as therapy is apparent. Although supplemental antioxidants prescribed in isolation have shown contradictory findings,[307,308] the synergistic effects of dietary antioxidants may be the key to prevent oxidative damage and inflammation.

Probiotics and prebiotics

The presence of dysbiosis in the intestinal bacteria flora has been noted for a role in the pathogenesis of NAFLD. The analyses of the gut microflora can provide insights into disease progression and correct probiotic and prebiotic supplementation.

In rats the probiotic MIYAIRI 588 *Clostridium butyricum* has beneficial effects in the prevention of NAFLD progression.[282] *Clostridium butyricum* is a butyric acid-producing Gram-positive anaerobe found in the soil and in the intestines of healthy animals and humans. Dietary supplementation of butyrate regulates energy homeostasis via its effects on glucose and lipid metabolism, controls fatty acid oxidation by regulating mitochondrial biogenesis, suppresses lipogenic gene expression, and inhibits reactive oxidative stress (ROS) and inflammation.

Fibre

There is currently a clinical trial studying the effect of prebiotic fibre on NAFLD at the University of Calgary.[309] Otherwise there are no human studies on the use of fibre and improved outcomes in NAFLD specifically. However, dietary supplementation with prebiotic fibres in rodent studies positively impacts NAFLD by modifying the gut microbiota, reducing body fat and improving glucoregulation.[310]

As a result of the link between NAFLD and insulin resistance, fibre intake may be of benefit. The American Gastroenterological Association has suggested fibre intake as a possible treatment option despite this lack of scientific validation.[311] Numerous studies have confirmed the efficacy of fibre intake in the regulation of obesity, insulin sensitivity, blood glucose regulation and the reduction of cardiovascular risk factors associated with the cluster of symptoms in the metabolic syndrome.[312–314] Fibre from wholefoods is recommended because of the beneficial health properties of other micronutrients, and a mix of both insoluble and soluble fibre should be encouraged.

Safe weight reduction through dietary modification

Obesity is the primary target in the treatment of NAFLD, thus weight loss is imperative for the resolution of pathology. Weight loss is beneficial in NAFLD as it addresses insulin resistance, hepatic free fatty acid supply and the production of inflammatory and fibrotic cytokines. Progressive weight loss has been shown to relieve many of the symptoms of NAFLD and NASH with improvements in abdominal pain, liver test results and blood chemistry.[315] Gradual weight loss is encouraged and the literature reports that a ten percent reduction[316] is necessary to improve transaminases and reduce steatosis, inflammation and fibrosis.[317]

DIETARY EXCLUSIONS

Fast food

A Swedish study[318] examined the impact of fast-food-based hyperalimentation (overeating) on alanine aminotransferase levels in 18 healthy participants. After 1 month of eating two fast-food meals per day, the participants increased their body weight by 5–15%. In addition, 13 developed pathological ALT abnormalities during the study period. The study also found that ALT elevations subsided during or within a few weeks of study completion. This suggests the importance of dietary modification and highlights the benefits that can be obtained quickly if poor eating habits are changed.

Processed carbohydrates and sugars

Consumption of carbohydrates and sugars unaccompanied by fibre, protein and good fats can exacerbate NAFLD due to lipogenesis which stimulates triglyceride synthesis.[319] Excessive consumption of sugars including fructose, especially in the form of soft drinks and fruit juices, has been linked to obesity, diabetes and metabolic syndrome. Fructose is believed to promote liver injury as the ATP depletion it induces mimics hepatic ischaemia and contributes to NAFLD by promoting hepatic necro-inflammation.[320] Excess fructose intake has also been found to aggravate the metabolic effects of copper deficiency.[321]

Copper and iron

Recent European research[322] resulted in the first report linking copper deficiency with the metabolic syndrome, insulin resistance and iron accumulation in NAFLD. A significant proportion of the 140 enrolled participants in this study were found to be copper deficient. Low copper status causes increased hepatic iron stores via decreased ferroportin-1 (FP-1) expression and ceruloplasmin ferroxidase action; iron export from the liver is thus blocked and contributes to hepatic iron deposition in NAFLD. The group with low serum and liver copper levels also presented with higher degrees of insulin resistance, as

SAMPLE DAILY DIET

BREAKFAST	
Mango and papaya lassi containing papaya, mango, natural yoghurt, water, honey and a splash of rosewater	NAFLD is characterised by inflammation thus the addition of fresh fruit, rich in anti-inflammatory and antioxidant constituents, will reduce inflammation. Probiotic-rich foods such as live yoghurt may help to improve gut flora. Overgrowth of gut microbiota is associated with NAFLD whereby liver injury may be partly caused by exposure to bacterial and fermentation agents produced by microflora which are metabolised in the liver.
SNACK	
Fresh pomegranate juice Walnuts (small handful)	Polyphenol-rich pomegranate juice, consumed over 12 weeks, has been shown to reduce elevated liver enzymes.[324] Consumption of antioxidant-rich walnuts is associated with more favourable lipid profile as well as reduced hepatic steatosis and inflammation.[325]
LUNCH	
Grilled salmon with Greek salad drizzled with olive oil	Polyunsaturated fatty acids, omega-3 fatty acids and monounsaturated fatty acids may play a protective role in NAFLD. Consumption of olive oil with omega-3 PUFAs has been shown to decrease serum liver enzyme activities and triglyceride levels.[326]
DINNER	
Stuffed mushrooms with basil pesto, feta, wild rice and salad	Compared with current dietary recommendations, even in the absence of weight loss, a Mediterranean style of diet reduces hepatic steatosis and improves insulin sensitivity in insulin-resistant people with NAFLD.[327] Appropriate consumption of complex carbohydrates, such as wholegrains, may prevent the development and/or progression of NAFLD as wholegrains are a source of antioxidants, vitamins, minerals and fibre.[328]

well as more prevalence of diabetes and metabolic syndrome. Accumulation of iron in the liver is responsible for oxidative damage and conversely reduced serum ferritin levels have been linked to reduced oxidative stress in the liver.[323]

NUTRITIONAL MEDICINE (SUPPLEMENTAL)

See 'Hepatobiliary nutritional objectives (nutrients)' and Table 11.5.

The role of supplemental nutritional medicine in the treatment of NAFLD focuses on control of fatty acid metabolism. However, as NAFLD is commonly regarded as the hepatic manifestation of the metabolic syndrome, the management of insulin resistance and blood glucose and lipid dysregularity associated with the metabolic syndrome is crucial. Specific nutritional supplements can also be introduced for their antioxidant and anti-inflammatory capabilities and play a role in the prevention of the progression of NAFLD to NASH and eventual cirrhosis or hepatocellular carcinoma. Almost all patients with liver disease and especially advanced liver disease have evidence of malnutrition,[329] thus supplementation is necessary to correct any vitamin or mineral deficiencies that may be contributing to the severity of any liver condition.

Nutritional medicine therapeutic objectives

- Promote optimal liver function and improve beta oxidation of fats (fatty acid metabolism) in the liver
- Address the metabolic syndrome picture (improve insulin resistance, regulate blood glucose, visceral adiposity, dyslipidaemia)
- Support any other associated endocrine dysfunction
- Reduce potential for fibrosis by reducing inflammation and oxidative damage
- Address chemical or drug toxicity that may be impeding optimal liver function
- Address deficiencies or requirements as noted in the literature.

Specific nutrients required

SAM-E

A SAM-e deficiency is believed to impair crucial functions of the liver and increase the liver's susceptibility to damage. SAM-e is regarded as the most important methyl donor in the human body and is required for the production of coenzyme Q10, carnitine, methylcobalamin and phosphatidycholine. Research indicates that SAM-e may upregulate and increase the antioxidant glutathione, reduce inflammation by downregulating TNF and upregulating interleukin 10 (IL-10), inhibit apoptosis of normal liver cells and stimulate apoptosis of carcinogenic hepatocytes.[330] In NAFLD, SAM-e has been found to protect against lipid peroxidation and decrease hepatocyte damage in steatohepatitis.[331,332]

BETAINE

Betaine is also a major methyl donor and a component of the metabolic cycle of methionine; research suggests it may decrease hepatic steatosis by increasing SAM-e.[333] Results from a human study on betaine supplementation in NASH suggest that betaine supplementation at 20 g daily for 1 year significantly improved the aminotransferase enzymes ALT and AST and biopsy revealed reduced fibrosis and fatty infiltration.[334]

ZINC

Zinc deficiency is thought to complicate many different liver diseases. No studies on the effects of zinc in NAFLD exist; however, in models of alcohol-induced steatosis and steatohepatitis zinc has demonstrated marked hepatoprotective action.[335,336] Both zinc deficiency and dysfunctional zinc metabolism have been linked to hepatic stress and inflammation.[337]

VITAMIN D

Deficiencies in vitamin D can result in insulin resistance, metabolic syndrome and NAFLD.[28]

Studies have shown that in individuals with obesity vitamin D levels are lower than for normal weight individuals, possibly sequestered in fat stores and therefore not bioavailable.[338] This deficiency might be exacerbated by inadequate input from sunlight and diet.[338] It has been estimated that vitamin D, via its receptor VDR, regulates over 200 genes involved in immune modulation, cell differentiation and proliferation, inflammation regulation, glucose and lipid metabolism; it is also an antifibrotic agent.[29,339] Barchetta et al showed that, independently from other metabolic parameters such as BMI, insulin resistance or adiponectin, liver VDR expression is inversely correlated with severity of NAFLD on histopathology.[340] Therefore encourage adequate exposure to sunlight. This will vary seasonally and geographically and will depend on skin pigmentation. Include foods high in vitamin D such as fatty fish and eggs and consider supplementation if deficient.

VITAMIN E

A 2012 review article concluded that vitamin E is only recommended in adults with NASH who do not have diabetes or cirrhosis, or an aggressive histology.[341] However, a 2015 meta-analysis concluded vitamin E significantly improved liver function and histological changes in patients with NAFLD/NASH.[342] Vitamin E significantly reduced aspartate transaminase (AST), alkaline phosphatase (ALP), inflammation and hepatocellular ballooning by −0.34 U/L compared with the control group. Vitamin E treatment in NASH showed reductions in AST of −13.91 U/L, ALT of −22.44 U/L, steatosis of −0.67 U/L, inflammation of −0.20 U/L and fibrosis of −0.30 U/L compared to controls.[342] Studies on children with NASH[343] demonstrate more promising results than studies on adults.[344] The mechanisms for therapeutic benefit of vitamin E in NAFLD and NASH include decreased NF-kB activation and inhibition of TNF production.[345]

CHROMIUM

Chromium deficiency has been reported to cause insulin resistance (IR), hyperglycaemia and hyperlipidaemia.[346] Chromium increases insulin receptor numbers, insulin binding to cells and insulin sensitivity.[347] Given the links between insulin resistance and NAFLD reported in the literature, chromium supplementation may improve the metabolic picture by reducing the severity of both metabolic syndrome and NAFLD pathogenesis.

MAGNESIUM

Magnesium deficiencies have been identified in the pathogenesis of both NAFLD and NASH as well as insulin resistance[348] and magnesium can improve insulin sensitivity in the metabolic syndrome.[349]

L-CARNITINE

Carnitine supplementation improves blood sugar control[350,351] and insulin sensitivity in patients with impaired glucose metabolism and plays a role in the metabolism of fatty acids.[352] Carnitine deficiency promotes an impairment of beta oxidation; this shifts hepatic fatty acid synthesis in favour of VLDL synthesis and encourages hepatic triglyceride synthesis.[353]

ALPHA LIPOIC ACID

Alpha lipoic acid's (ALA) activity exhibits free radical scavenging activity in both hydrophilic and lipophilic environments.[354] ALA can regenerate endogenous antioxidants and chelate metal ions.[355] It has suggested roles in cardiovascular disorders[356] and diabetes[357] and is also regarded as an anti-obesity agent because of its ability to suppress cAMP-activated protein kinase in the brain.[358] Given its success with the various metabolic dysfunctions that are linked to NAFLD, a role for its clinical use is evident.

TAURINE

Supplementation with taurine is associated with a reduction in increased serum cholesterol and triglycerides, increased liver lipid levels, increased serum and liver oxidation reactions, and arterial fat deposition, and increased serum and liver oxidation.[359]

ESSENTIAL FATTY ACIDS

Supplementation of omega-3 long-chain fatty acids with an antioxidant is beneficial in the treatment of NAFLD.[360] Research suggests that lower levels of hepatic omega-3 fatty acids may predispose the liver to steatosis by encouraging further lipid synthesis over oxidation and secretion.[361] The administration of 1000 mg/day of eicosapentaenoic docosahexaenoic acid for 1 year resulted in regression of steatosis in 46% of patients[362] and researchers concluded that prolonged supplementation with polyunsaturated fatty acids is beneficial in ameliorating fatty liver.

METHYL FACTORS (B_{12}, FOLIC ACID)

Folate and B_{12} supplementation has been found to improve insulin resistance, decrease homocysteine levels and improve endothelial dysfunction in a metabolic syndrome picture.[363] This suggests a role for methyl factors in the treatment of metabolic syndrome if associated with NAFLD. Both B_{12} and folate have a key role together in the synthesis of methionine from homocysteine. Current evidence[364] suggests folic acid acts as a methyl donor, reduces homocysteine levels and is involved in the synthesis of SAM-e. B_{12} is necessary for the metabolism of carbohydrates, fats and proteins and is involved in fatty acid synthesis, thus confirming its necessity as a supplement in NAFLD.

Dosage requirement

- SAM-e (S-adenosylmethionine: 200–400 mg b.i.d./t.d.s.
- Betaine: 10–20 g daily
- Zinc: 25–50 mg daily
- Vitamin D: 1000 IU daily
- Vitamin E: 1000 IU daily
- Chromium: 250 micrograms/day
- Magnesium: 250 mg b.i.d
- L-carnitine: 500 mg b.i.d. or 1000 mg/day
- Alpha lipoic acid: 300–600 mg/day
- Taurine: 500 mg t.d.s.
- Essential fatty acids: 1000 mg EPA/DHA/day

HERBAL MEDICINE

Herbal medicine therapeutic objectives

- Mediate and reduce oxidative stress and hepatic inflammation
- Improve overall liver function
- Promote effective hepatic detoxification (Phases I and II)
- Improve digestion and reduce any digestive disturbances associated with NAFLD
- Identify and treat underlying metabolic causes (obesity, metabolic syndrome, insulin resistance, dyslipidaemia)
- Support underlying metabolic processes.

Specific herbal medicine classes

The use of herbal medicine in the treatment of NAFLD encompasses the broad pathology of this condition and offers a unique treatment perspective to address and treat both the causes and the symptoms of NAFLD. Herbal medicine can be employed to reduce hepatic inflammation, improve insulin resistance and metabolism of fats, improve digestive symptoms associated with NAFLD and support the liver's detoxification processes.

Hepatobiliary antioxidant herbal medicines are agents that promote both Phase I and Phase II liver detoxification pathways. These herbal medicines are specifically indicated where there is evidence of hepatic dysfunction due to toxic burden. Such burden can result from environmental chemicals, heavy metals, food chemicals, drug use and chemicals released in the body during an infective process. Choleretics and cholagogues can improve hepatobiliary function through their ability to stimulate the production and release of bile. Both choleretics and cholagogues are also regarded as lipotrophic factors as they assist in the removal and prevent the deposition of fat in the liver via pathways of fatty acid metabolism. Hepatic anti-inflammatory medicines are a key component and are indicated in all cases of NAFLD owing to their ability to temper inflammation that leads to fibrosis and cirrhosis.

Digestive disturbances associated with NAFLD include burping, indigestion, reflux, flatulence, bloating and abdominal discomfort and intolerances to both fatty food and alcohol may be present. In this case, bitter digestives, carminatives and cholagogues are indicated. Herbal medicine can also be employed to manage metabolic dysfunction, insulin resistance and obesity. The vast therapeutic range of herbal medicine means that the practitioner can be guided by both the presenting symptoms and causes of NAFLD and can introduce the most appropriate herbal medicine depending on the specific presentation of the case.

Specific herbal medicines

SILYBUM MARIANUM (ST MARY'S THISTLE)

Silybum marianum has been used to treat liver conditions for thousands of years; in AD 77 Pliny the Elder reported it was 'excellent for carrying off the bile', and Culpeper suggested its effectiveness in removing spleen and hepatic obstructions.[365] The antioxidant activity of silymarin has been attributed to this constituent's ability to reduce free radical production, reduce lipid peroxidation and support liver detoxification.[366–370] Silymarin exhibits antifibrotic,[371–373] and anti-inflammatory activity,[40,366,374,375] and has demonstrated cytoprotective[376] and hepatocyte regenerative activity.

A 2005 pilot study[377] evaluated the effectiveness of silybin, vitamin E and phospholipids in NAFLD patients presenting with metabolic syndrome, liver fibrosis or the hepatitis C virus. Results from this preliminary study indicate that this silybin complex has therapeutic benefit in the treatment of NAFLD by reducing insulin resistance and liver fibrosis. A randomised clinical trial[378] assessed the use of silymarin on 50 patients with NAFLD, elevated liver enzymes and increased lipid accumulation detectable on sonography: 140 mg of silymarin was administered daily for 2 months. Results showed a statistically significant drop in both ALT and AST levels and researchers noted a role for silymarin in future treatment of NAFLD. A 2016 review looking at *Silybum marianum* and nutritional therapy for NAFLD (omega-3, vitamins E and D, antioxidants, *Silybum marianum*) showed that nutritional therapy is effective in modulating the molecular mechanisms that lead to fat accumulation, oxidative stress, inflammation and liver fibrosis in NAFLD patients.[379]

GLYCYRRHIZA GLABRA (LIQUORICE)

Liquorice root has a long history in the treatment of lung conditions, gastric disturbances and jaundice[380] and has been used in Europe since Greek, Roman and mediaeval times.[381] Culpeper suggested liquorice was a widely used remedy for coughs and lung complaints and the German Commission E monograph[382] suggests the use of liquorice for gastric and duodenal ulcers.

Glycyrrhizin is the biologically active form of liquorice in the bloodstream. It inhibits prostaglandin E2 production and demonstrates antioxidant activity through the induction of glutathione-S-transferase.[383] Antifibrotic actions have also been demonstrated in several rat models.[384,385] Both animal and human studies have demonstrated significant hepatoprotective action against cytoxicity in hepatocytes.[386,387] A study[388] on the use of liquorice in NAFLD found that 18 beta glycyrrhetinic acid prevented free-fatty-acid-induced lipid accumulation and cell apoptosis in human liver cells in vitro. Glycyrrhetinic acid significantly reduced free-fatty-acid-induced hepatic lipotoxicity by stabilising the integrity of lysosomes and mitochondria and by inhibiting enzyme activity. A role for the use of liquorice in the treatment of NAFLD is evident as free-fatty-acid-induced hepatic lipotoxicity plays a fundamental role in the pathogenesis of NAFLD.

Liquorice also inhibits the activity of the enzyme 11 beta hydroxysteroid dehydrogenase (11 beta HSD), which is responsible for the conversion of cortisol to cortisone.[389] Where central obesity is present, 11 beta HSD [type 1] is increased in adipose tissue[390] and increased cortisol in adipose tissue may be involved in the pathogenesis of the metabolic syndrome.[391]

PHYLLANTHUS ULMARIA (PHYLLANTHUS)

Phyllanthus ulmaria is a closely related species of *Phyllanthus amarus*, and it is a particularly useful herb for treating liver conditions. The benefits of *Phyllanthus* in the treatment of NAFLD originate from the herb's high antioxidant activity since hepatic oxidative stress is implicated in the pathogenesis of NAFLD. *Phyllanthus* has been tested both in vitro and in vivo and was found to alleviate steatohepatitis induced by methionine and choline deficiency by reducing oxidative stress, inflammation and lipid accumulation.[392]

COLEUS FORSKOHLII (COLEUS)

The insulin resistance and metabolic syndrome picture associated with NAFLD can be treated with coleus. Forskolin (diterpene) favourably alters body composition by decreasing body fat percentage and fat mass in overweight and obese men.[393] A study[394] on mildly overweight women concluded that a standardised coleus extract did not appear to promote weight loss but restricted weight gain. Forskolin may also contribute to weight loss via its ability to stimulate the thyroid,[395] cyclic AMP[396,397] and through insulin regulation.[398]

SALVIA MILTIORRHIZA (DAN SHEN)

Salvia miltiorrhiza is a traditional Chinese medicine (TCM) herb used in the treatment of both cardiovascular and liver disorders. There are no current human studies on the efficacy of dan shen in NAFLD; however, numerous rat studies demonstrate significant hepatoprotective[399] and antifibrotic[400–402] actions of the herb. A role for *Salvia miltiorrhiza* in the treatment of free fatty acid metabolism dysregulation and the closely associated metabolic syndrome may exist with animal studies demonstrating the herb has a hypolipidaemic[403] pharmacological action.

GYMNEMA SYLVESTRE (GYMNEMA)

Gymnema sylvestre has been used in India for over 2000 years in the treatment of diabetes mellitus.[404] It was first used by the Indian doctor Sushruta in the 6th century BC to treat diabetes; in his treatise Sushruta claimed 'it may be prognosticated that an idle man, who indulges in day sleep or follows sedentary pursuits or is in the habit of taking sweet liquids or cold and fattening food, will ere long fall an easy victim to this disease'.[405] Gymnema is useful in controlling hyperglycaemia[406] in diabetes by reducing blood glucose, glycosylated haemoglobin and glycosylated plasma protein. Gymnema enhances endogenous insulin production possibly by the regeneration of pancreatic beta cells in insulin-dependent diabetes mellitus.[407] Use of this herb to control fatty acid dysregulation and hypertriglyceridaemia may be beneficial due to gymnema's ability to reduce serum cholesterol and triglycerides[408] in hyperlipidaemic rats.

LIFESTYLE RECOMMENDATIONS

Dietary modification is the first line of treatment in the management of NAFLD and lifestyle modifications must be made to complement this approach. Physical activity improves insulin sensitivity[409] by preventing the induction of insulin resistance by lipids[410] and regulating the hepatic output of glucose. Exercise should include both aerobic and resistance training so excess kilojoules can be used and muscle mass increased to further improve insulin sensitivity. Weight loss can also result in changes to liver enzymes as research has demonstrated that weight loss through dietary restriction and physical activity can reduce aminotransferase levels.[411]

Cognitive behaviour therapy has been tested with success in the management of obesity and type 2 diabetes[412] and has been suggested as a management tool in NAFLD. A change in attitude is required in the physical, emotional, spiritual, familial, occupation, social and financial areas of a patient's life so that maximum benefit from any lifestyle changes implemented can be derived. Most of all, the patient should be encouraged to engage in self-care and reflection so that the importance of a simple healthy diet and lifestyle is understood on deeper levels.

CASE STUDY

OVERVIEW

A 55-year-old woman presented with fatigue, depression, dyspepsia, hypothyroidism and NAFLD. Her current medications are thyroxine 100 micrograms daily and atorvastatin 10 mg/day. Her doctor has recommended a 3-month dietary intervention for weight loss and blood sugar regulation to try to avoid medication for diabetes and hypertension.

CASE STUDY CONTINUED

CLINICAL EXAMINATION

BP: 140/90 mmHg, PR 80, Weight: 95 kg
Waist circumference: 92 cm

LABORATORY INVESTIGATIONS

ALT 60 U/L	(5–30)
AST 80 U/L	(10–35)
ALP 35 U/L	(20–35)
GGT 235 U/L	(5–35)
Triglycerides 1.9 mmol/L	(0.5–1.7)
HbA1c 6.2%	(normal range < 5.7%, prediabetic 5.7–6.4%)

Elevated LFTs (particularly ALT and GGT), raised triglycerides and dysglycaemia are typical of a diagnosis of NAFLD. A waist circumference of more than 80 cm, excess adipose tissue and sedentary lifestyle also suggest NAFLD. T2DM and CVD are both comorbidities in NAFLD. Elevated liver enzymes plus high GGT suggest alcohol abuse as well as fatty liver. Patient confirmed consumption of a bottle of wine a day.

TREATMENT PROTOCOL

INITIAL APPOINTMENT

Treatment objectives included:

- Encourage beneficial dietary and lifestyle changes to address dysglycaemia
- 20 minutes exercise a day of moderate exercise, consider weights
- Diet — low carbohydrate, higher protein, high fibre, healthy fats (omega-3), high antioxidant
- Alcohol cessation
- Adequate hydration with inclusion of green tea and dandelion root coffee
- Increase bitter and fermented foods
- Reduce OS and hepatic inflammation with antioxidant and anti-inflammatory — dietary, herbal and supplements
- Reduce the impact of the significant comorbid factor of hypertension with bergamot, garlic, hawthorn, vitamin E, magnesium and coenzyme Q10.

Specific medicines

- *Silybum marianum* standardised to contain 140 mg silybin, twice daily
- Chromium: 250 micrograms daily
- Magnesium: 600 mg daily
- Multivitamin, with vitamin B complex
- Fish oil EPA/DHA: 1000 mg twice daily

Herbal formula

Schisandra chinensis 1 : 2	25 mL
Galega officinalis 1 : 2	25 mL
Gymnema sylvestre 1 : 2	35 mL
Trigonella-foenum graecum 1 : 2	15 mL
Total	100 mL

7.5 mL twice daily before meals

SECOND APPOINTMENT

A month later patient was disappointed as had only lost 2 kg and 3 cm from waist circumference. Discussed the importance of exercise and exercise options. Patient is too self-conscious to join a gym and walking is painful but liked the idea of aqua aerobics and has a friend to go with.
Reinforced the need to eliminate or reduce alcohol for blood sugar regulation and liver health.
Repeated herbal formula.
Repeated specific medicines.

Additional specific medicines

Vitamin E: 500 IU daily
Coenzyme Q10: 150 mg daily.

THIRD APPOINTMENT

A month later patient was walking twice a week and attended one aqua aerobics class per week; and had reduced alcohol consumption by 50%; mood and energy were markedly improved. Weight loss was 4 kg and 3 cm from waist. Discussed health targets and deadline with GP to maintain motivation. Patient commited to elimination of alcohol, walking every morning for 30 minutes, two aqua aerobics classes a week, and improving breakfast quality to increase fibre, protein and reduce sugar.
Repeated herbal formula.
Repeated specific medicines.

FOURTH APPOINTMENT

A month later the patient was fully compliant with discussed plan and had lost a further 4 kg and 3 cm from waist. Mood was very good, and energy and sleep had improved. Discussed further dietary improvements and patient volunteered to increase exercise further.

OUTCOME

CLINICAL EXAMINATION

BP: 120/80, PR: 70, Weight: 85 kg
Waist circumference: 83 cm

Laboratory investigations

ALT 30 U/L	(5–30)
AST 35 U/L	(10–35)
ALP 28 U/L	(20–35)
GGT 70 U/L	(5–35)
Triglycerides 1.7 mmol/L	(0.5–1.7)
HbA1c 5.8%	(normal range < 5.7%, prediabetic 5.7–6.4%)

VIRAL HEPATITIS

Classification

Hepatitis can be classified as either acute or chronic. Acute hepatitis resolves within 6 months. For an infection to be classified as chronic it must have a duration of more than 6 months. Incidence of acute hepatitis results from infection with hepatitis viruses A, B, C, D or E; however, chronic hepatitis can only result from infection with hepatitis B or C.

Epidemiology

HEPATITIS A

Hepatitis A infection is considered to be a mild condition in children but middle-aged patients are more susceptible to severe hepatitis A virus (HAV) infections and experience more severe pathology.[413] However, studies also report that anti-HAV antibody prevalence is high in elderly populations, which explains the relatively low infection in this population.[414] The literature reports a decline in the number of hepatitis A virus (HAV) infections in the United States and this has been attributed to the implementation of vaccination programs.[415] HAV infection is the most common vaccine-preventable illness among travellers who move from low endemic zones like Europe, USA, Canada, Australia, New Zealand and Japan into high endemic areas in Africa, Asia, the Middle East and South America.[416]

HEPATITIS B

Chronic hepatitis B virus (HBV) infection affects approximately 375 million people worldwide. Current antiviral treatment effectively controls, but rarely clears, chronic HBV infection.[417] It is estimated that more than 1 million patients infected with HBV die from liver disease each year.[417,418] Current estimates suggest 3 million HIV-positive patients worldwide are infected with HBV.[419] Areas with the highest prevalence of HBV include the Middle East, Asia, sub-Saharan Africa and the Amazon basin; areas of low prevalence include Australia, North America and the United Kingdom.[416]

HEPATITIS C

The hepatitis C virus (HCV) was discovered in 1989 and previous to this was identified and classified as non-A, non-B hepatitis. Globally, an estimated 71 million people have chronic hepatitis C infection. According to the World Health Organization (WHO) regional data, the most affected areas are Eastern Mediterranean and European regions. Approximately 399 000 people die each year from hepatitis C-related liver diseases.[420] Factors associated with rapid disease progression include heavy alcohol intake, male gender and an older age of initial HCV infection.[421]

In the developing world, blood transfusions from unscreened donors and unsafe medical practice are the major modes of HCV transmission. Studies indicate that paid blood donors account for up to 63% of the blood supply in developing countries.[422] One Indian study reported that 95% of blood donors were screened for HIV, but only 6% were screened for HCV.[423]

HEPATITIS D

Hepatitis D or delta virus (HDV) is a defective RNA virus and requires co-infection with HBV for replication. This virus is the least common but is regarded as the most severe form of viral hepatitis.[424] In HBV cases, co-infection with HDV may increase the risk of severe disease progressions like cirrhosis or hepatocellular carcinoma.[425] HDV infection patterns are similar to infection patterns for HBV. This distribution in epidemic proportions is reported in the Mediterranean, the Amazon basin and Central Africa.[416] It has been estimated that about 15 million people are infected with HDV worldwide.[426]

HEPATITIS E

Hepatitis E virus (HEV) is an important global public health issue with an estimated 20 million infections and 70 000 deaths attributed to HEV genotypes 1 and 2 every year. However, the majority of infections are thought to remain asymptomatic.[427,428]

Aetiology

HEPATITIS A

The hepatitis A virus (HAV) is a highly contagious RNA picornavirus and is transmitted through the faecal–oral route, via person-to-person contact or through the ingestion of contaminated food.[429] Hepatitis A has an incubation period of 28 days and symptoms including fever, nausea, anorexia, jaundice, dark urine and abdominal pain may last for a period of 2 weeks to several months.[415]

HEPATITIS B

Hepatitis B virus (HBV) is an enveloped DNA virus with eight major genotypes (A–H). The virus is highly adaptive with drug resistance and vaccine-related mutations reported.[430,431] HBV infection occurs via blood and body fluids in adulthood through high-risk sexual activity or needle sharing.[432] In endemic areas, HBV transmission occurs from mother to child.[432]

HEPATITIS C

The hepatitis C virus (HCV) is a small RNA virus from the *Flaviviridae* family responsible for hepatitis C infection. HCV infection occurs primarily through the use of intravenous drugs and shared injection equipment.[433,434] Prior to 1990 the transfusion of blood and blood products was an acknowledged source of virus transmission.[413] The major mode of HCV transmission in children is via perinatal transmission. In women with detectable viraemia, the rate of mother-to-infant transmission is estimated to be 4–7%.[435] Transmission to female infants appears to be twice as high as transmission to male infants;[436] no reasons for this phenomenon have been given. HCV can be sexually transmitted with much less frequency than HIV or HBV; however, HIV infection facilitates the sexual transmission of HCV.[435]

HEPATITIS D

The hepatitis D virus (HDV) is a defective RNA virus and is one of the smallest viruses in the animal kingdom. HDV requires the presence of HBV to cause disease in humans and can be acquired either through the process of co-infection with HBV simultaneously or by superinfection in people already infected with HBV.[437] HDV infection has a similar clinical presentation to HBV infection. However, HDV can aggravate HBV infection and can increase the chance of serious liver damage.

HEPATITIS E

The family *Hepeviridae* is divided into two genera, *Orthohepevirus* (mammalian and avian HEV) and *Piscihepevirus* (trout HEV). *Orthohepevirus* from human, pig, wild boar, deer, mongoose, rabbit and camel can cause infection in humans. Human infections occur through the faecal–oral route and from undercooked meat, especially from swine, wild boar and wild deer. HEV can also be transmitted through blood. Blood transfusion screening for HEV is under serious consideration.[428]

The majority of infections are thought to remain asymptomatic[427] and usually self-limited but may persist and cause chronic hepatitis in immunocompromised patients such as in cases of organ transplant.[427,428] The most severe cases are in pregnant women infected with HEV genotype 1; these can result in high maternal, fetal and neonatal morbidity with mortality rates as high as 25%.[427,438]

Epidemics are noted in areas with both poor sanitation and substandard public health facilities.[438,439]

As hepatitis A, D and E are rare infections in Australia and are unlikely to present in a naturopathic clinic, attention will be focused on the pathogenesis and naturopathic treatment of hepatitis B and C.

Pathogenesis

HEPATITIS B

In the majority of adult patients, infection with HBV results in acute hepatitis that is self-limiting. This infection results in protective immunity and once resolved no further disease is evident. However, in 5–10% of the infected adult population the acute infection does not resolve[440] and chronic hepatitis B may result in either decompensated liver failure or hepatic carcinoma.

Research indicates that patients with chronic HBV infection lack the vigorous T-cell response necessary to control the infection.[441] Interferons α, β and γ and TNFα play a major role in viral clearance, while the destruction of infected cells by cytotoxic T-cells both contributes to viral clearance and is involved in subsequent liver damage.[442]

HEPATITIS C

Hepatitis C can present acutely or chronically if HCV replication persists. Approximately 20–40% of HCV infections are benign and self-limiting and clear within 6 months.[443] The spontaneous clearance of the virus is thought to be higher in symptomatic rather than asymptomatic cases and higher rates of clearance are reported in those patients with jaundice.[435] Acute HCV infection can progress to chronic hepatitis C in about 60–80% of cases.[444] (See Fig. 11.4.)

While acute HCV infection is characterised by a vigorous virus-specific immune response, chronic HCV infection is characterised by an impaired and dysfunctional immune response.[445–447] The immune system response in both acute and chronic cases causes damage to hepatic tissue in an attempt to destroy the virus. This cell damage and the cytotoxic chemicals produced by the immune system cause oxidative stress, which causes inflammation and fibrosis, accelerating liver disease through fibrosis to cirrhosis.[448,449]

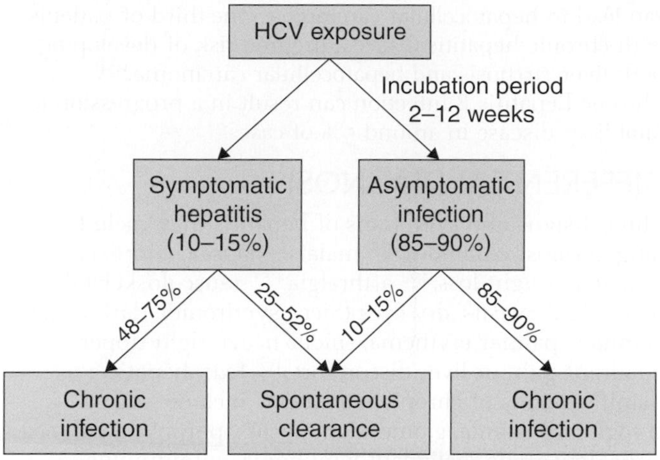

FIGURE 11.4 Outcome of HCV infection.

Source: Maheshwari, Anurag et al. Acute hepatitis C. The Lancet 372(9635): 321–332.

Following HCV exposure and resultant HCV infection, antibodies develop and target both the structural and the nonstructural regions of the virus.

The progression from acute to chronic and the failure of the immune system to irradicate the virus is due to the high rate of viral replication; research indicates that up to 10^{12} new viral particles are produced daily during the course of disease progression.[450]

SIGNS AND SYMPTOMS

Hepatitis B

Healthy adults who are exposed to the hepatitis B virus usually only suffer from a mild acute infection with the likelihood of chronic infection only about 5%. However, the likelihood of chronic infection in patients who are immunocompromised and in newborns is about 90%. Chronic infection usually results in normal liver enzymes, normal liver histology and, often, there are no symptoms reported.[451]

Hepatitis C

Most cases of acute hepatitis C are asymptomatic and symptoms including loss of appetite, weight loss and fatigue occur in less than 30% of patients. Such symptoms are often so mild that they do not interfere with the patient's normal daily routine.[452] Chronic hepatitis C progresses from acute hepatitis C infection in around 60–80% of cases and chronic infection can also be largely asymptomatic for many years.[444] The most common complaints in symptomatic patients are fatigue, abdominal pain, anorexia and weight loss. Jaundice is rare except in cases of advanced liver cirrhosis.[453]

Outcome of hepatitis infection

COMPLICATIONS

Although inflammation assists in the wound healing process, chronic inflammation from liver injury that persists over decades results in scarring, fibrosis and cirrhosis and can lead to hepatocellular carcinoma. One-third of patients with chronic hepatitis C face a lifetime risk of developing both liver cirrhosis and hepatocellular carcinoma.[454] Chronic hepatitis B infection can result in a progression to fatal liver disease in around 5% of cases.

DIFFERENTIAL DIAGNOSIS

Clinical signs and symptoms of hepatitis may include: fatigue (most common),[455] malaise, nausea, anorexia, pruritus, weight loss,[456] arthralgia,[455] musculoskeletal pain, night sweats, dry eyes (Sicca syndrome), dark urine, jaundice, palmar erythema, spider naevi, right upper quadrant pain or liver discomfort.[457] Extrahepatic manifestations of chronic hepatitis C include: mixed cryoglobulinaemia, glomerulonephritis, porphyria cutanea tarda, low-grade malignant lymphoma, autoimmune thyroiditis, lichen planus, Sjögren's syndrome, aplastic anaemia, polyarteritis nodosa, erythema nodosum, idiopathic pulmonary fibrosis[456] and diabetes mellitus.[457] Patients presenting with any of the above signs and symptoms should be referred to a general practitioner in all cases so that an accurate diagnosis can be made. The detection of antibodies will reveal the specific hepatitis infection and the genotype if relevant.

Clinicians are advised to build a solid symptom picture, refer at all times for a diagnosis and not to discount any complaint or symptom identified.

NATUROPATHIC DIAGNOSIS

Iridology

The liver region can be detected just before 8 o'clock on the right iris. Iridology cannot be used to diagnose cases of hepatitis but several iris and sclera signs will commonly present in cases of hepatitis. Tissue weaknesses in the liver area may present on the iris as lacunae, crypts, small lesions or psoric spots. White streaks in the hepatobiliary area indicate chronic inflammation; as the discolouration becomes duller, more chronicity is suggested. Grey streaks suggest a definite hypoactive stage of functioning, brown discolouration suggests toxic accumulation and black markings indicate a severely degenerated tissue and the advanced stages of chronic disease.

A brown or rust-coloured central or collarette heterochromia may also indicate liver dysfunction or may indicate a constitutional susceptibility. Yellow, brown or orange spots in the lymphatic zone of the iris and on the sclera also indicate liver congestion and toxicity.

Patients with hepatitis may also present with mental confusion and fogginess, difficulty concentrating, depression, irritability, anxiety and anger. In such cases, radii solaris may extend from the stomach and bowel area into the head area. All radii solaris indicate nerve damage in their origin and destination points and the organs they pass through may also demonstrate weakness or toxicity.

Nail analysis

Colour changes in the nail can be seen in cases of hepatitis. Jaundice is primarily responsible for yellow discolouration of the fingernails due to the build-up of bilirubin. Patients with chronic liver conditions may also present with Terry's nails. In this presentation, the nail turns white and has the appearance of ground glass. The nails are also referred to as either opaque or frosted. Terry's nails is thought to occur from an increase in connective tissue and a decrease in vascularity in the nail bed.[458] Any long-term systemic illness will result in nutritional deficiencies and such deficiencies present on the nail bed as Beau's lines. Beau's lines are transverse depressions that run across the fingernail. These lines will occur around the same spot in each nail and are indications that normal nail growth has been significantly disrupted.

Tongue analysis

When assessing the patient's tongue, it is also crucial that the whole mouth is investigated so that any other associated conditions can be identified and treated. Hepatitis patients may present with either oral thrush or mouth ulcers due to compromised immunity and poor nutrient status. An association between oral lichen planus (OLP) and HCV has also been reported in the literature.[459,460] Patients with hepatitis will often present with serrated edges along the sides of the tongue; this symptom was first noted in the literature in March 1835.[461] The tongue will often present with a white or yellow greasy coating. If interferon treatment has been started, then both lichenoid lesions and xerostomia (dry mouth) may be present.[462]

Urine and stool

In 94% of viral hepatitis cases, patients will present with dark urine. The bulk of patients with viral hepatitis will present with abdominal discomfort and diarrhoea.[448] Light or clay-coloured stools are a key feature of any viral hepatitis infection due to compromised liver function, a reduction in bile flow and a lack of bile salt excretion in the stool.

Investigations

Diagnosis is usually made on the basis of identifiable HCV exposure, unexplained increases in liver enzymes and the exclusion of other causes of acute liver disease. Polymerase chain reaction (PCR) testing for the HCV RNA virus can be used to detect HCV earlier than the serum antibody test, which relies on seroconversion.

Seroconversion usually occurs 4–10 weeks after exposure to HCV.[463] Antibody detection due to seroconversion is an unreliable method of identifying acute HCV infection as antibody appearance can be delayed in up to 30% of patients[464] and 10% of acutely infected patients lose HCV serological markers.[465]

Chronic HCV infection can remain asymptomatic for many years. However, some patients present with vague symptoms like fatigue, abdominal discomfort, nausea and pruritus. The diagnosis of chronic hepatitis C requires the presence of persistently elevated ALT and continuously positive PCR HCV RNA for 6 months or longer. In cases of chronic hepatitis, ALT values are usually mildly elevated and readings of up to 200 U/L can be seen (normal 0–40 U/L, this varies according to testing laboratory). There may be slight increases in values for GGT, AST, ALP and bilirubin. In chronic hepatitis C, values for ALT are usually higher than AST and GGT; ALP and bilirubin values can often be mildly elevated. Serum prothrombin time, albumin and haematological readings are usually normal until end-stage liver disease develops; in some cases serum albumin may be slightly decreased.

SPECIFIC NATUROPATHIC INVESTIGATIONS

The role of the naturopath is to investigate and document the signs and symptoms, refer to a general practitioner or liver specialist and use the detailed signs and symptoms to guide treatment and monitor progress. Monitoring key signs of quality of life such as fatigue and nausea are useful to direct therapy and support the patient.

Therapeutic considerations

CLINICAL DECISION MAKING AND RATIONALE

Advances in medicine now mean that most patients with HCV can be successfully treated. Genotype 3 remains difficult to treat in approximately 40% of cases. Treatment is, however, still costly and not available to people universally. For example, Egypt has the highest prevalence of hepatitis C virus (HCV) in the world, estimated nationally at 14.7%, mainly acquired iatrogenically.[466]

Therapeutic application

HISTORICAL PERSPECTIVE

The hepatitis B surface antigen (HBsAg) was first discovered in an Aboriginal Australian in 1963. However, infectious icterus has been recognised for around 2000 years.[442] After the discovery of both hepatitis A and B, there was clear evidence of further hepatitis cases not associated with HAV or HBV in around ten percent of cases.[467] These cases were given the classification non-A non-B hepatitis. The molecular identification of the hepatitis C virus was finally reported in 1988 and in 1989 the virus was renamed and published in the scientific literature. Effective treatment — direct-acting antivirals — available today has only been around since 2013. Before that the viral clearance rate was lower, especially for certain genotypes, and side effects were pronounced. Side effects included fatigue, myalgia, headaches, loss of appetite, depression, anxiety, forgetfulness, bone marrow suppression, thrombocytopenia and neutropenia. Because of the side effects, length of treatment and the lack of efficacy many patients declined treatment. As the side effects were so pronounced, often the patient's social and economic position prevented them from even considering treatment.

NATUROPATHIC PERSPECTIVE

The main role of the naturopath is to support the patient through diet and lifestyle while on direct-acting antiviral treatment. This is particularly true for patients with genotype 3 who have only a 75% clearance rate on direct-acting antiviral treatment.

When treating a patient with hepatitis it is important to remain educated in the latest clinical trends and stay familiar with evidence reported in the literature. A practitioner who engages in proactive self-education will be able to easily identify and address obstacles to cure and treat symptoms of the disease progression. It is important to maintain, where possible, written communication with the patient's specialist or general practitioner during their course of naturopathic treatment. Disease progression, treatment efficacy and patient response can be monitored quantitatively through liver biopsy results, liver function test results, full blood counts, tests for viral load and imaging studies.

The treatment of hepatitis centres on the need to treat the viral infection and reduce tissue damage from inflammation and oxidation that prevent the progression of the disease to fibrosis and sequelae to more serious pathology. Symptomatic treatment is also indicated and may provide the patient with marked improvements in quality of life. The treatment of chronic hepatitis B or C requires the following considerations:

- Assess the case presentation, consider differentials and refer for a diagnosis if one has not been provided. Pay particular attention to the patient's lifestyle history during case taking
- Identify any possible contraindications for treatment
- Reduce inflammation and oxidative damage to limit sequelae to more severe pathology
- Reduce symptoms of HCV infection — fatigue, depression, pruritus, gastrointestinal dysfunction, nausea
- Support optimal liver function through repair and protection of hepatocytes — improve organ integrity and function
- Address dietary and lifestyle concerns and limit any risk factors that hinder or obstruct the healing process.

NUTRITIONAL MEDICINE (DIETARY)

The role for the dietary treatment of hepatitis must primarily focus on ensuring adequate macronutrient and micronutrient intake.

As the liver coordinates nutrient metabolism, malnutrition in liver disease is common. Poor dietary intake of nutrients results from early satiety due to ascites, nausea, loss of appetite and the prescription of unpalatable diets prescribed by some dietitians and physicians.

Dietary therapeutic objectives

See 'Hepatobiliary nutritional objectives (dietary)' for an overview.

- Maintain adequate protein intake — required for healing and repair and immune system function
- Reduce intake of red meat to reduce iron intake — iron accumulation is associated with hepatic damage in chronic hepatitis C
- Increase intake of fresh fish and vegetarian sources of protein to ensure adequate protein intake
- Remove intake of processed foods, takeaway food and fatty cuts of red meat. These are high in fat and obesity has been linked to severity of disease progression

- Reduce intake of refined carbohydrates, avoid soft drinks or sugary fruit juices/cordials and do not add sugar to beverages or food
- Adjust diet to address poor appetite, early satiety and nausea — smaller more frequent meals will address these problems and stabilise blood sugars
- Improve digestion, reduce malabsorption and improve nutritional status — introduce dietary bitters and choleretics and suggest marinating animal protein
- Stabilise blood sugar levels with adequate fibre and protein intake to help avoid bingeing on fried carbohydrates and displacing beneficial nutrients and also to reduce the risk of insulin resistance and associated diabetes
- Avoid consumption of trans fatty acids to limit risk of further inflammation, oxidative stress and tissue damage
- Increase intake of dietary antioxidants with daily intake of fresh fruit and vegetables
- Drink dandelion and chicory root beverages.

Specific dietary treatments

DIETARY INCLUSIONS

Protein

The patient's weight and the degree of liver damage should be taken into consideration when calculating protein requirements in hepatitis. For stable liver disease and uncomplicated hepatitis, protein requirements range from 0.8 g to 1.0 g of protein per kg of body weight.[468] Protein intake at this level assists with tissue repair, immune function, nitrogen balance and blood sugar regulation.

Dietary restrictions in conventional medicine focus on protein restriction owing to concerns about hepatic encephalopathy. Protein requirements are lower where decompensated liver disease (unstable liver disease) is present. However, in stable hepatitis cases, protein intake should be encouraged and not be restricted due to concerns about hepatic encephalopathy.[15]

Dietary antioxidants

Oxidative mediated pathways are involved in the progression of persistent infection to fibrosis, cirrhosis and carcinogenesis, thus dietary antioxidants are crucial in the management of chronic hepatitis infection. Fruits and vegetables rich in vitamins E and C, selenium, carotenoids and anthocyanins are recommended for their powerful antioxidant activity and overall nutrient content. However, fruit consumption should remain at two pieces per day to avoid excessive sugar intake. Oxygen radical absorbance capacity (ORAC) measurements indicate that garlic, curly cabbage and Brussels sprouts are the strongest source of vegetable antioxidants.[20]

Foods for poor appetite, indigestion and nausea

Traditional foods that are noted for their beneficial effects on the liver include the bitter leaves of dandelion and chicory. These leaves will aid proper digestion by stimulating bile production and taken before a meal as a salad will help to stimulate the appetite. The bitter action will also assist if the patient complains of headaches or nausea. The addition of fresh parsley, beetroot, carrots, endive, limes and onion will stimulate the appetite, improve digestion and support liver function. The juice of half a lemon mixed with warm water and taken in the morning on an empty stomach before breakfast will also stimulate the appetite and improve digestive processes.

If indigestion is a problem, the inclusion of pineapple and papaya in the diet will assist with protein digestion. The use of fresh ginger in food will also calm the digestive system and added to hot water and taken as a tea, ginger will ease the nausea associated with hepatitis.

DIETARY EXCLUSIONS

Alcohol

Alcohol intake in patients with HCV has been associated with higher degrees of liver fibrosis, increased risk of cirrhosis and higher rates of mortality.[469] The consumption of alcohol and presence of fatty liver increases fibrosis in HCV patients, with higher fibrotic activity reported in obese and diabetic patients.[470] Alcohol is thought to precipitate fibrosis via upregulation of programmed hepatocyte death.[471] Stimulation of reactive oxygen species (ROS) production[472] and alcohol consumption have been linked to increases in hepatic iron stores which contribute to fibrosis.[473]

Fat intake and obesity

Steatosis has been associated with HCV infection and two major factors underlie the development of fatty liver in hepatitis. One type of steatosis is linked to viral replication and is mostly seen in patients with hepatitis genotype 3. Metabolic steatosis occurs in patients with fat accumulation and is independent of HCV infection.[474] Increases in body mass index contribute to the pathogenesis of steatosis and eventual fibrosis in chronic hepatitis C infection[475] and obesity can contribute to the progression of liver fibrosis in patients with hepatitis C.[476] Drastic changes in diet and lifestyle are required in HCV where obesity is apparent.

Iron

Test iron levels with a full iron study and if levels are elevated reduce sources in the diet. Iron accumulation in the liver plays a role in the severity of chronic HCV infection and fibrosis.[477] High plasma ferritin levels have been linked to increased free radical activity.[478] Increasing levels of serum iron have also been linked to greater amounts of hepatitis C viral RNA.[479] Abstinence from red meat, the introduction of a predominantly vegetarian diet and increased consumption of tannin-rich tea are suggested approaches for keeping iron levels of HCV patients in check.

Refined sugar and glycaemic control

An epidemiological link has been established between type 2 diabetes and HCV infection,[480] and cases of diabetes among people infected with

HCV are four times higher than in the general population.[481] Some researchers have suggested that HCV infection triggers autoimmune mechanisms that destroy pancreatic beta cells in susceptible people.[482] A low-GI diet should be followed and refined sugars and processed foods should be completely avoided to regulate blood sugars, avoid insulin resistance and prevent pancreatic damage.

SAMPLE DAILY DIET

BREAKFAST	
Immune-boosting juice: orange, beetroot, carrot, lemon, ginger Toast spread with beetroot, hummus and avocado	Fruits and vegetables are rich in immune-boosting substances and when consumed in a fresh juice provide a concentrated source of nutrients to support immunity. Betanin, a constituent found in beetroot juice, has been shown to protect against liver injury,[483] which may be useful in viral-induced hepatitis. Chickpeas in the hummus provide a source of protein, while beetroot and garlic in the hummus help to support immunity, with garlic functioning as an antiviral.
SNACK	
Fresh fruit and green tea	Fruit helps to support immunity while the green tea polyphenol, epigallocatechin-3-gallate has been shown to inhibit hepatitis C virus entry in vitro.[484]
LUNCH	
Vegetable spiced dhal	Dhal provides an easy-to-digest, nutritive meal. Curcumin within turmeric found in the dhal is a hepatic anti-inflammatory and may also help to inhibit viral entry into the liver cells.[485]
DINNER	
Chicken broth/congee made from shiitake mushrooms, garlic, leek, shallots, turmeric, rice or rice noodles	A broth provides an easy-to-digest nourishing meal to boost immunity. The allium family includes onions, garlic, leeks, shallots and chives and provides sulfur to enhance optimal liver function, while ginger contains gingerol, an antimicrobial and anti-inflammatory constituent to reduce hepatic inflammation.

NUTRITIONAL MEDICINE (SUPPLEMENTAL)

See 'Hepatobiliary nutritional objectives (nutrients)' and Table 11.5.

The role of supplemental nutritional medicine in the treatment of hepatitis focuses on reducing inflammation, improving overall liver function, reducing oxidative stress, improving mitochondrial function, restoring glutathione levels, reducing fibrosis and immune support.

Specific nutritional supplements can be introduced for their antioxidant and anti-inflammatory capabilities and play a role in preventing the progression of hepatitis to fibrosis, cirrhosis and hepatic carcinoma. Vitamin and mineral deficiencies are common in patients with chronic liver disease, thus supplementation is necessary to correct any deficiencies that may contribute to longstanding infection, inflammation and fibrosis.

NUTRITIONAL MEDICINE THERAPEUTIC OBJECTIVES

- Reduce and regulate hepatic inflammation
- Support overall liver function
- Reduce potential for fibrosis by reducing inflammation and oxidative damage
- Support both the immune and digestive systems by providing nutritional foundations
- Correct deficiencies or extra nutritional requirements resulting from infection and inflammation
- Support optimal nervous system functioning, thereby reducing depression, insomnia, fatigue and anxiety.

Specific nutrients required

VITAMIN E

Low serum and liver levels of vitamin E have been reported in patients with chronic HCV infection and have also been correlated with the degree of fibrosis.[486] Vitamin E supplementation in conjunction with conventional pharmacological therapy has been found to reduce total HCV viral load.[487] The hepatoprotective, anti-inflammatory and antifibrotic effects of a silybin phospholipids and vitamin E complex (SPV complex) has been reported.[488]

Vitamin E has also been studied for its antioxidant role in HBV. Andreone et al[489] conducted a 3-month trial on 22 HBV patients who did not respond to interferon treatment. They reported that five of the participants had a complete response to treatment where ALT levels normalise and HBV DNA was cleared from serum. They conducted a follow-up study on 32 chronic HBV patients and reported ALT normalisation in 47% and reduced HBV DNA in 53%.[490]

VITAMIN D

In osteodystrophy vitamin D levels and severity of liver disease were correlated with low bone mineral density.[491,492]

ZINC

The antioxidant activity of zinc can be related to its role as a component of superoxide dismutase (CuZnSOD) which is necessary for cellular defence against reactive oxygen species. Zinc also competes for binding sites with the pro-oxidant minerals iron and copper.[493] Serum and hepatic zinc are reduced in chronic HBV[494] and HCV[495] infection. Oral zinc supplementation is beneficial in chronic HCV infection by reducing serum ferritin and thus reducing oxidative stress and hepatic inflammation.[496] Zinc supplementation during interferon therapy has also demonstrated favourable results.[497]

SELENIUM

Selenium is required for the antioxidant activity of glutathione peroxidase. Low selenium levels have been directly associated with chronic liver pathologies[498] and variations in plasma glutathione peroxidase have been noted in chronic hepatitis C infection. A 3-year Chinese study revealed supplementation with table salt fortified with selenium lowered the incidence rate of infectious hepatitis,[499] and an inverse relationship between plasma selenium levels and hepatocellular carcinoma in chronic HBV and HCV patients has been reported.[500]

N-ACETYLCYSTEINE

N-acetylcysteine (NAC) is a precursor to glutathione and has been used historically in conventional medicine for the treatment of paracetamol poisoning. NAC is an antioxidant and anti-inflammatory derivative of the amino acid L-cysteine. NAC restores glutathione levels in the body by crossing the cell membrane and providing cysteine for glutathione synthesis.[501]

ALPHA LIPOIC ACID

Alpha lipoic acid is a beneficial compound in conditions where oxidative stress plays a major role. Alpha lipoic acid and dihydrolipoic acid have the ability to scavenge both hydrogen peroxide and superoxide.[502] Alpha lipoic acid also plays a role in carbohydrate metabolism via stimulation of glucose transport mechanisms[503] and this assists liver function and regulation of glycogenolysis, glycolysis and gluconeogenesis. This mechanism of action has further implications as diabetes mellitus[504] is frequently observed in patients with HCV.

FISH OILS

Depression is a noted symptom of chronic HBV and HCV infection. Supplementation with fish oils may be beneficial as people with depression have omega-3 fatty acid deficiencies and fish oil supplementation is beneficial in the treatment of depression.[505] Interferon can affect the metabolism of fats in the body and can significantly increase triglyceride levels. Concurrent fish oil supplementation with interferon therapy has been found to reduce both liver inflammation and raised levels of serum triglycerides and LDL cholesterol, while raising HDL cholesterol levels.[506]

TRYPTOPHAN

HCV patients have reduced serum tryptophan levels and frequently suffer from anxiety and depression, especially during interferon therapy.[507] Reduced serum tryptophan levels lowers 5HT synthesis in the brain and contributes to depression-related symptoms.[508]

Dosage requirement

- Vitamin E: 400–800 IU
- Vitamin D: 1000 IU per day
- Zinc: 50 mg/day
- Selenium: 150–400 micrograms/day
- N-acetylcysteine: 1800 mg/day
- Alpha lipoic acid: 200–600 mg/day
- Fish oils: 1000 mg DHA/1000 mg EPA/day
- Tryptophan: 50 mg t.d.s. (or 5HTP)

HERBAL MEDICINE

Herbal medicine therapeutic objectives

- Mediate and reduce hepatic inflammation
- Improve overall liver function
- Improve digestion and reduce any digestive disturbances associated with hepatitis
- Support the immune system in general
- Symptomatically reduce fatigue, nausea and depression and irritability associated with the infection and inflammation
- Protect the liver from fibrosis and cirrhosis and reverse where possible
- Prescribe herbal medicines in teas if indicated.

Specific herbal medicine classes

The use of herbal medicines in the treatment of chronic hepatitis centres on the need to support the liver and prevent the development of cirrhosis. Herbal medicines can be employed to reduce oxidative stress, hepatic inflammation and fibrosis. They can also support overall liver function, digestion, depression, sleep and quality of life. Hepatic anti-inflammatory, hepatoprotective and antioxidant medicines are key components and are indicated in all cases of hepatitis to reduce oxidative stress and inflammation and thus reduce the potential for fibrosis, cirrhosis and hepatocellular carcinoma. Digestive disturbances associated with hepatitis include nausea, indigestion, reflux, flatulence, bloating and abdominal discomfort. Bitter digestives, carminatives and gentle cholagogues are indicated for such disturbances.

To improve quality of life nervines, sedatives, thymoleptics and adaptogens can be prescribed as needed.

Specific herbal medicines

SILYBUM MARIANUM (ST MARY'S THISTLE)

Silymarin is the collective name for the flavolignans in *Silybum marianum* that are responsible for the hepatoprotective properties of the herb. Silymarin has been extensively researched for its protective effects on the liver and is one of the most studied herbal medicines for liver diseases.[509,510] Hepatoprotective effects are evident due to the herb's ability to scavenge and regulate the intracellular content of glutathione, stabilise cell membranes, stimulate hepatocyte regeneration and inhibit the transformation of hepatic stellate cells into fibroblasts thus reducing fibrosis.[511]

The herb demonstrates significant activity in the damage control and repair of chronic liver disease. However, its effect in the treatment of viral load in hepatitis is less studied. A systematic review on the use of complementary medicine in the treatment of chronic HCV reported that silymarin compounds were able to reduce liver transaminases in patients with chronic HCV infection but viral load and liver disease progression remained unaltered.[512] One study reported that administration of silymarin in a cohort of 83 HCV infected people achieved ALT normalisation in 15%.[513]

Studies have confirmed the antiviral action of silymarin in vitro.[39–42] Two main hypotheses explored to explain this effect are: (1) improved cellular response and (2) inhibition of viral function. A direct anti-HCV effect of silymarin was confirmed in a human trial using intravenous silybinin in a cohort of HCV interferon non-responders. In this study patients with a previous non-response to a full dose of interferon/ribavirin treatment were selected. Researchers reported an unexpected strong antiviral response after 7 days of silibinin infusions. They reported no serious adverse effects and that silibinin was well tolerated.[514] This study confirms previous work on the use of silymarin in vitro and is the first documentation of the antiviral properties of silibinin against HCV in humans.

The Hep573 Study administered a formulation containing 720 mg of silybinin and antioxidants (SOX) to 118 hepatitis C patients daily. Results of this trial showed significantly more ALT normalisation in the SOX group compared with the placebo or the silymarin-only groups after 24 weeks of treatment. Silymarin alone did not have an effect on liver inflammation or oxidative stress. It did reduce HCV RNA viral load even though this figure was not statistically significant.[515] These results suggest that the combination of silymarin and antioxidants may be beneficial in modifying necroinflammatory processes in chronic hepatitis C patients.

The use of herbal and nutritional herbal antioxidants combined has been assessed to verify whether supplementation can alter the course of chronic hepatitis C progression. One study[516] assessed oral treatment for 20 weeks with glycyrrhizin, *Schisandra*, silymarin, ascorbic acid, lipoic acid, L-glutathione and d-alpha-tocopherol. Intravenous preparations of glycyrrhizin, ascorbic acid, L-glutathione and B complex were administered daily for the first 10 weeks. Results indicated ALT normalisation in 44% of participants and a decrease in HCV viral load was noted in 25% of participants. Liver inflammation was reduced in 36% of participants and researchers noted a 58% improvement in patient quality of life.

SCUTELLARIA BAICALENSIS (BAIKAL SKULLCAP)

Scutellaria baicalensis has been used for thousands of years in traditional Chinese medicine, mainly for the treatment of inflammatory conditions including hepatitis. This herbal medicine has shown promising results in vitro with the active constituent wogonin demonstrating the suppression of HBV surface antigen production with no associated cytotoxicity.[517] Research corroborated this finding with wogonin displaying anti-hepatitis B virus activity in vitro and in vivo and indicated that wogonin could be developed as an anti-HBV drug.[518]

PHYLLANTHUS (PHYLLANTHUS)

Plants from the *Phyllanthus* genus are distributed throughout tropical and subtropical countries and have a strong traditional use in the treatment of chronic liver disease.[519] Early research highlighted some promising effects of *Phyllanthus niruri* (renamed *amarus*) on hepatitis B and woodchuck hepatitis B viruses both in vivo and in vitro.[520–522]

A 1988 study[523] generated much excitement when it reported that treatment with *Phyllanthus amarus* for 3 weeks resulted in a loss of the hepatitis B surface antigen (HBsAg) in more than half of the trial participants. However, a follow-up trial in 1990 by Leelarusamee et al[524] failed to reproduce these findings and in an effort to repeat the 1990 results Thyagarajan et al[525] obtained only 20% seroconversion rates in their second study. These initial promising results have not been replicated by other researchers.[526]

Further clinical trials in HBV patients have produced inconsistent findings. Zhang and colleagues[527] reported a significant reduction in HBeAg in the group treated with a whole plant extract of *Phyllanthus amarus* at 60 g of oral liquid per day and Zhu et al[528] reported similar findings with reductions in HBeAg in participants treated with 50 g of oral liquid per day prepared from the whole plant of *Phyllanthus urinaria*. A reduction in HBeAg indicates a reduction in multiplication of the virus. Berk et al[529] conducted a 10-day crossover trial on the efficacy of *Phyllanthus amarus* on levels of HBsAg, HBeAg and HBV DNA but reported no changes in outcome measures. Milne et al[530] assessed standardised extracts of geraniin from *Phyllanthus amarus* extract and used doses of 0.87 g per day (60 mg geraniin) in a randomised controlled trial conducted in New Zealand; however, no changes in serum levels of HBV or other biochemical liver markers were noted. The low methodological quality of the trials reporting favourable results has been noted.[531]

SHO-SAIKO-TO (TJ-9)

The traditional Japanese medicine Sho-saiko-to (TJ-9) has been used to treat hepatitis and has been widely studied in both animal and human trials. The main ingredients in this formulation are *Bupleurum chinensis*, *Scutellaria baicalensis* and *Glycyrrhiza glabra*. This formulation is recommended for the treatment of HBV and has demonstrated ability to reduce inflammation. A human study on both HBV and HCV patients found that 5.4 g of TJ-9 per day resulted in reductions in both ALT and AST.[532] Animal studies have confirmed that TJ-9 can reduce fibrosis by inhibiting hepatic stellate cells.[533] There have been about 10 case reports of interstitial pneumonia reported in the past decade associated with the use of TJ-9,[534,535] with some reports possibly linked to interferon therapy.[536]

GLYCYRRHIZA GLABRA (LIQUORICE)

Glycyrrhiza glabra has been used in Asian and European traditional medicine to alleviate peptic ulcer disease, constipation, cough and liver disorders.[537] Japanese researchers used the standardised extract, stronger neominophagen (SNMC) containing glycyrrhizin, cysteine and glycine as an established treatment for chronic hepatitis in animal studies. In one study, daily doses of 80 mg per day given intravenously for 2 weeks normalised elevated aspartate and alanine transaminase levels.[538] In vitro, glycyrrhizin modifies the expression of HBV-related antigens on hepatocytes and suppresses sialylation of the HBsAg.[539,540] Glycyrrhizin was given in combination with lamivudine intravenously and proved useful in the treatment of subacute hepatitis due to hepatitis B infection.[541]

Early human studies also showed promising results in the treatment of HCV. A retrospective Japanese trial noted administration of 100 mL of SNMC daily over a 10-year period in HCV patients resulted in a reduction of hepatocellular carcinoma over a 15-year period.[542] A 2006 study[543] reported that glycyrrhizin injection therapy significantly decreased the incidence of hepatocellular carcinoma in patients with IFN-resistant active chronic hepatitis C.

ASTRAGALUS MEMBRANACEUS (ASTRAGALUS)

Astragalus membranaceus is regarded as a Qi tonifying or adaptogenic herb in Chinese and Western herbal medicine. In Chinese medicine, astragalus is thought to affect both the spleen and the lung meridians. It is specifically indicated for spleen deficiency symptoms like diarrhoea, fatigue, poor appetite and spontaneous sweating.[544]

Most of the current research on the pharmacological actions of this herb focuses on its immune-stimulating polysaccharides. One study reported the immunomodulatory effect of astragalus on the Th1/Th2 balance in rats[545] and murine studies report that the hepatoprotective effects of saponins in *Astragalus radix* result from antioxidant and immune regulating activity.[546] Astragalus may also be of benefit in the treatment of chronic hepatitis as a combination extract of astragalus and *Salvia miltiorrhiza*, which has a demonstrated protective effect against chronic liver fibrosis.[547] Despite a small body of evidence-based research, the herb's traditional use in immune and adaptogenic support offers a more sound justification for use in chronic hepatitis.

OTHER IMPORTANT HERBAL MEDICINES

There is an array of herbal medicines that can offer benefit in the treatment of hepatitis and the reduction of symptoms from infection and inflammation. There is a paucity of current evidence-based scientific research that either supports traditional use or investigates herbal medicines within the context of traditional use. The available research merely scratches the surface of herbal medicines that have a history of reliability and efficacy.

Digestive problems respond exceptionally well to *Matricaria recutita* (chamomile). Depending on the stage and severity of liver disease, chamomile can be prescribed as an alcoholic extract or in most cases as a herbal tea. Chamomile offers digestive support due to its strong anti-inflammatory actions. *Foeniculum vulgare* (fennel) may also provide digestive support due to its ability to temper gas and indigestion. A fennel and liquorice tea combination can be used in conjunction with chamomile tea to reduce bloating and nausea associated with chronic hepatitis.

Lavandula angustifolia (lavender) tea is beneficial for the digestive system and in depression.

Achillea millefolia (yarrow) is much overlooked for the treatment of digestive concerns and can be of benefit if excessive sweating and fever are present. Hobbs[548] suggests this herb has energetic qualities similar to that of chamomile, possesses a bitter tonic quality and may improve fat digestion. In ancient legend, yarrow was used by Chiron the Centaur to cure the wound of Achilles; it was often called 'wound wort' or 'soldier's herb' due to its profound anti-inflammatory activity. *Melissa officinalis* (lemon balm) is a cooling herb and offers both digestive and nervous system support and, combined with *Passiflora incarnata* (passiflora) and taken as a tea, tempers the irritability and anxiety associated with hepatitis.

LIFESTYLE RECOMMENDATIONS

Lifestyle modifications are essential for long-term management and treatment of chronic hepatitis. Maintaining a healthy weight range is crucial in the treatment of hepatitis as being overweight has been implicated in more severe disease progression. Dietary modification plays a major role. However, exercise contributes to weight management and may also help to relieve anxiety and depression and improve vitality.

Patients should be advised to restrict the consumption of alcohol to reduce any unnecessary burden on the liver and because alcohol intake has also been implicated as an independent risk factor in the progression of HCV infection.[549] Smoking should be avoided as smoking reduces the liver's detoxification ability and can promote the progression to cirrhosis in chronic HBV[550] and HCV[551] infection. Unnecessary pharmaceutical drugs should be avoided and the intake of recreational drugs should be completely avoided.

Environmental and industrial toxins like solvents, pesticides and cleaning chemicals may exacerbate liver inflammation and hasten the progression towards fibrosis. These chemicals should be removed from the home and work environment and replaced with natural household cleaners. There are safe, homemade alternatives to the toxic household cleaning products on the market; a combination of vinegar, lemon, water, bicarbonate and salt is a useful and nontoxic household cleaner.

The proper disposal of personal hygiene products like razors, toothbrushes or tweezers that may come into contact with blood should also be discussed with the patient. This advice is usually made available in the literature provided by general practitioners or hepatitis advocacy groups. However, addressing these concerns is considered best practice from a naturopathic perspective. Proper education of family members and carers is also important to prevent the spread of the viruses.

Emotional support for the patient is important as depression and fatigue are symptoms of liver infection and inflammation and the side effects of drug therapy. It is essential that the naturopath maintains an up-to-date list of hepatitis support groups and support services and encourages the patient's interest and participation where appropriate. Support groups should encourage information sharing and an open, healthy and confidential dialogue between group members. Clinicians are advised to discourage patients from joining groups where negativity is rife and self-empowerment is discouraged.

CASE STUDY

OVERVIEW

A 65-year-old female presented with chronic hepatitis C. She had shared needles twice in her past, some 45 years ago. She has hepatitis C virus genotype 1a and was treated unsuccessfully with interferon monotherapy, then pegylated interferon and ribavirin, then pegylated interferon and ribavirin and boceprevir. Each of these treatments caused many side effects and it took her months to recover. She is soon to be placed on a 12-week trial of sofosbuvir and ledipasvir to clear the hepatitis C virus.

CLINICAL EXAMINATION

BP: 120/78 mmHg PR: 70, Weight: 65 kg

She has fatigue, back and joint pain, arthritis, brain fog and tinnitus

LABORATORY INVESTIGATIONS

ALT 130 U/L	(5–30)
AST 60 U/L	(10–35)
ALP 65 U/L	(20–35)
GGT 22 U/L	(5–35)
Albumin 44 g/L	(37–48)
Total bilirubin 16 μmol/L	(3–15)

TREATMENT PROTOCOL

INITIAL APPOINTMENT

- Prior to going on the direct-acting antiviral therapy, the focus is on enhancing her wellbeing, reducing oxidative stress and liver inflammation
- Reduce hepatic inflammation and improve liver function with *Silybum marianum*, *Schisandra chinensis*, *Curcuma longa* and *Andrographis paniculata*
- Support the immune system with *Andrographis paniculata*, *Astragalus membranaceus*, *Eleutherococcus senticosus*, zinc, vitamin C and selenium
- Enhance glutathione in the liver and reduce oxidative stress with *Silybum marianum*, *Camellia sinensis*, *Curcuma longa*, alpha lipoic acid, *Andrographis paniculata*, *Bacopa monniera*, selenomethionine, vitamin C, zinc, *Vitis vinifera* and lycopene

CASE STUDY CONTINUED

- Improve vitality and wellbeing with *Astragalus membranaceus*, *Centella asiatica*, activated coenzyme Q10 (ubiquinol).

HERBAL MEDICINE

Hepatoprotective supplement:

Silybum marianum 15 g standardised to contain 180 mg silybin.

Dose: 2 tablets b.i.d.

Antioxidant supplement:

Camellia sinensis 1 g
Curcuma longa 2 g (70 mg curcuminoids)
Silybum marianum 1 g, equiv silymarin 10 mg, equiv total silybin 4.29 mg
Vitis vinifera 3 g (20 mg procyanidins)
Selenomethionine 50 micrograms
Alpha lipoic acid 50 mg
Lycopene 20 mg
Elemental zinc 12.5 mg
Calcium ascorbate 100 mg

Dose: 2 tablets b.i.d.

Herbal formula

Astragalus membranaceus 1.2	30 mL
Andrographis paniculata 1.2	20 mL
Schisandra chinensis 1.2	20 mL
Bacopa monniera 1.2	30 mL
Centella asiatica 1.2	10 mL
Total	100 mL

Dose: 7 mL twice daily before meals

OUTCOME

While on direct-acting antiviral therapy, the emphasis is on maintaining the principles of a naturopathic diet as outlined in dietary inclusions in the hepatobiliary nutritional objectives. This was done by using herbs with vasodilatory effects to promote heart health such as *Achillea millefolium* and *Olea europea* and the nutrient-activated coenzyme Q10 to prevent pulmonary arterial hypertension, as well as the inclusion of vitamin D which may reduce the occurrence of drug resistance developing while on treatment.

After 6 months of naturopathic treatment her wellbeing had improved, she had diminished fatigue and brain fog, and her joint/back pain had improved.

All liver serum chemistry had normalised: ALT 30, AST 35, ALP 33, GGT 12, albumin 45 and bilirubin 8

She was in the best position to embark on the direct-acting antiviral therapy, which finally cleared the hepatitis C virus.

AUTOIMMUNE HEPATOBILIARY CONDITIONS

There are three autoimmune conditions that can affect the hepatobiliary system: autoimmune hepatitis (AIH), primary biliary cholangitis (PBC) and primary sclerosing cholangitis (PSC).

Autoimmune hepatobiliary conditions show similar signs and symptoms to other hepatobiliary diseases, with fatigue, nausea and upper right quadrant discomfort. Liver disease is confirmed with elevated liver enzymes and differentiated by the presence of specific autoimmune antibodies. Autoimmune hepatobiliary conditions are often accompanied by other autoimmune conditions.

Because of historic and current difficulty in accurate diagnosis it is generally accepted that the reported incidence and prevalence of autoimmune hepatitis are underestimated.[552]

The international incidence of AIH ranges from 0.67 to 2.0 per 100 000 people per year, and its prevalence ranges from 4.0 to 42.9 per 100 000 people. High prevalence is present in Alaska and Europe.[553]A 10-year study calculated that the mean annual incidence per 100 000 in Norway was 1.6 for PBC, 1.3 for PSC and 1.9 for AIH. The point prevalence per 100 000 on 31 December 1995 was 14.6, 8.5 and 16.9 for PBC, PSC and AIH, respectively.[554] The study calculated that the prevalence of PBC and AIH is of the same order of magnitude and about twice as high as that of PSC.[554]

A large epidemiological study of PBC in Italy and Denmark showed an annual incidence of PBC of 16.7 per million in Italy with a point prevalence of 160 per million in 2009.[555] In Denmark the incidence was 11.4 per million with a point prevalence of 11.5 per million in 2009.[555]The study showed a female-to-male ratio of 2.3 : 1 in Italy and 4.2 : 1 in Denmark. However, male sex was an independent predictor of all-cause mortality in both countries.[555]

Women are affected more often than men in AIH and PBC (70–80% of patients are women).[553] However, approximately 70% of patients with PSC are men, with a mean age of diagnosis around 40 years. Patients with PSC but without IBD are more likely to be women and to be older at diagnosis. Autoimmune hepatitis accounts for about 3% of liver transplantations in Europe, 4–6% in America and just 1% in Japan.[556]

An interesting study looking at neuroimaging changes in precirrhotic PBC patients suggests that the brain changes seen in PBC occur early in the pathological process, even before significant liver damage has occurred.[557] The study suggests that these changes are a result of cholestatic and/or inflammatory processes and cause the symptoms of fatigue and cognitive impairment.[557] The study calls for fast and efficacious treatment, especially when the first line of treatment fails to normalise brain function.[557]

CIRRHOSIS

Epidemiology

Cirrhosis is defined as a histological response to chronic liver injury and is an advanced stage of liver fibrosis that results in portal hypertension and hepatic insufficiency.

In 2010 cirrhosis accounted for one million deaths, or two percent of all deaths worldwide in that year.[558] This is an increase from 676,000 in 1980.

Classification

Cirrhosis can be classified as either compensated or decompensated and it can remain in a compensated state for years before the development and initiation of a decompensating event. Decompensated cirrhosis is characterised by the development of complications such as jaundice, ascites, encephalopathy, variceal haemorrhages or spontaneous bacterial peritonitis (Table 11.9).[559]

Aetiology

ALCOHOLIC LIVER DISEASE

Alcohol abuse represents a leading cause of cirrhosis, and liver regeneration is suppressed in alcoholic cirrhotic livers.[560,561] Alcohol consumption is related to cirrhosis due to its impact on reduced functionality of liver cells and alterations in the vascular system of the liver. Alcohol alters lipid and protein metabolism, stimulates collagen deposition and fibrosis, and inhibits liver cell regeneration. These processes result in scarring that distorts the liver's structure and impairs its function.

HEPATITIS B AND C

Concomitant viral hepatitis B or C infection with alcohol consumption can increase the risk of progression to cirrhosis and carcinoma.[562] However, infection with hepatitis B or C is acknowledged outright for its influence on cirrhotic pathogenesis.[563]

HELICOBACTER PYLORI INFECTION

The discovery of *Helicobacter hepaticus* as a causal agent of both hepatitis and hepato carcinoma in rodents[564] has led to interest in a role for *Helicobacter pylori* spp. in the aetiology of both cirrhosis and hepatocellular carcinoma. *H. pylori* infection is very common in patients with cirrhosis.[565] A role for *H. pylori* infection and increased ammonia production leading to hepatic encephalopathy[566] and gastroduodenal ulcers[567] has been suggested and bacteria have also been implicated in the progression of HCV to cirrhosis. Despite initial hypotheses and research, at this stage the relationship between *H. pylori* infection and cirrhosis is not aetiological and appears no more than an association.[568]

NASH

NAFLD can present as simple steatosis (fatty liver), which rarely has sequelae, or it can progress to steatosis with necroinflammation or fibrosis. If this progression is evident, the condition is referred to as NASH. Approximately 50% of NASH patients develop liver fibrosis, 15–30% develop cirrhosis and 3% can progress to liver failure.[348] Among NASH patients, obesity, diabetes and age over 40 years have been associated with an increased risk of liver fibrosis and progression to cirrhosis.[569]

TABLE 11.9 Signs and symptoms of decompensated cirrhosis

Sign/symptom	Causative factor
Anaemia	Microcytic anaemia from iron deficiency (ferritin and transferrin synthesised by liver). Macrocytic anaemia from folate and vitamin B_{12} deficiencies (storage in liver). Haemolytic anaemia due to impaired lipid synthesis in liver (red blood cell membrane abnormalities)
Ascites	Sinusoidal portal hypertension and systemic arterial vasodilation results in an increase in lymph formation and reduced lymph return
Caput medusae	Distended veins in the umbilical region as portal hypertension promotes reopening of the umbilical vein
Cirrhotic cardiomyopathy	Increase in cardiac output, defective heart contractility, reduced adrenergic function and impaired activity of the ventricular myocardium
Diabetes	Hypoglycaemia results from hepatocyte destruction, impaired glycogenolysis and gluconeogenesis
Dupuytren's contracture	Contraction of the palmar fascia with an inability to fully extend the fingers resulting from fibrosis and increased oxidative stress. May be more associated with alcoholic cirrhosis
Finger clubbing	Release of vascular endothelial growth factor (VEGF) at distal points. VEGF is induced by hypoxia and produces vascular hyperplasia, oedema and proliferation of fibroblasts and osteoblasts
Fetor hepaticus	Odour from dimethylsulfide resulting in portal blood shunting and liver failure
Gynaecomastia	Decreased clearance of androstenedione leading to increased serum oestrogens. SHBG levels are also increased, thus reducing free testosterone levels
Hepatic encephalopathy	Many factors implicated including alterations in neurotransmitter pathways, cerebral blood flow modulation, systemic inflammatory responses and ammonia build-up
Hepatopulmonary syndrome	Overproduction of nitric oxide, overexpression of endothelin B receptor and pulmonary arteriolar vasodilation and hypoxaemia
Hepatorenal syndrome	Progressive renal failure with vasoconstriction often secondary to acute hepatitis superimposed on cirrhosis. There are two types: type I and type II
Hyponatraemia	Results from hypersecretion of antidiuretic hormone and increased loss of sodium from diuretics and renal imbalances
Jaundice	Inability of hepatocytes to excrete bilirubin resulting in yellow skin, mucous membranes and sclera
Palmar erythema	Hyperoestrogenism resulting from liver failure to inactivate oestrogens
Pruritus	Elevated opioid peptides and bile acids
Spider angioma	Increased oestradiol with reduced liver clearance and hyperdynamic circulation in cirrhosis and other unknown reasons
Splenomegaly	Splenic congestion and portal hypertension and infiltration
Spontaneous bacterial peritonitis (SBP)	Gram-negative bacteria mostly *Escherichia coli*. Diagnosis positive for SBP if neutrophils > 250. Very poor prognosis if superinfection present
Varices	Portal hypertension and hyperdynamic circulation

Dong MH, Saab S. Complications of cirrhosis. Dis Mon 2008; 54(7):445–456; Ghassemi S, Guadalupe GT. Prevention and treatment of infections in patients with cirrhosis. Best Prac Res Clin Gastro 2007; 21(1):77–93; Ghosn SH, Kibbi AG. Cutaneous manifestations of liver diseases. Clin Dermatol 2008; 26:274–282; Lee RF, Glenn TK, Lee SS. Cardiac dysfunction in cirrhosis. Best Prac Res Clin Gas 2007; 21(1):125–140; Martinez-Lavin M. Exploring the cause of the most ancient clinical sign of medicine: finger clubbing. Semin Arthritis Rheum 2007; 36(6):380–385; McCormick PA, Murphy KM. Splenomegaly, hypersplenism and coagulation abnormalities in liver disease. Baillieres Best Pract Res Clin Gastroenterol 2000; 14(6):1009–1031; Narula HS, Carlson HE. Gynecomastia. Endocrinol Metab Clin N Am 2007; 36:497–519; Ruocco V, Psilogenis M, Schiavo AL. Dermatological manifestations of alcoholic cirrhosis. Clin Dermatol 1999; 17:463–468; Sandhu BS, Sanyal AJ. Management of ascites in cirrhosis. Clin Liv Dis 2005; 9:715–732; Sze D, Magsamen KE, McClenathan JH et al. Portal hypertensive hemorrhage from a left gastroepiploic vein caput medusa in an adhered umbilical hernia. J Vas Int Rad 2005; 16(2):281–285; Walshe JM. Foetor hepaticus. Lancet 1994; 343(8899):730; Yosipovitch G. Pruritus. Current Prob Derm 2003; 15(4):143–164.

Wilson's disease

Wilson's disease is an autosomal inherited disorder of copper metabolism resulting in the accumulation of copper in body tissues. The abnormal gene responsible for Wilson's disease was identified by three separate groups in 1993 and is located on chromosome 13.[570] Wilson's disease involves the impaired biliary excretion of copper which results in copper accumulation in the brain, liver and cornea. This excess copper results in excessive free radical damage. A striking feature of Wilson's disease is that patients will present with different clinical features; even patients within the same family present differently.[571]

Recognisable hallmarks of this disease include the presence of Kayser-Fleischer corneal rings, liver disease and neurological symptoms. Kayser-Fleischer rings are present in 95% of patients with neurological symptoms and 50–60% of patients without neurological symptoms and are not always obvious on inspection. Hepatic manifestations of Wilson's disease appear most commonly around the ages of 8 to 18 years and chronic liver disease can precede the development of neurological symptoms for years. Wilson's disease may also present similarly to chronic active hepatitis with patients reporting malaise, anorexia, fatigue and abdominal discomfort.[572]

The age at which Wilson's disease is diagnosed varies dramatically with reports ranging from 3 years to 61 years. It is considered rare, however, for Wilson's to manifest after the age of 40.[573] The clinical presentations of Wilson's also vary with age. Haemolysis is often reported between the ages of 7 and 14 years, chronic liver disease occurs around 18 years of age, and neurological symptoms can manifest between the ages of 14 and 40 with the median age 24 years. Neurological manifestations of Wilson's disease include the presence of tremor, dysarthria, headaches, dizziness, anxiety, speech and writing difficulty and convulsions.[574,575]

Haemochromatosis

Haemochromatosis is one of the most frequent genetic diseases found in white populations and affects 1 in 300 people of northern European descent. In 1996 the *HFE* gene was identified and associated with the manifestation of this disease.[576] This disease is an inherited disorder of iron metabolism and is characterised by the loading of iron into the parenchymal cells in the liver, heart and pancreas, resulting in iron overload and organ failure.

If left untreated, hereditary haemochromatosis can lead to cirrhosis, liver cancer, diabetes mellitus, cardiomyopathy, arthritis, hypopituitarism with hypogonadism and decreased life expectancy.[577] The excess iron associated with haemochromatosis generates high levels of ROS that the body's normal antioxidant defences are unable to handle. The generated ROS damage lipid membranes via the process of lipid peroxidation and as the liver attempts to repair damage to hepatocytes, fibrogenic pathways are initiated.[578]

Once hereditary haemochromatosis has been diagnosed, conventional treatment involves a course of iron depletion through twice weekly phlebotomy sessions and continued until serum ferritin levels are 50 micrograms/L. After this initial course of iron depletion, phlebotic maintenance should occur twice yearly and serum ferritin levels should remain around 50 micrograms/L.[579]

Pathogenesis

Liver fibrosis is a process characterised by nonparenchymal healing, with the replacement of damaged liver tissue with collagenous scar tissue and connective tissue. The fibrotic process is characterised by reduced activity of collagenase which is normally responsible for the degradation of fibrotic tissue. Collagen is predominantly secreted by hepatic myofibroblasts which are found in great numbers in areas of necroinflammation. These myofibroblasts secrete collagen and restrict collagenase activity.

Cirrhosis is an advanced stage of liver fibrosis and alterations in hepatic vasculature predominate. In the cirrhotic liver, myofibroblasts produce prolific extracellular matrix and this leads to central vein fibrosis, fibrous portal-tract expansion and capillarisation of the sinusoids. As a result, blood moves from the terminal portal veins and arteries to central veins and this leads to intrahepatic portal hypertension and compromised liver function. Cirrhosis can be either micronodular or macronodular. Micronodular cirrhosis presents as thin fibrotic nodules that surround regenerating hepatocytes, while in macronodular cirrhosis, fibrotic bands are thick and envelop portal tracts and hepatic venules. Fibrous septa develop in the liver as a result of angiogenesis and link the portal tracts to the central veins; these septa result in blood bypassing the lobular parenchyma. Venous occlusion also presents in cirrhosis and this leads to hypoxia and tissue ischaemia.[580,581]

COMPLICATIONS

Ascites

Ascites describes the accumulation of fluid within the peritoneal cavity. The most common cause of this condition is liver cirrhosis. However, other conditions such as cardiac failure, pancreatitis, malignancy and tuberculosis can also cause ascites.[582] Ascites develops as a result of portal hypertension, hypoalbuminaemia, the retention of sodium in the renal system and lymphatic congestion. Uncomplicated ascites is graded according to the severity of the presentation. Grade 1 ascites is mild and only detectable with the use of imaging studies. Grade 2 ascites involves moderate abdominal distension and grade 3 ascites involves severe abdominal distension.[583,584]

SIGNS AND SYMPTOMS OF DECOMPENSATED CIRRHOSIS

Portal hypertension

Portal hypertension describes an abnormal build-up of blood in the portal venous system as hepatic blood flow is

TABLE 11.10 Stages of hepatic encephalopathy

Stage	Symptom
1	Mild confusion, untidiness, slurred speech, irritability, reversal of sleep rhythm
2	Drowsiness, lethargy, personality changes, inappropriate behaviour, disorientation, lack of sphincter control
3	Inability to perform mental tasks, amnesia, fits of rage, confusion and incoherent speech
4	Coma

MacMath TL, Pons PT. Hepatic encephalopathy. J Emerg Med 1985; 3:401–407.

obstructed by fibrotic tissue. This build-up results from both an increase in intrahepatic vascular resistance and an increase in portal venous flow. Vascular resistance results from fibrotic architectural distortions and increased venous flow results from increased plasma volumes and hyperdynamic circulation. Portal hypertension is responsible for the migration from the preclinical to the more sinister state of clinical cirrhosis as it is a mechanism that contributes to the formation of both ascites and hepatic encephalopathy. As a result of the increased portal pressure, new blood vessels form; oesophageal varices represent the most important vessels as rupture results in a medical emergency and hospitalisation.[585]

Hepatic encephalopathy

There have been a number of theories presented to describe the aetiology and pathogenesis of hepatic encephalopathy (HE). However, the ammonia hypothesis remains the most reported theory.[586] Ammonia is usually produced in the gastrointestinal tract from the breakdown of proteins (amino, amino acids, purines and urea). Hyperammonaemia in cirrhosis is believed to promote the accumulation of glutamine in the astrocytes causing them to swell and altering neuropsychology.[587]

The GABA hypothesis suggests that in HE, GABA crosses the blood–brain barrier in patients with cirrhosis and increases natural benzodiazepines, interacts with ammonia and potentiates inhibitory postsynaptic potential.[588] The pathophysiology of HE is undoubtedly multifactorial as several neurotoxic compounds have been implicated in the pathogenesis of HE. Ammonia, benzodiazepines, inflammatory cytokines and neurosteroids are all thought to target the GABA-A receptor complex and promote symptoms of HE in cirrhosis patients.[589] Table 11.10 outlines the stages of hepatic encephalopathy development.

Hepatic osteodystrophy

Hepatic osteodystrophy (HO) is metabolic bone disease that can occur as a complication of liver disease and is often overlooked.[492] In a small study, 21 patients (29.2%) had normal bone mineral density (BMD) while 51 (70.8%) had low BMD. Of the 51 patients with low BMD, 36 (70.6%) had osteopenia and 15 (29.4%) had osteoporosis. Vitamin D levels and severity of liver disease were correlated with BMD.[491,492] Patients suspected of HO should be tested for BMD and vitamin D status and questioned about adequate dietary intake and weightbearing exercise.

DIFFERENTIAL DIAGNOSIS

Because of the progression from hepatitis infection to fibrosis, cirrhosis and eventual hepatocarcinoma (HCC) a differential diagnosis is essential to elicit the stage of disease progression. Cirrhosis needs to be differentially diagnosed from HCC so that the most effective conventional and complementary treatment can be administered. High serum concentrations of alpha-fetoprotein (AFP) may be indicative of HCC but AFP has a low diagnostic sensitivity and thus its use in early diagnosis is not favoured.[590] Although it would be rare for a patient to present with undiagnosed cirrhosis, the presence of ascites, hepatomegaly and varices needs to be identified and the patient referred for conventional diagnosis.

NATUROPATHIC DIAGNOSIS

Iridology

As with most other hepatobiliary conditions, the realm of iridology does not extend to the medical diagnosis of conditions or disease states. However, signs in the iris can present and direct a practitioner towards constitutional susceptibility and chronicity of any condition. Generally speaking, the presentation of iris signs will rely heavily on the chronicity and severity of the condition. A clinical study undertaken at the Bexel Irina Asian Hospital reported the most common iris signs in hepatobiliary conditions. Hardware and software used in this study were adapted to the dark, pigment-saturated type of irises of Asian people. The most common iris signs in hepatobiliary conditions were pigmentation of the autonomic nerve wreath, changes in the right iris between 7.30 and 8.10, a constricted autonomic nerve wreath in the liver region of the right iris and heterochromia.[591]

Nail analysis

Nail analysis in cirrhosis is important and is not limited to the realm of naturopathy alone as several nail signs form part of orthodox diagnosis of cirrhosis. Terry's nails were first reported in 1955[592] and display as white or the colour of ground glass and are due to connective tissue build-up and reduced vascularity of the nail bed.[593] Finger clubbing results from the release of vascular endothelial growth factor (VEGF) at distal points (fingers). VEGF is induced by hypoxia and produces vascular hyperplasia, oedema and proliferation of fibroblasts and osteoblasts.[594] Beau's lines may present with any condition where systemic metabolism and growth are interrupted. These lines can be a useful indicator for both clinical and subclinical signs of malnutrition.

For the most part, patients will present to a naturopath with a preexisting hepatobiliary diagnosis, thus nail signs become interesting confirmations of clinical pathology. Patients presenting with nail signs without a current medical diagnosis should be referred back to a general practitioner.

Tongue analysis

Tongue abnormalities associated with cirrhosis were first documented in the literature in 1957[595] and a characteristic swollen tongue with tooth imprints was reported. Practitioners are urged to consider the mouth during naturopathic assessment as cirrhosis can result in haemorrhagic changes, jaundiced mucosal tissues and gingival bleeding[596] within the oral cavity. Gustatory function is also impaired in cases of cirrhosis[597] and nutritional deficiencies may result in glossitis and cheilitis. Chronic disease states may also result in lowered immune function and opportunistic oral *Candida* infection. The smell of cigarettes or alcohol on the patient's breath are important clinical signs and should be addressed as a matter of urgency as the development of mouth or pharynx cancer is influenced by smoking, drinking and the presence of preexisting liver cirrhosis.[598]

Investigations

If cirrhosis is suspected, an initial evaluation of liver function will be completed. This evaluation should include a full blood count (particularly platelets) and a liver function test (serum bilirubin, aspartate aminotransferase (AST), alanine amino transferase (ALT), alkaline phosphatase (ALP), serum albumin and prothrombin time). When cirrhosis develops, liver tests may reveal impaired organ function causing low serum albumin, high globulins and raised serum bilirubin. Coagulation studies will reveal prolonged prothrombin time. Full blood count will reveal a decline in platelet count indicating progressive liver disease. Additionally, regular monitoring every 6 months of the liver tumour marker, alfa fetoprotein (AFP), is imperative in cirrhotics.

The interpretation of these tests is vital in the ongoing management of cirrhotic patients. It is important to ensure that the cirrhotic patient is reviewed by a hepatologist and monitored by their general practitioner in addition to naturopathic care. Table 11.11 outlines common findings through general laboratory markers in suspected cirrhosis patients.

TABLE 11.11 Common findings in suspected cirrhosis

Finding	Explanation
↑ ALT	Located in cytosol of hepatocytes, serum levels of ALT increase with liver damage
AST>ALT	Higher ratio used as a diagnostic tool for identifying cirrhosis in HCV patients and cirrhosis in general. Note that cirrhosis can exist in the presence of normal or near-normal transaminase levels
↑ Globulins	Failure of the liver to degrade immunoglobulins and shunting of blood carrying antigens to lymph tissue
↑ Bilirubin	Damaged hepatocytes cannot excrete bilirubin
↓ Albumin	Albumin is synthesised only in hepatocytes thus cirrhotic hepatic damage will result in decreased albumin synthesis
↓ Platelets	Due to splenic sequestration of platelets, reduced platelet production in bone marrow, reduced activity of thrombopoietin (TPO), increased pooling of platelets in spleen due to portal hypertension and increased destruction of platelets within the spleen
↑ Prothrombin time	Vitamin K dependent clotting factors are synthesised in the liver thus reducing prothrombin results in increased clotting time
AFP	AFP levels increase in presence of HCC

Afdhal N, McHutchison J, Brown R et al. Thrombocytopenia associated with chronic liver disease. J Hepatol 2008; 48:1000–1007; Li D, Mallory T, Satomura S. AFP-L3: a new generation of tumor marker for hepatocellular carcinoma. Clin Chimica Acta 2001; 313:15–19; Sheth SG, Flamm SL, Gordon FD et al. AST/ALT ratio predicts cirrhosis in patients with chronic hepatitis C virus infection. Am J Gastroenterol 1998; 93:44–48; Triger DR, Wright R. Hyperglobulinaemia is liver disease Lancet 1973; 301:1494–1496.

SPECIFIC NATUROPATHIC INVESTIGATIONS

There are no specific naturopathic investigations available to practitioners that bring any insight that cannot be deduced from good case taking skills. A functional liver detoxification profile (FLDP) may be of benefit, however, if cirrhosis is present: it is safe to assume that both Phase I and Phase II detoxification pathways will be impaired.

Clinicians are advised to pay particular attention to the manifestations of cirrhosis and monitor them closely. Assessing the patient's BMI will allow for the tracking and progression of cachexia. However, care should be taken if ascites is present as this will seemingly improve a patient's BMI. The patient's hair and nails should be assessed for signs of serious protein deficiency.

Clinicians are encouraged to make every reasonable effort to obtain the data needed to track the sequelae of disease progression. It is, however, important to remember that the patient may have been subjected to numerous invasive procedures during the course of conventional treatment, thus the clinician is urged to use discretion and common sense. Overall, naturopathic clinicians are advised to assess the patient holistically. The wellbeing of the patient should be considered at all times and suggestions and treatments should be offered to provide solutions to problems and not to verify evidence of disease progression that has already been determined through conventional methods.

Therapeutic considerations

CLINICAL DECISION MAKING AND RATIONALE

Although conventional medicine offers support for the treatment and management of cirrhotic complications, there is a distinct lack of conventional treatments available to patients that focus on repairing and protecting the liver once cirrhosis is present. Due to the risk of cirrhosis progressing to HCC, naturopathic treatment is important to minimise disease progression, improve liver function and improve the patient's quality of life.

The treatment of hepatitis centres on the need to minimise and prevent tissue damage from inflammation that promotes the progression of more sinister sequelae. Naturopathic treatment focuses on the protection of healthy hepatocytes and the repair of damaged hepatocytes. This is perhaps one of the more exciting ways that herbal medicine can be used as once liver cells are damaged, conventional medicine offers little in the way of treatment options designed to protect healthy and repair damaged hepatocytes.

Therapeutic application

HISTORICAL PERSPECTIVE

Nail clubbing and hepatic encephalopathy are two clinical manifestations of liver cirrhosis. However, they are not recent discoveries. Clubbing is regarded as the oldest clinical sign in medicine[594] and hepatic encephalopathy was noted in the literature in 1893 when Pavlov described the 'meat intoxication syndrome'. Researchers in Pavlov's team identified a causal relationship between the shunting of blood from the portal vein into the vena cava via the liver and the inability of the liver to metabolise ammonia. They identified increases in arterial blood ammonia levels in dogs after protein consumption and associated this with behavioural disturbances.[586]

NATUROPATHIC PERSPECTIVE

In the first instance, the cause of cirrhosis needs to be identified and appropriate naturopathic treatment strategies should be implemented. Factors associated with disease progression such as cigarette smoking, alcohol consumption and hepatitis infection need to be addressed. If relevant, treatment for any metabolic dysfunction is also highly indicated due to the links between NAFLD, metabolic syndrome and diabetes with cirrhosis. Symptomatic treatment is also highly indicated and will help to improve significantly the patient's qualify of life. Damage to the liver results in significant macronutrient and micronutrient deficiencies and ensuring patients receive adequate nutrition through the naturopathic diet is perhaps one of the simplest yet most rewarding approaches to treating the cirrhosis patient.

The treatment of cirrhosis requires the following considerations:

- Assess the case presentation and refer the patient for a diagnosis if one has not been provided
- Request copies of all laboratory investigations and imaging studies so that progress can be monitored and communication with general practitioners can be concise and precise
- Identify any possible contraindications for treatment
- Address the cause of cirrhosis and take steps to modify aetiological impact
- Reduce inflammation and fibrogenesis damage so as to limit sequelae to more severe pathology
- Address associated symptoms of cirrhosis — fatigue, depression, pruritus, gastrointestinal dysfunction, nausea
- Support optimal liver function through repair and protection of hepatocytes — improve organ integrity and function
- Provide dietary and lifestyle options which reduce discomfort and improve quality of life
- Address dietary and lifestyle concerns and limit any risk factors that hinder or obstruct the healing process.

NUTRITIONAL MEDICINE (DIETARY)

The role of dietary treatment and management of cirrhosis centres on preventing malnutrition.

The prevalence of malnutrition in cases of cirrhosis is well reported and protein calorie malnutrition (PCM) is common. Mechanisms for the malnutrition associated with cirrhosis include poor dietary intake due to loss of taste, unpalatable recommended diets, nausea and early satiety or infrequent feeding in hospital settings.[599]

There are several factors specifically associated with the process of malnutrition in cirrhosis. Glycogen stores and the process of gluconeogenesis is decreased in cirrhosis[600] and thus energy metabolism shifts from carbohydrate metabolism to fat oxidation. Insulin resistance is noted in both skeletal muscle and hepatocytes[601] and protein metabolism is impaired with protein requirements increasing due to decreased absorption and synthesis and increased degradation of protein. Low glycogen stores result in the use of body proteins in the process of gluconeogenesis and skeletal muscle degradation is increased and this results in muscle wasting.[602]

These processes are all amplified by hypermetabolism that significantly raises energy requirements and results in malnutrition if requirements are not met. Hypermetabolism is characterised by increased resting energy expenditure (REE)[603] and hypermetabolism in cirrhosis is well documented in the literature. The aetiology of hypermetabolism is unclear; however, it has been suggested as an extra-hepatic manifestation of chronic liver disease.[604] Malnutrition is an independent risk factor implicated in the long-term survival of cirrhosis patients[605] and the treatment of any patient with end-stage liver disease must involve significant dietary adjustment.

Dietary modification can limit the toxic load placed on the liver by poor food choices and it can improve the nutritional deficiencies that result from compromised liver functioning by making wise food choices. Dietary management must also take into account the patient's comfort levels and, in addition to improving the compromised nutritional status, must make eating and digestion nutritionally and emotionally rewarding.

Dietary therapeutic objectives

See 'Hepatobiliary nutritional objectives (dietary)' for an overview.

- Assess nutritional status and improve deficiencies in nutrient status with wise and manageable food choices
- Increase consumption of anti-inflammatory, bitter and raw foods to optimise liver function
- Support lipid metabolism and stabilise blood sugar levels if indicated

- Support optimal digestive and GIT function at all stages of disease progression
- Ensure a wide variety of food choices that are tasty, interesting and inspiring; the patient has enough to worry about. Tasteless food and a diet that centres on unnecessary restrictions are not the keys to healing
- Avoid alcohol as it promotes hepatocyte death and begin supplementation with vegetable juices
- Avoid food that places unnecessary stress on the liver (fats, sugars, additives and preservatives)
- Select vegetable proteins over animal proteins where possible but do not restrict protein intake as wound healing will be compromised
- Ensure dietary intake is adequate to avoid cachexia (common in cirrhosis)
- Encourage smaller, more frequent meals (five to seven per day is recommended)
- Reduce salt intake if ascites or oedema is present.

Specific dietary treatments

DIETARY INCLUSIONS

Protein

Protein is required for the synthesis of albumin, protease inhibitors, storage and iron binding proteins and coagulation factors and this occurs primarily in the liver. Protein degradation is evident even in early stages of liver disease while protein synthesis is impaired in late-stage liver disease and hepatic failure.[606] Protein energy malnutrition (PEM) is common in cirrhosis and occurs in 65–90% of cases.[607] It is usually clinically represented by reduced serum albumin levels and decreased skeletal muscle volume.

Patients with chronic liver disease present with increased concentrations of aromatic amino acids (AAAs) and decreased concentrations of branched chain amino acids (BCAAs). Amino acid supplementation with both types of amino acids is indicated in early-stage liver disease. However, late-stage disease may require supplementation with only branched chain amino acids to correct the ratio.[608,609]

Glucose production by glycogenolysis is reduced and glucose liver output is maintained by gluconeogenesis. The gluconeogenesis process drains the amino acid supply from peripheral tissues. The use of proteins for energy storage may explain the higher need for protein in cirrhosis patients.[610]

Energy and protein requirements for adults with uncomplicated cirrhosis are 100–125 kJ/kg/day and 0.8 g of protein/kg/day.[611,612] Adults with complicated cirrhosis should consume 100–170 kJ per kg of body weight per day with 1.0–1.5 g/kg protein per day to prevent muscle catabolism.[13]

Carbohydrate

Cirrhosis patients experience metabolic dysfunction characterised by insulin resistance in both the liver and muscle tissue, thus complex carbohydrates with a low glycaemic index should be chosen in the first instance. Refined carbohydrates and simple sugars should be avoided at all cost.

Vegetarian diet

The literature reports both favourable and unfavourable results[613,614] from the introduction of vegetarian diets in cirrhosis. As protein requirements in cirrhosis are high, the introduction of an unsupervised vegetarian diet that may lack essential amino acids is contraindicated. Vegetarian diets that are supervised and maintain the protein and total nutrient requirements needed to prevent malnutrition may be of use if patient compliance is high and quality of life is improved. In most cases, a diet rich in fresh vegetables and wholegrains that is predominantly vegetarian but contains high-quality protein from fish or lean turkey is recommended.

Coffee and coffee substitutes

Coffee consumption has been inversely associated with the risk of cirrhosis in several studies,[615,616] although consumption appears to be more beneficial in cases of alcoholic cirrhosis.[617] It is not clear whether the suggested hepatoprotective effects of coffee are related to caffeine or another chemical constituent.[618] The effects of coffee on the liver once decompensated cirrhosis is established have not been studied. Due to a lack of supportive data, coffee consumption should be moderated as unnecessary stresses on the liver should be avoided. Coffee substitutes like dandelion and chicory root beverages are a great alternative.

Other inclusions

Buckwheat is a nutritional food and is noted as a source of protein, lipids, vitamins and minerals. Its high rutin content results in antioxidant and capillary strengthening qualities.[619] Buckwheat is nutritious and highly digestible and should be included in the diet as a replacement for refined white flour. Buckwheat pancakes with fresh fruit are an ideal option for breakfast.

Carrots have been recognised for centuries as a liver friendly food and the hepatoprotective properties of *Daucus carota* have been noted in the literature.[620] Beetroot is another traditional food recognised for its healing properties for the liver and is a good source of the phytonutrient betaine, which has also been recognised for its hepatoprotective activity.[621] Carrots and beetroot can be grated and eaten as a salad, or juiced with green vegetables like spinach, celery, cabbage and cucumber to make liver-friendly juices. Vegetable juices are high in vitamins, minerals and antioxidant phytonutrients that are particularly beneficial in liver disease. The gentle cholagogue and choleretic action of fresh raw vegetables will also assist liver and digestive function. Oats are an extremely beneficial food as they are nutrient dense and contribute to blood sugar regulation.

DIETARY EXCLUSIONS

Sodium restriction

Patients with advanced cirrhosis have altered renal function and splanchnic circulation. These alterations result in abnormalities in extracellular fluid volume which contribute to the ascites and oedema commonly seen in cirrhosis patients. Urinary sodium excretion in cirrhosis patients can vary between 5 mEq/L and zero.[622] Some cirrhosis patients have moderately reduced urine sodium excretion and some experience severe sodium retention; with either presentation, sodium restriction is essential in the nutritional management of this condition. Patients should be discouraged from adding salt to food or consuming salt-containing electrolyte drinks. Takeaway foods need to be avoided due to their high salt content, as do soft drinks and any dehydrated foods in packets that water is added to. Patients need to be encouraged to eat food in its freshest state to avoid unnecessary salt consumption.

Salt and the human diet

The human diet was low in salt for around 5 million years; we relied on the salt that was naturally present in food to regulate fluid in our bodies. Humans started to add salt to food around 10 000 years ago. One thousand years ago salt intake in the Western diet rose to 5 g per day and in the 19th century European salt intake rose to a dramatic 18 g per day because of the consumption of salted meats. The introduction of refrigeration saw salt intake drop to around 10 g per day in the 20th century.[623] The commonly accepted level of salt consumed in Australia is 6 g of salt per day.[624] However, in a recent study using 24-hour urine collection, levels were found to be 50% higher at 9 g.[625] Foods with the highest salt content include bread, low-fibre cereals, hot dogs, sausages, savoury snack biscuits, canned soups, canned beans and spaghetti, and canned vegetables.[624] The judicious use of iodised salt may be applicable in cases of hypothyroidism.

Alcohol

The consumption of alcohol increases oxidative damage in the liver and has fibrosis-inducing effects in the presence of both hepatitis B and C. Alcohol consumption during interferon treatment may also worsen the treatment outcome.[626] A German study reported that daily intake of 80 g of alcohol was associated with a 2.3 times increased risk of death, the need for liver transplantation or cirrhosis in chronic hepatitis C patients.[627] Alcohol consumption should be completely excluded in all cases of hepatitis B, C, fibrosis and cirrhosis, and suitable alternatives like water with lime should be recommended.

NUTRITIONAL MEDICINE (SUPPLEMENTAL)

See 'Hepatobiliary nutritional objectives (nutrients)' and Table 11.5.

The role of supplemental nutritional medicine in the treatment of cirrhosis focuses on the correction of macronutrient and micronutrient deficiencies. As cirrhosis is closely linked to the metabolic syndrome, the management of blood sugar irregularities, insulin resistance and the prediabetic state is crucial. Nutritional supplements can also be introduced for their antioxidant, anti-inflammatory and antifibrotic action and will assist in the prevention of cirrhotic progression to hepatocellular carcinoma.

Nutritional medicine therapeutic objectives

- Correct macronutrient nutritional deficiencies contributing to cirrhotic malnutrition; ensure optimal protein intake
- Address micronutrient deficiencies or extra requirements as noted in the literature
- Promote optimal liver function: support detoxification, reduce inflammation, oxidation and cirrhotic progression
- Address associated metabolic syndrome picture.

Specific nutrients required

VITAMIN A

Hepatic vitamin A deficiency plays a role in hepatic fibrosis as decreased storage in hepatic stellate cells results in activation into myofibroblast-like cells and collagen synthesis.[628] Vitamin A deficiency in cirrhosis is also linked to an increased risk of HCC.[629]

VITAMIN E

Vitamin E is an important lipid-soluble antioxidant and inhibits lipid peroxidation. Decreased levels of vitamin E have been noted in chronic HCV infection, are inversely associated with fibrosis and have been noted in cirrhosis.[630]

ZINC

Poor zinc status is common in cirrhosis; low plasma levels reflect whole body deficiency.[631] Supplementation improves glucose and protein metabolism, appetite, membrane integrity, sensation of taste and immune function.[632]

SELENIUM

Selenium deficiencies have been reported in patients with hepatocellular injury and cirrhosis and deficiency may accelerate liver damage by decreasing the effect of glutathione peroxidase. Low selenium levels are also linked to carcinoma.[633]

PROBIOTICS

Bacterial infections are common complaints in patients with cirrhosis[634] and are associated with hepatic encephalopathy.[635] Compromised gut integrity has been linked to repeated bacterial infections in cirrhosis and altered gut microflora has been implicated in the pathogenesis of cirrhotic complications.[636] Probiotic supplementation is recommended to reduce the incidence of bacterial infection. Furthermore, the butyric acid resulting from probiotics is enormously beneficial for fatty liver.

BRANCHED CHAIN AMINO ACIDS

Cirrhotic patients present with high levels of aromatic amino acids (AAA) (tryptophan, phenylalanine and tyrosine) and low levels of branched chain amino acids (BCAA) (valine, isoleucine and leucine). BCAA supplementation corrects alterations in amino acid ratios, thus reducing malnutrition, and may improve hepatic encephalopathy.[612] Dosage recommendation is to take

SAMPLE DAILY DIET

BREAKFAST	
Beetroot, carrot and parsley juice Fruit salad with live yoghurt and natural muesli	Beetroot has been shown to be a hepatoprotective. Carrots are a rich source of beta-carotene which has been shown to reduce inflammation and oxidative stress, key features in cirrhosis. Fruit provides anti-inflammatory and antioxidant constituents while home-made muesli provides a source of fibre and B vitamins, the latter of which may be low due to insufficient storage by the compromised liver.
SNACKS	
Brazil nuts	Brazil nuts are a source of minerals. Selenium and zinc have been found to be low in individuals with liver disease, with levels being most profoundly decreased in patients with decompensated cirrhosis.
LUNCH	
Pumpkin, sweet potato and red lentil soup. Serve with a slice of sodium-reduced bread topped with tahini and avocado	Cirrhotic patients are almost always on a low-sodium diet if they have ascites, thus herbs and spices should be used to flavour food in place of sodium. Soups can be prepared without stock, using sweet vegetables such as sweet potato and pumpkin for flavour.
DINNER	
Herb-crusted John Dory served with steamed vegetables topped with pumpkin seeds	Fish provides a source of protein. Cirrhotic patients need adequate protein intake to prevent muscle wasting and catabolism. Zinc supplementation has resulted in improvements in liver functional reserve, hepatic encephalopathy and general nutritional status in individuals with cirrhosis, thus zinc-rich foods such as fish and pumpkin seeds should be encouraged.

Bémeur C, Butterworth RF. Nutrition in the management of cirrhosis and its neurological complications. J Clin Experiment Hepatol 2014; 4(2):141–150. Hammerich L, Tacke F. Eat more carrots? Dampening cell death in ethanol-induced liver fibrosis by β-carotene. Hepatobil Surg Nutr 2013; 2(5):248–251. Kujawska M, Ignatowicz E, Murias M et al. Protective effect of red beetroot against carbon tetrachloride- and N-nitrosodiethylamine-induced oxidative stress in rats. J Agric Food Chem 2009; 57(6):2570–2575. McClain CJ. Nutrition in patients with cirrhosis. Gastroenterol Hepatol 2016; 12(8):507–510. Somi MH, Rezaeifar P, Rahimi AO et al. Effects of low dose zinc supplementation on biochemical markers in non-alcoholic cirrhosis: a randomized clinical trial. Archives of Iranian Medicine 2012; 15(8):472–476. Thandassery RB, Montano-Loza AJ. Role of nutrition and muscle in cirrhosis. Curr Treat Options Gastroenterol 2016; 14(2):257–273.

either mixed combinations of amino acid formulations or individual amino acids at a minimum of 500 mg per amino acid per day. Ideally this is best supplemented with a late evening snack (see below).

OTHER CONSIDERATIONS

The addition of a late evening snack (LES) high in branched chain amino acids (BCAAs) is recommended for cirrhosis patients to improve energy malnutrition, correct amino acid imbalances and improve glucose tolerance.[637,638] BCAAs are found in all protein-containing foods, and eggs, poultry, meat and milk have significant BCAA content. Because of the high saturated fat content of such foods and the burden on the digestive system, it is advisable to use a BCAA supplement as a late evening snack in most instances.

Magnesium

Studies have shown that patients with cirrhosis have decreased total body magnesium levels due to poor absorption in the small intestine, enhanced urinary excretion and malnutrition.[639,640] Magnesium deficiency may play a role in the muscle cramps associated with cirrhosis and low magnesium levels also play a role in the development of insulin resistance.

Omega-3 fatty acids

Fish oils may also assist with cachexia associated with cirrhosis.

Dosage requirements

- Vitamin A: 2500 IU daily
- Vitamin E: 1000 IU daily
- Zinc: 25–50 mg daily
- Selenium: 150–400 micrograms daily
- Probiotics: 25–50 × 10^9 organisms per day
- Branched chain amino acids: 500 mg per amino acid per day
- Magnesium: 300 mg daily (divided doses for maximal absorption recommended)
- Omega-3 fatty acids: 6 g daily total fish oil content with a minimum of 600 mg EPA and 400 mg DHA.

HERBAL MEDICINE

Herbal medicine therapeutic objectives

- Reduce hepatic inflammation, oxidation and fibrosis
- Protect liver cells from damage and encourage the repair of damaged hepatocytes; improve overall liver function
- Improve appetite, support digestion and reduce associated nausea
- Support underlying metabolic disturbances: address the metabolic picture associated with end-stage liver disease
- Address depression, fatigue, sleep difficulties and any associated mental confusion/poor memory.

Herbal medicine classes

The use of herbal medicine in the treatment of cirrhosis centres on the need to reduce hepatic inflammation and fibrosis, protect hepatocytes and restore function to damaged hepatocytes, protect the liver from carcinogenesis, improve the metabolic state associated with the condition and support overall liver health. As treatment for established cirrhosis is limited, herbal medicines have much to offer.

Hepatobiliary antioxidant and anti-inflammatory herbal medicines will protect the liver from inflammation, oxidation and tissue necrosis and thus slow the progression from fibrosis to cirrhosis and eventual carcinoma. Herbal medicines that inhibit fibrogenesis play a key role in the reduction of this progression and are a priority. Herbal medicines that temper digestive disturbances are also indicated and carminatives, bitters, choleretics and cholagogues are indicated. The metabolic picture can also be addressed with specific herbal medicines.

As alcohol consumption is contraindicated in cirrhosis, tablet preparations of herbal medicines are preferred. However, the amount of alcohol in herbal tinctures and fluid extracts per dose is minimal and may be used in some cirrhotic patients.

Specific herbal medicines

SILYBUM MARIANUM (ST MARY'S THISTLE)

Silymarin is the collective name for the group of flavonolignans responsible for the hepatoprotective properties of *Silybum marianum*. *Silybum marianum* (milk thistle, St Mary's thistle) has been studied as an antioxidant, antifibrotic and anti-inflammatory agent both in animal models[641,642] and in humans.[643,644] Silybum is noted for its ability to scavenge and regulate the intracellular content of the antioxidant glutathione. Its ability to stabilise cell membranes and prevent toxins from entering hepatocytes has been reported, as has its ability to stimulate hepatocyte regeneration. One study[645] reported significant increases in survival in cirrhosis patients after daily administration of silymarin over 41 months compared with controls.

Silybum marianum is useful in the treatment and prevention of fibrosis and cirrhosis as it has demonstrated ability to inhibit the transformation of hepatic stellate cells (HSCs) into myofibroblasts in vitro, thereby potentially preventing the development of hepatic fibrosis. *Silybum marianum* is also indicated in the treatment of cirrhosis owing to its favourable activity on blood sugar regulation in diabetes and insulin resistance.[646]

SALVIA MILTIORRHIZA (DAN SHEN)

Salvia miltiorrhiza is a traditional Chinese medicine used to reduce blood stasis and improve circulation. Its effects on chronic liver disease have been researched in both in vivo and in vitro animal studies.[647,648] *Salvia miltiorrhiza* inhibits the activation and proliferation of hepatic stellate cells (HSCs) due to the activity of the constituents, protocatechuic aldehyde and salvianolic acid B.[649]

CENTELLA ASIATICA (GOTU KOLA)

Centella asiatica is a traditional Ayurvedic herbal medicine used to treat a wide range of indications. Studies in the late 1970s originally revealed the potential for the use of *Centella* in the prevention and treatment of liver cirrhosis.[650] More recent animal studies reveal *Centella asiatica* has a significant anti-liver fibrosis effect.[651] and can be used to treat drug-induced hepatic oxidative damage.[652] Such studies confirm traditional knowledge that observes both antifibrotic and fibrinolytic activity. *Centella asiatica* is also noted for its adaptogenic and nervine tonic activity,[653] which makes it a useful tonic for the cirrhosis patient who is suffering fatigue and depression.

SCUTELLARIA BAICALENSIS (BAIKAL SKULLCAP)

Scutellaria baicalensis is a traditional Chinese herbal medicine renowned for its anti-inflammatory and antioxidant activity.[654] Antifibrotic activity has been reported with one study[655] reporting that *Scutellaria baicalensis* inhibits liver fibrosis induced by bile duct ligation or carbon tetrachloride in rats. *Scutellaria baicalensis* has been noted for its hepatoprotective activity[656,657] and the Japanese herbal formula TJ-9 containing *Scutellaria baicalensis* and *Glycyrrhiza glabra* has a favourable effect on interleukin 12 production in hepatitis C-induced liver cirrhosis.[658] *Scutellaria* has potential as a botanical treatment for cirrhosis owing to its documented anticancer activity via its ability to inhibit human hepatoma cell lines.[659]

OTHER HERBAL CONSIDERATIONS

Apium graveolens (celery seed) and *Taraxacum officinale* (dandelion) taken as a gentle diuretic tea may assist with fluid build-up associated with ascites and oedema. *Camellia sinensis* (green tea) has been shown to protect the liver against drug-induced cirrhosis[660] and its antioxidant properties make it an essential herbal medicine that can be taken as a tea or as a tablet in combination with other herbal medicines like *Vitis vinifera* (grape seed), *Rosmarinus officinalis* (rosemary) and *Curcuma longa* (turmeric).

LIFESTYLE RECOMMENDATIONS

Any activity that adds insult and contributes to further toxic injury of the liver should be avoided at all cost. Spray paints, garden chemicals, glues, cleaning chemicals, room and bathroom air fresheners should all be avoided. Alcohol consumption and cigarette smoking are contraindicated at all times. Exercise will help regulate blood sugar, improve blood flow to the liver and assist with the management of stress or depression.

REFERENCES

[1] Jakoby WB. Detoxication: conjugation and hydrolysis. In: Arias IM, Jakoby WB, Popper H, et al, editors. The liver: biology & pathobiology. New York: Raven Press; 1988. p. 375–88.

[2] Grant DM. Detoxification pathways in the liver. J Inher Metab Dis 1991;14:421–30.

[3] Guengerich FP. Influence of nutrients and other dietary materials on cytochrome P-450 enzymes. Am J Clin Nut 1995;61(S3):651S–658S.

[4] Ingelman-Sundberg M, Rodriguez-Antona C. Pharmacogenetics of drug metabolizing enzymes: implications for a safer and more effective drug therapy. Philos Trans R Soc Lond B Biol Sci 2005;360:1563–70.

[5] Long A, Walker JD. Quantitative structure-activity relationships for predicting metabolism and modeling cytochrome p450 enzyme activities. Environ Toxicol Chem 2003;22(8):1894–9.

[6] Bymaster FP, Chao P, Schulze H, et al. Biopharmaceutical characterization, metabolism, and brain penetration of the triple reuptake inhibitor amitifadine. Drug metabolism letters. 2013;7(1):23–33.

[7] Li T, Chiang JYL. Rifampicin induction of CYP3A4 requires PXR crosstalk with HNF4α and co-activators, and suppression of SHP gene expression. Drug Metab Dispos 2006;34(5): 756–64.

[8] He N, Edeki T. The inhibitory effects of herbal components on CYP2C9 and CYP3A4 catalytic activities in human liver microsomes. Am J Ther 2004;11(3):206–12.

[9] Liska D, Lyon M, Jones DS. Detoxification and biotransformational imbalances. Explore 2006;2(2):122–40.

[10] Kiani J, Imam SZ. Medicinal importance of grapefruit juice and its interaction with various drugs. Nutr J 2007;6:33.

[11] Braun L. Drug interactions and complementary medicines: the evidence and mythology. International Evidence-Based Complementary Medicine Conference. Armidale, NSW, Australia: University of New England; 2009. p. 13–15.

[12] Pinninti NR, Mago R, de Leon J. Coffee, cigarettes and meds: what are the metabolic effects? Psychiatric Times 2005;22(6).

[13] Eghtesad S, Poustchi H, Malekzadeh R. Malnutrition in liver cirrhosis: the influence of protein and sodium. Middle East J Dig Dis 2013;5(2):65–75.

[14] Johnson TM, Overgard EB, Cohen AE, et al. Nutrition assessment and management in advanced liver disease. Nutr Clin Pract 2013;28(1):15–29.

[15] Bashir S, Lipman TO. Nutrition in gastroenterology and hepatology. Gastroenterology 2001;28(3):629–45.

[16] Fuhrman MP, Charney P, Mueller CM. Hepatic proteins and nutrition assessment. J Am Diet Assoc 2004;104(8):1258–64.

[17] Sulaberidze G, Okujava M, Liluashvili K, et al. Dietary fiber's benefit for gallstone disease prevention during rapid weight loss in obese patients. Georgian Med News 2014;231:95–9.

[18] Yasutake K, Kohjima M, Kotoh K, et al. Dietary habits and behaviors associated with nonalcoholic fatty liver disease. World J Gastroenterol 2014;20(7):1756–67.

[19] Gutteridge JM. Lipid peroxidation and antioxidants as biomarkers of tissue damage. Clin Chem 1995;41:1819–28.

[20] Boivin D, Lamy S, Dufour-Lord S, et al. Antiproliferative and antioxidant activities of common vegetables: a comparative study. Food Chem 2009;112:374–80.

[21] Suri S, Taylor MA, Verity A, et al. A comparative study of the effects of quercetin and its glucuronide and sulfate metabolites on human neutrophil function in vitro. Biol Pharm Bull 2008;76:645–53.

[22] Peterson J, Dwyer J. Flavonoids: dietary occurrence and biochemical activity. Nut Res 1998;18(12):1995–2018.

[23] Kaur G, Tirkey N, Chopra K. Beneficial effect of hesperidin on lipopolysaccharide-induced hepatotoxicity. Toxicology 2006;226:152–60.

[24] Middleton E. Effect of plant flavonoids on immune and inflammatory cell function. Adv Exp Med Biol 1998;439:175–82.

[25] Galvano F, La Fauci L, Lazzarino G, et al. Cyanidins: metabolism and biological properties. J Nut Biochem 2004;15:2–11.

[26] Youdim KA, McDonald J, Kalt W, et al. Potential role of dietary flavonoids in reducing microvascular endothelium vulnerability to oxidative and inflammatory insults. J Nut Biochem 2002;13:282–8.

[27] Eslamparast T, Eghtesad S, Poustchi H, et al. Recent advances in dietary supplementation, in treating non-alcoholic fatty liver disease. World J Hepatol 2015;7(2):204–12.

[28] Alvarez JA, Ashraf A. Role of vitamin D in insulin secretion and insulin sensitivity for glucose homeostasis. Inter J Endocrinol 2010;351–85.

[29] Eliades M, Spyrou E, Vitamin D. a new player in non-alcoholic fatty liver disease? World J Gastroenterol 2015;21(6):1718–27.

[30] Paolella G, Mandato C, Pierri L, et al. Gut–liver axis and probiotics: their role in non-alcoholic fatty liver disease. World J Gastroenterol 2014;20(42):15518–31.

[31] Leung C, Rivera L, Furness JB, et al. The role of the gut microbiota in NAFLD. Nat Rev Gastroenterol Hepatol 2016;13(7):412–25.

[32] Machado MV, Cortez-Pinto H. Diet, microbiota, obesity, and NAFLD: a dangerous quartet. Inter J Mol Sci 2016;17(4):481.

[33] Miele L, Valenza V, La Torre G, et al. Increased intestinal permeability and tight junction alterations in nonalcoholic fatty liver disease. Hepatology 2009;49(6):1877–87.

[34] Fromenty B, Pessayre D. Inhibition of mitochondrial beta oxidation as a mechanism of hepatotoxicity. Pharmacol Ther 1995;67:101–54.

[35] Luyckx FH, Lefebvre PJ, Scheen AJ. Non-alcoholic steatohepatitis: association with obesity and insulin resistance, and influence of weight loss. Diabetes Metab 2000;26:98–106.

[36] Martensson J. The effect of fasting on leukocycte and plasma glutathione and sulfur amino acids concentrations. Hepatology 1997;25:943–9.

[37] James OFW, Day CP. Nonalcoholic steatohepatitis (NASH): a disease of emerging identity and importance. J Hepatol 1998;29:495–501.

[38] Bemeur C, Butterworth RF. Reprint of: Nutrition in the management of cirrhosis and its neurological complications. J Clin Exp Hepatol 2015;5(Suppl. 1):S131–40.

[39] Ahmed-Belkacem A, Ahnou N, Barbotte L, et al. Silibinin and related compounds are direct inhibitors of hepatitis C virus RNA-dependent RNA polymerase. Gastroenterology 2010;138(3):1112–22.

[40] Polyak SJ, Morishima C, Shuhart MC, et al. Inhibition of T-cell inflammatory cytokines, hepatocyte NF-kappaB signaling, and HCV infection by standardized silymarin. Gastroenterology 2007;132(5):1925–36.

[41] Bonifaz V, Shan Y, Lambrecht RW, et al. Effects of silymarin on hepatitis C virus and haem oxygenase-1 gene expression in human hepatoma cells. Liver Int 2009;29(3):366–73.

[42] Wagoner J, Negash A, Kane OJ, et al. Multiple effects of silymarin on the hepatitis C virus lifecycle. Hepatology 2010;51(6):1912–21.

[43] Pincus MR, Tierno PM, Gleeson E, et al. Evaluation of liver function. In: Henry's clinical diagnosis and management by laboratory methods. 23rd ed. Elsevier; 2017. p. 289–305e3.

[44] Burke MD. Liver function: test selection and interpretation of results. Clin Lab Med 2002;22:377–90.

[45] Bhagavan NV. Enzymes III clinical applications. In: Medical biochemistry. Edinburgh: Academic Press; 2002. p. 121–32.

[46] Jacobson K, Witt-Sullivan HB. Interpreting abnormalities in routine liver biochemistry. Can Fam Physician 1992;561–6.

[47] Knight JA. Liver function tests: their role in the diagnosis of the hepatobiliary diseases. J Infus Nurs 2005;28(2):108–14.

[48] Kunutsor SK. Gamma-glutamyltransferase: friend or foe within? Liver Int 2016;36(12):1723–34.

[49] Pratt DS. Liver chemistry and function tests. In: Sleisenger and Fordtran's gastrointestinal and liver disease. 10th ed. Elsevier; 2016. p. 1243–1253e2.

[50] Pagana KD, Pagana TJ. Mosby's manual of diagnostic and laboratory tests. 2nd ed. St Louis: Mosby; 2002.
[51] Dufour DR, Lott JA, Nolte FE, et al. Diagnosis and monitoring of hepatic injury: recommendations for use of laboratory tests in screening, diagnosis and monitoring. Clin Chem 2000;46:2050–68.
[52] Hugenholtz GCC, Porte RTJ, Lisman T. The platelet and platelet function testing in liver disease. Clin Liver Dis 2009;13:11–20.
[53] Hoefs JC, Chen PT, Lizotte P. Noninvasive evaluation of liver disease severity. Clin Liver Dis 2006;10:535–62.
[54] Durand F, Valla D. Assessment of the prognosis of cirrhosis: Child–Pugh versus MELD. J Hepatol 2005;42:S100–7.
[55] Cuomo O, Perrella A. Arenga G. Model for end-stage liver disease (MELD) score system to evaluate patients with viral hepatitis on the waiting list: better than the Child–Turcotte–Pugh (CTP) system? Transplant Proc 2008;40:1906–9.
[56] Calès P, Boursier J, Oberti F, et al. FibroMeters: a family of blood tests for liver fibrosis. Gastroenterol Clin Biol 2008;32(6):40–51.
[57] Mikolasevic I, Orlic L, Franjic N, et al. Transient elastography (FibroScan®) with controlled attenuation parameter in the assessment of liver steatosis and fibrosis in patients with nonalcoholic fatty liver disease — where do we stand? World J Gastroenterol 2016;22(32):7236–51.
[58] Castera L, Forns X, Alberti A. Non-invasive evaluation of liver fibrosis using transient elastography. J Hepatol 2008;48:835–47.
[59] Jung KS, Kim SU. Clinical applications of transient elastography. Clin Mol Hepatol 2012;18(2):163–73.
[60] Shaheen AA, Wan AF, Myers RP. FibroTest and FibroScan for the prediction of hepatitis c related fibrosis: a systematic review of diagnostic test accuracy. Am J Gastroenterol 2007;102:2589–600.
[61] Enomoto M, Morikawa H, Tamori A, et al. Noninvasive assessment of liver fibrosis in patients with chronic hepatitis B. World J Gastroenterol 2014;20(34):12031–8.
[62] Lupsor Platon M, Stefanescu H, Feier D, et al. Performance of unidimensional transient elastography in staging chronic hepatitis C. Results from a cohort of 1202 biopsied patients from one single center. J Gastrointest Liver Dis 2013;22(2):157–66.
[63] Lukaczer D. Functional assessment of liver phase I and II detoxification. In: Pizzorno JE, Murray MT, editors. Textbook of natural medicine, vol. 1. 2nd ed. Edinburgh: Churchill Livingstone; 1999.
[64] Durantel D, Zoulim F. New antiviral targets for innovative treatment concepts for hepatitis B virus and hepatitis delta virus. J Hepatol 2016;64(1 Suppl.):S117–31.
[65] Tacke F, Kroy DC. Treatment for hepatitis B in patients with drug resistance. Ann Transl Med 2016;4(18):334.
[66] Wang YJ, Yang L, Zuo JP. Recent developments in antivirals against hepatitis B virus. Virus Res 2016;213:205–13.
[67] Wang HL, Lu X, Yang X, et al. Antiviral therapy in lamivudine-resistant chronic hepatitis B patients: a systematic review and network meta-analysis. Gastroenterol Res Pract 2016;2016:3435965.
[68] Tong S, Revill P. Overview of hepatitis B viral replication and genetic variability. J Hepatol 2016;64(1 Suppl.):S4–16.
[69] Ioannou GN, Beste LA, Chang MF, et al. Effectiveness of sofosbuvir, ledipasvir/sofosbuvir, or paritaprevir/ritonavir/ombitasvir and dasabuvir regimens for treatment of patients with hepatitis C in the Veterans Affairs National Health Care System. Gastroenterology 2016;151(3):457–471e5.
[70] Bertino G, Ardiri A, Proiti M, et al. Chronic hepatitis C: this and the new era of treatment. World J Hepatol 2016;8(2):92–106.
[71] Pawlotsky JM. NS5A inhibitors in the treatment of hepatitis C. J Hepatol 2013;59(2):375–82.
[72] Banerjee D, Reddy KR. Review article: safety and tolerability of direct-acting anti-viral agents in the new era of hepatitis C therapy. Aliment Pharmacol Ther 2016;43(6):674–96.
[73] Renard S, Borentain P, Salaun E, et al. Severe pulmonary arterial hypertension in patients treated for hepatitis C with sofosbuvir. Chest 2016;149(3):e69–73.
[74] Stedman C. Sofosbuvir, a NS5B polymerase inhibitor in the treatment of hepatitis C: a review of its clinical potential. Ther Adv Gastroenterol 2014;7(3):131–40.
[75] Asselah T, Thompson AJ, Flisiak R, et al. A predictive model for selecting patients with HCV genotype 3 chronic infection with a high probability of sustained virological response to peginterferon alfa-2a/ribavirin. PLoS ONE 2016;11(3):e0150569.
[76] Petersen J, Thompson AJ, Levrero M. Aiming for cure in HBV and HDV infection. J Hepatol 2016;65(4):835–48.
[77] Dalton HR, Kamar N. Treatment of hepatitis E virus. Curr Opin Infect Dis 2016;29(6):639–44.
[78] Almasio NL, Cottone C, D'Angelo F. Pegylated interferon therapy in chronic hepatitis C: lights and shadows of an innovative treatment. Dig Liv Dis 2007;39(Suppl. 1):S88–95.
[79] Wang YS, Youngster S, Grace M, et al. Structural and biological characterization of pegylated recombinant interferon alpha-2b and its therapeutic implications. Adv Drug Deliv Rev 2002;54:547–70.
[80] Nette T. Bear gallbladders to sell to not to sell. Wildlife Division. Nova Scotia, Canada: Department of Natural Resources; 2000.
[81] Lazaridis KN, Gores GJ, Lindor KD. Ursodeoxycholic acid mechanisms of action and clinical use in hepatobiliary disorders. J Hepatol 2001;35:134–46.
[82] Stokes CS, Gluud LL, Casper M, et al. Ursodeoxycholic acid and diets higher in fat prevent gallbladder stones during weight loss: a meta-analysis of randomized controlled trials. Clin Gastroenterol Hepatol 2014;12(7):1090–1100 e2. quiz e61.
[83] Krawczyk M, Miquel JF, Stokes CS, et al. Genetics of biliary lithiasis from an ethnic perspective. Clin Res Hepatol Gastroenterol 2013;37(2):119–25.
[84] Shaffer EA. Epidemiology of gallbladder stone disease. Best Pract Res Clin Gastroenterol 2006;20(6):981–96.
[85] Kalloo AN, Kantsevoy SV. Gallstones and biliary disease. Prim Care 2001;28(3):591–606.
[86] Weiss KM, Ferrell RE, Hanis CL, et al. Genetics and epidemiology of gallbladder disease in New World native peoples. Am J Hum Genet 1984;36(6):1259–78.
[87] Lammert F, Miquel JF. Gallstone disease: from genes to evidence based theory. J Hepatol 2008;48:S124–35.
[88] Sampliner RE, Bennett PH, Comess LJ. Gallbladder disease in Pima Indians: demonstration of high prevalence and early onset by cholecystography. N Engl J Med 1970;283:1358–64.
[89] Katsika D, Grjibovski A, Lammert F, et al. Genetic and environmental influences for gallstone disease related diagnoses: a Swedish twin study of 43,141 twin pairs. Hepatology 2005;41(5):1138–43.
[90] Shabanzadeh DM, Sorensen LT, Jorgensen T. Determinants for gallstone formation — a new data cohort study and a systematic review with meta-analysis. Scand J Gastroenterol 2016;51(10):1239–48.
[91] Grünhage F, Lammert F. Pathogenesis of gallstones: a genetic perspective. Best Pract Res Clin Gastroenterol 2006;20(6): 997–1015.
[92] Donovan JM. Physical and metabolic factors in gallstone pathogenesis. Gastroenterol Clin North Am 1999;28(1):75–97.
[93] Toouli J, Wright TA. Gallstones. Med J Aust 1998;169(3):166–71.
[94] Lee JY, Keane MG, Pereira S. Diagnosis and treatment of gallstone disease. Practitioner 2015;259(1783):15–19, 2.
[95] Vitek L, Carey MC. New pathophysiological concepts underlying pathogenesis of pigment gallstones. Clin Res Hepatol Gastroenterol 2012;36(2):122–9.
[96] Portincasa P, Moschetta A, Palasciano G. Cholesterol gallstone disease. Lancet 2006;368:230–9.
[97] Lin IC, Yang YW, Wu MF, et al. The association of metabolic syndrome and its factors with gallstone disease. BMC Fam Pract 2014;15:138.
[98] Cuevas A, Miquel JF, Soledad Reyes M, et al. Diet as a risk factor for cholesterol gallstone disease. J Am Coll Nutr 2004;23(3):187–96.
[99] Mendez-Sanchez N, Zamora-Valdes D, Chavez-Tapia NC, et al. Role of diet in cholesterol gallstone formation. Clin Chimica Acta 2007;376:1–8.
[100] Radmard AR, Merat S, Kooraki S, et al. Gallstone disease and obesity: a population-based study on abdominal fat distribution and gender differences. Ann Hepatol 2015;14(5):702–9.
[101] Tsai C, Leitzmann MF, Willett WC, et al. Weight cycling and risk of gallstone disease in men. Arch Intern Med 2006;166:2369–74.
[102] Tsai C, Leitzmann MF, Willett WC, et al. Glycemic load, glycemic index and carbohydrate intake in relation to risk of cholecystectomy in women. Gastroenterology 2005;129:105–12.
[103] De Santis A, Attili AF, Corradini SG, et al. Gallstones and diabetes: A case-control study in a free–living population sample. Hepatology 2003;25(4):787–90.

[104] Fazio S, Linton MF. The role of fibrates in managing hyperlipidaemia: mechanisms of action and clinical efficacy. Current Atheroscler Rep 2004;6(2):148–57.
[105] Grundy SM, Vega GL. Fibric acids: Effects on lipids and lipoprotein metabolism. Am J Med 1987;83(Suppl. 5B):9–20.
[106] Akin ML, Uluutku H, Erenoglu C, et al. Tamoxifen and gallstone formation in postmenopausal breast cancer patients: retrospective cohort study. World J Surg 2003;27:395–9.
[107] Heaton KW, Emmett PM, Symes CL, et al. An explanation for gallstones in normal weight women: slow intestinal transit. Lancet 1993;341:8–10.
[108] Fox JG, Dewhirst FE, Shen Z, et al. Hepatic *Helicobacter* species identified in bile and gallbladder tissue from Chileans with chronic cholecystitis. Gastroenterology 1998;114(4):755–63.
[109] Maurer KJ, Ihrig MM, Rogers AB, et al. Identification of cholelithogenic enterohepatic *Helicobacter* species and their role in murine cholesterol gallstone formation. Gastroenterology 2005;128:1023–33.
[110] Pandey M. *Helicobacter* species are associated with possible increase in risk of biliary lithiasis and benign biliary diseases. World J Surg Oncol 2007;5(94).
[111] Zhang FM, Yu CH, Chen HT, et al. *Helicobacter pylori* infection is associated with gallstones: epidemiological survey in China. World J Gastroenterol 2015;21(29):8912–19.
[112] Jonkers IJAM, Smelt AHM, Ledeboer M, et al. Gallbladder lowering therapy by bezafibrate and fish oil. Gut 2003;52:109–15.
[113] Chuang SC, Hsi E, Lee KT. Mucin genes in gallstone disease. Clin Chim Acta 2012;413(19–20):1466–71.
[114] Donovan JM. Pathogenesis of gallstones. In: Feldman M, LaRusso NF, editors. Gastroenterology and hepatology: the comprehensive visual reference. St Louis: Mosby; 1997.
[115] Portincasa P, Moschetta A, Petruzzelli M, et al. Symptoms and diagnosis of gallbladder stones. Best Pract Res Clin Gastroenterol 2006;20(6):1017–29.
[116] Malik AH, Malet P. Complications of cholelithiasis. In: Johnson LR, editor. Encyclopedia of gastroenterology. Edinburgh: Elsevier; 2003. p. 326–33.
[117] Jensen B. The science and practice of iridology, vol. 1. Escondido (CA): Bernard Jensen International; 1952.
[118] Hall D. Iridology: personality and health analysis through the iris. Melbourne (VIC): Nelson; 1980.
[119] Maciocia G. Tongue diagnosis in Chinese medicine. Rev ed. Seattle: Eastland Press; 1997.
[120] Choi EH, Lee N, Kim HJ, et al. *Schisandra fructus* extract ameliorates doxorubicin-induced cardiomycytes: altered gene expression for detoxification enzymes. Genes Nutr 2008;2:337–45.
[121] Houdart R, Perniceni T, Darne B, et al. Predicting colon bile duct lithiasis: determination and prospective validation of a model predicting low risk. Am J Surg 1995;170:38–43.
[122] Glenn F. Biliary tract disease since antiquity. Bull N Y Acad Med 1971;47(4):329–50.
[123] Gordon-Taylor G. On gallstones and their sufferers. Brit J Surg 1937;98(XXV):241–51.
[124] Moran S, Uribe M, Prado ME. Effects of fiber administration in the prevention of gallstones in obese patients on a reducing diet: a clinical trial. Rev Gastroenterol Mex 1997;62:266–72.
[125] Marcus SN, Heaton KW. Effects of a new, concentrated wheat fibre preparation in intestinal transit, deoxycholic acid metabolism and the composition of bile. Gut 1986;27:893–900.
[126] Gerhardt AL, Gallo NB. Full-fat rice bran and oat bran similarly reduce hypercholesterolemia in humans. J Nut 1998;128(5):865–9.
[127] Marlett JA, Hosig KB, Vollendorf NW, et al. Mechanism of serum cholesterol reduction by oat bran. Hepatol 1994;20(6):1450–7.
[128] Breneman JC. Allergy elimination diet as the most effective gallbladder diet. Ann Allergy 1968;26:83–7.
[129] Tsai C, Leitzmann MF, Willett WC, et al. Weight cycling and risk of gallstone disease in men. Arch Intern Med 2006;166:2369–76.
[130] Simon JA, Hudes ES. Serum ascorbic acid and gallbladder disease prevalence among US adults; the third national health and nutrition examination survey (NHANES III). Arch Int Med 2000;160:931–6.
[131] Mendez-Sanchez N, Gonzalez V, Aguayo P, et al. Fish oil (n-3) polyunsaturated fatty acids beneficially affect biliary cholesterol nucleation time in obese women losing weight. J Nutr 2001;131:2300–3.
[132] Tsai C, Leitzmann MF, Willett WC, et al. Long-term intake of trans-fatty acids and risk of gallstone disease in men. Arch Intern Med 2005;165:1011–15.
[133] Misciagna G, Centonze S, Leoci C, et al. Diet, physical activity and gallstones: a population based case controlled study in southern Italy. Am J Clinic Nutr 1999;69:120–6.
[134] Mathur A, Megan M, Al-Azzawi HH, et al. High dietary carbohydrates decrease gallbladder volume and enhance cholesterol crystal formation. Surgery 2007;141:654–9.
[135] Jamison J. Clinical guide to nutrition and dietary supplements in disease management. Edinburgh: Elsevier; 2003.
[136] Den Besten L, Connor WE, Bell S. The effect of dietary cholesterol on the composition of human bile. Surgery 1973;73:266–73.
[137] Dam H, Prange I, Jensen MK, et al. Studies on human bile: IV influence of ingestion of cholesterol in the form of eggs on the composition of bile in healthy subjects. Z Ernaehrungswiss 1971;10:178–87. [abstract cited].
[138] Lee DWT, Gilmore CJ, Bonorris G, et al. Effect of dietary cholesterol on biliary lipids in patients with gallstones and normal subjects. Am J Clin Nut 1985;42:412–20.
[139] Tuchweber B, Yousef IM, Ferland G, et al. Nutrition and bile formation. Nutr Res 1996;16(6):1041–80.
[140] Murray KP, Shin JH, Fox-Talbot MK, et al. Iron deficiency promotes cholesterol gallstone formation. Gastroenterology 1998;114(S1):A1307.
[141] Johnston SM, Murray KP, Martin SA, et al. Iron deficiency enhances cholesterol gallstone formation. Surgery 1997;122(2):354–62.
[142] Hall D. The natural health book. Melbourne (VIC): Nelson; 1976.
[143] Pitchford P. Healing with whole foods: Asian traditions and modern nutrition. 3rd ed. Berkeley (CA): North Atlantic Books; 2002.
[144] Higdon J. An evidence based approach to vitamins and minerals: health benefits and intake recommendations. New York: Thieme; 2003.
[145] Rajagopalan N, Lindenbaum S. The binding of Ca2+ to taurine and glycine conjugated bile salt micelles. Biochim et Biophys Acta 1982;711:66–74.
[146] Hafknscheid JCM, Hectors MPC. An enzymic method for the determination of the glycine/taurine ratio of conjugated bile acids in bile. Clin Chim Acta 1975;65:67–74.
[147] Segasothy M, Phillips PA. Vegetarian diet: panacea for modern lifestyle diseases? QJM 1999;92(9):531–44.
[148] Wu T, Zhang Z, Liu B, et al. Gut microbiota dysbiosis and bacterial community assembly associated with cholesterol gallstones in large-scale study. BMC Genom 2013;14:669.
[149] Gebhardt R. Anticholestatic activity of flavonoids from artichoke (*Cynara scolymus* L.) and of their metabolites. Med Sci Monit 2001;7(Suppl. 1):316–20.
[150] Vidyashankar S, Sambaiah K, Srinivasan K. Dietary garlic and onion reduce the incidence of atherogenic diet-induced cholesterol gallstones in experimental mice. Br J Nutr 2009;101(11):1621–9.
[151] Vidyashankar S, Sambaiah K, Srinivasan K. Regression of preestablished cholesterol gallstones by dietary garlic and onion in experimental mice. Metabolism 2010;59(10):1402–12.
[152] Toouli J, Jablonksi P, Watts JMcK. Dissolution of human gallstones: the efficacy of bile salt, bile salt plus lecithin and heparin solutions. J Surg Res 1975;19:47–53.
[153] Toouli J, Jabonski P, Watts JMcK. Gallstone dissolution in man using cholic acid and lecithin. Lancet 1975;306(7945):1124–6.
[154] Tuzhilin T. Treatment of patients with gallstones by lecithin. Am J Gastro 1976;65(3):231–5.
[155] Andrews WS, Pau CML, Chase P, et al. Fat soluble vitamin deficiency in biliary atresia. J Pediatr Surg 1981;16(3):284–90.
[156] Weiss RFW. Weiss's herbal medicine, classic edition. Stuttgart: Thieme; 2001.
[157] Mills SY. The essential book of herbal medicine. London: Arkana; 1991.
[158] Bartram T. Bartram's encyclopedia of herbal medicine. London: Robinson; 1998.
[159] Bohm K. Studies on the choleretic action of some drugs. Arzneim Forsch 1959;9:376–8.
[160] Jeon HJ, Kang HJ, Jung HJ, et al. Anti-inflammatory activity of *Taraxacum officinale*. J Ethnopharmacol 2008;115:82–8.

[161] Kirchhoff R, Beckers C, Kirchhoff GM, et al. Increase in choleresis by means of an artichoke extract. Phytomed 1994;1:107–15.
[162] Held C. Tagungsbericht con der. Deutschungarischen Phytopharmakon-Konferenxe. Budapest. 20 November 1991. Z Klin Med 1992;47:92–3. [abstract cited].
[163] Bundy R, Walker AF, Middleton RW, et al. Artichoke leaf extract (*Cynara scolymus*) reduces plasma cholesterol in otherwise healthy hypercholesterolemic adults: a randomized, double blind placebo controlled trial. Phytomed 2008;15:668–75.
[164] Srinivasan K, Sambalah K. The effect of spices on cholesterol 7 alpha-hydroxylase activity and on serum and hepatic cholesterol levels in the rat. Int J Vitamin Nutr Res 1991;61(4):364–9.
[165] Rasyid A, Lelo A. The effect of curcumin and placebo on human gall-bladder function: an ultrasound study. Aliment Pharmacol Ther 1999;13:245–9.
[166] Raysid A, Rashid A, Rahman ARA, et al. Effect of different curcumin dosages on human gall bladder. Asia Pac J Nut 2002;11(4):314–18.
[167] Marker RE, Turner DL. Sterols. CXV. Sapogenins. XLIV. The relation between diosgenin and cholesterol. J Am Chem Soc 1941;63(3):767–71.
[168] Oakenfull D, Sidhu GS. Could saponins be a useful treatment for hypercholesterolaemia? Eur J Clin Nutr 1990;44:79–88.
[169] Juarez-Oropeza MA, Diaz-Zagoya JC, Rabinowitz JL. In vivo and in vitro studies of hypocholesterolemic effects of diosgenin in rats. Int J Biochem 1987;19(8):679–83.
[170] Bartram T. Bartram's encyclopedia of herbal medicine. London: Robinson Publishing; 1998.
[171] O'Brien P, Carrasco-Pozo C, Speisky H. Boldine and its antioxidant or health-promoting properties. Chem Biol Interact 2006;159(1):1–17.
[172] Lanhers MC, Joyeux M, Soulimani R, et al. Hepatoprotective and anti-inflammatory effects of a traditional medicinal plant of Chile, *Peumus boldus*. Planta Med 1991;57(2):110–15.
[173] Kringstein P, Cederbaum AI. Boldine prevents human liver microsomal lipid peroxidation and inactivation of cytochrome P4502E1. Free Radic Biol Med 1995;18(3):559–63.
[174] Leitzmann MF, et al. Recreational physical activity and the risk of cholecystectomy in women. New Engl J Med 1999;341(11):777–84.
[175] Al Disi SS, Anwar MA, Eid AH. Anti-hypertensive herbs and their mechanisms of action: Part I. Front Pharmacol 2015;6:323.
[176] O'Grady JG, Lake JR, Howdle PD. Comprehensive clinical hepatology. London: Mosby Harcourt; 2000.
[177] Guyton AC. Textbook of medical physiology. 8th ed. Philadelphia: WB Saunders; 1991.
[178] Yokoyama S. Release of cellular cholesterol: molecular mechanism of cholesterol homeostastis in cells and in the body. Biochim et Biophys Acta 2000;1529:231–44.
[179] Yokayama S. HDL biogenesis and cellular cholesterol homeostasis. Ann Med 2008;40(S1):29–38.
[180] Friedman GD. Natural history of asymptomatic and symptomatic gallstones. Am J Surg 1993;165:399–404.
[181] Monson JRT, Duthie G, O'Malley K. Surgical emergencies. Edinburgh: Blackwell Science; 1999. p. 123.
[182] Chen LE, Haplin V, Whinney R. Acute cholecystitis. BMJ Clin Evid 2007;12:411.
[183] Ko CW, Lee SP. Gastrointestinal disorders of the critically ill. Biliary sludge and cholecystitis. Best Pract Res Clin Gastroenterol 2003;17(3):383–96.
[184] Ko CW, Lee SP. Gastrointestinal disorders of the critically ill. Biliary sludge and cholecystitis. Best Pract Res Clin Gastroenterol 2003;17(3):383–96.
[185] Indar AA, Beckingham IJ. Acute cholecystitis. BMJ 2002;325:639–43.
[186] Laria C, Arena L, Di Maio G, et al. Acute acalculous cholecystitis during the course of primary Epstein Barr virus infection: a new case and a review of the literature. Int J Infect Dis 2008;12:391–5.
[187] Prassoulia A, Panagiotoua J, Vakakib M, et al. Acute acalculous cholecystitis as the initial presentation of primary Epstein-Barr virus infection. J Ped Surg 2007;42:E11–13.
[188] Swisher SG, Schmit DJ, Hunt KK. Biliary disease during pregnancy. Am J Surg 1994;168:576.
[189] Ramin KD, Ramsey PS. Disease of the gallbladder and pancreas in pregnancy. Obstet Gynaecol Clin North Am 2001;28(3):571–80.
[190] Sharp HT. Gastrointestinal surgical conditions during pregnancy. Clin Obstet Gynecol 1994;37:306.
[191] Howard R. Acute acalculous cholecystitis. Am J Surg 1981;141:194.
[192] Brandt WE. Liver, biliary tree and gallbladder. In: Brandt WE, Helms CA, editors. Fundamentals of diagnostic radiology. 3rd ed. Lippincott Williams & Wilkins; 2007. p. 756–81.
[193] Apostolov E, Al-Soud WA, Nilsson I, et al. *Helicobacter pylori* and other *Helicobacter* species in gallbladder and liver of patients with chronic cholecystitis detected by immunological and molecular methods. Scand J Gastroenterol 2005;40(1):96–102.
[194] Chen DF, Hu L, Yi P, et al. *H. pylori* are associated with chronic cholecystitis. World J Gastroenterol 2007;13(7):1119–22.
[195] Pandey M, Shukla M. *Helicobacte*r species are associated with possible increase in risk of hepatobiliary tract cancers. Surg Oncol 2009;18(1):51–6.
[196] Jagannath SB, Singh KB, Cruz-Correa M, et al. A long-term cohort study of outcome after cholecystectomy for chronic acalculous cholecystitis. Am J Surg 2003;185:91–5.
[197] Thornell E, Jivegard L, Bukhave K, et al. Prostaglandin E2 formation by the gall bladder in experimental cholecystitis. Gut 1986;27:370–3.
[198] Hansel DE, Maitra A, Argani P. Pathology of the gallbladder: a concise review. Curr Diag Path 2004;10:304–17.
[199] Sharan F. Iridology. A complete guide to diagnosing through the iris and to related forms of treatment. Wellingborough: Thorsons Publishing Group; 1989.
[200] Gandolfi L, Torresan F, Solmi L, et al. The role of ultrasound in biliary and pancreatic disease. Eur J Ultrasound 2003;16:141–59.
[201] Yuso IF, Barkun JS, Barkun AN. Diagnosis and management of cholecystitis and cholangitis. Gastroenterol Clin N Am 2003;32:1145–68.
[202] Park MS, Yu JS, Kim YH, et al. Acute cholecystitis: comparison of MR cholangiography and US. Radiology 1998;209:781–5.
[203] Roe J. Clinical assessment of acute cholecystitis in adults. Ann Emerg Med 2006;48:101–3.
[204] Gruber PJ, Silverman RA, Gottesfeld S, et al. Presence of fever and leukocytosis in acute cholecystitis. Ann Emerg Med 1996;28:273–7.
[205] Rauws EAJ, Gouma DJ. Endoscopic and surgical management of bile duct injury after laparoscopic cholecystectomy. Best Pract Res Clin Gastroenterol 2004;18(5):820–46.
[206] Hale LP, Greer PK, Sempowski GD. Bromelain treatment alters leucocyte expression of cell surface molecules involved in cellular adhesion and activation. Cell Clin Immunol 2002;104(2):183–90.
[207] Maurer HR. Bromelain: biochemistry, pharmacology and medical use. Cell Mol Life Sci 2001;58(9):1234–45.
[208] Mozaffarian D, Pischon T, Hankinson SE, et al. Dietary intake of trans fatty acids and systemic inflammation in women. Am J Clin Nutr 2004;79(4):606–12.
[209] Kierstein S, Krytska K, Kierstein G, et al. Sugar consumption increases susceptibility to allergic airway inflammation and activates the innate immune system in the lung. J Allergy Clin Immunol 2008;121(2):S196.
[210] Schulze MB, Hoffmann K, Manson JE, et al. Dietary pattern, inflammation, and incidence of type 2 diabetes in women. Am J Clin Nutr 2005;82:675–84.
[211] Lopez-Garcia E, Schulze MB, Fung TT, et al. Major dietary patterns are related to plasma concentrations of markers of inflammation and endothelial dysfunction. Am J Clin Nutr 2004;80:1029–35.
[212] Gaby AR. Nutritional approaches to prevention and treatment of gallstones. Altern Med Rev 2009;14(3):258–67.
[213] Vidyashankar S, Sambaiah K, Srinivasan K. Dietary garlic and onion reduce the incidence of atherogenic diet-induced cholesterol gallstones in experimental mice. Br J Nutr 2009;101(11):1621–9.
[214] Kim YJ, Kim HJ, No JK, et al. Anti-inflammatory action of dietary fish oil and calorie restriction. Life Sci 2006;78(21):2523–32.
[215] Comalada M, Camuesco D, Saleta S, et al. In vivo quercitrin anti-inflammatory effect involves release of quercetin, which inhibits inflammation through down-regulation of the NF-KB pathway. Eur J Immunol 2005;35(2):584–92.
[216] Kim HP, Son KH, Chang H, et al. Anti-inflammatory plant flavonoids and cellular action mechanisms. J Pharmacol Sci 2004;96:229–45.
[217] Lee ES, Lee HE, Shin JY, et al. The flavonoid quercetin inhibits dimethylnitrosamine-induced liver damage in rats. J Pharm Pharmacol 2003;55:1169–74.
[218] Cushnie TP, Lamb AJ. Antimicrobial activity of flavonoids. Int J Antimicrob Agents 2005;26:343–56.

[219] Kim H, Kong H, Choi B, et al. Metabolic and pharmacological properties of rutin, a dietary quercetin glycoside, for treatment of inflammatory bowel disease. Pharm Res 2005;22(9):1499–509.
[220] Yang J, Guo J, Yuan J. In vitro antioxidant properties of rutin. LWT 2008;41:1060–6.
[221] Zielinska-Przyjemska M, Ignatowicz E. Citrus fruit flavonoids influence on neutrophil apoptosis and oxidative metabolism. Phytother Res 2008;22(12):1557–698.
[222] Son IS, Kim JH, Sohn HY, et al. Antioxidative and hypolipidemic effects of diosgenin, a steroidal saponin of yam (*Dioscorea* spp.), on high-cholesterol fed rats. Biosci Biotechnol Biochem 2007;71(12):3063–71.
[223] Yamaguchi Am Tazuma S, Ochi H, Chayama K. Choleretic action of diosgenin is based upon the increases in canalicular membrane fluidity and transporter activity mediating bile acid independent bile flow. Hepatol Res 2003;25(3):287–95.
[224] Bhandari MR, Kawabata J. Organic acid, phenolic content and antioxidant activity of wild yam (*Dioscorea* spp.) tubers. Nepal Food Chemistry 2004;88:163–8.
[225] Farombi EO, Britton G, Emerole G. Evaluation of antioxidant activity and partial characterisation of extracts from browned yam flour diet. Food Res Intern 2000;33:493–9.
[226] Accatino L, Pizarro M, Solis N. Effects of diosgenin, a plant-derived steroid, on bile secretion and hepatocellular cholestasis induced by estrogens in the rat. Hepatology 1998;28(1):129–40.
[227] Grieve M. A modern herbal. London: Jonathan Cape; 1979.
[228] Speroni R, Cervellati R, Govoni P, et al. Efficacy of different *Cynara scolymus* preparations on liver complaints. J Ethnopharmacol 2003;86:203–11.
[229] Aktay G, Delioman D, Ergun E, et al. Hepatoprotective effects of Turkish folk remedies on experimental liver injury. J Ethnopharmacol 2000;73:121–9.
[230] Holtmann G, Adam B, Haag S, et al. Efficacy of artichoke leaf extract in the treatment of patients with functional dyspepsia: a six-week placebo-controlled, double-blind, multicentre trial. Aliment Pharmacol Ther 2003;18:1099–105.
[231] Kraft K. Artichoke leaf extract: recent findings reflecting effects on lipid metabolism, liver, and gastrointestinal tracts. Phytomedicine 1997;4(4):369–78.
[232] Lopez-Molina D, Navarro-Martinez MD, Melgarejo FR, et al. Molecular properties and prebiotic effect of inulin obtained from artichoke (*Cynara scolymus* L.). Phytochemistry 2005;66:1476–84.
[233] Teitelbaum JE, Walker WA. Nutritional impact of pre and probiotics as protective gastrointestinal organisms. Ann Rev Nutr 2002;22:107–38.
[234] Monograph, *Matricaria chamomilla* (German chamomile). Alt Med Rev 2008;13(1):58–62.
[235] Ammon HPT, Kelber O, Okpanyi SN. Spasmolytic and tonic effect of Iberogast (STW 5) in intestinal smooth muscle. Phytomedicine 2006;13:SV67–74.
[236] Heinle H, Hagelauer D, Pascht U, et al. Intestinal spasmolytic effects of STW 5 (Iberogast) and its components. Phytomedicine 2006;13:75–9.
[237] Kelber O, Wittwew A, Lapke C, et al. Ex vivo/in vitro absorption of STW 5 (Iberogast) and its extract components. Phytomedicine 2006;13:107–13, SV.
[238] Schempp H, Weiser D, Kelber O, et al. Radical scavenging and anti-inflammatory properties of STW 5 (Iberogast) and its components. Phytomedicine 2006;13:SV36–44.
[239] Isetts BJ. Valerian. In: Tracy TS, Kingston RL, editors. Herbal products: toxicology and clinical pharmacology. 2nd ed. Totowa (NJ: Humana Press; 2007.
[240] Hazlelhoff B, Malingré TM, Meijer DK. Antispasmodic effects of valeriana compounds: an in-vivo and in-vitro study on the guinea-pig ileum. Arch Int Pharmacodyn Ther 1982;257(2): 274–87.
[241] Hoffman D. Complete illustrated guide to the holistic herbal. Dorset: Element Books; 1996.
[242] Oppenheimer A. Turmeric (curcumin) in biliary diseases. Lancet 1937;229:619–21.
[243] Coon JT, Ernst E. Herbal medicinal products for non-ulcer dyspepsia. Aliment Pharmacol Ther 2002;16(10):1689–99.
[244] Strimpakos AS, Sharma R. Curcumin: Preventative and therapeutic properties in laboratory studies and clinical trials. Antioxid Redox Signal 2008;10(3):511–35.
[245] Araujo CAC, Leon LL. Biological activities of *Curcuma longa*. Mem Inst Oswaldo Cruz 2001;96(5):723–8.
[246] Hemming JM, Guarraci FA, Firth TA, et al. Actions of histamine on muscle and ganglia of the guinea pig gallbladder. Am J Physiol 2000;279:G622–30.
[247] Moga MM. Alternative treatment of gallbladder disease. Med Hypotheses 2003;60(1):143–7.
[248] Kim HP, Son KH, Chang HW, et al. Anti-inflammatory plant flavonoids and cellular action mechanisms. J Pharmacol Sci 2004;96:229–45.
[249] Musso G, Gambino R, Cassader M. Recent insights into hepatic lipid metabolism in non-alcoholic fatty liver disease (NAFLD). Prog Lipid Res 2009;48:1–626.
[250] Ong JP, Pitts A, Younoss ZM. Increased overall mortality and liver related mortality in non-alcoholic fatty liver disease. J Hepatol 2008;49:608–12.
[251] Fazel Y, Koenig AB, Sayiner M, et al. Epidemiology and natural history of non-alcoholic fatty liver disease. Metab Clin Exp 2016;65(8):1017–25.
[252] Adams LA, Lindor KD. Nonalcoholic fatty liver disease. AEP 2007;17(11):863–9.
[253] Cave M, Deaciuc I, Mendez C, et al. Nonalcoholic fatty liver disease: predisposing factors and the role of nutrition. J Nut Bio 2007;18:184–95.
[254] de Alwis NMW, Day CP. Non-alcoholic fatty liver disease: the mist gradually clears. J Hepatol 2008;48:S104–12.
[255] Bondini S, Kleiner DE, Goodman Z, et al. Pathologic assessment of non-alcoholic liver disease. Clin Liv Dis 2007;11:17–23.
[256] Abdelmalek MF, Diehl AM. Nonalcoholic fatty liver disease as a complication of insulin resistance. Med Clin N Am 2007;91:1125–49.
[257] Samuel VT, Liu Z, Qu X, et al. Mechanism of hepatic insulin resistance in non alcoholic fatty liver disease. J Biol Chem 2004;279:32345–53.
[258] Marra F, Gastaldelli A, Baroni GS, et al. Molecular basis and mechanism of progression of non-alcoholic steatohepatitis. Trends Mol Med 2007;14(2):72–81.
[259] Girard J, Lafontan M. Impact of visceral adipose tissue on liver metabolism and insulin resistance. Part II: Visceral adipose tissue production and liver metabolism. Diabetes Metab 2008;34(5):439–45.
[260] Targer G, Bertolini L, Padovani R, et al. Relation of nonalcoholic steatohepatitis to early carotid atherosclerosis in healthy men: role of visceral fat accumulation. Diab Care 2004;27:2498–500.
[261] Loria P, Lonardo A, Bellentani S, et al. Non-alcoholic fatty liver disease (NAFLD) and cardiovascular disease: an open question. Nut Metab Cardio Dis 2007;17:684–98.
[262] Targher G. Non-alcoholic fatty liver disease as a determinant of cardiovascular disease. Atherosclerosis 2007;190:18–19.
[263] Johnson RJ, Segal M, Sautin Y, et al. Potential role of sugar (fructose) in the epidemic of hypertension, obesity/metabolic syndrome, diabetes, kidney disease and cardiovascular disease. Am J Clin Nutr 2007;86:899–906.
[264] Mayes PA. Intermediary metabolism of fructose. Am J Clin Nutr 1993;58:753S–65S.
[265] Ouyang X, Ciriloo P, Sautin Y, et al. Fructose consumption as a risk factor for non-alcoholic fatty liver disease. J Hepatol 2008;48:993–9.
[266] Goodman ZD, Ishak KG. Histopathology of hepatitis C virus infection. Semin Liv Dis 1995;15:70–81.
[267] Harrison SA. Insulin resistance among patients with chronic hepatitis C: aetiology and impact on treatment. Clin Gastroenterol Hepatol 2008;6(8):864–76.
[268] Rubbia-Brandt L, Quadri R, Abid K, et al. Hepatocyte steatosis is a cytopathic effect of hepatitis C genotype 3. J Hepatol 2000;33:106–15.
[269] Poustchi H, Negro F, Hui J, et al. Insulin resistance and response to therapy in patients infected with chronic hepatitis C virus genotypes 2 and 3. J Hepatol 2008;48:28–34.
[270] Adinolfi LE, Rinaldi L, Guerrera B, et al. NAFLD and NASH in HCV infection: prevalence and significance in hepatic and extrahepatic manifestations. Int J Mol Sci 2016;17(6).
[271] Cheung O, Sanyal AJ. Hepatitis C infection and nonalcoholic fatty liver disease. Clin Liv Dis 2008;12:573–85.
[272] Castera L, Hezode C, Roudot-Thoraval F, et al. Effect of anti-viral treatment of the evolution of liver steatosis in patients with

chronic hepatitis C: indirect evidence of a role of hepatitis C virus genotype 3 in steatosis. Gut 2004;53:406–12.
[273] Bjornsson E, Angula P. Hepatitis C and steatosis. Arch Med Res 2007;38:621–7.
[274] Lonardo A, Carani C, Carulli N, et al. 'Endocrine NAFLD' a hormonocentric perspective of non-alcoholic fatty liver disease pathogenesis. J Hepatol 2006;44:1196–207.
[275] Adams LA, Feldestein A, Lindor KD, et al. Nonalcoholic fatty liver disease among patients with hypothalamic and pituitary dysfunction. Hepatology 2004;39(4):909–14.
[276] Cerda C, Perez-Ayuso RM, Riquelme A, et al. Non alcoholic fatty liver disease in women with polycystic ovarian syndrome. J Hepatol 2007;47:412–17.
[277] Setji T, Holland N, Sanders L, et al. Non-alcoholic steatohepatitis and non-alcholic fatty liver disease in young women with polycystic ovarian syndrome. J Clin Endocrinol Metab 2006;91:1741–7.
[278] Michailov A, Kuneva T, Popov T. A comparative assessment of liver function in workers in the petroleum industry. Int Arch Occup Environ 1998;71:S46–9.
[279] Barberino JL, Carvahlo FM, Silvany-Neto AM, et al. Liver changes in workers at an oil refinery and in a reference population in the state of Bahia. Brazil Pan American J Pub Health 2005;17(1):30–7.
[280] Scorletti E, Byrne CD. Extrahepatic diseases and NAFLD: the triangular relationship between NAFLD, type 2-diabetes and dysbiosis. Dig Dis 2016;34(Suppl. 1):11–18.
[281] Boursier J, Mueller O, Barret M, et al. The severity of nonalcoholic fatty liver disease is associated with gut dysbiosis and shift in the metabolic function of the gut microbiota. Hepatology 2016;63(3):764–75.
[282] Endo H, Niioka M, Kobayashi N, et al. Butyrate-producing probiotics reduce nonalcoholic fatty liver disease progression in rats: new insight into the probiotics for the gut–liver axis. PLoS ONE 2013;8(5):e63388.
[283] Onyekwere CA, Ogbera AO, Samaila AA, et al. Nonalcoholic fatty liver disease: synopsis of current developments. Niger J Clin Pract 2015;18(6):703–12.
[284] Reddy JK, Rao MS. Lipid metabolism and liver inflammation. II. Fatty liver disease and fatty acid oxidation. Am J Physiol Gastrointest Liver Physiol 2006;290:G852–8.
[285] Diraison F, Moulin P, Beylot M. Contribution of hepatic de novo lipogenesis and reesterification of plasma non esterified fatty acids to plasma triglyceride synthesis during non-alcoholic fatty liver disease. Diabetes Metab 2003;29:478–85.
[286] Boden G. Free fatty acids (FFA), a link between obesity and insulin resistance. Front Biosci 1998;3:169–75.
[287] Seppala-Lindroos A, Vehkavaara S, Hakkinen AM, et al. Fat accumulation in the liver is associated with defects in insulin suppression of glucose production and serum free fatty acids independent of obesity in normal men. J Clin Endocrinol Metab 2002;87:3023–8.
[288] Leclercq IA, Farrell GC, Field J, et al. CYP2E1 and CYPP4a as microsomal catalysts of lipid peroxides in murine nonalcoholic steatohepatitis. J Clin Invest 2000;105:1067–75.
[289] Pessayre D, Fromenty B. NASH: a mitochondrial disease. J Hepatol 2005;42:928–40.
[290] Yuan M, Konstantopoulos N, Lee J, et al. Reversal of obesity and diet-induced insulin resistance with salicylates or targeted disruption of IKK–b. Science 2001;293:1673–7.
[291] Solga SF, Diehl AM. Non-alcoholic fatty liver disease: lumen–liver interactions and possible role for probiotics. J Hepatol 2003;38:681–7.
[292] Harrison SA, Diehl AM. Fat and the liver — a molecular overview. Sem Gastrointest Dis 2002;13:3–16.
[293] Wang YX, Wang LT, Gao YQ, et al. Epidemic survey of TCM syndrome typing and preliminary discussion on TCM etiology and pathogenesis of fatty liver. Zhongguo Zhong Xi Yi Jie He Za Zhi 2005;25(2):126–30. [Article in Chinese, abstract cited].
[294] Farrell GC, Larter CZ. Nonalcoholic fatty liver disease: from steatosis to cirrhosis. Hepatology 2006;43(2):S99–112.
[295] Adams LA, Angulo P. Role of liver biopsy and serum markers of liver fibrosis in non-alcoholic fatty liver disease. Clin Liver Dis 2007;11:25–35.
[296] Browning JD, Szczepaniak LS, Dobbins R, et al. Prevalence of hepatic steatosis in an urban population in the United States: impact of ethnicity. Hepatology 2004;40:1387–95.
[297] Trombini P, Piperno A. Ferritin, metabolic syndrome and NAFLD: Elective attractions and dangerous liaisons. J Hepatol 2007;46:549–52.
[298] Saadeh S, Younossi ZM, Remer EM, et al. The utility of radiological imaging in non-alcoholic fatty liver disease. Gastroenterology 2002;123:745–50.
[299] Toshimitsu K, Mastsuura B, Ohkubo I, et al. Dietary habits and nutrient intake of non-alcoholic steatohepatitis. Nutrition 2007;23:46–52.
[300] Westwater J, Fainer D. Liver impairment in the obese. Gastroenterology 1958;34(4):686–93.
[301] Adler M, Schaffer F. Fatty liver hepatitis and cirrhosis in obese patients. Am J Med 1979;67:811–16.
[302] Ludwig J, Viggiano TR, McGill DB, et al. Non-alcoholic steatosis. Mayo Clin Proc 1980;55:434–8.
[303] Gastrointestinal Expert Group. Therapeutic guidelines gastrointestinal version 4. North Melbourne (VIC): Therapeutic Guidelines Ltd; 2006.
[304] Angulo P. Current best treatment for non-alcoholic fatty liver disease. Expert Opin Pharmacother 2003;4:611–23.
[305] Tilg H, Diehl AM. Cytokines in alcoholic and nonalcoholic steatohepatitis. N Engl J Med 2000;343:1467–76.
[306] Morisco F, Vitaglione P, Amoruso D, et al. Foods and liver health. Mol Aspects Med 2008;29:144–50.
[307] Nobili V, Manco M, Devito R, et al. Effect of vitamin E on aminotransferase levels and insulin resistance in children with non-alcoholic fatty liver disease. Aliment Pharmacol Ther 2006;24(11–12):1553–61.
[308] Oliveira CPMS, da Costa Gayotto LC, Tatai C, et al. Vitamin C and vitamin E in prevention of nonalcoholic fatty liver disease (NAFLD) in choline deficient diet fed rats. Nutr J 2003;2:9.
[309] Lambert JE, Parnell JA, Eksteen B, et al. Gut microbiota manipulation with prebiotics in patients with non-alcoholic fatty liver disease: a randomized controlled trial protocol. BMC Gastroenterol 2015;15:169.
[310] Parnell JA, Raman M, Rioux KP, et al. The potential role of prebiotic fibre for treatment and management of non-alcoholic fatty liver disease and associated obesity and insulin resistance. Liver Int 2012;32(5):701–11.
[311] American Gastroenterological Association. American Gastroenterological Association medical position statement: nonalcoholic fatty liver disease. Gastroenterology 2002;123:1702–4.
[312] Davy BM, Melby CL. The effect of fiber-rich carbohydrates in features of syndrome X. J Am Diet Assoc 2003;103:83–6.
[313] Delzenne NM, Cani PD. A place for dietary fibre in the management of the metabolic syndrome X. Curr Opin Clin Nutr Metab Care 2005;8:636–40.
[314] Venn BJ, Mann JL. Cereal grains, legumes and diabetes. Eur J Clin Nutr 2004;58:1443–61.
[315] Eriksson S, Eriksson KF, Bondesso L. Nonalcoholic steatohepatitis in obesity: a reversible condition. Acta Med Scand 1986;220:83–8.
[316] Uneo T, Suguwara H, Sujaku K, et al. Therapeutic effects of restricted diet and exercise in obese patients fatty liver. J Hepatol 1997;27(1):103–7.
[317] Federico A, Trappoliere M, Loguercio C. Treatment of patients with non-alcoholic fatty liver disease: current views and perspectives. Dig Liver Dis 2006;38:789–801.
[318] Kechagias S, Arnerson A, Dahlqvist O, et al. Fast food based hyper-alimentation can induce rapid and profound elevation of serum alanine aminotransferase in healthy subjects. Gut 2008;57:649–54.
[319] Ouyang X, Cirillo P, Sautini Y, et al. Fructose consumption as a risk factor for non-alcoholic fatty liver disease. J Hepatol 2008;48:993–9.
[320] Cortez-Pinto H, Chatham J, Chacko VP, et al. Alterations in liver ATP homeostasis in human nonalcoholic steatohepatitis: a pilot study. JAMA 1999;282:1659–64.
[321] Fields M, Lewis CG. Dietary fructose but not starch is responsible for hyperlipidaemia associated with copper deficiency in rats: effect of high-fat diet. J Am Coll Nutr 1999;18:83–7.
[322] Aigner E, Theurl I, Haufe H, et al. Copper availability contributes to iron perturbations in human nonalcoholic fatty liver disease. Gastroenterology 2008;135:680–8.

[323] Yamamoto M, Iwasa M, Lwata K, et al. Restriction of dietary calories, fat and iron improves non-alcoholic fatty liver disease. J Gast Hep 2007;22(4):498–503.
[324] Ekhlasi G, Shidfar F, Agah S, et al. Effects of pomegranate and orange juice on antioxidant status in non-alcoholic fatty liver disease patients: a randomized clinical trial. Int J Vitam Nutr Res 2016;14:1–7.
[325] Gupta V, Mah X-J, Garcia MC, et al. Oily fish, coffee and walnuts: dietary treatment for nonalcoholic fatty liver disease. W J Gastroenterol 2015;21(37):10621–35.
[326] Sofi F, Giangrandi I, Cesari F, et al. Effects of a 1-year dietary intervention with n-3 polyunsaturated fatty acid-enriched olive oil on non-alcoholic fatty liver disease patients: a preliminary study. Int J Food Sci Nutr 2010;61:792–802.
[327] Ryan MC, Itsiopoulos C, Thodis T, et al. The Mediterranean diet improves hepatic steatosis and insulin sensitivity in individuals with non-alcoholic fatty liver disease. J Hepatol 2013;59:138–43.
[328] Ross AB, Godin JP, Minehira K, et al. Increasing whole grain intake as part of prevention and treatment of nonalcoholic fatty liver disease. Int J Endocrinol 2013;2013:585876.
[329] Hanje AJ, Fortune B, Song M, et al. The use of selected nutrition supplements and complementary and alternative medicine in liver disease. Nutr Clin Pract 2006;21:255.
[330] Purohit V, Abdelmalek MF, Barve S, et al. Role of S-adenosylmethionine, folate, and betaine in the treatment of alcoholic liver disease: summary of a symposium. Am J Clin Nut 2007;86(1):14–24.
[331] Song Z, Zhou Z, Chen T, et al. S-adenosylmethionine, cytokines and alcoholic liver disease. Alcohol 2002;27(3):185–92.
[332] Song Z, Zhou Z, Chen T, et al. SAM-e protects against acute alcohol induced hepatotoxicity in mice. J Nutr Biochem 2003;14(10):591–7.
[333] Bugianesi E, Marzocchi R, Villanova N, et al. Non-alcoholic fatty liver disease/non-alcoholic steatohepatitis (NAFLD/NASH): treatment. Best Pract Res Clin Gastroenterol 2004;18(6):1105–16.
[334] Abdelmalek MF, Angulo P, Jorgensen RA, et al. Betaine, a promising new agent for patients with nonalcoholic steatohepatitis: results of a pilot study. Am J Gastroenterol 2001;96:2711–17.
[335] Kang YJ, Zhou Z. Zinc prevention and treatment of alcoholic liver disease. Mol Aspects Med 2005;26:391–404.
[336] Lambert JC, Zhou Z, Wang L, et al. Prevention of alterations in intestinal permeability is involved in zinc inhibition of acute ethanol induced liver damage in mice. J Pharmacol Exo Ther 2003;305:880–6.
[337] McClain CJ, Antonow DR, Cohen DA, et al. Zinc metabolism in alcoholic liver disease. Alcohol Clin Exp Res 1986;10:582–9.
[338] Gallagher JC, Yalamanchili V, Smith LM. The effect of vitamin D supplementation on serum 25(OH)D in thin and obese women. J Ster Biochem Mol Biol 2013;136:195–200.
[339] Heer M, Egert S. Nutrients other than carbohydrates: their effects on glucose homeostasis in humans. Diabetes Metab Res Rev 2015;31(1):14–35.
[340] Barchetta I, Carotti S, Labbadia G, et al. Liver vitamin D receptor, CYP2R1, and CYP27A1 expression: relationship with liver histology and vitamin D3 levels in patients with nonalcoholic steatohepatitis or hepatitis C virus. Hepatology 2012;56(6): 2180–7.
[341] Pacana T, Sanyal AJ. Vitamin E and nonalcoholic fatty liver disease. Curr Opin Clin Nutr Metab Care 2012;15(6):641–8.
[342] Sato K, Gosho M, Yamamoto T, et al. Vitamin E has a beneficial effect on nonalcoholic fatty liver disease: a meta-analysis of randomized controlled trials. Nutrition 2015;31(7–8):923–30.
[343] Lavine JE. Vitamin E treatment of nonalcoholic steatohepatitis in children: a pilot study. J Pediatr 2000;136(6):734–8.
[344] Sanyal AJ, Mofrad PS, Contos MJ, et al. A pilot study of vitamin E versus vitamin E and pioglitazone for the treatment of nonalcoholic steatohepatitis. Clin Gastroenterol Hepatol 2004;2:1107–15.
[345] Hill DB, Devalaraja R, Joshi-Barve S, et al. Antioxidants attenuate nuclear factor-kappa B activation and tumor necrosis factor-alpha production in alcoholic hepatitis patient monocytes and rat kupffer cells, in vitro. Clin Biochem 1999;32:563–70.
[346] Aghdassi E, Salit IE, Mohemmed S, et al. W1818 chromium supplementation decreases insulin resistance and trunk fat. Gastroenterology 2008;134(4):A–722.
[347] Anderson RA. Chromium in the prevention and control of diabetes. Diabetes Metab 2000;26(1):22–7.
[348] Patrick L. Nonalcoholic fatty liver disease: relationship to insulin sensitivity and oxidative stress: treatment approaches using vitamin E, magnesium and betaine. Alt Med Rev 2002;7:276–91.
[349] Barbagallo M, Gupta RK, Bardicef M, et al. Altered ionic effects of insulin in hypertension: role of basal ion levels in determining cellular responsiveness. J Clin Endocrinol Metab 1997;82:1761–5.
[350] Grandi M, Pederzoli S, Sacchetti C. Effect of acute carnitine administration on glucose insulin metabolism in healthy subjects. Int J Clin Pharm Res 1997;17(4):143–7.
[351] Negro P. The effect of L-carnitine, administered via intravenous infusion of glucose on both glucose and insulin levels in healthy subjects. Drugs Exp Clin Res 1994;20(6):257–62.
[352] Molfino A, Cascino C, Ramaccini C, et al. L-carnitine administration improves insulin sensitivity in patients with impaired glucose metabolism. Eur J Invest Med 2008;19(8):S48.
[353] Allard JP. Other disease associations with non-alcoholic fatty liver disease (NAFLD). Best Prac Res Clin Gastroenterol 2002;16(5):783–95.
[354] Cremer DR, Rabeler R, Roberts A, et al. Long-term safety of alpha lipoic acid (ALA) consumption: a 2 year study. Reg Tech Pharm 2006;46:193–201.
[355] Biewenga GP, Haenen GR, Bast A. The pharmacology of the antioxidant lipoic acid. Gen Pharmacol 1997;29(3):315–31.
[356] Wollin SD, Jones PJ. Alpha-lipoic acid and cardiovascular disease. J Nutr 2003;133(11):3327–30.
[357] Ziegler D, Hanefeld M, Ruhnau KJ, et al. Treatment of symptomatic diabetic peripheral neuropathy with the antioxidant alpha-lipoic acid. A 3-week multicentre randomised controlled trial (ALADIN Study). Diabetologia 2005;38:1425.
[358] Kim MS, Park JY, Namkoong C, et al. Anti-obesity of alpha lipoic acid mediated by suppression of hypothalamic AMC activated protein kinase. Nat Med 2004;10(7):727–33.
[359] Militante D, Lobardini JB. Dietary taurine supplementation: hypolipidemic and antiatherogenic effects. Nut Res 2004;24:787–801.
[360] Allard JP, Aghdassi E, Saira M, et al. Nutritional assessment and fatty acid composition in non-alcoholic fatty liver disease (NAFLD): a cross sectional study. J Hepatol 2008;48:300–7.
[361] Araya J, Rodrogo R, Videla LA, et al. Increase in long chain polyunsaturated fatty acid ratio in relation to hepatic steatosis in nonalcoholic fatty liver disease patients. Clin Sci 2004;106:635–43.
[362] Capanni M, Calella F, Biagini MR, et al. Prolonged omega-3 polyunsaturated fatty acid supplementation ameliorates hepatic steatosis in patients with non-alcoholic fatty liver disease. Aliment Pharmacol Ther 2006;23(8):1143–51.
[363] Setola E, Monti LD, Galluccio E, et al. Insulin resistance and endothelial function are improved after folate and vitamin B12 therapy in patients with metabolic syndrome: relationship between homocysteine levels and hyperinsulinemia. Eur J Endocrinol 2004;151:483–9.
[364] Braun L, Cohen M. Herbs and natural supplements: an evidence-based guide. 2nd ed. Sydney: Elsevier; 2007.
[365] Luper S. A review of plants used in the treatment of liver disease part 1. Altern Med Review 1998;3:410–12.
[366] Aghazadeh S, Amini R, Yazdanparast R, et al. Anti-apoptotic and anti-inflammatory effects of *Silybum marianum* in treatment of experimental steatohepatitis. Exp Toxicol Pathol 2010;63(6):569–74.
[367] Gazák R, Purchartová K, Marhol P, et al. Antioxidant and antiviral activities of silybin fatty acid conjugates. Eur J Med Chem 2010;45(3):1059–67.
[368] Shaker E, Mahmoud H, Mnaa S. Silymarin, the antioxidant component and *Silybum marianum* extracts prevent liver damage. Food Chem Toxicol 2010;48(3):803–6.
[369] Velussi M, Cernigoi AM, De Monte A, et al. Long-term (12 months) treatment with an anti-oxidant drug (silymarin) is effective on hyperinsulinemia, exogenous insulin need and malondialdehyde levels in cirrhotic diabetic patients. J Hepatol 1997;26(4):871–9.
[370] Morazzoni P, Bombardelli E. *Silybum marianum* (*Carduus marianus*). Fitoterapia 1995;66(1):3–42.
[371] Basiglio CL, Sanchez Pozzi EJ, Mottino AD, et al. Differential effects of silymarin and its active component silibinin on plasma membrane stability and hepatocellular lysis. Chem Biol Interact 2009;179(2–3):297–303.

[372] Trappoliere M, Caligiuri A, Schmid M, et al. Silybin, a component of silymarin, exerts anti-inflammatory and anti-fibrogenic effects on human hepatic stellate cells. J Hepatol 2009;50(6):1102–11.
[373] Schuppan D, Jia JD, Brinkhaus B, et al. Herbal products for liver diseases: a therapeutic challenge for the new millennium. Hepatology 1999;30(4):1099–104.
[374] Morishima C, Shuhart MC, Wang CC, et al. Silymarin inhibits in vitro T-cell proliferation and cytokine production in hepatitis C virus infection. Gastroenterology 2010;138(2):671–81, 81.e1–2.
[375] El-Zayadi AR, Attia M, Badran HM, et al. Non-interferon-based therapy: an option for amelioration of necro-inflammation in hepatitis C patients who cannot afford interferon therapy. Liver Int 2005;25(4):746–51.
[376] Szilard S, Szentgyorgyi D, Demeter I. Protective effect of Legalon in workers exposed to organic solvents. Acta Med Hung 1998;45:249–56.
[377] Trappoliere M, Ferderico A, Tuccillo C, et al. Effects of a new pharmacological complex (silybin + vitamin E + phospholipids) on some markers of the metabolic syndrome and of liver fibrosis in patients with hepatic steatosis. Preliminary study. Minerva Gastroenterol Dietol 2005;51(2):193–9. [Article in Italian, abstract cited].
[378] Hajaghamohammadi AA, Ziaee A, Rafiei R. The efficacy of silymarin in decreasing transaminase activities in non-alcoholic fatty liver disease: a randomized controlled clinical trial. Hepat Mon 2008;88(33):191–5.
[379] Dongiovanni P, Lanti C, Riso P, et al. Nutritional therapy for nonalcoholic fatty liver disease. J Nutr Biochem 2016;29:1–11.
[380] Stickel F, Schuppan D. Herbal medicine in the treatment of liver diseases. Dig Liv Dis 2007;39:293–304.
[381] Fiore C, Eisenhut M, Ragazzi E, et al. Review: a history of the therapeutic use of liquorice. Eur J Ethnopharmacol 2005;99: 317–24.
[382] Blumenthal M, Goldberg A, Brinckmann J, editors. Herbal medicine expanded commission E monographs. Austin (TX): Integrative Medicine Communications; 2000.
[383] Van Rossum TG, Vulto AG, De Man RA, et al. Review article: glycyrrhizin as a potential treatment for chronic hepatitis C. Ailment Pharmacol Ther 1998;12:199–205.
[384] Wang JY, Guo JS, Li H, et al. Inhibitory effect of glycyrrhizin on NF-kappa B binding activity in CCL4-plus ethanol induced liver cirrhosis in rats. Liver 1998;18:180–5.
[385] Moro T, Shimoyama Y, Kushida M, et al. Glycyrrhizin and its metabolite inhibit Smad3-mediated type I collagen gene transcription and suppress experimental murine liver fibrosis. Life Sci 2008;83:531–9.
[386] Chan HT, Chan C, Ho JW. Inhibition of glycyrrhizic acid of aflatoxin B1 induced cytotoxicity in hepatoma cells. Toxicology 2003;188(2–3):211–17.
[387] Jeong HG, Kim JY. Induction of inducible nitric oxide synthase expression by 18b-glycyrrhetinic acid in macrophages. FEBS 2002;513:208–12.
[388] Wu X, Shang L, Gurley E, et al. Prevention of free fatty acid-induced hepatic lipotoxicity by 18 beta glycyrrhetinic acid through lysosomal and mitochondrial pathways. Hepatology 2008;47(6):1905–15.
[389] Whorwood CB, Sheppard MC, Stewart PM. Liquorice inhibits 11 beta-hydroxysteroid dehydrogenase messenger ribonucleic acid levels and potentiates glucocorticoid hormone action. Endocrinology 1993;132:2287–92.
[390] Paulsen SK, Pedersen SB, Fisker S, et al. 11 beta-HSD type 1 expression in human adipose tissue: impact of gender, obesity, and fat localization. Obesity (Silver Spring) 2007;15:1954–60.
[391] Matsuzawa Y. The metabolic syndrome and adipocytokines. FEBS Lett 2006;580(12):2917–21.
[392] Shen B, Yu J, Wang S, et al. *Phyllanthus urinaria* ameliorates the severity of nutritional steatohepatitis both in vitro and in vivo. Hepatology 2008;47:473–83.
[393] Godard MP, Johnson BA, Richmond SR. Body composition and hormonal adaptations associated with forskolin consumption in overweight and obese men. Obes Res 2005;13:1335–43.
[394] Henderson S, Magu B, Rasmussen C, et al. Effects of *Coleus forskohlii* supplementation on body composition and hematological profiles in mildly overweight women. J Int Soc Sports Nut 2005;2:54–62.
[395] Haye B, Aublin JL, Champion S, et al. Chronic and acute effects of forskolin on isolated thyroid cell metabolism. Mol Cell Endocrinol 1985;43(1):41–50.
[396] Gokmen-Polar Y, Coronel EC, Bahouth SW, et al. Insulin sensitizes beta-agonist and forskolin-stimulated lipolysis to inhibition by 2',5'-dideoxyadenosine. Am J Physiol Cell Physiol 1996;270:C562–9.
[397] Bdmaev V, Majeed M, Conte A, et al. Diterpene forskolin (*Coleus forskohlii*). A possible new compound for reduction of body weight increasing lean body mass. Piscataway (NJ): Sabinsa Corporation; 2000.
[398] Wiedenkeller DE, Sharp GW. Effects of forskolin on insulin release and cyclic AMP content in rat pancreatic islets. Endocrinology 1983;113:2311–13.
[399] Lin YL, Wu CH, Luo MH, et al. In vitro protective effects of salvianolic acid B on primary hepatocytes and hepatic stellate cells. J Ethnopharmacol 2006;105:215–22.
[400] Yang Y, Yang S, Chen M, et al. Compound astragalus and *Salvia miltiorrhiza* extract exerts anti-fibrosis by mediating TGF-/Smad signaling in myofibroblasts. J Ethnopharmacol 2008;118:264–70.
[401] Wasser S, Ho JMS, Ang HK, et al. *Salvia miltiorrhiza* reduces experimentally-induced hepatic fibrosis in rats. J Hepatol 1998;29:760–71.
[402] Li C, Lup J, Li L, et al. The collagenolytic effects of the traditional Chinese medicine preparation, han-dan-gan-le, contribute to reversal of chemical-induced liver fibrosis in rats. Life Sci 2003;72:1563–71.
[403] Ji W, Gong BQ. Hypolipidemic activity and mechanism of purified herbal extract of *Salvia miltiorrhiza* in hyperlipidemic rats. J Ethnopharmacol 2008;119:291–8.
[404] Shanmugasundaram KR, Panneezelvam CM, Samudram P, et al. The insulinotropic activity of *Gymnema sylvestra* an Indian medical herb used in controlling diabetes mellitus. Pharmacol Res Commun 1981;13(5):475.
[405] Shanmugasundaram KR, Panneerselvam C, Samudram P, et al. Enzyme changes and glucose utilization in diabetic rabbits: the effect of *Gymnema sylvestre*. J Ethnopharmacol 1983;7:205–34.
[406] Baskaran K, Ahamath BK, Shanmugasundaram M, et al. Antidiabetic effect of a leaf extract from *Gymnema sylvestris* in non insulin dependent diabetes mellitus patients. J Ethnopharmacol 1990;30:295–305.
[407] Shanmugasundaram ERB, Rajewsarf G, Baskaran K, et al. Use of gymnema leaf extract in the control of blood glucose in insulin dependent diabetes mellitus. J Ethnopharmacol 1990;30:281–94.
[408] Bishayee A, Chaterjee M. Hypolipidaemic and antiatherosclerotic effects of oral *Gymnema sylvestre* leaf extract in albino rats fed on a high fat diet. Phytother Res 1994;8:118–20.
[409] Bordenave S, Brandou F, Manetta B, et al. Effects of acute exercise on insulin sensitivity, glucose effectiveness and disposition index in type 2 diabetic patients. Diabetes Metab 2008;34:250–7.
[410] Schenk S, Cook JN, Kaufman AE, et al. Postexercise insulin sensitivity is not impaired after an overnight lipid infusion. Am J Physiol Endocrinol Metab 2005;288:E519–25.
[411] Ueno T, Sugawara H, Sujaku K, et al. Therapeutic effects of restricted diet and exercise in obese patients with fatty liver. J Hepatol 1997;27:103–7.
[412] Wilson GT, Brownell KD. Behavioral treatment for obesity. In: Fairburn CG, Brownell KD, editors. Eating disorders and obesity: a comprehensive handbook. 2nd ed. New York: Guilford Press; 2002. p. 524–8.
[413] Junaidi O, di Bisceglie AM. Ageing liver and hepatitis. Clin Geriatr Med 2007;23:889–903.
[414] Chien NT, Dundoo G, Horani MH. Seroprevalence of viral hepatitis in an older nursing home population. J Am Geriatr Soc 1999;47:1110–13.
[415] Koslap-Petraco MB, Shub M, Judelson R. Hepatitis A disease burden and current childhood cavvination strategies in the United States. J Ped Health Care 2008;22:3–11.
[416] Rafiq SM, Rashid H, Haworth E, et al. Hazards of hepatitis at the Hajj. Travel Med Infect Dis 2009;7(4):239–46.
[417] Zhang YY, Hu KQ. Rethinking the pathogenesis of hepatitis B virus (HBV) infection. J Med Virol 2015;87(12):1989–99.
[418] Jacob A, Kowdley KV. Epidemiology of hepatitis B — clinical implications. Med Gen Med 2006;8:13.
[419] Alter MJ. Epidemiology of viral hepatitis and HIV co-infection. J Hepatol 2006;44:S6–89.

[420] World Health Organization (WHO). Hepatitis C. 2017. Available from: www.who.int/mediacentre/factsheets/fs164/en/.
[421] Freeman AJ, Dore GJ, Law MG, et al. Estimating progression to cirrhosis in chronic hepatitis C virus infection. Hepatology 2003;34(4):809–16.
[422] Prati D. Transmission of hepatitis C virus blood transfusions and other medical procedures: a global review. J Hepatol 2006;45:607–16.
[423] Kapoor D, Saxena R, Sood B, et al. Blood transfusion practices in India: results of a national survey. Indian J Gastroenterol 2000;19:64–7.
[424] Koytak ES, Yurdaydin C, Glenn JS. Hepatitis D. Curr Treat Options Gastroenterol 2007;10:456–63.
[425] Fattovich G, Giustina G, Christensen E, et al. Influence of hepatitis delta virus infection on morbidity and mortality in compensated cirrhosis type B. European Concerted Action on Viral Hepatitis (Eurohep). Gut 2000;46:420–6.
[426] Farci P. Treatment of chronic hepatitis D: new advances, old challenges. Hepatology (editorial) 2006;44(3):536–9.
[427] Debing Y, Moradpour D, Neyts J, et al. Update on hepatitis E virology: implications for clinical practice. J Hepatol 2016;65(1):200–12.
[428] Khuroo MS, Khuroo MS. Hepatitis E: an emerging global disease — from discovery towards control and cure. J Viral Hepat 2016;23(2):68–79.
[429] Wasley A, Samandari T, Bell BP. Incidence of hepatitis A in the United States in the era of vaccination. JAMA 2005;294:194–201.
[430] Alavian SM, Keyvani H, Rezai M, et al. Preliminary report of hepatitis B virus genotype prevalence in Iran. World J Gastroenterol 2006;12:5211–13.
[431] Hollinger FB. Hepatitis B virus genetic diversity and its impact on diagnostic assays. J Viral Hepat 2007;14(Suppl. 1):11–15.
[432] Lavanchy D. Hepatitis B virus epidemiology, disease burden, treatment, and current and emerging prevention and control measures. J Viral Hepat 2004;11:97–107.
[433] Alter MJ. Epidemiology of hepatitis C. Hepatology 1997;26(Suppl. 1):62S–65S.
[434] Shepard CW, Finelli L, Alter MJ. Global epidemiology of hepatitis C virus infection. Lancet Infect Dis 2005;5:558–67.
[435] Maheshwari M, Ray S, Thuluvath PJ. Acute hepatitis C. Lancet 2008;372:321–32.
[436] European Paediatric Hepatitis C Virus (HCV) Network. A significant sex — but not elective caesarean section — effect on mother to child transmission of hepatitis C virus infection. J Infect Dis 2005;192:1872–9.
[437] Farci P. Delta hepatitis: an update. J Hepatol 2003;39(Suppl. 1):S212–19.
[438] Cowie BC, Adamopolous J, Carter K, et al. Hepatitis E infections, Victoria, Australia. Emerg Infect Dis 2005;11(3):482–4.
[439] Dalton BR, Bendall R, Ijaz S, et al. Hepatitis E: an emerging infection in developed countries. Lancet 2008;8:698–708.
[440] Hui CK, Lau GKK. Immune system and hepatitis B virus infection. Clin Virol 2005;34(Suppl. 1):S44–8.
[441] Webster GJ, Reignat S, Maini MK, et al. Incubation phase of acute hepatitis B in man: dynamic of cellular immune mechanisms. Hepatology 2000;32:1117–24.
[442] Shaw T, Locarnini SA. Hepatitis B. In: Encyclopedia of gastroenterology. Edinburgh: Elsevier; 2004. p. 315–22.
[443] Seeff LB. Natural history of chronic hepatitis C. Hepatology 2002;36:S35–46.
[444] Albert ML, Decalf J, Pol S. Plasmacytoid dendritic cells move down in the list of suspects: in search of the immune pathogenesis of chronic hepatitis C. J Hepatol 2008;49:1069–78.
[445] Koziel MJ. The role of immune responses in the pathogenesis of hepatitis C virus infection. J Viral Hep 1997;4(2):31–41.
[446] Ishii S, Koziel MJ. Immune responses during acute and chronic infection with hepatitis C virus. Clin Immun 2008;128:133–47.
[447] Dustin LB, Rice CM. Flying under the radar: the immunobiology of hepatitis C. Annu Rev Immunol 2007;25:71–9.
[448] Schuppan D, Krebs A, Bauer M, et al. Hepatitis C and liver fibrosis. Cell Death Differ 2003;10:S59–67.
[449] Gochee PA, Jonsoon JR, Clouston AD, et al. Steatosis in chronic hepatitis C: association with increased messenger RNA expression of collagen I, tumour necrosis factor-α and cytochrome P4502E1. J Gastro Hep 2003;18(4):386–92.
[450] Neumann AU, Lam NP, Dahari H, et al. Hepatitis C viral dynamics in vivo and the antiviral efficacy of interferon–alpha therapy. Science 1998;282:103–7.
[451] Wright TL, Lau JY. Clinic aspects of hepatitis B infection. Lancet 1993;342(8883):1340–4.
[452] Dickson RC. Clinical manifestations of hepatitis C. Clin Liver Dis 1997;1(3):569–85.
[453] Hoofnagle JH. Acute hepatitis C. In: Liang TJ, Hoofnagle JH, editors. Hepatitis biomedical research reports. San Diego: Academic Press; 2000. p. 71–83.
[454] Lauer GM, Walker BD. Hepatitis C virus infection. N Engl J Med 2001;345:41–52.
[455] Barrett S, Goh J, Coughlan B, et al. The natural course of hepatitis C virus infection after 22 years in a unique homogenous cohort: spontaneous viral clearance and chronic HCV infection. Gut 2001;49(3):423–30.
[456] Marcellin P. Hepatitis C: the clinical spectrum of the disease. J Hepatol 1999;31(Suppl. 1):9–16.
[457] Farrell GC. Chronic viral hepatitis. Med J Aust 1998;168(12): 619–26.
[458] Fawcett RS, Linford S, Stuhlberg DL. Nail abnormalities: clues to systemic disease. Am Fam Physician 2004;69(6):1417–22.
[459] Sugerman PB, Savage N. Oral lichen planus: causes, diagnosis and management. Aust Dent J 2002;47(4):290–7.
[460] Lodi G, Porter SR, Scully C. Hepatitis C virus infection: review and implications for the dentist. Oral Surg Oral Med Oral Pathol 1998;86:8–22.
[461] Bush F. Appearance of the tongue in hepatitis. Lancet 1835;602(23):871. (Letter to editor).
[462] Ojha J, Bhattacharyya I, Islam N, et al. Xerostomia and lichenoid reaction in a hepatitis C patient treated with interferon-alpha: a case report. Quintessence Int 2008;39(4):343–8.
[463] Mondelli MU, Cerino A, Cividini A. Acute hepatitis C diagnosis and management. J Hepatol 2005;42:S108–14.
[464] Farci P, Alter HJ, Wong D, et al. A long-term study of hepatitis C virus replication in non-A, non-B hepatitis. N Engl J Med 1991;325:98–104.
[465] Takaki A, Wiese M, Maertens G, et al. Cellular immune responses persist and humoral responses decrease two decades after recovery from a single-source outbreak of hepatitis C. Nat Med 2000;6:578–82.
[466] Mohamoud YA, Mumtaz GR, Riome S, et al. The epidemiology of hepatitis C virus in Egypt: a systematic review and data synthesis. BMC Infect Dis 2013;13:288.
[467] Feinstone SM, Kapikian AZ, Purcell RH, et al. Transfusion-associated hepatitis not due to viral hepatitis type A or B. N Engl J Med 1975;292:767–70.
[468] Hasse JM, Matarese LE. Medical nutrition therapy for liver, biliary system and exocrine pancreatic disorders. In: Mahan LK, Escott-Stump S, editors. Krause's food and nutrition therapy. St Louis: WB Saunders/Elsevier; 2008. p. 707–38.
[469] Regev A, Jeffers LJ. Hepatitis C and alcohol. Alcohol Clin Exp Res 1999;23:1543–51.
[470] Monto A, Alonzo J, Watson JJ, et al. Steatosis in chronic hepatitis C: relative contributions of obesity, diabetes mellitus, and alcohol. Hepatology 2002;36:729–36.
[471] Szabo G. Pathogenic interactions between alcohol and hepatitis C. Curr Gastroenterol Rep 2003;5(1):86–92.
[472] Rigamonti C, Mottaran E, Reale E, et al. Moderate alcohol consumption increases oxidative stress in patients with chronic hepatitis C. Hepatology 2003;38:42–9.
[473] Piperno A, Vergani A, Malosio I, et al. Hepatic iron overload in patients with chronic viral hepatitis: role of HFE gene mutations. Hepatology 1998;28(4):1105–9.
[474] Poynard T, Ratziu V, McHutchison J, et al. Effect of treatment with peginterferon or interferon alfa-2band ribavirin on steatosis in patients infected with hepatitis C. Hepatology 2003;38:75–85.
[475] Hourigan LF, Macdonald GA, Purdie D, et al. Fibrosis in chronic hepatitis C correlates significantly with body mass index and steatosis. Hepatology 2003;29(4):1215–19.
[476] Ortiz V. Contribution of obesity to hepatitis C-related fibrosis progression. Am J Gastroenterol 2002;97(9):2408–14.
[477] Olynyk JK, Reddy KR, Bisceglie AM, et al. Hepatic iron concentration as a predictor of response to interferon alpha

therapy in chronic hepatitis C. Gastroenterology 1995;108: 104–9.
[478] Farinati F, Cardin R, De Maria N. Iron storage, lipid peroxidation and glutathione turnover in chronic anti-HCV positive hepatitis. J Hepatol 1995;22:44956.
[479] Cotler SJ, Emond MJ, Gretch DR, et al. Relationship between iron concentration and hepatitis C virus RNA level in liver tissue. Clin Gastroenterol 1999;29:322–6.
[480] Fraser G, Harman I, Meller N, et al. Diabetes mellitus is associated with chronic hepatitis C but not chronic hepatitis B infection. Isr J Med Sci 1996;32:526–30.
[481] Custro N, Carroccio A, Ganci A, et al. Glycemic homeostasis in chronic viral hepatitis and liver cirrhosis. Diabetes Metab 2001;27:476–81.
[482] Noto H, Raskin P. Hepatitis C infection and diabetes. J Diabetes Comp 2006;20:113–20.
[483] Krajka-Kuźniak V, Paluszczak J, Szaefer H, et al. Betanin, a beetroot component, induces nuclear factor erythroid-2-related factor 2-mediated expression of detoxifying/antioxidant enzymes in human liver cell lines. Br J Nutr 2013;110(12):2138–49.
[484] Ciesek S, von Hahn T, Colpitts CC, et al. The green tea polyphenol, epigallocatechin-3-gallate, inhibits hepatitis C virus entry. Hepatology 2011;54(6):1947–55.
[485] Anggakusuma, Colpitts CC, Schang LM, et al. Turmeric curcumin inhibits entry of all hepatitis C virus genotypes into human liver cells. Gut 2014;63(7):1137–49.
[486] Jain SK, Pemberton PW, Smith A, et al. Oxidative stress in chronic hepatitis C: not just a feature of late stage disease. J Hepatol 2002;36:805–11.
[487] Look MP, Gerard A, Rao GS, et al. Interferon/antioxidant combination therapy for chronic hepatitis C — a controlled trial. Antiviral Res 1999;43(2):113–22.
[488] Falasca K, Ucciferri C, Mancino P, et al. Treatment with silybin-vitamin E-phospholipid complex in patients with hepatitis C infection. J Med Virol 2008;80(11):1900–6.
[489] Andreone P, Gramenzi A, Bernardi M. Vitamin E for chronic hepatitis B. Ann Intern Med 1998;128:156–7.
[490] Andreone P, Fiorino S, Cursaro C, et al. Vitamin E as treatment for chronic hepatitis B: results of a randomized controlled pilot trial. Antiviral Res 2001;49:75–81.
[491] Karoli Y, Karoli R, Fatima J, et al. Study of hepatic osteodystrophy in patients with chronic liver disease. J Clin Diag Res 2016;10(8):OC31–4.
[492] Goel V, Kar P. Hepatic osteodystrophy. Trop Gastroenterol 2010;31(2):82–6.
[493] Ho E. Zinc deficiency, DNA damage and cancer risk. J Nut Biochem 2004;15:572–8.
[494] Guumlr G, Bayraktar Y, Oumlzer D, et al. Determination of hepatic zinc content in chronic liver disease due to hepatitis B virus. Hepato-Gastroenterol 1998;45:472–6.
[495] Bode JC, Hanisch P, Henning H, et al. Hepatic zinc content in patients with various stages of alcoholic liver disease and in patients with chronic active and chronic persistent hepatitis. Hepatology 1998;8:1605–9.
[496] Himoto T, Hosomi N, Nakai S, et al. Efficacy of zinc administration in patients with hepatitis C virus-related chronic liver disease. Scand J Gastroenterol 2007;42(9):1078–87.
[497] Nagamine T, Takagi H, Takayama H, et al. Preliminary study of combination therapy with interferon-α and zinc in chronic hepatitis C patients with genotype 1b. Biol Trace Elem Res 2000;75(1–3):53–63.
[498] Czuczejko J, Zachara BA, Staubach-Topczewska E, et al. Selenium, glutathione and glutathione peroxidases in blood of patients with chronic liver diseases. Acta Biochim Pol 2003;50:1147–54.
[499] Yu SY, Li WG, Zhu YJ, et al. Chemoprevention trial of human hepatitis with selenium supplementation in China. Biol Trace Elem Res 1989;20(1–2):15–22.
[500] Yu MW, Horng IS, Hsu KH, et al. Plasma selenium levels and risk of hepatocellular carcinoma among men with chronic hepatitis. Am J Epidem 1999;150:367–74.
[501] Majano PL, Medina J, Zubia I, et al. N-Acetyl-cysteine modulates inducible nitric oxide synthase gene expression in human hepatocytes. J Hepatol 2004;40:632–7.
[502] Haenen G, Bast A. Scavenging of hypochlorous acid by lipoic acid. Biochem Pharmacol 1991;42:2244–6.
[503] Henrickson EJ, Jacob S, Streeper RS, et al. Stimulation by α-lipoic acid of glucose transport activity in skeletal muscle of lean and obese Zucker rats. Life Sci 1997;61(8):805–12.
[504] Narita R, Abe S, Kihara Y, et al. Insulin resistance and insulin secretion in chronic hepatitis C virus infection. J Hepatol 2004;41:132–8.
[505] Parker G, Gibson NA, et al. Omega-3 fatty acids and mood disorders. Am J Psychiatry 2006;163(6):969–78.
[506] Malaguarnera M, Restuccia N, Di Fazio I, et al. Fish oil treatment of interferon-alpha induced dyslipidaemia. Bio Drugs 1999;11(4):285–91.
[507] Zignego AL, Cozzi A, Carpenedo R, et al. HCV patients, psychopathology and tryptophan metabolism: analysis of the effects of pegylated interferon plus ribavirin treatment. Dig Liver Dis 2007;39(Suppl. 1):S107–11.
[508] Mann JJ. Neurobiology of suicidal behaviour. Nat Rev Neurosci 2003;4:819–28.
[509] Levy C, Seeff LD, Lindor KD. Use of herbal supplements for chronic liver disease. Clin Gastroenterol Hepatol 2004;2:947–56.
[510] Dhiman RK, Chawla YK. Herbal medicines for liver diseases. Dig Dis Sci 2005;50:1807–12.
[511] Fraschini F, Demartini G, Esposti D. Pharmacology of silymarin. Clin Drug Invest 2002;22(1):51–65.
[512] Mayer KE, Myers RP, Lee SS. Silymarin treatment of viral hepatitis: a systematic review. J Viral Hep 2005;12:559–67.
[513] El-Zayadi AR, Attia M, Badran HM, et al. Non interferon based therapy: an option for amelioration of necro-inflammation in hepatitis C patients who cannot afford interferon therapy. Liver Int 2005;25:746–51.
[514] Ferenci P, Scherzer TM, Kerschner H, et al. Silbinin is a potent antiviral agent in patients with chronic hepatitis C not responding to pegylated interferon/ribavirin therapy. Gastroenterology 2008;135(5):1561–7.
[515] Salmond SJ, George J, Strasser SI, et al The Hep573 study — a randomised controlled trial of complementary medicines in hepatitis C. Draft poster for the International Congress of Complementary Medicine Research; 29–31 March 2008.
[516] Melhem A, Stern M, Shibolet O, et al. Treatment of chronic hepatitis C virus infection via antioxidants. Results of a phase I clinical trial. J Clin Gastro 2005;39:737–42.
[517] Huang RL, Chen CC, Huang HL, et al. Anti-hepatitis B virus effects of wogonin isolated from *Scutellaria baicalensis*. Planta Med 2000;66(8):694–8.
[518] Guo Q, Zhao L, You Q, et al. Anti-hepatitis B virus activity of wogonin in vitro and in vivo. Antiviral Res 2007;74:16–24.
[519] Calixto JB, Santos ARS, Filbo VC, et al. A review of the plants of the genus *Phyllanthus*: their chemistry, pharmacology, and therapeutic potential. Med Res Rev 1998;18:225–58.
[520] Thyagarajan SP, Thiruneelakantan K, Subramanian S, et al. In vitro inactivation of HBsAg by *Eclipta alba hassk* and *Phyllanthus niruri* Linn. Indian J Med Res 1982;76:124–30.
[521] Venkateswaran PS, Millman I, Blumberg BS. Effects of an extract from *Phyllanthus niruri* on hepatitis B and woodchuck hepatitis B viruses: In vitro and in vivo studies. Proc Natl Acad Sci USA 1987;84:274–8.
[522] Jayaram S, Thyagarajan SP, Panchanadam M, et al. Anti-hepatitis B properties of *Phyllanthus niruri* Linn and *Eclipta alba hassk*: in vitro and in vivo safety studies. Biomedicine 1987;7:9–16.
[523] Thyagarajan SP, Subramanian S, Thirunalsundair T, et al. Effect of *Phyllanthus amarus* on chronic carriers of hepatitis B virus. Lancet 1988;2:764–6.
[524] Leelarasamee A, Trakulsomboon S, Maunwngyathi P, et al. Failure of *Phyllanthus amarus* to eradicate hepatitis B surface antigen from symptomless carriers. Lancet 1990;345:1600–1.
[525] Thyagarajan SP, Jayaram S, Valliammai T, et al. *Phyllanthus amarus* and hepatitis B. Lancet 1990;336:949–50.
[526] Berk L, de man RA, Scalm SW, et al. Beneficial effects of *Phyllanthus amaraus* for chronic hepatitis not confirmed. J Hepatol 1991;12:405–6.
[527] Zhang JL, He WN, Ye P. Clinical observations on *Phyllanthus amarus* for treating chronic hepatitis HBV infection. Chin J Int Trad West Med Liver Dis 1992;2:8–10.
[528] Zhu FM, Zhang JQ, Zhang XZ, et al. Observations on the effect of Fujian's *Phyllanthus amarus* treatment of HBV infection. Chin J Int Trad West Med Liver Dis 1992;2:10–11.

[529] Berk L, deMan RA, Schalm SW, et al. Beneficial effects of *Phyllantus amarus* for chronic hepatitis B, not confirmed. J Hepatol 1991;12:405–6.
[530] Milne A, Hopkirk N, Lucas CR, et al. Failure of New Zealand hepatitis B carriers to respond to *Phyllanthus amarus.* NZ Med J 1994;107:253.
[531] Martin KW, Ernst E. Antiviral agents from plants and herbs: a systematic review. Antivir Ther 2003;8:77–90.
[532] Hirayama C, Okumura M, Tanikawa K, et al. A multicentre randomised controlled trial of Sho Saiko To in chronic active hepatitis. Gastroenterol Jpn 1989;24(6):715–19.
[533] Shimizu I, Ma YR, Mizobuchi Y, et al. Effects of sho-saiko-to, a Japanese herbal medicine on hepatic fibrosis in mice. Hepatology 1999;29:142–60.
[534] Suzuki T, Higa M, Takahashi M, et al. A case of sho-Seiryu-to induced-pneumonia with a marked increase in peripheral eosinophils. Nihon Kokyuki Gakkai Zasshi 2006;4(8):578–82.
[535] Hatakeyama S, Tachibana A, Morita M, et al. Five cases of pneumonitis induced by sho-saiko-to. Hihon Kyobu Skikkan Gakkai Zasshi 1997;35(5):505–10.
[536] Ishizaki T, Sasaki F, Ameshima S, et al. Pneumonitis during interferon and/or herbal drug therapy in patients with chronic active hepatitis. Eur Resp J 1996;9(12):2831–5.
[537] Asl MN, Hosseinzadeh H. Review of pharmacological effects of *Glycyrrhiza* spp. and its bioactive compounds. Phytother Res 2008;22:709–24.
[538] Yamamura Y, Kotaki H, Tanaka N, et al. The pharmacokinetics of glycyrrhizin and its restorative effect on hepatic function in patients with chronic hepatitis and in chronically carbon-tetrachloride-intoxicated rats. Biopharm Drug Dispos 1997;18:717–25.
[539] Takahara T, Watanabe A, Shiraki K. Effects of glycyrrhizin on hepatitis B surface antigen: a biochemical and morphological study. J Hepatol 1994;21:601–9.
[540] Sato H, Goto W, Yamamura J, et al. Therapeutic basis of glycyrrhizin on chronic hepatitis B. Antivir Res 1996;30:171–7.
[541] Tandon A, Tandon BN, Bhujwala RA. Treatment of subacute hepatitis with lamivudine and intravenous glycyrrhizin: a pilot study. Hepatol Res 2001;20:1–8.
[542] Arase Y, Ikeda K, Murashima N, et al. The long-term efficacy of glycyrrhizin in chronic hepatitis C patients. Cancer 1997;79:1494–500.
[543] Ikeda K, Arase Y, Kobayashi M, et al. A long-term glycyrrhizin injection therapy reduces hepatocellular carcinogenesis rate in patients with interferon-resistant active chronic hepatitis C: a cohort study of 1249 patients. Dig Dis Sci 2006;51(3):603–9.
[544] Sinclair S. Chinese herbs: a clinical review of astragalus, ligusticum, and schizandrae. Alt Med Rev 1998;3(5):338–44.
[545] Kang H, Ahn KS, Cho C, et al. Immunomodulatory effect of astra-gali radix extract on murine TH1/TH2 cell lineage development. Biol Pharm Bull 2004;27:1946–50.
[546] Effects of astragalus (ASI, SK) on experimental liver injury. Yao Xue Xue Bao 1992;27(6):401–6. [Article in Chinese, abstract cited].
[547] Yang Y, Yang S, Chen M, et al. Compound astragalus and *Salvia miltiorrhiza* extract exerts anti-fibrosis by mediating TGF-beta/Smad signaling in myofibroblasts. J Ethnopharmacol 2008;118(2):264–70.
[548] Hobbs C. Foundations of health: the liver and digestive herbs. Capitola (CA): Botanica Press; 1992.
[549] McFarlane IG. Hepatitis C and alcoholic liver disease. Am J Gastro 1993;88:982–8.
[550] Pessione F, Ramond MJ, Njapoum C, et al. Cigarette smoking and hepatic lesions in patients with chronic hepatitis C. Hepatology 2001;34:121–5.
[551] Yu MW, Hsu FC, Sheen IS, et al. Prospective study of hepatocellular carcinoma and liver cirrhosis in asymptomatic chronic hepatitis B virus carrier. Am J Epidemiol 1997;145:1039–47.
[552] Francque S, Vonghia L, Ramon A, et al. Epidemiology and treatment of autoimmune hepatitis. Hepat Med 2012;4:1–10.
[553] Wang Q, Yang F, Miao Q, et al. The clinical phenotypes of autoimmune hepatitis: a comprehensive review. J Autoimmun 2016;66:98–107.
[554] Boberg KM, Aadland E, Jahnsen J, et al. Incidence and prevalence of primary biliary cirrhosis, primary sclerosing cholangitis, and autoimmune hepatitis in a Norwegian population. Scand J Gastroenterol 1998;33(1):99–103.
[555] Lleo A, Jepsen P, Morenghi E, et al. Evolving trends in female to male incidence and male mortality of primary biliary cholangitis. Sci Rep 2016;6:25906.
[556] Tanaka T, Sugawara Y, Kokudo N. Liver transplantation and autoimmune hepatitis. Intractable Rare Dis Res 2015;4(1):33–8.
[557] Grover VP, Southern L, Dyson JK, et al. Early primary biliary cholangitis is characterised by brain abnormalities on cerebral magnetic resonance imaging. Aliment Pharmacol Ther 2016;44(9):936–45.
[558] Mokdad AA, Lopez AD, Shahraz S, et al. Liver cirrhosis mortality in 187 countries between 1980 and 2010: a systematic analysis. BMC Med 2014;12:145.
[559] Schuppan D, Afdhal NH. Liver cirrhosis. Lancet 2008;371:838–51.
[560] Batey RG, Burns T, Benson RJ, et al. Alcohol consumption and the risk of cirrhosis. Med J Aust 1992;156:413–16.
[561] Horiguchia N, Ishacb EJN, Gao B. Liver regeneration is suppressed in alcoholic cirrhosis: correlation with decreased STAT3 activation. Alcohol 2007;51:271–80.
[562] Donato F, Tagger A, Gelatti U, et al. Alcohol and hepatocellular carcinoma: the effect of lifetime intake and hepatitis virus infections in men and women. Am J Epidemiol 2002;155:323–31.
[563] Perz JF, Armstrong GL, Farrington LA, et al. The contributions of hepatitis B virus and hepatitis C virus infections to cirrhosis and primary liver cancer worldwide. J Hepatol 2006;45:529–38.
[564] Ward JM, Fox JG, Anver MR, et al. Chronic active hepatitis and associated liver tumours in mice caused by a persistent bacterial infection with a novel *Helicobacter* species. J Natl Cancer Inst 1994;86:1222–7.
[565] Ponzetto A, Pellicano R, Leone N, et al. *Helicobacter* infection and cirrhosis in hepatitis C virus carriage: is it an innocent bystander or a troublemaker? Med Hypoth 2000;54:275–7.
[566] Farinati F, DeBona M, Floreani A, et al. *Helicobacter pylori* and the liver: any relationship? Ital J Gastroenterol Hepatol 1998;30:124–8.
[567] Ponzetto A, Fagoone S, Pellicano E. *Helicobacter pylori* and liver: development, endoscopic features. *Helicobacter pylori* infection, an actor with three roles? Dig Liver Dis 2001;34:399–402.
[568] Pellicano R, Menard A, Rizzetto M, et al. *Helicobacter* species and liver diseases: association or causation? Lancet Infect Dis 2008;8:254–60.
[569] Cortez-Pinto H, Camilo ME. Non-alcoholic fatty liver disease/non-alcoholic steatohepatitis (NAFLD/NASH): diagnosis and clinical course. Best Prac Res Clin Gastro 2004;18(6):1089–104.
[570] Bull PC, Thomas GR, Rommens JM, et al. The Wilson's disease gene is a putative copper transporting P-type ATPase similar to the Menkes gene. Nature Genet 1993;5:327–37.
[571] Ferenci D. Wilson's disease. Clin Liv Dis 1992;2(1):31–49.
[572] Bosworth BP, Landzberg BR. Neurological manifestations of gastrointestinal and hepatic diseases. Neurobiol Dis 2007;689–701.
[573] Gitlin N. Wilson's disease: the scourge of copper. J Hepatol 1998;28(4):734–9.
[574] Steindl P, Ferenci P, Dienes HP, et al. Wilson's disease in patients presenting with liver disease: a diagnostic challenge. Gastroenterology 1997;113:212–18.
[575] Stremmel W, Meyerrose KM, Niederau C, et al. Wilson's disease clinical presentation, treatment, and survival. Ann Intern Med 1991;115:720–6.
[576] Brissot P, Guyader D, Loreal O, et al. Clinical aspects of hemochromatosis. Transfus Sci 2000;23(30):193–200.
[577] Witte DL, Crosby WH, Edwards CQ. Practice guideline development task force of the college of American pathologists: hereditary hemochromatosis. Clin Chim Acta 1996;245:139–200.
[578] Pietrangelo A. Metals, oxidative stress, and hepatic fibrogenesis. Semin Liver Dis 1996;16:26–30.
[579] Bacon B, Powell LW, Adams PC, et al. Molecular medicine and haemochromatosis: at the crossroads. Gastroenterology 1999;116:193–207.
[580] Gieling RG, Bur AD, Mann DA. Fibrosis and cirrhosis reversibility: molecular mechanisms. Clin Liv Dis 2008;12:915–37.
[581] Pinzani M, Vizzutti F. Fibrosis and cirrhosis reversibility: clinical features and implications. Clin Liv Dis 2008;12:901–13.
[582] Sandhu BS, Sanyal AJS. Management of ascites in cirrhosis. Clin Liver Dis 2005;9:715–32.

[583] Rosner MH, Gupta R, Ellison D, et al. Management of cirrhotic ascites: physiological basis of diuretic action. Eur J Int Med 2006;17:8–19.
[584] Moore KP, Wong F, Gines P, et al. The management of ascites in cirrhosis: report on the consensus conference of the International Ascites Club. Hepatology 2003;38:258–66.
[585] de Franchis R, Primignani M. Natural history of portal hypertension in patients with cirrhosis. Clin Liv Dis 2001;5(3):645–63.
[586] Jalan R, Shawcross D, Davies N. The molecular pathogenesis of hepatic encephalopathy. Int J Biochem Cell Biol 2003;35:1175–81.
[587] Jalan R, Balata S, Olde Damink SWM, et al. Changes in neuropsychological function following hyperammonemia induced by a simulated bleed is mediated by increase in brain water. Hepatology 2001;35:67. [abstract].
[588] Albrecht J, Jones EA. Historical review: hepatic encephalopathy: molecular mechanisms underlying the clinical syndrome. J Neuro Sci 1999;170:138–46.
[589] Ahboucha S, Butterworth RF. The neurosteroid system: implication in the pathophysiology of hepatic encephalopathy. Neurochem Int 2008;52:575–87.
[590] Castaldo G, Orinai G, Lofrano MM, et al. Differential diagnosis between hepatocellular carcinoma and cirrhosis through a discriminating function based on results for serum analytes. Clin Chem 1996;42(8):1263–9.
[591] Canadian Neuro-Optic Research Institute (CNRI). Bexel Irina Asian Hospital Study of 352 Patients. STC Hospital sponsored clinical study — Korea. www.cnri.edu — unpublished data.
[592] Terry R. White nails in hepatic cirrhosis. Lancet 1955;263(6815):757–9.
[593] Smith KE, Fenske NA. Cutaneous manifestations of alcohol abuse. J Am Acad Dermatol 2000;43:1–16.
[594] Martinez-Lavin M. Exploring the cause of the most ancient clinical sign of medicine: finger clubbing. Semin Arthritis Rheum 2007;36(6):380–5.
[595] Pannhorst R, Hoffman H. Relation of liver diseases to changes in color of human tongue. Dtsch Med J 1957;8(5):232–6. [Article in German, English abstract cited].
[596] Golla K, Epstein JB, Cabay RJ. Liver disease: current perspectives on medical and dental management. Oral Surg Oral Med Oral Pathol Oral Radiol Endod 2004;98:516–21.
[597] Bloomfeld RS, Brevick G, Schiffman S, et al. Alterations of chemosensory function in end-stage liver disease. Physiol Behavior 1999;66(2):203–7.
[598] Keller AZ. Cirrhosis of the liver, alcoholism and heavy smoking associated with cancer of the mouth and pharynx. Cancer 2006;20(6):1015–22.
[599] O'Brien A, Williams R. Nutrition in end-stage liver disease: principles and practice. Gastroenterol 2008;134:1729–40.
[600] Changani KK, Jalan R, Cox IJ, et al. Evidence for altered hepatic gluconeogenesis in patients with cirrhosis using in vivo 31-phosphorus magnetic resonance spectroscopy. Gut 2001;49:557–64.
[601] Jessen N, Buhl ES, Schmitz O, et al. Impaired insulin action despite upregulation of proximal insulin signaling: novel insights into skeletal muscle insulin resistance in liver cirrhosis. J Hepatol 2006;45(6):797–804.
[602] Swart GR, van den Berg JWO, Wattinema DL, et al. Elevated protein requirements in cirrhosis of the liver investigated by whole body protein turnover studies. Clin Sci 1988;75:101–7.
[603] Schneeweis B, Graninger W, Ferenci P, et al. Energy metabolism in patients with acute and chronic liver disease. Hepatology 1990;11:387.
[604] Muller MJ, Bottcher J, Selberg O, et al. Hypermetabolism in clinically stable patients with liver cirrhosis. Am J Nutr 1999;69:1194.
[605] McCullough AJ, Tavill AS. Disordered energy and protein metabolism in liver disease. Semin Liv Dis 1991;11:265–77.
[606] O'Keefe SJ, Ogden J, Rund J. The use of 14C labelled phenylalanine to trace deranged aromatic amino acid metabolism in liver failure: a functional indicator with prognostic potential [abstract]. Gastroenterol 1989;96:A641.
[607] Moriwaki H, Miwa Y, Tajika M, et al. Branched-chain amino acids as a protein- and energy-source in liver cirrhosis. Biochem Biophys Res Comm 2004;313:405–9.
[608] Blonde-Cynober F, Ausse C, Cynober L. Abnormalities in branched chain amino acid metabolism in cirrhosis: influence of hormonal and nutritional factors and directions for future research. Clin Nutr 1999;18:5–13.
[609] Morgan TR, Moritz TE, Mendhall CL, et al. Protein consumption and hepatic encephalopathy in alcoholic hepatitis. VA Cooperative Study Group #275. J Am Coll Nutr 1995;14:152–8.
[610] Amodio P, Caregarol L, Pettenbl E, et al. Vegetarian diets in hepatic encephalopathy: facts or fantasies? Dig Liver Dis 2001;33:492–500.
[611] Swart GR, van den Berg JWO, van Vuure JK, et al. Minimum protein requirements in liver cirrhosis determined by nitrogen balance measurements at three levels of protein intake. Clin Nutr 1989;8:329–36.
[612] Kondrup J, Nielsen K. Protein requirement and protein utilization in patients with liver cirrhosis. Z Gastroenterol 1996;34:26–31.
[613] Bianchi GP, Marchesini G, Fabbri A, et al. Vegetable versus animal protein diet in cirrhotic patients with chronic encephalopathy: a randomized cross-over comparison. J Intern Med 1993;233:385–92.
[614] Shaw S, Worner TM, Lieber CS. Comparison of animal and vegetable protein sources in the dietary management of hepatic encephalopathy. Am J Clin Nutr 1983;38:59–63.
[615] Gallus S, Tavani A, Negri E, et al. Does coffee protect against liver cirrhosis? Ann Epidemiol 2002;12(3):202–5.
[616] Tverdal A, Skurtveit S. Coffee intake and mortality from liver cirrhosis. Ann Epidemiol 2003;13(6):419–23.
[617] Kendrick SFW, Day CP. A coffee with your brandy, Sir? J Hep 2007;46:980–2.
[618] Garattini S. Caffeine, coffee, and health. New York: Raven Press; 1993.
[619] Jiang P, Burczynski F, Campbell C, et al. Rutin and flavonoid contents in three buckwheat species *Fagopyrum esculentum*, *F. tataricum*, and *F. homotropicum* and their protective effects against lipid peroxidation. Food Res Int 2007;40(3):356–64.
[620] Bishayee A, Sarkar A, Chatterjee M. Hepatoprotective activity of carrot (*Daucus carota* L.) against carbon tetrachloride intoxication in mouse liver. J Ethno 1995;47(2):69–74.
[621] Vali L, Stefanovits-Banyai E, Szentmihalyi K, et al. Liver protecting effects of table beet (*Beta vulgaris* var. *rubra*) during ischemia reperfusion. Nutrition 2007;23(2):172–8.
[622] Cardenas A, Arroyo V. Mechanisms of water and sodium retention in cirrhosis and the pathogenesis of ascites. Best Pract and Res Clin Endo Metab 2003;17(4):607–22.
[623] Roberts WC. High salt intake, its origins, its economic impact, and its effect on blood pressure. Am J Cardiol 2001;88:1338–46.
[624] Grimes CA, Nowson CA, Lawrence M. An evaluation of the reported sodium content of Australian food products. Int J Food Sci Tech 2008;43(12):2219–29.
[625] Land M-A, Webster J, Christoforou A, et al. Salt intake assessed by 24 h urinary sodium excretion in a random and opportunistic sample in Australia. BMJ Open 2014;4:e003720. Available from:: http://bmjopen.bmj.com/content/4/1/e003720.
[626] Westin J. Moderate alcohol and fibrosis in chronic viral hepatitis. In Preedy VR, Watson RR, editors. Comprehensive handbook of alcohol related pathology. London: Elsevier; 2004. p. 833–43.
[627] Niederau C, Lange S, Heintges T, et al. Prognosis of chronic hepatitis C: results of a large, prospective cohort study. Hepatology 1998;28(6):1687–95.
[628] Leevy CM, Moroianu XA. Nutritional aspects of alcoholic liver disease. Clin Liv Dis 2005;9:67–81.
[629] Newsome PN, Beldon I, Moussa Y, et al. Low serum retinol levels are associated with HCC in patients with chronic liver disease. Ailment Pharmacol Ther 2000;14:1295–301.
[630] Di Sario Am, Candelaresi C, Omenetti A, et al. Vitamin E in chronic liver disease and liver fibrosis. Vitam Horm 2007;76:551–70.
[631] Bianchi GP, Marchesini G, Brizi M, et al. Nutritional effects of oral zinc supplementation in cirrhosis. Nut Res 2000;20(8):1079–89.
[632] Grungreiff K, Reinhold D. Liver cirrhosis and 'liver' diabetes mellitus are linked by zinc deficiency. Med Hypotheses 2005;64:316–17.
[633] Casaril M, Stanzial AM, Gabrielli GB, et al. Serum selenium in liver cirrhosis: correlation with markers of fibrosis. Clin Chim Acta 1989;182:221–8.
[634] Planas R, Balleste B, Alvarez MA, et al. Natural history of decompensated hepatitis C virus-related cirrhosis. J Hepatol 2004;40:823–30.

[635] Strauss E, Gomes de Sá Ribeiro F. Bacterial infections associated with hepatic encephalopathy: prevalence and outcome. Ann Hepatol 2003;2(1):41–5.
[636] Garcia-Tsao G, Wiest R. Gut microflora in the pathogenesis of the complications of cirrhosis. Best Prac Res Clin Gastroenterol 2004;18(2):353–72.
[637] Sakaida I, Tsuchiya M, Okamoto M, et al. Late evening snack and the change of blood glucose level in patients with liver cirrhosis. Hep Res 2004;30(1):67–72.
[638] Tsuchiya M, Sakaida I, Okamoto M, et al. The effect of a late evening snack in patients with liver cirrhosis. Hep Res 2005;31(2):95–103.
[639] Valta K, Valta P, Hockerstedt K, et al. Magnesium depletion in chronic terminal liver cirrhosis. Clin Transplant 2002;16:325–8.
[640] Cohen L. Magnesium and liver cirrhosis: a hypothesis. Magnesium 1985;4:1–4.
[641] Lieber CS, Leo MA, Cao Q, et al. Silymarin retards the progression of alcohol-induced hepatic fibrosis in baboons. J Clin Gastro 2003;37(4):336–9.
[642] Jeong DH, Lee GP, Jeong WI. Alterations of mast cells and TGF-beta 1 on silymarin treatment for CCl(4)-induced fibrosis. World J Gastroenterol 2005;11:1141–8.
[643] Saller R, Meier R, Brignoli R. The use of silymarin in the treatment of liver diseases' [Review]. Drugs 2001;61(14):2035–63.
[644] Rambaldi A, Jacobs BP, Iaquinto G, et al. Milk thistle for alcoholic and/or hepatitis B or C liver diseases — a systematic Cochrane Hepatobiliary Group Review with meta-analysis of randomised clinical trials. Am J Gastroenterol 2005;100:2583–91.
[645] Ferenci P, Dragosics B, Dittrich H, et al. Randomized controlled trial of silymarin treatment in patients with cirrhosis of the liver. J Hepatol 1989;9:105–13.
[646] Huseini HF, Larijani B, Heshmat R, et al. The efficacy of *Silybum marianum* (L.) Gaertn. (Silymarin) in the treatment of Type II diabetes: a randomized, double-blind, placebo-controlled, clinical trial. Phytother Res 2006;20:1036–9.
[647] Nan JX, Park EJ, Kang HC, et al. Anti-fibrotic effects of a hot-water extract from *Salvia miltiorrhiza* roots on liver fibrosis induced by biliary obstruction in rats. J Pharm Pharmacol 2001;53:197–204.
[648] She SF, Huang XZ, Tong GD. Clinical study on treatment of liver fibrosis by different dosages of Salvia injection. Zhongguo Zhong Xi Yi Jie He Za Zhi 2004;24:17–20. [Article in Chinese, English abstract cited].
[649] Tao LV, Xi-Xian Y. Comparison of protocatechuic aldehyde in Radix *Salvia miltiorrhiza* and corresponding pharmacological sera from normal and fibrotic rats by high performance liquid chromatography. World J Gastroenterol 2006;12(14):2195–200.
[650] Darnis F, Orcel L, de Saint-Maur PP, et al. Use of a triturated extract of *Centella asiatica* chronic hepatitic disorders. J Sem Hop 1979;55:1749–50. [Article in French, translated, abstract cited].
[651] Ming ZJ, Liu SZ, Cao L. Effect of total glucosides of *Centella asiatica* on antagonizing liver fibrosis induced by dimethylnitrosamine in rats. Zhongguo Zhong Xi Yi Jie He Za Zhi 2004;24(8):731–4. [Article in Chinese, English abstract cited].
[652] Flora SJ, Gupta R. Beneficial effects of *Centella asiatica* aqueous extract against arsenic-induced oxidative stress and essential metal status in rats. Phytother Res 2007;21(10):980–8.
[653] Thomsen M. Phytotherapy: desk reference. 2nd ed. Dee Why (NSW): Institut For Phytoterapi; 2001.
[654] Bochoráková H, Paulová H, Slanina J, et al. Main flavonoids in the root of *Scutellaria baicalensis* cultivated in Europe and their comparative antiradical properties. Phytother Res 2003;17(6):640–4.
[655] Nan JX, Park EJ, Kim YC, et al. *Scutellaria baicalensis* inhibits liver fibrosis induced by bile duct ligation or carbon tetrachloride in rats. J Pharm Pharmacol 2002;54(4):555–63.
[656] Zhang XP, Li ZF, Liu XG. Review in pharmacological study of baicalein. Chin Pharmacol Bull 2001;17(6):711–13. [Article in Chinese, English abstract cited].
[657] Lin CC, Shieh DE. In vivo hepatoprotective effect of baicalein, baicalin and wogonin from *Scutellaria rivularis*. Phytother Res 1996;10(8):651–4.
[658] Yamashiki M, Nishimura A, Huang XX, et al. Effects of the Japanese herbal medicine 'Sho-saiko-to' (TJ-9) on interleukin-12 production in patients with HCV-positive liver cirrhosis. Dev Immunol 1999;7(1):17–22.
[659] Chang WH, Chen CH, Lu FJ. Different effects of baicalein, baicalin and wogonin on mitochondrial function, glutathione content and cell cycle progression in human hepatoma cell lines. Plata Med 2002;86(2):128–32.
[660] Xiao J, Lu R, Shen X, et al. Green tea extracts protected against carbon tetrachloride-induced chronic liver damage and cirrhosis. Zhonghua Yu Fang Yi Xue Za Zhi 2002;36(4):243–6. [Article in Chinese English abstract cited].

The immune system

12

Leah Hechtman, Janet Schloss, Kathy Harris, Karen Bridgman

SECTION A: THE FUNDAMENTALS OF THE IMMUNE SYSTEM

OVERVIEW OF THE IMMUNE SYSTEM

Our immune system is a busy network of lymphoid tissue and organs, cells, humoral factors and cytokines.[1] How easily we are able to resist and recover from disease is largely due to how well our immune system is functioning. The immune system functions to protect us against the effects of the microbial pathogens that we face on a daily basis, as well as to help us to react against foreign substances and abnormal/cancer cells. The lymphatic system is highly important in terms of immunity as it functions to protect against invasion by facilitating specific immune responses against microbes or abnormal cells.[2] The lymphatic system comprises lymph, several lymphatic organs and tissues (such as the spleen and thymus) as well as the red bone marrow (Fig. 12.1).

LYMPHATIC VESSELS AND CIRCULATION

The lymphatic circulation relies on local pressure and contraction of the larger lymphatics as it does not contain a pump to move the lymph around. Lymph passes from the lymphatic capillaries into larger lymphatic vessels (similar to veins) and then into the lymph nodes which drain into the lymph trunks and pass into the thoracic left lymphatic duct and the right lymphatic duct. The lymph from the major portion of the thoracic duct flows through the thoracic duct while that from the right drains into the right lymphatic duct.[3] The lymphatic circulation is imperative for health and absence of disease. It has a series of one-way valves so the lymph can only move in one direction.

THE LYMPHATIC ORGANS AND TISSUES

The thymus gland

Described by the Roman anatomist Galen as the 'seat of courage', the thymus gland is the site of T-cell development, as well as regulation of the immune system where it optimises immune function, even in the sixth decade of life.[4] The thymus gland is located in the mediastinum and consists of two asymmetrical lobes; each lobe consists of a cortex and a medulla.[2] The cortex is home to small tightly packed lymphocytes (known as thymocytes), reticular epithelial cells and macrophages, while the medulla houses reticular cells and more densely proportioned lymphocytes. The reticular epithelial cells function to produce thymic hormones that in turn aid the maturation of T-cells. Anastasiadis and Ratnutunga[4] have suggested that loss of thymus function with age may be in some part related to the increased risk of infection and immune dysfunction seen in the elderly.

The lymph nodes

As with all the lymphatic organs and tissues, the lymph nodes participate in immune reactions, whereby they assist in the filtration of lymph, destroying unwanted substances so that the clean lymph can circulate to other areas of the body. The lymph nodes are 600 bean-shaped nodes[2] found on the lymphatic vessels; they are found in particularly large numbers near the groin and the mammary glands. The parenchyma of each lymph node may be divided into a superficial cortex and a deep medulla, of which the cortex can be further divided into an inner and an outer cortex. The outer cortex contains B lymphocytes while the inner cortex contains T lymphocytes.

Lymphatic nodules

The lymphatic nodules sound similar to the lymphatic nodes but differ. They are small oval nodules composed of lymphatic tissue that are found on the connective tissue of the mucous membranes in a wide array of bodily areas including the gastrointestinal tract and the respiratory tract.[2] Lymphatic nodules may occur by themselves (singular) or as multiple aggregations (e.g. the tonsils found in the pharyngeal region).

The spleen

The spleen is the body's largest filter of blood and is an oval-shaped mass of lymphatic tissue that can be found in the left upper quadrant of the body, connected to the stomach and under the diaphragm.[5]

The spleen functions to:[5]

- Filtrate blood
- Perform phagocytosis of erythrocytes

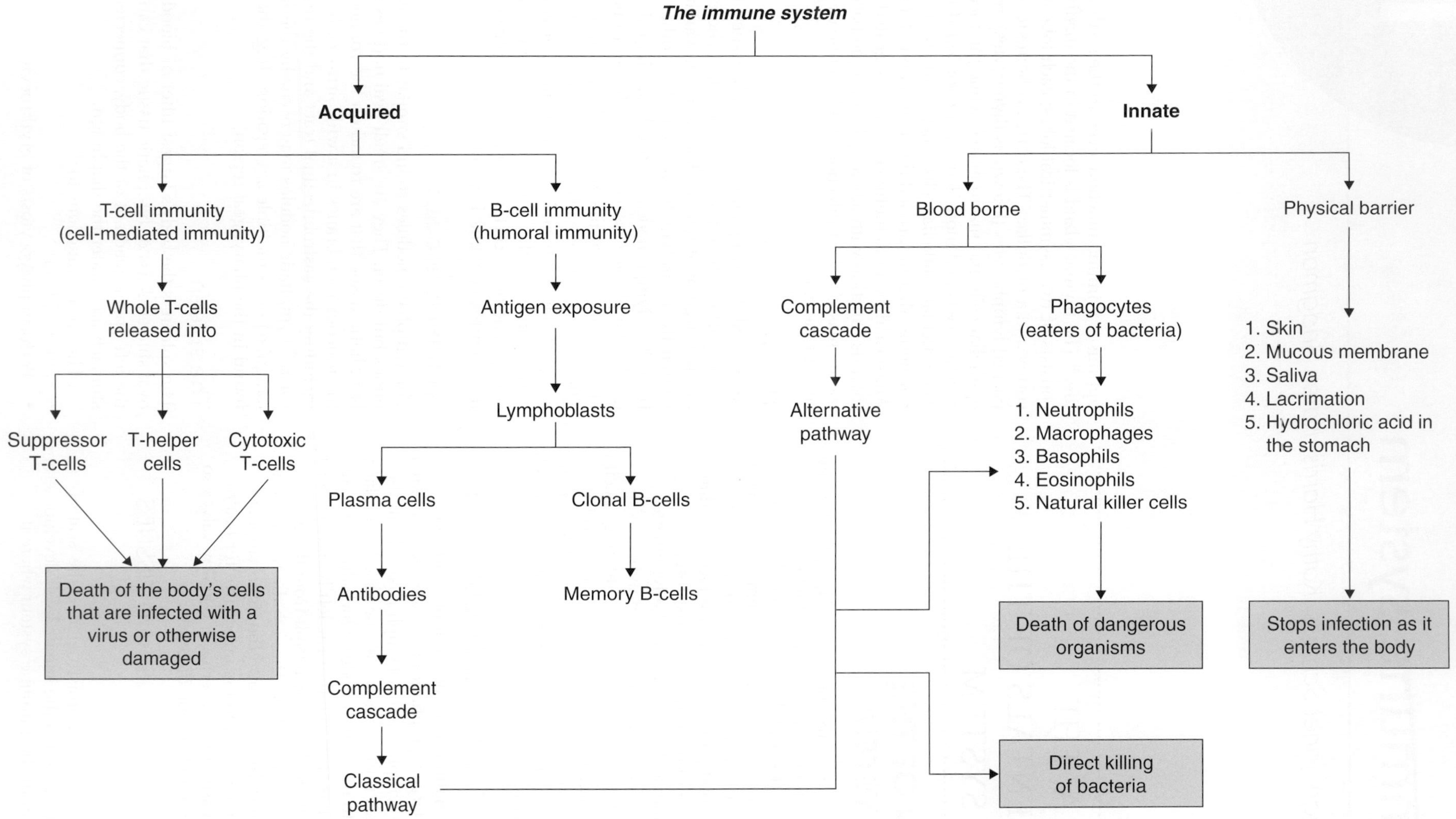

FIGURE 12.1 The immune system: flow chart.

- Recycle iron
- Capture and destroy pathogens
- Induce adaptive immune responses.

A capsule of dense, connective tissue can be found surrounding the spleen from which trabeculae stem inwards.[2] The spleen contains a number of blood vessels including small branches of arterioles that are enclosed in a protective covering of lymphoid tissue known as the white pulp; this consists of mostly lymphocytes and macrophages. The other parenchymal tissue of the spleen is called the red pulp and consists of red blood-filled venous sinuses; these function to filter blood, remove old erythrocytes and recycle iron. Blood flows into the spleen via the splenic artery entering the central arteries of the white pulp. From here the white pulp carries out a number of functions, as does the red pulp (detailed in Table 12.1).

A 'ruptured' spleen is something many people may have heard of, and often it requires the removal of the spleen. Considering the functions of the spleen, particularly the fact that it contains a quarter of the body's lymphocytes,[6] it is likely that some degree of immunity is likely to be compromised on removal. This is highlighted by Mebbius and Krall,[5] who acknowledge that the removal of the spleen in some humans leads to the inability to mount an appropriate immune response against certain bacteria. The body is highly adaptable, however, and other body structures (providing they are functioning correctly) can in part take over the job of the spleen.

The immune response to invaders can be divided into two parts:

1 Innate or nonspecific immunity — our primary defence system
2 Adaptive or specific/acquired immunity — our secondary defence system.

TABLE 12.1 The spleen

Area of the spleen	Description	Function
White pulp	Composed of lymphoid sheaths — lymphocytes and macrophages	• Lymphocytes (B-cells and T-cells) carry out immune functions • Splenic macrophages ingest blood-borne pathogens via phagocytosis
Red pulp	Consists of the venous sinuses and splenic cords (red blood cells, macrophages, lymphocytes, plasma cells and granulocytes)	• Macrophages remove old blood cells and platelets • Storage site of ⅓ of the body's platelets as well as storage of iron and erythrocytes • Haemopoiesis

Sources: Cesta MF. Normal structure, function, and histology of the spleen. Toxicol Pathol 2006; 34(5):455–465. Tortora GJ, Grabowski SR. Principles of anatomy and physiology. 9th edn. Biological Textbooks Wiley; 2000.

INNATE OR NONSPECIFIC IMMUNITY

The innate/nonspecific immunity functions immediately upon engagement with an invader; it comprises epithelial barriers, a cellular component (macrophages, polymorphonuclear leucocytes, natural killer (NK) cells, neutrophil, dendritic cells) and a non-cellular component with recognition molecules (C-reactive protein, serum amyloid protein, mannose-binding protein and complement). As mentioned, the innate immunity is immediate (and therefore not always specific); however, it helps to differentiate invading pathogens from host cells triggering phagocytosis and the elimination of the invader.

Innate defence mechanisms of the body can be split into two categories:

1 First-line defenders — skin and mucous membranes plus other fluids
2 Second-line defenders — antimicrobial proteins, natural killer cells and phagocytes and inflammatory responses.

First-line defenders

The first line of defence encompasses your skin and the mucous membranes — they function as your night club 'bouncers' and decide who can come into the body and who to turn away. Other first-line defence mechanisms your body uses to turn away pathogens include:

- Mucus (its stickiness functions like a trap)
- Urine (flushes toxins out of the body)
- Vomiting (expels microbes)
- Acidic vaginal secretions (prevent growth of certain bacteria).

Second-line defenders

If for some reason the first-line defenders have not done their job properly and the pathogens have entered the body, the second-line defenders come into play. These include the following.

(A) ANTIMICROBIAL PROTEINS

Antimicrobial proteins function to retard the growth of microbes. They include complement, interferons and transferrins. See Table 12.2.

TABLE 12.2 Antimicrobial proteins

Antimicrobial protein	Description	Defence function
Interferons	Proteins produced by infected lymphocytes, macrophages and fibroblasts	Interfere with virus replication
Complement	Normally inactive proteins found in blood and plasma membranes	Become activated and enhance immune, allergic and inflammatory reactions
Transferrins	Iron-binding proteins	Inhibit the growth of bacteria that use iron to grow

(B) NATURAL KILLER CELLS AND PHAGOCYTES

Natural killer cells

If the antimicrobial proteins have been ineffective against the invading pathogen they are attacked by the natural killer cells, a type of lymphocyte that as their name suggests, function to kill infectious pathogens as well as some tumour cells.

Phagocytosis

Two major cells, the neutrophils and the macrophages carry out phagocytosis — the process of ingesting microbial pathogens and other foreign matter. As well as being involved in nonspecific defence mechanisms, phagocytes are also highly involved in the immune response.

There are five stages to phagocytosis:

1 **Chemotaxis**: chemical attraction of phagocytes to a certain location in the body

↓

2 **Adherence**: the phagocyte attaches to the surface of the pathogen or foreign matter

↓

3 **Ingestion**: the phagocyte engulfs the pathogen/foreign matter

↓

4 **Digestion**: the phagocyte is transformed into a phagosome and merges with lysosomes to form a structure known as the phagolysosome. The lysosome provides lysozyme and digestive enzymes both of which help to break down the microbial cell, the phagocyte also forms potent oxidants in a process known as the 'oxidative burst'; it is here we can see the importance of good antioxidant intake to prevent free radical damage

↓

5 **Killing**: the oxidants and other chemicals secreted within the phagolysosomes kill the foreign pathogen; however, occasionally the pathogen may kill the phagocyte. In the case of a toxin such as brucellosis or Epstein-Barr virus (discussed later in this chapter) the pathogen may remain dormant for months or even years, waiting for the immune system to become compromised before it reactivates.

(C) INFLAMMATION

Inflammation is the body's nonspecific defence mechanism and a reaction to damaged cells. It is characterised by four cardinal signs: redness, pain, swelling and heat. Inflammation has three important stages: vasodilation of blood vessels and increased permeability of blood, phagocyte immigration and tissue repair. To understand the basis of what is happening at the most basic level in an immune/inflammatory condition it is good to have a general understanding of what is occurring at a cellular level during inflammation.

The inflammatory response

In response to injury a number of the body's cells (mast cells, basophils, platelets, macrophages and neutrophils) secrete histamine, which results in increased permeability and vasodilation of blood vessels. Vasodilation and increased permeability are good as they function to promote the flow of blood to the injury site providing nutrition to the damage area and also to clear out toxic debris. Polypeptides known as kinanes further instigate vasodilation and increased permeability.

Prostaglandins are released by damaged cells and may stimulate the movement of phagocytes to clear up the damage. Additionally, leukotrienes cause increased permeability and assist the phagocytes in adhering to the microbial pathogen. Complement, the antimicrobial protein discussed above, becomes active and stimulates various immune responses (for example destruction of bacteria, more histamine release).

ADAPTIVE ACQUIRED IMMUNITY

Adaptive/acquired immunity takes several days or weeks to develop; however, unlike innate immunity, adaptive immunity is extremely precise and exhibits an immunological memory whereby it cleverly remembers the invading pathogen. Thus, any subsequent exposure to this pathogen leads to a more vigorous and rapid response. With the help of other cells (for example macrophages), the lymphocytes recognise and destroy intruders such as viruses, toxins, cancer cells and the like; you might like to think of the lymphocytes as the security guards of the body and the intruders as robbers. Special lymphocytes known as T-cells (the security guards) destroy the intruding pathogens (the robbers) either by causing them to rupture or by releasing substances that kill their cells. Other special lymphocytes known as B-cells secrete antibodies that further destroy foreign substances in the body. Both the T-cells and the B-cells are produced from stem cells that originate in the red bone marrow.

In response to antigens the immune system must trigger a response. This can be cell mediated (involving T-cell immunity) or antibody/humoral mediated (involving B-cell immunity) See Table 12.3.

Fever

Fever is an abnormal rise in usual body temperature whereby the body's thermostat found in the hypothalamus

TABLE 12.3 Immune system response to antigens

Cell mediated	CD8 T-cells develop into cytotoxic/killer T-cells, responsible for killing and destroying pathogens involved in cell-mediated immune responses; these travel to sites of infections or where there is a tumour where they attack and eliminate the infected cells	Good for intracellular pathogens such as viruses, fungi, parasites, foreign tissue transplants, some cancer cells
Humoral/ antibody mediated	B-cells transform into plasma cells that secrete antibodies to inactivate the antigen. Involves memory T-cells which remember previous immune responses to a specific invader; when they come across that invader again they remember the immune response and initiate a rapid response to destroy the pathogen	Good for antigens and extracellular bacteria

resets itself; one situation in which fever may occur is in response to microbial infection and inflammation. The body is extremely clever and in response to invading bacteria, phagocytes arrive and engulf them; however, when the phagocytes ingest certain bacteria they trigger the release of certain cytokines such as interleukin-1 whose function it is to promote fever. Interleukin-1 travels to the hypothalamus stimulating the secretion of prostaglandins; it is these prostaglandins that reset the body's thermostat at a higher temperature.[2] At the first sign of a temperature many people will panic and try to suppress it; however, to a certain point fever is of benefit as it functions to:

- Kill and prevent many pathogens replicating
- Intensify the effects of interferon
- Enhance phagocyte activity
- Increase T-cell production
- Increase antibody production
- Increase cellular repair.

Though body temperature is increasing the patient will typically feel cold and complain of chills as a result of vasoconstriction. As core temperature and the temperature of the hypothalamic thermostat match, however, the chills disappear. Once the fever has dissipated and the thermostat is lowered, sweating and other means of cooling the body are used to bring the body back to the same lowered temperature of the hypothalamic thermostat.

Infection

Infections can be a predisposing or triggering factor for a number of conditions. In the naturopathic framework, it is essential to holistically consider potential pathogens that precipitated the patient's presentation. This section gives an overview of the main types of infections, and a number of specific infections that are associated with the development of chronic conditions. It is essential to thoroughly investigate and assess your patient's presentation. Chronic infection is a major underlying factor and successful treatment must ensure isolation of the pathogen and modification of treatment accordingly. Generally, treatment is required for an extended period of time to properly eradicate the infection and must deal with multiple factors including lifestyle, dietary, nutritional supplementation, herbal medicines and others.

Bacterial infections

Bacteria are microscopic, single-celled organisms that are found in all living material. They are extremely adaptable and can survive in most conditions. Bacteria are prokaryotes indicating that they do not have a distinct nucleus; rather, their DNA floats freely in the cell.

Bacteria may be classified according to Gram stain, shape, respiration, reproduction or grouping, as described in Table 12.4.

Examples of common bacterial infections include Enterobacteria such as salmonella, *Escherichia coli*, *Streptococcus pneumoniae*, gonorrhoea (*Neisseria gonorrhoeae*), listeriosis and meningococcal disease.

TABLE 12.4 Classification of bacteria

Classification	Features
Gram stain	Gram-positive/Gram-negative
Shape	Cocci (spheres), bacilli (rods), spirochetes (spirals), coccobacilli (between spheres and rods)
Respiration	Aerobes (require oxygen)/anaerobes (do not require oxygen)
Reproduction	Sporing/non-sporing
Grouping	Clusters (*Staphylococcus*), chains (*Streptobacillus*)

Viral infections

Viruses are minute organisms that are much smaller than bacteria and fungi. They are unable to reproduce on their own and so invade the host's cells, taking over so that they can replicate within them.

Viruses may be classified according to nucleic material, arrangement of nucleic acid or structure, as described in Table 12.5.

TABLE 12.5 Classification of viruses

Classification	Features
Nucleic material	DNA/RNA
Arrangement of nucleic acid	Single or double strand
Structure	Enveloped/non-enveloped

Examples of viral infections include hepatitis B, hepatitis C, herpes simplex virus (HSV), influenza virus, poliovirus, human immunodeficiency virus (HIV), human adenovirus type 1 and dengue virus type-2 (DEN-2) to name but a few. The majority of antibiotics are ineffective against viral infections and therefore should not be used.

Fungal infections

Fungal infections are seldom harmful except in the immune compromised such as cancer patients or in patients with AIDS.

Examples of fungal infections include *Candida albicans* and the *Aspergillus* spp.

SPECIFIC INFECTIONS

Epstein-Barr virus

Epstein-Barr virus (EBV) is a virus of the herpes family implicated in a number of conditions. Epstein-Barr virus has proved itself one of the most successful viruses due to its ability to stay in the body for life and is said to infect more than 90% of the general population's T and B lymphocytes before adulthood.[7] EBV is shed in the saliva, hence infection most commonly occurs as a result of contact with infectious saliva. The EBV replicates in the nasopharyngeal epithelium cells and then spreads to other structures such as the salivary glands where the virus replicates again, infecting the liver, spleen and B lymphocytes in peripheral blood.[8] EBV typically incubates for between 4 and 8 weeks and then symptoms present insidiously.[9] The most common clinical presentation of EBV is infectious mononucleosis, which presents with

TABLE 12.6 Complications of primary Epstein-Barr virus infection

Liver	Clinical jaundice (5%), abnormal liver function tests (80–90%), fulminant hepatitis (rare)
Respiratory	Respiratory tract obstruction, interstitial pneumonitis (rare)
Neurological	Encephalitis, acute cerebellar syndrome, aseptic meningitis, Guillain-Barré syndrome, cranial nerve palsy (especially VII), seizures
Spleen	Splenic rupture 0.1–0.5% spontaneous or after mild trauma, usually males, splenic infarction
Haematological	Thrombocytopenia, haemolytic anaemia, neutropenia, haemorrhage secondary to mucosal ulceration
Secondary infection	Streptococcal sore throat, sepsis in association with neutropenia
Renal	Haematuria, interstitial nephritis, glomerulonephritis (rare)
Immune	Depressed cell-mediated immunity
Cardiovascular	Myocarditis, pericarditis, arrhythmia, electrocardiogram change
Psychiatric	Depression, anxiety

Source: Macsween K, Crawford D. Epstein-Barr virus — recent advances. Lancet Infect Dis 2003; 3(3):131–140.

fever, sore throat and swollen lymph nodes with enlarged spleen and liver. However, other conditions such as multiple sclerosis,[10] rheumatoid arthritis, Burkitt's lymphoma, nasopharyngeal carcinoma and hairy cell leukaemia have all implicated EBV in their aetiology (see also Table 12.6). Symptoms associated with acute infection with EBV generally disappear within a few weeks however fatigue and malaise may persist for months.

EBV and autoimmunity

There is a large body of evidence that infection has a role in the pathogenesis of many human chronic autoimmune diseases. EBV has the unique ability to infect, activate and latently persist in B lymphocytes. When EBV infects resting B-cells in vitro, it drives them into activation and proliferation independently of T-cell help. Infection of B-cells from normal individuals in vitro results in the production of monoclonal autoantibodies reacting with antigens in multiple organs. This accounts for the transient appearance of autoantibodies during the course of infectious mononucleosis. Usually, the proliferating infected B-cells are eventually eliminated by EBV-specific cytotoxic CD8+ T-cells, but latently infected non-proliferating memory B-cells persist in the individual for life. Antigen-driven differentiation of latently infected memory B-cells into plasma cells may trigger entry into the lytic cycle with the production of infectious virus.

Cytomegalovirus

Human cytomegalovirus (CMV) is a betaherpes virus and the largest of the herpes viruses. It may be differentiated from other herpes viruses due to its salivary tropism, its slow replicative cycle in cellular cultures and its affinity of course for human beings.[11] The human cytomegalovirus is found in all populations and knows no seasonal variance.[12] The cytomegalovirus initially enters via the epithelium of the upper alimentary, respiratory or genitourinary tract.[13] It forms a lifelong bond with the human it infects, for once infected a person is always infected.[14] The human cytomegalovirus is typically asymptomatic but is associated with a wide range of diseases, particularly in those who are immune compromised. Infection with the human cytomegalovirus can occur via many mechanisms including sexual intercourse, salivary contact, breastfeeding, transfer via the placenta, blood transfusion and organ or stem cell transfusion.[15] Human cytomegalovirus infection is a major contributor to birth defects and in humans is thought to account for up to 8% of cases of mononucleosis.[16] Clinical presentation of symptoms of mononucleosis associated with cytomegalovirus infection is similar to that of Epstein-Barr virus and includes cervical lymphadenopathy, fever, myalgia, headache and rash.[13] However, it can be differentiated as it is unusual to see splenomegaly or tonsillopharyngitis with the human cytomegalovirus, though these commonly present with Epstein-Barr virus.[15]

Mycoplasma

Mycoplasma are the smallest self-replicating microorganisms. Structurally they are prokaryotes that contain no bacterial cell wall; they contain circular DNA and some ribosomes.[17] They can be found living within the mucus surfaces of the body including the respiratory and urogenital tracts, alimentary canal, joints and the eyes.[18] At least 15 mycoplasma substances have been identified in humans: some of the better known species include *Mycoplasma genitalium*, linked to urogenital infections, and *Mycoplasma pneumonia*, linked to a number of respiratory conditions. As with many of the microbial species discussed, the *Mycoplasma* spp. have been implicated in a number of disease states including fibromyalgia, chronic fatigue syndrome, HIV, various cancers, SLE (lupus) and Gulf War syndrome.

Enterovirus

The enteroviruses are one of the most common human viruses[19] and are a group of non-enveloped viruses that include the poliovirus, coxsackie A and B viruses, enterovirus 17 and the echoviruses[20] that belong to the Picornaviridae family. Structurally the enteroviruses are small with an RNA genome; however, over 64 different human enteroviruses have been identified. The enteroviruses cause degenerative changes to the cells of the body, but other disease presentations are thought to occur as a result of host immune response to infection. The enteroviruses have been linked to a number of other conditions, for example the coxsackie A virus 19 is linked to Guillain-Barré disease.[21] Other conditions linked to enteroviruses include type 1 diabetes mellitus and many diseases of autoimmune origin.[19] The virus typically infects the respiratory or gastrointestinal epithelium. Human transmission occurs primarily through the faecal–oral route or from respiratory secretions (e.g. saliva, sneezing).

Retrovirus

The retroviruses are a group of enveloped RNA-containing viruses that carry the enzyme reverse transcriptase inside their virions;[22] most other organisms store their genetic material in the form of DNA. The most well-known human retrovirus is HIV. Other retroviruses include HTLV-1 (human T-lymphotropic virus) that is implicated in adult T-cell leukaemia.[22]

Ross River fever

Ross River fever is a mosquito-borne alphavirus prevalent in Australia and Papua New Guinea. In Australia, between 1 January and 23 March 2010 there were 916 cases documented. This is substantially less than in the same period in 2008, which had already seen 2780 documented cases in the same 3-month period.[23] The majority of those infected with Ross River fever fall into the 25–44-year-old age group with no discrimination between male or female sex.[24] Risk of infection with Ross River fever increases in situations or periods that encourage mosquito breeding such as where there is increased rainfall and flooding; in Northern Australia most cases of Ross River fever occur between January and April.[24]

SYMPTOMS

The incubation period for Ross River fever ranges between 3 and 21 days.[24] Thus patients may typically present with symptoms as late as 3 weeks after the initial infection, underlining the importance of thorough questioning. The most common symptom of Ross River fever is acute arthralgia affecting the fingers, toes, hands, feet, elbows and knees that is usually symmetrical. Patients may also report tenderness, with limited range of movement, redness and swelling.[25] A high percentage of patients also experience malaise and fatigue.

Other common signs and symptoms include fever, muscle aches and pains, joint swelling, headache, rash and depression. Infection with Ross River fever in patients who present with acute polyarthritis and/or rash with a history of travel or residence in an infected area should be suspected and ascertained with appropriate serology. Question patients on their recent history of outdoor activities such as bush walking and camping, which are likely to increase the risk if undertaken in areas where there are infected mosquitos.

REDUCING RISK OF INFECTION FROM ROSS RIVER VIRUS

- Wear light, protective clothing
- Use mosquito repellents (essential oil combinations)
- Use mosquito coils/citronella candles
- Use mosquito nets/screens
- Remove water containers and other materials that may encourage mosquito breeding.

Legionnaires' disease

Legionellosis virus is found worldwide with the most common form to cause outbreaks being *Legionella pneumophilia*. The incidence rate for *Legionella* varies widely depending on the country's surveillance and reporting system. The most commonly reported cases have been in Europe, Australia and the USA where about 10–15 cases are detected per million of population. However, since many countries lack appropriate methods of diagnosis and insufficient reporting systems, the rate of cases of *Legionella* may be more prevalent in undeveloped countries.[26]

Legionella organisms are found naturally in the environment, such as in streams, rivers and mud.[27] However, under the right circumstances (warmth and moisture), they multiply within amoebae. Transmission of *Legionella* does not occur via person-to-person contact but rather through inhalation of contaminated aerosols (tiny droplets) during contact with contaminated vapour, usually from manufactured water systems[27] such as water pipes, shower heads and taps, air-conditioning units, cooling towers (respiratory equipment, spas and bath-houses).[28] Incubation of Legionnaires' disease is approximately 2–10 days. Clinical signs and symptoms manifest subsequently and include flu-like symptoms, fever, gastrointestinal symptoms such as diarrhoea, neurological disturbance such as confusion,[29] as well as headache, myalgia and anorexia.[27] Laboratory findings may show liver dysfunction and electrolyte disturbances including creatine kinase. The elderly, the immune-compromised and smokers are most at risk of pneumonia.[30]

Chlamydia

Chlamydia is a genus of Gram-negative, aerobic, obligate, intracellular pathogens which are reliant on the host's energy resources as they are unable to synthesise their own ATP.[31] Two main disease causing species of *Chlamydia* in humans are *Chlamydia trachomatis* and *Chlamydia pneumoniae*. *C. trachomatis* is the most commonly diagnosed bacterial sexually transmissible infection.[32] It is an intracellular bacterial pathogen that infects the genital and ocular mucosa of humans causing infections that can lead to pelvic inflammatory disease, infertility and eye infection. Other complications specific to pregnancy include ectopic pregnancy and premature rupture of membranes. *C. trachomatis* may be passed from mother to child during birth. It also affects males, and may result in urethritis, epididymitis and conjunctivitis.[33] Estimated incubation time for *C. trachomatis* is approximately 7–15 days.[33]

C. pneumoniae is transmitted via respiratory secretions infecting the respiratory system, contributing to respiratory tract infections such as bronchitis, sinusitis and pneumonia.[33] Because it can be asymptomatic a large number of those infected are not aware they have it; however, they can develop complications later on. It appears the chlamydial species may infect immune cells resulting in disrupted immune cell function contributing to the progression of several chronic inflammatory diseases. For example *Chlamydia pneumoniae* has been isolated from brain tissues of patients with degenerative neurological disorders such as Alzheimer's disease[34] as well as multiple sclerosis[35] and certain lymphomas.

Rickettsia

Rickettsia are intracellular, Gram-negative coccobacilli that lack flagella and multiply within eukaryotic cells. The defining trait of *Rickettsia* is that they cannot survive in their own environment; to live and reproduce they must do so inside the cell of another organism (the host). In humans they may be classified into three groups: the spotted fever group, the typhus group *Rickettsia*, and scrub typhus. *Rickettsia* may be transmitted to humans via ticks, through damaged skin via faeces from flies or lice, or through aerosol spray from animal faeces. The *Rickettsia* have an affinity for the endothelial cells infecting them causing the development of multi-systemic small vessel vasculitis affecting various organs of the body including the central nervous system, heart, lungs, skin, liver and kidneys.

SYMPTOMS

Symptoms will depend on the strain and of course the vital force of the patient. Despite the many different strains of *Rickettsia* (Table 12.7), after an incubation period they produce many similar symptoms including fever, headache, rash and myalgia. More serious manifestations may result in interstitial pneumonia, adult respiratory distress syndrome, meningoencephalitis, seizures, coma, hepatitis and renal failure.[36]

Brucella

Brucella are Gram-negative, aerobic or non-aerobic non-motile coccobacilli that can survive on bacteriological media or outdoors, though typically they are intracellular.[37] The *Brucella* spp. have been around for centuries having first been identified in 1886 from the spleen of a deceased soldier who had passed away after a febrile illness.[38] Brucellosis is an insidious disease; infection is largely thought to be transmitted to humans (who function as secondary hosts) via contact with animals (primary hosts). This may be via direct contact (e.g. abattoir workers) or via indirect contact with animal secretions containing the organism. *Brucella* may invade the host via respiratory or oral inhalation, as well as via the conjunctiva, from open wounds such as a cut, or even through unpasteurised dairy products such as cheese or uncooked meat.[39] In humans, four species of *Brucella* have been discovered to be pathogenic, namely *B. melitensis*, *B. abortus*, *B. suis* and *B. canis*. Of these, *B. melitensis* is the most commonly occurring; additionally, it is also the most serious.[38]

Symptoms may occur up to 8 weeks after the infection and while recognised as rarely being fatal, are associated with discomfort. Presentation may include: nonspecific flu-like symptoms for intermittent fever (increased in the evening to 38–41°C) with sweats, chills and fatigue. Hadda et al[40] note that brucellosis is a frequently missed cause of pyrexia, thus as a clinician it is important to consider this as a cause, particularly in patients who may have returned from international travel, as brucellosis is endemic in countries bordering the Mediterranean. Other symptoms include nausea, anorexia, back pain, headache and muscle pain as well as enlargement of the liver, spleen and exterior lymph nodes. More seriously, neurobrucellosis may occur. Perkins et al[38] have also noted that infection may be reactivated a year after the initial infection, presenting as chronic fatigue, depression, weight loss and arthritis. Because *Brucella* are intracellular microorganisms only a small number of antibiotics are effective at eradicating them. These antibiotics are usually used in combinations and include tetracycline, aminoglycosides, rifampicin and quinolones.

TABLE 12.7 Some rickettsioses discovered in Australia

Infection	Infecting organism	Area of Australia found
Queensland tick typhus, belongs to the spotted fever group	*Rickettsia australis*	East coast of Australia
Flinders Island spotted fever	*Rickettsia honei*	Tasmania, south Australia, Queensland, Torres Strait Islands
Scrub typhus	*Orientia tsutsugamushi*	Tropical Australia — Kimberley region of Western Australia, Northern Territory, far north Queensland, Torres Strait Islands
Q fever	*Coxiella burnetii*	New South Wales, Queensland
Endemic/ murine typhus	*Rickettsia typhi*	Western Australia, Victoria

Sources: Graves S, Stenos J. Rickettsioses in Australia. Ann N Y Acad Sci 2009; 1166:151–155. Graves S, Unsworth N, Stenos J. Rickettsioses in Australia. Ann N Y Acad Sci 2006; 1078:74–79.

Borrelia burgdorferi

Discovered in 1982, *Borrelia burgdorferi* is a species of highly motile, adaptable, spirochete bacteria transmitted in humans via infected ticks. It is the causative organism in Lyme disease in humans. Following its adhesion to a human, the infected tick attempts to draw blood. The *Borrelia burgdorferi* pathogen is typically housed in the gut of the tick and cleverly travels to the tick's salivary gland so that it can be transported into the human's blood through the tick's puncture wound; once there it localises in the host spreading through a number of tissues. After approximately 4–7 days, if the tick has not already been found and eliminated, enzyme degradation of the attachment joining the human and tick occurs, allowing the tick to freely detach itself from the human, but not before it takes one last big sip of blood.[41] Nau et al[42] have noted that transmission of *Borrelia burgdorferi* via a tick bite is rare in the first 24 hours; however, risk increases dramatically as adhesion time increases, thus removal of a tick as soon as one becomes aware of it would appear to be important.

Lyme disease commonly presents with a characteristic skin lesion erythema migrans, said to be the most clinically reliable symptom for diagnosis.[43] This may occur days or sometimes even weeks after the infected skin bite; following this a small red papule forms where the bite occurred, and as it grows bigger the centre clears to form a ring-like shape. In a percentage of people there is mild itching, burning or pain at the site.

Other skin manifestations include acrodermatitis chronica atrophicans and lymphocytosis benigna cutis, highly indicative of Lyme disease. The nervous system, heart, eyes and joints may also be affected by Lyme disease. Thus a range of signs and symptoms including intermittent oligoarticular arthritis, meningitis, cranial neuritis, radiculoneuropathy, encephalopathy, atrioventricular block, myopericarditis, neurological impairment and fatigue are all possible.[41]

Giardia lamblia

Giardia lamblia is a protozoan parasite that infects the small intestine of humans,[44] in particular the jejenum and duodenum.[45] Structurally, *Giardia lamblia* is a eukaryotic (unicellular) organism, which lacks mitochondria, nucleoli and perixosomes.

One of the most common sources of infection is oral consumption of contaminated water; however, it has also been noted that infection may occur as a result of person-to-person contact as well as contact with infected animals, in particular those that are domestic such as cats and dogs.[46] Severity of infection may differ according to the person's age, nutritional status, coexisting infection and of course the functioning of their immune system. For example, an immunocompromised 25-year-old with a history of frequent infections will likely present with more severe symptoms than a robust 25-year-old with no history of infection. The most important clinical signs to be aware of with giardiasis are watery diarrhoea, malabsorption, nausea, abdominal pain and subsequent weight loss;[47] human studies show clear impairment of the intestinal cells' digestive and absorptive functions.[48] Noteworthy and relevant when considering treatment options is the fact that infection with *Giardia lamblia* is associated with little to minimum inflammation of the mucosa.[45] Resolution of symptoms occurs in many, though chronic disease states may also occur.

The life cycle of *Giardia lamblia* can be split into two major stages:[49]

1 The proliferative trophozoite
2 The non-proliferative, infectious cyst.

Following ingestion of the parasite, excystation (the escape from the cyst) occurs in the upper part of the small intestine and the excyzoite is released. The infectious dose is low with only around 10–100 *Giardia* cysts required to cause infection. The excyzoite divides without DNA replication into four disease-causing trophozoites, which replicate in the lumen of the intestine. Once the *Giardia* cysts reach a certain concentration in the lumen symptoms occur, though interestingly this induction of symptoms typically occurs 6–15 days after infection, hence the importance of thorough questioning of a client's history including habits, such as kissing their dog or cat, recent holiday, contaminant water, etc. Concentration of *Giardia* cysts can be extremely high, with Roxström-Lindquist et al[45] noting that patients infected with *Giardia* may shed up to 1×10^8 of viable cysts per gram in their faecal matter.

Candida albicans

Candida albicans is the most prevalent fungal pathogen in human beings and a ubiquitous commensal in mammalian microbiome.[50] *Candida* is normally found in small amounts in the human body and is only considered a health issue if it becomes overgrown in certain areas, which is called candidiasis. There are several types of candidiasis that can cause discomfort and occasionally dangerous symptoms. These include:[51]

1 **Oral thrush/candidiasis or oropharyngeal or oesphageal candidiasis**: This involves a yeast infection in the mouth, throat or oesphageal area. It is most commonly found in infants, elderly, patients undergoing chemotherapy, and people with AIDS or other conditions that weaken the immune system. The most common symptoms include white spots inside the mouth and on the tongue, redness and soreness in the mouth area, sore throat and difficulty swallowing, and pain in the upper chest region.
2 **Genital candidiasis**: Is most commonly found in women with symptoms including extreme itching with soreness and redness in the vaginal area, white clumpy vaginal discharge that can look like cottage cheese and painful intercourse. In men, it is more likely to occur in men who were not circumcised. The symptoms include red rash on the penis and itching and burning on the tip of the penis.
3 **Nappy rash:** It is important to recognise that not all nappy rashes are caused by *Candida*. For it to be diagnosed as a candidiasis nappy rash, it will present with dark-red patches of skin in the area and folds of skin near the thighs with yellow, fluid-filled spots that can break open and become flaky.
4 **Invasive candidiasis or candidemia:** This form of candidiasis is where the *Candida* is found in the bloodstream and where it can spread to other parts of the body. Invasive candidiasis normally only occurs in a weakened immune state or if someone has come in contact with contaminated medical equipment. Symptoms are vague and can depend on the part of the body affected. Some symptoms including fever and chills continue after antibiotic treatment. This is a very serious condition that requires immediate medical treatment.

In addition to *Candida albicans* causing candidiasis, it has also been found to contribute to polymicrobial infections. Polymicrobial infections involving bacteria and *Candida albicans* are called trans-kingdom interactions, which can be either synergistic or antagonistic. This interaction can modulate the virulence and pathogenicity of both the bacteria and the *Candida* while impacting the pathogen-host immune response. Considering the rise in antibiotic and antifungal resistance, further research and understanding of trans-kingdom interactions is important in the context of pathogenesis, diagnosis and disease management.[52] The treatment for candidiasis is an anti-*Candida* diet and antifungal treatments.

Allergies

Allergies comprise of a set of highly prevalent diseases that in some cases can endanger people's lives.[53] Allergies are a common condition and for reasons still to be identified, seem to be increasing worldwide with unprecedented complexity and severity. The World Allergy Organization identified in 2011 that approximately 30–40% of the world population is now affected by one or more allergies. Children in particular bear the greatest burden of allergic diseases with the most common conditions including food allergies, eczema and asthma. As stated, the precise causes of this increase are still not fully understood but due to the increase, further research is being conducted.[54]

Allergies include the following conditions:[54]

- Allergic conjunctivitis
- Allergic rhinitis
- Allergy to drugs and biological agents
- Anaphylaxis
- Asthma
- Atopic eczema
- Food allergy
- Insect allergy
- Occupational allergy (different environments connected to occupations can cause an allergy response)
- Rhinosinusitis
- Sports and allergies (vigorous sports can trigger or exacerbate allergy syndromes)
- Urticaria and angio-oedema.

There are four types of allergic reactions.

TYPE 1 — ANAPHYLACTIC

Type 1 (anaphylactic) reactions are associated with the type I, IgE-mediated hypersensitivity reaction. The allergen interacts with IgE antibodies on the surface of mast cells and basophils and after re-exposure to the allergenic substance the mast cells and basophils secrete mediators such as histamine and leukotrienes that cause cutaneous (rash), respiratory (e.g. smooth muscle contraction of the lungs), cardiovascular and gastrointestinal signs and symptoms. Peanut allergy is a common food-related cause of lethal anaphylaxis.

TYPE 2 — CYTOTOXIC

Type 2 (cytotoxic) reactions involve IgG or IgM antibodies directing antigens against a person's blood cells or tissue cells.[2]

TYPE 3 — IMMUNE COMPLEX REACTIONS

Type 3 (immune complex) reactions: in the presence of specific antigen–antibody ratios (IgA or IgG) immune complexes escape from phagocytes but remain trapped in the blood vessels causing inflammation. This is often seen in rheumatoid arthritis patients who may show the presence of IgA and IgG antibodies.[55]

TYPE 4 — CELL-MEDIATED REACTIONS/ DELAYED HYPERSENSITIVITY REACTIONS

Type 4 reactions usually occur 12–72 hours after allergen exposure and are initiated by mononuclear leucocytes.[56]

There are a number of risk factors for allergic disease. The main risk factor is genetic or inherited allergies. Most allergic diseases are heterogenous and involve important gene–environmental interactions so understanding the human genome is important. This will determine the susceptibility for disease onset, phenotypes and sub-phenotypes, severity, and potential response to treatments. Many early genetic studies have given some insight but more research is being conducted due to emerging concepts and hypothesis. Epigenetic influences also play a major role which involves very complex aspects such as methylation of CpG islands in gene promoters, histone acetylation, phosphorylation and a large number of micro RNA which can influence transgenerational effects and gene–environmental interactions.

Other risk factors include environmental factors both indoor and outdoor, socio-economic factors, climate change and migration. Human development of new substances, changes in the earth's temperature, changes in air pollutants and the migration of people from one country to another which involves exposure to a different set of allergens such as pollens and diet are all involved in increasing the risk of people developing allergies.

A thorough history taking of the patient and understanding the immune response are all important aspects in identifying allergies and treatment options. However, not only are allergies on the rise, so are sensitivities, and recognising the difference is essential. This is related to food and beverages versus environmental exposure. The key difference between food allergies and food sensitivity/ intolerance is the body's response to ingestion. An allergy always involves an immune response whereas a sensitivity is largely triggered in the digestive system.

Treatment of allergies involves anti-allergy medication or herbs and decreasing exposure to the allergen. In addition, it will also involve symptomatic treatment which will be different in each individual.

Pathological testing for immune system

There are a number of laboratory tests for the immune system depending on what the doctors are looking at. To determine an immune condition, the tests outlined in Table 12.8 may be conducted.

ROLE OF THE NATUROPATH

Traditional interpretation

Though their origins may date back hundreds of years, HIV, cancer and autoimmune conditions are relatively newly characterised conditions and thus were undocumented by the Eclectics. Instead, the predominant conditions of the immune system the Eclectics dealt with were caused by illnesses such as the plague, tuberculosis, anthrax and leprosy. However, these conditions share a similarity with the immune conditions that contemporary herbalists help to manage in that they were all recognised to have a microbial origin; for example, the tuberculosis bacillus is implicated in tuberculosis and the bacillus *Mycobacterium leprae* in leprosy.

TABLE 12.8 General immune system pathology or other tests

Overview	Condition	List of pathology tests
General check		FBC — full blood count or complete blood count (CBC) ESR — erythrocyte sedimentation rate CRP — C-reactive protein
Allergies		Skin prick tests Allergen-specific IgE testing Total IgE testing Oral food challenge Patch testing
Atypical pneumonia/ chronic cough	Chronic coughs/pain/fatigue	Sputum mcs Mycobacterium tuberculosis *Legionella* Mycoplasma *Chlamydia* *Bordetella pertussis* Influenzas Adenovirus polymerase chain reaction (PCR) Q fever Mantoux
Autoimmune disease	General autoimmune check	Anti-nuclear antibody (ANA) test ESR CRP
	Addison's disease	Cortisol ACTH ACTH stimulation test Aldosterone Electrolytes Urea and creatine Glucose levels Renin Adrenal antibodies
	Inflammatory bowel disease (IBD), Crohn's disease, ulcerative colitis	Endoscopy Colonoscopy Comprehensive metabolic pain Faecal occult blood test or faecal immunochemical test Ova and parasite stool tests Calprotectin and lactoferrin CRP ESR
	Coeliac disease	Anti-tissue transglutaminase antibodies (anti-tTG, IgA or IgG) Deamidated gliadin peptide antibodies, IgA Anti-gliadin antibodies IgG and IgA *Less common* Anti-endomysial antibodies, IgA Anti-reticulin antibodies, IgA Anti-actin IgA
	Guillain-Barré syndrome	Anti-ganglioside antibodies
	Lupus (SLE)	ANA Urine analysis — for blood, protein or microscopic casts of kidney cells Rheumatoid factor (RF) Serum protein electrophoresis Complement C3, C4 Cryoglobulin
	Multiple sclerosis	Magnetic resonance imaging (MRI) scans Lumbar puncture — immunoelectrophoresis
	Rheumatoid arthritis	RF CCP antibodies — cyclic citrullinated peptide antibodies
	Scleroderma	ANA Scl-70 antibody Centromere antibody RNA POLIII antibody Lung function test Computed tomography (CT) X-rays Cardiac testing

Continued

TABLE 12.8 General immune system pathology or other tests—cont'd

Overview	Condition	List of pathology tests
Autoimmune disease (cont'd)	Sjögren's syndrome	ANA RF Anti-SS-A Anti-SS-B Polyclonal activation IgG
	Thyroid	Thyroid-stimulating hormone (TSH) FT4, FT3 Anti-thyroid peroxidase antibody TSH receptor antibodies Radioactive iodine uptake
	Type 1 diabetes mellitus	Blood glucose levels HbA1c GAD antibodies Oral glucose tolerance test Fructosamine Urine tests Cholesterol tests
Chronic fatigue syndrome		E/LFTs (EUC (electrolytes, urea, creatinine) and LFT (liver function test)) FBC ESR TSH Iron studies Urinalysis CMV, EBV Cortisol/ACTH HIV antibody test RF/CCP TB skin test ANA Lyme disease test MRI
Fungal infections	e.g. Candidiasis	Microscopic examinations Fungal culture
Gout		Uric acid
Hepatitis		E/LFT HAV-Ab IgM HBdAg HBV DNA HBeAg Anti-HCV HCV RNA Liver biopsy
HIV/AIDs		HIV antibody P24 protein testing HIV Western blot Multispot HIV-1/HIV-2 Viral load testing CD4 T-cell testing Genotype resistance testing
Influenza		Rapid influenza antigen test Direct fluorescent antibody (DFA) stain Viral culture RT-PCR Influenza A or B antibody test
Leukaemia		FBC Bone marrow aspiration/biopsy Flow cytometry Cytogenetic analysis and/or fluorescent in situ hybridisation (FISH) PCR Lumber puncture

TABLE 12.8 General immune system pathology or other tests—cont'd

Overview	Condition	List of pathology tests
Lymphomia/multiple myeloma		FBC Flow cytometry — CD markers Immunohistochemistry Chromosome studies Biopsy Bone marrow biopsy
Malaria		Malaria antigen PCR
Recurrent/persistent infections	Immune deficiency	FBC Immunoglobulins (IgA, IgG, IgM) Protein EPG HIV Fasting blood glucose (FBG) Complement Lymphocyte surface markers
Sexually transmitted infections	Gonorrhoea *Chlamydia* Syphilis Trichomonas Human papillomavirus (HPV) Genital herpes HIV Hepatitis	Swab of secretion or urine Swab Syphilis virus (blood) Lumbar puncture (spinal tap) Swab Urine or prostatic fluid Sampling of cells Swab See HIV See Hepatitis
Staph and MRSA		Culture Susceptibility testing
Travellers' diseases		Faecal testing — culture Faecal PCR Ova and parasite stool tests
Urinary tract infections		Urinalysis Urine culture
Vasculitis		FBC ESR CRP Creatinine E/LFT Urinalysis Anti-neutrophil cytoplasmic antibody Complement
Viruses	For fatigue and joint point	Ross River virus Epstein-Barr virus Barmah Forest virus Q fever Influenzas Any test for specific virus
Wilson's disease		Urine and blood copper Ceruloplasmin E/LFT Liver biopsy Genetic testing
Wound and skin infections		Gram stain Bacterial wound culture Antimicrobial susceptibility Potassium hydroxide preparation or KOH prep Fungal culture Acid-Fast Bacilli (AFB) culture and smear Blood culture Urine culture DNA or RNA testing

These conditions instigated a number of symptoms that were shown to involve the immune system including fever, chilliness, inflammation, the involvement of lymphatics and infection. The major herb detailed was *Echinacea* spp., prized by the Eclectics as 'it has not yet failed to antidote the most virulent organic infection to a greater or less degree'.[57] Also documented is the use of *Phytolacca decandra* for its effects on the lymphatic system and *Baptisia tinctoria* for its use in sepsis, likely to be as a result of its antiviral and immune-stimulating action. The choice of these herbs reveals the therapeutic goals associated with managing these types of immune conditions. The focus was to remove the offending pathogen. This idea is central to contemporary naturopathic management of immune conditions.

Modern interpretation

A healthy functioning immune system is crucial to overall health and wellbeing as it protects us against the multitude of pathogens we face on a daily basis. Naturopathy believes that the body is a self-regulating organism and thus the naturopath is merely the facilitator whose role it is both to enhance the proper functioning of the immune system so that it can ward off disease and also to protect and support it against further damage.

Modern naturopathy recognises a range of causative factors for conditions of the immune system and considers all causative triggers as potential treatment areas. These may include increased gut permeability, increased circulating immune complexes, food allergy or intolerance or underlying infective organism. Paramount to treatment is the understanding that the presence of microbial infection combined with a susceptible/vulnerable immune system precipitates immune-compromising events.

For a pathogen to become active or reactivate, the immune system must be compromised in some way. Compromising factors may include warmth, absence of good bacteria or the presence of sugar in the diet. As such, modern naturopathic management of the immune system focuses on a suitable range of modalities that enable stimulating, modulating or suppressing the immune system, depending on the individual's presentation.

The scope of modern naturopathic medicine for the management of the immune system may include:

- Herbal medicines: immune modulators, immune stimulants
- Therapeutic diets, e.g. avoiding dietary allergens
- Detoxification
- Nutritional therapies, for example immune stimulants such as vitamin C
- Physical therapies, for example balneotherapy.

Naturopathic treatment

NUTRITIONAL MEDICINE (DIETARY)

Specific dietary treatments

DIETARY INCLUSIONS

Antioxidant-rich foods

A diet rich in antioxidant foods helps to support a healthy immune system due to the ability of antioxidants to modify cell-mediated immune responses.[58] Antioxidants contain a rich array of phytochemicals that help to mediate oxidant-mediated tissue injury produced by the phagocytes as part of the body's defence against infection.

Protein

Inadequate protein in the diet is linked to dysfunction of the immune system. Adequate intake of dietary protein is imperative for healthy immune function.

Wholefood diet

A wholefood diet is one that is based upon fresh wholefoods that are as close to their natural state as possible. This ensures that the foods you eat retain a wide array of their nutrients and *prana*, or vital force. Another benefit of wholefoods is that they contain a range of nutrients found occurring naturally in their correct ratios, these nutrients work together synergistically to benefit the immune system. Refined foods on the other hand may have nutrients stripped out of them and then added back in; however, many as yet unidentified nutrients may be important for immune health and these will be left out. An example of a wholefood would be a fresh orange versus a cup of long-life reconstituted orange juice (probably lacking in vital force, bioflavonoids, fibre, etc).

DIETARY EXCLUSIONS

Sugar

Sugar is an immune suppressant with studies showing intake of sugar reduces the capacity of the white blood cells to function properly. Immune suppression has been shown to be at its highest 1–2 hours after consumption of sugar though immune suppression may still be evident 5 hours later. Further strengthening the argument for sugar reduction is the fact that many pathogens (for example, the fungus, *Candida*) thrive on sugar, leading to their increased virulence within the body.

Caffeine

Chronic and excessive intake of caffeine is likely to function as a stressor to the already depleted immune system. Furthermore, caffeine functions as a diuretic promoting the loss of much needed nutrients and therefore is not recommended where there is suboptimal immunity. Sources of caffeine include coffee, tea and energy drinks.

Preservatives, colourings, additives

Preservatives, colourings and additives are unnatural substances and foreign to the body and therefore should be avoided.

Nutritional supplementation

SPECIFIC NUTRIENTS REQUIRED

B complex

VITAMIN B_1

Deficiency of thiamine is associated with inhibition of humoral antibody formation.[59] Patients presenting with suboptimal immunity, under stress, taking the oral contraceptive pill or drinking excess alcohol may be at risk of B vitamin deficiencies. These stressors are likely to impact dramatically on the immune system.

Vitamin B_2

Similarly to vitamin B_1, vitamin B_2 is required for multiple bodily functions that are likely to directly and indirectly influence immune function. Directly, deficiency of vitamin B_2 is associated with disrupted tissue barriers to infection as well as inhibition of humoral antibody formation.[59]

Vitamin B_3

Deficiencies of vitamin B_3 have also been linked to disruption of the barriers to infection and inhibition of humoral antibody formation.[59]

Vitamin B_5

Vitamin B_5 is essential for life as a component of coenzyme A where it is involved in gene expression through replication of DNA and transcription of cell messages in cell signalling. Vitamin B_5 is involved in the synthesis of proteins, therefore any lack of vitamin B_5 will depress and interfere with production of proteins required for immunity.

Vitamin B_6

Vitamin B_6 is essential for healthy immune function and responses via its role in nucleic and protein biosynthesis. Deficiency of vitamin B_6 is associated with suppressed Th1 response with impaired antibody production, lymphocyte growth, decreased natural killer and T-cell activity (numbers and proliferation) as well as decreased IL-2 production.[60] Vitamin B_6 is also indispensable for humoral antibody responses from B lymphocytes of the bone marrow. Supplementation with vitamin B_6 restores Th1 immune response.[60]

Vitamin B_9

Similarly to vitamin B_6, folate plays an important role in the synthesis of nucleic acids and proteins; thus lack of folate will significantly impair immune function.[61] This manifests as impaired Th1 immune response with decreased circulating T lymphocytes, decreased natural killer cell activity, an increased CD4+/CD8+ ratio and decreased resistance to infection.[60]

Vitamin B_{12}

Vitamin B_{12} works together with vitamins B_6 and B_9 in the synthesis of nucleic acids and protein biosynthesis.[62] Vitamin B_{12} has been suggested to function as an immune modulator; individuals deficient in vitamin B_{12} show suppressed natural killer cell activity and abnormal CD4+/CD8+ ratio.

VITAMIN A

Vitamin A performs an important role in immunity through its modulating effects;[63] deficiency of vitamin A is associated with a number of immunological alterations including reduced function of neutrophils, macrophages and natural killer cells[64] as well as impaired antibody responses to challenge with protein antigens[65] and impairments in T- and B-cell function.[64] Vitamin A also maintains the health of the mucous membranes therefore lack of vitamin A is likely to result in reduced mucosal barrier function. Deficiency of vitamin A is associated with increased risk of a number of infectious conditions including HIV, measles and diarrhoeal disease.[66]

BETA-CAROTENE

Beta-carotene has demonstrated favourable effects on the immune system where it functions as an antioxidant to prevent damage in vitro to human lymphocytes following exposure to free radicals during response to infection.[67] Additionally other in vivo and in vitro studies show beta-carotene can increase B- and T-cell proliferation, increase helper T-cell lymphocytes, and protect phagocytic cells from auto-oxidative damage. Natural rather than synthetic beta-carotene should be used.

VITAMIN C

Decreased vitamin C leads to decreased phagocyte and immune function as well as increased risk of microbial infection. Supplementation with vitamin C has been shown to improve the function of the immune system and strengthen resistance to infection. Vitamin C is rapidly expended during infection or stress; high concentrations of vitamin C are found in the leucocytes,[68] the white blood cells that are involved in defending the immune system. Vitamin C exerts a broad range of immunological effects:

- Functions as an antioxidant; oxidative stress is linked to impaired immune responses[69]
- Stimulates the production of interferon[60]
- Stimulates monocyte movement[60]
- Has a role in lymphocyte proliferation[60]
- Has a role in natural killer cell activities[60]
- Enhances neutrophil chemotaxis and migration[70]
- Indirectly enhances immunity by regenerating vitamin E.

VITAMIN D

During the industrial revolution in the nineteenth century, rickets reached almost epidemic proportions in ill-fed children living in cities with little sunlight in northern European countries. A beneficial effect of sunlight and cod-liver oil was observed, but it was not until the 1930s that vitamin D was identified as the therapeutic element in those therapies.[71]

The classic function of vitamin D is to regulate calcium homeostasis and thus bone formation and resorption. However, less traditional functions of vitamin D have been demonstrated and include effects on the immune response. The identification of vitamin D receptors (VDRs) in peripheral blood mononuclear cells sparked the early interest in vitamin D as an immune system regulator.[72,73]

In humans, vitamin D is obtained by two distinct pathways: (1) vitamin D synthesis in the skin and (2) dietary intake. Sunlight catalyses the formation of cholecalciferol (vitamin D_3) from 7-dehydrocholesterol (pre-vitamin D_3) in the skin by photolysis-mediated cleavage of the B-ring in this molecule. In plants, ergocalciferol (vitamin D_2) is formed from ergocholesterol. Plant-based vitamin D_2 and animal vitamin D_3 enter the human body in the diet and are considered poorer forms and less than adequate for optimal daily requirements. Total body sun exposure easily provides the equivalent of an oral intake of 250 micrograms vitamin D.

TABLE 12.9 Vitamin D — Australian high-risk population groups with low serum 25OHD levels as reported in the literature

Highest risk groups	Prevalence of deficiency*
Residential care elderly in high-level care	55%
Residential care elderly in high- and low-level care	68–86%
Residential care elderly in low-level care	22%
Geriatric admissions to hospital	67%
Patients with hip fracture	61% 63%**
Dark-skinned women (particularly veiled)	>80%
Mothers of infants with rickets (particularly dark-skinned and veiled)	80%
Lower risk groups	
Community-dwelling elderly	17%
Women in winter:	
80+ years	22%
60–79 years	12%
20–59 years	8%

*Deficiency defined as either <25 or 28 nmol/L
**Deficiency defined as <50 nmol/L
Source: Nowson CA, Diamond TH, Pasco JA et al. Vitamin D in Australia — issues and recommendations. Aust Fam Phys 2004; (33):3.

Vitamin D is a potent immune modulator with countless studies highlighting this role. There is considerable evidence to support its prescription in a number of autoimmune conditions, cancer or HIV as is evident by the improvements in patient outcomes. Of most interest is the correlation between the incidence of autoimmune conditions with temperate influences — as is evident in multiple sclerosis. Furthermore, Th1 and Th2 cells are direct targets of $1,25(OH)_2D_3$.[74] As such, its prescription in abnormalities in immune function is both prudent and beneficial. See Table 12.9.

VITAMIN E

Vitamin E is a powerful antioxidant that plays an important role in maintaining the health of the immune system. Deficiency is associated with increased virulence of viral infections as well as impaired humoral and cell-mediated immunity presenting in humans with decreased T-cell mitogenesis, IL-2 production and phagocytic and chemotaxis function of the polymorphonuclear cells.[75]

A number of studies have investigated the immune-enhancing effects of vitamin E in the elderly population, as ageing is associated with a decline in immune function. In a small study, supplementation with vitamin E (800 mg/d dl-alpha-tocopheryl acetate for 1 month) in healthy elderly individuals has been shown to be beneficial in improving the immune response in a double-blind, placebo-controlled trial. The effect of vitamin E appeared to be mediated by a decrease in prostaglandin E2 (PGE2) and/or other lipid-peroxidation products.[76] In another small study with elderly patients administered 200 mg/d of vitamin E as alpha-tocopheryl it was again found to enhance immune parameters with significant improvement observed in several functions of lymphocytes, neutrophils and NK cells.[77] It is important to note that these studies have been conducted in small groups and over relatively short periods of time. It would be interesting to observe if even better results are seen when vitamin E is taken over a longer period of time.

SELENIUM

Selenium is an essential trace element found in high quantities within immune tissues such as the spleen and lymphatics.[78] Selenium functions as part of the selenoprotein enzymes to regulate immune function by influencing both innate and acquired immunity, and thus insufficient selenium will compromise both of these. Deficiency of selenium is associated with loss of immune competence and may result in:[60,79]

- Increased virulence of viruses which are usually harmless but due to lack of selenium mutate into more powerful and dangerous forms
- Decreased IgM and IgG titres
- Impaired neutrophil chemotaxis
- Impaired antibody production by lymphocytes.

However, subsequent supplementation with selenium produces profound results. Supplementation with selenium (200 micrograms/d) in patients replete of selenium was found to enhance response to antigen stimulation and lead to an increased ability to develop into cytotoxic lymphocytes and to destroy tumour cells.[80] Natural killer (NK) cell activity was also increased with the collected data indicating that the supplementation regimen resulted in a 118% increase in lymphocyte-mediated tumour cytotoxicity and an 82.3% increase in natural killer cell activity as compared with baseline value. In spite of these significant results plasma selenium did not increase, suggesting higher quantities may be required to increase selenium levels in those who are replete. Supplementation with selenium in patients with neck and head cancer during therapy (200 micrograms/day as sodium selenite) also produced positive results with regards to immune responses. A significantly enhanced cell-mediated immune responsiveness was demonstrated in the selenium group as reflected in the ability of the patients' lymphocytes to respond to stimulation with mitogen, to generate cytotoxic lymphocytes, and to destroy tumour cells. In contrast, those in the control group showed a decline in immune responsiveness during therapy.[81]

ESSENTIAL FATTY ACIDS

Essential fatty acids such as those found in fish oil are the gatekeepers of immune cell regulation and influence the behaviour of proteins involved in immune cell activation. Essential fatty acids are required for fuel for generation of energy of the cell and structurally as components of the

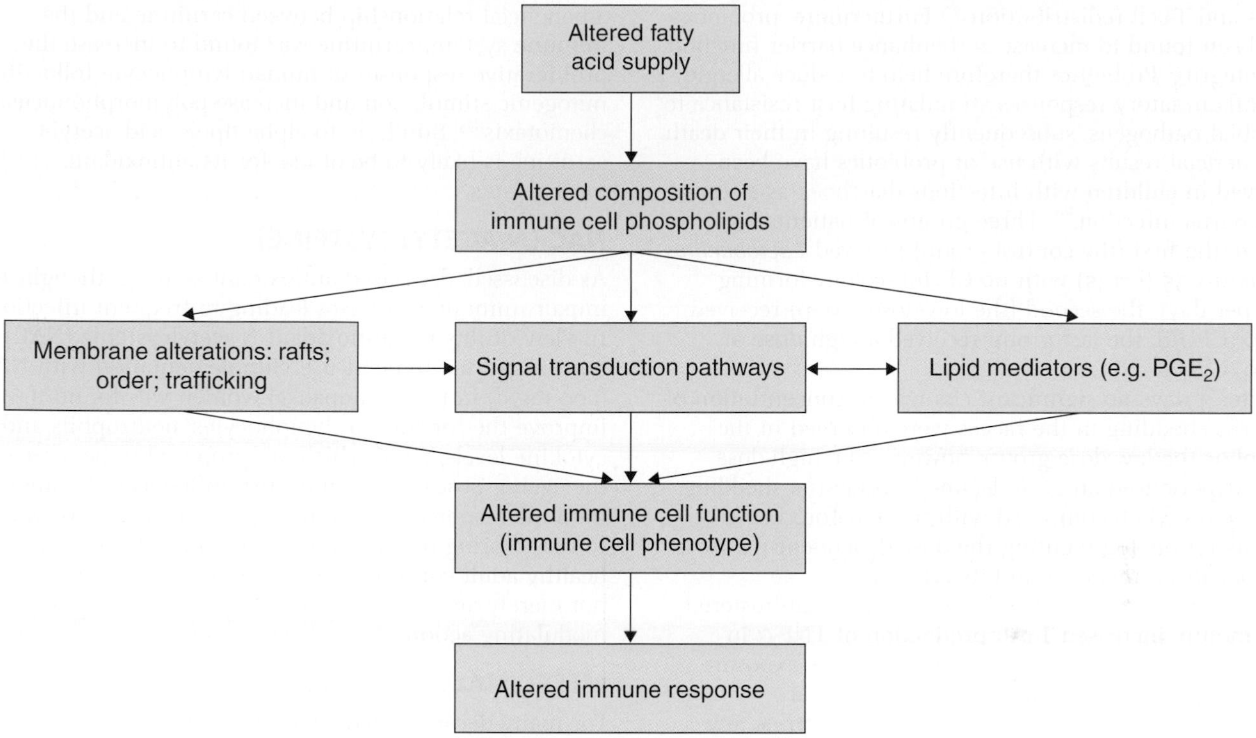

FIGURE 12.2 **Mechanisms by which an altered supply of fatty acids could affect immune responses.**
Source: Calder PC. Prostaglandins. Leukot Essent Fatty Acids 2008 Sep-Nov; 79(3-5): 101-8. Epub 23 Oct 2008.

cell membrane with alterations in the fatty acid composition of immune cells thought to influence T-cell reactivity and antigen presentation.[82] Fatty acids help to regulate gene expression and are precursors for synthesis of lipid mediators such as prostaglandins and leukotrienes. Increased membrane content of *n*-3 fatty acids results in a changed pattern of production of eicosanoids (involved in inflammation and immunity), resolvins and cytokines.[83] Mechanisms by which an altered supply of fatty acids could affect immune responses are shown in Fig. 12.2.[82]

ZINC

Zinc is highly important for immunity and influences both innate and acquired immunity. Zinc functions as a co-factor in the body for many immune-dependent responses including involvement in thymus hormone induction of T-cell function and IL-2 production. As an antioxidant zinc also protects against the free radical oxygen species that occur as a result of activated macrophages. Sergio also reports that zinc salts exhibit antiviral activity against more than 40 viruses.[84]

Given the actions of zinc upon the immune system it is not a surprise that deficiency is associated with impairment of immune function, including:[85]

- Macrophage function (phagocytosis, intracellular killing activity)
- Neutrophil functions (chemotaxis, generation of the oxidative burst)
- NK cell and complement activity
- T-cell lymphopenia
- Decreased lymphocyte response to mitogens
- Decreased CD4+ cells.

IRON

Adequate iron is critical for healthy immune function; deficiency is associated with impaired T-cell function and impaired IL-2 production.[86] Excessive iron is also deleterious to the immune system. As such, it is imperative to assess and investigate thoroughly prior to prescription.

COPPER

Suboptimal intake of copper is associated with compromised immune function as demonstrated by alterations in T-cell function.[87]

COENZYME Q10

Well known for its antioxidant effects, coenzyme Q10 also produces remarkable effects on the immune system. Supplementation with coenzyme Q10 (200 mg/d) has been shown to increase T4/T8 lymphocyte ratios[88] as well as IgG ratios in the blood.[89]

PROBIOTICS

A healthy gut function forms a protective barrier against antigens from food and microorganisms; however, this immunological protection is only possible if there are good indigenous microflora.

Probiotics have been shown to influence a number of components of immune response; they exhibit antimicrobial activity (such as reducing luminal pH, promoting secretion of antimicrobial peptides, inhibiting bacterial invasion, decreasing inflammation both local and systemic) as well as having immune modulating properties visible in their effects on the epithelial and dendritic cells, monocytes/macrophages and the B-lymphocytes, NK cells,

T-cells and T-cell redistribution.[90] Furthermore, probiotics have been found to increase and enhance barrier function and integrity. Probiotics therefore help to reduce allergic and inflammatory responses stimulating host resistance to microbial pathogens, subsequently resulting in their death.

Beneficial results with use of probiotics have been observed in children with infectious diarrhoea as a result of rotavirus infection.[91] Three groups of patients were formed: the first (the control group) received *Lactobacillus rhamnosus* 35 (Lcr35) with no CFU/d (colony-forming units per day); the second (the low-dose group) received 2×10^8 CFU/d; the last group received a high dose of 6×10^8 CFU/d.

After 3 days no significant changes in concentration of rotavirus shedding in the faeces were observed in the control or the low-dose group; however, the high-dose group experienced an 86% decline in rotavirus shedding after 3 days when compared with those before Lcr35 administration, highlighting the dose-dependent nature of *Lactobacillus rhamnosus* and its efficacy.

A patented strain of *Bacillus coagulans*, administered for 1 month, increased T-cell production of TNF-α in response to adenovirus and influenza A virus exposure suggesting increased immune response to viral challenge.[92] This same strain did not demonstrate any effects on other strains of the influenza virus, highlighting the fact that it is important to acknowledge that the potential of all strains differs; no extrapolation can be made comparing one strain to another as all are unique in their function and action in a particular diseased state.

While most probiotics are bacteria based, *Saccharomyces boulardii*, a yeast, has been found to be an effective probiotic in double-blind clinical studies.[93] One particularly defining feature of *Saccharomyces boulardii* is the fact that it is said to be resistant to the effects of antibiotics (unlike bacteria-based probiotics), and thus it produces good results for antibiotic-associated diarrhoea as well as recurrent *Clostridium difficile* intestinal infection.

PROTEIN

Impaired immunity is associated with protein deprivation producing particularly detrimental effects with regard to T-cell function and increased risk of infection; thus adequate protein is imperative for optimal immune function.[94] Intake is, of course, dependent on individual circumstances — clearly an individual with impaired renal clearance, for example, will not benefit from large amounts of protein.

ALPHA LIPOIC ACID

A number of microbial infective conditions are associated with widespread oxidative damage as a result of displacement of a balance between oxidants such as free radicals and antioxidants which may aid the progression of the diseased state, hence supplementation with antioxidants such as alpha lipoic acid has been recommended for many immune conditions, including HIV and hepatitis.

ACETYL-L-CARNITINE

Acetyl-L-carnitine is an antioxidant required for fatty acid transportation in the mitochondria. Early studies observed a beneficial relationship between carnitine and the immune system; carnitine was found to increase the proliferative responses of human lymphocyte following mitogenic stimulation and increase polymorphonuclear chemotaxis.[95] Similarly to alpha lipoic acid acetyl-L-carnitine is likely to be of use for its antioxidant mechanisms.

NAC (*N*-ACETYLCYSTEINE)

As discussed, decreased antioxidant status is thought to impair immune responses leading to frequent infections. In view of this the antioxidant *N*-acetylcysteine (NAC) has been suggested to be of use. Supplementation with NAC (600 mg/d) in postmenopausal women was found to improve the function of lymphocytes, neutrophils and cytokine levels, all of which are proposed to be affected by the ageing process, which in turn influences alterations in immune responses.[96] Supplementation with NAC was found to bring participants' values closer to those of healthy adult controls, the authors suggesting it possesses not merely an immune stimulating action but also a modulating action.

MEDICINAL MUSHROOMS

For many decades, medicinal mushrooms such as shiitake, reishi and turkey tail have been regarded as an ethnic medicine and have been widely used in diseases such as cancer. The active component of the mushrooms is a bioactive compound called polysaccharides or glycans which have been found to exhibit potential immunomodulating and anticancer properties. The glycans have been found to have two main actions: firstly, they are regarded as pathogen associated molecular pattern (PAMP)-like molecules which bind to particular receptors on the surface of immune cells which activates the signalling cascade. Secondly, they have been found to stimulate immune cell development.[97]

BIOFLAVONOIDS SUCH AS QUERCETIN

Quercetin and rutin are two flavonoids that are found in certain fruits and vegetables. They exhibit anti-inflammatory, antiviral and anticarcinogenic properties. Quercetin has also been found to attenuate lipid peroxidation, platelet aggregation and capillary permeability.[98]

RESVERATROL

Resveratrol has been found to strongly modulate the immune response including the activity of NK cells. Resveratrol can be found in many foods and beverages such as the skin of red grapes and red wine.[99]

Dosage requirements

Dosage requirements of specific nutrients are as shown in Table 12.10.

Herbal medicine

Some justifications for the use of herbal medicine are given in Table 12.11.

TABLE 12.10 Nutrient dosage requirements

Requirement	Justification	Therapeutic dose	Foods containing nutrient
Vitamin A	Immune-modulator, mucous membrane restorative, anti-infective agent. T-cell subpopulations, cytokines and antibody subclasses are all affected by vitamin A	10 000–50 000 IU/d	Kohlrabi, egg yolk, carrots, apricots, fish liver oils (e.g. cod)
Beta-carotene	Antioxidant, activates macrophages and lymphocytes, increases interferon activity, increases T- and B-cell proliferation, immune stimulant	10–40 mg/d	Carrots, broccoli, capsicum, papaya, sweet potatoes, red capsicums
Vitamin C	Antioxidant, immune stimulant, anti-infective, antiallergenic, enhances white blood cell function	250–2000 mg/d	Mango, guava, strawberries, blackcurrant, rosehips, sweet potatoes, paw paw, pineapple
Vitamin D	Potent immune modulator and other roles including calcium regulation	1000–4000 IU/d (blood tests depending)	Sunlight, cod liver oil, tinned salmon, tuna, sardines or mackerel, fortified foods
Vitamin E	Antioxidant, increases resistance to bacterial and viral infections, enhances immune parameters such as lymphocytes, neutrophils and natural killer cells	100–800 mg/d	Almonds, apricot oil, egg yolks, hazel nuts, wheatgerm, corn
Vitamin B_1	Required for humoral antibody formation	5–100 mg/d	Wholegrains, asparagus, beef, lamb, legumes, nuts, spirulina, wheatgerm
Vitamin B_2	Required for humoral antibody formation and tissue barriers to infection	10–100 mg/d	Almonds, eggs, milk, sprouts, wholegrains, asparagus, avocados, barley grass, beans, currants
Vitamin B_3	Required for humoral antibody formation and tissue barriers to infection	100–300 mg/d	Almonds, beef, chicken, eggs, legumes, peanuts, salmon, sardines, sunflower seeds
Vitamin B_5	Required for the synthesis of proteins and involved in gene expression through replication of DNA and transcription of cell messages in cell signalling	20–500 mg/d	Avocados, egg yolk, green vegetables, mushrooms, oranges, peas, sweet potatoes, wholegrains
Vitamin B_6	Vitamin B_6 is essential for healthy immune function and responses via its role in nucleic and protein biosynthesis. Deficiency is associated with immune dysregulation. Deficiency of vitamin B_6 is associated with decreased lymphocytes, impaired antibody responses and IL-2 production	10–100 mg/d	Avocados, bananas, brewers' yeast, oatmeal, egg yolk, chicken, mackerel, sunflower seeds, salmon, tuna, lentils, legumes
Vitamin B_9	Vitamin B_9 works in concert with vitamins B_6 and B_{12} in nucleic and protein biosynthesis. Deficiency is associated with immune dysregulation	1000–2000 micrograms/day	Barley, beans, sprouts, eggs, endive, green leafy vegetables
Vitamin B_{12}	Immune modulator, deficiency is associated with suppressed immune defence mechanisms	300–2000 micrograms/d	Egg yolk, salmon, sardines, bacterial synthesis in the gut
Essential fatty acids	Gatekeepers of immunity, required for structure and function of the immune cells, key roles in preventing inflammation	DHA/EPA: 1–3 g/d	Omega-3 fish oil
Coenzyme Q10	Influences host defence system, increases T4/T8 ratios of lymphocytes	30–300 mg/d	N/A
Selenium	Selenium is an antioxidant that has been linked to increased CD4T lymphocytes, enhanced T-cell functions and TNF-β induced increase in natural killer cell activity	100–300 micrograms/d	Brazil nuts, alfalfa, wholegrain cereals, meat, eggs, onion, garlic, broccoli
Iron	Key mineral for immune resistance	15–50 mg/d	Almonds, apricots, avocados, meat, parsley, oysters, pine nuts
Zinc	Key antioxidant with numerous fundamental roles in the immune system including antiviral activity	10–75 mg/d	Pumpkin seeds, sunflower seeds, egg yolks, seafood, oysters, beef

Continued

TABLE 12.10 Nutrient dosage requirements—cont'd			
Requirement	**Justification**	**Therapeutic dose**	**Foods containing nutrient**
Copper	Antioxidant required for healthy immune function	2–10 mg/d	Almonds, avocados, beans, mushrooms, sunflower seeds, wholegrains, water from copper pipes
Acetyl-L-carnitine	Antioxidant	400–2000 mg/d	Avocados, beef, chicken, fish
Alpha lipoic acid	Antioxidant that may help prevent disease progression as a result of oxidation	100–600 mg/d	Broccoli, potatoes, spinach, tomatoes
N-acetylcysteine	Antioxidant shown to improve white blood cell status	600 mg/d	Supplementation only
Probiotics	Influence a number of components of immune response including inflammation and allergy	Dependent on condition and strain	Yoghurt, supplements, fermented cabbage

IL-2, interleukin-2; DHA, docosahexaenoic acid; EPA, eicosapentaenoic acid; TNF-β, tumour necrosis factor beta
Sources: Folkers K, Morita M, McRee Jr J et al. The activities of coenzyme Q10 and vitamin B6 for immune responses. Biochem Biophys Re Commun 1993; 193(1):88–92. Harbige LS. Nutrition and immunity with emphasis on infection and autoimmune disease. Nutr Health 1996; 10 (4):285–312.

TABLE 12.11 Herbal medicine classes		
Class	**Example**	**Justification**
Antiallergic	*Scutellaria baicalensis* (skullcap)	Antiallergic herbs may be used to reduce the allergic response in the body. *Scutellaria baicalensis* is one such herb and is believed to inhibit histamine and leukotriene release from mast cells. It has traditionally been used in Japanese Kampo medicine in conditions that require the removal of excess heat.
Antibacterial	*Allium sativum* (garlic)	Antibacterial herbs such as *Allium sativum* exert a direct effect against pathogenic bacteria. It has demonstrated antibacterial action against a wide array of bacteria including methicillin-resistant *Staphylococcus aureus*.
Antibiotic	*Hydrastis canadensis* (goldenseal)	Antibiotic herbs such as *Hydrastis canadensis* function as natural antibiotics within the body. It contains a constituent known as berberine that is thought to kill a wide range of other types of germs, such as those that cause *Candida* (yeast) infections, viruses and various parasites such as tapeworms and *Giardia*.
Anticatarrhal	*Euphrasia* spp. (eyebright)	Anticatarrhal botanicals such as the *Euphrasia* spp. are those that help to counteract excess catarrh and congestion in the body. *Euphrasia* contains tannin constituents that help to bind catarrh, and exerts antimicrobial and anti-inflammatory properties also thought to be of use where there is congestion.
Antifungal	*Tabebuia avellanedae* (pau d'arco)	Antifungal herbs such as the *Tabebuia* spp. may be used in the immune system to exert direct effects against fungal pathogens. Two constituents, lapachol and β-lapachone, isolated from *Tabebuia avellanedae,* have been identified as being antifungal constituents within the *Tabebuia* spp. In vitro studies of *T. avellanedae* demonstrate broad-spectrum activity revealing it to be active against a number of the fungal strains. *T. avellanedae* showed best growth inhibition against *Aspergillus fumigatus*, *Cryptococcus neoformans*, *Microsporum gypseum*, *Penicillium purpurogenum*, *Saccharomyces cerevisiae* and *Trichophyton mentagrophytes*.
Antimicrobial	*Thymus vulgaris* (thyme)	Antimicrobial botanicals are those that elicit a general immune response against any microbial agents. For example *Thymus vulgaris* essential oil has been demonstrated for its efficacy against 15 strains of bacteria. Only a few species of bacteria were able to recover at least 50% of their metabolic function after contact with *Thymus vulgaris*; most of the strains were shown to have been inactivated almost completely. *Escherichia coli* O157:H7 was the most sensitive species, given that after contact with even the lowest concentration of oil cells could not be recovered.
Antioxidant	*Vitis vinifera* (grapeseed)	Antioxidant herbs such as *Vitis vinifera* are useful to prevent oxidative damage; oxidation is thought to impair immune responses leading to frequent infections.
Antipyretic	*Tanacetum parthenium* (feverfew)	Antipyretic herbs are those that reduce or prevent fever of infectious origin. The Eclectic physicians advocated the use of a warm infusion for its diaphoretic action to be used for intermittent fever.

TABLE 12.11 Herbal medicine classes—cont'd

Class	Example	Justification
Antiviral	*Hypericum perforatum* (St John's wort)	Antiviral herbal medicines elicit a direct immune response against viruses. For example, in vitro studies reveal the potential of *Hypericum perforatum* to exert anti-hepatitis B effects by preventing transcription of the hepatitis B virus.
Diaphoretic	*Achillea millefolium* (yarrow)	Diaphoretics such as *Achillea millefolium* may be used to induce therapeutic sweating during an infection, thus activating the immune system. This action may be used to help control fever.
Immuno-enhancing	*Andrographis panniculata* (andrographis)	Immune enhancers are those herbal medicines that stimulate one or more aspects of the immune reaction. For example, in vivo and in vitro studies reveal the ability of extracts of *Andrographis panniculata* to enhance immune function, possibly through modulation of immune responses altered during antigen interaction; *Andrographis panniculata* also appears able to reverse immune suppression induced by cyclophosphamide.
Immuno-modulatory	*Echinacea angustifolia* (echinacea)	Immune-modulators such as the *Echinacea* spp. are herbal medicines that modulate and balance the activity of the immune system.
Immune suppressant	*Hemidesmus indicus* (hemidesmus)	Immune suppressants such as *Hemidesmus indicus* are useful to depress an overactive immune system, such as in diseases of autoimmune origin.
Lymphatic	*Calendula officinalis* (calendula)	The lymphatic system is highly important for facilitating immune responses. Lymphatic tissue contains large numbers of lymphocytes, white blood cells involved in the immune response. Lymphatic herbs such as *Calendula officinalis* facilitate lymphatic circulation and aid in the removal of toxins from the body.

Sources: Cutler RR, Wilson P. Antibacterial activity of a new, stable, aqueous extract of allicin against methicillin-resistant *Staphylococcus aureus*. Br J Biomed Sci 2004; 61:1–4; 35:1630–2. Felter, HW and Lloyd, JU. King's American dispensatory, 18th edn. Rev 3. Portland 1905, reprinted 1983, Eclectic Medical Publications. Kim DS, Son EJ, Kim M et al. Antiallergic herbal composition from *Scutellaria baicalensis* and *Phyllostachys edulis*. Planta Med 2010; 76(7):678–682. Makino T, Hishida A, Goda Y et al. Comparison of the major flavonoid content of *S. baicalensis*, *S. lateriflora*, and their commercial products. J Nat Med 2008; 62(3):294–299. Marino M, Bersani C, Comi G. Antimicrobial activity of the essential oils of *Thymus vulgaris* L. measured using a bioimpedometric method. J Food Prot 1999; 62(9):1017–1023. Naik SR, Hule A. Evaluation of immunomodulatory activity of an extract of andrographolides from *Andographis paniculata*. Planta Med 2009; 75(8):785–791. Pang R, Tao J, Zhang S, et al. In vitro anti-hepatitis B virus effect of *Hypericum perforatum* L. J Huazhong Univ Sci Technolog Med Sci 2010; 30(1):98–102. Portillo A, Vila R, Freixa B, et al. Antifungal activity of Paraguayan plants used in traditional medicine. J Ethnopharmacol 2001; 76(1):93–98.

SECTION B: AUTOIMMUNE DISEASE

Epidemiology

Autoimmune disease (AD) is defined as a condition in which tissue injury and loss of function is caused by T-cell or antibody reactivity to self.[100] ADs rank as a major global health concern, along with cancer, cardiovascular disease and obesity-related disorders.[101] When ADs are considered as separate diseases, neither their incidence nor their prevalence is high; collectively, however, they are occurring in significant numbers which are increasing. ADs as a group affect approximately 8.5% of individuals worldwide.[102] The prevalence of some ADs, for example multiple sclerosis (MS) and type 1 diabetes, has dramatically increased in the developed world, correlating inversely with a prevalence of infectious diseases that has reciprocally diminished.[103] The prevalence of other ADs, such as rheumatoid arthritis (RA), seems to have declined since the 1960s, particularly in women. One theory links this to the more widespread use of oral contraceptives during the 1960s to 2000,[104] although there are data now that suggest the prevalence of RA is rising again.[105] While there are minimal data for developing countries, it is recognised that collectively, the population burden of ADs is large and underestimated.[106]

While ADs are underreported on death certificates, they represent the leading cause of death among middle-aged women[107] and they constitute one of the ten leading causes of death among US women younger than 65 years of age.[108] Premature coronary heart disease has emerged as a major cause of mortality in systemic ADs as the pathogenesis has a great deal in common with atherosclerosis, due to the inflammatory pathways.[109] In RA, life expectancy decrease is about 3–10 years. The other main causes of death in ADs are infectious, haematological, gastrointestinal and pulmonary complications.[105]

Classification

Although the definition of exactly what constitutes an AD varies, it is generally agreed that what differentiates an AD from other diseases is the production of autoantibodies which bind self-proteins, with consequent injury to tissues.[110] ADs can affect virtually any site in the body, and their clinical presentation varies widely. While there are many differences between them, there are many fundamental pathologies and genetic mechanisms that link all of them. ADs are associated with humoral and cellular immune system abnormalities and more than 80 have been described.[102] They fall into two categories: organ specific, such as type 1 diabetes, Graves' disease (GD) and myasthenia gravis (MG), and non-organ specific such as systemic lupus erythematosus (SLE), ankylosing spondylitis (AS) and rheumatoid arthritis (RA).

Aetiology

There is no single or simple model to explain what triggers immune system dysregulation and what sustains it. In an individual there will be various combinations of multiple predisposing, precipitating, excitatory and perpetuating factors that will interact in various complex ways. These include: genetic susceptibility; microbial agents past or present, acute or chronic, exogenous or endogenous; tissue damage; defects in various aspects of immune function; gender; dietary factors including food allergy or intolerances arising from loosening of tight junctions in the gut; intestinal dysbiosis; environmental factors; exposure to toxins, chemicals, drugs, radiation; occupation. In many patients who develop AD, one of these factors may drive the initial inflammatory attack on self-tissue, and this 'driver' may be referred to as the 'primary lesion' or the site/mechanism of initiation of the disease process.

GEOGRAPHICAL FACTORS

There are numerous variables in the geographic distribution of ADs, one being the level of sunlight, which has led to studies into the role that vitamin D levels may play. There is a decrease in some ADs in a north–south gradient in the northern hemisphere, for example MS prevalence is higher in North America and Canada than in Turkey; the prevalence of psoriasis in adults varies from 1.3–2.6% in the UK to 3.73–8.5% in Denmark and Norway, with Australia at 2.3–6.6%.[111] Roughly 1% of the population worldwide are affected with RA, with a higher prevalence in North America and northern Europe and a lower prevalence in southern Europe.[112] There seems to be a reciprocal south–north gradient in the prevalence of infectious diseases, and to coincide with that, SLE prevalence is higher in Spain and Greece than in Canada and Australia. However, there are disparities; for example, the prevalence of Sjögren's disease is much higher in the UK than in Denmark.[103]

GENETIC FACTORS

While there are predisposing genes that are a risk factor for developing AD, not all those who carry the gene(s) will develop the disease(s). It appears that less than one-third of the risk may be attributable to genetic predisposition, but this may change as knowledge of the genome increases. Numerous family studies have revealed that SLE and RA afflict family members at a greater rate than the general population; black North Americans are at higher risk for SLE than white North Americans. Genetic factors are claimed to contribute 50–60% of the risk of developing RA which is found at four times the expected rate in first-degree relatives of probands with seropositive disease. A family history of psoriasis is found in nearly 50% of cases and at least nine chromosomal loci have been identified that increase susceptibility.[112]

INFECTIVE TRIGGER

The risk factors for the occurrence and severity of ADs are many and complex but there is general agreement that infectious agents play a role in many. Some studies have shown that a broad exposure to a wealth of commensal, non-pathogenic microorganisms early in life is associated with protection against many ADs. For example Tobón and colleagues[105] found that a history of infections in infancy may protect against RA in adulthood. This has given credence to the 'hygiene hypothesis'.

ENVIRONMENTAL TRIGGERS

Environmental triggers also play a major role in disease expression, particularly when there are concomitant risk factors. Exposure to silica, including silicones in breast implants, organic solvents, mineral oils and other airborne toxins have been correlated with the occurrence of systemic scleroderma, SLE, autoimmune hepatitis, RA and small vessel vasculitis. People living within 50 metres of a road showed an increased risk of developing AD.[105] Smoking has been associated with an increased risk of developing RA, Crohn's disease (CD) and SLE and smoking is linked to worse outcomes in RA and CD.[113] Smoking may increase the production of rheumatoid factor (RF), which often precedes the clinical presentation of RA, especially in men.[112] The risk of developing RF-positive RA is substantially higher in smokers who carry two copies of shared-epitope genes.[105]

SEX HORMONES AND GENDER

Over 75% of patients with ADs are estimated to be women and AD is considered the fourth leading cause of disability for women.[114] Differences in AD manifestations by gender involve immunomodulation by sex hormones, non-hormonal factors encoded by genes on the X and Y chromosomes, infections more common in women and immunological phenomena unique to pregnancy. Hormones may play a role regulating the onset, severity and progression of the disease.

Systemic sclerosis and autoimmune thyroid disease (AITD) are highly prevalent among women. A systematic review showed a significant association between hormonal replacement therapy (HRT) exposure and increased risk of SLE.[114] AITD represents the main cause of hypothyroidism during pregnancy, ranging between 5 and 20% in prevalence with an average of 7.8%.

On the other hand, pregnancy may lead to remission of RA symptoms; a history of childbearing may protect against it; hormone replacement therapy (HRT) may decrease RA risk in women who carry the HLA-DRB1 gene.[105] RA and Sjögren's disease are more prevalent (66–90%) and more severe in women: *Proteus mirabilis* is one of the most common organisms in urinary tract infections and RA is associated with *Proteus* antibodies, thus could contribute to the higher incidence of RA in women, with a common onset post-partum.[115] MS sufferers also tend to go into remission during pregnancy, but this may be due to a change in the immune system rather than hormonal changes. SLE is more common in women, but more severe when it does occur in men, perhaps because the protective effect of testosterone is bypassed by some anomalies. Myasthenia gravis, type 1 diabetes and pernicious anaemia affect males and females equally. Ankylosing spondylitis is more common in men with only about 30% of cases being women.

OTHER FACTORS

Other major factors in the development and severity of ADs include low economic status, poor diet and psychological factors.[112] Patients with one organ-specific AD are at higher risk for another AD.[106]

Overview

Symptoms of an AD depend upon the organ(s) and tissues affected and range in severity from mildly debilitating to life-threatening. Autoantibodies may not be directly responsible for many of the manifestations of AD, but they are markers of disease, and it has been noted that autoantibodies may be found in serum samples many years before disease onset.[106]

Pathogenesis

When there is a prerequisite factor or factors in a person, there is a consequent abnormal responsiveness in some compartments of the immune system. This involves cell migration, antigen presentation, T-cell co-stimulation, T-cell activation and proliferation, cytokine release, T–B cell interaction and antibody production. A growing number of theories are being postulated about the details of the immune dysregulation as more T-cells and B-cells are identified. Regardless of the specific immune cells involved, the dysregulation induces cross-reaction with self-tissue and the inflammatory process is initiated, evolving typically in a step-wise pattern.

GENETIC SUSCEPTIBILITY

There are susceptibility alleles at the major histocompatibility complex (MHC) locus on chromosome 6 which display fragmented pieces of both self and non-self-antigens on the host cell's surface which probably account for about half of the genetic contribution to ADs. The main antigen-presenting proteins on the MHC are the human leucocyte antigens: locus A (HLA) class I and II. HLA class I molecules include HLA-A, -B, -C. They present peptides of only 8–9 amino acids in length and are expressed by nearly all nucleated cells in the body. They are concerned with alerting cytotoxic T lymphocytes to the presence of intracellular infections. HLA-B27 is the most common class I gene associated with ADs. Class II consists of HLA-DP, -DR, and -DQ; its products are expressed on many antigen-presenting cells including B lymphocytes, macrophages, dendritic cells, Langerhans' cells, and endothelial and other organ-specific antigen-presenting cells. Numerous other genes have more recently been implicated in affecting susceptibility including alleles at the CD152 (CTLA-4) locus as well as non-immune genes.[101]

Mutations in the methyl cycle rate-limiting enzyme MTHFR can result in hormonal and neurotransmitter imbalances and an accumulation of homocysteine which is associated with an increased risk for many ADs, including diabetes, autoimmune thyroid disease (AITD) such as Hashimoto's and Graves' disease, RA and vitiligo.[116]

In the pathogenesis of ADs, it is generally thought that the role of MHC class II proteins depends on the presentation to T-cells of a critical self-peptide, or there could be inherited poor functioning MHC class II molecules.[117] In the latter case, for example, T-cells which are known to be important in suppressing autoimmune reactions may be deficient in some way, such as those that express CD4, CD25 and Foxp3 proteins and regulatory T-cells (Tregs). However, many patients with the susceptibility-related MHC gene never develop any disease, and conversely individuals without it can develop the disease. It has been observed that in Japan there is a low frequency of the HLA alleles that increase the likelihood of type 1 diabetes and the incidence of the disease is low in that country.[118] It is interesting to note that genetically identical mice immunised in exactly the same way show great variability in their responses, indicating that there is a role for chance in an individual's immune reaction.[112]

MOLECULAR MIMICRY

Immunological cross-reactivity is a possible model for the pathogenesis of some ADs.[100] In this model, a microorganism or self-MHC antigen may act as the primary lesion. A microorganism exposure need not necessarily be a clinical infection, but it has presented to the immune system at some stage and left behind a clone of memory lymphocytes. The proteins of microorganisms provide many antigenic regions known as epitopes, and each microorganism might have many antigenic proteins, parts of which resemble human epitopes. It is known that each time a T-cell is activated by an antigen, it forms foreign-peptide self-MHC complexes and at the same time forms self-peptide self-MHC complexes. These are re-activated, perhaps many years later, by exposure to the same or an antigenically similar infection (second antigen). The activated T-cell provides co-stimulatory signals to B-cells which bind both microbial antigen and self-antigen, ingest, process and present epitopes of self-antigen, which can then be recognised by T-cells. These cross-reactive B-cells therefore contribute to a cascade of auto-reactivity. Upon this second exposure, the immune system continues reacting to self-components long after the pathogen has gone and the inflammatory process becomes self-sustaining.[101]

This model is known as 'molecular mimicry', a term introduced in 1968 by George Snell.[119] It is seen as a 'hit and run' process in which the microbial agent might be cleared, but elements of the immune response continue to assault the host.[120] The cross-reactivity leads to local or systemic tissue injury which subsequently releases more self-antigens, thereby inducing more antibodies, and the disease process compounds.

The self-MHC antigen complexes formed may be antigenically similar to a part of a microbe's amino acid sequence (homology) as can be seen in the two examples in Table 12.12.

There are residual parts of the sequence that are different, so the antigen and self-antigen are similar but not identical — similar enough to cross-react, yet different enough to break immunological tolerance. Perfectly identical structures might not lead to autoimmunity as they are more likely to be deleted or functionally silenced by tolerance mechanisms.

TABLE 12.12 Sequence similarities between human host proteins and microbial proteins

Human host protein microbial protein	Amino acid sequence (homology sequence in bold)	Residue	Autoimmune disease implicated
HLA-B27 *Klebsiella pneumoniae nitrogenase*	**QTDRED**L SR**QTDRED**E	70 KA186	*Klebsiella* has been associated with AS. Patients with AS have been shown to be positive for HLA-B27 in 90% of cases, while 7% of the general population share this.
A-gliadin Adenovirus 12 E1B	LGQGS**FRPSQ**QN LRRGM**FRPSQ**CN	206384	89% of patients with coeliac disease (HLA-DRB1, HLA-DQB1) and 17% of control patients were positive for Ad-12 infection.

AS, ankylosing spondylitis.
Source: Adapted from Oldstone MB. Molecular mimicry and immune-mediated diseases. Cell 1987; 50: 819–820.

TABLE 12.13 Pathogenic triggers to autoimmune diseases

Autoimmune disease	Related/triggering pathogen/s	Predisposing genetic factors
Ankylosing spondylitis (AS)	*Klebsiella pneumoniae*	HLA B27
Crohn's disease (CD)	*Mycobacterium avium paratuberculosis* *Saccharomyces cerevisiae, Escherichia coli* Mycoplasmas	CARD 15
Graves' disease	*Yersinia enterocolitica* *Helicobacter pylori*	HLA B8, HLA DRB1, DQB1
Multiple sclerosis (MS)	Epstein-Barr virus *Chlamydophila pneumoniae*	HLA DR2
Rheumatoid arthritis (RA)	*Proteus mirabilis* *Mycoplasma fermentans* or mitogen Epstein-Barr virus Chronic hepatitis C virus	HLA DRB1/DR4
Sjögren's syndrome	Epstein-Barr virus Coxsackie virus B Chronic hepatitis C virus	HLA B8 HLA DR3/W52
Systemic lupus erythematosus (SLE)	Epstein-Barr virus	HLA DR2
Type 1 diabetes	Coxsackie virus B Mumps Cytomegalovirus	HLA DR3/DR4
Ulcerative colitis (UC)	*Escherichia coli* Sulfate-reducing bacteria	HLA-DRB1; MUC-3

It has long been proposed that the number of memory CD8+ T-cells, which are generated by natural pathogen exposure or intentional vaccination to protect the host against specific viral infections, is inflexible, and that individual cells constantly compete for limited space so they displace previously generated ones. However, it is now known that they are not displaced and the compartment is able to grow in size with immunological experience. Auto-aggressive CD8+ memory T-cells reach a critical threshold with subsequent infections of pathogens sharing similar epitopes.[121] In order to induce AD, it seems that a sufficient number of auto-aggressive lymphocytes have to be generated to destroy the target tissue.[122] Thus, the patient's history of both infections and vaccinations influences their overall immune repertoire.

More recently it has been found that amino acid sequence homology may only be required for B-cell cross-reactivity in the humoral immune system. Because macrophages process antigens before presenting them to T-cells, homology would not be required for T-cell cross-reactivity, making it more likely to happen.

Molecular mimicry has been detected between pathogens and autoantigens recognised by antibodies or T-cells of patients with a broad variety of ADs, a sample of which can be seen in Table 12.13. However, there is no consistent firm proof for pathogens as inducers of ADs, except in acute rheumatic fever where *Streptococcus pyogenes* shares a structural similarity to *N*-acetyl-beta-D-glucosamine, and in Guillain-Barré syndrome where the association with *Campylobacter jejuni*, which shares a structural homology with the peripheral nerve GM1 ganglioside, could be convincingly reproduced in an animal model.[122]

MICROBIOME

The microbiome of the gut (the microorganisms, their genomes and surrounding habitat) is influenced by diet, infections, medications, stress and inheritance. Over the last decade computerised DNA sequencing technologies have allowed thousands of new microbial genomes to be identified and it is now accepted that many of these microbes accumulate and persist in body tissues and blood, some within a protective biofilm. Microbes impact many body processes and incrementally suppress innate immune defences. There is clear and increasing evidence that changes in the microbiota are associated with ADs.[123]

Evidence of particular pathogens in various ADs has been instrumental in enabling the health practitioner to implement a treatment protocol. *Klebsiella pneumoniae* organisms are likely triggers in AS and CD in genetically susceptible individuals. Patients from 16 different countries with AS showed high IgA antibody levels directed against *Klebsiella* which resemble HLA-B27.[124] *Helicobacter pylori* is considered a common denominator in more than 30 ADs, both organ specific and non-organ specific.[125] EBV and CMV are consistently associated with multiple ADs. *Proteus mirabilis* has been implicated in RA. *Escherichia coli* has been implicated in RA, CD and ulcerative colitis (UC).[126]

Mycobacterium avium subspecies *paratuberculosis* (MAP) appears to be linked to the aetiology of CD in genetically predisposed people via transmission through meat, dairy products and water. MAP is found in 30-50% of CD patients.[127] Other infectious causative agents studied in connection with CD include viruses, yeast, and bacteria including *Escherichia coli, Listeria monocytogenes, Chlamydia trachomatis, Pseudomonas maltophilia, Bacteroides fragilis* and *Mycobacterium kansasii.*

DEFECT IN HOMEOSTASIS

In some individuals there may be a lack of appropriate restoration to homeostasis within the central or peripheral tolerance mechanisms of the immune system. Critical to both central and peripheral tolerance is a process of negative selection in which T-cells that are strongly reactive to self-peptide–self-MHC complexes are eliminated and B-cells that are highly autoreactive are negatively selected in the spleen and deleted, unless they are needed for an inflammatory engagement.[128] An autoimmune-prone individual may have lax negative selection mechanisms, or an excess of apoptopic cells, or a problem in their clearance. Some individuals may have defects in multiple inhibitory pathways and thus be unable to suppress immune activation to resume homeostasis.

GUT EPITHELIAL BARRIER

While genetics predispose some people to AD and microbes and environmental factors can trigger and/or sustain the disease processes, the role of the gut must not be underestimated.

The intercellular tight junctions (TJs) in the intestines along with gut-associated lymphoid tissues (GALT) and the neuroendocrine network control the equilibrium between tolerance and immunity to non-self-antigens. In many cases, increased intestinal permeability seems to precede disease and causes an abnormality in antigen delivery that triggers the multiorgan process leading to the autoimmune response.[129]

Coeliac disease is the clearest example of the interplay between a genetic predisposition, an environmental trigger, gluten, and a highly specific humoral autoimmune response against tissue transglutaminase auto-antigen. After removing all traces of gluten from the patient's diet, symptoms resolve and autoimmune markers return to normal limits. Thus, the autoimmune process can be reverted once the interplay between genetic susceptibility and environmental trigger(s) can be prevented; that is, by re-establishing the intestinal barrier integrity and function. Several other ADs, including type 1 diabetes, inflammatory bowel disease (IBD), MS, atopic dermatitis, AS, Hashimoto's, autoimmune hepatitis and RA are characterised by increased intestinal permeability secondary to non-competent TJs that allow the passage of antigens from the intestinal flora, which then challenges the immune system to produce an immune response that can target any organ or tissue in genetically predisposed individuals.[130]

Zonulin, a protein excreted into the gut by enterocytes, is a known physiological modulator of TJs. Patients with coeliac disease are known to have increased zonulin levels which stimulate the opening of TJs and keep them open longer.[129] Zonulin production is known to be increased in other ADs such as type 1 diabetes. Once these TJs remain open, not only will substances leak out into the body, but zonulin can also signal to the cells to go into apoptosis. This will set up a vicious cycle of cell damage and cell death thus worsening the condition of the gut barrier. Zonulin production can be triggered by many things including intestinal exposure to bacteria such as *Vibrio cholerae, Shigella flexneri, Clostridium difficile* and enteropathogenic *Escherichia coli*[129] as well as increased emotional stress.[131]

Intestinal cells can be further damaged or destroyed by prolamins and agglutinins (two types of lectins in the seeds of grains, in some pseudograins, legumes and nightshades), saponins or other proteins that can be or become toxic in some people.[129]

DYSBIOSIS

A diverse colonic microbiota with abundant levels of *Faecalibacterium prausnitzii, Bifidobacterium species, Lactobacillus* species, *Akkermansia muciniphila* and many other beneficial microbes is needed in order to inhibit pathogens. Without such diversity the intestinal immune system becomes underdeveloped and certain functions such as macrophage phagocytes and immunoglobulin production are reduced.[113] Imbalance can contribute to intestinal wall hyperpermeability which in turn increases the antigen and endotoxin load. This can become a negative spiral and continue to exacerbate autoimmunity.

Analysis of the gut microflora in children with coeliac disease showed higher populations of Gram-negative bacteria such as *E. coli*, a greater diversity of pathogenic *Eubacteria* and increased *Bacteroides* counts along with low levels of *Lactobacilli*, *Bifidobacteria* and *Enterococci*.[132]

POOR LIVER DETOXIFICATION

When there is increased antigen load, reduced phagocytic capacity and subsequent increased endotoxin load in the blood from the digestive tract as autoimmunity progresses, the phagocytic Kupffer cells in the liver become overloaded. When this happens, they cannot effectively sequester all engulfed material and the risk of antigen or endotoxin spillover into the general circulation is substantially increased.[133] This then contributes to the sustaining factors of immune dysregulation.

OCCUPATION

Occupations that involve contact with the public have led to a possible hypothesis for the development of autoimmunity due to exposure to multiple infectious agents. For example, school teachers have been associated with ADs such as MS, Sjögren's disease, and systemic sclerosis, but not SLE.[134] It is postulated that exposure to some of the pathogens that are common in school-age children may be related to the development of these diseases. Other occupations in which there was found to be an increased risk of death from systemic ADs included receptionists and bank tellers. Occupations that involve exposure to chemicals and toxins are covered below.

CHEMICAL EXPOSURE

Ubiquitous synthetic compounds used in consumer products and industry such as stain- and water-resistant coatings for carpets and fabrics, fast-food contact materials, fire-resistant foams, paints and hydraulic fluids, bisphenol A in personal care products, triclosan and parabens in mouthwashes, makeup and more, are stable and persist in the environment, in wildlife and in humans globally. Many are both lipo- and hydrophobic and bind to proteins in serum. Their renal clearance is negligible and they are present in breast milk, liver, seminal fluid and umbilical cord blood. Such compounds are endocrine disrupters and are toxic to the immune system.[135] Organic pollutants such as these are commonly associated with autoimmune thyroiditis, and perhaps many other ADs, although more research is needed in this area.

Exposure to silica has been associated with systemic sclerosis, SLE and RA. Silica may promote autoimmunity by causing chronic inflammation and immune stimulation.[134] Solvents have been associated with ADs: mining machine operators, industrial machinery repairers, painters, coaters and decorators are associated with increased risk of SLE and systemic sclerosis. Firefighters, who are often exposed to a variety of chemicals such as polycyclic aromatic hydrocarbons, carbon monoxide, nitrogen dioxide, pesticides and benzene, have twice the risk of death from systemic sclerosis. The development of SLE has been associated with occupational exposure to metals, including mercury. Mercury exposure has also been linked to systemic sclerosis.[134]

People involved in farming occupations, especially crop farmers, have been found to be at increased risk of death from ADs, particularly RA, SLE and other systemic ADs.[134] Crop farmers are likely to be exposed to herbicides, fungicides, solvents, sunlight, silica and crop dusts. Farmers of all types are at more risk of type 1 diabetes.

IATROGENIC FACTORS

Drugs such as procainamide and hydralazine can induce a 'lupus-like response'; alpha- or beta-blockers may induce SLE; iodine may induce autoimmune thyroiditis; methyldopa may induce autoimmune haemolytic anaemia,[128] Hashimoto's thyroiditis may develop after treatment with IFN-α for hepatitis C.[136]

SIGNS AND SYMPTOMS

There is a vast range of ADs, so the signs and symptoms are many and varied depending on whether the disease is organ-specific or systemic, the stage of disease, the sustaining factors, and so on. General symptoms of being unwell could be due to AD, including but not limited to:

- Inflammation
- Fatigue, malaise
- Dizziness
- Intermittent low-grade fever
- Extreme sensitivity to cold in the extremities
- Sensitivity to light, sounds, tactile responses, smell
- Weakness and stiffness in muscles and joints
- Swelling in joints, arthralgia
- Neuralgia
- Skin changes
- Weight changes
- Gastrointestinal problems, especially food sensitivities
- Low or high blood pressure
- Irritability, anxiety or depression
- Hormonal changes or infertility
- Blood sugar irregularities
- A change in an organ or tissues
- Gait changes
- Vertigo
- Nutritional deficiencies.

COMPLICATIONS

Those suffering with AD often endure deterioration of kidney, heart and liver function, loss of other functions, disability, hospitalisations, outpatient visits, decreased productivity and impaired quality of life. They may have periods of remission where their active disease is quiescent, but they may suffer ongoing symptoms that have been caused by the inflammation as their disease has progressed. They will probably also suffer side effects of the drugs prescribed for their condition. Thus, quality of life can be severely compromised, and many patients die earlier than patients without AD.

DIFFERENTIAL DIAGNOSIS

Typically, multiple laboratory tests are needed and include basic studies like a complete blood count, comprehensive metabolic panel, inflammatory markers such as high-sensitivity CRP, fibrinogen and haptoglobin, ESR,

TABLE 12.14 Specific blood tests used in autoimmune disorders

Autoantibody	Rheumatoid arthritis	Sjögren's syndrome	Systemic lupus erythematosus	Ankylosing spondylitis
Rheumatoid factor (RF)	+ in 70%	+/−	+	Occasionally +
Antinuclear autoantibodies (ANA)	+ in 25–30%	+ in over 40–70%	+ in over 95%	
C-reactive protein (CRP)	H/L		N	
Erythrocyte sedimentation rate (ESR)	H		H	H
Anti-DNA antibodies	+/−	+/−	+	
IgA; IgM; IgG				H
Anticyclic-citrullinated-peptide (anti-CCP)	+ found up to 14 years before onset of disease			
Cardiolipin autoantibodies	+		+	
Antiscleroderma antibody (anti-SCL-70)		+/−		
Anti-Sjögren's syndrome A (anti-SSA)	+/−	+	+/−	

+antibody is present (positive); – antibody is not present; +/– antibody may or may not be present; H, high; N, normal; L, low

ferritin, ceruloplasmin, fibrinogen, haptoglobulin, immunological studies, including as appropriate, RF, anti-CCP, ANA, anti-dsDNA and organ-specific antibodies, although the presence of antibodies alone does not rule AD in or out, complement factors, immunoglobulins, cytokine analysis and HLA typing. See Table 12.14.

NATUROPATHIC DIAGNOSIS

Careful and thorough case taking in conjunction with laboratory testing can assist the naturopath in seeking confirmation of their provisional assessment of AD in patients displaying symptoms. If autoantibodies are not found, it may be worthwhile to retest at some future date, as some ADs go into remission from time to time. Serum genetic testing may be warranted as well as other inflammatory markers and other radiological investigations. Molecular faecal analysis of the microbiome is a useful adjunct.

The confirmation of the presence of autoantibodies and other markers of AD should lead the naturopath to search the case for all the factors that contributed to the aetiology and pathogenesis of the AD, an approach which is invaluable in designing an effective treatment protocol.

Investigations

Because AD is a complex, multifactorial disease, further investigations such as those below can assist the clinician in implementing a targeted and efficacious protocol for the patient. Such tests can also provide the patient with an understanding and education about their condition and thus keep them motivated to adhere to the recommendations provided.

SPECIFIC NATUROPATHIC INVESTIGATIONS

Thorough case history

By taking detailed notes on patients' history from birth, particularly infections, exposures and stressors, their symptoms, dietary habits and family health history, a skilled clinician may avoid the need to embark on a multitude of expensive tests in order to implement an effective treatment protocol. However, in some instances — for example, where a heavy metal or toxic overload is suspected, or where patient compliance is low and evidence is needed of the functional derangement in their system — one or more of the tests below may be warranted.

Zinc assessment

Immune function is dependent upon zinc status in both cellular and humoral immune responses. Low levels may contribute to a premature transition from Th1 activity to Th2. Zinc also promotes normal tissue repair.[137] Plasma zinc is the best determinate along with serum copper to accurately assess the balance between the two minerals.

Microbiome analysis

Until earlier this century, comprehensive stool analysis was undertaken to try to establish the 'good, the bad and the ugly' balance in the gut using culture techniques. The disadvantages of this method are firstly that the labs have been unable to successfully grow many members of the GIT ecosystem and further that the results have been reflective of changes (die-off) during shipping to the lab. Since the arrival of molecular technology to analyse microbial populations, there have been over 200 previously undescribed GIT species detected. Thus they provide a more accurate and comprehensive picture of the GIT ecosystem with no concerns over shipping time. These may be faecal testing, or as needed other sites in the body such as the oral mucosa and skin.

Precise identification of pathogenic species alongside a measure of the diversity of beneficial microbes helps the practitioner implement effective treatment strategies. Additional testing is available to ascertain levels of other key digestive markers present in the stool.

Heavy metal analysis

To determine toxic burden and mineral balances, a hair mineral analysis can be undertaken. It is particularly useful in identifying accumulation of heavy metals such as mercury and arsenic and monitoring the efficacy of detoxification of these toxins.

Urine toxic and essential elements

A pre- and post-provocation urinalysis test to determine toxic metal burden and, if desired, the status of essential elements. Agents such as ethylenediaminetetraacetic acid (EDTA), dimercaptosuccinic acid (DMSA), dimercaptopropane sulfonate (DMPS) or D-penicillamine are administered and net retention is measured over a 24-hour collection period. Essential element levels can be analysed in order to evaluate nutritional status and the efficacy of mineral supplementation during metal detoxification therapy.

Hepatic detox profile

A first morning urine test to assess chemical exposure and phase I and phase II detoxification without using challenge drugs. A sample is sent to the laboratory to test for urinary D-glucaric acid, a byproduct of phase I detoxification, and urinary mercapturic acids which are end product metabolites of conjugated xenobiotics.

Functional liver detoxification profile (fldp)

This assesses phase I and phase II detoxification pathways by using challenges (aspirin and paracetamol). Saliva and urine samples are collected at specific times by the patient and sent to the laboratory.

Therapeutic considerations

CLINICAL DECISION MAKING AND RATIONALE

ADs are among the most complex and difficult diseases to treat, but one of the diseases in which naturopaths can make an enormous difference to a patient's quality of life. By understanding and working with the aetiology, not just the symptomatology, of the particular AD that presents in the clinic, naturopaths provide a valuable holistic approach which works with the person in unique ways. This multi-faceted approach provides individualised support for the patient.

Thorough and detailed case taking is essential in order to determine the priorities in neutralising the disease cascade. Relevant testing should be undertaken to give a baseline level of the relevant markers of AD and the functioning of relevant organs, to allow the practitioner to monitor progress and adjust treatment accordingly. Specific causative factors must be identified for the individual patient as much as is reasonably possible. Particularly look for indications of problems in apparently unrelated systems or organs. Try to identify the process of the primary lesion: childhood illnesses, surgery, vaccinations, accidents or recurrent or chronic illnesses, especially in the respiratory, urinary or digestive systems.[133] Individualisation is critical.

Commonly, the patient will be under the care of a specialist and general practitioner concurrently, so it is important to keep the lines of communication open and keep other professionals informed of complementary treatment. Potential herb–drug–nutrient interactions need to be understood and the practitioner needs to differentiate between disease-related symptoms and drug side effects. One of the supports that the naturopath can offer is amelioration of drug side effects.

Inform the patient that this is a chronic condition and treatment will be step-wise and ongoing. Symptomatic relief will give encouragement to the patient to persist and motivate them to be compliant.

Holistically assess and provide guidance to the patient on ways of reducing current stressors in their environment: environmental, emotional, physical, mental and nutritional.

Therapeutic application

HISTORICAL PERSPECTIVE

The earliest understandings in immunology emerged in the late 19th century in the context of the battle to ward off infectious disease. It could be demonstrated that specific antibodies might be formed against such innocuous agents as egg albumin, bovine serum proteins and sheep red cells.[128] At the turn of the 20th century, cytotoxic antibodies against a variety of tissues were reported, including some animals that formed antibodies against their own spermatozoa which could destroy the sperm in vitro. When it was found that these antibodies seemed to have no effect in vivo, Paul Ehrlich, who played a major role in the early history of autoimmunity, convinced the world that a self-regulating mechanism would maintain equilibrium between the antibody and the antigen, a postulate that he named 'horror autoxicus': autoimmune disease was impossible.

During the late 1930s and 1940s a series of observations began to challenge this assumption. Antibodies formed in the apparent absence of antigens; there seemed to be a lack of relationship between immunity to certain viral diseases and the titre of antiviral antibodies. French immunologist Pierre Grabar in the mid-1900s saw the levels of autoantibodies as being derived from the endogenous physiological system of nutrition. He saw their primary role as 'opsonins': to identify and clutch onto protein molecules that should not be wandering around the body fluids, and present them to the active scavenger-defenders, the phagocytes, for destruction.[138] When these mechanisms failed, through toxic or viral action, there would be a breakdown in normal tolerance and a flood of autoantibodies.

Soon after an allograft rejection was observed in 1944, hypotheses emerged based on the self-non-self model of immunology, or 'immunological tolerance' theory. Dating from 1959, Burnet's 'clonal elimination' hypothesis suggested that at an early stage in fetal development, exposure to an antigen leads not to the usual stimulus to lymphocyte division by the body's defence mechanisms, but to elimination of the lymphocyte involved. All lymphocytes that could mount an attack on the body tissues should thus be removed.[139] This model is generally accepted now as providing the main basis for protection against autoimmune attack, although it is accepted that the immune system is far more complicated than this and there need to be mechanisms of tolerance that can operate continuously throughout life, not just during fetal development.

The year 1974 saw the discovery of the major histocompatibility complex (MHC), the most gene-dense region (over 3.5 million gene pairs) found on chromosome 6. Soon after that, in 1976, a theory of autoimmunity emerged, proposed by Ebringer, the 'cross-reactivity' theory: some bacterial antigens cross-react with the host HLA antigens (part of the MHC) because they are sufficiently similar; the immune system is provoked, then confused, and attacks both its own tissues and the antigen.[140] In 1979 Geczy and coworkers proposed the 'modifying factor theory' in which the HLA molecule is modified by a component of an antigen.

The last 60 years have seen an explosion in research into the complexities of the immune system, into immune modifying drugs, and into pathogens and genetics, although there is still much that is not understood. Steroidal drugs became widely available in the 1950s but in ensuing decades it was apparent that they were associated with a range of side effects. Medications to treat autoimmunity have increasingly focused on one single aspect of the immune system, often at the peril of the whole. Alongside this, there has been a tremendous amount of environmental change, and ever-increasing levels of toxins and stressors interlacing in people's lives. These toxins and stressors are potentially weakening immune systems in ways that can lead to or compound infection, inflammation and autoimmunity.

Research into complementary medicine has expanded also and there is a growing evidence-base to provide guidelines for therapy. Yet the modern naturopath still effectively employs traditional notions of treating the digestive system, eliminating toxicity, building the body's defences and attending to the diet.

ALLOPATHIC PERSPECTIVE

Patients with ADs are frequently prescribed anti-inflammatory drugs such as aspirin or non-steroidal anti-inflammatory drugs (NSAIDs) or corticosteroids in order to treat the symptoms. More recent pharmacological intervention has focused on the components of the immune system and the inflammatory response, in particular directed at suppressing the overactivity of T-cells and their adhesion to other cell types, or inhibitors of TNF-α or B-cell protein antibodies. For example, interferon, prescribed for some MS patients, causes a reduction in MHC class II presentation on antigen presentation cells, so reduces T-cell activity. In vitro and animal studies are investigating metformin to treat SLE by way of normalising T-cell metabolism through the dual inhibition of glycolysis and mitochondrial metabolism.

Biological response modifiers (BRMs) are TNF-α inhibitors and thus decrease the inflammatory expression of inducible nitric oxide synthase (iNOS) in macrophages and vascular endothelial cells. Newer biologicals are expensive and are targeted at B-cells; for example, rituximab which is a chimeric antibody against CD20, a protein expressed on B-cells. Low-dose naltrexone is sometimes employed in an attempt to improve the patient's quality of life in ADs such as MS, although its efficacy is not clearly established.

Even more recently, pharmacological studies have led to the development of agents that skew the balance of T-helper cells in favour of Th2 cell activity. This type of strategy runs the risk of suppressing the whole immune system. One of these drugs is glatiramer acetate which is used in MS, and seems to reduce the rate of relapse by about 30%.[141]

Occasionally, antimicrobial treatment may be administered as the understanding of the role of memory cells develops. Epidemiological and experimental evidence has been building an understanding of the role of memory B-lymphocyte reservoirs of infection of EBV in RA, SLE and MS. New antiviral therapies are being developed to target these viral memory cells.

Only recently, the scientific community publicly stated that they have gained insights on the importance of the intestinal resident flora for the host's health and disease.[142] Gut microbiota, they state, in fact plays a crucial role in modulating innate and acquired immune responses and thus interferes with the fragile balance of inflammation versus tolerance.

NATUROPATHIC PERSPECTIVE

The naturopath in the 21st century is able to build on their traditional roots and incorporate a deeper understanding of what initiates an autoimmune disease, what maintains and sustains it and what part memory cells, pathogens, genetics, gut and environment play in an individual's case. Each facet of the disease can then be targeted and this holistic approach to treatment can be very effective. The modern naturopath should be able to avoid 'healing crises' where 'things must get worse before they get better' by balancing, supporting and restoring the systems that are depleted and inflamed, all the while treating the whole person, individually. The naturopath needs to work alongside medications, be aware of any possible interactions and develop protocols to ameliorate some of their side effects, as the patient frequently seeks out a naturopath after diagnosis has been made and allopathic treatment has been implemented.

Whether the AD is organ specific or systemic, the goals of treatment are to address the cause and eliminate it if possible, to address the sustaining factors, to treat the symptoms, and to support the health of the whole person. If the naturopath can intervene early in an AD, they may be able to restore immunological homeostasis and correct immunological imbalance before the disease produces irreversible destruction. While treatment is underway, there will be times when the naturopath will need to put a hold on the treatment of the disease cascade and attend to acute infections, as it is very likely that these acute episodes will exacerbate the AD if they are not dealt with promptly. Meanwhile, a great deal of symptomatic relief can be given as well. Through dietary recommendations there is the potential to empower the patient to become an active participant in the therapeutic process.

Some general strategies for any stage of AD treatment include the following:

- Identify and eradicate as far as possible the precipitating factor(s) or primary lesion, whether infection(s), past or present, gut microbiome, toxic levels of chemicals, hormonal products, or heavy metals
- Down-regulate immunological memory, reduce the production of autoantibodies; increase circulating NK and NK T-cells
- Reduce inflammation
- Stimulate detoxification at tissue level
- Facilitate detoxification of any chemical, hormonal or heavy metal toxins
- Facilitate the removal of immune complexes especially by the spleen and Kuppfer cells so that the liver sequesters junk rather than presenting it to T-cells
- Remove any dietary allergens or intolerances, decrease zonulin production, heal tight junctions in the gut
- Support the organ(s) affected/involved
- Treat acute infections promptly and thoroughly
- Provide symptomatic relief
- Control or eliminate bowel flora dysbiosis
- Improve proteolytic function
- Restore nutritional deficiencies
- Address concomitant symptoms.
- Support the nervous system as necessary.
- Support the stress response and allostatic load.
- Treat any constipation.

NUTRITIONAL MEDICINE (DIETARY)

An inappropriate diet, in which foods are consumed that are difficult to digest for whatever reason, can derange immune function, causing cross-reaction between dietary proteins and self-tissue. Thus, it is important to assess any dietary factors that are contributing to immune system derangement and tissue inflammation and remove them. It is also important not to overload the system with processed foods, foods with chemical additives, or hormonal products. The focus needs to be on fresh, living, organic food as far as possible, with a balance of alkaline foods. Apart from such general guidelines, each person with AD will require individualised dietary advice dependent upon the predisposing, precipitating and sustaining factors in their case.

Dietary therapeutic objectives

Diet is critical in AD. There is no one-size-fits-all way of eating but it is almost certain that the patient with AD will need to make some quite drastic changes. The following dietary protocols have evidence behind them for various ADs:

- Gluten-free, grain-free, Paleo, Paleo autoimmune diets
- Plant-based, vegetarian, vegan, raw-foods, vegetable-juice diets
- GAPS (gut and psychology syndrome) diet
- SCD (specific carbohydrate diet)
- Low-sulfur diet
- IBD-AID (anti-inflammatory diet)
- Weston A Price Foundation diet
- Wahls protocol
- Mediterranean diet.

SPECIFIC DIETARY TREATMENTS

Dietary inclusions

ANTIOXIDANTS

Vegetables and fruits rich in antioxidants are crucial in the diet of the patient with AD in order to reduce oxidative stress. It should be kept in mind that the bioavailability of antioxidants may be impaired by one or many of several factors such as poor solubility, inefficient permeability, instability due to storage of food, first pass effect and gastrointestinal degradation.

Endogenous total antioxidant capacity (TAC) may be modulated by dietary ingestion of plant food. TAC has been found to be inversely associated with plasma levels of C-reactive protein (CRP), an inflammatory marker, in 243 non-diabetic participants.[143] Plasma carotenoid concentrations decline during the acute-phase response to infection and injury in the presence of increased levels of biomarkers of inflammation. A high intake of carotenoid-rich fruits and vegetables reduced CRP concentrations.[144] Lower serum concentrations of antioxidants were associated with an increased risk of RA in three studies.[145]

Fresh wheat grass juice squeezed from mature sprouts of wheat seeds (*Triticum aestivum*) is high in antioxidants and flavonoids. A small double blind RCT in patients with active distal UC who were given 100 cc of organic freshly squeezed wheatgrass juice daily for 1 month recorded significant reductions in the overall disease activity index and in the severity of rectal bleeding. One of the pathways to this improvement appeared to be the antioxidant properties of wheatgrass juice.[146]

FASTING AND VEGETARIAN OR VEGAN DIETS

A systematic review of over 30 studies showed a statistically and clinically significant beneficial long-term effect of fasting and vegetarian diets in the treatment of RA.[147] In one of the trials, patients with RA who fasted 7–10 days (partial fast), followed by 13 months on a vegetarian diet, had reduced pain, but not physical function or morning stiffness, immediately after intervention. Two other trials compared a 4-week elemental diet with an ordinary diet and reported no significant differences in pain, function or stiffness. The effects of vegan and elimination diets were uncertain. There were potential adverse effects, as there was a significantly higher total drop-out of 10% and a significantly higher weight loss in the diet groups compared with the control groups.[148]

A combination of fasting and vegetarian diets has been shown to reduce the ability of the urine to support the growth of *Proteus mirabilis*, which has been implicated in RA, and *Escherichia coli*, which has been implicated in RA, CD and UC.[126]

PROBIOTICS

Probiotics have the potential to modulate a predisposition to chronic inflammatory conditions and are an important part of therapy. Probiotics exert benefit both locally by attaching to epithelial barriers and stabilising the intestinal barrier, and systemically through inhibition of NF-kappaB, reduction of CD4 intraepithelial lymphocytes and modulation of apoptosis.[149] Recent studies have shown the effectiveness of *Saccharomyces cerevisiae var boulardii* in reducing IBD pathogenesis by trapping T-cells in mesenteric lymph nodes and exerting multiple anti-inflammatory mechanisms.[150] Also, in patients with CD, treatment with an adjunctive yeast preparation containing 1 g daily *Saccharomyces boulardii* and 1 g mesalazine two to three times daily resulted in a reduction of clinical relapses, which did not occur to the same extent when treated with mesalazine alone.[151] A multi-strain probiotic marketed asVSL#3 has been found to assist in inducing remission in patients with UC: at week 12, 43% of patients in the VSL#3 group were in remission versus 16% of controls ($P < 0.001$).[152] *Lactobacillus* GG was found to be equally effective as mesalazine in maintaining clinical remission in patients with UC and significantly more effective than mesalazine in prolonging the relapse-free time ($P < 0.05$).[153] Another study of patients with UC administered *Escherichia coli* Nissle 1917. After 12 months, the relapse rate was 25% in probiotic-treated teens versus 30% in the mesalazine group.[154]

OMEGA-3 FATTY ACIDS

A plethora of published literature supports the contention that omega-3 polyunsaturated fatty acids (PUFAs) have significant immunomodulatory and anti-inflammatory activity by modulating the type and amount of eicosanoids and cytokines[155] and by suppressing MHC class II expression.[156] Many studies have shown that the Mediterranean diet, which is high in oil-rich fish, olive oil and cooked vegetables, is protective against RA due to high omega-3 content. The best oily fish are sardines, herring, mackerel, salmon and tuna.

FIBRE

Soluble fibre, such as slippery elm, psyllium, vegetables and legumes, encourages healthy intestinal flora as well as keeping bowels regular. An open label, parallel-group, multicentre RCT of 102 patients with UC who were in remission tested the effects of psyllium seeds (*Plantago ovata*) compared with mesalazine (500 mg three times daily). Patients taking the psyllium (10 g twice daily) had a superior improvement in symptoms compared with the placebo group and it was concluded that psyllium may be as effective as mesalazine to maintain remission.[157]

FLAVONOIDS

Flavonoid-rich foods such as green tea, dark chocolate (in moderation), apples, cherries, berries, citrus, turmeric, ginger, broccoli and wheatgrass juice have the potential to modulate predisposition to chronic inflammatory conditions and can dramatically reduce inflammation. Their anti-inflammatory action is via inhibition of COX and LOX activities, eicosanoid biosynthesis, neutrophil granulation and prostaglandin synthesis inhibition.[158]

ALKALINE FOODS

Ensure a balance of alkaline foods such as fresh vegetables, sprouts, green tea and selected nuts and seeds, especially if the patient is on acidic medications such as NSAIDs. Highly acidic diets, especially those high in meat, poultry, dairy and grains, can exacerbate inflammation.

GARLIC

Garlic (*Allium sativum*) is antioxidant, immunomodulatory and antimicrobial (antibacterial, antifungal, antiparasitic and antiviral) and has demonstrated a protective effect against heavy metal poisoning, so is ideal to include in the diet of people with AD. Allicin is believed to be chiefly responsible for garlic's antimicrobial activity along with ajoene which may have greater antiviral activity. An open controlled trial of 30 patients with RA taking alisate, a garlic preparation produced in Russia, 300 mg twice daily for 4–6 weeks, compared with a control group who received conventional antirheumatic therapy, found that the alisate group achieved a good and partial response in 86.5% of cases.[159] Eating a fresh garlic clove or including 2–5 mg/day garlic oil will assist in acute infections.[160]

SPICES

Many spices have been found to be invaluable anti-inflammatories that are pharmacologically highly safe to consume and inexpensive. Turmeric powder when boiled in water for 10 minutes releases curcumin which can down-regulate NF-kappaB activation and the expression of COX-2, LOX, iNOS and other inflammatory markers, so is beneficial to include in the daily diet.[161] Curcumin also induces phase II liver detoxification and has antioxidant, antimicrobial and depurative activity.[162] Capsicum, especially hot, red chilli peppers, contains capsaicin which can suppress NF-kappaB activation.[161] Fennel and anise contain anethole which is antioxidant, inhibits lipid peroxidation, is a free radical scavenger, and anti-inflammatory. Fenugreek and wild yam roots contain diosgenin which has been shown to inhibit intestinal inflammation, suppress NF-kappaB activation and modulate the activity of LOX and COX-2 and has been found to induce apoptosis in human RA cells. Ursolic acid in rosemary has also been found to suppress NF-kappaB activation and thus LOX, COX-2 and iNOS expression. Ginger contains gingerol which is also anti-inflammatory.[161] Cumin, coriander, cinnamon and black pepper may also be useful, although there is insufficient research available to date.

PINEAPPLE AND PAPAYA

Fresh pineapple and papaya contain a variety of proteolytic enzymes including bromelain and papain which aid digestion and are anti-inflammatory. The anti-inflammatory action of bromelain appears to be mediated by decreasing levels of PGE2 and thromboxane, by modulation of some immune cell surface adhesion molecules and by increasing serum fibrinolytic activity, decreasing bradykinin levels thus reducing oedema and pain.[158] A clinical trial of patients with knee pain found significant improvement in symptoms and physical function from doses of 200–400 mg per day of bromelain.[158]

BRASSICA VEGETABLES

Broccoli sprouts, broccoli, Brussels sprouts and cauliflower are good sources of glucosinolates which are broken down to the isothiocyanate sulforaphane which induces phase II liver detoxification of xenobiotics and other toxins. They are also a good source of other nutrients including antioxidants.

Dietary exclusions

ALLERGENIC FOODS

Eliminate antigens such as dairy casein/lactose, wheat gliadin/gluten and yeast in an individual who is susceptible, as they are notorious for disturbing intestinal immunological function. Antigenic foods can exacerbate intestinal hyperpermeability which enables enteric antigens to penetrate the mucosa to an increased extent. Patients with CD on an elemental diet of predigested liquid free of antigenic challenge consisting of amino acids, dextrin, vitamins, oil and minerals experienced significantly greater improvement in symptoms than those on prednisolone.[163] CD patients who excluded cereals, dairy products, citrus and yeast experienced longer remission periods than those on corticosteroids.[164] A low-antigenic diet (dairy-free, gluten-free) which is rich in fish is protective against RA. In a trial with 110 patients with confirmed coeliac disease, the majority of patients' anti-*Saccharomyces cerevisiae* antibodies (ASCAs) disappeared during a gluten-free diet.[165] Eliminating cow's milk products caused symptomatic improvement in AS in one study.[166]

COW'S MILK

In addition to being a potential allergenic trigger for some individuals as discussed above, cow's milk may be a source of the pathogen *Mycobacterium avium* subspecies *paratuberculosis* (MAP), which has immune dysregulatory properties. MAP DNA has been detected in more than 90% of CD patients and may be implicated in other ADs such as Hashimoto's thyroiditis.[167] MAP seems to escape pasteurisation of cow's milk from cows with Johne's disease, a very prevalent disease that is similar to CD and is caused by MAP. MAP is environmentally persistent and is found in some water supplies as it is resistant to purification with chlorine, and in undercooked beef.[168] Should this organism be suspected of contributing to the pathogenesis of an AD, sources of it should be eliminated as far as possible, for example by reducing or eliminating dairy products or finding a source of MAP-free dairy products.

TRANS FATTY ACIDS

There is convincing evidence from observational studies and RCTs that trans fatty acids elevate inflammatory markers.[169] Low levels occur naturally in meat and milk from cows and sheep and variable amounts are produced by partial hydrogenation of vegetable oils or heating and frying oils at extreme temperatures. Foods highest in *trans* fats are doughnuts, margarine, potato chips, chicken nuggets, processed fish, sausage rolls, quiche, biscuits and shelf-stable cakes.[170]

STARCH

Klebsiella pneumoniae, likely triggers in some ADs such as AS and CD, use resistant starch processed to oligosaccharides by friendly bacteria as a major source of nutrition. While around 10% of patients with AS have overt IBD and 70% have subclinical terminal ileitis, many are asymptomatic, so testing for the presence of *Klebsiella pneumoniae* is advisable. If the organisms are present and the starch food source is removed, there will be a decrease in the number of organisms, thus a decrease in inflammation and permeability, reducing the stimulus for immune cross-reactivity, so symptoms will improve in some AD patients.[171] A significant result may take 4–6 months or more. Foods to reduce on the low-starch diet are: bread, potatoes, chips, rice, spaghetti, cereals, cakes and biscuits.

ALCOHOL

Alcohol increases oxidative damage to the liver and thus reduces its capacity to phagocytose immune complexes and to detoxify chemicals or xenobiotics. Alcohol is contraindicated during some drug therapy, such as interferon.

YEAST

Elevated anti-*Saccharomyces cerevisiae* antibodies (ASCAs) are found in about 65% of patients with CD. It is possible that removal of dietary baker's and brewer's yeast could be beneficial to some patients.

SULFUR-CONTAINING FOODS

Patients with active UC may have an overproduction of hydrogen sulfide due to an excess of sulfate-reducing bacteria (SRB). Hydrogen sulfide is toxic to the intestinal mucosa by competing with short-chain fatty acids. The modern diet in Western countries contains around six times the amount of sulfur as some rural diets such as in Africa. High-sulfur foods include eggs, dairy products, soy milk, mayonnaise, sulfated drinks such as wines, cordials and mineral water, garlic, onions, as well as foods with sulfur-containing additives such as dried fruits. Chronic UC patients who went on a low-sulfur diet for 12 months had a remarkable clinical improvement.[172]

Other dietary considerations

FOOD HYGIENE

Some harmful organisms can be found in foods, especially food from a *bain marie* which has been kept warm for hours. As discussed above, MAP organisms may be ingested in undercooked beef. Food is a potent source of some of the organisms that are associated with CD including adherent-invasive *Escherichia coli* (AIEC), bacterial flagellin, *Yersinia* spp., *Listeria* spp., *Klebsiella enterocolitica* and measles virus.

PATIENT'S HISTORY

A patient's dietary history, even as a baby, can illuminate some contributing factors to the development of AD. The introduction of gluten-containing foods to infants while breastfeeding appears to reduce the risk for coeliac disease in genetically susceptible infants. However, large

SAMPLE DAILY DIET

BREAKFAST	
Fruit salad comprised of kiwi fruit, papaya and pineapple served with a small quantity of coconut yoghurt and seed mix	A diet centred upon modulating autoimmunity should be gluten and dairy free, given the link between these components and active autoimmune disease and intestinal permeability. Kiwi, pineapple and papaya contain proteases (e.g. bromelain and papain). Proteases have pleiotropic immunological effects supporting an immunomodulatory potential for the intervention of inflammatory autoimmune diseases. Pumpkin and sunflower seeds are a source of zinc; zinc is required for optimum function of the tight junctions in the gut, reducing intestinal permeability which is linked to AI disease.
LUNCH	
Falafels with quinoa, tabouli and hummus. Serve with avocado, cold steamed broccoli, olives, tomatoes, carrots, and cucumber. Home-made dressing of olive oil, fresh garlic, lemon juice and pepper	A diet rich in plant polysaccharides and low in inflammatory fats and animal proteins has been hypothesised to favour pro-tolerogenic microbial species and promote gut immune regulation in individuals genetically at risk for autoimmune diseases such as type 1 diabetes.
DINNER	
Trout steamed with ginger, garlic, onion, lime juice, tamari and steamed rice. Ample green, yellow and orange vegetables, and a tablespoon of kimchi	Trout provides a source of omega-3 PUFAs which have been shown to down-regulate inflammation, a driver in autoimmune disease. Ginger is a digestive and also highly anti-inflammatory; a fermented food such as kimchi may be useful as a probiotic, but is also indicated due to other ingredients within the kimchi such as cruciferous vegetables which may also aid detoxification.
SNACKS	
1–2 pieces of at least 70% cocoa dark chocolate Vegetable juice with fresh turmeric added	Flavonol-rich dark chocolate exerts anti-inflammatory effects by increasing mRNA expression of the anti-inflammatory cytokine IL-10 Vegetable juice provides a concentrated source of antioxidant and anti-inflammatory constituents. Adding fresh turmeric further reduces inflammation and regulates the immune system due to curcumin inhibiting TNF-α-induced activation of NF-κB and COX-2.
BEVERAGES	
Purified water, green tea, herbal teas	Green tea is rich in polyphenols which may help to modulate chronic inflammatory diseases.

Sources: De Filippo C, Cavalieri D, Di Paola M et al. Impact of diet in shaping gut microbiota revealed by a comparative study in children from Europe and rural Africa. Proc Natl Acad Sci U S A 2010; 107:14691–14696. Roep BO, van den Engel NK, van Halteren AG et al. Modulation of autoimmunity to beta-cell antigens by proteases. Diabetologia 2002; 45(5):686–692. Wang X, Valenzano MC, Mercado JM et al. Zinc supplementation modifies tight junctions and alters barrier function of CACO-2 human intestinal epithelial layers. Dig Dis Sci 2013; 58(1):77–87.

amounts, as compared with small or medium amounts, increase the risk.[113]

NUTRITIONAL MEDICINE (SUPPLEMENTAL)

Nutritional medicine therapeutic objectives

It is important to correct any nutritional deficiencies resulting from dietary and lifestyle factors in an individual's case. Particularly address the deficiencies or requirements as noted in the literature, summarised in Table 12.15. Note the nutrients that are required when on drug therapy. Every patient with AD will be undergoing oxidative stress generated by the inflammatory processes and this needs substantial doses of antioxidants which can only be achieved by supplementation.

Specific nutrients required

See Table 12.15.

HERBAL MEDICINE

Herbal medicine therapeutic objectives

Multiple actions need to be employed when designing herbal formulas for the patient with AD, as summarised in Table 12.16. Because many patients will be taking prescribed medications, herb–drug interactions need to be checked. The patient will benefit from having an additional herbal formula to take when they get an acute infection from any source as most patients will experience a worsening of their AD symptoms after an acute infection that has not been effectively treated.

TABLE 12.15 Specific nutrients required

Requirement	Justification	Therapeutic dose	Food sources
Selenium	Inhibits the activation of NF-kappaB and therefore reduces IL-6 and TNF-α production. By restoring depleted hepatic and serum selenium levels CRP production is suppressed thereby attenuating the inflammatory process. It is a component of antioxidant enzyme glutathione peroxidase	200–400 micrograms/d	Alfalfa, Brazil nuts, cashew nuts, crab, eggs, garlic, kidney, liver, mackerel, tuna, oysters, wholegrain cereals, sesame and sunflower seeds, broccoli, onions
Zinc	Immune function depends on zinc status in both cellular and humoral immune responses: in the regulation of T lymphocytes, CD4 cells, NK T-cells, IL-2 and SOD. Low levels of zinc may contribute to a premature transition from efficient Th1-dependent cellular immune activity to Th2-dependent humoral immune function. Zinc promotes normal tissue repair and restores normal immune function without being an 'immune stimulant'. Low zinc levels may be associated with inflammatory conditions	10–75 mg/d elemental zinc	Beef, lamb, liver, egg yolks, ginger, herrings, oysters, sunflower and pumpkin seeds, wholegrains, yeast
Copper	Deficiency reduces antibody production, phagocytic activity, T-cell proliferation, and increases B-cell numbers. Copper is involved with zinc in SOD	2–5 mg/d	Almonds, pecans, legumes, buckwheat, dark chocolate, lamb, pork, organ meats, oysters, perch, prunes, sunflower seeds, wholegrain cereals
Iron	Low plasma iron selectively inhibits proliferation of Th1, and not Th2, cells and reduces cytotoxic activity of phagocytes	15–50 mg/d	Red meat, liver, red wine, apricots, parsley, pine nuts, soy beans, sunflower and pumpkin seeds, oysters, yeast
Magnesium	Deficiency increases eosinophils, IL-1, IL-6, TNF-α and histamine levels	300–600 mg/d	Almonds, cashews, cocoa, molasses, parsnips, soy beans, wholegrain cereals, kelp, eggs, seeds, leafy vegetables, mineral water
Vitamin A/ carotenoids	Potent immunomodulator: vitamin A metabolites modulate the Th1–Th2 balance and the differentiation of Treg cells. Deficiency reduces Ag-specific IgG and IgE, and Th2 cytokines. Carotenoids may scavenge peroxynitrite.	Vitamin A 10 000–25 000 IU/d Beta-carotene 10–40 mg/d	Carrots, sweet potatoes, cabbage, dark-green leafy vegetables, pumpkin, broccoli, peppers, green beans, melons, avocado, green olives, orange fruits, tomatoes, apricots
Vitamin B complex	Deficiency reduces antibody responses, lymphocyte proliferation. B_{12} is a potent nitric oxide scavenger. B_{12} deficiency depresses phagocyte functions	1–2 per day (dose-dependent)	Legumes, whole grains, nuts, beans, brewer's yeast, leafy green vegetables
Vitamin C	Antioxidant function protects phagocytes; deficiency of vitamin C lowers phagocyte activity and slows wound repair. Ascorbate may scavenge peroxynitrite and helps regenerate other antioxidants	250–5000 mg/d	Blackcurrant, broccoli, citrus fruits, strawberries, rosehips, guava, mangoes, pineapple
Vitamin D	Potent immunomodulator: selectively suppresses Th1 and not Th2 or CD8+ cell activity. Data have implicated vitamin D deficiency with MS, SLE and psoriasis and other ADs. Vitamin D receptors have been identified on almost all immune modulating cells	400–1600 IU/d Up to 5000 IU in extreme northern or southern latitudes	Vitamin D appears to be necessary as a supplement as fish liver oil, not just dietary. Synthesised by the action of sunlight on skin
Vitamin E	A potent chain-breaking antioxidant, so reduces oxidative stress; α-tocopherol, especially at high doses, decreases the release of proinflammatory cytokines; γ-tocopherol can scavenge peroxynitrite and decrease NF-kappaB activation and CRP levels; tocotrienols are reported to have a role in protecting cells from excitotoxicity	100–800 IU/d	Plant seeds and vegetable oils, walnuts, pecans, almonds, beef, corn, egg yolk, safflower, sunflower, wheatgerm

TABLE 12.15 Specific nutrients required—cont'd			
Requirement	**Justification**	**Therapeutic dose**	**Food sources**
Omega-3 polyunsaturated fatty acids	PUFAs, particularly EPA and DHA, have significant immunomodulatory and anti-inflammatory activities. In general, the consumption of fish oil upregulates apoptosis in lymphocytes, reduces lymphocyte proliferation, T-cell-mediated cytotoxicity, NK-cell activity, macrophage-mediated cytotoxicity and suppresses MHC class II expression, antigen presentation, and production of proinflammatory cytokines and adhesion molecule expression	3.1–8.4 g EPA + DHA have reported decreases in the production of ROS and superoxide	Fish, especially salmon, tuna, mackerel, cod and sardines, cod liver oil, mustard seed oil, linseed oil
Alpha lipoic acid	Inhibits production of NF-kappaB; scavenges peroxynitrite, is synergistic with other antioxidants	100–600 mg/d	Muscle meats, heart, kidney, liver, and to a lesser degree, fruits, vegetables, potatoes
Coenzyme Q10	Scavenges peroxynitrite. Stimulates mitochondrial function	30–300 mg/d	Nuts, seeds, broccoli, spinach, sardines
Probiotics	Some strains antagonise NF-kappaB activation, decrease TNF-α, IL-1, IL-8 and promote IL-10 and Treg cells. Several strains adhere to mucosal tissue and limit pathogen access to the epithelium. Some strains may be active secretors of antimicrobial agents	10^8–10^{10} cfu/d for most strains	Fermented cabbage and dairy milk, yoghurt
Flavonoids	Epicatechin, catechin and specific dimers regulate NF-kappaB cells while suppressing production of proinflammatory cytokines. Scavenge peroxynitrite, superoxide and nitric oxide allow regeneration of other antioxidants	4.2 mg — 3 g daily	Spirulina, cocoa, red wine, tea, red grapes, berries, apples, citrus fruits, spinach, red peppers, celery. Absorption rate may not be high

AD, autoimmune disease; cfu, colony forming unit; CRP, C-reactive protein; DHA, docosahexaenoic acid; EPA, eicosapentaenoic acid; MS, multiple sclerosis; PUFA, polyunsaturated fatty acid; ROS, reactive oxygen species; SLE, systemic lupus erythematosus; SOD, superoxide dismutase.
Sources: Ahmad R, Rasheed Z, Ahsan H. Biochemical and cellular toxicology of peroxynitrite: implications in cell death and autoimmune phenomenon. Immunopharmacol Immunotoxicol 2009; 31:388–396. Calder PC, Albers R, Antoine JM et al. Inflammatory disease processes and interactions with nutrition. Br J Nutr 2009; 101(Supplement):S1-45. Duntas LH. Selenium and inflammation: underlying anti-inflammatory mechanisms. Horm Metab Res 2009; 41(6):443–447. Munger KL, Zhang SM, O'Reilly E et al. Vitamin D intake and incidence of multiple sclerosis. Neurology 2004; 63(5):60–65. Stargrove MB, Treasure J, McKee DL. Herb, nutrient and drug interactions. Clinical implications and therapeutic strategies. Missouri: Mosby Elsevier; 2008. Clarke JO, Mullin GE. A review of complementary and alternative approaches to immunomodulation. Nutr Clin Prac 2008; 23(1):49–62.

TABLE 12.16 Herbal medicine classes		
Class	**Key herbs within class**	**Justification**
Immunomodulator	*Echinacea* spp., *Andrographis paniculata*, *Astragalus membranaceus*, *Eleutherococcus senticosus*, *Panax ginseng*, *Uncaria tomentosa* (POA type)	Eliminate pathogenic organisms by enhancing immunity; increase phagocytosis with echinacea.
Immunosuppressant	*Hemidesmus indicus*, *Tylophora indica*	Employed to suppress immune over-reactivity to help to break the vicious cycle. Best stopped during acute infections.
Adaptogen/tonic	*Astragalus membranaceus*, *Avena sativa*, *Centella asiatica*, *Codonopsis pilosula*, *Eleutherococcus senticosus*, *Ganoderma lucidum*, *Panax ginseng*, *Rehmannia glutinosa*, *Rhodiola rosea*, *Schisandra chinensis*, *Withania somnifera*	Adaptogens have a broad therapeutic activity and encourage the body to adapt better when under stress by providing resistance to the action of a wide variety of harmful factors. Many adaptogens are also immune modulating.
Anti-inflammatory	*Aesculus hippocastanum*, *Apium graveolens*, *Boswellia serrata*, *Bupleurum falcatum*, *Curcuma longa*, *Dioscorea villosa*, *Filipendula ulmaria*, *Glycyrrhiza glabra*, *Harpogophytum procumbens*, *Hemidesmus indicus*, *Salix* spp., *Tanacetum parthenium*, *Tylophora indica*, *Uncaria tomentosa* (POA type), *Vaccinium myrtillus*, *Zingiber officinale*	By choosing the appropriate anti-inflammatory herb(s) to control the release of inflammatory cytokines, to negate the depression of the adrenal gland caused by steroid hormones, and to down-regulate other inflammatory pathways, the progression of tissue destruction in ADs can be slowed or halted and symptoms of immune dysfunction can be reduced.
Antioxidant	*Astragalus membranaceus*, *Camellia sinensis*, *Curcuma longa*, *Ginkgo biloba*, *Rosmarinus officinalis*, *Schisandra chinensis*, *Silybum marianum*, *Thymus vulgaris*, *Vaccinium myrtillus*, *Vitus vinifera*	Antioxidant activity is fundamental to the treatment of all inflammatory disorders.

Continued

TABLE 12.16 Herbal medicine classes—cont'd

Class	Key herbs within class	Justification
Antiviral	*Hypericum perforatum, Thuja occidentalis*	When a patient with AD has a viral infection, choose the appropriate antiviral in an acute formula. If patient history indicates recurrent enveloped viral infections, *Hypericum* can be given as a prophylactic as there can be recurrent flare-ups.
Antibacterial	*Allium sativum* (allicin-releasing preparations), *Citrus* spp., *Hydrastis canadensis, Thymus vulgaris*	4–13 drops of citrus seed extract daily have been found to reduce faecal counts of *E. coli, Candida* spp., *Geotrichum* spp.
Antifungal	*Allium sativum* (allicin-releasing preparations), *Citrus* spp., *Tabebuia avellanedae, Thymus vulgaris*	When fungal infection is active in a patient with AD, it needs to be eliminated.
Antiparasitic	*Artemesia absinthium, Berberis vulgaris, Commiphora mol mol, Hydrastis canadensis, Stemona sessilifolia, Tabebuia avellanedae*	If parasites are contributing to dysbiosis in the gastrointestinal tract they need to be eliminated.
Bitter	*Andrographis paniculata, Artemisia absinthium, Berberis vulgaris, Gentiana lutea, Harpogophytum procumbens, Hydrastis canadensis, Tanacetum parthenium*	Bitter tonics have a long traditional use to assist in assimilation of food, especially in allergies, to cool the system, and to provide tone to the digestive tract. Pharmacological studies indicate that they increase gastric secretions and stimulate small intestinal enzymes.
Demulcent/gut mucous membrane healing	*Filipendula ulmaria, Hydrastis canadensis, Matricaria recutita, Ulmus rubra*	Intestinal wall integrity will be protective against overgrowth of pathogens and reduce the load of circulating endotoxins and antigen complexes.
Antiallergic	*Albizia lebbek, Scutellaria baicalensis, Tanacetum parthenium*	Allergies or food intolerances are implicated in some ADs. By down-regulating the allergic response with these herbs, along with their anti-inflammatory activity, disease progression can be halted or slowed.
Circulatory stimulant	*Capsicum* spp., *Ginkgo biloba, Xanthoxylum americanum*	These can diffuse heat throughout the body and improve blood flow to the gastrointestinal tract to improve absorption of nutrients and other herbal medicines. They can be useful in inflammatory conditions.
Nervine tonic	*Avena sativa, Centella asiatica, Hypericum perforatum, Melissa officinalis, Scutellaria lateriflora, Verbena* (vervain)	Patients with AD may experience some level of depression and exhaustion. Supporting the nervous system and brain chemistry can be useful.
Depurative	*Arctium lappa, Berberis aquifolium, Curcuma longa, Galium aparine, Hemidesmus indicus, Hydrastis canadensis, Solidago virgaurea, Tabebuia avellanedae, Taraxacum officinale, Urtica dioica*	Depuratives have been traditionally employed to effect a gradual change in chronic disease states, especially skin, joint and connective tissue disorders. They can also upregulate the P-gp pump at the tissue level to remove toxins.
Diuretic	*Aesculus hippocastanum, Apium graveolens, Arctostaphylos uva-ursi, Barosma betulina*	To reduce oedema and local swelling if present.
Liver detoxifier	*Curcuma longa, Rosmarinus officinalis, Schisandra chinensis, Silybum marianum*	Toxins such as xenobiotics, cigarette smoke and heavy metals are often involved in AD, so the liver needs to be supported, especially to upregulate phase II detoxification.
Hepatic	*Bupleurum falcatum, Cynara scolymus, Schisandra chinensis, Silybum marianum*	To improve liver function, in particular Kuppfer cells.
Other organ support	As indicated in the individual disease	See the relevant chapters.
Symptom management, for example analgesic	*Salix alba, Corydalis ambigua, Eschscholzia californica*	While anti-inflammatories are fundamental to assist in management of symptoms, in many ADs additional assistance may be required. *Salix alba* is a key herb in managing pain from arthritic conditions whereas *Corydalis* is indicated in inflammation in hollow organs such as the gastrointestinal tract; hypnotic analgesics such as *Eschscholzia* can be employed when pain is contributing to insomnia.

POA, pentacyclic oxindole alkaloids.

Immune function needs to be modulated, not in a reductionist way as in the allopathic medicine approach, but in a holistic way: by down-regulating immunological memory and breaking the vicious cycle of 'hit and run' aetiology. This can be achieved by using an immunosuppressant which should be stopped whenever the patient is experiencing any signs and symptoms of acute infections.

Further, whenever the 'primary lesion' can be identified it should be treated accordingly as if it was currently active in the patient. For example, in a patient with RA and a history of UTIs, treat with antibacterial herbs specific to the urinary tract and with cranberry, even though they may have no symptoms. In a patient with RA and a history of EBV, treat with a herb that is antiviral to enveloped viruses, such as *Hypericum perforatum*.[173]

The production of inflammatory cytokines including the interleukins and TNFs must be reduced in ADs. Withdrawal of the NSAID Vioxx from the market has led to an increased interest in natural anti-inflammatory treatments and there are many herbal medicines that have this capacity via many different pathways. The naturopath would choose from the vast array of anti-inflammatory herbs by understanding the mechanisms of inflammation in the individual patient. For example, herbs such as boswellia, turmeric, devil's claw and ginger reduce production of eicosanoids so can be prescribed in the same situations where the COX inhibitors are used. The advantage of the herbal medicines is that they are dual inhibitors of both COX and 5-LOX pathways, so are unlikely to have the side effects of the COX inhibitors.

The evidence base for herbal use in ADs is growing rapidly, albeit many studies are designed using multiple herbs or herb plus drug combinations. For example, a large study from Japan followed 258 patients for 3 years who had undergone surgery for CD.[174] Within 1 month of surgery, patients received either mesalazine (2250 to 3000 mg/day), azathioprine (50 to 100 mg/day) or the traditional herbal formula daikenchuto (7.5 to 15 g/day, comprising processed ginger 50%, *Panax ginseng* 30% and Japanese or Szechuan pepper 20% (*Zanthoxylum* species)) for at least a year. Forty-four needed reoperation with intestinal resection within 3 years due to disease recurrence. However, the rate was significantly lower in the herbal group than in the pooled non-herbal group. In another study, a herbal tablet comprising myrrh 100 mg, chamomile extract 70 mg and coffee charcoal 50 mg (4 tablets per day) was investigated for maintaining remission in UC, compared to mesalazine (500 mg/day).[175] While there was no significant difference between the two treatment groups in relapse rates, endoscopy or faecal biomarkers, the herbal preparation showed a good safety profile and tolerability along with good potential efficacy comparable to the gold standard therapy mesalazine.

Herbal medicine classes

See Table 12.16.

Specific herbal medicines

HEMIDESMUS INDICUS — HEMIDESMUS

Hemidesmus is a unique herb in its capacity for immune depression, although human clinical trials are needed. *Hemidesmus indicus* suppressed both the cell-mediated and humoral components of the immune system in a study of sheep red blood cells, skin allograft rejection and phagocytic activity of the reticuloendothelial system in mice.[176] When *Hemidesmus* was tested on human cell lines, it was found to inhibit NF-kappaB/DNA interactions with lower effects on cell growth, which indicates its potential effectiveness in ADs and inflammatory diseases.[177] Alteration of gene expression represents a very promising approach to controlling diseases in which genetic susceptibility exerts influence at either the causative level or as a sustaining/amplifying factor.

ECHINACEA SPP. — ECHINACEA

Echinacea is a major immune modulating herb and has great value during acute infections to prevent further immune dysregulation in patients with AD. It is also a valuable anti-inflammatory herb. There has been much controversy over the safety and value of echinacea in AD and there are some cases where echinacea might not suit the circumstances. However, in patients with AD whose NK cells and NK T-cells are deficient, such as in many patients with SLE, psoriasis and RA, echinacea could increase these vital cells. A study of mice with type 1 diabetes fed *Echinacea purpurea* found there was a substantial and significant increase in NK cell numbers.[178] Echinacea may stimulate phagocytic activity, especially macrophages. It seems to provide better direct clearance and inactivation of pathogenic organisms and better immune surveillance of new pathogens or other opportunistic pathogens. It may decrease the chronic presence of microorganisms.[179] A pilot study looked into the efficacy and safety of *Echinacea purpurea* extract (150 mg twice daily for 9 months) with or without steroids as compared to conventional steroid therapy alone in low-grade autoimmune uveitis in 51 patients.[180] The uveitis settled well in the echinacea group and they had greater time off steroids with no adverse reactions.

Traditionally, echinacea has been used fruitfully in both acute infections and for long-term immunomodulation.

UNCARIA TOMENTOSA (POA CHEMOTYPE) — CAT'S CLAW

Cat's claw protected cells against oxidative stress, and reduced inflammation in several in vivo studies. The mechanism of action may involve suppression of NF-kappaB cells.[181] A small 24-week double-blind placebo controlled trial with 40 patients with RA undergoing sulfasalazine or hydroxychloroquine treatment resulted in a modest reduction of the number of painful joints compared with placebo.[182]

HYPERICUM PERFORATUM — ST JOHN'S WORT

A great deal of research into hypericin's antiviral activity lends support for its efficacy against enveloped viruses that may be implicated in some ADs, such as herpes viruses, EBV, CMV, Ross River virus, hepatitis B and C, rubella virus, and many of the viruses that cause the common cold and influenza. The mode of action may be through inactivating free virions and interfering with the steps in the replication cycle.[183] St John's wort extract and hyperforin were both found to be effective in blocking inflammatory cytokines in beta cell lines in vitro.[184] As it also has antidepressant and nervine tonic activity, it may be an ideal adjunct to other herbal treatments for ADs, where herb–drug interactions are not problematic.

BOSWELLIA SERRATA — BOSWELLIA

Boswellia's anti-inflammatory action is very useful in ADs such as RA, CD and UC. Its mechanism of action is via a reduction in leukotriene production, by inhibiting 5-lipoxygenase (5-LOX) and other inflammatory mediators. After 6 months of treatment with *Boswellia* extract in an uncontrolled trial, patients with RA had reduced levels of C-reactive protein. A double-blind RCT with 102 patients with CD found no difference in CD activity index (CDAI) compared with mesalazine, and a reduction in both groups when compared with baseline.[185] As a result of its alleged safety, *Boswellia* was considered superior over mesalazine in terms of a risk–benefit evaluation.[158] In a small uncontrolled study six juvenile patients with moderate to severe CD took *Boswellia* (dose not stated) along with fish peptides, bovine colostrum and *Lactobacillus* GG, as well as a dairy-free, reduced grain and carrageenan diet. Within 2 months all patients went into remission and sustained remission for 18 months or more.[186]

Researchers compared administration of *Boswellia* (350 mg t.d.s. for 6 weeks) with sulfasalazine (1 g t.d.s. for 6 weeks) and found similar improvements in clinical, laboratory and histopathological parameters in patients with IBD. While 70% of the *Boswellia* patients went into remission, only 40% of the sulfasalazine patients went into remission.[187] It is thought that this is due in part to inhibition of NF-kappaB and down-regulation of the proinflammatory cascade.[149]

CURCUMA LONGA — TURMERIC

For centuries it has been known that turmeric exhibits anti-inflammatory activity and more recently its antioxidant, antimicrobial and depurative activity has been noted. The active constituent, curcuminoids which are known as curcumin, is a polyphenolic compound isolated from the rhizome that has traditionally been used for pain and wound-healing. Recent studies have shown that curcumin ameliorates MS, RA, psoriasis and IBD in human and animal models. It regulates inflammatory cytokines and NF-kappaB signalling pathways in immune cells.[188] A recent study states that up to 8 g/day of curcumin for 18 months is non-toxic to humans, but its utility is limited by its aqueous insolubility. The researchers used a heat-solubilised (curcumin or turmeric heated in boiling water for 10 minutes) form of curcumin which they found binds to proteins, thus inhibiting an autoantibody–antigen interaction. This preparation significantly decreased binding of autoantibodies from Sjögren's syndrome and SLE to their cognate antigens.[162] Other preparations combine curcumin with lecithin, or coconut oil and black pepper, to increase bioavailability.

Curcumin is a potent free radical scavenger in vivo. Studies have demonstrated that it is an inhibitor of NF-kappaB and leads to downstream regulation and inhibition of proinflammatory genes and cytokines including TNF-α and iNOS.[189] In a double-blind RCT multicentre trial with 89 patients with UC, 1 g of curcumin twice daily resulted in both clinical improvement and a statistically significant decrease in the rate of relapse.[190]

TANACETUM PARTHENIUM — FEVERFEW

Again, human trials are needed, but feverfew contains parthenolide which is the major sesquiterpene lactone, a powerful anti-inflammatory, which works by inhibiting the expression of proinflammatory cytokines including TNF-α, IL-1, IL-4, IL-8, IL-12 and NF-kappaB.[158]

Lifestyle recommendations

Many simple lifestyle changes can improve the quality of life of a patient with AD and the progression of the inflammation:

- Exercise regularly — gentle exercise such as walking, yoga, deep breathing, light aerobics, hydrotherapy, swimming
- Spend time in the natural sunlight early morning and late afternoon
- Be involved in the treatment plan and try to understand the facets of the disease
- Get enough sleep
- Reduce stress by practising relaxation techniques such as meditation or imagery
- Join a support group if appropriate.

CASE STUDY

OVERVIEW

ED, a 29-year-old nulliparous single woman presented with moderately severe thoracic pain which had been treated for over 4 years by an osteopath and occasional acupuncture treatment. She stated that her spine felt 'crunchy', with burning pain that was slightly better for anti-inflammatory medication. She also experienced stiffness in the cervical spine with no history of trauma. More recently she was experiencing right-sided sacroiliac pain. She had nausea and abdominal bloating, both of which were worse after having cow's milk, wheat, oats, legumes, soy milk, grapes, apples, corn, rice and alcohol. Her bowels were 'sluggish'. She had recurrent herpes simplex virus symptoms when she was stressed. Mild AS was diagnosed. She appeared to be quite despondent about having a potentially destructive disease at such a young age.

CLINICAL EXAMINATION

Weight: 47 kg
BP: 110/62 mmHg
PR: 78 bpm

CASE STUDY CONTINUED

LABORATORY INVESTIGATIONS

HLA B27 positive
Antigliadin antibodies negative
Rheumatoid factor negative
Antinuclear antibodies negative
ESR 36 (1–34)
IgA 3.99 (0.60–3.96)
IgG, IgE, IgM all in normal range
MRI showed desiccated discs, synovial arthritic changes in joints

MEDICATIONS

Celecoxib 100 mg b.i.d.
Escitalopram oxalate 10 mg once daily
Sulfasalazine 1 g b.i.d.

TREATMENT PROTOCOL

INITIAL APPOINTMENT

At the initial consultation, some of the pathogenesis of AS was explained to the patient, so that she could understand the contributing factors and the necessity to attempt to address the cause, in order to motivate her to persist with treatment. She stated that she would like to cease taking the sulfasalazine if possible over time.

HERBAL MEDICINE

Formula 1

See table.

Herbal medicine	Ratio	Quantity	Rationale
Echinacea spp.	1:2	60 mL	Enhance phagocytosis, enhance immune surveillance; resolve the presence of microorganisms; anti-inflammatory
Hypericum perforatum (high hypericin)	1:2	50 mL	Reduce the activity and recurrence of herpes simplex virus; nervine tonic to assist her mood and coping mechanisms
Rehmannia glutinosa	1:2	70 mL	Anti-inflammatory, adrenal tonic, adaptogen
Hydrastis canadensis	1:3	30 mL	Anti-inflammatory to the gut; mucus membrane trophorestorative; bitter; antibacterial
Total: 210 mL			

Adjunct

A separate 200 mL bottle containing *Hemidesmus* to be added at 2 mL per dose when she experiences no signs of acute infection in order to suppress the overactive elements in her immune system. It was explained to her why she needed to stop taking it during acute infections, and she was instructed to take extra measures to quickly treat any acute infections.

NUTRITIONAL MEDICINE

Dietary

Because she was taking an NSAID, there was an increased risk of gut permeability, and dairy and gluten allergies could be implicated.[191] She was advised, therefore, to continue to avoid cow's milk and wheat, plus a low-starch diet was implemented because her symptoms suggested that *Klebsiella pneumoniae*, or a similar starch-loving organism, may be involved. Foods that she was to eliminate were the following three food groups:

- Grains, cereals and roots. Anything made with, thickened with or mixed with: arrowroot, baking powder (usually contains wheat flour), barley, bran, burghul, bulgar, corn (maize), couscous, kazu, malt, modified starch, oats, polenta, rye, sago, semolina, sorghum, tapioca, wheat.
  - This included: bread, rolls, buns, croissants, breakfast cereals, muesli, cakes, biscuits, cookies, crackers, pastries, cream puffs, éclairs, pies, flans, quiches, pizzas, battered deep-fried foods, all pasta and noodles, dumplings, doughnuts, pancakes, all puddings, soufflés, custard-powder custards, white sauces, cheese sauces, gravies, sausages, meatloaf, rissoles or any meatballs and mixtures containing breadcrumbs or modified starch, sandwiches, most pâtés and relishes and chutneys, many pills and medications which contain maize starch or modified starch or cornflour.
- Lentils and pulses. Anything made with, thickened with or mixed with: adzuki beans, black-eyed beans, black fermented Chinese beans, borlotti beans, broad beans, chick peas, dhal, haricot beans, kidney beans, lentils, lima beans, mung beans, pinto beans, soya beans, split peas.
  - This included: baked beans, bean salads, soups, casseroles, soy meat substitutes, TVP (textured vegetable protein), bean sauces, soy sauce, tamari sauce, shoyu sauce.
- Bananas, unripe fruit.
  NB. Tofu may be low enough in starch to be tolerable.

Supplemental

- EPA/DHA supplement was prescribed at a dose of 3 g twice daily.
- Calcium supplement was prescribed due to reduced dietary intake.

LIFESTYLE/EDUCATION

She was advised to avoid cigarette smoking, including passive smoking, to continue to swim and to engage in gentle yoga and breathing exercises and to try to get sufficient sleep.

FOLLOW-UP

Her symptoms stabilised quite quickly but she mentioned that each time she ate potato products, her joints 'crunched' more, so she was advised to take potatoes out of her diet as

CASE STUDY CONTINUED

well. She was advised to increase her consumption of fish, spices, fresh garlic, fresh organic vegetables, sprouts, nuts and seeds and green tea. It was vital for her to focus on the foods that she could eat so that she did not lose any weight. While it was difficult for her at first, she experienced such an amelioration of her symptoms that she felt it was worth it. When she ate starchy foods, she did not feel well. She was able to reduce the sulfasalazine over a few months under her doctor's guidance, and *Boswellia* tablets (3–4 daily) were introduced as a substitute. It is now 5 years since treatment was implemented and she remains stable, with good management of her symptoms and no further progression of her disease.

SECTION C: INTRODUCTION TO CANCER

Epidemiology

In Australia the cancer statistics are not looking promising. Overall 1 in 3 men and 1 in 4 women in the country will be directly affected by cancer in the first 75 years of life. Cancer accounts for 29% of male deaths and 25% of female deaths in Australia each year. Despite the optimism generated by the media, the incidence of cancer in males and females over the last 30 years has been increasing. Only in lung cancer in males has the mortality rate been declining. Overall survival for all types of cancer after 5 years is 49.5% for males and 58.2% for females.[192]

ROLE OF THE NATUROPATH

Statistics show that 33–83% of people with cancer use complementary and alternative medicines (CAM) after diagnosis. The most likely users are educated women with breast cancer. Patients using CAM are more optimistic than others and the most common reason they choose to use CAM treatments is to provide hope for their wellbeing and survival.[193] In Europe, 48% of people with the diagnosis of cancer use herbal medicines.[194]

The most common scenario is that people combine conventional medicine and complementary therapies, where approximately 80% of people with cancer who use CAM are also undergoing conventional treatment. It is a lot more daunting with the fear component and the authoritative medical system to decide to try CAM alone when diagnosed (although a small number do so with some success).

Overview

Cancer is a disease that is gradually increasing in Western populations (despite the continuous series of supposed 'cures' we see paraded before us on news programs). It is still a disease primarily of older people but the figures show increasing rates in younger people. The primary medical treatments for cancer are surgery, radiotherapy and pharmaceuticals (chemotherapy) and overall medicine still has strong objections to any alternatives such as herbal medicines or nutritional supplements. This is despite increasing evidence that complementary medicines can significantly improve outcomes. However, as patients are more informed and specialists seek the best care for their patients, this response is changing.

Pathogenesis

THE CELL CYCLE

At a molecular level, cancer is a disease where regulation of the cell cycle goes awry and normal cell growth and behaviour are lost. Focusing on the role various therapies have on the cell cycle[195] can provide a basic molecular explanation for both medical treatments and (increasingly) herbal/nutritional support.

The cell cycle is an ordered series of events culminating in cell growth and division into two daughter cells (mitosis). Non-dividing cells are not considered to be in the cell cycle. When a cell is in any phase of the cell cycle other than mitosis, it is deemed to be in its interphase.

Briefly a cell cannot divide unless two processes alternate:

- The doubling of its genome (DNA) in the S phase (synthesis phase) of the cell cycle
- The halving of that genome during mitosis (the M phase) when the nuclear chromosomes separate and cytoplasmic division occurs.

The period between M and S is called G_1 (Gap 1); that between S and M is G_2 (Gap 2).

The cell cycle consists of: G_1 (growth and preparation of the chromosomes for replication), S (synthesis of DNA when DNA replication occurs), G_2 (preparation) for M (mitosis).

Chemical damage to DNA is itself not a mutagenic event, but if unrepaired can be converted to a mutagenic event during the process of DNA replication. Because DNA synthesis itself is a tightly controlled, highly coordinated process, delays in progression through the S phase as a consequence of DNA damage, or insufficient availability of protein or DNA precursors, frequently result in cell death, chromosomal abnormalities or mutations. Since these latter two events are closely associated with carcinogenesis, it is not surprising that many of the genes found to be damaged in cancer cells have actions that relate to cell cycle checkpoint control.

Regulation of the cell cycle

How cell division (and thus tissue growth) is controlled is a complex process. The following are some of the important features in regulation and places where errors can lead to cancer. The passage of a cell through the cell cycle is controlled by proteins in the cytoplasm, the cyclins and cyclin-dependent kinase (CDK), and their levels rise and fall through different stages. CDK and the cyclins are major control switches for the cell cycle, causing the cell to move from G_1 to S or G_2 to M.

One of the most frequently mutated genes in human solid tumours is the tumour suppressor gene *p53*. This gene (*p53*), which has been called 'the guardian of the genome', has among its functions the monitoring of the integrity of the genome and has the capacity either to delay replication until repair has been completed, or if damage is too extensive, to induce a series of events leading to the programmed death of the cell by the process called apoptosis.

Restriction point — p53

Restriction point — p53 is a protein that functions to block the cell cycle if the DNA is damaged. The levels of p53 are increased in damaged cells. The p53 protein senses DNA damage and can halt progression of the cell cycle in both G_1 and G_2, allowing time for the repair of DNA. The p53 protein is a key player in apoptosis, forcing severely damaged (or not repairable) cells to commit 'suicide'. For example p53 has the ability to evaluate the extent of damage to DNA caused by radiation. At low levels of radiation, producing damage that can be repaired, p53 triggers arrest of the cell cycle until the damage is repaired. At high levels of radiation, producing severely damaged DNA, p53 triggers apoptosis (assuming there are adequate functioning levels of p53). p53 qualifies as a tumour suppressor gene and more than half of all human cancers have p53 mutations and/or have no functioning p53 protein.

Cell cycle checkpoints

There are several cell cycle checkpoints in human (and mammalian) cells.[195]

1. A cell will enter and leave the cell cycle many times, temporarily or permanently. It mainly exits the cycle at G_1 and enters a stage called G_0 (G zero). At this point it is often called 'quiescent', a misnomer as it is in fact busy carrying out its functions in the organism, for example secretion, conducting nerve impulses or attacking pathogens. Often G_0 cells are terminally differentiated and will never re-enter the cell cycle but instead will carry out their function in the organism until they die. For other cells G_0 can be followed by re-entry into the cell cycle. Most of the lymphocytes in human blood are in G_0, however with proper stimulation such as an appropriate antigen, they can be stimulated to re-enter the cell cycle (at G_1) and proceed on to new rounds of alternating **S** phases and mitosis.

   G_0 represents not simply the absence of signals for mitosis but an active repression of the genes needed for mitosis. Cancer cells cannot enter G_0 and can therefore repeat the cell cycle, that is reproduce, indefinitely.
2. Cells have devised further elaborate checkpoints to prevent premature entry into the division cycle. The next significant checkpoint occurs in late G_1, approximately 4 hours prior to the cell's entry into the S phase. At this point cells possess multiple mechanisms to prevent inappropriate passage from G_1 into the S phase of the cycle where DNA synthesis occurs. The most dangerous DNA mutations occur in cells damaged in late G_1 and early S phase, after the p53 restriction point, thereby increasing the chance of proliferation and carcinogenesis.
3. There are also other cell cycle checkpoints which can be activated in the G_2 or M phase of the cell cycle in response to DNA damage.

Cancer cells, through alterations in the cell cycle, have significantly greater turnover rates than normal cells. They have gained the ability to become 'immortal' through various mechanisms including evading apoptosis and reactivating telomerase, thereby developing a greater ability to proliferate. (Telomerase is the enzyme, normally dormant in most mature cells, that restores DNA fragments to the end of the chromosome (the telomere), thus when activated it 'immortalises' the cell.) In these processes the cancer cells develop the ability for angiogenesis (to grow or parasitise their own blood supply), and by being able to evade the inhibition of surrounding tissue and becoming undifferentiated, they can metastasise to both neighbouring areas and distant sites in the body.

Aetiology

RISK FACTORS FOR ONCOGENESIS

The evolution of the normal cell to a malignant one involves many processes whereby genes involved in the normal homeostatic mechanisms suffer a series of mutational damages which result in the activation of genes (the oncogenes) that stimulate proliferation or protection against cell death. It also involves the inactivation of genes (tumour suppressor genes) which would normally inhibit proliferation. (Genes which are activated by mutation are called oncogenes; those inactivated by mutation are called tumour suppressor genes.) This damage can be the result of endogenous (internal) processes such as errors in replication of DNA or from attack by free radicals generated during metabolism (oxidation). DNA damage can also result from interactions with exogenous (external) agents such as ionising radiation and chemical carcinogens. Eventually an aspiring cancer cell faces two major challenges: it must overcome normal controls on apoptosis and become immortal, and it must obtain supplies of nutrients and oxygen to maintain this high rate of proliferation (angiogenesis).

The vast majority of mutations that give rise to cancer are not inherited and rise spontaneously as a consequence of chemical (or radiation) damage to DNA. However, because of the multiple checks and balances that exist in cells to limit inappropriate proliferation, malignant human cells must accumulate multiple mutations in crucial cellular genes to allow unchecked replication and invasion.

Even medical treatments used for cancer can cause the very problem that they are trying to fix. Ionising radiation can directly damage the DNA by causing single- and double-strand breaks to the DNA helix, and can also induce indirect damage as a consequence of radiolysis of water, yielding free radicals (oxidative) damage.[196] The double-strand breaks are the main problem because if both strands are damaged, the cell has no undamaged template that can provide the information necessary to reconstitute the strands.

The role of infection in oncogenesis

Other possible triggers for oncogenesis are infection by various organisms including viruses such as Epstein-Barr virus and hepatitis B and C viruses, and there is increasing interest in the role of more unusual organisms such as

Mycoplasma fermentans or *Chlamydia pneumoniae* in the development of oncogenesis. *H. pylori* is also considered a risk factor for gastric tumours.

From Huang et al 2001, 50 of 90 cases (56%) of gastric carcinoma were positive for mycoplasma. In other gastric diseases, the mycoplasma infection rate was 28% (18/49) in chronic superficial gastritis, 30% in gastric ulcer and 37% in intestinal metaplasia. In colon carcinoma, the mycoplasma infection rate was 55.1%, but it was only 20.9% in adenomatous polyps. Gastric and colon cancers with high differentiation had a higher mycoplasma infection rate than those with low differentiation. Mycoplasma infections were found in 50.9% of oesophageal cancers, 52.6% of lung cancers, 39.7% of breast cancers and 41% of gliomas.[197]

This can provide a real challenge to current medical thinking. If these organisms are shown to be present alongside the diagnosis of cancer, it may be more appropriate to prescribe specific antibiotics (e.g. doxocyclin) or antibiotic herbs rather than chemotherapy. In fact some antibiotics are considered chemotherapy agents — adriamycin and doxorubicin for example. While these are prescribed generically, perhaps the specific organism needs to be identified and the specific antibiotic prescribed.

Investigations

Correct diagnosis is a critical part of the successful management of any illness. For cancer and other life-threatening illnesses, it is even more important. Members of the medical profession are highly skilled diagnosticians and provide the best care within their scope of practice. With the current medical model being as fragmented and focused on key specificities, the collaboration with a CAM practitioner provides a holistic overview and treatment plan to complement care. CAM practitioners are skilled diagnosing where a person's health has become unbalanced and where this needs correcting. These polarities are both important if the person is to regain their health and quality of life. These parameters in the diagnosis of health and disease provide different types of information, and both are important as it is essential to have as much information as possible to be able to make informed choices about treatments.

With the medical model (and testing), it is important to be informed about the risks and benefits of the diagnostic procedures themselves as many of these can be quite invasive. While medical testing can be effective in diagnosing the detail of the cancer involved, the side effects (such as excess radiation from multiple CAT scans) can also involve increased future risk for iatrogenic cancer development. The risks and benefits need to be well thought through.

Diagnostic procedures with CAM are much less invasive and contain very little risk to the consumer, apart from the nonspecificity of the tests. This translates to the risk of missing an important diagnosis if the person doing the testing is not sufficiently competent (or sufficiently trained) for the task.

The following section describes some of the most common testing procedures for a selection of cancer types.

ALLOPATHIC INVESTIGATIONS

Biopsy

In diagnosing cancer, a sample of the tissue needs to be removed for examination under a microscope. Biopsies can be done in various ways:

- A needle is used to withdraw tissue or fluid from the area (fine-needle biopsy or large-gauge needle core biopsy)
- An endoscope (a thin, lighted tube) is used to look at areas inside the body and remove cells or tissues
- Surgery is used to remove part or all of the tumour and the tissue removed is sent for examination (excisional biopsy).

Tissue removed during a biopsy is sent to a pathology laboratory, where it is sliced into thin sections for viewing under a microscope in a histological (tissue) examination. The pathologist may also examine cytological (cell) material which is present in fluids — urine, CSF, sputum, peritoneal fluid, pleural fluid and cervical or vaginal smears.

While biopsies are considered important for accurate medical diagnosis, there is evidence to suggest that biopsies are safer if taken after the tumour has been removed (particularly in solid tumours) (excisional biopsies), rather than breaking the tumour capsule with the needle and risking spread.[198]

Tumour markers

Tumour markers are molecules that are found in abnormal amounts in the blood, urine or tissues of patients with cancer. Different tumour markers are found in different types of cancer and they may be used for diagnosis, to predict a patient's response to therapies (medical and CAM), check a patient's response to treatment, or determine if the cancer has returned. Overall they cannot be used alone to diagnose cancer and must be combined with other tests.

Ideally tumour markers can be used for one of four purposes:

1. Screening a healthy population or a high-risk population for the presence of cancer
2. Making a diagnosis of cancer or of a specific type of cancer
3. Determining the prognosis in a patient
4. Monitoring the course in a patient in remission or while receiving surgery, radiation, or chemotherapy.

However, because of their lack of sensitivity and specificity, medical tests generally do not meet these requirements totally.

Tumour antigens

Tumour antigens include markers defined by both monoclonal antibodies and the so-called oncofetal antigens. These are present in the embryo or fetus, and while they diminish to low levels in the adult, they can reappear in the tumour. In general, tumour markers are produced by the tumour itself or by the body in response to the presence of cancer or non-cancerous conditions.

Carcinoembryonic antigen (CEA)

Carcinoembryonic antigen (CEA) is a protein found in many types of cells but is associated with tumours and the developing fetus. It is found in the plasma membrane of tumour cells. Elevated levels are detected in a variety of cancers including colon, pancreatic, gastric, lung, ovarian and breast cancer. It is also detected in benign conditions including cirrhosis, inflammatory bowel disease, chronic lung disease and pancreatitis. It can be elevated in smokers and in a small percentage of the general healthy population. There is a significant body of research showing its prognostic value for colon cancer and the use of the marker with staging of the cancer.[199] The normal range for CEA in an adult non-smoker is less than 2.5 ng/mL and for a smoker less than 5.0 ng/mL.

Alphafetoprotein (AFP)

Alphafetoprotein (AFP) is a normal fetal serum glycoprotein synthesised by the liver, yolk sac and gastrointestinal tract that shares fetal origins with albumin. AFP is of importance in the diagnosis of hepatocellular carcinoma. It can also be elevated in normal pregnancy and benign liver disease such as hepatitis and cirrhosis. AFP can also be elevated in malignant pancreatic cancers, gastric cancers, colonic cancers and bronchogenic cancers not necessarily associated with liver metastases. Normal range is less than 10 micrograms/L.

CA125

CA125 is an antigen present in 80% of ovarian carcinomas, its level corresponding with the patient's clinical condition. For ovarian tumours it is more accurate than CEA. It is also elevated in other cancers including endometrial, pancreatic, lung, breast and colon cancer and in menstruation, pregnancy, endometriosis and other gynaecological and non-gynaecological conditions. Normal value varies between laboratories but is generally less than 35 U/mL.

CA19-9

CA19-9 is a monoclonal antibody generated against a colon carcinoma cell line to detect a monosialoganglioside found in patients with gastrointestinal adenocarcinoma. It is found to be elevated in 21–42% of cases of gastric cancer, 20–40% of colon cancer, and 71–93% of pancreatic cancer. Normal range is less than 40 U/mL.

CA15-3

An elevated CA15-3 in conjunction with high alkaline phosphatase has been shown to predict the chances of early recurrence in breast cancer.[200] Normal values can vary but should be less than 25 U/mL.

BRCA1 and *BRCA2*

BRCA1 and *BRCA2* are human tumour suppressor genes which produce proteins, called breast cancer type 1 susceptibility protein and breast cancer type 2 susceptibility protein. They are found in the cells of breast and other tissue, where they help repair damaged DNA and destroy the cell when DNA cannot be repaired. If *BRCA1* or 2 is damaged, the damaged DNA can let the cell duplicate without control, and turn into cancer. The position of a mutation in the *BRCA1* or *BRCA2* gene can reflect the relative incidences of breast and ovarian cancer within a family.

The *BRCA2* mutation carries an increased risk for cancers of the prostate, pancreas, gallbladder/bile duct and stomach, as well as for malignant melanoma. The *BRCA2* mutation also appears to confer higher risks for male breast cancer. *BRCA1* mutation confers a higher incidence of ovarian cancer than does *BRCA2* mutation. *BRCA1* is more associated with triple negative breast cancer and frequently appears in younger women. *BRCA2* is more common in postmenopausal women and is highly responsive to hormone treatments.

BRCA1 and BRCA2 proteins were also found to collaborate with one another on a common pathway of tumour suppression, through the S phase of the cell cycle.

Both *BRCA1* and *BRCA2* are sensitive to oxidative damage and particularly to radiation damage. Young women exposed to radiation particularly in the stage of breast development have a specifically increased risk of subsequent breast cancer as adults.[201]

Hypermethylation has been shown to inactivate the *BRCA* genes and has been found to be an issue particularly in oestrogen receptor (ERα) negative breast cancer.[201] Histone deacetylation is a contributing factor to the abnormal methylation and therefore damage in *BRCA1* and *BRCA2* genes in patients diagnosed with breast cancer.

Prostate-specific antigen (PSA)

Prostate-specific antigen (PSA) (normal 0–4 ng/mL) is a glycoprotein that is prostate specific, *not* cancer specific. A variety of conditions can raise PSA levels: prostatitis (prostate inflammation), benign prostatic hypertrophy (prostate enlargement) and prostate cancer. PSA levels tend to increase with age. Some prostate glands normally produce more PSA than others and the levels can vary with race: African Americans often have higher PSA levels; Asian men often have lower PSA levels. However, PSA is sensitive for the presence of prostate cancer as well as benign prostatic hypertrophy. Age-specific ranges for serum PSA are shown in Table 12.17.

Hormones

Hormones are produced by many tumours and may be natural products of their associated organ, or represent abnormal synthesis reflecting unregulated cancer cell metabolism, for example insulin production by islet cell tumour, calcitonin by medullary thyroid carcinoma and prolactin by pituitary tumours. Normal values of calcitonin in

TABLE 12.17 Age-specific reference ranges for serum PSA (ng/mL)

Age range (years)	Black	Caucasian	Japanese
40–49	0.0–2.0	0.0–2.5	0.0–2.0
50–59	0.0–4.0	0.0–3.5	0.0–3.0
60–69	0.0–4.5	0.0–4.5	0.0–4.0
70–79	0.0–5.5	0.0–6.5	0.0–5.0

men should be less than 13.8 ng/L, in women less than 6.4 ng/L. Normal levels for prolactin are less than 2–15 mg/L. Oestrogen is better measured by urinary metabolites.

Immunoglobulins

Production of a monoclonal immunoglobulin molecule (paraprotein) is characteristic of multiple myeloma. These paraproteins are usually complete antibody molecules but may include lambda or kappa chains of any immunoglobulin subtype.

Immunoglobulins are valuable in the staging and treatment of myeloma, the amount of paraprotein serving as an index of tumour volume. Response to treatment is indicated by a fall in paraprotein production, whereas a rise points to relapse.

Tumour grading

Tumour grading is a system used to classify cancer cells in terms of how abnormal they look under a microscope and how quickly the tumour is likely to grow and spread. Many factors are considered when determining tumour grade, including the structure and growth pattern of the cells. The specific factors used to determine tumour grade vary with each type of cancer.

Histological grade is a measure of differentiation and refers to how much the tumour cells resemble normal cells of the same tissue type (or otherwise); nuclear grade refers to the size and shape of the nucleus in tumour cells and the percentage of tumour cells that are dividing.

Tumour grade should not be confused with tumour/cancer staging. Cancer staging refers to the extent or severity of the cancer, based on factors such as the location of the primary tumour, tumour size, number of tumours, and the extent of lymph node involvement.

Medical diagnostic techniques

ULTRASOUND

Ultrasound, also called sonography, is an imaging technique in which high-frequency sound waves (above the human threshold) are bounced off tissues and internal organs, producing a picture called a sonogram. Ultrasound imaging is used to distinguish between solid tumours and fluid-filled cysts. Ultrasound can also be used to evaluate lumps that are hard to see on a mammogram. Ultrasound is sometimes used as part of other diagnostic procedures such as fine-needle aspiration (a needle biopsy), to accurately locate the site for testing.

Ultrasound is a relatively safe and non-invasive procedure. However, it is not as accurate for detecting microcalcification in breast cancer, a cluster of which indicates the greater likelihood of metastases, and therefore has an effect on prognosis.

MAMMOGRAMS

Mammography is an x-ray image of the breast. It is considered the first step in diagnosis of breast cancer. It is an uncomfortable technique and does pick up ductal carcinoma in situ (DCIS) in the earlier stages when it often manifests as just a thickening and does not form a lump. Some DCIS will resolve naturally and some will progress to invasive breast cancer but as this is difficult to determine, medical treatment is carried out routinely.

Younger women usually have denser breasts than older women. As a woman ages, the amount of glandular tissue normally decreases and the amount of fatty tissue increases. Because breast cancers tend to develop in the dense tissue of the breast, older women whose mammograms show more dense tissue have a higher risk of developing breast cancer. Abnormalities in dense breasts can be more difficult to detect on a mammogram, therefore this test may not be as useful in premenopausal women.

Mammograms are also better for detecting microcalcification. However, there are potentially risks involved with repeated mammograms as all radiation is cumulative. The results of a recent meta-analysis of seven early trials indicated that mammography screening may result in less benefit and more harm than previously reported — due to both the radiation received and the potential for overdiagnosis and therefore unnecessary treatment.[202]

CT

A CT scan (also called CAT scanning — computed axial tomography) is a diagnostic procedure that uses x-ray equipment to obtain cross-sectional pictures of the body. The CT computer gives pictures as detailed 3-D images of organs, bones and other tissues. It is used to detect or confirm the presence of a tumour and to provide information about the size and location of the tumour and whether it has spread. It can also help determine whether the cancer is responding to treatment. CT scans can have high diagnostic accuracy.

Occasionally the contrast agents used for imaging can cause allergic reactions such as itching or hives or more serious allergic reactions including shortness of breath and swelling of the throat or other parts of the body. However, the major risk of CT scanning involves the high doses of radiation received (one scan gives the equivalent radiation of 500 x-rays, and two or three CT scans (45 mSv) give the equivalent to the radiation levels at Hiroshima or Nagasaki — 40–50 mSv).[203] The practitioner and the patient need to weigh the risks with the potential diagnostic benefits.

MRI

In magnetic resonance imaging (MRI), a magnet linked to a computer creates detailed pictures of areas inside the body without the use of radiation. Each MRI produces hundreds of images of the appropriate body part from side-to-side, top-to-bottom and front-to-back. MRIs are very useful diagnostically, but there is a dearth of studies on the potential long-term risks of this procedure.

PET

The positron emission tomography (PET) scan creates computerised images of chemical changes that take place in tissue. The patient is given an injection of a substance that consists of a combination of a sugar and a small amount of radioactive material. The radioactive sugar can help in locating a tumour, because cancer cells take up or absorb sugar faster than other tissues in the body.

PET scans may be useful to determine whether a breast mass is cancerous. However, they are more accurate in detecting larger and aggressive tumours than they are in locating small (less than 8 mm) and/or less aggressive tumours. They may also detect cancer when other imaging techniques show normal results.

SENTINEL LYMPH NODE BIOPSY

A sentinel lymph node biopsy is a procedure in which a low-dose radioactive material is injected near the tumour. The injected substance, filtered sulfur colloid, is tagged with the radionuclide technetium-99m. Imaging is usually started within 5 minutes of injection and the node appears from 5 minutes to 1 hour (prior to the biopsy). About 15 minutes before the biopsy the physician injects a blue dye in the same manner. Then, during the biopsy, the physician visually inspects the lymph nodes for staining and uses a type of Geiger counter to assess which lymph nodes have taken up the radioactive tracer. One or several nodes may take up the dye and tracer — these nodes are the sentinel lymph nodes. The surgeon then removes these lymph nodes and sends them to be examined under a microscope.

The advantage of having this test is that it enables the surgeon to take out only the affected lymph nodes and one or two nodes after that, to ensure they are clear, and helps preserve the unaffected nodes. Without this test, most surgeons will do an 'axillary clearance' removing all the axillary lymph nodes whether they are affected by the cancer or not. An axillary clearance can create long-term problems with lymphoedema. The benefits of this test far outweigh the risk of the small dose of radiation.

TUMOUR STAGING

Staging is a description of the extent or severity of an individual's cancer based on the size of the original (primary) tumour and the extent of spread in the body (Table 12.18).

There are various ways to stage tumours, the common elements in most systems being:

- Location of the primary tumour
- Tumour size and the number of tumours
- Lymph node involvement
- Cell type and how closely the cancer cells resemble normal tissue
- Presence or absence of metastasis.

TABLE 12.18 Tumour staging

Stage	Definition
Stage 0	Carcinoma in situ (early cancer that is still confined to the layer of cells in which it began)
Stage I, stage II, and stage III	Higher numbers indicate more extensive disease: greater tumour size, and/or spread of the cancer to nearby lymph nodes and/or organs adjacent to the primary tumour
Stage IV	The cancer has spread to another organ

TAMOXIFEN SCREENING

A recently developed test can determine whether tamoxifen will be successful or not measuring a cytochrome P450 pathway, the CYP2D6. This can provide useful information for women with oestrogen receptor breast cancer who need to make decisions about their treatment. However, at this stage it is expensive and not covered by Medicare.[204]

A side effect of tamoxifen taken long term is the enhanced risk of developing endometrial lesions including cancer — with a poor clinical outcome. This appears to be mediated through oestrogenic and non-genomic pathways.[205]

Naturopathic investigations

CAM practitioners need effective methods of measuring parameters of health that they can then manipulate with the therapies that they use. These methods must be easy to access, relatively non-invasive and provide information that the practitioner can use, not only to determine the most appropriate treatment necessary but also to monitor the progress of the patient and their treatment.

The role of the naturopath in the treatment of cancer is to support healthy function of organs, improve quality of life and increase survival time. An effective approach should be based on knowledge of the function of all systems — with the means to test them. The systems requiring a testing method are mainly digestive, immune, lymphatic and endocrine systems and a measure is needed of oxidative stress levels, inflammation and the regulative abilities of the patient. These tests can give clear indications of the specific CAM treatments required and can then be used to monitor their success or otherwise.

Overall these tests can be used successfully to determine the functional state of the body and for monitoring the success or otherwise of both medical and CAM treatments. They can also help with decision making regarding choice of treatments, depending on the perceived severity of, and potentially correctable factors relating to, the condition.

BREAST SELF-EXAMINATION (BSE) AND CLINICAL BREAST EXAMINATION (CBE)

The sensitivity, specificity, and positive predictive values of CBE (and BSE with a person experienced in checking) are estimated at 40–69%, 88–99%, and 40–50%, respectively. CBE can find tumours that are node-negative and <2 cm diameter, when the chance of survival is greatest. CBE may also find tumours that cannot be seen with mammography (15% of palpable tumours).[206] Research indicates that 80–85% of tumours are discovered by the woman herself, practising BSE. These are then confirmed by other diagnostic procedures.

THERMOGRAPHY (INCLUDES BREAST SCREENING)

Thermography or thermal imaging is based on the principle that metabolic activity and vascular circulation in both precancerous tissue and the area surrounding a developing cancer are almost always higher than in normal tissue. Cancerous tumours require an ever-increasing supply of nutrients and therefore increase circulation to their cells either by parasitising local blood vessels or by the process of angiogenesis. This results in an increase in regional surface temperatures of the area. Using extremely sensitive infrared cameras and sophisticated computers to detect these changes and analyse them, high-resolution diagnostic images of these temperature variations are produced. Because of thermography's sensitivity, these temperature variations may be among the earliest signs of cancer (including breast cancer) and/or a precancerous state of the tissue. 'Hot' areas signify inflammation, whereas 'cold' areas are indicative of abnormal functioning tissue (such as tumours). Thermography is non-invasive, has little in the way of side effects and the images can be diagnostically very useful. It can provide a more accurate and safer alternative to mammography.

Thermography can image many parts of the body and is used for more than breast screening.

LIVE BLOOD ANALYSIS (LBA)

Live blood analysis (LBA) tests the digestive and immune system and can also detect any unusual pathogenic organisms such as *Mycoplasma fermentans* and cell wall deficient organisms. LBA is essentially a blood differential using living cells — it examines the morphology of cells and equates digestive system disorders to the abnormalities noted. It is also effective in recognising changes in white cell numbers and activity. If any pathogenic organisms are detected, this test can be followed up by nested PCR (polymerase chain reaction) for high definition of the microbes potentially causing infection. There is research to suggest that some oncogenes are activated by microorganisms such as *Mycoplasma fermentans.*[207] There is substantial research on viral triggers for oncogenesis.

CLOT RETRACTION TEST (CRT)

The clot retraction test (CRT) was originally developed as a bedside ESR in 1952 and later studies have shown a 95% sensitivity and specificity in neoplasm detection. Changes are seen often months prior to changes in routine pathology. The CRT indicates oxidative stress, inflammation and various systemic organ functions including lymphatic function and immune parameters. It also shows levels of heavy metals, parasites and, if there is sufficient glutathione, an indication of selenium adequacy.

URINARY TESTING FOR OESTROGEN METABOLITES

Oestrogens are known for their proliferative effects on oestrogen-sensitive tissues resulting in tumorigenesis. Results of experiments in multiple laboratories over the last 20 years have shown that a large part of the cancer-inducing effect of oestrogen involves the formation of agonistic metabolites of oestrogen, especially 16 alpha-hydroxyestrone (16α-OHE1) which contributes to breast cancer development. Other metabolites, such as 2-hydroxyestrone (2-OHE1) and 2-hydroxyestradiol are protective against the oestrogen-agonist effects of 16 alpha-hydroxyestrone, and inhibit breast cell proliferation. Measuring these metabolites is therefore an indication of the oestrogen problem. There is an ELISA test available that measures the ratio of 16α-OHE1 to 2-OHE1. For urine specimens a reference limit of greater than 2.0 is generally considered a normal value for the 2-OHE1/16α-OHE1 ratio. Although there are no published data on effects of high ratios, 8.0 seems to be a reasonable limit for how high the value might be allowed to rise before advising moderation of supplements such as I-3-C or DIM supplementation.[208] A 24-hour urine collection is a common procedure.

SALIVARY HORMONE TESTING

Salivary hormone testing measures the free and therefore biologically active form of several of the major hormones in saliva — oestriol, oestradiol, oestrone, progesterone, testosterone, DHEA and cortisol. They have been shown to be a reasonably accurate reflection of hormone levels present inside cells, where the hormone action takes place, whereas blood tests measure hormones outside the cells. Salivary testing is considered to be the gold standard for hormone analysis by the World Health Organization (WHO). However, there is some criticism of the validity of oestrogen and progesterone testing as the hormone levels fluctuate, especially in women with irregular periods. They can be useful at times if there is a perceived hormone imbalance but they need to be done weekly for 1 month for increased accuracy. However, even with oestrogen receptor tumours the hormone studies are often normal as it is the type of oestrogen that is the problem; urinary metabolites may be a more effective measure.

HAIR ANALYSIS FOR HEAVY METALS

Heavy metals can directly and indirectly damage DNA which correlates with an increased risk of cancer (called genotoxicity). There are possibly other non-genotoxic pathways that are due to irritation or immunotoxicity. A number of metals are known to be carcinogenic. These are mainly arsenic, beryllium, cadmium, nickel and hexavalent chromium. The usual target is the lungs, though arsenic has a unique association with skin cancers that has been recognised for many years. Plasma levels of minerals including Ca, Fe, K, Mg, Na and Zn were lower in cancer patients than in healthy volunteers.[209] High copper levels are found in breast cancer patients and frequently in non-Hodgkin's lymphoma patients, particularly in relapsing patients.[210,211]

The best way to test for heavy metals is with a hair analysis, where about a tablespoon of hair is taken from the back of the head then analysed. The hair must be clean, undyed and washed with a shampoo that does not contain metals such as zinc and selenium.

Therapeutic considerations

CLINICAL DECISION MAKING AND RATIONALE

There is increasing and substantial evidence that naturopaths and CAM practitioners have a critical role to play in prevention and support in the treatment of cancer patients. With their holistic, health-based philosophy and individualised approach, they offer a valuable tool, either standing alone or alongside Western medicine, in the treatment of one of our most common degenerative diseases. Their mode of diagnosis and treatment supporting the health of the person offers another perspective that research is increasingly supportive of in the 'fight' against cancer.

Using dietary and lifestyle changes, prescribing nutrient and herbal medicines naturopaths and CAM practitioners can not only make the medical treatments more effective, as well as reducing the potential pharmaceutical load for the patient, but they can also improve overall outcomes by improving the health of the person and their quality of life, and potentially reduce the chance of recurrence of the cancer.

Appendix 12.1 at the end of the book outlines the seven cluster events that trigger carcinogenesis and that can be targeted for treatment.

Therapeutic application

ALLOPATHIC PERSPECTIVE

Chemotherapy

Chemotherapy damages the DNA of the cell (generally while the cell is dividing) and forces growth arrest. Different drugs can affect different processes of the cell cycle. If the cell cannot repair itself, cell death will occur. Toxicities that occur with chemotherapeutic drugs also harm the faster dividing normal cells, such as those found in hair follicles, the bone marrow or the lining of the gastrointestinal tract (which is why the side effects commonly are alopecia, myelosuppression and gastrointestinal symptoms). The therapeutic index of a drug reflects the difference between its efficacy (tumour cell killing) versus its toxicity to normal cells.

Chemotherapy drugs have different mechanisms of action and different toxicity profiles and are divided into several groups based on how they affect:

- Specific chemical substances within cancer cells
- Cellular activities or processes the drug interferes with
- Specific phases of the cell cycle (which the drug affects).

Most chemotherapy is given as a combination of drugs that work together to kill cancer cells. Combining drugs that have different actions at the cellular level may help reduce the risk of the cancer developing resistance to one particular drug. The development of multidrug resistance (MDR) is a major concern with chemotherapy.

EFFECTIVENESS AND CONCERNS

Chemotherapy works best on cancers having a high proportion of rapidly dividing cells, such as leukaemias and lymphomas, but it is less effective on cancers characterised by a low proportion of dividing cells, such as solid tumours found in the colon, rectum, lung and breast. In these cancers, chemotherapy is used in conjunction with either radiation and/or surgery.

Chemotherapy resistance can occur if the cell repairs its DNA after the cytotoxic effects of the DNA damaging agents (instead of cell death) — leading to multidrug resistance.

Research increasingly shows that as a result of the DNA damage caused by chemotherapeutic agents patients surviving chemo- or radiotherapy are at an increased risk of iatrogenic cancer.[212] The chemotherapy drugs of most concern include alkylating agents such as cyclophosphamide which reacts with DNA in a similar manner to chemical carcinogens. Antibiotics (such as doxorubicin) interact with DNA and induce free-radical damage to the genome. The risk is proportional to the cumulative dose, with younger patients being more susceptible (they have more time for the iatrogenic diseases to develop). The most extensive data for increased risk have been accumulated in survivors of Hodgkin's disease in which the risk for developing secondary cancers was 17.6% compared with 2.6% in the general population. The most rapidly developing cancers were leukaemias, with the incidence maximum at 8 years post therapy, in contrast to solid tumours which usually first appear approximately 10 years post therapy and continue to increase in incidence with time. This is consistent with evidence that leukaemias require fewer mutations than do solid tumours.[213]

Interestingly, the *BRCA1* gene is essential for repair in response to DNA damage and is therefore protective, but it increases susceptibility to breast cancer when damaged and/or inactivated. Inactivation of *BRCA1* in mouse cells results in increased cell sensitivity to DNA-damaging agents.[214]

Chemotherapy reduces the white cell count (primarily neutrophils), making the recipient increasingly susceptible to severe infection. This has led to the introduction of more pharmaceuticals that raise the white cell count in patients receiving chemotherapy. The normal range for the white blood cell count varies between laboratories but is usually between 4300 and 10 800 cells per cubic millimetre of blood. This can be referred to as the leucocyte count and can be expressed in international units as 4.3 to 10.8×10^9 cells per litre.

Chemotherapy also includes drugs such as steroids (dexamethasone, prednisolone — to reduce the inflammation caused by the treatment), anti-oestrogens (tamoxifen) and aromatase inhibitors.

Targeted therapies

These days there is new research into chemotherapy and new types of drugs are being produced, such as signal transduction inhibitors, biological response modifiers and monoclonal antibodies. Trastuzumab (Herceptin®) is a monoclonal antibody that has received considerable press. Overexpresssion of the *HER2* oncogene occurs in 25–30% of human breast cancers and is associated with poor outcomes. It often occurs with oestrogen-receptor-negative disease, making these tumours resistant to hormonal therapies. Treatment is limited by both cardiotoxicity and acquired resistance.[215]

Unfortunately recent research is also showing that up to 70% of breast cancer patients are now developing (or have acquired) a resistance to trastuzumab. This translates into a large number of patients who have either stopped responding to trastuzumab, or who have lost the clinical benefits from this drug — leading to further research on supplementary drugs that may be able to be added to reduce this resistance — and increasing the pharmaceutical load even further.[216]

Interestingly research has been investigating the role of COX-2 inhibition in reducing trastuzumab resistance — with some success. While the majority of research has centred around COX-2 inhibitors such as celecoxib, a small paper looked at the role of conjugated linoleic acid (CLA) in reducing trastuzumab resistance, and showed positive results. CLA has been shown to have antitumour properties and to inhibit NF-kB activity and COX-2.[217]

On a dietary note, an interesting area of research with *HER2* activity supports the use of a Mediterranean diet as protective in breast cancer. Several studies on human breast cancer-derived cell lines showed that the polyphenols in extra virgin olive oil inhibited *HER2* activity by generating the degradation of the HER2 protein itself. Extra-virgin olive oil (EVOO) phenolics drastically down-regulated the HER2 protein and preferentially inhibited the proliferation of HER2-overexpressing breast cancer cells, and increased apoptosis. Its activity was unrelated to the antioxidant effects.[218]

A diet high in EVOO was found to act as a negative modulator of breast carcinogenesis and a predictor of a lower level of malignancy as well as drastically suppressing the expression of *HER2*, while synergistically enhancing the *HER2* down-regulatory effect of trastuzumab. No toxicities were reported with the high doses of EVOO.[219]

ISSUES WITH TRASTUZUMAB

There is an increasing ethical and economic dilemma with trastuzumab. It is an expensive medication for both patient and government. The side effects can be severe (usually cardiovascular). Perhaps this money would be better invested in breast cancer research or prevention, or spent on early detection programs, which will prevent recurring costs of treatment in future.[220] Prescribing *Crataegus monogyna* and coenzyme Q10 can normalise cardiac enzymes when on trastuzumab.

Angiogenesis inhibition

Angiogenesis is the process by which new blood capillaries form by sprouting from an existing small vessel. This process is of critical importance in tumours as their growth is limited by the available blood supply. It is therefore beneficial for tumours to induce the formation of a capillary network so that nutrients can be supplied directly to the tumour; in this way, tumour cells are said to parasitise the blood vessels of normal cells.

Angiogenesis inhibition should therefore limit tumour growth, and the search for antiangiogenic drugs is an active area in cancer research. Medically thalidomide is considered effective but this brings into question the potential side effects in women of reproductive age. There are effective alternatives that are worth considering, such as the cartilage remedies (shark, bovine and glucosamine and chondroitin sulfate), *Allium sativum*, selenium, *Camellia sinensis*, the isoflavones — genistein, diadzein and grapeseed (*Vinus vitifera*) etc. These specifically inhibit vascular endothelial growth factor and have direct activity against angiogenesis.[221]

Hormone therapies

Hormones, or hormone-like drugs, alter the action or production of female or male hormones. They have a different action to standard chemotherapy and can slow the growth of breast, prostate and endometrial cancers, which normally grow in response to hormone levels. Other cancers that may respond to oestrogen are melanomas and some lung cancers (oestrogen receptor positive).

Once again there are effective alternatives such as indoles, isothiocyanates and the ferments of soy or kudza — genistein and diadzein. *Curcuma longa* (turmeric) is also worth prescribing as it improves oestrogen dominance triggered by the environmental impact of chemicals.[222]

Appendixes 12.2 and 12.3 outline tamoxifen and indole applicability and inhibition of various pathways.

Aromatase inhibition needs to be considered: a study was conducted on dietary influences showing that safflower oil increases aromatase and omega-3 fatty acids decrease aromatase. The results showed that dietary fatty acids play a role in modifying steroid hormone action through modulating these steroid metabolising enzymes.[223]

Natural products that have aromatase inhibitory activity (and include those that will reduce COX-2 overexpression) are grape seed extract, *Viscum album, Garcinia mangostana, Camellia sinensis, Curcuma longa,* green leafy vegetables (kale is a good example), *Trifolium pratense, Glycyrrhiza glabra, Ginkgo biloba,* quercetin and phytooestrogens for example.[224]

Recent research shows a close link between overexpression of the inflammatory COX-2 pathways in increased aromatase catalysed oestrogen biosynthesis.[225] It therefore stands to reason that natural products that reduce the overexpression of these pathways will also act as aromatase inhibitors. However, to date, there has been very little research done on herbs and nutrients being used in this capacity.

Tumour vaccines

Researchers are developing vaccines that may encourage the patient's immune system to recognise cancer cells. These vaccines are used after the cancer is diagnosed, and can be made in various ways: from cells extracted from the tumour or from dendritic cells (from the patient).

Interleukin-2 (IL-2) is also often injected, which enhances T-cell immunity in cancer patients, and interleukin-12 (IL-12), which enhances the vaccine. The vaccines would be given to prevent the cancer from returning or to get the body to reject similar tumours.[226]

Radiotherapy

Radiation is used to treat 60% of cancer patients and is usually a local treatment. Radiotherapy uses x-rays, electron beams or radioactive isotopes (from naturally occurring radioactive elements such as radium, or from artificially produced radioactive isotopes of nonradioactive elements such as caesium) to shrink tumours, either by destroying cancer cells or by damaging them so much that they can no longer multiply. Radiation can be a useful cancer treatment because it kills cancer cells while causing less damage to normal cells. This occurs because the x-ray beams are shot from different angles to maximise radiation at the tumour site and minimise corollary damage. Healthy tissue is shielded from radiation as much as possible, usually with some form of 'lead apron'.

Radiation therapy works directly by damaging the DNA of cells, or indirectly by the ionisation of water, forming free radicals (hydroxyl radicals), which then damage the DNA. Most of the radiation effect is through free radical damage. Once a cancer cell's DNA is destroyed, it can no longer undergo replication and the cell dies.

Radiation is most effective when the cancer cell is actually dividing — when the cancer cell is in the M (mitosis) phase of its cell cycle — therefore cancers with rapidly dividing cells, such as leukaemia (cancer of the blood cells) and lymphoma (cancer of the lymph nodes) are more sensitive to radiation than cancers in which the cells divide more slowly.

The effectiveness of radiation is enhanced when it is used in combination with surgery, chemotherapy or hormone therapy.

TYPES OF RADIOTHERAPY

There are two basic types of radiotherapy, external beam (E(X)BRT or teletherapy) and internal (brachytherapy). In EBRT, radiation is delivered from a source outside the body.

Brachytherapy works by placing radioactive isotopes either close to, or inside the body. It can take the form of interstitial, intracavity, intraluminal, or as a radiopharmaceutical such as oral ingestion of iodine-131 (^{131}I) taken for thyroid cancer.

Side effects

Radiation therapy itself is painless. The most common side effects are fatigue, nausea, tiredness, and external skin discomfort (burns) and ulceration. Because radiation triggers an inflammatory response and swelling this is of particular concern in brain tissues.

The nature of the side effects depends on the site that receives the radiation and the treatment schedule (type of radiation, dose, fractionation, concurrent chemotherapy). Individuals vary in their reaction to radiation but doses are generally not individualised.

Medium- and long-term side effects

Medium- and long-term side effects may be minimal and depend on the tissue receiving treatment and the dose used. Fibrosis is common, and secondary malignancies occur in a minority of patients. Infertility can be an issue if the area to be irradiated is close to ovaries or testes.

What needs to be remembered (particularly from a medical/scientific perspective) is that all radiation received is cumulative over a lifetime. From a CAM perspective radiation damage to tissues may be partially corrected — depending on the dose and frequency.

A number of plants high in antioxidants and anti-inflammatory compounds have been shown to be efficacious in protecting against radiation damage; plants such as *Camellia sinensis, Curcuma longa, Nigella sativa, Crataegus microphylla* and *Angelica sinensis.*[227]

Retreatment

Retreatment of previously irradiated sites is also an issue, as all tissues have a maximum lifetime tolerance for radiation, so retreatment of a site which received a maximum safe dose years before can cause significant damage.

Limitations

One of the major limitations of radiotherapy is that the cells of solid tumours become deficient in oxygen (hypoxic) and the more hypoxic the tumours are, the more resistant they are to the effects of radiation, because oxygen 'fixes' or makes permanent the radiation damage to DNA.

Much research has been devoted to overcoming this problem, including the use of high-pressure oxygen tanks and blood substitutes that carry increased oxygen used concurrently.[228]

For radiation protection in healthy cells, think of the mushroom polysaccharides, the ginsengs and antioxidants, especially selenium. There is some debate that coenzyme Q10 may protect cancer cells from radiation (as well as normal cells), so for safety, avoid this until after the treatment.

Using calendula cream during radiotherapy may help reduce skin burning and ulceration. Several studies have compared it with trolamine for the prevention of acute dermatitis while undergoing radiotherapy for breast cancer and calendula cream has been shown to be very effective.[229] It is certainly a great deal more effective than the sorbolene cream often used in radiotherapy departments. Aloe vera gel could be considered as well as it has excellent properties for repairing damaged skin from burns, including radiation burns.[230]

Internally a mixture of vitamin E analogues — tocopherols and tocotrienols — has been shown to reduce the DNA damage caused by radiation.[231]

Surgery

Surgery can be a useful adjunct to all treatments for cancer if it is done appropriately. Removing the bulk of the tumour can assist the immune system to recover. However, this is only symptomatic treatment and is not dealing with the cause of the problem.

To minimise damage and to reduce the side effects of surgical procedures give vitamin C to improve liver metabolism and clearance of anaesthesia (but check blood clotting to ensure safety), arnica 30 for bruising and surgical shock, zinc and vitamin E to help with healing and reduction of scarring.

NATUROPATHIC PERSPECTIVE

Some in the medical profession criticise the use of nutritional and herbal remedies in treating people with cancer — either singly or in combination with allopathic medicine. One of the main issues is the divergent approach by both sides (and the philosophies behind these different approaches), which leads to a misunderstanding of the meaning of 'treatment' with cancer. The medical approach is primarily a disease-based approach, whereby an arsenal of toxic treatments is employed to 'kill' and remove the cancer. While this does have some uses and can kill the disease (cancer), it is limited by what it does not do — namely restore health.

Medical research is based on a disease model — both philosophically and practically — which produces a dilemma when exploring the benefit of dietary modifications to support a degenerative illness (i.e. cancer) with dietary intervention. Epidemiological evidence shows a strong association of dietary modifications with cancer, but is unable to show that these interventions will cure cancer. Dietary interventions can improve the health of a patient and the CAM clinician is best suited to this task. The CAM clinician places significant importance on restoring the health of the patient and sees dietary interventions as a foundational component to achieve this.

Nutritional medicine (dietary)

Hippocrates has been credited with saying 'Let your food be your medicine and your medicine be your food'.

According to meta-analyses of the research, up to 70% of cancer in Western populations can be attributed to diet and lifestyle, with exposure to tobacco products the major single contributor at 30%. The remaining increased risk appears to be associated with deficiencies in dietary factors, principally a lack of fruits and vegetables, which exert a protective role on cancer induction.[232] The main protective components in plants are the flavonoids which have major antioxidant and inflammatory effects.

Unfortunately with the increasing exposure to a range of exogenous agents, either chemical or physical, these environmental challenges can potentially damage DNA and trigger carcinogenesis. Spontaneous DNA damage does occur, which gives rise to mutations that can act as a molecular fingerprint indicating the specific exposure. Foods, specific nutrients (such as N-acetyl cysteine and glutathione) and plant medicines can assist with detoxification of these chemicals and improve immune function.

The cultural story

With the strong association of cancer with food choices, different cultures will therefore be prone to different cancers, and this has been shown to be the case. For example, the Japanese diet predisposes its citizens to a higher risk of stomach cancer from the irritant effect of pickled foods; in parts of Africa, the people are more prone to liver cancer from the aflatoxin component of the repeated ingestion of large amounts of peanuts — these being a major protein source.

To improve our health and to protect against the common cancers of Western society, we need to be aware of the common foods we consume that can potentially cause problems, and those that we need to eat more of for protection against degenerative disease (mainly foods that are high in antioxidants). We also need to be aware of the value of different approaches to dietary balance.

World Cancer Research Fund review

Every 10 years the World Cancer Research Fund conducts an international epidemiological review of guidelines for cancer prevention and produces a report that delineates the roles that various dietary factors may play in the process of carcinogenesis, along with the voluminous epidemiological literature that demonstrates associations of foods and/or nutrients with the prevention of cancer.

Based on this extensive review, a series of dietary recommendations for the prevention of cancer is developed for the report. In the 2007 report, the recommendations suggest that a plant-based diet that minimises consumption of red meat and processed meat and emphasises the consumption of a variety of vegetables, fruits and wholegrain cereals would decrease the risk of a variety of cancers. In fact the report shows that increasing the consumption of vegetables and fruits from 250 to (as little as) 400 g/d may be associated with a 23% decreased risk of cancer worldwide.[233]

Many 'diets': similar principles

There have been many diets and food programs written for different types of cancer. All have similar principles, although the details may vary somewhat. Overall, the basic diet for people with cancer is based on several consistent factors. These are:

- Lowering the animal protein component (NB: people with brain tumours need higher levels of proteins and fats — not necessarily animal — and ketogenic diets help shrink some brain tumours)
- Regulating/reducing chronic inflammation with foods, nutrients and herbs
- Manipulating fats (lipids) (regulating the inflammatory prostaglandin cascade)
- Reducing levels of free radical damage and oxidation with antioxidants (in vegetables and fruits, various nutrients and herbal medicines)
- Balancing hormones (oestrogen dominance is an increasing problem)
- Reducing chemical overload.

The role of refined 'sugars'

A 4-year study at the National Institute of Public Health and Environmental Protection in The Netherlands compared 111 biliary tract cancer patients with 480 controls. Cancer risk associated with the intake of sugars, independent of other energy sources, more than doubled for the cancer patients with the higher intake of sugars.[234]

An epidemiological study in 21 modern regions or countries that keep track of morbidity and mortality (e.g. Europe, North America, Japan) revealed that sugar intake is a strong risk factor that contributes to higher breast cancer rates, particularly in older women.[235]

Dietary regimens that have been shown to improve health in cancer patients

1 Macrobiotic
2 Budwig
3 Gerson
4 Dietary restriction (and timing of eating).

MACROBIOTIC DIET

Themacrobiotic diet was developed by George Ohsawa and Michio Kushi. The diet is predominantly vegetarian, organic, wholefoods diets. There is substantial evidence that the many dietary factors recommended by macrobiotics are associated with decreased cancer risk.

Women consuming a macrobiotic diet have lower circulating oestrogen levels, suggesting a lower risk of breast (and hormonal-based) cancer due in part to the high phyto-oestrogen content of the macrobiotic diet.[236]

The macrobiotic diet consists of 50–60% whole cereal grains (mainly brown rice), 25–30% vegetables (organically grown with minimal processing), 5–10% soups, including miso soup, and 5–10% legumes and sea vegetables. White meat, fish and fruit are recommended in limited amounts. Foods to avoid are potatoes, sweet potatoes, tomatoes, eggplants, peppers, asparagus, spinach, beets, zucchini, avocados, mayonnaise, red meat and tea, coffee.

Plenty of fresh air, exercise, meditation and the wearing of cotton (preferably organic) clothing are recommended and there are restrictions on watching television.

Macrobiotic research — positive

For over 25 years the researchers worked with people with a variety of incapacitating symptoms relating to exposures to common xenobiotics. A survey was conducted on 160 patients who complained of chemically-induced symptoms and were encouraged to incorporate a macrobiotic diet into their program. Questionnaires were sent to all.

Before the diet, many of these people felt they had done as much as they could in other ways to reduce their xenobiotic exposures and resulting symptoms.

Of 160 questionnaires, 56 (35%) were returned and of these, 39 (26%) were completed so they could be included in the study.

Results: Overall, those on the comprehensive program, which included inhalant injections, environmental controls and correction of nutrient deficiencies, reported lessened chemical sensitivity by an average of 76%. The participants felt that they were 59% less chemically sensitive directly due to the macrobiotic diet, and they felt that the macrobiotic diet provided additional unanticipated relief, and should therefore be considered for those with persistent symptoms triggered by chemical exposure.[237]

Macrobiotic research — concerns

Research has demonstrated concerns that the macrobiotic diet is very low in kilojoules, as most of the healthy adults reported having lost weight on the diet, and several cases of protein–calorie malnutrition were documented among infants and children (and adults) who were fed strict a macrobiotic diet.

In nutrient terms intakes of riboflavin, niacin, vitamin B_{12} and folate were below the RDA/RDI, calcium intakes in macrobiotic adults and children were 50–60% below RDA, iron intakes of macrobiotic women and children averaged 62–84% of the RDA but those of the men exceeded the RDA. Low B_{12} and scurvy were noted in some patients.

Results: It was felt by the researchers that there was a need to eat large amounts of food to gain correct nutrients and in the West, the cost of the special foods could be prohibitive.[238,239]

THE 'BUDWIG' DIET

The Budwig diet was developed by Dr Johanna Budwig with her extensive interest in the low ALA (alpha-linolenic acid) content of blood and the bioenergetic aspect of different foods.[240] From her research she concluded that photons of light could be captured and drawn into the body via the electron-dense essential fats such as ALA from flax oil.

The diet consists of flaxseed oil mixed with cottage cheese or quark (the 'spread'), rich in sulfur amino acids to increase uptake of the ALA, plus large amounts of organic fresh vegetables and fruit.

Recipe for the spread

Place 250 mL flaxseed oil into a bowl, add 450 g organic quark (or low-fat 1% cottage cheese) and 4 tablespoons (60 mL) raw honey. Blend or mix together and add just enough organic low-fat milk or filtered water to get the contents of the bowl to mix together.

In 5 minutes, a preparation of a custard-like consistency results that has no taste of the oil (and no oily 'ring' should be seen when you rinse out the bowl).

Organic yoghurt can be used in the proportions of 30 g of yoghurt to 1 tablespoon (15 mL) each of flaxseed oil and of honey and blend.

General rules for the Budwig diet

- Pure sugar is absolutely forbidden. If necessary grape juice or maple syrup may be added to sweeten. Minimal raw unheated honey is allowed.
- Forbidden foods: all animal fats — meat (unless organic or biodynamic), dairy (except the spread), all salad oils (including commercial mayonnaise), all butter, margarines, all preserved meats and fish, as the preservatives block the metabolism of flaxseed oil.
- Include: freshly squeezed organic vegetable juices are recommended — carrot, celery, beetroot. Occasional freshly squeezed apple or pear juice.
- Three times per day a warm (herb) tea is essential, such as peppermint, rosehip, grape tea, green tea, and this can be sweetened with a little raw honey if necessary.
- A minimum of 120 g of the spread must be consumed per day (throughout the day).
- All vegetables and dairy products should be organic or biodynamic.
- Keep all flaxseed oil in the refrigerator and use quickly — before it turns rancid. Rancid oil is detrimental for health so check and replace if in any doubt about its freshness.
- Flaxseed oil can be applied to the skin or used as a retention enema — 250 mL.
- The night meal must be eaten before 6 pm.

An advantage of the Budwig diet is that it can be manipulated to increase the proteins and fats (with the 'spread') in a healthy way and thus can be used as a safe ketogenic diet for people with brain tumours. It also allows for a little more organic animal/fish protein if necessary.

THE GERSON DIET

Thirty years of clinical experimentation led to a successful method for 'treating' advanced cancer.[241] There is a Gerson clinic in the USA that is still operating today and is run by Dr Max Gerson's children and grandchildren. The Gerson diet is based on the concepts that cancer patients have low immunoreactivity and generalised tissue damage, especially of the liver, and that when the cancer is destroyed, toxic degradation products appear in the bloodstream which can lead to coma and death from liver failure.

The diet consists of high-potassium foods (and low sodium) with no fats or oils, and minimal animal proteins. Foods encouraged are the juices of raw fruits and vegetables and of raw liver as these provide active oxidising enzymes which facilitate rehabilitation of the liver. Iodine and niacin supplementation are recommended. Caffeine enemas are recommended daily as these cause dilation of bile ducts, facilitating excretion of toxic cancer breakdown products by the liver and the dialysis of toxic products from blood across the colonic wall.

The Gerson diet must be used as an integrated whole. Parts of the therapy used in isolation will not be successful (as with other specific diets). Taken as a whole the Gerson diet has been very successful for many years, although it is difficult to follow.

Key points of the Gerson diet

- Thirteen glasses of the prescribed juices must be drunk every day. The juice must come from organic fruits and vegetables and one glass of the specified juice drunk every hour within 15 minutes of being made. 1 to 2 glasses of organic calf liver juice are included in the program
- All meals are vegetarian, made of organically grown fruits, vegetables and whole grains
- Supplements that need to be taken concurrently include Lugol's iodine, vitamin B_{12}, potassium, thyroid hormone, a crude liver extract with B_{12} (IM), and pancreatic enzymes
- Regular enemas are important, including coffee or chamomile enemas to remove toxins
- Food must be prepared without salt, spices, and no aluminium cookware or utensils used.

The Gerson diet research

The high potassium:sodium ratio of the Gerson dietary treatment for cancer can be expected to produce a substantial enhancement of aldosterone levels. Some tumours may be mineralocorticoid sensitive and host resistance to neoplastic invasion may be enhanced by mineralocorticoids. In this diet, potassium is high and further enhanced by supplementation and sodium is low. The diet is also high in antioxidants, low in saturated fats with high essential fatty acids. Thyroid function is maximised with Lugol's solution and thyroid extract. This can be particularly important with hormone-based cancer.[242]

DIETARY RESTRICTION — TIMING

Restricting the timing of eating proteins and fats can improve immune function and reduce inflammation. Glucocorticoid manipulation is a possibility where the timing of eating can alter the production of glucocorticoids. The eating pattern means that proteins and fats can only be eaten within a 6-hour timeframe. No alcohol or caffeine can be consumed as these stimulate adrenal function.

Dietary (kilojoule) restriction — undernutrition not malnutrition

Dietary (kilojoule) restriction has been researched as the basis for increased longevity and health. It has also been shown to suppress carcinogenesis generally, including the carcinogenic action of several classes of chemicals, such as polycyclic hydrocarbons (benzopyrenes and DMBA), and alkylating and methylating agents (e.g. diethylnitrosamine and methylazoxymethanol).

It inhibits several forms of radiation-induced cancers. The inhibitory action of dietary restriction on carcinogenesis is effective in many species, for a variety of tumour types, and for both spontaneous tumours and tumours caused by different types of tumour-inducing agents. Dietary restriction also retards noncancer ageing-associated pathologies, such as nephropathy, cardiomyopathy, gastric ulcers and cataracts.[243]

Nutrients that it is essential to maintain high levels of are selenium, zinc, copper and manganese, as well as the antioxidant vitamins A, C and E, beta-carotene and coenzyme Q10.

Food components of interest

Research has been conducted on many components of food and their role in the prevention of degenerative disease — including cancer. As it is perceived that the basis of most chronic disease is the result of the damage caused by an excess of inflammation and/or an excess of oxidation (these two vital processes are intricately intertwined), the components in foods and plants that regulate these processes are of great interest. Stimulating the immune system and regulating hormonal balance is also important. The main food components discussed here are:

1. Essential fatty acids that regulate inflammatory pathways
2. Phenolic compounds such as the important flavonoids which are antioxidant and anti-inflammatory
3. Polysaccharides (and oligosaccharides), which have immune stimulating properties
4. Phyto-oestrogens involved in regulating hormonal balance
5. Indoles and isothiocyanates (hormonal balance and liver detoxification)
6. Vitamin and mineral components, with multiple roles to play
7. Fibre components of food
8. Probiotics (the microbiome) and prebiotics such as inulin
9. Fermented foods and foods with high enzyme activity.

Nutritional medicine (specific foods)

CAMELLIA SINENSIS — GREEN TEA

Green tea contains catechins, principally epigallocatechin gallate (EGCG), which has been shown to have powerful antioxidant activity, as well as being anti-inflammatory and

SAMPLE DAILY DIET

BREAKFAST	
Smoothie: papaya, banana, spinach, avocado, flaxseed, low allergen protein powder and coconut water	A smoothie provides an easy to assimilate, nutrient-dense meal designed to boost immunity and energy while reducing inflammation. Folate-rich foods are involved in intestinal cell proliferation, the latter of which may be damaged after cytotoxic therapy for cancer resulting in increased intestinal permeability, thus foods containing folate should be emphasised to promote gut healing so absorption is not compromised. Flaxseed consumption may reduce cancer cell growth by preventing proliferation of tumours, thus is advocated, particularly if the cancer is hormone driven. A smoothie also provides a useful vehicle for individuals trying to gain weight prior to chemotherapy. In an attempt to reduce the impact of cancer-related anorexia it can be modified to include foods such as avocado and tahini to add nutrients and kilojoules, preventing weight loss.
LUNCH	
Pumpkin, spinach, tomato and mixed mushroom risotto served with a small quantity of fish	A plant-based diet is associated with reduced risk and a protective action against cancer. Diets rich in fruit, vegetables, wholegrains, and omega-3 fatty acid containing foods are rich in flavonoids that help protect against DNA damage and have been shown to reduce postcancer fatigue compared to those with diets containing low quantities of these foods. Aside from the protective action of phytochemicals in a plant-based diet, they are also rich in fibre, which itself is known to be protective against many cancers. As smell, taste and appetite may be affected, food should be modified with herbs for flavour as desired.
DINNER	
Mixed mushroom broth/soup made with ginger, broccoli, kombu, celery, sweet potato, carrot, Asian mushrooms, tofu	A broth or soup provides a nutritive, hydrating meal that is easy to consume, particularly if the patient has mouth/throat soreness resulting in difficulty swallowing. Ginger can be used to stimulate appetite and decrease nausea, particularly during chemotherapy, while Asian mushrooms such as shiitake are known to be chemoprotective due to their immune-modulating and antitumour properties. The addition of vegetables provides minerals and vitamins to nourish the immune system and aid liver detoxification from chemotherapy.
SNACK	
Fresh vegetable juice made with turmeric and black pepper Honey placed on the oral mucosa Ginger tea Green tea	Curcumin with turmeric has been shown to induce apoptosis and slow down cellular proliferation. Piperine in black pepper increases bioavailability of curcumin. Honey may reduce radiation-induced oral mucositis. Ginger may reduce nausea associated with chemotherapy. Polyphenols in green tea exhibit chemoprotective activity via mechanisms including anti-proliferative activity and suppression of angiogenesis.

Sources: Arslan M, Ozdemir L. Oral intake of ginger for chemotherapy-induced nausea and vomiting among women with breast cancer. Clin J Oncol Nurs 2015; 19(5):E92–97. Cho HK, Jeong YM, Lee HS et al. Effects of honey on oral mucositis in patients with head and neck cancer: a meta-analysis. Laryngoscope 2015; 125(9):2085–2092. Demark-Wahnefried W, Polascik TJ, George SL et al. Flaxseed supplementation (not dietary fat restriction) reduces prostate cancer proliferation rates in men presurgery. Cancer Epidem Biomark 2008; 17(12):3577–3587. George VC, Dellaire G, Rupasinghe HP. Plant flavonoids in cancer chemoprevention: role in genome stability. J Nutr Biochem 2016; 45:1–14. Jung YD, Ellis LM. Inhibition of tumour invasion and angiogenesis by epigallocatechin gallate (EGCG), a major component of green tea. Int J Exp Pathol 2001; 82(6):309–316. Souza NC, Simões BP, Júnior AA et al. Changes in intestinal permeability and nutritional status after cytotoxic therapy in patients with cancer. Nutr Cancer 2014; 66(4):576–582. Zick SM, Colacino J, Cornellier M et al.Fatigue reduction diet in breast cancer survivors: a pilot randomized clinical trial. Breast Cancer Res Treat 2017; 161(2):299–310. Zick SM, Sen A, Han-Markey TL et al. Examination of the association of diet and persistent cancer-related fatigue: a pilot study. Oncol Nurs Forum 2013; 40(1):E41–E49.

activating the p53 tumour suppressor gene to increase apoptosis (of abnormal cells).[244] Research into drinking green tea at concentrations normally consumed by humans (approximately 6 to 8 cups per day) blocked up to 87% of skin cancer, 58% of stomach cancer and 56% of lung cancer in mice.[245]

Green tea has had extensive research conducted on it and it shows up as a particularly useful beverage to assist in the maintenance of health and in the prevention of degenerative disease. Research has shown that it has anti-inflammatory and cancer chemopreventive effects in many animal tumour bioassays, cell culture systems and epidemiological studies. Supplementing with EGCG results in apoptosis of a variety of cancer cells, but not of normal cells, and shows a dose-dependent inhibition of cell growth at the G_0/G_1-phase arrest of the cell cycle.

Green tea has also been shown to trigger the induction of apoptosis in human epidermoid carcinoma (A431) cells, but not in normal human epidermal keratinocytes, which suggests that EGCG-caused cell cycle deregulation and apoptosis of cancer cells may be mediated through NF-kappaB inhibition (a major inflammatory pathway associated with the instigation and promotion of chronic diseases such as cancer).[246]

ASPALATHUS LINEARIS — ROOIBOS TEA

For similar properties to green tea without the caffeine, rooibos tea is worth considering.[247] It has high levels of antioxidant (aspathalin) that potentially lowers the risk of cancer as it has a regulating role in cell proliferation and apoptosis. Rooibos reduces age-related accumulation of lipid peroxidase and increases phase 2 activity in the liver, improving oxidative status. It also scavenges super oxide radicals and protects DNA.

Rooibos contains multiple flavonoids with significant anti-inflammatory activity. The polysaccharide component stimulates antibody production and immunity.[248]

Green bosch (unfermented rooibos tea) has higher antioxidant activity than the normal (red) fermented version, and research has shown it may be as — or even more — beneficial than green tea.[249]

ALLIUM FAMILY — GARLIC, ONIONS

Garlic has been shown to help destroy cancerous cells in much the same way as chemotherapeutic drugs, without the side effects. Ajoene (a major active ingredient) has been shown to be three times as toxic to malignant cells as normal cells. Garlic acts as a 'biological response modifier' that boosts immune function by boosting the anticancer activity of macrophages and T-cells. It also has major anti-infective properties and can reduce levels of fungal/yeast overproliferation.

Garlic and onions have more than 30 different anticancer substances that have been shown to reduce stomach cancer (maybe its antibiotic effect against *H. pylori*), as well as breast, skin, lung and liver cancer.

Research has shown that eating 85 g of garlic, onions, chives or spring onions daily reduces stomach cancer by 40%.[250]

POLYSACCHARIDES — MUSHROOMS

Polysaccharides are a structurally diverse group of biological macromolecules which are widely spread in nature. The main sources are mushrooms and algae but polysaccharides are in many plants. They are composed of repetitive structural features — polymers of monosaccharides joined by glycosidic linkages, and they present the highest capacity for carrying biological information because of their great structural variability. Many of these polysaccharides are biologically active antitumour and immunostimulant.

Mushrooms (high in plant polysaccharides) are undergoing scientific analyses and development to prevent and treat cancer. Two classes of polysaccharides in mushrooms are the primary focus of investigations:

- Beta-glucan polysaccharides, as biological response modifiers for the adjuvant treatment of many types of cancer
- Oligosaccharin-related oligosaccharides, for the prevention of sun-induced skin cancer.[251]

More than 50 mushroom species have yielded potential immunoceuticals, which exhibit significant anticancer activity in experimental model systems. Mushrooms also have powerful oxygen free radical scavenging (antioxidant) properties.

Mushrooms have long been valued as tasty, nutritious food by many societies and different cultures throughout the world. To the ancient Romans they were the 'food of the Gods', resulting from bolts of lightning thrown to the earth by Jupiter during thunderstorms; the Egyptians considered them as 'a gift from the God Osiris'; the Chinese viewed them as 'the elixir of life'. At least 182 genera of mushrooms contain biologically active polysaccharides including:

- Maitake — *Grifola frondosa*
- Reishi — *Ganoderma lucidum*
- Cordyceps — *Cordyceps sinensis*
- Coriolus — *Coriolus (Trametes) versicolor*
- Field mushroom — *Agaricus blazei*
- Shiitake — *Lentinus edodes*
- *Poria cocos.*

Mushroom research

Two polysaccharides from *Coriolus versicolor* — PSK (polysaccharide-K) and PSP (polysaccharide-P) — have demonstrated the most promise to date. These protein-bound polysaccharides have been used as a chemo-immunotherapy agent in the treatment of cancer in Asia for over 30 years. PSK and PSP were found to boost immune cell production, reduce the side effects of chemotherapy symptoms (when used as adjuvant therapies), and enhance tumour infiltration by immune cells.[252]

Impressive results have been obtained with orally administered extracts of *Agaricus blazei* in tumour-bearing animals where dramatic regression of tumours was demonstrated in multiple studies.[253]

A very interesting pilot study conducted at Houston Medical School in 2014, on women diagnosed with persistent HPV infection, showed that supplementing with a compound derived from mushrooms (e.g. *Ganoderma lucidum* Reishi) totally cleared the virus from the women in 6 months with a daily dose of 3 g. Phase II trials are underway.[254]

ALOE VERA — *ALOE BARBADENSIS*

Aloe vera is a plant high in polysaccharides. Aloe contains an important polysaccharide, acemannan, and active glycoprotein fractions (lectins). These are anti-inflammatory, chemotactic, antimicrobial and immune stimulant. Aloe vera juice (consumed orally) reduces tumour mass in some types of cancer, enhances the effectiveness of some of the pharmaceutical drugs used in chemotherapy against cancer, and inhibits metastasis.[255] Aloe vera juice has also been shown to stabilise blood glucose and repair digestive function.

HORMONAL BALANCING — PHYTO-OESTROGENS

Soy — Glycine max

The addition of soy products in the diet is a contentious issue. Soy contains phyto-oestrogens and genistein (a product of fermentation). Soy beans are a staple in Asian diets (especially Chinese and Japanese). The inclusion of soy has been shown to have protective effects. Singaporean Chinese women who eat twice as much soy protein as women consuming a Western (or other) diet have been shown to have 50% lower incidence of breast cancer. Typically about 85 g of soy beans was consumed per day and was consumed as soy milk, tofu, miso, tempeh, flour, beans (soy protein).[256,257]

Soy has been shown to protect against prostate cancer in men who eat it daily, specifically the soy ferments. Prostate cancer is lower in men who eat fermented soy protein regularly — it decreases dihydrotestosterone (DHT), the excess of which is a contributing factor in prostate disease.[258]

The ferments of soy (miso and tempeh) provide genistein and are perceived to be more protective. Genetically modified organism (GMO) soy products are best avoided as these may trigger major health problems.[259,260]

INDOLES AND ISOTHIOCYANATES

Indoles are naturally occurring compounds found in cruciferous vegetables and are known to stimulate detoxifying enzymes in the gut and liver. The main food sources are (raw) broccoli, Brussels sprouts, cabbage, cauliflower, collards, kale, kohlrabi, mustard greens, rapeseed, rutabaga and turnips. Research indicates their potential value as a chemopreventive agent for breast cancer through the oestrogen receptor (ER) modulating effect.[261,262] Indoles down-regulate the expression of the oestrogen-responsive genes and upregulate *BRAC1*. They inhibit expression of cycline-dependent kinase-6 and induce a G1 cell cycle arrest independent of (oestrogen receptor) ER signalling.

A randomised clinical trial showed that indoles can increase the 2-OH-oestrone:oestriol metabolite ratio, thereby decreasing the risk of ER-sensitive breast cancer and cervical cancer. Indoles can cause apoptosis of prostate cancer cells in vitro and hold promise for preventing cancer with a papilloma virus component and in various skin cancers. Indoles induce cytochrome P450 1A1, increasing the detoxification of liver and improving the metabolism of oestrogen.[263]

Indoles have a similar outcome to tamoxifen. There is evidence to support that indoles have a different mechanism of action than tamoxifen and that these two substances can be used synergistically.[264]

Doses: treatment and prevention of illness both use doses of 200–400 mg per day of Indole-3-carbinol. Supplemental indoles are contraindicated in pregnancy.[265]

Isothiocyanates act synergistically with indoles and prevent colon tumorigenesis by both stimulating apoptosis and enhancing intracellular defences against genotoxic agents. They both possess cancer chemopreventative properties.[266]

FIBRE IN FOODS

The fibre (soluble and insoluble) component of food plays a major protective role in the battle against cancer and degenerative disease. By speeding up the processing of food residues through the bowel and by supporting the bacteria that are beneficial to health, they reduce faecal mutagen/carcinogen concentrations, reduce the length of exposure of the mucosa to mutagens (increase bowel transit time), inhibit faecal mutagen synthesis by lowering the acidity (pH) and encourage the growth of the correct bowel flora.

Fibre (particularly soluble fibre) increases butyrate which is the energy source of the bowel bacteria and a major cancer-inhibiting metabolite. Fibre ferments to butyrate with the correct bacteria and in turn 'feeds' them. Dietary fibre-resistant starches are best for this — whole cereals, fruit and vegetables, green bananas (boiled) or the fibre 'supplements', slippery elm, psyllium, oat, rice, barley bran.

PROBIOTICS — LACTOBACILLI AND BIFIDOBACTERIA[267]

Along with fibre in the diet, adding the foods that provide the correct bowel bacteria also help to protect against cancer. These foods are sauerkraut, miso, yoghurts and kefirs (high in lactobacilli) and other traditional fermented foods. Foods high in inulin will assist in the establishment and maintenance of correct bowel microflora — the microbiome. Fermented foods such as kefir, sauerkraut, miso and fermented vegetables provide a bioavailable source of a range of lactobacilli.

INULIN (OLIGOSACCHARIDES)

In in vivo studies, the anticancer properties of prebiotic chicory inulin and oligofructose were shown in experimental models.[268] Inulin is useful in chemoprevention where cancer-inducing chemicals mimic the effect of toxic metabolites of certain food compounds in the intestine.

Some research has been conducted in genetically predetermined models, in which genes that protect against cancer have been removed (mice). Prebiotics (chicory fructans) and probiotics (lactobacilli or bifidobacteria) have been shown to be protective against colon cancer. Inulin promotes the growth of beneficial bacteria in the gut as it ferments to butyrate — an essential metabolite in the gut which is the preferred energy source for colonic epithelial cells, contributes to the maintenance of gut barrier functions and has both immunomodulatory and anti-inflammatory properties.[269]

NORMALISATION OF *BRCA1* AND *BRCA2* GENES

BRCA1 and *BRCA2* gene abnormalities can be a significant factor in the development of breast cancer when their normal protective mechanisms have been deregulated through epigenetic damage. This damage relates to hypermethylation and histone deacetylase (HDAC) activity. Therefore inhibitors of these mechanisms should improve outcomes, especially if diagnosed early and the appropriate dietary and supplemental changes instigated.

There are a variety of plant/food-based compounds that have been shown to be effective when converted by metabolism to intermediates that inhibit these processes.

Important are short chain fatty acids such as fibre in foods that metabolise to form butyrates in the gut (slippery elm is an example) and zinc is a cofactor in many reactions. Other dietary factors that can be converted by metabolism to compounds that inhibit HDAC and hypermethylation (or supplemented) are organic selenium and sulfur-based compounds (including garlic and the Allium family), indoles and sulforanes from the brassicas and polyphenols. Resveratrol has been shown to be particularly effective.[270]

Radiation damage is also a factor in generating dysregulation of these genes. Supplementing with analogues of vitamin E — tocopherols and tocotrienols have shown the ability to repair radiation-induced DNA damage.[271] Resveratrol,[272] ECGC (green tea) and curcumin are also showing promise.[273]

FERMENTED FOODS

Naturally fermented foods and beverages contain both functional and non-functional microorganisms. The functional organisms formed during food fermentation transform the compounds in food sources, enhancing the bioavailability of nutrients, and degrading toxic components and antinutritive factors. Fermentation also produces antioxidant and antimicrobial compounds, stimulates probiotic function and provides useful bioactive compounds, such as lactic acid bacteria and bifidobacteria. Health benefits of fermented foods are the synthesis of nutrients (such as B vitamins), and the prevention of cancer, cardiovascular disease, gastrointestinal disorders, allergic reactions and diabetes to name a few.[274]

While there are many fermented foods worldwide a couple are particularly worthy of mention.

Kefir

Kefir is a complex fermented dairy product created largely through the fermentation of milk by lactic acid bacteria and yeasts that exist in symbiotic association in a matrix of polysaccharides and proteins in kefir grains. It is a traditional food of the peoples of the Caucasus region. Kefir is a powerful probiotic that has antitumour, anticarcinogenic, antimicrobial and immunomodulatory activity. Kefir promotes the growth of bifidobacteria in the colon. It has been shown to exert antitumour and antiproliferative activity on a range of cancers including colon cancer and breast cancer.[275] It increases p53 expression and induces cell cycle arrest in the G1 phase in adult lymphoblastic leukaemia, inducing apoptosis of the cancer cells.[276]

Miso

Miso, a fermented soy product, has substantial research on its protective effects against a variety of cancers. The fermentation process produces compounds such as genistein and daidzein and it is these phytochemicals that have shown the greatest activity. Cancers reduced by regular ingestion of these fermented foods include breast cancer, prostate cancer, colon cancer, endometrial cancer[277] and lung cancer.[278]

ORGANIC FOODS

Food grown organically has higher levels of nutrients compared to non-organic food due to avoidance of herbicides, pesticides and other chemicals. Studies overall have shown much higher levels of minerals in organic foods and about twice the vitamin content.

One study showed that the total phenolic compounds (the anti-inflammatory flavonoids) and ascorbic acid content of various berries and corn grown by organic and sustainable agricultural methods was significantly higher, compared with those grown by conventional agricultural practices. This research also showed that freezing retained the phenolic compounds better than drying.[279]

SUMMARY OF FOODS

There are many bioactive plant substances available in fruits and vegetables such as the carotenoids, vitamins A, C and E and folate (in dark-green leafy vegetables). The substances include powerful anticancer substances such as the flavonoids and isothiocyanates found in cassava, garlic, onions, and purple, red and black fruits and vegetables — blueberries, eggplant, red cabbage, beetroot, dark-green vegetables, dark-yellow-orange vegetables. The cabbage family — broccoli, Brussels sprouts, cauliflower — are high in protective substances such as isothiocyanates, indoles and sulforane. Organic vegetable juices, drunk on a daily basis are an excellent way of consuming concentrated nutrients and antioxidants. The commonly prescribed ones are carrot, celery and beetroot (often with a little ginger root), green vegetable juices with mint for increased detoxification. *Chlorella* (algae) can be added to this as well for a real detoxification boost.

If a vegan diet is important, make sure the super food spirulina is eaten as well for the added protein and nutrients such as vitamin B_{12} (hard to get in vegan diets). Miso and tempeh (B_{12} is formed from a fermentation process) are also good sources of this critical nutrient. Vegans should have their zinc, iron and vitamin B_{12} levels checked annually as these are the nutrients most likely to be deficient.

Foods that are high in polysaccharides have been shown to enhance immune function. Mushrooms (shiitake, reishi, etc.) and aloe vera (drinking) gel are two on which much research has been conducted with positive results.

Eating at least five servings of vegetables and two servings of fruit per day is an excellent and tasty way to maintain health (a single serving is 100 g), and freshly ground flaxseeds for phyto-oestrogens and essential fatty acids could be included. Supplement with probiotics (e.g. yoghurt, kefir) to improve digestive function, so the nutrients in the food will be digested and absorbed, and therefore metabolised correctly. To feed the correct bowel bacteria, eat foods high in inulin such as Jerusalem artichoke, asparagus, garlic, leeks and onions, and what are today considered herbs (some would say weeds) chicory root and dandelion root and leaves. Chicory (the highest source) and dandelion roots were traditional casserole vegetables. The Australian bush food, the yam daisy or murnong, is also high in inulin. Having the correct bowel bacteria grows some of the critical B vitamins such as folic acid and B_{12}. Cooking will taste better for using lots of garlic, onions, ginger and turmeric. If the patient reacts adversely to garlic and onions, this is an indication that the sulfation pathway (the main detoxification pathway) in the liver is not functioning correctly and will need to be supported with nutrients and herbal medicines. Some salt is often necessary so use small amounts of unprocessed Celtic or macrobiotic sea salt which has a similar electrolyte profile to human blood, and therefore confers some health benefits.

Overall a diet that is protective against all cancers is one that is high in vegetables (particularly juiced) and low in fruit (be careful of sugars). It is also important to eat organic high-fibre foods (ideally consuming 30–35 g fibre per day), consume small amounts of animal (saturated) fat with high essential fatty acids, especially the omega-3 fatty acids. Balancing the ratio of essential fatty acids is increasingly important as many people have high levels of omega-6 fatty acids (from highly processed omega-6 oils such as safflower and sunflower oils). Higher levels of omega-6 in relation to omega-3 fatty acids are known to trigger an inflammatory response. The total fat intake should be less than 30% of kilojoules eaten. Extra virgin olive oil is a fat that has sustained the health of the Mediterranean people for millennia. It contains an omega-9 fatty acid and there is a place for it in healthy diets. For variety, organic cold-pressed macadamia oil, coconut oil and tea (seed) oil can also be beneficial in moderate doses, as these oils are high in antioxidants. They are also suitable for cooking (at medium temperatures), in preference to olive oil which has a low smoke point.

It is important to eat an adequate but lowish kilojoule diet — slightly less food per day correlates with increased longevity and less degenerative disease — avoid sugars and refined foods and minimise alcohol.[280]

Doses: folic acid and B_{12}. A placebo-controlled study with a dose-response suggests that based on the lymphocyte index, a level of 700 micrograms/day for folic acid and 700 micrograms/day for vitamin B_{12} improves genomic stability.[281]

NUTRITIONAL MEDICINE (SUPPLEMENTATION)

There are various nutrient deficiencies that have been shown to increase the risk of cancer growth. These are low levels of potassium, low magnesium and high sodium and low levels of selenium (and/or glutathione).[282] Zinc is important in accurate genetic copying of DNA and must be adequate for health. To improve cell membrane fluidity (permeability), vitamins A, C, E, beta-carotene, and the minerals selenium, organic germanium and magnesium are critically important.

It is important to reduce the exposure to excess oxidation and inflammation to reduce the risk of carcinogenesis. Exposure to chemicals such as those found in personal hygiene products, plastics, cleaning products and non-organic foods should be avoided as chemicals (and their residues) interfere with the optimal functioning of body systems. Eat organic food, remove household chemicals, reduce environmental chemicals, be aware of electromagnetic radiation (e.g. mobile phones and computers), avoid drinking from plastic bottles and so on.

Detoxification of the liver needs to be improved. The sulfation pathways in the liver, which are the major detoxification pathways, are also the pathways for correct oestrogen metabolism. It has been shown that increasing chemical exposure reduces the liver's ability to metabolise oestrogen correctly, with the result that (worldwide) humans are becoming increasingly 'oestrogenised', leading in turn to the increasing incidence of oestrogen-based cancers such as breast cancer.[283] Poor dietary habits and low nutrients exacerbate poor detoxification and compromise liver function even further.

Issues

Digestion and absorption are major issues: 70% of our immune function is in the digestive system as this is where our greatest environmental challenges occur. By eating food (foreign to the body), the digestive system is the organ with the greatest exposure to the external environment and must be functioning optimally to digest and absorb the required nutrients. The integrity of the gut-associated lymphoid tissues (GALT) is critical for immunity.

- Sugar consumption can be a significant dietary issue, so avoiding refined sugars is a common theme in cancer prevention.
- Improve cellular metabolism, respiration and regulate the energy source to promote healthy cells. Improve oxygenation, reduce oxidation and reduce toxicity.
- Regulate hormonal balance — for example, phyto-oestrogens soy (*Glycine max*), red clover (*Trifolium pratense*) and flaxseed (*Linum usitatissimum*). Many plants contain the balancing phyto-oestrogens
- Reduce inflammation — flavonoids, essential fatty acids.

Regulating the inflammatory process is critical in managing and improving health. There are many pathways that can be manipulated to do this. The main plant components that inhibit inflammation are the flavonoids such as quercetin, hesperidin and rutin. Nutrients such as zinc, vitamins A, C, E and B_6 and the essential fatty acids GLA, EPA and DHA are the food components regulating the inflammatory response. Many herbal plants have a high flavonoid content, for example *Ginkgo biloba, Zingiber officinalis, Curcuma longa, Tanacetum parthenium* and *Filipendula ulmaria.*

The balance of omega-6:omega-3 fatty acids (+DHA) is crucial in the management of inflammation. Today we consume excess omega-6 fatty acids but we have trouble metabolising them — and this excess is triggering increased inflammation. Consuming large amounts of polyunsaturated fatty acids is not necessarily healthy.

For most of humanity's existence prior to agriculture, the omega-6:omega-3 ratio would have been 1:1 to 3:1; today it is more likely to be 10:1 or higher. High dietary omega-6:omega-3 ratios are associated with increased risk for cardiovascular disease, some types of cancer, and tend to exacerbate many inflammatory responses.[284]

Doses

The general therapeutic dosage of fish oils for healthy persons for preventive purposes is 3000 mg per day (supplying 540 mg of EPA and 360 mg of DHA). The therapeutic dosage of fish oils for various conditions is generally higher and clinical trials have used doses of up to 34 000 mg per day. Dosages of 5000–15 000 mg per day are more commonly used.[285]

The World Health Organization and governmental health agencies of several countries recommend consuming 300–500 mg of total EPA plus DHA per day.

It is possible to obtain useful quantities of the active ingredients of fish oils, that is docosahexaenoic acid (DHA) and eicosapentaenoic acid (EPA), by including oily fish in the diet. The highest quantities of DHA and EPA are found in: herring (1600 mg DHA/EPA per 100 g), wild salmon (1200 mg DHA/EPA per 100 g), bluefish (1200 mg DHA/EPA per 100 g), tuna (500 mg DHA/EPA per 100 g), and cod (300 mg DHA/EPA per 100 g). Cod liver oil supplements contain approximately 33 mg of EPA and 30 mg DHA per mL. Due to concerns with pollution in the water and risk of mercury toxicity, it is often preferred to supplement for purity of active constituents. If this is chosen, careful selection of product is essential.

Specific nutrients

When prescribing the doses recommended, many of these are considerably higher than Australian Government recommendations. The doses for optimal nutrition supporting cancer are recommended.

ANTIOXIDANTS

Antioxidants are critically important in the maintenance of good immune function and protection against cancer. Excess oxidative stress damages immunity by activating various inflammatory chemicals such as cytokines, and high levels of free radicals and nitric oxide (NO) damage cellular macromolecules, such as lipids, proteins and DNA. Antioxidant supplementation reverses many immune deficiencies (including cancer), resulting in greater numbers of total lymphocytes and T-cells, increased NK cell activity, decreased lipid peroxidation and decreased inflammation.[286] The main antioxidant nutrients (both water soluble and fat soluble) are vitamins A, C D, E, coenzyme Q10 (ubiquinol), and the minerals selenium and zinc.

Oxidative stress is induced by a wide range of environmental factors including UV stress, pathogen invasion, allergies, environmental chemicals and oxygen shortage. Generation of reactive oxygen species (ROS) is characteristic of hypoxia. Of the ROS, hydrogen peroxide and the superoxide radical are both produced in a number of cellular reactions, and by various enzymes such as lipoxygenases, peroxidases, nicotinamide adenine dinucleotide phosphate (NADPH) oxidase and xanthine oxidase. The main cellular components susceptible to damage by free radicals are lipids (peroxidation of unsaturated fatty acids in membranes), proteins (denatured), carbohydrates and nucleic acids.

The formation of ROS is prevented by an antioxidant system with low molecular mass antioxidants (ascorbic acid, glutathione, tocopherols), enzymes regenerating the reduced forms of antioxidants, and ROS-interacting enzymes such as superoxide dismutase (SOD), peroxidases and catalases. In plant tissues many phenolic compounds (in addition to tocopherols) are potential antioxidants. Flavonoids, tannins and lignin precursors may work as ROS-scavenging compounds. Antioxidants act as a cooperative network, employing a series of interlocking reactions.[287]

VITAMIN A

Retinoids are vitamin A derivatives that are critical in the regulation of several physiological and pathological processes, including immune function and cancer development. They function as biological response modifiers. Evidence has been accumulated indicating that retinoids may exert beneficial effects in both immune-mediated disorders and tumours. In regard to cancer, retinoids directly target neoplastic cells by inducing differentiation, inhibiting cell growth or promoting apoptosis and being antiproliferative.[288] Retinoids are effective chemotherapeutic agents against skin, head, neck and liver cancers and are particularly effective against haemotological cancers.

Dose

Vitamin A inhibits the proliferation of many types of cancer cells. The recommended dosage of vitamin A for cancer patients is 100 000–300 000 IU per day. Thyroid cancer patients should not use supplemental vitamin A. This is far above the Australian Government recommendation of 2500 IU per day. Taking it as cod liver oil (naturally sourced), and zinc as a component retinol binding protein to transport vitamin A out of the liver will reduce the toxicity a little. In Australia a more realistic dose would be 25 000 IU.[289]

VITAMIN C

Vitamin C has been researched for many years and is well known as a nutritional supplement with antioxidant properties. In the research, vitamin C inhibited the expression of two categories of genes necessary for cell cycle progression, and was particularly useful in the S phase arrest of proliferative normal and tumour cells. Highest concentrations of vitamin C led to necrotic cell death and inhibited tumour regression. It has antiproliferative activity, more so at the elevated concentrations that could be obtained using IV injections.[290]

Dose

Avoid straight calcium ascorbate as it seems to alter calcium:magnesium balance, especially in the doses required here. Orally, mixed ascorbates or sodium ascorbate are better and doses vary but vitamin C needs to be taken 4 hourly to keep blood levels up. The standard dose is 1 teaspoon (1–2.5 g total vitamin C) powder/4 times per day. Ideally 18 g per day is recommended orally, but this may still not produce the optimal dose for the condition. IV dose is 30 g/3 times per week (if tolerated), but this must be supplemented by the oral dose in the intervening days. Ideally 50–100 g dose will give optimal blood levels. At concentrations above 1000 μmol/L, vitamin C is toxic to some cancer cells but not to normal cells in vitro.[291]

VITAMIN D

Vitamin D plays a major role in activating T-cells. Vitamin D receptors form the T-cell signalling device that enables T-cells to recognise a foreign pathogen and mobilise to fight it. It is important in regulating inflammation and infection. Calcitriol, the hormonal form of vitamin D, potentiates the activity of common anticancer drugs and the activity of the immune system, especially in breast cancer and prostate cancer.[292] Vitamin D reduces the reactive oxygen species (ROS), the major compounds involved in oxidation and inflammation.[293] Research shows that up to 86% of some population groups in Australia are vitamin D deficient (e.g. the elderly in residential care; see Table 12.9).[294]

Dose

The dosage of vitamin D needs to be 1500 IU per day but can be up to 3000 IU per day if bimonthly monitoring of blood levels is being undertaken to ensure no toxicity.[295]

VITAMIN E

Vitamin E is a major fat-soluble antioxidant. While there has been some debate about its effects with radiotherapy, there is extensive research for immune improvement, and for positive outcomes when prescribed in conjunction with chemotherapy. Vitamin E succinate (alpha-tocopherol succinate) has generated much interest as an adjunctive cancer therapy. It demonstrated growth inhibition of human B-cell lymphoma and oestrogen receptor-negative breast cancer cell lines in vitro. Vitamin E arrested tumour cells in the G_1 phase of the cell cycle, leading to apoptosis.[296] Vitamin E (200 mg daily), given together with 18 g/day omega-3 fatty acids from fish oil, prolonged the survival in patients with generalised malignancy in a randomised controlled trial. Improvement in T-helper/suppressor ratio was also noted with treatment.[297] The addition of vitamin E to either 5-fluorouracil or doxorubicin enhances the effect of these agents on human colon cancer cells.[298] Vitamin E (mixed tocopherols and tocotrienols) has been shown to reduce and help repair DNA damage from radiation in patients with the *BRAC1* and *BRAC2* genes.[299]

Dose

Vitamin E (alpha-tocopheryl) succinate is the preferred form and the dose recommended is 400–800 IU per day although much higher doses appear to be safe.[300]

ZINC

Zinc[301] is important because it affects multiple aspects of the immune system. Loss of zinc from biological membranes increases their susceptibility to oxidative damage and impairs their functioning. Zinc maintains a healthy immune system and helps the body to fight off a range of infections and protects against cancer. It specifically inhibits the growth of a range of viruses including Epstein-Barr virus as it complexes with proteins on critical nerve endings and surface proteins of viruses and interrupts nerve impulses, thus blocking the viruses from attaching to the cells. Zinc deficiency, particularly in the elderly, leads to depressed immunity with significantly increased susceptibility to cancer and an increase in morbidity and mortality.[302] Zinc protects against DNA damage. Zinc is also critical for neuropsychological functions and for normalising hormonal balance in both men and women. Up to 25% of the world's population may be deficient in zinc with varying levels found around the world, based on soil constituents, diet and environmental impact.[303]

Dose

Optimal daily allowance for zinc is 15–50 mg per day. It is better absorbed taken on an empty stomach but can make people feel nauseated so is best taken just before bed. When supplementing with zinc long term, support this with 10% copper.[304]

SELENIUM

Selenium is a crucial element in a number of central antioxidative systems. Its potential role in cancer has three aspects — prevention, improvement of prognosis in established disease, and as an adjuvant to conventional cancer therapy to reduce side effects.[305] Selenium has been shown to possess cancer-preventive activity in both animal models and humans, and it functions through various mechanisms. Selenium metabolites inhibit key attributes (proliferation, survival and matrix degradation) of endothelial cells critical for angiogenesis.[306] Selenoproteins inhibit the initiation phase of carcinogenesis, altering genes in a manner that leads to inhibition of cell proliferation and induction of apoptosis. The anticarcinogenic mechanisms of selenium compounds include effects on gene expression, DNA damage and repair, signalling pathways, regulation of cell cycle and apoptosis, prevention of metastases and angiogenesis. Among the naturally occurring organoselenium compounds, Se-methylselenocysteine is considered more effective than the more extensively studied forms, such as selenomethionine and sodium selenite.[307]

Dose

For preventive medicine, 200 micrograms/day selenium treatment has been shown to decrease total cancer incidence by a statistically significant 25%,[308] but for persons already diagnosed with cancer 400 micrograms was a more appropriate dose. Up to 400 micrograms per day has been prescribed for cancer patients, with no toxicity, although this would need to be monitored closely by a doctor. This dose is well above the Australian Government RDA of 200 micrograms per day.

THE ANTIOXIDANT DEBATE

There has been an ongoing heated debate for some years on the potential adverse effects of antioxidants and herbs prescribed for patients on chemotherapy and/or radiotherapy and there has been significant research on this issue.

There is some research that suggests antioxidants are best avoided concurrently with chemotherapy agents as chemotherapy employs a free radical mechanism to elicit its response. However, an adjunctive treatment can offer great promise in cancer therapy, as much published research indicates the cautious and judicious use of a number of antioxidants can be helpful in the treatment of cancer; both as sole agents and as adjuncts to standard radiation and chemotherapy protocols.[309]

It has been suggested that antioxidants might interfere with the oxidative mechanisms of alkylating agents as these drugs create substantial DNA damage, resulting in cell necrosis. The evidence, however, refutes this, as it indicates that a sizeable amount of chemotherapy damage is by different mechanisms which trigger apoptosis or cell death. Given this evidence, the argument that antioxidants are likely to interfere with most chemotherapy is too simplistic and probably untrue. Interactions between antioxidants and chemotherapeutics cannot be predicted solely on the basis of presumed mechanisms of action. Also many chemotherapeutic agents do not act via an oxidative mechanism (for example, 5-fluorouracil or tamoxifen).

A recent study was conducted on small-cell lung cancer in humans using a combination chemotherapy of cyclophosphamide, adriamycin (doxorubicin) and vincristine with radiation and a combination of antioxidants, vitamins, trace elements and fatty acids. The conclusion was 'antioxidant treatment, in combination with chemotherapy and irradiation, prolonged the survival time of patients' compared with expected outcome without the composite oral therapy.[310]

There is also a large body of evidence showing a positive effect of antioxidants in the period immediately following chemotherapy administration resulting in a higher percentage of successful outcomes.[309]

The research has highlighted what can be otherwise a difficult topic in the circumstances of the life-threatening nature of the disease. We all want our patients to get well in the best way possible. Antioxidants also reduce the side effects of chemotherapy, improve the quality of life of the patient and reduce the chance of recurrence. Selected antioxidants at specific doses also have cancer preventive effects if taken regularly.

HERBAL MEDICINE

Allopathic medicine uses plant derivatives. However, it is the plant alkaloids that have received the most attention, as these have powerful effects in the human body and are therefore used as forms of chemotherapy; for example, the vinca alkaloids (vincristine and vinblastine) from the periwinkle (*Catharanthus rosea*) and taxanes from the bark of the Pacific yew tree (*Taxus brevifolia*). Plant alkaloids are mitotic inhibitors. They can stop mitosis or inhibit enzymes for making proteins needed for reproduction of the cell. They are cell cycle specific and work during the M phase of the cell cycle.

But whether to use herbal (plant) medicines in combination with chemotherapy provokes a debate similar to that of the combination of antioxidants and chemotherapy or radiotherapy.[311]

Korean ginseng (*Panax ginseng*) has been extensively studied in Asia with approximately 1500 studies done, 500 on the pharmacological properties. Overall the research shows that Korean ginseng is an excellent adaptogen for the elderly, for debility and to enhance the body's capacity to cope with stress.

Large case-control studies in Korea found an inverse association of cancer and ginseng consumption, with the relative risk of cancer being 50% less in ginseng users. The risk profile showed a clear dose response relationship over time and with the particular type of ginseng (red ginseng powder). There was also a preventive effect after 1 year.

Concurrent use of *Panax ginseng* has been shown to improve outcomes with both chemotherapy and radiotherapy.[312] Ginsengosides have been shown to induce differentiation of cancer cells (only undifferentiated cells can spread), by reducing inflammation through inhibiting COX-2 expression, by upregulating transcription of superoxide dismutase and catalase (antioxidants), inducing the process of apoptosis, reducing the overexpression of growth factors, decreasing the expression of oncogenes, and inhibiting the process of proliferation by decreasing angiogenesis and cell adhesion (as effective as fluorouracil). Ginseng is also known as an immune-modulator as it lowers cortisol levels under stress and activates T-cells.[313]

Eleutherococcus senticosus (Siberian ginseng) and other ginsengs have similar properties.

Herbal medicines and multidrug resistance

There is substantial research being conducted on the inhibition of P-glycoprotein (P-gp) transporters and the development (or otherwise) of multidrug resistance (MDR) — the bane of chemotherapy. P-gp expression triggers cells to start producing increasing numbers of metabolic pumps to expel toxins from the cells, particularly chemotherapy drugs. Therefore inducers of P-gp are unfavourable to the outcomes, and inhibitors of P-gp are favourable. Multidrug resistance to chemotherapy caused by increased P-gp expression is common in cancer cell lines. The individual expression of P-gp can vary eightfold and is encoded by various genes; for example, the *MDR1* gene in breast cancer. Women who express the *MDR1* gene (and therefore higher levels of P-gp) are three times more likely to fail to respond to chemotherapy by developing multidrug resistance. Agents that induce P-gp transporters generate a poor response to chemotherapy, therefore agents that inhibit this activity (inhibit P-gp expression) are potentially useful in improving outcomes.[314]

There has been significant research on P-gp transporters and the effect of herbal medicines in inhibiting these. The herbs that inhibit P-gp expression may therefore have a role in reducing the risk of chemotherapy resistance, potentially leading to more effective therapies with less toxicity. Herbs (and nutrients) that inhibit P-gp include: *Curcuma longa* (turmeric), quercetin, *Camellia sinensis* (green tea), resveratrol (from grape skins), *Silybum marianum* (St Mary's thistle), and the berberine-containing herbs — *Hydrastis canadensis* (goldenseal), *Coptis chinensis* (goldthread). P-gp transport inhibitors are also found in grapefruit juice, apple juice, *Rosmarinus officinalis* (rosemary extract) and genistein (from soy).

By the same token, herbs that induce P-gp (such as *Hypericum perforatum* (St John's wort)) should be avoided.

Hypericum has been found to cause the increased clearance of irinotecan (and possibly paclitaxel and tamoxifen). Best practice therefore indicates that it is contraindicated for administration to patients who are undergoing chemotherapy.[315] Also avoid grapefruit juice while on chemotherapy with paclitaxel or tamoxifen as this can alter the dosage (through liver metabolism (3A4) pathways).

P53 SUPPRESSOR GENE

Agents that increase the expression of the *p53* tumour suppressor gene will improve outcomes in patients. *p53* is a major trigger for apoptosis and is inhibited in oncogenesis. The *p53* gene regulates genes important to the cells' response to chemotherapy, largely through the multidrug resistance gene (*MDR1*) expression in tumours. *MDR1* has also been shown to inactivate the *p53* tumour suppressor gene. The loss of functioning *p53* can reduce the body's ability to resist the growth of tumours (e.g. tamoxifen) and the loss of functional *p53* may induce P-gp expression and increase the development of multidrug resistance.

Research shows promise with herbal medicines that can inhibit these P-gp transporters and that can increase the activity of the *p53* gene. Herbs that increase *p53* and therefore apoptosis include: *Camellia sinensis* (green tea),[316] *Centella asiatica* (gotu kola),[317] *Glycyrrhiza glabra* (liquorice root), *Terminalia arjuna, Poria cocos* (mushroom polysaccharides),[318] *Artemesia annua* (Chinese wormwood), iscador (mistletoe preparation) and ginsengs.

COX (PROSTAGLANDIN) PATHWAYS

Research shows that substances that inhibit the COX pathways not only reduce inflammation but also may play a role in reducing P-gp expression. COX-2 inhibitors reduce inflammation and aromatase (for oestrogen receptor tumours). Grape seed, *Zingiber officinale* (ginger), *Allium sativum* (garlic), *Curcuma longa* (turmeric) and the salicylate containing herbs such as *Filipendula officinalis* (meadowsweet) and *Salix alba* (white willow) bark are effective at inhibiting these pathways. Specific COX-2 inhibitors are *Curcuma longa* (turmeric), ginseng, *Camellia sinensis* (green tea), as well as fish oils, quercetin and genistein (soy).[319]

CAMELLIA SINENSIS (GREEN TEA)

Catechins (in green tea) (epigallocatechin gallate (EGCG)) are powerful antioxidants and anti-inflammatories that activate the *p53* tumour suppressor gene. Green tea can be drunk along with chemotherapy and has synergistic activity. Green tea acts at different levels and via different mechanisms than chemotherapy. Green tea inhibits the COX-2 inflammatory pathways, promotes cell cycle arrest and increases apoptosis (activates *p53*). It disables the multiresistant pumps and is a major antioxidant.

CURCUMA LONGA (TURMERIC)

Apart from its activity as a P-gp inhibitor, it has been shown that curcumin works by way of another mechanism unrelated to P-gp. Some tumours produce high levels of glutathione S-transferase (GST), an antioxidant enzyme that helps protect the cells from oxidative injury by chemotherapy agents. Curcumin appears to inhibit this enzyme in vitro in cancer cells, potentiating the effects of the chemotherapy drug doxorubicin, even when P-gp levels are high. Compared with several other GST inhibitors (in vitro) in neoplastic cells, curcumin was by far the strongest inhibitor. Resistance to chemotherapy drugs is commonly associated with elevations in cellular levels of the inflammatory mediator nuclear factor kappaB (NFκB), a process that is inhibited by curcumin, reducing drug resistance in cancer cells.[320]

Curcuma plays many roles in improving the health of the person undergoing treatment for cancer. It reduces P-gp transporters, reduces MDR, reduces toxicity in the liver, as well as being antioxidant and anti-inflammatory through several pathways including COX-2.[321]

Integrated treatment: chemotherapy, nutrients and herbal medicines[322]

MELATONIN

Melatonin protects against many of the toxic effects of chemotherapy. Melatonin also helps with sleep, is an antidepressant, regulates oestrogen receptors and is a powerful antioxidant. Melatonin increases *p53* expression and modifies the inflammatory cytokines.[323]

Dose: Melatonin may only be prescribed in Australia by a registered medical practitioner, with a daily dose of 2 mg/day; however, recommended doses for chemotherapy adjuvant prescriptions are between 3 and 40 mg/day. It is best taken after the sun has set. Optimal dosage is achieved once the patient experiences a quality night's sleep.[324]

VITAMIN C

Vitamin C reverses vincristine resistance and improves the effectiveness of adriamycin, cisplatin, doxorubicin and paclitaxel (paclitaxel).[325]

QUERCETIN

Quercetin has been shown to inhibit adriamycin resistance in oestrogen receptor negative breast cancer and to potentiate the action of many chemotherapeutic drugs, while reducing side effects.

Dose: 2000 mg per day in divided doses, taken with bromelain to improve digestion.

GLUTATHIONE (AND SELENIUM)

Glutathione (and selenium) reduce the neurotoxicity, nephrotoxicity and myelosuppression of cisplatin and reduce damage to the brain, the kidneys and bone marrow.[326]

AGED GARLIC (*ALLIUM SATIVUM*)

Aged garlic (*Allium sativum*) protects the liver with methotrexate (along with folic acid).

CENTELLA ASIATICA (GOTU KOLA)

Centella asiatica (gotu kola) reduces chemotherapy resistance with vincristine and vinblastine.

CRATEGUS MONOGYNA (HAWTHORN) AND COENZYME Q10

Crategus monogyna (hawthorn) and coenzyme Q10 reduce heart damage from the side effects of herceptin and doxorubicin.

Dose of coenzyme Q10: 300–400 mg per day with food.[327]

INDOLES (BRASSICA FAMILY)

Indoles (brassica family) inhibit P-glycoprotein activity by inhibiting the binding specifically of doxorubicin and vinblastine, making these more effective. They also improve oestrogen metabolism and can enhance the oestrogen blocking effects of tamoxifen.

RHODIOLA ROSEA (RHODIOLA)

Rhodiola rosea protects the liver with adriamycin.

ROSMARINUS OFFICINALUS (ROSEMARY)

Rosmarinus officinalus reduces resistance to a broad range of compounds by increasing the intracellular accumulation of drugs such as doxorubicin, vinblastine (P-gp inhibitor). It also has antioxidant properties and is liver and brain protective.

WITHANIA SOMNIFERA (WITHANIA)

Withania somnifera reduces the leucopenia induced by cyclophosphamide and has an immunopotentiating and myeloprotective effect.

ASTRAGALUS MEMBRANACEUS AND PLATINUM-BASED CHEMOTHERAPY

A meta-analysis of 34 randomised studies was conducted involving 2815 patients. When taking a traditional *Astragalus* formula, 12 studies showed reduced risk of death at 12 months, 30 studies reported improved tumour response, two studies showed reduced risk of death at 24 months.

In four studies with 257 patients, a preparation of *Panax ginseng, Astragalus membranaceus, Eleutherococcus senticosus* and *Mylabirs cichoi* stabilised or improved patient performance. The conclusion from this research was that: '*Astragalus*-based Chinese herbal medicine may increase effectiveness of platinum-based chemotherapy when combined with chemotherapy'. The researchers found evidence that *Astragalus*-based Chinese herbal medicine may increase the effectiveness (by improving survival, tumour response and performance status) and reduce the toxicity of standard platinum-based chemotherapy for advanced non-small-cell lung cancer. *Astragalus* also potentiates therapeutic activity in chemotherapy (mitomycin, cisplatin, cyclophosphamide, fluorouracil) and radiotherapy.[328]

LIFESTYLE RECOMMENDATIONS

Reduce chemicals in the immediate environment

There are many ways to reduce chemicals in the immediate environment and awareness of where the chemicals are and how contact with them is made — and avoiding that contact as much as possible — is important. Eating organic or biodynamic food helps; filtering tap water (can add colloidal minerals to replace the minerals needed), or drinking rainwater (not in the middle of the city unless the tank has a diverter and it is well filtered). Use 'safe' cleaning materials such as the old favourites — bicarbonate of soda, white vinegar. A variety of environmentally sound 'mitts' that do not require chemicals at all for cleaning are also available.

Avoid pharmaceuticals when safe to do so (and get second opinions when they are prescribed as there are often alternatives). Avoid recreational drugs. Only use chemical-free cosmetics and creams — emu oil, rosehip oil and vitamin E oil make great moisturisers without the additional chemicals.

Check out occupational hazards and environmental hazards. It can be difficult to change occupation but it may be possible to minimise the exposure.

Sun exposure

Sun exposure for 20 minutes per day without sunglasses and sunscreen is best to assist with vitamin D absorption. Small doses of sunlight frequently are important — half an hour on face, arms and legs is the minimum, three times per week — or take a vitamin D supplement regularly. Sleep issues can be assisted with regular sunlight exposure to optimise circadian rhythm and melatonin secretion.

CASE STUDY

OVERVIEW

BS, a 3-year-old male presented accompanied by his mother. He had been breastfed for 14 months. The birth involved a long labour, and as the baby went into fetal distress, the mother had a Caesarean section. All his vaccinations were up to date including chickenpox and meningococcal disease.

He appeared a normal baby initially but started to develop a few mild symptoms such as speech delay, although this is improving, and he has a moderate stutter. At 12 months his right eye used to turn, but that has been fixed with an eye patch.

At 2 years old he had a severe viral infection with high temperatures and febrile convulsions for 4 to 5 days. One month later, his temperature rose, he started twitching and he had several seizures. Medically it was thought that he had brain inflammation. As the seizures did not improve he was referred to a neurologist.

A CT scan was performed that showed a posterior fossa brain tumour which was confirmed by MRI. This was diagnosed as an astrocytoma. The tumour was surgically removed but because of its position, not all of it could be removed.

Two weeks after surgery he had improved, but was still getting seizures every couple of days. He was prescribed carbamazepine 7 mL (140 mg b.i.d.).

The family refused chemotherapy and radiotherapy as treatment and decided to work with both his neurologist

CASE STUDY CONTINUED

(watchful waiting and regular testing) and to use complementary therapies.

Six months later another MRI was performed and some of the tumour was still visible.

As he had no further seizure activity and was lethargic, the carbamazepine dose was dropped to 2 mL. No further seizure activity was noted at this lower dose and his energy improved.

DIETARY

As his mother had already conducted her own research on diet and was very interested in nutrition, his diet was reasonably good for a child of his age.

Breakfast: semolina with eggs, almonds and goat's milk, cinnamon and brown sugar (1 teaspoon)
Morning snack: organic bread and butter, nuts
Lunch: goat's milk yoghurt, vegetable juice diluted, avocado, garlic and lemon juice
Dinner: vegetables, flaxseed oil with 2-minute noodles
Snacks: sultanas, chips home made with olive oil
Supplements: brewer's yeast, cod liver oil
Water: filtered
Other: organic food generally.

CLINICAL EXAMINATION

Weight: 13 kg
Height: 87 cm

He appeared a normal child, if quiet for his age.

LABORATORY INVESTIGATIONS

Blood tests (FBC, ESR) essentially normal
Blood group: O +ve

MEDICATIONS

Carbamazepine (carbamazepine) 2 mL

TREATMENT PROTOCOL

INITIAL APPOINTMENT

At the initial consultation, it was arranged for the boy to have a live blood analysis and a clot retraction test. These give an overall picture of the functional state of the body, can detect some pathogenic bacteria and have a cancer marker. In his case the marker was 1½ (out of a possible 4), indicating that the tumour was still relatively localised but he was at risk if it increased at all. He also showed a deficiency of glutathione (selenium deficiency). There was also evidence of inflammation, some lymphatic involvement and issues with digestion.

HERBAL MEDICINE

Herbal medicine	Ratio	Quantity	Rationale
Ginkgo biloba	1:2	25 mL glycetract	Promotes peripheral vasodilation, antioxidant, improves cerebral metabolism, reduces hypoxia, anti-inflammatory
Bacopa monnieri	1:2	25 mL glycetract	Anticonvulsant, improves memory and learning, antioxidant, adaptogenic
Melissa officinalis	1:2	25 mL glycetract	Spasmolytic, sedative, improves memory and concentration, digestive
Centella asiatica	1:2	25 mL glycetract	Cognitive enhancing and potent antioxidant for the central nervous system, adaptogenic, increases brain glutathione levels, digestive
Total: 100 mL			

Dose: 2 drops b.i.d. initially then gradually increase to 10 drops b.i.d. if no adverse reaction.

NUTRITIONAL MEDICINE

Dietary

Brain tumours of nervous system origin respond better to a diet that is more ketogenic[329] (as does epilepsy)[330] so his mother was advised that a higher fat and protein diet with small oily deep sea fish, nuts, organic eggs and flaxseed oil would be more appropriate. This also fitted with the blood type dietary principles as he was O positive, a blood group that generally requires more concentrated protein. It was suggested he avoid wheat as gluten fragments can trigger an inflammatory response in the gut and also cross blood–brain barrier.[331] He was already avoiding cow's milk and had been having goat's or sheep's milk yoghurt.

Supplemental

Vitamin C powder ⅛ tsp b.i.d.
Selenium drops (10 micrograms/drop) 1 drop b.i.d.
Concentrated fish oils liquid 5 mL b.i.d. with lecithin granules added to his breakfast
Slippery elm powder 1.25 g in water
Probiotic powder (children's formula)
Children's multivitamin 1 tablet/d
Epsom salts baths for relaxation and detoxifying

FOLLOW-UP

As his symptoms were relatively well controlled, the most obvious improvement was in his socialisation at preschool. He did not like all the supplements so his mother used to hide these in various foods such as smoothies, muesli, etc. His LBA and CRT results improved dramatically with the staging going down to ½.

After 12 months his mother stopped the carbamazepine, under medical supervision, and he has had no recurrence of the seizures for the last 6 years. He is still taking the herbs, although now they are a decoction of dried herbs. The formula has changed a little depending on his LBA and CRT results. From the initial testing, his selenium levels have normalised; however, low-dose supplementation is continuing

CASE STUDY CONTINUED

as a preventive. His levels of inflammation have reduced, his lymphatic and digestive systems are functioning normally. He has grown significantly and is doing well at school and now loves reading. His latest CRT result shows that the cancer marker has disappeared (previously it was ½ for several years). His LBA showed poor bile production so extra lecithin has been added to his diet, with the recommendation that he take his fish oil liquid at the same time.

He has been having annual MRIs to monitor the tumour. The parents have refused any further CT scans because of the potential radiation levels. The tumour has been shrinking slowly and for the last 2 years there has been no sign of it at all. The neurologist is not convinced, however, and says maybe it is still there, she 'just can't see it'. However, his mother is keeping him on a regular regimen of supplements including the fish oils, the herbal mixtures, selenium drops (3 drops b.i.d.) and vitamin C (500 mg b.i.d.). She adds olive leaf extract (3 mL b.i.d.) over the cold and flu season and his infection rate is very low. He is not taking any pharmaceutical medication. As his parents are vegetarian, it has been difficult to keep the protein levels higher, but they are aware of this and his condition has improved dramatically.

REFERENCES

[1] Parkin J, Cohen B. An overview of the immune system. Lancet 2001;357(9270):1777–89.
[2] Tortora GJ, Grabowski SR. Principles of anatomy and physiology. 9th ed. Biological Textbooks, Wiley; 2000.
[3] Mallick A, Bodenham AR. Disorders of the lymph circulation: their relevance to anaesthesia and intensive care. Br J Anaesth 2003;91(2):265–72.
[4] Anastasiadis K, Ratnutunga C. The thymus gland diagnosis and surgical management. Berlin Heidelberg: Springer-Verlag; 2007.
[5] Mebius RE, Kraal G. Structure and function of the spleen. Nat Rev Immunol 2005;5(8):606–16.
[6] Cesta MF. Normal structure, function, and histology of the spleen. Toxicol Pathol 2006;34(5):455–65.
[7] Gilden DH, Mahalingam R, Cohrs RJ, et al. Herpesvirus infections of the nervous system. Nat Clin Pract Neurol 2007;3(2):82–94.
[8] Bennett NJ, Steel RW Pediatric mononucleosis and Epstein-Barr virus infection. Medscape 2 November 2017.
[9] Dasco C. Epstein-Barr virus infection office practice of neurology. 2nd ed. USA: Elsevier; 2003. p. 481–2.
[10] Pender MP. Preventing and curing multiple sclerosis by controlling Epstein-Barr virus infection. Autoimmun Rev 2009;8(7):563–8.
[11] Mocarski ES, Courcelle CT. Cytomegalovirus and their replication. In: Knipe D, Howley P, editors. Fields virology. Philadelphia: Lippincott, Williams and Wilkins; 2001. p. 2629–73.
[12] Stagno S, Britt W. Cytomegalovirus infections, infectious diseases of the foetus and newborn infant. 6th ed. USA: Saunders; 2006. p. 739–81.
[13] Landolfo S, Gariglio M, Gribaudo G, et al. The human cytomegalovirus. Pharmacol Ther 2003;98(3):269–97.
[14] Revello M, Gerna G. Pathogenesis and prenatal diagnosis of human cytomegalovirus infection. J Clin Virol 2004;29(2):71–83.
[15] Gandhi M, Khanna R. Human cytomegalovirus: clinical aspects, immune regulation, and emerging treatments. Lancet Infect Dis 2004;4(12):725–38.
[16] Nesmith JD, Pass RF. Cytomegalovirus infection in adolescent. In: Overturf GD, Jacobs RF, editors. Adolescent medicine: state of the art reviews. Philadelphia: Hanley and Belfus; 1995. p. 79–90.
[17] Nijs J, Nicolson GL, De Becker P, et al. High prevalence of Mycoplasma infections among European chronic fatigue syndrome patients. Examination of four Mycoplasma species in blood of chronic fatigue syndrome patients. FEMS Immunol Med Microbiol 2002;34(3):209–14.
[18] Endresen GK. Mycoplasma blood infection in chronic fatigue and fibromyalgia syndromes. Rheumatol Int 2003;23(5):211–15.
[19] Palacios G, Oberste MS. Enteroviruses as agents of emerging infectious diseases. J Neurovirol 2005;11(5):424–33.
[20] Abzug MJ. The enteroviruses: an emerging infectious disease? The real, the speculative and the really speculative. Adv Exp Med Biol 2008;609:1–15.
[21] Hsiung GD, Wang JR. Enterovirus infections with special reference to enterovirus 71. J Microbiol Immunol Infect 2000;33(1):1–8.
[22] Pan H. Retroviruses. Encyclopedia of microbiology. USA: Elsevier; 2009. p. 519–34.
[23] Rulli N, Suhrbier A, Hueston L, et al. Ross River virus: molecular and cellular aspects of disease pathogenesis. Pharmacol Ther 2005;107(3):329–42.
[24] Australian Government Department of Health and Ageing. National notifiable diseases surveillance system. Available at: http://www9.health.gov.au/cda/source/cda-index.cfm.
[25] Harley D, Sleigh A, Ritchie S. Ross River virus transmission, infection, and disease: a cross-disciplinary review. Clin Microbiol Rev 2001;14(4):909–32.
[26] Sakamoto R. Legionnaire's disease, weather and climate. Bull World Health Organ 2015;93:435–6. doi.org/10.2471/BLT.14.142299.
[27] Diederen BMW. *Legionella* spp. and legionnaires' disease. J Infect 2008;56:1e12.
[28] Sasaki T, Matsumoto N, Nakao H, et al. An outbreak of Legionnaires' disease associated with a circulating bathwater system at a public bathhouse. I: a clinical analysis. J Infect Chemother 2008;14(2):117–22.
[29] Greig JE, Carnie JA, Tallis GF, et al. An outbreak of Legionnaires' disease at the Melbourne Aquarium, April 2000: investigation and case-control studies. Med J Aust 2004;180(11):566–72.
[30] Hilbi H, Jarraud S, Hartland E, et al. Update on Legionnaires' disease: pathogenesis, epidemiology, detection and control. Mol Microbiol 2010;76(1):1–11.
[31] Manavi K. A review on infection with *Chlamydia trachomatis*. Best Pract Res Clin Obstet Gynaecol 2006;20(6):941–51.
[32] Walker Hocking J, Regan J, et al. Chlamydia screening — Australia should strive to achieve what others have not. Med J Aust 2008;188(2):106–8.
[33] HealthVic. Chlamydia (genital infection). Available from; https://www2.health.vic.gov.au/public-health/infectious-diseases/disease-information-advice/chlamydia.
[34] Balin BJ, Little CS, Hammond CJ, et al. *Chlamydophila pneumoniae* and the etiology of late-onset Alzheimer's disease. J Alzheimers Dis 2008;13(4):371–80.
[35] Contini C, Seraceni S, Cultrera R, et al. *Chlamydophila pneumoniae* infection and its role in neurological disorders. Interdiscip Perspect Infect Dis 2010;2010:273573.
[36] Valbuena G, Walker D. Infection of the endothelium by members of the order Rickettsiales. Thromb Haemost 2009;102/6(Dec):1007–291.
[37] Whatmore AM. Current understanding of the genetic diversity of *Brucella*, an expanding genus of zoonotic pathogens. Infect Genet Evol 2009;9(6):1168–84.
[38] Perkins SD, Smither SJ, Atkins HS. Towards a *Brucella* vaccine for humans. FEMS Microbiol Rev 2010;34(3):379–94.
[39] Whatmore AM. Current understanding of the genetic diversity of *Brucella*, an expanding genus of zoonotic pathogens. Infect Genet Evol 2009;9(6):1168–84.
[40] Hadda V, Khilnani G, Kedia S. Brucellosis presenting as pyrexia of unknown origin in an international traveller: a case report. Cases J 2009;2:7969.
[41] Melski JW. Lyme borreliosis. Semin Cutan Med Surg 2000;19(1):10–18.
[42] Nau R, Christen HJ, Eiffert H. Lyme disease — current state of knowledge. Dtsch Arztebl Int 2009;106(5):72–81, quiz 82, I.
[43] Stanek G, Strle F. Lyme borreliosis. Lancet 2003;362(9396):1639–47.
[44] Adam R. The *Giardia lamblia* genome. Int J Parasitol 2000;30(4):475–84.
[45] Roxström-Lindquist K, Palm D, Reiner D, et al. Giardia immunity — an update. Trends Parasitol 2006;22(1):26–31.

[46] Thompson RCA. The zoonotic significance and molecular epidemiology of *Giardia* and giardiasis. Vet Parasitol 2004;126:15–35.
[47] Müller N, von Allme N. Recent insights into the mucosal reactions associated with *Giardia lamblia* infections. Int J Parasitol 2005;35(13):1339–47.
[48] Farthing MJ. The molecular pathogenesis of giardiasis. J Pediatr Gastroenterol Nutr 1997;24:79–88.
[49] Müller N, von Allmen N. Recent insights into the mucosal reactions associated with *Giardia lamblia* infections. Int J Parasitol 2005;35(13):1339–47.
[50] Noble SM, Gianetti BA, Withcley JN. *Candida albicans* cell-type switching and functional plasticity in the mammalian host. Nat Rev Microbiol 2017;15(2):96–108.
[51] What is candidiasis? WebMD. 2017. Available from: www.webmd.com/skin-problems-and-treatments/guide/candidiasis-yeast-infection#1.
[52] Allison DL, Willems HM, Jayatilake JA, et al. Candida–bacteria interactions: their impact on human disease. Microbiol Spectr 2016;4(3).
[53] Sanchez J, Cardona R, Caraballo L, et al. Allergen immunotherapy: mechanisms of action, and therapeutic and socioeconomic impact. Consensus of the Asociacion Colombiana de Alergia, Asma e Imunologia. Biomedica 2016;36(3):463–74.
[54] Pawanker R, Canonica GW, Hogate ST, et al, editors. White book on allergies. World Allergy Organization; 2011.
[55] Anzilotti C, Riente L, Pratesi F, et al. IgG, IgA, IgM antibodies to a viral citrullinated peptide in patients affected by rheumatoid arthritis, chronic arthritides and connective tissue disorders. Rheumatology (Oxford) 2007;46(10):1579–82.
[56] Abramson SL Delayed hypersensitivity reactions. Medscape; 23 December 2015.
[57] Ellingwood F. The Eclectic practice of medicine with especial reference to the treatment of disease. USA: 1910.
[58] Hughes DA. Effects of dietary antioxidants on the immune function of middle-aged adults. Proc Nutr Soc 1999;58(1):79–84.
[59] Dreizen S. Nutrition and the immune response — a review. Int J Vitam Nutr Res 1979;49(2):220–8.
[60] Wintergerst ES, Maggini S, Hornig DH. Contribution of selected vitamins and trace elements to immune function. Ann Nutr Metab 2007;51(4):301–23.
[61] Zimmermann M. Burgenstein's handbook of nutrition, micronutrients in the prevention and therapy of diseases. New York: Thieme; 2001.
[62] Pagana KD, Pagana TJ. Mosby's diagnostic and laboratory test references. USA: Elsevier; 2008. p. 483.
[63] Rumore MM. Vitamin A as an immunomodulating agent. Clin Pharm 1993;12(7):506–14.
[64] Stephensen CB. Vitamin A, infection, and immune function. Annu Rev Nutr 2001;21:167–92.
[65] Semba RD. Vitamin A, immunity, and infection. Clin Infect Dis 1994;19(3):489–99.
[66] Semba RD. Vitamin A and immunity to viral, bacterial and protozoan infections. Proc Nutr Soc 1999;58(3):719–27.
[67] Bendich A. Carotenoids and the immune response. J Nutr 1989;119(1):112–15.
[68] Muggli R. Vitamin C and the immune system. Encyclopedia of Immunology. USA: Elsevier; 1998. p. 2491–4.
[69] Bendich A. Antioxidant vitamins and human immune responses. Vitam Horm 1996;52:35–62.
[70] Muggli R. Vitamin C and the immune system. Encyclopedia of Immunology. UK: Elsevier; 1998. p. 2491–4.
[71] Bouillon R. Vitamin D: from photosynthesis, metabolism and action to clinical applications. In: DeGroot L, Jameson J, editors. Endocrinology. Philadelphia: Saunders; 2005. p. 1435–63.
[72] Bhalla AK, Amento EP, Clemens TL, et al. Specific high-affinity receptors for 1,25-dihydroxyvitamin D3 in human peripheral blood mononuclear cells: presence in monocytes and induction in T lymphocytes following activation. J Clin Endocrinol Metab 1983;57:1308–10.
[73] Provvedini DM, Tsoukas CD, Deftos LJ, et al. 1,25-dihydroxyvitamin D_3 receptors in human leucocytes. Science 1983;221:1181–3.
[74] Mahon BD, Wittke A, Weaver V, et al. The targets of vitamin D depend on the differentiation and activation status of CD4-positive T cells. J Cell Biochem 2003;89:922–32.
[75] Moriguchi S, Muraga M. Vitamin E and immunity. Vitam Horm 2000;59:305–36.
[76] Meydani SN, Barklund MP, Liu S, et al. Vitamin E supplementation enhances cell-mediated immunity in healthy elderly subjects. Am J Clin Nutr 1990;52(3):557–63.
[77] De la Fuente M, Hernanz A, Guayerbas N, et al. Vitamin E ingestion improves several immune functions in elderly men and women. Free Radic Res 2008;42(3):272–80.
[78] Rayman MP. The importance of selenium to human health. Lancet 2000;356(9225):233–41.
[79] Beck MA, Shi Q, Morris VC, et al. Rapid genomic evolution of a non-virulent Coxsackievirus B3 in selenium-deficient mice results in selection of identical virulent isolates. Nat Med 1995;1:433–6.
[80] Kiremidjian-Schumacher L, Roy M, Wishe HI, et al. Supplementation with selenium and human immune cell functions. II. Effect on cytotoxic lymphocytes and natural killer cells. Biol Trace Elem Res 1994;41(1–2):115–27.
[81] Kiremidjian-Schumacher L, Roy M, Glickman R, et al. Selenium and immunocompetence in patients with head and neck cancer. Biol Trace Elem Res 2000;73(2):97–111.
[82] Calder PC. The relationship between the fatty acid composition of immune cells and their function. Prostaglandins Leukot Essent Fatty Acids 2008;79(3–5):101–8.
[83] Calder PC. Fatty acids and immune function: relevance to inflammatory bowel diseases. Int Rev Immunol 2009;28(6):506–34.
[84] Sergio W. Zinc salts that may be effective against the AIDS virus HIV. Med Hypotheses 1988;26:251–3.
[85] Patrick L. Nutrients and HIV: part two — vitamins A and E, zinc, B-vitamins, and magnesium. Altern Med Rev 2000;5(1):39–51.
[86] Thibault H, Galan P, Selz F, et al. The immune response in iron-deficient young children: effect of iron supplementation on cell-mediated immunity. Eur J Pediatr 1993;152:120–4.
[87] Failla ML, Hopkins RG. Is low copper status immunosuppressive? Nutr Rev 1998;56(1/2):S59–64.
[88] Folkers K, Hanioka T, Xia LJ, et al. Coenzyme Q10 increases T4/T8 ratios of lymphocytes in ordinary subjects and relevance to patients having the AIDS related complex. Biochem Biophys Res Commun 1991;176(2):786–91.
[89] Folkers K, Morita M, McRee J Jr. The activities of coenzyme Q10 and vitamin B6 for immune responses. Biochem Biophys Res Commun 1993;193(1):88–92.
[90] Ng SC, Hart AL, Kamm MA, et al. Mechanisms of action of probiotics: recent advances. Inflamm Bowel Dis 2009;15(2): 300–10.
[91] Fang SB, Lee HC, Hu JJ, et al. Dose-dependent effect of *Lactobacillus rhamnosus* on quantitative reduction of faecal rotavirus shedding in children. J Trop Pediatr 2009;55(5):297–301.
[92] Baron M. A patented strain of *Bacillus coagulans* increased immune response to viral challenge. Postgrad Med 2009;121(2):114–18.
[93] Czerucka D, Piche T, Rampal P. Review article: yeast as probiotics — *Saccharomyces boulardii*. Aliment Pharmacol Ther 2007;26(6):767–78.
[94] Daly JM, Reynolds J, Sigal RK, et al. Effect of dietary protein and amino acids on immune function. Crit Care Med 1990;18(Suppl. 2):S86–93.
[95] De Simone C, Ferrari M, Lozzi A, et al. Vitamins and immunity: II. Influence of L-carnitine on the immune system. Acta Vitaminol Enzymol 1982;4(1–2):135–40.
[96] Arranz L, Fernández C, Rodríguez A, et al. The glutathione precursor *N*-acetylcysteine improves immune function in postmenopausal women. Free Radic Biol Med 2008;45(9):1252–62.
[97] Devi KS, Maiti TK. Immunomodulating and anti-cancer properties of pharmacologically relevant mushroom glycans. Recent Pat Biotechnol 2016;10(1):72–8.
[98] Li Y, Yao J, Han C, et al. Quercetin, inflammation and immunity. Nutrients 2016;8(3):167.
[99] Leischner C, Burkard M, Pfeiffer MM, et al. Nutritional immunology: function of natural killer cells and their modulation by resveratrol for cancer prevention and treatment. Nutr J 2016;15(1):47.
[100] Davidson A, Diamond B. General features of autoimmune disease. In: Rose NR, Mackey IR, editors. The autoimmune diseases. 4th ed. St Louis: Elsevier; 2006. p. 25–36.
[101] Rose NR, Mackay IR, editors. The autoimmune diseases. 5th ed. Academic Press; 2014.

[102] Cooper GS, Bynum ML, Somers EC. Recent insights in the epidemiology of autoimmune diseases: improved prevalence estimates and understanding of clustering of diseases. J Autoimmun 2009;33:197–207.

[103] Youinou P, Pers J-O, Gershwin ME, et al. Geo-epidemiology and autoimmunity. J Autoimmun 2010;34(3):J300–6.

[104] Doran MF, Crowson CS, O'Fallon WM, et al. The effect of oral contraceptives and estrogen replacement therapy on the risk of rheumatoid arthritis: a population based study. J Rheumatol 2004;31:207–13.

[105] Tobón GJ, Youinou P, Saraux A. The environment, geo-epidemiology, and autoimmune disease: rheumatoid arthritis. J Autoimmun 2010;35(1):10–11

[106] Scofield RH. Autoantibodies as predictors of disease. Lancet 2004;363(9420):1544–6.

[107] Cooper GS, Stroehla BC. The epidemiology of autoimmune diseases. Autoimmun Rev 2003;2(3):119–25.

[108] Walsh SJ, Rau LM. Autoimmune diseases: a leading cause of death among young and middle-aged women in the United States. Am J Pub Health 2000;90:1463–6.

[109] Abou-Raya A, Abou-Raya S. Inflammation: a pivotal link between autoimmune diseases and atherosclerosis. Autoimmun Rev 2006;5(5):331–7.

[110] Berkow R, Fletcher AJ New Jersey, USA: Merck & Company Inc; 1992.

[111] Parisi R, Symmons DP, Griffiths CE, et al. Global epidemiology of psoriasis: a systematic review of incidence and prevalence. J Invest Dermatol 2013;133(2):377–85.

[112] Koda-Kimble MA, Young LY, Alldredge BK, et al. Applied therapeutics: the clinical use of drugs. Philadelphia: Lippincott Williams & Wilkins; 2009.

[113] Calder PC, Albers R, Antoine JM, et al. Inflammatory disease processes and interactions with nutrition. Br J Nutr 2009; 101(Suppl.):S1–45.

[114] Anaya J-M, Ramirez-Santana C, Alzate MA, et al. The autoimmune ecology. Front Immunol 2016;7:139.

[115] Ebringer A, Wilson C. The use of a low starch diet in the treatment of patients suffering from ankylosing spondylitis. Clin Rheumatol 1996;15(Suppl.. 1):62–6.

[116] Brustolin S, Giugliani R, Félix TM. Genetics of homocysteine metabolism and associated disorders. Braz J Med Biol Res 2010;43(1):1–7.

[117] De Groot LJ. Graves' disease and the manifestations of thyrotoxicosis. The thyroid and its diseases. South Dartmouth, MA: Endocrine Education Inc.; 2008.

[118] Kawasaki E, Matsuura N, Eguchi K. Type 1 diabetes in Japan. Diabetologia 2006;49:828–36.

[119] Snell GD. The H-2 locus of the mouse: observations and speculations concerning its comparative genetics and its polymorphism. Folia Bioologica (Praha) 1968;14(5):335–58.

[120] Oldstone MB. Molecular mimicry and immune-mediated diseases. Cell 1987;50:819–20.

[121] Vezys V, Yates A, Casey KA, et al. Memory CD8 T-cell compartment grows in size with immunological experience. Nature Immunol 2009;457:196–9.

[122] Christen U, Hintermann E, Holdener M, et al. Viral triggers for autoimmunity: is the 'glass of molecular mimicry' half full or half empty? J Autoimmun 2010;34:38–44.

[123] Proal AD, Albert PJ, Marshall TG. The human microbiome and autoimmunity. Curr Opin Rheumatol 2013;25:234–40.

[124] Rashid T, Wilson C, Ebringer A. The link between ankylosing spondylitis, Crohn's disease, *Klebsiella*, and starch consumption. Clin Dev Immunol 2013;2013:872632.

[125] Smyk DS, Koutsoumpas AL, Mytilinaiou MG, et al. *Helicobacter pylori* and autoimmune disease: cause or bystander. World J Gastroenterol 2014;20(3):613–29.

[126] Kjeldsen-Kragh J, Kvaavik E, Bottolfs M, et al. Inhibition of growth of *Proteus mirabilis* and *Escherichia coli* in urine in response to fasting and vegetarian diet. APMIS 1995;103(11):818–22.

[127] Naser SA, Sagramsingh SR, Naser AS, et al. *Mycobacterium avium* subspecies *paratuberculosis* causes Crohn's disease in some inflammatory bowel disease patients. World J Gastroenterol 2014;20(23):7403–15.

[128] Mackay IR, Rose NR, editors. The autoimmune diseases. Academic Press; 2014.

[129] Fasano A. Leaky gut and autoimmune diseases. Clin Rev Allergy Immunol 2012;42(1):71–8.

[130] Fasano A. Zonulin, regulation of tight junctions, and autoimmune diseases. Ann N Y Acad Sci 2012;1258(1):25–33.

[131] Assimakopoulos SF, Papageorgiou I, Charonis A. Enterocytes' tight junctions: from molecules to diseases. World J Gastrointest Pathophysiol 2011;2(6):123–37.

[132] Di Cagno R, De Angelis M, De Pasquale I, et al. Duodenal and faecal microbiota of celiac children: molecular, phenotype and metabolome characterization. BMC Microbiol 2011;11:219.

[133] Bone K. Treating autoimmune disease. a phytotherapeutic perspective. Modern Phytotherapist 1994;1(1):1–8.

[134] Gold LS, Ward MH, Dosemeci M, et al. Systemic autoimmune disease mortality and occupational exposures. Arth Rheum 2007;56(10):3189–201.

[135] Melzer D, Rice N, Depledge MH, et al. Association between serum perfluorooctanoic acid (PFOA) and thyroid disease in the NHANES Study. Environ Health Perspect 2010.

[136] McLachlan SM, Rapoport B. Breaking tolerance to thyroid antigens: changing concepts in thyroid autoimmunity. Endocr Rev 2014;35(1):59–105.

[137] Stargrove MB, Treasure J, McKee DL. Herb, nutrient and drug interactions. St Louis: Mosby Elsevier; 2008.

[138] Graber P. Self and not-self in immunology. Lancet 1974;303(7870):1320–2.

[139] Mills SY. The essential book of herbal medicine. London: Arkana Penguin Books; 1991.

[140] Ebringer A, Cox NL, Abuljadayel I, et al. *Klebsiella* antibodies in ankylosing spondylitis and *Proteus* antibodies in rheumatoid arthritis. Br J Rheumatol 1988;27(Suppl.II):72–85.

[141] Fagan TF, Faustman DL. Sex differences in autoimmunity. Adv Mol Cell Biol 2004;34:295–306.

[142] Diamanti AP, Manuela Rosado M, Laganà B, et al. Microbiota and chronic inflammatory arthritis: an interwoven link. J Transl Med 2016;14:233.

[143] Brighenti F, Valtuena S, Pellegrini N. Total antioxidant capacity of the diet is inversely and independently related to plasma concentration of high-sensitivity C-reactive protein in adult Italian subjects. Br J Nutr 2005;93:619–25.

[144] Calder PC, Albers R, Antoine JM, et al. Inflammatory disease processes and interactions with nutrition. Br J Nutr 2009; 101(Suppl.):S1–45.

[145] Pattison DJ, Harrison RA, Symmons DP. The role of diet in susceptibility to rheumatoid arthritis: a systematic review. J Rheumatol 2004;31(7):1310–19.

[146] Ben-Arye E, Goldin E, Wengrower D, et al. Wheat grass juice in the treatment of active distal ulcerative colitis. Scan J Gastroenterol 2002;37(4):444–9.

[147] Müller H, de Toledo FW, Resch KL. Fasting followed by vegetarian diet in patients with rheumatoid arthritis: a systematic review. Scan J Rheumatol 2001;30(1):1–10.

[148] Hagen KB, Byfuglien MG, Falzon L, et al. Dietary interventions for rheumatoid arthritis. Cochrane Database Syst Rev 2009;(1):CD006400.

[149] Clarke JO, Mullin GE. A review of complementary and alternative approaches to immunomodulation. Nutr Clin Prac 2008;23(1):49–62.

[150] Pothoulakis C. Review article: anti-inflammatory mechanisms of action of *Saccharomyces boulardii*. Aliment Pharmacol Ther 2009;30:826–33.

[151] Guslandi M, Mezzi G, Sorghi M, et al. *Saccharomyces boulardii* in maintenance treatment of Crohn's disease. Dig Dis Sci 2000;45(7):1462–4.

[152] Sood A, et al. The probiotic preparation, *VSL#3* induces remission in patients with mild-to-moderately active ulcerative colitis. Clin Gastroenterol Hepatol 2009;7:1202–9.

[153] Zocco MA, dal Verme LZ, Cremonini F, et al. Efficacy of *Lactobacillus* GG in maintaining remission of ulcerative colitis. Aliment Pharmacol Ther 2006;23:1567–74.

[154] Henker J, Muller S, Laass MW, et al. *Probiotic Escherichia coli Nissle 1917 (EcN)* for successful remission maintenance of ulcerative colitis in children and adolescents: an open-label pilot study. Z Gastroenterol 2008;46:874–5.

[155] Simopoulos AP. Omega-3 fatty acids in inflammation and autoimmune diseases. J Am Coll Nutr 2002;21(6):495–505.

[156] Selmi C, Tsuneyama K. Nutrition, geoepidemiology, and autoimmunity. Autoimmun Rev 2010;9(5):A267–70.
[157] Fernández-Bañares F, Hinojosa J, Sánchez-Lombraña J, et al. Randomized clinical trial of *Plantago ovata* seeds (dietary fiber) as compared with mesalamine in maintaining remission in ulcerative colitis. Spanish Group for the Study of Crohn's Disease and Ulcerative Colitis (GETECCU). Am J Gastroenterol 1999;94(2):427–33.
[158] Yuan G, Wahlqvist ML, Guoqing H, et al. Natural products and anti-inflammatory activity. Asia Pac J Clin Nutr 2006;15(2):143–52.
[159] Denisov LN, Andrianova IV, Timofeeva SS. Garlic effectiveness in rheumatoid arthritis. Tereapevticheskii Arkhiv 1999;71(8):55–8.
[160] Braun L, Cohen M. Herbs and natural supplements: an evidence-based guide. Marrickville, NSW: Elsevier; 2010.
[161] Aggarwal BB, Kunnumakkara AB, Harikumar KB, et al. Potential of spice-derived phytochemicals for cancer prevention. Planta Med 2008;74(13):1560–9.
[162] Kurien BT, D'Souza A, Scofield RH. Heat-solubilized curry spice curcumin inhibits antibody-antigen interaction in in vitro studies: a possible therapy to alleviate autoimmune disorders. Mol Nutr Food Res 2010;54:1–8.
[163] Okada M, Yao T, Yamamoto T, et al. Controlled trial comparing an elemental diet with prednisolone in the treatment of active Crohn's disease. Hepatogastroenterology 1990;37(1):72–80.
[164] Riordan AM, Rucker JT, Kirby GA, et al. Food intolerance and Crohn's disease. Gut 1994;35(4):571–2.
[165] Mallant-Hent RC, Mary B, von Blomberg E, et al. Disappearance of anti-*Saccharomyces cerevisiae* antibodies in coeliac disease during a gluten-free diet. Eur J Gastroenterol Hepatol 2006;18(1):75–8.
[166] Appelboom T, Durez P. Effect of milk product deprivation on spondyloarthropathy. Ann Rheum Dis 1994;53(7):481–2.
[167] Sisto M, Cucci L, D'Amore M, et al. Proposing a relationship between *Mycobacterium avium* subspecies paratuberculosis infection and Hashimoto's thyroiditis. Scand J Infect Dis 2010;42:787–90.
[168] Greenstein RJ, Collins MT. Emerging pathogens: is *Mycobacterium avium* subspecies paratuberculosis zoonotic? Lancet 2004;364(9432):396–7.
[169] Willett WC. Trans fatty acids and cardiovascular disease — epidemiological data. Atheroscler Supp 2006;7(2):5–8.
[170] NSW Food Authority. Trans fatty acids survey; 2008. www.foodauthority.nsw.gov.au/_Documents/corporate_pdf/trans-fatty-acid-survey–FI037–0902.pdf.
[171] Rashid T, Ebringer A, Tiwana H, et al. Role of *Klebsiella* and collagens in Crohn's disease: a new prospect in the use of low-starch diet. Eur J Gastroenterol Hepatol 2009;21(8):843–9.
[172] Roediger WE. Decreased sulphur amino acid intake in ulcerative colitis. Lancet 1998;351(9115):1115.
[173] Dreyfus DH. Autoimmune disease: a role for new anti-viral therapies? Autoimmun Rev 2011;11(2):88–97.
[174] Kanazawa A, Sako M, Takazoe M, et al. Daikenchuto, a traditional Japanese herbal medicine, for the maintenance of surgically induced remission in patients with Crohn's disease: a retrospective analysis of 258 patients. Surg Today 2014;44(8):1506–12.
[175] Langhorst J, Varnhagen I, Schneider SB, et al. Randomised clinical trial: a herbal preparation of myrrh, chamomile and coffee charcoal compared with mesalazine in maintaining remission in ulcerative colitis — a double-blind, double-dummy study. Aliment Pharmacol Ther 2013;38(5):490–500.
[176] Atal CK, Sharma ML, Kaul A, et al. Immunomodulating agents of plant origin. 1: Preliminary screening. J Ethnopharmacol 1986;18(2):133–41.
[177] Lampronti I, Khan MT, Bianchi N, et al. Bangladeshi medicinal plant extracts inhibiting molecular interactions between nuclear factors and target DNA sequences mimicking NF-kappaB binding sites. Med Chem 2005;1(4):327–33.
[178] Delorme D, Miller SC. Dietary consumption of echinacea by mice afflicted with autoimmune (type 1) diabetes: Effect of consuming the herb on hemopoietic and immune cell dynamics. Autoimmunity 2005;38(6):453–61.
[179] Bone K. Autoimmune disease. A phytotherapeutic perspective. Townsend Letter for Doctors and Patients 1999;193(194):94–8.
[180] Neri PG, Stagni E, Filippello M, et al. Oral *Echinacea purpurea* extract in low-grade, steroid-dependent, autoimmune idiopathic uveitis: a pilot study. J Ocul Pharmacol Ther 2006;22(6):431–6.
[181] Bone K. Herbs for the treatment of chronic immune deficiency. Phytotherapist Perspective 2000;10(May).
[182] Mur E, Hartig F, Eibl G, et al. Randomized double blind trial of an extract from the pentacyclic alkaloid-chemotype of *Uncaria tomentosa* for the treatment of rheumatoid arthritis. J Rheumatol 2002;29(4):678–81.
[183] Kubin A, Wierrani F, Burner U, et al. Hypericin — the facts about a controversial agent. Curr Pharm Des 2005;11(2):233–53.
[184] Menegazzi M, Novelle M, Beffy P, et al. Protective effects of St John's wort extract and its component hyperforin against cytokine-induced cytotoxicity in a pancreatic beta-cell line. Int J Biochem Cell Biol 2008;40(8):1509–21.
[185] Gerhardt H, Seifert F, Buvari P, et al. Therapy of active Crohn disease with Boswellia serrata extract H15. Zeitschrift für Gastroenterologie 2001;39(1):11–17.
[186] Slonim AE, Grovit M, Bulone L. Effect of exclusion diet with nutraceutical therapy in juvenile Crohn's disease. J Am Coll Nutr 2009;28(3):277–85.
[187] Gupta I, Parihar A, Malhotra P. Effects of gum resin of *Boswellia serata* in patients with chronic colitis. Planta Med 2001;67:391–5.
[188] Bright JJ. Curcumin and autoimmune disease. Adv Exp Med Biol 2007;595:425–51.
[189] Rahman I, Biswas SK, Kirkham PA. Regulation of inflammation and redox signaling by dietary polyphenols. Biochem Pharmacol 2006;72:1439–52.
[190] Hanai H, Iida T, Takeuchi K. Curcumin maintenance therapy for ulcerative colitis: randomized, multicenter, double-blind, placebo-controlled trial. Clin Gastroenterol Hepatol 2006;4:1502–6.
[191] Panush RS, Stroud RM, Webster EM. Food-induced (allergic) arthritis. Inflammatory arthritis exacerbated by milk. Arth Rheum 1986;29(2):220–2226.
[192] Cancer Australia. All cancers in Australia. 2017. Available from: https://canceraustralia.gov.au/affected-cancer/what-cancer/cancer-australia-statistics.
[193] Richardson M, Sanders T, Lynn Palmer J, et al. Complementary/alternative medicine use in a comprehensive cancer centre and the implications for oncology. J Clin Onc 2000;18:2505–14.
[194] Molassiotis A, Panteli V, Patiraki E, et al. Complementary and alternative medicine use in lung cancer patients in eight European countries. Complement Ther Clin Prac 2006;12:34–9.
[195] Bertram J. The molecular basis of cancer. Mol Aspects Med 2000;21(6):167–223.
[196] Hall J, Angele S. Radiation, DNA damage and cancer. Mol Med Today 1999;5:157–64.
[197] Huang S, Li JY, Wu J, et al. Mycoplasma infections and different human carcinomas. World J Gastroenterol 2001;7(2):266–9.
[198] Hansen N, Hansen NM, Ye X, et al. Manipulation of the primary breast tumor and the incidence of sentinel node metastases from invasive breast cancer. Arch Surg 2004;139:634–40.
[199] MedicineNet.com. 2018. Available at: www.medicinenet.com/carcinoembryonic_antigen/article.htm#what_are_the_limitations_of_cea_testing.
[200] Keshaviah A, Dellapasqua S, Rotmensz N, et al. CA15-3 and alkaline phosphatase as predictors for breast cancer recurrence: a combined analysis of seven International Breast Cancer Study Group trials. Ann Oncol 2007;18(4):701–8.
[201] Scully R. Role of BRCA gene dysfunction in breast and ovarian cancer predisposition. Breast Cancer Res 2000;2:324–30.
[202] Gøtzsche PC, Nielsen M. Screening for breast cancer with mammography. Cochrane Database Syst Rev 2006;(4):CD001877.
[203] Brenner D, Hall E. Computed tomography — an increasing source of radiation exposure. N Engl J Med 2007;357:2277–84.
[204] Beveridge J, Beverage JN, Sissung TM, et al. CYP2D6 polymorphisms and the impact on tamoxifen therapy. J Pharm Sci 2007;96:2224–31.
[205] Hu R, Hilakivi-Clarke L, Clarke R. Molecular mechanisms of tamoxifen-associated endometrial cancer (review). Oncol Lett 2015;9(4):1495–501.
[206] Kearney A, Murray M. Breast cancer screening recommendations: is mammography the only answer? J Midwifery Womens Health 2009;54:393–400.
[207] Huang S, Li JY, Wu J, et al. Mycoplasma infections and different human carcinomas. World J Gastroenterol 2001;7(2):266–9.
[208] Lord R, Lord RS, Bongiovanni B, et al. Estrogen metabolism and the diet-cancer connection: rationale for assessing the ratio of

urinary hydroxylated estrogen metabolites. Alern Med Rev 2002;7(2):112–29.
[209] Qaisara P, Malik Salman A, Shah Munir H, et al. Statistical analysis of trace metals in the plasma of cancer patients versus controls. J Hazard Mater 2008;152(3):1215–21.
[210] Shah-Reddy I, Khilanani P, Bishop CR, et al. Serum copper levels in non-Hodgkin's lymphoma. Cancer 1980;45(8):2156–9.
[211] Mill O, Zowczak A, Iskra M, et al. Analysis of serum copper and zinc concentrations in cancer patients. Biol Trace Elem Res 2001;82(1–3):1–8.
[212] Fraser MC, Tucker MA. Second malignancies following cancer therapy. Semin Oncol Nurs 1989;5:43–55.
[213] Tucker MA, Coleman CN, Cox RS, et al. Risk of second cancers after treatment for Hodgkin's disease. N Engl J Med 1988;318:76–81.
[214] Chen HW, Lin RJ, Xie W, et al. Regulation of hormone-induced histone hyperacetylation and gene activation via acetylation of an acetylase. Cell 1999;1999(98):675–86.
[215] Nahta R, Esteva FJ. Trastuzumab: triumphs and tribulations. Oncogene 2007;26:3637–43.
[216] Ahmad S, Gupta S, Kumar R, et al. Herceptin resistance database for understanding mechanism of resistance in breast cancer patients. Sci Rep 2014;4:4483.
[217] Flowers M, Thompson P. *t10c12* Conjugated linoleic acid suppresses HER2 protein and enhances apoptosis in SKB23 breast cancer cells: possible role of COX-2. PLoS ONE 2009;4(4):e5342.
[218] Menendez J, Vasquez-Marin A, Garcia-Villalba R, et al. tabAnti-HER2 (*erb*B-2) oncogene effects of phenolic compounds directly isolated from commercial extra-virgin olive oil (EVOO). BMC Cancer 2008;8:377.
[219] Menendez J, Vellon A, Colomer R, et al. Oleic acid, the main monounsaturated fatty acid of olive oil, suppresses HER-2 neu (*erb*B-2) expression and synergistically enhances the growth inhibitory effects of trastuzumab (Herceptin) in breast cancer cells withbHER-2/neu oncogene amplification. Ann Oncol 2005;16:359–71.
[220] Dent R, Clemons M. Editorial. BMJ 2005;331:1202.
[221] Vance D, Vance R, Sagar S. Targeting angiogenesis with integrative cancer therapies. Integr Cancer Ther 2000;5:9.
[222] Verma SP, Goldin BR, Lin PS. The inhibition of the estrogenic effects of pesticides and environmental chemicals by curcumin and isoflavonoids. Environ Health Perspect 1998;106:807–12.
[223] Venkatraman J, Mamta Rao MS, Carol S, et al. Effect of dietary lipids on activities of hepatic steroid metabolising enzymes (5α-reductase and aromatase) and composition of microsomes. Nutr Res 1996;16(10):1749–59.
[224] Khan S, Zhao J, Khan I, et al. Potential ability of natural products as regulators of breast cancer associated aromatase promoters. Reprod Biol Endocrinol 2011;9:91.
[225] Harris R, Casto B, Harris Z. Cyclooxygenase-2 and the inflammogenesis of breast cancer. World J Clin Oncol 2014;5(4): 677–92.
[226] Nelson B. IL-2, regulator T cells and tolerance. J Immunol 2004;172:3983–8.
[227] Arora R, Gupta D, Chawla R, et al. Radioprotection by plant products: present status and future prospects. Phytother Res 2005;19:1–22.
[228] Bertram JS. The molecular biology of cancer. Mol Aspects Med 2000;21(6):167–223.
[229] Pommier P, Gomez F, Sunyach M, et al. Phase III randomized trial of *Calendula officinalis* compared with trolamine for the prevention of acute dermatitis during irradiation for breast cancer. J Clin Oncol 2004;22:1447–53.
[230] Saini DK, Saini MR. Evaluation of radioprotective efficacy and possible mechanism of action of aloe gel. Environ Toxicol Pharmacol 2011;31:427–35.
[231] Singh V, Beattie L, Seed T. Vitamin E: tocopherols and tocotrienols as potential radiation countermeasures. J Radiat Res 2013;54(6):973–88.
[232] Doll R, Peto R. The causes of cancer: quantitative estimates of avoidable risks of cancer in the United States today. J Natl Cancer Inst 1981;66:1191–308.
[233] World Cancer Research Fund and American Institute for Cancer Research. Food, nutrition, physical activity, and the prevention of cancer: a global perspective. 1997. American Washington DC: AIRC; 2007. Available from:: www.wcrf.org/sites/default/files/Second-Expert-Report.pdf.
[234] Moerman CJ, Bueno de Mesquita HB, Runia S, et al. Dietary sugar intake in the aetiology of biliary tract cancer. Int J Epidemiol 1993;22(2):207–14.
[235] Seeley S, Kushi LH, Cunningham JE, et al. Diet and breast cancer: the possible connection with sugar consumption. Med Hypotheses 1983;11(3):319–27.
[236] Kushi LH, Cunningham JE, Heber J, et al. The macrobiotic diet in cancer. J Nutr 2001;131:S3056–64.
[237] Rogers SA. Improvement in chemical sensitivity with the macrobiotic diet. J App Nutr 1996;48(3):85–92.
[238] Bowman BB, Kushner RF, Dawson SC, et al. Macrobiotic diets for cancer treatment and prevention. J Clin Oncol 1984;2:702–71.
[239] Dagnelie PC, van Staveren WA. Macrobiotic nutrition and child health: results of a population-based, mixed-longitudinal cohort study in the Netherlands. Am J Clin Nutr 1994;59(Suppl.): S1187–96.
[240] Budwig J. Flax oil as a true aid against arthritis, heart infarction, cancer and other diseases. Vancouver: Apple Publishing Co; 1994.
[241] Gerson M. The cure of advanced cancer by diet therapy: a summary of 30 years of clinical experimentation. Physiol Chem Phys 1978;10(5):449–64.
[242] McCarty M. Aldosterone and the Gerson diet — a speculation. Med Hypoth 1981;7:591–7.
[243] Hursting SD, Kari FW. The anti-carcinogenic effects of dietary restriction: mechanisms and future directions. Mutat Res 1999;443(1–2):235–49.
[244] Hofmann C, Sonenshein S. Green tea polyphenol epigallocatechin-3 gallate induces apoptosis of proliferating vascular smooth muscle cells via activation of p53. FASEB J 2003;17:702–4.
[245] Editorial. The potential of green tea against cancer. Environmental Nutrition 1994;3.
[246] Ahmad N, Gupta S, Mukhtar H. Green tea polyphenol epigallocatechin-3-gallate differentially modulates nuclear factor kappa B in cancer cells versus normal cells. Arch Biochem Biophys 2000;376:338–46.
[247] Na H, Na HK, Mossanda KS, et al. Inhibition of phorbolester induced COX-2 expression by some edible African plants. Biofactors 2004;21:149–53.
[248] Joubert E, Gelderblom WC, Louw A, et al. South African herbal teas: *Aspalathus linearis, Cyclopia* spp. and *Athrixia phylicoides* — a review. J Ethnopharmacol 2008;119:376–412.
[249] Villano D, Pecorari M, Testa M, et al. Unfermented and fermented rooibos teas (*Aspalathus linearis*) increase plasma total antioxidant capacity in humans. Food Chem 2010;123:679–83.
[250] Lau B. Garlic compounds modulate macrophage and T-lymphocyte functions. Molec Biol 1991;3:103–7.
[251] Borchers A, Borchers AT, Keen CL, et al. Mushrooms, tumors, and immunity: an update: review. Exp Biol Med 2004;229:393–406.
[252] Fisher M, Yang LX. Anticancer effects and mechanisms of polysaccharide-K (PSK): implications of cancer immunotherapy. Anticancer Res 2002;22:1737–54.
[253] Takaku T, Kimura Y, Okuda H. Isolation of an antitumor compound from *Agaricus blazei Murill* and its mechanism of action. J Nutr 2001;131:1409–13.
[254] Smith J Japanese mushroom extract could help treat HPV infections. Paper presented at the 11th International Conference of the Society for Integrative Oncology. Abstract 138. Presented October 26, 2014.
[255] Reynolds T, Dweek A. Aloe vera gel: a review update. J Ethnopharmacol 1999;68:3–37.
[256] Lee H. Dietary effects on breast cancer risk in Singapore. Lancet 1991;337:1197–200.
[257] Wu A, Wu AH, Koh WP, et al. Soy intake and breast cancer risk in Singapore Chinese health study. Br J Cancer 2008;99(1): 196–200.
[258] Messina J, Messina MJ, Persky V, et al. Soy intake and cancer risk: a review of the in vitro and in vivo data. Nutr Cancer 1994;21(2):113–31.
[259] Bouker K, Hilakivi-Clarke L. Genistein: does it prevent or promote breast cancer? Environ Health Perspect 2000;108:701–8.
[260] Shao Z, Shao ZM, Shen ZZ, et al. Genistein's "ER-dependent and independent actions" are mediated through ER pathways in

ER-positive breast carcinoma cell lines. Antican Res 2000;20(4):2409–16.
[261] Bell M, Bell MC, Crowley-Nowick P, et al. Placebo-controlled trial of indole-3-carbinol in the treatment of CIN. Gynecol Oncol 2000;78(2):123–9.
[262] Meng Q, Yuan F, Goldberg ID, et al. Indole-3-carbinol is a negative regulator of estrogen receptor-signaling in human tumor cells. J Nutr 2000;130:2927–31.
[263] Ge X, Yannai S, Rennert G, et al. 3,3′-Diindolylmethane induces apoptosis in human cancer cells. Biochem Biophys Res Commun 1996;228(1):153–8.
[264] Cover C, Hsieh SJ, Cram EJ, et al. Indole-3carbinol and tamoxifen cooperate to arrest the cell cycle of MCF-7 human breast cancer cells. Cancer Res 1999;54:1244–51.
[265] Indole-3-carbinol. Monograph. Alt Med Rev 2005;10(4):337–9.
[266] Bonnesen C, Eggleston IM, Hayes JD, et al. Dietary indoles and isothiocyanates that are generated from cruciferous vegetables can both stimulate apoptosis and confer protection against DNA damage in human colon cell lines. Can Res 2001;61:6120–30.
[267] Thomsen M. Probiotics — enhancing health with beneficial bacteria. Alt Comp Ther 2006;12:14–21.
[268] Femia A, Femia AP, Luceri C, et al. Antitumorigenic activity of the prebiotic inulin enriched with oligofructose in combination with the probiotics *Lactobacillus rhamnosus* and *Bifidobacterium lactis* on azoxymethane-induced colon carcinogenesis in rats. Carcinogenesis 2002;23:1953–60.
[269] Riviere A, Selak M, Lantin D, et al. Bifidobacteria and butyrate-producing colon bacteria: importance and strategies for their stimulation in the human gut. Front Microbiol 2016;7:979.
[270] Rajendran P, Williams DE, Emily Ho E, et al. Metabolism as a key to histone deacetylase inhibition. Crit Rev Biochem Mol Biol 2011;46(3):181–99.
[271] Singh P, Krishnan S. Vitamin E analogs as radiation response modifiers. Evid Based Complement Alternat Med 2015;2015:741301.
[272] Dobrzynska M. Resveratrol as promising natural radioprotector. A review. Rocz Panstw Zakl Hig 2013;64(4):255–62.
[273] Kma L. Plant extracts and plant-derived compounds: promising players in a countermeasure strategy against radiological exposure. Asian Pac J Cancer Prev 2014;15(6):2405–25.
[274] Tamang J, Shin D, Jung S, et al. Functional properties of microorganisms in fermented foods. Front Microbiol 2016;7:578.
[275] Khoury N, El-Hayek S, Tarras O, et al. Kefir exhibits anti-proliferative and pro-apoptotic effects on colon adenocarcinoma cells with no significant effects on cell migration and invasion. Int J Oncol 2014;45(5):2117–27.
[276] Rafie N, Golpour Hamedani S, Ghisvand R, et al. Kefir and cancer: a systemic review of the literature. Arch Int Med 2015;18(2):852–7.
[277] Myung S, Choi H, Kim S, et al. Soy intake and risk of endocrine-related gynaecological cancer: a meta-analysis. BJOG 2009;116(3):1697–705.
[278] Yang W, Va P, Wong M, et al. Soy intake is associated with lower lung cancer risk results from a meta-analysis of epidemiological studies. Am J Clin Nutr 2011;94(6):1575–83.
[279] Assami D, Asami DK, Hong YJ, et al. Comparison of total phenolic and ascorbic acid content of freeze dried and air dried marionberry, strawberry and corn, grown using conventional, organic and sustainable agriculture practices. J Agric Food Chem 2003;51: 1237–41.
[280] Donaldson M. Nutrition and cancer: a review of the evidence for an anticancer diet. Nutr J 2004;3:19–57.
[281] Fenech M. The role of folic acid and vitamin B12 in genomic stability of human cells. Mutat Res 2001;475(1–2):57–67.
[282] Schrauzer GN, White DA, Schneider CJ. Cancer mortality correlation studies. III. Statistical association with dietary selenium intakes. Bioinorg Chem 1977;7:35–56.
[283] Li Y, Burns K, Arao Y, et al. Differential estrogenic actions of endocrine-disrupting chemicals bisphenol A, bisphenol AF, and zearalenone through estrogen receptor α and β in vitro. Environ Health Perspect 2012;120:1029–35.
[284] Eaton SB, Eaton SB 3rd, Sinclair AJ, et al. Dietary intake of long-chain polyunsaturated fatty acids during the Paleolithic period. World Rev Nutr Diet 1998;83:12–23.
[285] Firshein R. The nutraceutical revolution. New York: Riverhead Books via Penguin Putnam; 1998. p. 75.
[286] Knight J. Review: free radicals, antioxidants and the immune system. Ann Clin Lab Sci 2000;30(2):145–58.
[287] Blokhina O, Virolainen E, Fagerstedt KV, et al. Antioxidants, oxidative damage and oxygen deprivation stress: a review. Ann Bot 2003;(Special no):179–94.
[288] Montrone M, Martorelli D, Rosato A, et al. Retinoids as critical modulators of immune functions: new therapeutic perspectives for old compounds. Endocr Metab Immune Disord Drug Targets 2009;9(2):113–31.
[289] Segala M, editor. Disease prevention and treatment. 3rd ed. Florida: Life Extension Media; 2000. p. 139.
[290] Belin S, Kaya F, Duisit G, et al. Antiproliferative effect of ascorbic acid is associated with the inhibition of genes necessary to cell cycle progression. PLoS ONE 2009;4(2):e4409.
[291] Padayatty SJ, Riordan HD, Hewitt SM, et al. Intravenously administered vitamin C as cancer therapy: three cases. CMAJ 2006;174(7):937–42.
[292] Cui Y, Rohan TE. Vitamin D, calcium, and breast cancer risk: a review. Cancer Epidemiol Biomarkers Prev 2006;15(8):1427–37.
[293] Weitsman G, Weitsman GE, Ravid A, et al. Vitamin D enhances caspase-dependent and -independent TNFalpha-induced breast cancer cell death: the role of reactive oxygen species and mitochondria. Int J Cancer 2003;106(2):178–86.
[294] Nowson CA, Diamond TH, Pasco JA, et al. Vitamin D in Australia — issues and recommendations. Aust Fam Phys 2004;33(3):133–8.
[295] Giovannucci E, Liu Y, Rimm EB, et al. Prospective study of predictors of vitamin D status and cancer incidence and mortality in men. J Natl Cancer Instit 2006;98(7):451–9.
[296] Turley JM, Fu TF, Ruscetti FW, et al. Vitamin E succinate induces Fas-mediated apoptosis in estrogen receptor-negative human breast cancer cells. Cancer Res 1997;57:881–90.
[297] Gogos CA, Ginopoulos P, Salsa B, et al. Dietary omega-3 polyunsaturated fatty acids plus vitamin E restore immunodeficiency and prolong survival for severely ill patients with generalized malignancy. Cancer 1998;82:395–402.
[298] Chinery R, Brockman JA, Peeler MO, et al. Antioxidants enhance the cytotoxicity of chemotherapeutic agents in colorectal cancer: a p53-independent induction of p21 via C/EBP-beta. Nat Med 1997;3(1233–1241).
[299] Singh P, Krishnan S. Vitamin E analogs as radiation response modifiers. Evid Based Complement Alternat Med 2015;2015:741301.
[300] Hathcock JN, Azzi A, Blumberg J, et al. Vitamins E and C are safe across a broad range of intakes. Am J Clin Nutr 2005;81(4): 736–45.
[301] Prasad AS. Zinc deficiency: has been known of for 40 years but ignored by global health organizations. BMJ 2003;326(7386): 409–10.
[302] Shankar AH, Prasad AS. Zinc and immune function: the biological basis of altered resistance to infection. Am J Clin Nutr 1998; 68(Suppl.):S447–63.
[303] Maret W, Sandstead HH. Zinc requirements and the risks and benefits of zinc supplementation. J Trace Elem Med Biol 2006;20(1):3–18.
[304] Russell RM. New micronutrient dietary reference intakes from the National Academy of Sciences. Nutr Today 2001;36: 163–71.
[305] Micke O, Schomburg L, Buentzel J, et al. Selenium in oncology: from chemistry to clinics. Molecules 2009;14(10):3975–88.
[306] Cheng J, Jiang C, Jiang W, et al. Selenium-induced inhibition of angiogenesis in mammary cancer at chemopreventive levels of intake. Mol Carcinogenesis 1999;26:213–25.
[307] El-Bayoumy K, Sinha R. Mechanisms of mammary cancer chemoprevention by organoselenium compounds. Review. Mutat Res 2004;551:181–97.
[308] Reid ME, Duffield-Lillico AJ, Slate E, et al. The nutritional prevention of cancer: 400 mcg per day selenium treatment. Nutr Cancer 2008;60(2):155–63.
[309] Lamson D, Lamson DW, Brignall MS, et al. Antioxidants in cancer therapy: their actions and interactions with oncologic therapies. Alternat Med Rev 1999;4(5):304–29.
[310] Jaakkola K, Lähteenmäki P, Laakso J, et al. Treatment with antioxidant and other nutrients in combination with chemotherapy and irradiation in patients with small-cell lung cancer. Anticancer Res 1992;12(3):599–606.

[311] Yarnell E, Abascal K. Can botanicals reduce multidrug resistance in cancer? Alternat Complement Ther 2002;8(6):336–40.

[312] Shin H, Shin HJ, Kim YS, et al. Enhancement of antitumor effects of paclitaxel (taxol) in combination with red ginseng acidic polysaccharide (RGAP). Planta Med 2004;70(11):1033–8.

[313] Cui Y, Shu XO, Gao YT, et al. Association of ginseng use with survival and quality of life among breast cancer patients. Am J Epidemiol 2006;163:645–53.

[314] Ratnasinghe D, Kasprzak BH, Taylor PR, et al. Cyclooxygenase-2, P-glycoprotein-170 and drug resistance: is chemoprevention against multidrug resistance possible? Anticancer Res 2001;21(3C):2141–7

[315] Hennessy M, Kelleher D, Spiers JP, et al. St John's wort increases expression of P-glycoprotein: implications for drug interactions. Br J Clin Pharmacol 2002;53:75–82.

[316] Huang Q, Wu L, Tashiro S, et al. Catechin, an ingredient of green tea protects murine microglia from oxidative stress-induced DNA damage and cell cycle arrest. J Pharmacol Sci 2005;98(1):16–24.

[317] Lee Y, Jin D, Kwon E, et al. Asiatic acid, a triterpene, induces apoptosis through intracellular Ca2+ release and enhanced expression of p53 in HepG2 human hepatoma cells. Cancer Lett 2002;186(1):83–91.

[318] Lemieszek M, Rzeski W. Anticancer properties of polysaccharides isolated from fungi of the Basidiomycetes class. Contemp Oncol (Pozn) 2012;16(4):285–9.

[319] Bemis DL, Capodice JL, Anastasiadis AG, et al. Zyflamend, a unique herbal preparation with nonselective COX inhibitory activity induces apoptosis of prostate cancer cells that lack COX-2 expression. Nutr Cancer 2005;52:202–12.

[320] Duke J. Turmeric, the queen of COX-2-inhibitors. Alternat Complement Ther 2007;13:229–34.

[321] Anuchapreeda S, Leechanachai P, Smith MM, et al. Modulation of P-glycoprotein expression and function by curcumin in multidrug-resistant human KB cells. Biochem Pharmacol 2002;64:573–82.

[322] Conklin K. Dietary antioxidants during cancer chemotherapy: impact on chemotherapeutic effectiveness and development of side-effects. Nutr Cancer 2000;37(1):1–18.

[323] Lissoni P, Tancini G, Barni S, et al. Treatment of cancer chemotherapy-induced toxicity with the pineal hormone melatonin. Support Care Cancer 1997;5(2):126–9.

[324] Blask DE, Dauchy RT, Sauer LA, et al. Putting cancer to sleep at night: the neuroendocrine/circadian melatonin signal. Endocrine 2005;27(2):179–88.

[325] Kurbacher CM, Wagner U, Kolster B, et al. Ascorbic acid (vitamin C) improves the antineoplastic activity of doxorubicin, cisplatin, and paclitaxel in human breast carcinoma cells in vitro. Cancer Lett 1996;103(2):183–9.

[326] Smyth JF, Bowman A, Parren T, et al. Glutathione reduces the toxicity and improves quality of life of women diagnosed with ovarian cancer treated with cisplatin: results of a double-blind, randomised trial. Ann Oncol 1997;8:569–73.

[327] Crane FL. Biochemical functions of coenzyme Q10. J Am Coll Nutr 2001;20(6):591–8.

[328] McCulloch M, See C, Shu X-J, et al. *Astragalus*-based Chinese herbs and platinum-based chemotherapy for advanced non-small-cell lung cancer: meta-analysis of randomized trials. J Clin Oncol 2006;24(3):419–30.

[329] Zhou W, Mukherjee P, Kiebish MA, et al. The calorie restricted ketogenic diet: an effective alternative diet for malignant brain cancer. Nutr Metab 2007;4:5.

[330] Bough H, Rho I. Anticonvulsant mechanisms of the ketogenic diet. Epilepsia 2007;48(1):43–58.

[331] Fasano A Celiac disease insights: clues to solving autoimmunity. Scientific American August 2009.

Ear, nose and throat

13

Annmarie Cannone

OVERVIEW OF EAR, NOSE AND THROAT

The areas of the ear, nose and throat are anatomically situated in the upper respiratory tract (URT). Collectively, these three structures fit under the term of otorhinolaryngology.

The nasal cavity in particular consists of finger-like protrusions called cilia. These cells constantly move in a swaying motion to filter out inspired air. Mucous membranes line these structures and provide moisture and also act as filters for inspired air.[1,2]

The throat acts as a passage way not only for food but also for inspired air to filter through to the lungs.[1,2]

The ears, despite being crucial for hearing, have a strong role in the maintenance of equilibrium.[1,2]

Anatomy of ear, nose and throat (upper respiratory tract)

EARS

The ears are divided into three regions (Fig. 13.1).

External ear: This portion of the ear is visible and is primarily involved with hearing. It is comprised of the pinna, also known as the auricle. The external auditory

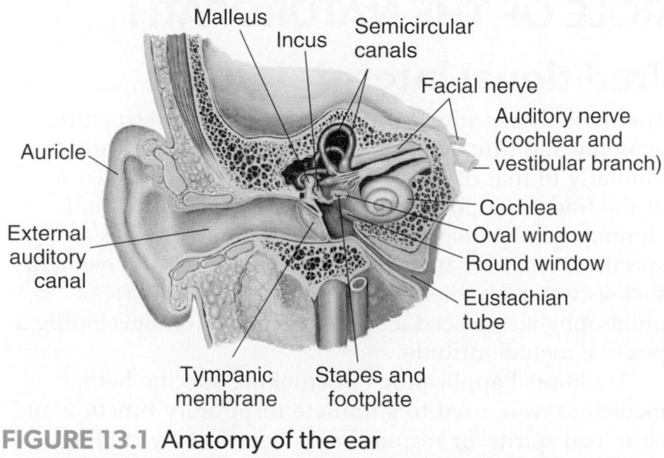

FIGURE 13.1 Anatomy of the ear

Source: Ball J, Dains J, Flynn J et al. Seidel's guide to physical examination. 8th edn. Copyright © 2015 by Mosby, an imprint of Elsevier Inc.

canal also constitutes the external ear.[1,2] This is a tube-like structure that leads to the middle ear. Sound waves enter this canal and hit the tympanic membrane (eardrum) and cause it to vibrate. The tympanic membrane is the structure that separates the external ear from the middle ear.[1,2]

Middle ear: Similarly to the external ear, the middle ear is also a primary structure for hearing. It is composed of a small chamber in the temporal bone called the tympanic cavity.[1,2] Three small bones, known collectively as the ossicles (malleus — hammer, incus — anvil and stapes — stirrup) transmit the vibrations of the tympanic membrane to the inner ear. The vibrations move from the malleus to the incus and then to the stapes.[1,2] The stapes presses against a membrane known as the oval window. Movement of the oval window sets the fluids contained in the inner ear in motion.[1,2] The eustachian tube connects the inner ear with the thorax. This structure is usually closed and opens briefly when we yawn or swallow. It has the primary function of maintaining and equalising pressure in the middle ear with atmospheric pressure. For as long as pressure in the ear is equalised, the tympanic membrane is able to vibrate freely.[1,2]

Inner ear: This area has primary involvement with hearing and maintaining equilibrium. It is comprised of bony, maze-like chambers, known as osseous labyrinths.[1,2] These chambers are filled with perilymph. The chambers are divided into the cochlea, the vestibule and the semicircular canals. The cochlea is comprised of the organ of Corti, which contains hair cells that act as hearing receptors and, when in motion, transmit impulses along the cochlear nerve to the auditory cortex of the brain, semicircular canal and vestibule. This is where equilibrium receptors are located and is where the interpretations of sound occur. These receptors are responsive to changes in direction of movement.[1,2] Within the semicircular canal, there is a receptor region composed of a tuft of hair cells covered in a gelatinous compound that has a crucial role for maintaining spatial orientation.[1,2]

The vestibule contains receptors known as maculae; these are essential to the body's sense of static equilibrium. As the head moves, small pieces of calcium salts known as otoliths move in a gel-like material in response to changes in the pull of gravity.[1,2] The otoliths pull on the gel, which in turn pulls on the hair cells in the maculae.[1,2]

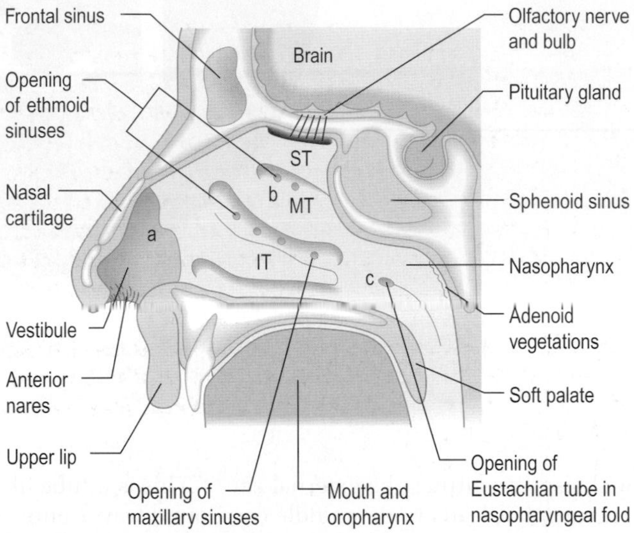

FIGURE 13.2 Anatomy of the nose

Source: Kumar P et al. Kumar and Clark's clinical medicine. 9th edn. Elsevier Ltd.

NOSE

The nose has two portions (Fig. 13.2).

External portion: consists of a supporting framework of bone and hyaline cartilage, which is covered with muscle and skin, and lined with mucous membranes.

Internal portion: is a large cavity (called the nasal cavity) that is lined with muscle and mucous membranes.[1,2] Anteriorly, the internal nose merges with the external nose, and posteriorly it opens into the pharynx.[1,2] Ducts from the paranasal sinuses and the nasolacrimal duct also open into the internal nose. The nasal cavity is divided into left and right sides by the nasal septum.[1,2] This part of the nose contains olfactory (smell) receptors.

The functions of the nose include to:

- Detect olfactory stimuli (smell)
- Moisten, warm and filter inhaled air
- Aid in speech.

THROAT

Pharynx: the pharynx is commonly known as the throat, and is a funnel-shaped tube found between the nasal cavity and the larynx, posterior to the oral cavity (Fig. 13.3).[1,2] The pharynx is divided into three regions, listed below from superior to inferior:

1. Nasopharynx: a passageway for air only
2. Oropharynx: a passageway for both air and food
3. Laryngopharynx: a passageway for both air and food.

The functions of the pharynx include:

- Passageway for air, food and drink
- Resonating chamber of speech sounds
- Location of tonsils
- Warming and moistening air.

Larynx: the larynx is commonly known as the voice box, and is located between the pharynx and the trachea. The larynx consists of nine pieces of cartilage. One of these, the thyroid cartilage, forms the laryngeal prominence, commonly known as the Adam's apple, which is located anteriorly and is larger in males than in females.

Another piece of cartilage, called the epiglottis, which is encased in a mucous membrane, closes off the passageway between the pharynx and the larynx during swallowing. This ensures food and drink do not move into the larynx and towards the lungs. Instead, food is directed into the oesophagus, an organ of the digestive system.

The larynx contains vocal folds (also known as vocal cords), which produce sounds as they vibrate when air passes by. The tension of the vocal folds is responsible for pitch — if they are pulled tight it leads to the production of sounds with a higher pitch, while decreased tension produces sounds with a lower pitch. The vocal folds are thicker and longer in men due to the effects of androgens, and as a result they vibrate more slowly and produce sounds with a lower pitch.

Although sound originates from the vocal cords, other structures are involved in converting this sound into recognisable speech. These include the pharynx, mouth, nasal cavity and paranasal sinuses (all of these act as resonating chambers), as well as the muscles of the pharynx, face, tongue and lips (help to make particular sounds and to enunciate words).

The functions of the larynx include:

- Passageway for air
- Production of speech sounds.

Tonsils and adenoids: both the tonsils and adenoids fit into the category of mucosa-associated lymphatic tissue, also known as MALT. There are five tonsils that form a ring at the junction of the oral cavity and the oropharynx and at the junction of the nasal cavity and nasopharynx. The tonsils function as part of the immune system to respond against inhaled or ingested foreign substances. The single pharyngeal tonsil, commonly known as the adenoid, is located in the posterior wall of the nasopharynx. The two palantine tonsils are situated in the posterior region, on either side of the oral cavity, and the paired lingual tonsils are located at the base of the tongue. Usually, both the palantine and lingual tonsils are removed during a tonsillectomy.[1,2]

ROLE OF THE NATUROPATH

Traditional interpretation

Traditionally not much was known about the structure, anatomy and functionality of the ears, nose and throat. Similarly to that of the lower respiratory tract, much of the traditional focus was around expectoration and elimination of foreign substances. Nature cure was a specific system for treating diseases with natural elements such as water, air, diet, herbs and sunshine. This philosophy also placed a strong emphasis on developing a positive mental attitude.

Traditional applications of smoking specific herbal medicines were used to stimulate respiratory function and clear 'bad spirits' or respiratory congestion. By ridding excess mucus and catarrh from the body it was believed that optimal health would be achieved.

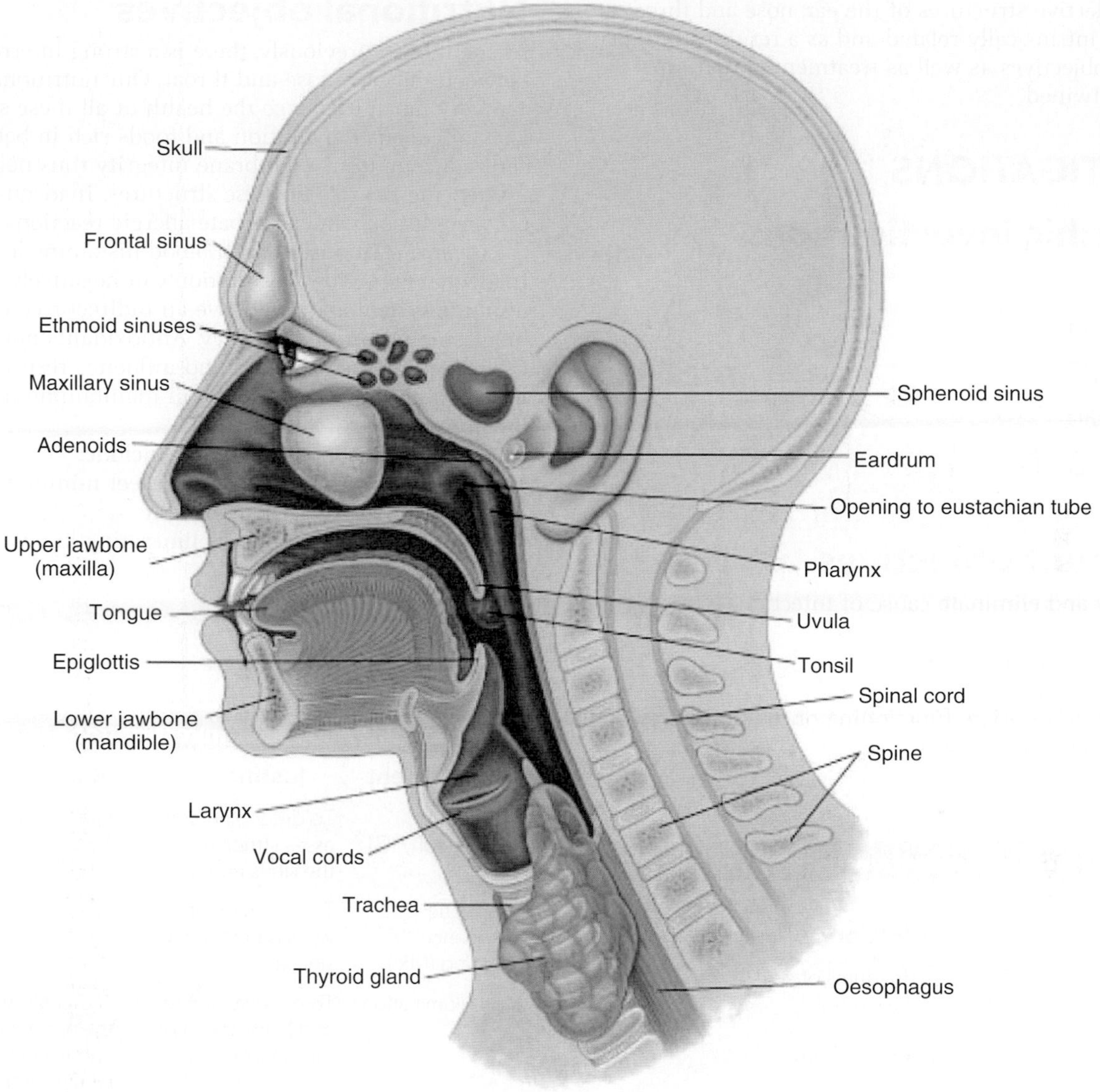

FIGURE 13.3 Anatomy of the throat

Source: From the Merck Manual Consumer Version (known as the Merck Manual in the US and Canada and the MSD Manual in the rest of the world), edited by R Porter. Copyright (2017) by Merck Sharp & Dohme Corp, a subsidiary of Merck & Co, Inc, Kenilworth, NJ. Available at http://www.merckmanuals.com/consumer. Accessed 28 July 2017.

Modern interpretation

As with all aspects of ill health, naturopathy has a strong focus on nurturing and supporting the innate ability of the body to heal itself. The greater understanding obtained through research has enabled the complex structures of the ear, nose and throat to be understood and supported accordingly. Determining the cause for lapses of ill health for these structures provides for effective and successful treatment.

Modern naturopathy understands there is a pathogenic role to the sub-optimal functioning of the upper respiratory tract. Through this knowledge, not only can there be appropriate management of symptoms but also the immune system can be supported and nurtured to allow for a reduction in the frequency, intensity and, ultimately, elimination of disease processes.

The modern naturopath understands the importance and role that nutritional, dietary and herbal medicine can play in supporting the eliminatory processes that occur, to reach a state of balance and restoration of function and health. Many symptoms such as mucus production are a sign of the body attempting to eliminate a pathogenic substance and as a result, treatment is focused around supporting and strengthening this.

The identification of causative factors, whether these are internal or external factors, plays a crucial role in restoring health. These factors can be related to poor hygiene; inability to adapt and cope with stress, thus placing further burden on the immune system; poor dietary choices; lack of hydration; or simply a compromised immune system thus contributing to allergies and intolerances.

The collective structures of the ear, nose and throat are very much intrinsically related and as a result of this, treatment objectives as well as treatment options are very much intertwined.

INVESTIGATIONS

Allopathic investigations

THE EAR

See Table 13.1.

THE NOSE

See Table 13.2.

THE THROAT

See Table 13.3.

Treatment objectives

- Identify and eliminate cause of infection
- Reduce inflammatory processes
- Provide symptomatic relief
- Reduce congestion
- Support appropriate functioning of the immune system
- Reduce allergic response.

TABLE 13.1 Allopathic investigations of the ear

Assessment	Justification	Reference ranges
Computed tomography (CT) scan	To assess structures of the ear and to reveal intratemporal or intracranial processes	n/a
Magnetic resonance imaging (MRI)	To assess structures of the ear and to reveal intratemporal or intracranial processes	n/a
Physical examination via otoscope	To inspect the health of the tympanic membrane (TM)	Swollen, inflamed and red TM indicates the presence of infection A pinkish/grey and somewhat translucent TM indicates the absence of infection
Audiometry and tympanometry	To assess the presence of auditory damage	Presence, diminished or absence of hearing
Discharge swab cultures	To determine and identify the presence of infection	Positive/negative
Tympanocentesis	To identify infection type	Positive/negative

Nutritional objectives

As mentioned previously, there is a strong interrelationship between the ears, nose and throat. Our nutritional status can very much influence the health of all these structures. Lack of adequate hydration and foods rich in beta-carotene can reduce mucous membrane integrity thus negatively influencing the role of these structures. Inadequate vitamin C consumption can exacerbate allergic reactions because of the inverse relationship with blood histamine levels.[3] Inadequate protein consumption can negatively impact the immune system and thus have an indirect role in increasing infection frequency. Antioxidants not only influence immune function and influence resistance to infection, they also have a role in maintaining mucous membrane integrity and health.

General nutritional objectives include:

- Increasing hydration levels to meet minimum standard of 30 mL per kg of body weight
- Identifying, avoiding and eliminating known dietary allergens

TABLE 13.2 Allopathic investigations of the nose

Assessment	Justification	Reference ranges
Computed tomography (CT) scan	To determine and asses structures of the sinus region	n/a
Magnetic resonance imaging (MRI)	To obtain greater visualisation of the sinuses	n/a
Transillumination	To observe airflow and illumination of the sinuses	A dull glow indicates the antrum is air filled and excludes sinusitis Diminished illumination indicates reduced airflow and confirms sinusitis
Nasal swab	To determine and identify the presence of infection	Positive/negative
Physical examination — palpation	To determine and localise the presence of sinus tenderness	Positive/negative for tenderness
Rhinomanometry	To measure the flow and pressure variations throughout the nasal cavities	Presence or obstruction of pressure and air flow
Acoustic rhinometry	To provide objective geometric study of the nasal cavities	Presence or absence of obstacles
IgE testing	To determine the presence of allergens	Positive/negative

TABLE 13.3 Allopathic investigations of the throat

Assessment	Justification	Reference ranges
Neck palpation	To determine the absence or presence of lymphadenopathy	Positive/negative for lymphadenopathy
Oral cavity inspection	To observe structures of the oral cavity	Presence or absence of ulcers, abnormal masses and exudates Swollen/inflamed tonsils and uvula Small patches of exudate on the palate can indicate oral thrush A large, white membrane covering the tonsils can indicate Epstein-Barr virus (EBV) A generalised red, swollen appearance with exudate can indicate *Streptococcus* infection
Oral cavity/throat swab	To determine the presence and nature of infection	Positive/negative
Full blood count	To determine if there is a causative nature such as leukaemia	*Haemoglobin (Hb):* Men: 130–180 g/L Women: 115–165 g/L *Red cell count (RCC):* Men: 4–5–6.5 × 10^{12}/L Women: 3.8–5–5.8 × 10^{12}/L *Packed cell volume (PCV):* Men: 0.40–0.54 Women: 0.37–0.47 *Mean cell volume (MCV):* 80–100 fL *Mean cell haemoglobin (MCH):* 27–32 pg *Mean cell haemoglobin concentration (MCHC):* 300–350 g/L *Reticulocyte count:* 10–100 × 10^9/L *Neutrophils:* 2–7.5 × 10^9/L *Lymphocytes:* 1–4 × 10^9/L *Monocytes:* 0.0–1 × 10^9/L *Eosinophils:* 0.0–0.5 × 10^9/L *Basophils:* 0.0–0.3 × 10^9/L *NRBC:* <1 × 100 WBC *Platelets:* 150–450 × 10^9/L
Fasting blood glucose test	To determine the presence of diabetes as a causative factor	3-6–6.0 mmol/L
Mononucleosis test	To determine the presence of antibodies, caused by Epstein-Barr virus	Positive/negative
Laryngoscopy	To observe the health of the larynx	Presence of obstructions, lesions, inflammation or swelling can indicate laryngitis

NRBC: nucleated red blood cells.

- Increasing nutrient-dense food and eliminating energy-dense food
- Increasing foods rich in beta-carotene, vitamin C, selenium and zinc
- Ensuring adequate dietary protein.

Specific herbal medicines

DISCUSSION AND APPLICATION

Before the development of diagnostic tools much of the role of the herbalist was to determine and eliminate symptoms. The causes of symptoms were not always known and, as a result, a strong focus developed on providing symptomatic relief for those suffering from upper respiratory tract infections. Today, much of what we can provide as naturopaths is based on traditional use of herbal medicine, combined with appropriate diagnostic tools to adequately treat the cause of the symptoms.

HERBAL MEDICINE CLASSES

Many of the herbal medicines used for the upper respiratory tract contain a combination of active constituents, which provide the herbal medicines with their synergistic effect. Many of the herbal medicines for the ear, nose and throat have combined antimicrobial, antiviral, anti-inflammatory and diaphoretic properties.

Demulcents

Demulcent herbal medicines have a specific anti-inflammatory and soothing property to mucous membranes and are used specifically for acute inflammatory conditions of the upper respiratory tract. Such herbal medicines include *Verbascum thapsus* (mullein) and *Althaea officinalis* (marshmallow). Generally, plants with a high mucilaginous property tend to be characterised as demulcents. Other examples include *Ulmus rubra* (slippery elm) and *Glycyrrhiza glabra* (liquorice).

The roots and leaves of marshmallow are rich in mucilage consisting of numerous polysaccharides such as L-rhamnose, D-galactose and D-galacturonic acid and D-glucaronic acid. In vitro studies have shown the polysaccharides to induce phagocytosis and reduce inflammation.[4]

Antimicrobials

Antimicrobials are herbal medicines that have a strong focus on eliminating certain microbes that may be causative of or exacerbate symptoms. Such herbal medicines include *Melaleuca officinalis* (tea tree), *Eucalyptus globulis* (eucalyptus), *Syzygium aromaticum* (clove), *Allium sativum* (garlic) and *Commiphora molmol (*myrrh).

Polyphenolic compounds and tannins are believed to enable the herbal medicine to exert broad-spectrum antimicrobial and antiviral activity. Examples of these compounds include protocatechuic acid, caffeic acid and rosmarinic acid found in *Melissa officinalis* (lemon balm). In garlic, sulfur compounds such as allicin, allylmethyl trisulfide and diallyl disulfide are responsible for its antibacterial, antiviral and antifungal activity.[4]

Analgesics

Analgesics provide symptomatic pain relief via their role in reducing swelling and inflammation. Such herbal medicines include *Matricaria chamomilla* (German chamomile), *Calendula officinalis* (calendula) and *Hypericum perforatum* (St John's wort).

The lipophilic triterpene alcohols, notably the esters of faradiol, found in the flowering heads of calendula, provide the plant with its anti-inflammatory properties.[4] The mechanism that causes this to occur is not yet fully understood.

Antiallergics

Many flavonoids, although they do exhibit effective antiallergic properties, tend to be not as effective as conventional antiallergic/antihistamine medications. They mostly contain pyrrolizidine alkaloids, which are toxic and can induce liver failure. In contrast, herbal medicines such as *Albizia lebbeck* (albizia) contain a combination of alkaloids, steroids, flavonoids and glycosides. In in vivo and in vitro tests these active constituents have displayed significant mast cell stabilisation effects similar to those of cromoglycate. Some studies have also reported 62% degranulation inhibition.[4]

Immunostimulants

Many compounds have been determined to have immunostimulant activity, with many constituents still yet to be investigated. The most commonly known compounds include caffeic acid derivatives such as echinosides, found in *Echinacea* spp. In addition a combination of alkylamides and polysaccharides are responsible for echinacea's immunomodulatory and immunostimulatory activity.[4] These compounds are thought to activate T- and B-cell leucocytes and have a specific influence on nonspecific cellular immunity.

Triterpenoid saponins such as astragalosides I–VIII and their acetyl derivatives, found in *Astragalus membranaceus* (astragalus), have been identified for their immunostimulant activity, specifically for use in colds and upper respiratory tract infections.[4]

HERBAL MEDICINE PREPARATIONS

Inhalations and essential oils

Vaporisers, nasal snuffs and other inhalant methods often contain ingredients from the *Melaleuca* family (tea tree), mint family (menthol content) or eucalyptus family (camphor content). Such preparations include peppermint, thyme, pine, lavender, lemon or eucalyptus essential oils. In addition, chamomile flowers (tea or essential oil) are used for allergic rhinitis because of their anti-inflammatory and antiallergic properties.

The use of essential oils in the form of inhalations proves to be quite effective for infants, children and the elderly. They can be used as decongestants, antispasmodics and expectorants. The essential oils 1,8 cineole, terpineol and α-pinene found in eucalyptus are responsible for its physiological activity.

Teas

Teas are used especially for colds and flu, temperature and throat problems; for example, lime flower, yarrow, elderflower and peppermint teas.

Gargles

Gargles of herbal medicines that are antibacterial and antimicrobial are used especially for URT infections/inflammation. They include myrrh, thyme, calendula and sage.

Nasal sprays

Nasal sprays can be made with essential oils and/or herbal preparations (best to use teas rather than tinctures or fluid extract):

- Saline preparation with tea tree nasal spray
- Chamomile flowers (tea or essential oil) for allergic rhinitis — anti-inflammatory, antiallergic.

Throat sprays

- Preparations made with antibacterial, antimicrobial herbal medicines, for example: myrrh, thyme, calendula, sage, clove

- Demulcent herbal medicines; for example, liquorice, marshmallow
- Astringent herbal medicines; for example, witch hazel, raspberry leaf.

Lozenges and cough drops

- Propolis, honey, ice cubes, zinc lozenges, liquorice, marshmallow, vitamin C.

Ear drops

A combination of the herbal medicines mentioned in the analgesic paragraphs can be used to provide symptomatic relief for those suffering from otitis media, particularly in children.

Onion compress (poultice)

Placing a warm compress of onion, wrapped in a linen cloth, directly below the temporomandibular joint (TMJ) may provide temporary symptomatic pain relief for otitis media sufferers.

Directions: Gently simmer ½ onion in ¼ cup of water for a few minutes. Wrap the simmered onion in several layers of cheesecloth and allow to cool so it doesn't burn the skin. Apply over the ear several times a day until the pain eases.

THE EARS

Otitis media

EPIDEMIOLOGY

Acute otitis media (AOM) is a common problem in early childhood; approximately two-thirds of children have at least one episode by the age of 3 years and 90% of children have at least one episode prior to the commencement of school. Peak age of prevalence is 6–18 months.[5]

AETIOLOGY AND PATHOGENESIS

Globally, otitis media is the second major cause of hearing loss.[6] In 2013, it was ranked fifth on the global burden of disease and affected over 1 billion people.[6] It is characterised by inflammation and moderate to severe bulging of the tympanic membrane (TM) with or without the presence of fluid exudate. Erythema is also a common sign of otitis media; however, this is not a main diagnostic sign as erythema of the TM can also be present in respiratory tract infections.[7]

Commonly, otitis media occurs as a result of a viral infection of the upper respiratory tract that contributes to inflammation and dysfunction of the eustachian tube.[7] The eustachian tube not only equalises air pressure within the ear, it also plays a role in draining nasopharynx secretions and protecting the ear from these secretions. When the eustachian tube is not functioning efficiently, these secretions easily enter the middle ear and cause infection.[8]

Symptoms of otitis media usually occur in the following sequence: congestion of the upper respiratory tract, usually as a result of a viral infection; swelling of the eustachian tube mucosa, resulting in narrowing of the tube which leads to an accumulation of fluid which, if contaminated by bacteria, can result in otitis media.

Research suggests the presence of bacterial biofilms in the middle ear may be a major contributing factor to the development of recurrent acute and chronic otitis media.[9]

Middle ear cultures have identified bacterial infections as the main cause of otitis media, with *Streptococcus pneumoniae* and *Haemophilus influenzae* being the most common bacterial causes, not only in children but in all age groups.[10]

Common causes include:

- Virus (25%)
- *Streptococcus pneumoniae* (35%)
- Non-typable strains of *Haemophilus influenzae* (25%)
- *Moraxella catarrhalis* (15%).

Aa noted, viral infections are usually precursors to the development of otitis media, with respiratory viral infections being the main viral contributor.[11] Rhinoviruses and influenza viruses have also been determined as being causative microbes.[11] Links have been established between an increase in the severity and intensity of otitis media and the presence of both viral and bacterial infections.[11,12]

SIGNS AND SYMPTOMS

The symptomatology of otitis media varies, depending on the degree and extent of the infection.[10–12] The most common symptoms include inflammation of the middle ear mucosa which can mostly be identified with redness of the tympanic membrane; this can result in erythema.[10–12] Other specific symptoms include ear pain/discomfort, vertigo, tinnitus, with the most severe sign being hearing loss.[10–12] Fever, lethargy and pallor are also associated nonspecific signs and symptoms.

ACUTE OTITIS MEDIA AND CHRONIC OTITIS MEDIA

Other than the aforementioned signs and symptoms, acute otitis media can be associated with discharge in the auditory canal, which may be as a secondary result of perforation to the tympanic membrane. As well as this, the pinna may become red and inflamed and the tympanic membrane can appear red and/or yellow.

With chronic otitis media, there is persistent inflammation and bulging of the tympanic membrane with chronic ear drainage and persistent feeling of the ears being blocked or full. Inflammation behind the ear can also be a sign of chronic otitis media.

Complications

If not treated appropriately and in a timely manner, over time otitis media, especially with recurrent bouts, can contribute to permanent hearing loss. This usually occurs as a result of scarring and erosion of the middle ear. If not treated at all, the infection can erode the mastoid and spread to the brain meninges and be life threatening.

DIFFERENTIAL DIAGNOSIS

Because the signs and symptoms of otitis media overlap with other infections and diseases of the auditory canal, it is imperative to rule these out initially.[13] Upon examination, otitis media needs to be distinguished from myringitis as well as inflammation of the external auditory meatus.[13] The most common differential diagnosis is serous tympanic effusion, which does not involve pain, erythema of the tympanic membrane or exudate in the tympanic cavity.[13] An accurate differential diagnosis is difficult to make during the initial phases of acute otitis media or during the recovery phase. It is much simpler to differentiate chronic otitis media from other conditions due to the nature of its symptomatology.[12]

NATUROPATHIC DIAGNOSIS

Because of the general acute nature of otitis media, naturopathic diagnosis relies on the diagnosis of allopathic medicine to form the framework of treatment objectives and treatment goals. Many of the diagnostic tools used are only accessible by the medical fraternity.

INVESTIGATIONS

See Table 13.1.

THERAPEUTIC CONSIDERATIONS

CLINICAL DECISION MAKING AND RATIONALE

As naturopaths, it is crucial to acknowledge and recognise when it is beneficial to refer the patient to a medical professional for further treatment. When determining the need for referral, it is important to combine the patient's symptom picture with the signs being exhibited. The length of time the patient has been experiencing symptoms and the degree of pain experienced can aid with this decision-making process.

It is crucial that all children below the age of 2 years who are experiencing a fever of 38°C and above are immediately referred to their medical practitioner for treatment. Recurrent and persistent otitis media may warrant referral to an otorhinolaryngologist for further investigation. The presence of any exudate in the middle ear means the patient should be referred on to a medical professional.

Much of what is achievable when treating otitis media is based on managing symptoms and providing a degree of symptomatic relief. In addition, immune support is encouraged to reduce the frequency of infections.

THERAPEUTIC APPLICATION

Depending on what has contributed to the otitis media, the initial treatment measure is to provide symptomatic relief through the use of non-steroidal anti-inflammatory medications and analgesics such as paracetamol. If there is an infectious component, antibiotics will be used. Common antibiotics include amoxicillin and cefalexin. Determining the cause of otitis media is crucial in preventing its recurrence as well as preventing the development into chronic otitis media. Promoting appropriate hygiene and immune supportive practices can be of great assistance in reducing the incidence of otitis media globally.
Appropriate and correct management of upper respiratory tract infections can be a large component in reducing the development and frequency of this commonly occurring condition.

Historical perspective

Until the 17th century, knowledge around ear diseases was limited. Prior to this time, otitis media was extremely common, particularly in the poorest of children. It wasn't until the 19th century that a greater understanding of the anatomy, function and diseases of the ears was developed and, as a result, various diagnostic tools and treatment options became available. Prior to the discovery of antibiotics, the treatment of ear infections and complications was centred around surgical drainage of the tympanic membrane. Today, some of these methods are still employed.

Otitis media usually occurs as a result of unresolved upper respiratory tract infections which occur with poor hygiene and a suboptimal immune system. Children from developing countries and those who are from lower socioeconomic regions of developed countries have a much higher incidence of otitis media compared to the remainder of the population.[6] This is a result of reduced access to healthcare services and poor hygiene practices which contribute to compromised immune systems.[6]

Naturopathic perspective

The naturopath's role is to identify and treat the cause of otitis media. Many cases of otitis are self-limiting, with the body being able to provide sufficient support via the immune system to eliminate the infection. With this in mind, symptomatic relief through herbal analgesics as well as immune support through nutrients can make a great impact not only on the recovery process but also in reducing the frequency and incidence of otitis media. Supporting the immune system will not only aid with relieving the otitis media, it will also provide a supportive framework for the body to efficiently ward off any future infections.

Nutritional medicine (dietary)

- The diet should be conducive and supportive to allow appropriate functioning of the immune system
- Easily digestible protein in the form of soups is recommended to support the immune system and provide nourishment, especially for children who tend to experience anorexia when they are unwell
- The diet should contain adequate amounts of fluid to improve the integrity of the mucous membranes
- Known allergens that may exacerbate inflammation and otitis media should be removed.

DIETARY EXCLUSIONS

Although not recent, research has indicated a direct correlation between food allergies and the recurrence of otitis media: 78% of children with recurrent otitis media have a food allergy.[14] When an elimination diet of the particular food allergen was conducted, 86% of participants noted an improvement in the frequency of otitis media.[14] When the offending food was reintroduced into the diet, there was a direct correlation with the increase in the incidence of otitis media in 96% of the studied participants.[14] Much of the research available, despite being outdated, does provide a link between dietary and environmental allergens and the development and recurrence of otitis media.[15]

The main offending allergens have been found to be dairy milk, in particular cow's milk, wheat, egg white, peanuts, soy, corn, tomatoes, chicken and apple.[16]

It is believed that an allergic reaction may contribute to a blockage of the eustachian tube by causing inflammation of the mucous membranes as well as swelling of the nose that leads to forced air and secretions in the middle ear.[17] The middle and inner ear are known to be immunologically responsive and this includes responsiveness to food hypersensitivities.[17]

SAMPLE DAILY DIET

BREAKFAST	
Stove-cooked rolled quinoa with ground cinnamon, filtered water, nut butter and poached apple	Cinnamon has been shown to aid with reducing inflammatory processes, with quinoa providing essential protein to aid with immune function
LUNCH	
Salmon fillet with sautéed garlic and spinach	Provides essential fatty acids in the form of omega-3 to enhance the body's ability to reduce inflammation. Garlic is a known antimicrobial and immune stimulant
DINNER	
Organic chicken soup with seasonal vegetables	Nutrient-dense, easily digestible and protein-rich meal to not only enhance fluid intake but also support and encourage appropriate immune function via consuming sufficient protein
SNACKS	
Poached pears and apples with cinnamon and nutmeg	Nutmeg and cinnamon have been used in traditional Ayurvedic medicine to aid with reducing inflammation
BEVERAGES	
Mineral water at least 1–2 L per day Chamomile, peppermint and elder tea	To ensure adequate hydration and protect the health of the mucous membranes

Nutritional medicine (supplemental)

NUTRITIONAL MEDICINE THERAPEUTIC OBJECTIVES

The main aim of nutritional supplementation is to:

- Improve and support the immune system
- Provide symptomatic relief by reducing inflammation
- Reduce the incidence and frequency of recurrence.

Vitamin D

Vitamin D has a strong influence on modulating the immune system and, as a result, may play a role in reducing the frequency and intensity of otitis media. During a single blind randomised trial 116 children who had a history of recurrent acute otitis media were supplemented with 1000 IU per day of vitamin D or placebo for 4 months. Episodes of acute otitis media were monitored for 6 months.[18] The incidence of acute otitis media was much lower in the treatment group than in those receiving the placebo ($p = 0.03$) and the best results were seen in those participants whose serum vitamin D was greater than 30 ng/mL ($p < 0.001$).[18] This study illustrates the role and importance of vitamin D in reducing the frequency of acute otitis media in children who suffer from vitamin D hypovitaminosis.

Zinc

Zinc plays a crucial and central role in the immune system. It is vital for the development and function of cells mediating nonspecific immunity, such as neutrophils and natural killer cells.[19] It also has a strong influence on the development of acquired immunity. In addition, it acts as an antioxidant. Deficiencies in zinc have been linked to reduced immune response, an altered host resistance to infections and increased tissue repair time.[19,20]

Various large and well-controlled trials have shown that supplementation with zinc displays a significant protective effect in reducing suppurative otitis media.[19–21] Participants with low serum zinc levels also had a higher incidence of mucoid otitis media than those with sufficient zinc levels.[20–22]

Antioxidants: vitamins C, A and E

Vitamin C

Vitamin C is essential for efficient functioning of the immune system. Ascorbic acid has been found to modulate T-cell gene expression, specifically influencing genes involved in immune system function.[23] It can also stimulate the production of interferon, a protein that stimulates the synthesis of the antibodies of IgG and IgM, as well as the humoral thymus factor.[23]

Vitamin A

Vitamin A is a fat-soluble vitamin that is essential for immune function, cellular differentiation, vision and reproduction. It has anti-inflammatory, anti-infective and antioxidant activities.[22,24] The retinoids are crucial for the maintenance and health of the respiratory epithelium and mucous membranes. It has been hypothesised that vitamin A deficiencies may influence the health of the eustachian tube, tympanic membrane and middle ear mucosa by affecting oxidant vs antioxidant levels, epithelial function and sub-epithelial oedema. A deficiency may also contribute to altered secretion of mucin and secretory immunoglobulins.[22,24]

Vitamin E

Vitamin E is a lipid-soluble antioxidant and has been found to optimise and enhance immune function. Because of its strong antioxidant role, it suppresses oxidative damage and has the ability to upregulate glutathione peroxidase.[13] It also has an influence on humoral antibody production and enhances resistance to bacterial infections as well as influencing T-lymphocyte and natural killer cell response.[23]

A small study investigated the role vitamins A, C and E have in the recurrence and incidence of acute otitis media. Twenty-three children aged between 2 and 7 years with recurrent otitis media and tonsillitis were studied to determine their antioxidant serum status.[20] The study group was compared to a control group of 29 in the same age group. It was found that those with recurrent otitis media had statistically significant ($p < 0.05$) lower serum levels of the above nutrients.[20] Glutathione peroxidase levels were also shown to be much lower, compared to the healthy control group.[20] Although the cohort was small, this study demonstrates the role these nutrients may have in reducing the incidence of recurrent otitis media.

Xylitol

Xylitol is a sugar alcohol and is commonly used as a natural sweetener. In vitro studies have demonstrated its ability to inhibit *S. pneumoniae*.[25] A Cochrane review was conducted to investigate the efficacy and safety of xylitol in children under 12 years of age who suffer from acute otitis media.[25] Four studies were identified and all were conducted in a Finnish day care centre.[25] Three out of the four studies concluded that xylitol at 8.4 g five times a day acted as a prophylactic to reduce the occurrence of acute otitis media by 25–40%.[25] (Children's dosages should be calculated using Clark's rule.)

Dosage requirements

The dosage requirements are based on the literature:
- Vitamin D: 1000 IU per day
- Zinc: 10–50 mg per day
- Vitamin A: 5000–20 000 IU per day
- Vitamin C: 500–2000 mg in divided dose daily
- Vitamin E: 200–800 IU per day
- Xylitol: 8.4 g five times daily.

Herbal medicine

Herbal medicine therapeutic objectives

- Modulate immune function and response
- Reduce inflammation
- Reduce pain and discomfort.

Limited research is available to determine the effective treatment of otitis media through the use of botanical medicine; however, traditional uses of certain herbal medicines and formulas are known.

Sinupret

Sinupret is a German-manufactured herbal combination formula used to treat upper respiratory tract infections. It contains extracts of five herbs: elderflowers (*Sambucus nigra*) 36 mg, primrose flowers with calyx (*Primula veris*) 36 mg, common sorrel (*Rumex acetosa*) 36 mg, vervain 36 mg (*Verbena officinalis*) and gentian (*Gentiana lutea*) 12 mg.

A controlled prospective study of Sinupret included 40 children hospitalised for acute otitis media. The mean age of the children was 4.5 years.[26] Treatment included conventional antibacterial therapy and nasal decongestants. The combined use of Sinupret enabled the exudate to disappear within 4.2 days compared to 7.7 days in the control group ($p < 0.01$).[26] The study demonstrated the possible use of this herbal combination with antibiotic treatment to reduce recovery time for children who suffer from acute otitis media.[26]

Verbascum thapsus (Mullein)

Mullein is known as a demulcent and has been used in chronic otitis media to reduce inflammation and thus reduce pain. It can provide effective symptomatic relief. Studies have not been conducted to assess the efficacy of mullein in isolation; however, studies have investigated the use of mullein in combination with other herbal preparations.

Otikon, a herbal preparation consisting of *Verbascum thapsus, Calendula officinalis, Allium sativum* and *Hypericum perforatum* in olive oil, has been studied in two randomised trials for its effectiveness. The dose used in both studies was 5 drops three times a day placed in the external ear canal.[27,28] Both studies found a statistically significant reduction in ear pain and provided sufficient analgesia within 3 days of treatment. This was reflected as a 95.9% improvement in symptoms.[27,28] This was compared to anaesthetic alone which provided only 84.7% relief, and anaesthetic with antibiotics which provided a 77.8% improvement in symptoms.[27,28]

Echinacea spp. (Echinacea)

Echinacea is one of the most commonly used herbal medicines because of its strong influence on immune modulation. It is also effective for upper respiratory tract infections.[29] A meta-analysis investigated the use of ethanolic extracts of echinacea for upper respiratory tract infections.[29] These infections included otitis media. In the participants who experienced a higher susceptibility, stress or a state of immunological weakness, echinacea halved the risk of recurrent upper respiratory tract infections. The recurrence of otitis media was also less frequent in the echinacea treatment group.[29]

Another study was conducted to assess the effectiveness of a novel herbal and nutritional formula called Imoviral Junior, in the treatment of recurrent respiratory tract infections, such as otitis media.[30] Imoviral contains echinacea, acerola (vitamin C), beta-glucan, zinc and arabinogalactan.[30] The study groups consisted of 37 children who suffered 19 episodes of inflammatory episodes such as tonsillitis and otitis media within a 6-month period prior to treatment.[30] After treatment with Imoviral, 77% of the children reported improvements in chronic episodes and a reduced frequency of acute episodes.[30] This study provides evidence for the possible use of echinacea combined with antioxidant nutrients to reduce the frequency and incidence of otitis media.[30]

Essential oils

Essential oils and volatile oils have been known to exert antimicrobial activity. The effects of basil oil (*Ocimum basilicum*) and components of essential oils such as thymol, carvacrol and salicylaldehyde have been compared to those of a placebo when placed in the ear canal of rats with experimentally induced acute otitis media caused by pneumococci or *H. influenzae*.[31] Applying the essential oils into the external ear canal of the rats was effective for the treatment of the above pathogens and reduced inflammation associated with otitis media. Studies are required in human participants; however, these initial results prove promising.[31]

An in vitro study investigated the effects of *Eucalyptus smithii* and *Juniperus communis* essential oils against bacterial biofilms from *S. aureus* and *P. aeruginosa*. The study found that the essential oils were able to interfere with the starting phases of biofilm production, as well as inhibit mature biofilms.[32] This study provides new perspectives for the treatment of otitis media and associated biofilm production.

LIFESTYLE RECOMMENDATIONS

As otitis media most commonly occurs in children aged between 6 months and 2 years, lifestyle recommendations can be limiting; however, certain strategies can be implemented to reduce the rate of contracting infections that may exacerbate otitis media.

- Ensure appropriate hygiene practices
- Reduce pathogenic exposure, especially if child attends day care
- Where appropriate, breastfeeding is encouraged as multiple studies have indicated a reduction in the incidence of otitis media in infants who are breastfed, as opposed to bottle fed
- Reduce exposure to any known allergens or triggers
- Encourage children to avoid touching their ears as this can cause a further infiltration of pathogens into the middle ear.

CASE STUDY

BC is a 4-year-old child who presented with recurrent acute otitis media. She was experiencing a painful ear that had not resolved in a couple of days. No fluid exudate had been noted. There had been a history of a recurrent sore throat.

Patient's diet consisted of cow's milk 3 times per day, copious amounts of cheese and refined carbohydrates, with limited water and protein other than dairy products.

PHYSICAL EXAMINATION RESULTS

Appeared to be fatigued. Lobule and helix appeared red and inflamed.

CASE STUDY CONTINUED

VITAL SIGNS

BP: Not conducted due to age
Temperature: 38°C
Pulse: 100 bpm
Respiratory rate: 23 resp/min
Height: 95 cm
Weight:13 kg
BMI: 14

HEAD AND NECK

Face: Pallor noted
Ears: Red and inflamed tympanic membrane on examination — right ear
Throat: Slightly inflamed tonsils

RESPIRATORY

Chest inspection: Normal
Palpation: Normal
Percussion: Normal
Auscultation: Normal

OTHER SYSTEMS

NAD

TREATMENT PROTOCOL

As the patient was suffering from acute otitis media, treatment initially focused on symptomatic relief, combined with immune support. The importance of monitoring symptoms and fever was discussed with the patient's mother and she was strongly advised to take her daughter to their GP if the fever had not reduced within the next 24–48 hours or if the right ear pain worsened.

Herbal medicine

Echinacea spp.: 20 mL
Calendula officinalis: 15 mL
Verbascum thapsus: 150 mL
Dose: Based on Clark's rule: 1 mL daily

Nutritional medicine

Dietary

A reduction and ultimately an avoidance of dairy milk and dairy products were strongly advised for the next 3 weeks. This was to prevent further congestion of the upper respiratory tract and, subsequently, the eustachian tube. It was recommended for BC to consume up to 500 mL of water per day. This could also be consumed in the form of chicken broth and soup. Increasing non-dairy forms of protein consumption was also advised. Refined carbohydrates were eliminated in the diet.

Supplemental

- Vitamin C (Mixed bioflavonoids): 1000 mg daily, consumed in divided doses
- Zinc: 5 mg twice daily

Special topic: Fever management

CHILDREN'S FEVER — DETECTING DANGER

In the past, doctors advised treating a fever on the basis of temperature alone, but now they recommend taking both the temperature and the child's overall condition into account.

Children whose temperatures are lower than 39°C usually do not require allopathic medication, unless they are uncomfortable. If an infant of 3 months or younger has a rectal temperature of 38°C or higher, seek medical assistance immediately.

For older children, take behaviour and activity level into account. Watching how a child behaves helps interpretation of the child's condition. The illness is unlikely to be serious if the child:

- Maintains social contact and activity
- Maintains their appetite (appetite normally reduces or wanes during fever)
- Is alert and responds to communication
- Is happy and smiling
- Has normal skin colour
- Looks well when their temperature comes down.

Detecting a child's fever

Tactile temperature detection does not give an accurate measure of a child's temperature. Temperature must be taken with a functional thermometer. Fever is confirmed if:

- 38°C measured rectally
- 37.5°C measured orally
- 37.2°C measured in an axillary position.

Medical intervention

The exact temperature that should trigger a call to the doctor depends on the age of the child, the illness and whether the child has other symptoms with the fever.

Doctor

Call the child's doctor if:

- an infant younger than 3 months old has a temperature of 38°C
- an older child has a temperature of higher than 40°C. If an older child has a fever of less than 40°C, call the doctor if the child also:
- refuses fluids or seems too ill to drink adequately
- has persistent diarrhoea or repeated vomiting
- has any signs of dehydration
- has a specific complaint (e.g. sore throat or earache)
- still has a fever after 24 hours in a child aged younger than 2 years or after 72 hours in a child aged 2 years or older
- has recurrent fevers, even if they only last a few hours each night.

Emergency

Seek emergency care if the child shows any of the following signs along with a fever:

- inconsolable crying for several hours
- extreme irritability
- lethargy and difficulty waking
- rash or purple spots that look like bruises on the skin (that were not there before the child got sick)
- blue lips, tongue and nails
- infant's soft spot on the head seems to be bulging outward
- stiff neck
- severe headache
- limpness and refusal to move
- difficulty breathing that does not get better when the nose is cleared
- leaning forward and drooling
- seizure.

Naturopathic intervention

Practical support

- Reduce the amount of clothing worn and use natural fibres to encourage sweating
- Sponge bath with lukewarm water
- Adjust room temperature as required
- Offer sufficient fluids to avoid dehydration — water, soup, broths, ice blocks/icy poles. Avoid all caffeine-containing beverages and soft drinks. Electrolyte drinks are often not necessary
- Support appetite as the child requests (within reason); however, avoid sugar and refined foods
- Encourage rest and sleep as needed
- Keep the child away from school until the temperature has been normal for at least 24 hours.

Herbal medicine support

Antipyretics

Otherwise known as febrifuges, antipyretics are herbal medicines that reduce or prevent fever. They are not to be confused with antihydrotic herbal medicines — herbs that reduce sweating. Antihydrotic herbal medicines are indicated in instances such as hot flushes in menopause, while antipyretics are herbal medicines that reduce *fever* often of infectious origin.

It is important to reflect on Thomsonian medicine — which encouraged fever as the body's natural way of eliminating toxins and eradicating infection. This process is still encouraged in herbal medicine; however, there can be instances where fever needs to be reduced — such as in children or in chronic or dire situations. Eventually you will be able to determine which instance requires reduction of fever and which does not. Interestingly, many of the medicines within this class exhibit multiple actions and most show immune stimulating effects, thus ensuring that you will both eradicate the condition and reduce the fever.

Important herbal medicines include:

Achillea millefolium (yarrow)
Andrographis panniculata (andrographis)
Baptisia tinctoria (wild indigo)
Melissa officinalis (lemon balm)
Rehmannia glutinosa (rehmannia)
Salix spp. (willow)
Scutellaria baicalensis (baikal skullcap).

Diaphoretics

Also known as sudorifics, diaphoretics are herbal medicines that promote sweating during a fever. It is this action that enables the medicines to control a fever. Please note that they are not to be confused with antipyretics, which reduce a fever.

Important herbal medicines include:

Achillea millefolium (yarrow)
Asclepias tuberosa (pleurisy root)
Eupatorium perfoliatum (bone set)
Hyssopus officinalis (hyssop)
Inula helenium (elecampane)
Mentha x piperita (peppermint)
Nepeta cataria (catmint)
Sambucus nigra (elderflower)
Solidago spp. (goldenrod)
Tilia spp. (lime or linden flowers)
Zingiber officinale (ginger).

THE NOSE

Sinusitis and allergic rhinitis

EPIDEMIOLOGY

Using data obtained from the 2014–2015 Australian Health Survey, it is estimated that 7.1 million Australians suffer from a chronic respiratory condition. This figure has increased by 400 000 since 1995. Of this number, 4.5 million Australians suffer from allergic rhinitis and 1.9 million suffer from chronic sinusitis.[33]

CLASSIFICATION

Sinusitis

Sinusitis is often classified as rhinosinusitis. Acute viral rhinosinusitis (the common cold) is the most common form of acute rhinosinusitis. Acute bacterial rhinosinusitis (ABRS) usually occurs as a complication of acute viral rhinosinusitis, but it can also occur with mechanical nasal obstruction (especially in children, where a foreign body should be excluded on initial history and examination, particularly if symptoms are unilateral), odontogenic infection, immunodeficiency and deficient mucociliary clearance mechanisms. Acute bacterial rhinosinusitis is usually caused by *Streptococcus pneumoniae* or *Haemophilus influenzae* and less frequently by *Moraxella catarrhalis* (the latter is more common in children under 6 years).[34] Occasionally, chronic sinusitis of the maxillary sinus results from a tooth infection.

Allergic rhinitis

Allergic rhinitis is classified as mild when these features are not present, or moderate to severe when one or more of these features are present. In paediatrics, persistent mouth breathing and dental crowding could be considered markers for severe disease.[34]

AETIOLOGY

Sinusitis

Sinusitis is usually caused by a viral or bacterial infection. Non-infectious causes of sinusitis include allergy, foreign body, deviated septum, tumour, polyps and trauma. Acute bacterial rhinosinusitis (ABRS) shares symptoms with the viral upper respiratory tract infection (URTI), including rhinorrhoea, nasal congestion, facial pressure and fever. Infections of the frontal sinuses typically present with greater intensity and severity and may require hospital admission. Bacterial infection typically follows the impairment of mucus clearance and the obstruction of sinus ostia caused by viral respiratory infection. The paranasal sinuses are ordinarily sterile. With infection, the most common microorganisms isolated from maxillary sinuses are *S. pneumoniae, Streptococci, Pneumococci, Haemophilus influenzae* and *Moraxella catarrhalis*.[35]

Chronic sinusitis can typically be attributed to a low-grade infection (such as *Mycoplasma* spp.) or an allergic background. In 25% of cases of chronic maxillary sinusitis there is an underlying dental infection. It is imperative to caution patients as although vasoconstrictors and antihistamines cause transient relief, their chronic use is contraindicated because there is usually a reflex reaction following continual administration.

Allergic rhinitis

Allergic rhinitis is an allergic reaction triggered by pollen, mould, animal dander, dust and other similar inhaled allergens. Environmental chemicals within buildings can induce lethargy, headache and blocked or runny nose as well as symptoms of chronic sinusitis. Particulate matter in polluted air and chemicals such as chlorine and detergents, which can normally be tolerated, can greatly aggravate the condition.

Seasonal allergic rhinitis/hay fever

Pollen seasons vary considerably in different parts of the world. Pollens that cause hay fever in the spring usually come from trees such as oak, elm, maple, alder, birch, juniper and olive; in the early summer, from grasses such as bluegrasses, timothy, redtop and orchard grass; and in the late summer, from ragweed. Often grasses pollinate for much longer, and there are other autumn weeds to consider. Occasionally, mould spores can cause seasonal allergy.

Perennial allergic rhinitis

Perennial (year-round) allergic rhinitis causes symptoms similar to those of seasonal allergic rhinitis, but the symptoms vary in severity, often unpredictably, throughout the year.

The allergen in a year-round allergy may be house dust mites, feathers, animal dander or moulds. Nasal congestion, which is common, may block the eustachian tubes in the ears, causing hearing problems, particularly in children. A doctor must distinguish perennial allergic rhinitis from recurring sinus infections (sinusitis) and growths inside the nose (nasal polyps). Sinusitis and nasal polyps could be complications of the allergic rhinitis.

Some people who experience chronic nasal inflammation, sinusitis, nasal polyps, negative skin test results and large numbers of eosinophils in their nasal secretions are prone to a severe reaction to aspirin or non-steroidal anti-inflammatory drugs.

People who have a chronically stuffy and runny nose but no sinusitis, nasal polyps or any demonstrable allergy may have a different condition — vasomotor rhinitis — which is not caused by allergy.

OVERVIEW

Sinusitis is an infection of the paranasal sinuses causing inflammation of the mucosal lining. Allergic rhinitis is the most common form of non-infectious rhinitis and is associated with an IgE-mediated immune response. It is often associated with ocular symptoms and with sinusitis. Allergic rhinitis and asthma often coexist and this association should be actively sought in the history and examination and, if indicated, the patient tested for reversible airway obstruction. Atopic dermatitis (eczema) is also commonly associated. Allergic rhinitis and rhinosinusitis are increasingly being regarded as interrelated and part of a spectrum of airway inflammatory disease. The severity of allergic rhinitis is classified according to the presence or absence of sleep disturbance; impairment of daily activities, leisure or sport; impairment of school or work; and troublesome symptoms.[34]

PATHOGENESIS

In acute sinusitis the infection lasts up to 4 weeks; in subacute sinusitis the infection lasts 4 weeks to 3 months; in recurrent sinusitis the infection is more than 3–4 episodes/year lasting at least 10 days, with no symptoms between episodes; and in chronic sinusitis the infection lasts more than 3 months. Most episodes of sinusitis-like symptoms are viral in origin and are a normal part of common cold and influenza-like illnesses. Viral sinusitis is generally self-limiting and does not require treatment.

When a person with a sensitised immune system inhales an allergen, such as pollen or dust, it triggers antibody production. These antibodies mostly bind to mast cells, which contain histamine. When the mast cells are stimulated by pollen and dust, histamine and other chemicals are released. This causes itching, swelling and excess mucus production.

Allergy

Allergic rhinitis has an obvious allergy component. Studies indicate that as many as 84% of cases of chronic sinusitis can be attributed to underlying allergies.[36,37] Patients with chronic sinusitis should be aggressively screened for environmental and food allergies by a number of assessments including radioallergosorbent test (RAST), IgE/IgG food allergy profiles, cytotoxic food allergy profiles and other assessments.

SIGNS AND SYMPTOMS

Sinusitis

Acute rhinosinusitis is characterised by nasal blockage (congestion or obstruction) or nasal discharge (anterior or posterior nasal drip) — with or without facial pain or pressure and reduction or loss of smell, and lasting for less than 12 weeks.[34]

Other important signs and symptoms include:

- Fever, chills and frontal headache
- History of acute viral respiratory infection, dental infection or nasal allergy
- Nasal congestion and purulent discharge
- Pain, tenderness, redness and swelling over the involved sinus
- Transillumination shows opaque sinus.

Chronic infection:

- May produce no symptoms other than mild postnasal discharge, a musty odour or a non-productive cough.

Allergic rhinitis

Once the pollen season starts, the nose, roof of the mouth, back of the throat and eyes itch gradually or abruptly. Watery eyes, sneezing and a clear watery discharge from the nose usually follow. Some people develop headaches, coughing and wheezing, become irritable and depressed, lose their appetite and have trouble sleeping. The inner eyelids and whites of the eyes may become inflamed (conjunctivitis). The lining of the nose may become swollen and bluish-red, leading to a runny nose and stuffiness. Seasonal allergic rhinitis is usually easy to recognise. Skin tests and the person's history of symptoms can help the naturopath determine which pollen is causing the problem.

Symptoms vary in severity from person to person. Very sensitive individuals can experience hives or other rashes. Allergic rhinitis is characterised by continuous or periodic nasal congestion, rhinorrhoea, sneezing, pruritus of the conjunctiva, nasal mucosa and oropharynx, allergic shiners and fatigue.

COMPLICATIONS

Sinusitis

Complications are potentially quite serious because of the anatomical relationship of the sinuses to the eyes and brain. These complications include orbital cellulitis, orbital abscess and potentially life-threatening intracranial complications such as cavernous sinus thrombosis, meningitis and brain abscess. Chronic sinusitis is defined by the presence of two major, or one major and two minor criteria. Non-infectious factors such as allergy and irritants appear to initially cause inflammation then bacteria may have some role in its persistence. Purulent nasal discharge, nasal congestion and/or facial pain or pressure for more than 5–7 days plus high fever (38.4°C or more), unilateral maxillary sinus tenderness, severe headache or worsening symptoms after initial improvement are signs of more serious infections and may need antibiotic therapy.[34]

Allergic rhinitis

Several disorders may be associated with allergies: comorbidities include eczema, asthma, depression and migraine. Allergic rhinitis is one of the main triggers of asthma.

DIFFERENTIAL DIAGNOSIS

Sinusitis

The diagnosis is primarily clinical. Definitive diagnosis is by endoscopy showing one or more polyps, mucopurulent discharge from the middle meatus, oedema or obstruction at the middle meatus.[34]

Allergic rhinitis

Allergic rhinitis is often associated with ocular symptoms and with sinusitis. Allergic rhinitis and asthma often coexist and this association should be actively sought in the history and examination and, if indicated, the patient tested for reversible airway obstruction. Atopic dermatitis (eczema) is also commonly associated with hay fever.[34]

NATUROPATHIC DIAGNOSIS

Naturopathic diagnosis needs to consider a complete holistic assessment. Relevant questions include discovering the long-term history regarding:

- Dental hygiene
- Allergy (food, chemical, airborne, environmental)
- Full dietary review
- Recent immunisations
- Potential occupational hazards
- Exposure to environmental chemicals
- Headache/migraines.

Referral to a relevant specialist for further investigations and assessment is warranted in cases of a chronic nature.

INVESTIGATIONS

See Table 13.2.

CT scan

CT has the ability to visualise the paranasal sinuses and the osteomeatal complex, the anatomical entity central to the diagnosis of ABRS. The changes seen in CT examination are not sufficiently specific for sinusitis, and CT should be used carefully and within the clinical context. When surgical management is being considered, as in cases of persistent infection or complicated infections, CT may be indicated in planning therapy. Coronal CT scan images of the sinuses can be very helpful for evaluating acute or chronic sinusitis.

Allergy testing

Allergy testing may be beneficial in determining the specific allergens. Tests may include investigations for food sensitivities. Allergy testing may reveal the specific allergens a person is sensitive to. Skin testing is the most common method of allergy testing and may include intradermal, scratch, patch or other tests. Less commonly, the suspected allergen is dissolved and dropped onto the lower eyelid as a means of testing for allergies. In some individuals who cannot undergo skin testing, the RAST blood test may be helpful in determining specific allergen sensitivity.

Nasal smear

A nasal smear can sometimes be helpful for establishing the diagnosis of allergic rhinitis. The presence of eosinophils is consistent with allergic rhinitis. Results are neither sensitive nor specific for allergic rhinitis and should not be used exclusively for establishing the diagnosis.

Radiographic studies

While radiographic studies are not needed to establish the diagnosis of rhinitis, they can be helpful for evaluating possible structural abnormalities or to help detect complications or comorbid conditions, such as sinusitis or adenoid hypertrophy.[38,39]

Specific naturopathic investigations

Because of the acute nature of the condition, additional investigations are often not required. In the incidence of repeated or chronic infections, referral for allergy studies is appropriate such as IgG/IgE food profiles and chemical sensitivities. Strong chronic infections warrant additional investigations for low-grade dormant pathogens such as *Mycoplasma* spp.

THERAPEUTIC CONSIDERATIONS

Clinical decision making and rationale

SINUSITIS

Antibiotics are the main initial treatment for suspected bacterial sinusitis. Antibiotic therapy for chronic rhinosinusitis has not been shown to improve outcomes in children, whereas the benefits of antibiotic therapy for adult chronic sinusitis have not been studied.[34] Antibiotics can shorten the duration of the illness, but spontaneous resolution or improvement of symptoms after 2 weeks was found to occur in 80% of patients given a placebo in controlled trials. Hence observation and supportive therapy are recommended for those patients with mild facial pain and fever less than 38.3°C. If symptoms are moderately severe after 5 days, intranasal corticosteroids, either as monotherapy or in conjunction with antibiotics, will give symptomatic relief. Antibiotic therapy, as well as intranasal corticosteroids, may be given to patients with severe rhinosinusitis symptoms (purulent nasal discharge, nasal congestion and/or facial pain or pressure) for more than 5–7 days plus any of the following features: high fever (38.4°C or more), unilateral maxillary sinus tenderness, severe headache or worsening symptoms after initial improvement.[34]

ALLERGIC RHINITIS

It is essential to reduce the exposure to the allergens. Even dietary allergens should be identified and eliminated. Treatment aims to reduce the impact of the allergen, by reducing exposure, reduce the immune response and generally improve the body's resistance. Symptoms control is essential.

THERAPEUTIC APPLICATION

Historical perspective

SINUSITIS

Surgical management of frontal sinusitis disease was first described in the 18th century. Knowledge of mucociliary function was absent and no regard was given to preserving frontal sinus function. The procedures were radical, highly invasive and disfiguring.[39] The surgical strategy was to remove all sinus mucosa from the major sinuses. Although the approach today is function-preserving, minimally invasive and non-disfiguring, the use of intranasal procedures should be a last resort.

ALLERGIC RHINITIS

Because of the mysterious nature of allergies, ancient people believed that reactions were curses brought about by evil spirits. Some practitioners, however, recognised the connection between allergic symptoms and plants or cats. Patients were often bled or given questionable medicines to combat allergies and asthma. In 1869 Charles Blackley performed the first allergy test on himself, by putting pollen directly into a cut in his skin. The term 'allergy' was coined by Von Pirquet in 1906 to describe disorders resulting from hyper-reaction to normally innocuous environmental agents. Initially the technique of allergen immunotherapy was crude, but with the subsequent key discovery of IgE, more accurate methods of diagnosis (such as RAST) were developed.[40]

Naturopathic perspective

In acute sinusitis, the immediate therapeutic goals are to re-establish drainage and clear the acute infection. This can be achieved by using any of the following measures:

- Local application of heat
- Local use of volatile oils and herbal medicines with antibacterial properties
- Immune system support through nutritional supplementation and herbal medicines
- Reduction in exposure to allergic potentials
- Avoidance of known pro-inflammatory dietary triggers or allergens.

In chronic sinusitis if associated with allergy and allergic rhinitis, long-term control will require strict avoidance of identified airborne or dietary allergens. In addition, correction of the underlying trigger/problem is essential for eradication of recurrence. These factors include inhaled allergens but also food allergies and sensitivities. Digestive disorders and bowel dysbiosis may also play a role and any imbalances need to be corrected. Depression, stress and other negative mental and emotional states lower the body's ability to fight infections and need to be addressed.

NUTRITIONAL MEDICINE (DIETARY)

Dietary therapeutic objectives

The diet should be highly nutritious yet easy to digest and not taxing on the digestive system. Any mucus-forming foods should be avoided. Specific nutritional supplementation may be used to assist the body in fighting the infection while reducing symptoms of inflammation, swelling and pain. Dietary triggers should be avoided.

Specific dietary treatments

Dietary inclusions

Patients should consume a nutrient-dense diet to facilitate and support the body's own healing mechanisms. It is recommended that patients increase the intake of fruits and vegetables, onions and omega-3 fatty acids while decreasing the intake of omega-6 and trans-fatty acids.[41]

The patient must ensure that they have adequate fluid intake to reduce inflammation and thin the mucus. This may include fresh vegetable juices, broths, soups, herbal teas and pure water. Heating liquids (herbal teas and broths) may further assist to help drain mucus.

Trial other dairy sources (sheep, goat, buffalo) and other milk replacements (soy, oat, almond) if cow's dairy aggravates presentation.

Dietary exclusions

Until appropriate dietary allergens can be ascertained, elimination of common food allergens should be encouraged while awaiting a more definitive diagnosis. These include dairy products (cow's and other milk sources), wheat, eggs, citrus, corn, peanuts, nuts and shellfish. Chickpeas have also been found to trigger allergic reactions in populations in which they are a staple food.

If a chronic picture is present, consider trialling a dairy- and salt-free diet for at least 3 months. Overall, reduce the intake of sugar, salt, saturated fats, cow's dairy and wheat until symptoms settle or definitive diagnosis of potential food allergens is confirmed.

NUTRITIONAL MEDICINE (SUPPLEMENTAL)

Nutritional medicine therapeutic objectives

- Nutritional repletion to support and optimise immune function
- Nutritional supplementation to reduce inflammation
- Symptomatic support as indicated
- Reduced frequency and intensity of episodes.

Specific nutrients required

Zinc

Zinc deficiency results in a decreased numbers of T-cells and natural killer cells that typically protect the body against infection. As a result, the respiratory system and body as a whole are more susceptible to invasion from disease-causing pathogens and less able to recover from illness. Zinc has potent antiviral properties and has been found to suppress inflammation in the respiratory tract caused by infection from human rhinovirus and other irritants.[43] It has been postulated, due to the favourable effect of zinc on resolution of symptoms associated with the common cold that it might also play a key role in ameliorating symptoms associated with allergic rhinitis as these two conditions share many common symptoms.

SAMPLE DAILY DIET

BREAKFAST	
Quinoa, cinnamon and pear cereal. Serve with almond milk	Quinoa is an ancient grain, revered by the Inca people. Quinoa has a warm, nutty flavour and provides a favourable alternative to wheat-based cereals, which may typically aggravate sinusitis and rhinitis. Quinoa contains a balanced amino acid profile and is the highest of all grain-like ingredients — it is actually a berry — in protein. Pears have a sweet, slightly sour flavour and are said to be useful in eliminating excess mucus from the body.[42] A sprinkle of cinnamon — a gentle, warming herb — provides flavour and aids digestion. The addition of almond milk (which can be made at home or may be purchased from the local healthfood store) provides a non-dairy replacement for milk that still provides optimal amounts of protein and calcium.
LUNCH	
Red lentil and vegetable dhal (made with spices such as mustard seeds, turmeric and garlic) served with basmati rice	Dhal provides an easy-to-digest meal in which a number of kitchen spices with therapeutic actions can be used. Many of these herbs have a warming nature that helps to liquefy mucus, aiding in its removal from the body; these include cumin, chilli and ajwain. Some of these herbs also have other specific medicinal actions useful for sinusitis and rhinitis; for example, mustard seeds display an antibacterial action and garlic is a natural antibiotic.
DINNER	
Steamed white fish in a turmeric base with an assortment of greens and ginger	Fish provides a good source of protein without being overly heavy in the body. The addition of turmeric, a powerful antioxidant and anti-inflammatory, and ginger in combination with steamed greens such as kale and spinach provides an excellent source of nutrients to further support immunity.
SNACKS	
Two kiwi fruit with 10 almonds	Kiwi fruit are rich in vitamin C, which prevents histamine secretion, a key player that presents in sinusitis and allergic rhinitis. The addition of almonds provides protein, good fats and a source of calcium.
BEVERAGES	
Warming antimicrobial tea made from: 4 tbsp freshly grated ginger root, 1 tbsp crushed black pepper corns, 8 sprigs of thyme, 12 fresh basil leaves	Crush all ingredients with mortar and pestle. Place in thermos with purified hot water and let it sit for 1 hour. Sip throughout the day.

Vitamin C and bioflavonoids

Vitamin C and its associated bioflavonoids prevent the production of histamine from white blood cells. It has been shown to reduce inflammation as well as reducing allergic responses, as a result of downregulating histamine production. Due to the nature of allergic rhinitis, through its mechanism of action, vitamin C may play a crucial role.[44]

A small, placebo-controlled, crossover study demonstrated that 2 g of vitamin C significantly decreased bronchial responsiveness to histamine challenge in patients with allergic rhinitis.[45]

Quercetin is a potent antioxidant that inhibits hyaluronidase and inflammatory processes while stabilising cell membranes. This results in prevention of mast cell and basophil degranulation. In a Japanese in vitro study, quercetin significantly inhibited antigen-stimulated histamine release from the mast cells of patients with allergic rhinitis.[46] The recommended dosage of quercetin is 250–600 mg, three times daily, 5–10 minutes before meals.[47]

Vitamin D

The mechanism by which vitamin D exerts its role in sinusitis and rhinitis is not entirely known. Vitamin D is able to exert many physiological processes in the body, one of which is its ability to modulate the immune system, possibly by affecting the balance between T helper subset 1 (Th1) and subset 2 (Th2) cytokines, favouring Th2 domination. Symptoms of sinusitis and rhinitis typically worsen in the winter, when there is more deficiency of vitamin D, and provide a theory behind the pathogenesis of vitamin D's role in these conditions.[50] Similarly, both sinusitis and rhinitis are characterised by inflammation, also seen in asthma, for which recent evidence supports the use of vitamin D.

A cross-sectional study conducted between 2012 and 2013 of 1833 Qatari children below the age of 16 found those with a vitamin D deficiency had a higher incidence and recurrence rate of allergic rhinitis than those whose vitamin D status was optimal ($p < 0.001$).[48]

Vitamin E

Vitamin E is a fat-soluble antioxidant that has been hypothesised to reduce immune allergic responses by modulating mast cells whose hyperactivity and accumulation in the tissues leads to increased production of inflammatory mediators implicated in the pathogenesis of allergic rhinitis.[49] In a double-blind placebo-controlled study of patients with allergic rhinitis, nasal symptom scores were found to be lower in patients supplementing with 800 mg/d of vitamin E in addition to their regular antiallergic treatment, in comparison to the placebo. While there was no effect noted with regards to ocular symptoms, the authors concluded that supplementation with vitamin E may be a useful addition to the treatment of patients with seasonal rhinitis.[49]

Supplementation with vitamin E has been demonstrated to relieve symptoms associated with seasonal allergic rhinitis. It has been shown to reduce the allergic response to known pathogens and airborne molecules.[44]

Vitamin A

Vitamin A has multiple roles in the immune system including increasing resistance to infection and enhancing the role of various white blood cells. Because of its immunomodulating role and its responsibility for maintaining the respiratory epithelial surfaces, vitamin A has been proposed as a treatment for sinusitis. Vitamin A assists the cilia, thus promoting the excretion of mucus from the nasal passages, and in rabbit studies retinoic acid (RA) has been shown to enhance ciliary ultrastructure in regenerated sinus mucosa; however, human clinical trials are lacking.

NAC (N-acetylcysteine)

Airway mucociliary clearance depends on the properties and volume of secreted mucus, ciliary function, and mucociliary interactions. In chronic sinusitis, mucus viscoelasticity is higher than the optimal values for mucociliary clearance. Mucolytic agents such as *N*-acetylcysteine (NAC) and proteolytic enzymes can reduce viscoelasticity and promote mucociliary clearance.[51] NAC is by far the more frequent prescription as the free sulfhydryl group of NAC interacts with the disulfide bonds of mucus glycoproteins, thereby breaking the protein network into less viscous strands. It can be taken orally, or as a 10% solution by dilution with saline.[52]

Proteolytic enzymes (bromelain)

Proteolytic enzymes include trypsin, chymotrypsin, serratia peptidase, bromelain and streptokinase. It is hypothesised that they may be able to break down complex proteins at the site of inflammation, exert some antimicrobial effect, or act directly on the naked peptide region of mucus glycoproteins.

Bromelain is a proteolytic enzyme from the pineapple fruit. Bromelain's systemic anti-inflammatory effects were tested in an older placebo-controlled trial in patients with sinusitis and resulted in improved breathing and decreased mucosal inflammation.[42] Bromelain may be beneficial due to its mucolytic and anti-inflammatory actions. The therapeutic dosage for allergic rhinitis ranges from 400 to 500 mg three times daily. Bromelain can be taken concurrently with quercetin. In one double-blind study, orally administered bromelain showed significant benefit in the treatment of chronic sinusitis by assisting in the breakdown of mucus.[47,53]

A prospective, open label observational pilot study included 12 patients suffering with or without nasal polyps associated with chronic rhinosinusitis who had undergone prior sinus surgery. A specific extract of bromelain tablets, 500 FIP, was prescribed for 3 months. It was found that supplementation with bromelain improved total symptom scores, total rhinoscopy scores and quality of life. The equivalent daily dose was 3000 FIP daily.[54] Although the sample size of this study was rather small, it does provide supportive evidence for the use of bromelain and further research is definitely required to further substantiate this evidence.

Dosage requirements

The dosage requirements listed below are based on adult doses reported in the literature:

- Zinc 30–50 mg/d
- Mixed flavonoids: 50 mg
- NAC: 600–15 000 mg/d
- Bromelain: 500–1000 mg/d with up to 2000 mg/d as needed
- Quercetin: 400–500 mg/d t.d.s.
- Vitamin A: 5000 IU/d or beta-carotene: 25 000 IU/d
- Vitamin C: 500 mg every 2 hours in the acute or 500 mg t.d.s. (up to bowel tolerance)
- Bioflavonoids: 1000 mg/d
- Vitamin D: 1000 IU/d (review pathology levels and increase as indicated, based on deficiency)
- Vitamin E: 250–800 IU/d.

HERBAL MEDICINE

Herbal medicine therapeutic objectives

Herbal therapeutics for acute and chronic presentations are similar. For acute presentations, the dose should be higher and given more frequently and treatment may need to be supplemented with diaphoretics if fever is present.

- Reduce the allergic response
- Support immune regulation and eradicate pathogen (if present)
- Treat any infection directly
- Reduce pain and inflammation
- Restore proper function to mucous membranes
- Reduce excessive secretions/clear mucus
- Control symptoms
- Remove causes
- Reduce exposure to aeroallergens (allergic)
- Seasonal rhinitis must be prophylactically treated for at least 6/52 prior to season.

Specific chronic objectives

- Depuratives for long-term elimination
- Consider environmental and dietary influences
- Consider topical applications/nasal sprays as chronic infections are difficult to treat and can be stubborn
- Avoidance of allopathic antihistamines and steroid-based decongestants as they further compromise immune function.

Herbal medicine classes

In both sinusitis and allergic rhinitis it is imperative to reduce the body's allergic response. Allergens such as animal dander and dust mites have been typically linked to these conditions, and the application of these herbs generally produces a reduction in symptoms such as sneezing, providing much needed relief for the patient. Additionally both conditions are characterised by inflammation, so this needs to be addressed with upper respiratory anti-inflammatory herbs to reduce inflammation.

Nasal congestion is a common complaint from sufferers of sinusitis and may be eased with the use of herbal medicines from the anticatarrhal class of botanicals that reduce the formation of mucus, the mucolytics, which dissolve mucus, as well as circulatory stimulants and lymphatic herbs. It is important to treat the infection and here the use of antiviral and antibacterial herbs is warranted. In the case of chronic conditions where the mucosa has withstood chronic stress it may be appropriate to improve the health of the mucosa with mucosal trophorestoratives. Where there is an immune challenging influence (for example leaky gut) this needs to be addressed with the appropriate herbal class. Finally, the immune-enhancing classes of herbs need to be given in order to support the function of the immune system.

Specific treatment includes immune-enhancing herbs such as *Echinacea* spp., *Andrographis paniculata* (andrographis) and *Picrorrhiza kurroa* (picrorrhiza) to support the immune system fighting the infection, antiviral and antibacterial herbs and essential oils, anticatarrhals including *Solidago virgaurea* (goldenrod) to reduce mucus secretions and *Hydrastis canadensis* (goldenseal) to restore balance to the mucous membranes. Antiallergic herbs including *Albizia lebbeck* (albizia) and *Scutellaria baicalensis* (baikal skullcap) are indicated in allergic sinusitis. Mucolytic herbs including *Allium sativum* (garlic) and *Armoracia* (horseradish) may be used to break up thick mucus and thereby ease congestion in the sinuses. Use of a humidifier with the essential oils of thyme, peppermint and eucalyptus is particularly beneficial. A stronger effect can be achieved by steam inhalation by placing the oils in a bowl of boiling water and inhaling the vapours. For chronic sinusitis it may be beneficial to add lymphatic herbs such as *Calendula officinalis* (marigold), *Phytolacca decandra* (poke root) and *Galium aparine* (cleavers).

Antiallergic herbs including *Albizia lebbeck* (albizia), *Scutellaria baicalensis* (baikal skullcap) and *Thylophora indica* (asthma weed) may tone down the allergic response, while anticatarrhal herbs such as *Euphrasia officinalis* (eyebright), *Solidago virgaurea* (goldenrod) and *Hydrastis canadensis* (goldenseal) may help reduce the excessive secretions from the mucous membranes. Respiratory demulcents contain mucilage and have soothing and anti-inflammatory effects and include *Althaea officinalis* (marshmallow), which is often given as a glycerol extract, *Ulmus rubra* (slippery elm), used in powder form, and *Plantago lanceolata* (ribwort).

Specific herbal medicines

Albizia lebbeck (albizia)

Albizia has been used for centuries in Ayurvedic medicine to aid with reducing symptoms such as runny nose, sneezing and coughing, which are often associated with sinusitis and allergic responses. It is classed as an antiallergic herbal medicine. In vitro and in vivo evidence of mast cell stabilisation with albizia provides a theoretical basis for its use in allergic conditions. Albizia combines well with other antiallergic, anti-inflammatory and anticatarrhal herbs such as feverfew, eyebright, ribwort and baikal skullcap (*Scutellaria baicalensis*).

An extract of albizia was used in already allergic rat models to determine its effect on histamine H1 receptor (H1R) and histidine decarboxylase (HDC) genes. The use of albizia was found to reduce the incidence of sneezing and nasal rubbing as well as suppressing H1R and HDC. As well as this, inflammatory cytokines such as IL-4, IL-5 and IL-13 were suppressed. This research provides a theoretical basis that albizia may positively affect the histamine cytokine network.[55]

The traditional dosage of albizia bark or bark powder for decoction or infusion is 3–6 g per day. The adult dosage is 3.5–8.5 mL per day (25–60 mL per week) of 1 : 2 liquid extract.[56]

Scutellaria baicalensis (baikal skullcap)

Flavonoids such as baicalin and baicalein obtained from baikal skullcap have been shown to have marked antiallergic activity. In many animal models, they have demonstrated antiallergic and antiasthmatic activity. They have also been found to inhibit histamine from peritoneal mast cells in rats.[57]

Scutellaria baicalensis is a traditional Chinese herb used to clear heat and dry dampness. Diseases with heat are associated with symptoms such as fever, irritability, thirst, cough and expectoration of thick, yellow sputum. Damp diseases may be associated with diarrhoea, a feeling of heaviness of the chest and painful urination.[58] From a modern perspective this suggests that baikal skullcap may be useful for infection and inflammation of the respiratory, digestive and urinary systems. Scientific investigations have indeed shown that baikal skullcap and its constituents have antibacterial, antiviral, anti-inflammatory, hepatoprotective and diuretic actions.[59]

Urtica dioica (stinging nettle)

Traditionally *Urtica dioica* has been used to treat allergies in the form of skin disorders[60] and asthma.[61] How *Urtica dioica* works in relation to rhinitis is unclear but it has been proposed that it is perhaps due to its anti-inflammatory action and its histamine content (it contains 6.1 ng per nettle hair).[62] Though no studies have been conducted on *Urtica dioica* and sinusitis, a randomised double-blind trial investigating the use of *Urtica dioica* for the management of allergic rhinitis produced positive results. Just over half of the patients taking 300 mg of freeze-dried *Urtica dioica* twice daily reported a reduction in symptoms associated with rhinitis.[63]

In vitro studies have demonstrated the ability of nettle to downregulate several key inflammatory cytokines that contribute to symptoms associated with seasonal allergies. It has also demonstrated the ability to inhibit histamine as well as to limit mast cell degranulation and inhibit prostaglandins that are associated with exacerbating the inflammatory response related to allergic reactions.[64]

Curcuma longa (turmeric)

Turmeric is known for its multiple health-restoring properties and it has been used in treating several diseases, including several respiratory disorders. The active component of turmeric is curcumin, a polyphenolic phytochemical, which displays anti-inflammatory, antiamyloid, antiseptic, antitumour and antioxidative properties. Curcumin was reported to have antiallergic properties with an inhibitory effect on histamine release from mast cells. The effectiveness of curcumin in allergy and asthma has been further investigated using a murine model of allergy. The results indicate a marked inhibition of allergic response in animals treated with curcumin, suggesting a major role for curcumin in reducing the allergic response.[65] Curcumin or turmeric extract may be beneficial in an overall antiallergic treatment of allergies including hay fever and asthma.

Amoracia rustica (horseradish)

Amoracia rusticana has traditionally been used for respiratory complaints and is well known for its pungent flavour and its decongestant action. *Amoracia rusticana* contains a wide array of constituents including mustard oil, mustard oil glycosides and sinigrin (which displays a mild antibiotic effect). Sulfur compounds within *Amoracia rusticana* appear to decrease the thickness of mucus by altering the structure of mucopolysaccharide constituents, reducing the sensation of congestion and catarrh. The German Commission E approves the internal use of *Amoracia rusticana* for the treatment of respiratory tract infections, noting its antimicrobial action. *Amoracia rusticana* also promotes perspiration making it useful in fevers, colds and flu.

A German study was conducted with 858 patients suffering with acute sinusitis and acute bronchitis. Participants were supplemented either with a herbal preparation containing horseradish and nasturtium or with antibiotics. The study concluded that the herbal preparation was comparable to antibiotic therapy in reducing the symptoms and progression of acute sinusitis and bronchitis.[66]

Allium sativum (garlic)

Garlic displays antioxidant and antimicrobial activity as well as anti-inflammatory, antiviral, antiparasitic, antibacterial and immune-stimulating actions, providing an argument for its use in the treatment of sinusitis and allergic rhinitis. Traditionally garlic has been used to treat colds, flu, rhinitis and coughs yet there appears to be a lack of clinical trials to support its use for this action, with the majority of evidence having been collected for its cardiovascular benefits.

Myrtol

Myrtol standardised is a phytotherapeutic extract (distillate) consisting mainly of three monoterpenes ([+] alpha-pinene, d-limonene and 1,8-cineole) and has been found to be more effective than a placebo in the treatment of acute non-purulent sinusitis as demonstrated by a multicentre randomised controlled trial involving 331 patients. The dosage of myrtol is 300 mg three to four times a day, and its safety has been established in long-term studies of bronchitis. The duration of treatment mentioned for sinusitis was 6 days.[67]

Aller-7

Aller-7 is a proprietary polyherbal complex containing *Terminalia bellirica* (myrobalan), *terminalia chebula* (terminalia), *Phyllanthus emblica* (emblic), *Albizia lebbeck* (albizia), *Zingiber officinale* (ginger), *Piper longum* (long pepper) and *Piper nigrum* (black pepper). It has been used in a multicentre clinical trial to determine its effectiveness in allergic rhinitis. A total of 171 patients suffering from allergic rhinitis participated in a double-blind, randomised, placebo-controlled study. The patients were aged between 18 and 59 years and for 12 weeks were supplemented with 660 mg of Aller-7 twice daily. The three major symptoms of sneezing, rhinorrhoea and nasal congestion were significantly reduced. Improvement was also observed in eosinophil count, mucociliary clearance time, and peak respiratory and nasal flow rate.[68] Although this study is not recent and more studies are required, Aller-7 may be an effective treatment for those suffering from allergic rhinitis.

Topical applications

Nasal spray

Version 1

Scutellaria baicalensis (baikal skullcap) — 2 mL (1:2)
Hydrastis canadensis (goldenseal) — 2 mL (1:3)
Euphrasia officinalis (eyebright) — 2 mL (1:2)
Mixed with: sea salt (¼ tsp), glycerin (5 mL), purified water (30 mL).

Version 2

Scutellaria baicalensis (baikal skullcap) — 1 mL (1:2)
Hydrastis canadensis (goldenseal) — 1 mL (1:3)
Euphrasia officinalis (eyebright) — 1 mL (1:2)
Matracaria chamomilla (chamomile) — 1 mL (1:2)
Mixed with: sea salt (½ tsp), warm purified water (½ cup)

LIFESTYLE RECOMMENDATIONS

Environmental

Environmental control requires the elimination of dust mites, use of air-filtering vacuum cleaners, installation of an air cleaner with a high-efficiency particulate air filter, and whatever methods are necessary to maintain the humidity under 50%. Some particularly sensitive patients may need to have all pets removed, along with carpeting and feather bedding.[69]

Heat applications

Local applications of heat have been shown to be effective in alleviating both short- and long-term symptoms of sinusitis.[70]

Saline washes

Ayurvedic practitioners recommend using a neti pot to gently irrigate the nasal passages with warm saline douches by placing the pot's spout in one nostril and letting the saline run out the other. The neti mechanically removes allergens such as pollen, dander and dust mites, thus relieving the trigger for the allergic rhinitis. Intranasal douche with saline water or herbal medicines (diluted) can be beneficial.

Other

- Rest, adequate sleep and stress reduction are essential
- Avoid anything that may aggravate the symptoms
- A hot Epsom salt bath, a steam bath or sauna twice a week in the evenings
- Encourage fresh air and exercise, walking, jogging, yoga
- Hot packs over the affected area
- Environmental chemicals within buildings can induce lethargy, headache and blocked or runny nose as well as symptoms of chronic sinusitis
- Inhalations either as chest liniments, snuffs, vaporisers, hot showers or similar should be encouraged as frequently as possible using essential oils such as eucalyptus, tea tree, peppermint, lavender and other menthol spp. Steam inhalation with or without essential oils can also be effective
- Reduce amount of time spent outside if it is a seasonal allergy especially
- Wash hair and change clothes after being outside to remove pollens that may enter the eye or nasopharyngeal areas
- Avoid smoking and passive smoking
- Investigate chronic sinusitis for abnormalities (polyps, growths, immune dysfunction, elevated CRP, etc.)
- Caution for secondary infection signs and symptoms — fever, chills, etc.

CASE STUDY

OVERVIEW

PH is a self-employed, 38-year-old successful chartered accountant. He is married with four children. Since he was a child, he has always suffered from seasonal allergic rhinitis; however, over the past few months, he has noticed an increase in the incidence and severity of his rhinitis. Simply walking outside causes an onset of sinus congestion, sinus headache and watery eyes.

He works long hours travelling up to 3 hours to and from work and between different offices. He is quite active and exercises at least 3 or 4 times per week. He has competed in

CASE STUDY CONTINUED

international touch football competitions; however, the severity of his rhinitis has prevented him from competing of late.

Mowing the lawns has become an issue and to do so, PH is required to wear a face mask and goggles. If he doesn't, he suffers from constant nasal congestion and headaches for a week after.

Due to his stress levels, sleep can be problematic at times and sinus congestion contributes to snoring and prevents him from having a restful night's sleep.

PH generally consumes a well-balanced diet but he does find it difficult to consume a sufficient amount of water and he often snacks on copious amounts of chocolate throughout the day. Breakfast tends to be non-existent. He consumes at least 2 or 3 cups of coffee per day usually with milk and 1 sugar.

PH enjoys dairy and consumes 3–4 servings per day.

CLINICAL EXAMINATION

GENERAL INSPECTION

Alert, cooperative.

Vital signs

BP: 120/85 mmHg sitting, 125/90 mmHg standing
Temperature: 37.0°C
Pulse: 75 bpm
Respiratory rate: 15 resp/min
Height: 1.65 m
Weight: 60 kg
BMI: 22

Face and neck

Marked tenderness in sinus and orbital regions
Sclera — bloodshot and watery
Bright redness of nasal mucosa

Respiratory

Chest inspection: Normal appearance
Percussion: Resonant all zones
Auscultation: Air entry all zones

INVESTIGATION RESULTS

Blood testing

All within normal range

Other

IgE: 200 kU/L (0–120)

TREATMENT PROTOCOL

Treatment was initially focused around immune support combined with symptomatic relief and long-term goals based around stress reduction strategies.

Herbal medicine

Because PH's rhinitis is triggered by environmental factors, symptomatic relief and immune support were the main focus.
Albizia lebbeck (albizia) 1 : 2: 60 mL
Scutellaria baicalensis (baikal skullcap) 1 : 2: 60 mL

CASE STUDY CONTINUED

Echinacea spp. (echinacea) 1 : 2: 80 mL
Dosage: 7.5 mL b.i.d.

Nutritional medicine

Dietary

The dietary focus was on eliminating dairy completely from the diet and substituting with almond milk.

Limiting coffee to once daily and consuming without milk or sugar.

Education around limiting refined carbohydrates and ensuring adequate protein consumed on a daily basis, to enhance and influence immune function.

Hydration was stressed and PH advised to consume at least 2 L of water per day and up to 3 L daily when exercising.

Supplemental

Vitamin C powder (mixed salts with bioflavonoids): 1000 mg t.d.s.
Zinc: 30 mg b.i.d.
Vitamin A: 2500 IU b.i.d.

Lifestyle/education

Nasal irrigation through the use of a neti pot to be done on a daily basis to aid with reducing bacterial overgrowth and preventing the reoccurrence of postnasal drip.

Hot compresses to the sinus region on a nightly basis.

Inhalation of essential oils of eucalyptus, tea tree and menthol up to three times daily to aid with nasal decongestion and reduce the incidence of sinus headaches. 3 drops of the essential oils added to a mug of hot water to aid with compliance.

Stress reduction strategies such as meditation and Pilates.

Education around sinus massage to ensure adequate drainage of the sinus region on a daily basis.

Acute rhinopharyngitis and influenza

EPIDEMIOLOGY

Influenza, commonly known as the flu, is highly contagious and accounts for 3500 deaths, 18 000 hospitalisations and 300 000 GP consultations each year in Australia. Ten per cent of work absenteeism is due to influenza.[71] In the first half of 2016 in Australia, there were 13 764 laboratory confirmed cases of influenza.[71]

CLASSIFICATION

Rhinosinusitis symptoms are classified as mild, moderate or severe, and acute or chronic. In acute rhinosinusitis symptoms are less than 12 weeks in duration, and in chronic rhinosinusitis the symptoms last longer than 12 weeks.[72] Picornaviruses are the most common cause of viral illness worldwide. Rhinoviruses (previously called coryzaviruses, muriviruses, enterovirus-like viruses, nasal secretion agents and Salisbury strains) are the most common cause of acute respiratory tract illness (ARTI) and upper respiratory tract infections (URTIs), traditionally defined as 'common colds'. Human rhinoviruses (HRVs) have been subclassified using tissue tropism and host range, antiviral susceptibility and phylogeny, and more than 100 varieties have been identified.

AETIOLOGY

Non-allergic or vasomotor rhinitis has no identified medical cause, although natural therapists believe it may be caused or exacerbated by diet. Rhinitis may also be drug-induced, rhinitis medicamentosus, caused by overuse of nasal sprays containing decongestants. Acute viral rhinopharyngitis, or acute coryza (common cold), is a highly contagious viral infectious disease of the upper respiratory system, primarily caused by picornaviruses (including rhinoviruses) or coronaviruses. Close proximity with someone suffering an acute cold, poor hygiene (not washing hands, sharing eating utensils), poor immunity and lack of vitamin D increase the risk of infection. Environmental chemicals within buildings can induce lethargy, headache and blocked or runny nose as well as symptoms of chronic sinusitis.

OVERVIEW

Rhinitis and sinusitis usually coexist and inflammation of the nasal mucosa and paranasal sinuses is concurrent in most individuals. The diagnosis is primarily clinical. Definitive diagnosis is by endoscopy showing polyps, mucopurulent discharge from the middle meatus, oedema or obstruction at the middle meatus.

PATHOGENESIS

The primary site of rhinovirus infection is in the nasal epithelium. After initial infection, the viral replication cycle begins within 8 to 12 hours. Virus may be detected in the nasal washings of volunteers 24 hours after inoculation and reach a maximum peak by the second or third day. The titres then start to decline and the virus is usually undetectable by the fifth day. Symptoms of cold appear one day after inoculation and peak on the third or fourth day. It is uncertain whether the development of rhinitis is due to the direct cytocidal effect of virus replication or through the release of mediators. Histamine has not been shown to play any role in the development of rhinitis. Following infection, a specific humoral response is found in both serum and nasal secretions. Serum-neutralising antibodies do not appear until 14 days after infection and thus recovery is probably not mediated by antibodies. Serum antibodies remain elevated for many years and are probably responsible for protecting the person against reinfection. However, local neutralising antibodies are lost after 2 years.[73]

SIGNS AND SYMPTOMS

Symptoms usually begin within 2 to 5 days after infection, although occasionally in as little as 10 hours after infection. The first indication of a cold is often a sore or scratchy throat. Other common symptoms are runny nose, congestion, sneezing and cough. These are sometimes accompanied by muscle aches, fatigue, malaise, headache, weakness or loss of appetite. The symptoms usually resolve spontaneously in 7–10 days but some can last for up to 3 weeks. The incubation period for influenza is usually 1–3 days and the illness commences abruptly with a fever, headache, shivering and generalised muscle aching. There may be a dry cough, sore throat, coryza, prostration, myalgia, headache and chills.

COMPLICATIONS

The common cold can lead to opportunistic co-infections or superinfections such as acute bronchitis, bronchiolitis, croup, pneumonia, sinusitis, otitis media or strep throat. People with chronic lung diseases such as asthma and COPD are especially vulnerable. Colds may cause acute exacerbations of asthma, emphysema or chronic bronchitis. Complications include secondary bacterial infection, pneumonia, encephalomyelitis (rare) and depression.[74]

DIFFERENTIAL DIAGNOSIS

Other disorders to be considered include allergic, gustatory rhinitis (vagally mediated), rhinitis medicamentosa (e.g. due to topical decongestants, antihypertensives, cocaine abuse), hormonal rhinitis (e.g. related to pregnancy, hypothyroidism, oral contraceptive use), anatomical rhinitis (e.g. deviated septum, choanal atresia, adenoid hypertrophy, foreign body, nasal tumour), immotile cilia syndrome (ciliary dyskinesis), cerebrospinal fluid leak, nasal polyps and granulomatous rhinitis (e.g. Wegener granulomatosis, sarcoidosis).[75] On day 3 of symptoms, if the patient has symptoms of only rhinitis — congestion, nasal obstruction and low-grade cough without any physical findings in the lungs — one can be fairly secure in diagnosing the common cold. If other symptoms such as wheezing or conjunctivitis or laryngitis or muscular aching have developed since the onset of symptoms, the common cold probably can be excluded.[76]

NATUROPATHIC DIAGNOSIS

Because of the acute nature of the presentation, clinical observation and examination are typically the only diagnostic strategies required.

INVESTIGATIONS

The advent of the new rapid influenza type A slide test has made confirmation of influenza much more accurate. The rapid test for respiratory syncytial virus (RSV) has improved diagnostic accuracy in the very young population and should be considered in any high-risk child younger than age 2 who has symptoms compatible with the common cold early in the course of an illness. This group has a high likelihood of progressing to bronchiolitis and croup.[76]

Specific naturopathic investigations

If repeated infections are present, holistic considerations need to be considered. Assessment of dietary, lifestyle, social, environmental, occupational, social, emotional and mental health should be employed.

THERAPEUTIC CONSIDERATIONS

Clinical decision making and rationale

The best way to avoid a cold is to avoid close contact with existing sufferers; to wash hands thoroughly and regularly; and to avoid touching the eyes, nose, mouth and face. Antibacterial soaps have no effect on the cold virus; it is the mechanical action of hand washing with the soap that removes the virus particles. As with hand washing with soap and water, alcohol gels provide no residual protection from reinfection.

Treatment of acute rhinosinusitis of any cause is targeted at symptom relief. Use of oral and topical nasal decongestants provides benefit for short-term use in adults; there is no evidence supporting their use in children. Studies of treatment with antihistamines alone for the common cold have shown no faster recovery, and only small benefit for sneezing and rhinorrhoea at the expense of sedation. In combination with decongestants, no effect was seen in small children, but some benefit in general recovery and nasal symptoms was noted in older children and adults. Intranasal ipratropium decreases rhinorrhoea, and may decrease sneezing and promote nasal drying.[35] The management of influenza includes bed rest, analgesics, high fluid intake and antiviral agents (neuraminidase inhibitors). Influenza vaccinations may offer some protection.[75]

THERAPEUTIC APPLICATION

Historical perspective

The common cold has intrigued physicians and the general public for centuries. In the early 1900s it was treated in the following way. The patient was put to bed, the bowels were relaxed and when the temperature was high, it was treated with antipyrine (a nasty chemical, dimethoxyquinazoline). Pain and other distressing symptoms were relieved by 'coryza' tablets containing a combination of morphia, atropia and caffeine. By 1930 an infectious cause for the common cold was being considered and in 1944 it was well established that the aetiological factor is a virus. With the introduction of sulfonamides in the late 1930s some clinicians claimed the drugs were effective against colds. Numerous articles about sulfa drugs in the literature of that time made such claims. The excitement about using antibiotics may have resulted from their effectiveness against pneumonia, a common disease of the time associated with high mortality.[74]

Naturopathic perspective

The primary therapeutic consideration is the status of the patient's immune system. If the patient's immune system is in good function, the illness will be short-lived. Enhancing general immune function may shorten the course of the disease. In cases of poor immune function, every effort should be made to strengthen the immune system by following the recommendations.

NUTRITIONAL MEDICINE (DIETARY)

Dietary therapeutic objectives

The diet should be highly nutritious yet easy to digest and not taxing on the digestive system. Any mucus-forming foods should be avoided. Specific nutritional supplementation may be used to assist the body in fighting the infection while reducing symptoms of inflammation, swelling and pain.

Specific dietary treatments

Dietary inclusions

The patient should eat as little as possible and increase the intake of fluids, drinking plenty of diluted vegetable juices, broths and herbal teas. Natural antibiotic foods such as garlic, onion and ginger should be encouraged either as a succus, in teas or in foods.

Fresh ginger root sliced with raw or manuka honey, cinnamon quills, lemon juice, +/− fresh chilli, onion succus and garlic in hot water will encourage the diaphoretic effect and assist in the body's ability to naturally eradicate the infection.

Herbal teas using the combination of yarrow, elder and peppermint (sambucus, achillea and mentha) can be beneficial to act as diaphoretics and be immune stimulating.

Warming spices of ginger, chilli, thyme and sage should be encouraged.

Dietary exclusions

Common allergens, especially dairy products that are also thought to exacerbate excessive mucus production, should be avoided.

SAMPLE DAILY DIET

BREAKFAST	
Freshly squeezed orange, carrot, beetroot and ginger juice. Add one serve of a good-quality protein powder to meet daily protein requirements	A vegetable juice provides a quick and easily absorbable source of nutrition to the immune compromised body. Vitamin C promotes the production of interferon, a protein that may help to reduce the duration of influenza. Carrots and beetroot are rich in carotenoids, which play an important role in immunity. Ginger is a gentle circulatory stimulant, and its warming nature is perfect for alleviating congestion and the flu.
LUNCH	
Clear broth with wakame, shiitake mushrooms and ginger	Wakame is a highly nutritious form of seaweed. In Chinese medicine it is said to transform and resolve phlegm and is particularly useful for coughs where there is green or yellow mucus.[42] The warmth of the broth and ginger heats the body, helping to clear the fever if present. Shiitake mushrooms are easy to prepare and contain a constituent known as interferon, which plays a key role in immunity.[42]
DINNER	
Green soup made from blended zucchini, spinach, watercress, garlic and onion	May be served with some crackers on the side if desired. The addition of a boiled egg if tolerated will increase daily protein intake. Garlic is a powerful immune booster with antiviral and antibiotic activity.
SNACKS	
Seasonal fruit	High in phytonutrients and antioxidants to boost health status.
BEVERAGES	
Hot water with lemon juice and manuka honey	

NUTRITIONAL MEDICINE (SUPPLEMENTAL)

Nutritional medicine therapeutic objectives

- Reduce inflammation
- Increase and support immune response
- Alleviate symptoms
- Prevent recurrence
- Address deficiencies.

Specific nutrients required

Nutrients should generally be taken in divided dosages throughout the day, especially during acute episodes.

Vitamin D

Vitamin D is emerging as a major vitamin, not just for healthy bones but also for general health and disease prevention. A recent meta-analysis of 18 randomised controlled trials found that supplemental cholecalciferol (vitamin D) significantly reduces *all cause* mortality. Vitamin D's final metabolic product is a potent, pleiotropic, repair and maintenance, seco-steroid hormone that targets more than 200 human genes in a wide variety of tissues. In other words, vitamin D has as many mechanisms of action as genes it targets. One of the most important genes vitamin D upregulates is cathelicidin, a naturally occurring broad-spectrum antibiotic (antimicrobial polypeptide). Natural vitamin D levels in humans living in a sun-rich environment are between 40 and 70 ng per mL, levels obtained by few modern humans. Assessing serum 25-hydroxy-vitamin D (25(OH)D) is the only way to make the diagnosis and to assure treatment is adequate and safe. Three treatment modalities exist for vitamin D deficiency: sunlight, artificial ultraviolet B (UVB) radiation and vitamin D_3 supplementation. Treatment of vitamin D deficiency in otherwise healthy patients with 2000–7000 IU vitamin D_3 per day should be sufficient to maintain year-round 25(OH)D levels between 40 and 70 ng per mL. Theoretically, pharmacological doses of vitamin D_3 (2000 IU per kg per day for 3 days) may produce enough of the naturally occurring antibiotic cathelicidin to cure common viral respiratory infections, such as influenza and the common cold.[77]

Vitamin C

A Cochrane systematic review of 30 trials published before 1992 found that vitamin C supplementation does not prevent colds, but that high-dose supplementation (1–2 g) at the onset of a cold reduces the duration of symptoms by approximately a half day.[78] Another review reached similar conclusions but pointed out small trials with a positive preventive effect and attributed this effect to the subset of patients tested: highly stressed individuals and participants with a low dietary intake of vitamin C, especially the elderly. The magnitude of the reduction of cold symptoms is greater in children and with larger doses (≥2 g/day). Analysis of 23 studies suggests that vitamin C in daily dosages of two or more grams is effective in managing the common cold. A review of 30 clinical trials confirmed that the duration of symptoms is reduced by vitamin C. A prophylactic effect has not been demonstrated in clinical trials.[46]

Zinc

Zinc plays an important role in cell-mediated immune functions and also functions as an antioxidant and anti-inflammatory agent. A Cochrane review conducted in 2013 found that supplementation within 24 hours of the onset of the common cold can reduce the rate of symptoms in otherwise healthy adults. Much of the data surrounds supplementing with more than 20 mg of zinc lozenges daily.[79] Zinc lozenges can also have a bad taste and cause nausea, significantly reducing patient compliance.[41] Differences in zinc preparations, including form (zinc gluconate versus zinc acetate), amount (elemental zinc per lozenge; ranges from 5 to 23 mg), and composition of the lozenge have been identified as possible explanations why study results are inconsistent.[80] A double-blind placebo-controlled trial involving 213 patients with common colds used an over-the-counter nasal zinc gel (Zicam), with statistically significant shortening of cold duration from 9 days to 2.3 days.[81] Please note use of Zicam products is inadvisable due to side effects of persistent anosmia.

Zinc has known immune-stimulant effects, and a randomised double-blind study from France found that the addition of minerals (zinc and selenium) to the nutritional regimen of institutionalised elderly people decreased the frequency of respiratory infections and increased antibody titres to influenza vaccine.[82] Other studies have confirmed that initiating zinc supplementation within 24 hours of onset of symptoms and continuing until symptoms resolve may reduce the symptoms or the mean duration of a cold by several days. In one study the duration was reduced nearly 50% (from 8.1 to 4.5 days)[81] while in another study zinc sulfate had no effect on the duration of cold symptoms but reduced their severity.[83] Giving zinc prophylactically for many months may significantly reduce the incidence of the common cold in children (dose from 13.3 to 15 mg daily).[84,85] A trial using a 15 mg dose in adults, however, was not better than a placebo in reducing the incidence or symptoms of the common cold.[86]

Essential fatty acids

A randomised, crossover, double-blind study found that a combination of 596 mg of linolenic acid (omega-6) and 855 mg of alpha-linolenic acid (omega-3) administered during two consecutive winters to children aged between 36 and 49 months with recurrent upper respiratory tract infections significantly decreased the number of episodes of infection and absences from school.[87] Nutrients are generally taken in divided dosages throughout the day, especially during acute episodes.

Dosage requirements

The dosage requirements listed below are based on adult doses that have been reported in the literature:

- Zinc: 20–60 mg/d
- Vitamin A: 15 000 IU/d or beta-carotene: 6 mg/d
- Vitamin C: 1–4 g/d in divided doses
- Vitamin D: 1000 IU/d
- Vitamin E: 400–800 IU/d
- Mixed flavonoids: 50 mg/d
- Essential fatty acids: omega-3 (1–2 g) + omega-6 (600 mg)/d.

HERBAL MEDICINE

Herbal medicine therapeutic objectives

The common cold and influenza are treated in a somewhat similar way. Influenza is more serious and intense and may require more vigorous treatment.

- Reduce pain
- Soothe inflamed mucous membranes
- Reduce excessive coughing
- Reduce excessive mucus production
- Facilitate expectoration
- Encourage or induce sweating
- Support immune system
- Reduce systemic inflammation
- Reduce risk of complications
- Modify fever and manage where necessary to fight invading pathogen.

Herbal medicine classes

The use of botanicals for the management of influenza helps to support the body's natural defences and at best results in a reduction in symptoms as well as the incidence and severity of influenza.

The use of immune stimulants and enhancers is the first line of treatment. These herbs enhance the function of the immune system, stimulating an immune response when required. Immune stimulants are typically given in conjunction with herbs from the antibacterial or antiviral classes. The choice of botanical will be dependent on whether the pathogen is antibacterial or antiviral in origin.

Typically in influenza the patient will experience high fever as the body tries to kill the offending pathogen. In these cases, the classes of herbs known as antipyretics and diaphoretics may be of use due to their respective ability to reduce fever and promote sweating during a fever, facilitating the healing process.

Treatment includes antiviral herbs such as *Hypericum perforatum*, antibacterial herbs including *Thymus vulgaris*, garlic, immune-enhancing herbs such as *Echinacea* spp., *Andrographis paniculata* and *Picrorrhiza kurroa*. Diaphoretics can be given as hot teas to reduce the fever. Diaphoretic herbs include *Mentha piperita* (peppermint), *Achillea millefolium* (yarrow), *Tilia* spp. (lime flowers), *Sambucus nigra* (elder) and *Zingiber officinale* (ginger). Some immune-stimulating herbs, including *Astragalus membranaceus*, and stimulating tonics such as *Panax ginseng* are traditionally contraindicated in the acute stage of infection. *Eleutherococcus senticosus* may be given with immune-stimulating herbs such as *Echinacea* spp. and *Andrographis paniculata* during acute infections. Anticatarrhal herbs help reduce the excessive mucus production and include *Euphrasia officinalis* (eyebright), *Sambucus nigra* (elder) and *Hydrastis canadensis* (goldenseal). Mucolytics, which make mucus easier to expectorate, may also be useful.

Specific herbal medicines

Echinacea spp. (echinacea)

Echinacea is one of the most widely used botanicals for the treatment of influenza. It has an affinity for the immune system, exerting upon it multiple actions including immune modulation, immune enhancing, antiviral and antibacterial activity. In a recent in vitro trial a commercial standardised extract of *Echinacea purpurea* was found to inactivate human H1N1-type1V, highly pathogenic avian 1V (HPA1V) as well as swine-origin 1V by interfering with the way in which the virus entered into cells. Additionally no signs of resistant variants were produced in comparison with Oseltamivir, which produced resistant viruses.[88]

Overall, clinical studies support the use of echinacea in the treatment of URTIs, including common cold, sinusitis, influenza and sore throat — especially if treatment is commenced early.[58]

A meta-analysis was conducted to determine the effectiveness of echinacea in the prevention and treatment of the common cold. It was shown that the prophylactic use of echinacea related to a lower rate of colds in comparison to a placebo,; however, the individual studies alone did not demonstrate these results. As a result, further research is required to determine the effectiveness of echinacea, with larger sample sizes.[89]

For the treatment of upper respiratory tract infections, the dose recommended most often by experts is 500–1000 mg three times daily, for 5–7 days. A total daily dose of 900 mg has been shown to be superior to 450 mg daily for the improvement of cold or flu symptoms. The recommended dose of expressed juice is 6–9 mL daily in divided doses, for 5–7 days, according to most experts. The recommended tincture dosage is 0.75–1.5 mL, gargled then swallowed, 2–5 times daily, for 5–7 days (daily dose should have equivalent of 900 mg dried echinacea root), according to most experts.[90] Echinacea is often combined with andrographis in fixed formulations in Australia.

Andrographis paniculata (andrographis)

Andrographis is an Ayurvedic herb that has traditionally been used for centuries to support the immune system. Andrographis contains the plant constituent andrographolide, a diterpene lactone thought to be responsible for much of andrographis's activity. In clinical trials andrographis has been found to decrease the duration and severity of the symptoms such as sore throat and nasal congestion associated with mild upper respiratory tract infections.[91] Results are believed to be best when treatment is started within the first 36–48 hours of symptoms.

Animal and laboratory studies show that andrographis may have a number of other potential therapeutic uses, including as an anti-inflammatory agent and as a treatment for chemically induced liver damage. It has also been studied in human clinical trials for the flu and familial Mediterranean fever. Preparations that contain 48–60 mg of andrographolide constituents have been taken in divided doses three or four times daily for respiratory infections. A 300 mg Kan Jang® tablet containing 4% andrographolides has been taken four times daily for cold treatment (for a total daily dose of 48 mg andrographolides). Lower daily doses, such as 200–300 mg, have been tested for respiratory infection prevention. Use appears to be safe for up to 2 weeks. Higher doses may be unsafe and cause side effects. Long-term use of andrographis preparations (beyond 2 weeks) has not been well studied. Doses of 500–3000 mg of andrographis leaf have been taken by mouth three times daily.[90]

Kan Jang®: *Eleuthorococcus senticosus* (Siberian ginseng) and *Andrographis paniculata* (andrographis)

More recently, andrographis has become popular in Scandinavia as a remedy for upper respiratory infections (URIs) and the flu. The most widely tested product is a product called Kan Jang® (Swedish Herbal Institute). This product is available with andrographis alone and in combination with *Eleutherococcus senticosus*. The combination product is highly controversial in Western herbal medicine as Siberian ginseng is known to be contraindicated in acute conditions.

Glycyrrhiza glabra (liquorice)

The use of glycyrrhiza can be traced back to ancient transcripts from Indian, Chinese and Egyptian medicine which describe its use for symptoms of viral respiratory infections. Glycyrrhizin, the main active constituent within *Glycyrrhiza glabra* root, is a triterpene glycoside that has been demonstrated to have powerful antiviral activity. This antiviral activity is postulated to be a result of two factors: immune modulation and the open effect on the host–virus interaction.[92] In vitro studies demonstrate the antiviral effects of glycyrrhizin on human lung epithelial cells and human lung fibroblasts from infection with the influenza A virus where it appears to inhibit uptake of the virus.

Astragalus membranaceus (astragalus)

Astragalus membranaceus is traditionally used as a tonic and treatment for colds and flu, either alone or in conjunction with other herbs. Astragalus is rich in polysaccharides, flavonoids and nutrients, all of which contribute to its immuno-supportive properties. Astragalus has been shown to activate and stimulate the proliferation of various immune cells, particularly CD8 and CD4 T-cells. A combination of *Echinacea purpurea, Astragalus membranaceus,* and *Glycyrrhiza glabra* has been further shown to have an additive (synergistic) effect on activation but not proliferation of T-cells.[93]

Olea europea (olive leaf)

Olive leaf extract contains phenolic compounds, specifically oleuropein, which have demonstrated potent antimicrobial, antioxidant and anti-inflammatory activity. Oleuropein and elenolic acid have been shown to have antiviral and antibacterial activity in vitro and in vivo.[94,95]

Baptisia tinctoria (baptisia)

A randomised double-blind placebo-controlled trial of 238 participants with acute cold symptoms showed that a formula of *Baptisia tinctoria, Echinacea purpurea* root and *Thuja occidentalis* leaf given daily for 7–9 days significantly reduced intensity and duration of symptoms compared with placebo. In subjects who suffered from moderate symptom intensity at baseline, at least 50% improvement by day 5 was experienced in 55.3% of the treatment group compared with 27.3% of the placebo group ($p = 0.017$). If patients with colds are able to start the application of the herbal remedy as soon as practical after the occurrence of the initial symptoms, the benefit would be expected to increase.[96]

Allium sativa (garlic)

A study found that an allicin-containing garlic supplement reduced the incidence and duration of the common cold in 146 volunteers. Subjects received one capsule daily for 12 weeks in 4 winter months, and symptoms were assessed via a symptom diary using a five-point scale. In the garlic supplemented group, 24 colds were reported compared with 65 in the placebo group; the treatment group experienced shorter duration of cold symptoms compared with placebo — 1.5 versus 5.0 days, respectively.[97]

Sambucus nigra (elder)

Sambucus nigra is a warming diaphoretic that was used traditionally by the eclectics and in folk medicine for the treatment of influenza. Modern studies confirm the use of *Sambucus nigra* for reduction of influenza-like symptoms (particularly in the early stages), with one small clinical trial providing efficacy for its use in influenza A and B infections.[98] It is believed that *Sambucus* renders viruses non-functional by staining and coating them.

Pelargonium sidoides (pelargonium)

Pelargonium root has been traditionally used for the symptomatic treatment of the common cold. It contains highly antioxidant oligomeric proanthocyanidins and oxygenated coumarins. A Cochrane review using specific extracts of pelargonium known as umckaloabo and kaloba found pelargonium root sped up the recovery from the common cold and reduced the frequency of symptoms. Although these results are positive, they were weak in comparison to placebo and as a result, further research is required to determine the effectiveness of pelargonium for use in the common cold.[99]

HERBAL MEDICINE — DECOCTION

An infusion of *Alchemilla millefolium* (yarrow), *Mentha x piperita* (peppermint) and *Sambucus nigra* (elderflower), drunk as hot as possible throughout the day, encourages diaphoretic potential and immune stimulation. Fresh sliced ginger and lemon juice (fresh) can be added to encourage diaphoretic effect and further stimulate immune response.

LIFESTYLE RECOMMENDATIONS

- Rest, adequate sleep and stress reduction are essential
- Fresh air and sunlight
- Gentle exercise as the body allows
- Encourage elimination through sweating
- Some people respond better when wearing synthetic fibres, which encourage the eliminatory response. In these situations it can be beneficial to increase heat throughout the night with added blankets to eliminate toxins during sleep. It is essential to bathe in the morning and wash bed linen and pyjamas
- Bathing 1–2 times per day to stimulate the lymphatic system
- Inhalations (vaporisers, personal inhalations, snuffs), using essential oils and steam to eradicate the infection and ease breathing
- Appropriate hygiene to prevent reinfection and infection of those around them.

CASE STUDY

OVERVIEW

JJ is a 40-year-old international banker. He works on average 13-hour days and is frequently flying overseas and interstate. Over the past 3 months, he has suffered frequent colds and flu with the most current incident causing him to reluctantly take a week off work. His symptoms usually commence with joint aches and pains, general malaise and fatigue, headaches and a productive cough. Currently, JJ is suffering from anorexia, a 39°C fever and pharyngitis together with a productive cough consisting of yellow/green sputum.

JJ's job is very stressful and he rates his stress levels 9/10. He has very limited time for relaxation and exercise. He consumes up to 5 espressos per day and at least two scotch on the rocks per evening.

CLINICAL EXAMINATION

General inspection

Fatigued, irritable and appears gaunt

CASE STUDY CONTINUED

Vital signs

BP: 140/90 mmHg
Temperature: 39°C
Pulse: 90 bpm
Respiratory rate: 18 resp/min
Height: 1.75 m
Weight: 80 kg
BMI: 26

Head and neck

Face: Unremarkable
Eyes: Darkened circles under eyes

Lymphatic

Neck: Cervical lymphadenopathy — small nodes in right

Respiratory

Throat: Inflamed pharynx
Chest inspection: Slight low-grade wheezing
Palpation: Trachea — midline
Supraclavicular/axillary nodes: Nil
Percussion: Resonant sounds — left/right lobes
Auscultation: Air entry all zones

Other systems

NAD, unremarkable

TREATMENT PROTOCOL

Immune support was the main focus of treatment together with acute symptomatic relief. Long-term strategies were to improve stress response to prevent further burden on immune function and as a result, limit the amount of influenza recurrences.

Herbal medicine

Echinacea spp. (echinacea blend) 1 : 2: 50 mL
Astragalus membranaceus (astragalus) 1 : 2: 50 mL
Pelargonium sidoides (pelargonium) 1 : 5: 70 mL
Eupatorium perfoliatum (bone set) 1 : 2: 30 mL
Dosage: 7.5 mL twice daily

Diaphoretic tea

Infusion of *Alchillea millefolium* (yarrow), *Mentha x piperita* (peppermint) and *Sambucus nigra* (elderflowers) drunk as hot as possible throughout the day.

Fresh sliced ginger and lemon juice (fresh) can be added to encourage diaphoretic effect and further stimulate immune response.

Nutritional medicine

Dietary

- Strictly avoid caffeine and alcohol consumption
- Avoid refined carbohydrates
- Ensure adequate hydration
- Promote stews, soups and bone broths to nourish and support the immune system

CASE STUDY CONTINUED

- Ensure consumption of stewed vegetables and fruit to promote adequate consumption of vitamins and minerals.

Supplemental

Vitamin C powder (mixed salts with bioflavonoids): ½–1 g q.i.d.
Zinc citrate 30 mg t.d.s. in acute, then reduced by 30 mg as infection resolves. Zinc lozenges can be used as an alternative if throat symptoms present.
Activated B vitamins 1 cap in the morning with food (stress history)
Magnesium citrate 300 mg b.i.d. (stress history).

Lifestyle/education

Encourage elimination through sweating — throughout the night especially.
Rest, adequate sleep and stress reduction are essential.
Inhalations (vaporisers, personal inhalations, snuffs), using essential oils and steam to eradicate the infection and ease breathing.
Appropriate hygiene to prevent reinfection and infection of others.

THE THROAT

See Table 13.3.

Pharyngitis and tonsillitis

EPIDEMIOLOGY

Tonsillitis and pharyngitis affect all ages but most cases are in the age group 5–15 years. Males and females are affected alike; transmission is person-to-person and favoured by crowding.

Group A beta-haemolytic streptococcus (GABHS) may account for 5–15% of pharyngitis cases in adults and 12–35% in school-age children.[35]

CLASSIFICATION

Chronic disease of the tonsils and adenoids includes adenoid vegetations, chronic tonsillitis and adenoiditis, hypertrophy of tonsils and adenoids, other chronic diseases (e.g. ulceration) and unspecified diseases of the tonsils and adenoids. Chronic pharyngitis encompasses chronic nasopharyngitis, chronic pharyngitis and chronic rhinitis. Acute pharyngitis includes acute sore throat (excluding abscess), acute laryngopharyngitis and chronic pharyngitis caused by streptococcal pharyngitis or viruses (excluding enteroviral vesicular, herpes simplex, infectious mononucleosis or influenza virus).

AETIOLOGY

Pharyngitis is predominantly viral in aetiology, accounting for as much as 65% of all cases in adults. Tonsillitis is due to *Streptococcus pyogenes* in approximately 20% of cases. In coxsackie virus infections sore throat is associated with pharyngeal vesicles (herpangina) or with hand and foot vesicles. Epstein-Barr virus infection is characterised by fatigue, functional impairment and cervical lymphadenopathy. Bacterial causes of sore throat include GABHS. Environmental chemicals within buildings can induce lethargy, headache and blocked or runny nose as well as symptoms of chronic sinusitis. Tonsillitis may be caused by group A streptococcal bacteria, resulting in strep throat. Viral tonsillitis may be caused by numerous viruses.

OVERVIEW

Attacks of acute tonsillitis and adenoiditis and tonsillar and adenoid hypertrophy are among the important health problems in preschool and school-age children. The social and physical morbidity these illnesses cause is significant. If they do not respond to medical treatment and disturb the life of the patient significantly, tonsillectomy may be performed.

PATHOGENESIS

The viruses gain access to the mucosal cells lining the nasopharynx and replicate in these cells. Damage to the host is often due to damage to the cell in which the virus is replicating. In bacterial infections, the bacterial cell attaches to the mucosal epithelial cells. Non-suppurative lesions resulting in rheumatic fever and glomerulonephritis may develop following strep throat infections. The course of viral acute rhinopharyngitis is generally self-limited in nature and mild in severity. Symptoms may persist for more than 1 week in more than 50% of cases, and for 2 weeks in 25%. The cause is most commonly rhinovirus and to a lesser extent coronavirus (typically in midwinter) and adenovirus (typically in spring to autumn). Although laboratory identification can be accomplished, the time required to identify the cause may exceed the duration of the illness and the yields may be highly variable.[35] Other common viruses include *Haemophilus influenzae*[100] and Epstein-Barr virus.[101] The most common bacterial pathogens cultivated from patients with peritonsillar abscess are beta-haemolytic streptococcus followed by mixed culture with or without anaerobes.[102]

The oxidation products produced during inflammation are involved in the tissue injury. The antioxidants play a role in neutralising the destruction of these oxidation products. Since chronic tonsillitis and adenoid hypertrophy are chronic inflammatory diseases in the oro- and nasopharynx, there is a significant possibility that the balance between oxidation products and antioxidants is involved in the appearance and the chronicity of these diseases in the pharynx. However, the role of oxidants and antioxidants in the pathogenesis of chronic tonsillitis and adenoid hypertrophy is not well defined.[103] It is, however, known that oxidants and antioxidants play a significant role in the pathogenesis of chronic tonsillitis and adenoid hypertrophy in children. These children are under significant oxidative stress; tonsillectomy and adenoidectomy can significantly decrease this stress in these patients, but do not normalise it completely.[102,104] Further studies are necessary to evaluate their possible therapeutic role in preventing recurrent tonsillitis and treating postoperative patients to help normalise their blood levels of antioxidants; in the meantime it seems justified to use antioxidant supplementation as part of the treatment of tonsillitis.

SIGNS AND SYMPTOMS

The cardinal feature of pharyngitis, sore throat, is also a feature of the common cold. In adenovirus infections it is usually accompanied by adenitis and conjunctivitis. The typical symptoms of streptococcal pharyngitis are sudden onset of sore throat accompanied by fever. In children, abdominal pain and vomiting are also reported. The physical findings may include pharyngeal erythema, tonsillar exudates and enlarged cervical lymph nodes. Fever, palatal petechiae and uvular swelling, none of which are specific for streptococcal infection, are also found. All of these historical and physical features are common to infections by other agents, including group C and group G streptococcus.

Tonsillitis is an infection of the tonsils. Symptoms of tonsillitis include a severe sore throat, painful/difficulty swallowing, coughing, headache, fever and chills. Tonsillitis is characterised by signs of red, swollen tonsils, which may have a purulent exudative coating of white patches. There may be enlarged and tender neck cervical lymph nodes.

COMPLICATIONS

It is vital to be aware of *Haemophilus influenzae* infection in children, especially those aged between 2 and 4 years, when the deadly problem of epiglottitis can develop suddenly. These patients present with a short febrile illness, respiratory difficulty (cough is not a feature) and are unable to swallow.[75]

Peritonsillar abscess may occur as a complication of an acute tonsillitis and involves pus collection in the loose connective tissue of the peritonsillar space. An abscess may develop lateral to the tonsil during an infection, typically several days after the onset of tonsillitis. This is termed a peritonsillar abscess (or quinsy). Rarely, the infection may spread beyond the tonsil resulting in inflammation and infection of the internal jugular vein giving rise to a spreading septicaemia infection.

DIAGNOSIS

At least 50% of sore throats, mainly pharyngitis, will be caused by a virus. A viral infection is supported by the presence of coryza prodromata, hoarseness and nasal stuffiness. It is difficult to distinguish clinically between bacterial and viral causes. The main issue is to determine whether the sore throat has a treatable cause by interpretation of the clinical and epidemiological data. Many cases of sore throat are caused by a virus and generally do not show marked inflammatory changes or purulent-looking exudates.[75]

DIFFERENTIAL DIAGNOSIS

Apart from acute epiglottitis it is important not to overlook carcinoma of the oropharynx or tongue, or acute leukaemia. The severe infections not to be missed include streptococcal pharyngitis with its complications, including quinsy, diphtheria and HIV infection. Bacterial causes include GABHS. The presence of cough and rhinorrhoea suggests a non-GABHS aetiology. Rheumatic fever must be differentiated from other diseases that affect the joints.[75]

NATUROPATHIC DIAGNOSIS

Because of the acute nature of the presentation, diagnosis is made on clinical observation and/or confirmation from the patient's general practitioner.

INVESTIGATIONS

Because a therapist may be unable to clinically distinguish GABHS from other causes of pharyngitis, a laboratory test will in some cases be necessary to confirm the diagnosis. A throat culture, consisting of a throat swab incubated on blood agar and confirming GABHS growth by the inhibitory effects of bacitracin, has been the standard for diagnosis; however, results of this culture are only available after 24–48 hours, with a delay in immediate and appropriate therapy. With this delay, the benefits of timely treatment, which include reducing risk of disease transmission, diminishing symptoms and speeding recovery, are jeopardised. Rapid antigen detection testing (RADT) for GABHS was developed to provide more immediate, albeit more costly results, with a demonstrated specificity exceeding 95% relative to blood agar culture. A clinical score based on the cumulative presence or absence of specific clinical features may be used to exclude or entertain the diagnosis of GABHS, thereby reducing the need for both throat cultures and unnecessary antibiotics.[35]

Specific naturopathic investigation

Because of the acute nature of the condition, further naturopathic assessments are often not required. Repeated infections of a chronic picture warrant further immunological studies and accurate assessment of immune suppressants or challenges.

THERAPEUTIC CONSIDERATIONS

Clinical decision making and rationale

In acute respiratory infection, the immediate therapeutic goals are to re-establish drainage and clear the acute infection. Various measures can be used: local application of heat, local use of volatile oils and botanicals with antibacterial properties, and immune system support. Because chronic sinusitis is often associated with allergy, long-term control depends on isolation and elimination of the food or airborne allergens and correction of the underlying problem that allowed the allergy to develop.[105]

GABHS is the only commonly occurring infection for which antibiotic therapy is beneficial; the goal is to expedite clinical recovery, decreasing the likelihood of suppurative complications (such as abscess), preventing acute rheumatic fever, and limiting transmission of the disease.[35]

Treatments of tonsillitis consist of pain management medications and lozenges. If bacteria cause the tonsillitis, then antibiotics are prescribed, with penicillin being most commonly used. Erythromycin is used for patients allergic to penicillin. In many cases of tonsillitis, the pain caused by the inflamed tonsils warrants the prescription of topical anaesthetics for temporary relief. Viscous lidocaine (lignocaine) solutions are often prescribed for this purpose. Ibuprofen or other analgesics can help to decrease the oedema and inflammation, which will ease the pain and allow the patient to swallow liquids sooner.

When a virus causes tonsillitis, the length of illness depends on which virus is involved. Usually, a complete recovery is made within 1 week; however, some rare infections may last for up to 2 weeks. Chronic cases may indicate tonsillectomy (surgical removal of tonsils) as a choice for treatment. Treatment of the viral or bacterial pharyngitis is aimed at eradication of the organism from the upper respiratory tract and soothing inflamed mucosa.

THERAPEUTIC APPLICATION

Historical perspective

Today there is a general agreement that tonsil and adenoid removal has little or no role to play in the long-term management of upper respiratory tract infections. However, in the past surgical excision of tonsils and adenoids was advocated to remove the septic focus. Only after the immunological aspects of the lymphatic system were recognised did the understanding that the tonsils may be related to long-term immunity in URTI develop. Naturopaths strongly believe that no organ or normal tissue should be removed unless absolutely necessary and all other options explored. Non-infectious pharyngitis may be related to poor posture and referral to osteopathic treatment may be necessary. The primary therapeutic consideration is the status of the patient's immune system. If the patient's immune system is in good function, the illness will be short-lived. Enhancing general immune function may shorten the course. In cases of poor immune function, every effort should be made to strengthen the immune system by following the recommendations given in Chapter 12.[105]

Naturopathic perspective

- Acute symptomatic relief is the prime objective in conjunction with immune support and eradication of immune suppressants
- Assessment of hepatobiliary and lymphatic health is essential, especially if there is a history of Epstein-Barr virus or other insidious viral infections that affect the long-term immune response and recovery
- Dietary exclusions may be warranted if associated negative effects are assessed.

NUTRITIONAL MEDICINE (DIETARY)

Dietary therapeutic objectives

The diet should be highly nutritious yet easy to digest and not taxing on the digestive system. Any mucus-forming foods should be avoided. Specific nutritional supplementation may be used to assist the body in fighting the infection while reducing symptoms of inflammation, swelling and pain. It has been found that low antioxidant levels in blood may predispose children to frequent upper respiratory tract infections by negatively influencing their immune system. Antioxidants and oxidation products have also been found in tonsil and adenoid tissues of patients with chronic adenotonsillitis indicating their association with this disease. During chronic inflammatory processes antioxidants decrease slowly when the level of oxidative stress they can neutralise is exceeded. Low antioxidant levels may be the result of chronic diseases. Free radical damage to the membrane lipids of leucocytes leads to increased permeability, and therefore decreases their immune function. DNA damage by free radicals decreases synthesis of certain critical factors by leucocytes and decreases the reproductive capacity of leucocytes. Low antioxidant levels in blood may predispose children to frequent upper respiratory tract infections by negatively influencing their immune system.[106] A recent investigation of 20 children with chronic adenotonsillitis and 19 children with adenotonsillar hypertrophy in whom adenotonsillectomy was performed strongly suggests that oxidants and antioxidants have an important role in the pathogenesis of adenotonsillar hypertrophy and chronic adenotonsillitis.[104]

Specific dietary treatments

Dietary inclusions

A diet rich in fruit and vegetables should be observed. The diet should consist of foods that are soft and easy to swallow. Increase fluids; drink plenty of diluted vegetable juices, broths, herbal teas. The patient should eat as little as possible.

A throat gargle of hot water mixed with a little salt and lemon juice may be used several times daily.

Dietary exclusions

During the acute phase, elimination of common food allergens such as cow's dairy (and other milks), wheat, eggs, citrus, soy, refined carbohydrates, gluten, corn and peanuts is indicated until a more definitive diagnosis can be made.[105]

It is beneficial to avoid sugar during the acute immune response and avoidance of all colourings/preservatives/additives is advisable. Anything which may aggravate the symptoms should be avoided.

Other dietary considerations

The diet should be light and easy to swallow. Mash or puree foods if swallowing is difficult.

NUTRITIONAL MEDICINE (SUPPLEMENTAL)

Nutritional medicine therapeutic objectives

Nutrients may be given to support the immune system, reduce inflammation and soothe the symptoms. Dietary and nutritional assessment may be given to reduce the risk of the condition becoming chronic. It is important to address specific nutritional deficiencies, to support the immune system, reduce inflammation, provide pain relief and reduce the risk of complications.

SAMPLE DAILY DIET

BREAKFAST	
Puréed vegetable soup with vegetarian protein included (lentils, brown rice, split peas). Added ginger for warmth, diaphoretic properties and circulatory stimulation	The inclusion of protein is essential to support the immune response. Puréeing enables easier swallowing.
LUNCH	
A bowl of freshly prepared steamed vegetables such as carrot, cabbage, cauliflower, squash and beans with silken tofu for protein	
DINNER	
Puréed vegetable soup with vegetarian protein included (lentils, brown rice, split peas). Added ginger for warmth, diaphoretic properties and circulatory stimulation	The inclusion of protein is essential to support the immune response. Puréeing enables easier swallowing.
SNACKS	
Fresh fruit	Can be stewed or puréed for easier swallowing and LSA or nut meal stirred through for added protein and essential fatty acid content.
BEVERAGES	
A glass of lukewarm water with half a freshly squeezed lime and a teaspoon of honey or a glass of fresh cold orange or lemon juice, diluted with water on 50 : 50 basis, as desired Juices of carrot, beetroot and cucumber, taken individually or in combination.	The formula proportion recommended, when used in combination, is 300 mL of carrot juice, 100 mL of beetroot juice and 100 mL of cucumber juice.

Specific nutrients required

Nutrients are generally taken in divided dosages throughout the day, especially during acute episodes.

Zinc

Zinc plays a critical role in the regulation and maintenance of host defence systems where it appears to interfere with the process of infection. A deficiency of zinc impairs antibody-mediated responses to infection, which play important roles in inhibiting the colonisation and phagocytosis of encapsulated bacteria.

In vitro studies suggest that poor zinc status damages the nonspecific barrier function of airway epithelial cells, which have the responsibility of removing aspirated bacteria from the respiratory tract.[107] Zinc prophylaxis has also been seen to reduce the incidence of *Streptococcus pneumoniae* tonsillitis in adult patients with sickle cell anaemia. This suggests that it may have a restorative effect on the barrier function of the respiratory mucous membranes as well as local antibody mediated responses.[9]

As zinc homeostasis is essential for immune function, oxidative stress and apoptosis, a study was conducted to determine the absence or presence of zinc and iron in tonsillar tissue obtained from patients who suffered from recurrent tonsillitis and tonsillar hypertrophy.[108] Both iron and zinc concentrations were significantly lower in the recurrent tonsillitis samples, with iron concentrations being higher than zinc, despite still being low. This study indicates the importance of zinc for potentially reducing the incidence of recurrent tonsillitis.[108]

Vitamin C and bioflavonoids

Suboptimal levels of vitamin C have been linked to poor immune status. Decreased numbers of lymphocyte CD8 and level of immunoglobulins G and M were observed in patients with chronic tonsillitis. The study authors concluded that decreased quantities of nutrients including vitamin C affects cell and humoral immunity level leading to disbacteriosis, decompensation of the disease and development of complications.[109] Additionally, clinical studies reveal that antioxidants such as vitamin C could play a significant role in the pathogenesis of chronic tonsillitis and adenoid hypertrophy in children. Children with these conditions are under significant oxidative stress and while tonsillectomy and adenoidectomy significantly decrease this oxidative stress they cannot normalise it completely, unlike antioxidants.[110]

Vitamin D

Vitamin D enhances immune mechanisms and inhibits respiratory inflammation. Deficiency of vitamin D has been linked to an increased rate of tonsillectomy and is also considered a risk factor for cancer later in life (breast, prostate, leukaemia, lymphoma). In addition, low vitamin D status is a risk factor for pre-eclampsia during pregnancy, which is also correlated with an increased risk of breast cancer.[111]

Vitamin D may have a preventive role in recurrent pharyngotonsillitis by inhibiting bacterial biofilm formation. Some data has indicated lower serum vitamin D levels in children who suffer from recurrent tonsillitis.[112] A study investigated the correlation between serum vitamin D levels and recurrent group A streptococcal tonsillopharyngitis in adults. The study indicated that serum vitamin D levels <25 ng/mL correlated with recurrent pharyngotonsillitis.[113] Although this is only one study, it does indicate the possible importance of vitamin D in the prevention of recurrent tonsillitis in those individuals with known deficiencies.

Vitamin E

Vitamin E plays a key role in immunity. Vitamin E levels along with other antioxidants have been found to be decreased in children with tonsillitis.[114] Vitamin E has been proposed as an alternative treatment for tonsillectomy due to its antioxidant action.[115]

Vitamin A or beta-carotene

Micronutrient deficiencies such as that of beta-carotene and infectious diseases often coexist and exhibit complex interactions leading to infection. Beta-carotene possesses immune-modulating activity and thus its presence or absence influences the susceptibility of a host to infectious diseases and the course and outcome of such diseases. Levels of beta-carotene have been found to be decreased in children with tonsillitis.[116]

Dosage requirements

The dosage requirements listed below are based on adult doses that are reported in the literature:

- Zinc: 30–60 mg daily
- Vitamin C: 1–2 g or more daily
- Vitamin D: 1000 IU daily
- Vitamin E: 400–800 IU daily
- Beta-carotene: 6 mg daily
- Mixed flavonoids: 50 mg.

HERBAL MEDICINE

Herbal medicine therapeutic objectives

- Modulating the immune response
- Allowing the body to fight the infection
- Minimising inflammation, pain and swelling
- Using lymphatic herbal medicines to improve lymphatic drainage
- After the acute infection is resolved, long-term treatment with immune-enhancing herbal medicines may be used to reduce the risk of recurrence.

Herbal medicine classes

Tonsillitis is characterised by infection, hence one of the first herbal classes required in an attempt to eliminate the infection will be those botanicals that display local and systemic antimicrobial activity to the upper respiratory tract. These include such herbs as *Comiphora molmol* (myrrh), *Thymus vulgaris* (thyme), *Salvia officinalis* (sage), *Baptisia tinctoria* (wild indigo), propolis and *Hydrastis canadensis* (goldenseal).

Of equal importance is the simultaneous need for improved immune system function. This may be achieved via the application of immune modulators and stimulants such as the *Echinacea* spp., which regulate the activity of the immune system. The tonsils are composed of lymphatic tissue, therefore lymphatic herbs are highly indicated. The choice of lymphatic herb will depend on whether the infection is acute or chronic.

Inflammation plays a significant role in the pain and discomfort experienced by the patient, hence the application of soothing, anti-inflammatory herbs such as *Glycyrrhiza glabra* (liquorice) and *Althaea officinalis* (marshmallow) will provide much-needed relief. In chronic conditions sustaining factors such as allergy need to be addressed. Additionally, adaptogens and tonics such as *Astragalus membranaceus* (astragalus) may also be beneficial to support the patient during stressful periods and assist in slowly rebuilding a compromised immune system.

See the relevant drug interactions table at the back of the book.

Specific herbal medicines

Echinacea spp. (echinacea)

Extracts of echinacea are one of the most popular herbs for upper respiratory tract infections. The objective of a 2006 Cochrane review was to assess whether there is evidence that echinacea preparations are 1) more effective than no treatment, 2) more effective than placebo, 3) similarly effective to other treatments in a) the prevention and b) the treatment of the common cold. All 16 trials except one were described as double blind. The majority had reasonable to good methodological quality. Three comparisons investigated prevention of colds and 19 comparisons tested treatment of colds. A variety of different echinacea preparations were used. None of the three comparisons in the prevention trials showed an effect over the placebo. Echinacea preparations tested in the clinical trials differed greatly. The authors concluded that there is some evidence that preparations based on the aerial parts of *Echinacea purpurea* might be effective for the early treatment of colds in adults but that the results are not fully consistent. They went on to state that beneficial effects of other echinacea preparations for preventive purposes might exist (and this is certainly the experience of herbalists) but have not been shown in independently replicated, rigorous randomised trials.[117] A more recent meta-analysis evaluating the effect of echinacea on the incidence and duration of the common cold examined 14 unique studies. This review found that echinacea decreased the odds of developing the common cold by 58% (p <0.001) and the duration of a cold by 1.4 days (p = 0.01).[106]

Pelargonium sidoides (pelargonium)

Research has shown that *Pelargonium sidoides* and its isolated constituents have moderate direct antibacterial potencies and notable immune modulatory capabilities. The immune modulatory activities are mediated mainly by the release of tumour necrosis factor alpha (TNF-α) and nitric oxides, the stimulation of interferon-beta, and the increase of natural killer cell activity. Further biological activities in vitro are improved phagocytosis, oxidative burst and intracellular killing of human peripheral blood phagocytes, and an inhibition of the interaction of group A streptococci and host epithelia. *P. sidoides* has been shown in placebo-controlled clinical trials and in several observational studies to be a successful treatment of the common cold, acute bronchitis and acute rhinosinusitis. In all controlled clinical trials, treatment with pelargonium was superior in efficacy, with a significant reduction of disease-specific symptoms compared with a placebo, and showed a very good tolerability.[116]

Commiphora molmol (myrrh)

Commiphora molmol is a member of the Burseraceae family. Its oleo-gum resin derived from the stems is the plant part used for the management of tonsillitis and pharyngitis. *Commiphora molmol* contains a multitude of active constituents including volatile oil, furanosesquiterpenes, resins, sterols and mucilage, responsible for its therapeutic actions within the body. *Commiphora molmol* displays antimicrobial, astringent, antiseptic and vulnerary action and produces a local stimulating effect on the mucous membranes of the respiratory tract and the tonsils, particularly when they appear pale in colour. The British Herbal Pharmacopoeia advocates the use of *Commiphora molmol* for the common cold and for mouth ulcers, gingivitis and pharyngitis as a mouth wash and gargle.[118]

Phytolacca decandra (poke root)

Phytolacca decandra is a member of the Phytolaccaceae family and is native to North America. The dried roots of *Phytolacca decandra* are used medicinally and contain triterpenoid saponin glycosides, alkaloids and tannins. *Phytolacca decandra* may be used in the respiratory system for inflammatory conditions of the upper respiratory tract and lymphadenitis.[118] Its use is particularly indicated in tonsillitis where it acts as a lymphatic and antiviral agent to remove lymphatic congestion and enhance the proper functioning of the immune system. Use of *Phytolacca decandra* should be avoided in young children due to its ability to cause an acute toxic reaction in a relatively small dose. Other gentler lymphatics may be used in its place.

Baptisia tinctoria (wild indigo)

The primary indication for recommendation of *Baptisia* is for infections of the upper respiratory tract. It contains a number of constituents including alkaloids, coumarins, resins and polysaccharides. *Baptisia tinctoria* is of marked value in many forms of malignant sore throat, particularly where there is tonsillitis, pharyngitis, gingivitis, acute catarrhal infection, offensive breath and fever, due to its antimicrobial and antiseptic activity. The British Herbal Pharmacopoeia recommends the use of *Baptisia tinctoria* for pharyngitis and acute catarrhal infections.[118]

Pseudowintera spp. (horopito)

Horopito is endemic to New Zealand and has been used by the indigenous Māori internally and topically for many centuries. It has traditionally been used for chest infections, colds and a range of skin conditions as well as for its antimicrobial activity. Research has suggested it contains anti-inflammatory, antifungal, antibacterial and analgesic properties. Its main biological active constituents are bicyclic sesquiterpene dialdehyde, polygodial, tannins and essential oils such as euogenol.[119] Because of its physiological activity, it may theoretically aid with reducing pain and inflammation associated with tonsillitis.

Leptospermum scoparium (manuka)

Manuka is native to New Zealand and, similar to horopito, has been used by the indigenous Māori for many years. It has been used for its effectiveness against a broad range of pathogens and acts as a mucous membrane tonic. It has antiseptic and astringent properties and can be used both topically and systemically. In vitro studies have indicated positive results with manuka being able to downregulate inflammation by specifically influencing TLR1/TLR2 signalling pathways.[120] The phenolic compounds of manuka are thought to have a positive impact on inflammation. Given the symptoms and causes of tonsillitis, manuka may prove to be an effective option for treatment.

Other

Herbal tea

Warm herbal teas can ease symptoms, including *Achillea millefolium* (yarrow), *Mentha x piperita* (peppermint), *Matracaria recutita* (chamomile), *Sambucus nigra* (elderflower).

Gargles

Throat gargles using herbal medicines (and others) that can eradicate the infection and provide mild anaesthetising effects are beneficial. Often practitioners encourage a swish and swallow approach to herbal formulations in lieu of secondary preparations. Examples: *Thymus vulgaris* (thyme), *Salvia officinalis* (sage), propolis, *Commiphora molmol* (myrrh), NaCl (table salt).

Topical applications

Topical applications can provide symptomatic relief including propolis, *Ulmus fulva* (slippery elm) paste, manuka honey.

LIFESTYLE RECOMMENDATIONS

- Rest, adequate sleep and stress reduction are essential. Resting the voice is essential as well
- A heating compress may be applied to the throat
- Anything which may aggravate the symptoms should be avoided
- Minimise exposure to inhaled irritants
- Avoid smoking and passive smoking.

Chronic picture

In an instance of repeated inflammation:

- Query lifestyle factors for pharyngitis (frequent speaking, singing)
- Query lymphatic health for tonsillitis.

CASE STUDY

OVERVIEW

RO is a 28-year-old school teacher who presents with recurrent and persistent tonsillitis. She is currently experiencing sore, inflamed tonsils and what she describes as a sore neck. RO feels generally unwell and run down and has experienced a low-grade fever for the past few days.

CASE STUDY CONTINUED

CLINICAL EXAMINATION

On examination she is experiencing inflamed palatine tonsils, with pustular exudate present on both tonsils. Her tongue is covered with a white, thin film. It has been suggested for RO to have a tonsillectomy due to having a recurrence of tonsillitis more than 4 times per year.

General inspection

General pallor and malaise and appears to be in a state of exhaustion

Vital signs

BP: 118/76 mmHg
Temperature: 38.5°C
Pulse: 85 bpm
Respiratory rate: 18 resp/min
Height: 1.65 m
Weight: 60 kg
BMI: 22

Head and neck

Face: Unremarkable

Lymphatic

Neck: Cervical lymphadenopathy — small, tender nodes on both left and right

Respiratory

Throat: Inflamed pharynx
Chest inspection: Normal
Palpation: Trachea — midline
Supraclavicular/axillary nodes: Nil
Percussion: Resonant sounds — left/right lobes
Auscultation: Air entry all zones

Other systems

NAD, unremarkable

TREATMENT PROTOCOL

The main initial focus of treatment was to support and improve immune function and response as well as providing symptomatic relief, especially during acute flare-ups. A secondary focus on stress response was also a component of the treatment protocol.

Herbal medicine

Herbal formulation

Echinacea spp. (echinacea premium blend)1 : 2: 70 mL
Thymus vulgaris (thyme)1 : 2: 30 mL
Leptospermum scoparium (manuka) 1 : 2: 50 mL
Astragalus membranaceus (astragalus) 1 : 2: 50 mL
Dosage: 7.5 mL twice daily

Gargle

Throat gargles consisting of warm water and NaCl (table salt) — ½ teaspoon as needed together with 2 drops each of eucalyptus and tea tree oil added to the solution. RO was instructed to use this throat gargle each morning and evening.

CASE STUDY CONTINUED

Throat spray

Throat spray consisting of per dose (4 sprays):

Althaea officinalis (marshmallow) extract equivalent to dry root 40 mg

Salvia fruticosa (sage) extract equivalent to dry herb 30 mg

Calendula officinalis (calendula) extract equivalent to dry flower 10 mg

Echinacea angustifolia (echinacea) extract equivalent to dry root 10 mg

Commiphora molmol (myrrh) stem bark oleoresin 1 mg

Syzygium aromaticum (clove) bud essential oil 1.25 μL

Nutritional medicine

Dietary

- Avoidance of dairy, refined carbohydrates and caffeine
- Promotion of adequate fluid consumption to ensure appropriate hydration and ensuring liquids are at room temperature
- Use of herbal teas consisting of yarrow, linden and peppermint to aid with fever resolution, with the addition of manuka honey for its antiseptic properties
- Encouragement to eat easily digested and absorbable foods. Examples include chicken vegetable soup, vegetable casseroles, stews and organic bone broths

Supplemental

- Vitamin C powder (mixed salts with bioflavonoids): 1 g q.i.d. in acute and then reduced to 1 g b.i.d.
- Zinc citrate (or as zinc lozenges): 30 mg t.d.s. in acute, then reduced to 30 mg daily
- Vitamin A: 5000 IU/day

Lifestyle/education

- Rest, adequate sleep
- Resting the voice
- A heating compress may be applied to the throat
- Minimise exposure to inhaled irritants
- Avoidance of smoking and passive smoking
- Avoidance of alcohol, recreational drugs
- Avoidance of intense exercise and social activity in the acute

Query lymphatic health and immunological function

- Referral for immunological studies and viral history (FBC, CRP, immunoglobulins, EBV, CMV) is imperative, especially when there is a history of recurrent and persistent tonsillitis
- Referral for food IgE/IgG profile

REFERENCES

[1] Tortora G, Derrickson B. Principles of anatomy and physiology. 11th ed. New Jersey: Wiley; 2006.

[2] Huether S, McCance K. Understanding pathophysiology. 4th ed. St Louis, Missouri: Mosby; 2008.

[3] Braun L, Cohen M. Herbs and natural supplements: an evidence based guide. 4th ed. Sydney: Elsevier; 2015. p. 1122.

[4] Heinrich M, Barnes J, Williamson E. Fundamentals of pharmacognosy and phytotherapy. London: Churchill Livingstone; 2008.

[5] Kong K, Coates H. Natural history, definitions, risk factors and burden of otitis media. Med J Aust 2009;191(9):39.

[6] Myburgh HC, van Zijl W, Swanepoel D, et al. Otitis media diagnosis for developing countries using tympanic membrane image-analysis. EBioMedicine 2016;(5):156–60.

[7] Ferri F. Ferri's clinical advisor. Philadelphia: Elsevier; 2017. p. 908–9.

[8] Bennett J, Dolin R, Blaser M. Mandell, Douglas and Bennett's principles and practice of infectious diseases. 8th ed. Philadelphia: Elsevier Saunders; 2015. p. 767–73.

[9] Post C. Direct evidence of bacterial biofilms in otitis media. Laryngoscope 2015;125(9):2003–14.

[10] Casey JR, Pichichero M. Changes in frequency and pathogenesis causing acute otitis media in 1995–2003. Paediatric Infec Dis J 2004;23:824–8.

[11] Chanmaitree T, Owen MJ, Howie VM. Respiratory viruses interfere with bacteriologic response to antibiotic in children with acute otitis media. J Infec Dis 1990;162:S46–9.

[12] Ruohala A, Meurman O, Nikkari S, et al. Microbiology of acute otitis media in children with tympanostomy tubes: prevalence of bacteria and viruses. Clin Infec Dis 2006;43:1417–22.

[13] Thomas J, Bermer R, Zahnert T, et al. Acute otitis media: a structured approach. Dtsch Arztebl Int 2014;111(9):151–60.

[14] Nsouli T, Nsouli S, Linde R, et al. Role of food allergy in serous otitis media. Ann Allergy 1994;73(3):215–19.

[15] James J. Common respiratory manifestations of food allergy: a critical focus on otitis media. Curr Allergy Asthma Rep 2004;4(4):294–301.

[16] Hurt DS. Association of otitis media with effusion and allergy as demonstrated by intradermal skin testing and eosinophil cationic protein levels in both middle ear effusions and mucosal biopsies. Laryngoscope 1996;106(9 Pt 1):1128–237.

[17] Ramakrishnan J. The role of food allergy in otolaryngology disorders. Curr Opin Otolaryngol Head Neck Surg 2010;18(3):195–9.

[18] Marchiso P, Consonni D, Baggi E, et al. Vitamin D supplementation reduces the risk of otitis media in otitis prone children. Paediatr Infect Dis J 2013;32(10):1055–560.

[19] Shankar A, Prasad A. Zinc and immune function: the biological basis of altered resistance to infection. Am J Clin Nutr 1998;68(2):S447–63.

[20] Cemek M, Dede S, Bayiroğlu F, et al. Oxidant and antioxidant levels in children with acute otitis media and tonsillitis: a comparative study. Int J Pediatr Otorhinolaryngol 2005;69:823–7.

[21] Elemraid M, MacKenzie J, Frazer W, et al. Nutritional factors in the pathogenesis of ear disease in children: a systematic review. Ann Trop Paed 2009;29:85–99.

[22] Lasisi A. Comparative analysis of middle ear immune response and micronutrient level between mucoid and purulent otitis media. J Otolaryngol Head Neck Surg 2009;38:477–82.

[23] Braun L, Cohen M. Herbs and natural supplements: an evidence-based guide. 4th ed. Sydney: Elsevier; 2015. p. 1104.

[24] Aladag I, Guven M, Eyibilen A, et al. Efficiency of vitamin A in experimentally induced acute otitis media. Int J Paediatr Otrorhinolaryngol 2007;71(4):623–8.

[25] Azarpazhooh A, Limeback H, Lawrence H, et al. Xylitol for preventing acute otitis media in children up to 12 years of age. Cochrane Database Syst Rev 2011;(11):CD007095.

[26] Subbotina M, Kunitsina M, Buksha I, et al. The use of Sinupret in the combined treatment of acute otitis media in children. Vestn Otorinolaryngol 2009;(2):43–5.

[27] Sarell EM, et al. Efficacy of naturopathic extracts in the management of ear pain associated with acute otitis media. Arch Pediatr Adolesc Med 2001;155(7):796–9.

[28] Sarell EM, et al. Naturopathic treatment for ear pain in children. Pediatrics 2003;111:e574–9.

[29] Schapowal A, Klein P, Johnston S. Echinacea reduces the risk of recurrent respiratory tract infections and complications: a meta-analysis of randomized controlled trials. Adv Ther 2015;32(3):187–200.

[30] Miretti A, Forti S, Tassone G, et al. Efficacy of complex herbal compound of *Echinacea angustifolia* (Imoviral Junior) in recurrent upper respiratory tract infections during paediatric age: preliminary results. Minerva Pediatr 2011;63(3):177–82.

[31] Kristinsson K, Magnusdottir A, Petersen H, et al. Effective treatment of experimental acute otitis media by application of volatile fluids into the ear canal. JID 2005;191:1876–80.
[32] Camporese A. In vitro activity of *Eucalyptus smithii* and *Juniperus communis* essential oils against bacterial biofilms and efficacy perspectives of complementary inhalation therapy in chronic and recurrent upper respiratory tract infections. Le Infezioni in Medicine 2013;2:117–24.
[33] Australian Institute of Health and Welfare. Chronic respiratory conditions including asthma and COPD; 2017. Available at www.aihw.gov.au/chronic-respiratory-conditions.
[34] eTG complete. eTG complete; 2009. http://online.tg.org.au/complete/.
[35] Mostov PD. Treating the immunocompetent patient who presents with an upper respiratory infection: pharyngitis, sinusitis, and bronchitis. Prim Care 2007;34(1):39–58.
[36] Gutman M, Torres A, Keen KJ, et al. Prevalence of allergy in patients with chronic rhinosinusitis. Otolaryngol Head Neck Surg 2004;130:545–52.
[37] Emanuel IA, Shah SB. Chronic rhinosinusitis: allergy and sinus computed tomography relationships. Otolaryngol Head Neck Surg 2000;123:687–91.
[38] Sheik J, Najib U. Rhinitis, allergic: differential diagnoses and workup. eMedicine 2009;11–12. Available from: www.medscape.com.
[39] Chiu AG. Frontal sinus surgery: its evolution, present standard of care, and recommendations for current use. Ann Otol Rhinol Laryngol 2006;196(Suppl.):13–19.
[40] Kim DS, Drake-Lee AB. Allergen immunotherapy in ENT: historical perspective. J Laryngol Otol 2003;117(12):940–5.
[41] Jaber R. Respiratory and allergic diseases: from upper respiratory tract infections to asthma. Prim Care 2002;29(2):231–61.
[42] Pitchford P, Healing with whole foods. Emeryville, CA: North Atlantic Books; 1993.
[43] Novick SG, Godfrey JC, Pollack RL, et al. Zinc-induced suppression of inflammation in the respiratory tract, caused by infection with human rhinovirus and other irritants. Med Hypotheses 1997;49(1):347–57.
[44] Dhanawat G. Rhinitis, sinusitis and ocular disease 2100. New approach to treat allergic rhinitis with vitamin E, cod liver oil and vitamin C with use of nasal steroid spray. World Allergy Organ J 2013;6(Suppl. 11):175.
[45] Bucca C, Rolla G, Oliva A, et al. Effect of vitamin C on histamine bronchial responsiveness of patients with allergic rhinitis. Ann Allergy 1990;65(4):311–14.
[46] Otsuka H, Inaba M, Fujikura T, et al. Histochemical and functional characteristics of metachromatic cells in the nasal epithelium in allergic rhinitis: studies of nasal scrapings and their dispersed cells. J Allergy Clin Immunol 1995;96(4):528–36.
[47] Jamison J. Clinical guide to nutrition and dietary supplements in disease management. Melbourne: Churchill Livingstone; 2003.
[48] Bener A, Ehlayel MS, Bener HZ, et al. The impact of vitamin D deficiency on asthma, allergic rhinitis and wheezing in children: an emerging public health problem. J Family Community Med 2014;21(3):154–61.
[49] Zingg J. Vitamin E and mast cells. Vitam Horm 2007;76:393–418.
[50] Wjist M, Hypponen E. Vitamin D serum levels and allergic rhinitis. Allergy 2007;62(9):1085–6.
[51] Majima Y. Mucoactive medications and airway disease. Paediatr Respir Rev 2002;3:104–9.
[52] Grandjean EM, Berthet P, Ruffmann R, et al. Efficacy of oral long-term N-acetylcysteine in chronic bronchopulmonary disease: a meta-analysis of published double-blind, placebo-controlled clinical trials. Clin Ther 2000;22:209–21.
[53] Ryan RE. A double-blind clinical evaluation of bromelains in the treatment of acute sinusitis. Headache 1967;7:13–17.
[54] Burrner L, Achilles N, Bohm M, et al. Efficacy and tolerability of bromelain in patients with chronic rhinosinusitis — a pilot study. B-ENT 2013;9(3):217–25.
[55] Nurul IM, Mizughuchi H, Shahriar M, et al. *Albizia lebbeck* suppresses histamine signaling by the inhibition of histamine H1 receptor and histidine decarboxylase gene transcriptions. Int Immunopharmacol 2011;11(11):1766–72.
[56] Bone K. Clinical applications of Ayurvedic and Chinese herbs. Australia: Phytotherapy Press; 1996.
[57] Mills S, Bone K. Principles and practice of phytotherapy. Edinburgh: Churchill Livingstone; 2013.
[58] Bensky D, Gamble A. Chinese herbal medicine: materia medica. Seattle: Eastland Press; 1986.
[59] Braun L, Cohen M. Herbs and natural supplements: an evidence-based guide. Sydney: Elsevier; 2015. p. 48–9.
[60] Felter HW, Lyodd JU. King's American dispensatory. 18th ed, rev 3. Portland: Eclectic Medical Publications; 1905. [reprinted 1983].
[61] Grieve M. A modern herbal. New York: Dover; 1971.
[62] Oliver F, Amon EU, Breathnach A, et al. Contact urticaria due to the common stinging nettle (*Urtica dioica*) — histological, ultrastructural and pharmacological studies. Clin Exp Dermatol 1991;16(1):1–7.
[63] Mittman P. Randomized, double-blind study of freeze-dried *Urtica dioica* in the treatment of allergic rhinitis. Planta Med 1990;56(1):44–7.
[64] Roschek B, Fink RC, McMichael M, et al. Nettle extract (*Urtica dioica*) affects key receptors and enzymes associated with allergic rhinitis. Phytother Res 2009;7:920–6.
[65] Kurup VP, Barrios CS. Immunomodulatory effects of curcumin in allergy. Mol Nutr Food Res 2008;52(9):1031–9.
[66] Goos KH, Albrecht U, Schneider B. On-going investigations on efficacy and safety profile of a herbal drug containing nasturtium herb and horseradish root in acute sinusitis, acute bronchitis and acute urinary tract infection in children in comparison with other antibiotic treatments. Arzneimittelforschung 2007;57(4):238–46.
[67] Federspil P, Wulkow R, Zimmermann T. [Effects of standardized Myrtol in therapy of acute sinusitis–results of a double-blind, randomized multicenter study compared with placebo]. Laryngorhinootologie 1997;76(1):23–7.
[68] Saxena Vs, Venkateshwarlu K, Nadig P, et al. Multicenter clinical trials in novel polyherbal formulation in allergic rhinitis. Int J Clin Pharmacol Res 2004;24(2–3):79–94.
[69] Evans R III. Environmental control and immunotherapy for allergic disease. J Allergy Clin Immunol 1992;90:462–8.
[70] Yerushalmi A, Karman S, Lwoff A. Treatment of perennial allergic rhinitis by local hyperthermia. Proc Natl Acad Sci USA 1982;79:4766–9.
[71] Australian Govrnment: Department of Health. Australian Influenza Surveillance Report; 2016 June: (2). Available from: www.health.gove.au/internet/main/publishing.nsf/Content/cda-surveil-ozflu-flucurr.htm/$File/Australian-Influenza-Surveillance-Reprt.pdf.
[72] Mozherenkov VP, Shubina LF. [Treatment of chronic conjunctivitis with Calendula]. Med Sestra 1976;35(4):33–4.
[73] Wong D. Virology online; 2009. Available from: http://virology-online.com/viruses/CORZA2.htm.
[74] Kirkpatrick GL. The common cold. Prim Care 1996;23(4):657–75.
[75] Murtagh JE. John Murtagh's general practice. 4th ed. Sydney: McGraw-Hill; 2007.
[76] Sheik J, Najib U. Rhinitis, allergic: differential diagnoses and workup. eMedicine 2009;2009:11–12. Available from: www.medscape.com.
[77] Cannell JJ, Hollis BW. Use of vitamin D in clinical practice. Altern Med Rev 2008;13(1):6–20.
[78] Hemila H, Chalker E, et al. Vitamin C for preventing and treating the common cold. Cochrane Database Syst Rev 2013;(1):CD000980.
[79] Singh M, Das RR. Zinc for the common cold. Cochrane Database Syst Rev 2013;(6):CD001364, 18.
[80] Hulisz D. Efficacy of zinc against common cold viruses: an overview. J Am Pharm Assoc (2003) 2004;44(5):594–603.
[81] Hirt M, Nobel S, Barron E. Zinc nasal gel for the treatment of common cold symptoms: a double-blind, placebo-controlled trial. Ear Nose Throat J 2000;79(10):778–80, 782.
[82] Prasad AS, Fitzgerald JT, Bao B, et al. Duration of symptoms and plasma cytokine levels in patients with the common cold treated with zinc acetate. A randomized, double-blind, placebo-controlled trial. Ann Intern Med 2000;133(4):245–52.
[83] Kurugol Z, Bayram N, Atik T. Effect of zinc sulfate on common cold in children: randomized, double blind study. Pediatr Int 2007;49(6):842–7.
[84] McElroy BH, Miller SP. Effectiveness of zinc gluconate glycine lozenges (Cold-Eeze) against the common cold in school-aged subjects: a retrospective chart review. Am J Ther 2002;9(6):472–5.

[85] McElroy BH, Miller SP. An open-label, single-center, phase IV clinical study of the effectiveness of zinc gluconate glycine lozenges (Cold-Eeze) in reducing the duration and symptoms of the common cold in school-aged subjects. Am J Ther 2003;10(5):324–9.
[86] Veverka DV, Wilson C, Martinez MA, et al. Use of zinc supplements to reduce upper respiratory infections in United States Air Force Academy Cadets. Complement Ther Clin Pract 2009;15(2):91–5.
[87] Venuta A, Spano C, Laudizi L, et al. Essential fatty acids: the effects of dietary supplementation among children with recurrent respiratory infections. J Int Med Res 1996;24(4):325–30.
[88] Pleschka S, Stein M, Schoop M, et al. Anti-viral properties and mode of action of standardized *Echinacea purpurea* extract against highly pathogenic avian influenza virus (H5N1, H7N7) and swine-origin H1N1(S-O1V). Virol J 2009;13(6):197.
[89] Karsch-Volk M, Barrett B, Linde K. Echinacea for preventing and treating the common cold. JAMA 2015;313(6):618–19.
[90] Natural Standard. Echinacea Professional Monograph; 2009. Natural Standard.
[91] Coon JT, Ernst E. *Andrographis paniculata* in the treatment of upper respiratory tract infections: a systematic review of safety and efficacy. Planta Med 2004;70(4):293–8.
[92] Wolkerstorfer A, Kurz H, Bachhofner N et al. Glycyrrhizin inhibits influenza A virus uptake into the cell. Antiviral Res 2009;83(2):171–8.
[93] Brush J, Mendenhall E, Guggenheim A, et al. The effect of *Echinacea purpurea, Astragalus membranaceus* and *Glycyrrhiza glabra* on CD69 expression and immune cell activation in humans. Phytother Res 2006;20(8):687–95.
[94] Soret MG. Antiviral activity of calcium elenolate on parainfluenza infection of hamsters. In: Hobby G, editor. Antimicrobial agents and chemotherapy. Bethesda: Williams & Wilkins; 1969. p. 160–6.
[95] Tranter HS, Tassou SC, Nychas GJ. The effect of the olive phenolic compound, oleuropein, on growth and enterotoxin B production by *Staphylococcus aureus*. J Appl Bacteriol 1993;74(3):253–9.
[96] Henneicke-von Zepelin H, Hentschel C, Schnitker J, et al. Efficacy and safety of a fixed combination phytomedicine in the treatment of the common cold (acute viral respiratory tract infection): results of a randomised, double blind, placebo controlled, multicentre study. Curr Med Res Opin 1999;15(3):214–27.
[97] Josling P. Preventing the common cold with a garlic supplement: a double-blind, placebo-controlled survey. Adv Ther 2001;18(4): 189–93.
[98] Zakay-Rones Z, Thom E, Wollan T, et al. Randomized study of the efficacy and safety of oral elderberry extract in the treatment of influenza A and B virus infections. J Int Med Res 2004; 32(2):132–40.
[99] Timmer A, Gunther J, Motschall E, et al. *Pelargonium sidoides* extract for treating acute respiratory tract infections (review). Cochrane Database Syst Rev 2013;(10):CD006323.
[100] Gaffney RJ, Cafferkey MT. Bacteriology of normal and diseased tonsils assessed by fine-needle aspiration: *Haemophilus influenzae* and the pathogenesis of recurrent acute tonsillitis. Clin Otolaryngol Allied Sci 1998;23(2):181–5.
[101] Dias EP, Rocha ML, Carvalho M, et al. [Detection of Epstein-Barr virus in recurrent tonsillitis]. Braz J Otorhinolaryngol 2009;75(1):30–4.
[102] Segal N, El Saied S, Puterman M. Peritonsillar abscess in children in the southern district of Israel. Int J Pediatr Otorhinolaryngol 2009;73(8):1148–50.
[103] Yilmaz T, Koçan EG, Besler HT. The role of oxidants and antioxidants in chronic tonsillitis and adenoid hypertrophy in children. Int J Pediatr Otorhinolaryngol 2004;68(8):1053–8.
[104] Kiroglu AF, Noyan T, Oger M, et al. Oxidants and antioxidants in tonsillar and adenoidal tissue in chronic adenotonsillitis and adenotonsillar hypertrophy in children. Int J Pediatr Otorhinolaryngol 2006;70(1):35–8.
[105] Pizzorno JE, Murray MT. Textbook of natural medicine. 3rd ed. Edinburgh: Elsevier; 2009.
[106] Yılmaz T, Koçan EG, Besler HT. The role of oxidants and antioxidants in chronic tonsillitis and adenoid hypertrophy in children. Int J Pediatr Otorhinolaryngol 2004;68(8):1053–8.
[107] Truong-Tran AQ, Carter J, Ruffin R, et al. New insights into the role of zinc in the respiratory epithelium. Immunol Cell Biol 2001;79:170–7.
[108] Somuk B, Sapmaz E, Solyalic H, et al. Evaluation of iron and zinc levels in recurrent tonsillitis and tonsillar hypertrophy. Am J Otolaryng 2016;37(2):116–19.
[109] Aleszczyk J. [Connection between changing the vitamin and immune status and the character of the throat microflora in patients with chronic tonsillitis]. Otolaryngol Pol 2003;57(2): 221–4.
[110] Prasad AS, Beck FW, Kaplan J, et al. Effect of zinc supplementation on incidence of infections and hospital admissions in sickle cell disease (SCD). Am J Hematol 1999;61:194–202.
[111] Grant WB. Tonsillectomy may be an indicator of low vitamin D status, a risk factor for cancer later in life. Cancer Causes Control 2009;20:1235–6.
[112] Esposito S, Lelii M, Vitamin D. and respiratory tract infections in childhood. BMC Infect Dis 2015;15:487.
[113] Nseir W, Mograbi J, Abu-Rahmeh Z, et al. The association between vitamin D levels and recurrent group A streptococcal tonsillopharyngitis in adults. Int J Infect Dis 2012;16(10):e735–8.
[114] Cemek M, Dede S, Bayiroğlu F, et al. Oxidant and antioxidant levels in children with acute otitis media and tonsillitis: a comparative study. Int J Pediatr Otorhinolaryngol 2005;69(6):823–7.
[115] Shukla GK, Sharma S, Shukla A, et al. Comparative status of oxidative damage and antioxidant enzymes in chronic tonsillitis patients. Boll Chim Farm 1998;137(6):206–9.
[116] Lizogub VG, Riley DS, Heger M. Efficacy of a *Pelargonium sidoides* preparation in patients with the common cold: a randomized, double blind, placebo-controlled clinical trial. Explore (NY) 2007;3(6):573–84.
[117] Linde K, Barrett B, Wolkart K, et al. Echinacea for preventing and treating the common cold. Cochrane Database Syst Rev 2006;(1):CD000530.
[118] British Herbal Medicine Association's Scientific Committee. British Herbal Pharmacopoeia; 1983. Barmouth: BHMA.
[119] Rasmussen P. *Pseudowintera* spp. (Horopito): a monograph. Aust J Herb Med 2014;26(4):150.
[120] Tomblin V, Ferguson L, Han D, et al. Potential pathway of anti-inflammatory effect by New Zealand honeys. Int J Gen Med 2014;7:149–58.

14 The respiratory system

Annmarie Cannone

OVERVIEW OF THE RESPIRATORY SYSTEM

During fetal life, from birth to maturity and throughout adult life, the respiratory system is intertwined with nutrition. An optimal respiratory system enables the body to obtain the oxygen required to meet its cellular demands for nutrients and to remove metabolic waste products. Optimal nutrition is essential for the formation, development, growth, maturity and protection of a healthy respiratory system. The respiratory structures include the nose, pharynx, larynx, trachea, bronchi, bronchioles, alveolar ducts and alveoli. Supporting structures include the skeleton and the muscles, especially the intercostals and abdominal muscles and the diaphragm. Within one month of conception, respiratory system structures are recognisable. The pulmonary system grows and matures during gestation and childhood. Ageing is associated with diminished lung integrity. Gas exchange is the major function of the respiratory system. The lungs enable the body to obtain the oxygen required to meet its cellular metabolic demands and to remove carbon dioxide produced by these processes. The cavities and tracts also function to filter, warm and humidify the inspired air; synthesise arachidonic acid; and convert angiotensin I to angiotensin II.[1]

Just like eating, breathing is an immunological event. Inspired air is laden with particles and microorganisms. The mucus in the airways keeps the airways moist and traps the particles and microorganisms from the air. Most cells that line the trachea, bronchi and bronchioles have cilia which constantly sweep the particles upward towards the pharynx. The epithelial surface of the alveoli contains macrophages which will engulf and destroy the foreign particles and microorganisms, and each time a person breathes, contaminated mucus passes into the digestive tract, to eventually be eliminated.

See Fig. 14.1 for an overview of the whole respiratory system.

Anatomy of the respiratory system

Structurally the respiratory system can be divided into two parts:

1 The upper respiratory system, consisting of the nose, pharynx and associated structures (such as sinuses). See Chapter 13 for detailed information on the upper respiratory tract
2 The lower respiratory system, consisting of the trachea, bronchi and lungs.

LOWER RESPIRATORY SYSTEM

Trachea

The trachea, commonly known as the windpipe, is found between the larynx and the bronchi, and is anterior to the oesophagus. It is about 12 cm long, 2.5 cm in diameter, and is kept open by 16–20 C-shaped rings of cartilage. This construction prevents the collapse of the trachea, especially during inspiration. The trachea is lined with pseudostratified ciliated columnar epithelium, which has a protective function and secretes mucus.

The functions of the trachea include the passage and filtration of air.

Bronchi

The trachea divides into right and left primary bronchi, which supply the right and left lung respectively. The bronchi are two short tubes, similar in structure to the trachea, which lead to and carry air into each lung. They are lined with pseudostratified ciliated columnar epithelium and, like the trachea, contain incomplete cartilage rings to hold them open.

On entering the lungs the primary bronchi divide into the secondary bronchi, which branch to form the tertiary bronchi; these divide to form the bronchioles, which divide repeatedly and terminate in very small tubes called the terminal bronchioles.

This gradual narrowing of the bronchi to bronchioles also involves a gradual reduction in the amount of cartilage, and a corresponding increase in the amount of smooth muscle tissue.

The epithelium gradually changes from pseudostratified ciliated columnar epithelium in the bronchi to non-ciliated simple cuboidal epithelium in the terminal bronchioles.

Lungs

The lungs are paired, cone-shaped, spongy organs, situated in the thoracic cavity. They are separated from each other

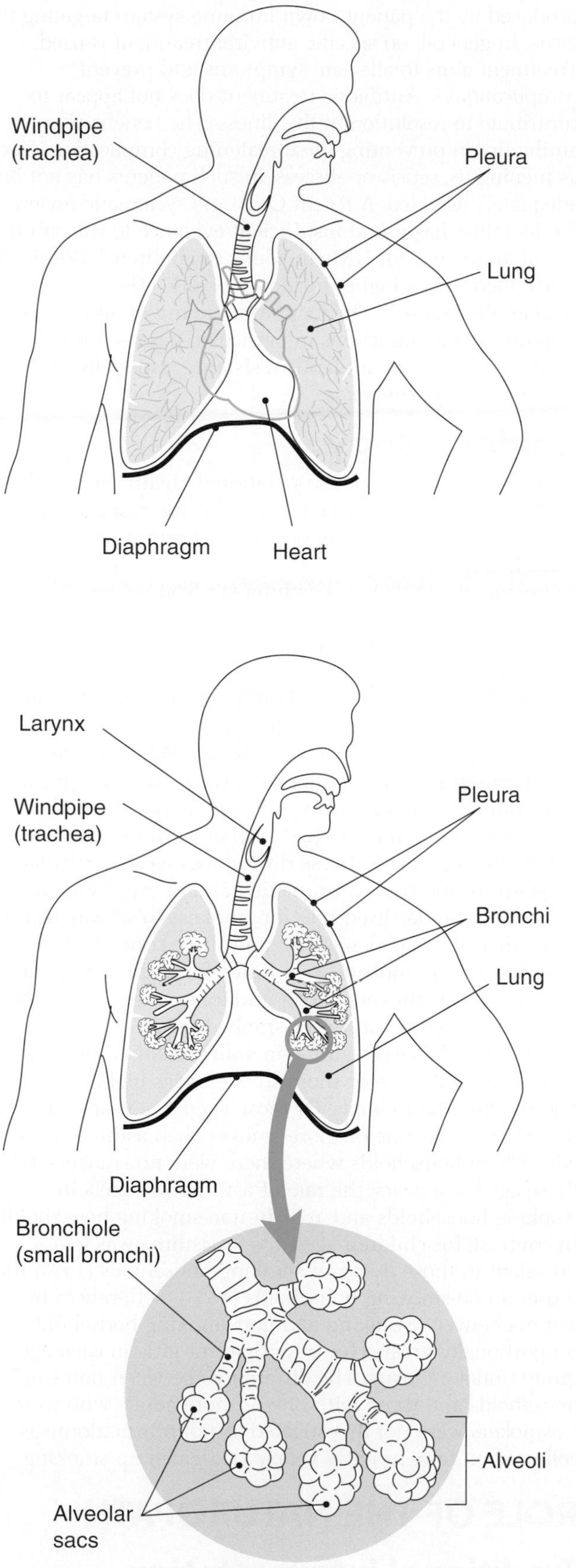

FIGURE 14.1 The respiratory system

by the mediastinum, which contains the heart and other structures.

Each lung is surrounded by a double-layered serous membrane called the pleural membrane. The two layers are the:

- *Parietal pleura*: this is the most superficial layer, and it lines the wall of the thoracic cavity
- *Visceral pleura*: this is the deepest layer, and it covers the lungs.

The space between the parietal and visceral pleura is called the pleural cavity, and it is filled with serous fluid. This fluid has a number of important functions:

- It reduces friction between the membranes so that they slide easily across each other during breathing
- It causes the two layers of membrane to adhere to one another, in much the same way as a thin film of water causes two flat sheets of glass to stick to one another. This essentially allows the lungs to adhere to the thoracic wall, so that if the thoracic cavity expands, the lungs expand also. This happens when we breathe
- Each lung has a number of lobes. The right lung has three lobes (superior, middle and inferior), while the left lung has two lobes (superior and inferior). The left lung is smaller than the right lung and contains a concavity called the cardiac notch, which is where the heart is located.

Alveoli

At the end of the numerous bronchioles are the tiny air sacs called alveoli that contribute to the spongy texture of the lungs. They have very thin walls that are just one cell thick. Each alveolus is supplied by numerous capillaries, to allow the exchange of gases (oxygen and carbon dioxide) between the air in the alveoli and the blood.

There are about 700 million alveoli in an adult's lungs, which have a total surface area of 50–80 square metres (about the size of a tennis court). This large surface area allows rapid and efficient gas exchange to take place between the air in the alveoli of the lungs and the nearby blood capillaries.

Each alveolus is lined by epithelium, and its underlying basement membrane.

There are two types of epithelial cells:

1. *Type I alveolar cells*: simple squamous cells that form an almost complete lining of the alveolar wall. These cells are the most numerous, and are the main site for gas exchange
2. *Type II alveolar cells*: also called septal cells, are dispersed between the type 1 alveolar cells. These cells secrete alveolar fluid that keeps the surface of the alveoli moist. Alveolar fluid also contains surfactant, a phospholipid/lipoprotein mixture that lowers the surface tension of the alveolar fluid and therefore reduces the tendency of the alveoli to collapse.

The alveoli also contain phagocytic cells, called alveolar macrophages, which remove dust and debris.

RESPIRATION

Respiration is the exchange of gases between the atmosphere, the blood and the cells of the body. Respiration takes place in three basic steps.

Pulmonary ventilation

Also called breathing, pulmonary ventilation is the inspiration (inflow) and expiration (outflow) of air between the atmosphere and the lungs.

External (pulmonary) respiration

External (pulmonary) respiration is the exchange of gases between the air spaces of the lungs and the blood in the pulmonary capillaries. In this step oxygen moves from the air spaces of the lungs into the blood, and carbon dioxide moves in the opposite direction.

Internal respiration

Internal respiration is the exchange of gases between the blood in systemic capillaries and tissue cells. In this step oxygen moves from the blood to the tissue cells, and carbon dioxide moves in the opposite direction.

RESPIRATORY INFECTIONS

Overview

The upper respiratory tract is lined by stratified squamous epithelium, and columnar, goblet and gland cells generally line the lower respiratory tract (LRT). There are normal flora occupying the upper respiratory tract and the evaluation of infections is complicated by the presence of colonising species, which may have no role in infection. Physiological mucus production may be altered here by nonspecific and non-infectious causes, further complicating diagnosis. Because the specific aetiological agent of an upper respiratory infection is often not identified, clinical judgment is required in the approach to their diagnosis and treatment. The causative agent of these infections is typically a virus.[2]

Management

The management of upper respiratory infections (URIs) is complicated by the confusing terminology that has arisen to define their anatomical locations, while ignoring their usually diffuse nature. The term URI has come to encompass multiple clinical entities including pharyngitis, sinusitis and bronchitis, as well as nonspecific respiratory infections, a designation that includes the common cold. The classification scheme based upon the predominant anatomical site of the presenting symptom complex tends to be poorly specific for directing therapy.[2]

Classification

Acute respiratory tract infections (ARTIs) range from minor (e.g. common cold) through to very serious conditions (e.g. severe acute respiratory syndrome). ARTIs are caused by over 200 viruses or bacteria. They are transmitted directly through person-to-person contact, either by airborne droplets from a sneeze or cough, or by direct contact with nasal or throat secretions, articles freshly soiled with secretions of the nose and throat, or by transmission via an object indirectly. For example, sore throat can either be a disease in itself, or result from other diseases, such as influenza and glandular fever. Uncomplicated ARTIs, such as the common cold and sore throat, recover spontaneously as a result of antibodies produced by the patient's own immune system targeting the virus. In general, no specific antiviral treatment is used. Treatment aims to alleviate symptoms and prevent complications.[3] Antibiotic treatment does not appear to contribute to resolution of the illness. The benefit of antibiotics in preventing life-threatening complications, such as meningitis, sepsis or abscess, in such patients has not been adequately assessed. A recent Cochrane systematic review of the literature has found insufficient evidence to warrant the use of antibiotics for URIs in adults or children.[4] Within this study, there was a higher incidence of side effects associated with antibiotic use.[4] The inappropriate use of antibiotics, for respiratory tract infections in particular, has been implicated in the emergence of antibiotic resistance, especially in *Streptococcus pneumoniae*.[2]

Epidemiology

According to the 2014–2015 National Health Survey,[5] 7.1 million Australians suffer from a chronic respiratory condition. The commonly occurring respiratory conditions include hay fever (15% of the population), chronic rhinosinusitis (15%) and asthma (10.8%).

The overall rate of respiratory conditions was higher for females (39%) than for males (36%). Recent respiratory illnesses were most prevalent in winter (25%) and spring (24%). They were less prevalent in summer (17%) and autumn (19%). There was little seasonal variability in asthma experienced as a recent illness. When age and sex standardised rates for adults were compared, the prevalence of respiratory conditions overall was higher in smokers (37%) and in ex-smokers (41%) than in those who had never smoked (36%). These differences were particularly apparent in the case of bronchitis and/or emphysema, where the standardised rate for smokers (9%) was nearly twice that of ex-smokers (5%) and three times that of those who had never smoked (3%). Rates for asthma were also higher among smokers (11%) and ex-smokers (11%) than among those who had never smoked (9%).

The prevalence of asthma in young children living in households with one or more smokers was higher than in non-smoking households. Of those aged 0–4 years, 13% in households with one or more smokers had asthma compared with 9% in households where there were no smokers. Of those aged 5–9 years, the rate of asthma was 22% in smoking households and 18% in non-smoking households. In contrast, for children aged 10–14, asthma was less prevalent in those living in smoking households (17%) than those in non-smoking households (20%). Differences in asthma between smoking and non-smoking households were proportionally greater for boys than for girls in each age group under 15 years. The differences between non-smoking households and those with one or more adults who were ex-smokers were not investigated as no information was collected on how recently people had given up smoking.

ROLE OF THE NATUROPATH

Traditional interpretation

The principles of naturopathic philosophy include identifying and treating the cause and the whole person using the innate healing power of the body. Prevention is the underlying philosophy of naturopathy and this underpins treatment objectives.

The respiratory system and its management was a subject of much interest to the traditional physicians of the past. Treatment of respiratory conditions with expectorants can be traced back to the 3rd century BC when Hippocrates used liquorice to manage coughs, asthma and other respiratory conditions.[6]

When treating the respiratory system, a strong focus was to encourage elimination. It was believed that by clearing excess mucus and catarrh optimal health would be achieved. Traditional applications of smoking specific herbal medicines were used to stimulate respiratory function and clear 'bad spirits' or respiratory congestion.

Culpeper, in the 17th century, also advocated the use of liquorice for conditions of the respiratory tract such as conjunctivitis and tuberculosis, stating:

> *Liquorice boiled in fair water, with some Maiden-hair and figs, makes a good drink for those that have a dry cough or hoarseness, wheezing or shortness of breath, and for all the griefs of the breast and lungs, phthisic or consumptions caused by the distillation of salt humours on them. The fine powder of Liquorice blown through a quill into the eyes that have a pin and web (as they call it) or rheumatic distillations in them, doth cleanse and help them. The juice of Liquorice is as effectual in all the diseases of the breast and lungs, the reins and bladder, as the decoction. The juice distilled in Rose-water, with some Gum Tragacanth, is a fine licking medicine for hoarseness and wheezing.*[7]

The prescriptions of the Eclectics, the forerunners of today's naturopaths, were designed to offer support to the respiratory system by nourishing the lungs and bronchi. They noted that the respiratory system regularly encountered 'excitants' such as pollutants, pollens and dust.

When treating the respiratory system the Eclectics considered there to be two main focuses: firstly, the condition of the secretion; and secondly, eliminating the offending pathogen and secretion from the body.

> *The condition of the secretions must be considered in every case. Elimination seldom receives sufficient attention in any disease. With the suppression of the secretions there is always a demand for increased elimination.*[8]

From this statement we can see that the Eclectics were fairly advanced in their way of thinking. Suppressed secretions, visible by such things as dry skin and constipation (when accompanied by respiratory disease), signified the possibility that the pathogen still remained at large within the body. Additionally, the nature of the secretion — for example, the yellow pus associated with conjunctivitis or the sputum of asthma so eloquently described by Thomas in 1907 as containing small, jelly-like balls floating in their mucin[9] — gave the Eclectics a good idea of firstly, which condition they were dealing with, secondly, the infective nature of the pathogen (e.g. bacterial), and thirdly, the preferential botanical, homeopathic or other agent to use to eliminate it.

To induce elimination the Eclectics favoured heating therapies such as footbaths laced with mustard that promoted sweating by the body.

> *Elimination at the onset of acute disease, has long been promptly and satisfactorily re-established by the use of hot foot baths, hot diaphoretic drinks and induced perspiration.*[8]

These heating therapies encouraged the body to sweat, stoking a fever, thereby killing the offending pathogen. Additionally the heat loosened and liquefied mucus in the system, allowing it to be more easily discharged from the body.

As for botanical treatment, the Eclectics employed respiratory sedatives and tonics and sedatives. Lobelia was considered by the Eclectic physicians to be one of the most important herbs for the respiratory system. The Eclectics used it to strengthen and relieve spasm in the respiratory system; however, use of this herb in modern times is scheduled. The Eclectics also advocated the use of agents that acted upon the mucous and serous membranes of the respiratory tract such as turpentine, though turpentine is not so commonly used today!

> *An extreme outpour of mucus whether from the bronchial tubes, from the stomach or from the intestinal canal, may be controlled often better with turpentine, than with other remedies. This may be given in doses of from two to five drops, on sugar slowly dissolved in the saliva within the mouth and the saliva swallowed.*[8]

Seemingly novel to use today, traditional applications of smoking the specific respiratory herbal medicines such as lobelia, belladonna and stramonium[10] or burning herbs in dishes, while inhaling the fumes, were commonplace to stimulate respiratory function and clear 'bad spirits' or respiratory congestion.

Modern interpretation

Naturopathy is the application of the principles of natural therapy within the context of modern scientific knowledge that evolved throughout the last half of the 20th century, building on nature cure, homeopathy and indigenous medicines from different parts of the world. Naturopathy is a philosophy and healthcare approach that takes into consideration one's view of life (spiritual and emotional), lifestyle and individual uniqueness. People are treated based on their own individual case rather than on generalisations. Three people suffering from influenza may receive three different treatment programs because of their individual circumstances of genetics, environment, beliefs, diet and lifestyle. Nutrition is of primary importance in naturopathy because food is considered not only nourishment, but also as medicine. Naturopathic medicine uses a wide array of methods to restore or maintain health and starts with the basics of the nature cure (air, water, light and earth). All naturopathic therapies aim to support the body's ability to fight infections and recover health. This also applies to the treatment of acute illnesses of the upper respiratory tract. A combination of therapies is selected that will enhance the body's capacity to fight bacteria and viruses, while also helping to remove cellular waste products.

Treatment objectives

- Improve the quality and quantity of air flow entering and exiting the respiratory tract (mouth, nasal passages and sinuses, pharynx/throat, larynx/trachea, bronchi, lungs)
- Improve gas exchange in the lungs
- Eradicate any infection
- Reduce inflammation
- Reduce allergic response
- Encourage expectoration: generally it is perceived that excessive mucus dampens and weakens respiratory function; however, expectoration needs to ensure that the requirements specific to the presenting patient are considered.

Nutritional medicine

The relationship between malnutrition and respiratory disease has long been recognised. Malnutrition adversely affects lung structure, elasticity and function; respiratory muscle mass, strength and endurance; lung immune defence; and control of breathing. Protein and iron deficiencies cause low haemoglobin resulting in diminished oxygen-carrying capacity of the blood. Calcium, magnesium, phosphorus and potassium deficiencies may compromise respiratory muscle function at the cellular level. Hypoproteinaemia is associated with pulmonary oedema, and adequate levels of proteins and phospholipids are essential for maintenance of surfactant, which is necessary for keeping the alveoli expanded. Vitamin C is necessary for collagen in the connective tissues of the respiratory system. Adequate water, glycoproteins, electrolytes and nutrients such as vitamin A are essential for the production of normal mucus. Antioxidants are also essential for a healthy mucous membrane.[1] Refer to Table 14.7 later in this chapter for a full discussion.

Herbal medicine

DISCUSSION AND APPLICATION

Herbal medicine and phytotherapy (modern herbal therapeutics) have a very long tradition in the treatment of respiratory tract diseases. Before health practitioners had reliable diagnostic instruments, diagnostics and therapy were based on symptoms and signs, of which the cough was one of the most important. A large number of herbal preparations are empirically used in the therapy of cough. The basic mechanism of action of herbal antitussives may be the same as those of orthodox antitussives, most of which originated from herbal predecessors. The mechanisms may include:[11]

- Central cough suppression — narcotic, non-narcotic
- Peripheral cough suppression — anaesthetic, depletion of substance P
- Receptor/sensory nerve suppressive effect
- Bronchodilator/sensory nerve suppressive effect
- Influence of mucociliary clearance
- Antibacterial, antiviral activity.

ACTIVE CONSTITUENTS

Herbal medicines for the respiratory system contain many active constituents and it is not always possible to identify a single active compound responsible for the clinical effect. It is likely that several compounds in combination provide a synergistic effect. The following is a brief discussion of some of the constituents found in the herbs used for disorders of the respiratory system.

Saponins

Saponins irritate vagal nerves by a reflex action leading to increased mucus secretion in the airways. Additionally, the breathing and cough centres are irritated, resulting in more frequent expectoration. However, higher doses of saponins can irritate the mucous membranes of the stomach and intestine leading to emesis, diarrhoea and bleeding. Saponin-containing herbs include *Hedera helix* (ivy leaves), *Primula veris* (primula) and *Thymus vulgaris* (thyme). *H. helix* leaf extract has been shown in double-blind trials to suppress the cough reflex in patients with chronic bronchitis. The antitussive activity of *H. helix* has been shown to be comparable to the cough-suppressive activity of ambroxol. The activity is thought to be based on a combined effect of the saponins, flavonoids and tannins.[11]

Alkaloids

The mechanism of action of some alkaloids, increasing the phlegm secretion by reflexive mechanism, is similar to saponins. The root of the South African plant *Uragoga ipecacuanhae* contains emetin and cephaeline with such expectorant activities. However, chronic administration and overdose may evoke arrhythmias, heart muscle impairment, and convulsions.[11]

Flavonoids

Flavonoids include flavanes (catechin), flavones (luteolin, apigenin, diosmin), isoflavones (genistein, daidazin), flavanols (rutin, quercetin, quercitrin, kaempferol, myricetin, hyperoside) and flavanones (hesperidin, naringenin). In the respiratory system, the flavonoids have been shown to have spasmolytic, anti-inflammatory, antibacterial, antiviral, antitussive and antiallergic activities. Flavonoid-containing herbs include *Hedera helix, Plantago lanceolata, Primula veris* and *Verbascum densiflorum.*[11]

Essential oils

Essential oils cause irritation in many tissues, including the airway epithelium, by direct stimulation of secreting cells which may accelerate the movement of ciliar epithelium. Essential oils also have antibacterial and anti-inflammatory effects. Essential oils used in the respiratory system include aniseed, fennel, thyme, pine and eucalyptus oils.[11]

Mucilage

Mucilaginous herbs reduce inflammation associated with dry irritating cough by providing a protective layer on its surface, which diminishes the irritation of cough receptors (rapidly adapting cough receptors, RARs) on myelinated fibres of vagal nerves as well as irritation of nerve endings of non-myelinated C-fibres. This leads to decreased irritation to cough induced by inflammatory mediators or foreign bodies on impaired mucous membrane. Mucilagenous herbs include *Ulmus fulva* (slippery elm), *Althaea officinalis* (marshmallow) and *Plantago lanceolata* (ribwort).[11]

HERBAL MEDICINE CLASSES

Expectorants

Expectorants facilitate the removal of mucus and other material from the lungs, bronchi and trachea. Expectorants promote drainage of mucus from the lungs by thinning the mucus and also lubricate the irritated respiratory tract. Expectorant comes from the Latin *expectorare,* to expel from the chest, originating from *ex-*, meaning out of and *pectus,* referring to the chest. Sometimes the term *expectorant* is incorrectly extended to any cough medicine. Expectorants are sometimes grouped into relaxing and stimulating expectorants while others are not specifically defined.

The plant expectorants can act in the following ways:[11]

- Secretolytic — secretolytic expectorants may increase mucus secretion by stimulating the serous cells of the submucosal glands. This leads to production of mucus with lower viscosity, making its removal easier by mucociliar clearance. Thin mucus can easily scavenge the bacterial and corpuscular particles, which are then expectorated faster
- Mucolytic — mucolytic expectorants may modulate the physical and chemical properties of mucus. This may lead to the fission of the disulfide bonds in the mucus glycoprotein chains, thereby decreasing its viscosity
- Secretomotoric — stimulating expectorants may work by increasing the cilia motion in the airway ciliar epithelium. This mechanism improves mucociliar clearance.

General expectorants include *Artemisia absinthium* (wormwood), *Plantago lanceolata* (ribwort), *Trifolium pratense* (red clover), *Verbascum thapsus* (mullein), *Viola odorata* (violet leaves), *Viola tricolor* (heartsease) and *Zingiber officinale* (ginger). Relaxing expectorants include *Adhatoda vasica* (adhatoda), *Euphorbia hirta* (euphorbia), *Glycyrrhiza glabra* (liquorice), *Marrubium vulgare* (white horehound), *Foeniculum vulgare* (fennel), *Pimpinella anisum* (anise) and *Thymus vulgaris* (thyme), while more stimulating expectorants include *Angelica archangelica* (archangelica), *Asclepias tuberosa* (pleurisy root), *Grindelia camporum* (grindelia), *Inula helenium* (elecampane), *Polygala tenuifolia* (polygala), *Thuja occidentalis* (thuja) and *Lobelia inflata* (lobelia — scheduled in Australia).

Anticatarrhals

Anticatarrhals counteract, or suppresses, catarrh. These medicinal plants reduce excessive secretions from mucous membranes. They also decrease nasal congestion and mucosal hypersensitivity and oedema. Anticatarrhals are traditionally divided into their site of action, either lower or upper, although there is much overlapping. Ephedra is often used for both, as is polygala. Anticatarrhals for the lower respiratory system include *Bryonia dioica* (bryony), *Polygala tenuifolia* (polygala), *Ephedra sinica* (ephedra) and *Verbascum thapsus* (mullein). Unfortunately ephedra is banned as a herbal medicine in many countries because of the general abuse of ephedrine. Anticatarrhals for the upper respiratory system include *Allium sativum* (garlic), *Berberis* spp. (barberry species), *Chamomilla recutita* (chamomile), *Euphrasia officinalis* (eyebright), *Hydrastis canadensis* (goldenseal), *Polygonum bistorta* (bistort), *Salvia officinalis* (sage), *Sambucus nigra* (elder flowers) *Mentha x piperita* (peppermint), *Nepeta hederacea* (ground ivy) and *Solidago virgaurea* (goldenrod). *Hydrastis canadensis* is particularly indicated where there is copious yellow to green discharge of a chronic nature and for postnasal drip. *Salvia officinalis* has a general drying effect on bodily secretions including the mucous membranes and may be indicated where secretions are particularly copious and watery.

Mucolytics

Mucolytics dissolve or thin mucus, allowing for removal by normal chest physiology. Herbal mucolytics include sulfur-containing herbs such as *Allium sativum* (garlic), *Armoracia rusticana* (horseradish) and *Allium cepa* (onions).

Antitussives

Antitussives relieve cough either through soothing (demulcents) or removing (expectorants) the irritation, or depressing the cough reflex. Antitussive herbs therefore include anticatarrhals, expectorants and demulcents: *Althaea officinalis* (marshmallow), *Bupleurum falcatum* (bupleurum), *Cimicifuga racemosa* (black cohosh), *Dioscorea* spp. (wild yam), *Glycyrrhiza glabra* (liquorice), *Humulus lupulus* (hops), *Inula helenium* (elecampane), *Prunus serotina* (wild cherry), *Schisandra chinensis* (schizandra) and *Thymus vulgaris* (thyme).

Respiratory spasmolytics (antispasmodics)

Respiratory spasmolytics or antispasmodics relax the bronchioles of the lungs. Common spasmolytics include *Adhatoda vasica* (adhatoda), *Inula helenium* (elecampane), *Thymus vulgaris* (thyme), *Grindelia camporum* (grindelia), *Euphorbia hirta* (euphorbia) and *Glycyrrhiza glabra* (liquorice).

Respiratory antiseptics

Respiratory antiseptics include *Thymus vulgaris* (thyme), *Inula helenium* (elecampane) and *Allium sativum* (garlic). Essential oils are generally viewed as more powerful antiseptics compared with herbal extracts. Essential oils and methanol extracts obtained from aerial parts of *Thymus vulgaris* and *Pimpinella anisum* seeds have been evaluated for their single and combined antibacterial activities against nine Gram-positive and Gram-negative pathogenic bacteria: *Staphylococcus aureus, Bacillus cereus, Escherichia coli, Proteus vulgaris, Proteus mirabilis, Salmonella typhi, Salmonella typhimurium, Klebsiella pneumoniae* and *Pseudomonas aeruginosa.* The essential oils and methanol extracts revealed promising antibacterial activities against most pathogens. Maximum activity of *Thymus vulgaris* and *Pimpinella anisum* essential oils and methanol extracts were observed against *Staphylococcus aureus, Bacillus cereus* and *Proteus vulgaris.* Combinations of essential oils and methanol extracts showed an additive action against most tested pathogens, especially *Pseudomonas aeruginosa.*[12] Respiratory antiseptics and medicinal plants which are used to fight infections include *Asclepias tuberosa* (pleurisy root), *Echinacea* spp. (echinacea), *Inula helenium* (elecampane), *Picrorhiza kurroa* (picrorhiza), *Salvia officinalis* (sage), *Solidago virgaurea* (goldenrod) and *Thymus vulgaris* (thyme).

Respiratory demulcents

Demulcent herbs contain mucilage and have a soothing and anti-inflammatory action on the respiratory mucosa. The major respiratory demulcent is *Althaea officinalis* (marshmallow root). Other respiratory demulcents include *Drosera longifolia* (sundew), *Glycyrrhiza glabra* (liquorice), *Plantago lanceolata* (ribwort), *Plantago major* (plantain), *Polygonum bistorta* (bistort), *Trigonella foenum-graecum* (fenugreek), *Verbascum thapsus* (mullein) and *Zingiber officinale* (ginger).

Diaphoretics

Diaphoretics induce therapeutic sweating during an infection which is thought to help activate the immune system. Sweating may also reduce excessive heat and inflammation. Diaphoretics include *Achillea millefolium* (yarrow), *Asclepias tuberosa* (pleurisy root), *Bryonia dioica* (bryony), *Capsicum* spp. (cayenne, chilli), *Eupatorium perfoliatum* (boneset), *Hyssopus officinalis* (hyssop), *Inula helenium* (elecampane), *Melissa officinalis* (lemon balm), *Mentha x piperita* (peppermint), *Nepeta cataria* (catmint), *Sambucus nigra* (elder flowers), *Tilia* spp. (lime tree), *Zanthoxylum clava-herculis* (prickly ash) and *Zingiber officinale* (ginger).

Mucous membrane trophorestoratives

Hydrastis canadensis (goldenseal) is known traditionally as a mucous membrane tonic or trophorestorative; that is, it is used to restore the healthy function of mucous membranes.

Antiallergic herbs

The main antiallergic herbs for the respiratory system are *Albizia lebbeck* (albizia), *Scutellaria baicalensis* (baikal skullcap) and *Tylophora indica* (asthma weed). Other antiallergic plant medicines include *Angelica sinensis* (dong quai), *Chamomilla recutita* (chamomile), *Paeonia lactiflora* (peony), *Picrorhiza kurroa* (picrorhiza), *Tanacetum parthenium* (feverfew) and *Curcuma longa* (turmeric).

INVESTIGATIONS

PATHOLOGY TESTS

Pathology tests are summarised in Table 14.1.

LUNG FUNCTION TESTS

Lung function tests are summarised in Table 14.2.

IMAGING STUDIES

Imaging studies are summarised in Table 14.3.

OTHER TESTS

Some of the other tests used are listed in Table 14.4.

Other investigations

Cough

Cough results from irritation of cough receptors located in the pharynx, larynx and bronchi, and this irritation could be due to infection, inflammation, tumour or foreign body. The duration, productiveness and characteristics of cough should be ascertained in order to work out its likely cause.

- Unproductive cough may be observed in certain viral respiratory infections and in interstitial (atypical) pneumonia caused by *Mycoplasma* or viruses (discussed later). Largely unproductive cough may be the only symptom in asthma, particularly in children. Cough in children occurring regularly after exercise or at night, is virtually diagnostic of asthma. Curiously, unproductive cough is frequently reported by patients taking ACE inhibitors for hypertension or heart failure. Tumours, especially lung carcinoma, can in later stages present with persistent cough
- Productive cough may occur in certain viral lower respiratory tract infections and especially infections of bacterial origin, such as acute bronchitis, bronchopneumonia, lobar pneumonia, lung abscess or bronchiectasis (a chronic bacterial infection leading to deformation and dilation of the bronchioles with accumulation of pus; frequently seen in association with the inherited condition cystic fibrosis). Productive cough is a main feature of chronic bronchitis (discussed later)
- Usually cough is not associated with pain, but painful cough may be seen in tracheitis (stretching of inflamed trachea during coughing) or pneumonia with pleurisy, as well as lung carcinoma with pleural involvement.

Coughs are often worse at night, possibly provoked by a change in temperature or humidity in the bedroom.

SPUTUM

Sputum (phlegm) is a mixture of excessive bronchial secretion and inflammatory exudate, and may be caused by inflammation or infection. The consistency and colour of the sputum can vary depending on the cause. *Mucoid* sputum may be caused by chronic irritation (e.g. dust,

TABLE 14.1 Pathology testing

Assessment	Justification	Reference ranges	
Blood gases	Arterial blood sample to evaluate blood pH, oxygen and carbon dioxide	pO_2: 11.0–13.5 kpa (80–100 mmHg) (varies with age) pCO_2: 4.6–6.0 kpa (35–45 mmHg) pH: 7.36–7.44 (36–44 nmol/L) Base excess: (–3) to (+3) mmol/L Alveolar-arterial pO_2 difference: <3.3 kPa (<25 mmHg) if $FiO_2 = 0.21$ (that is, room air)	
Full blood count	To assess for anaemia	Haemoglobin (Hb)	Men: 130–180 g/L Women: 115–165 g/L
		Red cell count (RCC)	Men: 4–5–6.5 × 10^{12}/L Women: 3.8–5–5.8 × 10^{12}/L
		Packed cell volume (PCV)	Men: 0.40–0.54 Women: 0.37–0.47
		Mean cell volume (MCV)	80–100 fL
		Mean cell haemoglobin (MCH)	27–32 pg
		Mean cell haemoglobin concentration (MCHC)	300–350 g/L
		Reticulocyte count	10–100 × 10^9/L
Iron studies	To assess for iron deficiency anaemia	Transferrin	1.7–3.0 g/L
		Total iron binding capacity (TIBC)	45–80 µmol/L
		Transferrin saturation	0.15–0.45 (15–45%)
		Serum iron	Iron: 10–30 µmol/L
		Ferritin (serum)	Adult female: 15–200 micrograms/L; following the menopause, levels progressively approach those for adult males Adult male: 30–300 micrograms/L
		Soluble transferrin receptor	Varies with method, age, gender and pregnancy
Cystic fibrosis (CF) testing	CF genetic mutations (ideal investigation) Other: sweat chloride, immunoreactive trypsin (IRT), stool trypsin	Positive genetic mutation confirms status The normal sweat chloride values are 10–35 milliequivalents per litre Immunoreactive trypsin (IRT) (trypsinogen test): 140–400 ng/L Stool trypsin confirms if positive	
Alpha-1 antitrypsin (AAT)	To determine if patient has AAT deficiency	100–300 mg/mL	
Sputum culture	To diagnose infective organism	Gram stain for bacteria and fungi; DFA for viruses (e.g. respiratory syncytial virus (RSV), influenza virus), *Legionella* spp., *Pneumocystis jiroveci*; acid fast stains for mycobacteria Aerobic culture on non-selective media; selective media if appropriate (e.g. *Legionella* spp.) Mycobacterial culture; prolonged culture for fungus; virus detection, culture Nucleic acid detection after amplification may be used for detection of *Legionella* spp., *Pneumocystis jiroveci*, mycobacteria, mycoplasma, *Chlamydia trachomatis* in bronchial washes or lavage specimens	
AFB smear and culture	To diagnose tuberculosis and non-tuberculosis mycobacteria (NTM)	Positive/negative	
Blood cultures	To diagnose bacteria, yeast, viral infections	Positive/negative	
Influenza testing	To diagnose influenza	Influenza A viral RNA detection Influenza B viral RNA detection	
Lung biopsy	To evaluate lung tissue for damage and for cancer	Postive/negative	

Continued

TABLE 14.1 Pathology testing—cont'd

Assessment	Justification	Reference ranges	
Sputum cytology	To evaluate lung cells for abnormal changes and for cancer	*Normal*: normal lung cells are present in the sputum sample *Abnormal*: abnormal cells are present in the sputum sample	
Fetal lung maturity (FLM)	Used to evaluate the lung maturity of a fetus and may include tests for lecithin/sphingomyelin (L/S) ratio, phosphatidylglycerol (PG), foam stability index (FSI) or lamellar body counts (LBC). May be used to determine age of gestation before caesarean delivery or when a pregnant woman is having symptoms of premature labour	TDx-FLM assay *Interpretation* Probable immaturity Transitional immaturity Transitional maturity Probable maturity	 *Ranges (mg surfactant/g albumin)* <24 24–39 40–54 >55
Drug screen	To detect presence of drug in overdose that may lead to decreased respiration or acute respiratory distress	Various	

Source: Huether SE, McCance K. Understanding pathophysiology. 4th edn. St Louis: Mosby; 2010.

TABLE 14.2 Lung function tests (pulmonary function tests, PFTs)

Assessment	Description	Measurements
Spirometry	Measures the amount and rate of air exhalation as a patient blows out through a tube. It is performed to evaluate narrowed or obstructed airways	**Lung function test** Forced vital capacity (FVC) Forced expiratory volume (FEV_1*) FEV_1 divided by FVC Forced expiratory flow 25–75% Peak expiratory flow (PEF) Maximum voluntary ventilation (MVV) Slow vital capacity (SVC) Total lung capacity (TLC) (VT) Functional residual capacity (FRC) Residual volume (RV) Expiratory reserve volume (ERV) RV divided by TLC ratio
Air flow with a peak flow meter	Measures the rate of exhalation. Patients with asthma can use it at home to help monitor their condition	Peak flow readings are often classified into three zones of measurement: green, yellow or red A peak flow reading in the green zone signifies the asthma is under good control A peak flow reading in the yellow zone is cautionary. This indicates that the respiratory airways of the body are narrowing A peak flow reading in the red zone indicates severe respiratory narrowing; this is dangerous and typically the patient will need to go to hospital or doctor immediately
Lung volume	The quantity of air a person takes into their lungs and how much is left in the lungs after exhalation. Helps evaluate the elasticity of the lungs, the movement of the rib cage, and the strength of the muscles associated with respiration	As above
Diffusing capacity measurement	Assesses the transfer of oxygen from the lung air sacs to the bloodstream by evaluating how much carbon monoxide is absorbed when a small quantity is inhaled (not enough to harm)	As above

*FEV_1 = forced expiratory volume in 1 second.

smoke), viral infections and bronchial asthma, and is usually clear, whitish or grey (in heavy smokers it can be brown to blackish). *Purulent* sputum is yellowish or greenish and is an indication of bacterial involvement. Mucopurulent sputum has components of both. *Rusty* sputum is a characteristic finding in bacterial lobar pneumonia and its colour is derived from altered blood (discussed later). *Pink frothy sputum* (fluid mixed with air and a small amount of blood) is found in severe pulmonary oedema, for example caused by left-sided heart failure.

Blood-stained sputum is called *haemoptysis*, and all grades of severity may occur, from slight blood streaking to massive haemorrhage. It should not be confused with haematemesis, which is the vomiting of blood from the GI tract. Haemoptysis always demands an aetiological explanation. Important causes include: bronchial/lung tumours, pulmonary infarction (due to pulmonary embolism), bronchiectasis, pulmonary tuberculosis, lobar pneumonia and sometimes acute and chronic bronchitis.

If appropriate inspect the sample of patient sputum after asking them to expectorate. A small amount of sputum is normal in every individual, light yellow or clear in colour and with no odour. Table 14.5 describes sputum appearance in different respiratory conditions.

CHEST PAIN

The lungs (except in the trachea and large bronchi) and the visceral pleura have no pain fibres, whereas the parietal pleura, chest wall and mediastinal structures are sensitive to pain. The common types and causes of pain are:

- Pleuritic pain is caused by two rough pleural surfaces rubbing together such as in pleural inflammation (pleurisy) or pulmonary infarction with plural involvement. It is described as unilateral, sharp, stabbing and worse on deep inspiration, coughing or sneezing. The pain may interfere with breathing ('I have to catch my breath')
- Pain due to chest wall involvement is usually caused by localised muscle strain (pulled muscle as in sport activities or even violent coughing) or by trauma (chest blow, especially if associated with rib fractures), and it is difficult to distinguish from pure pleuritic pain on clinical grounds alone. However, these pains are often worse on palpation, percussion, twisting/turning, bending or rolling over in bed (an uncommon feature of other diseases). Bornholm disease (epidemic pleurodynia) is thought to be a viral infection (coxsackie viruses have been implicated) of the intercostal muscles and produces very severe pain in the epigastrium or lower anterior chest. It is more

TABLE 14.3 Imaging studies

Assessment	Justification
Chest x-ray	Used to look at lung structure and chest cavity
Computed tomography (CT) scan	Used for more detailed evaluation of lung structure
Magnetic resonance imaging (MRI)	Used to look at detailed pictures of organs and vessels in the chest
Ultrasound	Used to detect fluid between the pleural membranes
Nuclear lung scanning	Used to help detect pulmonary embolism and, rarely, to evaluate the effectiveness of lung cancer treatment
Positron emission tomography (PET) scan	Used to help diagnose lung cancer

TABLE 14.5 Sputum colours

Sputum colour	Condition
Mucoid (clear whitish-grey)	Viral respiratory infections, asthma (may be thick and gel-like), dust inhalation
Yellow or green	Bacterial infection
Rusty or blood-tinged (haemoptysis)	Pneumococcal pneumonia, pulmonary infarction, tuberculosis, cancer, sometimes chronic bronchitis
Blackish	Heavy smokers, coal miners
Pink and frothy	Pulmonary oedema

TABLE 14.4 Other relevant assessments

Assessment	Justification	Reference ranges	
Electrocardiogram (ECG)	To review heart rhythm, to determine if heart disease may be affecting breathing	Multiple variations discussed thoroughly in Chapter 20	
Sleep studies	Usually performed at special sleep centres to help determine whether a person is breathing normally during sleep	Apnoea hypopnoea index (AHI) sometimes also called the respiratory distress index (RDI)	
		AHI	RATING
		<5	Normal
		5–15	Mild
		15–30	Moderate
		>30	Severe

common in children and usually associated with fever, headache, sore throat and malaise. No treatment is needed and the disease subsides spontaneously within a few days, but may be a diagnostic challenge. Severe constant pain not related to breathing usually indicates malignant disease involving the chest wall. Costochondritis is an inflammation of the rib cartilage (usually more than one) that presents with sharp chest pain which worsens on pressure and movement. The cause is unknown but the condition may follow a blow to the chest, unusual physical activity or upper respiratory infection. It is a benign condition that results in complete recovery in a couple of days
- Mediastinal pain is deep, dull and poorly localised and can result from cancer of the lung, presumably from involvement and pressure on mediastinal structures such as lymph nodes, trachea and oesophagus.

ALTERATIONS IN BREATHING

Normal breathing (eupnoea) is rhythmic and effortless. It produces a soft rustling sound as air rushes into the lungs, with little noise produced on expiration. These are called vesicular breath sounds. These sounds tend to be louder in children than adults. When there is an airway obstruction, such as in asthma, chronic bronchitis and emphysema, the intensity of vesicular sounds diminishes.[13] The main alterations of breathing patterns include the following.

Hyperpnoea

Hyperpnoea is increased volume of breathing, but appropriate to circumstances, for example exercise, metabolic acidosis (e.g. in diabetes).

Hyperventilation

Hyperventilation is volume disproportionate to metabolic carbon dioxide production, and with associated sensations, for example tingling in fingers and lips, dizziness, blurring of vision. It is often caused by severe anxiety/panic attacks.

Tachypnoea

Tachypnoea is increased rate of shallow breathing found in restrictive lung disorders with decreased lung compliance (e.g. pulmonary fibrosis, pulmonary oedema) or in conditions associated with pleuritic pain (e.g. lobar pneumonia).

Dyspnoea

Dyspnoea (breathlessness) is breathing accompanied by conscious effort (laboured breathing); it is a subjective sensation of uncomfortable breathing frequently described by patients as air hunger or shortness of breath.

Dyspnoea is a complex phenomenon with different mechanisms:

- Increased airflow resistance (asthma, chronic bronchitis, emphysema)
- Increased lung stiffness (pulmonary fibrosis, pulmonary congestion/oedema, pneumonia)
- Lung reflexes going through the respiratory centre (pulmonary oedema, pulmonary embolism)
- Central mechanisms (anxiety).

Adventitious (added) sounds are sounds superimposed on the breath sounds. These include:

Wheeze

Wheeze is a high-pitched musical whistling sound, best heard during expiration, and sometimes on inspiration, and have a hissing quality. It is a characteristic symptom in diseases causing bronchoconstriction (especially bronchial asthma and chronic obstructive bronchitis). Low-pitched wheezes may have a snoring quality and may originate in larger airways, while high-pitched ones come from smaller airways and have a whistly quality.[13] Wheeze should be distinguished from stridor.

Stridor

A loud, harsh and continuous sound produced by partial obstruction of the upper airways (larynx and trachea) due to inflammation and oedema (e.g. in acute epiglottitis in children caused by *H. influenzae* or inhaled foreign body, or oedema of the glottis/larynx in acute anaphylactic reaction to bee sting or injected drugs). It is mainly heard on inspiration and, at times, during expiration.[13]

Crackles

Moist, inspiratory discontinuous bubbling sounds caused by opening of closed airways filled with secretion. Fine crackles are heard during late inspiratory patterns and occur in moderate pulmonary oedema, pneumonia or lung fibrosis. Coarse crackles are early inspiratory and can be heard in bronchitis and resolving pneumonia. Depending on the condition, wheezes and crackles can be heard concurrently.[13]

Pleural rub

Pleural rub is produced by inflamed surfaces of the pleura rubbing together. This sound resembles that of bending new leather. This occurs during the end of inspiration and the beginning of expiration. The sounds are also associated with pleural pain.[13]

CYANOSIS

Cyanosis is bluish discolouration of the skin or mucous membranes caused by an excess of reduced haemoglobin (without oxygen) in the blood. Certain conditions can be responsible for cyanosis and it is useful to distinguish between peripheral and central cyanosis.

Peripheral cyanosis

Peripheral cyanosis is associated with stasis of blood (congestion) in peripheral tissues when more oxygen is extracted from blood, leading to accumulation of deoxygenated haemoglobin. The most common causes are right ventricular failure and venous thrombosis/insufficiency when cyanosis is most visible on the legs (e.g. around the ankles). This is a localised phenomenon and, not surprisingly, oedema (swelling) is usually noted due to increased capillary hydrostatic pressure.

TABLE 14.6 Changes in lung sounds with pulmonary disease

Lung disease	Breath sounds	Adventitious lung sounds
Pneumonia	Bronchial or absent	Inspiratory crackles
Atelectasis (patent bronchus)	Harsh vesicular/ bronchial	Late inspiratory crackles
Atelectasis (obstructed bronchus)	Absent or diminished vesicular	None
Pneumothorax	Absent or barely heard vesicular	None
Emphysema	Diminished vesicular	Wheezes and crackles
Chronic bronchitis	Vesicular	Crackles and wheezes
Pulmonary fibrosis	Harsh vesicular	Inspiratory crackles
Pulmonary oedema	Diminished vesicular	Inspiratory crackles
Pleural effusion	Diminished vesicular or even absent	None, possible friction rub depending on amount of fluid
Asthma	Diminished vesicular	Wheezes

Central cyanosis

Central cyanosis results from generalised arterial hypoxaemia (reduced saturation of blood with oxygen) and affects all skin but it is usually more readily seen on mucous membranes (lips, mouth, tongue) as they are thinner than the skin. Central cyanosis indicates impaired gas exchange and oxygenation of blood in the lungs, and may be caused by certain lung disorders (e.g. chronic obstructive pulmonary disease [COPD], status asthmaticus, lobar pneumonia) or left ventricular failure with congestion and oedema in the lungs. In rare instances central cyanosis may be caused by abnormal shunting and mixing of blood in the heart (e.g. inborn hole in the heart such as ventricular septal defect). Serious central cyanosis may be seen in intoxication with drugs that can cause depression of the respiratory centre in the brain (e.g. heroin overdose).

Changes in lung sounds with pulmonary disease are summarised in Table 14.6 and useful nutritional supplements are described in Table 14.7.

Allopathic treatment

The severity of symptoms of respiratory disease depends very much on the disease. Common symptoms include dyspnoea, which usually occurs with exercise and can interfere with daily activities. In severe cases: shortness of breath can occur while resting, cough with or without the

TABLE 14.7 Nutritional medicine

Requirement	Justification	Dose
Vitamin A	Vitamin A is a fat-soluble nutrient that exerts an anti-inflammatory action in the lungs. Vitamin A is essential for preserving the integrity of the mucous membranes and the lung epithelium in particular, maintenance of the lung tissue and lung cell repair. Vitamin A appears to protect against tissue pathologies in the upper and lower respiratory tract; however, more studies are required to determine the mechanism by which this occurs	15 000–50 000 IU/d
Vitamin C	Free radical scavenger, which may play a role in the modulation of airway inflammation. Prevents histamine secretion and increases histamine detoxification. Immune boosting action, essential for fighting infection, etc. associated with respiratory diseases. High doses are found in the fluid lining the respiratory tract	500 mg/d–10 000 mg/d (orally, in divided doses)
Vitamin D_3	Vitamin D inhibits pulmonary inflammatory responses while enhancing defence mechanisms against respiratory pathogens. Deficiency increases the risk of upper respiratory tract infections and tuberculosis and decreases the FEV_1 in asthma and wheezing diseases	600–4000 IU/d**General recommendation is between 1000 and 4000 IU/day; however, in strong deficiency states (proven by blood tests), increasing the dose is recommended
Vitamin E	Lipid-soluble antioxidant that reacts with peroxyl radicals to terminate membrane lipid peroxidation. Found in the fluid that lines the respiratory tract. Dietary vitamin E has been shown to be associated with lower lung cancer risk	100–800 IU/d10 mg/d to decrease lung cancer risk (from diet)
Magnesium	Bronchodilator of airway smooth muscle inhibits cholinergic neuromuscular transmission and stabilises mast cells and T-lymphocytes as well as being anti-inflammatory	500 mg/d

Continued

TABLE 14.7 Nutritional medicine—cont'd

Requirement	Justification	Dose
Zinc	Zinc is essential for multiple cellular functions including immunity where it functions as an intracellular signal molecule for immune cells. In the respiratory system, zinc is required for the maintenance of healthy mucous membranes. Beneficial therapeutic response of zinc supplementation has been observed in respiratory conditions such as tuberculosis, pneumonia and acute lower respiratory tract infection	30–60 mg/d
Quercetin	Flavonoid with antioxidant and anti-inflammatory activity. Quercetin forms a strong matrix by reinforcing collagen. Quercetin may assist in reducing inflammation and maintaining the health of nasal mucosa by effecting mast cell proliferation and secretory granule development. It blocks substances involved in allergies by preventing the release of histamine from the basophils and mast cells. In a Japanese study of mast cells taken from the nasal mucosa of individuals with perennial rhinitis, quercetin significantly inhibited antigen-stimulated histamine release between 46% and 96%	600–1500 mg/d
Bromelain	Bromelain has been found to be an effective mucolytic agent in respiratory tract diseases such as sinusitis, asthma and COPD due to its anti-inflammatory, immune-modulating and antiasthma actions. (However, note that bromelain allergy can itself cause respiratory symptoms such as bronchospasm, difficulty breathing, etc.)	300–1600 mg/d
Omega-3 fatty acids (DHA/EPA)	Numerous applications for the management of respiratory diseases including modulators of chronic inflammation, correcting altered fatty acid metabolism in cystic fibrosis and possible role in modulation of infectious processes and impaired pulmonary blood flow	EPA: 300–900 mg DHA: 200–400 mg Total of 3–6 g of fatty acids
Selenium	Selenium influences the way in which the body fights infection by enhancing the activity of certain white blood cells that protect the body against viruses and bacteria. Through its antioxidant action selenium protects against free radicals that damage lung tissue and enzymes	100–400 micrograms/day
Probiotics	Probiotics exert a beneficial effect in the prevention and treatment of allergic respiratory conditions such as allergic rhinitis through modification of the systemic and local immune system via gut ecosystem	5–45 billion CFU
Coenzyme Q10	As an antioxidant and to reduce histamine release	90–500 mg/d
R-alpha lipoic acid	Anti-inflammatory, antioxidant, immune stimulating — especially beneficial if environmental toxins are problematic. Best to be prescribed with vitamin E and other nutrients if antioxidant recycling is the focus	100–600 mg/d
N-acetylcysteine (NAC)	Mucolytic, glutathione precursor and specifically improves lung function and symptom control in conditions such as asthma, COPD and acute bronchitis. It is typically prescribed in cases of excessive mucus and catarrh	400–1800 mg/d

Sources: Baybutt R, Agostino M. Vitamin A and emphysema. Vitamins and Hormones 2007;75:385–401; Bromelain Natural Standard Research Collaboration. Natural Standard Monographs. Available from: www.naturalstandard.com; Hughes DA, Norton R. Vitamin D and respiratory health. Clin Exper Immunol 2009;158(1):20–5; Knapp HR. Omega-3 fatty acids in respiratory diseases: a review. J Am Coll Nutr 1995 Feb;14(1):18–23; Kupcayk M, Kuna P. Mucolytics in acute and chronic respiratory tract disorders. II. Uses for treatment and antioxidant properties. Pol Merkuriusz Lek 2002;1269:248–52; Oseiki H, Eddey S. The power of clinical nutrition in cardiovascular and respiratory conditions. Australia: Bioconcepts Publishing; 2009; Prasad AS. Zinc role in immunity, oxidative stress and chronic inflammation. Curr Opin Clin Nutr Metab Care 2009 Nov;12(6):646–52; Roswall N, Olsen A, Christensen J et al. Source-specific effects of micronutrients in lung cancer prevention. Lung Cancer 2010 Mar;67(3):275–81.

production of sputum, haemoptysis, chest pain, noisy breathing, either wheeze or stridor; somnolence; loss of appetite; weight loss and cyanosis. Investigation tests used include chest x-ray, pulmonary function test, computed tomography scan, culture of microorganisms from secretions such as sputum, bronchoscopy, and biopsy of the lung or pleura; ventilation-perfusion scan and ultrasound scanning can be useful to detect fluid such as pleural effusion. Treatment of respiratory disease depends on the particular disease, the severity of disease and the patient. Lifestyle factors such as regular exercise and healthy nutrition are important in preventing and treating respiratory disease. Vaccination can prevent some respiratory diseases. Commonly used medications include corticosteroids, bronchodilators, antibiotics, anticoagulants, cancer chemotherapy and immune suppressants. In addition patients may be treated by physiotherapy, oxygen, mechanical ventilation, liquid ventilation, surfactant replacement therapy, radiotherapy and surgery.

A note about research and the placebo

Placebo treatment has been reported to improve subjective and objective measures of disease in up to 30–40% of patients with a wide range of clinical conditions. A review of eight clinical trials on the effects of antitussive medicines on cough associated with acute upper respiratory tract infection shows that 85% of the reduction in cough was related to treatment with a placebo, and only 15% attributable to the active ingredient. Treatment with a cough medicine can be viewed as consisting of three components: pharmacological, physiological (demulcent) and placebo. The placebo effect is related to belief in the effectiveness of the treatment and this idea must in some way influence the central control of cough. Studies on the placebo effect of analgesics indicate that the placebo effect may be mediated by endogenous opioid neurotransmitters and this may explain the analgesic potency of opioid medicines such as morphine. With active pharmacological ingredients contributing only 15% to the effects of cough treatment it seems reasonable to conduct more research on the other components of treatment such as placebo.[14]

Potential interactions between drugs and herbs commonly used to treat the respiratory system are listed in in the drug interactions table at the back of the book.

Special topic: Coughs and herbal medicines

The most common cause of cough is an acute respiratory infection, whether a URTI or acute bronchitis. Persistent coughing with a URTI is usually due to the development of sinusitis with a postnasal drip. Cough is also the cardinal symptom of bronchitis. Other causes of a non-productive cough include inhaled irritants, inhaled foreign body, bronchial neoplasm, pleurisy, interstitial lung disorders, tuberculosis, whooping cough, gastro-oesophageal reflux disorder (GORD) and hiatus hernia. Postnasal drip is the commonest cause of a persistent or chronic cough, especially causing nocturnal cough due to secretions (mainly from chronic sinusitis) tracking down the larynx and trachea during sleep. Cough is also a feature of smokers, who often have a morning cough with little sputum. Causes of productive cough include chronic bronchitis, bronchiectasis, pneumonia, asthma, bronchial carcinoma, lung abscess and tuberculosis. Bronchial carcinoma must not be overlooked. A worsening cough is the commonest presenting problem. Certain pharmaceutical drugs may also cause coughing. Blood-stained sputum (haemoptysis), which varies from small flecks of blood to massive bleeding, requires thorough investigation. Often the diagnosis can be made by chest x-ray. The commonest causes are URTI and acute bronchitis followed by chronic bronchitis. Other causes include bronchiectasis, pneumonia, tuberculosis, neoplastic disease, pulmonary infarction, foreign body, cardiac disorders and anticoagulant therapy.[15]

HERBAL COUGH MEDICINES

Most popular cough medicines throughout the world are based on herbal extracts with the addition of flavourings including honey and syrup. The following herbs are some of the most popular used in herbal cough mixtures in Western herbal medicine.

Althaea officinalis (marshmallow)

Marshmallow is used to soothe sore throats, laryngitis, tonsillitis and cough. The marshmallow root contains mucilage, starch, pectin, flavonoids and minerals. The antitussive activity of *A. officinalis* has been found to be comparable to the activity of peripherally active antitussive dropropizine.[16]

Foeniculum vulgare (fennel)

Fennel is traditionally used in the treatment of digestive complications (dyspepsia, flatulence), and for stimulation of lactation. Fennel seed contains 2–6% essential oil with anethole as the main compound (50–70%). Fennel seeds also contain creosol and α-pinene, which probably have secretomotoric activity, increase the motility of cilia in the ciliar epithelium in the airways, thereby promoting the expulsion of phlegm and expectoration.[16]

Inula helenium (elecampane)

Elecampane contains sesquiterpene lactones (bitter substances) and eudesmanolides (alantolactone, isoalantolactone and others). The mixture of alantolactones is also known as helenin or elecampane camphor. Elecampane root contains about 50% of complex carbohydrates known as fructooligosaccharides (FOS), including 20–44% of inulin. Other components include triterpenes, sterols, inulin and other saccharides. The root extract is used to dilute viscose phlegm in conditions with impaired expectoration.[16]

Plantago lanceolata (ribwort)

Ribwort contains the glycosides, aucubin and catalpol, and the flavonoids apigenin and luteolin, mucilage, tannins, pectins and saponins. Ribwort is mainly used to stimulate expectoration. It also has a protective effect on the mucous membranes and has anti-inflammatory activities. For accentuation of expectorant effect, ribwort may be combined with fennel, primula and thyme.[16]

Primula veris (cowslip)

Primula is traditionally used for bronchitis and cough. It contains mainly saponins and flavonoids. Primula is expectorant and secretolytic and is indicated in dry airway inflammation, laryngitis and bronchitis.[16]

Thymus vulgaris (thyme)

The therapeutic effect of thyme is due to an essential oil containing thymol, thymol methylether, p-cymol, carvacrol, α-pinene, linalol, borneol and cineol. In addition, thyme contains tannins, organic acids, saponins and flavonoid glycosides. Thyme is antibacterial, expectorant and bronchodilating and is recommended for inflammation with insufficient excretion of secretions and in spastic bronchitis.[16]

Verbascum thapsus (mullein)

Mullein contains mainly mucilage, iridoids (aucubins, catalpols), saponins and the flavonoids apigenin, luteolin, kaempferol and rutin. Mullein is an expectorant used for dry inflammation of the respiratory tract with a non-productive cough. The mucilage provides a protective layer on the mucous membranes leading to a decreased irritation of the cough receptors.[16]

ASTHMA

Epidemiology

There is a global health concern regarding the rising incidence and prevalence of asthma and associated allergic disorders.[17] The prevalence of asthma in Australia is 14% in children and 6–7% in adults. For reported asthma, the sexes are almost equally affected. Asthma is the fourth commonest condition by prevalence and twentieth by incidence, making it the ninth leading cause of disease burden. The prevalence of current asthma is about 10% in Australian adults (16 years and over), and about 11% in children. Asthma frequently presents in childhood, but can occur for the first time at any age. While there is concern about the over-diagnosis of asthma in children, there is evidence of under-diagnosis of asthma in older people. More boys than girls have asthma. However, after teenage years, asthma is more common in women than in men. Asthma is more common among Indigenous Australians, particularly adults, than among other Australians.

There is a strong link between asthma and allergy: more than 80% of people with asthma have evidence of allergic sensitisation. Around 40% of children who have asthma live with smokers and are likely to be exposed to passive smoke. There is little seasonal variability in asthma experienced as a recent illness. When age and sex standardised rates for adults were compared, the prevalence of respiratory conditions overall was higher in smokers (37%) and in ex-smokers (41%) than in those who had never smoked (36%). These differences were particularly apparent in the case of bronchitis and/or emphysema, where the standardised rate for smokers (9%) was nearly twice that of ex-smokers (5%) and three times that of those who had never smoked (3%). Rates for asthma were also higher among smokers (11%) and ex-smokers (11%) than among those who had never smoked (9%). The prevalence of asthma in young children living in households with one or more smokers was higher than in non-smoking households. Of those aged 0–4 years, 13% in households with one or more smokers had asthma compared with 9% in households where there were no smokers. Of those aged 5–9 years, the rate of asthma was 22% in smoking households and 18% in non-smoking households. In contrast, for children aged 10–14, asthma was less prevalent in those living in smoking households (17%) than those in non-smoking households (20%). Differences in asthma between smoking and non-smoking households were proportionally greater for boys than for girls in each age group under 15 years.[18]

By far the most common LRT allergic condition is asthma. According to medical research the incidence of the condition has risen dramatically over the last 25 years. Consequently the numbers of individuals with the condition seeking help from a naturopath is increasing.

Classification

Asthma severity is defined by the intensity of treatment required to achieve good asthma control. Mild asthma is asthma that can be well controlled with short-acting β_2-agonists alone or with low-dose inhaled corticosteroids. Severe asthma is asthma that requires high-intensity treatment (high-dose inhaled corticosteroids plus long-acting β_2-agonist, with or without other therapy) to maintain good control, or where good control is not achieved despite high-intensity treatment. The severity and treatment should be reviewed at least annually. Terminology is confusing because the term 'severity' may also be applied to the severity of an attack or acute exacerbation. Asthma may be severe due to persistent problems interfering with management despite appropriate intervention (e.g. smoking, poor adherence), persistent comorbidities (e.g. sinusitis, psychosocial problems) or treatment-resistant asthma.[19]

Aetiology

The risk factors for persistent wheezing and predisposition to asthma include maternal history of asthma, family history of asthma or atopy, eczema, hay fever, increased IgE levels, maternal smoking or any exposure to smoke, pets, carpeting, severe and persistent symptoms at a young age, those born prematurely and frequent symptoms in the first year of life. Antibiotic use in the first year of life is associated with the development of atopy and asthma later in life. It therefore has been postulated that antibiotics have an immunomodulating action on the Th1 response mediated through changes in bowel flora that could program the development of asthma. A 2001 placebo-controlled, clinical trial published in *The Lancet* addressed this immunomodulating effect.[20] *Lactobacillus rhamnosus* or placebo was given prenatally to mothers (who had at least one first-degree relative with atopic eczema, allergic rhinitis or asthma) and to their babies during infancy for 6 months. The frequency of atopic eczema in the intervention group was half that of the control group. The number of children who developed asthma (six) was too low, however, to draw statistically significant conclusions from this study. Nutritional variables, such as decreased fresh fruit and vegetable intake and decreased omega-3 or omega-6 ratios, may play a role in the increase in atopic disorders including asthma worldwide.[21] Several studies have shown that oxidative stress is a consequence of the inflammatory process in asthma and is associated with increased bronchial hyperactivity.[22]

Overview

Asthma is a chronic inflammatory disorder of the airways characterised by variable airway obstruction and airway hyperresponsiveness in which the prominent clinical manifestations include wheezing and shortness of breath. Among children, it is the most common chronic disease and a leading cause of disability.[22]

In a person with asthma, the airways narrow in response to stimuli that do not affect the airways in normal lungs. The narrowing can be triggered by many stimuli. In an asthma attack, the smooth muscles of the bronchi go into spasm, and the tissues lining the airways swell from inflammation and secrete mucus into the airways. These actions narrow the diameter of the airways (a condition called bronchoconstriction); the narrowing requires the person to exert more effort to move air in and out.

Pathogenesis

The pathogenesis of asthma includes activated lymphocytes, eosinophilic airway inflammation, mucus hyperproduction and airway hyperresponsiveness leading to airflow obstruction. This is associated with contraction of the airway smooth muscle and swelling of the airway wall due to smooth muscle hypertrophy and hyperplasia, inflammatory cell infiltration, oedema, goblet cell and mucous gland hyperplasia, mucus hypersecretion, protein deposition including collagen, and epithelial desquamation.

Certain cells in the airway, particularly the mast cells, are thought to be responsible for initiating the airway narrowing. Mast cells throughout the bronchi release substances such as histamine and leukotrienes that cause smooth muscle to contract, mucus secretion to increase, and certain white blood cells to migrate to the area. Mast cells can be triggered to release these substances in response to something they recognise as foreign (an allergen), such as pollen, house dust mites or animal dander. However, asthma is also common and severe in many people without defined allergies. When someone with asthma exercises or breathes cold air, a similar reaction occurs. Stress and anxiety also can trigger mast cells to release histamine and leukotrienes. Eosinophils, another type of cell found in the airways of people with asthma, release additional substances including leukotrienes and other materials, contributing to airway narrowing.[23]

COMMON TRIGGERS

- House dust mites
- Feathers
- Cockroaches (and their excrement)
- Animal dander
- Exercise
- Pollens
- Smoke
- Cold air
- Sulfites (food preservatives and naturally occurring).

Anything that can be done to reduce exposure to these triggers can reduce the number or severity of the attacks.

Signs and symptoms

The clinical features of asthma are wheeze, intermittent shortness of breath, chest tightness and dry cough.

Asthma attacks vary in frequency and severity. Some people with asthma are symptom free most of the time, with an occasional, brief, mild episode of shortness of breath. Others cough and wheeze most of the time and have severe attacks after viral infections, exercise or exposure to allergens or irritants. Crying or hearty laughing may also bring on symptoms.

Asthma attack

- Initial symptoms include shortness of breath, coughing or chest tightness; also itching of the chest or neck, especially in children
- Sudden wheezing which is particularly noticeable when the person breathes out
- It may come on slowly with gradually worsening symptoms
- It may last minutes or hours or days
- A dry cough at night or while exercising may be the only symptom
- During the acute, anxiety and sweating are common.

Severe attack

- Limited speech without stopping for breath
- Wheezing often diminishes due to reduced airflow
- Confusion, lethargy and cyanosis may develop and are signs that emergency intervention is required
- Usually a person recovers completely, even from a severe asthma attack.

Types of asthma

Early-onset (atopic) asthma (extrinsic asthma)

Early-onset asthma is the most common type of asthma. It presents as a hereditary tendency to be hypersensitive to certain allergens and to readily produce large quantities of IgE antibodies. It typically has its onset in childhood and generally occurs in atopic individuals who readily form IgE antibodies to commonly encountered allergens. The classic naturopathic triad of asthma, eczema and hay fever is typical with a strong family history presentation. Fortunately in these types, complete remission of asthma is common among young children; however, asthma or hay fever may continue into adulthood and be passed on generationally.

In these types, it is unusual for a single allergen to be the sole cause of asthma. The cluster of allergens generally enter the bronchi with the inspired air and are derived from organic material such as pollen, mite-containing house dust, cockroaches, feathers, animal dander and fungal spores. Much less frequently, similar effects may be produced by ingested allergens derived from certain foods such as fish, eggs, milk, yeasts and wheat, nuts and peas, which presumably reach the bronchi via the bloodstream. The reaction that eventuates is an anaphylactic antigen-antibody reaction (type I hypersensitivity), which causes the release of pharmacologically active substances (e.g. histamine, leukotrienes, prostaglandins), which provoke mucus secretion, bronchial constriction and an allergic inflammatory reaction.

FEATURES

- Sudden onset with wheezing and dyspnoea
- Minimal or absent respiratory symptoms in between episodes
- Known triggers will precipitate an episode but can be spontaneous
- Duration and severity of attacks vary.

Late-onset (non-atopic) asthma (intrinsic asthma)

External allergens are not the cause of aggravation of this asthma, rather triggering mechanisms are non-immune and include:

- Exposure to cold air
- Strong scents
- Dust and tobacco smoke
- Respiratory viral infections
- Physical exertion
- Emotional stress.

Pathological findings include occlusion of bronchi and bronchioles by thick mucus, inflammatory infiltrate, patchy necrosis and shedding of epithelial cells, hypertrophy of smooth muscle in bronchial wall, hypertrophy of submucosal mucous glands and increased number of mucus-producing goblet cells in bronchial epithelium.

FEATURES

- Primarily occurs in adults
- Chest tightness, wheeze, breathlessness on exertion are common
- Nightly spontaneous cough and wheeze can occur (often relates to environmental triggers)
- Chronic picture unless controlled appropriately
- Severe episodes can occur and present with cough and excessive mucus.

Complications

Factors that are known to be associated with an increased risk of adverse outcomes include low lung function (increased risk of exacerbations and accelerated decline in lung function), smoking (increased risk of accelerated decline in lung function, and need for higher corticosteroid doses), high doses of inhaled corticosteroids (increased risk of adverse effects such as dysphonia, oral candidiasis, osteoporosis, cataract, glaucoma) and over- or under-use of therapy. Other factors predictive of poorer clinical outcomes include increased airway hyperresponsiveness and sputum eosinophilia, which may be identified during specialist referral.[24]

Diagnosis

Important history and examination points: a definite diagnosis of asthma can be difficult to obtain in young children; it is therefore important that alternative diagnoses are carefully considered and regular assessment carried out. In children of school age and above, response to bronchodilators, peak expiratory flow (PEF) variability or tests of bronchial hyperreactivity may confirm the diagnosis.

Differential diagnosis

Breathlessness may be caused by COPD, cardiac failure, hyperventilation/dysfunctional breathing, vocal cord dysfunction, lack of fitness, obesity, pulmonary hypertension, large airway stenosis, pulmonary fibrosis, lung cancer, pleural effusion or bronchiectasis. A wheeze could be caused by COPD, large airway stenosis, inhaled foreign body, vocal cord dysfunction or bronchiectasis. Chest tightness may be caused by gastro-oesophageal reflux or ischaemic heart disease; a dry cough by rhinitis, COPD, gastro-oesophageal reflux, foreign body or lung cancer; and sputum production may be caused by COPD (chronic bronchitis), bronchiectasis, foreign body, lung cancer or rhinosinusitis.[19]

Naturopathic diagnosis

Naturopathic diagnosis bases its philosophy on contributing or causative factors that aggravate the presentation. Fundamentally it relies on the allopathic diagnosis as a base and then expands its considerations to incorporate and consider other causes — dietary, lifestyle, occupational, exercise, social, environmental and emotional factors are all considered.

Investigations

Measures include peak expiratory flow (PEF) and forced expiratory volume in 1 second (FEV_1). Diagnosis of asthma is confirmed if there is more than 20% diurnal variation in PEF on 3 days in a week for 2 weeks measured over a period of time (percentage peak flow variability = [highest–lowest]/highest × 100); or a change in FEV_1 of 15% and 200 mL or more; or PEF 20% and 60 L/minute or more increase after short-acting β_2-agonist (e.g. salbutamol 2.5 mg by nebuliser or 400 micrograms by metered-dose inhaler [MDI] plus spacer); or increase after trial of steroids (e.g. prednisolone 30 mg daily for 14 days); or decrease after 6 minutes of exercise (running).

SPECIFIC NATUROPATHIC INVESTIGATIONS

Dietary and lifestyle assessment

Comprehensive dietary and lifestyle evaluation for a comprehensive weekly assessment to ascertain triggers.

IgG/IgE FOOD PROFILE

Definitive assessment of potential food allergy or intolerance triggers is essential to ascertain dietary influence. It is imperative that thorough assessment of the patient's current dietary intake be assessed to enable correct assessment selection, as food reactions will generally only be strongly positive to foods that are currently consumed.

IgE/IgG INHALANT ALLERGY PANEL

To assess influence of chemical or environmental impact; to assess impact of grasses, weeds, trees, moulds and indoor allergens (including animal and insect [cockroaches, mites]).

ALCAT FOOD/CHEMICAL INTOLERANCE ASSESSMENTS

To assess influence of chemical or environmental impact. Specific food additives and food colouring testing can be performed as well as assessment against pharmacoactive agents, environmental chemicals and moulds.

GI PROFILE OR DIGESTIVE ANALYSIS

To assess digestive health and ensure that appropriate microflora colonisation is present in order to protect and restore immune function. To assess optimal digestive processes and nutritional absorption. Hypochlorhydria, lactase insufficiency and other gastrointestinal disorders have also been associated with asthma.

Therapeutic considerations

CLINICAL DECISION MAKING AND RATIONALE

Good asthma control aims to:

- Improve quality of life
- Maintain lung function
- Minimise medication adverse effects
- Reduce risk of morbidity, hospitalisation or death from asthma
- Reduce risk factors
  - Personal and family history of atopy
  - Exposure to environmental allergens, occupational sensitivities and respiratory viruses, smoking and passive smoke
- Assess and treat external influences
  - Digestive function and sufficient hydrochloric acid and digestive enzymes
  - Allergy or intolerance
  - Emotional stressors
  - Exercise patterns
  - Temperament/personality type.

Therapeutic application

HISTORICAL PERSPECTIVE

For the last 30 years pharmaceutical therapy of asthma has consisted primarily of five classes of drugs: β_2-agonists, anticholinergics, methylxanthines, cromones and corticosteroids. The first four of these classes have origins in herbal treatments going back 5000 or 6000 years.[25] Current initial allopathic treatment includes the prescription of a short-acting β_2-agonist via spacer device. Dose is 1–2 inhalations up to every 4 hours. Failure to obtain relief from an inhaler may be a medical emergency.[24]

NATUROPATHIC PERSPECTIVE

As with many complex diseases, the initial cause or causes of asthma (e.g. hypochlorhydria) may initiate a sequence of events that becomes self-propagating (e.g. hypochlorhydria-induced food allergies leading to increased intestinal permeability and then to increased susceptibility to food allergy). Effective treatment requires control of both the initiating cause or causes and the induced physiological abnormalities. Many studies have demonstrated the protective effect of breastfeeding in the prevention of asthma.[23]

A recent international review shows that the prevalence of asthma and other allergic disorders is increasing worldwide. The report questions the roles played by established risk factors such as dust mites, air pollution and smoking in the rising prevalence of asthma. The report recommends expanding the research focus to include the study of other factors (e.g. increased rates of immunisations and the disappearance of measles, hepatitis A and tuberculosis) that may program the initial susceptibility to sensitisation or contribute to the development of asthma independent of atopic sensitisation.[26]

Asthma is a complex immune disorder. It appears as if Th1/Th2 balance is an important aetiological factor. An excessive Th2 response encourages IgE release, which leads to the production of a raft of inflammatory mediators. This provides us with an important lead to possible naturopathic treatment. For example, we can dampen an excessive Th2 response with the herbal medicine *Tylophora indica* (tylophora), and dampen IgE release with *Albizia lebbeck* (albizia) and *Scutellaria baicalensis* (baikal skullcap).

Allergies and sensitivities to chemicals are major factors in childhood asthma. The predisposition to allergy is often developed, however, long before a child is born. Apart from hereditary influences, a child's health may be compromised if either parent has poor nutritional status or is exposed to toxins pre conception. It is therefore important to ensure optimum nutrition, health and fitness in both parents at least 6 months before conception. During pregnancy use only fresh, natural and unprocessed organic food if possible. Intake of common allergenic foods should be eliminated or reduced. The mother should eat fish or take a purified fish oil supplementation during pregnancy and lactation. Breastfeeding may reduce the incidence and severity of asthma. The first year of a child's life is critical in terms of chemical exposure. A baby's liver is immature and unable to detoxify many compounds. Good digestion is also essential and adequate sleep. Stress is known to exacerbate asthma and measures should be taken to decrease stress. Supplementation with nutrients and herbal medicines, especially the adaptogens, may increase a person's resilience to stress.[23]

Nutritional medicine (dietary)

SPECIFIC DIETARY TREATMENTS

Dietary inclusions

An Italian cross-sectional study involving 18 737 children aged 6–7 years found that an increased intake of citrus and kiwi fruits (rich in vitamin C) was a highly significant protective factor for wheezing over 12 months.[27]

Some primary dietary inclusions are:

- Increased intake of fresh fruits and vegetables, nuts, seeds, wholegrains
- Increased intake of garlic, onions, horseradish, ginger and chilli
- General wholefood diet
- Adequate fluid intake — juices, broths, soups, herbal teas.

Dietary exclusions

A carefully planned elimination diet may be used to determine food allergies. The foods most commonly associated with asthma are cow's milk, eggs, chocolate, soy, corn, rice and apple. However, a wide range of foods and food chemicals may be implicated.[23] Delayed reactions may occur in people with salicylate sensitivity. Foods high in salicylates include chocolate, banana, tomato sauces, citrus, milk and food colourings. It is thought that up to 20% of people have varying levels of aspirin sensitivity.[28] Dehydration may exacerbate exercise-induced asthma. Excess salt intake also may correlate with increased bronchial reactivity, and increased salt intake was found to correlate with increased bronchial hyperresponsiveness to metacholine in a case-controlled study.[29]

Some primary exclusions are:

- Red meat — arachadonic acid link to series 2 prostaglandins and leukotrienes (transient airway hyperresponsiveness)
- Sugar, salt, saturated fats, cow's dairy, wheat, processed foods, additives, preservatives, colourings — especially tartrazine (yellow food dye)
- Avoiding very cold fluids
- Avoiding all dietary sources of MSG and its derivatives
- Avoiding dietary sources of sulfites (220) — alcohol, dried fruits, pre-prepared salads.

Caffeine avoidance is controversial for asthma patients. Practitioners must be aware that eliminating caffeine may exacerbate bronchoconstriction, because of the bronchodilatory effects of xanthines. As such, careful consideration and observation of patients are recommended.

Nutritional medicine

Nutritional medicine therapeutic objectives

Nutritional variables, such as decreased fresh fruit and vegetable intake and decreased omega-3 to omega-6 ratios, may play a role in the increase in atopic disorders including asthma worldwide.[30] Several studies have shown that oxidative stress is a consequence of the inflammatory process in asthma and is associated with increased bronchial hyperactivity.[18]

Antioxidant intake through food, however, has decreased and may be playing a role in the increased asthma prevalence worldwide. Vitamin E is a potent antioxidant and an elevated dietary intake of vitamin E has been positively correlated with lung function in older adults and with decreased levels of serum IgE and diminished atopy in a random sample of 2633 adults.[19] Selenium is an essential co-factor of the enzyme glutathione peroxidase, which plays a major role in fighting oxidative stress. A number of studies have reported a decrease in blood levels of glutathione peroxidase in asthmatic patients.[18]

The high levels of omega-6 fatty acids (from meat and vegetable oil) and low levels of omega-3 fatty acids (from nuts, seeds, legumes and fatty fish intake) in the Western diet are theoretically problematic, because such a profile may lead to an increase in prostaglandin E2 levels, which

SAMPLE DAILY DIET

BREAKFAST	
Fresh fruit salad using 2–4 pieces of seasonal fruit (e.g. kiwi, mango, guava, strawberries)	These fruits contain high amounts of vitamin C, bioflavonoids and antioxidants that are required to improve respiratory measures and prevent histamine secretion. Serve with 2–3 tablespoons of linseed, sunflower and almond (LSA) mix and tahini to meet protein requirements.
LUNCH	
Falafel served with tabouli, hummus and tahini on a mountain bread wrap	Chickpeas found in falafel and hummus provide a good source of vegetarian protein. Tahini provides a quality source of calcium that may also help to reduce asthma symptoms. In addition to being a source of flavonoids, the parsley found in tabouli also contains vitamins A and C, both highly indicated for their immune-enhancing properties in asthma.
DINNER	
Poached salmon with Chinese greens and sesame seeds	Salmon is a good source of omega-3 fatty acids known to have anti-inflammatory and immune-modulating effects in asthma. Dark-green leafy vegetables protect the lungs[13] and are a prime source of magnesium, which is a well-known bronchodilator. Steaming ensures minimal nutrient losses and the addition of sesame seeds provides another good non-dairy source of calcium.
SNACKS	
Smoothie made from papaya, goat's milk and flaxseed oil	Goat's milk provides a dairy alternative in asthma and is usually well tolerated by asthmatics. The addition of papaya further aids in the digestion of the goat's milk as papaya contains papain, an enzyme that aids digestion of proteins. The addition of flaxseed oil provides a source of fatty acids, which reduce muscle spasm constriction associated with asthma.
BEVERAGES	
Liquorice tea, fenugreek tea	Provide a soothing, anti-inflammatory and demulcent action, reducing irritation of the bronchi. Reduce mucus production.

eventually promotes the synthesis of IgE that sets the stage for atopy and inflammation. Also, omega-3 polyunsaturated fatty acids, which are present in fish oils, are metabolised into less bronchoconstricting and inflammatory mediators than omega-6 polyunsaturated fatty acids.[19] Two studies have shown that high levels of fatty fish intake correlate with improved lung function in adult smokers[31] and in children.[32]

The International Study of Asthma and Allergies in Childhood and the TRANSFAIR study (which examined the intake of fatty acids in Western Europe) concluded that there was a positive association between the intake of trans-fatty acids (found in margarine and hydrogenated vegetable oils in biscuits, crackers, commercial breads, cakes and chips) and the prevalence of symptoms of asthma, allergic rhinoconjunctivitis and atopic eczema.[25]

An Australian study conducted in an area with a high prevalence of childhood asthma found that consumption of high levels of linoleic acid (omega-6 polyunsaturated fatty acid) significantly increased the risk of developing childhood asthma.[33]

Magnesium is used as a bronchodilator in the emergency treatment of asthma. Elevated magnesium intake in food is correlated with decreased airway reactivity to metacholine challenge, and people with asthma have reduced levels of erythrocyte magnesium.[19]

Diminished zinc levels were found in a subset of patients with asthma; zinc deficiency may lead to a shift in the Th1/Th2 (the two types of T-helper cells) response, favouring the Th2 response characteristic of asthma.[19]

Specific nutrients required

B VITAMINS

The causative link between B vitamin deficiency and the development of atopic conditions and asthma has long been investigated. Much of the most recent evidence is around B_9 and B_{12} polymorphisms and an increased risk for the development of self-reported asthma. Studies have indicated that polymorphisms in each of these B group vitamins were associated with shortness of breath; however, they did not affect lung function or atopy.[34] The causative relationship is believed to be related to methylenetetrahydrofolate reductase (MTHFR) polymorphisms being correlated with elevations in IgE levels. As with B_9 and B_{12}, B_6 is involved in cellular development and regulation, and deficiencies have been linked to a reduced incidence of allergic reactions and asthma diagnosis.[35] The mechanism of action is yet to be determined and the B group vitamins have mostly been effective in asthma incidence reduction when deficiencies have been present.

VITAMIN C

Vitamin C supports immunity and decreases inflammation and studies have shown that supplementation with 2 g of vitamin C prior to exercise may protect from exercise-induced asthma. The requirement for vitamin C is increased by stress, smoking, pollution and alcohol consumption. Low intake of vitamin C and manganese is associated with a five-fold increase in bronchial reactivity.[23] There is a strong theoretical basis for the use of vitamin C in asthma; however, recent research is inconclusive and further randomised controlled trials are required.

FLAVONOIDS

Flavonoids appear to be key antioxidants in the treatment of asthma. Various flavonoids, including quercetin, have been shown to inhibit histamine release from mast cells and basophils when stimulated by antigens and other ligands. Flavonoids also inhibit phospholipase A2 in neutrophils, lipoxygenase, anaphylactic contraction of smooth muscle, phosphodiesterase in the lung (resulting in increased cAMP levels), biosynthesis of SRS-A and calcium influx.[19]

MAGNESIUM

It has been proposed that magnesium is able to induce bronchial smooth muscle relaxation in a dose-dependent manner, possibly by inhibiting calcium reflux into cytosole, histamine release from mast cells and/or acetylcholine release from cholinergic nerve endings.[36] There is also evidence to indicate lower levels of magnesium in erythrocytes in asthmatics. The use of magnesium sulfate intravenously resulted in the improved management of moderate to severe bronchial asthma with respect to improvement in pulmonary function and reductions in the number of hospital admissions.[36] Although there seems to be some evidence linking magnesium intake and red blood cell levels of magnesium to lung function, the author of a review found only one randomised, double-blind, placebo-controlled clinical trial in which magnesium (400 mg/day) supplementation was added to a low-magnesium diet for 3 weeks. A high magnesium intake was associated with improvement in symptom scores, although not in objective measures of airflow or airway reactivity in these stable asthmatic participants.[19]

OMEGA-3 FATTY ACID

Children who regularly eat fish have a lower risk of developing asthma, and may experience fewer attacks. A study of 468 children by the Sydney Royal Prince Alfred Institute of Respiratory Medicine found that children who eat fresh oily fish, including salmon, tuna and mackerel, at least once a week may avoid asthma. It was found that two out of four children prone to asthma did not suffer attacks if they included oily fish in their diet. However, eating tinned oily fish such as tuna or salmon, or fish fingers made no difference to asthma risk and researchers believe this is due to processing.[32]

Exercise-induced asthma (EIA) occurs in up to 90% of individuals with asthma and approximately 10% of the general population without asthma. Treatment of EIA almost exclusively involves the use of pharmacological medications. However, there is accumulating evidence that a dietary excess of salt and omega-6 fatty acids, and a dietary deficiency of antioxidant vitamins and omega-3 fatty acids, can modify the severity of EIA.[37]

A patented extract of New Zealand green-lipped mussels known as lyprinol/omega XL, which is rich in omega-3 fatty acids, was studied for its effect on airway inflammation and bronchoconstriction in asthmatics. Twenty asthmatics participated in the randomised, double-blind cross-over trial for 8 weeks supplementing with 8 capsules per day or placebo.[38] Each capsule contained approximately 72 mg EPA and 48 mg DHA with a total of 50 mg lonega-3 (n-3) per capsule. Supplementation resulted in attenuation of airway inflammation and reductions in bronchoconstriction as well as a statistically significant reduction in the use of rescue medication and bronchodilators. The researchers concluded that green-lipped mussels may have beneficial effects by serving as a pro-resolving agonist and/or inflammatory antagonists.[38]

COENZYME Q10 (CoQ10)

Excess oxygen free radicals are known to be part of the pathogenesis of asthma[39] and the modulation of antioxidant defences by antioxidant supplementation may be beneficial. CoQ10 levels and other antioxidants have been found to be reduced in asthmatics compared with controls[40,41] and supplementation with antioxidants including CoQ10 has been shown to decrease both oxidative stress and asthma symptoms.[42,43] In a case report of a patient with chronic asthma treated with glucocorticoid for 45 years, symptoms of glucocorticoid-induced myopathy were attenuated by the administration of CoQ10.[44] This report suggests that CoQ10 may decrease some long-term side effects in glucocorticoid-treated asthmatics, in addition to providing the aforementioned antioxidant protection. In a 1-year double-blind trial involving 322 patients with congestive heart failure, supplementation with CoQ10 at a dose of 2 mg/kg/day for 1 year decreased episodes of cardiac asthma compared with a placebo (p <0.001).[43] Long-term administration of corticosteroids in asthma patients has been shown to result in mitochondrial dysfunction and oxidative damage of mitochondrial and nuclear DNA. An open, cross-over, randomised clinical study with 41 bronchial asthma patients has shown that CoQ10 supplementation may reduce the dosage of corticosteroids needed to control symptoms in these patients. A reduction in the dosage of corticosteroids required by the patients following antioxidant supplementation was observed, indicating lower incidence of potential adverse effects of the drugs, decreased oxidative stress.[41]

Dosage requirements

The dosage requirements listed below are based on adult doses that are reported in the literature.

- High-strength B complex: 1–2 tablets/d
- Pyridoxine (vitamin B_6): 25–50 mg b.i.d.
- Vitamin C (as ascorbic acid): 2000–3000 mg/d in divided doses
- Quercetin: 600 mg/d
- Vitamin D: 1000 IU/d
- Magnesium: 250 mg/d t.d.s.
- Mixed flavonoids: 50 mg/d
- Zinc: 20–40 mg/d
- CoQ10: 150 mg/d
- Omega-3: 1–2 g/d
- EPA: 17.0–26.8 mg/per kg of body weight
- DHA: 7.3–11.5 mg/per kg of body weight.

HERBAL MEDICINE

Herbal medicine therapeutic objectives

- Reduce the allergic response
- Reduce bronchorestriction
- Support the immune regulation
- Reduce inflammation
- Reduce excessive secretions.

Herbal medicine classes

Asthma is characterised by chronic inflammation of the airways and thus requires the use of botanical classes of herbs with specific demulcent and anti-inflammatory actions that reduce irritation and soothe the inflamed bronchi. Antiallergic herbs reduce airway sensitivity, toning down the allergic response to triggered allergens such as carpet and pollen, while bronchodilators reduce bronchoconstriction and spasm. The presence of tenacious, mucoid sputum requires the application of stimulating and warming expectorants to aid in its removal as well as anticatarrhal herbs which may help reduce excessive secretions from the mucous membranes. Other classes of herbs unrelated to the respiratory system such as nervines and adaptogens may also be used, particularly if stress is a causative factor. Immune modulators should always be given, particularly if attacks are regular and there is concurrent infection.

Antiallergic herbs including *Albizia lebbeck* (albizia), *Scutellaria baicalensis* (baikal skullcap) and *Thylophora indica* (asthma weed) may tone down the allergic response, while anticatarrhal herbs such as *Euphrasia officinalis* (eyebright), *Solidago virgaurea* (goldenrod) and *Hydrastis canadensis* (goldenseal) may help reduce the excessive secretions from the mucous membranes. Respiratory demulcents contain mucilage and have soothing and anti-inflammatory effects and include *Althaea officinalis* (marshmallow) which is often given as a glycerol extract, *Ulmus rubra* (slippery elm) used in powder form and *Plantago lanceolata* (ribwort).

Specific herbal medicines

TYLOPHORA INDICA (TYLOPHORA)

Tylophora indica, also known as asthma weed or *Tylophora asthmatica,* is a twining perennial plant belonging to the Asclepiadaceae family. The leaves of tylophora contain several alkaloids including tylophorine, tylophorinine, tylophorinidine, isotylocrebrine and septicine, flavonoids, sterols and tannins. The alkaloids tylophorine and tylophorinine are highest in the leaves during flowering periods, with levels up to 0.5%. Tylophora is traditionally used in the treatment of bronchial asthma, bronchitis and rheumatism. Two early, positive, double-blind studies reported on the use of tylophora for a short period (6–7 days) with long-lasting effects for 4–12 weeks. Two other small cross-over double-blind studies showed a positive effect on night symptoms, peak expiratory flow rate and ventilatory capacity. Recent studies suggest that its action may be due to immunosuppressive activities. There have been five clinical trials examining the benefits of tylophora in asthma. The dosages and preparations varied greatly. In one trial the participants chewed one fresh leaf daily; in the second trial an ethanol tincture was used; in the third they were given pure alkaloids extracted from tylophora; and in the last two, they were given dried powder. While four of the trials demonstrated a moderate benefit, the fifth trial could not demonstrate any statistical difference between tylophora and placebo.[45,46] One double-blind randomised trial with a well-designed placebo (containing ipecac to reproduce some nausea) and involving 135 patients did not demonstrate any significant effect of the plant. Tylophora's mechanism of action seems to be through direct stimulation of the adrenals and increasing cyclic AMP levels.[19] A systematic review of these five trials concluded that the efficacy of tylophora in the treatment of asthma is inconclusive.[47] To avoid the side effects caused by chewing the fresh leaf, tylophora is best taken as a 1:5 tincture at a dose of 1–2 mL/day for short-term treatment of up to 4 weeks at a time or as a solid dose (extract equivalent to 200–400 mg dry leaf).

BOSWELLIA SERRATA (FRANKINCENSE GUM RESIN)

The resin of *Boswellia serrata*, known in India as salai guggul, contains boswellic acids, which have been shown to inhibit leukotriene synthesis. Activation of transcription factor NF-kappaB is elevated in several chronic inflammatory diseases and is responsible for the enhanced expression of many proinflammatory gene products. Acetyl-11-keto-beta-boswellic acid (AKBA) inhibits NF-kappaB activity.[48] Only one clinical trial examining the efficacy of boswellia for asthma has been published on MedLine. In a double-blind randomised clinical trial of 80 adult patients with bronchial asthma, boswellia significantly improved the forced expiratory volume (FEV) compared with a placebo ($p <0.0001$). Twenty-three (23) males and 17 females in the age range 18–75 years having a mean duration of bronchial asthma of 9.58 +/− 6.07 years were treated with a preparation of boswellia resin, 300 mg thrice daily for a period of 6 weeks. A total of 70% of patients showed improvement of disease as evidenced by the disappearance of physical symptoms and signs such as dyspnoea and rhonchi, a decrease in the number of attacks and an increase in FEV, and decreases in eosinophilic count and ESR. The control group of 40 patients (16 males and 24 females in the age range 14–58 years with a mean asthma duration of 32.95 +/− 12.68 years), were treated with lactose 300 mg thrice daily for 6 weeks. Only 27% of patients in the control group showed improvement.[48]

COLEUS FORSKOHLII (COLEUS)

Coleus contains small amounts of a potent substance called forskolin. Forskolin increases the levels of cyclic AMP causing bronchodilation. Forskolin has been found to stabilise basophils and mast cells, thus decreasing the release of histamine and other inflammatory compounds. In a small (16 patients) randomised trial, a coleus-containing capsule resulted in measurable bronchodilation in patients with asthma.[19]

EPHEDRA SINECA (MA HUANG)

Chinese herbalists traditionally used ma huang in the early stages of respiratory infections and for the short-term treatment of certain kinds of asthma, eczema, hay fever, narcolepsy and oedema. Ephedra is a scheduled herb in many countries including Australia.

GINKGO BILOBA (GINKGO)

Although mostly known for improving cognitive function in early multi-infarct dementia and Alzheimer's disease, ginkgo is also known for its antiasthmatic properties. Ginkgo inhibits platelet-activating factor (PAF), a potent mediator of the allergic and inflammatory reaction in asthma. A placebo-controlled study showed a significant clinical improvement in FEV_1 at 8 weeks when using a concentrated ginkgo leaf liquor (15 g three times a day).[49] The usual dose is 120 mg standardised extract (24% ginkgoflavones) daily.

GLYCYRRHIZA GLABRA (LIQUORICE)

Liquorice's expectorant properties are used in bronchitis and asthma. Liquorice is an anti-inflammatory herb with mineralocorticoid and glucocorticoid effects. Many in vitro studies have demonstrated that liquorice inhibits 11-β-dehydrogenase, blocking the conversion of cortisol to cortisone. Liquorice also has PAF-inhibiting, antitussive and expectorant activities.[19]

PICRORHIZA KURROA (PICRORHIZA)

Picrorhiza is a small perennial herb which grows in the alpine Himalayas at 3000–5000 metres. The root and rhizomes were often used as substitutes for gentian. It is an ingredient of many Ayurvedic remedies used for the treatment of liver ailments and immune disorders. The effects of aerosol doses of the antiallergic compound disodium cromoglycate (DSCG) have been compared with oral doses of picrorhiza root in guinea pigs. The antiallergic mast cell stabilising effect of picrorhiza was confirmed in later in vitro and in vivo studies. Picrorhiza also enhances the bronchodilating effects of sympathicomimetic amines used as asthma drugs. The adult dosage of the powdered root used in trials or recommended in texts varies from 400 to 1500 mg per day, although daily doses as high as 3.5 g have been recommended for the treatment of fevers. The corresponding range for a 1:2 extract is about 1–4 mL per day (7–28 mL/week). The intense bitterness of picrorhiza makes use of tablets or capsules preferable unless the bitter tonic action is also required.[45]

SCUTELLARIA BAICALENSIS (BAIKAL SKULLCAP)

Baicalein is a bioflavone found within the roots of baikal skullcap and is known to reduce eotaxin production in human fibroblasts. However, its role in reducing airway inflammation is not entirely known. An in vivo study assessed the benefits of baicalein in asthma induced rat models.[50] The study found baicalein was able to reduce perivascular and peribronchial infiltration of inflammatory cells as well as inhibiting TNF-α and IL-4 and 13. It was also found to restore airway injury and restore mitochondrial function.[50] Human clinical trials are required to further assess the benefits on baicalein in asthmatic subjects.

LIFESTYLE RECOMMENDATIONS

Avoid asthma triggers

- Allergens — animal dander, dust mites, airborne moulds and pollen (do regular cleaning)
- Respiratory viral infections
- Aspirin, NSAIDs and salicylates
- Nonspecific irritants — cigarette smoke, dust, odours, irritant fumes, changes in temperature, humidity, atmospheric pressure
- Psychological — crying, screaming, hard laughing
- Reduce stress and learn ways to deal with stress.

Other

- Keep bedroom temperature stable
- Patients should try to avoid substances or conditions that may precipitate reactions. These include additives and contaminants such as dyes, flavourings and preservatives, moulds, dust mites, animal fur and various industrial or agricultural chemicals
- Low stomach acid, lactase insufficiency and other gastrointestinal disorders have also been associated with asthma
- Certain drugs and neurochemicals including caffeine, theobromine, alcohol, histamine, tryptamine, tyramine, dopamine phenylethylamine and serotonin may also be implicated[20]
- Massage may help reduce anxiety in asthmatic children and their parents and improve respiratory capacity
- Specific exercises and especially special breathing exercises may be beneficial:
  - Yoga may be beneficial for asthma. Yoga combines meditation, breathing techniques and postural exercises
  - Plenty of fresh air
  - Exercise — walking, jogging
  - Russian Buteyko breathing technique
  - Qigong and tai chi.
- Rest, adequate sleep and stress reduction are essential
- Exposure to house dust mites can be reduced by removing wall-to-wall carpets and keeping the relative humidity low (preferably below 50%) in the summer by using air conditioning. Special pillow and mattress covers can help reduce exposure to these mites
- Cats and dogs must be removed to significantly decrease animal dander
- Irritating fumes such as cigarette smoke should also be avoided
- In some people with asthma, aspirin and other non-steroidal anti-inflammatory drugs trigger attacks
- Tartrazine, a yellow colouring used in some drug tablets and food, may also bring on an attack
- Sulfites commonly added to foods as a preservative may trigger attacks after a susceptible person eats from a salad bar or drinks beer or red wine.

CASE STUDY

OVERVIEW

FC is a 33-year-old female and is currently a stay-at-home mother, looking after 2 children under the age of 4 years. She has been experiencing wheezing and dyspnoea lately and finds her high stress and anxiety levels exacerbate these symptoms. She has commenced a full-time tertiary education course and is finding it difficult to cope with studying and other day-to-day activities. She is unable to exercise on a regular basis due to her poor respiratory function.

FC finds that certain foods exacerbate her asthma but is unable to accurately pinpoint what foods may further contribute to her symptoms. During spring her asthma is exacerbated as she also suffers from hay fever.

She also experiences frequent colds and flu and her immune function tends to be under stress on a regular basis.

FC eats well and attempts to eat a predominately organic and wholefood diet. Full-fat dairy is eaten on a daily basis and she drinks up to 3 cups of coffee per day.

As a child, FC suffered from eczema; however, this has been relatively resolved since improving her diet.

Pulmonary mucus is produced on a daily basis and the FC advises she feels congested on a daily basis.

CLINICAL EXAMINATION

General inspection

Alert, cooperative

Vital signs

BP: 120/70 mmHg sitting/standing
Temperature: 36.5°C
Pulse: 70 bpm
Respiratory rate: 14 resp/min
Height: 1.65 m
Weight: 58 kg
BMI: 21 kg/m^2

Respiratory

Chest inspection: Barrel chest
Palpation: Trachea — midline
Supraclavicular/axillary nodes — nil
Percussion: Resonant all zones
Auscultation: Wheezing on exhalation in both right and left lung bases

TREATMENT PROTOCOL

Because of the possible correlation between dietary allergens and triggers it is essential to identify and eliminate all triggers. Symptomatic relief is the main focus and priority of treatment, along with reducing hyperresponsiveness to environmental and dietary triggers.

HERBAL MEDICINE

Verbascum thapsus (mullein): 60 mL
Glycyrrhiza glabra (liquorice) STD Ext: 40 mL
Calendula officinalis (calendula): 40 mL

CASE STUDY CONTINUED

Scutellaria baicalensis (baikal skullcap): 60 mL
Dose: 7.5 mL twice daily

NUTRITIONAL MEDICINE

Dietary

- Eliminate caffeine and dairy consumption
- Ensure adequate hydration
- Encourage consumption of adequate protein to support immune processes
- Promote consumption of monounsaturated and polyunsaturated fatty acids to aid with reducing inflammatory cytokines.

Supplemental

Vitamin C + bioflavonoids: 1 g b.i.d.
Zinc citrate: 30 mg 1 capsule twice daily
Concentrated omega liquid (EPA, DHA): ½ teaspoon b.i.d.: 1.6 g omega-3 (70%) 35% EPA (813 mg), 25% DHA (563 mg).

LIFESTYLE

- Stress and anxiety management discussion with suggestions
- Refrain from pushing herself with exercise and encourage yoga and Pilates as gentler forms of exercise
- Avoid substances, situations or conditions that aggravate reactions — foods, excessive exercise, dust mites, chemicals; avoid allergens, nonspecific irritants and strong changes in temperature.

EDUCATION

Avoid

- Food sources of preservatives, colourings, additives, especially MSG, tartrazine and food dyes
- Household triggers and cleaning regimens.

REFERRAL

- Referral for IgG/IgE food profile
- Referral for vitamin D and red cell zinc — potential prescription (results depending).

PNEUMONIA

Epidemiology

There is a lack of detailed information pertaining to the incidence of pneumonia in Australia. This is in part because pneumonia is commonly a complication of influenza, though hospitalisations of patients suffering from influenza — which then progresses to pneumonia — are usually recorded as just a single case of influenza. Thus the estimated burden of pneumonia is actually thought to be much higher than current statistics suggest.

In New South Wales, the Northern Territory, South Australia, Queensland and Western Australia in the period between July 2002 and June 2005 there were 7378 hospitalisations for influenza and 223 863 for influenza and pneumonia combined. Of the latter, 16 680 (7%) were identified as occurring in Aboriginal and Torres Strait Islander peoples.[51]

In the United States community-acquired pneumonia (CAP) requiring hospital admission occurs in about 258 per 100 000 population per year, rising to 962 per 100 000 among those aged 65 years or over. Mortality rates in recent years appear to have increased. Mortality averages 14%, but is less than 1% for those not requiring admission to hospital.[52]

Classification

Pneumonia is usually classified according to where it was contracted, that is community or hospital acquired; or if the patient was immunosuppressed. Community-acquired pneumonia (CAP) is commonly defined as an acute infection of the lower respiratory tract occurring in a patient who has not resided in a hospital or healthcare facility in the previous 14 days.

Aetiology

Community-acquired pneumonia occurs in people who are not or have not been in hospitalised recently, and who are not institutionalised or immune-compromised. CAP is usually caused by *Streptococcus pneumoniae*, which is now becoming resistant to antibiotics.[15]

It is particularly dangerous in the elderly and often occurs in immune-compromised people — particularly those who abuse recreational drugs or alcohol. It can also occur in healthy individuals but will typically indicate immune-compromisation following an insult to the host defence mechanisms: viral infection (especially influenza), cigarette smoke and other noxious fumes, impairment of consciousness (which depresses the gag reflex, allowing aspiration), neoplasms, and hospitalisation. In immunocompetent, non-elderly adults, cigarette smoking is the strongest independent risk factor for invasive pneumococcal disease.[53]

Overview

Pneumonia is inflammation of lung tissue. It usually presents as an acute illness with cough, fever and purulent sputum plus physical signs and x-ray changes if consolidated.

Pneumonia has a number of pathogenic triggers including:

- Viral (influenza) — most common
- Mycoplasma
- Bacterial
- Bacterial + viral
- Chlamydia
- Other including Legionnaire's and toxin exposures.

Pathogenesis

Pneumonia usually begins as a colonisation of the mucosa of the nasopharynx followed by spread into the lower respiratory tract. The airway distal to the larynx is normally sterile due to several protective mechanisms, both mechanical and humoral. The mucus-covered ciliated epithelium that lines the lower respiratory tract propels sputum to the larger bronchi and trachea, evoking the cough reflex. The respiratory secretions contain substances that exert nonspecific antimicrobial actions: α_1-antitrypsin, lysozyme and lactoferrin. At the level of the alveoli, potent defence mechanisms are present including alveolar macrophages, a rich vasculature capable of rapidly delivering lymphocytes and granulocytes, and an efficient lymphatic drainage network.[54]

The immunoglobulin respiratory system defences are the strongest protector from developing pneumonia or other conditions. Immunoglobulin A (IgA) is present in high concentrations in the upper respiratory tract and immunoglobulin G (IgG) is present in high concentrations in the lower respiratory tract. Both work together to neutralise bacterial and viral toxins, agglutinate bacteria and reduce bacterial attachment to mucosal surfaces.

PRIMARY SIGNS AND SYMPTOMS

The initial presentation can be misleading, especially when the patient presents with constitutional symptoms such as fever, malaise and headache, rather than respiratory symptoms. A cough, although usually present, can be relatively insignificant in the total clinical picture.

Pneumonia patients usually present with the following symptoms:

- 90% with cough
- 66% with dyspnoea (breathlessness, shortness of breath)
- 66% with sputum production
- 50% with pleuritic chest pain, myalgia, arthralgias, night sweats and absence of sore throat and rhinorrhoea
- Fever greater than 37.8°C
- Pulse more than 100 beats/minute
- Raised respiratory rate
- The elderly patient may present with confusion.

TYPES OF PNEUMONIA

Mycoplasmal pneumonia

Mycoplasma are bacteria that lack cell walls. *Mycoplasma pneumoniae* is the most frequent cause of community-acquired, non-pyogenic pneumonia. Slow recovery is the general rule, but the course is quite variable. Repeated infections often extending over a number of months can present themselves. *Mycoplasma* is a common cause of chronic fatigue syndrome and other fatigue-based conditions. It is imperative that successful eradication of the condition is ensured.

SIGNS AND SYMPTOMS

- Most commonly occurs in children or young adults — its development does not necessarily indicate the same warning triggers for other types of pneumonia
- Insidious onset over several days
- Headache and malaise are common early symptoms
- Non-productive cough
- Minimal physical findings
- Temperature generally <39°C
- Blood results: white blood cell count is normal or slightly elevated
- X-ray: pneumonia pattern consists of white patches.

Bacterial: streptococcal pneumonia

Streptococcus pneumoniae is the most common bacterial pneumonia and the most common cause of pneumonia requiring hospitalisation. It is imperative that the correct diagnosis and assessment of severity is made with the patient's doctor before treatment is commenced. Care must be taken especially for elderly or immunocompromised patients. It is typically preceded by an upper respiratory infection and the patient will present with sudden onset of shaking, chills, fever and chest pain.

While antibiotic therapy is frequently administered, there are a number of reports suggesting that most bacterial pneumonias are resistant to antibiotic therapy (most commonly penicillin-resistant and macrolide-resistant). Thus the use of natural medicines has become more common in the treatment of these patients. At times natural medicines may be prescribed as an adjunct to antibiotic treatment to stimulate and support the immune system's response to the prescription and increase therapeutic effect.

SIGNS AND SYMPTOMS

- Blood: leucocytosis
- Sputum: Gram-positive diplococci are present in the sputum smear (caution: this should be confirmed with blood culture as the nasopharynx naturally habitats *Pneumococcus* spp.). Sputum is pinkish or blood-specked at first, then becomes rusty at the height of the infection, and finally yellow and mucopurulent during resolution
- Physical assessment: initially chest inspiration is diminished on the involved side, breath sounds are suppressed and fine inspiratory crackles are heard. Later classic signs of consolidation appear (bronchial breathing, crepitant crackles, dullness)
- X-ray: lobar or segmental consolidation.

Viral pneumonia

Viral pneumonia is one of the most common presentations due to its associated progression from simple influenza. Presentation is as a typical influenza onset — fever, myalgia and headache — and as pneumonia develops patients exhibit signs and symptoms (and x-ray findings) similar to mycoplasma infections.

COMPLICATIONS

Complications associated with pneumonia include bacteraemia, pleurisy, empyema, lung abscess and acute respiratory distress syndrome.

DIFFERENTIAL DIAGNOSIS

Correct diagnosis of the type of pneumonia is the primary requirement. This is best achieved through sputum and/or blood culture. A blood culture is typically a more accurate method of diagnosis than sputum culture because 15–25% of all cultures are positive early in the disease, regardless of whether the patient has a bacterial pneumonia or not.[54]

CAP should be considered when a patient presents with two or more of the following symptoms: fever; rigors; new-onset cough; change in sputum colour if there is a chronic cough; chest discomfort; dyspnoea.[52]

Differential diagnoses include acute exacerbation of chronic bronchitis, tuberculosis, acute bronchitis, common cold, influenza, lung cancer and cardiac failure and hyperventilation secondary to metabolic acidosis in sepsis.

NATUROPATHIC DIAGNOSIS

Naturopathic diagnosis relies on effective investigations from the traditional medical community. As a priority, determine the pathogen responsible for the infection. Then modify treatment accordingly. If treatment is able to be specific with respect to herbal medicine prescriptions, clinical outcome is greater.

Naturopathic considerations will acknowledge:

- Severity of infection
- Current lifestyle and potential triggers
- Current immune system challenges
- Identification and acknowledgment of stressors (emotional, social, nutritional, physical, environmental, other).

Naturopathic diagnosis sees low-grade infections as a primary trigger for the development of pneumonia. If the patient presents with a severe resistant case, further investigations are warranted. Consideration of DNA testing for underlying infections should be considered.

DNA TESTING

DNA testing uses polymerase chain reaction (PCR) technology to detect certain pathogenic and opportunistic microorganisms present in blood. PCR, whether in a single assay or multiple assay (multiplex PCR) has allowed single detection or simultaneous detection and differentiation of multiple species of organisms in which the level of sensitivity and specificity is still unmatched by any other laboratory procedures. PCR assay has made it possible for clinicians to rapidly screen individuals for potentially pathogenic organisms such as *Mycoplasma*. Community-acquired respiratory tract infections, and in particular atypical pneumonia, may be caused by either *Chlamydia pneumoniae* or *Mycoplasma pneumoniae*. One form possibly results in the need for hospitalisation whereas the other may be responsible for long-lasting disease. Rapid identification is recommended in order to administer the specific treatment required. DNA for PCR analysis is extracted from both the RBC and WBC blood components, not just white cell nuclei as in other procedures.

INVESTIGATIONS

- Chest x-ray is the cardinal investigation. However, x-ray is a poor guide to the likely pathogen
- Blood cultures are the most specific diagnostic test for the causative organism, but are positive in only about 10% of patients admitted to hospital
- Viral immunofluorescence testing of a nasopharyngeal aspirate is rapid and useful if it detects influenza or respiratory syncytial virus. Virus detection does not preclude a secondary bacterial invader.[52]

SPECIFIC NATUROPATHIC INVESTIGATIONS

Unless a chronic picture presents, general investigations are sufficient. In the event of chronic relapsing pneumonia, referral for DNA (PCR) testing and other investigations to ascertain reduced immune function are warranted. These must include allergy testing, coeliac screen, HIV testing, toxin exposure and similar.

Therapeutic considerations

ALLOPATHIC TREATMENT

Medical treatment includes analgesia for pleuritic chest pain, for example paracetamol or non-steroidal anti-inflammatory drugs (NSAIDs) and oral antibiotic regimen. Early antibiotic use reduces morbidity and mortality and reduces risk of complications; however, resistance is increasing. CAP is common, and many patients will recover with a simple oral antibiotic regimen, or even without antibiotics. However, a small proportion are at significant risk of death.[52]

CLINICAL DECISION MAKING AND RATIONALE

- Assessment of the severity of the presentation must be the prime objective. If the patient is frail, elderly or severely immunocompromised, only support the patient's care with strict direction from the patient's general practitioner
- Appropriate assessment to ascertain specificity of infection is essential to direct treatment appropriately
- Review causative factors for reduced immune response to initiate infection
- Assess and recommend modifications to diet, lifestyle, social activities and occupational practices as necessary.

Therapeutic application

HISTORICAL PERSPECTIVE

Pneumonia has been recognised as a disease entity since remote times, with definitions of the condition traceable in ancient Greek, Roman and Arabic writings. Identification of *Streptococcus pneumoniae* as the most common causative agent was only achieved about 120 years ago. Although the introduction of antibiotics has obviously greatly improved the treatment of pneumonia, the disease is still associated with considerable morbidity and mortality.[55]

NATUROPATHIC PERSPECTIVE

Pneumonia presents following significant stress that causes immune depletion. Thorough investigation and assessment to determine causative factor/s are essential for optimal long-term support and benefit.

Initial treatment should focus on the following aspects:

- Avoidance of smoking and exposure to chemicals that aggravate recovery (active and passive)

- Rest, sleep and recuperation — full recovery requires total commitment to getting well
- Sufficient emotional and psychological support for optimal recovery
- Sufficient dietary support (hydration and food) for optimal recovery
- Nutritional supplementation to address deficiencies and optimise immune responsiveness to eradicate infection
- Herbal prescriptions to eradicate infection and restore respiratory function.

NUTRITIONAL MEDICINE (DIETARY)

Dietary therapeutic objectives

- Support immune response with appropriate dietary sources of required nutrients
- Control symptoms by eliminating aggravating dietary triggers
- Elimination diet to accurately assess dietary influences
- Avoid all immune suppressant foods.

Specific dietary treatments

DIETARY INCLUSIONS

- Increase intake of fresh fruits and vegetables
- Increase intake of garlic, onions, horseradish, ginger and chilli
- General wholefood diet
- Adequate fluid intake — juices, broths, soups, herbal teas.

DIETARY EXCLUSIONS

- Sugar, salt, saturated fats, cow's dairy, wheat, processed foods, additives, preservatives, colourings.

SAMPLE DAILY DIET

BREAKFAST	
Chicken and basmati rice congee/kanji	'Congee', as it is called in Asia, or 'kanji', as it is known in India, is a watery gruel with a similar consistency to porridge or soup and is considered to be a therapeutic food. It provides a warm and easy-to-digest meal. Typically no spices or salt are added and although it may appear bland, it prevents the body from being overwhelmed by overly rich foods and an excess of flavours, a favourable approach when the person is unwell. The chicken provides a valuable source of protein, required to stimulate the immune system, while the basmati rice provides carbohydrate to be used for energy. Basmati rice has a lower glycaemic index than other forms of rice and thus prevents spikes in blood sugar. It is also considered a 'lighter' rice (i.e. it is easily digestible) and is highly indicated for damp conditions, particularly where there is stagnation.[29] Vegetables may be added to the congee if tolerated by the patient.
LUNCH	
Bowl of lightly steamed seasonal vegetables (choose from broccoli, carrot, zucchini, squash, pumpkin, sweet potato, snow peas). Serve with a small (100–150 g) piece of steamed white fish	The assortment of vegetables provides a variety of immune-boosting vitamins and minerals while the fish provides a much-needed source of protein to aid the functioning of the immune system.
DINNER	
Dinner should be the lightest meal of the day so as not to tax the body. For severe conditions the breakfast congee or a broth may be repeated. For mild conditions a home-made mixed vegetable soup or some poached or stewed fruit will suffice	
SNACKS	
Only as needed to enable immune recovery	If chosen, should be low carbohydrate and adhere to recommendations above. Suggestions include puréed vegetable and lentil soup or stewed pear with LSA and tahini.
BEVERAGES	
Adequate hydration is essential for recovery. Ensure that water needs are met — aim for at least 30 mL/kg and increase with sweating	Diaphoretic herbal teas can be encouraged to support the immune response.

NUTRITIONAL MEDICINE (SUPPLEMENTAL)

Nutritional medicine therapeutic objectives

- Supplement with nutrients to assist with improving the respiratory tract response to eradicating pathogen
- Prescribe appropriate nutrients to support immune response
- Control symptoms
- Support respiratory tract drainage
- Prevent recurrence by increasing nutritional status of the patient
- Support causative trigger by addressing underlying deficiency.

Specific nutrients required

VITAMIN A

Adequate vitamin A is required to maintain the epithelial lining of the respiratory tract. Deficiency of vitamin A may render the body vulnerable to infection which can easily progress to pneumonia.[56] Vitamin A may be more beneficial when combined with zinc. A study of 2482 children aged 6 months to 3 years revealed that those children given initial high doses of vitamin A followed by 4 months of elemental zinc (10 mg/day for infants and 20 mg/day for children older than 1 year) had a reduced incidence of pneumonia that was not present in the group given only vitamin A.[57]

A randomised double-blind trial of 189 children with measles (average age 10 months) in South Africa evaluated the efficacy of vitamin A in reducing complications. Providing 400 000 IU (120 mg retinyl palmitate), half on admission and half a day later, reduced the death rate by more than 50% and the duration of pneumonia, diarrhoea and hospital stay by 33%.[58]

VITAMIN C

In the early part of the twentieth century, before the advent of effective antibiotics, many controlled and uncontrolled studies demonstrated the efficacy of large doses of vitamin C, but only when started on the first or second day of infection. If administered later, vitamin C tended only to lessen the severity of the disease. Researchers also demonstrated that in pneumonia white cells take up large amounts of vitamin C.[59]

Vitamin C supplementation may be beneficial in elderly patients with pneumonia. In a double-blind study 57 elderly patients hospitalised for severe acute bronchitis and pneumonia were given either 200 mg/day of vitamin C or a placebo. Patients were assessed by clinical and laboratory methods (vitamin C levels in the plasma, white blood cells and platelets; sedimentation rates; and white blood cell counts and differential). Patients receiving the modest dosage of vitamin C demonstrated substantially increased vitamin C levels in all tissues even in the presence of an acute respiratory infection. Using a clinical scoring system based on major symptoms of respiratory infections, results indicated that the patients receiving the vitamin C fared significantly better than those on the placebo. The benefit of vitamin C was most obvious in patients with the most severe illness, many of whom had low plasma and white blood cell vitamin C levels on admission.[60]

A Cochrane review assessing five trials found preventive or therapeutic benefits of vitamin C against pneumonia; however, another study which assessed hospital-acquired pneumonia showed no benefit. The review indicated an 80% reduction in pneumonia incidence in the prophylactic vitamin C group.[61] Although the studies reviewed produced positive results, they were conducted in extreme conditions and this makes it difficult to extrapolate the information for the general population. The use of vitamin C for pneumonia needs to be further investigated to meet a definitive conclusion for its use in pneumonia.[61] However, due to its low side effect profile, Vitamin C may be beneficial in those pneumonia patients who have low plasma vitamin C levels.

BIOFLAVONOIDS

In animal models the flavonoid fisetin was found to significantly reduce lung myeloperoxidase levels and gene expression of inflammatory mediators, highlighting the potential use as nutraceuticals in the treatment of pulmonary inflammatory diseases.[62]

ZINC

Zinc is required for multiple cellular tasks, and the immune system particularly depends on a sufficient availability of this essential trace element. Low zinc status, perhaps in part because low zinc status impairs immunity, may be a risk factor for pneumonia. Low zinc status decreases resistance to pathogens and is associated with increased incidence and duration of pneumonia, increased use and duration of antimicrobial treatment and increased overall mortality in the elderly.[63]

A parallel, double-blind, randomised controlled trial was conducted on 120 children aged between 3 and 60 months suffering from pneumonia. The children received 5 mL of zinc gluconate every 12 hours or a placebo along with the common antibiotic.[64] The primary outcome of the study was recovery from pneumonia.[64] Zinc supplementation was able to improve the recovery time from pneumonia and aid in symptomatic resolution, when combined with antibiotic therapy at the onset of hospital admission.[64]

BROMELAIN

Bromelain increases CD2-mediated T-cell activation and enhances antigen-independent binding to monocytes. Bromelain also increases interferon (IFN)-gamma-dependent and tumour necrosis factor alpha (TNF-α) in peripheral blood monocytes leading to immunomodulatory effects.[65]

VITAMIN E

Vitamin E is a fat-soluble antioxidant that has been shown to repair mucous membrane tissues and assist in the function of the cilia in clearing excessive mucus from the respiratory system. It increases humoral antibody production, resistance to bacterial infections, cell-mediated immunity, the T-lymphocyte response, TNF production and natural killer cell activity, thereby playing a role in immunocompetence.[66]

Dosage requirements

The dosage requirements listed below are based on adult doses that are reported in the literature:

- Vitamin A: 50000 IU/day for 1 week or beta-carotene: 30 mg/day and then reduce
- Vitamin C: 500 mg every 2 hours up to bowel tolerance (vitamin C in doses >2000 mg/day may cause nausea and diarrhoea)
- Vitamin E: 200 IU/t.d.s.
- Bioflavonoids: 1000 mg/day
- Zinc: 30–60 mg/day
- Bromelain 500–750 mg t.d.s. between meals.

HERBAL MEDICINE

Herbal medicine therapeutic objectives

Herbal medicine treatment aims at treating the infection, supporting the immune system, reducing inflammation, reducing excessive secretions and alleviating the cough.

- Determine the causative agent and use appropriate immune modulation
- Control symptoms
- Dietary exclusions — elimination diets may be best determinant
- Support respiratory tract drainage
- Promote drainage by the use of local heat, massage and expectorants.

Herbal medicine classes

Pneumonia signifies the presence of a severely compromised immune system and thus the first herbal classes that need to be employed are those that stimulate and support the immune system. Known as the immune enhancers, it is these herbs that stimulate a specific immune response when required. The causative infectious organism — whether of viral, bacterial, fungal or parasitic origin — also needs to be considered and then eradicated with the use of herbs with known actions against that particular pathogen. Herbal classes to consider include the lower respiratory antimicrobials, antivirals, antibacterials and antifungals.

Given that pneumonia is characterised by inflammation of the lungs, anti-inflammatory herbs with an affinity for the lower respiratory tract need to be chosen. The fluid that fills the infected lung/s indicates the use of several herbal classes including the mucolytics to break down the excess mucus and the expectorants to facilitate the removal of mucus from the lungs.

Where fever management is deemed necessary diaphoretic herbs may be employed to promote sweating. Lastly, to soothe the respiratory tract and any cough that accompanies pneumonia, soothing anti-inflammatory and demulcent herbs should be employed in conjunction with antitussives.

Specific herbal medicines

There is no specific herb for the treatment of pneumonia itself as a whole, rather herbal medicine offers a range of botanicals with different actions to support the body so that it can use its own innate intelligence to fight off the disease itself.

DROSERA SPP. (SUNDEW)

The Eclectics used *Drosera* spp. traditionally for expulsive or explosive spasmodic cough, with dryness of the air passages, whooping cough and uncontrollable irritating cough.[14] While scientific studies are lacking, we know that *Drosera* contains the active constituent known as plumbagin that has been found to inhibit bacteria that cause pneumonia. *Drosera* also functions as cough suppressant; constituents within *Drosera* known as naphthoquinones are thought to be responsible for its cough-suppressing action.[67]

ASCLEPIUS TUBEROSA (PLEURISY ROOT)

Asclepius tuberosa is a perennial native to the southern US. As its name suggests, the root is the part used and functions as an expectorant to promote the expulsion of phlegm.[68] No clinical studies have been found detailing the efficacy of *Asclepius* specifically in pneumonia; however, traditionally *Asclepius tuberosa* root was considered to be a primary lung tonic and was used by Native Americans for respiratory complaints including pneumonia.[59]

In the convalescing stage of pneumonia, and other respiratory lesions, when suppression of the expectoration and dyspnoea threaten, small doses at frequent intervals may correct the trouble. In *dry asthma* with fever, but lacking the spasmodic element, 5-drop doses of specific asclepias should do good service. As a remedy for dry and constricted *cough* it may be given in small amounts, preceded half an hour beforehand by specific lobelia in doses of 1 or 2 drops. In *catarrhal troubles* specific asclepias, well diluted, are useful as a local remedy when used early in the disease. It, as well as *Euphrasia* and *matricaria* (*Chamomilla*), is among our best drugs for snuffles, or *acute nasal catarrh of infants*. In *phthisis* it is valuable to alleviate the distressing cough and to allay irritability of the mucus surfaces, and is not without good effects on the circulation and the stomach, through its subtonic action. It is an excellent remedy for ordinary colds. It is, in fact, one of our best drugs for catarrhal conditions, whether of the pulmonary or gastrointestinal tract, especially when produced by recent colds.[67]

PRUNUS SEROTINA (WILD CHERRY)

Prunus serotina belongs to the Rosaceae family and is native to North America. It contains several constituents of which, for its antitussive action, prunasin, a cyanogenic glycoside derived from the inner bark, is most important.[68] No clinical studies have been found detailing the use of *Prunus* in isolation for the management of pneumonia; however, traditionally it was used by both the Eclectics and Native Americans for persistent cough and pneumonia:[67]

> *It [Prunus] is, therefore, valuable in all those cases where it is desirable to give tone and strength to the system, without, at the same time, causing too great an action of the heart and blood vessels, as, during convalescence from pleurisy, pneumonia, acute hepatitis, and other inflammatory and febrile diseases. Its chief property is its power of relieving irritation of the mucus surfaces, making it an admirable remedy in many gastro-intestinal, pulmonic, and urinary troubles.*

Prunus is indicated for dry and irritable coughs, particularly where the condition is chronic.

LIFESTYLE RECOMMENDATIONS

- Avoid smoking and passive smoking
- Promote expectoration with postural drainage:
  - Training of patient (and family member) will enable this to be achieved multiple times per day in the acute
  - Consider having patient attend clinic regularly in conjunction with intercostal massage and chest liniment application
  - Lymphatic drainage
- Inhalations and chest rubs using essential oils of peppermint, eucalyptus, lavender and tea tree as frequently as possible:
  - Drops on the shower floor
  - Oil burners in room
  - Chest liniments
- Keep warm and away from draughts.

Mustard poultice 1 × day

Consider using a mustard poultice if mucus is very stubborn and thick.

100 g freshly ground mustard seeds mixed with warm water (45°C) into a thick paste. Spread paste onto a cloth that is to be applied to the skin. Lay a dampened gauze on skin and then apply poultice — never directly to skin. Apply for 1 minute and then remove.

CASE STUDY

OVERVIEW

KM is a 21-year-old university student who has been bothered by a cold for most of the first semester of this year. She had been getting several colds a year though they usually did not last as long as her current one. She had the usual symptoms: sore throat, lymphadenopathy, blocked sinuses, hacking cough with moderate quantities of yellow sputum. Two days ago her cough became considerably worse. Sputum amount increased and was purulent. She had a temperature of 38.4°C and complained of pain in her left side on breathing. Respiration was shallow. She felt weak and ached all over and suffered from anorexia. Yesterday she was getting ready to go to her final exam when she collapsed in her room. Her roommate and some friends brought her to the local GP. The GP listened to her breath sounds and diagnosed pneumonia with exhaustion. She was sent to have a CXR, sputum culture and blood test. KM's diagnosis was confirmed and her GP prescribed doxycycline and bed rest.

CLINICAL EXAMINATION

Physical examination

Pale, fatigued and overstressed. Her exam and study regimen appears to be quite taxing on her.

Family history

Unremarkable.

CASE STUDY CONTINUED

Social history

Socialises regularly and parties with drugs and alcohol on a regular basis. Smokes 1–1.5 packets of 8 mg cigarettes per day to keep her weight down and to manage her stress levels. She takes ecstasy on weekends with friends and binge drinks most weekends. Her drink of choice is vodka and tonic but she often shares cocktails or champagne with her girlfriends.

Dietary history

Often skips breakfast relying on coffee (no milk or sugar) and cigarettes to keep her going. She sometimes forgets to eat lunch or may have a salad sandwich. Dinner consists of pasta and tomato sauce. She rarely eats vegetables or fruit unless they are mixed into things and rarely cooks for herself. She lives with two school friends close to the university campus and is a member of the university gym which she attends most days to swim in the indoor swimming pool.

INVESTIGATIONS

CXR results

Area of uniform opacity confined within the boundaries of the left lower lobe. Slight loss of volume and air-filled bronchi can be seen within the affected lobe.

Sputum culture

Streptococcus pneumoniae +++

Laboratory results

Test	Result	Normal range
WBC	21.1 × 103/mm^3	5–10 × 10^3
ESR	74 mm/hr	2–20
CRP	162 mg/L	0–25

Anthropometric measurements

Weight: 48.2 kg
Height: 1.63 m
BMI: 18.2 kg/m^2

TREATMENT PROTOCOL

KM's presentation was concerning as there were obvious triggers that had prompted her pneumonia infection. Consideration of the following salient aspects included:

Health influence	Relevant treatment objective
Presentation	KM requires acute management to eradicate the pneumonia infection and rebuild her body for optimal recovery. Long-term considerations require acknowledgment and appropriate treatment. Treatment was structured on a priority basis
Lifestyle and social	Refrain from alcohol, smoking and recreational drugs Referral to university counsellor for long-term support and recovery

CASE STUDY CONTINUED

Health influence	Relevant treatment objective
Psychological	Concern regarding KM's potential eating disorder and low BMI. Referral letter to GP to discuss management was conducted and discussion with KM planned at follow-up appointment
Financial	Due to study commitment and financial pressures, prescription was limited and adjusted accordingly
Dietary	Poor dietary intake warranted query regarding potential disordered eating behaviour. Dietary modifications (acute) to support recovery are essential

Herbal medicine

Inula helenium (elecampane): 60 mL
Hydrastis canadensis (goldenseal) 1 : 3: 40 mL
Thymus vulgaris (thyme): 30 mL
Echinacea spp. (echinacea blend): 70 mL
Grindelia camporum (grindelia): 20 mL

Dose: 5 mL q.i.d. in the acute with reduction to 5 mL t.d.s. in approximately 3–4 days and maintained until follow-up appointment (2 weeks post).

Other

Mustard poultice 1 × day

Consider using a mustard poultice (see above) if mucus is very stubborn and thick.

Nutritional medicine

Dietary

KM was sent to stay at her parents and they were contacted and encouraged to help KM to adopt the following dietary suggestions:

- Avoid all immune-suppressant foods (sugar, refined foods, caffeine, alcohol)
- Increase intake of fresh fruits and vegetables
- Increase intake of garlic, onions, horseradish, ginger and chilli
- General wholefood diet
- Adequate fluid intake — juices, broths, soups, herbal teas.

Supplemental

Vitamin C + bioflavonoids: 1 g q.i.d.
NAC: 250 mg q.i.d.
Probiotic (multistrain): 45×10^9 b.i.d.

Lifestyle/Education

- Avoid smoking and passive smoking
- Avoid recreational drugs
- Promote expectoration with postural drainage
- Inhalations (steam) and chest rubs using essential oils (respiratory blend)
- Keep warm and away from draughts
- Sleep, rest and recuperation
- No exercise in the acute stage.

BRONCHITIS

NOTE: A general summary of the differences between acute and chronic bronchitis is included in this section; however, a full discussion regarding chronic bronchitis can be found in the next topic, chronic obstructive pulmonary disease (COPD).

Classification and aetiology

Bronchitis is classified as acute or chronic bronchitis.

ACUTE BRONCHITIS

Acute bronchitis is an acute infectious disease causing inflammation of the bronchi. It usually occurs in previously well individuals and it is associated with a normal chest radiograph (although rarely undertaken). Infective organisms can only be identified in up to a third of cases. The viruses most commonly implicated are influenza A and B, parainfluenza, coronavirus, rhinovirus and respiratory syncytial virus. Bacterial causes are rare and include *Chlamydia pneumoniae, Bordetella pertussis* and *Mycoplasma pneumoniae.* Non-infectious causes of acute cough include allergy, asthma, environmental exposures, heart failure, gastro-oesophageal reflux and tumour. Bacterial infection causes fewer than 10% of the cases of infectious bronchitis; only *Bordetella pertussis, Mycoplasma pneumoniae* and *Chlamydia pneumoniae* have been identified as primary agents.

Other factors which can predispose to this kind of bacterial infection include cold, damp, dust and cigarette smoking.

CHRONIC BRONCHITIS

Strict diagnostic criterion for diagnosis of chronic bronchitis is: productive cough on most days on at least 3 consecutive months for more than 2 successive years, provided other causes of productive cough such as bronchiectasis and untreated chronic asthma have been excluded.

Overview

Acute bronchitis is an acute infectious disease causing inflammation of the bronchi.

Pathogenesis

ACUTE BRONCHITIS

Respiratory viruses appear to be the most common cause of acute bronchitis with fewer than 10% of patients having a bacterial infection. The organism responsible for acute bronchitis is rarely identified in clinical practice because viral cultures and serological assays are not routinely performed. There is mucosal injury, epithelial cell damage, and the release of pro-inflammatory mediators. Transient airflow obstruction and transient bronchial hyperresponsiveness can be seen in approximately 40% of previously healthy individuals with an acute viral respiratory tract infection.[69]

CHRONIC BRONCHITIS

Chronic bronchitis appears to develop in response to long-continued exposure to various types of irritants on the bronchial mucosa in susceptible individuals.

These irritants are:

- Cigarette tobacco smoke (the most important irritant); however, for unknown reasons only about 15% of smokers develop clinically significant chronic bronchitis
- Dust
- Smokes and fumes occurring at workplace in certain industries (cadmium is especially toxic)
- General atmospheric pollution in industrial cities and towns particularly with sulfur dioxide, nitrogen oxides and particulates from burning fossil fuels (increasingly important problem).

In susceptible individuals these irritants, directly or through the autonomic nervous system, induce hypersecretion of mucus, cause hypertrophy of mucous glands, and lead to the formation of new mucus-secreting goblet cells in the bronchial mucosa. *Infection* usually with *Streptococcus pneumoniae* (pneumococcus) and/or *Haemophilus influenzae* is very important in aggravating the established condition, but it is not essential for development/progression of the condition. In other words chronic bronchitis is not a chronic bacterial infection. It is now known that many exacerbations of chronic bronchitis are due to upper respiratory viral infections (e.g. rhinoviruses) and to environmental factors such as exposure to *dampness, fog* and *sudden temperature changes.* Pathologically, there is mucosal oedema with infiltration with macrophages and neutrophils, hypertrophy of bronchial glands, hypertrophy/hyperplasia of bronchial smooth muscle and permanent structural damage (scarring) of the airway walls that reduce the calibre of the air passages.

A major proportion of airflow obstruction in chronic bronchitis is not due to bronchial smooth muscle contraction and is thus *irreversible* unlike the airflow obstruction in chronic asthma. Air becomes trapped in the alveoli because the degree of obstruction is greater during expiration. Overdistension of the alveoli results and disruption of their walls may occur (*emphysema*).

Signs and symptoms

Acute bronchitis

The first symptom is an irritating, unproductive cough accompanied by upper retrosternal discomfort or burning pain caused by tracheitis. When the bronchi become involved there is also a sensation of tightness in the chest, and breathlessness with wheeze may be present. The sputum is at first scanty, mucoid, viscid and difficult to produce, and occasionally may be streaked with blood.

After 1–2 days it becomes mucopurulent and more copious. As the infection extends down the bronchial tree there may be associated pyrexia of 38–39°C. In the vast majority of cases recovery takes place spontaneously over the next 4–8 days without the patient ever becoming seriously ill.[15]

Occasionally breathlessness and productive cough increase when the infection reaches the smaller bronchi and bronchioles ('bronchiolitis') and the condition becomes indistinguishable from bronchopneumonia. Persistent fever suggests this complication.

Cough-variant asthma may be difficult to distinguish from uncomplicated acute bronchitis, which may also be associated with transient bronchial hyperresponsiveness but typically resolves after 2–3 weeks. Acute bronchitis is a self-limited respiratory disorder, and when the cough persists for >3 weeks, other diagnoses must be considered.

Chronic bronchitis

The main feature is repeated attacks of productive cough, usually after colds during the winter months, but eventually cough is present all the year round.

Morning cough with large amounts of sputum is characteristic, especially in heavy smokers (smoking reduces ciliary clearance of mucus).

Sputum may be mucoid (whitish) and tenacious and occasionally streaked with blood (haemoptysis); purulent sputum was thought to be an indication of bacterial infection, but this may not be the case in all patients.

Wheeze, breathlessness and tightness in the chest are almost always found; central cyanosis due to impaired gas exchange and hypoxaemia may follow when the mucous membranes of the lips and tongue appear bluish.

For reasons not entirely clear, the patients tend to be obese.

Clinical pattern often referred to as the blue and bloated type may be seen in late stage of chronic bronchitis; these patients are cyanosed and bloated from obesity and right-sided heart failure (see below) with consequent peripheral oedema. They may appear drowsy due to the effect of retained carbon dioxide (hypercapnia) on the CNS.

Complications

Acute bronchitis

Although a single episode of bronchitis usually is not cause for concern, it can lead to pneumonia in some people. Older adults, infants, smokers and people with chronic respiratory disorders or heart problems are at greatest risk of getting pneumonia. Other complications include emphysema, right-sided heart failure and pulmonary hypertension.

Chronic bronchitis

Pulmonary hypertension is due to reflex closure of pulmonary arterioles in hypoventilated areas of the lungs as well as to destruction of the pulmonary vascular bed by associated emphysema.

Right ventricular failure (cor pulmonale) is a final consequence of the pulmonary hypertension and the major cause of death in these patients.

Differential diagnosis

Acute bronchitis

The diagnosis of acute bronchitis is established in a patient who has the sudden onset of cough, with or without sputum expectoration, and without evidence of pneumonia, the common cold, acute asthma or an acute exacerbation of chronic bronchitis.[70] Pneumonia is a relatively frequent and important cause of cough that must be excluded as a diagnosis because it may be associated with significant mortality.[2]

Chronic bronchitis

Emphysema, bronchiectasis, carcinoma, chronic obstructive pulmonary disease (COPD) — see next topic for full discussion.

Naturopathic diagnosis

Acute bronchitis

Due to the nature of this condition, diagnosis is based on clinical presentation.

Chronic bronchitis

It is largely clinical when the above-mentioned criteria are met. Consideration of lifestyle factors, dietary and general nutritional status is essential. See next topic for full discussion.

Investigations

Acute bronchitis

Rarely necessary as diagnosis is generally made on clinical grounds in primary care. Influenza virus is likely if acute bronchitis occurs during an outbreak or epidemic of influenza. C-reactive protein (CRP) is generally not elevated and chest radiograph is generally normal.

Chronic bronchitis

X-ray of the lungs usually produces no characteristic abnormalities.

Pulmonary function tests are abnormal — TLC and RV are reduced, forced expiratory volume in one second (FEV_1), peak expiratory flow (PEF) and VC are also reduced, which is consistent with airflow obstruction. These findings are not substantially improved by inhaled bronchodilators although most patients report subjective improvement.

In more advanced stages hypoxaemia (reduction of PO_2) can be found, later on followed by hypercapnia (a rise in PCO_2).

Exercise test (e.g. distance walked in 10 minutes, number of stairs the patient can climb in a continuous attempt) is a valuable estimate of everyday disability.

SPECIFIC NATUROPATHIC INVESTIGATIONS

As this is an acute condition, further investigations are unnecessary. If a chronic picture eventuates, immunological studies and investigations into immune onslaughts and environmental influences are required.

Therapeutic considerations

ALLOPATHIC TREATMENT

Treatment guidelines derived from the available evidence recommend against routine antibiotic therapy for uncomplicated acute bronchitis. A systematic review found antibiotic therapy for acute bronchitis offers only modest benefit. Antibiotic therapy is, however, recommended for acute bronchitis caused by pertussis. A Cochrane review of antibiotics for pertussis[71] found that short-term therapy with azithromycin (3 days), clarithromycin (7 days) or erythromycin (7 days) was as effective as long-term therapy with erythromycin in eradicating infection from the nasopharynx with fewer side effects in the short-term treatment. Although antibiotics were effective in eliminating *B. pertussis*, they did not alter the subsequent clinical course of the illness. There is insufficient evidence to determine the benefit of prophylactic treatment of pertussis contacts. Bronchodilators may be beneficial in individuals who demonstrate airflow obstruction. Symptomatic therapy, including inhaled bronchodilators for those who show evidence of airway obstruction and antitussives for those who have chest discomfort or sleep disturbance from cough, may be added.[2]

CLINICAL DECISION MAKING AND RATIONALE

Acute bronchitis

- It is essential to control symptoms, improve the immune response and eradicate the infection
- Identification of known causes of triggers is essential for successful outcome. For example, smoking must be prevented
- Dietary exclusions are essential if they are known to aggravate the patient or if a definitive diagnosis has been made. In the short term, elimination of known immune suppressant foods such as sugar is required
- During acute infection it is important to give frequent dosages of all prescriptions (especially herbal medicines).

Chronic bronchitis

- Reduction of bronchial irritation is achieved through stopping smoking (the only measure that can slow down progression of the disease), avoidance of dusty and smoke-laden atmospheres and even a change of occupation if necessary
- Treatment of bacterial respiratory infection (if identified) is very important; the vast majority of bacterial infections are caused by *Streptococcus pneumoniae* and *Haemophilus influenzae* which respond to many broad-spectrum antibiotics; however, this type of treatment does not significantly alter the course of the disease
- It is useful to try to stimulate expectoration by giving the patient plenty of fluids, hot drinks or inhalations of steam
- Bronchodilator medications can be tried, and their value in each particular case should be assessed. In general they are much less effective than in bronchial asthma, but they still improve symptoms and exercise tolerance
- The type of chronic inflammation found in chronic bronchitis does not respond well to corticosteroids in

contrast to bronchial asthma, but nevertheless inhaled steroids may be tried to assess their effectiveness in individual patients

- In case of severe exacerbations, hospital treatment is necessary with bronchodilator therapy, intravenous rehydration, oxygen therapy and massage (tapotement and percussion) to assist expectoration
- See next topic for full discussion.

Therapeutic application

HISTORICAL PERSPECTIVE

Chronic bronchitis was first named and described in 1808. The disease has of course been known since earliest times and was traditionally described as a disease of excessive phlegm. Traditional remedies included garlic, pepper, cinnamon, turpentine, coffee, ipecac and potassium nitrate. Many modern bronchodilator drugs are derived from the traditional folk remedies including ephedrine, atropine and methylxanthines.[72]

NATUROPATHIC PERSPECTIVE

Naturopathy recognises that eradicating the causative infective trigger and supporting the body's ability to fight infection are the primary goals in acute bronchitis. Stress, depression and other negative emotions may play a significant role in allowing the immune system to become overwhelmed with the infection and interfere with patient recovery. Lack of sleep, poor nutrition, mould or living in damp environments, lack of exercise and relaxation, and pollution may also increase an individual's susceptibility to contracting acute bronchitis and affect their recovery. For patients suffering from chronic bronchitis, it is important to acknowledge that their lifestyle and dietary choices will significantly affect the successful outcome of treatment.

NUTRITIONAL MEDICINE (DIETARY)

Dietary therapeutic objectives

The diet should be highly nutritious yet easy to digest and not taxing on the digestive system. Any mucus-forming foods should be avoided. Specific nutritional supplementation may be used to assist the body in fighting the infection while reducing symptoms of inflammation, swelling and pain.

Specific dietary treatments

DIETARY INCLUSIONS

- Increase intake of fresh fruits and vegetables
- Increase intake of garlic, onions, horseradish, ginger and chilli
- General wholefood diet
- Adequate fluid intake — water, herbal teas, juices, broths.

DIETARY EXCLUSIONS

- Sugar, salt, saturated fats, cow's dairy, wheat, processed foods, additives, preservatives, colourings
- Avoid known allergens/intolerances as necessary.

SAMPLE DAILY DIET

BREAKFAST	
Toast of high-quality, stoneground bread (such as rye, spelt, millet). Spread with nut butter made from almonds, Brazil nuts and cashews and topped with alfalfa sprouts	Essential fatty acids, protein content and taste achieved by nut butter.
LUNCH	
Vegetable stew made with an assortment of seasonal vegetables, spiced appropriately. Protein selection from steamed white fish or grilled lamb tenderloin	Vegetables provide a range of vitamins and minerals that will enhance the immune system. Stewing allows the vegetables to be partially broken down allowing for easier assimilation. Heavy foods and poor absorption can further create more mucus in the body.
DINNER	
Chicken and vegetable soup	The humble chicken soup or congee for respiratory complaints is not just a myth. Researchers in the US have found that the ingredients in chicken soup help to inhibit neutrophils (white blood cells that stimulate the production of mucus), which are released in great numbers by viral infections.
SNACKS	
Baked apple in skin stuffed with walnuts, cinnamon and ginger	
BEVERAGES	
Optimal hydration to thin the mucus chosen from pure water, herbal teas and fresh vegetable juices	

NUTRITIONAL MEDICINE (SUPPLEMENTAL)

Nutritional medicine therapeutic objectives

- Improve and stimulate the immune response to eradicate the pathogen
- Restore mucous membrane integrity of the bronchi to eliminate mucus and catarrh.

Specific nutrients required

VITAMIN C

Studies have shown a reduction of at least 80% in the incidence of pneumonia and bronchitis in patients taking vitamin C group[73] and one randomised trial reported substantial treatment benefit from vitamin C in elderly UK patients hospitalised with pneumonia or bronchitis. A total of 57 elderly patients admitted to hospital with acute respiratory infections (bronchitis and bronchopneumonia) received either 200 mg vitamin C per day or placebo. This relatively modest oral dose led to a significant increase in plasma and white cell vitamin C concentration even in the presence of acute respiratory infection. Using a clinical scoring system based on major symptoms of the respiratory condition, patients supplemented with the vitamin fared significantly better than those on the placebo. This was particularly the case for those commencing the trial most severely ill, many of whom had very low plasma and white cell vitamin C concentrations on admission.[74]

VITAMIN D

Vitamin D deficiency is associated with an increased susceptibility to respiratory infections, but there are no studies on its use for acute bronchitis. Increasing evidence is emerging to support the role of vitamin D in immunity. Vitamin D deficiency has been shown to increase the risk of upper respiratory tract infections. Deficiency has also been found to decrease the forced expiratory volume in 1 s (FEV_1) in asthma and wheezing diseases, hence the benefits of supplementation in bronchitis. Vitamin D appears capable of inhibiting pulmonary inflammatory responses while enhancing innate defence mechanisms against respiratory pathogens.[75] Population-based studies showing an association between circulating vitamin D levels and lung function provide strong justification for its application in bronchitis and other respiratory diseases.

ZINC

Zinc is essential for proper respiratory function via the role it plays in maintaining phagocytic and natural killer cell function as well as cellular and humoral immunity. In the respiratory system, zinc functions firstly as an antioxidant and secondly as an antiapoptotic agent.[76] Supplementation is likely to be beneficial; however, no clinical studies have been reported for acute bronchitis.

VITAMIN A

Vitamin A is a primary component of the body's immune system. A diet with suboptimal levels of vitamin A has been linked with an increased risk of chronic bronchitis.[77]

VITAMIN E

Vitamin E plays a key role in immune responses where it has been shown to enhance humoral and cell-mediated immunity.

SELENIUM

Selenium enhances the activity of white blood cells that protect against certain viruses and bacteria. Through its action as an antioxidant it protects against free radicals which damage lung tissue and are known to be involved in the pathogenesis in many chronic diseases.

MAGNESIUM

Magnesium plays a key role in reducing spasm and constriction of the respiratory muscles via its role as a bronchodilator. Magnesium has also been shown to inhibit cholinergic neuromuscular transmission and stabilises mast cells and T-lymphocytes, thus providing a rationale for its use.

Dosage requirements

The dosage requirements listed below are based on adult doses that are reported in the literature:

- Vitamin A: 20 000 IU twice daily for 1 month, then to 15 000 daily
- Vitamin C: 500–1000 mg every 3 hours up to bowel tolerance
- Vitamin D: 1000 IU daily
- Calcium: 1000 mg/d
- Magnesium: 500 mg/d
- Zinc: 30–50 mg/d
- Vitamin E: 400 IU/d
- Selenium: 150 micrograms/day.

HERBAL MEDICINE

Herbal medicine therapeutic objectives

ACUTE BRONCHITIS

During the dry, unproductive cough phase demulcents are used to moisten and cool the mucous membrane and anticatarrhals are used when the sputum is copious. The implications of this are that it is likely that as the condition changes in character the formula should change slightly to meet the changing treatment goals.

In effect this will mean that in the initial dry phase demulcents (along with immune modulators, diaphoretics, expectorants, antimicrobials and antitussives) will be used. As the condition progresses to a more copious mucus output, the need for demulcents will lessen and the need for anticatarrhals will increase. It is also likely at this time that diaphoretics will probably no longer be required (i.e. the feverish, hot stage has passed). Be alert to the changing treatment goals and respond accordingly with the appropriate herbs that represent the actions required to meet these changing treatment goals.

Acute bronchitis needs to be treated using frequent doses of herbal therapeutics:

- Support the immune system
- Reduce the infection and inflammation
- Ease excessive cough
- Clear mucus secretions and improve expectoration.

CHRONIC BRONCHITIS

- As above
- Main aim to reduce the activity of the mucus secreting glands and goblet cells. Excessive mucus coats bronchial walls and clogs bronchioles, giving poor clearance ability.

Herbal medicine classes

Herbal therapeutics for acute bronchitis include the following:

- Immune-enhancing herbs are paramount for conditions such as bronchitis where the immune system is compromised. They may work to both modulate and stimulate immune system function or by balancing the activity of the immune system. The immune enhancers are an extremely important class of herbs for the management of bronchitis, particularly for preventing the progression of acute bronchitis into chronic bronchitis.
- Depending on the source of infection (bacterial/viral) either an antibacterial or antiviral botanical specific for the respiratory system will need to be used. These agents elicit a specific immune response to bacterial- or viral-infection-causing pathogens.
- Bronchitis is characterised by inflammation of the bronchial tree that results in pain and irritation for the patient, hence the benefits of applying bronchial anti-inflammatory herbs and soothing demulcents which have a specific affinity for the bronchi. These herbs help to reduce inflammation, easing the discomfort of the patient.
- Increased mucus production highlights the possible application of three classes of herbs, the mucolytics, the anticatarrhals and the expectorants. Anticatarrhal herbs reduce the formation of mucus, while mucolytics aid in the breakdown of mucus, making it easier to remove. The application of expectorant herbs facilitates the coughing up of residue (and hence aids in its removal from the body). Diaphoretic herbs (also known as sudorifics) may also be used to promote sweating such as in the case of fever associated with bronchitis.
- Antitussive herbs should be used to provide relief from cough, and mucous membrane tonics and trophorestoratives may be used to heal the compromised respiratory lining.

Specific herbal medicines

ADHATODA VASICA (ADHATODA)

Adhatoda has many common names, including bansa and basuti in Hindi and vasaka and amalaka in Sanskrit. Adhatoda, also known as Malabar nut tree, grows as a multi-branched, dense shrub that can be found throughout the plains and foothill regions of India. It has white flowers and opposite ascending branches with long, dark green leaves. The leaves and roots are used medicinally. Scientific interest has focused on vasicine, one of the major alkaloids in adhatoda, from which the mucolytic drug bromhexine was developed. Adhatoda leaves contain quinazoline alkaloids (0.5–2%), including vasicine (45–95%), vasicinine, vasicinone, oxyvasicinine, deoxyvasicine, deoxyvasicinone and vasicinol. Vasicinone and oxyvasicinine are auto-oxidation products.

Adhatoda has expectorant, bronchodilator, mucolytic, antispasmodic, anti-inflammatory, antiasthmatic and oxytocic properties. It is indicated for respiratory diseases including asthma, acute and chronic bronchitis, bronchiectasis and emphysema. It is also used for post-partum haemorrhage, and to assist uterine involution, as well as for dyspepsia and, locally, for gum disease. The usual adult dosage is 1–2 g daily although the dried leaf has been administered in powder form in doses of 30 g. Fresh leaves of bansa juice are normally given at doses of 10–20 mL once or twice a day. An overdose, however, can cause nausea or occasional vomiting. Adhatoda is contraindicated in pregnancy due to its oxytocic activity.

Vasicine has been the focus of much research and is the raw product from which the drug bromhexine was developed. Studies have demonstrated that vasicine and vasicinone both have bronchodilatory activity. Antitussive activity was not observed, but vasicine increased ciliary movement and inhibited bronchial secretions in isolated tissue. When given orally, however, adhatoda extract had a marked antitussive activity (comparable to codeine) against coughing induced by peripheral irritant stimuli. It was one-quarter as active as codeine in preventing coughing induced by the electrical stimulation of tracheal mucosa. The bioavailability of vasicine can be increased by the addition of *Piper longum* (long pepper).

There have only been a small number of clinical studies of adhatoda extract. Early, uncontrolled clinical studies in India found that adhatoda extract provided good relief of acute bronchitis especially where the sputum was thick and tenacious. The extract relieved the cough and thinned the sputum in patients with chronic bronchitis and provided mild relief for asthma sufferers. More recently a randomised double-blind clinical trial reported that a herbal formulation containing adhatoda, echinacea, eleutherococcus and liquorice significantly improved the symptoms of uncomplicated upper respiratory disease compared with placebo.[78]

PELARGONIUM SIDOIDES (PELARGONIUM)

Research has shown that *Pelargonium sidoides* and its isolated constituents have moderate direct antibacterial potencies and notable immune modulatory capabilities. The immune modulatory activities are mediated mainly by the release of tumour necrosis factor alpha (TNF-α) and nitric oxides, the stimulation of interferon-beta, and the increase of natural killer cell activity. Further biological activities in vitro are improved phagocytosis, oxidative burst and intracellular killing of human peripheral blood phagocytes, and an inhibition of the interaction of group A streptococci and host epithelia. *P. sidoides* has been shown in placebo-controlled clinical trials and in several observational studies to be a successful treatment of the common cold, acute bronchitis and acute rhinosinusitis. In all controlled clinical trials, treatment with pelargonium was superior in efficacy, with a significant reduction of disease-specific symptoms compared with placebo, and showed a very good tolerability.[79]

ALTHAEA OFFICINALIS (MARSHMALLOW)

Traditionally *Althaea officinalis* root was used to treat respiratory complaints such as hoarseness as well as mucous membrane disorders including catarrh and pneumonia. It contains mucilage, which helps coat the throat and act as a cough suppressant. *Althaea* in a combined herbal preparation in conjunction with dry ivy leaf extract (main active ingredient), decoction of thyme and aniseed, and mucilage of marshmallow root were investigated in an open clinical trial.[80] A total of 62 patients with a mean age of 50 years (range 16–89 years) were treated. The patients had either an irritating cough in consequence of common cold ($n = 29$), bronchitis ($n = 20$) or respiratory tract diseases with formation of viscous mucus ($n = 15$). The mean daily intake the patients ingested was 10 mL (range 7.5–15 mL) of syrup with the mean duration of treatment 12 days (range 3–23 days).

At the end of the final visit all patients showed an improvement in symptoms as compared with baseline. Doctors and patients assessed efficacy as good or very good in 86% and 90% of the cases, respectively, highlighting the efficacy of these botanicals for alleviation of cough in respiratory conditions such as bronchitis.

LIFESTYLE RECOMMENDATIONS

- Avoid cough suppressants
- Use foot baths and hot packs to stimulate circulation (especially for chronic presentations)
- Use inhalations and chest rubs
- Keep warm and away from draughts
- Use postural drainage/physiotherapy
- Assess and remove household and environmental triggers
- Avoid smoking and passive smoking.

CASE STUDY

OVERVIEW

KB is a 37-year-old account executive who has come to see you because of acute bronchitis. Her doctor recently diagnosed her condition but she has refused to take allopathic medications. She is experiencing tightness in the chest as well as a tickling, non-productive cough that keep her awake at night. Her cough is starting to get more productive.

She has been under significant amounts of stress at work and has neglected her health, diet and lifestyle.

CLINICAL EXAMINATION

General inspection

Alert, cooperative, fatigued.

Vital signs

BP: 115/75 mmHg sitting/standing
Temperature: 38.3°C
Pulse: 88 bpm (usually 70 bpm)
Respiratory rate: 17 resp/min
Height: 1.60 m
Weight: 60 kg
BMI: 23.4 kg/m^2

CASE STUDY CONTINUED

Respiratory

Throat: Mild pharyngitis
Chest inspection: Unremarkable
Palpation: Trachea — midline
Supraclavicular/Axillary nodes — nil
Percussion: Resonant all zones
Auscultation: Adventitious sounds (crackles) — mild — confirming bronchitis

SUMMARY OF FINDINGS

- Fever
- Malaise
- Mild rhinorrhoea
- Dyspnoea
- Myalgia/arthralgia
- Adventitious sounds (crackles).

TREATMENT PROTOCOL

Due to the acute nature of the presentation and the patient's avoidance of antibiotic therapy, treatment was more aggressive and comprehensive to successfully eradicate the infection. Sleep was deemed a priority for successful recovery; hence multiple herbal medicine prescriptions were made. Expectoration was stimulated throughout the day and relaxation at night.

HERBAL MEDICINE

Day formula

Euphorbia hirta (euphorbia): 20 mL
Inula helenium (elecampane): 60 mL
Thymus vulgaris (thyme): 30 mL
Echinacea spp. (echinacea blend): 70 mL
Plantago lanceolata (ribwort): 40 mL
Dose 5 mL t.d.s.

Night formula

Prunus serotina (wild cherry bark): 50 mL
Glycyrrhiza glabra (liquorice): 30 mL
Althaea officinalis (marshmallow) — Glycetract: 30 mL
Dose 5 mL before bed shaken thoroughly and repeat doses as required throughout the night (maximum 20 mL during the night)

Diaphoretic tea

Infusion of *Alchemilla millefolium* (yarrow), *Mentha x piperita* (peppermint) and *Sambucus nigra* (elderflower) drunk as hot as possible throughout the day.

Fresh sliced ginger and lemon juice (fresh) can be added to encourage diaphoretic effect and further stimulate immune response.

NUTRITIONAL MEDICINE

Dietary

KB was advised to avoid dairy products, refined foods and sugar, caffeine and soft drinks. She was encouraged to drink warm herbal teas (as above) and warm drinks of lemon juice with manuka honey.

CASE STUDY CONTINUED

She was encouraged to eat as appetite encouraged and to ensure that food was easy to swallow and digest — soups, stews, broths, casseroles.

Supplemental

Vitamin C powder (mixed salts with bioflavonoids): 1 g q.i.d. in acute and then reduced to 1 g b.i.d.
Zinc citrate (or as zinc lozenges): 30 mg t.d.s. in acute, then reduced to 30 mg
NAC: 250 mg t.d.s.

LIFESTYLE/EDUCATION

- Rest, adequate sleep and stress reduction are essential
- Encourage elimination through sweating — throughout the night especially
- Keep warm and away from draughts
- Postural drainage with essential oils and steam inhalations
- Appropriate hygiene to prevent reinfection and infection of others.

CHRONIC OBSTRUCTIVE PULMONARY DISEASE (COPD)

Epidemiology

COPD develops over many years and is mainly found to affect middle-aged and older people while asthma affects people of all ages. The prevalence of COPD increases with age and mostly occurs in people aged 55 and over.[81] According to the 2014–15 Australian Health Survey, the prevalence of COPD in Australians aged 45 and over was 5.1%, an estimated 460 400 people. The prevalence did not differ significantly between males and females.[82]

COPD affects an estimated 8.8% of Indigenous Australians aged 45 and over. This equates to approximately 10 300 people; however, the statistics are believed to be underreported in this demographic.[83] COPD prevalence in Indigenous Australians is 2.5 times higher than the prevalence for other Australians.

Aetiology

A substantial body of evidence indicates that tobacco smoke is the most important risk factor for COPD (80–90% of patients in Western societies), although other environmental, occupational and genetic (e.g. α1-antitrypsin deficiency) factors are also involved.[84]

Overview

Chronic obstructive pulmonary disease (COPD) is a disease of the lungs in which the airways become narrowed. This leads to a limitation of the flow of air to and from the lungs causing shortness of breath. In contrast to asthma, the limitation of airflow is poorly reversible and usually gets progressively worse over time.

CLASSIFICATION OF COPD SEVERITY

See Table 14.8.

Pathogenesis

Airway obstruction can be due to loss of supporting elastic recoil from the lung tissue and/or luminal narrowing as a result of airway wall thickening.[85] The pathogenesis of COPD is strongly linked to the effects of cigarette smoke, with chronic lung inflammation being a characteristic feature in all stages of COPD, even the early stages. Systemic markers of inflammation, particularly C-reactive protein, fibrinogen and tumour necrosis factor alpha, have recently been shown to be significantly increased in plasma and associated with reduced lung function, functional capacity and energy metabolism in patients with stable COPD, compared with healthy patients. These studies suggest that COPD is a complex multicomponent disease that affects both the lungs and the organs outside the lungs. Indeed, COPD patients commonly have comorbid medical conditions, such as cardiovascular disease, lung cancer, muscle wasting, diabetes and depression, which are likely to impact quality of life, increase hospitalisation and reduce survival. Referral for advice or specialist investigation may be appropriate at any stage of the disease. Long-term oxygen therapy, ventilatory support (non-invasive ventilation and conventional invasive mechanical ventilation) and surgical approaches (bullectomy, lung volume reduction surgery and lung transplantation) can improve lung function, symptoms and possibly also survival. These forms of intervention are usually reserved for patients with more severe disease and those with respiratory failure, who are unlikely to be routinely managed by primary care clinicians.[75]

TABLE 14.8 Classification of COPD severity

Factor	Mild	Moderate	Severe
Spirometry findings: postbronchodilator FEV_1	60% to 80% predicted	40% to 59% predicted	Less than 40% predicted
Functional assessment (activities of daily living)	Few symptoms No effect on daily activities Breathless on moderate exertion	Increasing dyspnoea Breathless on the flat Increasing limitation of daily activities	Dyspnoea on minimal exertion Daily activities severely curtailed

Source: Bellamy D, Smith J. Role of primary care in early diagnosis and effective management of COPD. Int J Clin Pract 2007;61(8):1380–9.
FEV_1 = forced expiratory volume in 1 second

Signs and symptoms

Symptoms of COPD include breathlessness, cough, sputum production, recurrent respiratory infection and wheezing. Typically breathlessness, which may be the patient's only symptom, initially occurs only on exertion but worsens insidiously over several years.[75]

Complications

The most common cause of COPD exacerbations is bacterial and viral infection. Chronic bacterial contamination of the airway is common in COPD and may be an important part of the pathogenic process even when the disease is stable. Hypoxaemic patients with COPD may develop pulmonary hypertension, which may be present for years without causing symptoms. In some patients it leads to the development of the clinical syndrome of cor pulmonale and heart failure.[75]

Diagnosis

The diagnosis of COPD requires lung function assessments. Correct identification of patients with COPD has proved difficult in general practice. Patients are often unwilling to report symptoms, which may play a part in the apparent underdiagnosis of COPD. Patients often accept their symptoms as part of ageing or a consequence of smoking, making them less likely to report symptoms. COPD is often not diagnosed until there are clinical symptoms and the disease is moderately advanced. Early diagnosis of COPD is recommended in any patient over the age of 35 who has chronic cough (present intermittently or every day throughout the day), chronic sputum production, shortness of breath (dyspnoea), frequent winter 'bronchitis' or wheeze and/or a history of exposure to disease risk factors (particularly tobacco smoke, occupational dusts and chemicals, and smoke from home cooking and heating fuels).

A detailed medical history (including the presence of allergic airways disease and other comorbid disease, for example heart disease and rheumatic disease, family history of COPD, pattern of symptom development, history of exacerbations and hospitalisation as a result of respiratory disorder, and impact of disease on the patient's lifestyle) is particularly useful for a new patient who may have COPD because it may aid in the development of specific management strategies at the outset.[59]

Differential diagnosis

There is an overlap of chronic bronchitis, emphysema and asthma within COPD. Chronic bronchitis, airway narrowing and emphysema are independent effects of cigarette smoking, and may occur in various combinations. Asthma is by definition associated with reversible airway obstruction. Patients with asthma whose airway obstruction is completely reversible do not have COPD.[75]

Naturopathic diagnosis

Because of the aetiology of COPD, a holistic assessment is essential; however, diagnosis considers the aetiological parameters paramount to the development of the condition.

Investigations

SPIROMETRY

Spirometry is the best screening tool for COPD and is sensitive enough to detect COPD in its early stages, long before disabling effects are apparent. It should, therefore, be used to confirm the presence of the disease in any patient thought to be at risk of COPD. Spirometry is a simple technique to assess lung function in terms of maximal volume of air forcibly exhaled from the point of maximal inspiration (forced vital capacity (FVC)) and the volume of air exhaled during the first second of this manoeuvre (forced expiratory volume in 1 s (FEV_1)). It is suggested that a postbronchodilator FEV_1 of <80% predicted together with an FEV_1/FVC ratio of <70% is indicative of airflow limitation that is not fully reversible.[59]

OTHER MARKERS OF COPD

FEV_1 does not fully reflect the burden of a multi-component disease such as COPD and other markers, such as the level of breathlessness, exacerbations and hospitalisation, can provide a more complete picture of how the disease is affecting any given individual. Peak flow monitoring is not generally recommended in COPD; however, this may be useful in differential diagnosis of patients with asthma and in COPD patients with comorbid asthma.

SPECIFIC NATUROPATHIC INVESTIGATIONS

Because of the aetiology of COPD, a holistic assessment is essential. Repeated infections warrant consideration into immunological status, though extended investigations may not be required.

Therapeutic considerations

CLINICAL DECISION MAKING AND RATIONALE

COPD is both preventable and treatable. While COPD management previously focused on the reduction and control of symptoms, it is now appreciated that improving the health status and quality of life, preventing disease progression, preventing and treating exacerbations and complications, and reducing mortality are equally important.

Therapeutic application

ALLOPATHIC PERSPECTIVE

The GOLD guidelines have proposed four main components of COPD management:

1. Assessing and monitoring disease
2. Reducing the risk factors
3. Managing stable COPD
4. Managing exacerbations.

These goals can be achieved by the initiation of comprehensive management initiatives for COPD that include advice and support for smoking cessation, early diagnosis, education and self-management, timely implementation of effective management strategies and multidisciplinary pulmonary rehabilitation programs.[59]

Pharmacological treatment strategies

Several pharmacological interventions are currently recommended for the management of COPD, including bronchodilators, glucocorticosteroids and vaccines. Bronchodilators and glucocorticosteroids have been shown to improve and prevent symptoms, reduce the frequency and severity of exacerbations, improve exercise tolerance and improve health status; they are, therefore, the most commonly used drugs in COPD.[59] Short acting β_2-agonists (salbutamol, terbutaline) or the anticholinergic drug ipratropium bromide (Atrovent) may relieve wheeze and shortness of breath. For more severe symptoms, longer acting β_2-agonists including salmeterol and formoterol (eformoterol) may be initiated.

HISTORICAL PERSPECTIVE

One of the earliest descriptions of the disease is believed to be a 1679 case of voluminous lungs. In 1789, Matthew Baillie illustrated an emphysematous lung. Dr René Laennec, best known as the man who invented the stethoscope, used the term 'emphysema' in his 1837 treatise on respiratory illnesses. He noted that patients suffering from the condition had lungs that did not collapse when autopsied, due to mucus congestion. The term chronic obstructive pulmonary disease (COPD) was first used in 1965 by William Briscoe. Since then, COPD has become the preferred term used to describe this condition, although occasionally terms like chronic obstructive lung disease (COLD) or chronic obstructive airway disease (COAD) are used.[86]

NATUROPATHIC PERSPECTIVE

Smoking cessation programs

Smoking cessation is the most effective way to reduce the risk of developing COPD. Furthermore, smoking cessation has beneficial effects that extend beyond COPD-specific mortality, such as reducing deaths from cardiovascular diseases and lung cancer.[87]

Pulmonary rehabilitation

Pulmonary rehabilitation intervention is designed to optimise physical and social performance using comprehensive multidisciplinary programs that combine exercise training with pharmacological therapy, nutritional assistance and patient education.[59]

NUTRITIONAL MEDICINE (DIETARY)

Dietary therapeutic objectives

Apart from smoking cessation, a diet high in fruits and vegetables may help prevent COPD. Higher levels of antioxidant nutrients (vitamins C and E, selenium and beta-carotene) as measured by dietary assessment and serum biomarkers are associated with better lung function (i.e. FEV_1). Malnutrition is common among patients with COPD and seems to correlate with the severity of the condition.[19]

Specific dietary treatments

Dietary counselling and food fortification can improve symptoms and general health status for patients with COPD who are at risk of malnutrition. A total of 59 COPD outpatients were randomised to receive dietary counselling and advice on food fortification or to receive a dietary advice leaflet only. After a 6-month intervention period, the participants were followed for 6 months. Daily kilojoule and protein intake was significantly greater in the intervention group than in controls. The intervention group gained about 2 kg in the first 6 months and maintained that gain, while the comparison group steadily lost about 3 kg over the 12-month study. In terms of symptoms and functional outcomes, intervention patients had significantly better scores on the St George's Respiratory Questionnaire, the Short Form-36 health change score and the Medical Research Council dyspnoea score, than did controls. Many of the beneficial changes persisted during the follow-up period. The Activities of Daily Living score was also better in the intervention group than in controls, although the difference fell short of statistical significance. By contrast, the dietary intervention appeared to have no impact on respiratory function or on respiratory and skeletal muscle strength. Dietary counselling and food fortification resulted in weight gain and improvements in outcome in nutritionally at-risk outpatients with COPD, both during and beyond the intervention period.[88]

DIETARY INCLUSIONS

Fresh seasonal fruit and vegetables should make up a large percentage of the diet. A number of publications corroborate the notion that people who have a diet rich in fruit and vegetables have a lower risk of poor respiratory health. This effect is most likely due to the increased levels of antioxidants.[23]

A case-controlled study involving Japanese participants with COPD found that increased intake of dietary soy-containing products (e.g. bean sprouts and tofu) was associated with a decreased risk of COPD and respiratory symptoms such as breathlessness.[89] Whether this result can be extrapolated for the Australian population remains to be seen.

For optimal nutrition the diet should be predominantly based on fresh wholefoods. Kitchen herbs with therapeutic action such as the antioxidant and anti-inflammatory action displayed by *Curcuma longa* (turmeric) should be consumed when possible.

DIETARY EXCLUSIONS

Foods with known detrimental effects on the immune system and body as a whole should be avoided. These include such things as refined sugar and grains, fast foods, processed foods such as biscuits, jams and cakes, saturated fats, take-away, soft drinks and alcohol. Additionally, foods that promote mucus production in the body such as dairy products (e.g. milk, cheese and ice cream) and wheat also need to be avoided.

SAMPLE DAILY DIET

BREAKFAST	
Poached eggs (free range and organic where possible) with rocket, fresh basil and oregano salad. Drizzle with olive oil and season with freshly ground pepper. Serve with salt-reduced baked beans. NOTE: For underweight patients requiring extra kilojoules add ½–1 avocado	Eggs provide a prime source of protein and good fats, while the olive oil adds additional kilojoules. Baked beans add fibre and provide much-needed energy for the lung muscles. Lung muscles of patients with COPD require 10 times more kilojoules than those of the average individual. Underweight patients with COPD are recommended to consume a high protein/high good fats diet to first keep up their kilojoule requirements and second reduce carbon dioxide production and thus pressure on the lungs.
LUNCH	
Baked sweet potato stuffed with tuna in olive oil, corn and chives	Serve with a side salad containing your choice of the following: alfalfa or snowpea sprouts, cherry tomatoes, cucumber, grated carrot, grilled eggplant, sliced raw mushrooms, avocado and lettuce. Dress salad with flaxseed oil, balsamic vinegar and sesame seeds. Sweet potato is a good source of complex carbohydrates, beta-carotene and vitamin C. Tuna satisfies protein requirements, while the salad ingredients provide much-needed vitamins and minerals to enhance immunity.
DINNER	
Grilled rainbow trout with oven-roasted vegetables (beetroot, pumpkin, zucchini, potato). Serve with basil and garlic pesto	Rainbow trout is a good source of omega-3 fatty acids that are recognised to have numerous roles in the body, the anti-inflammatory and immune-modulating benefits being the most beneficial for COPD. The addition of roasted vegetables provides a spectrum of vitamins and minerals while basil and garlic are both antibacterial, useful if there is any infection in the body.
SNACKS	
Banana smoothie made with banana, good-quality protein powder and almond milk	For underweight patients requiring additional kilojoules tahini or flaxseed oil may be added to the smoothie.
BEVERAGES	
30 mL/kg body weight of pure water daily to ensure mucus stays viscous and is easy to expel. Add sliced lime/lemon if flavour is required	

Other dietary considerations

Evidence from several studies suggests that a low-fat, high-carbohydrate diet, compared with a high-fat, low-carbohydrate diet, worsens exercise performance and lung function in patients with COPD.[19]

NUTRITIONAL MEDICINE (SUPPLEMENTAL)

Nutritional medicine therapeutic objectives

- Reduce inflammation
- Ease breathing
- Reduce the risk of infections
- Protect against the effects of long-term use of glucocorticoid therapy such as osteoporosis.

Specific nutrients required

ESSENTIAL FATTY ACIDS

Most epidemiological data point to the protective effects of diets high in fish oil and magnesium.[19] Fish contains n-3 polyunsaturated fatty acids, principally eicosapentaenoic acid and docosahexaenoic acid (DHA), which are known to interfere with the body's inflammatory response and may be of benefit in chronic inflammatory conditions. Among omega-3 fatty acids from fish, it is the level of DHA (not EPA) as measured in the plasma of 2349 smokers and ex-smokers that was inversely related to the odds of having COPD, as established clinically and by spirometry.[90] In a later study, the relation between the dietary intake of omega-3 fatty acids and chronic obstructive pulmonary disease in 8960 current or former smokers participating in a population-based study of atherosclerosis was analysed. After control for pack-years of smoking, age, sex, race, height, weight, energy intake and educational level, docosahexaenoic acid was inversely related to the risk of COPD in a quantity-dependent fashion. The adjusted odds ratio for the highest quartile was 0.66 for chronic bronchitis (95% confidence interval, 0.52 to 0.85; p <0.001 for linear trend across the range of intake value), 0.31 for physician-diagnosed emphysema (95% confidence interval,

0.18 to 0.52; *p* for linear trend, 0.003), and 0.50 for spirometrically detected COPD (95% confidence interval, 0.32 to 0.79; *p* for linear trend, 0.007). It can be concluded from this study that a high dietary intake of omega-3 fatty acids may protect cigarette smokers against COPD.[91]

In 2012–2013, several observational studies emerged, which demonstrated that circulating omega-3 PUFA levels in COPD were inversely associated with systemic inflammation and positively associated with clinical outcomes.[92] However, a recent systematic review has found limited evidence to support the use of omega-3 in COPD.[93] Large-scale clinical trials using omega-3 PUFAs alone are yet to be conducted and are required to determine accurate dosing and benefits of omega-3 supplementation.

ANTIOXIDANTS

The substantial increase in the prevalence of asthma over the past 20 years may be partially explained by the reduced dietary intake of antioxidant nutrients like beta-carotene and vitamins A, C and E, as well as the mineral co-factors essential for antioxidant defence mechanisms such as zinc, selenium and copper.[54] However, a study found no benefit from supplementation with alpha-tocopherol or beta-carotene on the symptoms of chronic obstructive pulmonary disorder but did support the beneficial effect of dietary intake of fruits and vegetables rich in these compounds.[94]

VITAMIN A

Vitamin A exhibits specific therapeutic effects upon the respiratory system, via its anti-inflammatory action upon the lungs and its preservation of the mucous membranes and lung epithelium. Further studies are required to determine the exact mechanism by which vitamin A protects tissue pathologies in the respiratory system.

VITAMIN C

Vitamin C is highly indicated for the management of COPD due to its multiple therapeutic applications with regards to respiratory health. Aside from its immune-modulating role and its antioxidant activity, subjects who consume high doses of vitamin C have been shown to have larger forced expiratory volume in one second (FEV_1) and forced vital capacity (FVC) than their counterparts.[95] Long-term vitamin C intake is associated with better lung function.

BIOFLAVONOIDS

Flavonoids assist with free radical scavenging properties and enhance the use of vitamin C in the body. A higher flavonoid (catechin, flavonol and flavone) intake is associated positively with FEV_1 and inversely with chronic cough.[96]

VITAMIN E

Though no studies have been found highlighting a direct benefit between vitamin E supplementation and COPD, chronic oxidant burden and depletion of endogenous antioxidants have been proposed to play a key role in the pathogenesis of chronic obstructive pulmonary disease (COPD), hence the benefits of supplementation with vitamin E. Intake of vitamin E (75 mg/d) in combination with beta-carotene (15 mg/d) and vitamin C (650 mg/d) in Mexican workers exposed to high levels of ozone was associated with reduced bronchoconstriction.[97]

SELENIUM

Higher intake of antioxidants such as selenium is associated with better lung function.[98] It appears that antioxidants such as selenium play a role in host defence against oxidative lung damage. Antioxidants such as selenium are also said to alter the function of macrophages and thus influence their role in immunity and inflammation.

ZINC

As previously discussed zinc plays a role in multiple enzyme systems and cellular functions, particularly those that influence immunity, as zinc functions as an intracellular signal molecule for immune cells. COPD patients could be susceptible to develop zinc deficiency due to immune dysfunction and the fact that COPD increases the possibility of infection.

MAGNESIUM

Serum magnesium levels are decreased by diuretics and oral corticosteroids. Routine serum magnesium determinations are indicated in patients with COPD who are taking diuretics or oral steroids because of the potential negative effects of hypomagnesaemia on respiratory function.[19]

N-ACETYLCYSTEINE

N-acetylcysteine (NAC) is a specially modified form of the dietary amino acid cysteine. NAC has been used as a mucolytic in the treatment of chronic bronchitis. It also increases the level of the potent antioxidant, glutathione, and has an inhibitory effect on bacterial adherence to the oropharynx. NAC is a safe supplement, and a recent meta-analysis of eight double-blind placebo-controlled trials demonstrated that NAC (at a dosage of 400–1200 mg/day for a duration of 3–6 months) reduced the number of acute exacerbations by 23% as compared with a placebo in patients with chronic bronchitis. An even larger European systematic review confirmed the beneficial effect of NAC in patients with chronic bronchitis and confirmed its safety for up to 24 weeks. The dose used in the trials ranged between 400 and 1200 mg a day. NAC is contraindicated in patients taking nitrates because it may worsen nitrate-induced headaches.[19]

Systematic reviews assessing the benefit of NAC have found it to be beneficial at high doses of 1200 mg/day in preventing COPD exacerbations, whereas lower doses did not provide much benefit. This indicates there is very much a dose-dependent relationship between NAC and COPD.[99]

COENZYME Q10

Coenzyme Q10, or ubiquinone, is involved in electron transfer in the inner mitochondrial membrane. A small, open trial found coenzyme Q10 serum levels to be decreased in patients with COPD. Eight patients with COPD received supplementation with 90 mg of coenzyme Q10 for 8 weeks. The study suggests that CoQ10 has a favourable effect on muscular energy metabolism in patients with chronic lung diseases who have hypoxaemia at rest and/or during exercise.[100]

AMINO ACIDS

Abnormal plasma amino acid profiles have been reported in patients with COPD. Patients who are underweight with low muscle mass have been shown to have a deficiency in branched chain amino acids.[101]

Dosage requirements

The dosage requirements listed below are based on adult doses that are reported in the literature:

- Fish oils: 1–6 g total fish oils/d (EPA 800–1000 mg, DHA 300 mg)
- Vitamin A: 50000 IU/d
- Vitamin C: 500–1000 mg t.d.s. up to bowel tolerance
- Bioflavonoids: 50 mg/d
- Vitamin E: 1000 IU/d
- Selenium: 150 micrograms/d
- Zinc: 50 mg/d
- Magnesium: 500 mg/d
- NAC: 1200 mg/d
- Coenzyme Q10: 90–150 mg/d
- Complete protein powder or amino acid combination: 1–2 serves/d depending on BMI.

HERBAL MEDICINE

- ↓ Mucus + remove from the body
- Relieve symptoms such as coughing
- Improve immune function and prevent secondary infection
- Reduce inflammation, irritation and regeneration and repair mucosal lining.

Herbal medicine classes

Excessive mucus secretion from the tracheobronchi dominates COPD and hence the use of stimulating expectorants and mucolytics is essential to remove mucus from the body as well as reduce symptoms such as cough while simultaneously promoting better quality of life for the patient.

Immune supportive herbs are also essential as they help to maintain and support the immune system, which is typically under extreme stress and at risk of secondary infection (in particular lung infection such as pneumonia). To optimise lung function, bronchodilators which reduce constriction of the bronchi are required.

The application of anti-inflammatory herbal medicines helps to reduce chronic inflammation due to irritants such as cigarette smoke. Demulcent herbs will also help to soothe and reduce irritation and inflammation. Botanicals that display antioxidant qualities such as *Vitis vinifera* (grapeseed) may also be warranted, particularly if patients continue to engage in detrimental immune compromising activities such as smoking and drinking alcohol.

Mucosal trophorestoratives will also be required to aid in the regeneration and repair of the disrupted mucosal lining. Antimicrobial herbs may be indicated if infection is present. Common infective agents associated with COPD include *S. pneumoniae* and *H. influenzae*.

Circulatory and cardiac herbs support and maintain a healthy cardiovascular system and may be required to prevent and adequately treat other secondary issues associated with COPD.

Nervines and adaptogens may also be required for psychological and physiological support. While a number of classes of herbs have been listed, it is heartening to know that many of the herbs required for the conditions of the respiratory tract have multiple actions, therefore designing a formula that encompasses all the actions and herbal classes above is not impossible.

Specific herbal medicines

HYPERICUM PERFORATUM (ST JOHN'S WORT)

Depression is a common concern in patients with COPD, perhaps due in part to the pain experienced as well as the loss of quality of life. As a result, those herbs which display antidepressant and nervine activity are highly indicated. St John's wort has multiple therapeutic applications in the management of COPD. Firstly, it fits the criteria as an antidepressant, making it ideal to manage depression associated with COPD. Secondly, it is a potent antiviral and thus may be used if infection is of viral origin. Thirdly, Remotiv, a standardised extract of *Hypericum perforatum* (St John's wort), is being trialled as a supportive remedy during smoking cessation therapy. This offers patients an effective supportive aid in which patients may stop smoking.

COLEUS FORSKOHLII (COLEUS)

Coleus forskohlii is an Ayurvedic herb that contains forskolin, a diterpene that displays bronchodilator and antiallergic activity. Forskolin activates the adenylate cyclase and raises cyclic AMP levels in a variety of tissues. Animal and in vivo studies reveal promising results. Forskolin inhibits the immunological release of leukotrienes and histamine, relaxing airway smooth muscle and preventing bronchospasm.[102] This provides a rationale for its use as a bronchodilator in the management of COPD. Additionally enticing is the fact that forskolin also displays a positive inotropic effect on the myocardium.[45] This makes it a key herb in the COPD patient who requires concurrent cardiovascular support.

THYMUS VULGARIS (THYME)

Thymus vulgaris is a powerful expectorant with mucolytic and antibacterial activity. It has been noted that the tar obtained from smoking often precipitates in the respiratory tract, disabling the cilia on the epithelium and inhibiting the self-cleaning of bronchia.[103] Herbal expectorants such as *Thymus* work by increasing the secretion of the mucosa and hence facilitate coughing up the secrete residual. Expectorant herbs appear to work primarily by influencing the gastric mucosa and following a reflex stimulation that results in the bronchial glands increasing their secretions. Volatile-oil type expectorant herbs such as *Thymus* display a direct stimulatory effect on the bronchial glands by means of local irritation. These actions provide an explanation for the use of *Thymus vulgaris* as a preferable botanical for the management of COPD.

A 3-month, double-blind trial of 246 individuals with chronic bronchitis found that long-term treatment with essential oil monoterpenes helped prevent the typical worsening of chronic bronchitis that occurs during the winter and was well tolerated.[104]

INULA HELENIUM (ELECAMPANE)

Inula helenium is a member of the Compositae family and contains mucilage, volatile oils, inulin and sterols. *Inula helenium* may be employed in respiratory conditions that require botanicals with an antitussive, bactericidal or gentle stimulating expectorant action. The fact that *Inula helenium* has these actions has led to it being employed for the management of respiratory conditions for centuries. Herbalists throughout the Middle Ages prescribed it for coughs and bronchitis while Nicholas Culpeper speaks on *Inula helenium* as follows:[7]

> *The fresh roots of Elecampane preserved with sugar, or made into a syrup or conserve, are very effectual to help the cough, shortness of breath, and wheezing in the lungs. The dried root made into powder, and mixed with sugar, and taken, serves to the same purpose...*

Although no clinical studies have been conducted on *Inula helenium*'s efficacy in COPD, its actions above and the context in which it was used historically provide a rationale for its application in COPD.

POLYGALA TENUIFOLIA (CHINESE SENEGA)

Polygala tenuifolia, known in Chinese as Yuan zhi, is native to China and Japan where it is dispensed for catarrh in the chest.[68] *Polygala tenuifolia* is a stimulating expectorant highly indicated in chronic bronchitis, particularly where there is cough with sputum. It contains triterpenoid saponin glycosides (tenuigenin A and tenuigenin B), resins and fatty acids among other constituents.

ESSENTIAL OILS

Inhalations of essential oils such as eucalyptus and peppermint may aid with loosening mucus, dilate airways and as a result, allow the patient to breathe with greater ease.

LIFESTYLE RECOMMENDATIONS

- Moderate exposure to sunlight and gentle weight-bearing exercise are recommended
- Reduction (and ultimately) the cessation of smoking is imperative as smoking further negatively impacts lung, immune function and total bodily functioning
- Physiotherapy and breathing exercises are useful due to their ability to provide pulmonary rehabilitation
- In patients who continue to smoke, regular exercise may help to allay decline in lung function.[105]

CASE STUDY

OVERVIEW

KR, a 56-year-old man, presents with shortness of breath on exertion. He is a car mechanic and runs his own successful car repair business. He lives with his wife. His son is 29 and his daughter, aged 26, recently moved out of home as she just got married. Both he and his wife noticed that he was getting short of breath while dancing at his daughter's wedding. KR does no regular exercise and is a heavy drinker (5–10 beers per night) and smoker (1–2 packets of cigarettes per day since he was 16 years of age — i.e. 40 years). He has a smoker's cough on waking, producing white to yellow sputum. He has a history of chronic bronchitis but has not been properly monitored or treated.

He does not get short of breath when lying flat, sleeps with one pillow and has never woken in the middle of the night feeling breathless or short of breath. He is unaware of his blood pressure as the last time he saw a doctor was years ago. He has no previous cardiovascular history; however, his father died of a myocardial infarction at age 52 and his brother at age 54. Diet is predictably poor consisting of lots of takeaway foods, butter, fried foods, red meat and saturated fats. System review is otherwise unremarkable. He has seen his GP but is waiting for his appointment to the cardiologist and respiratory specialist.

CLINICAL EXAMINATION

General inspection

Alert, cooperative, obese

Vital signs

BP: 135/90 mmHg (standing)
Temperature: 36.9°C
Pulse: 78 bpm, regular rhythm
Respiratory rate: 18 resp/min
Height: 1.84 m
Weight: 105 kg
BMI: 31 kg/m^2

Cardiovascular

Pulses: Peripheral — present, JVP — not raised, carotids — unremarkable
Praecordium: Apex beat — not displaced, parasternal heave — nil, thrills — nil
Auscultation: Heart sounds — dual, murmurs — nil

Respiratory

Chest inspection: Barrel chest
Palpation: Trachea — midline
Supraclavicular/axillary nodes — nil
Percussion: Hyperresonant
Auscultation: Occasional moist crackles bilateral bases, occasional polyphonic expiratory wheeze

CASE STUDY CONTINUED

INVESTIGATION RESULTS

Blood testing

Lipids

Cholesterol: 6.0 (3.9–5.5)
Triglycerides: 3.2 (0.5–2.0)

LFT

All within range but upper levels.

TREATMENT PROTOCOL

Because of the comprehensive nature of this presentation, strong referral and intercommunication were essential. Compliance concerns were paramount, however. The severity of his presentation was explained to the patient and he agreed to all recommendations.

HERBAL MEDICINE

Liquid formulation

Adhatoda vasica (adhatoda): 30 mL
Inula racemosa (inula): 70 mL
Inula helenium (elecampane): 40 mL
Coleus forskohlii (coleus): 80 mL
Dose: 7.5 mL b.i.d. standard adult dose, calculated based on weight to increase to 12 mL b.i.d. (NB: Dose reduced as he lost weight.)

Adjunct

Hypericum perforatum (St John's wort) standardised tablet preparation (Ze 117): 1 tab t.d.s.

NOTE: Prescription was supported until medications were implemented from specialist. They were then reviewed for potential interactions.

NUTRITIONAL MEDICINE

Dietary

High essential fatty acid, low refined carbohydrate, optimal protein diet was recommended. It was advised to encourage high sources of antioxidants from fresh fruits and vegetables.

Protein was calculated at 1.0 g/kg body weight (slight increase for immune system repair from standard 0.8 g/kg). Vegetarian and fish sources of protein were encouraged where possible. Saturated fat consumption was discouraged.

Weight loss was recommended and the patient was asked to maintain a diet and lifestyle assessment with changes systematically introduced as treatment progressed. It was discussed that future referral to a dietitian might be required if compliance or response was poor.

Avoidance of alcohol and caffeine was recommended.

Supplemental

Coenzyme Q10: 150 mg b.i.d.
NAC: 250 mg b.i.d.
Selenium: 250 micrograms/day
Vitamin A: 5000 IU b.i.d.
Vitamin E: 400 IU b.i.d.

CASE STUDY CONTINUED

Vitamin C + bioflavonoids: 1 g b.i.d.
Zinc: 25 mg b.i.d.
Concentrated omega liquid (EPA, DHA): ½ teaspoon b.i.d.: 1.6 g omega-3 [70%]; 35% EPA [813 mg], 25% DHA [563 mg]

NOTE: Doses above are standard adult doses but were adjusted and calculated based on his weight of 105 kg and reduced as he lost weight.

LIFESTYLE

- Avoidance of smoking and passive smoke exposure. It was discussed that due to the extended history of smoking, sudden stopping of smoking was to be avoided as this could exacerbate the patient's health considerably. Reduction was to be encouraged and referral to psychologist/hypnotherapist was organised to plan to reduce and stop smoking over the next month
- Essential oil inhalations (shower, vaporiser, snuffs) at a minimum of 2 × day with respiratory blend of essential oils
- Moderate exposure to sunlight and gentle weight-bearing exercise
- Avoidance of substances or conditions that aggravate reactions
- Change of household cleaning products to reduced chemical forms.

EDUCATION

- Household triggers and cleaning regimens
- Weight balance, energy expenditure vs energy intake, exercise.

FURTHER INVESTIGATIONS

- Vitamin D — potential prescription (results depending)
- Repeat cholesterol (with full profile) — fasting
- MTHFR and homocysteine — fasting
- hs-CRP, Apo-A
- Insulin, fasting glucose, HbA1c
- TSH, urinary iodine, thyroid antibodies
- CXR, ECG, stress test and other investigations as recommended by the cardiologist.

REFERRAL

- Referral to quit smoking (hypnotherapist/psychologist). Patient chose this option as a starting place with discussion of alternative options
- Referral to physiotherapist for regular postural drainage and education classes with wife to assist long term
- Referral to personal trainer to implement weight loss program in conjunction with healthcare team.

MULTIDISCIPLINARY HEALTH TEAM

Regular intercommunication with healthcare team consisting of:

- General practitioner
- Respiratory physician
- Cardiologist
- Physiotherapist
- Personal trainer
- Hypnotherapist/psychologist.

Special topic: pleurisy

PLEURISY

The incidence of pleurisy is not entirely known. The condition usually occurs as a result of other infections or secondary to lower respiratory tract infections such as pneumonia, bronchitis and tuberculosis. As a result of this, the epidemiology of pleurisy varies in accordance with the underlying aetiology.

Pleurisy, also known as pleuritis, is characterised by inflammation of the pleura and describes the chest pain syndrome characterised by a sharp pain in the chest cavity that worsens with inspiration. There are essentially two layers of pleura: one covers the lungs, known as visceral pleura, and the other covers the inner wall of the chest, known as parietal pleura. In order for these two layers to not rub against each other and cause friction, the layers are lubricated by pleural fluid. When infection or inflammation is present, the amount of pleural fluid increases and can result in pleural effusion.

Pleurisy tends to occur as a result of underlying pneumonia (viral or bacterial), pulmonary infarction, tumour infiltration or connective tissue diseases such as systemic lupus erythematosus. Inhaled or chemical exposure such as ammonia can also contribute to pleurisy. In severe cases, pulmonary embolism, pneumothorax and trauma such as fractures to the ribs or pleural cavity can also exacerbate pleurisy.

Signs and symptoms

The signs and symptoms of pleurisy are very distinctive and the pain in the chest tends to be very sharp and is aggravated by breathing, particularly inspiration. Other signs and symptoms include:

- Sudden pain onset
- Pain usually localised without radiation
- Sharp knife-like pain
- Continuous pain with sharp exacerbations
- Associated symptoms such as dyspnoea, cough and haemoptysis.

Complications

- Long-standing pleurisy can result in rapid shallow breathing as the body attempts to obtain as much oxygen as possible. This is known as dyspnoea and can result in cyanotic changes if not corrected.
- Pleural effusion occurs as a complication of untreated pleurisy and there are several categories including:
  - Uncomplicated pleural effusion doesn't contain infective pathogens and very rarely results in long-term and permanent pulmonary issues
  - Complicated pleural effusion contains infective and inflammatory pathogens and if unresolved, can result in fibrotic damage to the lungs and can impair lung function and negatively affect inspiration
  - Transudative pleural effusion rarely requires drainage and often occurs as a result of congestive heart failure
  - Exudative pleural effusion contains excess protein, blood or inflammatory cytokines and pathogens. It quite often requires drainage and is often associated with pneumonia or lung cancer.

Treatment

Much of what can be offered through naturopathic treatment is based around symptomatic relief and quite often treatment will be combined with pharmaceutical medication, as an adjunct. If pleurisy has progressed to complicated effusion it is strongly recommended the patient exclusively seeks assistance from their medical professional as it can progress to a life-threatening situation.

In general, if COPD and pneumonia are treated effectively, pleurisy will not result; however, in some instances it does.

Treatment objectives include:

- Reducing inflammation
- Providing symptomatic relief
- Improving immune response

Much of what can be offered is through lifestyle advice and includes:

- Ensuring adequate rest and relaxation
- Reducing exposure to stress
- Reducing exposure to airborne pathogens
- Ensuring adequate sleep on a nightly basis.

PULMONARY SARCOIDOSIS

Epidemiology

The incidence of sarcoidosis in Australia is not known but data obtained about a population in southeastern Australia showed that, between 2000 and 2005, 4.4–6.3 patients per 100 000 were affected.[106] Sarcoidosis can occur in any age group; however, it mostly affects people in their late 20s to early 40s.[107]

Aetiology

The aetiology of sarcoidosis is not completely understood but advances in research over the last decade have allowed for the immunopathogenesis to be understood in greater detail.[108]

The development of sarcoidosis is contributed to by an inflammatory response to an environmental antigen in a genetically susceptible person. Known triggers can include mould, mildew and toxic airborne chemicals, *Propionibacterium acnes* and mycobacteria; tobacco smoking is inversely correlated with sarcoidosis.[108,109]

Pathogenesis

Sarcoidosis is a granulomatous disease and is characterised by clusters of histocytes, known as granulomas. These granulomas form when the immune system is attempting to ward off foreign pathogens or materials and isn't successful in doing so. The granulomas present in sarcoidosis are non-necrotising.[108,109]

Epidemiological data suggest certain occupations are more susceptible to the development of sarcoidosis and the triggering antigen varies depending on ethnicity, geographic location and individual genetic background.[108,109]

Once the antigen enters the host, the molecule or pathogen is phagocytosed by antigen-presenting cells (APCs), namely macrophages or dendritic cells.[108,109] The APCs process the antigen and present it via human leukocyte antigen (HLA) class II molecules to a restricted set of T-cell receptors on naïve T lymphocytes, primarily of the CD4+ class. The immune reaction converts T lymphocytes to Th1, followed by cellular recruitment, proliferation and differentiation leading to the formation of the sarcoid granuloma.[108,109]

The pathogenesis of this disease tends to involve the interplay between antigen, HLA class II molecules and T-cell receptors. It is the combination of these three factors that influences the development of sarcoidosis.[108,109] The granulomas present within sarcoidosis are characterised by a core of monocyte-derived epitheliod histocytes and multinucleated giant cells. A multitude of chemokines and cytokines have also been associated with the development of granulomas in sarcoidosis.[108,109]

Research is still ongoing in this area and it is not completely understood whether or not one or multiple exogenous antigens contribute to the aetiological development of this disease.[108,109] It has been hypothesised that recurrent granulomatous inflammation may be due to failure of immune regulatory mechanisms to limit the duration of the inflammatory process and response. It has been reported that serum amyloid A protein is deposited within the granuloma and it is this protein that has the ability to elicit an immune response and trigger cytokine release thus perpetuating the disease process.[110] A defective ability of T lymphocytes, namely of T-reg cells to function correctly, has been shown to negatively influence the disease process and contribute to an increase in disease flare-ups and increased granuloma formation.[108–110]

In most cases, the granulomas present are self-limiting; however, in some instances, if the granulomas do not heal, the tissue affected can become inflamed and subsequently local fibrosis may occur.[107]

Of those diagnosed with sarcoidosis, 90% will be diagnosed with pulmonary sarcoidosis. The pathogenesis follows the same pathway as previously mentioned; however, alveolar macrophages become activated. The localised cellular response that contributes to the disease process includes interleukin-1, interleukin-2, B-cell growth factor, B-cell differentiation, fibroblast growth factor and fibronectin.[107]

Signs and symptoms

The signs and symptoms related to pulmonary sarcoidosis are not very specific to the disease itself and are very much interrelated with other diseases. As a result of this, a definitive diagnosis can take many years to determine. In order for sarcoidosis to be ruled out as a cause of the signs and symptoms, patients tend to experience the following symptoms for greater than three months:[109]

- Fever
- Dyspnoea
- Recurrent cough
- Chest discomfort
- Chest crackles
- Chronic low-grade fever
- Fatigue and malaise
- Weight loss
- Anorexia
- Weakness.

Complications

In half of the diagnosed cases, the disease is not severe and tends to resolve without treatment. In the other half of the diagnosed cases, early or late respiratory complications can be experienced. Early complications include respiratory insufficiency by bronchial airway obstruction. The most commonly occurring latent complication includes pulmonary fibrosis.[111] As a result of this, COPD and fibrosis of the proximal bronchi can occur. In severe cases, cor pulmonale (right-sided abnormal enlargement of the heart as a result of lung dysfunction) can also occur.[111]

Haemoptysis usually only occurs as a result of fibroemphysematous (abnormal increase in size of air spaces resulting in laboured breathing and increased susceptibility to infection) lesions. Respiratory complications account for half of the 5% of deaths due to sarcoidosis. Usually, respiratory complications can be visible in radiographic imaging during stages III and IV of the disease.[111]

Differential diagnosis

Due to the complications related to sarcoidosis, many of the symptoms resemble commonly occurring obstructive airway diseases such as asthma, bronchitis and pneumonia. In many instances, further investigation is not warranted unless the patient has been experiencing chronic symptoms for greater than 3 months.[112]

Other specific disorders to be excluded are:

- Tuberculosis
- Atypical mycobacteria
- Fungal infection such as aspergillosis, blastomycosis and histoplasmosis
- Brucellosis
- Mycoplasmal infection
- Syphilis
- Wegener's granulomatosis
- Sjögren's syndrome
- Hodgkin's and non-Hodgkin's lymphoma.

Diagnosis

Diagnosis is primarily determined based upon chest imaging, biopsy and exclusion of other granulomatous disorders. Sarcoidosis is most often suspected when hilar adenopathy (bilateral enlargement of the lymph nodes of the pulmonary hila) is detected on a chest x-ray. If an x-ray is not definitive, which quite often is not, pulmonary biopsy of the affected site is often conducted.[108,109] To determine the severity of sarcoidosis, pulmonary function tests and exercise pulse oximetry are conducted.[108,109]

Naturopathic diagnosis

Because of the acute and chronic nature of sarcoidosis, the need for a naturopathic diagnosis is not warranted as diagnosis is based on the results obtained from thorough investigations by the patient's general practitioner.

TABLE 14.9 Sarcoidosis x-ray criteria

Stage	Definition	Incidence of spontaneous remission
0	Normal chest x-ray	–
I	Bilateral hilar, paratracheal and mediastinal lymphadenopathy without parenchymal infiltrates	60–80%
II	Bilateral hilar and mediastinal adenopathy with interstitial infiltrates (usually in upper lung fields)	50–65%
III	Diffuse interstitial infiltrates without hilar adenopathy	<30%
IV	Diffuse fibrosis, often associated with fibrotic appearing conglomerate masses, traction bronchiectasis and traction cysts	0%

Source: From the Merck Manual Professional Version (known as the Merck Manual in the US and Canada and the MSD Manual in the rest of the world), edited by R Porter. Copyright (2017) by Merck Sharp & Dohme Corp, a subsidiary of Merck & Co, Inc, Kenilworth, NJ. Available at http://www.merckmanuals.com/professional. Accessed 30 May 2017.

Investigations

CHEST X-RAY

A chest x-ray is conducted to determine the presence or absence of hilar adenopathy. The x-ray screen can also roughly predict the likelihood of spontaneous remission in patients with pulmonary involvement. The staging of sarcoidosis is based on the x-ray criteria listed in Table 14.9.

BIOPSY

Endobronchial ultrasound-guided transbronchial needle aspiration of mediastinal or hilar lymph node has a reported diagnostic yield of 90%. It is usually the main diagnostic tool for patients with intrathoracic involvement. The biopsy can also aid with determining if there is a pathogenic role in the development of sarcoidosis.[108,109]

FULL BLOOD COUNT AND BLOOD PARAMETERS

A full blood count is conducted to determine or exclude presence of infection and in many instances neutrophilia and eosinophilia are present.[108,109] Erythrocyte sedimentation rate (ESR) and C-reactive protein (CRP) are predictors of inflammation and an elevation of these markers can be nonspecific indicators of inflammation.[108,109]

SPIROMETRY

Spirometry is conducted to determine the extent to which the granulomas have affected lung function and capacity. Those with stage III–IV sarcoidosis tend to have diminished lung function that is unable to be reversed.

SPECIFIC NATUROPATHIC INVESTIGATIONS

Naturopathic investigations are very much limited to allopathic investigations. In some instances, it is beneficial to determine if there is a presence of environmental or toxic exposure that may be further contributing to the progression of the disease. This can be determined through hair tissue mineral analysis as a certain toxic load can exacerbate sarcoidosis.

Therapeutic considerations

CLINICAL DECISION MAKING AND RATIONALE

Much of what can be done for those suffering from sarcoidosis is based around symptomatic relief and immune support. Treatment should aim to:

- Improve and maintain quality of life
- Support and improve immune function
- Support and improve lung function
- Eliminate known triggers that exacerbate symptoms
- Avoid known causative factors.

Therapeutic application

HISTORICAL PERSPECTIVE

Much of the treatment is based around downregulating the immune response as well as preventing inflammation. Many of the pharmaceuticals that have been used don't actually enhance and modulate the immune system but rather suppress it.

The use of corticosteroids in sarcoidosis has been known since 1948. Within the allopathic paradigm, corticosteroids are inexpensive, widely available and effective. They have the ability to downregulate many facets of the immune system and immune response. The downside to this, however, is that the toxicity profile of corticosteroids in those with sarcoidosis has not been extensively studied.[113,114]

For pulmonary sarcoidosis, prednisone is often prescribed at a dose of 20–40 mg daily but to date no studies have determined the optimal dosing ranges required for treatment. What has been determined is that higher doses of corticosteroids don't offer additional benefit for pulmonary sarcoidosis.[113,114]

Methotrexate is a cytotoxic medication and is commonly used for the treatment of sarcoidosis. The typical dose tends to be 10–20 mg transdermally, once weekly.[113,114]

NATUROPATHIC PERSPECTIVE

The primary goal in treating sarcoidosis is to provide the patient with better quality of life. Those with chronic pulmonary sarcoidosis tend to have extensive fibrosis of the lungs and as a result, fatigue, malaise and dyspnoea tend to be quite common.

The roles of the naturopath are to support and improve immune function to subsequently prevent the progression of sarcoidosis. Much of what we can achieve is through downregulating inflammatory cascades as well as providing immunomodulators to enhance immune function and to promote appropriate functioning of T-helper cells to therefore reduce the generation of granulomas, and subsequently fibrosis.

Lung function is almost always compromised in sarcoidosis and with the assistance of pulmonary restorative herbs, quality of life can be enhanced. Much of the treatment provided through herbal and nutritional medicine will be taken in conjunction with corticosteroids and at times, with cytotoxic medications. As a result, it is crucial to prevent any negative nutrient–drug interactions.

NUTRITIONAL MEDICINE (DIETARY)

Dietary inclusions

The role that diet plays in the development and progression of sarcoidosis is yet to be determined; however, from knowing the role the immune system plays in this disease process it is essential the diet consists of:

- Nutrient-dense foods such as fresh fruit and vegetables. Organic where possible to reduce toxic burden
- Sulfur-containing herbs and vegetables such as garlic and onion to aid with immune function
- Essential fatty acids to downregulate inflammatory cascades
- Mixed bioflavonoids and vitamin C to support immune function.

Dietary exclusions

As inflammation is a major factor in the development of sarcoidosis, it is crucial to avoid all foods and beverages that may contribute to inflammation. This includes:

- Limiting red meat to a maximum serving of once weekly to ensure avoidance of pro-inflammatory sources
- Avoiding refined carbohydrates and sugar to reduce burden on immune system
- Eliminating known foods that can contribute to mucus formation such as milk, cheese and all dairy products
- Eliminating alcohol to reduce burden on immune system and prevent further development of inflammation.

SAMPLE DAILY DIET

BREAKFAST	
Poached, organic egg with wilted greens and mushrooms on sourdough bread	To ensure adequate protein consumption to facilitate immune function and lung restoration.
LUNCH	
Organic whole chicken soup with seasonal vegetables and shitake and reishi mushrooms	To support appropriate immune function by providing sufficient protein and essential nutrients for immune health.
DINNER	
Lemon and herb marinated Atlantic salmon with seasonal salad and olive oil vinaigrette	To facilitate the downregulation of inflammatory cytokines by consuming a balanced ratio of MUFAs and PUFAs.
SNACKS	
Almond chia pudding with mixed berries	Antioxidant and PUFA rich.
BEVERAGES	
Ensure adequate hydration of 30 mL per kg of body weight	To lubricate and ensure the health of mucous membranes.

NUTRITIONAL MEDICINE (SUPPLEMENTAL)

Nutritional medicine therapeutic objectives

- Support and enhance immune function
- Reduce incidence of recurrent infection
- Reduce inflammation by reducing inflammatory cytokines.

Specific nutrients required

BIOFLAVONOIDS — QUERCITIN AND VITAMIN C

Vitamin C and its associated bioflavonoids, especially quercitin, have been known to display powerful antioxidant properties, as well as having immunomodulatory and anti-inflammatory roles. As sarcoidosis is predominately a pro-inflammatory state, the roles of these antioxidants have been studied in such patients.[115]

A study conducted to determine the antioxidant status of sarcoidosis patients found a significant reduction in plasma levels of vitamin C, quercetin and glutathione compared to those levels of healthy patients. Severe forms of sarcoidosis displayed a trend towards even lower glutathione levels thus possibly indicating the correlation with greater oxidative stress as the disease progresses. Because of the decline in antioxidant levels, reactive oxygen species (ROS) are significantly elevated and promote inflammation of the lungs by activating NF-K β and activator protein 1 that induce pro-inflammatory markers and cytokines.[116,117]

The same study found quercetin to downregulate pro-inflammatory cytokines such as TNF-α and IL-8 production in LPS-induced sarcoidosis patients. Although this was an ex vivo study, it supports the use and significant role such antioxidants can play in patients with sarcoidosis. Randomised clinical trials are warranted to provide solid evidence for these data.[115]

PROBIOTICS

Probiotic strains have been used for many years for their role in influencing and enhancing immune function. Specific strains that have been studied for their immunomodulatory properties include *Lactobacillus rhamnosus GG, Lactobacillus casei Shirota, Lactobacillus johnsonii La1, Bifidobacterium lactis DR 10* and *Saccharomyces cerevisiae boulardii.* These strains have been shown to enhance nonspecific cellular immune responses characterised by activation of macrophages, natural killer cells, antigen-specific cytotoxic T lymphocytes and the release of various cytokines.[118] The role of these probiotic strains provides a theoretical basis for their use in patients suffering from sarcoidosis due to their immune incompetent state.

ZINC

Because the immune system is highly proliferative, it is very susceptible to zinc deficiency. Zinc plays a crucial role in both innate and adaptive immunity. It has the ability to modulate the production of cytokines and interleukins thus influencing inflammation.[119] When there is a zinc deficiency, T-cells become vulnerable and their development and functionality become affected. Every aspect of the immune system relies on zinc in one way or another.[119] Insufficient zinc will not provide for a properly developed and functioning immune system and as a result, susceptibility to infection and diseases increases.[119] The use of zinc in patients with sarcoidosis not only provides for improvements in immune system functionality but can also aid with reducing inflammation and, as a result, may reduce the production of fibrotic tissue within the lungs.

OMEGA-3

Over the years, the role of omega-3 fatty acids in reducing inflammation has been mixed, with research both proving and disproving its role in downregulating inflammatory cytokines; however, recent research is showing its positive role in this area.[120,121]

Doses greater than 2 g per day of omega-3 fatty acids have been shown to reduce IL-6 and TNF-α in both healthy and unhealthy participants.[121] The use of 2.5 g of omega-3 fatty acids daily showed a 12% reduction in IL-6, compared to a 36% increase in this inflammatory marker in the placebo group.[120] This research suggests omega-3 fatty acids can be of benefit in reducing inflammatory cytokines in those suffering from sarcoidosis.

Special topic: Vitamin D and sarcoidosis

Hypercalcaemia occurs in 4–11% of patients with existing sarcoidosis. The reason behind this is still not entirely known, with more research being required. However, because of this risk factor, the use of vitamin D supplementation has been very much discouraged in these patients and research to date has been conflicting. In order to determine if vitamin D does indeed increase the risk of hypercalcaemia in patients with sarcoidosis, a small randomised controlled trial was conducted.[122]

Twenty-seven participants were randomised into either placebo or control group. The treatment group, whose serum vitamin D was <50 nmol/L, received 50 000 IU of vitamin D per week for 4 weeks followed by 50 000 IU per month for 11 months.[122] Although the sample size was small, and larger scale studies are warranted, the study concluded that supplementation with vitamin D did not alter urine or serum levels of calcium, thus it did not have an influential role on the development of hypercalcaemia. This research suggests vitamin D can be supplemented in patients with sarcoidosis without having a negative influence on calcium status.[122]

Dosage requirements

The dosage requirements are based on the literature and evidence provided:

- Vitamin C combined with mixed bioflavonoids: 1–2 g in divided doses daily
- Multistrain probiotic: 30 billion daily
- Zinc: 30–60 mg in divided doses daily
- Omega-3 fatty acid- EPA/DHA: 2.5 g in divided doses daily.

HERBAL MEDICINE

Herbal medicine therapeutic objectives

- Enhance immune function
- Reduce incidence of infection
- Improve lung function and capacity
- Reduce side effect profile of pharmaceutical medication.

The pathogenesis of sarcoidosis is still under much investigation and as a result, the role of botanical medicine is very much unknown. Due to this, the use of botanical medicine is based on historical uses and on the knowledge we have of the herbal medicines' phytotherapeutic and pharmacodynamic roles.

ECHINACEA SPP.

Echinacea has long been used for its immunomodulatory and immunostimulatory role. Patients who experience sarcoidosis experience poor immune function and, as a result, are highly susceptible to develop recurrent upper respiratory and lower respiratory tract infections.[123] Experimental studies suggest echinacea's role doesn't entirely stimulate the immune system but rather, it modulates and corrects the immune system function. In other experimental and clinical trials, it has been shown to reduce inflammation by downregulating IL-2, IL-6 and TNF-α.[123] It has also exerted both antiviral and antibacterial functions.[123] The multifunctional role of echinacea proves it to be a beneficial herbal medicine in the relief of symptoms and preventing the relapse of sarcoidosis in those who are affected.[123]

VERBASCUM THAPSUS (MULLEIN)

Mullein has been used for centuries for its topical and systemic emollient and demulcent roles. It is believed to have a specific role on the respiratory system, particularly the lungs by having a positive influence on the mucus membranes and alveoli. Its traditional use has been based on the herb's ability to aid with the restoration of lung function, which is crucial for pulmonary sarcoidosis.

THYMUS VULGARIS (THYME)

Thyme has traditionally been used for its role in relieving symptoms and conditions of the lower respiratory tract. It can be orally ingested and used as a gargle to reduce bacterial and viral infections of the respiratory tract.[124] It has also proven in in vivo studies to have antispasmodic and anti-inflammatory actions[124] and has displayed broad-spectrum antimicrobial roles, which may benefit those with recurrent pulmonary sarcoidosis due to infection.

GLYCYRRHIZA GLABRA (LIQUORICE)

Although specific research for the use of liquorice in sarcoidosis is lacking, there is sufficient information available to support the use of liquorice for its anti-inflammatory properties.[124] Beta-glycyrrhetinic acid, a major metabolite of glycyrrhizin (GL), is largely mediated by cortisol.[124] There is a synergistic effect between GL and other chemical constituents of liquorice in suppressing the expression of nitric oxide, an inflammatory mediator. It has also been shown to attenuate pro-inflammatory cytokines and may be a useful and an effective adjunct to treatment, especially when the aim of treatment is to downregulate inflammation.[124]

LIFESTYLE RECOMMENDATIONS

Depending on the severity of pulmonary sarcoidosis, many lifestyle changes are required to ensure improved quality of life and reduced rates of relapses. Such recommendations include:

- Avoid smoking and being exposed to passive smoke
- Avoid exposure to pathogens
- Eliminate exposure to known toxins that exacerbate the condition such as workplace and household chemicals
- Always wear a mask if exposed to pathogens or known toxins
- Use a humidifier to reduce exposure to mould, mildew, dust and other airborne particles.

CASE STUDY

JT is a 56-year-old male who presented to clinic with stage III pulmonary sarcoidosis. His presenting complaint was recurrent respiratory tract infections and frequent (monthly) hospitalisation due to lowered immunity. He currently works as a truck driver; however, he was previously a mechanic but changed jobs due to the progression of his sarcoidosis.

He is very immunocompromised and any exposure to others with a cold/flu causes him to become hospitalised. He is unable to exercise and walking up and down the hallway of home tends to exhaust him.

JT's diet consists of refined carbohydrates, 2–3 cups of coffee per day, and limited water and protein consumption.

Strong history of antibiotic use due to recurrent infections. However, oral antibiotics are no longer effective and IV antibiotics are required upon admission to hospital.

CLINICAL EXAMINATION

General inspection

Appeared fatigued, dyspnoeic and was struggling to speak due to reduced oxygen capacity. Walking into the clinic appeared to tire him.

Vital signs

BP: 160/90 mmHg (medicated)
Temperature: 38°C
Pulse: 110 bpm
Respiratory rate: 12 resp/min

CASE STUDY CONTINUED

Height: 1.65 m
Weight: 65 kg
BMI: 23 kg/m^2

Head and neck

Face: NAD
Ears: NAD
Throat: NAD

Respiratory

Chest inspection: Normal
Palpation: Normal
Percussion: Normal
Auscultation: Very faint crackles
Chest x-ray: Fibrotic changes in the upper zone of left lung

Other systems

Musculoskeletal: Degeneration of lumbar and thoracic spine upon BMD
Vitamin D: 40 ng/mL
Full blood count: Recurrent neutrophilia

Medication

Prednisone: 25 mg daily
Rosuvastatin: 20 mg daily
Pantoprazole: 40 mg daily
Candesartan: 16 mg daily

TREATMENT PROTOCOL

Because of the severity of JT's sarcoidosis, treatment was focused around providing a better quality of life and reducing the frequency of hospital admission. Treatment objectives were:

- Improve immune function
- Reduce frequency of hospital admission
- Improve quality of life.

HERBAL MEDICINE

Echinacea spp.: 60 mL
Astragalus membranaceus: 60 mL
Thymus vulgarus: 60 mL
Verbascum thapsus: 40 mL
Dose: 7.5 mL twice daily

NUTRITIONAL MEDICINE

Dietary

Nutritional counselling was provided and patient was educated around differences between each of the macronutrients and each of their sub-classes. Patient was advised to:

- Increase omega-3 fatty acid consumption to at least 2 servings of fresh fish per week
- Avoid refined carbohydrates and substitute with complex carbohydrates
- Increase protein consumption to at least 0.8 g per kg of body weight daily
- Increase water consumption to 0.30 mL per kg of body weight daily

CASE STUDY CONTINUED

- Reduce and eventually eliminate coffee consumption
- Avoid alcohol consumption.

Supplemental

- Vitamin C (mixed bioflavonoids): 2 g daily, consumed in divided doses
- Zinc: 30 mg twice daily
- Omega-3 (EPA/DHA) : 1.5 g twice daily
- Vitamin D: 3000 IU daily for the next month

FOLLOW-UP

After 6 months of treatment, JT was only hospitalised once and he was able to commence exercising and walk up hills with ease. His quality of life had improved dramatically and, in conjunction with his specialist, his prednisone dose was reduced. He was able to live a normal life and his immune system was functioning correctly and he was able to be exposed to pathogens without his own immune system becoming compromised.

REFERENCES

[1] Mueller D. Medical nutrition therapy for pulmonary disease. In: Mahan LK, Escott-Stump S, editors. Krause's food and nutrition therapy. 12th ed. St Louis: Saunders Elsevier; 2008. p. 899–920.
[2] Mostov PD. Treating the immunocompetent patient who presents with an upper respiratory infection: pharyngitis, sinusitis, and bronchitis. Prim Care 2007;34(1):39–58.
[3] Wu T, Yang X, Zeng X, et al. Traditional Chinese medicine in the treatment of acute respiratory tract infections. Respir Med 2008;102(8):1093–8.
[4] Arroll B, Kenealy T. Antibiotics for the common cold and acute purulent rhinitis. Cochrane Database Syst Rev 2005;(3):CD000247.
[5] Australian Bureau of Statistics (ABS). National Health Survey: first results, 2014–15. Cat. no. 4364.0.55.001. Canberra: ABS; 2015.
[6] Castleman M. The new healing herbs. Hinkler Books; 2003.
[7] Culpeper N. Culpeper's complete herbal.1653. Available from: www.bibliomania.com/2/1/66/113/frameset.html.
[8] Ellingwood F. The Eclectic practice of medicine with especial reference to the treatment of disease. 1910.
[9] Thomas R. The Eclectic practice of medicine. 1907. Available from: www.henriettesherbal.com/eclectic/thomas/asthma.html.
[10] Thomas R. The Eclectic practice of medicine. Part II, p. 42. 1907. Available from: www.swsbm.com/EclecticMed/Eclectic%20 Medicine_Part_2.pdf.
[11] Franova S, Nosalova G, Mokry J. Phytotherapy of cough. In: Khan MTH, Ather A, editors. Advances in phytomedicine, vol. 2. US: Elsevier; 2006.
[12] Al Bayati FA. Synergistic antibacterial activity between *Thymus vulgaris* and *Pimpinella anisum* essential oils and methanol extracts. J Ethnopharmacol 2008;116(3):403–6.
[13] Huether SE, McCance K. Understanding pathophysiology. 4th ed. St Louis: Mosby; 2010. p. 714–47.
[14] Eccles R. The powerful placebo in cough studies? Pulm Pharmacol Ther 2002;15(3):303–8.
[15] Murtagh J. John Murtagh's general practice. 4th ed. Sydney: McGraw-Hill; 2007.
[16] Franova S, Nosalova G, Mokry J. Phytotherapy of cough. In: Khan MTH, Ather A, editors. Advances in phytomedicine, vol. 2. US: Elsevier; 2006. p. 111–31.
[17] Pawankar R, Canonica GW, Holgate ST, et al. Allergic diseases and asthma: a major global health concern. Curr Opin Allergy Clin Immunol 2012;12:39–41.
[18] ABS. National Health Survey: asthma and other respiratory conditions, Australia. Cat. no. 4373.0. Canberra: ABS; 1995.
[19] Jaber R. Respiratory and allergic diseases: from upper respiratory tract infections to asthma. Prim Care 2002;29(2):231–61.
[20] Marko K, Salminen S, Arvilommi H, et al. Probiotics in primary prevention of atopic disease. A randomized placebo controlled trial. Lancet 2001;357:1076–9.
[21] Black PN, Sharpe S. Dietary fat and asthma: Is there a connection? Eur Respir J 1997;10(1):6–12.
[22] Sahiner U, Birben E, Erzurum S, et al. Oxidative stress in asthma. World Allergy Organ J 2011;4(10):151–8.
[23] Braun L, Cohen M. Herbs and natural supplements: an evidence-based guide. 3rd ed. Sydney: Elsevier; 2010.
[24] Therapeutic Guidelines Limited. eTG complete. http:// online.tg.org.au/complete/.
[25] Cockcroft DW. Pharmacologic therapy for asthma: overview and historical perspective. J Clin Pharmacol 1999;39(3):216–22.
[26] Cannell JJ, Hollis BW. Use of vitamin D in clinical practice. Altern Med Rev 2008;13(1):6–20.
[27] Forestiere F, Pistelli R, Sestini P, et al. Consumption of fresh fruit rich in vitamin C and wheezing symptoms in children. SIDRIA Collaborative Group, Italy (Italian Studies on Respiratory Disorders in Children and the Environment). Thorax 2000;55(4):283–8.
[28] Perry CA, Dwyer J, Gelfand JA, et al. Health effects of salicylates in foods and drugs. Nutr Rev 1996;54(8):225–40.
[29] Zimmerman M. Burgerstein's handbook of nutrition: micronutrients in the prevention and therapy of disease. New York: Thieme; 2001.
[30] Black PN, Sharpe S. Dietary fat and asthma: Is there a connection? Eur Respir J 1997;10(1):6–12.
[31] Britton J. Dietary fish oil airways obstruction. Thorax 1995;50(Suppl. 1):S11–15.
[32] Hodge L, Salome CM, Peat JK, et al. Consumption of oily fish and childhood asthma risk. Med J Aust 1996;164(3):137–40.
[33] Haby MM, Peat JK, Marks GB, et al. Asthma in preschool children: prevalence and risk factors. Thorax 2001;56(8):589–95.
[34] Thuesen BH, Husemoen LL, Ovesen L, et al. Atopy, asthma and lung function in relation to folate and vitamin B(12) in adults. Allergy 2010;Nov(11):1146–54.
[35] Sharma S, Litonjua A. Asthma, allergy, and responses to methyl donor supplements and nutrients. J Allergy Clin Immunol 2014;133(5):1246–54.
[36] Hossein S, Pegah A, Said A, et al. The effect of nebulized magnesium sulfate in the treatment of moderate to severe asthma attacks: a randomized clinical trial. Am J Emerg Med 2016;34:883–6.
[37] Mickleborough T, Gotshall R. Dietary components with demonstrated effectiveness in decreasing the severity of exercise-induced asthma. Sports Med 2003;33(9):671–81.
[38] Mickelborough T, Vaughn C, Shei R, et al. Marine lipid fraction PCSO-524 (lyprinol omegal XL) of the New Zealand green lipped mussel attenuates hyperpnea-induced bronchoconstriction in asthma. Respir Med 2013;107(8):1152–63.
[39] Florence TM. The role of free radicals in disease. Aust NZ J Ophthalmol 1995;23(1):3–7.
[40] Gazdik F, Gvozdjakova A, Horvathova M, et al. Levels of coenzyme Q10 in asthmatics. Bratisl Lek Listy 2002;103(10):353–6.
[41] Gvozdjakova A, Kucharska J, Bartkovjakova M, et al. Coenzyme Q10 supplementation reduces corticosteroids dosage in patients with bronchial asthma. Biofactors 2005;25(1–4):235–40.
[42] Miller AL. The etiologies, pathophysiology and alternative/ complementary treatment of asthma. Altern Med Rev 2001;6(1):20–47.
[43] Morisco C, Trimarco B, Condorelli M. Effect of coenzyme Q10 therapy in patients with congestive heart failure: a long term multicenter randomized study. Clin Investig 1993;71(Suppl. 8): S134–6.
[44] Mitsui T, Umaki Y, Nagasawa M, et al. Motor neuron involvement in patient with long term corticosteroid administration. Intern Med 2003;42(9):862–6.
[45] Bone K. Clinical applications of Ayurvedic and Chinese herbs. Warwick, Qld: Phytotherapy Press; 1996.
[46] Bone K, Morgan M. Tylophora: Indian lobelia. MediHerb Professional Review 1995;(47).
[47] Huntley A, Ernst E. Herbal medicines for asthma: a systematic review. Thorax 2000;55(11):925–9.

[48] Gupta I, Gupta V, Parihar A, et al. Effects of *Boswellia serrata* gum resin in patients with bronchial asthma: results of a double-blind, placebo-controlled, 6-week clinical study. Eur J Med Res 1998;3(11):511–14.
[49] Li MH, Zhang HL, Yang BY. [Effects of ginkgo leave concentrated oral liquor in treating asthma.] Zhongguo Zhong Xi Yi Jie He Za Zhi 1997;17(4):216–18.
[50] Mabalirajan U, Ahmad T, Rehman R, et al. Baicalein reduces airway injury in allergen and IL-13 induced airway inflammation. PLoS ONE 2013;8(4):e62916.
[51] Australian Government. Communicable diseases intelligence: Influenza and pneumonia. Australian Government Department of Health and Ageing; 2008. p. 32. Available from: www.health.gov.au/internet/publications/publishing.nsf/Content/cda-cdi32suppl.htm~cda-cdi32suppl-results.htm~cda-cdi32suppl-results-flu.htm.
[52] Johnson PD, Irving LB, Turnidge JD. Community-acquired pneumonia. Med J Aust 2002;176(7):341–7.
[53] Nuorti JC, Butler JC, Farley MM, et al. Cigarette smoking and invasive pneumococcal disease. N Engl J Med 2000;342:681–9.
[54] Pizzorno JE, Murray MT. Textbook of natural medicine. 3rd ed. Edinburgh: Elsevier; 2009.
[55] Blasi F, Aliberti S, Pappalettera M, et al. 100 years of respiratory medicine: pneumonia. Respir Med 2007;101(5):875–81.
[56] Kirchmann G, Kirchmann J. Nutrition almanac. 4th ed. New York: McGraw-Hill; 1996.
[57] Bhandari N, Bahl R, Taneja S, et al. Effect of routine zinc supplementation on pneumonia in children aged 6 months to 3 years: randomised controlled trial in an urban slum. BMJ 2002;324(7350):1358.
[58] Hussey GD, Klein M. A randomized, controlled trial of vitamin A in children with severe measles. N Engl J Med 1990;323(3):160–4.
[59] Murray MT. Pneumonia: bacterial, mycoplasmal, and viral. In: Pizzorno JE, Murray MT, editors. Textbook of natural medicine. 3rd ed. Philadelphia: Elsevier; 2009.
[60] Hunt C, Chakravorty NK, Annan G. The clinical and biochemical effects of vitamin C supplementation in short-stay hospitalized geriatric patients. Int J Vitam Nutr Res 1984;54(1):65–74.
[61] Hemila H, Louhiala P. Vitamin C for preventing and treating pneumonia. Cochrane Database Syst Rev 2013;(8):CD005532.
[62] Geracts L, Haegens A, Brauers K, et al. Inhibition of LPS induced pulmonary inflammation by specific flavonoids. Biochem Biophys Res Commun 2009;382(3):598–603.
[63] Barnet JB, Hamer DH, Meydhani SN. Low zinc status: a new risk factor for pneumonia in the elderly? Nutr Rev 2010;68(1):30–7.
[64] Qasemsadeh M, Fathi M, Tashvighi M, et al. The effect of adjuvant zinc therapy on recovery from pneumonia in hospitalized children: a double-blind randomized controlled trial. Scientifica (Cairo) 2014;2014:Article 694193.
[65] Bromelain Natural Standard Research Collaboration. Natural Standard Monographs. Available from: www.naturalstandard.com.
[66] Meydani M. Vitamin E. Lancet 1995;345(8943):170–5.
[67] Felter HW, Lloyd JU. King's American dispensatory. 18th ed. Cincinnatti, USA: Ohio Valley Co; 1898. 3rd revision, 2 volumes.
[68] Chevallier A. The encyclopaedia of medicinal plants. Dorling Kindersley; 1996.
[69] Braman SS. Chronic cough due to chronic bronchitis: ACCP evidence-based clinical practice guidelines. Chest 2006;129(Suppl. 1):S104–15.
[70] Irwin RS, Baumann MH, Bolser DC, et al. Diagnosis and management of cough executive summary. Chest 2006;129(Suppl. 1):1S–23S.
[71] Altunaiji S, Kukuruzovic R, Curtis N, et al. Antibiotics for whooping cough (pertussis). Cochrane Database Syst Rev 2007;(3):CD004404.
[72] Ziment I. History of the treatment of chronic bronchitis. Respiration 1991;58(Suppl. 1):37–42.
[73] Hemila H, Douglas RM. Vitamin C and acute respiratory infections. Int J Tuberc Lung Dis 1999;3(9):756–61.
[74] Hunt C, Chakravorty NK, Annan G, et al. The clinical effects of vitamin C supplementation in elderly hospitalised patients with acute respiratory infections. Int J Vitam Nutr Res 1994;64(3):212–19.
[75] Hughes DA, Norton R. Vitamin D and respiratory health. Clin Exp Immunol 2009;158(1):20–5.
[76] Zalewski PD, Truong-Tran AQ, Grosser D, et al. Zinc metabolism in airway epithelium and airway inflammation: basic mechanisms and clinical targets. A review. Pharmacol Ther 2005;105:127–49.
[77] Morabia A, Sorenson A, Kumanyika SK, et al Vitamin A, cigarette smoking, and airway obstruction. Am J Resp Dis 1989;140(5):1312–16.
[78] Narimanian M, Badalyan M, Panosyan V, et al. Randomized trial of a fixed combination (KanJang) of herbal extracts containing *Adhatoda vasica, Echinacea purpurea* and *Eleutherococcus senticosus* in patients with upper respiratory tract infections. Phytomedicine 2005;12(8):539–47.
[79] Lizogub VG, Riley DS, Heger M. Efficacy of a *Pelargonium sidoides* preparation in patients with the common cold: a randomized, double blind, placebo-controlled clinical trial. Explore (NY) 2007;3(6):573–84.
[80] Büechi S, Vögelin R, von Eiff MM, et al. Open trial to assess aspects of safety and efficacy of a combined herbal cough syrup with ivy and thyme. Forsch Komplementarmed Klass Naturheilkd 2005;12(6):328–32.
[81] Australian Institute of Health and Welfare. Chronic respiratory conditions including asthma and COPD. 2017. Available from: www.aihw.gov.au/chronic-respiratory-conditions.
[82] ABS. National Health Survey: first results, 2014–15. Cat no. 4364.0.55.001. Canberra: ABS; 2016.
[83] ABS. Australian Aboriginal and Torres Strait Islander Health Survey: first results, Australia, 2012–13. ABS cat. no. 4727.0.55.001. Canberra: ABS; 2013.
[84] Therapeutic Guidelines Limited. eTG complete. Available from: http://online.tg.org.au/complete/.
[85] Bellamy D, Smith J. Role of primary care in early diagnosis and effective management of COPD. Int J Clin Pract 2007;61(8):1380–9.
[86] Mandal A. History of chronic obstructive pulmonary disease. New Medical Life Sciences, 2016. Available from: www.news-medical.net/health/History-of-Chronic-Obstructive-Pulmonary-Disease.aspx.
[87] Pride NB. Smoking cessation: effects on symptoms, spirometry and future trends in COPD. Thorax 2001;56:ii7–10.
[88] Weekes CE, Emery PW, Elia M. Dietary counselling and food fortification in stable COPD: a randomised trial. Thorax 2009;64(4):326–31.
[89] Hirayama F, Lee AH, Binns CW, et al. Soy consumption and risk of COPD and respiratory symptoms: a case-control study in Japan. Respir Res 2009;10:56.
[90] Shahar E, Boland LL, Folsom AR, et al. Docosahexaenoic acid and smoking-related chronic obstructive pulmonary disease. The Atherosclerosis Risk in Communities Study Investigators. Am J Respir Crit Care Med 1999;159(6):1780–5.
[91] Shahar E, Folsom AR, Melnick SL, et al. Dietary n-3 polyunsaturated acids and smoking-related chronic obstructive pulmonary disease. Am J Epidemiol 2008;168(7):796–801.
[92] Wood LG. Omega-3 polyunsaturated fatty acids and chronic obstructive pulmonary disease. Curr Opin Clin Nutr Metab Care 2015;18(2):128–32.
[93] Atlantis E, Cochrane B. The association of dietary intake and supplementation of specific polyunsaturated fatty acids with inflammation and functional capacity in chronic obstructive pulmonary disease: a systematic review. Int J Evid Based Healthc 2016;14(2):53–63.
[94] Rautalahti M, Virtamo J, Haukka J, et al. The effect of alpha-tocopherol and beta-carotene supplementation on COPD symptoms. Am J Respir Crit Care Med 1997;156(5):1447–52.
[95] Britton JR, Pavord ID, Richards A, et al. Dietary antioxidant vitamin intake and lung function in the general population. Am J Respir Crit Care Med 1995;151:1138–87.
[96] Tabak C, Arts IC, Smit HA, et al. Chronic obstructive pulmonary disease and intake of catechins, flavonols, and flavones: the MORGEN study. Am J Respir Crit Care Med 2001;164:61–4.
[97] Romieu I, Meneses F, Ramirez M, et al. Antioxidant supplementation and respiratory functions among workers exposed to high levels of ozone. Am J Respir Crit Care Med 1998;158:226–32.

[98] Hu G, Cassano PA. Antioxidant nutrients and pulmonary function: the Third National Health and Nutrition Examination Survey (NHANES III). Am J Epidemiol 2000;151(10):975–81.
[99] Braun L, Cohen M. Herbs and natural supplements: an evidence based guide. 4th ed. Sydney: Elsevier; 2015. p. 644–5.
[100] Fujimoto S, Kurihara N, Hirata K, et al. Effects of coenzyme Q10 administration on pulmonary function and exercise performance in patients with chronic lung diseases. Clin Investig 1993;71(Suppl. 8):S162–6.
[101] Yoneda T, Yoshikawa M, Fu A, et al. Plasma levels of amino acids and hypermetabolism in patients with chronic obstructive pulmonary disease. Nutrition 2001;17:95–9.
[102] Kreutner W, Chapman RW, Gulbenkian A, et al. Bronchodilator and antiallergy activity of forskolin. Eur J Pharmacol 1985;111(1):1–8.
[103] Bylka W, Matławska I, Witkowska-Banaszczak E. [Expectorant herbal medicines in respiratory tract diseases in tobacco smokers] [Article in Polish]. Przegl Lek 2005;62(10):1182–4.
[104] Meister R, Wittig T, Beuscher N, et al. Efficacy and tolerability of myrtol standardized in long-term treatment of chronic bronchitis. A double-blind, placebo-controlled study. Study Group Investigators. Arzneimittelforschung 1999;49(4):351–8.
[105] Weiss RF. Weiss's herbal medicine. Classic ed. USA: Thieme; 2001.
[106] Gillman A, Steinfort C. Sarcoidosis in Australia. Intern Med J 2007;37(6):356–9.
[107] Better Health Channel. Sarcoidosis. 2014. Available from: www.betterhealth.vic.gov.au.
[108] Baughman RP, Culver DA, Judson MA. A concise review of pulmonary sarcoidosis. Am J Respir Crit Care Med 2011;183:573–81.
[109] Iannuzzi M, Birendra S. Merck Manual Professional Version. Sarcoidosis. Available from: www.merckmanuals.com/professional/pulmonary-disorders/sarcoidosis/sarcoidosis.
[110] Chen ES, Song Z, Willett MH, et al. Serum amyloid A regulates granulomatous inflammation in sarcoidosis through toll like receptor-2. Am J Respir Crit Care Med 2010;181:360–73.
[111] Nunes H, Maurer C, Naccache JM, et al. Severe pulmonary sarcoidosis. Ann Med Interne (Paris) 2001;152(2):96–102.
[112] Laohaburanakit P, Chan A. Obstructive sarcoidosis. Clin Rev Allergy Immunol 2003;25(2):115–29.
[113] Wijsenbeek M, Culver D. Treatment of sarcoidosis. Clin Chest Med 2015;36:751–67.
[114] Coker RK. Management strategies for pulmonary sarcoidosis. Ther Clin Risk Manag 2009;5:575–84.
[115] Boots AW, Drent M, Swenne E, et al. Antioxidant status associated with inflammation in sarcoidosis: a potential role for antixodiants. Respir Med 2009;103:364–72.
[116] McNee W. Oxidative stress and lung inflammation in airways disease. Eur J Pharmacol 2001;429:195–207.
[117] Rehman I. Oxidative stress, transcription factors and chromatin remodeling in lung inflammation. Biochem Pharmacol 2002;64:935–42.
[118] Ashraf R, Shah NP. Immune system stimulation by probiotic micro-organisms. Crit Rev Food Sci Nutr 2014;54(7):938–56.
[119] Bonaventura P, Benedetti G, Albarede F, et al. Zinc and its role in immunity and inflammation. Autoimmun Rev 2015;14:277–85.
[120] Kiecolt-Glaser JK, Belury MA, Andridge R, et al. Omega-3 supplementation lowers inflammation in healthy middle-aged and older adults: a randomised controlled trial. Brain Behav Immun 2012;26:988–95.
[121] Kiecolt-Glaser JK, Belury MA, Andridge R, et al. Omega-3 supplementation lowers inflammation and anxiety in medical students: a randomized controlled trial. Brain Behav Immun 2011;25:1725–34.
[122] Bolland M, Wilsher M, Grey A, et al. Randomised controlled trial of vitamin D supplementation in sarcoidosis. BMJ 2013;3:1–8.
[123] Bennett J, Dolin R, Blaser M. Mandell, Douglas and Bennett's principles and practice of infectious diseases. 8th ed. Elsevier; 2015. p. 601–2.
[124] Braun L, Cohen M. Herbs and natural supplements: an evidence-based guide. 4th ed. Sydney: Elsevier; 2015. p. 982–5.

15 The musculoskeletal system

Leah Hechtman, Lisa Costa-Bir, Bradley McEwen

SECTION A

OVERVIEW OF THE MUSCULOSKELETAL SYSTEM

The term 'musculoskeletal system' refers to the integration of the skeletal system and the muscular system. The musculoskeletal system is a relatively broad and perhaps deceiving term as this system encompasses not only the skeleton and the muscles but also a group of smaller subsystems, namely the tendons, ligaments, joints, cartilage and other connective tissue structures. Together these systems work as a whole, providing the basic functions of the musculoskeletal system that are essential to life (Table 15.1 and Fig. 15.1).

The musculoskeletal system is the largest collective system within the body. In healthy human adults the musculoskeletal system makes up about half of the total body weight (though it is slightly less in women).[1] With assistance from the nervous system, the human body's ability to maintain posture and carry out a range of voluntary movements is a result of the complex interplay that occurs between the joints, muscles, bones, tendons and ligaments of the musculoskeletal system.

The skeletal muscles generate forces that are relayed to the joints and bones which in turn produce movement. It is this functional role of production in movement that leads to the musculoskeletal system being referred to as the body's primary locomotive system; this system plays an important role by providing stability, support and protection against any demands that might upset balance in the body.

The skeletal system

The adult human skeleton consists of 206 bones and accounts for between 12% and 15% of total body weight.[2] When the skeleton first forms it is made of flexible cartilage, but within a few weeks, it begins the process of ossification, where cartilage is replaced by hard deposits of calcium phosphate and stretchy collagen. It takes about 20 years for this process to be completed.

TABLE 15.1 Overview of the musculoskeletal system

Component	Definition
Bursa	A fluid sac between the muscles and bones that forms in areas of friction
Cartilage	The protective gel-like substance that lines the joints and the intervertebral disc
Joint	The place of union between two or more bones
Ligament	A fibrous band of tissue that connects bone to bone
Skeletal muscle	A form of striated muscle tissue that assists the skeleton with movement
Skeleton	The supporting internal structure of the human body composed of bone and cartilage that protects and supports the soft organs, tissues and other parts
Tendon	A fibrous band of tissue that connects muscle to bone

FUNCTIONS OF THE SKELETAL SYSTEM

Protection of the vital organs

One of the most important functions of the skeletal system is to protect the vital organs of the body. Some examples of this important function include the skull (cranium) forming a protective cage around the brain, the pelvic cavity protecting the bladder and the ribcage protecting the heart and lungs.

Support

The skeleton forms the framework of the human body where it provides structure and a frame for the organs and tissues of the body. In this way, it can be compared with the scaffolding on a new building. By providing a structural framework, the body is able to maintain posture and form, playing a key role in providing stability and support.

Body movement

The body is able to move because of the interaction between the skeletal system, the muscles and nervous system.

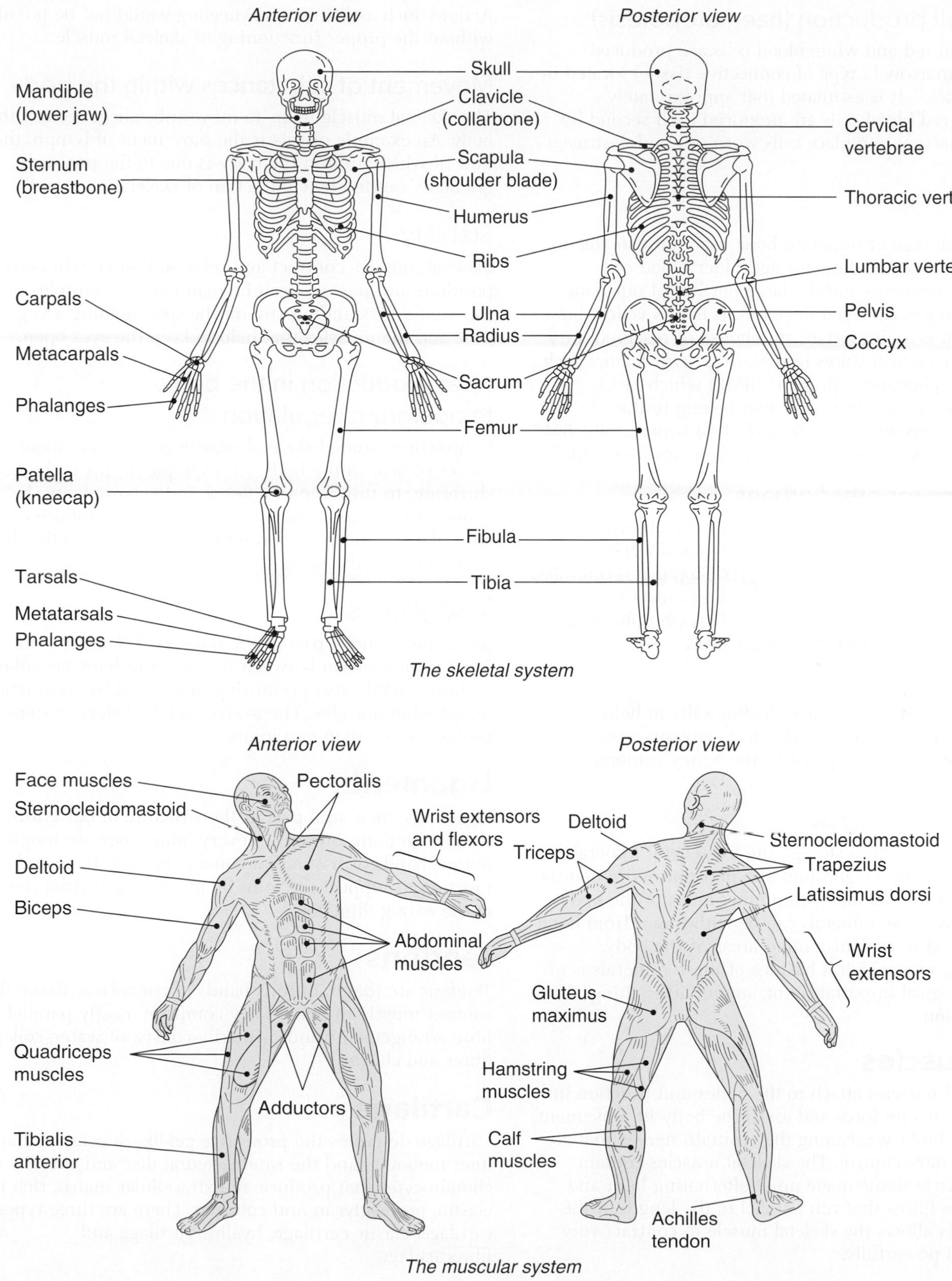

FIGURE 15.1 The musculoskeletal system — muscles and skeletal system.

Blood cell production (haematopoiesis)

Platelets and red and white blood cells are produced by the red marrow (a type of connective tissue) located in specific bones.[3] It is estimated that approximately 2.6 million red blood cells are produced each second by the bone marrow to replace cells worn out and destroyed by the liver.[4]

Storage

As well as storage of minerals, bone tissue is also able to store triglycerides. As humans age, older blood cell production decreases and the large portion of our bone marrow changes from red to yellow. It is this yellow bone marrow that is an important storehouse of reserved fatty acids. The bone also stores important growth factors such as bone morphogenetic proteins (BMP) which are multifunctional growth factors that belong to the transforming growth factor beta (TGF-β) superfamily. BMP signalling plays a critical role in cartilage development.[5]

Assistance for other organs

The kidney is regulated to inhibit phosphate reabsorption and the synthesis of 1,25(OH)(2)D (a form of vitamin D) by the release of fibroblast growth factor-23 (FGF-23) that is controlled by the bones. Disorders of increased FGF-23 function are associated with rickets or osteomalacia, hypophosphataemia and inappropriately low 1,25(OH)(2)D levels.[6]

Protection

The bones absorb and release alkaline salts to help maintain a systemic pH. While this is advantageous, it comes partly at the expense of the bones' mineral stores.[7]

Mineral homeostasis

Bone tissue serves as a storage site for several minerals including calcium, magnesium and phosphorus. When the supply of these minerals within other areas of the body becomes low, these minerals can be withdrawn from bone into the blood to replenish other areas of the body. Maintaining physiological balance of these minerals is of crucial biological importance for, among other things, bone mineralisation.

The muscles

The skeletal muscles attach to the bones and function in unison to generate force and assist the body in movement. They are voluntary, meaning they contain nerves that are under voluntary control. The skeletal muscles contain striated muscle tissue made up of alternating light and dark muscle fibres that run parallel to the length of the muscle. This allows the skeletal muscle to contract very quickly and powerfully.

FUNCTIONS OF THE SKELETAL MUSCLES

Body movement

Similarly to the bones, the skeletal muscles are required to help the body move. By contracting and relaxing, the muscles help to bend the skeleton into various positions. Actions such as lifting and kneeling would not be possible without the proper functioning of skeletal muscle.

Movement of substances within the body

The skeletal muscle helps to move substances around the body. An example of this is the movement of lymph, the flow of which around the body is due to the pressure gradients exerted by contraction of skeletal muscles.[3]

Stability

Skeletal muscles contract and relax so that certain body positions and postures can be maintained. Examples of this would be standing still on the spot, holding a yoga pose and the muscles that help to keep the eyes open.

Heat production in the body/ temperature regulation

Contracting striated skeletal muscle generates a major source of heat in the body. An example of this is the body shivering. In this scenario, flexor and extensor muscles simultaneously and involuntary contract to produce a muscular tremor in response to a cold stimuli so that heat is produced in the body.[8]

The joints

Joints are a crucial part of the musculoskeletal system and function as a union between two or more bony articular surfaces[9] while also permitting movement by contraction of opposing muscles. The average adult skeletal system contains more than 200 joints.

Ligaments

Ligaments are a vital part of the structure of our entire skeleton and are present in every joint. They are tough, fibrous bands of tissue that connect bone to bone and function to support the joint by preventing it from moving in the wrong direction.

Tendons

Tendons are tough, fibrous bands of connective tissue that connect muscle to bone. They comprise mostly parallel fibre arrangements and primarily consist of water, collagen fibres and elastin.[10]

Cartilage

Cartilage describes the protective gel-like substance that lines the joints and the intervertebral disc and consists of chondrocytes that produce an extracellular matrix rich in elastin, proteoglycan and collagen. There are three types of cartilage: elastic cartilage, hyaline cartilage and fibrocartilage.

Bursa

Bursa are fluid-filled sacs which sit between the muscles and bones and form in areas that are susceptible to friction, such as the knee joint. They function to decrease friction and act as a protective cushion.

ROLE OF THE NATUROPATH

Traditional interpretation

The treatment of musculoskeletal deficits is one of the most compelling matters that have engaged the attention of naturopaths throughout history. Understanding and acknowledging the efforts of the practitioners before our time helps to maintain continuity between contemporary treatments and those of our ancestors.

The early naturopathic doctors advocated a prescription of exercise, sunshine, fresh air, good nutrition, prayer, constructive thinking, meditation and a positive mental attitude for good health. They believed a routine with all these things in balance would provide the basic framework for good health.

Rheumatoid arthritis, degenerative arthritis and gout all feature prominently in Ellingwood's materia medica, yet find themselves not classified per se as conditions of the musculoskeletal system. Rather, they are neatly placed into the category of 'constitutional diseases' suggesting that the Eclectics may have believed these conditions were caused as a result of one's constitution.

Like most present-day naturopaths, the physicians of the past used a multifaceted approach in their management of musculoskeletal disorders, not relying solely on botanicals or diet alone. Heat therapies, including hot baths, hot water bottles, hot bricks and warm ironed flannel, were all promoted as aids for rheumatic conditions due to their ability to promote free perspiration and promote total bone metamorphosis. Topical heating liniments (similar to those that we use today) containing wintergreen oil, mustard oil and salicyclic acid also featured.

Dietary manipulation featured prominently in the traditional teachings of the Eclectics. Those who were 'careless in their diet' were said to be commonly afflicted with arthritis and it was recommended that they should avoid nitrogenous foods as well as coffee and tea, suggesting that the Eclectics had some idea that toxicity, food intolerance and/or inflammation were causative or worsening factors in the pathogenesis of musculoskeletal disorders. Those afflicted with chronic rheumatism were advised to refrain from tea and coffee and to omit meat from the diet. A vegetable diet with plenty of pure water was advocated, showing that these recommendations for rheumatic conditions are congruent with present-day naturopathic teachings.

This is very much in line with Ayurvedic medicine, which teaches that many arthritic disorders come from an accumulation of 'ama' (toxicity) in the joints. Ama is a byproduct of weak digestion ('agni'). This ancient Ayurvedic link between arthritis and the gut is fascinating, given that present-day medicine has also observed a link between food intolerances/sensitivities and disorders of the musculoskeletal system/aggravation of symptoms.

Our ancient forebears were remarkably intelligent and insightful and many of the issues that plagued them are still of concern to us today. Cod liver oil, a rich source of vitamin D, was used traditionally to treat and prevent rickets, a condition resulting from prolonged vitamin D deficiency. Physicians of the 1840s spoke of its effects on bone health, stating 'whether the disease of rickets be in its most severe form, with swollen joints and crooked legs, or at its commencement, the cod liver oil will supersede every other means of cure'.[11] Today vitamin D deficiency is still a concern and many naturopaths will recommend cod liver oil as recommended centuries before.

Central to the traditional approach to the musculoskeletal system was the belief that conditions of this system were characterised by an accumulation of toxins and wastes unable to be or improperly eliminated by the body. This resulted in toxaemia and subsequent breakdown of the body. Toxicity as a causative factor is noted by Ellingwood, who states: '[muscular rheumatism] is undoubtedly an indirect or remote result of autotoxemia'.[12]

Because of this toxicity, prescription was generally geared towards the botanical classes of medicines known as 'depuratives', with the main treatment objective being cleansing and detoxifying of the body. Ellingwood highlights the efficacy of treatment with depuratives in relation to rheumatoid arthritis, stating: 'I believe that those patients have obtained the best results who have persisted for a long period in the use of the botanic alteratives [such as *Rumex crispus*] and antirheumatic remedies, in the form of infusions or decoctions, conjoined with a strict attention to diet and hygienic surroundings'.[12]

Modern interpretation

Modern naturopathic treatment of the musculoskeletal system is still based upon the traditional naturopathic principles of 'Primum No Nocere' (First Do No Harm), 'Tolle Causam' (Treat the Cause) and 'Vis Mediatrix Naturae' (The Healing Power of Nature). Taking on the traditional knowledge passed on by the Eclectics discussed above, it builds on the knowledge that toxicity plays a key role in the pathogenesis of the diseased state, discovering other possible causative factors for conditions of the musculoskeletal system that include gender, genetics, environmental triggers, increased intestinal permeability, autoimmune disease, increased circulating immune complexes, excessive inflammatory processes and oxidative stress.

The modern naturopathic approach to the musculoskeletal system brings with it many advances, including the benefits of technology in the guise of clinical laboratory and pathology testing. A more complex understanding of how botanical and nutritional supplements (and their active constituents) work on a biochemical level is also of benefit. Our knowledge of the pathophysiology of diseases as well as the science of naturopathy has also advanced profoundly. While *Curcuma longa* has been used for inflammatory conditions of the musculoskeletal system in Ayurvedic medicine for centuries, it has only recently been discovered that many of its anti-inflammatory effects are caused by its active constituent curcumin. By knowing more about how our medicines work we can work towards advances in the treatment of patients and hence better results.

Like their forebears, modern naturopathic physicians use a variety of modalities in the management of the musculoskeletal system, including diet, detoxification, botanicals, nutritionals and physical therapy techniques. They may also work concurrently with other healthcare professionals who specialise in the management of musculoskeletal disorders, such as osteopaths, chiropractors and massage therapists. The modern naturopath recognises that the musculoskeletal system is central to the patient's wellbeing and that a healthy and optimally functioning musculoskeletal system is vital for good health and an important determinant of quality of life. While there is a greater understanding of how the musculoskeletal system works and the causative factors influencing musculoskeletal conditions, modern naturopaths validate the work of their forebears by using similar treatment modalities in their management of musculoskeletal conditions. An example of this is the use of the botanical *Salix alba*, which was recommended by first-century Western physician Dioscorides for pain and inflammation[13] and is still in use today for the same purpose.

The naturopathic physician realises that the musculoskeletal system can reflect changes in and produce changes in other body systems, hence it should come as no surprise that the musculoskeletal system will reflect many internal illnesses and may aggravate or accelerate the process of disease in another body system. This is central to naturopathic philosophy, which recognises that the human body is an integrated, whole organism in which no part functions independently. Abnormalities in the structure or function of one part of the body may unfavourably influence other parts and, eventually, the body as a whole. An example of this is small intestine bacterial overgrowth which occurs in the gastrointestinal system but is linked to the pathogenesis of rheumatoid arthritis, a condition of the musculoskeletal system.

Musculoskeletal disorders constitute a problem of major public health importance. About half the adult population is reported to experience some sort of musculoskeletal symptoms and 39–45% have long-lasting problems. The course of musculoskeletal disorders is marked by periods of remission and exacerbation with most individuals not experiencing complete resolution of their symptoms and disabilities.[14] Musculoskeletal pain is one of the most significant occupational health hazards for healthcare professionals. For instance, the prevalence of general musculoskeletal pain among dentists had been found to vary between 64% and 93%, with the most commonly cited regions of pain being the back (36.3–60.1%) and neck (19.8–85%).[15] Furthermore, physical, mental and emotional stress plays an important role in the aetiology of musculoskeletal conditions. Upper extremity musculoskeletal disorders are common in office workers with shoulder, elbow and hand/wrist disorders associated with poor mental health, such as somatic symptoms, anxiety/insomnia, social dysfunction and depression. Anxiety/insomnia was strongly correlated with shoulders, elbows and hands/wrists symptoms.[16] Melancholic depression has been associated with a higher prevalence of musculoskeletal pain in comparison with atypical depression.[17]

In summary, the modern naturopath considers a few key areas, as the inner environment and metabolism equals a healthy musculoskeletal system:

- Assessment of toxin build-up
- Support to remove wastes and toxins in blood, lymphatic system, gastrointestinal tract, liver and the urinary system, especially the kidneys
- Is there an underlying infective origin?
- Assessment of inflammatory markers and markers of autoimmunity
- Pain relief
- Investigation and correction of any nutritional deficiencies
- Investigation for food allergies and/or intolerances
- Improve digestive function and nutrient absorption
- Dietary modifications as necessary
- Assessment of weight, weight management program may be required if overweight or obese
- Improvement of the function of the affected joints, e.g. range of movement
- Improvement of quality of life
- Chronic diseases require long-term treatment.

Nutritional requirements

Specific nutritional objectives are listed in Table 15.2.

Herbal medicine classes

Herbal medicine classes used for the musculoskeletal system are listed in Table 15.3.

Investigations

Investigations used for the musculoskeletal system are listed in Table 15.4.

Potential interactions

See the interactions tables at the back of the book.

TABLE 15.2 Nutritional requirements

Requirement	Reason	Therapeutic dose	Dietary source
Boron	Trace mineral involved in the development and maintenance of healthy bones. Boron is involved in the efficient absorption of calcium in the body and also activates vitamin D	2–7 mg/day, UL 9.6 mg/day	Almonds, hazelnuts, peanut butter, apples, pears, prunes, raisins, soy milk
Calcium	Required for the development and maintenance of the skeleton as well as proper neuromuscular function. Stored in the bones where it provides structure and strength. Other functions include nerve conduction, cell signalling, cell membrane function and protein metabolism	1000–2000 mg/day (in divided doses)	Tinned sardines and salmon (with the bones), almonds, dairy products (milk, yoghurt, cheese), tahini, sesame seeds, leafy green vegetables (spinach, broccoli, bok choy), dried figs
Copper	Cross-links proteins such as collagen and elastin contributing to the structure of the extracellular matrix. Like zinc, it is an important component of metalloenzymes and dietary deficiency results in peroxidise damage to the joints due to decreased concentrations of the cytosolic antioxidant enzyme superoxide dismutase	2–5 mg/day	Beans, lentils, Brazil nuts, crab, lobster, mussels, prawns
Magnesium	Enhances calcium and phosphate absorption and deposition. Increases the strength of bones and is required for mineralisation of the teeth and bones. Magnesium is also involved in nerve conduction, regulation of vascular tone, ATP production and the synthesis and metabolism of protein and DNA	300–1000 mg/day (in divided doses e.g. 300 mg t.d.s.)	Eggs, cocoa, almonds, brewers yeasts, cashews, green leafy vegetables, kelp, wheat bran, wheatgerm, buckwheat
Manganese	Co-factor in the formation of bone cartilage and bone collagen, as well as in bone mineralisation. The synthesis of proteoglycans is dependent on manganese. Manganese is also a component of manganese superoxide dismutase (MnSOD)	100–2600 micrograms/day UL 11 mg/day	Almonds, beans, coconuts, corn, kelp, sunflower seeds, legumes, walnuts, wholegrains
Selenium	Powerful antioxidant and component of a family of four enzymes, the glutathione peroxidases 1–4 which are involved in catalysing, reducing and deactivating free radicals and other potential oxidants. Glutathione peroxidases can downregulate the expression of inflammatory genes. Constituent of selenoprotein P, which scavenges peroxynitrite, an inflammatory agent produced in inflamed joints. Selenium is also involved in immune modulation and thyroid hormone metabolism	200–250 micrograms/day	Brazil nuts, fish, shellfish, lentils and pulses, kidney and liver (choose organic)
Zinc	Necessary for the creation of the collagen that forms a framework for mineralisation. Important component of metalloenzymes. Dietary deficiency results in peroxidise damage to the joints due to decreased concentrations of the cytosolic antioxidant enzyme superoxide dismutase. Zinc is also involved in general growth and development, immune modulation, cell membrane activity and nerve transmission	10–75 mg/day	Pumpkin seeds, sunflower seeds, oysters, wholegrains, beef, baked beans, cashews, egg yolks, ginger, herring, liver (organic), milk, lamb
Vitamin C	Water-soluble vitamin that reduces oxidative damage and is essential for the hydroxylation of proline in precollagen to form collagen. Maintains the integrity and stability of connective tissue. Vitamin C is also involved in immune modulation, metabolism of cholesterol and neurotransmitters. Stores are used up in conditions where there is oxidative stress	250–5000 mg/day (in divided doses)	Kiwi fruit, guava, papaya, mangoes, strawberries, acerola cherries

Continued

TABLE 15.2 Nutritional requirements—cont'd			
Requirement	**Reason**	**Therapeutic dose**	**Dietary source**
Vitamin D	Assists with calcium and phosphorus absorption, both of which are vital for the normal development of bones. Inadequate vitamin D is associated with impaired intestinal calcium absorption and must be corrected for ingested calcium to be effective. Vitamin D is also involved in differentiation, proliferation, modulation of the immune system and maintains muscle strength and integrity	600–5000 IU/day based on blood levels*	Synthesised by the action of sunlight on fish liver oils such as cod, tuna; also found in egg yolks, sprouted seeds and milk
Vitamin E	Fat-soluble vitamin that inhibits the release of arachidonic acid from phospholipids and reduces eicosanoid formation, reducing inflammation and pain. Reactive oxygen species (ROS) are formed in the tissues and have been identified in the pathogenesis of many musculoskeletal disorders. Antioxidants such as vitamin E have been found to scavenge free radicals such as ROS. Vitamin E is also involved in immune regulation, modulation of vascular function and promotes wound healing	100–600 IU/day	Almonds, wheatgerm, safflower, egg yolks, corn, beef, nuts
Vitamin K (phytomenadione)	Facilitates calcium's incorporation into the bones' hydroxyapatite crystals. Vitamin K plays an essential role as a coenzyme during the synthesis of the biologically active form of a number of proteins involved in bone metabolism (osteocalcin found in bone and matrix Gla protein) and blood coagulation	1 microgram/kg of body weight	Broccoli, eggs, kale, kelp, spinach, beans, cabbage, lettuce, soybeans and soybean oil
Omega-3 fatty acids	Analgesic and anti-inflammatory. Replace arachidonic acid in the inflammatory cell membranes providing an anti-inflammatory action that is linked to the production of alternative eicosanoids, the reduction of pro-inflammatory cytokines and leukotrienes, as well as inhibiting the activation of T lymphocytes and of catabolic enzymes. Omega-3 is also involved in cholesterol metabolism, endothelial function, neurotransmission, cell signalling and membrane function and structure	800–2700 mg/day DHA 3000–5000 mg/day EPA	Pilchards, salmon, trout, herring, mackerel and vegetarian sources such as chia seeds, flaxseeds and walnuts
Cod liver oil	Anti-inflammatory action and may be used to reduce dose of NSAIDs. Source of vitamin D to further assist with bone health	1–10 g/day (150 mg EPA, 70 mg DHA)	Supplementation only
Bromelain	Contains proteolytic enzymes that have been found to be analgesic, which directly influence pain mediators such as bradykinin. Blocks pro-inflammatory metabolites and assists in preventing and reducing oedema at inflammation sites. Increases serum fibrinolytic activity and decreases PGE_2 and thromboxane A_2 thereby reducing inflammation. Stimulates monocytes to secrete cytokines and induces phagocytosis by white blood cells	160–1000 mg/day	Stem and fruit of the pineapple plant
Quercetin	Flavonoid with antioxidant and anti-inflammatory activity. Quercetin forms a strong matrix by reinforcing collagen. In rats, quercetin has been found to inhibit the proliferation, differentiation and mineralisation of osteoblastic cells. Quercetin also has immune modulating, antihistamine and neuroprotective properties	300–2000 mg/day	Red wine, grapefruit, onions, apples, black tea and in lesser amounts, in leafy green vegetables and beans. Quercetin is also found in medicinal plants including *Ginkgo biloba*, *Hypericum perforatum* (St John's wort), *Sambucus* spp. (elderberry) and many other herbs

TABLE 15.2 Nutritional requirements—cont'd

Requirement	Reason	Therapeutic dose	Dietary source
Glucosamine	A naturally occurring substance found in the joints. Assists in the production of proteoglycans, hyaluronic acid and mucopolysaccharides, constituents that produce joint tissue such as tendons. Glucosamine also has anti-inflammatory properties	1500 mg/day (500 mg t.d.s.)	Does not appear in significant amounts in most diets; however, it is found in the shells of crustaceans
Methyl-sulfonyl-methane (MSM)	Hypothesised to stabilise cell membranes, slowing or stopping leakage from injured cells and to scavenge hydroxyl-free radicals which trigger inflammation thus inhibiting degenerative changes that may occur in osteoarthritis	3–6 g/day MSM should be taken for at least 3 months	Green plant foods and vegetables. It is easily destroyed when foods are processed
S-adenosylmethionine (SAMe)	Incorporates sulfate groups into proteoglycans which help to maintain cartilage and protect joints. SAMe is also involved in the synthesis of glutathione, protein and neurotransmitters and is involved in methylation	200–1600 mg/day (in divided doses, e.g. 200–400 mg b.i.d.–t.d.s.)**	Supplementation only

*General recommendation is between 1000 and 4000 IU/day; however, in strong deficiency states (proven by blood tests), increasing the dose is recommended.

**Ensure that you assess the patient's methylation prior to prescribing.

Sources:[56,106,107,560,695–702]

TABLE 15.3 Herbal medicine classes

Class	Example	Justification
Analgesics and anodynes (provide pain relief)	*Corydalis ambigua* (corydalis)	*Corydalis ambigua* is a bitter, warming herb with a long history of use in traditional Chinese medicine as a pain reliever. The rhizome is the plant part favoured and is said to have between 1% and 10% of the analgesic potency of opium. *Corydalis ambigua* is widely stocked in the modern naturopathic dispensary as a first-line analgesic, but despite its popularity there has been little in the way of modern clinical studies. In one small pilot study undertaken on patients taking 3.25 g/day of *Corydalis yanhusuo* (said to be interchangeable with *Corydalis ambigua*) in combination with *Angelicae dahuricae*, pain intensity was significantly decreased and the level at which patients reported cold-induced pain to be bothersome was reduced ($p < 0.01$ for both). A dose-related analgesic effect was also observed
	Salix alba (white willow bark)	*Salix alba* is the bark of the young, 2–3-year-old branches of the willow tree and is well known as the botanical precursor of aspirin. It possesses anti-inflammatory and analgesic properties attributable to one of its pharmacologically active constituents, the salicylates found within its bark. ESCOP and the Commission E approve the use of willow bark for diseases accompanied by rheumatic ailments. The *British Herbal Pharmacopoeia* indicates its use for arthritic conditions. See also the section on analgesia
Antimicrobials	*Hypericum perforatum* (St John's wort)	Infections are believed to contribute to the maturation of the immune system from the innate to the adaptive phases and may take part in the induction of autoimmune conditions such as rheumatoid arthritis. Common infective agents include cytomegalovirus and Epstein-Barr virus. St John's wort contains two bioactive components — hypericin and hyperforin — both of which have been identified as powerful antiviral agents. St John's wort also has anxiolytic, antidepressant, anti-inflammatory and analgesic properties
Anti-inflammatories	*Curcuma longa* (turmeric)	Turmeric has been used in Ayurvedic medicine for the management of inflammatory conditions for centuries. Curcumin is a lipophilic polyphenol and is the active constituent found within turmeric deemed responsible for a wide array of its pharmacological actions. Several modes of action have been found for its anti-inflammatory effects on the body, including inhibition of: arachidonic acid metabolism, the enzymes lipoxygenase 5-LOX and cyclooxygenase-2 (COX-2), inducible nitric oxide synthase (iNOS), inflammatory cytokines such as TNF-α, interleukins (IL)-1, -2, -6, -8 and -12, monocyte chemoattractant protein (MCP) and migration inhibitory protein. Turmeric also has immune modulating, wound healing and hepatoprotective actions

Continued

TABLE 15.3 Herbal medicine classes—cont'd

Class	Example	Justification
Antirheumatics	*Zingiber officinale* (ginger)	Ginger is a powerful anti-inflammatory that has traditionally been used in Ayurvedic and Tibb medicine for rheumatic disorders. It appears to inhibit prostaglandins and leukotriene biosynthesis due to its ability to dually inhibit eicosanoid elevated prostaglandins and leukotrienes, both of which are characteristic of rheumatic disorders. Ginger also has analgesic, antiplatelet, antioxidant, antispasmodic and antiemetic properties
COX/and or lipoxygenase inhibitors	*Boswellia serrata* (boswellia/ frankincense)	Boswellia, also known as frankincense, has a long history of use, having been mentioned in the Bible as one of the gifts brought to the baby Jesus by the three kings. The active constituents within boswellia are known as boswellic acids (α and β boswellic acid) and have been found to inhibit prostaglandin and leukotriene biosynthesis, 5-lipoxygenase (LOX) and cyclooxygenase (COX). In modern times *Boswellia* extracts have shown efficacy in treating musculoskeletal disorders such as rheumatoid arthritis and osteoarthritis of the knee
Steroidal anti-inflammatories	*Glycyrrhiza glabra* (liquorice)	Steroidal anti-inflammatories help to inhibit steroidal pathways of inflammation. The roots and stolons of liquorice contain glycyrrhizin, a triterpenoid saponin that displays steroid-like activity and has a long history of use as an anti-inflammatory agent. Liquorice also has antioxidant, antispasmodic, lipid-lowering and hepatoprotective properties
Circulatory stimulants	*Capsicum* spp.	Capsaicin (8-methyl-*N*-vanillyl-6-noneamide) is the pungent active constituent found within *Capsicum* spp. It may be taken systemically or applied topically to enhance circulation and blood flow time and hence nutrient flow. Capsaicin also promotes the release of the neurotransmitter substance P, which after repeated applications has been found to reduce an individual's perception of pain (as it depletes sensory neurons of substance P) and has been postulated to be beneficial in fibromyalgia and osteoarthritis. The Commission E approves the use of cayenne for painful muscle spasms in areas of shoulder, arm and spine of adults and children
Connective tissue regenerators	*Centella asiatica* (gotu kola)	One of the primary mechanisms of action of *Centella* is the stimulation of type I collagen production, which ultimately aids in the repair of connective tissue. Triterpenoid compounds have been identified as important constituents within *Centella* that contribute to its regenerative effects on the connective tissue; these include asiaticoside, madecassoside, centelloside and asiatic acid. In a rat model madecassoside orally administered substantially attenuated type II collagen-induced arthritis. The underlying mechanisms of action may be mainly through regulating the abnormal humoral and cellular immunity as well as preventing joint destruction
Depuratives	*Urtica dioica* (nettle)	Traditionally, urtica was recommended to manage musculoskeletal complaints though perhaps in a different carrier than most naturopaths use today! Grieve says: 'The nettle beer made by cottagers is often given to their old folk as a remedy for gouty and rheumatic pains'. Modern-day naturopaths still use depuratives such as urtica to improve detoxification and elimination, thus helping to reduce accumulated metabolic waste products in the body. Urtica may be used systemically as well as topically, providing there is no known allergy to nettle
Diuretics	*Apium graveolens* (celery)	From a naturopathic perspective, accumulation of waste substances in the body is believed to contribute to arthritis and rheumatism, hence the excretion of these wastes through the urine will be beneficial. The seeds of celery's wild ancestors, which originated around the Mediterranean, were widely used as a diuretic and for gout. Celery is also high in sodium and potassium which contributes to its ability to increase urinary output, thereby removing waste. Celery also has anti-inflammatory and potential antioxidant properties
Immune modulators	*Hemidesmus indicus* (hemidesmus)	*Hemidesmus indicus* is an Ayurvedic herb that has been used to treat rheumatic disorders. It suppresses both the cell-mediated and humoral components of the immune system. This activity suggests it would be of benefit in autoimmune disorders
Musculoskeletal spasmolytic	*Matricaria recutita* (chamomile)	Chamomile is one of the most well recognised and used herbs. Over 120 constituents have been identified in the chamomile flower, including bisabolol, spiroethers and apigenin. Some of these have been studied with respect to their spasmolytic activities. Although the spasmolytic activity of chamomile preparations is widely acknowledged, the mechanisms underlying smooth muscle relaxation remain unclear. Clinical studies reveal cAMP-PDE inhibition by chamomile infusions as a likely mechanism underlying the spasmolytic activity, but other mechanisms may also be concurrent

Sources: [232,238,464,583,590,703–711]

TABLE 15.4 Investigations

Assessment	Normal adult values	Implication
Antinuclear antibodies (ANA)	Negative/positive The normal titre (a metric used to measure the presence and amount of antibodies in blood) of ANA is 1:40	An ANA test is performed if autoimmune conditions affecting the musculoskeletal system are suspected. A low titre of 1:40 is considered to be weak and clinically insignificant. Elevated levels (positive result) are common in systemic lupus erythematosus (SLE), Sjögren's syndrome, rheumatoid arthritis and scleroderma. A negative result excludes lupus in 90% of cases. A speckled pattern may be associated with specific rheumatic disorders such as SLE, SLE overlap syndromes, mixed connective tissue disease and Sjögren's syndrome
Antibodies to extractable nuclear antigens (ENA): Antibody to Sm Antibody to nRNP Antibody to SSA Antibody to SSB Antibody to Scl-70 Antibody to Jo-1	Detected/not detected	The presence of antibodies against extractable nuclear antigen is highly suggestive of systemic rheumatic disease. Defined antigen specificities include: RNP — mixed connective tissue disease; Sm — highly specific for SLE; Ro (SS-A) — subacute cutaneous lupus, associated with recurrent abortion, congenital heart block and Sjögren's syndrome; La (SS-B) — Sjögren's syndrome; and Scl 70 — scleroderma
Anti-DNA antibodies	Detected/not detected	Anti-DNA antibodies are the serological hallmark of SLE and unique markers of the immunological disturbances critical to disease pathogenesis. Anti-DNA autoantibodies deposit in the tissue to incite inflammation and damage as well as to induce cytokine production
Cyclic citrullinated peptide antibodies (CCPA)	Detected/not detected	CCPA is considered the most promising diagnostic and prognostic rheumatoid arthritis marker. The sensitivity of CCPA is comparable to that of the rheumatoid factor, while its specificity for this disease is much higher. CCPA detection may be very useful for diagnostics of early seronegative rheumatoid arthritis, differential diagnosis between rheumatoid arthritis and other rheumatic diseases and for the prognosis of severe erosive articular lesion. High levels may indicate that the patient is at increased risk for damage to the joints. It is typically positive in >60% of rheumatoid arthritis patients. Presence confirms aggressive type of rheumatoid arthritis
HLA-B27 antigen	Detected/not detected	Human leucocyte antigens (HLAs) are proteins that help the body's immune system tell the difference between its own cells and foreign, harmful substances. Signifies the possibility of autoimmune disease
C-reactive protein (CRP) test	<5.0 mg/L	C-reactive protein (CRP) is an acute-phase protein that plays a major role in the regulation of the inflammatory response. The level of CRP rises when there is inflammation throughout the body thus it may be used as a tool to confirm the pathogenesis of autoimmune disease and inflammatory responses
Serum uric acid	Female: 0.15–0.40 mmol/L Male: 0.20–0.45 mmol/L	Serum uric acid measures the amount of urate in the blood. Hyperuricaemia is the primary risk factor for the development of gout. However, in the first attacks serum uric acid is often under the upper limit of normal
Rheumatoid factor (RF)	<30 IU/L	Rheumatoid factors are autoantibodies (usually IgM) and are used to help diagnose rheumatoid arthritis and to distinguish it from other forms of arthritis and other conditions that cause similar symptoms of joint pain, inflammation and stiffness. RF is negative in 30% of patients early in illness; if initially negative, it can be repeated 6–12 months after disease onset. RF can be positive in numerous other conditions including lupus, scleroderma, Sjögren's syndrome, various viral, parasitic or bacterial infections. It is not an accurate measure of disease progression
Complement levels	Normal/decreased	Complement levels are of nine major complement proteins associated with some diseases. Decreased amounts may be associated with lupus, Gram-negative septicaemia and shock, as well as malaria. They play a role in the development of inflammation. The test is often used to monitor patients with SLE and other autoimmune diseases. Although it can point to a number of conditions, a decreased complement level can point towards SLE. Complement levels are normal or elevated in rheumatoid arthritis
Cryoglobulins	Positive/negative	Abnormal proteins in the blood that will precipitate when the body temperature drops below normal, causing blockage of the blood vessels. Seen in SLE

Continued

TABLE 15.4 Investigations—cont'd

Assessment	Normal adult values	Implication
Creatine kinase (CK)	Neonate: 70–380 U/L; adult female: 30–180 U/L; adult male: 60–220 U/L	Elevation of CK with CKMB as >5% of CK indicates a myocardial origin of CK. CK levels may also be increased with skeletal muscle injury (e.g. after intramuscular injection or excessive exercise), in myositis, myopathy, rhabdomyolysis or hypothyroidism
Immunoglobulins IgG, IgA and IgM	IgG: 6.5–16.0 IgA: 0.6–4.0 IgM: 0.5–3.0	Elevated levels signify humoral immunodeficiency. Immunoglobulins are often high in rheumatoid arthritis
Mycoplasma, *Chlamydia*, *Borrelia* or other infective organisms	Detected/not detected	Presence is strongly associated as a contributing/causative factor for a number of conditions. DNA panel of assessment may be more appropriate in long-term patients
Cytomegalovirus IgG/IgM	Detected/not detected	Detection is consistent with past exposure to cytomegalovirus, implicated in autoimmune conditions such as rheumatoid arthritis
Epstein-Barr virus antibodies	Detected/not detected	Epstein-Barr virus (EBV) is known to infect human B lymphocytes and epithelial cells, creating a reservoir in these cells. EBV has been implicated in systemic lupus erythematosus and rheumatoid arthritis
Liver function tests — serum alkaline phosphatase	Adult (non-pregnant) 25–100 U/L	Alkaline phosphatase (ALP) is an enzyme found in high levels in bone and liver. Raised levels of ALP in the presence of a musculoskeletal condition may indicate a disorder of the bone. Elevated serum ALP is often seen in active rheumatoid arthritis and polymyalgia rheumatica
Thyroid function tests: Thyroid-stimulating hormone (TSH) Thyroxine (free T4) Triiodothyronine (T3)	TSH: 0.4–4.0 mU/L. Thyroxine (free T4): 10–25 pmol/L Triiodothyronine (T3): 4.0–8.0 pmol/L	It has been suggested that some fibromyalgia patients have thyroid hormone resistance (also called type II hypothyroidism) and that this is the main factor leading to symptoms of fibromyalgia
Thyroid antibodies	Antithyroglobulin antibodies, antithyroid peroxidase antibodies	The frequency of rheumatic diseases appears to be higher in patients with autoimmune thyroid disease. The presence of thyroid antibodies confirms autoimmune involvement in the pathogenesis of the disease. Often seen in fibromyalgia
Ferritin	Adult female: 15–200 micrograms/L; following the menopause, levels progressively approach those for adult males. Adult male: 30–300 micrograms/L	Ferritin is a protein found in all cells, especially in those involved in the synthesis of iron compounds, iron metabolism and iron storage. Ferritin concentrations increase in response to infection, trauma and acute inflammation. High serum transferring saturation or ferritin levels occur in haemochromatosis which may be seen in arthritis. Anaemia (normochromic and normocytic) is common in rheumatoid arthritis and has been found to be proportional to the rate of inflammation
Platelets (thrombocytes)	$150–400 \times 10^9/L$	Thrombocytopenia (low number of platelets) is common in SLE because of the autoimmune mechanism. Thrombocytosis (high number of platelets) is common in rheumatoid arthritis
Leucocyte (white cell count) (WCC)	$4.0–11.0 \times 10^9/L$	Leucopenia (low white blood cells) is seen in SLE and Sjögren's syndrome due to autoimmune mechanism. Leucocytosis (high white blood cells) is seen in rheumatoid arthritis and reflects the degree of inflammation
Neutrophils (granulocytes)	$2.0–7.5 \times 10^9/L$	Neutropenia (low number of neutrophils) is seen in SLE. Neutrophilia (high neutrophils) is seen in rheumatoid arthritis
Lymphocytes	$1.5–4.0 \times 10^9/L$	Lymphopenia is seen in SLE because of lymphocytotoxic antibodies
Haemoglobin	130–180 g/L (adult male) 115–165 g/L (adult female)	Slightly decreased haemoglobin seen in rheumatoid arthritis
Erythrocyte sedimentation rate (ESR)	*Child:* 2–15 mm in 1 h *Adult female:* 17–50 years: 3–19 mm in 1 h 51–70 years: <20 mm in 1 h >70 years: <35 mm in 1 h *Adult male:* 17–50 years: 1–10 mm in 1 h 51–70 years: <14 mm in 1 h >70 years: <30 mm in 1 h	The ESR reflects an increase in the plasma concentration of acute-phase proteins, especially fibrinogen. This test shows the presence of inflammation in the body. A rising ESR can mean an increase in inflammation. ESR will be raised in rheumatoid arthritis but not in osteoarthritis. It is a nonspecific indicator of inflammatory and neoplastic disease; C-reactive protein is a more sensitive early indicator of an acute-phase response. It can be used to diagnose and monitor temporal arteritis and polymyalgia rheumatica

TABLE 15.4 Investigations—cont'd

Assessment	Normal adult values	Implication
Bone mineral density (dual-energy x-ray absorptiometry (DEXA/DXA) scanning)	Bone mineral density (BMD) is expressed in terms of a T-score, representing the number of standard deviations from a young healthy patient's mean BMD Normal bone density: T-score greater than −1 Osteopenia (low bone mass): T-score between −1 and −2.5 Osteoporosis: T-score less than −2.5	DEXA/DXA scanning is considered to be the gold standard for diagnosis of osteoporosis and is used to predict the risk of fracture by measuring bone mineral density. DEXA should be undertaken every 2 years unless there is accelerated bone loss (for example as a side effect of medication use) in which case it should be undertaken on a yearly basis
X-rays, MRI	Various findings	Can detect a number of musculoskeletal diseases such as degenerative processes, loss of cartilage, narrowing of joint space or presence of tophi and other abnormalities
Synovial fluid analysis (joint fluid)	Various findings	May show diseases such as infection or crystals of uric acid in joints
Methylenetetrahydrofolate reductase (MTHFR) polymorphisms — C677T and A1298C	Heterozygous/homozygous/compound heterozygous or negative for these polymorphisms	Heterozygous, homozygous and compound heterozygous MTHFR polymorphisms have been associated with increased risk of chronic disease

Sources: Kumar P, Clark M. Clinical medicine. 3rd edn. Edinburgh: Baillière Tindall; 1994. Liu M, Dai Y, Yao X et al. Anti-rheumatoid arthritic effect of madecassoside on type II collagen-induced arthritis in mice. Int Immunopharmacol 2008; 8:1561–1566. Pamuk ON, Cakir N. The frequency of thyroid antibodies in fibromyalgia patients and their relationship with symptoms. Clin Rheumatol 2007; 26:55–59. Rindfleisch A, Muller D. Diagnosis and management of rheumatoid arthritis. Am Fam Physician 2005; 72(6):1037–1047. Sambrook PN, Seeman E, Phillips SR et al. Preventing osteoporosis: outcomes of the Australian Fracture Prevention Summit. Med J Aust 2002; 176:S1–S16. Symbion Pathology laboratory report.

SECTION B

OSTEOARTHRITIS

Osteoarthritis (OA) is a degenerative joint disease characterised by changes in all joint tissues, including bone, cartilage and synovium (Fig. 15.2). This degeneration leads to chronic pain and loss of function.[18] The term osteoarthritis comes from a combination of two Greek words, 'osteo' meaning bone and 'arthro' meaning joint, thus indicating the body parts involved in this condition. It is considered a 'wear and tear' disease process, which affects individuals as they age or those who stress particular joints, such as the hands of an artist, the knees of a runner or the back of someone with a sedentary lifestyle or one who frequently self-initiates joint adjustments.

It is important to remember that those who enable self-initiated 'adjustments' place extra wear and tear on their joints. They receive a pseudo-endorphin rush on release of the tension and create a vicious cycle whereby the muscles perpetuate the tension and the symptomatic relief.

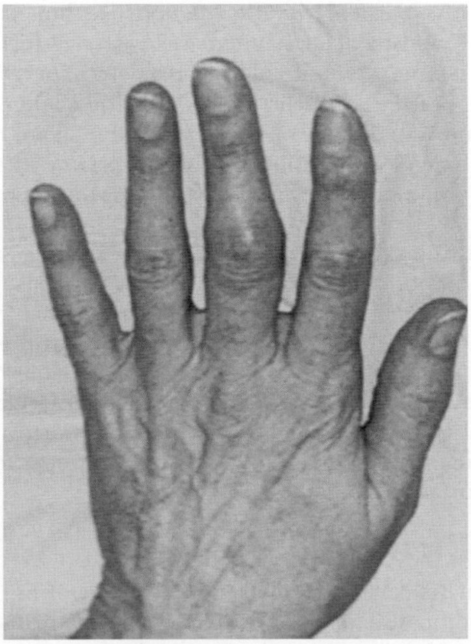

FIGURE 15.2 Osteoarthritis.

Firestein GS, Budd RC, Sergent JS et al. Kelley's textbook of rheumatology. 8th edn. WB Saunders; 2008.

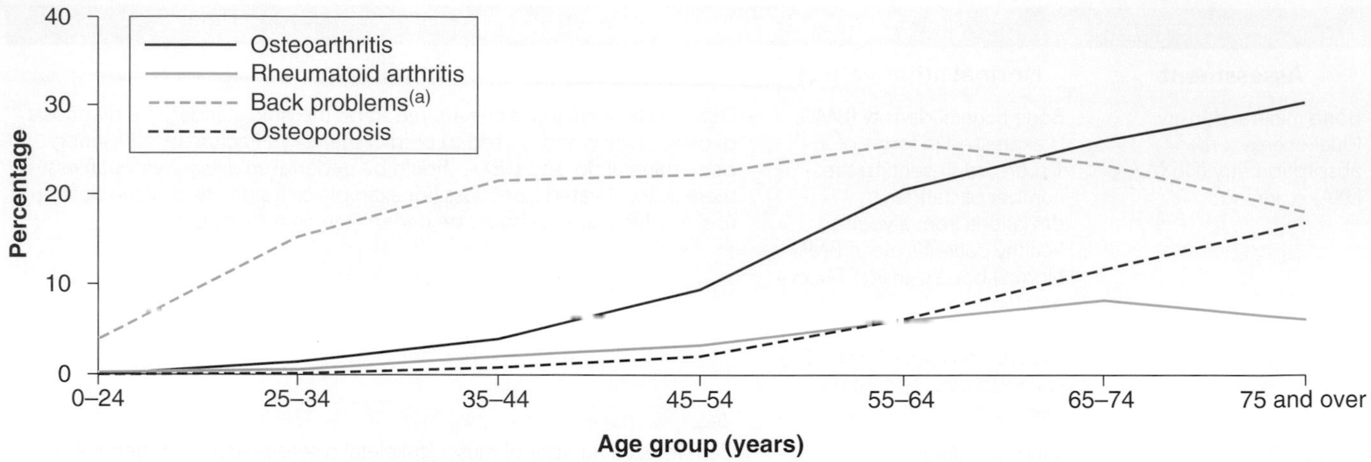

(a) Includes back pain, back problems and disc disorders

FIGURE 15.3 Musculoskeletal conditions by age, 2004–05.

Australian Bureau of Statistics. National Health Survey: a summary of results, 2004–05. Cat. no. 4364.0. Canberra: ABS; 2005.

Epidemiology

Osteoarthritis is the most common form of arthritis and a leading cause of chronic disability in Western society affecting millions of people.[18] Osteoarthritis is the most common musculoskeletal disorder[19] and is a major cause of pain and disability in the elderly.[19] It has been suggested that by 2020 the prevalence of osteoarthritis will have doubled[20] due to increased life expectancies as well as the growing incidence of obesity, which is known to increase the risk of osteoarthritis.

Women have been found to have a higher risk of osteoarthritis, particularly after menopause, but the prevalence of osteoarthritis increases with age for both men and women.[19] Radiological prevalence surveys reveal the presence of visible osteoarthritic changes on x-ray in more than 50% of people over the age of 65 years and the changes are visible in almost everyone after 85 years, although not everyone will be symptomatic (Fig. 15.3).[19]

Interestingly, but in line with current knowledge, women are more likely than men to use vitamins, minerals or herbal treatments for arthritis or osteoporosis.[21] Hip and knee replacements have been suggested as the most cost-effective intervention replacements available[19] but surely prevention is better? Hip and knee replacements are commonly performed for patients with osteoarthritis[19] — the role of preventive medicine would appear to be very important (Fig. 15.4).

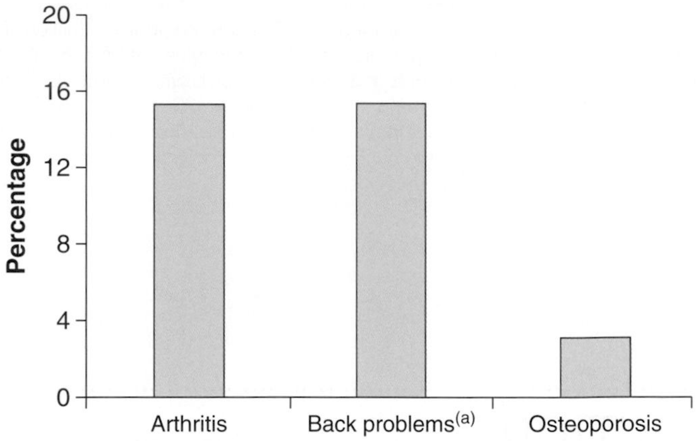

(a) Includes back pain, back problems and disc disorders

FIGURE 15.4 Prevalence of musculoskeletal conditions, 2004–05.

Australian Bureau of Statistics. National Health Survey: a summary of results, 2004–05. Cat. no. 4364.0. Canberra: ABS; 2005.

Classification

Osteoarthritis can be divided into two categories: primary/idiopathic osteoarthritis (i.e. osteoarthritis of unknown origin) or secondary arthritis (as a result of another factor, such as trauma or misalignment). Despite the different classifications, the radiological pathological and clinical findings are generally the same. Osteoarthritis may also be divided into smaller subclassifications according to, for example, the site or the number of joints involved.[22–24]

- Classification according to site — which location of the body does the arthritis present in? For example, is it in the knee, hip, elbow, hand or all joints?
- Classification according to number of joints involved — how many joints are affected? Osteoarthritis may be polyarticular (affecting many joints) or monoarticular (affecting one joint).

Aetiology

AGE

Osteoarthritis is one of the most frequent and disabling diseases of the elderly.[18] It is unusual for a patient to present with osteoarthritis before the age of 40 years old[25]

American College of Rheumatology (ACR) diagnostic criteria for osteoarthritis

ACR CRITERIA FOR THE CLASSIFICATION AND REPORTING OF OSTEOARTHRITIS OF THE HAND[22]

1. Hand pain, aching, or stiffness
2. And at least three of the following four features:
   - Hard tissue enlargement of two or more of 10 selected joints
   - The second and third distal interphalangeal (DIP), the second and third proximal interphalangeal and the first carpometacarpal joints of both hands
   - Hard tissue enlargement of two or more DIP joints
   - Fewer than three swollen metacarpophalangeal joints
   - Deformity of at least one of the 10 selected joints.

NB: This classification method yields a sensitivity of 94% and a specificity of 87%.

ACR CRITERIA FOR THE CLASSIFICATION AND REPORTING OF OSTEOARTHRITIS OF THE HIP[23]

1. Hip pain
2. And at least two of the following three features:
   - ESR <20 mm/h
   - Radiographic femoral or acetabular osteophytes
   - Radiographic joint space narrowing (superior, axial and/or medial).

Note: This classification method yields a sensitivity of 89% and specificity of 91%.

ACR CRITERIA FOR THE CLASSIFICATION AND REPORTING OF OSTEOARTHRITIS OF THE KNEE[24]

Clinical and laboratory

Knee pain plus at least five of nine:

- Age >50
- Stiffness <30 min
- Crepitus
- Bony tenderness
- Bony enlargement
- No palpable warmth
- ESR <40 mm/h
- Rheumatoid factor <1 : 40
- Synovial fluid signs of osteoarthritis (clear, viscous or white blood cell count <2000/mm^3).

92% sensitive, 75% specific.

Clinical and radiographic

Knee pain plus at least one of three:

- Age >50
- Stiffness <30 min
- Crepitus

plus osteophytes.

91% sensitive, 86% specific.

Clinical*

Knee pain plus at least three of six:

- Age >50
- Stiffness <30 min
- Crepitus
- Bony tenderness
- Bony enlargement
- No palpable warmth.

95% sensitive, 69% specific.

*Alternative is four of six, which is 84% sensitive and 89% specific.

and thus increasing age has been identified to be a strong risk factor for osteoarthritis of all joints,[26,27] but it is important to acknowledge that osteoarthritis does not affect all ageing people, hence there are numerous other factors at play than just the ageing process.

GENETIC ALTERATIONS/HEREDITABILITY

Genetics have been observed to play a role in the risk of developing osteoarthritis in a number of studies though the mechanism is unknown. As early as 1941 Stecher[28] observed that Heberden's nodules in osteoarthritic fingers were more likely to occur in twins than in the general population. A genetic influence of up to 65% was observed in another study undertaken on 500 female twins aged between 45 and 70 years screened for osteoarthritis of the knees and hands.[29] Heritability of hip OA has been estimated to be around 40–60%.[18] Correlations of osteoarthritic disease were found to be significantly higher in identical twins than non-identical twins. Similarly, primary polyarticular osteoarthritis in a Dutch family has been linked to microsatellite markers on chromosome 2q and appears to be passed on in an autosomal dominant fashion.[30] More research needs to be undertaken to further elucidate the relationship between genetic alterations and predisposition to osteoarthritis.

OBESITY

Obesity is a major risk factor for osteoarthritis, particularly of the knee[31,32] and hip.[33] Excess weight places increased load on the joints of the body and the increased presence of macrophages in the adipose tissue increases inflammation.

MECHANICAL STRESS/OCCUPATION

Mechanical stress, such as heavy lifting (approximately 10–20 kg over 10 + years), has been clearly shown to increase the risk of developing osteoarthritis of the hip. Farmers have been shown to have an increased risk of osteoarthritis of the hips after being in their occupation for 10 or more years.[34] Moderate evidence also exists for a relationship between kneeling, heavy lifting and knee osteoarthritis.[35]

MISALIGNMENT

Misalignment of the knee/hip/ankle has been suggested to influence the risk of osteoarthritis[36] and is associated with structural loss and acceleration of cartilage loss due to the increased load placed on the various structures of the body.[37,38] Legs that are different lengths may also increase the risk of osteoarthritis. People with a difference in the length of their legs of at least 2 cm were almost twice as likely as those with legs of equal length to have osteoarthritis of the knee as diagnosed by radiography.[39]

JOINT TRAUMA/INJURY

Trauma or injury which compromises the integrity of the structures within the joint has also been suggested to influence the aetiology of osteoarthritis.[40] In a cohort prospective study involving 1321 participants, median age 22 years, Gelber et al[41] examined the relationship between injuries in young adults and risk of later hip or knee osteoarthritis. Over a follow-up of 36 years, 141 participants reported joint injuries and 96 developed osteoarthritis. It was concluded that young adults with knee injuries are at considerably increased risk of osteoarthritis later in life. This is an interesting finding because prevention of osteoarthritis is usually targeted at older people. This leads to the question of whether prevention of osteoarthritis, or at least putting in place prevention programs, should start when we are in our younger years, particularly in those with a positive family history of osteoarthritis.

NUTRITION

Nutritional status and subsequent deficiencies and excesses of certain nutrients have been found to be associated with risk of osteoarthritis. These factors are discussed in more detail later in this chapter.

SEX HORMONES

A deficiency of oestrogen has been related to osteoarthritic alterations in articular tissues, including increased joint laxity, alterations in the extracellular matrix and increased fat mass and leptin,[42] which promotes the breakdown of cartilage. Herrero-Beaumont et al[42] note that oestrogen effects are dose-dependent; thus administering high doses of oestrogen is not necessarily the best option given the link between high-dose oestrogen and the breakdown of cartilage and ligaments.

Overview

See Table 15.5.

TABLE 15.5 Potential causes of secondary osteoarthritis

Developmental	Congenital hip dislocation Legg–Calves–Perthes disease Epiphyseal dysplasias
Mechanical	Hypermobility syndromes (Ehlers–Danlos, hyperlaxity syndromes) Leg length discrepancy Malalignment
Trauma (acute or chronic	Accidental Sports injury Occupational Iatrogenic (postsurgical)
Metabolic	Haemochromatosis Wilson's disease Mucopolysaccharidoses Amyloidosis Ochronosis Gout Pseudogout Calcium crystal deposition
Endocrine	Acromegaly Hyperparathyroidism Hypothyroidism
Inflammatory	Any systemic rheumatic disease Septic arthritis
Miscellaneous	Haemophilias Paget's disease Osteonecrosis Neuropathic arthropathy

Source: Mandl L. Epidemiology of osteoarthritis. In: Sharma L, Berenaum F, eds. Osteoarthritis: a companion to rheumatology. Edinburgh: Elsevier; 2007. pp. 1–14.

Pathogenesis

Osteoarthritis is a degenerative disease characterised by gradual loss of joint function. In a healthy joint, the articular cartilage forms a thin layer covering the joints and overlaying the subchondral bone, preventing friction.[25] Cartilage is composed of chondrocytes surrounded by an extracellular matrix made up of water, proteoglycans and collagen.[25] In a healthy person these allow the cartilage to be resilient when placed under force, such as running or jumping. In osteoarthritis, proteolytic enzymatic destruction leads to loss of proteoglycans and loss of cartilage, leaving the cartilage weak and more susceptible to stressors.

Fibrillation,[43] a process by which numerous small cracks and fissures develop on the articular cartilage, occurs and results in breakdown or complete erosion of cartilage so that pieces of cartilage start to break off into the synovial fluid, leaving the subchondral bone exposed. Inflammatory mediators ensue as phagocytic synovial cells ingest breakdown products and produce pro-inflammatory cytokines such as interleukin 1 (IL-1) and tumour necrosis factor alpha (TNF-α),[44] which appear to be the principal mediators of joint destruction. These cytokines downregulate extracellular matrix protein biosynthesis while simultaneously activating matrix metalloproteinase gene expression. This causes extracellular matrix degradation.

The exposed subchondral bone is now without the cushioning of the cartilage and grinds against the joint surface, losing its ability to move smoothly. It also loses its shape, thickening at the rim of the joint and developing cysts.[45] In an attempt to repair the loss and damage, irregular bony outgrowths known as osteophytes, which are said to be the radiological hallmark of osteoarthritis,[46] form in the margins of the joints to add stability, but these too may break off.

SIGNS AND SYMPTOMS

Clinical features of osteoarthritis include:

- Pain — may be exacerbated by activity, usually relieved by rest[25]
- Bony enlargement of the joint (Heberden's or Bouchard's nodes)
- Joint swelling
- Tenderness around/on the joint area
- Limited range of movement/loss of function[25]
- Stiffness[25]
- Cracking (crepitus)
- Usually presents in an asymmetrical manner
- Typically affected joints include the distal and proximal interphalangeal joints in the hand, hips and knees[25]
- Deformity of joints
- Weakness of the surrounding muscles (e.g. quadriceps in osteoarthritis of the knee).

COMPLICATIONS

Constant swelling, inflammation and bony expansion around the joints results in pain and deformity, impairing normal function. Loss of function causes atrophy of surrounding muscular tissue due to lost mobility. Some studies report a reduction or loss of quality of life.[47] In some situations complete replacement of the joint may be required (artificial joint replacement surgery).

DIFFERENTIAL DIAGNOSIS

Differential diagnoses for osteoarthritis are exhaustive, but the most usual considerations include:

- Rheumatoid arthritis (note that rheumatoid arthritis is symmetrical)
- Pseudo gout
- Psoriatic arthritis
- Ankylosing spondylitis
- Calcium pyrophosphate deposition disease
- Arthritis associated with inflammatory bowel disease
- Reactive arthritis
- Sarcoidosis.

NATUROPATHIC DIAGNOSIS

Fundamentally, diagnosis is achieved from allopathic considerations and elimination of other more complicated conditions. Naturopathic diagnosis considers a few additional key areas:

- Digestive function for nutritional absorption (check for gluten intolerance and inflammatory bowel diseases such as Crohn's disease and ulcerative colitis)
- Nutritional intake of bone-building nutrients (e.g. minerals and cofactors)
- Investigate and correct any nutritional deficiencies found
- Medication or drug side effects that compromise bone health
- Hormonal status of patient and implications for bone mineralisation
- Weight balance (both current and historical)
- Exercise and lifestyle history to assess impact of bone mineralisation and bone degeneration
- Emotional health and wellbeing (correlating with neurotransmitter synthesis, especially dopamine and endorphin production).

Investigations

No single laboratory marker has been identified to diagnose osteoarthritis. Blood tests tend to be normal (unless there is another concurrent disease state) as do inflammatory markers. As a result, osteoarthritis is typically diagnosed based upon clinical presentation, history and radiological findings.

RADIOGRAPHY FOR OSTEOARTHRITIS

Radiography is the most common imaging technique used to diagnosis osteoarthritis and reveals anatomical changes such as damage to cartilage indirectly through joint space narrowing as well as damage to bone in the form of osteophytes and subchondral sclerosis. Radiography may be used to confirm clinical findings and rule out other pathologies, but it must be noted that radiography findings do not always correlate well with severity of symptoms expressed by the subject as cartilage is not always directly visualised in the initial stages of the disease.[20,48]

SPECIFIC NATUROPATHIC INVESTIGATIONS

Bone resorption assay

Serial bone scans are costly and do not indicate present bone activity. Also, they can only detect changes in bone density over long periods of time, often up to 12 months. The bone resorption assay, however, detects biochemical markers which reflect present remodelling activity. It measures the deoxypyridinoline fragment of type I collagen breakdown from a single urine specimen. This is the fragment that contains the cross-linking point and has been demonstrated to be more specific to bone resorption than breakdown fragments measured in some earlier types of assays.

Nutrient and toxic elements

A review of nutritional and toxic elements is essential to assess bone mineralisation requirements and to determine whether toxic elements are present that negatively affect nutrient repletion or useability. The medium assessed is dependent on the health of the patient, but as a general rule, erythrocyte measurements are best for nutrients (except selenium which is best via whole blood). Toxic elements are best assessed via whole blood for current exposure, urine for active chelation and hair for storage status.

Essential fatty acids

This assessment enables a thorough review of essential fatty acid status of the patient to support individualised and specific prescription of essential fatty acids. When incorporated into the cell membranes of the body, omega-3 and omega-6 fatty acids function as precursors for eicosanoids that control a host of cellular functions and responses. The balance between the pro-inflammatory and anti-inflammatory eicosanoids is influenced in large part by the balance of fatty acids we consume. Since inflammation is an integral component of osteoarthritis, nutrients that counteract inflammation can have profound health benefits.

Therapeutic considerations

CLINICAL DECISION MAKING AND RATIONALE

When presented with a patient with osteoarthritis, a few key areas, as mentioned in the section on naturopathic diagnosis, should be considered. Assessment of these factors will enable a holistic and thorough treatment protocol to be achieved. Osteoarthritis frequently prompts generalised treatment approaches that do not factor in the multiple causative variables for each individual.

A few important points for consideration include:

- Severity of degenerative process and presentation
- Duration of condition
- Lifestyle influences including exercise, physical activity, occupation (past and present), home environment, social activities
- Impact on quality of life including emotional and mental wellbeing
- Compounding factors including weakness of surrounding muscle, deformity and restriction of movement
- Age and hormonal status
- Weight of patient
- Nutritional status
- Degree of inflammation
- Other health implications.

Therapeutic application

HISTORICAL PERSPECTIVE

The Eclectics advocated the use of 'alterative herbs'[12] (botanicals that cleanse and purify the blood) for the treatment of osteoarthritis symptoms, suggesting they believed that toxicity in some part influenced the aetiology of osteoarthritis. Interestingly, the vehicle the botanicals were delivered in differed from that of today, being a syrup consisting of corydalis, capsicum and stillingia (an alterative)[12] taken over a long period of time and suggested to favourably influence some cases of osteoarthritis. This effect was probably due to a mixture of the analgesic, circulatory stimulant and alterative actions displayed by the aforementioned herbs. The use of echinacea was also suggested to be of benefit in some cases, probably because of its depurative and immune supportive actions.[12]

From a lifestyle perspective, the Eclectics favoured exercise and massage, suggesting that prolonged inactivity worsened symptoms.[12] A liberal diet was also prescribed, but it was noted that an excess of nitrogenous food as well as tea and coffee should be avoided. Noteworthy is the observation that vegetarians were less likely to be afflicted with osteoarthritis than meat eaters, once again implying that acid-promoting foods were likely to influence the pathogenesis of osteoarthritis.

NATUROPATHIC PERSPECTIVE

The modern naturopathic perspective encourages and has developed from the Eclectic perspective. It continues the principles of herbal alteratives and depuratives to support in the clearance of residual eliminatory wastes. It expands on this principle and recognises that all eliminatory pathways should be supported — digestive, renal/urinary, skin, blood and hepatic. This is exemplified by the concurrent dual actions of most musculoskeletal herbal medicines that are applicable for both skin and musculoskeletal conditions.

This principle is supported and expanded through nutrition — both dietary and supplemental — and encouraged with various lifestyle practices as well. It is essential that impact and wear and tear of the joints is reduced/avoided.

NUTRITIONAL MEDICINE (DIETARY)

Dietary therapeutic objectives

- Investigate and correct any nutritional deficiencies with diet or nutritional supplements.
- Bone matrix building should be supported and encouraged with wholefood dietary principles, encouraging optimal nutrient density and absorption.
- Foods that aggravate inflammation (specific to the patient) should be avoided. Modifications to the diet should be nutritionally sound and balanced.
- Fresh fruits and vegetables rich in antioxidants should be encouraged to prevent oxidation, reduce inflammation and protect against further degradation of the joint, bone and surrounding tissues.
- Saturated, trans or oxidised fats that may contribute to pro-inflammatory pathways and subsequent symptomatology should be avoided.
- Plants of the Solanaceae family should be reduced or eliminated. This includes tomatoes, potatoes, eggplant, capsicum and tobacco.
- Abundant consumption of flavonoid-rich berries or extracts should be encouraged.
- All simple, processed or concentrated carbohydrates must be avoided.
- Complex carbohydrate, high-fibre foods should be emphasised.

SPECIFIC DIETARY TREATMENTS

Dietary inclusions

NUTRIENT-RICH DIET

Bone, cartilage and ligament are living entities reliant on regular sources of nutrition; without a constant supply of nutrients required to support the matrix, breakdown will take place. Taking this into consideration a diet that encompasses a range of fresh wholefoods with plenty of variation and seasonal produce is likely to be high in the wide range of nutrients required to maintain the matrix and is thus likely to be most beneficial.

ANTIOXIDANTS FROM FRUIT, ESPECIALLY VITAMIN C

Vitamin C functions as an antioxidant but is also required for the development of normal cartilage. It should therefore come as no surprise that a diet that contains optimal amounts of fruit rich in vitamin C has been found to exert a protective effect, reducing the risk of osteoarthritis of the knee. In one study, 293 people with no history of osteoarthritis were followed up after 10 years; those with higher dietary intake of vitamin C were noted to have a reduction in bone size and the number of bone marrow lesions, both important in the pathogenesis of knee osteoarthritis.[49] This study builds on results from the Framingham Osteoarthritis Cohort Study, in which it was found that although dietary vitamin C did not appear to protect against the development of osteoarthritis, intake was associated with a reduced risk of progression in the disease process.[50] Foods rich in vitamin C include rosehips, blackcurrants, mango, kiwi and citrus fruits.

The Framingham Osteoarthritis Cohort Study[50] also suggested that dietary vitamin E and beta-carotene reduced the risk of progression of knee osteoarthritis, although these results were less convincing than those for vitamin C and have not been replicated in later studies.[49,51] It has been noted that fat-soluble vitamins such as vitamin E may not have the same access to certain tissues as the water-soluble vitamins,[52] providing a possible explanation for these less then convincing results. Certainly it appears that people with osteoarthritis may require additional antioxidants such as vitamin E, with Kowsari et al.[53] noting that many arthritis patients appeared to be marginally deficient in certain nutrients, some of which, such as vitamin E, might relate to immunological events that play a part in the pathogenesis of osteoarthritis. Vitamin E has been found to inhibit the development of osteoarthritis in rats fed a vitamin E-rich diet.[54]

ANTI-INFLAMMATORY DIET

Osteoarthritis is characterised by inflammation, therefore it is logical to assume that a diet rich in anti-inflammatory constituents is likely to bring some benefits. There is good evidence that supplementary omega-3 fatty acids alleviate the progression of osteoarthritis, so plentiful amounts of foods containing these fats, such as oily fish and nuts and seeds, should be included in the diet both for their lubricating effects in the body and their anti-inflammatory and antioxidant action. A number of herbs and spices show great benefit in the management of osteoarthritic symptoms. Turmeric and ginger both exhibit anti-inflammatory properties and should be included in the diet. Ginger as a tea is highly indicated, particularly if there is a coating on the tongue.

Dietary exclusions

SATURATED FAT OR PRO-INFLAMMATORY FOODS

While a diet with optimal amounts of omega-3 fatty acids is likely to be beneficial in osteoarthritis, a diet high in saturated fat is likely to produce opposite effects, contributing to inflammation in the body. In mice given a diet high in fats with a high content of saturated fat, such as pork fat, the development of spontaneous osteoarthritis was greatly favoured.[55] Further adding to the argument is that a diet high in saturated fat is associated with increased risk of obesity, which in turn is a risk factor for the development of osteoarthritis; with this in mind, saturated fat and processed foods should be kept to a minimum.

NUTRITIONAL MEDICINE (SUPPLEMENTAL)

Nutritional medicine therapeutic objectives

- Address deficiencies of nutrients (and cofactors) that support bone mineralisation and support of the joint capsule and surrounding tissues
- Increase anti-inflammatory and antioxidant nutrients to prevent and address symptoms or progressive degenerative effects
- Support the manufacture of glycoproteins and glycosaminoglycans
- Stimulate the production of the extracellular matrix by chondrocytes
- Suppress inflammatory mediators (e.g. collagenase, hyaluronidase)
- Inhibit cartilage degeneration.

Specific nutrients required

B COMPLEX (ALL B VITAMINS INCLUDING B_1, B_2, B_3, B_5, B_6, FOLATE/FOLINIC ACID/L-5MTHF, B_{12})

The B vitamins are very important in health and wellbeing and none more so than in osteoarthritis. Thiamine, riboflavin and pyridoxine have been noted for their ability to reduce sensitivity to painful stimuli[58] and thus may be useful to help relieve pain associated with osteoarthritis. Fursultiamine, a thiamine derivative, has also been shown to enhance the effects of glucosamine and chondroitin in experimental osteoarthritis in animal studies,[59] further suggesting a role for the B vitamins.

Although the mechanism of action of vitamin B_3 is unknown, in the form of niacinamide the vitamin shows great potential in reducing symptoms associated with osteoarthritis. In a double-blind, placebo-controlled pilot study involving 72 patients with osteoarthritis randomised for treatment with niacinamide or an identical placebo for 12 weeks, those in the niacinamide group experienced substantial benefits compared with the placebo group, with improvements in the global impact of osteoarthritis, joint flexibility, reduced inflammation and a reduction in standard anti-inflammatory medications all noted.[60] Dysfunctional pantothenic acid (B_5) metabolism has also been suggested to contribute to the pathogenesis of osteoarthritis and benefits have been documented with daily supplementation, although once pantothenic acid is removed, symptomatology appears to return.[61] When using folinic acid or L-5MTHF, consider the methylation status of the patient. Also investigate MTHFR (C677T, A1298C).

BORON

Boron is essential for healthy bones and joints. The incidence of arthritis is noted to be higher in countries

SAMPLE DAILY DIET

BREAKFAST	
Fresh papaya with a squeeze of lemon/lime Millet cereal made with mixed berries and almond milk	Papaya is a source of vitamin C as well as proteolytic enzymes. Both have been shown to be beneficial for the relief of osteoarthritis symptoms. Millet is a nutritious grain rich in B vitamins, which have multiple actions with regards to joint health (see B vitamin explanation). Mixed berries provide an easily assimilated source of antioxidants; free radical damage has been observed to contribute to joint damage.
LUNCH	
Miso soup served with soba noodles, tofu, grated ginger, shitake mushrooms and wakame	Dried shitake mushrooms are a rich source of vitamin D (1600 IU/40 micrograms)[56] important for the normal turnover of articular cartilage, while ginger is a warming circulatory stimulant and anti-inflammatory with proven benefits in osteoarthritis due to its ability to suppress prostaglandin synthesis through inhibition of cyclooxygenase-1 and cyclooxygenase-2. Wakame is a highly nutritious sea vegetable with optimal amounts of omega-3 fatty acids and various other nutrients, such as the B vitamins, important for joint health.
DINNER	
Salmon and sweet potato patties with dill yoghurt, served with baby spinach, cucumber and walnut salad	Salmon is a prime source of omega-3 fatty acids shown to downregulate prostaglandins, preventing inflammation associated with arthritis. Sweet potato is a source of vitamin C, which plays an important role in osteoarthritis as an antioxidant and for the synthesis of connective tissue.
SNACKS	
Trail mix made from a mixture of raw almonds, sunflower seeds, pumpkin seeds, cashews and dried cranberries Kiwi fruit	Contains a number of nutrients required for joint health as well as anti-inflammatory constituents. Rich source of vitamin C.
BEVERAGES	
Fresh ginger tea Green tea	Use a 2-inch (5 cm) piece of ginger or ginger powder. Make in a teapot or cup covered with a saucer to prevent therapeutic oils from escaping. The oils stimulate the circulation and are anti-inflammatory. Epigallocatechin-3-gallate from green tea may inhibit the degradation of cartilage.[57]

where less than 1 mg/day of boron is consumed daily and is lower in countries where boron consumption is high.[62] Decreased quantities of boron are found in bones adjacent to joints with osteoarthrosis and in bones from fracture patients.[63] This is thought to be a result of increased turnover of bone close to the arthritic joint.

CALCIUM

Bone resorption has been found to be increased in women with osteoarthritis of the knee.[64] This alteration in calcium regulation suggests that extra supplementation with calcium is required to prevent osteoporosis and other conditions in which calcium depletion plays a role.

COPPER

Articular cartilage is dependent upon a regular supply of copper.[65] Copper functions as an antioxidant and cofactor in many enzyme systems, including the enzyme lysyl oxidase, which has been observed to be essential for the formation of pyridoline cross-links between collagen fibrils.[65] Copper helps to modulate the extracellular matrix by upregulating collagen anabolism in human articular chondrocytes and promoting the cross-linking of elastin,[66] assisting with the structure of connective tissue. Decreased levels of copper and a deficiency of lysyl oxidase have been suggested to cause inadequately cross-linked proteins,[66] which results in fragile cartilage[65] susceptible to the degeneration we know to be synonymous with osteoarthritis.

ESSENTIAL FATTY ACIDS (EPA, DHA, GLA)

Few clinical trials have assessed the efficacy of essential fatty acids in the management of symptoms of osteoarthritis, but many patients still continue to use them with great success. Omega-3 fatty acids have been shown to reduce in mRNA levels for various proteins known to be important in the pathology of osteoarthritis.[67] A combination of eicosapentaenoic acid (EPA) and conjugated linoleic acid (CLA) has been shown to reduce excessive prostaglandin levels in cultured human arthritic chondrocytes; excessive prostaglandin is known to promote inflammation, thus worsening symptoms of osteoarthritis.[68] Pathological changes in indicators of degradation and inflammation in human osteoarthritic cartilage have also been shown to be abrogated following exposure to omega-3 fatty acids.[69] Human clinical trials are required to further confirm the efficacy of essential fatty acids in osteoarthritis.

GLUCOSAMINE

Glucosamine is one the most popular supplements for the management of osteoarthritic symptoms.[70] Natural glucosamine is an endogenous amino sugar found in and around the cartilage, where it is required for the manufacture of glycoproteins and glycosaminoglycans. The majority of the glucosamine we get from supplements is derived from marine exoskeletons (chitin in crustacean shells).

Glucosamine has been shown to exert beneficial effects for the relief of osteoarthritis symptoms in a number of clinical trials. It is thought to stimulate the metabolism of articular cartilage, thus alleviating pain. Two studies involving a total of 218 patients evaluated the efficacy of glucosamine therapy in comparison to ibuprofen, a non-steroidal anti-inflammatory drug (NSAID) and found that supplementation with glucosamine sulfate (500 mg t.d.s.) was just as efficacious as ibuprofen.[71] Long-term use of glucosamine (1–3 years) has also been suggested to help prevent the need for joint replacement. Bruyere et al[72] conducted an 8-year observational study on patients with knee osteoarthritis and found that people taking glucosamine sulfate were 57% less likely to require total joint replacement than those given the placebo. Pavelka et al[73] also observed significant benefits, finding that administration of glucosamine sulfate (1500 mg/day) seemed to slow down the progression of osteoarthritis affecting the knee over a 3-year period. The consequences of these results are significant given the economic, psychological and physical costs for people with osteoarthritis.

Despite the many positive results there are also conflicting results. For example, the Glucosamine/Chondroitin Arthritis Intervention Trial (GAIT), a large (n = 1583), high-quality, National Institutes of Health-funded, multicentre randomised controlled trial showed no significant difference between use of glucosamine and placebo. This study has been criticised, however, for its methodological flaws and high drop-out rate (up to 25% of people), as well as the fact that it used glucosamine hydrochloride rather than glucosamine sulfate.[74] There is much debate on the efficacy and value of glucosamine hydrochloride and whether it is comparable to glucosamine sulfate. A clinical study undertaken over a 6-week period by Zhang et al[75] found glucosamine hydrochloride to be just as effective as glucosamine sulfate, but the sample size and time period of this study are perhaps too small and short to form a real conclusion. A Cochrane review has also suggested that brand may play a large part in the efficacy of products[76] with the Rotta preparation showing glucosamine to be superior to placebo but non-Rotta brands shown to be inferior. If this is true, then it may provide an explanation as to why such large discrepancies exist in clinical studies; it also suggests that we should question whether all brands are equally effective. Clearly, in the prescription of glucosamine it is essential to scrutinise preparations to ensure the best clinical outcome.

The results of studies investigating the use of glucosamine for osteoarthritis of the knee are summarised in Table 15.6.

CHONDROITIN

Chondroitin is a sulfated glycosaminoglycan found within the extracellular matrix of the cartilage. In supplement form it is derived from either bovine or shark sources, but the majority of studies revealing beneficial results have been undertaken using Condrosulf® which is of bovine origin. Chondroitin is thought to exert its effects in osteoarthritis via a number of mechanisms, including:

- Stimulation of production of the extracellular matrix by chondrocytes[77]
- Suppression of inflammatory mediators (e.g. collagenase, hyaluronidase)
- Inhibition of cartilage degeneration
- Anti-inflammatory action.

Uebelhart et al[78] conducted a randomised, double-blind placebo-controlled study investigating the effects of intermittent treatment with chondroitin sulfate on osteoarthritis of the knee. Patients were randomised into two groups receiving either 800 mg chondroitin sulfate or placebo per day for two periods of 3 months during 1 year. Chondroitin administered in this manner was found to improve pain and function compared with placebo, revealing it to have a carryover effect of approximately 3 months, which would be useful for those with milder symptoms. Beneficial results have also been observed in earlier studies. Kahan et al[79] conducted a study investigating the long-term effects of chondroitin 4 and 6 sulfate on knee osteoarthritis in which 622 patients were randomly assigned either 800 mg/day of chondroitin sulfate or placebo over a 2-year period. At the end of the study joint width space was found to be minimised in those patients taking chondroitin, suggesting a beneficial effect; furthermore, pain was also significantly reduced. A 2015 Cochrane systematic review was conducted on the effects of chondroitin sulfate in the treatment of osteoarthritis. Forty-three randomised controlled trials including 4962 participants treated with chondroitin and 4148 participants given placebo or another control (non-steroidal anti-inflammatory drugs, analgesics, opioids) were included in the systematic review. The majority of trials were in knee osteoarthritis as well as hip and hand osteoarthritis. The length of trial duration varied from 1 month to 3 years. Compared to placebo, participants treated with chondroitin achieved statistically significant and clinically meaningful better pain scores in studies that ran for less than 6 months. Chondroitin improved knee pain by 20%. Chondroitin slightly slowed down the narrowing of joint space on x-rays of the affected joint. People who took chondroitin had 0.18 mm less reduction

TABLE 15.6 Glucosamine in osteoarthritis of the knee

Author	Study design	Number of participants	Duration	Site of osteoarthritis	Dose	Results
Bruyere et al 2004	Two 3-year, randomised, placebo-controlled, prospective, independent studies	414 (319 postmenopausal women)	3 years	Knee	Glucosamine sulfate 1500 mg/day or placebo	After 3 years, postmenopausal participants in the glucosamine sulfate group showed no joint space narrowing whereas participants in the placebo group experienced narrowing. After 3 years the WOMAC Index showed an improvement in the glucosamine sulfate group and a trend for worsening in the placebo group
Pavelká et al 2002	Randomised, placebo-controlled, double-blind	202	3 years	Knee	Glucosamine sulfate 1500 mg/day or placebo	Significant final differences on the Lequesne Index and the WOMAC Index and pain, function and stiffness subscales for glucosamine. Long-term treatment with glucosamine sulfate slowed the progression of knee osteoarthritis, possibly determining disease modification
Bruyere et al 2003	Prospective placebo-controlled	212	3 years	Knee	Glucosamine sulfate 1500 mg/day or placebo	In patients with mild OA glucosamine sulfate use was associated with a trend towards a significant reduction in joint space narrowing
Reginster et al 2001	Double-blind, randomised, placebo-controlled	212	3 years	Knee	Glucosamine sulfate 1500 mg/day or placebo	Improvement in WOMAC compared with placebo. Pain and function were significantly improved by glucosamine
Herrero-Beaumont et al 2007	Randomised, double-blind, placebo-controlled	318	6 months	Knee	Glucosamine sulfate 1500 mg/day or placebo	More effective than placebo at improving symptoms. Paracetamol was used as a side comparator and although paracetamol also had a higher responder rate compared with placebo, it failed to show significant effects on the algofunctional indices

WOMAC Index is a self-administered questionnaire and assesses the three dimensions of pain, joint stiffness and disability in knee and hip osteoarthritis using 24 questions. WOMAC = Western Ontario and McMaster Universities Arthritis Index

Sources: Bruyere O, Honore A, Ethgen O et al. Correlation between radiographic severity of knee osteoarthritis and future disease progression. Results from a 3-year prospective, placebo-controlled study evaluating the effect of glucosamine sulfate. Osteoarthr Cartil 2003; 11:1–5. Bruyere O, Pavelka K, Rovati LC et al. Glucosamine sulfate reduces osteoarthritis progression in postmenopausal women with knee osteoarthritis: evidence from two 3 year studies. Menopause 2004; 11:138–143. Herrero-Beaumont G, Ivorra JA, Del Carmen Trabado M et al. Glucosamine sulfate in the treatment of knee osteoarthritis symptoms: a randomized, double-blind, placebo-controlled study using acetaminophen as a side comparator. Arthritis Rheum 2007; 56(2):555–567. Pavelká K, Gatterova J, Olejarova M et al. Glucosamine sulfate use and delay of progression of knee osteoarthritis. A 3-year, randomized, placebo-controlled, double-blind study. Arch Intern Med 2002; 162:2113–2123. Reginster JY, Deroisy R, Rovati LC et al. Long-term effects of glucosamine sulfate on osteoarthritis progression: a randomised, placebo-controlled clinical trial. Lancet 2001; 357:251–256.

in minimum joint space width than those who took placebo. Chondroitin was found to have little or no difference in adverse events versus other agents.[80]

While not wanting to detract from these favourable results, it is important to acknowledge that a number of the clinical trials assessing the efficacy of chondroitin in osteoarthritis have received financial gains and sponsorship from the industry. McAlindon et al[81] conducted a quality assessment on chondroitin and observed that in some trials manufacturers assisted with methodology and design, including data collection and randomisation. Taking this into account, it is clear that unbiased human clinical trials are required to determine the effects of chondroitin in osteoarthritis before efficacy may be properly determined.

Some studies supporting the beneficial effects of chondroitin sulfate in osteoarthritis are summarised in Table 15.7.

TABLE 15.7 Beneficial effects of chondroitin sulfate in osteoarthritis

Author	Type of study	Length of study	Location of osteoarthritis	Dose	Improvements observed in chondroitin group
Verbruggen et al 1998	Randomised, placebo-controlled, double-blind	36 months	Interphalangeal finger joints	Condrosulf (400 mg t.d.s.) versus placebo	Decreased number of new erosive arthritic finger joints
Bucsi and Poor 1998	Randomised, placebo-controlled, double-blind	6 months	Knee	800 mg/day (Condrosulf) or placebo	Lequesne's Index decreased Spontaneous joint pain decreased Improvements also seen in walking time
Michel et al 2005	Randomised, double-blind, controlled pilot	12 months	Knee	800 mg/day (Condrosulf) or placebo	Reduction in pain Increased joint mobility capacity Possible ability to stabilise joint space width and modulate bone and joint metabolism
Kahan et al (2009)	Randomised, placebo-controlled, double-blind	24 months	Knee	800 mg/day	Reduction in pain Reduction in minimum joint space width

Sources: Bucsi L, Poor G. Efficacy and tolerability of oral chondroitin sulfate as a symptomatic slow-acting drug for osteoarthritis (SYSADOA) in the treatment of knee osteoarthritis. Osteoarthr Cartil 1998; 6:31–36. Kahan A, Uebelhart D, De Vathaire F et al. Long-term effects of chondroitin 4 and 6 sulfate on knee osteoarthritis: the study on osteoarthritis progression prevention, a two-year, randomized, double-blind, placebo-controlled trial. Arthritis Rheum 2009; 60:524–533. Michel BA, Stucki G, Frey D et al. Chondroitins 4 and 6 sulfate in osteoarthritis of the knee a randomized controlled trial. Arthritis Rheum 2005; 52:779–786. Verbruggen G, Goemaere S, Veys EM. Chondroitin sulfate: S/DMOAD (structure/disease modifying anti-osteoarthritis drug) in the treatment of finger joint OA. Osteoarthr Cartil 1998; 6(Suppl. A):37–38.

TABLE 15.8 Possible modes of action of glucosamine and chondroitin in osteoarthritis

Glucosamine	Chondroitin
Provides substrate	Provides substrate
Increases proteoglycan synthesis	Increases proteoglycan synthesis by chondrocytes
Inhibits cytokines (IL-1α)	Inhibits cytokines
Inhibits proteases (matrix metalloproteinase and collagenase)	Inhibits proteases (collagenase)
Reduces prostaglandin E_2 production	Increases viscosity of synovial fluid
Interferes with binding of NF-κB in chondrocytes	Increases bone mineralisation and repair

Source: Huskisson EC. Glucosamine and chondroitin for osteoarthritis. J Int Med Res 2008; 36(6):1161–1179.

GLUCOSAMINE AND CHONDROITIN IN COMBINATION

Many preparations contain a combination of glucosamine and chondroitin. The specific actions thought to be caused by each constituent are summarised in Table 15.8.

GREEN-LIPPED MUSSEL

The knowledge that green-lipped mussel may have some benefits as an adjuvant therapy for the modern treatment of mild to moderate osteoarthritis symptoms first became apparent when the coastal-dwelling Māori population who consumed a diet rich in green-lipped mussels were observed to have a lower incidence of osteoarthritis than their inland dwelling relatives. They have been suggested to work via inhibition of 5-lipoxygenase,[82] but their anti-inflammatory action has also been attributed to omega-3 fatty acid content. Results from human clinical trials have been inconsistent, with a 2006 systematic review by Cobb and Ernst[83] suggesting it was an ineffective product, while in contrast a 2008 systematic review by Brien et al[84] suggested possible benefit. A multicentre trial conducted by Cho et al[82] in which 60 patients with symptomatic osteoarthritis of the knee and hip were given green-lipped mussel (Lyprinol) showed beneficial results within 1 month, with 53% of patients reporting significant relief. At 2 months, 80% of patients reported pain relief and improvement of joint function. Noting its traditional application and the high percentage of the population with osteoarthritis, further research assessing the efficacy of the green-lipped mussel appears warranted.

S-ADENOSYLMETHIONINE (SAMe)

The exact mechanism by which *S*-adenosylmethionine (SAMe) exerts its effects in osteoarthritis is undetermined but includes anti-inflammatory mechanisms and analgesic effects via inhibition of cyclooxygenase.[85] In-vitro studies on human chondrocyte articular differentiation also suggest that SAMe has positive effects on proteoglycans[86] (components of cartilage) and may thus assist in the regeneration of cartilage tissue, preventing osteoarthritis. In a long-term multicentre open trial involving 108 patients, the efficacy and tolerance of SAMe were studied for 2 years in patients with osteoarthritis of the knee, hip and spine.[87] The patients received 600 mg of SAMe daily for the first 2 weeks and thereafter 400 mg daily (equivalent to two tablets of 200 mg each) until the end of the 2-year treatment. Improvements with supplementation of SAMe were visible after the first weeks of treatment and continued up to the end of the study. Detailed laboratory tests carried out at the start and after 6, 12, 18 and 24 months of treatment showed no pathological changes, suggesting that SAMe postponed degenerative changes associated with osteoarthritis. As a positive side effect, SAMe also improved feelings of depression associated with osteoarthritis.

A meta-analysis undertaken by Soeken et al[88] found SAMe to be as effective as NSAIDs in reducing pain and improving functional limitation in patients with osteoarthritis without the adverse effects often associated with NSAID therapies. As yet, the majority of studies undertaken on SAMe have involved small sample groups so further studies of better quality are required.

VITAMIN C

Vitamin C is required both structurally and functionally in the management of osteoarthritis. Structurally, vitamin C plays an essential role in the synthesis of collagen, an important protein that makes up joint cartilage, and functionally vitamin C is an antioxidant, protecting against the effects of reactive oxygen species known to play a role in the pathogenesis of osteoarthritis.

VITAMIN D

Vitamin D is involved in the normal turnover of articular cartilage and is seemingly important in the management and prevention of osteoarthritis. Low dietary vitamin D has been shown on numerous occasions to increase susceptibility to osteoarthritis in a number of sites in the body. In a study of 1104 elderly men in the Osteoporotic Fractures in Men Study, those with a deficiency of vitamin D were twice as likely to have prevalent radiographic hip osteoarthritis as well as slower walking time and more hip pain[89] than those with adequate levels. Results from the Rotterdam study produced similar results, with low dietary vitamin D intake observed to increase the risk of progression of radiographic osteoarthritis of the knee in both male and female participants.[90] Furthermore, a Tasmanian study found that sunlight exposure and serum 25(OH)D levels were both associated with decreased knee cartilage loss.[91] Clearly, adequate levels of vitamin D are crucial for cartilage health. Supplementation with vitamin D to enhance skeletal health and improve vitamin D status in those with deficiency appears warranted and may prevent and/or retard cartilage loss, thus protecting against the development and worsening of osteoarthritis.

VITAMIN E

Several small studies conducted in the late 1970s and early 1980s showed benefit from vitamin E supplementation in participants with osteoarthritis. In one 10-day study approximately half of the 29 patients taking vitamin E 600 mg (900 IU/day) experienced a reduction in pain compared with only 4% of those receiving placebo.[92] Beneficial results were also observed by Blankenhorn,[93] who conducted a 6-week double-blind, placebo-controlled trial in which 56 people with osteoarthritis taking vitamin E 400 mg (600 IU/day) experienced significant improvement in every efficacy measured. Following these results, a number of studies undertaken produced conflicting results, stating vitamin E to be ineffective in certain types of osteoarthritis,[94,95] but a 6-month study which compared 400 mg (600 IU/day) of oral vitamin E versus 1500 mg/day glucosamine sulfate once again found vitamin E to be just as effective as glucosamine for reducing symptoms associated with osteoarthritis of the knee.[96] Vitamin E has been suggested to exert analgesic,[97] anti-inflammatory[97] and beneficial immunological effects in osteoarthritis. Vitamin E is also warranted for its antioxidant action: participants with osteoarthritis have been shown to exhibit higher free radical production.[98]

ZINC

Articular cartilage is dependent upon a regular supply of zinc where it helps to maintain connective tissue and functions as an antioxidant and inflammatory mediator. Production of free radicals have been found in the synovial fluid of those with arthritis, where they contribute to joint damage. Levels of the antioxidant enzyme zinc-copper superoxide dismutase (ZnCuSOD) have been found to be increased, suggesting increased requirements.[99]

DOSAGE REQUIREMENTS

The dosage requirements listed below are based on adult doses that have been reported in the literature.

- B complex (all B vitamins) high-dose combination, preferably activated forms:
  - Thiamine 20–40 mg/day
  - Riboflavin 20–50 mg/day. Riboflavin 5′-Phosphate 20–40 mg/day
  - Niacinamide acid 50–100 mg as a base dose
    - Additional 900–4000 mg/day[100]
  - Pantothenic acid 150–300 mg as a base dose
    - Additional 1000–5000 mg/day[100]
  - Pyridoxine 50–100 mg/day. Pyridoxal 5′-phosphate 20–50 mg/day
  - Folic acid 500–1000 micrograms/day. Choose folinic acid or MTHF 500 micrograms/day if MTHFR polymorphism. When using folinic acid or MTHF, consider the methylation status of the patient. Also investigate MTHFR (C677T, A1298C)[101]
  - Hydroxo- or methylcobalamin 500–1000 micrograms/day determined by the methylation status of the patient
  - Choline 50–100 mg/day
  - Inositol 50–100 mg/day
  - Biotin 250–500 micrograms/day
- Boron 6 mg/day[102]
- Chondroitin 800–1200 mg/day
- Copper 2–4 mg/day (in ratio to zinc)
- Calcium 1000–2000 mg/day
- Glucosamine 1500 mg/day
- Magnesium 150–850 mg/day
- SAMe 600–1200 mg/day[87,103,104]
- Vitamin C 1000–3000 mg/day
- Vitamin D 400–1600 IU[105]
- Vitamin E 600 mg (900 IU)/day[92]
- Zinc 20–50 mg/day (ensure zinc to copper ratio is 1 : 1)
- EFAs: 800–2700 mg/day DHA,[106] 3000–5000 mg/day EPA.[107]

HERBAL MEDICINE

Herbal medicine therapeutic objectives

- To reduce joint pain
- To reduce inflammation

- To reduce oxidative stress
- To increase circulation to the joints
- To relieve pain of entrapped nerves where applicable
- To reduce the effects of stress and nourish the nervous system where necessary.

Herbal medicine classes

- Analgesic
- Anodyne
- Anti-inflammatory (TNF-α, NF-κB, interleukins, prostaglandins)
- Antioxidant
- Antirheumatic
- COX and/or lipoxygenase inhibitor
- Circulatory stimulants
- Musculoskeletal spasmolytics
- Adaptogens, nervines, sedative/relaxant herbal medicines as necessary
- Topical herbal classes
  - Analgesic
  - Anti-inflammatory
  - Musculoskeletal spasmolytic
  - Rubefacient/irritant.

Specific herbal medicines

APIUM GRAVEOLENS (CELERY)

Despite a lack of proper clinical trials, *Apium graveolens* is one of the most popular herbs for the management of osteoarthritic symptoms, at least from a consumer perspective.[108] It contains apiin, a constituent that has been found to exert an anti-inflammatory action[109] likely to be beneficial in osteoarthritis.

BOSWELLIA SERRATA (BOSWELLIA)

The oleogum resin of *Boswellia serrata*, an Ayurvedic herb, possesses specific anti-inflammatory, anti-arthritic and analgesic activity.[110] *Boswellia serrata* contains alpha and beta boswellic acid, both of which have been shown to prevent inflammation by inhibiting 5-lipoxygenase and cyclooxygenase and possibly other factors such as cytokines (interleukins and TNF-α) and the complement system.[111] This action is proposed for the therapeutic action of *Boswellia serrata* in osteoarthritis.

Boswellia serrata has displayed efficacy in a number of human clinical trials, particularly those that involve osteoarthritis of the knee. In one such trial involving 30 patients given *Boswellia serrata* or placebo, the *Boswellia* group reported a reduction in knee pain, increased knee flexion, the ability to walk further and a reduction in the frequency of swelling in the knee joint, although no radiological changes were noted.[110] 5-Loxin, an extract of *Boswellia serrata* and lipoxygenase inhibitor enriched with 30% 3-*O*-acetyl-11-keto-beta-boswellic acid (AKBA) administered to participants over approximately 3 months was found to prevent the breakdown of cartilage in osteoarthritic patients as well as inducing clinically and statistically significant improvements in pain scores and physical functioning scores, some as early as 7 days after initial supplementation.[112]

Five studies of three different extracts from *Boswellia serrata* and their effects in osteoarthritis were included in a Cochrane systematic review. Moderate-quality evidence from two studies (85 participants) indicated that 90 days treatment with 100 mg of enriched *Boswellia serrata* extract improved symptoms compared to placebo. Mean pain was 40 points on a 0 to 100 point VAS scale (0 is no pain) with placebo; enriched *Boswellia serrata* reduced pain by a mean of 17 points (95% confidence interval (CI), 8 to 26). Physical function was 33 points on the Western Ontario and McMaster Universities Osteoarthritis Index (WOMAC) 0 to 100 point subscale (0 is no loss of function) with placebo; enriched *Boswellia serrata* improved function by 8 points (95% CI, 2 to 14). Possible benefits of other *Boswellia serrata* extracts over placebo were confirmed in moderate-quality evidence from two studies (97 participants) of enriched *Boswellia serrata* 100 mg plus non-volatile oil and low-quality evidence from small single studies of a 999 mg daily dose of *Boswellia serrata* extract and 250 mg daily dose of enriched *Boswellia serrata*.[113]

The general dose of *Boswellia* is between 600 and 3000 mg gum resin per day or equivalent and it is generally regarded as a safe herb with minimal side effects.

CAPSICUM SPP. (CAYENNE, CHILLI)

Capsaicin, the active constituent within *Capsicum* spp., has been suggested to be useful in the management of arthritis.[114] Capsaicin works by depleting levels of substance P,[114] high levels of which are thought to be a marker for pain and chronic inflammation. In animal studies, capsaicin has been shown to function as an anti-inflammatory[115] in rats with arthritis. Capsaicin also functions as a circulatory stimulant, aiding the flow of nutrients to areas of the body that need it.

CORYDALIS AMBIGUA (CORYDALIS)

Corydalis ambigua is indicated for pain associated with osteoarthritis due to its analgesic[116] and sedative/tranquillising[116] action. As yet, there have been limited human clinical studies investigating the efficacy of *Corydalis ambigua* and none specifically directed at its use for osteoarthritis, but results achieved in clinical practice allow for therapeutic recommendation for application of this botanical.

CURCUMA LONGA (TURMERIC)

Curcumin is a curcuminoid and an active constituent found within turmeric. Turmeric has a long history of safe use as food and it has long been used as an anti-inflammatory treatment in traditional Chinese and Ayurvedic medicine.[117] Data from in-vivo and in-vitro studies suggest curcumin to have specific benefits in the management of osteoarthritis. Curcumin has been shown to protect human chondrocytes via its antioxidant action, scavenging reactive oxygen and nitrogen species in vitro, inhibiting IL-1β-induced nitric oxide production in bovine and human chondrocytes and human cartilage explants and displaying IL-1β-induced superoxide dismutase activity in bovine chondrocytes in monolayers.[118] Via its anti-inflammatory action, curcumin also inhibits NF-κB-dependent gene transcription in chondrocytes, COX-2, but not COX-1, gene expression in IL-1β-treated bovine chondrocytes in monolayers, IL-6 and IL-8 gene expression by bovine and human chondrocytes and IL-6, IL-8 and prostaglandin E_2 (PGE_2) production by human chondrocytes and cartilage explants.[118] Curcumin also modulates the expressions of phospholipase A2 and various transcription factors involved in energy metabolism such as signal transducer and activator of transcription, peroxisome proliferator-activated receptor-γ (PPAR-γ), activator protein-1 and cAMP responding element binding protein.[117]

Daily supplementation of 120 mg of curcuminoids for 4 weeks ($n = 34$) was as effective as 75 mg of diclofenac sodium ($n = 39$) in suppressing the synthesis of COX-2 in monocytes in the synovial fluid of patients suffering from mild-to-moderate osteoarthritis diagnosed using the criteria of the American College of Rheumatology.[119] A systematic review and meta-analysis found that 8–12 weeks of standardised turmeric extracts (typically 1000 mg/day of curcumin) reduced arthritis symptoms (mainly pain and inflammation-related symptoms) and resulted in similar improvements of the symptoms as ibuprofen and diclofenac sodium. Turmeric is better tolerated than ginger and pepper due to being less hot and spicy.[117] A randomised double-blind study compared the effects of curcumin (4 × 500 mg/day; $n = 52$) with those of ibuprofen (2 × 400 mg/day; $n = 55$) in patients who were over 50 years of age, had severe knee pain and their radiography showed the presence of osteophytes. The main outcomes were improvement in pain on level walking, pain on stairs and functions of knee assessed by time spent during 100-metre walk and going up and down a flight of stairs. Both the groups showed improvements in all assessments. The curcumin group was statistically better in patient satisfaction, timed walk or stair climbing and pain during walking or stair climbing.[120] Patients were randomly assigned into *Curcuma* extracts (1500 mg/day; $n = 171$) and ibuprofen groups (1200 mg/day; $n = 160$) for 4 weeks. The mean of all WOMAC scores at weeks 0, 2 and 4 showed significant improvement when compared with the baseline in both groups. The 6-minute walk distance was 310 metres and 304 metres in the *Curcuma* and ibuprofen groups, respectively.[121] A study examined the effects of Meriva (curcumin plus phosphatidylcholine for better bioavailability). Patients ($n = 100$) with mild osteoarthritis were recruited. They were already under various treatments. The control group ($n = 50$) continued with only the current treatment but Meriva (2 × 500 mg/day totalling 200 mg curcumin) was added to the study group ($n = 50$). After 8 months, WOMAC scores for pain significantly reduced in the Meriva group from 16.6 to 7.3 ($p < 0.05$), with no significant change in the control group. The scores for stiffness in the Meriva group significantly reduced from 7.4 to 3.2 ($p < 0.05$), whereas there was no change in the control group. The scores of physical function in the Meriva group significantly reduced from 56.6 to 22.8 ($p < 0.05$). There was no significant improvement in the control group. The mean treadmill test distances changed from 82.3 to 156 m/6 minutes in the control group but the increase was much greater in the treatment group (from 77.3 to 344 m/6 minutes). All the inflammatory markers (IL6, IL1β, VCAM-1, sCD40L, ESR) were significantly decreased ($p < 0.05$) in the study group but not in the control group. Furthermore, negative effects on social function caused by osteoarthritis significantly decreased in the Meriva group in addition to improvements in wellbeing and emotional function, whereas there was no significant change in the control group.[122]

A combination extract of turmeric and *Boswellia* was investigated in the management of osteoarthritis. After 3 months, the treatment group showed significant improvements in the pain-free walking time, degree of pain before and after passive and active movement tenderness and grade of knee effusion compared to placebo. This result was attributed to the reduction in inflammation indicated by CD4+ and CD45RO+ T-cells and serum Fas ligand, as well as oxidative stress indicated by serum nitrite/nitrate and superoxide dismutase levels in the patients. Another trial compared the effects of the combination of 700 mg turmeric and 300 mg *Boswellia* extract ($n = 14$) and 200 mg celecoxib ($n = 14$) for 12 weeks. The number of patients suffering from moderate-to-severe joint pain and joint line tenderness was reduced in the treatment group compared to the placebo group.[119]

A pilot randomised double-blind placebo-control parallel-group clinical trial was conducted among patients with mild-to-moderate knee OA. Patients were assigned to curcuminoid complex (curcuminoids 500 mg and 5 mg Bioperine; $n = 19$) or matched placebo ($n = 21$) for 6 weeks. WOMAC scores revealed a significant reduction in the global ($p < 0.001$) as well as all subscale ($p < 0.001$ for pain and physical function and $p = 0.043$ for stiffness) scores in the curcuminoid group by the end of the 6-week trial.[123]

A study investigated the effects of 1000 mg *Curcuma longa* extract ($n = 29$), 1500 mg glucosamine ($n = 28$), the combination of both ($n = 24$) and placebo ($n = 29$) on osteoarthritis for 42 days. *Curcuma longa* extract alone was more effective in improving all WOMAC subscales and total score, clinician global impression of change, joint tenderness, crepitation, effusion and limitation to movement than the combination and placebo group. The number of patients needing paracetamol and cases of adverse reaction were also the lowest in the group taking *C. longa* extract alone.[119]

ESCHSCHOLZIA CALIFORNICA (CALIFORNIAN POPPY)

Pain is a key feature of osteoarthritis and significantly affects quality of life for many sufferers therefore anything that can provide pain relief is likely to be well received. *Eschscholzia californica* has mild sedative and analgesic effects[124,125] and thus may be used to reduce and relieve pain associated with arthritis. Animal studies support the indication of a peripheral but not a central analgesic effect.[125]

GUAIACUM OFFICINALE (GUAIACUM)

Guaiacum officinale contains anti-inflammatory constituents[126] and is advocated by the *British Herbal*

Pharmacopoeia for chronic rheumatic conditions.[127] Despite its recognition as an anti-inflammatory in conditions affecting the musculoskeletal system there has been little in the way of clinical trials assessing efficacy. Nevertheless, the resin of *Guaiacum officinale* is sold as part of a combination of herbs that includes *Salix alba, Cimicifuga racemosa, Smilax* and poplar bark in a proprietary product known as Reumalex®. In a small, randomised placebo-controlled study involving 82 people undertaken over 2 months, Reumalex was found to exert mild analgesic effects in those with arthritic pain compared with placebo.[128]

HARPAGOPHYTUM PROCUMBENS (DEVIL'S CLAW)

Harpagophytum procumbens has been used successfully for the treatment of osteoarthritis of the spine, knee and hip, with Chrubasik et al[129] noting that at least 60% of patients given a water extract of *Harpagophytum procumbens* reported benefit to some extent. In those who responded to treatment, pain was reduced by approximately 80% after 2–3 months,[130] probably as a result of the anti-inflammatory and analgesic effects of the herb. A systematic review undertaken by Gagnier et al[131] further confirms the efficacy of *Harpagophytum procumbens,* as does the monograph of the European Scientific Cooperative on Phytotherapy (ESCOP),[132] which advocates the use of *Harpagophytum procumbens* for osteoarthritis. The active constituent within *Harpagophytum procumbens* believed to be in some part responsible for its effects is an iridoid glycoside called harpagoside. The strongest evidence is for administration of >50 mg of harpagoside/day. Daily doses of *Harpagophytum procumbens,* standardised to 50 mg or 100 mg harpagoside, may be better than placebo for short-term improvements in low back pain and may reduce the use of rescue medication.[133]

SALIX SPP. (WILLOW BARK)

The analgesic effects of *Salix* spp. have been known for centuries; it has even been suggested that Hippocrates recommended *Salix* spp. in the form of a decoction for rheumatic pain. A double-blind placebo-controlled study undertaken by Schmid et al[134] investigated the efficacy of 240 mg/day salicin or placebo in participants with osteoarthritis of the knee or hip and observed a reduction in pain just 2 weeks into treatment in comparison with placebo. In the control group the pain actually increased. Daily doses of *Salix alba,* standardised to 120 mg or 240 mg salicin, reduced low back pain better than placebo. Research indicates that white willow bark is probably better than placebo for short-term improvements in low back pain and rescue medication.[133]

*URTICA URENS/DIOICA/*SPP. (NETTLE)

Extracts of *Urtica* spp. have been suggested to inhibit the transcription factor NF-κB, which is known to be pro-inflammatory and thus unwanted where there is osteoarthritis.[135] In vitro, hox alpha, a stinging needle extract acid, has also been found to suppress the effects of inflammatory mediators which would typically contribute to upregulation of matrix metalloproteinase.[136] There is also evidence to suggest that *Urtica* leaf placed directly on the affected area may relieve symptoms of pain associated with osteoarthritis.[137]

ZANTHOXYLUM CLAVA-HERCULIS (PRICKLY ASH)

The bark of the southern prickly ash, *Zanthoxylum clava-herculis,* was noted by the Eclectics to be a gentle circulatory stimulant valued for its therapeutic action in rheumatic complaints due to its eliminative action.[138] Felter states that the tincture made from the prickly ash berries is the best drug that can be given for 'chronic muscular rheumatism' as well as having benefits in lumbago and myalgia.[139]

ZINGIBER OFFICINALE (GINGER)

The rhizome of *Zingiber officinale* has been used extensively in traditional Ayurvedic and Tibb medicine systems for its beneficial actions in arthritis. *Zingiber officinale* displays anti-inflammatory and analgesic actions useful in the management of osteoarthritic symptoms. Gingerols found in *Zingiber officinale* are a type of oleresin shown to inhibit a number of pro-inflammatory mediators including COX-1[140] and COX-2,[141] as well as leukotriene and prostaglandin synthesis. Altman and Marcussen[142] observed that internal supplementation with *Zingiber officinale* reduced symptoms associated with osteoarthritis of the knee, although those in the *Zingiber* group experienced more side effects (gastrointestinal disturbance) than those in the placebo group. Haghighi et al[143] found *Zingiber officinale* to be efficacious for primary knee osteoarthritis, particularly with regard to pain, but in contrast to the previous study, Haghighi et al reported minimal side effects.

A double-blind, placebo-controlled, cross-over study investigated the effects of ginger on osteoarthritis of the hip or knee. There were three treatment periods of 3 weeks each, with either 170 mg ginger extract, ibuprofen 400 mg or placebo administered t.d.s. (equivalent to 510 mg ginger, 300 mg ibuprofen per day). Of the 56 patients, 20 had primarily osteoarthritis of the hip and 36 of the knee. The ginger-treated group reported significantly less pain compared with the placebo group for the first period before cross-over, but not after cross-over, while the ibuprofen group showed a stronger reduction in pain. A ranking of efficacy of the three treatment periods found that ibuprofen>ginger extract>placebo was found for visual analogue scale of pain ($p < 0.00001$). This study showed a better effect of both ibuprofen and ginger extract than placebo (Chi-square, $p < 0.05$).[144]

Forty-three patients with confirmed osteoarthritis (knee and hip) were included in a randomised controlled study. A group of 21 patients was given ginger 340 mg daily for 4 weeks. Another group (positive control) of 22 patients received 100 mg diclofenac daily for the same period. Both groups also received 1000 mg glucosamine daily. Ginger was found to be as effective as diclofenac but safer in treating osteoarthritis, being without effect on the stomach mucosa. The increased mucosal prostaglandins synthesis in the ginger group supports an increased mucosa-protective potential.[145]

HOPS, ROSEMARY EXTRACT AND OLEANOLIC ACID COMBINATION

An 8-week observational trial investigated the efficacy of Meta050 (a proprietary, standardised combination of reduced iso-alpha-acids from hops, rosemary extract and oleanolic acid) on pain in patients with rheumatic disease (osteoarthritis, rheumatoid arthritis and fibromyalgia). Patients were given 440 mg Meta050 3 times a day for 4 weeks. The dosage was then changed to 880 mg twice a day for the subsequent 4 weeks. Pain and condition-specific symptoms were assessed using a standard visual analogue scale (VAS) and an abridged arthritis impact measurement scale (AIMS2). Following treatment, a statistically significant decrease in pain of 50% and 40% was observed in arthritis patients using the VAS ($p < 0.0001$) and AIMS2 ($p < 0.0001$), respectively.[146]

OTHER PREPARATIONS

Topical creams, ointments and rubefacients

Topical therapies have been used for centuries for the management of aches and pains associated with musculoskeletal conditions. A number of botanicals exert a rubefacient action when applied topically. These oils cause irritation and reddening to the applied area, resulting in the blood vessels of the area dilating and causing warming effect, while also improving blood flow, circulation and nutrition to the area.

Common rubefacients include:

- *Brassica alba/nigra* (mustard seeds)
- *Capsicum* spp. (chilli)
- *Gaultheria procumbens* — volatile oil (wintergreen)
- Menthol oils — *Gaultheria procumbens* (volatile oil), *Mentha* × *piperita* (peppermint).

A systematic review investigated the effects of topical creams for treating osteoarthritis. Arnica gel was compared to ibuprofen. The effect on pain was measured (higher scores mean more severe pain). After 3 weeks of treatment, people who applied arnica rated their pain to be 3.8 points lower than people who applied ibuprofen. Physical function was then investigated (lower scores mean better function). People who applied arnica rated their physical function to be 0.4 points lower than people who applied ibuprofen. Comfrey extract cream was compared to placebo. After 3 weeks of treatment, people who applied comfrey rated their pain to be 16.3 points lower (20.08 to 12.58 points lower) than people who applied placebo.

After another 3 weeks of treatment, people who applied comfrey rated their pain to be lower by 20.9 points from baseline and people who applied placebo rated their pain to be lower by 4.6 points from baseline on a scale of 0 to 100.[147] Furthermore, *Symphytum officinale* (comfrey root extract) ointment was better than placebo ointment for short-term improvements in pain as assessed by VAS. Aromatic lavender essential oil applied by acupressure may reduce subjective pain intensity and improve lateral spine flexion and walking time compared to untreated participants.[148]

LIFESTYLE RECOMMENDATIONS

There is good evidence to support a number of lifestyle recommendations in the management of symptoms associated with osteoarthritis.

Time outs

Regular 'time outs' to de-stress, rest and recuperate.

Appropriate footwear

Appropriate footwear is extremely important in reducing the risk of osteoarthritis as well as relieving the symptoms. Osteoarthritis of the knee is more common in women and the effect of style of shoe has been investigated and proposed as an influence. Studies show that high heels alter the forces acting at the knee and can contribute to joint changes.[149] Even shoes with moderately high heels (4 cm) have been found to significantly increase the knee torques thought to be relevant in the development and/or progression of knee osteoarthritis. Thus wearing shoes with high heels should be avoided, particularly in those with preexisting osteoarthritis.[150] The addition of heel and sole supports as a treatment for osteoarthritis of the knee has been investigated in numerous studies and found to reduce pain,[151,152] signifying benefits for the patient.

Exercise

Although many patients express concern that exercise may further contribute to their symptoms, exercise appears to be valuable in the management of osteoarthritic symptoms, reducing pain and disability provided no trauma is incurred.[153] Varied exercise is to be recommended, including muscle stretching and strengthening. A 2008 Cochrane review of 32 studies found there to be platinum level evidence that land-based therapeutic exercise provides benefit in terms of reduced knee pain and improved physical function for people with knee osteoarthritis.[154] A Cochrane review also suggested aquatic exercise to be beneficial for osteoarthritis of the knee and hips.[155] Clearly, exercise should be gentle and suitable for the individual's ability and constitution.

Maintenance of healthy body weight

Acknowledging the strong link that exists between obesity and osteoarthritis suggests maintenance of a healthy body weight to be imperative; notably, however, the focus should be on fat loss rather than just weight loss. It is important to note that many studies have obtained impressive results in reducing the risk of osteoarthritis and increasing function with even minor amounts of weight/fat loss,[156] emphasising that obesity is a very modifiable risk factor of osteoarthritis. In one study, weight reduction of 10% resulted in a 28% improvement in joint function in overweight females with osteoarthritis of the knee.[157]

Massage

A clinical study in patients with osteoarthritis of the knee who were receiving massage twice weekly reported improvements in pain, stiffness, physical function and range of movement.[158] Thus regular massage can be seen as beneficial in relieving symptoms associated with osteoarthritis, but what can you do if you cannot afford two massages a week? In Ayurveda, daily self-massage of the whole body (known as *abhyanga*) is recommended to keep the joints mobile and relieve symptoms of osteoarthritis. The type of oil chosen is dependent on one's constitution, but cured black sesame oil is generally suitable for all constitutions and is said to penetrate through seven layers of the skin. The oil is heated by placing the jar of oil in a dish of warm water and when warm it is applied directly onto the body. For osteoarthritis, special attention should be paid to gently massaging the affected joints. For the time-poor, the whole massage can be done in 10 minutes; for others, more time can be spent on individual areas of the body. Oil may be left on (particularly good for those with dry skin) or washed off, but a thin film of oil is considered beneficial, therefore shower with warm rather than hot water.

CASE STUDY

OVERVIEW

AB, a 55-year-old married man, attended the clinic with osteoarthritis of the neck, hands and knees. X-ray diagnosis of osteoarthritis 2 years prior to this appointment. He attended the clinic due to the pain getting worse. He suffered general muscle stiffness in the morning and after periods of inactivity. There was tenderness on palpation and moderate pain on passive motion. Stiffness improves after moderate activity.

AB has been driving buses for 20 years. He tends to drive 8–10 hours per day 5 days a week. He has two 30-minute breaks throughout the day when he will have an early lunch and a mid-afternoon snack before the afternoon busy school/work period. His diet was a diet typical of his generation. He had cornflakes with milk for breakfast with a mug of coffee with milk and 1 sugar. Lunch was 1–2 salad sandwiches with chicken or ham on white bread. Morning tea break consisted of a chocolate muffin and a small cappuccino. He had steak and vegetables (peas, corn, carrot, potato) for dinner with a cup of tea (with milk). He didn't drink much water as he feared having to stop frequently while driving the bus. He consumed 2–3 beers on a Sunday afternoon with friends. Every second Saturday he consumed 2–3 beers while watching a football game at a local club match.

His stress levels ranged 7–8/10 on weekdays and 6/10 on weekends. His sleep averaged 6–7 hours per night weeknights and he slept in for an extra hour on Sundays. He woke refreshed except when the stress levels were at 8/10.

CLINICAL EXAMINATION

General inspection

Generally happy, pleasant person. Appeared to have something on his mind.

CASE STUDY CONTINUED

Vital signs

BP 138/95 mmHg
Pulse 78 BPM
Temperature 37.3°C
Height 1.78 m
Weight 86 kg
BMI 27.14 kg/m^2
Dryness around the finger nails. Hands trembled bilaterally after 6 seconds. White spots and mild vertical ridging on most nails
Slowed capillary return
Scalloping around the edge of the tongue

Musculoskeletal

Joints	ROM normal in all joints except neck, hands and knees: ↓ ROM. General muscle stiffness in the morning and after periods of inactivity. Stiffness improves after moderate activity.
Neck	Pain worse for movement and stress/tension
Hands	Pain in both hands with the pain worse in the left hand. Pain worse from stress and work.
Knees	Pain in knees, worse in the left knee.

INVESTIGATION RESULTS

X-ray — neck, hands and knee

No fractures or dislocations noted. Osteophyte formation in both hands and both knees with the left side being worse. Joint effusion in both knees with narrowing of the joint space. There was narrowing of the joint space in the neck.

Blood testing

Mildly elevated LFT, particularly ALP and homocysteine. Vitamin D (25(OH)D) level was 68 nmol/L.

TREATMENT PROTOCOL

This case was a classic presentation of osteoarthritis. Years of wear and tear of driving a bus exacerbated his condition. Treatment considered the following variables in development of a program:

- Nutritional intake of bone-building nutrients
- Correction of nutritional deficiencies
- Reduce inflammation and oxidative stress
- Reduce pain
- Digestive function for nutritional absorption
- Weight balance (both current and historical) as he was overweight
- Exercise and lifestyle to assess impact of bone mineralisation and bone degeneration. Most of his day is sitting and driving.

INVESTIGATIONS

The following investigations were ordered:

- Bone mineral density
- Reassess vitamin D in 3 months
- Liver function test
- Cholesterol profile.

CASE STUDY CONTINUED

INITIAL APPOINTMENT

HERBAL MEDICINE

Herbal medicine	Quantity	Justification
Salix alba	40 mL	Anti-inflammatory, anti-arthritic and analgesic activity
Harpagophytum procumbens	40 mL	Anti-inflammatory
Curcuma longa	50 mL	Anti-inflammatory, antioxidant, hepatic
Uncaria tomentosa	40 mL	Anti-inflammatory, anti-arthritic and analgesic activity
Withania somnifera	40 mL	Adaptogen, nervine
Zingiber officinale	10 mL	Circulatory stimulant, anti-inflammatory
Total	220 mL	

Dose: 10 mL in water before breakfast and before dinner (can take a 5 mL extra dose during the day if there is an elevation in pain)

NUTRITIONAL MEDICINE

Dietary

- Increasing hydration and reducing alcohol and caffeine was vital to success of treatment. Water intake was required to be increased to a minimum of 2.6 L/day (aim for 30 mL per kg body weight/day).
- Bone matrix building was supported and encouraged with wholefood dietary principles encouraging optimal nutrient density and absorption.
- Almonds, Brazil nuts, cashews and walnuts were added as a snack while driving. They were added for their mineral content (calcium, magnesium, selenium, zinc).

CASE STUDY CONTINUED

- Pro-inflammatory foods were avoided.
- Fish was added twice per week in the place of steak. He was to expand on his range of vegetables, especially broccoli.
- Food allergies and intolerances were investigated. Potential problem foods were removed from the diet.
- He reduced saturated fat content and included foods that had a low-medium glycaemic index to maintain his energy throughout the day.

Supplemental

- Omega-3: high-potency, concentrated formula: 1200 mg EPA and 800 mg DHA t.d.s.
- Glucosamine 1500 mg b.i.d. and chondroitin 500 mg b.i.d.
- Magnesium 200–300 mg t.d.s.
- Manganese 5 mg b.i.d.
- Zinc 25 mg b.i.d.
- High-potency B complex (activated forms) 1 capsule with breakfast and 1 capsule with lunch
- Glutamine 5000 mg in water b.i.d.
- Lysine 1000 mg in water b.i.d.
- Inositol 1000 mg in water b.i.d.

LIFESTYLE/EDUCATION

As he was overweight (and had gained 5 kg in the last year), he was encouraged to increase his physical activity to reduce his weight. The physical activity was to be daily. Commencing with a mild walk 20 minutes per day (in the evening) for the first week. The duration of walking in the second week was increased to 30 minutes per day and slightly more strenuous. From the third week onwards, a 10-minute walk was added to the morning. Stress management techniques, particularly time outs, were suggested to improve his quality of life. The time outs were to be performed at times he felt his stress levels were increasing.

GOUT

Epidemiology

The incidence and prevalence of gout is increasing dramatically (Fig. 15.5). Gout typically occurs more frequently in men and when compared with women, men have a 4–9-fold increased risk of developing the condition.[159] Gout is also suggested to be the most common type of inflammatory joint disease diagnosed in men over 40.[160] The prevalence of gout is 3.9% in the US, 0.9% in France, 1.4–2.5% in the UK, 1.4% in Germany; in New Zealand the prevalence of gout is 3.2% European and 6.1% Māori.[161] Studies show that certain ethnic groups, such as the Polynesians, have an increased risk of gout.[162]

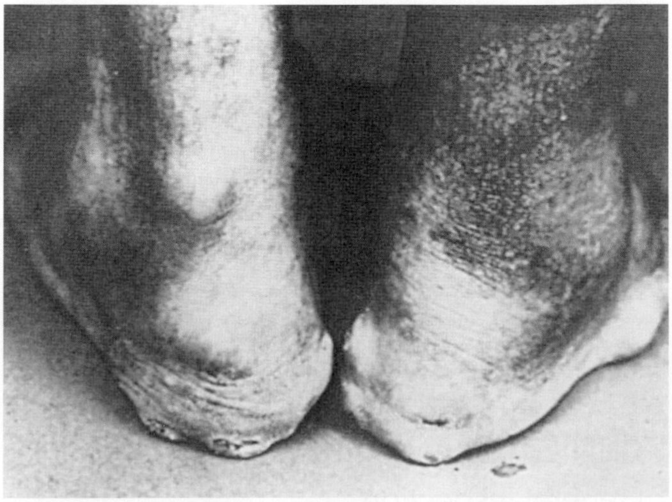

FIGURE 15.5 Gout.
Firestein GS, Budd RC, Sergent JS et al. Kelley's textbook of rheumatology. 8th edn. WB Saunders; 2008.

Classification

Classification systems consider two main variables: causative factors and duration of presentation.

CAUSATIVE FACTORS

Gout can be classified as either primary or secondary:

- In primary gout the underlying dysfunction causing the hyperuricaemia is unknown or the main manifestation of the dysfunction is the gout.[163] Primary gout accounts for the majority of cases seen in clinic.
- Secondary gout refers to disorders where gout occurs as a known consequence of other factors, for example use of certain drugs or as a result of another disorder such as renal failure.
  See Table 15.9.

DURATION OF PRESENTATION[164]

Acute gout

The first attack of gout is usually monoarticular and acute, most often in the big toe or other part of the foot. The joint is usually very painful, red and swollen, subsiding over a period of days to a week or two if untreated. Acute attacks can be severe and may mimic septic arthritis, with fever, malaise, leucocytosis and raised inflammatory markers. The peak incidence is in the age group 40–60 years and anyone with an attack before the age of 30 requires further investigation for an underlying cause (excessive alcohol and purine intake, enzyme defect, increased cell turnover or renal disease).

A diagnosis of gout as the cause of an acutely inflamed joint in a child is not tenable, unless the individual has a genetic defect in urate metabolism.

Subacute gout

Subsequent attacks can involve more joints and have more systemic features, including fever. These attacks may be of limited severity and may be separated by long intervals of relatively normal joint function. The attack may not be recognised as gout and may be thought to be a sprain or another injury.

Chronic gout

Eventually, recurrent attacks may fail to resolve completely and slowly lead to a crippling destructive arthritis. Chronic gout may be pauci- or polyarticular. Gouty tophi are frequently seen at this stage and are usually present on the elbows (olecranon bursae), knees (prepatellar bursae) and the peripheral joints such as the toes and fingers.

The symmetrical involvement of the small joints of both hands can mimic rheumatoid arthritis or psoriatic arthritis. Complicating this latter situation is the fact that elevated uric acid levels are common in psoriasis.

Asymptomatic hyperuricaemia

Asymptomatic hyperuricaemia may be present from birth in those with an enzyme deficiency, but otherwise tends to occur in at-risk males from puberty onwards and in women after menopause. It may be present for the life of the individual, or lead to an attack of gout or manifestations of nephrolithiasis.

Aetiology

GENETICS

It has become apparent that genetics are involved in the aetiology of gout. A number of studies have pointed out the possibility of hereditary tendencies, with specific gene polymorphisms observed to cause enzyme defects. For example, a deficiency of hypoxanthine guanine phosphoribosyltransferase 1 (HPRT1) has been shown to cause overproduction of uric acid.[165] Similarly, excess activity of the enzyme phosphoribosylpyrophosphate synthetase (PRPS1),[166,167] an X chromosome-linked disorder of purine metabolism, also causes overproduction of uric acid.

As mentioned above, specific ethnic groups have also been identified to have increased genetic risk. For example, Taiwanese people have been shown to have a gene polymorphism of monamine oxidase A suggested to be responsible for their predisposition to hyperuricaemia and gout,[168] while the high prevalence of gout in the Māori population has been suggested to be caused by a genetic variation in the renal urate transporter SLC2A9.[169]

OBESITY

A small pilot study undertaken by Dessein and colleagues[170] suggests that obesity increases serum urate and decreases renal clearance, increasing the risk of gout. Fat loss in obese patients has been linked to a decrease in uric acid levels[171] and therefore is likely to reduce the risk of gout.

COMORBIDITIES

Gout is associated with metabolic syndrome and is a risk factor for cardiovascular disease.[172,173]

Patients with diabetes, chronic kidney disease, hypertension and hyperlipidaemia have also been suggested to be at increased risk of gout.[174]

AGE/SEX

Risk of gout increases with age for both men and women.[175] While gout affects more men overall, in women gout typically presents after menopause as the fall in oestrogen (which functions to increase excretion of uric acid) and results in more uric acid in the blood.[163]

MEDICATIONS

Gout has been linked to the use of a number of medications. These medications may inhibit uric acid excretion or the way in which the kidneys excrete uric acid (Table 15.10). Examples include low-dose aspirin[176] and diuretics. The latter are an important cause of secondary hyperuricaemia, which occurs due to volume depletion and reduced renal tubular secretion of uric acid.[163]

DIET

Intake of purine-rich foods (discussed in more detail later in this chapter) is associated with increased incidence of gout in men.[177] Beer and liquor (but not wine) consumption is also associated with increased serum urate levels.[178]

TABLE 15.9 The ACR/EULAR gout classification criteria*

	Categories	Score
Step 1: Entry criterion (only apply criteria below to those meeting this entry criterion) **Step 2:** Sufficient criterion (if met, can classify as gout without applying criteria below) **Step 3:** Criteria (to be used if sufficient criterion not met)	At least 1 episode of swelling, pain, or tenderness in a peripheral joint or bursa. Presence of MSU crystals in a symptomatic joint or bursa (i.e. in synovial fluid) or tophus	
Clinical Pattern of joint/bursa involvement during symptomatic episode(s) ever†	Ankle *or* midfoot (as part of monoarticular or oligoarticular episode without involvement of the first metatarsophalangeal joint)	1
	Involvement of the first metatarsophalangeal joint (as part of monoarticular or oligoarticular episode)	2
Characteristics of symptomatic episode(s) ever • Erythema overlying affected joint (patient-reported or physician-observed) • Can't bear touch or pressure to affected joint • Great difficulty with walking or inability to use affected joint	One characteristic Two characteristics Three characteristics	1 2 3
Time course of episode(s) ever Presence (ever) of ≥2, irrespective of anti-inflammatory treatment: • Time to maximal pain <24 hours • Resolution of symptoms in ≤14 days • Complete resolution (to baseline level) between symptomatic episodes	One typical episode Recurrent typical episodes	1 2
Clinical evidence of tophus Draining or chalk-like subcutancous nodule under transparent skin, often with overlying vascularity, located in typical locations: joints, ears, olecranon bursae, finger pads, tendons (e.g. Achilles)	Present	4
Laboratory Serum urate: measured by uricase method Ideally should be scored at a time when the patient is not receiving urate-lowering treatment and it is >4 weeks from the start of an episode (i.e. during intercritical period); *if* practicable, retest under those conditions. The highest value irrespective of timing should be scored	<4 mg/dL (<0.24 mmol/litre)‡ 5–8 mg/dL (0.36–<0.48 mmol/litre) 8 –<10 mg/dL (0.48 –<0.60 mmol/litre) ≥10 mg/dL (≥0.60 mmol/litre)	−4 2 3 4
Synovial fluid analysis of a symptomatic (ever) joint or bursa (should be assessed by a trained observer)§	MSU negative	−2
Imaging¶ Imaging evidence of urate deposition in symptomatic (ever) joint or bursa: ultrasound evidence of double-contour sign# *or* DECT deposition**	Present (either modality)	4
Imaging evidence of gout-related joint damage: conventional radiography of the hands and/or feet demonstrates at least 1 erosion††	Present	4

*A web-based calculator can be accessed at: http://goutclassificationcalculator.auckland.ac.nz and through the American College of Rheumatology (ACR) and European League Against Rheumatism (EULAR) websites.
†Symptomatic episodes are periods of symptoms that include any swelling, pain and/or tenderness in a peripheral joint or bursa.
‡If serum urate level is <4 mg/dL (<0.24 mmoles/litre), *subtract 4 points*; if serum urate level is ≥4 –<6 mg/dL (≥0.24 –<0.36 mmoles/litre), score this item as 0.
§If polarising microcopy of synovial fluid from a symptomatic (ever) joint or bursa by a trained examiner fails to show monosodium urate monohydrate (MSU) crystals, *subtract 2 points*. If synovial fluid was not assessed, score this item as 0.
¶If imaging is not available, score these items as 0.
#Hyperechoic irregular enhancement over the surface of the hyaline cartilage that is independent of the insonation angle of the ultrasound beam (note: false-positive double-contour sign [artifact] may appear at cartilage surface but should disappear with a change in the insonation angle of the probe).
**Presence of colour-coded urate at articular or periarticular sites. Images should be acquired using a dual-energy computed tomography (DECT) scanner, with data acquired at 80 kV and 140 kV and analysed using gout-specific software with a 2-material decomposition algorithm that colour-codes urate. A positive scan is defined as the presence of colour-coded urate at articular or periarticular sites. Nailbed, submillimetre, skin, motion, beam hardening and vascular artifacts should not be interpreted as DECT evidence of urate deposition.
††Erosion is defined as a cortical break with sclerotic margin and overhanging edge, excluding distal interphalangeal joints and gull wing appearance.
Source: Neogi T, Jansen TL, Dalbeth N et al. 2015 Gout Classification Criteria: an American College of Rheumatology/European League Against Rheumatism collaborative initiative. Arth Rheumatol 2015; 67(10):2557–2568.

TABLE 15.10 Drugs that increase/decrease urate concentrations

Drugs that raise serum urate concentrations	Drugs that lower serum urate concentrations
Diuretics	Ascorbic acid
Tacrolimus	Benzbromarone
Cyclosporin	Calcitonin
Ethambutol	Citrate
Pyrazinamide	Oestrogens
Cytotoxic chemotherapy	Fenofibrate
Ethanol	Losartan
Salicylates (low dose)	Probenecid
Levodopa	Salicylates (high dose)
Ribavirin and interferon	Sulfinpyrazone
Teriparatide	

Source: Richette P, Barden T. Gout. Lancet 2010; 375:318–328.

TRAUMA

Trauma and irritation have been suggested to play some part in the locality of gout crystals. The thumbs and the big toe are both common sites for crystal deposition and are both sites of mechanical stress.

Overview

Although the exact metabolic defect in gout is unknown in the majority of cases, gout is one of the most controllable metabolic diseases. The increased serum uric acid level observed in primary idiopathic gout can be divided into three categories:

- Majority: increased synthesis of uric acid
- Less than 30%: reduced ability to excrete uric acid
- Minority: overproduction of uric acid, as well as underexcretion of uric acid.

THE CLASSIC GOUT PICTURE

The classic description of gout was by an English physician, Sydenham, who suffered from gout in 1683. Little has changed in the clinical picture of gout in more than 300 years. Sydenham's classic description was as follows:

> *The victim goes to bed and sleeps in good health. About two o'clock in the morning he is awakened by a severe pain in the great toe; more rarely in the heel, ankle, or instep. The pain is like that of a dislocation and yet parts feel as if cold water were poured over them. Then follows chills and shivers and a little fever. The pain which at first was moderate, becomes more intense. With its intensity the chills and fever increase. After a time this comes to a height, accommodating itself to the bones and ligaments of the tarsus and metatarsus. Now it is a violent stretching and tearing of the ligaments — now it is a gnawing pain and now a pressure and tightening. So exquisite and lively meanwhile is the feeling of the part affected, that it cannot bear the weight of bedclothes nor the jar of a person walking in the room. The night is passed in torture, sleeplessness, turning the part affected and perpetual change of posture; the tossing about of the body being as incessant as the pain of the tortured joint and being worse as the fit comes on. Hence the vain effort by change of posture, both in the body and the limb affected, to obtain an abatement of pain.*[179]

Subsequent attacks are common, with the majority having another attack within a year. However, nearly 7% never have a second attack. Chronic gout is extremely rare nowadays because of the advent of dietary therapy and drugs that lower uric acid levels. Some degree of kidney dysfunction occurs in nearly 90% of patients with gout and there is a higher risk of kidney stones.

Pathogenesis

Gout is monosodium urate (MSU) deposition disease. It occurs when patients have had, at some time, urate concentrations sufficiently elevated (usually >0.46 mmol/L) for the solubility coefficient of sodium urate to be exceeded long enough for crystals to form in tissues. At the time of presentation with gout or renal stones the plasma urate may be misleadingly 'normal'.[164]

The condition is caused by altered metabolism of purines, the end product of which is uric acid. As a result of an inability to excrete uric acid (90% of patients) and/or the overproduction of uric acid (10% of patients) hyperuricaemia occurs.[180] When uric acid levels are exceeded, monosodium urate crystal deposition occurs in various areas of the body, such as the joints, kidneys and soft tissues.[181]

URIC ACID METABOLISM

Uric acid is formed in the liver from dietary and endogenous purine precursors. A purine-free diet reduces urate excretion by 40%, so diet is a significant source of the urate precursors. Urate is eliminated by the kidneys (two-thirds) and the digestive system (one-third). Renal excretion is inhibited by some organic anions and drugs which compete for active transport of uric acid into the tubules. These include diuretics (the most important cause of secondary gout in the middle-aged and the elderly), low-dose aspirin and cyclosporin. Other drugs enhance urate excretion by blocking reabsorption in the renal tubule. Any drug or condition which causes a rapid rise or lowering of serum urate levels can precipitate an attack of acute gout.[164]

Almost all of the plasma urate is filtered at the glomerulus: only the small amount bound to protein is not filtered. Renal excretion is peculiar in that about 80% of the filtered uric acid is reabsorbed in the proximal tubule of the nephron. Actually, the distal tubule secretes most of the uric acid found in the urine. Distal to this site, some post-secondary reabsorption occurs.[182]

Uric acid is a highly insoluble molecule and at pH 7.4 and body temperature, the serum is saturated at 6.4–7 mg/100 mL. Although higher concentrations do not necessarily result in urate deposition (some unknown factor in serum appears to inhibit urate precipitation), the chance of an acute attack is greater than 90% when the level is above 9 mg/100 mL.[179]

SIGNS AND SYMPTOMS

Gout attacks in men and women have been observed to share the same symptoms but may present differently in their location. In the male patient gout will typically present with an acute rapid development of pain, swelling and tenderness, most commonly affecting the metatarsophalangeal joint of the large toe, though other joints including the knees, fingers, wrists and olecranon bursae may be affected.[183] A 10-year study observing the differences between presentation of gout in men and women noted that in women gout presented most commonly in the hands, tarsal joints, knees and ankles and tended to be polyarticular; few women got an initial attack of gout affecting the metatarsophalangeal joint of the large toe.[184]

Overlying erythema[185] and limited range of motion usually accompanies pain and swelling; systemically there may also be fever, chills and fatigue.[186] Tophaceous gout, chronic polyarticular arthritis, urate nephrolithiasis and interstitial nephropathy are also manifestations of gout, though these are more associated with chronic attacks.[187] Most commonly, the first attack of gout will usually occur at night.[188]

Preliminary criteria for the classification of gout according to the American College of Rheumatology include:[189]

- Monosodium urate monohydrate microcrystals in joint fluid during attack
- More than one attack of acute arthritis
- Maximum inflammation developed in 1 day
- Monoarthritis attack
- Redness observed or swollen
- First metatarsophalangeal joint painful or swollen
- Unilateral first metatarsophalangeal joint attack
- Unilateral tarsal joint attack
- Tophus (proven or suspected) — aggregated deposits of monosodium urate monohydrate (tophi) chiefly in and around the joints of the extremities but also in subcutaneous tissue, bone, cartilage and other tissues
- Hyperuricaemia
- Asymptomatic swelling within a joint on x-ray
- Subcortical cysts without swelling on x-ray
- Joint fluid culture negative for organisms during attack.

COMPLICATIONS

Left untreated, constant hyperuricaemia results in recurrent attacks of gout,[190] leading to a destructive form of arthritis known as tophaceous gout. This is characterised by large, tophaceous deposits into the joints and surrounding tissues[191] and causes chronic inflammation pain and damage and erosion to the affected joints. Tophaceous deposits (known as tophi) may cause ulceration[186] and have also been found in the cornea of the eye. They may also cause conjunctivitis, uveitis or scleritis.[192]

Complications of gout may also affect the kidneys, resulting in uric acid calculi, chronic urate nephropathy and acute uric acid nephropathy.[193] More seriously, in men, gout is associated with an increased risk of mortality from death from all causes.[194]

DIFFERENTIAL DIAGNOSIS

Acute gout

- Infective/septic arthritis
- Bursitis, cellulitis, tenosynovitis
- Other crystal arthropathy — 'pseudogout' caused by calcium pyrophosphate dihydrate crystal deposition, apatite or brushite arthritis or periarthritis
- Traumatic arthritis
- Haemarthrosis
- Rheumatoid arthritis with palindromic onset
- Reactive arthritis
- Spondyloarthritis with peripheral joint involvement
- Psoriatic arthritis
- Sarcoid arthritis
- Rheumatic fever.

Chronic gout

- Nodular rheumatoid arthritis
- Psoriatic arthritis
- Osteoarthritis with Heberden's and Bouchard's nodes
- Sarcoid arthritis
- Xanthomatosis.

NATUROPATHIC DIAGNOSIS

Naturopathic diagnosis sees gout as a preventable disease whereby simple dietary and lifestyle changes can modify even the most chronic picture. As such, diagnosis relies on allopathic determinants. Diagnosis will also consider the health and functioning of additional body systems such as the hepatobiliary, digestive and renal/urinary.

Investigations

PRIMARY INVESTIGATIONS

The patient with suspected gout requires:

- Plasma urate assay (this may be normal in acute gout)
- Aspiration, where possible, of an affected joint, bursa or tophus (to obtain a firm diagnosis by detection of urate crystals using compensated polarised light microscopy)
- A search for secondary causes, including impaired renal clearance of urate and increased cell turnover, as appropriate.

ADDITIONAL INVESTIGATIONS

Plain radiography

In patients with the very first manifestations of gout, no radiographic findings are present. Typical plain radiographic features of chronic gout include visualisation of tophi as soft-tissue or intraosseous masses and the presence of a non-demineralising erosive arthropathy with erosions that are well defined with sclerotic or overhanging margins.

The joint space is usually preserved until late in the disease and other features such as periosteal new bone formation, extraarticular erosions, intraosseous calcifications, joint space widening and subchondral collapse may be present. Radiographic abnormalities are most frequently present in the feet, particularly in the first metatarsal phalangeal joint.

Radiographic damage is a late feature of chronic gout, typically occurring 15 years after onset of the disease and is virtually always present in patients with subcutaneous tophi. Oblique projections may enhance observation of small erosions.

CT scan

CT allows excellent visualisation of tophi. MSU crystals obtained from tophi measurements are possible with this assessment. Use of CT may assist in differentiating tophi from other subcutaneous nodules. CT has the potential to play a role in clinical assessment of chronic gout in a number of situations; in assessing complications of gout, in guiding aspiration, in assisting with non-invasive diagnosis of subcutaneous nodules, in identification of deep intra-articular tophi and in evaluation of bone erosion associated with gout.

MRI

Although findings are not specific for the diagnosis of gout, MRI allows early detection of tophi and bone erosion in patients with gout. Synovial involvement may also be appropriately evaluated with MRI. The relative lack of specificity of MRI and the technique's high cost, however, limit its role in routine clinical assessment of gout.

Ultrasonography

The impact of ultrasonography has been highlighted in a study of 35 patients with asymptomatic hyperuricaemia.[195] Small tophaceous deposits were found in 12 (34%) of these patients and an increased power-Doppler signal was observed in 8 (23%) patients, suggesting on-site inflammation. This study using ultrasonography is the first to bridge the gap between asymptomatic hyperuricaemia and symptomatic deposition of urate, namely gout. Imaging showing crystal deposition and inflammation may support starting early treatment strategies.

Synovial fluid analysis

This involves aspiration of the fluid from the inflamed gouty joint to look for monosodium uric acid crystals under a microscope.

Measurement of urinary uric acid levels over 24 hours

This test determines the presence of hyperuricaemia and whether it is caused by urate overproduction or underexcretion.

SPECIFIC NATUROPATHIC INVESTIGATIONS

There are no specific naturopathic investigations available to assess the presence of gout. Supportive listening, case taking and observational skills will usually confirm a diagnosis in conjunction with pathology results. As the disease reflects dietary and lifestyle affluence excessive assessments are typically unnecessary, although the following functional tests may be applicable.

Functional liver detoxification profile

Suboptimal liver function may indicate build-up of toxicity in the body. Excess strain on the liver is likely to indicate that there is also excess burden on the kidneys.

Essential fatty acids

Essential fatty acids (EFAs) analysis and/or omega-3 index should be carried out because EFAs can be used to downregulate inflammation in gout; deficiency will prevent this from happening.

Hair mineral analysis

Hair mineral analysis is a useful tool to measure minerals and toxic metals. Some toxic metals (e.g. lead) are indicated in the aetiology of gout.

Metabolic profile

Recent research has linked the incidence of gout with insulin resistance and metabolic syndrome. As such, it is beneficial to organise an assessment of fasting blood glucose levels, insulin and HbA1c, liver function test, urea, electrolytes and creatinine, with potential 2-hour glucose tolerance test in cases of suspected obesity. Weight, height, BMI and waist-to-hip ratio are important assessment strategies.

Therapeutic considerations

CLINICAL DECISION-MAKING AND RATIONALE

The management of gout involves providing rapid pain relief, preventing further attacks if possible, preventing the formation of gouty tophi and destructive arthritis and dealing with any associated medical conditions such as alcoholism, hyperlipidaemia, hypertension, obesity and glucose intolerance/insulin resistance.

Most important is patient education about the need for additional treatment if alcohol and dietary modification fail to bring about a normal urate level. Compliance to dietary and lifestyle modifications is crucial. The emphasis should be on lifelong therapy and anything that will ensure compliance and adherence.

Acute gout

Initially, gout may subside spontaneously in less than a week, but the patient will usually seek help. Anti-inflammatory herbal medicines and nutrients are essential in full doses and increased frequency to reduce inflammation and pain relatively quickly.

Intercritical gout

The name intercritical gout is given to the asymptomatic interval between (even severe) recurrent attacks of acute gout. Most untreated patients will have a second attack within 2 years. Eventually, these recurrent acute attacks occur more frequently, with longer duration and become polyarticular. This period between acute attacks is the opportunity to establish the diagnosis, try to correct the reversible causes, correct any nutritional deficiencies and institute urate-lowering therapy with appropriate prophylaxis to avoid an acute exacerbation.

Chronic gout

Chronic gout is usually difficult to treat and requires strict compliance and adherence to treatment suggestions and prescriptions. The prescriptions are adjusted for gouty flare ups using the acute dosage prescribing. Dietary and lifestyle modifications have to be followed strictly.

There is no asymptomatic period in which to commence urate-lowering therapy. The patient may be unwilling to take allopurinol because of previous experience of having had acute attacks precipitated by its inappropriate use without colchicine or NSAID cover. It is usually vital to resolve the inflammation if possible, before very slowly introducing additional treatment measures.

Hyperuricaemia

Treatment for hyperuricaemia is unnecessary unless the patient has symptoms (or has the potential to develop severe adverse effects from the underlying condition). In general, asymptomatic hyperuricaemia in patients on thiazide diuretics, or with high cell turnover from underlying disorders, are less likely to develop gout or renal complications than those with a family history of gout. When gout does arise, usually in elderly hyperuricaemic patients, it may present as acute inflammation in joints already affected by arthritis, for instance Heberden's nodes. If the hyperuricaemia is due to medications, it is logical to try to correct it by stopping or changing the medications before a problem arises.

Therapeutic application

HISTORICAL PERSPECTIVE

Descriptions of gout, particularly that afflicting the joints of the big toe, can be traced back as far as Hippocrates' time where he described the condition as the 'disease of kings'.[196] Herbal compendiums from the 16th and 17th centuries[197] tell of kitchen remedies for painful gout-afflicted joints, including the wrapping of gout-affected limbs in cloths soaked in a mixture of *Trigonella foenum-graecum* (fenugreek) and the juice of *Brassica oleracea* (cabbage), while *Avena sativa* (oats) was consumed to remove the sludge associated with gout of the feet.

Furthermore, the herbals tell of the benefits of *Hypericum perforatum*, consumed as a wine to ease gout affecting the feet while *Thymus vulgaris* (thyme) was administered in the form of a vinegar to expel the slime that caused gout.

Of the Eclectic physicians, Ellingwood favoured the use of the botanical *Colchicum autumnale*, suggested to be a 'magical eliminative' for the treatment of gout.[198] *Zingiber officinale* was also used for 'old and gouty individuals',[138] probably because of its gentle circulatory stimulant effects. A mixture of capsicum, syrup of orange peel, sodium bromide, sodium iodide and morphine was also said to be excellent for pain relief during gout.[198] Noting the influence of diet in the aetiology of gout, Thomas[199] recommended reducing the quantity consumed at meals, noting: 'Everybody eats more than is necessary past the age of 40 anyway'. As expected and in line with modern naturopathic treatment, meat, liquor and sweet wines were forbidden, while a diet rich in fruit (but not that which was high in sugar such as bananas) and vegetables (but not that which was acidic) was favoured, in particular celery, cabbage, lettuce and turnip.

NATUROPATHIC PERSPECTIVE

The naturopathic approach for chronic gout does not differ substantially from the standard medical approach:

- Dietary modifications are paramount. If the patient commits to dramatic dietary changes, it is likely to significantly positively affect their uric acid levels. Investigate and correct any nutritional deficiencies.
- Lifestyle modifications are additionally important. Exercise and physical activity are strong preventers of gout.
- Weight loss is essential. Determine the patient's ideal body weight (using BMI and waist-to-hip ratio) and direct and support a weight loss and weight management program.
- Control alcohol consumption.
- Determine and eliminate dietary triggers, e.g. food allergies and intolerances that may exacerbate their condition.
- Supplement with nutritionals and prescribe herbal medicines to prevent further attacks and reduce uric acid levels.
- Address lead toxicity, or any other heavy metal toxicity, if present.

NUTRITIONAL MEDICINE (DIETARY)

Dietary therapeutic objectives

- Avoid consumption of alcohol.
- Avoid high purine-containing foods (e.g. organ meats, meat, yeast, poultry). Protein intake may require adjustment and should be calculated at 0.8 g/kg body weight. Urinary 24-hour uric acid levels can be used to monitor compliance with a purine-free diet.
- Avoid saturated and trans fatty acids. Encourage cold-pressed oils and other essential fatty acids, particularly omega-3.
- Avoid refined carbohydrates and encourage complex carbohydrates. Include low-medium glycaemic index foods.
- Balance dietary intake with energy expenditure and dietary requirements for healthy living.
- Provide foods that reduce weight (if indicated), increase metabolism and support healthy weight management.
- Achieve ideal body weight.
- Investigate and correct nutritional deficiencies.
- Ensure hydration is sufficient and optimal for hydration and elimination.

- Liberal amounts (250–500 g/day) of cherries and other anthocyanoside-rich (i.e. red-blue) berries (or extracts) should be consumed.
- Cease consumption of coffee, tea and other caffeinated beverages due to diuretic effect on body fluid distribution and volume.

Specific dietary treatments

DIETARY INCLUSIONS

Low-fat dairy products

A diet high in dairy was initially thought to increase the risk of gout, but present-day clinical studies link a diet with optimal amounts of low-fat dairy products with reduced risk of gout.[177] The inclusion of dairy as a dietary treatment may be seen as controversial by some, so when choosing dairy products it is important to choose sensibly; low-fat ice cream is unlikely to provide the same benefits as natural biodynamic yoghurt.

Fresh fruit and vegetables

A diet rich in fruit and vegetables has been suggested to reduce the frequency of gout[200] and reduce the severity of other chronic diseases. Vitamin C-rich foods in particular appear to be of great benefit.[201] Foods rich in vitamin C include kiwi fruit, mangoes, guava and berries.

Cherries

Consumption of cherries has been suggested to be efficacious for treating manifestations of gout. Plasma urate, antioxidant and inflammatory markers were measured in 10 healthy women who consumed two servings (280 g) of cherries after an overnight fast.[202] A decrease in plasma urate after cherry consumption was observed, as was a decrease in inflammatory indices. The decrease seen in plasma urate supports the reputation for cherries as an effective anti-gout remedy. The reductions in inflammatory indices also suggest that constituents within cherries may be anti-inflammatory.

Nuts, seeds and legumes

Nuts, legumes and wholegrains have been suggested to be healthy choices for the comorbidities of gout and may also help to prevent insulin resistance.[201]

DIETARY EXCLUSIONS

Purines — animal-derived

Consumption of animal-derived purine-rich foods, such as seafood and red meat, has been shown to increase the risk of gout.[177] This risk is thought to increase by 21% for every additional serving of meat consumed.[177] Risk is also likely to be greater in those with preexisting gout as renal urate clearance is likely to already be compromised. Interestingly and very noteworthy is the fact that moderate intake of purine-rich vegetables such as peas, beans, lentils, spinach, mushrooms and cauliflower does not appear to increase the risk of gout.[177]

Foods high in purine include:

- Processed meats
- Organ meats/offal
- Red meats
- Shellfish/crustaceans
- Yeast (brewer's and baker's)
- Oily fish — herring, sardines, mackerel and anchovies
- Red wine
- Port.

Soft drinks

Data from the large Health Professionals Follow-up Study (HPFS) suggest that consumption of sugar-sweetened soft drinks and fructose is associated with increased risk of gout in males.[203] Data from other surveys have suggested a link between sweetened soft drinks, fructose and hyperuricaemia.[204] In both studies diet soft drinks were not associated with risk, but from a naturopathic perspective these are not deemed favourable if there is presence of artificial sweetener. Something to note is that the consumption of energy drink acutely increases platelet aggregation and mean arterial pressure while decreasing endothelial function in healthy young adults.[205] Increased platelet aggregation has been implicated in cardiovascular disease and inflammation.

Alcohol

In those with a diagnosis or predisposition to gout, intake of alcohol should be avoided. Alcohol is associated with increased serum uric acid[56] as well as increased risk of gout. A 12-year prospective study undertaken by Choi et al[206] observed that risk varies according to choice of alcoholic beverage; beer in particular increases risk more than spirits, whereas moderate wine drinking does not increase the risk at all.

Saturated fat

Many foods high in saturated fat are highly inflammatory in the body and are undesirable where there is gout. In addition, a number of chronic diseases in which excessive intake of saturated fat is thought to play a part have been found to be associated with gout, including metabolic syndrome and cardiovascular disease.

NUTRITIONAL MEDICINE (SUPPLEMENTAL)

Nutritional medicine therapeutic objectives

- Investigate and address nutritional deficiencies that precipitate unhealthy dietary practices and cravings.
- Support optimal weight balance and management.
- Provide symptomatic relief and reduce inflammation, pain and oxidative stress.
- Improve circulation.
- Improve liver and kidney function.
- Support optimal clearance of uric acid and other metabolites through the body.

Specific nutrients required

BROMELAIN

Bromelain is a proteolytic enzyme that may assist in reducing pain, swelling and inflammation associated with soft-tissue injury/trauma, thus suggesting a promising role in the treatment of gout. Bromelain exhibits significant analgesic,[207] anti-inflammatory[207] and anti-oedematous[208]

SAMPLE DAILY DIET

BREAKFAST	
Fresh fruit salad containing 1 kiwi fruit, 12 cherries and strawberries served with LSA and raw nuts and seeds Celery and ginger juice	Vitamin C has been shown to reduce levels of urate by decreasing production of uric acid therefore foods rich in vitamin C such as cherries, strawberries and kiwi fruit are all advocated. Vitamin C is also a powerful antioxidant which may hypothetically assist in reducing damage associated with articular inflammation. Cherries have been shown to be particularly beneficial for gout, with consumption (at least 12 fresh cherries) associated with reduced risk of gout flares. Celery is an alkalising diuretic which may aid clearance of toxins while ginger assists in reducing inflammation.
LUNCH	
Spinach, watercress, zucchini and potato soup with white beans Rice toast with avocado, lemon and salt and pepper	Animal protein should be replaced with vegetarian sources of protein to reduce risk of gout attack. A 12-year prospective study observed that each additional serving of meat per day increased the risk of gout by 21%, whereas each additional weekly seafood serving increased risk by 7%. Moderate intake of purine-rich vegetables was not associated with an increased risk of gout. Potassium-rich foods such as spinach and avocado are promoted to reduce acidity in the body.
DINNER	
Sweet potato and white bean chilli	A high prevalence of metabolic syndrome exists in patients with gout, compared with in non-gout patients thus a diet that is blood sugar balancing and anti-inflammatory is imperative. Meals should be wholefood and high in fibre, with foods with known benefits for blood sugar control such as cinnamon promoted.
SNACK	
Fresh seasonal fruit and vegetables, e.g. carrot sticks 8–16 cups of water during flares Cherry juice concentrate	Anti-inflammatory Aids removal of uric acid from the body Reduced risk of gout

Sources: Beyl RN Jr, Hughes L, Morgan S. Update on importance of diet in gout. Am J Med 2016; 129(11):1153–1158. Choi K, Atkinson K, Karlson EW et al. Purine-rich foods, dairy and protein intake, and the risk of gout in men. N Engl J Med 2004; 350(11):1093–1103. Johnson R, Rideout B. Uric acid and diet — insights into the epidemic of cardiovascular disease. N Engl J Med 2004; 350:1071–1073. Juraschek,SP, Miller ER, Gelber AC. Effect of oral vitamin C supplementation on serum uric acid: a meta-analysis of randomized controlled trials. Arthritis Care Res (Hoboken) 2011; 63(9):1295–1306. Zhang Y, Neogi T, Chen C et al. Cherry consumption and decreased risk of recurrent gout attacks. Arthritis Rheum 2012; 64(12):4004–4011.

actions, decreasing oedema and neutrophil migration to sites of acute inflammation,[209] stimulating monocytes (white blood cells) to secrete cytokines (immune-modulating agents) while also inducing phagocytosis (the process used to destroy dead or foreign cells) by white blood cells. As yet no studies have been found assessing the individual efficacy of bromelain in a clinical trial in patients with gout, but these actions warrant further investigation.

QUERCETIN

Quercetin has been suggested to be beneficial in the management of gout because of its ability to inhibit xanthine oxidase.[210] In addition, quercetin inhibits leukotriene synthesis,[211] reducing inflammation and has antihistamine and antioxidant properties.

VITAMIN C

Megadoses of vitamin C are probably contraindicated in individuals with gout, as vitamin C may increase uric acid levels in a small number of individuals, but vitamin C has been clinically proven to reduce serum uric acid levels in relatively low doses.[212] Data from a 20-year prospective study indicate that risk of gout decreases with increased vitamin C intake (1500 mg/day or more), independent of dietary and other risk factors for gout, such as BMI, age, hypertension, diuretic use and alcohol use.[213]

ESSENTIAL FATTY ACIDS (EPA, DHA, GLA)

As yet there are no published data examining the use of essential fatty acids for the management of gout in humans, but several animal and experimental studies have examined the relationship between essential fatty acids and xanthine oxidase and urate crystal formation. A recent study undertaken by Kawai et al[214] observed that partially hydrogenated fish oil administered daily to rats depressed the activity of xanthine dehydrogenase, positively affecting serum and urinary uric acid. Tate et al[215] observed that in rats induced with urate crystals and fed a diet enriched with GLA and EPA, the enriched GLA diet suppressed cellular inflammation (leucocyte accumulation, crystal phagocytosis, lysosomal enzyme activity) but showed little effect in reducing fluid/exudate. On the other hand, the EPA-enriched diet suppressed the fluid phase but not the cellular phase of inflammation. Essential fatty acids have proven anti-inflammatory effects in humans for a number of conditions and their therapeutic use in gout deserves more research.

GLUCOSAMINE, CHONDROITIN AND GREEN-LIPPED MUSSEL

Crystalline deposits have been found in gout-affected joints where they detrimentally affect the articular cartilage. Glucosamine and chondroitin are well known for their chondro-protective effects and glucosamine has been suggested to stimulate the regeneration of cartilage following experimentally induced damage,[216] while chondroitin inhibits cartilage breakdown and stimulates production of the extracellular matrix. While no clinical studies have been undertaken assessing the effects of glucosamine and chondroitin in gout, their application is likely to help protect the joints and surrounding tissue from gout-induced damage.[217] Similarly, while no studies have been undertaken assessing the efficacy of green-lipped mussel in gout, it displays anti-inflammatory activity specific to the musculoskeletal system and thus may be useful in reducing swelling and inflammation with gout.

B COMPLEX (ALL B VITAMINS INCLUDING B_1, B_2, B_3, B_5, B_6, FOLATE, B_{12})

Supportive literature on the prescription of B vitamins is limited, but as B vitamins are water soluble it is beneficial to maintain supplementation until the condition is treated and reversed. Of importance, high doses of nicotinic acid are contraindicated (>50 mg/day) as it competes with uric acid for excretion.[179] After reviewing the patient, activated B vitamins may be used, especially if a MTHFR polymorphism has been found. A significant association between hyperuricaemia (> or = 7 mg/dL) and MTHFR 677T allele carriers was observed in a Japanese study.[218] When using folinic acid or MTHF, consider the methylation status of the patient.

DOSAGE REQUIREMENTS

The dosage requirements listed below are based on adult doses that have been reported in the literature.

- Bromelain 200–400 mg two–three times daily between meals[219]
- Quercetin 200–400 mg two–three times daily between meals[219]
- Vitamin C 500 mg/day for 2 months[212]
- EFAs:
  - DHA 800-2700 mg/day[106]
  - EPA 3000-5000 mg/day EPA[107]
- Glucosamine: 1500 mg/day
- Chondroitin: 800–1200 mg/day
- Green-lipped mussel: 1500–3000 mg in acute followed by 500–2000 mg as maintenance
- B complex (all B vitamins) high-dose combination, preferably activated forms
  - Thiamine 20–40 mg/day
  - Riboflavin 20–50 mg. Riboflavin-5-phosphate sodium 20–40 mg
  - Niacinamide 50–100 mg/day; nicotinic acid up to maximum 50 mg/day
  - Pantothenic acid 150–300 mg/day
  - Pyridoxine 50–100 mg/day (pyridoxyl-5-phosphate 20–60 mg/day)
  - Folic acid/folinic acid/MTHF 500–1000 micrograms/day. When using folinic acid or MTHF, consider the methylation status of the patient. Also investigate MTHFR (C677T, A1298C)
  - Hydroxo- or methylcobalamin 500–1000 micrograms/day determined by the methylation status of the patient
  - Choline 50–100 mg/day
  - Inositol 50–100 mg/day
  - Biotin 250–500 micrograms/day.

HERBAL MEDICINE

Herbal medicine therapeutic objectives

- To reduce joint pain
- To reduce inflammation and oxidative stress, particularly around the joints
- To increase circulation to the joints
- To remove wastes and eliminate toxins
- Kidney and liver support if indicated
- To reduce the effects of stress and nourish the nervous system where necessary.

Herbal medicine classes

It is advantageous to select the herbal medicines that will increase excretion of urates from the kidneys. The primary modern herbal medicines that adhere to the traditional concept include *Apium graveolens* (celery seed), *Taraxacum officinale* folia (dandelion leaf) and *Urtica dioica* folia (nettle leaf). Additional anti-inflammatory herbal medicines may be indicated as well in aggravated cases.

- Anti-inflammatory
- Antioxidant
- Antirheumatic
- Circulatory stimulant
- Diuretic: anti-gout and general
- Renal tonics
- Analgesic/anodyne if indicated
- Hepatobiliary/GI tract support if indicated
- Other classes include adaptogens and nervine, antispasmodic, sedative/relaxant herbal medicines as necessary.

Specific herbal medicines

AGROPYRON REPENS (COUCH GRASS)

The rhizome of *Agropyron repens* is a diuretic and was favoured by the Eclectic physicians for its effects on renal secretion in gout.[138] The impaired ability of the kidneys to clear uric acid from the body has been identified as a cause of gout,[219] and *Agropyron repens* through its action as a diuretic promotes the removal of toxic build-up via the kidneys. From a naturopathic perspective this toxic build-up is thought to contribute to the pathogenesis of gout. As yet there are no pharmacological and clinical studies examining the action of *Agropyron repens* in the treatment of gout, but its traditional application and mechanism of action provide a rationale for its use as an adjuvant therapy.

ANTHOCYANIDINS, PROANTHOCYANIDINS AND ANTHOCYANOSIDE EXTRACTS (E.G. *VACCINIUM MYRTILLUS*)

Anthocyanidins, proanthocyanidins and anthocyanoside are powerful flavonoids that display significant antioxidant and anti-inflammatory activity within the body. Clinical studies[220,221] suggest that flavonoids may inhibit the activity of xanthine oxidase, an enzyme that produces uric acid and reactive oxygen species during the breakdown of purines. Not only does xanthine oxidase increase uric acid in the body, it may also promote free radicals, causing damage to surrounding tissues.[222]

Botanicals such as *Vaccinium myrtillus* (bilberry) and *Vitis vinifera* (grape seed),[223] which contain optimal amounts of flavonoids, may be useful in the management of gout and are likely to inhibit the action of xanthine oxidase, thus reducing uric acid while simultaneously preventing inflammation and free radical damage. As yet there have been no human clinical trials accessing the efficacy of botanicals such as these in the management of gout, but in mice pre-treated with oxonate to induce hyperuricaemia, administration with procyanidins from grape seeds was found to reduce serum uric acid levels and decrease hepatic xanthine oxidase activity.[220]

APIUM GRAVEOLENS (CELERY)

Apium graveolens is a mild diuretic[224] and was traditionally used to help relieve rheumatic complaints.[225] Like *Agropyron repens* discussed above, the role of *Apium graveolens* as a diuretic is likely to involve the promotion of renal excretion of uric acid. *Apium graveolens* has also been identified as containing over 25 anti-inflammatory constituents,[226] which are also likely to be of benefit in reducing inflammation associated with gout.

BOSWELLIA SERRATA (BOSWELLIA)

Leukotrienes are eicosanoid inflammatory mediators derived from arachidonic acid via lipoxygenase enzyme[227] that have been found to contribute to inflammation in the body. Elevated levels of leukotrienes have been identified in the tissues or exudates of those with gout[227,228] and have been suggested to exist in significantly greater quantities than is found in the synovial fluid of patients with rheumatoid arthritis or osteoarthritis,[229] revealing the extent of their activity. *Boswellia serrata* is a well-known inhibitor of pro-inflammatory mediators in the body, including leukotrienes, via inhibition of 5-lipoxygenase.[230,231] This inhibition appears to be the mechanism by which *Boswellia serrata* exerts its anti-inflammatory and anti-arthritic activity and provides a rationale for its use in gout and other disorders characterised by inflammation.

CURCUMA LONGA (TURMERIC)

Curcumin is the most abundant polyphenol in *Curcuma longa* and has been identified to have a range of actions that may be useful in gout, including antioxidant and anti-inflammatory[232] activity. Curcumin has also been shown to inhibit xanthine dehydrogenase/oxidase,[233] the enzyme that converts xanthine to uric acid and promotes oxidation in the body, further heightening the benefits for its application in gout. As yet there has been little in the way of human clinical trials assessing the efficacy of curcumin in human musculoskeletal system conditions.

GUAIACUM OFFICINALE (GUAIACUM)

The resin or wood of *Guaiacum officinale* has been employed medicinally for the management of gout for hundreds of years. Murrell[234] documents its use for the management of 'chronic gouty affections' as early as the late 1800s and this application is further confirmed by Grieve,[225] who writes of its ability in helping to relieve pain and inflammation associated with gout not only during but also between attacks, suggesting a prophylactic action. The action of *Guaiacum officinalis* appears to be multifaceted: when consumed warm as a decoction, it acted as an 'acrid stimulant, increasing heat of body and circulation', but when taken cool, it functioned as a diuretic. Both actions are seemingly useful in gout to eliminate toxic matter from the body.

HARPAGOPHYTUM PROCUMBENS (DEVIL'S CLAW)

Harpagophytum procumbens displays significant anti-inflammatory[235] and analgesic activity, highlighting its use for pain and inflammation associated with gout. The efficacy of oral *Harpagophytum procumbens* was investigated in one study involving a small group of patients with gout or rheumatic pain given 1230 mg/day dried root extract versus a second group who were given phenylbutazone for just under a month.[236] *Harpagophytum procumbens* was found to be more efficacious than phenylbutazone for management of gout and rheumatic pain, with significantly fewer side effects. Acknowledging the latter, more clinical trials are welcomed to further confirm the benefits of *Harpagophytum procumbens* in gout.

JUNIPERUS COMMUNIS (JUNIPER)

Traditional use of *Juniperus communis* berries for the treatment of gout can be traced back as far as 1590 to one of the most important herbals of the 16th and 17th century, the book of Matthiolus which suggests the consumption of juniper berries cooked in wine to rid oneself of gout, as well as the application of juniper oil to affected joints to ease pain and irritation.[197] The sixteenth-century physician Leonhart Fuchs, described as one of the original fathers of botany, also suggests *Juniper communis* for the management of gout, advocating the internal consumption of whole juniper berries to 'expel slime' associated with gout.[197] In modern medicine no clinical trials could be found examining the therapeutic use of *Juniperus communis* in gout.

SALIX SPP. (WILLOW BARK)

The *Salix* species have been a popular remedy treatment of gout for centuries. Records of its use can be found in at least five of the most important herbal books of the 16th and 17th centuries. Its bark and leaves were cooked in water and soaked in rags that were then applied to affected gouty joints.[197]

In modern-day medicine, *Salix* spp. have been studied and have been shown to exhibit anti-inflammatory and analgesic activities in musculoskeletal disorders such as osteoarthritis and back pain.[237] While there have been no clinical trials examining the efficacy of willow bark in gout, its therapeutic activity in other musculoskeletal conditions provides a rationale for its use in gout.

TARAXACUM OFFICINALE FOLIA (DANDELION LEAF)

Taraxacum officinale was traditionally used for the management of gout.[238] It contains sesquiterpene lactones that are thought to exert both anti-inflammatory[238] and diuretic[238,239] actions likely to be useful in the resolution of gout symptoms. It is the leaf of *Taraxacum officinale* rather than the root that is most useful in gout because of its diuretic action. In a recent pilot study,[240] intake of an ethanolic extract of dandelion leaf significantly increased urinary frequency and excretion in human participants. Although there are no studies pertaining specifically to gout, one can hypothesise that this fast-acting, diuretic effect of *Taraxacum officinale* folia would increase urinary output of uric acid and would thus be beneficial in gout.

URTICA URENS/DIOICA SPP. (NETTLE)

Urtica spp. were traditionally applied externally to help relieve gout, particularly that affecting the feet.[197] *Urtica dioica* has been suggested to exert a specific analgesic[241] action in those with joint pain and is also often used as a depurative/alterative. Nettle is also a diuretic and is thus likely to be useful in increasing the urinary output of uric acid.

ZANTHOXYLUM CLAVA-HERCULIS (PRICKLY ASH)

Zanthoxylum clava-herculis is a gentle circulatory stimulant, useful where there is sluggish circulation.[138] It may be used as an adjuvant for the treatment of gout due to its ability to stimulate blood flow and nutrition as well as the movement of toxins as a result of its alterative action.[198] The Eclectics report of its use in rheumatism, where it was teamed with colchicum (used for gout).[198]

ZINGIBER OFFICINALE (GINGER)

Recent studies have confirmed the knowledge of the Eclectics with a constituent found within *Zingiber officinale* shown to inhibit urate-induced crystal formation. This constituent is 6-shogaol, which has been found to exhibit a number of actions that would be useful in the management of gout, including anti-inflammatory and analgesic activities.[242] In a study involving mice injected with urate crystals into their joints, following administration with 6-shogaol, reductions in paw volume, lysosomal enzymes, lipid peroxidation and pro-inflammatory cytokine TNF-α were observed.[243] The authors suggest that 6-shogaol can be regarded as a useful tool for the treatment of acute gouty arthritis.

LIFESTYLE RECOMMENDATIONS

Cold applications

Local ice therapy may be useful as an adjuvant therapy during attacks of gout by reducing pain.[244,245]

Exercise and a healthy lifestyle

There is a reduced risk of gout in men who are more physically active, maintain ideal body weight, consume diets rich in fruit and limit meat and alcohol.[246] Lower BMI is also associated with reduced risk of comorbidities associated with gout, such as metabolic syndrome.

Stress management

Stress management techniques and time outs are highly suggested in inflammatory conditions. Time outs can provide brief pain relief and should be practised daily.

CASE STUDY

OVERVIEW

SR is a 32-year-old male presenting with gout. He is a very busy executive of a young company and works long hours to maintain its success. There is a lot of pressure to keep the company performing as it is a unique enterprise with businesses overseas copying his successful business program. He had been suffering from gout for the past year. He first noticed the pain in his right toe after a busy week 3 months earlier; it was made worse by the bed sheets or when he wore tighter socks. He describes the pain as sharp and like 'acid crystals' digging in. When there is an attack, he has to have his foot outside the bed and wear loose socks. Sometimes he has to apply ice for 15 minutes to help reduce pain.

His energy levels range from 5/10 weekdays to 7–8/10 on weekends. He sleeps 5–6 hours per night and wakes relatively refreshed. Throughout the day he gets tight neck and shoulder muscles.

PAST HISTORY

Generally, he has been well. His childhood was healthy. He has a good immune system where he might get 1 cold per year that he gets over very quickly.

DIET

- Red meat: 6 nights a week (steak for dinner Sunday to Friday). Every second Wednesday he has a steak lunch meeting
- White meat: 6 days a week (Monday to Saturday for lunch), e.g. chicken and turkey with tomato, capsicum and cheese
- Fish: once a month
- Sweets: Strong sugar cravings. Most days he will consume a piece of cake with cream
- Dairy products: high consumption of cheese (with most meals), milk, ice-cream and cream
- Vegetables: peas, corn, carrots, adds tomato-based sauces to his steaks
- Fruit: 1–2 apples per week
- Alcohol: 2–3 beers most nights (helps him to relax)
- Water: 500 mL/day
- Coffee: Averages 5 per day

CLINICAL EXAMINATION

Blood pressure 150/98 mmHg
Pulse 86 BPM

CASE STUDY CONTINUED

Weight 1.70 m
Height 82 kg
BMI 28.37 kg/m^2
Face: red and dry, vertical line between the eyebrows
Eyes: stye in the left eye. This occurs 5–6 times per year and can last 1–2 weeks
Tongue: scalloping and a mild quiver
Nails: vertical ridging, redness around the nails.

TREATMENT PROTOCOL

HERBAL MEDICINE

Herbal medicine	Extract	Quantity	Justification
Curcuma longa	1:2	60 mL	Antioxidant, anti-inflammatory
Withania somnifera	2:1	50 mL	Adaptogen, nervine
Apium gravelolens	1:2	40 mL	To reduce uric acid and alkalise the body fluids
Taraxacum officinale root	1:1	60 mL	Hepatic, digestive tonic
Zingiber officinale	1:5	10 mL	Anti-inflammatory activity, circulatory stimulant — aid in transport of active constituents to target organs
TOTAL		220 mL	

Dose: 7.5 mL b.i.d. in water.

NUTRITIONAL MEDICINE

Dietary

The diet was reviewed for nutritional deficiencies, food allergies and intolerances. Recommendations included:

- Investigate and correct any nutritional deficiencies
- Encourage vegetarian sources of protein
- Avoid animal-derived protein sources except low-fat dairy products (minimal)
- Encourage fresh fruit and vegetable consumption — especially cherries
- Increase water intake (minimum 30 mL/kg body weight per day)
- 30 mL of sour cherry juice in a glass of water once daily
- Maintain balanced blood sugar levels (chromium, magnesium, zinc)
- Reduce sugar, caffeine and refined carbohydrates
- Avoid alcohol and soft drinks
- Avoid caffeinated beverages in all forms
- Avoid saturated and trans fatty acids
- Reduce/avoid pro-inflammatory foods or any identified food allergens and intolerance.

CASE STUDY CONTINUED

Supplemental

- Bromelain 200–400 mg 2–3 times daily between meals
- Quercetin 400–500 mg 2–3 times daily between meals
- Zinc 25 mg b.i.d.
- High-potency omega-3: EPA 600 mg and DHA 200 mg t.d.s.
- Glucosamine 1500 mg/day and chondroitin 500–750 mg/day
- Green-lipped mussel 500 mg b.i.d.
- B complex (all B vitamins) high-dose combination, in activated forms: 1 capsule with breakfast and 1 capsule with lunch
- Taurine 1000 mg in water b.i.d.
- Inositol 1000 mg in water b.i.d.

LIFESTYLE/EDUCATION

- Weight management was encouraged with education regarding optimal lifestyle and exercise changes to encourage reaching and maintaining healthy weight range.
- A daily walk of 15–20 minutes was encouraged during the day to 'clear the mind'.
- Stress management and relaxation exercises were suggested.
- A time out of 15 minutes was suggested every morning before work and in afternoon to reduce stress levels.

FOLLOW-UP

Mild improvement in pain was noted after 2 weeks. After 4 weeks, there was further reduction in pain. His energy on weekdays improved from 5/10 to 6–7/10 and improved on weekends from 7–8/10 to 8/10. He now sleeps 6 hours per night and wakes more refreshed. Throughout the day he still gets tight neck and shoulder muscles but not to the same extent.

FIBROMYALGIA

Epidemiology

Fibromyalgia is a multifaceted condition and presents with a variety of symptoms (Fig. 15.6). It occurs considerably more frequently in women, with a female to male ratio of 9:1 observed.[247] Fibromyalgia most commonly presents between the ages of 20 to 50 years, increasing in severity with age until around 70 years when symptoms start to reduce.[248] A 2009 review by Spaeth[249] suggests that fibromyalgia affects approximately 2–3% of the general population; however, others have suggested an even higher incidence, estimating that the condition may affect between 2 and 13% of the population.[179] In a survey undertaken involving five European countries, 4.7% of the population was found to be affected by fibromyalgia,[250]

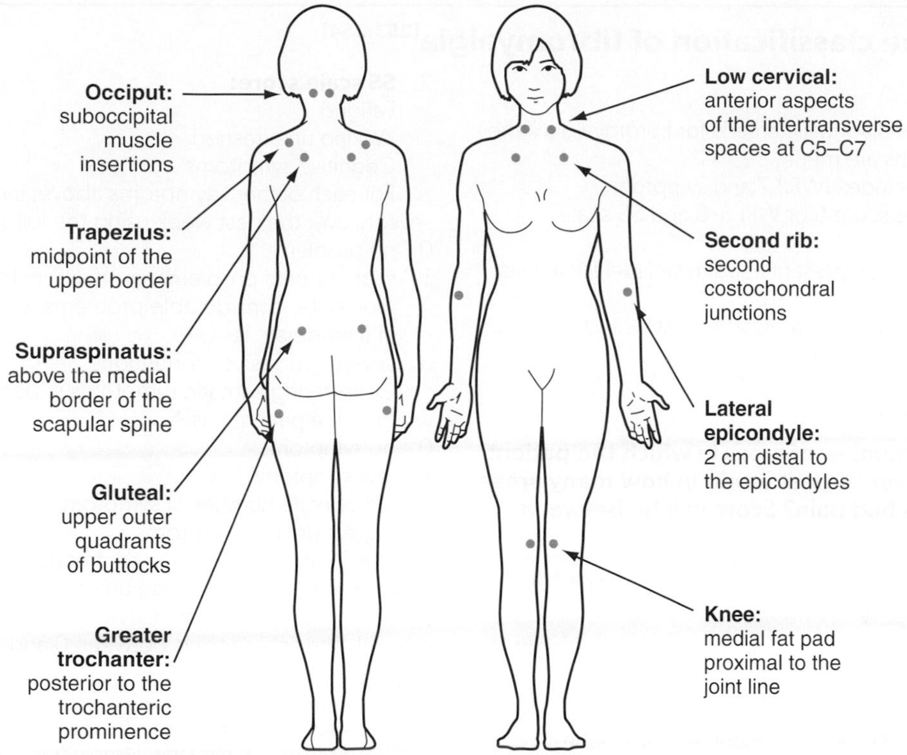

FIGURE 15.6 Fibromyalgia.

Rakel RE. Textbook of family medicine. 7th edn. Saunders: 2007.

and slightly higher figures were observed for women in an American survey (5%),[251] leading to speculation that the incidence of fibromyalgia may be increasing.

Classification

Classification of fibromyalgia is based upon the criteria proposed by the American College of Rheumatology 2010 (below). While these criteria have been criticised and suggested as less than ideal for individual patient diagnosis,[252] as yet no other universal means of classification has been decided upon.

Aetiology

A number of different mechanisms have been proposed as to the aetiology of fibromyalgia. As yet, why fibromyalgia occurs remains a mystery and from the variety of symptoms that present in clinic one could hypothesise there actually may not be one single causative factor.

CENTRAL NERVOUS SYSTEM ABNORMALITIES

Central nervous system dysfunction is a key feature in fibromyalgia,[255] in which the spinal and cerebral cortex's ability to process pain becomes altered. In response to chronic pain the brain becomes 'rewired' and small amounts of pain begin to present as large amounts of pain when in fact it is the same identical repeated painful stimulation. This is termed 'central sensitisation' and describes the overreaction/exaggeration of the central nervous system to pain (hyperalgesia).[256]

ALTERED NEUROTRANSMITTERS

Alterations in the serotonergic system of patients with fibromyalgia have been observed[257] as have lower levels of serotonin in the body. These are likely to contribute to the depressed mood and pain so frequently seen in fibromyalgia patients, as serotonin promotes natural opiate pain control.[258] Disruptions in dopamine D_2 receptor function[259] and decreased quantities of dopamine have also been observed in patients with fibromyalgia.[260] Dopamine is known to play a key role in perception of pain and modulation of analgesia within the body and thus its deficiency can be hypothesised to contribute to the pain and decreased wellbeing experienced in fibromyalgia.

DYSREGULATION OF THE HYPOTHALAMIC–PITUITARY–ADRENAL AXIS

Alterations in the hypothalamic–pituitary–adrenal (HPA) axis are known to exist in patients with fibromyalgia and have been suggested to contribute to many of the symptoms experienced.[261] Currently, it is unclear whether HPA dysfunction precedes fibromyalgia or if fibromyalgia occurs as a result of altered HPA axis activity.

Criteria for the classification of fibromyalgia[253,254]

CRITERIA

A patient satisfies diagnostic criteria for fibromyalgia if the following 3 conditions are met:

1. Widespread pain index (WPI) 7 and symptom severity (SS) scale score 5 or WPI 3–6 and SS scale score 9.
2. Symptoms have been present at a similar level for at least 3 months
3. The patient does not have a disorder that would otherwise explain the pain.

ASCERTAINMENT

1. **WPI: note the number of areas in which the patient has had pain over the last week. In how many areas has the patient had pain? Score will be between 0 and 19.**

Neck	Upper arm, left	Hip (buttock, trochanter), left	Jaw, left
Upper back	Upper arm, right	Hip (buttock, trochanter), right	Jaw, right
Lower back	Lower arm, left	Upper leg, left	Chest
Shoulder girdle, left	Lower arm, right	Upper leg, right	Abdomen
Shoulder girdle, right		Lower leg, left	
		Lower leg, right	

2. **SS scale score:**
   Fatigue
   Waking unrefreshed
   Cognitive symptoms

For each of the 3 symptoms above, indicate the level of severity over the past week using the following scale:

0 no problem
1 slight or mild problems, generally mild or intermittent
2 moderate, considerable problems, often present and/or at a moderate level
3 severe: pervasive, continuous, life-disturbing problems

Considering somatic symptoms in general, indicate whether the patient has:*

0 no symptoms
1 few symptoms
2 a moderate number of symptoms
3 a great deal of symptoms

The SS scale score is the sum of the severity of the 3 symptoms (fatigue, waking unrefreshed, cognitive symptoms) plus the extent (severity) of somatic symptoms in general. The final score is between 0 and 12.

*Somatic symptoms that might be considered: muscle pain, irritable bowel syndrome, fatigue/tiredness, thinking or remembering problem, muscle weakness, headache, pain/cramps in the abdomen, numbness/tingling, dizziness, insomnia, depression, constipation, pain in the upper abdomen, nausea, nervousness, chest pain, blurred vision, fever, diarrhoea, dry mouth, itching, wheezing, Raynaud's phenomenon, hives/welts, ringing in ears, vomiting, heartburn, oral ulcers, loss of/change in taste, seizures, dry eyes, shortness of breath, loss of appetite, rash, sun sensitivity, hearing difficulties, easy bruising, hair loss, frequent urination, painful urination and bladder spasms.

IMMUNE DYSREGULATION

Immune dysregulation has been identified in fibromyalgia though why it occurs is unclear. Disruption of the HPA axis and alterations in the sympathetic nervous system[262] and even vaccination[263] have been proposed as being involved.

INFECTION

Goldenberg[264,265] conducted a number of surveys to assess the possibility of fibromyalgia occurring as a result of underlying chronic viral infection. Patients were asked if they remembered or believed that any event preceded the onset of fibromyalgia. It was found that viral illness, such as upper respiratory tract symptoms, featured in 10% of cases. Results in a second survey were more significant with 55% of participants noting their illness began with a viral syndrome or an upper respiratory tract infection. Further studies have suggested that a number of infective agents may be involved in the development of fibromyalgia/fibromyalgia symptoms. These include the hepatitis B[266] and C[267] viruses, HIV[268] and mycoplasma, but as yet no single infectious agent has been identified.[263] As such, it is imperative that a thorough screening is conducted on any patient suspected of or diagnosed as having fibromyalgia.

GENDER/HORMONES

Fibromyalgia affects significantly more women than men and thus gender and the sex hormones have been suggested to play a part in the pathophysiology. Pamuk and Cakir[269] observed a positive relationship between the menstrual cycle and onset of menopause in influencing pain and the severity of other fibromyalgia-related symptoms, but in contrast Okifuji and Turk[270] found no relationship between the sex hormones and pain in regularly menstruating women with fibromyalgia syndrome.

THYROID FUNCTION

Considerable evidence indicates that inadequate thyroid hormone regulation due to hypothyroidism or cellular resistance to thyroid hormone is the underlying mechanism of the two main features of fibromyalgia: chronic widespread pain and abnormal tenderness.

GENES/FAMILIAL TENDENCY

Fibromyalgia displays a familial trend, as shown in the study conducted by Arnold et al[271] who observed that first-degree relatives of people with fibromyalgia had an eightfold risk of also developing fibromyalgia. Symptoms associated with fibromyalgia were also observed to have a genetic background in the Finnish Twin Cohort study,[272] strengthening the argument of those who have suggested that there may be genetic polymorphism involvement in the pathophysiology of fibromyalgia.

STRESS

Not surprisingly, stress (physical, psychological or physiological) has been suggested to play a causative role in the pathogenesis of fibromyalgia. Onset of fibromyalgia has been observed to follow a stressful or traumatic event (Box 15.1).[273]

SUBSTANCE P

Substance P is an amino acid involved in the transmission of pain from the periphery to the central nervous system. It has been suggested to be a biological marker of chronic pain states.[274] Elevated quantities of substance P have been observed in the cerebrospinal fluid of people with fibromyalgia, sometimes as much as three times the normal amount.[275]

Overview

Fibromyalgia is a pattern of symptoms culminating with neurogenic pain dysfunction.

Pathogenesis

SIGNS AND SYMPTOMS

The cardinal symptoms of fibromyalgia have been described as chronic widespread pain and tenderness on multiple soft-tissue sites of the body.[276] A plethora of other symptoms, however, also commonly present, including anxiety, depression, disturbed sleep, chronic fatigue, irritable bowel syndrome, headaches, poor memory, concentration problems/cognitive dysfunction, tingling, numbness and premenstrual syndrome.[277] Other less specific symptoms include stiffness, coldness, sicca symptoms, exercise intolerance and dysmenorrhoea.

The associated symptoms and conditions of fibromyalgia are described in Fig. 15.7.[252]

BOX 15.1 Stressors capable of triggering fibromyalgia and related conditions

- Peripheral pain syndromes
- Infections (e.g. parvovirus, Epstein-Barr virus, Lyme disease, Q fever)
- Physical trauma (e.g. motor vehicle accidents)
- Psychological stress/distress
- Hormonal alterations (e.g. hypothyroidism)
- Drugs
- Vaccines
- Certain catastrophic events (war, but not natural disasters)

Source: Clauw D. Fibromyalgia: an overview. Am J Med 2009; 122(12, Suppl. 1):S3–S13.

COMPLICATIONS

Physically, fibromyalgia is unlikely to result in any life-threatening complications, but it is acknowledged that it is a disabling, painful condition that impacts greatly on a person's quality of life. Results from a focus study of female patients with fibromyalgia revealed that many women felt socially isolated and that their condition disrupted relationships with family and friends.[277] Because of their symptoms the women experienced a reduction in their ability to go about their activities of daily living and were less able to participate in leisure or physical activities because of unpredictable and fluctuating symptoms. Many reported a loss of their career or inability to progress in careers or education.

Goldenberg[252] notes that patients with fibromyalgia who are led to believe their condition is associated with trauma and similar conditions are more likely to assume a sick role and as such this is understandable. Instead of taking this approach he emphasises the importance of reassuring the patient and educating them on their condition and what they can do to ease symptoms and benefit themselves. He cites the example of White et al[278] who observed that patients with fibromyalgia experienced a reduction in symptoms and significant health improvements after a diagnosis of fibromyalgia. The way we present a diagnosis of a condition to a client and the subsequent treatment plan is thus an important consideration in naturopathic clinical practice and may influence the outcome.

DIFFERENTIAL DIAGNOSIS

Differential diagnosis of fibromyalgia is not straightforward because of the multitude of symptoms that present as well as their presence in many other conditions. In addition, while fibromyalgia is a condition in its own right, it may also overlap with other conditions. Taking this into account, it is imperative that a thorough naturopathic case history and physical examination is taken.

The differential diagnosis of fibromyalgia includes a number of conditions, including viral infections, osteoporosis, rheumatoid arthritis, systemic lupus erythematosus, polymyalgia rheumatica, myositis myopathies, ankylosing spondylitis, neuropathies, chronic fatigue syndrome and myofascial pain syndrome (Table 15.11). Differential diagnosis must also include hypothyroidism and malignancies, both of which may also mimic fibromyalgia.[248]

NATUROPATHIC DIAGNOSIS

Naturopathic diagnosis considers all aetiological aspects and aims to define the causative agent/s or promoters of

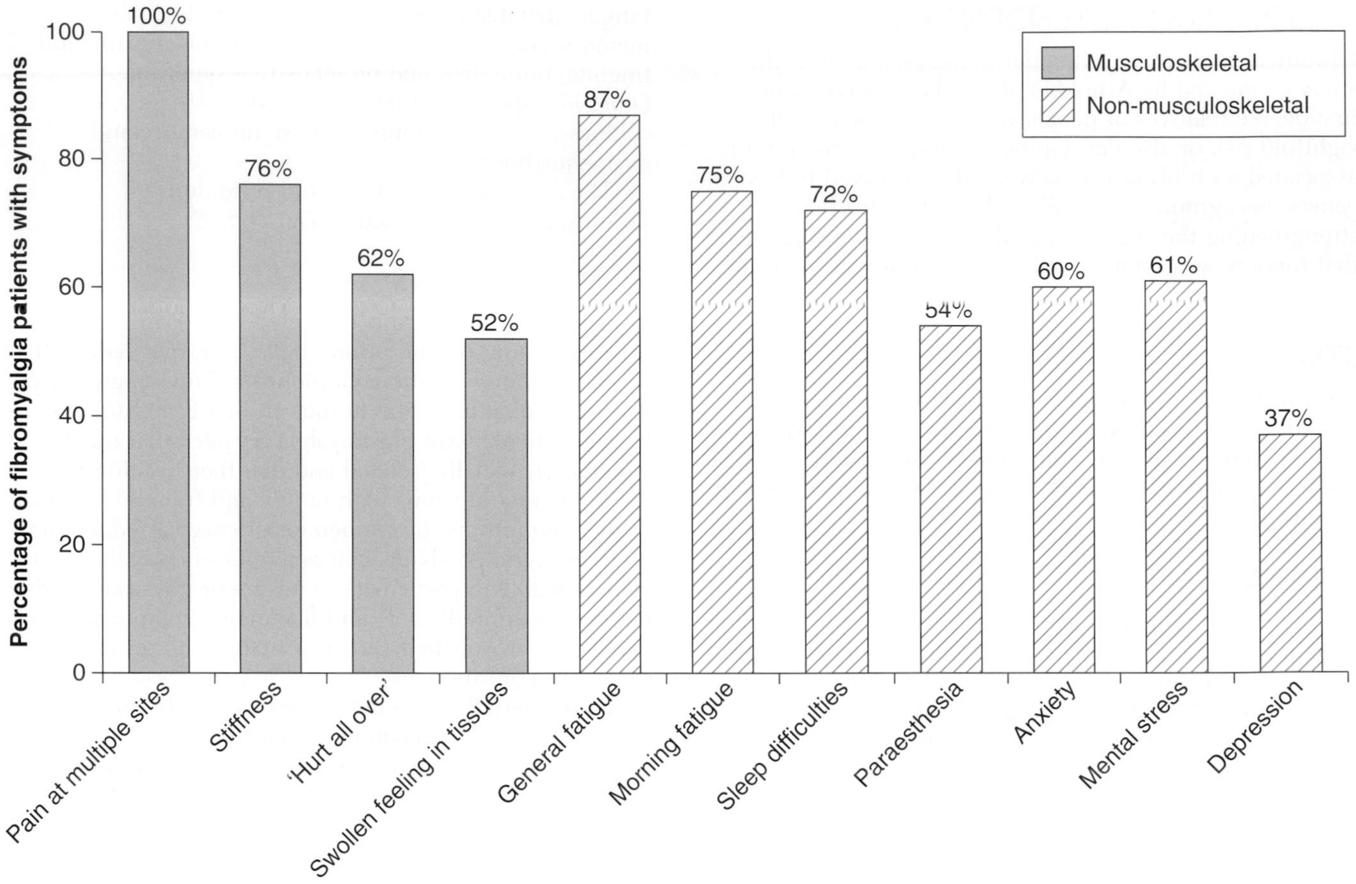

FIGURE 15.7 Associated symptoms and conditions of fibromyalgia.

Goldenberg D. Diagnosis and differential diagnosis of fibromyalgia. Am J Med 2009; 122(12):Suppl 1: S14–S21.

the condition. While medical diagnosis is incorporated, naturopathic diagnosis considers a wider scenario, paramount for holistic review and assessment. Because chronic fatigue syndrome is considered a diagnosis of exclusion, the naturopathic framework reviews the diagnosis of fibromyalgia as limiting. However, the criteria proposed by the American College of Rheumatology sheds light on the diagnosis of fibromyalgia. This is especially because of the multifaceted nature of the disease presentation. Thorough investigation is essential for the diagnosis in order to accurately ascertain a full picture of the patient's health.

Investigations

THOROUGH INVESTIGATIONS

Although there is no specific marker for fibromyalgia, essential investigations include a number of assessments to eliminate contributing factors or other conditions, including:[276]

- Full blood count (FBC)
- Electrolytes, urea, creatinine (EUC)
- Liver function test (LFT)
- Erythrocyte sedimentation rate (ESR)
- C-reactive protein (CRP)
- Thyroid-stimulating hormone (TSH) (±fT3, fT4)
- Reverse T3
- Thyroid antibodies (and antinuclear antibodies)
- Coeliac profile
- Iron studies
- Red cell magnesium
- Red cell or plasma zinc
- Serum copper
- Vitamin D
- Serum calcium
- MTHFR (C677T and A1298C)
- Parathyroid hormone (PTH)
- Rheumatoid factor (RF)
- Epstein-Barr virus (EBV)
- Cytomegalovirus (CMV)
- HIV
- *Mycoplasma, Chlamydia* and *Borrelia* DNA PCR
- Fasting glucose, insulin
- 24-hour urinary cortisol
- Reproductive hormone assessment (as indicated).

Examination of tender points, both through palpation and patient involvement, is an essential component of a thorough investigation.

TABLE 15.11 Differential diagnosis of fibromyalgia

Condition	Distinguishing feature from fibromyalgia
Rheumatoid arthritis	Joint swelling, deformities, elevated ESR, CRP
Systemic lupus erythematosus	Rash, multisystemic inflammation, elevated ESR, ANA
Polymyalgia rheumatica	Age ≥60 years, severe stiffness when inactive, elevated ESR
Myositis, myopathies	Weakness, elevated muscle enzymes
Ankylosing spondylitis	Back, neck immobility, elevated ESR, abnormal x-rays
Hypothyroidism	Abnormal thyroid function assessments
Neuropathies	Weakness, loss of sensation, abnormal EMG, NCV
Myofascial pain syndrome	Abrupt onset, pain is characteristically regional
Chronic fatigue syndrome	Conditions can overlap and are frequently misdiagnosed in both aspects. It is imperative to organise a thorough assessment to eliminate other contributing factors. CFS is a diagnosis of exclusion and typically does not present with the extent of trigger point tenderness. Other signs and symptoms are similar

ANA, antinuclear antibodies; CFS, chronic fatigue syndrome; CRP, C-reactive protein; EMG, electromyography; ESR, erythrocyte sedimentation rate; NCV, nerve conduction velocity.
Adapted from: Adams N, Sim J. An overview of fibromyalgia syndrome: mechanisms, differential diagnosis and treatment approaches. Physiotherapy 1998; 84(7):304–318. Goldenberg D. Diagnosis and differential diagnosis of fibromyalgia. Am J Med 2009; 122(12, Suppl. 1):S14–S21.

SPECIFIC NATUROPATHIC INVESTIGATIONS

Fibromyalgia Impact Questionnaire (FIQ)

The Fibromyalgia Impact Questionnaire is a useful tool to evaluate the overall symptomatology of fibromyalgia. (See Appendix 15.1 later in the book for the full questionnaire.)

Functional assessments

ADRENAL HORMONE PROFILE

This monitors the level of the stress hormones cortisol and DHEA-S. Altered cortisol is seen in fibromyalgia and may influence symptoms such as fatigue.

FOOD PROFILE TABLE/FOOD SENSITIVITY

This profiles common foods that the patient may be sensitive to. A number of food sensitivities have been shown to exacerbate fibromyalgia symptoms.[279] Once the food sensitivities or intolerances have been identified they are to be eliminated from the diet. Retesting is suggested for food sensitivities to investigate other potential sensitivities that may have been previously masked.

Therapeutic considerations

CLINICAL DECISION MAKING AND RATIONALE[252]

Summarised in Fig. 15.8.

History taking

Capturing the symptoms in a time-efficient manner:

- Symptom survey questionnaire
- Patient-generated lists of symptoms experienced (to be handed to practitioner)
- Associated dysfunction: sleep, irritable bowel, irritable bladder, depression
- Contextual information
- Comorbidities.

Physical examination

Screening musculoskeletal examination:

- Range of movement and swelling
- Tender points (see Fig. 15.9 for appropriate tender points examination)
- General check-up.

Management

The explanation: physiological; informative analogies.

Positive messages

- Not organ- or life-threatening
- Lifestyle adjustments
- Aerobic fitness
- Leisure activities
- Diet
- Caffeinated and sugar-sweetened beverages
- Self-management courses
- Support groups
- Improve sleep hygiene
- Interpretation of investigations.

Treatment

- Pain relief
- Symptomatic management
- Neurotransmitter support
- HPA axis support.
- Potential referral to psychologist.

Attention to comorbidities

- Assess and consider comorbidities.

Less used formal interventions

- Psychotherapy
- Cognitive behavioural therapy.

Therapeutic application

HISTORICAL PERSPECTIVE

Fibromyalgia is a relatively new term, first used in the early 1970s,[280] so it should come as no surprise that there is no mention of it in the texts of the Eclectics. In saying

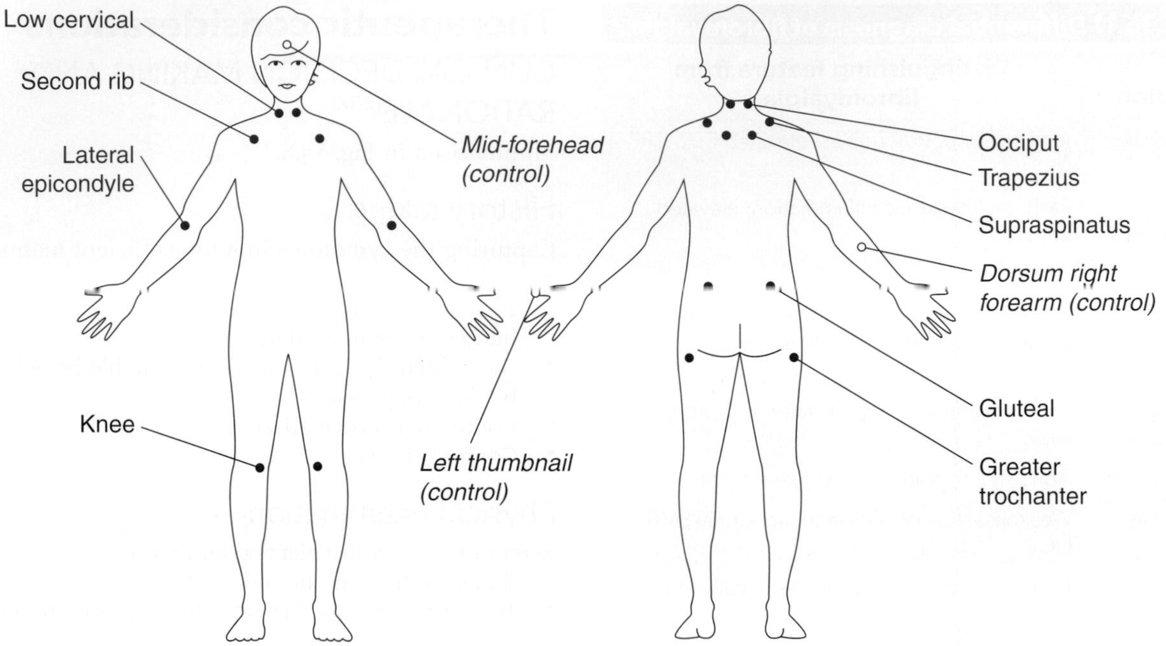

FIGURE 15.8 Symptoms and conditions for fibromyalgia.

Goldenberg D. Diagnosis and differential diagnosis of fibromyalgia. Am J Med 2009; 122(12):Suppl 1: S14–S21.

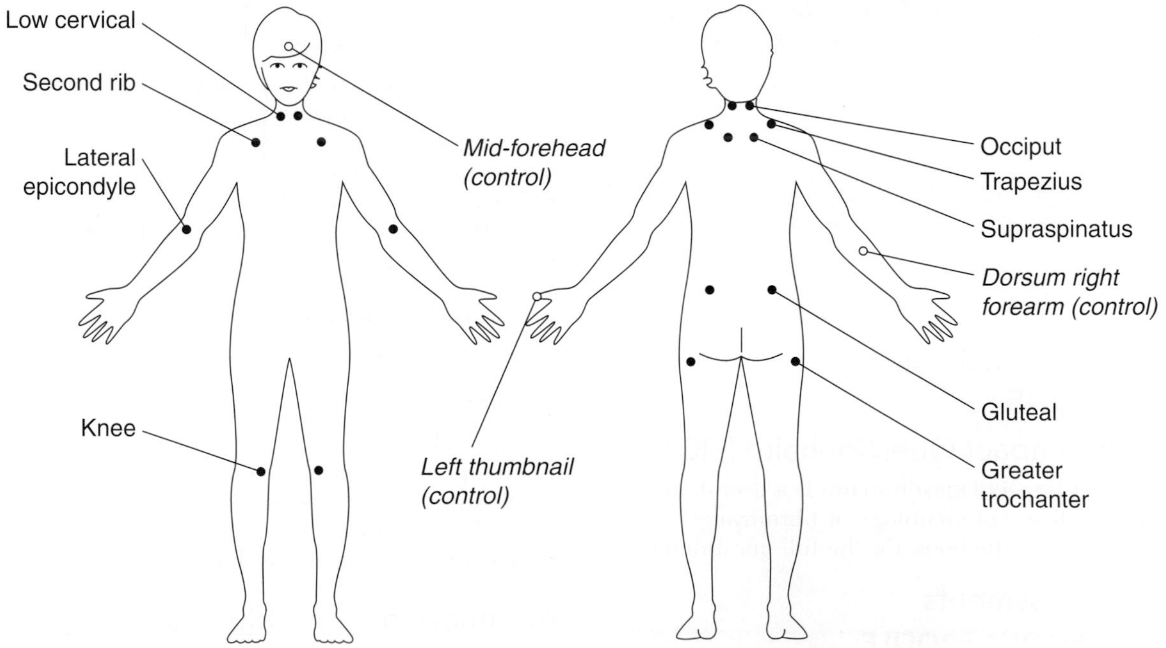

FIGURE 15.9 Tender points examination.

Goldenberg D. Diagnosis and differential diagnosis of fibromyalgia. Am J Med 2009; 122(12):Suppl 1: S14–S21.

this, while fibromyalgia is a new term it does not necessarily appear to be a new condition. Mention of other conditions with very similar symptoms can be traced back to at least 1592 to French physician Guillaume de Baillou, who is famous for the initial terminology of muscular rheumatism.[280] By the early 1800s descriptions of rheumatism had become more clearly defined, with articular rheumatism and muscular rheumatism separated into two very different conditions. Articular rheumatism was classified as a deforming rheumatism (such as osteoarthritis), while muscular rheumatism was known as a non-deforming soft-tissue disorder (such as fibromyalgia). The description of muscular rheumatism that can be found in the Eclectic texts is likely to be a collective reference to fibromyalgia. Thomas[199] describes 'myalgia/muscular rheumatism' as a 'painful affection of the muscles and their attachments, the fasciae and periosteum', a description seemingly characteristic of fibromyalgia.

For the treatment of muscular rheumatism (aka fibromyalgia) the Eclectics prescribed the internal use of cimicifuga for its effects upon the muscular system and gelsenium for its action upon the nerves and elimination channels.[12] In line with present-day research, the Eclectics suggested a vegetarian diet with ample fresh water and optimal elimination.

NATUROPATHIC PERSPECTIVE

The pain of fibromyalgia can be explained as a biological warning system that alerts a person to conditions that are threatening to the integrity of their tissues. Pain is normally felt when neural receptors in tissues have become sensitised by inflammation during the healing process. The pain system can become dysfunctional, however, as a warning either through lack of responsiveness, as seen when nerves are damaged by physical trauma or disease, or through inappropriate hyperresponsiveness, as seen in fibromyalgia. In the latter situation, pain is experienced under conditions of mundane stretch and pressure that offer no threat to the tissues and in the absence of the factors operating in other conditions.

Fibromyalgia can be likened to an alarm that has become oversensitive and is generating its unpleasant signal/s under conditions that offer no threat. The warning is unpleasant but offers no useful information. If the alarm cannot be fixed simply or replaced, as is the case in fibromyalgia, one must examine ways of muting its warning and becoming less distracted by its unpleasant and unwanted presence.

The patient should be reassured that the problem, while difficult to resolve entirely, is neither organ-threatening nor life-threatening. Within the above interpretative framework of pain dysfunction, a reduction in situational stresses that are personally and therefore physiologically challenging can be advocated, to the extent that this is possible. Improving general health through increased general fitness, recreational exercise and leisure activities can also foster a more comfortable equilibrium. Exercise prescriptions should be directed towards aerobic fitness and should be encouraged in spite of moderate fatigue. A social dimension to exercise can have a positive effect upon participation and continuation. Attention to diet and avoidance of excess caffeine may be helpful. Mutual support from those similarly affected can have a positive effect.[281]

NUTRITIONAL MEDICINE (DIETARY)

Dietary therapeutic objectives

- Investigate and correct any nutritional deficiencies
- Avoid caffeine in any form — coffee, tea, cola, chocolate, energy drinks and supplements containing caffeine (e.g. weight loss formulas, energy supplements)
- Avoid glutamate-containing foods, such as MSG
- Avoid aspartate-containing foods, such as aspartame and other artificial sweeteners
- Reduce foods high in salt and abstain from adding salt to cooking
- Avoid foods which have been proven to produce an IgG or IgE response in the body
- Encourage general wholefood principles
- Encourage adequate hydration (e.g. 30 mL per kg body weight).

Specific dietary treatments

DIETARY INCLUSIONS

Antioxidants

A number of small studies have suggested that a diet that is rich in plant antioxidants may reduce symptoms associated with fibromyalgia.[282–284] These types of foods primarily reflect a vegan/vegetarian diet based upon raw foods made up largely of such things as berries, fruits, vegetables, salads, grains, roots, barley grass, nuts and germinated seeds and sprouts. A diet such as this is typically rich in anti-inflammatory and health-promoting constituents such as quercetin, beta-carotene, lignans, vitamins C and E and lycopene, and omits coffee, tea and salt. In general terms it is comparable to a naturopathic detoxification diet. Patients following these types of diet have experienced positive results, with patients in one study reporting perceived improvement in their health as well as a reduction in joint stiffness and pain, highlighting the profound role that diet can play in fibromyalgia.[282]

It is worth noting, however, that following completion of these studies, all patients resumed their former omnivorous diet. This highlights the difficulties faced by patients with regards to compliance and motivation when undertaking a therapeutic diet. It also highlights the need for proper education on the benefits of such a diet and the constant support and motivation that must be conveyed by the practitioner to the patient. Given the difficulty faced by patients to continue this type of diet, a diet based upon fresh, whole foods[179] with moderate amounts of good-quality protein and essential fatty acids and one that is devoid of symptom triggers (discussed below) should suffice.

DIETARY EXCLUSIONS

Potential dietary links to central sensitisation and fibromyalgia have been suggested.[285] In particular, glutamate, aspartate and substance P are thought to enhance transmission of pain signals in patients with fibromyalgia,[285,286] so excessive intake of foods containing glutamates and aspartates should be reduced or avoided. These foods may include many items that commonly feature in the average person's diet, including MSG (a source of glutamate), soft drinks containing aspartame (a source of aspartate), food colouring, chocolate, cow's milk, caffeine and shellfish.[279]

NUTRITIONAL MEDICINE (SUPPLEMENTAL)

Nutritional medicine therapeutic objectives

- Investigate and correct nutritional deficiencies
- Support neurochemistry to alleviate symptoms and address deranged pain pathways

SAMPLE DAILY DIET

BREAKFAST	
Chia porridge with fresh seasonal fruit	A wholefood diet[287] is advocated. This ensures removal of excitotoxins/additives in particular glutamates, aspartame and altered proteins (like gelatin, hydrolysed isolates). The latter compounds appear to have a 'pro-algesic' action and removal is suggested to be beneficial in reducing pain associated with fibromyalgia.
LUNCH	
Zucchini pasta with brown lentils and a rocket, spinach and cashew pesto	Magnesium is found in leafy greens and nuts while zinc is found in nuts and legumes. Low zinc and magnesium may support excitotoxicity thus the diet should contain foods that provide optimal levels of both nutrients. A raw vegan diet is associated with reduced pain and joint stiffness.
DINNER	
Ginger and pumpkin dhal	Non-coeliac gluten sensitivity may be an underlying cause of fibromyalgia syndrome thus a gluten-free diet is advocated. Anti-inflammatory spices such as ginger and turmeric may be useful to downregulate inflammation.

Sources: Isasi C, Colmenero I, Casco F et al. Fibromyalgia and non-celiac gluten sensitivity: a description with remission of fibromyalgia. Rheumatol Int 2014; 34(11):1607–1612. Kaartinen K, Lammi K, Hypen M et al. Vegan diet alleviates fibromyalgia symptoms. Scand J Rheumatol 2000; 29(5):308–313. Pitchford P. Healing with whole foods. Berkeley. CA: North Atlantic Books; 1993.

- Support neurotransmitter synthesis for optimal serotonin, endorphin and encephalin synthesis
- Reduce inflammation and oxidative stress
- Alleviate pain
- Antispasmodic nutrients for muscular cramps (e.g. magnesium, calcium)
- Normalise circadian rhythm with specific nutritional strategies.

Specific nutrients required

5-HTP, TRYPTOPHAN

Dodabhoy and Clauw[288] note that any type of compound that simultaneously raises both serotonin and noradrenaline will be beneficial in the management of pain associated with fibromyalgia. Low levels of serotonin and its precursor L-tryptophan have been observed in the cerebrospinal fluid of patients with fibromyalgia, suggesting dysfunction in serotonin synthesis or metabolism.[289] Given that serotonin plays a key role in the regulation of pain and mood supplementation, serotonin precursors such as 5-hydroxytryptophan and L-tryptophan may be useful in reducing symptoms associated with fibromyalgia.

A double-blind placebo-controlled study involving 50 patients with fibromyalgia administered 100 mg of 5-hydroxytryptophan three times daily for 1 month and produced beneficial results with few side effects.[290] Similarly efficacious results were reported in an open study where improvements in the number of tender points, anxiety, pain intensity, quality of sleep and fatigue[291] were reported. 5-hydroxytryptophan is well absorbed from an oral dose, with approximately 70% reaching the bloodstream,[292] but only 1% of L-tryptophan is converted to serotonin, the rest being utilised for protein synthesis.[293] If L-tryptophan is prescribed, it is essential that concurrent B complex is taken to ensure optimal conversion through the serotonin pathway.

B COMPLEX (ALL B VITAMINS INCLUDING B_1, B_2, B_3, B_5, B_6, FOLATE, B_{12})

Supplementation with the B vitamins is crucial in the management of fibromyalgia. The B vitamins are involved in numerous enzyme systems within the body and their inability to maintain their roles within the body is sure to be missed. A number of studies have observed alterations in the metabolism of thiamine (vitamin B_1) in people with fibromyalgia.[294,295] Thiamine (as with all the other B vitamins) is required for energy metabolism and this alteration in the metabolism of thiamine will influence the fatigue experienced by fibromyalgia subjects. Similarly, nicotinic acid (vitamin B_3) is required for the conversion of L-tryptophan into serotonin, so deficiency of nicotinic acid will therefore result in less conversion of the much-needed serotonin in fibromyalgia. Increased concentrations of homocysteine have been found in the cerebrospinal fluid of patients with fibromyalgia. A deficiency of B vitamins is linked to hyperhomocysteinaemia.[296]

An intravenous protocol known as the Myers' cocktail has been used successfully to reduce symptoms associated with fibromyalgia in a number of patients.[297] Referral to an integrative GP trained in intravenous prescriptions is required.

As discussed, it has also been shown that people with fibromyalgia process pain differently due to central sensitisation. Vitamin B_{12} has been referred to as the 'analgesic vitamin'[298] because of its ability to relieve pain. Although no studies could be found with regard to the efficacy of vitamin B_{12} therapy in fibromyalgia patients, supplementation may be beneficial where indicated.

HIGH-POTENCY MULTIVITAMIN AND MINERAL FORMULA

A high-potency multivitamin and mineral formula is suggested to provide extra nutritional support. Many patients with fibromyalgia show some signs of nutritional deficiency.

CALCIUM

Calcium ions play an important role in the physiology of muscular contraction as well as the nervous system and thus it is logical to acknowledge that alterations in the concentration of calcium ions may be involved in the pathogenesis of fibromyalgia because of the physical manifestations that present with fibromyalgia, such as muscular spasm. Plasma levels of calcium in fibromyalgia patients have often been observed to be in the normal range, but in some studies[299] intracellular calcium concentrations in fibromyalgia patients have been found to be significantly reduced in comparison to those of healthy controls, backing up results from hair mineral analysis[300] which show high levels of calcium in the hair of fibromyalgia patients. These results provide a link to calcium's role in muscular hypertonus associated with fibromyalgia and are a subsequent indication for supplementation where required.

COENZYME Q10

Both abnormal mitochondria and oxidative stress have been implicated to play a role in fibromyalgia.[255,301] Coenzyme Q10 (ubidecarenone and ubuiqinol) is a powerful antioxidant and an essential electron carrier in the mitochondrial respiratory chain; alterations and dysfunction of coenzyme Q10 distribution in the blood have been observed in patients with fibromyalgia and thus supplementation has been deemed beneficial.[302] In an open pilot study designed to evaluate the potential benefits of coenzyme Q10 combined with *Ginkgo biloba* extract in people with fibromyalgia syndrome, those receiving 200 mg/day of coenzyme Q10 in combination with *Ginkgo biloba* reported substantial improvements in quality of life scores, with 64% claiming benefits in the way they felt.[303]

EFAs (EPA AND DHA), FLAXSEED OIL

The therapeutic effects of omega-3 fatty acids are well known, particularly with regard to musculoskeletal health and include anti-inflammatory and analgesic actions. Moreover and particularly relevant to fibromyalgia, omega-3 fatty acids have been suggested to influence plasma cortisol, modulating the stress response.[304] The relationship between omega-3 fatty acids and fibromyalgia has not received as much attention as other musculoskeletal disorders such as rheumatoid arthritis. Nevertheless, they appear beneficial. In an open, uncontrolled single-blind study involving 12 female patients given high doses of omega-3 fatty acids for 1 month, statistically significant changes were observed for tender point counts, pain severity, fatigue and depression.[305] A case report by Ko et al[304] also reports beneficial results, revealing a considerable reduction in tender points following supplementation with 2400 mg/day DHA and EPA for 7 months, though it is noted for analgesia that this is a conservative dose and that doses of 7500 mg/day DHA/EPA may be used.

Quality of omega-3 fatty acids is imperative and high-quality brands with higher EPA/DHA content are recommended. Only omega-3 fatty acids should be consumed, as omega-6 fatty acids may promote inflammation in the body[306] and may be counterproductive to what is hoped to be achieved.

ACETYL-L-CARNITINE

Fibromyalgia is linked to a number of metabolic dysfunctions, including mitochondrial dysfunction.[307,308] Acetyl-L-carnitine is well known for its effects on mitochondrial function and energy production, but it may also help to relieve pain. In a multicentre randomised clinical trial evaluating the efficacy of acetyl-L-carnitine in patients with overt fibromyalgia, supplementation with acetyl-L-carnitine was found to reduce pain as well as improve mental health status.[309]

MAGNESIUM

Magnesium plays an important role in the pathophysiology of fibromyalgia, with serum magnesium levels found to be decreased in people with fibromyalgia.[310] Magnesium used in combination with malic acid in patients with fibromyalgia for a 2-month period was found to reduce muscle pain, myalgia and tender point index (on average from 19 to 8).[311] This is not surprising given the multifaceted role of magnesium in the body, which includes ATP production, muscle relaxant and analgesic activity.

S-ADENOSYLMETHIONINE (SAMe)

SAMe exerts anti-inflammatory, antidepressant and analgesic effects,[312] making it useful in the management of fibromyalgia. In clinical trials, SAMe has produced mixed results. In a 6-week trial of patients with fibromyalgia given 800 mg/day orally of SAMe benefits were observed in clinical disease activity, pain experienced during the last week, fatigue, morning stiffness and mood in the SAMe group compared with placebo, but tender point score and muscle strength did not change between groups.[312] In contrast, Volkmann et al[313] found no benefits, although it should be noted they used a considerably shorter time frame (10 days), lower dose (600 mg/day) and different mode of administration (IV). This emphasises the importance of correct dosing and time periods for therapeutic effects to be seen.

ANTIOXIDANTS — VITAMINS C AND E AND BIOFLAVONOIDS

While the aetiology of fibromyalgia is undetermined, an imbalance between antioxidants and oxidative stress in favour of oxidative stress has been suggested to play a role in the pathogenesis. Certainly in clinical studies total antioxidant capacity of plasma has been found to be significantly lower in patients with fibromyalgia in comparison to control groups.[314,315] Supplementation with antioxidants that control reactive oxygen species in the body (thus preventing oxidative stress and subsequent inflammation), such as vitamins C and E, have been suggested and appear highly warranted. Bioflavonoids should be taken with vitamin C to enhance its absorption.

VITAMIN D

A number of patients with fibromyalgia are found to be vitamin D deficient[316,317] and this may affect the severity of their symptoms, particularly given the role of vitamin D in muscle health. Armstrong et al[317] found that fibromyalgia patients deficient in vitamin D also scored higher in depression and anxiety scores than those with normal levels. Surprisingly, in the latter study no relationship was noted with vitamin D deficiency and musculoskeletal symptoms.

Fibromyalgia has been suggested to be associated with increased risk of osteoporosis in women.[318] A small study undertaken by Al-Allaf et al[319] revealed that premenopausal women with fibromyalgia appear at increased risk of developing osteoporosis or osteomalacia than their age-matched counterparts. Given the role of vitamin D in bone health, it would appear that the application of vitamin D in patients with fibromyalgia would be multifunctional.

ZINC

Serum zinc has been found to be reduced in patients with fibromyalgia[310,320] and in one study investigators found a significant correlation between serum zinc level and the number of tender points in patients.[310] As yet, there has been little research investigating the role of zinc in fibromyalgia, but results from the latter study provide rationale for further investigations to be undertaken to ascertain its role, independent of its antioxidant function.

DOSAGE REQUIREMENTS

The dosage requirements listed below are based on adult doses that have been reported in the literature.

- B complex (all B vitamins) high-dose combination, preferably activated forms:
  - Thiamine 50–100 mg/day (at least 50 mg of vitamin B_1 per tablet[179])
  - Riboflavin 50–100 mg/day. Riboflavin sodium phosphate 20–40 mg
  - Niacinamide/nicotinic acid 50–100 mg/day
  - Pantothenic acid 150–300 mg/day
  - Pyridoxine 20–60 mg/day. Pyridoxyl phosphate 20–60 mg/day
  - Folic acid 500–1000 micrograms/day. Folinic acid/ MTHF 500–1000 micrograms/day. Investigate MTHFR.[101] Assess methylation status before supplementing with MTHF
  - Cyanocobalamin 5000–10 000 micrograms/day. Methylcobalamin 5000 micrograms/day[179]
  - Choline 150–300 mg/day
  - Inositol 150–300 mg/day
  - Biotin 500 micrograms/day
- Vitamin C 1000–3000 mg/day[179]
- Vitamin D 1000–15000 IU/day (dependent on pathology results)
- Vitamin E 800–1600 IU/day[179]
- 5-hydroxytryptophan 300–400 mg/day[321]
- SAMe 800 mg/day
- Coenzyme Q10 (ubidecarenone and ubuiqinol) 300 mg/ day
- Coenzyme Q10 200 mg/day in combination with 200 mg extract of *Ginkgo biloba* for 3 months[322]
- Acetyl-L-carnitine 1500 mg/day (NB 500 mg of this was done intramuscularly in this study)[309]
- Magnesium 300–600 mg/day (with 2400 mg/day, as malate in this study)[311]
  - Typical dose should encourage minimum of 1000 mg/day
- Calcium 2000 mg/day.[179]

HERBAL MEDICINE

Herbal medicine therapeutic objectives

Herbal medicines can support the patient and provide symptomatic alleviation. Expect that the patient will require to take their prescription for months or even years to resolve the impact of this disease (Table 15.12).

Specific herbal medicines

ANDROGRAPHIS PANICULATA (ANDROGRAPHIS)

The suggestion that an infective agent may be involved in the pathogenesis of fibromyalgia highlights the need for the use of botanicals with known immune-enhancing actions. One such herb is *Andrographis paniculata*, an Ayurvedic herb traditionally indicated for infectious illnesses and febrile diseases and shown to exert anti-inflammatory,[323] antimicrobial[324] and immune-stimulating[325] actions, all likely to be useful in fibromyalgia. The mechanism by which *Andrographis* exerts its effects on the immune system is unclear, but it is known that the diterpene constituent andrographolide, which is deemed responsible for a wide array of the plant's pharmacological actions, prevents oxygen free radical production by neutrophils as well as the binding of nuclear factor B to DNA in vitro, disabling the activity of a number of inflammatory proteins such as cyclooxygenase-2.[323,326]

GLYCYRRHIZA GLABRA (LIQUORICE)

Reductions in cortisol have been noted in people with fibromyalgia as compared with healthy people.[327] Low cortisol states and fibromyalgia have been observed to share many of the same features, including fatigue and muscular aches. *Glycyrrhiza glabra*, via its ability to increase cortisol, provides adrenal support, helping to lessen fatigue while also increasing the body's resistance to stress via its action as an adaptogen.

HYPERICUM PERFORATUM (ST JOHN'S WORT)

As discussed earlier, depression is common in people with fibromyalgia and may be caused by low serotonin levels. People with both fibromyalgia and depression have been shown to have poorer outcomes than those with just fibromyalgia.[328]

Hypericum perforatum has been found to inhibit the reuptake of dopamine, serotonin and noradrenaline as well as having the ability to downregulate beta-adrenergic receptors, upregulate serotonin receptors and mildly

TABLE 15.12 Therapeutic objectives for herbal medicines in fibromyalgia

Treatment goal	Action required	Herbal medicine
Internal treatments		
Modify immune response	Antimicrobial — e.g. mycoplasma, virus	*Allium sativum* *Andrographis paniculata* *Arctostaphylos uva-ursi* *Astragalus membranaceus* *Calendula officinalis* *Commiphora mol-mol* *Echinacea* spp./*radix* *Hydrastis canadensis* *Hypericum perforatum* *Uncaria tomentosa*
Modify immune response	Immune modulator	*Andrographis paniculata* *Astragalus membranaceus* *Baptisia tinctoria* *Bupleurum falcatum* *Codonopsis pilosula* *Echinacea* spp. *Hemidesmus indicus* *Picrorrhiza kurroa* *Rehmannia glutinosa* *Tabebuia avellanedae* *Uncaria tomentosa*
Serotonin/dopamine modulation	5HT antagonism	*Zingiber officinale*
Serotonin/dopamine modulation	HPA modulator	*Panax ginseng* *Vitex agnus-castus*
Serotonin stimulation	Antidepressant	*Hypericum perforatum*
Reduce inflammation	Anti-inflammatory	*Apium graveolens* *Boswellia serrata* *Bupleurum falcatum* *Curcuma longa* *Glycyrrhiza glabra* *Rehmannia glutinosa* *Tanacetum parthenium* *Zingiber officinale*
Thyroid modulation (if indicated)	Thyroid stimulant	*Coleus forskholii* *Fucus vesiculosus* *Withania somnifera*
Blood sugar modulation (if indicated)	Blood sugar modulator	*Codonopsis pilosula* *Galega officinalis* *Gymnema sylvestre*
Relieve symptomatic effects of pain and discomfort	Analgesic/anodyne	*Anemone pulsatilla* *Corydalis ambigua* *Eschscholzia californica* *Gaultheria procumbens* (volatile oil) *Harpagophytum procumbens* *Humulus lupulus* *Matricaria recutita* *Passiflora incarnata* *Piper methysticum* *Piscidia erythrina* *Salix* spp.

Continued

TABLE 15.12 Therapeutic objectives for herbal medicines in fibromyalgia—cont'd		
Treatment goal	**Action required**	**Herbal medicine**
Improve circulation	Circulatory stimulation	*Angelica archangelica* *Brassica alba/nigra* *Capsicum* spp. *Cinnamomum zeylanicum* *Juniperus communis* *Rosmarinus officinalis* *Urtica urens/dioica/*spp. *Zanthoxylum clava-herculis* *Zingiber officinale*
Improve cerebral circulation	Cerebral circulatory stimulant	*Ginkgo biloba* *Zingiber officinale*
Reduce musculoskeletal spasm	Musculoskeletal spasmolytic	*Cimicifuga racemosa* *Dioscorea* spp. *Glycyyrhiza glabra* *Lavandula officinalis* (volatile oil) *Matricaria recutita* *Piper methysticum* *Valeriana officinalis/edulis* *Viburnum opulus* *Viburnum prunifolium* Rubefacients
Reduce disordered response of HPA axis	Tonic	*Eleutherococcus senticosus* *Panax ginseng* *Withania somnifera*
Improve responsiveness of adrenal glands, alleviate adrenal exhaustion	Adrenal tonic/adrenorestorative	*Glycyrrhiza glabra* *Rehmannia glutinosa*
Reduce disordered response of HPA axis	Adaptogen	*Centella asiatica* *Eleutherococcus senticosus* *Glycyrrhiza glabra* *Panax ginseng* *Rehmannia glutinosa* *Schisandra chinensis* *Withania somnifera*
Reduce stress	Nervine	*Avena sativa* *Centella asciatica* *Hypericum perforatum* *Lavandula officinalis* *Matricaria recutita* *Passiflora incarnata* *Piper methysticum* *Piscidia erythrina* *Scutellaria lateriflora* *Valeriana officinalis* *Verbena officinalis*

TABLE 15.12 Therapeutic objectives for herbal medicines in fibromyalgia—cont'd

Treatment goal	Action required	Herbal medicine
Improve quality of sleep	Sedative/relaxant	*Anemone pulsatilla* *Apium graveolens* *Cimicifuga racemosa* *Corydalis ambigua* *Eschscholzia californica* *Humulus lupulus* *Matricaria recutita* *Melissa officinalis* *Passiflora incarnata* *Piper methysticum* *Piscidia erythrina* *Scutellaria lateriflora* *Valeriana officinalis* *Verbena officinalis* *Viburnum opulus* *Withania somnifera* *Zizyphus spinosa*
Topical treatments		
Relieve symptomatic effects	Rubefacient	*Arnica montana* *Brassica alba, B. nigra* *Capsicum* spp. *Cinnamomum camphora* (volatile oil) *Eucalyptus* spp. (volatile oil) *Gaultheria procumbens* (volatile oil) *Juniperus communis* (volatile oil) *Mentha × piperita* (volatile oil) *Rosmarinus officinalis* (volatile oil) *Salvia officinalis* (volatile oil) *Thymus vulgaris* (volatile oil) *Zingiber officinale*
Relieve symptomatic effects	Topical musculoskeletal spasmolytic	*Lavandula officinalis* (volatile oil) *Matricaria recutita* (volatile oil) *Mentha × piperita* (volatile oil) *Piper methysticum*
Relieve symptomatic effects	Topical analgesic	Menthol oils — *Gaultheria procumbens* (volatile oil), *Mentha × piperita* *Arnica montana* *Capsicum frutescens* *Harpagophytum procumbens* *Matricaria recutita*

HPA, hypothalamic–pituitary–adrenal axis.
Source: Grassi W, De Angelis R, Lamanna G, Cervini C. The clinical features of rheumatoid arthritis. Eur J Radiol 1998; 27(Suppl. 1): S18–S24.

inhibit monoamine oxidases, leading to increased serotonin, dopamine and noradrenaline.[329] Aside from its antidepressant effects, *Hypericum perforatum* also exhibits analgesic effects, suggested to occur via inhibition of prostaglandin synthesis.[330] These actions are all likely to be beneficial in fibromyalgia.

Symptoms of fibromyalgia have been conventionally managed with drugs such as tricyclic antidepressants and anticonvulsants. One of the great benefits of *Hypericum perforatum*, aside from its efficacy, is the low incidence of side effects that occur with supplementation. A 2008 Cochrane review found *Hypericum perforatum* to be effective in major depression and to be more effective than standard antidepressants with fewer side effects.[331] As yet there is a scarcity of clinical trials assessing the efficacy of *Hypericum perforatum* in the management of fibromyalgia symptoms, but from the literature reviewed it is clear that it has considerable therapeutical potential in the management of fibromyalgia symptoms and is deserving of further research. Caution the use of *Hypericum* with some medications.

PANAX GINSENG (KOREAN GINSENG)

In the ancient Chinese system of medicine, *Panax ginseng* has been regarded as a revered tonic and restorative, useful for conditions where there is lack of vitality and debility. Several pharmacological studies have investigated the effects of *Panax ginseng*, revealing it to possess potent adaptogenic activity, thought to occur as a result of corticosteroid-like activity.[332] This ability to increase resistance to a range of stressors is highly important in fibromyalgia, where the body is in a dysfunctional state and is under constant stress.

PIPER METHYSTICUM (KAVA)

Anxiety is a common finding in fibromyalgia[333,334] and may impact substantially on quality of life. *Piper methysticum* (kava) is one of the most researched botanicals for alleviation of generalised anxiety and most importantly for the patient it appears to work fairly quickly. Sarris et al[335] conducted a 3-week placebo-controlled double-blind crossover clinical study involving 60 people with elevated stable anxiety. They were given five tablets daily containing *Piper methysticum* (each containing 3.2 g, standardised to 50 mg of kavalactones) or placebo. In this study kava was found to exert significant anxiolytic and antidepressant action and was deemed to be just as effective in people with anxiety and depression as in those with anxiety on its own. Similarly beneficial results were observed in a systematic review of herbal medicines for the treatment of anxiety conducted by Ernst,[336] in which 11 randomised controlled trials were reviewed, assessing the efficacy of *Piper methysticum* for management of anxiety. *Piper methysticum* was shown beyond reasonable doubt to instigate anxiolytic effects in humans with little in the way of side effects.

REHMANNIA GLUTINOSA (REHMANNIA)

Rehmannia glutinosa has been revered in traditional Chinese medicine as a yin tonic and for its wide range of pharmacological actions upon the systems of the body.[337] Stress has been suggested to be a risk factor in fibromyalgia,[338] as continuous stress placed upon an overwhelmed body leaves the body open to chronic illness.[339] Harris[340] notes that *Rehmannia glutinosa* is particularly useful when the body is under stress and that this is probably because of the adaptogen and adrenal restorative effects *Rehmannia* exerts upon the body.

RHODIOLA ROSEA (RHODIOLA)

Rhodiola rosea has been shown to exert anxiolytic[341] and antidepressant[342] effects in human clinical trials and thus it is likely to be well utilised in the fibromyalgia patient who presents with depression and/or anxiety. *Rhodiola rosea* also exerts significant activity as an adaptogen. Olsson et al conduced a randomised, double-blind, placebo-controlled, parallel-group study assessing the efficacy of *Rhodiola rosea* administered to people with stress-related fatigue. They found that *Rhodiola rosea* increased energy and mental performance (in particular concentration) while decreasing cortisol response to awakening stress in burnout patients with fatigue syndrome.[343] This action provides further rationale for the therapeutic application of *Rhodiola rosea* in fibromyalgia.

VALERIANA OFFICINALIS (VALERIAN)

Sleep disruption in patients with fibromyalgia is common, with as many as 99% of patients reporting poor sleep quality.[344] Adequate sleep is imperative when one considers the healing that occurs during sleep as well as the fact that lack of sleep is associated with worsening of fibromyalgia symptoms.[345] As yet, there have been no studies assessing the efficacy of *Valeriana officinalis* in fibromyalgia, but given the links between lack of sleep and increased severity of symptoms *Valeriana officinalis* and other herbal sedatives may offer a gentle way in which to promote better quality and quantity of sleep without severe side effects.

The mechanism by which *Valeriana officinalis* exerts its effects is unknown and widely debated. Valerian contains valerenic acid, which is suggested to be responsible for its sedative activity. Valerenic acid has been shown to modulate,[346] inhibit and potentiate[347] GABA(A)receptors. GABA is involved in the relaxation response.

Valerian also contains terpene derivatives called valepotriates, but while these constituents were initially thought to be responsible for the action of *Valeriana officinalis*, we now know they degrade easily and are thus unlikely to be responsible for the sedative effects of the plant.

A review by Koetter suggests that *Valeriana officinalis* may also function like adenosine, an inhibitory neuromodulator that induces sleep. Koetter[348] provides in-vitro and animal research suggesting *Valeriana officinalis* to be an adenosine A1 receptor agonist, which in animal studies increases slow-wave activity in the cortex and hippocampus. A systematic review and meta-analysis undertaken by Bent et al[349] reviewing 16 studies involving a total of 1093 patients found *Valeriana officinalis* to be effective in improving sleep quality without providing a groggy sensation the next morning. While the results of this review were positive, the authors noted that most studies were of poor methodological quality.

VIBURNUM OPULUS (CRAMP BARK)

As fibromyalgia is characterised by widespread pain with palpable tender spots in numerous parts of the body, botanicals that help to ease this pain, cramping, restless legs and the stiffness associated with fibromyalgia[350] are imperative to improve the patient's quality of life. *Viburnum opulus* is a Native American herb that is useful for cramps and spasms of all kinds.[138] Because of its musculospasmolytic activity it provides relief from the muscular tension and soreness synonymous with fibromyalgia. The actions of *Viburnum opulus* have been known for centuries; the Eclectics advocated its use for pain in the thighs and back and bearing down, expulsive pains.[138] Despite this, sadly there have been no clinical trials examining its efficacy in easing the symptoms of fibromyalgia, although its therapeutic action and traditional application make it the primary herb for fibromyalgia, particularly in conjunction with St John's wort.

VIBURNUM PRUNIFOLIUM (BLACK HAW)

As with *Viburnum opulus* above, *Viburnum prunifolium* is well regarded in traditional medicine for its antispasmodic and relaxant actions.[351,352] Although no published clinical studies could be found examining the therapeutic effects of *Viburnum prunifolium* in humans, much less in fibromyalgia, its antispasmodic and relaxant actions make it highly useful in fibromyalgia to ease spasm and subsequently pain. The bark of *Viburnum prunifolium* displays a particularly affinity for the female reproductive system and is commonly used for gynaecological conditions, particular menstrual cramping and pain. *Viburnum prunifolium* was prized by the Eclectic physicians who used it for dysmenorrhoea, severe lumbar and bearing-down pains, as well as for intermittent, painful contractions of the pelvic tissues.[138] Two constituents of *Viburnum prunifolium* — scopoletin and esculetin — have been noted to instigate an antispasmodic action on the muscle of the uterus[353] and are likely to be responsible for its relaxant action on the female reproductive system. *Viburnum prunifolium* would seem likely to be useful in women presenting with concurrent fibromyalgia and reproductive complaints.

VITEX AGNUS-CASTUS (CHASTE TREE)

Vitex agnus-castus is a well-known modulator of the hypothalamic–pituitary–adrenal (HPA) axis and is thus likely to be useful in patients with fibromyalgia, where the HPA axis is known to be altered. *Vitex agnus-castus* may also be useful because of its dopaminergic action, as low dopamine has been found in fibromyalgia. Furthermore, it may also be useful in its role as a cycle regulator in women with menstrual disturbance associated with fibromyalgia. The ability of *Vitex agnus-castus* to modulate progesterone may also indirectly lead to an elevation in mood as progesterone is a natural antidepressant.[354]

WITHANIA SOMNIFERA (ASHWAGANDHA)

Fibromyalgia has been suggested to occur as a result of a failure of the body to adapt to a hostile environment[355] and brings with it a range of symptoms, including fatigue, pain and anxiety.[356] The application of a gentle, regenerating botanical such as *Withania somnifera* would seem to be indicated.

Withania somnifera is valued in Ayurvedic medicine for its gentle 'rasayana' (rejuvenating) and revitalising effects on the body, particularly where there is debility and fatigue.[357] In animal studies,[358] *Withania somnifera* has proved itself to be an adaptogen, which has been suggested to exert an 'anti-stress' action. In humans, naturopathic management of anxiety using *Withania somnifera* (300 mg b.i.d. standardised to 1.5% with anolides, prepared from root) in combination with a standard multivitamin, dietary advice and breathing techniques was found to reduce anxiety and improve quality of life. Results were more significant than in a comparison group of participants receiving psychotherapy, breathing techniques and a placebo.[359]

ZINGIBER OFFICINALE (GINGER)

Zingiber officinale is well known for its warming, stimulating action on the body's circulatory system and less known for its effects as an anxiolytic. Gingerols and galanolactone constituents within *Zingiber officinale* appear to be antagonistics of the serotonin 5-HT_3 receptor,[360] resulting in an anxiolytic action. As yet, this anxiolytic activity has been observed in rats[361] but has not been tested in humans. The possibility of *Zingiber officinale* being used in the management of anxiety in patients with fibromyalgia is an exciting potential area for research.

ZIZYPHUS SPINOSA (ZIZYPHUS)

Stress, anxiety and nervous tension can be associated with lack of sleep[362] and this lack of sleep may in part influence the severity of symptoms of people with fibromyalgia. *Zizyphus spinosa* has been used in traditional Chinese medicine for anxiety and sleeplessness,[363] being said to quieten the spirit and replenish the body during sleep.[364] Since both anxiety and sleep disorders commonly present in fibromyalgia, application of *Zizyphus spinosa* is likely to be helpful. Interestingly, the seeds and leaves of *Zizyphus spinosa* have been shown to inhibit central nervous system function, whereas the fruit appears to have a gentle sedative effect, promoting sleep.[365]

LIFESTYLE RECOMMENDATIONS

Exercise

Exercise is essential to improve mental and emotional wellbeing; increase circulation, relieve tension and support bone health through weight-bearing exercises. It is beneficial to recommend a staggered introduction to exercise, particularly if the person is sedentary or has low physical activity levels and encourage the patient to pace themselves and slowly increase intensity and duration over time.

Physical treatment

Massage and manipulative therapies such as chiropractic or osteopathic treatments are essential to ensure correct posture and body structure. Regular massage can alleviate pain and discomfort. Other physical therapies should be trialled and assessed for efficacy.

CASE STUDY

OVERVIEW

KC is a 24-year-old female personal assistant who presented to the clinic with a diagnosis of fibromyalgia. The muscle pain and stiffness is 8/10 most days. Her symptoms presented a year after she suffered glandular fever (Epstein-Barr virus). She presents as stressed (8/10), tense, anxious and fatigued (energy level 4/10 most days). She is ambitious and has worked hard to get to the position of personal assistant to a high-level executive. She worries that if she doesn't keep performing at the high level expected she will lose her job. During the consultation she talks about her ongoing stress levels since the age of 15 years. Her stress levels further increased around the time of her Year 12 exams but she won't discuss the situation any further.

Her symptoms can be exacerbated by emotional stress, poor sleep and exposure to dampness and cold weather. She read about MTHFR on social media and was tested. She was found to be MTHFR C677T Heterozygous. Her mother and aunt have diagnosed hypothyroidism.

CLINICAL EXAMINATION

BP 109/73 mmHg
Temperature 37.3°C
Pulse 78 bpm
Respiratory rate 18 resp/min

CASE STUDY CONTINUED

Height 1.74 m
Weight 60 kg
BMI 19.82 kg/m^2
Face: pale. Darkness under the eyes
Tongue: scalloping around the edges. Tongue quivered.
Nails: dryness around the nails. White spots on several nails with moons only on the thumbs. Slow capillary return.

Blood testing

FBC: All within normal range
LFT: All normal range
Electrolytes: All within normal range
Iron studies: Within normal range with serum iron at the lower end of normal range
CRP: Within normal range
Rheumatoid factor: Negative
Antinuclear antibody: Negative
CRP: Normal range
MTHFR: C677T Heterozygous

TREATMENT PROTOCOL

FURTHER INVESTIGATIONS

Referral for a number of additional assessments was conducted to establish contributing or causative factors that exacerbated or caused the presentation. These included:

- Thyroid-stimulating hormone (TSH) (fT3, fT4)
- Reverse T3
- Thyroid antibodies
- Coeliac profile
- Red cell magnesium
- Red cell or plasma zinc
- Serum copper
- Vitamin D
- Fasting glucose and HbA_{1c}
- Epstein-Barr virus (EBV) (to confirm history)
- Cytomegalovirus (CMV)

INITIAL APPOINTMENT

HERBAL MEDICINE

Herbal medicine	Extract	Quantity	Justification
Rhodiola rosea	1:2	70 mL	Adpatogen, adrenal tonic, anti-inflammatory
Corydalis ambigua	1:2	50 mL	Analgesic, anti-inflammatory
Passiflora incarnata	1:2	50 mL	Musculoskeletal spasmolytic, nervine, sedative
Withania somnifera	1:1	40 mL	Adaptogen, nutritive, nervine tonic
Zingiber officinale	1:5	10 mL	Circulatory stimulant, anxiolytic
TOTAL		220 mL	

Dose: 7.5 mL b.i.d. An extra dose of 5 mL may be taken when muscle pain/tension is worse.

CASE STUDY CONTINUED

NUTRITIONAL MEDICINE

Dietary

- Investigate and correct nutritional deficiencies
- Avoid caffeine in any form — coffee, tea, cola, chocolate
- Avoid artificial sweeteners, flavours, colours, preservatives and glutamate-containing foods such as MSG
- Avoid foods that have shown potential allergy/intolerance effects
- Encourage general wholefood principles
- Encourage adequate hydration (aim for greater than 30 mL/kg body weight per day)
- Optimise protein intake as her protein needs were insufficient in her current diet. Protein needs were calculated as 1.0 g/kg.

Supplemental

- High-dose B complex in activated form: 1 capsule with breakfast and 1 capsule with lunch
- Magnesium 200 mg t.d.s.
- Vitamin C (buffered) 500 mg b.i.d.
- Zinc 25–30 mg b.i.d.
- Omega-3 EPA 600 mg and DHA 400 mg t.d.s.
- Glutamine 5000 mg in water t.d.s.
- Taurine 500 mg in water t.d.s.
- Inositol 2000 mg in water t.d.s.

LIFESTYLE/EDUCATION

Exercise

She was prescribed stretching exercises each day in the evening for the first 2 weeks. After 2 weeks, she was to continue with the stretching exercises and start going for short walks. In the long term, she was to increase the grading of the exercise, for example increase the length of time and the environment in which she walked (from flat surfaces to hills).

Massage

She had a light massage weekly to relieve the muscular tension. Weekly massages were chosen due to the stiffness and tenderness of the muscles and to alleviate her concerns about the massage making them worse. Aerobic exercise was added in the second week to improve circulation and reduce stress. She could use local applications of heat if required.

Stress management

A 15-minute time out was encouraged daily at work to improve her focus and reduce stress levels. On weekends, her time outs were longer as she could sit in the local park and do deep breathing exercises without the worries of work affecting her. For the second week onwards, a time out for 15–20 minutes twice daily was recommended.

FOLLOW-UP

After 2 weeks, her muscular pain and stiffness had decreased from an 8/10 to 7/10. Her energy levels had increased from 4/10 to 6/10 and she slept slightly better. Her anxiety levels remained the same. After 4 weeks, she had a further reduction in muscular pain and stiffness to a level of 6/10. Her energy levels remained at 6/10 but she felt she got more work completed.

OSTEOPOROSIS

Epidemiology

Osteoporosis has been found to occur more frequently in women (5%) than men (1%) and has been found to be associated with increasing age, the greatest prevalence being seen in the age group 75 years and older. These results were found to be highest in women, with 26% of women reporting osteoporosis in the age group 75 years and older. The prevalence of osteoporosis in 2009 was estimated to be 10%, but in the absence of interventions it is expected to increase to 13.2% by 2021.[366] In 2001 an osteoporotic fracture was estimated to occur every 8.1 minutes; by 2021 this figure is expected to increase to one fracture every 3.7 minutes.[367] Osteoporotic fractures are a large cause of mortality and morbidity. (See Fig. 15.10.)

Classification

Osteoporosis is a systemic disease characterised by low bone mass and microarchitectural deterioration of the bone tissue leading to an increase in bone fragility.[368] Osteoporosis may be classified as either primary or secondary. Primary osteoporosis accounts for the majority of cases seen in clinical practice; secondary osteoporosis occurs as a result of certain medications (e.g. corticosteroids) or conditions (e.g. hyperthyroidism).

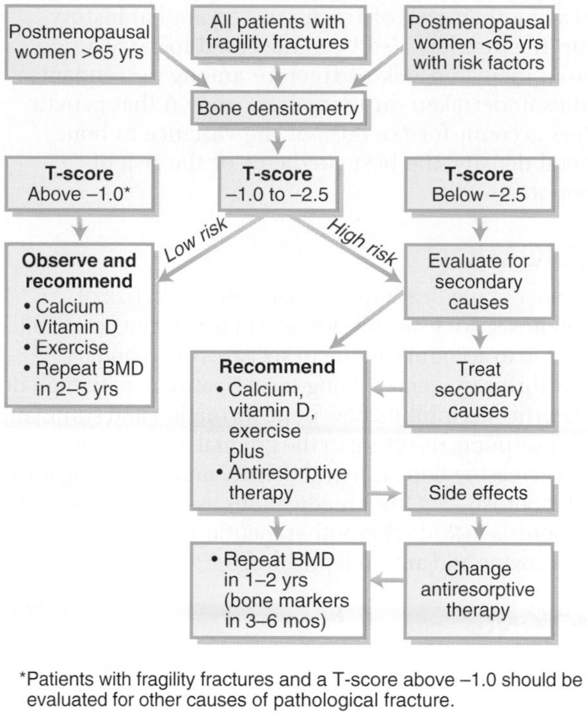

FIGURE 15.10 Osteoporosis.

Kronenberg H, Melmed S, Polonsky K et al. Williams textbook of endocrinology. 11th edn. Saunders: 2008.

Aetiology

AGE

Osteoporosis is the greatest cause of fracture in older people. It is a major cause of injury, long-term disability and death in older people.[369] After midlife, bone loss occurs at a rate of 1% per year in both men and women.[370] This explains why osteoporosis is primarily diagnosed in older adults. The risk of fracture in women with osteoporosis increases from 15% in those aged 60–64 years up to 71% for those aged greater than 80 years. Although there is a much lower incidence in men, there is a similar age-related increase in the risk of fracture, that risk being 1.6% in men aged 60–64 years up to 19% for men aged greater than 80 years.[369]

Adult peak bone mass is usually achieved by the age of 30 and the bone-building years before the age of 18 are especially important. It has thus been suggested that the time to prevent osteoporosis is really during adolescence.[371]

ALCOHOL

Heavy intake of alcohol is associated with osteoporosis.[372] Not only does it cause depletion of nutrients required for bone health (e.g. the B vitamins) it is also known to disrupt calcium and bone homeostasis, leading to reduced bone mineral density and risk of fracture.

LOW BODY WEIGHT

Young women with low BMI but with normal menstruation, hormonal profile and negative for anorexia nervosa may be at increased risk of osteoporosis. A study undertaken by Galusca et al[373] noted that women with constitutional thinness typically had a high incidence of low bone mass associated with small bone size, overall diminished breaking strength but normal bone turnover.

DECLINE IN SEX STEROID HORMONES

In postmenopausal women reduced levels of oestrogen and the lack of control of parathyroid hormone have been recognised as underlying the development of osteoporosis. Low oestrogen results in increased bone resorption; bone loss increases to 2% every year for up to 14 years in women at menopause.[374] It has also been observed that in women, by the age 65, calcium absorption is 50% of adolescent absorption levels.[375] Changes in male sex hormones are also thought to contribute to osteoporosis in men.[376,377]

Three main considerations for the decline in sex steroid hormones for women are:

- Early menopause without hormone replacement therapy (HRT) or oral contraceptives
- History of amenorrhoea (due to anorexia nervosa, hyperprolactinaemia or exercise-induced amenorrhoea), infrequent menses, late menstrual onset, anovulation
- Premenopausal hypogonadism.

GENETICS

A family history of osteoporosis is considered to be a significant risk factor for osteoporosis.[378–380] In one study, premenopausal daughters of women with postmenopausal osteoporosis were also found to have reduced bone mass increasing their risk of fractures.[380] Familial history of hip fracture has also been observed to carry a twofold increased risk of fracture among descendants.[381] Studies undertaken on twins have shown that genetic factors account for 60–80% of the variance in bone mineral density, the best predictor of the risk of osteoporosis.[382]

MEDICATION

A number of medications are associated with risk of osteoporosis. For example, long-term use of glucocorticoids is estimated to account for one in six cases of secondary osteoarthritis in men.[383] Long-term treatment with high-dose glucocorticoids inhibits new bone formation and stimulates bone resorption, resulting in the gradual loss of bone over time, decreasing bone mineral density and increasing the risk of osteoporosis.[384] Other medications associated with risk of osteoporosis include chemotherapeutic agents, excess levothyroxine and antiepileptic drugs.[372]

SMOKING

Smoking is associated with sustained decreased bone mass and increased fracture risk. A meta-analysis undertaken by Ward and Klesges[385] estimated that smoking increased the lifetime risk of developing a vertebral fracture by 13% in women and 32% in men; smoking was also estimated to increase lifetime hip fracture risk by 31% in women and 40% in men.

SEDENTARY LIFESTYLE

An increasingly sedentary lifestyle has been suggested as a significant contributing factor for the increased prevalence of osteoporosis, as lack of movement results in reduced bone density. Prolonged bed rest may also contribute.

VITAMIN D AND CALCIUM DEFICIENCY

Both calcium and vitamin D are required for the structure and support of the skeletal system; insufficiency may result in bone loss, thus increasing the risk of fracture. These are discussed in more detail further in this chapter. Of importance it is essential to consider inadequate calcium and vitamin D intake during pregnancy and nursing as a prime contributing or causative factor. With each pregnancy, nutrient levels will decline if not properly addressed through diet and/or supplementation.

LIFESTYLE AND ENVIRONMENT

Lack of exposure to sunlight for vitamin D absorption is an essential consideration. To ensure optimal absorption and utilisation, cholesterol, liver and kidney health should be assessed to ensure appropriate hydroxylation is achieved.

DIGESTIVE HEALTH

Calcium absorption is dependent on the ionisation of calcium in the digestive system. It is first solubilised and ionised by stomach acid and then absorbed, primarily in the small intestine. It has been suggested that over 40% of postmenopausal women are deficient in hydrochloric acid, thus contributing to ineffective solubilisation and ionisation and thus absorption.

Osteoporosis is a well-known extraintestinal manifestation of inflammatory bowel diseases. It is more common in Crohn's disease compared to ulcerative colitis. It has been estimated that osteopenia in ulcerative colitis is found in about 35% of the patients and osteoporosis in about 15%, based on DXA scans. In patients with ulcerative colitis, poor nutrition and malabsorption (particularly of calcium, vitamin D and K) can be caused by lack of appetite, insufficient diet and diarrhoea. Inflammatory bowel disease associated inflammatory cytokines, such as IL-1, IL-6 and TNF-α, have been shown to directly affect bone metabolism.[368]

OTHER

Other causes of osteoporosis include:[372]

- Gastrointestinal disease (malabsorption, post-gastrectomy)
- Glucocorticoid excess (exogenous or endogenous)
- Hypercalciuria
- Hypogonadism (including androgen deprivation therapy)
- Other endocrine diseases (e.g. hyperparathyroidism, hyperthyroidism)
- Malignancy (e.g. multiple myeloma, leukaemia)
- Mastocytosis
- Rheumatoid arthritis
- Chronic obstructive pulmonary disease.

Overview

Osteoporosis is the most common bone disease and is characterised by low bone mass and deterioration of the bone tissue that occurs as the result of a disproportional relationship between bone resorption and bone deposition, specifically increased osteoclast resorption coupled with decreased osteoblast reformation.[386] It may be compounded by excessive bone resorption after peak mass has been achieved[387] as well as poor bone mass acquisition during adolescence, as bone mass increases rapidly from puberty until the mid-20s–30s when peak bone mass is achieved.[387]

PATHOGENESIS

Both men and women lose bone mass as age progresses after the mid-30s, but this loss is accelerated in some women because of the deficiency of oestrogen that occurs at menopause. As a result, the bones become fragile and porous, increasing susceptibility to fracture and other complications such as shrinkage of vertebrae.

SIGNS AND SYMPTOMS

Osteoporosis has been described as the 'silent disease' because of its insidious presentation. Back pain or fracture may be the first sign that osteoporosis is present, but by the time it gets to this stage the condition is actually well established. It is important to acknowledge that in osteoporosis bone may be so fragile that a fracture may occur just by bending, coughing or lifting something.

Other symptoms that may result due to vertebral osteoporosis include:

- Stooped posture
- Dowager's hump
- Loss of height
- Kyphosis (spinal deformity)[45]
- Protruding abdomen.[45]

Subsequent investigations may reveal low bone mass and microarchitectural deterioration of bone tissue.

COMPLICATIONS

Complications of osteoporosis include chronic pain, restricted movement, fractures, disability and reduced quality of life.[388] Risk of mortality from fractures is high, with a small sample study of the Australian population showing that in older women and men, all low-trauma fractures were associated with increased mortality risk for 5–10 years. Subsequent fracture was associated with increased mortality risk for an additional 5 years.[389] Approximately 50% of fracture-related deaths in women are due to hip fractures, 28% to clinical vertebral fractures and 22% to other fractures. In individuals who have experienced hip fractures, 20% die within the next year and 20% will require permanent nursing home care.

DIFFERENTIAL DIAGNOSIS

Because of osteoporosis presenting as a deterioration of bone mineral density, a number of differentials must be considered:

- Ageing (especially postmenopause)
- Immobilisation
- Nutritional causes: calcium or vitamin D deficiency, or both
- Malnutrition, malabsorption
- Postgastrectomy
- Scurvy
- Total parenteral nutrition
- Pregnancy and lactation
- Aluminium toxicity
- Corticosteroid excess
- Cushing's syndrome or disease
- Steroid therapy
- Other endocrine disorders — hypogonadism (e.g. Klinefelter's syndrome, Turner's syndrome, early oophorectomy), thyrotoxicosis, acromegaly, hyperparathyroidism, hypopituitarism, type 2 diabetes
- Inherited bone matrix abnormalities — homocysteinuria, Marfan's syndrome, Ehlers–Danlos syndrome, osteogenesis imperfecta, Menkes' syndrome
- Rheumatoid arthritis
- Ankylosing spondylitis
- Malignancy — lymphoma, leukaemia, multiple myeloma, Waldenström's macroglobulinaemia, systemic mastocytosis, carcinomatosis
- Heparin therapy (chronic)
- Chronic obstructive pulmonary disease
- Chronic acidosis (especially renal tubular acidosis, metabolic acidosis secondary to high-protein diet)
- Alcoholism
- Hepatic insufficiency, cirrhosis (alcoholic or other)
- Methotrexate
- Chronic anticonvulsant therapy
- Chronic renal failure (renal osteodystrophy)
- Paget's disease (with predominantly lytic lesions)
- Juvenile (idiopathic)
- Cystic fibrosis
- Riley–Day syndrome
- Hypophosphatasia
- Female distance runners
- Smoking.

NATUROPATHIC DIAGNOSIS

All postmenopausal women and postandropausal men should be assessed for risk factors associated with osteoporosis. This should include:

1. Thorough medical history
2. Physical examination:
   (a) Include height, weight and BMI. Height variables of greater than 3.5–4 cm may be associated with verterbral compression and increased fracture risk
   (b) Routine annual height measurement should be mandatory for all people over 50
   (c) Excessive kyphosis of the thoracic spine, dowager's hump, dental caries, tooth loss, receding gums and back pain should raise suspicion of osteoporosis
3. Laboratory assessments
4. Risk assessment considering all aetiological factors.

Genetics, lifestyle factors and hormonal status are the major factors that influence the balance between bone resorption and bone formation. As such, diagnosis needs to consider all of these variables thoroughly. No one risk factor or combination of risk factors will accurately predict which patients will or will not experience osteoporosis or osteoporotic fractures. The more risk factors present, the greater the potential for lower bone mass and the higher the risk of fracture.

Risk factors are important guides in the clinical assessment of osteoporosis risks that contribute to optimal preventive strategies. Important risk factors that contribute to a holistic diagnosis include:

- Assessment of medical conditions for contributing or causative factors
- Assessment of current or historical medication use
- Consideration of various endocrine disorders, malignancies and/or collagen metabolism disorders
- Assessment of genetic influences — highest incidence is found in Caucasians, slender physical frame, those with a strong family history, especially first-degree relatives
- Assessment of nutritional status, including cholesterol, calcium, vitamin D and other bone nutrients (e.g. magnesium, manganese, silica, zinc, vitamin K).

Investigations

DUAL-ENERGY X-RAY ABSORPTIOMETRY (DEXA) SCANNING

Dual-energy x-ray absorptiometry (DEXA or DXA) scanning is considered to be the gold standard for diagnosis of osteoporosis and is used to predict the risk of fracture by measuring bone mineral density. DEXA should be undertaken every 2 years for these with suspected osteoporosis or women postmenopause and men >55 years unless there is accelerated bone loss (for example as a side effect of medication use), in which case it should be undertaken on a yearly basis.[367]

Bone mineral density is expressed in terms of a 'T-score,' representing the number of standard deviations from a young healthy patient's mean bone mineral density:[367]

- Normal bone density: T-score greater than −1
- Osteopenia (low bone mass): T-score between −1 and −2.5
- Osteoporosis: T-score less than −2.5.

SPECIFIC NATUROPATHIC INVESTIGATIONS

Osteoporosis Risk Assessment (NTx)

The Osteoporosis Risk Assessment (NTx) is a urine test which detects the risk of osteoporosis by measuring the rate of bone resorption via the excretion of cross-linked *N*-telopeptides (NTx), a breakdown product of type 1 bone collagen. Quantitative measures of NTx provide an indicator of human bone resorption well before significant changes are obvious on bone mineral density scans.

The NTx marker can also be used to monitor the efficacy of antiresorptive therapies such as hormone replacement (HRT) and/or calcium supplementation in postmenopausal women, individuals with osteoporosis and those with Paget's disease.

Female hormonal profile (saliva)

Female hormone profile monitors changes in hormone status over the course or part of the menstrual cycle, by measuring the sex hormones. This test is a more accurate representation of hormone status in the body and may be useful to measure levels of declining steroid hormones such as oestrogen. A blood test measuring female hormonal profile can be used to support the findings of the saliva test.

2 and 16 urinary oestrogen metabolites

This test monitors oestrogen metabolism in men and women. A high ratio indicates an oestrogen-deficient state, which may indicate an increased risk of osteoporosis.

Liver function test

Although a liver function test is used to screen for, detect, evaluate and monitor liver inflammation and damage, it can also be performed to measure bone issues indirectly. For example, alkaline phosphatase (ALP) is an enzyme found in high levels in bone and liver with smaller amounts found in the intestines. When a liver function test is conducted and the other liver function enzymes such as bilirubin, gamma-glutamyl transferase (GGT), alanine aminotransferase (ALT) or aspartate aminotransferase (AST) are normal, this suggests that the ALP might be coming from bone. Conversely, if the other liver function enzymes are also raised, this usually indicates liver dysfunction or disease. ALP can also be raised in bone diseases such as Paget's disease (where bones become enlarged and deformed), healing fractures and vitamin D deficiency.

Bone resorption assay (urine)

The bone resorption assay detects biochemical markers that reflect present remodelling activity — the deoxypyridinoline fragment of type I collagen breakdown from a single urine specimen. This is the fragment that contains the cross-linking point and has been demonstrated to be more specific to bone resorption than breakdown fragments measured in some earlier assays.

Fat-soluble vitamin profile

This profile assesses levels of all fat-soluble vitamins. This assessment is not crucial if blood levels of vitamin D are assessed, but the additional evidence of other fat-soluble vitamin status is beneficial when considering the building blocks of steroid hormone synthesis.

Therapeutic considerations

CLINICAL DECISION MAKING AND RATIONALE

- Assess age and hormonal impact
- Assess dietary and nutritional status (deficiencies and excesses)
- Investigate food allergies and intolerances
- Assess heavy metals, e.g. lead
- Assess exercise and lifestyle practices
- Consider alternative contributors to presentation
- Focus on prevention of deterioration with education regarding supportive strategies.

Therapeutic application

HISTORICAL PERSPECTIVE

Osteoporosis is an ancient disease with mention of this condition traced back 3000 years to the Biblical references of King David who stated 'My strength failed and my bones are consumed', 'My bones wasted away through my anguished roaring all day long'.[390] Of course, whether or not this really refers to osteoporosis is debatable. There is certainly no mention of osteoporosis as a condition in the texts of the Eclectics, although it may have been defined by some other name. The Eclectics did, however, document a number of botanicals used for the healing of fractures. *Eupatorium perforatum* (boneset) was used for deep-seated aching pains in the muscles and the periosteum[138] (the outer lining of the bones). *Symphytum officinale* (comfrey) was favoured by Eclectic physician Felter as a vulnerary and for its ability to promote the quick healing of fractured bones.[138]

NATUROPATHIC PERSPECTIVE

Osteoporosis is a preventable disease that requires optimal and healthy dietary and lifestyle habits. Supporting and promoting healthy bones should be a base skill for all men and women. Education needs to focus on understanding and encouraging a few key areas:

- Lifestyle practices and exercise habits that prevent skeletal fragility and deterioration of microarchitecture

- Lifestyle practices that prevent or reduce the risk of fractures
- Nutritional modifications (dietary and supplemental) that preserve bone mass and strength and improve muscle integrity.

Dietary calcium is obviously of paramount importance, but it is essential to acknowledge the multifactorial nature of the condition and consider all variables, including hormonal, environmental, dietary, lifestyle, exercise, medication and other factors. In addition, bone mineralisation comprises multiple nutrients and their cofactors.

NUTRITIONAL MEDICINE (DIETARY)

Dietary therapeutic objectives

- Investigate and correct nutritional deficiencies
- Avoid dietary factors that inhibit absorption and promote calcium excretion: salt, sugar, animal protein, soft drinks, coffee, alcohol, tannin-containing beverages (tea, red wine)
- Increase food sources that optimise nutrients for bone building
- Increase consumption of green leafy vegetables and fermented soy products
- Support dietary combinations that encourage nutrient absorption
- Encourage wholefood dietary principles that provide optimal nutrient levels
- Increase water intake for fluid optimisation.

Specific dietary treatments

DIETARY INCLUSIONS

Fresh wholefood diet

Bone is living tissue and reliant on a constant supply of varied nutrients, including calcium, magnesium, vitamin K, boron, manganese and zinc. A diet that contains a variety of fresh wholefoods will provide the required nutrition to the bones and surrounding tissues not only to make them stronger but also to assist in quick healing if fracture is sustained. For this reason, a balanced diet based upon the principles of variety and wholefoods is recommended.

Fruit and vegetables

Fruits and vegetables contain an array of nutrients required for bone health, including antioxidants (such as vitamin C) as well as minerals calcium, magnesium and potassium,[391] which may assist with acid–alkaline balance, shown to be important in osteoporosis.[392] A number of studies examining the effects of osteoporosis have observed the link between a diet rich in fruit and vegetables and bone health; in the Framingham osteoporosis cohort study each extra serving of fruit or vegetables was associated with a 1% increase in bone mineral density.

Vegetarian diet

Vegetarians, and particularly vegans, may be at greater risk of lower bone mineral density and fracture. A large study identified lower intakes of protein, vitamin B_{12}, vitamin D and retinol (vitamin A) in both lactoovovegetarians and vegans relative to meat eaters, with these nutrients being particularly low in vegans. In addition, calcium was found to be lower in vegans than in lactoovovegetarians or in meat eaters. Therefore, careful selection of foods and the use of supplements can help ensure healthy bone status to reduce fracture risk. However, it is noted that a vegetarian diet with high intakes of fruit and vegetables tends to provide higher intakes of vitamin C, potassium, magnesium, carotenoids, flavonoids and other phytonutrients. These antioxidant and anti-inflammatory nutrients have been shown to protect bone.[393]

Prunes

Daily intake of approximately 100 mg/day of *Prunus domestica* (prunes/dried plums) has been shown to have beneficial effects on bone.[394] Consumption of prunes daily by postmenopausal women significantly increased serum markers of bone formation, total alkaline phosphatase (ALP), bone-specific alkaline phosphatase and insulin-like growth factor-I by 12, 6 and 17%, respectively over a 3-month period.[395]

Soybean isoflavones

Inconsistent results have been seen with regard to the benefits of soybean isoflavones and their relationship with bone health. The collective sum of these data, however, suggests that diets rich in phytoestrogens have bone-sparing effects in the long term.[396,397] As such, it is recommended to encourage a more traditional approach to soy consumption, focusing on fermented sources of soy as opposed to some of the heavily processed products currently available.

Dietary fatty acids

Consumption of dietary fatty acids has been suggested to influence bone in many ways, including effects on osteoblastogenesis, osteoblast activity, calcium balance, membrane function and reducing inflammatory cytokines such as interleukin-1 (IL-1), IL-6 and TNF-α.[398] Findings from observational and randomised controlled trials suggest that higher fatty fish intake is linked with reduced risk of fragility fracture. Human studies support a greater intake of total PUFAs, total omega-3 fatty acid for higher bone mineral density and reduced risk of fragility fracture.[399] In the Framingham Osteoporosis Study, greater than or equal to 3 servings of fatty fish per week was protective against 4-year loss of femoral neck BMD and dietary ALA was associated with lower risk of hip fracture.[400] More research is required.

Calcium and magnesium food sources

Adequate intake of calcium is central to the prevention of osteoporosis, but in numerous countries many women and men, as well as children and adolescents, do not get the recommended daily intake of calcium required. Dairy products, such as yoghurt and milk, should not be used to make up the majority of calcium requirements in the diet as they do not contain optimal amounts of magnesium and other bone-building nutrients. Calcium in isolation can inhibit the absorption and metabolism of magnesium, so foods that are naturally high in calcium as well as other bone-building nutrients (e.g. magnesium and zinc), such as almonds, leafy green vegetables and tahini, should be included in the diet.

Protein

Early studies suggested that a diet high in protein was linked with loss of urinary calcium and risk of fractures,[401] but studies now suggest that dietary protein may actually be favourable in helping to prevent fractures and thus risk of osteoporosis.[402,403] Protein has been shown to increase insulin-like growth factor-I,[404] which provides a source of nutrition to the bones. Clearly, moderate protein is important for healthy bones and this word 'moderate' should be emphasised; there is a fine line between over- and underconsumption of protein and each appears to affect bone negatively. Thus moderate intake of protein would appear to be the sensible approach and best in osteoporosis. In view of this it is prudent to recommend calculating a patient's protein requirements (e.g. 0.8–1.0 g per kg body weight/day) and prescribing protein from both animal and vegetarian sources in a balanced manner.

DIETARY EXCLUSIONS

Sodium

Although sodium is required by the body, a high intake of salt has been linked to osteoporosis[405–407] and may occur as a result of increased calcium excretion in urine.[406,408] Many processed foods contain high levels of sodium (for example breakfast cereal) and a reduction in salt intake can be achieved easily by reducing processed and prepackaged foods and swapping to a wholefood diet. Small changes, such as replacing salt used in cooking with fresh herbs, will also help. Something to note is that although Himalayan salt and Celtic sea salt are healthier alternatives to table salt, they still contain sodium. Therefore, their consumption should be limited in people with osteoporosis and other bone disorders.

Caffeinated beverages including coffee and tea

Consumption of coffee and tea has been linked to increased risk of osteoporosis. Moderation appears to be the key when it comes to drinking coffee or tea, as daily intake of caffeine of approximately 330 mg or more (equivalent to 2–4 cups of coffee) is associated with an increased risk of osteoporotic fractures, especially in women with a low intake of calcium.[409–411] An intake in excess of 4 cups of tea is also associated with increased risk of hip fractures. It is important to also acknowledge the potential negative health effects of decaffeinated preparations (unless water decaffeinated) as well as the impact of the tannin content in tea on digestive function and absorption of nutrients due to the binding nature of tannins.

Carbonated beverages

Consumption of carbonated drinks that contain phosphoric acid has been associated with reduced bone mineral density, particularly in association with low calcium intake.[412–414] A short-term intervention study of healthy young men following a 10-day period of high intake of cola (2.5 L) in combination with a low-calcium diet was found to induce increased bone turnover compared with a high intake of milk (2.5 L) with a low-calcium diet. This study suggests that the consumption of cola and other soft drinks in combination with a low calcium intake may negatively affect bone health.[415] Furthermore, in the Framingham Osteoporosis Study, the intake of cola but not other soft drinks was associated with lower bone mineral mass in women but not men.[412]

Saturated fat

Recent studies in rats observed that those fed a high-fat diet experienced significant bone loss due to resorptive changes in trabecular architecture.[416] Studies are yet to be undertaken in humans, but if positive they may provide a link between obesity and osteoporosis.

NUTRITIONAL MEDICINE (SUPPLEMENTAL)

Nutritional medicine therapeutic objectives

- Provide symptomatic relief from pain and inflammation
- Investigate and correct nutritional deficiencies and provide bone-building nutrients
- Support renal and hepatobiliary function to optimise vitamin D hydroxylation and activation
- Optimise digestive function by increasing HCl and enzyme release to increase nutrient absorption
- Investigate for food intolerances or allergies that may lead to nutritional deficiencies or absorption issues
- Investigate the digestive system for potential conditions that may alter absorption of nutrients, e.g. coeliac disease, Crohn's disease
- Reduce weight if overweight or obese
- Stabilise collagen structures
- Improve hormonal receptor activity (sex dependent)
- Reduce oxidation.

Specific nutrients required

B COMPLEX (ALL B VITAMINS INCLUDING B_1, B_2, B_3, B_5, B_6, FOLATE, B_{12})

Evidence highlights the importance of the B vitamins in osteoporosis, which is no surprise when one considers their vast therapeutic actions and applications within the body. The Rotterdam Study revealed that increased dietary intake of riboflavin and pyridoxine was associated with higher femoral neck bone density,[417] while in other studies low serum folate and pyridoxine have been associated with an altered cancellous bone structure.[418] Vitamin B_{12} is thought to stimulate osteoblast activity and bone formation.[391] A meta-analysis of 7475 individuals in 4 prospective studies showed a 4% lower fracture risk for each 50 pmol/L increase in vitamin B_{12} concentration (RR: 0.96; 95% CI: 0.92, 1.00). Among older adults in the Framingham Osteoporosis Study, plasma vitamin B_{12} concentrations <200 pg/mL (148 pmol/L) compared with higher concentrations were significantly associated with lower BMD. In NHANES III participants, BMD was lower and osteoporosis significantly more likely ($P < 0.01$) with increasing serum methylmalonic acid (MMA), a functional indicator of vitamin B_{12} inadequacy.[400] Deficiency of vitamin B_{12} is also associated with a decreased bone mass through increased osteoclast formation. This is believed to be caused by increased methylmalonic acid and homocysteine levels,[419] leading to risk factors for reduced

SAMPLE DAILY DIET

BREAKFAST	
Green smoothie: banana, avocado, kale, flaxseed	Banana, avocado and kale are all rich in magnesium, calcium, potassium and vitamin K. High consumption of plant-based foods is recommended due to their low acid load and high potassium content. Low acid load is correlated with lower bone resorption and higher BMD. Unlike spinach, kale exhibits excellent absorbability for its calcium.
LUNCH	
Sardines with tahini, zucchini pasta	Sardines consumed with the bone are a source of calcium and omega-3 fatty acids. By consuming them with plenty of vegetables, low acid load of the diet is maintained, reducing leaching of minerals from the bone to maintain homeostasis.
DINNER	
Turmeric tempeh with broccoli and bok choy	Observational and epidemiological studies suggest that dietary intake of fermented soy products can attenuate menopause-induced osteoporotic bone loss by decreasing bone resorption and stimulating bone formation. Plant proteins are favoured over animal proteins as animal proteins are associated with increased fracture risk. Tempeh is an excellent source of vitamin K_2 which is required for bone health. Curcumin is highly antioxidant and reduces osteoclastogenesis as a result of increased antioxidant activity and impaired RANKL signalling.
SNACK	
6 prunes Kiwi fruit	Daily consumption of 50 g of dried plum (equivalent to 5–6 dried plums) for 6 months was shown to be as effective in preventing bone loss in older, osteopenic postmenopausal women, compared to the placebo group. Kiwi fruit is rich in vitamin C, magnesium, calcium and vitamin K, all of which are required for bone health.

Sources: Heaney RP, Weaver CM. Calcium absorption from kale. Am J Clin Nutr 1990; 51(4):656–657. Hooshmand S, Arjmandi BH. Viewpoint: dried plum, an emerging functional food that may effectively improve bone health. Ageing Res Rev 2009; 8(2):122–127. Wynn E, Krieg MA, Lanham-New SA et al. Postgraduate Symposium: Positive influence of nutritional alkalinity on bone health. Proc Nutr Soc 2010; 69(1):166–173.

bone mineral density and increased fracture risk.[419] Hyperhomocysteinaemia occurs as a result of decreased quantities of B vitamins (especially B_6, folate and B_{12}) and has been linked to osteoporosis[420] and increased risk of hip fractures.[421] It appears to disturb cross-linking of collagen by accumulating in the bone-stimulating osteoclasts towards bone resorption.[422]

BORON

Boron is a trace element thought to play an important role in bone health, preventing the loss of calcium stores from the bone, reducing magnesium excretion via the urine and inhibiting bone demineralisation.[423] Although there is plenty of information available about the effect of boron on bone health, little has been published in the way of human clinical trials.

CALCIUM

Approximately 99% of the body's calcium stores are found within the skeleton, where it forms the structure of the bone.[375] A number of studies have been undertaken to assess the efficacy of calcium supplementation in osteoporosis. A meta-analysis carried out by Tang et al[424] in 2007 involving 29 randomised trials found good evidence to support the use of calcium, or calcium in combination with vitamin D supplementation, over a treatment period of approximately 3.5 years in the preventive treatment of osteoporosis in people aged 50 years or older. The authors suggest for best therapeutic effect a minimum dose of 1200 mg/day of calcium and 800 IU/day of vitamin D should be taken. In 2008, Reid et al[425] repeated this meta-analysis, but focused on hip fractures. In stark contrast to the earlier meta-analysis, they found that calcium supplementation (in isolation) actually increased the risk of hip fractures. With such results it is understandable that there is some confusion. Does calcium increase or decrease risk of fractures? Looking in detail at these studies, it can be seen that there is actually only one randomised controlled trial and one observational study suggesting that calcium may increase hip fractures. The numerous studies reporting a beneficial effect as presented in the meta-analysis by Tang et al would appear to far outweigh these. This does, however, bring up an interesting point: should vitamins and minerals be taken in isolation? It is known that the many vitamins and minerals work synergistically; perhaps calcium also is one of the major players?

Another important point to consider is the form of calcium prescribed. There are many different forms of calcium for the practitioner to choose from, each with its own positives and negatives. Some forms of calcium are absorbed better than others. For example, research in women with postmenopausal osteoporosis found that calcium citrate had a better bioavailability than calcium carbonate.[426] Factors such as these may explain the variation in results seen in clinical trials. As noted by Shangraw,[427] the solubility of many calcium salts is dependent upon pH. Thus the type of calcium used, the condition of the patient and the time of administration should all be considered. Calcium citrate may be taken without food and may be useful for patients with achlorhydria or those who are taking histamine-2 blockers or protein-pump inhibitors.[375] Calcium carbonate, on the other hand, is not recommended for patients with achlorhydria and should be consumed with meals[427] as absorption of calcium is increased in an acidic environment (such as when the stomach is breaking down food). Calcium supplements that dissolve slowly and are taken on an empty stomach are likely to be insoluble.

Absorption of calcium appears to be best when taken in a dose of 500 mg/day or less.[428] Most importantly, when choosing a calcium supplement the elemental content (rather than the total) content is the most important consideration.

ESSENTIAL FATTY ACIDS (EPA, DHA, GLA)

Inflammatory mediators such as PGE_2, leukotriene B_4, IL-1 and TNF have all been shown to promote the resorption of bone.[429] Omega-3 fatty acids, however, display an inhibitory role against these agents[306] and may thus prevent the resorption of bone, playing a key role in regulating the activity of osteoblasts and osteoclasts.

A randomised, double-blind, placebo-controlled trial investigated the effects of omega-3 PUFA supplementation on bone turnover markers and red blood cell (RBC) fatty acid levels in older postmenopausal women. One hundred and twenty-six postmenopausal women (mean age 75±7 years) were treated with omega-3 PUFA (1200 mg EPA/DHA/day, $n = 85$) or placebo (olive oil, $n = 41$) for 6 months. All women received 315 mg calcium citrate and 1000 IU cholecalciferol. Bone-specific alkaline phosphatase and osteocalcin decreased in the omega-3 PUFA group ($P < 0.05$). Bone turnover decreased with omega-3 PUFA, but not statistically compared to placebo. RBC DHA increased in the omega-3 PUFA group, compared to no change in the placebo group ($P < 0.001$). The ratio of DHA+EPA:arachidonic acid increased by 42 % in the omega-3 PUFA group and by 5% in the placebo group ($P < 0.001$). Short-term omega-3 PUFA supplementation increased RBC concentrations of DHA and omega-3:omega-6 ratios.[430]

GLUCOSAMINE, CHONDROITIN AND GREEN-LIPPED MUSSEL

Glucosamine is well known for its effects in the treatment of arthritic symptoms and it also appears to be beneficial in osteoporosis. In-vitro studies reveal the ability of glucosamine sulfate to increase alkaline phosphatase activity (a marker for osteoblast formation), collagen synthesis, osteocalcin secretion and mineralisation in osteoblastic cells. Glucosamine also exerts anti-inflammatory effects against inflammatory mediators, protecting against catabolism in osteoblasts.

The beneficial effects of chondroitin and green-lipped mussel on the health of the joints have been previously discussed in the section on osteoarthritis. For these reasons, chondroitin and green-lipped mussel should be recommended in osteoporosis, recalling that the joints function as the union between two or more bones. If the joints are not strong and durable they will not be able to support the bones.

MAGNESIUM

Magnesium is the second most abundant intracellular cation found within the vertebrate body,[431] where it is involved in a number of activities supporting bone strength, preservation and remodelling. While much is made of the relationship between calcium and osteoporosis, magnesium has not received the same degree of exposure. Given its role in the bone as well as the fact that deficiency is associated with a number of conditions including osteoporosis,[431] its importance should not be underestimated.

The average dietary intake of magnesium is low and magnesium is believed to be excreted rapidly. This suggests that a large percentage of the population is deficient. In one study, magnesium levels in red blood cells were found to be significantly lower in postmenopausal women with osteoporosis than in those who did not have osteoporosis.[432]

Magnesium supplementation in people with osteoporosis has produced promising results; Aydin et al[433] observed that short-term oral administration of magnesium citrate (1830 mg/day for 1 month) suppressed bone turnover in a small study involving 10 postmenopausal osteoporotic women. In a review, Dreosti[434] reports on magnesium supplementation for 2 years in Israeli postmenopausal women diagnosed with osteoporosis. Trabecular bone density increased (up to 8%) and bone loss was arrested in 87% of women. In some cases, both an increase in bone density and arrested bone loss occurred. In comparison, the control group lost on average 1% of bone density per year. Similar benefits were reported in another study of postmenopausal women in Czechoslovakia. After 2 years of supplementation with magnesium, nearly 65% were classified totally free of pain and with no further deformity of vertebrae, with the condition in the remainder either arrested or slightly improved.

As yet, the majority of these studies have been undertaken in women, but given the growing number of men diagnosed with osteoporosis, trials assessing the effects of magnesium in men with low bone mass are welcomed.

SILICA

In animals, deficiency of silica is associated with malformations in the skull and peripheral bones, poorly formed joints, reduced contents of cartilage, collagen and alterations in the mineral balance of the femur and vertebrae of the body.[435] Hence supplementation in osteoarthritis, which is synonymous with many of these same features would appear logical. A number of human studies examining supplementation with silica have displayed positive results, revealing silica to increase bone mineral density within the spine,[436] femur[437] and hips;[438,439] although the latter is only in premenopausal women not postmenopausal, it may be suggestive of an interaction between silica and oestrogen.[440] The exact mechanism by which silica exerts its effects in the bone is undetermined but appears to be in some part due to synthesis or stabilisation of collagen.[440]

ZINC

Lower levels of zinc have been found in vegetarian and vegan diets. Lower serum and bone zinc have been noted in patients with osteoporosis. In a 2-year controlled trial, postmenopausal women were randomly assigned to treatment with calcium plus copper and zinc compared with calcium plus corn starch, with usual daily zinc intakes <8.0 mg. The patients benefited from the copper and zinc supplements. Although zinc is found in nuts, beans and wholegrains, the phytate in these foods makes zinc less bioavailable than it is from animal-based sources. Higher intakes of these foods may be needed to meet dietary requirements. The US Food and Nutrition Board recommends at least 50% more zinc for those who obtain it from vegetarian sources. Supplementation may be required.[400]

VITAMIN C

Vitamin C plays an important structural role within the bone,[441] where it is required for the collagen linking that occurs in fibrils of the bone. Vitamin C also encourages the activity of alkaline phosphatase, required for the formation of osteoblasts. Studies have shown that both dietary vitamin C and vitamin C from supplements is associated with a beneficial effect on levels of bone density in postmenopausal women,[442,443] especially when used concurrently with calcium supplements. As expected, vitamin C also exerts a protective role in males, with intake associated with lower 4-year bone loss in elderly men.[444] In the Framingham Study, people in the highest tertile of total vitamin C intake had significantly fewer hip fractures ($P = 0.04$) and non-vertebral fractures ($P = 0.05$) compared to those in the lowest tertile of intake. People in the highest category of supplemental vitamin C intake had significantly fewer hip fractures ($P = 0.02$) and non-vertebral fractures ($P = 0.07$) compared to non-supplement users.[445]

VITAMIN D

Adequate vitamin D intake is an integral component of osteoporosis management because of its key role in maintaining the physiology of the bone. Vitamin D assists calcium and phosphorus absorption, both of which are vital for the normal development of bones. Vitamin D insufficiency has been found in those with fractures. In one study 96% of women with a hip fracture were also found to have insufficient vitamin D levels.[446]

Vitamin D deficiency has many serious consequences for overall health and wellbeing. It is associated with muscle weakness, predominantly of the proximal muscle groups, manifested by feelings of heaviness in the legs, tiring easily, difficulty in escalating stairs and rising from a chair or seated position. Supplementation with vitamin D has been found to improve muscle strength, walking distance, functional ability and body sway in elderly people with vitamin D deficiency and muscle weakness. These findings and the observed improvements in bone density after vitamin D supplementation, provide an explanation for the association between vitamin D supplementation and fewer falls and non-vertebral fractures in elderly people.[447]

The protective effects of vitamin D have undergone much study. Results from a Cochrane systematic review found that vitamin D supplementation, while unlikely to prevent a fracture when given alone, was likely to reduce fractures in institutionalised older people when given together with calcium.[448]

A meta-analysis of primary prevention high-quality trials published in 2005 found that oral cholecalciferol (D_3) in a daily dose of 700–800 IU or intermittently 100 000 IU every 4 months with or without calcium, should reduce both hip and non-vertebral fracture risk significantly compared with placebo in ambulatory or institutionalised elderly persons.[449]

Another meta-analysis, this time involving nine studies and assessing the effect of vitamin D on the risk of falls and fractures, revealed a trend towards a reduction in the risk of falls among participants given vitamin D compared with placebo.[450] Other studies reveal that vitamin D (1000 IU) taken with calcium can slow or prevent bone loss in osteoporosis.[451]

A 5-year Australian study of 120 community-dwelling women found that the addition of vitamin D (1000 IU) to calcium (1200 mg) lowered parathyroid hormone levels and maintained bone mineral density of the hip at 3, 7 and 5 years. The authors concluded that vitamin D has long-term beneficial effects on bone density in elderly women living in a sunny climate, probably mediated by a long-term reduction in bone turnover rate.[452]

VITAMIN K

Phylloquinone (vitamin K_1) is the major type of dietary vitamin K and is consumed in the diet especially from green leafy vegetables, whereas menaquinone-4 (vitamin K_2) is the major form of vitamin K in the tissues, including bone. Vitamin K_2 is synthesised by bacteria in the intestines. A number of foods also contain vitamin K_2, notably natto (fermented soy beans), cheese and curds, with natto being the richest source of vitamin K known.[453] Vitamin K_2 regulates bone remodelling, an important process necessary to maintain adult bone. Bone remodelling involves removal of old or damaged bone by osteoclasts and its replacement by new bone formed by osteoblasts.[454] Vitamin K_2 is a cofactor of gamma-carboxylase. Gamma-carboxylase converts the glutamic acid (Glu) residue in osteocalcin molecules to gamma-carboxyglutamic acid (Gla) that is essential for gamma-carboxylation of osteocalcin. Vitamin K_2 sustains lumbar BMD and prevents osteoporotic fractures in patients with age-related osteoporosis. It prevents vertebral fractures in patients with glucocorticoid-induced osteoporosis, increases the metacarpal BMD in the paralytic upper extremities of patients with cerebrovascular disease and sustains the lumbar BMD in patients with liver-dysfunction-induced osteoporosis. Vitamin K deficiency may contribute to osteoporotic fractures.[455] A randomised clinical intervention study was conducted among 325 postmenopausal women receiving either 45 mg/day of vitamin K_2 (MK-4, menatetrenone) or placebo for 3 years. The daily dose of MK-4 was given as a 15 mg capsule 3 times daily, preferably after a meal. Bone mineral content and hip geometry were assessed by DXA. Bone strength indices were calculated from DXA-BMD, femoral neck width and hip axis length. The bone mineral content of the femoral neck in the MK-4 group decreased at a significantly lower rate than in the placebo group. A statistically significant effect of vitamin K treatment was observed on the serum concentrations of carboxylated osteocalcin and under-carboxylated osteocalcin. Total osteocalcin and bone-specific alkaline phosphatase, markers of bone formation, were also significantly higher in the MK-4 group as compared to placebo.[456] High-dose vitamin K is needed to prevent fractures in postmenopausal women with osteoporosis.[453]

VITAMIN E

Oxidative stress has been suggested to play a role in the pathogenesis of osteoporosis and has been found to be increased in both men[457] and women[458] with osteoporosis. Vitamin E is known for its antioxidant action and ability to scavenge free radicals. In elderly men, high oxidative stress is associated with reduced bone mineral density, which is more pronounced in individuals with low serum levels of the antioxidant vitamin E.[459] Animal studies have indicated that vitamin E may be able to improve bone material and structure,[460] so studies in humans, which are currently lacking, are warranted to further investigate the protective effects of vitamin E in bone health.

DOSAGE REQUIREMENTS

The dosage requirements listed below are based on adult doses that have been reported in the literature.

- B complex (all B vitamins) high-dose combination, preferably activated forms:
  - Thiamine 20–50 mg/day
  - Riboflavin 50 mg/day. Riboflavin 5′-phosphate 20–50 mg/day
  - Niacinamide/nicotinic acid 50–150 mg/day
  - Pantothenic acid 150–250 mg/day
  - Pyridoxine 50–100 mg/day. Pyridoxal 5′-phosphate 20–50 mg/day
  - Folic acid 500–1000 micrograms/day as folinic acid or L-5MTHF determined by the methylation status of the patient
  - Hydroxo- or methylcobalamin 500–1000 micrograms/day determined by the methylation status of the patient
  - Choline 150 mg/day
  - Inositol 150 mg/day
  - Biotin 500 micrograms/day
- Boron 3–5 mg/day[179]
- Calcium 800–2000 mg/day (estimate dietary intake and supplement the difference to reach the total)
- Vitamin K (especially K_2) 150–400 micrograms/day with some studies going up to the dose of 45 mg/day (however, use caution with high doses until research supports the higher dosage range)[453]
- Essential fatty acids: 1000–2000 mg/day DHA and EPA[461]
- Glucosamine 1500 mg/day
- Chondroitin 800–1200 mg
- Green-lipped mussel 1500–3000 mg in acute condition followed by 500–2000 mg as maintenance
- Magnesium 400–800 mg/day[179]
- Silica 28 mg/day for 4 weeks[436]
- Vitamin D 800–5000 IU/day (consider higher — depending on pathology results)
- Vitamin C at least 750 mg/day
- Vitamin E 600 mg (900 IU)/day.[92]

HERBAL MEDICINE

Herbal medicine therapeutic objectives

- Provide symptomatic relief from pain and inflammation
- Reduce oxidative stress
- Increase circulation, remove wastes and eliminate toxins
- Support renal and hepatobiliary function to optimise vitamin D hydroxylation and activation
- Optimise digestive function, increase HCl and enzyme release to increase nutrient absorption
- Improve hormonal receptor activity (sex dependent).

Herbal medicine classes

- Analgesic/anodyne
- Anti-inflammatory and antirheumatic
- Antioxidant
- Circulatory stimulant
- Nutritive/bone builder
- Depuratives and alteratives
- Renal tonics
- Hepatics and hepatotrophorestoratives
- Digestive tonics — bitters, GI tract anti-inflammatory, GI tract demulcent, GI tract antiseptic, HCl balancer, mucous membrane trophorestoratives
- Oestrogen or testosterone receptor modulating
- Antioxidant/flavonoid-rich — proanthocyanidin- and anthocyanidin-rich herbal medicines.

Specific herbal medicines

APIUM GRAVEOLENS (CELERY)

Apium graveolens has been used traditionally to neutralise the body of acidity and to ease rheumatic pain.[462] The latter action makes it particularly useful for rheumatic pain associated with osteoporosis. As yet there are no human studies examining the effects of *Apium graveolens* in osteoporosis in human clinical studies, however recent research[392] suggests the benefits of nutritional alkalinity on bone health. The Western diet is thought to increase risk of osteoporosis due to the excess of acidic foods, therefore *Apium graveolens*, which is generally considered to be an alkalising herb, could be beneficial in this way.

BOSWELLIA SERRATA (BOSWELLIA)

It has been suggested that increased pro-inflammatory cytokines in the body, such as IL-1, IL-6 and TNF-α, are associated with decreased bone mass and greater fracture risk, but the totality of evidence is limited.[463] If inflammation is an important risk factor for osteoporosis then use of botanicals such as *Boswellia serrata* would surely be useful; *Boswellia serrata* displays anti-inflammatory actions and has been observed to be clinically effective in a number of inflammatory conditions.[464] It also exhibits analgesic[465] effects specific to the musculoskeletal system and thus may be useful in relieving pain associated with osteoporosis.

CAPSICUM SPP. (CAYENNE, CHILLI)

Capsaicin is an alkaloid and the irritant constituent within chilli and cayenne that has been found to modulate perception of pain by depleting stores of substance P from within small nociceptor sensory neurons.[466] As yet there are no clinical trials examining the efficacy of *Capsicum* spp. in the treatment of pain associated with osteoporosis, but its mode of action and the results seen in clinical practice suggest it may be useful, particularly in those that present with cold, damp constitutions, who would benefit from its warming circulatory stimulant action.

CORYDALIS AMBIGUA (CORYDALIS)

Pain is a common symptom in osteoporosis, probably caused by osteoporotic bone fractures and musculoskeletal malfunctioning. *Corydalis ambigua* displays analgesic properties and thus may be useful to ease pain associated with osteoporosis. The rhizome of *Corydalis ambigua*, as one component of a traditional Chinese medicine formulation known as 'Gusong II', has been used successfully to inhibit bone resorption and decrease urinary excretion of calcium in menopausal osteoporosis.[467] Because of the other herbs used in this formulation, it is impossible to reach conclusions on the individual action of *Corydalis ambigua* with regard to bone resorption in osteoporosis, but as an adjuvant it appears to be a useful botanical to ease symptoms associated with osteoporosis.

CURCUMA LONGA (TURMERIC)

The nuclear transcription factor NF-κB acts to regulate DNA and when improperly activated it has been shown to mediate inflammation and has been linked to several inflammatory disorders as well as osteoporosis. Curcumin, the active constituent within *Curcuma longa*, exerts significant anti-inflammatory and antioxidant actions and has been shown in experimental studies to block the pathway that activates NF-κB, thereby preventing inflammation.[468] Curcumin has also been observed to prevent osteoclastogenesis,[468] and osteoclast differentiation and activation[469] a process linked with bone loss, further highlighting a possible role in the management of osteoporosis. There are very few clinical studies in humans investigating the effect of curcumin on osteoporosis. Because osteoporosis is asymptomatic and does not directly lead to mortality, clinical research may need to focus on fracture risk.[469]

DIOSCOREA SPP. (WILD YAM)

Dioscorea villosa contains lycoside and steroidal saponins, including diosgenin and dioscin, alkaloids, tannins and phytosterols constituents.[470] Interestingly, another name for this botanical is 'rheumatism root',[470] which suggests an effect on the musculoskeletal system. *Dioscorea villosa* has been proposed to have an oestrogenic effect because of the theoretical ability of its steroidal saponins to bind to oestrogen receptors.[470] As a result of this action it may be used by herbalists in menopausal/postmenopausal women to support oestrogen levels, thus minimising the bone loss associated with hormonal changes in menopause. Although no studies have been undertaken examining the effects of *Dioscorea* spp. in isolation to reduced loss of bone mass, as part of a formulation known as 'Drynol Cibotin', *Dioscorea* in combination with seven other botanicals (used in traditional Chinese medicine for the management of osteoporosis) has been found to increase cell proliferation and inhibit apoptosis in osteoblasts.[471]

ESCHSCHOLZIA CALIFORNICA (CALIFORNIAN POPPY)

As the body becomes more kyphotic, other tissue structures, such as the muscles and ligaments, adapt to support the body. Usually, this is beyond their normal role and results in great pain. Pain may also be experienced where fractures occur. As yet there have been no clinical studies assessing *Eschscholzia californica* for relief of osteoporotic pain, but this herb has demonstrated analgesic effects[125] in other conditions and thus may be useful as an analgesic in osteoporosis. Where a patient presents with concurrent anxiety, which is not uncommon due to the fear of possible fracture and the impact of the condition on quality of life,[472] *Eschscholzia californica* is also indicated for its anxiolytic action.

HARPAGOPHYTUM PROCUMBENS (DEVIL'S CLAW)

Bone pain has been suggested to be the most common symptom in patients with osteoporosis[473] and any botanicals that assist in relieving pain associated with osteoporosis are likely to be well received by the patient, particularly as herbal analgesics are unlikely to come with the same side effects as mainstream analgesics. *Harpagophytum procumbens* has been used successfully in a number of musculoskeletal disorders, including acute lower back pain, probably because of its analgesic, anti-inflammatory and antirheumatic actions. This suggests a possible role for its application in pain associated with osteoporosis, particularly back pain associated with vertebral osteoporosis.[474] The anti-inflammatory actions of Devil's claw include the reduction of inflammatory cytokines (IL-6, IL-1β and TNF-α), PGE2, COX-2 inhibition and NO and the modulation of arachidonic acid metabolism and eicosanoid biosynthesis.[475]

SALIX SPP. (WILLOW BARK)

Extracts of various *Salix* species have been recommended for rheumatic complaints and pain disorders[476] and because of its anti-inflammatory and mild analgesic effects it may be useful in relieving symptoms such as pain associated with osteoporosis. Results from a study undertaken with a specific *Salix* extract indicate that it might exert its analgesic effects via inhibition of pro-inflammatory cytokines as well as inhibition of COX-2-mediated PGE_2 release, however this appears to occur through compounds other than salicin or salicylate.[477]

ZANTHOXYLUM CLAVA-HERCULIS (PRICKLY ASH)

Zanthoxylum clava-herculis is a gentle circulatory stimulant that contains alkaloids, lignans, tannins, resins and volatile oil.[478] It may be useful in osteoporosis because of its ability to stimulate blood flow. Increased blood flow to osteoporotic areas of the body ensures supply of oxygen and much needed nutrients to the bones and joints to aid in their growth and repair.

ZINGIBER OFFICINALE (GINGER)

Like *Zanthoxylum clava-herculis* above, *Zingiber officinale* may be useful in osteoporosis because of its circulatory stimulant action, whereby it increases blood flow around the body, assisting in the flow of nutrients and the removal of wastes. Ginger also has anti-inflammatory, antiplatelet and carminative effects.[479] The anti-inflammatory effects of ginger include modulation of leukotriene and prostaglandin synthesis and inhibition of NF-κB. Ginger may also be useful for chronic pain management in clinical practice.[475]

LIFESTYLE RECOMMENDATIONS

Exercise

Exercise prior to puberty has a positive association with bone growth compared with children of the same age who did not exercise. Additionally, exercise during adulthood has been shown to prevent bone loss.[480] Two types of exercises are especially important for maintaining bone density:

- Weight-bearing exercises in which bones and muscles work against gravity[481]
- Resistance training in which muscular strength is used to improve muscle mass and bone strength.[482]

Numerous studies suggest exercise to be beneficial in osteoporosis, but some may be better than others. For example, a meta-analysis involving eight studies assessing walking for preservation of bone mineral density in postmenopausal women found it useful for preserving bone mass at the neck but not at the spine.[483] Yoga has been found to have a positive effect on pain, physical functions, social functions, general health perception and balance in postmenopausal women with osteoporosis.[484] Tai chi may positively affect risks associated with low bone density, such as reduced fall frequency, musculoskeletal strength and neuromuscular coordination.[485,486]

Sunlight

Sunlight exposure for vitamin D synthesis should be appropriate for skin type, with protection advised against skin cancers while ensuring adequate exposure for vitamin D.

Acupuncture and cupping

Treatment with acupuncture/cupping therapy three times a week for 3 months was found to improve quality of life in patients with osteoporosis.[487]

Smoking

Cessation of smoking is recommended to preserve bone mineral density. Ex-smokers experience reduced risk of fractures compared with those who actively smoke, but still have more risk than those who have never smoked.[385]

CASE STUDY

OVERVIEW

DJ, a 48-year-old woman, presented to the clinic with early osteoporosis (diagnosed via bone mineral density). Her mother and aunt have osteoporosis. Menarche was 16 years of age. She typically has low physical activity levels as a result of working in an office. She works in finance and there is pressure in the office for all staff to reach their KPIs earlier than required. Her stress levels at work (9/10) can seep into her personal life where she finds it hard to wind down and relax. Analysis of her diet shows low intake of calcium, magnesium, zinc and protein. Upon further questioning, she revealed that she competed in a number of sports in her teenage years. She felt a lot of pressure to perform at a high level. She was conscious of her body image and weight around that time due to competition of the sports she was playing and athletics and competing with other girls about appearance. There was a culture of bullying and exclusion if girls didn't conform to the group.

Her previous history showed low immunity in her 20s. She was later diagnosed with postviral syndrome.

CLINICAL EXAMINATION

BP 120/82 mmHg
Pulse 70 bpm
Height 1.72 m
Weight 64 kg
BMI 21.63 kg/m^2
Nails indicated marked calcium deficiencies as they had several white dots on the thumb, index and middle finger nails. The nails were weak and easily chipped.
Her face was pale and dry. There were 2 vertical lines between the eye brows.
She had pale conjunctiva.

TREATMENT PROTOCOL

Initial consultation was to reduce her stress levels and increase her bone mineral density.

PATHOLOGY

- Repeat bone mineral density in 3 months
- Vitamin D level
- Liver function test
- Urea, electrolytes, creatinine, eGFR
- Cholesterol (total cholesterol, HDL, LDL, VLDL).

OTHER

- Diet diary to investigate her diet deeper for nutritional deficiencies and to review her diet from her 20s and 30s to assess nutritional status
- Assessment of lifestyle exposure to heavy metals.

CASE STUDY CONTINUED

INITIAL APPOINTMENT

HERBAL MEDICINE

Herbal medicine	Extract	Quantity	Justification
Passiflora incarnata	1:2	60 mL	Nervine, analgesic
Harpagophytum procumbens	1:2	80 mL	Analgesic, anti-inflammatory, antirheumatic
Taraxacum officinale (root)	1:2	40 mL	Hepatic, cholagogue, digestive tonic
Glycyrrhiza glabra	1:1	30 ml	Adaptogen, anti-inflammatory, hepatic
Zingiber officinale	1:5	10 mL	Circulatory stimulant, anti-inflammatory, carminative
TOTAL		220 mL	

Dose: 7.5 mL b.i.d.

NUTRITIONAL MEDICINE

Dietary

- 1 heaped teaspoon of *Curcuma longa* mixed into natural yoghurt daily.
- Avoid dietary factors that promote calcium excretion: salt, sugar, animal protein, soft drinks, coffee, alcohol, tannin-containing beverages (tea, red wine).
- Investigate food allergies and intolerance and appropriately modify the diet.
- Investigate and correct nutritional deficiencies.
- Increase food sources that optimise nutrients for bone building — especially calcium-rich foods.
- Increase consumption of green leafy vegetables, cashews, almonds, Brazil nuts, walnuts to increase mineral intake for bone mineral density (calcium, magnesium, manganese, potassium, zinc).
- Encourage wholefood dietary principles that provide optimal nutrient levels.

Supplemental

- Boron 3 mg/day
- Calcium 500 mg t.d.s.
- Magnesium 250 mg t.d.s.
- Zinc 25 mg t.d.s.
- Vitamin D 1000 IU t.d.s.
- Vitamin K2 180 micrograms t.d.s.
- Omega-3 EPA 600 mg t.d.s. and DHA 400 mg t.d.s.
- Glutamine 5000 mg in water b.i.d.
- Taurine 500 mg b.i.d. (to increase calcium absorption).

LIFESTYLE/EDUCATION

- Movement and stretching to be encouraged, e.g. yoga.

CASE STUDY CONTINUED

- A 15–20 minute walk daily to increase muscle strength, increase circulation and to destress.
- Daily exposure to sunlight before 10 am or after 4 pm (minimum of 20 minutes per day).
- A time out for 15 minutes per day to manage stress. This can be increased to twice per day. It was suggested that she took a time out any time she feels stressed.

FOLLOW-UP

After 4 weeks, she felt her stress levels at work had decreased from 9/10 to 7–8/10. She was not taking her work stress home with her as often. She mentioned that her muscular aches had reduced from 8/10 to 6/10. When asked why she didn't discuss this at the initial consultation, she replied that she had the muscular aches for over 10 years and it was a 'normal part of life'.

RHEUMATOID ARTHRITIS

Epidemiology

Gender may be an influential factor as rheumatoid arthritis occurs more frequently in women than men with a ratio of approximately 1 : 3. Genetic and hormonal factors have been suggested to account for this difference.[488] Although rheumatoid arthritis can occur in younger people, its prevalence generally increases with age.

Classification

Rheumatoid arthritis (RA) is a chronic inflammatory disease characterised by joint swelling, joint tenderness and destruction of synovial joints (see Fig. 15.11), leading to severe disability and premature mortality.[489] See the following three boxes for more details.[489–491]

Royal Australian College of General Practitioners clinical guidelines for the diagnosis of rheumatoid arthritis

Rheumatoid arthritis is suspected if the following signs and symptoms are present:

- Morning stiffness in and around the joints, lasting for longer than 30 min
- Tenderness and swelling of three or more joints, including the elbows, wrists, hands, knees, ankles or feet, present for at least 6 weeks
- Symmetrical involvement of metacarpophalangeal or metatarsophalangeal joints; that is, both hands or both feet
- Positive blood test for rheumatoid factor and/or anti-CCP (anticyclic citrullinated peptide) antibodies
- Other causes ruled out (for example, infection).

Royal Australian College of General Practitioners. Rheumatoid arthritis clinical guidelines. Melbourne: RACGP; 2008. Available from: www.racgp.org.au/Content/NavigationMenu/ClinicalResources/RACGPGuidelines/Arthritis/RAguideline.pdf.

2010 American College of Rheumatology/European League Against Rheumatism classification criteria for rheumatoid arthritis

A. Joint distribution (0–5)	
1 large joint (e.g. shoulders, elbows, hips, knees and ankles)	0
2–10 large joints (as above)	1
1–3 small joints (e.g. metacarpophalangeal joints, proximal interphalangeal joints, second through fifth metatarsophalangeal joints, thumb interphalangeal joints and wrists)	2
4–10 small joints (as above)	3
>10 joints (at least 1 of the involved joints must be a small joint; the other joints can include any combination of large and additional small joints, as well as other joints not specifically listed elsewhere (e.g. temporomandibular, acromioclavicular, sternoclavicular)	5
B. Serology (0–3)	
Negative rheumatoid factor (RF) AND negative anticitrullinated protein antibody (ACPA)	0
Low positive RF OR low positive ACPA	2
High positive RF OR high positive ACPA	3
C. Symptom duration (0–1)	
<6 weeks	0
≥6 weeks	1
D. Acute phase reactants (0–1)	
Normal CRP AND normal ESR	0
Abnormal CRP OR abnormal ESR	1
E. Duration of symptoms*	
<6 weeks	0
≥6 weeks	1

*Duration of symptoms refers to patient self-report of the duration of signs or symptoms of synovitis (e.g. pain, swelling, tenderness) of joints that are clinically involved at the time of assessment, regardless of treatment status.

Classification criteria for RA (score-based algorithm: add score of categories A–D. A score of ≥6/10 is needed for classification of a patient as having definite RA.

Adapted from Aletaha D, Neogi T, Silman AJ et al. 2010 Rheumatoid arthritis classification criteria. Arthritis Rheum 2010; 62(9): 2569–2581.

American College of Rheumatology criteria for rheumatoid arthritis

Criteria	Definitions
Morning stiffness	Morning stiffness in and around the joints lasting at least 1 h before maximal improvement
Arthritis of three or more joint areas	Soft-tissue swelling or fluid (not bony overgrowth alone) observed by a physician in at least three joint areas simultaneously; the 14 possible joint areas (right or left) are: Proximal interphalangeal Metacarpophalangeal Wrist Elbow Knee Ankle Metatarsophalangeal
Arthritis of hand joints	At least one of wrist, metacarpophalangeal joint or proximal interphalangeal joint swollen as above
Symmetrical arthritis	Simultaneous involvement of the joint areas above on both sides of the body (bilateral involvement of proximal interphalangeal, metacarpophalangeal or metatarsophalangeal joints is acceptable without absolute symmetry)
Rheumatoid nodules	Subcutaneous nodules, over bony prominences or extensor surfaces or in juxta-articular regions, observed by a physician
Serum rheumatoid factor	Demonstration of abnormal amounts of serum rheumatoid factor by any method that has been positive in <5% of normal control subjects
Radiographic changes	Radiographic changes typical of rheumatoid arthritis on postero-anterior hand and wrist radiographs; changes must include erosions or unequivocal bony decalcification localised or most marked adjacent to the involved joints (osteoarthritis changes alone do not qualify)

For classification purposes, patients are said to have rheumatoid arthritis if they satisfy at least four of the above seven criteria. The first three criteria must be present for at least 6 weeks.

Brooks PM. Rheumatoid arthritis: aetiology and clinical features. Medicine 2006; 10(34):379–382.

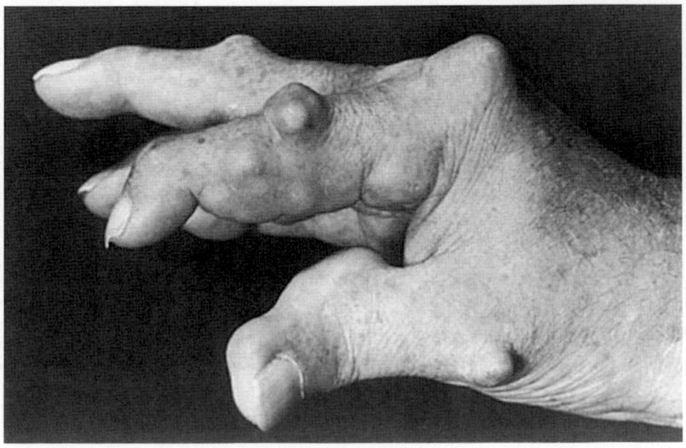

FIGURE 15.11 Rheumatoid arthritis.

Ferri's clinical advisor 2011. Mosby: 2010. From Canoso JJ. Rheumatology in primary care. Philadelphia: Saunders; 1997.

Aetiology

AUTOIMMUNITY

It is generally accepted that rheumatoid arthritis is an autoimmune condition, where the body's own immune system attacks itself due to a loss of ability to recognise self proteins from non-self proteins.[492] Autoimmunity and the overall systemic and articular inflammatory load drive the destructive progression of rheumatoid arthritis.[489] The T-cells appear to play a large part in this, driving the immune system to induce inflammation in the peripheral tissues (Fig. 15.12). For many years, rheumatoid arthritis was thought to primarily be a T-helper 1 (Th1)-mediated inflammatory autoimmune disease, but more recently B-cells have also been implicated in the pathogenesis, and rheumatoid arthritis is now suggested to occur as an abnormal interaction between the two.[493] The presence of autoantibodies, including IgM rheumatoid factor (RF) and anti-citrullinated protein antibodies (ACPA), would seem to confirm the autoimmune component of rheumatoid arthritis.

ALTERED BOWEL FLORA AND SMALL INTESTINAL BACTERIAL OVERGROWTH (SIBO)

Rheumatoid arthritis has been linked to alterations in normal gut physiology. Changes in small intestine microflora have been observed, including the presence of small intestinal bacterial overgrowth (SIBO),[494] and disease activity appears to be higher in patients with SIBO than in patients without. Patients with rheumatoid arthritis have also been observed to have a high rate of elevated faecal bacteria such as *Clostridium perfringens*[495] in comparison with healthy controls. Interestingly, alteration of the faecal bowel flora as a result of a raw vegan diet has been shown to result in reduced disease activity.[496]

PERMEABLE DIGESTIVE SYSTEM

The intestinal mucosa has been suggested to be abnormally permeable (increased intestinal permeability, colloquially known as 'leaky gut') and a site of absorption of antigens in rheumatoid arthritis.[497]

CIGARETTE SMOKING

Cigarette smoking appears to increase the risk of developing rheumatoid arthritis.[498–500] Polycyclic hydrocarbons from constituents of cigarette smoke appear able to induce pro-inflammatory cytokines from fibroblast-like synoviocytes in rheumatoid arthritis patients.[501]

DIET/FOOD ALLERGIES

Diet has been suggested to play a role in the development of inflammatory arthritis, particularly the presence of lectins.[492] While diet appears to play a role, the mechanisms by which it does so remain undetermined.

GENETICS

Genetic/hereditary susceptibility has been suggested to largely influence the development of rheumatoid arthritis. Analysis of British and Finnish populations suggest it may account for up to 60% of cases.[502] While one single gene has not been found that causes rheumatoid arthritis, a sequence polymorphism in the *HLA-DR B1* gene appears to be a strong genetic risk factor in several ethnic groups,[503,504] although clearly genetics alone do not completely explain the occurrence of the disease. Decreased activity of 5, 10-methylenetetrahydrofolate reductase (MTHFR) has been associated with rheumatoid arthritis.[505] A meta-analysis demonstrated that the MTHFR C677T polymorphism was involved in the genetic susceptibility of rheumatoid arthritis in Asian people, whereas the MTHFR A1298C polymorphism was associated with genetic susceptibility to rheumatoid arthritis in the overall population.[506] Research indicates that MTHFR polymorphism was associated with higher levels of TNF-α as well as high levels of homocysteine. Elevated homocysteine is commonly found in patients with rheumatoid arthritis. This may be partially responsible for the high rate of cardiovascular complications.[505] Research is indicating that patients with MTHFR polymorphism may not respond to or benefit from methotrexate treatment.[507]

MICROBIAL INFECTION

A number of studies have implicated microbial infection in the development of rheumatoid arthritis with a range of infective agents (in particular viruses) observed in patients, these include parvovirus B19, rubella, the hepatitis B and C viruses, Epstein-Barr virus,[508] cytomegalovirus[509] and mycoplasma.[510]

VACCINATION

Vaccination has also been noted as a trigger in some individuals.[511]

Overview

Rheumatoid arthritis is a classic example of a multifactorial disease in which an assortment of genetic and environmental factors contribute to the disease process. These are elaborated on and discussed throughout.

Pathogenesis

The pathogenesis of rheumatoid arthritis is an undetermined process, although it is known that it involves a complex interaction between inflammatory mediators, cytokines, growth factors, chemokines, adhesion molecules and the matrix metalloproteinases,[512] which appear to activate immune cells, transforming the synovium into an invasive structure known as the pannus.[512]

The synovium thickens substantially and there is oedema[512] (contributing to the stiffness seen in rheumatoid arthritis), increased vascularity, with increased proliferation and infiltration of macrophages, lymphocytes and plasma cells, sometimes with necrosis within the synovia.[386] Angiogenesis is active and leads to new blood vessels proliferating to provide for the hypertrophic synovium. The

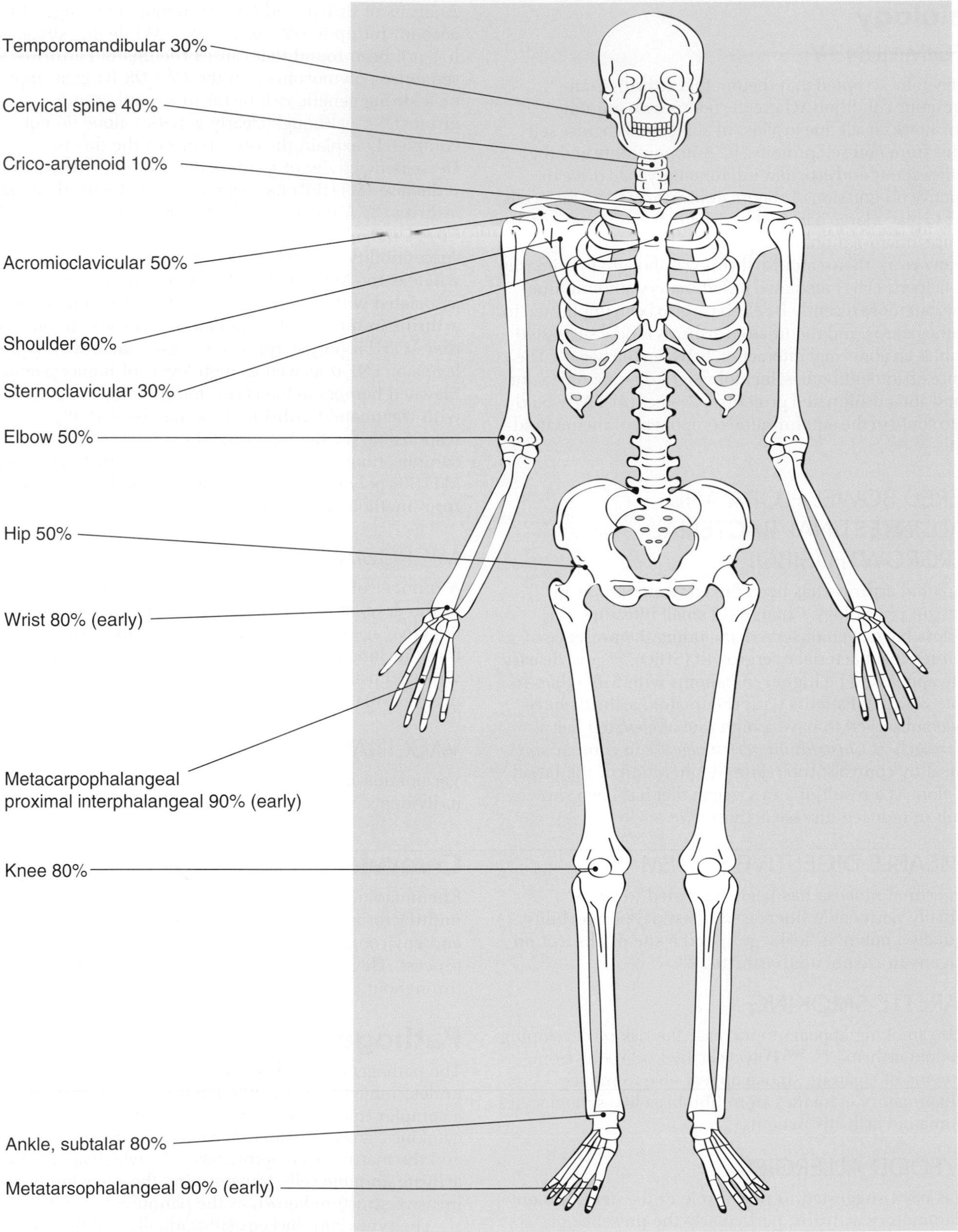

FIGURE 15.12 Involvement of joint sites in established rheumatoid arthritis.

Brooks PM. Rheumatoid arthritis: aetiology and clinical features. Medicine 2006; 10(34):379–382.

thickened synovium fills the joint spaces, invading the surfaces of the articular cartilage, subchondral bones, ligaments and tendons, causing destruction largely mediated by cytokine-induced degradative enzymes, notably the matrix metalloproteinases.[513] By invading and covering the musculoskeletal structures the pannus prevents synovial fluid from nourishing the articular cartilage and surrounding tissues and this results in erosion of the cartilage and bone and its subsequent destruction.

Activated T lymphocytes[514] and B lymphocytes[515] have both been implicated in rheumatoid arthritis, although the exact mechanism by which they function and the way in which they interact together in rheumatoid arthritis remains unclear.

SIGNS AND SYMPTOMS

Symptoms of rheumatoid arthritis include:

- Joint pain and swelling usually in the hands, knees and wrists (look for symmetry)
- Pain typically worse upon waking in the morning
- Stiffness
- Swelling
- Inflammation
- Warmth felt at and around joints
- Tenderness
- Limited or loss of range of movement (ROM)
- Fatigue
- Rheumatoid nodules (symmetrical polyarthritis lumps that appear under the skin near the joints).

COMPLICATIONS

The complications of rheumatoid arthritis are many and affect multiple body systems. Chronic inflammation of the joints leads to disability, deformity and may impact greatly on a person's quality of life. A number of comorbidities and increased mortality are also associated with rheumatoid arthritis. In particular, cardiovascular disease is associated with the disease as some studies have suggested that patients with rheumatoid arthritis have a two- to four-fold higher risk of developing a myocardial infarction than those without rheumatoid arthritis.[516,517]

Acknowledging the wide array of complications that may occur in rheumatoid arthritis (Table 15.13), it is prudent to maintain a holistic approach to patient assessment and care.

TABLE 15.13 Rheumatoid arthritis: extraarticular manifestations

Constitutional	Fever Asthenia Weight loss Malaise Anorexia
Cardiovascular	Vasculitis Pericardial inflammation Myocarditis Mitral valve disease Conduction defects
Respiratory	Pleural effusions Pulmonary nodules Interstitial fibrosis Pneumonitis Arteritis
Ophthalmic	Keratoconjunctivitis sicca Episcleritis Scleritis Conjunctivitis
Neurological	Compression neuropathy Mononeuritis multiplex Cervical myelopathy Central nervous system disease (stroke, seizure)
Skin	Distal leg ulcers Palmar erythema Cutaneous vasculitis
Haematological	Anaemia Thrombocytosis Granulocytopenia Eosinophilia Cryoglobulinaemia Hyperviscosity
Renal	Glomerulonephritis Vasculitis Secondary amyloidosis
Rheumatoid nodules	Subcutaneous Lung parenchymal
Hepatobiliary	Elevated liver enzymes

Source: Grassi W, De Angelis R, Lamanna G et al. The clinical features of rheumatoid arthritis. Eur J Radiol 1998; 27(Suppl. 1):S18–S24.

DIFFERENTIAL DIAGNOSIS[512,518]

Please see the comparison chart of differentiating patient presentations in Fig. 15.13.

Spondyloarthropathies

- Ankylosing spondylitis
- Enteric infections
- Inflammatory bowel disease
- Psoriatic arthritis
- Reiter's arthritis
- Whipple's disease.

Infectious causes

- Acute rheumatic fever
- Bacterial endocarditis
- Gonococcal arthritis
- Lyme disease
- Viral infections (parvovirus B19, HIV, hepatitis C).

Metabolic and endocrine causes

- Arthritis of thyroid disease
- Gout
- Haemochromatosis
- Haemoglobinopathies
- Pseudogout.

Patterns of illness

	1 Rheumatoid arthritis	2 Ankylosing spondylitis	3 Reiter's syndrome or Reactive arthritis	4 Psoriatic arthropathy	5 Arthritis of inflammatory bowel disease	6 Systemic lupus erythematosus	7 Fibrositis syndrome	8 Degenerative joint disease (osteoarthritis)	9 Gout (uratic)	10 Pseudogout (chondrocalcinosis)
Distribution of synovitis	Polyarticular symmetrical great and small joints including wrist and elbow	Axial-spinal and SIJ and ribs, usually spares small joints	Greater joints, IP toes, LE > UE	Polyarticular asymmetrical DIP, great and small joints, IP toes	Greater joints, LE > EU	Same as RA	Nonarticular, nonobjective	Polyarticular symmetrical great and small joints with DIP, CMC and lumbar spine, spares wrist and elbow	MTP 1 tarsus, ankle, knee	Knees, ankles, wrists, elbows
Persistence	+++	+++	+6 months	+++	+3 months	None, brief and episodic	+++	+++	Episodic attacks 1 week	Episodic attacks 1 week
Inflammation present	+++	+++	++	++	++	+	–	–	++	+
Rheumatoid factor	+ 80%	–	–	–	–	+15%	–	–	–	–
Antinuclear antibody	+ 20%	–	–	–	–	+>95%	–	–	–	–
SF	I	I	I	I	I	N to I	N of present	N	I MSU crystals	I CPPD crystals
SF complement	Low	N to high	N to high	N to high	N to high	Low		Low	N	N
Extraarticular features	Nodules, gel reaction	Heel pain, irritus	Keratodermia, geographic tongue, conjunctivitis urethritis, heel pain, Achilles tendinitis	Psoriasis vulgaris of skin or nails	Chronic ulcerative colitis, Crohn's disease, erythema nodosum	Skin, vascular, renal, pleuropulmonary, CNS, discoid lupus	Multiple tender points in muscle, chronic headache, irritable bowel	None	Tophi	None (calcific deposits in joint cartilage on x-ray)
Classic deformity	Ulnar deviation and volar subluxation	Stiffened posture, rigid neck, ribs and spine, kyphosis	None	Deflexed DIP joints, occasional mutilating	None	None occasional ulnar deviation MCP	None	Heberden's nodes, Bouchard's nodes, Bunions, exostoses	None	None; DJD is frequent
Hypertrophic change on x-ray	–	– Joints + periosteum	–	–	–	–	–	+++	–	+ DJD frequently
Erosive change on x-ray	+++	+	+ –	++	+	–	–	+	+	+
Ankylosis of joints on x-ray	+ –	+++	+ –	+ –	+	–	–	+	–	–
Sacroiliac erosions on x-ray	–	+95%	+ –	+30%	+30%	–	–	–	–	–
Psoriasis vulgaris	–	–90%	–	+99%	–	–	–	–	–	–
HLA-B27	6–8%	+94%	+60%	+30%	20%	6–8%	6–8%	6–8%	6–8%	6–8%
Anti-DNA	–	–	–	–	–	+ frequent	–	–	–	–

SIJ = sacroiliac joint; IP = interphalangeal; LE = lower extremities; UE = upper extremities; DIP = distal interphalangeal; RA = rheumatoid arthritis; CMC = carpometacarpal; MTP = metarsophalangeal; SF = synovial fluid; I = inflammatory; MSU = monosodium urate; CPPD = calcium pyrophosphate dihydrate; CNS = central nervous system; MCP = metacarpophalangeal; DJD = degenerative joint disease; HLA = human leucocyte antigen; N = similar to serum values.

FIGURE 15.13 Differentiating patient presentations.

Source: Mackenzie AH. Differential diagnosis of rheumatoid arthritis. Am J Med 1988; 85:(Suppl. A4).

Connective tissue diseases

- Acute relapsing symmetric seronegative synovitis
- Dermatomyositis
- Polymyalgia rheumatica
- Polymyositis
- Scleroderma
- Still's disease
- Systemic lupus erythematosus.

Other diseases that can mimic rheumatoid arthritis

- Amyloidosis
- Angio-immunoblastic lymphadenopathy
- Arthritis associated with oral contraceptives
- Malignancy
- Sarcoidosis.

NATUROPATHIC DIAGNOSIS

Naturopathic diagnosis relies on medical interpretation to conclude assessment, but it delves deep into causative and contributing factors. Consideration centres around a few key areas:

- Epigenetics, genetic susceptibility and ensuring that genes are not 'switched on'
- Abnormal bowel permeability, increased intestinal permeability, dysbiosis and SIBO
- Abnormal antibodies and immune complexes (investigate all options)
- Microbial hypotheses and underlying or triggering infection
- Decreased hormonal levels or hormonal imbalance (especially DHEA and cortisol)
- Food allergies — IgG or IgE response
- Free radical damage, oxidative stress and oxidation
- Dietary and nutritional deficiencies
- Lifestyle factors.

Investigations

The investigations used are summarised in Table 15.14.

RHEUMATOID FACTOR

While considered a primary diagnostic marker, rheumatoid factor is also associated with a number of other conditions (Table 15.15).

OTHER

The following additional medical professional tools are highly beneficial for both diagnosis and management of patients:

- DASS 28 Assessment Table (see Appendix 15.2)
- Health Assessment Questionnaire (HAQ-DI)© (see Appendix 15.3)
- Functional Assessment of Chronic Illness Therapy — Fatigue (see Appendix 15.4).

These tools are commonly used by medical professionals to measure joint function, quality of life and disease activity for people with rheumatoid arthritis. They are especially beneficial to use on a regular basis to ensure that changes and developments are acknowledged, with the modification of treatment protocols.

SPECIFIC NATUROPATHIC INVESTIGATIONS

Complete digestive stool analysis

This provides an overview of the components of digestion, absorption, intestinal function and microbial flora, as well as identifying pathogenic bacteria, parasites and yeasts. Useful due to the link between rheumatoid arthritis, GI tract pathogens and altered bowel permeability.

Intestinal permeability

This is a non-invasive method for assessing gastrointestinal mucosal integrity. Altered intestinal permeability has been linked to rheumatoid arthritis.

Functional liver detoxification profile

This supports accurate identification of the individual's detoxification profile and assists in the direction of treatment. It is particularly good when patients are taking medications that may impact liver function (e.g. methotrexate).

Essential fatty acids

EFAs provide the substrate for eicosanoids (prostaglandins) which play a vital role in the regulation of inflammatory conditions such as rheumatoid arthritis. A meta-analysis of studies of patients with long-standing rheumatoid arthritis indicated that omega-3 fish oil supplementation at doses supplying at least 2900 mg/day (EPA and DHA) decreased tender joint count and duration of morning stiffness. Omega-3 supplements can suppress production of pro-inflammatory lipids (PGE2 and leukotriene B4) and pro-inflammatory cytokines (TNF-α and interleukin-1β). An Australian RCT found that EPA was positively associated with time to remission (American College of Rheumatology criteria). Additionally, a one unit increase in plasma phospholipid EPA (as % of total fatty acids) was associated with a 12.2% increase in the probability of remission at any time during the study period ($P = 0.02$). Plasma phospholipids EPA+DHA was positively associated with time to remission.[519]

Therapeutic considerations

CLINICAL DECISION MAKING AND RATIONALE

Although current drug therapy may be effective in providing short-term benefit, it does not provide long-term benefits to patients with rheumatoid arthritis. There are numerous studies indicating that long-term health effects from medications and progression of disease degrades the body and shortens lifespan.

TABLE 15.14 Investigations for rheumatoid arthritis

Assessment	Justification
Antinuclear antibodies (ANA)	Elevated levels (positive result) suggest RA (as well as other conditions)
Antibodies to extractable nuclear antigens (ENA)	To eliminate other musculoskeletal conditions
HLA B27 antigen	Assesses autoimmune component
Erythrocyte sedimentation rate (ESR)	ESR will be increased in RA due to inflammation
C-reactive protein (CRP)	Assess inflammatory impact of condition
Rheumatoid factor (RF)	Diagnose RA and to distinguish it from other forms of arthritis and other conditions that cause similar symptoms of joint pain, inflammation and stiffness
The amount of RF in blood can be measured in three additional assessments:	
1. Agglutination tests	The most common method mixes the patient's blood with tiny latex beads covered with human antibodies (IgG). The latex beads clump or agglutinate if rheumatoid factor (IgM RF) is present. However, this method does not detect the presence of IgG or IgA RF
2. Nephelometry test	This method mixes the patient's blood with antibodies that cause the blood to clump if RF is present. A light is passed through the tube containing the mixture and an instrument measures how much light is blocked by the mixture. Higher levels of RF create a cloudier sample and allow less light to pass through, measured in units. This method will detect all isotypes of RF. The presence of RF is not diagnostic of RA because of its lack of specificity for RA
3. Cyclic citrullinated peptide antibodies	Diagnostic and prognostic rheumatoid arthritis marker. Anticyclic citrullinated peptide antibodies (anti-CCP)-ELISA determination in early arthritis may be a good predictor of disease persistence and radiographic joint damage. The detection of anti-CCP antibody before the onset of the RA and the high concentration of autoantibodies in synovial fluid suggest a possible pathogenetic role of citrullination. The high specificity of anti-CCP antibody, its ability to identify patients with early RA and distinguish it from other types of arthritis potentially make it a key serological marker in the near future
Iron studies (ferritin especially)	Anaemia (normochromic and normocytic) is common in RA and has been found to be proportional to the rate of inflammation. Serum iron level and total iron-binding capacity are usually low
CMV, EBV, HIV	Assess for causative viral infection
Complement levels	Complement levels are normal or elevated in RA
Immunoglobulins IgG, IgA and IgM	Immunoglobulins are often high in elevated rheumatoid arthritis
Serum alkaline phosphatase (ALP)	Elevated serum ALP is often seen in active RA
Full blood count (FBC)	Assess for thrombocytosis, leucocytosis, neutrophilia or haemoglobin fluctations (reduced) commonly seen in RA patients Anaemia, usually normocytic and normochromic or hypochromic is present Decreased erythropoiesis is also commonly present
Coeliac screen	Assess for autoimmune tendency
Vitamin D 25(OH)0 + 1,25(OH)2D	Assess nutrient level to determine impact on immune derangement and musculoskeletal health
Mycoplasma, *Chlamydia* and *Borrelia* DNA PCR	Assess for triggering infection
Magnetic resonance imaging (MRI)	Currently, MRI is the best imaging modality to detect erosions. Specially designed MRI equipment called extremity MRI depicts soft-tissue changes and damage to cartilage and bone even better and at an earlier stage than does computed tomography. However, its cost precludes its widespread use
Ultrasound	Special ultrasound techniques called power Doppler ultrasonography (PDUS) or quantitative ultrasound (QUS) may be helpful in RA. Doppler ultrasound can aid in the initial diagnosis of RA even in the presence of minimal radiographic data on presentation. PDUS may be reliable for monitoring inflammatory activity in the joint

TABLE 15.14 Investigations for rheumatoid arthritis—cont'd

Assessment	Justification
Imaging studies	Plain radiography of affected joints is essential in the evaluation of patients. The earliest changes occur in the wrists or feet and consist of soft-tissue swelling and juxtaarticular demineralisation. Later, the diagnostic changes of uniform joint-space narrowing are evident and erosions develop. The erosions are often first evident at the fifth metatarsal head or ulnar styloid and at the juxtaarticular margins, where the bony surface is not protected by cartilage. These changes frequently take several years to develop
Synovial fluid	Confirmation of RA and to assess severity of condition

RA, rheumatoid arthritis; RF, rheumatoid factor.
Sources: Khurana R, Berney S. Clinical aspects of rheumatoid arthritis. Pathophysiology 2005; 12(3):153–165. Rindfleisch A, Muller D. Diagnosis and management of rheumatoid arthritis. Am Fam Physician 2005; 72(6):1037–1047.

TABLE 15.15 Other conditions associated with raised rheumatoid factor

Category	Diseases
Rheumatic diseases	Rheumatoid arthritis, systemic lupus erythematosus, scleroderma, mixed connective tissue diseases, Sjögren's syndrome
Viral infections	Acquired immunodeficiency syndrome, mononucleosis, hepatitis, influenza and many others; after vaccination (may yield falsely elevated titres of antiviral antibodies)
Parasitic infections	Trypanosomiasis, kala-azar, malaria, schistosomiasis, filariasis and others
Chronic bacterial infections	Tuberculosis, leprosy, yaws, syphilis, brucellosis, subacute bacterial endocarditis, salmonellosis
Neoplasms	Lymphoma, myeloma, postirradiation or chemotherapy
Other hyperglobulinaemic states	Hypergammaglobulinaemic purpura, cryoglobulinaemia, chronic liver disease, sarcoid, other chronic pulmonary diseases

Source: Cope AP. T cells in rheumatoid arthritis. Arthritis Res Ther 2008; 10(Suppl. 1):S1.

Rheumatoid arthritis is a multifactorial condition that requires a comprehensive therapeutic approach focusing on reducing factors involved in the disease process:

- Intestinal permeability
- Poor digestive microflora balance and diversity
- Circulating immune complexes
- Immune dysfunction
- Free radicals, oxidative stress and oxidation
- Hormonal imbalance
- Dietary and nutritional deficiencies
- Epigenetic and genetic influences — triggers for switching on the process.

Of prime importance is the control of inflammation, which is best achieved primarily through dietary modification and the prescription of herbal medicines and nutritional supplementation. Joint regeneration should be encouraged, with supplementation and modified lifestyle practices and supervised exercise programs.

Therapeutic application

HISTORICAL PERSPECTIVE

Rheumatoid arthritis has been treated since the time of the Eclectics, who used a wide range of herbs and techniques to resolve this complex disease. *Cimicifuga racemosa* was suggested for rheumatoid and myalgic pain and was considered to be a chief remedy for these conditions, because of its anodyne activity,[138] although analgesics such as *Corydalis* also featured. Depuratives such as *Iris versicolor*, *Phytolacca decandra* and *Rumex crispus* were also advocated, probably for their ability to improve elimination.[12] External heating applications were thought to be beneficial and the Eclectics suggested immersing the joints in hot water and salt, wrapping them in flannel and then surrounding them by hot bricks or hot water bottles. The Eclectics also favoured balneotherapy advocating courses of hot baths at springs, Turkish baths and hot air treatment, all with good results.

NATUROPATHIC PERSPECTIVE

The naturopathic approach must be aggressive, with increasing treatment intensity based on the patient's presentation. Naturopathic measures may be sufficient if the presentation is mild–moderate, but co-managed care in conjunction with various medications is often indicated as the disease progresses and develops. If medication is taken, modifications to treatment may be required to reduce the side effects of the drugs.

Dietary modification is paramount to the success of treatment and thus compliance and patient motivation are the most important aspects of the patient–practitioner relationship. Symptomatic relief can also be attained through the use of standard physical therapy techniques (i.e. exercise, heat, cold, massage, diathermy, lasers and paraffin baths), anti-inflammatory botanicals and nutrients and, in appropriate patients, bowel detoxification. Additional supportive measures will address the areas clearly outlined in clinical decision making and rationale.

Psychological aspects need to be addressed. Evidence is gathering that underscores the importance of the psychological makeup of the patient with rheumatoid arthritis. Also salient is the patient's style of coping as well as the support given by the patient's social circles, belief systems and relationship with the practitioner.

NUTRITIONAL MEDICINE (DIETARY)

Dietary therapeutic objectives

Dietary modification is cardinal to effective treatment outcome. The Western diet is one of the most strongly suggestive triggers for the development of rheumatoid arthritis and a wholefood diet is imperative for optimal health and disease treatment and prevention.

General principles include:

- Investigate and address nutritional deficiencies
- Avoid sugar, red meat, refined carbohydrates, processed foods, chemicals, additives, preservatives, artificial colours, saturated and trans fats
- Investigate for food intolerances and allergies. Once the offending foods have been found, they are to be eliminated from the diet
- Encourage fresh fruits and vegetables for antioxidant sources, complex carbohydrates, wholegrains and fibre, cold-pressed vegetarian sources of essential fatty acids
- Encourage organic foods when possible
- Encourage vegetarian or pesco-vegetarian dietary practices.

It is imperative to avoid food allergies (both IgE and IgG).

Specific dietary treatments

DIETARY INCLUSIONS

Anti-inflammatory diet

McCann[520] suggests that nutritional therapy for rheumatoid arthritis should include anti-inflammatory nutrients with a minimum amount of meat and plenty of fish, wholegrains, fruits and vegetables. This supports results from other reviews, which suggests that a diet based on the principles of the traditional Mediterranean diet (i.e. one that is rich in fish, plant foods and olive oil) is protective against the development of rheumatoid arthritis,[521,522] which is likely to be a result of its low saturated fat content and high levels of antioxidants.[523]

Antioxidant-rich diet

In patients with rheumatoid arthritis, antioxidant status has been found to be lower than that in healthy controls,[524] thus intake of foods rich in antioxidants (such as fruit and vegetables) are suggested to prevent damage to joints as a result of free radicals and oxidative stress. Diets that are low in fruits and vegetables including vitamin C are associated with increased risk of developing rheumatoid arthritis.[525,526]

Fasting/vegetarian/vegan diet

A number of studies have observed beneficial effects in patients who regularly undertake partial/full fasting,[527,528] but it has been observed that many patients will relapse once food is reintroduced. This prompted Kjeldsen-Kragh et al[529] to investigate the effects of fasting in 27 individuals with rheumatoid arthritis following a vegan/vegetarian diet. The participants undertook a partial fast lasting between 7 and 10 days and were then administered a gluten-free, vegan diet for 3.5 months, though the diet gradually changed to a lacto-vegetarian diet towards the completion of the study. After just 1 month, there was improvement in the number of tender joints, swollen joints, pain, duration of morning stiffness, grip strength and inflammatory laboratory markers such as ESR, CRP and WBC. These benefits were still present 1 year later when the group was reassessed.

A 2009 Cochrane review suggests that fasting followed by a vegetarian diet/Cretan Mediterranean diet may improve pain when compared with an ordinary diet.[530] Any fasting regimen requires careful consideration of the patient's health and regular monitoring.

Omega-3 fatty acids

Clinical trials show that dietary omega-3 fatty acids (in particular eicosapentaenoic acid) have numerous beneficial effects for rheumatoid arthritis, including reductions in inflammation and pain (Fig. 15.14). Patients with rheumatoid arthritis should aim to consume omega-3 fatty acids on a daily basis. Fish with high omega-3 content include salmon, rainbow trout, sardines and mackerel.[531] As previously mentioned, omega-3 was positively associated with time to remission.[519]

A light diet

From an Ayurvedic perspective, when symptoms are exacerbated and the disease is at its most chronic, the food consumed should be light, little and liquid (e.g. ginger tea, gruels, soups) so as to reduce the load and toxic burden of the body.[532]

DIETARY EXCLUSIONS

Pro-inflammatory foods

Dietary intake of alcohol and coffee and their relationship with rheumatoid arthritis have produced mixed results, with some studies showing increased risk of rheumatoid arthritis[533] and others showing no or decreased risk.[534,535] From a naturopathic perspective, alcohol is nutrient depleting and since many people with rheumatoid arthritis are already nutrient deficient alcohol should be avoided. In addition, coffee and alcohol are acidic and thus promote inflammation in the body, which of course is undesirable in rheumatoid arthritis which is characterised by inflammation. For the same reasons, heavily processed and refined foods should also be avoided.

Allergenic foods

Dietary manipulation and exclusion may give benefit to some patients, as food sensitivities have been linked to rheumatic disorders, being suggested to evoke specific immune responses and immunological reactions.[536] Dairy products, tomatoes, corn, wheat and meat products[537] have all been implicated and food testing may be indicated to check for individual intolerances/sensitivities and subsequently elimination/exclusion diets implemented to remove the offending food(s) if indicated.

Meat

Pattison et al[538] observed that high consumption of red meat and total protein was associated with increased risk for inflammatory polyarthritis, but contradictory results were seen in a later study by Benito-Garcia et al[539] who

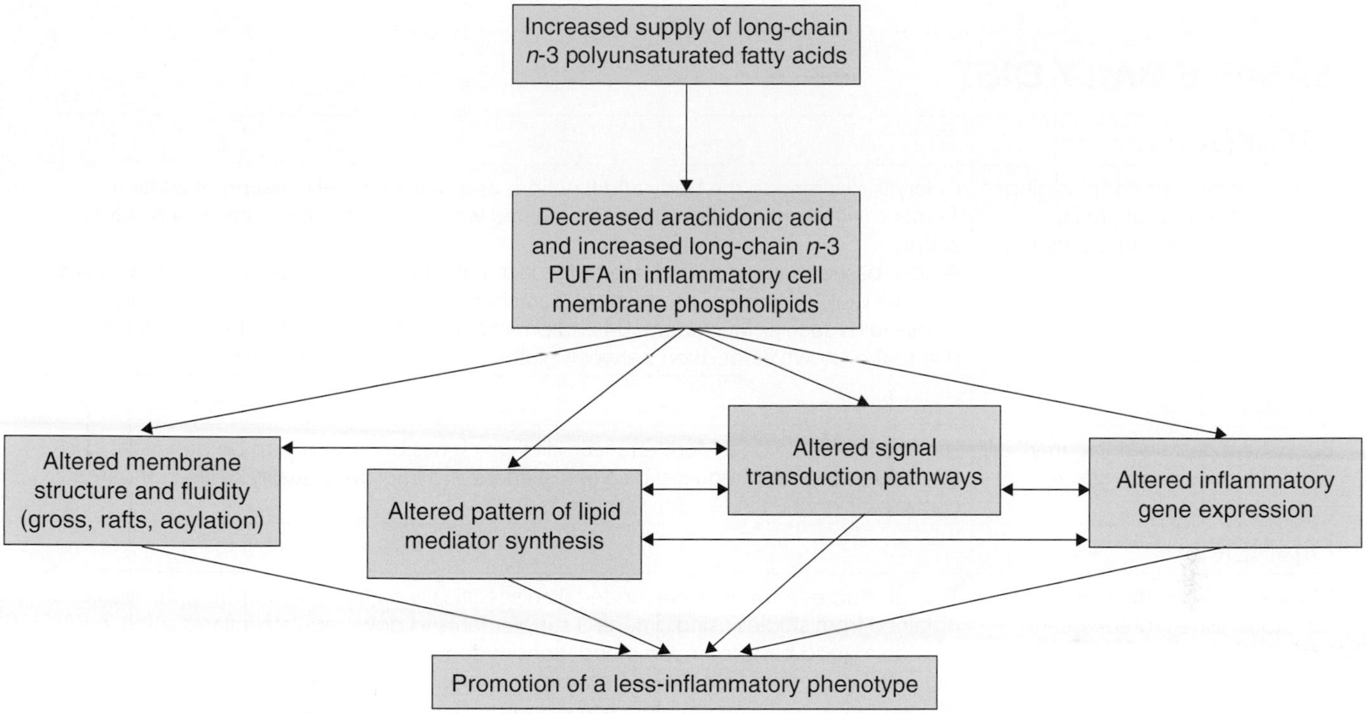

FIGURE 15.14 Mechanisms by which n-3 PUFA can affect inflammatory cell activity.
Source: Calder PC. Session 3: Joint Nutrition Society and Irish Nutrition and Dietetic Institute Symposium on 'Nutrition and autoimmune disease'. PUFA, inflammatory processes and rheumatoid arthritis. Proc Nutr Soc. 2008; 67(4):409–418. Reproduced by permission.

were unable to confirm an association between protein or meat and risk for rheumatoid arthritis. While meat may not increase risk of rheumatoid arthritis, it may influence symptoms: high intake of meat and its byproducts has been hypothesised to increase inflammation associated with rheumatoid arthritis.[540] Nitrates used to preserve meats may also increase inflammation.

NUTRITIONAL MEDICINE (SUPPLEMENTAL)

Nutritional medicine therapeutic objectives

- Investigate and address nutritional deficiencies
- Reduce inflammation
- Reduce pain
- Modulate autoimmunity
- Eliminate past or present infections
- Aid detoxification and elimination
- Reduce GI tract permeability
- Balance and replace GI tract microflora
- Improve liver function
- Treat hormonal imbalances (if appropriate)
- Reduce oxidative stress
- Support emotional and mental health and address historical effects of stress.

Specific nutrients required

B COMPLEX (ALL B VITAMINS INCLUDING B_1, B_2, B_3, B_5, B_6, FOLATE, B_{12})

Vitamin B_6 deficiency affects both humoral and cell-mediated immune responses. Deficiency is associated with immunological changes observed in patients with rheumatoid arthritis.[541]

Deficient vitamin B_6 status has been observed in two separate studies of people with rheumatoid arthritis (in particular, plasma levels of pyridoxal-5′-phosphate (PLP), the active form of vitamin B_6). This is thought to occur as a result of TNF-α production.[542] Concurrent supplementation with folic acid in patients taking methotrexate, a folate antagonist used in rheumatoid arthritis, is also necessary and reduces the side effects from methotrexate-induced toxicity which may occur as a result of folate depletion.[543,544] Additionally, patients with MTHFR may not respond to methotrexate therapy.[507] Folic acid supplementation has also been suggested to be beneficial to reduce the risk of hyperhomocysteinaemia and cardiovascular disease, which is common and accelerated in rheumatoid arthritis.[543,545] Folinic acid or MTHF may be used in the place of folic acid in patients with MTHFR. Decreased serum vitamin B_{12} has been observed in people with rheumatoid arthritis,[546,547] but other studies have shown no relationship between vitamin B_{12} and rheumatoid arthritis,[548] suggesting the importance of screening for vitamin B_{12}.

BROMELAIN

Bromelain is an enzyme derived from pineapple that displays anti-inflammatory and analgesic actions[549] upon the structures of the musculoskeletal system. In combination with other proteolytic enzymes it has been shown to reduce levels of TGF-β in people with

SAMPLE DAILY DIET

BREAKFAST	
Celery, carrot, turmeric plus ginger Quinoa porridge with chia, walnuts, cherries and blueberries	Celery is alkalising to the body and functions as a diuretic for elimination of wastes. Turmeric is immune regulating and, combined with ginger, provides anti-inflammatory activity. A plant-based diet is favoured due to the fact that it reduces exogenous arachidonic acid from the diet, decreasing production of arachidonic acid-derived pro inflammatory eicosanoids such as leukotriene B4 and prostaglandin E2. Meals should be gluten free due to the known association between gluten and autoimmune disease.
LUNCH	
Buckwheat pasta with creamy avocado and spinach sauce	Lunch is modelled on a Mediterranean diet which has been shown to be beneficial in RA. Participants reported reduced pain and stiffness and improved quality of life compared to controls.
DINNER	
Mackerel salad with cucumber, tomatoes, olives, green beans, broccoli	Though studies have not been undertaken specifically on fish consumption, the results obtained from studies using omega-3 supplements to downregulate inflammation in RA provide a good basis for recommendations to consume oily fish. Epidemiological studies suggest a protective association between consumption of fish high in omega-3 fatty acids and risk of RA, and a recent meta-analysis found that omega-3 fatty acid supplementation reduced the need for NSAIDs in RA patients. Sashimi style, steaming or poaching the fish is recommended rather than frying, to minimise production of free radicals.
SNACK	
Seasonal fruit and raw nuts and seeds	Provide protection from oxidative stress and inflammation.

Sources: Lee YH, Bae SC, Song GG. Omega-3 polyunsaturated fatty acids and the treatment of rheumatoid arthritis: a meta-analysis. Arch Med Res 2012; 43(5):356–362. McKellar G, Morrison E, McEntegart A et al. A pilot study of a Mediterranean-type diet intervention in female patients with rheumatoid arthritis living in areas of social deprivation in Glasgow. Ann Rheum Dis 2007; 66(9):1239–1243. Skoldstam L, Hagfors L, Johansson G. An experimental study of a Mediterranean diet intervention for patients with rheumatoid arthritis. Ann Rheum Dis 2003; 62(3):208–214.

rheumatoid arthritis.[550] In a small, uncontrolled clinical study involving 29 people (26 of whom had rheumatoid arthritis), approximately 72.5% experienced resolution or reduction in soft-tissue swelling following ingestion of bromelain.[551] Further, high-powered studies are required to confirm the results of this study.

COPPER

Copper is a component of superoxide-dismutase enzyme, an antioxidant system within the body, including around the joints. Decreased dietary copper is likely to lead to a reduction in intracellular copper, contributing to reduction in antioxidant defence mechanisms. In open studies, intraarticular (of superoxide dismutase) and intramuscular (of copper) administration has been found to induce remission of rheumatoid arthritis.[552] Whether this effect can be extrapolated to supplementation with copper remains to be seen.

Lysyl oxidase, a copper-dependent amine oxidase, plays an essential role in the biogenesis of connective tissue matrices by crosslinking the extracellular matrix proteins, collagen and elastin.[553]

DIGESTIVE ENZYMES

Abnormalities in gut function including altered antigen handling of food by the gut, elevation of cross-reactive food antibodies in proximal gut secretions,[554] gastritis and achlorhydria[555] have all been noted in people with rheumatoid arthritis. Supplementation with digestive enzymes helps to support healthy digestive function and aid in the digestion of fats, proteins, carbohydrates and fibre when the body's own enzymes are lacking. Digestive enzymes are particularly relevant if the patient has a diet that is typically low in foods with natural enzymes (because of a predominance of processed, refined foods).

ESSENTIAL FATTY ACIDS

Gamma linolenic acid (GLA)

The evidence on gamma linolenic acid (GLA) is not as strong as it is for omega-3, but for vegetarians it provides a possible alternative. A meta-analysis conducted by Cameron et al found that borage, blackcurrant and evening primrose oils containing GLA doses equal to or higher than 1400 mg/day were beneficial in the alleviation of rheumatic complaints, whereas lower doses (approximately 500 mg) were ineffective.[556]

Eicosapentaenoic acid (EPA) and docosahexaenoic acid (DHA)

The essential fatty acids eicosapentaenoic acid (EPA) and docosahexaenoic acid (DHA) also appear to be useful in rheumatoid arthritis because of their ability to inhibit the metabolism of arachidonic acid to inflammatory eicosanoids, reduce gene expression of cyclooxygenase-2 (COX-2) but not COX-1, reduce gene expression of inflammatory cytokines and cartilage-degrading proteinases as well as affect signalling pathways for transcription factors (e.g. NF-κB) and reduce lymphocyte proliferation.[557] Furthermore, they may also exert immune specific mechanisms relevant to rheumatoid arthritis, such as antigen presentation, T-cell reactivity and inflammatory cytokine production.[531] (See Fig. 15.15.)

There is a wealth of data to support the efficacy of omega-3 fatty acids in reducing pain, number of tender joints, duration of morning stiffness, use of non-steroidal anti-inflammatory drugs and improving physical performance in patients with rheumatoid arthritis as shown in Tables 15.16 and 15.17.[106] Vegetarian sources of omega-3 include flaxseed/linseed, walnut and algal oil.[558]

GLUCOSAMINE, CHONDROITIN AND GREEN-LIPPED MUSSEL

Inflammation of the lining of the joint in rheumatoid arthritis erodes articular cartilage, resulting in joint deformity. While glucosamine and chondroitin have been studied extensively for their role in joint health related to osteoarthritis, the same cannot be said for rheumatoid arthritis. However, given that both glucosamine and chondroitin function to provide a substrate for matrix synthesis and repair, their application in rheumatoid arthritis is likely to be helpful in an attempt to conserve articular cartilage. Similarly, while there is a lack of studies investigating the efficacy of green-lipped mussel and resolution of symptoms in rheumatoid arthritis, its anti-inflammatory action and the therapeutic benefits observed with its application in osteoarthritis suggest that it too may be useful in reducing inflammation of the joint tissue.

QUERCETIN

Quercetin exerts antioxidant, antihistamine and anti-inflammatory effects likely to be useful in rheumatoid arthritis. In animal and experimental studies, quercetin has been observed to inhibit a number of inflammatory processes associated with arthritis, including neutrophil activation, synoviocyte proliferation and angiogenesis.[559]

MANGANESE

Manganese is required both structurally and functionally for management of rheumatoid arthritis. Firstly, from a structural perspective, manganese is required for the production of proteoglycans that make up the cartilage and connective tissue. Secondly, as a component of the enzyme manganese superoxide dismutase, manganese functions as a powerful antioxidant,[560] highly important in protecting the joints against the excess generation of reactive oxygen species and oxidative stress seen in rheumatoid arthritis patients.

S-ADENOSYLMETHIONINE (SAMe)

Cartilage and tendon extracellular matrices are composed of, among other things, collagens, elastin and proteoglycans. In experimental studies

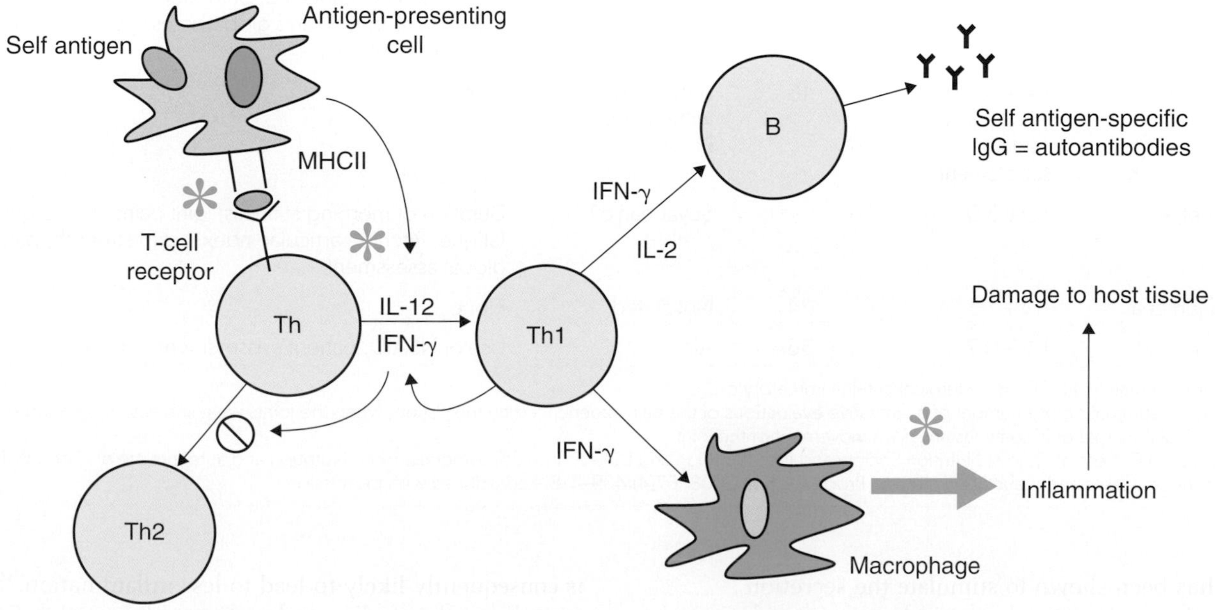

FIGURE 15.15 Anti-inflammatory and immune modulating effects of omega fatty acids.

Source: Calder PC. Session 3: Joint Nutrition Society and Irish Nutrition and Dietetic Institute Symposium on 'Nutrition and autoimmune disease'. PUFA, inflammatory processes and rheumatoid arthritis. Proc Nutr Soc 2008; 67(4):409–418. Reproduced with permission.

TABLE 15.16 Benefit of omega-3 fatty acids — meta-analysis

Reference	Dose of EPA+DHA(g/d)	Duration (weeks)	Placebo	Clinical outcomes improved with long-chain omega-3 PUFAs
Kremer et al	1.8 + 1.2	12	Paraffin oil	No. of tender joints; duration of morning stiffness
Kremer et al	2.7 + 1.8	14	Olive oil	No. of tender joints; no. of swollen joints; time to fatigue; physician's global assessment
Cleland et al	3.2 + 2.0	12	Olive oil	No. of tender joints; grip strength
van der Tempel et al	2.0 + 2.3	12	Coconut oil	No. of swollen joints; duration of morning stiffness
Kremer et al	1.7 + 1.2	24	Olive oil	No. of tender joints; no. of swollen joints; grip strength; physician's global assessment
Kremer et al	3.5 + 2.4	24	Olive oil	No. of tender joints; no. of swollen joints; grip strength; physician's global assessment; duration of morning stiffness
Tullekan et al	2.0 + 1.3	12	Coconut oil	No. of swollen joints; joint pain
Skoidstarn et al	1.8 + 1.2	24	Mixed oils	No. and severity of tender joints; physician's global assessment; use of NSAID
Esperson et al	2.0 + 1.2	12	Mixed oils	No. of severity of tender joints
Nielsen et al	2.0 + 1.2	12	Vegetable oil	No. of tender joints; duration of morning stiffness
Kjeldsen-Kragh et al	3.8 + 2.0	16	Maize oil	No. and severity of tender joints; duration of morning stiffness
Lau et al	1.7 + 1.1	52	Air	Use of NSAID
Geusens et al	1.7 + 0.4	52	Olive oil	Physician's pain assessment; patient's global assessment; use of NSAID and/or disease-modifying antirheumatic drugs
Kremer et al	4.6 + 2.5	26–30	Maize oil	No. of tender joints; duration of morning stiffness; physician's assessment of pain; physician's global assessment; patient's global assessment
Volker et al	Total 40 mg/kg (approx 2.2–3.0)	15	Mixed oils	No. of swollen joints; duration of morning stiffness; patient's assessment of pain; patient's global assessment; physician's global assessment; health assessment by questionnaire
Adam et al	Approx 2.4 + 1.8	12	Maize oil	No. of swollen joints; no. of tender joints; patient's global assessment; physician's global assessment; patient's assessment of pain
Remas et al	1.4 + 0.2 (+0.5 γ-inolenic acid) in a liquid supplement	16	Liquid supplement without added PUFA	None
Berbert et al	Total 3.0		Soyabean oil	Duration of morning stiffness; joint pain; time to onset of fatigue; Ritchie's articular index*; grip strength, patient's global assessment
Sundrarjun et al	1.9 + 1.5	24	Not stated	None
Galarraga et al	1.5 + 0.7	36	Air	Use of NSAID; patient's assessment of pain

Approx, approximately; NSAID, non-steroidal anti-inflammatory drug.
*Based on the summation of a number of quantitative evaluations of the pain experienced by the patient when the joints were subjected to pressures exerted over the articular margin or in some instances on movement of the joint.
Source: Calder PC. Session 3: Joint Nutrition Society and Irish Nutrition and Dietetic Institute Symposium on 'Nutrition and autoimmune disease'. PUFA, inflammatory processes and rheumatoid arthritis. Proc Nutr Soc 2008; 67(4):409–418. Reproduced with permission.

SAMe has been shown to stimulate the secretion and synthesis of proteoglycans in human articular cartilage[561] as well as reverse the damaging effects of tumour necrosis factor in the cultured synovial cells of rabbits.[562] SAMe may also reduce nitric oxide levels, which is consequently likely to lead to less inflammation.[563] The majority of the studies undertaken with regard to SAMe and arthritis have examined the effects of SAMe and osteoarthritis, but there is no reason that SAMe should not exert the same chondroprotective/restorative effects in

TABLE 15.17 Summary of the results of placebo-controlled studies using dietary long-chain omega-3 PUFAs (in the form of fish oil) in patients with rheumatoid arthritis

Outcome	No. of studies	No. of patients		Significance of effect of omega-3 PUFAs: *p* value
		Control	Omega-3 PUFAs	
Patient-assessed pain	13	247	254	0.03
Physician-assessed pain	3	61	62	0.45
Duration of morning stiffness	8	150	156	0.003
No. of painful and/or tender joints	10	210	215	0.003
Ritchie articular index*	4	68	67	0.40
NSAID consumption	3	79	77	0.01

NSAID, non-steroidal anti-inflammatory drug.
*Based on the summation of a number of quantitative evaluations of the pain experienced by the patient when the joints were subjected to pressures exerted over the articular margin or in some instances on movement of the joint.
Source: Calder PC. Session 3: Joint Nutrition Society and Irish Nutrition and Dietetic Institute Symposium on 'Nutrition and autoimmune disease'. PUFA, inflammatory processes and rheumatoid arthritis. Proc Nutr Soc 2008; 67(4):409–418. Reproduced with permission.

patients with rheumatoid arthritis. Further studies are required to assess the mechanism by which SAMe regenerates cartilage and following these, its efficacy in rheumatoid arthritis.

SELENIUM

The antioxidant action of selenium is well used in rheumatoid arthritis[564] due to the increased free radical production and oxidative stress suggested to occur as a result of disruptions of immunoregulatory cytokine production,[565] in particular through the phagocytic activity of the polymorphonuclear leucocytes.[566] Selenium deficiency is common among people with rheumatoid arthritis[565,567] and selenium deficiency has even been suggested to be a possible risk factor for rheumatoid factor-negative rheumatoid arthritis.[568] A double blind study investigating the efficacy of selenium-enriched yeast (200 micrograms/day) in patients with rheumatoid arthritis over a 3-month period found that symptoms such as painful, swollen and stiff joints improved in both the selenium group and the placebo, allowing no real conclusion to be made.[569] Selenium is also involved in immune regulation and thus may be useful in correcting the autoimmune aspect of rheumatoid arthritis.

VITAMIN A

Structurally, vitamin A is required for cell differentiation and maturation[570] as well as for the healthy maintenance of cartilage. For example, the epiphyseal cartilage cells cannot achieve their growth, development and replacement without vitamin A. Vitamin A levels have been found to be reduced in people with rheumatoid arthritis,[571] which is significant given the actions of vitamin A in the body. Antioxidant status has been shown in numerous studies to be diminished in people with rheumatoid arthritis, which in turn results in tissue damage and inflammation, highlighting the importance of supplementation with antioxidants such as vitamin A, particularly if patients are taking conventional medicines.[572] Vitamin A also helps to regulate the immune system[570] further highlighting its importance in rheumatoid arthritis.

VITAMIN C

In a similar manner to vitamin A, vitamin C is required in rheumatoid arthritis for its antioxidant and structural effects. As an antioxidant, vitamin C may help to minimise tissue damage and inflammation as a result of free radicals and oxidative stress. Structurally, vitamin C is in high demand as articular cartilage is dependent upon a regular supply to make collagen and elastin. It is also required for glycosaminoglycan synthesis.[570] Deficiency of vitamin C is likely to lead to weak and diminished joint cartilage. Adequate vitamin C is thus required to aid in its repair and regeneration and prevent damage from reactive oxygen species.

VITAMIN D

Vitamin D is likely to be useful in rheumatoid arthritis specifically for its role as an immunoregulator. In-vitro data suggest that vitamin D helps to regulate the production of the matrix metalloproteinases by chondrocytes and that vitamin D receptor lignans may be able to partially control the development of rheumatoid arthritis.[573] Certainly greater intake of vitamin D is associated with reduced risk of rheumatoid arthritis, while low vitamin D has been suggested to be associated with higher disease activity.[574] Participants with rheumatoid arthritis administered a high dose of 1 alpha(OH)D3 experienced a significant clinical improvement, thought to occur as a result of vitamin D's immunomodulatory action.[575]

VITAMIN E

Lipid vitamins such as vitamin E are found within the synovial fluid of joints and decreased levels have been found in patients with rheumatoid arthritis, suggesting increased needs by the body.[576] Early studies observed vitamin E (1200 mg (1800 IU)/day) to exert a mild analgesic effect in participants with rheumatoid arthritis already taking antirheumatic drugs, although in this study no differences in inflammation or antioxidant parameters were seen.[577] As with a number of the nutrients discussed before, vitamin E also functions as an antioxidant and immune enhancer/modulator. Theoretically, both are likely to be useful in the management of rheumatoid arthritis. In spite of these actions there have been few studies showing beneficial effects of vitamin E in rheumatoid arthritis. The quality and methodology of studies performed may partly influence this.

ZINC

The matrix metalloproteinases are a family of zinc-dependent proteinases that are involved in cartilage breakdown in rheumatoid arthritis. Low levels of zinc have been observed in people with rheumatoid arthritis.[578–580] This is problematic as zinc is a component of the antioxidant enzyme superoxide dismutase and deficiency of this enzyme is likely to leave the joint susceptible to damage from oxidation.[581] It is not known whether deficiency of zinc contributes to disease activity by compromising cellular immune function, but rheumatoid arthritis has been suggested to cause zinc deficiency as a result of chronic inflammation as well as the use of certain medications.[560]

Preliminary studies have shown benefit in patients with rheumatoid arthritis taking zinc sulfate (220 mg three times daily, equivalent to 50 mg elemental zinc three times daily); zinc-treated patients reported improvements with regard to joint swelling, morning stiffness, walking time and the patient's own impression of overall disease activity.[582]

DOSAGE REQUIREMENTS

The dosage requirements listed below are based on adult doses that have been reported in the literature.

- B complex (all B vitamins) high-dose combination, preferably activated forms:
  - Thiamine 20–40 mg/day
  - Riboflavin 50 mg/day. Riboflavin 5′ phosphate 20–40 mg
  - Niacinamide/nicotinic acid 50–100 mg/day
  - Pantothenic acid 150–300 mg/day
  - Pyridoxine 50–100 mg/day. Pyridoxal-5-phosphate 20–60 mg/day
  - Folate 500–1000 micrograms/day as folinic acid or L-5MTHF determined by the methylation status of the patient
  - Additional folic acid 5 mg/day or folinic acid (2000 micrograms/day+) if taking methotrexate
  - Consider testing for methylenetetrahydrofolate reductase (MTHFR) polymorphism (C677T or A1298C). If positive for C677T or A1298C polymorphism, MTHF is the preferred form of folate
  - Hydroxo- or methylcobalamin 500–1000 micrograms/day determined by the methylation status of the patient
  - Choline 250–500 mg/day
  - Inositol 250–500 mg/day
  - Biotin 250–500 micrograms/day
  - If positive for MTHFR C677T or A1298C polymorphism, a higher dose of biotin is required for the metabolism of folate and it derivatives
  - Bromelain 200–400 mg/day
- Digestive enzymes: Specific for each patient but may be from porcine (e.g. pepsin 100 mg t.d.s.) or vegetarian sources
- GLA 1400 mg/day
- DHA 1200–2500 mg/day[531]
- EPA 1700–4600 mg/day[531]
- Copper 1 mg/day[219]
- Glucosamine 1500 mg/day
- Chondroitin 800–1200 mg/day
- Green-lipped mussel 1500–3000 mg in acute followed by 500–2000 mg as maintenance
- Quercetin 600–1200 mg/day
- Manganese 15 mg/day[219]
- SAMe 600–1200 mg/day
- Selenium 200 micrograms/day[219]
- Vitamin A 5000–10,000 IU/day (caution dose during pregnancy, <8000 IU/day)
- Vitamin C 1000–3000 mg/day[219]
- Vitamin D 1000–4000 IU (may need to be increased in conjunction with medical assistance to 50000 IU/day) (pathology dependent)
- Vitamin E 1200 mg (1800 IU)/day (divided doses)
- Zinc 45–80 mg/day[219]
- Glutamine 5000 mg BD
- Probiotics (multi-strain) 45–90 billion organisms/day. Can increase dosage (e.g. 45–90 billion 2–3 times daily) if there is digestive involvement (e.g. increased intestinal permeability, Crohn's disease, ulcerative colitis)

HERBAL MEDICINE

Herbal medicine therapeutic objectives

MEDICATION EFFECTS

Patients with a history of corticosteroid use (e.g. prednisone) and those being weaned off corticosteroids should be prescribed *Bupleurum falcatum, Glycyrrhiza glabra, Rehmannia glutinosa* and *Panax ginseng*, which prevent and/or reverse the adrenal gland atrophy induced by these drugs.

GENERAL APPROACH

Rheumatoid arthritis is a multifactorial condition and, as it is complex, all of these factors will be taken into account but not all factors will be required for every patient. Because of the underlying pathogenesis, treatment is focused on the following areas:

- Genetic factors — adaptogens (adrenal restoratives to reduce aggravating stimulation of genetic predisposition)
- Abnormal bowel permeability — mucous membrane trophorestoratives, astringents, demulcents
- Dysbiosis and small intestinal bacterial overgrowth (SIBO) — pre- and probiotics, antimicrobial/antiseptic, mucous membrane trophorestoratives. The specific class depends on the pathogen (e.g. anthelmintic, antiviral)
- The presence of abnormal antibodies and immune complexes — immune modulators, immune enhancers, immune depressants. The specific class depends on the antibodies and immune complexes involved and the pathogen (e.g. anthelmintic, antiviral)

- Microbial hypotheses — antimicrobial/antiseptics, immune modulators, immune enhancers, immune depressants. The specific class depends on the pathogen (e.g. anthelmintic, antiviral)
- Decreased dehydroepiandrosterone (DHEA) levels — HPA modulators, adaptogens, adrenal restoratives.

STANDARD PROTOCOL

A standard protocol for the patient should include:

- Eliminate past or present infections — antimicrobial/antiseptics, immune modulators, immune enhancers, immune depressants. The specific class depends on the pathogen (e.g. anthelmintic, antiviral)
- Modulate autoimmunity — immune modulators, immune enhancers, immune depressants
- Use depuratives to aid detoxification and elimination — depuratives/alteratives, lymphatics
- Reduce GI tract permeability — mucous membrane trophorestoratives, astringents, tonics, demulcents
- Balance and replace GI tract microflora — prebiotics and probiotics, antimicrobial/antiseptics, mucous membrane trophorestoratives. The specific class depends on the pathogen (e.g. anthelmintic, antiviral)
- Improve liver function — hepatotonics, hepatoprotectives, hepatotrophorestoratives, choleretics, cholagogues
- Treat hormonal imbalances if appropriate — HPA modulators, adaptogens, adrenal restoratives
- Reduce inflammation with anti-inflammatory remedies — steroidal anti-inflammatories, general anti-inflammatories
- Reduce oxidative stress — antioxidants, anti-inflammatories
- Reduce pain with specific analgesics — analgesics, anodynes.

Specific herbal medicines

APIUM GRAVEOLENS (CELERY)

Apium graveolens has been traditionally favoured for its beneficial effects in rheumatism.[583] It contains the constituent apiin, known to exert an anti-inflammatory action,[109] which may in part explain its therapeutic effects. Another possible mechanism may be its diuretic action[584] as diuretics encourage the elimination of acidic metabolic wastes from the body and acidic metabolites have been linked to inflammation.

BOSWELLIA SERRATA (BOSWELLIA)

Boswellia serrata has displayed anti-inflammatory activity in a number of inflammatory conditions via its action on cyclooxygenase and 5-lipoxygenase and is thus likely to be useful in rheumatoid arthritis,[464] particularly where it may enable patients to reduce the dose of their medication. A double-blind pilot study conducted by Sander et al observed that the resin extract of *Boswellia serrata* (3600 mg/day) in addition to current therapy (e.g. NSAIDs) showed promise for the treatment of polyarthritis. While no significant changes were noted between the groups, more of those in the *Boswellia* group were able to reduce their dose of NSAIDs, signifying possible clinical benefits.[585]

BUPLEURUM FALCATUM (BUPLEURUM)

Bupleurum is a well-known Chinese herb with an affinity for the liver. In traditional Chinese medicine *Bupleurum* root is said to disperse liver energy, clear heat and relieve congestion.[586] This cooling action is likely to be useful in rheumatoid arthritis, where heat in the joints caused by inflammation is often reported. *Bupleurum* exerts an anti-inflammatory and hepatoprotective action.[587,588] In addition, it may be useful for patients taking medications that affect liver function, for example methotrexate.

CORYDALIS AMBIGUA (CORYDALIS)

Rheumatoid arthritis is characterised by intermittent flare-ups of joint pain.[589] These may be so painful as to significantly alter quality of life. *Corydalis ambigua* has been reported to have analgesic activity[590] but as yet no clinical trials have been conducted assessing its use in reducing pain associated with rheumatoid arthritis. Its documented actions and the effects observed in clinical practice provide a basis for its use as an effective analgesic in rheumatoid arthritis.

CURCUMA LONGA (TURMERIC)

Curcumin, the active constituent of *Curcuma longa*, is a powerful antioxidant and anti-inflammatory substance. Curcumin has been shown in experimental studies to prevent experimentally induced rheumatoid arthritis[591] and to exert an antiproliferative action in the synovial fibroblasts obtained from patients with rheumatoid arthritis.[592] Curcumin decreases levels of cyclooxygenase-2 (COX-2) mRNA and prostaglandin E_2, which are critical mediators of inflammation,[592] and displays significant protective effects specific to the joint tissue.[593] *Curcuma* also mediates inflammatory transcription factors, cytokines, redox status, protein kinases and enzymes that all promote inflammation.[594,595] The cumulative evidence collected suggests that curcumin is likely to be beneficial in rheumatoid arthritis.

ECHINACEA SPP. (ECHINACEA)

Immunoregulatory strategies have been suggested to be the treatment of the future with respect to modulating autoimmune diseases,[596] thus echinacea, which has well documented actions on the immune system as a modulator may well be useful in rheumatoid arthritis. Echinacea's proposed immunostimulant action has led some proponents to question the safety of its use in rheumatoid arthritis, given the presence of a seemingly already overstimulated immune system. Rather than simply stimulating the immune system, however, echinacea appears to have a regulating/modulating effect. There have been a few isolated cases in which echinacea has been reported to induce an autoimmune state,[597] but one cannot also deny the cases where echinacea has been prescribed beneficially.

As yet, no studies have examined the use of echinacea in rheumatoid arthritis, but a study was found assessing the efficacy of echinacea in mice with autoimmune diabetes.[596] *Echinacea* spp. substantially stimulated the production and number of natural killer cells. This study further highlights the role of the natural killer cells in autoimmunity.

Dysfunction of natural killer cells has been linked to a number of autoimmune disorders.[596] Further studies, preferably in humans, are required to examine the safety and mechanism of *Echinacea* spp. in people with rheumatoid arthritis.

ESCHSCHOLZIA CALIFORNICA (CALIFORNIAN POPPY)

Eschscholzia californica has been traditionally used for its analgesic action and its ability to alleviate pain and produce calm sleep.[138] The importance of pain relief in rheumatoid arthritis has already been discussed and as sleep is also usually disturbed the sedative action of *Eschscholzia californica* may also be useful. Rheumatoid arthritis patients often report sleep that is of poor quality which may be influenced by pain associated with the disease or other factors such as stress. It is important to note the importance of optimal quality and quantity of sleep; disrupted sleep is associated with increased perception of pain and disease progression as well as decreased quality of life and outcome measures.[598,599]

GUAIACUM OFFICINALE (GUAIACUM)

Guaiacum officinale is an alterative and diuretic herb prized by the Eclectics for its effects in chronic rheumatism and was traditionally administered as a compound decoction or syrup[138] to reduce inflammation. Guaiacum is also highly antiseptic, leading to its traditional use for rheumatic sore throat and rheumatic pharyngitis. The Eclectics suggested this may precede an attack of acute inflammatory rheumatism, with the tonsils suggested to be the foci of infection.[139] This suggests that *Guaiacum officinale* may also be useful when rheumatoid arthritis as a result of an infective origin is indicated.

HARPAGOPHYTUM PROCUMBENS (DEVIL'S CLAW)

Harpagophytum procumbens displays anti-inflammatory and subsequently analgesic activity in the musculoskeletal system. Although it has been studied primarily for osteoarthritis, its actions and the therapeutic benefits observed in clinical studies pertaining to osteoarthritis suggest it may be of some use in rheumatoid arthritis, particularly as harpagoside, the active constituent within *Harpagophytum procumbens*, has been shown to inhibit arachidonic acid metabolism and interact with eicosanoid biosynthesis to produce anti-inflammatory effects.[600] In-vitro studies also reveal that *Harpagophytum procumbens* demonstrates antioxidant properties; free radicals and oxidative stress are known to produce damage to the joints, hence the antioxidant action demonstrated by *Harpagophytum procumbens* has also been suggested to contribute to its anti-inflammatory and analgesic action.[601]

HEMIDESMUS INDICUS (HEMIDESMUS)

The persistent activation of the immune system in rheumatoid arthritis leads to autoimmunity, known to play a key role in the pathogenesis of rheumatoid arthritis.[602] *Hemidesmus indicus* is an Ayurvedic herb used in traditional medicine for rheumatic complaints,[603] and it may be useful in rheumatoid arthritis for its depressant action upon the immune system.[604] Experimental studies have revealed the ability of *Hemidesmus indicus* to suppress both cell-mediated and humoral aspects of the immune system.[604] *Hemidesmus indicus* works well in combination with *Echinacea* spp. for management of the autoimmune aspect of rheumatoid arthritis.

REHMANNIA GLUTINOSA (REHMANNIA)

The root of *Rehmannia glutinosa* has been used in traditional Chinese medicine as an immune suppressant,[238] thus in a similar manner to *Hemidesmus indicus* above it is useful in rheumatoid arthritis to suppress the overactive immune system. Beneficial results have been observed in uncontrolled trials of participants with rheumatoid arthritis using *Rehmannia glutinosa*, but well-designed trials remain scarce.[238]

SALIX SPP. (WILLOW BARK)

Willow bark has been used for centuries for its anti-inflammatory and pain-relieving effects, which probably occur as a result of its salicylate content. These actions make it highly useful for the pain and inflammation associated with rheumatoid arthritis, so much so that the German Commission E, *British Herbal Compendium* and ESCOP all document its efficacy for use in rheumatic ailments.[239] A small double-blind, placebo-controlled study undertaken by Biegert et al[605] conducted to assess the efficacy of *Salix alba* in rheumatoid arthritis (240 mg/day of salicin) observed a reduction in pain in those patients with rheumatoid arthritis compared with the placebo group, but the result was not significant. A large, better designed trial is required for a more accurate analysis to be made.

SMILAX ORNATA (SARSAPARILLA)

Smilax ornata is a diuretic[13] and alterative herb. These actions led to *Smilax* being prized by the Eclectic physicians for its ability to promote the elimination of toxic matter and wastes in rheumatic conditions.[138] Build-up of toxins in the body is linked to inflammation and likely to exacerbate symptoms in rheumatoid arthritis.

UNCARIA TOMENTOSA (CAT'S CLAW)

A randomised 52-week, two-phase study investigated the effect of a purified extract from cat's claw in patients with active rheumatoid arthritis. Twenty-four weeks of treatment with the cat's claw extract resulted in a reduction of the number of painful joints compared to placebo (by 53.2% vs 24.1%; $p = 0.044$). Patients receiving the cat's claw extract only during the second phase experienced a reduction in the number of painful ($p = 0.003$) and swollen joints ($p = 0.007$) compared to the values after 24 weeks of placebo.[606]

URTICA URENS/DIOICA SPP. (NETTLE)

Urtica spp. has been used in traditional Chinese medicine for rheumatism and inflammatory conditions,[607] but it has yet to be studied in patients with rheumatoid arthritis, which is surprising since it possesses diuretic,[138] anti-inflammatory and alterative effects, actions seemingly useful in rheumatoid arthritis. In-vitro studies observe the ability of hox alpha, a specific *Urtica* extract to prevent the upregulation of matrix metalloproteinase in human chondrocytes, leading to a reduction in the degradation of the extracellular matrix characteristic in rheumatoid arthritis.[136] Other extracts have been shown to decrease the production of TNF-α and T-cell inducers.[608] These actions are especially relevant in rheumatoid arthritis where disrupted T-cell function and TNF-α are implicated in the pathogenesis of rheumatoid arthritis.

ZANTHOXYLUM CLAVA-HERCULIS (PRICKLY ASH)

Zanthoxylum clava-herculis was traditionally used for rheumatic complaints because of its eliminative action[138] and was said to be useful in chronic muscular rheumatism as well as for lumbago and myalgia.[139] It would be used as an adjuvant herb for the management of symptoms associated with rheumatoid arthritis, although as yet there have been no clinical studies assessing its efficacy for this purpose.

ZINGIBER OFFICINALE (GINGER)

Zingiber officinale is a warming botanical useful in rheumatoid arthritis as an anti-inflammatory[609] and antirheumatic.[609] Given these actions, it can be assumed that *Zingiber officinale* would reduce inflammation and thus pain associated with rheumatoid arthritis. Furthermore, because of its action as a circulatory stimulant, *Zingiber officinale* promotes blood flow, bringing much-needed nutrition and oxygen to the joints and surrounding tissues, thus assisting in their maintenance and functionality.

LIFESTYLE RECOMMENDATIONS

Tai chi and yoga

Tai chi has been used as a therapeutic preventive of arthritis in Chinese culture for centuries and in clinical trials has been found to increase range of motion in patients with rheumatoid arthritis.[610] Gentle forms of yoga may also be helpful, with small studies showing that yoga undertaken 2–3 times a week by people with rheumatoid arthritis may decrease perception of pain and disability index[611] as well as reducing dose of medication.[612]

Balneotherapy (spa therapy or mineral baths)

Balneotherapy involves bathing in an indoor pool filled with mineral water at a temperature between 31 and 36°C, using mineral packs and mud compresses. A number of studies have been conducted using this therapy in patients with rheumatoid arthritis and it appears to soothe pain and improve joint motion.[613,614] A Cochrane review,[615] however, while acknowledging the beneficial effects observed in a number of studies, suggests that because of methodological errors better-quality studies should be undertaken. Water exercise therapy also appears to be beneficial in people with rheumatoid arthritis.[616]

Shoe wear

Supportive shoe wear is recommended for patients with rheumatoid arthritis to reduce force and impact on their joints. A Cochrane review observed that extra-depth shoes and moulded insoles may decrease pain on weight-bearing activities such as standing, walking and stair-climbing, but found there to be insufficient evidence to support hand and wrist splinting.[617]

Pain management techniques

Pain is a cardinal feature in patients with rheumatoid arthritis, but many patients are reluctant to take medication for fear of addiction, side effects and drug interactions.[618] Non-pharmacological methods of pain management offer an alternative means of pain relief and one that is in the control of the patient themselves. These include such things as visualisation, meditation, deep breathing and yoga nidra, all of which are good for stress management. Stress, both psychological and physiological, has been found to have a role in exacerbations of rheumatoid arthritis.

Counselling

Referral to a counsellor is specifically indicated to support the patient's emotional and mental wellbeing.

CASE STUDY

OVERVIEW

GH, a 42-year-old female, attends the clinic with a diagnosis of rheumatoid arthritis (diagnosed 3 years ago). She is a secretary and has recently noticed that the pain in her hands has gotten worse. The pain is in both hands and she rates it as an 8/10. She gets early morning bilateral stiffness in the hands, knees, back and shoulders. The stiffness lasts around 60 minutes after rising in the morning and can occur after any prolonged inactivity. The joints swell with the pain, become tender and limit the range of motion. She has generalised fatigue (energy 5–6/10) and weakness in the afternoon. She occasionally has a low-grade fever. She has sluggish circulation where she gets fluid around the ankles and in her fingers most weeks. The fluid in her fingers exacerbates her symptoms. She has a new online business that she works on the weekends. This business adds to her fatigue. She wishes to leave her secretarial job and work full-time with her online business.

Her appetite can be low some days. She may forget to eat a meal from time to time due to lack of appetite. She sometimes gets bloating after meals containing wheat, gluten and dairy. Her childhood was relatively healthy. During her teenage years (14–17 years) she had frequent colds (3 or 4 per year) that took extra time for her 'to get over'.

Breakfast
2 pieces of toast with butter and strawberry jam. Instant coffee with milk
Morning tea
Instant coffee with milk. 2–3 chocolate biscuits
Lunch
Chicken salad. Instant coffee with milk
Afternoon tea
Instant coffee with milk. Chocolate muffin or blueberry muffin
Dinner
Stir fry vegetables. 1 × cup of tea with milk

CASE STUDY CONTINUED

CLINICAL EXAMINATION

Weight 64 kg
Height 1.59 m
BMI 25.32 kg/m^2
Blood pressure 117/78 mmHg
Pulse 72 BPM
Face: dry and red complexion
Eyes: pale conjunctiva
Nails: dryness around the nails

TREATMENT PROTOCOL

INVESTIGATIONS

- Liver function test
- Full blood count
- Urea, electrolytes, creatinine
- Plasma zinc

TREATMENT

INITIAL APPOINTMENT

HERBAL MEDICINE

Herbal medicine	Extract	Quantity	Justification
Taraxacum officinale (root)	1:2	40 mL	Hepatic, cholagogue, digestive tonic
Harpagophytum procumbens	1:2	50 mL	Anti-inflammatory
Calendula officinalis	1:2	30 mL	Lymphatic, immune-regulating, vulnerary, gastrointestinal antiseptic
Uncaria tomentosa	1:2	50 mL	Supportive of healthy digestive ecology, gastrointestinal antimicrobial, anti-inflammatory and antiseptic
Passiflora incarnata	1:2	40 mL	Analgesic, nervine
Zingiber officinale	1:5	10 mL	Anti-inflammatory, circulatory stimulant, carminative
TOTAL		220 mL	

Dose: 5 mL in water t.d.s.

SYMPTOM RELIEF

HERBAL MEDICINE

Herbal medicine	Extract	Quantity	Justification
Corydalis ambigua	1:2	40 mL	Analgesic, anti-inflammatory
Salix alba	1:2	30 mL	Analgesic, anti-inflammatory
Cucuma longa	1:2	40 mL	Analgesic, anti-inflammatory
TOTAL		110 mL	

Dose: 5 mL in water as required, up to 4 times daily.

NUTRITIONAL MEDICINE

Dietary

- The diet was assessed for nutritional deficiencies and steps were taken to correct any deficiencies.
- Allergies and intolerances were investigated. Her diet diary confirmed reactions to wheat, gluten-containing foods and dairy.
- Strict dietary recommendations were suggested. The patient was placed on an anti-inflammatory diet that avoided gluten-containing grains, sugar, refined carbohydrates, caffeine, alcohol, red meat, processed foods, chemicals, additives, preservatives, saturated and trans fats.
- She was encouraged to increase fresh organic fruits and vegetables, complex carbohydrates, wholegrains and fibre, cold-pressed vegetarian sources of essential fatty acids and follow a pesco-vegetarian diet.
- Hydration (30 mL per kg body weight) and protein (1.0 g per kg body weight) were calculated and optimised.
- Simple, easily digested food was recommended initially to ensure that her digestive system could digest and assimilate her intake.

Supplemental

- Probiotics (multi-strain) 45–90 billion organisms in the evening
- Magnesium 200 mg t.d.s.
- Zinc 30 mg t.d.s. with food
- Glucosamine 1500 mg b.i.d.
- Chondroitin 400 mg b.i.d.
- Green-lipped mussel 500 mg t.d.s. in acute flare-ups followed by 500 mg b.i.d. as maintenance
- Omega-3: EPA 600 mg t.d.s. DHA 400 mg t.d.s. Can take an extra EPA 300 mg and DHA 200 mg in acute flare-up
- Glutamine 2500 mg in water b.i.d.
- Glycine 2000 mg in water b.i.d.
- Lysine 1000 mg in water b.i.d.

LIFESTYLE/EDUCATION

She was prescribed time outs for 10 minutes twice per day, once in the morning and once in the mid-afternoon. When she worked on her online business, it was suggested that she took regular breaks; for example, 5 minutes every hour, to reduce her stress and the stress on her hands. A mindfulness app for her phone was investigated.

For physical activity, she was to start walking 10–15 minutes per day to improve her circulation, reduce the excess fluid and to destress.

CASE STUDY CONTINUED

During acute inflammation, passive range-of-motion exercises were performed to help prevent flexion contractures. Range-of-motion exercises of the hands were done in warm water as the heat improves muscle function by reducing stiffness and muscle spasm.

FOLLOW-UP

After 4 weeks she felt that her stress levels had slightly reduced. One day a week the office is very busy where she does more work. On those days the pain remained at 8/10. She found a mindfulness app for her phone that she used daily. She was able to concentrate more on her online business and it was already gaining momentum.

After 8 weeks, the pain in her hands had reduced and she felt more energy. She had less muscular tension in her neck and shoulders. Her appetite increased and her craving for biscuits had gone.

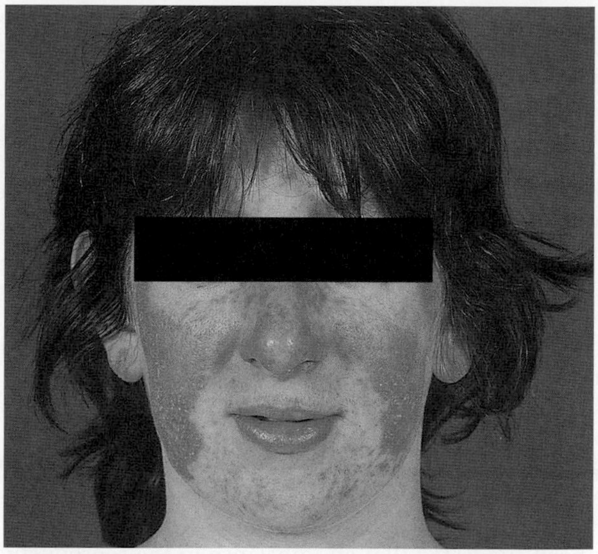

FIGURE 15.16 Systemic lupus erythematosus (SLE).
Source: Walker B et al. Davidson's principles and practice of medicine, 22nd edn. © 2014, Elsevier Limited. All rights reserved.

SYSTEMIC LUPUS ERYTHEMATOSUS

Epidemiology

Systemic lupus erythematosus (SLE) is an autoimmune condition[619] that primarily affects adults (Fig. 15.16), but SLE may also present in juveniles. The condition occurs frequently in women between the ages of 20 and 40 years and world prevalence has a female-to-male ratio of approximately 10 : 1.[620] Research is showing a genetic link of SLE.[621,622]

Classification

According to the American College of Rheumatology 1997 criteria,[623] a patient may be classified as having systemic lupus erythematosus if they have four or more of the following signs/symptoms:

- Malar rash
- Discoid rash
- Photosensitivity
- Oral ulcers
- Arthritis involving two or more peripheral joints (usually non-erosive)
- Serositis
- Pleuritis or pericarditis
- Renal disorder
- Neurological disorder (e.g. seizures in the absence of any other disorder)
- Haematological disorder (e.g. haemolytic anaemia with reticulocytes, leucopenia, thrombocytopenia)
- Immunological disorder (e.g. anti-DNA antibodies, positive finding of antiphospholipid antibodies)
- Positive finding of antinuclear antibodies (ANA).

Aetiology

AUTOIMMUNITY

Systemic lupus erythematosus is a chronic, systemic disorder characterised by widespread inflammation affecting multiple body systems. It is one of the most clinically and serologically diverse of the autoimmune diseases.[624] It is recognised as an autoimmune condition in which the body's own immune system attacks itself. This is visible through the high concentration of antinuclear antibodies that usually present in laboratory testing.

GENDER

Female sex is considered to be the biggest risk factor for SLE, with incidence and prevalence rates for men approximately 1/10th of those of women.[625]

GENETICS

Genetic susceptibility plays a strong role in the aetiology of SLE, with a high prevalence observed in identical twins as well as first-degree relatives of people with the condition. Human leucocyte antigen (HLA)-DR2 and -DR3 regions are the most closely linked genes to SLE,[626] but at least 100 different genes have been implicated in the pathogenesis.[627] With genetics in mind, patients with a Northern European ancestry were significantly associated with photosensitivity (odds ratio = 1.64) and discoid rash (odds ratio = 1.93).[624]

Research is suggesting that genetic background, including HLA class II, is important for the induction of certain autoantibodies that contribute to the clinical heterogeneity and variation in disease outcomes among patients with SLE.[624] MTHFR polymorphisms were found to increase the risk of thrombosis in patients with lupus. MTHFR polymorphisms also resulted in decreased ability to metabolise and reduce plasma homocysteine.[628]

INFECTION

Microbial infection has also been hypothesised to be involved in the pathogenesis of SLE. A number of viruses have been implicated, including Epstein-Barr virus, parvovirus and cytomegalovirus.[629–631] Increased viral load and numbers of latently infected peripheral B-cells as well as impaired functional T-cell responses have been observed in participants with SLE compared with controls. These viruses have been hypothesised to trigger autoimmunity via structural or functional molecular mimicry, cross-reacting with proteins to modulate antigen processing, activation or apoptosis of B- and T-cells, macrophages or dendritic cells.[632]

HORMONAL

The fact that SLE occurs more frequently in women than in men suggests there may be a hormonal element. SLE has been observed to flare up during pregnancy as well as 2 weeks before the menstrual period and during the child-bearing years. Although women with SLE have not been found to have excess oestrogen, alterations in their metabolism of oestrogen have been observed. In men it has been suggested that an imbalance in the reproductive hormones, such as oestrogens and androgens, may increase risk of SLE.[633]

FOOD ALLERGIES

Early reports suggested that food allergies may act as a triggering factor for SLE.[634] This is not a surprise when one considers that food allergies have been linked with other autoimmune disorders. Patients should be tested for food allergies/sensitivities if food hyperreactivity is suspected.

OCCUPATIONAL EXPOSURE

Epidemiological and experimental research suggests a potential link between occupational exposure to such things as crystalline silica, solvents and pesticides and subsequent risk of SLE. For example, occupational exposure to crystalline silica has been suggested to promote or accelerate development of SLE,[635–637] requiring some other factor to break immune tolerance or initiate autoimmunity. The specific manifestation of this effect may depend on underlying differences in genetic susceptibility or other environmental exposure.

EXPOSURE TO ULTRAVIOLET RADIATION

Sunlight increases the number of apoptotic cells in the skin and blood; this could exacerbate SLE by increasing the release of intracellular nuclear antibodies, leading to the generation of more antibodies, which ultimately precipitates the disease. Ultraviolet radiation (e.g. from sun exposure, tanning beds and even light bulbs)[638] may induce or exacerbate skin lesions in patients with SLE.

MEDICATION

Systemic lupus erythematosus may be induced by the use of certain drugs (for example hydralazine or procainamide) and typically manifests with the same symptoms and laboratory findings as idiopathic SLE. Drug-induced lupus erythematosus, however, is recognised as not being 'true' SLE as it typically resolves once exposure to the offending drug stops.[639,640]

Overview

SLE is a chronic inflammatory autoimmune disease affecting multiple organ systems, with 50% of patients displaying neuropsychiatric involvement.[641] It is considered to be in a family of rheumatic disorders that includes rheumatoid arthritis, scleroderma, polymyositis and Sjögren's syndrome. The incidence of SLE has tripled over the past 40 years from 1.51 people per 100 000 to 5.56 people per 100 000.[641]

SLE predominantly affects the central nervous system (CNS), with peripheral nervous system involvement less common. The most common neurological problems are headaches and migraines, which may relate to intracranial hypertension with an increase in platelet aggregation and thrombosis of the cerebral venous system, followed by immune complex deposition with the arachnoid villi.[641] The second most common features are seizures, which may be wrongly diagnosed as an isolated epileptic syndrome. Psychiatric disturbances include mood fluctuations or psychosis, with dementia as a long-term complication. It appears as if these neurological symptoms relate to the infiltration of inflammatory cells into small blood vessels in the brain with necrotic changes to vessel walls.[641]

Pathogenesis

Systemic lupus erythematosus is recognised as an autoimmune disorder that occurs as a result of abnormalities in the function of T-cells, B-cells and cells of the monocytic lineage.[642] Mok and Lau[643] note that in SLE the loss of immune tolerance, increased antigenic load, uncontrolled and excessive T-cell help, unsuppressed B-cells and the shifting of T-helper 1 (Th1) to Th2 immune responses result in B-cell hyperactivity and the production of pathogenic autoantibodies. These pathogenic autoantibodies are the key feature of this disease and, coupled with impaired complement activation and defective clearance of apoptotic cells, lead to tissue injury and damage and widespread inflammation as they attack the body.

Numerous antibodies have been identified with SLE:[641]

- Antinuclear antibodies (ANA) — these are the hallmark of SLE
- Anti-DNA antibodies — these may contribute to the disease and are sometimes found in normal individuals and those with rheumatoid arthritis and Sjögren's syndrome
- Anti-double stranded DNA (anti-dsDNA) antibodies are classic biomarkers of lupus disease activity that have been shown in some, but not all, studies to be predictors of outcome in lupus nephritis studies[624]
- Anti-snRNP antibodies which direct themselves against ribonucleoproteins but are also associated with other rheumatic diseases
- Antiribosomal antibodies which have been linked with the CNS involvement
- Antiphospholipid antibodies, which may be of IgG, IgM or IgA isotypes and form a part of the circulating antibodies directed at phospholipids.

GENERATION OF ANTIBODIES

Several putative mechanisms are involved:

- Defects in the basic processes involved in the normal transformation of a B lymphocyte into an antibody-secreting plasma cell
- Genetic factors point to defects in multiple genes on chromosome 1 in regions bearing loci that encode for immunological proteins
- Apoptosis, DNA and SLE-related antibodies — normal healthy individuals have small quantities of circulating DNA and RNA but the levels in SLE patients are much higher. It is thought that SLE patients have a greater rate of apoptosis, which leads to an ineffective clearance by phagocytes. The immune system then regards these unprocessed DNA fragments as foreign antigens and anti-DNA antibodies are generated.

CYTOKINES

Cytokine production in people with SLE differs markedly from that in unaffected individuals, with interleukins 6, 8 and 10 (IL-6, IL-8, IL-10) increased by a factor of 10, indicating a major imbalance between pro-inflammatory and anti-inflammatory cytokines.

COMPLEMENT AND SLE

Complement has long been implicated in SLE. It appears that patients with SLE have an inherited complement deficiency and that this, coupled with deficient clearance of apoptotic cells helps to generate the abnormalities in circulating nucleosomes leading to antibody production. Complement levels are a classic biomarker of lupus disease activity that have been shown in some, but not all, studies to be predictors of outcome in lupus nephritis studies.[624]

INTERFERON AND LUPUS

Increased levels of IFNα were first reported in patients with lupus nearly 40 years ago. Serum from patients with lupus has been found to contain an IFN-inducing factor. Immune complexes of anti-dsDNA antibodies and DNA have been found to induce IFNα production in normal peripheral blood mononuclear cells which could then induce the differentiation of peripheral blood monocytes into dendritic cells. This gene signature is characterised by the highly coordinated upregulation of type I IFN-inducible inflammatory cytokines, chemokines and other genes whose expression levels are closely correlated with clinical and laboratory measures of SLE.[624]

SIGNS AND SYMPTOMS

A number of different signs and symptoms may present in SLE, as summarised in Table 15.18.

COMPLICATIONS

Complications associated with SLE are many and depend upon the areas of the body affected:

- Kidneys — lupus nephritis is a major cause of morbidity and mortality affecting up to 60% of patients and may result in loss of kidney function if left untreated[644]
- Cardiovascular system — patients with SLE are 5–6 times more likely to have a significant coronary event (e.g. myocardial infarction) compared with the general population[645]
- Neurological system — patients with SLE may develop neuropsychiatric manifestations including cognitive dysfunction, depression, anxiety, seizures and psychosis.

QUALITY OF LIFE

Health-related quality of life is significantly lower in patients with SLE when compared with the general population.[646]

MORBIDITY

Although survival rates for lupus have increased, death still occurs prematurely in many patients, with mortality

TABLE 15.18 Signs and symptoms in systemic lupus erythematosus

Body system	Effects
Systemic	Fatigue, malaise, weight loss
Integumentary	Malar butterfly erythema (fixed erythema, flat or raised, over the malar eminences, tending to spare the nasolabial folds), discoid rash (erythematous raised patches with adherent keratotic scaling and follicular plugging: atrophic scarring may occur in older lesions), photosensitivity, alopecia due to hair follicles being plugged with keratin
Musculoskeletal	Joint pain, arthritis, myalgia, arthrosis, Jaccoud's arthropathy, tendonitis
Neurological	Headaches, depression, seizures, migraines
Immunological	Mouth ulcers, lymphadenopathy
Circulatory/vascular	Raynaud's phenomenon
Cardiovascular	Accelerated atherosclerosis, pericarditis, myocarditis, pericardial effusion, stroke, myocardial infarction, stroke
Renal	Nephritis, persistent proteinuria
Pulmonary	Pleurisy, inflammation of lung lining, pleural effusion, (chest pain, cough, breathlessness)
Gastrointestinal	Abdominal pain, dyspepsia
Haematological	Anaemia, leucopenia, thrombocytopenia, thrombosis

rates observed to be three times those of an age- and sex-matched population in most studies.[647]

DIFFERENTIAL DIAGNOSIS

There are a vast number of differential diagnoses possible due to the myriad of symptoms and multiple organ involvement. Important considerations include:

- Undifferentiated connective tissue disease
- Fibromyalgia with positive ANA
- Sjögren's syndrome
- Vasculitis
- Early-stage rheumatoid arthritis
- Drug-induced lupus
- Idiopathic thrombocytopenia purpura
- Antiphospholipid syndrome
- Multiple sclerosis
- Sarcoidosis
- Bacterial endocarditis.

NATUROPATHIC DIAGNOSIS

Diagnosis considers the autoimmunity aspect to be paramount to the presentation and potential treatment. It is essential to ensure that a holistic assessment is conducted that combines thorough case taking, physical assessment, psychological review and dietary and lifestyle analysis.

Investigations

General investigations are summarised in Table 15.19.

SPECIFIC NATUROPATHIC INVESTIGATIONS

Specific investigations are summarised in Table 15.20.

Therapeutic considerations

CLINICAL DECISION MAKING AND RATIONALE

Due to autoimmunity, it is essential to consider all triggering variables for thorough and holistic assessment and treatment. Key areas include:

- Triggering infection identification
- Query parasitic infestation in GI tract
- Assess GI tract function, presence of dysbiosis, SIBO or flora imbalances
- Assess GI tract integrity and intestinal wall damage
- Assess exposure to xenobiotic toxins

TABLE 15.19 Investigations for systemic lupus erythematosus

Assessment	Justification
Antinuclear antibodies (ANA)	Confirm SLE diagnosis
Antibodies to extractable nuclear antigens (ENA)	Confirm SLE and exclude other conditions
Anti-DNA antibodies	Anti-DNA antibodies are the serological hallmark of SLE and unique markers of the immunological disturbances critical to disease pathogenesis. Anti-DNA antibodies deposit in the tissue to incite inflammation and damage as well as induce cytokine production
HLA B27 antigen	Assesses autoimmune component
Anti-phospholipid antibodies	Associated with an increased risk of thrombosis
Erythrocyte sedimentation rate (ESR)	High levels can indicate increased inflammation and infection
C-reactive protein (CRP)	Assess inflammatory impact of condition
Rheumatoid factor (RF)	Distinguish from other forms of arthritis and other conditions that cause similar symptoms of joint pain, inflammation and stiffness. Can be positive in SLE
CMV, EBV, HIV	Assess for causative viral infection
Complement levels	Complement levels are decreased in SLE
Iron studies	Iron-deficiency anaemia is common in SLE patients
Red cell vitamin B_{12} and folate	Anaemia is common in SLE patients
Full blood count (FBC)	Assess for thrombocytopenia, leucopenia, neutropenia, lymphopenia or haemoglobin/Hct fluctations (reduced)
Coeliac screen	Assess for autoimmune tendency
Vitamin D	Assess nutrient level to determine impact on immune derangement and musculoskeletal health
Mycoplasma, *Chlamydia* and *Borrelia* DNA PCR	Assess for triggering infection
Observe renal involvement Creatinine (plasma) Blood urea nitrogen (BUN) Albumin (plasma/serum)	 Increases if kidney filtering function is impaired Increases if kidney filtering function is impaired Decreased if protein in urine is present

TABLE 15.20 Specific naturopathic investigations	
Genetic diagnostic testing	Preventive genetic diagnostic testing focuses on individual risk profiles, in combination with traditional risk factors and the familial medical history. This helps to explain why individuals are affected differently by the same environmental factors. The knowledge of genetic factors makes preventive medicine easier in that, for example, if the polymorphism result indicates an increased risk for developing SLE, the patient needs regular screening and a nutritional optimisation plan. Most importantly, it helps the practitioner determine a suitable treatment plan tailored to the patient's individual genetic needs. Also test for MTHFR to assess folate metabolism, methylation issues, metabolic issues and comorbidities
Intestinal permeability	Also referred to as a 'leaky gut' test, is a precise and non-invasive method for assessing gastrointestinal mucosal integrity. Damage to the lining of the GI tract (small and large intestine) is common in people with autoimmune conditions
Essential fatty acids profile	EFAs provide the substrate for eicosanoids (prostaglandins) that play a vital role in the regulation of inflammatory conditions
Baseline hormone profiles	These profiles help to identify if hormonal imbalance is causing SLE. Results obtained from the test make it possible for practitioners to individualise treatment in order to establish optimal hormone balance
IgE/IgG food sensitivity profiles	Identifies food sensitivities in the patient with SLE, food sensitivities have been linked to the aetiology of SLE

- Improve proteolytic function and protein digestion
- Assess severity of autoimmunity
- Assess hormonal involvement
- Assess neurotransmitter balance
- Consider emotional, stress and mental impact (historically and currently).

Therapeutic application

NATUROPATHIC PERSPECTIVE

- Assess and thoroughly investigate. Ensure that all considerations are acknowledged
- Modulate autoimmunity
- Reduce inflammation, oxidative stress and oxidation
- Protect the central nervous system
- Encourage appropriate eliminatory pathways
- Address and treat current or subclinical infections
- Ensure dietary and lifestyle practices are conducive to healing and wellbeing.

NUTRITIONAL MEDICINE (DIETARY)

Dietary therapeutic objectives

- Investigate and correct nutritional deficiencies
- Support nutritional requirements with a balanced diet
- Check diet for food intolerances and remove foods found to cause intolerance or allergy
- Encourage antioxidant-rich fruits and vegetables
- Encourage an organic/biodynamic wholefood diet
- Ensure protein needs are met and balanced — vegetarian sources are generally encouraged as well as small quantities of well-digested animal sources. Premarinating fish and meats will assist as will consuming digestive bitters and bitter foods with each meal
- Encourage optimal digestive processes with conscious eating and consideration of slow cooking, regulated eating and calculated portion so as not to overburden the body
- Avoid pro-inflammatory foods.

Specific dietary treatments

DIETARY INCLUSIONS

Anti-inflammatory diet

One of the primary goals in systemic lupus erythematosus is to reduce inflammation. As such, a diet that contains optimal amounts of anti-inflammatory constituents is likely to be most beneficial. Supplementation with fish oils, which are well known for their anti-inflammatory and immune regulatory effects, have shown to be of benefit in SLE. Omega-3 from dietary sources such as salmon, anchovies, sardines, flaxseeds, chia seeds and walnuts should be encouraged.

Antioxidants

A diet rich in antioxidants, espcecially vitamin C, is required in SLE to reduce inflammation and prevent damage from free radicals to the various body systems. A Japanese study found that dietary vitamin C intake may prevent reoccurrence of active lupus, possibly because of its antioxidant and immune properties.[648]

Alkalising diet/wholefoods diet

Although unproven, an alkalising diet is likely to be useful in SLE because of its ability to minimise inflammation in the body. A diet based upon a variety of fresh wholefoods will be nutrient dense, thus providing an array of nutrients required for total health.

DIETARY EXCLUSIONS

Inflammatory foods

Due to the presence of inflammation, foods that promote inflammation in the body should be omitted. These include such things as heavily processed and refined foods, sugar, alcohol and coffee.

Allergenic foods

Patients with SLE may be more prone to food allergies, with a number of case studies reporting remission in symptoms following food elimination diets.[649–651] Food sensitivity testing should be employed and the offending agent(s) removed.

Kidney burden

High-protein diets and any substances that place burden on the kidneys should be avoided if lupus nephritis is present, but it is important to recognise that adequate protein is still required for growth and repair and immune functions.

NUTRITIONAL MEDICINE (SUPPLEMENTAL)

Nutritional medicine therapeutic objectives

- Investigate and correct any nutritional deficiencies. A multivitamin mineral supplement may be required due to poor gastrointestinal status
- Investigate food allergies and intolerances and remove offending foods
- Modulate autoimmunity and support optimal immune function
- Eradicate underlying infection
- Reduce inflammation, oxidative stress and oxidation
- Protect the CNS and support optimal function
- Provide adrenal restorative nutrients to reduce the impact of stress.

Specific nutrients required

B COMPLEX (ALL B VITAMINS INCLUDING B_1, B_2, B_3, B_5, B_6, FOLATE, B_{12})

The B vitamins are involved in numerous systems within the body and reveal positive therapeutic benefits when administered to patients with SLE. Leung[652] suggests that SLE is influenced by vitamin B_5 deficiency and reports of the administration of high-dose vitamin B_5 (10000 mg/day) in 12 women with SLE in combination with other B vitamins (vitamin B_1 500 mg/day, vitamin B_6 200 mg/day, vitamin B_{12} 2000 micrograms/day), as well as 2000 mg/day of vitamin C and two tablets of Super B and two tablets of multivitamins with minerals) over a 2-year period. Within 1 month all patients showed a varying degree of improvement, particularly the symptom of fatigue. Follow-up revealed the incidence of fever to be reduced and no major flares were noted. In many cases, the original SLE medications could gradually be reduced. The authors advised that the vitamins and dosages be revised according to the needs of the individual patient. Complications of SLE such as pernicious anaemia may also respond well to B vitamin supplementation, in particular vitamin B_{12}. The B vitamins (in particular vitamins B_3, B_6, folate and B_{12}) may also be useful for cardiovascular disease associated with SLE, as homocysteine has been found to be elevated in patients with SLE in a number of studies. Nicotinic acid

SAMPLE DAILY DIET

BREAKFAST	
Smoothie: papaya, coconut milk and flaxseed smoothie	An anti-inflammatory, immune-regulating diet is suggested for SLE due to its autoimmune nature. Papaya contains papain, a natural anti-inflammatory enzyme, as well as vitamin C. Vitamin C intake via food has been inversely associated with risk for developing active SLE. Flaxseed has been noted to be reno-protective in individuals with SLE.
LUNCH	
GF tabouli made with quinoa, hummus, falafels, olives and cabbage	Dysbiosis is noted in individuals with SLE leading to an altered microbiome being heavily indicated in the pathogenesis of SLE. Taking this into account, a plant-based diet with ample fibre and prebiotics in conjunction with fermented foods is recommended to improve the microbiome composition and also to protect against CVD, a leading cause of death in SLE.
DINNER	
Steamed snapper with Asian greens, fresh turmeric and ginger	Snapper is a source of omega-3 fatty acids, which exhibit anti-inflammatory and immune-regulating properties that may be useful in SLE. Asian greens provide a source of cruciferous vegetables to assist with excretion of oestrogen from the body. Oestrogen is known to have a stimulating action on the immune system and is implicated in the pathogenesis of autoimmune disease.
SNACK	
Cashews with chia pudding	Provides essential fatty acids and calcium.

Sources: Clark WF, Kortas C, Heidenheim AP et al. Flaxseed in lupus nephritis: a two-year nonplacebo-controlled crossover study. J Am Coll Nutr 2001; 20(2 Suppl):143–148. Hevia A, Milani C, López P et al. Intestinal dysbiosis associated with systemic lupus erythematosus. mBio 2014; 5(5):e01548–14. Minami Y, Sasaki T, Arai Y et al. Diet and systemic lupus erythematosus: a 4 year prospective study of Japanese patients. J Rheumatol 2003; 30(4):747–754.

therapy has also been suggested for hard-to-treat dyslipidaemia in patients with SLE.[653] In patients with MTHFR polymorphisms, folinic acid or 5-MTHF are prescribed instead of folic acid due to lower enzyme activity. Dyslipidaemia is common in patients with SLE and may put patients at greater risk of cardiovascular disease.

BROMELAIN

As yet there are no human studies assessing the effects of bromelain in patients with SLE; however, in-vitro studies reveal bromelain to exert anti-inflammatory[209] effects that may be useful in SLE due to the widespread systemic inflammation[654] that is characteristic of this condition.

DIGESTIVE ENZYMES

Altered intestinal permeability is a common feature of autoimmune conditions and may occur as a result of undigested food that travels into the bloodstream. Digestive enzymes contain a range of enzymes used to support healthy digestion by aiding digestion of fats, proteins, carbohydrates and fibre.

ESSENTIAL FATTY ACIDS (EPA, DHA, GLA)

Essential fatty acids have many properties likely to be of benefit in SLE, including immune regulatory and anti-inflammatory properties. Oral supplementation with omega-3 fatty acids has been found to have positive effects in SLE patients. In a 6-month study, positive effects were seen while supplementing with a fairly low dose of omega-3 fatty acids (3000 mg/day of fish oil, providing 1800 mg/day EPA and 1200 mg/day DHA). Benefits were observed not only in terms of disease activity but also in terms of improved endothelial function and reduced oxidative stress.[655] Acknowledging the relationship between cardiovascular disease and SLE, the benefits seen in terms of vascular protection from this study are encouraging. A 6-month, randomised, single-blind, placebo-controlled, parallel-group pilot study of omega-3 oil in SLE was conducted. Patients were randomised to receive fish oil (6 capsules/day equalling 2.25 g EPA and 2.25 g DHA) or visually identical placebo (6 capsules/day purified (refined, not extra-virgin) olive oil) in addition to their background therapies. The energy/fatigue subscale of the Rand SF-36 produced a trend in improvement for the fish oil group ($p = 0.092$). Emotional wellbeing also showed a trend for improvement in the fish oil group ($p = 0.070$). Erythrocyte sedimentation rate, a measure of systemic inflammation, showed a significant reduction in the fish oil group compared to the placebo group ($p = 0.008$).[656]

GLUCOSAMINE, CHONDROITIN AND GREEN-LIPPED MUSSEL

Joint inflammation is common if not universal in patients with SLE. It is estimated that up to 90% of patients will present with complaints of arthralgia, arthritis and/or tendinitis.[657] Any joint may be affected, although typically the smaller joints are the most problematic. As yet there have been no clinical studies assessing the effects of glucosamine, chondroitin or green-lipped mussel in SLE, but in view of their respective anti-inflammatory and chondro-protective properties they are likely to be useful in patients who present with joint pain. Given the association between SLE and conditions such as arthritis deformans and rheumatoid-like non-erosive hand deformities (Jaccoud's syndrome),[658] the application of one or a combination of glucosamine/chondroitin/green-lipped mussel would appear imperative as a preventive.

QUERCETIN

There have been no human clinical studies investigating the effects of quercetin in SLE, but it is well known that quercetin possesses strong antioxidant and anti-inflammatory capabilities that are undoubtedly of benefit in the condition. These two actions appear to be closely intertwined. Quercetin scavenges oxidants such as tumour necrosis factor that would otherwise promote inflammation within the body. It also possesses anti-coagulative[659] and anti-atherogenic[660] properties that may be useful in SLE due to the high rates of premature atherosclerosis[661,662] and cardiovascular symptoms that present in patients.

MAGNESIUM

The high prevalence of generalised musculoskeletal complaints in SLE suggests that magnesium would be of benefit due to its fundamental role in enzyme function, anti-inflammation, muscle contraction and relaxation, where it aids in the relief of magnesium-related deficiency symptoms such as muscular aches, spasms and cramps.

MANGANESE

Reactive oxygen species are implicated in the pathogenesis of SLE and thus manganese in the form of the antioxidant enzyme manganese superoxide dismutase (MnSOD) may help to protect against damage induced by these free radicals. Low serum levels of manganese have been found in the serum of patients with SLE[663] and it has been suggested that patients with the condition may benefit from supplementation with manganese.[664] Specific genetic polymorphisms of manganese superoxide dismutase have been theorised to occur in people with SLE, but Yen et al[665] could not find proof of this in their study.

SAMe

T-cell DNA methylation levels decrease with age, activating genes implicated in lupus-like autoimmunity. Maintenance of DNA methylation depends on DNA methyltransferase 1 (Dnmt1) and intracellular *S*-adenosylmethionine (SAMe) levels, so if there is a deficiency of SAMe there is an increased risk of lupus occurring.[666] Furthermore, SAMe exerts an anti-inflammatory effect, an action likely to be of use in reducing inflammation and arthritis-like symptoms in SLE. The antidepressant action of SAMe may also be useful for patients who exhibit signs of depression.

SELENIUM

Selenium is a trace mineral that displays antioxidant, anti-inflammatory and immunological properties of use in SLE. As yet no studies have been undertaken in humans, but in New Zealand Black × New Zealand White (NZB/NZW) F mice, which spontaneously develop an autoimmune disease resembling human SLE, those administered selenium were found to have higher natural killer cell activity and improved survival rates than controls.[667] Human clinical studies appear warranted given these results.

VITAMIN A

The use of vitamin A in SLE is controversial due to the lack of published data available in humans, but high-dose vitamin A treatment (100 000 IU/day for 2 weeks) in people with SLE resulted in an enhancement of antibody-dependent cell-mediated cytotoxicity, natural killer activity and blastogenic response to mitogens.[668] Vitamin A is involved in immune regulation and is also an antioxidant, providing an explanation for these effects.

VITAMIN C

Increased oxidative stress and impaired antioxidant status have been found in SLE,[669] so it is not surprising that vitamin C in its role as an antioxidant has been found to decrease lipid peroxidation in patients with SLE.[670]

VITAMIN D

Vitamin D exerts a significant immunoregulatory role within the body and exerts effects upon T-cells, B-cells and dendritic cells[671] known to be involved in the pathogenesis of SLE. Discovery of the relationship between vitamin D and autoimmune disorders such as SLE has prompted much investigation. Deficiency of vitamin D has been found to be extremely common in patients with SLE,[672,673] prompting some to suggest that vitamin D deficiency may be a possible aetiological factor for autoimmune diseases. Certainly it has been observed that patients with SLE have many factors that put them at risk of vitamin D deficiency, including use of steroids, hydroxychloroquine and anti-vitamin D antibodies,[674] and thus supplementation with vitamin D is advised in an attempt to regulate the immune system.

VITAMIN E

Vitamin E (536 mg (800 IU)/day) functions as an antioxidant and has been found to decrease lipid peroxidation in participants with SLE.[670] Vitamin E has also been suggested to be able to suppress autoantibody production in patients with SLE consuming vitamin E (150–300 mg (224–448 IU)/day) in combination with prednisolone via a mechanism independent of antioxidant activity.[675] Other studies suggest that high doses of vitamin E (603–1072 mg (900–1600 IU)/day) appear to be most useful for clearing rashes associated with SLE.[676]

ZINC

Zinc is required in SLE for its immunoregulatory effects, but high doses have been cautioned against for fear of stimulating an already overactive immune system. The addition of zinc is of further benefit for its antioxidant, anti-inflammatory and tissue healing effects, also useful in SLE.

DOSAGE REQUIREMENTS

The dosage requirements listed below are based on adult doses that have been reported in the literature.

- B complex (all B vitamins) high-dose combination, preferably activated forms.
  - Thiamine 20–40 mg/day
  - Riboflavin 50 mg/day. Riboflavin 5′ phosphate 20–40 mg
  - Niacinamide 500–1000 mg/day
  - Pantothenic acid 150–300 mg/day
  - Pyridoxine 50–100 mg/day. Pyridoxal-5-phosphate 20–60 mg/day
  - Folate 500–1000 micrograms/day as folinic acid or L-5MTHF determined by the methylation status of the patient
  - Additional folic acid 5 mg/day or folinic acid/MTHF (2000 micrograms/day) if taking methotrexate — as methotrexate works by antagonising folate, vitamin B9 supplementation may cause treatment failure; such supplementation must be coordinated with the prescribing physician
  - Cyanocobalamin 500–1000 micrograms/day. Methylcobalamin 500–1000 micrograms/day
  - Choline 150–250 mg/day
  - Inositol 150–250 mg/day
  - Biotin 250–500 micrograms/day
- Bromelain 200–400 mg/day
- Digestive enzymes: Specific for each patient but may be from porcine (e.g. pepsin 100 mg t.d.s.) or vegetarian sources
- EFAs: 3000 mg/day of fish oil, providing 1800 mg/day EPA and 1200 mg/day DHA (divided doses e.g. 600 mg EPA and 400 mg DHA t.d.s.)
- Glucosamine 1500 mg/day
- Chondroitin 800–1200 mg/day
- Green-lipped mussel 1500–3000 mg in acute followed by 500–2000 mg as maintenance
- Quercetin 600–1200 mg/day
- Magnesium 500–800 mg/day (e.g. 300 mg t.d.s.)
- Manganese 15 mg/day
- SAMe 600–1200 mg/day (e.g. 200–400 mg b.i.d. or t.d.s.)
- Selenium 70–200 micrograms/day[677]
- Vitamin A 5000 IU/day[677]
- Vitamin C 500–2000 mg/day[670] (divided doses e.g. 500 mg q.i.d., 1000 mg b.i.d., 500 mg t.d.s.)
- Vitamin D 1000–5000 IU (pathology-dependent) (depending on dosage, do divided doses twice or three times daily, e.g. 3000 IU b.i.d.)
- Vitamin E 800 IU/day[670]
- Zinc 45–75 mg/day
- Glutamine 2000 mg b.i.d.
- Probiotics (multi-strain) 45–90 billion organisms/day (e.g. 45 billion 1–2 times daily).

HERBAL MEDICINE

Herbal medicine therapeutic objectives

- To modulate immune function through immunodepressants and immunomodulators
- To reduce the presence of microorganisms/infective agents through antimicrobials and treatment specific to the infective agent (e.g. antiviral, antibacterial)
- To control or eliminate dysbiosis, reduce abnormal intestinal permeability, repair intestinal wall damage through mucous membrane trophorestoratives, astringents, demulcents

- To reduce the impact of xenobiotic toxins by supporting the liver with hepatics, hepatotrophorestoratives, bitters
- To improve proteolytic function through digestive bitters
- To reduce inflammation through anti-inflammatories, steroidal anti-inflammatory agents
- To reduce oxidative stress through antioxidant and anti-inflammatory herbals
- To regulate hormonal factors and support the stress response through adaptogens, adrenal restoratives
- To protect the CNS through antioxidants and neuroprotection
- To eliminate and support clearance of toxins through lymphatics, diuretics, bitters, hepatics, blood tonics, immunomodulators, circulatory stimulants.

Specific herbal medicines

BOSWELLIA SERRATA (BOSWELLIA)

Inflammation is chronic in SLE, but one would think that the addition of *Boswellia serrata* would be likely to reduce leukotrienes and other inflammatory mediators because of its ability to inhibit the enzyme 5-lipoxygenase, resulting in reduced inflammation. The effects of *Boswellia serrata* are additionally useful in autoimmune conditions, where it has been found to possess anti-complementary activity. In vitro, boswellic acids inhibited C3-convertase of the classical complement pathway, suggesting a possible mechanism by which it exerts its effect on autoimmune disorders.[678] Clinical testing in people with SLE is needed.

CURCUMA LONGA (TURMERIC)

Curcumin has been shown to inhibit a range of autoimmune diseases by regulating inflammatory cytokines such as IL-1β, IL-6, IL-12, TNF-α and IFN-γ and associated JAK-STAT, AP-1 and NF-κB signalling pathways in immune cells,[679] so it may also show promise in inhibiting SLE. In-vitro studies reveal that heat-solubilised curcumin/turmeric can significantly decrease binding of autoantibodies from SLE patients by up to 52–70%, but as yet there have been few human clinical trials, largely due to the aqueous insolubility of curcumin. Nevertheless, these results show great promise for the effects of administering curcumin in patients with SLE.[680] Additionally useful are the antioxidant properties of curcumin, which may assist in preventing the oxidation and modification of proteins implicated in SLE.[680]

ECHINACEA SPP. (ECHINACEA)

Systemic lupus erythematosus is an autoimmune condition so is likely to be aided by botanicals such as echinacea that act to regulate an overactive immune system. Although echinacea is thought to have a stimulating action upon the immune system it is perhaps better to consider it as an immune modulator or regulator. This action is visible in a study by Neri et al in patients with low-grade, steroid-dependent autoimmune uveitis. Patients in the echinacea group received echinacea (150 mg twice a day) as add-on therapy while the other group were treated with conventional medicine alone.[681] Those who did not receive echinacea required a longer treatment period with steroids, with a steroid-off time of 121 and 87 days. No adverse reactions were recorded from commercial-grade echinacea. The authors concluded that echinacea appears safe and effective in the control of low-grade autoimmune idiopathic uveitis. As yet there are no clinical studies assessing the effects of echinacea in SLE and thus further studies are required to assess its efficacy.

GINKGO BILOBA (GINKGO)

Protection of the CNS is a prime treatment objective in SLE. Ginkgo is known for its neuroprotective properties, which are probably a result of its significant antioxidant activity. Raynaud's phenomenon commonly manifests in SLE and describes a cutaneous symptom in which the blood vessels spasm in response to stress, cold stimuli (e.g. a change in weather), moisture or vibration.[682] The closure of the blood vessels leads to cyanosis and poor circulation in the fingers, toes and, more uncommonly, the nose and ears; pain and numbness are commonly experienced.[683] *Ginkgo biloba* is an effective peripheral circulatory stimulant that has displayed promising results for patients with Raynaud's phenomenon. Supplementation with Seredrin, a *Ginkgo biloba* extract, administered to patients over a 10-week period was found to significantly reduce the number of attacks experienced by patients per week from 13.2 (±16.5) to 5.8 (±8.3), a reduction of approximately 56%, whereas placebo reduced the number by only 27%.[684]

GLYCYRRHIZA GLABRA (LIQUORICE)

Glycyrrhiza glabra contains many properties that may be useful in patients presenting with SLE, including its use as an adrenal tonic and anti-inflammatory properties. Corticosteroids are commonly prescribed in SLE because of their anti-inflammatory action, but long-term use is associated with adrenal insufficiency as the body's own natural corticosteroid production reduces or stops all together. *Glycyrrhiza glabra* contains glycyrrhizic acid, the active constituent that inhibits the enzyme 11-beta-hydroxysteroid dehydrogenase, thus slowing/preventing cortisol breakdown.

HARPAGOPHYTUM PROCUMBENS (DEVIL'S CLAW)

Harpagophytum procumbens is a popular anti-inflammatory and analgesic botanical that may be useful in treating inflammation and rheumatism associated with SLE. It appears to be well tolerated long term,[685] which is beneficial since many medications (such as corticosteroids) prescribed for SLE have multiple side effects when prescribed long term.

HEMIDESMUS INDICUS (HEMIDESMUS)

Hemidesmus is well regarded for autoimmune conditions such as SLE due to its immune-suppressant properties. It combines well with echinacea for treatment of autoimmune disorders.

HYPERICUM PERFORATUM (ST JOHN'S WORT)

Hypericum perforatum is a botanical with multiple applications in SLE due to its antidepressant, antiviral, anxiolytic and nervine actions. Mood disorders such as anxiety and depression[686–688] are more common in patients with SLE than in the general population, which is hardly surprising given the enormity of the disease. *Hypericum perforatum* is well known for its anxiolytic and antidepressant effects but as yet no studies can be found examining its effects in patients with SLE suffering from anxiety and/or depression. Because of its action on the nervous system, *Hypericum perforatum* should be considered in patients with SLE who present with depression, anxiety or inability to cope with stressors. Given that viral infection has been hypothesised to be involved in the pathogenesis of SLE, the addition of *Hypericum perforatum* may also be useful because of its antiviral properties. It is essential to assess for any photosensitivity which can aggravate or compound the presentation. Specific extracts with reduced hyperforin concentration may be most applicable. Caution concomitant use with medications due to enhancement of cytochrome P450 enzyme pathway.

REHMANNIA GLUTINOSA (REHMANNIA)

As with *Glycyrrhiza glabra, Rehmannia glutinosa* is well utilised in SLE because of its adrenal restorative action. In traditional Chinese medicine it has been used in autoimmune conditions because of its proposed immunomodulating effects. *Rehmannia glutinosa* is also regarded as a kidney tonic and has been used in Chinese medicine (in combination with a number of other herbs) for nephritis associated with SLE.[238] Further well-designed human clinical trials are warranted to confirm the multifaceted action of *Rehmannia glutinosa* in SLE.

SALIX SPP. (WILLOW BARK)

As yet there have been no studies assessing the effects of *Salix* spp. in SLE, but the German Commission E highlights its use for inflammation, headaches and fever, all of which may be present in SLE. The *British Herbal Compendium* reports analgesic properties and advocates its use for rheumatic and arthritic conditions,[609] which the joint complaints associated with SLE could be likened to. The efficacy of *Salix* is suggested to be a result of the salicylates found within its bark.

ZINGIBER OFFICINALE (GINGER)

The effects of *Zingiber officinale* are yet to be studied in SLE but it is likely to be useful for its anti-inflammatory, circulatory stimulant and antirheumatic properties. *Zingiber officinale* exerts a warming, pungent action that may help to relieve symptoms associated with Raynaud's phenomenon and ease joint pain and stiffness. *Zingiber officinale* has been found to be effective in a number of inflammatory conditions where it helps to relieve rheumatic muscular pain and thus may ease pain associated with SLE.

LIFESTYLE RECOMMENDATIONS

Avoiding triggers (e.g. sunlight)

A number of patients with lupus complain of increased photosensitivity, so preventive measures such as staying out of the sun or wearing protective clothing will help. Interestingly, Lehmann and Homey[689] have noted that patients may not be aware of the detrimental effects of sunlight on their disease as the development of skin lesions after UV injury is typically delayed, starting from a few days up to 3 weeks after the irradiation, though the lesions may persist for many months.

Smoking cessation

Smoking is associated with numerous health risks, especially increased risk of vascular complications such as venous thrombosis associated with lupus, so quitting is imperative.

Stress management techniques

Chronic stress worsens the quality of life in patients with lupus and may worsen clinical symptomatology perceived by patients,[690] so techniques that assist in the management of stress may be helpful.[691] Cognitive behavioural technique has been found to reduce psychological stress in patients with lupus,[692] while exercise may improve cardiovascular fitness, reduce metabolic abnormalities, fatigue and depression, and improve quality of life.[693] Interestingly, Wittmann et al[694] note that patients who recognise personal growth in response to the illness may experience reduced suffering, so this is something that may be useful for practitioners to foster with patients. Massage and yoga are useful in managing stress.

CASE STUDY

OVERVIEW

GR, a 58-year-old female, presented with systemic lupus erythematosus and Sjögren's syndrome. Her diagnosis was 8 years ago. She suffers from joint pain, swelling and stiffness, 'butterfly' malar rash, along with fatigue and dry skin. Her joint stiffness can last for 20–30 minutes in the morning. Exposure to the sun may bring on lupus skin lesions on her face, arms and chest. She presents with dry mouth and dry eyes that burn, itch and feel gritty most days. She finds sexual intercourse uncomfortable at times due to vaginal dryness. She has a cough every month that may persist for up to a week. The cough normally resolves on its own. One to two times per month she suffers from a headache that leaves her feeling fatigued. A year ago she noticed that her hair is thinning. The thinning hair concerns her and causes her some stress. When she feels stressed she gets tingling in her hands. Her concentration is 'foggy' several times per week. She needs to sit down and relax to bring her focus back. She gets mouth ulcers 1–3 times per month and her glands can become swollen 1–2 times per month.

Her diet is average. She feels nauseous when she eats too fast. When she eats bread and milk she feels bloated. The bloating subsides 30 minutes later. She feels constipated and finds it difficult to defecate. She feels better after a bowel movement.

She suffered from asthma during her childhood. Her asthma improved by her mid-20s. However, she does get out of breath easily when she exerts herself, even walking up stairs.

CASE STUDY CONTINUED

CLINICAL EXAMINATION

- BP 138/95 mmHg
- Pulse 79 BPM
- Height 1.66 m
- Weight 60 kg
- BMI 21.77 kg/m^2
- Face: dry with malar rash
- Skin: dry skin with dry red lumps on the back of the arms
- Tongue: dry, scalloping, central crack and a mild quiver
- Nails: mild vertical ridging, lack of moons, white spots on index and middle fingers

FURTHER TESTING

- Full blood count (checking for leucocytopenia, thrombocytopenia)
- Urea, electrolytes, creatinine
- Iron studies
- Urinalysis: for protein, blood, creatinine

TREATMENT PROTOCOL

INITIAL APPOINTMENT

Herbal medicine

Herbal medicine	Extract	Quantity	Justification
Passiflora incarnata	1:2	50 mL	Nervine, analgesic
Uncaria tomentosa	1:2	60 mL	Adaptogen, anti-inflammatory, analgesic
Ginkgo biloba	STD ext	40 mL	Antioxidant, CNS protective
Harpagophytum procumbens	1:2	60 mL	Anti-inflammatory, analgesic
Zingiber officinale	1:5	10 mL	Anti-inflammatory, circulatory stimulant, carminative
TOTAL		220 mL	

Dosage: 7.5 mL b.i.d.

Acute flare-up formula

Herbal medicine	Extract	Quantity	Justification
Withania somnifera	1:2	30 mL	Adaptogen, nervine
Salix alba	1:2	40 mL	Anti-inflammatory, analgesic
Corydalis ambigua	1:2	40 mL	Anti-inflammatory, analgesic
TOTAL		110 mL	

5 mL in water as required, up to 4 times daily

CASE STUDY CONTINUED

NUTRITIONAL MEDICINE

Dietary

She was advised to improve her intake of protein (1.0 g per kg body weight per day), hydration (30 mL per kg body weight per day) and organic fruits and vegetables (following a Mediterranean-style diet) as much as possible. Her fluid intake was to be as regular as possible to maintain moisture in the mouth and throat. She added a smoothie a day with a scoop of protein powder, chia seeds, blueberries, coconut flakes and LSA (linseed, sunflower, almond powder). When nutritional deficiencies were found they were corrected with specific foods.

Supplemental

- High-potency B complex (activated): 1 capsule with breakfast and 1 capsule with lunch
- Probiotics (multi-strain) 45 billion organisms twice per day
- Zinc 30 mg b.i.d.
- Magnesium 200 mg t.d.s.
- Selenium 150 micrograms/day
- Vitamin B_6 — Pyridoxyl-5-phosphate 50 mg daily
- Quercetin 500 mg t.d.s.
- Bromelain 200 mg t.d.s.
- Omega-3 EPA 600 mg and DHA 400 mg t.d.s.
- Glutamine 5000 mg in water b.i.d.
- Glycine 2000 mg in water b.i.d.
- N-acetylcysteine 1000 mg in water b.i.d.

LIFESTYLE/EDUCATION

Avoid direct sunlight and unnecessary UV exposure. Stress management techniques were suggested including finding a hobby. She was to have a time out for 10 minutes in the morning and 10 minutes in the afternoon/evening.

FOLLOW-UP

After 4 weeks, her energy levels had slightly improved. She noticed that her hair was stronger, which made her happier. The time outs and her new hobby of painting had improved her stress levels.

After 8 weeks, her energy further improved. Her mouth didn't feel as dry and she had fewer mouth ulcers during the last 4 weeks. She continued painting and was excited that she had sold three paintings.

REFERENCES

[1] Wackerhage H, Rennie M. How nutrition and exercise maintain the human musculoskeletal mass. J Anat 2006;208:451–8.

[2] Watkins J. Structure and function of the musculoskeletal system. Champaign, IL: Human Kinetics; 1999.

[3] Tortora JG, Grabowski SR. Principles of anatomy and physiology. 9th ed. New York: John Wiley; 2000.

[4] France R. Introduction to sports medicine and athletic training. New York: Thomas Delmar Learning; 2004.

[5] Chen D. Bone morphogenetic proteins. Growth Factors 2004;22:233–41.

[6] McKay CP, Portale A. Emerging topics in paediatric bone and mineral disorders. Semin Nephrol 2009;29:370–8.

[7] Krieger NS, Frick KK, Bushinsky DA. Mechanism of acid-induced bone resorption. Curr Opin Nephrol Hypertens 2004;13:423–36.

[8] Jansky L. Contribution of striated muscles to heat production. Experientia 1977;33:1123–4.
[9] Clarkson H. Musculoskeletal assessment: joint range of motion and manual muscle strength. 2nd ed. Philadelphia: Lippincott Williams & Wilkins; 2000.
[10] Weintraub W. Tendon and ligament healing: a new approach to sports and overuse injury. New Mexico: Paradigm Publications; 2003.
[11] Carpenter KJ. Early ideas on the nutritional significance of lipids. J Nutr 1998;128:423s–426s.
[12] Ellingwood F. The Eclectic practice of medicine with especial reference to the treatment of disease; 1910. Available from: www.henriettesherbal.com/eclectic/ellingwood1/index.html.
[13] Castleman M. The new healing herbs, the classic guide to natures best medicines. Heatherton, Victoria: Hinkler Books; 2001.
[14] Wiitavaara B, Fahlström M, Mats Djupsjöbacka M. Prevalence, diagnostics and management of musculoskeletal disorders in primary health care in Sweden — an investigation of 2000 randomly selected patient records. J Eval Clin Pract 2017;23(2):325–32.
[15] Vijay S, Ide M. Musculoskeletal neck and back pain in undergraduate dental students at a UK dental school — a cross-sectional study. Br Dent J 2016;221(5):241–5.
[16] Alavi SS, Makarem J, Abbasi M, et al. Association between upper extremity musculoskeletal disorders and mental health status in office workers. Work 2016;55(1):3–11.
[17] Korniloff K, Mauno Vanhala MD, et al. Musculoskeletal pain in melancholic and atypical depression. Pain Med 2017;18(2):341–7.
[18] Castaño-Betancourt MC, Evans DS, Ramos YFM, et al. Novel genetic variants for cartilage thickness and hip osteoarthritis. PLoS Genet 2016;12(10):e1006260.
[19] March LM, Bagga H. Epidemiology of osteoarthritis in Australia. Med J Aust 2004;180:S6–10.
[20] Hunter D, Lo G. The management of osteoarthritis: an overview and call to appropriate conservative treatment. Rheum Dis Clin North Am 2008;34:689–712.
[21] Australian Bureau of Statistics. National health survey. Canberra: Australian Bureau of Statistics; 2004–2005.
[22] Altman R, Alarcon G, Appelroth D, et al. The American College of Rheumatology criteria for the classification and reporting of osteoarthritis of the hand. Arthritis Rheum 1990;33:1601–10.
[23] Altman R, Alarcon G, Appelroth D, et al. The American College of Rheumatology criteria for the classification and reporting of osteoarthritis of the hip. Arthritis Rheum 1991;34:505–14.
[24] Altman R, Alarcon G, Appelroth D, et al. The American College of Rheumatology criteria for the classification and reporting of osteoarthritis of the knee. Arthritis Rheum 1986;29:1039–49.
[25] Dieppe PA, Lohmander LS. Pathogenesis and management of pain in osteoarthritis. Lancet 2005;365:965–73.
[26] Felson DT, Zhang Y. An update on the epidemiology of knee and hip osteoarthritis with a view to prevention. Arthritis Rheum 1998;41:1343–55.
[27] Felson DT, Lawrence RC, Dieppe PA, et al. Osteoarthritis: new insights. Part 1: the disease and its risk factors. Ann Intern Med 2000;133:635–46.
[28] Stecher RM. Heberden's nodes. Heredity in hypertrophic arthritis of the finger joints. Am J Med Sci 1941;201:801.
[29] Spector TD, Cicuttini F, Baker J, et al. Genetic influences on osteoarthritis: a twin study on women. BMJ 1996;312:94.
[30] Loughlin J. Genetic epidemiology of primary osteoarthritis. Curr Opin Rheumatol 2001;13:111–1116.
[31] McAlindon T, Zhang Y, Hannan M, et al. Are risk factors for patellofemoral and tibiofemoral knee osteoarthritis different? J Rheumatol 1996;23:332–7.
[32] Spector TD, Hart DJ, Doyle DV. Incidence and progression of osteoarthritis in women with unilateral knee disease in the general population: the effect of obesity. Ann Rheum Dis 1994;53:565.
[33] Cooper C, Inskip H, Croft P, et al. Individual risk factors for hip osteoarthritis: obesity, hip injury and physical activity. Am J Epidemiol 1998;147:516–22.
[34] Jensen LK. Hip osteoarthritis: influence of work with heavy lifting, climbing stairs or ladders, or combining kneeling/squatting with heavy lifting. Occup Environ Med 2008;65:6–19.
[35] Jensen LK. Knee osteoarthritis: influence of work involving heavy lifting, kneeling, climbing stairs or ladders, or kneeling/squatting combined with heavy lifting. Occup Environ Med 2008;65:72–89.
[36] Zhang Y, Jordan J. Epidemiology of osteoarthritis. Rheum Dis Clin North Am 2008;34:515–29.
[37] Cerejo R, Dunlop DD, Cahue S, et al. The influence of alignment on risk of knee osteoarthritis progression according to baseline stage of disease. Arthritis Rheum 2002;46:2632–6.
[38] Felson DT, McLaughlin S, Goggins J, et al. Bone marrow edema and its relation to progression of knee osteoarthritis. Ann Intern Med 2003;139:330–6.
[39] Golightly YM, Allen KD, Renner JB, et al. Relationship of limb length inequality with radiographic knee and hip osteoarthritis. Osteoarthr Cartil 2007;15:824–9.
[40] Hanlon CR, Estes W. Osteoarthritis aggravated by trauma. Am J Surg 1949;78:556–69.
[41] Gelber AC, Hochberg MC, Mead LA, et al. Joint injury in young adults and risk for subsequent knee and hip osteoarthritis. Ann Intern Med 2000;133:321–8.
[42] Herrero-Beaumont G, Blas-Roman JA, Castañeda S, et al. Primary osteoarthritis no longer primary: three subsets with distinct etiological, clinical and therapeutic characteristics. Semin Arthritis Rheum 2009;39:71–80.
[43] Martel-Pelletier J. Pathophysiology of osteoarthritis. Osteoarthr Cartil 2004;12:S31–3.
[44] Fernandes JC, Martel-Pelletier J, Pelletier JP. The role of cytokines in osteoarthritis pathophysiology. Biorheology 2002;39(1–2):237–46.
[45] Kumar P, Clark M. Clinical medicine. 3rd ed. Edinburgh: Baillière Tindall; 1994.
[46] Goldrick S. Role of bone in osteoarthritis pathogenesis. Med Clin North Am 2009;93(1):25–31.
[47] Abramson SB, Attur M, Yazici Y. Prospects for disease modification in osteoarthritis. Nat Clin Pract Rheumatol 2006;2(6):304–12.
[48] Vincent T, Watt F. Osteoarthritis. Medicine (Baltimore) 2010;38(3):151–6.
[49] Wang Y, Hodge AM, Wluka AE, et al. Effect of antioxidants on knee cartilage and bone in healthy, middle-aged subjects: a cross-sectional study. Arthritis Res Ther 2007;9(4):R66.
[50] McAlindon TE, Jacques P, Zhang Y, et al. Do antioxidant micronutrients protect against the development and progression of knee osteoarthritis? Arthritis Rheum 1996;39:648–56.
[51] Wluka AE, Stuckey S, Brand C, et al. Supplementary vitamin E does not affect the loss of cartilage volume in knee osteoarthritis: a 2 year double blind randomized placebo controlled study. J Rheumatol 2002;29:2585–91.
[52] Darlington LG, Stone TW. Antioxidants and fatty acids in the amelioration of rheumatoid arthritis and related disorders. Br J Nutr 2001;85(3):251–69.
[53] Kowsari B, Finnie SK, Carter RL, et al. Assessment of the diet of patients with rheumatoid arthritis and osteoarthritis. J Am Diet Assoc 1983;82(6):657–9.
[54] Kaiki G, Tsuji H, Yonezawa T, et al. Osteoarthrosis induced by intra-articular hydrogen peroxide injection and running load. J Orthop Res 1990;8:731–40.
[55] Wilhelmi G. [Potential effects of nutrition including additives on healthy and arthrotic joints. I. Basic dietary constituents] [Article in German]. Z Rheumatol 1993;52(3):174–9.
[56] Rayman M, Pattison DJ. Dietary manipulation in musculoskeletal conditions. Best Pract Res Clin Rheumatol 2008;22:535–61.
[57] Rasheed Z, Anbazhagan AN, Akhtar N, et al. Green tea polyphenol epigallocatechin-3-gallate inhibits advanced glycation end product-induced expression of tumor necrosis factor-alpha and matrix metalloproteinase-13 in human chondrocytes. Arthritis Res Ther 2009;11(3):R71.
[58] França DS, Souza AL, Almeida KR, et al. B vitamins induce an antinociceptive effect in the acetic acid and formaldehyde models of nociception in mice. Eur J Pharmacol 2001;421:157–64.
[59] Kobayashi T, Notoya K, Nakamura A, et al. Fursultiamine, a vitamin B_1 derivative, enhances chondroprotective effects of glucosamine hydrochloride and chondroitin sulfate in rabbit experimental osteoarthritis. Inflamm Res 2005;54(6):249–55.
[60] Jonas WB, Rapoza CP, Blair WF. The effect of niacinamide on osteoarthritis: a pilot study. Inflamm Res 1996;45(7):330–4.

[61] Anand JC. Pantothenic acid and osteoarthrosis. Lancet 1963;282(7318):1168.
[62] Newnham RE. Essentiality of boron for healthy bones and joints. Environ Health Perspect 1994;102(Suppl. 7):83–5.
[63] Helliwell TR, Kelly SA, Walsh HP, et al. Elemental analysis of femoral bone from patients with fractured neck of femur or osteoarthrosis. Bone 1996;18(2):151–7.
[64] Hunter DJ, Hart D, Snieder H, et al. Evidence of altered bone turnover, vitamin D and calcium regulation with knee osteoarthritis in female twins. Rheumatology (Oxford) 2003;42(11):1311–13116.
[65] Goggs R, Vaughan-Thomas A, Clegg PD, et al. Nutraceutical therapies for degenerative joint diseases: a critical review. Crit Rev Food Sci Nutr 2005;45(3):145–64.
[66] Héraud F, Savineau C, Harmand MF. Copper modulation of extracellular matrix synthesis by human articular chondrocytes. Scand J Rheumatol 2002;31(5):279–84.
[67] Zainala Z, Longmana AJ, Hursta S, et al. Relative efficacies of omega-3 polyunsaturated fatty acids in reducing expression of key proteins in a model system for studying osteoarthritis. Osteoarthr Cartil 2009;17(7):896–905.
[68] Shen CL, Dunn DM, Henry JH, et al. Decreased production of inflammatory mediators in human osteoarthritic chondrocytes by conjugated linoleic acid. Lipids 2004;39:161–6.
[69] Curtis CL, Rees SG, Little CB. Pathologic indicators of degradation and inflammation in human osteoarthritic cartilage are abrogated by exposure to n-3 fatty acids. Arthritis Rheum 2002;46:1544.
[70] Kirkham SG, Samarasinghe RK. Review article: glucosamine. J Orthop Surg (Hong Kong) 2009;17:72–6.
[71] Ruane R, Griffiths P. Glucosamine therapy compared with ibuprofen for joint pain. Br J Community Nurs 2002;7(3): 148–52.
[72] Bruyere O, Pavelka K, Rovati LC, et al. Total joint replacement after glucosamine sulfate treatment in knee osteoarthritis: results of a mean 8 year observation of patients from two previous 3 year randomised placebo controlled trials. Osteoarthr Cartil 2008;16(2):254–60.
[73] Pavelka K, Gatterova J, Olejarova M, et al. Glucosamine sulfate use and delay of progression of knee osteoarthritis. A 3-year, randomized, placebo-controlled, double-blind study. Arch Intern Med 2002;162:2113–23.
[74] Clegg DO, Reda DJ, Harris CL, et al. Glucosamine chondroitin sulfate and the two in combination for painful knee osteoarthritis. N Engl J Med 2006;354:795–808.
[75] Zhang WB, Zhuang CY, Li JM, et al. [Efficacy and safety evaluation of glucosamine hydrochloride in the treatment of osteoarthritis]. Zhonghua Wai Ke Za Zhi 2007;45(14):998–1001.
[76] Towheed T, Maxwell L, Anastassiades TP, et al. Glucosamine therapy for treating osteoarthritis. Cochrane Database Syst Rev 2005;(2):CD002946.
[77] Kubo M, Ando K, Mimura T, et al. Minireview: chondroitin sulfate for the treatment of hip and knee osteoarthritis: current status and future trends. Life Sci 2009;85:477–83.
[78] Uebelhart D, Malaise M, Marcolongo R, et al. Intermittent treatment of knee osteoarthritis with oral chondroitin sulfate: a one-year, randomized, double-blind, multicenter study versus placebo. Osteoarthr Cartil 2004;12(4):269–76.
[79] Kahan A, Uebelhart D, De Vathaire F, et al. Long-term effects of chondroitins 4 and 6 sulfate on knee osteoarthritis: the study on osteoarthritis progression prevention, a two-year, randomized, double-blind, placebo-controlled trial. Arthritis Rheum 2009;60:524–33.
[80] Singh JA, Noorbaloochi S, MacDonald R, et al. Chondroitin for osteoarthritis. Cochrane Database Syst Rev 2015;(1):CD005614.
[81] McAlindon T, LaValley MP, Gulin JP, et al. Glucosamine and chondroitin for treatment of osteoarthritis: a systematic quality assessment and meta-analysis. JAMA 2000;283(11):1.
[82] Cho SH, Jung YB, Seong SC, et al. Clinical efficacy and safety of Lyprinol, a patented extract from New Zealand green-lipped mussel (*Perna canaliculus*) in patients with osteoarthritis of the hip and knee: a multicenter 2-month clinical trial. Eur Ann Allergy Clin Immunol 2003;35(6):212–2116.
[83] Cobb CS, Ernst E. Systematic review of a marine nutriceutical supplement in clinical trials for arthritis: the effectiveness of the New Zealand green-lipped mussel *Perna canaliculus*. Clin Rheumatol 2006;25(3):275–84.
[84] Brien S, Prescott P, Coghlan B, et al. Systematic review of the nutritional supplement *Perna Canaliculus* (green-lipped mussel) in the treatment of osteoarthritis. QJM 2008;101:167–79.
[85] Rutjes AW, Nüesch E, Reichenbach S, et al. S-adenosylmethionine for osteoarthritis of the knee or hip. Cochrane Database Syst Rev 2009;(4):CD007321.
[86] Harmand MF, Vilamitjana J, Maloche E, et al. Effects of S-adenosylmethionine on human articular chondrocyte differentiation. An in vitro study. Am J Med 1987;83(5A):48–54.
[87] König B. A long-term (two years) clinical trial with S-adenosylmethionine for the treatment of osteoarthritis. Am J Med 1987;83(5A):89–94.
[88] Soeken KL, Lee WL, Bausell RB, et al. Safety and efficacy of S-adenosylmethionine (SAM-e) for osteoarthritis. J Fam Pract 2002;51(5):425–30.
[89] Chaganti RK, Parimi N, Cawthon P, et al. Association of 25-hydroxyvitamin D with prevalent osteoarthritis of the hip in elderly men: the osteoporotic fractures in men study. Arthritis Rheum 2010;62(2):511–5114.
[90] Bergink AP, Uitterlinden AG, Van Leeuwen JP, et al. Vitamin D status, bone mineral density and the development of radiographic osteoarthritis of the knee: the Rotterdam Study. J Clin Rheumatol 2009;15(5):230–7.
[91] Ding C, Cicuttini F, Parameswaran V, et al. Serum levels of vitamin D, sunlight exposure and knee cartilage loss in older adults: the Tasmanian older adult cohort study. Arthritis Rheum 2009;60(5):1381–9.
[92] Machtey I, Ouaknine L. Tocopherol in osteoarthritis: a controlled pilot study. J Am Geriatr Soc 1978;26(7):328–30.
[93] Blankenhorn G. Clinical effectiveness of vitamin E in activated arthroses. A multi center placebo-controlled double-blind study. Z Orthop 1986;124:340–3.
[94] Chrubasik S. Vitamin E for rheumatoid arthritis or osteoarthritis: low evidence of effectiveness. Z Rheumatol 2003;62(5):491.
[95] Brand C, Snaddon J, Bailey M, et al. Vitamin E is ineffective for symptomatic relief of knee osteoarthritis: a six month double blind, randomised, placebo controlled study. Ann Rheum Dis 2001;60(10):946–9.
[96] Haflah NH, Jaarin K, Abdullah S, et al. Palm vitamin E and glucosamine sulfate in the treatment of osteoarthritis of the knee. Saudi Med J 2009;30(11):1432–8.
[97] Miehle W. Vitamin E in active arthroses and chronic polyarthritis. What is the value of alpha-tocopherol in therapy? Fortschr Med 1997;115(26):39–42.
[98] Surapaneni KM, Venkataramana G. Status of lipid peroxidation, glutathione, ascorbic acid, vitamin E and antioxidant enzymes in patients with osteoarthritis. Indian J Med Sci 2007;61(1):9–14.
[99] Ostałowska A, Kasperczyk S, Kasperczyk A, et al. Oxidant and anti-oxidant systems of synovial fluid from patients with knee post-traumatic arthritis. J Orthop Res 2007;25(6):804–12.
[100] Berkson D. Osteoarthritis, chiropractic and nutrition: osteoarthritis considered as a natural part of a three stage subluxation complex: its reversibility: its relevance and treatability by chiropractic and nutritional correlates. Med Hypotheses 1991;36(4):356–67.
[101] McEwen BJ. Methylenetetrahydrofolate reductase (MTHFR): mythology or polymorphism(ology)? Adv Integr Med 2016;3(3):79–81.
[102] Newnham RE. Essentiality of boron for healthy bones and joints. Environ Health Perspect 1994;102(Suppl. 7):83–5.
[103] Caruso I, Pietrogrande V. Italian double-blind multicenter study comparing S- adenosylmethionine, naproxen and placebo in the treatment of degenerative joint disease. Am J Med 1987;83:66–71.
[104] Montrone F, Fumagalli M, Sarzi Puttini P, et al. Double-blind study of S-adenosyl-methionine versus placebo in hip and knee arthrosis. Clin Rheumatol 1985;4:484–5.
[105] Jamison J. Osteoarthritis clinical guide to nutrition and dietary supplements in disease management. Edinburgh: Churchill Livingstone; 2003. p. 363–71.
[106] Goldberg RJ, Katz J. A meta-analysis of the analgesic effects of omega-3 polyunsaturated fatty acid supplementation for inflammatory joint pain. Pain 2007;129:210–23.
[107] Proudman S, Cleland S, James M. Dietary omega-3 fats for treatment of inflammatory joint disease: efficacy and utility. Rheum Dis Clin North Am 2008;34:469–79.

[108] Zochling J, March L, Lapsley H, et al. Use of complementary medicines for osteoarthritis — a prospective study. Ann Rheum Dis 2004;63(5):549–54.

[109] Mencherini T, Cau A, Bianco G, et al. An extract of *Apium graveolens* var. dulce leaves: structure of the major constituent, apiin and its anti-inflammatory properties. J Pharm Pharmacol 2007;59(6):891–7.

[110] Kimmatkar N, Thawani V, Hingorani L, et al. Efficacy and tolerability of *Boswellia serrata* extract in treatment of osteoarthritis of knee — a randomized double blind placebo controlled trial. Phytomedicine 2003;0(1):3–7.

[111] Ammon HP. Boswellic acids in chronic inflammatory diseases. Planta Med 2006;72(12):1100–16.

[112] Sengupta K, Alluri KV, Satish AR, et al. A double blind, randomized, placebo controlled study of the efficacy and safety of 5-Loxin for treatment of osteoarthritis of the knee. Arthritis Res Ther 2008;10(4):R85.

[113] Cameron M, Chrubasik S. Oral herbal therapies for treating osteoarthritis. Cochrane Database Syst Rev 2014;(5):CD002947.

[114] Cordell GA, Araujo OE. Capsaicin: identification, nomenclature and pharmacotherapy. Ann Pharmacother 1993;27(3):330–6.

[115] Colpaert FC, Donnerer J, Lembeck F. Effects of capsaicin on inflammation and on the substance P content of nervous tissues in rats with adjuvant arthritis. Life Sci 1983;32:1827–34.

[116] Zhu XZ. Development of natural products as drugs acting on central nervous system. Mem Inst Oswaldo Cruz 1991;86(Suppl. 2):173–5.

[117] Daily JW, Yang M, Park S, et al. Efficacy of turmeric extracts and curcumin for alleviating the symptoms of joint arthritis: a systematic review and meta-analysis of randomized clinical trials. J Med Food 2016;19(8):717–29.

[118] Henrotin Y, Clutterbuck AL, Allaway D, et al. Biological actions of curcumin on articular chondrocytes. Osteoarthr Cartil 2010;18(2):141–9.

[119] Chin K-Y. The spice for joint inflammation: anti-inflammatory role of curcumin in treating osteoarthritis. Drug Des Devel Ther 2016;10:3029–42.

[120] Kuptniratsaikul V, et al. Efficacy and safety of *Curcuma domestica* extracts in patients with knee osteoarthritis. J Altern Complement Med 2009;15(8):891–7.

[121] Kuptniratsaikul V, Dajpratham P, Taechaarpornku W, et al. Efficacy and safety of *Curcuma domestica* extracts compared with ibuprofen in patients with knee osteoarthritis: a multicenter study. Clin Interv Aging 2014;9:451–8.

[122] Belcaro G, Cesarone MR, Dugall M, et al. Efficacy and safety of Meriva®, a curcumin-phosphatidylcholine complex, during extended administration in osteoarthritis patients. Altern Med Rev 2010;15(4):337–44.

[123] Panahi Y, Rahimnia AR, Sharafi M, et al. Curcuminoid treatment for knee osteoarthritis: a randomized double-blind placebo-controlled trial. Phytother Res 2014;28(11):1625–31.

[124] Rolland A, Fleurentin J, Lanhers MC, et al. Behavioural effects of the American traditional plant *Eschscholzia californica*: sedative and anxiolytic properties. Planta Med 1991;57(3):212–16.

[125] Rolland A, Fleurentin J, Lanhers MC, et al. Neurophysiological effects of an extract of *Eschscholzia californica* Cham. (Papaveraceae). Phytother Res 2001;15(5):377–81.

[126] Duwiejua M, Zeitlin IJ, Waterman PG, et al. Anti-inflammatory activity of *Polygonum bistorta, Guaiacum officinale* and *Hamamelis virginiana* in rats. J Pharm Pharmacol 1994;46(4):286–90.

[127] The british herbal pharmacopoeia, vol. 1. Bournemouth: British Herbal Medicine Association; 1990.

[128] Mills SY, Jacoby RK, Chacksfield M, et al. Effect of a proprietary herbal medicine on the relief of chronic arthritic pain: a double-blind study. Br J Rheumatol 1996;35:874–8.

[129] Chrubasik S, Thanner J, Künzel O, et al. Comparison of outcome measures during treatment with the proprietary *Harpagophytum* extract Doloteffin in patients with pain in the lower back, knee or hip. Phytomedicine 2002;9:181–94.

[130] Crubasik J, et al. Evidence of effectiveness of herbal antiinflammatory drugs in the treatment of painful osteoarthritis and chronic low back pain. Phytother Res 2007;21:675–83.

[131] Gagnier JJ, Chrubasik S, Manheimer E. *Harpagophytum procumbens* for osteoarthritis and low back pain: a systematic review. BMC Complement Altern Med 2004;4:13.

[132] ESCOP Monograph. *Harpagophyti radix*, Fascicule 2; 1996. Available from: http://www.escop.com/.

[133] Oltean H, Robbins C, van Tulder MW, et al. Herbal medicine for low-back pain. Cochrane Database Syst Rev 2014;(12):CD004504.

[134] Schmid B, Ludtke R, Selbmann HK, et al. Efficacy and tolerability of a standardized willow bark extract in patients with osteoarthritis: randomized placebo-controlled, double blind clinical trial. Phytother Res 2001;15:344–50.

[135] Riehemann K, Behnke B, Schulze-Osthoff K. Plant extracts from stinging nettle (*Urtica dioica*), an antirheumatic remedy, inhibit the proinflammatory transcription factor NF-kB. FEBS Lett 1999;442:89–94.

[136] Schulze-Tanzil G, de SP, Behnke B, et al. Effects of the antirheumatic remedy hox alpha — a new stinging nettle leaf extract — on matrix metallo-proteinases in human chondrocytes in vitro. Histol Histopathol 2002;17:477–85.

[137] Randall C, Randall H, Dobbs F, et al. Randomized controlled trial of nettle sting for treatment of base-of-thumb pain. J R Soc Med 2000;93:305–9.

[138] Felter HW, Lloyd JR. Kings American dispensatory. Portland OR: Eclectic Materia Medica Publications; 1898.

[139] Felter HW. The Eclectic materia medica, pharmacology and therapeutics. Portland, OR: Eclectic Materia Medica Publications; 1922.

[140] Koo LK, Ammit AJ, Tran VH, et al. Gingerols and related analogues inhibit arachidonic acid-induced human platelet serotonin release and aggregation. Thromb Res 2001;103:387–97.

[141] Tjendraputra E, Tran VH, Liu-Brennan D, et al. Effect of ginger constituents and synthetic analogues on cyclooxygenase-2 enzyme in intact cells. Bioorg Chem 2001;29:156–63.

[142] Altman RD, Marcussen KC. Effects of a ginger extract on knee pain in patients with osteoarthritis. Arthritis Rheum 2001;44:2531–8.

[143] Haghighi A, Tavalaei N, Owli N. Effects of ginger on primary knee osteoarthritis. Int J Rheumatol 2006;1(1):3–7.

[144] Bliddal H, Rosetzsky A, Schlichting P, et al. A randomized, placebo-controlled, cross-over study of ginger extracts and ibuprofen in osteoarthritis. Osteoarthritis Cartilage 2000;8(1): 9–12.

[145] Drozdov VN, Kim VA, Tkachenko EV, et al. Influence of a specific ginger combination on gastropathy conditions in patients with osteoarthritis of the knee or hip. J Altern Complement Med 2012;18(6):583–8.

[146] Lukaczer D, Darland G, Tripp M, et al. A pilot trial evaluating Meta050, a proprietary combination of reduced iso-alpha acids, rosemary extract and oleanolic acid in patients with arthritis and fibromyalgia. Phytother Res 2005;19(10):864–9.

[147] Cameron M, Chrubasik S. Topical herbal therapies for treating osteoarthritis. Cochrane Database Syst Rev 2013;(5):CD010538.

[148] Oltean H, Robbins C, van Tulder MW, et al. Herbal medicine for low-back pain. Cochrane Database Syst Rev 2014;(12):CD004504.

[149] Kerrigan DC, Todd MK, Riley PO. Knee osteoarthritis and high-heeled shoes. Lancet 1998;351(9113):1399–401.

[150] Kerrigan DC, Johansson JL, Bryant MG, et al. Moderate-heeled shoes and knee joint torques relevant to the development and progression of knee osteoarthritis. Arch Phys Med Rehabil 2005;86(5):871–5.

[151] Keating EM, Faris PM, Ritter MA, et al. Use of lateral heel and sole wedges in the treatment of medial osteoarthritis of the knee. Orthop Rev 1993;22(8):921–4.

[152] Tohyama H, Yasuda K, Kaneda K. Treatment of osteoarthritis of the knee with heel wedges. Int Orthop 1991;15:31–3.

[153] Bosomworth NJ. Exercise and knee osteoarthritis: benefit or hazard? Can Fam Physician 2009;55(9):871–8.

[154] Fransen M, McConnell S. Exercise for osteoarthritis of the knee. Cochrane Database Syst Rev 2008;(4):CD004376.

[155] Bartels EM, Lund H, Hagen KB, et al. Aquatic exercise for the treatment of knee and hip osteoarthritis. Cochrane Database Syst Rev 2007;(4):CD005523.

[156] Cicuttini FM, Baker JR, Spector TD. The association of obesity with osteoarthritis of the hand and knee in women: a twin study. J Rheumatol 1996;230:1221–6.

[157] Christensen R, Astrup A, Bliddal B. Weight loss: the treatment of choice for knee osteoarthritis? A randomized trial. Osteoarthritis Cartilage 2005;13(1):20–7.

[158] Perlman AI, Sabina A, Williams AL, et al. Massage therapy for osteoarthritis of the knee: a randomized controlled trial. Arch Intern Med 2006;166(22):2533–8.
[159] Tausche AK, Jansen TL, Schröder HE, et al. Gout — current diagnosis and treatment. Dtsch Arztebl Int 2009;106(34–35):549–55.
[160] Nuki G. Gout. Medicine (Baltimore) 2002;30(9):71–7.
[161] Neogi T, Jansen TL, Dalbeth N, et al. 2015 Gout Classification Criteria: an American College of Rheumatology/European League Against Rheumatism collaborative initiative. Arthritis Rheumatol 2015;67(10):2557–68.
[162] Simmonds HA, McBride MB, Hatfield PJ, et al. Polynesian women are also at risk for hyperuricaemia and gout because of a genetic defect in renal urate handling. Br J Rheumatol 1994;33(10):932–7.
[163] Richette P, Barden T. Gout. Lancet 2010;375:318–28.
[164] eTG complete. Therapeutic Guidelines Ltd; 2006.
[165] Kelley W, Rosenbloom F, Henderson F, et al. A specific enzyme defect in gout associated with over-production of uric acid. Proc Natl Acad Sci USA 1967;57:1735–9; 277:441–50.
[166] García-Pavía P, Torres RJ, Rivero M, et al. Phosphoribosylpyrophosphate synthetase overactivity as a cause of uric acid overproduction in a young woman. Arthritis Rheum 2003;48(7):2036–41.
[167] Becker MA, Losman MJ, Itkin P, et al. Gout with superactive phosphoribosylpyrophosphate synthetase due to increased enzyme catalytic rate. J Lab Clin Med 1982;99(4):495–511.
[168] Tu HP, Ko AM, Wang SJ, et al. Monoamine oxidase A gene polymorphisms and enzyme activity associated with risk of gout in Taiwan aborigines. Hum Genet 2010;127(2):223–9.
[169] Hollis-Moffatt JE, Xu X, Dalbeth N, et al. Role of the urate transporter SLC2A9 gene in susceptibility to gout in New Zealand Maori, Pacific Island and Caucasian case-control sample sets. Arthritis Rheum 2009;60(11):3485–92.
[170] Dessein P, Shipton E, Stanwix A, et al. Beneficial effects of weight loss associated with moderate calorie/carbohydrate restriction and increased proportional intake of protein and unsaturated fat on serum urate and lipoprotein levels in gout: a pilot study. Ann Rheum Dis 2000;59:539–43.
[171] Yamashita S, Matsuzawa Y, Tokunaga K, et al. Studies on the impaired metabolism of uric acid in obese subjects: marked reduction of renal urate excretion and its improvement by a low-calorie diet. Int J Obes 1986;10:255–64.
[172] Keenan RT, Pillinger MH. Hyperuricemia, gout and cardiovascular disease — an important 'muddle'. Bull NYU Hosp Jt Dis 2009;67(3):285–90.
[173] Gaffo AL, Edwards NL, Saag KG. Gout. Hyperuricemia and cardiovascular disease: how strong is the evidence for a causal link? Arthritis Res Ther 2009;11(4):240.
[174] Weaver AL. Epidemiology of gout. Cleve Clin J Med 2008;75(Suppl. 5):S9–12.
[175] Bhole V, de Vera M, Rahman MM, et al. Epidemiology of female gout: 52-year follow-up of a prospective cohort. Arthritis Rheum 2010;62(4):1069–76.
[176] Caspi D, Lubart E, Graff E, et al. The effect of mini-dose aspirin on renal function and uric acid handling in elderly patients. Arthritis Rheum 2000;43:103–8.
[177] Choi H, Atkinson K, Karlson E, et al. Purine-rich foods, dairy and protein intake and the risk of gout in men. N Engl J Med 2004;350:1093–103.
[178] Choi H, Curhan G. Beer, liquor and wine consumption and serum uric acid level: the Third National Health and Nutrition Examination Survey. Arthritis Rheum 2004;51:1023–9.
[179] Pizzorno J, Murray M. Textbook of natural medicine. 4th ed. Oxford: Elsevier; 2012.
[180] Nuki G. Gout medicine 2006;34(10):417–23.
[181] Eggebeen AT. Gout: an update. Am Fam Physician 2007;76(6):801–8.
[182] Nutrition Foundation. Nutrition reviews' present knowledge in nutrition. 5th ed. Washington, DC: Nutrition Foundation; 1984. p. 740–56.
[183] Grahame R, Scott JT. Clinical survey of 354 patients with gout. Ann Rheum Dis 1970;29:461–8.
[184] Meyers OL, Montegudo FS. A comparison of gout in men and women. A 10-year experience. S Afr Med J 1986;70:721–3.
[185] Schlesinger N. Diagnosis of gout. Minerva Med 2007;98(6):759–67.
[186] Schlesinger N. Diagnosis of gout: clinical, laboratory and radiologic findings. Am J Manag Care 2005;11(Suppl. 15):S443–50; quiz S465–468.
[187] Luk AJ, Simkin PA. Epidemiology of hyperuricemia and gout. Am J Manag Care 2005;11(Suppl. 15):S435–42; quiz S465–468.
[188] Tausche AK, Jansen TL, Schröder HE, et al. Gout — current diagnosis and treatment. Dtsch Arztebl Int 2009;106(34–35):549–55.
[189] Wallace SL, Robinson H, Masi AT, et al. Preliminary criteria for the classification of the acute arthritis of primary gout. Arthritis Rheum 1977;20:895–900.
[190] Doherty M. New insights into the epidemiology of gout. Rheumatology (Oxford) 2009;48(Suppl. 2):ii2–iii8.
[191] Baer A. Treatment of gout and hyperuricemia. In: Bittar EE, Bittar N, editors. Principles of medical biology, vol. 8, Part 3. London: Elsevier; 1997. p. 723–35.
[192] Berman EL. Clues in the eye: ocular signs of metabolic and nutritional disorders. Geriatrics 1995;50(7):34–6, 43–4.
[193] Kim KY, Ralph Schumacher H, Hunsche E, et al. A literature review of the epidemiology and treatment of acute gout. Clin Ther 2003;25(6):1593–617.
[194] Kim SY, De Vera MA, Choi HK. Gout and mortality. Clin Exp Rheumatol 2008;26(5 Suppl. 51):S115–9.
[195] Puig JG, de Miguel E, Castillo MC, et al. Asymptomatic hyperuricemia: impact of ultrasonography. Nucleosides Nucleotides Nucleic Acids 2008;27:592–5.
[196] Star VL, Hochberg MC. Prevention and management of gout. Drugs 1993;45:212–22.
[197] Adams M, Berset C, Kessler M, et al. Medicinal herbs for the treatment of rheumatic disorders — a survey of European herbals from the 16th and 17th century (Review). J Ethnopharmacol 2009;121:343–59.
[198] Ellingwood F. The American materia medica, therapeutics and pharmacognosy. Portland, OR: Eclectic Medical Publications; 1919.
[199] Thomas R. The Eclectic practice of medicine. Portland, OR: Eclectic Medical Publications; 1907.
[200] Johnson R, Rideout B. Uric acid and diet — insights into the epidemic of cardiovascular disease. N Engl J Med 2004;350:1071–3.
[201] Choi HK. A prescription for lifestyle change in patients with hyperuricemia and gout. Curr Opin Rheumatol 2010;22(2):165–72.
[202] Jacob RA, Spinozzi GM, Simon VA, et al. Consumption of cherries lowers plasma urate in healthy women. J Nutr 2003;133:1826–9.
[203] Choi HK, Curhan G. Soft drinks, fructose consumption and the risk of gout in men: prospective cohort study. BMJ 2008;336(7639):309–12.
[204] Choi JW, Ford ES, Gao X, et al. Sugar-sweetened soft drinks, diet soft drinks and serum uric acid level: the Third National Health and Nutrition Examination Survey. Arthritis Rheum 2008;59(1):109–16.
[205] Worthley MI, Prabhu A, De Sciscio P, et al. Detrimental effects of energy drink consumption on platelet and endothelial function. Am J Med 2010;123(2):184–7.
[206] Choi HK, Atkinson K, Karlson EW, et al. Alcohol intake and risk of incident gout in men: a prospective study. Lancet 2004;363(9417):1277–81.
[207] Leipner J, Iten F, Saller R. Therapy with proteolytic enzymes in rheumatic disorders. Biodrugs 2001;15:779–89.
[208] Maurer HR. Bromelain: biochemistry, pharmacology and medical use. Cell Mol Life Sci 2001;58:1234–45.
[209] Fitzhugh DJ, Shan S, Dewhirst MW, et al. Bromelain treatment decreases neutrophil migration to sites of inflammation. Clin Immunol 2008;128(1):66–74.
[210] Jamison J. Quercetin. Clinical guide to nutrition and dietary supplements in disease management. Edinburgh: Churchill Livingstone; 2003. p. 633–6.
[211] Formica J, Regelson W. Review of the biology of quercetin and related bioflavonoids. Food Chem Toxicol 1995;33(12):1061–80.
[212] Huang HY, Appel LJ, Choi MJ, et al. The effects of vitamin C supplementation on serum concentrations of uric acid: results of a randomized controlled trial. Arthritis Rheum 2005;52:1843–7.
[213] Choi HK, Gao X, Curhan G. Vitamin C intake and the risk of gout in men: a prospective study. Arch Intern Med 2009;169(5): 502–7.
[214] Kawai Y, Takahashi S, Satoh A, et al. Decreased activity of xanthine dehydrogenase and serum uric acid in rats fed partially hydrogenated fish oil. Nutr Res 1993;13(11):1325–30.

[215] Tate GA, Mandell BF, Karmali RA, et al. Suppression of monosodium urate crystal-induced acute inflammation by diets enriched with gamma-linolenic acid and eicosapentaenoic acid. Arthritis Rheum 1988;31:1543–50.

[216] Kelly GS. The role of glucosamine sulfate and chondroitin sulfates in the treatment of degenerative joint disease. Altern Med Rev 1998;3(1):27–39.

[217] Kubo M, Ando K, Mimura T, et al. Chondroitin sulfate for the treatment of hip and knee osteoarthritis: current status and future trends. Life Sci 2009;85(13–14):477–83.

[218] Itou S, Goto Y, Suzuki K, et al. Significant association between methylenetetrahydrofolate reductase 677T allele and hyperuricemia among adult Japanese subjects. Nutr Res 2009;29(10):710–15.

[219] Murray M, Pizzorno J. Encyclopedia of natural medicine. 2nd ed. New York: Little Brown; 2003.

[220] Wang Y, Zhu JX, Kong LD, et al. Administration of procyanidins from grape seeds reduces serum uric acid levels and decreases hepatic xanthine dehydrogenase/oxidase activities in oxonate-treated mice. Basic Clin Pharmacol Toxicol 2004;94(5):232–7.

[221] Nagao A, Seki M, Kobayashi H. Inhibition of xanthine oxidase by flavonoids. Biosci Biotechnol Biochem 1999;63(10):1787–90.

[222] Lespade L, Bercion S. Theoretical study of the mechanism of inhibition of xanthine oxidase by flavonoids and gallic acid derivatives. J Phys Chem B 2010;114(2):921–8.

[223] Nassiri-Asl M, Hosseinzadeh H. Review of the pharmacological effects of *Vitis vinifera* (grape) and its bioactive compounds. Phytother Res 2009;23(9):1197–204.

[224] Scientific Committee of the British Herbal Medicine Association. British herbal pharmacopeia. Bournemouth: British Herbal Medicine Association; 1983.

[225] Grieve M. A modern herbal. London: Jonathon Cape; 1979.

[226] Duke J. The green pharmacy herbal handbook: your comprehensive reference to the best herbs for healing. Emmaus, PA: Rodale Press; 2000.

[227] Ford-Hutchinson AW. Leukotrienes: their formation and role as inflammatory mediators. Fed Proc 1985;44(1 Pt 1):25–9.

[228] Goetzl EJ, Payan DG, Goldman DW. Immunopathogenetic roles of leukotrienes in human diseases. J Clin Immunol 1984;4(2):79–84.

[229] Rae SA, Davidson EM, Smith MJ. Leukotriene B4, an inflammatory mediator in gout. Lancet 1982;2(8308):1122–4.

[230] Safayhi H, Boden SE, Schweizer S, et al. Concentration-dependent potentiating and inhibitory effects of Boswellia extracts on 5-lipoxygenase product formation in stimulated PMNL. Planta Med 2000;66(2):110–1113.

[231] Safayhi H, Mack T, Sabieraj J, et al. Boswellic acids: novel, specific, nonredox inhibitors of 5-lipoxygenase. J Pharmacol Exp Ther 1992;261(3):1143–6.

[232] Jurenka JS. Anti-inflammatory properties of curcumin, a major constituent of *Curcuma longa*: a review of preclinical and clinical research. Altern Med Rev 2009;14:141–53.

[233] Lin JK, Shih CA. Inhibitory effect of curcumin on xanthine dehydrogenase/oxidase induced by phorbol-12-myristate-13-acetate in NIH3T3 cells. Carcinogenesis 1994;15(8):1717–21.

[234] Murrell W. The use of *Guaiacum* in the treatment of chronic gouty affections. Lancet 1896;147(3797):1592.

[235] Lanhers M-C, Fleurentin J, Mortier F, et al. Anti-inflammatory and analgesic effects of an aqueous extract of *Harpagophytum procumbens*. Planta Med 1992;58:117–23.

[236] *Harpagophyti radix*. ESCOP monographs: the scientific foundation for herbal medicinal products. 2nd ed. Exeter, UK: European Scientific Cooperative on Phytotherapy and Thieme; 2003. p. 233–40.

[237] Gagnier JJ, van Tulder MW, Berman B, et al. Herbal medicine for low back pain: a Cochrane review. Spine 2007;32(1):82–92.

[238] Natural Standard Research Collaboration. Natural standard monographs. Online. Available from: www.naturalstandard.com.

[239] Blumenthal M, Busse WR. The complete German Commission E monographs, therapeutic guide to herbal medicines. Austin, TX: American Botanical Council, Integrative Medicine Communications; 1998.

[240] Clare BA, Conroy RS, Spelman K. The diuretic effect in human subjects of an extract of *Taraxacum officinale* folium over a single day. J Altern Complement Med 2009;15(8):929–34.

[241] Randall C, Meethan K, Randall H, et al. Nettle sting of *Urtica dioica* for joint pain — an exploratory study of this complementary therapy. Complement Ther Med 1999;7:126–31.

[242] Suekawa M, Ishige A, Yusas K, et al. Pharmacological actions of pungent constituents, (6)-gingerol and (6)-shogaol. J Pharmacobio-Dyn 1984;7:836–48.

[243] Sabina EP, Rasool M, Mathew L, et al. 6-Shogaol inhibits monosodium urate crystal-induced inflammation — an in vivo and in vitro study. Food Chem Toxicol 2010;48(1):229–35.

[244] Schlesinger N. Response to application of ice may help differentiate between gouty arthritis and other inflammatory arthritides. J Clin Rheumatol 2006;12(6):275–6.

[245] Schlesinger N, Detry MA, Holland BK, et al. Local ice therapy during bouts of acute gouty arthritis. J Rheumatol 2002;29(2):331–4.

[246] Williams PT. Effects of diet, physical activity and performance and body weight on incident gout in ostensibly healthy, vigorously active men. Am J Clin Nutr 2008;87(5):1480–7.

[247] Bartels EM, Dreyer L, Jacobsen S, et al. Fibromyalgia, diagnosis and prevalence. Are gender differences explainable? Ugeskr Laeger 2009;171(49):3588–92.

[248] Chong YY, Ng BY. Clinical aspects and management of fibromyalgia syndrome. Ann Acad Med Singapore 2009;38(11):967–73.

[249] Spaeth M. Epidemiology, costs and the economic burden of fibromyalgia. Arthritis Res Ther 2009;11(3):117.

[250] Branco JC, Bannwarth B, Failde I, et al. Prevalence of fibromyalgia: a survey in five European countries. Semin Arthritis Rheum 2010;39(6):448–53.

[251] Lawrence RC, Felson DT, Helmick CG, National Arthritis Work Group, et al. Estimates of the prevalence of arthritis and other rheumatic conditions in the United States. Part II. Arthritis Rheum 2008;58:26–35.

[252] Goldenberg D. Diagnosis and differential diagnosis of fibromyalgia. Am J Med 2009;122(12, Suppl. 1):S14–21.

[253] Wolfe F, Smythe HA, Yunus MB, et al. The American College of Rheumatology 1990 criteria for the classification of fibromyalgia. Report of the Multicenter Criteria Committee. Arthritis Rheum 1990;33(2):160–72.

[254] Wolfe F, Clauw DJ, Fitzcharles MA, et al. The American College of Rheumatology Preliminary diagnostic criteria for fibromyalgia and measurement of symptom severity. Arthritis Care Res (Hoboken) 2010;62(5):600–10.

[255] Staud R, Rodriguez ME. Mechanisms of disease: pain in fibromyalgia syndrome. Nat Clin Pract Rheumatol 2006;2(2):90–8.

[256] Meeus M, Nijs J, et al. Chronic musculoskeletal pain in patients with chronic fatigue syndrome: a systematic review. Eur J Pain 2007;11(4):377–86.

[257] Russell IJ, Vaeroy H, Javors M, et al. Cerebrospinal fluid biogenic amine metabolites in fibromyalgia/fibrositis syndrome and rheumatoid arthritis. Arthritis Rheum 1992;35:550e6.

[258] Marchard S. Physiology of pain mechanisms: from the periphery to the brain. Rheum Dis Clin North Am 2008;34(2):285–309.

[259] Malt EA, Olafsson S, Aakvaag A, et al. Altered dopamine D2 receptor function in fibromyalgia patients: a neuroendocrine study with buspirone in women with fibromyalgia compared with female population based controls. J Affect Disord 2003;75:77–8.

[260] Wood PB, Holman AJ. An elephant among us: the role of dopamine in the pathophysiology of fibromyalgia. J Rheumatol 2009;36(2):221–4.

[261] Crofford LJ, Pillemer SR, Kalogeras KT, et al. Hypothalamic–pituitary–adrenal axis perturbations in patients with fibromyalgia. Arthritis Rheum 1994;37:1583–92.

[262] Carvalho LS, Correa H, Silva GC, et al. May genetic factors in fibromyalgia help to identify patients with differentially altered frequencies of immune cells? Clin Exp Immunol 2008;154(3):346–52.

[263] Ablin JN, Shoenfeld Y, Buskila D. Fibromyalgia, infection and vaccination: two more parts in the etiological puzzle. J Autoimmun 2006;27(3):145–52.

[264] Goldenberg DL. Fibromyalgia and other chronic fatigue syndromes: is there evidence for chronic viral disease? Semin Arthritis Rheum 1988;18(2):111–20.

[265] Goldenberg DL. Fibromyalgia and its relation to chronic fatigue syndrome, viral illness and immune abnormalities. J Rheumatol 1989;19:91–3.
[266] Adak B, Tekeoglu I, Ediz L, et al. Fibromyalgia frequency in hepatitis B carriers. J Clin Rheumatol 2005;11:157–9.
[267] Buskila D, Shnaider A, Neumann L, et al. Fibromyalgia in hepatitis C virus infection. Another infectious disease relationship. Arch Intern Med 1997;157:2497–500.
[268] Simms RW, Zerbini CA, Ferrante N, et al. Fibromyalgia syndrome in patients infected with human immunodeficiency virus. The Boston City Hospital Clinical AIDS team. Am J Med 1992;92:368–74.
[269] Pamuk ON, Cakir N. The variation in chronic widespread pain and other symptoms in fibromyalgia patients. The effects of menses and menopause. Clin Exp Rheumatol 2005;23(6):778–82.
[270] Okifuji A, Turk D. Sex hormones and pain in regularly menstruating women with fibromyalgia syndrome. J Pain 2006;7(11):851–9.
[271] Arnold LM, Hudson JI, Hess EV, et al. Family study of fibromyalgia. Arthritis Rheum 2004;50:944–52.
[272] Markkula R, Järvinen P, Leino-Arjas P, et al. Clustering of symptoms associated with fibromyalgia in a Finnish twin cohort. Eur J Pain 2009;13(7):744–50.
[273] Demitrack MA, Crofford LJ. Evidence for and pathophysiologic implications of hypothalamic-pituitary-adrenal axis dysregulation in fibromyalgia and chronic fatigue syndrome. Ann N Y Acad Sci 1998;1:684–97.
[274] Dadabhoy D, Clauw DJ. Therapy insight: fibromyalgia — a different type of pain needing a different type of treatment. Nat Clin Pract Rheumatol 2006;2(7):364–72.
[275] Evengard B, Nilsson CG, Lindh G, et al. Chronic fatigue syndrome differs from fibromyalgia. No evidence for elevated substance P levels in cerebrospinal fluid of patients with chronic fatigue syndrome. Pain 1998;78(2):153–5.
[276] Ablin J, Neumann L, Buskila D. Pathogenesis of fibromyalgia — a review. Joint Bone Spine 2008;75(3):273–9.
[277] Arnold LM, Crofford LJ, Mease PJ, et al. Patient perspectives on the impact of fibromyalgia. Patient Educ Couns 2008;73(1):114–20.
[278] White KP, Nielson WR, Harth M, et al. Does the label 'fibromyalgia' alter health status, function and health service utilization? A prospective, within-group comparison in a community cohort of adults with chronic widespread pain. Arthritis Rheum 2002;47:260–5.
[279] Deuster PA, Jaffe RM. A novel treatment for fibromyalgia improves clinical outcomes in a community-based study. J Musculoskelet Pain 1998;6(2):133–49.
[280] Inanici F, Yunus MB. History of fibromyalgia: past to present. Curr Pain Headache Rep 2004;8(5):369–78.
[281] eTG complete, Therapeutic Guidelines, Ltd, eTG29; November 2009.
[282] Hänninen, Kaartinen K, Rauma AL, et al. Antioxidants in vegan diet and rheumatic disorders. Toxicology 2000;155(1–3):45–53.
[283] Kaartinen K, Lammi K, Hypen M, et al. Vegan diet alleviates fibromyalgia symptoms. Scand J Rheumatol 2000;29(5):308–13.
[284] Donaldson MS, Speight N, Loomis S. Fibromyalgia syndrome improved using a mostly raw vegetarian diet: an observational study. BMC Complement Altern Med 2001;1:7.
[285] Holton KF, Kindler LL, Jones KD. Potential dietary links to central sensitization in fibromyalgia: past reports and future directions. Rheum Dis Clin North Am 2009;35(2):409–20.
[286] Ozgocmen S, Ozyurt H, Sogut S, et al. Current concepts in the pathophysiology of fibromyalgia: the potential role of oxidative stress and nitric oxide. Rheumatol Int 2006;26(7):585–97.
[287] Pitchford P. Healing with whole foods. Berkeley. CA: North Atlantic Books; 1993.
[288] Dodabhoy D, Clauw DJ. Therapy insight: fibromyalgia — a different type of pain needing a different type of treatment. Nat Clin Pract Rheumatol 2006;2(7):364–72.
[289] Clauw DJ, Williams DA. Relationship between stress and pain in work-related upper extremity disorders: the hidden role of chronic multisystem illnesses. Am J Ind Med 2002;41(5):370–82.
[290] Caruso I, Sarzi Puttini P, Cazzola M, et al. Double-blind study of 5-hydroxytryptophan versus placebo in the treatment of primary fibromyalgia syndrome. J Int Med Res 1990;18(3):201–9.
[291] Sarzi Puttini P, Caruso I. Primary fibromyalgia syndrome and 5-hydroxy-L-tryptophan: a 90-day open study. J Int Med Res 1992;20(2):182–9.
[292] Birdsall TC. 5-hydroxytryptophan: a clinically-effective serotonin precursor. Altern Med Rev 1998;3(4):271–80.
[293] Juhl JH. Fibromyalgia and the serotonin pathway. Altern Med Rev 1998;3(5):367–75.
[294] Eisinger J, Plantamura A, Ayavou T. Glycolysis abnormalities in fibromyalgia. J Am Coll Nutr 1994;24(2):144–8.
[295] Wolfe F, Ross K, Anderson J, et al. Aspects of fibromyalgia in the general population: sex, pain threshold and fibromyalgia symptoms. J Rheumatol 1995;22:151–6.
[296] Regland B, Andersson M, Abrahamsson L, et al. Increased concentrations of homocysteine in the cerebrospinal fluid in patients with fibromyalgia and chronic fatigue syndrome. Scand J Rheumatol 1997;26(4):301–7.
[297] Gaby AR. Intravenous nutrient therapy: the 'Myers' cocktail'. Altern Med Rev 2002;7(5):389–403.
[298] Dordain G, Aumaitre O, Eschalier A, et al. Vitamin B_{12}, an analgesic vitamin? Critical examination of the literature. Acta Neurol Belg 1984;84(1):5–11.
[299] Magaldi M, Moltoni L, Biasi G, et al. Role of intracellular calcium ions in the physiopathology of fibromyalgia syndrome. Boll Soc Ital Biol Sper 2000;76(1–2):1–4.
[300] Ng S. Hair calcium and magnesium levels in patients with fibromyalgia: a case center study. J Manipulative Physiol Ther 1999;22(9):586–93.
[301] Cordero MD, De Miguel M, Moreno Fernandez AM, et al. Mitochondrial dysfunction and mitophagy activation in blood mononuclear cells of fibromyalgia patients: implication in the pathogenesis of the disease. Arthritis Res Ther 2010; 12(1):R17.
[302] Cordero MD, Moreno-Fernández AM, deMiguel M, et al. Coenzyme Q10 distribution in blood is altered in patients with fibromyalgia. Clin Biochem 2009;42(7–8):732–5.
[303] Lister RE. An open, pilot study to evaluate the potential benefits of coenzyme Q10 combined with *Ginkgo biloba* extract in fibromyalgia syndrome. J Int Med Res 2002;30(2):195–9.
[304] Ko GD, Nowacki NB, Arseneau L, et al. Omega-3 fatty acids for neuropathic pain: case series. Clin J Pain 2010;26(2):168–72.
[305] Ozgocmen S, Catal SA, Ardicoglu O, et al. Effect of omega-3 fatty acids in the management of fibromyalgia syndrome. Int J Clin Pharmacol Ther 2000;38:362–3.
[306] Simopoulos AP. Essential fatty acids in health and chronic disease. Am J Clin Nutr 1999;70(Suppl. 3):560S–569S.
[307] Yunus MB, Kalyan-Raman UP, Kalyan-Raman K. Primary fibromyalgia syndrome and myofascial pain syndrome: clinical features and muscle pathology. Arch Phys Med Rehabil 1988;69(6):451–4.
[308] Park JH, Niermann KJ, Olsen N. Evidence for metabolic abnormalities in the muscles of patients with fibromyalgia. Curr Rheumatol Rep 2000;2(2):131–40.
[309] Rossini M, Di Munno O, Valentini G, et al. Double-blind, multicenter trial comparing acetyl 1-carnitine with placebo in the treatment of fibromyalgia patient. Clin Exp Rheumatol 2007;25(2):182–8.
[310] Sendur OF, Tastaban E, Turan Y, et al. The relationship between serum trace element levels and clinical parameters in patients with fibromyalgia. Rheumatol Int 2008;28(11):1117–21.
[311] Abraham G, Flechas J. Management of fibromyalgia: rationale for the use of magnesium and malic acid. J Nutr Environ Med 1992;3(1):49.
[312] Jacobsen S, Danneskiold-Samsøe B, Andersen RB, et al. adenosylmethionine in primary fibromyalgia. Double-blind clinical evaluation. Scand J Rheumatol 1991;20(4):294–302.
[313] Volkmann H, Nørregaard J, Jacobsen S, et al. Double-blind, placebo-controlled cross-over study of intravenous S-adenosyl-L-methionine in patients with fibromyalgia. Scand J Rheumatol 1997;26(3):206–11.
[314] Altindag O, Celik H. Total antioxidant capacity and the severity of the pain in patients with fibromyalgia. Redox Rep 2006;11(3):131–5.
[315] Akkuş S, Naziroğlu M, Eriş S, et al. Levels of lipid peroxidation, nitric oxide and antioxidant vitamins in plasma of patients with fibromyalgia. Cell Biochem Funct 2009;27(4):181–5.
[316] Huisman AM, White KP, Algra A, et al. Vitamin D levels in women with systemic lupus erythematosus and fibromyalgia. J Rheumatol 2001;28(11):2535–9.

[317] Armstrong DJ, Meenagh GK, Bickle I, et al. Vitamin D deficiency is associated with anxiety and depression in fibromyalgia. Clin Rheumatol 2007;26(4):551–4.

[318] Swezey RL, Adams J. Fibromyalgia: a risk factor for osteoporosis. J Rheumatol 1999;26(12):2642–4.

[319] Al-Allaf AW, Mole PA, Paterson CR, et al. Bone health in patients with fibromyalgia. Rheumatology (Oxford) 2003;42(10): 1202–6.

[320] Eisinger J. Reactive oxygen species, antioxidant status and fibromyalgia. J Musculoskelet Pain 1998;5:5–15.

[321] Nicolodi M, Sicuteri F. Fibromyalgia and migraine, two faces of the same mechanism. Serotonin as the common clue for pathogenesis and therapy. Adv Exp Med Biol 1996;398:373–9.

[322] Lister RE. An open, pilot study to evaluate the potential benefits of coenzyme Q10 combined with *Ginkgo biloba* extract in fibromyalgia syndrome. J Int Med Res 2002;30(2):195–9.

[323] Shen YC, Chen CF, Chiou WF. Andrographolide prevents oxygen radical production by human neutrophils: possible mechanism(s) involved in its anti-inflammatory effect. Br J Pharmacol 2002;135:399–406.

[324] Singha PK, Roy S, Dey S. Antimicrobial activity of *Andrographis paniculata*. Fitoterapia 2003;74(7–8):692–4.

[325] Calabrese C, Berman SH, Badish JG, et al. A phase I trial of andrographolide in HIV positive patients and normal volunteers. Phytother Res 2000;14:333.

[326] Wikman G. Effect of andrographolide and Kan Jang — fixed combination of extract SHA-10 and extract SHE-3 — on proliferation of human lymphocytes, production of cytokines and immune activation markers in the whole blood cells culture. Phytomedicine 2002;9:598–605.

[327] Izquierdo Alvarez S, Bancalero Flores JL, et al. [Evaluation of urinary cortisol levels in women with fibromyalgia]. Med Clin (Barc) 2009;133(7):255–7.

[328] Lange M, Krohn-Grimberghe B, Petermann F. [Fibromyalgia: influence of depressive symptoms on the outcome after rehabilitation] [in German]. Rehabilitation (Stuttg) 2009;48(5):298–305.

[329] Müller WE, Rolli M, Schäfer C, et al. Effects of hypericum extract (LI 160) in biochemical models of antidepressant activity. Pharmacopsychiatry 1997;30(Suppl. 2):102–7.

[330] Bukhari IA, Dar A, Khan RA, et al. Antinociceptive activity of the methanolic extracts of St Johns wort (*Hypericum perforatum*) preparation. Pak J Pharm Sci 2004;17(2):13–119.

[331] Linde K, Berner MM, Kriston L. St John's wort for major depression. Cochrane Database Syst Rev 2008;(4):CD000448.

[332] Nocerino E, Amato M, Izzo AA. The aphrodisiac and adaptogenic properties of ginseng. Fitoterapia 2000;71(Suppl. 1): S1–5.

[333] Shuster J, McCormack J, Pillai Riddell R, et al. Understanding the psychosocial profile of women with fibromyalgia syndrome. Pain Res Manag 2009;14(3):239–45.

[334] Gormsen L, Rosenberg R, Bach FW, et al. Depression, anxiety, health-related quality of life and pain in patients with chronic fibromyalgia and neuropathic pain. Eur J Pain 2010;14(2):127, e1–e8.

[335] Sarris J, Kavanagh DJ, Byrne G, et al. The Kava Anxiety Depression Spectrum Study (KADSS): a randomized, placebo-controlled crossover trial using an aqueous extract of *Piper methysticum*. Psychopharmacology (Berl) 2009;205(3):399–407.

[336] Ernst E. Herbal remedies for anxiety — a systematic review of controlled clinical trials. Phytomedicine 2006;13(3):205–8.

[337] Zhang RX, Li MX, Jia ZP. *Rehmannia glutinosa*: review of botany, chemistry and pharmacology. J Ethnopharmacol 2008;117(2):199–214.

[338] Martinez-Lavin M. Biology and therapy of fibromyalgia. Stress, the stress response system and fibromyalgia. Arthritis Res Ther 2007;9(4):216.

[339] Chrousos GP, Gold PW. The concepts of stress and stress system disorders. Overview of physical and behavioral homeostasis. JAMA 1992;267:1244–52.

[340] Harris K. Managing menopause naturally. Haberfield, NSW: KC Media Products; 2002.

[341] Bystritsky A, Kerwin L, Feusner JD. A pilot study of *Rhodiola rosea* (Rhodax) for generalized anxiety disorder (GAD). J Altern Complement Med 2008;14(2):175–80.

[342] Darbinyan V, Aslanyan G, Amroyan E, et al. Clinical trial of *Rhodiola rosea* L. extract SHR-5 in the treatment of mild to moderate depression. Nord J Psychiatry 2007;61(5):343–8.

[343] Olsson EM, von Schéele B, Panossian AG. A randomised, double-blind, placebo-controlled, parallel-group study of the standardised extract shr-5 of the roots of *Rhodiola rosea* in the treatment of subjects with stress-related fatigue. Planta Med 2009;75(2):105–12.

[344] Theadom A, Cropley M, Humphrey KL. Exploring the role of sleep and coping on quality of life in fibromyalgia. J Psychosom Res 2007;62(2):145–51.

[345] Bigatti SM, Hernandez AM, Cronan TA, et al. Sleep disturbances in fibromyalgia syndrome: relationship to pain and depression. Arthritis Rheum 2008;59(7):961–7.

[346] Trauner G, Khom S, Baburin I, et al. Modulation of GABAA receptors by valerian extracts is related to the content of valerenic acid. Planta Med 2008;74(1):19–24.

[347] Khom S, Baburin I, Timin E, et al. Valerenic acid potentiates and inhibits GABA(A) receptors: molecular mechanism and subunit specificity. Neuropharmacology 2007;53(1):178–87.

[348] Koetter U. Valerian and hops: synergy, mode of action clinical evidence. Botanical medicine from bench to bedside. Mary Ann Liebert, Inc; 2009. pp. 154–66.

[349] Bent S, Padula A, Moore D, et al. Valerian for sleep: a systematic review and meta-analysis. Am J Med 2006;119(12):1005–12.

[350] Wolfe F, Ross K, Anderson J, et al. The prevalence and characteristics of fibromyalgia in the general population. Arthritis Rheum 1995;38:19–28.

[351] American Herbal Pharmacopoeia. American Herbal Pharmacopoeia and Therapeutic Compendium, Black Haw Bark *Viburnum prunifolium*. Analytical, quality control and therapeutic monograph. Santa Cruz, CA: American Herbal Pharmacopoeia; 2000. p. 1–17.

[352] British Herbal Pharmacopoeia. *Viburnum prunifolium*. Bournemouth: British Herbal Medical Association; 1983. p. 23.

[353] Dog TL, Micozzi M. Menstrual cramps. Women's health in complementary and integrative medicine. Elsevier Churchill Livingstone; 2005. p. 42–50.

[354] Lee J. Natural progesterone. 2nd ed. Bristol: John Carpenter; 1999.

[355] Martinez-Lavin M, Vargas A. Complex adaptive systems allostasis in fibromyalgia. Rheum Dis Clin North Am 2009;35(2):285–98.

[356] Fibromyalgia: poorly understood; treatments are disappointing. Prescrire Int 2009;18(102):169–73.

[357] Rege NN, Thatte UM, Dahanukar SA. Adaptogenic properties of six rasayana herbs used in Ayurvedic medicine. Phytother Res 1999;13(4):275–91.

[358] Bhattacharya SK, Muruganandam AV. Adaptogenic activity of *Withania somnifera*: an experimental study using a rat model of chronic stress. Pharmacol Biochem Behav 2003;75(3):547–55.

[359] Cooley K, Szczurko O, Perri D, et al. Naturopathic care for anxiety: a randomized controlled trial. PLoS ONE 2009;4(8):e6628.

[360] Huang QR, Iwamoto M, Aoki S, et al. Anti-5-hydro-xytryptamine effect of galanolactone, diterpenoid isolated from ginger. Chem Pharm Bull 1991;39:397–9.

[361] Vishwakarma SL, Pal SC, Kasture VS, et al. Anxiolytic and antiemetic activity of *Zingiber officinale*. Phytother Res 2002;16(7):621–6.

[362] Ford DE, Kamerow DB. Epidemiologic study of sleep disturbances and psychiatric disorders. JAMA 1989;262:1479–84.

[363] Koetter U, Barrett M, Lacher S, et al. Interactions of magnolia and ziziphus extracts with selected central nervous system receptors. J Ethnopharmacol 2009;124(3):421–5.

[364] Benskey D, Clavery S, Stoger E. Chinese herbal materia medica. 3rd ed. Portland, OR: Eastland Press; 2004. p. 470–3.

[365] Wu SX, Zhang JX, Xu T, et al. Effects of seeds, leaves and fruits of *Ziziphus spinosa* and jujuboside A on central nervous system function. Zhongguo Zhong Yao Za Zhi 1993;18(11):685–7, 703–704.

[366] Chen JS, Hogan C, Lyubomirsky G, et al. Management of osteoporosis in primary care in Australia. Osteoporos Int 2009;20(3):491–6.

[367] Sambrook PN, Seeman E, Phillips SR, et al. Preventing osteoporosis: outcomes of the Australian Fracture Prevention Summit. Med J Aust 2002;176:S1–16.

[368] Piodi LP, Poloni A, Ulivieri FM, et al. Managing osteoporosis in ulcerative colitis: something new? World J Gastroenterol 2014;20(39):14087–98.

[369] Nowson CA. Prevention of fractures in older people with calcium and vitamin D. Nutrients 2010;2(9):975–84.
[370] Jones G, Nguyen T, Sambrook P, et al. Progressive loss of bone in the femoral neck in elderly people: longitudinal findings from the Dubbo osteoporosis epidemiology study. BMJ 1994;309:691–5.
[371] Schettler AE, Gustafson EM. Osteoporosis prevention starts in adolescence. J Am Acad Nurse Pract 2004;16(7):274–82.
[372] Binkley N. A perspective on male osteoporosis. Best Pract Res Clin Rheumatol 2009;23:755–68.
[373] Galusca B, Zouch M, Germain N, et al. Constitutional thinness: unusual human phenotype of low bone quality. J Clin Endocrinol Metab 2008;93(1):110–1117.
[374] Ahlborg H, Johnell O, Turner C, et al. Bone loss and bone size after menopause. N Engl J Med 2003;349:32.
[375] Straub DA. Calcium supplementation in clinical practice: a review of forms, doses and indications. Nutr Clin Pract 2007;22(3):286–96.
[376] Legrand E, Hedde C, Gallois Y, et al. Osteoporosis in men: a potential role for the sex hormone binding globulin. Bone 2001;29(1):90–5.
[377] Khosla S, Amin S, Orwoll E. Osteoporosis in men. Endocr Rev 2008;29(4):441–64.
[378] Robitaille J, Yoon PW, Moore CA, et al. Prevalence, family history and prevention of reported osteoporosis in U.S. women. Am J Prev Med 2008;35(1):47–54.
[379] Jouanny P, Guillemin F, Kuntz C, et al. Environmental and genetic factors affecting bone mass. Similarity of bone density among members of healthy families. Arthritis Rheum 1995;38:61–7.
[380] Seeman E, Hopper JL, Bach LA, et al. Reduced bone mass in daughters of women with osteoporosis. N Engl J Med 1989;320:554–8.
[381] Ferrari S. Human genetics of osteoporosis. Best Pract Res Clin Endocrinol Metab 2008;22(5):723–35.
[382] Ralston SH, de Crombrugghe B. Genetic regulation of bone mass and susceptibility to osteoporosis. Genes Dev 2006;20(18):2492–506.
[383] Seeman E, Melton LJ 3rd, O'Fallon WM, et al. Risk factors for spinal osteoporosis in men. Am J Med 1983;75:977–83.
[384] Olney RC. Mechanisms of impaired growth: effect of steroids on bone and cartilage. Horm Res 2009;72(Suppl. 1):30–5.
[385] Ward KD, Klesges RC. A meta-analysis of the effects of cigarette smoking on bone mineral density. Calcif Tissue Int 2001;68(5):259–70.
[386] Cotran R, Kumar V, Robbins S. Pathological basis of disease. 4th ed. Philadelphia: WB Saunders International; 1989.
[387] Kenny A. Osteoporosis, pathogenesis, diagnosis and treatment in older adults. Rheum Dis Clin North Am 2000;26(3):569–91.
[388] Australian Institute of Health and Welfare. Arthritis and musculoskeletal conditions in Australia. Publication No. PHE 67. Canberra: AIHW; 2005.
[389] Bliuc D, Nguyen ND, Milch VE, et al. Mortality risk associated with low-trauma osteoporotic fracture and subsequent fracture in men and women. JAMA 2009;301(5):513–21.
[390] Ben-Noun LL. What was the disease of the bones that affected King David? J Gerontol A Biol Sci Med Sci 2002;57(3):M152–4.
[391] Tucker KL. Osteoporosis prevention and nutrition. Curr Osteoporos Rep 2009;7(4):111–1117.
[392] Wynn E, Krieg MA, Lanham-New SA, et al. Postgraduate Symposium: positive influence of nutritional alkalinity on bone health. Proc Nutr Soc 2010;69(1):166–73.
[393] Tucker KL. Vegetarian diets and bone status. Am J Clin Nutr 2014;100(Suppl. 1):329S–35S.
[394] Arjmandi BH, Khalil DA, Lucas EA, et al. Dried plums improve indices of bone formation in postmenopausal women. J Womens Health Gend Based Med 2002;11(1):61–8.
[395] Hooshmand S, Arjmandi BH. Viewpoint: dried plum, an emerging functional food that may effectively improve bone health. Ageing Res Rev 2009;8(2):122–7.
[396] Yamori Y, Moriguchi EH, Teramoto T, et al. Soybean isoflavones reduce postmenopausal bone resorption in female Japanese immigrants in Brazil: a ten-week study. J Am Coll Nutr 2002;21(6):560–3.
[397] Setchell KD, Lydeking-Olsen E. Dietary phytoestrogens and their effect on bone: evidence from in vitro and in vivo, human observational and dietary intervention studies. Am J Clin Nutr 2003;78(Suppl. 3):S593–609.
[398] Maggio M, Artoni A, Lauretani F, et al. The impact of omega-3 fatty acids on osteoporosis. Curr Pharm Des 2009;15(36):4157–64.
[399] Longo AB, Ward WE. PUFAs, Bone mineral density and fragility fracture: findings from human studies. Adv Nutr 2016;7(2):299–312.
[400] Tucker KL. Vegetarian diets and bone status. Am J Clin Nutr 2014;100(Suppl. 1):329S–35S.
[401] Feskanich D, Willett WC, Stampfer MJ, et al. Protein consumption and bone fractures in women. Am J Epidemiol 1996;143:472–9.
[402] Munger RG, Cerhan JR, Chiu BC. Prospective study of dietary protein intake and risk of hip fracture in postmenopausal women. Am J Clin Nutr 1999;69:147–52.
[403] Hannan MT, Tucker KL, Dawson-Hughes B, et al. Effect of dietary protein on bone loss in elderly men and women: The Framingham Osteoporosis Study. J Bone Miner Res 2000;15:2504–12.
[404] Dawson-Hughes B. Interaction of dietary calcium and protein in bone health in humans. J Nutr 2003;133:852S–854S.
[405] He FJ, MacGregor GA. A comprehensive review on salt and health and current experience of worldwide salt reduction programmes. J Hum Hypertens 2009;23(6):363–84.
[406] Caudarella R, Vescini F, Rizzoli E, et al. Salt intake, hypertension and osteoporosis. J Endocrinol Invest 2009;32(Suppl. 4):15–20.
[407] Cappuccio FP, Kalaitzidis R, Duneclift S, et al. Unravelling the links between calcium excretion, salt intake, hypertension, kidney stones and bone metabolism. J Nephrol 2000;13(3):169–77.
[408] Woo J, Kwok T, Leung J, et al. Dietary intake, blood pressure and osteoporosis. J Hum Hypertens 2009;23(7):451–5.
[409] Kiel DP, Felson DT, Hannan MT, et al. Caffeine and the risk of hip fracture: the Framingham Study. Am J Epidemiol 1990;132(4):675–84.
[410] Hallström H, Wolk A, Glynn A, et al. Coffee, tea and caffeine consumption in relation to osteoporotic fracture risk in a cohort of Swedish women. Osteoporos Int 2006;17(7):1055–64.
[411] Hernandez-Avila M, Colditz GA, Stampfer MJ, et al. Caffeine, moderate alcohol intake and risk of fractures of the hip and forearm in middle-aged women. Am J Clin Nutr 1991;54(1): 157–63.
[412] Tucker KL, Morita K, Qiao N, et al. Colas, but not other carbonated beverages, are associated with low bone mineral density in older women: The Framingham Osteoporosis Study. Am J Clin Nutr 2006;84(4):936–42.
[413] American Academy of Pediatrics Committee on School Health. Soft drinks in schools. Pediatrics 2004;113(1):152–4.
[414] Mahmood M, Saleh A, Al-Alawi F, et al. Health effects of soda drinking in adolescent girls in the United Arab Emirates. J Crit Care 2008;23(3):434–40.
[415] Kristensen M, Jensen M, Kudsk J, et al. Short-term effects on bone turnover of replacing milk with cola beverages: a 10-day interventional study in young men. Osteoporos Int 2005;16(12):1803–8.
[416] Patsch JM, Kiefer FW, Varga P, et al. Increased bone resorption and impaired bone microarchitecture in short-term and extended high-fat diet-induced obesity. Metabolism 2011;60(2):243–9.
[417] Yazdanpanah N, Zillikens MC, Rivadeneira F, et al. Effect of dietary B vitamins on BMD and risk of fracture in elderly men and women: the Rotterdam study. Bone 2007;41(6):987–94.
[418] Holstein JH, Herrmann M, Splett C, et al. Low serum folate and vitamin B-6 are associated with an altered cancellous bone structure in humans. Am J Clin Nutr 2009;90(5):1440–5.
[419] Vaes BL, Lute C, Blom HJ, et al. Vitamin B(12) deficiency stimulates osteoclastogenesis via increased homocysteine and methylmalonic acid. Calcif Tissue Int 2009;84(5):413–22.
[420] McLean RR, Hannan MT. B vitamins, homocysteine and bone disease: epidemiology and pathophysiology. Curr Osteoporos Rep 2007;5(3):112–1119.
[421] Petramala L, Acca M, Francucci CM, et al. Hyperhomocysteinemia: a biochemical link between bone and cardiovascular system diseases? J Endocrinol Invest 2009;32(Suppl. 4):10–14.
[422] Herrmann M, Peter Schmidt J, Umanskaya N, et al. The role of hyperhomocysteinemia as well as folate, vitamin B(6) and B(12) deficiencies in osteoporosis: a systematic review. Clin Chem Lab Med 2007;45(12):1621–32.
[423] Palacios C. The role of nutrients in bone health, from A to Z. Crit Rev Food Sci Nutr 2006;46(8):621–8.

[424] Tang B, Eslick G, Nowson C, et al. Use of calcium or calcium in combination with vitamin D supplementation to prevent fractures and bone loss in people aged 50 years and older: a meta-analysis. Lancet 2007;370:657–66.
[425] Reid H, Bolland M, Grey A. Effect of calcium supplementation on hip fracture. Osteoporos Int 2008;19:1119–23.
[426] Heller HJ, Greer LG, Haynes SD, et al. Pharmacokinetic and pharmacodynamic comparison of two calcium supplements in postmenopausal women. J Clin Pharmacol 2000;40:1237–44.
[427] Shangraw RF. Factors to consider in the selection of a calcium supplement. Public Health Rep 1989;104(Suppl.): 46–50.
[428] Harvey JA, Zobitz MM, Pak CY. Dose dependency of calcium absorption: a comparison of calcium carbonate and calcium citrate. J Bone Miner Res 1988;3:253–8.
[429] Watkins BA, Lippman HE, Le Bouteiller L, et al. Bioactive fatty acids: role in bone biology and bone cell function. Prog Lipid Res 2001;40:125–48.
[430] Dong H, et al. Effects of omega-3 polyunsaturated fatty acid supplementation on bone turnover in older women. Int J Vitam Nutr Res 2014;84(3–4):124–32.
[431] Rude RK, Singer FR, Gruber HE. Skeletal and hormonal effects of magnesium deficiency. J Am Coll Nutr 2009;28(2):131–41.
[432] Odabasi E, Turan M, Aydin A, et al. Magnesium, zinc, copper, manganese and selenium levels in postmenopausal women with osteoporosis. Can magnesium play a key role in osteoporosis? Ann Acad Med Singapore 2008;37(7):564–7.
[433] Aydin H, Deyneli O, Yavuz D, et al. Short-term oral magnesium supplementation suppresses bone turnover in postmenopausal osteoporotic women. Biol Trace Elem Res 2010;133(2):136–43.
[434] Dreosti IE. Magnesium status and health. Nutr Rev 1995;53(Suppl.): S23–7.
[435] Martin KR. The chemistry of silica and its potential health benefits. J Nutr Health Aging 2007;11(2):94–7.
[436] Reffitt et al. (unpub 2002) as cited in Jugdaohsingh R. Silicon and bone health. J Nutr Health Aging 2007;11(2):99–110.
[437] Eisinger J, Clairet D. Effects of silicon, fluoride, etidronate and magnesium on bone mineral density: a retrospective study. Magnes Res 1993;6(3):247–9.
[438] Jugdaohsingh R, Tucker KL, Qiao N, et al. Silicon intake is a major dietary determinant of bone mineral density in men and pre-menopausal women of the Framingham Offspring Cohort. J Bone Miner Res 2004;19:297–307.
[439] Macdonald HM, Hardcastle AE, Jugdaohsingh R, et al. Dietary silicon intake is associated with bone mineral density in premenopausal women and postmenopausal women taking HRT. J Bone Miner Res 2005;20:S393.
[440] Jugdaohsingh R. Silicon and bone health. J Nutr Health Aging 2007;11(2):99–110.
[441] Schaafsma A, de Vries PJ, Saris WH. Delay of natural bone loss by higher intakes of specific minerals and vitamins. Crit Rev Food Sci Nutr 2001;41(4):225–49.
[442] Hall SL, Greendale GA. The relation of dietary vitamin C intake to bone mineral density: results from the PEPI study. Calcif Tissue Int 1998;63(3):183–9.
[443] Morton DJ, Barrett-Connor EL, Schneider DL. Vitamin C supplement use and bone mineral density in postmenopausal women. J Bone Miner Res 2001;16:135–40.
[444] Sahni S, Hannan MT, Gagnon D, et al. High vitamin C intake is associated with lower 4-year bone loss in elderly men. J Nutr 2008;138(10):1931–8.
[445] Sahni S, Hannan MT, Gagnon D, et al. Protective effect of total and supplemental vitamin C intake on the risk of hip fracture–a 17-year follow-up from the Framingham Osteoporosis Study. Osteoporos Int 2009;20(11):1853–61.
[446] LeBoff MS, Hawkes WG, Glowacki J, et al. Vitamin D-deficiency and post-fracture changes in lower extremity function and falls in women with hip fractures. Osteoporos Int 2008;19(9):1283–90.
[447] Janssen HC, Samson MM, Verhaar HJ. Vitamin D deficiency, muscle function and falls in elderly people. Am J Clin Nutr 2002;75(4):611–15.
[448] Avenell A, Gillespie WJ, Gillespie LD, et al. Vitamin D and vitamin D analogues for preventing fractures associated with involutional and post-menopausal osteoporosis. Cochrane Database Syst Rev 2009;(2):CD000227.
[449] Bischoff-Ferrari HA, Willett WC, Wong JB, et al. Fracture prevention with vitamin D supplementation: a meta-analysis of randomized controlled trials. JAMA 2005;293(18):2257–64.
[450] Jackson C, Gaugris S, Sen SS, et al. The effect of cholecalciferol (vitamin D3) on the risk of fall and fracture: a meta-analysis. QJM 2007;100(4):185–92.
[451] Nowson CA, Margerison C. Vitamin D intake and vitamin D status of Australians. Med J Aust 2002;177:149–52.
[452] Zhu K, Devine A, Dick IM, et al. Effects of calcium and vitamin D supplementation on hip bone mineral density and calcium-related analytes in elderly ambulatory Australian women: a five-year randomized controlled trial. J Clin Endocrinol Metab 2008;93(3):743–9.
[453] Iwamoto J, Vitamin K. therapy for postmenopausal osteoporosis. Nutrients 2014;6(5):1971–80.
[454] Myneni VD, Mezey E. Regulation of bone remodeling by vitamin K2. Oral Dis 2017;23(8):1021–8.
[455] Iwamoto J, et al. Effects of vitamin K2 on osteoporosis. Curr Pharm Des 2004;10(21):2557–76.
[456] Knapen MH, Schurgers LJ, Vermeer C. Vitamin K2 supplementation improves hip bone geometry and bone strength indices in postmenopausal women. Osteoporos Int 2007;18(7):963–72.
[457] Yalin S, Bagis S, Polat G, et al. Is there a role of free oxygen radicals in primary male osteoporosis? Clin Exp Rheumatol 2005;23(5):689–92.
[458] Sendur OF, Turan Y, Tastaban E, et al. Antioxidant status in patients with osteoporosis: a controlled study. Joint Bone Spine 2009;76(5):514–18.
[459] Ostman B, Michaëlsson K, Helmersson J, et al. Oxidative stress and bone mineral density in elderly men: antioxidant activity of alpha-tocopherol. Free Radic Biol Med 2009;47(5):668–73.
[460] Mehat MZ, Shuid AN, Mohamed N, et al. Beneficial effects of vitamin E isomer supplementation on static and dynamic bone histomorphometry parameters in normal male rats. J Bone Miner Metab 2010;28(5):503–9.
[461] Seaman D. Health care for our bones: a practical nutritional approach to preventing osteoporosis. J Manipulative Physiol Ther 2004;27(9):591–5.
[462] Ellingwood F. Ellingwood's therapeutist, vol. 2. Portland, OR: Eclectic Materia Medica Publications; 1908.
[463] McLean RR. Proinflammatory cytokines and osteoporosis. Curr Osteoporos Rep 2009;7(4):134–9.
[464] Ernst E. Frankincense: systematic review. BMJ 2008;337:a2813.
[465] Menon MK, Kar A. Analgesic and psychopharmacological effects of the gum resin of *Boswellia serrata*. Planta Med 1971;19(4):333–41.
[466] Hayman M, Ka P. Capsaicin: a review of its pharmacology and clinical applications. Curr Anaesth Crit Care 2008;19(5–6):338–43.
[467] Weibin S, Hao Z, Ning D, et al. Clinical biochemical observation on the treatment of postmenopausal osteoporosis with Gusong II. Chin J Integr Med 1998;4(1):9–11.
[468] Bharti AC, Takada Y, Aggarwal BB. Curcumin (diferuloylmethane) inhibits RANK ligand-induced NF-K B activation in osteoclast precursors and suppresses osteoclastogenesis. J Immunol 2004;172:5940–7.
[469] Peddada KV, Peddada KV, Shukla SK, et al. Role of curcumin in common musculoskeletal disorders: a review of current laboratory, translational and clinical data. Orthop Surg 2015;7(3):222–31.
[470] Romm A. Botanical medicine for women's health. St Louis: Elsevier Churchill Livingstone; 2010. p. 550–611.
[471] Wegiel B, Persson JL. Effect of a novel botanical agent Drynol Cibotin on human osteoblast cells and implications for osteoporosis: promotion of cell growth, calcium uptake and collagen production. Phytother Res 2010;24(Suppl. 2):S139–47.
[472] Gold DT. The clinical impact of vertebral fractures: quality of life in women with osteoporosis. Bone 1996;18(3, Suppl. 1):S185–9.
[473] Gennari C. Analgesic effect of calcitonin in osteoporosis. Bone 2002;30(Suppl. 5):S67–70.
[474] Brendler T, Gruenwald J, Ulbricht C, Natural Standard Research Collaboration, et al. Devil's claw (*Harpagophytum procumbens* DC): an evidence-based systematic review by the Natural Standard Research Collaboration. J Herb Pharmacother 2006;6(1):89–126.

[475] Ghasemian M, Owlia S, Owlia MB. Review of anti-inflammatory herbal medicines. Adv Pharmacol Sci 2016;2016:9130979.
[476] Chrubasik S, Eisenberg E, Balan E, et al. Treatment of low back pain exacerbations with willow bark extract: a randomized double-blind study. Am J Med 2000;109(1):9–14.
[477] Fiebich BL, Chrubasik S. Effects of an ethanolic salix extract on the release of selected inflammatory mediators in vitro. Phytomedicine 2004;11(2–3):135–8.
[478] Chevallier A. Encyclopedia of medicinal plants. London: Dorling Kindersley; 2001.
[479] McEwen BJ. The influence of herbal medicine on platelet function and coagulation: a narrative review. Semin Thromb Hemost 2015;41(3):300–14.
[480] Guadalupe-Grau A, Fuentes T, Guerra B, et al. Exercise and bone mass in adults. Sports Med 2009;39(6):439–68.
[481] Zehnacker CH, Bemis-Dougherty A. Effect of weighted exercises on bone mineral density in post-menopausal women. A systematic review. J Geriatr Phys Ther 2007;30(2):79–88.
[482] Suominen H. Muscle training for bone strength. Aging Clin Exp Res 2006;18(2):85–93.
[483] Martyn-St James M, Carroll S. Meta-analysis of walking for preservation of bone mineral density in postmenopausal women. Bone 2008;43(3):521–31.
[484] Tüzün S, Aktas I, Akarirmak U, et al. Yoga might be an alternative training for the quality of life and balance in postmenopausal osteoporosis. Eur J Phys Rehabil Med 2010;46(1):69–72.
[485] Lui PP, Qin L, Chan KM. Tai Chi Chuan exercises in enhancing bone mineral density in active seniors. Clin Sports Med 2008;27(1):75–86, viii.
[486] Wayne PM, Kiel DP, Krebs DE, et al. The effects of Tai Chi on bone mineral density in postmenopausal women: a systematic review. Arch Phys Med Rehabil 2007;88(5):673–80.
[487] Zhao R, Liu ZL, Wang JM, et al. Combination of acupuncture with cupping increases life quality of patients of osteoporosis. Zhongguo Zhen Jiu 2008;28(12):873–5.
[488] Van Vollenhoven RF. Sex differences in rheumatoid arthritis: more than meets the eye. BMC Med 2009;7:12.
[489] Aletaha D, Neogi T, Silman AJ, et al. 2010 Rheumatoid Arthritis Classification Criteria. Arthritis Rheum 2010;62(9): 2569–81.
[490] Brooks PM. Rheumatoid arthritis: aetiology and clinical features. Medicine (Baltimore) 2006;10(34):379–82.
[491] Royal Australian College of General Practitioners. Rheumatoid arthritis clinical guidelines. Melbourne: RACGP; 2008. Available from: www.racgp.org.au/Content/NavigationMenu/ClinicalResources/RACGPGuidelines/Arthritis/RAguideline.pdf.
[492] Cordain L, Toohey L, Smith MJ, et al. Modulation of immune function by dietary lectins in rheumatoid arthritis. Br J Nutr 2000;83(3):207–17.
[493] Gorman C, Cope A. Immune-mediated pathways in chronic inflammatory arthritis. Best Pract Res Clin Rheumatol 2008;22(2):221–38.
[494] Henriksson AE, Blomquist L, Nord CE, et al. Small intestinal bacterial overgrowth in patients with rheumatoid arthritis. Ann Rheum Dis 1993;52(7):503–10.
[495] Shinebaum R, Neumann Cooke EM, Wright V. Comparison of faecal flora in patients with rheumatoid arthritis and controls. Br J Rheumatol 1987;26:329–33.
[496] Peltonen R, Nenonen M, Helve T, et al. Faecal microbial flora and disease activity in rheumatoid arthritis during a vegan diet. Br J Rheumatol 1997;86:64–6.
[497] Jenkins RT, Rooney PJ, Jones DB, et al. Increased intestinal permeability in patients with rheumatoid arthritis: a side effect of oral nonsteroidal anti-inflammatory drug therapy? Br J Rheumatol 1987;26(2):103–7.
[498] Alamanos Y, Drosos AA. Epidemiology of adult rheumatoid arthritis. Autoimmun Rev 2005;4(3):130–6.
[499] Klareskog L, Stolt P, Lundberg K, et al. New model for an etiology of rheumatoid arthritis: smoking may trigger HLA-DR (shared epitope)-restricted immune reactions to autoantigens modified by citrullination. Arthritis Rheum 2006;54:38–46.
[500] Sugiyama D, Nishimura K, Tamaki K, et al. Impact of smoking as a risk factor for developing rheumatoid arthritis: a meta-analysis of observational studies. Ann Rheum Dis 2010;69(1):70–81.
[501] Onozaki K. Etiological and biological aspects of cigarette smoking in rheumatoid arthritis. Inflamm Allergy Drug Targets 2009;8(5):364–8.
[502] MacGregor AJ, Snieder H, Rigby AS, et al. Characterizing the quantitative genetic contribution to rheumatoid arthritis using data from twins. Arthritis Rheum 2000;43:30–7.
[503] Kochi Y, Suzuki A, Yamada R, et al. Genetics of rheumatoid arthritis: underlying evidence of ethnic differences. J Autoimmun 2009;32(3–4):158–62.
[504] Pratt AG, Isaacs JD, Mattey DL. Current concepts in the pathogenesis of early rheumatoid arthritis. Best Pract Res Clin Rheumatol 2009;23(1):37–48.
[505] Shaker OG, et al. Methylene tetrahydrofolate reductase, transforming growth factor-β1 and lymphotoxin-α genes polymorphisms and susceptibility to rheumatoid arthritis. Rev Bras Reumatol Engl Ed 2016;56(5):414–20.
[506] Cen H, Huang H, Zhang LN, et al. Associations of methylenetetrahydrofolate reductase (MTHFR) C677T and A1298C polymorphisms with genetic susceptibility to rheumatoid arthritis: a meta-analysis. Clin Rheumatol 2017;36(2):287–97.
[507] Lima A, Bernardes M, Azevedo R, et al. Moving toward personalized medicine in rheumatoid arthritis: SNPs in methotrexate intracellular pathways are associated with methotrexate therapeutic outcome. Pharmacogenomics 2016;17(15):1649–74.
[508] Toussirot E, Roudier J. Pathophysiological links between rheumatoid arthritis and the Epstein-Barr virus: an update. Joint Bone Spine 2007;74(5):418–26.
[509] Belin V, Tebib J, Vignon E. Cytomegalovirus infection in a patient with rheumatoid arthritis. Joint Bone Spine 2003;70(4):303–6.
[510] Kawahito Y, Ichinose S, Sano H, et al. *Mycoplasma fermentans* glycolipid-antigen as a pathogen of rheumatoid arthritis. Biochem Biophys Res Commun 2008;369(2):561–6.
[511] Symmons D, Chakravarty K. Can immunisation trigger rheumatoid arthritis? Ann Rheum Dis 1993;52:843–4.
[512] Khurana R, Berney S. Clinical aspects of rheumatoid arthritis. Pathophysiology 2005;12(3):153–65.
[513] Feldman M, Taylor P. Rheumatoid arthritis: pathogenic mechanisms and therapeutic targets. Drug Discov Today Dis Mech 2004;1(3):289–95.
[514] Cope AP. T cells in rheumatoid arthritis. Arthritis Res Ther 2008;10(Suppl. 1):S1.
[515] Silverman GJ, Carson DA. Roles of B cells in rheumatoid arthritis. Arthritis Res Ther 2003;5(Suppl. 4):S1–6.
[516] Del Rincon ID, Williams K, Stern MP, et al. High incidence of cardiovascular events in a rheumatoid arthritis cohort not explained by traditional cardiac risk factors. Arthritis Rheum 2001;44:2737–45.
[517] Grassi W, De Angelis R, Lamanna G, et al. Cardiovascular morbidity and mortality in women diagnosed with rheumatoid arthritis. Circulation 2003;107:1303–7.
[518] Mackenzie AH. Differential diagnosis of rheumatoid arthritis. Am J Med 1988;85:Suppl–A4.
[519] Proudman SM, et al. Plasma n-3 fatty acids and clinical outcomes in recent-onset rheumatoid arthritis. Br J Nutr 2015;114(6):885–90.
[520] McCann K. Nutrition and rheumatoid arthritis. Explore (NY) 2007;3(6):616–18.
[521] Pérez-López FR, Chedraui P, et al. Cuadros effects of the Mediterranean diet on longevity and age-related morbid conditions. Maturitas 2009;64(2):67–79.
[522] Aho K, Heliovaara M. Risk factors for rheumatoid arthritis. Ann Med 2004;36:242–51.
[523] Sköldstam L, Hagfors L, Johansson G. An experimental study of Mediterranean diet intervention for patients with rheumatoid arthritis. Ann Rheum Dis 2003;62:208–14.
[524] Bae S, Kim S, Sung M. Inadequate antioxidant nutrient intake and altered plasma antioxidant status of rheumatoid arthritis patients. J Am Coll Nutr 2003;22:311–15.
[525] Cerhan JR, Saag KG, Merlino LA, et al. Antioxidant micronutrients and risk of rheumatoid arthritis in a cohort of older women. Am J Epidemiol 2003;157:345–54.
[526] Harrison B, Thomson W, Symmons D, et al. The influence of HLA-DRB1 alleles and rheumatoid factor on disease outcome in an inception cohort of patients with early inflammatory arthritis. Arthritis Rheum 1999;42:2174–83.

[527] Muller H. Fasting followed by vegetarian diet in patients with rheumatoid arthritis: a systematic review. Scand J Rheumatol 2001;30:1–10.
[528] Abendroth A, Michalsen A, Lüdtke R, et al. Changes of intestinal microflora in patients with rheumatoid arthritis during fasting and a Mediterranean diet. Eur J Integr Med 2008;1(Suppl. 1):25.
[529] Kjeldsen-Kragh J, Borchgrevink CF, Laerum E, et al. Controlled trial of fasting and one-year vegetarian diet in rheumatoid arthritis. Lancet 1991;338(8772):899–902.
[530] Hagen KB, Byfuglien MG, Falzon L, et al. Dietary interventions for rheumatoid arthritis. Cochrane Database Syst Rev 2009;(1):CD006400.
[531] Calder PC. Session 3: Joint Nutrition Society and Irish Nutrition and Dietetic Institute Symposium on 'Nutrition and autoimmune disease' PUFA, inflammatory processes and rheumatoid arthritis. Proc Nutr Soc 2008;67(4):409–18.
[532] Svoboda RE. Prakriti: your Ayurvedic constitution. 2nd ed. Twin Lakes: Lotus Tree Press; 1998.
[533] Heliövaara M, Aho K, Knekt P, et al. Coffee consumption, rheumatoid factor and the risk of rheumatoid arthritis. Ann Rheum Dis 2000;59(8):631–5.
[534] Källberg H, Jacobsen S, Bengtsson C, et al. Alcohol consumption is associated with decreased risk of rheumatoid arthritis: results from two Scandinavian case-control studies. Ann Rheum Dis 2009;68(2):222–7.
[535] Karlson EW, Mandl LA, Aweh GN, et al. Coffee consumption and risk of rheumatoid arthritis. Arthritis Rheum 2003;48(11): 3055–60.
[536] Henderson CJ, Panush R. Diets, dietary supplements and nutritional therapies in rheumatic diseases. Rheum Dis Clin North Am 1999;25(4):937–68.
[537] Dugowson CE. Rheumatoid arthritis. In: Goldman MB, Hatch MC, editors. Women and health. San Diego, CA: Academic Press; p. 674–85.
[538] Pattison DJ, Symmons DP, Lunt M, et al. Dietary risk factors for the development of inflammatory polyarthritis: evidence for a role of high level of red meat consumption. Arthritis Rheum 2004;50:3804–12.
[539] Benito-Garcia E, Feskanich D, Hu FB, et al. Protein, iron and meat consumption and risk for rheumatoid arthritis: a prospective cohort study. Arthritis Res Ther 2007;9(1):R16.
[540] Grant WB. The role of meat in the expression of rheumatoid arthritis. Br J Nutr 2000;84:589–95.
[541] Rall LC, Meydani SN. Vitamin B6 and immune competence. Nutr Rev 1993;51(8):217–25.
[542] Roubenoff R, Roubenoff RA, Selhub J, et al. Abnormal vitamin B6 status in rheumatoid cachexia. Association with spontaneous tumor necrosis factor alpha production and markers of inflammation. Arthritis Rheum 1995;38(1):105–9.
[543] Whittle SL, Hughes RA. Folate supplementation and methotrexate treatment in rheumatoid arthritis: a review. Rheumatology (Oxford) 2004;43(3):267–71.
[544] Baggott JE, Morgan SL. Folic acid supplements are good (not bad) for rheumatoid arthritis patients treated with low-dose methotrexate. Am J Clin Nutr 2008;88(2):479–80, author reply 480.
[545] Szekanecz Z, Kerekes G, Dér H, et al. Accelerated atherosclerosis in rheumatoid arthritis. Ann N Y Acad Sci 2007;1108:349–58.
[546] Segal R, Baumoehl Y, Elkayam O, et al. Anemia, serum vitamin B_{12} and folic acid in patients with rheumatoid arthritis, psoriatic arthritis and systemic lupus erythematosus. Rheumatol Int 2004;24(1):14–119.
[547] Vreugdenhil G, Wognum AW, van Eijk HG, et al. Anaemia in rheumatoid arthritis: the role of iron, vitamin B_{12} and folic acid deficiency and erythropoietin responsiveness. Ann Rheum Dis 1990;49(2):93–8.
[548] Pitcher CS, Lindsay DJ, Hill AG. Absorption of vitamin B_{12} in rheumatoid arthritis. Ann Rheum Dis 1970;29(5):533–6.
[549] Klein G, Kullich W. Reducing pain by oral enzyme therapy in rheumatic diseases. Wien Med Wochenschr 1999;149(21–22):577–80.
[550] Desser L, Holomanova D, Zavadova E, et al. Oral therapy with proteolytic enzymes decreases excessive TGF-beta levels in human blood. Cancer Chemother Pharmacol 2001;47(Suppl.):S10–15.
[551] Cohen A, Goldman J. Bromelains therapy in rheumatoid arthritis. Pa Med J 1964;67:27–30.
[552] Aaseth J, Haugen M, Førre O. Rheumatoid arthritis and metal compounds — perspectives on the role of oxygen radical detoxification. Analyst 1998;123(1):3–6.
[553] Smith-Mungo LI, Kagan HM. Lysyl oxidase: properties, regulation and multiple functions in biology. Matrix Biol 1998;16(7):387–98.
[554] Hvatum M, Kanerud L, Hällgren R, et al. The gut–joint axis: cross reactive food antibodies in rheumatoid arthritis. Gut 2006;55(9):1240–7.
[555] Henriksson K, Uvnäs-Moberg K, Nord CE, et al. Gastrin, gastric acid secretion and gastric microflora in patients with rheumatoid arthritis. Ann Rheum Dis 1986;45(6):475–83.
[556] Cameron M, Gagnier JJ, Little CV, et al. Evidence of effectiveness of herbal medicinal products in the treatment of arthritis. Part 2: Rheumatoid arthritis. Phytother Res 2009;23(12):1647–62.
[557] Hurst S, Zainal Z, Caterson B, et al. Dietary fatty acids and arthritis. Prostaglandins Leukot Essent Fatty Acids 2010;82(4–6):315–3118.
[558] Lane K, Derbyshire E, Li W, et al. Bioavailability and potential uses of vegetarian sources of omega-3 fatty acids: a review of the literature. Crit Rev Food Sci Nutr 2014;54(5):572–9.
[559] Jackson JK, Higo T, Hunter WL, et al. The antioxidants curcumin and quercetin inhibit inflammatory processes associated with arthritis. Inflamm Res 2006;55(4):168–75.
[560] Zimmermann M. Burgenstein's handbook of nutrition, micronutrients in the prevention and therapy of diseases. New York: Thieme; 2001.
[561] Harmand MF, Vilamitjana J, Maloche E, et al. Effects of S-adenosylmethionine on human articular chondrocyte differentiation. An in vitro study. Am J Med 1987;83:48S–54S.
[562] Gutierrez S, Palacios I, Sanchez-Pernaute O, et al. SAM-e restores the changes in the proliferation and in the synthesis of fibronectin and proteoglycans induced by tumour necrosis factor alpha on cultured rabbit synovial cells. Br J Rheumatol 1997;37:27–31.
[563] Hosea Blewett HJ. Exploring the mechanisms behind S-adenosylmethionine (SAM-e) in the treatment of osteoarthritis. Crit Rev Food Sci Nutr 2008;48(5):458–63.
[564] Ryan-Harshman M, Aldoori W. The relevance of selenium to immunity, cancer and infectious/inflammatory diseases. Can J Diet Pract Res 2005;66(2):98–102.
[565] Yazar M, Sarban S, Kocyigit A, et al. Synovial fluid and plasma selenium, copper, zinc and iron concentrations in patients with rheumatoid arthritis and osteoarthritis. Biol Trace Elem Res 2005;106(2):123–32.
[566] Tarp U. Selenium and the selenium-dependent glutathione peroxidase in rheumatoid arthritis. Dan Med Bull 1994;41(3):264–74.
[567] Köse K, Doğan P, Kardas Y, et al. Plasma selenium levels in rheumatoid arthritis. Biol Trace Elem Res 1996;53(1–3):51–6.
[568] Knekt P, Heliövaara M, Aho K, et al. Serum selenium, serum alpha-tocopherol and the risk of rheumatoid arthritis. Epidemiology 2000;11(4):402–5.
[569] Peretz A, Siderova V, Nève J. Selenium supplementation in rheumatoid arthritis investigated in a double blind, placebo-controlled trial. Scand J Rheumatol 2001;30(4): 208–12.
[570] Sowers M, Lachance L. Vitamins and arthritis: the roles of vitamins A, C, D and E. Rheum Dis Clin North Am 1999;25(2):315–32.
[571] Honkanen V, Konttinen YT, Mussalo-Rauhamaa H. Vitamins A and E, retinol binding protein and zinc in rheumatoid arthritis. Clin Exp Rheumatol 1989;7(5):465–9.
[572] Jaswal S, Mehta HC, Sood AK, et al. Antioxidant status in rheumatoid arthritis and role of antioxidant therapy. Clin Chim Acta 2003;338(1–2):123–9.
[573] Adorini L. Immunomodulatory effects of vitamin D receptor ligands in autoimmune diseases. Int Immunopharmacol 2002;2(7):1017–28.
[574] Cutolo M, Otsa K, Uprus M, et al. Vitamin D in rheumatoid arthritis. Autoimmun Rev 2007;7(1):59–64.
[575] Andjelkovic Z, Vojinovic J, Pejnovic N, et al. Disease modifying and immunomodulatory effects of high dose 1 alpha (OH) D3 in rheumatoid arthritis patients. Clin Exp Rheumatol 1999;17:453–6.
[576] Honkanen V, Konttinen YT, Mussalo-Rauhamaa H. Vitamins A and E, retinol binding protein and zinc in rheumatoid arthritis. Clin Exp Rheumatol 1989;7(5):465–9.
[577] Edmonds SE, Winyard PG, Guo R, et al. Putative analgesic activity of repeated oral doses of vitamin E in the treatment of rheumatoid

arthritis. Results of a prospective placebo controlled double blind trial. Ann Rheum Dis 1997;56(11):649–55.
[578] Zoli A. Serum zinc and copper in active rheumatoid arthritis: correlation with interleukin 1β and tumour necrosis factor α. Clin Rheumatol 1998;17(5):378–82.
[579] Helliwell M, Coombes EJ, Moody BJ, et al. Nutritional status in patients with rheumatoid arthritis. Ann Rheum Dis 1984;43:386–90.
[580] Kremer JM, Bigaouette J. Nutrient intake of patients with rheumatoid arthritis is deficient in pyridoxine, zinc, copper and magnesium. J Rheumatol 1996;23(6):990–4.
[581] Fang YZ, Yang S. Wu G Free radicals, antioxidants and nutrition. Nutrition 2002;18:872–9.
[582] Simkin PA. Oral zinc sulfate in rheumatoid arthritis. Lancet 1976;2(7985):539–42.
[583] Greive M. A modern herbal; 1931. Available from: http://botanical.com/index.html.
[584] Mahran GH, Kadry HA, Isaac ZG, et al. Investigation of diuretic drug plants. Phytochemical screening and pharmacological evaluation of *Anethum graveolens* L, *Apium graveolens* L, *Daucus carota* L. and *Eruca sativa* mill. Phytother Res 2006;5(4):169–72.
[585] Sander O, Herborn G, Rau R. Is H15 (resin extract of *Boswellia serrata*, 'incense') a useful supplement to established drug therapy of chronic polyarthritis? Results of a double-blind pilot study [in German]. Z Rheumatol 1998;57:11–116.
[586] Moga MM. Alternative treatment of gallbladder disease. Med Hypotheses 2003;60(1):143–7.
[587] Abe H, Sakaguchi M, Odashima S, et al. Protective effect of saikosaponin-d isolated from *Bupleurum falcatum* L. on CC14-induced liver injury in the rat. Naunyn Schmiedebergs Arch Pharmacol 1982;320(3):266–71.
[588] Abe H, Sakaguchi M, Yamada M, et al. Pharmacological actions of saikosaponins isolated from *Bupleurum falcatum*. 1. Effects of saikosaponins on liver function. Planta Med 1980;40(4):366–72.
[589] Watkins KW, Shifren K, Park DC, et al. Age, pain and coping with rheumatoid arthritis. Pain 1999;82(3):217–28.
[590] Yuan CS, et al. Effects of *Corydalis yanhusuo* and *Angelicae dahuricae* on cold pressor-induced pain in humans: a controlled trial. J Clin Pharmacol 2004;44:1323–7.
[591] Funk JL, Oyarzo JN, Frye JB, et al. Turmeric extracts containing curcuminoids prevent experimental rheumatoid arthritis. J Nat Prod 2006;69:351–5.
[592] Park C, Moon DO, Choi IW, et al. Curcumin induces apoptosis and inhibits prostaglandin E(2) production in synovial fibroblasts of patients with rheumatoid arthritis. Int J Mol Med 2007;20(3):365–72.
[593] Henrotin Y, Clutterbuck AL, Allaway D, et al. Biological actions of curcumin on articular chondrocytes. Osteoarthr Cartil 2010;18(2):141–9.
[594] Shehzad A, et al. Curcumin in inflammatory diseases. Biofactors 2013;39(1):69–77.
[595] Bright JJ. Curcumin and autoimmune disease. Adv Exp Med Biol 2007;595:425–51.
[596] Delorme D, Miller SC. Dietary consumption of Echinacea by mice afflicted with autoimmune (type I) diabetes: effect of consuming the herb on hemopoietic and immune cell dynamics. Autoimmunity 2005;38(6):453–61.
[597] Kocaman O, Hulagu S, Senturk O. Echinacea-induced severe acute hepatitis with features of cholestatic autoimmune hepatitis. Eur J Intern Med 2008;19(2):148.
[598] Wolfe F, Michaud K, Li T. Sleep disturbance in patients with rheumatoid arthritis: evaluation by medical outcomes study and visual analog sleep scales. J Rheumatol 2006;33(10):1942–51.
[599] Boomershine CS. Effective rheumatoid arthritis treatment requires comprehensive management strategies. Arthritis Res Ther 2009;11(6):138.
[600] Loew D, Mollerfeld J, Schodter A, et al. Investigations on the pharmocokinetic properties of *Harpagophytum* extracts and their effects on eicosanoid biosynthesis in vitro and ex vivo. Clin Pharmacol Ther 2001;69:356–64.
[601] Grant L, McBean DE, Fyfe L, et al. The inhibition of free radical generation by preparations of *Harpagophytum procumbens* in vitro. Phytother Res 2008;23(1):104–10.
[602] Maciejewska RH, Jüngel A, Gay RE, et al. Innate immunity, epigenetics and autoimmunity in rheumatoid arthritis. Mol Immunol 2009;47(1):12–18.
[603] Deepak D, Srivastava S, Khare A. Pregnane glycosides from *Hemidesmus indicus*. Phytochemistry 1997;44(1):145–51.
[604] Atal CK, Sharma ML, Kaul A, et al. Immunomodulating agents of plant origin. I: preliminary screening. J Ethnopharmacol 1986;18(2):133–41.
[605] Biegert C, Wagner I, Ludtke R, et al. Efficacy and safety of willow bark extract in the treatment of osteoarthritis and rheumatoid arthritis: results of 2 randomized double-blind controlled trials. J Rheumatol 2004;31(11):2121–30.
[606] Mur E, Hartig F, Eibl G, et al. Randomized double blind trial of an extract from the pentacyclic alkaloid-chemotype of uncaria tomentosa for the treatment of rheumatoid arthritis. J Rheumatol 2002;29(4):678–81.
[607] Zhang Q, Li L, Liu L, et al. Effects of the polysaccharide fraction of *Urtica fissa* on castrated rat prostate hyperplasia induced by testosterone propionate. Phytomedicine 2008;15(9):722–7.
[608] Broe J, Behnke B. Immunosuppressant effect of IDS 30, a stinging nettle leaf extract, on myeloid dendritic cells in vitro. J Rheumatol 2002;29:659–66.
[609] Bradley PR, editor. British herbal compendium, vol. 1. Bournemouth: British Herbal Medicine Association; 1992.
[610] Han A, Robinson V, Judd M, et al. Tai chi for treating rheumatoid arthritis. Cochrane Database Syst Rev 2004;(3):CD004849.
[611] Bosch PR, Traustadóttir T, Howard P, et al. Functional and physiological effects of yoga in women with rheumatoid arthritis: a pilot study. Altern Ther Health Med 2009;15(4):24–31.
[612] Badsha H, Chhabra V, Leibman C, et al. The benefits of yoga for rheumatoid arthritis: results of a preliminary, structured 8-week program. Rheumatol Int 2009;29(12):1417–21.
[613] Sukenik S, Neumann L, Flusser D, et al. Balneotherapy for rheumatoid arthritis at the Dead Sea. Isr J Med Sci 1995;31(4):210–2114.
[614] Sukenik S, Neumann L, Buskila D, et al. Dead Sea bath salts for the treatment of rheumatoid arthritis. Clin Exp Rheumatol 1990;8(4):353–3517.
[615] Verhagen AP, Bierma-Zeinstra SM, Cardoso JR, et al. Balneotherapy for rheumatoid arthritis. Cochrane Database Syst Rev 2003;(4):CD000518.
[616] Danneskiold-Samsøe B, Lyngberg K, Risum T, et al. The effect of water exercise therapy given to patients with rheumatoid arthritis. Scand J Rehabil Med 1987;19(1):31–5.
[617] Egan M, Brosseau L, Farmer M, et al. Splints/orthoses in the treatment of rheumatoid arthritis. Cochrane Database Syst Rev 2003;(1):CD004018.
[618] Fitzcharles MA, DaCosta D, Ware MA, et al. Patient barriers to pain management may contribute to poor pain control in rheumatoid arthritis. J Pain 2009;10(3):300–5.
[619] The Australasian Society of Clinical Immunology and Allergy (ASCIA). Systemic lupus erythematosus. Available from: www.allergy.org.au/patients/autoimmunity/systemic-lupus-erythematosus-sle.
[620] Manson J, Rahman A. Systemic lupus erythematosus. Orphanet J Rare Dis 2006;1:6.
[621] Segasothy M, Phillips P. Systemic lupus erythematosus in Aborigines and Caucasians in central Australia: a comparative study. Lupus 2001;10:439–44.
[622] Bossingham D. Systemic lupus erythematosus in the far north of Queensland. Lupus 2003;12:327–31.
[623] Albilia JB, Lam DK, Clokie CM, et al. Systemic lupus erythematosus: a review for dentists. J Can Dent Assoc 2007;73(9):823–8.
[624] Smith MF, et al. Biomarkers as tools for improved diagnostic and therapeutic monitoring in systemic lupus erythematosus. Arthritis Res Ther 2009;11(6):255.
[625] Pons-Estel GJ, Alarcón GS, Scofield L, et al. Understanding the epidemiology and progression of systemic lupus erythematosus. Semin Arthritis Rheum 2010;39(4):257–68.
[626] Simard JF, Costenbader KH. What can epidemiology tell us about systemic lupus erythematosus? Int J Clin Pract 2007;61(7):1170–80.
[627] Tsao BP. Update on human systemic lupus erythematosus genetics. Curr Opin Rheumatol 2004;16:513–21.

[628] Kaiser R, et al. Genetic risk factors for thrombosis in systemic lupus erythematosus. J Rheumatol 2012;39(8):1603–10.
[629] Poole BD, Templeton AK, Guthridge JM, et al. Aberrant Epstein-Barr viral infection in systemic lupus erythematosus. Autoimmun Rev 2009;8(4):337–42.
[630] Niller HH, Wolf H, Minarovits J. Regulation and dysregulation of Epstein-Barr virus latency: implications for the development of autoimmune diseases. Autoimmunity 2008;41(4):298–328.
[631] Hayashi T, Lee S, Ogasawara H, et al. Exacerbation of systemic lupus erythematosus related to cytomegalovirus infection. Lupus 1998;7(8):561–4.
[632] Francis L, Perl A. Infection in systemic lupus erythematosus: friend or foe? Int J Clin Rheumatol 2010;5(1):59–74.
[633] Walker SE. Estrogen and autoimmune disease. Clin Rev Allergy Immunol 2011;40(1):60–5.
[634] Anderson JA, Weiss L, Rebuck JW, et al. Hyperreactivity to cows' milk in an infant with LE and tart cell phenomenon. J Pediatr 1974;84:59–67.
[635] Parks CG, Cooper GS, Nylander-French LA, et al. Occupational exposure to crystalline silica and risk of systemic lupus erythematosus: a population-based, case-control study in the southeastern United States. Arthritis Rheum 2002;46(7): 1840–50.
[636] Finckh A, Cooper GS, Chibnik LB, et al. Occupational silica and solvent exposures and risk of systemic lupus erythematosus in urban women. Arthritis Rheum 2006;54(11):3648–54.
[637] Parks CG, Cooper GS. Occupational exposures and risk of systemic lupus erythematosus: a review of the evidence and exposure assessment methods in population- and clinic-based studies. Lupus 2006;15(11):728–36.
[638] Klein R, Sayre R, Dowdy J, et al. The risk of ultraviolet radiation exposure from indoor lamps in lupus erythematosus. Autoimmun Rev 2009;8(4):320–4.
[639] Vedove CD, Del Giglio M, Schena D, et al. Drug-induced lupus erythematosus. Arch Dermatol Res 2009;301(1): 99–105.
[640] Marzano AV, Vezzoli P, Crosti C. Drug-induced lupus: an update on its dermatologic aspects. Lupus 2009;18(11):935–40.
[641] Scolding NJ, Joseph FG. The neuropathology and pathogenesis of systemic lupus erythematosus. Neuropathol Appl Neurobiol 2002;28:173–89.
[642] Perl A. Pathogenic mechanisms in systemic lupus erythematosus. Autoimmunity 2010;43(1):1–6.
[643] Mok CC, Lau CS. Pathogenesis of systemic lupus erythematosus. J Clin Pathol 2003;56:481–90.
[644] Navaneethan SD, Viswanathan G, Strippoli GF. Treatment options for proliferative lupus nephritis: an update of clinical trial evidence. Drugs 2008;68(15):2095–104.
[645] Full LE, Ruisanchez C, Monaco C. The inextricable link between atherosclerosis and prototypical inflammatory diseases rheumatoid arthritis and systemic lupus erythematosus. Arthritis Res Ther 2009;11(2):217.
[646] Mok CC, Ho LY, Cheung MY, et al. Effect of disease activity and damage on quality of life in patients with systemic lupus erythematosus: a 2-year prospective study. Scand J Rheumatol 2009;38(2):121–7.
[647] Borchers AT, Keen CL, Shoenfeld Y, et al. Surviving the butterfly and the wolf: mortality trends in systemic lupus erythematosus. Autoimmun Rev 2004;3(6):423–53.
[648] Minami Y, Sasaki T, Arai Y, et al. Diet and systemic lupus erythematosus: a 4 year prospective study of Japanese patients. J Rheumatol 2003;30(4):747–54.
[649] Cooke HM, Reading CM. Dietary intervention in systemic lupus erythematosus: 4 cases of clinical remission and reversal of abnormal pathology. Int Clin Nutr Rev 1985;5:166–76.
[650] Diumenjo MS, Lisanti M, Vallés R, et al. [Allergic manifestations of systemic lupus erythematosus.]. Allergol Immunopathol (Madr) 1985;13(4):323–6.
[651] Rea WJ, Brown OD. Mechanisms of environmental vascular triggering. Clin Ecol 1985;3:122–8.
[652] Leung LH. Systemic lupus erythematosus: a combined deficiency disease. Med Hypotheses 2004;62(6):922–4.
[653] Ardoin SP, Sandborg C, Schanberg LE. Management of dyslipidemia in children and adolescents with systemic lupus erythematosus. Lupus 2007;16(8):618–26.
[654] Munoz LE, Janko C, Chaurio RA, et al. IgG opsonized nuclear remnants from dead cells cause systemic inflammation in SLE. Autoimmunity 2010;43(3):232–5.
[655] Wright SA, O'Prey FM, McHenry MT, et al. A randomised interventional trial of omega-3-polyunsaturated fatty acids on endothelial function and disease activity in systemic lupus erythematosus. Ann Rheum Dis 2008;67(6):841–8.
[656] Arriens C, Hynan LS, Lerman RH, et al. Placebo-controlled randomized clinical trial of fish oil's impact on fatigue, quality of life and disease activity in systemic lupus erythematosus. Nutr J 2015;14:82.
[657] Amissah-Arthur MB, Gordon C. GPs have key role in shared care of patients with SLE. Practitioner 2009;253(1724):19–24.
[658] Van Vugt RM, Derksen RH, Kater L, et al. Deforming arthropathy or lupus and rhupus hands in systemic lupus erythematosus. Ann Rheum Dis 1998;57(9):540–4.
[659] Bucki R, Pastore J, Giraud F, et al. Flavonoid inhibition of platelet proagulant activity and phosphoinositide synthesis. J Thromb Haemost 2003;1:1820–8.
[660] De Whalley CV, Rankin S, Hoult JR, et al. Flavonoids inhibit the oxidative modification of low density lipoproteins by macrophages. Biochem Pharmacol 1990;39:1743–50.
[661] Von Feldt JM. Premature atherosclerotic cardiovascular disease and systemic lupus erythematosus from bedside to bench. Bull NYU Hosp Jt Dis 2008;66(3):184–7.
[662] Bruce IN. Not only ... but also': factors that contribute to accelerated atherosclerosis and premature coronary heart disease in systemic lupus erythematosus. Rheumatology (Oxford) 2005;44(12):1492–502.
[663] Yilmaz A, Sari RA, Gundogdu M, et al. Trace elements and some extracellular antioxidant proteins levels in serum of patients with systemic lupus erythematosus. Clin Rheumatol 2005;24(4):331–5.
[664] Watts D. The nutritional relationship of manganese. J Orthomol Med 1990;5(4):219–22.
[665] Yen JH, Chen CJ, Tsai WC, et al. Cytochrome P450 and manganese superoxide dismutase genes polymorphisms in systemic lupus erythematosus. Immunol Lett 2003;90(1):19–24.
[666] Li Y, Liu Y, Strickland FM, et al. Age-dependent decreases in DNA methyltransferase levels and low transmethylation micronutrient levels synergize to promote overexpression of genes implicated in autoimmunity and acute coronary syndromes. Exp Gerontol 2009;45(4):312–22.
[667] O'Dell JR, McGivern JP, Kay HD, et al. Improved survival in murine lupus as the result of selenium supplementation. Clin Exp Immunol 1988;73(2):322–7.
[668] Gergely P, Csáky L, González-Cabello P. Immunological effects of retinoids. Tokai J Exp Clin Med 1990;15(2–3):235–9.
[669] Bae SC, Kim SJ, Sung MK. Impaired antioxidant status and decreased dietary intake of antioxidants in patients with systemic lupus erythematosus. Rheumatol Int 2002;22(6):238–43.
[670] Tam LS, Li EK, Leung VY, et al. Effects of vitamins C and E on oxidative stress markers and endothelial function in patients with systemic lupus erythematosus: a double blind, placebo controlled pilot study. J Rheumatol 2005;32(2):275–82.
[671] Kamen DL, Aranow C. The link between vitamin D deficiency and systemic lupus erythematosus. Curr Rheumatol Rep 2008;10(4):273–80.
[672] Borba VZ, Vieira JG, Kasamatsu T, et al. Vitamin D deficiency in patients with active systemic lupus erythematosus. Osteoporos Int 2009;20(3):427–33.
[673] Damanhouri LH. Vitamin D deficiency in Saudi patients with systemic lupus erythematosus. Saudi Med J 2009;30(10):1291–5.
[674] Barnes TC, Bucknall RC. Vitamin D deficiency in a patient with systemic lupus erythematosus. Rheumatology 2004;43:393–4.
[675] Maeshima E, Liang XM, Goda M, et al. The efficacy of vitamin E against oxidative damage and autoantibody production in systemic lupus erythematosus: a preliminary study. Clin Rheumatol 2007;26(3):401–4.
[676] Ayers S, Mihan R. Is vitamin E involved in the autoimmune mechanism? Cutis 1978;21:321–5.
[677] Brown AC. Lupus erythematosus and nutrition: a review of the literature. J Ren Nutr 2000;10(4):170–83.
[678] Kapil A, Moza N. Anticomplementary activity of boswellic acids — an inhibitor of C3-convertase of the classical complement pathway. Int J Immunopharmacol 1992;14(7):1139–43.

[679] Bright JJ. Curcumin and autoimmune disease. Adv Exp Med Biol 2007;595:425–51.
[680] Kurien BT, D'Souza A, Scofield RH. Heat-solubilized curry spice curcumin inhibits antibody-antigen interaction in in vitro studies: a possible therapy to alleviate autoimmune disorders. Mol Nutr Food Res 2010;54(8):1202–9.
[681] Neri PG, Stagni E, Filippello M, et al. Oral *Echinacea purpurea* extract in low-grade, steroid-dependent, autoimmune idiopathic uveitis: a pilot study. J Ocul Pharmacol Ther 2006;22(6):431–6.
[682] Wigley FM. Clinical practice. Raynaud's phenomenon. N Engl J Med 2002;347:1001–8.
[683] Luks A, Grissom C, Jean D, et al. Can people with Raynaud's phenomenon travel to high altitude? Wilderness Environ Med 2009;20(2):129–38.
[684] Muir AH, Robb R, McLaren M, et al. The use of *Ginkgo biloba* in Raynaud's disease: a double-blind placebo-controlled trial. Vasc Med 2002;7(4):265–7.
[685] Grant L, McBean DE, Fyfe L, et al. A review of the biological and potential therapeutic actions of *Harpagophytum procumbens*. Phytother Res 2007;21(3):199–209.
[686] Philip EJ, Lindner H, Lederman L. Relationship of illness perceptions with depression among individuals diagnosed with lupus. Depress Anxiety 2009;26(6):575–82.
[687] Kozora E, Ellison MC, West S. Depression, fatigue and pain in systemic lupus erythematosus (SLE): relationship to the American College of Rheumatology SLE neuropsychological battery. Arthritis Rheum 2006;55(4):628–35.
[688] Bachen EA, Chesney MA, Criswell LA. Prevalence of mood and anxiety disorders in women with systemic lupus erythematosus. Arthritis Rheum 2009;61(6):822–9.
[689] Lehmann P, Homey B. Clinic and pathophysiology of photosensitivity in lupus erythematosus. Autoimmun Rev 2009;8(6):456–61.
[690] Peralta-Ramírez MI, Jiménez-Alonso J, Godoy-García JF, Group Lupus Virgen de las Nieves, et al. The effects of daily stress and stressful life events on the clinical symptomatology of patients with lupus erythematosus. Psychosom Med 2004;66(5):788–94.
[691] Bricou O, Taïeb O, Baubet T, et al. Stress and coping strategies in systemic lupus erythematosus: a review. Neuroimmunomodulation 2006;13(5–6):283–93.
[692] Navarrete-Navarrete N, Peralta-Ramírez MI, Sabio-Sánchez JM, et al. Efficacy of cognitive behavioural therapy for the treatment of chronic stress in patients with lupus erythematosus: a randomized controlled trial. Psychother Psychosom 2010;79(2):107–15.
[693] Carvalho MR, Sato EI, Tebexreni AS, et al. Effects of supervised cardiovascular training program on exercise tolerance, aerobic capacity and quality of life in patients with systemic lupus erythematosus. Arthritis Rheum 2005;53(6):838–44.
[694] Wittmann L, Sensky T, Meder L, et al. Suffering and posttraumatic growth in women with systemic lupus erythematosus (SLE): a qualitative/quantitative case study. Psychosomatics 2009;50(4):362–74.
[695] Galarraga B, Ho M, Youssef HM, et al. Cod liver oil (n-3 fatty acids) as an non-steroidal anti-inflammatory drug sparing agent in rheumatoid arthritis. Rheumatology (Oxford) 2008;47:665–9.
[696] Gruenwald J, Graubaum HJ, Harde A. Effect of cod liver oil on symptoms of rheumatoid arthritis. Adv Ther 2002;19:101–7.
[697] Walker AF, Bundy R, Hicks SM, et al. Bromelain reduces mild acute knee pain and improves well-being in a dose-dependent fashion in an open study of otherwise healthy adults. Phytomedicine 2002;9:681–6.
[698] Notoya M, Tsukamoto Y, Nishimura H, et al. Quercetin, a flavonoid, inhibits the proliferation, differentiation and mineralization of osteoblasts in vitro. Eur J Pharmacol 2004;485:89–96.
[699] Shaik YB, Castellani ML, Perrella A, et al. Role of quercetin (a natural herbal compound) in allergy and inflammation. J Biol Regul Homeost Agents 2006;20:47–52.
[700] Braun L, Cohen M. An evidence-based guide to herbs and natural supplements. Edinburgh: Elsevier, Churchill Livingstone; 2007.
[701] Brien S, Prescott P, Bashir N, et al. Systematic review of the nutritional supplements dimethyl sulfoxide (DMSO) and methylsulfonylmethane (MSM) in the treatment of osteoarthritis. Osteoarthr Cartil 2008;16:1277–88.
[702] Kim LS, Axelrod LJ, Howard P, et al. Efficacy of methylsulfonylmethane (MSM) in osteoarthritis pain of the knee: a pilot clinical trial. Osteoarthr Cartil 2006;14:286–94.
[703] Bone K. Clinical applications of Ayurvedic and Chinese herbs, monographs for the Western practitioner. Warwick, Queensland: Phytotherapy Press; 1996.
[704] Blumenthal M, Goldberg A, Brinckmann J. Herbal medicine: the expanded commission E monographs. Newton, MA: Integrative Medicine Communications; 2000.
[705] World Health Organization (WHO). WHO Monographs on selected medicinal plants, vol. 1. Geneva: WHO; 1999.
[706] Srivastava KC, Mustafa T. Ginger (*Zingiber officinale*) in rheumatism and musculoskeletal disorders. Med Hypotheses 1992;39:342–8.
[707] Jetty Lee Y, Kim M, Yoon S-W, et al. Short-term control of capsaicin on blood and oxidative stress in rats in vivo. Phytother Res 2003;17:454–8.
[708] Keital W. Capsicum pain plaster in chronic non-specific low back pain. Arzneimittelforschung 2001;51:896–903.
[709] Liu M, Dai Y, Yao X, et al. Anti-rheumatoid arthritic effect of madecassoside on type II collagen-induced arthritis in mice. Int Immunopharmacol 2008;8:1561–6.
[710] Atal CK, Sharma ML, Kaul A, et al. Immunomodulating agents of plant origin. I: Preliminary screening. J Ethnopharmacol 1986;18:133–41.
[711] Maschi O. Inhibition of human cAMP-phosphodiesterase as a mechanism of the spasmolytic effect of *Matricaria recutita* L. J Agric Food Chem 2008;56:5015–20.

16 The dermatological system

Matthew J. Leach

SECTION A

OVERVIEW OF THE DERMATOLOGICAL SYSTEM

Anatomy

The integumentary system, which includes the skin, nails, hair, mucous membranes, and associated exocrine glands, is the largest system in the body in terms of surface area. The skin, in particular, is comprised of three main parts — the epidermis, the dermis and the subcutaneous layer (hypodermis) (Fig. 16.1). The most superficial layer, the epidermis, varies in thickness from 0.10 to 4.5 mm and consists of four to five organised layers of keratinocytes, or keratin-containing epithelial cells.[1] The epidermis also contains a number of specialised cells, including Langerhans cells (for immunity), Merkel cells (for the reception of touch) and melanocytes (for melanin production).

The second layer of the skin, the dermis, is composed of connective tissue and elastic fibres, and is subdivided into the papillary layer and reticular layer. The papillary layer contains sensory neurons, capillaries and lymphatic vessels that supply the epidermis, and also tactile corpuscles for the reception of light touch.[1] The deeper layer of the dermis, the reticular layer, contains many of the integumentary accessory structures, including the sebaceous (oil) glands, sudoriferous (sweat) glands, hair follicles, tactile corpuscles (for the reception of light touch) and lamellated corpuscles (for the reception of vibration and deep pressure).

The deepest layer of the skin, the subcutaneous layer, comprises connective tissue and adipose (fat) tissue. Large blood vessels are located in the superficial subcutaneous layer, and capillaries are located in the deeper portion.[2]

Physiology

While the skin and its associated structures are important for aesthetic purposes and for the creation of individual identity, other functions of the integumentary system are of far greater importance. These functions centre around four key roles — protection, sensation, homeostasis and nutrition. Details of these functions are outlined in Box 16.1.

Symptomatology

The skin and associated structures are continuously exposed to the external environment, and as a result are particularly prone to pathophysiological changes, including injury, infection and inflammation. These functional changes may manifest locally as erythema, heat, pain, pruritus, immobility, skin lesions, ulceration, pigment changes, bleeding and exudation which, if left untreated or poorly managed, may lead to scarring, contracture formation, disfigurement and/or amputation. Apart from these physical implications, these complications also impact negatively on an individual's self-image and psychological wellbeing.

ROLE OF THE NATUROPATH

The traditional naturopathic interpretation of chronic skin conditions is that they represent an inner disharmony whereby the body is unable to clear toxins. This explains why 'blood-cleansing' herbal medicines have traditionally been used in naturopathy to treat skin conditions. This theory of toxic accumulation has led many naturopaths to use potent and extreme detoxification herbs to manage skin complaints, often with strong reactions. External applications have similarly been applied, particularly for symptomatic relief of itchy, inflamed, and infected or bruised integumentary conditions, with much more soothing outcomes for patients. Traditionally, a patient with a skin condition was treated in a holistic manner, with assessment of their diet, digestion and lifestyle. This traditional treatment approach has continued to the modern day, although internal medicines have been used with a more gentle approach.

The modern naturopathic practitioner will almost certainly be exposed to a range of acute and chronic dermatological disorders in clinical practice. The role of the naturopath in the treatment of these conditions may vary from a primary care responsibility, to a complementary role, depending on patient preference, the nature and severity of the complaint, and the types of health practitioners involved. Regardless of the role the practitioner adopts, the principles of the discipline should always govern the naturopath's approach to treatment.

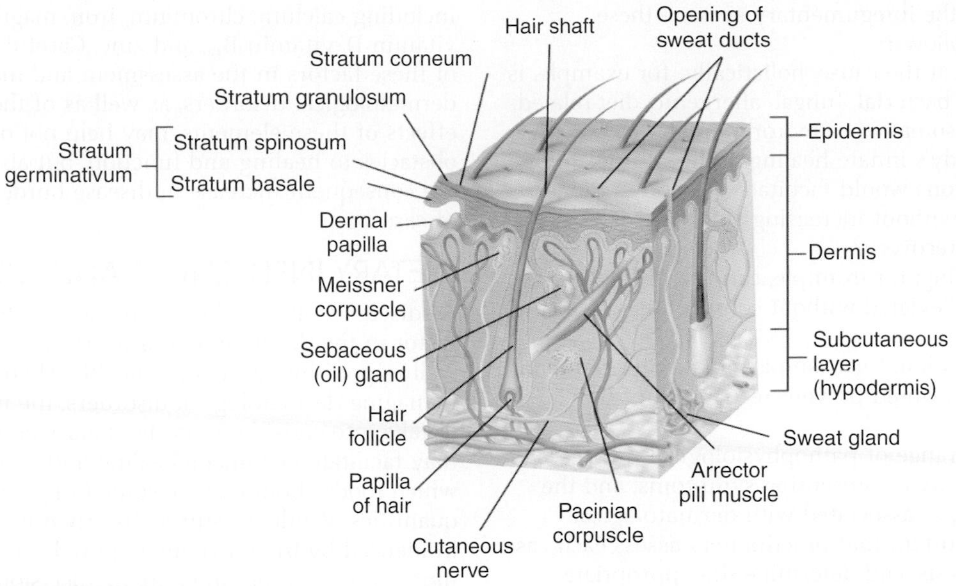

FIGURE 16.1 Anatomical structure of the skin.

Stanworth DR, Humphrey JH, Bennich H et al. Lancet 1967; ii, 330.

BOX 16.1 Functions of the integumentary system

Protection

PHYSICAL BARRIER

The tight network of keratinocytes within the epidermis acts as a physical barrier, which protects the body and underlying structures from toxins, pathogens, noxious agents, abrasive stress and fluid loss. Sensible perspiration further protects the body through an irrigation effect, which dilutes toxins and facilitates their removal. In contrast, cerumen (earwax) from the external auditory canal of the ear traps foreign material, thus preventing the material from damaging the tympanic membrane (eardrum). The secretion of melanin from epidermal melanocytes also protects cells and underlying tissues from the harmful effects of ultraviolet radiation.

CHEMICAL BARRIER

Various secretions from the exocrine glands of the integumentary system, including by-products of these secretions, lower the pH of the skin to protect it against microbial growth. The sebum from sebaceous glands and a peptide from sweat add to these antimicrobial effects.[2]

IMMUNITY

In addition to the nonspecific defences highlighted above, the skin also plays an important role in immune surveillance, with the assistance of Langerhans cells. These cells remove antigenic material located in the epidermis, and present the antigens to T-cells, which activate a cell-mediated immune response.[2] While Langerhans cells provide some protection to the body, they are susceptible to the damaging effects of ultraviolet light.[1]

Sensation

DETECTION OF STIMULI

The presence of nerve endings and sensory receptors throughout the epidermal and dermal layers of the skin permit the detection of both pleasant and noxious stimuli, including the reception of light touch (tactile corpuscles), normal touch (Merkel cells), vibration and deep pressure (lamellated corpuscles).[2]

Homeostasis

BODY TEMPERATURE

Insensible and sensible perspiration facilitate the loss of heat energy through convection and evaporation, which assists in the reduction of core body temperature. Conversely, the presence of adipose tissue in the subcutaneous layer and the process of piloerection (which contributes to goose bumps) insulate the skin from unnecessary heat loss. Together, these actions assist in maintaining the core temperature of the body.

EXCRETION

The sudoriferous glands eliminate water, electrolytes (including sodium, chloride and potassium), protein, fatty acids and some waste products (such as urea and ammonia) onto the surface of the epidermis.

Nutrition

SYNTHESIS OF VITAMIN D

Exposing the skin to ultraviolet radiation catalyses the conversion of 7-dehydrocholesterol (normally present in the epidermis) to the previtamin cholecalciferol (vitamin D_3).

STORAGE OF LIPIDS

The adipocytes in the dermis and subcutaneous layer of the skin store lipids, as well as lipid-soluble vitamins.

With reference to the integumentary system, these principles are as follows:

- Identify and treat the cause, holistically; for example, is the cause viral, bacterial, fungal, allergenic, diet-related, genetic, psychosomatic or environmental?
- Support the body's innate healing ability; for example, what interventions would facilitate the body's innate healing ability without increasing suffering or compromising recovery?
- Alleviate suffering; for example, can the presenting symptoms be alleviated without compromising healing or recovery?
- Focus on prevention; for example, what education and/or interventions would prevent recurrence of the disease?

Because of the range of pathophysiological processes involved, the diversity of presenting symptoms, and the number of aetiologies associated with dermatological disorders, it is important that practitioners assess each case on an individual basis, and determine the appropriate course of treatment accordingly.

The modern naturopath draws largely on the traditional interpretation of the underlying cause of skin disorders, blending this with their scientific understanding of elimination pathways, immunological disorders and inflammatory cascades. However, this concept of treating skin conditions both internally and externally continues to be used by the modern naturopath. Indeed, the concept of blood-cleansing herbs remains, with the terms 'depuratives' or 'alteratives' being used in its place.

Specific nutritional objectives

POTENTIAL DEFICIENCIES AND REQUIREMENTS

A fundamental role of the naturopath in managing integumentary system complaints is to explore whether nutritional deficiency is an aetiological factor in the disease and, if so, to determine what conditions may have contributed to the actual or perceived nutritional deficit. This is particularly important as nutritional deficiencies may contribute to, exacerbate or prolong a number of dermatological disorders. Before a practitioner can investigate the aetiology of the disorder, however, they must first be aware of the nutrients that are essential for integumentary health. The nutrients that are primarily responsible for maintaining skin and mucous membrane integrity and defence include arginine, ascorbic acid, copper, glycine, leucine, lysine, pantothenic acid, protein, silicon, vitamins A and E, and zinc. If a deficiency in one or more of these key nutrients is identified, the cause of the deficit needs to be explored. Factors that may reduce circulating levels of these nutrients include age, gender, diet, lifestyle, comorbidities and metabolic, enzymatic and absorption defects.

Another factor that may contribute to a nutritional deficiency, or compound an existing deficit, is pharmaceutical therapy. Drugs prescribed for the management of dermatological complaints may reduce serum or tissue levels of essential micronutrients, including calcium, chromium, iron, magnesium, vitamin D, vitamin B_{12}, and zinc. Careful consideration of these factors in the assessment and management of dermatological disorders, as well as of the composite effects of these elements, may help not only to minimise obstacles to healing and function, but also to reduce the consequent increase in disease burden and cost of care.

DIETARY INFLUENCES AND OBJECTIVES

As discussed above, dietary intake may be a contributing factor in the development of nutritional deficiencies, as well as poor integumentary health. Therefore, when managing dermatological disorders, the naturopath needs to take into consideration the dietary components that may facilitate or impede healing and, in effect, determine which foods should be consumed in greater or lesser quantities. While a naturopath's treatment decision will be influenced by the nutrients required for optimal skin and mucous membrane function, the decision will also be affected by patient preference and functional capacity, the aetiology of the condition, and the principles of the discipline. To determine an appropriate dietary plan, the clinician needs to consider the following treatment objectives:

- Identify and eliminate components of the diet that contribute to or exacerbate the dermatological disorder (i.e. food additives, allergens)
- Identify and maximise components of the diet that facilitate integumentary healing and function (i.e. bioflavonoids, antioxidants)
- Prioritise dietary choices according to patient preference, budget and functional capacity in order to maximise treatment compliance.

Specific herbal medicine classes

Herbal medicine plays a pivotal role in the naturopathic management of dermatological disorders. The modes of action that are particularly relevant to this system include those described below.

ADAPTOGENIC HERBAL MEDICINES

Adaptogenic herbal medicines assist in the ability to cope with stressors, either external or internal. As stress can play an important role in the recovery from many integumentary conditions, the adaptogenics are an important class of herbs to include in the treatment plan. Examples of adaptogenic herbs that may be used for this purpose are *Asparagus racemosus, Astragalus membranaceus, Centella asiatica, Eleutherococcus senticosus, Glycyrrhiza glabra, Panax ginseng, Rehmannia somnifera, Rhodiola rosea, Schisandra chinensis* and *Withania somnifera.*

ALTERATIVE (OR DEPURATIVE) HERBAL MEDICINES

Alterative (or depurative) herbs assist in the cleansing and detoxification processes of the body. These herbs have an extensive history of use for dermatological conditions;

however, they should be given in small incremental doses in order to prevent an exacerbation of the condition. Examples of such herbs include *Arctium lappa, Berberis aquifolium, Gallium aparine, Iris versicolor, Rumex crispus* and *Urtica dioica.*

ANTIALLERGIC HERBAL MEDICINES

Antiallergic herbal medicines modulate the release of chemical mediators from mast cells, such as histamine and leukotrienes, and can reduce distress, discomfort and scratch-induced skin trauma. Herbs that may be indicated in allergic skin disorders include *Albizia lebbeck, Perilla frutescens, Scutellaria baicalensis* and *Tanacetum parthenium.*

ANTI-INFLAMMATORY HERBAL MEDICINES

Anti-inflammatory herbal medicines modulate the destructive effects of chronic inflammation and can help relieve associated discomfort, as well as facilitate tissue repair. Examples of dermatological anti-inflammatory herbs include *Aloe barbadensis, Calendula officinalis, Glycyrrhiza glabra, Hydrastis canadensis, Matricaria recutita* and *Urtica dioica.*

ANTIBACTERIAL HERBAL MEDICINES

Antibacterial herbal medicines inhibit bacterial replication and prevent unwanted tissue destruction, inflammation and pain. Examples of antibacterial herbs include *Echinacea* spp., *Hydrastis canadensis, Scutellaria baicalensis, Tabebuia avellanedae* and *Thymus vulgaris.*

ANTIPRURITIC HERBAL MEDICINES

Antipruritic herbal medicines reduce pruritus and can lessen individual distress, as well as the likelihood of skin trauma and associated infection from scratching. *Smilax ornata, Mentha x piperita* and *Piper methysticum* are examples of antipruritic herbs used in cutaneous disorders.

ANTIFUNGAL HERBAL MEDICINES

Antifungal herbal medicines inhibit fungal growth and can prevent unnecessary tissue destruction, inflammation and pain. Herbs with reported antifungal activity include *Calendula officinalis, Tabebuia avellanedae* and *Thymus vulgaris.*

ANTIVIRAL HERBAL MEDICINES

Antiviral herbal medicines inhibit viral replication and can prevent needless tissue destruction, inflammation and pain. Herbs with reported antiviral activity include *Hypericum perforatum, Melissa officinalis* and *Thuja occidentalis.*

ASTRINGENT HERBAL MEDICINES

Astringent herbs assist with the contraction of mucous membranes (when applied topically), and are particularly useful in facilitating the wound-healing process. Examples of such herbs are *Calendula officinalis, Commiphora mol mol, Euphrasia officinalis, Glechoma hederacea, Hamamelis virginiana* and *Myrica cerifera.*

CIRCULATORY STIMULANT HERBAL MEDICINES

Circulatory stimulant plant extracts both stimulate and improve peripheral circulation, thereby enhancing the integumentary health of these areas. Examples of herbs used for this purpose are *Capsicum* spp., *Ginkgo biloba, Zanthoxylum clava-herculis* and *Zingiber officinale.*

DEMULCENT OR MUCILAGINOUS HERBAL MEDICINES

Demulcent or mucilaginous herbal medicines soothe irritated or inflamed tissues; this not only reduces individual distress and discomfort, but also protects the skin from the external environment. Herbs with demulcent activity include *Althaea officinalis, Glycyrrhiza glabra, Plantago lanceolata, Stellaria media* and *Verbascum thapsus.*

IMMUNOMODULATING HERBAL MEDICINES

Immunomodulating herbal medicines, which promote nonspecific and specific resistance, can reduce the risk and/or severity of local and systemic infection, as well as the sequelae of pain, malaise and tissue destruction. Examples of immunostimulant plant extracts include *Andrographis paniculata, Astragalus membranaceus, Echinacea* spp., *Eleutherococcus senticosus, Panax ginseng* and *Withania somnifera.*

LYMPHATIC HERBAL MEDICINES

Lymphatic herbal medicines improve the flow of lymphatic fluid or increase lymphatic drainage, allowing for a greater flow of nutrients to, and elimination from, the integumentary tissues. Examples of these herbs include *Baptisia tinctoria, Calendula officinalis, Echinacea* spp., *Galium aparine, Iris versicolor* and *Phytolacca decandra.*

VULNERARY HERBAL MEDICINES

Vulnerary herbal medicines facilitate wound healing, and help to reduce pain, disability and risk of infection. Herbs with vulnerary activity include *Aloe barbadensis, Calendula officinalis, Centella asiatica, Hypericum perforatum* and *Matricaria recutita.*

Allopathic treatment

An allopathic approach to disorders of the integumentary system is typically determined following the acquisition of a detailed history and physical examination, which may or may not include the use of appropriate diagnostic tests and procedures. The treatment plan often focuses on the relief of symptoms, and the elimination of the perceived cause of the condition, such as an infectious agent, allergen or undesirable immune–inflammatory activity. Examples of medications typically prescribed for common dermatological disorders are listed in the interactions tables at the back of the book, together with possible interaction effects between these drugs and naturopath-prescribed herbs and nutrients.

ANTIBIOTICS

Oral and/or topical antibiotics are often prescribed for bacterial skin infections, such as impetigo, wound infection, cellulitis, erysipelas, skin abscess and folliculitis. These agents may inhibit bacterial replication (i.e. bacteriostatic effects) or destroy bacteria (i.e. bactericidal effects) depending on the mode of action; such actions may include impairment of bacterial cell membrane permeability, inhibition of protein synthesis, or destruction of bacterial DNA. Examples of antibiotics prescribed for bacterial skin infection include cefalexin, erythromycin, fusidic acid, metronidazole and mupirocin.

ANTIFUNGALS

Oral and/or topical antifungal agents are often indicated for fungal skin infections, including tinea, onychomycosis and candidiasis. These agents act by interfering with fungal cell-wall permeability, which leads to growth inhibition or cell death.[3] Clotrimazole, ketoconazole, miconazole and tolnaftate are examples of agents prescribed for fungal skin infections.

ANTIHISTAMINES

Antihistamines may be prescribed for the treatment of generalised pruritus and urticaria. These agents act by blocking histamine (H_1) receptors, thus preventing histamine-induced effects, such as pruritus and urticaria.[3] Antihistamines administered for cutaneous disorders may include fexofenadine, loratadine, pheniramine, promethazine and trimeprazine.

ANTIVIRALS

Oral and/or topical antiviral agents are often indicated when a viral infection is present, such as herpes simplex virus or herpes zoster virus. These agents inhibit viral synthesis by inhibiting viral DNA polymerase,[3] which is required for viral replication. Antiviral agents that may be prescribed for herpes infection include aciclovir, famciclovir and valaciclovir.

CORTICOSTEROIDS

Oral and/or topical corticosteroids are generally indicated for inflammatory and pruritic skin disorders, such as eczema, dermatitis and psoriasis. These agents act similarly to endogenous glucocorticoids, in that they stabilise leucocyte lysosomal membranes, inhibit histamine activity, reduce capillary wall permeability and oedema formation, and inhibit macrophage accumulation.[3] Betamethasone, hydrocortisone, prednisolone and triamcinolone are examples of corticosteroid medications that may be administered for skin inflammation and pruritus.

IMMUNOMODULATORS

Immunomodulators may be prescribed in severe inflammatory or autoimmune skin disorders, such as psoriasis and dermatitis. Immunomodulators act by interfering with various immune response pathways, therefore attenuating the cascade of events leading to skin irritation and inflammation.[3] These agents include cyclosporine A, tacrolimus and pimecrolimus.

RETINOIDS

Retinoids are generally indicated for disorders of keratinisation, such as psoriasis and acne. The actual mode of action of these agents is not clear, but it is suggested that retinoids reduce sebum production and inflammation, and modulate cell differentiation and proliferation.[3] Acitretin, isotretinoin, tazarotene and tretinoin are examples of retinoid agents prescribed for acne and psoriasis.

SECTION B

DERMATITIS/ECZEMA

Epidemiology

Atopic dermatitis affects 12% of children and 3% of adults.[4] In contrast, contact dermatitis affects 1–10% of the population, and can develop at any age.[5] While infective dermatitis may also occur at any age, nummular and stasis dermatitis are most likely to occur in middle-aged patients and elderly women, respectively.[6]

Classification

Dermatitis is defined as a superficial inflammation of the skin. The terms 'dermatitis' and 'eczema' are synonymous, and will therefore be used interchangeably throughout this chapter. The severity of the condition can be defined as acute, subacute or chronic, while the origin of dermatitis can be classified as exogenous or endogenous. Endogenous forms include atopic, seborrhoeic, nummular and stasis dermatitis, and exogenous forms include contact and infective dermatitis.

Aetiology

There are myriad factors that may contribute to the pathogenesis of eczema, and not surprisingly, there are numerous classifications of the condition. The range of exogenous factors includes, but is not limited to, topical drugs, plants, cosmetics, metal compounds, dyes, detergents, chemicals, latex, wool, synthetic fibres, mineral oils, urine, saliva, and bacterial or fungal pathogens.[6] Exposure to these agents can produce physiological effects ranging from skin damage and irritation (e.g. irritant contact dermatitis), to hypersensitivity reactions (e.g. allergic contact dermatitis), depending on individual susceptibility, the concentration of the agent and the duration of exposure.[5,7]

A number of endogenous factors also play a role in the development of eczema. These include immunological abnormalities (e.g. family history of atopic disease), environmental elements (e.g. food allergies) and emotional influences (e.g. stress).[7] Patients with endogenous eczema may also demonstrate reduced ceramide content of the stratum corneum, immunoglobulin E (IgE) dysregulation, reduced production of antimicrobial peptides from

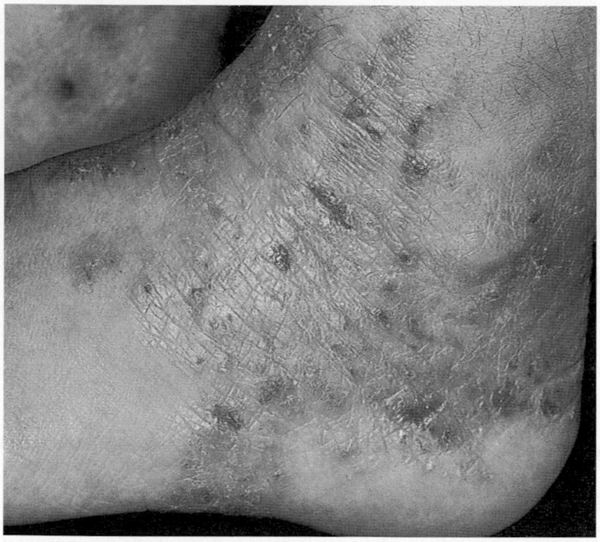

FIGURE 16.2 Atopic dermatitis.

keratinocytes, impaired cellular immunity, and decreased ß-adrenergic and increased α- adrenergic/cholinergic reactivity.[4] In contact dermatitis, a range of environmental factors may further increase an individual's susceptibility to the condition, including excessive exposure to water, excessive heat, sweating, low humidity, and mechanical stress, such as repeated handwashing.[5]

Signs and symptoms

The clinical manifestations of dermatitis, such as erythema, heat and pruritus, are largely attributed to the underlying inflammatory process of the disease. While these symptoms are common across all subtypes of dermatitis, there are some distinct differences. Acute dermatitis, for example, is associated with oedema, vesicle formation, exudation, pain and impaired function. Subacute dermatitis, on the other hand, manifests as erosions, crusting, scaling and exfoliation, whereas chronic dermatitis appears as dryness, scaling, thickening and hardening of the skin[8] (Fig. 16.2). Regardless of the subtype, the presence of these symptoms will almost certainly contribute to irritability, sleep disturbance, negative self-esteem and self-image, and a subsequent decline in health-related quality of life.[9]

Complications

The possible clinical complications of this condition can be physical, psychological or behavioural. Physical complications such as infection (bacterial, fungal and viral infections are common) can be severe if left untreated. Allergy to prescribed medications (both oral and topical) can occur, as individuals with such conditions tend to have strong allergic tendencies, and therefore caution should be exercised when prescribing. The psychological and behavioural effects of dermatitis can be due to the location of lesions (i.e. highly visibility to others), sleep deprivation caused by overnight scratching, lack of concentration (due to itching) and reduced self-esteem.

Differential diagnosis

The diagnosis of dermatitis and its specific subgroup (e.g. contact dermatitis) is important, as it can give added information about the cause of the condition. Dermatitis should be differentiated from other skin conditions (e.g. psoriasis, lichen simplex chronicus), immunological conditions (e.g. dermatitis herpetiformis, dermatomyositis), infectious conditions (e.g. *Candida*, dermatophytes, herpes simplex), malignant skin lesions and a number of metabolic diseases (e.g. phenylketonuria, tyrosinaemia, histidinaemia, zinc deficiency, pyridoxine and niacin deficiency).

Naturopathic diagnosis

NAIL ANALYSIS

The general quality of the fingernails should be assessed and any suspicions of protein deficiency or inadequate intake of vitamins and minerals should be addressed in a nutritional analysis. Pitting (i.e. appearance of small pin pricks in the nail) and flaking of the nails are common in patients with psoriasis, and this should be kept in mind as a differential diagnosis. The lanula of the nail, which should be visible, can provide information on hydrochloric acid levels and metabolic activity. White spots or markings are common in patients with dermatitis and can denote zinc deficiency.

INSPECTION AND PALPATION OF THE SKIN

Inspection of the skin should be conducted under natural light, with close attention paid to the following aspects:

- Colour — general pigmentation, widespread colour change, pallor, erythema, cyanosis and jaundice
- Temperature — note particularly heated, inflamed red areas, as these have the possibility of being infected
- Moisture — dermatitis-affected areas are likely to be very dry, but it is important to take note of the patient's unaffected skin in order to make comparisons, and to look for indications of essential fatty acid deficiencies. Also look for any areas of pus or infection
- Texture
- Thickness
- Oedema.

The more detail that is reported in the patient's case notes during the physical examination, the greater is the possibility for both the practitioner and the patient to note any positive or negative effects of treatment over time. Photographs of lesions can be a reliable method for monitoring clinical progress but it is important that the patient provides express permission for the taking of such photographs.

Investigations

There are no specific laboratory investigations for endogenous forms of dermatitis as the diagnosis of these conditions is generally based on the patient's clinical presentation and family history.[6] In exogenous forms of eczema, however, the suspected antigen may be identified using allergy skin testing. In this investigation, the skin of the patient is exposed to a number of suspected allergens, which can be administered topically as a patch test, injected intraepidermally as a prick-puncture test, or introduced intradermally. While these tests can rapidly detect the presence of immunoglobulin E (IgE) mediated allergies, they are not capable of detecting non-IgE-mediated allergies, and may yield false-positive results in some individuals.[10]

In very young patients or those with widespread dermatitis, radioallergosorbent testing (RAST) and enzyme-linked immunosorbent assay (ELISA) are appropriate alternatives to allergy skin testing.[11] Both these procedures quantify the presence of IgE in patient serum but, unlike skin testing, can only detect a limited number of IgE-mediated allergies. Thus, in some cases, the results of RAST and ELISA may be misleading.

The eosinophil count is another test for detecting allergic disease. These white blood cells play a key role in the phagocytosis of antigen–antibody complexes, and proliferate in the presence of allergies. However, the eosinophil count can also rise in the presence of parasitic infection, myeloproliferative disorders, rheumatoid arthritis and Hodgkin's disease[11] — because of this, the eosinophil count cannot conclusively confirm or refute allergy as a cause of eczema.

SPECIFIC NATUROPATHIC INVESTIGATIONS

An investigation used in the detection of delayed food sensitivity reactions is immunoglobulin G4 (IgG4) food antibody testing. While this test reveals whether an immunological response to a food component has occurred, it is not indicative of food allergy or intolerance,[12] and therefore may not be an appropriate measure of these conditions.

Functional profiles, including intestinal permeability assessment or comprehensive digestive stool analysis, may also be used to support or dismiss suspicions of leaky gut syndrome or intestinal dysbiosis as potential causes of eczema.

Therapeutic considerations

Even though dermatitis appears to be a relatively benign disorder, the condition can be a manifestation of several severe disease states. Therefore, to minimise patient harm, and to ensure the patient receives the most appropriate treatment, the practitioner should consider the following differential diagnoses when performing a clinical assessment of dermatitis: scabies, mycosis (fungal infection), pellagra, cutaneous T-cell lymphoma, Wiskott–Aldrich syndrome, erysipelas and acrodermatosis enteropathica. In the event that a serious disease state may be associated with the condition, the practitioner should refer the patient to their general practitioner for further review.

CLINICAL DECISION MAKING AND RATIONALE

Naturopathic treatment of dermatitis centres on finding and treating the cause of the condition. As dermatitis is primarily an idiopathic response to a stressor, the cause can be difficult to identify quickly. Hence the role of the naturopath is to continuously assess and reassess the treatment protocol, often beginning with a broad approach to treatment and, over time, narrowing down to more specific objectives. Severe cases of dermatitis may require the naturopath to work closely with the patient's general practitioner and/or specialist, and for the patient to be treated with the use of both naturopathic and allopathic medicines. The naturopathic practitioner should discuss the signs and symptoms of infection with the patient (or the patient's primary care giver) to ensure that any infection is treated promptly.

Therapeutic application

NATUROPATHIC PERSPECTIVE

There are a number of modifiable risk factors associated with the pathogenesis of dermatitis. As such, it is critical that practitioners focus their attention on the first naturopathic principle highlighted in Section A of this chapter (i.e. identify and treat the cause). A comprehensive assessment of the patient's medical, family, environmental and clinical history, in conjunction with an elimination diet and/or food and lifestyle diary, will assist the practitioner in correctly identifying the triggers of dermatitis, and therefore help to minimise disease recurrence, as well as unnecessary physical and emotional distress to the patient. As these dietary and lifestyle changes can cause significant stress to both the patient and their primary care giver/family, it is important to assist the patient by providing detailed examples of food substitutes and suppliers. If allergies to dust and animal dander are present, detailed information on ways to reduce exposure to these allergens is essential to ensure long-term treatment objectives are met. Attending to the first naturopathic principle, followed by the selection of appropriate interventions to support the body's innate healing ability will, in effect, address both the third (alleviate suffering) and fourth (prevention) principles of care.

As the identification of triggers can be a lengthy process, the use of short-term measures to reduce inflammation, itching and dryness can help foster patient compliance with dietary and lifestyle changes. This can also reduce associated psychological and behavioural effects of the condition. Supportive strategies include topical applications such as creams, compresses and ointments.

Due to the nature of dermatitis (especially when chronic), the naturopathic therapeutic approach can take time. This aspect should be discussed openly with the patient to ensure that they have realistic expectations of improvement. A combination of physical and emotional support is vital in the naturopathic approach to treatment. The extent of the emotional impact of this condition should not be underestimated. If the naturopathic practitioner is not comfortable counselling the patient, referral to another healthcare practitioner may be required.

NUTRITIONAL MEDICINE (DIETARY)

Therapeutic objectives

The dietary approach to dermatitis should focus on two key goals: to exclude factors known to trigger or exacerbate the condition; and to maximise intake of nutrients with anti-inflammatory, antiallergic and vulnerary effects. To achieve these goals, appropriate objectives for the dietary management of dermatitis should be followed. Drawing from the nutritional goals highlighted in Section A of this chapter, these objectives include:

1. Identify and eliminate foods that may contribute to or exacerbate eczema
2. Increase consumption of seafood to increase omega-3 fatty acid, selenium, vitamin D and zinc intake
3. Increase consumption of fruits and vegetables to augment ascorbic acid, bioflavonoid, iron, vitamin A and vitamin E intake
4. Increase consumption of low-allergenic nuts and seeds to improve iron, niacin, selenium, vitamin E, omega-3 fatty acid and zinc intake
5. Increase lean meat consumption to elevate iron, niacin, selenium, vitamin E and zinc intake.

Specific treatments

To address objective one, the practitioner will need to commence an elimination or oligoantigenic diet. This diet will assist the clinician in establishing whether any dietary components are responsible for the pathogenesis of the dermatitis. While there are many variations to the elimination diet in terms of complexity, content and duration, the diet should always aim to minimise patient uncertainty in order to maximise compliance. A simple approach to the elimination diet is to have a patient avoid all potentially allergenic foods for a minimum of one week, including cow's milk products, eggs, wheat, rye, barley, peanuts, corn, shellfish, bananas, apples, oranges, potatoes, parsley, carrots and soya beans, and any foods containing artificial colours, flavours or preservatives. After this 1-week elimination period, the patient can reintroduce a new food every 2 days and monitor the recurrence of dermatitis-related signs and symptoms. The presence or absence of any adverse reactions during these oral food challenges should be recorded in a food and lifestyle diary, and reviewed at the next naturopathic consultation. The foods identified as being associated with dermatitis should then be eliminated from the diet. For a more in-depth discussion of the elimination diet, see Chapter 10.

The effectiveness of elimination diets in the treatment of eczema has been investigated in a number of prospective studies and systematic reviews.[13–15] The majority of these studies have shown that the elimination of specific food allergens from the diet effectively reduces the severity of eczema when the food allergy has been confirmed. There is little evidence, however, to support the use of elemental or general elimination diets, possibly because the presence of food allergy had not been established in these studies.

An example of a daily diet that complies with the dietary treatment objectives for individuals with dermatitis or eczema is given below.

NUTRITIONAL MEDICINE (SUPPLEMENTAL)

Therapeutic objectives

In the event that an individual is unable to comply with dietary recommendations, where nutritional deficiency is unlikely to be adequately addressed by diet alone, or where higher than normal doses of nutrients are required, a practitioner may consider nutritional supplementation. When nutritional supplementation is warranted, the following objectives for treating dermatitis or eczema need to be considered:

1. Reduce tissue levels of arachidonic acid and proinflammatory cytokines by increasing serum and tissue levels of ascorbic acid, bioflavonoids, omega-3 fatty acids, selenium, vitamin D and vitamin E
2. Improve skin integrity and/or facilitate wound healing by increasing serum and tissue levels of ascorbic acid, bioflavonoids, iron, omega-3 fatty acids, vitamin A, vitamin E and zinc
3. Support local and systemic immunity by increasing serum and tissue levels of ascorbic acid, iron, selenium, vitamin A, vitamin D, vitamin E and zinc
4. Resolve intestinal dysbiosis by improving the numbers of beneficial intestinal flora.

Specific nutrients required

VITAMIN A

Vitamin A is necessary for epithelial cell differentiation, collagen synthesis, phagocytosis, antibody production and intercellular adhesion.[16] A Cochrane review of one placebo-controlled trial on vitamin A and dermatitis concluded there was insufficient evidence to support or refute the use of topical vitamin A preparations in napkin dermatitis.[17] The number of case reports associating topical vitamin A preparations with contact dermatitis should also highlight to practitioners the need for caution when using topically administered vitamin A.

VITAMIN C

Vitamin C has long been promoted as an anti-inflammatory agent. The findings of an open-label, randomised controlled trial of 64 obese adults lend support to this claim, which showed statistically significant reductions in C-reactive protein (CRP) and interleukin 6 (both markers of acute inflammation) in participants receiving vitamin C supplementation (500 mg b.i.d. for 8 weeks) versus those receiving placebo.[18] The effect of ascorbic acid on atopic dermatitis is also unclear. While several recent studies have reported an inverse relationship between plasma vitamin C levels and either the presence of eczema[19] or the severity of atopic dermatitis in adolescents/adults,[20] other studies have indicated a positive association between perinatal vitamin C intake and risk of atopic eczema in infants at 2 years of age.[20,21] These conflicting findings indicate that the effectiveness of

SAMPLE DAILY DIET

BREAKFAST	
Pancakes/pikelets (gluten-free [GF], egg free) made from a buckwheat base, serve with fresh fruit and a carrot, celery and ginger juice (or use NUDIE brand from the supermarket if you don't have a juicer)	Gluten and egg are both common food triggers for worsening eczema/dermatitis thus should be avoided. Flours containing gluten can be replaced with quinoa and/or buckwheat while eggs can be replaced with egg replacers such as flaxseed or chia seed. Pikelets can be made ahead of time, frozen and then popped in the toaster to reheat. Serve with antioxidant- and anti-inflammatory-rich fruit and maple syrup or honey to sweeten. A vegetable juice provides a concentrated source of nutrients in an easy-to-assimilate form that aids detoxification. Carrots are a source of carotenoids. In mice studies, consumption of beta-carotene was shown to protect against atopic dermatitis. The addition of celery acts as a diuretic to help remove accumulation of wastes, while ginger functions as a gentle anti-inflammatory.
LUNCH	
GF wrap containing avocado, shredded slow-cooked lamb and grated carrot. Serve with roasted pumpkin and sweet potato Punnet of blueberries	The composition of intestinal bacteria impacts food sensitisation in the gastrointestinal tract as well as pathogenesis of eczema. Avocado and sweet potato are both excellent sources of prebiotics. Consumption of prebiotics may reduce severity of atopic dermatitis. This is due to their ability to provide fuel for intestinal microflora thereby improving the intestinal environment. Adequate fibre is essential and provided through the vegetables and fruit. Fibre promotes bowel frequency, important since retention of faecal matter may result in reabsorption of toxins that may then be released through the skin.
DINNER	
Salmon patties with GF pasta (vegetable-based sauce made with cooked tomatoes, mushrooms and grated zucchini and carrots)	Omega-3 fatty acids found in oily fish such as salmon displace arachidonic acid, reducing inflammatory mediators seen in atopic dermatitis. Consumption of fish during the first year of life has been found to reduce the risk of eczema in children. A tomato-based sauce (with additional carrots) provides beta-carotene, a precursor to vitamin A. Many drugs that reduce eczema severity are based on vitamin A analogues.
SNACKS	
Fresh fruit Rice crackers (unflavoured)	Fresh fruit (provided there is no intolerance) may be used to boost the immune system. Rice crackers are considered to be low-allergen and suitable for most children with atopic dermatitis.

Hiragun M, Hiragun T, Oseto I et al. Oral administration of β-carotene or lycopene prevents atopic dermatitis-like dermatitis in HR-1 mice. J Dermatol 2016 Oct; 43(10):1188–1192; Osborn DA, Sinn JKH. Prebiotics in infants for prevention of allergy. Cochrane Database Syst Rev 2013; 2:CD006474; Shibata R, Kimura M, Takahashi H et al. Clinical effects of ketose, a prebiotic oligosaccharide, on the treatment of atopic dermatitis in infants. Clin Exp Allergy 2009; 39(9):1397–1403; Zhang GQ, Liu B, Li J et al. Fish intake during pregnancy or infancy and allergic outcomes in children: a systematic review and meta-analysis. Pediatr Allergy Immunol 2016 Sep 3.

ascorbic acid supplementation in atopic disease requires further investigation.

VITAMIN D

Vitamin D may modulate the pathogenesis of atopic dermatitis via anti-inflammatory (i.e. decreasing IL-2 and IL-4 production) and immunomodulatory (i.e. increasing epidermal antimicrobial peptides, inhibiting Th1 cell proliferation, reducing interferon-γ secretion) effects, and by improving stratum corneum barrier formation (i.e. increasing. synthesis).[22] The findings of a meta-analysis of four high-quality RCTs lend support to this argument, finding vitamin D supplementation (i.e. oral cholecalciferol or sun exposure) to be significantly more effective than controls in reducing the severity of atopic dermatitis symptoms in children and adults.

VITAMIN E

The anti-inflammatory effect of vitamin E has been demonstrated in a number of studies; this activity may be attributed to the inhibition of cytokine-triggered activation of NF-κB.[23] There is emerging clinical evidence to suggest that this activity may translate into clinical improvements in patients with dermatitis. In a double-blind, randomised placebo-controlled trial involving 70 participants with mild to moderate atopic dermatitis, significantly greater improvements in the subjective symptoms and severity of atopic dermatitis were observed in patients receiving vitamin E supplementation (400 IU/day for 4 months) when compared to patients receiving placebo.[24]

IRON

Iron deficiency can occur during periods of inflammation, a condition known as 'anaemia of inflammation'. This reduction in iron levels may also mimic chronic inflammation.[25] This suggests that iron may play an important role in inflammatory dermatoses. Indeed, a cohort study of 157 mother–child pairs revealed a marginally significant increase in the risk of doctor-diagnosed eczema among children whose mothers had low maternal iron status at delivery.[26] While iron deficiency or anaemia should always be corrected, more research is required to investigate the therapeutic effects of iron for the patient with dermatitis.

SELENIUM

Selenium inhibits nuclear factor-κB activation in vitro,[27] suggesting a possible anti-inflammatory effect for the mineral. A cohort study of 834 mother–infant pairs also revealed an inverse association between hair-mineral selenium levels in infants and mothers, and risk of atopic dermatitis in infants.[28] While these findings suggest a possible role for selenium in the management of dermatitis, a double-blind RCT of 60 adults with atopic eczema found 600 micrograms/day selenium for 12 weeks did not have a significant effect on the severity of eczema when compared with placebo.[29]

ZINC

Children with atopic dermatitis demonstrate significantly lower hair zinc levels when compared with healthy controls.[30] The findings of a comparative study of 101 children (aged 2–14 years) indicate that zinc supplementation may improve hair zinc levels as well as eczema severity and pruritus.[30] However, the results of a double-blind, placebo-controlled trial of 50 children aged 1–16 years showed that oral zinc sulfate (185.4 mg/day for 8 weeks) was no more effective than placebo at reducing the severity of atopic eczema.[31] These conflicting findings indicate that more research is required to determine the effectiveness of zinc for dermatitis.

ESSENTIAL FATTY ACIDS

Omega-3 fatty acids have been shown to reduce inflammatory markers in epidemiological, observational and clinical study populations.[32] A Cochrane systematic review of three RCTs (involving patients with atopic dermatitis) indicates fish oil may be more effective than placebo in improving participant-rated symptom scores and the total area affected, but no more effective than placebo in reducing the need for prescribed medication for symptomatic relief. Changes in physician-rated symptom scores were inconclusive due to inconsistencies across the studies.[33]

PROBIOTICS

Lactobacilli spp. exhibit both local and systemic anti-inflammatory and immunomodulatory effects. A meta-analysis of 25 RCTs found probiotic supplementation to be significantly more effective than controls in reducing the severity of atopic dermatitis in both children and adults; the effectiveness of probiotics in infants with atopic dermatitis was inconclusive.[34]

QUERCETIN

Quercetin demonstrates anti-inflammatory activity in vitro. In particular, it inhibits nitric oxide production and nuclear factor-κB activation.[35] The bioflavonoid also inhibits the proinflammatory cytokines IL-1β, IL-6 and TNF-α, as well as increasing IL-10 in vivo.[36] While data from pilot studies suggest quercetin supplementation may reduce nickel patch-induced contact dermatitis and ultraviolet (UV) B-induced skin erythema,[37] evidence from well-designed clinical studies is lacking.

Dosage requirements

The dosage requirements listed below are based on adult doses used in clinical trials. Where clinical data are absent or insufficient, the doses are based on those reported in the literature.[38–40]

- Ascorbic acid 250 mg b.i.d.
- Iron 15 mg/day (if indicated on pathology investigations)
- *Lactobacilli rhamnosus* probiotic 1×10^9 colony forming units (cfu)/g b.i.d.
- Quercetin 500 mg b.i.d.
- Selenium 200 micrograms/day
- Vitamin A 5000 IU/day
- Vitamin D 400–1000 IU/day
- Vitamin E 400–800 IU/day
- Zinc 25–60 mg/day.

HERBAL MEDICINE

Therapeutic objectives

The integration of herbal medicine within a naturopathic treatment plan allows a practitioner to deliver a more targeted approach to eczema. Furthermore, when herbal medicine is integrated appropriately (i.e. without compromising the principles of naturopathic care), the treatment approach will be delivered more holistically. In order for practitioners to safely and effectively manage dermatitis using herbal medicine, the following treatment objectives should be considered:

1. Identify and treat the cause of dermatitis to prevent exacerbation and recurrence
2. Manage inflammation to minimise unnecessary discomfort and tissue destruction
3. Reduce mast cell activity to decrease pruritus and associated scratch-induced skin trauma
4. Facilitate wound healing to reduce pain, disability and risk of infection
5. Enhance specific and nonspecific immunity to prevent wound infection
6. Manage associated symptoms of dermatitis to reduce discomfort and improve wellbeing.

Herbal medicine classes

The herbal medicine classes that are indicated for the management of eczema are antiallergic, anti-inflammatory, antipruritic, demulcent and vulnerary.

Specific herbal medicines

There are many herbs that demonstrate at least one of the aforementioned actions. However, it would not be useful for a busy practitioner if all these herbs were listed. Instead, only those herbs that have been investigated clinically, or that exhibit several of the activities mentioned above, are listed here.

ALBIZIA LEBBECK (ALBIZIA)

Albizia lebbeck has been used traditionally as an antiallergic, antimicrobial and anti-inflammatory, although there is currently a lack of clinical studies investigating the role of *Albizia* in eczema.

ALOE BARBADENSIS (ALOE)

Aloe barbadensis exhibits vulnerary, anti-inflammatory, immunostimulant and antibacterial effects, suggesting a possible role in inflammatory dermatoses. Emerging clinical evidence indicates that *Aloe* may be beneficial to patients with dermatitis. In one RCT of 66 infants, *Aloe* cream (administered 3 times a day for 10 days) was found to be as effective as calendula cream in reducing the severity of nappy dermatitis, but less effective than calendula in reducing the number of rash sites.[41] Notwithstanding, the effectiveness of *Aloe* versus placebo for the treatment of dermatitis warrants further exploration.

ARCTIUM LAPPA (BURDOCK)

Arctium lappa has been prescribed traditionally as a depurative for various chronic skin disorders. While experimental data indicate that burdock also exhibits anti-inflammatory, antimicrobial and antioxidant effects in vivo,[42] clinical studies are required to confirm the use of this herb for dermatitis.

AZADIRACHTA INDICA (NEEM)

Azadirachta indica has demonstrated significant anti-inflammatory activity in rats, immunomodulatory activity in mice, and a wide spectrum of antimicrobial effects in vitro.[43,44] While these experimental findings support the traditional actions of neem leaf, the clinical efficacy of *Azadirachta* in dermatitis remains unclear. Please note that neem is restricted in Australia for internal usage — guidelines specify that usage is restricted to form (only neem seed oil in concentrations ≤1%) and application (topical application only).

MATRICARIA RECUTITA (CHAMOMILE)

Matricaria recutita demonstrates anti-inflammatory, immunostimulant, antibacterial and mild sedative properties. The efficacy of topically applied Kamillosan, a chamomile ointment, has been examined in a number of comparative trials, and found to be more effective than 0.5% hydrocortisone cream and placebo in patients with atopic dermatitis after 2 weeks;[45] as effective as 0.25% hydrocortisone and superior to 0.75% fluocortin butyl ester and 5% bufexamac in patients suffering from eczema of the hands, forearms and lower legs after 3–4 weeks;[46] and superior to 0.1% hydrocortisone acetate and Kamillosan ointment base in patients with experimentally induced toxic contact dermatitis.[47] However, these results should be interpreted with caution given the methodological limitations of these trials.

CENTELLA ASIATICA (GOTU KOLA)

Centella asiatica has traditionally been used for its vulnerary and anti-inflammatory activity. A constituent of gotu kola, madecassol, has been shown to decrease the severity of acute radiation dermatitis in rats when compared with controls, possibly via an anti-inflammatory effect.[48] An open trial of 20 patients found that the topical application of a *C. asiatica* extract and essential oil formulation for 6 weeks prevented wound infection (a complication of dermatitis) in 75% of contaminated wounds, while healing 64% of all acute and chronic wounds.[49] Even so, the methodological limitations of this study and the paucity of clinical data on the efficacy of gotu kola in persons with dermatitis indicate that further research is needed.

ECHINACEA SPP. (ECHINACEA)

Echinacea spp. exhibits anti-inflammatory, immunostimulant and antibacterial effects. While data from animal studies indicate that topical applications of *Echinacea purpurea* may facilitate skin healing, there is insufficient evidence to support or refute the effectiveness of *Echinacea* in dermatitis.

GLYCYRRHIZA GLABRA (LIQUORICE)

Glycyrrhiza glabra has traditionally been administered for its anti-inflammatory and demulcent activity. A double-blind RCT of 60 patients with atopic dermatitis found the topical application of 2% liquorice gel was more effective than 1% liquorice gel in reducing erythema, oedema and pruritus scores over 2 weeks ($p < 0.05$).[50] Whether the oral administration of liquorice offers any long-term clinical benefit to patients with eczema, however, requires further investigation.

HYPERICUM PERFORATUM (ST JOHN'S WORT)

Hypericum perforatum demonstrates vulnerary, anti-inflammatory and analgesic properties. In a double-blind RCT of 21 patients suffering from mild to moderate atopic dermatitis, *Hypericum* cream applied twice daily for 4 weeks significantly reduced the intensity of eczematous lesions ($p < 0.05$), as well as skin colonisation with *Staphylococcus aureus* ($p = 0.06$), when compared with placebo.[51] It is not clear, however, whether these effects can be replicated with orally administered St John's wort.

Topical application

A suitable herbal formula for the management of dermatitis is listed below. These extracts should be reduced by half over low heat, and poured while hot into 100 g organic cream base. The cream should be applied to lesions twice daily.

Herbal medicine	Quantity	
Matricaria recutita	1:2 liquid extract	20 mL
Glycyrrhiza glabra	1:1 liquid extract	15 mL

LIFESTYLE RECOMMENDATIONS

Myriad modifiable exogenous and endogenous factors can be associated with the pathogenesis of dermatitis. As such, lifestyle modification may greatly reduce the incidence and severity of the condition. The avoidance of topical applications such as cosmetics, moisturisers, medications, perfumes, plant extracts and mineral oils, for instance, may eliminate some of the more common exogenous triggers of eczema. With regard to clothing, cotton textiles should replace wool and synthetic fibres, non-colour-fast dyes should be avoided, and an additional rinse cycle during washing should be employed to minimise exposure to laundry detergents. Exposure to latex, cleaning agents, aerosols and other household chemicals should also be avoided.

Reduction of stress

Perceived stress is associated with a significantly greater risk of atopic dermatitis, as demonstrated in a survey of 33,018 Korean adults.[52] Thus, effective stress-management strategies may be essential in the treatment of eczema by helping individuals cope with major life events.

One potentially useful treatment option may be massage. To illustrate, in one controlled clinical trial of 20 children with atopic eczema, parent-administered massage, 20 minutes/day for 4 weeks, significantly ($p < 0.05$) reduced redness, scaling, lichenification, excoriation and pruritus compared with the control group, which significantly improved only on the scaling measure.[53]

Relaxation techniques may be another useful treatment strategy for eczema. An RCT of 25 patients with atopic dermatitis found progressive muscle relaxation led to significantly greater improvements in anxiety, pruritus and loss of sleep, but not disease area or severity, when compared with control.[54]

The effect of other stress-reduction techniques in the amelioration of eczema, such as tai chi, yoga and meditation, however, is not yet clear. As a final control measure, exposure to frequently ringing mobile phones and video gaming should be minimised, as these technologies have been found to increase stress and to aggravate symptoms of eczema.[55]

CASE STUDY

OVERVIEW

The parents of CP, a 3-year-old girl, presented to the clinic complaining of a rash to the child's face, anterior neck, wrists and ankles, which had been present for the past 6 months. The parents stated that CP regularly complained of itchy skin, which led to irritability and broken sleep most nights. The pruritus and flare-up of the lesions were aggravated by scratching, wool and oranges, and ameliorated by German chamomile cream. Apart from eczema, CP had no medical or surgical history. CP used a children's multivitamin once daily. The parents were distressed by the condition, and wanted CP's skin to appear normal again.

CASE STUDY CONTINUED

CLINICAL EXAMINATION

On examination, the lesions to the abovementioned regions were pink, dry, scaly and lichenified. There was no exudate, oedema, vesicles or pain, but excoriations were evident.

TREATMENT PROTOCOL

INITIAL APPOINTMENT

The overall treatment goal established for CP was that the severity of lesion flare and pruritus would decrease by 50% within 1 month. In order to achieve this goal, the following interventions were necessary.

HERBAL MEDICINE

Continue applying German chamomile cream to the lesions twice daily.

NUTRITIONAL MEDICINE

Dietary

One-week elimination diet (as previously outlined), after which a new food should be reintroduced every 2 days; at least seven servings of fruit and vegetables daily (excluding oranges, corn, bananas, apples, potatoes, parsley and carrots); at least five servings of wholegrain cereals daily (excluding wheat, rye, corn and barley); one to two servings of nuts and seeds daily (excluding peanuts and other potentially allergenic nuts); lean lamb/poultry 3 times a week; seafood 3 times a week (excluding shellfish); and avoid food containing artificial colours, flavours and preservatives.

SUPPLEMENTAL

Continue the children's multivitamin one tablet daily; commence *Lactobacilli rhamnosus* probiotic 1×10^9 cfu/g b.i.d.

LIFESTYLE/EDUCATION

Minimise exposure to cosmetics, moisturisers, perfumes, plant extracts, mineral oils, wool, synthetic fibres, non-colour-fast dyes, latex, cleaning agents, aerosols and other household chemicals; include an additional rinse cycle during laundry washing to minimise exposure to laundry detergents; massage child's back and neck with cold-pressed organic flaxseed oil every night for 20 minutes prior to settling; increase parental bonding activities, such as reading, playing and drawing, to reduce emotional stress in the child.

FOLLOW-UP

CP was reviewed once a fortnight to maintain patient compliance with the management plan, clinical progress and monitoring of prescribed interventions.

PSORIASIS

Epidemiology

Between 1% and 5% of the population are affected by psoriasis.[6] While the condition can occur at any age, the disorder has a propensity to peak around adolescence (16–22 years) and later in adulthood (57–60 years).[6]

Classification

Psoriasis is an inherited skin disorder characterised by chronic inflammation, and epidermal thickening, hyperplasia and hyperkeratosis. The condition can manifest as one of two types. Type 1 occurs in early adulthood (typically the second to third decade of life), and is the more severe form of the disease. This form is often resistant to therapy, and is associated with a family history of the condition. In contrast, type 2 psoriasis often occurs in the fifth to sixth decade of life, is less severe, and is not associated with a family history of the disorder.[56] In addition to these two classifications are several subtypes of psoriasis, including the plaque, guttate, pustular and erythrodermic variants.

Aetiology

GENETIC PREDISPOSITION

The aetiology of psoriasis remains uncertain, although a genetic predisposition to psoriasis is evident, with a positive family history being common among sufferers.[6] Indeed, in a survey of 1376 Italian patients with psoriasis, a positive family history of the disease was reported by 46% of individuals.[57]

DEFECTS IN CELLULAR PROLIFERATION

Defects in cellular proliferation are also apparent. A reduction in intraepidermal cyclic adenosine monophosphate (cAMP), for instance, can result in increased proteinase activity, and keratinocyte proliferation. Reduced cAMP levels are also associated with increased arachidonic acid production, leukotriene B-4 activation, neutrophil degranulation and epidermal inflammation.[58] These cellular defects increase the skin's susceptibility to chronic plaque formation.

DIGESTIVE FACTORS

Factors that may contribute to changes in the levels of these chemical messengers include incomplete protein digestion, bowel toxaemia and impaired hepatic function. Inadequate protein digestion, for instance, increases levels of undigested amino acids in the bowel lumen which, on exposure to intestinal flora, may form toxic polyamines, which have been shown to reduce cAMP production.[59,60] The presence of gut-derived toxins from intestinal bacteria and fungi, on the other hand, raises levels of cyclic guanidine monophosphate (cGMP), which in effect increases cellular proliferation.[59] Even though impaired liver function and the accumulation of these toxins might contribute to and/or exacerbate the symptoms of psoriasis, clinical data supporting these three theories are lacking.

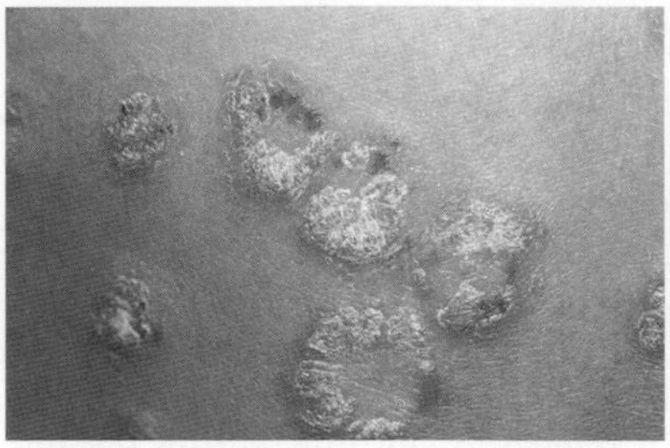

FIGURE 16.3 Psoriatic plaques.

INTRINSIC AND EXTRINSIC FACTORS

A number of intrinsic and extrinsic factors can also trigger the onset and relapse of psoriasis. Of the intrinsic triggers, emotional stress is considered to be a key exacerbating factor.[56] How stress affects psoriasis is explored later in this chapter. Alcohol, epidermal trauma, sunburn, β-haemolytic streptococcal infection, gluten, viral infection and medications, including β-adrenergic blockers, angiotensin-converting enzyme inhibitors, terbinafine, non-steroidal anti-inflammatory drugs, lithium, chloroquine and interferon-α,[6,56] are among the many extrinsic factors associated with psoriasis.

Pathogenesis and differential diagnosis

Each subtype of psoriasis manifests as a different cluster of signs and symptoms. The most common subtype, plaque psoriasis, generally presents on the scalp, trunk and limbs as demarcated, erythematous and thickened plaques covered with fine silvery scales (Fig. 16.3). Pruritus and nail pitting often accompany this subtype. Guttate psoriasis, on the other hand, manifests as distinct, scaly, erythematous, droplet-like lesions to the scalp, face, ears, trunk and proximal extremities. The pustular variant may be generalised or localised to the palmar or plantar surfaces, manifesting as erythematous, pustule-studded lesions, together with pyrexia and malaise. The other major variant, erythrodermic psoriasis, is a dermatological emergency, presenting as malaise, extensive and severe erythema and exfoliation, and reduced skin function.[8,56,61] In a small proportion of psoriasis cases, patients may also develop psoriatic arthritis, a condition closely resembling rheumatoid arthritis.

Naturopathic diagnosis

NAIL ANALYSIS

The general quality of the fingernails needs to be assessed and any suspicions of protein deficiency or inadequate intake of vitamins and minerals should be addressed. Pitting (i.e. the appearance of small pin pricks in the nail) and flaking of the nails are common in patients with psoriasis, and can be present on both fingernails and toenails. Similarly, 'oil drop' stippling is common — this appears as yellowish-brown spots under the nail plate. The lunula of the nail, which should be visible, can provide information about hydrochloric acid levels and metabolic activity; for instance, small or poorly visible lunula may be indicative of hypochlorhydria. White spots or markings are common in patients with psoriasis due to their high skin cell turnover rate, and can denote zinc deficiency.

TONGUE ANALYSIS

There is no 'skin' area of the tongue, although useful information can still be obtained regarding general health and the function of other organs of the body. Of particular note is the area at the rear of the tongue (which denotes the bladder, kidneys and intestines), as this can give information about the sluggishness of the digestive system. Attention should also be paid to the tip of the tongue (the heart area of the tongue), which can denote emotional stress (especially if it is very red in comparison to the other areas). This would be a pertinent finding as psoriasis is commonly exacerbated by stress.

INSPECTION AND PALPATION OF THE SKIN

Inspection of the skin should be conducted under natural light with close attention paid to the following aspects:

1. Colour — general pigmentation, widespread colour change, pallor, erythema, cyanosis and jaundice
2. Temperature — psoriatic lesions are commonly warmer than the surrounding skin (particularly plaque psoriasis). This should be noted, as a reduction in the level of heat is a sign of healing (even if the size of the lesion remains the same)
3. Moisture — psoriatic lesions tend to be very dry and scaly, while pustular psoriasis lesions contain moist pockets of pus. If a patient does not have pustular psoriasis and there is pus present on a lesion, this may be a sign of infection and requires prompt treatment
4. Texture — psoriatic lesions are clearly demarcated from the surrounding skin, due largely to a change in skin texture. The size of the lesions should be measured and noted (or photographed, with the patient's express consent) to enable ongoing evaluation of treatment efficacy
5. Thickness — the thickness of the plaque lesions is important, as this can change and can be used as an indicator of improvement, regardless of whether the size of the lesion changes
6. Oedema.

The more detail that is reported in the patient's case notes during the physical examination, the greater is the possibility for both the practitioner and the patient to note any positive or negative effects of treatment over time. Photographs of lesions can be a reliable method for monitoring clinical progress also, but it is important that the patient provides express permission for the taking of such photographs.

Investigations

Due to the distinguishing characteristics of psoriatic lesions, diagnosis is generally based on clinical presentation alone. Where the clinician is in doubt, however, a biopsy of the lesion may be performed. Histological findings from the biopsy that may indicate the presence of psoriatic disease include: evidence of inflammatory cells within the dermis and epidermis; increased mitosis of fibroblasts, keratinocytes and endothelial cells; and acanthosis (thickening of the skin).[62]

A liver function test (LFT) provides information about liver function (i.e. total protein, albumin, bilirubin, ammonia) and hepatocyte integrity (i.e. alkaline phosphatase (ALP), γ-glutamyl transpeptidase (GGT), alanine amino transferase (ALT), aspartate amino transferase (AST)). While an abnormal LFT, such as elevated blood ammonia, might point to impaired hepatic detoxification as a contributing factor in psoriasis, ammonia levels are unlikely to rise above the normal range in mild-to-moderate liver disease.[11]

Specific naturopathic investigations

Practitioners may choose to complete a comprehensive digestive stool analysis (CDSA), liver function test (LFT) and/or functional hepatic detoxification profile (FHDP) in order to isolate a possible cause of the psoriasis. A CDSA, for instance, can provide information on enzymatic digestion, fatty acid absorption, microbiological balance and metabolic markers of disease, helping to establish whether incomplete protein digestion, intestinal dysbiosis, candidiasis, and subsequent bowel toxaemia, are contributing factors in the pathogenesis of psoriasis.

A more specific and sensitive measure of liver detoxification is the functional hepatic detoxification profile (FHDP). This test measures the rate of phase I and II liver detoxification following caffeine, aspirin and paracetamol challenge. Findings from the FHDP, such as a reduction in the rate of substance clearance, may help a clinician determine whether a patient is able to effectively clear toxic metabolites from the blood,[63] including those that may be implicated in the pathogenesis of psoriasis.

Therapeutic considerations

Even though the characteristic appearance of psoriatic lesions somewhat defines the disease, it is important to recognise that a number of other conditions may present in a similar way. Conditions that practitioners should consider in their differential diagnoses include seborrhoeic dermatitis, secondary syphilis, fungal infections, lichen planus, pityriasis rosea, contact dermatitis and squamous cell carcinoma. In the event that a potentially serious condition is suspected, the patient should be referred to their general practitioner for further review.

CLINICAL DECISION MAKING AND RATIONALE

The naturopathic practitioner needs to consider both the physical and emotional therapeutic aspects of the psoriasis patient. This approach differs significantly from conventional treatment, which primarily relies on providing patients with short-term symptomatic relief. The traditional view of treatment should also be taken into account. This involves considering the concepts of internal blood heat, internal damp heat, liver stagnation and vital energy deficiency. The use of cooling or bitter herbs has an important role to play here, as does an emphasis on an anti-inflammatory diet.

PHYSICAL

Clear discussions regarding the signs of improvement (even slight changes in the thickness or nature of the lesions) can help foster continued patient compliance with treatment. Care must be taken to highlight that chronic conditions take time to improve.

As psoriasis is a chronic condition, it is important to discuss with patients the long-term effects of using conventional topical treatments, such as topical steroid applications. The benefit of substituting these agents with naturopathic alternatives may be significant.

EMOTIONAL

Psoriasis is known to be exacerbated by stress, and thus it is vital that the practitioner discusses with the patient strategies for stress management. It is also important for the practitioner to be aware of the emotional and social implications of having a condition that may be clearly visible to others. The patient may have feelings of shame and anger about their condition, which can impact on their relationships with others. If the naturopath does not feel secure in their ability to discuss the emotional aspects of the patient's condition, referral to a counsellor or psychologist may be of benefit to the patient.

Therapeutic application

NATUROPATHIC PERSPECTIVE

The management of psoriasis is relatively more complicated than the other conditions detailed in this chapter, because of the genetic aetiology of the disease and the fact that this cause is not amenable to naturopathic treatment. Notwithstanding, a practitioner may still be able to attend to the first principle of naturopathic care by addressing other potential causes or triggers of the disease, as listed above. Identifying and resolving the aetiology of psoriasis may in effect reduce the frequency and severity of exacerbations, and help to address the fourth principle of care, prevention. The selection of appropriate interventions that target both the cause of the disease and future exacerbations should, as a result, reduce immediate and long-term suffering, and therefore help to improve patient wellbeing and quality of life.

NUTRITIONAL MEDICINE (DIETARY)

Therapeutic objectives

The dietary approach to psoriasis should focus on three fundamental goals: to eliminate foods that aggravate psoriasis; to incorporate foods that facilitate gastrointestinal and hepatic function; and to maximise intake of nutrients with anti-inflammatory, antioxidant and vulnerary effects. To achieve these goals, appropriate objectives for the dietary management of psoriasis should be followed. Drawing from the nutritional goals outlined in Section A of this chapter, these objectives include:

1. Reduce intake of gluten-containing foods
2. Increase intake of fibre to facilitate bowel motility, elimination and repair
3. Increase intake of filtered water to support bowel elimination
4. Increase consumption of fruits and vegetables to augment ascorbic acid, β-carotene, fibre, folic acid and vitamin E intake
5. Increase consumption of seafood to increase omega-3 fatty acid, selenium, vitamin B_{12}, vitamin D and zinc intake
6. Increase consumption of low-allergenic nuts and seeds to improve folic acid, omega-3 fatty acid, selenium, vitamin E and zinc intake.

Specific dietary treatments

When considering the dietary management of psoriasis, naturopaths should first focus on the elimination of foods that aggravate the condition. One dietary component that may exacerbate psoriasis is gluten. It is believed that gluten sensitivity may trigger the condition by stimulating the release of cytokines from T-cells, and by increasing small intestine permeability and superantigen uptake.[64] The association between gluten and psoriasis is partly supported by findings from a review of several small, predominantly case-based, studies; these studies suggest that in patients with psoriasis, who are antigliadin antibody (AGA) positive, a gluten-free diet may help to reduce psoriasis area and severity.[65] Notwithstanding, these studies are not designed to demonstrate causation; consequently, the effectiveness of gluten-free diets for psoriasis remains inconclusive.

Given that the aforementioned wholegrain foods are good sources of both insoluble and soluble fibre, elimination of these foods means that alternative sources of fibre will need to be sought in order to facilitate gastrointestinal and hepatic function. Psyllium, fruits, vegetables, legumes, nuts and seeds, for example, contain adequate sources of insoluble and soluble fibre which, when combined with 6–8 glasses of filtered water a day may reduce colon pH and microbial overgrowth, bowel transit time and bowel toxaemia. Improvements in psoriasis symptoms may also be aided by consuming foods listed under objectives 4, 5 and 6 above, as these foods contain nutrients, flavonoids and essential fatty acids that can modulate inflammation and oxidative stress. In fact, a multicentre, case-control study involving 316 patients with psoriasis and 366 controls found the consumption of fresh fruit, carrots, tomatoes and β-carotene significantly reduced the odds of developing psoriasis ($p < 0.05$), while green vegetable intake demonstrated a marginally significant risk reduction ($p = 0.05$).[66]

An example of a daily diet that complies with the dietary treatment objectives for individuals with psoriasis follows.

SAMPLE DAILY DIET

BREAKFAST	
Quinoa porridge with papaya and live yoghurt	A gluten-free diet has been shown to decrease psoriasis severity, improving skin lesions. Quinoa/rice can be used as a GF alternative to oats or wheat-based cereals. The addition of live yoghurt provides probiotic strains useful since dysbiosis is implicated in the pathogenesis of psoriasis.
LUNCH	
Vegetable and red lentil dhal (with emphasis on ample ginger, turmeric) with rice	Dhal provides a wholefood plant-based meal option. A wholefood plant-based diet has been proposed to be beneficial to individuals with psoriasis, since there is decreased intake of arachidonic acid and consequently a reduction in inflammatory eicosanoid formation, which is otherwise seen in high concentrations in psoriatic lesions. Ginger and turmeric further help to downregulate inflammation.
DINNER	
Baked salmon cooked in a parcel with lemon slices, herbs, sliced leek, thinly sliced potato, olive oil, salt and pepper. Serve with steamed broccoli and zucchini	Diets rich in omega-3 polyunsaturated fatty acids from fish oil have been associated with improvement of psoriasis in clinical trials. Patients can be oriented to eat oily fish rich in omega-3 due to its immune regulating and anti-inflammatory action.
SNACK	
Mixed nuts and pumpkin seeds	Vitamin E and the minerals manganese, zinc, and selenium help to decrease oxidative stress and the production of reactive oxygen species implicated in psoriasis. Nuts are an excellent source of these nutrients as well as fatty acids.

Bhatia BK, Millsop JW, Debbaneh M et al. Diet and psoriasis: part 2. Celiac disease and role of a gluten-free diet. J Am Acad Dermatol 2014; 71(2):350–358; Fry L, Baker BS, Powles AV et al. Psoriasis is not an autoimmune disease? Exp Dermatol 2015 Apr; 24(4):241–244.

NUTRITIONAL MEDICINE (SUPPLEMENTAL)

Therapeutic objectives

In the event that an individual is unable to comply with the dietary recommendations, where nutritional deficiency is unlikely to be adequately addressed by diet alone, or where higher than normal doses of nutrients are required, a practitioner may consider nutritional supplementation. When nutritional supplementation is warranted, the following objectives for treating psoriasis need to be considered:

1. Support local and systemic immunity by increasing serum and tissue levels of ascorbic acid, selenium, vitamin A, vitamin B_{12}, vitamin D, vitamin E and zinc
2. Reduce tissue levels of arachidonic acid and proinflammatory cytokines by increasing serum and tissue levels of ascorbic acid, omega-3 fatty acids, selenium, vitamin B_{12}, vitamin D and vitamin E
3. Improve skin integrity and/or facilitate wound healing by increasing serum and tissue levels of ascorbic acid, omega-3 fatty acids, vitamin A, vitamin E and zinc
4. Reduce oxidative stress by increasing serum and tissue levels of ascorbic acid, omega-3 fatty acids, selenium, and vitamin E.

Specific nutrients required

VITAMIN A

Vitamin A is necessary for normal epithelial cell differentiation, collagen synthesis, phagocytosis, antibody production and intercellular adhesion.[16] A systematic review of six RCTs concluded that oral retinoids at 75 mg/day were moderately effective at reducing the surface area and severity of psoriasis when compared with placebo.[67] However, the agents examined in this review were synthetic, and thus the findings may not be representative of the effects of β-carotene or natural vitamin A. The evidence is also more than a decade old, highlighting the need for an updated review of the evidence of effectiveness of vitamin A in psoriasis.

VITAMIN C

Vitamin C has long been promoted as an anti-inflammatory agent. The findings of an open-label, randomised controlled trial of 64 obese adults lend support to this claim, which showed statistically significant reductions in C-reactive protein (CRP) and interleukin 6 (both markers of acute inflammation) in participants receiving vitamin C supplementation (500 mg b.i.d for 8 weeks) versus those receiving placebo.[18] However, it is uncertain whether vitamin C demonstrates any clinical benefit in psoriasis, due to a lack of clinical evidence in this area.

VITAMIN D

Vitamin D downregulates the expression of tissue necrosis factor-α (TNF-α), IL-6, IL-1 and IL-8 in monocytes in patients with type 2 diabetes,[22] indicating a possible anti-inflammatory and immunomodulatory effect. Vitamin D may also help to reduce keratinocyte proliferation and increase cell differentiation.[67] In terms of clinical evidence, a Cochrane review of 30 RCTs found topical vitamin D analogues to be significantly more effective than placebo in improving psoriasis, including investigator and patient assessment of overall global improvement, total severity scores, and psoriasis area and severity indices. However, these findings should be interpreted with caution given the very high level of heterogeneity found in the meta-analysis.[68] The evidence of effectiveness for oral vitamin D and psoriasis is less convincing due to the low number of studies, high-risk of bias, and inconsistencies in findings.[69]

VITAMIN E

The anti-inflammatory effect of vitamin E has been demonstrated in a number of studies; this activity may be attributed to the inhibition of cytokine-triggered activation of NF-κB.[23] Even so, there is a paucity of clinical evidence to support the administration of vitamin E in psoriasis. Clinical studies have also failed to demonstrate a significant difference in plasma vitamin E levels between those with psoriasis and healthy controls.[70]

VITAMIN B_{12}

Vitamin B_{12} has been shown in vitro to stimulate helper and suppressor T-cell activity,[71] while also suppressing T-cell cytokine production.[72] Patients with psoriasis demonstrate lower plasma vitamin B_{12} levels than controls although plasma vitamin B_{12} levels do not correlate with psoriasis severity.[73] In a small RCT of 13 patients with plaque psoriasis, the application of a vitamin B_{12} and avocado-oil cream for 12 weeks was shown to be as effective as calcipitriol treatment in reducing the severity of psoriasis.[74] However, these results should be interpreted with caution given the small sample size, inadequate control and the confounding effect of the avocado oil.

FOLIC ACID

Folic acid levels have been shown to be lower in patients with psoriasis relative to healthy controls[73] although evidence of an association between folic acid levels and psoriasis area and severity is inconsistent.[73,75] One factor that may contribute to lower plasma folate levels in psoriasis sufferers is the use of folate antagonists, such as methotrexate. Even so, clinical trials have found folate antagonists to be effective at improving the symptoms of psoriasis.[76] Therefore, given that folic acid may reduce the effectiveness of folate antagonist drugs,[77] and that there is insufficient evidence to support the use of folate therapy in psoriasis, folic acid supplementation is not recommended in this condition.

SELENIUM

Selenium inhibits nuclear factor-κB activation in vitro,[27] suggesting a possible anti-inflammatory effect for the mineral. While selenium is also an integral component of the body's antioxidant system, there is conflicting evidence regarding the effect of selenium supplementation on plasma and epidermal glutathione enzyme activity. Regardless of the mechanism of action, a double-blind controlled trial has shown that 600 micrograms of selenium for 12 weeks had no significant effect on the severity of psoriasis when compared with placebo.[78] While more recent studies suggest selenium may be beneficial in psoriasis, these studies did not use mono-preparations of selenium; thus the results of these studies are confounded by the effects of the other treatment(s). Consequently, further research in this area is still needed.

ZINC

Zinc may play a preventive role in the pathogenesis of psoriasis via reductions in oxidative stress.[79] Although some studies demonstrate lower serum zinc levels in patients with psoriasis relative to age- and sex-matched controls,[79] the evidence is not consistent.[80,81] Clinical studies have also failed to demonstrate a benefit of oral zinc supplementation in persons with psoriasis.[82,83]

ESSENTIAL FATTY ACIDS

Omega-3 fatty acids have been shown to reduce inflammatory markers in epidemiological, observational and clinical study populations.[32] While RCTs have reported significant improvements in the surface area and severity of both guttate and plaque psoriasis following intravenous administration of omega-3 polyunsaturated fatty acids,[84,85] evidence for the effectiveness of orally administered omega-3 fatty acids/fish oil is weak due to methodological limitations and/or confounding by concomitant treatment effects.[69]

Dosage requirements

The dosage requirements listed below are based on adult doses used in clinical trials. Where clinical data are absent or insufficient, however, the doses are based on those reported in the literature.[38–40]

- Ascorbic acid 500 mg b.i.d.
- Fish oil 6 g/day (equivalent to 720 mg docosahexaenoic acid (DHA) and 1080 mg eicosopentanoic acid (EPA))
- Vitamin A 5000 IU/day
- Vitamin B_{12} 250–1000 micrograms/day with a multi-B vitamin
- Vitamin D_3 400–1000 IU/day
- Vitamin E 400–800 IU/day

HERBAL MEDICINE

Therapeutic objectives

The integration of herbal medicine within a naturopathic treatment plan enables a practitioner to deliver a more targeted approach to psoriasis. Furthermore, when herbal medicine is integrated appropriately (i.e. without compromising the principles of naturopathic care), the treatment approach will be delivered more holistically. In order for practitioners to safely and effectively manage psoriasis using herbal medicine, the following treatment objectives should be considered:

1. Identify and treat the triggers of psoriasis to prevent exacerbation and recurrence
2. Manage inflammation to minimise unnecessary discomfort and tissue destruction
3. Improve gastrointestinal function to minimise microbial overgrowth, enhance protein digestion, and reduce bowel toxaemia

4 Facilitate detoxification and liver function to assist with the elimination of accumulated waste products
5 Facilitate lesion healing to reduce pain, disability and risk of infection
6 Enhance specific and nonspecific immunity to prevent wound infection
7 Manage associated symptoms of psoriasis to reduce discomfort and improve quality of life.

Herbal medicine classes

The herbal medicine classes that are indicated for the management of psoriasis are: adaptogenic, anti-inflammatory, antioxidant, digestive, depurative, hepatic and vulnerary.

The primary objective in the use of topically applied herbal medicines is to provide symptomatic relief. This can be achieved by administering anti-inflammatory and vulnerary herbs (e.g. *Aloe vera, Chamomilla recutita* and *Glycyrrhiza glabra*). The application of such topical creams or ointments throughout the day can greatly assist in reducing dryness, itching and inflammation of the lesions.

Orally administered herbal medicines aim to treat the underlying causes of the condition (see 'Therapeutic objectives'). For example, antioxidant herbs may provide support by countering the oxidation caused by the absorption of free radicals from bowel toxaemia. Anti-inflammatory herbs are of particular use as they can be used to substitute conventional steroidal anti-inflammatories, and help to provide relief from painful, inflamed lesions. Depurative and hepatic herbs aim to assist with the detoxification processes of the body. However, it is important to note that if these herbs are not given in small incremental doses, exacerbation of psoriasis can occur, potentially decreasing patient compliance and trust. Digestive herbs aim to improve digestion and to help regulate bowel habits (hence assisting in the elimination of toxins). The importance of adaptogenic herbs is not to be underestimated, as they can play a pivotal role in addressing the underlying stress response of the patient.

Specific herbal medicines

There are many herbs that demonstrate at least one of the aforementioned actions. However, it would not be useful for a busy practitioner if all these herbs were listed. Instead, only those herbs that have been investigated clinically, or that exhibit several of the activities mentioned above, are listed here.

ALOE BARBADENSIS (ALOE)

Aloe barbadensis exhibits vulnerary, anti-inflammatory, antioxidant, antinociceptive, immunomodulatory, vulnerary and antibacterial effects.[86] In spite of these favourable effects, the evidence of effectiveness of aloe in psoriasis is inconsistent. In a systematic review of three double-blind RCTs, aloe gel/cream was found to be superior to placebo in one trial (n = 60), inferior to placebo in another trial (n = 40), and as effective as triamcinolone acetonide in the third trial (n = 80), for changes in the psoriasis area and severity index.[87] Differences in aloe dose and formulation and study design may explain these disparate findings.

ARCTIUM LAPPA (BURDOCK)

Arctium lappa has been prescribed traditionally as a laxative and depurative for various chronic skin disorders. Clinical research suggests burdock may also possess anti-inflammatory and antioxidant effects, with one RCT finding burdock root tea to be more effective than boiled water at reducing serum high-sensitivity C-reactive protein, interleukin-6 and indicators of oxidative stress (i.e. total antioxidant capacity, superoxide dismutase) in patients with knee osteoarthritis.[88] However, whether these effects translate into clinical improvements in patients with psoriasis is as yet unknown.

AZADIRACHTA INDICA (NEEM)

Azadirachta indica is another depurative herb that has demonstrated significant anti-inflammatory activity in rats, immunomodulatory activity in mice, and a wide spectrum of antimicrobial effects in vitro.[43,44] Clinical evidence indicates that neem leaf may also be effective in psoriasis. In a double-blind, placebo-controlled trial of 44 patients with plaque psoriasis, the oral administration of an aqueous extract of neem leaves 3 times daily for 4 weeks, together with twice daily application of 5% coal tar ointment, was found to be significantly more effective than placebo or coal tar alone at reducing psoriasis surface area and severity ($p < 0.001$).[89] For safety reasons, it is important to note that the use of *Azadirachta* is restricted in Australia, including the form (only neem seed oil in concentrations ≤1%) and the route (topical application only).

BERBERIS AQUIFOLIUM (OREGON GRAPE)

Berberis aquifolium was traditionally prescribed for psoriasis because of its depurative, anti-inflammatory, antimicrobial and antipsoriatic activity. These effects have been supported by findings from an RCT, in which Oregon grape ointment was found to be effective at improving cellular cutaneous immune mechanisms, as well as reducing keratinocyte hyperproliferation.[90] In terms of clinical outcomes, a review of four RCTs suggests Oregon grape ointment/cream may be more effective than controls, and as effective as topical pharmaceuticals in improving psoriatic symptoms and quality of life in persons with psoriasis.[87]

MATRICARIA RECUTITA (CHAMOMILE)

Matricaria recutita demonstrates a range of effects that may be useful in the treatment of psoriasis, including anti-inflammatory, immunostimulant, antibacterial, vulnerary and mild sedative properties. Nevertheless, the clinical effectiveness of chamomile in psoriasis is unclear.

CENTELLA ASIATICA (GOTU KOLA)

Centella asiatica has traditionally been used for its vulnerary, depurative, and anti-inflammatory activity. While the extract has been shown to inhibit keratinocyte proliferation in vitro,[91] the clinical effectiveness of gotu kola in psoriasis is not certain and thus, clinical research is warranted.

COLEUS FORSKOHLII (COLEUS)

Coleus forskohlii exhibits both anti-inflammatory and digestive effects, and has been claimed to improve psoriasis by elevating cAMP levels. However, research is needed to validate this claim.

ECHINACEA SPP. (ECHINACEA)

Echinacea spp. exhibit anti-inflammatory, immunostimulant, depurative and antibacterial effects. While data from animal studies indicate that topical applications of *Echinacea purpurea* may facilitate wound healing, the clinical effect of *Echinacea* in psoriasis is not yet clear.

GLYCYRRHIZA GLABRA (LIQUORICE)

Glycyrrhiza glabra has traditionally been administered for its anti-inflammatory, laxative and demulcent activity. In support of these effects, a pilot open-label, parallel-group trial of 40 patients with palmar and/or plantar psoriasis found *Glycyrrhiza glabra* cream (in combination with milk proteins) plus corticosteroid cream to be significantly more effective than corticosteroid cream alone in improving psoriasis desquamation, surface area and subjective symptoms.[92] Given the limitations of the study design, and the confounding effects of the other constituents within the liquorice-based cream, the effectiveness of liquorice for psoriasis remains inconclusive.

HYDRASTIS CANADENSIS (GOLDENSEAL)

Hydrastis canadensis has a long history of use as a depurative, bitter tonic, antimicrobial, vulnerary and anti-inflammatory agent. Experimental studies indicate that berberine, an alkaloid of goldenseal, may reduce the symptoms of psoriasis by decreasing both prostaglandin E_2 levels[93] and keratinocyte hyperproliferation.[94] Even so, there is a paucity of clinical data to support these findings.

SILYBUM MARIANUM (ST MARY'S THISTLE)

Silybum marianum demonstrates both antioxidant and hepatic activity. While these effects are important in the overall management of psoriasis, there is a dearth of clinical evidence to support the administration of St Mary's thistle in this disorder.

SMILAX ORNATA (SARSAPARILLA)

Smilax ornata is a herb that possesses anti-inflammatory and depurative activity. While a number of open trials predating 1942 suggested that orally administered sarsaparilla root may improve the symptoms of psoriasis,[44] there have been no recent controlled trials to support these claims.

WITHANIA SOMNIFERA (ASHWAGANDHA)

Withania somnifera has traditionally been administered for the management of psoriasis, possibly because of its anti-inflammatory and immunomodulating effects. Even though these actions have been demonstrated in experimental studies,[95,96] there is insufficient clinical data to support the use of ashwagandha in psoriasis at present.

ZINGIBER OFFICINALE (GINGER)

Zingiber officinale was traditionally prescribed as a digestive and circulatory stimulant, for the purpose of increasing the bioavailability of simultaneously administered herbs. Even though ginger has been shown to increase drug absorption and plasma half-life in rabbits,[97] clinical evidence is lacking.

LIFESTYLE RECOMMENDATIONS

Stress

Stress is often implicated in the pathogenesis of psoriasis. In fact, the majority of psoriasis sufferers believe that stress is an exacerbating or a causal factor of the disease.[98,99] In support of this belief, a 3-year study of 95 patients with non-progressive psoriasis found stressful life events often preceded a rise in cortisol levels by an average of 2 weeks. This was followed by the development of an infectious illness 4 weeks later and, after another 2 weeks, the eruption of psoriasis.[100] While this proposition requires further investigation using larger samples, the positive effect of stress-reduction strategies on psoriasis outcomes lends further support to the stress–psoriasis hypothesis. In an RCT of 37 patients who were undergoing phototherapy or photochemotherapy for psoriasis, audiotape-guided mindfulness meditation significantly increased the rate of resolution of psoriatic lesions when compared with a non-tape control.[101] It is possible that other stress-reduction strategies may also be useful in the management of psoriasis, including yoga, tai chi, guided imagery and progressive muscle relaxation.

Alcohol

Some people may turn to alcohol in an attempt to manage psychological stress, but alcohol consumption may elevate histamine levels[64] and, in effect, aggravate psoriasis. In fact, studies demonstrate a significant association between alcohol intake and psoriasis surface area and severity,[102,103] particularly among male sufferers. Even though abstinence or moderation of alcohol intake may help to reduce the severity of psoriasis, evidence from intervention studies is lacking.

Sunlight exposure

Some patients with psoriasis may be advised to increase their level of sunlight exposure to accelerate recovery. However, while a number of clinical trials have shown ultraviolet B (UVB) radiation and a combination of ultraviolet A (UVA) radiation and the photosensitising agent psoralen to be effective in reducing the surface area of psoriasis,[67] the evidence for natural sunlight is less convincing. Studies have shown that a combination of sunlight and psoralen is more effective than natural sunlight and placebo at reducing psoriasis surface area,[67] but these studies pre-date 1982 and have major methodological limitations.

Carbon arc lamps have been used since the early 19th century in an attempt to harness the benefits obtained from natural sunlight.[104] Indeed, studies conducted on the type of ultraviolet (UV) radiation at the Dead Sea (which has a long history of popularity with psoriatic patients) showed that, due to the geographic location, there is a greater amount of the therapeutic long UVB rays,[105] giving scientific validation to the positive results found by patients undergoing treatment in the area.

Modern UV therapy uses lamps that concentrate the presence of the long UVB rays (narrow-band UVB 311 nm lamps) and have strict filters for the more harmful UV rays, thus providing a more effective and safe form of phototherapy for the psoriasis patient. A number of clinical trials have shown UVB radiation and a combination of UVA radiation and the photosensitising agent psoralen to be effective at reducing the surface area of psoriasis.[106] Many practitioners are concerned about the increased exposure to UV radiation and the possible long-term side effects of photoageing and skin cancer. However, a review of available literature from 1966 to 2002 showed that there was no increased risk of skin cancer among patients undertaking UVB therapy.[107] As the new form of narrow-band UVB therapy has only been in wide use for less than 20 years, and because the latency period for developing skin cancer can be 20 years or longer, further longitudinal studies need to be conducted.

CASE STUDY

OVERVIEW

TA, a 25-year-old male, presented to the clinic with psoriasis. The psoriasis had been present for the past 7 years, although short periods of remission occurred infrequently. He reported that his father also had the condition. He obtained moderate relief from 0.05% betamethasone cream applied twice daily, although he was reluctant to continue using the steroid cream because of its skin thinning effect. He also self-administered one multivitamin tablet a day and 1 g of fish oil twice daily. Although he did not smoke and was of normal weight (body mass index (BMI) 22), he enjoyed two glasses of red wine every night after work. TA's medical history was otherwise unremarkable.

CLINICAL EXAMINATION

On examination, demarcated, erythematous and thickened plaques covered with fine silvery scales were present on the anterior and posterior torso, and bilaterally on the elbows, knees and shoulders. These lesions were accompanied by moderate pruritus and desquamation, which often worsened when TA was emotionally stressed.

TREATMENT PROTOCOL

INITIAL APPOINTMENT

The overall treatment goal for TA was to reduce the surface area of psoriatic lesions by 25% within 1 month. In order to achieve this goal, the following interventions were implemented.

HERBAL MEDICINE

Administer the herbal complex listed below and apply 10% *Berberis aquifolium* cream to lesions t.d.s.

CASE STUDY CONTINUED

Herbal medicine	Quantity	
Azadirachta indica	1 : 2 liquid extract [In Australia, this herb should be substituted with *Hydrastis canadensis* 1 : 3 liquid extract, 15 mL]	15 mL
Smilax ornata	1 : 2 liquid extract	30 mL
Zingiber officinale	1 : 2 liquid extract	10 mL

Dose: 2.5 ml t.d.s. before meals.

NUTRITIONAL MEDICINE

Dietary

Consume at least three servings of fresh fruit, four servings of vegetables (particularly tomatoes, carrots, sweet potato and pumpkin), five servings of wholegrain cereals (excluding wheat, rye, oats, barley and triticale), and one to two servings of nuts and seeds daily. Consume lean pork/poultry 3 times a week, lean seafood 3 times a week (excluding shellfish) and drink 6–8 glasses of filtered water daily.

Supplementation

Continue multivitamin one tablet daily (which provided vitamin A 5000 IU and vitamin D_3 400 IU); increase fish oil to 3 g b.i.d.

LIFESTYLE/EDUCATION

Walk 20–30 minutes/day; perform mindfulness meditation, relaxation, guided imagery, yoga or tai chi for 30 minutes/day; reduce alcohol intake to 1 glass/day, with a view to limiting intake to 1 glass every 2–3 days if psoriasis symptoms improve.

FOLLOW-UP

TA was reviewed once a month to monitor compliance with the management plan, assess clinical progress, and evaluate the effectiveness of the prescribed interventions.

ACNE

Epidemiology

Most individuals will be affected by acne at some time in their life. In fact, 80–85% of people will be affected by the condition to some degree between the ages of 11 and 30 years.[108] While the vulgaris, conglobata and fulminant variants of acne are most likely to affect adolescent males, the excorié, rosacea, cosmetica, mature-onset and pyoderma faciale variants of acne are more prevalent among women.[108]

Classification

Acne is a skin disorder that affects the pilosebaceous units (acne vulgaris) and/or the underlying blood vessels (rosacea) of the skin. Acne vulgaris, rosacea, acne fulminans, pyoderma faciale, acne excorié, mature-onset form, acne conglobata, neonatal and infantile acne are some of the variants of the disease. Each of these variants can be further classified as mild, moderate or severe.

Aetiology

There are a number of processes that may be responsible for the pathogenesis of acne and a number of modifiable and non-modifiable triggers of acne have been reported in the literature

NON-MODIFIABLE FACTORS

In adolescents, puberty and genetics play an integral role. This may be because androgen, sebum and growth hormone levels peak during the adolescent period.[109] Elevated androgen levels may increase sebum production and abnormal follicular keratinisation and desquamation, leading to the formation of follicular plugs and the subsequent blockage of the pilosebaceous unit, resulting in the formation of comedones.[108] The positive correlation between androgen levels (including free testosterone, total testosterone and dehydroepiandrosteron sulfate) and acne severity is partly supported by a case-control study comparing 141 woman with acne vulgaris to 73 healthy women.[109] Hormone fluctuations during pregnancy and menstruation may also exacerbate the disease.[6]

The abovementioned effects, together with the proliferation of the bacterium *Propionibacterium acnes*, may further facilitate the development of acneiform lesions. *P. acnes* may be a particularly important trigger in the pathogenesis of acne, as the bacterium promotes inflammatory activity by releasing chemotactic factors and proteases, while also hydrolysing sebum into proinflammatory free fatty acids.[8,108] In rosacea, it is believed that an underlying vascular defect may be responsible,[8] although the actual aetiology of this disorder remains elusive.

MODIFIABLE FACTORS

The modifiable factors of acne development include topical agents (i.e. cosmetics, creams), medications (i.e. steroids, anticonvulsants), occlusive objects (i.e. helmets, shirt collars), and perspiration.[6,110] In rosacea, common triggers include sun exposure, cold or hot weather, wind, hot baths, exercise, emotional stress, alcohol, spicy foods, cosmetics and hot drinks.[5,6] The ingestion of foods with a high glycaemic index (GI) may also contribute to the pathogenesis of acne, which is discussed in more detail below.

Pathogenesis

In most cases, acne is confined to the face, upper back and chest, where pilosebaceous units are most numerous, except for rosacea, which is often localised to the face. In mild cases of acne, lesions may be limited to open (blackheads) and closed (whiteheads) comedones, and papules (Fig. 16.4). In more severe cases, inflamed papules, pustules, nodules and cysts may develop, which may lead to scarring.[8,108] The presence of these lesions, as well as scarring, can result in significant psychological distress for the patient and their family.

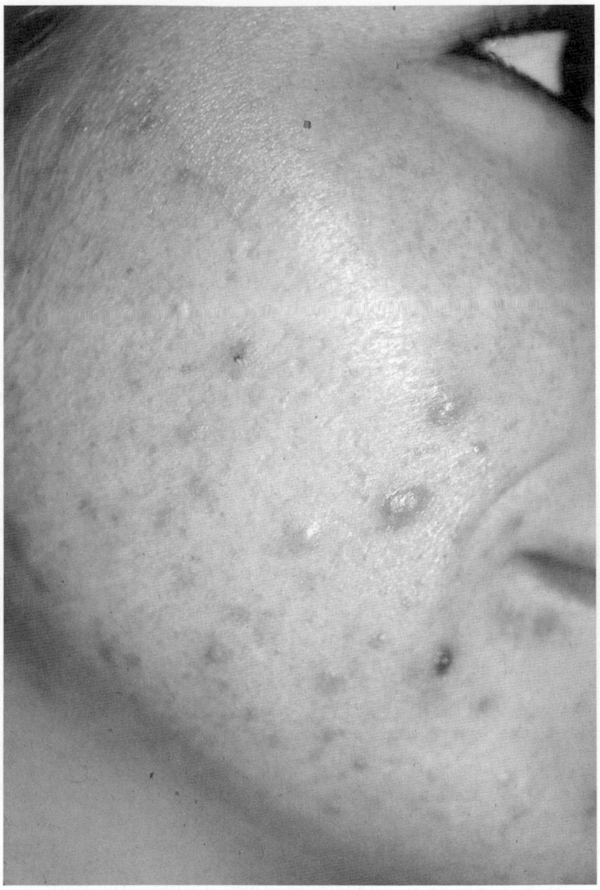

FIGURE 16.4 Acne vulgaris to face.

Systemic manifestations may also present in variants such as acne fulminans, with symptoms including pyrexia, malaise, arthralgia, myalgia, leucocytosis and weight loss.[108] In rosacea, acneiform lesions may be accompanied by facial erythema, oedema and telangiectasia.[6]

Complications

Complications of acne can be psychological, emotional or physical in nature. Psychological and emotional effects can include depression, anxiety and reduced self-esteem due to socialisation difficulties related to personal appearance. Unfortunately, the added stress caused by the psychological impact of this condition can lead to an increase in acne severity.

Physical scarring of the skin can range from being non-existent to severe. The amount of scarring is linked to the severity of the acne, and the level of dermal involvement. The following categories have been developed to define the severity further:

- Type 1: comedomal, no scarring present
- Type 2: papular, mild scarring
- Type 3: pustular, moderate scarring
- Type 4: nodulocystic, severe scarring.

Differential diagnosis

A differential diagnosis should be made to ensure that the correct therapeutic objectives and outcomes are met. Acne vulgaris should be differentiated from rosacea (previously called 'acne rosacea') and perioral dermatitis. Rosacea and perioral dermatitis can be distinguished from acne vulgaris by comparing the following features:

- Form of lesion: acne vulgaris lesions are follicular (commonly forming pustular comedones); rosacea has a greater vascular involvement (erythema and telangiectasia) and can also have a glandular component (hyperplasia of the nose, leading to rhinophyma). Perioral dermatitis lesions have a more eczematous appearance (small, dry, inflamed lesions)
- Distribution of lesions: acne vulgaris can be widespread across the whole face, chest, back, neck and shoulders. Rosacea usually affects the central part of the face (primarily across the cheeks and nose). Perioral dermatitis is primarily located around the mouth and eyes
- Age of patient: patients with rosacea are commonly older than patients with acne vulgaris or perioral dermatitis.

Naturopathic diagnosis

NAIL ANALYSIS

The general quality of the patient's fingernails needs to be assessed. Any suspicions of protein deficiency or inadequate intake of vitamins and minerals should be addressed in a detailed nutritional analysis. The following abnormal signs may be present in acne vulgaris:

- Hard/thick nails — overconsumption of protein and/or fat
- Soft/thin nails — overconsumption of alcohol, coffee and/or sugar
- Peeling nails — overconsumption of fruit, soft drinks, chemicals, drugs and medication; lack of essential fatty acids, and high levels of stress
- Brittle nails — lack of essential fatty acids, and a diet rich in refined carbohydrates and stimulants.

INSPECTION AND PALPATION OF THE SKIN

Inspection of the skin should be conducted under natural light, with close attention paid to the following aspects:

- Colour — general pigmentation, widespread colour change, pallor, erythema, cyanosis and jaundice
- Temperature — take particular note of heated, inflamed red areas, as these may be infected
- Moisture — affected areas are likely to be either dry or oily. It is important to take note of unaffected skin in order to make comparisons, and to look for indications of essential fatty acid deficiencies. Also look for areas of pus or infection, and note their severity
- Texture — look at the general texture of the skin, especially for signs of scarring, and the severity of this
- Thickness — pay attention to the height or thickness of comedones
- Area of distribution — note the areas affected (e.g. back, neck, cheeks, forehead). Make detailed notes on the number of comedones in each area, for comparison at future appointments
- Oedema — look for signs of oedema (especially if cystic comedones are present) as this can assist in identifying signs of severe infection.

The more detail that is reported in the patient's case notes during the physical examination, the greater is the possibility for both the practitioner and the patient to note any positive or negative effects of treatment over time. Photographs of lesions can be a reliable method for monitoring clinical progress also, but it is important that the patient provides express permission for the taking of such photographs.

Investigations

A diagnosis of acne can only be determined by clinical examination, as there are no specific tests for diagnosing this condition. Attempts to isolate a physiological cause of the condition may also prove futile, as most patients with acne demonstrate normal androgen levels,[108] and *P. acnes* is a normal resident of human skin. However, this should not prevent practitioners from attempting to identify triggers of the disease, as highlighted below.

SPECIFIC NATUROPATHIC INVESTIGATIONS

Naturopathic practitioners may find benefit in referring the patient for a liver function test (LFT), a comprehensive digestive stool analysis (CDSA) and/or a functional liver detoxification profile (FLDP). These tests can provide detailed, useful information about the patient's digestive and detoxification abilities, two areas that are commonly underactive in patients with acne.

Therapeutic considerations

Even though the presence of acneiform lesions may be highly indicative of one of many variants of acne, it is important to recognise that a number of other conditions may also present in a similar way, which may require a different approach to treatment. Conditions that may be mistaken for acne include folliculitis, Favre–Racouchot syndrome, seborrhoeic dermatitis, lupus erythematosus, perioral dermatitis and adverse drug reactions. In the event that a serious disease state may be mimicking acne, the practitioner should refer the patient to their general practitioner for further review.

CLINICAL DECISION MAKING AND RATIONALE

It is important that the naturopathic practitioner consider the many social, psychological and emotional implications of this condition, as well as the more obvious physical effects. Primary to the naturopathic approach is addressing the underlying causes of the condition (e.g. bowel function, emotional stressors and hormone involvement). By ensuring that all aspects of the condition are considered, the overall health and wellbeing (both in the short term and the long term) of the patient will be the best possible. As practitioners are often treating young adults with this condition, the use of herbal medicines that effect hormonal cascades should be considered with due care and attention (e.g. *Vitex agnus-castus*).

Therapeutic application

NATUROPATHIC PERSPECTIVE

Many of the factors contributing to the development of acneiform lesions are neither modifiable nor reliably detected with conventional pathology tests, which may limit how a naturopath manages the disease. In other words, some practitioners may find it difficult to address the first naturopathic principle (i.e. identifying and treating the cause of the acne). Despite these concerns, a comprehensive assessment of the patient's medical, environmental, family and clinical history can assist the practitioner in identifying a number of triggers of acne, and therefore help to minimise disease severity or recurrence, as well as unnecessary physical and emotional distress to the patient. This can include addressing the primary hormone imbalance and exacerbating factors such as insulin resistance, infection and inflammation. Attending to the first naturopathic principle then selecting appropriate interventions to support the body's innate healing ability will, in effect, address both the third (alleviate suffering) and fourth (prevention) principles of care.

NUTRITIONAL MEDICINE (DIETARY)

Therapeutic objectives

The dietary approach to acne should focus on three essential goals: to eliminate foods that are comedogenic or aggravate acne; to incorporate foods that facilitate normal skin function; and to maximise intake of nutrients with anti-inflammatory and vulnerary effects. To achieve these goals, appropriate objectives for the dietary management of acne should be followed. Focusing on the nutritional goals highlighted in Section A of this chapter, these objectives include:

1. Identify and eliminate foods that may contribute to or exacerbate acne
2. Reduce consumption of refined, processed and sweetened foods as these may elevate serum insulin levels
3. Increase fibre intake to improve glycaemic control
4. Increase consumption of seafood to increase niacin, omega-3 fatty acid, selenium, vitamin D and zinc intake
5. Increase consumption of fruits and vegetables to augment ascorbic acid, vitamin A and vitamin E intake
6. Increase consumption of low-allergenic nuts and seeds to improve niacin, selenium, vitamin E, omega-3 fatty acid and zinc intake
7. Increase lean meat consumption as this will improve niacin, selenium, vitamin E and zinc intake
8. Increase wholegrain consumption as this will improve fibre, selenium, vitamin E and zinc intake.

Specific treatments

The identification and elimination of dietary triggers should be the primary goal of acne management. Thus, foods that promote or exacerbate acne, particularly rosacea, should be eliminated, including alcohol, spicy foods and hot beverages.

Other dietary considerations

Individuals with acne should be encouraged to minimise the consumption of foods with a high GI. The chronic consumption of high-GI foods promotes hyperinsulinaemia and insulin resistance, which in turn increase free levels of insulin growth factor and androgens. Elevated levels of these hormones can lead to increased keratinocyte proliferation and sebum production, and subsequent acne formation.[111] This theory is partly supported by a number of small RCTs in which adolescents with acne following a 10–12 week, low-GI/low glycaemic-load diet demonstrated a significant reduction in androgen levels/markers, acne severity and inflammatory lesion counts compared with those consuming a high-GI diet.[112,113] Individuals who present with acne should therefore be encouraged to substitute high GI foods (e.g. refined, sweetened and highly processed products) with foods that have a low GI (e.g. wholegrains, fruits with edible skins) or are high in protein (e.g. eggs, lean meat).

An example of a daily diet that complies with the dietary treatment objectives for individuals with acne is given below.

NUTRITIONAL MEDICINE (SUPPLEMENTAL)

Therapeutic objectives

In the event that an individual is unable to comply with dietary recommendations, where nutritional deficiency is unlikely to be adequately addressed by diet alone, or where higher than normal doses of nutrients are required, a practitioner may consider nutritional supplementation. When nutritional supplementation is warranted, the following objectives for treating acne need to be considered:

- Reduce tissue levels of arachidonic acid and proinflammatory cytokines by increasing serum and tissue levels of ascorbic acid, omega-3 fatty acids, selenium, vitamin D and vitamin E
- Support local and systemic immunity by increasing serum and tissue levels of ascorbic acid, selenium, vitamin A, vitamin E and zinc
- Improve glycaemic control by increasing serum and tissue levels of niacin and zinc
- Improve skin integrity and/or facilitate lesion healing, by increasing serum and tissue levels of ascorbic acid, omega-3 fatty acids, vitamin A, vitamin E and zinc.

Specific nutrients required

VITAMIN A

Vitamin A is necessary for collagen synthesis, phagocytosis, antibody production, epithelial cell differentiation, and intercellular adhesion.[16] Clinical evidence indicates that patients with acne have significantly lower plasma concentrations of vitamin A than healthy controls.[114] While a number of clinical studies indicate that topical vitamin A formulations (in combination with other plant extracts/constituents and

SAMPLE DAILY DIET

BREAKFAST	
Pear, cinnamon and chia seed porridge with almond milk	High levels of insulin and an increased insulin growth factor 1 (IGF-1) as a result of high glycaemic load cause increased production of androgen hormones and sebum associated with acne, thus breakfast should be geared around low-GI foods. Pears and chia seeds are low GI and high in fibre, resulting in blood sugar stability, particularly when combined with cinnamon which has also been shown to help regulate blood sugar levels.
LUNCH	
Vietnamese salad: marinated tempeh with cucumber, carrot, bean sprouts, mint, lime and garlic. Serve with a small quantity of basmati rice (low GI)	Leucine-rich meat and insulinotrophic dairy proteins are also linked to acne. These can be replaced with vegetarian proteins such as tempeh and dairy alternatives. Consumption of refined high-GI foods is linked to the pathogenesis of acne, thus should be replaced with wholefood carbohydrates such as wholegrains, quinoa, millet and buckwheat. Herbs and spices such as basil and garlic should be used abundantly in the diet to stimulate the immune system and for their antimicrobial action.
DINNER	
Fish and vegetable pie topped with mashed sweet potato	Omega-3 fatty acids have the ability to lower IGF-1 levels, suggesting that they may have a beneficial effect in treatment of acne. EPA can inhibit production of leukotriene B4 which is involved in sebum production. The vegetables in this meal provide fibre. A high-fibre diet may also improve acne. Fibre binds to hormones and wastes, assisting their removal from the body. Fibre may also help to balance blood sugar levels assisting with glycaemic load.
SNACK	
Trail mix made from pumpkin and sunflower seeds and dried coconut Fresh fruit plus raw vegetables with guacamole	Zinc is a micronutrient that is essential for the development and functioning of the human skin. It has been shown to be bacteriostatic against *Propionibacterium acnes*, to inhibit chemotaxis and to reduce production of pro-inflammatory cytokine — tumour necrosis factor α. Consumption of fruits and vegetables is associated with downregulation of the nutrient-sensitive kinase, mammalian target of rapamycin complex 1 (mTORC1) involved in signalling of growth factors such as insulin and leucine.

Kucharska A, Szmurło A, Sińska B. Significance of diet in treated and untreated acne vulgaris. Postępy Dermatol Alergol 2016; 33(2):81–86; Mahmood SN, Bowe WP. Diet and acne update: carbohydrates emerge as the main culprit. J Drugs Dermatol 2014 Apr; 13(4):428–435; Melnik B. Dietary intervention in acne: attenuation of increased mTORC1 signaling promoted by Western diet. Dermatoendocrinol 2012 Jan 1; 4(1):20–32.

antimicrobial ingredients) may be effective at reducing the severity of acne vulgaris and the number of acne lesions in patients with mild-to-moderate acne after 12 weeks of therapy,[115,116] these studies have major methodological limitations (i.e. no control group or comparison with an active medication, and the confounding effects of other constituents within the vitamin A formulations); thus the effectiveness of vitamin A for acne remains inconclusive.

VITAMIN C

Vitamin C has long been promoted as an anti-inflammatory agent. The findings of an open-label, randomised controlled trial of 64 obese adults lend support to this claim, which showed statistically significant reductions in C-reactive protein (CRP) and interleukin 6 (both markers of acute inflammation) in participants receiving vitamin C supplementation (500 mg b.i.d for 8 weeks) versus those receiving placebo.[18] In addition to this anti-inflammatory effect, vitamin C may also reduce cutaneous lipid peroxidation and *P. acnes* replication.[117] In terms of clinical evidence, a double-blind RCT of 50 participants with acne vulgaris found the topical application of 5% sodium L-ascorbyl-2-phosphate (a stable vitamin C derivative) lotion twice daily for 12 weeks significantly reduced investigator global assessment score, participant global assessment score and acne lesion counts when compared with placebo.[118] Further research is needed to corroborate this evidence.

VITAMIN E

The anti-inflammatory effect of vitamin E has been demonstrated in a number of studies; this activity may be attributed to the inhibition of cytokine-triggered activation of NF-κB.[23] Plasma concentrations of vitamin E have also been found to be significantly lower in patients with acne as compared with healthy controls,[114] although there is insufficient evidence to date to suggest that vitamin E supplementation improves acne.

VITAMIN B_3

Niacinamide reduces inflammatory mediator release,[119] and in experimental studies with human subjects, has been shown to decrease inflammatory activity and trans-epidermal water loss, as well as increase corneocyte surface area and maturity and stratum corneum thickness.[120] While evidence is lacking for the oral administration of vitamin B_3, several controlled clinical trials have shown topical 4% niacinamide gel to be as effective as antibiotic gel at reducing the number and severity of acneiform lesions.[121,122]

SELENIUM

Selenium inhibits nuclear factor-κB activation in vitro,[27] suggesting a possible anti-inflammatory effect for the mineral. However, whether these actions affect the clinical outcomes of acne is unclear.

ZINC

Zinc deficiency adversely effects immune function, including phagocytosis, natural killer cell activity, and the oxidative burst,[13] indicating that zinc may play an important role in modulating immune activity. Importantly, zinc ascorbate solution demonstrates antimicrobial activity against *Propionibacterium* strains in study participants.[123] While a systematic review of the literature indicates that orally and topically administered zinc may be effective at reducing the severity of acne,[124] findings from trials have been inconsistent; more research needs to be conducted in this area.

PROBIOTICS

Lactobacilli spp. exhibit both local and systemic anti-inflammatory and immunomodulatory effects. Lending support to these effects are the findings of a prospective, open-label study, which found probiotic supplementation, when used together with oral minocycline (an antibiotic) to be more effective than probiotic or minocycline alone in reducing acne lesion count after 8 and 12 weeks in 45 women with acne vulgaris.[125] However, given the low methodological quality of this study, no firm conclusions can yet be made regarding the effectiveness of probiotics for acne.

ESSENTIAL FATTY ACIDS

Omega-3 fatty acids have been shown to reduce inflammatory markers in epidemiological, observational and clinical study populations.[32] The translation of these effects into clinical outcomes has been demonstrated in a 10-week RCT of 45 patients with mild-to-moderate acne, with omega-3 fatty acids (2 g EPA and EPA) shown to be as effective as gamma-linoleic acid at reducing acne lesion counts and acne severity; no such changes were seen in the no-treatment group.[126] Notwithstanding, the absence of a suitable control group limits the conclusions that can be drawn from this study.

Dosage requirements

The dosage requirements listed below are based on adult doses used in clinical trials. Where clinical data are absent or insufficient the dosages are based on those reported in the literature.[38–40]

- Ascorbic acid 500 mg b.i.d.
- Fish oil 3 g/day (equivalent to 360 mg DHA and 540 mg EPA)
- *Lactobacillus* spp. probiotic 1 × 10^9 cfu/g daily
- Niacinamide 12 mg/day with a multi-B-vitamin complex
- Selenium 200 micrograms/day
- Vitamin A 5000 IU/day
- Vitamin E 400–800 IU/day
- Zinc 25–60 mg.

HERBAL MEDICINE

Therapeutic objectives

The integration of herbal medicine within a naturopathic treatment plan allows a practitioner to deliver a more targeted approach to acne. Furthermore, when herbal medicine is integrated appropriately (i.e. without compromising the principles of naturopathic care), the treatment approach will be delivered more holistically. Thus, in order for practitioners to safely and effectively manage acne using herbal medicine, the following treatment objectives should be considered:

- Identify and treat the cause of acne to minimise exacerbation and recurrence
- Manage inflammation to minimise unnecessary discomfort and tissue destruction
- Facilitate wound healing to reduce pain, scarring and risk of infection
- Enhance specific and nonspecific immunity to prevent wound infection
- Reduce microbial replication to prevent unwanted tissue destruction, inflammation, pain and scarring
- Normalise androgen production to control keratinocyte proliferation and sebum production
- Manage associated symptoms of acne to reduce discomfort and improve wellbeing.

Herbal medicine classes

The herbal medicine classes that are indicated for the management of acne are the antiandrogens, anti-inflammatories, antibacterials, immunostimulants and vulneraries.

Specific herbal medicines

There are many herbs that demonstrate at least one of the abovementioned actions. However, it would not be useful for the busy practitioner to list all of these herbs here. Therefore, only those herbs that have been investigated clinically or that exhibit several of the abovementioned activities are listed below.

COMMIPHORA MOL MOL (MYRRH)

Commiphora mol mol exhibits a number of important actions, including anti-inflammatory, vulnerary and antimicrobial activity. Clinically, a small RCT in 20 patients with nodulocystic acne demonstrated that oral Gugulipid extract (equivalent to 25 mg guggulsterone), administered twice daily for 3 months was as effective as oral tetracycline at reducing the number of inflamed acneiform lesions.[127] Larger studies are needed to corroborate these findings.

ECHINACEA SPP. (ECHINACEA)

Echinacea spp. exhibit anti-inflammatory, immunostimulant and antibacterial effects. While *Echinacea purpurea* demonstrates bacteriocidal activity against *P. acnes* in vitro, and inhibits *P. acnes*-induced secretion of pro-inflammatory cytokines from skin fibroblasts,[128] human clinical trials are required to confirm these results.

GLYCYRRHIZA GLABRA (LIQUORICE)

Glycyrrhiza glabra demonstrates anti-inflammatory, mild antiandrogenic and immunomodulatory activity, as well as antimicrobial activity against *P. acnes* in vitro.[129] While these properties are desirable, there is currently insufficient clinical evidence to support the administration of liquorice in acne.

MELALEUCA ALTERNIFOLIA (TEA TREE)

Melaleuca alternifolia essential oil was traditionally applied as an anti-inflammatory, antimicrobial and antiseptic agent among Indigenous Australians. Experimental data have since shown that *P. acnes* is particularly sensitive to the effects of tea tree oil,[130] which suggests a possible role for tea tree oil in the treatment of acne. A review of five controlled trials reported that the topical application of 5% tea tree oil gel/extract was significantly more effective than placebo and 2% erythromycin gel, as effective as 5% *Lactobacillus* fermented *Chamaecyparis obtusa*, and less effective than 5% benzoyl peroxide, at reducing the number of inflamed acneiform lesions or total lesion count.[131]

VITEX AGNUS-CASTUS (CHASTE TREE)

Vitex agnus-castus has been shown to reduce serum luteinising hormone and testosterone levels in murine models.[132] This action may provide some explanation for the outcomes of an earlier controlled trial in 161 patients with acne, which found chaste tree treatment for 12 weeks was significantly superior to placebo in improving the signs of acne.[133] However, apart from the lack of adequate detail, more clinical data are needed to corroborate these findings.

ZINGIBER OFFICINALE (GINGER)

Zingiber officinale was traditionally prescribed as a digestive and circulatory stimulant for the purpose of increasing the bioavailability of simultaneously administered herbs. Even though ginger has been shown to increase drug absorption and plasma half-life in rabbits,[97] clinical evidence is lacking.

LIFESTYLE RECOMMENDATIONS

The appearance, location and potential outcomes of acne, such as scarring, can adversely affect the psychological wellbeing of sufferers, and add additional stress to an individual's life. As well as being a negative consequence of acne, stress may also play a role in the pathogenesis of the disease. A prospective cohort study in 94 Singaporean secondary school students showed that psychological stress is positively correlated ($p = 0.029$) with the severity of acne vulgaris, especially in males.[134] However, there are inconsistencies in the evidence, with another study comparing 40 individuals with acne to 40 healthy controls finding no association between intensity of stress and acne severity.[135] Notwithstanding, strategies that help individuals to reduce their level of psychological stress may be helpful in the resolution of acne. In support of this statement, an RCT involving 30 dermatology patients with acne vulgaris showed that 6 weeks of biofeedback-assisted relaxation and cognitive imagery was significantly more effective than attention-comparison and medical control at reducing acne severity.[136] Other interventions that may generate similar benefits in acne sufferers include mindfulness meditation, relaxation, guided imagery, yoga and tai chi.

CASE STUDY

OVERVIEW

BV, a 17-year-old male, presented to the clinic with severe acne, which had been present for the past 4–5 years. He has applied 5% benzoyl peroxide to the lesions twice daily for most of that period, which had reduced the severity of the inflammation but not the number of lesions. Apart from the benzoyl peroxide, BV did not self-administer any other prescribed, over-the-counter medications or illicit drugs. However, over the past 4 years, BV had completed several courses of tetracyclines and tretinoin for the acne, which had minimal effect. His diet was high in saturated fat, salt and added sugars, and low in micronutrients, due to the frequent consumption of takeaway and processed snack foods. Due to the demands of school studies, he had little time to engage in sports or regular physical activity, although he walked to and from school daily, which amounted to 50 minutes/week.

CLINICAL EXAMINATION

There were multiple open and closed comedones, inflamed papules and pustules present on the majority of the face and upper back. However, there was no evidence of cysts, scarring, underlying erythema or oedema. He was normotensive (116/72 mmHg), a non-smoker, a non-drinker and slightly overweight (BMI 27).

TREATMENT PROTOCOL

INITIAL APPOINTMENT

The primary treatment goal for BV was to reduce the number of inflamed acneiform lesions by 50% within 4 weeks. In order to achieve this goal, the following interventions were implemented.

HERBAL MEDICINE

Administer the herbal complex listed below before meals, and apply 5% *Melaleuca alternifolia* gel to the lesions 3 times daily.

CASE STUDY CONTINUED

Herbal medicine	Quantity	
Echinacea purpurea	1:2 liquid extract	30 mL
Commiphora mol mol	1:5 liquid extract	10 mL
Zingiber officinale	1:2 liquid extract	10 mL

Dose: 2.5 mL t.d.s.

NUTRITIONAL MEDICINE

Dietary

Commence a low-GI diet by avoiding refined, sweetened and highly processed foods, and consume at least three servings of fresh fruit daily (preferably with the skin intact); one to two servings of nuts and seeds daily; at least four servings of vegetables daily; at least five servings of wholegrain cereals daily; lean meat 3 times a week; lean seafood 3 times a week; and 6–8 glasses of filtered water daily.

Supplemental

Zinc 25 mg b.i.d.

LIFESTYLE/EDUCATION

Perform relaxation, mindfulness meditation, yoga, tai chi and/or guided imagery for 30 minutes/day; walk for at least 20–30 minutes/day.

FOLLOW-UP

The patient was reviewed once a fortnight to monitor compliance with the management plan, assess clinical progress and to evaluate the effectiveness of the prescribed interventions.

SKIN INFECTIONS

Epidemiology

While skin infections can affect persons of all ages, some infections are more prevalent among certain groups of individuals. Children, for instance, are particularly susceptible to a number of bacterial skin infections, such as impetigo and erysipelas, as well as the viral infections molluscum contagiosum, measles and chickenpox. The elderly, on the other hand, are particularly prone to chronic wound infections and cellulitis.

Classification

The invasion and proliferation of pathogenic microorganisms within the integumentary system can result in one of many different types of skin infection. These infections can be acute, subacute or chronic, depending on the period of onset and the duration of illness. Skin infections can also vary in severity, ranging between mild, moderate and severe.

Aetiology

From a biomedical viewpoint, microorganisms are believed to be the principal cause of skin infections. Bacterial invasion and proliferation can be attributed to the development of abscesses, cellulitis, wound infections, scalded skin syndrome, folliculitis, acne, impetigo and erysipelas. Fungal infections, on the other hand, are responsible for conditions such as candidiasis, tinea, onychomycosis and blastomycosis. Viruses are another leading cause of skin infection, which can result in cold sores, shingles, warts, chickenpox, measles and molluscum contagiosum.

Pathogenesis

Given the range of skin infections that can present in clinical practice, this section highlights the clinical manifestations that typically present in viral, fungal, and bacterial skin infections.

A pathognomonic feature of localised viral skin infections is vesicle formation. These clear, fluid-filled lesions often have an erythematous base, and may present on the lips (cold sores) or along a unilateral dermatome (shingles). Local viral infections may also manifest as papules, or solid raised lesions, as in warts and molluscum contagiosum. In fungal skin infections, patients may present with localised pruritus (candidiasis or tinea), scaling (tinea), maceration (tinea or candidiasis), thickened/discoloured nails (onychomycosis) and/or localised papules and pustules (candidiasis or tinea). The manifestations of bacterial infections, however, are somewhat more complex to characterise, as patients may present with any number or variation of signs and symptoms, including erythema (cellulitis or erysipelas), pain (abscesses), exudation (wound infection), blisters (impetigo) and/or papules (folliculitis). More generalised symptoms associated with skin infections can include pyrexia, lymphadenopathy and malaise.[8]

Complications

Complications of skin infections can be diverse and can include the following.

- Bacterial conditions: glomerulonephritis (impetigo), scarring (chronic wound infections), time in isolation leading to social and emotional complications (impetigo), septicaemia (cellulitis and wound infections), hair loss (folliculitis)
- Fungal conditions: hyper-/hypopigmentation (tinea), folliculitis (candidiasis, tinea), scarring and secondary bacterial infections from excessive scratching (tinea), vaginitis (candidiasis), nail loss (onychomycosis), secondary bacterial infection (onychomycosis), permanent lung damage, meningitis (blastomycosis)
- Viral conditions: scarring (measles, chickenpox), post-herpetic neuralgia (shingles), deafness (due to secondary middle ear infections caused from measles and chickenpox), meningitis (measles, chickenpox), oral ulceration (chickenpox, herpes zoster (see Fig. 16.5)), temporary blindness (shingles).

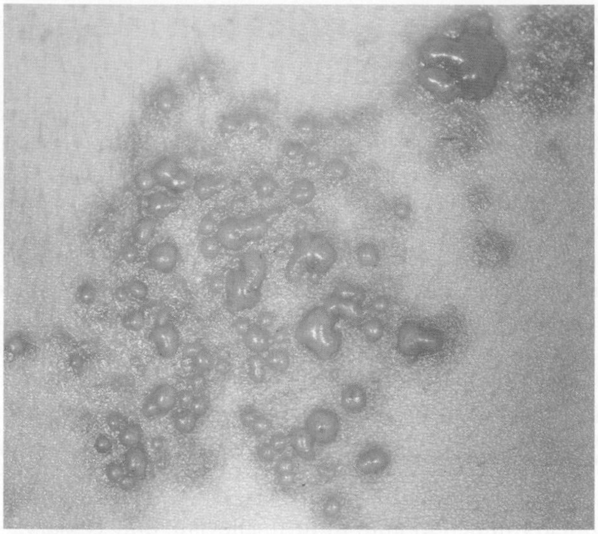

FIGURE 16.5 Lesions of herpes zoster.

Differential diagnosis

BACTERIAL CONDITIONS

- Impetigo versus herpes, ecthyma, tinea and psoriasis
- Cellulitis versus deep vein thrombosis (DVT). Differentiate by noting the temperature of the skin (typically normal or cool in DVT, but raised in cellulitis), the presence of lymphadenopathy (not present in DVT) and skin colour (typically normal or cyanotic in DVT and red in cellulitis).

FUNGAL CONDITIONS

- Tinea versus candidiasis, seborrhoeic dermatitis, intertrigo, psoriasis, erythrasma
- Candidiasis versus bacterial vaginosis, trichomoniasis, cervical inflammation, vaginal allergies, spermicide allergies, detergent allergies, normal vaginal discharge, *Chlamydia* and gonorrhoea
- Onychomycosis versus psoriasis, paronychia, nail trauma, malignancy, endocrine disease, lichen planus and atopic eczema
- Blastomycosis versus boils, carbuncles, chronic fatigue syndrome and histoplasmosis.

VIRAL CONDITIONS

- Molluscum contagiosum versus varicella, basal cell carcinoma, lichen planus, *Chlamydia*, genital herpes and gonorrhoea
- Measles versus rubella, erythema infectiosum, exanthem subitum, infectious mononucleosis and dengue fever
- Chickenpox versus Stevens–Johnson syndrome (SJS), herpes virus, contact dermatitis, scabies, atopic dermatitis, smallpox, and hand, foot and mouth disease
- Herpes versus impetigo, varicella, scabies, trauma, cervicitis, chickenpox, shingles, tonsillitis and vulvar cancer.

Naturopathic diagnosis

INSPECTION AND PALPATION OF THE SKIN

Inspection of the skin should be conducted under natural light with close attention paid to the following aspects:

- Colour — general pigmentation, widespread colour change, pallor, erythema, cyanosis and jaundice
- Temperature — particularly take note of heated, inflamed red areas as these may be infected
- Moisture — look for areas of pus or infection, note their severity, and treat accordingly
- Texture — look at the general texture of the skin, especially for signs of scarring, and the severity of this
- Thickness — pay attention to the height or thickness of any rash or lesion
- Area of distribution — note the areas affected (e.g. back, thorax, abdomen, face, limbs), and make detailed notes on the number and nature of the condition/lesions in each area
- Oedema — look for signs of oedema (especially if cystic lesions or cellulitis is present).

The more detail that is reported in the patient's case notes during the physical examination, the greater is the possibility for both the practitioner and the patient to note any positive or negative effects of treatment over time. Photographs of lesions can be a reliable method for monitoring clinical progress also, but it is important that the patient provides express permission for the taking of such photographs.

Investigations

Many infectious skin disorders can be diagnosed by clinical examination alone. Where there is uncertainty, however, a number of laboratory investigations can be conducted to assist the clinician in supporting or refuting a diagnosis. Microbiological examination of fungal, parasitic and bacterial specimens, for instance, can be performed within the clinic, and can provide rapid results.[137] In this procedure, a skin lesion is scraped or swabbed, mounted on a slide and examined under a microscope to detect the presence of abnormal cells/organisms, such as hyphae (in fungal disease), bacteria or parasites. Unfortunately, this test lacks specificity and may not be useful for differentiating between certain disorders, particularly those of viral origin.

A more sensitive diagnostic method, which can be used to identify organisms more definitively, is bacterial, viral and fungal culture.[137] Similar to microscopy, lesions are swabbed or scraped, but instead of mounting the specimen, the sample is immersed in an appropriate transport medium and, at a pathology laboratory, is cultured in a suitable growth medium to allow sufficient numbers of the organism to be isolated, identified and quantified. A drawback of this test, however, is that bacterial, viral and fungal cultures can take up to 1, 28 and 42 days, respectively, to yield results.[138]

A test that is relatively more costly to conduct in some instances, but has comparatively higher specificity and a shorter test time, is microorganism detection via polymerase chain reaction (PCR) culture or nucleic acid amplification.[138] In this test, deoxyribonucleic acid (DNA) is extracted from the collected specimen and rapidly amplified using DNA polymerase. Sufficient copies of the pathogen's DNA are then produced so that the pathogen can be isolated and identified.

Therapeutic considerations

As previously discussed, a number of pathological microorganisms may be responsible for skin infections, including viruses, fungi and bacteria. However, not everyone who is exposed to these pathogenic agents will develop a skin infection, which suggests that a deeper underlying cause may be responsible. In some situations, skin trauma may be the cause of cutaneous infections, including injury from shaving, intravenous drug abuse, gardening and insect/animal bites. In many cases, however, impaired immune function is likely to be the reason why microbial exposure progresses to a local or systemic skin infection. An individual's susceptibility to these infections may also be increased in the presence of diabetes, immunosuppression, peripheral vascular disease, malnutrition, HIV infection and poor hygiene. For viral infections such as herpes, stress, malaise, febrile illness and UV radiation may also be implicated.[8]

Even though many skin infections appear relatively benign, such as cold sores, warts and folliculitis, sites of skin infection can be complicated by secondary infection, and in some cases may lead to systemic infection and death. The correct identification and treatment of these conditions is therefore critical in reducing a patient's risk of death and disability. Hence, other conditions that may present similarly to skin infection, yet require a distinctly different approach to treatment, should not be overlooked. Examples of such conditions include bullous pemphigoid, contact dermatitis, dermatitis herpetiformis, pityriasis rosea, psoriasis, pyoderma gangrenosum, systemic lupus erythematosus and urticaria.

CLINICAL DECISION MAKING AND RATIONALE

It is essential that naturopathic practitioners refer patients for further testing or examination if they are not confident of providing a clear diagnosis, if severe signs of infection or DVT are present, or if they are concerned about the presentation. Practitioners must also be aware of occupational, health and safety guidelines surrounding infectious conditions, to ensure the wellbeing of their patients and the workplace. Practitioners must also consider legal and ethical decisions regarding sexually transmittable infections and other infectious conditions.

The emotional, psychological and physical implications of the aforementioned conditions should be considered, ensuring a holistic approach to treatment is maintained. This is especially important when treating patients with chronic or long-term infectious conditions.

Therapeutic application

NATUROPATHIC PERSPECTIVE

The four principles of naturopathic medicine, as outlined in Section A of this chapter, provide a useful framework for the management of skin infections. To address the first of these principles, the clinician needs to identify and treat the cause of the infection, including the predisposing factors of infection and the pathological agents involved. This will enable the practitioner to deliver more effective and appropriate care for the patient. In addition, the naturopath needs to incorporate interventions that support the body's innate healing ability, including strategies that improve skin integrity, as well as specific and nonspecific immunity. This two-pronged approach creates an environment that is incompatible with microbial growth, which may not only hasten recovery, but also prevent secondary infection and, in turn, alleviate unnecessary suffering.

NUTRITIONAL MEDICINE (DIETARY)

Therapeutic objectives

The dietary approach to skin infection should focus on three essential goals: to incorporate foods that facilitate normal skin function; to eliminate foods that compromise immune function; and to maximise the intake of nutrients with vulnerary effects. To achieve these goals, appropriate objectives for the dietary management of skin infection should be followed. Drawing from the nutritional goals highlighted in Section A of this chapter, these objectives include:

1. Reduce consumption of refined, processed and high-fat foods as these may reduce micronutrient stores and/or compromise immune function
2. Increase consumption of fruits and vegetables to augment ascorbic acid, β-carotene and bioflavonoid intake
3. Increase consumption of low-allergenic nuts and seeds to improve copper and zinc intake
4. Increase consumption of seafood to increase copper, lysine, selenium and zinc intake
5. Increase wholegrain consumption to increase lysine, selenium and zinc intake
6. Increase lean meat consumption to increase lysine and zinc intake.

SPECIFIC TREATMENTS

Adherence to a well-balanced diet, with a specific focus on nutrient density and diversity, should satisfy the abovementioned dietary objectives. Avoiding pre-prepared, processed and takeaway meals, and focusing on the preparation and consumption of wholefoods, will also help to reduce the intake of sodium, added sugar and saturated fat. The latter is particularly important, as it has been observed that high-fat diets suppress immune function,[139] chiefly T-cell-mediated immunity.[140] One approach that can help lower the consumption of these components within the diet, but at the same time elevate micronutrient intake, and thus facilitate immune function, is to increase fruit and vegetable intake[141] to at least two and five servings a day, respectively. Consuming a diverse range of nuts, wholegrain cereals, lean meats and seafood will further improve micronutrient intake, as well as protein ingestion, which is essential for cell division, immunity, and the production of collagen, keratin and elastin for skin integrity.

An example of a daily diet that complies with the dietary treatment objectives for individuals with skin infections is given below.

NUTRITIONAL MEDICINE (SUPPLEMENTAL)

Therapeutic objectives

In the event that an individual is unable to comply with dietary recommendations, where nutritional deficiency is unlikely to be adequately addressed by diet alone, or where higher than normal doses of nutrients are required, the practitioner may consider nutritional supplementation. When nutritional supplementation is warranted, the following objectives for treating skin infections need to be considered:

1. Support local and systemic immunity by increasing serum and tissue levels of ascorbic acid, quercetin, selenium, vitamin A and zinc
2. Reduce microbial load/proliferation by increasing serum and tissue levels of copper, lysine, quercetin, vitamin A and zinc
3. Facilitate lesion healing by elevating serum and tissue levels of ascorbic acid, vitamin A, vitamin E and zinc
4. Improve skin integrity by increasing serum and tissue levels of ascorbic acid, copper, lysine, vitamin A and zinc.

SAMPLE DAILY DIET

BREAKFAST	
Juice: carrot, orange and ginger juice Probiotic-rich yoghurt with fresh fruit salad and seed mix — pumpkin and sunflower	A juice provides a variety of vitamins such as beta-carotene and vitamin C to boost immunity against microbial infection, as well as promote skin health and detoxification of microbes from the body. The ginger functions to reduce inflammation while also acting as an antimicrobial. Cutaneous microbiota are known to induce inflammation and may influence the activity of skin diseases; additionally, dysbiosis has been implicated in dermatological diseases. Fermented dairy products, such as yoghurt, are a natural source of probiotics and work simultaneously modulating the gastrointestinal tract microbiota while also modifying skin disease. Pumpkin seeds provide a source of zinc for skin healing and repair.
LUNCH	
Chicken and vegetables with buckwheat pasta with pesto (pesto made from basil, garlic, parmesan)	The pasta provides a good source of fibre and B vitamins. Basil and garlic are both powerful antimicrobials that can be used to support the immune system and also provide antibacterial/fungal/viral activity.
DINNER	
Homemade 'healthy' fried rice made with corn, carrot, peas, broccoli, onion, mushrooms, tamari and ginger Serve with homemade tamari, honey, garlic and ginger organic chicken strips	Traditional eclectic understanding of skin disease centred upon the concept of disordered elimination and detoxification channels; this dinner provides an assortment of vegetables high in fibre to promote elimination channels in the bowel as well as from the *Allium* and cruciferous family to promote liver detoxification due to their sulfur content. The addition of chicken provides a low-allergen protein to support healthy immune function as well as detoxification.
SNACKS	
Fresh fruit — kiwifruit, strawberries, mango, lychees Hummus made with garlic, serve with sweet potato wedges	These fruits are high in vitamin C and bioflavonoids, helping improve the immune response against infection. They also provide fibre to improve elimination and act as a fuel source for gut bacteria. Garlic is an immunostimulant, prebiotic and antimicrobial. Sweet potato provides beta-carotene for skin healing.
BEVERAGES	
Drink 6–8 glasses of filtered water a day	If not contraindicated, the individual should aim to drink 6–8 glasses of filtered water daily. This helps ensure that the patient is adequately hydrated; it also assists in the detoxification processes of the body.

Specific nutrients required

VITAMIN A

Vitamin A is necessary for phagocytosis, antibody production, lymphocyte activity, collagen synthesis, epithelial cell differentiation and intercellular adhesion,[16] and thus, it may be useful as a treatment for infectious skin conditions. Retinoic acid and retinol, for instance, have both been observed in vitro to inhibit the growth of human papilloma virus infected keratinocytes.[142] Two small clinical trials in healthy human volunteers have also shown topical retinaldehyde to exhibit antibacterial activity against Gram-negative bacteria, but not against Gram-positive bacteria or *Candida*.[143] While these findings highlight the potential use of vitamin A in the treatment of warts and bacterial skin infections, more research needs to be conducted.

VITAMIN C

Ascorbic acid plays an important role in immunomodulation, influencing natural killer cell activity, lymphocyte proliferation and chemotaxis.[144] Vitamin C is also responsible for the biosynthesis of collagen, which is essential for maintaining skin integrity. In terms of effectiveness, however, there is a paucity of evidence supporting the use of vitamin C in skin infections. For herpes labialis, there is limited evidence. In one RCT of 32 patients with recurrent mucocutaneous herpes, for instance, topical ascorbic acid solution, applied every 30 minutes for 24 hours, was found to significantly reduce viral load ($p < 0.01$) and eschar duration ($p < 0.01$) when compared with placebo.[145] Whether these effects apply to orally administered vitamin C warrants further investigation.

COPPER

Copper is a cofactor for lysyl oxidase, which is responsible for the cross-linking of collagen and elastin in connective tissue, and therefore, plays an important role in the maintenance of skin integrity. Copper also acts as an antimicrobial, with copper complexes demonstrating bacteriostatic activity against Gram-positive and Gram-negative bacteria, and fungistatic action against yeast and mould.[146] In a 14-day prospective, multi-centred, randomised, comparative, open-label trial, of which 149 adults with active HSV-1 and HSV-2 lesions were recruited, topical Dynamiclear™ (copper sulfate pentahydrate and *Hypericum perforatum*) was found to be more effective than 5% acyclovir in reducing HSV symptoms (i.e. acute pain, erythema and vesiculation) with fewer adverse effects.[147] As it is not possible to separate the effects of copper from *Hypericum*, it remains uncertain as to whether copper alone is effective in improving skin infection.

SELENIUM

Selenium plays an important immunomodulatory role via its influence on cellular adherence, cell migration, phagocytosis, cytokine secretion, and the oxidative burst;[148] these effects may offer some benefit to patients with skin infections. In a double-blind randomised study of 60 cancer patients with secondary lymphoedema, sodium selenite application in combination with physical therapy for 3 weeks prevented the development of erysipelas; this effect was maintained throughout the 3-month follow-up period. By contrast, 50% of patients in the control group developed the condition over the same period.[149] A number of studies have also compared the clinical efficacy of 2.5% selenium sulfide shampoo with that of conventional antifungal agents in patients with tinea versicolor,[150–153] but results have been inconsistent.

ZINC

Zinc (gluconate) may play a part in improving cutaneous immune activity by upregulating the cutaneous antimicrobial peptides, human beta-defensin-2 and psoriasin.[154] Adding to this, zinc (acetate) demonstrates antimicrobial activity against *Propionibacterium* strains in study participants.[123] Despite these favourable effects, most research on zinc and skin infection has focused on herpes simplex virus infection. In several controlled clinical trials it has been observed that topically applied zinc oxide/zinc sulfide significantly reduces the recurrence, severity and duration of herpes labialis infection.[155,156] It should be noted, however, that these effects are not necessarily representative of orally administered zinc, which requires further investigation.

LYSINE

Lysine is required for the biosynthesis of collagen and protein. This amino acid has also been shown to inhibit replication of the herpes simplex virus in vitro,[157] particularly when the arginine/lysine ratio favours lysine.[158] A Cochrane review of interventions for the prevention of herpes simplex labialis identified only one RCT for lysine, which found lysine to be no more effective than placebo in preventing herpes labialis.[157] While a number of controlled trials not meeting the Cochrane review inclusion criteria have also investigated the clinical efficacy of orally administered L-lysine for herpes infection, the results have been inconsistent.[158–164] As such, it is uncertain whether lysine offers any clinical benefit to patients with herpes simplex virus infection.

PROBIOTICS

Lactobacilli spp. exhibit both local and systemic immunomodulatory effects. However, there is insufficient clinical evidence to support the administration of probiotics in cutaneous infections.

QUERCETIN

Quercetin demonstrates immunostimulant and antiviral activity in vitro, inducing interferon-γ production while inhibiting interleukin-4 synthesis.[165] The effect of this bioflavonoid in human skin infections, however, has not been adequately explored.

Dosage requirements

The dosage requirements listed below are based on adult doses used in clinical trials. Where clinical data are absent or insufficient the doses are based on those reported in the literature.[38,39,166]

- Ascorbic acid 500 mg b.i.d.
- Copper 2 mg/day
- Lysine 500 mg b.i.d.
- Quercetin 500 mg b.i.d.
- Selenium 200 micrograms/day
- Vitamin A 5000 IU/day
- Zinc 15–60 mg/day.

HERBAL MEDICINE

Therapeutic objectives

The integration of herbal medicine within a naturopathic treatment plan allows the practitioner to deliver a more targeted approach to skin infections. Furthermore, when herbal medicine is integrated appropriately (i.e. without compromising the principles of naturopathic care), the treatment approach will be delivered more holistically. Thus, in order for practitioners to safely and effectively manage skin infections using herbal medicine, the following treatment objectives should be considered:

1. Identify and treat the cause of the skin infection to minimise unnecessary discomfort and tissue destruction
2. Enhance specific and nonspecific immunity to control microbial proliferation
3. Inhibit microbial replication to prevent unwanted tissue destruction, inflammation, pain and scarring
4. Facilitate wound healing to reduce pain, disability and risk of secondary infection
5. Manage associated symptoms of skin infection to reduce discomfort and improve wellbeing.

Herbal medicine classes

The herbal medicine classes that are indicated for the management of skin infections are antibacterials, antifungals, antimicrobials, antiparasitics, antiseptics, antivirals, immunostimulants and vulneraries.

Specific herbal medicines

There are many herbs that demonstrate at least one of the actions mentioned above. However, it would not be useful for the busy practitioner to list all these herbs here. Therefore, only those herbs that have been investigated clinically or that exhibit several of the abovementioned actions are listed below.

ANDROGRAPHIS PANICULATA (ANDROGRAPHIS)

Andrographis paniculata has been traditionally used as an immunostimulant and antimicrobial agent. While the herb has been observed to inhibit the growth of herpes simplex virus type 1,[167] *Bacillus subtilis, Staphylococcus aureus, Escherichia coli, Pseudomonas aeruginosa* and *Candida albicans*,[168] the effectiveness of *Andrographis* in cutaneous disorders requires investigation.

ALLIUM SATIVUM (GARLIC)

Allium sativum has a long history of use as an antimicrobial and immunomodulatory agent, with the herb having been shown to improve macrophage, natural killer cell and T-lymphocyte function in vitro, and to modulate immunoglobulin production, cytokine secretion and phagocytosis in vitro.[169] In terms of antimicrobial effects, allicin, a key constituent of garlic, has been shown to exhibit antibacterial activity against a wide range of Gram-negative and Gram-positive bacteria; antifungal activity against *Candida albicans*; and antiparasitic and antiviral activity.[170] Ajoene, another compound isolated from garlic, also demonstrates antifungal activity. In two small randomised trials, 0.6% and 1% ajoene gel was found to be as effective as 1% terbinafine cream in improving the healing rate of tinea corporis, tinea cruris and tinea capitus.[171,172] Whether these effects are representative of whole garlic extract, however, warrants further investigation.

AZADIRACHTA INDICA (NEEM)

Azadirachta indica has demonstrated immunomodulatory activity in mice,[43] and a wide spectrum of antimicrobial affects in vitro.[44] A single application of neem seed extract shampoo also demonstrates antiparasitic activity against all stages of head lice in children, although it is unclear how this effect compares with control agents.[173] The body of clinical evidence for neem leaf and cutaneous infections is therefore currently limited. For safety reasons, it is important to note that the use of *Azadirachta* is restricted in Australia, including the form (neem seed oil in concentrations ≤1% only) and the route (topical application only) of administration.

ECHINACEA SPP. (ECHINACEA)

Echinacea spp. exhibit immunostimulant, antiviral, antibacterial and vulnerary effects. In relation to the integumentary system, *Echinacea pallida* has been shown to inhibit herpes simplex virus type 1 and type 2 replication in vivo;[174] however, the effectiveness of *Echinacea purpurea* extract in patients with genital herpes has been observed to be no more effective than placebo.[175] The clinical effectiveness of *Echinacea* in other cutaneous infective disorders also requires investigation.

EUGENIA CARYOPHYLLATA (*SYZYGIUM AROMATICUM*) (CLOVES)

Eugenia caryophyllata has demonstrated antibacterial, fungicidal and antiviral activity in vitro, including activity against herpes simplex virus type 1 and type 2,[176] *Staphylococcus epidermidis, Escherichia coli, Candida albicans*[177] and *Staphylococcus aureus*.[178] Nonetheless, there is insufficient clinical evidence to support the use of cloves for skin infections.

GLYCYRRHIZA GLABRA (LIQUORICE)

Glycyrrhiza glabra demonstrates immunomodulatory and antimicrobial activity. More specifically, constituents of liquorice have been shown to inhibit herpes simplex type 1 replication in vivo,[179] and methicillin-susceptible and methicillin-resistant *Staphylococcus aureus* proliferation and pathogenicity in vitro.[180] Even so, the clinical effectiveness of liquorice in skin infections remains uncertain.

MELALEUCA ALTERNIFOLIA (TEA TREE)

Melaleuca alternifolia was traditionally used as an antibacterial, fungicidal, antiviral and antiseptic agent among Indigenous populations. The effect of tea tree oil in fungal and viral skin infections, in particular, has received the most attention from investigators to date. Two RCTs, for instance, observed that 10–50% tea tree oil was significantly more effective than placebo at reducing symptom severity of tinea pedis, although the reported effect of the oil on mycological cure rate was inconsistent.[181,182] In 117 patients with distal subungual onychomycosis, the topical application of 100% tea tree oil for 6 months was found to be as effective as 1% clotrimazole at improving symptom resolution and mycological culture cure.[183] For herpes labialis, a pilot trial in 20 patients suggested that 6% tea tree oil may greatly reduce time to re-epithelialisation, even though the effect on culture cure was not found to be significantly different from placebo.[184]

MELISSA OFFICINALIS (LEMON BALM)

Melissa officinalis has been traditionally prescribed for its antibacterial and antiviral activity. Experimental studies indicate that the aqueous extract of *Melissa officinalis* is particularly effective against herpes simplex virus type 1.[185] This activity is partly supported by findings from an RCT in 66 patients with recurrent herpes labialis. The authors observed that 1% lemon balm cream applied to the lesions four times daily for 5 days significantly reduced lesion size, severity of symptoms and duration of healing when compared with placebo.[186]

ZINGIBER OFFICINALE (GINGER)

Zingiber officinale was traditionally prescribed as a digestive and circulatory stimulant, for the purpose of increasing the bioavailability of simultaneously administered herbs. The essential oil of ginger also demonstrates virucidal activity against aciclovir-resistant herpes simplex virus type 1,[187] although clinical evidence of this effect is lacking.

LIFESTYLE RECOMMENDATIONS

As highlighted previously, there are a number of factors that can increase an individual's susceptibility to infection. One of these risk factors is emotional stress. Experimental studies have demonstrated that exposure to psychological stress elevates endogenous glucocorticoid production, resulting in decreased synthesis of epidermal antimicrobial peptides,[188] interferon-β and interferon-γ.[189] It has been observed that reduced expression of the latter impairs the host's ability to control herpes simplex virus replication, resulting in prolongation of the infectious period.[189] These impairments in nonspecific immunity are further compounded by changes in skin integrity, with psychological stress contributing to a reduction in epidermal cell proliferation and differentiation, and corneodesmosome density and size.[190] Stress therefore compromises the ability of the integumentary system to protect the body against pathogenic invasion.

Stress reduction

Given the reported association between stress and immune function, it would be reasonable to assume that the prevention and management of skin infection should incorporate appropriate strategies to combat stress. Even so, evidence to date is somewhat limited. A systematic review of sixteen studies (including RCTs, controlled trials and retrospective case-control studies) indicated tai chi may be effective in improving cell-mediated immunity (including lymphocyte and natural killer cell activity), and antibody response (including IgG and IgA concentration), although the effects on clinical outcomes were inconclusive.[191] Another study involving 62 HIV-positive men showed that 10 weeks of a cognitive–behavioural stress-management intervention significantly reduced herpes simplex virus type 2 antibody titres when compared with a waiting list control group, suggesting that the intervention group had greater cellular control over HSV infection.[192] While there is theoretical justification for using stress-reduction techniques in the management of skin infection, there is limited clinical evidence to support their use.

CASE STUDY

OVERVIEW

PM, a 32-year-old female, presented to the clinic seeking treatment for herpes labialis. The lesions had been recurrent over the past 9 months, with outbreaks occurring every 2–3 months. The lesions were preceded by tingling, and once manifested were painful and itchy. The duration from tingling to full epithelialisation was approximately 2 weeks. She stated that the lesions manifested only when she was overly stressed, and were temporarily relieved by ice. The patient's medical and surgical history was unremarkable, although the patient did self-administer a daily vitamin B complex capsule for stress. She was of normal weight (BMI 24) and was a non-smoker, and consumed 2–3 glasses of white wine most weekends.

CLINICAL EXAMINATION

Two crops of three vesicles on the left superior and left inferior lips, along the vermillion border. Underlying erythema and mild oedema evident, and mild submandibular lymphadenopathy and malaise.

TREATMENT PROTOCOL

INITIAL APPOINTMENT

Following the completion of a comprehensive clinical assessment, the overall treatment goal for the patient was to prevent further outbreaks of herpes simplex over the next 6 months. In order to achieve this goal, the following interventions were implemented.

HERBAL MEDICINE

A suitable immunostimulant herbal formula for the management of skin infections is listed below. The

CASE STUDY CONTINUED

recommended adult dose for this oral formula is 5 mL b.i.d. before meals.

Herbal medicine	Quantity	
Echinacea purpurea	1:2 liquid extract	35 mL
Andrographis paniculata	1:2 liquid extract	30 mL
Zingiber officinale	1:2 liquid extract	5 mL

NUTRITIONAL MEDICINE

Dietary

Maintain a well-balanced diet by consuming at least seven servings of fruit and vegetables daily; five servings of wholegrain cereals daily; lean beef/lamb/poultry/pork 3 times weekly; and lean seafood 3 times weekly. Reduce the consumption of arginine-rich foods, such as nuts, seeds and chocolate, to increase the dietary lysine:arginine ratio.

Supplemental

Lysine 1000 mg b.i.d., and apply zinc acetate, zinc oxide or zinc sulfide solution to the lesions every 2 hours until resolved.

LIFESTYLE/EDUCATION

Walk for 20–30 minutes/day; perform tai chi, relaxation, guided imagery or yoga for 30 minutes/day.

FOLLOW-UP

Review the patient once a fortnight to monitor patient compliance with the management plan, clinical progress and the effectiveness of the prescribed interventions.

LEG ULCERATIONS

Epidemiology

Leg ulcers affect around 0.6% of the Western population,[193] and are most prevalent in females and the elderly, with incidence increasing with advancing age.

Classification

Leg ulceration is defined as a chronic, often recurring, wound of the lower leg, which has been present for more than 4 weeks.

Aetiology

There are many underlying causes of leg ulceration. Factors that contribute to the development of leg ulcers, however, vary according to ulcer type. The most common aetiologies are chronic venous insufficiency, arterial insufficiency and neuropathy. Less common causes include lymphoedema, trauma, pressure, malignancy and infection.

VENOUS ULCERS

Venous leg ulceration can be attributed to events that damage vein or valve integrity. Deep vein thrombosis, congenital defects, lower leg fractures or surgery, pregnancy and leg trauma are examples of such events. Subsequent damage to the venous system can lead to venous insufficiency, initiating the development of venous hypertension, endothelial dysfunction, tissue destruction and ulceration.[193]

ARTERIAL ULCERS

Arterial ulceration is primarily caused by atherosclerotic changes to the arteries, although it can be attributed to other disorders such as thalassaemia, sickle cell disease, vasculitis and thromboangiitis.[194] The risk factors that contribute to the development of atherosclerosis are the same as those that play a role in the pathogenesis of coronary heart disease, including smoking, sedentary lifestyle, obesity, high sodium intake, dyslipidaemia, diabetes, hypertension and family history.[194]

NEUROPATHIC ULCERS

The underlying cause of neuropathic ulceration is peripheral neuropathy, which is often associated with diabetes mellitus, but can also be attributed to alcoholism, leprosy, chemotherapy, nutritional deficiencies, autoimmune disorders, heavy metal toxicity, ischaemia or nerve injury.[195] The absent or impaired sensation to the foot makes it difficult for individuals to identify when an injury occurs, and thus undetected skin changes can rapidly become chronic ulcers.

SIGNS AND SYMPTOMS

Every aetiology of leg ulceration is closely associated with a characteristic set of clinical manifestations. Venous leg ulcers, for example, are generally sloughy, shallow, have moderate exudate, and are located in the gaiter area of the leg (Fig. 16.6). Symptoms of venous insufficiency, such as ochre pigmentation, varicose veins and leg oedema, may also accompany these ulcers.[193]

Arterial ulcers, on the other hand, are painful, have minimal exudate and demarcated borders, and are located

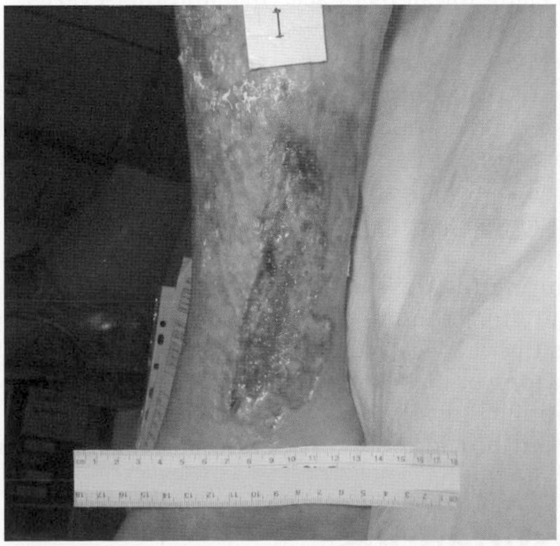

FIGURE 16.6 Venous leg ulcer of the left lateral gaiter area.

in the distal lower leg, foot and/or toes. In these ulcers, signs of arterial insufficiency may be present, including faint pedal pulses, absence of lower limb hair, cool skin temperature, and pale, dusky skin tone.[194]

Neuropathic ulcers differ again, in that they give minimal to no pain, and are often located on the toes and sole of the foot. The presence of paraesthesia and altered sensation, as well as warm skin temperature, may further support a neuropathic aetiology.

In addition to these physical manifestations, leg ulceration is associated with significant psychosocial and financial implications, including depression, anxiety, social isolation, immobility and unemployment.[193]

DIFFERENTIAL DIAGNOSIS

Leg ulceration has a number of differential diagnoses depending on the age of the patient.

- Children: scalded skin syndrome, physical abuse, ulcerating impetigo, cutaneous vasculitis and epidermolysis bullosa
- Adults: syphilis, lupus vulgaris/tuberculous, yaws (a tropical skin infection due to *Treponema pertenue*), pyoderma gangrenosum, ulcerating impetigo, physical abuse, squamous skin carcinoma and systemic lupus erythematosus.

Naturopathic diagnosis

INSPECTION AND PALPATION OF THE SKIN

Inspection of the skin should be conducted under natural light with close attention paid to the following aspects:

- Colour — general pigmentation, widespread colour change, pallor, erythema, cyanosis and jaundice
- Temperature — note in particular any heated, inflamed, red areas, as these may be infected
- Moisture — inspect for signs of dehydration (e.g. dry, cracked, flaky skin), and look for areas of pus or infection; note their severity, and treat/refer accordingly
- Texture — look at the general texture of the skin, especially for signs of scarring, and the severity of this
- Thickness — pay attention to the depth of the ulcer
- Area of distribution — note the area(s) affected, and make detailed notes on the number and nature of the ulcer(s) in each area, and their diameter
- Oedema — look for signs of oedema, both proximal to the ulcer and on peripheral areas of the limbs.

The more detail that is reported in the patient's case notes during the physical examination, the greater is the possibility for both the practitioner and the patient to note any positive or negative effects of treatment over time. Photographs of ulcers can be a reliable method for monitoring clinical progress also, but it is important that the patient provides express permission for the taking of such photographs.

Investigations

A number of diagnostic investigations can be used to determine the aetiology of a leg ulcer. These tests can assist the practitioner in making a decision about the most appropriate course of treatment.

CONTINUOUS WAVE DOPPLER ULTRASONOGRAPHY

The ankle brachial pressure index (ABPI) is a useful screening tool for arterial insufficiency. A hand-held, continuous-wave Doppler probe is used to measure the systolic blood pressure at the feet/ankles and the arms. A ratio closest to 1.0 indicates that the two blood pressures are similar, while an ABPI below 0.8 is suggestive of arterial impairment of the lower extremities,[196] and an index above 1.3 indicates non-compressible arteries, often of diabetic origin.[197]

VENOUS DUPLEX IMAGING

A more advanced diagnostic method is venous duplex imaging, which uses ultrasound to assess blood flow direction and velocity.[198] This non-invasive test can also be used to identify incompetent valves and to visualise areas of narrowing or occlusion.[198] Such information is particularly useful in detecting the presence of chronic venous insufficiency.

ELECTRONEUROGRAPHY

For neuropathic ulceration, the presence of neuropathy can be confirmed using electroneurography, or nerve conduction studies. In this procedure, electrodes are placed on the skin surface over the nerve of interest and a stimulus applied. The time required for the impulse to travel from the proximal electrode to the distal electrode is measured in metres per second. A significant decrease in the conduction velocity of the nerve can indicate peripheral nerve injury or disease, such as diabetic neuropathy.[198]

SKIN BIOPSY

To rule out dysplasia as the cause of ulceration, skin biopsy may be performed, whereby a small sample of the lesion or wound is excised and microscopically examined. Cancerous lesions that may manifest as chronic leg ulcers include basal cell carcinoma and squamous cell carcinoma.[6]

CULTURE AND SENSITIVITY

For recalcitrant wounds or suspected wound infection, the ulcer can be wiped with a sterile swab, which is then sent to a pathology laboratory in an appropriate transport medium. By culturing the specimen in a suitable growth medium, sufficient numbers of the organisms can be isolated, so that the type and quantity of bacteria present, as well as the antibiotics the bacterial strains are sensitive or resistant to, can be determined.[198]

Therapeutic considerations

There are a number of factors that are associated with delayed wound healing, and these should be borne in mind when developing an overall plan of care. Factors suspected of delaying wound closure include cigarette smoking, alcohol, advancing age, malnutrition and psychosomatic stress.[199] Certain interventions are also known to have adverse effects on wound healing, including corticosteroids, radiotherapy and immunosuppressive agents. Diabetes is another condition that may contribute to the development of ulceration, as well as to delays in wound closure, due to ischaemic, neuropathic and/or structural changes. A condition closely associated with the pathogenesis of type 2 diabetes is obesity, which may also compromise wound closure by increasing tissue tension, reducing vascular perfusion and tissue oxygenation, and increasing the risk of infection.[200]

CLINICAL DECISION MAKING AND RATIONALE

It is vital that the naturopathic practitioner work with other members of the patient's healthcare team (e.g. general practitioner, community nurse, physiotherapist) to ensure that the patient receives the best possible outcome.

If the ulceration is a secondary condition, it is important that the practitioner assist the patient to address the primary condition (e.g. diabetes). Patients with serious circulatory conditions should be referred to their general practitioner for further testing.

Therapeutic application

NATUROPATHIC PERSPECTIVE

Once the aetiology of the wound has been identified, an overall plan of care can be developed. When constructing the care plan the four naturopathic principles for managing integumentary system disorders highlighted earlier in this chapter should be borne in mind. To elaborate, the management of leg ulceration should identify and address all factors contributing to the pathogenesis of ulceration, including any factor known to delay wound healing. Addressing these factors should, in theory, reduce the risk of ulcer recurrence, and therefore accomplish the role of prevention. The treatment approach should also facilitate wound healing without causing unnecessary discomfort or burden for the individual. This approach should consider not only oral and topically administered therapies, but also appropriate lifestyle interventions.

NUTRITIONAL MEDICINE (DIETARY)

Therapeutic objectives

Given that nutritional deficiencies can contribute to the pathogenesis of leg ulceration, as well as delays in wound healing, a detailed dietary plan is fundamental to the successful management of this condition. Appropriate objectives for the dietary management of leg ulceration should therefore be followed. Focusing on the nutritional goals highlighted in Section A of this chapter, these objectives include:

1. Reduce sodium, saturated fat, and sugar intake as these may contribute to or exacerbate arterial insufficiency and advanced glycation end products
2. Increase fibre intake to improve glycaemic control, attenuate atherogenesis and reduce venous hypertension
3. Increase fruit and vegetable consumption as this will augment ascorbic acid, β-carotene, pantothenic acid, silicon and vitamin E intake
4. Increase nut and seed consumption as this will improve arginine, copper, leucine, pantothenic acid, vitamin E and zinc intake
5. Increase wholegrain consumption as this will increase arginine, leucine, lysine, pantothenic acid, silicon, vitamin E and zinc intake
6. Increase lean meat consumption as this will improve glycine, leucine, lysine, vitamin E and zinc intake
7. Increase seafood consumption as this will augment copper, glycine, leucine, lysine, pantothenic acid and zinc intake.

Specific treatments

Adherence to a well-balanced diet, with a particular focus on diversity and nutrient density, should satisfy the above dietary objectives. For example, avoiding processed, takeaway and pre-prepared meals, and focusing on the preparation and consumption of wholefoods will help to reduce the intake of sodium, saturated fat and added sugar. Consuming a diverse range of nuts, wholegrain cereals, lean meats and seafood, on the other hand, will increase micronutrient intake, as well as protein ingestion, which is essential for cell division, immunity, and the production of collagen, keratin and elastin for skin integrity. The increased consumption of wholegrain cereals, and fruits and vegetables will also help to increase fibre intake.

An example of a daily diet that complies with the dietary treatment objectives for individuals with leg ulceration is given below.

NUTRITIONAL MEDICINE (SUPPLEMENTAL)

Therapeutic objectives

In the event that an individual is unable to comply with dietary recommendations, where nutritional deficiency is unlikely to be adequately addressed by diet alone, or where higher than normal doses of specific nutrients are required, the practitioner may consider nutritional supplementation. When nutritional supplementation is warranted, the following objectives for managing leg ulceration need to be considered:

1. Facilitate collagen formation by increasing serum and tissue levels of ascorbic acid, β-carotene, copper, glycine, lysine and silicon
2. Aid protein synthesis by increasing serum and tissue levels of arginine, lysine and zinc
3. Facilitate angiogenesis by increasing serum and tissue levels of ascorbic acid, copper and vitamin E
4. Support local and systemic immunity by increasing serum and tissue levels of arginine, ascorbic acid, β-carotene, pantothenic acid and zinc
5. Facilitate cell proliferation by increasing serum and tissue levels of arginine, β-carotene and pantothenic acid.

SAMPLE DAILY DIET

BREAKFAST	
Immune boosting juice: carrot, celery, ginger and turmeric Sardines on toast	Ginger and turmeric are anti-inflammatory spices that can be used to manage chronic inflammation, reducing tissue destruction. Both ginger and turmeric are antimicrobial, helping to prevent wound infection, while ginger also functions as a circulatory stimulant to aid venous flow for improved nutrient transfer to the area. Leg ulcers are commonly seen in individuals with diabetes; thus adding a source of protein and healthy fats in the form of the sardines to have in combination with the juice helps to ensure stable blood sugar levels.
LUNCH	
Sweet potato and carrot soup with a garlic, pumpkin seed and rocket pesto Serve with toast	Sweet potato and carrots provide a source of beta-carotene to aid skin healing and repair. The garlic in the pesto provides immune and antimicrobial properties designed to stimulate the immune system and prevent infection, while the addition of the pumpkin seeds provides a source of zinc which is required for collagen synthesis, wound healing and immunity.
DINNER	
Shakshuka (eggs, poached in a spicy tomato, onion and garlic sauce with crumbled feta and parsley)	Eggs provide an easy-to-digest protein. Adequate protein is required to obtain the amino acids such as glycine and leucine which are involved in synthesis of collagen. The addition of onions and garlic provides immune support and prevents microbial replication, while a small quantity of chilli improves circulation, reducing discomfort.
SNACK	
Ample fresh fruit and vegetables Oat and cinnamon slice	Fresh fruit and vegetables stimulate immune function and aid wound healing and repair. Oats are a source of silica which is required for collagen synthesis.

Specific nutrients required

β-CAROTENE AND VITAMIN A

β-carotene and vitamin A are necessary for epithelial cell differentiation, collagen synthesis, phagocytosis, antibody production and intercellular adhesion.[16] A double-blind RCT of 40 patients who had undergone photorefractive keratectomy showed that retinol palmitate 25 000 IU and α-tocopherol 230 mg, administered 3 times daily for 30 days and twice daily for 60 days, significantly decreased corneal re-epithelialisation time when compared with controls ($p = 0.03$).[201] Even so, the clinical effect of vitamin A or β-carotene in chronic wounds requires investigation.

VITAMIN B_5

Pantothenic acid promotes fibroblast proliferation and improves the wound-breaking strength of surgical wounds in rabbits.[202] A double-blind RCT has demonstrated that a combination of pantothenic acid 200 mg/day and ascorbic acid 1 g/day for 21 days increased fibroblast proliferation in acute tattoo resections.[203] However, there is insufficient clinical evidence to support the use of vitamin B_5 in chronic leg ulceration.

VITAMIN C

Ascorbic acid is responsible for angiogenesis and immunomodulation, as well as the synthesis of collagen, which is a key component of connective tissue. In spite of these actions, there is inconclusive evidence to support the administration of vitamin C alone in chronic wounds, with two controlled trials on ascorbic acid and pressure ulceration[204,205] demonstrating conflicting results. While more recent trials suggest multi-nutrient supplements may facilitate healing of chronic wounds, it is not possible to separate the effects of vitamin C from the other nutrients in these formulations.

VITAMIN E

Vitamin E is claimed to promote wound healing and angiogenesis, as well as reduce scarring,[206] although the specific mechanisms of action are not clear. The effect of vitamin E on skin ulcers is also uncertain, with only one randomised controlled trial identified. This study of 27 patients with systemic sclerosis-associated digital ulcers found alpha-tocopherol gel applied twice a week resulted in a significantly greater reduction in ulcer healing time and ulcer pain than standard ulcer care.[207] Further investigation should determine whether these effects can be demonstrated with supplemental vitamin E.

COPPER

Copper is required for angiogenesis, and is a cofactor for two important enzymes, including tyrosinase for melanin formation, and lysyl oxidase for the cross-linking of collagen and elastin in connective tissue.[166] Despite these important effects, and the number of experimental studies that have investigated the role of copper in wound healing, there is a paucity of clinical evidence to support these data, and thus more research is required.

SILICA

Silica is needed for the enzyme prolyl hydroxylase, which is responsible for collagen synthesis.[208] While there are several non-adherent, silicon-containing dressings available on the market, it is not yet clear if silicon in either topical or oral form has any effect on wound healing in humans.

ZINC

Zinc is involved in protein synthesis, nonspecific and specific immunity, and wound healing. Despite these effects, a Cochrane review of six RCTs found orally administered zinc sulfate to be no more effective than placebo in facilitating healing of arterial and venous leg ulcers.[209] It could be argued that topical applications of zinc may be more effective than oral zinc in facilitating wound healing due to its localised anti-inflammatory, autodebridement and anti-infective activity.[210] Notwithstanding, a systematic review of eight RCTs found little difference in wound healing rates between venous leg ulcers treated with topical zinc versus other dressings;[211] however, given the methodological limitations of the included studies, more evidence is required to either confirm or refute the effectiveness of topical zinc in leg ulceration.

ARGININE

Arginine plays an important role in wound healing by promoting cell proliferation, collagen synthesis and antioxidant enzyme activity, and by reducing pro-inflammatory cytokine levels in the wound bed.[212] Even though numerous animal studies have demonstrated that arginine may facilitate wound healing, there is limited clinical evidence to support these data. In a small randomised controlled trial, arginine supplementation at a dosage of 4.5 g daily for 3 weeks was found to be as effective as a 9 g daily dose of arginine, but more effective than historical controls, in improving the rate of wound healing in 23 inpatients with stage II, III or IV pressure ulceration.[213] Notwithstanding, the methodological limitations of this study prevent any firm conclusions from being made. Also, the findings of this study do not shed any light on the wound healing effects of arginine in chronic leg ulceration. While a number of trials do suggest that multi-nutrient supplements containing arginine may facilitate the healing of chronic wounds, it is not possible to separate the effects of arginine from the other nutrients in these formulations; consequently, the clinical effectiveness of arginine for leg ulceration remains unclear.

GLYCINE

Glycine is a major component of collagen, and plays an important role in protein synthesis. However, there is insufficient clinical evidence to support the use of supplemental glycine alone in leg ulceration.

LEUCINE

Leucine plays an important role in collagen synthesis. Nonetheless, there is insufficient clinical evidence to support the use of supplemental glycine alone in chronic wounds.

LYSINE

Lysine is required for the formation of collagen and protein. Lending support to the wound healing effect of lysine are the findings of a double-blind randomised controlled trial of 50 hospitalised patients with decubitus ulcers; the trial found the topical application of lysine hyaluronate for 15 days to be significantly more effective than sodium hyaluronate in reducing ulcer size.[214] While these effects are promising, they do not shed any light on the clinical effectiveness of supplemental lysine for leg ulceration.

Dosage requirements

The dosage requirements listed below are based on adult doses used in clinical trials. Where clinical data are absent or insufficient the doses are those reported in the literature.[38,39,166]

- Arginine 500 mg b.i.d.
- Ascorbic acid 250 mg q.i.d.
- β-carotene 15 mg b.i.d.
- Copper 2 mg/day
- Glycine 500 mg b.i.d.
- Leucine 500 mg b.i.d.
- Lysine 500 mg b.i.d.
- Pantothenic acid 100 mg b.i.d.
- Silica 25 mg/day
- Vitamin E 400–800 IU/day
- Zinc 25–80 mg/day

HERBAL MEDICINE

Therapeutic objectives

The integration of herbal medicine within a naturopathic treatment plan allows the practitioner to deliver a more targeted approach to leg ulceration. Furthermore, when herbal medicine is integrated appropriately (i.e. without compromising the principles of naturopathic care), the treatment approach will be delivered more holistically. Thus, in order for practitioners to safely and effectively manage leg ulceration using herbal medicine, the following treatment objectives should be considered:

1. Identify and treat the cause of leg ulceration to prevent unnecessary delays in wound healing as well as ulcer recurrence
2. Enhance specific and nonspecific immunity to prevent wound infection
3. Manage chronic inflammation to minimise unnecessary discomfort and tissue destruction
4. Reduce microbial replication to prevent unwanted tissue destruction, inflammation, pain and scarring
5. Facilitate wound healing to reduce pain, disability and risk of infection
6. Manage associated symptoms of leg ulceration to reduce discomfort and improve wellbeing.

Herbal medicine classes

The herbal medicine classes that are indicated for the management of leg ulceration are anti-inflammatories, antibacterials, demulcents, immunostimulants, venotonics and vulneraries. Definitions of these terms can be found in Section A of this chapter. The term 'venotonic', which is not listed in Section A, is defined as an agent that improves venous tone or integrity. These agents are specifically indicated for chronic venous insufficiency. While there are a number of additional approaches that need to be considered in the management of other leg ulcer types, it is beyond the scope of this chapter to discuss these. A more detailed approach to these underlying conditions, such as diabetes and peripheral vascular disease, can be found elsewhere in this book.

Specific herbal medicines

There are many herbs that demonstrate at least one of the actions mentioned above. However, it would not be useful for the busy practitioner to list all these herbs here. Instead, only those herbs that have been investigated clinically or that exhibit several of the abovementioned activities are listed below.

AESCULUS HIPPOCASTANUM (HORSE CHESTNUT)

Aesculus hippocastanum demonstrates venotonic, anti-inflammatory, and anti-oedemic activity. A Cochrane review of 17 RCTs found oral horse chestnut seed extract (HCSE), standardised to 100–150 mg/day aescin, was superior to placebo in all placebo-controlled trials, and at least equally effective as reference medications (in four out of five studies) at reducing lower leg volume, oedema, calf and ankle circumference, pain and pruritus.[215] In relation to leg ulceration, an RCT involving 54 patients with venous leg ulceration showed that 12 weeks of oral HCSE treatment (standardised to 150 mg/day aescin) significantly reduced the percentage of wound slough ($p = 0.045$) and the number of dressing changes ($p = 0.009$) compared with placebo.[216] However, there was no significant difference between groups with regard to changes in wound surface area, depth, volume, pain or exudation, possibly due to the insufficient power of the trial.

ALOE BARBADENSIS (ALOE)

Aloe barbadensis exhibits vulnerary, anti-inflammatory, immunostimulant and antibacterial effects. Nonetheless, there is conflicting evidence to support the use of *Aloe* in wound care. For instance, aloe vera gel was found to be no more effective than saline-soaked gauze dressings in 30 patients with pressure ulceration[217] or simple dressings in 90 women with caesarean-section incisions.[218] Yet, aloe gel dressings were associated with a significantly faster rate of wound healing in 17 patients who had undergone facial dermabrasion[219] and 60 patients with chronic ulcers[220] when compared with controls. The inconsistencies in the evidence highlight the need for further scientific investigation.

CALENDULA OFFICINALIS (CALENDULA)

Calendula officinalis displays vulnerary, anti-inflammatory, immunostimulant and antibacterial activity. A systematic review of six RCTs found only weak evidence to support the topical administration of *Calendula* in acute and chronic wounds, suggesting that further investigation is needed.[221]

CENTELLA ASIATICA (GOTU KOLA)

Centella asiatica exhibits vulnerary, venotonic and peripheral vasodilatory effects. Despite the number of experimental studies supporting the wound-healing effect of gotu kola, few clinical data are available. In one open-label trial of 20 patients, topical application of a *C. asiatica* extract and essential oil formulation for 6 weeks prevented wound infection in 75% of contaminated wounds, while healing 64% of all acute and chronic wounds.[49] In an RCT involving 200 diabetic patients with chronic infective wounds, oral *C. asiatica* extract (equivalent to 300 mg asiaticoside daily) was found to be more effective than placebo at improving wound contraction, but less effective than placebo in facilitating granulation tissue formation.[222]

MATRICARIA RECUTITA (CHAMOMILE)

Matricaria recutita demonstrates anti-inflammatory, immunostimulant, antibacterial and mild sedative properties. Two controlled trials have found chamomile extract, when applied 2 to 3 times daily for 2 weeks, to be significantly more effective than controls at reducing wound healing time in post-dermabrasion of the arm,[223] and in peristomal skin breakdown.[224] However, the effect of chamomile extract in these acute wounds cannot be extrapolated to chronic leg ulcers, and therefore, warrants further investigation.

ECHINACEA SPP. (ECHINACEA)

Echinacea spp. exhibit anti-inflammatory, immunostimulant and antibacterial effects. While data from animal studies indicate that topical applications of *Echinacea purpurea* may facilitate wound healing, there is a paucity of clinical evidence to support these data.

HYDRASTIS CANADENSIS (GOLDENSEAL)

Hydrastis canadensis displays vulnerary, anti-inflammatory, immunostimulant and antibacterial activity. However, there is a paucity of experimental and clinical data to support the administration of goldenseal in leg ulceration.

HYPERICUM PERFORATUM (ST JOHN'S WORT)

Hypericum perforatum demonstrates vulnerary, anti-inflammatory and analgesic properties. A double-blind RCT of 144 patients with incisional wounds from caesarean section found *H. perforatum* ointment, applied 3 times daily for 16 days, greatly improved wound healing at day 10, scar formation at day 40, and symptoms of wound pain and pruritus when compared with placebo ointment and no treatment.[225] While these findings support the wound healing effects of St John's wort for acute wounds, the effects of hypericum on chronic wound or leg ulcer healing is not yet known.

ZINGIBER OFFICINALE (GINGER)

Zingiber officinale has been traditionally prescribed as a digestive and circulatory stimulant, for the purpose of increasing the bioavailability of simultaneously administered herbs. Even though ginger has been shown to increase drug absorption and plasma half-life in rabbits,[97] clinical evidence is lacking.

LIFESTYLE RECOMMENDATIONS

The management of leg ulceration would not be complete without due consideration of appropriate lifestyle interventions. These interventions are important not only in facilitating wound closure, but also in addressing the many factors that impede wound healing. The cessation of smoking and a reduction in alcohol intake, for instance, can resolve two common risk factors that are associated not only with the pathogenesis of arterial insufficiency and ulceration, but also with delays in wound healing. As for venous insufficiency, the oedema and leg pain associated with this condition may be managed through appropriately applied compression therapy, massage and leg elevation.[193] For all skin disorders, it is also critical that normal skin function is maintained through appropriate hygiene practices, adequate hydration and suitable clothing.

Physical activity

Physical activity plays an important role in wound management. Apart from facilitating weight loss where being overweight or obesity is an associated risk factor, exercise may also improve arterial perfusion, tissue oxygenation, venous return and wound healing. A small 12-week RCT of 13 older adults with active venous leg ulceration reported higher rates of completely healed ulcers and greater reductions in ulcer area in those participating in a home-based progressive resistance exercise program compared to those receiving usual care; however, the differences between groups were not statistically significant, possibly because the study was underpowered.[226] Much larger trials are needed to determine whether these trends towards improvement translate into significant improvements in wound healing.

Stress

The adverse effects of stress on ulcer healing may also be addressed through the implementation of suitable stress-management strategies, including meditation, tai chi, yoga, music therapy, aromatherapy and progressive muscle relaxation. Apart from relaxation, guided imagery[227] and biofeedback,[228] however, there is a dearth of evidence linking stress reduction to improvements in wound healing.

CASE STUDY

OVERVIEW

HS, a 76-year-old female, presented to the clinic requesting treatment advice for a leg ulcer. Apart from being prescribed aspirin 100 mg/day and sotalol 320 mg in the morning for the management of atrial fibrillation, she self-administered paracetamol 1000 mg at night. She did not smoke or consume alcohol, but was obese (BMI 33). She had received wound care from a district nursing service twice weekly for the last 12 months, but due to the slow rate of wound healing is seeking alternative options to facilitate wound closure.

CLINICAL EXAMINATION

The patient reports a history of atrial fibrillation, eczema, lymphoedema and a two-vessel cardiac angioplasty. On closer examination, the patient is found to have a shallow (1 mm) venous ulcer to the right medioposterior gaiter. The ulcer is predominantly sloughy (89%), causes little pain (pain score 3/10) and is surrounded by macerated tissue. The wound has been active for the past 12 months, and is one of eight ulcer episodes that have developed over the last 5 years.

TREATMENT PROTOCOL

INITIAL APPOINTMENT

The overall treatment goal for HS was to completely heal the leg ulcer within 6 months. In order to achieve this goal, the following interventions were implemented.

HERBAL MEDICINE

A suitable herbal formula for the management of venous leg ulceration is listed below. The recommended adult dose for this oral formula is 7.5 mL b.i.d. before meals.

Herbal medicine	Quantity	
Aesculus hippocastanum	1:2 liquid extract	30 mL
Echinacea purpurea	1:2 liquid extract	30 mL
Centella asiatica	1:2 liquid extract	30 mL
Zingiber officinale	1:2 liquid extract	10 mL

Apply 10% *Calendula officinalis* ointment to the wound edges during dressing changes or, if the nursing service agrees, to the wound surface.

NUTRITIONAL MEDICINE

Dietary

Consume at least seven servings of fruit and vegetables, five servings of wholegrain cereals and one to two servings of nuts and seeds daily; as well as lean beef/lamb/poultry/pork 3 times weekly and lean seafood 3 times weekly.

Supplemental

Administer a nutritional supplement that provides at least 30 mg β-carotene, 1000 mg ascorbic acid, 400 IU α-tocopherol and 200 mg pantothenic acid as a daily dose.

CASE STUDY CONTINUED

LIFESTYLE/EDUCATION

Walk 20–30 minutes every second day, increasing the duration and frequency of walking when exercise tolerance improves; elevate legs above heart level for a total of 2 hours during waking hours; avoid prolonged periods of standing; perform relaxation and guided imagery techniques for 30 minutes every 1–2 days.

FOLLOW-UP

Review the wound and the patient once a month so that compliance with the management plan, clinical progress and the effectiveness of the prescribed interventions can be monitored.

URTICARIA

Epidemiology

This self-limiting condition can affect individuals of all ages, and may first appear in childhood or at any time during adulthood.[8]

Classification

Urticaria, or hives, is a transient, immunological condition that affects the dermal layer of the skin. A more severe form of the condition is angio-oedema, which involves both the dermis and the subcutaneous layer of the skin. Depending on the duration of the condition, urticaria may be defined as acute (<6 weeks) or chronic (>6 weeks), with acute urticaria representing 70% of all urticaria cases.[6] (See Fig. 16.7.)

Aetiology

Urticaria is generally triggered by an allergic or non-allergic cause, such as insect bites and stings, medications and foods. Medications often implicated in urticaria include penicillins, cephalosporins, aspirin, opiates, non-steroidal anti-inflammatory drugs (NSAIDs), vaccines, blood products and anaesthetics. Food triggers can include seafood, eggs, cow's milk, tree nuts, wheat, spices, bananas, apples, oranges, potatoes, parsley, carrots, beans and food additives.[5] In all cases, these factors trigger cutaneous mast cell degranulation, resulting in the release of histamine and inflammatory cytokines, causing capillary vasodilation and increased vascular permeability, and the subsequent manifestation of histamine- and inflammation-related effects,[8] as detailed below.

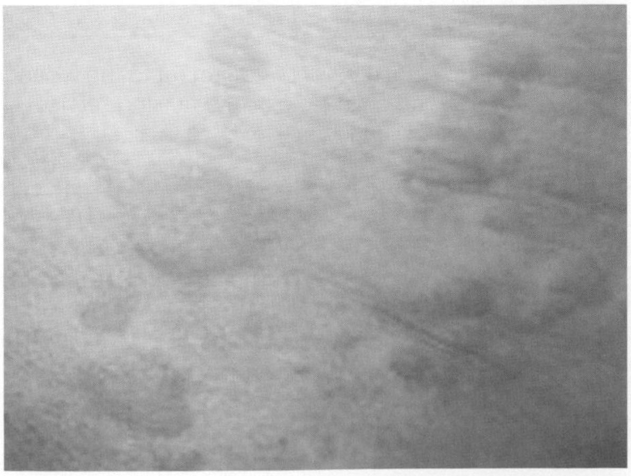

FIGURE 16.7 Urticaria.
Source: © DermNet New Zealand

NON-ALLERGIC TRIGGERS

Apart from the primary causes highlighted above, there are a number of additional factors that may contribute to the development of urticaria. These non-allergic triggers of mast cell degranulation include emotional stress, heat, extreme cold, fever, perspiration, exercise, sunlight, water, alcohol, pressure and friction, including stroking or rubbing of the skin.[61] Even though the underlying mechanisms of these physical urticarias remain poorly elucidated, the existence of mast cells with heightened sensitivity to environmental stimuli may be a causal factor.[228]

Urticaria can also be triggered by *Candida* sensitivity, menstruation and viral infection.[8,229] Elevated progesterone levels may be a contributing factor in the pathogenesis of menstrual- and/or pregnancy-induced urticaria,[8] although the evidence for such a relationship is weak.

SIGNS AND SYMPTOMS

The clinical manifestations of urticaria can be grouped into local and systemic symptoms. Locally, urticaria presents as a triad of signs and symptoms, which include pruritus, erythema, and a circumscribed area of oedema known as 'wheals'. In most cases, these symptoms resolve within 24 hours.[8] Systemic manifestations can include malaise, dizziness, vomiting, diarrhoea, wheezing, abdominal pain and arthralgia.[8] Collectively, these symptoms can have a profound effect on individual wellbeing due to sleep deprivation, poor self-image and self-esteem, depression and anxiety.

Complications

Complications can occur due to the allergic aspect of this condition. If the patient shows signs of anaphylaxis, or severe allergic reactions, immediate medical assistance is required.

Differential diagnosis

While urticaria may appear to be a relatively benign disorder, the condition can be associated with several severe disease states. As such, the practitioner should consider the following differential diagnoses when completing a clinical assessment of urticaria: mastocytosis, vasculitis, erythema multiforme, bullous pemphigoid, viral infection, rubella, hepatitis, Schnitzler's syndrome, Muckle–Wells syndrome and infectious mononucleosis.[8,61]

Naturopathic diagnosis

INSPECTION AND PALPATION OF THE SKIN

Inspection of the skin should be conducted under natural light with close attention paid to the following aspects:

- Colour — general pigmentation, widespread colour change, pallor, erythema, cyanosis and jaundice
- Temperature — palpate the lesions to feel for raised temperature
- Moisture — inspect the lesions for the level of moisture/dryness, and note this; if pus is present, treat accordingly
- Texture — look at the general texture of the skin and compare this with the lesions
- Thickness — pay attention to the height of the lesions
- Area of distribution — note the area(s) affected, and make detailed notes on the number and nature of the lesion(s) in each area, and their general diameter
- Oedema — look for signs of oedema, both proximal to the lesions and in any surrounding areas.

The more detail that is reported in the patient's case notes during the physical examination, the greater is the possibility for both the practitioner and the patient to note any positive or negative effects of treatment over time. Photographs of lesions can be a reliable method for monitoring clinical progress also, but it is important that the patient provides express permission for the taking of such photographs.

Investigations

SPECIFIC NATUROPATHIC INVESTIGATIONS

There are no specific diagnostic investigations for urticaria. The cause of the condition, however, may be detected using one of a number of tests.

Immunoglobulin G4 (IgG4) food antibody testing indicates that an immunological response to a food component has occurred. However, the test is not indicative of food allergy or intolerance,[12] and therefore, may not be an appropriate measure in these conditions.

Immunoglobulin E (IgE) specific tests are another method of identifying allergies. Dermatological investigations, for instance, expose the skin of the patient to a number of suspected allergens. These diluted allergens can be administered topically as a patch test, injected intraepidermally as a prick-puncture test, or introduced intradermally. While these tests can be used to rapidly detect the presence of IgE-mediated allergies, they do not detect non-IgE-mediated allergies, and therefore may yield false-positive results in some individuals.[10] These tests are preferred over radioallergosorbent testing (RAST) and enzyme-linked immunosorbent assay (ELISA), however, as they are relatively less expensive and produce more immediate results.[6,11]

The eosinophil count is another test for detecting allergic disease. These white blood cells play a key role in the phagocytosis of antigen–antibody complexes, and proliferate in the presence of allergies. However, the eosinophil count can also rise in the presence of parasitic infection, myeloproliferative disorders, rheumatoid arthritis and Hodgkin's disease,[11] and therefore this measure does not conclusively confirm or refute allergy as a cause of urticaria.

Therapeutical considerations

CLINICAL DECISION MAKING AND RATIONALE

Consideration of the underlying cause of the condition is of primary importance, with a secondary focus on providing symptomatic relief for the patient. This will ensure that the patient is more likely to be compliant with any recommended dietary and lifestyle changes.

Therapeutic application

NATUROPATHIC PERSPECTIVE

The four naturopathic principles for treating integumentary system disorders, as highlighted in Section A of this chapter, are fundamental to the management of urticaria. The first principle, in particular, is of primary importance, as the identification and elimination of factors contributing to the pathogenesis of urticaria should minimise recurrence, as well as mitigate unnecessary physical and emotional distress to the patient. A comprehensive assessment of the patient's medical, family, environmental and clinical history, in conjunction with an elimination diet and/or food and lifestyle diary, will assist the practitioner in correctly identifying the triggers of urticaria. When medications or serious disease states are associated with the condition, the practitioner should refer the patient to their prescribing clinician or general practitioner for review.

NUTRITIONAL MEDICINE (DIETARY)

Therapeutic objectives

The dietary approach to urticaria should focus on two key goals: to exclude factors known to trigger or exacerbate the condition; and to maximise intake of nutrients with desirable therapeutic effects. To achieve these goals, appropriate objectives for the dietary management of urticaria should be followed. Drawing from the nutritional goals highlighted in Section A of this chapter, these objectives include:

1. Identify and eliminate artificial food colours, flavours and preservatives that may contribute to or exacerbate urticaria
2. Identify and eliminate foods that may trigger or aggravate urticaria
3. Increase consumption of seafood to increase vitamin B_{12} and omega-3 fatty acid intake
4. Increase consumption of fruits and vegetables to augment ascorbic acid, β-carotene, bioflavonoid and vitamin E intake
5. Increase consumption of low-allergenic nuts and seeds to improve niacin, omega-3 fatty acid and vitamin E intake
6. Increase lean meat consumption to improve niacin, vitamin B_{12} and vitamin E intake.

Specific treatments

To address objectives 1 and 2 above, the practitioner will need to commence an elimination or oligoantigenic diet. This diet will assist the clinician in establishing whether any dietary components are responsible for the pathogenesis of urticaria. While there are many variations to the elimination diet in terms of complexity, content and duration, the diet should always aim to minimise patient uncertainty, and maximise patient compliance. A simple approach to the elimination diet is to have a patient avoid all potentially allergenic foods for a minimum of 1 week, including cow's milk products, eggs, wheat, rye, barley, peanuts, corn, shellfish, bananas, apples, oranges, potatoes, parsley, carrots and soya beans, and any foods containing artificial colours, flavours or preservatives. After a 1-week elimination period, the patient can reintroduce a new food every 2 days and monitor the recurrence of urticarial symptoms. The presence or absence of any adverse reactions during this time should be recorded in a food and lifestyle diary, and reviewed at the next naturopathic consultation. The foods identified as being associated with urticaria should then be eliminated from the diet.

Other dietary considerations

Despite the long history of use of elimination diets in naturopathic practice, few studies have explored the clinical efficacy of these diets in urticaria. Several studies indicate that elimination diets may be helpful in improving the symptoms of chronic urticaria,[230,231] however not all studies report promising results.[232] These inconsistent findings do not allow any firm conclusions to be drawn about the effectiveness of elimination diets for urticaria.

An example of a daily diet that complies with the dietary treatment objectives for patients with urticaria is given below.

NUTRITIONAL MEDICINE (SUPPLEMENTAL)

Therapeutic objectives

In the event that an individual is unable to comply with dietary recommendations, where nutritional deficiency is unlikely to be adequately addressed by diet alone, or where higher than normal doses of nutrients are required, the practitioner may consider nutritional supplementation. When nutritional supplementation is warranted, the following objectives for treating urticaria need to be considered:

1. Reduce histamine release or mast cell activity by increasing serum and tissue levels of ascorbic acid, bioflavonoids, niacinamide, omega-3 fatty acids and vitamin E, and by consuming probiotics
2. Reduce tissue levels of arachidonic acid and proinflammatory cytokines by increasing serum and tissue levels of ascorbic acid, bioflavonoids, niacinamide, omega-3 fatty acids and vitamin E
3. Improve skin integrity by increasing serum and tissue levels of ascorbic acid, bioflavonoids, omega-3 fatty acids and vitamin E.

SAMPLE DAILY DIET

BREAKFAST	
Sweet potato toast (made by cutting sweet potato thinly and putting in the toaster) topped with ricotta and cinnamon	A gluten-free diet reduces the inflammation associated with urticaria, helping to decrease production of anti-IgE receptor antibodies. Instead of gluten-containing breads, sweet potato can be thinly sliced and used as a nutrient-rich bread alternative.
LUNCH	
Pumpkin and sage risotto	A pseudoallergen-free diet has been shown to reduce medication use and improve symptoms of urticaria. All vegetables are permitted on a pseudoallergen-free diet with the exception of artichokes, peas, mushrooms, rhubarb, spinach, tomatoes and tomato sauces, olives and peppers. Clients can improvise with other vegetables and grains which are less allergenic.
DINNER	
Miso-roasted chicken with ginger Asian-style stir-fried vegetables and rice noodles	Fish and crustaceans are prohibited on a pseudoallergen-free diet; however, other animal proteins such as lamb and chicken are permitted. Ample vegetables should be consumed to provide anti-inflammatory constituents to downregulate inflammatory mediators.
SNACK	
Pumpkin seeds with natural live yoghurt	Chronic urticaria is associated with disturbed intestinal permeability because a defective mucosal barrier promotes exposure to luminal content, triggering an immunological response that promotes intestinal inflammation. Pumpkin seeds are rich in zinc. Zinc modulates tight junctions in the gut while probiotics may help to ameliorate mucosal barrier dysfunction.

Michielan A, D'Incà R. Intestinal permeability in inflammatory bowel disease: pathogenesis, clinical evaluation, and therapy of leaky gut. Mediators Inflamm 2015; 2015:628157.

Specific nutrients required

VITAMIN C

Ascorbic acid levels were found to be inversely related to blood histamine levels in two small human studies,[233,234] although whether this is associated with improvements in the incidence or symptoms of urticaria is not yet certain.

VITAMIN E

Vitamin E has been shown to reduce wasp-venom-induced histamine and prostaglandin D_2 in vitro,[235] as well as serum IgE levels and associated pruritus in study participants.[24] However, the clinical effects of vitamin E supplementation in urticaria have not yet been established.

VITAMIN B_3

Niacinamide reduces inflammatory mediator release and mast cell histamine release in vivo.[119] However, the clinical effect of supplemental niacin in urticaria has not been explored.

VITAMIN B_{12}

Low vitamin B_{12} levels have been demonstrated in patients with chronic spontaneous urticaria relative to the general population.[236] Furthermore, when patients with urticaria are administered weekly intramuscular injections of 1000 micrograms vitamin B_{12} (as reported in two separate studies), the majority demonstrated symptomatic relief.[237,238] Even so, there is no recent evidence from well-designed RCTs to support these dated findings, demonstrating a need for current research.

PROBIOTICS

Lactobacilli spp., particularly *Lactobacillus brevis*, when consumed for 4 weeks, reduced IgE production and histamine secretion in mice.[239] However, there is no clinical evidence to show that probiotics reduce the incidence or severity of urticaria.

ESSENTIAL FATTY ACIDS

Omega-3 fatty acids have been shown to reduce inflammatory markers in epidemiological, observational and clinical study populations,[32] while α-linolenic acid has been shown in vitro to reduce histamine content as well as histamine release from antigen-stimulated cells.[240] Nevertheless, there is a paucity of clinical data to support the administration of omega-3 fatty acids in urticaria.

QUERCETIN

Quercetin has been shown in vitro and in vivo to reduce histamine release from mast cells.[36] However, whether this impacts on the clinical outcomes of urticaria requires further investigation.

RUTIN

Rutin inhibits histamine release from activated mast cells in vitro,[241] but whether rutin demonstrates symptomatic improvement in patients with urticaria is unclear.

Dosage requirements

The dosage requirements listed below are based on adult doses used in clinical trials. Where clinical data are absent or insufficient, the doses are based on those reported in the literature.[38,39,166]

- Ascorbic acid 250 mg q.i.d.
- Fish oil 3 g/day (equivalent to 720 mg DHA and 1080 mg EPA)
- *Lactobacillus* spp. probiotic 1×10^9 cfu/g daily
- Niacinamide 12 mg/day
- Quercetin 500 mg b.i.d.
- Rutin 500 mg b.i.d.
- Vitamin B_{12} 250–1000 micrograms/day
- Vitamin E 400–800 IU/day

HERBAL MEDICINE

Therapeutic objectives

The integration of herbal medicine within a naturopathic treatment plan allows the practitioner to deliver a more targeted approach to urticaria. Furthermore, when herbal medicine is integrated appropriately (i.e. without compromising the principles of naturopathic care), the treatment approach will be delivered more holistically. Thus, in order for practitioners to safely and effectively manage urticaria using herbal medicine, the following treatment objectives should be considered:

1. Identify and treat the cause of urticaria to prevent exacerbation and recurrence
2. Manage inflammation to minimise unnecessary discomfort and tissue destruction
3. Reduce mast cell activity to decrease pruritus and oedema, and associated scratch-induced skin trauma
4. Manage associated symptoms of urticaria to reduce discomfort and improve wellbeing.

Herbal medicine classes

The herbal medicine classes that are indicated for the management of urticaria are the antiallergics, anti-inflammatories, antipruritics and demulcents.

Specific herbal medicines

There are many herbs that demonstrate at least one of the above actions. It would not be useful to the busy practitioner if all these herbs were listed here. Instead, only those herbs that have been investigated clinically or that exhibit several of the abovementioned activities are listed below.

ALOE BARBADENSIS (ALOE)

Aloe barbadensis, particularly the constituent alprogen, inhibits histamine and leukotriene release from activated guinea-pig lung mast cells.[242] Extracts of aloe vera gel have also demonstrated lipo-oxygenase and cyclo-oxygenase inhibition in several animal models,[243] which supports the traditional use of the herb as an anti-inflammatory agent. However, whether these effects have any relevance to humans requires further investigation.

GLYCYRRHIZA GLABRA (LIQUORICE)

Glycyrrhiza glabra has traditionally been administered for its anti-inflammatory and demulcent activity. However, the clinical effectiveness of this herb in the management of urticaria has not yet been investigated.

MATRICARIA RECUTITA (CHAMOMILE)

Matricaria recutita, when administered orally as an ethyl acetate extract or essential oil, exhibits antipruritic activity in vivo,[244] and as an aqueous extract inhibits IL-1β, IL-6 and TNF-α in vitro (all biomarkers of inflammation).[245] While there is some clinical evidence to corroborate traditional claims of an anti-inflammatory effect and, more importantly, to support the effectiveness of topically applied chamomile in inflammatory dermatoses, there is a paucity of clinical data to justify the administration of oral or topical chamomile in urticaria.

PERILLA FRUTESCENS (PERILLA)

Perilla frutescens, although traditionally consumed as a food, dose-dependently inhibits histamine release from rat peritoneal mast cells when administered intraperitoneally as a hot-water extract,[246] and suppresses percutaneous anaphylaxis in rats when administered orally as a decoction.[247] More importantly, the antiallergic effects of *Perilla* have been supported by findings from a double-blind RCT in 29 participants with seasonal allergic rhinoconjunctivitis. In this trial, patients receiving orally administered rosmarinic acid-enriched *Perilla* extract reported a significant reduction in lacrimation, itchy eyes, itchy nose, and the numbers of neutrophils and eosinophils in nasal fluid when compared with controls.[248] However, whether these antiallergic effects apply to urticaria remains unclear.

SCUTELLARIA BAICALENSIS (BAIKAL SKULLCAP)

Scutellaria baicalensis was traditionally prescribed as an anti-inflammatory and antiallergic agent. The extract of *Scutellaria baicalensis* has been shown to reduce the passive cutaneous anaphylaxis reaction in vivo, inhibit histamine release in vitro, and restore IL-8 and TNF-alpha expression and inhibit mitogen-activated protein kinase expression in vitro.[249] The constituents of baikal skullcap, including baicalein and wogonin, have also demonstrated a range of anti-inflammatory effects in vivo and in vitro. Clinical trials are needed to determine whether these effects translate into clinical benefits in persons with urticaria.

TANACETUM PARTHENIUM (FEVERFEW)

Tanacetum parthenium dose-dependently inhibits histamine release from anti-IgE-stimulated rat peritoneal mast cells in vitro,[250] while also exhibiting anti-inflammatory effects in various animal models.[251] Even though these findings support the traditional actions of the herb, clinical trial data are needed to confirm these antiallergic and anti-inflammatory effects.

ZINGIBER OFFICINALE (GINGER)

Zingiber officinale was traditionally prescribed as a digestive and circulatory stimulant for the purpose of increasing the bioavailability of simultaneously administered herbs. Even though ginger has been shown to increase drug absorption and plasma half-life in rabbits,[97] clinical evidence is lacking.

LIFESTYLE RECOMMENDATIONS

In addition to the dietary factors listed above, a number of lifestyle activities may also be implicated in the development or exacerbation of urticaria. Modification of these lifestyle factors may, therefore, help to minimise urticarial pathogenesis and recurrence.

Alcohol and smoking

Case reports have suggested that cigarette and cannabis smoking may be associated with type 1 allergic reactions in susceptible individuals.[252] In an epidemiological study of 3027 Chinese patients with urticaria, alcohol consumption was identified as a trigger of wheals in 56% of patients;[253] this may be because alcohol increases the risk of hypersensitivity reactions by elevating serum IgE levels.[254] A reduction in alcohol intake and cessation of smoking may be instrumental in reducing the incidence of urticaria in susceptible individuals.

Stress

Another potential trigger of hives is stress. In a case-control study comparing 45 patients with chronic urticaria to 45 age- and sex-matched healthy controls, patients with urticaria demonstrated much higher rates of stress (as measured by the presumptive stressful life events scale) and greater systemic inflammation (as measured by IL-18 and high-sensitivity CRP).[255] These findings suggest that stress management strategies may play an important role in managing urticaria. In fact, a systematic review of the literature on psychological treatment for urticaria indicates that hypnosis and relaxation may be effective at reducing urticarial wheals,[256] although further investigation is still needed in this area.

Other strategies

Other strategies that may provide control over potential triggers of urticaria include wearing clothing made of natural fibres, avoiding extreme ambient temperatures, minimising sun exposure and avoiding strenuous exercise.

CASE STUDY

OVERVIEW

SA, a 27-year-old female, presented to the clinic complaining of a raised red rash that had been recurring every 2–3 weeks for the past 8 months. She reported intense pruritus to the face and anterior chest while the urticaria was present, which was ameliorated by betamethasone cream, and exacerbated by scratching and emotional stress. The urticaria generally lasted for 24–48 hours, and was often accompanied by malaise, irritability and diarrhoea. She stated that the urticaria was becoming increasingly unbearable, and was seeking relief from the condition.

CLINICAL EXAMINATION

Multiple raised wheals with surrounding erythema were evident on the face and anterior chest, together with signs of

CASE STUDY CONTINUED

excoriation from scratching. She had a history of asthma and anxiety, for which she self-administered a salbutamol inhaler 2 puffs p.r.n., betamethasone cream daily, and alprazolam 0.5 mg at night. She did not smoke or consume alcohol, was afebrile (36.6°C), and was of normal weight (BMI 23).

TREATMENT PROTOCOL

INITIAL APPOINTMENT

The overall treatment goal for SA was to decrease the frequency and severity of urticaria by 50% within 1 month. In order to achieve this goal, the following interventions were implemented.

HERBAL MEDICINE

Apply 10% *Matricaria recutita* ointment to lesions 3 times daily.

A suitable herbal formula for the management of urticaria is listed below. The recommended adult dose for this oral formula is 5 mL t.d.s. Note that *Perilla* seed extract has been omitted from this formula as it is currently unavailable as a liquid extract in Australia.

Herbal medicine	Quantity	
Tanacetum parthenium	1 : 5 tincture	20 mL
Matricaria recutita	1 : 2 liquid extract	20 mL
Scutellaria baicalensis	1 : 2 liquid extract	50 mL
Zingiber officinale	1 : 2 liquid extract	10 mL

NUTRITIONAL MEDICINE

Dietary

Commence a 1-week elimination diet, as detailed earlier in this chapter, after which a new food should be reintroduced every 2 days; consume at least seven servings of fruit and vegetables daily (excluding corn, bananas, apples, oranges, potatoes, parsley and carrots); consume at least five servings of wholegrain cereals daily (excluding wheat, rye, corn and barley); consume one to two servings of nuts and seeds daily (excluding peanuts and other potentially allergenic nuts); consume lean lamb/poultry 3 times weekly; consume lean seafood 3 times weekly (excluding shellfish); and avoid food containing artificial colours, flavours and preservatives.

Supplemental

Administer a nutritional supplement that provides at least 1000 mg ascorbic acid, 12 mg niacinamide, 400 IU α-tocopherol, 1000 mg rutin, 1000 mg quercetin and 250 micrograms vitamin B_{12} as a daily dose.

Lifestyle/education

Walk 20–30 minutes/day; perform relaxation, guided imagery, yoga or tai chi for 30 minutes/day; limit sun exposure to less than 10 minutes/day, avoiding exposure between 10 am and 3 pm; wear clothing made of natural fibres such as cotton.

CASE STUDY CONTINUED

FOLLOW-UP

Review patient once a fortnight to monitor compliance with the management plan, clinical progress, and the effectiveness of the prescribed interventions.

REFERENCES

[1] Herbal and nutritional protocols for common conditions. 6th ed. Warwick, Queensland: Phytotherapy Press; 2010.
[2] Ernst E, Pittler MH, Wider B, editors. The desktop guide to complementary and alternative medicine. An evidence-based approach. 2nd ed. Edinburgh: Mosby Elsevier; 2006.
[3] Longmore JM, Wilkinson IB, Baldwin A, et al. Oxford handbook of clinical medicine. 9th ed. Oxford: Oxford University Press; 2014.
[4] Ring J. Atopic dermatitis. Heidelberg: Springer Cham; 2016.
[5] Tofte S. Eczematous disorders. In: Bobonich MA, Nolen ME, editors. Dermatology for advanced practice clinicians. Philadelphia: Wolters Kluwer; 2015.
[6] Porter R, Kaplan J, editors. Merck manual: Professional edition. Kenilworth, NJ: Merck Sharp & Dohme; 2016. Available from:: www.merckmanuals.com/professional/dermatologic-disorders/dermatitis/atopic-dermatitis-eczema.
[7] Graham-Brown R, Harman K, Johnston G. Dermatology: Lecture notes. 11th ed. Chichester: John Wiley & Sons; 2017.
[8] Griffiths CEM, Barker J, Bleiker T, et al. Rook's textbook of dermatology. 9th ed. Chichester: John Wiley; 2016.
[9] Lewis-Jones S. Quality of life and childhood atopic dermatitis: the misery of living with childhood eczema. Int J Clin Pract 2006;60(8):984–92.
[10] Asero R, Ballmer-Weber BK, Beyer K, et al. IgE-Mediated food allergy diagnosis: current status and new perspectives. Mol Nutr Food Res 2007;51(1):135–47.
[11] Pagana KD, Pagana TJ, Pagana TN. Mosby's diagnostic and laboratory test reference. 12th ed. St Louis, MO: Elsevier Mosby; 2015.
[12] Stapel SO, Asero R, Ballmer-Weber BK, et al. Testing for IgG4 against foods is not recommended as a diagnostic tool. EAACI Task Force Report. Allergy 2008;63(7):793–6.
[13] Norrman G, Tomicic S, Bottcher MF, et al. Significant improvement of eczema with skin care and food elimination in small children. Acta Paediatr 2007;94(10):1384–8.
[14] Fiocchi A, Bouygue GR, Martelli A, et al. Dietary treatment of childhood atopic eczema/dermatitis syndrome (AEDS). Allergy 2004;59(S78):78–85.
[15] Bath-Hextall FJ, Delamere FM, Williams HC. Dietary exclusions for established atopic eczema. Cochrane Database Syst Rev 2008;(1): Article No. CD005203.
[16] Leach MJ. A critical review of natural therapies in wound management. Ostomy Wound Manage 2004;50(2):36–51.
[17] Davies MW, Dore AJ, Perissinotto KL. Topical vitamin A, or its derivatives, for treating and preventing napkin dermatitis in infants. Cochrane Database Syst Rev 2005;(4): Article No. CD004300.
[18] Ellulu MS, Rahmat A, Patimah I, et al. Effect of vitamin C on inflammation and metabolic markers in hypertensive and/or diabetic obese adults: a randomized controlled trial. Drug Des Devel Ther 2015;9:3405–12.
[19] Amin MN, Liza KF, Sarwar MS, et al. Effect of lipid peroxidation, antioxidants, macro minerals and trace elements on eczema. Arch Dermatol Res 2015;307(7):617–23.
[20] Shin J, Kim YJ, Kwon O, et al. Associations among plasma vitamin C, epidermal ceramide and clinical severity of atopic dermatitis. Nutr Res Pract 2016;10(4):398–403.
[21] Laitinen K, Kalliomaki M, Poussa T, et al. Evaluation of diet and growth in children with and without atopic eczema: follow-up study from birth to 4 years. Br J Nutr 2005;94(4):565–74.
[22] Kim G, Bae JH. Vitamin D and atopic dermatitis: A systematic review and meta-analysis. Nutrition 2016;32(9):913–20.

[23] Wang Y, Park NY, Jang Y, et al. Vitamin E γ-tocotrienol inhibits cytokine-stimulated NF-κB activation by induction of anti-inflammatory A20 via stress adaptive response due to modulation of sphingolipids. J Immunol 2015;195(1):126–33.

[24] Jaffary F, Faghihi G, Mokhtarian A, et al. Effects of oral vitamin E on treatment of atopic dermatitis: A randomized controlled trial. J Res Med Sci 2015;20(11):1053–7.

[25] David V, Martin A, Isakova T. Inflammation and functional iron deficiency regulate fibroblast growth factor 23 production. Kidney Int 2016;89(1):135–46.

[26] Nwaru BI, Hayes H, Gambling L, et al. An exploratory study of the associations between maternal iron status in pregnancy and childhood wheeze and atopy. Br J Nutr 2014;112(12):2018–27.

[27] Vunta H, Davis F, Palempalli UD, et al. The anti-inflammatory effects of selenium are mediated through 15-deoxy-delta12,14-prostaglandin J2 in macrophages. J Biol Chem 2007;282(25):17964–73.

[28] Yamada T, Saunders T, Kuroda S. Cohort study for prevention of atopic dermatitis using hair mineral contents. J Trace Elem Med Biol 2013;27(2):126–31.

[29] Fairris GM, Perkins PJ, Lloyd B, et al. The effect on atopic dermatitis of supplementation with selenium and vitamin E. Acta Derm Venereol 1989;69(4):359–62.

[30] Kim JE, Yoo SR, Jeong MG, et al. Hair zinc levels and the efficacy of oral zinc supplementation in patients with atopic dermatitis. Acta Derm Venereol 2014;94(5):558–62.

[31] Ewing CI, Gibbs AC, Ashcroft C, et al. Failure of oral zinc supplementation in atopic eczema. Eur J Clin Nutr 1991;45(10):507–10.

[32] Ticinesi A, Meschi T, Lauretani F. Nutrition and inflammation in older individuals: focus on vitamin D, n-3 polyunsaturated fatty acids and whey proteins. Nutrients 2016;8(4):186.

[33] Bath-Hextall FJ, Jenkinson C, Humphreys R, et al. Dietary supplements for established atopic eczema. Cochrane Database Syst Rev 2012;(2):CD005205.

[34] Kim SO, Ah YM, Yu YM, et al. Effects of probiotics for the treatment of atopic dermatitis: a meta-analysis of randomized controlled trials. Ann Allergy Asthma Immunol 2014;113(2):217–26.

[35] Hamalainen M, Nieminen R, Vuorela P, et al. Anti-inflammatory effects of flavonoids: genistein, kaempferol, quercetin, and daidzein inhibit STAT-1 and NF-κB activations, whereas flavone, isorhamnetin, naringenin, and pelargonidin inhibit only NF-κB activation along with their inhibitory effect on iNOS expression and NO production in activated macrophages. Mediators Inflamm 2007;45673.

[36] Karuppagounder V, Arumugam S, Thandavarayan RA, et al. Molecular targets of quercetin with anti-inflammatory properties in atopic dermatitis. Drug Discov Today 2016;21(4):632–9.

[37] Weng Z, Zhang B, Asadi A, et al. Quercetin is more effective than cromolyn in blocking human mast cell cytokine release and inhibits contact dermatitis and photosensitivity in humans. PLoS ONE 2012;7(2012):e33805.

[38] Braun L, Cohen M. Herbs and natural supplements: an evidence-based guide. 3rd ed. Marrickville, NSW: Elsevier; 2015.

[39] Kroner Z. Vitamins and minerals. Santa Barbara, California: Greenwood; 2011.

[40] Osiecki H. The nutrient bible. 9th ed. Eagle Farm, Queensland: Bio Concepts Publishing; 2014.

[41] Panahi Y, Sharif MR, Sharif A. A randomized comparative trial on the therapeutic efficacy of topical aloe vera and *Calendula officinalis* on diaper dermatitis in children. ScientificWorldJournal 2012;2012:810234.

[42] Chan YS, Cheng LN, Wu JH, et al. A review of the pharmacological effects of *Arctium lappa* (burdock). Inflammopharmacology 2011;19(5):245–54.

[43] Beuth J, Schneider H, Ko HL. Enhancement of immune responses to neem leaf extract (*Azadirachta indica*) correlates with antineoplastic activity in BALB/c-mice. In Vivo 2006;20(2):247–51.

[44] Bone K. A clinical guide to blending liquid herbs. St Louis, MO: Churchill Livingstone; 2003.

[45] Patzelt-Wenczler R, Ponce-Poschl E. Proof of efficacy of Kamillosan® cream in atopic eczema. Eur J Med Res 2000;5(4):171–5.

[46] Aertgeerts P, Albring M, Klaschka F, et al. Comparative testing of Kamillosan cream and steroidal (0.25% hydrocortisone, 0.75% fluocortin butyl ester) and non-steroidal (5% bufexamac) dermatologic agents in maintenance therapy of eczematous diseases. Z Hautkr 1985;60(3):270–7.

[47] Nissen HP, Biltz H, Kreysel HW. Profilometry, a method for the assessment of the therapeutic effectiveness of Kamillosan ointment. Z Hautkr 1988;63(3):184–90.

[48] Chen YJ, Dai YS, Chen BF, et al. The effect of tetrandrine and extracts of *Centella asiatica* on acute radiation dermatitis in rats. Biol Pharm Bull 1999;22(7):703–6.

[49] Morisset R, Cote N, Panniset J, et al. Evaluation of the healing activity of *Hydrocotyle* tincture in the treatment of wounds. Phytother Res 1987;1(3):117–21.

[50] Saeedi M, Morteza-Semnani K, Ghoreishi MR. The treatment of atopic dermatitis with liquorice gel. J Dermatolog Treat 2003;14(3):153–7.

[51] Schempp CM, Windeck T, Hezel S, et al. Topical treatment of atopic dermatitis with St John's wort cream — a randomized, placebo controlled, double blind half-side comparison. Phytomedicine 2003;10(Suppl. 4):31–7.

[52] Park H, Kim K. Association of perceived stress with atopic dermatitis in adults: a population-based study in Korea. Int J Environ Res Public Health 2016;13(8):760.

[53] Schachner L, Field T, Hernandez-Reif M, et al. Atopic dermatitis symptoms decreased in children following massage therapy. Pediatr Dermatol 1998;15(5):390–5.

[54] Bae BG, Oh SH, Park CO, et al. Progressive muscle relaxation therapy for atopic dermatitis: objective assessment of efficacy. Acta Derm Venereol 2012;92(1):57–61.

[55] Kimata H. Enhancement of allergic skin wheal responses in patients with atopic eczema/dermatitis syndrome by playing video games or by a frequently ringing mobile phone. Eur J Clin Invest 2003;33(6):513–17.

[56] Weller RB, Hunter HJA, Mann MW. Clinical dermatology. 5th ed. Chichester: John Wiley & Sons; 2015.

[57] Altobelli E, Petrocelli R, Marziliano C, et al. Family history of psoriasis and age at disease onset in Italian patients with psoriasis. Br J Dermatol 2007;156(6):1400–1.

[58] Thomas J, Kumar P, Balaji SR, et al, editors. Textbook of psoriasis. New Delhi, India: Jaypee Brothers; 2016.

[59] Pizzorno JE, Murray MT. Textbook of natural medicine. 4th ed. St Louis, Missouri: Churchill Livingstone; 2013.

[60] Clo C, Caldarera CM, Tantini B, et al. Polyamines and cellular adenosine 3′:5′-cyclic monophosphate. Biochem J 1979;182(3):641–9.

[61] Habif TP. Clinical dermatology: a colour guide to diagnosis and therapy. 6th ed. Philadelphia, PA: Elsevier; 2016.

[62] Weinberg JM. Psoriasis. In: Hall JC, editor. Sauer's manual of skin diseases. 10th ed. Philadelphia, PA: Lippincott Williams & Wilkins; 2010.

[63] Liska D, Lyon M, Jones DS. Detoxification and biotransformational imbalances. Explore (NY) 2006;2(2):122–40.

[64] Wolters M. Diet and psoriasis: experimental data and clinical evidence. Br J Dermatol 2005;153:706–14.

[65] Bhatia BK, Millsop JW, Debbaneh M, et al. Diet and psoriasis, part II: celiac disease and role of a gluten-free diet. J Am Acad Dermatol 2014;71(2):350–8.

[66] Naldi L, Parazzini F, Peli L, et al. Dietary factors and the risk of psoriasis. Results of an Italian case–control study. Br J Dermatol 1996;134(1):101–6.

[67] Griffiths CEM, Clark CM, Chalmers RJG, et al. A systematic review of treatments for severe psoriasis. Health Technology Assessment Monograph. Norwich: HMSO; 2000.

[68] Mason AR, Mason J, Cork M, et al. Topical treatments for chronic plaque psoriasis. Cochrane Database Syst Rev 2013;(3):CD005028.

[69] Millsop JW, Bhatia BK, Debbaneh M, et al. Diet and psoriasis, part III: role of nutritional supplements. J Am Acad Dermatol 2014;71(3):561–9.

[70] Kokcam I, Naziroglu M. Antioxidants and lipid peroxidation status in the blood of patients with psoriasis. Clin Chim Acta 1999;289(1–2):23–31.

[71] Sakane T, Takada S, Kotani H, et al. Effects of methyl-B_{12} on the in vitro immune functions of human T lymphocytes. J Clin Immunol 1982;2:101–9.

[72] Yamashiki M, Nishimura A, Koska Y. Effects of methylcobalamin (vitamin B_{12}) on in vitro cytokine production of peripheral blood mononuclear cells. J Clin Lab Immunol 1992;37:173–82.
[73] Brazzelli V, Grasso V, Fornara L. Homocysteine, vitamin B12 and folic acid levels in psoriatic patients and correlation with disease severity. Int J Immunopathol Pharmacol 2010;23(3):911–16.
[74] Stucker M, Memmel U, Hoffmann M, et al. Vitamin B_{12} cream containing avocado oil in the therapy of plaque psoriasis. Dermatology 2001;203:141–7.
[75] Malerba M, Gisondi P, Radaeli A, et al. Plasma homocysteine and folate levels in patients with chronic plaque psoriasis. Br J Dermatol 2006;155(6):1165–9.
[76] Flytstrom I, Stenberg B, Svensson A, et al. Methotrexate vs. ciclosporin in psoriasis: effectiveness, quality of life and safety. A randomized controlled trial. Br J Dermatol 2008;158(1):116–21.
[77] Baran W, Batycka-Baran A, Zychowska M, et al. Folate supplementation reduces the side effects of methotrexate therapy for psoriasis. Expert Opin Drug Saf 2014;13(8):1015–21.
[78] Fairris GM, Lloyd B, Hinks L, et al. The effect of supplementation with selenium and vitamin E in psoriasis. Ann Clin Biochem 1989;26(1):83–8.
[79] Sheikh G, Masood Q, Majeed S, et al. Comparison of levels of serum copper, zinc, albumin, globulin and alkaline phosphatase in psoriatic patients and controls: a hospital based case control study. Indian Dermatol Online J 2015;6(2):81–3.
[80] Kreft B, Wohlrab J, Fischer M, et al. Analysis of serum zinc level in patients with atopic dermatitis, psoriasis vulgaris and in probands with healthy skin. Hautarzt 2000;51(12):931–4.
[81] Ozturk G, Erbas D, Gelir E, et al. Natural killer cell activity, serum immunoglobulins, complement proteins, and zinc levels in patients with psoriasis vulgaris. Immunol Invest 2001;30(3):181–90.
[82] Burrows NP, Turnbull AJ, Punchard NA, et al. A trial of oral zinc supplementation in psoriasis. Cutis 1994;54(2):117–18.
[83] Leibovici V, Statter M, Weinrauch L, et al. Effect of zinc therapy on neutrophil chemotaxis in psoriasis. Isr J Med Sci 1990;26(6):306–9.
[84] Grimminger F, Mayser P, Papavassilis C, et al. A double-blind, randomized, placebo-controlled trial of n-3 fatty acid based lipid infusion in acute, extended guttate psoriasis. Rapid improvement of clinical manifestations and changes in neutrophil leukotriene profile. Clin Investig 1993;71(8):634–43.
[85] Mayser P, Mrowietz U, Arenberger P, et al. Omega-3 fatty acid-based lipid infusion in patients with chronic plaque psoriasis: results of a double-blind, randomized, placebo-controlled, multicenter trial. J Am Acad Dermatol 1998;38(4):539–47.
[86] Miroddi M, Navarra M, Calapai F. Review of clinical pharmacology of *Aloe vera* L. in the treatment of psoriasis. Phytother Res 2015;29(5):648–55.
[87] Deng S, May BH, Zhang AL, et al. Plant extracts for the topical management of psoriasis: a systematic review and meta-analysis. Br J Dermatol 2013;169(4):769–82.
[88] Maghsoumi-Norouzabad L, Alipoor B, Abed R. Effects of *Arctium lappa* L. (burdock) root tea on inflammatory status and oxidative stress in patients with knee osteoarthritis. Int J Rheum Dis 2016;19(3):255–61.
[89] Pandey SS, Jha AK, Kaur V. Aqueous extract of neem leaves in treatment of psoriasis vulgaris. Ind J Dermatol Venereol Leprol 1994;60(2):63–7.
[90] Augustin M, Andrees U, Grimme H, et al. Effects of *Mahonia aquifolium* ointment on the expression of adhesion, proliferation, and activation markers in the skin of patients with psoriasis. Forsch Komplementarmed 1999;6(Suppl. 2):19–21.
[91] Sampson JH, Raman A, Karlsen G, et al. In vitro keratinocyte antiproliferant effect of *Centella asiatica* extract and triterpenoid saponins. Phytomedicine 2001;8(3):230–5.
[92] Cassano N, Mantegazza R, Battaglini S, et al. Adjuvant role of a new emollient cream in patients with palmar and/or plantar psoriasis: a pilot randomized open-label study. G Ital Dermatol Venereol 2010;145(6):789–92.
[93] Kuo CL, Chi CW, Liu TY. The anti-inflammatory potential of berberine in vitro and in vivo. Cancer Lett 2004;203(2):127–37.
[94] Muller K, Ziereis K, Gawlik I. The antipsoriatic *Mahonia aquifolium* and its active constituents. II. Antiproliferative activity against cell growth of human keratinocytes. Planta Med 1995;61(1):74–5.
[95] Rasool M, Varalakshmi P. Suppressive effect of *Withania somnifera* root powder on experimental gouty arthritis: an in vivo and in vitro study. Chem Biol Interact 2006;164(3):174–80.
[96] Rasool M, Varalakshmi P. Immunomodulatory role of *Withania somnifera* root powder on experimental induced inflammation: an in vivo and in vitro study. Vascul Pharmacol 2006;44(6):406–10.
[97] Okonta JM, Uboh M, Obonga WO. Herb–drug interaction: a case study of effect of ginger on the pharmacokinetic of metronidazole in rabbit. Indian J Pharm Sci 2008;70(2):230–2.
[98] O'Leary CJ, Creamer D, Higgins E, et al. Perceived stress, stress attributions and psychological distress in psoriasis. J Psychosom Res 2004;57(5):465–71.
[99] Zachariae R, Zachariae H, Blomqvist K, et al. Self-reported stress reactivity and psoriasis-related stress of Nordic psoriasis sufferers. J Eur Acad Dermatol Venereol 2004;18(1):27–36.
[100] Weigl BA. The significance of stress hormones (glucocorticoids, catecholamines) for eruptions and spontaneous remission phases in psoriasis. Int J Dermatol 2000;39(9):678–88.
[101] Kabat-Zinn J, Wheeler E, Light T, et al. Influence of a mindfulness meditation-based stress reduction intervention on rates of skin clearing in patients with moderate to severe psoriasis undergoing phototherapy (UVB) and photochemotherapy (PUVA). Psychosom Med 1998;60(5):625–32.
[102] Behnam SM, Behnam SE, Koo JY. Alcohol as a risk factor for plaque-type psoriasis. Cutis 2005;76(3):181–5.
[103] Kirby B, Richards HL, Mason DL, et al. Alcohol consumption and psychological distress in patients with psoriasis. Br J Dermatol 2008;158(1):138–40.
[104] Diffey B, Farr PM. An appraisal of ultraviolet lamps used for the phototherapy of psoriasis. Br J Dermatol 1987;117:49–56.
[105] Kudish AI, Abels D, Harari M. Ultraviolet radiation properties as applied to photoclimatherapy at the Dead Sea. Int J Dermatol 2003;42:359–65.
[106] Almutawa F, Thalib L, Hekman D, et al. Efficacy of localized phototherapy and photodynamic therapy for psoriasis: a systematic review and meta-analysis. Photodermatol Photoimmunol Photomed 2015;31(1):5–14.
[107] Lee E, Koo J, Berger T. UVB phototherapy and skin cancer risk: a review of the literature. Int J Dermatol 2005;44:355–60.
[108] Paller AS, Mancini AJ. Hurwitz clinical pediatric dermatology: a textbook of skin disorders of children and adolescence. 5th ed. New York: Elsevier; 2016.
[109] Alan S, Cenesizoglu E. Effects of hyperandrogenism and high body mass index on acne severity in women. Saudi Med J 2014;35(8):886–9.
[110] Feldman S, Carrecia RE, Barham KL, et al. Diagnosis and treatment of acne. Am Fam Physician 2004;69:2123–30.
[111] Cordain L. Implications for the role of diet in acne. Semin Cutan Med Surg 2005;24(2):84–91.
[112] Kwon HH, Yoon JY, Hong JS, et al. Clinical and histological effect of a low glycaemic load diet in treatment of acne vulgaris in Korean patients: a randomized, controlled trial. Acta Derm Venereol 2012;92(3):241–6.
[113] Smith R, Mann N, Makelainen H, et al. A pilot study to determine the short-term effects of a low glycemic load diet on hormonal markers of acne: a nonrandomized, parallel, controlled feeding trial. Mol Nutr Food Res 2008;52(6):718–26.
[114] El-Akawi Z, Abdel-Latif N, Abdul-Razzak K. Does the plasma level of vitamins A and E affect acne condition? Clin Exp Dermatol 2006;31(3):430–4.
[115] Veraldi S, Barbareschi M, Guanziroli E. Treatment of mild to moderate acne with a fixed combination of hydroxypinacolone retinoate, retinol glycospheres and papain glycospheres. G Ital Dermatol Venereol 2015;150(2):143–7.
[116] Lee HE, Ko JY, Kim YH. A double-blind randomized controlled comparison of APDDR-0901, a novel cosmeceutical formulation, and 0.1% adapalene gel in the treatment of mild-to-moderate acne vulgaris. Eur J Dermatol 2011;21(6):959–65.
[117] Klock J, Ikeno H, Ohmori K, et al. Sodium ascorbyl phosphate shows in vitro and in vitro efficacy in the prevention and treatment of acne vulgaris. Int J Cosmet Sci 2005;27(3):171–6.
[118] Woolery-Lloyd H, Baumann L, Ikeno H. Sodium L-ascorbyl-2-phosphate 5% lotion for the treatment of acne vulgaris: a randomized, double-blind, controlled trial. J Cosmet Dermatol 2010;9(1):22–7.

[119] Namazi MR. Nicotinamide: a potential addition to the anti-psoriatic weaponry. FASEB J 2003;17:1377–9.
[120] Mohammed D, Crowther JM, Matts PJ, et al. Influence of niacinamide containing formulations on the molecular and biophysical properties of the stratum corneum. Int J Pharm 2013;441(1–2):192–201.
[121] Khodaeiani E, Fouladi RF, Amirnia M, et al. Topical 4% nicotinamide vs. 1% clindamycin in moderate inflammatory acne vulgaris. Int J Dermatol 2013;52(8):999–1004.
[122] Weltert Y, Chartier S, Gibaud C, et al. Double-blind clinical assessment of the efficacy of a 4% nicotinamide gel (Exfoliac NC Gel) versus a 4% erythromycin gel in the treatment of moderate acne with a predominant inflammatory component. Nouv Dermatol 2004;23(7):385–94.
[123] Iinuma K, Noguchi N, Nakaminami H, et al. Susceptibility of *Propionibacterium acnes* isolated from patients with acne vulgaris to zinc ascorbate and antibiotics. Clin Cosmet Investig Dermatol 2011;4:161–5.
[124] Brandt S. The clinical effects of zinc as a topical or oral agent on the clinical response and pathophysiologic mechanisms of acne: a systematic review of the literature. J Drugs Dermatol 2013;12(5):542–5.
[125] Jung GW, Tse JE, Guiha I, et al. Prospective, randomized, open-label trial comparing the safety, efficacy, and tolerability of an acne treatment regimen with and without a probiotic supplement and minocycline in subjects with mild to moderate acne. J Cutan Med Surg 2013;17(2):114–22.
[126] Jung JY, Kwon HH, Hong JS, et al. Effect of dietary supplementation with omega-3 fatty acid and gamma-linolenic acid on acne vulgaris: a randomised, double-blind, controlled trial. Acta Derm Venereol 2014;94(5):521–5.
[127] Thappa DM, Dogra J. Nodulocystic acne: oral gugulipid versus tetracycline. J Dermatol 1994;21(10):729–31.
[128] Sharma M, Schoop R, Suter A, et al. The potential use of echinacea in acne: control of *Propionibacterium acnes* growth and inflammation. Phytother Res 2011;25(4):517–21.
[129] Nam C, Kim S, Sim Y, et al. Anti-acne effects of Oriental herb extracts: a novel screening method to select anti-acne agents. Skin Pharmacol Appl Skin Physiol 2003;16(2):84–90.
[130] Raman A, Weir U, Bloomfield SF. Antimicrobial effects of tea-tree oil and its major components on *Staphylococcus aureus, Staph. epidermidis* and *Propionibacterium acnes*. Lett Appl Microbiol 1995;21(4):242–5.
[131] Hammer KA. Treatment of acne with tea tree oil (melaleuca) products: a review of efficacy, tolerability and potential modes of action. Int J Antimicrob Agents 2015;45(2):106–10.
[132] Nasri S, Oryan S, Rohani AH, et al. The effects of *Vitex agnus-castus* extract and its interaction with dopaminergic system on LH and testosterone in male mice. Pak J Biol Sci 2007;10(14):2300–7.
[133] Amann W. Improvement of acne vulgaris following therapy with. *Agnus castus* (Agnolyt). Ther Ggw 1967;106:124–6.
[134] Yosipovitch G, Tang M, Dawn AG, et al. Study of psychological stress, sebum production and acne vulgaris in adolescents. Acta Derm Venereol 2007;87(2):135–9.
[135] Rokowska-Waluch A, Pawlaczyk M, Cybulski M. Stressful events and serum concentration of substance p in acne patients. Ann Dermatol 2016;28(4):464–9.
[136] Hughes H, Brown BW, Lawlis GF, et al. Treatment of acne vulgaris by biofeedback relaxation and cognitive imagery. J Psychosom Res 1983;27(3):185–91.
[137] Burg G, Kempf W, Kutzner H, editors. Atlas of dermatopathology: practical differential diagnosis by clinicopathologic pattern. Chichester, West Sussex: John Wiley & Sons; 2015.
[138] Turgeon ML. Linne & Ringsrud's clinical laboratory science: concepts, procedures, and clinical applications. 7th ed. St Louis, Missouri: Elsevier; 2016.
[139] Plat J, Mensink RP. Food components and immune function. Curr Opin Lipidol 2005;16(1):31–7.
[140] Han SN, Leka LS, Lichtenstein AH, et al. Effect of a therapeutic lifestyle change diet on immune functions of moderately hypercholesterolemic humans. J Lipid Res 2003;4(12):2304–10.
[141] Epstein LH, Gordy CC, Raynor HA, et al. Increasing fruit and vegetable intake and decreasing fat and sugar intake in families at risk for childhood obesity. Obes Res 2001;9(3):171–8.
[142] Pirisi L, Batova A, Jenkins GR, et al. Increased sensitivity of human keratinocytes immortalized by human papillomavirus type 16 DNA to growth control by retinoids. Cancer Res 1995;52(1):187–93.
[143] Pechere M, Germanier L, Siegenthaler G, et al. The antibacterial activity of topical retinoids: the case of retinaldehyde. Dermatology 2002;205(2):153–8.
[144] Wintergerst ES, Maggini S, Hornig DH. Immune-enhancing role of vitamin C and zinc and effect on clinical conditions. Ann Nutr Metab 2006;50(2):85–94.
[145] Hovi T, Hirvimies A, Stenvik M, et al. Topical treatment of recurrent mucocutaneous herpes with ascorbic acid-containing solution. Antiviral Res 1995;27(3):263–70.
[146] Rodriguez-Arguelles MC, Lopez-Silva EC, Sanmartin J, et al. Copper complexes of imidazole-2-, pyrrole-2- and indol-3-carbaldehyde thiosemicarbazones: inhibitory activity against fungi and bacteria. J Inorg Biochem 2005;99(11):2231–9.
[147] Clewell A, Barnes M, Endres JR, et al. Efficacy and tolerability assessment of a topical formulation containing copper sulfate and *Hypericum perforatum* on patients with herpes skin lesions: a comparative, randomized controlled trial. J Drugs Dermatol 2012;11(2):209–15.
[148] Huang Z, Rose AH, Hoffman PR. The role of selenium in inflammation and immunity: from molecular mechanisms to therapeutic opportunities. Antioxid Redox Signal 2012;16(7):705–43.
[149] Kasseroller R. Sodium selenite as prophylaxis against erysipelas in secondary lymphedema. Anticancer Res 1998;18(3C):2227–30.
[150] Ansarin H, Ghaffarpour G. Comparison of effectiveness between ketoconazole 2% and selenium sulfide 2.5% shampoos in the treatment of tinea versicolor. Iran J Dermatol 2005;8(2):21.
[151] del Palacio Hernanz A, Delgado Vicente S, Menendez Ramos F, et al. Randomized comparative clinical trial of itraconazole and selenium sulfide shampoo for the treatment of pityriasis versicolor. Rev Infect Dis 1987;9(Suppl. 1):S121–7.
[152] Hull CA, Johnson SM. A double-blind comparative study of sodium sulfacetamide lotion 10% versus selenium sulfide lotion 2.5% in the treatment of pityriasis (tinea) versicolor. Cutis 2004;73(6):425–9.
[153] Sanchez JL, Torres VM. Double-blind efficacy study of selenium sulfide in tinea versicolor. J Am Acad Dermatol 1984;11(2 Pt 1):235–8.
[154] Poiraud C, Quereux G, Knol AC, et al. Human beta-defensin-2 and psoriasin, two new innate immunity targets of zinc gluconate. Eur J Dermatol 2012;22(5):634–9.
[155] Iraji F, Faghihi G. A randomized double-blind placebo-controlled clinical trial of two strengths of topical zinc sulfate solution against recurrent herpes simplex. Arch Iran Med 2003;6(1):13–15.
[156] Godfrey HR, Godfrey NJ, Godfrey JC, et al. A randomized clinical trial on the treatment of oral herpes with topical zinc oxide/glycine. Altern Ther Health Med 2001;7(3):49–56.
[157] Chi CC, Wang SH, Delamere FM, et al. Interventions for prevention of herpes simplex labialis (cold sores on the lips). Cochrane Database Syst Rev 2015;(8):CD010095.
[158] Griffith RS, DeLong DC, Nelson JD. Relation of arginine–lysine antagonism to herpes simplex growth in tissue culture. Chemotherapy 1981;27(3):209–13.
[159] DiGiovanna JJ, Blank H. Failure of lysine in frequently recurrent herpes simplex infection. Treatment and prophylaxis. Arch Dermatol 1984;120(1):48–51.
[160] McCune MA, Perry HO, Muller SA, et al. Treatment of recurrent herpes simplex infections with l-lysine monohydrochloride. Cutis 1984;34(4):366–73.
[161] Milman N, Jessen O, Scheibel J. Lysine therapy of recurrent herpes simplex labialis. Ugeskr Laeg 1979;141(43):2960–2.
[162] Simon CA, Van Melle GD, Ramelet AA. Failure of lysine in frequently recurrent herpes simplex infection. Arch Dermatol 1985;121(2):167–8.
[163] Milman N, Scheibel J, Jessen O. Lysine prophylaxis in recurrent herpes simplex labialis: a double-blind, controlled crossover study. Acta Derm Venereol 1980;60(1):85–7.
[164] Griffith RS, Walsh DE, Myrmel KH, et al. Success of l-lysine therapy in frequently recurrent herpes simplex infection. Treatment and prophylaxis. Dermatologica 1987;75(4):183–90.
[165] Nair MP, Kandaswami C, Mahajan S, et al. The flavonoid, quercetin, differentially regulates Th-1 (IFNgamma) and Th-2 (IL4) cytokine

gene expression by normal peripheral blood mononuclear cells. Biochim Biophys Acta 2002;1593(1):29–36.
[166] Higdon J. An evidence-based approach to vitamins and minerals: health benefits and intake recommendations. 2nd ed. Stuttgart, Germany: Thieme; 2012.
[167] Aromdee C, Suebsasana S, Ekalaksananan T, et al. Stage of action of naturally occurring andrographolides and their semisynthetic analogues against herpes simplex virus type 1 in vitro. Planta Med 2011;77(9):915–21.
[168] Singha PK, Roy S, Dey S. Antimicrobial activity of *Andrographis paniculata*. Fitoterapia 2003;74(7–8):692–4.
[169] Arreola R, Quintero-Fabian S, Lopez-Roa RI. Immunomodulation and anti-inflammatory effects of garlic compounds. J Immunol Res 2015;2015:401630.
[170] Ankri S, Mirelman D. Antimicrobial properties of allicin from garlic. Microbes Infect 1999;1(2):125–9.
[171] Ledezma E, Lopez JC, Marin P, et al. Ajoene in the topical short-term treatment of tinea cruris and tinea corporis in humans. Randomized comparative study with terbinafine. Arzneimittelforschung 1999;49(6):544–7.
[172] Ledezma E, Marcano K, Jorquera A, et al. Efficacy of ajoene in the treatment of tinea pedis: a double-blind and comparative study with terbinafine. J Am Acad Dermatol 2000;43(5 Pt 1):829–32.
[173] Abdel-Ghaffar F, Al-Quraishy S, Al-Rasheid KA, et al. Efficacy of a single treatment of head lice with a neem seed extract: an in vivo and in vitro study on nits and motile stages. Parasitol Res 2012;110(1):277–80.
[174] Schneider S, Reichling J, Stintzing FC, et al. Anti-herpetic properties of hydroalcoholic extracts and pressed juice from *Echinacea pallida*. Planta Med 2010;76(3):265–72.
[175] Vonau B, Chard S, Mandalia S, et al. Does the extract of the plant *Echinacea purpurea* influence the clinical course of recurrent genital herpes? Int J STD AIDS 2001;12(3):154–8.
[176] Tragoolpua Y, Jatisatienr A. Anti-herpes simplex virus activities of *Eugenia caryophyllus* (Spreng.) Bullock & S.G. Harrison and essential oil, eugenol. Phytother Res 2007;21(12):1153–8.
[177] Fu Y, Zu Y, Chen L, et al. Antimicrobial activity of clove and rosemary essential oils alone and in combination. Phytother Res 2007;21(10):989–94.
[178] Perez C, Anesini C. Antibacterial activity of alimentary plants against *Staphylococcus aureus* growth. Am J Chin Med 1994;22(2):169–74.
[179] Sabouri Ghannad M, Mohammadi A, Safiallahy S, et al. The effect of aqueous extract of *Glycyrrhiza glabra* on herpes simplex virus 1. Jundishapur J Microbiol 2014;7(7):e11616.
[180] Rohinishree YS, Negi PS. Effect of licorice extract on cell viability, biofilm formation and exotoxin production by *Staphylococcus aureus*. J Food Sci Technol 2016;53(2):1092–100.
[181] Satchell AC, Saurajen A, Bell C, et al. Treatment of interdigital tinea pedis with 25% and 50% tea tree oil solution: a randomized, placebo-controlled, blinded study. Australas J Dermatol 2002;43(3):175–8.
[182] Tong MM, Altman PM, Barnetson RS. Tea tree oil in the treatment of tinea pedis. Australas J Dermatol 1992;33(3):145–9.
[183] Buck DS, Nidorf DM, Addino JG. Comparison of two topical preparations for the treatment of onychomycosis: *Melaleuca alternifolia* (tea tree) oil and clotrimazole. J Fam Pract 1994;38(6):601–5.
[184] Carson CF, Ashton L, Dry L, et al. *Melaleuca alternifolia* (tea tree) oil gel (6%) for the treatment of recurrent herpes labialis. J Antimicrob Chemother 2001;48(3):450–1.
[185] Astani A, Reichling J, Schnitzler P. *Melissa officinalis* extract inhibits attachment of herpes simplex virus in vitro. Chemotherapy 2012;58(1):70–7.
[186] Koytchev R, Alken RG, Dundarov S. Balm mint extract (Lo-701) for topical treatment of recurring herpes labialis. Phytomedicine 1999;6(4):225–30.
[187] Schnitzler P, Koch C, Reichling J. Susceptibility of drug-resistant clinical herpes simplex virus type 1 strains to essential oils of ginger, thyme, hyssop, and sandalwood. Antimicrob Agents Chemother 2007;51(5):1859–62.
[188] Aberg KM, Radek KA, Choi EH, et al. Psychological stress downregulates epidermal antimicrobial peptide expression and increases severity of cutaneous infections in mice. J Clin Invest 2007;117(11):3339–49.
[189] Ortiz GC, Sheridan JF, Marucha PT. Stress-induced changes in pathophysiology and interferon gene expression during primary HSV-1 infection. Brain Behav Immun 2003;17(5):329–38.
[190] Choi EH, Brown BE, Crumrine D, et al. Mechanisms by which psychologic stress alters cutaneous permeability barrier homeostasis and stratum corneum integrity. J Invest Dermatol 2005;124(3):587–95.
[191] Ho RT, Wang CW, Ng SM. The effect of t'ai chi exercise on immunity and infections: a systematic review of controlled trials. J Altern Complement Med 2013;19(5):389–96.
[192] Cruess S, Antoni M, Cruess D, et al. Reductions in herpes simplex virus type 2 antibody titers after cognitive behavioral stress management and relationships with neuroendocrine function, relaxation skills, and social support in HIV-positive men. Psychosom Med 2000;62(6):828–37.
[193] Leach MJ. Making sense of the venous leg ulcer debate: a literature review. J Wound Care 2004;13(2):52–7.
[194] Grey JE, Harding KG, Enoch S. ABC of wound healing: venous and arterial leg ulcers. BMJ 2006;332:347–50.
[195] Marsden K, Tuck S, Meeking D. Diabetes and foot disease. In: Shaw K, Cummings MH, editors. Diabetes: chronic complications. 3rd ed. Chichester: John Wiley & Sons; 2012.
[196] Goldstein D, Vogel K, Mureebe L, et al. Differential diagnosis: assessment of the lower extremity ulcer — is it arterial, venous, neuropathic? Wounds 1998;10(4):125–31.
[197] Lopez A, Phillips T. Venous ulcers. Wounds 1998;10(5):149–57.
[198] Van Leeuwen AM, Bladh ML. Davis's comprehensive handbook of laboratory and diagnostic tests with nursing implications. 6th ed. Philadelphia, PA: FA Davis; 2015.
[199] Vileikyte L. Stress and wound healing. Clin Dermatol 2007;25(1):49–55.
[200] Wilson JA, Clark JJ. Obesity: impediment to wound healing. Crit Care Nurs Q 2003;26(2):119–32.
[201] Vetrugno M, Maino A, Cardia G, et al. A randomised, double masked, clinical trial of high dose vitamin A and vitamin E supplementation after photorefractive keratectomy. Br J Ophthalmol 2001;85(5):537–9.
[202] Aprahamian M, Dentinger A, Stock-Damge C, et al. Effects of supplemental pantothenic acid on wound healing: experimental study in rabbit. Am J Clin Nutr 1985;41(3):578–89.
[203] Vaxman F, Olender S, Lambert A. Effect of pantothenic acid and ascorbic acid supplementation on human skin wound healing process. Eur Surg Res 1995;27(3):158–66.
[204] Taylor T, Rimmer S, Day B, et al. Ascorbic acid supplementation in the treatment of pressure sores. Lancet 1974;2(7880):544–6.
[205] ter Riet G, Kessels AG, Knipschild PG. Randomized clinical trial of ascorbic acid in the treatment of pressure ulcers. J Clin Epidemiol 1995;48(12):1453–60.
[206] Baumann L. Cosmeceuticals and cosmetic ingredients. New York: McGraw-Hill; 2014.
[207] Fiori G, Galluccio F, Braschi F, et al. Vitamin E gel reduces time of healing of digital ulcers in systemic sclerosis. Clin Exp Rheumatol 2009;27(3 Suppl. 54):51–4.
[208] Ducheyne P, Healy KE, Hutmacher DW, et al, editors. Biomaterials: metallic, ceramic and polymeric biomaterials, vol. 1. Amsterdam, Netherlands: Elsevier; 2011.
[209] Wilkinson EAJ. Oral zinc for arterial and venous leg ulcers. Cochrane Database Syst Rev 2014;(9):CD001273.
[210] Lansdown AB, Mirastschijski U, Stubbs N, et al. Zinc in wound healing: theoretical, experimental, and clinical aspects. Wound Repair Regen 2007;15(1):2–16.
[211] O'Connor S, Murphy S. Chronic venous leg ulcers: is topical zinc the answer? A review of the literature. Adv Skin Wound Care 2014;27(1):35–44.
[212] Khalin I, Kocherga G. Arginine glutamate improves healing of radiation-induced skin ulcers in guinea pigs. Int J Radiat Biol 2013;89(12):1108–15.
[213] Leigh B, Desneves K, Rafferty J, et al. The effect of different doses of an arginine-containing supplement on the healing of pressure ulcers. J Wound Care 2012;21(3):150–6.
[214] Felzani G, Spoletini I, Convento A, et al. Effect of lysine hyaluronate on the healing of decubitus ulcers in rehabilitation patients. Adv Ther 2011;28(5):439–45.
[215] Pittler M, Ernst E. Horse-chestnut seed extract for chronic venous insufficiency. Cochrane Database Syst Rev 2012;(2):CD003230.

[216] Leach MJ, Pincombe J, Foster G. Clinical efficacy of horsechestnut seed extract in the treatment of venous ulceration. J Wound Care 2006;15(4):159–67.
[217] Thomas D, Goode P, LaMaster K, et al. Acemannan hydrogel dressing versus saline dressing for pressure ulcers. Adv Wound Care 1998;11(6):273–6.
[218] Molazem Z, Mohseni F, Younesi M, et al. *Aloe vera* gel and cesarean wound healing; a randomized controlled clinical trial. Glob J Health Sci 2015;7(1):203–9.
[219] Fulton J. The stimulation of postdermabrasion wound healing with stabilized *Aloe vera* gel–polyethylene oxide dressing. J Dermatol Surg Oncol 1990;16(5):460–7.
[220] Avijgan M, Kamran A, Abedini A. Effectiveness of *Aloe vera* gel in chronic ulcers in comparison with conventional treatments. Iran J Med Sci 2016;41(3):S30.
[221] Leach MJ. *Calendula officinalis* for wound healing: a systematic review. Wounds 2008;20(8):236–43.
[222] Paocharoen V. The efficacy and side effects of oral *Centella asiatica* extract for wound healing promotion in diabetic wound patients. J Med Assoc Thai 2010;93(Suppl. 7):S166–70.
[223] Glowania H, Raulin C, Swoboda M. The effect of chamomile on wound healing — a controlled clinical–experimental double-blind study. Z Hautkr 1987;62(17):1267–71, 1262.
[224] Dabirian A, Charosai F, Alavi Majd H, et al. Comparing between the healing effects of chamomile solution and topical steroid on peristomal skin wound. Faculty Nurs Midwifery Q 2006;15(50):39.
[225] Samadi S, Khadivzadeh T, Emami A, et al. The effect of *Hypericum perforatum* on the wound healing and scar of cesarean. J Altern Complement Med 2010;16(1):113–17.
[226] O'Brien J, Edwards H, Stewart I, et al. A home-based progressive resistance exercise programme for patients with venous leg ulcers: a feasibility study. Int Wound J 2013;10(4):389–96.
[227] Broadbent E, Kahokehr A, Booth RJ, et al. A brief relaxation intervention reduces stress and improves surgical wound healing response: a randomised trial. Brain Behav Immun 2012;26(2):212–17.
[228] Rice B, Kalker AJ, Schindler JV, et al. Effect of biofeedback-assisted relaxation training on foot ulcer healing. J Am Podiatr Med Assoc 2001;91(3):132–41.
[229] Kasperska-Zajac A, Brzoza Z, Rogala B. Sex hormones and urticaria. J Dermatol Sci 2008;52(2):79–86.
[230] Guida B, De Martino CD, De Martino SD, et al. Histamine plasma levels and elimination diet in chronic idiopathic urticaria. Eur J Clin Nutr 2000;54(2):155–8.
[231] Bunselmeyer B, Laubach HJ, Schiller M, et al. Incremental build-up food challenge — a new diagnostic approach to evaluate pseudoallergic reactions in chronic urticaria: a pilot study: stepwise food challenge in chronic urticaria. Clin Exp Allergy 2009;39(1):116–26.
[232] Hsu ML, Li LF. Prevalence of food avoidance and food allergy in Chinese patients with chronic urticaria. Br J Dermatol 2012;166(4):747–52.
[233] Johnston CS, Martin LJ, Cai X. Antihistamine effect of supplemental ascorbic acid and neutrophil chemotaxis. J Am Coll Nutr 1992;11(2):172–6.
[234] Johnston CS, Solomon RE, Corte C. Vitamin C depletion is associated with alterations in blood histamine and plasma free carnitine in adults. J Am Coll Nutr 1996;15(6):586–91.
[235] Gueck T, Aschenbach JR, Fuhrmann H. Influence of vitamin E on mast cell mediator release. Vet Dermatol 2002;13(6):301–5.
[236] Wu CH, Eren E, Ardern-Jones MR, et al. Association between micronutrient levels and chronic spontaneous urticaria. Biomed Res Int 2015;2015:926167.
[237] Simon SW. Vitamin B_{12} therapy in allergy and chronic dermatoses. J Allergy 1951;22:183–5.
[238] Simon SW, Edmonds P. Cyanocobalamin (B_{12}): comparison of aqueous and repository preparations in urticaria: possible mode of action. J Am Geriatr Soc 1964;12:79–85.
[239] Segawa S, Nakakita Y, Takata Y, et al. Effect of oral administration of heat-killed *Lactobacillus brevis* SBC8803 on total and ovalbumin-specific immunoglobulin E production through the improvement of Th1/Th2 balance. Int J Food Microbiol 2008;121(1):1–10.
[240] Kawasaki M, Toyoda M, Teshima R, et al. Effect of alpha-linolenic acid on the metabolism of omega-3 and omega-6 polyunsaturated fatty acids and histamine release in RBL-2H3 cells. Biol Pharm Bull 1994;17(10):1321–5.
[241] Chen S, Gong J, Liu F, et al. Naturally occurring polyphenolic antioxidants modulate IgE-mediated mast cell activation. Immunology 2000;100(4):471–80.
[242] Ro JY, Lee BC, Kim JY, et al. Inhibitory mechanism of aloe single component (alprogen) on mediator release in guinea pig lung mast cells activated with specific antigen–antibody reactions. J Pharmacol Exp Ther 2000;292(1):114–21.
[243] Vazquez B, Avila G, Segura D, et al. Antiinflammatory activity of extracts from *Aloe vera* gel. J Ethnopharmacol 1996;55(1):69–75.
[244] Kobayashi Y, Takahashi R, Ogino F. Antipruritic effect of the single oral administration of German chamomile flower extract and its combined effect with antiallergic agents in ddY mice. J Ethnopharmacol 2005;101(1–3):308–12.
[245] Drummond EM, Harbourne N, Marete E, et al. Inhibition of proinflammatory biomarkers in THP1 macrophages by polyphenols derived from chamomile, meadowsweet and willow bark. Phytother Res 2013;27(4):588–94.
[246] Makino T, Furuta Y, Wakushima H, et al. Anti-allergic effect of *Perilla frutescens* and its active constituents. Phytother Res 2003;17(3):240–3.
[247] Makino T, Furuta A, Fujii H, et al. Effect of oral treatment of *Perilla frutescens* and its constituents on type-I allergy in mice. Biol Pharm Bull 2001;24(10):1206–9.
[248] Takano H, Osakabe N, Sanbongi C, et al. Extract of *Perilla frutescens* enriched for rosmarinic acid, a polyphenolic phytochemical, inhibits seasonal allergic rhinoconjunctivitis in humans. Exp Biol Med 2004;229(3):247–54.
[249] Jung HS, Kim MH, Gwak NG, et al. Antiallergic effects of *Scutellaria baicalensis* on inflammation in vivo and in vitro. J Ethnopharmacol 2012;141(1):345–9.
[250] Hayes NA, Foreman JC. The activity of compounds extracted from feverfew on histamine release from rat mast cells. J Pharm Pharmacol 1987;39(6):466–70.
[251] Jain NK, Kulkarni SK. Antinociceptive and anti-inflammatory effects of *Tanacetum parthenium* L. extract in mice and rats. J Ethnopharmacol 1999;68(1–3):251–9.
[252] Stockli SS, Bircher AJ. Generalized pruritus in a patient sensitized to tobacco and cannabis. J Dtsch Dermatol Ges 2007;5(4):303–4.
[253] Zhong H, Song Z, Chen W, et al. Chronic urticaria in Chinese population: a hospital-based multicenter epidemiological study. Allergy 2014;69(3):359–64.
[254] Gonzalez-Quintela A, Vidal C, Gude F. Alcohol, IgE and allergy. Addict Biol 2004;9(3–4):195–204.
[255] Varghese R, Rajappa M, Chandrashekar L, et al. Association among stress, hypocortisolism, systemic inflammation, and disease severity in chronic urticaria. Ann Allergy Asthma Immunol 2016;116(4):344–8.
[256] Buffet M. Management of psychologic factors in chronic urticaria. When and how? Ann Dermatol Venereol 2003;130(Spec. 1): 1S145–59.

17

The urinary system

Leah Hechtman, Teresa Mitchell-Paterson

SECTION A

OVERVIEW OF THE URINARY SYSTEM

The urinary system (also known as the renal system) is made up of the two kidneys, the two ureters, the urinary bladder and the urethra (see Fig. 17.1). The function of the urinary system is to act as a filter, storage and transport system for urine. In this section the anatomy, physiology and functions of each of the components of the urinary system are discussed in detail.

The kidneys

The kidneys are two bean-shaped organs that lie in a retroperitoneal position between the twelfth thoracic vertebra (T12) and the third lumbar vertebra (L3). The right kidney lies slightly lower than the left one as it is crowded by the liver. A healthy adult kidney should be 3 cm thick, 10–12 cm long, 5–7 cm wide and weigh approximately 150 g. The ureters, nerves, blood and lymphatic vessels leave and enter at the centre of the concave border of each kidney, called the renal hilus (see Fig. 17.2). Each kidney is surrounded by three layers of supportive tissue: the renal capsule (a deep fibrous layer), the adipose capsule (a fatty cushioning mass) and the renal fascia (a thin superficial layer that anchors the kidney to surrounding structures).

Within the kidney there are two distinct regions: the renal cortex (superficial and light in colour) and the renal medulla (deep to the cortex and reddish brown in colour). The renal medulla contains the renal pyramids (cone-shaped tissue), which can number from 8 to 18, depending on the size of the kidney. The renal pyramids face internally (with the base facing outward) so that their apices or papillae (nipples) point towards the renal hilus. They are formed of bundles of nephrons (microscopic urine filtering and collecting tubules).

The kidneys are highly vascularised organs, receiving a quarter of the resting cardiac output (approximately 1200 mL) per minute via the left and right renal arteries. This blood is filtered by the nephrons, which are made up of a renal corpuscle (which filters the blood) and a tubule (which allows for the reabsorption of fluid into the bloodstream, and secretion of waste, drugs and extra ions into the fluid to be excreted). The urine drains from the microscopic nephron tubules to the papillary ducts and then into the cup-like minor and major calyces, before being funnelled into the renal pelvis and finally exiting the kidney to the ureter.

FUNCTION OF THE KIDNEYS

The kidneys perform the primary functions of the urinary system.[1]

Excretion of waste and foreign substances

The production of urine in the kidneys allows waste products such as ammonia, urea, bilirubin and creatinine to be excreted from the body. Foreign substances such as environmental toxins and drugs can also be eliminated in urine.

Vitamin D hydroxylation and calcium maintenance

The kidneys maintain calcium levels via the hydroxylation of inactive vitamin D and the production of the active form of vitamin D, 1,25-dihydroxy vitamin D (calcitriol), in the proximal tubule (see Fig. 17.3).

Erythropoietin and red blood cells

The kidneys are involved in red blood cell production via the production of erythropoietin (see Fig. 17.1).

Maintenance of blood osmolarity

A constant blood osmolarity of approximately 290 mOsm/L is maintained due to the regulation of solutes conserved or excreted in urine.

Regulation of the ionic composition of blood

The calcium, chloride, phosphate, potassium and sodium ion levels in the blood are all regulated by the kidneys.

Regulation of blood pH

The pH of the blood (7.35–7.45) is regulated through the excretion of hydrogen ions into and the conservation of bicarbonate ions in the urine.

Regulation of blood volume and pressure

The elimination of fluids from the body in the form of urine and the conservation of fluids in the body aid in the

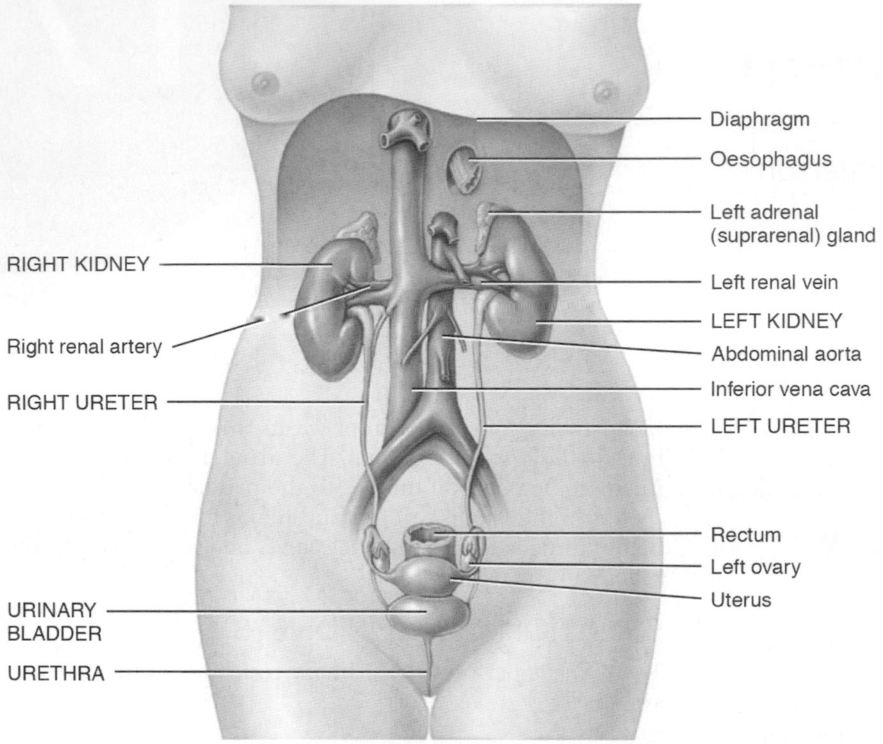

(a) Anterior view

Functions of the urinary system

1. The kidneys regulate blood volume and composition, help regulate blood pressure, synthesise glucose, release erythropoietin, participate in vitamin D synthesis, and excrete wastes by forming urine.
2. The ureters transport urine from the kidneys to the urinary bladder.
3. The urinary bladder stores urine.
4. The urethra discharges urine from the body.

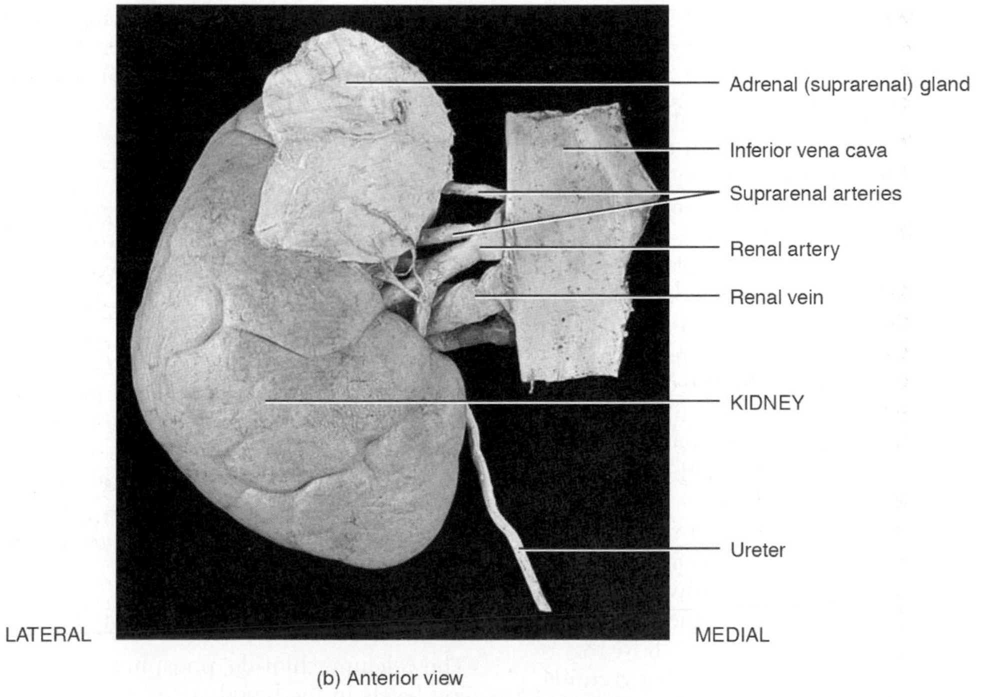

(b) Anterior view

FIGURE 17.1 Diagram showing urinary system (including kidneys, ureters, urinary bladder and urethra [men and women])

Republished with permission of John Wiley & Sons from Tortora G, Derrickson B. Principles of anatomy and physiology. 12th edn. New York: Wiley; 2009.

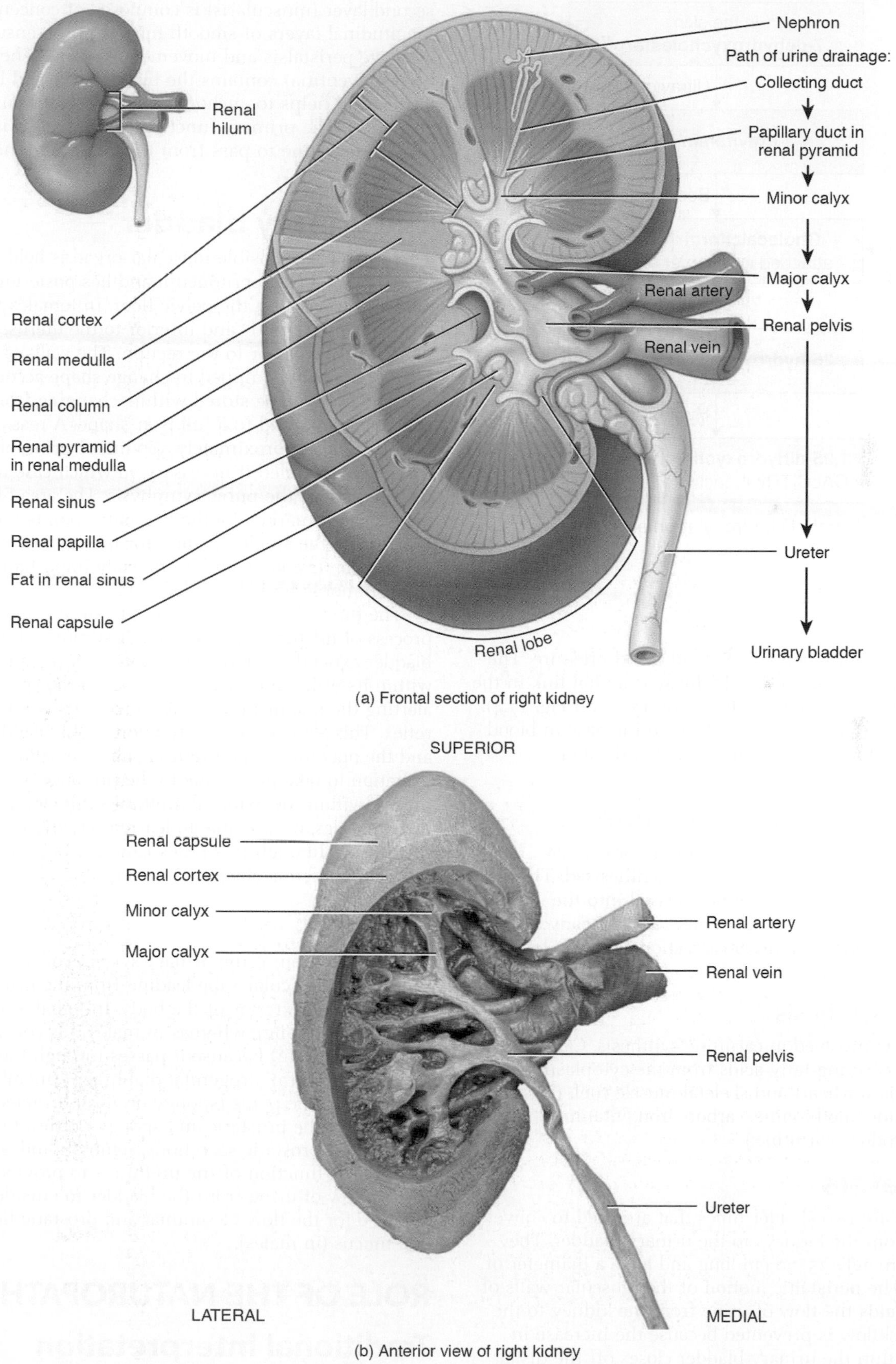

FIGURE 17.2 Detailed diagram of the kidney, showing the renal cortex and medulla, the renal pyramids, the nephrons (with a closer view of the renal corpuscle and tubule), also showing the papillary ducts, minor and major calyces and renal pelvis

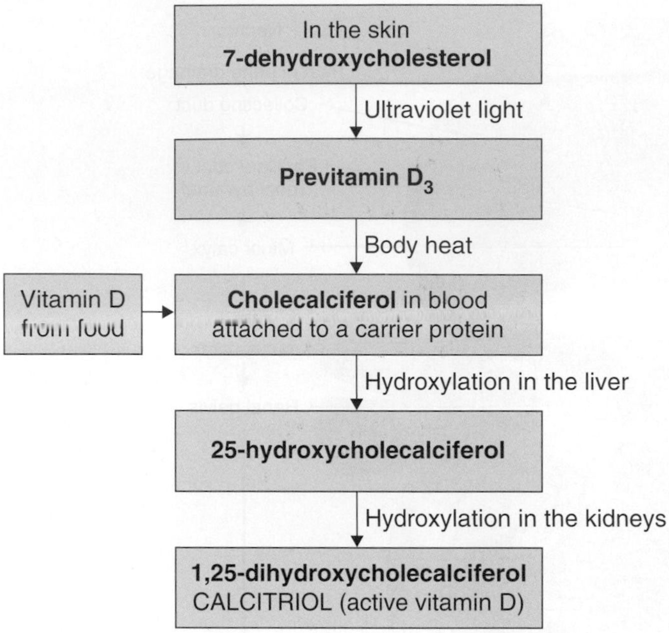

FIGURE 17.3 Vitamin D hydroxylation and calcium maintenance

regulation of both blood volume and blood pressure. The renin-angiotensin-aldosterone pathway is a vital link in the blood pressure regulatory system (Box 17.1 and Fig. 17.4). An increase in renin release leads to an increase in blood pressure, due to an increase in sodium and water reabsorption in the renal tubules.

Regulation of blood glucose levels

Glutamine is used by the kidneys in the process of gluconeogenesis, in which glucose is synthesised. The glucose thus formed can then be released into the bloodstream to aid in the maintenance of a steady blood glucose level. Glucose counter-regulation can then be achieved.

Carnitine synthesis

The kidney is involved in carnitine synthesis. Carnitine is involved in carrying fatty acids from the cytoplasm to the mitochondria for heart and skeletal muscle fuel. (The body requires lysine, methionine, carbon, iron, vitamin B_6 and niacin to produce carnitine.)

The ureters

The ureters are two slender tubes that are used to convey the urine from the kidneys to the urinary bladder. They are approximately 25–30 cm long and have a diameter of 1–10 mm. The peristaltic motion of the muscular walls of the ureters aids the flow of urine from the kidney to the bladder. Backflow is prevented because the increase in pressure within the urinary bladder closes off the distal ends of the ureters. The ureters are made up of three layers. Mucus secreted from the internal wall (mucosa) of the ureters prevents any contact with the urine. The second layer (muscularis) is composed of concentric and longitudinal layers of smooth muscle fibres, ensuring effective peristalsis and movement of urine. The third layer (adventitia) contains the blood, nerve and lymphatic vessels and helps to anchor the ureters to the surrounding structures. The primary function of the ureters is as a conduit for urine to pass from the kidneys to the urinary bladder.

The urinary bladder

This smooth, collapsible muscular organ is held in position by the folds of the peritoneum and lies posterior to the pubic symphysis on the pelvic floor. In females it is anterior to the uterus and inferior to the uterus, and in males it lies anterior to the rectum. The walls of the bladder are well equipped to change shape according to the volume of urine stored within, changing from a collapsible pyramid to a full pear shape. A reasonably full bladder holds approximately 500 mL of urine, although this can be doubled if necessary, in which case it can be palpated above the pubic symphysis. The area of the bladder floor marked by the two entry points for the ureters and the single opening for the urethra is known as the trigone (triangle), and is clinically important as this site commonly harbours infection.

The function of the bladder is to store urine until the process of micturition is desired or stimulated. When the bladder expands to above 200–400 mL stretch receptors within its walls send nerve impulses to the spinal cord, alerting the micturition centre to trigger the micturition reflex. This leads to the contraction of the bladder walls and the opening of the urethral sphincter, allowing urination to take place. Due to the presence of skeletal muscle within the external urethral sphincter and pelvic floor muscles, we are able to learn as children to control this reflex, although this reflex can only be held for a limited period once begun.

Urethra

This final section of the urinary system consists of a small, thin-walled muscular tube leading from the urinary bladder to the exterior of the body. In females it is quite short (3–4 cm long), whereas in males it is considerably longer (15–25 cm) because it passes through the prostate (prostatic urethra), urogenital diaphragm (membranous urethra) and the penis (spongy urethra). In males there are openings in the prostatic and spongy urethra to allow for the entry of prostatic secretions, seminal fluid, sperm and mucus. The function of the urethra is to provide a passage for the flow of urine from the bladder to outside the body, and also for the flow of seminal and prostatic fluid, sperm and mucus (in males).

ROLE OF THE NATUROPATH

Traditional interpretation

The flow and properties of urine have been a target of interest for numerous ancient healing traditions throughout the world, including the Egyptian, Babylonian and Indian

BOX 17.1 Renal hormonal control

The renin–angiotensin–aldosterone system is a series of reactions designed to help regulate blood pressure.

1. When blood pressure falls (for the systolic pressure, to ≤100 mmHg), the kidneys release the enzyme renin into the bloodstream.
2. Renin splits angiotensinogen, a large protein that circulates in the bloodstream, into pieces. One piece is angiotensin I.
3. Angiotensin I, which is relatively inactive, is split into pieces by angiotensin-converting enzyme (ACE). One piece is angiotensin II, which is highly active.
4. Angiotensin II, a hormone, causes the muscular walls of the small arteries (arterioles) to constrict, increasing the blood pressure. Angiotensin II also triggers the release of the hormone aldosterone from the adrenal glands.
5. Aldosterone causes the kidneys to retain salt (sodium) and excrete potassium. The sodium causes water to be retained, thus increasing blood volume and blood pressure.

Normally, whenever a change (e.g. increased activity or a strong emotion) causes a transient increase in blood pressure, one of the body's compensatory mechanisms is triggered to counteract the change and keep the blood pressure at normal levels. For example, an increase in the amount of blood pumped out by the heart, which tends to increase blood pressure, causes dilation of the blood vessels and an increase in the kidneys' excretion of salt and water, which tends to reduce blood pressure.

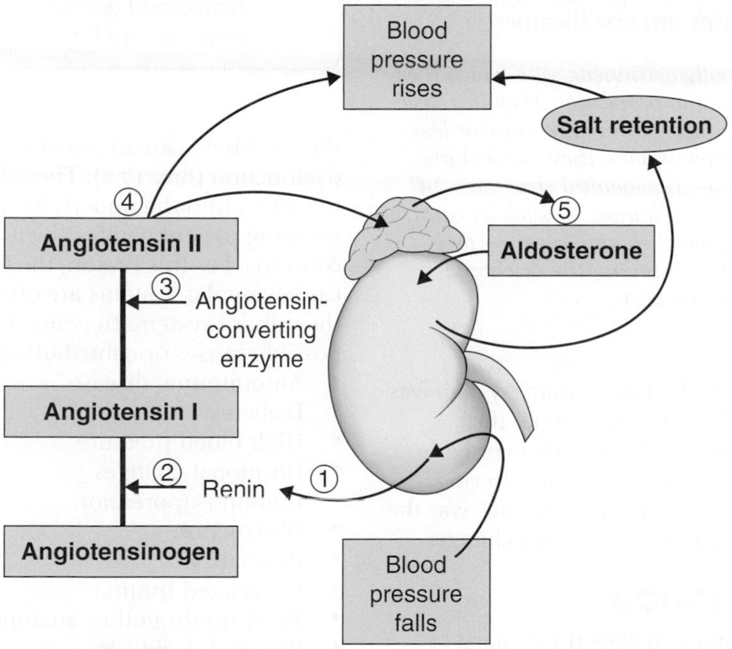

FIGURE 17.4 Blood pressure regulation

Adapted from Tortora G, Derrickson B. Principles of anatomy and physiology. 12th edn. New York: John Wiley & Sons, 2009.

traditions.[2] Hippocratic (468–377 BC) medicine had a wealth of knowledge of the urinary tract, with the code of medicine even stating 'I will not cut, even for the stone, but will leave such procedures to the practitioners of that craft'.[2] This implies that there were physicians who specialised in the treatment of urinary stones, with the Hippocratic writings placing emphasis on the colour, sediment, odour, quality and consistency of the urine. Physicians such as Ammonius, Celsus and Aretaeus (1st century AD), who came from the Hippocratic and Alexandrian schools, wrote in detail about techniques for the removal of urinary stones via surgery and with herbs. Bladder and kidney diseases and their symptoms were widely discussed and written about by early physicians. For example, Galen described difficulty of urination as having three stages: dysuria (stage 1), the mildest, slight difficulty urinating; stranguria (stage 2), the urine is excreted in drops; and ischuria (stage 3), no urine is passed.[2]

Tibetan medicine (8th century AD) placed great emphasis on the observation of urine, this adding to the general health picture or 'constitution' of the patient:

> *Wind urine is like water with big bubbles. Bile urine is red yellow with much steam and a strong smell. Phlegm urine is white having little vapour or smell.*
>
> ***The 'three roots' from Padma Karpo's Commentary on the Four Tantras.***[3]

Avicenna (Abou Ali Sina, 980–1037 AD), in his medicinal and philosophical masterpiece, *al-Qanun* (*The Cannon of*

Medicine) devoted a whole section to the practice of urinoscopy, giving great detail about the examination of the quantity, colour, foam, texture, odour, clarity and presence of sediment in the urine (similar to the Hippocratic writings).[4] Diseases were classified according to the results of the physician's urinoscopy. Avicenna's writings had a lasting impact on the diagnostic techniques used by physicians throughout Europe via the medical school at Salerno. Physicians in the later Middle Ages continued to use uroscopy as a central part of their practice. Indeed, the most common portrayal of a physician during this time was that of one holding a 'urine glass' in their hand.[5]

The 17th century brought scientific discoveries of the components of urine, tests to determine specific gravity and microscopic examination. This led physicians, over time, to lose the traditional skills of urinoscopy and become more reliant on the new method of diagnosis. However, traditional herbs continued to be used to provide symptomatic relief, as seen in Cook's (1869)[6] description of the benefits of *Arctostaphylos uva-ursi* (bearberry):

> *These leaves are principally astringent, with which they combine mild tonic and soothing properties. They increase the flow of urine; and while their powers are more or less expended upon all mucous membranes, they particularly show their influence upon the urino-genital structures. In chronic and sub-acute mucus discharges — such as catarrh of the bladder, leucorrhea, gonorrhea, and gleet — they serve an admirable purpose in lessening the discharge gradually, and giving tone to the parts.*
>
> ***Cook W***

Key to the traditional approach to the urinary system was the belief that it provided vital information about the patient's health and disease process. The ability to provide symptomatic relief to patients, who were often suffering from extreme pain or were in a very debilitated state, was the driving force behind the use of herbs and dietary changes.

Modern interpretation

The modern naturopath continues to view the urinary system as a key indicator of health. However, the traditional knowledge of urinoscopy has largely been exchanged for the analysis and interpretation of laboratory tests. Fortunately, traditional knowledge of a large number of urinary herbs continues to provide practitioners with many herbal tools for the treatment of a wide variety of urinary conditions. A holistic approach to the treatment of these conditions continues, with an emphasis on diet, lifestyle factors, and the use of symptomatic and preventive medication (particularly herbs). For example, bearberry (as mentioned by Cook in 1869[6]; see above) continues to be used by modern practitioners, for conditions similar to those Cook cites, thus continuing the long tradition of the use of urinary herbs. An exception to the continued treatment of urinary conditions is the use of herbs for the treatment of urinary stones. This is no longer commonplace as allopathic methods of treatment are preferred to ensure patient safety.

The knowledge of dietary influences on renal health (e.g. protein and potassium) ensures that the modern naturopath can work alongside other health practitioners in the combined care of patients with acute and chronic renal dysfunction (Box 17.2). The role of the naturopath is always to seek to find the underlying cause of disease, while also ensuring patient comfort by addressing symptomatic concerns. For this reason, the immune, nervous and cardiovascular systems are often treated concurrently with the urinary system. In general, there are a number of possible causes or contributing factors to consider:[7]

- Autoimmune disease
- Diabetes
- High blood pressure
- Hormonal changes
- Immunosuppression
- Obstruction
- Pregnancy
- Sex-related trauma
- Short urethra/other anatomical causes of infection
- Bacterial dysbiosis.

BOX 17.2 Warning signs when treating urinary and renal complaints

There is potential for complications when treating the urinary/renal system so the following warning signs must be considered and immediate referral made to a medical practitioner to ensure that the health of the patient is protected:

- Temperature under 38.3°C: lower urinary tract infection or temperature above 38.3°C: upper urinary tract infection
  - burning or difficulty during urination
  - more frequent urination (especially at night)
  - passage of blood in the urine
  - puffiness around the eyes
  - swelling of the hands and feet
  - pain in the small of the back just below the ribs that is not aggravated by movement
  - high blood pressure
  - undiagnosed headaches.

INVESTIGATIONS

UREA AND ELECTROLYTES (U AND E)

This test is conducted if an imbalance of the electrolytes or acid–base balance is suspected. This test should also be requested if the patient is medicated with angiotensin-converting enzyme (ACE) inhibiters or diuretic medication, and has renal and/or cardiac disease. The interpretation of the results of this test is summarised in Table 17.1.

BLOOD UREA NITROGEN (BUN)

The amount of urea nitrogen in the blood is an indirect, rough measurement of renal function and glomerular filtration rate. The BUN test also has a role in assessing liver function. Urea is formed in the liver as an end product of protein metabolism and digestion. The urea is deposited in the blood and then transported to the

TABLE 17.1 Urea and electrolytes (U and E): test interpretation*

Test category	Normal range	Clinical significance
Sodium	Serum: 135–144 mmol/L Urine: 75–300 mmol/24 hours	The concentration of sodium is closely related to the patient's level of hydration. High serum levels (hypernatraemia) may occur with dehydration. Low serum levels (hyponatraemia) can result from fluid retention (e.g. renal and cardiac disease). High urinary levels increase urinary calcium, increasing the risk of developing calculi
Potassium	Serum: 3.8–5.1 mmol/L Urine: 40–100 mmol/24 hours (varies with diet)	The monitoring of potassium levels is indicated in patients on diuretic medication and those with renal disease or gastrointestinal tract fluid losses (e.g. diarrhoea). Increased levels can indicate acidosis, renal failure and mineralocorticoid deficiency. Decreased levels are found with some diuretic medications (e.g. thiazide diuretic therapy), gastrointestinal conditions (e.g. vomiting and diarrhoea), alkalosis and mineralocorticoid excess
Chloride	Serum: 95–110 mmol/L	Chloride assessment is indicated in patients who are suspected to have an acid–base disturbance (e.g. metabolic alkalosis). High levels (hyperchloraemia) are associated with hypernatraemia caused by bicarbonate loss, or renal tubular acidosis. Low levels (hypochloraemia) are associated with hyponatraemia and metabolic alkalosis
Bicarbonate	Serum: 22–32 mmol/L	Bicarbonate testing is indicated too for suspected acid–base disorders and renal tubular acidosis. High levels are associated with metabolic alkalosis and low levels are associated with acidosis
Urea	Serum: neonate 1.0–4.0 mmol/L adult 3.0–8.3 mmol/L Urine: 420–720 mmol/24 hours	The urea level is an indication of renal function. Increased levels are associated with reduced glomerular filtration (due to renal disease), bleeding into the gastrointestinal tract and hypercatabolic conditions. Decreased levels are common in pregnancy, decreased protein intake, severe liver disease and water retention
Creatine	Serum : 44–133 mmol/L	
eGFR	Serum : > 90 mL/min/1.73m^3	

*Reference ranges are from The Royal College of Pathologists of Australia. RCPA manual. Available from: www.rcpa.edu.au/Library/Practising-Pathology/RCPA-Manual/Home

TABLE 17.2 Blood urea nitrogen (BUN): normal findings

Age group	Normal range
Adult	10–20 mg/dL or 3.6–7.1 mmol/L (SI units)
Elderly	May be slightly higher than adult levels
Child	5–18 mg/dL
Infant	5–18 mg/dL
Newborn	3–12 mg/dL
Critical value	>100 mg/dL indicates serious impairment of kidney function

kidneys for excretion. Therefore, the BUN is related to the metabolic function of the liver and the excretory function of the kidneys. A large number of renal diseases cause an inadequate excretion of urea, and thus the concentration in the blood rises above normal (Table 17.2). Patients with severe liver disease will have a decreased BUN. The BUN is less accurate than the creatinine clearance (see below) as an indicator of renal disease.

GLOMERULAR FILTRATION RATE (GFR)

The GFR is used to categorise the state of health of the kidneys. If the filtering function of the kidneys is reduced, the blood levels of a urinary analyte rise. Increased levels indicate reduced glomerular filtration rate (common in renal disease).

- Decreased renal function: GFR <50%
- Insufficient renal function: GFR <75%
- Renal failure: GFR <85%
- Chronic renal failure: GFR <20 mL/min
- End-stage renal disease: GFR <90%.

CREATININE CLEARANCE RATE

Creatinine is a byproduct of muscle breakdown, and is excreted via the kidneys. Serum, urine and total clearance levels are measured to assess glomerular health; that is, to determine the GFR. The clinical significance of and normal ranges for serum, urine and total clearance of creatinine are given in Table 17.3.

GLUCOSE

It is important to monitor glucose levels (preferably after fasting) to ensure that renal health has not led to secondary effects on glucose metabolism. If readings are abnormal,

TABLE 17.3 Creatinine: normal levels in serum and urine, and total clearance rate*		
Test category	**Normal range**	**Clinical significance**
Serum	Child (<12 years): 0.04–0.08 mmol/L Adult female: 0.05–0.11 mmol/L Adult male: 0.06–0.12 mmol/L	If the filtering function of the kidneys is reduced, the blood levels of creatinine rise. Increased levels indicate reduced glomerular filtration rate (common in renal disease). Reduced levels are common in patients with reduced muscle mass (e.g. elderly patients). (Creatinine clearance is the preferred test in early-stage renal disease)
Urine	Child: 0.07–0.19 mmol/24 hours/kg Adult female: 5–16 mmol/24 hours Adult male: 9–18 mmol/24 hours *Note*: 24-hour collection depends on age, gender, muscle mass and amount of meat in diet	Urine creatinine is tested in conjunction with other tests to determine the total creatinine clearance and for comparison with other urinary analytes
Creatinine clearance rate	1.5–2.3 mL/second (corrected for body surface area)	This test is more sensitive than serum creatinine for the detection of early glomerular dysfunction. High values can indicate muscular dystrophies, hyperthyroidism and starvation. Low values indicate renal insufficiency and hypothyroidism *Note*: Creatinine clearance may not decrease until one-third of the glomeruli cease to function

*Reference ranges are from The Royal College of Pathologists of Australia. RCPA manual. Available from: www.rcpa.edu.au/Library/Practising-Pathology/RCPA-Manual/Home

follow-up insulin, HbA1c and glucose tolerance testing may be required (see Chapter 21).

RED BLOOD CELL (RBC) PARAMETERS

Because of the role of the kidneys in erythropoietin synthesis and subsequent RBC production, close monitoring of RBC parameters is essential. Failing renal health can present with signs and symptoms of anaemia that cannot be misinterpreted. Typical presentation begins with falling haemoglobin levels, followed by falling haematocrit readings, and eventually a change in the mean corpuscular haemoglobin concentration (MCHC) (which can be seen as a change in the colour of the RBCs) and mean corpuscular volume (MCV). Long-term anaemia will present with an increased RBC distribution width (RDW) due to the reduction in the capacity for RBC production.

SERUM ALBUMIN

Serum albumin is the most abundant protein in human blood plasma. It is produced in the liver as pre-proalbumin and has a serum half-life of approximately 20 days. Its main role is to maintain oncotic pressure (colloid osmotic pressure), which is a form of osmotic pressure that pulls water into the circulatory system (capillaries). Hypoalbuminaemia can be caused by excess excretion from the kidneys, whereas hyperalbuminaemia is typically a sign of severe or chronic dehydration.

ANTINUCLEAR ANTIBODIES (ANA) AND EXTRACTABLE NUCLEAR ANTIGENS (ENA)

Tests for ANA and ENA are performed if autoimmune conditions affecting the kidney are suspected. The ENA is of use in identifying systemic lupus erythematosus (SLE) that has a kidney involvement, as anti-double-stranded DNA (anti-ds-DNA) elevations are common in such cases. A positive ANA test indicates an autoimmune condition, and in such cases further testing is required.

URINALYSIS

Urinalysis consists of the physical, chemical and microscopic examination of the urinary byproducts of metabolism (Table 17.4):

- Physical assessment: an evaluation of the colour, clarity, odour and concentration of the urine
- Chemical assessment: an evaluation of nine substances that provide valuable information about health and disease
- Microscopic examination: identification and counting of the types of cells, casts, crystals and other components present in the urine (e.g. mucus or bacteria).

Dipstick testing within a clinical setting can provide fast results for the patient and clinician. Most dipsticks test for the following: pH, protein, glucose, ketones, bilirubin, haemoglobin, nitrites, leucocyte esterase, urobilinogen and specific gravity. By comparing the test dipstick with the control, a fast analysis of the test urine can be made.

Patients taking a urine sample should follow the instructions given, as the timing and manner in which the sample is taken and stored can influence the test results.

URINE MICROSCOPY, CULTURE AND SENSITIVITIES (URINE M/C/S)

This test is conducted if a urinary tract infection is suspected. Normally the urine does not contain significant numbers of microorganisms such as yeasts and bacteria. Urine is collected midstream (MSU) and the sample cultured to determine the type of microorganisms that are the cause of infection. The most commonly identified microorganism is *Escherichia coli*. Others that are commonly identified include

Klebsiella spp., *Proteus* spp., *Saprophyticus* spp. and *Staphylococcus* spp., and yeasts of the *Candida* genus.

URINE PROTEIN (TOTAL)/URINE ALBUMIN

These tests are conducted if kidney disease is suspected, or for monitoring previously diagnosed kidney disease. If the blood levels of protein are high (see Table 17.4) then, even with normal kidney function, low levels of protein can enter the urine. Kidney disease is suspected when blood levels remain normal but there is still protein in the urine. This is due to possible damage of the glomerular filtration within the nephrons of the kidneys, as normal functioning kidneys retain or reabsorb proteins. Albumin protein molecules are normally detected in the early stages of kidney disease due to their relatively small size, with the amount increasing according to the level of damage. Later

TABLE 17.4 Urinalysis: clinical significance of results*

Test category	Normal result	Clinical significance
Appearance	Clear	Cloudy urine can indicate the presence of pus, RBCs, bacteria or the ingestion of certain foods (e.g. fats, urates and phosphates)
Colour	Amber yellow (depends on concentration)	Dark red: bleeding from kidneys Bright red: bleeding from lower urinary tract Dark yellow to brownish: suggestive of urobilinogen or bilirubin Green: infection *Note*: Some foods, such as beetroot and rhubarb, and some medications can affect the colour of urine
Odour	Aromatic	Strong, sweet smell of acetone (pear drops): diabetes Foul odour: infection
pH	4.6–8 (average 6)	Acid–base imbalance affects the pH of urine. Overly acidic or alkaline urine is associated with the formation of kidney stones
Specific gravity	Newborn: 1.002–1.020 Adult: 1.005–1.030	Note that specific gravity decreases with age. Normal adult levels generally fall in the range 1.010–1.025
Protein	0–8 mg/dL 50–80 mg/24 hours (at rest) <250 mg/24 hours (during exercise)	Protein levels are a sensitive indicator of kidney function. Normal results show little or no protein in the urine. A high level of protein in the urine is one of the key indicators of kidney disease
Bilirubin	None	Conjugated bilirubin is water soluble and can be excreted via the urine if blood levels are high. This normally indicates a blockage or obstruction of the biliary ducts
Urobilinogen	0.01–1.0 Ehrlich units/mL	Absence: may be due to complete obstructive jaundice or treatment with broad-spectrum antibiotics Low levels: congenital enzymatic jaundice (hyperbilirubinaemia syndromes) or medication that decreases urine pH Elevated levels: can indicate haemolytic anaemia or liver disease
Ketones	None	Ketones are produced when fat, not glucose, is used as the body's main source of energy. This may be an indication of diabetes, starvation, insulin overdose or severe stress
Nitrites	None	The presence of nitrites in the urine indicates a urinary tract infection. Gram-negative bacteria (e.g. *Escherichia coli*) convert nitrates to nitrites, and thus a positive result confirms the presence of bacteria in the urinary tract
Leucocyte esterase	Negative	This enzyme is released by white blood cells. A positive result is an indication of a urinary tract infection
Crystals	None	The presence of crystals indicates kidney stone formation has occurred or is imminent
Casts	None	These are clumps of material or cells that form in the distal and collecting tubules of the kidney. The clumps are tube shaped, thus the name 'casts'. Different types of cast indicate different conditions
Glucose	Fresh specimen: none 24-hour specimen: 50–300 mg/24 hours	Normally, all the glucose is reabsorbed by the proximal renal tubules. Glucose appears in the urine when the blood glucose level exceeds the capability of the renal system to reabsorb the glucose (about 180 mg/dL). The presence of glucose in the urine is known as glycosuria, and this may indicate diabetes mellitus, kidney disease (which affects the renal tubules) or other causes of glucose intolerance. The diagnosis must be confirmed by further testing (e.g. fasting glucose, glucose tolerance test, further kidney function testing) *Note*: Glycosuria is not always abnormal. It can occur immediately after eating large amounts of carbohydrates

Continued

TABLE 17.4 Urinalysis: clinical significance of results*—cont'd

Test category	Normal result	Clinical significance
White blood cells (WBCs)	0–4 per low power field	The presence of ≥5 WBCs in the urine indicates a urinary tract infection involving the kidneys or bladder, or both *Note*: Vaginal discharge may contaminate the specimen and give misleading results
WBC cast	None	These are clumps of WBCs that form in the distal and collecting tubules of the kidney. The clumps are tube shaped, thus the name 'casts'. WBC casts are indicative of inflammation or infection and can indicate pyelonephritis (direct infection of the kidney) and other kidney disease
Red blood cells (RBCs)	≤2	The presence of RBCs in the urine is known as haematuria, which can be microscopic or gross. The most common causes of RBCs in the urine are disease of the bladder, ureter or urethra
RBC cast	None	These are clumps of red blood cells that form in the distal and collecting tubules of the kidney. The clumps are tube shaped, thus the name 'casts'. RBC casts are highly indicative of glomerular damage

*Reference ranges are from The Royal College of Pathologists of Australia. RCPA manual. Available from: www.rcpa.edu.au/Library/Practising-Pathology/RCPA-Manual/Home
Source: Blann A. Why do we test for urea and electrolytes? Nurs Times 2014; 110(5):19–21.

in the disease process larger proteins, such as globulins, may be detected. Thus a urine albumin test can be requested separately to a total urine protein test, in order to monitor early signs of kidney disease in patients with diabetes or high blood pressure.

Diagnosing poor renal health

The signs and symptoms of poor renal health are as follows:

- Proteinuria (microalbuminaemia)
- Uraemia
- Bone pain, altered height or bone mass
- Altered lipid and amino acid levels
- Unbalanced calcium/phosphorus ratio
- Abnormal bun/creatinine ratio (normal bun/creatinine ratio is 10:1; creatinine doubles when renal function decreases by 50%)
- Presence or history of urinary tract infections
- Frequent weight shifts
- Leg cramps
- Weakness, pallor, anaemia
- Itching and dry skin
- Loss of appetite
- Difficulty sleeping
- Serum creatinine >1.7 mg/dL (chronic kidney disease)
- Protein energy malnutrition (PEM) or wasting.

Specific nutritional objectives

To ensure optimal renal function and urinary system health a number of nutritional objectives need to be considered. Overall, the nutritional approach to treatment aims to reduce the burden on the urinary system while maintaining an emphasis on its role as a key elimination organ. Dietary control is often required, both to manage urinary symptoms and to prevent further damage to the function of the system as a whole. Such dietary restriction can often be difficult for the patient to implement and maintain, and therefore patient education is key to ensuring positive long-term health outcomes.

The nutritional requirements for maintaining a healthy urinary system are listed in Table 17.5.

PROTEIN CALCULATIONS

Protein requirements are typically calculated according to growth stage of and the energy expended by an individual. With respect to renal function, a number of additional considerations are required. It is important to ensure that the amount of dietary (and supplemental) protein is calculated for each individual patient, first based on renal function, and second on their energy output. The calculation and prescription of protein requirements are summarised in Table 17.6.

Because of the potential aggravation of protein on renal function, communication and direction from the patient's medical practitioner/nephrologist should always be encouraged.

Herbal medicines

There is an array of herbal medicine classes that are specific to the urinary system. This enables practitioners to target the urinary organs and structures, ensuring the best possible health outcomes for the patient. General herbal classes can also be used for urinary conditions (e.g. immunomodulators) depending on the nature of the presenting complaint. The classes of herbal medicines specific to this system aim to provide symptomatic relief (e.g. urinary demulcents), treat the underlying cause (e.g. urinary antiseptics), prevent further complications (e.g. bacteriostatics) and tonify the kidneys (renal tonics) (Table 17.7).

Potential interactions

Potential interactions between herbs and nutrient supplements, and pharmaceutical drugs used for conditions of the urinary system, are summarised in the interactions tables at the back of the book.

TABLE 17.5 Nutritional requirements

Nutrient	Justification	Therapeutic range	Food sources
B complex	B vitamins are water soluble and are cleared readily. Seek medical advice if patient has failing renal function. Food sources of nutrients may be more appropriate than supplementation	Vitamin B_1: 25–150 mg Vitamin B_2: 25–200 mg Vitamin B_3: 25–50 mg Vitamin B_5: 25–500 mg Vitamin B_6: 10–150 mg Vitamin B_9: 500–1000 micrograms Vitamin B_{12}: 500–1000 micrograms	**Vitamin B_1:** fortified cereals and flours, rice bran, wheatgerm, brewer's yeast, oat bran, pork, wholegrains, trail mix snacks, sunflower seeds, pine nuts, soya milk, sesame seeds, raw peanuts, pistachio nuts, buckwheat, wheat bran, rolled oats, wholemeal pastas, whey powder, lima beans, pinto beans, mung beans, peas, egg yolks, cornmeal, Brazil nuts, lentils, broad beans Note: cooking may remove up to 85% of thiamine content of food. **Vitamin B_2:** liver, beef, fortified cereals, poultry, wild rice, dairy products, brewer's yeast, whey powder, fresh wheatgerm, almonds, mushrooms, egg yolk, Swiss and cheddar cheese, millet, soya beans, parsley, cashew nuts, rice bran, lentils, sesame and sunflower seeds, rye, broccoli, mung beans, avocado, asparagus, dark leafy greens **Vitamin B_3:** liver, red meat, salmon, tuna, chicken, halibut, white fish, fortified cereals and milks, wheatgerm, peanuts, legumes, brewer's yeast, organ meats, mushrooms, brown rice, bulgur wheat, sesame and sunflower seeds, wholemeal pasta, buckwheat, dried peaches **Vitamin B_5:** peanuts, liver, kidney, avocado, hazelnuts, mushrooms, sunflower seeds, brewer's yeast **Vitamin B_6:** muesli, wholegrains, fortified cereals, liver, sunflower seeds, lentils, kidney beans, avocado, peas, nuts, chicken, beef, kidney, fish, legumes, bananas, kale, spinach, turnip greens, sweet red capsicum, potatoes, Brussels sprouts, sweet potatoes, cauliflower, leek **Vitamin B_9:** liver, wheatgerm, asparagus, lettuce, dark leafy green vegetables, enriched cereals, lentils, legumes, orange juice, broccoli, nuts **Vitamin B_{12}:** liver, kidney, poultry, crustaceans, fish, fortified cereals, eggs, dairy products
Vitamins B_6, B_9 (folic acid) and B_{12}	Homocysteine levels increase as renal failure progresses, contributing to increased cardiovascular risk for patients. Patients require supplementation to replace B vitamin losses during dialysis treatment	Vitamin B_6: 10–150 mg Vitamin B_9: 500 micrograms Vitamin B_{12}: 50–200 micrograms	Vitamin B_6: brewer's yeast, wheatgerm, tuna, chicken, egg yolk, legumes, mackerel, sunflower seeds Vitamin B_9: organ meats, green leafy vegetables, brewer's yeast, wheatgerm, blackeyed peas Vitamin B_{12}: meat, fish, eggs, cheese, milk, oysters
Vitamin C	To assist with immune function and to help prevent and fight bacterial infection. In chronic renal failure vitamin C can aid in reducing oxidative stress caused by decreased renal function	250–5000 mg/day	Acerola cherries, guava, red and green capsicum (peppers), parsley, broccoli, kale leaves
Vitamin D	Used for immune modulation in kidney disease associated with an autoimmune response. Also used to supplement vitamin D levels in patients with reduced renal production of calcitriol	400–1600 IU/day	Butter, oily fish, cheese, eggs
Vitamin E	To reduce oxidative damage due to reduced renal function, enhance immune function and reduce inflammation. Patients on haemodialysis may benefit from supplementation	100–800 IU/day Haemodialysis 500 IU/day	Wheatgerm, almonds, sunflower seeds, walnuts, cashews, avocado, brown rice, olive oil, oily fish, green vegetables
Coenzyme Q10 (CoQ10)	To reduce oxidative damage and aid creatinine clearance in patients with chronic renal failure on dialysis	50 mg t.d.s.	Almonds, broccoli, mackerel, organ meats, rice bran, sesame seeds, sardines

Continued

TABLE 17.5 Nutritional requirements—cont'd

Nutrient	Justification	Therapeutic range	Food sources
Calcium	Calcium levels are often reduced in patients with kidney disease, particularly if it is chronic in nature. Renal calculi caused by calcium oxalate require calcium supplementation/intake to be closely monitored. Calcium (carbonate/acetate) supplementation may be prescribed to aid phosphate binding	1000–2000 mg/day	Kelp, Swiss cheese, cheddar cheese, carob flour, almonds, brewer's yeast, parsley, Brazil nuts, tofu, dried figs, spinach, yoghurt, milk
Magnesium	Magnesium can aid in the prevention and treatment of renal calculi (500 mg/day), aid in the utilisation of calcium and prevent muscle cramping (common in dialysis patients)	300–600 mg/day	Kelp, wheat bran, wheatgerm, almonds, cashews, blackstrap molasses, brewer's yeast, buckwheat, Brazil nuts
Phosphorus	Serum phosphate levels rise as renal disease progresses. Strict monitoring and control are necessary to avoid hyperphosphataemia-induced hyperparathyroid disease		Soft drinks (carbonated), brewer's yeast, bran cereals, nuts and seeds, dried peas, beans and legumes, sardines, cheese, milk, dairy products
Potassium	Potassium levels should be monitored and dietary changes made accordingly. This is particularly important if the patient is using diuretic medication or is undergoing dialysis		Dulse, kelp, sunflower seeds, wheatgerm, almonds, raisins, parsley, Brazil nuts, peanuts, dates, dried figs, avocado, pecans, garlic, spinach
Sodium	Sodium levels need to be monitored and controlled due to the influence of this ion on fluid retention	In renal conditions <2 g/d is advisable	Processed, preserved and packaged foods; olives, seaweeds, cheese, potato chips, tinned vegetables/soup, bread, sandwich meats, salami
Zinc	Zinc is indicated to reduce stone formation/size, and to improve immune function and tissue health	25–50 mg/day	Sesame seeds, pumpkin seeds, sunflower seeds, walnuts, almonds, homemade muesli, dhal, oysters, meat, fish, chicken, eggs, wholegrains
Essential fatty acids	ω3 essential fatty acids are used to reduce inflammation and oxidative damage, and to aid in balancing high-density lipoprotein/low-density lipoprotein (HDL/LDL) ratios	EPA: 3–8 g DHA: 2–4 g	Cod liver oil, mustard seed oil, tuna, salmon, mackerel, cod, sardines
Protein	Protein intake should be modified according to the level of renal function. High protein intake places an increased burden on kidney function due to the increase in urea, phosphate, sulfate and nitrogenous compounds formed	Protein intake should be calculated according to body weight depending on renal health	Legumes, lean cuts of meat, fish, chicken (organic), cheese, milk, eggs, bread, nuts and seeds, tofu, tempeh
Probiotics	Probiotics, particularly *Lactobacillus* spp., can aid in restoring balance to intestinal and vaginal microorganism growth. This is associated with a reduced risk of urinary tract infections	Multistrain probiotics: 25×10^9/day to 75×10^9/day	Fermented cabbage, miso, yoghurt, kefir

Source: Braun L, Cohen M. Herbs and natural supplements: an evidence-based guide. 4th edn. Vol 2. Chatswood NSW: Churchill Livingstone; 2014.

TABLE 17.6 Calculation of protein requirements according to growth stage and energy expenditure

Health status	Daily protein calculation (all ranges are dependent on the level of activity of the individual)
Healthy adult	0.8–1.2 g protein/kg body weight
Sedentary adult	0.8 g protein/kg body weight
Active adult	1.0–1.2 g protein/kg body weight
Sedentary adolescent	1.2–1.4 g protein/kg body weight
Active adolescent	1.8–2.0 g protein/kg body weight
Endurance athlete	1.2–1.4 g protein/kg body weight
Resistance training (muscle building)	1.4–1.8 g protein/kg body weight (maximum of 2.0 g protein/kg body weight in loading period)
Acute renal failure	0.6–0.8 g protein/kg body weight (acute); increase to 1.2 g protein/kg body weight during recovery
Chronic and end-stage renal failure	Non-dialysed patients: 0.6 g protein/kg body weight
Haemodialysis	1.2 g protein/kg body weight
Peritoneal dialysis	1.2–1.5 g protein/kg body weight
Kidney transplant	1.3–2.0 g protein/kg body weight (while on immunosuppressive medications), then follow with normal adult recommendations

TABLE 17.7 Discussion and application

Class	Example	Justification
Anti-inflammatory (urinary)	*Agropyron repens* (couch grass)	Traditionally used in European and British traditions for urinary tract infections, gout, kidney and bladder inflammation and calculi. This herb is listed by the German Commission E to be used for the treatment of inflammatory diseases of the urinary tract, and for the prevention of kidney gravel. The British Herbal Pharmacopoeia notes the use of couch grass for cystitis with inflammation or irritation of the urinary tract. Further clinical studies need to be conducted on this herb to determine the mechanism of action.
Antilithic	*Crataeva nurvala* (crataeva)	This Ayurvedic herb has a long history of use and was cited in the old samhitas Charak (210 BC–170 AD) and Sushrata (176–340 AD) for the treatment of urinary calculi. Clinical studies on rats have shown a reduction in the formation of calcium oxalate kidney stones after administration of a crataeva decoction. Oral administration of the sterol luprol (a key constituent of the crataeva bark) demonstrated a reduction in tubular damage and crystal deposition in the kidneys of rats.
Antiseptic (urinary)	*Arctostaphylos uva-ursi* (bearberry)	This Native American herb contains the glycoside arbutoside, which is hydrolysed in the gut, glucuronidated in the liver, and then excreted via the kidneys, where it decomposes spontaneously in a sufficiently alkaline environment (in urine with pH >7) releasing hydroquinone. Hydroquinone acts as a direct antimicrobial agent on bacteria within the urinary system. Other urinary antiseptics work in a similar manner, by delivering the active antimicrobial action directly to the site of action.
Bacteriostatic (inhibition of bacterial adhesion)	*Vaccinium macrocarpon* (cranberry)	*Vaccinium macrocarpon* was initially used by the Native American healing tradition for the treatment of bladder and kidney disease. Clinical trials have since shown its efficacy in reducing bacterial adhesion (particularly *E. coli*) to the bladder and urethra lining. This is largely thought to be due to the presence of proanthocyanidins (PACs), rather than the previous hypothesis of lowering the pH of urine (acidification). It is used widely for the prevention of urinary tract infections, with new research suggesting wider use for *H. pylori* induced gastrointestinal conditions.
Bladder tonic	*Crataeva nurvala* (crataeva)	The Ayurvedic tradition of use includes disorders of the urinary system including urinary stones and inflammation. Clinical research conducted on patients with urinary incontinence, pain and retention of urine associated with benign prostatic hyperplasia (BPH) has shown that crataeva can help to reduce symptoms and improve bladder tone. A small trial on a product with crataeva and horsetail (*Equisetum arvense*) showed significant ($p \leq 0.05$) reduction in incontinence associated with activity over a 3-month trial period.
Demulcent (urinary)	*Zea mays* (corn silk)	*Zea mays* and other urinary demulcents are high in mucopolysaccharides. Their mechanism of action is still unclear; however, they are thought to reduce inflammation of the urinary tract epithelium via a reflex action within the gastrointestinal system. This increase in mucus production can help to provide symptomatic relief of pain and burning for the patient.

Continued

TABLE 17.7 Discussion and application—cont'd		
Class	Example	Justification
Diuretic/ aquaretic	*Apium graviolens* (celery seed)	There is some debate about the nomenclature of this herb class, as they are considered by some to be aquaretic medicines (rather than diuretic) due to their promotion of fluid loss without marked change to electrolyte balance. A more complete understanding of their mechanism of action requires further study. The increased loss of fluid from the kidneys aids in the removal of bacteria, and can assist in the passing of urinary stones.
Renal tonic	*Solidago* spp. (golden rod)	Renal tonics, such as golden rod, help to improve the function and tone of the kidneys and are listed by the German Commission E for the treatment of inflammatory conditions of the lower urinary tract, urinary calculi and kidney gravel.
Renal protective	*Rheum palmatum* (Chinese rhubarb)	Renal protective or antinephrotoxic herbs provide a unique action of protecting the kidneys from damage and improving renal function. Chinese rhubarb has a long history of traditional use for nephritic disease. Animal studies have shown *Rheum palmatum* can improve glomerular filtration rates, reduce proteinuria and glomerulosclerosis.

SECTION B

URINARY TRACT INFECTIONS (CYSTITIS)

Epidemiology

Urinary tract infection (UTI) is a major source of disease (see Fig. 17.5). It causes substantial suffering for the patient and, especially if not treated properly, may — in extreme cases — cause substantial kidney damage in adults; however in children this has not been proven.[8] Recurrent kidney infection can cause abscess formation, disseminated intravascular coagulation, acute respiratory distress syndrome and sepsis. It is thought that the long-term consequences of poor management can result in systemic pathophysiological processes via a complex set of pathways that affect the homoeostasis of the body.[9] It is therefore important to diagnose a UTI early and treat patients with acute UTI adequately.

Although UTIs can occur in both men and women, they are approximately 50 times more common in adult women than adult men. This may be because women have a shorter urethra that may allow bacteria to ascend more easily into the bladder. In males, incidence generally indicates an anatomical abnormality, a prostate infection or rectal intercourse.

UTIs in women are very common.

There are 6 categories of UTIs: *uncomplicated infection,* which resolves quickly with no damage to the urinary system; *complicated infection* where obstruction, renal calculi or reflux can occur; *isolated infection* which is a one-off infection or may recur after 6 months; *unresolved infection* where therapy fails; *reinfection* where the pathogenic organism recurs after two weeks; and *relapse,* where the same microorganism reinfects within two weeks (difficult to differentiate between the latter two).[10]

- UTIs account for 25% of bacterial infections among women
- 50–60% of all women will experience a UTI in their lifetime
- Isolated infections will occur in 20–40% of healthy women
- Symptomatic infection of the bladder (lower UTI) has been estimated to occur in up to 50–60% of women at some stage during their lives.[10,11]

In children, UTI occurs more commonly in girls. Approximately 10% of Australian girls will have had a UTI by adulthood, commonly the onset is after the age of 2. However, the reverse is true of boys: 2–3% will have a UTI during childhood and of that 2–3%, 60% will be before the age of 2.[12]

SPECIFIC SUBPOPULATIONS AT INCREASED RISK OF DEVELOPING A UTI

Other groups include:

- Infants
- Pregnant women
- The elderly
- Patients with spinal cord injuries and/or catheters
- Patients with diabetes
- Patients with multiple sclerosis
- Patients with human immunodeficiency virus (HIV) infection or acquired immune deficiency syndrome (AIDS)
- Patients with underlying urological abnormalities.[13]

Classification

The term 'urinary tract infection' refers to the presence of a certain threshold number of bacteria in the urine (usually >100 000/mL). The term covers the conditions cystitis (bacteria in the bladder), urethral syndrome and pyelonephritis (infection of the kidneys). Lower UTIs involve the bladder, whereas upper UTIs also involve the kidneys (pyelonephritis). Bacterial cystitis (also called acute cystitis) can occur in men and women.

The majority of infections begin in the urethra and ascend to the bladder (cystitis). Because of the risk of infection reaching the kidneys it is vital that herbal treatment yields quick results, particularly in acute

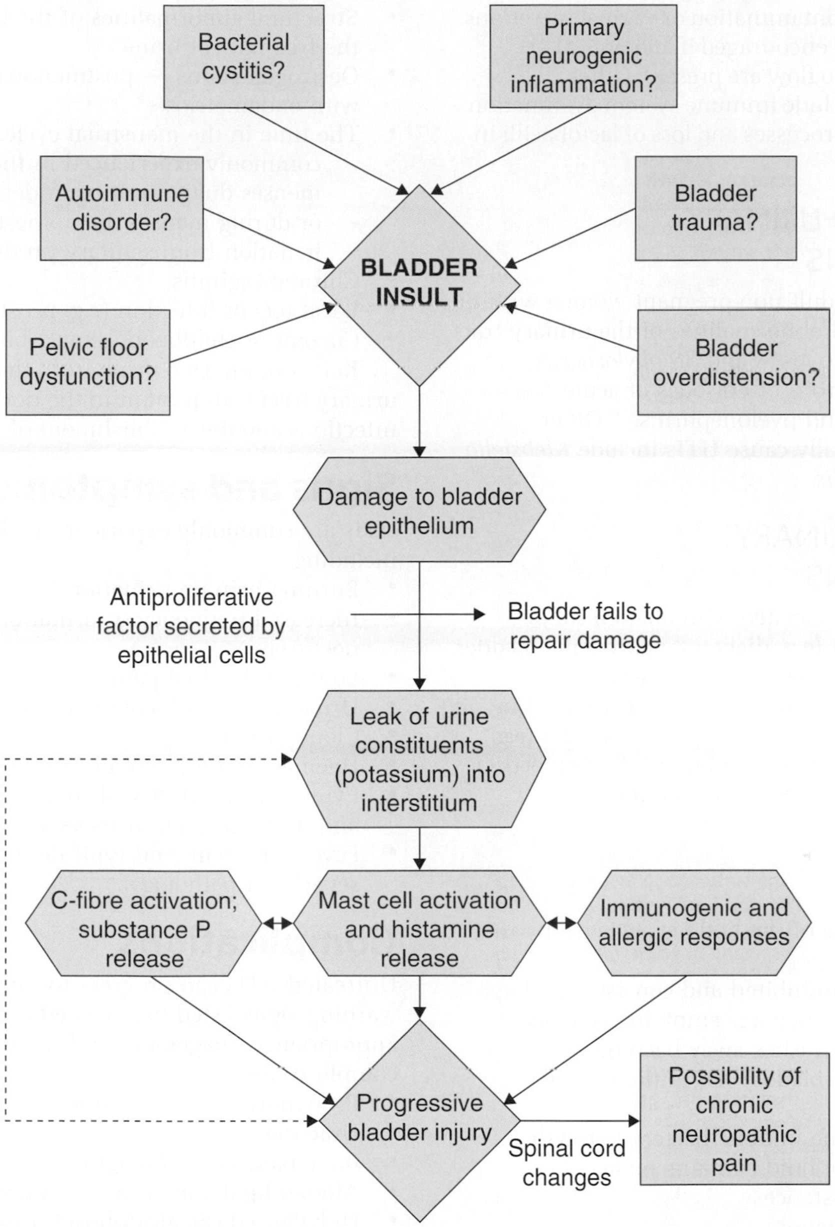

FIGURE 17.5 Urinary tract infections (cystitis)

infection. The indications for urgent medical referral are given in Box 17.3.

Aetiology

Most UTIs arise from the 'ascending' route of infection. The first step is colonisation of the periurethral tissues by uropathogenic organisms, followed by the passage of bacteria through the urethra. Infection arises from bacterial proliferation (growth) within the otherwise sterile urinary tract.

Urine is sterile until it reaches the urethra, which transports it from the bladder to the urethral opening. Bacteria can enter the body and reach the urinary tract through the urethral opening. These bacteria are most

BOX 17.3 Urinary tract infection: indications for urgent medical referral

If any of the following are relevant to your patient, medical referral is required:

- Significant results are not obtained within 12–24 hours
- The condition worsens
- Kidney pain is present
- High fever, nausea and/or vomiting eventuate
- Blood in the urine.

commonly from faecal contamination or vaginal secretions. Ascending infections are encouraged if anatomical or functional obstructions to flow are present. Other compounding factors include immune system dysfunction, allergy or autoimmune processes and loss of lactobacilli in the vaginal flora.[10]

UNCOMPLICATED URINARY TRACT INFECTIONS

These mainly occur in adult non-pregnant women with no functional or anatomical abnormalities of the urinary tract. *Escherichia coli* causes 70–95% and *Staphylococcus saprophyticus* causes 5–10% of episodes of acute uncomplicated cystitis and pyelonephritis.[14] Other organisms that occasionally cause UTIs include *Klebsiella* spp. and *Proteus mirabilis*.

COMPLICATED URINARY TRACT INFECTIONS

Complicated UTIs are associated with anatomical or functional abnormalities (e.g. diabetes, neurogenic bladder, nephrolithiasis) that increase the risk of serious complications or treatment failure. *E. coli* is isolated in 20–50% of cases, but other Gram-negative bacteria (e.g. *Proteus, Klebsiella*), enterococci and group B streptococci (*Streptococcus agalactiae*) are more common in complicated UTI.[10,14]

Pathogenesis

The antibacterial defence of the body is achieved by the following:

- Urine flow that is uninhibited and consists of a large volume, and complete bladder emptying is allowed:
  - the flow of urine washes away bacteria
  - the surface of the bladder has antimicrobial properties
  - the pH of the urine inhibits bacterial growth
  - in males, prostatic fluid contains many antimicrobial substances
- Optimal immune function:
  - the body rapidly secretes white blood cells to control bacteria if present.

Many factors are associated with an increased risk of bladder infection:

- Sexual activity pre-menopausal (spermicides, condoms, pre and post-coitus voiding)
- The age of the first UTI (more prevalent in early-onset UTI)
- Maternal history of UTIs
- Those with diabetes type 2 have a higher risk
- Excessive cleansing, douching, wiping techniques (unsubstantiated)[10]
- Faecal contamination
- Vaginal infection secretions
- Pregnancy (twice as frequent)
- Homosexual activity (in males)
- Poor hygiene of either sexual partner
- Contraceptive pill (oestrogen changes)
- Mechanical trauma or irritation
- Structural abnormalities of the urinary tract that block the free flow of urine
- Oestrogen status — postmenopausal women, women with endometriosis
- The time in the menstrual cycle:
  - commonly experienced in the luteal phase prior to menses due to oestrogen deficiency
  - or during menses due to oestrogen deficiency, irritation from sanitary products or poor hygiene
- Chronic vaginitis
- Local foci of infection (e.g. prostate, kidneys)
- Current or childhood sexual abuse.

Reflux of infected urine from the bladder into the upper urinary tract is important in the development of kidney infections and the establishment of recurrent infections.

Signs and symptoms

UTIs are commonly experienced with symptoms including:

- Burning pain on urination (dysuria)
- Increased frequency of urination, polyuria and/or nocturia
- Lower abdominal pain
- Urine that is dark coloured and has a strong odour
- Cloudy urine
- Haematuria (occasionally)
- Pyuria (urine white cell count greater than 10000/mL) and bacteriuria on urinalysis
- Fever can occur, and typically indicates increasing severity of pathology.

Complications

Untreated UTIs can progress to involve the kidneys. The warning signs listed below need careful consideration, and appropriate management and referral to prevent complications:

- Proteinuria (microalbuminaemia)
- Uraemia
- Bone pain, altered height or bone mass
- Altered lipid and amino acid levels
- Unbalanced calcium/phosphorus ratio
- Abnormal bun/creatinine ratio (normal ratio is 10:1; creatinine doubles when renal function decreases by 50%)
- Presence or history of UTIs
- Frequent weight shifts
- Leg cramps
- Weakness
- Pallor, anaemia
- Itching and dry skin
- Loss of appetite
- Difficulty sleeping
- Serum creatinine >1.7 mg/dL (chronic kidney disease)
- Protein energy malnutrition (PEM) or wasting.

Differential diagnosis

Urethral syndrome

Urethral syndrome (frequency and dysuria) is used to describe approximately 50% of women with these complaints who have either no bacterial growth or counts of <100 000 colony forming units (cfu)/mL on repeated urine cultures.

PYELONEPHRITIS

Pyelonephritis most commonly occurs as a result of UTIs, particularly in the presence of transient (occasional) or persistent backflow of urine from the bladder into the ureters or kidney pelvis (vesicoureteric reflux). Signs and symptoms include, in addition to those of a UTI, flank pain or back pain, fever, chills with shaking, and feeling generally unwell.

Acute pyelonephritis

Acute pyelonephritis can be severe in the elderly, in infants and in people who are immunosuppressed (e.g. those with cancer or AIDS). Although most people who present to the doctor or hospital have symptomatic UTIs, some can be asymptomatic and only those who are at high risk of developing further infections (pregnant women and the elderly) may require treatment. Some people have recurrent UTIs, with an average of two to three episodes a year. Children typically present with a high fever and systemic symptoms such as lethargy (tiredness), vomiting and poor feeding.

Interstitial cystitis

Interstitial cystitis is a chronic inflammatory condition of the bladder. There is often a long history of frequency, urinary discomfort and urgency in the absence of proven infection. Pain is usually suprapubic, although urethritis, loin pain and dyspareunia are also common. Patients with this condition also tend to have a higher incidence of inflammatory bowel disease, systemic lupus erythematosus, irritable bowel syndrome and fibromyalgia.

Endometriosis

Patients with recurrent UTIs should be properly screened for endometriosis in case potential endometrial cells are covering the bladder and causing recurrent irritation. For a full discussion see Chapter 18.

Sexually transmitted infections (STIs)

Young women who present with acute pain on urination or difficulty in urinating usually have either acute cystitis or acute urethritis caused by *Chlamydia trachomatis, Neisseria gonorrhoeae* or herpes simplex virus. Vaginitis caused by *Candida* spp. or *Trichomonas* can also involve dysuria. These infections can usually be differentiated on the basis of presenting symptoms, physical examination and urine analysis. A urine culture and vaginal culture may also be needed.

Naturopathic diagnosis

Due to the infective nature of UTIs, naturopaths interpret UTIs as a sign of lowered immunity, stress and hygiene concerns.

Investigations

The diagnosis of a UTI is often vague, as clinical symptoms and the presence of significant amounts of bacteria in the urine typically show poor correlation. Therefore, the diagnosis is often made on urinary findings and clinical presentation (signs and symptoms).

URINALYSIS

Urinalysis is the first investigation that should be conducted. Initial assessment using a dipstick in a clinical setting can be beneficial, but is potentially imprecise. A urinalysis is a group of tests that detect and semiquantitatively measure various compounds that are eliminated in the urine. These compounds include the byproducts of normal and abnormal metabolism as well as cells (including bacteria) and cell fragments. Midstream urine collection is preferred for accuracy of findings, 'clean catch'.[10]

A complete urinalysis consists of:

- Physical examination: to evaluate the colour, clarity and concentration of the urine
- Chemical examination: to test chemically for nine substances that provide valuable information about health and disease
- Microscopic examination: to identify and count the type and number of cells, casts, crystals and other components (bacteria, mucus) present in the urine. A microscopic examination is typically performed if there is an abnormal finding on the physical or chemical examination, or if specifically requested. Microscopic examination of the infected urine can show high levels of white blood cells (WBCs) and bacteria.

Dipstick methods

Dipsticks are invaluable for a qualitative and rough quantitative analysis. Typically, they provide information on pH, protein, glucose, ketones, bilirubin, haemoglobin, leucocyte esterase, nitrite and urobilinogen. Some dipsticks also allow for the detection of WBCs and bacteria (including semiquantitative cultures).

The dipstick is used to test for the presence of leucocyte esterase, with or without urinary nitrite and pyuria. However, there are problems with the sensitivity and specificity of the test. Using a dipstick may produce a false-negative result if bladder bacteria have not had enough time to produce a sufficient amount of nitrite to be detected in the test. The accuracy of the test is also altered if the individual is eating a vegetable-free diet or is using a diuretic.

Nitrite tests are also frequently negative, even in the presence of two bacteria, *Staphylococcus saprophyticus* and *Enterococcus* spp. Thus, a more accurate assessment would rely on the results of the leucocyte esterase test than on the nitrite test.

Urine culture

A urine culture is often done when the history and physical examination suggest that something more sinister is occurring. If a recent UTI has been treated and the symptoms are recurring, a culture would identify the possibility of a resistant pathogen. The urine culture is used to determine the quantity and type of bacteria involved. In more than 95% of UTIs, a single bacterial species is the problem. When mixed bacterial species are grown, the probability of contamination is high. *Staphylococcus epidermidis*, diphtheroids and lactobacilli are commonly found in the distal urethra, but rarely cause UTIs.

OTHER CONSIDERATIONS

Intravenous pyelogram

Those with recurrent urinary tract infections should undergo an intravenous pyelogram (urogram) to determine if a structural abnormality is present. Alternatively, cystourethroscopy or an ultrasound scan should be considered.

Pelvic examination

A pelvic examination is indicated if the history is consistent with vaginitis or cervicitis, or if there is confusion regarding the diagnosis.

SPECIFIC NATUROPATHIC INVESTIGATIONS

Naturopathic investigations include determining dietary triggers for UTIs and significant consideration of lifestyle influences. Complete history taking is typically the first objective, followed by in-clinic urinalysis/dipstick testing and referral for further investigations.

The examination and assessment should include:

- A thorough physical examination to assess the abdominal, renal and surrounding musculoskeletal areas
- Urinalysis/dipstick testing (midstream urine collection) in the clinic and referral for full urinalysis, as required
- Comprehensive assessment including questions pertaining to:
  - sexual activities (including contraception, lubricants, recent sexual practices and sexual hygiene)
  - hygiene and toilet habits
  - washing detergents, toiletries, cleaning products, toilet paper
  - sanitary products, menstrual timing and menstrual history
  - tight clothing and underwear material.

Therapeutic considerations

CLINICAL DECISION MAKING AND RATIONALE

The main treatment objectives include the following:

- Appropriately manage and care for the patient to prevent the development of the condition
- Support and enhance the immune response of the patient
- Encourage protective measures to reduce bacterial colonisation and prevent reoccurrence
- Encourage adequate hydration to increase urinary elimination and flushing of the bladder and urethral opening
- Promote pH changes that inhibit growth of the infective organism
- Prevent bacterial adherence to the endothelial cells of the bladder.

Appropriate patient care

While urinary tract infections are typically benign conditions, it is important to monitor patients closely and address abnormalities or concerns immediately. Patients should notify their practitioner immediately if there is any change in their condition. The practitioner is encouraged to retest further urine cultures if the first sample was positive, to assess the patient's progress and therapeutic outcome. This is best done 1–2 weeks following treatment initiation.

Increasing urinary output and hydration

Patients should be encouraged to increase their fluid intake to >2 L/day. Fluids that should be encouraged include pure water, herbal teas and fresh vegetable juices. Patients should be advised to avoid soft drinks, concentrated fruit juices/drinks, coffee, tea and alcohol.

Enhancing immune function

General immune-stimulating initiatives should be encouraged, with dietary, nutritional supplemental, lifestyle and herbal modifications.

MEDICAL MANAGEMENT

The development of antimicrobial therapy was the defining moment of 20th century medicine, and one of the key innovations in medical history. However, widespread use of certain antimicrobial agents, most notably amoxicillin and trimethoprim/sulfamethoxazole (TMP/SMX), has resulted in the development of resistance to these agents, which has been accompanied by a decrease in their clinical and bactericidal efficacy. Other treatments which may be considered include three days of trimethoprim, trimethoprim or a fluoroquinolone such as ciprofloxacin. Note that fluoroquinolones are not commonly used due to possible increased resistance of bacteria to this class of medication.[15]

The initial treatment of a UTI is typically a urine alkalinising agent to relieve symptoms, in conjunction with a high fluid intake and complete bladder emptying. Over-the-counter methenamine (hexamine) hippurate is available from pharmacies and is often the first line of treatment.[16] If there is no amelioration of symptoms or if the UTI perpetuates, treatment is then by antibiotics. Commonly used antibiotics are cefalexin, trimethoprim or trimethoprim + sulfamethoxazole. Prophylactic antibiotic prescriptions are commonly given to patients with chronic relapsing UTIs (including children), and intravaginal oestrogen may be prescribed for postmenopausal women. There does not seem to be a standard protocol for the duration, specific drug treatment or dose recommendations for intravaginal oestrogen therapies.[15]

Therapeutic application

NATUROPATHIC PERSPECTIVE

UTIs plagued mankind long before bacteria were recognised as the causative agents of disease and before urology became an established medical specialty. In 2005, Nickel[17] published a comprehensive review of the recorded medical history of UTIs, from their first description in ancient Egyptian papyri up to the present day. He concluded that, before the recognition of the bacterial origin of UTIs, treatment was predominantly palliative. A summary of the understanding and treatment of UTIs is given below.

- The Ebers papyrus from ancient Egypt provided detailed descriptions and a classification of urinary diseases, and recommended treatment approaches ranging from herbal treatments and bed rest, to invasive procedures, including surgery for stones, abscesses and retention. Treatments were generally recommended to ameliorate urinary symptoms, but no insight into the pathological mechanisms was given
- Hippocrates believed that disease was caused by disharmony of the four humours, and accordingly diagnosed urinary disorders
- Roman medicine further expanded the conservative approach (bed rest, diet, narcotics and herbs) advocated by Greek physicians, while also improving invasive techniques (surgical lithotomy for stones and catheterisation for retention)
- The Arabian physician Aetius refined uroscopy and created a detailed classification and interpretation of urinary disease based on this technique
- There were no major advances in the Middle Ages, although existing therapies were refined and treatments for gonococcal urethritis were described in detail
- The early 19th century provided vivid and detailed descriptions of UTIs. However, this was before the knowledge that UTIs are caused by microorganisms. Management included hospitalisation, bed rest, attention to diet, plasters, narcotics, herbal enemas and douches, judicious bleeding (direct bleeding, cupping and leeches), and surgery for stones, abscess and retention
- The discovery of microorganisms as the aetiological agents of infectious diseases in general and inflammation associated with urinary diseases in particular provided an impetus for physicians to critically examine management approaches and develop evidence-based strategies for the treatment of UTIs. Various antibacterial agents (e.g. hexamine, mercurochrome, hexylresorcinol, methylene blue, pyridium, acriflavin and mandelic acid) showed promise in laboratory studies but their efficacy in clinical investigations was disappointing
- Finally, in 1937, Helmholtz (in the *Journal of Urology*) showed that sulfanilamide was effective as an antimicrobial agent in UTIs, and so began the modern era of antimicrobial therapy.[17]

NUTRITIONAL MEDICINE (DIETARY)

Therapeutic objectives

1. Optimise digestive function and microflora colonisation with urinary specific probiotics
2. Avoid suspected and known food allergens
3. Encourage digestive immunity and immune-stimulating foods
4. Optimise hydration and flushing through the bladder and urethral opening (aim to drink 30 mL/kg body weight)
5. Balance pH with specific berry juices (cranberry and blueberry)
6. Encourage antioxidant-rich foods to increase immune support and response
7. Reduce immune-suppressant foods such as sugar and refined carbohydrates
8. Reduce urinary irritant substances such as caffeinated beverages (coffee, tea, cocoa, coke), alcohol and spicy foods.

Specific treatments

DIGESTIVE MICROFLORA

As the primary cause of UTIs stems from stool bacteria, it is understandable that dietary modifications can enable significant reduction in infection risk and amelioration of symptoms. Modification of stool composition and digestive health is undoubtedly a positive health influence.

A study highlighted various dietary protective factors found in berries and fermented foods. A higher intake of foods containing flavonoids, vitamin C (berries) and probiotics was found to decrease complications from urinary tract infection, particularly in subgroups of pregnant females, neurogenic bladder, catheterisation, HIV and immune-compromised patients.[18]

Therefore, it is prudent to increase probiotic and prebiotic foods to support this objective. Common probiotic-containing foods include yoghurt and kefir (fermented milk) and prebiotic foods include miso paste and umeboshi paste.

Members of the *Allium* family, such as garlic (*Allium sativum*) and onion (*Allium cepa*), have been shown to produce antimicrobial activity against a number of microorganisms, including *E. coli*, *Proteus* spp., *Klebsiella pneumoniae*, *Staphylococcus* spp. and *Streptococcus* spp.[19]

Overconsumption of sugar and other refined carbohydrates will disturb the microflora balance and will foster unhealthy organism inhabitation of the digestive and urinary system.

General support of optimal digestive function is to be encouraged, with a dietary focus on wholegrains, complex carbohydrates, fibre, adequate fresh vegetables and fruits, cold-pressed oils, fermented dairy products and sufficient protein to enable appropriate immune response.

AVOIDANCE OF DIETARY TRIGGERS

Common dietary allergens will undoubtedly reduce the ability of the immune system to fight the infection. Therefore, it is essential to remove any allergens from the diet, particularly in a patient suffering recurrent infections.

DIETARY INCLUSIONS

- Prebiotic and probiotic foods, such as yoghurt, kefir, sauerkraut, miso, umeboshi and oats

- Liberal amounts of immune-stimulating foods, such as garlic and onions
- A large amount of fluids (at least 2 L/day) — remember to consider the quality of water and its source
- 0.5 L/day of unsweetened cranberry juice or 0.25 L/day of blueberry juice (see the full discussion in the herbal medicine section, below).

DIETARY EXCLUSIONS

- All simple sugars
- Refined carbohydrates
- Full-strength fruit juice
- Food allergens
- Caffeinated beverages
- Alcohol.

NUTRITIONAL MEDICINE (SUPPLEMENTAL)

Therapeutic objectives

- Rebalance microflora colonies in the bladder
- Stimulate immunity to eradicate infection
- Support tissue integrity and tissue repair
- Provide antioxidant nutrients to support immune function
- Prevent adhesion of pathogenic organisms to uroepithelial cells.

Specific nutrients required

PROBIOTICS

The human body contains probiotic species throughout, the quantity and species being determined by location and

SAMPLE DAILY DIET

BREAKFAST	
Wholegrain, untoasted and unsweetened muesli with natural nuts and seeds sprinkled throughout. Fresh mixed berries and natural, unsweetened yoghurt. Cinnamon and vanilla extract used to sweeten as desired	The muesli provides complex carbohydrates, essential fatty acids and protein to stabilise blood sugars, provide optimal nutrition and foster appropriate digestive health. Mixed berries are an excellent source of antioxidant nutrients and will support and regulate the pH of the urine. Yoghurt will provide dietary probiotics to regulate digestive microflora and reduce transference of unhealthy bacteria to the urinary system. Cinnamon can act as a mild anti-inflammatory and astringent, and will also reduce sugar requirements for the meal.
LUNCH	
Mixed vegetable salad, yoghurt and garlic dressing, chickpeas, sunflower seeds and brown rice	Vegetables are chosen for fibre content to support digestive health, yoghurt for probiotic content, garlic for immune support, chickpeas for easily digestible protein and vegetarian fibre, sunflower seeds for added protein and essential fatty acids, and brown rice for fibre, complex carbohydrates and to complete the protein requirements with the other vegetarian protein foods.
DINNER	
Mixed vegetables stir fried with two cloves of garlic and half an onion	Onions and garlic are included to support immune response and to reduce infection.
Protein options to add to the stir-fried vegetables	Organic lean chicken breast (excellent protein for immune support); tofu (especially if postmenopausal, for added phyto-oestrogen content); fresh salmon (for added essential fatty acid content to reduce inflammation).
SNACKS	
Mixed vegetable juice (celery, carrot, beetroot, ginger, spinach)	This combination of vegetables provides a gentle diuretic, extra hydration and highly absorbable nutrients. If the patient agrees, juiced garlic is a beneficial inclusion for immune stimulation and support.
Trail mix (pumpkin seeds, sunflower seeds, flax seeds, almonds, cashews)	This is a great source of protein, vitamins and minerals, although care should be taken to ensure that all nuts and seeds are raw (unroasted), unsalted and fresh. If the patient has a known nut allergy, avoidance/extreme caution of all nuts is advised.
BEVERAGES	
Mixed vegetable juice (celery, carrot, beetroot, ginger, spinach)	Herbal teas such as corn silk, dandelion leaf and nettle leaf provide diuretic support and hydration. Chamomile can offer mild sedation and pain relief. The patient should aim to drink 8–12 glasses/day of pure water.

system. As research into this area has evolved it has become possible to identify and isolate species with greater specificity. The bladder has been shown to contain several species of probiotics that we know of (*Lactobacillus iners, L. crispatus, L. gasseri* or *L. jensenii,* which maintain the acidic pH).[19,20] Microbiome changes occur in various health states and diseases and within ethnic groups.[21] The urethra contains 10^1–10^2 *E. coli,* which typically are from transference from the large intestine. The vagina ecology is dominated by *Lactobacillus* spp., which adhere to the uroepithelial cells and inhibit the adherence of pathogenic organisms.[21] This is especially beneficial as studies have shown that women with recurrent UTIs have increased uropathogens on the introitus and vagina.[22]

Microbiological and clinical studies on the use of *Lactobacillus* spp. in treating UTIs have shown promising results,[23] with *L. rhamnosus* and *L. reuteri* [*fermentum*] being found to be the most effective.[23,24] The results also indicate that probiotic treatment is especially effective in the prevention of UTIs, probably due to its effects on pH regulation and inhibition of adherence.

In view of the above, daily dietary supplementation with natural yoghurt and other fermented dairy products is advisable, with probiotic supplementation as necessary. In severe UTIs, topical preparations of probiotic powders mixed with natural yoghurt and vitamin E oil often provide the most rapid resolution of the infection and symptomatic relief. A typical recipe for such a preparation is as follows:

- 1 teaspoon of probiotic powder containing multiple *Lactobacillus* spp., especially *L. acidophilus, L. rhamnosus, L. reuteri* and *L. casei. Bifidobacterium* spp. have also been shown to inhibit various gastrointestinal tract colonisations, such as those by *E. coli,* and therefore provide additional support
- 1 tablespoon of unsweetened, natural yoghurt (full-fat)
- 1 vitamin E capsule broken open and mixed with oil into a paste.

The mixture is applied topically, being inserted into the vagina if required. For optimal results the mixture can be syringed into the vagina and left in situ overnight.

VITAMIN C

Vitamin C is an essential nutrient, as humans are one of the few animal species that cannot synthesise it endogenously. Although the vitamin is found widely in fruit and vegetables, up to 100% can be destroyed during cooking and storage because it is sensitive to light, heat, oxygen and alkaline environments. Therefore supplementation for therapeutic purposes is advisable.

Vitamin C is an important biological antioxidant and has been a popular nutritional supplement for decades. It is an electron donor (reducing agent or antioxidant), and this accounts for most of its biochemical and molecular functions. It is involved in many biochemical processes, such as collagen biosynthesis and immune stimulation. In vivo and in vitro studies have provided evidence of immunostimulatory effects of vitamin C, generally at doses above the recommended daily intake (RDI). Vitamin C favourably modulates lymphocytes and phagocytes, regulates natural killer cells, and under certain conditions can influence antibody and cytokine synthesis.[25] It is these roles of vitamin C that are involved in maintaining the normal tissue of the bladder and urethra.

Vitamin C is a known urinary acidifier, and this may prove beneficial in some types of UTI. Clinical studies indicate that the therapeutic dose required is 4–12 g taken in divided doses every 4 hours.

BIOFLAVONOIDS

Bioflavonoids act synergistically with vitamin C, and these two nutrients are often found together in foods. Bioflavonoids have the following effects on vitamin C:

- Improve the absorption of vitamin C
- Extend the activity of vitamin C
- Prevent oxidation of vitamin C
- May partially substitute for vitamin C in its biological functions.

Therefore, it is prudent to co-supplement bioflavonoids and vitamin C in order to enhance the efficacy of the prescription and outcome.

VITAMIN A

Vitamin A is a fat-soluble vitamin that is found in high amounts in liver (especially in the livers of animals living in cold climates, such as polar bears). Vitamin A plays a role in the health of skin, mucous membranes and connective tissue, and in supporting the immune system functions and protecting against infection.

It is advisable to co-supplement vitamin A with zinc in initial prescriptions, and then to reduce zinc supplementation as zinc repletion occurs. The rationale for this is that, in zinc deficiency, the level of vitamin A is reduced in the plasma and elevated in the liver, because zinc is required for the absorption, transport and use of vitamin A.

Β-CAROTENE

In cases where vitamin A supplementation is inadvisable (due to the high storage capacity of the liver for this vitamin and the subsequent toxic risk), long-term β-carotene supplementation may be preferred. β-carotene is a vitamin A precursor; it has antioxidant effects and plays a role in disease prevention.

VITAMIN E

Vitamin E is a fat-soluble vitamin. Its main role is as an antioxidant. In addition, it supports the integrity of the mucous membranes and the recovery of other body tissues. It prevents the oxidation of vitamin A in the gastrointestinal tract and at storage sites during transport. It has also been shown to protect against some of the effects of vitamin A toxicity.

ZINC

Zinc is an essential trace element for all forms of life. More than 85% of total body zinc is found in skeletal muscle and bone. The biological function of zinc can be catalytic, structural or regulatory.

Zinc is a component of various enzymes that help maintain the structural integrity of proteins and regulate gene expression. Zinc metalloenzymes include ribonucleic acid polymerases, alcohol dehydrogenase, carbonic anhydrase and alkaline phosphatase.[26]

One of the major roles of zinc is to enhance the immune response and support effective elimination of pathogens. It has been shown to increase resistance to infection and increase white blood cell numbers and activity.

It is important to monitor the dose of zinc correctly, as high doses (>80 mg/day long term) have been associated with increased urinary physiology (including UTIs) and associated hospital admissions.[26]

D-MANNOSE

D-mannose is a naturally occurring simple sugar contained in cranberry juice. It inhibits adherence of pathogenic organisms to the uroepithelial cells. It has a specific affinity for *E. coli*, and appears to bind directly to the glycoprotein of the pathogen (lectin projection), forming a D-mannose–*E. coli* complex that is unable to adhere to the bladder wall and is effectively eliminated through urination.[27] Supplementation with D-mannose typically leads to symptom alleviation within a few days.

Dosage requirements

All the doses listed below are adult doses reported in the literature:

- Probiotics: multi-species (high in *Lactobacilli* spp. where possible), ½ teaspoon 3–4 times daily (30–50 × 10^7 organisms per teaspoon)
- Vitamin C: 5 g/d maximum in divided doses (up to bowel tolerance)
- Bioflavonoids: 1000 mg/day
- Vitamin A: 25 000 IU/day (short term 1–2 weeks ensure patient is not pregnant)
- β-carotene: 30 mg/day
- Vitamin E: 500 IU/day
- Zinc: 30–60 mg/day
- D-mannose: 500 mg every 2 hours for 5 days.

HERBAL MEDICINE

Before antibiotics, there were herbal medicines, and these continue to be used today as an effective treatment option for UTIs. Herbal medicines are particularly useful for recurrent infections, as they have an important preventive effect. The herbal medicines most commonly used in UTIs are given in Table 17.8.

TABLE 17.8 The major herbal medicines used in urinary tract infections

Name	Main constituent(s)	Main action in urinary tract
Barosma betulina (Buchu)	Flavonoids, terpenoids, mucilage	Antibacterial
Agropyron repens (Couch grass)	Terpenoids, glycosides, mucilage	Potentially prevents bacterial adhesion, soothing
Althaea officinalis (Marshmallow)	Mucilage	Soothing
Apium graveolens (Celery)	Terpenoids	Aquaretic, anti-inflammatory
Arctostaphylos uva-ursi (Uva ursi)	Arbutin	Antibacterial
Betula spp. (Birch)	Salicylates, terpenoids	Aquaretic, anti-inflammatory
Chimaphila umbellata (Pipsissewa)	Arbutin	Antibacterial
Crataeva nurvala (Crataeva)	Lupeol	Tonic
Equisetum arvense (Horsetail)	Saponins, alkaloids	Aquaretic
Glycyrrhiza glabra (Liquorice)	Glycyrrhizin, flavonoids	Anti-inflammatory, soothing
Hydrastis canadensis (Goldenseal)	Alkaloids, hydrastine, berberine	Antibacterial, immunostimulant
Juniperus communis (Juniper)	Terpenoids	Anti-inflammatory, antimicrobial, aquaretic
Levisticum officinale (Lovage)	Coumarins	Aquaretic
Piper methysticum (Kava)	Kava lactones, resin	Sedative, nervine
Populus tremuloides (White poplar)	Glycosides	Anti-inflammatory
Scutellaria spp. (Skullcap)	Flavonoids	Sedative, nervine
Solidago virgaurea (Goldenrod)	Saponins, flavonoids, glycosides	Aquaretic, anti-inflammatory
Taraxacum officinalis (Dandelion [leaf])	Glycosides, terpene lactones	Aquaretic, diuretic
Vaccinium macrocarpon (Cranberry)	Proanthocyanidins	Prevents bacterial adhesion, antiseptic
Zea mays (Corn silk)	Mannose, mucilage	Potentially prevents bacterial adhesion, aquaretic, soothing

Source: Adapted from Abascal K, Yarnell E. Botanical medicine for cystitis. Alt Comp Ther 2008; 14203:69–77.

Therapeutic objectives

1. Prevent adherence of bacteria to the urethra and bladder
2. Increase diuresis to flush out the urethra and bladder
3. Eradicate pathogens through antimicrobial and antibacterial actions
4. Increase the immune response
5. Tonify, heal and reduce inflammation of the urethra and bladder.

Herbal medicine classes

- Bladder tonics
- Diuretics
- Urinary demulcents
- Urinary antiseptics
- Urinary tract astringents
- Immune stimulants
- Antibacterials
- Antimicrobials
- Lymphatics.

Specific herbal medicines

DIURETIC HERBAL MEDICINES

Herbal medicines used for their diuretic properties are listed in Table 17.9. A discussion of whether these medicines are true diuretics or are, in fact, aquaretics is given in Box 17.4.

Solidago spp. (goldenrod)

Solidago extracts are used as adjunct therapy in patients with lower UTIs.[28] No single active constituent has been isolated from the plant; rather, multiple compounds are likely to contribute to its actions. Scientific research is limited, with minimal human trials. However, the little research that has been conducted remains promising, and historical and clinical evidence is strong, as goldenrod exhibits consistent diuretic effects.[25]

ANTIMICROBIAL AND ANTI-ADHESION HERBAL MEDICINES

Vaccinium macrocarpon Ait/(cranberry) *fructus*

Fructus is a native North American bog plant of the Ericaceae family. Cranberries (particularly in the form of juice) have been used widely for several decades for the prevention and treatment of UTIs, and a number of clinical trials have shown them to be highly effective.[29,30] Cranberry is non-toxic and is safe in pregnancy and lactation, given that it is routinely consumed as a food in such situations without ill effects.[30] Cranberries comprise

BOX 17.4 Aquaretic or diuretic?

The term 'diuretic' may be an incorrect description for these herbal medicines. Some herbalists believe that plants traditionally referred to as diuretics may not act by interfering with the renal handling of ions, but instead may act to increase blood flow to the kidneys and thereby raise the glomerular filtration rate (i.e. have an aquaretic action). Whether they are aquaretics or diuretics, these agents can benefit patients with UTIs, as increased urine flow helps wash bacteria out of the urinary bladder.

TABLE 17.9 Diuretic herbal medicines

Potency	Latin name (common name)	Part used	Family	Miscellaneous notes	Commission E approved for diuresis
Strong	*Solidago* spp. (goldenrod)	Herba	Asteraceae	Anti-inflammatory	Yes
	Levisticum officinale W Koch (lovage)	Radix	Apiaceae	Mild risk of photosensitivity	Yes
	Betula spp. (birch)	Folium	Betulaceae	Antimicrobial, anti-inflammatory	Yes
	Petroselinum crispum (Mill) Nyman ex AW Hill (parsley)	Radix, fructus	Apiaceae	Antispasmodic, anti-inflammatory	Yes (root only)
	Aplum graveolens L (celery)	Fructus	Apiaceae	Antispasmodic	No
Medium	*Taraxacum officinale* Weber ex FH Wigg (dandelion)	Folium	Asteraceae	Bitter digestive tonic	No
	Ononis campestris Koch and Ziz (restharrow)	Radix	Fabaceae	Aqueous extracts only	Yes
	Urtica dioica L (stinging nettle)	Folium	Urticaceae	Anti-inflammatory, radix for BPH	Yes
Mild	*Parietaria judaica* L (pellitory-of-the-wall)	Herba	Urticaceae		No
	Galium aparine L (cleavers)	Herba	Rubiaceae		No
	Equisetum arvense L (horsetail)	Herba	Equisetaceae	Commission E also approves topical use for wounds and internal use for post-traumatic oedema	Yes
	Chimaphila umbellata L WPC Barton (pipsissewa)	Herba	Ericaceae	Demulcent, mild antimicrobial	No

BPH benign prostatic hyperplasia
Source: Reprinted with permission of Springer Nature. From Yarnell W. Botanical medicines for the urinary tract. World J Urol 2002; 20:285–93.

nearly 90% water, but also contain various organic substances such as quinic acid, malic acid and citric acid, as well as glucose and fructose (Table 17.10).

Until recently, it was suggested that the quinic acid caused large amounts of hippuric acid to be excreted in the urine, which then acted as an antibacterial agent (Box 17.5).[31] However, it has since been demonstrated that cranberries prevent bacteria (particularly *E. coli*) from adhering (sticking) to the uroepithelial cells that line the wall of the bladder.[32] It is now known that two chemicals, both found in cranberry, mediate the adhesion of bacteria to the uroepithelial cells that line the wall of the bladder — fructose, which inhibits adherence of type 1 (mannose specific) fimbriated *E. coli*; and proanthocyanidins, which inhibit the adherence of type 1 and P-fimbriated (α-galactose-(1-4) specific) *E. coli*.[33] Although many juices contain fructose, only cranberries and blueberries contain the polymeric compound.[34] Blueberries exhibit similar constituents (*Vaccinium angustifolium* Ait and other species) to cranberries, and show similar anti-adhesion activity.[34] Cranberry has also been shown to inhibit binding of *E. coli* to intestinal mucosa and binding of *Helicobacter pylori* to gastric mucosa.[35,36]

There have been an astounding number of studies on the efficacy of cranberry juice in treating UTIs as evidenced in the Cochrane review referred to above.[30] This meta-analysis of the results of thirteen RCTs with 9 parallel and 4 cross-over trials concluded that cranberry products significantly reduce the incidence of UTIs in women with recurrent UTIs, girls and pregnant females (relative risk [RR] 0.49; 95% CI: 0.34 to 0.73) compared with a placebo/control.[30]

Based on the literature, to achieve positive effects from cranberry juice requires a daily intake of 250–300 mL at least three times daily (ideally 2 L/day). This can be unpalatable, expensive or inconvenient for some and, depending on the quality of the cranberry juice, potentially ineffective or harmful. Most cranberry juices on the market contain one-third cranberry juice mixed with water and sugar. As sugar is detrimental to the immune

TABLE 17.10 Composition of raw cranberries and cranberry juice (per 100 g/mL)

Ingredient	Raw cranberries	Cranberry juice
Water (%)	87.32	87.13
Calories	46	46
Total carbohydrate (g)	11.97	12.2
Sugars (g)	4.27	12.1
Dietary fibre (g)	3.6	0.1
Protein (g)	0.46	<0.1
Fat (g)	0.13	<0.1
Minerals		
Sodium (mg)	2	2
Potassium (mg)	80	77
Calcium (mg)	8	8
Iron (mg)	0.2	0.25
Vitamins		
Vitamin C (mg)	14	9.3
Thiamin (mg)	0.012	0.009
Riboflavin (mg)	0.020	0.018
Niacin (mg)	1.101	0.019
Vitamin B_6 (mg)	1.057	0.052
Folate (micrograms)	1	1
Vitamin A IU	63	45
Vitamin E IU	1.32	1.20
Vitamin K (phylloquinone) micrograms	5.0	5.1
pH	Not analysed	2.5

Note: loss of some nutrient quantity in extracted form
Jepson RG, Williams G, Craig JC. Cranberries for treating urinary tract infections. Cochrane Database Syst Rev 2012; Oct 17:CD001321.

BOX 17.5 Evidence for cranberry as a urine acidifier

In 1923, Blatherwick and Long reported that the pH was lowered for two healthy volunteers by eating prunes and cranberries. They noted the following in the urine: a decrease in pH, an increase in titratable acidity, no significant changes in phosphorus excretion, an increase in ammonia output, a marked decrease in total nitrogen, and a very large increase in organic acids and hippuric acid. Subsequently, in 1933, Fellers et al evaluated the effects of cranberries in six men aged 22–27 years. The men consumed 100–300 g/day of cranberries. The titratable acidity, organic acids, hippuric acid, hydrogen ion concentration and ammonia were increased in the urine. The amount of hippuric acid recovered from the urine was proportional to the weight of cranberries consumed. The hippuric acid in the urine was largely voided over a 24-hour period after the ingestion of cranberries. The origin of most of the hippuric acid in the urine was quinic acid. The investigators found that an ordinary serving of 56–140 g of cranberry sauce (equivalent to 22–54 g of fresh cranberries) produced only very slight increases in urinary acidity. Later, in 1995, Bodel et al evaluated the effects of a cranberry juice cocktail consisting of one part juice from pressed cranberries and two parts water. Participants consumed up to 4 L of the cocktail daily. The urine was only slightly more acidic, with the pH change ranging from +0.1 to –0.5. None of the urine samples possessed antibacterial activity against *Escherichia coli* at the pH at which they were voided.

Blatherwick NR, Long ML. Studies of urinary tract acidity. II. The increased acidity produced by eating prunes and cranberries. J Biol Chem 1923; 57:815–18; Bodel PT, Cotran R, Kass EH. Cranberry juice and the antibacterial action of hippuric acid. J Lab Clin Med 1995; 54:881–8; Fellers CR, Redmon BC, Parrott EM. Effect of cranberries on urinary acidity and blood alkali reserve. J Nutr 1933; 6:455–63.

system, the use of sweetened cranberry juice cannot be recommended. Fresh cranberry (unsweetened or sweetened with apple or grape juice) or blueberry juice is preferred.

Cranberry tablets are also available and have been proven to be the most effective clinically and the most economical for the patient.[33] In one randomised controlled study 150 sexually active women aged 21–72 years were studied to assess the relative cost-effectiveness and efficacy of cranberry tablets and cranberry juice. Women were assigned to one of three groups of prophylaxis: placebo juice + placebo tablets, placebo juice + cranberry tablets, or cranberry juice + placebo tablets. Tablets were taken twice daily, and juice 250 mL t.d.s. Both cranberry juice and cranberry tablets statistically significantly decreased the number of patients experiencing at least one symptomatic UTI a year (to 20% and 18%, respectively) compared with placebo (to 32%) (p <0.05). Total antibiotic consumption was less annually in both treatment groups compared with placebo. Cost-effectiveness ratios demonstrated that cranberry tablets were twice as cost-effective as organic juice for prevention.[33]

A summary of the evidence regarding the use of cranberries is given in Table 17.11.

Arctostaphylos uva-ursi (bearberry)

Most research on *Arctostaphylos uva-ursi* (bearberry or upland cranberry) has focused on its urinary antiseptic component, arbutin, which typically makes up 6.3–9.6% of the leaves. In the body, arbutin is hydrolysed to hydroquinone and glucose. Hydroquinone is most effective in an alkaline urine. However, crude plant extracts are more effective medicinally than isolated arbutin.[37]

A double-blind study of the use for 1 month of an *A. uva-ursi* extract, standardised to arbutin and methylarbutin, in women with recurrent cystitis (defined as three or more infections in the previous year), found that *A. uva-ursi* prevented further episodes of cystitis in the year following the study. In contrast, 23% of women in a placebo group experienced at least one further episode of cystitis in the same period. The difference between the two groups was both statistically and clinically significant, and no side effects were noted in either group.[38] A more recent study suggests it is better suited as prophylactic treatment and for relief of mild symptoms. To be avoided in pregnancy.[38]

Punica granatum (pomegranate)

Punica granatum has a demonstrated antimicrobial activity (folia) in both aqueous and ethanolic extracts. The evidence suggests both aqueous and ethanolic solutions are effective against *E coli*, and ethanolic solutions against *Staphylococcus*. The ethanolic extract was also effective against *Candida albicans*, which makes this form of phytotherapy useful in the treatment of UTIs.[39]

DEMULCENT HERBAL MEDICINES

A number of the diuretic herbal medicines also exhibit demulcent properties; that is, they soothe irritated urothelial surfaces. Such demulcent medicines include:

- *Agropyron repens* (couch grass)
- *Althaea officinalis* (marshmallow)
- *Ulmus* spp. (slippery elm)
- *Zea mays* (corn silk).

While scientific research on these medicines is limited, traditional application warrants these prescriptions. They are highly safe, soothing and restorative additions to the holistic herbalist's armamentarium.

PRIMARY PROTOCOL

Cranberry

A number of effective cranberry tablets are available on the market. According to the results of trials, the most

TABLE 17.11 Findings from clinical studies on the use of cranberry supplementation in UTIs

Study	Summary of findings
Foxman (2015)	Review: Occurrence of UTIs in female study among women, undergoing gynaecological surgery with catheterisation, use of cranberry extract capsules postoperative reduced incidence of UTIs by 50%.
Huddleston (2015)	Review: Cranberry juice and extract did not reduce frequency of recurrent urinary tract infections in women; however there were multiple methodological flaws. Observed benefit in women > 50 years.
Maki (2016)	Double blind, placebo-controlled, multicentre clinical trial. Cranberry juice reduced the number of clinical UTI episodes in women with UTI history.
Liska DJ (2016)	Primary use of cranberry in healthy women has suggested positive results in the reduction of UTIs. Meta-analysis of prevention is conflicting; considerations for future research are methodology, heterogeneity, population groups, pathology, physiology and weight of summary risk estimates.
Kennedy (2016)	Multinational, cross-sectional study in the use of herbal medicines including cranberry in pregnancy. Generally considered safe in non-pregnant females, with paucity of studies in pregnancy. However, no negative outcomes determined for the fetal development in a large retrospective cohort study of 68 522 women of whom 919 were using cranberry during pregnancy.

Sources: Foxman B, Cronenwett AEW, Spino C et al. Cranberry juice capsules and urinary tract infection after surgery: results of a randomized trial. Am J Obstet Gynecol 2015; 213(2):194. e.8; Huddleston S, Ludwig MJ. Does cranberry juice or cranberry extract reduce the frequency of recurrent urinary tract infections in women? Evidence-Based Practice 2015; 18(3):7–8; Kennedy DA, Lupattelli A, Koren G et al. Safety classification of herbal medicines used in pregnancy in a multinational study. BMC Complementary and Alternative Medicine 2016; 16:102; Liska DJ, Kern HJ, Maki KC. Cranberries and urinary tract infections: how can the same evidence lead to conflicting advice? Adv Nutr 2016; 7:498–506; Maki KC, Kaspar KL, Khoo C et al. Consumption of cranberry juice beverage lowered the number of clinical urinary tract infection episodes in women with a recent history of urinary tract infection. Am Soc Nutr 2016; 103(6) :1434–42.

TABLE 17.12 Composition of example herbal formula for UTIs

Constituent	Dilution	Amount	Action
Agathosma betulina (buchu)	1:2	40 mL	Antimicrobial, urinary antiseptic
Arctostaphylos uva-ursi (bearberry)	1:2	40 mL	Antimicrobial, anti-adhesion
Solidago spp. (goldenrod)	1:2	40 mL	Anti-inflammatory, diuretic
Calendula officinalis (calendula)	1:2	40 mL	Lymphatic, immune stimulant, mucous membrane tonic
Crataeva nurvala (crataeva)	1:2	60 mL	Bladder tonic
Total		220 mL	

Sources: Stothers LA. Randomized trial to evaluate effectiveness and cost effectiveness of naturopathic cranberry products as prophylaxis against urinary tract infection in women. Can J Urol 2002; 9(3):1558–1562; Wang CH, Fang CC, Chen NC et al. Cranberry-containing products for prevention of urinary tract infections in susceptible populations: a systematic review and meta-analysis of randomized controlled trials. Arch Intern Med 2012; 172(13):988–96.

effective formulation provides 400–800 mg/day of 25:1 dry concentrate (based on fresh weight), which is equivalent to 10–20 g/day of fresh berries.

The dosage is as follows:

- Acute UTI: 2 tablets t.d.s. or q.i.d.
- Subacute UTI: 1 tablet t.d.s. or q.i.d.
- Prophylaxis: 1 tablet b.i.d.

Herbal formula

The composition of the herbal formula is given in Table 17.12. The dosage is as follows:

- Acute UTI: 5 mL 3–5 times daily
- Subacute UTI: 5 mL b.i.d. or t.d.s.

LIFESTYLE RECOMMENDATIONS

Sexual and personal health

Patients should be encouraged to modulate sexual hygiene practices and consider the following key objectives:

- Urinate after intercourse. In cases of recurrent infection, women can use a douche of *Hydrastis canadensis* (goldenseal) and *Calendula officinalis* (calendula), or tea tree (diluted) washes
- Avoid toxic lubricants, flavoured or scented condoms, and wash diaphragms thoroughly. In cases of recurrent infection, consider alternative contraception to diaphragm
- In recurrent infection or infection from cross-contamination, encourage the use of condoms
- In postmenopausal women, encourage the use of condoms with a natural lubricant, such as Sylk (pH regulated to 4.5–4.7) or natural yoghurt
- Use unperfumed toilet paper
- Women should be encouraged to wipe away from the vagina and urethra after passing a stool
- Review toiletries to ensure the patient uses natural alternatives that are unscented and non-irritating.

CASE STUDY

OVERVIEW

AR is a 30-year-old female who presents with dysuria with pain and urgency. She has had several bouts of cystitis in the past and states that this current one feels the same. The onset was 24 hours ago. Initially there was mild urgency with some discomfort (1/10; 1 being little pain and 10 being unbearable). However, it is now at 3/10 and she is concerned as she understands that there are potential complications should this condition be left untreated for too long. Of note is that she had not seen her partner for 3 weeks as he was away on business and she describes her sexual activity as very active over the weekend when he returned. She is not on the oral contraceptive pill and her form of contraception is spermicide and condoms.

HISTORY

AR is a marathon runner. Her diet consists of high glycaemic sports drinks, foods and gels pre, during and post training sessions, with little to no water. Her usual diet is high carbohydrate. Breakfast varies with egg, white bread and margarine, sometimes grain breads and occasionally wheat biscuits and skim milk. She enjoys a large watermelon juice or a skim milk-based smoothie with berries and a little protein powder at times for morning tea or a black double shot coffee. Lunch may be Thai food, Chinese or a stir fry, all of which she likes smothered with sweet sauces. Dinner varies; however, it is a copy of lunch, possibly with the occasional roast dinner when she visits her mother.

She enjoys her running sessions and also completes two to three weight training sessions a week. She presents with bloating, flatulence and occasional diarrhoea at times although she is unaware of the triggers. Her energy levels are high during the day at 8/10 which is useful as she is a personal trainer; however, she states she crashes at 6–7 pm, may have a micro sleep and then stay awake until 12 pm. She finds it hard to get back to sleep and feels sluggish on rising in the morning. Her family history is of cardiovascular disease though both parents smoked from an early age.

CLINICAL EXAMINATION

AR has mounting suprapubic pain, with some tenderness. On observation of a urine sample the urine appears slightly cloudy with a mild odour. She states that she thinks the toilet tissue after wiping has a slight pink tinge.

INVESTIGATION RESULTS

Urinary dipstick analysis

Odour: mild
Colour: dark yellow

CASE STUDY CONTINUED

Leucocytes: ++
Nitrite: NAD
Urobiligen: NAD
Protein: +
pH: 8 (possible due to increased urinary alkaliser)
Haemoglobin: ++
Specific gravity: 1.020
Ketone: NAD
Bilirubin: +
Glucose: negative
Bacterial activity: ≥100 000 cfu/mL

Urine culture

E. coli: positive
Proteus spp.: negative
Klebsiella spp.: negative
Pseudomonas spp.: negative
Enterococcus: negative
Staphylococcus spp.: positive

TREATMENT PROTOCOL

INITIAL APPOINTMENT

Combined herbal medicine and lactobacillus

Cranberry tablets containing:
Vaccinum macrocarpon: 10.8 g equiv proanthocyanidins 18 mg
Punica granatum: 3.75 equiv punicalagins 150 mg
Vitamin D: 12.5 micrograms equiv 500 IU
Lactobacillus plantarum: 12.5 billion CFU
Dosage:
Acute UTI: 1 tablet t.d.s. or q.i.d.
Subacute UTI: 1 tablet b.i.d.
Prophylaxis: 1 tablet. q.i.d.

Herbal formula with the following composition (total 200 mL):
Echinacea blend (echinacea): 1 : 2, 60 mL (antimicrobial, immune enhancing)
Zea mays (corn silk): 1 : 1, 60 mL (anti-inflammatory, diuretic, demulcent)
Solidago spp. (goldenrod): 1 : 2, 40 mL (anti-inflammatory, diuretic)
Arctostaphylos uva-ursi (bearberry): 1 : 2, 60 mL (astringent, diuretic, urinary antiseptic).
Dosage:
Acute UTI: 5 mL 3–5 times daily
Subacute UTI: 5 mL b.i.d. or t.d.s.

NUTRITIONAL MEDICINE

Dietary

Increase hydration: aim to drink 2–2.5 L/day pure water (calculated on basis of 30 mL/kg body weight)
Increase herbal teas such as *Urtica dioica* folia (nettle) and *Calendula officinalis* (calendula)
Avoid soft drinks (diet coke), fruit juices and caffeinated beverages
Avoid sugar and refined carbohydrate.
Encourage prebiotic and probiotic foods (e.g. yoghurt, kefir, miso).

CASE STUDY CONTINUED

Nutritional supplementation

Ensure adequate probiotic strain
Topical application of probiotic (1 teaspoon) mixed into natural yoghurt as required, for pain relief
500 mg vitamin C with bioflavonoids every hour until symptoms subside, then 1 g t.d.s. for remainder of week
Zinc 25 mg b.i.d.

LIFESTYLE/EDUCATION

- Sexual hygiene education, including postcoital urination, and discussion about contraception and spermicidal and condom use
- Hygiene and washing education.

FOLLOW-UP

All symptoms settled within 24 hours and resolved in 2 days. The protocol was continued over a period of a week with all other lifestyle guidelines. The urinary care tablets were continued for 1 month. AR was cautioned to be aware of acute onset and to reintroduce prescriptions at the onset should symptoms recur in the future.

ENURESIS

Enuresis (bed-wetting) is typically a condition of childhood, but it can and does affect people of all ages (see Fig. 17.6). Incontinence (generally perceived as the adult presentation) is covered in greater detail in Chapters 18 and 19.

Epidemiology

Nocturnal enuresis is a common paediatric problem and was first documented as early as 1550 BC.[40] It occurs worldwide in all cultures and races, and has been problematic from antiquity to the present day. Epidemiological studies have reported prevalence rates of 3.8% to 25%, depending on patient age, country of nationality and the definition used.[40]. In Australia enuresis occurs in approximately 20% of 5-year-olds, 10% of 10-year-olds and may resolve by 14% in each of the ensuing years. Only 34% of families with children who suffer nocturnal enuresis seek medical advice.[41,42]

Classification

Enuresis is not often considered to be technically a disease of the urinary organs, but rather a psychological condition that affects the urinary system. Night-time bed-wetting (or nocturnal enuresis (NE) or sleep-wetting) is involuntary urination while asleep. It is normal in infancy, but can be a source of embarrassment when it persists into school age or the teen years. The aetiology of EN is elusive but is no doubt linked to the urological system with further possible links to genetic, psychosocial, hormonal and neurodevelopmental factors.[43]

Enuresis can be primary or secondary, and nocturnal or diurnal. Nocturnal and diurnal enuresis can further be classified into monosymptomatic and polysymptomatic enuresis (see Fig. 17.7).

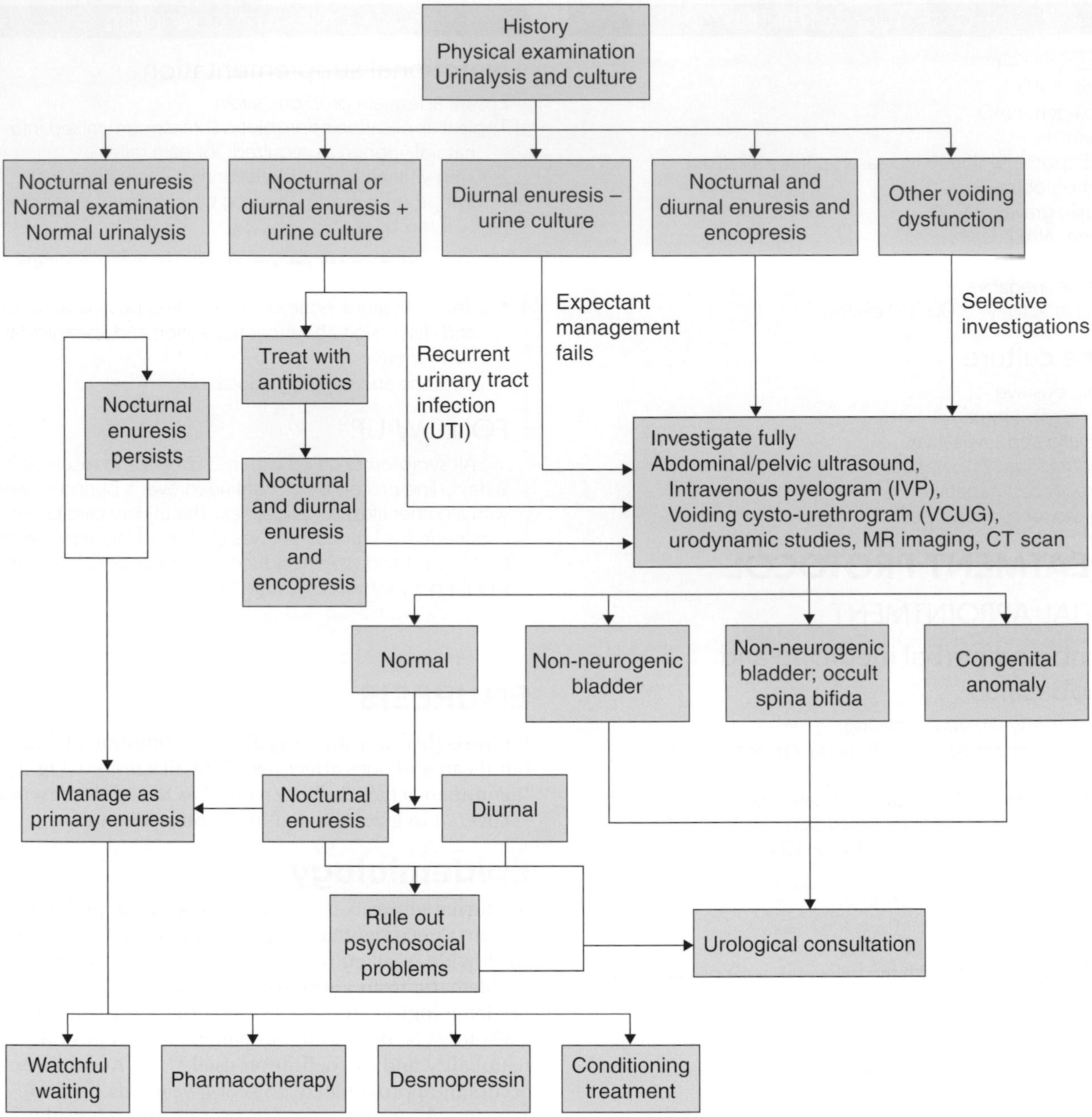

FIGURE 17.6 Enuresis

Chin AI, Lerman SE. Bedwetting. In Encyclopedia of infant and early childhood development. London: Academic Press; 2008.

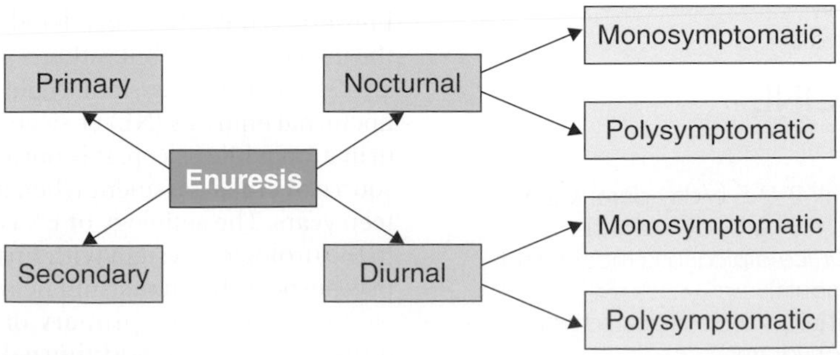

FIGURE 17.7 Classification of enuresis

Chin AI, Lerman SE. Bedwetting. In Encyclopedia of infant and early childhood development. London: Academic Press; 2008.

PRIMARY ENURESIS

Primary enuresis refers to wetting in a person who has never been dry for at least 6 months. Primary enuresis describes one of the following conditions where:

- The child has never been dry at night
- The child does not sleep dry without being taken to the toilet by another person
- The child has some dry nights, but continues to average at least two wet nights a week, with no long periods of dryness.

SECONDARY ENURESIS

Secondary enuresis refers to wetting that begins after at least 6 months of dryness. Secondary enuresis is often, but not always, caused by emotional stress.

NOCTURNAL ENURESIS

Nocturnal enuresis refers to wetting that usually occurs during sleep (night-time incontinence).

DIURNAL ENURESIS

Diurnal enuresis refers to wetting when awake (daytime incontinence).

Aetiology

Children usually achieve night-time dryness by developing one or both of two abilities, as outlined in Box 17.6. The persistence of nocturnal enuresis in children probably has many causes. Multiple theories have been proposed including: genetic predisposition; physiological problems, including low functional bladder capacity and bladder instability; increased night-time urine production due to behavioural or endocrine factors; and delay of maturation. Ultimately, nocturnal enuresis is a problem of too great a urine production relative to bladder capacity. The reason for this is hypothesised to be related to problems with arousal, small bladder capacity and large overnight urine production, attention-deficit hyperactivity disorder (ADHD), constipation, encopresis, developmental problems, male gender and young age.[44]

Pathogenesis

In an Australian study,[45] 2856 parents of primary school children (47.4% girls) aged 7.3 ± 1.3 years (mean ± standard deviation) completed a questionnaire (overall response rate 35%). The results showed that daytime incontinence, symptoms of bladder dysfunction, encopresis, social concerns, delayed age at walking and emotional stressors were positively associated with moderate frequency of enuresis. Age-adjusted independent risk factors for moderate nocturnal enuresis were male gender, encopresis, emotional stressors, daytime incontinence, social concerns and voiding frequency.

A summary of risk factors for nocturnal enuresis is given in Table 17.13.

Signs and symptoms

- Night-time bed-wetting
- Encopresis
- Daytime incontinence.

BOX 17.6 Normal regulation of urine

Children usually achieve night-time dryness by developing one or both of two abilities. There appear to be some hereditary factors in how and when these develop.

One factor is a hormone cycle in which a minute burst of antidiuretic hormone happens daily at about sunset, reducing kidney output of urine well into the night, so that the bladder does not fill until morning. This hormone cycle is not present at birth. Many children develop it between the ages of 2 and 6 years, others between 6 years and the end of puberty, and a few not at all.

The other factor is the ability to awaken before urinating. For some children this is a natural extension of learning to be aware of and control their bladder while awake. For others, a variety of factors suppress or disrupt this awareness when asleep, and they are unlikely to develop it. Taking children to use the toilet while not fully awake can prolong dependence, by encouraging them to urinate while nearly asleep.

TABLE 17.13 Risk factors for nocturnal enuresis stratified by severity (adjusted odds ratios)

	OR (95% CI)		
Risk factor	Severe enuresis	Moderate enuresis	Mild enuresis
Male gender	2.0 (1.3–3.1)	1.8 (1.1–3.1)	2.1 (1.6–2.8)
Encopresis	2.7 (1.6–4.4)	2.1 (1.1–4.3)	1.6 (1.0–2.4)
Emotional stressor	1.2 (0.5–2.7)	2.3 (1.2–4.2)	1.3 (0.9–2.0)
Daytime incontinence	4.8 (2.9–7.9)	2.6 (1.3–5.2)	3.0 (2.1–4.2)
Social concerns	0.7 (0.3–1.8)	2.4 (1.2–4.5)	1.3 (0.9–1.8)
Bladder dysfunction	3.6 (2.4–5.3)	2.4 (1.4–4.4)	2.0 (1.5–2.7)

Complications

- Psychological trauma
- Missed diagnosis
- Reduced growth due to sleep irregularities.

Differential diagnosis

- Urinary tract infection
- Insulin dependent diabetes
- Renal disease
- Psychological trauma/stress
- Allergies and intolerances
- Respiratory concerns (sleep apnoea)
- Obesity.

Investigations

- Urinalysis and culture:
  - to enable identification of underlying infection
  - to assess for potential glucose elevations
- General pathology (FBC, U+E = urea and electrolytes):
  - to assess and eliminate underlying pathology and ensure general health and wellbeing
- Blood glucose:
  - to eliminate diabetes (only if urinalysis is positive or if blood is already being drawn)
- Physical examination:
  - thorough neurological and abdominal examination, and referral to a general practitioner for genitourinary examination
  - signs of sexual abuse should be reviewed and referred appropriately.

SPECIFIC NATUROPATHIC INVESTIGATIONS

IgG food allergy testing

The immunoglobulin G (IgG) radioallergosorbent test (RAST) measures IgG4 antibodies for specific antigens using the enzyme-linked immunosorbent assay (ELISA) technique. The test is very sensitive and is useful for the identification of food sensitivities. It tests blood IgG4 reactions to 90 or so different foods. The results of this test should be interpreted with caution. Food sensitivities are graded from 1+ to 4+. Many 1+ and 2+ foods can be kept in the diet if rotated regularly with other less allergenic foods. If these foods produce symptoms, however, they should be avoided for a period of time. Foods that elicit a 3+ or 4+ result should be avoided until the underlying causes have been established and rectified.

The naturopathic framework considers enuresis to be a stress reaction of the body. It is hypothesised that the consumption of food substances to which a person is intolerant or allergic will contribute to perpetuating a stress reaction in the body and will thus exacerbate enuresis reactions.

Stool tests

If the patient does not improve and underlying digestive health is compromised, the naturopath may consider further investigations to assess digestive health. The expectation would be that a presentation of encopresis would warrant such investigation. A functional stool analysis may be crucial to understanding the function of the gastrointestinal tract. This test is a comprehensive stool test that is designed to identify pathogenic and commensal microbiota, as well as exogenous bacteria and parasites. The test also measures markers of digestion and maldigestion, together with certain markers of disease activity, such as blood, pus, mucus, WBCs and lactoferrin.

Functional bladder capacity diary

The approximate functional bladder capacity can be ascertained by the child (and parent) keeping a fluid intake/output diary, as illustrated in Table 17.14.

TABLE 17.14 Example of a fluid intake/output diary

Time	Fluid intake	Food intake	Urine output	Stool output
8 am	100 mL water	1 cup cereal with ½ cup milk	75 mL	1 full bowel movement
12 am	Nil	Nil	Accident (full bladder volume)	Nil

Source: Chin AI, Lerman SE. Bedwetting. In Encyclopedia of infant and early childhood development. London: Academic Press; 2008, pp. 156–64.

Therapeutic considerations

CLINICAL DECISION MAKING AND RATIONALE DETERMINE THE CAUSE

See Fig. 17.8.

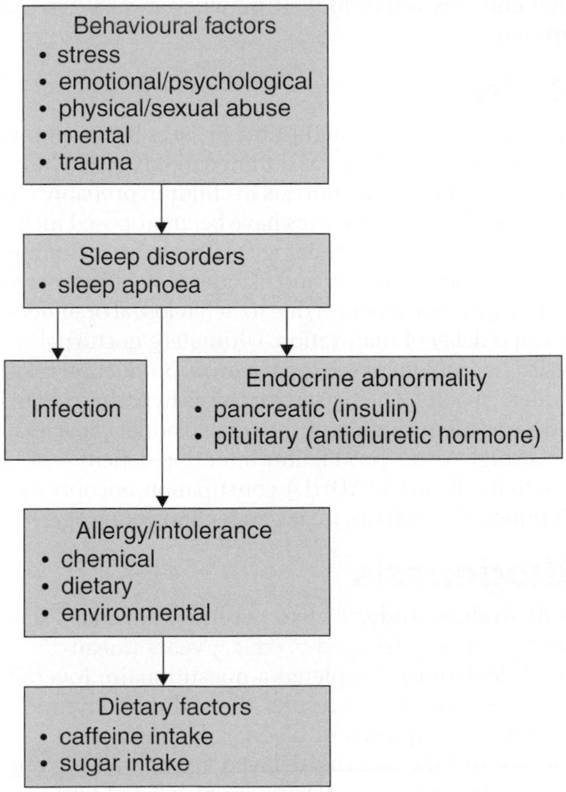

FIGURE 17.8 Flow chart of clinical decision-making process

OPTIMISE RESPIRATORY HEALTH

Snoring needs to be eliminated, as it has been noted that children who habitually snore more often have primary nocturnal enuresis.[46] Therefore, determining the cause of snoring may reduce associated symptoms. Causes of snoring include dietary allergens, environmental moulds and respiratory abnormalities. Further assessment and appropriate treatment are required.

Obesity

Studies have suggested that there is a high rate of obesity in children with dysfunctional voiding, especially nocturnal enuresis. Guven et al.[47] found that 38% of children with a body mass index (BMI) in the 85th percentile or above suffered from nocturnal enuresis, and 62% had dysfunctional voiding. Therefore, optimising a child's weight to within the healthy weight range is prudent for successful clinical outcome.

Therapeutic application

ALLOPATHIC PERSPECTIVE

The most commonly used and effective treatment for enuresis is the bed-wetting alarm. This is recommended as the primary treatment selection. The response to this approach is best in children aged >5 years who have been attending school for at least 3 months.

Drug prescriptions, including desmopressin, require a specialist's consideration due to potential safety concerns and negative outcomes. Recently it has been suggested that tricyclic antidepressants (TCAs) should no longer be used for the treatment of childhood enuresis.

Commonly used treatments for nocturnal enuresis are listed in Box 17.7.

Naturopathic perspective

NUTRITIONAL MEDICINE (DIETARY)

Therapeutic objectives

1 Regulate and optimise fluid intake throughout the day and reduce at night
2 Eliminate known triggers and known diuretic substances
3 Eliminate allergens and foods to which the patient is intolerant.

BOX 17.7 Common behavioural and pharmacological treatments for nocturnal enuresis

Behavioural

- Fluid intake regulation
- Bladder training
- Bed-wetting alarm
- Motivational therapy
- Hypnotherapy
- Acupuncture

Pharmacological

- Desmopressin
- Imipramine
- Anticholinergic drugs

Chin AI, Lerman SE. Bedwetting. In Encyclopedia of infant and early childhood development. London: Academic Press; 2008.

Specific treatments

DIETARY INCLUSIONS

Although fluid restriction is often recommended, it has not been shown to be effective, and could place the child at risk of dehydration. More effective is a redistribution of fluid intake to decrease nocturnal polyuria. The patient should still aim to drink the optimal fluid intake. Water intake is best calculated as 30 mL/kg of body weight.

DIETARY EXCLUSIONS

- Avoid all known allergens and foods to which the patient is intolerant
- Avoid preservatives, colourings, additives and flavourings
- Pay attention to the monosodium glutamate (MSG; INS 621) and nitrites content (common in processed meats, such as sausage, and smoked foods)
- Avoid caffeine and other stimulants
- Reduce intake of sugar, refined carbohydrates and other refined products.

NUTRITIONAL MEDICINE (SUPPLEMENTAL)

Therapeutic objectives

There is little research evidence to support nutritional prescriptions as a treatment for enuresis. Therefore, dietary supplements should only be prescribed if dietary intake is inadequate, or if indicated by the clinical assessment and review.

Specific nutrients required

PROBIOTICS

As indicated above, probiotics may be beneficial for supporting the micro-ecology of the urinary and digestive systems if UTIs are frequent or if encopresis is present.

DOSAGE

Multi-strain (with a high *Lactobacillus* spp. content where possible), ½ teaspoon b.i.d. (30–50 × 10^7 organisms per teaspoon). It is essential that all prescriptions are calculated using Clark's rule, to ensure safety when prescribing for children.

HERBAL MEDICINE

Therapeutic objectives

1 Improve bladder control and regulate urine release
2 Emotional and nervine support if emotional factors are aggravating the condition.

Herbal medicine classes

See Table 17.15.

URINARY SYSTEM

- Urinary antiseptics: these are used if infection is detected in the urinalysis
- Urinary demulcents: these are used to soothe the uroepithelial tissue after infection or to soothe irritation from incomplete voiding, strained voiding or voiding throughout the night

SAMPLE DAILY DIET

BREAKFAST	
Oat porridge with natural yoghurt, fresh fruit, sprinkling of LSA (linseed, sunflower and almond meal) and cinnamon; served with fresh mixed vegetable and fruit juice	Oat porridge provides wholegrain complex carbohydrates to support energy throughout the day and is a prebiotic food source that will encourage healthy gastrointestinal tract bacteria. Natural yoghurt is a healthy source of probiotics. LSA contains essential fatty acids for cognitive support and protein for balancing blood sugar levels. Fresh juice can encourage the use of diuretic vegetables such as celery, beetroot and carrot, which will further support phased diuretic objectives.
LUNCH	
Sandwiches with homemade dips, cold meats and salad vegetables	Avoid pre-prepared dips and purchased cold meats due to the potential preservatives and nitrite content which can irritate both mood and the bladder.
DINNER	
Homemade pizza with char-grilled vegetables, fetta and homemade sauce	Homemaking the pizza base and sauce ensures avoidance of preservatives, colourings and additives. Involving children in cooking encourages their interest in meals, and pizza is a child-friendly selection in this regard.
SNACKS	
Homemade tahini and carob fudge	A healthier alternative to chocolate and provides added protein. In addition, carob is astringent and so can reduce bladder irritation.
Yoghurt with nuts, seeds and fresh fruit	For the provision of probiotics.
BEVERAGES	
Optimal pure water intake (calculated as 30 mL/kg body weight), in preference to all other fluids	Fresh lemon and lime slices, fresh mint leaves or small quantities of fresh fruit juices can be added for taste as required. Avoidance of all caffeinated beverages is essential.

TABLE 17.15 Composition of example herbal formula for enuresis

Constituent	Dilution	Amount	Action
Zea mays (corn silk)	1:1	20 mL	Urinary diuretic and demulcent
Chamomilla recutita (chamomile)	1:2	30 mL	Mild sedative, nervine tonic
Melissa officinalis (lemon balm)	1:2	20 mL	Nervine tonic, mood relaxant, mild anxiolytic
Crataeva nurvala (crataeva)	1:2	30 mL	Bladder tonic
Total		100 mL	

- Diuretics: when phased throughout daylight hours in conjunction with modification of hydration these herbal medicines enable the regulation of bladder voiding during the day and reduce the need to urinate throughout the evening and during sleep. They also stimulate the bladder receptors to trigger acknowledgment of the need to void, thus supporting the child's awareness of the need to urinate
- Bladder tonics: these tonify the bladder after irritation or infection, and reduce incontinence.

NERVOUS SYSTEM

- Antidepressants or anxiolytics: these are indicated if emotional triggers perpetuate the enuresis or if the child is of an anxious nature
- Nervines: these are best used when sleep irregularities are present that affect enuresis, if stress and anxiety perpetuate the presentation or if the child is emotionally affected
- Adaptogens: these are used if stress contributes to the presentation.

LIFESTYLE RECOMMENDATIONS

Motivational therapy

Motivational therapy promotes behaviour modification by making the child responsible for their enuresis and rewarding their successes. The therapy requires that the parents and child develop a positive relationship with respect to enuresis, and that a good rapport is established between the clinician and the family. Although it is difficult to assess the success of motivational therapy, in monosymptomatic nocturnal enuresis it has been estimated to be as high as 40–54%.[48]

Hypnotherapy

Hypnotherapy has been shown to be successful in a number of cases. The premise is to train the patient to wake up when they need to urinate during the night. It also aims to educate the patient to perceive that the bladder will be able to hold more urine, and that they will be able to control their own urination. A clinical trial has shown that three 30-minute sessions of hypnotherapy produce a similar response rate as imipramine (a tricyclic antidepressant), and a greater response rate at 6 months (68% compared with 24%).[49] It was also noted that hypnotherapy is more effective in children over 7 years old. The National Institute for Health and Care Excellence (NICE) 2016 guideline suggests priority should be given for research in the area of treatment.[50]

Strategies to avoid

The literature shows that the following strategies should be avoided:

- Punishment
- Taking the child to the toilet during the night without fully waking them
- Waking the child during the night before wetting has occurred (to resolve bed-wetting)
- Prolonged use of nappies or pull-ups.

General recommendations

- Reduce exposure to toxins, heavy metals and cigarette smoke, as these have been shown to irritate the kidneys and bladder
- Encourage optimal weight, regular exercise and spending time outdoors
- Ensure that psychological health is addressed, and refer as necessary to a psychologist, counsellor or similar.

CASE STUDY

OVERVIEW

DN, a nine-year-old boy, presents at clinic with enuresis since attempting removal of night-time nappies and potty training at 2 years of age. He only achieves complete night time dryness twice a week at most and this has not been sequential and is not predictable by temperament or food intake. His mother has indicated that evening fluid intake may have an impact.

He is asking to go to school camp for a period of a week during the school holidays (3 months hence); his mother is obviously concerned. This has spurred the child on to be motivated to do whatever is necessary to help himself before his trip. He presents as quite a nervous child and does not like the school toilets, often withholding drinks and urination practice during the day to avoid the toilets. Therefore, when he arrives home after school he is thirsty and drinks copious amounts of fruit juice, which his mother waters down by

CASE STUDY CONTINUED

50%. He also is constipated and may empty his bowels three to four times a week and again resist the urge while at school.

The family are mostly vegetarian, he has a good appetite, eats regularly and the content of the food is high fibre: wholegrain cereal with soy milk, wholegrain (often non-wheat) sandwiches for lunch with cheese, vegan sausage or egg and salad, fruit during recess and occasionally chips and mini biscuits. He eats home-cooked vegetarian wholewheat pasta, lasagna, or brown rice and lentil curry, occasionally white fish, baked potato or sweet potato wedges with skin on and vegetables. DN is not a fan of yoghurt, however will attempt it with added fruit. He is likely achieving close to the recommended fibre intake for his age at 24 g per day.[51]

Naturopathic physical examination sees distinct iridology nerve rings 6–7, tremulous tongue, with white coat and bitten nails.

He is not on any medication and does not take supplements.

No medical tests or blood tests have been performed except a microscopic urine analysis which was NAD. He is not showing symptoms of diabetes or renal disease.

PRIMARY NOCTURNAL ENURESIS

TREATMENT PROTOCOL

Initial appointment

The focus of the appointment was to discuss a strategy for daytime toileting, hydration, herbal support for neurogenic disposition and magnesium for nervous system support, with additional short-term probiotic and prebiotic assistance for bowel relief, encouraging natural transit time and ease of defecation. Referral was written for support for both parents and child to a paediatric psychologist specialising in this field.

Dietary

- Optimise daytime hydration at recess and lunch time (with support of teachers), quantity determined using 35 mL per kg of body weight, more if perspiring and exercising
- Increase dietary sources of magnesium foods
- Reduce intake of fruit juices and encourage a titrated reduction to 25% juice 75% water
- Optimise intake of yoghurt — add stewed fruit such as prunes and kiwi fruit to assist with bowel function.

Herbal formula for enuresis of neurogenic origin (GABAnergic modulation; see Table 17.15)

Herbal formula

Passiflora incarnata: 1.0 g
Matricaria chamomilla: 750 mg
Magnesium amino acid chelate as magnesium biglycinate: 600 mg (equiv 60 mg)
Alpha-casozepine milk protein: 100 mg

½ metric teaspoon in the morning and one flat teaspoon before bed in juice for first month

Reduced to ½ metric teaspoon morning and evening thereafter

CASE STUDY CONTINUED

Nutritional supplement support

As above — child dose magnesium biglycinate dependent on weight of child

Probiotic children's multiflora probiotic with *Lactobacillus, Bifidobacterium lactis, Lactobacillus rhamnosus*, oligofructose ⅔ teaspoon in water first thing in the morning before food.

Lifestyle education

- Educate parents to discuss treatment protocol with teachers to engage their support
- Discuss the importance of early morning defecation and time and space to allow for this to happen in a busy lifestyle
- Encourage child to speak with psychologist to overcome daytime voiding and defecation issues.

REFERRAL

Paediatric psychologist

FOLLOW-UP

Two-week follow-up saw 4 dry nights per week. One month follow-up saw one to two enuresis episodes, and at 3 months there was total resolution of the condition. The teachers at his school were very supportive and encouraged timed voiding and 'quiet whisper', indicators for defecation times, to avoid embarrassment.

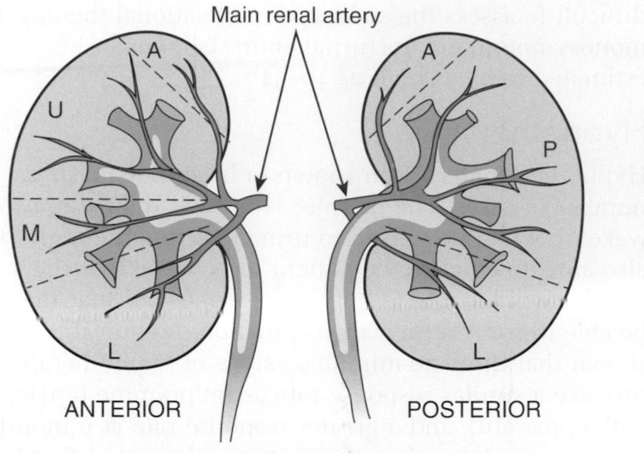

FIGURE 17.9 Diagram of arterial supply of the kidneys. A, apical; U, upper; M, middle; L, lower; P, posterior. Brenner BM. Brenner and Rector's the kidney. 8th edn. Saunders; 2007.

RENAL FAILURE

Naturopathic practitioners do not have sufficient training to support patients with significant renal pathology. The inclusion of this condition in this chapter is primarily to alert practitioners to the factors they should bear in mind within their own practice. It is prudent to co-manage patients in a holistic manner with the patient's urologist/nephrologist, general practitioner, dietitian and other members of the healthcare management team.

It is essential that practitioners are not overzealous with their support and deviate too extensively from the guidelines given below. At all times caution must be employed and immediate referral for appropriate management ensured. The recommendations given here are of a general nature to ensure that the practitioner remains respectfully cautious at all times. Herbal medicines are to be avoided at all times unless specific and individual approval has been provided by the patient's specialist. In these instances, liquid herbal medicines are best avoided due to their alcohol content, and tablet prescription or teas used instead. It is essential that readers do not misinterpret this statement and assume that herbal medicines in these forms are appropriate for all patients. Herbal prescriptions should be avoided at all times.

Epidemiology

One in ten Australians is at risk of developing chronic kidney disease, with 3 to 5 times higher rates in Indigenous populations.[52,53] and one in seven Australians over age 25 years has at least one clinical sign of existing chronic kidney disease (CKD) (e.g. reduced kidney function, presence of proteinuria or haematuria).[54,55] The prevalence of the disease is similar for males (10.3%) and females (9.5%). In those aged 18–54 years the rate is 6%, for those aged 65–74 it is 21%, and in those aged 75 and over it is more than 42%.[56] Furthermore, proteinuria is found in 2.4% of the total Australian population, and the incidence is four times higher in people with diabetes and five times higher in those with high blood pressure.[57] The Australian Diabetes Obesity and Lifestyle Study (AusDiab) suggests approximately 6 million Australians demonstrate at least one of the major risk factors for the disease. This equates to 1.4 million adults.[57]

Classification

Renal failure can present as acute or chronic forms. A brief differentiation is given in Box 17.8.

Aetiology

Kidney disease is primarily caused by one of three conditions:[54]

- Diabetes (31%)
- Nephritis or inflammation of the kidney (25%)
- Hypertension (16%).

Chronic renal disease, irrespective of the cause, typically progresses to end-stage renal failure over time. There are a number of variables that influence this progression and, of these, dietary factors appear to be the most compounding. Dietary modifications to restrict protein, phosphates and sodium all produce positive outcomes, even when other considerations are disregarded. Therefore, it is prudent to modify the diet as a primary intervention.

Additional triggers include:

- Infection
- Hypertension (especially when mismanaged or undiagnosed for an extended period of time)

BOX 17.8 Forms of renal failure

Acute renal failure	Chronic renal failure
High blood pressure	Oedema
Abnormal urinalysis	Polyneuropathy
Anaemia	Signs of fluid overload, including abnormal heart and lung sounds
Reduced kidney functioning: azotaemia (accumulation of nitrogenous wastes such as creatinine and urea)	A urinalysis may show blood, casts, protein or some other abnormality.
	Findings on kidney or abdominal ultrasound scan, computed tomography (CT) or intravenous pyelogram (IVP) are nonspecific.
	A chest x-ray may show fluid overload.
	A kidney biopsy may show one of the forms of chronic glomerulonephritis or nonspecific scarring of the glomeruli
	Oedema
	Other abnormalities:
	Urine specific gravity
	Urine concentration test
	Uric acid, urine
	Total protein
	Urine RBC
	Urine protein
	Creatinine clearance
	Urine creatinine
	Complement component 3; Complement
	BUN
	Antiglomerular basement membrane
	Albumin

- Immunological reactions (autoimmune processes against kidney tissue)
- Cadmium poisoning
- Exposure to organic solvents, including xylene, toluene and others
- Medication abuse, including analgesics and recreational drugs.

RISK FACTORS

- Hypertension: higher systolic readings are an independent risk factor for CKD. Absolute risk appears to be low in end-stage renal disease in those with mild hypertension at 0.34%. This highlights the need for appropriate blood pressure management.[58]
- Diabetes: approximately 25–45% of diabetic patients will develop CKD. Metabolic syndrome is a further independent risk factor; it is not known whether the syndrome furthers the prediction above that of the individual risk factors (e.g. hypertension as listed here).[56]
- Alcohol: there is an association between chronic alcohol consumption and hypertension; however the impact of consumption and progression has yet to be defined.[56]
- Cigarette smoking: a meta-analysis from 17 observational and case-controlled studies associated smoking with CKD. The risk factors are >20 cigarettes per day and age >40 years.[56]
- Obesity: 20.5% of Australians are obese.[56]
- Family history: a genetic predisposition to chronic kidney disease increases a person's risk to 20% if either a first- or second-degree relative has the disease.[56]
- Age: due to the ageing processes, the risk of kidney disease increases after the age of 50 years.
- Aboriginal and Torres Strait Islander descent: there is a greater prevalence (eightfold) of chronic kidney disease in some Indigenous Australian communities due to the high incidence of risk factors such as diabetes, high blood pressure and lack of health education.[56] Other contributory factors in this group are poor nutrition, high alcohol use, streptococcal throat and skin infections, socioeconomic disadvantage resulting in low levels of education, high unemployment, low income, crowded living conditions and low birth-weight babies. The incidence of kidney failure is increasing in the Aboriginal population at a faster rate than in non-Aboriginal Australians.[56]
- Benign prostatic hypertrophy: in men aged 50 years and older there was a reported 2.4% prevalence.[52]
- Other relevant risk factors for the general population are socioeconomic status (low income), kidney stones, cardiovascular disease, rheumatoid arthritis and cancer.[56]

Investigations

All the investigations listed in the first section of this chapter are relevant. They include:

- Electrolytes (U and E)
- Blood urea nitrogen (BUN)
- Glomerular filtration rate (GFR)
- Creatinine
- Albumin
- Uric acid
- Full blood count (FBC)
- Glucose
- Urinalysis, including culture, microscopy, albumin, protein and creatinine.

SPECIFIC NATUROPATHIC INVESTIGATIONS

Heavy metal testing

Heavy metal testing is beneficial to eliminate potential exposure to toxins such as cadmium, which is a known nephrotoxic. The test can be done using one of three different specimens — hair, blood or urine. The clinician can determine which is most appropriate based on presentation and need.

Hair analysis

There is a long history of the use of hair in detecting chronic exposure to toxic heavy metals in humans and animal models. Heavy metals concentrate in hair to levels that are several hundredfold above the concentrations found in blood. If the level of any toxic heavy metal is elevated in the hair, there is reason to investigate the origin of exposure. High levels in hair may reflect early chronic exposure before other signs and symptoms appear. However, a confounder is poor growth of hair due to illness, which may provide a false-positive result because of higher concentrations in the hair provided.

Blood assessment

Erythrocyte and whole blood levels are good indicators of body pools of both essential elements and toxic elements. These levels typically reflect current exposure rather than storage. Regulating agencies have deemed whole blood to be the correct specimen to use when assessing *current* exposure to aluminium, arsenic, cadmium, lead and mercury. Some elements can accumulate in tissues and cause toxic effects.

Urine assessment

Urine testing is primarily used to monitor levels of toxic metals and for special mineral uptake testing. Consecutive urine tests can be used to assess 6–8 hour profiles in patients receiving oral or intravenous metal chelating agents to mobilise toxic elements from body pools. Alternatively, 24-hour collection profiles may be used, with or without administration of chelating agents, to assess the rate of excretion of the elements concerned. The total output of urine over 24 hours is collected, and the daily output of nutrient and/or toxic element is determined.

Therapeutic considerations

CLINICAL DECISION MAKING AND RATIONALE

When treating renal failure, it is important to acknowledge that a number of key treatment objectives should be considered due to the essential functions of the kidneys in maintaining the health of the body system:

- Biochemical control
- Anaemia control
- Antihypertensive agents
- Bone disease
- Vitamin and mineral deficiencies
- Water-soluble vitamins (vitamin C, vitamin B complex)
- Vitamin D_3
- Calcium
- Potassium
- Infection risk
- Malnutrition
- Depression.

If renal failure reaches a critical level, other treatment options will need to be considered. These include haemodialysis or peritoneal dialysis, or transplant.

Naturopathic perspective

NUTRITIONAL MEDICINE (DIETARY)

Therapeutic objectives

1. Encourage a clean, wholefood diet that optimises nutritional intake and reduces harmful effects to the renal system
2. Eliminate all irritant and toxic substances that interfere with renal function.

Specific treatments

DIETARY INCLUSIONS

- Ensure hydration is optimal and appropriately calculated based on kidney function and body weight (30 mL/kg)
- Monitor serum potassium levels and encourage intake through food sources as necessary
- Eat 5–6 smaller meals throughout the day to stabilise the metabolism and prevent malnutrition. This also reduces the burden on the renal system
- Optimise fibre and complex carbohydrates in the diet to stabilise and optimise digestive function and bowel transit time
- Encourage calcium and potassium food sources.

DIETARY EXCLUSIONS

- Reduce the diet sodium content to <2 g/day (depending on blood pressure)
- Eliminate all caffeinated beverages (tea, coffee, cola drinks, chocolate), refined sugars, soft drinks, other carbonated beverages and alcohol
- Reduce phosphate intake to <5–10 mg/kg body weight.

OTHER DIETARY CONSIDERATIONS

Protein

Protein requirements are typically determined depending on growth stage and energy expended. With respect to renal function, a number of additional considerations are required. Ensure that dietary (and supplemental) protein is adjusted for each patient, based first on renal function and second on energy output (Table 17.16). Due to the potential aggravation of therapies on renal function, communication with and direction from the patient's medical practitioner/nephrologist should always be encouraged.

Protection from malnutrition should always be considered. Protein selection should focus on vegetarian sources where possible, with reduced animal sources.

TABLE 17.16 Daily dietary protein in health and in renal failure

Health status	Daily protein calculation (ranges are dependent on level of activity)
Healthy adult	0.8–1.2 g protein/kg body weight
Acute renal failure	0.6–0.8 g protein/kg body weight (acute) Then increase to 1.2 g protein/kg body weight in recovery
Chronic and end-stage renal failure	Non-dialysed patients: 0.6 g protein/kg body weight
Haemodialysis	1.2 g protein/kg body weight
Peritoneal dialysis	1.2–1.5 g protein/kg body weight
Kidney transplant	1.3–2.0 g protein/kg body weight (while on immunosuppressive medication), then follow with normal adult recommendations

Macronutrient and micronutrient requirements

The nutrient requirements for adults with renal disease depend on the stage of disease, as outlined in Table 17.17. Familiarity with nutritional terminology and calculations is required to work with this information.

NUTRITIONAL MEDICINE (SUPPLEMENTAL)

Therapeutic objectives

- Supplementation aims to address deficiencies caused by reduced renal function
- Oversupplementation is best avoided; prescriptions should solely focus on need rather than perceived need.

Specific nutrients required

B VITAMINS

All water-soluble vitamins should be encouraged. However, the B vitamins are particularly important due to their role in red blood cell formation. The reduction in erythropoietin synthesis in patients with renal failure can induce anaemia, and B vitamins can assist in both red blood cell parameters and improvements in symptoms. Patients on frusemide may lose water-soluble nutrients; however, caution is needed with supplementation of B vitamins. Foods containing B vitamins may be a more prudent option. In trials frank B vitamin therapy in homocystinaemia and end-stage renal disease, although beneficial for lowering homocystinaemia, worsened atrial size and left ventricular diastolic function.[59]

VITAMIN C

Vitamin C is another water-soluble vitamin that is reduced in failing renal function. In erythropoietin deficiency and subsequent anaemia, vitamin C has been shown to potentiate the mobilisation of iron from inert tissue stores, and to facilitate the incorporation of iron into protoporphyrin.[60] It is also advisable to prescribe vitamin C for patients taking diuretic prescriptions such as frusemide, due to the loss of water-soluble nutrients.

IRON

If the patient is anaemic and laboratory indices suggest an iron deficiency, supplemental iron should be prescribed. The prescription should be for easily absorbable forms in small doses throughout the day, which should be taken concurrently with vitamin C to increase absorption.

COENZYME Q10

In a 2015 study CoQ_{10} supplementation at doses as high as 1800 mg per day were found to be safe in all participants and well tolerated in most. Short-term daily CoQ_{10} supplementation decreased plasma isofuran concentrations in a dose-dependent manner. CoQ_{10} supplementation may improve mitochondrial function and decrease oxidative stress in patients receiving haemodialysis.[61]

OTHER ANTIOXIDANTS

Antioxidants are potent supportive nutrients that reduce the oxidation associated with the progression of renal disease and complications such as hyperlipoproteinaemia and cardiovascular diseases. A number of experimental models have been tested, but no clinical trials have been conducted that clearly indicate safety of prescription. Therefore, prescription should be assessed on an individual basis according to renal function.

VITAMIN D

Because of the role of the kidneys in the hydroxylation of vitamin D into its active form, vitamin D deficiencies are common in renal disease. It is important to note that blood levels reflect the liver level of vitamin D (25-hydroxycholecalciferol) and not the active form, which has gone through an additional hydroxylation process (1,25-dihydroxycholecalciferol). Therefore, it is prudent to

TABLE 17.17 Nutrient requirements for adults with renal disease

Stage of renal health	Energy	Protein	Fluid	Sodium	Potassium	Phosphorus
Impaired renal function	30–35 kcal/kg IBW	0.6–1.0 g/kg IBW	Ad libitum	2–3 g/day	Ad libitum or increased with diuretics	0.8–1.2 g/day or 8–12 mg/kg IBW
Haemodialysis	35 kcal/kg IBW	1.2 g/kg IBW	750–1000 mL/day + urine output	2–3 g/day	2–3 g/day or 40 mg/kg IBW	0.8–1.2 g/day or <17 mg/kg IBW
Peritoneal dialysis	30–35 kcal/kg IBW	1.2–1.5 g/kg IBW	Ad libitum (minimum of 2 L/day urine output)	2–3 g/day	3–4 g/day	0.8–1.2 g/day
Transplant (early)	30–35 kcal/kg IBW	1.3–2.0 g/kg IBW	Ad libitum	Variable	Variable (monitor with medication)	1.2 g/day + calcium 1.2 g/day
Transplant (≥6 weeks after)	Achieve or maintain IBW	1.0 g/kg IBW	Ad libitum	Variable	Variable	Calcium 1.2 g/day

IBW, ideal body weight.
Source: Mahan LK, Escott-Stump S. Krause's food and nutrition therapy. 13th edn. Oxford: Saunders Elsevier; 2012.

order a laboratory test to determine the level of the active form. As vitamin D is fat soluble, it should be prescribed only if deficiency is present, and referral for injection should be considered in cases of severe deficiency.

CALCIUM

Because of the vitamin D deficiencies that are commonly present in renal disease, and the role of this vitamin in calcium absorption and use, calcium deficiencies are common. It is advisable to take a preventive approach, depending on the severity of the deficiency. Only modest prescriptions should be given, and dietary sources encouraged where possible.

POTASSIUM

The interplay between sodium and potassium is complex so potassium supplementation should only be considered if serum levels fall too low. Potassium-rich food sources should be encouraged as a safer, easier prescription.

Dosage requirements

It is important to consider patients with renal failure carefully. At all times, it is imperative that practitioners liaise closely with the patient's renal physician to ensure that prescriptions for vitamins and other supplements are approved and safe.[62]

Note: practitioners are required to assess dosages carefully and take into account recommendations provided in Box 17.9.

The doses listed below are based on adult doses reported in the literature.

- B complex (preferably in its activated form). Assess suitability and discuss with specialist before supplementing: 1 capsule/day
- Specific quantities of each B vitamin:
  - vitamin B_1 25 mg
  - vitamin B_2 25 mg
  - vitamin B_3 20–30 mg
  - vitamin B_5 25 mg
  - vitamin B_6 10–50 mg
  - vitamin B_9 500–1000 micrograms
  - vitamin B_{12} 500–1000 micrograms

  The upper end of the recommended range should be prescribed when there is anaemia. In such cases, divided doses are the most efficacious for a positive clinical outcome
- Vitamin C: 250 mg taken 3–5 times daily until 4000 mg has been administered, followed by a maintenance dose of 1000 mg/day (in divided doses) and encouragement to eat fresh fruit and vegetables
- Iron: 12–24 mg t.d.s. or q.i.d. (preferably in iron amino acid chelate form)
- Coenzyme Q10: 100–200 mg/day
- Alpha lipoic acid: 200–300 mg/day
- Vitamin E: 400 IU/day
- Vitamin D: 1000–5000 IU/day; the dose should be calculated according to the deficiency shown by pathology results
- Calcium: 500–1000 mg/day; the dose should be calculated according to the deficiency shown by pathology results.

BOX 17.9 Supplement dosage requirements in renal failure

In a patient with diminished renal function, doses may be altered by reducing the dose or by extending the interval between doses. The following points should also be noted:

- Where no modification of the dose or interval is required, normal therapeutic doses are indicated
- It is best to refrain from hyperdosing due to the potential for harm. At all times consider and adhere to dose ranges and maintain care and caution
- Spacing prescriptions throughout the day is often advisable, as this reduces the load on the kidneys with regard to clearance
- The use of quality products free from excipients (or reduced excipients) is particularly important to reduce potential impact on the kidneys.

HERBAL MEDICINE

Herbal medicines are best avoided due to their potential for harm in renal disease.

LIFESTYLE RECOMMENDATIONS

- Activity should be regulated according to the patient's energy, health and wellbeing
- Avoidance of exposure to all environmental toxins should be encouraged, to protect renal function and reduce the burden of clearance. Common sources of such toxins include:
  - chemicals in toiletries, cleaning products and household products
  - hair dyes and make-up are common sources of heavy metals
  - passive or personal smoking
  - recreational drug use
  - non-organic foods.

REFERENCES

[1] Tortora G, Derrickson B. Principles of anatomy and physiology. 12th ed. New York: Wiley; 2009.

[2] Neuburger M. The early history of urology. Bull Med Libr Assoc [Reisman D, trans] 1937;23(3).

[3] Ware EW. A brief history of urology at Baylor University Medical Center. Proc (Bayl Univ Med Cent) 2003;16(4):430–4.

[4] Micozzi M. Fundamentals of complementary and integrative medicine. 4th ed. St Louis, MI: Saunders; 2011.

[5] Smith RD. Avicenna and the Canon of Medicine: a millennial tribute. West J Med 1980;1133(4):367–70.

[6] Cook W. The physiomedical dispensatory. Cincinnati, OH: WmH Cook; 1869.

[7] Osiecki H, Meeke F. The digestive and the renal systems. Eagle Farm Qld: Bio Concepts Publishing; 2005.

[8] Toffolo A, Ammenti A, Montini G. Long-term clinical consequences of urinary tract infections during childhood: a review. Acta Paediatr 2012;101(10):1018–31.

[9] Eckardt KU, Coresh J, Devuyst O, et al. Evolving importance of kidney disease: from subspecialty to global health burden. Lancet 2013;382(9887):158–69.

[10] Al-Badr A, Al-Shaikh G. Recurrent urinary tract infections management in women: a review. Sultan Qaboos Univ Med J 2013;13(3):359–67.

[11] Kelly J. Clinical syndromes of urinary tract infection. Curr Ther 1977;38(7):15–21.
[12] Kennedy S. UTI in children. Part 1 How to treat. Australian Doctor; 2009. Available from: www.australiandoctor.com.au/cmspages/getfile.aspx?guid=265a608d-cbf0-451e-b65e-50d2716356da.
[13] Foxman B. Epidemiology of urinary tract infections: incidence, morbidity and economic costs. Am J Med 2002;8(113 Suppl. 1A):S5–13.
[14] Fihn SD. Clinical practice. Acute uncomplicated urinary tract infection in women. N Engl J Med 2003;349(3):259–66.
[15] Kodner CM. Recurrent urinary tract infections in women: diagnosis and management. Am Fam Physician 2010;82(6):638–43.
[16] eMIMS Cloud. Hexamine hippurate. MIMS Australia; 2016.
[17] Nickel JC. Management of urinary tract infections: historical perspective and current strategies: Part 1 Before antibiotics. J Urol 2005;173:21–6.
[18] Posadas R, Monroy-Torres R, Naves-Sanchez J. Intake of vitamin C, probiotics, flavonoids and nutritional status in pregnant women with urinary tract infection. Immunol Endocr Metab Agents Med Chem 2014;14(1):40–5.
[19] Raghuwanshi S, Misra S, Bisen PS. Indian perspective for probiotics: a review. Indian J Diary Sci 2014;68(3):1–12.
[20] Ravel J, Gajer P, Abdo Z, et al. Vaginal microbiome of reproductive-age women. Proc Natl Acad Sci U S A 2010;108(S1):4681–7.
[21] Kovachev SM. Obstetric and gynecological diseases and complications resulting from vaginal dysbacteriosis. Microb Ecol 2014;68(2):173–84.
[22] Grin PM, Kowalewska PM, Ahazzanie W, et al. *Lactobacillus* for preventing recurrent urinary tract infections in women: meta-analysis. Can J Urol 2013;20(1):6607–14.
[23] Abad CL, Safdar N. The role of *Lactobacillus* probiotics in the treatment or prevention of urogenital infections — a systematic review. J Chemother 2009;21(3):243–52.
[24] Rath S, Padhy RN. Monitoring in vitro antibacterial efficacy of 26 Indian spices against multidrug resistant urinary tract infecting bacteria. Integr Med Res 2014;3(3):133–41.
[25] Braun L, Cohen M. Herbs and natural supplements: an evidence-based guide, vol. 2. 4th ed. Chatswood, NSW: Churchill Livingstone; 2014.
[26] Johnson AR, Munoz A, Gottlieb JL, et al. High dose zinc increases hospital admissions due to genitourinary complications. J Urol 2007;177(2):639–43.
[27] Kranjcec B, Papes D, Altara S. D-mannose powder for prophylaxis of recurrent urinary tract infections in women: a randomized clinical trial. World J Urol 2014;32(1):79–84.
[28] Blumenthal M, Busse WR, Goldberg A. The complete German Commission E monographs. Boston, MA: American Botanical Council, Austin and Integrative Medicine Communications; 1998.
[29] United States Department of Agriculture. Basic report: 09078 cranberries, raw; 2016. Available from: https://ndb.nal.usda.gov/ndb/foods/show/2191?manu=&fgcd=.
[30] Jepson RG, Williams G, Craig JC. Cranberries for treating urinary tract infections. Cochrane Database Syst Rev 2012;doi:10.1002/14651858.CD001321.pub5.
[31] Mills S, Bone K. Principles and practice of phytotherapy. Sydney: Churchill Livingstone; 2000.
[32] Stapleton AE, Dziura J, Hooton TM. Recurrent urinary tract infection and urinary *Escherichia coli* in women ingesting cranberry juice daily: a randomized controlled trial. Mayo Clin Proc 2012;87(2):143–50.
[33] Gupta A, Swivedi M, Mahdi AA, et al. Inhibition of adherence of multi-drug resistant *E. coli* by proanthocyanidin. Urol Res 2011;40(2):143–50.
[34] Gonzalez de Llano D, Esteban-Fernandez A, Sanchez-Patan F, et al. Anti-adhesive activity of cranberry phenolic compound and their microbial-derived metabolites against uropathogenic *Escherichia coli* in bladder epithelial cell cultures. Int J Mol Sci 2015;16(6):12119–30.
[35] Ofek I, Goldhar J, Zafriri D, et al. Anti-*Escherichia coli* adhesion activity of cranberry and blueberry juices. N Engl J Med 1991;324(22):1599.
[36] Shmuely H, Domniz N, Yahav J. Non-pharmacological treatment of *Helicobacter pylori*. World J Gastro Pharm 2016;7(2):171–8.
[37] Pizzorno JE, Murray MT. Textbook of natural medicine. 3rd ed. Philadelphia, PA: Elsevier; 2006.
[38] EMA. Assessment report on *Arctostaphylos uva-ursi* (L.); 2012. Spreng., folium, European Medicine Agency EMA/HMPC/573462/2009 Rev.1.
[39] Rawat S, Ishaq F, Khan A. Antimicrobial effects of drugs, medicinal plant extracts and essential oils against pathogenic bacteria causing urinary tract infection. Global J Biotech Biochem 2013;8(1):15–24.
[40] Culbert TP, Banez GA. Wetting the bed: integrative approaches to nocturnal enuresis. Explore (NY) 2008;4(3):215–20.
[41] Franco I, Austin PF, Bauer SB. Pediatric incontinence: evaluation and clinical management. West Sussex, UK: Wiley Blackwell; 2015.
[42] Caldwell PHY, Hodson E, Craig JC, et al. Bedwetting and toileting problems in children. MJA Practice Essentials, Paediatrics. Med J Aust 2005;182(4):190–5.
[43] Caldwell P, Deshpande A. Nocturnal enuresis in children and adolescents. How to treat. Australian Doctor; 2012. Available from: www.australiandoctor.com.au/cmspages/getfile.aspx?guid=a09a805c-1e6a-403c-bd94-70ba0cf8b84c.
[44] Butler RJ, Robinson JC, Holland P, et al. Investigating the three systems approach to complex childhood nocturnal enuresis—medical treatment interventions. Scand J Urol Nephrol 2004;38:117.
[45] Sureshkumar P, Jones M, Caldwell PHY, et al. Risk factors for nocturnal enuresis in school age children. J Urol 2009;182(6):2893–9.
[46] Jeyakumar A, Rahman SI, Armbrecht ES, et al. The association between sleep-disordered breathing and enuresis in children. Laryngoscope 2012;122(8):1873–7.
[47] Guven A, Giramonti K, Kogan BA. The effect of obesity on treatment efficacy in children with nocturnal enuresis and voiding dysfunction. J Urol 2007;178(4):1458–62.
[48] Meltem E, Unsal O, Ozgul Y, et al. Motivation therapy in children with primary monosymptomatic nocturnal enuresis. Haseki Tip Bulteni 2016;(54):1.
[49] Banerjee S, Srivastav A, Palan BM. Hypnosis and self-hypnosis in the management of nocturnal enuresis: a comparative study with imipramine therapy. Am J Clin Hypn 1993;36(2):113–19.
[50] National Institute for Health and Care Excellence (NICE). Clinical guideline: Bedwetting in under 19s (CG111). NICE; 2010.
[51] National Health and Medical Research Council. Nutrient reference values for Australia and New Zealand: Dietary fibre; 2014. Available from: www.nrv.gov.au/nutrients/dietary-fibre.
[52] Australian Institute of Health and Welfare. Chronic kidney disease; 2016. Available from: www.aihw.gov.au/chronic-kidney-disease/.
[53] Johnson DW, Jones GRD, Mathew TH, et al. Chronic kidney disease and measurement of albuminuria or proteinuria: a position statement. Med J Aust 2012;197(4):224–5.
[54] McDonald S, Chang S, Excell L. The Thirtieth ANZDATA Registry Report. Adelaide, SA: Australia and New Zealand Dialysis and Transplant Registry; 2007.
[55] Johnson D. Risk factors for early chronic kidney disease. KHA-CARI guidelines. Kidney Health Australia; 2012.
[56] Australian Institute of Health and Welfare (AIHW). Chronic kidney disease in Australia. AIHW Cat. No. PHE 68. Canberra: AIHW; 2005.
[57] Atkins RC, Briganti EM, Zimmet PZ, et al. Brief report. Association between albuminuria and proteinuria in the general population: the AusDiab Study. Nephrol Dial Transplant 2003;18:2170–4.
[58] Briganti EM, Shaw JE, Chadban SJ, et al. Untreated hypertension among Australian adults: the 1999–2000 Australian Diabetes, Obesity and Lifestyle Study (AusDiab). Med J Aust 2003;179(3):135–9.
[59] Rafeq Z, Roh JD, Kaufman J, et al. Adverse myocardial effects of B vitamin therapy in subjects with chronic kidney disease and hyperhomocystinaemia. Nutr Metab Cardiovasc Dis 2013;23(9):836–42.
[60] Macdougall IC. Metabolic adjuvants to erythropoietin therapy. Miner Electrolyte Metab 1999;25:357–64.
[61] Yeung CK, Billins FT, Claessens AJ. Coenzyme Q10 dose-escalation study in hemodialysis patients: safety, tolerability, and effect on oxidative stress. BMC Nephrol 2015;16:183.
[62] Mahan LK, Escott-Stump S. Krause's food and nutrition therapy. 13th ed. Oxford: Saunders Elsevier; 2012.

18

The female reproductive system

Leah Hechtman

SECTION A

OVERVIEW OF THE FEMALE REPRODUCTIVE SYSTEM

The reproductive system of the female is made up of a series of organs unique to the female, sitting within the pelvic cavity. As a whole, these organs work closely together and with other systems of the body, such as the endocrine system, to ensure the functions of menstruation, conception, pregnancy and childbirth through production of the female gamete (ova), sexual intercourse, while also providing a nourishing environment for fertilisation of the ova and sperm, housing the baby during gestation and, finally, enabling childbirth.

The female reproductive system can be divided into two parts: the internal structures (the uterus, ovaries, fallopian tubes, vagina and mammary glands) and the external structures (the labia majora, labia minora, vulva, Cowper's glands and clitoris; see Fig. 18.1).

The uterus (the womb)

> *The womb is the field of generation; and if this field be corrupted it is in vain to expect any fruit though it be ever so well sown.*
>
> ***Aristotle***[1]

The uterus is a pear-shaped and -sized organ found sitting deep within the pelvic cavity. As suggested by Aristotle, the uterus is the site of regeneration, for without it pregnancy could not occur. The uterus has other important roles within the body, including migration of sperm,[2] implantation of the fertilised ovum,[2] nourishment of the fetus and embryo,[2] as well as being the site of menstruation[3] and a supportive structure to other organs in the body such as the bowel and bladder.

The uterus can be divided into three parts: the fundus, the body and the cervix (which is the neck of the uterus which opens into the vagina), as well as three layers: the perimetrium, the endometrium and the myometrium. The perimetrium is the outer layer and functions to cover the urinary bladder and the rectum. The myometrium is the middle layer and is composed of three layers of smooth muscle fibres. The female reproductive condition known as adenomyosis occurs within this tissue.[4] The endometrium is the inner layer, and consists of a single layer of simple columnar epithelium that sits on top of connective tissue known as stroma. The endometrium can be further divided into two layers: the functional layer, which is shed during menstruation, and the basal layer, which does not shed and from which the functional layer is formed each time menstruation occurs.

The endometrium undergoes changes according to the stage of the menstrual cycle. During the proliferative phase, the endometrium proliferates and increases in blood vessels. During the secretory phase the endometrium becomes thick and highly vascular in preparation for the embryo. If fertilisation does not occur, menstruation occurs due to shedding of the endometrium.

The ovaries

The ovaries are a pair of glands that sit within the pelvis on either side of the uterus and are implicated in many female reproductive disorders, including ovarian cysts and polycystic ovaries. Each ovary resembles an unshelled almond in terms of size and shape, and contains the immature/unfertilised female egg, known as the oocyte, that will be stored and released into the fallopian tubes during ovulation. The ovaries also function to secrete sex hormones such as testosterone (which is then converted to oestrogen), progesterone, inhibin and relaxin.

Each ovary consists of seven parts:

- The ovarian surface epithelium — a layer of simple epithelium that covers the surface of the ovary[5] also known as the 'germinal' epithelium[6]
- The tunica albuginea — made up of dense connective tissue
- The ovarian cortex — also made up of dense connective tissue that contains the ovarian follicles
- The ovarian medulla — made up of loose connective tissue, blood vessels, lymphatics and nerves

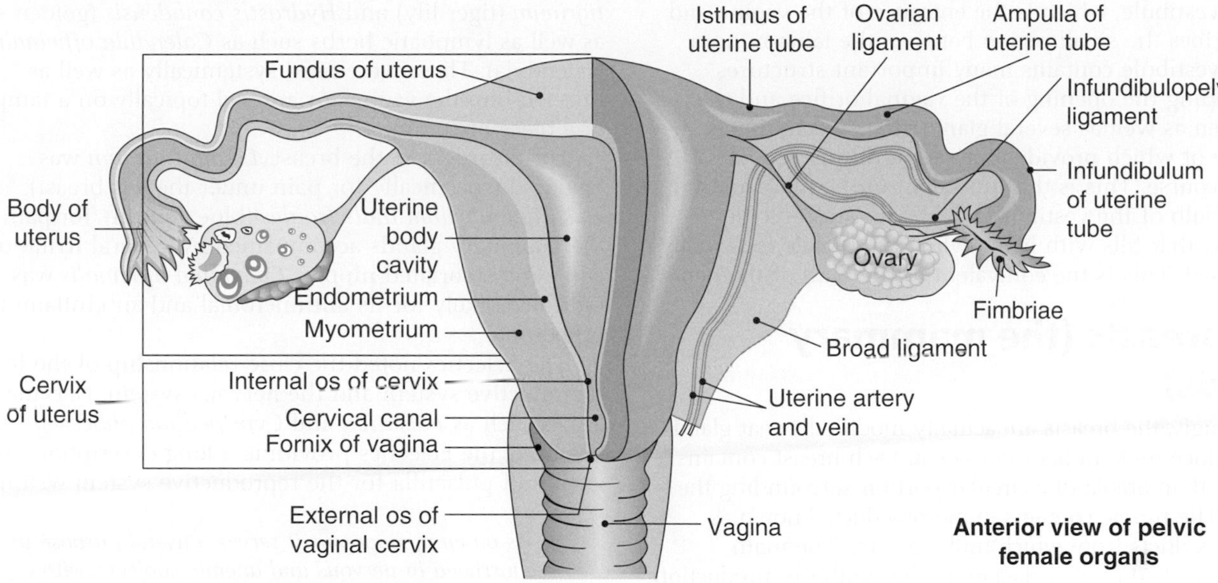

FIGURE 18.1 The female reproductive system.

Source: Katz V. Comprehensive gynecology. 5th edn. Maryland Heights: Mosby; 2007.

- Ovarian follicles — fluid-filled structures in which the oocytes grow and develop, found within the ovarian cortex
- A mature (Graafian) follicle — a single, large fluid-filled cavity into which the developed and matured oocyte known as the secondary oocyte is released (this is called ovulation)
- The corpus luteum — 'the yellow structure' formed from the follicle following ovulation that produces progesterone and other hormones until it degenerates (if pregnancy does not occur) into the corpus albicans, white fibrous tissue.

The fallopian tubes

The fallopian tubes are a pair of 10 cm long tubes[3] that extend from the uterus and play a very important role in conception and fertilisation of an egg by sperm. They act as a transport system conveying the fertilised ova and secondary oocytes from the ovaries to the uterus. At the end of each fallopian tube is a funnel-shaped portion known as the infundibulum, and from this a fringe of finger-like projections hang facing the ovary. Despite their small size, the detailed transport mechanisms taking place within the fallopian tubes at an organ level are quite outstanding. Each fallopian tube is composed of three layers, each with its own function. Cilia of ciliated columnar epithelium and secretory cells line the internal layer. The cilia function to promote the transport of the secondary oocytes through the fallopian tubes, while the secretory cells contain microvilli that provide nutrition for the ovum.[3] The middle layer of the fallopian tubes is known as the muscularis and, as the name suggests, is composed of muscle that produces peristaltic contractions to further move the oocyte or fertilised ovum closer to the uterus. The serosa makes up the outer layer.

The vagina

The vagina is a tubular organ located below the urethral opening. It is lined with mucous membranes that contain large amounts of glycogen. Glycogen breaks down to produce lactic acid and thus an acidic environment is created within the vagina that serves as a protective mechanism to minimise microbial infection, although it may still occur as in the case of vaginitis. The vagina has many functions: as an exit for the baby during birth, as the site of insertion for the penis during sexual intercourse (and for the possibility of conception), and as a channel for menstrual blood.

The vulva

The vulva refers to the external genitalia of the female and includes:

- The mons pubis, the mound of fatty tissue that sits in front of the vagina and is covered in pubic hair. The mons pubis serves as a cushion for the pubic symphysis.
- The labia majora, which comprise two longitudinal pieces of skin and fatty tissue covered in pubic hair. They contain sweat and oil glands. This is the female equivalent of the scrotum.
- The labia minora, which sit in the middle of the labia majora and are two smaller longitudinal folds of skin. They contain oil glands but no sweat glands, pubic hair or fatty tissue. This is the female equivalent of the penile urethra.
- The clitoris, which is located at the anterior junction of the labia minora.[3] It contains erectile tissue and numerous nerve endings that upon stimulation may result in sexual pleasure for the woman. This is the female equivalent of the penis.

- The vestibule, which is the entrance of the vagina and describes the small region between the labia minora. The vestibule contains many important structures including the opening of the vaginal orifice and the hymen as well as several glands that secrete mucus, some of which provide lubrication during sexual intercourse. This is the equivalent to the male urethra.
- The bulb of the vestibule, which contains erectile tissue, that fills with blood when the female is sexually aroused. This is the equivalent to the bulb of the penis.

The breasts (the mammary glands)

Interestingly, the breasts are actually modified sweat glands that produce milk, rather than sweat. Each breast contains a nipple and an areola (the circular portion surrounding the nipple). The nipple contains numerous ducts known as lactiferous ducts from which milk appears. The main function of the breasts is lactation: the synthesis, production and ejection of milk. They may also experience dysfunction, as in the case of mastalgia, and other breast disorders.

ROLE OF THE NATUROPATH

Traditional interpretation

Disorders of the reproductive system apparently also afflicted our female ancestors, and botanical treatments for endometriosis, dysmenorrhoea, amenorrhoea, metrorrhagia and menorrhagia are all documented within the texts of the Eclectics. The Eclectics favoured the use of female restoratives and reproductive tonics such as *Viburnum prunifolium* (black haw), *Packera aurea* (life root) and *Aletris farinosa* (true unicorn root) to regulate the workings of the reproductive system.[7] *Viburnum* spp.[7] were also employed for their antispasmodic effects, particularly in the uterus where they reduced cramping and thus pain, making them ideal as uterine relaxants in conditions such as dysmenorrhoea.

Antiseptics such as *Thuja occidentalis* (thuja) were included for their ability to mop up catarrhal diseases of the female generative organs such as leucorrhoeal discharge[8] while astringents and anti-haemorrhagics such as *Trillium erectum* (Beth root) and *Hydrastis canadensis* (golden seal) were employed successfully in menorrhagia, uterine haemorrhage and metrorrhagia.[8] The Eclectics also noted *Hydrastis canadensis* to be particularly useful in fungoid endometritis and lacerated cervix.

In uterine disorders, botanicals such as *Mitchella repens* and *Actaea racemosa* were thought to be effective remedies due to their regulating function. Emmanogogues such as *Ruta graveolens* (rue)[9] were used chiefly for their action upon the uterus, although the dose-dependence of rue was noted, large doses seemingly thought to be poisonous. The warming, circulatory stimulant action of *Zingiber officinale* (ginger) appeared to reduce pain associated with menstruation, and the Eclectics suggested it for the 'pangs of menstruation'.[8]

For eruptions and inflammatory conditions of the vulva and vagina, the Eclectics favoured the use of *Lilium tigrinum* (tiger lily) and *Hydrastis canadensis* (golden seal) as well as lymphatic herbs such as *Calendula officinalis* (calendula). These were used systemically as well as injected into the vagina, or applied topically on a tampon or a piece of cotton.

For disorders of the breast, *Lilium tigrinum* was favoured (specifically for pain under the left breast),[7] as was *Caulophyllum thalictroides* (blue cohosh) 'for pain in the mammary glands accompanied by general irritation', while for excoriated nipples *Calendula officinalis* was indicated, likely for its antimicrobial and anti-inflammatory properties.

The Eclectics noted the close relationship of the female reproductive system and the nervous system. Nervine tonics such as *Pulsatilla* and *Cypripedium pubescens* were favoured, the Eclectics providing a long description on the virtues of pulsatilla for the reproductive system writing:

> *As an emmenagogue, it serves a useful purpose in amenorrhoea in nervous and anemic subjects, with chilliness a prominent symptom. When menstruation is suppressed, tardy or scanty from taking cold, or from emotional causes, pulsatilla is the remedy. In dysmenorrhoea, not due to mechanical causes, and with the above-named nervous symptoms, no remedy is more effective. Leucorrhoea, with a free, thick, milky, or yellow, bland discharge and pain in the loins, and particularly in scrofulous individuals, calls for pulsatilla. It is a remedy for mild forms of hysteria, where the patient is weak and weeps easily, has fears of impending danger, and passes large quantities of clear, limpid urine, and menstruation is suppressed. The long-continued use of pulsatilla as an intercurrent remedy, is accredited with curative effects in uterine colic, but it is of no value during an attack. Pulsatilla frequently proves a good remedy in ovaritis and ovaralgia with tensive, tearing pain.*[8]

Notably absent from Felter and Lloyd's work are *Vitex agnus-castus*, *Angelica sinensis* and *Tribulus terrestris*, three herbs favoured in modern naturopathic medicine of the female reproductive system. *Angelica sinensis* and *Tribulus terrestris* originate from Asia and India, respectively, and reflect advances in modern-day naturopathic medicine. *Vitex agnus-castus* has a lengthy heritage, with usage dating back to the time of Hippocrates (460–377 BC), who wrote 'If blood flows from the womb, let the woman drink dark wine in which the leaves of the chaste tree have been steeped.' Use for gynaecological conditions is also noted in the works of Pliny and Dioscorides (1st century AD), as well as Theophrastus (3rd century AD). 'The trees furnish medicines that promote urine and menstruation.' wrote Pliny, 'They encourage abundant rich milk.'

Modern interpretation

Female reproductive complaints are commonly seen in many modern naturopathic clinics and a number of naturopathic approaches (for example vitamin and mineral therapy) have proven very useful in maintaining the health of the female reproductive system and reducing symptoms.

One of naturopathic medicine's greatest virtues and of particular benefit to gynaecology is its concern with treating the cause rather than merely suppressing symptoms. Many female patients will have an extensive history of complaints that they have simply just accepted. Here the naturopath's role is as an educator, teaching the patient about the internal workings of their body and the causative factors contributing to their individual condition.

Knowledge on the structure, function and workings of the female reproductive structures and hormones continues to grow. We are now aware of the link between the pituitary and the female reproductive system and what each hormone does in the body. Our knowledge of botanicals and supplements and the effects they exert in the female reproductive system has also developed. Similarly, our knowledge on the healing power of certain foods (for example the brassica family) and the mechanisms through which they exert an influence on the female reproductive structures of the body continues to grow.

While the development of society has brought with it many benefits for treatment of the female reproductive system (e.g. laboratory testing for hormones, testing procedures to visibly observe cysts on the ovaries) it also has some drawbacks. Xeno-oestrogens, a gift of the modern era, are known to be prime endocrine disruptors and their detrimental effects on the female reproductive system are becoming increasingly recognised. Environmental factors[10,11] such as xeno-oestrogens are just one causative factor linked to dysfunction of the female reproductive system. Others include:

- Obesity[12]
- Liver dysfunction
- Hormonal imbalance
- Stress
- Oxidative damage[13–15]
- Immune disruption[16]
- Nutrient deficiency
- Inflammation[13]
- Genetics[17]
- Infectious pathology such as pelvic inflammatory disease or vaginitis[18]
- Hygienic behaviours[19]
- Hypothalamic–pituitary–ovarian (HPO) axis dysfunction.

Naturopathic medicine is non-invasive and gentle on the body. The naturopath works as facilitator, gently guiding the body back to homeostasis, restoring balance, always acknowledging the body's own innate ability to heal itself. This, as with all the bodily systems, encompasses a multifaceted approach. Individualised treatment is paramount, and will typically use herbal medicines and nutrient supplementation.

Central to the core of naturopathic philosophy is the liver and associated pathways. Optimal hepatobiliary function and detoxification mechanisms are imperative. A balanced diet that minimises exposure to xeno-oestrogens, saturated and trans fatty acids, alcohol and refined sugars is also important, given the links between diet, nutritional deficiency and disorders of the female reproductive system.

Specific nutritional objectives

A number of nutrients have been identified as useful for the regulation and healthy function of the female reproductive structures (Table 18.1). Some of these have an affinity for specific reproductive structures or the manufacture of sex hormones; others have been identified as potential deficiencies and thus increased requirements. As always, application is dependent upon the individual's constitution and their disease manifestation.

TABLE 18.1 Specific nutritional objectives

Nutrient	Justification	Therapeutic dosage	Dietary source
Vitamin A	Displays immune,[20] regulatory,[20] antioxidant[21] and tissue repair functions specific to the female reproductive system. Cofactor of 3β-dehydrogenase in steroidogenesis; deficiencies may result in impaired enzyme activity[22] and thus low oestrogen. May be indicated where there is menorrhagia[23]	10 000–20 000 IU/day	Kohlrabi, egg yolk, carrots, apricots, fish liver oils (e.g. cod)
Vitamin B_1	Coenzyme in the body with essential roles in metabolism and ATP production; as part of the enzyme thiamine pyrophosphatase vitamin B_1 is found in the plasma membrane of epithelial cells in the uterus where it is suggested to be controlled by oestrogen and progesterone[24] Oral contraceptive may deplete levels of vitamin B_1[25]	5–150 mg/day	Legumes, wheatgerm, wholegrains, nuts
Vitamin B_2	Cofactor in numerous enzyme systems within the body. Maintains mucosal and epithelial tissues[25] (both of which are found making up the reproductive organs). Required for activation of vitamin B_6 and folic acid, both of which play important roles within the female reproductive system.[25] Oral contraceptive pill may increase requirements[26]	10–200 mg/day	Avocados, beans, sprouts, broccoli, eggs, milk

Continued

TABLE 18.1 Specific nutritional objectives—cont'd

Nutrient	Justification	Therapeutic dosage	Dietary source
Vitamin B_3	Required for energy production and involved in synthesis of certain hormones such as oestrogen, progesterone and testosterone	5–500 mg/day	Almonds, chicken, eggs, legumes, salmon, sardines
Vitamin B_5	Required for steroid hormone production	20–500 mg/day	Avocados, egg yolk, sweet potato, green vegetables, mushrooms
Vitamin B_6	Crucial cofactor in many cellular processes of the female reproductive system including hormone synthesis. Required for synthesis of prostaglandins[25] and maintenance of normal intracellular magnesium concentration.[27] Indirect effects on oestrogen[28]	50–500 mg/day[29] (however check for neuralgia regularly)	Chicken, egg yolk, legumes, salmon, tuna, walnuts
Folic acid	May be decreased where there is blood loss due to menorrhagia, therefore requirements may need to be increased.[30] Requirements may be increased if taking the oral contraceptive pill[26]	1000–5000 micrograms/day	Leafy green vegetables, lentils, eggs, beans
Vitamin B_{12}	Vitamin B_{12} is required for erythropoiesis mechanisms, such as DNA replication and cell proliferation. Requirements may increase in the presence of menorrhagia	300–1000 micrograms/day	Salmon, sardines, egg yolk, oysters, bacterial synthesis in the gut
Choline	Required for conjugation of oestrogen	1000–3500 mg/day	Egg yolk, lecithin, beans
Vitamin C	Antioxidant, found maintaining the ovaries, important factor in uterine oestrogen binding.[31] Immune stimulant for infective conditions of the female reproductive system such as vaginitis. May be decreased where there is blood loss due to menorrhagia, therefore requirements may need to be increased[30]	250–5000 mg/day	Blackcurrants, kiwi, mangoes, guava, rosehips, strawberries, parsley, citrus fruits
Bioflavonoids	Enhances the absorption of vitamin C. May reduce heavy bleeding,[32] therefore possible role in female reproductive conditions characterised by heavy bleeding	1000 mg/day	Citrus fruits, buckwheat, vegetables
Vitamin D	Necessary for the synthesis of specific vaginal structural proteins, such as cytokeratins. Deficiency results in a reduction of cytokeratins resulting in loss of epithelial structural integrity and desquamation.[33] Deficiency of vitamin D is seen in a number of female patients with reproductive complaints.[33,34] Key roles include immunity, bone health and mood	400–1600 IU/day. Dose may be increased in instances of deficiency as evidenced by pathology investigations	Synthesised by the action of sunlight on fish liver oils such as cod, tuna, also found in egg yolks, sprouted seeds and milk
Vitamin E	Required for hormonal balance and immunity. In the form of an antioxidant it regulates the arachidonic acid cascade to eicosanoid production[35] by reducing prostaglandin formation.[36] Maintains the health of the ovaries[25]	100–800 IU/day (natural mixed forms)	Almonds, wheatgerm, safflower, egg yolks, corn, beef, nuts
Chromium	Component of glucose tolerance factor, required for blood sugar regulation	100–300 micrograms/day	Apples, asparagus, oysters, prunes, cheese
Iron	May be indicated where there is menorrhagia such as in fibroids or endometriosis due to possible anaemia	10–75 mg/day	Red meat, apricots, oysters, sunflower seeds, pumpkin seeds, pine nuts
Zinc	Numerous roles within the female reproductive system including antioxidant, tissue repair, immune response and hormone and inflammation regulation	10–60 mg/day	Beef, baked beans, wholegrains, oysters, pumpkin seeds, cashews, sunflower seeds

TABLE 18.1 Specific nutritional objectives—cont'd			
Nutrient	**Justification**	**Therapeutic dosage**	**Dietary source**
Manganese	Antioxidant and blood sugar modulation	2–15 mg/day	Almonds, carrots, broccoli, sunflower seeds, walnuts, legumes, whole grains
Magnesium	Significant effects in the female reproductive system via numerous pathways. Roles in cell membrane stability, vascular contraction, sedation of neuromuscular excitability, reduced perception of pain, mood improvement,[37] reduced fluid retention and anxiety associated with premenstrual symptoms[38,39]	300–800 mg/day	Green leafy vegetables, cocoa, almonds, brewers yeasts, cashews, kelp, wheat bran, wheatgerm, buckwheat, nuts and seeds
Calcium	Bone health (important during menopause), involved in muscular contraction therefore may reduce menstrual cramps, low levels observed in the week of menstruation	1000–2000 mg/day	Almonds, dairy products, figs, salmon and sardines (with bones), tahini, sesame seeds, molasses, green leafy vegetables
Potassium	Maintains fluid balance	3–8 g/day	Vegetables, sardines, avocado, banana, dates, citrus fruits
Selenium	Selenium is a potent antioxidant. Reactive oxygen species (ROS) are indicated in female reproductive disorders. Oestrogen deficit following menopause may cause a decrease in selenium status in postmenopausal women, accelerating the process of ageing[40,41]	100–300 micrograms/ day	Almonds, beans, coconuts, corn, kelp, sunflower seeds, legumes, walnuts, whole grains
Silica	Repair of scar tissue, reduce adhesion formation	20–30 mg/day	Barley, oats, wholegrain cereals, root vegetables
Omega-3 fatty acids	Precursors of eicosanoids. Useful in female reproductive disorders characterised by inflammation[42] due to anti-inflammatory activity, also influences immune cell regulation, and the behaviour of proteins involved in immune cell activation	500–1080 mg/day EPA[43] 300–720 mg/day DHA[43] 165–350 mg/day GLA	Pilchards, salmon, trout, herring, salmon, mackerel
Coenzyme Q10	Minimises oxidative damage and necessary for cellular metabolic processes and ATP production	30–300 mg/day	Almonds, broccoli, mackerel, sardines, salmon, sesame seeds
Lipoic acid	Blood sugar regulation	100–600 mg/day	
N-acetyl-cysteine (NAC)	Antioxidant (reactive scavenging species) implicated in many reproductive disorders. Insulin-sensitising effect (therefore useful for polycystic ovary syndrome (PCOS))[44] May decrease testosterone and free androgen index values in PCOS patients.[44] Possible therapeutic use in postmenopausal women as antioxidants such as NAC are potent inhibitors of osteoclast differentiation and function[45]	100–1500 mg/day[25] 1800 mg/day for PCOS effects, this was increased to 3000 mg/ day for morbidly obese patients[44]	Supplements only
Phyto-oestrogens (e.g. isoflavones, coumestans, lignans and flavonoids)	Help to modulate oestrogen in the body	20–160 mg/day	Red clover, linseed, soybeans, alfalfa, chickpeas
Indole-3-carbinol	Hormone regulation. Can shift oestrogen metabolism towards less oestrogenic metabolites	200–400 mg/day[46]	The Brassica family (broccoli, Brussels sprouts, etc.)

Continued

TABLE 18.1 Specific nutritional objectives—cont'd

Nutrient	Justification	Therapeutic dosage	Dietary source
Probiotics	Found in healthy vaginal microbiota, depleted levels in bacterial vaginosis. Use intravaginally and orally to improve vaginal flora and treat and prevent urogenital infections such as bacterial vaginosis[47]	Strain-dependent Multi-strains are advisable and doses should be between 25 and 100 × 10^9/day in divided doses. Topical application is advisable for some conditions Most promising strains appear to be *Lactobacillus acidophilus* or combination of *Lactobacillus rhamnosus* GR-1 and *Lactobacillus fermentum* RC-14 1.6 × 10^9/day[48,49]	Natural yoghurt, fermented foods, supplements

Specific herbal medicine classes

The specific herbal medicine classes used are listed in Table 18.2.

Investigations

ALLOPATHIC TESTING

Investigations used allopathically for female reproductive system disorders are summarised in Table 18.3.

TABLE 18.2 Specific herbal medicine classes

Class	Example	Justification
Adaptogen	*Panax ginseng* (Korean ginseng)	Adaptogens provide fortification in times of fatigue and exhaustion by supporting the stress response and are highly indicated in conditions of the female reproductive system due to the exacerbating effects of stress. A standardised extract of *Panax ginseng* given to symptomatic menopausal women for 4 months was found to improve quality of life. Although no reduction was seen with regards to hot flushes, significant benefits were experienced with regards to increased feelings of wellbeing and health subscales in favour of *Panax ginseng* compared with the placebo. This may be due to its adaptogenic action[50]
Adrenal tonic	*Glycyrrhiza glabra* (liquorice)	Adrenal tonics support the healthy functioning of the adrenal glands. This is imperative as, among other things, elevated cortisol may lead to insulin resistance and hyperprolactinaemia. *Glycyrrhiza glabra* affects cortisol metabolism by inhibiting 11β-hydroxysteroid dehydrogenase. It may be necessary to prescribe an alternative adrenal tonic in those patients with fluid retention, because of the mineralocorticoid effects of *Glycyrrhiza glabra*
Anodynes/ analgesics	*Corydalis ambigua* (corydalis)	Anodynes and analgesics are those herbs that relieve pain in the female reproductive system (e.g. period pain). Traditionally used as an alterative and tonic,[8] *Corydalis ambigua* contains tetrahydropalmatine (THP), an alkaloid which has been found to possess not only analgesic activity, but also sedative–tranquillising actions. THP appears to affect the dopamine pathways of the body: (–)-THP is a dopamine receptor antagonist while (+)-THP is a selective dopamine depletor[51]
Anti-androgenic	*Glycyrrhiza glabra* (liquorice)	Anti-androgen herbs are those that block the effects of androgens (steroid hormones responsible for male characteristics). The anti-androgenic action of *Glycyrrhiza glabra* occurs via the blockage of several enzymes involved in the synthesis of androgens and oestrogens. These include stimulation of aromatase activity, blockage of 17β-hydroxysteroid dehydrogenase and C17,20 lyase, as well as 5α- and 5β-reductase activity,[52] making it useful in conditions of the female reproductive tract characterised by increased androgens such as PCOS

TABLE 18.2 Specific herbal medicine classes—cont'd

Class	Example	Justification
Anticystic	*Thuja occidentalis* (thuja)	Cysts are a common occurrence in many female reproductive conditions including PCOS and ovarian cysts. The Eclectics valued *Thuja occidentalis* for its astringent and antiseptic[9] action, using it for 'restrained haemorrhages occasioned by malignant growths'.[8] While no clinical trials exist examining the efficacy of *Thuja occidentalis* in relation to the reduction or removal of cysts from the female reproductive system, thuja contains a powerful essential oil which displays potent immunomodulating and antiviral activity[53] and in clinical practice appears to exert anticystic activity
Antidepressant	*Hypericum perforatum* (St John's wort)	The antidepressant classes of botanicals are those that alleviate depression. *Hypericum perforatum* has been shown to be of use in mood disorders associated with female reproductive system including menopause and premenstrual tension.[54] In one small study, menopausal women supplementing with *Hypericum perforatum* experienced improved mood.[55] Sexual wellbeing also improved
Anti-haemorrhagic	*Capsella bursa-pastoris* (shepherd's purse)	The anti-haemorrhagic herbs such as *Capsella bursa-pastoris* are essential in female reproductive conditions where there is excessive or heavy bleeding, such as during menopause or with fibroids. *Capsella bursa-pastoris* has traditionally been indicated for this situation. The Eclectics prized it for 'Chronic hemorrhages and menorrhagia with too frequent and long continued, or constant, colorless discharge'[8]
Anti-hydrotic	*Salvia officinalis* (sage)	Hot flushes are caused by declining levels of oestrogen and increasing luteinising hormone.[28] *Salvia officinalis* was used traditionally by the Eclectics to treat hyperhidrosis. When taken warm, the Eclectics found that it produced free sweating, while when taken cold it restrained excessive sweating.[9] In modern times, *Salvia officinalis* given in combination with a cooling herb (*Medicago sativa*, alfalfa) to menopausal women resulted in a reduction in hot flushes and night sweats in approximately 67% of women[56]
Anti-inflammatory	*Angelica sinensis* (dong quai)	The anti-inflammatory herbs such as *Angelica sinensis* are specific for reducing inflammation within the female reproductive system. The root of *Angelica sinensis* has been used for centuries to regulate the workings of the female menstrual cycle and it is indicated for dysmenorrhoea, irregular menstruation, amenorrhoea and menopause
Anti-mastalgia	*Vitex agnus-castus* (chaste tree berry)	Mastalgia is a common premenstrual syndrome and is associated with latent hyperprolactinaemia.[57] *Vitex agnus-castus* is approved by the German Commission E for the treatment of mastalgia.[58] Diterpene constituents within *Vitex agnus-castus* exert a dopaminergic effect by binding to dopamine receptors in the hypothalamus and anterior pituitary, preventing the release of prolactin
Anti-prostaglandins	*Tanacetum parthenium* (feverfew)	Overproduction of certain prostaglandins within the body have been linked to disorders of the female reproductive system.[59,60] Anti-prostaglandin herbs such as *Tanacetum parthenium* have been found to inhibit prostaglandin biosynthesis[61] and thus may be effective in female reproductive conditions where there is pain and inflammation
Astringent	*Trillium erectum* (Beth root)	The astringents promote healing and reduce discharges. *Trillium erectum* is a fast-acting astringent with an affinity for the mucous membranes and the uterus. The astringent effects of *Trillium erectum* are gentle and thus it does not cause excessive dryness. The Eclectics favoured its use therapeutically where there was excessive menstruation[62]
Blood sugar modulators	*Gymnema sylvestre* (gymnema)	Blood sugar modulators such as *Gymnema sylvestre* are well regarded for their hypoglycaemic effects. They may be used to help to manage blood sugar abnormalities such as insulin resistance and metabolic syndrome associated with female reproductive conditions such as PCOS
Blood tonic	*Panax notoginseng* (Tienchi ginseng)	Herbs that prevent blood stasis such as *Panax notoginseng* are useful in female reproductive conditions such as congestive dysmenorrhoea. Clinical studies[63] reveal *Panax notoginseng* to exert significant anticoagulant and antiplatelet activities. This provides a rationale for its traditional application in Chinese medicine, where it has been used for its effects on the blood to disperse blood clots, promote circulation of blood and eliminate stasis[64]

Continued

TABLE 18.2 Specific herbal medicine classes—cont'd

Class	Example	Justification
Emmenogogue	*Mentha pulegium* (pennyroyal)	*Mentha pulegium* has a long history of use as an emmenogogue. The Eclectics describe its use for obstructive and painful menstruation and for its action of diminishing excessive amounts of blood in the uterus.[62] Safety of using this class should be considered at all times
Female tonic	*Asparagus racemosus* (shatavari)	Shatavari is an Ayurvedic herb that has long been used in traditional Indian medicine as a rejuvenating female tonic. Shatavari nourishes and rejuvenates the female tissues, improving fertility, promoting menses and sexual appetite. While the mechanism by which shatavari works has not been well established, the steroidal saponins within shatavari are thought to impart hormone-like activity. These constituents appear to interact with the hypothalamus or pituitary, the result of which has a regulating and tonifying effect on the reproductive system[28]
HPO modulator	*Vitex agnus-castus* (chaste tree berry)	Disruption of the hypothalamic–pituitary–adrenal axis is associated with many female reproductive conditions. *Vitex agnus-castus* has been used for centuries for female reproductive complaints and is known to modulate hypothalamic pituitary function. This makes it a useful botanical for disorders of the hypothalamic pituitary axis
Hypothyroid	*Fucus vesiculosus* (bugleweed)	The endocrine system and the female reproductive system are closely associated. Disorders in one may influence the other. In some females, hypothryoidism is associated with the development of enlarged multicystic ovaries,[65,66] hence acknowledging the role of the endocrine system within female reproductive complaints is imperative. *Fucus vesiculosus* helps to regulate the function of the thyroid gland and may be useful in patients suffering from hypothyroidism
Liver detoxicant	*Schisandra chinenesis* (schisandra)	Liver detoxification is highly important in naturopathic treatment of female reproductive complaints. If detoxification mechanisms are impaired, circulating hormones and toxins are unable to be broken down and slowly increase within the body. *Schisandra chinensis* works on both phase 1 and phase 2 detoxification, improving enterohepatic recycling of toxins/hormones and thus promoting clearance from the body
Lymphatic	*Calendula officinalis* (calendula)	*Calendula officinalis* is a herb with lymphatic properties. Lymphatic vessels exist in many areas of the female reproductive system including the corpeus luteum[67] and aid the clearance of lymphatic congestion, stimulating drainage and eliminating wastes
Mucous membrane tonic	*Hydrastis canadensis* (golden seal)	Mucous membrane tonics such as *Hydrastis canadensis* enhance the health of mucous membranes such as those found in the vagina. Traditionally, *Hydrastis canadensis* was used as a healing agent for cervical erosion and for vaginal and uterine discharge[9]
Nervine	*Melissa officinalis* (melissa)	Nervine herbs function to support the body and balance the nervous system. *Melissa officinalis* exerts a soothing and calming effect on the body; its gentle nature makes it ideal as an adjuvant in female reproductive conditions where it helps to restore the nervous system, relieving tension and unrest
Prolactin reducing	*Vitex agnus-castus* (chaste tree berry)	Hyperprolactinaemia is the excessive production of prolactin. *Vitex agnus-castus* has a modulating effect on prolactin secretion from the pituitary gland and has been shown to lower serum prolactin[68]
Tissue restorative	*Centella asiatica* (gotu kola)	Herbs that promote tissue repair and healing are important, particularly in female reproductive conditions where there is scarring and adhesions. While no studies have been undertaken on *Centella asiatica*'s actions in specific female reproductive complaints such as endometriosis, the fact that it stimulates type 1 collagen production[69] provides a rationale for its use
Uterine tonics	*Angelica sinensis* (dong quai)	Uterine tonics such as dong quai are those herbs that strengthen, tone and normalise the activity of the uterus

PCOS, polycystic ovary syndrome.

TABLE 18.3 Investigations

Test category	Normal result	Clinical significance
Blood glucose (fasting)	Venous plasma or serum Fasting: 3.0–5.4 mmol/L >2 h post-prandial 'Random': 3.0–7.7 mmol/L	Detection of hyperglycaemia and hypoglycaemia Diagnosis and as a screening test for diabetes mellitus Monitoring glycaemic control Useful diagnostic tool for PCOS (may be elevated)
Lipid panel	Cholesterol (serum/plasma): optimal level <4.0 mmol/L HDL: female population reference range: 1.0–2.2 mmol/L. Therapeutic targets: >1.0 LDL: Population reference range: 2.0–3.4 mmol/L. Therapeutic targets: <2.5 mmol/L Triglycerides: <1.7 mmol/L (fasting)	Lipids may be elevated in some female reproductive conditions (e.g. PCOS[70]) NB. Triglycerides may be elevated with oral contraceptive use
Vitamin B_{12} (serum)	Generally 120–680 pmol/L	Levels may be reduced in female reproductive complaints characterised by menorrhagia due to folate deficiency or megaloblastic anaemia due to vitamin B_{12} deficiency
Folate (red cell and serum)	Red cell: 360–1400 nmol/L Serum: 7–45 nmol/L.	Levels may be reduced in female reproductive complaints characterised by menorrhagia due to megaloblastic anaemia
Vitamin D (25-hydroxy)	General consensus is that readings should be >100 nmol/L but many labs use the range 51–160 Mild deficiency: 25–50 nmol/L Moderate deficiency: 12.5–25 nmol/L Severe deficiency: <12.5 nmol/L	Essential to assess for deficiency; however, assesses post-liver hydroxylation only
Vitamin D (1,25-dihydroxy)	35–120 pmol/L	Assesses usable vitamin D levels in the body post liver and kidney hydroxylation
Iron studies	Ferritin: 15–200 micrograms/L Iron: 10–30 μmol/L Iron-binding capacity: 45–80 μmol/L Transferrin saturation: 0.15–0.45 (15–45%) Transferrin: 1.7–3.0 g/L	Levels may be reduced in female reproductive complaints characterised by menorrhagia Suspected iron deficiency, iron overload, acute iron poisoning (see iron toxicity). The assessment of iron deficiency or overload may be complicated by the presence of an acute phase response or hepatocellular disease. In general, serum ferritin is the preferred test for the assessment of iron deficiency, however levels may be normal (up to 100 micrograms/L) when iron deficiency coexists with an acute phase response. Soluble transferrin receptor levels are more useful, as they are not affected in an acute phase response; levels are normal in anaemia of chronic disease uncomplicated by iron deficiency. An alternative approach to the patient with suspected iron deficiency and/or chronic inflammatory disease is to assess the haemoglobin response to iron therapy
Dehydroepiandrosterone sulfate (DHEA-S)	Age dependent Adult female, premenopausal: 2.0–11.0 μmol/L	Investigation of infertility, hirsutism and virilisation in females May be elevated in PCOS. Useful to assess for deficiency in oopause or menopause
Free androgen index (FAI)	0.3–4.0% (FAI = total testosterone/ SHBG × 100)	Increased in PCOS
Testosterone	0.2–1.8 nmol/L	May be increased in PCOS
Sex hormone binding globulin (SHBG)	30–110 nmol/L	Increased in PCOS or when androgen response is greater When SHBG levels are increased beyond what is expected, there is likely to be less free testosterone available to the tissues than is indicated by the total testosterone. If SHBG concentrations are decreased, more of the total testosterone is 'bioavailable' (not bound to SHBG)
Androstenedione (AD)	Serum: 3.5–9.0 nmol/L	Investigation of female hirsutism (it is elevated in 60% of the cases) and virilisation AD may be elevated in PCOS, congenital adrenal hyperplasia, and tumours of the adrenals or gonads AD is not helpful in separating adrenal from gonadal causes of excess androgen secretion

Continued

TABLE 18.3 Investigations—cont'd		
Test category	**Normal result**	**Clinical significance**
Follicle-stimulating hormone (FSH)	Method-dependent, and related to menstrual cycle in females Basal 2.0–13.0 U/L Mid-cycle peak 8.0–25.0 U/L Postmenopausal 25.0–150.0 U/L	Useful to assess cycle health and predict or diagnose menopause Levels are increased when pituitary secretion occurs in the absence of feedback inhibition by gonadal androgens or oestrogens (primary gonadal hypofunction, postmenopausal state, castration) Increased levels may also be seen with pituitary gonadotroph tumours, although some tumours secrete only the α subunit Levels are decreased if ovarian or testicular failure is due to pituitary or hypothalamic disease
Luteinising hormone (LH)	Levels will be dependent on the method used, the age, stage of the menstrual cycle and whether the patient is postmenopausal. LH secretion is pulsatile and single results may be misleading Basal 2.5–13.0 U/L Mid-cycle peak 18.0–95.0 U/L Postmenopausal 18.0–80.0 U/L	Useful to assess cycle health and eliminate pathology. Investigation of female infertility to distinguish primary gonadal failure from pituitary/hypothalamic failure Identification of ovulation in the investigation of menstrual cycle disturbances and female infertility. LH peak occurs just prior to, and identifies, ovulation High levels are found in primary gonadal failure Low levels occur with hypothalamic failure (responds to gonadotrophin-releasing hormone) and pituitary failure (no response) PCOS is associated with an increased LH/FSH ratio. If amenorrhoea is due to undiagnosed pregnancy, spuriously elevated results may be obtained using older assay methods which show cross-reactivity with hCG
Progesterone (P4)	Follicular phase: 0.1–4.3 nmol/L Luteal phase: 5.8–96.0 nmol/L Midluteal phase: 9.2–117.0 nmol/L Postmenopausal: 0.0–2.7 μmol/L 5–16 weeks' gestation: 37.0–205.0 nmol/L	Useful to assess cycle health and eliminate pathology NB: Imperative to know the day of the cycle to assess correctly; best assessed 7 days post ovulation (i.e. generally day 21 but highly individual) Failure of progesterone levels to increase in the latter part of the menstrual cycle indicates an anovulatory cycle or corpus luteum inadequacy
Oestradiol (E2)	Early follicular phase: <400 pmol/L Preovulatory phase: 600–2500 pmol/L Luteal phase: 150–1700 pmol/L Postmenopausal: <200 pmol/L	Useful to assess cycle health and eliminate pathology Diagnosis of precocious puberty Monitoring of oestrogen therapy is only possible if the drug being administered is oestradiol Monitoring ovulation induction in in-vitro fertilisation Assessment of women with suspected hypothalamic or pituitary disease Increased levels indicate an endogenous or exogenous source of increased oestradiol NB Imperative to know the day of the cycle to assess correctly; best assessed on day 3
Prolactin (total)	Female: 85–500 mIU/L	Assessment of patients with a suspected pituitary tumour; investigation of infertility, amenorrhoea, galactorrhoea and impotence Increased levels are found in patients with prolactinomas and hypothalamic disorders, which may be associated with the amenorrhoea–galactorrhoea syndrome Some drugs cause increased levels, e.g. phenothiazines, metoclopramide and oestrogens Increased levels occur during normal pregnancy and lactation Some methods may give falsely high values due to macroprolactin variants NB: Essential to get patient to sit for 15–20 min prior to blood draw to ensure accuracy of reading. Physiological causes of increased prolactin (e.g. stress, strenuous exercise, pregnancy, breast palpation, nipple stimulation) should be avoided prior to collection of specimen
Anti-Müllerian hormone	<10.0 pmol/L: Suggestive of failing ovulatory reserve >20.0 pmol/L: Indicates the possibility of: 1. PCOS 2. increased risk of ovarian hyperstimulation syndrome in a stimulated cycle 3. in postmenopausal females — granulosa cell tumour	Useful to assess ovarian reserve in patients suspected of premature or early menopause or to confirm fertility status

TABLE 18.3 Investigations—cont'd

Test category	Normal result	Clinical significance
Human chorionic gonadotrophin (hCG) (plasma, serum or urine)	<5 mIU/L (non-pregnant)	The reference interval in pregnancy varies with gestational age Qualitative test: diagnosis of pregnancy including ectopic pregnancy Quantitative test: diagnosis of threatened abortion or ectopic pregnancy (sequential tests may be needed) Monitoring hCG-producing tumours (e.g. hydatidiform mole, uterine choriocarcinoma, gonadal and extragonadal germ cell tumours): an assay that detects the free β subunit as well as the whole molecule is required and is also suitable for pregnancy-related applications If pregnancy occurs the test becomes positive 6–10 days following ovulation The normal doubling time for the hormone in early pregnancy is 36 h. Low levels for gestational age and/or a low rate of increase may indicate threatened abortion or ectopic pregnancy High levels for gestational age may indicate molar pregnancy Increased levels in a patient with a history of an hCG-producing tumour indicate residual or recurrent tumour

TABLE 18.4 Naturopathic investigations

Baseline hormone profile	This test provides valuable information on female hormonal status and the potential impact this may have on physical and emotional health. Tests levels of oestrone, oestradiol, oestriol, progesterone, testosterone and DHEA-S
Functional liver detoxification profile	This provides an indication of an individual's detoxification status and is useful where there is hormonal imbalance to provide information addressing how well the liver is coping with breaking down and removing hormones from the body
Vitamins, mineral and antioxidants	This test measures the status of a number of nutrients. Nutritional deficiency may aggravate a number of female reproductive conditions
Oestrogen profile	This measures oestrogen metabolites and the ratios of 'good' and 'bad' oestrogens
Female hormone profile	This includes a number of tests to evaluate risk factors for women, including metabolic syndrome profile, essential fatty acid profile, serum peroxides and oestrogen profile
DNA/oxidative stress marker	Reactive oxygen species and free radical species are implicated in many female reproductive disorders. This test may provide a recommendation to increase antioxidants to support female reproductive health and wellbeing

NATUROPATHIC INVESTIGATIONS

Investigations used naturopathically for female reproductive system disorders are summarised in Table 18.4.

SECTION B

THE MENSTRUAL CYCLE

The female reproductive cycle encompasses the cyclical changes and the complex interplay that occurs between the ovaries, uterus and hormones. At 20 weeks of fetal life, the female embryo contains more oocytes than at any other time in her life. Multiple sources suggest that the maximal oogonial content of the gonad at this time is between 6 and 7 million. Approximately a million follicles are present at the time of her birth and about 300 000 are left at the time of menarche. She then will lose 20–30 follicles each cycle. It is believed that approximately 360–400 of these follicles over 30 years will mature and be released by the body, with the remainder being lost from each cycle. From this point in time germ cell content will irretrievably decrease until menopause, when her stores of oocytes will be finally exhausted.

The average duration of a female's menstrual cycle may vary depending on her individual make-up and the health of her reproductive system. A 28-day cycle (±7 days) is considered normal and is used as an example to show the stages of the menstrual cycle (Fig. 18.2).

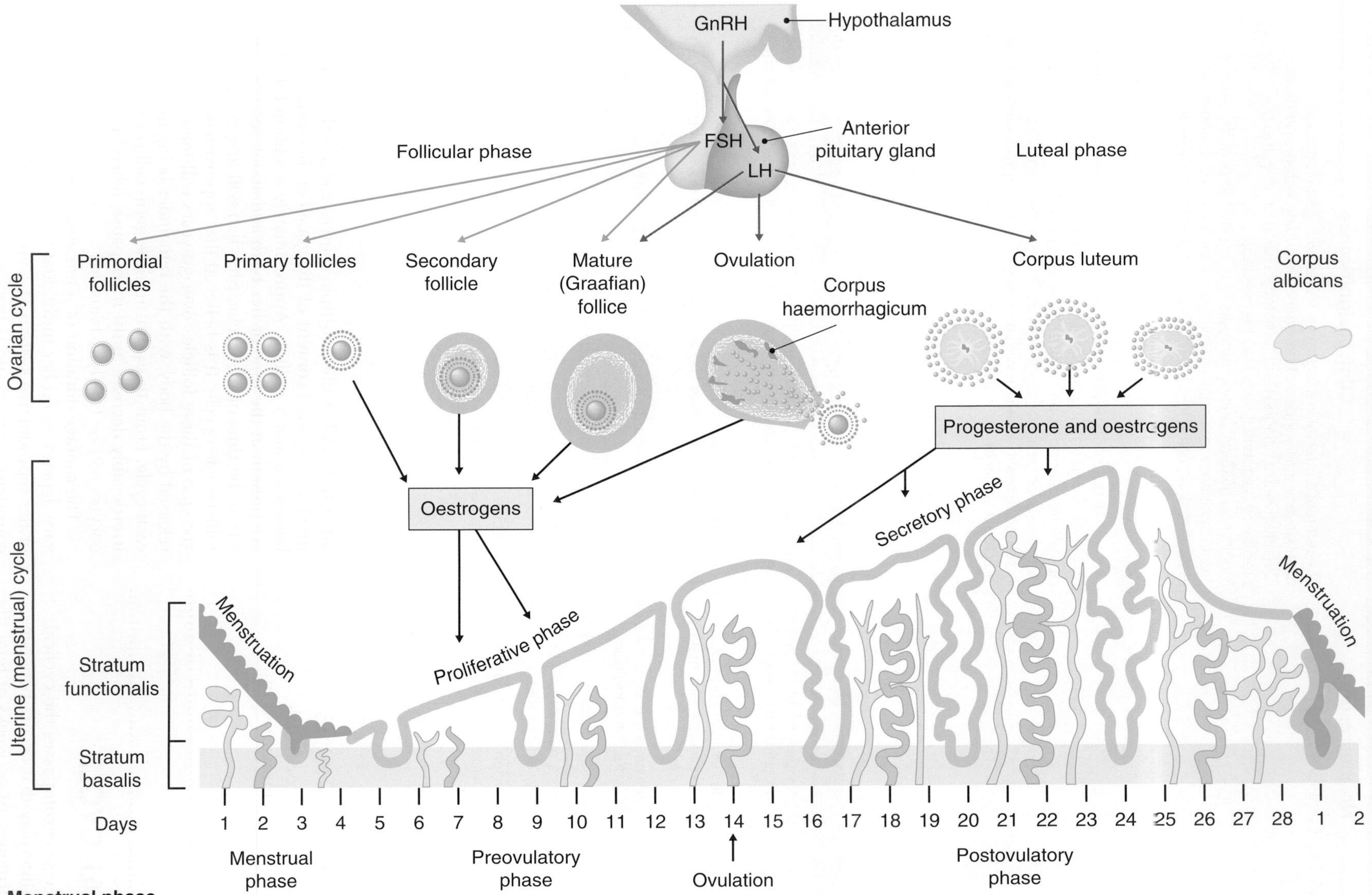

Menstrual phase
First day is considered beginning of 28-day cycle
Preovulatory phase (before egg is released)
Lasts from day 6 to day 13 (most variable timeline)
Ovulation (egg is released)
Typically occurs on day 14. Please note that many women experience this on different days and that is okay!
Postovulatory phase (after egg is released)
Typically lasts 12–16 days

FIGURE 18.2 Phases of the female reproductive cycle.

Source: Tortora JG, Grabowski SR. Principles of anatomy and physiology. 12th edn. New York: John Wiley; 2009. Republished with permission of John Wiley & Sons Inc.

The physiology of menstruation

A regular menstrual pattern requires a functioning reproductive hormone feedback system, which includes the hypothalamus, anterior pituitary gland, ovaries and normal uterine and vaginal anatomy.

The menstrual cycle is 'switched on' when the hypothalamus secretes gonadotrophin-releasing hormone (GnRH), which in turn initiates the release of follicle-stimulating hormone (FSH) from the anterior pituitary. FSH in turn stimulates the growth of a cohort of ovarian follicles (approximately between 20 and 30 per cycle), the granulosa cells of which produce increased amounts of the hormone oestradiol which in turn triggers a surge of luteinising hormone (LH) that causes the dominant follicle to ovulate.

As a result of the stimulation by oestradiol, the endometrium thickens in preparation for implantation of an embryo, should fertilisation and pregnancy occur. The dominant follicle resolves to become the corpus luteum, which then produces progesterone and oestradiol.

If pregnancy does not occur, the corpus luteum becomes non-functional and stops producing hormones, causing the breakdown of the endometrium and menstrual bleeding begins.

MENSTRUAL PHASE (DAYS 1–5)

The menstrual phase typically refers to the first 5 days of the menstrual cycle. In the ovaries approximately 20–30 secondary follicles per ovary are stimulated by the release of FSH, while in the uterus, declining levels of progesterone and other hormones stimulate a chain of events that result in the release of the menstrual flow. During menstruation, the endometrium (uterine lining) that had built up during the previous cycle is shed. The bloody tissue of the endometrium provides an excellent environment for the implantation of a fertilised egg; however, the hormone progesterone is necessary to maintain the thickness of the endometrium. When implantation does not take place, the levels of progesterone drop. As a result, the endometrium can no longer be maintained and it is shed. Menstrual flow comprises blood, mucus, tissue fluids and epithelial cells from the stratum functionalis. This flow exits the body from the uterus out through the vagina, in the process known as menstruation.

THE PROLIFERATIVE PHASE/PRE-OVULATION (DAYS 6–13)

The uterus is now in the proliferative phase. In response to exposure from oestrogen the lining of the endometrium starts to thicken again, reforming the stratum functionalis.

Low progesterone levels also permit the pituitary gland to begin secreting another important hormone — follicle-stimulating hormone (FSH). As the name implies, FSH stimulates the ovary to begin selection of another egg for ovulation during the new cycle. Between 20 and 30 follicles begin to grow towards maturity with the presence of FSH. Each egg is encased in its own follicle, which is a fluid-filled sac in the ovary.

Development of the dominant follicle

By approximately the 8th day of the cycle FSH causes one of the many follicles to become 'dominant' and to fully develop the egg inside. This Graafian follicle secretes oestrogen and inhibin, which results in a decrease in the amount of FSH. The remaining follicles then disintegrate and the dominant follicle continues to grow until it is ready for ovulation, forming a blister bulge on the surface of the ovary.

Oestrogen and cervical fluid

During the development of the Graafian follicle, the increase in oestrogen causes the body to build up the endometrium again in anticipation of possible implantation by a fertilised ovum during the new cycle. At this time, increased oestrogen levels are also causing glands around the cervix to secrete cervical fluid. Cervical fluid has several purposes in human reproduction:

- It is a natural lubricant
- It provides nutrients for sperm to live
- It provides sperm a means to travel to the fallopian tubes.

Cervical fluid is what enables conception to take place — without it, sperm would die within a few hours and would not be able to reach the ovum in the fallopian tube. Early in the fertile phase, cervical fluid will be sticky and opaque, but as ovulation approaches, it normally becomes clear, stretchy, and even watery, like raw eggwhite. Eggwhite-quality cervical fluid indicates the most fertile time of the cycle and precedes the release of the follicle.

LUTEINISING HORMONE AND OVULATION (DAY 14)

When oestrogen levels reach their highest level, they cause the pituitary gland to secrete high levels of luteinising hormone (LH). It is this hormone which causes the dominant ovarian follicle to release the ovum in the process of ovulation. Ovulation normally occurs within 12–36 h of this surge of LH.

The secondary oocyte is swept into the fallopian tube, and travels to the uterus through the action of the cilia. Its life depends on a chance encounter with a travelling sperm that just happens to be in the area, for unless they meet the oocyte will die.

THE LUTEAL PHASE (DAYS 15–28)

For approximately 2 weeks after ovulation, progesterone is released by what used to be the ovarian follicle, now called the corpus luteum, while it is attached to the ovarian wall. Progesterone causes the endometrium to remain conducive to the implantation of a fertilised ovum. It also causes the woman's temperature to rise perceptibly, typically by 0.2°C. It is this rise in temperature that is used to identify ovulation by women practising fertility awareness.

Progesterone also causes oestrogen levels to drop, resulting in a drying up of cervical fluid. This period of the cycle is known as the 'luteal phase' and, when followed by menstruation, its length is usually fairly consistent, normally lasting between 12 and 16 days.

The ruptured Graafian follicle transforms into the corpus haemorrhagicum (very much like a blood clot) and forms part of the corpus luteum, which releases progesterone, oestrogen, relaxin and inhibin, helping to maintain the thickened uterine lining. When fertilisation occurs, it normally takes place in the fallopian tube and life begins. The fertilised egg then travels to the uterus where it implants into the thickened endometrium. The first thing the fertilised ovum does after implantation is secrete hCG (human chorionic gonadotrophin), which in turn causes the corpus luteum to continue secreting progesterone. The progesterone keeps the endometrium thickened and prevents menstruation and miscarriage.

If fertilisation does not take place, the corpus luteum degrades and the drop in progesterone and other hormones stimulates the release of the menstrual flow as described and the cycle starts again. If the blastocyst (5–6 day old embryo) does implant, pregnancy occurs.

HORMONE ORDER

A useful clinical tip is to remember the order of hormones in the body with the following mnemonic:[71]

- **F**ollicle-stimulating hormone
- **O**/Estrogen
- **L**uteinising hormone
- **O**vulation
- **P**rogesterone.

Menstruation

The purpose of menstruation is uncertain and is associated with many myths and superstitions throughout history. It occurs solely in primates and involves regular partial endometrial shedding and remodelling. It is accompanied by endometrial transudation and bleeding and has the potential to be a high-risk process for the individual.

Menstruation probably has its evolutionary origins in egg-laying, placentation, parturition and postpartum uterine involution. The range of species in which it occurs includes humans, great apes, higher primates, elephant shrew and some species of bats. Technically, it occurs in mammals who meet the following criteria:

- Have invasive deciduate placentation
- Have the capacity to involute and remodel the uterus especially after birth and miscarriage
- Are able to support the development of spiral arterioles and distinct stratification of the endometrium
- Have spontaneous cyclical decidualisation of the endometrium pre-implantation.

WHAT IS NORMAL?

The normal menstrual cycle in humans is defined as 28 days (±7 days) in length, 4–7 days (±2 days) in duration, with a blood loss of 30–40 mL (mean) with an upper limit of 60–80 mL. Each month will likely produce minor monthly variations due to various factors, but most women maintain consistency month to month based on their genetics and hormonal status.

VARIATIONS IN BLOOD LOSS VOLUME

It has been suggested that in historical terms women bled for less time (approximately one day) and that over time this has increased. Apparently, the volume of blood has remained the same but duration has extended to approximately 4 days. Studies that have measured blood loss have demonstrated that patients with menorrhagia have a considerable increase in menstrual blood flow during the first 3 days (up to 92% of their total menses being lost at this time). This finding suggests that the mechanisms responsible for cessation of menstruation are as effective in women who have menorrhagia as in normal women, despite the very high blood loss.

MENORRHAGIA — HOW MUCH IS TOO MUCH?

Objective menorrhagia is measured menstrual blood loss of 80 mL or more per cycle. Objective menstrual blood loss measurements are rarely performed outside clinical research. The alkaline haematin method is a useful research tool, but women on the whole find it inconvenient and distasteful to collect soiled sanitary wear for analysis. The PBAC or pictorial blood loss assessment chart has been used as an alternative. However, there have been difficulties with validation, and there is evidence that it offers no benefit in the objective diagnosis of menorrhagia. More commonly the diagnosis of menorrhagia is based on the woman's subjective assessment of her periods. This in turn will be affected by a woman's perception of what is normal, and tolerance of her menstrual symptoms.

ABNORMAL UTERINE BLEEDING

Some common causes of abnormal uterine bleeding are listed in Tables 18.5[72] and 18.6.[73]

TABLE 18.5 Common causes of irregular bleeding at various age groups

Age				
15–20	20–30	30–45	45–55	55+
Sexually transmitted infection, cervicitis (especially *Chlamydia*) Cervical ectropion			HRT Endometrial cancer	
		Endometrial polyps Endometrial hyperplasia Uterine fibroids		
Intrauterine device (IUD)/intrauterine system (IUS)				
Pregnancy and complications, miscarriage, ectopic pregnancy Contraceptive steroid (especially progestogens) Endometriosis				
Trauma, surgery				

Source: Adapted from Read C, May T, Stellingwerff M. Irregular vaginal bleeding. In: How to treat yearbook. Australian Doctor; 2007.

TABLE 18.6 Possible causes of menorrhagia or abnormal uterine bleeding

Cause	Possible aetiology
Anovulation	Excessive oestrogen; failure of midcycle surge of luteinising hormone; hypothyroidism; hyperprolactinaemia; polycystic ovarian disease, ovarian cysts
Mechanical causes	Uterine polyps, uterine fibroids, uterine cancer, intrauterine devices (IUDs), atopic pregnancy, pregnancy, endometriosis and endometritis
Intrauterine structural defects	Fibroids; polyps; cancer; ectopic pregnancy; intrauterine devices
Blood disorders (systemic coagulopathy component that may cause abnormal uterine bleeding)	1. Platelet abnormalities: thrombocytopenias, thrombocytopathies, von Willebrand's disease, leukaemias 2. Coagulation factor deficiencies: congenital deficiencies (mostly autosomal recessive); afibrinogenaemia; deficiencies of Factors II, V, VII, VIII, IX, X, XI, XIII and Factors V and VIII combined; carriers of X-linked deficiencies (FVIII, FIX); acquired deficiencies; liver dysfunction; vitamin K deficiency; anticoagulant use (heparin, warfarin, aspirin)

Source: Fraser I, Bonnar J, Peyvandi F. Requirements for research investigations to clarify the relationships and management of menstrual abnormalities in women with hemostatic disorder. Fertil Steril 2005;84:1360–5.

MENSTRUAL BLOOD

It has been known for some time that blood does not account for all of the menstrual discharge. A very detailed study of menstrual discharge collected directly from the uterus found menstrual haemoglobin concentrations to be between 4.0 and 5.0 g/100 mL (i.e. approximately 35% of venous concentrations on days 1–2 of the cycle.[74,75] About 50–60% of total menstrual flow is believed to be endometrial transudate (mean total flow = 60–80 mL).

It is not known whether or not the fallopian tubes secrete enough fluid to make a significant contribution. Cervical and vaginal secretions make some contribution to the fluid (approximately 1–5%) absorbed by sanitary pads or tampons but these components are likely to be small and are likely to only be a considerable component in the last few days of menses when most of the endometrial lining has been shed (Fig. 18.3). This possibly accounts for the high total fluid to blood loss ratio observed in oral contraceptive users.[75]

MENSTRUAL TERMINOLOGY

Unfortunately there is much ambiguity and confusion regarding definitions. Each country has varied interpretations for commonly used words to describe menstrual factors. As such, there are countless papers trying to develop consistency. Table 18.7 gives a summary of some currently accepted definitions.

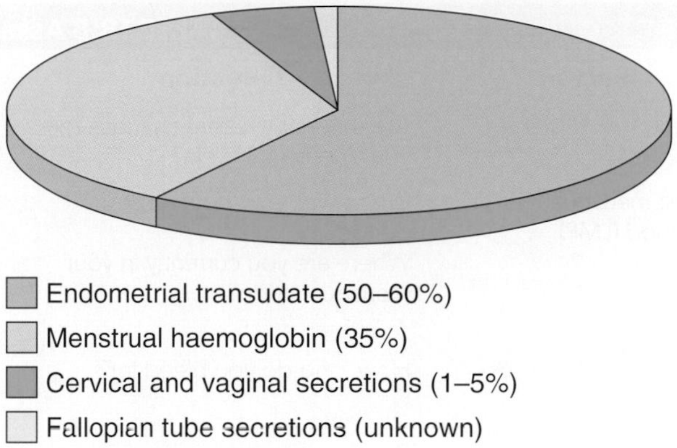

FIGURE 18.3 Menstrual blood composition.

Source: Katz V. Comprehensive gynecology. 5th edn. Maryland Heights: Mosby; 2007.

TABLE 18.7 Menstrual terminology

Amenorrhoea	Absence of menses Primary: menstruation cycles never start; secondary: menstruation cycles cease
Anovulation	Absence of ovulation
Dysfunctional uterine bleeding (DUB)	Abnormal uterine bleeding without any demonstrable organic cause
Dysmenorrhoea	Painful menstruation
Hypomenorrhoea	Scant, regular menstruation (<10 mL)
Intermenstrual bleeding	Variable amounts of bleeding occurring between regular menses
Menometrorrhagia	Irregular heavy bleeding
Menorrhagia	Prolonged excessive menstrual bleeding (>80 mL)
Metrorrhagia	Irregular/frequent intervals with excessive flow and duration
Oligomenorrhoea	Infrequent menstrual cycles (>35 days)
Polymenorrhoea	Frequent menses (<21 days)

Assessing the menstrual cycle

To thoroughly assess a patient's menstrual cycle, the questions listed in Table 18.8 can be asked to elucidate aspects of concern. Please note that this is not a diagnostic system but can provide clues and insights for the practitioner.

TABLE 18.8 Assessing the menstrual cycle

Factor	Question	Explanation
Recent changes	Are there any recent changes to your menstrual cycle?	A general question can often elucidate varying responses that can prompt alternative enquiry
Last menstrual period (LMP)	When was your last menstrual period? Where are you currently in your menstrual cycle?	It is essential to ask the patient what day of their cycle they are currently as it both prompts explanation of how to determine the day and also elucidates the patient's awareness of their cycle Any bleeding in a postmenopausal women is considered an emergency and requires immediate referral
Duration of menses	How long do you bleed for?	Bleeding for greater than 7 days per cycle warrants investigation. Bleeding shorter than 2 days may indicate anovulatory bleeding and warrants further investigation. Shorter cycles should beckon enquiry as to flow quantity to eliminate anovulatory cycles
Duration of cycle	How many days in your entire cycle? Are you aware of the duration of your follicular and/or luteal phase?	Cycles shorter than 21 days or longer than 35 days warrant further investigation Follicular phase should be 10–16 days and luteal phases need to be 10–16 days but typically are 12–14 days in length It is important to establish with patients what day 1 constitutes (first day full bleed, not spotting) as this can confuse practitioners otherwise
Colour	What colour is your menstrual blood?	Healthy menstrual flow is believed to be bright red in colour. This is due to haemoglobin percentage and ease of flow. A healthy menstruation is bright red in colour from start to finish. Darkened red/burgundy hues are typically associated with increased inflammation and prostaglandin synthesis. As the colour darkens, increased oxidation of haemoglobin is likely suggesting stagnation of menstrual flow Tampon users will likely experience dark-brown bleeds at the start and end of the bleed Darker blood can be a sign of endometriosis (especially very dark brown or extremely dark red). Dark blood which is thick, brown or 'looks old' can indicate sluggish menstrual flow Pale, thin blood can be an indicator of perimenopausal transition as women often experience bleeds that are pale pink in colour. Alternatively it can indicate poorly regulated hormonal balance
Consistency	Is the bleed watery, thin or thick?	Watery bleeds are synonymous with perimenopausal transition as hormone insufficiencies are likely to have reduced endometrial lining build-up. Alternatively, they can occur postsurgical in procedures such as terminations or D and Cs for the same reason. Thicker bleeds are often associated with increased endometrial lining which can correlate with endometriosis or other similar conditions
Clotting	Do you experience any clots in your menstrual blood? If so, what size are they? How frequently do you experience them? Do you experience any pain when you pass the clots?	Small clots are considered a normal component of menstrual bleeds. They generally indicate excessive blood flow and are formed when anticlotting factors normally present in the menstrual blood are unable to keep the blood in a fluid state because of the volume of blood lost As the clot size increases a few considerations should be taken: Iron status — deficiency correlates with increased clot formation due to interrelationship with haemoglobin Presence of endometriosis — increased endometrial tissue presence increases coagulation of bleeds and increases consistency. Endometriosis patients will likely experience blood clotting and as the disease increases in severity, so too do the size and intensity of their blood clots. Most will complain of needing to 'pass' their blood clots with much pain and discomfort Coagulation disorders

TABLE 18.8 Assessing the menstrual cycle—cont'd

Factor	Question	Explanation
Menstrual flow	How heavy is your menstrual flow? How often do you need to change your pad/tampon/other? What strength of sanitary item do you use (light, regular, heavy)? Do you ever experience flooding or need to use multiple sanitary items at the same time?	Menstrual flow is highly subjective and there are countless studies that suggest that women are unable to accurately assess their menstrual loss
Sanitary use	Do you use pads, tampons or other?	Tampon users are likely to have increased pain and spasm due to muscular contraction to keep the tampon in place as well as theoretical concerns about chemicals included in tampon production. Tampon users are also likely to perpetuate retrograde blood flow or contain menstrual blood within the vaginal cavity. As such, oxidation will increase thus causing a brown discolouration of menstrual flow Sanitary pad users are likely to be more attuned to subtle changes in menstrual flow, have reduced menstrual cramping and make more accurate assessments of blood loss volume Other sanitary items such as menstrual cups should be asked about to assess impact on any menstrual irregularity
Spotting	Do you experience any spotting? If so, when does it occur? What colour is it?	Spotting around ovulation or post intercourse can be a sign of endometriosis or other pathology. Referral is warranted Spotting prior to full menstrual initiation (day 1) can indicate waning progesterone levels to sustain the luteal phase
Pain	Do you experience any pain with menses? If so, where is it located? When in your cycle do you experience it? On a scale of 1–10 how severe is the pain? Do you need to take any medication to relieve the pain?	Pain severity can indicate underlying pathologies that may warrant further investigation. Endometriosis pain scales are good assessment strategies (see Appendix 18.2 at the end of the book)
Dyspareunia	Do you experience pain during or after sexual intercourse?	Dyspareunia can indicate presence of endometriosis. It is important to ask for further information to assess if pain is associated with friction (dryness — menopause) or deep pain (endometriosis) or other
Dyschezia	Do you experience sharp pain when passing a bowel movement?	This may indicate endometriosis if other factors are present
Digestive effects	Do you experience any bowel changes prior to or during your menses?	Constipation prior to menses and diarrhoea during menses can indicate hormonal displacement
PMS	Do you experience any premenstrual symptoms? Mood changes Cravings or appetite changes Fluid retention or weight changes Breast symptoms Pain, cramping Headaches or migraines Hot flushes Acne or skin changes Libido changes	Classification and clarification of PMS symptoms will enable the practitioner to more accurately determine the cause of the presentation and direct treatment accordingly
Hot flushes	Do you experience hot flushes? If so, when in your cycle?	Oestrogen displacement experienced premenopausally can present with hot flushes prior to menses in the oopause period Oestrogen displacement experienced in the endometriosis patient may present with hot flushes either at ovulation, implantation (if pregnant) or premenstrually due to fluctuations and variations in oestrogen usability

Continued

TABLE 18.8 Assessing the menstrual cycle—cont'd

Factor	Question	Explanation
Ovulation awareness	Are you aware of your ovulation changes?	Fertile quality cervical fluid can be typically detected 3–5 days prior to ovulation. Consistency changes progress the fluid to eggwhite consistency typically 24 h prior to ovulation
Parity or gravida	Have you been pregnant previously?	Parity refers to how many pregnancies a patient has had and how many liveborn children she has Gravida refers to how many pregnancies she has had regardless of whether she has delivered the child or not
Contraception history	What form of contraceptives have you used?	It is important to pay attention to any contraceptives with hormonal involvement such as contraceptive pill, implants or others due to their subsequent effects on the menstrual cycle Diaphragm use can correlate with menstrual changes, especially if the patient previously used their diaphragm during menses or developed infections
Current method of contraception	What form of contraceptive do you use? If condoms, do you use lubricants?	Contraceptive choices can influence menstruation. Hormonal modulators such as the contraceptive pill significantly change the quality of menstrual flow. Condoms, spermicide and lubricants can cause allergic reactions, affect fertility and contribute to confusion when assessing menstrual flow
Discharge	Are you aware of any discharge changes? Odour? Redness? Itch?	Enquiry can provide useful information to assess for thrush or STIs
Thrush	Do you experience thrush? If so, is it cyclical?	Cyclical thrush is diagnostic of oestrogen displacement commonly occurring in endometriosis — especially when occurring premenstrually. Alternatively, it can indicate allergy to contraceptive or cross-contamination between sexual partners
Urinary tract infection (UTI)	Do you experience UTIs? If so, are they cyclical? Do you experience pain on urination?	Cyclical UTIs are diagnostic of oestrogen displacement commonly occurring in endometriosis — especially when occurring premenstrually
Libido	How would you rate your libido? Has this changed recently?	Loss of hormones at any stage but especially prior to menopause can reduce libido and may be a warning sign
Breast changes	Do you notice any breast changes throughout the cycle? Discharge?	Breast changes can indicate hormonal fluctuations or may indicate underlying pathologies that warrant further investigation. It is imperative that patients conduct breast self-examination on the same day of their menstrual cycle (monthly). The best time has been reported to be on day 7 of the cycle due to reduced hormonal stimulation and gives most accurate findings

PREMENSTRUAL SYNDROME (PMS)

Epidemiology

Premenstrual syndrome affects millions of Australian women each year. As many as 85%[76] of menstruating women report having one or more premenstrual symptoms; a further 7% experience incapacitating symptoms that may be severe enough to impair daily function and experience a more severe form of premenstrual syndrome known as premenstrual dysphoric disorder (PMDD) (Fig. 18.4).[77] Studies estimate that the incidence of PMS peaks among women aged 25–40,[76] but also acknowledge that adolescents frequently suffer the effects of PMS. A meta-analysis of 17 studies using international data from 1996 to 2011 estimated the global prevalence of PMS at 48%.[78]

A cross-sectional study published in 1997 undertaken on Australian women (aged between 18 and 45 years) involving 310 general practices sought to investigate the prevalence of PMS and the means of treatment used.[79] A premenstrual assessment form was administered to all the women participating in the study in which they recorded their responses to 10 common premenstrual symptoms. Between 11% and 32% of the women reported severe changes during the premenstrual phase on each of the 10 symptoms; the highest rates were observed for affective symptoms. Many of the women who completed the survey were fairly proactive in terms of their approach to treatment, with 85% reporting they had tried treatments (sometimes multiple) to help relieve premenstrual symptoms. Of these treatments, painkillers, rest, increasing fluids and exercise all featured prominently, having been tried by at least one-third of women. The treatments women nominated as most effective included dietary

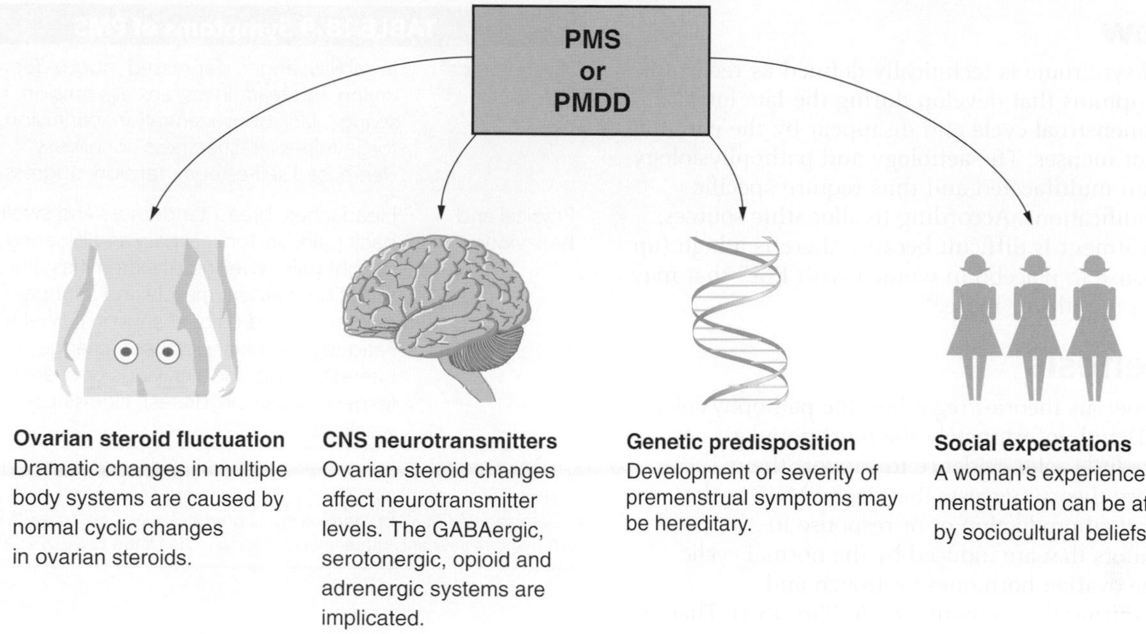

FIGURE 18.4 Premenstrual syndrome/premenstrual dysphoric disorder (PMS/PMDD).

Source: Adapted from Katz V. Comprehensive gynecology. 5th edn. Maryland Heights: Mosby; 2007.

changes, evening primrose oil, vitamins (including B_6) and exercise. Half of the women had sought help for their symptoms in the past, primarily from their general practitioner. Approximately 45% acknowledged they would like further assistance in helping to relieve symptoms associated with PMS. In Australia, women aged 34–39 with PMS and/or dysmenorrhoea were significantly more likely to use CAM practitioners frequently compared to women without PMS and/or dysmenorrhoea. The modalities favoured by this group of women were massage therapists, naturopaths/herbalists, acupuncturists, osteopaths and alternative health practitioners. Use of vitamins/dietary supplements, acupuncture, homeopathy, yoga/mind body practices and massage was found to be satisfactory as treatment in more than half of PMS sufferers who used these treatments.[80] A 2014 prospective cohort study of 9671 Australian women found that PMS and dysmenorrhoea are common among young women. Eighty per cent of the women reported experiencing PMS at one point or another during the 13 year follow-up and it tended to be a long-lasting problem for many women. Sixty per cent of women experienced dysmenorrhoea over the duration of the study, but for most women it was not a long-term condition. The study found a correlation between smoking and illicit drug use in women with persistent PMS, and smoking and obesity in women with dysmenorrhoea.[81]

Classification

Premenstrual syndrome is characterised by recurring somatic and psychological symptoms during the luteal phase of the menstrual cycle that are mostly relieved within a few days of menstruation. The psychological symptoms include irritability, mood swings, anxiety, depression and general dysphoria, associated with a sense of loss of control and being unable to cope. Physical symptoms include bloating, headaches and breast discomfort. There may also be exacerbation of chronic conditions such as epilepsy, migraine or asthma. Approximately 50% of women suffer from a moderate degree of premenstrual symptoms and/or disability, and 5% suffer severely. The latter group may satisfy DSM-5 diagnostic criteria for premenstrual dysphoric disorder (PMDD).

Aetiology

Many different aetiologies have been proposed for the symptoms of PMS; however, none have been definitively established as a dominant cause. The true aetiology of PMS is the consequence of complex and poorly understood interactions between ovarian hormones, endogenous opioid peptides, neurotransmitters, prostaglandins and the circadian, peripheral, autonomic and endocrine systems.[82]

Possible influences include:[82,83]

- Hormonal imbalance, specifically excess oestrogen, prostaglandin deficiency or excess, or low progesterone level during the luteal phase of the cycle, endogenous hormone allergy, hyperprolactinaemia
- Abnormal neurotransmitter response to ovarian signalling
- Disordered aldosterone function leading to sodium and water retention
- Endogenous opiates, serotonin deficiency, psychogenic
- Abnormal hypothalamic–pituitary–adrenal (HPA) axis function, leading to deficient adrenal hormone secretion
- Nutritional deficiency including magnesium, vitamin B_6 (pyridoxine)
- Carbohydrate intolerance, hypoglycaemia
- Environmental factors including stress.

Overview

Premenstrual syndrome is technically defined as recurrent signs and symptoms that develop during the late luteal phase of the menstrual cycle and disappear by the end of the full flow of menses. The aetiology and pathophysiology of PMS remain multifaceted and thus require specific treatment modifications. According to allopathic sources, evaluating treatment is difficult because there is a high (up to 40%) response to placebo in women with PMS that may continue for 3 months or more.[84]

Pathogenesis

There are numerous theories regarding the pathophysiology of PMS/PMDD and unfortunately the most popular therapies have little solid evidence to support them.

The primary theory suggests that PMS/PMDD is the result of abnormal production of or response to neurotransmitters that are induced by the normal cyclic changes of the ovarian hormones oestrogen and progesterone during the menstrual cycle (Box 18.1). There is evidence to support a role for several neurotransmitters: serotonin, noradrenaline, opioids and gamma-aminobutyric acid. Individual biological, genetic and psychological factors as well as sociocultural conditions may also play a role in the aetiology of the symptoms as well as their severity.

BOX 18.1 Action of female hormones

Oestrogen

Oestrogen excess/hypersensitivity may contribute to:

- Excess stimulation of the central nervous system, producing anxiety and irritability
- Increased cramping and contractions of the uterus
- Sodium retention, resulting in weight gain, water retention and bloating
- Potential histamine release, promoting allergy and skin issues
- Minor increase in prolactin, which can produce breast tenderness or pain, depression and dysphoria
- Increase in production of prostaglandins which can heighten pain, redness and swelling.

Progesterone

Relative progesterone excess may contribute to:

- Fatigue and depression
- Decreased libido
- Aldosterone formation and renin stimulation leading to water retention
- Hyperinsulinaemia
- Sedation
- Symptoms of excess corticosteroids.

Adapted from Mayo JL. Premenstrual syndrome: a natural approach to management. Applied Nutritional Science Reports 1999; 5(6).

SIGNS AND SYMPTOMS

Up to 150 different symptoms have been associated with PMS, ranging from psychological symptoms such as irritability, mood swings and depression, to physiological symptoms such as bloating, breast tenderness and headache (Table 18.9).

TABLE 18.9 Symptoms of PMS

Psychological	Irritability, anger, depressed mood/depression, crying and tearfulness, anxiety, tension, mood swings, lack of concentration, confusion, forgetfulness, restlessness, loneliness, decreased self-esteem, tension, aggression
Physical and behavioural	Headaches, breast tenderness and swelling, back pain, abdominal pain and bloating, weight gain, swelling of extremities, fluid retention, nausea, muscle and joint pain, pelvic discomfort and pain, change in bowel habits Fatigue, insomnia, dizziness, changes in sexual interest/libido, food cravings or overeating (especially carbohydrates), clumsiness, weakness

Adapted from Dickerson L, Mazyck P, Hunter M. Premenstrual syndrome. Am Fam Physician 2003;67:1743–52. Direkvand-Moghadam A, Sayehmiri K, Delpisheh A, et al. Epidemiology of premenstrual syndrome (PMS) — a systematic review and meta-analysis study. J Clin Diagn Res 2014;8(2):106–9.

COMPLICATIONS

The primary complication is the misdiagnosis or progression to PMDD. Differentiating between PMS and PMDD is defined by the timing of symptoms and is summarised below.

Diagnosis

Diagnosis of PMS is usually made through the association of the symptoms attributed to PMS with their occurrence during the luteal phase of the menstrual cycle. It is essential to use a menstrual cycle diary to ascertain this information accurately as recalled information is less accurate.

DIAGNOSTIC CRITERIA

Premenstrual syndrome (PMS)[85,86]

NATIONAL INSTITUTE OF MENTAL HEALTH

A 30% increase in the intensity of symptoms of premenstrual syndrome (measured using a standardised instrument) from cycle days 5 to 10 as compared with the 6-day interval before the onset of menses and documentation of these changes in a daily symptom diary for at least two consecutive cycles.

UNIVERSITY OF CALIFORNIA AT SAN DIEGO

At least one of the following affective and somatic symptoms during the five days before menses in each of the three previous cycles:

- Affective symptoms: depression, angry outbursts, irritability, anxiety, confusion, social withdrawal
- Somatic symptoms: breast tenderness, abdominal bloating, headache, swelling of extremities
- Symptoms relieved from days 4 through 13 of the menstrual cycle.

DSM-5 CRITERIA: PREMENSTRUAL DYSPHORIC DISORDER (PMDD)[87]

A In most menstrual cycles during the past year, five (or more) of the following symptoms were present for most of the time during the last week of the luteal phase, began to remit within a few days after the onset of the follicular phase, and were absent in the week after menses.

B At least one of the following 4 symptoms must be present with at least one of the symptoms being 1, 2, 3, or 4
  1 Markedly depressed mood, feelings of hopelessness, or self-deprecating thoughts
  2 Marked anxiety, tension, or feelings of being 'keyed up' or 'on edge'
  3 Marked affective lability (e.g. mood swings, feeling suddenly sad or tearful or increased sensitivity to rejection)
  4 Persistent and marked anger or irritability, or increased interpersonal conflicts

C At least one of the following symptoms must also be present. The total number of symptoms from criteria B and C must be 5 or more
  1 Decreased interest in usual activities (e.g. work, school, friends, hobbies)
  2 Subjective sense of difficulty in concentrating
  3 Lethargy, easy fatiguability, or marked lack of energy
  4 Marked change in appetite, overeating, or specific food cravings
  5 Hypersomnia or insomnia
  6 A subjective sense of being overwhelmed or out of control
  7 Other physical symptoms, such as breast tenderness or swelling, headaches, joint or muscle pain, a sensation of 'bloating,' or weight gain

  NB: In menstruating females, the luteal phase corresponds with the period between ovulation and the onset of menses, and the follicular phase begins with menses. In nonmenstruating females (e.g. those who have had a hysterectomy), determining the timing of the luteal and follicular phases may require measurement of circulating reproductive hormones.

D The symptoms are associated with clinically significant distress or interfering with work or school, or with usual social activities and relationships with others (e.g. avoidance of social activities, decreased productivity and efficiency at work or school).

E The disturbance is not merely an exacerbation of the symptoms of another disorder, such as major depressive disorder, panic disorder, persistent depressive disorder (dysthymia), or a personality disorder (although it may occur with any of these disorders).

F Criterion A should be confirmed by prospective daily ratings during at least two consecutive symptomatic cycles. (The diagnosis may be made provisionally before this confirmation.)

G The symptoms are not attributable to the physiological effects of a substance (e.g. a drug abuse, a medication, other treatment) or another medical condition (e.g. hyperthyroidism).

An algorithm for use in differentiating PMS from PMDD is given in Fig. 18.5.[76]

DIFFERENTIAL DIAGNOSIS[76]

- Affective disorder (e.g. depression, anxiety, dysthymia, panic)
- Anaemia
- Anorexia or bulimia
- Chronic medical conditions (e.g. diabetes mellitus)
- Dysmenorrhoea
- Endometriosis
- Hypothyroidism
- Oral contraceptive pill use
- Perimenopause
- Personality disorder
- Substance abuse disorders.

NATUROPATHIC DIAGNOSIS

Naturopathic diagnosis is paramount for successful treatment outcomes due to its validation and understanding of potential mechanisms of action causing the presentation. The most definitive categorisation continues to be the classification outlined in Table 18.10[89] as expertly defined and discussed by Ruth Trickey.[28]

Investigations

Because there is no biochemical marker for PMS/PMDD, the diagnosis is usually made on the basis of a patient's history.

SPECIFIC NATUROPATHIC INVESTIGATIONS

Menstrual charting

Prospective daily charting of symptoms over two full menstrual cycles is highly desirable for assessment, and is valuable as a means of differentiating premenstrual syndrome from premenstrual exacerbation of concurrent depression or anxiety, or symptoms associated with low oestrogen during the menses.

Other

Other extensive investigations can be considered if patient improvement is poor or if the practitioner requires more definitive understanding of the bodily processes. These may include:

- Hormone profile to assess hormonal status
- Metabolic profile including lipids and sugars
- Full endocrine review including thyroid profile
- Hepatobiliary function to assess function and detoxification ability
- Amino acid profile or organic acid profile for neurotransmitter synthesis and production
- Methylation and nutritional biochemical screening.

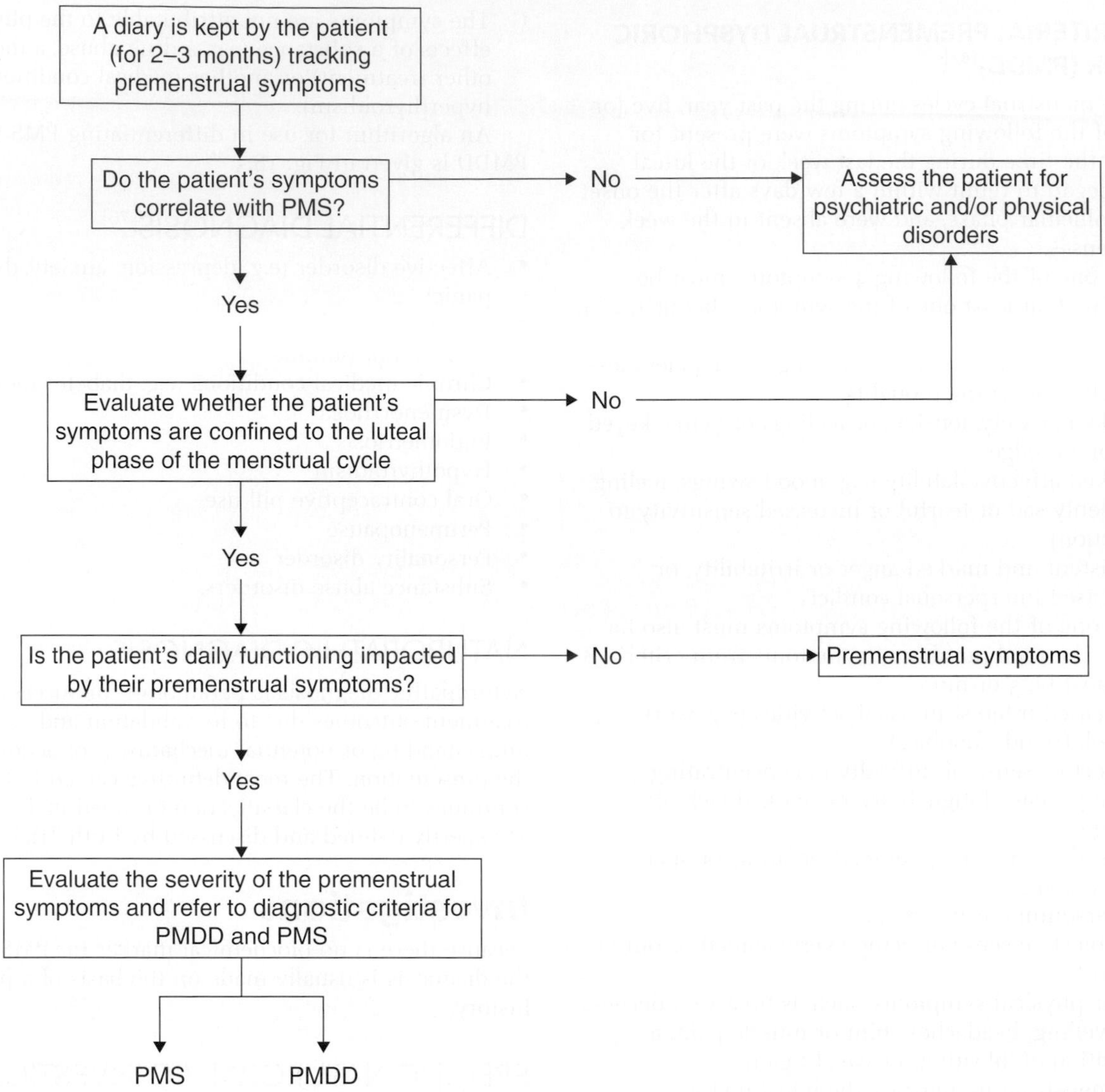

FIGURE 18.5 Algorithm for use in differentiating premenstrual symptoms, premenstrual syndrome (PMS) and premenstrual dysphoric disorder (PMDD).

Source: Adapted from Dickerson LM, Mazyck PJ, Hunter MH. Premenstrual syndrome. Am Fam Physician 2003; 67(8):1743–1752.

TABLE 18.10 PMS categories

Pattern	Possible aetiology	Characteristics
PMS-A (Anxiety)	Oestrogen excess and/or progesterone insufficiency potentially due to poor hepatic clearance or receptor insensitivity HPA-related diminished stress response Neurotransmitter-related effects from normal hormonal changes associated with menstruation	Anxiety, insomnia/dysomnia, irritability, emotional lability, palpitations, stress-induced sweating
PMS-C (Carbohydrate craving)	Possibly enhanced insulin-binding effects	Sugar cravings, increased appetite, headache, hypoglycaemia, palpitations, increased sweating
PMS-D (Depression)	Oestrogen leading to increased neurotransmitter degradation	Depression, despair, crying, feelings of hopelessness, fatigue, insomnia, apathy, low libido
PMS-H (Hyperhydration)	Possible effects on increased aldosterone in the late luteal phase due to excess oestrogen May relate to increased cortisol production from poor HPA regulation	Oedema of hands and feet (can extend up limbs), weight gain, bloating, breast tenderness and/or swelling, nipple sensitivity

Source: Adapted from Romm A. Botanical medicine for women's health. Churchill Livingstone; 2010.

TABLE 18.11 Naturopathic management of PMS/PMDD

Stage of treatment	Practitioner directed	Patient directed
Step 1	Evaluation of symptoms and correct diagnosis. If concerned, referral to GP to rule out psychiatric or other medical conditions Recommend specific dietary and lifestyle modifications (outlined below)	Completion of menstrual diary for at least 2–3 cycles Education, rest, dietary and lifestyle modifications Establish regular exercise and stress reduction techniques
Step 2	Referral for additional investigations to assess specificity of presentation (if required) Implementation of specific herbal and nutritional prescriptions based on interpreted presentation	Continuation of menstrual diary Continuation of previous recommendations Begin new prescriptions
Step 3	If after at least three complete menstrual cycles the patient is not experiencing a significant improvement or complete resolution of symptoms, work to identify additional causative factors as detailed above or change the treatment program	Possible referral for counselling and psychological support if emotional symptoms do not abate
Step 4	If patient does not improve at any stage of if they worsen, referral to medical practitioner to implement SSRI treatment may be warranted	

SSRI, selective serotonin reuptake inhibitor.

Therapeutic considerations

CLINICAL DECISION MAKING AND RATIONALE

The naturopathic approach to PMS should consider treatment implementation in a systematic manner, trialling lifestyle and dietary measures first and then implementing additional strategies sequentially. This is essential as most patients can alleviate symptoms easily with earlier interventions and may not require a comprehensive treatment program (Table 18.11).

Therapeutic application

HISTORICAL PERSPECTIVE

Although interest in the aetiology of premenstrual syndrome is a relatively new modern phenomenon, it appears that premenstrual syndrome itself is in actual fact not a modern condition. Examining the detailed writings of the Eclectic physicians it can be seen that many of the same symptoms reported by women today were observed in women of the early 1800s. Dysmenorrhoea appears to have been especially problematic, with a number of herbs described for this condition. These include *Pulsatilla*, which appears to be one of the best broad-spectrum botanicals for the management of premenstrual syndrome, with the Eclectics suggesting its use for dysmenorrhoea due to emotional causes as well as menstrual headache, swollen breasts, ovarian pain and low libido.[8] Other botanicals advocated for relief of dysmenorrhoea include primrose and *Piper methysticum*; the latter said to be especially useful for neuralgic or spasmodic dysmenorrhoea. In addition, viburnum due to its antispasmodic activity was favoured for neuralgic and spasmodic forms of dysmenorrhoea, while the circulatory stimulants *Zanthoxylum clava-herculis* and *Zingiber officinale* also lent their uses. The berries and bark of *Zanthoxylum clava-herculis* was favoured for neuralgic dysmenorrhoea with marked pain and hypersensitivity, while *Zingiber officinale* consumed as a beer (see recipe below) or wine was used to relieve the 'pangs of disordered menstruation'.

> *Ginger Beer — A good ginger beer may be prepared as follows: Take of white sugar, 2 pounds; lemon juice or cream of tartar, 14 drachms; honey, 12½ drachms; bruised ginger, 13 drachms; water, 2 gallons. Boil the ginger in 2 pints of the water for 3 hour; add the sugar, lemon juice, and honey, with the remainder of the water, and strain; when cold, add the white of an egg, and 24 minims of essence of lemon; let it stand for 4 days, and then bottle.*[8]

Analgesics such as *Piscidia piscipula* were suggested for female disorders, being found to be useful in alleviating neuralgic and other forms of dysmenorrhoea and in various pelvic neuroses, while for irregular menstruation *Tanacetum parthenium* was prized. *Hypericum* was used for menorrhagia, hysteria and nervous affections with depression, while *Ignatia*, observed to be for females only, was useful for women with menstrual disorders with colic-like pains, heavy dragging of the ovaries and an abnormally large and heavy womb. Last but by no means least is the use of *Vitex agnus-castus*; although documented by both Dioscorides (AD 77) and Hippocrates (4th century BC) for its value in uterine diseases,[88] it strangely finds no mention in the botanical literature of Kings.

ALLOPATHIC PERSPECTIVE

Although PMS has been a well-defined clinical entity for more than 60 years, some physicians still argue about its existence. As a result many women suffering from PMS do not receive proper treatment and have needed to seek assistance from alternative medicine practitioners.

Because no single treatment is universally effective for PMS/PMDD, many have doubted the existence of this disorder and criticised attempts to help women with their premenstrual symptoms. However, in the past 15 years there have been hundreds of prospective randomised clinical trials of various therapies, which have led to an evidence-based approach to the treatment of PMS/PMDD.

Non-pharmacological

Medicine takes the approach that initial treatment should focus on non-pharmacological methods including modification of lifestyle, exercise, relaxation techniques and cognitive behavioural therapy (CBT). The general approach is that if CBT is accessible and acceptable to the patient, it should be first-line treatment.

Pharmacological

Pharmacological treatment is only recommended for patients with disabling symptoms if the above-mentioned non-pharmacological methods fail. These include oral contraceptive containing drospirenone, or with a selective serotonin reuptake inhibitor (Table 18.12).

Oral contraceptive

The only oral contraceptive that has been subjected to a randomised controlled trial for treating PMS is one that combines ethinyloestradiol and drospirenone.

TABLE 18.12 Prescription medications commonly used in the treatment of premenstrual syndrome

Drug class and representative agents	Dosage*	Recommendations for use	Side effects
Androgens			
Danazol	100 to 400 mg twice daily	Prescribed to address mastalgia in luteal phase	Weight gain, decreased breast size, deepening of voice Monitor lipid profile and liver function
Diuretics			
Spironolactone	25 to 100 mg/day during luteal phase	Effective treatment to address bloating and breast tenderness	Antioestrogenic effects, hyperkalaemia
GnRH agonists			
Leuprolide		Prescribed to alleviate physical and behavioural symptoms of PMS. Marked side effects and limitations due to cost	Hypoestrogenic side effect, including atrophic vaginitis, hot flushes, cardiovascular effects and osteoporosis
Goserelin	3.6 mg SC every month		
Naferelin	400 micrograms intranasally twice daily		
NSAIDs			
Naproxen sodium	275 to 550 mg twice daily	Useful to assist with physical symptoms; however, other NSAIDs are equally effective	Nausea, gastric ulceration, renal dysfunction Use with caution in women with preexisting gastrointestinal or renal disease
SSRIs			
Fluoxetine Sertraline Paroxetine Fluvoxamine Citalopram	10 to 20 mg/day 50 to 150 mg/day 10 to 30 mg/day 25 to 50 mg/day 20 to 40 mg/day	Fluoxetine labelled as treatment for PMDD; however, all options are effective agents to alleviate behavioural and physical symptoms of PMS and PMDD Can be prescribed for use either as a daily medication or during the luteal phase (14 days pre menstruation)	Insomnia, drowsiness, fatigue, nausea, nervousness, headache, mild tremor, sexual dysfunction

SSRIs = selective serotonin reuptake inhibitors; PMDD = premenstrual dysphoric disorder; NSAID = non-steroidal anti-inflammatory drug; GnRH = gonadotrophin-releasing hormone; IM = intramuscularly; SC = subcutaneously.
*Taken orally unless otherwise indicated.
Note: these doses are normal doses, they are not necessarily the maximum doses seen in practice.
Source: Adapted from Dickerson L, Mazyck P, Hunter M. Premenstrual syndrome. Am Fam Physician 2003;67:8.

Drospirenone is a progestogen derived from spironolactone. Other more widely used combined oral contraceptive formulations contain 19-nortestosterone derivatives.

Selective serotonin reuptake inhibitors

Selective serotonin reuptake inhibitors (SSRIs) are highly effective in treating the symptoms of PMS, as shown by a comprehensive meta-analysis. Fluoxetine and sertraline are most commonly used, but other SSRIs are also effective. No difference in efficacy between SSRIs has been shown.

Intermittent dosing, limited to the 2-week interval before the expected next period, may be associated with less adverse effects and be more acceptable to patients. However, an intermittent regimen is not as effective as a continuous regimen. If the woman's pattern of symptoms is more suggestive of premenstrual exacerbation of a comorbid depressive or anxiety disorder, a continuous regimen would usually be more appropriate.

NATUROPATHIC PERSPECTIVE

Important considerations include:

- Metabolism and function of oestrogen and progesterone
- Deficient corpus luteum production
- Alterations or imbalances of the circulating ratios of oestrogen and progesterone based on the time of the month, thus aggravating the target tissues of these hormones
- Enterohepatic circulation and excretion of oestrogen
- Hormonal and neuroendocrine factors, including prolactin, prostaglandins and endorphins.

When adapting the naturopathic classification of PMS patterns, we can see that treatment can be modified as shown in Table 18.13.

TABLE 18.13 Treatment objectives for the PMS categories listed in Table 18.10

Pattern	Treatment objective
PMS-A (Anxiety)	Support oestrogen clearance and metabolism Support HPA axis and reduce cortisol secretion Regulate neurotransmitter production
PMS-C (Carbohydrate craving)	Improve insulin sensitivity and blood glucose control Regulate progesterone and dopamine inter-relationship
PMS-D (Depression)	Support and regulate oestrogen and progesterone ratio
PMS-H (Hyperhydration)	Support oestrogen clearance and metabolism Support fluid regulation and release Support HPA axis and reduce cortisol secretion

Adapted from Romm A. Botanical medicine for women's health. Churchill Livingstone; 2010.

NUTRITIONAL MEDICINE (DIETARY)

Dietary therapeutic objectives

- Adopt a low GI/GL/low Food Insulin Index (FII) diet and encourage regular small meals to stabilise blood sugar levels
- Eliminate sugar and refined carbohydrates
- Eliminate caffeine completely (all methyl-xanthines — coffee, tea (black, oolong, green; see Box 18.2), chocolate and other caffeine-containing beverages)
- Increase vegetarian protein intake and ensure complete protein intake is met
- Increase fibre and vegetable consumption, especially brassica family to assist with clearance of endogenous oestrogen (thyroid function dependent)
- Reduce animal proteins and follow a vegetarian or predominantly vegetarian diet
- Reduce exposure to exogenous oestrogens
- Avoid all soy products with suspected oestrogen dominance
- Reduce intake of saturated, trans and hydrogenated fats
- Reduce salt and alcohol intake.

Specific dietary treatments

A 2015 case-control study in Iran found that the Western dietary pattern is associated with an increase in the incidence of PMS.[90] Specific dietary factors are discussed below.

DIETARY INCLUSIONS

Fruit and vegetables

Fresh fruit and vegetables provide an array of nutrients required for a healthy reproductive system. In particular the brassica family (e.g. cabbage, Brussels sprouts, cauliflower, broccoli) are extremely useful in premenstrual syndrome to help conjugate oestrogen.[28] Try not to

BOX 18.2 Caffeine content of tea

- Black, white or green tea and oolong tea all contain caffeine and tannins
- Black tea is rolled, fermented and dried. This leads to oxidation and condensation making it less antioxidant but more astringent
- Green tea is heat-treated and rapidly dried, then rolled. It contains higher levels of antioxidants
- White tea is the uncured and un-oxidised tea leaf. It contains buds and young tea leaves, with higher caffeine than older leaves, suggesting the caffeine content of white teas may be higher than that of green teas. White tea also contains higher levels of theanine (an amino acid that has relaxing and mood enhancing properties)
- Oolong tea is semi-fermented and is therefore in between black and green teas.

overcook vegetables so that nutrients are retained, steaming and stir-frying are ideal.

Tryptophan-rich foods

Depletion of tryptophan has been shown to increase aggression in women during the premenstrual phase[91] thus foods rich in tryptophan should be encouraged. These include turkey, bananas, cottage cheese, pumpkin seeds, sesame seeds, legumes and dairy products.[25]

Fibre

Excess or unopposed oestrogen has been implicated in premenstrual syndrome. A diet high in fibre has been suggested to assist with excretion of oestrogen, though as yet there have been no studies assessing this in individuals with PMS.[83]

DIETARY EXCLUSIONS

Caffeine

Consumption of caffeine-containing beverages has been strongly related to prevalence of PMS[92,93] with the author from one study suggesting that women with PMS may even self-medicate with caffeine in response to PMS, thereby exacerbating their symptoms.[94] This relationship between caffeine and symptomatology appears to be dose dependent, with more severe symptoms experienced among those women who consumed more caffeine.[95] A recent prospective study on coffee and caffeine intake in the Nurses Health Study II did not find any association between total caffeine intake and PMS[96] Until further conclusive evidence is available, and due to the exacerbation of PMS symptoms demonstrated in some studies, the removal of coffee from the diet is highly recommended. Furthermore, caffeine increases calcium excretion, which is undesirable given the desirable effects of calcium in the amelioration of PMS (discussed in more detail in 'Calcium' below). Patients must be questioned on all forms of caffeine present in the diet, including coffee, tea, cola drinks, cocoa and energy drinks.

Saturated fats and deep-fried foods

Nutritional factors undoubtedly influence the aetiology of PMS. One such example is saturated fats and deep-fried foods. Both are highly inflammatory in the body and therefore should be avoided, particularly as low-grade inflammation has been linked to menstrual symptoms.[97] A study undertaken in Japanese women observed that those with the high intakes of fat (including saturated fat) experienced higher menstrual distress symptom scores, in particular higher scores with regards to pain associated with premenstrual syndrome.[98] Aside from their pro-inflammatory action, these types of foods are usually highly processed and provide little in the way of nutrients.

Sugar

A strong relationship exists between craving of sugar and the end of the menstrual cycle, with it being observed that cravings for sweets tend to increase around this time.[99,100] Consumption of foods high in sugar or with a sweet taste have been associated with higher prevalence of PMS[101] and thus they need to be regulated in the diet and consumed appropriately (i.e. fruit instead of lollies). A large number of sugary foods are devoid of any nutrients (e.g. lollies, fizzy drinks, fruit juices) and their consumption thus replaces an opportunity when more nutritious food could have been consumed. Sugar cravings should be supported with relevant nutrients (for example, chromium) and appropriate dietary protocols (for example, protein with each meal and a low glycaemic diet).

Sodium

A diet high in sodium in patients with fluid retention related to PMS is likely to further upset fluid balance. Patients must be advised on hidden sodium such as that found in processed, packaged foods and soft drinks.

Wheatgerm extract

A small triple-blind clinical trial in Iran showed that supplementing with 400 mg of wheatgerm extract (3 times per day, from mid cycle until day 5 of menstruation, resulted in a decrease in the severity of PMS symptoms.[102] Anaylsis of the results from the same cohort found a significant reduction in pain in dysmenorrhoea.[103] Wheatgerm contains vitamin B_6, vitamin E, calcium, magnesium and essential fatty acids, all of which have been identified as beneficial in the treatment and management of PMS (see below).

NUTRITIONAL MEDICINE (SUPPLEMENTAL)

Nutritional medicine therapeutic objectives

- Regulate hormonal synthesis and metabolism
- Improve oestrogen clearance through digestive and hepatobiliary pathways
- Regulate neurotransmitter production and interrelationship with hormones
- Regulate blood sugar levels, appetite and relieve cravings
- Relieve fluid retention and other symptoms including headaches, premenstrual pain, mastalgia and acne
- Improve circadian rhythm to regulate sleep patterns and subsequent effects on HPA and HPO axes.

Specific nutrients required

B COMPLEX

B complex is essential for supporting energy levels and the body's response to stress. Whenever carbohydrates are consumed, B vitamins are used in the process. They are regularly lost due to their water-soluble make-up and are required to supplement on a daily basis. The oral contraceptive pill decreases levels of several B vitamins[104] and thus if patients are taking the oral contraceptive it is important that B vitamins are replenished. A 2011 case-controlled study from the Nurses Health Study II cohort (n = 3025) found that intake of vitamin B_1 and B_2 from food sources is inversely associated with PMS

SAMPLE DAILY DIET

BREAKFAST	
Porridge with sliced banana and pumpkin seeds Celery and ginger juice	Oats are a source of B vitamins. A lower risk of PMS in women with high intakes of vitamin B_1 and B_2 from food sources has been noted; this may be due to the fact that thiamine is a precursor to GABA while vitamin B_2 is needed to activate vitamin B_6, which is a cofactor in the generation of serotonin from the amino acid tryptophan. Vitamin B_1 rich foods are also advocated because of the role of vitamin B_1 in carbohydrate metabolism and muscle tonus, the latter of which assists in reducing dysmenorrhea. Celery is a diuretic and may be useful in PMS-H by assisting with removing excess fluid. Ginger is a powerful anti-inflammatory that has been shown to reduce dysmenorrhoea when taken at least 3 days before menses begins.
LUNCH	
Salad: Rocket, radicchio, broccoli, Brussels sprouts, new potatoes, avocado, tinned salmon dressed with apple cider vinegar and lemon juice	Bitter greens can be used to stimulate bile flow and liver function reducing constipation while cruciferous vegetables are advocated to assist in removal of excess oestrogen from the body due to their indole-3 carbinol content as well as their fibre. Leafy greens and tinned salmon are an excellent source of calcium. Lower levels of calcium are seen in women with PMS; however, supplementation at relatively low doses is associated with improved mood and concentration providing a rationale for increased dietary calcium.
DINNER	
Roast vegetable salad with baby spinach, olives, quinoa and grilled salmon	Magnesium has been reported to reduce anxiety related to PMS and may assist in reducing fluid retention. Omega-3 fatty acids have been shown to reduce dysmenorrhoea via the suppression of prostaglandin synthesis; they may also assist with regulating mood.
SNACK	
Sweet potato wedges dusted with cinnamon	Ingestion of carbohydrates increases the plasma ratio of tryptophan to other large neutral amino acids resulting in increased serotonin synthesis. Cravings for sweets may be related to drops in serotonin that occur in some women premenstrually.

Sources: Abdollahifard S, Koshkaki AR, Moazamiyanfar R. The effects of vitamin B1 on ameliorating the premenstrual syndrome symptoms. Global J Health Sci 2014; 6(6):144–153. Boyle NB, Lawton CL, Dye L. The effects of magnesium supplementation on subjective anxiety Magnes Res 2016; 29(3):120–125. Chen CX, Barrett B, Kwekkeboom KL. Efficacy of oral ginger (*Zingiber officinale*) for dysmenorrhea: a systematic review and meta-analysis. Evid Based Complement Alternat Med 2016; 2016:6295737. Chocano-Bedoya PO, Manson JE, Hankinson SE et al. Dietary B vitamin intake and incident premenstrual syndrome. Am J Clin Nutr 2011; 93(5):1080–1086. Fathizadeh N, Ebrahimi E, Valiani M et al. Evaluating the effect of magnesium and magnesium plus vitamin B6 supplement on the severity of premenstrual syndrome. Iran J Nurs Midwifery Res 2010; 15(Suppl1):401–405. Møller SE. Serotonin, carbohydrates, and atypical depression. Pharmacol Toxicol 1992; 71 Suppl 1:61–71. Shobeiri F, Araste FE, Ebrahimi R et al. Effect of calcium on premenstrual syndrome: a double-blind randomized clinical trial. Obstet Gynecol Sci 2017; 60(1):100–105.

incidence. By comparison, supplemental intake of these vitamins, as well as other B vitamins, was associated with an increased risk of PMS.[105]

VITAMIN B_1

Dysmenorrhoea is a common complaint associated with PMS, but vitamin B_1 may be useful as it has been observed to be more effective than placebo at reducing dysmenorrhoea.

In a crossover study [106] involving 556 Indian female adolescents administered vitamin B_1 100 mg/day for 3 months, those consuming vitamin B_1 experienced a reduction in pain compared with a significantly increased proportion of women in the placebo group. After completion of the study at 3 months 87% of women in the vitamin B_1 group reported no pain.

A double-blind placebo-controlled clinical trial of 80 students with PMS showed that supplementation with 100 mg of vitamin B_1 twice daily during the week before menstruation for three consecutive cycles significantly decreased the severity of PMS symptoms. The placebo group also showed a significant decrease in severity of symptoms, but less than those of the treatment group.[107]

VITAMIN B_2

Vitamin B_2 is required for the function of flavin adenine dinucleotide and flavin mononucleotide, two cofactors crucial for many body functions, including the generation of energy from food.[108] Vitamin B_2 is also required for neurotransmitter function and is involved in adrenal and hormone function. Vitamin B_2 is required for the activation of vitamin B_6, which is crucial to prevent PMS.[108] Tyrer[94] notes that the oral contraceptive pill may decrease levels of vitamin B_2. Thus in women taking the oral contraceptive pill in the absence of supportive diet, supplementation would appear necessary.

VITAMIN B$_3$

Vitamin B$_3$ is required for over 200 enzyme systems in the body,[108] many of which are likely to influence the female reproductive system. Vitamin B$_3$ increases conversion of fatty acids to prostaglandin E1,[109] is required for neurotransmitter production and is vital for synthesis of various hormones including the sex hormones.

VITAMIN B$_5$

Vitamin B$_5$ is required to support adrenal function and protects against the effects of stress. As with the other B vitamins it is involved in the release of energy from food.

VITAMIN B$_6$

Vitamin B$_6$ is perhaps the most well-known B vitamin for the relief and management of PMS. It functions to modulate the production of the neurotransmitters GABA and serotonin, both of which have key roles in mood (pain, anxiety, depression) and may assist in the relief of fluid retention associated with PMS. Vitamin B$_6$ is also important for magnesium transportation in the cell membrane,[39] thus inadequate levels of vitamin B$_6$ will impact magnesium functions in the body. A review of nine studies, representing a total of 940 women with PMS, found that vitamin B$_6$ improved symptoms.[110] Four studies showed an improvement in feelings of depression associated with PMS, particularly that associated with high oestrogen/progesterone oral contraceptive pill use. There is controversy over the appropriate dose of vitamin B$_6$ to use for PMS due to risk of peripheral neuropathy, but supplements containing pyridoxine hydrochloride, the form of vitamin B$_6$ usually found in supplements, are sold in Australia with doses of 200 mg/day recommended. A small double-blind randomised controlled trial on 76 students showed that combining vitamin B$_6$ (40 mg) with calcium supplementation (500 mg) led to an increased positive effect on decreasing PMS symptoms compared to vitamin B$_6$ supplementation alone.[111]

VITAMINS B$_9$ AND B$_{12}$

Folate and B$_{12}$ work synergistically in all chemical reactions and primarily regulate correct cellular replication. They are involved in growth, development, energy release from food and in the activity of serotonin and other neurotransmitters and cell membrane stability, thus they may influence PMS via these pathways.

CALCIUM

Alterations in calcium metabolism have been suggested for a number of the symptoms experienced by women with PMS.[112,113] Certainly, Shamberger[114] observed low levels of calcium in the red blood cells and hair of patients with PMS. Low calcium levels are associated with a range of mental symptoms (also synonymous with PMS), including agitation and irritability. Changes in extracellular calcium metabolism have also been hypothesised to stimulate the neuromuscular junctions. This is compounded by the fact that many women do not consume the recommended daily intake of calcium.

Supplementation with elemental calcium 1000 mg/day when taken for at least 3 months appears to be useful for reducing symptoms associated with PMS. A small study involving 33 women given calcium carbonate (1000 mg/day) for 3 months followed by 3 months of a placebo was conducted to assess the efficacy in symptoms associated with PMS.[113] Calcium supplementation was associated with a reduction of premenstrual complaints during the luteal and menstrual phases of the cycle, with 73% of women reporting a reduction in symptoms (particularly fluid retention and pain). These results are confirmed by a double-blind study undertaken on female college students in their early twenties with PMS by Ghanbari et al.[115] The women were given 1000 mg/day of calcium carbonate in two divided doses or placebo for 3 months. On completion of the study it was observed that calcium supplements reduced early fatiguability, changes in appetite, and depression in women with PMS compared with the placebo group. A recent clinical trial conducted on 210 students comparing the effects of daily calcium carbonate (500 mg) supplementation vs vitamin B$_1$ (100 mg) supplementation found that both supplements reduced the physical intensity of PMS symptoms; however, calcium supplementation was more effective for reducing psychological symptoms.[116] Calcium carbonate has been shown to be poorly absorbed, thus it would be interesting to observe effects in future studies administering other forms of calcium such as amino acid chelate.

CHROMIUM

Chromium may be indicated to support blood sugar levels and reduce sugar cravings.

ESSENTIAL FATTY ACIDS (EFAs)

Essential fatty acids may be effective in treating menstrual-related pain. In a recent RCT 120 women were treated with either 1 or 2 g EFAs or placebo. Each gram of EFA in the treatment groups consisted of 210 mg of gamma linolenic acid, 175 mg of oleic acid, 345 mg of linoleic acid, 250 mg of other polyunsaturated acids and 20 mg of vitamin E. Supplements were taken nightly for 15 consecutive days, starting on the 15th day of the cycle, over a period of 6 months. Statistically significant reductions in severity of PMS started to appear after 3 months of treatment. The placebo group also demonstrated reductions. However, reductions in the treatment groups were bigger, and dose dependent. Prolonged use of the treatment for 6 months resulted in better clinical improvement than at 3 months.[117] A trial comparing the effectiveness of fish oil supplementation with ibuprofen for primary dysmenorrhoea found that supplementation with 1 g of fish oil on all days of the menstrual cycle had a higher efficacy than 400 mg of ibuprofen administered at the start of the pain (and in 8-hour intervals thereafter if required). The study consisted of 120 participants aged 18–22 years, randomly assigned to one of the two treatment groups. The EFA/DHA content of the fish oil was not specified.[118]

EVENING PRIMROSE OIL (GLA)

Evening primrose oil (*Oenothera biennis*) is commonly used for relief from PMS symptoms. It is believed that many women with PMS are deficient in linolenic acid, which is necessary for prostaglandin formation; hence the proposed mechanism of action. In spite of this observation and its popularity there is inconclusive clinical evidence to support the use of evening primrose oil in PMS as the majority of trials undertaken have been of poor methodological quality.[119,120] However, a modest beneficial effect cannot be eliminated entirely. Further studies with bigger sample sizes are required to determine the true efficacy of evening primrose oil. As we await improved clinical trials, it is beneficial to prescribe a comprehensive essential fatty acid profile of EPA, DHA and GLA.

IRON

Iron levels need to be checked and amended if required in patients with PMS, particularly those who complain of fatigue, heavy or long periods or consume little or no red meat. Iron deficiency and subsequent anaemia are likely to compound symptoms such as fatigue or depression associated with PMS.

MAGNESIUM

Magnesium is required in neuromuscular contraction, neurotransmitter function and cell membrane stability, and there are multiple ways in which it may influence PMS. Magnesium (200 mg/day) appears to assist in fluid retention associated with PMS. In a double-blind placebo-controlled, crossover study in which 38 women were administered magnesium as oxide, fluid retention in the second but not the first month of use was significantly reduced; no significant effects on mood-related symptoms were reported.[38] A randomised, double-blind, crossover study examining the effects of magnesium oxide (200 mg/day) in combination with vitamin B_6 (50 mg/day) found the combination to be useful for reducing anxiety-related premenstrual symptoms (nervous tension, mood swings, irritability or anxiety). There was also a non-significant trend with regards to reduced cravings.[39] A later study of 150 women treated over 2 months involved the randomised allocation of the participants to one of three groups: (1) magnesium supplementation only (250 mg/day); (2) magnesium (250 mg/day) and B_6 (40 mg/day) and (3) placebo group. Magnesium combined with B_6 was shown to be more effective than magnesium alone or placebo in lowering severity of PMS symptoms. Studies have indicated that at least 2 months is required for the therapeutic effects of magnesium to be effective.[39A] Acknowledging the short time period of the first study (1 month) and the form of magnesium used, one can hypothesise better results may be seen over a longer period of time with a better absorbed form of magnesium such as amino acid chelate. It is not stated what form of magnesium was used in the second trial. A case control study of the Nurses' Health Study II cohort assessing mineral intake via participant questionnaires found that magnesium intake was unrelated to PMS.[39B]

TRYPTOPHAN OR 5-HTP

Worsening mood swings in premenstrual dysphoria have been linked to a decline in brain serotonin function.[121] Tryptophan is the precursor to serotonin, and depletion of tryptophan has been shown to increase aggression in women during the premenstrual phase.[91] Supplementation with tryptophan (6 g/day) from the time of ovulation to the third day of menstruation has been found to reduce premenstrual symptoms of mood swings, tension and irritability in women with PMDD over a 3-month period.[122]

VITAMINS E AND D

Vitamin E is a fat-soluble vitamin and thus helps to regulate steroid hormone synthesis. In addition, it is a potent antioxidant that sacrifices itself in any oxidation reaction within the body. An early randomised, double-blind study tested the efficacy of vitamin E (400 IU/day) in women with PMS versus placebo over three cycles and observed a significant improvement in certain affective and physical symptoms in those women treated with D-alpha-tocopherol, while no benefits were noted in the placebo.[123] In a randomised double-blind controlled study 86 women were treated with vitamin D (200 mg daily), vitamin E (100 mg daily) or placebo for 2 months. PMS symptoms significantly decreased in all 3 groups.[124] A prospective cohort study (n = 401) based on the Nurses' Health Study II found no relation between plasma 25-hydroxyvitamin D levels and risk of PMS.[125] These findings are supported by a 2016 case-control study of 82 women in Iran.[126]

ZINC

Zinc is an essential cofactor for more than 200 enzymes,[25] including the metalloenzymes and metalloenzyme complexes. It is an important factor in the metabolism of neurotransmitters and prostaglandins, including dopamine, through its role in the metabolism of melatonin. Zinc levels have been observed to drop during the luteal phase and may be further aggravated by elevated levels of copper,[127] hence the benefits of supplementation. A small case-control study of 48 students found that higher serum zinc levels and total antioxidant capacity are associated with a lowered risk of PMS.[128] Acne and skin disturbances associated with the menstrual period may also respond well to zinc.

DOSAGE REQUIREMENTS

The dosage requirements listed below are based on adult doses that have been reported in the literature and clinical review:

- B complex (all B vitamins) high-dose combination, preferably activated forms
  - Thiamine 20–40 mg/day (100 mg/day for 3 months may be indicated)/day
  - Riboflavin 20–40 mg/day
  - Niacinamide 50–100 mg/day
  - Pantothenic acid 150–300 mg/day
  - Pyridoxine 50–100 mg/day
  - Folate as folinic acid or L5MTHF 500–1000 micrograms/day
  - Hydroxo or methyl cobalamin 500–1000 micrograms/day
  - Choline 50–100 mg/day
  - Inositol 50–100 mg/day
  - Biotin 250–500 micrograms/day

- Calcium 1200–1600 mg/day
- Chromium 200–600 micrograms/day
- Magnesium 400–800 mg/day
- Evening primrose oil (EPO) 2.5–5 g/day
- Iron 25–80 mg/day (depending on pathology results)
- Tryptophan 2.5 g/day or 5-HTP 50–400 mg/day
- Omega-3 fish oils 1080 mg/day EPA, 720 mg/day DHA
- Vitamin E 400 IU/day
- Zinc 50 mg/day.

HERBAL MEDICINE

Herbal medicine therapeutic objectives

- Regulate hormonal synthesis and metabolism
- Improve oestrogen clearance through digestive and hepatobiliary pathways
- Regulate neurotransmitter production and interrelationship with hormones
- Regulate blood sugar levels, appetite and relieve cravings
- Relieve fluid retention and other symptoms including headaches, premenstrual pain, mastalgia and acne
- Improve circadian rhythm to regulate sleep patterns and subsequent effects on HPA and HPO axes.

Herbal medicine classes

Herbal medicine classes used for PMS are listed in Table 18.14.

TABLE 18.14 Herbal medicine classes used for PMS

Class	Action
Hormonal modulators	Hormone modulation to regulate cascades and alleviate subsequent symptoms
Thymoleptics, nervine tonics, anxiolytics	Mood stabilisation and improvement
Adaptogens and adrenal restoratives	Improve stress response, stabilise HPA axis, reduce cortisol
Bitters, digestives	Improve protein digestion and digestive clearance of hormone metabolites, clear acne
Bulk laxatives	Improve clearance of hormone metabolites
Hepatics, cholagogues	Improve synthesis and metabolism of hormones and assist with clearance of hormone metabolites, clear acne
Diuretics	Relieve fluid retention
Spasmolytics	Relieve headaches and dysmenorrhoea
Lymphatics	Relief from mastalgia and other breast symptoms

Specific herbal medicines

VITEX AGNUS-CASTUS (CHASTE TREE BERRY)

Vitex agnus-castus has been used for gynaecological complaints for centuries; it contains a number of active constituents, including flavonoids, iridoids, alkaloids and volatile oils.[129] The mode of action of *Vitex agnus-castus* is undetermined but appears multifaceted. Low doses have been shown to increase luteinising hormone while decreasing follicle-stimulating hormone, working indirectly on progesterone.[83] Dopaminergic compounds present in *Vitex agnus-castus* are thought to be the most clinically important compounds for improvement of many symptoms of PMS because they reduce secretion of prolactin.[130]

Treatment with *Vitex agnus-castus* for PMS has been shown to be of benefit in a number of studies. A large study involving 1634 women with PMS given *Vitex agnus-castus* over three menstrual cycles reported a decrease in number of symptoms (and in some cases cessation of complaints) in 93% of patients.[130]

Berger et al[131] observed beneficial results with a specific extract of *Vitex agnus-castus* Ze 440 which was administered to women with PMS. Modified menstrual distress scores reduced by 42.5% by the end of the treatment period and while symptoms gradually returned after treatment cessation, interestingly a difference from baseline remained up to three cycles thereafter. Schellingberg[132] also demonstrated benefits with the same *Vitex* extract (Ze 440) administered over three cycles. Improvements were seen with regard to irritability, mood alteration, anger, headache and breast fullness. Furthermore, over half the women had a 50% or greater improvement in their symptoms. A 2012 randomised, placebo-controlled, double-blind study in Iran of 128 women suffering from PMS found that treatment with 40 drops of *Vitex* extract per day, 6 consecutive days prior to menstruation, resulted in significant improvements in PMS symptom severity ratings. It is interesting to note that improvements were also shown in the placebo group (although less significant than the *Vitex* group) indicating the psychological factors involved in PMS. The study duration for this trial was over six menstrual cycles.[133] A 2013 systematic review of clinical trials found that in one study that *Vitex agnus-castus* (20–40 mg/day) was more effective for physical symptoms in PMDD, while fluoxetine may be more effective for psychological symptoms in PMDD.[134] A second study showed that fluoxetine outperformed *Vitex* on all endpoint measurements in PMDD participants. *Vitex*, however, did show improvements and was associated with fewer side effects. *Vitex* was shown to be superior than placebo, pyridoxine and magnesium for alleviating total PMS symptoms, and psychological and physical sub clusters of symptoms.[134] Given the common side effects of fluoxetine, such as painful or enlarged breasts[135] and tiredness (symptoms that may already be present in PMS!), it would appear that *Vitex agnus-castus* may be a better option. The German Commission E approves the use of chaste tree berry for irregularities of the menstrual cycle, cyclical breast discomfort and premenstrual disturbances. A 2013 open-label clinical observation of 100 women who suffered from migraines during PMS, found that treatment with 40 mg/day of *Vitex agnus-castus* resulted in 66% of participants reporting a dramatic reduction in overall PMS symptoms, 42% of patients experienced a greater than 50% reduction in frequency of monthly migraine attacks and 57% of patients experienced a greater than 50% reduction in monthly days with headache.[136] A 2014 study of 69 Japanese women with PMS, aged 18–44 years, with treatment of 20 mg/day of *Vitex agnus-castus* showed a significant decrease in PMS symptoms after the first cycle, and symptoms continued to diminish for the next two cycles, with no substantial side effects reported.[137] These results are confirmed by a clinical trial of 105 nursing students in Iran suffering from mild to severe PMS. After administration of 20 mg *Vitex agnus-castus* extract daily over 3 months, 70% of participants experienced complete relief from their symptoms, the other participants experiencing statistically significant improvement in their symptoms.[138] A study in Russia of 121 patients with PMS aged 18–45 found that administration of 40 mg of dry extract of fruits of *Vitex agnus-castus* (1 tablet 20 minutes before breakfast daily during three menstrual cycles) resulted in a statistically significant reduction in physical and psychological symptoms of PMS.[139]

HYPERICUM PERFORATUM (ST JOHN'S WORT)

There is evidence that the serotonergic system plays a role in the pathogenesis of PMS, with some studies showing reduced serotonin in the luteal phase of the menstrual cycle. Furthermore, a number of PMS symptoms such as anxiety and depression are linked to alterations in the serotonergic system.

Hypericum perforatum has been shown to have profound benefits in the management of depression through its influence on the serotonergic system; therefore logically it may also be beneficial in PMS. A double-blind placebo-controlled study involving 36 women aged 18–45 years with regular menstrual cycles (25–35 days) with mild PMS administered *Hypericum perforatum* found it more effective than placebo treatment for the most common physical and behavioural symptoms associated with PMS, including physical symptoms (food craving, swelling) and behaviours (crying, fatigue, headaches, insomnia, poor coordination).[140] Pain-related symptoms only appeared to show improvement at the end of the treatment period, suggesting longer supplementation might be required to observe benefits in this category. Surprisingly, in this study mood-related symptoms (anxiety, depression, mood swings) did not show statistical benefit when compared with placebo, but fewer women reported these symptoms while taking *Hypericum perforatum* than with placebo treatment. Again, a longer treatment period may be required to observe significant changes in relation to mood.

In their study, Hicks et al[141] observed a non-significant trend in favour of *Hypericum perforatum* for relief of symptoms (in particular anxiety) associated with PMS. While the results from this study were statistically insignificant (therefore still clinically relevant) the authors hypothesise the possibility that this non-significant finding was the result of insufficient statistical power in the study, rather than a lack of efficacy of *Hypericum perforatum*.

An RCT study of 170 women with PMS found that those receiving *Hypericum perforatum* had a 40% reduction in PMS scores compared to baseline and the control group. The biggest improvements were seen in crying scores (71%) and depression (52%). The treatment group (n = 85) received 2680 micrograms hypericin tablets/day over 8 weeks (2 cycles) while the control group (n = 85) received placebo (2 cellulose tablets/day).[142]

ACTAEA RACEMOSA (BLACK COHOSH)

Actaea racemosa was traditionally used by the Eclectic physicians for female reproductive complaints synonymous with PMS, such as dysmenorrhoea, amenorrhoea and mastodynia, but in modern-day Australia *Actaea racemosa* is more commonly thought of as a botanical used for management of menopausal complaints. In Germany, *Actaea racemosa* is officially approved to be sold for the reduction of PMS symptoms.[143] This, combined with its traditional application, warrants clinical studies to assess its efficacy in PMS.

TARAXACUM OFFICINALE (FOLIA) (DANDELION LEAF)

Taraxacum officinale is a gentle herbal diuretic that may be used to help increase urinary output[144] and thus assist in the relief of fluid retention, a common symptom associated with PMS. *Taraxacum officinale* also contains significant amounts of minerals, including potassium, which may help to replenish potassium lost during diuresis.

WITHANIA SOMNIFERA (ASHWAGANDHA)

Stress is known to influence menstrual cycle function[145] and it is also likely to aggravate symptoms associated with PMS. How stress exerts these changes is unknown but has been proposed to in part involve alterations in the normal function of the HPA axis[146] (explaining why *Vitex agnus-castus* can be so useful because of its ability to regulate the hypothalamus). *Withania somnifera* is a gentle, rejuvenating tonic and adaptogen that helps the body to adapt to stressful situations. *Withania* may be used to enhance physical and mental health, particularly where there is debility,[147] stress and anxiety. A study of individuals with anxiety disorders administered *Withania somnifera* demonstrated reduced anxiety compared with placebo just 2 weeks after treatment began.[148] Since women with PMS often report symptoms of depletion such as anxiety and fatigue, supplementation with *Withania somnifera* may be of benefit.

PAEONIA LACTIFLORA (PEONY)

Paeonia lactiflora is a Chinese herb that exhibits anti-inflammatory, analgesic and antispasmodic[149] properties likely to be of use in PMS. The root of *Paeonia californica* is commonly boiled and used in a tea by the Chumash (traditional North American) community to help relieve menstrual-related cramps.[150] Anti-inflammatory constituents within *Paeonia lactiflora* such as paeonolide, a monoterpenoid, function by inhibiting the effects of platelet-activating factor, a pro-inflammatory agent.[125]

CROCUS SATIVUS STIGMA (SAFFRON)

A small double-blind, randomised placebo-controlled study of 78 PMS patients in Iran found that 30 mg of *C. sativus* per day (15 mg morning and evening) was effective in relieving the symptoms of PMS. It is hypothesised that the antidepressant effects of *C. sativus* might be the mechanism of action through which the results are achieved, due to the overlap between the symptoms of depression and PMS.[151] Similar results were achieved in another study using 30 mg of dried extract of saffron stigma once a day as the intervention over two menstrual cycles resulting in significant reduction in severity of PMS symptoms over time.[152] Saffron has also been shown to be effective in improving fluoxetine-induced sexual dysfunction in women. A small ($n = 34$) clinical trial of women with major depression who were being treated with 40 mg/day fluoxetine showed that 30 mg/day of saffron over 4 weeks improved sexual problems including arousal, lubrication and pain scores.[153]

GINKGO BILOBA

A 2009 randomised placebo controlled trial of *G. biloba* treatment (40 mg leaf extracts) in 85 women showed significant improvements in PMS symptoms. Both the placebo and the treatment groups showed improvements; however, the treatment group showed a significantly higher decrease in symptom severity than the placebo group.[154]

FOENICULUM VULGARE (FENNEL)

Treatment using 30 drops of fennel extract administered every 8 hours over 3 days of menstruation showed reduction in the severity of PMS symptoms compared to placebo in a randomised placebo controlled study in 250 women. Fennel produces a hormonal effect through its inhibitory effect on oxytocin and prostaglandin E2.[155] Another trial ($n = 68$) comparing the effects of fennel seed extract (46 mg of hydro-alcoholic fennel fruit extract) and vitamin E (100 IU) supplementation (administered every 6 hours for 3 days after the start of the menstrual cycle, for two consecutive cycles) on dysmenorrhoea showed that the pain intensity in the fennel extract group was significantly reduced, and still significant but less so for the vitamin E group. By the second cycle, 50% of participants in the fennel extract group, 25% in the vitamin E group and 4.8% in the placebo group were suffering no pain.[156] In a 2014 clinical trial involving 105 students with mild to moderate dysmenorrhoea, both treatment groups receiving fennel extract (30 drops every 4 h, 1 day before the start of the cycle until the third day) and *Vitex agnus-castus (*40 drops once a day in the morning) had higher effects on pain scores than mefenamic acid (250 mg every 4 h). All treatments were administered 1 day before the start of the cycle until the third day. The trial duration was for 3 cycles, one without any treatment, and the other two in one of the treatment groups.[157] A clinical trial administering 30 mg fennel extract every 4 hours (3 days before menstruation until the fifth day of the cycle) over 3 cycles showed a reduction in dysmenorrhoea symptoms, and a decrease in menstruation duration in participants.[158]

TRIGONELLA FOENUM-GRAECUM (FENUGREEK SEED)

A recent double-blind, randomised placebo controlled trial on the effects of fenugreek seed on pain severity in dysmenorrhoea in a group of 101 students in Iran showed that supplementation with fenugreek seed powder (900 mg three times daily for the first 3 days of menstruation) for two consecutive menstrual cycles resulted in significantly reduced pain severity. The duration of the pain was also decreased in the second cycle in the treatment group. Women in the treatment group also experienced improved symptoms of dysmenorrhoea including fatigue, headache, nausea, vomiting, lack of energy, syncope. Fenugreek has an antispasmodic effect on the gastrointestinal system, and its diuretic properties decrease pelvic hyperaemia, both of which might explain its effectiveness in dysmenorrhoea.[159]

MATRICARIA CHAMOMILA (CHAMOMILE)

A study comparing the effects of chamomile extract (100 mg three times a day) and mefenamic acid (250 mg three times per day) on the intensity of PMS symptoms found that intensity of emotional and psychological symptoms was significantly reduced in the chamomile group compared to the mefenamic acid group. Physical symptom reduction was not significantly different between the two groups. The study was conducted on 90 students. Interventions were administered from day 21 until the next onset of the menstruation period, over two cycles. A significant decrease in mastalgia was found in the chamomile group in the same study.[160]

ZINGIBER OFFICINALE (GINGER)

A clinical trial involving 70 participants found that intervention with ginger (250 mg DBS, 7 days before menstruation until 3 days after start of menstruation) resulted in a significant decrease in total PMS symptom severity, mood and physical and emotional symptoms.[161] Ginger inhibits the metabolism of cyclooxygenase and lipoxygenase, preventing the production of prostaglandins. In an older study of 150 students with primary dysmenorrhoea, treatment with ginger rhizome powder (250 mg), ibuprofen (400 mg) or mefenamic acid (250 mg) showed that ginger was as effective as the other treatments. All treatment groups received the same treatment protocol: administered four times a day for 3 days from the start of the menstrual period, over one cycle only.[162]

CURCUMA LONGA (TURMERIC)

A recent RCT involving a small number of women ($n = 70$) showed that treatment with 100 mg curcumin over three menstrual cycles (administered two times daily, 7 days before the start of menstruation and 3 days after the start) significantly increased brain-derived neurotrophic factor (BDNF) (which has been shown to have more alterations during the late luteal phase in women who suffer from PMS compared to those who don't) and decreased PMS symptoms during all three cycles, compared to placebo.[163,164] Curcumin demonstrates a neuroprotective effect by its ability to modulate levels of BDNF, noradrenaline (norepinephrine), dopamine, and serotonin. Curcumin's antidepressant activity via serotonin regulation might explain its role in attenuating PMS symptoms, particularly mood and behavioural symptoms. The anti-inflammatory effects of curcumin are another mechanism of action in its ability to improve PMS symptoms.

CINNAMOMUM ZEYLANICUM (CINNAMON)

A trial on the use of cinnamon (420 mg TBS) compared to ibuprofen (400 mg t.d.s.) over a 24-hour period found that while both groups showed reduction in pain scores in dysmenorrhoea compared to placebo, cinnamon was not as effective as ibuprofen.[165] For some women, this might still be a viable option given the side effects of NSAIDs.

LIFESTYLE RECOMMENDATIONS

Lifestyle changes are recommended for all women experiencing PMS. Often simple implementation provides significant reduction of symptoms.

Exercise

There is a paucity of research assessing the effects of exercise in PMS, but it is known that for many women, regular exercise will promote good mental health and reduce premenstrual symptoms such as fluid retention. It is important to exercise for pleasure rather than until exhaustion, so as to not deplete the body. Beneficial forms include yoga, belly dancing and Pilates to increase circulation to the abdominal area.

Stress

Stress has been implicated in premenstrual symptoms such as mastodynia, and so managing stress is critical for healthy reproductive function. Relaxation and adequate, good-quality sleep may also be effective treatment for physical and emotional premenstrual symptoms.[166]

Menstrual diary

Recording details of cycle, temperature, cervical mucus and symptoms in a diary can help patients recognise patterns in their menstrual cycle. It enables greater awareness of where a patient is during their menstrual cycle so that they can prepare for changes and acknowledge an awareness of their emotional shifts.

Heat therapy

Although unsubstantiated by research, a hotwater bottle, wheatbag or warm bath with Epsom salts may help to ease menstrual cramping and pain by aiding circulation and relieving congestion to the pelvic area. Alternatively, topical application of peppermint essential oil is beneficial (must be applied with a carrier oil).

Emotional

There are significant emotional fluctuations throughout the menstrual cycle. It is beneficial for women to connect to their emotional fluctuations through their cycle. The luteal phase can provide an optimal time for inward reflection and creative stimulation. Often PMS symptoms are more pronounced in those who deny themselves quiet time to reflect and process their emotions. Progressive relaxation and guided imagery are positive suggestions to support this time.

CASE STUDY

OVERVIEW

GY presented with extreme PMS symptoms post ovulation (i.e. entire luteal phase). Symptoms included marked breast tenderness, swelling and nipple sensitivity. As her cycle continued and menses grew closer, the symptoms worsened significantly. In addition, she was aware of bloating, abdominal distension and mild dysmenorrhoea 1–2 days prior to bleeding commenced.

She experienced such pronounced symptoms that simple airflow aggravated her breast pain and she had to own different bras of various cup sizes to accommodate her breast growth. Her breast enlargement increased by 1–2 cup sizes in the last 3 days of her cycle. She explained that any contact with her breasts caused discomfort, which affected her relationship with her husband significantly. Her mood deteriorated as her pain increased as well.

Her diet revealed intriguing findings. She drank between 10 and 12 cups of tea per day (strong black tea with skim milk and 1 sugar). A typical 150 mL cup of tea contains from 30 to 100 mg of caffeine, depending on how long the tea is infused and whether you brew with loose leaves or teabags (strong loose-leaf tea yields the most caffeine). GY preferred to leave the teabag in her mug and explained that her mug was a larger type that contained approximately 400 mL. As such, her daily caffeine intake was calculated as 77–267 mg per cup of tea with an expected daily intake based on 11 cups of 770–2937 mg.

In keeping with the systematic approach of treatment for PMS, GY was told that her caffeine intake had to reduce significantly as all other treatments would be negatively impeded with this excessive intake. She considered her options carefully and made a decision to cease all caffeine intake. Hydration calculation was explained to GY and explanation of the importance of fluid regulation. She was guided through caffeine withdrawal over 2 weeks.

All symptoms cleared within one cycle, never to return.

POLYCYSTIC OVARY SYNDROME (PCOS)

Epidemiology

Polycystic ovary syndrome (PCOS) is a heterogeneous endocrine disorder that potentially affects about one in seven women worldwide, making it one of the most common endocrine disorders in women of reproductive age.[167] (See Fig. 18.6.) According to the latest European Society of Human Reproduction and Embryology (ESHRE) guidelines, prevalence is between 6 and 10% based on the National Institute of Health criteria and as high as 15% when the broader Rotterdam criteria are applied.[168]

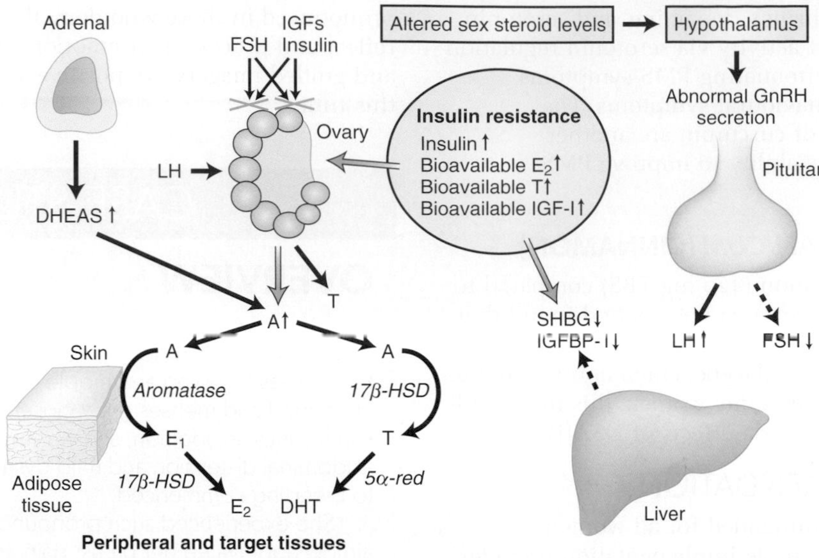

FIGURE 18.6 Polycystic ovary syndrome (PCOS).

Source: Kronenberg H. Williams textbook of endocrinology. 11th edn. Philadelphia: Saunders; 2007. Figure 16-32.

TABLE 18.15 Revised 2003 ESHRE/ASRM criteria for the diagnosis of PCOS

Presence of two of the following three criteria: 1. Oligo-anovulation 2. Clinical or biochemical evidence of hyperandrogenism 3. Polycystic ovaries on ultrasound examination. Exclusion required for elevated androgens of late-onset congenital adrenal hyperplasia, androgen-secreting tumours and Cushing's syndrome and for oligo/anovulation exclusion of thyroid disorder and elevated prolactin.

Sources: ESHRE/ASRM. ESHRE/ASRM Rotterdam Consensus Meeting Revised 2003 on diagnostic criteria and long-term health risks related to polycystic ovarian syndrome (PCOS). Hum Reprod 2004;19:41–7. ESHRE/ASRM. Revised 2003 consensus on diagnostic criteria and long-term health risks related to polycystic ovarian syndrome. Fertil Steril 2004;81:19–25.

Classification

At a consensus meeting between the American Society of Reproductive Medicine (ASRM) and ESHRE in 2003, a unifying definition of PCOS was proposed, encompassing a description of the morphology of the polycystic ovary, ovulatory disorder and hyperandrogenism[169,170] (Table 18.15). Because PCOS is a syndrome, no single diagnostic criterion is sufficient for clinical diagnosis.

Since the publication of the revised consensus statement for the definition of PCOS one study found a 14% prevalence of PCOS in the heterosexual subfertile population and 32% in lesbian women.[171]

The definition and diagnosis of PCOS remains controversial, and prevalence figures depend on which definition is used. The Rotterdam definition from 2003 is still the most widely accepted. The National Institute of Health definition (1990) is still the strictest, while the Rotterdam (2003) incorporates a wider spectrum of symptoms. The Androgen and PCOS Society has proposed a further definition which concentrates on androgen excess. There have been calls to change the name of PCOS as is it found to be confusing to patients with the syndrome and healthcare providers.[172]

Aetiology

The aetiology of this heterogeneous condition remains obscure and its phenotype expression varies.[168]

OBESITY

Obese women with PCOS are less likely to conceive than their lean counterparts.[173] Obesity is common in PCOS, often with a central distribution of adiposity. Central obesity appears to be particularly detrimental to ovarian function because it is associated with higher levels of fasting insulin, LH, oestrone and androstenedione than the same body mass with a peripheral fat distribution.[174] Obesity has both PCOS-independent and PCOS-synergistic effects on the metabolic and endocrinological profile.[173] Hyperinsulinaemia associated with obesity is the mechanism by which adiposity impacts on ovarian function in PCOS.[173] Elevated leptin levels have also been implicated because they appear to decrease aromatase activity in granulosa cells.[173]

INSULIN RESISTANCE

Although most women with PCOS tend to be obese, not all are. Both obese and non-obese women with PCOS are more insulin resistant and exhibit greater hyperinsulinaemia than women without PCOS of the same weight and age.[175]

ENVIRONMENTAL TOXINS

Studies have found significantly higher serum levels of perfluorinated compounds, polychlorinated biphenyls (PCBs), bisphenol A (BPA), pesticides and polycyclic aromatic hydrocarbons among women with PCOS compared with control groups. As yet, a causative relationship has not been established, but it is hypothesised that exposure to EDCs may worsen symptoms or contribute to the development of PCOS in genetically predisposed individuals. Higher levels of BPA exposure can lead to hyperandrogenism and hyperinsulinaemia which might be linked with PCOS development. It seems that a mother's exposure to BPA during pregnancy might lead to PCOS development in female offspring.[176–178]

Overview

Polycystic ovary syndrome is a persisting challenge for clinicians and researchers who try to elucidate its origins and distinguish primary pathological changes from secondary environmental disruptions.[179]

The major endocrine disruption is excessive androgen secretion or activity, and a large proportion of women also have abnormal insulin activity.[179,180] It has potentially profound implications for women with regard to anovulatory infertility and symptoms related to excess androgen production,[181] both having considerable psychological, social and economic consequences.[182]

Pathogenesis

POTENTIAL GENETIC DETERMINANTS OF PCOS

The ovarian androgen production in women with PCOS is due to the increased ovarian theca cell androgenic enzymatic activity of 3β-hydroxysteroid dehydrogenase (HSD) 17α-hydroxylase/C17,20 lyase, a product of CYP17.[181,183] This theca cell dysfunction may well explain the intra-ovarian hyperandrogenism, however granulosa and follicular abnormalities are potentially responsible for the ovulatory disorder.[181] Abnormalities of granulosa cell inhibin secretion appear to accentuate theca androgen secretion.[184] In addition, increased granulosa cell anti-Müllerian hormone (AMH) secretion and decreased secretion of oocyte-derived growth differential factor-9 (GDF-9) are also documented with PCOS.[185]

The commonly associated metabolic derangement of insulin resistance in PCOS is believed to be due to impairment of ovarian insulin signal transduction,[175] augmenting cytochrome P450scc, the rate-limiting step in ovarian steroidogenesis, and cytochrome P450c17α, the androgenic enzyme 17α-hydroxylase/C17,20 lyase.[181,183] Genetic abnormalities to produce these altered enzymatic activities have been difficult to determine; both post-translational regulation of C17,20 lyase by serine phosphorylation and mutations of CYP21 are mechanisms that have been demonstrated,[186] and an increased prevalence of tandem repeats in the gene promoter of the androgen-binding, sex hormone-binding globulin have been associated with PCOS.[187]

As insulin resistance is a common finding with women with PCOS,[181] investigations of the insulin receptor have found evidence of a link between mutations of the insulin receptor gene, *19p13.3*, and androgen levels in Caucasians.[188] In addition, a susceptibility to PCOS has been mapped to a locus in close proximity to the insulin receptor, D19S884 at *19p13.2*.[189] Elevated plasminogen activator inhibitor-1 (PAI-1) has been associated with increased miscarriage and cardiovascular risk factors in women with PCOS.[190] A 4G5G polymorphism in the promoter region of the *PAI-1* gene has been identified in women with PCOS and hypothesised as the cause of the increased metabolic sequelae of PCOS.[191]

It would appear that there are many genetic polymorphisms in women with PCOS and, hence, the influence of an adverse environment (whether antenatal, due to excess exposure to androgens in childhood or adulthood due to obesity) upon the genetic predisposition leads to the appearance of the PCOS phenotype.[181]

ANDROGEN ABNORMALITIES

Between 60 and 80% of women with PCOS have high concentrations of circulating testosterone[192] and approximately 25% have high concentrations of DHEA-S,[193] resulting in some investigators surmising that uncontrolled steroidogenesis may be the primary abnormality in this disorder.[167] Polycystic ovaries have a thickened thecal layer, and thecal cells derived from these ovaries secrete excessive androgens in vitro under basal conditions in response to LH stimulation.[194] The excessive secretion persists in cultured cells, suggesting a genetic association, but up to now none of the genes associated with steroid biosynthesis have been linked to PCOS through relevant polymorphisms or mutations.[195] However, increased expression and activity of thecal cell steroidogenic enzymes in patients with PCOS has been documented and this hyperactivity might be caused by a disturbance of intracellular signalling pathways that have not previously been implicated in the pathogenesis of PCOS.[167]

ABNORMALITIES OF FOLLICULOGENESIS

The phase of early follicular development up to an average follicular diameter of 5 mm is normal in PCOS.[173] Thereafter follicular maturation is disturbed, resulting in premature arrest of follicular growth.

Polycystic ovaries have two to six more primary, secondary and small antral follicles than do healthy ovaries.[196] The mechanism that determines excess numbers of follicles is unknown, but several lines of evidence indicate abnormal androgen signalling.[167] As defined by stringent consensus criteria, 90–100% of women with PCOS have polycystic ovaries[197] and several studies have reported a positive correlation between follicle number and serum testosterone and androstenedione concentrations in these women.[167]

Administration of dihydrotestosterone to female rhesus monkeys induces a polycystic ovary-like morphology, including increased ovarian volume and increased follicle numbers, suggesting a direct action on cells.[198] In addition, a polymorphism in the androgen receptor that affects the potency of its activity has been implicated in PCOS.[199] Another theory of increased follicular number in PCOS could be due to the very slow growth of the follicles creating a 'stockpiling' effect.[167] This slow growth might be mediated by deficient growth signals from the oocyte[200] or by the inhibitory effect of excess AMH.[201]

In anovulatory women with PCOS, antral follicle growth stops when the follicle is less than 10 mm in diameter, which is the stage just before the emergence of the dominant follicle.[167] Follicular arrest is associated with excessive stimulation of follicular cells by insulin, LH or both, in addition to a hyperandrogenic environment.[159] Insulin enhances the responsiveness of granulosa cells to LH, and in the ovaries of hyperinsulinaemic women with PCOS, arrested follicles show signs of premature luteinisation.[illegible] Granulosa cells from women with PCOS also seem to be selectively insulin resistant, whereby insulin-stimulated glucose metabolism is impaired but insulin resistant-stimulated steroidogenesis is normal, suggesting that deficient energy activity within the follicle contributes to anovulation.[167]

GONADOTROPHIN ABNORMALITIES

It has been postulated that relative FSH deficiency in PCOS is instrumental to the failure of follicular development.[203] This might be secondary to increased inhibin production or the result of hypothalamic–pituitary feedback by increased ovarian steroid concentrations.[173]

The role of inhibin in the pathogenesis of PCOS is still unclear. Inhibins are dimeric glycoproteins produced in the ovary and are known modulators of pituitary FSH secretion and ovarian steroidogenesis.[204] Inhibin-B selectively inhibits FSH secretion and studies evaluating inhibin-B concentrations in the serum or follicular fluid of women with PCOS have reported raised inhibin-B concentrations. Lockwood et al[205] hypothesised that abnormal pulsatility of inhibin-B in women with PCOS, together with high ambient levels of inhibin-B produced by a large cohort of small follicles, is instrumental in perpetuating the process of abnormal folliculogenesis.

Overall, these data suggest the presence of a defect of the hypothalamic–pituitary axis in PCOS, which is further supported by evidence of increased pituitary sensitivity to stimulation with corticotrophin-releasing factor, resulting in an excessive adrenocorticotropic hormone and cortisol response in women with PCOS.[206] However, high concentrations of androgens desensitise the hypothalamus to negative feedback by progesterone, suggesting that the abnormalities of gonadotrophin release in PCOS are secondary to abnormal steroid release by the ovaries or adrenal glands.[207]

THECA CELL FUNCTION

Histology reveals that polycystic ovaries are associated with an increase in the size of theca cells that envelop the follicle.[208] The theca cells of women with ovulatory and anovulatory PCOS hypersecrete androgens secondary to increased activity of P450c17, the key regulatory enzyme of androgen biosynthesis, which is modulated by serine phosphorylation.[173] Excessive serine phosphorylation targets the insulin receptor, creating a downstream effect of insulin receptor signalling and thereby abnormal insulin action on glucose metabolism.[175]

Insulin in turn acts synergistically with LH in stimulating androgen production in theca cells.[209] Although there is good evidence that the increased activity of P450c17 is induced by genetic factors, the abnormalities in proliferation and atresia of follicles also contribute to the excess of androgen production, or might reflect an additional or alternative pathogenic pathway.[210]

GRANULOSA CELL FUNCTION

The granulosa cells of women with PCOS and anovulation show evidence of increased aromatase activity response to both FSH and LH stimulation, resulting in enhanced oestrogen and progesterone synthesis.[173] This increase in aromatase activity is likely to be secondary to insulin, which stimulates oestradiol and progesterone production both independent of and synergistic with gonadotrophins.[210]

The increased levels of circulating oestrogen produce a tonic effect on LH production and give negative feedback to FSH secretion, thus perpetuating the cycles of abnormal folliculogenesis, abnormal steroidogenesis and abnormal gonadotrophin secretion.[173]

LH-INDUCED MATURATION ARREST

There is evidence for a premature response of the granulosa cells of small antral follicles to LH stimulation.[173] This might be due to abnormalities in LH secretion or to an augmentation of the LH stimulus through hyperinsulinaemia and/or hyperandrogenaemia.[173] A study investigating the preincubation with insulin reported significantly increased cellular responsiveness to subsequent LH stimulation with oestradiol and progesterone production.[202] This study also demonstrated that in ovulatory women (with both polycystic or normal ovaries) granulosa cells responded once a follicle had reached 9.5–10 mm in diameter. By contrast, in anovulatory women with polycystic ovaries, granulosa cells derived from follicles as small as 4 mm showed LH responsiveness.[202]

As in-vitro studies have highlighted the gonadotrophic properties of insulin, some authors have proposed that hyperinsulinaemia induces premature maturation of granulosa cells in vivo in anovulatory women with PCOS.[211,212] This premature response is detrimental to further follicular maturation because it suppresses granulosa cell growth and aromatase activity, increases progesterone production and, ultimately, induces cessation of normal follicular development and failure of dominance.[173,211,212]

INSULIN ACTION ABNORMALITIES

Women with PCOS appear to have a level of peripheral insulin resistance that is much like women with type 2 diabetes, which is characterised by a 35–40% decrease in insulin-mediated uptake.[213] Normoglycaemic women with PCOS display both fasting and glucose-challenged hyperinsulinaemia and a β-cell compensation that is inadequate for their degree of peripheral insulin resistance, suggesting that they are at higher risk of type 2 diabetes.[213,214]

Insulin resistance may contribute to hyperandrogenism and gonadotrophin abnormalities through several mechanisms.[167] High concentrations of insulin reduce circulating SHBG, thereby increasing the bioavailability of testosterone,[167] and might also serve as a cofactor to stimulate ovarian and adrenal androgen biosynthesis, thereby contributing to abnormal gonadotrophin concentrations.[215]

Acting on the liver, insulin inhibits the production of SHBG and IGF-1-binding protein (IGFBP-1), resulting in increased bioavailability of these substances.[208] In the ovary, increased IGF-1 is secreted by granulosa cells and acts in both an autocrine and a paracrine manner to modulate the stimulatory effects of gonadotrophins during many phases of follicular development.[216] In theca cells, IGF-1 may indirectly augment androgen production by increasing mRNAs for LH receptors and enzymes involved in steroidogenesis.[208] Post receptor signal abnormalities have been demonstrated in women with PCOS, but the abnormality is extrinsic to the receptor and specific and different tissues.[208]

Insulin resistance in PCOS is characterised by selective-tissue insulin sensitivity, in which some tissues seem highly resistant (i.e. skeletal muscle) and others sensitive (i.e. adrenal and ovary).[167] In affected tissues, metabolic pathways are generally resistant to stimulation by insulin, but mitogenic or steroidogenic pathways are not.[217]

GROWTH FACTORS

Growth differentiation factor 9 (GDF-9) is an oocyte-derived growth factor that is selectively expressed in developing oocytes.[185] Its essential role in folliculogenesis has been demonstrated in transgenic mice where GDF-9 deficiency blocked follicular development beyond the primary, one-layer follicle stage.[218] Perhaps even more striking was the complete lack of atresia. The authors concluded that GDF-9 deficiency resulted in arrested folliculogenesis before the granulosa cells gained competence to initiate apoptosis.[218] Studies of GDF-9 mRNA expression in normal human ovaries, polycystic ovaries and in ovaries from women with PCOS demonstrated reduced levels in growing oocytes in polycystic ovaries and PCOS ovaries.[173] The authors hypothesised that aberrant expression of GDF-9 might contribute to the pathogenesis of abnormal follicular development in this group of women.[173]

Epidermal growth factor (EGF) and its analogue transforming growth factor alpha (TGF-α), which works through the EGF receptor, are also implicated in the abnormal ovarian function of women with PCOS.[173] Physiological levels of EGF and TGF-α appear to be important for normal follicle maturation and alterations in local expression might be detrimental.[219] Studies in rodents and humans demonstrated a potent inhibition of FSH-induced oestrogen production in granulosa cells by EGF and TGF-α.[173] Granulosa cells from ovulatory polycystic ovaries and from ovaries in women with PCOS have been shown to express significantly higher levels of EGF receptors than granulosa cells from normal ovaries.[220]

The cytokine tumour necrosis factor α (TNF-α), has also been shown to be a local regulator of ovarian function, exerting an influence on apoptosis, steroidogenesis and follicle maturation.[173] Evidence for abnormal TNF-α production in women with PCOS was reported by Amato et al[221] where higher levels of TNF-α were found in the serum and follicular fluid of women with PCOS than normal ovulating women. In the same study, TNF-α concentrations were inversely associated with oestradiol levels.[221]

ATTENUATED APOPTOSIS

The majority of human follicles do not reach a stage of final maturation but face elimination by atresia. The process of follicle apoptosis is tightly regulated and influenced by endocrine, paracrine and autocrine factors.[173] The increased number of viable primary and secondary follicles in the polycystic ovary indicated the process of apoptosis is attenuated.[222]

Some factors implicated in chronic anovulation are listed in Table 18.16.

TABLE 18.16 Factors implicated in chronic anovulation

Factor	Abnormality	Consequence
FSH	Relative deficiency	Inadequate follicle stimulation
LH	Hypersecretion	Hyperandrogenaemia Follicle growth arrest
Insulin	Hypersecretion	Hyperandrogenaemia Follicle growth arrest
Androgens	Hypersecretion	Abnormal gonadotrophin release Follicle growth arrest
Oestrogens	Hypersecretion	Suppression of FSH secretion Increased (tonic) LH secretion
Inhibin B	Hypersecretion	Suppression of FSH secretion
Apoptosis	Attenuated	Increased cohort of small follicles active in steroidogenesis
Growth factors	Aberrant expression	Abnormal apoptosis Follicle growth arrest Suppression of oestrogen synthesis

Source: van der Spuy ZM, Dyer SJ. The pathogenesis of infertility and early pregnancy loss in polycystic ovarian syndrome. Best Pract Res Clin Obstet Gynaecol 2004;18(5):755–71.

SIGNS AND SYMPTOMS

The features of PCOS can be divided into three categories: clinical, endocrine and metabolic (Table 18.17).[223]

The first signs of PCOS may be an early andrenarche with an early appearance of pubic hair.[224] Although PCOS is not diagnosed until 2–3 years after menarche, it has been suggested that its origins lie in childhood or fetal life, since it has been demonstrated in animal studies that excess exposure to androgens in utero produces PCOS-like features.[225–227] Due to the family clustering of PCOS cases,

TABLE 18.17 Classification of the features of PCOS

Clinical	The clinical features include menstrual abnormalities, hirsutism, acne, alopecia, anovulatory infertility and recurrent miscarriages
Endocrine	The endocrine features include elevated androgens, luteinising hormone (LH), oestrogen, and prolactin
Metabolic	The metabolic features include insulin resistance, obesity, lipid abnormalities, and an increased risk of impaired glucose tolerance (IGT) and type 2 diabetes mellitus[223]

Source: Durant E, Leslie NS. Polycystic ovarian syndrome: a review of current knowledge. Journal Nurse Practitioners 2007 March:180–185.

it is believed that there is a genetic predisposition to PCOS whereby genomic variants act under the influence of genetic factors.[181,184]

Hyperandrogenism

Hyperandrogenism is the most constant and prominent component of PCOS, but reliable detection of this feature is not straightforward, and indices vary considerably dependent on age, body weight and ethnic origin.[167] Hyperandrogenism is assessed by clinical features, biochemical indices, or both. Clinically, hyperandrogenism is diagnosed by the most subjective assessment of cutaneous manifestations of excessive androgen activity, such as hirsutism, acne (especially in young women) and female pattern baldness (especially in older women).[209] Hirsutism is the most common of these symptoms, being present in about 60% of women with PCOS,[192] although rarely present in Asian women.[228]

Chronic anovulation

The major clinical signs of chronic anovulation are oligomenorrhoea or amenorrhoea.[167] Oligomenorrhoea is defined as less than eight periods per year, or cycles that are longer than 35 days, and amenorrhoea is absence of menstruation for more than 3 months without pregnancy.[167]

Polycystic ovaries on ultrasound

The morphological features of the polycystic ovary can be identified on ultrasound examination and include hyperechogenic stromal enlargement and multiple small follicles 2–8 mm in diameter arranged around the periphery or distributed through the stroma.[229]

Polycystic ovaries on transvaginal ultrasound are defined as the presence of 12 or more follicles measuring 2–9 mm in diameter, or increased ovarian volume (>10 mL) in the follicular phase.[167] Although there are other characteristic features, priority has been given to follicle number and ovarian volume because both have the advantage of being measured in real time and are regarded as key consistent features of polycystic ovaries.

Hyperinsulinaemia

The severity of hyperinsulinaemia that is manifested in adulthood in over 50% of even normal weight women with PCOS is influenced by both genetic and environmental factors, particularly obesity.[181,230] The manifestation of the phenotype of PCOS is said to be due to the development of insulin resistance due to the deposition of adipose tissue, even if a woman has a genetic or environmental predisposition to PCOS.[181] Hence it is possible for a woman to have a PCOS phenotype but by subsequent weight loss she may lose some of the features of PCOS and hence not express the PCOS phenotype.[231,232]

Hirsutism, acne, seborrhoea and alopecia

Women with PCOS have a higher incidence of all of these cutaneous symptoms compared with women with normal ovaries.[208]

Metabolic symptoms

A large proportion (40–60%) of women with PCOS will be obese, and a greater proportion (40–80%) will demonstrate insulin resistance.[208] While most obese patients are insulin-resistant, this feature is also a characteristic of lean PCOS patients.[208]

Recognised phenotypes in PCOS

The phenotypes for PCOS based on the Rotterdam Criteria are listed in Table 18.18.

COMPLICATIONS

The potential health consequences of PCOS are a lifelong issue (Table 18.19). There is little doubt that the prevalence of impaired glucose tolerance and diabetes mellitus is increased substantially in women with PCOS,[167] although the magnitude of the increase depends on the prevalence of obesity in the population, and racial influences are evident.[232] Conversion rates of glucose tolerance from normal to abnormal are accelerated in PCOS[233] and up to 10% of women with this disorder develop diabetes in the third or fourth decade.[233] The evidence for cardiovascular risks is less clear, although cardiovascular risk factors are substantially increased, including hyperlipidaemia, hyperandrogenaemia, hypertension, markers of a prothrombotic state, and markers of inflammation.[234]

There have been reports of an increased prevalence of metabolic syndrome in women with PCOS.[167] However, whether this increase is caused by a feature specific to PCOS or is merely a consequence of adiposity is unclear.[167] An increase in central fat, hyperinsulinaemia, glucose tolerance, increased blood pressure and other isolated features of metabolic syndrome are more common in women with PCOS than they are in the general population.[167]

PCOS has significant implications for women with regard to their reproductive potential: increased risk of anovulatory infertility, increased risk of miscarriage and increased risk of pregnancy complications.[181]

Physical symptoms associated with PCOS have been shown to cause a reduction in psychological wellbeing and sexual satisfaction.[235] This may result in feelings of frustration and anxiety and have negative impact on

TABLE 18.18 Phenotypes for PCOS based on the Rotterdam criteria

	Severe PCOS	Hyperandrogenism and chronic anovulation	Ovulatory PCOS	Mild PCOS
Periods	Irregular	Irregular	Normal	Irregular
Ovaries on ultrasonography	Polycystic	Normal	Polycystic	Polycystic
Insulin concentration	Increased	Increased	Increased	Normal
Risks	Potential long term	Potential long term	Unknown	Unknown
Prevalence of affected women	61%	7%	16%	16%

Source: Norman RJ, Dewailly D, Legro RS, et al. Polycystic ovarian syndrome. Lancet 2007;370:685–97.

TABLE 18.19 Lifelong health complications in PCOS

	Prenatal or childhood	Adolescence, reproductive years	Postmenopausal
Reproductive	Premature adrenarche Early menarche	Menstrual irregularity Hirsutism Acne Infertility Endometrial cancer Miscarriage Pregnancy complications	Delayed menopause
Metabolic	Abnormal fetal growth	Obesity Impaired glucose tolerance Insulin resistance Dyslipidaemia Type 2 diabetes	Obesity Impaired glucose tolerance Insulin resistance Dyslipidaemia Type 2 diabetes
Other		Sleep apnoea Fatty liver Depression	

Source: Norman RJ, Dewailly D, Legro RS, et al. Polycystic ovarian syndrome. Lancet 2007;370:685–97.

health-related quality of life.[235] The common physical manifestations in PCOS (including hirsutism, acne, obesity and male pattern balding) are associated with a decrease in health-related quality of life particularly in areas concerning social and emotional functioning, decreased sexual self-worth and sexual satisfaction, and increased emotional distress.[235] The physical symptoms that are associated with PCOS do not account alone for the increase in mood disturbances observed among patients with PCOS.[236]

A recent study reported a high incidence of depression and other mood disturbances in young women with PCOS.[237] Excess weight and difficulties losing weight were of particular concern. A high incidence of anxiety and eating disorders was also detected in this longitudinal study.[237]

The abnormal hormonal concentrations characteristic of PCOS might predispose women with this disorder to development of endometrial cancer, although data to support this finding are not very convincing.[238] The number of menstrual cycles is less important than the avoidance of endometrial hyperplasia, and intermittent induction of menstruation prevents abnormal uterine proliferation.[167]

DIFFERENTIAL DIAGNOSIS

The ESHRE/ASRM group proposed that PCOS be diagnosed after other conditions that are known to mimic or cause the features of PCOS be excluded. These include:[167]

- Congenital adrenal hyperplasia
- Cushing's syndrome
- Androgen-secreting tumours
- Hyperandrogenism
- Hyperprolactinaemia
- Insufficient follicle-stimulating hormone for ovulation.

NATUROPATHIC DIAGNOSIS

Naturopathic diagnosis relies on pathology and radiological results to interpret the severity of the presentation. It considers a holistic framework for the patient which includes the following variables.

PCOS confirmatory findings

- Ultrasound findings
- Hormone results
- Physical manifestation of androgenisation
- Menstrual history.

Risk of metabolic syndrome

- Blood sugar and insulin status
- Waist-to-hip ratio
- Body mass index (BMI)
- Lipid profile
- Cardiovascular risk
- Hepatobiliary health (confirmed with pathology and radiological investigations).

Investigations

OVERVIEW

Biochemical evaluation

- Female hormone profile: LH, FSH, oestradiol, progesterone, prolactin, BHCG, 17OH progesterone
- Androgen profile: free and bound testosterone, free androgen index (FAI), SHBG, DHEA-S, androstenedione
- Metabolic profile: fasting GTT, insulin, fasting glucose, HbA1c, HOMA
- Lipid profile: triglycerides, HDL, LDL, vLDL, total cholesterol, apolipoproteins, lipoproteins
- Thyroid panel: TSH, T3, T4, reverse T3, thyroid antibodies, urinary iodine or spot iodine.

Radiological studies

- Transabdominal and transvaginal ultrasound.

FAMILY HISTORY

Because of its genetic and metabolic implications, clinical investigation of PCOS should include examination of family history of diabetes mellitus, cardiovascular disease and hyperlipidaemia, possibly with assessment of relevant risk factors in siblings and older family members.[167]

Lifestyle issues, including a history of diet and exercise, should be investigated.

Clinical measurements might include calculation of BMI and relative waist circumference (waist-to-hip ratio).

Symptoms usually begin at menarche and manifest after puberty. Other causes should be assessed for those women who have a history of regular menstrual cycles and who then develop irregular cycles.

The family history often includes female relatives with irregular menstruation, severe acne, excess hair growth, and difficulty becoming pregnant.

Health-related quality of life is generally worse in women with PCOS than in women without the disorder.[167] A questionnaire of health-related quality of life specific for women has been developed for this purpose.[239]

DEVELOPMENTAL HISTORY

Women with PCOS usually report a history of menarche around 12–13 years of age and never develop a consistent pattern of regular menses.[223] Male hair patterns and skin changes often appear at the same time as secondary sex characteristics. The male hair patterns may include hair growth on the chin, cheek, sideburns, neck, chest, breast, upper arms and between the umbilicus and the pubic triangle.[223] Occasionally male pattern alopecia occurs. Acne can vary from mild to severe.[240]

POLYCYSTIC OVARIES ON ULTRASONOGRAPHY

High-frequency vaginal probes and image enhancing software are currently used in women with suspected PCOS to determine follicular phase ovarian follicle number (12 or more follicles measuring 2–9 mm in diameter) and ovarian volume (>10 mL).

The assessment of PCOS in adolescent girls should be done by transabdominal ultrasonography with measurement of ovarian volume only, because the criterion based on follicles is much less reliable by the abdominal route, especially in obese individuals.[241] The adult upper healthy threshold volume of 10 mL seems to be appropriate for postmenarchal adolescents.[242] Measurement of serum anti-Müllerian hormone (AMH), which is secreted by granulosa cells of developing follicles, is emerging as a potential surrogate for ultrasonography, as values correlate closely with antral follicle count in pilot investigations.[243] This assay is not valid for women older than 35 years but for others it may facilitate the diagnosis of PCOS in circumstances where ultrasonography is inappropriate or unavailable.[167]

HYPERANDROGENISM

Biochemically, hyperandrogenism is most commonly assessed by measurement of serum testosterone (T), and sex hormone-binding globulin (SHBG), followed by calculation of the free or bioavailable (free and weakly bound to albumin) fraction by the free androgen index (T/SHBG × 100) or the mass action equation, respectively.[244] The mass action equation is regarded as the method of choice to calculate free serum testosterone, if reliable assays are used and normative data specific to each assay are developed.[244]

The concentrations of other serum androgens, such as androstenedione or the adrenal androgen prasterone sulfate (known as DHEA-S) are often high in women with PCOS, but their measurement is of little value in the average clinical setting.[167]

Unfortunately, serum analysis fails to measure the biochemical hyperandrogenism of PCOS in about 20–40% of patients.[244] Most commercial assays for total serum testosterone are not designed or validated for detection within the normal range for women[167,244] raising concerns about their real diagnostic value. Moreover, the range that is considered healthy for women by commercial laboratories is very broad and has been shown to include many hyperandrogenic women, even those with severe hirsutism.[245]

LH/FSH RATIO

A hallmark of PCOS is an elevated LH/FSH ratio of 2 : 1 or 3 : 1. If a woman is having regular cycles, then testing on day 3 of the menstrual cycle is recommended. An increased LH/FSH ratio of greater than 2 : 1 is present in 60–70% of women with PCOS and is more likely to occur in non-obese women.[246] If the woman is experiencing oligomenorrhoea, an ovulatory LH surge should be ruled out by ascertaining whether a menstrual cycle occurred approximately 14 days after the test was performed.[246]

METABOLIC PROFILE

Women with PCOS are at risk of metabolic syndrome and diabetes.[240] A fasting lipid profile (cholesterol, triglycerides, HDL/LDL ratio, HDL cholesterol, LDL cholesterol) should be obtained to assess for cardiovascular risk. A fasting glucose tolerance test or HbA1c and insulin combination is recommended to assess for insulin resistance or type 2 diabetes.

Lipid profile typically produces the following parameters:

- Elevated total cholesterol
- Elevated triglycerides
- Elevated low-density lipoproteins (LDL)
- Low high-density lipoproteins (HDL)
- Low apoprotein A-12.

It is recommended that repeated measurements of glucose and lipid status should take place more regularly in women with PCOS than in women without the syndrome, because conversion from a healthy to a pathological state happens more frequently in the disorder.[233]

SPECIFIC NATUROPATHIC INVESTIGATIONS

Some specific naturopathic investigations are listed in Table 18.20.

Therapeutic considerations

CLINICAL DECISION MAKING AND RATIONALE

When presented with a PCOS patient, it is important to consider their presentation in significant detail and assess the accuracy of the findings. The diagnosis is frequently given with either limited findings or a comprehensive picture. Thorough assessment is imperative to determine the depth of treatment required.

Therapeutic application

ALLOPATHIC PERSPECTIVE

Oral contraceptive pill

COSMETIC ISSUES

Ovarian suppression through oral contraceptives is widely prescribed for hirsutism and acne, especially in the

TABLE 18.20 Specific naturopathic investigations for PCOS

Assessment	Justification
Dietary and lifestyle assessment	Assess patient's lifestyle practices and dietary choices. Encourages the patient to take responsibility for and awareness of their health choices. Enables practitioner to assess level of sedentary behaviour and scale of carbohydrate consumption
Hip-to-waist ratio and BMI	Assess extent of weight imbalance
Female hormone profile (saliva)	Female hormone profiles can monitor changes in hormonal status over the course of the menstrual cycle by measuring the sex hormones via saliva samples (which are collected on specific days of the month). Oestrone, oestradiol, oestriol, progesterone, testosterone and DHEA-S can be assessed
2 and 16 urinary oestrogen metabolite	The 2 and 16 urinary oestrogen metabolism test may be a useful tool in determining patients with a high risk of hormonal imbalance. Oestrogens are metabolised in two ways: the first pathway (2-hydroxyoestrone) is protective while the second pathway (16α-hydroxyoestrone) is more potent. This test identifies which is the dominant pathway (2 or 16) for oestrogen metabolism. The aim is to ensure that the ratio between 2 : 16 pathways is maintained at the ideal 2.0
Adrenal hormone profile	An adrenal hormone profile that measures cortisol and DHEA-S over a 24-h period may be a useful test for women with PCOS if stress and anxiety are also present
Cardiovascular health profile	As PCOS could be associated with cardiovascular disease, it may be prudent to suggest a serum cardiovascular health profile to analyse risk factors for cardiovascular disease. Parameters such as cholesterol, lipoproteins, triglycerides, fibrinogen, C-reactive protein, homocysteine, lipid peroxidises, vitamin E, magnesium, coenzyme Q10, insulin, total testosterone, free androgen index, sex hormone-binding globulin and ferritin are measured
Detoxification profile	Detoxification capacity profile (saliva/urine) to assess the liver's phase I and phase II detoxification capacity. Saliva and urine are analysed for metabolites of the three compounds to determine how well the liver can convert and clear toxins from the body. Adequate liver function is important to PCOS as the liver is responsible for SHBG production and for metabolising hormones such as oestrogen and testosterone
Metabolic syndrome profile	As metabolic syndrome is associated with the aetiology of PCOS, a metabolic syndrome profile (serum/plasma) that compiles several laboratory markers for this condition could be undertaken. Analytes reported include HDL cholesterol, triglycerides, glucose, insulin, asymmetric dimethylarginine and the AA/EPA ratio
Thyroid profile	To eliminate adjunct endocrine abnormalities
Salivary adrenal stress profile	Assess impact of stress on deterioration of endocrine function and stability

adolescent population.[167] The combined oral contraceptive pill (OCP), particularly when combined with cyproterone acetate, has significant beneficial effects in the improvement of hirsutism, acne lesion counts and sebum secretion.[247] However, side effects such as tiredness, reduced libido, and changes in liver function are common.[167] Laser electrolysis alone or in combination with topical application of eflornithine cream to retard hair growth can be effective to reduce hirsutism.[248] Insulin-sensitising agents such as metformin and thiazolidinediones might be useful in the treatment of hirsutism and acne because insulin resistance affects both disorders, but recommendations of these drugs for cosmetic purposes are premature.[167] Topical minoxidil 2–5% is regarded as an effective treatment for androgenic alopecia.[249]

Spironolactone, an anti-androgen, acts via blockade of the androgen receptor by competing for the receptor with dihydrotestosterone and has been used to improve hirsutism.[181]

MENSTRUAL IRREGULARITY

The use of the combined OCP is the most common allopathic treatment for symptoms of PCOS because it interferes with androgen activity via several mechanisms, including reduced androgen production, increased hepatic SHBG synthesis and competitive binding to androgen receptors by some progestogens.[167] However, the potential long-term metabolic side effects of combined OCPs in women with PCOS are being debated, especially since women with this disorder have a propensity for development of obesity and metabolic abnormalities.[167] Treatments that couple combined OCP with insulin sensitisers, anti-androgens or both are emerging as treatment options with potential benefits on metabolic abnormalities.[167]

Anti-oestrogen treatment

The commonest and first-line method for inducing ovulation in World Health Organization (WHO) group II anovulatory women, after the exclusion of hyperprolactinaemia, is clomiphene citrate. The mechanism of action is by the blocking of the negative feedback effect of oestrogen on the anterior pituitary, stimulating an increased secretion of gonadotrophins, thus augmenting follicular selection and stimulation.[181] Clomiphene citrate is effective in inducing ovulation in type 2 anovulatory women in approximately 80% of cases and pregnancy in approximately 50% after six cycles.[250] The reason for the disparity between ovulation and pregnancy is due to the anti-oestrogenic effect of the clomiphene citrate acting on both endometrial and ovarian levels, in addition to the development of a hostile cervical mucus.[181] With clomiphene citrate the miscarriage rate is not altered, the multiple-pregnancy rate is 6–8% and ovarian hyperstimulation syndrome is rare.[250]

Some women with PCOS are resistant to clomiphene citrate and do not ovulate at all, or fail to achieve pregnancy despite ovulation.[167] Factors that affect resistance to clomiphene citrate or failure to achieve pregnancy are, in order of importance, hyperandrogenaemia, obesity, ovarian volume and menstrual dysfunction.[167]

Aromatase inhibitors

Like clomiphene citrate, aromatase inhibitors reduce oestrogen stimulation of the hypothalamic–pituitary axis, but do so by reducing oestrogen biosynthesis. A randomised controlled trial has shown that there is less ovarian stimulation with the aromatase inhibitor letrozole than with clomiphene citrate, which might contribute to the lower rate of multiple pregnancies.[251] However, there is concern about the possibility of fetal abnormalities as a result of aromatase inhibition.[167]

Insulin sensitisers

In the view of hyperinsulinaemia that is intrinsic to the pathogenesis of PCOS, insulin sensitisers are frequently employed to induce ovulation.[181] Thiazolidinediones and D-chiro-inositol have been shown to increase ovulation and reduce hyperandrogenism in women with PCOS, but metformin remains the most commonly used agent.[167] Metformin is not approved by the US Food and Drug Administration (FDA) to induce ovulation and the best possible dose is unknown.[167] A recent meta-analysis, reported in a Cochrane review of 13 studies of anovulatory women with PCOS, the majority of whom had fasting insulin, demonstrated no effect on pregnancy rate when compared with placebo, but the combination of metformin and clomiphene citrate in clomiphene-resistant women led to a significant improvement in pregnancy rate.[252]

Gonadotrophin therapy

Gonadotrophin therapy is often used as a second-line therapy in anovulatory women with PCOS if they are either resistant to ovulation induction with anti-oestrogen treatment or fail to conceive.[181] However, women with PCOS are particularly sensitive to gonadotrophin therapy and have a significant chance of multiple follicle development and cycle cancellation.[253]

Statin therapy

Statins are showing promise in treatment of PCOS. They act by selectively inhibiting 3-hydroxy- 3-methylglutaryl-coenzyme A (HMG-CoA), the rate-limiting enzyme in the cholesterol biosynthesis pathway. In addition to lipid reduction, they target underlying stimulation of thecal androgen production and steroidogenesis. They also express antioxidant, anti-inflammatory and antiproliferative effects. The use of statins in the medical treatment of women with PCOS appears to have pleotropic cardiometabolic benefits, but further studies of longer duration are needed to confirm the whole spectrum of their clinical implication in this group. This therapy remains controversial due to the potential side effects. Statin therapy is not recommended in women who are planning pregnancy.[254,172]

Ovarian drilling

Laparoscopic ovarian diathermy or 'ovarian drilling' with either laser surgery or electrosurgery has been shown to be effective in the induction of ovulation in addition to a fall in serum androgens and LH in women with PCOS.[255] The mechanism of the effect of ovarian drilling is believed to be due to the damage to the ovarian androgen-producing tissue leading to a correction in the pituitary–ovarian feedback mechanism.[181] There are risks associated with the operation and development of intrapelvic adhesions.[167]

Infertility

Women with PCOS have an increased incidence of WHO group II anovulatory infertility.[181] Methods employed to induce ovulation consist of weight loss, anti-oestrogens, insulin sensitisers, gonadotrophins and laparoscopic 'ovarian drilling'.

HISTORICAL PERSPECTIVE

It is unclear whether polycystic ovary syndrome existed in the time of the Eclectic physicians as without the modern knowledge and technology we have today it is unlikely that the Eclectics would have been able to see the pearl-like cysts that appear on the ovaries. In saying this there are mentions of herbs for symptoms synonymous with PCOS in the texts of the Eclectics. For example, a number of botanicals are suggested for amenorrhoea. These include *Thuja occidentalis*, which was also favoured for its antiseptic action and ability to remove congestion in the ovaries. Other botanicals such as *Actaea racemosa* (described an as efficient agent for the restoration of suppressed menses) and *Caulophyllum thalictroides* (used for its effects on congested reproductive organs) were also promoted for their hormone-regulating effects.[8]

NATUROPATHIC PERSPECTIVE

The naturopathic approach considers that the patient's compliance and willingness to partake in their healing is paramount to the success of treatment. There are countless cases of patients normalising their abnormalities with weight loss, exercise and dietary modifications. These areas are priorities for the long-term successful normalisation of hormone cascades. If a patient expects 'a cure in a bottle', her recovery will be very challenging for both clinician and patient.

When developing a treatment plan, the naturopath will need to consider a few key areas to determine the extent of recommendations required. These include:

- Severity of findings on ultrasound
- Hormonal involvement: hormone levels through pathology investigations
- Menstrual impact: duration of amenorrhoea or infertility
- Physical manifestation of androgenisation
- Risk for metabolic syndrome and compounding factors.

NUTRITIONAL MEDICINE (DIETARY)

Dietary therapeutic objectives

- Aim to consume a diet of 30% complex carbohydrates, 40% protein and 30% lipids
- Avoid alcohol, caffeine and nutritional stressors
- Improve weight balance and advise to stabilise weight as required
- Reduce insulin resistance, stabilise blood sugar levels and avoid fluctuations that compound PCOS presentation by avoiding refined carbohydrates and sugar
- Support and prevent metabolic syndrome and associated compounding factors by supporting lipid profile through cardiovascular system and liver health.

Specific dietary treatments

DIETARY MODIFICATIONS

It is generally accepted that changes in diet can produce a profound and beneficial effect with regards to symptomatology and coexisting conditions (e.g. subfertility or amenorrhoea). The optimal diet for individuals with PCOS is recognised as not just being one that reduces symptomatology and assists with weight loss (in those that are overweight) but also one that protects against the associated pathologies of cardiovascular disease, diabetes, impaired fertility and certain cancers.

Anti-inflammatory hypocaloric diet

A study of 100 overweight and obese women with PCOS who went on an anti-inflammatory hypocaloric diet with physical activity for 12 weeks, resulted in significant improvements in body composition, hormones and menstrual cyclicity, blood pressure, glucose homeostasis, dyslipidaemia, CRP and serum amyloid A (SAA) (surrogate measures of cardiovascular risk). There was a clinically relevant weight loss that was associated with a reduced prevalence of type 2 diabetes mellitus and metabolic syndrome in the general population and improved fertility outcomes in PCOS. Sixty-three per cent of the women regained menstrual cyclicity and there was a 12% spontaneous pregnancy rate within the 12 weeks. The diet was a Mediterranean-inspired low glycaemic load (GL) anti-inflammatory diet based on combinations of nutrients, encouraging the consumption of legumes, fish and low-fat dairy products in a Mediterranean context. The dietary composition was 25% proteins, 25% fat, and 50% carbohydrates. Diets were designed as reduced-energy, low-fat, low-saturated fat, and moderate-to-high fibre diets.[256]

DASH diet

In another study, 60 women with PCOS were randomly assigned to a control diet or the DASH diet. Both diets consisted of 50–55% carbohydrate, 15–20% protein and 25–30% total fat, while the DASH diet was high in vegetables, fruits, wholegrains and low-fat dairy products, and low in saturated fats, cholesterol, refined grains and sweets. After 3 months the DASH diet was associated with significant weight loss and reduced BMI. There was also a significant reduction in serum androstenedione, and an increase in antioxidant status and sex hormone binding globulin.[257] A study by Frary et al[258] on the effects of dietary carbohydrates in PCOS concluded that it is energy restriction and weight loss in PCOS which improves ovulation rates, conception hyperandrogenaemia, glucose and insulin levels, insulin resistance and satiety hormones.

The composition of the diet is less important, so long as the weight loss is achieved.

Low starch and low dairy products

An 8-week dietary intervention trial of 24 women with PCOS showed that a low starch/low dairy diet improved weight parameters, inulin sensitivity, testosterone levels and hirsutism. The diet included lean animal protein (meat and poultry), fish and shellfish, eggs, non-starchy vegetables, low-sugar fruits (e.g. berries, apples, oranges, plums), avocado, olives, nuts and seeds, and oils (olive and coconut). Participants were instructed to exclude all grains, beans, dairy products (other than 30 g full fat cheese per day to assist with compliance), and sugar (including fruit juice from concentrate, raw turbinado sugar, evaporated cane juice, high-fructose corn syrup, honey, or agave nectar) because of their insulinaemic properties.[259]

Advanced glycation end products (AGEs)

Advanced glycation end products (AGEs) are highly reactive molecules that may induce structural and vascular changes. AGEs are formed by non-enzymatic reactions of sugars with proteins, nucleic acids and lipids. Women with PCOS tend to have higher levels of AGEs, and increased expression of AGEs as pro-inflammatory receptors in the ovarian tissue has been observed in PCOS. AGEs are associated with ovulatory dysfunction. Uncooked animal-derived foods are the major source of AGEs and thermal processing accelerates AGE formation. Diets containing high protein and fat have higher amounts of the AGEs in comparison to carbohydrate-rich diets. Cooking methods also affect dietary AGEs content in a diet — food prepared at low temperature with high moisture and brief heating time has fewer AGEs. The use of acidic marinades such as lemon juice and vinegar during cooking significantly reduces the AGE content in the diet. The highest level of AGEs per gram of food is present in dry-heat processed foods such as chips, crackers and cookies, which is due to the presence of oil, butter, cheese, nuts and eggs as ingredients in these foods. Dry-heat processing also accelerates dietary AGE formation in lean red meats and poultry due to presence of reactive amino-lipids and reducing sugars (fructose as well as glucose-6-phosphate). Fruits, vegetables, low fat milk, grains and legumes have the lowest dietary AGE content. It is advised to reduce consumption of foods containing high levels of AGEs for general wellbeing, but also for women with PCOS due to the AGEs' inflammatory inducing properties, and to improve ovulatory dysfunction. Increased AGEs are also associated with obesity and insulin resistance in PCOS.[254,260,261]

DIETARY INCLUSIONS

Low GI diet

In acknowledging that insulin resistance and compensatory hyperinsulinaemia are key features of PCOS, following a low glycaemic diet is highly recommended.[262] The glycaemic index (GI) is a classification index of carbohydrate foods based on postprandial glucose response (i.e. it ranks carbohydrate-rich foods in terms of their blood glucose raising potential). As yet, few studies have shown the efficacy of a low GI diet in PCOS, but results seen in patients with diabetes, combined with the observed link between PCOS and insulin, suggest it would be logical to advocate a low GI diet, not only to improve symptoms of PCOS but also to prevent long-term complications of cardiovascular disease and diabetes.

Newer dietary modifications that use the Food Insulin Index (FII) as opposed to the glycaemic index or glycaemic load are therapeutically more appropriate. See Chapter 21 for more information.

DIETARY EXCLUSIONS

Caffeine

Women with PCOS need to keep their caffeine intake to a minimum as caffeine may impact negatively on female reproduction. This is especially relevant to women with PCOS hoping to conceive as a number of clinical studies have shown that excess intake of caffeine may impair fertility.

Saturated fats and deep-fried foods

Women with PCOS are at risk of metabolic syndrome and cardiovascular disease and need to keep saturated fat and deep-fried foods to a minimum. These foods have been linked directly to increased risk of cardiovascular disease and metabolic syndrome. Typically, these foods are also deficient in nutrients.

Sugar

Sugar in all its forms needs to be minimised in the patient with PCOS. Sugar contributes to elevated blood sugar, contributing to symptomatology. Sugar-containing foods include fruit which should be kept to a maximum of two pieces daily. Fruit chosen should be low GI (i.e. a cup of berries instead of a cup of pineapple). If sugar is consumed, a protein component should also be included to ensure stable blood sugar levels.

Refined carbohydrates

Like sugar, refined carbohydrates such as white bread, lollies and pasta (which are ultimately broken down to sugar), aggravate PCOS by causing elevated levels of glucose and insulin. A high GI diet (i.e. one high in refined carbohydrates and sugars) has been found to worsen postprandial insulin resistance.[263]

NUTRITIONAL MEDICINE (SUPPLEMENTAL)

Nutritional medicine therapeutic objectives

- Stabilise reproductive hormones
- Reduce cyst formation and normalise ovulation timing
- Support and prevent metabolic syndrome and associated compounding factors by supporting lipid profile through cardiovascular system and liver health
- Improve weight balance and moderate weight as required
- Stabilise blood sugar levels and reduce insulin resistance
- Support adrenal function and reduce impact of cortisol and prolactin to hormone balance.

SAMPLE DAILY DIET

BREAKFAST	
Oats with cinnamon and blueberries	Cinnamon has been shown to improve menstrual cyclicity in women with PCOS and may reduce insulin resistance in individuals with PCOS by increasing phosphatidylinositol 3-kinase activity in the insulin signalling pathway, potentiating insulin action. Both consumption of oats and blueberries is associated with increased insulin sensitivity.
LUNCH	
Quinoa with cinnamon, lentils and rocket	Improved menstrual regularity is noted when following a low-glycaemic index diet in PCOS. While some studies favour a reduced dietary ratio of carbohydrates to proteins, adequate carbohydrate from wholefood sources is imperative for normal pituitary pulsing of LH and FSH as well as manufacture of T3. Low carbohydrate diets may reduce levels of T3, problematic since T3 is required for ovulation to take place. Recommendations in PCOS are to increase wholegrain intake and to avoid refined carbohydrates. Examples of wholegrain foods include brown rice and quinoa.
DINNER	
Home-made coleslaw made from red cabbage, white cabbage and grated carrot dressed with apple cider vinegar Serve with brown lentil burgers and hummus	Women with PCOS have elevated circulating serum CRP levels and their endometrium demonstrates altered expression of genes important to the immune system and inflammation. Since lower vegetable consumption has been observed in individuals with PCOS ample antioxidant and anti-inflammatory vegetables should be consumed to downregulate inflammation. Replacing animal protein with protein from vegetable sources is associated with a lower risk of ovulatory infertility, thus this may also be a useful consideration in PCOS. Consumption of vinegar may help to restore ovulatory function through improving insulin sensitivity in PCOS patients.
SNACK	
Celery boats with ABC (almond, Brazil and cashew nut) spread Pumpkin seeds Spearmint tea	Low GI, fibre rich snack Zinc may help to reduce alopecia and hirsutism thus zinc-rich foods should be promoted. Displays anti-androgenic activity.

Specific nutrients required

B COMPLEX

All the B vitamins are essential for healthy function as they are required as a cofactor in numerous enzyme pathways, for metabolic functions as well as for energy production. They are especially important to assist with the breakdown of carbohydrates to energy, to help support the stress response as well as reduce elevated homocysteine levels in women with PCOS taking metformin.[264]

VITAMIN B_1

Thiamine, via its role in the enzyme system thiamine pyrophosphate, is required for almost every cellular reaction in the body; hence any deficiency will impact the whole body. Thiamine plays a key role in the metabolism of carbohydrates and fats[108] thus it may be useful to improve insulin sensitivity. Patients with a history of oral contraceptive use are at risk of thiamine deficiency, so supplementation may be required to restore levels. Increased glucose metabolism results in increased requirements of thiamine by the body.[265] Thiamine deficiency also leads to impaired glucose tolerance.

VITAMIN B_2

Riboflavin also plays a key role in metabolism via its role in the flavin adenine dinucleotide/flavin mononucleotide system, which is required for normal carbohydrate metabolism.

VITAMIN B_3

Vitamin B_3 is required for a multitude of functions within the body and has been used successfully to treat symptoms synonymous with PCOS, including elevated LDL cholesterol, triglycerides and lipoprotein.

VITAMIN B_5

Vitamin B_5 is required for the breakdown of fats and carbohydrates via its function in coenzyme A.

VITAMIN B_6

Pyridoxine has been shown to reduce elevated homocysteine associated with metformin therapy[264] and additionally is recommended to stabilise hormone cascades.

VITAMIN B_9

Supplementation with folic acid has been shown to reduce elevated levels of homocysteine in patients with PCOS.[266] Since homocysteine is a marker for cardiovascular disease homocysteine should be screened for in all patients with PCOS. Supplementation with 5 mg folate/day for 8 weeks in overweight or obese women with PCOS reduced plasma homocysteine and serum CRP levels compared to placebo and treatment with 1 mg folate/day. There was also an increase in total antioxidant capacity and glutathione levels.[267]

VITAMIN B_{12}

Vitamin B_{12} (2000 micrograms/day) has been shown to reduce elevated homocysteine associated with metformin therapy.[264]

CHROMIUM

Chromium has been shown to improve insulin sensitivity in patients with PCOS. Lydic et al observed that 1000 micrograms/day of chromium picolinate given to 5 patients with PCOS over a 2-month period improved glucose disposal.[268] These results are especially exciting when we consider that the patients did not implement any changes in diet. If we assume that their diets were suboptimal, even more profound results may be possible with implementation of a low-GI diet with adequate protein. A more recent RCT of 85 women showed that supplementation with 1000 micrograms of chromium picolinate daily (in 5 divided doses of 200 micrograms each) over 6 months resulted in a significant reduction in BMI and fasting serum insulin. After 5 months menstrual cycles were more regulated and there was an increased chance of ovulation in the intervention group.[269]

ESSENTIAL FATTY ACIDS (EFAs)

Essential fatty acids have shown beneficial effects with regard to improved insulin sensitivity and anti-inflammatory properties. Non-alcoholic fatty liver disease has been linked to PCOS but supplementation with omega-3 fatty acids has been shown to have a beneficial effect on liver fat content and other cardiovascular risk factors in women with PCOS. Supplementation with omega-3 fatty acids (4 g/day of omega-3 fatty acids in the form of 4 × 1000 mg capsules of 56% docosahexaenoic acid and 27% eicosapentaenoic acid) has been shown to decrease liver fat, triglycerides and blood pressure in women with PCOS over an 8-week period.[270]

Studies have produced mixed results however with regards to EFAs and reproductive or metabolic abnormalities in PCOS and further rigorous trials are needed to establish efficacy in areas such as insulin regulation.[271]

MAGNESIUM

Low serum and body magnesium levels have been found in individuals with PCOS irrespective of steroid hormone concentrations compared with that of controls.[272] Given that hypomagnesaemia has been proposed as a possible underlying common mechanism of insulin resistance in a number of conditions, supplementation with magnesium would appear to be beneficial.

CONTROLLED-RELEASE ALPHA LIPOIC ACID

Alpha lipoic acid is a potent antioxidant that has been demonstrated to improve glycaemic control and improve insulin sensitivity[273] thus suggesting benefits for PCOS. Supplementation (600 mg twice daily) in lean, non-diabetic patients with PCOS over a period of approximately 4 months has been found to improve insulin sensitivity by 13.5% and lower triglycerides.[274] Two patients not taking the oral contraceptive pill experienced an increase in the number of menstrual cycles. Interestingly in this study treatment with alpha lipoic acid was not associated with an increase in plasma antioxidant capacity or a reduction in plasma lipid oxidation.

VITAMIN E

Oxidative stress and depletion of antioxidants have been suggested to play a role in the pathogenesis of PCOS by contributing to ovarian mesenchymal hyperplasia. Vitamin E via its antioxidant properties has been observed in experimental studies[275] to inhibit these free pro-oxidant constituents, counteracting this growth and highlighting the protective role of vitamin E in PCOS.

ZINC

Zinc plays a key role in modulating insulin in the body. Clinical studies assessing the effects of zinc supplementation (30 mg/day for 1 month) in obese individuals with insulin resistance have shown improvements in insulin sensitivity[276] while a cohort study observed that higher intakes of zinc were associated with a decreased risk of type 2 diabetes.[277] Acknowledging that zinc is involved in a number of enzyme systems within the body, its role in insulin sensitivity is likely to be only one of many ways in which zinc can favourably impact the pathogenesis of PCOS. For example, supplementation with zinc may also be useful for managing concurrent symptoms, such as acne associated with PCOS.

VITAMIN D

There is some evidence to suggest that vitamin D supplementation might be beneficial in PCOS for improved follicular development and regulation of the menstrual cycle; however, further rigorous trials are needed.[278] One study showed that 8 weeks of vitamin D_3 supplementation increased circulating soluble receptors for AGEs, which bind circulating AGEs. This is one mechanism by which vitamin D exerts a protective effect in PCOS.[279] Vitamin D deficiency is common in women with PCOS; some estimates indicate that 70–85% of women with PCOS may be vitamin D deficient, which may contribute to insulin resistance and obesity.[271] Studies have found that 8 weeks of supplementation with vitamin D (50 000 IU/day) and calcium (1000 mg/day) together had beneficial effects on inflammatory markers, total antioxidant capacity, serum insulin levels, insulin resistance markers, insulin sensitivity markers, triglyceride levels and VLDL-cholesterol levels in overweight vitamin D deficient women with PCOS. The results were significantly greater than treatment with either vitamin D or calcium alone.[280,281] Low levels of 25(OH) vitamin D have been associated with increased levels of autoimmune thyroid disease in PCOS.[282]

INOSITOL

Two isomers of inositol (myo-inositol and D-chiro-inositol) are mediators of insulin action. Myo-inositol is a nutrient belonging to vitamin B complex and is found in various foods. The highest concentrations are found in fresh fruits and vegetables, beans, grains, nuts and seeds. Especially high contents are found in almonds, walnuts and Brazil nuts, and oats and bran contain higher concentrations than other grains.[283] It can also be produced endogenously from glucose. There is some evidence to suggest that it may help to regulate metabolic factors in women with PCOS.[271] Myo-inositol potentially improves the metabolic profile in PCOS via improved insulin resistance, whereas D-chiro-inositol seems to have a positive effect on hyperandrogenism, although studies in D-chiro-inositol have produced mixed results.

SELENIUM

In a randomised double-blind placebo-controlled trial consisting of 64 women with PCOS, women were assigned to either the intervention group ($n = 32$) which received 200 micrograms selenium daily, or the control group ($n = 32$) which received placebo, for 8 weeks. Results showed that the pregnancy rate was higher in the intervention group, and alopecia and acne were decreased compared to the control group. The selenium group also showed decreased DHEA and CRP levels and decreased hirsutism.[275]

DOSAGE REQUIREMENTS

The dosage requirements listed below are based on adult doses that have been reported in the literature and clinical review:

- B complex (all B vitamins) high-dose combination, preferably activated forms
  - Thiamine 20–40 mg/day
  - Riboflavin 20–40 mg/day
  - Niacinamide 50–100 mg/day
  - Pantothenic acid 150–300 mg/day
  - Pyridoxine 20–60 mg/day
  - Folate as folinic acid or L-5MTHF 500–1000 micrograms/day
  - Hydroxo- or methylcobalamin 500–1000 micrograms/day
  - Choline 50–100 mg/day
  - Inositol 50–100 mg/day
  - Biotin 250–500 micrograms/day
- Chromium 250–750 micrograms/day
- Essential fatty acids: 4 g/day total omega-3 fatty acids (56% DHA and 27% EPA)[270]
- Magnesium 250–750 mg/day
- R-alpha lipoic acid 1200 mg/day
- Vitamin E 400–800 IU/day
- Zinc 30–60 mg/day
- Vitamin D 0.5 micrograms/200 IU (RDI). Up to 6000 IU/day to correct a deficiency[284]
- Myo-inositol 4g/day[271]
- Selenium 200 micrograms/day[275].

HERBAL MEDICINE

Herbal medicine therapeutic objectives

- Improve cell sensitivity to insulin and reduce resistance
- Restore HPA axis communication and reduce cortisol secretion
- Improve female hormone profile and reduce androgen levels
- Reduce cortisol and prolactin levels (if elevated)
- Support optimal hepatobiliary function to address lipid profile abnormalities.

Herbal medicine classes

Herbal medicine classes used to treat PCOS are listed in Table 18.21.

Specific herbal medicines

ACTAEA RACEMOSA (BLACK COHOSH)

Polycystic ovary syndrome is characterised by altered luteinising hormone secretion and thus may be assisted with *Actaea racemosa*, which is known to reduce LH and subsequently androgens.[28] A prospective, randomised controlled study investigated the role of *C. racemosa* (Klimadynon, Bionorica) in women with PCOS. The trial involved 100 women. The intervention group ($n = 50$) received *C. racemosa* 20 mg daily for 10 days, starting on the second day of their cycle, for three consecutive cycles.

TABLE 18.21 Herbal medicine classes used to treat PCOS

Class	Action
Adaptogen and adrenal restorative	Improve stress response; improve HPA axis and subsequent steroid hormone pathway
Hormonal modulator	Herbal medicine specific to each hormonal requirement should be prescribed to modify the cascades and hormonal balance; for example, FSH stimulation, LH depression, androgen depression
Hypolipidaemic	Reduce lipids and improve cholesterol synthesis, metabolism and subsequent steroid hormone pathway; regulate glycaemic control
Hypoglycaemic	Stabilise glycaemic control and optimise pancreatic function; weight reduction
Hepatic, cholagogue	Improve hepatobiliary function for cholesterol synthesis and metabolism, hormone regulation and secretion
Lymphatic and anticystic	Assist in reduction of cyst formation and support elimination of wastes

The control group received 50 mg clomiphene citrate twice daily, for 5 days starting on the second day of their cycle, for three consecutive cycles. The results showed significant positive changes in LH levels and FHS/LH ratio in the *C. racemosa* group. Progesterone levels were increased from the first treatment cycle (indicating improved ovulation), as was endometrial thickness.[285] A 2014 study of 194 patients found that administering clomiphene citrate in conjunction with *C. racemosa* improved ovulation outcomes and pregnancy rates. All patients were administered 150 mg clomiphene per day from days 3–7 of their cycle. In addition, the intervention group was administered 120 mg *C. racemosa* (Klimadynon, Bionorica) per day, from day 1 until the day of the pregnancy test or the start of the next cycle. Both groups received luteal phase support in the form of oral utrogestan (micronised progesterone) (50 micrograms per day) starting from the second day after hCG injection (Pregnyl) until the start of menstruation, a negative pregnancy test or the end of 12 weeks' gestation. Administration of *C. racemosa* was associated with lower mid-cycle LH, higher serum oestradiol and progesterone in the second half, as well as significantly thicker endometrium and shorter cycles.[286]

CINNAMOMUM SPP. (CINNAMON)

Managing insulin resistance and subsequently compensatory hyperinsulinaemia associated with PCOS is imperative to aid the resolution of the syndrome as well as to prevent complications such as development of type 2 diabetes. *Cinnamomum* spp. contains polyphenols found to stimulate autophosphorylation of the insulin receptor and inhibit protein tyrosine phosphatase I,[287] thereby improving insulin sensitivity. Wang et al[287] conducted a small pilot study involving 15 women with PCOS with either oligomenorrhoea or amenorrhoea. The women each received one capsule containing 333 mg of cinnamon extract to be taken three times daily for 8 weeks. Following oral administration of *Cinnamomum* spp. extract there was a significant reduction in fasting glucose as well as insulin resistance thought to be mediated through an increase in glucose utilisation. This highlights the efficacy of *Cinnamomum* spp. for management of insulin resistance associated with PCOS and provides a rationale for further studies using a larger sample to be conducted. A study of 45 women with PCOS found that *Cinnamomum* spp. supplementation (1.5 g/day, 500 mg t.d.s. for 6 months) improved the frequency of menstrual cycles compared to placebo. The study did not find any changes in measures of insulin resistance or serum androgen levels in either the intervention or placebo groups.[288]

GLYCYRRHIZA GLABRA (LIQUORICE)

Excess androgens are characteristic of PCOS so anti-androgen botanicals such as *Glycyrrhiza glabra* are indicated. *Glycyrrhiza glabra* affects androgen metabolism by blocking the effects of 17β-hydroxysteroid dehydrogenase and C17,20 lyase while stimulating the effects of aromatase, reducing serum testosterone.[289] Because of this it may be particularly useful as an adjuvant therapy of hirsutism associated with PCOS.[289]

GYMNEMA SYLVESTRE (GYMNEMA)

Acknowledging the link between PCOS and insulin resistance, administration with *Gymnema sylvestre*, a botanical that displays blood sugar-regulating properties, is highly indicated. As yet, no studies could be found assessing the effects of *Gymnema* in PCOS, but *Gymnema* has demonstrated efficacy in a number of human clinical trials in patients with diabetes, where it has been shown to reduce blood sugar, therefore it is likely to be of help in PCOS.[290]

PAEONIA LACTIFLORA (PEONY)

Paeonia has been shown to positively influence low progesterone, reduce elevated androgens (testosterone) and acts to modulate oestrogen and prolactin.[28]

Administration of a traditional herbal medicine called shakuyaku-kanzo-to, a decoction of *Glycyrrhiza glabra* and *Paeonia lactiflora*, has undergone a substantial amount of research particularly with regard to PCOS patients with infertility. Shakuyaku-kanzo-to has been found to lower plasma testosterone levels in 18/20 patients[291] and increase fertility, resulting in successful conception, as well as reducing LH:FSH ratios.[292]

PHYTOLACCA AMERICANA (PHYTOLACCA)

Phytolacca americana is a botanical native to North America that has traditionally been used for its effects on the mucous membranes, particularly where there is ulceration and hard, lymphatic enlargements.[8] In Western herbal medicine *Phytolacca americana* may be used for ovarian pain and infection where its lymphatic properties assist in the removal of wastes[129] such as the cysts in PCOS.

SCHISANDRA CHINENSIS (SCHISANDRA)

Schisandra chinensis works on both phase 1 and phase 2 liver metabolism where it promotes detoxification and healthy liver function. Liver support is required in PCOS to aid the clearance of sex hormones from the body and to prevent them from recirculating within the body. *Schisandra chinensis* functions as an adaptogen which is also likely to be helpful since stress is involved in the aetiology of PCOS.

THUJA OCCIDENTALIS (THUJA)

As yet there are no clinical trials assessing the effects of *Thuja occidentalis* in PCOS, but traditionally it has been used for its ability to remove growths from the body and assist in the clearance of catarrhal diseases of the female reproductive organs.[8] Thuja is described by the Eclectics as efficacious for removing fungus granulations (hardened, small masses of tissue) and was documented to destroy them in some instances. For this reason many practitioners choose to administer *Thuja occidentalis* as an adjuvant herb in PCOS, where it appears to exert a cyst-reducing action.

TRIBULUS TERRESTRIS (TRIBULUS)

Tribulus assists the PCOS patient by stimulating the release of FSH. When you consider a PCOS patient it is beneficial to reflect on the acronym provided in the discussion on menstruation — FELOP. This acronym supports the explanation that to initiate ovulation, the body's production of FSH needs to be stimulated to reduce the raised LH/FSH ratio.

Results of human and animal clinical trials support the FSH-stimulating prescription. In one study, 750 mg active furastanol (TLSE) per day for 5 days was given to women and was shown to increase FSH and oestradiol when compared with baseline women. The steroidal saponins are thought to bind to and stimulate (weakly) the hypothalamic oestrogen receptor sites.[293]

NB: Tribulus leaf standardised extract (TLSE) is a product obtained from the aerial parts of *Tribulus terrestris*, which contain mainly saponins of the furostanol type (not less than 45%, calculated as protodioscin). It was developed in Bulgaria from Mediterranean varieties of *Tribulus*. *Tribulus* concentrated extract equivalent to fucosterol saponins (protodiosci) is recommended generally in lieu of liquid preparations to obtain the sufficient doses required.

VITEX AGNUS-CASTUS (CHASTE TREE BERRY)

Since hypothalamic–pituitary–ovarian imbalance is implicated in PCOS, *Vitex agnus-castus*, which is an HPO regulator, is likely to be of benefit. A number of patients with PCOS also display hyperprolactinaemia[294] and an altered response to progesterone,[295] therefore the progesterogenic activity of *Vitex agnus-castus* and its ability to regulate prolactin will further assist in the management of PCOS symptoms. A 2016 study ($n = 70$) found that a combined low-dose oral contraceptive and *Vitex agnus-castus* were both as effective in normalising the menstrual cycle and reducing DHEA-S. Neither of the treatments had any effect on testosterone or prolactin levels.[296]

TRIGONELLA FOENUM-GRAECUM (FENUGREEK SEED)

An open-label non-randomised trial of 50 women with PCOS demonstrated that administration of a novel fenugreek seed extract enriched in furostanolic saponins resulted in a significant reduction in cyst size (with 36% of participants showing complete dissolution of the cysts) and the normalisation of regular menstrual cycles. The novel extract (1 g/day) was administered daily over a period of 3 months. Results showed significant increases in LH and FSH compared to baseline.[297] This is a preliminary study in a very specific formula and results are very promising. Further research is required.

CAMELLIA SINENSIS (GREEN TEA)

Green tea may have an anti-androgen effect due to the actions of epigallocatechins which inhibit the 5-alpha-reductase conversion of normal testosterone into DHT.[298] As yet no randomised controlled trials have been conducted into the effectiveness of green tea in androgen dependent conditions.

LIFESTYLE RECOMMENDATIONS

Smoking

Encourage patients who smoke to stop smoking.

Weight management

Clinically, there are two types of PCOS patients — those who are overweight and those who are normal weight. Dr John Eden, a reproductive endocrinologist at the Royal Hospital for Women Sydney, believes that women with PCOS could have a more direct evolutionary advantage in some special circumstances. The premise is that in times of starvation, survival of the species requires that some women can ovulate when their weight is optimal or even lower than optimal. As such, it is theorised that optimal weight is a crucial component for ideal ovulation.

Weight loss

The association between excessive weight, hyperandrogenaemia, impaired glucose tolerance, menstrual abnormalities and infertility emphasises the need to address lifestyle issues in women with PCOS, particularly nutrition and exercise.[167] Realistic and achievable weight loss can be set to improve an individual's reproductive and metabolic fitness because only a small (2–5%) reduction of body weight can greatly improve these indices.[299]

A small reduction in body weight was sufficient to restore ovulation and increase insulin sensitivity by 71% in obese anovulatory women.[300] Weight loss also increases SHBG concentration, reduces testosterone concentration and androgenic stimulation of the skin, improves menstrual function and conception rates and reduces miscarriage rates.[301] Although drugs to increase insulin sensitivity in diabetics are used to treat women with PCOS, weight reduction is more effective and should be the initial treatment of obese women with this disorder.[302] Although acute weight loss can be achieved with severe kilojoule restriction, long-term weight management is rare, and acute weight loss potentially has dangerous effects for reproduction.[303]

Exercise

Encourage and recommend daily exercise of a minimum of 30 minutes per day to assist weight loss and provide stress relief. Exercise is associated with lower depression in women with PCOS and being more active may offer mental health benefits in managing PCOS. Women with PCOS are more likely to express a lack of confidence about maintaining physical activity.[304] Prescription and advice need to be individualised and supportive.

Stress management

Due to the interaction between endocrine pathways and subsequent effects of stress on HPA/HPO axes, it is imperative to recommend stress management practices. Exercise may be the best recommendation due to its dual benefit, but meditation, yoga, breathing exercises and sufficient sleep and rest are also beneficial recommendations.

A 2011 Cochrane review found evidence that a healthy lifestyle (healthy diet, exercise and maintaining a healthy weight) reduces body weight and abdominal fat, reduces testosterone and improves hair growth and insulin resistance in women with PCOS.[305] An 8-week mindfulness stress management program in women with PCOS significantly reduced stress, anxiety and depression scores, lowered salivary cortisol levels, and increased life satisfaction and quality of life scores in the intervention group ($n = 23$) versus the control group ($n = 15$). The program included 30 minutes of daily mindfulness breathing exercises and diaphragm breathing exercises.[306]

CASE STUDY

OVERVIEW

KJ, a 31-year-old woman, presented with amenorrhoea for the previous 9 months. Her contraceptive history showed contraceptive pill usage from the age of 16 to 25, with subsequent introduction of depot medroxyprogesterone acetate (DMPA) (age 25–27) and then etonogestrel implant from age 27 to 30. She embarked on treatment as she wished to conceive within the next year but wanted to get her health sorted over the next few months.

Menarche was at 14 years and initial contraceptive pill was for androgenisation (acne and hirsutism) and eventually followed for contraceptive purposes.

On presentation she was still experiencing periodic cystic acne primarily on her back and shoulders as well as simple acne on her nose, forehead and chin.

CLINICAL EXAMINATION

- Height 162 cm
- Weight 76 kg
- BMI 29 (overweight)

TREATMENT PROTOCOL

INITIAL APPOINTMENT

Initial appointment consisted of assessment and referral for pathology investigations. Patient was also requested to complete a dietary and lifestyle diary. Education focused on the importance of dietary and lifestyle modifications that will be required with specific mention of weight modifications.

SECOND APPOINTMENT

Follow-up appointment was held 1 week later.

INVESTIGATIONS

Referral for assessments following the initial appointment revealed the following.

Transabdominal and transvaginal ultrasound

Polycystic ovaries (both right and left) — ovarian volume greater than 8 cm^3, number of follicles in left ovary >6 mm, in left ovary >5 mm, increased echogenicity of cervical OS.

CASE STUDY CONTINUED

Lipid profile

- Elevated total cholesterol 6.2 mmol/L
- Elevated triglycerides 2.3 mmol/L
- Elevated LDL 3.7 mmol/L
- Low HDL 0.9 mmol/L

Others

- FBC: NAD
- Vitamin D (25-hydroxy): 27 nmol/L
- Urinary iodine: 44 micrograms/L
- Hormone profile: androstenedione: 9.1 nmol/L
- FAI: 5.4%
- SHBG: 134 nmol/L
- FSH: 2.1 U/L
- LH: 18.0 U/L
- P4: 0.2 nmol/L
- PRL: 499 mIU/L
- Sugar profile: fasting glucose: 6.1 mmol/L
- HbA1c: 5.9%
- Insulin: 14 U/L
- Iron studies: ferritin 74 microgram/L
- TSH: 1.94 mIU/L

HERBAL MEDICINE

Herbal medicine	Ratio	Quantity	Justification
Gymnema sylvestre	1:1	80 mL	Blood sugar-regulating, pancreatic trophorestorative
Paeonia lactiflora	1:2	70 mL	Hormonal modulation, reduction of androgens
Glycyrrhiza glabra	STD ext	30 mL	Blood sugar-regulating, hormonal modulation, reduction of androgens
Vitex agnus-castus	1:2	40 mL	Hormonal modulator, cycle stimulant, lower prolactin and balance progesterone

TOTAL: 220 mL. Dose: 7.5 mL b.i.d.

ADJUNCT

Tribulus terrestris (tribulus) extract equivalent to dry herb (aerial parts) standardised to contain furostanol saponins as protodioscin 110 mg (9.0 g). Dose: 1 tab b.i.d. Justification: FSH stimulation to initiate cycle.

NUTRITIONAL MEDICINE

Dietary

- Consume a diet of 30% complex carbohydrates, 40% protein and 30% lipids
- Avoid alcohol, caffeine, and nutritional stressors
- Encourage dietary sources of essential fatty acids
- Follow insulin resistance dietary principles and avoid refined carbohydrates and sugar
- Increase consumption of cinnamon, fibre and flaxseed oil in the diet.

CASE STUDY CONTINUED

SUPPLEMENTAL

Nutrient	Dosage	Justification
Chromium	800 micrograms/day	Improved insulin sensitivity, weight loss and blood sugar regulation
Alpha lipoic acid	400 mg/day initially and increased to 600 mg/day	Blood sugar regulation, protection against diabetic complications, antioxidant
B complex (activated forms)	2 caps b.i.d.	Metabolism of carbohydrates, glucose metabolism, management and prevention of complications, hormonal regulation
Magnesium	1000 mg/day in divided doses	Improved insulin signalling and blood sugar regulation, energy production, lipid lowering
Zinc	60 mg/day	Hormonal regulation, clearance of acne
Vitamin D_3	5000 IU/day	To address deficiency and use positive blood sugar, mood and immune effects
Iodine	300 micrograms/day	Address deficiency and support thyroid function and metabolism

Lifestyle/education

- Daily exercise of 60 minutes per day
- Reduce stress in life and ensure 8 h of sleep per night.

UTERINE FIBROIDS

Epidemiology

Uterine fibroids, or leiomyomas, are the most common benign tumours in women in their reproductive years, and the most common tumours of the female reproductive tract.[307] A review by Okolo[307] reports on early studies which suggested that 1 in 4 women of reproductive age may have fibroids (diagnosed clinically), but it has been suggested that fibroids are typically underreported as many individuals remain asymptomatic. Histology has revealed more than double that clinical incidence. Clearly, the actual prevalence of fibroids is likely to be much higher.[308] This is further confirmed by autopsy reports which reveal that 1 in 2 women have uterine fibroids when examined postmortem (see Fig. 18.7).[309] Recent literature has estimated the prevalence of uterine fibroids as high as affecting 70%–80% of women over their lifetime.[310] In the US they account for 30% of all hysterectomies among women aged 18–44.[311]

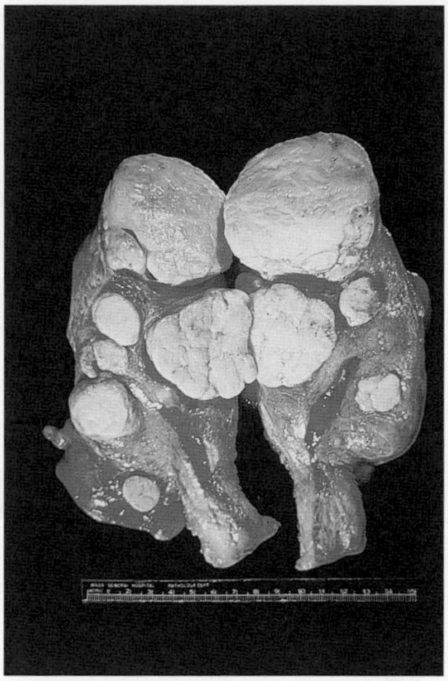

FIGURE 18.7 Uterine fibroids.

Source: Katz V. Comprehensive gynecology. 5th edn. Maryland Heights: Mosby; 2007.

Classification

On the basis of mitotic count, nuclear atypia and other morphological features, uterine smooth muscle tumours can be classified as leiomyomas, smooth muscle tumours of uncertain malignant potential (STUMPs) or leiomyosarcomas (LMSs).

Uterine fibroids are classified according to their location (see Fig. 18.8 and Table 18.22).

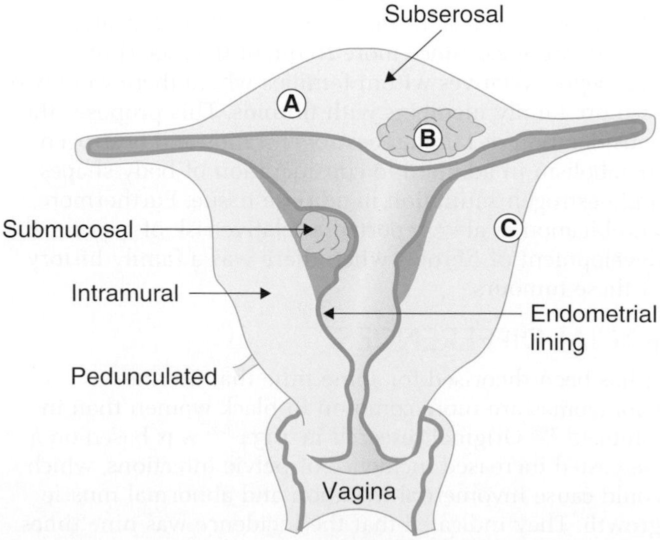

FIGURE 18.8 Location of uterine fibroids. **A**, **B** and **C** represent common locations requiring a combination of descriptive terms.

Source: Stewart E. Uterine fibroids. Lancet 2001; 357:293–298.

TABLE 18.22 Uterine fibroid classification according to location

Submucosal	Just under the endometrium
Intramural	Within the uterine muscle wall
Subserosal	From the outer wall of the uterus
Interligamentous	In the cervix between the two layers of the broad ligament
Pedunculated	On a stalk, either submucosal or subserous

TABLE 18.23 Factors that affect the risk of uterine fibroid tumours

Increased risk	Decreased risk
40 years or older	Smoking
Black race	In excess of five pregnancies
Family history of uterine fibroid tumours	Postmenopausal
Nulliparity	Oral contraceptive use over a prolonged period
Obesity	Use of depot medroxyprogesterone acetate

Source: Adapted from Evans P, Brunsell S. Uterine fibroid tumours: diagnosis and treatment. Am Fam Physician 2007;10(75):1503–8.

Aetiology

See Table 18.23 for summation.

FAMILY HISTORY

Vikhlyaeva et al[312] reported a familial predisposition in uterine leiomyomas. In their overview, they indicated that fibroids were 2.2 times more frequent (p <0.001) in first-degree relatives within families where there were two or more family members with fibroids. This proposes the consideration of familial oestrogen ratios and oestrogen metabolism in addition to consideration of body shapes and oestrogen saturation in adipose tissue. Furthermore, Lumbiganon et al[313] reported a relative risk of 3.47 for the development of fibroids when there was a family history of these tumours.

RACIAL DIFFERENCES

It has been theorised for some time that uterine leiomyomas are more common in black women than in white.[314–316] Original research in 1934[317] was based on a suggested increased incidence of pelvic infections, which could cause myometrial irritation and abnormal muscle growth. They indicated that the incidence was nine times higher in black versus white women. In 1996, Kjerrulff et al[318] studied 409 black women undergoing hysterectomy for non-cancerous conditions and compared the findings with those of 836 white women also undergoing hysterectomy for similar indications. They reported that 89% of the black women had fibroids compared with 59% of the white women. They also discovered that the black women having hysterectomies had significantly larger and a greater number of fibroids and that the fibroids caused significantly greater pelvic pain and significantly worse anaemia compared with the white women. Fibroids were also diagnosed and operated on at a younger age in significantly more black compared with white women. However, another study concluded that in both black and white populations women develop uterine fibroid tumours before menopause and that uterine fibroid tumours develop in black women at earlier ages than in white women.[319]

RADIATION

Review of those exposed to atomic bomb radiation indicates that there is an increased incidence of fibroids. Two papers[320,321] reported a dose–response relationship between the incidence of fibroids and atomic bomb radiation exposure. Both studies reviewed 1190 Hiroshima atomic bomb survivors using ultrasound and reported a significant dose–response relationship for the prevalence of uterine leiomyomas.

ENVIRONMENTAL TOXINS

Neonatal exposure to endocrine-disrupting compounds can reprogram normal physiological responses and increase disease susceptibility, including uterine fibroids, later in life.[322] A study of 495 women found significantly higher urinary concentrations of certain nonpersistant chemicals (BPA, phthalates, benzophenone-type UV filters) in those with fibroids compared to those without; however, an elevated odds ratio of association was not established.[323] An exploratory study found that persistent organic pollutant levels, in particular polychlorinated biphenyls (PCBs) may be associated with fibroids. The association is stronger with PCB levels in visceral fat: the same association was not found with serum levels.[324]

A prospective cohort study of US female nurses (the Nurses' Health Study II) assessed air pollution exposure and found that while there was no direct association with increased risk of uterine fibroids for exposures of PM10 (less than 10 microns) or PM10–2.5 (between 10 and 2.5 microns), chronic exposure to PM2.5 (2.5 microns) may be associated with a modest increased risk.[325]

NULLIPARITY

There is a definite association between nulliparity and the incidence of fibroids and this is confirmed in countless studies and research papers. Fibroids are believed to be significantly less common in parous women and more common in women who have undergone termination of pregnancy.[313,326,327]

The relative risk of fibroids has been shown to decrease with an increasing number of term pregnancies. The risk is one-quarter in women with five term pregnancies (live births and stillbirths) compared with women with no term pregnancies.[328] There was no reduction in risk reported with incomplete pregnancies but in fact a small, although not significant, increase in risk.[328] Interestingly, in one paper, Parazzini et al[326] showed that the risk of fibroids was also reduced with the number of induced abortions but not with the number of spontaneous abortions. They also showed that a history of infertility increased the relative risk of fibroid development two-fold in comparison with women who did not report such a history.

The underlying risk factor between parity and fibroid development is most probably the continuous oestradiol secretion, uninterrupted by pregnancy and lactation, or the increased number of menstrual cycles in a reproductive life. It is an increased number of cycles rather than an increase in serum oestradiol concentration per cycle that is the risk factor, as it has been shown that women with fibroids have circulating oestradiol concentrations similar to those of women who do not have fibroids.[329]

OBESITY

Weight is strongly related to the risk of developing uterine fibroids. Women weighing 70 kg or more have an almost three-fold risk of developing fibroids compared with women weighing less than 50 kg.[309] There are two possible reasons for this weight-related risk:

- There is an increased peripheral conversion by fat aromatase of circulating androgens to oestrogen in obese women
- In such women, there is a decrease in the hepatic production of sex hormone-binding globulin (SHBG), a carrier for oestrogen. This lowered concentration of SHBG may result in higher levels of 'free', physiologically active oestrogen.[330]

Therefore, obesity confers a relative hyperoestrogenic state, which may predispose to fibroid growth.

ACCESS TO HEALTHCARE

There is another opinion that factors such as greater access to healthcare, higher education, frequent Pap smears and increased use of the combined oral contraceptive (COC) pill are all suggestive of greater investigation and detection thus highlighting the increased incidence in this population.

Overview

Uterine fibroids, or leiomyomas, are the most common tumours in women during the reproductive years. In most countries, they are the most frequent indication for hysterectomy in premenopausal women and therefore present a major public health issue.

Although often asymptomatic, up to 50% of uterine fibroids cause symptoms severe enough to warrant therapy, and surgery is the standard treatment. Fibroid growth is stimulated by oestrogen and gonadotrophin-releasing hormone agonists, which induce a state of hypoestrogenism.[331]

The cause of uterine fibroids remains poorly understood. Increases in local oestradiol concentration within the fibroid itself may play a role in the cause and growth. Concentrations of oestrogen receptors in fibroid tissue are higher than in the surrounding myometrium but lower than in the endometrium.

Pathogenesis

Leiomyomas are the most common female reproductive tract tumours. They are probably of unicellular origin[332] and their growth rate is influenced by oestrogen, growth hormone and progesterone.[333] They consist of smooth muscle cells and connective tissue. Although studies have not clarified the exact process, uterine fibroid tumours arise during the reproductive years and tend to enlarge during pregnancy and regress after menopause. The use of oestrogen agonists is associated with an increased incidence of fibroid tumours,[334] and growth hormone appears to act synergistically with oestradiol in affecting the growth of fibroid tumours. Conversely, progesterone appears to inhibit their growth. As fibroids often demonstrate a growth spurt in the perimenopausal years, it is likely that during oopause the oestrogen displacement from the anovulatory cycles stimulates their growth.

SIGNS AND SYMPTOMS

The majority of fibroids are asymptomatic, but symptoms that are encountered include:

- Vague feeling of discomfort, pressure, congestion, bloating, heaviness in abdomen
- Abdominal enlargement
- Pelvic or urinary obstructive symptoms such as dyspareunia or polyuria
- Backache
- Abnormal bleeding: menorrhagia, metrorrhagia (occurs in >30% of women with fibroids)
- Pregnancy loss (miscarriage)
- Infertility.

COMPLICATIONS

Menorrhagia and anaemia

Abnormal bleeding is the most common presenting symptom for both premenopausal and postmenopausal women with myomas. There is no bleeding pattern that is diagnostic of myomas. Premenopausal women can have regular or irregular bleeding and can develop menorrhagia and/or metrorrhagia, although characteristically most myomas cause menorrhagia.[335]

Submucosal tumours are often cited as a cause of menorrhagia, but there is no evidence that the endometrium over submucosal tumours differs from that overlying other areas of the uterus.[336]

Thirty per cent of women with fibroids have been reported to have menstrual abnormalities, most often menorrhagia.[337] Menorrhagia can be underestimated or ignored and it is imperative that clinicians consider the physical, nutritional, emotional, mental and social impact of heavy blood loss. Because of the potential for metrorrhagia, the impact of menstrual loss cannot be understated.

Fibroid-related menorrhagia can be torrential, causing a rapid fall in haemoglobin levels. The major medical consequence of menorrhagia is anaemia (Hb <100 g/L).

Menorrhagia is the most common cause of anaemia in developed countries and is believed to be higher in women with fibroid-associated menorrhagia than in menorrhagia due to other causes.[338]

Women who have menorrhagia are often concerned about failure of their sanitary items, making them housebound on their heaviest days. They often prefer loss of income to social embarrassment. This causes considerable disruption to their lifestyles.

Cancer development?

Fibroid progression to cancer growth is highly controversial and debatable with a number of conflicting studies. In most women it is highly unlikely and is believed to be of concern in those with significant infiltrate and endometrial hyperplasia. In patients with significantly enlarged fibroids, rapidly growing fibroids or those with endometrial hyperplasia it is imperative to regularly assess lactate dehydrogenase (LDH) as a predictive warning sign for cancer development or infiltration.

DIFFERENTIAL DIAGNOSIS

- Ovarian neoplasm
- Endometrial carcinoma
- Fallopian tube or ovarian region abscess
- Tubo-ovarian inflammatory mass
- Diverticulum from the colon (inflammatory mass)
- Pelvic kidney
- Endometriosis
- Adenomyosis
- Congenital anomalies
- Uterine sarcoma
- Pelvic adhesions
- Retroperitoneal tumours.

NATUROPATHIC DIAGNOSIS

Naturopathic practitioners will rely on allopathic diagnosis in the first instance. In addition, it is important to consider a number of holistic considerations to review and prepare management of the patient.

Oestrogen exposure

Uterine fibroids do not have hyper- or hyposecretion of reproductive hormones, but have hyperactivity of oestrogen receptors coupled with a genetic predisposition.[339] The relevance of the endocrine changes is confirmed by the clinical effectiveness of hormonal treatments. In order to establish the correct treatment approach in gynaecological disorders, it is important to understand the endocrine pathophysiology and thoroughly assess endocrine disruptors throughout the woman's life. Furthermore, genetic influences and predispositions cannot be underestimated. Review of the extent of oestrogen exposure throughout the lifetime of the patient is beneficial (Table 18.24).

TABLE 18.24 Oestrogen exposure

Endogenous sources	Early age menarche Parity (or gravida) and age of earliest conception Cycle details — length of follicular vs luteal phase duration Obesity — especially location and weight distribution
Exogenous sources	Environmental exposure (plastics, pesticides, tap water) Synthetic hormone exposure (OCP, HRT) Dietary (dairy, meat, processed soy products)

Current and previous health

- Hepatobiliary health and oestrogen clearance and metabolism
- Hypertension and lipid profile
- Pelvic inflammatory disease
- IUD use (especially older copper-based types).

GENETICS

- Maternal oestrogen metabolism and clearance especially preconceptually, during pregnancy and as she matured
- Body shape and weight distribution
- Genetic predisposition to nutritional pathway defects or polymorphisms. Oestrogen (*ERβ* TC genotype) and progesterone (*PGR* GA/AA genotype) receptor gene polymorphisms have been found to be strongly correlated with uterine fibroid onset and development[340]
- Cancer genetics.

Investigations

Investigations for uterine fibroids are listed in Table 18.25.

SPECIFIC NATUROPATHIC INVESTIGATIONS

Case taking

Thorough medical history is essential, with appropriate menstrual cycle questioning to accurately assess and determine reproductive health. Assessment considering the variables discussed in the section on naturopathic diagnosis should be encouraged and include oestrogen (endogenous and exogenous), current and previous health and genetics.

Menstrual symptom diary

Use of a menstrual symptom diary (see Appendix 18.1 at the end of the book) is beneficial to assess the woman's cycle holistically and comprehensively. Symptothermal charting is also beneficial to assess follicular phase length compared with luteal phase. This is not imperative in considering the development of the disease but would provide information as to risk factor history. Historical review would be more appropriate. A menopausal symptom chart is also beneficial for perimenopausal patients.

Female hormone profile (saliva)

Female hormone profiles can monitor changes in hormonal status over the course of the menstrual cycle by

TABLE 18.25 Investigations used for uterine fibroids

Assessment	Comment and indication
FBC and iron studies	Essential to eliminate concurrent anaemia
LFT	Essential to assess abnormal cell growth and cancer risk (specifically LDH)
Cancer markers (CA125, CA19)	Controversial, assess cancer risk
Pelvic palpation	Presumptive diagnosis as uterus will often feel enlarged or with irregular edges. Formal diagnosis requires further investigation to eliminate other conditions
Transvaginal and transabdominal ultrasonography	Lowest sensitivity and specificity, noninvasive nature and cost-efficiency. Evaluates size and position of tumours. It is important to compare and contrast previous ultrasound reports at the same time of the menstrual cycle
Magnetic resonance imaging (MRI)	Preferred when precise myoma mapping is required (usually for surgical purposes), but it is the most expensive modality for evaluating fibroid tumours. Evaluates size and position of tumours
Sonohysterography	Used to evaluate the extent of submucosal fibroid tumours, but relatively invasive
Hysteroscopy	Used to evaluate the extent of submucosal fibroid tumours, but relatively invasive
Laparoscopy	Increased visualisation for submucosal pedunculated, intramural and subserous fibroids, invasive. Important if visibility is obstructed or compromised

measuring the sex hormones via saliva samples (which are collected on specific days of the month). Oestrone (E1), oestradiol (E2), oestriol (E3), progesterone (P4), testosterone (TT) and DHEA-S can be assessed (Table 18.26).

2 and 16 urinary oestrogen metabolism

The 2 and 16 urinary oestrogen metabolism test may be a useful tool in determining patients with a high risk of hormonal imbalance. Oestrogens are metabolised in two ways: the first pathway (2-hydroxyoestrone) is protective while the second pathway (16α-hydroxyoestrone) is more potent. This test identifies which is the dominant pathway (2 or 16) for oestrogen metabolism. The aim is to ensure that the ratio between the two pathways is maintained at the ideal 2.0 (Table 18.27).

Adrenal hormone profile

An adrenal hormone profile that measures cortisol and DHEA-S over a 24-h period may be useful due to adrenal involvement in steroid hormone synthesis and potential dysregulation of the HPA/HPO axis.

THERAPEUTIC CONSIDERATIONS

Clinical decision making and rationale

The notion that naturopathic treatment can shrink fibroids is simplistic and often unrealistic. Having said that, although it is important not to encourage unrealistic expectations, nevertheless shrinkage can occur with some patients. Arrested growth and symptomatic alleviation are achievable and more likely. It is important to acknowledge the patient's age and proximity to menopause, as fibroid size will naturally begin to reduce as endogenous production of oestrogen declines.

Most women seek naturopathic treatment as an alternative option to surgical procedures and to delay menopause for as long as possible. In these instances, it is beneficial to review fibroid growth regularly (approximately every 3 months) with repeat transabdominal and transvaginal ultrasounds. As previously stated, comparative assessments on the same day of the menstrual cycle are essential for optimal review and consideration. It is also beneficial to synchronistically review and assess liver function tests to review LDH in cautionary patients, and to assess FSH in those close to menopause.

TABLE 18.26 Oestrogen fluctuations through the cycle

	Follicular pg/mL	Luteal	Postmenopause pg/mL
Total oestrogen	70–400	70–700 pg/mL	<60
Oestradiol (E2)	50–300	200–400 pg/mL	<50
Oestrone (E1)	10–150	16–170 pg/mL	<20
Oestriol (E3)	5–50	10–60 pg/mL	<30
Progesterone	<1	5–25 ng/mL	<1

Source: Adapted from Lord RS, Brailley JA. Laboratory evaluations for integrative and functional medicine. 2nd edn. Metametrix Institute; 2008.

TABLE 18.27 Expected values for first morning urine oestrogen metabolites

Analyte	Premenopause	Postmenopause	Postmenopause with HRT
Oestrogen metabolite ratio (2OHE/16OHE)		>2.0 (healthy pre- and postmenopausal women)	
Urinary oestrogen metabolites (UEM) Index	4–110	5–18	6–158
16OHE[1]	3–30	2–8	5–25
2OHE[1]	3–40	2–10	10–75

Source: Adapted from Lord RS, Brailley JA. Laboratory evaluations for integrative and functional medicine. 2nd edn. Metametrix Institute; 2008.

TABLE 18.28 Recommended treatment options for women with uterine fibroid tumours

Patient characteristics	Treatment options
Asymptomatic women	Observation
Symptomatic women who require preservation of fertility	Non-surgical treatment or myomectomy
Symptomatic women who require preservation of the uterus but no preservation of fertility	Non-surgical treatment, uterine artery embolisation, myolysis or myometctomy
Women who have had a previous pregnancy that was complicated by uterine fibroid tumours and who wish to conserve their fertility	Myomectomy
Women with distortion of the uterus who are infertile	Myomectomy
Women with severe symptoms that require decisive treatment	Hysterectomy

Source: Adapted from Evans P, Brunsell S. Uterine fibroid tumours: diagnosis and treatment. Am Fam Physician 2007;10(75):1503–8.

Therapeutic application

HISTORICAL PERSPECTIVE

Fibroids appear to have been common at the time of the Eclectics, with a range of botanicals detailed to deal with their management. Astringents such as *Hydrastis canadensis* (golden seal)[8] and *Geranium maculatum* (geranium)[9] were used to help relieve haemorrhage, while *Gossypii radicis* cortex (cotton root bark) was regarded as an efficient remedy for the reduction of uterine subinvolution and fibroids. *Actaea racemosa* was used for ovarian pains of a dull aching character, dragging pains in the womb with a sense of soreness,[9] while *Caulophyllum thalictroides* (blue cohosh) was used for uterine inflammation and full and congested lymphatic tissues.[8]

ALLOPATHIC PERSPECTIVE

Surgery

Fibroids have traditionally been treated surgically, and they are the major reason for hysterectomy (Tables 18.28 and 18.29). In Australia, 21.7% of hysterectomies are reported to be performed because of fibroids, the prevalence of hysterectomy in Australia being 3.97 per 1000 women.[309] Hysterectomy is one of the most common surgical procedures performed in Australia.[341]

TABLE 18.29 Comparison of treatment options for women with uterine fibroid tumours

Treatment	Description	Advantages	Disadvantages	Fertility preserved?
Myomectomy	Endoscopic or surgical removal of tumours	Symptoms can be resolved with fertility preserved; perioperative morbidity is similar to that with hysterectomy	The number and extent of the tumours determine the success of the procedure; fibroids reoccur at a rate of 15–30% after five years	Yes
Gonadotrophin-releasing hormone agonists	Preoperative treatment to decrease size of tumours before hysterectomy, myomectomy, or myolysis	Reduces operative and recovery time and decreases blood loss	Increased risk of recurrence with myometcomy; long-term treatment is associated with menopausal symptoms, bone loss and high costs	Dependent on subsequent procedure
Uterine artery embolisation	Interventional radiological procedure to occlude uterine arteries	A short hospital stay of only 24–36 hours. Procedure is minimally invasive, avoiding larger surgery	Pain after the procedure may require extended hospitalisation; 17% chance of symptom recurrence at 30 months	No (limited experience)

TABLE 18.29 Comparison of treatment options for women with uterine fibroid tumours—cont'd

Treatment	Description	Advantages	Disadvantages	Fertility preserved?
Hysterectomy	Surgical removal of the uterus (transabdominal, transvaginal, or laparoscopic)	Definitive procedure for women who do not require preservation of fertility. Transvaginal procedure is associated with greater patient satisfaction and less pain, fever and blood loss than abdominal procedure	Surgical risks	No
Myolysis	In situ elimination of tumours by laser, heat or cryotherapy	Rapid recovery time with minimal blood loss. Procedure is straightforward and quick	Risk of recurrence is unknown; vaginal bleeding may be prolonged; delay in reduction of size of uterus	Unknown

Source: Adapted from Evans P, Brunsell S. Uterine fibroid tumours: diagnosis and treatment. Am Fam Physician 2007; 75(10):1503–1508.

TABLE 18.30 Alternatives to surgery for uterine fibroid tumours

Treatment	Benefit	Potential side effects	Negative
Gonadotrophin-releasing hormone (GnRH) agonists	Well-established therapy causing amenorrhoea and a rapid reduction in the size of the tumour	Significant side effects resulting from hypoestrogenism (e.g. hot flushes, vaginal dryness, bone demineralisation)	Best suited for women in the perimenopausal or preoperative periods. Not used for long-term treatment
Hormone therapy (cyclic or non-cyclic oestrogen–progestogen combinations)		Hormonal interference	Considered ineffective in alleviating the symptoms of fibroid tumours and limiting tumour growth
Mifepristone (RU486)	Reduced tumour size and improvement in symptoms	Folate deficiency	Legalities are complicated
Depot medroxyprogesterone acetate	Improvement in bleeding after treatment	Hormonal interference, long-term studies required	

Sources: Myers ER, Barber MD, Gustilo-Ashby T et al. Management of leiomyomata: what do we really know? Obstet Gynecol 2002; 100:8–17. Steinauer J, Pritts EA, Jackson R et al. Systematic review of mifepristone for the treatment of uterine leiomyomata. Obstet Gynecol 2004; 103:1331–1336.

Some women will need to undertake surgery for effective curative potential. Surgery is assessed and determined by the size, number and location of fibroids:

- Hysteroscopic resection
- Laparoscopic surgery for subserous and pedunculated fibroids
- Laparoscopy assisted vaginal hysterectomy
- Myomectomy
- Supracervical hysterectomy
- Uterine embolisation.

Medical treatments

Some alternatives to surgery that are available are listed in Table 18.30.

NATUROPATHIC PERSPECTIVE

At the heart of naturopathic treatment is consideration of the production and metabolism of oestrogen and its subsequent relationship with the hepatobiliary system. Conversion of oestrogen to oestrone and finally to oestriol is essential to reduce the oestrogen stimulation on the uterus and subsequent effects on fibroid growth. (See Figs 18.9 and 18.10.)

Reduced environmental and dietary exposure to exogenous oestrogens is additionally beneficial and should be encouraged. Dietary changes will improve a number of factors, including general health and wellbeing and fibroid-specific health concerns. Nutritional repletion from lost nutrients is best achieved through supplementation. Repletion of pathways will enable both symptomatic and functional amelioration. Herbal prescriptions provide strong symptomatic support and improvement in system health — both reproductive and secondary systems. Lifestyle changes include emotional support — crucial for those suffering from emotional distress associated with menorrhagia — as well as stress management useful to regulate hormonal cascades and axes.

NUTRITIONAL MEDICINE (DIETARY)

Dietary therapeutic objectives

- Encourage an anti-inflammatory diet to reduce compounding inflammatory mediators that aggravate the development of the fibroid. This includes dietary modifications

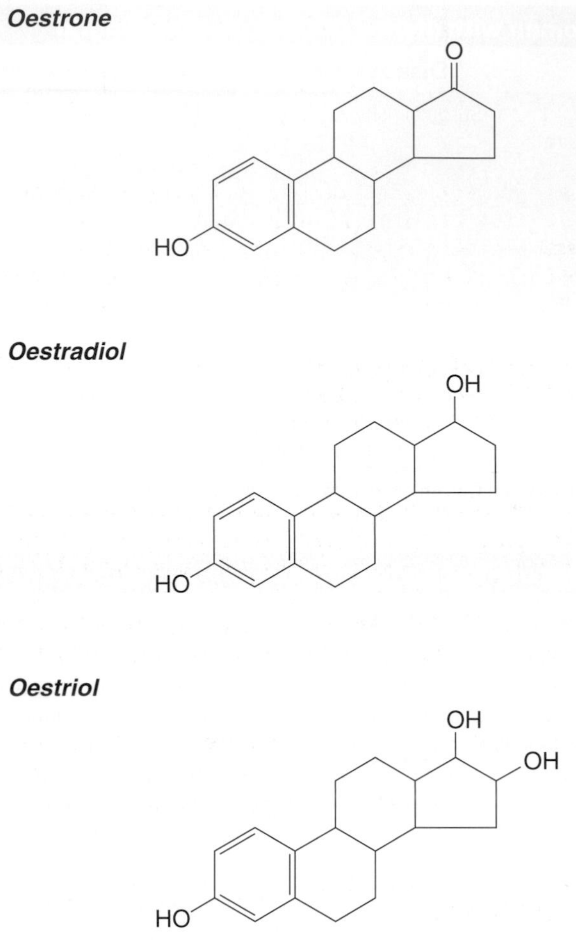

FIGURE 18.9 The oestrogens.

- Include: wholefood dietary principles, fresh organic fruits and vegetables, cold-pressed oils, oily fish, nuts and seeds (fresh)
- Exclude: red meat, processed foods, refined carbohydrates, sugar, excessive starches, dairy products, caffeine, saturated fats and deep-fried food
- Achieve a healthy body weight and weight distribution. Stored oestrogen is a compounding factor to the progression of the disease and aggravation of symptoms. Associated dietary modifications are crucial to assist this objective
- Promote oestrogen balance by increasing phyto-oestrogen food sources, excluding exogenous dietary sources of oestrogens, and increase brassica family vegetables.

Specific dietary treatments

DIETARY INCLUSIONS

Phyto-oestrogens

Phyto-oestrogens have a similar structure to human oestrogens and may act as weak oestrogens or anti-oestrogens within the body. Because of this unique function there is much debate on whether phyto-oestrogens may or may not be used therapeutically in women with fibroids, for if they do indeed promote oestrogen in the body then their use would be cautioned due to the relative excess of oestrogen already present in the body. It has been observed that phyto-oestrogens do not appear to exert an oestrogenic effect on the uterus (except when used by postmenopausal women at 150 mg/day isoflavones), instead they appear to oppose the effects of oestrogen, seemingly making them suitable for use by women with fibroids.[342] This view is supported by the results of an experimental study which found that genistein, a soy-derived phyto-oestrogen, inhibits oestradiol-induced leiomyoma cell proliferation.[343] A recent study showed that genistein inhibited fibroid tumour cell growth in vivo.[344]

Phyto-oestrogen-rich food sources that should be encouraged in the diet of women with or at risk of fibroids include flaxseed (whole seeds, meal and oil); whole soybeans and fermented soy sources including tempeh; alfalfa; and sesame seeds.

Fibre

High-fibre foods are beneficial to assist in bowel elimination and clearance of oestrogens. Fibre assists with the clearance of metabolites and assists with elimination through defecation. In addition, fibre sources can assist in regulating bowel transit time and relief of GI tract symptoms commonly experienced by those with fibroids, including bloating and flatulence.

Soluble fibre

Soluble fibres are found in fruits, grains (such as oats and barley) and legumes. These fibres absorb water and often become slimy and sticky. Fibres that are soluble include gums, pectin, mucilage and some hemicelluloses. Soluble fibre has the following actions in the body:

- Delays GI tract transit by decreasing stomach emptying and the transit of chyme
- Delays glucose absorption
- Reduces blood cholesterol and may reduce the risk of heart disease
- Prevents constipation by softening the stool and acting as a bulking agent.

Insoluble fibre

Insoluble fibres are found in wheatbran, wholegrain breads and cereals and vegetables. These fibres do not absorb water like soluble fibres. Fibres that are insoluble include cellulose, many hemicelluloses and lignins. Insoluble fibre has the following actions in the body:

- Accelerates GI tract transit (by accelerating the movement of chyme through the intestines)
- Prevents constipation, haemorrhoids, and possibly bowel cancer
- Increases faecal weight
- Reduces starch breakdown
- Delays glucose absorption and starch breakdown.

Fruit and vegetables, phytochemicals

Case control and cohort studies have demonstrated a protective effect of consumption of fruits and green vegetables.[345–347] Dietary phytochemicals may offer

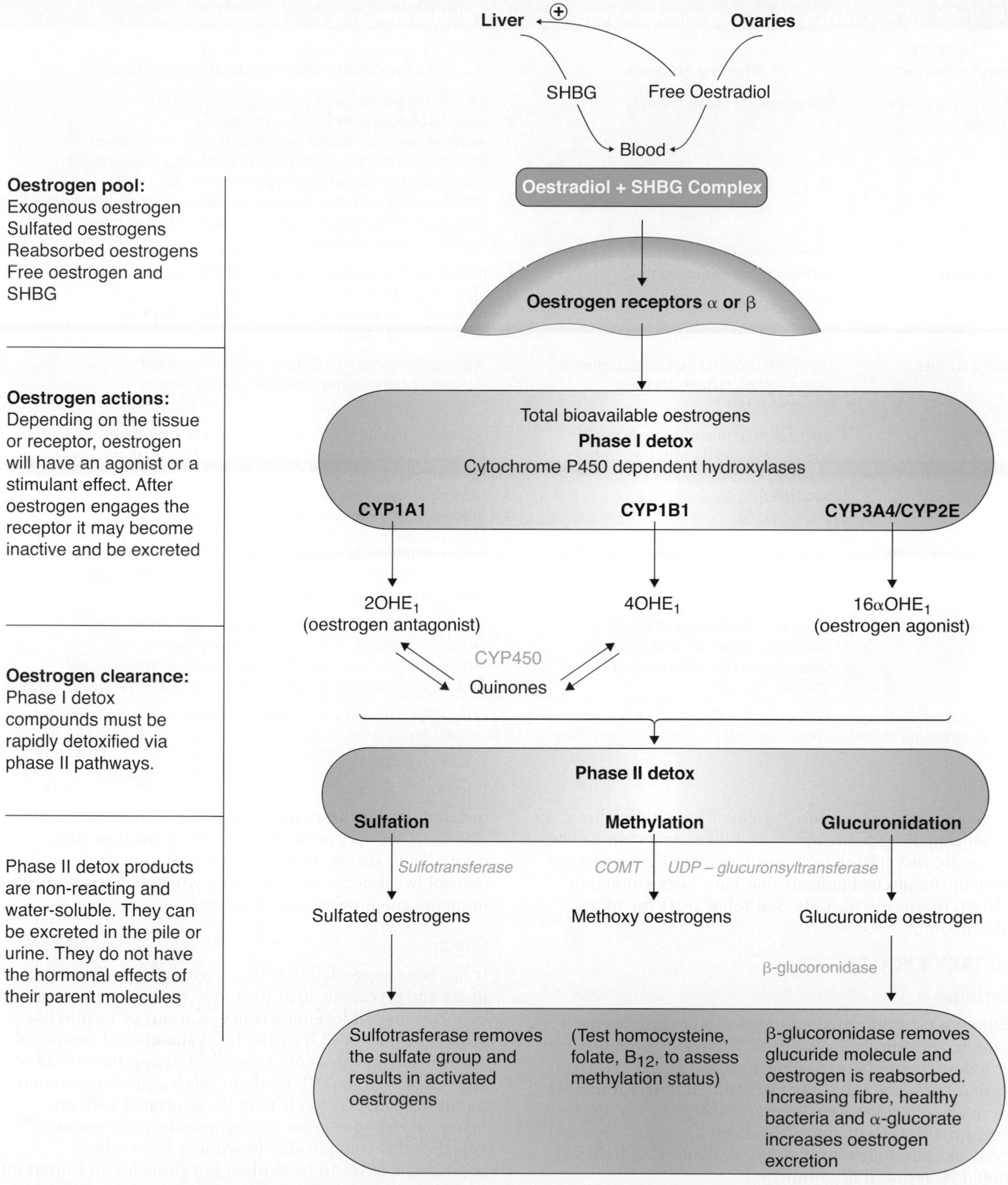

FIGURE 18.10 Oestrogen metabolism.

Source: Adapted from Lord RS, Brailley JA, Laboratory evaluations for integrative and functional medicine. 2nd edn. Metametrix Institute; 2008.

TABLE 18.31 Therapeutic effects of dietary phytochemicals on uterine fibroids

Dietary phytochemicals	Dietary sources	Therapeutic effects on uterine fibroids
Epigallocatechin gallate	Green tea (*Camellia sinensis*)	1. Inhibits the proliferation of leiomyoma cells. 2. Induces apoptosis in leiomyoma cells. 3. Reduces the volume and weight of tumours of female mice. 4. Reduces the incidence and size of spontaneously occurring leiomyomas of the oviduct in Japanese quail. 5. Reduces uterine fibroid volume, fibroid-specific symptom severity, induces significant improvement in health-related quality of life in premenopausal women.
Curcumin	Turmeric (*Curcuma longa*)	1. Inhibits uterine leiomyoma cell proliferation. 2. Induces apoptosis in leiomyoma cells. 3. Inhibits fibronectin production in leiomyoma cells. 4. Acts as PPARγ ligand.
Isoliquiritigenin	Licorice (*Glycyrrhiza uralensis*), shallot (*Allium ascalonicum*), soybean (*Glycine max*)	1. Induces the growth inhibition of leiomyoma cells. 2. Induces apoptosis in uterine leiomyoma cells.
Genistein	Soybeans (*G. max*), lupine (*Lupinus* spp.), fava bean (*Vicia faba*), kudzu (*Pueraria lobata*), psoralea (*Psoralea corylifolia*)	1. Stimulates leiomyoma cell proliferation at low concentration. 2. Inhibits leiomyoma and myometrial cell proliferation at high concentration. 3. Increases caspase activity. 4. Induces apoptosis in myometrial and leiomyoma cells. 5. Downregulates activin A, Smad3, and other TGF-γ pathway genes in human uterine leiomyoma cells. 6. Reduces the incidence and size of spontaneously occurring leiomyomas of the oviduct in Japanese quail.
Resveratrol	More than 70 species of plants, including mulberries and peanuts. Grapevines (*Vitis vinifera*) are the main sources	1. Inhibits proliferation of human uterine leiomyoma cells. 2. Induces apoptosis in human uterine leiomyoma cells. 3. Induces cell cycle arrest in human uterine leiomyoma cells. 4. Reduces collagen types I and III in human uterine leiomyoma cells.

Source: Islam MS, Akhtar MM, Ciavattini A et al. Use of dietary phytochemicals to target inflammation, fibrosis, proliferation, and angiogenesis in uterine tissues: promising options for prevention and treatment of uterine fibroids? Mol Nutr Food Res 2014; 58(8):1667–1684.

preventive and therapeutic benefits through the alteration of cell signalling pathways.[348,349] Epigallocatechin gallate, curcumin, resveratrol, isoliquiritigenin and genistein are some of the phytochemicals that have been studied in relation to uterine fibroids. See Table 18.31 for more information.

DIETARY EXCLUSIONS

Caffeine

Although no studies have proved a direct link between caffeine and fibroids, Wise et al[350] have suggested that in high doses, caffeine may induce stress-like effects in the pituitary adrenal axis, thus increasing the risk of uterine leiomyomas via increased secretion of prolactin. Coffee (>1 cup) and caffeine have also been linked to increased levels of early follicular phase oestradiol.[351] Caffeine should be reduced or eliminated.

SATURATED FATS AND DEEP-FRIED FOODS

Saturated fats and deep-fried foods are highly inflammatory within the body and tend to be deficient in health-promoting nutrients. Many come packaged in plastics, promoting xeno-oestrogens within the body which are likely to negatively affect oestrogen production and metabolism. Furthermore, Pizzorno and Murray[342] note that saturated fats prevent the body from converting oestradiol (a strong form of oestrogen) to oestrone and oestriol (weak form of oestrogen), which is likely to further influence the progression of fibroids.

Sugar

It has been suggested that foods with a high glycaemic index and glycaemic load (GL) may promote tumorigenesis by increasing endogenous concentrations of insulin-like growth factor I (IGF-I) or the bioavailability of oestradiol. A recent prospective cohort study studying the effects of high dietary GI and GL foods in Black American women found that high GI foods may be associated with an increased risk of uterine leiomyomas in some women.[352] Whether this is applicable to women from other populations is yet to be studied but provides an important consideration.

Alcohol

A recent Japanese study demonstrated a link between higher intake of alcohol and higher prevalence of uterine fibroids.[353] Furthermore, excess load placed on the liver is likely to put stress on detoxification systems that

SAMPLE DAILY DIET

BREAKFAST	
Orange, grapefruit and pomelo fruit salad with flaxseeds, sesame seeds and walnuts	A diet low in fruits and vegetables has been associated with an increased risk of developing fibroids suggesting a protective effect of fruit and vegetables. Moreover, women who consume more citrus fruits are less likely to develop fibroids, possibly due to the antiproliferative effect of flavonoids. The flavones apigenin and luteolin can induce inhibition of uterine fibroid growth by promoting apoptosis.
LUNCH	
Stir fry made with cruciferous vegetables, fresh turmeric and tofu	High intake of cabbage and broccoli is associated with reduced incidence of fibroids. Additionally, a plant-based diet has been hypothesised to decrease risk of uterine leiomyomas by reducing the bioavailability of endogenous hormones as well as reducing inflammation since the development of uterine leiomyomas may be triggered, at least in part, by a chronically active inflammatory immune system. Experimental data showed that curcumin inhibits uterine leiomyoma cell proliferation via regulation of apoptotic pathway.
DINNER	
Black bean tacos with tomato, corn and coriander	The incidence of uterine fibroids has been shown to be greater in populations who consume more red meats such as beef and ham thus a treatment strategy that excludes red meat and excessive animal fat is suggested. A high-fibre diet may assist with removal of oestrogen from the body.
SNACK	
Green tea Fresh fruit	Green tea extract has been shown to significantly reduce uterine fibroid volume and fibroid-specific symptom severity. Protective against fibroids.

Sources: Kim D-I, Lee T-K, Lim I-S et al. Regulation of IGF-I production and proliferation of human leiomyomal smooth muscle cells by *Scutellaria barbata D. Don* in vitro: isolation of flavonoids of apigenin and luteolin as acting compounds. Toxicol Appl Pharmacol 2005; 205(3):213–224. Malik M, Mendoza M, Payson M et al. Curcumin, a nutritional supplement with antineoplastic activity, enhances leiomyoma cell apoptosis and decreases fibronectin expression. Fertil Steril 2009; 91:2177–2184. Parazzini F, Di Martino M, Candiani M et al. Dietary components and uterine leiomyomas: a review of published data. Nutr Cancer 2015; 67(4):569–579. Roshdy E, Rajaratnam V, Maitra S et al. Treatment of symptomatic uterine fibroids with green tea extract: a pilot randomized controlled clinical study. Int J Women's Health 2013; 5:477–486. Shen Y, Wu Y, Lu Q et al. Vegetarian diet and reduced uterine fibroids risk: a case-control study in Nanjing, China. J Obstet Gynaecol Res 2016; 42(1):87–94. Wise LA, Palmer JR, Harlow BL et al. Risk of uterine leiomyomata in relation to tobacco, alcohol and caffeine consumption in the Black Women's Health Study. Hum Reprod 2004; 19:1746–1754. Wise LA, Radin RG, Palmer JR et al. Intake of fruit, vegetables, and carotenoids in relation to risk of uterine leiomyomata. Am J Clin Nutr 2011; 94(6):1620–1631.

may be better utilised breaking down hormones from the body.

NUTRITIONAL MEDICINE (SUPPLEMENTAL)

Nutritional medicine therapeutic objectives

Address obvious and subtle deficiencies that aggravate the presentation:

- Alleviate anaemia: improve iron stores and red blood cell health
- Reduce inflammation and oxidation
- Support optimal hepatobiliary function for oestrogen metabolism and clearance
- Support hormonal cascades and regulation of oestrogen balance
- Support nutritional requirements for healthy mucous membranes and surrounding tissue
- Provide symptomatic relief and improve circulation to reproductive tissues.

Specific nutrients required

B COMPLEX

B vitamins are required for numerous functions that may indirectly help manage fibroids. Several of the B vitamins are required for liver detoxification which enables oestrogen conjugation and excretion through hepatic clearance. They are also required for red blood cell production and reduction of anaemia risk.

ESSENTIAL FATTY ACIDS (EFAs)

Essential fatty acids are able to affect biosynthetic pathways responsible for prostaglandin synthesis and steroidogenesis, both of which have multiple roles in the maintenance of healthy reproductive function.[354] Essential fatty acids may also help to reduce inflammation via their anti-inflammatory effects thereby helping to ease pain.

IRON

Excessive and prolonged vaginal bleeding occurs in many women with fibroids, contributing to the risk of iron-deficiency anaemia.[355] All women who report long or excessive bleeds should undertake laboratory testing to assess iron levels. Where necessary, supplementation to restore healthy iron levels is warranted.

ANTIOXIDANTS

The conversion of oestradiol via 4-hydroxylation stimulates an oxidant stress response induced by free radicals. Antioxidant prescriptions are imperative to protect the hyperresponsive fibroid and uterine tissue.

ZINC

In some literature, fibroids are linked with an increased risk of endometrial cancer[356] hence the importance of immune and antioxidant-regulating nutrients such as zinc. Zinc is also required for healthy reproductive functioning and hormonal balance.

SELENIUM

Selenium is an essential trace mineral with powerful immunomodulating and antioxidant properties. Early studies have shown that levels of selenium were decreased in individuals with gynaecological cancer including endometrial, ovarian and cervical cancer.[357] Given the increased risk of endometrial cancer in the presence of fibroids, the protective anticancer[358] properties of selenium would appear necessary in patients with fibroids.

VITAMIN E

Vitamin E (300 mg/day) has been used to treat fibroids during pregnancy.[359] High rates of lipid peroxidation and decreased levels of vitamin E have been observed in patients with fibroids, hence the benefits of supplementation.[360]

VITAMIN D

Recent research has indicated an association between low vitamin D status and increased risk for uterine fibroids. A 2012 study of women 154 women in North Africa showed that lower serum vitamin D levels were significantly associated with the occurrence of uterine fibroids.[361] This was followed by a study of 1036 women in the USA (620 blacks and 416 whites) which supported these results.[362] Similar results were found in a study of 384 infertile Italian women.[363] In contrast to these results, an analysis of 3590 women in the National Health and Nutritional Examination Survey (NHANES 2001–2006) found no relationship between vitamin D status and risk of uterine fibroids; however, a probabilistic analysis (correcting for outcome misclassification) indicated that vitamin D deficiency was associated with uterine fibroids in white women, but not in black women.[364] Vitamin D has been shown in vitro to inhibit myometrial and leiomyoma cell growth,[365] and more recently an in-vivo study showed that treatment with vitamin D significantly reduced tumour size,[366] indicating a promising role for vitamin D not only in prevention of uterine fibroids but also potentially in treatment. A correlation has been found in vitro between reduced levels of vitamin D receptor (VDR) and upregulation of oestrogen and progesterone receptors in uterine fibroids.[367] Vitamin D-related genetic variants have been found to be associated with uterine fibroids — notably polymorphisms rs12800438 near DHCR7 (involved in vitamin D metabolism) and rs6058017 in ASIP (involved in skin pigmentation).[368] These variants might explain the differences seen in the increased rates of fibroids in black women compared to white women.

DOSAGE REQUIREMENTS

The dosage requirements listed below are based on adult doses that have been reported in the literature and clinical review:

- B complex (all B vitamins) high-dose combination, preferably activated forms
  - Thiamine 20–40 mg/day
  - Riboflavin 20–40 mg/day
  - Niacinamide/nicotinic acid 50–100 mg/day
  - Pantothenic acid 150–300 mg/day
  - Pyridoxine 20–60 mg/day
  - Folate as folinic acid or L-5MTHF 500–1000 micrograms/day
  - Hydroxo- or methylcobalamin 500–1000 micrograms/day
  - Choline 50–100 mg/day
  - Inositol 50–100 mg/day
  - Biotin 250–500 micrograms/day
- Essential fatty acids: 3 g/day total omega-3 fatty acids (45% DHA and 55% EPA)
- Iron 25–100 mg/day (blood results dependent)
- Zinc 60 mg/day
- Selenium 200–250 micrograms/day
- Vitamin E 800 IU/day in divided doses.
- Vitamin D 0.5 micrograms/200 IU (RDI). Up to 6000 IU/day to correct a deficiency[284]

HERBAL MEDICINE

Herbal medicine therapeutic objectives

- Assist to reduce symptoms of menorrhagia, metrorrhagia, anaemia, pain and inflammation
- Reduce oxidation triggered through oestrogen conversion
- Modulate HPA/HPO axis by regulating communication from steroid hormone synthesis
- Support oestrogen conversion and clearance of metabolites
- Support hormone excretion and biotransformation
- Improve uterine tone and circulation
- Arrest fibroid growth and shrink tumour where possible.

Herbal medicine classes

Herbal medicine classes used for uterine fibroids are listed in Table 18.32.

Specific herbal medicines

ACHILLEA MILLEFOLIUM (YARROW)

Menorrhagia is a common symptom associated with fibroids, hence the benefits of a botanical such as *Achillea*

TABLE 18.32 Herbal medicine classes used for uterine fibroids	
Class	**Action**
Cholagogue, hepatic	Regulate and support hormone metabolism, transformation and elimination. Support steroid hormone pathways
Hormonal modulator (includes phyto-oestrogen herbal medicines)	Regulate hormonal cascades, protect against oestrogen displacement issues
Uterine tonic	Reduce menorrhagia, improve integrity of uterine tonicity
Uterine astringent	Reduce menorrhagia, improve integrity of uterine tonicity
Circulatory stimulant (uterine)	Improve circulation to uterine tissues and relieve congestion, relieve pain
Lymphatic	Improve circulation to uterine tissues and relieve congestion, assist with oestrogen clearance from oestrogen tissues
Uterine spasmolytic	Relieve spasm and pain
Analgesic	Relieve spasm and pain
Blood tonic	Address anaemia and support blood building

millefolium that displays astringent[369] and anti-haemorrhagic[28] properties useful for reducing excess bleeding associated with fibroids. According to the literature, the pharmacological effects of *Achillea millefolium* are mainly due to its essential oil components, proazulenes and other sesquiterpene lactones, dicaffeoylquinic acids and flavonoids,[370] but whether these constituents are responsible for its astringent and antihaemorrhagic effects is unknown. As yet there has been little in the way of studies investigating its effects for relief of symptoms associated with fibroids.

ALCHEMILLA VULGARIS (LADIES' MANTLE)

Alchemilla vulgaris has been used for centuries in Europe where it is favoured for its coagulation, astringent and styptic properties.[371] These actions make it extremely useful for the treatment of excessive menstrual bleeding associated with fibroids. To date there are no clinical studies assessing the efficacy of *Alchemilla vulgaris* in fibroids.

CALENDULA OFFICINALIS (CALENDULA)

Calendula officinalis was traditionally used for all uterine and vaginal abrasions and ecchymosed tissues, probably because of its anti-inflammatory and antimicrobial properties.[8] Its lymphatic properties may be used to eliminate wastes from the body; Trickey[28] suggests *Calendula officinalis* may be used to help reduce the size of fibroids.

CAPSELLA BURSA-PASTORIS (SHEPHERD'S PURSE)

Capsella bursa-pastoris is a popular and efficacious botanical for the treatment of excessive bleeding associated with fibroids due to its astringent properties. It was used traditionally by the Eclectic physicians for chronic menorrhagia where there was too frequent and too long continued or constant, but almost colourless, menstrual flow.[8] There is little in the way of modern clinical research assessing the efficacy of *Capsella bursa-pastoris*, but renowned physician Rudolf Weiss advocates its use for persistent uterine bleeding or haemorrhage due to myoma (fibroid tumour).[372]

CHAMAELIRIUM LUTEUM (FALSE UNICORN ROOT)

Chamaelirium luteum is a plant with a long history of use by Native American populations for female reproductive disorders. It contains steroidal saponins and glycosides and functions as a uterine and ovarian tonic.[129]

Chamaelirium luteum may be used to help with the common symptoms of pelvic pressure having traditionally been used for 'pelvic fullness and heaviness, as if congested, with bearing-down sensation, as if the parts were about to fall out'. Note: It is important to respect the endangered species status of *Chamaelirium luteum* and consider alternatives where possible.

CINNAMOMUM SPP. (CINNAMON)

Cinnamomum spp. act as a gentle, warming circulatory stimulant that may be used to ease pelvic stagnation and aid in the removal of the fibroid. The tincture of the bark was traditionally used in uterine haemorrhage and menorrhagia, its most direct action being said to be upon the uterine muscular fibres, where it caused contraction and arrested bleeding.

In addition, cinnamon is used in traditional Chinese medicine in the patented formula 'Cinnamon and Peony', which has been shown to be effective both traditionally and in a number of trials. Referral to traditional Chinese medicine texts is advisable for a comprehensive discussion.

DIOSCOREA VILLOSA (WILD YAM)

Dioscorea villosa is a North American plant that was traditionally used for painful periods and ovarian pain.[129] In the early 1930s diosgenin, a saponin precursor[372] within *Dioscorea villosa*, was said to exert a progesterogenic effect. As yet no clinical studies have been able to confidently prove the progesterogenic effect of *Dioscorea villosa*, but many practitioners use *Dioscorea villosa* to great effect to regulate hormones in their patients and assist in the regulation of excessive oestrogen.

MITCHELLA REPENS (SQUAW VINE)

Mitchella repens is considered an ovarian and uterine tonic. The Eclectics suggested it for uterine disorders to help alleviate painful menstruation and relieve congestion in the pelvic organs, and traditionally used it as a female regulator.[7]

RUBUS IDAEUS (RASPBERRY LEAF)

Rubus idaeus has been used for centuries to strengthen and tone the uterus as well as for its effects as an astringent.[8] It contains polypeptides, flavonoids and tannins,[129] the latter likely to be responsible for its astringent effects.

VITEX AGNUS-CASTUS (CHASTE TREE BERRY)

Prolactin has been suggested to be a mitogenic growth factor for human leiomyoma and myometrial cells[373] hence the benefits of administering a dopamine agonist and subsequent inhibitor of prolactin such as *Vitex agnus-castus*. *Vitex agnus-castus* is commonly used for hormonal regulation, but as yet no clinical studies could be found assessing its effects for the management of fibroids.

ACTAEA RACEMOSA (BLACK COHOSH)

An RCT of 62 women in China compared the effects of black cohosh root extract (Remifemin, 40 mg/day) and tibolone (2.5 mg/day) in menopausal women with fibroids. Tibolone is administered as an effective alternative to hormone therapy, as it regulates the expression of oestrogen, progesterone and androgenic activity. Results after 3 months showed a notable difference between the two groups. Black Cohosh produced significant reduction in the volume and diameter of fibroids and has been shown to provide relief from menopausal symptoms.[374]

LIFESTYLE RECOMMENDATIONS

Specific recommendations include the following key areas:

- Weight balance and loss as required to reduce adipose impact on hormonal metabolism
- Exercise and stretching to improve circulation to pelvic region and support healthy weight balance
- Assessment of sanitary products to consider impact of chemicals (see section on 'Endometriosis' for a full discussion)
- Castor oil packs for pain relief as required.

CASE STUDY

OVERVIEW

TT was a 49-year-old woman who presented with marked uterine fibroid. Recent ultrasound and hysteroscopy in the gynaecology department revealed an intramural fibroid that was palpable at rest. She experienced significant menorrhagia, metrorrhagia, dysmenorrhoea and associated anaemia.

History revealed that she had used the combined oral contraceptive from age 24 until 47 with a 2-year gap for the pregnancy, birth and breastfeeding of her daughter. As a teenager, she experienced strong menorrhagia and dysmenorrhoea, hence the prescription. In addition, she had been a cigarette smoker from 18 to 38 years old (again with a break for the pregnancy, birth and breastfeeding period). Menarche occurred at 11 years old. Patient attended for consultation and she did not wish to undergo surgical

CASE STUDY CONTINUED

hysterectomy as per advice of her gynaecologist. Her gynaecologist was aware she was due to begin treatment, and had approved treatment pending regular 6-weekly LDH review and bimonthly ultrasound. Close communication between patient, gynaecologist, GP and myself was conducted throughout treatment.

CLINICAL EXAMINATION

- Height 165 cm
- Weight 73 kg
- BMI 26.8 (overweight) — central adiposity primarily

TREATMENT PROTOCOL

INVESTIGATIONS

Referral for assessments revealed:

- LFT: NAD (LDH WNL)
- Lipid profile: total cholesterol: 5.2 mmol/L
- Triglycerides: 1.8 mmol/L
- Elevated LDL: 3.0 mmol/L
- Low HDL: 1.2 mmol/L
- FBC: Marked anaemia
- Vitamin D (25-OH): 34 nmol/L
- Hormone profile: FSH: 4.0 U/L (day 3)
- Sugar profile: fasting glucose: 4.7 mmol/L
- Iron studies: ferritin: 3 microgram/L
- TSH: 2.14 mIU/L

HERBAL MEDICINE

Herbal medicine	Ratio	Quantity	Justification
Alchemilla vulgaris	1:2	50 mL	Astringent, hormonal regulating
Urtica dioica (leaf)	1:2	40 mL	Nutritive, circulatory stimulant
Calendula officinale	1:2	40 mL	Lymphatic, immune regulating, anti-inflammatory
Mitchella repens	1:2	50 mL	Uterine tonic, relieve congestion
Zingiber officinale	1:2	10 mL	Warming circulatory stimulant
Vitex agnus-castus	1:2	30 mL	Hormonal regulator

TOTAL: 220 mL. Dose: 7.5 mL b.i.d.

NUTRITIONAL MEDICINE

Dietary

- Patient had self-initiated a vegetarian diet 2 days prior to consultation due to her research. We discussed the importance of protein balance and reduction of excessive saturated fats and balanced her vegetarian intake
- Anti-inflammatory dietary principles were encouraged
- Exclusion of: red meat, processed foods, refined carbohydrates, sugar, excessive starches, dairy products, caffeine, alcohol, saturated fat and deep-fried food

CASE STUDY CONTINUED

- Dietary sources of essential fatty acids and vegetarian protein were encouraged
- Iron absorption, major food sources and food combining for optimal iron absorption was discussed
- Avoidance of food sources of xeno-oestrogens, increase of brassica vegetables and dietary phyto-oestrogens such as flaxseed (whole seeds, meal, and oil); whole soybeans and fermented soy sources including tempeh; alfalfa and sesame seeds.

Supplemental

Nutrient	Dosage	Justification
B complex (activated forms)	2 caps b.i.d.	Metabolism of carbohydrates, glucose metabolism, management and prevention of complications, hormonal regulation
Iron	48–96 mg/day (cycle day dependent)	Address deficiency and increase dosage 2 days prior to expected bleed and continue during bleed and for 3 days post
Vitamin E	500 IU b.i.d.	Mucous membrane integrity, hormonal regulation, oestrogen regulation, antioxidant
Selenium	200 micrograms/day	Antioxidant and cancer protection
Concentrated fish oil supplementation	1 cap b.i.d. total: EPA: 650 mg, DHA: 450 mg, Other omega-3 fats: 180 mg	Hormonal regulation, anti-inflammatory, regulation of prostaglandin synthesis
Zinc	60 mg/day	Hormonal regulation, antioxidant
Vitamin D_3	5000 IU/day	To address deficiency and utilise positive blood sugar, mood and immune effects

LIFESTYLE/EDUCATION

- Castor oil packs as required
- Heat packs as required
- Daily exercise as possible
- Avoidance of exogenous oestrogen sources
- Replacement of sanitary items with organic sanitary pads to reduce impact from chemical exposure
- Menstrual symptom diary was used to assess progress comprehensively.

ENDOMETRIOSIS

Epidemiology

Estimates of the frequency of endometriosis (Fig. 18.11) vary widely, as few well-conducted studies have reported data on the prevalence of endometriosis and no data are available on the frequency of the onset of the disease in a given period (its incidence) in women without a previous diagnosis.[375]

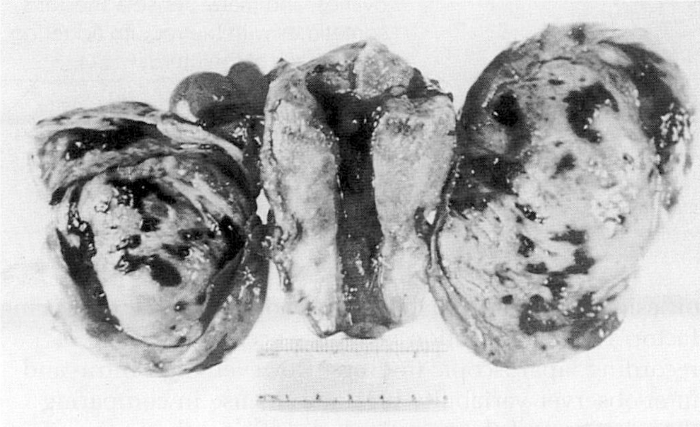

FIGURE 18.11 Endometriosis.

Source: From Katz V. Comprehensive gynecology. 5th edn. Maryland Heights: Mosby, 2007.

Studies that have analysed the frequency of endometriosis in women who underwent surgery for fibroids have suggested a prevalence of the condition of about 10%,[376] but women with fibroids share the same risk factors with endometriosis.[377]

The exact prevalence of endometriosis is unknown but estimates range from 2 to 10% within the general female population but up to 50% in infertile women.[378,379] The general consensus is that it occurs in 10% of women.

In part, these large variations can be explained by differences in the indications for laparoscopy and laparotomy, or merely by the differing degrees of attention paid by surgeons to the accurate identification of endometriotic lesions and by selective mechanisms drawing patients with suspected endometriosis towards specialised centres. It is worth noting that there are no published studies on representative samples of the general population. In general, it is difficult to compare estimates of prevalence because the published studies include women with different conditions, and are conducted in centres that apply different diagnostic criteria and exhibit different levels of clinical interest in endometriosis.

Classification

Endometriosis is most commonly found in the pelvis. The American Society for Reproductive Medicine (ASRM) classification is currently the most widely used staging system.[380] Point scores are assigned based on the number

TABLE 18.33 Stages of endometriosis

Stage	Disease	Description
I	Minimal	A few superficial implants
II	Mild	More and slightly deeper implants
III	Moderate	Many deep implants, small endometriomas on one or both ovaries, and some filmy adhesion
IV	Severe	Many deep implants, large endometriomas on one or both ovaries, and many dense adhesions, sometimes with the rectum adhering to the back of the uterus

Source: From the MSD Manual Professional Version (known as the Merck Manual in the US and Canada and the MSD Manual in the rest of the world), edited by R Porter. Copyright (2017) by Merck Sharp & Dohme Corp, a subsidiary of Merck & Co, Inc, Kenilworth, NJ. Available at http://www.msdmanuals.com/professional. Accessed 20 February 2018.

of lesions and their bilaterality. Lesion size is also a scoring factor. This classification is a fairly accurate method of recording laparoscopic findings. However, high intra- and inter-observer variability precludes its use in comparing the outcomes of therapeutic studies.[381] Further, this staging system does not correlate well with pain and dyspareunia[382] and fecundity rates cannot be predicted accurately.[383]

The stages of endometriosis are summarised in Table 18.33.

Diagnosis

Endometriosis diagnosis is based on the woman's history, symptoms and signs; the diagnosis is corroborated by physical examination and imaging techniques, and finally proven by histology of either a directly biopsied vaginal lesion, from a scar, or of tissue collected during laparoscopy. The visual recognition of endometriosis during laparoscopy alone is of limited value as it has a high false-positive rate. On the other hand, diagnosis during laparoscopy is dependent on the ability of the surgeon to recognise peritoneal disease in all its different appearances. If the surgeon performing the laparoscopy is not familiar with these appearances, endometriosis may be missed and left untreated — you see only what you recognise. This is especially relevant in deep infiltrating disease, where sometimes endometriosis is hidden beneath the peritoneal surface.[384]

Aetiology

The aetiological risk factors for endometriosis are summarised in Box 18.3.

AGE

Pelvic endometriosis is rare before the menarche and tends to decrease after the menopause.[375] Studies conducted in women under 50 suggested that the frequency of endometriosis increased with age until menopause, but more recent studies have not confirmed this.[376]

BOX 18.3 Aetiological risk factors

Genetic factors
- Ten-fold excess in female relatives compared with husband's female relatives
- High concordance rates in identical twins (compared with dizygous twins)

Hormonal factors
- Occur in reproductive years
- Proximity of cases to the ovaries

Peritoneal environment
- Aberrations in immunologically competent cells in peritoneum
- Growth factors

Retrograde menstruation
- Menorrhagia
- Cervical stenosis

Age
- Incidence peaks at 40–44 years

Other factors
- Angiogenesis
- Neurogenesis (PGP9.5)

Different selection criteria can explain some of these discrepancies. For instance, more young women now have undergone laparoscopy for infertility than was the case 20 years ago, when laparotomy was necessary to diagnose endometriosis.[375] However, there is no definitive relationship between age at diagnosis and severity of the disease.[375]

SOCIAL CLASS AND RACE

A greater frequency of endometriosis among women of higher social class has been reported.[385] However, this might be the result of a diagnostic 'bias'; that is, greater attention is paid to pelvic pain or infertility in women of higher social class.[375]

The same diagnostic bias might explain the higher frequency of the disease reported among white women.[375] Data on the prevalence in different races often do not take into account the reason for admission for surgical procedures, which might be selectively associated with a higher or lower likelihood of the disease being diagnosed.[375]

MENSTRUAL AND REPRODUCTIVE FACTORS

Epidemiological studies in the USA and Italy have suggested that women with early menarche, short and heavy menstrual cycles are at a higher risk of endometriosis.[386,387] This could be explained as a higher likelihood of pelvic contamination from menstrual endometrial material — the reflux hypothesis.[376]

Obstetric history, clinical and epidemiological data suggest that parity is inversely associated with the risk of endometriosis[376] but, unlike most clinical data, the few available epidemiological data have not generally shown any relationship between age at first pregnancy, spontaneous abortion and endometriosis.[386]

FAMILY HISTORY

It is suggested that the risk of endometriosis is higher in women whose mother or sisters have the disease.[388,389] In 1980, Simpson et al reported a six-fold risk of endometriosis in sisters of affected women. Women with an affected sibling or mother were found to be more likely to have severe than mild or moderate endometriosis.[389] Similar findings were observed in studies in the UK and Norway.[390,391] These findings, however, should be considered cautiously because information bias cannot be excluded. Cases of endometriosis might tend to recall a family history of the disease more accurately than controls.[375]

The 5–8% risk observed for first-degree relatives is more consistent with polygenic/multifactorial tendencies than with a single mutant gene (25 or 50%).[388] It is assumed that more than a single gene is involved or that multiple alleles exist at a single locus.[388] One or more Mendelian forms could coexist but polygenic inheritance is obligatory if endometriosis is assumed to be a single entity. Additional support for polygenic inheritance is the increased severity in familial cases.[388] As predicted, the greater the severity of a polygenic disorder, the greater the underlying genetic liability. Thus, the higher the proportion of affected relatives, the greater the likelihood that the proband has severe endometriosis.[388] In a study of 28 370 monozygotic or dizygotic female twins, 1228 female twins reported a history of endometriosis, and analysis showed that both genetic and unique, non-shared, environmental factors influenced the aetiology of endometriosis. The study supports the hypothesis that there is a strong genetic influence on phenotypic manifestations of endometriosis.[392]

GENETIC FACTORS

Of interest are studies exploring whether endometriosis is associated with perturbation of a hypothesised candidate gene or one of its polymorphisms.[388] Association between endometriosis and various phase I (aryl hydrocarbon receptor, CYPIAI, *N*-acetyltransferase 2) and phase II (GSTs, *N*-acetyltransferase 2) liver detoxification enzymes has been explored in several studies, but the elucidation of underlying genes and molecular mechanisms giving rise to endometriosis remains unclear.[388]

Polymorphisms in genes encoding cytokines or immunomodulating proteins have also been proposed to be implicated in the pathogenesis of endometriosis. Women with endometriosis diverge in their expression of several genes including heat-shock proteins, fibronectin, elastase and Toll-like receptors (TLRs) which play an important role in innate immunity.[393] Research suggests that TLR signalling is closely related with the pathogenesis of autoimmune diseases. Toll-like receptor-4 A896G (D299G) polymorphism was found to be associated with endometriosis.[394] Adhesion formation may be caused by an imbalance between fibrin-forming and fibrin-dissolving activities in the peritoneum. In a study evaluating plasminogen activator inhibitor-1 (PAI-1) genotypes in a group of women with and without endometriosis, 4G/4G and 4G/5G PAI-1 genotypes were particularly prevalent in infertile women with endometriosis compared to fertile women. Women with endometriosis and adhesions had higher peritoneal fluid concentrations of PAI- 1 compared to women with endometriosis but no adhesions. It has been hypothesised that the persistence of a fibrin matrix in the peritoneal cavity could allow menstrually deposited endometrial fragments to initiate endometriosis as a result of hypofibrinolysis.[395] A meta-analysis which combined results from a genomewide association study and replication studies showed that of the nine loci found to be associated with endometriosis in at least one of the studies, six (rs12700667 on 7p15.2, rs7521902 near WNT4, rs10859871 near VEZT, rs1537377 near CDKN2B-ASI, rs7739264 near ID4, and rs13394619 in GREBI) were statistically significant genome-wide, and two (FNI and intergenic 2p14) showed borderline statistically significant genome-wide association with moderate/severe disease.[396] One small study showed a locus near the vezatin (VEZT) gene to be statistically significantly associated with endometriosis in the general population.[397] A study showed associations at the IL1A locus were stronger in moderate/severe endometriosis than in all endometriosis cases, supporting the evidence for a link between inflammatory responses and the pathogenesis of endometriosis.[398]

DIOXIN EXPOSURE

Recent studies have suggested that exposure to dioxins might be a cause of endometriosis.[399] Should this finding be confirmed, it suggests that other environmental factors, as well as hormonal ones, might be associated with the risk of endometriosis.[375]

Chemicals in tampons include 2,3,7,8-tetra-chlorodibenzo-*p*-dioxin (TCDD) caused by bleached rayon, aluminium, alcohol and additives which also produce TCDD. TCDD and other dibenzodioxins and furans are ubiquitous environmental contaminants. In the past, bleaching of wood pulp products with chlorine gas had the potential to result in generation of additional dioxins. Given the widespread low-level background contamination of our environment with dioxins, it may be possible for rayon-containing tampons, as well as bleached or unbleached all-cotton tampons, to contain extremely low levels of some dioxins.[400] However, the author concluded that notwithstanding the possible influence of heavy TCDD contamination on endometriosis in some populations, there is no credible evidence that tampons, whether rayon or cotton, bleached or unbleached, contribute to endometriosis.[400] Nor is there any credible evidence that exposure to the potential low levels of dioxins in tampons would contribute to human exposure.[400]

Furthermore, in-utero dioxin exposure has been shown to cause progesterone resistance and a transgenerational risk of endometriosis.[401] This compounds the endometriosis risk and presentation for up to three generations.

TAMPON USAGE

There are several theories concerning the cause of endometriosis, the most popular of which is the premise that retrograde menstruation results in endometrial seeding of the peritoneal cavity. The possibility that tampon use might increase retrograde menstruation has been suggested; however, women with endometriosis do not appear to use tampons more than general population controls and retrograde menstruation is believed to occur in most women, whether or not they use tampons.[402] As this study is dated, newer research to confirm or dispute this finding is required.

IMMUNE FACTORS

Some epidemiological data have also linked the risk of endometriosis with the frequency of immune disorders.[403,404] In particular, in the Endometriosis Family Study, the prevalence of rheumatoid arthritis, systemic lupus erythematosus, hypo- or hyperthyroidism, and multiple sclerosis was higher in women with endometriosis than in controls.[375] An association with non-Hodgkin lymphomas and endometriosis has also been suggested.[405]

Overview

Endometriosis occurs when pieces of the womb lining, or endometrium, are found outside the womb (Box 18.4). This tissue behaves in the same way as it does in the womb — growing during the menstrual cycle in response to oestrogen in anticipation of an egg being fertilised and shedding as blood when there is no pregnancy. However, when it grows outside the womb, it is trapped and cannot leave the body as menstruation. Some women experience no symptoms, but for many it is very incapacitating, causing severe pain. The tissue can also stick to other organs, sometimes leading to infertility. It afflicts approximately 10% of women. The cause is poorly understood and there is no cure. Symptoms are traditionally treated with pain medication, hormone drugs or surgery.

Endometriosis is defined as the presence of functional endometrial glands and stoma outside the uterine cavity.[406] Women with endometriosis present with characteristic signs and symptoms: dysmenorrhoea, dyspareunia, chronic pelvic pain or subfertility.[406] Although endometriosis is a benign disorder, it does exhibit a cellular proliferation, cellular invasion and neoangiogenesis.[407] It develops predominantly in women of reproductive age and regresses after menopause or ovariectomy.[406] A growing body of evidence indicates that a combination of genetic, hormonal, immunological and anatomical factors contributes to the formation and development of the ectopic foci of endometriosis.[406]

The prevalence of endometriosis in women with pelvic pain and/or infertility is estimated to be between 20 and 90%.[382,408] In asymptomatic women having tubal ligation, its prevalence has been reported to be between 3 and 30%.[409,410] The high variability reported in prevalence may be explained by the heterogeneity of the population studies and by selection bias.[407] However, based on the few reliable data it has been suggested that the prevalence of the condition in an unselected population of premenopausal women is around 6–10%.[411,412]

Although there is no consistent information on the incidence of the disease, temporal trends suggest an increase in women of reproductive age.[375] This can partly be explained by changing reproductive habits.[375] Numerous epidemiological studies have indicated that nulliparous women and women reporting short and heavy menstrual cycles are at an increased risk of developing endometriosis.[375]

BOX 18.4 Summary of endometriosis

Definition: Endometrial tissue, composed of endometrial-type glandular tissue and stroma, is found outside the uterine cavity. Occurs almost exclusively in women in the reproductive years.

Incidence:

- 4–10% of all women
- 25–50% of women with infertility
- 5–25% of women admitted with pelvic pain
- 7% of women with pelvic masses.

DISTRIBUTION

- Uterosacral ligaments 63%
- Ovaries
  - Superficial 56%
  - Deep 20%
- Ovarian fossa 33%
- Anterior vesical pouch 22%
- Pouch of Douglas 19%
- Intestines 5%.

Pathogenesis

Despite being one of the most frequently encountered gynaecological diseases, the pathophysiology of endometriosis remains controversial. Although various theories have been proposed to explain the pathogenesis of endometriosis, no single theory has been found to account for the location of ectopic endometrium in all cases of endometriosis.[407] The following theories have been put forward.

TRANSPLANTATION THEORY

1 Retrograde menstruation (occurs in up to 90% of women)

2 Lymphatic dissemination
3 Blood vessel dissemination
4 Direct implantation.

METAPLASIA

Controversial and not accepted by all as possible, let alone probable.

INDUCTION

A substance in the retrograde menstrual flow that induces endometriosis.

The following theories provide an overview of current opinion in research.

Peritoneal fluid

The pathogenesis of endometriosis is believed to be strongly related to the peritoneal fluid constituents. Evidence suggests that laparoscopy, when performed during menses, can indicate that blood can be found in the peritoneal fluid in 75–90% of women with patent fallopian tubes.[413–415] Furthermore, viable endometrial cells recovered from the peritoneal fluid during menses can be grown in cell culture and can attach to and penetrate the mesothelial surface of the peritoneum.[416–418] Of interest, experimental endometriosis can be induced in non-human primates after surgically inducing peritoneal menstruation or retroperitoneal injection of menstrual endometrium and in women who receive peritoneal injections of their menstrual tissue.[419–421]

The peritoneum is the most extensive serous membrane in the human body. It contains 5–20 mL of straw-coloured fluid (peritoneal fluid) and the volume depends on various physiological conditions such as follicular activity, corpus luteum vascularity and hormone production. It is believed to arise from plasma or ovarian exudate.[422]

Peritoneal fluid contains a number of important substances, including steroid hormones, cytokines, growth factors and angiogenic factors.[422] These substances are then circulated throughout the abdominal cavity and are believed to be important for the spread of pelvic infection or postoperative adhesion formation. Cells within the peritoneal fluid include macrophages, granulocytes, lymphocytes, mesothelial cells and endometrial cells. It is the macrophage concentration that is highest during menstruation and is also believed to contribute to inflammation, adhesion formation, infertility and endometriosis.[422]

Endometrial cells are present in peritoneal fluid commonly from retrograde menstrual flow. They are common in women both with and without endometriosis; however, theories centralise around various chemicals that enable adherence to the serosa. It is believed that the peritoneal cavity and its fluid contents may be a powerful yet overlooked component of the regulatory systems within the body.[423]

In situ development theory

According to this theory, ectopic endometrium develops in situ from local tissues, including germinal epithelium of the ovary and remnants of the Müllerian and Wolffian ducts.[406] In a broader context, this theory also implies that peritoneal endometriosis results from in situ metaplasia of totipotential mesothelial cells.[424] The fact that endometriosis mostly occurs when endometrium is present, and that it is seldom seen in men, weakens the power of the concept of metaplasia to explain endometriosis.[406] As such, the metaplasia theory links more appropriately with a deranged autoimmune response that allows proliferation of ectopic endometrium in external places to the uterus.

Coelomic metaplasia theory

The basis of this theory is the observation from embryological studies that peritoneal mesothelium, the Müllerian ducts, and the germinal epithelium of the ovary are all derived from coelomic wall epithelium.[425] The hypothesis is that these tissues retain the capacity for further differentiation or that the peritoneal mesothelium and germinal epithelium contain undifferentiated cells capable of developing into functioning endometrium. The coelomic metaplasia theory can explain the occurrence of endometriosis in nearly all its unusual distal sites as coelomic epithelium can be found in the thoracic cavity, umbilicus and limb buds.[426] However, experimental proof that differentiated peritoneal cells can undergo further differentiation to produce endometriosis spontaneously or by being induced is lacking.[426]

A firm scientific basis for the concept of coelomic metaplasia has yet to be established and clinical observations have cast further doubt on the validity of this theory.[426] Endometriosis would be expected to occur in women without a uterus and men if peritoneal epithelium could undergo metaplasia.[427] The occurrence of endometriosis in men, however, has been reported in only a few cases of men receiving high-dose oestrogen therapy for prostatic carcinoma.[426,427] Despite the contribution of coelomic tissue to the development of peritoneum and pleura, endometriosis is located primarily in the pelvis and not uniformly distributed in other sites where the coelomic membrane is present (such as the abdominal and thoracic cavities).[407,426] In light of these observations and the lack of experimental evidence supporting the de novo formation of endometriosis by metaplasia, this theory is unlikely to be an explanation for the histogenesis of endometriosis in most women.[426]

The retrograde transplantation theory

According to this theory, endometriosis is a consequence of endometrial fragments through the fallopian tubes during menstruation, with subsequent implantation and growth on and into the peritoneum and ovary.[428]

The reflux implantation theory is based on the assumption that retrograde menstruation takes place and that viable endometrial cells reach the abdominal cavity and implant.[406] Although Sampson based this theory largely on clinical and anatomical observations rather than on experimental evidence, a large body of evidence has been provided over the years to make this a plausible suggestion.

Sampson's reflux implantation theory is also supported by the distribution of lesions in the abdominal cavity,[429] the demonstration of the viability of shed menstrual endometrium in tissue culture,[430] the high prevalence of pelvic endometriosis in girls with congenital menstrual outflow obstruction[431] and by obstruction of antegrade menstruation thus forcing retrograde menstruation to take place.[432] The last observation points to the fact that increased retrograde shedding of menstrual endometrium increases the likelihood of endometriosis.[406] This is supported by the fact that menstruations are often longer and heavier in women with endometriosis.[387]

However, Sampson's hypothesis supporting retrograde menstruation as the phenomenon responsible for endometriosis does not explain why the process — a physiological occurrence — does not result in the disease in all women.[375] From a pathogenic perspective, it is important to note that in the last few years, in patients with endometriosis, specific constitutive and/or acquired molecular alterations of eutopic and/or ectopic endometrium favouring its implantation have been identified for all the processes potentially involved in the phenomenon.[433] Molecules involved in apoptosis, adhesion molecules, growth and angiogenic factors, matrix metalloproteinases (MMPs) and the mechanisms involved in the escape from the immune system have been recognised as qualitatively or quantitatively different in eutopic and/or ectopic endometrium of women with endometriosis compared with the endometrium of disease-free women.[375] These alterations, which might affect the physiological activity of endometrium, are thought to explain why only some women develop the disease.[375]

Two aspects should be considered in this context: endometriosis itself favours a peritoneal inflammatory situation that could contribute to the maintenance of the disease.[434] Therefore, it is possible that many of the molecular alterations found in the ectopic endometrium of women with endometriosis — but also even in eutopic endometrium and/or systemically — are actually a consequence of the peritoneal inflammation rather than the cause of the disease.[375]

It has been hypothesised that some of the endometrial changes involved in implantation might depend on particular predisposing genes.[435] In endometriosis, the initial genetic event might involve genes that regulate cellular attachment (e.g. matrix metalloproteinases and integrins), unscheduled persistence (e.g. leucocytes or a cytokine receptor), or steroid responsiveness (e.g. hormone responsiveness).[375] The outcome would be refluxed endometrial cells that would adhere more readily to cellular surfaces within the peritoneal cavity.[375] Additional somatic mutations might arise as a second event.[375] These genes could involve inefficient metabolism of chemicals and/or toxins or tumour suppressor genes or cell cycle regulators that might confer upon cells the invasive features causing a more severe disease.[375] Both genetic events might be somatic and, therefore, acquired after birth in one or few cells, or the initial genetic event might be germline and every single cell be susceptible to the same likelihood of a second mutation.[375] Determination of the number and location of genes that are presumably pivotal for endometriosis is the subject for current research.

Immunological factors

The occurrence of retrograde menstruation has been demonstrated to be a near universal phenomenon consistent with the transplantation and induction theories of endometriosis.[426] The difference in the observed prevalence of endometriosis and the occurrence of retrograde menstruation are probably caused by additional factors that are responsible for the variable development and expression of endometriosis after initiation of the implants.[436] The immune response has been suggested as one of the factors that is involved with the attachment or clearance of refluxed endometrial tissue fragments.[436] Alterations in the immune response may prevent satisfactory disposal of menstrual debris, possibly increasing the chances of endometriosis development.[426] The nature and degree of impairment could account for the variable presentation of endometriosis. Alternatively, excessive menstrual reflux may overwhelm the capacity of an intact immune system to remove endometrial tissue or suppress its growth.[426]

The theory of an altered immune system and endometriosis suggests that changes in cell-mediated immunity and/or humoral immunity may contribute to the development of the disease.

CELL-MEDIATED IMMUNITY

Impairment of the cell-mediated immune response is thought to have a permissive effect on the implantation of refluxed endometrial cells, thereby increasing the chance of endometriosis development.[426] In women with endometriosis, a proliferation of peripheral blood lymphocytes in response to endometrial antigen and cells has been reported.[437] A decreased destruction of endometrial cells has also been suggested because the cytotoxic effect of peripheral blood lymphocytes against autologous endometrial cells is decreased in women with endometriosis.[437]

NATURAL KILLER (NK) CELLS

Natural killer (NK) cells have also been shown to be altered in women with endometriosis. NK cells are large granular lymphocytes that are cytotoxic to cells with an undefined target molecule and cells coated with antibody. Both peripheral and peritoneal cells from women with endometriosis display decreased cytotoxicity to autologous and heterologous endometrium compared with those of controls,[438] and peritoneal NK cell cytotoxicity has been shown to be inversely correlated with more severe stages of the disease.[439] Therefore it is postulated that the decrease in NK cell cytotoxicity to retrogradely shed endometrial tissue may allow for the establishment of this tissue in the peritoneal cavity.[436]

The observed decrease in NK activity appears to be a qualitative defect rather than a result of reduced numbers.[438] The decrease in NK activity has been reported to correlate with increasing oestradiol concentrations.[440] It is interesting to note that women with advanced endometriosis treated with gonadotrophin-releasing hormone (GnRH) agonists had an increase in NK-cell activity in peripheral blood mononuclear cells, which may be due to a direct effect of GnRH agonists or which may be indirect, via the lowering of serum oestradiol levels.[441] The cause of reduced NK activity is unknown.[437] Increased concentrations of transforming growth factor-β (TGF-β), IL-1 and tumour necrosis factor-α (TNF-α) in the peritoneal fluid of women with endometriosis have been reported.[442–444] TGF-β, however, inhibits NK activity, whereas IL-1 and TNF-α are expected to increase NK activity.[426]

Despite several studies reporting abnormal NK-cell activity in women with endometriosis, the clinical relevance of these results in relation to the development of endometriosis has been challenged.[445] More conclusive data are required to attribute a role to NK-cell activity in the development of endometriosis.[426]

In addition, both peritoneal fluid and sera from women with endometriosis have been shown to reduce NK-cell activity.[446] The constituents of the fluids responsible for this suppression have been hypothesised to be products of monocytes or macrophages.[446] Monocyte and macrophage products are known modulators of both immune and non-immune cells.[446] In particular, peritoneal macrophages have shown to be increased in total number, concentration and activational status in women with endometriosis.[447]

Associated with the increase in activational status of the macrophage is an increase in the release of their products such as growth factors and cytokines.[336] The postulated role of these macrophage products includes stimulation of endometrial cell proliferation,[448] and implantation of endometrial cells or tissue,[449] increased tissue modelling through regulation of matrix metalloproteinases,[450] and increased angiogenesis of the ectopic endometrial tissue.[451] Thus activated macrophages, through the liberation of cytokines and growth factors, could potentially contribute to early establishment of the disease at several foci.[436]

The possibility of a regulatory role for T-cells in the development of endometriosis has been suggested.[452] In women with mild endometriosis, quantification of T-cell subsets revealed a decrease in suppressor T-cell activity. In women with severe endometriosis, the decrease in suppressor T-cell activity was accompanied by an increase in helper T-cell activity.[452] These changes in the regulatory T-cells were suspected to have a role in the transition from mild to severe endometriosis.[453] Other conflicting results, however, show no change in the total number of peripheral lymphocytes or the percentage of T-cell subsets.[454] It is premature to conclude that altered T-cell responses in women with endometriosis are a causative factor until more rigorous data from well-designed human studies are available.[426]

HUMORAL-MEDIATED IMMUNITY

In addition to alterations in cell-mediated immunity, abnormalities in B-cell function and a high incidence of abnormal autoantibodies in women with endometriosis have been reported in several studies.[426] Antibodies to endometrial tissue may facilitate the growth of endometriosis by blocking the recognition sites required for T-cell-mediated destruction. Despite the detection of high levels of anti-endometrial antibodies (in particular, immunoglobulin G and immunoglobulin A) in sera, peritoneal fluid and endometrial tissue of women with endometriosis,[455] no correlation between antibody titres and disease severity was observed.[456] The suggestion of endometriosis as an autoimmune disease or part of a more generalised autoimmune syndrome has yet to be proved.[426]

AUTOIMMUNITY

There is debate as to whether endometriosis is truly an autoimmune disease. However, there are data currently available that strongly suggest that there are at least some very important similarities between endometriosis and such autoimmune diseases such as rheumatoid arthritis, Crohn's disease and psoriasis.[436] For example, increased inflammation, elevated levels of tissue remodelling components, altered apoptosis and increased local and/or systemic levels of cytokines.[436] In addition, like classical autoimmune diseases, endometriosis has been associated with polyclonal B-cell activation, immunological abnormalities in T- and B-cell functions, increased apoptosis, tissue damage, multi-organ involvement, familial occurrence, involvement of environmental cofactors, female preponderance and association with other autoimmune diseases (Table 18.34).[436] Endometriosis is associated with infertility and recurrent pregnancy loss, which might be explained by the presence of autoantibody abnormalities.[457] There is a higher risk of infertility associated with endometriosis in women aged less than 35 years old. This study was based on the Nurses' Health Study II cohort.[458]

However, for a disease to be truly autoimmune, it should be manifested in normal animals after adaptive transfer of immunoglobulin from the blood of affected tissues of subjects with the autoimmune disease.[436] To date, no such studies have been performed.[436]

TABLE 18.34 Common characteristics between autoimmune diseases and endometriosis
Tissue damage
Polyclonal B lymphocyte activity
T-lymphocyte immunological abnormalities
B-lymphocyte immunological abnormalities
Associated autoimmune diseases
Preponderance of females
Multiorgan involvement
Familial occurrence
Possible environmental factors
Possible genetic basis
Altered apoptosis

Source: Nothnick WB. Treating endometriosis as an autoimmune disease. Fertil Steril 2001;76(2):223–31

IATROGENIC

The iatrogenic introduction of endometrium to ectopic sites by mechanical transplantation has been suggested as another mechanism of endometriosis development.[426] Findings of endometriosis in episiotomy and laparotomy scars after gynaecological procedures support this theory.[459] The prospect of surgically transplanted endometrium has been demonstrated in animals and humans.[426] In women undergoing hysterectomy, cyclic bleeding occurred from excised endometrium that was intentionally implanted at the vaginal apex for psychological reasons.[426] The iatrogenic transplantation of endometrial tissue cannot account for most women with endometriosis.[426]

THE INDUCTION THEORY

The induction theory of endometriosis is a combination of the transplantation and coelomic metaplasia theories. This theory assumes that degenerating menstrual endometrium releases endogenous factors, which subsequently induce a metaplastic process in the serosal epithelium of ovaries and in the serosal cells of mesothelium, resulting in endometrial tissue.[460] To meet the criteria of endometriosis, both endometrial glands and stroma must be present in the ectopic lesion.[406] The reports supporting this theory have provided evidence that endometrium-like epithelium and glands are formed as a result of induction but unfortunately no direct evidence showing the formation of endometrial stroma has been reported.[406]

LYMPHATIC AND VASCULAR DISSEMINATION

Dissemination of endometrial cells through lymphatic or vascular channels has long been thought plausible.[407] To explain the occurrence of endometriosis at distant, non-contiguous sites, Halban[461] postulated that viable endometrial cells gain entry into open basal lymph and blood vessels and are embolised to ectopic sites. Similar mobilisation of endometrial cells might occur during surgical curettage of the endometrial cavity.[407]

EMBRYONIC CELL RESTS

The embryonic cell rests theory suggests that functioning endometrium can be formed by the activation of cell rests. This is based on the assumption that in areas adjacent to the Müllerian ducts, rudimentary duplications of the Müllerian system might be present, allowing cells of Müllerian origin to develop into functioning endometrium, particularly in peritoneal pockets or defects at the base of the broad ligaments.[407]

However, such incidental cell rests have not been demonstrated in the pelvis or thoracic cavity.[310] In addition, if this theory were correct, it would be expected to find endometriosis immediately after menarche, when hormonal stimulation is initiated.[310] By contrast, endometriosis has its highest incidence in women 25 years or older.[462]

DIRECT EXTENSION

The direct extension theory suggests that endometriosis arises from the invasion of endometrium through the uterine musculature.[426] This theory was based on the observation that glandular structures of adenomyosis were in direct contact with eutopic endometrium.[463] No conclusive evidence of the progression of endometrial invasion through the myometrium into the pelvis to present as endometriotic implants has been reported.[426]

ENDOMETRIOSIS LESION FORMATION: EVADING THE DEFENCE MECHANISM IN THE ABDOMINAL CAVITY

It was first reported that menstrual effluent evokes an inflammatory response when it arrives in the abdominal cavity and attracts large numbers of polymorphonuclear neutrophils (PMNs) and, subsequently, phagocytic and chemotactic leucocytes from the circulation.[464]

Prior to the onset of menstruation a marked influx of bone marrow-derived cells is observed. Approximately 70% of these cells are CD56+ natural killer (NK) cells, 20% are CD14+ macrophages and 10% CD3+ T-cells.[465] It is possible that the regurgitated menstrual effluent also contributes to the increased numbers of endometrial cells in the peritoneal cavity.

The physiological role of the inflammatory response is to clear the ectopic cells and tissue from the abdomen.[406] It appears that this is not a very effective system and microscopic endometriosis is probably intermittently present in all women with patent fallopian tubes and menstrual cycles.[406] Longer menstrual periods and heavier menstrual blood flow will result in larger amounts of endometrial tissue in the abdominal cavity, which increases the risk of developing symptomatic endometriosis.[406] Larger tissue fragments, and not individual cells or glands, have the capacity to develop into endometriotic lesions.[466]

The eutopic endometrium of women with endometriosis was also shown to be more resistant to lysis by NK cells than the eutopic endometrium of controls,[442] suggesting that endometrial tissue from endometriosis patients resides longer in the abdominal cavity.

The presence of substance A (a cytokine, a macrophage product, an angiogenic factor) has been studied in the peritoneal fluid of women with endometriosis.[406] Evidence supports the notion that protein factors present in the peritoneal fluid are able to affect processes in the peritoneum.[406] Dunselman and co-workers demonstrated that small proteins (<40 kDa) could be readily exchanged between the vasculature and the peritoneal fluid.[467] Thus, if the concentration of a certain factor is elevated in the peritoneal fluid, it might reach the circulation.[406] This suggests that factors present in the peritoneal fluid, which are basically exudates from peripheral blood, can also enter or re-enter the circulation and exert their influence on endometriotic lesions in a systemic way.[406]

MECHANISMS OF ADHESION

Cell adhesion molecules, most notably the integrins and cadherins, are the main mediators of cell–cell and cell–matrix adhesion and their expression might be important for the initial adhesion of the exfoliated tissue.[468]

Many studies have also investigated the expression pattern of integrins under physiological conditions in eutopic endometrium and in the pathological endometriotic tissue.[469] Numerous members of the integrin family are expressed by the endometrium throughout the menstrual cycle.[375] Integrins have been shown to form cell-surface complexes with MMPs to facilitate matrix degradation and motility, thereby facilitating directed cellular invasion.[470] Differences in the expression patterns of specific integrins between endometrial and endometriotic tissue might be of relevance because an aberrant cell–matrix interaction might allow glandular structures to grow deeply into the stroma, which would not otherwise be possible.[468]

Recently, however, hyaluronic acid and CD44 have been implicated in the interaction of peritoneal mesothelium with endometrial cells.[471] Peritoneal mesothelium produces hyaluronic acid that is expressed along the cell membrane of peritoneal mesothelial cells, contributes to the pericellular matrix, and is a major component of the extracellular matrix ground substance. CD44 is the principal receptor for hyaluronic acid. Endometrial stromal and epithelial cells express CD44. Further research is required to assess whether hyaluronic acid/CD44 binding is involved in the initial adherence of endometrium to peritoneal mesothelium.[375]

GROWTH AND SURVIVAL OF ECTOPIC CELLS

The demonstration of alterations in factors affecting endometrial proliferation suggests that aberrant growth contributes to the development of endometriosis.[375] Endometriosis requires oestrogen for its continued growth and, if deprived of this hormone, it tends to regress.[375] Aromatase is a cytochrome P450 enzyme that catalyses the rate-limiting step in oestrogen biosynthesis, the conversion of androgens to oestrogens.[383] Endometriotic cysts and extra-ovarian endometriotic implants express high levels of aromatase.[375] Prostaglandin E_2 (PGE_2) was identified as the most potent inducer of aromatase activity in endometriotic cells and oestrogen, in turn, was found to upregulate PGE_2 formation by stimulating cyclooxygenase type 2 enzyme.[375] Thus, a positive feedback loop for continuous local oestrogen and PGE_2 production is established in the pathological tissue itself.[375] These findings suggest that the aberrant expression of aromatase in endometriotic tissue might be involved in the pathogenetic mechanisms of endometriosis, promoting survival and growth of the lesion.[472]

Moreover, endometriosis tissue is often deficient in 17β-hydroxysteroid dehydrogenase type 2, which normally converts the strong oestrogenic compound 17β-oestradiol into the weakly oestrogenic oestrone.[406] Consequently, this protective mechanism, which lowers oestradiol levels, is lost in endometriosis tissue.[406] The higher oestradiol level of menstrual effluent in women with endometriosis than in controls conforms to this hypothesis.[406]

Together with steroid hormones, specific growth factors have been also demonstrated to favour endometriotic cell proliferation.[473] Basic fibroblast growth factor (bFGF) is constitutively present in the human endometrium and, as a result of its mitogenic and angiogenic activities, is probably involved in determining endometrial tissue modifications during the menstrual cycle.[474] Study results have speculated that, in women with endometriosis, oestrogens could indirectly influence bFGF expression by modulating the transcription of its antisense RNA.[475]

STEROID RESPONSIVENESS AND RECEPTOR CONTENT

The action of progesterone is mediated by its cognate receptors, which belong to the nuclear hormone receptor family.[375] Two progesterone receptor (PR) isoforms have recently been identified: namely PR-A and PR-B.[375] Although the exact functions of each of these isoforms are still unclear, there is increasing evidence that they are functionally different.[375] PR-B tends to be a stronger activator of progesterone target genes, whereas PR-A has been shown to act as a dominant repressor of PR-B.[375] PR-A also decreases the response to other steroid hormones such as androgen and oestrogen. PR isoforms have differential target gene specificity and might interact differently with a given promoter.[476] Therefore, it is conceivable that the alteration in the ratio of PR-A to PR-B in certain target tissues modifies the overall progesterone action via differential regulation of specific progesterone response genes.[477]

There is some evidence to suggest that endometriosis is characterised by a resistance to progesterone.[375] Attia et al have shown that only PR-A transcripts are present in endometriotic tissue sample, whereas both PR-A and PR-B transcripts are readily detectable in all eutopic samples.[477] Thus, progesterone resistance in endometriotic tissue might be accounted for by the presence of the inhibitory PR isoform PR-A and the absence of the stimulatory isoform PR-B.

An in-vitro study found that pro-inflammatory cytokines produced by epithelial cells can reduce expression of PR-B in adjacent stromal cells, resulting in a diminished progesterone response.[476] Notably, the reduced endometrial expression of PR-B induced by pro-inflammatory cytokines results in an altered PR-A/PR-B ratio, which mimics the in-vivo ratio observed in the eutopic endometrium of patients with endometriosis.[478] Osteen et al also found that inappropriate TGF-β signalling arises as a consequence of reduced progesterone responsiveness, a situation that might allow epithelial and/or immune pathways of paracrine communication to dominate stromal cells in the endometrium of women with endometriosis.[476] A complex array of locally produced factors may also act in concert to regulate MMP expression in response to progesterone.[476] In women with endometriosis, reduced responsiveness to progesterone results in altered expression of local cytokines and growth factors and thus dysregulated MMP expression.[476]

INVASION

Early lesion formation is an invasive event that requires breakdown of the extracellular matrix (ECM).[406] The ECM consists of collagens, proteoglycans and glycoproteins, including fibronectin and laminin.[406] Remodelling and breakdown of the ECM is mainly regulated by MMPs, the involvement of which was suspected after collagen breakdown products were found in the peritoneal fluid of patients with mild endometriosis.[479] MMPs have been implicated in the pathogenesis of endometriosis.[375]

MMPs play a pivotal role in the cyclic changes of growth and tissue breakdown that occur in the endometrium and, as expected, are under the regulation of oestrogen and progesterone.[379] For the most part, MMPs are synthesised during the proliferative phase and are thought to be stimulated by oestrogen.[476] Conversely, progesterone decreases the transcription and secretion of MMPs.[480]

Peritoneal invasion by endometrial tissue is thought to be dependent on MMPs and their specific tissue inhibitors (TIMPs).[375] This group of enzymes is important for the control of extracellular matrix turnover.[375] Recent reports suggest that eutopic endometrium from patients with endometriosis might be more invasive and prone to peritoneal implantation as a result of altered production of these proteolytic enzymes.[375,481] Abnormal expression of specific members of the MMP and TIMP families has been identified in both eutopic endometrium of affected women and in ectopic endometrium.[482] Moreover, expression patterns of both MMPs and TIMPs in endometriotic tissue appear to vary from eutopic tissue patterns, indicating that the cellular mechanisms regulating these factors might be defective in diseased tissue.[483] The exact mechanisms that lead to the aberrant expression of MMPs and TIMPs in endometriosis have yet to be defined.[375]

ACQUISITION OF BLOOD SUPPLY - VEGF AND ENDOMETRIOSIS

Vascularisation of endometriotic implants is probably one of the most important factors in the process of invasion of other tissues by endometrial cells.[484] The peritoneal environment is highly angiogenic, and increased activity and increased amounts of angiogenic factors have been demonstrated in peritoneal fluid from women with endometriosis.[375] Laparoscopic examination of endometriotic tissue has demonstrated this tissue-deriving blood from the surrounding peritoneum.[375]

In the endometrium, angiogenesis is regulated by many angiogenic and angiostatic factors, of which vascular endothelial growth factor (VEGF)-A appears to be the most important. In the proliferative phase of the menstrual cycle, oestradiol triggers VEGF-A expression in endometrial epithelial cells and stromal fibroblasts; this is further enhanced during the secretory phase.[485] Prior to menstruation, the endometrium as a result of vasoconstriction becomes hypoxic, which enhances the production of VEGF-A in the endometrial tissue even further.[485]

Elevated levels of VEGF are associated with increased blood vessel development and vascular permeability. It is expressed during the menstrual cycle as it facilitates follicle maturation and corpus luteum development post ovulation. The growing endometrium supports strong VEGF vascularisation to prepare for implantation. This results in increasing levels of inflammation, hypotension, and leakage of fluid and protein from vasculature.

BACTERIAL CONTAMINATION — ENDOMETRIAL MICROBIOTA

Endometriosis is a chronic inflammatory disease involving secondary inflammatory mediators.[486–489] Primary inflammatory mediators, e.g. bacterial endotoxin or lipopolysaccharide (LPS), trigger the secretion of various secondary inflammatory mediators, such as cytokines, chemokines, and growth factors, by mature/activated macrophages in the pelvis.[490] Results from several studies point to bacterial contamination of the endometrium as a potential new factor in the establishment of endometriosis.

A novel study demonstrated for the first time that menstrual blood of women with endometriosis is more contaminated with *E. coli* than that of control women and corresponds to higher levels of endotoxin in the menstrual fluid and consequently in the peritoneal fluid due to reflux of menstrual blood into the pelvis.[491] This may promote Toll-like receptor 4 (TLR4)-mediated growth of endometriosis, as evidenced by the increased endometrial cell growth in response to LPS and abrogation of these LPS-mediated effects by anti-TLR4 antibody. The concept of 'bacterial contamination hypothesis' for the development of endometriosis via LPS/TLR4-mediated engagement of innate immune response is suggested.[491]

The same authors identified that pathogenic genera including *Gardnerella*, *Entercoccus*, *Streptococcus* and *Staphylococcus* were predominantly identified in endometrial smears of women diagnosed with endometriosis followed by other taxa including *Actinomyces*, *Corynebacterium*, *Fusobacterium*, *Prevotella*, *Propionibacterium* compared to *Lactobacillus* spp.[492] In another study, Streptococcaceae and Staphylococcaceae spp. were significantly increased in the cystic fluid obtained from women with ovarian endometrioma.[493]

Women with a history of gynaecological infection are twice as likely to develop endometriosis[494] and are shown to have relief of endometriosis symptoms by prescribing antibiotics.[495]

When we consider the impact of oestrogen on the proliferation of endometriosis, it can be presumed that an additive effect would be possible of increased oestrogen and bacterial contamination. Khan et al demonstrated that in addition to the individual action of 17β-oestradiol (E2) and lipopolysaccharide (LPS) in promoting inflammatory response and growth of endometriosis, an additive effect between E2 and LPS might be involved in further worsening of pelvic inflammation and growth of endometriosis.[496] If we consider the internal milieu of the pelvic environment, a substantial amount of E2 and endotoxin in the pelvis of women with endometriosis may jointly trigger this detrimental effect.[491,497]

METHYLATION AND INFLAMMATION

The importance of optimising methylation cannot be underestimated. A recent study highlighted that endometriosis promotes a chronic inflammatory picture which can lead to potential epigenetic modification programming within the eutopic endometrium. Aberrant regulation of gene transcription and post-translational regulatory mechanisms through noncoding RNAs likely contribute to development of progesterone resistance and heightened response to oestrogen, which are two key characteristics of the eutopic endometrium of women with endometriosis.[498] In addition, the chronic inflammatory picture leads to hypersensitisation in areas of pain perception which perpetuates the cycle.

SPECIFIC ENDOMETRIOSIS LOCATIONS

Ovarian endometriosis

Different models have been proposed to explain the pathogenesis of typical ovarian endometriosis. The formation of typical chocolate cysts might be due to:

- Inversion and progressive invagination of the ovarian cortex after the accumulation of menstrual debris derived from bleeding of superficial endometriotic implants, which are located on the ovarian surface and adherent to the peritoneum[375]
- Secondary involvement of functional ovarian cysts by endometrial implants located on the ovarian surface[375]
- Metaplasia of the coelomic epithelium covering the ovary.

Deep rectovaginal endometriosis

There are two hypotheses for this form of endometriosis:

- An adenomyotic nodule that originates by modifications of Müllerian rests and progresses into endometriotic glands by a process of metaplasia[375]
- The natural evolution of peritoneal endometriosis of the pouch of Douglas as a consequence of its secondary infiltration.[375]

SIGNS AND SYMPTOMS

A significant number of women with endometriosis remain asymptomatic, while some exhibit excruciating presentations. Common signs and symptoms include those listed in Table 18.35.

Cyclic pain

Cyclic pain is pain that accompanies bleeding at the time of menstruation. This could involve the bladder (haematuria), bowel (haematochezia and dyschezia), or rarely, bleeding at uncommon sites such as the umbilicus, abdominal wall, perineum, lung or brain.[383]

TABLE 18.35 Symptoms of endometriosis

Menstrual	Cyclic pain Dysmenorrhoea Mittelschmerz (pain on ovulation) Heavy or long uncontrollable menstrual periods with small or large blood clots Premenstrual spotting Metrorrhagia Menstrual spotting post intercourse
Reproductive	Chronic pelvic pain Dyspareunia Infertility Hot flushes prior to menstruation Hot flushes at ovulation Hot flushes at conception and/or implantation Vaginal thrush (especially premenstrually)
Urinary	Dysuria and/or haematuria Urinary tract infections (especially premenstrually
Digestive	Dyschezia and/or haematochezia Nausea Abdominal bloating Flatulence Diarrhoea (especially with menses) Constipation (especially premenstrually) Vomiting
Neurological	Headaches Chronic fatigue Fainting Dizzy spells
Psychological	Depression Anxiety
Musculoskeletal	Pain in legs and thighs Back pain
Endocrinological	Hypoglycaemia
Haematological	Anaemia (especially iron deficiency)

Chronic pelvic pain

Defined as pain of greater than 6-month duration and not cyclical in nature.[499] An important point to remember is that the degree of visible endometriosis has no correlation with the degree of pain or symptomatic impairment. However, pain does appear to correlate with depth of tissue infiltration.[500] Midline disease is generally believed to be more painful than lateral disease.[383]

Acute exacerbations

These are believed to be caused by chemical peritonitis due to leakage of old blood from an endometriotic cyst. Recently, with conscious laparoscopic pain mapping, painful lesions were found to involve peripheral spinal nerves rather than autonomic nerves.[501]

Dysmenorrhoea

Secondary dysmenorrhoea occurs twice as often in women with endometriosis as in controls.[383] Pain frequently commences prior to menses and can last up to one week after menses. Endometriosis should be considered in a patient presenting with significant dysmenorrhoea.[383]

Dyspareunia

Deep dyspareunia may be due to scarring of the uterosacral ligaments, nodularity of the rectovaginal septum, cul-de-sac obliteration and/or uterine retroversion.[383] All of these may also lead to chronic backache. These symptoms are exaggerated during menses. Women with deep infiltration of the uterosacral ligaments were shown to have the most severe impairment of sexual function.[502]

Dyschezia and/or haematochezia

Through contiguous spreading, endometriosis may invade the rectovaginal septum and the interior rectal wall.[383] It may also involve the upper rectum and sigmoid colon. Cyclical rectal bleeding (haemochezia) is pathognomonic of endometriosis.[383] The ileum, appendix and caecum may also be involved, leading to intestinal obstruction.[283] Uterine serosa can also be affected promoting an inflammatory response causing obliteration of the cul-de-sac and form dense adhesions between the posterior vaginal wall or cervix and the anterior rectum, resulting in dyschezia and an alteration of bowel habits.[383]

Dysuria and/or haematuria

Through affected uterine serosa, vesicular lesions may provoke an inflammatory response and scarring that cause the bladder to adhere anteriorly. Interference in the genitourinary tract by endometriosis can affect the bladder, ureters and kidneys by invasion, compression and scarring.[383]

COMPLICATIONS

Making a diagnosis of endometriosis purely on presenting symptoms is difficult as there is considerable overlap with other conditions.[499] This often results in a delay in diagnosis of greater than 5 years.[503] This is important when one considers that endometriosis is a progressive disease that worsens over time.[382] The delay in diagnosis may also result in associated psychological morbidity.[504]

Complications that can arise from endometriosis include:

- Adhesion formation
- Pelvic cysts
- Endometriomas
- Ruptured endometriomas
- Bowel and ureteral obstruction resulting from pelvic adhesions
- Peritonitis from bowel perforation.

The prevalence of endometriosis in infertile women is estimated to range between 30% and 50%.[505] The most obvious causes in moderate or severe disease are the simple mechanical effects of endometriotic adhesions or ovarian cysts on fertility.[506] However, infertile patients with much milder forms of the disease are also seen. Although some specialists argue that these two findings may be casual rather than causal, others have cited evidence suggesting the possible involvement of endocrine abnormalities (e.g. attenuation of the luteinising hormone (LH) surge), luteinised unruptured follicle syndrome, defects in the luteal phase or abnormalities in peritoneal fluid (e.g. altered levels of prostanoids, cytokines, growth factors or interleukins).[506] Such changes could affect the environment within the fallopian tube or the pelvis, thus affecting the oocytes in some way.[506] Immune system deficiencies in patients with endometriosis could affect implantation, and this and oocyte defects may increase the rate of miscarriage.[506]

The infertility caused by pelvic endometriosis can also contribute to the development of mental disorders. In 2001, Bergqvist and Theorell[507] compared infertile women with endometriosis to fertile women and found that 50% of the women in the former group had looked for psychiatric help, or expressed a need for such help, within the preceding 4 weeks. In this study there was no correlation between infertility and psychiatric symptoms.

In 2006, Lorençatto et al[508] evaluating 100 Brazilian women with endometriosis, identified depression in 86% of those with chronic pelvic pain, compared with 38% of those without such pain.

In 1995, Waller and Shaw[509] found that women with mild symptomatic endometriosis presented with greater depression and more often suffered from sexual dysfunction. These results differ from those obtained in a study conducted by Renaer et al,[510] who demonstrated higher anxiety levels in the women with endometriosis-related pain.

MANIFESTATIONS

Peritoneal endometriosis

Superficial endometriosis has multiple appearances on laparoscopy. The classic lesion has a puckered, blue-black powder burn appearance.[511] Other appearances, including the microscopic, early or subtle (popular or glandular, vesicular) haemorrhagic (red vesicular or flame like) and fibrotic (from white to black pigmented) lesions, supposedly represent the evolution of a superficial implant.[511]

Neoangiogenesis and adhesion formation are typical features in the early, active implant.[511] Stromal vascularisation is highest in the red, non-fibrotic lesions, less frequent in the typical black lesions and scarce in the white lesions.[511] It is believed that the red lesions are early and very active, the black lesions are advanced and active and the white lesions are healed or inactive.[512]

Endometriomas

Endometriomas (endometrial cysts of the ovary) represent a superficial haemorrhagic and adhesive type of endometriosis.[511] The 'cyst'-like structures contain a thick 'chocolate-like' substance formed from old blood.[511] More than 90% of ovarian endometriomas are pseudocysts formed by the invagination of the ovarian cortex, which is sealed off by adhesions.[511] The site of invagination is characterised by fibrosis, retraction of the cortex, islands of glandular endometriotic tissue and organised blood clots.[511]

Imaging has become an important tool for the diagnosis of the ovarian endometrioma. Lesions on the ovary can vary in size from spots to large endometriomas.[383] The classic lesion is a chocolate cyst of the ovary that contains old blood that has undergone haemolysis.[383] Once intracystic pressure rises, the cyst perforates, spilling its contents within the peritoneal cavity. This can cause severe abdominal pain, typically associated with endometriosis exacerbations. The inflammatory response causes adhesions that further increase the morbidity of the disease.[383]

DIFFERENTIAL DIAGNOSIS

Given the nonspecific symptoms of endometriosis, the differential diagnosis is lengthy. The possibility of malignancy must be considered (Table 18.36).

NATUROPATHIC DIAGNOSIS

As the condition presents significant complications, it is likely that the patient will present with a formal diagnosis that the naturopath will be able to use. There are some patients who have not been diagnosed and benefit from thorough case taking and assessment. As such, please review the section below as often the extensive nature of the naturopathic consultation can elucidate undiagnosed presentations.

TABLE 18.36 Differential diagnosis of endometriosis by symptom

Dysmenorrhoea	Generalised pelvic pain
Primary Secondary adenomyosis myomas infection cervical stenosis	Pelvic adhesions, neoplasms, ovarian torsion, pelvic inflammatory disease, non-gynaecological causes, physical or sexual abuse
Dyspareunia	**Infertility**
Insufficient arousal causes diminished lubrication or diminished expansion of the vagina Gastrointestinal causes (e.g. constipation, irritable bowel syndrome, diarrhoea) Infection Urinary causes (e.g. urethral syndrome, interstitial cystitis) Musculoskeletal causes (e.g. pelvic relaxation, levator spasm) Pelvic vascular congestion	Anovulation Cervical factors (e.g. mucus, sperm, antibodies, stenosis) Luteal phase deficiency Male factor infertility Tubal disease or infection

Source: Adapted from Mounsey AL, Wilgus A, Slawson DC. Diagnosis and management of endometriosis. Am Fam Physician 2006.

Investigations

Although definitive diagnosis is only achieved from laparoscopic investigation, a number of other assessments can be beneficial in earlier stages.

LAPAROSCOPY

The 'gold standard' for diagnosing endometriosis in the abdomen and pelvis is the visual identification of characteristic lesions at laparoscopy.[499] Endometriosis has been described as protean in appearance.[383] The classic lesions are blue-black or have a powder-burned appearance.[383] However, the lesions can be red, white or non-pigmented.[383] Peritoneal defects and adhesions are also indicative.[383] However, the use of laparoscopy for the diagnosis of endometriosis is increasingly criticised for its invasiveness, limited reproducibility and gasbell artifacts.[511]

Laparoscopy is used to investigate the cause of disease in the interior of the abdominal or pelvic cavities with use of a long tube known as a laparoscope which has a small camera attached to it, via a small incision usually through the navel. Considered to be the gold standard by some in evaluation of pelvic pain associated with endometriosis, adhesions and pelvic congestion[513] as well as ovarian cysts and chronic pelvic inflammatory disease, however a 1993 review found that fewer than 50% of women with chronic pelvic pain were helped by diagnostic and operative laparoscopy.[514]

PHYSICAL EXAMINATION — PERFORMED BY GP

Clinical signs on examination can be difficult for a clinician to elicit.[499] Endometriotic nodules on the uterosacral ligaments or in the recto-vaginal septum can be found and a clinician may find them easier to feel on a combined vaginal–rectal examination.[499] These are most reliably palpated if the examination is undertaken during menstruation.[383] The uterus may be fixed in retroversion, owing to adhesions.[383] In some cases, endometriosis invading through the vaginal mucosa may be visible on speculum examination.[499]

LABORATORY STUDIES

CA125 (serum anticancer antigen 125)

CA125 is a marker for serous carcinoma, especially carcinoma of the ovary, but elevations are also seen in peritoneal disease of any cause. It is considered a primary initial investigation for women with endometriosis. It is raised in some women with endometriosis, particularly if they are more advanced, but according to some sources, the test remains nonspecific.[499] It is important to remember that elevations can occur with other reproductive pathologies; however, it is generally agreed that low levels are conducive with endometriosis pathology. If levels are elevated, all patients should undergo a transvaginal and transabdominal ultrasound to exclude other pathologies. In extreme elevations, referral for laparoscopic investigations is essential.

Reference range

The normal values for CA125 vary slightly among individual laboratories. In most laboratories, the normal value is less than 35 U/mL. In the patient who is being evaluated for a pelvic mass, a CA125 level greater than 65 is associated with malignancy in approximately 90% of cases. However, without a demonstrable mass, the association is much weaker.

CA125 and cancer

Although CA125 is a useful test in monitoring women who are being treated for ovarian cancer, a single CA125 test is not considered to be a useful screening test for cancer. Some women with ovarian cancer (up to 20%) never have elevated CA125 levels, while most women who do have elevated CA125 levels do not have cancer. In fact, because CA125 can be elevated in so many non-cancerous conditions, only about 3% of women with elevated CA125 levels have ovarian cancer.

Other potential markers have been assessed including the following.

Serum protein, PP14

Another serum protein, PP14, has been evaluated as a marker for endometriosis.[426] PP14 levels correlate with the severity of endometriosis and decrease during suppressive medical treatment of endometriosis.[515] In one paper, the sensitivity and specificity of PP14 in the diagnosis of endometriosis were 59% and 96%, respectively.[515]

Serum anti-endometrial antibodies

Serum anti-endometrial antibodies also have been evaluated as a test for endometriosis.[499] Elevation of anti-endometrial antibodies is usually observed in the presence of endometriosis.[426] The reported sensitivity and specificity of anti-endometrial antibodies are 83% and 79%, respectively.[516] In another study, anti-endometrial antibodies could not be found using several different detection methods used previously in other studies.[517] The clinical applicability of testing anti-endometrial antibodies remains to be determined.[426]

Gene expression analysis

Gene expression analysis is also beginning to identify potential markers for endometriosis in peripheral blood samples as well as in endometriotic lesions.[518] There is nothing conclusive at this stage.

TRANSVAGINAL ULTRASOUND

Transabdominal and transvaginal ultrasound are not considered optimal for diagnosis; however, they can detect large masses so are considered a useful alternative to exclude alternative pathologies or assist in the diagnosis of endometriosis if greater than stage 3.

Transvaginal ultrasound is not useful in the diagnosis of peritoneal endometriosis although it is useful for diagnosing endometriomas and disease infiltrating the bladder.[519] Transrectal ultrasound is a useful tool in diagnosing deep infiltrating disease in the recto-vaginal septum.[520]

MAGNETIC RESONANCE IMAGING (MRI)

Magnetic resonance imaging (MRI) has been shown to be of use in diagnosing the extent of deep nodular disease, particularly in the recto-vaginal septum.[521] However, the cost-effectiveness of this imaging modality for endometriosis has yet to be justified for use as a routine tool.[383]

OTHER

Vaginal lesions may be visually confirmed on speculum examination, in the bladder at cystoscopy or in the bowel mucosa at sigmoidoscopy.[499] It is considered good clinical practice to confirm a visual diagnosis with histological confirmation of at least one lesion.[522] However, negative histology does not exclude the diagnosis.[499] Histopathology is also recommended for atypical lesions to exclude malignancy and to differentiate from other possible benign lesions.[511] Disease sites and depths should be mapped and recorded to allow for adequate reassessment of the disease at subsequent laparoscopy if necessary.[522]

SPECIFIC NATUROPATHIC INVESTIGATIONS

Clinical assessment

A thorough clinical history that includes a detailed reproductive health history is an important naturopathic investigative tool. However, making a diagnosis purely on presenting symptoms is difficult as there is considerable overlap with other conditions. Please refer to extensive discussion in the previous section on menstruation for a full review. It is beneficial to use these questions regularly to assess progress and development of treatment.

Endometriosis pain journal

Appendix 18.2 at the end of the book provides a useful template that can be used with endometriosis patients. When used with patients, it provides a thorough review of the severity and impact of their individual disease process.

MTHFR

Folate metabolism is crucial for the correct replication of every cell in the body — including those within the uterus. Elimination of folate defects is essential to eliminate contributing factors.

Coeliac profile and gene screen

Due to immune irregularities that predispose the development of this condition, it is beneficial to eliminate compounding factors that may contribute to the disease progression and development.

Comprehensive digestive stool analysis

It is important to eliminate a concurrent digestive infection that is contributing to the pathogenesis and symptomatology.

Cytokine panel

It is useful to assess a cytokine panel to review potential interleukin fluctuations that are suggestive of a compounding variable such as an infection, parasite or histamine hypersensitivity.

Vitamin D and liver function test

Due to the conflicting research available regarding vitamin status and liver function (see below in nutrient discussion), it is imperative to assess the patient holistically and obtain both 25-hydroxyvitamin-D3 as well as a 1,25-dihydroxyvitamin-D3 in conjunction with a liver function test before prescribing vitamin D supplementation or considering its impact.

Therapeutic considerations

CLINICAL DECISION MAKING AND RATIONALE

The naturopathic approach considers multiple variables in its holistic assessment including the following key areas:

- Reduction of inflammation and identification and eradication of pathogen contributing to proliferation and sequelae
- Methylation function to reduce inflammation and cytokine levels
- Steroid hormone responsiveness and receptor activity
- Endogenous and exogenous exposure to oestrogen causing displacement issues
- Environmental toxin exposure, toxic burden and hepatobiliary clearance
- Hepatobiliary function, lipid profile and hormone synthesis
- Immune modulation, consideration of factors that compound autoimmune predisposition or immune hyper reactivity
- Level of oxidation, prooxidant factors in diet and lifestyle and antioxidant status
- Microflora status of digestive and reproductive systems
- Digestive health, function and nutrient absorption and assimilation
- Patient desire for outcome — symptomatic or goal oriented (i.e. fertility)
- Factors that impede menstrual flow and contribute to menstrual retrograde (i.e. sexual intercourse, sanitary items)
- Circulatory and lymphatic activity within reproductive organs and surrounding tissues, impediments to circulation throughout the body and blood cleansing through hepatobiliary channels.

Therapeutic application

HISTORICAL PERSPECTIVE

Endometriosis is an antique condition, having been described in 1960 by a German physician named Daniel Shroen.[523] While the condition was not defined during the time of the Eclectics, women presented with endometriosis-like presentations such as strong dysmenorrhoea, menorrhagia with clotting, dyspareunia, infertility and others. A wide range of botanicals were available for its management. For example, for pain relief anodynes and analgesics such as *Corydalis ambigua* were suggested for dysmenorrhoea,[8] while *Piscidia piscipula* was used in female disorders for its profound effects in alleviating neuralgic and other forms of dysmenorrhoea as well as other pelvic neuroses.[8] As well as *Corydalis ambigua*, a number of other botanicals are detailed for relief from particular types of dysmenorrhoea. These include *Tanacetum parthenium* applied as fomentation for painful dysmenorrhoea[8] and *Piper methysticum* for spasmodic dysmenorrhoea.[9] Circulatory stimulants such as *Zingiber officinale* were used to help relieve the pangs of disordered and painful menstruation[8] as was *Cinnamomum zeylanicum*, said to combine well with *Viburnum prunifolium*.

Acknowledging the role of the nervous system, *Anemone pulsatilla* was suggested for irregular menstruation to promote a normal and regular flow in combination with nervous system derangement[7] while *Hypericum perforatum* appeared useful for menorrhagia, hysteria, nervous affections with depression, haemoptysis and other haemorrhages.[8] Antispasmodics such as *Dioscorea villosa* and the viburnums were highlighted for their ability to help relieve pain or spasms;[8] *Viburnum prunifolium* in particular enjoys a long description in King's where it is described as a uterine sedative and tonic, being best for atonic states of the female reproductive organs (see modern description). *Calendula* was strongly endorsed for endometriosis, while for relief from excessive bleeding a number of botanicals are mentioned, however of these, King's suggests that *Achillea millefolium* is one of the best agents for the relief of menorrhagia.[8]

ALLOPATHIC PERSPECTIVE

In the treatment of endometriosis, diverse therapeutic approaches, including no treatment, medical treatment, surgical treatment, and a combination of medical and surgical treatment, have been used to address the clinical consequences (i.e. pain, infertility and pelvic masses).[426] The use of analgesia (e.g. non-steroidal anti-inflammatory drugs, NSAIDs) is also considered in patients with pain. Although there are reports of shortcomings in the classification system on which the studies evaluating treatment outcome are based, a clinician's decision making regarding treatment must be made with the available data. Most importantly, initial assessment of the reproductive goals of the patient is essential before initiating treatment. Moreover, a clear understanding of the treatment options and the desired end point can facilitate the formulation of a treatment plan to address the individual needs of each patient.

In most cases, women who reach the gynaecology clinic will already have been treated with NSAIDs in primary care. Although there is some evidence that these drugs reduce endometriosis-related pain,[499] the majority of women presenting to the gynaecologist in secondary care will report little benefit from this therapy.

MEDICAL THERAPY

Medical treatment consists of hormonal therapy that most commonly includes combination oral contraceptives, high-dose progestogen danazol and GnRH agonists.[426] The basis of pharmacological therapy is that endometriosis implants are capable of responding to hormones. These medications interrupt the cycle of stimulation and bleeding of ectopic endometrial tissue and induce atrophy of the implants, decreasing pain and the inflammatory response that may cause fibrosis and adhesions.[426] Unfortunately, current medical therapy is not definitive in the treatment of endometriosis because fibrosis and adhesions cannot be removed and recurrence of endometriosis may occur after cessation of treatment.[426]

Combined oral contraceptive pills (COCs), danazol, progestational agents and GnRH analogues form the mainstay of medical therapy. All these therapies have similar clinical efficacy in terms of reduction in pain-related symptoms and duration of relief. NSAIDs have not been shown to have any benefit in placebo-controlled trials.[524] In a systematic review, aromatase inhibitors were shown to have promising results for pain relief when combined with either progestogen COCs or GnRH analogues.[525] However, the authors concluded that the strength of this inference was limited due to lack of sizeable trials.[525]

COCs act by ovarian suppression and continuous progestogen administration.[383] All progestational agents act by decidualisation and atrophy of the endometrium.[383] GnRH analogues produce a hypogonadotrophic–hypogonadic state by downregulation of the pituitary gland. Currently, goserelin and leuprolide acetate are the commonly used agonists. Danazol acts by inhibiting the midcycle follicle-stimulating hormone (FSH) and luteinising hormone (LH) surges and preventing steroidogenesis in the corpus luteum.[383] It is the most extensively studied agent for endometriosis.[383] There are a number of side effects associated with medical treatments and these should be discussed with the patient prior to administration.

SURGICAL CARE

Surgical care can be broadly classified as conservative when reproductive potential is retained, semi-conservative when reproductive ability is eliminated but ovarian function is retained, and radical when the uterus and ovaries are removed. Age, desire for future childbearing, and deterioration of quality of life are the main considerations when deciding on the extent of surgery.

Conservative surgery

With conservative surgery, the aim is to destroy visible endometriotic implants and lyse peritubal and periovarian adhesions that are a source of pain and may interfere with ovum transport. The laparoscopic approach is the method of choice for treating endometriosis conservatively.[526] Ablation can be performed with laser or electrodiathermy.[383] Overall, the recurrence rate is 19% and is similar for all techniques.[527] Ovarian endometriomas can be treated by drainage or cystectomy.[383] Laparoscopic cystectomy was found to yield better pain relief and pregnancy rates than drainage.[528]

The absolute benefit for women undergoing surgical ablation of endometriosis is 30–40% over women having only diagnostic laparoscopy, in the short term.[383] This benefit reduced over time, and re-operation rate is as high as 50%.[529] In cases of rectovaginal endometriosis, significant short-term pain relief was reported by up to 80%, but at 1-year follow-up, 50% required analgesics or hormones for pain relief.[383]

Tubal flushing with oil-soluble media has been shown to improve pregnancy rates in women with endometriosis-associated infertility.[530]

Presacral neurectomy is used to relieve severe dysmenorrhoea.[383] Vascular injury to the middle sacral artery and vein is a potential complication, and some authors advocate prophylactic ligation.[383] Also, constipation is a long-term adverse effect (94%) of this procedure and should be considered while deciding whether to perform this procedure.[383]

Semi-conservative surgery

The indication for this type of surgery is mainly in women who have completed their childbearing, are too young to undergo surgical menopause, and are debilitated by the symptoms.[383] Such surgery involves hysterectomy and cytoreduction of pelvic endometriosis. Ovarian endometriosis can be removed surgically because one tenth of functioning ovarian tissue is all that is needed for hormone production.[383] Patients who undergo hysterectomy with ovarian conservation have a six-fold higher rate of recurrence compared with women who undergo oophorectomy.[531]

Medical therapy in women who have completed childbearing is equally efficacious for symptom suppression.[383]

Radical surgery

This involves total hysterectomy with bilateral oophorectomy and cytoreduction of visible endometriosis.[383] Adhesiolysis is performed to restore mobility and normal intrapelvic organ relationships.

Ureteric obstruction may warrant surgical release or excision of a damaged segment. Bowel obstruction may require a resection anastomosis or a wedge resection if the obstruction is confined to the anterior rectosigmoid.[383]

Endometriosis may recur in 15% of women after extirpative surgery, irrespective of whether hormone replacement therapy is given postoperatively.[532]

Comparison of medical and surgical therapy

In women who wish to preserve their reproductive potential, the rates of recurrent pain symptoms are 44% with surgical management and 53% with medical management.[533,534]

INFERTILITY

Surgery is usually the treatment of choice for endometriosis-associated infertility.[426] The advantage of surgical therapy in the treatment of infertility is the opportunity to remove adhesions and restore normal anatomy.[426] In contrast to medical treatment, a period of contraception is not required.[426] This provides the older infertility patients a time saving of up to 6 months, during which time fertility may decrease.[426] In general, within 1–2 years after surgical therapy for endometriosis, a pregnancy rate of approximately 65% can be expected.[426] Recurrence of endometriosis implants after surgery was reported for 28% of patients within 18 months and 40.3% after 5 years.[535]

In patients with minimal or mild endometriosis, laparoscopic treatment has been used frequently because treatment can be accomplished easily during diagnostic laparoscopy.[426] However, the ablation or removal of endometriosis implants potentially can increase the risk for postsurgical adhesion formation.[426] The decision to treat minimal or mild endometriosis has been based on the nature and location of the lesions, on the potential of the disease to become more advanced, and on the presence of pain symptoms.[426] In light of the difficulties in evaluating the data in the literature, the lack of rigorous clinical studies showing an improvement in fertility, and the variable length of follow-up in infertility studies, the conventional wisdom has been that surgical treatment for minimal or mild endometriosis does not confer an advantage over expectant management.[426]

In the presence of moderate or severe endometriosis, surgery has been advocated as the treatment of choice for endometriosis-associated infertility[426] due to the usual anatomical distortion associated with moderate or severe endometriosis.[426]

However, prospective randomised studies and systematic reviews assessing the effect of surgically corrected endometriosis on fecundity have been limited, sometimes contradictory and at best have demonstrated a modest effect (especially with minimal–mild endometriosis).[526–538]

Although laparoscopy is valued for its accurate and extensive diagnostic capabilities, it is an invasive procedure requiring general anaesthetic and hospitalisation.[539] Apart from general feelings of pain and discomfort, there is a risk of injury to abdominal vessels and bowel and the reported mortality rate due to surgical complications is between 3 and 7 deaths per 100 000 laparoscopies.[540]

NATUROPATHIC PERSPECTIVE

When presented with an endometriosis patient it is imperative to first assess the patient's goals for treatment. Occasionally the patient desires symptomatic support only and does not wish to make significant changes for successful modification of disease process. Assessment and discussion at the beginning of treatment can dispel myths and empower the patient to hope for more than natural alternatives to pharmaceutical analgesics and regular D and Cs.

The severity of presentation varies dramatically. It is expected that as women delay child-rearing mild endometriosis is generally expected. Severe cases tend to additionally associate with genetic influences and other variables. Thorough review using the endometriosis pain journal (Appendix 18.2 at the end of the book) can elucidate the extent of the presentation. It is useful to substantiate subjective interpretation with laboratory and surgical findings.

When presented with a patient immediately post laparoscopy and surgical ablation, practitioners are advised to focus treatment that aggressively prevents recurrence. If endometriosis is currently active, treatment should provide symptomatic relief in conjunction with disease reduction strategies and prevention of disease progression.

Endometriosis is not a condition to treat lightly. Optimal outcome is achieved with holistic consideration of all variables, comprehensive nutritional and herbal prescription, and dietary and lifestyle modifications. Simple strategies show limited effectiveness and maintain patient reliance on treatment rather than changing disease progression and development.

In consideration of clinical rationale, the following areas are comprehensively addressed concurrently:

- Reduction of inflammation
- Regulate methylation
- Improvement of hormone cascades and receptor responsiveness
- Avoidance of compounding oestrogen interferences
- Avoidance of environmental toxins and support of elimination
- Support of hepatobiliary function to support toxin clearance, lipid metabolism, hormone synthesis and metabolism
- Antioxidant supplementation
- Immune modulation
- Microflora recolonisation
- Improvement to digestive function
- Improvement of lymphatic and circulatory function
- Lifestyle and dietary changes
- Symptomatic support — reduce pain, reduce endometrial tissue displacement.

NUTRITIONAL MEDICINE (DIETARY)

Dietary therapeutic objectives

- Avoid exogenous oestrogen sources which compound hormone cascades
- Avoid endocrine disrupting chemicals. Organochlorines, such as those found on non-organic fruits and vegetables, have been positively associated with the risk for endometriosis[541]
- Encourage antioxidant foods such as fresh fruits and vegetables
- Encourage optimal microflora colonisation with pre and probiotic foods such as fermented sources
- Encourage immune building foods such as garlic, onion and fresh herbs
- Reduce immune aggravating foods such as sugar and refined carbohydrates
- Decrease proinflammatory foods such as saturated, trans and oxidised fat sources, A1 cow's milk dairy products, gluten containing foods
- Increase essential fatty acids for dietary sources of omega-3 fatty acids such as EPA and DHA for anti-inflammatory benefit
- Encourage indole-3-carbinole (I3C) food sources such as cruciferous vegetables to assist liver detoxification
- Avoid contributing factors such as caffeine and alcohol.

Specific dietary treatments

DIETARY INCLUSIONS

Antioxidant-rich foods

Oxidative stress is not the underlying cause of endometriosis; however. it plays a role in ectopic endometrial tissue implantation and is thought to promote angiogenesis and the growth and proliferation of endometrial lesions.[542] Peritoneal fluid containing ROS-generating iron, macrophages, and environmental contaminants such as PCBs may disrupt the balance between ROS and antioxidants, resulting in increased proliferation of tissue and adhesions. The evidence linking endometriosis and infertility to endogenous pro-oxidant imbalance promotes the use of antioxidants in therapy.[543] A study undertaken on Mexican women observed that women with endometriosis had lower antioxidant intakes than women without.[21] Following administration of a diet rich in antioxidants, antioxidant status in women with endometriosis improved; this is significant given that oxidative stress has been identified in women with endometriosis and is likely to aggravate inflammation and pathology. By naturopathic standards these types of inclusions in the diet are not difficult to follow comprising:

- Vitamin A (1050 micrograms retinol equivalents) (administered via vitamin A-rich vegetables, e.g. carrot, broccoli, chard)
- Vitamin C (500 mg) (administered via vitamin C-rich fruits, e.g. guava, oranges)
- Vitamin E (20 mg) (in the form of sunflower seeds and peanuts)
- Fresh fruits and vegetables.

A 2004 study[544] undertaken on Italian women with endometriosis observed that high intake of green vegetables and fresh fruit appeared to protect against endometriosis. This may be due to increased antioxidants, fibre or other factors. The brassica vegetables (e.g. Brussels sprouts, cabbage, broccoli) should all be encouraged in endometriosis due to their indole-3-carbinol content. Conversely there was an increase in risk in the prevalence of endometriosis in those who consumed a high intake of beef and other red meat as well as ham,[429] possibly due to its pro-inflammatory nature. A study showed that resveratrol was effective in reducing the size of endometrial implants, as well as the levels of vascular endothelial growth factor (VEGF) in the plasma and peritoneal fluid in a rat model. It increased suppression of VEGF in endometrial tissue and favoured histological changes in the focal point of the disease after treatment.[545] This further supports the role of antioxidants in the prevention and management of endometriosis, although further human trials are needed.

Omega-3 fatty acids

Omega-3 fatty acids should be encouraged in the diet. A study comparing 64 endometriosis patients with 74 healthy controls found that the levels of serum fatty acids did not appear to be significant marker for endometriosis; however, the ratio of omega-3 to omega-6 was associated with the severity of the illness.[546] This study supports findings of an early animal study which found that an improved ratio of omega-3 to omega-6 suppressed the thickening of the interstitium, an active site for inflammation in endometriosis.[547]

In another large study,[548] it was found that trans fats were linked to increased endometriosis risk and omega-3-rich food linked to lower risk. This study — which is the largest to have investigated the link between diet and endometriosis risk and the first prospective study to identify a modifiable risk factor for the condition — found that while the total amount of fat in the diet did not matter, the type of fat did. Women who ate the largest amount of long-chain omega-3 fatty acids were 22% less likely to be diagnosed with endometriosis than those who ate the least and that those who ate the most trans fats had a 48% increased risk, compared with those who ate the least.

The findings from 70 709 American nurses followed for 12 years, published in *Human Reproduction*,[548] not only suggested that diet may be important in the development of endometriosis, but also provided more evidence that a low-fat diet is not necessarily the healthiest and further bolstered the case for eliminating trans fats from the food supply.

In the study, the researchers collected information from 1989 to 2001 on 70 709 women enrolled in the US Nurses' Health Study II cohort. They used three food-frequency questionnaires spaced at 4-year intervals to record the women's usual dietary habits over the preceding year. They categorised consumption of the various types of dietary fat into five levels and related that information to later confirmed diagnoses of endometriosis. A total of 1199 women were diagnosed with the disease by the end of the study. The results were adjusted to eliminate any influence on the findings from factors such as total kilojoule intake, body mass index, number of children borne and race.

In the study, the highest contributor to endometriosis was mayonnaise and full-fat salad dressing, followed by fatty fish such as tuna, salmon and mackerel. The major sources of trans fats in this study were fried restaurant foods, margarine and crackers.

Anti-inflammatory foods

Given the widespread inflammation that occurs in endometriosis, foods with known anti-inflammatory effects should be consumed. These include turmeric, ginger, raw fresh nuts and seeds, oily fish, cold-pressed oils and antioxidant-rich foods. Recommending a formalised anti-inflammatory diet may be beneficial; however, it is best to individually assess the patient.

Fibre

Adequate fibre is also encouraged; fibre encourages the excretion of oestrogens[549] by binding to the oestrogen and aiding its removal via the bowel.

Nutrient-dense foods

A large prospective cohort study collected data from 70 617 women in the Nurses' Health Study II, between 1991 and 2005. A total of 1383 laparoscopically diagnosed cases of endometrioses were observed. The researchers found that intake of folate, vitamin C and vitamin E from food sources was inversely associated with endometriosis risk. There was no relationship between intake of these nutrients from supplements and endometriosis.[550] This might indicate that it is not necessarily the antioxidant content of these nutrients which is beneficial but other factors present in dietary patterns rich in these nutrients. A study of the relation between green vegetable and fruit intake and endometriosis found that green vegetable and fruit intake was inversely associated with endometriosis risk.[551] However, in a more recent case-controlled study, no association was found between vegetables and endometriosis risk, and an increased risk was found with number of servings per day of fruit.[552]

DIETARY EXCLUSIONS

Soy products

Endometriosis is considered an oestrogen-displacement condition. This is why the excessive consumption of soy, which may aggravate oestrogen receptor sites, is not recommended. While patients may be familiar with soy-containing products such as tofu, miso, tempeh or soy milk, many may not realise that the use of soy in processed foods is widespread. Textured soy protein may be found in hamburgers, sausages and other processed meat products, while soy protein isolate is often found in cheese, cereals, ice-cream, muesli and energy bars.[553] Lecithin is a common mixing ingredient that enables oil and water to coexist, hence its inclusion in chocolate (as a replacement for cocoa butter), packaged cakes and biscuits, mayonnaise and salad dressings. It is thus important to educate patients on foods that may contain 'hidden' soy as well as the benefits of a wholefood diet. Fermented soy products in small quantities are permissible if an individual's health allows.

Lecithin debate

There is much contention about advocating the prescription of lecithin for supporting liver function and the liver's role in the treatment of endometriosis. Lecithin is one of the richest sources of two key nutrients — choline and inositol. Both are considered lipotrophic factors and are supportive for liver detoxification. Lecithin is derived from soy or egg, but most of the lecithin available — both supplemental and food sources — is derived from soy. It is imperative to differentiate from the literature findings that are often based on egg-derived sources, as soy sources can be problematic for this complicated condition.

Caffeine

A case-control study observed that caffeine consumption of 300 mg/day or more was associated with increased prevalence of minimal or mild endometriosis among infertile women.[462] A significant increase in the risk of infertility due to tubal disease or endometriosis was also found for women consuming high amounts of caffeine.[554]

The consumption of caffeine has been extensively analysed, as it acts on the hepatic production of sex hormone-binding globulin (SHBG), reducing testosterone bioavailability, and inhibits aromatase, an enzyme involved in the conversion of androgens to oestrogens.[555]

A 2014 meta-analysis of the data found no evidence for an association between coffee/caffeine intake and endometriosis risk.[556] The inconsistency between studies might be due to the fact that caffeine intake cannot be compared across studies, as this is seldom measured — the amount of caffeine is dependent on the processing of the beans and preparation style, and types of coffee consumed might yield different results.

Saturated fats and deep-fried foods

Trans fats aggravate inflammation by increasing circulation of inflammatory markers and constituents thought to be involved in the pathogenesis of endometriosis, they also offer little in the way of good nutrition. As mentioned above for omega-3 fatty acids, consumption of palmitic acid, a saturated fat found primarily in animal fat, as well as trans fatty acids have both been associated with an increased risk of endometriosis.[557] It is prudent to discourage a high intake of saturated fats as it is also associated with an increased risk of other benign or malignant gynaecological conditions.[558,559]

Sugar

Careful consideration should be paid to quantity of sugar consumed by the patient. Sugar is an immune depressant, is highly inflammatory and provides little in the way of nutrition and thus is unlikely to benefit the endometriosis patient.

Alcohol

The role of alcohol in endometriosis is controversial.[560] Early studies[561] found a positive association between infertility, endometriosis and moderate intake of alcohol. However a more recent study[544] found no association between intake of alcohol and endometriosis.

Although specific literature for endometriosis is limited, due to the increased incidence in the perimenopausal age group the following information is pertinent. Cross-sectional[562] and acute experimental studies[563] in premenopausal women demonstrate that alcohol consumption is significantly associated with increased serum oestradiol. A 3-month interventional study in 34 premenopausal women found that moderate alcohol consumption (30 g/day) resulted in significant increases in plasma and urinary oestrogens within various menstrual cycle phases.[564] Other interventional studies have also found significant increases in plasma oestradiol following moderate alcohol consumption, although only within oral contraceptive users.[565,566]

Serum oestrone was unaffected by alcohol consumption in some studies,[565,567] leading to speculation that the alcohol-mediated decrease in the hepatic NAD/NADH ratio could result in reduced oxidation of oestradiol to oestrone.[565,568]

From a naturopathic perspective, while alcohol may or may not cause endometriosis it is likely to aggravate symptoms. A moderate intake of alcohol is related to increased levels of oestrogens[569] and alcohol depresses

SAMPLE DAILY DIET

BREAKFAST	
Smoothie: 2 cups of spinach, 1 ripe banana, raw almonds, sunflower seeds, chia seeds and ½ avocado	All meals should be gluten free due to the inflammatory nature of gluten. Painful symptoms of endometriosis may reduce following a GF diet for at least one year duration. Spinach, banana, nuts and seeds and avocado also supply magnesium. Magnesium inhibits the biosynthesis of F2 alpha prostaglandin, and has a role in myometrial relaxation and vasodilation assisting to reduce pain. Sunflower seeds are a source of vitamin B_6. Vitamin B_6 is involved in the production of E2 prostaglandin which assists with smooth muscle relaxation.
LUNCH	
Lemon broccoli and cannellini bean risotto	Cruciferous vegetables are recommended to support excretion of oestrogen and provide fibre. Excess oestrogen stimulates the formation of large amounts of prostaglandins leading to inflammation and pain.
DINNER	
Trout with lemon, baked Brussels sprouts, peas and macadamias	Oily fish and omega-3 fatty acids may assist in reducing inflammation. It has been proposed that omega-3 improves endometriosis-related symptoms, selectively modulating biosynthesis and biochemistry activity of specific prostaglandins involved in pelvic pain.
SNACK	
Small amounts of fresh fruit, increased quantities of fresh vegetables	Endometriosis is associated with a chronic inflammatory response within the peritoneal cavity promoting cell adhesion and activation of macrophages. For this reason ample vegetables (and small amounts of fresh fruit), which contain antioxidants and anti-inflammatory constituents, are suggested.

Sources: Manta L, Suciu N, Toader O et al. The etiopathogenesis of uterine fibromatosis. J Med Life 2016; 9(1):39–45. Marziali M, Venza M, Lazzaro S et al. Gluten-free diet: a new strategy for management of painful endometriosis related symptoms? Minerva Chir 2012; 67(6):499–504. Sesti F, Pietropolli A, Capozzolo T et al. Hormonal suppression treatment or dietary therapy versus placebo in the control of painful symptoms after conservative surgery for endometriosis stage III-IV. A randomized comparative trial. Fertil Steril 2007; 88(6):1541–1547.

immunity and results in valuable nutrients including B vitamins being lost. Furthermore, noting the importance of healthy liver function in endometriosis, the added strain that alcohol puts on the liver is likely to compound symptoms and the disease process further.

Gluten free

Avoidance of gluten-containing foods is advisable. A gluten-free diet has been shown to improve symptoms in 75% of endometriosis sufferers.[570]

Dairy free (A1 milk)

Avoidance of A1 dairy products is encouraged. In one study, A1 casein induced an inflammatory response in the digestive system compared to A2 casein.[571]

NUTRITIONAL MEDICINE (SUPPLEMENTAL)

Nutritional medicine therapeutic objectives

- Improve hormone cascades and receptor responsiveness
- Improve methylation function
- Reduce inflammation
- Address infective trigger and support optimal immune function
- Avoid compounding oestrogen interferences
- Support hepatobiliary function to support toxin clearance, lipid metabolism, hormone synthesis and metabolism
- Antioxidant supplementation
- Microflora recolonisation
- Improve digestive function
- Improve lymphatic function specific to pelvic region
- Provide symptomatic support — decrease inflammation, reduce pain, reduce endometrial tissue displacement.

Specific nutrients required

B COMPLEX

The B vitamins play an important role in endometriosis as they participate in numerous essential metabolic functions including energy metabolism, cellular growth and DNA and neurotransmitter production, all of which are required for good health. The B vitamins as a whole are required for healthy liver detoxification so that oestrogen and other substances may be broken down and excreted by the body. Phase 1 detoxification is in part reliant upon flavin adenine dinucleotide (part of vitamin B_2) and niacinamide adenine dinucleotide (part of vitamin B_3) while phase 2 liver detoxification is reliant upon vitamins B_6, B_9 and B_{12}.

Without adequate intakes of these B vitamins, normal detoxification processes cannot occur and oestrogen may be recirculated. As well as their uses in concert, the B vitamins also have individual functions. For example vitamin B_1 (100 mg/day) has been shown to be effective in treating dysmenorrhoea,[97] while vitamin B_6 is required for hormone and prostaglandin synthesis.[25] As yet there are no studies assessing the effects of the B vitamins in endometriosis but because the B vitamins are involved indirectly in so many metabolic processes and often require the presence of another B vitamin to function properly, adequate intake of all the B vitamins is imperative. Anaylsis in the Nurses' Health Study II cohort found that dietary intake of vitamin B_1 from food sources was associated with a 16% lower risk for endometriosis and B_9 a 21% decreased risk. Intake of B_3, B_6 and B_{12} from food sources was not associated with endometriosis diagnosis risk.[550]

CALCIUM

Unfortunately there is a paucity of studies assessing the therapeutic action of calcium specifically in endometriosis patients. As calcium is involved in healthy neuromuscular function[106] it should be given in combination with magnesium to help provide relief from spasm and cramps. Calcium deficiency is associated with muscular and premenstrual cramping. Supplementation has been observed to reduce pain associated with premenstrual syndrome[572] so may produce similar benefits in endometriosis though this is yet to be trialled. Calcium intake from food sources (but not total calcium intake) was inversely related to endometriosis in the Nurses' Health Study II cohort. Furthermore, calcium intake from dairy sources only was unrelated to endometriosis in this cohort.[573]

COENZYME Q10

Oxidative stress has been implicated in the chain of events leading up to endometriosis where reactive oxygen species have been suggested to control and worsen severity and progression of the disease[13] hence the benefits of proven antioxidants such as coenzyme Q10. Coenzyme Q10 is a powerful antioxidant that exhibits marked effects on reproductive organs and patients notice significant changes in menstrual flow and colour from supplementation within one cycle provided that the dose is sufficient (between 200 and 300 mg/day). Significant co-anti-inflammatory results are also clinically achievable quickly, with long-term responses producing significant reduction in pathology. It is especially important to note that the colour and consistency changes of menstrual blood are significantly influenced by oxidation of haemoglobin.

ESSENTIAL FATTY ACIDS (EFAs)

In vitro, animal[574] and a prospective human study[557] all suggest that omega-3 fatty acids are likely to be of benefit in endometriosis, but as yet there has been little research undertaken in the way of clinical trials. In-vitro studies show that omega-3 fatty acids suppress the survival of endometrial cells.[575] An animal study found that omega-3 levels influence immune, angiogenic and proliferative factors which are implicated in the establishment of endometriosis.[576] Given this, and the effects omega-3 fatty acids have with regards to prostaglandin metabolism and also inflammation, and knowing that these have been implicated in the aetiology of endometriosis it is logical to think that omega-3 fatty acids may help to reduce the inflammatory response and modulate cytokine function. Omega-3 fatty acids (1080 mg/day EPA, 720 mg/day DHA and 1.5 mg vitamin E over 2 months) have also been found useful for dysmenorrhoea,[31] which is a common symptom experienced in endometriosis. They may also be useful in providing relief from coexisting symptoms.

IRON

As a result of extensive blood loss and likelihood of menstrual clotting, assessment and treatment of iron deficiency is imperative. It is important to remember that iron-deficiency anaemia presents with menorrhagia and as the deficiency worsens, menstrual flow increases, thus exacerbating endometriosis presentation. It is important to measure iron levels before treating. Overproduction and increased levels of iron in the peritoneal fluid due to retrograde menstruation may lead to oxidative stress. Endometrial cells are estimated to be found in the peritoneal cavity of 59–79% of menstruating women, however only a small portion of women develop endometriosis. It is hypothesised that that impairment or efficacy of protective mechanisms against elevated iron levels might be responsible for this difference. Iron overload causes increased proliferation of endometrial lesions and progression of the disease.[577]

MAGNESIUM

As yet no controlled trials can be found assessing the effects of magnesium in endometriosis but a Cochrane review found magnesium[110] to be effective in reducing pain associated with menstrual cramping. This is significant as pain and cramping are common in both dysmenorrhoea and endometriosis. With regards to dysmenorrhoea it appears that magnesium needs to be taken for at least 5 months for full benefit to be observed. Magnesium also supports numerous other pathways that sustain and renew the body in endometriosis, including neurotransmitter and energy production, and lower levels of inflammatory markers including interleukin-6 and tumor necrosis factor α-R2. Magnesium has also been shown to relax smooth muscles and as a result may influence endometriosis through its effect on retrograde menstruation. A prospective cohort study (the Nurses' Health Study II) investigated the relationship between dairy intake and endometriosis. Magnesium content in dairy was extrapolated and an inverse relationship was found between magnesium intake from food sources and endometriosis risk.[573]

PROBIOTICS

Ensuring that there is healthy intestinal flora in patients with endometriosis is paramount. Many endometriosis patients experience abdominal bloating and distension as well as digestive discomfort. These symptoms correlate with hormonal fluctuations during women's cycles and affect nutrient absorption and aggravate symptomatology. The use of probiotics assists in eliminating bad bacteria that would otherwise be recycled back into the body contributing to the oestrogen excess observed in endometriosis patients.[578]

The gut microbiota is not only essential for a physiological gastrointestinal function, but acts as a central regulator of a variety of inflammatory and proliferative conditions as well as affecting oestrogen metabolism and stem cell homeostasis. Laschke and Menger hypothesise that there may be a direct link between pathological changes of the gut microbiota and the onset and progression of endometriosis.[579] A randomised, double-blind, placebo-controlled trial of *Lactobacillus gasseri* OLL2809 showed significant reduction in pain in treatment group after 12 weeks.[577]

SELENIUM

Selenium is a powerful antioxidant that carries out its functions through its incorporation into selenoproteins, which play a key role in antioxidant protection, influencing inflammatory and immune responses.[580] It upregulates Treg cells,[581] supports the corpus luteum and progesterone secretion/production[582] and is depleted in SIBO. Via its action on the liver, selenium also assists with the detoxification of oestrogens. Studies have shown that there are lower tissue levels in women with endometriosis.[583]

SILICA

Silica is required for the healthy development and functioning of connective tissues, particularly skin, tendons and bone. Inflammation results in adhesions that result in pain; scar endometriosis may occur in the presence of surgical scar tissue (e.g. in the case of hysterectomy or a caesarean section).[584] The importance of healthy connective tissue is paramount.

VITAMIN A AND BETA-CAROTENE

Beta-carotene is involved in the normal regulation of cell replication and differentiation in the human endometrium as well as healthy immune function and as an antioxidant. Experimental studies have suggested that beta-carotene inhibits the oestrogenic activity of 17β-oestradiol and genistein in cancer cells,[585] thus it may be interesting to see if the same is true of endometrial cells, particularly as a number of studies have pointed to a link between ovarian endometriosis and an increased incidence of both ovarian cancer and endometrial polyps.[586,587] As an antioxidant, particularly one that is proposed to have chemoprotective properties,[588] beta-carotene is likely to be of use.

VITAMIN C

A number of alterations in the immune system have been observed in individuals with endometriosis. These include increased numbers of peritoneal macrophages and local cytokines which modulate the growth of endometrial tissue as well as decreased T-cell reactivity and NK-cell cytotoxicity which leads to increased chance of abnormal endometrial implantation.[589] Vitamin C is well regarded for its effects on the immune system, where it appears able to function as an immune enhancer and stimulant system. As yet, there are few trials examining the effects of vitamin C in terms of its effects on immunity in women with endometriosis, but it is likely to be useful. Vitamin C is also likely to be useful in endometriosis due to its antioxidant abilities; women with endometriosis have been observed to have increased oxidative stress[590] but less in the way of antioxidant reserves. Analysis in the Nurses' Health Study II cohort found that dietary intake of vitamin C from food sources was associated with a 19% lower risk for endometriosis diagnosis.[550]

VITAMIN D

Vitamin D plays a key role in regulation of the immune system and so may be useful in the management of endometriosis. As one possible reason for endometriosis may involve a defective immune system[591] (resulting in the inability to recognise and eliminate endometrial tissue), vitamin D may be of use. Deficiency of vitamin D may also cause increases in inflammatory mediators, as the transport protein (D-binding protein) transforms into macrophage-activating factor if not used. Vitamin D-binding protein, specifically the GC*2 allele, has been found to be 3 times higher in women with endometriosis compared to those without. The GC*2 allele does not convert readily to a potent macrophage factor (unlike the GC*1 allele). It is speculated that the inability to sufficiently activate macrophage's phagocytotic function in women carrying the GC*2 polymorphism might allow endometriotic tissues to implant in the peritoneal cavity.[592] Vitamin D supplementation has been associated with reduction in pain scores in primary dysmenorrhoea through interference with prostaglandin synthesis (Fig. 18.12). The endometrium expresses vitamin D receptors and 1α-hydroxylase and there is an upregulation of vitamin D enzymes and receptors in the eutopic endometrium of women with endometriosis.[593] These factors all point to an interesting relationship between vitamin D and endometriosis. Larger clinical trials are needed to establish the possible effects of vitamin D exposure on endometriosis.

A large prospective cohort study which included 1385 women with endometriosis showed that women consuming more than three servings of dairy per day had an 18% lower risk of being diagnosed with endometriosis than women who consumed two servings per day.[573] The study also found that predicted plasma 25-hydroxyvitamin-D3 level was inversely associated with endometriosis which is in contrast to previous studies, possibly due to previous small sample sizes and the nature of the studies.

VITAMIN E

Vitamin E is highly recommended in endometriosis due to its antioxidant and anti-inflammatory properties.[594] Women with endometriosis have been shown to have a lower overall intake of vitamin E as well as lower levels of vitamin E within their peritoneal fluid. Lower levels of afamin, a specific carrier protein of vitamin E in extravascular fluids, were found in women with endometriosis.[595] There appears to be a strong association between vitamin E deficiency and endometriosis. In-vitro studies reveal vitamin E to have a protective effect on the

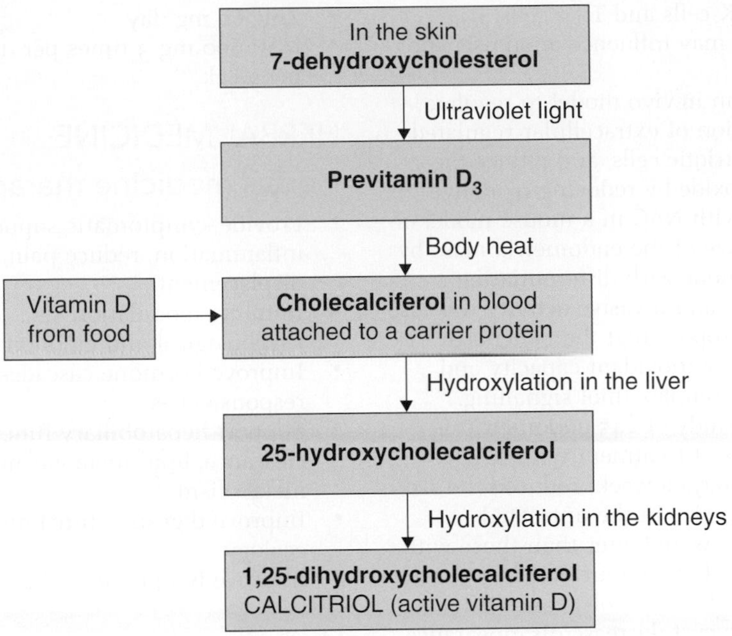

FIGURE 18.12 Vitamin D synthesis.

endometrium, helping to inhibit the proliferation of endometrial cells.[464] Activated macrophages as well as other pro-oxidants cause widespread oxidation in the peritoneal cavity, contributing to the excessive growth of endometrial cells and while antioxidants such as vitamin E usually function to offset this, vitamin E levels have been observed to be low in the lipoproteins of the peritoneal fluid.[596] Thus low levels in peritoneal fluid or deficiency in vitamin E may lead to unrestrained oxidative damage and promote abnormal endometrial growth.

Vitamin E may also be useful to prevent endometrial adhesions. This action is thought to be primarily through reduction of series 2 prostaglandins and better removal of pelvic debris by white blood cells. As yet the majority of studies have been undertaken in animals and have produced mixed results. Kagoma et al[597] observed a statistically significant decrease in the incidence and degree of adhesions in vitamin E-supplemented animals, but these same results were not reproduced by Sanfilippo et al,[598] who noted a trend towards less fibrosis and found no reduction in adhesion formation. It is important to acknowledge that, aside from the ethical issues of using animal test subjects, the latter studies are dated and were undertaken in animals, thus true extrapolation for humans is not possible. Further studies in humans are required to elucidate the true nature of vitamin E with regard to the prevention of endometrial adhesions, but it does appear to be useful due to its antioxidant function. Analysis in the Nurses' Health Study II cohort found that dietary intake of vitamin E from food sources was associated with a 30% lower risk for endometriosis diagnosis.[550]

VITAMIN K

Vitamin K is required in endometriosis to regulate blood clotting. Endometriosis patients can experience significant and painful menstrual clotting that can be related to various haematological factors. Vitamin K catalyses the carboxylation of a number of protein factors involved in blood clotting including prothrombin, forming the calcium-binding sites on glutamyl side-chains in the protein. As vitamin K regulates all eight clotting factors (including prothrombin, factors VII, IX and X and proteins S and C), it is a beneficial supportive nutrient for these patients.

Vitamin K is typically provided in sufficient quantities from bacteria in the GI tract and dietary sources, but in those with proven clotting abnormalities supplementation may be appropriate.

ZINC

Zinc is a key nutrient in endometriosis and oversees many functions. Zinc functions as an antioxidant, helping to mediate oxidative stress. It is also an anti-inflammatory agent, preventing the generation of inflammatory cytokines.[599] Zinc is also highly important for healthy immune regulation and may be useful to help to heal damaged endometrial tissue. Given that inflammation, oxidative stress and immune dysfunction all play a role in endometriosis, zinc would appear to be an important nutrient for the management of endometriosis. Zinc status should be assessed in all patients and corrected where necessary. A small 2014 study showed that women with endometriosis had lower serum zinc levels than healthy controls. While the authors identified a reasonable connection between a zinc deficiency and the ability of endometriotic cells to develop invasive features, no conclusion can be drawn as to whether zinc deficiency contributes to the initiation of endometriosis, or endometriosis causes a zinc deficiency.[600]

N-ACETYL CYSTEINE (NAC)

NAC downregulates NF-kB and reduces inflammatory cytokines. It is a precursor to glutathione which upregulates he activity of NK cells and Treg cells. It reduces oxidative stress and may influence apoptosis and angiogenesis favourably.[601]

NAC has been found in an in-vivo model to regulate cell proliferation and activation of extracellular regulated kinase (ERK 1/2) in endometriotic cells, and reduce the production of hydrogen peroxide by reducing oxidative stress.[602] Supplementation with NAC in a mouse model of endometriosis reduced the size of the endometria mass by replacing proliferative behaviour with differentiating behaviour. The inflammatory and invasive activity was also decreased. The researchers propose that the beneficial effects of NAC are beyond its antioxidant capacity and may be related to its role in complex thiol signalling.[603]

An observational cohort study of 145 endometriosis patients found that 3 months of treatment with NAC (600 mg t.d.s., 3 consecutive days a week) reduced the size of the cysts (vs an increase in size in the untreated patients). Results of the study were better than those with normal hormonal treatments. Twenty-four of the NAC-treated patients (vs 1 within controls) cancelled scheduled laparoscopy due to cyst decrease/disappearance and/or relevant pain reduction, or pregnancy.[604]

Specific nutrients required

DOSAGE REQUIREMENTS

The dosage requirements listed below are based on adult doses that have been reported in the literature and clinical review:

- B complex (all B vitamins) high-dose combination, preferably activated forms
  - Thiamine 20–40 mg/day
  - Riboflavin 20–40 mg/day
  - Niacinamide/nicotinic acid 50–100 mg/day
  - Pantothenic acid 150–300 mg/day
  - Pyridoxine 20–60 mg/day
  - Folate as folinic acid or L-5MTHF 500–1000 micrograms/day (increase in instances of MTHFR polymorphism)
  - Hydroxo or methylcobalamin 500–1000 micrograms/day
  - Choline 50–100 mg/day
  - Inositol 50–100 mg/day
  - Biotin 250–500 micrograms/day
- Calcium 500–1000 mg/day
- Coenzyme Q10 100–400 mg/day
- Essential fatty acids: 1080 mg/day EPA (over 2 months[31]), 720 mg/day DHA (over 2 months[31]), 165–350 mg/day GLA
- Iron 5–80 mg/day (if indicated on pathology)
- Magnesium 500–1000 mg/day
- Probiotics 25–50 × 10^{12}
- Selenium 100–250 micrograms/day
- Silica 20–30 mg/day
- Vitamin A 5000–10 000 IU or beta-carotene 6 mg daily
- Vitamin C 500–3000 g/day in divided doses
- Vitamin D 1000 IU minimum (dose should be calculated based on deficiency)
- Vitamin E 400–600 IU/day[31]
- Vitamin K 100–300 micrograms/day
- Zinc 60 mg/day
- NAC 600 mg 3 times per day, for 3 consecutive days per week[604]

HERBAL MEDICINE

Herbal medicine therapeutic objectives

- Provide symptomatic support — decrease inflammation, reduce pain, reduce endometrial tissue displacement
- Immune modulation
- Psychological and emotional support as stress relief
- Improve hormone cascades and receptor responsiveness
- Support hepatobiliary function to support toxin clearance, lipid metabolism, hormone synthesis and metabolism
- Improve digestive function and support optimal ecology
- Improve lymphatic and circulatory function.

Herbal medicine classes

Herbal medicine classes used for endometriosis are listed in Table 18.37.

TABLE 18.37 Herbal medicine classes used for endometriosis

Class	Action
Analgesic	Symptomatic pain relief
Antispasmodic	Symptomatic pain relief
Anti-inflammatory	Symptomatic pain relief, reduction in oxidation
Immunomodulator	Modulate immune response
Hormonal modulator	Stabilise hormonal cascades and regulate hormonal secretion Improve oestrogen metabolism, regulate oestrogen-to-progesterone ratio
Uterine tonic	Reduce endometrial tissue size and impact, improve uterine health
Hepatic, cholagogue	Support hepatic clearance of oestrogen metabolites and hormonal synthesis, support clearance of environmental toxins
Bitter	Encourage and support GI tract microecology
Lymphatic	Improve pelvic circulation and immunological function
Adaptogen, thymoleptic	Support patient emotionally and reduce impact of excessive cortisol production both on immune irregularities, HPA negative impact and inflammation

Specific herbal medicines

ALCHEMILLA VULGARIS (LADIES' MANTLE)

Menorrhagia is a common occurrence in women with endometriosis and may impact negatively on a woman's quality of life in many ways. Excessive blood flow may cause iron deficiency and subsequently fatigue and/or may cause discomfort, pain and embarrassment due to unforeseen flooding. *Alchemilla vulgaris* is a herbaceous perennial native to Europe that has been used traditionally for its beneficial effects on the female reproductive system. It displays astringent and coagulant[605] properties likely to be responsible for its ability to reduce the excessive bleeding that occurs with endometriosis. Trickey[28] reports a study in which *Alchemilla vulgaris* was administered to young females with menorrhagia approximately 10–15 days before their next expected period; this was found to reduce bleeding and the length of the menstrual cycle.

ANEMONE PULSATILLA (PASQUE FLOWER)

Anemone pulsatilla is a uterine tonic traditionally used by the Eclectics[7] for female reproductive disorders, particularly those that presented with nervous system alterations such as hysteria or melancholy. *Anemone pulsatilla* was said to quickly restore normal and regular menstrual flow. In addition, reproductive complaints such as loss of strength, chilliness, headaches and gastric involvement were also alleviated. It also provides marked antispasmodic and analgesic actions, which can assist in reducing pain, especially during menses.

CALENDULA OFFICINALIS (CALENDULA)

Calendula officinalis is detailed in the Eclectic texts for the treatment of endometriosis.[8] Modern research studies reveal *Calendula officinalis* to be an anti-inflammatory agent (thought to occur because of its triterpenoid content) and to enhance the immune response. Via its lymphatic and antiseptic action[129] it helps to cleanse and remove wastes from the endometrium. Animal studies have also revealed that it contains antispasmolytic constituents that may be additionally useful in endometriosis.[606] The antimicrobial properties may aid any associated endometriosis genitourinary infections and this may assist with reducing general immune activation and response.[607] To date no studies have been conducted on the effects of *Calendula officinalis* in individuals with endometriosis.

CHAMAELIRIUM LUTEUM (FALSE UNICORN ROOT)

Chamaelirium luteum or helonias root, as it was traditionally named, is a valuable botanical for the female reproductive system. The Eclectics used it for female reproductive conditions characterised by aching and propulsive pain due to its effects as a uterine tonic.[9] Modern research has demonstrated that *Chamaelirium luteum* contains steroidal saponins likely to influence this herb's tonifying effects on the ovaries and uterus. As mentioned in the section on fibroids, this herb is endangered so replacement with *Dioscorea villosa* (wild yam) or *Asparagus racemosus* (shatavari) is advised where possible.

CINNAMOMUM SPP. (CINNAMON)

Cinnamon-based herbals are a gentle, warming group of circulatory stimulants that have shown efficacy in a number of conditions. The cinnamon species, *Cinnamomum zeylanicum*, is perhaps the most widely used in Western herbal medicine. *Cinnamomum zeylanicum* may be used in endometriosis to help alleviate stasis and cramping due to its ability to enhance blood flow to the pelvic region. This is likely to help prevent the pain many women experience. Although unsubstantiated by clinical research, *Cinnamomum* was administered traditionally by the Eclectic physicians for uterine haemorrhage and menorrhagia in sweetened water to be taken frequently (every 5–20 minutes) and was believed to work upon the uterine muscular fibres, causing contraction and arresting bleeding.[8]

DIOSCOREA VILLOSA (WILD YAM)

Dioscorea villosa is a deciduous perennial vine used traditionally for 'dysmenorrhoea as a result of spasmodic irritation of the mucous membrane of the cervix uteri'.[8] It contains steroidal saponins, phytosterols, alkaloids and tannins and displays antispasmodic and anti-inflammatory properties that may be of use in endometriosis to help relieve disabling cramps in the pelvic area as well as aches around the rest of the body such as the back. *Dioscorea villosa* has been used traditionally in the Americas for painful periods.[129]

REHMANNIA GLUTINOSA (REHMANNIA)

Rehmannia glutinosa is a traditional Chinese herb that may be useful in endometriosis due to its tonic and anti-inflammatory properties. In their review Zhang et al suggest that *Rehmannia glutinosa* may also exert pharmacological actions upon the liver, the nervous system and the endocrine system,[608] although these are extrapolations from animal studies. Furthermore, given the proposed immune disruption that occurs in endometriosis, *Rehmannia glutinosa* may help to regulate the immune system. Zhang et al propose it to have both immune-enhancing and suppressive constituents. According to traditional Chinese teachings, *Rehmannia glutinosa* has an enriching effect upon the blood,[608] which may also be useful given the depletion that may occur with loss of blood from endometriosis.

ASPARAGUS RACEMOSUS (SHATAVARI)

Asparagus racemosus is a botanical native to India where it has been used in Ayurvedic medicine for a wide array of conditions, including those pertaining to female gynaecology. It is a beneficial alternative to *Chamaelirium luteum*, especially in instances of aggravated oestrogen displacement. Common presentations warranting prescription will include hot flushes (especially prior to menses), dry mucous membranes and emotional lability, especially in the premenstrual window. Additionally, shatavari supports and increases diminishing libido.

SILYBUM MARIANUM (ST MARY'S THISTLE)

The liver is required to conjugate oestrogens and other endogenous and exogenous substances such as xeno-oestrogens and dioxins and aid in their removal from the body to prevent recirculation and build-up. This is particularly crucial in endometriosis where a number of studies[11,609] have observed a link between environmental toxicants such as polychlorinated biphenyls and their role as potential contributory agents in the development of endometriosis. *Silybum marianum* has been shown to exert significant hepatoprotective properties and may thus help to protect against the effects of environmental toxins such as dioxins. Furthermore, although unproven, the antioxidant properties of *Silybum marianum* are likely to help protect the liver against the effects of oxidative damage. Liver tumours have been known to occur as a result of endometriosis.[610]

VIBURNUM OPULUS (CRAMP BARK)

The bark of *Viburnum opulus* may be used medicinally in endometriosis to help relieve muscular cramping and pain associated with menstruation due to the herb's antispasmodic properties. It contains a range of constituents, including coumarins, hydroquinones, tannnins and resin.[129] A study undertaken in the 1970s observed that viopudial, a constituent from within *Viburnum opulus* exerted antispasmodic activity,[611] however since then little has been published with regards to this action.

VIBURNUM PRUNIFOLIUM (BLACK HAW)

Viburnum prunifolium is a North American botanical, the roots and stem barks of which are prized for their spasmolytic action and their subsequent ability to ease cramps and spasms associated with disruptions in the normal menstrual cycle. This action is similar to that of *Viburnum opulus* discussed above, but *Viburnum prunifolium* is believed to have a more specific action on the uterus.[129]

The Eclectics observed that *Viburnum prunifolium* appeared to improve uterine and ovarian circulation, promoting pelvic nutrition. As a relaxant of pelvic tissues in the presence of congestion or where there was haemorrhage, painful, cramping menstruation with engorged tissues, *Viburnum prunifolium* was favoured. They noted that it combined beautifully with *Cinnamomum zeylanicum*.[9] *Viburnum prunifolium* contains iridoid glycosides that have been identified as responsible for its relaxant and antispasmodic properties, though it has been suggested that other mechanisms of action (e.g. through Ca^{2+} channel interactions) may also play some role.[612] Given that dysmenorrhoea and pain are common complaints in patients with endometriosis, administration of *Viburnum prunifolium* may be of assistance.

VITEX AGNUS-CASTUS (CHASTE TREE BERRY)

Vitex agnus-castus has been used for centuries for the treatment of female reproductive disorders and is used in modern medicine for the treatment of infertility and anovulatory cycles to name but a few conditions. As yet there are no studies assessing the effects of *Vitex agnus-castus* in endometriosis, but the herb is still used by many practitioners for its ability to regulate hormonal balance and improve the oestrogen-to-progesterone imbalance implicated in endometriosis.

CURCUMA LONGA (TURMERIC)

Curcumin has been shown in vitro to inhibit endometrial carcinoma cell migration and invasion by inhibiting the expression and activity of MMP-2 and -9 through regulation of the ERK signalling pathway.[613] Matrix metalloproteinases (MMPs) have been found to be elevated in endometriosis in vivo. Curcumin was shown to repress the MMP activity, thereby delaying endometriosis development and progression to the point where the authors proposed that there was a therapeutic potential of curcumin as an anti-endometriotic drug. They showed that curcumin downregulated NF-kB and promoted apoptosis.[614] A further in-vitro study showed that curcumin is able to suppress the proliferation of endometrial cells by reducing oestradiol which has been found to be a regulator of endometriosis.[615] Immunologically, it supports glutathione production[616] and Treg cells.[617] Curcumin also acts in the liver to assist phase I and II detoxification, thereby regulating the clearance of oestrogen, which potentiates further growth and development of the ectopic endometrium.[618] Curcumin shows promise in the prevention and management of endometriosis, however further rigorous human trials are warranted.

CAMELLIA SINENSIS (GREEN TEA)

In-vitro and in-vivo studies have shown that epigallocatechin-3-gallate (ECGC) can inhibit the development, growth and spread of endometriosis. ECGC has a strong anti-angiogenetic effect, and is a powerful antioxidant, inhibiting adhesion of endometriotic lesions and reducing their size.[619–623] Further human trials are needed before clinical effectiveness can be ascertained.

BERBERINE-CONTAINING HERBS INCLUDING *HYDRASTIS CANADENSIS* (GOLDEN SEAL), *BERBERIS VULGARIS* (BARBERRY)

A number of studies have shown that the phytochemical berberine is beneficial for endometriosis patients. It has been shown to neutralise the bacterial toxin LPS;[624] inhibit the release of inflammatory cytokines;[625] address SIBO (small intestinal bacterial overgrowth) which affects microflora status;[626] and repair intestinal permeability.[627]

LIFESTYLE RECOMMENDATIONS

Smoking

Some studies have suggested that heavy smokers are at decreased risk of endometriosis.[386] This finding can be explained in terms of the recognised anti-oestrogenic effects of smoking. Available data on the relationship between smoking and endometriosis risk are, however, limited and controversial.[560] It is not advisable to encourage patients to smoke regardless as oxidation is a crucial factor in the development and progression of the disease.

Exercise

Regular physical activity might be linked with lower levels of oestrogens and reduced endometriosis risk, but data on this issue are limited.[560] A systematic review and meta-analysis suggest that physical activity may reduce the risk of endometriosis, but did not conclusively support the hypothesis. This may be explained by variation in study design and choice of controls across studies.[628]

Sanitary products

Patients should be encouraged to use sanitary pads (or similar) and avoid the use of tampons where possible. A risk assessment study of dioxins in sanitary pads produced in Japan found that the daily exposure volumes were 1600 to 29 000 times lower than the tolerable daily intake.[629]

Sexual intercourse

Patients should be advised to refrain from sexual intercourse during menses due to potential links with retrograde blood flow.

Environmental impact

As environmental toxins are linked to endometriosis, a thorough environmental exposure history should be performed to identify possible toxins. Assessment for heavy metals, pesticides, solvents, phthalates and parabens is beneficial and every patient should be educated on how to avoid hormone-disrupting chemicals in food, water, air and personal care products.

Physical support

Patients should be referred to a physiotherapist with expertise and additional qualifications as a pelvic floor specialist.

CASE STUDY

OVERVIEW

AL was a 30-year-old woman who presented with severe endometriosis. She experienced extreme pain and very large clots, especially on days 1–4, and bled heavily for 7 days. She had had four previous laparoscopies that had ameliorated symptoms for 1–2 months with endometrial tissue recurring shortly after ablation. She had tried the combined oral contraceptive pill but it had caused significant emotional lability so had ceased. She was reluctant to continue having repeated surgeries and refused hysterectomy recommendation from one surgeon so was looking for alternatives.

In addition she had marked digestive insufficiencies and suffered from regular bloating, flatulence and loose bowel movements.

Lengthy discussion and investigation ensued revealing a number of marked concerns:

CASE STUDY CONTINUED

Assessment	Result	Treatment strategy
Liver function test (LFT)	Gilbert's syndrome (elevated bilirubin) Other LFT within normal limits	Avoidance of all alcohol (including alcoholic herbal medicines), liver support. Explained liver relationship with endometriosis and anaemia
Lipid profile	Total cholesterol: 3.2 mmol/L Triglycerides: 1.0 mmol/L Elevated low-density lipoproteins (LDL): 2.5 mmol/L Low high-density lipoproteins (HDL): 0.8 mmol/L	Low cholesterol profile thus insufficient building blocks for steroid hormone synthesis. Liver relationship acknowledged
FBC	Marked anaemia	Consistent with menorrhagia and MTHFR homozygosity
Vitamin D (25-hydroxy)	18 nmol/L	Consistent with poor liver function (Gilbert's syndrome), ethnicity (darker skin) and sunlight exposure
Hormone profile (serum)	SHBG: 72 nmol/L (Day 3) FSH: 5.0 U/L (Day 3) LH: 3.9 U/L (Day 3) P4: 36 nmol/L (Day 21) PRL: 312 mIU/L (Day 3) E2: 200 nmol/L (Day 3)	Confirmation of ovulation, all hormones NAD
Iron studies	Ferritin: <2 micrograms/L (marked anaemia)	Consistent with menorrhagia and poor liver function (Gilbert's syndrome)
MTHFR	Homozygous for C677T allele	Consistent with endometriosis and cellular proliferation
Serum B_{12}	150 pmol/L	Consistent with endometriosis cellular proliferation and related to MTHFR homozygosity
Coeliac gene screen	Homozygous for DQ2 allele	Related to immune irregularity and autoimmune tendency. Advised immediate referral to GP and gastroenterologist for confirmation

CASE STUDY CONTINUED

TREATMENT

Treatment was structured based on findings and consisted of the following.

HERBAL MEDICINE

No liquid herbal prescriptions while bilirubin level was elevated. Tablet preparation included:

- *Vitex agnus-castus* (chaste tree berry) — extract equivalent to dry fruit: 500 mg 1 tab b.i.d. for hormonal regulation
- Curcumin extract 500 mg/cap, 2 caps b.i.d.
- Berberine extract 500 mg/d, 1 cap b.i.d.

NUTRITIONAL MEDICINE

Dietary

The patient was a vegetarian already for religious reasons. She was advised to avoid all gluten-containing foods (follow-up revealed coeliac disease). She was advised to avoid sugar, processed foods, caffeine, alcohol and all phyto-oestrogen sources until her symptoms had stabilised. She was recommended to eat antioxidant foods, fermented food to support microflora colonisation, immune-building foods and digestive restorative foods such as slippery elm.

Supplemental

We discussed the important of high-dose nutrients through repletion period of 3 months and then review of health and nutrient markers to assess dose adjustment. She agreed to take vitamin D and fish oil supplementation regardless of animal origin.

Nutrient	Dosage	Justification
B complex (activated forms)	2 caps b.i.d.	Hormonal regulation and address anaemia, address MTHFR polymorphism with additional folinic acid
Folinic acid	500 micrograms b.i.d.	Support of MTHFR polymorphism
Iron	48–96 mg/day (cycle day dependent)	Address deficiency and increase dosage 2 days prior to expected bleed and continue during bleed and for 3 days post. Deficiency was believed to be as pronounced due to both excessive bleeding and coeliac disease (later confirmed) which inhibited absorption. Furthermore ferritin storage was compromised due to poor liver health
Vitamin E	500 IU b.i.d.	Mucus membrane integrity, hormonal regulation, oestrogen regulation, antioxidant

CASE STUDY CONTINUED

Nutrient	Dosage	Justification
Selenium	250 micrograms/day	Antioxidant and cancer protection, reduce inflammation
Concentrated fish oil supplementation	1 cap b.i.d. total: EPA 650 mg, DHA 450 mg, other omega-3s 180 mg	Hormonal regulation, anti-inflammatory, regulation of prostaglandin synthesis
Zinc	60 mg/day	Hormonal regulation, antioxidant
Vitamin D_3	1000 IU/day for week 1 and increasing to a maximum of 5000 IU/day after 5 weeks	To address deficiency and utilise positive immune regulatory effects. Staggered dosage was to allow the liver to reduce bilirubin and improve function for greater conversion
Coenzyme Q10	200–300 mg/day	Potent reproductive antioxidant to reduce endometrial lining migration and proliferation
Probiotic (multistrain)	25×10^9 CFU b.i.d.	Address digestive insufficiency, alleviate digestive symptoms and improve nutrient absorption
NAC	500 mg t.d.s.	Reduce angiogenesis, antioxidant, reduce cyst formation

LIFESTYLE/EDUCATION

- Endometriosis pain journal was used to assess progress comprehensively
- Castor oil or heat packs as required
- Avoidance of intercourse during menses
- Avoidance of exogenous oestrogen sources
- Replacement of sanitary items with organic sanitary pads to reduce impact from chemical exposure.

PELVIC INFLAMMATORY DISEASE (PID)

Epidemiology

According to the Centers for Disease Control and Prevention (CDC) in the USA, the rate of diagnosis of PID in hospital and ambulatory settings has been steadily declining since 2005. Several factors might be contributing to this decline including increases in *Chlamydia* and gonorrhoea screening coverage, more sensitive diagnostic technologies, and availability of single-dose therapies that increase adherence to treatment.[630] Accurate estimates are, however, difficult to obtain due to incomplete and untimely conventional non-electronic reporting methods and because many cases of silent and smouldering PID occur and are discovered only when the patient develops chronic complications of this process.[631] In addition, unlike gonorrhoea or HIV, PID is not notifiable to health authorities so for this reason exact figures on incidence and prevalence are not available.

In England, 50 000–75 000 cases are diagnosed annually, one-third of which occur in women between the ages of 16 and 24. An unknown proportion (perhaps as much as 70%) of incident cases remain undiagnosed.[632] Long-term sequelae, including chronic pelvic pain, ectopic pregnancy, tubal factor infertility,[631] and implantation failure in in-vitro fertilisation attempts may occur in up to 25% of patients, ultimately affecting approximately 11% of reproductive-aged women.[633] More than 100 000 women are estimated to become infertile each year as a result of PID.[633] (See Fig. 18.13.)

A number of factors contribute to the difficulty in determining the actual worldwide incidence and prevalence of PID, including lack of patient recognition of disease, difficulties in access to care, the often subjective method of disease diagnosis, lack of diagnostics and laboratory facilities in many developing countries, and underfunded and overstretched public health systems.[631,634]

The annual rate of PID in high-GNP countries has been reported to be as high as 10–20 per 1000 women of reproductive age.[631] Public health efforts employed in Scandinavia to decrease the prevalence of sexually transmitted infections (STIs) have been quite effective.[635] In Sweden alone, strategies increasing the awareness of STIs have produced a 40% decrease in the number of women being discharged from hospital for acute salpingitis between 1974 and 1984.[636]

Classification

To expedite treatment and maximise compliance, the diagnosis of PID in emergency departments and clinics is often based on clinical criteria, with or without additional

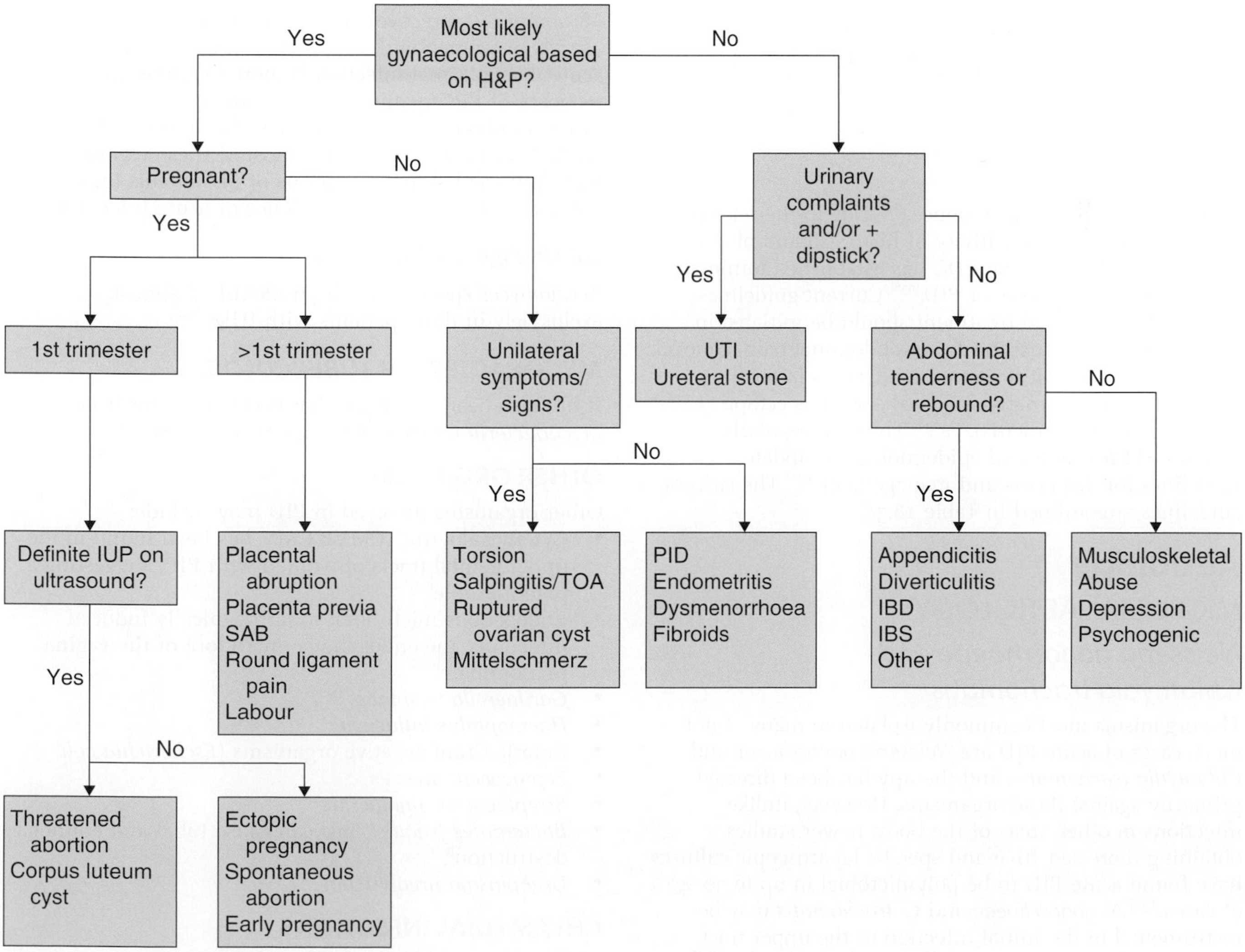

FIGURE 18.13 Pelvic inflammatory disease.

Source: Katz V. Comprehensive gynecology. 5th edn. Maryland Heights: Mosby; 2007. Figure 23-4.

TABLE 18.38 Current CDC guidelines for PID, stratifying diagnostic criteria into three groups

Group 1	Minimum criteria: empirical treatment indicated if no other aetiology explains findings Lower abdominal tenderness Bilateral adnexal tenderness Cervical motion tenderness
Group 2	Additional criteria improving diagnostic specificity include the following: Oral temperature >38.3°C Abnormal cervical or vaginal mucopurulent secretions Elevated erythrocyte sedimentation rate Elevated C-reactive protein Laboratory evidence of cervical infection with *N. gonorrhoeae* or *C. trachomatis* (culture or DNA probe)
Group 3	Specific criteria for PID based on procedures that may be appropriate for some patients are as follows: Laparoscopic confirmation Transvaginal ultrasonography (or MRI) showing thickened, fluid-filled tubes with/without free pelvic fluid or tubo-ovarian complex Endometrial biopsy showing endometritis

Source: Centers for Disease Control and Prevention, Workowski KA, Berman SM. Sexually transmitted diseases treatment guidelines; 2006. MMWR Recomm Rep 2006;55(RR–11):1–94.

laboratory and imaging evidence.[637] Due to the relatively poor specificity and sensitivity of historical and physical examination findings, the CDC has established minimal criteria for the diagnosis of PID.[638] Current guidelines suggest that empirical treatment should be initiated in women at risk who exhibit lower abdominal pain, adnexal tenderness and cervical motion tenderness (after the exclusion of an alternative diagnosis such as ectopic pregnancy or appendicitis).[631,638] The CDC regularly reviews STI research and epidemiology to update guidelines for diagnosis and management.[631] The current guidelines are outlined in Table 18.38.

Aetiology

MICROBIAL AETIOLOGY

Neisseria gonorrhoeae and *Chlamydia trachomatis*

The organisms most commonly isolated in many, if not most, cases of acute PID are *Neisseria gonorrhoeae* and *Chlamydia trachomatis*, and therapy has been directed primarily against these organisms. However, unlike infections in other areas of the body, newer studies obtaining more sensitive and specific laparoscopic cultures have found acute PID to be polymicrobial in up to 30–40% of cases.[631] *N. gonorrhoeae* and *C. trachomatis* may be instrumental in the initial infection of the upper tract, with anaerobes, facultative anaerobes and other bacteria increasingly isolated as inflammation increases and abscesses form.[631]

Predominant STIs

The microbiology of PID has also been found to reflect both the predominant STIs prevalent within a specific population and also less common organisms seen in specific populations. A 2006 cross-sectional study examined the role of HSV-2 and *Trichomonas vaginalis* in PID.[639] In this study of 736 women, those with *T. vaginalis* demonstrated a four-fold increase in the histological evidence of acute endometritis. Co-infection of HSV-2 with *N. gonorrhoeae, C. trachomatis* and bacterial vaginosis was also associated with histological evidence of acute endometritis.[639] HSV-2 was demonstrated to be associated with fallopian tube inflammation and lower tract ulcerations that may contribute to disruption of the endocervical canal mucus barrier.[639]

MYCOPLASMA GENITALIUM

M. genitalium has been isolated in the endometrium and fallopian tubes of women with PID.[640] Culture, serological and experimental lines of evidence suggest some role for genital *Mycoplasma.* Patients with PID frequently have *M. hominis* (55–70%) isolated from the cervix.[641] However, *M. hominis* was recovered from the tubal area in only 4–17% of women with PID.[641] Serological evidence of acute mycoplasmal infection is more common than recovery of the organism from the tubal area.[641] Increases in IgG antibody to *M. hominis* have been identified in 10–30% of patients with PID; most of these women also had significant serum elevations of *M. hominis* IgM antibody, which is further evidence of acute infection.[641]

ACTINOMYCES SPECIES

Actinomyces species have been identified almost exclusively in those patients with IUDs.[642]

MYCOBACTERIUM TUBERCULOSIS

It has also been suggested that PID may result from *Mycobacterium tuberculosis* in endemic areas.[643]

OTHER ORGANISMS

Other organisms involved in PID may include:

- Cytomegalovirus (CMV): CMV has been found in the upper genital tracts of women with PID, suggesting a potential role[631]
- Endogenous microflora: in iatrogenically induced infections, the endogenous microflora of the vagina predominate[631]
- *Gardnerella vaginalis*[631]
- *Haemophilus influenzae*
- Enteric Gram-negative organisms (*Escherichia coli*)
- *Peptococcus* species
- *Streptococcus agalactiae*
- *Bacteroides fragilis*: This can cause tubal and epithelial destruction[631]
- *Ureaplasma urealyticum.*

CHLAMYDIAL INFECTIONS

Chlamydia trachomatis infection is the most prevalent bacterial STI recognised throughout the world.[644] It is approximately three to four times more common than

N. gonorrhoeae and the proportion of PID attributed to *Chlamydia* is higher than that attributed to the gonococcus.[644] Chlamydiae are small, intracellular bacteria that need living cells to multiply. There are 18 distinct serotypes of *C. trachomatis*, with serotypes D to K causing sexually transmitted genital infections and neonatal infections.[645] *C. trachomatis* is the major cause of mucopurulent cervicitis and PID in women.[646] Chlamydial cervicitis is usually asymptomatic, but clinical findings may include cervical oedema and a mucopurulent discharge.[641] *Chlamydia* and *N. gonorrhoeae* may occur as coinfecting organisms.[644] Urethritis is often associated with chlamydial cervicitis.[644] Chlamydial cervicitis may be associated with at least three types of complications: (1) ascending infection from intraluminal spread of organisms from the cervix, producing PID; (2) ascending infection during pregnancy, resulting in premature rupture of the membranes, chorioamnionitis, premature delivery, puerperal and neonatal infections; and (3) the development of cervical neoplasia.[645] Fitz-Hugh–Curtis syndrome (perihepatitis) may also develop in association with chlamydial infections.[644]

C. trachomatis has been isolated from the cervix of 5–56% of women with PID.[641] Two recent studies used DNA detection of *C. trachomatis* and *N. gonorrhoeae*.[647] *C. trachomatis* was isolated from the fallopian tubes of about one-third of all women with the organism in the cervix and from 10% of all women with PID.[641] A complicating finding is that chlamydiae, in contrast to gonococci, can remain in the fallopian tube area for months and years after an initial infection.[641] Women with chlamydial salpingitis may develop progressive tubal damage caused by persistent infection if it is not effectively treated.[641]

GONORRHOEA

Between 10% and 19% of women with *N. gonorrhoeae* in the cervix have signs of PID.[648] Gonococcal virulence factors may explain why only some women develop PID.[641]

Gonorrhoea is caused by a Gram-negative diplococcus.[644] Humans are the only natural host for *N. gonorrhoeae*.[644] The urogenital tract is most frequently infected because of the organism's predilection for columnar or pseudostratified epithelium. In women, the endocervix is the most common site of gonorrhoea infection.[644] The majority of these infections are asymptomatic. Because of the asymptomatic nature of these infections, gonococcal cervicitis may go untreated and result in serious complications, such as disseminated gonococcal disease and acute PID. PID occurs in approximately 15% of women with untreated gonococcal cervicitis.[644]

Overview

Pelvic inflammatory disease (PID) is an infectious and inflammatory disorder of the upper female reproductive tract, including the uterus, fallopian tubes, and adjacent pelvic structures.[649] The terminology is not consistent, however, and many other terms are commonly used to describe the different manifestations of pelvic infection, including endometritis, salpingitis, salpingo-oophoritis, adnexitis, parametritis, pyosalpinx, tubo-ovarian abscess, tubo-ovarian complex, pelvic peritonitis, perihepatitis and peri-appendicitis.[649] PID is usually the result of infection ascending from the endocervix. While sexually transmitted infections such as *Chlamydia trachomatis* and *Neisseria gonorrhoeae* have been identified as causative agents,[650] *Mycoplasma genitalium* and other organisms have also been implicated.[651] The presentation varies from acute asymptomatic disease that requires admission to hospital, to asymptomatic damage that is only discovered later when infertility is investigated. Delays of only a few days in receiving appropriate treatment markedly increase the risk of sequelae, which include infertility, ectopic pregnancy and chronic pelvic pain.[652] The psychological consequences of pelvic infections can be devastating, especially because most patients are young.

Pathogenesis

NORMAL VAGINAL FLORA

The vagina normally contains a predominance of facultative lactobacilli and numerous but low concentrations of other facultative and anaerobic bacteria.[653] It is unclear whether the high endocervix normally supports a flora or if the recovery of bacteria from the cervix represents vaginal contamination.[641] Bacteria are not recovered by culture from normal endometrium and fallopian tubes, although it is possible that due to the opening of the cervix during menstruation, retrograde menstrual flow may facilitate ascent of microorganisms. Intercourse may contribute to the ascent of infection due to rhythmic mechanical uterine contractions. Bacteria may be carried along with sperm into the uterus and tubes. Factors important for the dissemination of organisms from the cervicovaginal flora to the uterus and fallopian tubes are not well understood, but data collected in several studies suggest that most cases of PID occur in two stages, with the first stage involving acquisition of a vaginal or cervical infection. The second stage of upper female genital tract infection occurs by direct ascent of microorganisms from the vagina and cervix.[631] Although the exact mechanism of ascent is unknown, studies have suggested that a number of factors may be involved. Alterations in the cervicovaginal microenvironment may result from antibiotic treatment and STIs that can disrupt the balance of endogenous flora, causing normally non-pathogenic organisms to overgrow and ascend.[631]

BACTERIAL VAGINOSIS

The relation between bacterial vaginosis (BV) associated organisms and their causative role in the aetiology of PID has been debated for some time; however, controversy still remains.[646] It is known that, epidemiologically, BV is the most common lower genital tract infection in women of reproductive age, and those women who have BV are more likely to have upper genital tract infection compared with those without.[654] Weisenfield et al[655] have also demonstrated that one in seven women with BV have evidence of subclinical PID and its related consequences on endometrial biopsy.

While studies have demonstrated a potential role of BV with both clinical signs of PID and histological endometritis,[656,657] Hillier et al[658] found that in 178 women with clinically suspected PID, the clinical entity of BV was not associated with endometritis on a multivariate analysis. They did, however, find that the presence of anaerobic Gram-negative rods was associated with endometritis via biopsy.[658] This is subsequent to stratifying for gonorrhoea and *Chlamydia*, and for possible contamination. This may suggest that invasion of the upper genital tract by BV microorganisms is a greater risk for histological endometritis compared with BV per se.[646]

Cervicitis is a common infection that is often the source of microbes that cause PID.[641] A reduction in the prevalence of cervicitis probably reduces the rate of PID.[641] Endometritis diagnosed by plasma cells within the endometrium is present in approximately 50% of women with cervicitis.[659] Infection within columnar cervical epithelial cells also often produces erythema, oedema and bleeding of the cervix.[641] *C. trachomatis* and *N. gonorrhoeae* are the most common organisms causing cervicitis and together they can be isolated in more than one half of the women with the infection.[660] The cause of infection in the remaining women is unknown, although *Mycoplasma genitalium* also causes a proportion of cervicitis.[661]

SPONTANEOUS PID

Spontaneous PID is limited to menstruating women. Women who develop PID with *N. gonorrhoeae* or *C. trachomatis* usually experience the onset of pain within 7 days of their menstrual period.[662] This observation suggests that PID caused by these bacteria is influenced by menses, possibly related to the opening of the cervix during menstruation with retrograde menstrual flow that may facilitate ascent of microorganisms.[631] The growth of *N. gonorrhoeae*, particularly the virulent transparent gonococcal phenotypes, may be stimulated during the secretory phase of the cycle just before menstruation.[663] The bacteriostatic effect of the cervical mucus on bacteria, which is greatest during the ovulatory phase of the cycle, is at its minimum before the onset of menses.[664] Cervical mucus provides a functional barrier against upward spread; however, the efficacy of this mechanism may be decreased by hormonal changes that occur during ovulation and menstruation. Gonococci,[662] *C. trachomatis*[665] and other bacteria appear to attach to sperm, and it is even possible that sperm can act as vectors to carry these bacteria into the uterus and fallopian tubes.[641] Intercourse may contribute to the ascent of infection due to rhythmic mechanical uterine contractions.[631]

INFECTIVE PATHWAY

The route by which the pathogens gain access to the upper female tract has only recently been explored. Menstruation, sperm and trichomonads have all been shown to be important in the transportation of pathogens into the salpinx.[666] The usual infection ascends along the mucosa from the cervix into the endometrium and to the fallopian tubes.[641] After bacteria reach the uterus, they may be transported to the fallopian tubes by contiguous spread or carried by ciliary motion.[641] Endometritis appears to be an intermediate level of infection between cervicitis and salpingitis.[641] Women with endometritis have an increased rate of abnormal vaginal bleeding and uterine tenderness.[641] Endosalpingitis is initiated after organisms reach the fallopian tube and attach to the mucosa.[641]

MICROBIAL AND HOST FACTORS

In the upper tract, a number of microbial and host factors appear to play a role in the degree of host inflammation and resultant scarring.[631] A cytokine response of INF-γ and various interleukins occurs with experimental *C. trachomatis* infection.[667] With acute infection, 60% of the lymphocytes were cytotoxic lymphocytes, which together with finding porforin, indicates activation of cytotoxic lymphocytes.[667] Repetitive infection may produce the severe permanent tubal damage by the immunopathogenic lymphocyte response.[641] The importance of cytotoxic lymphocytes is furthered by the observation that chlamydial salpingitis occurs more frequently among humans with human leucocyte antigen 31 (HLA-31).[668] HLA-31 is an MHC class I molecule that presents cytoplasmically processed antigen to cytotoxic lymphocytes. The impact of genetics on infection is complex. This class II molecule HLA DRA 0301 was associated with both chlamydial and gonococcal cervicitis and infertility, suggesting host genetics can increase both susceptability and disease severity.[669]

ANTIBODY RESPONSE

Local and serum IgA, IgM and IgG class antibodies are made in response to chlamydial infection. Partial protection against reinfection has been observed, but this protection appears short and serotype-specific.[670] Antibody appears to play a small role compared with cell-mediated immune responses in the resolution of infection.[641] While *C. trachomatis* screening control programs drive the prevalence and rate of PID down, a dichotomy may exist where such control programs might not allow the development of protective antibody to *C. trachomatis*, which might limit tubal damage.[670]

SPREAD OF INFECTION

Uterine infection is usually limited to the endometrium, but may be more invasive in a gravid or postpartum uterus.[631] Tubal infection initially affects the mucosa, but acute, complement-mediated transmural inflammation may develop rapidly and increase in intensity with subsequent infections.[631] Inflammation may extend to uninfected parametrial structures, including the bowel.[631] Infection may extend by spillage of purulent materials from the fallopian tubes or via lymphatic spread beyond the pelvis to produce acute peritonitis and acute perihepatitis (Fitz-Hugh–Curtis syndrome).[631]

RISK FACTORS

Risk factors for PID include multiple sexual partners, a history of prior STIs and a history of sexual abuse.[671]

Frequent vaginal douching has also been implicated.[672] Surgical procedures, such as endometrial biopsy, curettage and hysteroscopies break the cervical barrier, predisposing women to ascending infections.[631]

SEXUALLY TRANSMITTED INFECTIONS

As STIs are the commonest aetiological agents for PID, risk factors for developing PID can be related to those associated with the acquisition of STIs. STI acquisition is associated with early coitarche, young age and high-risk sexual behaviours (including multiple sexual partners).[646] The PID rate in 15- to 19-year-old women is approximately three times that in 20 to 24-year-old women and is approximately twice the PID rate of that for 25- to 29-year-old women.[673] The 16- to 19-year-old group are vulnerable, largely due to sexual behaviour; however, there may be also a degree of host susceptibility.[646] This is subsequent to those of a young age having large ectopias, increased permeability of cervical mucus and a decreased concentration of chlamydial antibodies and increased risk-taking behaviours.[674] Factors that may enhance or inhibit the development of acute salpingitis are listed in Table 18.39.

CONTRACEPTIVES

Debate continues to surround the use of contraception, including the intrauterine device (IUD), the oral contraceptive pill (OCP) and barrier methods, and the risk of developing PID.[675] A meta-analysis recently published addresses the issue of the IUD.[678] The authors found a relative risk of 3.3 in women using the IUD. This risk appears to be in the first few weeks after IUD insertion, reflecting iatrogenic ascension of pathogens into the upper genital tract. Women with a non-medicated IUD are two to three times more likely to develop PID than non-users.[676] Non-medicated IUDs annually cause acute salpingitis among 1–2% of users.[677] An IUD's tail, particularly a multifilament tail, is capable of assisting movement from the cervicovaginal area to the uterus.[678] The tail acts as a reservoir for bacteria through colonisation on the surface.[679] IUDs may also increase infection rate by promoting anaerobic bacterial growth, by producing micro-ulcers or by producing a chronic inflammatory reaction of the endometrium or the fallopian tube.[641] Progesterone dampens an immunology response and in preliminary studies progesterone IUDs appear to have a low PID rate.[641] However, large, well-controlled studies are needed of progesterone users.

Evidence that barrier methods reduce the risk of contracting PID, and indeed STIs in general, is conflicting.[646] This is possibly secondary to misclassification of proper condom use, or over-reporting of reliable use.[680] Interestingly, results from the PEACH study found that those women who used condoms inconsistently were at an increased risk of upper genital tract infections.[669] Conversely, they observed a trend towards reduced upper genital tract infections in those women who reported consistent use of barrier contraception compared with no contraception at all. The CDC recommends that spermicides and condoms containing nonoxynol-9 should be avoided, as a number of African studies have demonstrated that nonoxynol-9 can cause vaginal lesions and may increase the risk of HIV transmission.[641]

Oral contraceptive pills (OCPs) have been found to have differing effects on PID risks.[631] Previous studies have shown that OCP use has been associated with a reduction in the incidence of PID, even PID of chlamydial origin.[681] These findings, were based on older, higher hormonal doses of OCP.[646] This is contradictory to the findings that oral contraceptives are thought to increase the risk of endocervical infection, probably by increasing the zone of cervical ectopy.[682] Recent data from the PID Evaluation and Clinical Health study have addressed these inconsistencies.[672] They have found that OCP use does not reduce the risk of upper genital tract disease; but that women tended to have a reduced clinical severity of the disease. They go on to say that OCPs have been found to decrease the risk of symptomatic PID, possibly by increasing cervical mucus viscosity, decreasing menstrual anterograde and retrograde flow and modifying local immune responses, which may mask clinical recognition of PID.[682]

TABLE 18.39 Factors that enhance or inhibit the development of acute salpingitis

Enhancing factors	Inhibitory factors
N. gonorrhoeae *C. trachomatis* Cervicitis Endometritis Bacterial vaginosis Vaginal douching Non-medicated intrauterine device Oral contraceptives (controversial) Cigarette smoking High-risk sexual behaviour Early coitarche Inconsistent or no barrier protection use Surgical procedures	Cervical mucus Bactericidal antibodies Oral contraceptives (controversial)

Source: Adapted from Eschenbach DA. Acute pelvic inflammatory disease. Global Library Women's Medicine; 2008. doi 10.3843/GLOWM.1002

VAGINAL DOUCHING

Although a relationship between vaginal douching and PID has been suspected for some time, there have been difficulties interpreting this relationship, as studies have been retrospective and unable to demonstrate cause and effect.[683]

Douching three or more times a month with commercial products was associated with a three-fold increased rate of PID when demographic variables, gonorrhoea and *Chlamydia* infection were controlled in a multivariate analysis.[683] However, a subsequent prospective study of over 1100 women found no increase in incidence of PID among women who douche.[684] Interestingly, they found no association of the clinical entity of BV with douching and PID, furthering the debate surrounding the causative role of BV-associated microorganisms in the aetiology of PID.[684] Douching was usually undertaken as a habit and not in response to symptoms of infection.[641]

UNTREATED MALE SEXUAL PARTNERS

Untreated males with urethral *N. gonorrhoeae* and *C. trachomatis* infection are an important source of the initial and subsequent episodes of PID.[641] In one study, over 80% of male sexual partners had not been treated for gonorrhoea when the woman presented with PID.[685] About one-half of the male contacts with gonorrhoea were asymptomatic, and 40% of asymptomatic men had urethral *N. gonorrhoeae*.[641] The men remained asymptomatic for as long as 180 days after the women were treated.[641] Symptomatic non-gonococcal urethritis and asymptomatic chlamydial urethritis are also common among male contacts of patients with PID.[641] Therefore, examination and treatment of male sexual partners is crucial to decreasing the recurrence of PID.

SURGICAL PROCEDURES

It has been reported that cervical vaginal microorganisms are pushed into the endometrium by surgical procedures, including IUD insertion, dilation and curettage, hysterosalpingography and induced abortion.[641] Such procedures occurred before the onset of PID in 12% of cases.[686] PID has been reported in 1.5% of women within the first 3 months of IUD insertion.[687] Induced abortion led to PID in up to 20% of women with untreated *C. trachomatis* and bacterial vaginosis.[688]

SEX DURING MENSES

Sex while menstruating, or just afterwards, has also been linked to PID.[646] Indeed, endometritis is more common in women during, or just following, their period.[689] This is probably due to loss of the cervical plug, or possible hormonal changes affecting immune function. In addition, cigarette smoking has also been linked to PID. The postulated mechanisms include possible immune compromise, or smoking decreasing the activity of oestrogen.[646]

HIV

Women with human immunodeficiency virus (HIV) infection may have increased rates of PID.[641] The seroprevalence of HIV was higher in a US study[690] and in one Kenyan study[691] among those with PID compared with controls without PID. HIV patients with PID appear to have more pelvic abscesses and more frequently require surgery than PID patients without HIV.[692]

SIGNS AND SYMPTOMS

The following clinical features are suggestive of a diagnosis of PID:

- Lower abdominal pain and tenderness
- Deep dyspareunia
- Abnormal vaginal or cervical discharge
- Cervical excitation and adnexal tenderness motion
- Fever (>38°C).

Clinical symptoms and signs, however, lack sensitivity and specificity (the positive predictive value of a clinical diagnosis is 65–90% compared with laparoscopic diagnosis).[650]

COMPLICATIONS

Recurrent infection

A subsequent episode occurs in up to 25% of women after an episode of PID.[693] The frequency of infertility and other sequelae markedly increases after multiple infections, so attempts should be made to reduce subsequent PID through education, treatment of male sexual partners and close follow-up.[641] Women with sexually transmitted organisms tend to re-acquire these organisms, which further contribute to recurrent PID.[641] The high subsequent tubal infection rate may be related to the susceptibility of damaged fallopian tube mucosa to recurrent infection and perhaps to unrecognised persistent infection.[641]

Ectopic pregnancy

The number of ectopic pregnancies reported in the United States doubled in the 1980s but has decreased since 1990.[694] Between 1930 and 1980, the frequency of ectopic pregnancy after PID increased, perhaps related to antibiotic therapy.[641] Antibiotics reduce the total tubal occlusion rates but they do not reverse all tubal damage sustained before therapy.[641] Tubal damage causes the majority of tubal pregnancies.[695] Tubal damage from prior PID is observed in about 50% of women with an ectopic pregnancy.[673] Tubal entrapment of the ovum or slowed tubal transit time from damaged cilia presumably accounts for the tubal rather than intrauterine implantation of the pregnancy.

Westrom has estimated that among women who have had at least one episode of PID, there will be a six- to ten-fold increase in the rate of ectopic pregnancy; approximately 18% will have chronic abdominal or pelvic pain.[673] The risk of an ectopic pregnancy is about 7 times greater in women after PID than in women without prior PID.[673] Ectopic pregnancy rates increase with the severity of the tubal damage and with the number of episodes of PID.[696] The impact of ectopic pregnancy on subsequent infertility is considerable; only about one-half of women with an ectopic pregnancy ever conceive again.[641] If a pregnancy occurs following an ectopic pregnancy, the rate of another ectopic pregnancy is about 20%.[696]

Chronic abdominal pain

Chronic abdominal pain lasting longer than 6 months occurred in 17–18% of women after one or more episodes of PID, compared with 2–5% of women who have never had PID.[697] Chronic pain is present in 12% after one episode, 30% after two episodes and more than 60% after three or more episodes.[697] The pain is often constant, interferes with work, and results in increased physician visits, hospitalisations and abdominal operations.[698] Increased pain with menses and with intercourse also is common.[698] The theory that the pain is related to residual pelvic pathology is strengthened by an increased rate of infertility and dyspareunia among women with pain after PID.[641] Many of the hysterectomies and salpingo-oophorectomies after PID are performed because of chronic pain.[641]

Infertility

Infertility is one of the most common and dreaded consequences of PID. PID is a major cause of infertility, with the cost of infertility resulting from PID in the USA estimated to be approximately US$60 billion annually, ten times the cost of treating acute PID.[641]

The fallopian tube plays an important role in transport and nutritional support of the gametes and early conceptus.[644] After ovulation, the oocyte is swept into the tubal ostia by beating cilia. Oocytes then travel to the ampulla, where fertilisation occurs and zygote cleavage begins. Through the actions of the muscular myosalpinx and cilia, the oocyte and then the zygote are transported to the uterus. Compromised tubal function can occur after external or internal injury. Pelvic infection is a major cause of tubal subfertility.[695] Regardless of the initiating pathogen, a mixed microbial infection usually results. Infection frequently leads to intraluminal damage, destroying epithelium necessary for normal gamete transport and interaction. Hydrosalpinges often develop and may further interfere with reproduction. Hydrosalpinges interfere with fertility because of the mechanical closure of the distal tube as well as possible reflux of fluid from the hydrosalpinx into the tube and uterus.[644]

The severity of tubal subfertility after pelvic infection depends on the number and severity of episodes.[641] For example, infertility resulting from tubal occlusion occurs in 8% of women with one episode, 23% of women with two episodes and 43% of women with three episodes of PID.[652,699] The frequency of tubal occlusion also is related to the type and severity of PID and to age.[641] Tubal disease from prior salpingitis is present in 15–40% of infertile women in developed countries[700] and up to 65% of infertile women in developing countries.[701] Infertility is more common when PID is caused by organisms other than gonococci.[699,702] Infertility is more common after laparoscopically documented severe tubal infection (21%) than after moderate (16%) or mild (6%) tubal infection.[652,702] Older women are more likely than young women to develop tubal occlusion after PID.[703] Tubal infertility is also increased among women with >3 days of pain before treatment.[652]

DIFFERENTIAL DIAGNOSIS

Pelvic inflammatory disease should be one of the most important diagnoses in sexually active young women with pelvic pain but other conditions that may mimic PID should be kept in mind. These may be divided into gynaecological and non-gynaecological conditions (Table 18.40).[704] Many may present with peritonism and as a surgical emergency.[704]

TABLE 18.40 Pelvic inflammatory disease differential diagnosis

Gynaecological conditions	Non-gynaecological conditions
Ectopic pregnancy	Appendicitis
Septic abortion	Urinary tract infections or renal stones
Endometriosis	Gastroenteritis
Torsion of an ovarian cyst, haemorrhagic corpus luteum, rupture of an ovarian cyst	Inflammatory bowel disease
Mittelschmerz pain	Functional pain of 'unknown origin'
Cervicitis	Cholecystitis
Spontaneous abortion	Diverticulitis
Adnexal tumours	

Source: Khan ZE, Rizvi JH. Pelvic inflammatory disease and pelvic abscesses. Rev Gynecol Perin Pract 2006;6(3–4):185–91.

NATUROPATHIC DIAGNOSIS

Patients can present with a variety of symptoms, and significant variation may be seen in described symptoms, ranging from lower abdominal pain to dysuria. Women may be asymptomatic or seriously ill. Symptoms occur most commonly early in the menstrual cycle or at the end of menses, which has been attributed to low progesterone levels at this time, with consequent thinning of the cervical mucosal barrier.[631]

Lower abdominal pain is present in more than 90% of documented cases and is by far the most common presenting symptom.[631] Usually pain is described as dull, aching or crampy, bilateral, and constant; it begins a few days after the onset of the last menstrual period and tends to be accentuated by motion, exercise or coitus.[631] Pain may be exacerbated by movement or sexual activity (dyspareunia).

Pain from PID usually lasts less than 7 days; if pain lasts longer than 3 weeks, the likelihood that PID is the correct diagnosis declines substantially.[631] Abnormal vaginal discharge is present in approximately 75% of cases.[705] Unanticipated vaginal bleeding, often postcoital, coexists in about 40% of cases.[631] Temperature higher than 38°C (30%), nausea and vomiting manifest late in the clinical course of the disease.[631]

Investigations

PHYSICAL

The diagnosis of acute PID is primarily based on historical and clinical findings.[631] This is imprecise, with no single piece of historical, physical, or laboratory information found to be specific or sensitive for the disease.[646] A large number of patients may present atypically and exhibit no or few symptoms; however, more than one-quarter of these patients meet objective criteria for upper tract infection on laparoscopic examination.[631] The sensitivity of the pelvic examination is only 60%.[631] The physical examination usually reveals lower abdominal tenderness, cervical motion tenderness, and uterine or adnexal tenderness. Rebound tenderness and involuntary guarding may be noted and suggest associated peritonitis.

One large multicentre trial found adnexal tenderness to be the most sensitive physical examination finding (95% sensitive, $p < 0.001$).[706] Mucopurulent cervicitis is common, and, if absent, it provides a significant negative predictive value (NPV).[631] Adnexal fullness or disproportionate unilateral adnexal tenderness may indicate the development of a tubo-ovarian abscess.[631] Molander et al[707] found three variables to be significant predictors of the diagnosis: adnexal tenderness ($p < 0.001$), fever ($p < 0.001$) and an elevated sedimentation rate (ESR) ($p < 0.001$). In this study, these variables correctly classified 65% of patients with laparoscopically documented PID (95% CI 61–99%).

Right upper quadrant tenderness, especially if associated with jaundice, may indicate associated Fitz-Hugh–Curtis syndrome. A prospective cohort study in 117 incarcerated adolescents documented a 4% incidence of Fitz-Hugh–Curtis syndrome in those with mild-to-moderate PID.[708]

For the diagnosis of PID in sexually active young women, the CDC recommends uterine/adnexal tenderness or cervical motion tenderness as the minimal clinical criteria.

No single test is highly specific and sensitive for PID. Laboratory evaluation of any woman of child-bearing age in the emergency department should always include a pregnancy test. The possibility of septic abortion and ectopic pregnancy must be considered. Additional criteria may be used to enhance the specificity of the minimum criteria:

- Temperature higher than 38.3°C
- Abnormal cervical or vaginal mucopurulent discharge
- Presence of white blood cells (WBCs) on saline microscopy of vaginal secretions
- Elevated erythrocyte sedimentation rate
- Elevated C-reactive protein level
- Laboratory documentation of cervical infection with *N. gonorrhoeae* or *C. trachomatis*.

Urinalysis should be performed to help exclude urinary tract infections. A positive urinalysis does not exclude PID, because any inflammatory process in the contiguous pelvis can produce white blood cells in the urine.

Blood cultures are not helpful in the diagnosis of PID.

Microbiological diagnosis

STIs have been implicated as the causative factor in PID in a large proportion of cases. Sampling of the lower genital tract to identify pathogens is therefore essential, with multiple site sampling increasing the diagnostic yield.[646] Unfortunately, sampling of the upper genital tract is invasive, and not always practical or indicated. As such, a negative result from the lower genital tract does not preclude the diagnosis. Some important organisms to be tested will be discussed.

The standard for diagnosis of chlamydial infections remains isolation by tissue culture.[644] Rapid diagnostic tests have become broadly available commercially. These include a monoclonal antibody and enzyme-linked immunosorbent assay. A newer method of detection, the nucleic acid amplification test (NAAT), is now the test of choice for diagnosing chlamydial infections.[659] The NAAT is more sensitive than culture or antigen tests. The three commercial tests available utilise either the polymerase chain reaction, ligase chain reaction or transcription-mediated amplification method to identify chlamydial DNA.[644] With the use of these newer tests, it has become clear that older tests most likely underestimated the true prevalence of chlamydial infections. An additional advantage of these tests includes their use with a first-void urine specimen or with vaginal or vulvar swabs, therefore avoiding a pelvic examination.[644] The nucleic acid amplification tests are more expensive than antigen tests but should still be considered the test of choice because they will detect many more infected individuals.[644]

Some clinicians treating patients with infertility believe that it is also worthwhile to determine whether antibodies to *C. trachomatis* are present in the serum by measuring IgG antibodies to this organism. Studies such as that by Dabeekausen et al[709] found a good correlation between the presence of antibodies to *Chlamydia* and the presence of tubal adhesions or obstruction. Their study demonstrated that chlamydial antibody testing was more accurate than hysterosalpingogram in predicting tubal factor infertility.[709] However, current practice is to use hysterosalpingograms and cervical cultures as primary screening tests for tubal infertility, rather than chlamydial antibody testing.[644]

In the USA, chlamydial genital infections occur frequently among sexually active adolescents and young adults and often are asymptomatic. Consideration should be given to screening sexually active adolescents for chlamydial infections during routine annual examinations, even if symptoms are not present.[710] Screening women aged 20–24 should also be considered, particularly for those who have new or multiple sex partners and who do not consistently use barrier contraceptives.[644] The goals of early and aggressive screening are to reduce the most serious sequelae of *C. trachomatis* infections in women, including PID, ectopic pregnancy and infertility.[644] A recent investigation of patients in a health maintenance organisation demonstrated that screening and treatment of cervical infection can reduce the likelihood of PID.[710]

Because gonococcal infections among women are often asymptomatic, an important component of gonorrhoea control in the USA continues to be a screening of women at high risk for STIs.[710] The standard diagnostic test is a culture.[644] The CDC recommends that all gonorrhoea cases should be diagnosed or confirmed by culture to facilitate antibiotic susceptibility testing.[710]

The diagnosis of pelvic tuberculosis may be confirmed by histology, culture or by direct visualisation via laparoscopy.[644] Hysterosalpingogram also may show findings strongly suggestive of tuberculosis PID. The radiographic criteria for the diagnosis of pelvic tuberculosis by hysterosalpingogram have been described by Klein and associates as follows: calcified lymph nodes, irregular calcifications in the adnexal areas, obstruction of the fallopian tube in the zone of transition between the isthmus and the ampulla, multiple constrictions along the course of the fallopian tube, endometrial adhesions or deformity or obliteration of the endometrial cavity in the absence of a history of curettage or abortion, and vascular or lymphatic extravasation of contrast material.[711]

Imaging studies

A number of procedures can be performed to improve the diagnosis of PID and its complications.[631] These procedures are not necessary, nor are they indicated, in the management of every case of presumptive PID. However, due to the difficulty of definitive clinical diagnosis and the number of important surgical and gynaecological emergencies that may have similar presentations, they can be employed by the clinician.[631]

TRANSVAGINAL ULTRASONOGRAPHY

Helpful findings include thickened (>5 mm), fluid-filled fallopian tubes and free pelvic fluid in acute, severe PID. These findings alone do not demonstrate adequate specificity to make a definitive diagnosis of PID. However, pelvic abscesses may be seen as complex, adnexal masses with multiple internal echoes.[631]

In the individual who appears toxic or has asymmetrical pelvic findings, ultrasonography is an important diagnostic tool for the identification of a tubo-ovarian abscess.[704] Ultrasonography has been shown to demonstrate as many as 70% of adnexal masses missed on physical examination.[631] Pelvic ultrasonography is also useful in evaluating the possibility of ectopic pregnancy in those patients whose differential diagnosis includes both entities.[631] Ultrasonography can also be helpful in evaluating other entities in the differential diagnosis, including haemorrhagic ovarian cyst, ovarian torsion, endometrioma and appendicitis.[631]

COMPUTED TOMOGRAPHY (CT)

Computed tomography (CT) may be used in the differential diagnosis of PID. CT findings in PID include obscuration of the pelvic fascial planes, cervicitis, oophoritis, salpingitis, thickening of the uterosacral ligaments and the presence of simple or complex pelvic fluid or abscess collections.

MAGNETIC RESONANCE IMAGING (MRI)

Although the specificity (95%) and sensitivity (95%) of MRI are relatively high, it is costly and rarely indicated in acute PID.[631] If used in the management of PID, MRI can demonstrate thickened, fluid-filled tubes with or without free pelvic fluid or tubo-ovarian complex.[712]

Procedures

ENDOMETRIAL BIOPSY

Endometrial biopsy can be used to determine the histopathological diagnosis of endometritis.[646] Endometritis is uniformly associated with salpingitis.[689] Endometrial biopsy is approximately 90% specific and sensitive.[689] The procedure is performed with an endometrial suction pipette/curette and is well tolerated.[631] Specimens for culture may also be obtained during the procedure, but these are frequently contaminated with vaginal flora.[631]

LAPAROSCOPY

Laparoscopy is traditionally referred to as the 'gold standard' in the diagnosis of PID.[646] It is significantly more specific and sensitive than clinical criteria alone. The minimum criteria to diagnose PID laparoscopically include tubal wall oedema, visible hyperaemia of the tubal surface and the presence of exudate on the tubal surfaces and fimbriae.[631] Pelvic masses consistent with tubo-ovarian abscess or ectopic pregnancy can be directly visualised.[631] Hepatic abscess exudate and/or adhesions may be visible. Material can be obtained for definitive culture and histological studies. However, the procedure is expensive and invasive, exhibits inter-observer variability, and requires an operating room and anaesthesia.[707] Findings on laparoscopy do not necessarily correlate with the severity of illness, as only the surfaces of structures are visible.[646] Laparoscopy may not fully define PID in up to 20% of cases.[646]

Specific naturopathic investigations

A thorough clinical history and a physical examination that includes abdominal palpation would be indicated, however, due to the nature of this condition, *immediate* referral to a GP is required for suspected cases.

In addition, the patient's risk factors and history should be assessed for likelihood of infection with a sexually transmitted organism. The patient should be questioned about any new sexual partner, method of contraception and recent medical procedures. The source, severity and characteristics of the pelvic/abdominal pain should be evaluated.

Therapeutic considerations

CLINICAL DECISION MAKING AND RATIONALE

PID presents a clinical complexity due to the multiple microbial infections associated with the development of the disease. Many of these strains are antibiotic resistant thus increasing the tendency for high recurrence rate. It is the repeated infections that contribute to the devastating long-term clinical presentation with significant secondary repercussions.

Immediate treatment of PID addresses the relief of acute symptoms, eradication of current infection, and minimalisation of the risk of long-term sequelae.[631] From a public health perspective, treatment is aimed at the expeditious eradication of infection to reduce the risk of transmission of infection to new partners. It is also imperative to identify and treat current and recent partners to prevent the spread of STIs.[646] Early patient diagnosis and treatment appear to be critical in the preservation of fertility.[646]

Therapeutic application

ALLOPATHIC PERSPECTIVE

Antibiotics

Because of diagnostic difficulties and the potential for serious sequelae, the CDC advises that physicians should maintain a low threshold for aggressive patient treatment, with overtreatment preferred to no or delayed treatment.[710] Treatment initiated in the emergency department, clinic or surgery setting should be expeditiously begun and includes empirical broad-spectrum antibiotics to cover the full complement of common causes.[710] All regimens must thus be effective against Gram-negative facultative organisms, anaerobes and streptococci, as well as *C. trachomatis* and *N. gonorrhoeae*.

A number of studies (1992–2006) have demonstrated effectiveness of a variety of parenteral and oral regimens in both the elimination of acute symptoms and microbiological cure.[713] Only a single, large, randomised multicentre clinical study has effectively compared inpatient and outpatient oral and parenteral antibiotic regimens in the documented elimination of endometrial and tubal infection.[714] This study found no differences in outcome between inpatient and outpatient management in the study population.

Surgical care

Patients who do not improve in 72 hours are re-evaluated for possible laparoscopic or surgical intervention and to reconsider other possible diagnoses. Laparoscopic pelvic lavage, abscess drainage and lysis of adhesions may be necessary.[631]

Most tubo-ovarian abscesses (60–80%) resolve with antibiotic administration.[631] If patients do not respond appropriately, laparoscopy may be useful to identify loculations of pus requiring drainage.[631] An enlarging pelvic mass may indicate bleeding secondary to vessel erosion or a ruptured abscess. Unresolved abscesses may be drained percutaneously via posterior colpotomy, or via CT or ultrasonographic guidance, laparoscopically or by laparotomy.

The advantages of laparoscopy include direct visualisation of the pelvis and more accurate bacteriological diagnosis if cultures are obtained.[631] However, laparoscopy is not always available in acute PID.[646] In addition, this procedure is costly and requires general anaesthesia.[646] It should be used if the diagnosis is in doubt. However, if operative laparoscopy is used early in the course of the disease, copious irrigation and separation of thin adhesions by blunt dissection may prevent later sequelae.[631]

Laparotomy is usually reserved for surgical emergencies, such as abscesses that have ruptured, abscesses that have not responded to medical management and laparoscopic drainage, or in those who are not candidates for laparoscopic management.[631] Treatment may involve unilateral salpingo-oophorectomy or hysterectomy and bilateral salpingo-oophorectomy, depending on the intraoperative findings and the patient's desire for fertility maintenance.[631]

HISTORICAL PERSPECTIVE

Infectious disorders of the reproductive system such as PID were rife in the time of the Eclectics. Lack of knowledge on the manner in which sexually transmitted infections spread, poor hygiene and unprotected intercourse are all likely to have contributed and influenced the progression of many such conditions. The Eclectics used a variety of antimicrobial botanicals to eradicate the infective organisms. *Piper methysticum* is said to have been useful in relieving gonorrhoea[9] as were *Petroselinum sativum, Phytolacca americana, Commiphora myrrha* and *Hydrastis canadensis*[8] and since *N. gonorrhoeae* is implicated in PID these same types of botanicals may have been used for PID. To improve immunity and due to its anti-infective nature the Eclectics may have used *Echinacea,* highlighting its use for leucorrhoea 'in all of which there is a run-down condition of the system with fetid discharge'.[9] Lastly *Calendula officinalis* received strong endorsement where it was used as an interuterine wash for vaginitis, all uterine and vaginal abrasions ulcerations and leucorrhoea.[8]

NATUROPATHIC PERSPECTIVE

Due to the highly infectious nature of this condition and the high risk for recurrence and secondary concerns such as infertility, naturopathic treatment cannot be the sole treatment approach. It is essential to work in conjunction with a patient's GP and provide supportive immunological treatment. It is naïve to rely on naturopathic means of treatment as a sole treatment strategy.

If provided in conjunction with allopathic treatment, the naturopathic approach focuses on a few key aspects:

- Appropriately manage and care for patient to prevent development of condition
- Support and enhance the immune response of the patient
- Symptomatic relief from pain, discharge, bleeding, fever or other
- Reduction in inflammation and oxidation
- Microflora stabilisation and repletion in both the GI tract and reproductive systems
- Education for sexual health and contraceptive choices in the acute stage
- Conservation and support of fertility if required as well as co-management with other health professionals
- Encourage protective measures to reduce bacterial colonisation and prevent recurrence
- Encourage adequate hydration to increase urinary elimination.

NUTRITIONAL MEDICINE (DIETARY)

Dietary therapeutic objectives

- Avoidance of all pro-inflammatory foods
- Avoidance of all immune-suppressant foods including refined carbohydrates and sugar
- Encourage optimal hydration to support urinary eliminatory pathways
- Encourage adequate protein to support the immune response and repair and healing of tissues

- Encourage antioxidant and nutrient-rich fresh fruits and vegetables that support the healing process
- Encourage fermented foods and pre- and probiotic food sources to support gastrointestinal and reproductive microecology
- Encourage essential fatty acid-rich food sources to reduce inflammation
- Encourage immune-stimulating foods and those with antimicrobial constituents such as garlic and onion; and high essential oil culinary herbal medicines including thyme and oregano.

Specific dietary treatments

DIETARY INCLUSIONS

Anti-inflammatory foods

Given that PID is characterised by infection and inflammation, functional foods that are anti-infective, enhance the immune system and are anti-inflammatory are most indicated. The foods that fit into these categories include fresh fruit (not in excess due to sugar content), vegetables, various herbs and spices, nuts, seeds and oily fish. Adequate protein is also required to ensure a proper immune response.

DIETARY EXCLUSIONS

Sugar

Sugar consumption is known to impair the immune system. Murray[715] notes that glucose and vitamin C appear to compete for the same transport sites into white blood cells, thus excess sugar leads to a reduction in vitamin C subsequently reducing white blood cell function. Given these findings, sugar intake in all its forms (even juice and nectar, etc.) should be reduced.

NUTRITIONAL MEDICINE (SUPPLEMENTAL)

Nutritional medicine therapeutic objectives

- Support the immune response to eradicate infection
- Improve the immune system's response to the pathogen and protect the individual from repeated infection
- Reduce inflammation and oxidation
- Support and improve the integrity of the mucous membranes in reproductive tract
- Recolonise and support gastrointestinal and reproductive microecology
- Provide symptomatic relief from pain, discharge and discomfort.

SPECIFIC NUTRIENTS REQUIRED

Beta-carotene

Beta-carotene functions as an antioxidant and may be used to enhance the immune system by activating macrophages and lymphocytes and promoting interferon activity.[25] The ovary contains substantial quantities of beta-carotene,[342] which is likely to help protect against the oxidative and inflammatory damage that ensues in PID.

SAMPLE DAILY DIET

BREAKFAST	
Chicken congee with black rice, ginger and shiitake	Congee provides a restorative breakfast option with ginger and shiitake mushrooms used for their immune and anti-inflammatory properties. Organic chicken provides a protein source for optimal immune function as well as a source of zinc which may function as an antimicrobial.
LUNCH	
Roast pumpkin, carrot, oregano and garlic risotto	Provides a wide variety of vegetables to assist with immune function, in particular it is beta-carotene rich for antioxidant activity. Garlic and oregano exhibit powerful immune stimulant and anti-microbial properties.
DINNER	
Sweet potato and chickpea dhal with a side of sauerkraut	Dhal provides a range of anti-inflammatory and antioxidants constituents due to high use of herbs and spices such as cumin, turmeric, ginger, onion and garlic. Chickpeas provide a vegetarian source of protein to support the immune response. Sauerkraut provides a fermented food which may assist in providing additional support for reproductive microecology.
SNACK	
Fresh fruit	Immune support and prebiotic

Bromelain

Bromelain is a crude, aqueous extract from the stems and immature fruits of the pineapple plant. It has been suggested to be of benefit in inflammatory diseases[716] due to its anti-inflammatory activity where it has been shown to decrease neutrophil migration to inflammation sites.[716] Given the anti-inflammatory action of bromelain it may thus be of use in PID to counteract the widespread inflammation synonymous with this condition. Reducing inflammation is imperative in PID as inflammation may contribute to further serious complications; for example, inflammation of the fallopian tubes is linked to infertility and risk of ectopic pregnancy. Also likely to be of use is bromelain's ability to function as an immune modulator and its ability to enhance wound healing.[717] Bromelain's fibrinolytic activity is likely to assist in the prevention of pelvic scarring.

Probiotics

Symptoms such as abnormal vaginal discharge or bleeding, itching and odour signify the presence of genital infection and are common in patients with PID.[718] Probiotics have been used successfully in infectious female reproductive disorders including urogenital infections such as bacterial vaginitis,[47] and thus may be useful in PID. Given that many patients will be administered antibiotics, the argument for probiotics is further heightened. Further studies are required to elucidate specific doses and strains.

Preparation options

Daily dietary supplementation with natural yoghurt and other fermented dairy products is advisable, with probiotic supplementation recommended in addition. In most cases, topical preparations of probiotic powders mixed with natural yoghurt and vitamin E oil are often the fastest strategies and provide symptomatic relief (Box 18.5).

BOX 18.5 Probiotic recipe

- 1 tspn of probiotic powder containing multiple *Lactobacilli* strains, especially *L. acidophilus*, *L. rhamnosus*, *L. reuteri* and *L. casei*. *Bifidobacterium* strains have been shown to inhibit various GI tract colonisations such as *E. coli*, therefore providing additional support.
- 1 tablespoon of unsweetened, natural yoghurt (full-fat)
- 1 vitamin E capsule broken open and oil mixed into paste.

Apply topically and insert into the vagina as required. Mixture can be syringed into the vagina as well and kept internally overnight for optimal results.

Vitamin A

Vitamin A displays immune,[719] regulatory,[719] antioxidant[21] and tissue-repair functions relevant to management of PID. It also plays a key role in maintaining healthy mucous membranes, including those found in the female reproductive tract such as the vagina.

Vitamin C

Vitamin C is an immune stimulant and thus is critical to enhance the immune system's defence against the invading organisms implicated in PID. It is an anti-inflammatory and helps to decrease tissue destruction and support collage tissue repair. All of these roles combined help prevent the spread of infection, especially as a lack of vitamin C is associated with an increased susceptibility to infection.[358] It has also been shown to help to prevent pelvic scarring due to its fibrinolytic properties.[342]

Vitamin E

Vitamin E maintains the health of the ovaries[25] and is critical for healthy immune function. As an antioxidant it is likely to help protect the female structures from free radical damage caused by inflammation from PID.

Zinc

Zinc is a key mineral required to mount healthy defence mechanisms such as in the presence of infection implicated in pelvic inflammatory disease. The antimicrobial properties of zinc are broad spectrum and include action against *Chlamydia trachomatis*[720] and *Candida albicans*.[721] Deficiency of zinc is associated with increased risk of infection.[722]

Dosage requirements

The dosage requirements listed below are based on adult doses that have been reported in the literature and clinical review:

- Vitamin A 10000–20000 IU or beta-carotene 6 mg/day
- Vitamin E 400–800 IU/day
- Vitamin C 500 mg 4–6 times/day for the first week then decrease over 3 days to 250 mg t.d.s.
- Bromelain 250 mg four times/day for the first week and three times/day for 6 weeks
- Zinc 30–75 mg/day (higher in the acute)
- Probiotics: multistrain (with high *Lactobacillus* spp. where possible), ½ tspn 3–4 times per day (30–50 × 10^9 organisms per teaspoon).

HERBAL MEDICINE

Herbal medicine therapeutic objectives

- Improve the immune system's response to fight the pathogen and protect the individual from repeated infection
- Reduce inflammation and oxidation
- Support and improve the integrity of the mucous membranes in reproductive tract
- Recolonise and support gastrointestinal and reproductive microecology
- Provide symptomatic relief from pain, discharge and discomfort.

Herbal medicine classes

Herbal medicine classes used are listed in Table 18.41.

Specific herbal medicines

ALLIUM SATIVUM (GARLIC)

Given the infectious origin of PID, botanicals such as *Allium sativum* that display a natural antibiotic[723] activity and eliminate and/or reduce infection are required. *Allium sativum* has been used medicinally for thousands of years to improve general immunity and displays antibacterial, antiviral, antifungal and anti-protozoal properties relevant to the treatment of PID.

Pelvic inflammatory disease may involve multimicrobial aetiology, though the most common infective agents are *Chlamydia trachomatis* and *N. gonorrhoeae*,[718] hence the benefits of a broad-spectrum antimicrobial botanical. While no studies could be found specifically assessing the efficacy of *Allium sativum* in PID, its antimicrobial activity displayed in vitro against a wide range of other pathogens including *Brucella abortis*, *Staphylococcus aureus*, *Streptococcus viridans*, *Proteus vulgaris*, *Escherichia coli*, *Salmonella enteritidis*,

TABLE 18.41 Herbal medicine classes

Class	Action
Immune stimulants	Immune stimulants are beneficial to support the immune response and eradicate the pathogen. In addition, they can assist the effectiveness of antibiotic therapy and support the body's ability to respond effectively
Antimicrobial	Antimicrobial herbal medicines specifically target the pathogen and may be antibacterial, antiviral or other. The greater the specificity of the herbal medicine to the specific pathogen, the greater the outcome
Mucous membrane trophorestoratives	Restoration of the delicate mucous membranes within the vagina and reproductive organs is paramount to support an effective attack against the pathogens. Pathogenic infiltration can cause significant damage to the tissues and increase susceptibility to repeated infections
Lymphatic	Lymphatic herbal medicines provide immune support by encouraging lymphatic clearance and circulation to the area
Analgesic	Analgesic herbal medicines provide symptomatic pain relief that is much needed in acute presentations. Important considerations include *Anemone erythrina* or *Corydalis ambigua*
Anti-inflammatory	Reduction in inflammation allows greater healing of tissues and recovery

Klebsiella pneumonia and *Candida albicans*[723] provides a basis for its use in PID.

ARCTOSTAPHYLOS UVA-URSI (UVA URSI)

Arctostaphylos uva-ursi is a urinary antiseptic and anti-inflammatory that displays antimicrobial properties. It contains a constituent known as arbutin, a hydroquinone derivative. The antimicrobial action of *Arctostaphylos uva-ursi* is associated with the aglycone hydroquinone released from arbutin.[724] As well as arbutin, *Arctostaphylos uva-ursi* also contains tannins, phenolic acids, flavonoids such as quercetin as well as traces of volatile oil. In-vitro studies demonstrate *Arctostaphylos uva-ursi* to be antimicrobial, demonstrating bacteriostatic activity against *Proteus vulgaris, E. coli, Ureaplasma urealyticum, Mycoplasma hominis, Staphylococcus aureus, Pseudomonas aeruginosa,* Friedländer's pneumonia, *Enterococcus faecalis, Streptococcus* strains and *Candida albicans,* thus it may be useful to eliminate infective organisms in PID.[724]

BERBERIS AQUIFOLIUM (OREGON GRAPE)

Berberis aquifolium is an evergreen shrub that contains isoquinoline alkaloids including berberine.[129] Berberine has been demonstrated in vitro to be potent against a wide array of pathogens including bacteria, fungi, protozoans, viruses and, most importantly *Chlamydia,*[725] a common infective organism implicated in PID. It is important to note that berberine upregulates Pgp and as such is not absorbed from the GI tract. It is consequently a great antimicrobial for surfaces it can touch, such as the skin or GI tract, but is ineffective for the uterus, kidneys, lungs, etc. Thus topical application is advisable for efficacy of outcome. All other alkaloids included in Oregon grape can still be used as a mucous membrane tonic.

CALENDULA OFFICINALIS (CALENDULA)

Calendula officinalis, also known as marigold, is a colourful herb whose principal constituents include triterpenoids, flavonoids,[726] resins, glycosides, volatile oil and carotenes. *Calendula officinalis* displays anti-inflammatory[724] activity as well as antibacterial, antiviral, anti-protozoal[726] effects in vitro that may be of use in PID. The German Commission E[724] advocates the use of *Calendula officinalis* for internal inflammations and also reports clinical studies demonstrating antiviral and immune-stimulating activity; though unresearched, this immunostimulant activity (whereby polysaccharides within *Calendula* stimulate the immune system) is likely to be of particular value in PID to restore healthy immune function. Furthermore, because *Calendula officinalis* has been shown to aid internal wound-healing in vivo it may be of use to aid in the repair of reproductive tissue.

HYDRASTIS CANADENSIS (GOLDEN SEAL)

Hydrastis canadensis is a native American herb with immune-stimulant properties.[727] It contains alkaloid constituents including berberine, beta-hydrastine, canadine and canadaline. As discussed above, berberine has been found to exert broad-spectrum antimicrobial activity against a wide range of microorganisms including *Chlamydia,* although topical application is advised for positive outcome.[725] In-vitro studies also reveal the ability of *Hydrastis canadensis* to modify responses from lipopolysaccharide-stimulated macrophages during stimulation, hypothetically suggesting that it may work by reducing pro-inflammatory responses, thus indirectly leading to limited clinical symptoms during infection.[727] *Hydrastis canadensis* is also a powerful mucous membrane tonic and may help to restore health to the mucus-producing cells that line the female reproductive tract.

MELALEUCA ALTERNIFOLIA (TEA TREE)

Melaleuca alternifolia is a native Australian plant prized for its antimicrobial and anti-inflammatory effects.[728] Aboriginal Australians tell of healing lakes, which were in fact lagoons into which *Melaleuca alternifolia* leaves had fallen and decayed over time, a testament to its therapeutic and healing properties.[728] The oil of the plant is typically used and, as with *Allium sativum,* has been observed to demonstrate broad-spectrum activity against bacteria, viruses, fungi and protozoa. The mechanism of action of *Melaleuca alternifolia* appears to be dependent upon its target; against many bacteria it inhibits respiration while encouraging loss of intracellular material whereas against fungi it may also inhibit respiration and alter the cell membrane.[728]

THYMUS VULGARIS (THYME)

Thymus vulgaris is an evergreen herb whose flowering tops[129] may be used to enhance the immune response to invaders. The key constituents of *Thymus vulgaris* include essential oils such as thymol and carvacrol, as well as glycosides, flavonoids, alcohols, saponins and tannins.[729] *Thymus vulgaris* displays antimicrobial activity against a range of pathogens including bacteria such as *Staphylococcus aureus* and funguses such as *Candida albicans*.[729] As yet there are no studies assessing its effects in PID, but the antimicrobial activity displayed by *Thymus vulgaris* against the pathogens discussed above suggest it would be useful in eliminating the infective organisms implicated in PID.

Lifestyle recommendations

GENERAL RECOMMENDATIONS

Smoking, alcohol and recreational drugs should all be avoided due to their compounding effects on immune function and increase to oxidation and inflammation.

EDUCATION

Patients should be thoroughly educated about safe sex practices and potential warning signs for PID.

DOUCHING

Douching is no longer recommended and herbal douches are also questionable due to disturbance to the vaginal ecology and the ability for douching to enable greater travel of organisms through the genital tract.

SITZ BATHS

Traditionally, sitz baths have been an important component of the naturopathic treatment of PID. The contrast sitz bath is primarily used to increase pelvic circulation, bring an influx of macrophages to the area and provide decongestion of the pelvic inflammatory reaction.[730]

STI PREVENTION AND SAFE SEX PRACTICES

It is imperative to advise female patients who are not in monogamous relationships to maintain barrier methods of contraception, especially condoms. Condoms are preferential to diaphragms due to greater protection in the vaginal cavity thus reducing risk of infection considerably. Most male carriers are silent carriers with no obvious infection signs or symptoms, thus contributing to the increasing incidence of PID in the female population.

SEXUAL INTERCOURSE

It is inadvisable to allow sexual practices during active infection. Additional research suggests that sex during menses is also concerning if a condom is not used due to loss of the cervical plug and transport potential for pathogens through blood. Furthermore, the endometrial layer is believed to provide additional protection and this is obviously thinned and partially removed during menses.

CASE STUDY

OVERVIEW

BB, a 28-year-old woman, presented with lower abdominal pain, diarrhoea and abnormal vaginal discharge. On discussion she explained that she had been sexually experimental of late and had slept with three partners in the past 2 weeks. No barrier methods had been used as she was taking the COC.

Clinical examination revealed fever (38.6°C) and marked abdominal tenderness. Discussion revealed dyspareunia and spotting post intercourse.

The patient was immediately referred to the GP at the practice who referred for pathology and diagnosed PID secondary to *Chlamydia* infection. She was prescribed 1 week's prescription of doxycycline. Review was planned for one week's time or if symptoms aggravated.

Supportive treatment was advised and included the following.

HERBAL MEDICINE

Herbal medicine	Ratio	Quantity	Justification
Arctostaphylos uva-ursi	1:2	60 mL	Antimicrobial
Calendula officinalis (60% alc)	1:2	50 mL	Immune stimulant, lymphatic
Echinacea spp.	1:2	70 mL	Immune stimulant
Hydrastis canadensis	1:3	40 mL	Immune stimulant, mucus membrane trophorestorative

TOTAL: 220 mL. Dose: 7.5 mL t.d.s. (away from antibiotic prescription).

NUTRITIONAL MEDICINE

Dietary

- Avoidance of all immunosuppressant foods including refined carbohydrates and sugar
- Encourage optimal hydration to support urinary eliminatory pathways
- Encourage adequate protein to support the immune response and repair and healing of tissues
- Encourage antioxidant and nutrient-rich fresh fruits and vegetables that support the healing process
- Encourage fermented foods and pre- and probiotic food sources to support gastrointestinal and reproductive microecology
- Encourage essential fatty acid-rich foods sources to reduce inflammation
- Encourage immunostimulating foods and those with antimicrobial constituents such as garlic and onion; and high essential oil culinary herbal medicines including thyme and oregano.

CASE STUDY CONTINUED

Supplemental

- 1 tspn of probiotic powder containing multiple *Lactobacillus* strains, especially *L. acidophilus*, *L. rhamnosus*, *L. reuteri* and *L. casei*. *Bifidobacterium* strains have been shown to inhibit various GI tract colonisations such as *E. coli*, therefore providing additional support
- 1 tablespoon of unsweetened, natural yoghurt (full-fat)
- 1 vitamin E capsule broken open and oil mixed into paste Apply topically and inserted into the vagina as required.

Mixture can be syringed into the vagina as well and kept internally overnight for optimal results.

Internal prescriptions

- Vitamin A 10 000 IU t.d.s.
- Vitamin E 500 IU b.i.d.
- Vitamin C 500 mg 4–6 times/day for the first week
- Zinc 25 mg t.d.s.
- Probiotics: multistrain, ½ tspn 3–4 times per day (45 × 10^9 organisms per teaspoon) (antibiotic-resistant preparation).

LIFESTYLE/EDUCATION

- Avoidance of all sexual activity
- Education regarding contraception and safe sex practices
- Avoidance of alcohol, smoking, recreational drugs.

MENOPAUSE

Epidemiology

All women who live beyond the age of 55 will experience menopause, but each experience will be unique. The age at which the menopause starts varies according to the individual woman (Fig. 18.14). In 1978 the mean age of menopause in healthy Australian women was 50.4 years.[731] This is in line with contemporary figures which estimate that the average age of menopause is 51 (±5 years).[732] It is likely that the average Australian woman who reaches 50 years of age will experience approximately another 27–32 years of postmenopausal life. In fact the World Health Organization estimates that by 2030 there will be around 1.2 billion postmenopausal women, with 47 million women entering life post menopause every year.[732]

Premature menopause (menopause that occurs before the age of 40) affects up to 1%[733] of women, and usually occurs as a result of medical intervention or premature ovarian failure. Caucasian populations appear to be more prone to premature ovarian failure when compared with other ethnicities, including Chinese (0.5%) and Japanese (0.1%).[734]

Classification

PERIMENOPAUSE

Perimenopause is a time of intermittent symptoms of the menopause that first become apparent as egg numbers in the ovaries fall far enough to cause shortening of the menstrual cycle, particularly the follicular phase, and accompanied by elevation of serum FSH when measured during menstruation. As it progresses, menstrual cycles can shorten considerably, while becoming interspersed unpredictably by unusually long cycles, sometimes producing cystic follicles and even anovulatory dysfunctional bleeding, as well as episodes of hot flushes. Though fertility is low, there is still the chance that a woman may conceive.[735]

Last menstrual period (between Menopause transition and Postmenopause)

	Reproductive			Menopause transition		Postmenopause	
Reproductive stage	Early	Peak	Late	Early	Late	Early	Late
				Perimenopause			
Menstrual cycle	Variable or regular	Regular		Cycle length variable, 1 or 2 missed cycles per year	3 or more missed cycles	None	
Age (duration)	Puberty to mid-40s			Mid-40s to mid-50s (4 years)		Mean of 51 years to death	
Steroid hormones	Oestradiol 50 to 200 pg/mL Testosterone 400 pg/mL			Same or slightly higher Same		40 pg/mL same	0–15 pg/mL same
Pituitary hormones	FSH 10 mIU/mL day 2–4 LHH 10 mIU/mL day 2–4			Same or higher Same or higher		>100 mIU/mL >100 mIU/mL	

FIGURE 18.14 Menopause.

Source: Rakel D. Integrative medicine. 2nd edn. 2007 Philadelphia: Saunders; 2007.

OOPAUSE

Oopause is a new term for the normal cessation of female fertility up to 10 years before the menopause. It occurs in some women after the age of 33 and for most women by 45. It is different to perimenopause as it reflects failing ovarian function; however, regular menstruation may still be occurring.

If pregnancies are attempted through the oopausal transition, a woman who has had no prior reproductive disturbance will typically experience recurrent miscarriages before developing otherwise unexplained infertility. If she undertakes in-vitro fertilisation/assisted reproductive technology (IVF/ART) she typically experiences unexplained implantation failure of apparently satisfactory embryos then, in turn, a decreased rate of forming blastocysts, defective cleavage and failure of fertilisation.

MENOPAUSE (NATURAL)

Menopause is technically defined as the last natural menstrual period (so often a retrospective diagnosis). It is the natural state a woman is in after the ovaries have stopped ovulating because of depletion of eggs. The normal age of menopause is between 40 and 55 years, with an average in Western societies of 50–51 years.

Natural menopause may be diagnosed after 12 months of amenorrhoea, a result of loss of follicular ovarian activity and in the absence of another pathological cause.[736]

PREMATURE MENOPAUSE

Premature menopause is defined when menopause occurs before the age of 40.

PRIMARY OVARIAN FAILURE

Primary ovarian failure occurs when the ovaries are unable to produce enough follicles because of a problem in the ovary itself. This results in depletion of eggs before the age of 40 years (known as premature menopause, a cause of secondary amenorrhoea). It can also occur before the age puberty is expected (causing failure of puberty to happen, including primary amenorrhoea). It can sometimes occur in spite of good numbers of primordial follicles that (inexplicably, so far) do not develop. It may occur as a result of a mosaicism for Turner syndrome,[737] mumps ovaritis[737] or spontaneously due to an abnormal karyotype involving the X chromosome or in women with a normal 46,XX karyotype[738] as well as in the presence of autoimmune disease and other rare conditions.[738]

ARTIFICIAL MENOPAUSE

Artificial menopause may occur at any age and may occur as a result of chemotherapy or radiation for cancer therapy, or as a result of surgery (e.g. hysterectomy or other surgical intervention).[739]

Aetiology

Menopause is inevitable for those that reach the age, but a number of risk factors have been identified linked to earlier onset.

SMOKING

A number of studies[739,740] have linked smoking to risk of early menopause and smoking has been suggested to cause destruction of the ovarian follicles. One study showed a dose-dependent response, with 14+ cigarettes daily observed to promote earlier onset of menopause by 2 years, but less than 13 cigarettes and ex-smokers were found to experience menopause at the same time as non-smokers.[741,742] A 2014 systematic review and meta-analysis supported these results and smoking remains associated with an earlier age of natural menopause after adjusting for confounding factors. The same association was not found in ex-smokers who had a similar age of menopause onset.[743]

RACE/ETHNICITY

Both race and ethnicity have been determined as major factors with regards to onset of menopause.

For example, in one study,[744] in spite of only compromising 10% of the study sample, black women were found to experience menopause at a lower age (49.3 years) than white women (51.2 years).

GENETICS

Genetic factors have been suggested to influence the onset of menopause as seen in studies observing mothers and daughters, and twin and sib-pairs.[745,746]

OTHER

Other factors suggested to influence age at menopause as a result of oocyte depletion include living at higher altitudes, education, occupation, age at menarche, parity (how many pregnancies a woman has had), age at last pregnancy and if there has been use of oral contraceptives.[737,743]

A recent systematic review and meta-analysis of 22 studies found that low and moderate levels of alcohol consumption might be associated with later onset of menopause compared to no alcohol consumption. The association was weak and further investigation is required.[747]

Overview

Menopause is a universal phenomenon in women who reach the relevant age (commonly 51 years). With the increase in life expectancy, women may spend nearly half their lives in a postmenopausal state and will experience the short-term and long-term effects of menopause.

Although universal, menopausal symptoms vary widely between women and across cultures. Some women 'sail through it' and some experience severe and debilitating symptoms. Twelve months without a period is the commonly accepted rule for diagnosing menopause.

Pathogenesis

Natural menopause occurs when the body's natural secretion of progesterone, testosterone and oestrogen (in the form of oestradiol) is reduced due to the diminishment of the ovarian follicles,[736] preventing the endometrium from proliferating, resulting in no shedding of the uterus.

Prior to menopause, oestradiol is the strongest and principal form of oestrogen in the body; however, following menopause oestrone becomes the dominant form of oestrogen in the body.[748] Follicle-stimulating hormone and luteinising hormone levels begin to increase due to the diminished levels of the ovarian hormones, leading to an irregular menstrual cycle. For many women the cycle may become unpredictable,[735] and may be longer or heavier. Eventually women begin to notice that they skip cycles until they stop all together.

SIGNS AND SYMPTOMS

Menopausal symptoms can occur in perimenopausal women who still have a regular bleeding pattern, as well as in women with menstrual cycle disturbance or amenorrhoea. Dysfunctional heavy or infrequent and/or irregular uterine bleeding is common in response to the wide fluctuations of oestradiol production in the perimenopause. Ongoing significant bleeding should be investigated before commencing treatment in any form.

Many women navigating their way through the climacteric report a range of different symptoms; in fact, an estimated 85% report more than one symptom, leading 10% of women to seek help from their healthcare professional.[749] Irregularity in the menstrual cycle is usually the first sign during the fourth and fifth decade and marks the entry into perimenopause.

Vasomotor symptoms such as hot flushes are one of the most common complaints, particularly among Australian women. These occur due to temperature alterations as a result of gonadal hormone changes[750] and may be described as a 'transient warming sensation', 'increased perspiration', 'flushing' or 'intense heat spreading over the body'.[750] Highlighting just how commonplace hot flushes are, a 9-year longitudinal study undertaken in a small sample of Melbourne women observed that only 17% of women in the sample did not suffer from hot flushes during their transition period. In this group hot flushes were associated with women who had high FSH and low oestradiol levels, low exercise levels and were smokers.[751]

Urogenital symptoms such as vaginal dryness, atrophic vagina, vaginal/bladder infections and painful sexual intercourse may occur due to loss of oestrogen and androgen sensitisation in the vaginal tissue.[736] This loss of steroid hormones causes irritation and soreness, and its prevalence postmenopause is thought to be close to 50%. A range of other symptoms including increased visceral fat in the subcutaneous area,[752] loss of muscle mass and strength,[752] loss of bone density,[752] sleep disturbance, urinary leakage, severe tiredness, brain fog, depressive symptoms, joint pain, palpitations, insomnia and mood swings, loss of hair and diminished libido may also be experienced.[753]

Common symptoms are listed in Box 18.6.

BOX 18.6 Common symptoms of menopause

- Atrophic vaginitis
- Bladder infections
- Body aches
- Cognitive changes
- Hair loss
- Hot flushes
- Increased facial hair
- Irregular bleeding (perimenopause)
- Mood changes
- Sleep disturbances
- Urinary incontinence

COMPLICATIONS

Menopause may be a risk factor for a number of conditions including:

- *Osteoporosis:* The loss of oestrogen that occurs at menopause results in accelerated bone resorption and rapid decline in bone density hence women undergoing the menopausal transition are at increased risk of osteoporosis.
- *Breast cancer*: Later onset of menopause has been linked to increased risk of breast cancer; early studies showed that women who experienced a natural menopause at age 55 or older had double the breast cancer risk experienced by those whose menopause occurred before age 45.[754]
- *Cardiovascular disease*: Several studies have observed a link between increased risk of cardiovascular disease following menopause where among other things women have been found to experience a unique increase in lipids at the time of the menopause.[755] It is important to note that most of the risk factors for cardiovascular disease are able to be modified through changes in diet, lifestyle and exercise.

DIFFERENTIAL DIAGNOSIS

- Pregnancy: exclude as a reason for amenorrhoea[756]
- Pituitary dysfunction
- Uterine cancer
- Polycystic ovary syndrome: exclude as a reason for amenorrhoea
- Hyperthyroidism:[756] may experience hot flushes and anxiety, also associated with the menopausal transition
- Hypothyroid:[756] may experience weight gain, fatigue, or constipation synonymous with menopause.

NATUROPATHIC DIAGNOSIS

Naturopathic diagnosis of menopause will primarily involve detailed questioning about the quality and quantity of a woman's menstrual cycle, coexisting symptoms (e.g. hot flushes) and will also take into account the woman's age and family history. The naturopathic practitioner may ask a patient to observe her vaginal mucus and record her symptoms using a chart such as that found in Appendix 18.3 at the end of the book. Laboratory testing may be ordered, but is typically not useful, as diagnosis can usually be made on the patient's age and symptoms alone.

TABLE 18.42 Investigations used for menopause

Laboratory investigations	Full blood count, blood chemistry panel, lipid panel, thyroid function + antibodies, homocysteine, C-reactive protein and lipoproteins, vitamin D
Hormonal assessment	FSH is diagnostic. Ensure assessment is conducted on day 3 of cycle (if menstruating to assess perimenopausal status) or when periods are delayed to assess menopause timing. AMH can assess ovarian reserve — best if combined with follicle count on ultrasound
Breast examination and screening mammography	To assess for breast changes. Ensure patient is aware of self-examination techniques and has regularly performed breast self-examination so can detect changes
Pelvic examination	To assess for vaginal atrophy or other complications
Bone density testing	Eliminate osteoporosis or osteopenia, establish benchmark reading postmenopause or eliminate existing osteopenia or osteoporosis
Papanicolaou smear	Assess cervical health and cancer risk
Electrocardiogram	Assess cardiovascular health
Colonoscopy	If required, to eliminate GI tract changes
Weight assessment	Height, weight, BMI, waist-to-hip ratio
hCG	Eliminate pregnancy as cause of amenorrhoea
General physical examination	Vaginal thinning, hair loss, facial hair, abdominal adiposity
Cancer markers	Controversial assessment for prediction of cancers

Investigations

ALLOPATHIC INVESTIGATIONS

Investigations used are summarised in Table 18.42.

Specific naturopathic investigations

Specific naturopathic investigations are listed in Table 18.43.

Therapeutic considerations

CLINICAL DECISION MAKING AND RATIONALE

Menopause is a time when many cardiovascular risks emerge, namely central adiposity, increased insulin resistance and dyslipidaemia. Dietary modification and an appropriate exercise regimen will almost certainly be necessary for weight control and optimisation of the lipid profile. In addition, a few key treatment strategies will be beneficial including herbal medicines, nutritional supplementation, stress management and other strategies.

Some patients will feel sufficiently supported through naturopathic measures, but some will choose to combine treatments with hormone replacement therapy (HRT) prescriptions. It is beneficial to understand the function and effect of these on the body.

Therapeutic application

HISTORICAL PERSPECTIVE

Historically, menopause was a natural and welcome end to a woman's childbearing years and in many developing countries it is still viewed in this way.[757] The early French physicians were responsible for the term the 'menopause' but they believed that once this menopausal period was over, a new stage of renewed life and vigour were to follow.[758] In stark contrast, in the modern Western world menopause is often viewed as a deficiency disease characterised by loss. This representation is believed to have been started in the 1930s[757] thus thankfully it is likely that the Eclectics would not have viewed menopause in this way.

The use of botanicals in the climacteric does not receive as much mention as that of individual symptoms such as dysmenorrhoea, but the Eclectics make mention of homeopathics such as *Sanguinaria canadensis* (blood root),[759] highlighted for its efficacy in easing vasomotor disturbances such as hot flushes. *Actaea racemosa* is described as a utero-ovarian tonic and a remedy for atony of the reproductive tract, particularly that of the female, where it restored suppressed menses when there was a disordered action or lack of functional power in the uterus. *Hydrastis canadensis* was deemed useful in climacteric haemorrhage (flooding) due to its effect on the circulation, while *Salvia officinalis* (sage) may have been used for its efficacy in restraining exhausting sweats. *Leonurus cardiaca* (motherwort) was recommended for wakefulness, restlessness, disturbed sleep and an irritable, excitable, enfeebled state of the nervous system, while *Leonurus cardiaca* was also deemed to be useful for general debility, nervousness from irregular menstruation and palpitation of the heart and amenorrhoea. *Pulsatilla* was prized for its wide application to assist in issues with the reproductive organs, including nervousness and despondency, sadness, unnatural fear, tendency to weep, morbid mental excitement, marked depression of spirits; pain, with debility, nervousness, headache, insomnia and nervous exhaustion.

TABLE 18.43 Specific naturopathic investigations for menopause

Detailed history and case taking	The level of detail achieved from thorough case taking cannot be overestimated. Review all past and present health aspects and consider environmental, occupational, social, emotional, nutritional, psychological and physical aspects
Menopausal symptom diary	See Appendix 18.3; enables holistic review of symptomatology and progression with treatment
Cardiovascular risk profile	Blood pressure, lipid profile, homocysteine, diabetes screen
Baseline female hormone profile	Saliva test in which oestrone (E1), oestradiol (E2), oestriol (E3), progesterone (P4), testosterone (TT) and DHEA-S levels may be determined
Adrenal hormone profile	Measures stress hormones cortisol and DHEA-S, over the course of a day, determining adrenal function in patients presenting with symptoms such as anxiety, depression, mood swings, insomnia, headaches, low energy, stress, hormonal imbalance and poor immune function. Altered levels of cortisol and DHEA-S are indicative of acute and/or chronic mental and/or physical stress
Women's health profile	Assesses risk factors associated with genetics, biochemical imbalances and environmental influences for women of all ages
2 and 16 urinary oestrogen metabolites	Monitors oestrogen metabolism, thus helping to determine risk of hormone imbalance
Functional liver detoxification profile	The functional liver detoxification profile is used to identify how well the patient's detoxification mechanisms are functioning; inadequate detoxification signifies risk of increased toxic load on the body. Properly functioning detoxification mechanisms will ensure that the body is better able to cope with menopause
Thyroid hormonal profile and reverse T3	Thyroid function declines as women get older and an underactive thyroid is common in menopausal and postmenopausal women
Osteoporosis risk assessment	The osteoporosis risk assessment (NTx) is a urine test which measures the risk of osteoporosis by detecting the rate of bone resorption (breakdown) well before significant changes are obvious on bone mineral density scans. Risk of osteoporosis increases at menopause

ALLOPATHIC PERSPECTIVE

The 'treatment' of menopause from an allopathic perspective is largely based upon attempts to alleviate symptoms. Hormone replacement therapy, initially popular, fell from grace after the Women's Health Initiative observed that the conjugated equine oestrogen administered to women was found to increase risk of stroke and venous thromboembolic events.[760] Its prescription is still recommended and involves short-term (1–5 years) HRT for the primary indication of menopause symptoms, using a combination of oestrogen and a progestogen. It is prescribed in the form of creams, pills, sprays, implants and patches. Oestrogen (in women who have undergone a hysterectomy) or oestrogen with progestogen (in women with an intact uterus) has been suggested to be the primary means of treatment for management of vasomotor symptoms such as hot flushes.[761] If a patient wishes to take (or is taking) conventional HRT it is worth discussing alternative options, including bioidentical hormones and other non-equine-derived hormonal replacements.

Each individual will need to decide if they wish to take:

- Natural hormone replacement therapy (nHRT) (bioidentical hormone therapy)
- Conventional hormones (cHRT) (standard HRT)
- Condition-specific non-oestrogen pharmaceuticals
- Selective noradrenaline reuptake inhibitors (SSRIs) and other non-hormonal medications such as gabapentin and clonidine, typically suggested for treating hot flushes in women where HRT is inappropriate (e.g. women with risk of breast or other oestrogen-sensitive cancers, endometrial hyperplasia or undiagnosed uterine bleeding).

Currently available HRT schedules are described in Table 18.44.

NATUROPATHIC PERSPECTIVE

When approaching a patient who is going through or has recently transitioned through the menopause, it is important to focus on three key areas:

- Symptomatic support
- Treatment for any disease processes present
- Prevention of any future disease processes.

Symptomatic support prevails when the patient presents, but holistic thought requires practitioners to consider other processes currently occurring and those potentially expected.

NUTRITIONAL MEDICINE (DIETARY)

Dietary therapeutic objectives

- Dietary objectives that offer prevention and protection from cancer (especially breast and colorectal), Alzheimer's disease, cardiovascular disease, diabetes and other chronic health problems
- Support the skeletal system and encourage dietary sources of calcium and other bone nutrients
- Encourage optimal digestive processes with fibre-rich foods
- Encourage phyto-oestrogen food sources

TABLE 18.44 Current HRT schedule

	Ultra-low dose	Low dose	Medium dose	High dose
Progestogen				
Progestogen: continuous				
Norethisterone	350 micrograms	350 micrograms	350–700 micrograms	700 micrograms
Medroxyprogesterone acetate	2.5 mg	2.5 mg	2.5–5 mg	5 mg
Dydrogesterone	5 mg	5 mg	5 mg	5 mg
Progestogen: cyclical				
Norethisterone	0.7 mg on days 1–12 of calendar month	0.7 mg on days 1–12 of calendar month	0.7–2.5 mg on days 1 to 12 of calendar month	2.5 mg on days 1–12 of calendar month
Medroxyprogesterone acetate	5 mg on days 1–12 of calendar month	5–10 mg on days 1–12 of calendar month	5–10 mg on days 1–12 of calendar month	10 mg on days 1–12 of calendar month
Dydrogesterone	10 mg on days 1–12 of calendar month	10 mg on days 1–12 of calendar month	10 mg on days 1–12 of calendar month	10 mg on days 1–12 of calendar month
Oestrogen				
Transdermal patch (doses expressed as release rate per 24 h)				
Oestradiol		25–37.5 micrograms	50–75 micrograms	100 micrograms
Transdermal gel				
Oestradiol 1 mg/g			1 mg	
Oral				
Conjugated oestrogens	0.3 mg on alternate days	0.3 mg	0.625 mg	1.25 mg
Oestradiol	1 mg on alternate days	1 mg	2 mg	
Oestradiol valerate	1 mg on alternate days	1 mg	2 mg	

Source: Adapted from eTG complete, Therapeutic guidelines Ltd; Nov 2009.

- Adopt general wholefood dietary principles such as high in fruit, vegetables, wholegrains, vegetarian protein, nuts, seeds, legumes
- Avoid saturated, trans and hydrogenated fats; simple and refined carbohydrates, sugar and processed foods. A cross-sectional study of postmenopausal women in China found that those consuming a predominantly whole plant food diet had lower depression scores (26% reduction), whereas processed food intake was positively associated with perceived stress and depression (79.3% increased risk), and negatively associated with self-esteem scores.[762]
- Dietary modifications to prevent weight gain and reduce central adiposity.

Specific dietary treatments

DIETARY INCLUSIONS

Phyto-oestrogens

A diet rich in phyto-oestrogens has been promoted to help reduce symptoms of menopause. A 12-week study observed the effects of a diet rich in phyto-oestrogens as compared with a regular omnivorous diet in women with menopausal complaints.[763] The phyto-oestrogen group replaced a quarter of their daily kilojoule intake with miso, flaxseed and tofu. Serum levels of phyto-oestrogens increased significantly in the group consuming a diet rich in phyto-oestrogens, while they remained the same in the test group. Menopausal symptomatology decreased in both groups, but when the groups were analysed separately the phyto-oestrogen group was found to experience improvement with regard to hot flushes and vaginal dryness; levels of sex hormone-binding globulin were also increased in the phyto-oestrogen group. These results have been supported by meta-analyses of the data.[764,765] Reviews of 16 or 17 double-blind studies quantified the effect and found that in terms of the reported frequency and severity of hot flushes, isoflavones were 25–26% more effective than placebo, and they achieved 57% of the potency of oestrogen.[766,767]

One type of phyto-oestrogens — the soy-isoflavones — are found as a staple in the traditional Asian diet. Phyto-oestrogens such as isoflavones are believed to compete with oestrogen for the same receptors, thus exerting oestrogenic effects.[768] Soy foods can potentially reduce ischaemic heart disease in postmenopausal women, and soy protein directly lowers blood LDL cholesterol concentrations. Soy isoflavones improve endothelial function and can possibly slow the progression of

TABLE 18.45 Phyto-oestrogen sources

Lignans	Coumestrol	Phytosterols	Isoflavones
Linseeds	Soy sprouts	Olives	Soy beans
Rye	Alfalfa	Sunflower oil	Alfalfa
Millet	Red clover	Soy beans	Red clover
Sesame seeds	Green beans	Pumpkin kernels	Parsley
Sunflower seeds	Mung beans		Chick peas
Seaweeds	Red beans		Mung beans
Buckwheat	Split peas		Wholegrains
Wholegrains	Cow peas		
Fruits/veg	Olives		

NB: Lignans are formed from the action of bowel bacteria on most high-fibre foods, such as wholegrains.

subclinical atherosclerosis.[769] Isoflavones are found in legumes, lentils, beans such as kidney beans, lima beans, broad beans and chickpeas, but the richest source are soybeans which contain 2–4 mg of isoflavones per gram of protein (Table 18.45).[770] As noted by Vincent and Fitzpatrick[770] isoflavones found in supplement form lack the protein, lipids and other phytochemicals found in the whole soybean, thus it is logical to assume they may not work in the same manner when separated from synergistic constituents.

Soy constituents

Soybeans are noteworthy for their high protein content, approximately 38%. They also contain 18% fat, primarily polyunsaturated fats and only a small amount of saturated fats. Thirteen per cent of the soybean is made up of soluble carbohydrates (sucrose, stachyrose, raffinose and others), 15% insoluble carbohydrates (dietary fibre) and 14% moisture, ash and miscellaneous compounds.[342]

Flaxseed

Flaxseed is a rich source of dietary lignans and isoflavones. A number of studies have reviewed its efficacy for menopausal women with mixed results. One study assessed the daily consumption of two slices of bread containing 25 g of flaxseed (46 mg lignans) versus wheat bran (<1 mg lignans; control) every day for 12 consecutive weeks. Both groups experienced a reduction in the quantity of hot flushes, suggesting that flaxseed-enriched bread was no more effective than control for reducing hot flushes.[771] However, another small pilot study involving 30 women examined the effect of 40 g/day of crushed flaxseed over a 6-week period added to the daily diet.[772] On average, the mean decrease in hot flush scores after flaxseed therapy was 57%, while the mean reduction in daily hot flush frequency decreased from 7.3 to 3.6 following flaxseed therapy. A 2013 systematic review of the literature found little evidence to support the use of flax in alleviating vasomotor symptoms of menopause; however, it did find an association with a lower risk of breast cancer.[773]

From a naturopathic perspective, flaxseed is best consumed fresh from flaxseeds that are freshly crushed and stored appropriately. As a polyunsaturated fatty acid, flaxseed is highly unstable and oxidises easily when exposed to light or high temperatures. Flaxseed when provided in cooked foods such as bread or muffins may not provide substantial health-promoting properties. This is important to note, as most studies use bread sources as their chosen delivery source. Heating of flaxseed at high temperatures (as is the case when it is found in bread or a muffin) results in it becoming rancid, particularly when it then sits on the bakery shelf for a number of days.

Daily dietary flaxseed may also help to protect against cardiovascular disease, the risk of which is increased at onset of menopause. Studies have shown that a daily intake of flaxseed (30–40 g/day) improves lipid profiles in menopausal women.[774,775]

Calcium-rich foods

Bone mineral density decreases at menopause, thus patients' diets should be screened for adequate intake of calcium and other bone-building nutrients.

Dried plums (prunes)

Studies have shown that consumption of prunes improves bone mineral density in postmenopausal women. One study used 100 g/day in conjunction with 400 mg calcium and 400 IU vitamin D (in both the control and intervention groups),[776] while another study showed that 50 g of prunes per day (5–6 prunes) over 6 months was as effective as 100 g/day in preventing bone loss in older osteopenic postmenopausal women.[777]

DIETARY EXCLUSIONS

Caffeine

Given the effects of caffeine on the bones and the decreased bone mineral density that typically occurs at around the time of menopause, caffeine intake should be minimised. Acknowledging the deleterious effects of caffeine on the adrenal glands the argument to exclude it from the diet is further heightened.

Refined sugar

Sugary foods are usually devoid of nutrients and may promote the presence of *Candida*. In addition, since risk of diabetes and metabolic syndrome increases at onset of menopause, sugar should be avoided.

Spicy foods

Chilli and other spicy foods may cause heat in the body, aggravating symptoms of hot flushes.

NUTRITIONAL MEDICINE (SUPPLEMENTAL)

Nutritional medicine therapeutic objectives

- Support for secondary production of hormone production
- Nutrient prescriptions that offer prevention and protection from cancer (especially breast and

SAMPLE DAILY DIET

BREAKFAST	
Oats with prunes, sunflower seeds and flaxseed	Flaxseed consumption has been shown to reduce hot flush frequency and intensity, including night sweats. Daily consumption of prunes has been shown to improve bone mineral density in postmenopausal women.
LUNCH	
Seaweed with salmon sashimi, avocado, sesame seeds, millet and edamame Miso soup	Seaweed and sesame seeds are sources of lignans which are a phyto-oestrogen source. A diet rich in phyto-oestrogens may reduce signs and symptoms associated with peri-menopause. In addition, soy isoflavones improve endothelial function and possibly slow the progression of subclinical atherosclerosis. Wholegrain foods rich in lignans such as millet have been shown to help reduce cholesterol and increase urinary enterodiol excretion.
DINNER	
Tempeh burger with lettuce, grated carrot, sauerkraut and beetroot hummus	Dietary inclusion of whole soy foods containing approximately 60 mg/d of isoflavones has been shown to improve bone health. In particular it resulted in increasing serum osteocalcin, a marker of bone formation, in postmenopausal women as well as reducing bone turnover during early menopause, in part due to a reduction in urinary deoxypyridinoline, a marker of bone reabsorption.
SNACK	
Green smoothie with tahini	Green leafy vegetables and tahini are an excellent source of plant-based calcium, magnesium and vitamin K, all of which can be used to support bone health and reduce risk of osteoporosis which accelerates at peri-menopause.

Sources: Durazzo A, Carcea M, Adlercreutz H et al. Effects of consumption of whole grain foods rich in lignans in healthy postmenopausal women with moderate serum cholesterol: a pilot study. Int J Food Sci Nutr 2014; 65(5):637–645. Hooshmand S, Kern M, Metti D et al. The effect of two doses of dried plum on bone density and bone biomarkers in osteopenic postmenopausal women: a randomized, controlled trial. Osteoporos Int 2016; 27(7):2271–2279. Messina M. Soy foods, isoflavones, and the health of postmenopausal women. Am J Clin Nutr 2014; 100 Suppl 1:423S–4230S.

colorectal), Alzheimer's disease, cardiovascular disease, diabetes and other chronic health problems
- Specific nutrients to stabilise blood sugar levels, reduce lipidaemia, improve cognition and improve antioxidant status in the body
- Specific nutrients to support the skeletal system and bone nutrient status
- Nutrient prescriptions to support healthy weight balance and reduce central adiposity
- Antioxidants — oxidative stress plays an important role in the ageing process. The decline of antioxidant levels in the body combined with the loss of oestrogen is associated with many of the consequences of menopause, including heart disease, vasomotor disturbances and osteoporosis.[778] The following antioxidants have been found to be beneficial to women in the perimenopausal and postmenopausal phases: vitamin C, vitamin E, phytoestrogens, melatonin, *Curcuma longa* (turmeric), grape polyphenols and lycopene.

Specific nutrients required

B COMPLEX

Adequate intake of the B vitamins is particularly important during menopause due to the physiological stress placed on the body, as the transitional changes that occur at menopause are many. Decline in sex hormone production may influence changes in mood, libido, cognitive function as well as the occurrence and severity of menopausal symptoms such as hot flushes and disordered sleep.

The B vitamins are required for numerous functions within the body. Each has its own individual function as well as working synergistically with the other B vitamins. For example, vitamin B_1 is required for cardiovascular health and brain and nervous system function. It may also help to counteract fatigue, a common complaint in menopausal patients. Vitamins B_2 and B_5 are required for healthy adrenal gland function, critical during menopause.

Vitamin B_3 is important for cellular health, metabolism and energy production. Vitamin B_3 dilates blood vessels improving circulation to the heart, improving nutrition and oxygen while also lowering blood pressure. Plasma levels of homocysteine tend to be lower in women at reproductive age than in those who are postmenopausal suggesting that the increased risk of cardiovascular disease documented in postmenopausal women may be related to the increase in homocysteine levels. Vitamin B_6 in conjunction with vitamins B_9 and B_{12} work together to reduce elevated levels of homocysteine. Low intake of these vitamins increases homocysteine in the blood; high levels of homocysteine in the blood are associated with an increased risk of heart attack and stroke. Vitamin B_6 is involved in the balance of adequate glutathione/glutathione disulfide levels which is important in menopause and postmenopause. Vitamins B_1, B_2, B_3 and B_6 are required for generating neurotransmitters which may impact on the mood and cognitive function aspects of menopause.[779]

CALCIUM

Calcium requirements increase at menopause due to bone mineral density loss, which typically accelerates around the time of menopause. Many women are unable to obtain the recommended daily intake of calcium through diet alone and thus supplementation may be required. Supplementation with calcium (in combination with vitamin D) has been demonstrated to reduce bone loss in peri- and postmenopausal women while the placebo group actually lost total bone mineral density at a rate of about 0.4% per year.[780]

A recent study on the effects of 3 years of supplementation of vitamin D (400–1200 IU) and calcium 1–1.5 g) in 77 women with postmenopausal osteoporosis showed that the treatment was associated with favourably altered bone mineral and organic matrix properties.[781]

ESSENTIAL FATTY ACIDS

An essential fatty acid supplement containing 400 mg fish oil (30% EPA and 20% DHA), 100 mg oil of borage (20% GLA) and a mixture of vitamin E (13.5 IU), policosanols and lipoic acid (25 mg) taken twice daily has shown promise in reducing the incidence of hot flushes in menopausal women.[782] The mechanism by which this occurs is unclear but may involve the influence of omega-3 fatty acids on neuronal membranes and/or the modulation of the neurotransmitter function and the serotonergic system. Omega-3 fatty acids are also likely to help manage coexisting symptoms of cardiovascular disease that may typically present with menopause. Essential fatty acids might also be expected to play a role in modulating cognitive and mood symptoms in menopause; however, a recent study of 1616 women in the Multi-Ethnic Study of Atherosclerosis (MESA) cohort found that among women who were not on HRT, higher intakes of EPA and DHA were associated with increased risk of depressive symptoms. For women on HRT, no association was seen.[783] These results are contradictory to those found in a 2016 study,[784] which showed that in postmenopausal women on HRT, low erythrocyte levels of omega-3 were correlated with higher Depression Inventory scores, whereas no association was found in women who were not on HRT. Further research is required.

PROBIOTICS

The healthy vagina typically contains lactobacilli that help to protect against pathogens, but in response to hormonal changes occurring at menopause, including changes in the micro-anatomical features of the vaginal epithelium and in particular decreased oestrogen secretion, genitourinary atrophy may occur. The combination of the decline in oestrogen and atrophy leads to decreased glycogen levels and subsequent depletion of lactobacilli and a rise in vaginal pH, creating the perfect environment for enterobacteria to colonise the vagina. The result of this is an increased risk of vaginal infection.[785] A predominance of lactobacilli and low bacterial diversity is associated with a decrease in vaginal dryness in menopause. Women who are on HRT have been demonstrated to have levels of *Lactobacillus* species similar to premenopausal women.[785]

Randomised controlled studies assessing the efficacy of probiotic supplementation on menopausal women have produced favourable results. Petricevic et al[786] observed that oral application of lactobacilli (2.5×10^9 CFU each of *L. rhamnosus* GR-1 and *L. reuteri* RC-14) once daily for 2 weeks resulted in a substantial improvement in the vaginal flora of postmenopausal women. Interestingly, three individuals from the control group had progressed to bacterial vaginosis by the end of the study compared with none in the probiotics group, highlighting the efficacy of probiotics to raise vaginal flora quality and improve urogenital health. Data are promising regarding the treatment with probiotics for menopause symptoms, however a Cochrane review found that there is not significant evidence for or against the use of probiotics for bacterial vaginosis symptoms.[787]

VITAMIN A

In conjunction with other antioxidants, vitamin A protects cardiovascular function and improves immune function. As oestrogen depletes, vitamin A oversees the health of the mucous membranes throughout the body but is especially beneficial for vaginal integrity.

VITAMIN C

Oxidative stress occurs during menopause and is related to the loss of oestrogens that previously exerted a protective and antioxidant action on low-density lipoproteins.[14] Vitamin C has been shown to improve endothelial function in healthy postmenopausal oestrogen-deficient women[788] and may also improve bone mineral density in postmenopausal women through its ability to stimulate procollagen, enhance collagen synthesis and stimulate alkaline phosphatase activity, a marker for osteoblast formation.[789]

VITAMIN D

Vitamin D is highly indicated in menopause due to its role in maintaining skeletal health. At menopause women typically experience a rapid decline in the sex steroids, with low levels of oestrogen leading to increased bone resorption and subsequent bone loss, increasing the risk of fracture. Taking calcium has been shown to be useful in helping to maintain bone density, but the addition of vitamin D combined with calcium not only enhances calcium absorption and bone mineralisation[790] but also enhances muscle health, stimulates bone maturation, matrix formation, bone remodelling and osteoclast cell activity,[791] helping to prevent osteoporosis.

Prevention of fractures has been observed at serum levels above 75 nmol/L,[792] so why is it that vitamin D deficiency has suddenly become so prevalent in Australia? One factor can be linked to modernisation. In their review,

Borradale and Kimlin[791] note that wild-caught fish have four times the amount of vitamin D than farmed fish, but a vast percentage of the fish found in supermarkets is actually farmed rather than wild. Another influencing factor may be the large quantity of time many of us spend indoors rather then in the sun and the increase of sunscreen use. Because food contains relatively small quantities of vitamin D combined with the fact that despite a sunny climate in Australia, vitamin D deficiency is still prevalent, supplementation may be necessary, particularly for women entering the menopausal transition. In view of this it is imperative to properly screen patients prior to, during and post menopause.

VITAMIN E

Vitamin E is an antioxidant with an affinity for the female reproductive system. It has been shown to be efficacious for the treatment of hot flushes by reducing their frequency and severity after only 1 month of administration.[793] Vitamin E may also be useful for lubricating the vagina,[794] which can often become dry during menopause due to hormonal decline.

ZINC

Zinc plays a key role in the female reproductive system, but oestrogen deficiency/decline in the menopausal woman has been suggested to increase urinary loss of zinc from the body leading to zinc deficiency,[795] hence the benefits of supplementation. Zinc levels are also noted to be reduced in postmenopausal women with osteoporosis and osteopenia when compared with controls.[796]

DOSAGE REQUIREMENTS

The dosage requirements listed below are based on adult doses that have been reported in the literature and clinical review:

- B complex (all B vitamins) high-dose combination, preferably activated forms (Note: It is essential to warn patients of potential side effects from activated forms of B vitamins (especially activated B_3). When taken on an empty stomach, within 10 minutes the patient can experience marked redness, heating and flushing which can appear to feel like a hot flush. The inclusion of a full meal (preferably with high protein and essential fatty acids) prior to taking activated B vitamins can slow down absorption and thus prevent this flush response.)
  - Thiamine 20–40 mg/day
  - Riboflavin 20–40 micrograms/day
  - Niacinamide 50–100 mg/day
  - Pantothenic acid 150–300 mg/day
  - Pyridoxine 20–60 mg/day
  - Folate as folinic acid or L-5MTHF 500–1000 micrograms/day
  - Hydroxo or methylcobalamin 500–1000 micrograms/day
  - Choline 50–100 mg/day
  - Inositol 50–100 mg/day
  - Biotin 250–500 micrograms/day
- Calcium 1000–2000 mg/day (bone mineral density results dependent)
- Essential fatty acids: 500–1000 mg/day EPA, 350–700 mg/day DHA, 150–300 mg/day GLA
- Probiotics: minimum of 2.5×10^9 CFU each of *L. rhamnosus* GR-1 and *L. reuteri* RC-14[786] or preferably a multistrain probiotic of at least $25–50 \times 10^9$ CFU
- Vitamin A 15 000–20 000 IU/day
- Vitamin C 1000 mg/day, preferably in divided doses for optimal utilisation
- Vitamin D minimum 800 IU/day should be taken for bone health in menopause.[797] Dose should be calculated and based on pathology interpretation
- Vitamin E 400 IU/day[793]–800 IU/day in divided doses[761]
- Zinc 25–50 mg/day.

HERBAL MEDICINE

Herbal medicine therapeutic objectives

- Relief from symptoms that aggravate and indicate lowered hormone levels
- Prevention of cardiovascular disease
- Prevention of cancers
- Prevention of atrophic states including incontinence, pelvic laxity, sexual debility and dryness to mucous membranes
- Optimise digestive function to nutrient absorption
- Support bone building.

Herbal medicine classes

Herbal medicine classes used in menopause are listed in Table 18.46.

Specific herbal medicines

ACTAEA RACEMOSA (BLACK COHOSH)

Actaea racemosa is one of the most widely used botanicals for the relief of vasomotor symptoms associated with menopause and in Germany it is approved as a non-prescription medicine for treatment of hot flushes.[798] Its mode of action is undetermined, but it appears to be multifaceted, including decreasing luteinising hormone, thus reducing hot flushes[799] as well as the ability to act as a selective oestrogen receptor modifier depending on the tissue receptor.[800]

A systematic review conducted by Shams et al[798] assessed the effects of *Actaea racemosa* for treatment of vasomotor symptoms and identified nine trials of use, of which seven were able to be used in a meta-analysis. The trials included healthy perimenopausal women between the ages of 40 and 60 years and concluded that preparations containing *Actaea racemosa* improved overall climacteric symptoms by 26%. An additional finding relevant to herbalists was the fact that *Hypericum perforatum* appeared to complement the effects of *Actaea racemosa*, thus using together may be useful.[801]

Wuttke et al[802] conducted a study on the benefits of a *Actaea racemosa* preparation (CR BNO 1055) versus oestrogen or placebo therapy in 97 menopausal women and found *Actaea racemosa* to be as effective as conjugated oestrogens in reducing climacteric complaints, when compared with the placebo group. Of note is the fact

TABLE 18.46 Herbal medicine classes used in menopause

Symptomatic	
Adaptogen, adrenal restorative Nervine Sedative, hypnotic Antidepressant, anxiolytic Emollient, vulnerary Antihydrotic Bladder tonic Cognitive enhancer	To support patient through transition, HPA modulation, reduction in cortisol secretion To support stress recovery To assist in regulating circadian rhythm To support mood and address anxiety or depression Address mucous membrane dryness Alleviate hot flushes and associated perspiration Improve bladder tonicity To improve cognition
Endocrine	
Phyto-oestrogen Hypoglycaemia Hormonal modulator	To regulate and support hormonal cascades Weight stabilisation, prevention of diabetes Regulation of hormonal cascades
Cardiovascular	
Hypolipidaemic Hepatic, cholagogue Hypotensive Antidysrhythmic Cardiac tonic	To improve lipid profile and increase steroid hormone synthesis for secondary production To regulate and support cardiac function
Skeletal	
Nutritive Phyto-oestrogen	To improve bone mineral density
Immune	
Antioxidant Hepatic, cholagogue	Reduce oxidation and prevent pro-oxidant pathways Assist with clearance of oestrogen metabolites
Gastrointestinal	
Bulk laxatives Bitters	Regulate bowel transit time, encourage clearance of cholesterol fragments Improve nutrient absorption and protein assimilation

that *Actaea racemosa* significantly increased superficial vaginal cells, reducing atrophy. The oestrogenic effects of *Actaea racemosa* in the vagina are important as they both promote lubrication and stimulate acidity of the vaginal milieu, reducing the risk of vaginal infections as a lower pH prevents ascending infections. A recent small RCT ($n = 54$) found that the use of black cohosh extract (40 mg/day) was not superior to placebo for relieving moderate to severe menopausal symptoms in Thai women.[803] These results are in contradiction to an earlier RCT of 84 postmenopausal women in Iran, which found that treatment with 6.5 mg daily of dried black cohosh root extract over 8 weeks resulted in a reduction of vasomotor, psychiatric, physical and sexual symptoms.[804] A 2012 Cochrane review on the safety and efficacy of black cohosh for the treatment of menopausal symptoms found that there was insufficient evidence to support its use;[805] however, a re-analysis of the Cochrane review by Beer et al[806] suggested that there is a standardised mean difference of 0.385 (p <0.0001) in favour of black cohosh for the management of menopausal symptoms. Further rigorous studies are warranted.

Given the decreased bone mineral density that typically occurs around this time it is interesting to note that *Actaea racemosa* exerts beneficial effects with regard to bone metabolism by stimulating osteoblast activity, and is thus likely to be useful in the prevention of osteoporosis.[807]

Actaea racemosa has been implicated in a few, but serious, cases of hepatotoxicity, but a recent study undertaken on women given *Actaea racemosa* over a 12-month period observed no significant changes with regards to total hepatic perfusion and liver functions, suggesting that intake of *Actaea racemosa* for 1 year by healthy postmenopausal women with no evidence of liver disease does not seem to affect the liver.[808]

DIOSCOREA VILLOSA (WILD YAM)

Dioscorea villosa is commonly found in many menopause preparations where it may be used to help relieve symptoms such as hot flushes and headaches associated with menopause.[809] It contains various steroidal saponins, including diosgenin, that have been claimed to influence endogenous steroidogenesis,[810] but as yet this is purely hypothetical as there have been no well-designed studies on the efficacy of internal preparations of *Dioscorea villosa* in the management of menopausal symptoms. Nevertheless, beneficial results are often observed in clinical practice.

HUMULUS LUPULUS (HOPS)

Humulus lupulus is native to Eurasia but has also been introduced to other temperate regions including Australia.[811] In-vitro studies reveal *Humulus lupulus* to contain a substance known as 8PN which has been described as one of the most powerful plant-derived oestrogenic substances known; 8PN has been shown to mimic the action of 17β-oestradiol (though at a lesser degree), so it is logical to think that *Humulus lupulus* may be used efficaciously to manage symptoms related to postmenopausal oestrogen deficiency.[811] A prospective, randomised, double-blind, placebo-controlled study conducted over 12 weeks with 67 menopausal women (aged between 45 and 60 years) administered a hop extract standardised on 8PN observed a favourable effect on vasomotor symptoms (such as hot flushes) and other menopausal discomforts.[812] A 2010 pilot study however did not find a significant advantage of 8PN over placebo in the first 16 weeks of treatment, but after this time frame the difference became significant (as a result of the decreasing effect of placebo).[813] In addition, *Humulus lupulus* may also be beneficial for its sedative properties for menopausal women experiencing sleep disorders, a common cause of complaint in menopause.

LEONURUS CARDIACA (MOTHERWORT)

The German Commission E advocates the use of *Leonurus cardiaca* for palpitations, anxiety or other nervous disorders, while the Eclectics suggested its use for nervousness from irregular menstruation as well as disturbed sleep.[7] For these reasons it is a useful botanical to give during the time of menopause for women who experience symptoms such as these. Furthermore, acknowledging the increasing cardiovascular risk for many women as they progress towards menopause, the administration of *Leonurus cardiaca* may be additionally useful due to its simple heart tonic effects.[7]

PANAX GINSENG (KOREAN GINSENG)

Panax ginseng has been suggested to have oestrogenic and adaptogenic properties[814] and thus may be of use in menopause. A double-blind placebo-controlled trial revealed the ability of *Panax ginseng* to improve quality of life (depression, wellbeing, health) in symptomatic, postmenopausal women over a 4-month period, but there was only a slight improvement for symptomatic relief (e.g. hot flushes), suggesting that *Panax ginseng*, despite its proposed hormonal effects, may not use these when it exerts its effects in menopause.[50] Similar results with regard to this non-hormone-modulated mechanism of action of *Panax ginseng* were seen in another study in which *Panax ginseng* was administered to women with climacteric symptoms over a 1-month period. The herb was found to improve a number of symptoms related to the menopause, in particular fatigue, insomnia and depression. The mechanism of action in this case appeared to be brought about in part by the effect of *Panax ginseng* on stress-related hormones, as evidenced by its ability to instigate a decrease in cortisol/DHEA-S ratio.[814]

A 2016 systematic review of the trials found positive evidence for the use of *Panax ginseng* in sexual function and arousal, and in hot flush scores in menopausal women. Specific results on hot flush frequency, hormone levels or endometrial thickness were inconclusive due to risk of bias in the trials.[815]

PIPER METHYSTICUM (KAVA KAVA)

Anxiety is a common complaint in menopause[816] and is likely to impact substantially on quality of life. *Piper methysticum* is a botanical from the Pacific islands that has anxiolytic and sedative actions thought to be in part due to its active constituents, the kavalactones.[817] *Piper methysticum* may be useful to help relieve neuro-vegetative complaints associated with menopause, such as anxiety and sleeplessness. Researchers studying the combined use of hormone replacement therapy and *Piper methysticum* extract have found it to be effective against menopausal anxiety, with *Piper methysticum* appearing to accelerate resolution of psychological symptoms.[816]

SALVIA OFFICINALIS (SAGE)

Herbal teas (at least 1 L) or tablets containing *Salvia officinalis* have been reported to be useful in hyperhidrosis[818] and may also be useful for menopause where night sweats and hot flushes typically exist. Despite its popularity for hot flushes and the like there has been relatively little in the way of clinical studies. One study used a combination of *Salvia officinalis* and *Medicago sativa* (alfalfa — an energetically cooling herb) for the treatment of hot flushes in 30 menopausal women and found that hot flushes and night sweating completely disappeared in 20 women: four women showed good improvement and the other six showed a reduction in symptoms, suggesting these two herbs may be effective for treating menopausal symptoms.[56]

An 8-week clinical trial of menopausal women conducted in eight practices in Switzerland showed that daily treatment with a tablet of fresh sage leaves (equivalent 3400 mg tincture of fresh sage leaves) resulted in a significant decrease in the incidence of hot flushes. The incidence decreased by 50% after 4 weeks, and by 64% within 8 weeks. The mean number of mild, moderate, severe, and very severe flushes decreased by 46%, 62%, 79%, and 100% over 8 weeks, respectively.[819]

ASPARAGUS RACEMOSUS (SHATAVARI)

Asparagus racemosus is an Ayurvedic herb that contains steroidal saponins and sapogenin,[820] which may be useful in menopause. Shatavari is believed to control all three *doshas* (the constitutions that make up the body) while rejuvenating the blood and female reproductive organs as well as increasing sexual secretions. Shatavari is especially useful for conditions characterised by excess *pitta* (excess heat) and may help menopausal complaints such as hot flushes.[821]

TRIFOLIUM PRATENSE (RED CLOVER)

Trifolium pratense is one of the most widely researched botanicals for menopausal health. It contains isoflavones thought to act as agonist/antagonists on oestrogenic receptors.[768] These include genistein, biochanin A, daidzein and formononetin. A meta-analysis observed a reduction in hot flush frequency in individuals given *Trifolium pratense* compared with placebo, suggesting that isoflavones in red clover may be useful for treating hot flushes in menopausal women.[822] *Trifolium pratense* also appears to be of benefit for the vaginal atrophy and atrophic vaginitis that may present with menopause, negatively affecting a woman's sexual life. In a prospective, randomised double-blind trial postmenopausal women supplementing with an extract of *Trifolium pratense* (80 mg isoflavones) for 90 days reported improved vaginal and sexual wellbeing, with women reporting a decrease in vaginal dryness, dyspareunia as well as an improved libido.[823] This was further evidenced by vaginal sampling, which displayed a significant improvement of the karyopyknotic, cornification and basal cell maturation index. A recent meta-analysis of standardised extract of *Trifolium pretense* (Promensil) at 80 mg dosage found a statistical and clinically significant benefit in the treatment of hot flushes in menopause.[824]

VITEX AGNUS-CASTUS (CHASTE TREE BERRY)

Vitex agnus-castus has a long history of use for female reproductive disorders but has only been used since the

20th century for menopausal complaints. In 1930 Gerhaud Madhaus included *Vitex agnus-castus* in his manual for menopausal complaints[825] and this was further emphasised by a 1972 report suggesting that *Vitex agnus-castus* was efficacious for menopausal bleeding and complaints.[88] *Vitex agnus-castus* exerts dopaminergic activity and has an affinity for opioid receptors, which may in part influence its effects in menopause.[88] In spite of these examples, clinical studies have not demonstrated a link between intake of *Vitex agnus-castus* and reduced vasomotor symptoms of menopause such as hot flushes,[826] although PMS symptoms such as anxiety and hydration in late perimenopausal women appear to be relieved in women taking *Vitex agnus-castus*.[88] The use of *Vitex agnus-castus* in menopause warrants further study, as does the use of *Vitex agnus-castus* essential oils (using the berry or the leaf) as some positive results have been observed in menopausal women administering them in a variety of methods.[825,827]

LEPIDIUM MEYENII (MACA)

Maca is a South American plant of the Brassica family and has been used traditionally as an adaptogenic plant to manage anaemia, infertility and female hormone balance. A systematic review of its use in the treatment of menopausal symptoms found limited evidence of its effectiveness due to the small number of trials, small sample sizes and average methodological quality of the studies.[828] A 12-week trial of 29 menopausal women in Hong Kong showed that 3.3 g of maca per day reduced symptoms of depression and lowered diastolic blood pressure as compared to placebo.[829]

LIFESTYLE RECOMMENDATIONS

Weight stabilisation

As a woman approaches her menopausal transition the body often lays down extra adipose tissue in the abdominal region regardless of dietary or lifestyle modifications. This is often seen as a protective mechanism for future hormone release or as an indication of deteriorated systems. For optimal prevention of disease complications it is beneficial to regulate weight gain and support patients to reach and sustain their ideal body weight.

Exercise

Exercise is a crucial component for successful treatment. It has been shown to:

- Decrease bone loss and improve bone mineralisation
- Decrease lipid levels
- Improve cardiovascular function
- Improve circulation
- Improve oxygen and nutrient utilisation in all tissues
- Improve stress-handling ability
- Increase endurance and energy levels
- Increase self-esteem, mood, and frame of mind
- Reduce blood pressure
- Provide relief from hot flushes
- Improve antioxidant status.

Acupuncture

A systematic review and meta-analysis of the data found that acupuncture treatment is associated with a significant reduction in sleep disturbances in peri and postmenopausal women.[830]

CASE STUDY

OVERVIEW

AC was a 54-year-old woman who had experienced her last menstrual period 13 months prior and had recently been confirmed as progressing through menopause. Her FSH was 72 U/L at her last blood test. Vitamin D had reduced to 49 nmol/L with total cholesterol reading of 5.9 nmol and LDL 4.0 nmol/L.

She was concerned about recent diagnosis of osteopenia and had come to seek support for health, long-term health and wellbeing. She had experienced anxiety (normal thyroid function) and mild urinary incontinence since her oestrogen had reduced.

TREATMENT PROTOCOL

HERBAL MEDICINE

Herbal medicine	Ratio	Quantity	Justification
Cynara scolymus	1:2	70 mL	Hypolipidaemic, hepatic, support secondary production of hormones
Crataeva nurvala	1:2	80 mL	Bladder tonic
Actaea racemosa	1:2	30 mL	Hormonal support — selective oestrogen receptor modifier
Hypericum perforatum	STD ext	30 mL	Thymoleptic, anxiolytic

TOTAL: 220 mL. Dose: 7.5 mL b.i.d.

NUTRITIONAL MEDICINE

Dietary

- Support the skeletal system and encourage dietary sources of calcium and other bone nutrients. Lengthy discussion about calcium absorption, forms and food strategies
- Encourage optimal digestive processes with fibre-rich foods
- Encourage phyto-oestrogen food sources — fermented sources, sprouts, flaxseeds especially
- Adopt general wholefood dietary principles such as high in fruit, vegetables, wholegrains, vegetarian protein, nuts, seeds, legumes
- Avoid saturated, trans and hydrogenated fats; simple and refined carbohydrates, sugar and processed foods.

CASE STUDY CONTINUED

Supplemental

Nutrient	Dosage	Justification
B complex	1 cap/day	Hormonal support, neurotransmitter production, cardiovascular protection (homocysteine)
Calcium	1200 mg/day in divided doses	Address deficiency and treat osteopenia
Vitamin E	500 IU b.i.d.	Mucous membrane integrity, hormonal regulation, oestrogen regulation, antioxidant
Concentrated fish oil supplementation	1 cap b.i.d. total: EPA 650 mg, DHA 450 mg, other omega-3s 180 mg	Hormonal regulation, anti-inflammatory, regulation of prostaglandin synthesis
Vitamin D_3	5000 IU/day	To address deficiency and use positive mood and immune effects
Zinc	50 mg/day	Prevent progression to osteoporosis, reproductive hormone regulation

LIFESTYLE/EDUCATION

- Daily exercise — focusing on weight-bearing exercises
- Avoidance of exogenous oestrogen sources
- Menopausal symptom diary was used to assess progress comprehensively
- Vitamin D absorption discussion, sunlight education.

REFERENCES

[1] Gomel V. The uterus and fertility. Fertil Steril 2008;89(1):1–16; Aristotle as cited in Taylor E.
[2] Taylor E, Gomel V. The uterus and fertility. Fertil Steril 2008;89(1):1–16.
[3] Tortora JG, Grabowski SR. Principles of anatomy and physiology. 9th ed. New York: John Wiley; 2000.
[4] Benagiano G, Brosens I, Carrara S. Adenomyosis: new knowledge is generating new treatment strategies. Womens Health (Lond) 2009;5(3):297–311.
[5] Auersperg N, Wong AS, Choi KC, et al. Ovarian surface epithelium: biology, endocrinology, and pathology. Endocr Rev 2001;22(2):255–88.
[6] Nishida T, Nishida N. Reinstatement of 'germinal epithelium' of the ovary. Reprod Biol Endocrinol 2006;4:42.
[7] Ellingwood F. The American materia medica, therapeutics and pharmacognosy. Portland, OR: Eclectic Medical Publications; 1919.
[8] Felter HW, Lloyd JR. King's American dispensatory. Portland, OR: Eclectic Materia Medica Publications; 1898.
[9] Felter HW. The Eclectic materia medica, pharmacology and therapeutics. Portland, OR: Eclectic Materia Medica Publications; 1922.
[10] Maffini MV, Rubin BS, Sonnenschein C, et al. Endocrine disruptors and reproductive health: the case of bisphenol-A. Mol Cell Endocrinol 2006;254–255:179–86.
[11] Rier S, Foster WG. Environmental dioxins and endometriosis. Semin Reprod Med 2003;21(2):145–54.
[12] Pandey S, Bhattacharya S. Impact of obesity on gynecology. Womens Health (Lond) 2010;6(1):107–17.
[13] Ngô C, Chéreau C, Nicco C, et al. Reactive oxygen species controls endometriosis progressiion. Am J Pathol 2009;175(1):225–34.
[14] Agarwal A, Gupta S, Sharma RK. Role of oxidative stress in female reproduction. Reprod Biol Endocrinol 2005;14(3):28.
[15] Agarwal A, Allamaneni SS. Role of free radicals in female reproductive diseases and assisted reproduction. Reprod Biomed Online 2004;9(3):338–47.
[16] Rier SE. Environmental immune disruption: a comorbidity factor for reproduction? Fertil Steril 2008;89(Suppl. 2):e103–8.
[17] Prapas N, Karkanaki A, Prapas I, et al. Genetics of polycystic ovary syndrome. Hippokratia 2009;13(4):216–23.
[18] Biggs WS, Williams RM. Common gynecologic infections. Prim Care 2009;36(1):33–51, viii.
[19] Zhang XJ, Shen Q, Wang GY, et al. Risk factors for reproductive tract infections among married women in rural areas of Anhui Province, China. Eur J Obstet Gynecol Reprod Biol 2009;147(2):187–91.
[20] Sawatsri S, Desai N, Rock JA, et al. Retinoic acid suppresses interleukin-6 production in human endometrial cells. Fertil Steril 2000;73(5):1012–19.
[21] Mier-Cabrera J, Aburto-Soto T, Burrola-Méndez S, et al. Women with endometriosis improved their peripheral antioxidant markers after the application of a high antioxidant diet. Reprod Biol Endocrinol 2009;28(7):54.
[22] Lithgow DM, Politzer WM. Vitamin A in the treatment of menorrhagia. S Afr Med J 1977;51(7):191–3.
[23] Brabin L, Brabin BJ. The cost of successful adolescent growth and development in girls in relation to iron and vitamin A status. Am J Clin Nutr 1992;55(5):955–8.
[24] Bucci M, Murphy CR. Hormonal control of enzyme activity during the plasma membrane transformation of uterine epithelial cells. Cell Biol Int 2001;25(9):859–71.
[25] Osiecki H. The nutrient bible. 6th ed. Eagle Farm, QLD: Bioconcepts Publishing; 2004.
[26] Vitamins and the pill. Can Med Assoc J 1974;111(3):211. [No authors listed] Editorial.
[27] Abraham GE, Lubran MM. Serum and red cell magnesium levels in patients with premenstrual tension. Am J Clin Nutr 1981;34:2364.
[28] Trickey R. Women, Hormones and the menstrual cycle. 2nd ed. Crows Nest, Aust: Allen & Unwin; 2003.
[29] Dennehy CE. The use of herbs and dietary supplements in gynecology: an evidence-based review. J Midwifery Womens Health 2006;51(6):402–9.
[30] Akhmeteli KT, Eradze TsSh, Tushurashvili PR, et al. Vitamins C, B_{12} and folic acid in latent iron deficiency. Georgian Med News 2005;128:109–11.
[31] Harel Z, Biro F, Kollar L, et al. Supplementation with vitamin C and/or vitamin $B_{(6)}$ in the prevention of Depo-Provera side effects in adolescents. J Pediatr Adolesc Gynecol 2002;15(3):153–8.
[32] Mukherjee GG, Gajaraj AJ, Mathias J, et al. Treatment of abnormal uterine bleeding with micronized flavonoids. Int J Gynaecol Obstet 2005;89(2):156–7.
[33] Peacocke M, Djurkinak E, Thys-Jacobs S. Treatment of desquamative inflammatory vaginitis with vitamin D: a case report. Cutis 2008;81(1):75–8.
[34] Hahn S, Haselhorst U, Tan S, et al. Low serum 25- hydroxyvitamin D concentrations are associated with insulin resistance and obesity in women with polycystic ovary syndrome. Exp Clin Endocrinol Diabetes 2006;114:577–83.
[35] Seibal MM. The role of nutrition and nutritional supplements in women's health. Fertil Steril 1999;72(4):579–91.
[36] Ziaei S, Zakeri M, Kazemnejad A. A randomized controlled trial of vitamin E in the treatment of primary dysmenorrheal. BJOG 2005;112:466–9.

[37] Fachinetti F, Borella P, Sances G, et al. Oral magnesium successfully relieves premenstrual mood changes. Obstet Gynecol 1991;78:177.
[38] Walker AF, De Souza MC, Vickers MF, et al. Magnesium supplementation alleviates premenstrual symptoms of water-retention. J Womens Health 1998;7:1157.
[39] De Souza MC, Walker AF, Robinson PA, et al. A synergistic effect of a daily supplement for 1 month of 200 mg magnesium plus 50 mg vitamin B_6 for the relief of anxiety-related premenstrual symptoms: a randomized, double-blind, crossover study. J Womens Health Gend Based Med 2000;9(2):131–9.
[39A] Fathizadeh N, Ebrahimi E, Valiani M, et al. Evaluating the effect of magnesium and magnesium plus vitamin B6 supplement on the severity of premenstrual syndrome. Iran J Nurs Midwifery Res 2010;15(Suppl. 1):401–5.
[39B] Chocano Bedoya PO, Manson JE, Hankinson SE, et al. Intake of selected minerals and risk of premenstrual syndrome. Am J Epidemiol 2013;177(10):1118–27.
[40] Massafra C, Felice CD, Gioia D, et al. Variations in erythrocyte antioxidant glutathione peroxidase activity during the menstrual cycle. Clin Endocrinol (Oxf) 1998;49:63–7.
[41] Ha EJ, Smith AM. Plasma selenium and plasma and erythrocyte glutathione peroxidase activity increase with estrogen during the menstrual cycle. J Am Coll Nutr 2003;22:43–51.
[42] Gorjão R, Azevedo-Martins AK, Rodrigues HG, et al. Comparative effects of DHA and EPA on cell function. Pharmacol Ther 2009;122(1):56–64.
[43] Harel Z, Biro FM, Kottenhahn RK, et al. Supplementation with omega-3 polyunsaturated fatty acids in the management of dysmenorrhoea in adolescents. Am J Obstet Gynecol 1996;174(4):1335–8.
[44] Fulghesu AM, Ciampelli M, Muzj G, et al. N-acetyl-cysteine treatment improves insulin sensitivity in women with polycystic ovary syndrome. Fertil Steril 2002;77:1128–35.
[45] Sanders KM, Kotowicz MA, Nicholson GC. Potential role of the antioxidant N-acetylcysteine in slowing bone resorption in early post-menopausal women: a pilot study. Transl Res 2007;150(4):215.
[46] Reed GA, Peterson KS, Smith HJ, et al. A phase I study of indole-3-carbinol in women: tolerability and effects. Cancer Epidemiol Biomarkers Prev 2005;14(8):1953–60.
[47] Abad CL, Safdar N. The role of lactobacillus probiotics in the treatment or prevention of urogenital infections — a systematic review. J Chemother 2009;21(3):243–52.
[48] Reid G, Beuerman D, Heinemann C, et al. Probiotic *Lactobacillus* dose required to restore and maintain a normal vaginal flora. FEMS Immunol Med Microbiol 2001;32:37–41.
[49] Falagas ME, Betsi GI, Athanasiou S. Probiotics for the treatment of women with bacterial vaginosis. Clin Microbiol Infect 2007;13(7):657–64.
[50] Wiklund IK, Mattsson LA, Lindgren R, et al. Effects of a standardized ginseng extract on quality of life and physiological parameters in symptomatic postmenopausal women: a double-blind, placebo-controlled trial. Swedish Alternative Medicine Group. Int J Clin Pharmacol Res 1999;19(3):89–99.
[51] Zhu XZ. Development of natural products as drugs acting on central nervous system. Mem Inst Oswaldo Cruz 1991;86(Suppl. 2):173–5.
[52] Armanini D, Castello R, Scaroni C, et al. Treatment of polycystic ovary syndrome with spironolactone plus liquorice. Eur J Obstet Gynecol Reprod Biol 2007;131(1):61–7.
[53] Naser B, Bodinet C, Tegtmeier M, et al. *Thuja occidentalis* (*Arbor vitae*): a review of its pharmaceutical, pharmacological and clinical properties. Evid Based Complement Alternat Med 2005;2(1):69–78.
[54] van Die MD, Bone KM, Burger HG, et al. Effects of a combination of *Hypericum perforatum* and *Vitex agnus-castus* on PMS-like symptoms in late-perimenopausal women: findings from a subpopulation analysis. J Altern Complement Med 2009;15(9):1045–8.
[55] Grube B, Walper A, Wheatley D. St John's wort extract: efficacy for menopausal symptoms of psychological origin. Adv Ther 1999;16(4):177–86.
[56] De Leo V, Lanzetta D, Cazzavacca R, et al. Treatment of neurovegetative menopausal symptoms with a phytotherapeutic agent (abstract only). Minerva Ginecol 1998;50(5):207–11.
[57] Wuttke W, Jarry H, Christoffel V, et al. Seidlová-Wutt Chaste tree (*Vitex agnus-castus*) — pharmacology and clinical indications. Phytomedicine 2003;10(4):348–57.
[58] Blumenthal M, Goldberg A, Brinckmann J, editors. Herbal medicine. Expanded Commission E Monographs. Integrative Medicine, Communications. Newton, MA: Integrative Medicine Communications; 2000.
[59] Mannix LK. Menstrual-related pain conditions: dysmenorrhea and migraine. J Womens Health (Larchmt) 2008;17(5):879–91.
[60] Wu MH, Shoji Y, Chuang PC, et al. Endometriosis: disease pathophysiology and the role of prostaglandins. Expert Rev Mol Med 2007;9(2):1–20.
[61] Collier HO, Butt NM, McDonald-Gibson WJ, et al. Extract of feverfew inhibits prostaglandin biosynthesis. Lancet 1980;2(8200):922–3.
[62] Cook W. The physiomedical dispensatory. Portland, OR: Eclectic Materia Medica; 1869.
[63] Lau AJ, Toh DF, Chua TK, et al. Antiplatelet and anticoagulant effects of *Panax notoginseng:* comparison of raw and steamed *Panax notoginseng* with *Panax ginseng* and *Panax quinquefolium.* J Ethnopharmacol 2009;125(3):380–6.
[64] The State Pharmacopoeia Commission of People's Republic of China. Pharmacopoeia of the People's Republic of China, vol. 1. Beijing: Chemical Industry Press; 2000.
[65] Panico A, Lupoli GA, Fonderico F, et al. Multiple ovarian cysts in a young girl with severe hypothyroidism. Thyroid 2007;17(12):1289–93.
[66] Kubota K, Itho M, Kishi H, et al. Primary hypothyroidism presenting as multiple ovarian cysts in an adult woman: a case report. Gynecol Endocrinol 2008;24(10):586–9.
[67] Xu F, Stouffer RL. Existence of the lymphatic system in the primate corpus luteum. Lymphat Res Biol 2009;7(3):159–68.
[68] Kilicdag EB, Tarim E, Bagis T, et al. Fructus agni casti and bromo-criptine for treatment of hyperprolactinemia and mastalgia. Int J Gynaecol Obstet 2004;85:292–3.
[69] MacKay D, Miller AL. Nutritional support for wound healing. Altern Med Rev 2003;8(4):359–77.
[70] Dewailly D, Hieronimus S, Mirakian P, et al. Polycystic ovary syndrome (PCOS). Ann Endocrinol (Paris) 2010;71:8–13.
[71] Wechsler T. Taking charge of your fertility. Rev ed. USA: Quill; 2002.
[72] Read C, May T, Stellingwerff M. Irregular vaginal bleeding. In: how to treat yearbook. Australian Doctor; 2007.
[73] Fraser I, Bonnar J, Peyvandi F. Requirements for research investigations to clarify the relationships and management of menstrual abnormalities in women with hemostatic disorder. Fertil Steril 2005;84:1360–5.
[74] Ebert R, Nold B. Gerinnungsphysiologische studien am mestrualblut. Schweiz Med Wochenschr 1956;36:999.
[75] Fraser IS, McCarron G, Markham R, et al. Blood and total fluid content of of menstrual discharge. Obstet Gynecol 1985;65(2):194–8.
[76] Dickerson L, Mazyck P, Hunter M. Premenstrual syndrome. Am Fam Physician 2003;67:1743–52.
[77] Vigod SN, Ross LE, Steiner M. Understanding and treating premenstrual dysphoric disorder: an update for the women's health practitioner. Obstet Gynecol Clin North Am 2009;36(4):907–24, xii.
[78] Direkvand-Moghadam A, Sayehmiri K, Delpisheh A, et al. Epidemiology of premenstrual syndrome (PMS) — a systematic review and meta-analysis study. J Clin Diagn Res 2014;8(2):106–9.
[79] Campbell EM, Peterkin D, O'Grady K. Sanson-Fisher premenstrual symptoms in general practice patients. Prevalence and treatment. J Reprod Med 1997;42(10):637–46.
[80] Fisher C, Adams J, Hickman L, et al. The use of complementary and alternative medicine by 7427 Australian women with cyclic perimenstrual pain and discomfort: a cross-sectional study. BMC Complement Altern Med 2016;16(1):1.
[81] Ju H, Jones M, Mishra GD. Premenstrual syndrome and dysmenorrhea: symptom trajectories over 13 years in young adults. Maturitas 2014;78(2):99–105.
[82] Mayo JL. Premenstrual syndrome: a natural approach to management. Applied Nutritional Science Reports 1999;5(6).
[83] Girman A, Lee R, Kliger B. An integrative medicine approach to premenstrual syndrome. Am J Obstet Gynecol 2003;188(Suppl.): S56–65.

[84] eTG complete, Therapeutic guidelines Ltd; Nov 2009.
[85] ACOG Practice Bulletin. Clinical management guidelines for obstetrician-gynecologists. Number 15, April 2000. Premenstrual syndrome. Obstet Gynecol 2000;95:1–9.
[86] Kessel B. Premenstrual syndrome. Advances in diagnosis and treatment. Obstet Gynecol Clin North Am 2000;27:625–39.
[87] American Psychiatric Association. Diagnostic and statistical manual of mental disorders. 5th ed. Washington, DC: American Psychiatric Association; 2013. p. 717–18.
[88] van Die MD, Burger HG, Teede HJ, et al. *Vitex agnus-castus* (chaste-tree/berry) in the treatment of menopause-related complaints. J Altern Complement Med 2009;15(8):853–62.
[89] Romm A. Botanical medicine for women's health. Churchill Livingstone; 2010.
[90] Farasati N, Siassi F, Koohdani F, et al. Western dietary pattern is related to premenstrual syndrome: a case–control study. Br J Nutr 2015;114(12):2016–21.
[91] Bond AJ, Wingrove J, Critchlow DG. Tryptophan depletion increases aggression in women during the premenstrual phase. Psychopharmacology (Berl) 2001;156(4):477–80.
[92] Rossignol AM. Caffeine-containing beverages and premenstrual syndrome in young women. Am J Public Health 1985;75(11):1335–7.
[93] Rossignol AM, Bonnlander H. Caffeine-containing beverages, total fluid consumption, and premenstrual syndrome. Am J Public Health 1990;80(9):1106–10.
[94] Rossignol AM, Bonnlander H, Song L, et al. Do women with premenstrual symptoms self-medicate with caffeine? Epidemiology 1991;2(6):403–8.
[95] Rossignol AM, Bonnlander H. Caffeine-containing beverages, total fluid consumption, and premenstrual syndrome. Am J Public Health 1990;80(9):1106–10.
[96] Purdue-Smithe AC, Manson JE, Hankinson SE, et al. A prospective study of caffeine and coffee intake and premenstrual syndrome. Am J Clin Nutr 2016;104(2):499–507.
[97] Puder JJ, Blum CA, Mueller B, et al. Menstrual cycle symptoms are associated with changes in low-grade inflammation. Eur J Clin Invest 2006;36(1):58–64.
[98] Nagata C, Hirokawa K, Shimizu N, et al. Soy, fat and other dietary factors in relation to premenstrual symptoms in Japanese women. BJOG 2004;111(6):594–9.
[99] Cohen IT, Collins A, Eneroth P, et al. Food cravings, mood, and the menstrual cycle. Horm Behav 1987;21(4):457–70.
[100] Rodin J, Mancuso J, Granger J, et al. Food cravings in relation to body mass index, restraint and estradiol levels: a repeated measures study in healthy women. Appetite 1991;17:177–85.
[101] Rossignol AM, Bonnlander H. Prevalence and severity of the premenstrual syndrome. Effects of foods and beverages that are sweet or high in sugar content. (Abstract only). J Reprod Med 1991;36(2):131–6.
[102] Ataollahi M, Akbari AA, Mojab F, et al. The effect of wheat germ extract on premenstrual syndrome symptoms. Iran J Pharm Res 2015;14(1):159–66.
[103] Atallahi M, Akbari SA, Mojab F, et al. Effects of wheat germ extract on the severity and systemic symptoms of primary dysmenorrhea: a randomized controlled clinical trial. Iran Red Crescent Med J 2014;16(8):e19503.
[104] Tyrer LB. Nutrition and the pill (Abstract only). J Reprod Med 1984;29(Suppl. 7):547–50.
[105] Chasan-Taber L, Chocano-Bedoya PO, Manson JE, et al. Dietary B vitamin intake and incident premenstrual syndrome. Am J Clin Nutr 2011;93(5).
[106] Proctor ML, Farquhar CM. Dysmenorrhoea. Clin Evid 2007;2007:pii: 0813.
[107] Abdollahifard S, Koshkaki AR, Moazamiyanfar R. The effects of vitamin B_1 on ameliorating the premenstrual syndrome symptoms. Glob J Health Sci 2014;6(6):144.
[108] Reavley N. The new encyclopedia of vitamins minerals & supplements. Bookman Press; 1998.
[109] Horrobin DF. The role of essential fatty acids and prostaglandins in the premenstrual syndrome (Abstract only). J Reprod Med 1983;28(7):465–8.
[110] Proctor ML, Murphy PA. Herbal dietary therapies for primary and secondary dysmenorrhoea (Cochrane Review). The Cochrane Library, Issue 2. Oxford: Update Software; 2002.
[111] Masoumi SZ, Ataollahi M, Oshvandi K. Effect of combined use of calcium and vitamin B_6 on premenstrual syndrome symptoms: a randomized clinical trial. J Caring Sci 2016;5(1):67.
[112] Thys-Jacobs S, McMahon D, Bilezikian JP. Cyclical changes in calcium metabolism across the menstrual cycle in women with premenstrual dysphoric disorder. J Clin Endocrinol Metab 2007;92(8):2952–9.
[113] Thys-Jacobs S, Ceccarelli S, Bierman A, et al. Calcium supplementation in premenstrual syndrome. J Gen Intern Med 1989;4:181–3.
[114] Shamberger RJ. Calcium, magnesium, and other elements in the red blood cells and hair of normals and patients with premenstrual syndrome. Biol Trace Elem Res 2003;94(2):123–9.
[115] Ghanbari Z, Haghollahi F, Shariat M, et al. Effects of calcium supplement therapy in women with premenstrual syndrome. Taiwan J Obstet Gynecol 2009;48(2):124–9.
[116] Samieipour S, Kiani F, Babaei Heydarabadi A, et al. Comparing the effects of vitamin B1 and calcium on premenstrual syndrome (PMS) among female students, Ilam-Iran. International Journal of Pediatrics 2016;4(9):3519–28.
[117] Rocha Filho EA, Lima JC, Neto JS, et al. Essential fatty acids for premenstrual syndrome and their effect on prolactin and total cholesterol levels: a randomized, double blind, placebo-controlled study. Reprod Health 2011;8(1):1.
[118] Zafari M, Behmanesh F, Agha Mohammadi A. Comparison of the effect of fish oil and ibuprofen on treatment of severe pain in primary dysmenorrhea. Caspian J Intern Med 2011;2(3):279–82.
[119] Douglas S. Premenstrual syndrome. Evidence-based treatment in family practice. Can Fam Physician 2002;48:1789–97.
[120] Kwan I, Onwude JL. Premenstrual syndrome. Clin Evid 2007;2007:pii: 0806.
[121] Eriksson O, Wall A, Marteinsdottir I, et al. Mood changes correlate to changes in brain serotonin precursor trapping in women with premenstrual dysphoria. Psychiatry Res 2006;146(2):107–16.
[122] Monograph. Altern Med Rev 2006;11(1):52–6. [No authors listed] L-Tryptophan.
[123] London RS, Murphy L, Kitlowski KE, et al. Efficacy of alpha-tocopherol in the treatment of the premenstrual syndrome. J Reprod Med 1987;32(6):400–4.
[124] Dadkhah H, Ebrahimi E, Fathizadeh N. Evaluating the effects of vitamin D and vitamin E supplement on premenstrual syndrome: a randomized, double-blind, controlled trial. Iran J Nurs Midwifery Res 2016;21(2):159.
[125] Bertone-Johnson ER, Hankinson SE, Forger NG, et al. Plasma 25-hydroxyvitamin D and risk of premenstrual syndrome in a prospective cohort study. BMC Womens Health 2014;14(1):1.
[126] Rajaei S, Sene AA, Norouzi S, et al. The relationship between serum vitamin D level and premenstrual syndrome in Iranian women. Int J Repro Biomed 2016;14(10):665.
[127] Chuong CJ, Dawson EB. Zinc and copper levels in premenstrual syndrome. Fertil Steril 1994;62(2):313–20.
[128] Fathizadeh S, Amani R, Haghighizadeh MH, et al. Comparison of serum zinc concentrations and body antioxidant status between young women with premenstrual syndrome and normal controls: a case-control study. Int J Reprod Biomed (Yazd) 2016;14(11):699.
[129] Chevallier A. Encylopedia of medicinal plants. Dorling Kindersley; 2001.
[130] Loch EG, Selle H, Boblitz N. Treatment of premenstrual syndrome with a phytopharmaceutical formulation containing *Vitex agnus-castus*. J Womens Health Gend Based Med 2000;9(3):315–20.
[131] Berger D, Schaffner W, Schrader E, et al. Efficacy of *Vitex agnus-castus* L. extract Ze 440 in patients with pre-menstrual syndrome (PMS). Arch Gynecol Obstet 2000;264(3):150–3.
[132] Schellenberg R. Treatment for the premenstrual syndrome with agnus castus fruit extract: prospective, randomised, placebo controlled study. BMJ 2001;322(7279):134–7.
[133] Zamani M, Neghab N, Torabian S. Therapeutic effect of *Vitex agnus-castus* in patients with premenstrual syndrome. Acta Med Iran 2012;50(2):101.
[134] van Die MD, Burger HG, Teede HJ, et al. *Vitex agnus-castus* extracts for female reproductive disorders: a systematic review of clinical trials. Planta Med 2013;79(07):562–75.
[135] Better Health Channel. Premenstrual syndrome (PMS); 2017. Available from: www.betterhealth.vic.gov.au/health/ConditionsAndTreatments/premenstrual-syndrome-pms.

[136] Ambrosini A, Di Lorenzo C, Coppola G, et al. Use of *Vitex agnus-castus* in migrainous women with premenstrual syndrome: an open-label clinical observation. Acta Neurol Belg 2013;113(1):25–9.
[137] Momoeda M, Sasaki H, Tagashira E, et al. Efficacy and safety of *Vitex agnus-castus* extract for treatment of premenstrual syndrome in Japanese patients: a prospective, open-label study. Adv Ther 2014;31(3):362–73.
[138] Ibrahim RM, Soliman SM, Mahmoud HM. Effect of *Vitex agnus castus* (VAC) on premenstrual syndromes among nursing students. J Am Sci 2012;8(4):144–53.
[139] Ledina AV, Prilepskaya VN. Improvement of quality of life of women with a premenstrual syndrome as estimate of efficiency of herbal medical treatment on the basis of *Vitex agnus castus*. Middle East J Sci Res 2013;17(4):472–6.
[140] Canning S, Waterman M, Orsi N, et al. The efficacy of *Hypericum perforatum* (St John's wort) for the treatment of premenstrual syndrome: a randomized, double-blind, placebo-controlled trial. CNS Drugs 2010;24(3):207–25.
[141] Hicks SM, Walker AF, Gallagher J, et al. The significance of 'nonsignificance' in randomized controlled studies: a discussion inspired by a double-blinded study on St John's wort (*Hypericum perforatum* L.) for premenstrual symptoms. J Altern Complement Med 2004;10(6):925–32.
[142] Ghazanfarpour M, Kaviani M, Asadi N, et al. *Hypericum perforatum* for the treatment of premenstrual syndrome. Int J Gynecol Obstet 2011;113(1):84–5.
[143] Bendich A. The potential for dietary supplements to reduce premenstrual syndrome (PMS) symptoms. J Am Coll Nutr 2000;19(1):3–12.
[144] ESCOP. 'Taraxaci herba' and 'Taraxaci radix.' Monographs on the medicinal uses of plant drugs; 1997. Exeter, UK. European Scientific Cooperative on Phytotherapy as cited in Blumenthal M. The complete German commission E monographs. Austin: American Botanical Council; 1998.
[145] Allsworth JE, Clarke J, Peipert JF, et al. The influence of stress on the menstrual cycle among newly incarcerated women. Womens Health Issues 2007;17(4):202–9.
[146] Allsworth JE, Clarke J, Peipert JF, et al. The influence of stress on the menstrual cycle among newly incarcerated women. Womens Health Issues 2007;17(4):202–9.
[147] Kulkarni SK, Dhir A. *Withania somnifera:* an Indian ginseng. Prog Neuropsychopharmacol Biol Psychiatry 2008;32(5):1093–105.
[148] Andrade C, Aswath A, Chaturvedi SK, et al. A double-blind placebo-controlled evaluation of anxiolytic efficacy of an ethanolic extract of *Withania somnifera.* Indian J Psychiatry 2000;42:295–301; as cited in Kulkarni SK, Dhir A. *Withania somnifera:* an Indian ginseng. Prog Neuropsychopharmacol Biol Psychiatry 2008;32(5):1093–105.
[149] Ren ML, Zhang X, Ding R, et al. Two new monoterpene glucosides from *Paeonia lactiflora* Pall. J Asian Nat Prod Res 2009;11(7):670–4.
[150] Adams JD Jr, Garcia C. Women's health among the Chumash. Evid Based Complement Alternat Med 2006;3(1):125–31.
[151] Agha-Hosseini M, Kashani L, Aleyaseen A, et al. *Crocus sativus* L.(saffron) in the treatment of premenstrual syndrome: a double-blind, randomised and placebo-controlled trial. BJOG 2008;115(4):515–19.
[152] Beiranvand SP, Beiranvand NS, Moghadam ZB, et al. The effect of *Crocus sativus* (saffron) on the severity of premenstrual syndrome. Eur J Intern Med 2016;8(1):55–61.
[153] Kashani L, Raisi F, Saroukhani S, et al. Saffron for treatment of fluoxetine-induced sexual dysfunction in women: randomized double-blind placebo-controlled study. Hum Psychopharmacol 2013;28(1):54–60.
[154] Ozgoli G, Selselei EA, Mojab F, et al. A randomized, placebo-controlled trial of *Ginkgo biloba* L. in treatment of premenstrual syndrome. J Altern Complement Med 2009;15(8):845–51.
[155] Delaram M, Heydarnejad MS. Herbal remedy for premenstrual syndrome with fennel (*Foeniculum vulgare*) — randomized, placebo-controlled study. Age (Dordr) 2011;55(5.6):57–63.
[156] Moslemi L, Bekhradi R, Moghaddam G. Comparative effect of fennel extract on the intensity of primary dysmenorrhea. Afr J Pharm Pharmacol 2012;6(24):1770–3.
[157] Zeraati F, Shobeiri F, Nazari M, et al. Comparative evaluation of the efficacy of herbal drugs (fennelin and vitagnus) and mefenamic acid in the treatment of primary dysmenorrhea. Iran J Nurs Midwif Res 2014;19(6):581–4.
[158] Ghodsi Z, Asltoghiri M. The effect of fennel on pain quality, symptoms, and menstrual duration in primary dysmenorrhea. J Pediatr Adolesc Gynecol 2014;27(5):283–6.
[159] Younesy S, Amiraliakbari S, Esmaeili S, et al. Effects of fenugreek seed on the severity and systemic symptoms of dysmenorrhea. J Reprod Infertil 2014;15(1):41–8.
[160] Sharifi F, Simbar M, Mojab F, et al. Comparison of the effects of *Matricaria chamomila* (chamomile) extract and mefenamic acid on the intensity of premenstrual syndrome. Complement Ther Clin Pract 2014;20(1):81–8.
[161] Khayat S, Kheirkhah M, Behboodi Moghadam Z, et al. Effect of treatment with ginger on the severity of premenstrual syndrome symptoms. ISRN Obstet Gynecol 2014;792708.
[162] Ozgoli G, Goli M, Moattar F. Comparison of effects of ginger, mefenamic acid, and ibuprofen on pain in women with primary dysmenorrhea. J Altern Complement Med 2009;15(2):129–32.
[163] Khayat S, Fanaei H, Kheirkhah M, et al. Curcumin attenuates severity of premenstrual syndrome symptoms: a randomized, double-blind, placebo-controlled trial. Complement Ther Med 2015;23(3):318–24.
[164] Fanaei H, Khayat S, Kasaeian A, et al. Effect of curcumin on serum brain-derived neurotrophic factor levels in women with premenstrual syndrome: a randomized, double-blind, placebo-controlled trial. Neuropeptides 2016;56:25–31.
[165] Jaafarpour M, Hatefi M, Khani A, et al. Comparative effect of cinnamon and Ibuprofen for treatment of primary dysmenorrhea: a randomized double-blind clinical trial. J Clin Diagn Res 2015;9(4):QC4–7.
[166] Goodale IL, Domar AD, Benson H. Alleviation of premenstrual syndrome symptoms with the relaxation response. Obstet Gynecol 1990;75:649–55.
[167] Norman RJ, Dewailly D, Legro RS, et al. Polycystic ovarian syndrome. Lancet 2007;370:685–97.
[168] ESHRE. Consensus on women's health aspects of polycystic ovary syndrome (PCOS). Hum Reprod 2012;27(1):14–24.
[169] ESHRE/ASRM. ESHRE/ASRM Rotterdam Consensus Meeting Revised 2003 on diagnostic criteria and long-term health risks related to polycystic ovarian syndrome (PCOS). Hum Reprod 2004;19:41–7.
[170] ESHRE/ASRM. Revised 2003 consensus on diagnostic criteria and long-term health risks related to polycystic ovarian syndrome. Fertil Steril 2004;81:19–25.
[171] Azziz R, Woods KS, Reyna R. The prevalence of polycystic ovarian syndrome in an unselected population. J Clin Endocrinol Metabol 2004;89:2745–9.
[172] Rooney S, Pendry B. Phytotherapy for polycystic ovarian syndrome: a review of the literature and evaluation of practitioners' experiences. J Herb Med 2014;4(3):159–71.
[173] van der Spuy ZM, Dyer SJ. The pathogenesis of infertility and early pregnancy loss in polycystic ovarian syndrome. Best Pract Res Clin Obstet Gynaecol 2004;18(5):755–71.
[174] Norman RJ, Davies MJ, Lord J, et al. The role of lifestyle modification in polycystic ovarian syndrome. Trends Endocrinol Metab 2002;13:251–7.
[175] Dunaif A. Insulin resistance and the polycystic ovarian syndrome: mechanism and implications for pathogenesis. Endocr Rev 1997;18:774–800.
[176] Palioura E, Kandaraki E, Diamanti-Kandarakis E. Endocrine disruptors and polycystic ovary syndrome: a focus on bisphenol A and its potential pathophysiological aspects. Horm Mol Biol Clin Investig 2014;17(3):137–44.
[177] Rutkowska A, Rachoń D. Bisphenol A (BPA) and its potential role in the pathogenesis of the polycystic ovary syndrome (PCOS). Gynecol Endocrinol 2014;30(4):260–5.
[178] Merkin SS, Phy JL, Sites CK, et al. Environmental determinants of polycystic ovary syndrome. Fertil Steril 2016;106(1):16–24.
[179] Carmina E, Rosato F, Janni A, et al. Extensive clinical experience: relative prevalence of different androgen excess in 950 women referred because of clinical hyperandrogenism. J Clin Endocrinol Metab 2006;91:2–6.

[180] Ehrmann DA. Polycystic ovarian syndrome. N Engl J Med 2005;352:1223–36.
[181] Hart R, Norman R. Polycystic ovarian syndrome-prognosis and outcomes. Best Pract Res Clin Obstet Gynaecol 2006;20(5):751–78.
[182] Azziz R, Marin C, Hoq L, et al. Health care-related economic burden of polycystic ovarian syndrome during the reproductive life span. J Clin Endocrinol Metab 2005;90:4650–8.
[183] Nelson VL, Qin Kn KN, Rosenfield RL. The biochemical basis for increased testosterone production in theca cells propagated from patients with polycystic ovarian syndrome. J Clin Endocrinol Metab 2001;86:5925–33.
[184] Diamanti-Kandarkis E, Pipieri C. Genetics of polycystic ovarian syndrome: searching for the way out of the labyrinth. Hum Reprod Update 2005;11:631–43.
[185] Teixeira Filho FL, Baracat EC, Lee TH. Aberrant expression of growth differentiation factor-9 in oocytes of women with polycystic ovary syndrome. J Clin Endocrinol Metab 2002;87:1337–44.
[186] Witchel SF, Aston CE. The role of heterozygosity for CYP21 in the polycystic ovarian syndrome. J Pediatr Endocrinol Metab 2000;(Suppl. 13):1315–17.
[187] Xita N, Tsatsoulis A, Chatzikryiakidou A, et al. Association of the (TAAA)n repeat polymorphism in the sex hormone-binding globulin (SHBG) gene with polycystic ovarian syndrome and relation to SHBG serum levels. J Clin Endocrinol Metab 2002;87:3708–20.
[188] Ukkola O, Rankinen T, Gagnon J, et al. A genome-wide linkage scan for steroids and SHBG levels in black and white families: the HERITAGE Family Study. J Clin Endocrinol Metab 2002;87:3708–20.
[189] Urbank M, Woodroffe A, Ewens KG, et al. Candidate gene region for polycystic ovarian syndrome (PCOS) on chromosome 19p13.2. J Clin Endocrinol Metab 2005;90:6623–9.
[190] Glueck CJ, Wang P, Goldenberg N, et al. Pregnancy outcomes among women with polycystic ovarian syndrome treated with metformin. Hum Reprod 2002;17:2858–64.
[191] Diamanti-Kandarkis E, Palioniko G, Alexandraki K, et al. The prevalence of 4G5G polymorphism of plasminogen activator inhibitor-1 (PAI-1) gene in polycystic ovarian syndrome and its association with plasma PAI-1 levels. Eur J Endocrinol 2004;150:793–8.
[192] Chang WY, Knochenhaur ES, Bartolucci AA, et al. Phenotypic spectrum of polycystic ovary syndrome: clinical and biochemical characterisation of the three major subgroups. Fertil Steril 2005;83:1717–23.
[193] Kumar A, Woods KS, Bartolucci AA, et al. Prevalence of adrenal androgen excess in patients with polycystic ovarian syndrome (PCOS). Clin Endocrinol (Oxf) 2005;62:644–9.
[194] Gilling-Smith C, Willis DS, Beard RW, et al. Hypersecretion of androstenedione by isolated thecal cells from polycystic ovaries. J Clin Endocrinol Metab 1994;79(4):1158–65.
[195] Escobar-Morreale HF, Luque-Ramirez M, San-Millan JL. The molecular-genetic basis of functional hyeprandrogenism and the polycystic ovarian syndrome. Endocr Rev 2005;26:251–82.
[196] Webber LJ, Stubbs S, Stark J, et al. Formation and early development of follicles in the polycystic ovary. Lancet 2003;362:1017–21.
[197] Welt CK, Gudmundsson JA, Arason G, et al. Characterising discrete subsets of polycystic ovarian syndrome as defined by the Rotterdam criteria: the impact of weight on phenotype and metabolic disorder. J Clin Endocrinol Metab 2006;91:4842–8.
[198] Vendola KA, Zhou J, Adesanya OO, et al. Androgens stimulate early follicular growth in the primate overy. J Clin Invest 1998;101:2622–9.
[199] Misfud A, Ramirez S, Yong EL. Androgen receptor gene CAG trinucleotide repeast in anovulatory infertility and polycystic ovaries. J Clin Endocrinol Metab 2000;85:3484–8.
[200] Maciel GA, Baracat EC, Benda JA. Stockpiling of transitional and classic primary follicles of women with polycystic ovarian syndrome. J Clin Endocrinol Metab 2004;89:5321–7.
[201] Jonard S, Dewailly D. The follicular excess in polycystic ovaries, due to intra-ovarian hyperandrogensim, may be the main culprit for follicular arrest. Hum Reprod Update 2004;10:107–17.
[202] Willis DS, Watson H, Mason HD, et al. Premature response to luteinising hormone of granulosa cells from anovulatory women with polycystic ovarian syndrome: relevance to mechanism of anovulation. J Clin Endocrinol Metab 1998;83:3983–91.
[203] Fauser BC, Van Heusden AM. Manipulation of human ovarian function: physiological concepts and clinical consequences. Endocr Rev 1997;18:71–106.
[204] Magoffin DA, Jakimuik AJ. Inhibin A and inhibin B and activin A concentrations in follicular fluid from women with polycystic ovarian syndrome. Hum Reprod 1998;13:2693–8.
[205] Lockwood GM, Muttukrishna S, Groome NP, et al. Mid-follicular phase pulses of inhibin B are absent in polycystic ovarian syndrome and are initiated by successful laparoscopic ovarian diathermy: a possible mechanism regulating emergence of the dominant follicle. J Clin Endocrinol Metab 1998;83:1730–5.
[206] Lanzone A, Petraglia F, Fulghesu AM, et al. Corticotropin-releasing hormone induces an exaggerated response of adrenocorticotropic hormone and cortisol in polycystic ovarian syndrome. Fertil Steril 1995;63:1195–9.
[207] Blank SK, McCartney CR, Marshall JC. The origins and sequelae of abnormal neuroendocrine function in polycystic ovarian syndrome. Hum Reprod Update 2006;12:351–61.
[208] Norman RJ, Hickey T, Moran L, et al. Polycystic ovarian syndrome-diagnosis and etiology. Int Congr Ser 2004;1266:225–32.
[209] Barnes RB. The pathogenesis of polycystic ovary syndrome: lessons from ovarian stimulation studies. J Endocrinol Invest 1998;21(9):567–79.
[210] Franks S, Mason H, White D, et al. Etiology of anovulation in polycystic ovarian syndrome. Steroids 1998;63:306–7.
[211] Hillier SG. Current concepts of the roles of follicle stimulating hormone and luteinising hormone in folliculogenesis. Human Repro 1994;9:188–91.
[212] Yong EL, Baird DT, Yates R, et al. Hormonal regulation of the growth and steroidogenic function in human granulose cells. J Clin Endocrinol Metab 1992;74:842–9.
[213] Dunaif A, Segal KR, Shelley DR, et al. Evidence for distinctive and intrinsic defects in insulin action in polycystic ovarian syndrome. Diabetes 1992;41:1257–66.
[214] Ehrmann DA, Sturis J, Byrne MM, et al. Insulin secretory defects in polycystic ovarian syndrome. Relationship to insulin sensitivity and family history of non-insulin dependent diabetes mellitus. J Clin Invest 1995;96:520–7.
[215] Willis D, Mason H, Gilling-Smith C, et al. Modulation by insulin of follicle stimulating hormone and luteinsing hormone actions in human granulose cells of normal and polycystic ovaries. J Clin Endocrinol Metab 1996;81:302–9.
[216] Giudice LC. Growth factor action on ovarian function in polycystic ovary syndrome. Endocrinol Metab Clin North Am 1999;vi:325–39.
[217] Diamanti-Kandarkis E, Papvassiliou AG. Molecular mechanisms of insulin resistance in polycystic ovarian syndrome. Trends Mol Med 2006;12:324–32.
[218] Dong J, Albertini DF, Nishimori K, et al. Growth differentiation factor-9 is required during early ovarian folliculogenesis. Nature 1996;383:531–5.
[219] Maruo T, Laoag-Fernandez JB, Takekida S, et al. Regulation of granulose cell proliferation and apoptosis during follicular development. J Gynaecol Endocrinol 1999;13:410–19.
[220] Almahbobi G, Misajon A, Hutchinson P, et al. Hyperexpression of epidermal growth factor receptors in granulose cells from women with polycystic ovarian syndrome. Fertil Steril 1998;70:750–8.
[221] Amato G, Conte M, Mazziotti G, et al. Serum and follicular fluid cytokines in polycystic ovarian syndrome during stimulated cycles. Obstet Gynecol 2003;101:1177–82.
[222] Homberg R, Amsterdam A. Polycystic ovary syndrome: loss of the apoptotic mechanism in the ovarian follicles? J Clin Endocrinol Metab 1998;21:552–7.
[223] Durant E, Leslie NS. Polycystic ovarian syndrome: a review of current knowledge. J Nurse Pract 2007;3:180–5.
[224] Lucky AW, Rosenfield RL, McGuire J. Adrenal androgen hyperesponsiveness to adrenocorticotropin in women with acne and/or hirsutism: adrenal enzyme defects and exaggerated andrenarche. J Clin Endocrinol Metab 1986;62:840–8.
[225] Abbott DH, Barnett DK, Bruns CM, et al. Androgen excess fetal programming of female reproduction: a developmental aetiology for polycystic ovary syndrome? Hum Reprod Update 2005;11:357–74.

[226] Abbott DH, Dumesic DA, Franks S. Development origin of polycystic ovarian syndrome- a hypothesis. J Endocrinol 2002;174:1–5.
[227] Robinson JE, Birch RA, Taylor JA. In utero programming of sexually differentiated gonadotrophin releasing hormone (GnRH) secretion. Domest Anim Endocrinol 2002;23:43–52.
[228] Carmina E, Koyama T, Chang L, et al. Does ethnicity influence the prevalence of adrenal hyperandrogenism and insulin resistance in polycystic ovarian syndrome? Am J Obstet Gynecol 1992;167:1807–12.
[229] Adams J, Franks S, Polson DW, et al. Multifollicular ovaries: clinical and endocrine features and response to pulsatile gonadotrophin releasing hormone. Lancet 1985;2:1375–9.
[230] Kiddy DS, Hamilton-Fairly D, Bush A. Improvment in endocrine and ovarian function during dietary treatment of obese women with polycystic ovarian syndrome. Clin Endocrinol (Oxf) 1992;36:105–11.
[231] Crosignani PG, Colombo M, Vegetti W. Overweight and obese anovulatory patients with polycystic ovaries: parallel improvements in anthropometric indices, ovarian physiology and fertility rate induced by diet. Hum Reprod 2003;18:1928–32.
[232] Boudreaux MY, Talbot EO, Kip KE, et al. Risk of T2DM and impaired fasting glucose among PCOS subjects: results of an 8 year follow-up. Curr Diab Rep 2006;6:77–83.
[233] Ehrmann DA, Barnes RB, Rosenfield RL, et al. Prevalence of impaired glucose tolerance and diabetes in women with polycystic ovary syndrome. Diabetes Care 1999;22:141–6.
[234] Orio F, Palomba S, Colao A. Cardiovascular risk in women with polycystic ovary syndrome. Fertil Steril 2006;86(Suppl. 1):S20–1.
[235] Hahn S, Janssen OE, Tan S, et al. Clinical and psychological correlates of quality-of-life in polycystic ovary syndrome. Eur J Endocrinol 2005;153:853–60.
[236] Himelein MJ, Thatcher SS. Polycystic ovary syndrome and mental health: a review. Obstet Gynecol Surv 2006;61:723–32.
[237] Kerchner A, Lester W, Stuart SP, et al. Risk of depression and other mental health disorders in women with polycystic ovary syndrome: a longitudinal study. Fertil Steril 2009;91(1):207–11.
[238] Hardiman P, Pillay OC, Atiomo W. Polycystic ovary syndrome and endometrial carcinoma. Lancet 2003;361:1810–12.
[239] Guyatt G, Weaver B, Cronin L, et al. Health related quality of life in women with polycystic ovary syndrome, a self-administered questionnaire, was validated. J Clin Epidemiol 2004;57:1279–87.
[240] Sherif K. Polycystic ovary syndrome in primary care. Female Patient 2006;31(1):25–9.
[241] Balen AH, Laven JS, Tan SL, et al. Ultrasound assessment of the polycystic ovary: international consensus definitions. Hum Reprod Update 2003;9:505–18.
[242] Bridges NA, Cooke A, Healy MJ, et al. Standards for ovarian volume in childhood and puberty. Fertil Steril 1993;60:456–60.
[243] Pigny P, Jonard S, Robert Y, et al. Serum anti-Müllerian hormone as a surrogate for antral follicle count for definition of the polycystic ovarian syndrome. J Clin Endocrinol Metab 2006;91:941–5.
[244] Vermeulen A, Verdonck L, Kauffman JM. A critical evaluation of simple methods for the estimation of free testosterone in serum. J Clin Endocrinol Metab 1999;84:3666–72.
[245] Ayala C, Steinberger E, Smith KD, et al. Serum testosterone levels and reference ranges in reproductive-age women. Endocr Pract 1999;5:322–9.
[246] American Association of Clinical Endocrinologists. American Association of Clinical Endocrinologists position statement on metabolic and cardiovascular consequences of polycystic ovary syndrome. Endocrinol Pract 2005;11(2):125–34.
[247] Archer JS, Chang RJ. Hirsutism and acne in polycystic ovary syndrome. Best Pract Res Clin Obstet Gynaecol 2004;18:737–54.
[248] Shapiro J, Lui H. Treatments for unwanted facial hair. Skin Ther Lett 2005;10:1–4.
[249] Ellis JA, Shapiro R, Harrap SB. Androgenic alopecia: pathogenesis and potential for therapy. Exp Rev Mol Med 2002;2002:1–11.
[250] Messinis IE. Ovulation induction: a mini review. Hum Reprod 2005;20:2688–97.
[251] Fatemi HM, Kolibianakis E, Tournaye H, et al. Clomiphene citrate versus letrozole for ovarian stimulation: a pilot study. Reprod Biomed Online 2003;7:543–6.
[252] Lord JM, Flight IH, Norman RJ. Insulin-sensitising drugs (metformin, troglitazone, rosiglitazone, pioglitazone, D-chiro-inositol) for polycystic ovary syndrome. Cochrane Database Syst Rev 2003;(3):CD003053.
[253] Nugent D, Vandekerckhove P, Hughes E, et al. Gonadotrophin therapy for ovulation induction in sub-fertility associated with polycystic ovary syndrome. Cochrane Database Syst Rev 2000;(4):CD000410.
[254] Bargiota A, Diamanti-Kandarakis E. The effects of old, new and emerging medicines on metabolic aberrations in PCOS. Ther Adv Endocrinol Metab 2012;3(1):27–47.
[255] Farquhar C, Lilford R, Majoribanks J, et al. Laparoscopic 'drilling' by diathermy or laser for ovulation induction in anovulatory polycystic ovary syndrome. Cochrane Database Syst Rev 2005;(3):CD001122.
[256] Salama AA, Amine EK, Salem HA, et al. Anti-inflammatory dietary combo in overweight and obese women with polycystic ovary syndrome. N Am J Med Sci 2015;7(7):310.
[257] Azadi-Yazdi M, Karimi-Zarchi M, Salehi-Abargouei A, et al. Effects of dietary approach to stop hypertension diet on androgens, antioxidant status and body composition in overweight and obese women with polycystic ovary syndrome: a randomised controlled trial. J Hum Nutr Diet 2017;30:275–83.
[258] Frary JM, Bjerre KP, Glintborg D, et al. The effect of dietary carbohydrates in women with polycystic ovary syndrome. Minerva Endocrinol 2014;10(10).
[259] Phy JL, Pohlmeier AM, Cooper JA, et al. Low starch/low dairy diet results in successful treatment of obesity and co-morbidities linked to polycystic ovary syndrome (PCOS). J Obes Weight Loss Ther 2015;5(2):259.
[260] Garg D, Merhi Z. Advanced glycation end products: link between diet and ovulatory dysfunction in PCOS? Nutrients 2015;7(12):10129–44.
[261] Palimeri S, Palioura E, Diamanti-Kandarakis E. Current perspectives on the health risks associated with the consumption of advanced glycation end products: recommendations for dietary management. Diabetes Metab Syndr Obes 2015;8:415–26.
[262] Marsh K, Brand-Miller J. The optimal diet for women with polycystic ovary syndrome? Br J Nutr 2005;94:154–65.
[263] Brynes AE, Edwards MC, Ghatei MA, et al. A randomised four-intervention crossover study investigating the effect of carbohydrates on daytime profiles of insulin, glucose, non-esterified fatty acids and triacylglycerols in middle-aged men. Br J Nutr 2003;89:207–18.
[264] Kilicdag EB, Bagis T, Tarim E, et al. Administration of B-group vitamins reduces circulating homocysteine in polycystic ovarian syndrome patients treated with metformin: a randomized trial. Hum Reprod 2005;20(6):1521–8.
[265] Thornalley PJ. The potential role of thiamine (vitamin B_1) in diabetic complications. Curr Diabetes Rev 2005;1(3):287–98.
[266] Kazerooni T, Asadi N, Dehbashi S, et al. Effect of folic acid in women with and without insulin resistance who have hyperhomocysteinemic polycystic ovary syndrome. Int J Gynaecol Obstet 2008;101(2):156–60.
[267] Bahmani F, Karamali M, Shakeri H, et al. The effects of folate supplementation on inflammatory factors and biomarkers of oxidative stress in overweight and obese women with polycystic ovary syndrome: a randomized, double-blind, placebo-controlled clinical trial. Clin Endocrinol (Oxf) 2014;81(4):582–7.
[268] Lydic ML, McNurlan M, Bembo S, et al. Chromium picolinate improves insulin sensitivity in obese subjects with polycystic ovary syndrome. Fertil Steril 2006;86(1):243–6.
[269] Ashoush S, Abou-Gamrah A, Bayoumy H, et al. Chromium picolinate reduces insulin resistance in polycystic ovary syndrome: randomized controlled trial. J Obstet Gynecol Res 2016;42(3):279–85.
[270] Cussons AJ, Watts GF, Mori TA, et al. Omega-3 fatty acid supplementation decreases liver fat content in polycystic ovary syndrome: a randomized controlled trial employing proton magnetic resonance spectroscopy. J Clin Endocrinol Metab 2009;94(10):3842–8.
[271] Mansour A, Hosseini S, Larijani B, et al. Nutrients as novel therapeutic approaches for metabolic disturbances in polycystic ovary syndrome. EXCLI J 2016;15:551–64.
[272] Muneyyirci-Delale O, Nacharaju VL, Dalloul M, et al. Divalent cations in women with PCOS: implications for cardiovascular disease. Gynecol Endocrinol 2001;15(3):198–201.

[273] Singh U, Jialal I. Alpha-lipoic acid supplementation and diabetes. Nutr Rev 2008;66(11):646–57.
[274] Masharani U, Gjerde C, Evans JL, et al. Effects of controlled-release alpha lipoic acid in lean, nondiabetic patients with polycystic ovary syndrome. J Diabetes Sci Technol 2010;4(2):359–64.
[275] Duleba AJ, Foyouzi N, Karaca M, et al. Proliferation of ovarian theca-interstitial cells is modulated by antioxidants and oxidative stress. Hum Reprod 2004;19(7):1519–24.
[276] Marreiro DN, Geloneze B, Tambascia MA, et al. Effect of zinc supplementation on serum leptin levels and insulin resistance of obese women. Biol Trace Elem Res 2006;112:109–18.
[277] Sun Q, van Dam RM, Willett WC, et al. Prospective study of zinc intake and risk of type 2 diabetes in women. Diabetes Care 2009;32(4):629–34.
[278] Fang F, Ni K, Cai Y, et al. Effect of vitamin D supplementation on polycystic ovary syndrome: a systematic review and meta-analysis of randomized controlled trials. Comp Ther Clin Pract 2017;26:53–60.
[279] Irani M, Minkoff H, Seifer DB, et al. Vitamin D increases serum levels of the soluble receptor for advanced glycation end products in women with PCOS. J Clin Endocrinol Metab 2014;99(5):E886–90.
[280] Foroozanfard F, Jamilian M, Bahmani F, et al. Calcium plus vitamin D supplementation influences biomarkers of inflammation and oxidative stress in overweight and vitamin D-deficient women with polycystic ovary syndrome: a randomized double-blind placebo-controlled clinical trial. Clin Endocrinol (Oxf) 2015;83(6):888–94.
[281] Asemi Z, Foroozanfard F, Hashemi T, et al. Calcium plus vitamin D supplementation affects glucose metabolism and lipid concentrations in overweight and obese vitamin D deficient women with polycystic ovary syndrome. Clin Nutr 2015;34(4):586–92.
[282] Muscogiuri G, Palomba S, Caggiano M, et al. Low 25 (OH) vitamin D levels are associated with autoimmune thyroid disease in polycystic ovary syndrome. Endocrine 2016;53(2):538–42.
[283] Porcaro G, Bizzarri M, Monastra G, et al. Strategies for the treatment of polycystic ovary syndrome (PCOS) women: the role of myoinositol (MI) and d-chiro-inositol (DCI) between diet and therapy. In: Cobbs B, editor. Polycystic ovary syndrome (PCOS): clinical aspects, potential complications and dietary management. Hauppauge, NY: Nova Science Publishers; 2016.
[284] Holick MF, Binkley NC, Bischoff-Ferrari HA, et al. Evaluation, treatment, and prevention of vitamin D deficiency: an Endocrine Society clinical practice guideline. J Clin Endocrinol Metab 2011;96(7):1911–30.
[285] Kamel HH. Role of phyto-oestrogens in ovulation induction in women with polycystic ovarian syndrome. Eur J Obstet Gynecol Reprod Biol 2013;168(1):60–3.
[286] Shahin AY, Mohammed SA. Adding the phytoestrogen *Cimicifugae racemosae* to clomiphene induction cycles with timed intercourse in polycystic ovary syndrome improves cycle outcomes and pregnancy rates — a randomized trial. Gynecol Endocrinol 2014;30(7):505–10.
[287] Wang JG, Anderson RA, Graham GM 3rd, et al. The effect of cinnamon extract on insulin resistance parameters in polycystic ovary syndrome: a pilot study. Fertil Steril 2007;88(1):240–3.
[288] Kort DH, Lobo RA. Preliminary evidence that cinnamon improves menstrual cyclicity in women with polycystic ovary syndrome: a randomized controlled trial. Am J Obstet Gynecol 2014;211(5):487.e1–e6.
[289] Armanini D, Mattarello MJ, Fiore C, et al. Liquorice reduces serum testosterone in healthy women. Steroids 2004;69(11–12):763–6.
[290] Leach MJ. *Gymnema sylvestre* for diabetes mellitus: a systematic review. J Altern Complement Med 2007;13(9):977–83.
[291] Takahashi K, Yoshino K, Shirai T, et al. Effect of a traditional herbal medicine (shakuyaku-kanzo-to) on testosterone secretion in patients with polycystic ovary syndrome detected by ultrasound. (Abstract only). Nippon Sanka Fujinka Gakkai Zasshi 1988;40(6):789–92.
[292] Takahashi K, Mutiara S, Kita N, et al. Odd variation of 75 g oral glucose tolerance test results in a Japanese patient with polycystic ovary syndrome: a case report. Arch Gynecol Obstet 2007;275(5):405–9.
[293] Milanov S, Maleeva E, Taskov M, et al. MBI: Medicobiologic Information; 1985; 4:27.
[294] Bracero N, Zacur H. Polycystic ovary syndrome and hyperprolactinemia. Obstet Gynecol Clin North Am 2001;28(1):77–84.
[295] Shayya R, Chang RJ. Reproductive endocrinology of adolescent polycystic ovary syndrome. BJOG 2010;117(2):150–5.
[296] Shahnazi M, Khalili AF, Hamdi K, et al. The effects of combined low-dose oral contraceptives and vitex agnus on the improvement of clinical and paraclinical parameters of polycystic ovarian syndrome: a triple-blind, randomized, controlled clinical trial. Iran Red Crescent Med J 2016;18(12).
[297] Swaroop A, Jaipuriar AS, Gupta SK, et al. Efficacy of a novel fenugreek seed extract (trigonella foenum-graecum, Furocyst™ in polycystic ovary syndrome (PCOS). Int J Med Sci 2015;12(10):825.
[298] Grant P, Ramasamy S. An update on plant derived anti-androgens. Int J Endocrinol Metab 2012;10(2):497–502.
[299] Moran LJ, Brinkworth G, Noakes M, et al. Effects of lifestyle modification in polycystic ovary syndrome. Reprod Biomed Online 2006;12:569–78.
[300] Huber-Buchbolz MM, Carey DG, Norman RJ. Restoration of reproductive potential by lifestyle modification in obese polycystic ovary syndrome: role of insulin sensitivity and luteinising hormone. J Clin Endocrinol Metab 1999;84:1470–4.
[301] Moran LJ, Noakes M, Clifton PM, et al. Dietary composition in restoring reproductive and metabolic physiology in overweight women with polycystic ovary syndrome. J Clin Endocrinol Metab 2003;88:812–19.
[302] Knowler WC, Barrett-Connor E, Fowler SE, et al. Reduction in the incidence of type II diabetes with lifestyle intervention or metformin. N Engl J Med 2002;346:393–403.
[303] Tsagareli V, Noakes M, Norman RJ. Effect of a very low calorie diet on in vitro fertilisation outcomes. Fertil Steril 2006;86:227–9.
[304] Banting LK, Gibson-Helm M, Polman R, et al. Physical activity and mental health in women with polycystic ovary syndrome. BMC Womens Health 2014;14(1):51.
[305] Moran LJ, Hutchison SK, Norman RJ, et al. Lifestyle changes in women with polycystic ovary syndrome. Cochrane Database Syst Rev 2011;(2):CD007506.
[306] Stefanaki C, Bacopoulou F, Livadas S, et al. Impact of a mindfulness stress management program on stress, anxiety, depression and quality of life in women with polycystic ovary syndrome: a randomized controlled trial. Stress 2015;18(1):57–66.
[307] Okolo S. Incidence, aetiology and epidemiology of uterine fibroids. Best Pract Res Clin Obstet Gynaecol 2008;22(4):571–88.
[308] Cramer SF, Patel A. The frequency of uterine leiomyomas (Abstract only). Am J Clin Pathol 1990;94(4):435–8.
[309] Vollenhoven B. Introduction: the epidemiology of uterine leiomyomas. Baillières Clin Obst Gynaecol 1998;12(2):169–76.
[310] Katz TA, Yang Q, Treviño LS, et al. Endocrine-disrupting chemicals and uterine fibroids. Fertil Steril 2016;106(4):967–77.
[311] Wise LA, Laughlin-Tommaso SK. Epidemiology of uterine fibroids: from menarche to menopause. Clin Obstet Gynecol 2016;59(1):2–4.
[312] Vikhlyaeva EM, Khodzhaeva ZS, Fantschenko ND. Familial predisposition to uterine leiomyomas. Int J Gynecol Obstet 1995;51:127–31.
[313] Lumbiganon P, Rugpao S, Phandhu-fung S, et al. Protective effect of depot-medroxyprogesterone acetate on surgically treated uterine leiomyomas: a multicentre case-control study. Br J Obstet Gynaecol 1995;103:909–18.
[314] Marsh EE, Ekpo GE, Cardozo ER, et al. Racial differences in fibroid prevalence and ultrasound fibdings in asymptomatic young women (18–30): a pilot study. Fertil Steril 2013;99:1951–7.
[315] Chibber S, Mendoza G, Cohen L, et al. Racial and ethnic differences in uterine fibroid prevalence in a diverse cohort of young asymptomatic women (18–30 yo). Fertil Steril 2016;106(3):Supp:e97.
[316] Moorman PG, Leppert PL, Myers ER, et al. Comparison of characteristics of fibroids in African American and white women undergoing premenopausal hysterectomy. Fertil Steril 2013;99(3):768–76.
[317] Witherspoon JT, Butler VW. The etiology of uterine fibroids, with special reference to the frequency of their occurrence in the Negro: an hypothesis. Surg Gynecol Obstet 1934;58:57–61.
[318] Kjerulff KH, Langenberg P, Seidman JD, et al. Uterine leiomyomas. Racial differences in severity, symptoms and age at diagnosis. J Reprod Med 1996;41:483–90.

[319] Day Baird D, Dunson DB, Hill MC, et al. High cumulative incidence of uterine leiomyoma in black and white women: ultrasound evidence. Am J Obstet Gynecol 2003;188(1):100–7.
[320] Kawamura S, Kasagi F, Kodama K, et al. Prevalence of uterine myoma detected by ultrasound examination in the atomic bomb survivors. Radiat Res 1997;147:753–8.
[321] Kodama K, Fujiwara S, Yamada F, et al. Profiles of non-cancer diseases in atomic bomb survivors. World Health Stat Q 1996;49:7–16.
[322] Yang Q, Diamond MP, Al-Hendy A. Early life adverse environmental exposures increase the risk of uterine fibroid development: role of epigenetic regulation. Front Pharmacol 2016;7.
[323] Pollack AZ, Louis GB, Chen Z, et al. Bisphenol A, benzophenone-type ultraviolet filters, and phthalates in relation to uterine leiomyoma. Environ Res 2015;137:101–7.
[324] Trabert B, Chen Z, Kannan K, et al. Persistent organic pollutants (POPs) and fibroids: results from the ENDO study. J Expo Sci Environ Epidemiol 2015;25(3):278–85.
[325] Mahalingaiah S, Hart JE, Laden F, et al. Adult air pollution exposure and risk of uterine leiomyoma in the Nurses' Health Study II. Epidemiology 2014;25(5):682.
[326] Parazzini F, Negri E, La Vecchia C, et al. Reproductive factors and risk of uterine fibroids. Epidemiology 1996;7:440–2.
[327] Samadi AR, Lee NC, Flanders D, et al. Risk factors for self-reported uterine fibroids: a case control study. Am J Public Health 1996;86:858–62.
[328] Ross RK, Pike MC, Vessey MP, et al. Risk factors for uterine fibroids: reduced risk associated with oral contraceptives. Br Med J 1986;293:359–63.
[329] Spellacy WN, Le Maire WJ, Buhi WC, et al. Plasma growth hormone and estradiol levels in women with uterine myomas. Obstet Gynecol 1972;40:829–34.
[330] Shikora SA, Niloff JM, Bistrian BR, et al. Relationship between obesity and uterine leiomyomata. Nutrition 1991;7:251–5.
[331] Lethaby A, Vollenhoven B, Sowter MC. Pre-operative GnRH analogue therapy before hysterectomy or myomectomy for uterine fibroids (Review). Cochrane Database Syst Rev 2001;(2):CD000547.
[332] Hashimoto K, Azuma C, Kamiura S, et al. Clonal determination of uterine leiomyomas by analyzing differential inactivation of the X-chromosome-linked phosphoglycerokinase gene. Gynecol Obstet Invest 1995;40:204–8.
[333] Evans P, Brunsell S. Uterine fibroid tumours: diagnosis and treatment. Am Fam Physician 2007;10(75):1503–8.
[334] Chalas E, Constantino JP, Wickerham DL, et al. Benign gynecologic conditions among participants in the Breast Cancer Prevention Trial. Am J Obstet Gynecol 2005;192:1230–7.
[335] Ryan GL, Syrop CH, Van Voorhis BJ. Role, epidemiology and natural history of benign uterine mass lesions. Clin Obstet Gynecol 2005;48(2):312–24.
[336] Lumsden MA, Wallace EM. Clinical presentation of uterine fibroids. Baillières Clin Obstet Gynecol 1998;12:177–95.
[337] Buttram VC, Reiter RC. Uterine leiomyomata: etiology, symptomatology and management. Fertil Steril 1981;36:433–45.
[338] Fraser I, McCarr G, Markham R, et al. Measured menstrual blood loss in women with menorrhagia associated with pelvic disease or coagulation disorder. Obstet Gynecol 1986;9:630–3.
[339] Petraglia F, Musacchio C, Luisi S, et al. Hormone-dependent gynaecological disorders: a pathophysiological perspective for appropriate treatment. Best Pract Res Clin Obstet Gynaecol 2008;22(2):235–49.
[340] Veronica M, Ali A, Venkateshwari A, et al. Association of estrogen and progesterone receptor gene polymorphisms and their respective hormones in uterine leiomyomas. Tumour Biol 2016;37(6):8067–74.
[341] Renwick M, Sadhowsky K. Variations in surgery rates. Australian Institute of Health. Health Services Series 2. Canberra: AGPS; 1991.
[342] Pizzorno J, Murray M. Textbook of natural medicine. 4th ed. Churchill Livingstone; 2012.
[343] Miyake A, Takeda T, Isobe A, et al. Repressive effect of the phytoestrogen genistein on estradiol-induced uterine leiomyoma cell proliferation. Gynecol Endocrinol 2009;25(6):403–9.
[344] Castro L, Gao X, Moore AB, et al. A high concentration of genistein induces cell death in human uterine leiomyoma cells by autophagy. Expert Opin Environ Biol 2016;5(Suppl. 1).
[345] He Y, Zeng Q, Dong SY, et al. Associations between uterine fibroids and lifestyles including diet, physical activity and stress: a case-control study in China. Asia Pac J Clin Nutr 2013;22(1):109–17.
[346] Wise LA, Radin RG, Palmer JR, et al. Intake of fruit, vegetables, and carotenoids in relation to risk of uterine leiomyomata. Am J Clin Nutr 2011;94(6):1620–31.
[347] Shen Y, Wu Y, Lu Q, et al. Vegetarian diet and reduced uterine fibroids risk: a case–control study in Nanjing, China. J Obstet Gynecol Res 2016;42(1):87–94.
[348] Islam MS, Akhtar MM, Ciavattini A, et al. Use of dietary phytochemicals to target inflammation, fibrosis, proliferation, and angiogenesis in uterine tissues: promising options for prevention and treatment of uterine fibroids? Mol Nutr Food Res 2014;58(8):1667–84.
[349] Islam MS, Segars JH, Castellucci M, et al. Dietary phytochemicals for possible preventive and therapeutic option of uterine fibroids: signaling pathways as target. Pharmacol Rep 2017;69(1):57–70.
[350] Wise LA, Palmer JR, Harlow BL, et al. Risk of uterine leiomyomata in relation to tobacco, alcohol and caffeine consumption in the Black Women's Health Study. Hum Reprod 2004;19(8):1746–54.
[351] Lucero J, Harlow BL, Barbieri RL, et al. Early follicular phase hormone levels in relation to patterns of alcohol, tobacco, and coffee use. Fertil Steril 2001;76(4):723–9.
[352] Radin RG, Palmer JR, Rosenberg L, et al. Dietary glycemic index and load in relation to risk of uterine leiomyomata in the Black Women's Health Study. Am J Clin Nutr 2010;91(5):1281–8.
[353] Nagata C, Nakamura K, Oba S, et al. Association of intakes of fat, dietary fibre, soya isoflavones and alcohol with uterine fibroids in Japanese women. Br J Nutr 2009;101(10):1427–31.
[354] Wathes DC, Abayasekara DR, Aitken RJ. Polyunsaturated fatty acids in male and female reproduction. Biol Reprod 2007;77(2):190–201.
[355] Gupta S, Jose J, Manyonda I. Clinical presentation of fibroids. Best Pract Res Clin Obstet Gynaecol 2008;22(4):615–26.
[356] Fortuny J, Sima C, Bayuga S, et al. Risk of endometrial cancer in relation to medical conditions and medication use. Cancer Epidemiol Biomarkers Prev 2009;18(5):1448–56.
[357] Sundström H, Ylikorkala O, Kauppila A. Serum selenium and thromboxane in patients with gynaecological cancer. Carcinogenesis 1986;7(7):1051–2.
[358] Zimmermann M. Burgensteins handbook of nutrition. New York: Theime; 2001.
[359] Fruscella L, Ciaglia EM, Danti M, et al. [Vitamin E in the treatment of pregnancy complicated by uterine myoma] [Article in Italian]. (Abstract only). Minerva Ginecol 1997;49(4):175–9.
[360] Poliakova VA, Vinokurova EA, Suplotov SN, et al. [Evaluation of the rate of lipid peroxidation and antioxidant defense in blood during gynecological laparoscopic operations] [Article in Russian]. (Abstract only). Klin Lab Diagn 2009;6:37–9.
[361] Sabry M, Halder SK, Allah AS, et al. Serum vitamin D3 level inversely correlates with uterine fibroid volume in different ethnic groups: a cross-sectional observational study. Int J Womens Health 2013;5:93–100.
[362] Baird DD, Hill MC, Schectman JM, et al. Vitamin D and the risk of uterine fibroids. Epidemiology 2013;24(3):447–53.
[363] Paffoni A, Somigliana E, Vigano P, et al. Vitamin D status in women with uterine leiomyomas. J Clin Endocrinol Metab 2013;98(8):E1374–8.
[364] Mitro SD, Zota AR. Vitamin D and uterine leiomyoma among a sample of US women: findings from NHANES, 2001–2006. Reprod Toxicol 2015;57:81–6.
[365] Bläuer M, Rovio PH, Ylikomi T, et al. Vitamin D inhibits myometrial and leiomyoma cell proliferation in vitro. Fertil Steril 2009;91(5):1919–25.
[366] Halder SK, Sharan C, Al-Hendy A. 1, 25-dihydroxyvitamin D3 treatment shrinks uterine leiomyoma tumors in the Eker rat model. Biol Reprod 2012;86(4):116.
[367] Al-Hendy A, Diamond MP, El-Sohemy A, et al. 1, 25-dihydroxyvitamin D3 regulates expression of sex steroid receptors in human uterine fibroid cells. J Clin Endocrinol Metab 2015;100(4):E572–82.
[368] Wise LA, Ruiz-Narváez EA, Haddad SA, et al. Polymorphisms in vitamin D-related genes and risk of uterine leiomyomata. Fertil Steril 2014;102(2):503–10.
[369] Blumenthal M. The Complete German Commission E Monographs. Integrative Medicine Communications; 2000.

[370] Nemeth E, Bernath J. Biological activities of yarrow species (*Achillea* spp.). Curr Pharm Des 2008;14(29):3151–67.

[371] Natural Medicines. Natural Standard monographs; 2018. Available from https://naturalmedicines.therapeuticresearch.com/.

[372] Weiss RF. Weiss's herbal medicine. Classic ed. New York: Georg Thieme verlag; 2001.

[373] Nowak RA, Mora S, Diehl T, et al. Prolactin is an autocrine or paracrine growth factor for human myometrial and leiomyoma cells. Gynecol Obstet Invest 1999;48(2):127–32.

[374] Ross SM. Efficacy of a standardized isopropanolic black cohosh (*Actaea racemosa*) extract in treatment of uterine fibroids in comparison with tibolone among patients with menopausal symptoms. Holist Nurs Pract 2014;28(6):386–91.

[375] Vigano P, Parazzini F, Somigliana E, et al. Endometriosis: epidemiology and aetiological factors. Best Pract Res Clin Obstet Gynaecol 2004;18(2):177–200.

[376] Gruppo Italiano per lo studio dell'endometriosi. Prevalence and anatomical distribution of endometriosis in women with selected gynacaelogical conditions: results from a multicentric Italian study. Hum Reprod 1994;9:1158–62.

[377] Parazzini F, La Vecchia C, Negri E, et al. Epidemiologic characteristics in women with uterine fibroids. A case-control study. Obstet Gynecol 1988;72:853–7.

[378] Eskenazi B, Warner ML. Epidemiology of endometriosis. Obstet Gynecol Clin North Am 1997;24:235–58.

[379] Meuleman C, Vandenabeele B, Fieuws S, et al. High prevalence of endometriosis in infertile women with normal ovulation and normospermic partners. Fertil Steril 2009;92:68–74.

[380] American Society for Reproductive Medicine. Revised American Society for Reproductive Medicine classification of endometriosis. Fertil Steril 1997;67(5):817–21.

[381] Hornstein MD, Gleason RE, Orav J, et al. The reproducibility of the revised American Fertility Society classification of endometriosis. Fertil Steril 1993;59(5):1015–21.

[382] Konincks PR, Meuleman C, Demeyre S, et al. Suggestive evidence that pelvic endometriosis is a progressive disease, whereas deeply infiltrating endometriosis is associated with pelvic pain. Fertil Steril 1991;55:759–65.

[383] Kapoor D, Davila W. Endometriosis. eMedicine Specialties. 2017. Available from: http://emedicine.medscape.com/article/271899-overview.

[384] Dunselman GA, Vermeulen N, Becker C, et al. ESHRE guideline: management of women with endometriosis. Hum Reprod 2014;29(3):400–12.

[385] Neme RM, Andrade DC, Brestia M, et al. Epidemiological study on the risk factors of pelvic endometriosis in Brazil. Fertil Steril 2002;77:537.

[386] Cramer DW, Wilson E, Stillman RJ, et al. The relation of endometriosis to menstrual characteristics, smoking and exercise. JAMA 1986;255:1904–8; Cited in: Vigano P, Parazzini F, Somigliana E, et al. Endometriosis: epidemiology and aetiological factors. Best Pract Res Clin Obstet Gynaecol 2004;18(2):177–200.

[387] Darrow SL, Vena JE, Batt RE, et al. Menstrual cycle characteristics and the risk of endometriosis. Epidemiology 1993;4:135–42.

[388] Bishoff F, Simpson JL. Genetics of endometriosis: heritability and candidate genes. Best Pract Res Clin Obstet Gynaecol 2004;18(2):219–32.

[389] Simpson JL, Elias S, Malinak LR, et al. Heritable aspects of endometriosis. Am J Obstet Gynecol 1980;137:237.

[390] Coxhead D, Thomas EJ. Familial inheritance of endometriosis in a British population. A case control study. J Obstet Gynecol 1993;13:42–4.

[391] Moen MH, Magnus P. The familial risk of endometriosis. Acta Obstetrics et Gynaecologica Scandinavia 1993;72:560–4.

[392] Saha R, Pettersson HJ, Svedberg P, et al. Heritability of endometriosis. Fertil Steril 2015;104(4):947–52.

[393] Kajihara H, Yamada Y, Kanayama S, et al. New insights into the pathophysiology of endometriosis: from chronic inflammation to danger signal. Gynecol Endocrinol 2011;27(2):73–9.

[394] Latha M, Vaidya S, Movva S, et al. Molecular pathogenesis of endometriosis; Toll-like receptor-4 A896G (D299G) polymorphism: a novel explanation. Genet Test Mol Biomarkers 2011;15(3):181–4.

[395] Augoulea A, Alexandrou A, Creatsa M, et al. Pathogenesis of endometriosis: the role of genetics, inflammation and oxidative stress. Arch Gynecol Obstet 2012;286(1):99–103.

[396] Rahmioglu N, Nyholt DR, Morris AP, et al. Genetic variants underlying risk of endometriosis: insights from meta-analysis of eight genome-wide association and replication datasets. Hum Reprod Update 2014;20(5):702–16.

[397] Pagliardini L, Gentilini D, Sanchez AM, et al. Replication and meta-analysis of previous genome-wide association studies confirm vezatin as the locus with the strongest evidence for association with endometriosis. Hum Reprod 2015;30(4):987–93.

[398] Sapkota Y, Low SK, Attia J, et al. Association between endometriosis and the interleukin 1A (IL1A) locus. Hum Reprod 2015;30(1):239–48.

[399] Konincks PR, Braet P, Kennedy SH, et al. Dioxin pollution and endometriosis in Belgium. Hum Reprod 1994;9:1001–3.

[400] Scialli AR. Tampons, dioxins, and endometriosis. Reprod Toxicol 2001;15(3):231–8.

[401] Bruner-Tran KL, Gnecco J, Ding T, et al. Exposure to the environmental endocrine disruptor TCDD and human reproductive dysfunction: translating lessons from murine models. Reprod Toxicol 2017;68:59–71.

[402] Lamb K, Berg N. Tampon use in women with endometriosis. J Commun Health 1985;10(4):215–22.

[403] Sinaii N, Cleary SD, Ballweg ML, et al. High rates of autoimmune and endocrine disorders, fibromyalgia, chronic fatigue syndrome and atopic diseases among women with endometriosis. Hum Reprod 2002;17:2715–24.

[404] Smith SK. The aetiology of endometriosis. Hum Reprod 1994;9:1274.

[405] Olson JE, Cerhan JR, Janney CA, et al. Psotmenopausal cancer risk after self-reported endometriosis diagnosis in the Iowa women's health study. Cancer 2002;94:1612–18.

[406] Nap AW, Groothius PG, Demir AY, et al. Pathogenesis of endometriosis. Best Pract Res Clin Obstet Gynaecol 2004;18(2):233–44.

[407] Gazvani R, Templeton A. New considerations for the pathogenesis of endometriosis. Review article. Int J Gynaecol Obstet 2002;76:117–26.

[408] Farquhar CM. Extracts from the 'clinical evidence.' Endometriosis. Br Med J 2000;320:1149–52.

[409] Balasch J, Creus M, Fabregues F, et al. Visible and non-visible endometriosis at laparoscopy in fertile and infertile women and in patients with chronic pelvic pain: a prospective study. Hum Reprod 1996;11:387–91.

[410] Waller KG, Lindsay P, Curtis P, et al. The prevalence of endometriosis in women with infertile partners. Eur J Obstet Gynecol 1993;48:135–9.

[411] Hummelshoj L, Prentice A, Groothuis P. Update on endometriosis. Womens Health 2006;2(1):53–6.

[412] Leibson CL, Good AE, Hass SL, et al. Incidence and characterisation of diagnosed endometriosis in a geograhically defined population. Fertil Steril 2004;82(2):314–21.

[413] Halme J, Becker S, Wing R. Accentuated cyclic activation of peritoneal macrophages in patients with endometriosis. Am J Obstet Gynecol 1984;148:85–90.

[414] Liu DT, Hitchcock A. Endometriosis: its association with retrograde menstruation, dysmenorrhoea, and tubal pathology. Br J Obstet Gynaecol 1986;93:859–62.

[415] Blumenkrantz MJ, Gallagher N, Bashore RA, et al. Retrograde menstruation un women undergoing chronic peritoneal dialysis. Obstet Gynecol 1981;57:667–70.

[416] Kruitwagen RFPM, Poels LG, Willemsen WN, et al. Endometrial epithelial cells in peritoneal fluid during the early follicular phase. Fertil Steril 1991;55:297–303.

[417] Palmer JR, Driscoll SG, Rosenberg L, et al. Oral contraceptive use and risk of gestational trophoblastic tumours. J Natl Cancer Inst 1999;91:635–40.

[418] Geraedts JP, Harper J, Braude P, et al. Preimplantation genetic diagnosis (PGD), a collaborative activity of clinical genetic departments and IVF centres. Prenat Diagn 2001;21:1086–92.

[419] Speroff L, Fritz MA. Clinical gynecologic endocrinology and infertility. 7th ed. USA: Lippincott, Williams & Wilkins; 2005. p. 1103.

[420] D'Hooge TM, Bambra CS, Xiao L, et al. Intrapelvic injection of menstrual endometrium causes endometrosis in baboons. Am J Obstet Gynecol 1995;173:125–34.

[421] Ridley J, Edwards IK. Experimental endometriosis in the human. Am J Obstet Gynecol 1958;76:783–90. Cited in Speroff L, Fritz MA. Clinical gynecologic endocrinology and infertility. 7th ed. USA: Lippincott, Williams & Wilkins; 2005. p. 1104.
[422] Markham R. Peritoneal fluid: physiology and biochemistry, Lecture handout 3rd March. Sydney, Australia: Dr Robert Markham; 2009.
[423] Cicinelli E, Einer-Jensen N, Hunter RH, et al. Peritoneal fluid concentrations of progesterone in women are higher close to the corpus luteum compared with elsewhere in the abdominal cavity. Fertil Steril 2009;92(1):306–10.
[424] Haney AF. Aetiology and histogenesis of endometriosis. Prog Clin Biol Res 1990;323:1–18.
[425] Novak E. Pelvic endometriosis. Am J Obstet Gynecol 1931;22:826–37.
[426] Kim AH, Adamson GD. Benign gynaecology: endometriosis. Global Library Women's Medicine; 2008.
[427] Schrodt GR, Alcorn MD, Ibanez J. Endometriosis of the male urinary system: a case report. J Urol 1980;124:722.
[428] Sampson JA. The development of the implantation theory for the origin of endometriosis. Am J Obstet Gynecol 1940;40:549–57; Cited in: Vigano P, Parazzini F, Somigliana E, et al. Endometriosis: epidemiology and aetiological factors. Best Pract Res Clin Obstet Gynaecol 2004;18(2):177–200.
[429] Jenkins S, Olive DL, Haney AF. Endometriosis: pathogenic implications of the anatomic distribution. Obstet Gynecol 1986;67(3):335–8.
[430] Koks CAM, Dunselman GAJ, De Goeij AFPM, et al. Evaluation of a menstrual cup to collect shed endometrium for in vitro studies. Fertil Steril 1997;68:560–4.
[431] Sanfilippo JS, Watkins NG, Schneider KN, et al. Endometriosis in association with uterine anomaly. Am J Obstet Gynecol 1986;154:39–43. Cited in: Nap AW, Groothius PG, Demir AY, et al. Pathogenesis of endometriosis. Best Pract Res Clin Obstet Gynaecol 2004;18(2):233–44.
[432] D'Hooghe TM, Bambra CS, Suleman MA, et al. Development of a model of retrograde menstruation in baboons (*Papia anubis*). Fertil Steril 1994;62:635–8.
[433] Oral E, Arici A. Pathogeneisis of endometriosis. Obstet Gynecol Clin North Am 1997;24:219–33.
[434] Lebovic DI, Mueller MD, Taylor RN. Immunobiology of endometriosis. Fertil Steril 2001;75:1–110.
[435] Simpson JL, Faridech ZB, Kamat A, et al. Genetics of endometriosis. Obstet Gynecol Clin North Am 2003;30:21–40.
[436] Nothnick WB. Treating endometriosis as an autoimmune disease. Fertil Steril 2001;76(2):223–31.
[437] Steele RW, Dmowski WP, Marmer DJ. Immunologic aspects of human endometriosis. Am J Reprod Immunol 1984;6:33–6.
[438] Wilson TJ, Hertzog PJ, Angus D, et al. Decreased natural killer cell activity in endometriosis patients: relationship to disease pathogenesis. Fertil Steril 1994;62:1086–8.
[439] Ho HN, Chao KH, Chen HF, et al. Peritoneal natural killer cytotoxicity and CD25+CD3+ lymphocyte subpopulation are decreased in women with stage III-IV endometriosis. Hum Reprod 1995;10:2671–5.
[440] DiStefano G, Provinciali M, Muzzioll M, et al. Correlation between oestradiol serum levels and NK cell activity in endometriosis. Ann N Y Acad Sci 1994;741:197–201.
[441] Hsu C, Lin Y, Wang S, et al. Immunomodulation in women with endometriosis receiving GnRH agonist. Obstet Gynecol 1997;89:993–8.
[442] Oosterlynck DJ, Cornillie FJ, Waer M, et al. Women with endometriosis show a defect in natural killer activity resulting in a decreased cytotoxicity to autologous endometrium. Fertil Steril 1991;56:45–51.
[443] Fakih H, Baggett B, Holtz G, et al. Interleukin-1: a possible role in the infertility associated with endometriosis. Fertil Steril 1987;47:213–17.
[444] Halme J. Release of tumour necrosis factor-alpha by human peritoneal macrophages *in vivo* and *in vitro*. Am J Obstet Gynecol 1989;161:1718–25.
[445] Hill JA. Immunology and endometriosis. Fertil Steril 1992;58:262–8.
[446] Oosterlynck DJ, Mueleman C, Waer M, et al. Immunosuppressive activity of peritoneal fluid in women with endomedtriosis. Obstet Gynecol 1993;82:206–12.
[447] Dunselman GAJ, Hendrix MGR, Bouckaert PXJ, et al. Functional aspects of peritoneal macrophages in endometriosis of women. J Reprod Fertil 1988;82:707–10.
[448] Hammond MG, Oh ST, Anners J, et al. The effect of growth factors on the proliferation of human endometrial stromal cells in culture. Am J Obstet Gynecol 1993;168:1131–6.
[449] Iwabe T, Harada T, Tsudo T, et al. Tumour necrosis factor-α promotes proliferation of endometriotic stromal cells by inducing interleukin-8 gene and protein expression. J Clin Endocrinol Metab 2000;85:824–9.
[450] Osteen KG, Keller NR, Feltus FA, et al. Paracrine regulation of matrix metalloproteinase expression in the normal endometrium. Gynecol Obstet Invest 1999;48(Suppl.):2–13.
[451] Taylor RN, Ryan IP, Moore ES, et al. Angiogenesis and macrophage activation in endometriosis. Ann N Y Acad Sci 1997;828:194–207.
[452] Cunningham DS, Hansen KA, Coddington CC. Changes in T-cell regulation of responses to self antigens in women with pelvic endometriosis. Fertil Steril 1992;58:114–17.
[453] Kim DH, Chi JS, Kim JK, et al. Environmental factors in development of endometriosis. Kor J Obstet Gynecol 1998;41(3):746–56.
[454] Gleicher N, Dmowski WP, Siegel I, et al. Lymphocyte subsets in endometriosis. Obstet Gynecol 1984;63:463–7.
[455] Mathur S, Peress MR, Williamson HO, et al. Autoimmunity to endometrium and ovary in endometriosis. Clin Exper Immunol 1982;50(2):259–66.
[456] Evers JLH, Dunselman GAJ, Vanderlinden PJO. Markers for endometriosis. Clin Obstet Gynecol 1993;7:715–18.
[457] Muse K. Endometriosis and infertility. In: Wilson E, editor. Endometriosis. New York: Alan R Liss Inc; 1987.
[458] Prescott J, Farland LV, Tobias DK, et al. A prospective cohort study of endometriosis and subsequent risk of infertility. Hum Reprod 2016;31(7):1475–82.
[459] Wittich AC. Endometriosis in an episiotomy scar: review of the literature and report of case. J Am Osteopath Assoc 1982;82:22–3.
[460] Ohtake H, Katabuchi H, Matsuura K, et al. A novel in vitro experimental model for ovarian endometriosis: the three dimensional culture of human ovarian surface epithelial cells in collagen gels. Fertil Steril 1999;71:50–5.
[461] Halban J. Hysteroadenosis mctaplastica. Wien Klin Wochenschr 1924;37:1205–6.
[462] Berube S, Marcoux S, Maheux R, et al. Characteristics related to the prevalence of minimal or mild endometriosis in infertile women. Epidemiology 1998;9:504–10.
[463] Cullen TS. Adenomyoma of the uterus. Philadelphia: WB Saunders; 1908. Cited in: Kim AH, Adamson GD. Benign gynaecology: endometriosis. Global Library Women's Medicine; 2008.
[464] Haney AF, Muscato JJ, Weinberg JB. Peritoneal fluid cell populations in infertility patients. Fertil Steril 1981;35:696–8.
[465] Jones RK, Bulmer JN, Searle RF. Phenotypic and functional studies of leucocytes in human endometrium and endometriosis. Hum Reprod Update 1998;4:702–9.
[466] Nap AW, Groothuis PG, Demir AY, et al. Tissue integrity is essential for ectopic implantation of human endometrium in the chicken chorioallantoic membrane. Hum Reprod 2003;18:30–4.
[467] Dunselman GAJ, Bouckaert PXJM, Evers JLH. The acute-phase response in endometriosis of women. J Reprod Fertil 1988;83:803–8.
[468] Beliard A, Donnez J, Nisolle M, et al. Localization of laminin, fibronectin, E-cadherin, and integrins in endometrium and endometriosis. Fertil Steril 1997;67:266–72.
[469] van der Linden PJ, de Goeij AE, Dunselman GA, et al. Expression of cadherins and integrins in human endometrium throughout the menstrual cycle. Fertil Steril 1995;63:1210–16.
[470] Brooks PC, Sromblad S, Sanders LC, et al. Localization of matrix metalloproteinase MMP-2 to the surface of invasive cells by interaction with integrin alphav beta3. Cell 1996;85:683–93.
[471] Dechaud H, Craig A, Monotoya-Rodriguez IA, et al. Mesothelial cell-associated hyaluronic acid promotes adhesion of endometrial cells to mesothelium. Fertil Steril 2001;76:1012–18.

[472] Zeitoun KM, Bulun SE. Aromatase: a key molecule in the pathophysiology of endometriosis and a therapeutic target. Fertil Steril 1999;72:961–9.
[473] Gazvani R, Templeton A. Peritoneal environment, cytokines and angiogenesis in the pathophysiology of endometriosis. Reproduction 2002;123:217–26.
[474] Fujimoto J, Hori M, Ichigo S, et al. Expression of basic fibroblast growth factor and its mRNA in uterine endometrium during the menstrual cycle. Gynecol Endocrinol 1996;10:193–7.
[475] Mihalich A, Reina M, Mangioni S, et al. Different basic fibroblast growth factor and fibroblast growth factor-antisense expression in eutopic endometrial stromal cells derived from women with and without endometriosis. J Clin Endocrinol Metab 2003;88:2853–9.
[476] Osteen KG, Bruner-Tran KL, Eisenberg E. Reduced progesterone action during endometrial maturation: a potential risk factor for the development of endometriosis. Fertil Steril 2005;83(3):529–37.
[477] Attia GR, Zeitoun K, Edwards D, et al. Progesterone receptor isoform A but not B is expressed in endometriosis. J Clin Endocrinol Metab 2000;85:2897–902.
[478] Igarashi TM, Bruner-Tran KL, Yeaman GR, et al. Reduced expression of progesterone receptor-B in the endometrium of women with endometriosis and in cocultures of endometrial cells exposed to 2,3,7,8-tetrachlorodibenzo-p-dioxin. Fertil Steril 2005;84(1):67–74.
[479] Spuijbroek MDEH, Dunselman GAJ, Menheere PPAC, et al. Early endometriosis invades the extracellular matrix. Fertil Steril 1992;58:929–33.
[480] Salamonsen LA, Butt AR, Hammond FR, et al. Production of endometrial matrix metalloproteinases, but not their tissue inhibitors, is modulated by progesterone withdrawal in an in vitro model for menstruation. J Clin Endocrinol Metab 1997;82:1409–15.
[481] Martelli M, Campana A, Bischof P. Secretion of matrix metalloproteinases by human endometrial cells in vitro. J Reprod Fertil 1993;98:67–76.
[482] Chung HW, Lee JY, Moon HS, et al. Matrix metalloproteinase-2, membranous type 1 matrix metalloproteinase, and tissue inhibitor of metalloproteinase-2 expression in ectopic and eutopic endometrium. Fertil Steril 2002;78(4):787–95.
[483] Sharpe-Timms KL. Endometrial anomalies in women with endometriosis. Ann N Y Acad Sci 2001;943:131–47.
[484] McLaren J. Vascular endothelial growth factor and endometriotic angiogenesis. Hum Reprod Update 2000;6:45–55.
[485] Matsuzaki S, Canis M, Murakami T, et al. Immunohistochemical analysis of the role of angiogenic status in the vasculature of peritoneal endometriosis. Fertil Steril 2001;76(4):712–16.
[486] Halme J, Hammond M, Hulka J, et al. Retrograde menstruation in healthy women and in patients with endometriosis. Obstet Gynecol 1984;64:151–4.
[487] Nisolle M, Casanas-Roux F, Donnez J. Immunohistochemical analysis of proliferative activity and steroid receptor expression in peritoneal and ovarian endometriosis. Fertil Steril 1997;68:912–19.
[488] Khan KN, Kitajima M, Hiraki K, et al. Immunopathogenesis of pelvic endometriosis: role of hepatocyte growth factor, macrophages and ovarian steroids. Am J Reprod Immunol 2008;60:383–404.
[489] Harada T, Iwabe T, Terakawa N. Role of cytokines in endometriosis. Fertil Steril 2001;76:1–10.
[490] Halme J, Becker S, Haskill S. Altered maturation and function of peritoneal macrophages: possible role in pathogenesis of endometriosis. Am J Obstet Gynecol 1987;156:783–9.
[491] Khan KN, Kitajima M, Hiraki K, et al. *Escherichia coli* contamination of menstrual blood and effect of bacterial endotoxin on endometriosis. Fertil Steril 2010;94:2860–3.e1–3.
[492] Khan KN, Fujishita A, Kitajima M, et al. Intra-uterine microbial colonization and occurrence of endometritis in women with endometriosis. Hum Reprod 2014;29:2446–56.
[493] Khan KN, Fujishita A, Masumoto H, et al. Molecular detection of intrauterine microbial colonization in women with endometriosis. Eur J Obstet Gynecol Reprod Biol 2016;199:69–75.
[494] Lin W-C, Chang CY-Y, Hsu Y-A, et al. Increased risk of endometriosis in patients with lower genital tract infection — a nationwide cohort study. Medicine (Baltimore) 2016;95(10):1–8.
[495] Cicinelli E, Trojano G, Mastromauro M, et al. Higher prevalence of chronic endometritis in women with endometriosis: a possible etiopathogenetic link. Fertil Steril 2017;108(2):289–95.
[496] Khan KN, Kitajima M, Inoue T, et al. 17β-Estradiol and lipopolysaccharide additively promote pelvic inflammation and growth of endometriosis. Reprod Sci 2015;22(5):585–94.
[497] Khan KN, Masuzaki H, Fujishita A, et al. Association of interleukin-6 and estradiol with hepatocyte growth factor in peritoneal fluid of women with endometriosis. Acta Obstet Gynecol Scand 2002;81(8):764–71.
[498] Ahn SH, Singh V, Tayade C. Biomarkers in endometriosis: challenges and opportunities. Fertil Steril 2017;107(3):523–32.
[499] Barton-Smith P, Ballard K, Kent ASH. Endometriosis: a general review and rationale for surgical therapy. Rev Gynaecol Perin Pract 2006;6:168–76.
[500] Konincks PR, Martin DC. Deep endometriosis: a consequence of infiltration or retraction or possibly adenomyosis externa? Fertil Steril 1992;58(5):924–8.
[501] Demco L. Mapping the source and character of pain due to endometriosis by patient-assisted laparoscopy. J Am Assoc Gynecol Laparosc 1998;5(3):241–5.
[502] Ferrero S, Esposito F, Abbamonte LH. Quality of sex life in women with endometriosis and deep dyspareunia. Fertil Steril 2005;83(3):573–9.
[503] Trelour SA, Martin NG, Kennedy SH, et al. Characteristics and symptoms in 3895 women diagnosed with endometriosis in an Australian epidemiological study. In: Ninth World Congress on Endometriosis; 2005: 85. Barton-Smith P, Ballard K, Kent ASH. Endometriosis: a general review and rationale for surgical therapy. Rev Gynaecol Perin Pract 2006;6:168–76. Cited in:.
[504] Ballard K, Lowton K, Wright J. What's the delay? A qualitative study of women's experiences of reaching a diagnosis of endometriosis. Fertil Steril 2006;86(5):1296–301.
[505] Practice Committee of the American Society for Reproductive Medicine. Endometriosis and infertility. Fertil Steril 2004;82:S40–5.
[506] Ledger WL. Endometriosis and infertility: an integrated approach. Int J Gynecol Obstet 1999;64(Suppl. 1):33–40.
[507] Bergqvist A, Theorell T. Changes in quality of life after hormonal treatment of endometriosis. Acta Obstet Gynecol Scand 2001;80(7):628–37.
[508] Lorençatto C, Petta CA, Navarro MJ, et al. Depression in women with endometriosis with and without chronic pelvic pain. Acta Obstet Gynecol Scand 2006;85(1):88–9.
[509] Waller KG, Shaw RW. Endometriosis, pelvic pain, and psychological functioning. Fertil Steril 1995;63(4):796–800.
[510] Renaer M, Vertommen H, Nijs P, et al. Psychological aspects of chronic pelvic pain in women. Am J Obstet Gynecol 1979;134:75–80.
[511] Brosens I, Puttemens P, Campo R, et al. Diagnosis of endometriosis: pelvic endoscopy and imaging techniques. Best Pract Res Clin Obstet Gynaecol 2004;18(2):285–303.
[512] Brosens I. Is mild endometriosis a progressive disease? Hum Reprod 1994;9:2209–11.
[513] Sharma D, Dahiya K, Duhan N, et al. Diagnostic laparoscopy in chronic pelvic pain. Arch Gynecol Obstet 2011;283(2):295–7.
[514] Howard FM. The role of laparoscopy in chronic pelvic pain: promise and pitfalls. Obstet Gynecol Surv 1993;48(6):357–87.
[515] Telimaa S, Kauppila A, Rönnberg L, et al. Elevated serum levels of endometrial secretory protein PP14 in patients with advanced endometriosis: suppression by treatment with danazol and high-dose medroxyprogesterone. Am J Obstet Gynecol 1989;161:866–71.
[516] Wild RA, Hirisave V, Bianco A, et al. Endometrial antibodies versus CA-125 for the detection of endometriosis. Fertil Steril 1991;55:90–4.
[517] Switchenko AC, Kauffman RS, Becker M. Are there antiendometrial antibodies in sera of women with endometriosis? Fertil Steril 1991;56:235–41.
[518] Hornung D, Xo H, Rehbein M, et al. A new diagnostic tool? CCR1 mRNA expression in peripheral blood leucocytes of patients with and without endometriosis is significantly differently expressed. Eur J Obstet Gynecol Reprod Biol 2004;125(Suppl. 1):S35.
[519] Moore J, Copely S, Morris J, et al. A systematic review of the accuracy of ultrasound in the diagnosis of endometriosis. Ultrasound Obstet Gynecol 2002;20(6):630–4.
[520] Chapron C, Vieira M, Chopin N, et al. Accuracy of rectal endoscopic ultrasonography and magnetic resonance imaging in the diagnosis of rectal involvement for patients presenting with deeply

infiltrating endometriosis. Ultrasound Obstet Gynecol 2004;24(2):175–9.
[521] Bazot M, Nassar J, Derai E, et al. Value of sonography and MR imaging for the evaluation of deep pelvic endometriosis. J Radiol 2005;86(5 Pt 1):461–7.
[522] Kennedy S, Bergqvist A, Chapron C, et al. ESHRE guide for the diagnosis and treatment of endometriosis. Hum Reprod 2004;20(10):2698–704.
[523] Signorile PG, Baldi A. Endometriosis: new concepts in the pathogenesis. Int J Biochem Cell Biol 2010;42(6):778–80.
[524] Allen C, Hopewell S, Prentice A, et al. Nonsteroidal anti-inflammatory drugs for pain in women with endometriosis. Cochrane Database Syst Rev 2009;CD004753.
[525] Nawathe A, Patwardhan S, Yates D, et al. Systematic review of the effects of aromatase inhibitors on pain associated with endometriosis. Br J Obstet Gynaecol 2008;115(7):818–22.
[526] Cook AS, Rock JA. The role of laparoscopy in the treatment of endometriosis. Fertil Steril 1991;55(4):663–80.
[527] Revelli A, Modotti M, Ansaldi C, et al. Recurrent endometriosis: a review of biological and clinical aspects. Obstet Gynecol Surv 1995;50(10):747–54.
[528] Beretta P, Franchi M, Ghezzi F, et al. Randomized clinical trial of two laparoscopic treatments of endometriomas: cystectomy versus drainage and coagulation. Fertil Steril 1998;70(6):1176–80.
[529] Vercellini P, Crosignani PG, Abbiati A, et al. The effect of surgery for symptomatic endometriosis: the other side of the story. Hum Reprod Update 2009;15(2):177–88.
[530] Johnson NP. A review of the use of lipiodol flushing for unexplained infertility. Treat Endocrinol 2005;4(4):233–43.
[531] Namnoum AB, Hickman TN, Goodman SB, et al. Incidence of symptom recurrence after hysterectomy for endometriosis. Fertil Steril 1995;64(5):898–902.
[532] Redwine DB. Endometriosis persisting after castration: clinical characteristics and results of surgical management. Obstet Gynecol 1994;83(3):405–13.
[533] Sutton CJ, Pooley AS, Ewen SP, et al. Follow-up report on a randomized controlled trial of laser laparoscopy in the treatment of pelvic pain associated with minimal to moderate endometriosis. Fertil Steril 1997;68(6):1070–4.
[534] Walker KG, Shaw RW. Gonadotrophin-releasing hormone analogues for the treatment of endometriosis: long-term follow-up. Fertil Steril 1993;59(3):511–15.
[535] Gordts S, Boeckx W, Brosens I. Microsurgery of endometriosis in infertile patients. Fertil Steril 1991;42:520.
[536] Parrazini F. Ablation of lesions or no treatment in minimal-mild endometriosis in infertile women: a randomised trial. Hum Reprod 1999;14:1332–4.
[537] Olive DL, Pritts EA. The treatment of endometriosis: a review of the evidence. Ann N Y Acad Sci 2002;955:217–22.
[538] Hughes E, Ferdorkow D, Collins J, et al. Ovulation suppression versus placebo in the treatment of endometriosis. In: Lilford R, Hughes E, Vandekerckhove P, editors. Subfertility module of the Cochrane Database Systematic Reviews. British Medical Journal Publishing Group; 1996.
[539] Jacobson TZ, Barlow DH, Koninckx PR, et al. Laparoscopic surgery for subfertility associated with endometriosis. Cochrane Database Syst Rev 2002;(4):CD001398.
[540] Chapron C, Querleu D, Bruhat MA, et al. Surgical complications of diagnostic and operative gynaecological laparoscopy: a series of 29966 cases. Hum Reprod 1998;13:867–72.
[541] Louis GM, Chen Z, Peterson CM, et al. Persistent lipophilic environmental chemicals and endometriosis: the ENDO Study. Environ Health Perspect 2012;120(6):811.
[542] Harlev A, Gupta S, Agarwal A. Targeting oxidative stress to treat endometriosis. Expert Opin Ther Targets 2015;19(11):1447–64.
[543] Sekhon LH, Agarwal A. Endometriosis and oxidative stress. In: Studies on women's health. Humana Press; 2013. p. 149–67.
[544] Parazzini F, Chiaffarino F, Surace M, et al. Selected food intake and risk of endometriosis. Hum Reprod 2004;19:1755–9.
[545] Ergenoğlu AM, Yeniel AÖ, Erbaş O, et al. Regression of endometrial implants by resveratrol in an experimentally induced endometriosis model in rats. Reprod Sci 2013;20(10):1230–6.
[546] Khanaki K, Nouri M, Ardekani AM, et al. Evaluation of the relationship between endometriosis and omega-3 and omega-6 polyunsaturated fatty acids. Iran Biomed J 2012;16(1):1.
[547] Netsu S, Konno R, Odagiri K, et al. Oral eicosapentaenoic acid supplementation as possible therapy for endometriosis. Fertil Steril 2008;90(4):1496–502.
[548] Missmer SA, Chavarro JE, Malspeis S, et al. A prospective study of dietary fat consumption and endometriosis risk. Hum Reprod 2010;25(6):1528–35.
[549] Rose DP, Lubin M, Connolly JM. Effects of diet supplementation with wheat bran on serum estrogen levels in the follicular and luteal phases of the menstrual cycle. Nutrition 1997;13(6):535–53.
[550] Darling AM, Chavarro JE, Malspeis S, et al. A prospective cohort study of vitamins B, C, E, and multivitamin intake and endometriosis. J Endometr 2013;5(1):17–26.
[551] Parazzini F, Chiaffarino F, Surace M, et al. Selected food intake and risk of endometriosis. Hum Reprod 2004;19(8):1755–9.
[552] Trabert B, Peters U, De Roos AJ, et al. Diet and risk of endometriosis in a population-based case–control study. Br J Nutr 2011;105(03):459–67.
[553] Patisaul HB, Jefferson W. The pros and cons of phytoestrogens. Front Neuroendocrinol 2010;31(4):400–19.
[554] Grodstein F, Goldman MB, Ryan L, et al. Relation of female and infertility to consumption of caffeinated beverages. Am J Epidemiol 1993;137:133–6.
[555] Wedick NM, Mantzoros CS, Ding EL, et al. The effects of caffeinated and decaffeinated coffee on sex hormone-binding globulin and endogenous sex hormone levels: a randomized controlled trial. Nutr J 2012;11:86.
[556] Chiaffarino F, Bravi F, Cipriani S, et al. Coffee and caffeine intake and risk of endometriosis: a meta-analysis. Eur J Nutr 2014;53(7):1573–9.
[557] Missmer SA, Chavarro JE, Malspeis S, et al. A prospective study of dietary fat consumption and endometriosis risk. Hum Reprod 2010;25(6):1528–35.
[558] Chiaffarino F, Parazzini F, La Vecchia C, et al. Diet and uterine myomas. Obstet Gynecol 1999;94:395–8.
[559] La Vechia C, Decarli A, Franceschi S. Dietary factors and the risk of breast cancer. Nutr Cancer 1987;10:205–18.
[560] Missmer SA, Cramer DW. The epidemiology of endometriosis. Obstet Gynecol Clin North Am 2003;30:1–19.
[561] Grodstein F, Goldman MB, Cramer DW. Infertility in women and moderate alcohol use. Am J Public Health 1994;84(9):1429–32.
[562] Muti P, Trevisan M, Micheli A, et al. Alcohol consumption and total estradiol in premenopausal women. Cancer Epidemiol Biomarkers Prev 1998;7(3):189–93.
[563] Mendelson JH, Lukas SE, Mello NK, et al. Acute alcohol effects on plasma estradiol levels in women. Psychopharmacology (Berl) 1988;94:464–7.
[564] Reichman ME, Judd JT, Longcope C, et al. Effects of alcohol consumption on plasma and urinary hormone concentrations in premenopausal women. J Natl Cancer Inst 1993;85:722–7.
[565] Sarkola T, Makisalo H, Fukunaga T, et al. Acute effect of alcohol on estradiol, estrone, progesterone, prolactin, cortisol, and luteinizing hormone in premenopausal women. Alcohol Clin Exp Res 1999;23:976–82.
[566] Eriksson CJ, Fukunaga T, Lindman R. Sex hormone response to alcohol. Nature 1994;369:711.
[567] Dorgan JF, Reichman ME, Judd JT, et al. The relation of reported alcohol ingestion to plasma levels of estrogens and androgens in premenopausal women [Maryland, United States]. Cancer Causes Control 1994;5:53–60.
[568] Mendelson JH, Lukas SE, Mello NK, et al. Acute alcohol effects on plasma estradiol levels in women. Psychopharmacology (Berl) 1988;94:464–7.
[569] Ginsburg ES. Estrogen, alcohol and breast cancer risk. J Ster Biochem Mol Biol 1999;69:299–306.
[570] Marziali M, Venza M, Lazzaro S, et al. Gluten-free diet: a new strategy for management of painful endometriosis related symptoms? Minerva Chir 2012;67(6):499–504.
[571] Ho S, Woodford K, Kukuljan S, et al. Comparative effects of A1 versus A2 beta-casein on gastrointestinal measures: a blinded randomised cross-over pilot study. Eur J Clin Nutr 2014;68(9):994–1000.
[572] Fugh-Berman A, Kronenberg F. Complementary and alternative medicine (CAM) in reproductive age women: a review of randomized controlled trials. Reprod Toxicol 2003;17:137–52.

[573] Harris HR, Chavarro JE, Malspeis S, et al. Dairy-food, calcium, magnesium, and vitamin D intake and endometriosis: a prospective cohort study. Am J Epidemiol 2013;177(5):420–30.
[574] Covens AL, Christopher P, Casper RF. The effect of dietary supplementation with fish oil fatty acids on surgically induced endometriosis in the rabbit. Fertil Steril 1988;49:698–703.
[575] Gazvani MR, Smith L, Haggarty P, et al. High omega-3:omega-6 fatty acid ratios in culture medium reduce endometrial-cell survival in combined endometrial gland and stromal cell cultures from women with and without endometriosis. Fertil Steril 2001;76(4):717–22.
[576] Attaman JA, Stanic AK, Kim M, et al. The anti-inflammatory impact of omega-3 polyunsaturated fatty acids during the establishment of endometriosis-like lesions. Am J Reprod Immunol 2014;72(4):392–402.
[577] Itoh H, Uchida M, Sashihara T, et al. *Lactobacillus gasseri* OLL2809 is effective especially on the menstrual pain and dysmenorrhea in endometriosis patients: randomized, double-blind, placebo-controlled study. Cytotechnology 2011;63(2):153–61.
[578] Pizzorno J, Murray M. Textbook of natural medicine. 3rd ed. St Louis: Elsevier; 2006.
[579] Laschke MW, Menger MD. The gut microbiota: a puppet master in the pathogenesis of endometriosis? Am J Obstet Gynecol 2016;215(1):68.e1–e4.
[580] Turner RJ, Finch JM. Selenium and the immune response. Proc Nutr Soc 1991;50(2):275–85.
[581] Xue H, Wang W, Li Y, et al. Selenium upregulates $CD4^{=}CD25^{=}$ regulatory T cells in iodine-induced autoimmune thyroiditis model of NOD.H-2^{h4} mice. Endocr J 2010;57(7):595–601.
[582] Ceko MJ, Hummitzsch K, Hatzirodos N, et al. X-ray fluorescence imaging and other analyses identify selenium and GPX1 as important in female reproductive function. Metallomics 2015;7(1):71–82.
[583] Guerrero HCA, Montenegro BL, Diaz DLJ, et al. Endometriosis and deficienct intake of antioxidants molecules related to reipheral and peritoneal oxidative stress. Ginecol Obstet Mex 2006;74(1):20–8.
[584] Shelat VG, Low CH. Scar endometriosis. Aust N Z J Surg 2009;79(4):311–12.
[585] Hirsch K, Atzmon A, Danilenko M, et al. Lycopene and other carotenoids inhibit estrogenic activity of 17beta-estradiol and genistein in cancer cells. Breast Cancer Res Treat 2007;104(2):221–30.
[586] Van Gorp T, Amant F, Neven P, et al. Endometriosis and the development of malignant tumours of the pelvis. A review of literature. Best Pract Res Clin Obstet Gynaecol 2004;18(2):349–71.
[587] Kontoravdis A, Augoulea A, Lambrinoudaki I, et al. Ovarian endometriosis associated with ovarian cancer and endometrial-endocervical polyps. J Obstet Gynaecol Res 2007;33(3):294–8.
[588] Czeczuga-Semeniuk E, Wolczynski S. Identification of carotenoids in ovarian tissue in women (Abstract only). Oncol Rep 2005;14(5):1385–92.
[589] Berkkanoglu M, Arici A. Immunology and endometriosis. Am J Reprod Immunol 2003;50(1):48–59.
[590] Van Langendonckt A, Casanas-Roux F, Donnez J. Oxidative stress and peritoneal endometriosis. Fertil Steril 2002;77(5):861–70.
[591] Kyama CM, Debrock S, Mwenda JM, et al. Potential involvement of the immune system in the development of endometriosis. Reprod Biol Endocrinol 2003;1:123.
[592] Faserl K, Golderer G, Kremser L, et al. Polymorphism in vitamin D-binding protein as a genetic risk factor in the pathogenesis of endometriosis. J Clin Endocrinol Metab 2011;96(1):E233–41.
[593] Sayegh L, Fuleihan GE, Nassar AH. Vitamin D in endometriosis: a causative or confounding factor? Metabolism 2014;63(1):32–41.
[594] Cheung JP, Tsang HH, Cheung JJ, et al. Adjuvant therapy for the reduction of postoperative intra-abdominal adhesion formation. Asian J Surg 2009;32(3):180–6.
[595] Seeber BE, Czech T, Buchner H, et al. The vitamin E–binding protein afamin is altered significantly in the peritoneal fluid of women with endometriosis. Fertil Steril 2010;94(7):2923–6.
[596] Murphy AA, Santanam N, Parthasarathy S. Endometriosis: a disease of oxidative stress? Semin Reprod Endocrinol 1998;16(4):263–73.
[597] Kagoma P, Burger SN, Seifter E, et al. The effect of vitamin E on experimentally induced peritoneal adhesions in mice. Arch Surg 1985;120(8):949–51.
[598] Sanfilippo JS, Booth RJ, Burns CD. Effect of vitamin E on adhesion formation (Abstract only). J Reprod Med 1995;40(4):278–82.
[599] Prasad AS. Impact of the discovery of human zinc deficiency on health. J Am Coll Nutr 2009;28(3):257–65.
[600] Messalli EM, Schettino MT, Mainini G, et al. The possible role of zinc in the etiopathogenesis of endometriosis. Clin Exper Obstet Gynecol 2014;41(5):541–6.
[601] Mokhtari V, Afsharian P, Shahhoseini M, et al. A review on various uses of N-acetyl cysteine. Cell J (Yakhteh) 2017;19(1):11–17.
[602] Ngô C, Chéreau C, Nicco C, et al. Reactive oxygen species controls endometriosis progression. Am J Pathol 2009;175(1):225–34.
[603] Pittaluga E, Costa G, Krasnowska E, et al. More than antioxidant: N-acetyl-L-cysteine in a murine model of endometriosis. Fertil Steril 2010;94(7):2905–8.
[604] Porpora MG, Brunelli R, Costa G, et al. A promise in the treatment of endometriosis: an observational cohort study on ovarian endometrioma reduction by N-acetylcysteine. Evid Based Complement Alternat Med 2013;240702.
[605] National Standards monograph. Accessed online at http://naturalstandard.com.
[606] Bashir S, Janbaz KH, Jabeen Q, et al. Studies on spasmogenic and spasmolytic activities of *Calendula officinalis* flowers. Phytother Res 2006;20:906–10.
[607] Safdar W, Majeed H, Naveed I, et al. Pharmacognostical study of the medicinal plant *Calendula officinalis* L.(family Compositae). Int J Cell Mol Biol 2010;1:108–16.
[608] Zhang RX, Li MX, Jia ZP. *Rehmannia glutinosa*: review of botany, chemistry and pharmacology. J Ethnopharmacol 2008;117(2):199–218.
[609] Porpora MG, Medda E, Abballe A, et al. Endometriosis and organochlorinated environmental pollutants: a case-control study on Italian women of reproductive age. Environ Health Perspect 2009;117(7):1070–5.
[610] Khan A, Craig M, Jarmulowicz M, et al. Liver tumours due to endometriosis and endometrial stromal sarcoma. HPB (Oxford) 2002;4(1):43–5.
[611] Nicholson JA, Darby TD, Jarboe CH. Viopudial, a hypotensive and smooth muscle antispasmodic from Viburnum opulus. Proc Soc Exp Biol Med 1972;140(2):457–61.
[612] Cometa MF, Parisi L, Palmery M, et al. In vitro relaxant and spasmolytic effects of constituents from *Viburnum prunifolium* and HPLC quantification of the bioactive isolated iridoids. J Ethnopharmacol 2009;123(2):201–7.
[613] Chen Q, Gao Q, Chen K, et al. Curcumin suppresses migration and invasion of human endometrial carcinoma cells. Oncol Lett 2015;10(3):1297–302.
[614] Jana S, Rudra DS, Paul S, et al. Curcumin delays endometriosis development by inhibiting MMP-2 activity. Indian J Biochem Biophys 2012;49:342–8.
[615] Zhang Y, Cao H, Yu Z, et al. Curcumin inhibits endometriosis endometrial cells by reducing estradiol production. Iran J Reprod Med 2013;11(5):415–22.
[616] El-Ashmawy IM, Ashry KM, El-Nahas AF, et al. Protection by turmeric and myrrh against liver oxidative damage and genotoxicity induced by lead acetate in mice. Basic Clin Pharmacol Toxicol 2006;98(1):32–7.
[617] Cony Y, Wang L, Konrad A, et al. Curcumin induces the tolerogenic dendritic cell that promotes differentiation of intestine-protective regulatory T cells. Eur J Immunol 2009;39(11):3134–46.
[618] Harris T, Vlass AM. Can herbal medicines improve cellular immunity patterns in endometriosis. Med Aromat Plants 2015;4(184).
[619] Laschke MW, Schwender C, Scheuer C, et al. Epigallocatechin-3-gallate inhibits estrogen-induced activation of endometrial cells in vitro and causes regression of endometriotic lesions in vivo. Hum Reprod 2008;23(10):2308–18.
[620] Ricci AG, Olivares CN, Bilotas MA, et al. Natural therapies assessment for the treatment of endometriosis. Hum Reprod 2013;28(1):178–88.
[621] Wang CC, Xu H, Man GC, et al. Prodrug of green tea epigallocatechin-3-gallate (Pro-EGCG) as a potent anti-angiogenesis agent for endometriosis in mice. Angiogenesis 2013;16(1):59–69.

[622] Xu H, Becker CM, Lui WT, et al. Green tea epigallocatechin-3-gallate inhibits angiogenesis and suppresses vascular endothelial growth factor C/vascular endothelial growth factor receptor 2 expression and signaling in experimental endometriosis in vivo. Fertil Steril 2011;96(4):1021–8.
[623] Xu H, Lui WT, Chu CY, et al. Anti-angiogenic effects of green tea catechin on an experimental endometriosis mouse model. Hum Reprod 2009;24(3):608–18.
[624] Chu M, Ding R, Chu Z, et al. Role of berberine in anti-bacterial as a high-affinity LPS antagonist binding to TLR4/MD-2 receptor. BMC Complement Altern Med 2014;14:89.
[625] Kumar R, Nair V, Gupta YK, et al. *Berberis aristata* ameliorates adjuvant-induced arthritis by inhibition of NF-κB and activating nuclear factor-E2-related factor 2/hem oxygenase (HO)-1 signaling pathway. Immunol Invest 2016;45(6):473–89.
[626] Chedid V, Dhalla S, Clarke JO, et al. Herbal therapy is equivalent to rifaximin for the treatment of small intestinal bacterial overgrowth. Glob Adv Health Med 2014;3(3):16–24.
[627] Gu L, Li N, Gong J, et al. Berberine ameliorates intestinal epithelial tight-junction damage and down-regulates myosin light chain kinase pathways in a mouse model of endotoxinemia. J Infect Dis 2011;203(11):602–1612.
[628] Ricci E, Viganò P, Cipriani S, et al. Physical activity and endometriosis risk in women with infertility or pain: systematic review and meta-analysis. Medicine (Baltimore) 2016;95(40): e4957.
[629] Ishii S, Katagiri R, Kataoka T, et al. Risk assessment study of dioxins in sanitary napkins produced in Japan. Regul Toxicol Pharmacol 2014;70(1):357–62.
[630] Centers for Disease Control and Prevention (CDC). 2015 sexually transmitted diseases surveillance [Internet]. CDC; 2016. Available from: https://www.cdc.gov/std/stats15/womenandinf.htm.
[631] Shepherd SM. Pelvic inflammatory disease. eMedicine; 2010. Available from: http://emedicine.medscape.com/article/256448.
[632] Price MJ, Ades AE, Welton NJ, et al. Proportion of pelvic inflammatory disease cases caused by *Chlamydia trachomatis*: consistent picture from different methods. J Infect Dis 2016;214(4):617–24.
[633] Romero R, Espinoza J, Mazor M. Can endometrial infection/ inflammation explain implantation failure, spontaneous abortion, and preterm birth after in vitro fertilization? Fertil Steril 2004;82(4):799–804.
[634] Low N, Broutet N, Adu-Sarkodie Y, et al. Global control of sexually transmitted infections. Lancet 2006;368(9551):2001–16.
[635] Sorbye IK, Jerve F, Staff AC. Reduction in hospitalized women with pelvic inflammatory disease in Oslo over the past decade. Acta Obstet Gynecol Scand 2005;84(3):290–6.
[636] Eggar M, Low N, Davey Smith G, et al. Screening for Chlamydial infections and the risk of ectopic: ecological study. Br Med J 1998;316:1776–80.
[637] Hack JB, Hecht C. Emergency physicians' patterns of treatment for presumed gonorrhoea and *Chlamydia* in women: one centre's practice. J Emerg Med 2009;37(3):257–63.
[638] Centers for Disease Control and Prevention, Workowski KA, Berman SM. Sexually transmitted diseases treatment guidelines; 2006. MMWR Recomm Rep 2006;55(RR–11):1–94.
[639] Cherpes TL, Wiesenfeld HC, Melan MA, et al. The associations betweeen pelvic inflammatory disease, *Trichomonas vaginalis* infection, and positive herpes simplex virus type 2 serology. Sex Transm Dis 2006;33:747–52.
[640] Ross JD. Is *Mycoplasma genitalium* a cause of pelvic inflammatory disease? Infect Dis Clin North Am 2005;19(2):407–13.
[641] Eschenbach DA. Acute pelvic inflammatory disease. Global Library Women's Medicine; 2008.
[642] Viberga I, Odlind V, Lazdane G, et al. Microbiology profile in women with pelvic inflammatory disease in relation to IUD use. Infect Dis Obstet Gynaecol 2005; 13(4):183–90.
[643] Avan BI, Fatmi Z, Rashid S. Comparison of clinical and laparascopic features of infertile women suffering from genital tuberculosis (TB) or pelvic inflammatory disease (PID) or endometriosis. J Pak Med Assoc 2001;51(11):393–9.
[644] Rhoton-Vlasak A. Infections and infertility. Prim Care Update Ob Gyns 2000;7(5):200–6.
[645] Paavonen J. *Chlamydia trachomatis* infection from diagnosis to treatment and prevention. In: Kempers RD, Cohen JC, Haney AF, et al, editors. Fertility and reproductive medicine. Amsterdam: Elsevier; 1998.
[646] Barrett S, Taylor C. A review on pelvic inflammatory disease. Review-continuing education. Int J STD AIDS 2005;16:715–21.
[647] Ness RB, Trautmann G, Richter HE, et al. Effectiveness of treatment strategies of some women with pelvic inflammatory disease: a randomized trial. Obstet Gynecol 2005;106:573–80.
[648] Moller BR, Mardh P-A, Akrons S, et al. Infection with *Chlamydia trachomatis*, *Mycoplasma hominis*, and *Neisseria gonorrhoeae* in patients with acute pelvic inflammatory disease. Am Ven Dis 1981;8:198–205.
[649] Paavonen J. Pelvic inflammatory disease. Medicine (Baltimore) 2005;33(10):43–6.
[650] Bevan CD, Johal BJ, Mumtaz G, et al. Clinical, laparoscopic and microbiological findings in acute salpingitis: a report on a United Kingdom cohort. Br J Obstet Gynaecol 1995;102:407–18.
[651] Baveja G, Saini S, Sangwan K, et al. A study of bacterial pathogens in acute pelvic inflammatory disease. J Commun Dis 2001;33:121–5.
[652] Hillis SD, Joesoef R, Marchbanks PA, et al. Delayed care of pelvic inflammatory disease as a risk for impaired fertility. Am J Obstet Gynecol 1993;168:1503–9.
[653] Hillier SL, Krohn MA, Rabe LK, et al. The normal vaginal flora, H2O2-producing lactobacilli and bacterial vaginosis in pregnant women. Clin Infect Dis 1993;16(Suppl. 4):S273–5.
[654] Yudin MH, Hillier SL, Weisenfield HC. Vaginal polymorphonuclear leucocytes and bacterial vaginosis as markers for histological endometritis among women without symptoms of pelvic inflammatory disease. Am J Obstet Gynecol 2003;188:318–23.
[655] Weisenfeld HC, Hillier SL, Krohn MA, et al. Lower genital tract infection and endometritis: insight into subclinical pelvic inflammatory disease. Obstet Gynecol 2002;100:456–63.
[656] Korn AP, Bolan G, Padian N, et al. Plasma cell endometritis in women with symptomatic endometritis. Am J Obstet Gynecol 1995;85:387–90.
[657] Paavonen J, Tiesala K, Heinonen PK, et al. Microbiological and histological findings in acute pelvic inflammatory disease. Br J Obstet Gynaecol 1978;94:454–60.
[658] Hillier SL, Kiviat NB, Hawes SE, et al. Role of BV-associated micro-organisms in endometritis. Am J Obstet Gynecol 1996;175:435–41.
[659] Paavonen J, Kiviat N, Brunham RC, et al. Prevalence and manifestation of endometritis among women with cervicitis. Am J Obstet Gynecol 1985;152:280–5.
[660] Brunham RC, Paavonen J, Stevens CE, et al. Mucopurulent cervicitis: the ignored counterpart in women of urethritis in men. N Engl J Med 1984;311:1–6.
[661] Manhart LE, Critchlow CW, Holmes KK, et al. Mucopurulent cervicitis and *Mycoplasma genitalium*. J Infect Dis 2003;187:650–7.
[662] James AN, Knox JM, Williams PR. Attachment of gonococci to sperm: influence of physical and chemical factors. Br J Vener Dis 1976;52:128–35.
[663] Draper DL, James JF, Brooks GF, et al. Comparison of virulence markers of peritoneal and fallopian tube isolates with endocervical *N. gonorrhoeae* isolates from women with acute salpingitis. Infect Immun 1980;27:88888.
[664] Zucherman H, Kahane A, Carmel S. Antibacterial activity of human cervical mucus. Gynecol Invest 1975;6:265–71.
[665] Wolner-Hanssen P, Mardh P-A. In vitro tests of adherence of *Chlamydia trachomatis* to human spermatozoa. Fertil Steril 1984;42:102–7.
[666] Pizzorno J, Murray M. Textbook of natural medicine. 3rd ed. St Louis: Elsevier; 2006.
[667] Van Voorhis WC, Barrett LK, Cosgrove Sweeney C, et al. Analysis of lymphocyte phenotype and cytokine activity in the inflammatory infiltrates of the upper genital tract of female macaques infected with *Chlamydia trachomatis*. J Infect Dis 1996;174:647–51.
[668] Kimani J, Maclean IW, Bwayo JJ, et al. Risk factors for *Chlamydia trachomatis* pelvic inflammatory disease among sex workers in Nairobi, Kenya. J Infect Dis 1996;173:1437–44.
[669] Ness RB, Brunham RC, Shen C, et al; PID Evaluation Clinical Health (PEACH) study investigators. Associations among human leucocyte antigen (HLA) class II DQ variants, bacterial sexually transmitted diseases, endometritis, and fertility among women

with clinical pelvic inflammatory disease. Sex Transm Dis 2004;31:301–4.
[670] Brunham RC, Pourbohloul B, Mak S, et al. The unexpected impact of a *Chlamydia trachomatis* infection control program on susceptibility to reinfection. J Infect Dis 2005;192:1836–44.
[671] Champion JD, Piper J, Shain RN, et al. Minority women with sexually transmitted diseases: sexual abuse and risk for pelvic inflammatory disease. Res Nurs Health 2001;24(1):38–43.
[672] Ness RB, Soper DE, Holley RL, et al. Hormonal and barrier contraception and risk of upper genital tract disease in the pelvic inflammatory disease evaluation and clinical health study. Am J Obstet Gynecol 2001;185:121–7.
[673] Weström L. Incidence, prevalence, and trends of acute pelvic inflammatory disease and its consequences in industrialized countries. Am J Obstet Gynecol 1980;138:880–92.
[674] Washington A, Aral S, Wolner-Hanssen P, et al. Assessing risk for pelvic inflammatory disease and its sequelae. JAMA 1991;266:2581–6.
[675] Gareen IF, Cleveland S, Morgenstern H. Intrauterine devices and pelvic inflammatory disease: meta-analyses of published studies 1974–1990. Epidemiology 2000;11:589–97.
[676] Senanayake P, Kramer DG. Contraception and the etiology of pelvic inflammatory disease: new perspectives. Am J Obstet Gynecol 1980;138:852–7.
[677] Daling JR, Weiss NS, Voigt LF, et al. The intrauterine device and primary tubal infertility. N Engl J Med 1992;326:203–4.
[678] Tatum HJ, Schmidt FA, Phillips D, et al. The Dalkon shield controversy: structural and bacteriological studies of IUD tails. JAMA 1975;231(7):711–17.
[679] Banks HL, Williamson HO. Scanning electron microscopy of Dalkon shield tails. Fertil Steril 1983;40(3):334–7.
[680] Ellish NJ, Weisman CS, Celentaro D, et al. Reliability of partner reports of sexual history in a heterosexual population at a sexually transmitted disease clinic. Sex Transm Dis 1996;23:446–52.
[681] Wolner-Hanssen P, Eschenbach DA, Paavonen J, et al. Decreased risk of symptomatic chlamydial pelvic inflammatory disease associated with oral contraceptive use. JAMA 1990;263:54–9.
[682] Cottingham J, Hunter D. *Chlamydia trachomatis* and oral contraceptive use: a quantitative review. Genitourin Med 1992;68:209–16.
[683] Wolner-Hanssen P, Eschenbach DA, Paavonen J, et al. Association between vaginal douching and acute pelvic inflammatory disease. JAMA 1990;263:1936–41.
[684] Ness RB, Hillier SL, Kip KE, et al. Douching, pelvic inflammatory disease, and incident gonococcal and chlamydial genital infection in a cohort of high-risk women. Am J Epidemiol 2005;161:186–95.
[685] Eschenbach DA, Buchanan TM, Pollock HM, et al. Polymicrobial etiology of acute pelvic inflammatory disease. N Engl J Med 1975;293:166–71.
[686] Weström L, Mardh PA. Chlamydial salpingitis. Br Med Bull 1983;39:145–7.
[687] Gareen IF, Cleveland S, Morgenstern H. Intrauterine devices and pelvic inflammatory disease: meta-analyses of published studies 1974–1990. Epidemiology 2000;11:589–97.
[688] Giertz G, Kallings I, Nordenvall M, et al. A prospective study of *Chlamydia trachomatis* infection following legal abortion. Acta Obstet Gynecol Scand 1987;66:107–11.
[689] Ross JD. What is endometritis and does it need treatment? Sex Transm Infect 2004;80:252–3.
[690] Safrin S, Dattel BJ, Hauer L, et al. Seroprevalence and epidemiologic correlates of human immunodeficiency virus infections in women with acute pelvic inflammatory disease. Obstet Gynecol 1990;75:666–70.
[691] Cohen C, Sinei S, Reilly M, et al. Effect of human immunodeficiency virus type I infection upon acute salpingitis: a laparoscopic study. J Infect Dis 1998;178:1352–6.
[692] Irwin KI. Potential for bias in studies of the influence of human immunodeficiency virus infection on the recognition, incidence, clinical course, and microbiology of pelvic inflammatory disease. Obstet Gynecol 1994;84:463–8.
[693] Falk V. Treatment of acute non-tuberculous salpingitis with antibiotics alone and in combination with glucocorticoids. A prospective double blind controlled study of the clinical course and prognosis. Acta Obstet Gynecol Scand 1965;44(Suppl. 6):3–118. Cited in: Eschenbach DA. Acute pelvic inflammatory disease. Global Library Women's Medicine; 2008.
[694] Centers for Disease Control and Prevention. Ectopic pregnancy — United States, 1990–1992. MMWR Morb Mortal Wkly Rep 1995;44:46.
[695] Khalaf Y. Tubal subfertility. Br Med J 2003;327:610–13.
[696] Joesoef R, Westrom L, Reynolds G, et al. Recurrence of ectopic pregnancy: the role of salpingitis. Am J Obstet Gynecol 1991;165:46–50.
[697] Weström L, Svensson L, et al. Chronic pain after acute pelvic inflammatory disease. In: Belfort P, editor. Advances in gynecology and obstetrics. Proceedings of the XIIth World Congress of Gynecology and Obstetrics, Rio de Janeiro. 1988. p. 265.
[698] Adler MW, Belsey EH, O'Connor BH. Morbidity associated with pelvic inflammatory disease. Br J Vener Dis 1982;58:151–4.
[699] Khatamee MA. Infertility: a preventable epidemic? Int J Fertil 1988;34:246–51.
[700] Hull MG, Glazener CM, Kelly NJ, et al. Population study of causes, treatment, and outcome of infertility. Br Med J 1985;291:1693–7.
[701] Cates W, Rolfs RT Jr, Aral SO. Sexually transmitted diseases, pelvic inflammatory disease, and infertility: an epidemiologic update. Epidemiol Rev 1990;12:199–220.
[702] Weström L. Effect of acute pelvic inflammatory disease on fertility. Am J Obstet Gynecol 1975;121:707–13.
[703] Westrom L. Incidence, prevalence, and trends of acute pelvic inflammatory disease and its consequences in industrialized countries. Am J Obstet Gynecol 1980;138:880–4.
[704] Khan ZE, Rizvi JH. Pelvic inflammatory disease and pelvic abscesses. Rev Gynecol Perin Pract 2006;6(3–4):185–91.
[705] Patton DL, Esquenazi B, Shevchuk M, et al. Association between *Chlamydia trachomatis* and abnormal uterine bleeding. Am J Reprod Immunol 2007;57(5):361–6.
[706] Peipert JF, Ness RB, Blume J, et al. Clinical predictors of endometritis in women with symptoms and signs of pelvic inflammatory disease. Am J Obstet Gynecol 2001;184(5):856–63.
[707] Molander P, Finne P, Sjöberg J, et al. Observer agreement with laparoscopic diagnosis of pelvic inflammatory disease using photographs. Obstet Gynecol 2003;101(5 Pt 1):875–80.
[708] Risser WL, Risser JM, Benjamins LJ, et al. Incidence of Fitz-Hugh-Curtis syndrome in adolescents who have pelvic inflammatory disease. J Pediatr Adolesc Gynecol 2007;20(3):179–80.
[709] Dabeekausen YA, Evers JL, Land JA, et al. *Chlamydial trachomatis* antibody testing is more accurate than hysterosalpingography in predicting tubal factor infertility. Fertil Steril 1994;61:833–7.
[710] Centers for Disease Control and Prevention. CDC guidelines for treatment of sexually transmitted diseases: recommendations and reports. MMWR Recomm Rep 1998;47:49–87.
[711] Klein TA, Richmond JA, Michell DR Jr. Pelvic tuberculosis. Obstet Gynecol 1976;48:99–104.
[712] Tukeva TA, Aronen HJ, Karjalainen PT, et al. MR imaging in pelvic inflammatory disease: comparison with laparoscopy and US. Radiology 1999;210(1):209–16.
[713] Haggerty CL, Ness RB. Newest approaches to treatment of pelvic inflammatory disease: a review of recent randomized clinical trials. Clin Infect Dis 2007;44(7):953–60.
[714] Ness RB, Soper DE, Holley RL, et al; for the Pelvic Inflammatory Disease Evaluation and Clinical Health (PEACH) Study Investigators. Effectiveness of inpatient and outpatient treatment strategies for women with pelvic inflammatory disease: results from the Pelvic Inflammatory Disease Evaluation and Clinical Health (PEACH) randomized trial. Am J Obstet Gynecol 2001;186:929–37.
[715] Murray M. The immune factor. Canada: Mind Publishing Inc; 2001.
[716] Fitzhugh DJ, Shan S, Dewhirst MW, et al. Bromelain treatment decreases neutrophil migration to sites of inflammation. Clin Immunol 2008;128(1):66–74.
[717] Maurer HR. Bromelain: biochemistry, pharmacology and medical use. Cell Mol Life Sci 2001;58(9):1234–45.
[718] Crossman SH. The challenge of pelvic inflammatory disease. Am Fam Physician 2006;73(5):859–64.
[719] Sawatsri S, Desai N, Rock JA, et al. Retinoic acid suppresses interleukin-6 production in human endometrial cells. Fertil Steril 2000;73(5):1012–19.
[720] Greenberg SB, Harris D, Giles P, et al. Inhibition of *Chlamydia trachomatis* growth in McCoy, HeLa, and human prostate cells by

zinc (Abstract only). Antimicrob Agents Chemother 1985;27(6):953–7.

[721] Böhler K, Meisinger V, Klade H, et al. Zinc levels of serum and cervicovaginal secretion in recurrent vulvovaginal candidiasis. Genitourin Med 1994;70(5):308–10.

[722] Saper RB, Rash R. Zinc: an essential micronutrient. Am Fam Physician 2009;79(9):768–72.

[723] Adetumbi MA, Lau BH. *Allium sativum* (garlic) — a natural antibiotic. Med Hypotheses 1983;12(3):227–37.

[724] Blumenthal M, editor. The complete German Commission E monographs. Austin: American Botanical Council; 1998.

[725] Berberine. Altern Med Rev 2000;5(2):175–7. [No authors listed].

[726] Basch E, Bent S, Foppa I, Natural Standard Research Collaboration, et al. Marigold (*Calendula officinalis* L.): an evidence-based systematic review by the Natural Standard Research Collaboration. J Herb Pharmacother 2006;6(3–4):135–59.

[727] Clement-Kruzel S, Hwang SA, Kruzel MC, et al. Immune modulation of macrophage pro-inflammatory response by goldenseal and Astragalus extracts. J Med Food 2008;11(3):493–8.

[728] Carson CF, Hammer KA, Riley TV. *Melaleuca alternifolia* (tea tree) oil: a review of antimicrobial and other medicinal properties. Clin Microbiol Rev 2006;19(1):50–62.

[729] Basch E, Ulbricht C, Hammerness P, et al. Thyme (*Thymus vulgaris* L.), thymol. J Herb Pharmacother 2004;4(1):49–67.

[730] Pizzorno J, Murray M. Textbook of natural medicine. 4th ed. Churchill Livingstone; 2012.

[731] Walsh RJ. The age of the menopause of Australian women. Med J Aust 1978;2(5):181–2, 215.

[732] World Health Technical Report Series. Research on the menopause in the 1990s. World Health Organization Geneva; 1996.

[733] Woad KJ, Watkins WJ, Prendergast D, et al. The genetic basis of premature ovarian failure. Aust N Z J Obstet Gynaecol 2006;46:242–4.

[734] Luborsky JL, Meyer P, Sowers MF, et al. Premature menopause in a multi-ethnic population study of the menopause transition. Hum Reprod 2003;18(1):199–206.

[735] Hardman SM, Gebbie AE. Hormonal contraceptive regimens in the perimenopause. Maturitas 2009;63(3):204–12.

[736] Nelson H. Menopause. Lancet 2008;371(9614):760–70, 1.

[737] Vermeulen A. Environment, human reproduction, menopause, and andropause. Environ Health Perspect 1993;101(Suppl. 2):91–100.

[738] Cooper AR, Baker VL, Sterling EW, et al. The time is now for a new approach to primary ovarian insufficiency. Fertil Steril 2011;95(6):1890–7.

[739] Northrupp C, Lindquist O, Bengtsson C. The effect of smoking on menopausal age. Maturitas 1979;1(3):171–3.

[740] Midgette AS, Baron JA. Cigarette smoking and the risk of natural menopause. Epidemiology 1990;1(6):474–80.

[741] Kinney A, Kline J, Levin B. Alcohol, caffeine and smoking in relation to age at menopause. Maturitas 2006;54(1):27–38.

[742] Parente RC, Faerstein E, Celeste RK, et al. The relationship between smoking and age at the menopause: a systematic review. Maturitas 2008;61(4):287–98.

[743] Schoenaker DA, Jackson CA, Rowlands JV, et al. Socioeconomic position, lifestyle factors and age at natural menopause: a systematic review and meta-analyses of studies across six continents. Int J Epidemiol 2014;43(5):1542–62.

[744] Bromberger JT, Matthews KA, Kuller LH, et al. Prospective study of the determinants of age at menopause. Am J Epidemiol 1997;145:124–33.

[745] Voorhuis M, Onland-Moret NC, van der Schouw YT, et al. Human studies on genetics of the age at natural menopause: a systematic review. Hum Reprod Update 2010;16(4):364–77.

[746] Kevenaar ME, Themmen AP, Rivadeneira F, et al. A polymorphism in the AMH type II receptor gene is associated with age at menopause in interaction with parity. Hum Reprod 2007;22(9):2382–8.

[747] Taneri PE, Kiefte-de Jong JC, Bramer WM, et al. Association of alcohol consumption with the onset of natural menopause: a systematic review and meta-analysis. Hum Reprod Update 2016;22(4):516–28.

[748] Cui J, Yong S, Li R. Estrogen synthesis and signaling pathways during ageing: from periphery to brain. Trends Mol Med 2013;19(3):197–209.

[749] Woods NF, Mitchell ES. Symptoms during the perimenopause: prevalence, severity, trajectory, and significance in women's lives. Am J Med 2005;118(Suppl. 12B):14–24.

[750] Deecher DC, Dorries K. Understanding the pathophysiology of vasomotor symptoms (hot flushes and night sweats) that occur in perimenopause, menopause, and postmenopause life stages. Arch Womens Ment Health 2007;10(6):247–57.

[751] Guthrie JR, Dennerstein L, Taffe JR, et al. Hot flushes during the menopause transition: a longitudinal study in Australian-born women. Menopause 2005;12(4):460–7.

[752] Maltais ML, Desroches J, Dionne IJ. Changes in muscle mass and strength after menopause. J Musculoskelet Neuronal Interact 2009;9(4):186–97.

[753] MacBride MB, Rhodes DJ, Shuster LT. Vulvovaginal atrophy. Mayo Clin Proc 2010;85(1):87–94.

[754] Trichopoulos D, MacMahon B, Cole P. Menopause and breast cancer risk. J Natl Cancer Inst 1972;48(3):605–13.

[755] Matthews KA, Crawford SL, Chae CU, et al. Are changes in cardiovascular disease risk factors in midlife women due to chronological ageing or to the menopausal transition? J Am Coll Cardiol 2009;54(25):2366–73.

[756] Martin KA, Manson JE. Approach to the patient with menopausal symptoms. J Clin Endocrinol Metab 2008;93(12):4567–75.

[757] Singh A, Kaur S, Walia I. A historical perspective on menopause and menopausal age (Abstract only). Bull Indian Inst Hist Med Hyderabad 2002;32(2):121–35.

[758] Stolberg M. [From 'anni climacterici' to 'menopause.' The historical roots of the concept of 'climacteric']. (Abstract only). Wurzbg Medizinhist Mitt 2005;24:41–50.

[759] Boericke W. Boericke's Materia Medica; 1901. Excerpt: The tinctures.

[760] The Women's Health Initiative Steering Committee. Effects of conjugated equine estrogen in postmenopausal women with hysterectomy. The Women's Health Initiative randomized controlled trial. JAMA 2004;291:1701–12.

[761] Umland EM. Treatment strategies for reducing the burden of menopause-associated vasomotor symptoms. J Manag Care Pharm 2008;14(Suppl. 3):14–19.

[762] Liu ZM, Ho SC, Xie YJ, et al. Associations between dietary patterns and psychological factors: a cross-sectional study among Chinese postmenopausal women. Menopause 2016;23(12):1294–302.

[763] Brzezinski A, Adlercreutz H, Shaoul R, et al. Short-term effects of phytoestrogen-rich diet on postmenopausal women. Menopause 1997;4(2):89–94.

[764] Chen MN, Lin CC, Liu CF. Efficacy of phytoestrogens for menopausal symptoms: a meta-analysis and systematic review. Climacteric 2015;18(2):260–9.

[765] Franco OH, Chowdhury R, Troup J, et al. Use of plant-based therapies and menopausal symptoms: a systematic review and meta-analysis. JAMA 2016;315(23):2554–63.

[766] Taku K, Melby MK, Kronenberg F, et al. Extracted or synthesized soybean isoflavones reduce menopausal hot flash frequency and severity: systematic review and meta-analysis of randomized controlled trials. Menopause 2012;19(7):776–90.

[767] Li L, Lv Y, Xu L, et al. Quantitative efficacy of soy isoflavones on menopausal hot flashes. Br J Clin Pharmacol 2015;79(4):593–604.

[768] Carroll D. Nonhormonal therapies for hot flashes in menopause. Am Fam Physician 2006;73:457–64, 467.

[769] Messina M. Soy foods, isoflavones, and the health of postmenopausal women. Am J Clin Nutr 2014;100(Suppl. 1):423S–430S.

[770] Vincent A, Fitzpatrick L. Soy isoflavones: are they useful in menopause? Mayo Clin Proc 2000;75(11):1174–84.

[771] Simbalista RL, Sauerbronn AV, Aldrighi JM, et al. Consumption of a flaxseed-rich food is not more effective than a placebo in alleviating the climacteric symptoms of postmenopausal women. J Nutr 2010;140(2):293–7.

[772] Pruthi S, Thompson SL, Novotny PJ, et al. Pilot evaluation of flaxseed for the management of hot flashes. J Soc Integr Oncol 2007;5(3):106–12; Summer.

[773] Dew TP, Williamson G. Controlled flax interventions for the improvement of menopausal symptoms and postmenopausal bone health: a systematic review. Menopause 2013;20(11):1207–15.

[774] Lucas EA, Wild RD, Hammond LJ, et al. Flaxseed improves lipid profile without altering biomarkers of bone metabolism in

postmenopausal women. J Clin Endocrinol Metab 2002;87(4):1527–32.
[775] Patade A, Devareddy L, Lucas EA, et al. Flaxseed reduces total and LDL cholesterol concentrations in Native American postmenopausal women. J Womens Health (Larchmt) 2008;17(3):355–66.
[776] Hooshmand S, Saadat R, Chai SC, et al. Comparative effects of dried plum and dried apple on bone in postmenopausal women. Br J Nutr 2016;106(6):923–30.
[777] Hooshmand S, Kern M, Metti D, et al. The effect of two doses of dried plum on bone density and bone biomarkers in osteopenic postmenopausal women: a randomized, controlled trial. Osteoporos Int 2016;27(7):2271–9.
[778] Doshi SB, Agarwal A. The role of oxidative stress in menopause. J Midlife Health 2013;4(3):140–6.
[779] Wakeman MP. An open label pilot study to evaluate the effectiveness of a proprietary krill oil formulation in the relief of troublesome symptoms of the menopause. Int J Sci Res 2016;5(8).
[780] Di Daniele N, Carbonelli MG, Candeloro N, et al. Andreoli effect of supplementation of calcium and vitamin D on bone mineral density and bone mineral content in peri- and post-menopause women; a double-blind, randomized, controlled trial. Pharmacol Res 2004;50(6):637–41.
[781] Paschalis EP, Gamsjaeger S, Hassler N, et al. Vitamin D and calcium supplementation for three years in postmenopausal osteoporosis significantly alters bone mineral and organic matrix quality. Bone 2017;95:41–6.
[782] Campagnoli C, Abbà C, Ambroggio S, et al. Polyunsaturated fatty acids (PUFAs) might reduce hot flushes: an indication from two controlled trials on soy isoflavones alone and with a PUFA supplement. Maturitas 2005;51(2):127–34.
[783] Colangelo LA, Ouyang P, Golden SH, et al. Do sex hormones or hormone therapy modify the relation of n-3 fatty acids with incident depressive symptoms in postmenopausal women? The MESA Study. Psychoneuroendocrinology 2017;75:26–35.
[784] Jin Y, Park Y. Effects of hormone therapy on the association between erythrocyte levels of n-3 polyunsaturated fatty acids and depression in postmenopausal women. J FASEB 2016; 30(1):Supp.
[785] Muhleisen AL, Herbst-Kralovetz MM. Menopause and the vaginal microbiome. Maturitas 2016;91:42–50.
[786] Petricevic L, Unger FM, Viernstein H, et al. Randomized, double-blind, placebo-controlled study of oral lactobacilli to improve the vaginal flora of postmenopausal women. Eur J Obstet Gynecol Reprod Biol 2008;141(1):54–7.
[787] Senok AC, Verstraelen H, Temmerman M, et al. Probiotics for the treatment of bacterial vaginosis. Cochrane Database Syst Rev 2009;(4):CD006289.
[788] McSorley PT, Young IS, Bell PM, et al. Vitamin C improves endothelial function in healthy estrogen-deficient postmenopausal women. Climacteric 2003;6(3):238–47.
[789] Morton DJ, Barrett-Connor EL, Schneider DL. Vitamin C supplement use and bone mineral density in postmenopausal women. J Bone Miner Res 2001;16(1):135–40.
[790] Geusens P. Strategies for treatment to prevent fragility fractures in postmenopausal women. Best Pract Res Clin Rheumatol 2009;23(6):727–40.
[791] Borradale D, Kimlin M. Vitamin D in health and disease: an insight into traditional functions and new roles for the 'sunshine vitamin.'. Nutr Res Rev 2009;22(2):118–36.
[792] Bischoff-Ferrari HA, Dawson-Hughes B. Where do we stand on vitamin D? Bone 2007;41(1 Suppl. 1):S13–19.
[793] Ziaei S, Kazemnejad A, Zareai M. The effect of vitamin E on hot flashes in menopausal women. (Abstract only). Gynecol Obstet Invest 2007;64(4):204–7.
[794] Gladstar R. Herbal healing for women. New York: Simon & Schuster; 1993.
[795] Herzberg M, Lusky A, Blonder J, et al. The effect of estrogen replacement therapy on zinc in serum and urine. Obstet Gynecol 1996;87:1035–40.
[796] Mutlu M, Argun M, Kilic E, et al. Magnesium, zinc and copper status in osteoporotic, osteopenic and normal post-menopausal women. J Int Med Res 2007;35(5):692–5.
[797] Tang B, Eslick G, Nowson C, et al. Use of calcium or calcium in combination with vitamin D supplementation to prevent fractures and bone loss in people aged 50 years and older: a meta-analysis. Lancet 2007;370:657–66.
[798] Shams T, Setia MS, Hemmings R, et al. Efficacy of black cohosh-containing preparations on menopausal symptoms: a meta-analysis. Altern Ther Health Med 2010;16(1):36–44.
[799] Borrelli F, Ernst E. *Cimicifuga racemosa*: a systematic review of its clinical efficacy. Eur J Clin Pharmacol 2002;58:235–41.
[800] Bodinet C, Freudenstein J. Influence of marketed herbal menopause preparations on MCF-7 cell proliferation. Menopause 2004;11:281–9.
[801] Chung DJ, Kim HY, Park KH, et al. Black cohosh and St John's wort (GYNO-Plus®) for climacteric symptoms. Yonsei Med J 2007;48(2):289–94.
[802] Wuttke W, Seidlová-Wuttke D, Gorkow C. The *Cimicifuga* preparation BNO 1055 vs conjugated estrogens in a double-blind placebo-controlled study: effects on menopause symptoms and bone markers. Maturitas 2003;14(44 Suppl. 1):S67–77.
[803] Tanmahasamut P, Vichinsartvichai P, Rattanachaiyanont M, et al. *Cimicifuga racemosa* extract for relieving menopausal symptoms: a randomized controlled trial. Climacteric 2015;18(1):79–85.
[804] Mohammad-Alizadeh-Charandabi S, Shahnazi M, Nahaee J, et al. Efficacy of black cohosh (*Cimicifuga racemosa* L.) in treating early symptoms of menopause: a randomized clinical trial. Chin Med 2013;8(1):20.
[805] Leach MJ, Moore V. Black cohosh (*Cimicifuga* spp.) for menopausal symptoms. Cochrane Database Syst Rev 2012;(9):CD007244.
[806] Beer AM, Osmers R, Schnitker J, et al. Efficacy of black cohosh (*Cimicifuga racemosa*) medicines for treatment of menopausal symptoms — comments on major statements of the Cochrane Collaboration report 2012 "black cohosh (*Cimicifuga* spp.) for menopausal symptoms (review)". Gynecol Endocrinol 2013;29(12):1022–5.
[807] Wuttke W, Gorkow C, Seidlová-Wuttke D. Effects of black cohosh (*Cimicifuga racemosa*) on bone turnover, vaginal mucosa, and various blood parameters in postmenopausal women: a double-blind, placebo-controlled, and conjugated estrogens-controlled study. Menopause 2006;13(2):185–96.
[808] Nasr A, Nafeh H. Influence of black cohosh (*Cimicifuga racemosa*) use by postmenopausal women on total hepatic perfusion and liver functions. Fertil Steril 2009;92(5):1780–2.
[809] National Standards monograph. Accessed from http://www.naturalstandard.com.
[810] Komesaroff PA, Black CV, Cable V, et al. Effects of wild yam extract on menopausal symptoms, lipids and sex hormones in healthy menopausal women. Climacteric 2001;4(2):144–50.
[811] Chadwick LR, Pauli GF, Farnsworth NR. The pharmacognosy of *Humulus lupulus* L. (hops) with an emphasis on estrogenic properties. Phytomedicine 2006;13(1–2):119–31.
[812] Heyerick A, Vervarcke S, Depypere H, et al. A first prospective, randomized, double-blind, placebo-controlled study on the use of a standardized hop extract to alleviate menopausal discomforts. Maturitas 2006;54(2):164–75.
[813] Erkkola R, Vervarcke S, Vansteelandt S, et al. A randomized, double-blind, placebo-controlled, cross-over pilot study on the use of a standardized hop extract to alleviate menopausal discomforts. Phytomedicine 2010;17(6):389–96.
[814] Tode T, Kikuchi Y, Hirata J, et al. Effect of Korean red ginseng on psychological functions in patients with severe climacteric syndromes. Int J Gynaecol Obstet 1999;67(3):169–74.
[815] Lee HW, Choi J, Lee Y, et al. Ginseng for managing menopausal woman's health: a systematic review of double-blind, randomized, placebo-controlled trials. Medicine (Baltimore) 2016;95(38):e4914.
[816] De Leo V, la Marca A, Morgante G, et al. Evaluation of combining kava extract with hormone replacement therapy in the treatment of postmenopausal anxiety. Maturitas 2001;39(2):185–8.
[817] Singh YN, Singh NN. Therapeutic potential of kava in the treatment of anxiety disorders. CNS Drugs 2002;16(11):731–43.

[818] Togel B, Greve B, Raulin C. Current therapeutic strategies for hyperhidrosis: a review. Eur J Dermatol 2002;12(3):219–23.
[819] Bommer S, Klein P, Suter A. First time proof of sage's tolerability and efficacy in menopausal women with hot flushes. Adv Ther 2011;28(6):490–500.
[820] Goyal RK, Singh J, Lal H. *Asparagus racemosus* — an update. Indian J Med Sci 2003;57(9):408–18.
[821] Svoboda R. Ayurveda for women. A guide to vitality and health. New Delhi: New Age Books; 1999.
[822] Coon JT, Pittler MH, Ernst E. *Trifolium pratense* isoflavones in the treatment of menopausal hot flushes: a systematic review and meta-analysis. Phytomedicine 2007;14(2–3):153–9.
[823] Chedraui P, Hidalgo L, San Miguel G, et al. Red clover extract (MF11RCE) supplementation and postmenopausal vaginal and sexual health. Int J Gynaecol Obstet 2006;95(3):296–7.
[824] Myers SP, Vigar V. Effects of a standardised extract of *Trifolium pratense* (Promensil) at a dosage of 80 mg in the treatment of menopausal hot flushes: a systematic review and meta-analysis. Phytomedicine 2017;24:141–7.
[825] Lucks BC, Sørensen J, Veal L. *Vitex agnus-castus* essential oil and menopausal balance: a self-care survey. Complement Ther Nurs Midwifery 2002;8(3):148–54.
[826] van Die MD, Burger HG, Bone KM, et al. *Hypericum perforatum* with *Vitex agnus-castus* in menopausal symptoms: a randomized, controlled trial. Menopause 2009;16(1):156–63.
[827] Chopin Lucks B. *Vitex agnus-castus* essential oil and menopausal balance: a research update. Complement Ther Nurs Midwifery 2003;9(3):157–60.
[828] Lee MS, Shin BC, Yang EJ, et al. Maca (*Lepidium meyenii*) for treatment of menopausal symptoms: a systematic review. Maturitas 2011;70(3):227–33.
[829] Stojanovska L, Law C, Lai B, et al. Maca reduces blood pressure and depression, in a pilot study in postmenopausal women. Climacteric 2015;18(1):69–78.
[830] Chiu HY, Hsieh YJ, Tsai PS. Acupuncture to reduce sleep disturbances in perimenopausal and postmenopausal women: a systematic review and meta-analysis. Obstet Gynecol 2016;127(3):507–15.

SAMPLE DAILY DIET

Polcystic ovary syndrome (PCOS)

Akdoğan M, Tamer MN, Cüre E, et al. Effect of spearmint (*Mentha spicata* Labiatae) teas on androgen levels in women with hirsutism. Phytother Res 2007;21(5):444–7.
He LX, Zhao J, Huang YS, et al. The difference between oats and beta-glucan extract intake in the management of HbA1c, fasting glucose and insulin sensitivity: a meta-analysis of randomized controlled trials. Food Funct 2016;7(3):1413–28.
Jamilian M, Foroozanfard F, Bahmani F, et al. Effects of zinc supplementation on endocrine outcomes in women with polycystic ovary syndrome: a randomized, double-blind, placebo-controlled trial. Biol Trace Elem Res 2016;170(2):271–8.
Kort DH, Lobo RA. Preliminary evidence that cinnamon improves menstrual cyclicity in women with polycystic ovary syndrome: a randomized controlled trial. Am J Obstet Gynecol 2014;211(5):487.e1–e6.
Moran LJ, Ko H, Misso M, et al. Dietary composition in the treatment of polycystic ovary syndrome: a systematic review to inform evidence-based guidelines. J Acad Nutr Diet 2013;113(4):520–45.
Riley JK, Jungheim ES. Is there a role for diet in ameliorating the reproductive sequelae associated with chronic low-grade inflammation in polycystic ovary syndrome and obesity? Fertil Steril 2016;106(3):520–7.
Shishehgar F, Ramezani Tehrani F, Mirmiran P, et al. Comparison of dietary intake between polycystic ovary syndrome women and controls. Glob J Health Sci 2016;8(9):54801.
Stull AJ. Blueberries' impact on insulin resistance and glucose intolerance. Antioxidants (Basel) 2016;5(4):pii: E44.
Ullrich IH, Peters PJ, Albrink MJ. Effect of low-carbohydrate diets high in either fat or protein on thyroid function, plasma insulin, glucose, and triglycerides in healthy young adults. J Am Coll Nutr 1985;4(4):451–9.
Wang JG, Anderson RA, Graham GM 3rd, et al. The effect of cinnamon extract on insulin resistance parameters in polycystic ovary syndrome: a pilot study. Fertil Steril 2007;88(1):240–3.
Wu D, Kimura F, Takashima A, et al. Intake of vinegar beverage is associated with restoration of ovulatory function in women with polycystic ovary syndrome. Tohoku J Exp Med 2013;230(1):17–23.

19 The male reproductive system

Daniel Robson, Leah Hechtman

SECTION A

OVERVIEW OF THE MALE REPRODUCTIVE SYSTEM

The reproductive system is one of the most important systems in the body — without it, we could not reproduce. The external structures of the male reproductive system include the penis and scrotum. The internal structures include the vas deferens, testes (testicles), urethra, prostate gland and seminal vesicles. Sperm, which carries the man's genes, is made in the testes and stored in the seminal vesicles. During ejaculation, sperm is transported in a fluid (semen) through the urethra.

The male reproductive organs perform the following functions:

- Produce, maintain and transport sperm (the male reproductive cells) and protective fluid (semen)
- Discharge sperm within the female reproductive tract during sex
- Produce and secrete male sex hormones, which are responsible for maintaining the male reproductive system.

Anatomy

SCROTUM

The scrotum is a small pouch-like structure, composed of skin and superficial fascia that hangs from the penis. The scrotum houses the testicles and regulates their temperature via its muscular contraction. It thus plays a vital role in the production of viable, healthy sperm. Fig. 19.1 shows the male reproductive system.

TESTICLES

The testicles are a pair of oval-shaped glands that sit within the scrotum. Each male has two testicles weighing approximately 10–15 g each.[1] The production of sperm occurs within the seminiferous tubules, which are found within the testicles. Also important within the testicles is the production of the male sex hormone testosterone, which is synthesised from cholesterol. Testosterone is secreted by a cluster of cells called the Leydig cells, which are located close to the seminiferous tubules.

EPIDIDYMIS

The epididymis lies to the posterior of each testis. It contains a tightly coiled structure known as the ductus epididymis, which functions as a storage site for the sperm, and also as a transporter, projecting the sperm into the vas deferens.

VAS DEFERENS

The vas deferens is a continuation of the tail of the epididymis, and its function is to store sperm (sometimes for several months) and to transport sperm from the epididymis to the urethra.

EJACULATORY DUCTS

The ejaculatory ducts are small ducts (approximately 2.5 cm long)[1] that eject sperm just prior to ejaculation.

SEMINAL VESICLES

The seminal vesicles are a pair of tubular glands that secrete an alkaline fluid to neutralise the acidic environment of the male reproductive system. Seminal vesicle secretions constitute more than half the volume of semen.[1]

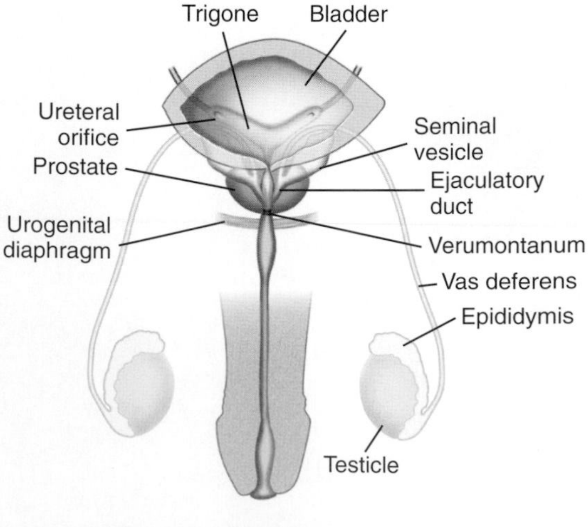

FIGURE 19.1 The male reproductive system

Mandell G, Bennett J, Dolin R. Mandell, Douglas, and Bennett's principles and practice of infectious diseases. 7th edn. Churchill Livingstone; 2009.

PROSTATE GLAND

The prostate is a doughnut-sized gland that is shaped like a walnut. The prostate gland secretes a milky, acidic fluid that assists in semen coagulation after ejaculation. The fluid makes up approximately 25% of the volume of semen, and contains several constituents, including citric acid, acid phosphatase and prostate-specific antigen (PSA).[1]

URETHRA

The urethra is a long tube that functions as a passage for both sperm and urine. The urethra passes through a number of the male reproductive structures, including the penis and prostate gland.

COWPER'S GLANDS (BULBOURETHRAL GLANDS)

These are a pair of glands, the size of a pea, that sit just above the bulb of the penis. During sexual arousal, the Cowper's glands secrete an alkaline fluid that neutralises the acidic environment of the urethra, protecting the sperm. In addition, these glands secrete mucus to lubricate the tip of the penis and the urethra during intercourse. This is to prevent damage to the sperm during ejaculation.

SEMEN

Semen is a sticky, milky, alkaline fluid consisting of a mixture of sperm and the secretions from the Cowper's glands, the prostate gland, the seminal vesicles and the seminiferous tubules. Seminal fluid has many functions, including functioning as a transporter, being a source of nutrition for the sperm, and protecting the sperm from damage.

PENIS

The penis is the external male copulatory organ. It is cylindrical in shape when flaccid. It can be divided into three regions: the body, the root and the glans penis (the head). The body of the penis is composed of three cylindrical masses of tissue bound together by fibrous tissue and covered with skin. The lateral two masses are known as the corpora cavernosa, and the third mass, which lies between the other two, is called the corpus spongiosum. The three masses consist of erectile tissue with numerous blood vessels. Upon sexual stimulation, the arteries supplying the penis fill with blood, resulting in the penis lengthening and stiffening. As more blood fills the tissue chambers, the veins that carry the blood away from the penis are compressed. When there is equilibrium between the flow of blood in the dilated veins and the flow in the veins carrying the blood away, an erection occurs.

The root of the penis begins directly under the Cowper's glands and consists of a number of structures, including the bulb of the penis and the crura of the penis (singular 'crus'). The crura are attached to the ischial and inferior pubic rami, and are covered by the ischiocavernosus muscle. Contraction of these muscles assists with ejaculation.

Lastly, the glans penis is the mushroom-shaped head of the penis that supports the foreskin (if still attached). It contains the distal urethra and forms an opening (the external urethral orifice) for the excretion of urine and semen.

ROLE OF THE NATUROPATH

Traditional interpretation

At first it may appear that the Eclectic physicians largely neglected treatment of the male reproductive system. However, a closer look reveals descriptions of botanicals for the treatment of male reproductive dysfunctions documented under 'Special genitourinary remedies'.[2] The treatment of the male reproductive system was not dissimilar from that of today, with the Eclectics favouring male reproductive tonics, nervines and aphrodisiacs. One well-used botanical was *Serenoa repens* (saw palmetto), which was favoured for its use as a male reproductive tonic. Not only was it indicated therapeutically for dysfunctions of the prostate, but it was also prized for its use in impotence, infections, sexual perversion, sexual neurasthenia and its overall effect on the male reproductive structures:[2]

> *It is demanded in enlarged prostate, with throbbing, aching, dull pain, discharge of prostatic fluid, at times discharge of mucus, also of a yellowish, watery fluid, with weakened sexual power, orchialgia, epididymitis and orchitis, when associated with enlarged prostate ... In the treatment of impotence in young men who have been excessive in their habits, or have masturbated, it can be relied upon with positiveness. It will overcome the excitability from exhaustion and increase sexual power in those newly married who, having been anxious concerning their sexual strength or ability, have become suddenly almost entirely impotent after marriage.*

The Eclectics advocated the use of male tonic herbs in combination with nervine tonics such as *Avena sativa* (oats), believing them to enhance the action of each other:

> *It,* [Serenoa] *combined with a direct nerve tonic, such as* Avena sativa *in doses of fifteen drops, or the one one-hundredth of a grain of phosphorus, will establish a cure. It will relieve any undue irritation, due to excess and exhaustion, that may be present in any part of the genito-urinary apparatus.*[2]

This addition of the nervine class of herbs signifies that the Eclectics acknowledged the important role of the nervous system in male reproductive system dysfunction.

The use of botanicals for the treatment of sexually transmitted infections was largely confined to the treatment of men. The Eclectic physician Jones (1911)[3] set aside a chapter entitled 'Special Remedies for the Male Organs of Generation', which deals largely with sexually transmitted infections such as syphilis and gonorrhoea, which were likely to have been pressing concerns to males of the time. Although late-onset hypogonadism had not yet been identified as an entity, Ellingwood seemed to have some inkling of the condition, suggesting the use of *Delphinium staphisagria*:

> *I have used it to good advantage with Avena and saw palmetto in impotence, especially that occurring in men who have been excessive and dissipated in their habits, appearing usually about the age of forty-five.*[2]

Noticeably absent from the materia medica are *Tribulus terrestris* and *Panax ginseng*, which commonly feature in modern-day formulas for treating dysfunction of the male reproductive system. Coming from countries outside North America, these botanicals are likely to have been unknown to the Eclectics of the time, and thus provide an insight into the development of and advances in modern naturopathic medicine for the male reproductive system.

Modern interpretation

Men's health is a growing area of healthcare, and a range of factors have been identified as contributing to disorders of the male reproductive system. These include:

- Hormone imbalance
- Oxidative stress
- Immune suppression
- Inability to manage stress
- Environmental factors
- Nutrient deficiency/excess
- Iatrogenic causes
- Inflammation
- Obesity
- Endothelial dysfunction.

These factors are well within the domain and expertise of the modern naturopath. Taking the role of facilitator, the modern naturopath works to restore the body to its natural balance, while acknowledging that men have distinctly different needs to women and thus treating accordingly.

The modern naturopath uses a wide variety of therapeutic modalities, including diet, herbs and supplements, either as preventive therapy or as restoratives (see Table 19.2 later in this chapter). This approach follows on the work of the Eclectics, with herbs such as *Serenoa repens* continuing to be used, and acknowledges the close relationship that the reproductive system has with the other systems of the body, particularly the cardiovascular, nervous and immune systems. Knowledge of the complex workings of the reproductive system allows for greater specificity of application of therapeutic modalities. In addition, the availability of other herbal medicine systems, including Ayurveda and traditional Chinese medicine, allows for a more diverse selection of herbs from which to choose.

The naturopathic approach encourages preventive medicine, within which functional assessments are considered imperative for long-term health. To this end testing, including the baseline male hormone profile (see later in this chapter), can provide an analysis of hormone status. Preventive PSA testing may be warranted in men with a family history of prostate cancer or based on symptom presentation; however, its role as a general prostate cancer screening tool is controversial, with conflicting positions held by relevant international professional bodies.[4]

INVESTIGATIONS

An overview of the laboratory investigations used in evaluating male reproductive system dysfunction and an interpretation of the results obtained are given in Table 19.1.

Prostate-specific antigen (PSA) testing

The role of PSA testing as a general screening tool for early identification of prostate cancer is an area of controversy.[5] While increasing PSA levels are associated

TABLE 19.1 Investigations in male reproductive system dysfunction

Test category	Normal result*	Clinical significance
Total testosterone	8–35 nmol/L	Low levels may be implicated in erectile dysfunction, low libido and late-onset hypogonadism
Free testosterone	170–519 pmol/L	Low levels may be implicated in erectile dysfunction, low libido and late-onset hypogonadism
Dihydrotestosterone	1–2.5 nmol/L	Main androgen and active form of testosterone
Sex hormone binding globulin (SHBG)	10–50 nmol/L	Changes can be associated with hypogonadism
Follicle-stimulating hormone (FSH)	1.0–5.0 U/L	In the presence of low testosterone, an increased value is indicative of primary testicular failure and a normal or low value is indicative of secondary hypogonadism
Luteinising hormone (LH)	2.0–10 U/L	In the presence of low testosterone, an increased value is indicative of primary testicular failure. A normal or low value is indicative of secondary hypogonadism
Prostate-specific antigen (PSA)	0.0–4.0 ng/mL#	PSA is organ specific, not pathology specific. Raised levels may be seen in prostate cancer, benign prostatic hyperplasia or prostatitis

Source: Tortora G, Grabowski S. Principles of anatomy and physiology. 9th edn. New York: Biological Sciences Textbooks/Wiley; 2000.
*Age-specific ranges refer to adult male. Ranges vary depending on the pathology service provider.
#PSA testing is an area of controversy. See the text discussion for more information.

with higher risks of prostate cancer, it is also a marker of prostate volume (as in benign prostatic hyperplasia [BPH]), and prostatitis.[5] Screening of the general male population is known to increase prostate cancer diagnosis and diagnosis of more localised disease; however, concerns surround its impacts on over-diagnosis and associated over-treatment of prostate cancer, with resulting increased patient morbidity.[5]

There is no consensus on the use of PSA testing in men without a history of prostate cancer. Most professional bodies agree that PSA testing should only be done in men who are well informed about the risks and benefits associated with it.[4] The suggested minimum age at which to start testing PSA levels of well-informed men of average risk varies among associations. Most suggest 50–55 as the earliest age; however, some suggest a single baseline test at age 40 to establish prostate cancer risk.[4] Advice as to when to stop PSA screening is also variable, with an age cut-off of 69–75 suggested, or less than 10–15 year life expectancy.[4]

In men who are at high risk of prostate cancer most associations agree that PSA testing should be offered at a younger age. A higher risk of prostate cancer exists for African American men, having a family history of prostate cancer (especially if the family member was diagnosed before age 65), or having the *BRCA1* or *BRCA2* mutation.[6]

In regards to interpreting a raised PSA, no specific PSA level is indicative of prostate cancer. PSA is a continuous parameter; increased levels are associated with a higher likelihood of diagnosing prostate cancer,[5] but it can still be present in men with low PSA values.[5] The traditional PSA threshold for triggering a biopsy is 4.0 ng/mL; however, results from the Prostate Cancer Intervention vs Observation Trial (PIVOT) suggest that this threshold could be increased to at least 10 ng/mL, as the greatest benefit to prostate cancer treatment was seen in this trial at baseline PSA levels of 10–20 ng/mL.[6]

A free/total (f/t) PSA ratio may be used in men with a PSA less than 10 ng/mL to help differentiate between BPH and prostate cancer. A lower f/t PSA is indicative of a greater probability of prostate cancer, with 56% of men with a f/t PSA less than 0.10 having prostate cancer diagnosed on biopsy, compared to only 8% with a f/t PSA more than 0.25.[5]

In addition to the above investigations, the following functional tests are sometimes used by naturopathic practitioners.

Specific naturopathic assessments

MALE HORMONE PROFILE

A male hormone profile may be indicated to assess the balance and metabolism of the male sex hormones. The test includes both total and calculated free testosterone, luteinising hormone (LH), follicle-stimulating hormone (FSH), prolactin, inhibin and sex hormone binding globulin (SHBG).

Androgen metabolism is assessed by measuring the level of oestradiol, which is reflective of aromatase activity, and thus may have bearing on reproductive health.

NUTRIENT AND TOXIC ELEMENT PROFILE

Toxic elements and selenium are measured in whole blood, and other trace elements, such as magnesium, potassium, chromium and zinc, are measured in erythrocytes. Zinc status is important in relation to prostate health and testosterone deficiency; however, reliable means of assessing status at this stage are unavailable.[7] Screening for toxic elements may be of value as heavy metal accumulation can impact upon male reproductive function.

DNA/OXIDATIVE STRESS MARKER

Reactive oxygen species and free radical species are implicated in many male reproductive disorders, and an assessment of these assists in determining accurate prescriptions of antioxidants.

FATTY ACID PROFILE

As the prostate and other structures of the reproductive system are composed of glandular tissue, a plasma fatty acid profile is of benefit to assess dietary adequacy of essential fatty acids and to evaluate the level of arachidonic acid (involved in the inflammatory prostaglandin pathway).

CARDIOVASCULAR HEALTH PROFILE

As male reproductive health is intricately related to cardiovascular health, it may be indicated to obtain a serum cardiovascular health profile in order to identify risk factors for cardiovascular disease. Measures of cholesterol, lipoproteins, triglycerides, fibrinogen, C-reactive protein (CRP), homocysteine, lipid peroxidises, vitamin E, magnesium, coenzyme Q10 (CoQ10), insulin and ferritin may be of value.

URINARY OESTROGEN METABOLISM

The urinary oestrogen metabolism test can be used to determine whether a patient has a high risk of hormone imbalance. Oestrogens are metabolised in two ways: the first pathway (2-hydroxyoestrone) is protective, while the second pathway (16α-hydroxyoestrone) is more potent. The test identifies which is the dominant pathway (2 or 16) for oestrogen metabolism. The aim is to ensure that the ratio between pathway 2 and pathway 16 is maintained at the ideal value of 2.0. A low ratio (reduced 2-hydroxy metabolite production) indicates a state of oestrogen excess, which may be a contributing factor to oestrogen-dependent cancers, such as prostate cancer.

DETOXIFICATION CAPACITY PROFILE

The detoxification capacity profile is used to assess the phase I and phase II detoxification capacity of the liver and is useful where there is a hormone imbalance. Saliva and urine are analysed for the metabolites of three compounds to determine how well the liver can convert and clear toxins from the body. Adequate liver function may have bearing on hormonal balance, as the liver is responsible for hormone production and metabolism.

See Table 19.2.

TABLE 19.2 Key herbal medicines in male reproductive health

Example	Justification
Serenoa repens (saw palmetto)	*Serenoa repens* has been used traditionally for disorders of the male reproductive tract including those that are prostate related. The lipidosterolic extracts of *Serenoa repens* have demonstrated evidence of 5α-reductase and α-receptor inhibition activity, and anti-inflammatory activity. It has an evidence base either individually or in combination with other treatments for treating male lower urinary tract symptoms attributed to benign prostatic hypertrophy, chronic bacterial prostatitis, and chronic prostatitis/chronic pelvic pain syndrome.
Eurycoma longifolia (tongkat ali)	Traditionally reputed as a male reproductive tonic, improving libido, erectile function, stamina and endurance. Evidence supports its use in treating symptoms associated with late-onset hypogonadism. It has demonstrated testosterone-enhancing and erection-promoting properties.
Panax ginseng (Korean ginseng)	Widely reputed as adaptogen and male reproductive tonic. Has demonstrated efficacy in improving erectile dysfunction, potentially via nitric oxide upregulating activity of ginsenosides.
Pinus pinaster (maritime pine)	Pine bark extracts demonstrate antioxidant, anti-inflammatory, cardiovascular protective and neuroprotective properties. In combination with L-arginine, it has demonstrated efficacy in treating erectile dysfunction and male lower urinary tract symptoms by increasing endogenous nitric oxide production and therefore improving vascular perfusion to the male genitourinary organs.
Withania somnifera (ashwagandha)	Traditionally indicated as an aphrodisiac, adaptogen and rejuvenating male tonic. Has demonstrated testosterone-elevating and fertility-enhancing properties in stressed infertile men, and improves physical performance.
Tribulus terrestris (tribulus)	Demonstrated to improve libido and sexual function in both men and women. May improve erectile function. Generally considered to be androgenic, although results from studies are unclear. Likely impacts sexual function by endothelial and nitric oxide (NO) dependent mechanisms and a possible androgen receptor modulating activity.
Vaccinium macrocarpon (cranberry)	Demonstrates urinary antiseptic and anti-inflammatory activity. Has been shown to improve lower urinary tract symptoms in men diagnosed with benign prostatic hyperplasia and non-bacterial prostatitis.
Crocus sativus (saffron)	Has a diverse application in male reproductive health, demonstrating antidepressant, anxiolytic, antioxidant and anti-inflammatory properties. Traditionally used to improve libido and erectile function. Clinical trial evidence supports its use in erectile dysfunction and SSRI-induced sexual dysfunction in men.
Linum usitatissimum (flaxseeds/ linseeds)	Has a clinical application as part of the treatment of male lower urinary tract symptoms. Has been shown to reduce proliferation rates of benign prostate epithelium and prostate cancer. Constituents demonstrate weak oestrogen receptor binding capacity and possible 5-α reductase inhibiting activity.
Urtica dioica radix (nettle root)	Demonstrates improvements in male lower urinary tract symptoms. Mechanisms of action suggested to include aromatase inhibition and antiproliferative effects on prostate epithelial cells and inhibition of SHBG binding.
Silybum marianum (milk thistle)	Typically thought of in relation to liver disease, has been shown recently to effectively relieve male lower urinary tract symptoms, reduce PSA and improve objective urinary measures. Mechanisms of action suggested are prostate anti-inflammatory, antioxidant and pro-apoptotic properties. ER-β agonist and ER-α antagonist activity in the prostate epithelium has also been demonstrated.
Mucuna pruriens (velvet bean)	Traditionally indicated as a restoring and invigorating male reproductive tonic, renowned for improving libido and erectile function. In men treated for infertility, has been demonstrated to increase testosterone.
Secale cereale, *Phleum pratense* and *Zea mays* (flower pollen extract)	Numerous studies demonstrate efficacy in treating obstructive and irritative symptoms attributed to benign prostatic enlargement. Also shown to improve pain, urinary and sexual dysfunction symptoms associated with chronic prostatitis/chronic pelvic pain syndrome. May improve recovery of sexual and urinary function following prostate surgery. Phytosterols and secalosides in the extract are attributed with anti-inflammatory and antiproliferative effects in the prostate and smooth muscle function altering effects in the bladder and urethra.

Sources: [83, 85, 86, 114, 115, 117, 124, 125, 128, 129, 131, 132, 141, 144–146, 148–151, 215, 234, 239, 241, 348–351, 353–355, 357, 358, 458, 465, 466, 470, 471]

Nutritional medicine

Key nutritional supplements indicated in male reproductive health conditions are summarised in Table 19.3.

POTENTIAL INTERACTIONS

The potential interactions between herbal medicines and dietary supplements and pharmaceutical drugs are summarised in the interactions tables at the back of the book.

SECTION B

MALE LOWER URINARY TRACT SYMPTOMS

Lower urinary tract symptoms (LUTS) are commonly experienced in men, having significant impact on health-related quality of life.[8] LUTS is the preferred term for describing the constellation of symptoms and signs experienced by ageing men historically

TABLE 19.3 Key nutritional supplements in male reproductive health

Nutrient	Role in treating male reproductive health conditions	Therapeutic dose	Dietary sources
Zinc	Necessary for normal prostate structure, immunity, inflammation and hormonal regulation. Required for healthy formation and maturation of sperm. Deficiency results in decreased testosterone. Supplementation shown to improve symptoms in chronic bacterial prostatitis, chronic prostatitis/chronic pelvic pain syndrome (CP/CPPS). Corrects low testosterone and erectile dysfunction (ED) in end-stage renal disease.	20 mg–60 mg/day	Seafood (oysters and shellfish), meat, liver, eggs, nuts, seeds, legumes and wholegrains
Selenium	An important antioxidant found in high concentrations in the male reproductive system, where it has roles in male fertility and prostate health. In combination treatment, supplementation reduces CP/CPPS symptoms, improves urinary symptoms in lower urinary tract symptoms (LUTS) and reduces prostate inflammation.	50 micrograms–200 micrograms day	Brazil nuts, meat, fish eggs, wholegrains and dairy products
Lycopene	Accumulates at high concentrations in the prostate gland demonstrating antioxidant and anti-inflammatory activity. Shown to arrest prostate volume and PSA increases in benign prostatic enlargement. In combination products, shown to reduce prostate inflammation, improve LUTS and symptoms of CP/CPPS.	5 mg–15 mg/day	Tomatoes and tomato products, red capsicum, guava, watermelon, pink or red grapefruit and papaya
β-sitosterol	Supplementation improves urinary symptoms, maximum urinary flow rate, and postvoid residual urine in LUTS.	30 mg–135 mg/day	Vegetable oils, nuts, seeds and avocado
L-arginine	Semi-essential amino acid required for nitric oxide synthesis and therefore vascular function. Supplementation shown to improve erectile function, and LUTS. Concurrent treatment with pycnogenol likely to result in better outcomes.	460 mg–5000 mg/day	Animal protein, nuts, seeds, algae, soy protein and rice protein
Quercetin	Anti-inflammatory and antioxidant improving pain and quality of life in CP/CPPS. As a component of treatment, improved efficacy of antibiotic treatment in chronic bacterial prostatitis.	500 mg twice/day	Onion, black tea, apples, blackcurrant, red leaf lettuce and asparagus

Continued

TABLE 19.3 Key nutritional supplements in male reproductive health—cont'd

Nutrient	Role in treating male reproductive health conditions	Therapeutic dose	Dietary sources
Vitamin D	Deficiency associated with LUTS, increased PSA, increased prostate size, erectile dysfunction and hypogonadism. Treatment with synthetic vitamin D_3 analogue arrested benign prostatic enlargement.	1500–2000 IU/day to maintain blood levels	Produced endogenously in response to UVB exposure. Dietary sources include fatty fish, butter, eggs, fortified foods, mushrooms
Magnesium	Serum magnesium correlated to testosterone levels. Supplementation shown to increase free and total testosterone in young healthy men.	100 mg–500 mg/day	Dark-green leafy vegetables, legumes, nuts, cocoa, wholegrain cereals
L-carnitine (as acetyl-L-carnitine and/or propionyl-L-carnitine)	Low serum carnitine in renal disease correlated with low free testosterone. Supplementation improves sexual function in late-onset hypogonadism (LOH) associated with renal disease. Improves ED in diabetic men. Improves effectiveness of PDE-5 inhibitors in ED treatment.	250 mg–4000 mg/day	Dietary sources of carnitine include animal protein, avocado and tempeh
Vitamin E	Important antioxidant involved in cardiovascular disease protection. Improved efficacy of PDE-5 inhibitors in the treatment of ED.	300 mg α-tocopherol/day	Cold pressed Vegetable oils, nuts, seeds, spinach, kale, sweet potato, egg yolk, liver, soya beans
Inositol	Appears to improve nitric oxide signalling and endothelial function and reduce oxidative stress. Supplementation with folic acid improved erectile function in diabetic men.	4000 mg/day	Citrus fruit, legumes, brewer's yeast, wholegrains and animal protein
Co-enzyme Q10	Improves vascular endothelial function, relevant in ED treatment. Improves ED when caused by Peyronie's disease.	100 mg–300 mg daily	Animal protein, broccoli, cauliflower, nuts and soy
Vitamin B_6	With folic acid, improved responsiveness to PDE-5 inhibitors in diabetics homozygous or heterozygous for MTHFR 677T.	50–100 mg/day	Animal protein, wholegrains, legumes, eggs, vegetables and nuts
Folate	With vitamin B_6, improved responsiveness to PDE-5 inhibitors in diabetics homozygous or heterozygous for MTHFR 677T.	400 micrograms–15 mg/day	Legumes, fresh green leafy vegetables, asparagus, broccoli, sprouts, nuts, fortified cereals and organ meats
Niacin	High-dose monotherapy improved ED in men with hyperlipidaemia. Combination treatment has improved ED in diabetic men and men with arterial ED.	20 mg–200 mg/day. 1500 mg nicotinic acid has been used in ED, however such doses are associated with side effects	Animal protein, almonds, eggs, legumes, tofu, tempeh

Sources: [7, 69, 78, 87, 106, 108, 111, 112, 114, 115, 117, 118, 120, 121, 142–144, 214, 224, 225, 233, 329, 334–337, 339–343, 379, 447, 450–452, 456, 472–487]

ascribed to an enlarged prostate caused by benign prostatic hyperplasia (BPH).[9] A growing body of research now demonstrates that a number of non-prostate related pathologies can be implicated in male LUTS.[10,11] The modern view of male LUTS emphasises a need to move away from a prostate-centric perspective in evaluating and managing these symptoms.[8]

Three broad categories of male LUTS exist; storage (irritative), voiding (obstructive) and postmicturition symptoms.[9] Storage (irritative) symptoms include urgency, frequency, nocturia and incontinence (including urge incontinence). Voiding (obstructive) symptoms include hesitancy, poor urinary flow, intermittency, straining and terminal dribble. Postmicturition symptoms are typified by postvoid dribble and a sense of incomplete emptying.[9]

Classification

Previously considered to be the primary reason for the development of LUTS in ageing men, benign prostatic hyperplasia (BPH; previously known as benign prostatic hypertrophy), is now recognised to be only one of a number of equally important pathological and functional causes of LUTS that typically develop as men age.[8] Bladder dysfunction manifested as overactive bladder (OAB)[12] or underactive bladder (UAB),[13] and nocturnal polyuria, are now recognised as important contributors to male LUTS.[8] Additionally, numerous other urological and non-urological conditions (such as neurological disease, renal disease, diabetes, sleep apnoea and urinary tract infections) can give rise to LUTS[8] and as such must be considered in evaluation and treatment by the naturopathic clinician.

BPH is a histological, not a clinical, diagnosis, and is characterised pathologically by a proliferation, but not increased size of, epithelial cells and stromal cells originating from the periurethral area and transition zones of the prostate gland.[14] Benign prostatic enlargement (BPE), while related to BPH, technically refers to the finding of an enlarged prostate gland, either palpable on digital rectal examination (DRE) or observed on prostate imaging.[15] Bladder outlet obstruction (BOO), a potential consequence of BPE caused by BPH, describes the physical means by which an enlarged prostate gives rise to LUTS.[14]

Bladder dysfunction giving rise to male LUTS may be due to either overactive bladder (OAB), or underactive bladder (UAB). OAB is a clinical diagnosis, comprising of the storage symptoms of LUTS, of which urinary urgency is predominant.[16] It has been defined by the International Continence Society as 'urinary urgency, usually accompanied by frequency and nocturia, with or without urgency urinary incontinence, in the absence of a urinary tract infection or other obvious pathology'.[16] It can occur either independently, or in combination with BPE.[17]

Conversely, underactive bladder (UAB) describes symptoms resulting from ineffective bladder smooth muscle contraction, or detrusor underactivity (DU), a common yet poorly understood clinical entity contributing to or independently responsible for LUTS presenting in ageing men.[18] Clinical features are those of impaired bladder emptying, such as weak stream, intermittency, straining and a feeling of incomplete voiding,[19] which are on clinical grounds difficult to differentiate from BOO caused by BPE.[13]

Nocturnal polyuria, a potential cause of nocturia, is defined by a normal 24-hour urinary output, but with increased urine output at night of more than 20% of total 24-hour urinary output in young adults, and 33% for adults over 65.[20] It represents a disruption to the normal circadian pattern of urine production, where urine output is normally decreased during sleep hours in an age-dependent manner.[20]

Epidemiology

A large study of men in eight Asian countries and Australia found that the prevalence of LUTS increased with advancing age, with 18%, 29%, 40% and 56% of men in their 40s, 50s, 60s and 70s respectively, reporting moderate to severe symptoms.[21]

BPH, as defined histologically and an important cause of LUTS, is virtually nonexistent before the age of 30. Its prevalence is seen to increase rapidly during the 4th decade, peaking at 88% of men aged in their 80s.[15] Prostate volume, as an indicator or BPH, has been shown to increase from 25 mL in men aged 30–39, to 35–45 mL for men aged 70–79.[15]

Bladder dysfunction in the form of OAB affects 11.8–14.3% of men, with an age-associated increase observed.[22] UAB, resulting from detrusor underactivity (DU) has been estimated to affect 9–28% of men under 50, increasing to 48% of men over 70, although epidemiological data are limited.[13] Nocturnal polyuria is thought to affect at least 40% of men aged between 50 and 78, with prevalence increasing to 56.9% of men between 70 and 78.[20]

Overview

Trouble-free micturition is dependent upon the normal functioning of two discreet processes, the filling and storage of urine in the bladder, and bladder emptying or voiding. Bladder filling and storage of urine require normal bladder compliance; that is, the capacity to accommodate increasing volumes of urine at low bladder smooth muscle (detrusor muscle) tone. This is accompanied by appropriate bladder sensation. For filling to occur the bladder outlet must be closed at rest and maintain closure with increased intra-abdominal pressure.[23]

For bladder emptying to occur successfully, the bladder smooth muscle must be able to contract with enough force and duration. At the same time, smooth muscle of the bladder neck and proximal urethra, and skeletal muscle of the proximal urethra (intramural striated sphincter) and external urethral sphincter must be sufficiently relaxed. Passage through the urethra must then be free of any anatomical obstructions.[23]

Pathophysiology or dysfunction affecting either, or a combination, of these processes can then result in LUTS.[23]

Pathogenesis

Lower urinary tract symptoms (LUTS) in men have a multifactorial aetiology, of which benign enlargement of the prostate gland is one possible important causal factor.[8] Others include bladder dysfunction such as OAB and UAB, and nocturnal polyuria,[8] all of which can contribute independently or in combination with each other.

PATHOPHYSIOLOGY OF LUTS CAUSED BY BPH

Benign prostatic hyperplasia is a consequence of increased cell proliferation and/or decreased cell apoptosis[14]

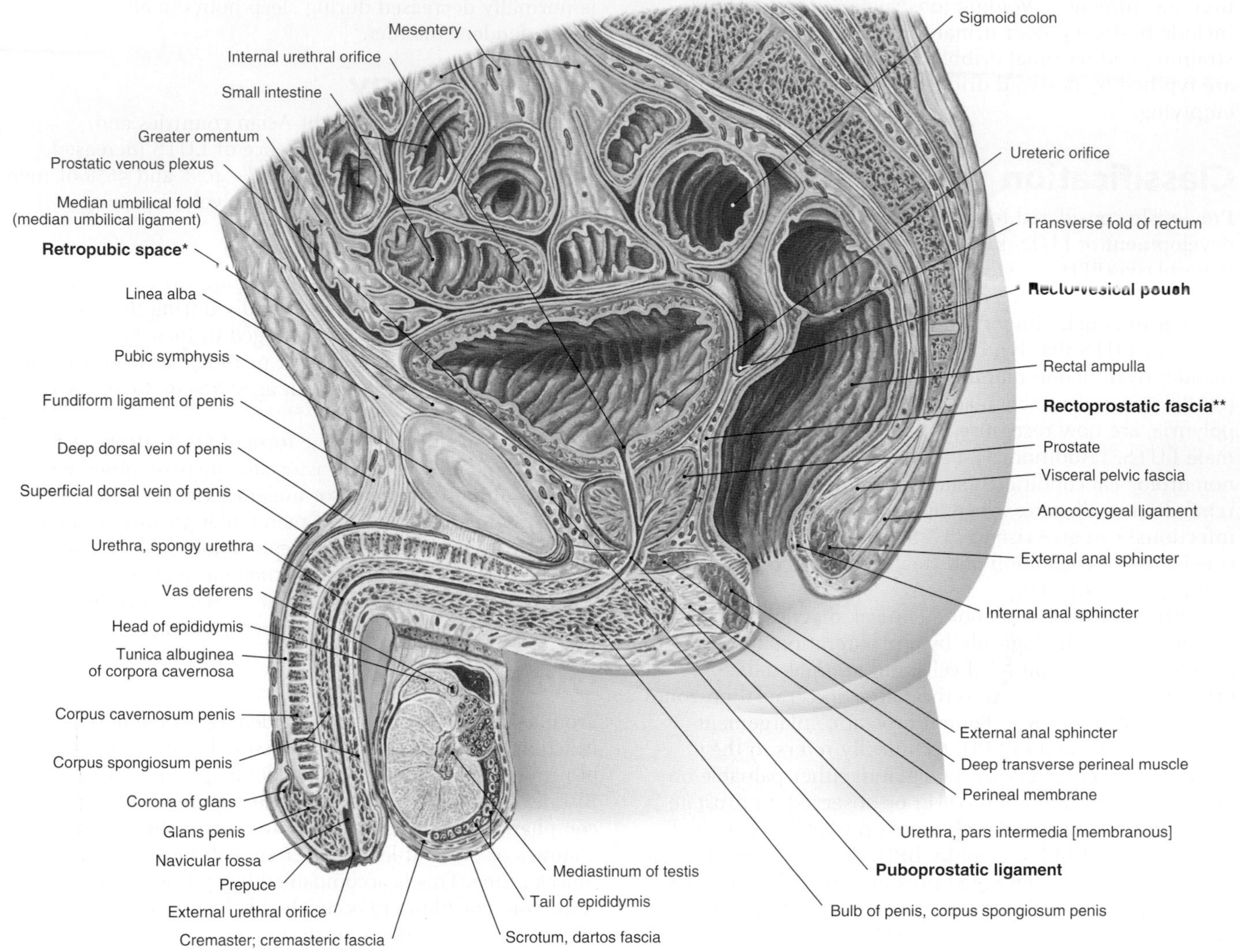

FIGURE 19.2 Anatomy and spatial relationship of the prostate gland to the lower urinary tract

Source: Paulsen F, Waschke J. Sobotta atlas of human anatomy. 15th edn. 2011 © Elsevier GmbH, Urban & Fischer, Munich.

affecting epithelial and stromal cells of the periurethral area of the prostate, with resultant microscopic and macroscopic nodules in the prostate gland.[15] This process generally begins in the transition zone around the urethra, with extension proximally into the periurethral zone.[14] Overall, BPH tissue is comprised of approximately 20% epithelial elements and 80% stromal, with around 50% of the stromal component being smooth muscle.[24] Compression of the prostatic urethra occurs due to nodular growth enlargement of the prostate transition zone being constrained by the outer prostatic capsule.[14] The result is an impact upon urine flow causing bladder outlet obstruction (BOO), and thus LUTS.[25]

THE ROLE OF PROSTATE SMOOTH MUSCLE

Smooth muscle makes up a significant volume of the hyperplastic prostate gland,[15] contributing around 50% of the stromal component.[24] Sympathetic nervous system innervation to the stroma regulates smooth muscle cell tone and helps to coordinate prostate gland secretions.[26] The most abundant adrenoreceptors in prostate smooth muscle are the α_{1A} adrenoreceptors, which mediate active smooth muscle tension,[15] while elastic elements in the stroma and extra cellular matrix (ECM) contribute to passive tissue force independent of smooth muscle contraction.[15] Alpha$_{1A}$ adrenoreceptors are expressed generally in prostate stromal cells, and in addition to regulating smooth muscle tone, appear to also play a role in stimulating prostate growth.[26] Normal prostatic smooth muscle tone and growth also appear to be regulated by nitric oxide (NO), with neural nitric oxide synthase (nNOS) and endothelial nitric oxide synthase (eNOS) both being identified in prostate tissue.[26] Evidence suggests that older men, and those with an enlarged prostate, demonstrate less

NOS expression in the prostate.[26] These newer understandings of the role of the NO-cGMP (nitric oxide-cyclic guanosine monophosphate) pathway have resulted in the use of PDE5-Is as a therapeutic strategy in the treatment of LUTS in men.[27]

BLADDER INVOLVEMENT IN LUTS

Lower urinary tract symptoms in men may simply be a result of outflow obstruction due to BPE or active compression of the prostatic urethra by prostate smooth muscle; or it may be due to bladder dysfunction, either secondary to changes caused by BPE, or as a primary source of urinary symptoms independent of prostate pathology. Obstruction of the prostatic urethra by an enlarged prostate can drive adaptive changes to the bladder that contribute to LUTS, even when relief of prostate-induced obstruction (such as prostate surgery) is achieved.[15] The response of the bladder detrusor muscle to urinary obstruction includes smooth muscle cell hypertrophy and phenotype changes, the associated intra- and extracellular changes of which lead to an instability of the detrusor muscle and impaired capacity for contractility. An increase in collagen deposition in the detrusor muscle results in trabeculation (thickening) limiting bladder compliance.[15] It has been suggested that bladder distension secondary to BOO may cause a type of ischaemia-reperfusion injury to the bladder, driving changes to bladder biochemistry, histology and neural pathways resulting in micturition problems.[28] Of particular relevance in this model is the role of oxidative stress, which experimentally has been shown to cause changes to detrusor muscle contraction and C fibre activation, that could plausibly result in both overactive and underactive detrusor activity.[29] Short-term bladder ischaemia has been shown to result in smooth muscle instability and overactivity. Long-term ischaemia has been shown to result in smooth muscle underactivity as a consequence of exhausted smooth muscle energy, inflammation, fibrosis and degeneration.[30]

Independent of BOO, bladder dysfunction either as OAB or UAB may be a primary cause of LUTS, to the extent that some authors have suggested that the bladder is the central organ involved.[12] Symptoms of bladder dysfunction overlap with other causes of LUTS and in older men often occur alongside BPH.[17] Storage LUTS, especially urgency and urge incontinence, are well correlated to detrusor muscle overactivity;[16] however, not with BPH.[12] In the case of UAB, impaired detrusor contractility results in prolonged and incomplete bladder emptying,[31] leading to symptoms such as decreased and/or interrupted stream, hesitancy, incomplete bladder emptying, straining and/or decreased sensation.[19] While common, the extent to which detrusor underactivity contributes to male LUTS is unclear due to overlap between presenting symptoms of BOO caused by BPE, and its frequent coexistence with BPE.[13] Thus bladder dysfunction is an important consideration in men with LUTS, especially when therapeutic response to prostate-targeted therapy is unsuccessful.

Aetiology

The cause of hyperplasia of prostate tissue is currently unknown, although it appears likely that a multitude of factors such as inflammation, hormonal changes and growth factor dysregulation converge to create a cycle of dysregulated cell growth and cell death that results in overall growth of the prostate gland. Alterations in growth factors, inflammatory mediators and steroid hormones appear to be involved.

GROWTH FACTORS

Growth in cell numbers is a consequence of an imbalance between cell proliferation and cell death. An imbalance of growth factors resulting in abnormal apoptosis and/or cell proliferation appears to be involved in prostate cell hyperplasia, and demonstrates a complex interplay between the hormonal and inflammatory environment of the prostate.[15,32,33] Transforming growth factor beta 1 (TGF-β1) is of particular interest, being considered to be involved in BPH development because of its role in inducing fibroblast differentiation into myofibroblasts and its role in stromal cell remodelling.[32] It is also an inhibitor of epithelial cell growth, this action perhaps being downregulated or lost in BPH.[15] Insulin-like growth factor II (IGF-II), along with dihydrotestosterone (DHT) concentrations, has been found to be higher in periurethral stromal cells of BPH patients, and animal studies demonstrate that decreasing androgen receptor (AR) expression also decreases insulin-like growth factor 1 (IGF-I) in prostate stromal cells.[32] Other growth factors of interest that have been implicated in BPH include fibroblast growth factor (FGF), transforming growth factor (TGF), epidermal growth factor (EGF) and keratinocyte growth factor.[15,32]

ROLE OF HORMONES

Androgens

The role that androgens have in BPH is complex. While it is evident that they play a role, it is likely to be a permissive rather than causative one.[15] Androgens are needed for normal cell proliferation and differentiation, essential for the growth and development of the prostate.[15] The prostate gland is unique in that it continues to respond to androgens throughout the lifecycle, an ability that is lost in other androgen-dependent organs such as the penis.[15] Evidence for androgen involvement in BPH is supported by the observation that androgen deprivation, either in the form of castration, endocrine disorders or antiandrogenic medication, can prevent the development of BPH, or can reduce prostate volumes in men with already enlarged prostates.[15,34]

A consistent correlation between serum testosterone (total, free/bioavailable) and prostate volume on the International Prostate Symptom Score (IPSS) has, however, not been found.[15,35] (See Box 19.1.) This may be because the predominant androgen present in the prostate is dihydrotestosterone (DHT),[36] formed mostly locally by the conversion of testosterone in prostate stromal cells by 5-α reductase type 2,[15] and to a smaller extent by epithelial cells by 5-α reductase type 1.[34] Its central role is in

BOX 19.1 The International Prostate Symptom Score (IPSS)

Patient name: Date:	Not at all	Less than 1 time in 5	Less than half the time	About half the time	More than half the time	Almost always	YOUR SCORE
1. Incomplete emptying Over the past month, how often have you had a sensation of not emptying your bladder completely after you finish urinating?	0	1	2	3	4	5	
2. Frequency Over the past month, how often have you had to urinate again less than two hours after you have finished urinating?	0	1	2	3	4	5	
3. Intermittency Over the past month, how often have you found you stopped and started again several times when you urinated?	0	1	2	3	4	5	
4. Urgency Over the past month, how often have you found it difficult to postpone urination?	0	1	2	3	4	5	
5. Weak stream Over the last month, how often have you had a weak urinary stream?	0	1	2	3	4	5	
6. Straining Over the past month, how often have you had to push or strain to begin urination?	0	1	2	3	4	5	
	None	**Once**	**Twice**	**3 times**	**4 times**	**5 times or more**	**YOUR SCORE**
7. Nocturia Over the past month, how many times did you most typically get up each night to urinate from the time you went to bed until the time you got up in the morning?	0	1	2	3	4	5	
Total IPSS							
Quality of life due to urinary symptoms	**Delighted**	**Pleased**	**Mostly satisfied**	**Mixed**	**Mostly unhappy**	**Unhappy**	**Terrible**
If you were to spend the rest of your life with your urinary condition just the way it is now, how would you feel about that?	0	1	2	3	4	5	6

Grading of patient severity is done by adding up the total scores for questions 1–7.

0–7 = mildly symptomatic

8–19 = moderately symptomatic

20–35 = severely symptomatic

The quality of life score is measured separately, and is an attempt to capture the overall impact of symptoms on quality of life.

Source: Barry MJ, Fowler FJ, O'Leary MP et al. The American Urological Association Symptom Index for Benign Prostatic Hyperplasia. The Journal of Urology, Elsevier, February 2017.

supporting prostate growth; stimulating cell proliferation, differentiation and androgen-regulated gene transcription.[36] Its androgenic properties are more potent than that of testosterone, having a higher affinity for the androgen receptor (AR), and forming a more stable androgen-receptor complex.[15] Higher serum levels of DHT have been observed in men with BPH compared to unaffected men, and higher DHT/testosterone ratio has been associated with a higher prevalence of BPH.[34] Studies exploring the relationship between intraprostatic DHT and BPH have, however, been conflicting, with older cadaver-based studies finding a positive association, but more recent studies on living men finding no significant relationship.[36]

Inhibition of testosterone conversion to DHT is the target for current therapies used to treat BPH, the 5-α reductase inhibitors finasteride (targeting type 2 receptors) and dutasteride (targeting type 1 and 2 receptors) demonstrating efficacy in reducing intraprostatic DHT and improving LUTS.[34] Interestingly, dual inhibition of type 1 and type 2 5-α reductase with dutasteride in BPH, compared to only targeting type 2 5-α reductase with finasteride, demonstrates greater clinical efficacy.[15] This suggests that extraprostatic DHT has a role in BPH as type 1 5-α reductase is predominantly present in tissues such as the skin and liver,[15] and is only present in the prostate to a small extent in epithelial cells.[34] It may also point to a role for prostate epithelial cells in promoting stromal cell hyperplasia via a paracrine mechanism.[34]

It may be that the role of androgens in BPH relates to the androgen receptor (AR), a higher androgen concentration and AR concentration being found in primitive BPH nodules in the periurethral area of the transition zone compared to other prostate regions.[34] Some preliminary evidence also points to androgen receptor genetic polymorphisms perhaps playing a role, although the evidence is at this stage conflicting.[25]

Oestrogen

As well as being a target for androgens, the prostate is an important target for oestrogens.[25] Of the endogenous oestrogens produced in men — oestrone (E1), oestradiol (E2) and oestriol (E3) — E2 is considered the most potent.[25] In men, about 80% of oestradiol (E2) is a result of the conversion of testosterone via aromatase, with another 20% being produced mostly by Leydig cells.[37] Prostatic production of oestrogen has been suggested to be involved in prostate hyperplasia, with reduced aromatase expression demonstrating a decline in prostate proliferation.[25] In canine models of BPH, oestrogen treatment stimulates stromal proliferation and also induces the AR, appearing to act synergistically with androgens to promote experimental BPH.[15]

Numerous studies have shown a relationship between serum oestrogens and prostate volume, and the development of BPH and LUTS.[25] In men with larger prostate volumes, higher oestradiol in peripheral circulation has been found.[15] Prostate volume was correlated positively with serum oestradiol levels in the Olmsted County Study in men with above median serum testosterone, but not with below median testosterone.[38]

The role of oestrogen receptors is likely to be important in BPH, as oestrogen receptors (ER-α and ER-β) are expressed in prostate tissue.[15] The oestrogenic response is determined by the expression of the type of oestrogen receptor. ER-α stimulation is associated with a stromal proliferative response and promotes epithelial squamous metaplasia and epithelial dysplasia. ER-β stimulation has an antiproliferative response, stimulating differentiation and generally promoting antioxidant and anti-inflammatory effects.[15] BPH has been correlated with an increased expression of ER-α and reduced ER-β, seen mostly in stromal cells and detected also in epithelial cells.[39] Polymorphisms of the gene responsible for encoding ER-β (*ESR2*) have also recently been found to be increased in men with BPH.[40]

INFLAMMATION

A growing body of evidence now substantiates the role of inflammation in LUTS, particularly relating to the pathogenesis and progression of BPH.[41]

Prostate tissue derived from patients with BPH, even in the absence of symptoms, demonstrates infiltration with markedly increased populations of T and B lymphocytes, macrophages and mast cells. The presence of $CD4^+$ T-helper cells is increased by up to 28 times in the BPH-affected prostate, and has been demonstrated to directly stimulate the proliferation of prostate stromal and epithelial cells, and to increase IL-15 production.[33]

Other products of prostate inflammation identified in BPH tissues have demonstrated interactions with epithelial and stromal cells indicating the propensity to stimulate prostatic hyperplasia, promote angiogenesis and inhibit apoptosis. Interleukin 8 (IL-8) is of particular interest, as it demonstrates powerful growth factor activity for prostate stromal and epithelial cells, is produced by BPH epithelial and stromal cells, and its presence in seminal plasma is a reliable biomarker for prostate inflammation in BPH and chronic prostatitis/chronic pelvic pain syndrome (CP/CPPS).[33] Other inflammatory biomarkers found in BPH tissue have demonstrated hyperplasia inducing characteristics. These include the interleukins IL-1α, IL-2, IL-4, IL-6, IL-17; interferon gamma (IFN-γ); and fibroblast growth factor 2 (FGF-2).[33] Interleukin 1β (IL-1β) and C-reactive protein (CRP) have been shown to inhibit prostate cell apoptosis, which may also be involved.[33] Prostatic cells also release mediators stimulating their own growth, inflammation therefore perpetuating a cycle of progressive tissue hyperplasia.[42]

In the bladder, animal studies have demonstrated that increased detrusor muscle contractions can be by direct bladder irrigation with oxidants (H_2O_2), the effects of which are diminished by antioxidants.[43] Elevated urinary cytokines, chemokines and growth factors have also been seen in OAB patients compared to controls, supporting the role of inflammation in bladder dysfunction.[43]

Two large longitudinal studies have demonstrated that the extent or presence of chronic prostate inflammation at baseline can predict IPSS, clinical progression and the need for invasive therapy 4 years later.[41] In the Medical Therapy of Prostatic Symptoms (MTOP) study, acute urinary retention, which is an indicator of BPH progression, occurred only in men who demonstrated prostate inflammation at baseline.[41] Systemic inflammation has also been shown to be associated with BPH, with higher serum C-reactive protein (CRP) shown to be correlated with an increased prevalence of BPH, but not intensity of LUTS.[33] In another study, higher serum CRP was associated with the persistence of urgency symptoms in men undergoing current medical BPH treatment.[44]

PELVIC ISCHAEMIA

A growing body of evidence points to the role of pelvic ischaemia-induced structural and functional changes to the lower urinary tract organs having a significant role in the development of LUTS in ageing men.[29,30,43] Ischaemia has been observed experimentally to induce inflammatory and free radical induced alterations to bladder structure, smooth muscle function, increased collagen deposition, and impairment of the NO/cGMP pathway.[30] In the prostate, ischaemia-induced alterations in prostate structure and function with increased fibrosis, reduced cGMP, increased contractile sensitivity[30] and upregulation of growth factor secretion by prostate stromal cells have been observed.[45]

Clinically, colour Doppler ultrasonography has demonstrated significantly reduced vascular perfusion to both the bladder neck and the prostate in elderly patients with LUTS (both male and female) compared to younger healthy controls.[46] Daily and nightly micturition frequency was also correlated negatively with urinary bladder perfusion.[46] Reduced vascular perfusion of the prostate transition zone has also been found in men with histological BPH, compared to healthy men and men with prostate cancer.[45] In men with LUTS, a lower bladder filling capacity and lower urinary tract vascular perfusion was found compared to healthy men.[47] Treatment with α-blockers for 5 weeks resulted in markedly improved vascular perfusion and bladder filling capacity, further supporting the LUTS ischaemia hypothesis, but also demonstrating that measures to improve vascular perfusion may improve LUTS.[47]

ASSOCIATED CONDITIONS

While evidence for causation is at this stage limited, a growing body of evidence demonstrates associations between metabolic syndrome, obesity, cardiovascular disease (CVD) and erectile dysfunction with the presence of male LUTS, suggesting roles in contribution, or commonalities in aetiology. Inflammation, derangements in vascular function, hormonal alterations and autonomic overactivity are likely mechanisms by which these conditions may be involved in LUTS.

Metabolic syndrome

A large body of cross-sectional epidemiological evidence supports an association between metabolic syndrome and LUTS in men. Two recent systematic reviews and meta-analyses found that having metabolic syndrome was associated with a higher total prostate volume (especially in the transition zone),[48,49] annual prostate growth rate and serum PSA.[49] The number of metabolic syndrome components present also has a positive association with BPH/BOO, with central obesity and hypertriglyceridaemia being the most predictive.[50] Obesity, waist circumference and low serum HDL cholesterol have also been found to predict for increased prostate volume.[48] In women, metabolic syndrome has been associated with OAB,[51] indicating that the impact of metabolic syndrome on LUTS is not necessarily confined to effects on the prostate.

While longitudinal studies demonstrating causation are at this stage limited, plausible causative mechanisms for the role of metabolic syndrome in LUTS exist. As metabolic syndrome is known to cause sympathetic overactivity, it could influence storage symptoms of LUTS via stimulation of detrusor smooth muscle contractions.[50] Metabolic syndrome may also contribute to prostate gland changes via inflammatory mechanisms as metabolic syndrome has been demonstrated to increase prostate histological inflammation.[50] Inflammatory driven alterations to bladder smooth muscle is also a means by which metabolic syndrome may contribute to bladder dysfunction.[51]

Obesity

Obesity as determined by most anthropometric measures has been shown to be associated with an increased prevalence and severity of LUTS.[52] Obese men were twice as likely to report LUTS than non-obese men, and have been shown to be 3.5 times more likely to have prostate enlargement.[52] Degree of adult weight gain has been shown to increase the risk of developing LUTS, and to increase the risk of LUTS progression.[53] For men undergoing prostate surgery as a treatment strategy for LUTS, an incomplete recovery of both total IPSS and storage IPSS 6–12 months postoperatively was associated with a waist circumference greater than 102 cm.[54] Mechanisms by which obesity may promote LUTS are by increasing systemic inflammation and oxidative stress, and potentially altering oestrogen–testosterone balance via increasing aromatisation of testosterone to oestrogen in adipose tissue.[52]

Cardiovascular disease

Men with moderate to severe LUTS were found to have a more than five-fold increase in the risk of a Framingham CVD risk score of ≥10%.[55] Framingham risk score was also associated with higher voiding IPSS and worse sexual function.[55] A recent cross-sectional study found that having moderate to severe LUTS carried an adjusted odds ratio of 1.81 for CVD; however, on longitudinal analysis, no causative association was seen.[56] A higher degree of carotid intima-media and carotid-femoral pulse-wave velocity indicating systemic arterial stiffness and atherosclerotic changes was associated with LUTS in both men (presumed to be caused by BPH) and women (diagnosed as OAB).[57] The presence of atherosclerosis was also shown to be associated with a lower maximum flow rate and voided volume, and higher urinary frequency in men with LUTS.[58]

With regards to hypertension a positive association has been reported with IPSS, obstructive urinary symptoms, intermittency, weak stream and straining symptoms in a retrospective study of men who had undergone TURPS for BPH and LUTS.[59] In an earlier study, hypertension was shown to be more prevalent with the degree of frequency and nocturia symptoms. In this study, α-blockers generally improved storage and voiding symptoms; however their effect on storage symptoms was greater in hypertensive patients.[60]

Erectile dysfunction

An epidemiological link between ED and LUTS is well established. A shared pathogenesis of reduced NO tissue availability, increased Rho-kinase activity, increased autonomic sympathetic activity, pelvic atherosclerosis and sex hormone alterations may be the uniting mechanisms between these two conditions in men.[61] In men with ED aged over 50, the presence of LUTS had a strong correlation with ED, exceeding that of age. Storage symptoms, as opposed to voiding symptoms, demonstrated a stronger correlation with ED, suggesting that the shared common underlying disruption of impaired smooth muscle relaxation, occurring in the corpora cavernosa and detrusor muscle, unites these symptoms.[61] In younger men, LUTS was a single predictor of ED. Combination with cardiovascular risk factors increased its severity.[61]

Pathogenesis

SIGNS AND SYMPTOMS

Lower urinary symptoms may be classified as storage (irritative), voiding (obstructive) or postmicturition.[9] Storage symptoms include urgency, frequency, nocturia and incontinence (including urge incontinence). Voiding (obstructive) symptoms include hesitancy, poor urinary flow, intermittency, straining and terminal dribble. Postmicturition symptoms are typified by postvoid dribble and a sense of incomplete emptying.[9]

COMPLICATIONS

Bladder outlet obstruction secondary to BPH can lead to acute urinary retention, renal insufficiency and renal failure, recurring urinary tract infections, bladder stones, haematuria and bladder failure.[14]

DIFFERENTIAL DIAGNOSIS

Numerous pathological processes, including those beyond the genitourinary tract, can produce urinary symptoms and must therefore be considered in the differential diagnosis of male LUTS.

Conditions other than BPH/BPE and bladder dysfunction that can give rise to urinary symptoms include prostate cancer, urinary tract infections (UTIs), bladder tumour, bladder stones, prostatitis and urethral stricture.[8] Neuropathic voiding dysfunction is an important consideration, as neurological disease or injury (centrally and peripherally) can cause various patterns of urinary dysfunction. Differentials in this category include but are not limited to stroke, brain tumour, Parkinson's disease, multiple sclerosis, spinal cord injury and diabetic peripheral neuropathy.[23]

Conditions that can alter urine output should also be considered, such as diabetes mellitus or insipidus, kidney disease, heart failure and sleep apnoea.[8]

NATUROPATHIC DIAGNOSIS

A thorough medical history is essential to explore potential differential diagnoses, and to identify common comorbidities that may be related to the presentation. The use of a validated symptom questionnaire such as the International Prostate Symptom Score (IPSS) is recommended, as it provides a means to quantify and specifically identify symptoms and impact upon quality of life. This can then be used during follow-up consultations to objectively assess therapy efficacy.[8]

Specific questioning about sexual function should always be included, due to the well-established association between erectile dysfunction and male LUTS.[62] Questioning about sleep quality is also important, as nocturia can be influenced by insomnia, sleep apnoea and restless legs syndrome.[20] Conversely, disruptions to sleep by nocturia and urgency can have significant impacts upon patient quality of life.[17] Questioning about bowel function is relevant, due to associations between OAB and chronic constipation and faecal incontinence.[17]

The use of frequency-volume charts (FVC) or bladder diaries, where urine volume and time of voiding are recorded, can be valuable in assessing storage (irritative) symptoms, especially nocturia.[8] If used, voiding diaries should be recorded for a duration of at least 3 days to avoid sampling errors.[8]

Investigations

PHYSICAL EXAMINATION

General screening observations such as blood pressure, weight, height, BMI and abdominal circumference are of value to evaluate associated comorbidities. A focused physical examination to assess the suprapubic area for signs of bladder distension and a neurological examination for sensory and motor deficits are often undertaken.[8] A suitably qualified practitioner should perform a digital rectal examination to help determine prostate cancer, and to evaluate prostate volume which can help guide treatment choices.[8] The external genitalia should also be examined to look for evidence of urethral discharge, penile cancer, meatal stenosis and phimosis.[8]

Urinary dipstick analysis is necessary in the initial consultation, paying particular attention to the presence of blood, protein, ketones, glucose, leucocytes and nitrites. This is important to screen for urinary tract infection, diabetes mellitus, renal disease and haematuria.[8]

LABORATORY STUDIES

PSA testing is performed if a diagnosis of prostate cancer will change management. The benefits and risks of testing are discussed with the patient. Serum PSA has been demonstrated to predict for prostate volume, with a PSA of more than 1.5 ng/mL predicting a prostate volume of more than 30 mL.[63] It has also been shown to be a strong predictor for clinical progression, benign prostatic obstruction (BPO), and can predict the risk of requiring BPE surgery and the occurrence of acute urinary retention.[8] Thus PSA testing can be helpful in ascertaining prostate involvement in male LUTS.

Postvoid residual (PVR) urine assessment may be used to help diagnose bladder outlet obstruction (BOO), although it does not differentiate BPE from detrusor muscle underactivity.[63] It can however help identify patients at risk of acute urinary retention.[63]

Uroflowmetry is a non-invasive urodynamic test that evaluates lower urinary tract function. It can be useful for monitoring treatment effects and if used, should be performed prior to treatment. However, its value as a diagnostic test is limited.[63]

Imaging may be performed to evaluate prostate volume as this can predict symptom progression and development of complications. Prostate volume measurements are also used to guide treatment decisions.[63] Imaging of the bladder may be performed to evaluate bladder wall thickness and weight as part of the diagnosis of BOO. Imaging of the upper urinary tract is generally not performed, except in men with large postvoid residual urine, haematuria or history of kidney stones.[63]

Urethrocystoscopy is indicated in men who present with LUTS and haematuria (gross or microscopic), urethral stricture or its risk factors, or a history of bladder cancer.[8]

Urodynamic studies such as filling cystometry, pressure flow studies and videourodynamics are able to identify the functional or condition cause for LUTS such as BOO/BPO, detrusor muscle underactivity or overactivity, and poor bladder compliance. Due to their invasive nature, they are generally only performed if prior conservative treatment approaches have not been effective, or before surgical treatment.

Assessment of renal function by serum creatinine or estimated glomerular filtration rate is indicated, as renal disease has been associated with LUTS, and can be a complication of comorbidities such as cardiovascular disease and diabetes.[63] Other relevant investigations relate to the identification of modifiable related comorbidities such as cardiovascular disease and metabolic syndrome. Therefore glucose studies (HbA1c, fasting blood glucose, glucose tolerance) and blood lipids (total cholesterol, LDL cholesterol, HDL cholesterol, triglycerides) should be performed. Assessment of serum circulating 25-hydroxyvitamin D (25(OH)D) would also be appropriate for those at risk of vitamin D deficiency due to a correlation between vitamin D deficiency and male LUTS.[64]

SPECIFIC NATUROPATHIC INVESTIGATIONS

Nutrient and toxic element profile

Toxic elements and selenium are measured in whole blood, and other trace elements such as magnesium, potassium, chromium and zinc are measured in erythrocytes. There may also be some value in screening for toxic elements.

Male hormone profile

A male hormone profile is indicated to assess male hormone balance and metabolism. The test includes both total and free testosterone, oestradiol, LH, FSH, prolactin, inhibin and SHBG.

Cardiovascular health profile

As male LUTS are associated with cardiovascular disease, a serum cardiovascular health profile may be of value to analyse risk factors for cardiovascular disease. Important parameters to be measured and assessed are cholesterol, lipoproteins, triglycerides, fibrinogen, CRP, homocysteine, lipid peroxidises, vitamin E, magnesium, CoQ10, insulin and ferritin.

Urinary oestrogen metabolism

The urinary oestrogen metabolism test may be beneficial where BPH is present to assess the oestrogen fraction present to influence treatment choices and goals.

Detoxification capacity profile

The detoxification capacity profile is used to assess the phase I and phase II detoxification capacity of the liver. Saliva and urine are analysed for metabolites of three compounds to determine how well the liver can convert and clear toxins from the body. Adequate liver function may have some bearing where BPH is present, as the liver has a role in hormone production and metabolism.

Metabolic syndrome profile

As metabolic syndrome is associated with the aetiology of BPH, a metabolic syndrome profile (serum and plasma) that includes several laboratory markers for this condition can be undertaken. Analytes reported include HDL cholesterol, triglycerides, glucose, insulin, asymmetric dimethylarginine and the arachidonic acid/eicosapentaenoic acid (AA/EPA) ratio.

Therapeutic considerations

ALLOPATHIC TREATMENT

Alpha-1 blockers such as alfuzosin, doxazosin, tamsulosin and terazosin are considered first-line drug treatment options for male LUTS, demonstrating efficacy in managing storage and voiding LUTS, and having a rapid onset of action.[63] Their mode of action is considered to be due to smooth muscle relaxation in the prostate, via inhibition of noradrenaline binding to smooth muscle cells.[24] They may also work via improving blood flow to the lower urinary tract.[47] Side effects include asthenia, dizziness, orthostatic hypotension and ejaculatory dysfunction.[63]

5α-reductase inhibitors (finasteride and dutasteride) are used in men with moderate to severe LUTS with an enlarged prostate (>40 mL) and/or a PSA more than 1.4–1.6 ng/mL.[63] Their effect on symptoms is considered slow acting, with clinical improvement over placebo seen after 6–12 months.[63] Their mode of action is by blocking the conversion of testosterone to dihydrotestosterone (DHT), inducing apoptosis of prostate epithelial cells and reducing prostate volumes and PSA.[63] Need for surgery and the risk of acute urinary retention have been shown to be reduced by 5α-reductase inhibitors. Side effects include sexual dysfunction such as reduced libido, erectile dysfunction, ejaculatory disorders and gynaecomastia.[63]

Phosphodiesterase-5 inhibitors (PDE5-Is) such as tadalafil have been demonstrated to be effective in improving LUTS, demonstrating activity in promoting smooth muscle relaxation, improving oxygenation and modification to neural activity to the lower urinary tract, and reducing prostate inflammation.[27] They are likely to be particularly well indicated where erectile dysfunction is also present.[27] Side effects include flushing, gastro-oesophageal reflux, headache and nasal congestion.[63]

Other medications used in male LUTS include antimuscarinics (anticholinergics) where OAB is considered to be involved[65] or desmopressin as an antidiuretic.[63]

SURGICAL TREATMENT

Refractory urinary retention and high-pressure chronic urinary retention are indicators for prostate surgery. Other indicators are recurrent UTI, recurrent gross haematuria, bladder calculi, renal insufficiency or large bladder diverticula that are demonstrated to be secondary to BPE/BOO.[65]

Surgical treatment options include transurethral resection of the prostate (TURP) and transurethral incision of the prostate (TUIP). TURP is the standard procedure used for men with prostate volumes 30 mL to 80 mL, and involves removal of prostate tissue from the transition zone obstructing the urinary tract.[63] TUIP involves incision of the bladder outlet without any removal of prostate tissue and is used where prostate volumes are smaller than 30 mL. Improvements in symptoms and urodynamic parameters are considered significant and sustained. Complications include perioperative mortality, bleeding, TUR-syndrome, acute urinary retention, clot retention and urinary tract infection.[63] Urinary incontinence, urinary tract infections, bladder neck contracture, urethral stricture, retrograde ejaculation and erectile dysfunction are potential long-term complications of the procedures.[63]

In the case of large prostate glands (80–100 mL), open prostatectomy is used. Open prostatectomy is considered to be the most effective surgical procedure in managing BPO-caused LUTS; however, it is associated with significant potential complications. In the short term these include mortality (less than 0.25%) and significant bleeding. Long-term risks include urinary incontinence, bladder neck contracture and urethral stricture.[63]

Other surgical approaches to BPH include transurethral microwave therapy, which has demonstrated similar efficacy to TURP but with reduced morbidity; transurethral needle ablation of the prostate (TUNA), again with similar symptom improvement to TURP with lower morbidity, laser treatment and prostatic stents.[63]

Therapeutic application

HISTORICAL PERSPECTIVE

Traditional treatment of LUTS centred on the use of male tonics and prostatic anti-inflammatories. Highly prized and recommended in high doses by Ellingwood was *Serenoa repens*, which was not so much recommended for a hypertrophied prostate but rather for prostatic irritation and relaxation of the prostate tissue. Interestingly, the Eclectics noted that *S. repens* appeared to be able to enlarge wasted organs such as the testicles, yet paradoxically to reduce enlarged organs such as the prostate. Thus *S. repens* may have regulating action on the male genitourinary structures, particularly as it was also noted to increase bladder tone and relieve pain. Given the multifaceted actions of *S. repens* and its apparent affinity for all things prostate, it appears the Eclectics may have prescribed this herb in isolation for the treatment of BPH.

NATUROPATHIC PERSPECTIVE

The initial priority is to identify symptoms and symptom severity, and impact upon quality of life. Thorough evaluation to identify likely cause(s) of LUTS, contributing factors and associated comorbidities is essential.

Treatment should focus on:

- Symptomatic alleviation
  - In relation to identified or clinically suspected BPE, reducing prostate smooth muscle spasm, inflammation, hyperplasia and oxidative stress
  - Where bladder dysfunction is identified or suspected, soothing bladder irritability and inflammation and improving bladder tone
- Improving lower urinary tract vascular perfusion
- Prostate hormone modulation
  - Reduce excessive conversion of testosterone to DHT via modification of the 5α-reductase pathway; reduce conversion of testosterone to oestradiol via modification of the aromatase pathway, and modification of oestrogen and DHT receptor binding
- Support optimal cardiovascular health, body weight, physical activity and blood sugar regulation
- Address sexual dysfunction if present.

NUTRITIONAL MEDICINE (DIETARY)

Therapeutic objectives

Dietary management of male LUTS aims to:

- Include dietary components demonstrated to improve LUTS and/or shown to be protective against LUTS development
- Limit or exclude components demonstrated to exacerbate LUTS and/or to increase the risk of LUTS development
- Support optimal health and address identified nutritional risks
- Address associated comorbidities such as cardiovascular disease, metabolic syndrome, obesity, type 2 diabetes mellitus and erectile dysfunction.

Overall diet quality

The overall diet should support optimal health, paying particular attention to cardiovascular disease, metabolic syndrome, and obesity prevention and management. A Mediterranean-style diet provides an appropriate basis as it is rich in dietary components likely to be of benefit in men with LUTS, such as tomato products as a source of lycopene,[66] vegetables and fruit,[67] legumes,[68] and nuts and seeds as a source of β-sitosterol,[69] zinc and selenium.[69] It also limits those that may be problematic such as saturated fat[70] and animal protein.[71] It is also well validated as both protective and able to treat associated comorbidities such as metabolic syndrome, obesity,[72] cardiovascular disease[73] and erectile dysfunction.[74] Controversial in relation to LUTS risk is the regular inclusion of alcohol;[75] however, this can be adapted for the purposes of the male client with LUTS. Regular inclusion of soy products[76] is an ideal overall dietary approach for patients with or at risk of LUTS.

Fruit and vegetables

Of the epidemiological evidence for a protective role of a dietary component in male LUTS, vegetable consumption is one of the most consistent. A recent 4-year prospective study of Chinese men aged over 65 years found that high levels of fruit and vegetable intake (>350 g/1000 kcal/day) were associated with a basal IPSS lower by 17.3% compared to moderate fruit and vegetable consumption (250–350 g/1000 kcal/day).[67] In particular, intake of dark and leafy vegetables >50 g/1000 kcal/day reduced the risk of LUTS progression and risk of symptomatic BPH after 4 years by 37.2% and 34.3% respectively.[67] Ten-year prior total and dark-yellow vegetable intake was also shown to be associated with reduced risk of BPH surgery in an Australian case-control study,[70] and reduced risk of developing BPH (physician diagnosis and IPSS) was seen with increased vegetable consumption 7 years prior.[66] In an Italian case-control study, soups, pulses, cooked vegetables and citrus fruit were found to be protective against BPH surgery.[68]

Individual nutrients found abundantly in vegetables and fruits have been found to be associated with lower LUTS risk, although the evidence is less consistent than that for whole fruit and vegetables.

Dietary intake of the carotenoids α-carotene, β-carotene and cis β-carotene were associated with a reduced risk of surgically treated BPH in an Italian case-control study, and vitamin C intake also tended towards a reduced risk.[77] Dietary consumption of lycopene slightly reduced risk of BPH development 7 years later,[66] and increased circulating levels of vitamin E, lycopene, selenium and antioxidants were inversely associated with LUTS.[78] Contradicting these observations, a 7-year longitudinal study failed to associate the consumption of vitamin C, vitamin E, β-carotene, α-carotene, β-cryptoxanthin, lycopene or lutein/zeaxanthin with reduced LUTS progression or LUTS remission.[79]

Dietary fat

Evidence exists for a role of dietary fat in male LUTS, although to date it is somewhat contradictory, making it difficult to develop clear recommendations.

Total fat and polyunsaturated fat were shown to be associated with increased risk of developing BPH in a 7-year longitudinal study.[66] An earlier Italian study, however, identified an inverse association between dietary polyunsaturated fatty acids, linoleic and linolenic acid with BPH.[80]

A cross-sectional, case-control study found that butter and margarine consumption was positively associated with histologically confirmed BPH, with seed oils also marginally positively associated. The same study found that olive oil consumption was not associated with BPH.[81] High-fat dairy food intake 10 years prior was associated with an increasing trend for BPH;[70] however, in a later cross-sectional study low dairy consumption was associated with increased LUTS.[82]

While the evidence is unclear, at this stage it would be sensible to advise limitation of animal fats (such as butter, full-fat dairy products, fatty meat products, lard etc), and refined sources of omega-6 PUFAs such as margarines, sunflower, safflower and grapeseed oils. Inclusion of monounsaturated oils such as olive or macadamia oil, unrefined sources of omega-6 PUFAs such as nuts and seeds, and sources of omega-3 fats such as fatty fish, linseeds and chia seeds should be encouraged.

Dietary protein

Evidence for the role of protein intake in male LUTS is also contradictory. A large 8-year study of men with LUTS found a positive association between protein consumption and BPH, with animal protein sources having a marginally stronger association than vegetable protein.[71] In another longitudinal study, protein intake was found to be protective, although men eating red meat at least once daily had a 38% increased risk of BPH.[66] An Italian case-control study found that increased consumption of eggs and poultry was associated with increased BPH risk[68] and conversely, an Australian study found that men consuming more than 146 g/day of meat 10 years previously had lower risk of BPH development.[70]

Again, a sensible approach to advising dietary protein is warranted in male BPH patients. Due to the protective role of vegetables in LUTS, vegetarian sources of protein such as legumes, including soy, nuts and seeds, should be emphasised. Inclusion of seafood sources of protein is also warranted due to the cardiovascular and anti-inflammatory benefits of omega-3 PUFAs.

Dietary carbohydrates

A single Italian case-control study found that increased starch intake was associated with increased BPH although it was acknowledged by the researchers that this association had not been previously noted in studies involving populations typically consuming lower levels of starch.[80] It was also noted that sources of starch in this group were dominated by white bread, pasta and rice,[80] its relevance to wholegrain starch sources therefore being unknown. For this reason it is suggested that a sensible approach to carbohydrates is taken, with wholegrain sources being preferenced.

Dietary inclusions

LINUM USITATISSIMUM (FLAXSEEDS/LINSEEDS)

Flaxseeds are an important dietary inclusion in men with LUTS, studies on the minimally processed food and flaxseed lignan extracts suggesting benefits on LUTS and objective measures of prostate health and urinary function.[83–85] Flaxseed lignans, predominantly the phyto-oestrogen secoisolariciresinol diglucoside (SDG), are thought to be important active components involved in flaxseed's therapeutic activity. SDG's metabolites, enterodiol and enterolactone, have weak oestrogen-binding capacity, and have been suggested to demonstrate 5-α reductase inhibiting activity.[85]

Consumption of 30 g ground flaxseeds (equivalent to approximately 210 mg SDG)[84] daily in combination with a low-fat diet (20% total energy, exclusive of fat from flaxseed and fish) for 6 months, was shown to significantly reduce PSA by 31% (8.47 ±3.82 to 5.72 ± 3.16 ng/mL) and the proliferation rate of benign epithelium as assessed on repeat biopsy.[83] Total cholesterol was also shown to reduce significantly by 12%. No changes in total testosterone were seen with treatment, although in a previous study of men with prostate cancer significant reductions were seen in total testosterone with the same treatment protocol.[83]

Supplementation with flaxseed extract for 4 months, delivering 300 mg or 600 mg SDG daily, was shown to significantly improve IPSS and quality of life, and non-significantly improve maximum urinary flows and postvoid residual urine in men with LUTS. Due to a strong placebo response, only quality of life measures in the men taking 600 mg SDG daily were significantly improved compared to the control.[85] Similarly, a more recent study supplementing 100 mg or 200 mg SDG daily for 8 weeks resulted in significant improvements in total IPSS, and obstructive and irritative symptoms from baseline.[84] A strong placebo response, however, meant that significant differences were not seen between treatment groups.[84]

While the results from controlled trials on flaxseed and male LUTS have delivered unclear outcomes, the low cost and additional cholesterol-lowering[83] and prostate cancer risk-lowering benefits,[86] make flaxseeds an important dietary inclusion in men with LUTS. It is suggested that minimally processed ground flaxseeds are used, as opposed to flaxseed supplements, as flaxseed as a whole food is a significant source of β-sitosterol,[69] also shown to be potentially beneficial in male LUTS.[87]

PUMPKIN SEEDS

Pumpkin seeds have a long tradition for treating urinary disorders, with both pumpkin seed extracts and pumpkin seed oil having been subjected to clinical trials assessing efficacy in treating male LUTS. Pumpkin seeds contain sterols, including Δ5-sterols and Δ7-sterols, which are considered potentially important. Compared to other plant medicines used to treat male LUTS, Δ7-sterols are unique to pumpkin seeds[88] and have been suggested to competitively inhibit DHT receptor binding due to a molecular similarity to DHT.[89] A 5α-reductase inhibition mechanism has also been suggested by some authors.[89]

Pumpkin seed oil (ProstaFit® pumpkin seed oil 360 mg and vitamin E 30 mg) twice daily significantly improved IPSS from a baseline of 14.50 ± 5.36, to 11.90 ± 4.09 and 9.24 ± 3.60 at 3 and 6 months respectively.[90] Uroflowmetry was shown to improve by 31%, with no changes reported in prostate volume or PSA.[90]

A four-arm study compared 320 mg/day pumpkin seed oil, saw palmetto oil (320 mg/day) or combined pumpkin seed oil 320 mg/saw palmetto oil 320 mg, to placebo in 62 men with LUTS.[91] All active treatment arms saw significant reductions in IPSS, pumpkin seed oil demonstrating a reduction of 33.8% and 58.0% at 3 months and 12 months respectively. Maximum urinary flow rate improved significantly in the pumpkin seed oil and saw palmetto oil groups, but not the combined treatment group. Prostate specific antigen (PSA) declined significantly only in the combination treatment arm, by 58.3% and 41.7% at 3 months and 12 months respectively.[91] All active treatment groups reported a gradual decline in prostate volume over the treatment period; however, these were not statistically significant.[91]

More recently, a large placebo-controlled study demonstrated improvements in IPSS over 12 months with 10 g pumpkin seeds daily or 1000 mg pumpkin seed extract daily. Declines in IPSS were 5.4 ± 5.1 and 4.2 ± 5.4 in the wholeseed and seed extract respectively, although this was not significantly different to the placebo arm that resulted in similar improvements (4.2 ± 5.6).[88]

Given the long tradition of use in male LUTS, and encouraging studies demonstrating efficacy of pumpkin seeds/extracts in the trials discussed, the inclusion of pumpkin seeds as a daily dietary inclusion appears warranted as a low-cost, low-risk treatment option in men with LUTS.

SOY ISOFLAVONES

Epidemiological evidence suggests a protective role for dietary isoflavones in male LUTS. Soybeans and products derived from soybeans (such as tofu, tempeh) are the most notable sources of isoflavones,[92] containing predominantly genistein, daidzein and glycitein.[93] Small amounts of isoflavones can also be found in other legumes, grains and vegetables.[92]

In a cross-sectional study of 2000 Chinese men, total daily dietary intake of isoflavones demonstrated an inverse association with LUTS severity.[76] In a small sample of men with LUTS attributed to BPH, lower prostate concentrations of genistein were found compared to men without BPH.[94] Prostate genistein levels were also negatively correlated to prostate volume.[95] A number of mechanisms may explain the possible protective role of isoflavones in male LUTS. In addition to anti-inflammatory and antioxidant activity,[93] soy isoflavones have demonstrated 5α-reductase inhibition, aromatase inhibition and oestrogen receptor antagonism.[96]

Based on the above observations, soy products and soy isoflavone supplements are often recommended as part of a strategy for managing LUTS in men. Clinical trial evidence supporting this recommendation is, however, limited. In a prospective, double-blind, placebo-controlled pilot study, 40 mg soy isoflavones daily for 12 months, while significantly improving IPSS, peak urine flow rate and postresidual urine, was no better than the placebo group, who also saw significant improvements in these measures. An exception was a marginal significant difference between the peak urine flow rate and incomplete emptying subscore in the IPSS (from the 6th to the 12th month) where soy isoflavones were marginally superior.[96]

Seoritae (*Glycine max*) is a black soybean used in traditional Korean cuisine, differentiated from other black soybeans by a bluish colour extending throughout the bean. Seoritae contains a high concentration of isoflavones and anthocyanins,[97] and researchers explored the therapeutic effect of seoritae extract (4200 mg) in a placebo-controlled clinical trial in men with mild to moderate LUTS.[97] Twelve weeks treatment resulted in significant improvements in IPSS, storage, voiding and quality of life subscores in the treatment group only. No changes were seen in maximum urinary flow rate, postvoid residual urine or PSA levels in either group.[97]. Therapeutic activity was attributed to the isoflavones and anthocyanins present in the bean.[97] A previous animal study demonstrated that seoritae extract could reduce prostate weight, oxidative stress and 5α-reductase activity.[98]

Considering the available epidemiological and clinical evidence for soy isoflavones in male LUTS, and the body of evidence supporting a cardiovascular, cholesterol lowering, blood sugar regulating[99] and prostate cancer risk reducing[100] benefit of soy consumption, regular inclusion of soy products is justified as a dietary strategy for managing male LUTS and its comorbidities.

Dietary exclusions

ALCOHOL

Curtailing alcohol consumption is commonly recommended as a measure to control male LUTS; however, the evidence for its role appears to be contradictory.

A recent longitudinal study of 9712 Korean men, with an average follow-up of 27.9 months, found that consumption of <29 g/day alcohol reduced the likelihood of developing moderate to severe LUTS. Consumption of 30 g or more daily was, however, associated with an increased chance of developing moderate to severe LUTS.[101] In another study, alcohol consumption over a 3-year period was found to be unrelated to LUTS deterioration.[102]

A meta-analysis pooling the results of 12 studies using BPH as a primary outcome found that 36 g or more of alcohol daily was associated with a 35% reduced likelihood of BPH.[75]. Definitions of BPH used in the studies varied, although most involved BPH surgery, findings of an enlarged prostate, or changes on uroflowmetry.[75]

Of four studies evaluated in the meta-analysis using LUTS as a primary outcome measure (as determined by IPSS), three demonstrated that alcohol consumption was associated with a significantly increased likelihood of LUTS, while one demonstrated reduced LUTS.[75] While these findings appear to contradict each other, they possibly reflect the difference between how alcohol modifies pathological changes to the genitourinary tract, specifically those leading to BPH, and how it modifies urinary symptoms. In the case of defined BPH, either by surgery or physical findings, the observation of an inverse relationship may indicate a protection against the pathological changes to the prostate that then go on to cause BPH, a mechanism involving moderation of cardiovascular risk factors being the most obvious.[75] Where LUTS have been used as the defined endpoint, what we are seeing is perhaps how alcohol contributes to symptoms, rather than the pathological process underlying them. As alcohol is a diuretic[75] it stands to reason that LUTS, especially storage LUTS,[63] can be acutely exacerbated by its consumption.

On this basis, it is suggested that the naturopathic clinician individualise advice regarding alcohol depending on how patient's symptoms respond to its ingestion. Storage symptoms such as urgency, frequency and nocturia are likely to be the symptoms most exacerbated.[63] For men whose symptoms are not worsened, consuming <30 g/day of alcohol without episodic heavy drinking is likely to be of benefit to cardiovascular and overall health of the patient,[103] and may potentially alter the pathological process underlying the development of LUTS.

CAFFEINE

As part of a strategy for symptom management, caffeinated beverages should generally be avoided, particularly for those men experiencing storage (irritative) symptoms.

Longitudinal data from the Boston Area Community Health Cohort found that consumption of more than two cups of coffee daily at baseline compared to none, was associated with greater odds of LUTS progression particularly in storage (irritative) symptoms (OR 2.09).[104] A small controlled crossover study of 9 women and 3 men with overactive bladder symptoms demonstrated that 4.5 mg/kg caffeine in water, compared to water alone, acutely increased urgency and frequency symptoms, and decreased the sensation threshold during bladder filling.[105] Voided urine volume and flow rate were also increased.[105]

NUTRITIONAL MEDICINE (SUPPLEMENTAL)

Therapeutic objectives

- Supplement with specific nutrients demonstrated to relieve symptoms and modify long-term consequences of BPH/BPE and BOO
- Reduce lower urinary tract inflammation and oxidative stress
- Supplement to address identified related comorbidities such as cardiovascular disease, metabolic syndrome and erectile dysfunction, as shared pathophysiology is likely.

Specific nutritional supplementation

ZINC

Zinc is a popularly recommended nutritional supplement in the management of LUTS/BPH/BPE in men. The basis for this is its well-established high concentration in the prostate gland and physiological role in prostate structure and function.[106] Zinc is essential for maintaining acinar and ductal epithelium structure and integrity, regulating conversion of testosterone to DHT, supporting immunological and inflammatory defences in the prostate, and regulating prostate epithelial growth and apoptosis.[106]

Despite the known physiological roles of zinc in prostate health, no study to date has been performed assessing the therapeutic role of zinc supplementation in BPH/LUTS in men. Additionally, epidemiological research provides unexpected correlations. Results from a recent meta-analysis suggest that higher serum zinc is associated with increased BPH,[106] reflecting an earlier study in which prostate tissue levels of zinc were seen to be elevated in BPH.[107] Higher dietary zinc, in cross-sectional studies, has also been associated with increased BPH.[77,81] A longitudinal study, however, contradicted these findings, demonstrating a weak reduction in BPH risk with higher dietary zinc.[66]

SAMPLE DAILY DIET

BREAKFAST	
Scrambled tofu with turmeric, spinach, stone-ground bread and green tea	Soy-containing foods are a source of the isoflavones genistein and daidzein. Isoflavones have been shown to help improve a number of BPH symptoms including postresidual voiding and urine flow rate.* Green tea is highly antioxidant and its catechin, ECG, may help modulate the production of androgens via inhibition of 5-alpha reductase, thereby reducing the conversion of normal testosterone into the more potent DHT.†
SNACK	
Fruit salad with 3 tbsp crushed flaxseeds	Dietary flaxseed improves LUT symptoms and QOL in men with BPH.‡
LUNCH	
Lentil and vegetable bolognaise in a cooked tomato-based sauce	Vegetables contain a range of antioxidant and anti-inflammatory constituents designed to protect against BPH. In the Prostate Cancer Prevention Trial consumption of at least four servings of vegetables was associated with significantly lower risk of BPH compared with those who ate less than one serving daily.§ Cooked tomato-based products are an excellent source of lycopene which has been shown to help inhibit BPH progression and reduce symptoms.¶ Lentils are an additional source of isoflavones.
SNACK	
Fresh watermelon juice + pumpkin, sunflower and Brazil nut seed mix	Watermelon is a source of lycopene. Sunflower and pumpkin seeds contain zinc. Brazil nuts contain selenium. Zinc and selenium are found in high concentrations within the prostate gland; however, significant deficiency of zinc has been in seen in males with BPH# and low serum selenium has been hypothesised to increase risk of BPH.**
DINNER	
Marinated tempeh, rice served with cruciferous vegetables drizzled in pumpkin seed oil	Consumption of pumpkin seed oil improves prostate symptom scores and QOL.†† Soy-containing foods are a source of the isoflavones genistein and daidzein. Isoflavones have been shown to help improve a number of BPH symptoms including postresidual voiding and urine flow rate.

*Wong WC, Wong EL, Li H et al. Isoflavones in treating watchful waiting benign prostate hyperplasia: a double-blinded, randomized controlled trial. J Altern Complement Med 2012 Jan;18(1):54–60.
†Grant PI, Ramasamy S. An update on plant derived anti-androgens. Int J Endocrinol Metab 2012 Spring;10(2):497–502.
‡Simons R, Sonawane N, Verbruggen M et al. Efficacy and safety of a flaxseed hull extract in the symptomatic management of benign prostatic hyperplasia: a parallel, randomized, double-blind, placebo-controlled, pilot study. J Med Food 2015 Feb;18(2):233–40.
§Espinosa G. Nutrition and benign prostatic hyperplasia. Curr Opin Urol 2013 Jan;23(1):38–41.
¶Ilic D. Lycopene for the prevention and treatment of prostate disease. Recent Results Cancer Res 2014;202:109–14.
#Christudoss P, Selvakumar R, Fleming JJ et al. Zinc status of patients with benign prostatic hyperplasia and prostate carcinoma. Indian J Urol 2011 Jan;27(1):14–18.
**Eichholzer M, Steinbrecher A, Kaaks R et al. Effects of selenium status, dietary glucosinolate intake and serum glutathione S-transferase α activity on the risk of benign prostatic hyperplasia. BJU Int 2012 Dec;110(11 Pt C):E879–85.
††Hong H, Kim CS, Maeng S. Effects of pumpkin seed oil and saw palmetto oil in Korean men with symptomatic benign prostatic hyperplasia. Nutr Res Pract 2009 Winter;3(4):323–7.

Given the above conflict between available evidence and common clinical naturopathic practice, it is clear that recommending zinc supplementation as a specific strategy for management of BPH/LUTS in men is premature. However, as summarised below, zinc supplementation may have a role in management of comorbidities often related to BPH/LUTS such as metabolic syndrome, hyperglycaemia and cardiovascular disease, and may form part of the holistic management of a patient with LUTS.

SELENIUM

Selenium may be potentially useful in male LUTS as an antioxidant, particularly considering its role as a key component of glutathione peroxidase[108] and the implicated role of oxidative stress in male LUTS.[109] In epidemiological research increased serum selenium levels have been associated with a reduced risk of BPH[108] and LUTS.[78]

At this stage, no human research has been performed exploring the therapeutic role of selenium monotherapy in male LUTS. Its supplementation with *Serenoa repens* and lycopene in animal and human studies, however, suggests synergistic anti-inflammatory, antioxidant, growth factor inhibition and pro-apoptotic properties.[110,111] These are explored in further detail later in this section in relation to the therapeutic application of *Serenoa repens*.

LYCOPENE

Epidemiological studies suggest both dietary intake and serum concentrations of lycopene are inversely associated with the risk of developing BPH/LUTS.[66,78] Lycopene demonstrates both antioxidant and anti-inflammatory activity, and has been shown to accumulate at high concentrations in the prostate gland.[111]

Clinically, evidence exists for lycopene supplementation in improving both subjective and objective measures of urinary function in men with histologically diagnosed BPH. Compared to placebo, 15 mg lycopene daily for 6 months arrested progression of prostate enlargement and significantly reduced serum PSA.[112] Comparatively, prostate volume in the placebo group was shown to increase by an average 9.6 mL. While both placebo and treatment groups experienced significant improvements in total and obstruction-related symptoms of the IPSS, the effect in the treatment group was significantly greater.[112]

In combination with *Serenoa repens* and selenium, lycopene appears to have synergistic anti-inflammatory, antioxidant, growth factor inhibition and pro-apoptotic properties.[110,111]

Achieving lycopene intake at therapeutic doses through dietary measures is easily managed by the consumption of tomato products. For example, half a cup of canned tomatoes contains approximately 17 mg lycopene.[69]

β-SITOSTEROL

β-sitosterol is a common phytosterol distributed in plant foods,[113] high amounts being found in vegetable oils, nuts, seeds and avocado.[69]

A systematic review of available double-blind placebo-controlled trials found that β-sitosterol supplementation demonstrates significant improvements in urinary symptoms, maximum urinary flow rate, and postvoid residual urine in men with LUTS attributed to BPH. IPSS and quality of life scores were also shown to improve by 35% and 31% respectively.[87]

Combined results of supplements using nonglucosidic β-sitosterol were shown to improve maximum urinary flow rate (Q_{max}) by 53%, and postvoid residual urine (PVR) by 46%. Prostate volume, however, was not found to be altered. Dosages of β-sitosterol used ranged from 30 mg to 135 mg daily for a treatment duration of 4–26 weeks.[87]. It is worth noting that 100 g of pistachio nuts contain approximately 198 mg β-sitosterol, indicating that obtaining therapeutic doses of this nutrient is plausible via dietary means.

PYCNOGENOL® AND L-ARGININE

With growing evidence that LUTS may share a vascular aetiology with erectile dysfunction[28] and accumulating evidence for the role of phosphodiesterase-5 inhibitors for the treatment of LUTS,[27] it is plausible that other agents impacting upon endothelial function could be well indicated in this condition. Pycnogenol®, in combination with L-arginine, has been previously shown to be effective in treating erectile dysfunction.[114–116] Its mechanism of action has been attributed to a synergism between the two, whereby L-arginine provides a substrate for NO, and Pycnogenol® upregulates endothelial NO synthase, thereby increasing endogenous NO production and vasodilation.[115]

This novel clinical application of Pycnogenol® and L-arginine has very recently been supported by a small, open label randomised study, whereby 60 mg Pycnogenol® and 575 mg L-arginine (as aspartate) were taken by men aged 55–80 with LUTS and erectile dysfunction. Sixteen weeks of treatment significantly improved total IPSS, storage and voiding subscores of the IPSS, quality of life, overactive bladder symptom score (OOBSS) and sexual function as determined by IIEF5.[117]

QUERCETIN

Quercetin may have a role in the treatment of BPH, due to its apparent ameliorating effect on prostate inflammation and oxidative stress in patients with chronic prostatitis/chronic pelvic pain syndrome, and the evidence that prostate inflammation is likely to be involved in the pathogenesis of BPH.[118] In BPH, an unspecified dose of quercetin was compared to placebo, and shown to improve maximal urine flow rate by 3.2 mL/s, and IPSS by 4.6 points after 3 months of treatment.[119]

VITAMIN D

Supplemental vitamin D may be of benefit in LUTS in men, although studies are limited to synthetic vitamin D analogues, and epidemiological evidence suggesting that serum vitamin D is correlated with LUTS.

A recent 4-year prospective study found that for men with 25(OH)D ≤60 nmol/L, increasing serum levels of 25(OH)D were associated with reduced IPSS and reduced risk of moderate/severe LUTS 4 years later.[64] In a recent cross-sectional study, vitamin D deficiency (<20 ng/mL) was correlated with a higher prostate volume (42 vs 28 mL), PSA (3.28 vs 2.55 ng/mL), IPSS (4.47 vs 1.98) and reduced maximum urinary flow rate (13.44 vs 29.98 mL/s) compared to non-deficient men.[120] While studies on vitamin D supplementation in LUTS have not yet been performed, treatment with a synthetic vitamin D_3 analogue for 12 weeks has been demonstrated to arrest prostate growth in men with BPE.[121] This evidence, and epidemiological evidence for deficiency contributing to LUTS, suggests that treatment with vitamin D in men at risk of or identified as vitamin D deficient, may be of value in male LUTS.

TABLE 19.4 Nutritional supplementation for associated comorbidities in male LUTS

Nutrient	Supportive evidence
Zinc	Zinc plays a significant role in the treatment of hyperglycaemia and dyslipidaemia and therefore may be indicated where type 2 diabetes or metabolic syndrome is a contributing factor.
Essential fatty acids (EPA/DHA)	EPA and DHA supplementation may improve insulin resistance, blood lipids and hypertension. Protection against vascular disease and vascular death has been reported. Improvements in vascular endothelial function have been reported.
Magnesium	Has demonstrated benefits in improving insulin sensitivity, triglycerides, diastolic and systolic blood pressure.
Chromium	Numerous human studies demonstrate beneficial effects of chromium supplementation, particularly in the form of chromium picolinate, on glycaemic control and blood lipids in patients with type 2 diabetes. Negative effects on insulin sensitivity have, however, been seen in non-obese, non-diabetic patients, suggesting that chromium supplementation is best avoided in this group.
Coenzyme Q10	Demonstrates improvements in cardiovascular function, improving vascular endothelial function, blood pressure, blood lipids, antioxidant status and blood glucose control.

Sources: [343–346, 448, 453, 488–499]

Additional nutritional supplement considerations relate to specific management of associated comorbidities as indicated, and are summarised in Table 19.4.

Dosage requirements

The doses listed below are based on adult doses reported in the literature pertaining to male reproductive health.

- Zinc: 20 mg–100 mg/day
- Selenium: 50 micrograms–200 micrograms day. Care should be taken not to exceed this dose, as cardiovascular benefits of selenium have demonstrated a narrow therapeutic range[122]
- Lycopene 5 mg–15 mg/day. Higher doses if used as a monotherapy
- β-sitosterol: 30 mg–135 mg/day
- L-arginine: 460 mg–5000 mg/day combined with Pycnogenol®
- Pycnogenol®: 60 mg–120 mg/day combined with L-arginine
- Quercetin: 500 mg twice/day
- Vitamin D: The Endocrine Society recommends supplementing 6000 IU/day in adults who are vitamin D deficient for 8 weeks to achieve a 25(OH)D blood level of above 75 nmol/L. 1500–2000 IU/day is then suggested to maintain blood levels[123]
- Essential fatty acids (fish oil): 1100 mg–5600 mg EPA and DHA/day
- Coenzyme Q10: 100–300 mg daily
- Magnesium:100 mg–500 mg/day
- Chromium: 200 micrograms–500 micrograms/day.

HERBAL MEDICINE

Therapeutic objectives

1. Relieve urinary symptoms by reducing BOO (if present) with specific prostate anti-inflammatory, androgen/oestrogen modulating, pro-apoptoptic and antiproliferative activity
2. Relieve irritative symptoms by reducing bladder and genitourinary hyperactivity
3. Improve bladder tone where UAB is present or suspected
4. Reduce genitourinary inflammation
5. Reduce genitourinary oxidative stress
6. Improve lower urinary tract vascular perfusion.

Herbal medicine classes

PROSTATE TONICS

Where prostate involvement is suspected or demonstrated in male LUTS, herbal remedies that have prostate-centred activity are well indicated. Those shown to be efficacious appear to exert their effects via local androgen/oestrogen modulating, anti-inflammatory, antiproliferative and pro-apoptotic activity in the prostate. Those demonstrating these properties and primarily used as prostate tonics are *Serenoa repens* (saw palmetto),[124] *Urtica* spp. (nettle radix)[125] and *Pygeum africanum* (pygeum),[126] although the use of pygeum at this stage is discouraged due to significant sustainability issues.[127] Other medicines with specific prostate-modifying activity that may be considered here are pollen extract (Cernilton®)[128] and *Silybum marianum* (milk thistle).[129] Species within the *Epilobium* genus (willow herb), especially *Epilobium parviflorum* (small-leafed willow herb), also have a traditional application in treating male LUTS symptoms attributed to benign prostate enlargement and associated bladder and kidney disease.[130]

URINARY DEMULCENTS

Soothing urinary demulcents such as *Agropyron repens* (couch grass), *Crataeva nurvala* (crataeva), *Althaea officinalis* (marshmallow leaf) and *Solidago virgurea* (golden rod) are specifically indicated when irritative urinary symptoms are present such as frequency, urgency and nocturia. *Crataeva nurvala* specifically has a reputation of being able to improve bladder tone, and is also indicated where urinary incontinence is present.

URINARY ASTRINGENTS

Patients with BPE can develop haematuria,[15] thus urinary astringents with a reputation for controlling bleeding from the genitourinary tract are well indicated. *Equisetum arvense* (horsetail), *Plantago lanceolata* (ribwort), *Plantago major* (greater plantain) and *Achillea millefolium* (yarrow) are important considerations in this situation.

URINARY ANTISEPTICS

Historically men with BPE have been considered at increased risk of urinary tract infections, particularly where increased postvoid residual urine is present, although evidence of this association to date is lacking.[15] Regardless, the inclusion of urinary antiseptics as a component of herbal formula is traditionally indicated, and may have therapeutic benefits. Those to consider are *Arctostaphylos uva-ursi* (bearberry), *Barosma betulina* (buchu), *Juniperus communis* (juniper), *Piper methysticum* (kava) and *Vaccinium macrocarpon* (cranberry).

CIRCULATORY TONICS/STIMULANTS

Given the identification of a role for pelvic ischaemia in male LUTS,[29,30,43] a place for herbal medicines with a reputation for improving circulation, especially to the genitourinary organs, may be indicated. Here, remedies used for the treatment of erectile dysfunction may be worthy of consideration due to a potential shared pathophysiology.[61] Of particular note would be *Pinus pinaster* (maritime pine bark) and *Crocus sativus* (saffron). *Pinus pinaster* has demonstrated benefits in improving erectile dysfunction via an endothelial-based mechanism[114] and has also demonstrated efficacy in male LUTS.[117] *Crocus sativus* has demonstrated efficacy in improving erectile dysfunction,[131] has noted anti-inflammatory and antioxidant properties, and a traditional use in cardiovascular disease.[132] Other circulatory stimulants such as *Ginkgo biloba* (ginkgo), *Zanthoxylum clava-herculis* (prickly ash), *Rosmarinus officinalis* (rosemary) and *Zingiber officinale* (ginger) may also be indicated based upon the individual therapeutic context.

ANTI-INFLAMMATORIES AND ANTIOXIDANTS

There is considerable evidence that inflammation[41] and oxidative stress[109] play a role in the development of male LUTS. Herbal remedies that have shown efficacy in this condition such as *Serenoa repens,* pollen extract and *Silybum marianum* have demonstrated prostate anti-inflammatory and/or antioxidant activity, suggesting that other herbal extracts sharing these properties may also have a role in treating male LUTS. *Curcuma longa* (turmeric), *Camellia sinensis* (green tea), *Pinus pinaster* (maritime pine bark), *Vaccinum myrtillus* (bilberry) and *Vitis vinifera* (grape seed and skin extract) have in animal models of BPH, all demonstrated potential therapeutic activity.[89,133–136] This preliminary evidence suggests a potential novel approach in the management of male LUTS when clinically indicated.

Specific herbal medicines

SERENOA REPENS (SAW PALMETTO)

Extracts of *Serenoa repens* are one of the most widely researched and dispensed herbal medicines for the treatment of male LUTS. Its actions in alleviating male LUTS are thought to involve inhibition of prostate hyperplasia through androgen-mediated and inflammatory-mediated mechanisms, and to potentiate smooth muscle relaxation in the prostate. This is likely to be achieved via 5α-reductase and α-receptor inhibition, androgen receptor binding modulation, eicosanoid synthesis inhibition[124] and pro-apoptotic activity,[111] of which there is evidence for *Serenoa repens* extracts.

Three main meta-analyses to date have evaluated the evidence for *Serenoa repens* in the management of male LUTS. The first conducted in 2004 by Boyle et al, an update of a previous meta-analysis conducted in 2000 by the same authors, limited evaluation to 17 trials (14 randomised clinical trials and three open label studies) using Permixon®, a hexane-derived lipidosterolic extract.[137] The conclusions of this meta-analysis were that Permixon® treatment resulted in a mean reduction in IPSS of 4.78, improvement in peak urinary flow rate of 2.22 mL/s (1.02 mL/s more than placebo), and a reduction in the mean number of nocturnal voids by 1.01 (0.38 greater effect than placebo).[137]

However, a more recent updated Cochrane review evaluating 32 randomised controlled trials concluded that *Serenoa repens* was not better than placebo for treating BPH-related urinary symptoms.[138] The previous version of the review published in 1998 had concluded that treatment with *Serenoa repens* was associated with mild improvements in urinary symptoms; however, the inclusion of two high-quality trials performed since then[139,140] resulted in the changed finding.[138] The strongest criticisms of this meta-analysis centre on the pooling of results from different *Serenoa repens* extracts, with acknowledgment (as is the case in general with herbal medicine research) that compositional variation exists between products regarding extraction methods and the resulting constituents present, and therefore therapeutic efficacy of the resulting medicines.[141] Indeed, the high-quality trials, failing to demonstrate superiority of *Serenoa repens* over placebo, used either CO_2[139] or ethanol derived extracts (both with high fatty acid concentrations), as opposed to hexane derived extracts, that have been the subject of a greater number of human clinical trials.[124] Hexane derived lipidosterolic extracts have also demonstrated superior in-vitro 5α-reductase inhibiting activity, fibroblast proliferation inhibiting activity, and anti-inflammatory activity compared to other commercial single extracts available, and as such have been suggested to be the preferred choice for practitioners recommending *Serenoa repens* products.[124]

On this basis, the most recent review and meta-analysis evaluating *Serenoa repens,* like Boyle et al in 2004, limited analysis to studies using a lipidosterolic extract obtained by hexane extraction (Permixon®). When Permixon® was compared to placebo, overall significant improvements in nocturia (– 0.31 nocturnal voids than placebo), and maximum urinary flow rate (Q_{max}) (3.37 mL/s greater than placebo) were found.[141] When compared to the allopathic treatments tamsulosin and finasteride, Permixon® treatment was found to demonstrate similar improvements in IPSS and quality of life scores, but with less adverse effects on sexual function.[141] Q_{max} was however slightly improved with finasteride treatment compared to

Permixon®. Combining Permixon® and tamsulosin was also shown to result in small but significant improvements in IPSS scores compared to either treatment alone.[141]

While the findings of the two meta-analyses limited to a specifically well-characterised hexane-derived liposterolic extract make a case for *Serenoa repens* in the treatment of male LUTS, the improvements demonstrated compared to placebo are quite modest, and arguably, of limited clinical value. It may be, however, that combination treatment of *Serenoa repens* with selenium and lycopene supplementation may improve therapeutic efficacy. Preliminary in-vitro and in-vivo animal studies suggest that anti-inflammatory and antioxidant activity, reduction of growth factor expression, and improvement in histological changes are enhanced more by this combination than *Serenoa repens* alone.[110,111] Testosterone stimulated BPH in rats was also better prevented by *Serenoa repens,* lycopene and selenium combination, compared to *Serenoa repens* monotherapy, through growth factor inhibition and pro-apoptotic mechanisms.[111]

In human trials, 12-month treatment of male LUTS with *Serenoa repens* 320 mg (CO_2 lipidic extract containing 85% fatty acids sterols), lycopene 5 mg and selenium 50 micrograms (Profluss®) was compared with tamsulosin, or a combination of Profluss® and tamsulosin.[142] At 6 and 12 months, combination Profluss® with tamsulosin resulted in a significantly greater improvement in IPSS compared to either treatment alone. At 12 months, Q_{max} was significantly more improved with combined Profluss® and tamsulosin treatment compared to monotherapy, and improvement in postvoid residual was significantly better in the tamsulosin and combination group, compared to the Profluss® only group. The percentage of men with at least a 3-point decrease in IPSS (considered to be clinically significant) was 53.7%, 51.3% and 71.6% in the Profluss®, tamsulosin and Profluss®/tamsulosin groups respectively, the difference between combination treatment being significantly better than either treatment alone.[142]

Profluss® has also been evaluated regarding its effects on histological prostate inflammation in men with LUTS associated with bladder outlet obstruction, with or without high-grade prostate intraepithelial neoplasia (HGPIN) and/or atypical small acinar proliferation (ASAP). After 6 months of treatment with Profluss®, the group with BPH and HGPIN/ASAP had significantly less extension of prostate inflammation, and a lower grading of prostate inflammation when compared to control. In the group with BPH but no HGPIN/ASAP, 3 months treatment with Profluss® resulted in a non-significant smaller extension of inflammation and no change in prostate inflammation grading. Both BPH groups saw significant reductions in inflammatory cell infiltrates compared to the control, and in the group with HGPIN/ASAP, a significant reduction in serum PSA levels was also seen.[143]

These studies suggest that *Serenoa repens,* when combined with lycopene and selenium treatment, is able to moderate prostate inflammation in men with BPH,[143] and result in similar impacts on urinary symptoms as tamsulosin.[142] This combination may also be superior to *Serenoa repens* monotherapy in moderating prostate inflammation, as demonstrated by the in vitro and animal studies mentioned earlier, and a clinical trial in men with Category IIIa (inflammatory) chronic prostatitis/chronic pelvic pain syndrome, where Profluss® was able to improve symptom scores and markers of prostate inflammation significantly more than *Serenoa repens* alone.[144] More research is needed, however, to compare this approach to placebo treatment, as neither of the above studies used a controlled placebo group.

For the naturopathic practitioner, the findings of well-designed clinical trials[139,140] failing to demonstrate the therapeutic efficacy for *Serenoa repens,* should help to inform our prescribing of this popular medicinal herb in male LUTS. The alternative positive (albeit modest) findings of two meta-analyses limiting evaluation specifically to hexane-derived high fatty acid extracts[137,141] underscores that, if recommending commercial *Serenoa repens* products for male LUTS, products that either use this validated extract, or that closely match it (being high in the free fatty acid compounds thought to be important in its therapeutic activity), is most likely to result in therapeutic outcomes. Additionally, it appears that combination treatment, particularly with selenium and lycopene supplementation, may result in better outcomes overall.

POLLEN EXTRACTS

Pollen extracts have been shown to be of benefit in LUTS in men diagnosed with BPH. Cernilton, a proprietary extract produced from the machine collected pollen of *Secale cereale, Phleum pratense* and *Zea mays* is the most widely studied pollen extract for prostate-related disorders and is thought to act via anti-inflammatory and antiproliferative mechanisms in the prostate, and to potentially alter smooth muscle function in the bladder and urethra. These effects have been attributed to the phytosterols and secalosides present.[145]

A systematic review of trials evaluating the effect of Cernilton on LUTS attributed to BPH, found that pollen extract can improve IPSS, obstructive urinary symptoms, irritative symptoms, and nocturia by 55%, 63%, 68% and 36.5% respectively.[128] Most men treated (78%) reported symptom improvement.[128] Objective measures of urinary function demonstrated an improvement of 36.5% in postvoid residual urine (PVR) in two of the placebo-controlled trials evaluated;[128] however, improvements in urinary flow rates were not observed.[128] Study duration ranged between 12 and 24 weeks, and dosage 126 mg Cernilton 2–3 times daily.[128]

A more recent placebo-controlled trial was performed evaluating the effects of Cernilton extract on LUTS and sexual dysfunction following TURP for BPH.[146] Following TURP, 10–30% of men continued to experience LUTS, the degree of histological prostatitis being a predictor for worse post-surgery outcomes.[146] Treatment with 70 mg twice daily for at least 3 months following surgery resulted in improved LUTS and sexual function, dependent on the severity of histological prostatitis at baseline. Men with the most severe histological prostatitis saw significant differences in storage symptoms, quality of life and IEFF-5 compared to placebo, whereas in those with moderate prostatitis only IEFF-5 scores improved. Those men with mild prostatitis saw no significant benefits over placebo.

The evidence for bee pollen in treating male LUTS, as opposed to using a proprietary pollen extract, is limited to a single small placebo-controlled trial. Benefits were demonstrated on objective urinary measures; however, not on subjective symptoms due to a profound reduction of the IPSS in the placebo group.[147] Treatment for 12 weeks with 320 mg of bee pollen extract resulted in a significant improvement in maximum flow rate (Q_{max}) by 4.5 mL/s from baseline; however, compared to placebo this was not significant. Postvoid residual urine (PVR) also improved (– 7.6 mL ± 14.4 mL), although this was not significantly different to the placebo or a lower dose of extract (160 mg) where PVR actually appeared to increase.[147]

URTICA DIOICA RADIX (NETTLE ROOT)

Nettle root is commonly recommended in the treatment of LUTS associated with BPH, having been subjected to many, mostly open label studies since the late 1970s.[125] The majority of these trials have demonstrated improvements in male LUTS, using a number of different outcome measures.[125]

The mechanisms by which nettle root is thought to improve LUTS in men have been explored in a number of in vitro studies. Extracts (particularly lignans found in the root) have demonstrated inhibition of SHBG binding to prostate receptors and steroid hormones, suggesting a mechanism of action involving displacement of steroid hormones from SHBG, and prevention of SHBG interaction with prostate receptors.[125] Extracts have also demonstrated aromatase inhibition and antiproliferative effects on prostate epithelial cells in vitro.[125]

In a 6-month, double-blind, randomised, placebo-controlled, partial crossover comparative trial in 620 men with LUTS, 120 mg nettle root extract (as liquid extract) three times daily resulted in significant improvements in IPSS, peak flow rate, postvoid residual volume (PVR) and prostate volume.[148] In the treatment group, IPSS declined from 19.8 to 11.8, significantly more than placebo where IPSS reduced from 19.2 to 17.7. A significantly increased peak flow rate of 8.2 mL/s, decrease in PVR from 73 mL to 36 mL, and decrease in prostate volume from 40.1 mL to 36.3 mL was seen in the treatment group, with no changes in PVR and prostate volume reported for placebo.[148] In an open label extension of the trial, all participants who chose to continue were treated with nettle root extract and evaluated at 18 months. Patients initially receiving active treatment maintained all improvements reported, and in those who crossed over from the placebo group, improvements in all variables were reported to be to the same extent as those seen in the treatment arm of the double-blind trial period.[148]

SILYBUM MARIANUM (MILK THISTLE)

While not typically considered among herbalists as a treatment for male LUTS, a placebo-controlled clinical trial has demonstrated the efficacy of *Silybum marianum* (milk thistle) extract, in combination with selenium supplementation, in relieving LUTS and improving objective measures of urinary function.[149] Six months treatment with silymarin 570 mg and selenium 240 micrograms (as L-selenomethionine) resulted in significant improvements in the total IPSS (– 3.385 ± 3.075); and irritation (– 1.769 ± 1.704), obstruction (– 1.615 ± 2.210) and quality of life (– 0.731 ± 0.724) subscores compared to placebo.[149] Total PSA levels were shown to decrease insignificantly in the treatment group, whereas in the placebo group, PSA levels increased by 7.3%. Measures of bladder volume, urinary flow rate and postvoid residual urine were also improved in the treatment group.[149]

The role of *Silybum marianum* in male LUTS may be due to anti-inflammatory,[150] antioxidant and pro-apoptotic properties of silymarin in the prostate,[129] as suggested by animal studies demonstrating a protective effect against testosterone-induced BPH. It has also been suggested in animal models that silymarin demonstrates SERM activity, acting as an ER-β agonist and downregulator of ER-α in the prostate epithelium.[129]

CRANBERRY (*VACCINIUM MACROCARPON*)

Cranberry may be useful in men with LUTS who present with obstructive and irritative urinary symptoms, as demonstrated in a placebo-controlled trial of men with BPH, elevated PSA and histopathologically confirmed non-bacterial chronic prostatitis.[151] Improvements in IPSS and quality of life scores were seen after taking 1500 mg cranberry fruit powder (223 mg organic acids, 1.65 mg anthocyanins, 29.5 mg condensed tannins, 52 mg total phenols) daily for 6 months.[151] Significant improvements compared to placebo were also seen in frequency, intermittency, urgency, weak stream, straining and nocturia. A significant reduction in total PSA levels was also demonstrated, as were objective urinary parameters (urinary flow rate, prostate bladder voiding and postvoid residual volumes) which were improved in more than 70% of the men.[151]

PYGEUM AFRICANUM (PYGEUM)

Pygeum africanum is native to South Africa, where it was traditionally used to treat 'old man's disease', probably a reference to its effects on LUTS. Active constituents are largely unknown; however, those proposed to be responsible are phytosterols such as β-sitosterol[126] and N-butylbenzene-sulfonamide, found in vitro to demonstrate androgen receptor antagonist activity.[152]

In vitro and in vivo animal studies suggest that *Pygeum africanum* extract minimises prostate stromal cell proliferation through interactions with epidermal growth factor (EGF), basic fibroblast growth factor (bFGF) and insulin-like growth factor (IGF-1).[126] It also appears to target bladder function, having been shown to mitigate BOO or ischaemia-induced changes to the bladder, restoring smooth muscle contractility.[126]

In human studies, a Cochrane review of 18 clinical trials found moderate to large improvements in urological symptoms and flow measures with *Pygeum africanum* treatment of male LUTS. Pooled analysis of five double-blind placebo-controlled trials found residual urine volume was reduced by 24%, peak urine flow increased by 23%, and nocturia reduced by 19%.[153]

Pygeum africanum is currently listed on Appendix II of the Convention on International Trade in Endangered Species of Wild Fauna and Flora (CITES) and has been since 1995. Global demand for *Pygeum africanum* is high, and is likely to increase.[154] Despite this, and the economic viability of *Pygeum africanum* bark cultivation, the majority of exported bark is sourced from material harvested from wild trees,[127] mostly using unsustainable methods such as ring barking, tree felling or excessive bark stripping.[155] Currently separate supply chains for cultivated material do not exist, thus preventing the conscious consumer from choosing only cultivated sources of the bark.[127] While the available evidence supports the efficacy of *Pygeum africanum* for treating male LUTS, until verifiable cultivated sources are available, practitioners should avoid recommending *Pygeum africanum* products.

LIFESTYLE RECOMMENDATIONS

Physical activity

Current evidence supports an association between physical activity and lower urinary tract symptoms in men. Increased leisure and home time physical activity has been shown to be associated with a reduction in LUTS, with the greatest association being seen in irritative urinary symptoms and in obese men.[156] Men who engaged in more than 1 hour a week of physical activity had a 13% and 34% less chance of reporting nocturia or severe nocturia respectively.[157] For men already with LUTS, a daily energy expenditure during leisure and physical activity of less than 140 kcal was associated with LUTS deterioration over a 3-year period.[102]

At this stage, no intervention studies evaluating physical activity as a treatment for LUTS/BPH in men have been performed; however, given the associated conditions of cardiovascular disease, metabolic syndrome, obesity with LUTS, and evidence for a vascular and inflammatory aetiology, exercise therapy is likely to prove to be beneficial in these patients.

Pelvic floor exercises

Men who performed pelvic floor exercises daily for 12 weeks immediately following transurethral resection of the prostate had a greater improvement in IPSS and quality of life score compared to men who did not do pelvic floor exercises.[158] Significant differences were seen between the two groups in regards to the storage symptoms score, but not voiding scores and postvoid residual urine measures did not differ between the two groups.[158]

In men with OAB symptoms without BOO who were taking α-blockers, behavioural treatment that involved pelvic floor muscle exercises, urge suppression techniques and delayed voiding was shown to reduce urinary frequency, nocturia and urinary incontinence.[159] Compared to antimuscarinic therapy, behavioural modification demonstrated greater reductions in nocturia episodes.[159]

These studies suggest that pelvic floor exercises can form an important part of managing storage symptoms in male LUTS.

CASE STUDY

OVERVIEW

Patrick, a 62-year-old male, presents with an increasing need to urinate during the night. For the past 3 years he has needed to get up 1 or 2 times a night to urinate; however, during the past 6 months this has increased to 3 times most nights. During the past 6 months he has also started experiencing difficulty initiating urination, having to strain on most occasions. He has also noticed that the force of his stream has decreased, and he sometimes feels like he has not completely emptied his bladder. He finds that during the day he needs to urinate frequently, and on a couple of occasions has experienced urinary incontinence. He does not experience any pain associated with urination and has not had a urinary tract infection before that he is aware of. Patrick filled out an IPSS questionnaire, the total score being 18 (moderately symptomatic).

Patrick experiences erectile dysfunction, which he says has become progressively evident over the past 3–5 years. He is not particularly concerned about this, as he has not been in a steady sexual relationship since the death of his wife 7 years previously. He does use the services of a sex worker from time to time, in which case he has been prescribed Cialis (tadalafil) 10 mg once daily for on demand use, which he finds effective enough.

Patrick's diet is based heavily on animal protein. Breakfast is either a bowl of toasted muesli with a banana and full-cream milk, or bacon and eggs with two slices of white bread. Lunch is usually a ham, cheese and tomato sandwich, again with white bread. His evening meal typically consists of meat (either steak, lamb chops or sausages) with some vegetables which are usually mashed potato and steamed carrots, broccoli and cauliflower. Snacks are either a piece of fruit, or a couple of sweet biscuits.

Patrick drinks 4–6 cups of coffee a day, and typically has a beer most evenings. Occasionally he gets together with his friends for a few drinks, but finds that these days he can only cope with 2–3 beers at the most before he feels he has had enough.

Patrick walks his dog most mornings, which is at a brisk pace for at least 45 minutes. His exercise tolerance he feels is quite good for his age.

Patrick has high blood pressure, which is currently medicated with olmesartan medoxomil (20 mg once daily). Systems review was otherwise unremarkable.

Physical examination findings were as follows.

- The patient looks well
- Pulse: 60 bpm regular
- Respiratory rate: 12 respirations/minute
- Temperature: 36.6°C
- Blood pressure: 130/85 mmHg
- Weight: 69 kg
- Height: 1.65 m
- Body mass index (BMI): 25.34 kg/m^2
- Pelvic examination: No bladder distension present
- Conjunctiva: pink
- Nails: Some longitudinal ridging, otherwise NAD
- Capillary refill: 2 seconds
- Random blood glucose: 6.8 mmol/L

CASE STUDY CONTINUED

Patrick recently saw his general practitioner in relation to his urinary symptoms, who undertook a digital rectal examination and noted an enlarged, non-tender prostate gland. Examination of the external genitalia revealed no abnormalities. Investigations were undertaken with the relevant findings being:

- Prostate specific antigen (PSA): 2.6 ng/mL (predictive of an enlarged prostate)
- Urine microbiological examination:
  - Glucose: Nil
  - Protein: Nil
  - Blood: Nil
  - Leucocytes: Nil
  - Culture: No organisms cultured
  - No other abnormalities detected
- 25-OH vitamin D: 43 nmol/L (moderate deficiency)
- HbA1c: 5.6 % (normal)
- Full blood count: NAD
- Kidney function: NAD
- Total cholesterol: 6.7 mmol/L (elevated)
- HDL cholesterol: 0.9 mmol/L (low)
- LDL cholesterol: 4.5 mmol/L (high)
- Triglycerides: 2.9 mmol/L (high)

INITIAL TREATMENT

The initial treatment was aimed at relieving urinary symptoms by limiting or eliminating exacerbating factors (such as caffeine and alcohol), and using medicines targeting prostate enlargement and bladder overactivity. Addressing underlying cardiovascular risk factors (hypercholesterolaemia, hypertension and overweight) and vitamin D deficiency was also a priority, with emphasis placed on dietary and lifestyle modifications.

HERBAL MEDICINE

- Herbal tea 200 g
  - *Hibiscus sabdariffa* 100 g
  - *Althaea officinalis* leaf 40 g
  - *Agropyron repens* 40 g
  - *Rosmarinus officinalis* 20 g
  - Dose: 3–4 rounded tablespoons per pot of hot water Drink throughout the day
- Extract of *Secale cereale*, *Phleum pratense* and *Zea mays* pollen (63 mg), 2 tablets twice daily.

NUTRITIONAL MEDICINE (DIETARY)

- Eliminate processed cereal for breakfast. Replace with oats either as porridge or soaked overnight in calcium-fortified soy milk and/or yoghurt. Top with blueberries/raspberries and two tablespoons of ground flaxseeds (as a source of lignans)
- Incorporate regular consumption of nuts and seeds, especially unsalted pistachios, Brazil nuts and pumpkin seed kernels. Aim for at least a big handful daily
- Incorporate soy products daily, ideally tempeh (due to higher isoflavones) or tofu. Replace cow's milk with a minimally processed soy milk alternative. Already marinated tofu, fried and with either a salad or lightly steamed vegetables can serve as a quick meal

CASE STUDY CONTINUED

- Replace bread with a wholegrain sourdough. Reserve bacon for occasional use and instead have eggs with a fresh green salad, fried mushrooms, tomatoes and avocado
- Incorporate tomato-based dishes regularly. Aim for the equivalent of half a cup of canned tomatoes daily
- Incorporate legume-based meals at least 2–3 times weekly in place of red meat
- Aim to eat fish at least 2–3 times a week

NUTRITIONAL MEDICINE (SUPPLEMENTAL)

- Vitamin D_3: 6000 IU daily for at least 8 weeks or until deficiency is corrected. Maintain vitamin D levels with 2000 IU daily
- Coenzyme Q10: 150 mg daily
- Selenium (as selenomethionine): 200 micrograms daily
- Pycnogenol 60 mg: 1 capsule daily
- L-arginine powder. Dissolve ¼ to ½ teaspoon into water or juice and take daily with Pycnogenol

LIFESTYLE EDUCATION

- Restrict or eliminate caffeinated and alcoholic beverages due to their exacerbating effect on storage LUTS
- If alcoholic beverages are to be consumed, avoid drinking in the evening
- Avoid drinking fluid within 2 hours going to bed
- Practise pelvic floor exercises as outlined in Dorey, 2013.[160] Contract and relax the pelvic floor paying attention to breathe deeply, and avoiding tension of the buttocks. Introduce exercises gradually, aiming for 3 contractions of 10 seconds each in a lying, sitting and standing position. These should be performed twice daily.

FOLLOW-UP CONSULTATION (4 WEEKS LATER)

Patrick reported that he had noticed improvements in relation to urgency, frequency and nocturia episodes. He had not had any episodes of urinary incontinence since the last consultation, which he admitted probably had a lot to do with limiting coffee, which he had reduced to 1–2 cups in the morning. He had also dramatically reduced his alcohol intake, which he felt was likely improving his nocturia episodes. Obstructive urinary symptoms (straining, reduced stream and incomplete bladder emptying), however, had not changed much. Discussed that these symptoms were likely related to BOO, and as such were likely to be the slowest to respond to therapy. Patrick reported that his GP wished him to start on statin therapy to control his hyperlipidaemia, but Patrick wanted to try something natural to see if that could help first.

ADDITIONAL RECOMMENDATIONS

NUTRITIONAL MEDICINE (SUPPLEMENTAL)

- Chinese red yeast rice powder, 2 g daily in food.

CASE STUDY CONTINUED

FOLLOW-UP CONSULTATION (4 WEEKS LATER)

Patrick was continuing to notice improvements in his urinary symptoms, with urgency, frequency and nocturia episodes being much reduced, to the point where he was not so bothered by them. Obstructive symptoms (straining, reduced stream and incomplete bladder emptying) were still present; however, he had noticed that some improvement was beginning to occur. Patrick was also surprised to report that he had noticed improvements in erectile function.

PROSTATITIS

Prostatitis is a broad and somewhat confusing term used to describe several conditions of varying clinical features, pathophysiology and aetiology, the common element of which is the presence of genital and pelvic pain accompanied by urinary symptoms.[161]

Epidemiology

Prostatitis as an umbrella diagnosis is one of the most common urological conditions in men, with an overall international prevalence estimated to be 7.1%.[162] In men younger than 50 years old, prostatitis is the most common urological diagnosis; and in men over 50, it is the third most common following benign prostatic hyperplasia and prostate cancer.[162]

Classification

The National Institutes of Health classification has been accepted internationally and includes four syndromes:[163]

- Category I — acute bacterial prostatitis. Characterised by acute infection of the urinary tract by well-recognised uropathogenic bacteria
- Category II — chronic bacterial prostatitis. Persistent bacterial infection of the prostate characterised by recurrent urinary tract infections caused by the same organism
- Category III — chronic prostatitis/chronic pelvic pain syndrome. Characterised by chronic pelvic pain symptoms in the absence of urinary tract infection. The symptoms include characteristic urogenital pains, voiding and sexual dysfunction that substantially reduce the patient's quality of life. Two subsets have been identified:
  - Category IIIA — inflammatory chronic prostatitis/chronic pelvic pain syndrome. Associated with leucocytes in the expressed prostatic fluid, post-prostate massage urine or seminal fluid
  - Category IIIB — non-inflammatory chronic prostatitis/chronic pelvic pain syndrome. Characterised by the absence of leucocytes in the expressed prostatic fluid, post-prostate massage urine or seminal fluid
- Category IV — asymptomatic inflammatory prostatitis. Occurring in patients who have no symptoms but who have documented inflammation in prostatic tissue, prostatic secretions or semen. Typically, this is identified during evaluation of other genitourinary tract issues such as infertility.

Acute bacterial prostatitis

Acute bacterial prostatitis (ABP) is a relatively rare cause of prostatitis, accounting for approximately 5% of cases. It is characterised by an acute urinary tract infection involving the prostate gland.[164]

AETIOLOGY

Infection is typically with Gram-negative Enterobacteriaceae family bacteria originating from the gastrointestinal flora,[165] with *Escherichia coli* accounting for 65–80% of infections.[162] Other organisms include *Pseudomonas aeruginosa*, *Proteus mirabilis*, *Serratia* spp., *Klebsiella* spp. and *Enterobacter aerogenes*.[162] Gram-positive bacteria, predominantly *Enterococci*, have also been implicated,[162] as have *Cryptococcus* spp., *Histoplasma* spp. and *Mycobacterium tuberculosis* in men who are immune compromised.[166]

The implicated organism infects the prostate by urethral ascension; reflux into the prostatic ducts by contaminated urine, direct introduction by urethral instrumentation or transrectal biopsy; or by seeding from the circulatory or lymphatic system.[166]

RISK FACTORS

Risk factors for ABP are sexual transmission from an infected partner,[165] unprotected anal intercourse and prolonged catheterisation and instrumentation.[167] Other cited risk factors are those that contribute to bacterial colonisation such as intraprostatic ductal reflux, phimosis, redundant foreskin, other infections of the genitourinary tract such as urinary tract infection and epididymitis, transurethral surgery and recent transrectal prostate needle biopsy.[167] Disorders that increase the risk of urinary stasis such as urethral stricture and an enlarged prostate are also potential risk factors.[164]

COMPLICATIONS

ABP is associated with serious complications such as septicaemia, prostatic abscess, systemic inflammatory response syndrome,[165] pyelonephritis and epididymitis.[167] 10% of patients with ABP will also go on to develop chronic bacterial prostatitis (CBP), and 10% will develop chronic prostatitis/chronic pelvic pain syndrome (CP/CPPS).[165] Some of the modifiable factors that increase the risk of progression to either CBP or CP/CPPS are the presence of diabetes, the use of urethral catheterisation as opposed to suprapubic catheterisation (which is protective) during ABP treatment, and shorter duration of antibiotic therapy.[164]

SIGNS AND SYMPTOMS

The clinical features of ABP are those typical of a urinary tract infection such as frequency, dysuria and urinary urgency. Systemic symptoms such as malaise, fever, chills and sweats are also usually present.[166] Perineal, rectal and pelvic pain and obstructive urinary symptoms such as weak stream, dribbling and hesitancy suggest prostate gland involvement.[166] The presence of fever is also highly predictive, with 90% of men with urinary tract infection and fever having prostate infection.[165]

On physical examination, the patient with ABP will generally appear unwell. They may present as systemically toxic with fever, flushing, tachycardia, tachypnoea and possibly hypotension.[162] Palpation of the abdomen often reveals suprapubic tenderness, and digital rectal examination reveals a hot, boggy and extremely tender prostate.[162] If practitioners are qualified to perform a digital rectal examination, cautious palpation of the prostate when ABP is suspected is recommended due to the risk of precipitating abrupt clinical decompensation.[166]

DIFFERENTIAL DIAGNOSES

- Prostate cancer[167]
- Urethritis[167]
- Pyelonephritis.

INVESTIGATIONS

Patients must be referred for urinalysis and urine cultures, with confirmation of a urinary tract infection necessary for the diagnosis of ABP. Postvoid residual urine measurements are performed to identify urinary retention as this is not always evident.[166] Where sepsis is suspected, blood cultures are indicated, and imaging of the prostate may be performed where prostatic abscess is suspected.[166]

Chronic prostatitis

Both chronic bacterial prostatitis (CBP) and chronic prostatitis/chronic pelvic pain syndrome (CP/CPPS) present very similarly, with differentiation only occurring on investigational finding.[168]

Chronic bacterial prostatitis (Category II)

Chronic bacterial prostatitis (CBP) is a relatively uncommon cause of prostatitis symptoms, accounting for only 5% of cases.[161] It is characterised by recurring urinary tract infections often with the same organism, with which during asymptomatic periods, the offending organism is present in prostatic secretions.[166]

AETIOLOGY

Like ABP, most infections are caused by *E. coli*, which accounts for 80% of infections.[169] Other implicated organisms include *Pseudomonas aeruginosa, Proteus mirabilis, Klebsiella* spp., *Enterobacter* spp.,[166] *Trichomonas* spp., *Candida* spp., *Chlamydia trachomatis, Ureaplasma urealyticum* and *Mycoplasma hominis*.[169]

In some cases, CBP may follow from ABP.[165] Routes of infection may be from ascending urethral infection, reflux of microbe-contaminated urine into prostatic ducts, lymphogenous or direct migration of gastrointestinal bacteria, or spread from the circulation.[169]

RISK FACTORS

CBP can be a consequence of ABP.[165] The risk of progression to CBP is increased in diabetics, the use of urethral catheterisation during ABP treatment, and shorter duration of antibiotic therapy for ABP.[164]

High-pressure dysfunctional voiding patterns secondary to anatomical or neurophysiological urinary obstruction could also have a role in CBP, resulting in reflux of bacteria-contaminated urine into prostatic ducts, causing recurring prostate infection. The reflux of urine in the prostate can also cause development of prostatic calculi. Calculi can then serve as a nidus for refluxed bacteria in protected aggregates, providing a source for persistent or recurrent prostatic and urinary infection despite adequate antibiotic therapy.[162]

SIGNS AND SYMPTOMS

Clinical presentation is difficult to differentiate from those presenting with CP/CPPS.[168] Symptoms include genital, ejaculatory and abdominal pain, with associated lower urinary tract symptoms (LUTS) and sexual dysfunction.[161,170] The patient may also present with intermittent episodes resembling acute bacterial prostatitis, but typically without a fever, and for which antibiotic treatment brings about resolution.[166]

DIFFERENTIAL DIAGNOSIS

- Prostate cancer[169]
- Benign prostatic enlargement[169]
- Ureteral stricture[169]
- Urethritis[169]
- Urinary tract obstruction[169]
- Anorectal abscess[169]
- Sexually transmitted infection.

COMPLICATIONS

CBP is associated with impaired fertility and higher rates of premature ejaculation.[166] While acute infection of the prostate is potentially life threatening, chronic infection of the prostate is not associated with increased mortality.[169]

INVESTIGATIONS

Diagnosis is based upon culture and microscopy results of specimens derived from the '4 glass test' or '2 glass test', which are used to identify and localise the site of infection and inflammation.[168] Transrectal ultrasound may also be indicated to identify prostatic calcification, which can be a source of recurrent infection.[166]

Chronic prostatitis/chronic pelvic pain syndrome (Category III)

CP/CPPS is defined by the presence of chronic pelvic pain lasting for at least 3 months without any other identifiable pathology. It is typically characterised by genital, ejaculatory and abdominal pain, with associated lower urinary tract symptoms (LUTS) and sexual dysfunction.[161,170] The diagnosis of CP/CPPS is by far the largest contributor to prostatitis, accounting for at least 95% of cases.[161] The severity of symptoms and impact on daily living is profound, being similar to that experienced by men with myocardial infarct, angina and active Crohn's disease.[162]

AETIOLOGY

CP/CPPS is a diagnosis of exclusion, characterised in many ways by what it is not. It is not an acute or chronic/recurrent infection of the prostate gland or urinary tract with typical urological pathogens.[170] It is somewhat of an enigma, with the term 'prostatitis' adding to the confusion for patients and clinicians alike, as the cause of pelvic pain, lower urinary tract symptoms and sexual dysfunction for a patient diagnosed with chronic prostatitis may or may not involve the prostate gland at all, and will have numerous possible aetiologies.

INFLAMMATION

The term prostatitis implies prostatic inflammation; however, the evidence for an inflammatory cause in CP/CPPS is mixed.

The presence of prostate inflammation as indicated by prostate biopsy has only been found in one-third of men diagnosed with CP/CPPS,[171] suggesting that not all men with symptoms actually have prostate inflammation. The presence of white blood cells (WBCs) in prostatic fluid and seminal plasma is used to differentiate inflammatory (Category IIIA) from non-inflammatory (Category IIIB) presentations. This distinction may be erroneous given that WBCs in the prostatic fluid and seminal plasma have also been found in asymptomatic men as well as those with a diagnosis.[172] WBCs in EPS, VB3 or seminal plasma also fail to correlate with National Institutes of Health (NIH) prostatitis symptoms.[172]

There is evidence, however, that in some men at least, inflammation of the prostate or male accessory glands could have a role to play. Studies have demonstrated the presence of elevated pro-inflammatory cytokines in the seminal plasma and expressed prostatic secretions of men diagnosed with CP/CPPS. Interleukin 6 (IL-6), interleukin 8 (IL-8), interferon gamma (INFγ),[173] macrophage inflammatory protien-1-α (MIP-1-α), tumour necrosis factor α (TNF-α), interleukin 1β (IL-1β) and epithelial neutrophil activating factor-78 (ENA-78) have been demonstrated to be elevated in CP/CPPS, with TNF-α, IL-1β, and ENA-78 elevated in Category IIIA.[174] MIP-1-α was also shown be associated with National Institutes of Health Chronic Prostatitis Symptom Index (NIH-CPSI) scores and pain.[174]

AUTOIMMUNITY

It is plausible that an autoimmune pathogenesis may be involved in some men presenting with CP/CPPS.

Prostate stromal cells have been demonstrated to act as antigen presenting cells and express toll-like receptors (TLRs). When triggered by TLR agonists such as a virus or bacteria, prostate stromal cells produce pro-inflammatory cytokines such as IL-6, and chemokines such as C-X-C motif chemokine 10 (CXCL10) and IL-8. IL-8 and CXCL10 are able to recruit inflammatory cells, thus having the capacity to induce and maintain prostatic inflammation.[175]

In animal models of prostatitis, significant intraprostatic inflammation associated with a T-cell and antibody response to prostate autoantigens can be induced by immunising rats and mice with prostate gland extracts or prostate antigens. The non-obese diabetic (NOD) mouse, prone genetically to develop autoimmune disease that is organ specific (such as type 1 diabetes, thyroiditis, orchitis), also develops spontaneous auto-immune prostatitis.[175]

In human studies, men with CP/CPPS have demonstrated an increased T-cell response to seminal plasma compared to controls, and have been demonstrated to have autoantibodies to human seminal vesicle secretory protein 2 (SVS2). Prostatic antigens have also been shown to provoke an elevated lymphoproliferative response in men with CP/CPPS.[174]

It has been suggested that an initial infection, or intraprostatic reflux of urine or semen, in a genetically or hormonally susceptible individual, could provide the trigger that precipitates an autoimmune prostatitis.[175]

MICROBIAL INVOLVEMENT

While the diagnosis of Category III CP/CPPS is differentiated by the absence of a urinary tract infection, there is evidence implicating a pathogenic or microbial aetiology in some cases. This may be due to infection with a difficult to culture organism such as *Chlamydia trachomatis* or *Ureaplasma urealyticum,* genitourinary dysbacteriosis, or persistent inflammation following a resolved infection.

The similar symptomatology of CP/CPPS with bacterial prostatitis and urinary tract infection has fuelled the hypothesis that CP/CPPS may be the result of a persistent infection of the prostate with difficult-to-culture organisms.[170] Numerous studies have been conducted, with a number of possible organisms implicated; however, no clear aetiopathological agent has been identified at this stage.

Reports have implicated *Chlamydia trachomatis* as an aetiological agent in some men with chronic prostatitis. *Chlamydia trachomatis* has been identified in prostate tissue specimens, semen, prostatic fluid, early morning urine, and urethral cultures in up to 56% of men with a diagnosis of CP/CPPS.[162] In men previously diagnosed with CP/CPPS, polymerase chain reaction (PCR) testing of semen found that 36.6% of men with Category IIIA had either *Chlamydia trachomatis, Ureaplasma urealyticum* or both; and 36% of men diagnosed with Category IIIB had either *Chlamydia trachomatis* or *Ureaplasma urealyticum.*[176] However, other studies have failed to support these findings, with many unable to culture or detect *Chlamydia trachomatis* in prostate tissue samples, urethral or prostate specimens.[162] Where *C. trachomatis* has been identified, however, targeted antimicrobial therapy has resulted in clinical improvements.[177]

Ureaplasma urealyticum, a common intracellular organism, has also been reported in numerous studies to be found in prostate tissue and prostate secretions in men diagnosed with CP/CPPS.[162] Treatment with antimicrobials specific to this organism when identified has also demonstrated both microbial clearance and symptom improvement.[177]

Other organisms that have been inconsistently implicated are Gram-positive organisms such as *Staphylococcus saprophyticus*, haemolytic streptococci, *Staphylococcus aureus* and other coagulase negative *Staphylococcus*. When the microorganism has been localised to the prostate, eradication with antimicrobial therapy has demonstrated good clinical outcomes.[162]

Some researchers have suggested that the reason the evidence has been inconsistent regarding microbial involvement in CP/CPPS is that, rather than a specific pathogen being implicated as a causative agent in this condition, genitourinary dysbacteriosis may instead be the underlying cause.[178]

Studies have shown that men with CP/CPPS have a greater diversity of bacteria in expressed prostatic secretions (EPS), seminal fluid, prostate tissue[179] and midstream urine samples[180] compared to healthy controls. The most common bacteria found in the semen of healthy men and men with CP/CPPS were coryneforms, lactobacilli, coagulase negative staphylococci, micrococci and streptococci.[181] In men with CP/CPPS, Enterobacteriaceae, *Staphylococcus aureus* and enterococci were identified in the semen, whereas they were not present in controls.[181] Midstream urine samples in men with CP/CPPS demonstrated a higher representation of Clostridia and Bacteroidia, and less Bacilli than controls.[180] Differences in genitourinary microbiome were also seen according to clinical presentation and symptom severity.[180]

Of particular interest to some researchers have been the coryneforms, with some suggesting that they may be an overlooked pathogen in this condition.[162] Coryneforms are present in both healthy men and men with CP/CPPS and as such most species are considered to be commensal flora.[179] Phenotypic differences have however been demonstrated in the coryneforms isolated from men with CP/CPPS compared to those found in healthy controls. Expression of secretory inhibitor of lysozyme (SIL) and secretory inhibitor or platelet microbicidal protein (SIPMP) was significantly higher in the coryneforms found in men with CP/CPPS.[182] These compounds inhibit aspects of host innate immunity, suggesting a pathogenic interaction with the host.[182] Similarly, the same researchers found that flora present in the seminal fluid of men with CP/CPPS demonstrate a higher anticomplement activity than those found in healthy controls.[181] Complement is involved in phagocytosis and killing of bacteria in the urinary tract, again demonstrating a propensity of the genitourinary flora of men with CP/CPPS to inhibit innate immune defences of the host.[181]

These data suggest that rather than a specific pathogen being implicated in CP, a microecological disorder of the genitourinary microbiota may instead have an aetiological role.

GASTROINTESTINAL MICROBIOTA

More recently, differences in gastrointestinal tract (GIT) microbiota have been demonstrated in men with CP/CPPS. These differences were characterised by lower microbiome diversity, and under-representation of Prevotella compared to controls. A duration of CP/CPPS symptoms for longer than 48 months predicted less microbiome diversity when compared to men who had symptoms for less than 48 months.[183] The difference in gut microbiome seen here may simply relate to the prolonged courses of antibiotics that CP/CPPS patients are often subjected to, or may relate to the bidirectional relationship altered gut microbiome has with visceral pain perception, autoimmunity and psychological disturbances.[183] Low representation of Prevotella has also been associated with other inflammatory diseases such as type 1 diabetes mellitus and non-alcoholic fatty liver disease, and is seen to be dominant in the digestive tracts of those who consume a high-fibre and high vegetable diet.[183]

NEURAL SENSITISATION

Men with CP/CPPS demonstrate changes in nervous system function that could be contributing factors to their pain symptoms. It has been suggested that the central sensitisation hypothesis for chronic pain may in some way explain the pain experience of men with CP/CPPS.[174] In this theory, an increase in neuron excitability and synaptic efficiency occurs in central nociceptive pathways precipitated by an initial nociceptor (pain) stimulus. The consequence is that even with removal of a pain stimulus or low nociceptor stimulation, or non-noxious stimulation such as touch and pressure, pain perception continues.[184] Altered pain perception has been demonstrated in men with CP/CPPS, with a higher pain intensity observed with thermal stimuli applied to the perineum when compared to controls.[174] Lower pressure pain thresholds for genitopelvic and non-genitopelvic muscle sites compared to controls have also been demonstrated, suggesting an overall lower pain threshold.[185] Expansion of areas where pain is perceived is also a feature of central sensitisation,[184] and this phenomenon is observed by practitioners working with men who have CP/CPPS.[174]

PELVIC FLOOR MUSCLE DYSFUNCTION

It has been demonstrated that pelvic floor muscle dysfunction is a feature in most patients with CP/CPPS, and could in fact be the primary source of pain symptoms in some men.

Dysfunction is characterised by increased muscle spasm, muscle tone and pain in the levator ani, coccygeus, psoas and groin muscles;[186] inhibited capacity for conscious relaxation and contraction of the pelvic floor;[187] and reduced pelvic floor muscle mobility.[188] Painful myofascial trigger points have been identified in men with CP/CPPS, the majority having myofascial tenderness in the puborectalis/pubococcygeus (90.3%), rectus abdominis (55.6%) and external oblique (52.8%) muscles.[189] Palpation of trigger points is able to elicit referred pain at pain sites experienced by the men as part of their CP/CPPS presentation. For example, in men who experienced penile pain as a part of their syndrome, 97% and 78.8% experienced penile pain from palpation of puborectalis/pubococcygeus and the rectus abdominis trigger points respectively; and for men who experienced pain in the perineum, 76.8% and 51.8% experienced perineum pain from palpation of the rectus abdominis and adductor magnus respectively.[189]

DYSFUNCTIONAL VOIDING AND INTRAPROSTATIC REFLUX

In men with CP/CPPS, urodynamic studies have confirmed a decrease in maximal flow rates and obstructive flow patterns, which may be a consequence of anatomical or neurophysiological abnormalities.[162] Vesicourethral dyssynergia has been demonstrated on video-urodynamic studies and changes in the preprostatic sphincter have been shown on ultrasound studies. Dyssynergic voiding can lead to a chronic neuromuscular state and neuropathic pain, or can contribute to urinary reflux into the prostate.[162] Refluxing urine, while providing a means for bacterial colonisation of the prostate in the case of CBP, also contributes to inflammation of the prostate from chemical irritation.[162] Refluxed urine can also contribute to prostatic calcification, which in men with CP/CPPS has been found to be highly prevalent.[190] Prostatic calcification in CP/CPPS has been associated with duration of symptoms, prostate inflammation and colonisation of the prostate by both uropathogenic and non-uropathogenic bacteria.[190]

PSYCHOLOGICAL

There is a significant body of research demonstrating that mental health, coping strategies and relationships influence the intensity of symptoms and overall quality of life measures of men with CP/CPPS.[191] Men with CP/CPPS also experience increased psychiatric comorbidities[191] and report higher rates of poor relationship functioning.[192] A history of sexual, physical or emotional abuse is also associated with an increased likelihood of reporting CP/CPPS symptoms.[174]

Depression and anxiety are present in more men with CP/CPPS compared to unaffected men. Depression has been found to affect 12–24% of men with CP/CPPS.[192,193] Anxiety disorder is also more frequent, with 60% of men with CP/CPPS having a diagnosis of anxiety disorder compared to 15% of unaffected men.[191] Anxiety disorder was reported to be 2.1 times more prevalent 2 years prior to diagnosis than controls,[194] suggesting that anxiety disorder may be involved in causation in some cases.

Severity of symptoms is impacted upon by psychological and relationship factors. Pain catastrophising and a feeling of helplessness were shown to be present in 25% of men with CP/CPPS,[192] and along with depression severity,[192,195,196] have been shown to be associated with increased pain intensity and lower quality of life.[191] Spousal support is also a significant factor in how symptoms are experienced. Where a spouse engages the patient in distraction strategies (e.g. involving in other activities) less pain and disability are experienced.[197] On the other hand, an increased solicitous response by a spouse (such as encouraging to rest) is associated with greater pain and disability.[197] It is thought that solicitous responses to a partner's pain can act to reinforce pain behaviours, and that encouraging patients to engage in activities that can distract from the pain experience may be more beneficial.[197]

Not surprisingly, stress appears to influence symptoms, having an association with exacerbated pain and diminished quality of life in CP/CPPS.[191] Perceived stress in the 6 months following a healthcare consultation increased the pain and disability experienced 12 months later.[191] Endocrinological alterations involving the hypothalamus-pituitary-adrenal axis have been demonstrated in men with CP/CPPS, with a blunted ACTH response to stress, and elevated serum cortisol levels on awakening compared to controls.[174]

OTHER ASSOCIATED CONDITIONS AND CONSEQUENCES

Chronic pain syndromes

In men with CP/CPPS, a higher prevalence of other chronic pain syndromes such as irritable bowel syndrome (IBS), chronic fatigue syndrome (CFS) and fibromyalgia-like symptoms have been reported.[174] A recent longitudinal population-based study found that prior diagnosis with IBS was two-fold higher in men with CP/CPPS than in controls.[198] CFS has also been reported to be more than twice as prevalent in CP/CPPS patients, and a high reported history (21%) of musculoskeletal, rheumatological or connective tissue disease has also been found.[199]

These links may be explained by the central sensitisation hypothesis, with these conditions being associated with an exaggeration of pain perception.[199] In the case of IBS, an anatomical overlap between peripheral nerves that innervate the bowel and urinary system may contribute to pain perception and dysfunction in one system, while stimulus may originate in the other.[198] These conditions could also share common links via hypothalamic-pituitary-adrenal axis dysfunction, inflammation and immunological mechanisms.[174]

Male factor infertility

CP/CPPS may result in detrimental effects on male fertility. Alterations in sperm concentration, sperm morphology, sperm motility, acrosome functionality, and increased DNA fragmentation have been found in men with CP/CPPS.[200] Genitourinary inflammation and associated elevations in oxidative stress are likely to be involved.[200]

Prostate cancer

A positive association has been demonstrated in a number of studies between prostatitis and prostate cancer. A meta-analysis of 20 available case control studies found that men with prostatitis were 1.5 times more likely to also have prostate cancer;[201] however, because studies failed to differentiate between prostatitis classifications, interpretation of these results is difficult. A lack of longitudinal studies in this meta-analysis means that a causal relationship between prostatitis and prostate cancer cannot be inferred.[201] A more recent Finnish longitudinal study comparing men who reported prostatitis symptoms and prostate cancer at 15 years follow-up (again without differentiation of prostatitis classification) failed to demonstrate a statistically significant relationship.[202]

Cardiovascular disease

Increased self-reported cardiovascular disease has been found in men with CP/CPPS.[203] Bladder pain syndrome/interstitial cystitis, a chronic pain condition considered to overlap in many ways with CP/CPPS,[162] has also been found to increase the risk of developing later coronary heart disease.[204] These observations are supported by a small study exploring cardiovascular function in men with CP/CPPS that found increased vascular arterial stiffness and vascular endothelial dysfunction evident in comparison to healthy controls.[205] While this research is preliminary, it suggests that cardiovascular disease risk could be increased in these patients. It may also point to a vascular/endothelial mechanism involved in pain experienced by men with CP/CPPS.

CLINICAL PRESENTATION

Pelvic or genital pain is the most predominant symptom in men with CP/CPPS.[162] Most frequently it is located in the perineum, testicles, pubis and penis.[161,206] Pain may also be experienced in the rectum, upper thighs, inguinal, lower back and retropubic areas.[161,162] Pain with or following ejaculation, and pain on urination, are also common.[206] Ejaculatory pain is the most prominent and disruptive symptom for many men, and possibly represents the most discriminating symptom in this condition.[162] Pain intensity has been shown to be the biggest predictor for quality of life in these men.[196]

Storage and obstructive urinary symptoms such as frequency, urgency, incomplete bladder emptying, poor or variable urinary flow are also present in many patients.[161,162] Disturbances in sexual function such as premature ejaculation, erectile dysfunction, haematospermia, prostatorrhoea, and reduced libido can also occur;[161,207] however they are not considered to be pathognomonic.[162]

To be defined as chronic, symptoms are present for at least 3 months. The impact of symptoms on daily function and quality of life can be significant, having been shown to be similar to that experienced by patients with myocardial infarct, angina and active Crohn's disease.[162]

EVALUATION OF PATIENTS PRESENTING WITH CHRONIC PROSTATITIS

Validated tools for assessment are available that can be used by the naturopathic practitioner to quantify symptoms and impact on quality of life, direct treatment approach, and more objectively measure response to therapy. The National Institutes of Health Chronic Prostatitis Symptom Index (NIH-CPSI) addresses the three most important symptom areas experienced by men with CBP and CP/CPPS (pain, urinary function and quality of life) and has been well validated for use in clinical practice (see Box 19.2).[163]

An assessment of sexual functioning is also appropriate, as while disruption to function may be part of the clinical presentation for patients, they may not volunteer this information. The use of a sexual functioning questionnaire (such as the Brief Sexual Function Inventory)[208] may be useful in this context. Otherwise direct questions regarding sexual function, especially as it pertains to ejaculation (pain, premature ejaculation), libido, ability to attain and maintain an erection, and ability to reach climax are relevant.

PHYSICAL EXAMINATION

Physical examination findings in patients with both CBP and CP/CPPS are similar, and fairly unremarkable with the exception of pain.[162] No physical examination finding is in itself pathognomonic; however, value lies in excluding other diagnoses that can give rise to similar symptoms. Vital signs must be taken to assess for signs of systemic infection (hyperthermia, tachycardia, tachypnoea and hypotension) which would be indicative of acute bacterial prostatitis.[162]

Examination should focus on the genitourinary system, with consideration for differential diagnoses. A suitably qualified clinician should perform a digital rectal examination, which may reveal a normal prostate, or one that is enlarged and 'softer than normal'.[162] Examination of the pelvic floor muscles lateral and anterior to the prostate may reveal muscle spasm and trigger points that on palpation can reproduce the patient's pain.[170] Anal sphincter tone may also be increased. Examination and palpation of external genitalia, groin, perineum and coccyx can help to identify areas of pain and discomfort.[209]

A urine dipstick analysis should be performed to screen for the presence of urinary tract infection which, if present, would be suggestive of acute or chronic bacterial prostatitis.

INVESTIGATIONS

A urinalysis and midstream culture is essential for the differentiation of CP/CPPS from acute and chronic bacterial prostatitis.[162] Other recommended investigations include the 4-glass test or 2-glass test for further localisation and differentiation between bacterial and inflammatory chronic prostatitis (see Box 19.3).[206] Measurement of postvoid residual urine (typically by transabdominal ultrasonography), and uroflowmetry measurement of urinary flow rate are also highly recommended to assess urinary symptoms.[162] Urodynamics may be performed to assess for causes for the symptoms such as detrusor vesical neck or external sphincter dyssynergia, urethral obstruction, or fibrosis and hypertrophy of the vesical neck.[162]

Investigations that are generally not recommended for most men presenting with chronic prostatitis symptoms, but may be indicated in specific clinical situations, include cystoscopy (lower urinary tract endoscopy), semen analysis and culture, transrectal ultrasound of the prostate and pelvic imaging, assessment for sexually transmitted infection or urethral culture, serum PSA and prostate biopsy.[162]

DIFFERENTIAL DIAGNOSIS

Numerous differential diagnoses exist for CP/CPPS, which is essentially a diagnosis of exclusion. Any condition that

BOX 19.2 The National Institutes of Health Chronic Prostatitis Symptoms Index

Pain or discomfort

1. In the last week, have you experienced any pain or discomfort in the following areas?

	Yes	No
a. Area between recturm and testicles (perineum)	☐$_1$	☐$_0$
b. Testicles	☐$_1$	☐$_0$
c. Tip of the penis (not related to urination)	☐$_1$	☐$_0$
d. Below your waist, in your pubic or bladder area	☐$_1$	☐$_0$

2. In the last week, have you experienced:

	Yes	No
a. Pain or burning during urination?	☐$_1$	☐$_0$
b. Pain or discomfort during or after sexual climax (ejaculation)?	☐$_1$	☐$_0$

3. How often have you had pain or discomfort in any of these areas over the last week?

☐$_0$ Never
☐$_1$ Rarely
☐$_2$ Sometimes
☐$_3$ Often
☐$_4$ Usually
☐$_5$ Always

4. Which number best describes your AVERAGE pain or discomfort on the days that you had it, over the last week?

☐	☐	☐	☐	☐	☐	☐	☐	☐	☐	☐
0	1	2	3	4	5	6	7	8	9	10
NO PAIN										PAIN AS BAD AS YOU CAN IMAGINE

Urination

5. How often have you had a sensation of not emptying your bladder completely after you finished urinating, over the last week?

☐$_0$ Not al all
☐$_1$ Less than 1 time in 5
☐$_2$ Less than half the time
☐$_3$ About half the time
☐$_4$ More than half the time
☐$_5$ Almost always

6. How often have you had to urinate again less than two hours after you finished urinating, over the last week?

☐$_0$ Not at all
☐$_1$ Less than 1 time in 5
☐$_2$ Less than half the time
☐$_3$ About half the time
☐$_4$ More than half the time
☐$_5$ Almost always

Impact of symptoms

7. How much have your symptoms kept you from doing the kinds of things you would usually do, over the last week?

☐$_0$ None
☐$_1$ Only a little
☐$_2$ Some
☐$_3$ A lot

8. How much did you think about your symptoms, over the last week?

☐$_0$ None
☐$_1$ Only a little
☐$_2$ Some
☐$_3$ A lot

Quality of life

9. If you were to spend the rest of your life with your symptoms just the way they have been during the last week, how would you feel about that?

☐$_0$ Delighted
☐$_1$ Pleased
☐$_2$ Mostly satisfied
☐$_3$ Mixed (about equally satisfied and dissatisfied)
☐$_4$ Mostly dissatisfied
☐$_5$ Unhappy
☐$_6$ Terrible

Scoring the NIH-Chronic Prostatitis Symptom Index domains

Pain: Total of items 1a, 1b, 1c, 1d, 2a, 2b, 3 and 4 = ______

Urinary symptoms: Total of items 5 and 6 = ______

Quality of life impact: Total of items 7, 8 and 9 = ______

Interpretation

Pain severity categorisation is based on

CPSI Question 4; mild 0–3; moderate 4–6; severe 7–10 and

CPSI pain domain; mild 0–7; moderate 8–13; severe 14–21

For assessment of clinical response to treatment, an improvement in the total score by 6 points is considered clinically relevant

Source: © National Institutes of Health, US Department of Health and Human Services.

BOX 19.3 The '4-glass' and '2-glass' tests for differentiating chronic prostatitis

The differentiation of Categories II (chronic bacterial prostatitis) and Category III (chronic prostatitis/chronic pelvic pain syndrome), and further sub-categorisation of Category III into either inflammatory (IIIA) or non-inflammatory (IIIB) CP/CPPS relies upon results obtained from either the 4-glass or the 2-glass test. Both of these tests are used to localise and identify infection and inflammation in the male genitourinary tract.

In the 4-glass test, samples derived from the first voided urine (VB1), midstream urine (VB2), expressed prostatic secretions (EPS) and post prostatic massage urine (VB3) undergo microscopy and culturing for the presence of bacteria and white blood cells. The VB1 represents the urethral sample; VB2 the bladder sample; and the EPS and VB3 the prostate sample. A 10-fold increase of uropathogenic bacteria in the EPS or VB3 compared to the VB1 and VB2 is diagnostic of Category II, chronic bacterial prostatitis. The absence of uropathogenic bacteria, but presence of excessive white blood cells in the EPS or VB3, is indicative of Category IIIA CP/CPPS. Where uropathogenic bacteria and excessive white blood cells are absent in EPS and VB3 samples a diagnosis of Category IIIB CP/CPPS is made.

A simpler and cheaper alternative often used by urologists is the 2-glass test, where samples are derived from two urine samples; one midstream urine sample, and then one following prostate massage. Both samples undergo microscopy (for presence of white blood cells) and culture. A positive culture of uropathogenic bacteria from either the pre or post massage urine is diagnostic for Category II chronic bacterial prostatitis. An absence of uropathogenic bacteria determines a Category III classification. Category IIIA chronic prostatitis is differentiated by the presence of white blood cells in the post prostatic massage urine sample, and absence in the midstream sample. Category IIIB chronic prostatitis has neither white blood cells nor uropathogenic bacteria in pre or post prostate massage urine.

Source: Gill BC, Shoskes DA. Bacterial prostatitis. Curr Opin Infect Dis 2016 Feb;29(1):86–91; Krieger JN, Nyberg L, Nickel JC. NIH consensus definition and classification of prostatitis. JAMA 1999;281(3):236–7.

can cause pelvic pain and/or LUTS must be considered. This can include but is not limited to:[210]

- Benign prostatic enlargement
- Bacterial prostatitis
- Prostate cancer
- Prostatic abscess
- Prostatic cyst
- Testicular cancer
- Inflammatory bowel disease
- Radiculopathies
- Urolithiasis
- Urethral cancer
- Urethral diverticula
- Carcinoma in situ of the urinary bladder
- Urethritis
- Seminal vesiculitis
- Sexually transmitted infection.

Therapeutic considerations

ALLOPATHIC TREATMENT APPROACHES

Acute bacterial prostatitis

Acute bacterial prostatitis is a serious infection with potentially life-threatening complications such as septicaemia, necessitating management with appropriate antibiotic therapy by a medical practitioner.

Unlike in chronic bacterial prostatitis (discussed below), an acutely inflamed prostate does not represent the same barriers to prostate penetration of antimicrobials. As a consequence, most antibiotics are able to reach necessary intraprostatic concentrations to be effective.[166] Patients presenting with a clinical picture of sepsis or systemic inflammatory response syndrome require hospitalisation and typically IV antibiotic therapy.[166] Initial broad-spectrum IV antibiotics are usually followed by at least 4 weeks of oral antibiotics.[168] Urinary retention is treated with catheterisation,[168] with suprapubic catheterisation demonstrating less progression to chronic prostatitis.[164]

Chronic bacterial prostatitis

Allopathic treatment with antibiotics in CBP is the mainstay treatment, and is justified based on the confirmed presence of uropathogenic bacteria. Antibiotics suitable for the job in this circumstance are however limited, due to the difficulty of an antimicrobial agent achieving sufficient concentrations at the target sites (prostate tissue, ducts and intracellular compartments).[177] Many barriers must be crossed to reach the site of infection, and to do this the antimicrobial must be sufficiently lipophilic. An effective antimicrobial must also be active at a higher pH, as the infected prostate is an alkaline environment.[177] Fluoroquinolones, trimethoprim and macrolides are the few agents able to penetrate the prostate sufficiently, and have higher efficacy with increasing pH, thus making them particularly suitable. Fluoroquinolones are considered first-choice agents in chronic bacterial prostatitis.[177] In men infected with *E. coli* and other enterobacteria, 28 days treatment with fluoroquinolones typically results in a cure rate of 60–80%.[168]) In situations of bacterial resistance to fluoroquinolones, trimethoprim in combination with sulfamethoxazole is used.[168] In special situations such as chlamydial infection, macrolides and tetracyclines are the prescribed agents.[177]

In cases of recurrence of bacterial prostatitis, prophylactic antibiotics are typically prescribed; however, evidence of efficacy for this approach is currently lacking.[177]

Even with treatment with optimal antibiotic agents, recurrence occurs in 25–50% of cases. The development of antibiotic resistance is also of increasing concern.[166]

Chronic prostatitis/chronic pelvic pain syndrome

Due to the heterogeneous nature of the condition, and the enigmatic nature of CP/CPPS, allopathic treatment options that have been demonstrated to be effective are limited.

Most men diagnosed with CP/CPPS are prescribed prolonged courses of antibiotics such as tetracycline, quinolone, levofloxacin and ciprofloxacin.[211] This is despite the fact that few randomised trials of antibiotic treatment have been conducted in these patients, and the majority have failed to demonstrate a clinical benefit.[211] In the case of organisms not typically thought to be uropathogenic being cultured from prostate-specific specimens, treatment with fluoroquinolone antibiotics and resulting eradication of the organism have resulted in both short- and long-term successful treatment comparable to that seen for antibiotic treatment in men where known uropathogens were cultured.[212] Some patients with negative prostatic specimen cultures do however report symptom improvement with antibiotic treatment. It has been suggested that this may be due to the anti-inflammatory actions of some antibiotics.[170] Based on this evidence, the current recommendations are that antibiotics should not be used as a primary treatment option in CP/CPPS.[209]

Other allopathic treatments are aimed at reducing symptoms associated with the syndrome. These include α-blockers (terazosin, tamsulosin, alfuzosin, doxazosin and silodosin) for treating voiding symptoms, and anti-inflammatories such as the COX-2 inhibitor celecoxib and the mast cell inhibitor pentosan polysulfate.[211] Hormonal therapy is sometimes prescribed, with mepartricin (a drug that reduces prostate oestrogen) potentially improving NIH-CPSI scores, and 5α-reductase inhibitors, that have demonstrated no significant benefit.[209]

Therapeutic application

HISTORICAL PERSPECTIVE

Prostatitis was generally considered to be a fairly serious condition. However, in 1919, Jones stated 'elderly men died from want of better treatment'.[3] Thankfully, in modern times this has changed. The Eclectics prescribed a range of different modalities for the management of prostatitis, including the internal consumption of ammonia, and heat therapy in the form of warm compresses applied to the inflamed prostate gland. Jones also used food as medicine, suggesting that flaxseed tea be drunk freely in order to render the urine bland and non-irritating.[3] The Eclectics also dispensed botanicals, including *Serenoa repens*, which was indicated for an 'enlarged prostate, with throbbing, aching, dull pain, discharge of prostatic fluid, at times discharge of mucus, also of a yellowish, watery fluid, with weakened sexual power'.[2] Other botanicals documented for use in prostatitis are likely to be unfamiliar to modern naturopaths. These include *Delphinium staphisagria* which was thought to 'arrest excessive prostatic discharge and mucopurulent discharges from the urethra', and *Chimaphila*, a diuretic and astringent specific for chronic prostatic irritation and chronic prostatitis.[2]

NATUROPATHIC PERSPECTIVE

Acute bacterial prostatitis

ABP is a serious infection, with potentially life-threatening complications, with which allopathic treatment is well indicated and effective. As such, the role of the naturopathic clinician in this case is a supportive one, with prompt referral for allopathic medical management being the primary objective when ABP is suspected based on clinical grounds. Where adjuvant naturopathic treatment is practical and appropriate and does not disrupt allopathic approaches, the following therapeutic objectives should be considered:

1 Acute immune system support
2 Improve efficacy of allopathic treatment
   – Reduce infection recurrence
3 Reduce side effects of allopathic treatment
4 Adjuvant antimicrobial support to the genitourinary tract.

NUTRITIONAL MEDICINE (DIETARY)

Nutritional support for acute bacterial prostatitis should be consistent with that given for acute infections. An emphasis should be placed upon the maintenance of adequate hydration and electrolyte balance, and a focus upon simple, minimally processed, easy-to-digest foods.

NUTRITIONAL MEDICINE (SUPPLEMENTAL)

Therapeutic objectives

1 Acute immune support
2 Improve efficacy of allopathic treatment
   – Reduce infection recurrence
3 Reduce side effects of allopathic treatment.

Specific nutrients required

The following nutritional supplements may improve the efficacy of allopathic antibiotic treatment, as extrapolated from research in chronic bacterial prostatitis and discussed further in this chapter:

- Zinc (elemental) 50 mg daily
- Selenium (elemental) 50–200 micrograms daily
- Quercetin 50–500 mg twice daily
- Lycopene 15 mg daily.

PROBIOTICS

The use of a probiotic demonstrated to reduce antibiotic associated side effects and to beneficially alter a disrupted gastrointestinal microbiota composition is indicated as a supportive measure when ABP is diagnosed. A well-indicated probiotic in this instance is *Lactobacillus rhamnosus* GG,[213] readily available as a probiotic yoghurt and as a nutritional supplement in many countries. Supplementation should occur at least during antibiotic treatment, and also following, for best outcomes.

HERBAL MEDICINE

Herbal medicine therapeutic objectives

1 Acute immune support
2 Improve efficacy of allopathic treatment
  – Reduce infection recurrence
3 Adjuvant genitourinary antimicrobial support
4 Symptom management.

Herbal medicines shown to reduce bacterial reoccurrence in CBP are worthy of inclusion here, and include *Serenoa repens* (saw palmetto), *Arctostaphylos uva-ursi* (bearberry), *Urtica dioica* radix (nettle root) and *Curcuma longa* (turmeric).[214,215] *Allium sativum* (garlic) may be also well indicated.[216]

Treatment should otherwise be targeted towards acute immune support, especially making use of *Echinacea* spp. (Echinacea) or *Andrographis paniculata.* Urinary antiseptics such as *Barosma betulina* (buchu), *Juniperus communis* (juniper) and *Vaccinium macrocarpon* (cranberry) may also be of value.

Symptomatic relief may be achieved with the use of urinary tract demulcents such as *Agropyron repens* (couch grass), *Crataeva nurvala* (crataeva) and *Althaea officinalis* (marshmallow leaf); and analgesics such as *Piper methysticum* (kava), *Piscidia erythrina* (Jamaican dogwood), *Corydalis ambigua* (corydalis), *Anemone pulsatilla* (pasque flower) and *Eschscholzia californica* (Californian poppy).

Chronic bacterial prostatitis (Category II) and chronic prostatitis/chronic pelvic pain syndrome (Categories IIIA and IIIB)

Chronic bacterial prostatitis and chronic prostatitis/chronic pelvic pain syndrome overlap considerably. The two conditions are difficult to distinguish on clinical grounds, and are only differentiated by laboratory testing.[168] The finding that non-uropathogenic bacteria may have a role in Category III CP/CPPS,[181] or that uropathogenic organisms can sometimes be identified with more sensitive investigations,[162,176] helps to further blur the line between the two classifications. As such, the following section on therapeutics will address the treatment of 'chronic prostatitis' more broadly, and make reference to specific categories and sub-categories as relevant.

The naturopathic practitioner is reminded that chronic prostatitis is a heterogeneous condition, with various potential aetiologies present, and combinations of symptom expression possible. Only a small number of patients presenting with chronic prostatitis will have a demonstrated urogenital infection, although many will be led to believe that they do, and will have been subjected to months/years of antibiotic treatment with the hopes of eradicating the elusive infection. It is also possible, as discussed in previous sections, that a patient diagnosed with chronic prostatitis may not have any prostate gland involvement, and rather be experiencing a more systemic chronic pain syndrome, or myofascial pain syndrome originating in the pelvic floor, or extension of pain and subsequent urinary dysfunction via central sensitisation mechanisms as a consequence of pain and dysfunction in the gastrointestinal tract.

TABLE 19.5 Diagnostic criteria for UPOINT phenotypes

Domain	Diagnostic criteria
Urinary	Bothersome irritative or obstructive urinary symptoms NIH-CPSI urinary score >4 Elevated postvoid urine
Psychological	Clinical depression Anxiety/stress Catastrophising (verbalised helplessness and hopelessness)
Organ specific (bladder or prostate)	Specific prostate tenderness Symptom relief with voiding Leucocytosis in prostatic fluid Haematospermia Extensive prostatic calcification
Infection	Positive cultures of prostate fluid in absence of UTI Documented successful response to antimicrobial therapy Previous history of UTI
Neurological/ systemic	Clinical evidence of central neuropathy Pain outside pelvis Systemic pain syndrome (irritable bowel syndrome, fibromyalgia, chronic fatigue syndrome)
Tenderness	Palpable tenderness and/or painful muscle spasm or trigger points in abdomen and/or pelvic floor
Sexual	Erectile dysfunction Orgasmic dysfunction Sexual desire impairment

Source: adapted from [218,219]

Therefore, individualised care is the key. UPOINT, a validated clinical tool that phenotypes patients with CP/CPPS, has been shown to result in better therapeutic outcomes over monotherapy.[217] UPOINT categorises patients into one or more of six domains: Urinary, Psychosocial, Organ-specific, Infection, Neurological/Systemic and Tenderness (muscle).[218] The number of domains present correlates with chronic prostatitis symptom severity.[218] A seventh category (Sexual) has been suggested to be included.[219] While this was not shown to correlate with symptom severity or quality of life,[220] for clinical evaluation and treatment purposes considering a sexual domain is of value.

Phenotyping patients based upon specific diagnostic criteria (outlined in Table 19.5) is then used to guide treatment choices, with treatment targeted to address the specific domain(s) identified in an individual patient.

NUTRITIONAL MEDICINE (DIETARY)

Therapeutic objectives

1 Support optimal health and prevent nutritional deficiencies

2 Include dietary components demonstrated to reduce prostate inflammation
3 Support optimal gastrointestinal microbiotia
4 Eliminate aggravating factors
5 Reduce inflammation
6 Reduce cardiovascular disease risk.

At this stage, there is little evidence available exploring specific dietary approaches as part of the management of both CBP and CP/CPPS. However, knowledge of aetiological factors, and limited research on specific nutrients, can guide us as to an appropriate therapeutic approach.

One study demonstrated that for men with Category IIIA and IIIB CP/CPPS, following a list of extensive lifestyle rules for 3 months that included general dietary advice to increase fruit and vegetable consumption, increase dietary fibre, and to follow a 'balanced' diet (carbohydrate 50%, fat 30%, protein 20%), resulted in substantial improvements in the NIH-CPSI.[221]

A Mediterranean, predominantly plant-based diet, rich in vegetables, fruit and wholegrains, and deriving protein from legumes, nuts, seeds and seafood, provides an appropriate base for a CP/CPPS dietary approach. Such an approach is validated to protect against associated comorbidities such as cardiovascular disease[73] and erectile dysfunction.[74] A wholefood, plant-based dietary approach is also ideal for supporting optimal gastrointestinal microbiota[222] found to be disrupted in men with CP/CPPS.[183]

Dietary inclusions

Dietary sources of specific nutrients demonstrated to have a therapeutic effect in CBP and CP/CPPS should be regularly included. Dietary intake of zinc from both plant (pumpkin seeds, sunflower seeds, sesame seeds and Brazil nuts) and animal sources should be given attention, due to zinc's antimicrobial role in the prostate[223] and capacity to improve symptoms in both CBP[224] and CP/CPPS.[225] Dietary sources of selenium such as Brazil nuts should also be regularly included due to selenium's role in reducing prostate inflammation.[143] Similarly, dietary sources of lycopene in the form of tomatoes, particularly processed tomato products such as tomato paste, should be regularly included due to documented antioxidant and anti-inflammatory activities in the prostate[226] and animal research suggesting benefit in CBP.[227]

Other foods found to have a beneficial effect on prostate and lower urinary tract health should also be included, such as flaxseeds/linseeds,[83] soy[76] and pumpkin seed kernels.[88] Ensuring adequate hydration and including fibre sources such as psyllium are also likely to improve symptoms.[228]

Dietary exclusions

FOOD SENSITIVITIES

Food sensitivity has been reported as a potential contributor to symptoms in men with CP/CPPS, with 43.5% of men reporting that certain ingested substances could worsen pain, frequency and urgency symptoms. The most commonly reported aggravating foods were 'spicy' foods, coffee, hot peppers, alcoholic beverages, tea and chilli.[228] Thus exploration of potential dietary triggers can be of particular value in managing CP/CPPS symptoms.

NUTRITIONAL MEDICINE (SUPPLEMENTAL)

Consideration of the UPOINT clinical phenotype can help to guide nutritional and herbal medicine prescription decisions.

Where confirmed CBP is present (i.e. uropathogenic microorganisms are cultured from prostatic specimens), the naturopathic clinician is safe to attempt primary management if appropriate as, unlike ABP, CBP is not

SAMPLE DAILY DIET

BREAKFAST	
Salmon fillet with avocado and a carrot and ginger juice	Reducing inflammation reduces pain associated with CP/CPPS. Salmon and avocado are rich in PUFAs which are known to be anti-inflammatory, particularly to the urogenital tract; ginger is also anti-inflammatory. Carrot is a source of carotenoids including lycopene which has an affinity for the prostate gland. Beta-carotene rich carrots and antimicrobial ginger both assist in supporting immune function, helping to reduce infection, if the CP/CPPS is of infective origin.
LUNCH	
Spaghetti with garlic and basil pesto	Garlic has antibacterial and anti-inflammatory properties that may help to reduce CP/CPPS.* Additionally, it is a powerful antifungal and immune stimulant. CP/CPPS that does not resolve with antibiotics may be of fungal origin; therefore including antifungal foods in the diet may assist with amelioration of symptoms.
DINNER	
Turmeric-crusted cod with garlic-roasted beetroot and carrots and gluten-free tabouli	Some forms of CP/CPPS are auto-immune driven, thus gluten-free grains are suggested to reduce inflammation and reduce intestinal permeability.
BEVERAGE	
Golden milk chai	Contains turmeric which is immune-regulating and anti-inflammatory.

*Sohn DW, Han CH, Jung YS et al. Anti-inflammatory and antimicrobial effects of garlic and synergistic effect between garlic and ciprofloxacin in a chronic bacterial prostatitis rat model. Int J Antimicrob Agents 2009 Sep;34(3):215–19.

associated with increased mortality.[169] However in this case antibiotic treatment is justified, as 28-day treatment with an appropriately chosen antibiotic can bring about clinical resolution in many cases.[168] However relapse rates are common and antibiotic resistance is of a growing concern.[166] The naturopathic clinician in this case can play an important role in improving allopathic treatment responses.

Therapeutic objectives

When CBP is confirmed, therapeutic objectives include:

1 Use specific antimicrobial treatment targeting the genitourinary tract
2 Improve efficacy of antibiotic treatment
3 Reduce side effects of antibiotic treatment
4 Reduce progression to CP/CPPS
5 Support optimal immune function and address impediments to the immune response.

In the case of CP/CPPS, and also appropriate for CBP, therapeutic objectives include:

1 Treat prostatitis pain symptoms, identifying where possible if originating from the prostate, bladder, urethra, pelvic floor musculature or gastrointestinal tract
2 Relieve irritative and obstructive urinary symptoms
3 Reduce genitourinary inflammation, especially of the prostate and/or bladder
4 Reduce oxidative stress
5 Manage psychological contributing factors such as depression, anxiety and stress
6 Manage sexual dysfunction if present.

SPECIFIC TREATMENTS

Combination herbal/nutritional supplements for CBP

A combination herbal and probiotic supplement (Lactorepens®) containing *Serenoa repens* 320 mg, *Lactobacillus sporogenes* 200 mg (strain not specified) and arbutin 100 mg was taken once daily for 30 days in combination with a 21-day course of a fluoroquinolone antibiotic (prulifloxacin 600 mg daily). The combined treatment significantly reduced infection recurrence rate at 2 months compared to antibiotic monotherapy (7.8% vs 27.6%). NIH-CPSI total and all sub scores (pain, urinary, quality of life) were significantly more improved in the combination group at 2, 4 and 6 months compared to antibiotic treatment only, and the number of patients who had CBP symptoms 6 months after treatment was much lower with the combination treatment (6.5%) compared to antibiotic-only treatment (26.3%).[215]

Similarly, less bacterial recurrence and better symptom resolution was achieved with combined herbal medicine treatment containing *Serenoa repens* 160 mg (30% fatty acids and sterols), *Urtica dioica* 120 mg (0.4% β-sitosterol), quercetin 100 mg and curcumin 200 mg taken for 14 days with prulifloxacin 600 mg. At 1 month after treatment only 10% of the combined herbal and antibiotic group had bacterial recurrence, compared to 41% of the antibiotic-only group. Symptoms of CBP at 1 month and 6 months after treatment were 10.4% and 9.4% respectively in the combination group, compared to 73% and 78.4% of the antibiotic-only group.[214]

Zinc

Zinc supplementation is a consideration in the case of both confirmed CBP and CP/CPPS. Among its many functions, zinc has an antimicrobial role in the prostate as a component of prostate antibacterial factor (PAF), and is important for acinar and ductal cell stability.[223] It has also been found to be lowered in prostate specimens in men with CP (category not specified) as demonstrated in a recent meta-analysis.[223] A Chinese study reported improvements in pain, urinary symptoms and quality of life in men with CBP supplemented with oral zinc in combination with antibiotics.[224] In men with Category III CP/CPPS, 220 mg zinc sulfate in combination with the alpha blocker prazosin taken for 12 weeks, was shown to result in significantly greater decreases in both total and pain scores of the NIH-CPSI compared to prazosin therapy alone.[225]

Quercetin

A key nutritional supplement in the management of patients with CP/CPPS is quercetin. In these men it has demonstrated the capacity to significantly relieve pain, presumably via anti-inflammatory and antioxidant mechanisms.[118]

Treatment with 500 mg twice daily for 1 month in men with Category IIIa and IIIb CPPS reduced total average NIH-CPSI scores from 21.0 to 13.1. Improvements in symptoms were seen in the pain (10.3 reduced to 6.2) and quality of life domain scores (8 reduced to 4.9). No significant improvements were seen in urinary symptoms. A 25% (clinically meaningful) response was observed in 67% of men in the treatment group, compared to 20% of men in the placebo group. White blood cell counts in prostatic secretions were also seen to be significantly reduced with quercetin treatment compared to placebo.[118]

A follow-up open label study performed by the same authors combined the same dose of quercetin with bromelain and papain (amounts not specified) for 1 month. Similar results were seen with symptom improvement. Oxidative stress in the prostate, assessed using prostatic fluid isoprostane levels as a surrogate, were found to reduce significantly.[118] It is suggested that patients trial quercetin for at least 6 weeks, with symptom improvement sometimes occurring within days. If a symptom response occurs within 6 weeks, continued improvement over a 3-month period can be expected.[229]

Antioxidants

Measures to reduce oxidative stress are an important consideration in the management of CBP and CP/CPPS. Men with inflammatory CP/CPPS have evidence of elevated systemic and seminal fluid oxidative stress, indicated by increased diene conjugates in sperm and seminal plasma, increased urinary 8-isoprostanes (indicative of lipid peroxidation), and reduced total spermatozoa antioxidant status and seminal plasma total antioxidant activity.[230] Men with CP/CPPS also demonstrate a higher frequency of manganese superoxide dismutase (MnSOD) polymorphism and reduced seminal and systemic super oxide dismutase (SOD) and glutathione peroxidase (Gsh-Px).[231] In CBP, higher levels of systemic oxidative stress are seen compared to healthy controls.[232] Considering this, and the impact inflammation has on oxidative stress, supplementation with agents that exert antioxidant activity in the male genitourinary tract should be considered.

A combination of lycopene (1.5 mg), epigallocatechin gallate (green tea extract, 250 mg), ellagic acid (pomegranate extract, 250 mg), selenium (82.5 micrograms) and zinc (20 mg) was supplemented daily for 6 months in men with NIH Category IIIA CP/CPPS and compared to placebo. The pain subscore of the NIH-CPSI was reduced from a baseline of 11.8 to 9.9 after treatment. Leucocytes in semen and expressed prostatic secretions were significantly reduced, and improvements in semen parameters (increased progressive motility and reduction in atypical forms) were also seen.[233] The reduction in the pain domain score, while statistically significant, is not likely to have a clinically significant impact. To achieve this, a three-point reduction in the pain domain score of the NIH-CPSI is needed.[234] Therefore, as a stand-alone therapy this supplement approach is not likely to be adequate; however, it may be useful as part of a multimodality treatment.

Selenium

As an ingredient in herb/nutrient combination products discussed elsewhere in this chapter, selenium supplementation has demonstrated efficacy in CP/CPPS symptom management,[144,233] and in reducing prostate inflammation.[143,233] Its role in chronic prostatitis is likely to be related to its immune modulating and antioxidant properties.[144] In a rat study, pre-treatment with oral selenium reduced the development of bacterial prostatitis, reduced prostate inflammation and improved the efficacy of antibiotic treatment.[235]

Lycopene

Human studies evaluating lycopene in chronic prostatitis are limited to combination therapy with other nutrients and herbs, where it has demonstrated efficacy in reducing CP/CPPS symptoms[144,233] and clinical and histological markers of prostate inflammation.[143,233] Lycopene demonstrates antioxidant and anti-inflammatory activity,[226] supporting its therapeutic role in prostatitis. In a rat model of chronic bacterial prostatitis, oral treatment with a combination of lycopene and ciprofloxacin was more effective at reducing prostate inflammation, and prostate and urinary bacteria growth than ciprofloxacin alone.[227]

DOSAGE REQUIREMENTS

The doses listed below are based on adult doses reported in the literature:

- Quercetin: 50 mg to 500 mg twice/day. Higher dose used for CP/CPPS
- Zinc: 20 mg–100 mg/day
- Selenium: 50 micrograms–200 micrograms daily. Care should be taken not to exceed this dose as cardiovascular benefits of selenium have demonstrated a narrow therapeutic range[122]
- Lycopene 5 mg–15 mg/day.

HERBAL MEDICINE

Therapeutic objectives

As per nutritional medicine (supplemental) objectives.

Herbal medicine classes

IMMUNE STIMULANTS/TONICS

If the involvement of infection has been demonstrated, or is suspected based upon a history of urinary tract infection preceding the onset of symptoms, immune system stimulants/tonics are well indicated. These include *Echinacea* spp. (echinacea), *Andrographis paniculata* (andrographis), *Tinospora cordifolia* (guruchi) and *Astragalus membranaceus.*

URINARY ANTISEPTICS

Urinary antiseptics including *Arctostaphylos uva-ursi* (bearberry), *Barosma betulina* (buchu), *Juniperus communis* (juniper) and *Vaccinium macrocarpon* (cranberry) are indicated if infection has been demonstrated or is suspected based on history. Specifically, arbutin derived from *Arctostaphylos uva-ursi* has been shown as part of a supplement combination to improve microbial clearance in combination with antibiotic treatment.[215]

Although not generally considered a urinary antiseptic, but well known as an antimicrobial agent, oral *Allium sativum* (garlic) extract demonstrated in an animal model of bacterial prostatitis both antimicrobial and anti-inflammatory properties. In this study, it was also shown to improve the efficacy of antibiotic treatment.[216]

It is also plausible that urinary antiseptics may have a role in modulating a disrupted genitourinary microbiota, which appears to be a feature in CP/CPPS.[178]

URINARY DEMULCENTS

Soothing urinary demulcents such as *Agropyron repens* (couch grass), *Crataeva nurvala* (crataeva), *Althaea officinalis* (marshmallow leaf) and *Solidago virgaurea* (goldenrod) are specifically indicated when irritative urinary symptoms are present such as frequency, urgency and pain on urination.

Male reproductive tonics

Of specific value where prostate inflammation is apparent are *Serenoa repens* (saw palmetto) and *Urtica* spp. (nettle radix). Where sexual dysfunction is present, consider adjuvant approaches that directly address the presenting dysfunction, although treating underlying prostate inflammation (if present) and pelvic/genitourinary muscle dysfunction will likely improve sexual dysfunction symptoms also. It is possible that endothelial dysfunction has a role in CP/CPPS, suggested by the correlation with cardiovascular abnormalities.[205] Thus, if erectile dysfunction is present, treating with agents that can improve endothelial function such as *Pinus pinaster* (maritime pine bark) may be well indicated. *Crocus sativus* (saffron) is also very well indicated here because of its demonstrated benefits in treating erectile dysfunction[131] and also its antidepressant, anxiolytic, antioxidant, anti-inflammatory and analgesic properties.[132]

Other male reproductive tonics that are potentially well indicated are *Mucuna pruriens* (velvet bean), *Withania somnifera* (withania) and *Panax ginseng* (Korean ginseng). *Mucuna pruriens* is traditionally indicated for improving ejaculation control and erectile dysfunction, and has demonstrated a capacity to reduce male reproductive oxidative stress.[236,237]

Analgesics

Pain is the predominant symptom that predicts quality of life in patients with chronic prostatitis, and thus effective pain management is a major priority in any herbal prescription. Managing pain effectively at the outset will help to allow other therapeutic strategies to work, breaking the cycle of pain catastrophising that is often a feature in chronic prostatitis. *Piper methysticum* (kava), *Piscidia erythrina* (Jamaica dogwood), *Corydalis ambigua* (corydalis), *Anemone pulsatilla* (pasque flower), *Eschscholzia californica* (Californian poppy) and *Crocus sativus* (saffron) are all worthy of consideration here.

Nervines and adaptogens

Anxiety and depression are often present in men with CP/CPPS[191] and contribute to the severity of symptoms and lower quality of life.[191,192,195,196] Therefore, it is important that the therapeutic strategy employed addresses any presenting mood disorder and helps to improve stress resilience. Nervines that may be well indicated in CP/CPPS include *Crocus sativus* (saffron), *Leonurus cardiaca* (motherwort), *Lavandula officinalis* (lavender), *Hypericum perforatum* (St John's wort) and *Avena sativa* (green oats). Ideal adaptogens include *Withania somnifera* (withania) and *Panax ginseng* (Korean ginseng).

Muscle relaxants

Smooth muscle and skeletal muscle spasm are likely implicated in CP/CPPS symptoms, both at the level of urinary control and the pelvic floor musculature.[162,186] Herbal medicines with a reputation for being muscle relaxants may be well indicated. These include *Piper methysticum* (kava), *Viburnum opulus* (cramp bark), *Valeriana officinalis* (valerian) and *Lobelia inflata* (lobelia).

SPECIFIC HERBAL MEDICINES

Serenoa repens (saw palmetto)

Saw palmetto is a common treatment recommendation for prostatitis symptoms based on its traditional application as a prostate-specific male genitourinary tonic and its role in managing urinary symptoms associated with bladder outlet obstruction. Modern in vitro and in vivo evidence demonstrates that *Serenoa repens* has anti-inflammatory properties targeting the prostate,[238] predominantly by inhibiting prostaglandin and leukotriene synthesis and modifying histamine-induced capillary permeability.[144]

As a monotherapy, *Serenoa repens* has demonstrated mixed results in clinical trials evaluating its role in CP/CPPS. More than 60% of patients experienced a moderate/marked improvement (greater than or equal to 50% improvement) in subjective global assessment scores and NIH-CPSI scores after taking an unspecified dose of saw palmetto extract (Permixon®) for 18 months. Urinary symptoms (as assessed by IPSS), quality of life and mean peak flow rate also improved.[239] A prospective, 1-year trial comparing saw palmetto to finasteride in Category III CP/CPPS found that 325 mg of an unspecified *Serenoa repens* extract failed to demonstrate any prolonged improvements in NIH-CPSI scores. Initial improvements were seen at 3 months in NIH-CPSI pain and quality of life domains; however, these were not maintained by the 6- and 12-month follow-up period.[240]

Combined treatment with other prostate-specific nutrients may improve *Serenoa repens* efficacy. Eight-week treatment with Profluss®, a proprietary combination of *Serenoa repens* extract 320 mg, selenium 50 micrograms and lycopene 5 mg, was found to reduce the total NIH-CPSI score by more than 50% in men with Category IIIA CP/CPPS. This was compared to 320 mg *Serenoa repens* monotherapy treatment, resulting in a smaller yet still clinically significant reduction of symptom scores by 26%. Urinary symptoms were reduced in both groups, again more so with combination treatment, demonstrating a 50% reduction in IPSS scores compared to a little under 11% in the saw palmetto only group. Measurable improvements in mean peak flow rate were also demonstrated with combination treatment, but not saw palmetto monotherapy.[144]

This same nutraceutical combination was shown in a more recent study to reduce histological prostate inflammation and inflammatory infiltrates — B lymphocytes (CD20), T lymphocytes (CD3, CD8) and macrophages (CD68) — in men with lower urinary tract symptoms associated with BPH after 3–6 months of treatment.[143]

As a component of a herbal and nutraceutical approach, *Serenoa repens* may help to improve bacterial clearance and symptoms in chronic bacterial prostatitis when taken with antibiotics.[214,215]

Flower pollen extracts

Flower pollen extracts have been shown in numerous cohort studies and two randomised placebo-controlled studies to demonstrate clinical improvement in men with CP/CPPS.[145]

Studies support its use in targeting pain, urinary and sexual dysfunction symptoms associated with CP/CPPS. The proprietary extract Cernilton® has been the most extensively researched of available extracts, being produced from the machine-collected pollen of *Secale cereale*, *Phleum pratense* and *Zea mays*. Phytosterols and secalosides present in the extract are thought to be involved in the therapeutic activity of the product, which appears to exert anti-inflammatory and antiproliferative effects, and to potentially alter smooth muscle function in the bladder and urethra.[145] Other proprietary extracts (Prostat/Poltit[241] and Deprox 500[242]) have also been studied.

Treatment for 12 weeks with two capsules of Cernilton (Cernitin T60 60 mg, Cernitin GBX 3 mg) taken every 8 hours, in men with NIH Category III CP/CPPS, resulted in significant reductions in the NIH-CPSI total score by 8.72 points, which was significantly more than placebo.[234] Significant improvements were also seen in the pain and quality of life domains, but not in micturition or sexual function. A minimum 25% reduction in NIH-CPSI scores (considered clinically significant) occurred in 76.5% of the treatment group compared to 42.6% of placebo group.[234]

A study using the proprietary pollen extract Prostat/Poltit found that 74 mg 3 times daily for 6 months in men with Category IIIA and IIIB CP/CPPS resulted in significant improvements in pain, voiding and storage symptoms compared to placebo. Sexual function was also seen to improve; with low libido, erectile dysfunction, premature ejaculation and delayed ejaculation all reducing in frequency in the treatment group.[241]

A more recent study evaluating Deprox 500®, a combination of pollen extract (500 mg) and unspecified amounts of B vitamins (B_1, B_2, B_6, folate, B_{12}), found that two tablets daily for 4 weeks demonstrated significant improvements in total NIH-CPSI scores, pain and quality of life when compared to ibuprofen. The improvement seen in total scores was quite profound, a reduction from 24.9 at baseline to 12.8 after 4 weeks. Significant differences in reduction in pain and improvement in quality of life were seen depending on CP/CPPS categorisation, with men in Category IIIB (non-inflammatory) having an even greater improvement.[242] These results were consistent with a previous open label study with the same product and for the same duration.[243]

Cranberry (*Vaccinium macrocarpon*)

Cranberry may be useful in men with chronic prostatitis who present with obstructive and irritative urinary symptoms. Cranberry prevents adherence of pathogenic strains of *E. coli* to the bladder epithelium and appears to exert anti-inflammatory activity;[151] both these properties may be useful in the management of CBP or CP/CPPS.

Men with histopathologically confirmed non-bacterial chronic prostatitis, lower urinary tract symptoms, BPH and elevated PSA had significantly improved IPSS and quality of life scores after taking 1500 mg cranberry fruit powder (223 mg organic acids, 1.65 mg anthocyanins, 29.5 mg condensed tannins, 52 mg total phenols) daily for 6 months. Significant improvements compared to placebo were seen in frequency, intermittency, urgency, weak stream, straining and nocturia. Objective urinary parameters (average urinary flow rate, prostate bladder voiding and postvoid residual volumes) were also significantly improved in more than 70% of the men.[151]

LIFESTYLE RECOMMENDATIONS

Comprehensive lifestyle changes

Evidence exists for patients with Category IIIA and IIIB CP/CPPS deriving benefit from extensive dietary, sexual habit and lifestyle modification. Men were asked to follow a set of lifestyle 'rules' for 3 months (Box 19.4) aimed at reducing risk factors identified after systematic review of available literature. Men who followed the rules had a substantial reduction in total NIH-CPSI scores, from 22.1 at the beginning of the intervention period to 8.1 at the end. This is in contrast to the control group who had a reduction in NIH-CPSI scores from 21.9 pre-treatment to 17.6 post-treatment.[221]

While any one of the interventions, or combination of, could be responsible for the clinical response seen in patients, the rules are quite rational, and should be fairly simple to implement for most patients, making it a viable treatment approach in this patient group.

BOX 19.4 Lifestyle 'rules' for CP/CPPS

- Avoid consumption of all kinds of alcoholic beverages
- Avoid consumption of spicy foods, pepper, chilli and coffee
- Diet 50% carbohydrate, 30% fat, 20% protein
- Increase fruit, vegetables and foods rich in fibre
- Avoid having 2 ejaculations during the same day
- Avoid a period of sexual abstinence longer than 4 days
- Try not to delay ejaculation in both intercourse and masturbation
- Do not practise interrupted coitus as a contraceptive method
- Walk and practise relaxing sports activities (swimming, jogging, free exercises)
- Avoid sedentary activities and sitting positions for a long time
- Use a doughnut-shaped cushion if seated for a long time
- Avoid sports that can be traumatic to your prostate (cycling, motorcycling, horse riding etc)
- Avoid wearing tight underpants or trousers
- Take frequent hot baths or bidets during which you relax and release your pelvic muscles

Exercise

An inverse association has been demonstrated between total leisure time physical activity and risk of CP/CPPS, with moderate and high-intensity exercise showing similar associations.[244]

In patients who have CP/CPPS, an 18-week program consisting of 40 minutes fast-paced walking and postural muscle and isometric strengthening exercises, resulted in significant improvements in total NIH-CPSI scores and sub scores (pain, urinary symptoms, quality of life); anxiety and depression. The control group, undertaking flexibility and motion exercises performed 3 times weekly, also experienced significant improvements in all measures with the exception of urinary symptoms, although pain and total NIH-CPSI scores were more improved with aerobic exercise.[245]

PELVIC FLOOR PHYSICAL THERAPY

For effective multimodality treatment of men with CP/CPPS, a relationship with a skilled physical therapist is

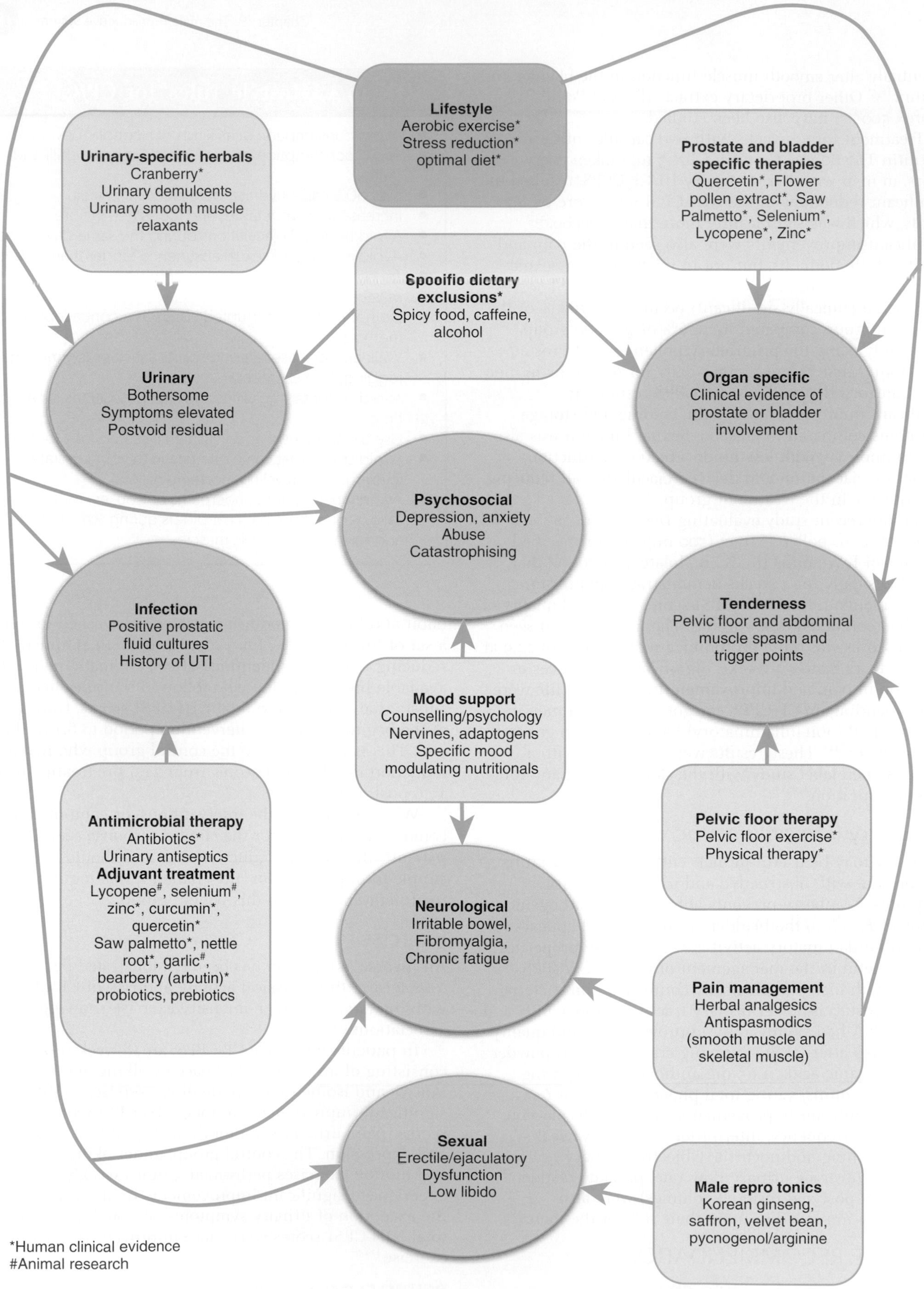

FIGURE 19.3 A therapeutic approach to CP/CPPS

Source: Adapted from Shoskes DA, Nickel JC. Classification and treatment of men with chronic prostatitis/chronic pelvic pain syndrome using the UPOINT system. World J Urol 2013;31:755–760.

extremely advantageous. As discussed previously, many patients with CP/CPPS have pelvic floor muscle dysfunction that contributes to their symptoms. Treatment with pelvic floor physical therapy, in numerous clinical studies, has been shown to effectively treat most of the symptoms associated with CP/CPPS.

Pelvic floor biofeedback re-education with a pelvic floor physical therapist has been shown to effectively manage CP/CPPS symptoms. Over 6–8 treatment sessions, 97% of men had a reduction in the total NIH-CPSI by an average 12.2 points. Sessions involved instruction on constriction and relaxation of the pelvic floor musculature, supported with practitioner verbal guidance and biofeedback measurements from a rectal EMG probe. The majority of men also experienced improvements in micturition, pain and quality of life scores, and a reduction in resting tone of the levator ani muscle.[246]

Myofascial physical therapy has also been demonstrated to improve symptoms of CP/CPPS. Patients received 1 hour sessions for 10 weeks involving comprehensive and targeted myofascial trigger point release and connective tissue manipulation to the abdominal wall, back, buttocks and thighs; and transrectal treatment of pelvic floor soft tissues. Patients were also taught pelvic floor drops, home exercises and stretches as deemed appropriate. Global response assessment in men with CP/CPPS indicated 64% as markedly or moderately improved from myofascial physical therapy. A high response was also seen from the control group in this study, with 40% of men markedly or moderately improved from non-individualised global therapeutic massage.[247]

A comprehensive multi-practitioner administered myofascial release, education in self-administered trigger point release, and paradoxical relaxation training program has demonstrated improvements in pain, micturition and quality of life scores. Overall a 30% reduction in total NIH-CPSI scores was seen, with 60% of participants having a greater than 6-point reduction.[248] A very similar program, incorporating practitioner administered myofascial release and paradoxical relaxation training for 1 month, also demonstrated improvements in sexual dysfunction as well as pain symptoms in men with CP/CPPS. In this program 47% of men had a greater than 50% improvement in ejaculatory pain and difficulty achieving an erection symptoms, and 52% of men had a greater than 50% improvement in difficulty maintaining erections and achieving ejaculation symptoms.[249]

CASE STUDY

OVERVIEW

Steven, a 23-year-old male, presents with premature ejaculation. He is currently in a monogamous heterosexual relationship, having been sexually active with his current partner for about 6 months. He has been experiencing early ejaculation since his first sexual relationship of 3 months, which ended 12 months previously, and during masturbation. Currently ejaculation occurs within 30 seconds of vaginal

CASE STUDY CONTINUED

penetration, with an aching pain also felt in his perineum and lower back when he ejaculates. This pain has been noticed for the past 8 months during both self-stimulated and partnered ejaculations. He reports a low interest in engaging in sexual activity, predominantly due to fear and embarrassment about his sexual performance, but also due to the discomfort it causes him. He does not however experience any difficulties attaining or maintaining an erection.

In addition to perineal pain on ejaculation, Steven experiences what he describes as a 'dull burning' most of the time, experienced around his testicles, perineum and sometimes his inner thighs. This pain is relieved with warm baths, which he has most days to relieve the pain.

Steven also experiences urinary urgency and frequency. He says he does not have difficulty initiating urination, although when he does urinate it is typically only small quantities. He finds he also has to urinate frequently during the night. He also reports a burning pain felt in his penis on urination on most occasions. He says that his urine looks and smells normal. Urinary symptoms have been present for the past 9 months or so, with varying degrees of intensity. He has not ever had a urinary tract infection that he is aware of.

Steven reports that he tends to suffer from anxiety and also experiences low self-confidence which he says has been present since adolescence. He has been previously treated by a psychologist and over the years has learnt mindfulness meditation but has fallen out of practice.

Systems review reveals that Steven tends to be constipated (type 1–2 on the Bristol Stool Chart when constipated), passing a stool once every 2–3 days. Stools are otherwise normal. He does experience some abdominal bloating and distension, especially when he is feeling 'backed up'.

On most weekends Steven goes out drinking with friends, although he curtails his drinking to a maximum of 4–6 beers as he finds his urinary symptoms are worsened by alcohol. On 2 or 3 nights during the week he will have up to 2 beers in the evening.

Exercise is fairly infrequent. He sometimes walks to work; however, most days he catches the bus. He says that he currently feels unfit and would like to improve his fitness level.

Steven's diet consists mostly of easy-to-prepare meals. A typical breakfast consists of cornflakes with cow's milk and a teaspoon of sugar. Lunch is typically a ham, cheese and tomato sandwich on wholemeal bread. The evening meal is usually sausages, a lamb chop or beef steak with mashed potato and carrots, beans, peas and corn. Fish is consumed irregularly. Beans and legumes are irregularly consumed, although his partner is exploring the idea of adopting a vegetarian diet so they have had chickpea curry once or twice lately which he is quite fond of. Snacks are typically a packet of potato crisps or the occasional piece of fruit.

Steven drinks 1 or 2 coffees in the morning, but avoids drinking more as he notices that this worsens his urinary symptoms. Otherwise he drinks either water (when he remembers), apple juice with breakfast, and the occasional soft drink on his lunch break at work.

Steven does not currently take any prescription medications. He takes a multivitamin supplement and two fish oil capsules daily when he remembers. He has no allergies that he is aware of.

CASE STUDY CONTINUED

Six months previously Steven was referred to a urologist in relation to his urinary and ejaculatory symptoms. Digital rectal examination revealed a normal-sized prostate that was tender to palpate and increased anal sphincter tone. Midstream and post massage urine were negative for cultured organisms and white blood cells. Postvoid residual was normal. His urologist diagnosed chronic prostatitis and suggested a 28-day trial of ciprofloxacin which resulted in no noticeable improvement in symptoms.

Physical examination findings were as follows:

- The patient looks well
- Pulse: 92 bpm regular
- Respiratory rate: 16 respirations/minute
- Temperature: 36.7°C
- Blood pressure: 147/75 mmHg
- Height: 1.72 m
- Weight: 65 kg
- Body mass index (BMI): 21.9 kg/m^2
- Conjunctiva: pink
- Nails: evidence of chewing, however otherwise NAD
- Capillary refill: within 2 seconds
- Random blood glucose: 4.8 mmol/L
- Urine:
  Urine was pale coloured, clear with little odour
  Urinary dipstick analysis:
  - Leucocytes: Nil
  - Nitrites: Nil
  - Protein: Nil
  - pH: 5
  - Specific gravity: 1.005
  - Blood: Nil
  - Urobilinogen: Nil
  - Bilirubin: Nil
  - Ketones: Nil
  - Glucose: Nil
- Pelvic and abdominal examination were unremarkable

TREATMENT PROTOCOL

INITIAL APPOINTMENT

Initial treatment was aimed to address the presenting complaint of premature ejaculation and to specifically relieve urinary and ejaculatory pain. The patient was counselled that his sexual difficulties were likely related to his diagnosis of chronic prostatitis, the connection to which he was not aware of at the time. Discussed that treating the chronic prostatitis was therefore likely to bring about improvements in sexual and urinary function. Discussion was also had around sexual practices, especially how taking the emphasis away from penetrative sex and towards other mutually pleasurable foreplay activities may help to disperse his performance anxiety, and also help his partner achieve sexual satisfaction independent of successful penetrative sex. We also discussed how fostering a healthy sexual relationship with himself through focused masturbation practices could help to improve his sexual performance. Issues around shame and a conditioning to rush when masturbating (to avoid getting caught) were discussed as potential contributors to early ejaculation.

Initial recommendations were as follows:

CASE STUDY CONTINUED

HERBAL MEDICINE

- Herbal complex 200 mL
  Serenoa repens 90 mL
  Leonurus cardiaca 80 mL
  Crocus sativus (1:20) 20 mL
  Anemone pulsatilla 10 mL
  Dose: 5 mL taken in water or juice 3 times daily
- *Mucuna pruriens* powder: Take 1 flat teaspoon twice daily in milk or water

NUTRITIONAL MEDICINE (DIETARY)

- Encourage general wholefood diet principles
- Avoid urinary irritants such as coffee and alcoholic beverages. Preferentially choose water as a beverage as opposed to high-sugar beverages such as juice and soft drink
- Preference a piece of fruit or mixed raw nuts and seeds as snacks. In particular, include 3 Brazil nuts daily as a significant dietary source of selenium
- Introduce rolled oats as an alternative breakfast, either cooked as porridge or soaked overnight in milk as a Bircher muesli
- Add blueberries or raspberries as a source of prebiotic and antioxidant polyphenols, and 1–2 tablespoons of ground flaxseeds as a prebiotic food and source of anti-inflammatory omega-3 PUFAs and phytoestrogen lignans
- Consume a probiotic yoghurt containing *Lactobacillus rhamnosus GG* daily
- Encourage tomato-based meals, particularly the addition of salt-free tomato paste concentrate to savoury meals as a dietary source of lycopene
- Incorporate vegetarian sources of protein, introducing legume-based meals such as chickpea curry, minestrone soup with mixed beans, and tofu stir fry. Aim for at least 2–3 vegetarian meals per week
- Eat fresh green salad with a healthy protein such as canned tuna, sardines, chickpeas or three bean mix for lunch. Otherwise, fill out sandwich with salad vegetables, marinated tofu or humus.

NUTRITIONAL MEDICINE (SUPPLEMENTAL)

1. Combined quercetin 600 mg and bromelain 200 mg: 2 tablets daily
2. Zinc 30 mg (as amino acid chelate): 1 tablet daily
3. Lactulose: 1 teaspoon daily gradually increased to 1 tablespoon daily. Suggested as a prebiotic and also as a laxative to improve bowel regularity.

LIFESTYLE EDUCATION

- Minimise urinary irritants such as caffeinated beverages and alcohol
- Exercise. Aim for at least 30 minutes daily such as walking to and from work most days. Incorporate some moderate to high-intensity exercise (such as cycling, jogging) at least 3 times a week
- Practise pelvic floor exercises. Contract and relax the pelvic floor following the exercises outlined in Dorey, 2013[160] paying attention to breathing deeply, and avoiding tension of the buttocks. Introduce exercises

CASE STUDY CONTINUED

gradually aiming for 3 contractions of 10 seconds each in a lying, sitting and standing position. These should be performed twice daily. Reduce frequency of exercises, duration of contraction or number of contractions if any exacerbation of pelvic pain is experienced, gradually building back up again as tolerated

- Practise masturbation with awareness. Ensuring adequate privacy and time; masturbate using mindfulness principles, with an awareness of body sensations, breathing rate, muscles contracted and pressure and speed of stimulation, especially when reaching the point of climax. With this awareness, practise deep slow breathing, relaxation of contracted muscles, slowing stroke rate and altering stimulation pressure. When feeling close to ejaculation rest until control is regained, when masturbation can continue. Contracting and relaxing the pelvic floor can help to regaining control. Once control is regained, masturbation can continue, repeating the above until completion is desired. If any exacerbation of symptoms is experienced, reduce frequency and duration of masturbation exercises, gradually building back up as tolerated.

FOLLOW-UP CONSULTATION 3 WEEKS LATER

Steven reported significant improvements in perineum, testicular and upper thigh pain within 2 weeks of starting treatment. Pain on ejaculation was also noticeably improved. He was still experiencing frequency and urgency; however, pain on urination was noticeably better. He had enthusiastically taken on the dietary recommendations, and both he and his partner were enjoying eating more vegetarian meals. He had noticed that his bowel frequency had also increased and his stools had softened.

Steven had begun walking to work, and incorporating an early morning jog 2 or 3 times weekly. While his fitness noticeably had a lot to be desired, he felt that the increase in exercising was improving his self-confidence.

Ejaculation time was still shortened; however, both he and his partner were feeling less tension around this as they were enjoying exploring alternative ways of sexual intimacy. Steven was engaging in masturbation awareness exercises and felt that during these sessions his time to ejaculation was better, and he was becoming more aware of how his body tried to 'rush' him to ejaculation.

ADDITIONAL RECOMMENDATIONS

Address urinary symptoms and continue to support lifestyle changes already suggested.

A herbal tea was prescribed to relieve irritative urinary symptoms. It contained:

Althaea officinalis (marshmallow leaf) 20 g
Agropyron repens (couch grass) 20 g
Hibiscus sabdariffa (roselle) 30 g
Avena sativa (green oats) 30 g

Directions: Infuse 6 rounded tablespoons in a large teapot of hot water. Allow to cool and drink throughout the day

CASE STUDY CONTINUED

THIRD CONSULTATION (4 WEEKS LATER)

Pain symptoms had reduced to a slight perineum discomfort following ejaculation and upon urination after ejaculating. Frequency and urgency symptoms were noticeably improved, with nocturia episodes limited to 1–2 times a night.

Steven had noticed that during masturbation he was much improved at prolonging the time to ejaculation. During vaginal penetration, ejaculation time was still sooner than he would prefer, however he felt he was getting better control, and was typically able to last between 1 and 2 minutes before ejaculating. Steven expressed confidence he was continually improving, and that with changes in the ways he and his partner were intimate, this was also less of an issue for the time being.

Steven reported that his self-confidence continued to improve, and that his management of anxiety was profoundly better than it had ever been. He attributed this to a continued increase in aerobic exercise frequency to jogging 3–4 times weekly.

ERECTILE DYSFUNCTION

Epidemiology

Erectile dysfunction (ED) is defined as the consistent or recurrent inability to attain and/or maintain a penile erection sufficient for sexual activity that persists for 3 months or more.[250] Overall, worldwide prevalence rates of ED are 10–20%.[251] Age is significantly correlated to ED prevalence, with 1–10% of men under 40 years affected, up to 15% of 40–49-year-olds, 20–40% of 60–69-year-olds and 50%–100% of men in their 80s and 90s.[252] It has been projected that as many as 322 million men worldwide will have ED by 2025.[253]

Classification

For classification of male erectile dysfunction see Box 19.5.

PSYCHOGENIC

It was once thought that psychogenic factors accounted for most presentations of ED; however this perspective has now altered to acknowledge that in most cases, ED is a mixed condition of both psychological and physical causes.[254] When significant psychological or interpersonal distress is present with a presentation of ED, psychogenic ED is often diagnosed. It may be general and represent an overall lack of arousability, or situational, such as related to a specific sexual partner or performance anxiety.[254,255]

How psychological factors impact upon erectile function is complex. Behaviourally, negative thoughts, low self-confidence and performance anxiety can all lead to reduced erectile function, and depression is known to negatively affect subjective sexual arousal.[256] Biologically, dysregulation of the HPA axis occurs in major depressive disorder, with the effect of excess catecholamines impeding the cavernosal muscle relaxation needed for penile tumescence. Psychological factors may also

BOX 19.5 Classification of erectile dysfunction

Organic

I. Vasculogenic
   A. Arteriogenic
   B. Cavernosal
   C. Mixed
II. Neurogenic
III. Anatomical
IV. Endocrinological

Psychogenic

I. Generalised
   A. Generalised unresponsiveness
      1. Primary lack of sexual arousability
      2. Ageing-related decline in sexual arousability
   B. Generalised inhibition
      1. Chronic disorder of sexual intimacy
II. Situational
   A. Partner-related
      1. Lack of arousability in specific relationship
      2. Lack of arousability owing to sexual object preference
      3. High central inhibition owing to partner conflict or threat
   B. Performance-related
      1. Associated with other sexual dysfunction (e.g. rapid ejaculation)
      2. Situational performance anxiety (e.g. fear of failure)
   C. Psychological distress or adjustment related
      1. Associated with negative mood state (e.g. depression) or major life stress (e.g. death of partner)

Source: Lue TF. Physiology of penile erection and pathophysiology of erectile dysfunction. In Wein W, Kavoussi L, Partin A. Campbell-Walsh urology. 11th edn. Philadelphia: Elsevier; 2016. pp. 612–42.

contribute to organic ED pathophysiology. Mental stress has been demonstrated to contribute to endothelial dysfunction, systemic inflammation, blood glucose dysregulation and atherosclerosis, which are all recognised contributing factors in ED.[256]

VASCULAR ERECTILE DYSFUNCTION

Vascular ED occurs due to either an arterial insufficiency (arteriogenic) or inflow problem, or a venous insufficiency (venogenic) or outflow problem.[257]

Arteriogenic ED is seen in men who have arterial occlusive disease that prevents enough blood from entering the penis during excitation.[254] In most men with arteriogenic ED, reduced penile perfusion occurs as a consequence of atherosclerosis.[254] Otherwise, damage to the hypogastric-cavernous-helicine arterial tree secondary to pelvic trauma or pelvic irradiation can be the cause of the reduced penile perfusion.[254]

Endothelial cells, which line the arteries, also play a major role in erectile function. These cells express nitric oxide synthase (NOS), which in turn produces NO, a potent mediator of smooth muscle relaxation and subsequent erections.[257] Impairment in endothelial-dependent vasodilation is thought to result from low-grade inflammation accompanying metabolic syndrome, obesity and diabetes, and is considered the common link between ED and coronary artery disease.[258]

Venogenic ED occurs when there is a failure of venous occlusion preventing outflow of blood from the penis.[254] Instead of the cavernous sinuses trapping blood from arterial inflow, they passively emit blood into the systemic circulation. Venogenic ED is multifactorial, with degenerative changes to the tunica albuginea as a consequence of Peyronie's disease, diabetes or traumatic injury (penile fracture) resulting in impairment of subtunical and emissary vein compression.[254] Inadequate sinusoidal expansion with resulting impaired subtunical venule compression can be the result of insufficient trabecular smooth muscle relaxation. Venous leakage may also be the result of structural alterations of the cavernous smooth muscle, trabeculae and endothelium.[254]

NEUROGENIC ERECTILE DYSFUNCTION

Neurogenic ED refers to ED induced by a disease or dysfunction affecting the central nervous system, cavernous or pudendal nerves: 10–19% of ED is estimated to have a primarily neurogenic cause.[254]

Pathology affecting areas of the brain involved in sexual drive and erection (medial preoptic area of the hypothalamus, paraventricular nucleus of the hypothalamus and hippocampus) such as Parkinson's disease, stroke and temporal lobe epilepsy can often induce ED. Brain tumours, dementias and brain trauma can also be associated.[254]

Disorders at the spinal cord level (spinal cord injury, multiple sclerosis, disc herniation and tumours) disrupt erectile function by impacting upon afferent and efferent neural pathways. The position of the lesion and the extent of neural pathway disruption determine the impact.[259]

Damage to the peripheral nerves by a disease process such as diabetes[260] or pelvic trauma or surgery such as radical prostatectomy can also be a cause of ED through disruption of the hypogastric plexus or the cavernous nerves.[254]

ENDOCRINOLOGICAL

Erectile dysfunction can occur as a consequence of a number of hormonal alterations. It is considered one of the most important symptoms required for diagnosis of late-onset hypogonadism, characterised by low circulating levels of androgens.[261] Any other dysfunction affecting the hypothalamic-pituitary axis, hyperprolactinaemia and thyroid disease (underactive or overactive thyroid) can also result in erectile dysfunction.[254]

Aetiology

Organic, physiological, endocrine and psychogenic factors are involved in the ability to attain and maintain an erection, and thus the aetiology of ED is typically multifactorial, as almost any disease that can alter the nervous, vascular or hormone systems may affect erectile function.

Pathogenesis

PSYCHOLOGICAL FACTORS

Depression is the most consistent mental health condition correlated with ED, with a bidirectional cause and effect relationship demonstrated by numerous longitudinal studies.[256,262,263]

For men with major depressive disorder, a 3.2 fold greater risk of developing ED was found compared to men who were not depressed. Treatment with pharmacological therapy for depression was shown in this group to reduce the risk of developing ED, even with agents that were of a high risk of causing ED as a side effect. Men who did not receive pharmacological therapy were 3.9 times more likely to develop ED; 3.6 times more likely if treated with high-risk medications; and 2.5 times more likely if taking medications that were of low risk.[256] However an earlier Finnish study's findings contradicted these findings, demonstrating that antidepressant treatment increased the rate of ED in depressed men, with 4.5 times the rate of depressed men having ED 5 years later if treated with antidepressants, and a 1.2 times higher rate of ED if untreated, compared to men who were not depressed.[262]

AGE

The prevalence of ED increases with advancing age. A peak in ED prevalence of 64% of men aged over 70 years compared to an overall prevalence of 30% of 40–79-year-olds was seen in the European Male Aging Study (EMAS).[264]

Ageing is associated with changes that independently contribute to ED risk; however, increasing morbidities also associated with age such as cardiovascular disease, diabetes, hypertension, chronic kidney disease, depression and polypharmacy will also contribute to ED via a multitude of mechanisms.[265]

Ageing is associated with a number of impairments to the vascular mechanisms enabling erection to occur. This is seen as a consequence of increased age-associated atherosclerosis in the arterial bed of the penis.[265] Impaired vasodilation and sinusoidal smooth muscle relaxation are also seen to occur, as a result of endothelial dysfunction from reduced endothelial and neuronal nitric oxide synthase (eNOS and nNOS) activity and availability.[265]

The structure of the penis changes with ageing. The percentage of smooth muscle cells (measured using computerised image analysis) was seen to differ depending on age, with reduced levels associated with older men.[266] Corporal fibrosis occurs with ageing due to increased collagen fibre deposition.[265] These changes in the smooth muscle component, elastic fibres or collagen types provoke mechanical changes in the ageing penis, thereby reducing its compliance and elasticity. This impacts upon compression of emissary veins against the tunica albuginea resulting in corporeal venous leakage and therefore compromised erectile function.[265]

Hormonal changes such as age-associated androgen deficiency may also be a contributor to erectile function decline[267] and are discussed in detail elsewhere in this chapter.

DIABETES

Diabetic men are more likely to develop erectile dysfunction, as demonstrated by the MMAS finding of a relative risk of 1.83 for treated and untreated diabetic men compared to men without diabetes.[268] A recent cross-sectional study found that men with erectile dysfunction were at 2.2 times higher odds of having undiagnosed diabetes.[269] More severe ED in diabetic men is associated with older age, duration of diabetes, poor glycaemic control and the presence of microvascular disease and cardiovascular disease.[270]

How diabetes contributes to ED is multifactorial. Diabetes is associated with endothelial dysfunction, macrovascular and microvascular complications, peripheral neuropathy and nephropathy, all of which can contribute to the development of pathological changes impacting upon erectile function.[260]

CARDIOVASCULAR DISEASE

A large body of evidence demonstrates that cardiovascular health is inextricably linked to erectile function. Both conditions share common risk factors of hypertension, diabetes mellitus, hypercholesterolaemia, smoking and obesity.[254,271] Numerous studies have identified a high prevalence of ED in men with peripheral, cerebral and coronary vascular diseases,[254] and common pathophysiological links of endothelial dysfunction, chronic inflammation and androgen deficiency have been identified.[258]

The relationship between cardiovascular disease and vascular ED has been suggested to be manifestations of the same pathophysiological vascular changes. Evidence for this exists in the capacity of ED to predict for future cardiovascular disease, as demonstrated by a meta-analysis of cohort studies finding the presence of ED increased future cardiovascular events by 42%, myocardial infarct by 62% and cerebrovascular events by 39%.[272] In younger men, the presence of ED carried a higher risk of developing CVD than the risk seen in older men, suggesting a more aggressive pathophysiology in this age group.[272] In men with chronic coronary syndrome who had ED, onset of sexual dysfunction preceded coronary artery disease presentation in 93% of cases, occurring on average 2 years before.[273]

Extent of vascular disease has also been shown to be related to ED prevalence, with a greater atherosclerotic burden likely to impact upon the small vessels supplying the penis. Men presenting with more atherosclerosis manifested as acute coronary syndrome (ACS) with two or more vessels affected, or chronic coronary syndrome (CCS), had a similar prevalence of ED (55% and 65% respectively). This was higher than men presenting with ACS and only one coronary vessel affected who had an ED prevalence similar to that of the control group (22% and 24% respectively).[273]

The close links between ED and cardiovascular disease (CVD) and the capacity of ED to predict for future coronary artery disease is thought to relate in part to the smaller size of penile arteries (1–2 mm) compared to that of coronary arteries (3–4 mm) thus being more sensitive to impacts upon alterations in blood flow.[258] ED and CVD are both associated with endothelial dysfunction characterised by impaired NO bioavailability and inflammation.[258] Lower brachial artery flow mediated vasodilation (FMD), and elevated high sensitivity C-reactive protein (hs-CRP), used as markers for endothelial dysfunction and chronic inflammation respectively, have been shown to be correlated to erectile dysfunction in young men (under 40 years) who had ED of unknown aetiology.[258] Other markers of systemic inflammation (C-reactive protein, intercellular adhesion molecule-1, interleukin(IL)-6, IL-10, IL-1β and tumour necrosis factor α) have been shown to be elevated in men with ED, with increased expression of inflammatory markers also associated with onset and severity.[258] Chronic systemic inflammation also contributes to endothelial dysfunction and leads to increased thrombosis development.[258]

Thus, the presence of ED, especially in younger men, could serve as a barometer of cardiovascular health and should prompt the clinician to further assess cardiovascular risk.

METABOLIC SYNDROME

A recent meta-analysis of eight available observational studies demonstrated a 2.6 fold increase in ED risk associated with metabolic syndrome.[274] Individual components of the metabolic syndrome have also been found to be independently associated with ED, with elevated fasting blood sugar having the highest impact (OR 2.07), followed by waist circumference (OR 1.71) and hypertension (OR of 1.53).[274] Increased cholesterol, triglycerides and BMI were demonstrated to predict for future ED in the 25-year longitudinal Rancho Bernardo Study.[275]

The contribution of metabolic syndrome to ED is complex, and can be related to individual effects and interactions between its components. Fundamentally, it impacts upon cardiovascular risk and atherosclerosis, endothelial dysfunction, systemic inflammation[274] and hypogonadism,[276] all of which are pathophysiological pathways identified in erectile dysfunction development.

OBESITY

Moderate to severe and complete ED prevalence has been positively associated with BMI greater than 30.0 kg/m^2, high body weight, and total body fat percentage.[271] In men with ED, having a BMI greater than 25 kg/m^2 was associated with a higher prevalence of a vasculogenic cause for the ED as determined by penile duplex parameters, with 59.3% of overweight men and 23.1% of lean men having vasculogenic ED.[277]

Similarly to metabolic syndrome, the ways in which obesity impacts upon erectile dysfunction risk are complex. A vascular aetiology through its contribution to endothelial dysfunction and increasing cardiovascular risk, increased systemic inflammation, and metabolic aberrations such as insulin resistance and hypogonadism, are all potential mechanisms by which erectile function is altered.[278,279]

SMOKING

Current smokers, and ex-smokers, are at a 51% and 20% increased risk respectively of developing erectile dysfunction compared to men who have never smoked.[280] Duration of being a smoker, and number of cigarettes smoked daily, is also a determinant of ED risk as indicated in a meta-analysis of mostly cross-sectional studies.[281] Each 10 cigarettes smoked daily increases ED risk by 14% above nonsmoker levels, and each 10 years smoking increases risk by 15%.[281]

Smoking impacts upon erectile function directly by diminishing neuronal and endothelial derived NO synthase mediated vasodilation, and inhibition of NO in the corpora cavernosum.[282] Disinhibition of Rho-associated kinase (ROK) activity also promotes vasoconstriction, and smoking-induced calcification of vascular elastin fibres promotes arterial stiffness.[282] Smoking also contributes to comorbidities independently associated with ED such as atherosclerosis, arterial-insufficiency and type 2 diabetes.[282]

IATROGENIC CAUSES

Radical prostatectomy (RP) as a treatment for prostate cancer commonly results in ED, with reported incidences of ED following RP varying between 14% and 90%.[283] Damage to the cavernous nerves and/or pudendal arteries resulting in a neurogenic and/or arterial insufficiency is the primary reason for ED in this case.[283] An obligatory neural dormancy following prostate removal may also contribute to secondary erectile tissue damage with losses in smooth muscle and increases in collagen within the corpora cavernosa leading to veno-occlusive dysfunction, further impacting upon post RP erectile function.[283] A number of factors can impact upon erectile function in these men such as age, pre-surgery erectile function, surgical approach, and burden of urinary symptoms.[283,284] A bilateral or unilateral nerve sparing (NS) RP is the current approach of choice; however, depending on cancer characteristics, some men will still undergo non-NS procedures. Also, while NS techniques, especially bilateral NS radical prostatectomy (BLNSRP), are related with better recovery of erectile function, they still can result in high levels of erectile dysfunction.[283,284] One study showed that 12 months following nerve-sparing surgery, 66% of men were still found to have severe ED, compared to 85% of men who had non-nerve-sparing surgery and 39% of men before surgery.[284] Maximum recovery of erectile function after RP can take at least 24 and sometimes 48 months, with very few men expecting to achieve erectile function equivalent to pre-surgery status.[283] Evidence from current literature stresses the importance of early intervention in ED of any form in order to preserve endothelial, smooth muscle and neural function and to prevent corporal fibrosis.[283]

Pelvic radiotherapy as a treatment for prostate cancer or other pelvic cancers can result in ED. In men treated for prostate cancer with external beam radiotherapy, incidence of ED is 30–40%.[285] Rates increase within 1–2 years of treatment, appearing to plateau at 3 years post treatment as a consequence of radiation therapy's progressive effects.[285] Damage to the blood vessels and nerves supplying the penis and damage to the pelvic musculature are likely to be implicated.[286] Radiation dose to the penile bulb is also likely to be an important determinant of erectile function outcomes, due to the bulb's close proximity to the prostate and vascular and nerve supply.[286] Cardiovascular health prior to radiotherapy is also likely to impact ED development. In men who had a combination of hypertension, diabetes and hyperlipidaemia, ED incidence 4 years post treatment was 75%, compared to 44% for men with no vascular comorbidities. The number of comorbidities also made a difference, with the more present, the higher the prevalence of ED.[287]

Surgery for BPH has been documented to be associated with ED; however, this association is considered controversial due to the scarcity of high-level evidence. A recent systematic review of this topic suggested that neither bipolar transurethral resection of the prostate (B-TURP), modified transurethral resection of the prostate (M-TURP), holmium laser enucleation of the prostate (HoLEP) nor greenlight photoselective vaporisation of the prostate (PVP) predicted the development of erectile dysfunction.[288]

Another important iatrogenic consideration is the contribution of medication side effects in the development of ED. The contribution of medications can be complicated by the fact that often the conditions they treat (such as cardiovascular disease and depression) are also aetiological factors in ED. Ageing, also an aetiological factor in ED, is associated with polypharmacy, increasing the risk of medication side effects being involved.[265] Commonly implicated medicines include but are not limited to antihypertensive agents such as thiazide diuretics, β-adrenergic blockers and aldosterone receptor antagonists (spironolactone); antidepressants such as selective serotonin reuptake inhibitors (SSRIs), tricyclics and monoamine oxidase inhibitors; anxiolytics such as benzodiazepines, antipsychotics including both typical and atypical antipsychotics; and antiandrogens such as androgen receptor antagonists, 5α-reductase inhibitors and luteinising hormone releasing hormone agonists.[265] It is imperative that routine evaluation of medication history be performed when considering the ED aetiology of an individual patient.

CYCLING

Bicycle riding has been suggested to be a risk factor in the development of ED in some men; however, this association is controversial given the cardiovascular benefits and therefore benefits on erectile function that result from increased physical activity.

ED risk is hypothesised to be increased as a result of compression and strain of the pudendal nerves and arteries from excessive perennial pressure.[289,290] A recent systematic review suggested that the evidence was not sufficient enough to discourage cycling as a measure to reduce the risk of ED; however some men, especially those who experience genital numbness in relation to cycling, may be at increased risk of ED and benefit from modifying cycling frequency, technique and saddle style.[290]

PENILE CONDITIONS

Peyronie's disease

Peyronie's is a disorder of the penis affecting around 9% of men.[291] It is characterised by the formation of a mostly collagen-containing inelastic fibrous plaque on the tunica albuginea, which leads to a progressive curvature, bending, shortening or narrowing of the penis.[292] The result is varying degrees of intercourse difficulty due to the extent of penile deformity and mild to moderate penile pain.[293] It is a condition that can be implicated in erectile dysfunction, with 20% of men with Peyronie's having ED.[291] This is thought to result from progression of fibrosis into the corporeal smooth muscle and the media of penile arteries, leading to a veno-occlusive and/or vasculogenic ED, with psychogenic factors also arising as a consequence of the penile deformity.[291]

The cause of Peyronie's is currently unknown, although the most often cited explanation for plaque formation in the tunica albuginea is tissue damage from repetitive mechanical stress and microvascular damage during intercourse, leading to an abnormal inflammatory wound healing response.[292] The tendency to develop Peyronie's has been suggested to have a genetic basis, with gene expression patterns bearing similarity to patients with Dupuytren's disease.[294] Peyronie's has also been associated with higher rates of cigarette smoking, diabetes mellitus, hypertension and autoimmune disease, suggesting a vascular or inflammatory aetiology.[295]

Priapism

Priapism is characterised by a persistent, usually painful, erection of the penis, unrelated to sexual stimulation or desire, and which is not relieved by ejaculation.[296] It is the result of the persistent engorgement of the corpora cavernosa of the penis originating from a disturbance in the mechanisms that control normal penile detumescence.[296] Priapism is a urological emergency that requires prompt medical management due to the risks of permanent ED and penile necrosis if left untreated.[296] Its aetiology is frequently idiopathic, but it is also associated with a number of medical conditions and pharmacological agents, with intracavernosal treatment of ED being involved in many adult cases. Other causes include sickle cell anaemia, leukaemia and trauma.[296]

Overview

The importance of erectile function for men and their partners is shaped and informed by a number of different factors. Thus the assessment and treatment of erectile dysfunction can present numerous challenges to the health professional.

In simplistic terms, erection is a neurovascular reflex event, modified by the endocrine and central nervous systems.[297] (See Box 19.6.) Its initiation can be via the stimulation of afferent receptors in the penis, but it can also be stimulated by imagination, tactile, visual and olfactory stimuli.[297] The satisfaction derived from a sexual experience is however perceived not by

BOX 19.6 The physiology of an erection

With sexual stimulation, neurotransmitter release from cavernous nerve terminals triggers smooth muscle relaxation of the erectile tissue (corpora cavernosa and corpus spongiosum) and the arterioles and arteries supplying it. Consequently, there is an increase in blood flow to the erectile tissue, and expansion of the sinusoidal spaces where incoming blood can collect. Sinusoidal expansion results in compression of the subtunical venous plexuses between the peripheral sinusoids and the tunica albuginea surrounding the corpora cavernosa, therefore reducing venous outflow. As the tunica albuginea is stretched to capacity, emissary veins between the inner and outer circular layers are also compressed, further decreasing venous outflow. As a result of the restricted venous outflow, intracavernosus pressure increases to about 100 mmHg, raising the penis from a dependent position to its erect state. Reflex contraction of the ischiocavernosus muscle with sexual stimulation contributes further to increase intracavernosal pressure (200 mmHg or more) and therefore penile rigidity.

Neurophysiology

The penis is innervated by autonomic (sympathetic and parasympathetic) and somatic (motor and sensory) nerves.

Sensory nerve fibres transmitting sensory information from receptors in the glans, penile skin, urethra and corpus cavernosum converge to form the dorsal nerve, which then form the pudendal nerve, entering the spinal cord at S2–S4. Motor neurons of the pudendal nerve innervate the bulbospongiosus and ischiocavernosus muscles, contributing to erection by contraction of the ischiocavernosus muscle, and ejaculation by contraction of the bulbospongiosus muscle.

The cavernous nerves are branches of the pelvic plexus supporting autonomic fibre innervation to the penis. Sympathetic and parasympathetic fibres in the cavernous nerves regulate blood flow into the corpus cavernosum during erection and detumescence, with parasympathetic stimulation primarily responsible for erection, and the sympathetic pathway for detumescence.

Erection is primarily initiated by release of nitric oxide (NO) from nonadrenergic/noncholinergic neurotransmission, and maintained by NO release from the endothelium. Acetylcholine release from parasympathetic nerve terminals also contributes indirectly to erection via presynaptic inhibition of adrenergic neurons, and stimulation of NO release from endothelial cells.

NO increases cyclic guanosine monophosphate (cGMP) and cyclic adenosine monophosphate (cAMP) production, which in turn relaxes smooth muscle in arteries, arterioles and cavernous smooth muscle, thereby increasing blood flow into erectile tissues. NO is produced from the oxidation of L-arginine, the reaction catalysed by nitric oxide synthase (NOS). Three isoforms of NOS have been identified, neuronal (nNOS), endothelial (eNOS) and inducible (iNOS) which are all expressed in the corpus cavernosum.

The erection is maintained until ejaculation, which usually leads to detumescence. Detumescence after erection likely results from a combination of cessation of NO release, the breakdown of cGMP by phosphodiesterases, and sympathetic nerve excitation with ejaculation. Noradrenaline released by sympathetic fibres in the penis is the primary agent responsible for smooth muscle contraction in the penis and penile arteries, its actions supported by neuropeptide Y also released at sympathetic nerve terminals. The result is contraction of trabecular smooth muscle, which allows blood to be released via re-opened venous channels, and consequently penis flaccidity.

Additional neurotransmitters and neuromodulators expressed in penile tissues and/or the nerves that supply them suggested to be involved in erectile function include vasoactive intestinal polypeptide, calcitonin gene-related peptide, and substance P. These mediators demonstrate pro-erectile properties by promoting endothelial NO synthesis. In addition to noradrenaline and neuropeptide Y, mediators involved in opposing erection by promoting contraction of cavernous smooth muscle are endothelin-1, prostaglandin I_2, prostaglandin $F_{2\alpha}$ and thromboxane A_2.

Centrally, the hypothalamic and limbic pathways play an important role in the integration and control of sexual and reproductive functions. The hypothalamic medial preoptic area (MPOA) and paraventricular nucleus (PVN) are considered key CNS structures involved in controlling erection and sexual function. Stimulation of the MPOA elicits an erectile response via parasympathetic nerves of the pelvic and cavernous nerves. The PVN of the hypothalamus contributes oxytocinergic fibres to the brainstem and spinal cord, the release of oxytocin having erection-promoting properties. Neurons in the PVN also express NOS, the inhibition of which prevents oxytocin-induced erections. This suggests that NO activity plays an important role centrally as well as peripherally in erectile function.

Sources: Awad A, Alsaid B, Bessede T et al. Evolution in the concept of erection anatomy. Surg Radiol Anat 2011 May;33(4):301–12; Kim ED. Erectile dysfunction. Medscape 2016. Available from: http://emedicine.medscape.com/article/444220-overview#showall; Lue TF. Physiology of penile erection and pathophysiology of erectile dysfunction. In Wein W, Kavoussi L, Partin A. Campbell-Walsh urology. 11th edn. Philadelphia: Elsevier; 2016. pp. 612–42.

the penis, but subjectively by the mind, which in turn is influenced by both conscious and unconscious processes.[297]

Signs and symptoms

A consistent or recurrent inability to attain and/or maintain a penile erection sufficient for sexual activity that persists for 3 months or more is the definition and primary symptom of ED,[250] except in the case of trauma or surgically induced ED where the time interval does not apply.[298] Lower urinary tract symptoms (LUTS) including weak or intermittent urinary stream, straining, hesitancy, terminal dribbling, incomplete emptying, urgency, frequency, urge incontinence and nocturia can often coexist with ED.[62]

Complications

Erectile dysfunction can often predict future cardiovascular events and the presentation of coronary heart disease, and is also associated with an increased risk of all-cause mortality.[272]

Depression can develop as a result of ED, while ED can also develop secondary to depression.[262,263] Performance anxiety during sexual encounters is also reported in men with ED.[299]

Partners of men with ED are obviously impacted, with increased prevalence of sexual dysfunction reported in some studies.[298]

Differential diagnosis

ED is an accompanying symptom in a number of conditions, and a common side effect of some medications as discussed previously. Differential diagnoses in a presentation of erectile dysfunction should therefore include the following.

Vascular disease

- Atherosclerosis[273]
- Peripheral vascular disease[254]
- Coronary artery disease[27]
- Hypertension[300]
- Blood vessel and nerve trauma (e.g. from bicycle riding).[289]

Systemic disease

- Type 2 diabetes mellitus[300]
- Scleroderma[300]
- Renal failure[254]
- Liver cirrhosis[300]
- Haemochromatosis.[300]

Neurological disease

- Temporal lobe epilepsy[254]
- Cerebrovascular events[254]
- Alzheimer's disease/dementia[287]
- Brain injury[254]
- Multiple sclerosis[287]
- Guillain–Barr syndrome[300]
- Spinal cord disorders such as injury, disc prolapse or tumour[254]
- Depression.[300]

Respiratory disease

- Chronic obstructive pulmonary disease[301]
- Obstructive sleep apnoea.[302]

Endocrine conditions

- Hyperthyroidism[254]
- Hypogonadism[303]
- Hypopituitarism.[300]

Male reproductive conditions

- Prostatitis.[161]

Nutritional states

- Malnutrition.[300]

Haematological disease

- Sickle cell anaemia[300]
- Leukaemias.[300]

Fig. 19.4 illustrates an algorithm for diagnostic evaluation of erectile dysfunction.

Naturopathic diagnosis

Because of the nature of the condition, diagnosis is made on the patient's objective assessment of their erectile difficulties. Thorough evaluation and diagnosis by a medical practitioner is warranted because of the numerous underlying pathologies that can give rise to ED.

Goal-directed assessment is an important element in initiating management of ED. The patient and partner (if applicable) should both be involved in clinical decisions, recognising that patient preferences and expectations regarding management can vary greatly. Partner interviews have been shown to impact diagnosis and treatment in 58% of cases.[304] Given the relationship ED has with chronic disease highly prevalent in the community and its capacity for predicting future cardiovascular events and all-cause mortality, screening of all men as a routine part of history taking is likely to have high value in early identification and treatment of both sexual dysfunction and its related conditions.

Medical history

A thorough sexual history must be conducted, in a manner that is sensitive to the patient's ethnic, cultural and personal background. Involving a partner (if applicable) is preferable. Avoid making assumptions about sexual orientation and relationship dynamics such as monogamy.[298] Determine the specific nature of the problem, being sure to differentiate erectile dysfunction from other sexual difficulties such as libidinal, ejaculatory and orgasmic disorders. Ascertain the presence of decreased arousal and whether this precedes erectile symptoms or is incidental to it. Obtain specific information about severity, onset, duration and impact upon the patient and partner(s). Ask specifically about speed of onset (i.e. gradual or rapid), and any precipitating events such as a traumatic sexual event, relationship stress, stressful life events or physical trauma. Determine the quality (in relation to rigidity and duration) of morning and masturbation-induced erections and ascertain if the erectile difficulties are consistent with all sexual partners. Question specifically if any genital pain or change in genital shape is present. Identify if any previous attempts have been made to treat the problem.[250,305,306]

Take a detailed medical history with particular enquiry into the presence of lower urinary tract symptoms (LUTS) due to their high prevalence associated with ED.[62] Detailed enquiry into the presence of cardiovascular disease and risk factors (hyperlipidaemia, hypertension, coronary vascular disease), metabolic syndrome, diabetes mellitus, neurological disease, renal and thyroid disorders is essential. Exploration of symptoms suggestive of hypogonadism (detailed further in this chapter) is also necessary. Explore any history of pelvic or penile trauma and medical interventions (such as pelvic surgery or radiotherapy) that may have preceded onset of ED.[298,306]

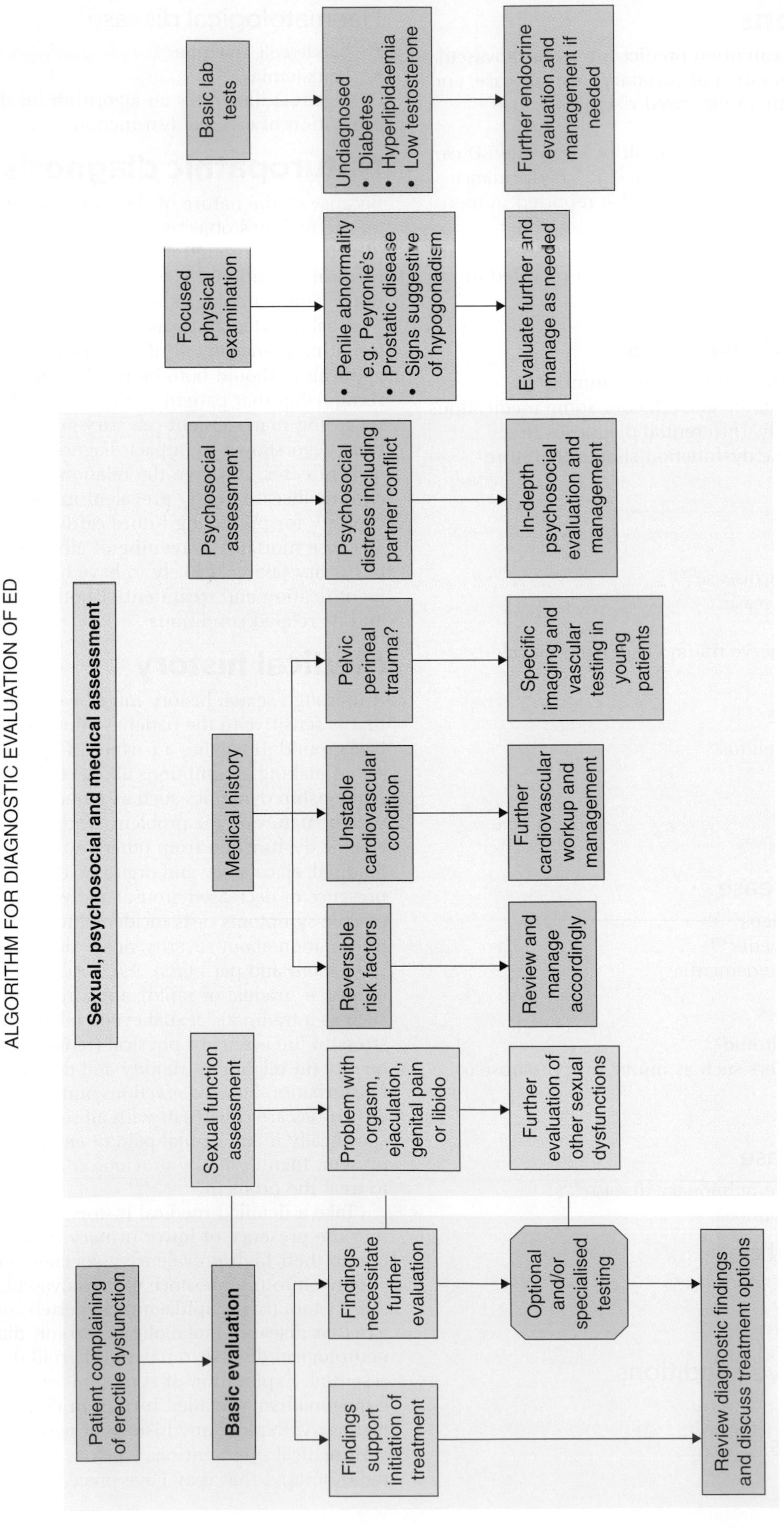

FIGURE 19.4 Algorithm for diagnostic evaluation of ED
Wein AJ. Campbell-Walsh urology. 9th edn. Saunders; 2007.

Enquire about any altered genital or perianal sensations. Ask questions relating to pelvic floor muscle function with specific questions relating to the presence of any urinary or bowel incontinence.[307]

Consideration of psychological and psychiatric history, specifically the presence of depression, anxiety or psychiatric illness is important, as is exploration of the role of emotional stressors and interpersonal relationships.[298]

A detailed medication history is essential, as is enquiry into lifestyle factors such as smoking, physical activity, alcohol consumption and substance use/abuse.[250]

As a part of developing a detailed history, validated questionnaires such as the International Index of Erectile Function (IIEF) or its abbreviated form the IIEF-5 can be useful to assess domains of sexual function, provide a measure of ED severity and assess the impacts of intervention strategies (see Box 19.7).[298,306]

PSYCHOGENIC VERSUS ORGANIC FACTORS

Psychogenic ED is generally characterised by a sudden onset with complete and immediate loss of sexual function, although this may vary depending on the partner and circumstances.[305] The presence of morning erections is considered to be suggestive of a psychogenic cause, although the evidence for this is variable.[305] Organic ED is usually more gradual in onset, with incremental progression of dysfunction, except in the case of ED caused by an immediate traumatic event. Erections are usually not observed with organic ED, even in the most stimulatory sexual encounters.[308]

Physical examination

Comprehensive evaluation consists of examination relevant to cardiovascular, neurological, endocrine and genitourinary systems. Physical examination in men with ED necessitates examination of the genitalia, with referral to an appropriate medical professional if the naturopathic physician is not qualified to do so. This should include examination of the penis for any related abnormalities such as Peyronie's plaques, deformity and micropenis; the testes to assess for their presence, size and position in relation to endocrinological abnormalities (such as hypogonadism); and testing of the bulbocavernosus reflex (by squeezing the glans penis with simultaneous digital palpation of the bulbocavernosus muscle via the anus) for evaluation of the presence of peripheral neuropathy involvement.[298]

Assessment of BMI and waist circumference, blood pressure, heart rate and pedal and femoral pulses can help to ascertain the presence of vascular causes.[298] Observation

BOX 19.7 The abridged International Index of Erectile Function (IIEF-5)

Over the past 6 months:

1. How do you rate your **confidence** that you could get and keep an erection?	Very low 1	Low 2	Moderate 3	High 4	Very high 5
2. When you had erections with sexual stimulation, **how often** were your erections hard enough for penetration?	Almost never/never 1	A few times (much less than half the time) 2	Sometimes (about half the time) 3	Most times (much more than half the time) 4	Almost always/always 5
3. During sexual intercourse, **how often** were you able to maintain your erection after you had penetrated (entered) your partner?	Almost never/never 1	A few times (much less than half the time) 2	Sometimes (about half the time) 3	Most times (much more than half the time) 4	Almost always/always 5
4. During sexual intercourse, **how difficult** was it to maintain your erection to completion of intercourse?	Extremely difficult 1	Very difficult 2	Difficult 3	Slightly difficult 4	Not difficult 5
5. When you attempted sexual intercourse, **how often** was it satisfactory for you?	Almost never/never 1	A few times (much less than half the time) 2	Sometimes (about half the time) 3	Most times (much more than half the time) 4	Almost always/always 5

*The IIEF-5 score is the sum of the ordinal responses to the five items; thus, the score can range from 5 to 25.

Source: Reprinted by permission from Macmillan Publishers Ltd. Rosen RC, Cappelleri JC, Smith MD et al. Development and evaluation of an abridged, 5-item version of the International Index of Erectile Function (IIEF-5) as a diagnostic tool for erectile dysfunction. Int J Impot Res 2000 Jan 12;11(6):319–26.

of reduced facial, pubic and axillary hair may suggest hypogonadism,[309] and hypo- or hyperthermia, tachycardia or bradycardia may suggest thyroid abnormalities. Clinic random blood glucose measurement and urinary dipstick analysis can be used to screen for hyperglycaemia and glucosuria.

Investigations

Routine laboratory tests are necessary to identify modifiable and aetiological factors in an individual patient's presentation. This should include assessment of hyperglycaemia by fasting glucose and haemoglobin A1c (HbA1c), and evaluation of blood lipids.[250] Serum total testosterone obtained with more than one morning sampling, from which calculated free testosterone can be derived (in combination with sex hormone binding globulin and albumin), can be used to screen for hypogonadism,[303] especially in the presence of suggestive symptoms, signs and risk factors such as low sexual desire, diminished morning erections and obesity.[303] Depending on the clinical context, thyroid-stimulating hormone, luteinising hormone, follicle-stimulating hormone, prolactin, urinalysis and prostate-specific antigen may also be indicated.[250,298]

Specialised diagnostic evaluation of ED may be indicated in complex clinical presentations such as in the case of primary ED in an adolescent or young adult or patients with penile deformities.[306] These include but are not limited to vascular investigations such as dynamic infusion cavernosometry and cavernosography (DICC), intracavernous injection pharmacotesting (ICI) and ICI and colour duplex ultrasonography.[298] Neurophysiological investigations such as nocturnal penile tumescence and rigidity studies (NPTR) and bulbocavernosus reflex latency may be indicated.[298]

SPECIFIC NATUROPATHIC INVESTIGATIONS

A male hormone profile may be useful to assess the balance and metabolism of male hormones. It includes both total and free testosterone, oestradiol, free androgen index (bioavailable testosterone) and SHBG.

Cortisol and DHEA-S (saliva)

In combination with a comprehensive case history, salivary cortisol and DHEA-S testing may have some clinical utility to assess hypothalamic–pituitary–adrenal adaptation to psychological stress. A high cortisol/DHEA ratio is related to chronic stress and depression,[310] lower levels of DHEA-S in relation to cortisol suggesting a more detrimental stress response due to DHEA-S's protective and regenerative role. Elevations in salivary cortisol have been associated with both CVD risk factors and metabolic risk factors.[311]

Cardiovascular health profile

A serum cardiovascular health profile may be appropriate to analyse risk factors for cardiovascular disease, which is intricately associated with ED. Parameters measured include cholesterol, lipoproteins, triglycerides, fibrinogen, CRP, homocysteine, lipid peroxidises, vitamin E, magnesium, CoQ10, insulin, total testosterone, free androgen index, SHBG and ferritin.

Metabolic syndrome profile

As metabolic syndrome is associated with the aetiology of ED, a metabolic syndrome profile (serum/plasma) that compiles several laboratory markers for this condition can be undertaken. Analytes reported include HDL cholesterol, triglycerides, glucose, insulin, asymmetric dimethylarginine and the AA/EPA ratio.

Therapeutic considerations

CLINICAL DECISION MAKING AND RATIONALE

The understanding and management of ED have evolved greatly, as evidenced by the increased recognition of the organic aetiologies of this condition.[308] The current availability of effective and safe oral drugs for ED, in conjunction with the tremendous media interest in the condition, has increased the number of men seeking help for ED. The primary goal of the management strategy for a patient with ED is to cure the patient's symptoms by adopting both a symptomatic and a holistic approach. Because ED may be associated with modifiable or reversible factors, these may be modified prior to, or in conjunction with, specific therapeutic options. Identification and appropriate management of any underlying pathology such as cardiovascular disease, diabetes mellitus, metabolic syndrome or hypogonadism are an essential component in the therapeutic approach to the patient with ED.

Patients may be using pharmacological therapy for ED and, if so, it is the practitioner's responsibility to be fully informed of potential risks and benefits of combining therapy. For the most part, advantages for the patient can be expected, in that more immediate results may be seen with on-demand therapy such as phosphodiesterase-5 (PDE-5) inhibitors, and potentially more sustained results seen with complementary approaches and lifestyle changes.

Psychosexual counselling is often appropriate as even when aetiology is organic there can be coexisting psychosocial factors. Interventions such as anxiety management and cognitive and/or behaviour therapy may therefore be necessary.

GOAL-DIRECTED TREATMENT

It is imperative to determine what the patient (and partner if applicable) actually wants or expects to accomplish through treatment.[308] Patients vary in their level of acceptance of their sexual disorder, and some may not wish to attempt more invasive therapies, which will typically be the motivation for seeing a naturopathic clinician for ED. However, depending on the extent of the issue and the underlying cause, invasive intervention may be the best option and realistic discussion about this should occur.

Therapeutic application

HISTORICAL PERSPECTIVE

When the member is no way stirred and can never perform the action of coition, this is a sign of frigidity of nature, but when it is stirred and yet cannot become erect, it is a sign of witchcraft.

Malleus Maleficarum, 1487[312]

Thankfully, by the time of the Eclectics people had become more advanced in their way of thinking! Given the sensitive nature of ED, the Eclectics surprisingly provided substantial documentation on their treatment of the condition. Jones likens the male suffering from ED to a man with 'lost manhood' and nervous debility, stating:

> *When we have nervous irritable patients, who imagine they are not competent to perform the duties of a husband, have lost confidence in themselves, have the discharge, too soon, more or less leaking of semen at stool and with the least sexual excitement, they are frequently called impotent — and they think they are — when they are only neurasthenic.*[3]

The understanding that the nervous system influences ED was not lost to the Eclectics. Gentle nervine tonics such as *Turnera diffusa* were valued in the treatment of sexual impotence[2] as was *Avena sativa*, which was prescribed as first-line treatment by the homeopath Jones, who suggested 20 drops after each meal and a little with water before bed.[3] Male tonics such as *Serenoa repens* were also well used. Ever popular, although a surprising choice for use in ED, was echinacea, which was thought to be an efficient remedy for impotence, though why is not explained. The sixth decimal of selenium was suggested for erections that were too slow and weak, or where the patient felt he was cross and weak afterwards, or if prostatic fluid oozed out while sitting or walking.

As for diet, drinking tea and coffee was believed to weaken the nerves, resulting in the escape of the semen[3] and without abstinence from these it was believed that a patient would not be cured.

ALLOPATHIC MEDICINE

The centrepieces of allopathic ED treatment are the phosphodiesterase-5 (PDE-5) inhibitors such as sildenafil citrate (Viagra), vardenafil hydrochloride (Levitra) and tadalafil (Cialis). The PDE-5 enzyme is predominantly expressed in the smooth muscle of the corpus cavernosum. It hydrolyses cyclic guanosine monophosphate (cGMP), which is the intracellular mediator of the nitric oxide signalling pathway. NO causes relaxation of smooth muscle, enabling the vasodilation necessary for erection to occur. PDE-5 inhibitors prevent the breakdown of cGMP, thereby permitting the biological cascade of events that is required for normal erectile function.[298] PDE-5 inhibitors can cause adverse events related to vasodilation and vasorelaxation in other parts of the body that express PDE-5. Headache, flushing and dyspepsia have been reported and all PDE-5 inhibitors have been shown to potentiate the hypotensive effects of organic nitrates. The drugs are therefore contraindicated in patients taking organic nitrates, and they should be used with caution in patients taking α-blockers due to concerns about additive hypotensive actions.[298] While the majority of men achieve successful intercourse (70%) with the use of PDE-5 inhibitors, efficacy in some populations, such as diabetic men, is significantly less (40–50%).[313]

Androgen replacement therapy is often an option where testosterone deficiency is identified in association with ED. It is recognised that androgen replacement may offer other potential benefits besides sexual function, including improvements in quality of life, osteoporosis, metabolic syndrome, type 2 diabetes mellitus and obesity, which may be related to decreased androgen levels.[314–316] However, there are potential risks with such therapy, including prostate disease.[317]

Second-line allopathic therapy, when oral treatments and other approaches are unsuccessful, includes localised treatments such as intracavernosal injections, intraurethral suppositories and vacuum constriction devices.

Alprostadil (synthetic prostaglandin E1) is the most commonly prescribed injectable agent for localised treatment of ED. It is often used as a monotherapy, or in combination with papavarine and phentolamine.[298] All agents act as vasodilators, inducing corporeal smooth muscle relaxation. Alprostadil achieves this via activation of intracellular adenylate cyclase, thereby stimulating cyclic adenosine monophosphate (cAMP). Priapism and penile fibrosis have been reported with its use, but at lower incidences than with other agents. Penile pain is however a commonly reported adverse event.[298] Combination therapy improves efficacy rates; however penile fibrosis prevalence is increased in relation to papaverine.[318]

Intraurethral administration of synthetic prostaglandin E1 is sometimes used as a less invasive means of administering local vasodilators than intracavernosal injection. Absorption occurs via the mucous lining of the urethra, into the corpus spongiosum surrounding it, then into the corpus cavernosa.[298] Individual anatomical variability and technical procedure of administration result in variable efficacy of this technique,[298] having a lower clinical success than intracavernosal injections.[318] Side effects experienced can be penile pain, dizziness and urethral bleeding.[318]

A non-pharmacological therapy that has been used for many years is the vacuum constriction device. This is a mechanical device designed to draw venous blood into the penis, at which point a constriction band is applied at the base to retain it. There is a learning curve with this device, and adverse events can include bruising, petechiae, unnatural erection, numbness and trapped ejaculation.[298]

Surgical implantation of a penile prosthesis is considered a more permeant treatment for ED, particularly for men who do not respond to pharmacotherapy. Patients report a high level of satisfaction; however, they are restricted to an unnatural erectile response. Complications include mechanical failure and infection.[318]

NATUROPATHIC PERSPECTIVE

The management of ED is commonly treated initially with a combination of herbal medicines, nutritional supplements, dietary modifications and counselling, along with modification of lifestyle habits. It is recommended that patients are counselled to modify any detrimental behaviours (e.g. cigarette smoking, excessive alcohol consumption, recreational drug use, sedentary behaviour) in order to improve their sexual ability and to prevent the ED from worsening.

Primary considerations in the treatment of ED are:

- Specific attention given to identified organic or functional factors such as cardiovascular disease and associated compromised peripheral circulation, atherosclerosis and endothelial dysfunction; metabolic syndrome, diabetes and androgen deficiency
- Psychological factors such as anxiety and depression, whether considered to be causative of or consequential to the ED.

NUTRITIONAL MEDICINE (DIETARY)

Therapeutic objectives

1. Support optimal health and address any specific nutritional risks
2. Include dietary components demonstrated to improve cardiovascular function and improve erectile function
3. Include foods that support cardiovascular function and avoid those that aggravate or compound aggravating factors
4. Include antioxidant foods and those that support vascular integrity
5. Support optimal body weight with appropriate dietary modifications
6. Ensure that blood sugar levels are regulated by adoption of a low glycaemic index diet, minimising refined and high glycaemic index carbohydrates. Level of intervention will be dictated by indicators of blood sugar control.

Specific treatments

DIETARY INCLUSIONS

Wholefood, high antioxidant, plant-based diet

Because of the well-established link between cardiovascular health and ED, and the capacity of ED to predict for future cardiovascular events, adoption of a dietary approach that reduces the risk of CVD is essential. Low-grade subclinical inflammation leads to altered endothelial function and oxidative stress, resulting in atherosclerosis. A diet rich in antioxidants and anti-inflammatory constituents is necessary to protect the vasculature from oxidative damage, and thus could be a prophylactic tool for preventing smooth muscle dysfunction and fibrosis in ED.[319]

A cross-sectional study demonstrated a link between diet quality and risk of erectile dysfunction, with degree of adherence to the Mediterranean diet (characterised by a diet high in vegetables, legumes, cereals, fruit, nuts and fish; and low in meat, poultry and dairy) being associated with lower ED risk.[320] In this study, the dietary components found to be most protective were vegetables, fruit, nuts and a higher monounsaturated to saturated fat ratio.[320] In men with ED, who were overweight with or without metabolic syndrome, adherence to a dietary pattern consistent with the Mediterranean diet, in conjunction with other lifestyle modifications including moderate exercise for 30 minutes at least 5 times weekly, resulted in improvements in erectile function.[321] Restoration of normal erectile function was more likely to occur in participants who achieved a 5% reduction in body weight, increased monounsaturated fat intake to more than 10% total energy, reduced saturated fat intake to less than 10% total energy, increased fibre intake to more than 15 g per 1000 kcal, and increased exercise to more than 4 hours/week. Sixty per cent of participants who achieved all of these goals experienced a restoration of erectile function.[321] In men with metabolic syndrome and ED, following this style of diet increased the average IIEF-5 score by 3, with 13 of the 35 men in the treatment group achieving normal erectile function.[74] This was accompanied by improvements in endothelial function measurements, reduction in inflammation (as measured by CRP) and improvements in other metabolic syndrome risk factors (HDL and LDL cholesterol, triglycerides, plasma glucose and insulin).[74]

Low glycaemic index diet

Considering that risk of ED is associated with elevated fasting glucose and diabetes mellitus, optimal blood sugar management is a priority in these patients. Adopting low glycaemic index dietary strategies is a validated measure to improve long-term and short-term glycaemic control,[322] and can also be an effective approach in facilitating weight loss.[323]

Nuts and seeds

Nuts should be recommended as a daily inclusion in men with ED. Daily nut consumption (28 g) has been shown in a meta-analysis of longitudinal studies to lower the risk of cardiovascular mortality by 39%, primarily by reducing the risk of coronary artery disease deaths.[324] Nut consumption has also been demonstrated to result in favourable effects on glycaemic control[324] and to correlate with a lower incidence of ED.[320]

As a therapeutic intervention, inclusion of 100 g daily of pistachio nuts for 3 weeks has been shown to result in profound improvements in erectile function as measured by IIEF-15 scores, which increased from a baseline of 36 to 54.2.[325] All 5 domains of the IIEF-15 increased, the erectile function domain increasing from a baseline of 12.1 to 21.4. These improvements were accompanied by an increase in peak systolic velocity (PSV) measurements, indicating improved penile vascular perfusion, and favourable changes in HDL, LDL and total cholesterol.[325] The effect of the pistachios on erectile function was attributed to improvements in endothelial function, reductions in oxidative stress and as a significant dietary source of L-arginine which is a NO precursor essential for vasodilation.[325]

Alcohol

Historically, alcohol has been thought to have detrimental effects upon sexual performance and previous advice has been for men with ED to avoid alcohol consumption. The relationship between alcohol and ED in available epidemiological studies is however unclear. A meta-analysis of available cross-sectional studies suggests that a J-shaped relationship of alcohol consumption with

ED exists.[326] That is, 'low or moderate levels' of alcohol demonstrate a protective relationship compared to abstinence, whereas 'high levels' of consumption increase risk.[326] What the thresholds of alcohol are that define 'low or moderate levels' and 'high levels' in relation to ED risk appear to be dependent on the population studied. In a population of Chinese men, not more than one standard drink per week was protective against ED compared to abstainers, whereas more than three standards drinks was associated with increased risk.[327] In contrast, 11–23 standard drinks a week was protective in a Belgian population, whereas more than this was associated with an increased risk.[328] These cross-sectional findings have not, however been validated by longitudinal studies, which thus far have failed to demonstrate a protective or detrimental effect of chronic alcohol consumption upon the risk of developing ED.[326]

Given that cardiovascular disease is a major risk factor for the development of ED, it seems reasonable to inform our recommendations surrounding alcohol on the relationship it has with CVD. Similar to the relationship described with ED, a J-shaped curve describing risk of ischaemic heart disease (IHD) with alcohol consumption exists when compared to alcohol abstainers.[103] Drinkers who consume an average <30 g/day of alcohol without episodic heavy drinking enjoy the lowest IHD risk when compared to those who abstain or consume larger quantities.[103] Thus it would be appropriate to advise men with ED to limit alcohol consumption to <30 g daily and to avoid episodic heavy drinking, recommendations in line with reducing risk of IHD.[103]

SAMPLE DAILY DIET

BREAKFAST	
Smoothie: banana, parsley, spinach, avocado, water, rice protein powder	Spinach and parsley are a source of nitrates, the reduction of which provides a natural means of generating nitric oxide (NO) availability in the body. NO is essential for genital blood flow.
SNACK	
Pistachio nuts and a piece of seasonal polyphenol-rich fruit	Consumption of 100 g of pistachio nuts has been shown to improve erectile function in men after 3 weeks.* Higher total intake of fruit, a major source of anthocyanins and flavanones, is associated with a 14% reduction in risk of ED.†
LUNCH	
Salmon with quinoa with roasted vegetables and salad	A Mediterranean-style diet is associated with improvements in ED. A Mediterranean diet that is prevalent in oily fish, wholegrains and vegetables but low in red and processed meat and refined grains is more represented in participants without ED‡ and has been shown to reduce deterioration of sexual function because of a reduction in inflammation. Dietary habits that reduce low-grade clinical inflammation counteract a pro-inflammatory state that results in endothelial dysfunction and a decrease in the availability and activity of NO.
SNACK	
Brazil nuts and oat muesli bar	Brazil nuts are a rich source of selenium which is required for testosterone production. Stress plays a part in ED with higher morning cortisol levels associated with ED;§ oats are a nervous system trophorestorative, rich in B vitamins which may help adaptation to stress.
DINNER	
Mussels with garlic and chilli	Mussels are a source of zinc which is required for manufacture of testosterone. Testosterone regulates nearly every component of erectile function, and is involved with coordinating penile erection with sex, modulating the timing of the erectile process, as well as sexual desire. Zinc deficiency is linked to increased conversion of testosterone to oestrogen via the aromatase enzyme. Elevated oestrogen increases the incidence and severity of erectile dysfunction.¶,#

*Aldemir M1, Okulu E, Neşelioğlu S et al. Pistachio diet improves erectile function parameters and serum lipid profiles in patients with erectile dysfunction. Int J Impot Res 2011 Jan–Feb;23(1):32–38.
†Cassidy A, Franz M, Rimm EB. Dietary flavonoid intake and incidence of erectile dysfunction. Am J Clin Nutr 2016 Feb;103(2):534–541.
‡Esposito K, Giugliano F, Maiorino MI et al. Dietary factors, Mediterranean diet and erectile dysfunction. J Sex Med 2010 Jul;7(7):2338–2345.
§Kalaitzidou I, Venetikou MS, Konstadinidis K et al. Stress management and erectile dysfunction: a pilot comparative study. Andrologia 2014 Aug; 46(6):698–702.
¶Schulster M, Bernie AM, Ramasamy R. The role of estradiol in male reproductive function. Asian J Androl 2016 May–Jun;18(3):435–440.
#El-Sakka AI. Impact of the association between elevated oestradiol and low testosterone levels on erectile dysfunction severity. Asian J Androl 2013 Jul;15(4):492.

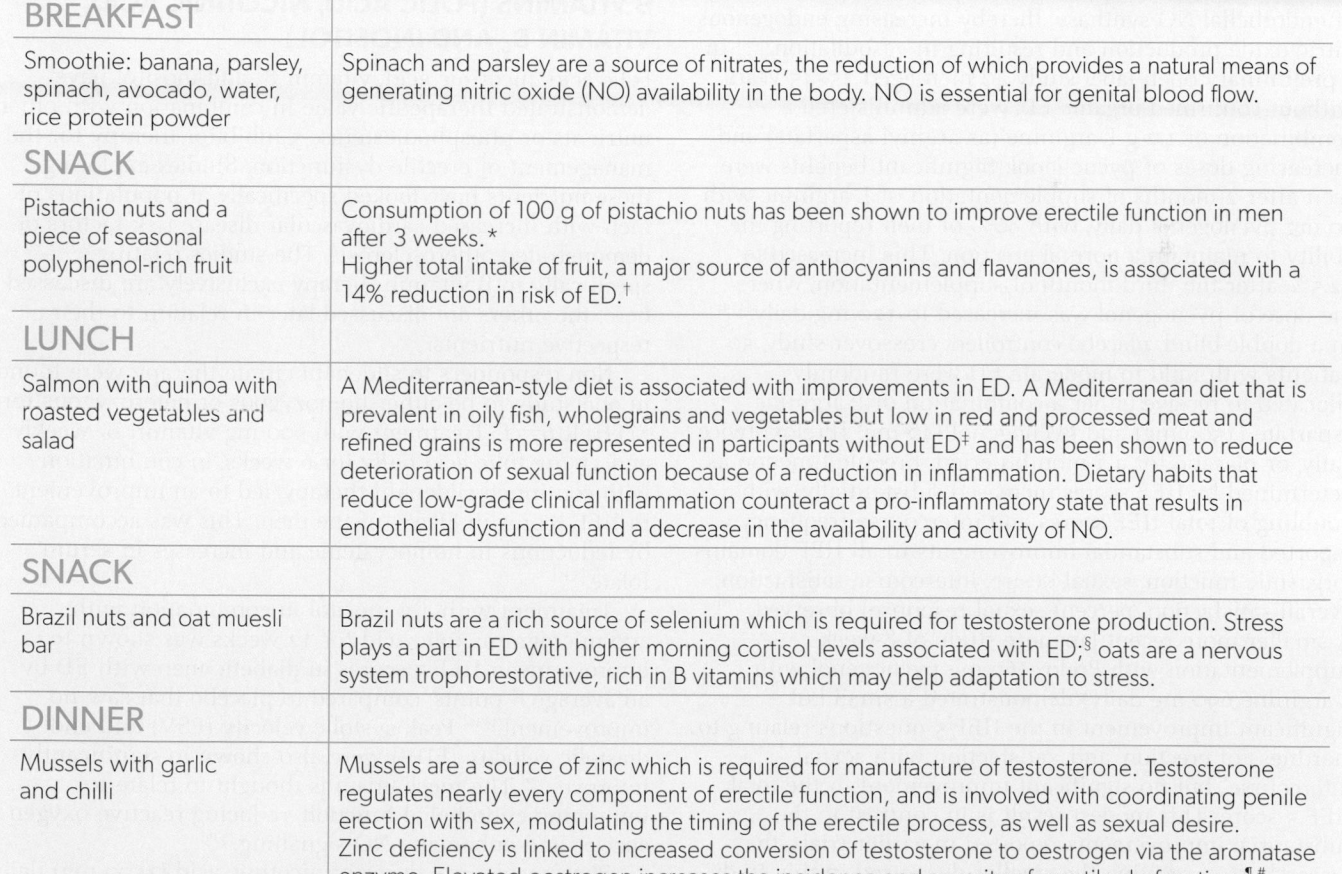

NUTRITIONAL MEDICINE (SUPPLEMENTAL)

Therapeutic objectives

1. Improve erectile function with specific evidence-based nutritional supplementation
2. Provide vascular support and optimise cardiovascular function
3. Support optimal sex hormone balance, specifically androgen production
4. Support optimal blood sugar management
5. Reduce oxidative stress and inflammation
6. Provide nutrients to support optimal mood and address mood disorders if indicated.

Specific nutrients required

PYCNOGENOL (FRENCH MARITIME BARK EXTRACT) AND L-ARGININE

Pycnogenol (French maritime bark extract) is most effective when combined with L-arginine, as the two appear to work synergistically, with L-arginine providing a substrate for NO, and pycnogenol upregulating the activity of endothelial NO synthase, thereby increasing endogenous nitric oxide production and resulting in vasodilation.[114] In a preliminary open label study 40 men aged 25–45 years, without confirmed organic ED, were administered a combination of 1.7 g L-arginine (as arginyl aspartate) and increasing doses of pycnogenol. Significant benefits were seen after 2 months of supplementation of L-arginine with 80 mg pycnogenol daily, with 80% of men reporting the ability to maintain a normal erection. This increased to 92.5% after the third month of supplementation, where the dose of pycnogenol was increased to 120 mg daily.[114] In a double-blind, placebo-controlled, crossover study, 50 patients with mild to moderate ED were randomly allocated to receive either a combination of L-arginine aspartate (1500 mg) and pycnogenol (40 mg) (Prelox) twice daily, or placebo for a 1-month period. Erectile function as determined by IIEF scores increased substantially, with a doubling of total IIEF scores and intercourse frequency reported and substantial improvements in all IIEF domains (orgasmic function, sexual desire, intercourse satisfaction, overall satisfaction, percent sexual response) observed.[115] A smaller more recent Japanese study of 8-week supplementation with Prelox (60 mg pycnogenol with L-arginine 690 mg daily) demonstrated a small but significant improvement in the IIEF-5 questions relating to 'hardness of erection' and 'satisfaction with sexual intercourse', but no significant improvement in the total IIEF-5 score. This modest result is in contrast to the substantial improvements reported in earlier trials, the researchers suggesting the smaller dose used in this study may have been responsible for this.[116]

L-ARGININE

L-arginine as a monotherapy appears to have limited value as a treatment for ED; however, studies using it in combination with other nutritional supplements or herbal extracts have demonstrated better efficacy and are discussed in association with those nutrients. High dose supplementation (5 g) daily for 6 weeks resulted in subjective improvements in erectile function in 31% of supplemented men,[329] whereas a study using a smaller dose (1500 mg) for a shorter duration (17 days) demonstrated no significant improvement in erectile function.[330]

VITAMIN E

Vitamin E has been shown in animal studies to ameliorate ED in diabetic,[331] hypertensive[332] and aged rat models.[333] This appears to be due to its antioxidant activity, whereby it enhances levels of circulating nitric oxide and superoxide dismutase (SOD). Human research into the benefits of vitamin E for erectile dysfunction is limited to a small prospective study of men identified as 'non-responders' to phosphodiesterase-5 inhibitor therapy. One-month treatment with 300 mg α-tocopherol in combination with sildenafil or vardenafil resulted in subjective improvements in erectile function in 8 of the 9 men studied, with 5 of the men having an increase in the IIEF-5 score.[334]

B VITAMINS (FOLIC ACID, NICOTINIC ACID, VITAMIN B_6 AND INOSITOL)

Folic acid, nicotinic acid, vitamin B_6 and inositol have demonstrated therapeutic value in combination with other nutrients or phosphodiesterase-5 inhibitor therapy for the management of erectile dysfunction. Studies exploring these nutrients have looked specifically at populations of men with increased cardiovascular disease risk factors or demonstrated atherosclerosis. The studies relating specifically to B vitamin therapy exclusively are discussed here; the others are discussed later in relation to their respective nutrients.

Non-responders to sildenafil citrate therapy were found in one study to be either homozygous or heterozygous for MTHFR 677T. Treatment with 600 mg vitamin B_6 weekly and 15 mg folic acid daily for 6 weeks, in combination with continued sildenafil therapy, led to an improvement in IIEF scores in 88.9% of the men. This was accompanied by reductions in homocysteine and increases in serum folate.[335]

Treatment with 4 g inositol in combination with 400 micrograms folic acid for 12 weeks was shown to improve mean IIEF-5 scores in diabetic men with ED by an average 8 points, compared to placebo that saw no improvement.[335] Peak systolic velocity (PSV) and end diastolic velocity (EDV) were also shown to significantly improve.[336] The mechanism is thought to relate to improving endothelial function, reducing reactive oxygen species and enhancing NO signalling.[336]

Pharmacological doses of nicotinic acid (1500 mg) daily for 12 weeks demonstrated improvements in total and erectile function domain scores of the IIEF in patients with moderate to severe ED with dyslipidaemia.[337] Frequency of penetration and frequency of maintained erections after penetration scores were specifically improved in these men.[337] Improvements in function were not however demonstrated in men with mild or mild-moderate erectile dysfunction.[337] The dose of nicotinic acid used in this study was associated with side effects, with flushing and skin itchiness occurring in 36.3% and 32.5% of participants respectively.[337]

L-CARNITINE

Propionyl-L-carnitine, in combination with other nutrients or PDE-5 inhibitors, has been indicated therapeutically for the treatment of ED. It increases mitochondrial and endothelial function, acts as an antioxidant and reduces damage to DNA.[338] A combination of 250 mg propionyl-L-carnitine, 2500 mg L-arginine and 20 mg niacin was found to result in a mean improvement of 5.7 points on the IIEF-5 questionnaire in diabetic men with ED after 3 months of treatment.[339] Forty-six per cent of the men were observed to experience substantial erectile function improvement, and 37% experienced a small positive change in function.[339]

This same supplement combination has been shown to improve efficacy of PDE-5 inhibitors in various populations of men with increased cardiovascular risk. In men who had ED of arterial origin, and who were poor responders to sildenafil therapy, combined supplement and sildenafil treatment for 8 weeks resulted in significantly improved treatment efficacy.[340] Sixty-eight per cent of the men were considered responders (as defined by an increase in IIEF-5 score by 5 points) to combined supplement and sildenafil treatment compared to 45% who responded to sildenafil on its own, or 32% who responded to the supplement on its own.[340] Combined treatment also resulted in a quicker maximum therapeutic effect at 3 weeks.[340]

Similarly, on-demand use of sildenafil for the treatment of sexual dysfunction as a complication of prostatectomy was more effective when given in combination with 2 g acetyl-L-carnitine and 2 g propionyl-L-carnitine daily for 4 months.[341]

COENZYME Q10

Coenzyme Q10 supplementation has been demonstrated to improve outcomes in men with Peyronie's disease. Treatment with 300 mg coenzyme Q10 daily for 24 weeks in men with early chronic Peyronie's disease resulted in improvements in erectile function as measured by the IIEF-5, reduced pain, reduced mean plaque size and mean penile curvature.[342] In the treatment group, only 13.6% of patients had a progression of their condition, compared to 56.1% in the placebo group.[342] The effect of coenzyme Q10 in this condition is thought to be as an antioxidant, as plaque formation of the corpora tunica is postulated to be a consequence of oxidative stress.[342] Coenzyme Q10 also demonstrates properties that are of relevance in addressing aetiological factors involved in ED. Vascular endothelial function,[343] blood pressure,[344] blood lipids[345] and blood glucose control[346] have all been demonstrated to be improved with coenzyme Q10 supplementation, suggesting a role in ED beyond that where Peyronie's is the cause.

Additional supplementation may be targeted towards addressing aetiological factors such as cardiovascular disease, metabolic syndrome, diabetes and depression where indicated. Suggestions are made below (Table 19.6); however, the clinician is directed to relevant chapters of this text for comprehensive coverage.

TABLE 19.6 Nutritional supplementation for associated comorbidities of erectile dysfunction

Nutrient	Supportive evidence
Zinc	Zinc supplementation in zinc deficiency has been shown to improve erectile function and correct low testosterone in patients with end-stage renal disease. Zinc plays a significant role in the treatment of hyperglycaemia and dyslipidaemia. Zinc also demonstrates a role as an adjunct treatment of depression which may be indicated as part of the management of ED.
Selenium	Selenium supplementation has been demonstrated to have beneficial effects on cardiovascular disease risk and blood glucose control. Where male LUTS co-exists with ED, supplementation may confer additional benefits.
Essential fatty acids (EPA/DHA)	EPA and DHA supplementation may improve insulin resistance, blood lipids and hypertension. Protection against vascular disease and vascular death has been reported. Improvements in vascular endothelial function have been reported.
Vitamin D	Deficiency of vitamin D has been associated with ED and derangements in endothelial function. A case study demonstrated improvements in ED with correction of deficiency. Deficiency is associated with low testosterone, which supplementation has been shown to correct. Higher vitamin D status is associated with a more favourable lipid profile, including HDL cholesterol, triglycerides, lower waist circumference, serum glucose and lower risk of metabolic syndrome.
Magnesium	Magnesium has demonstrated benefits in improving insulin sensitivity, triglycerides, and diastolic and systolic blood pressure.
Chromium	Numerous human studies demonstrate beneficial effects of chromium supplementation, particularly in the form of chromium picolinate, on glycaemic control and blood lipids in patients with type 2 diabetes. Negative effects on insulin sensitivity have, however, been seen in non-obese, non-diabetic patients, suggesting that chromium supplementation is best avoided in this group.
B complex	An association between low vitamin B_{12} and folate and increased rates of depression is evident. Long-term B vitamin supplementation rather than short term may be of benefit in depression; however evidence is inconsistent.

Sources: [110, 111, 122, 443, 445, 447, 448, 453, 474, 479, 488–498, 500–505]

DOSAGE REQUIREMENTS

The doses listed below are based on adult doses reported in the literature:

- L-arginine: 690 mg–5000 mg/day (best combined with pycnogenol, higher doses if monotherapy)
- Pycnogenol: 60 mg–120 mg/day
- Vitamin E: 300 mg α-tocopherol/day
- Inositol: 4000 mg/day
- Propionyl-L-carnitine: 250 mg–2000 mg/day
- Acetyl-L-carnitine: 2000 mg/day
- Coenzyme Q10: 100–300 mg daily. Higher dose used where Peyronie's is present
- Zinc: 20 mg–100 mg/day
- Selenium: 50 micrograms–200 micrograms daily. Care should be taken not to exceed this dose, as cardiovascular benefits of selenium have demonstrated a narrow therapeutic range[122]
- Vitamin D: The Endocrine Society recommends supplementing 6000 IU/day in adults who are vitamin D deficient for 8 weeks to achieve a 25(OH)D blood level of above 75 nmol/L. 1500–2000 IU/day is then suggested to maintain blood levels[123]
- Magnesium:100 mg–500 mg/day
- Chromium: 200 micrograms–600 micrograms/day
- Essential fatty acids (fish oil): 1100 mg–5600 mg EPA and DHA/day
- B complex
  - vitamin B_1: 50–100 mg/day
  - vitamin B_2: 50 mg/day
  - vitamin B_3: 20–200 mg/day. 1500 mg doses have been used in ED; however, such doses are associated with side effects
  - vitamin B_5: 50–200 mg/day
  - vitamin B_6: 50–100 mg/day
  - vitamin B_9: 400 micrograms-15 mg/day. High doses can mask vitamin B_{12} deficiency
  - vitamin B_{12}: 125–2000 micrograms/day.

HERBAL MEDICINE

Therapeutic objectives

1. Improve erectile function with specific evidence-based herbal medicines
2. Support optimal sexual function with male reproductive tonics
3. Regulate and balance male hormone profile, using androgenic herbal medicines if indicated
4. Support optimal cardiovascular health, manage risk factors, and improve vascular tone and cardiac function
5. Promote optimal peripheral circulation
6. Reduce oxidative stress and inflammation
7. Support an optimal stress response and vitality
8. Support optimal mood and treat anxiety and depression (if present).

Herbal medicine classes

MALE TONICS

Herbal medicines form an important component of the naturopathic treatment approach to ED, especially in the form of male tonic herbal medicines. Specific male tonics include *Panax ginseng* (Korean ginseng), *Serenoa repens* (saw palmetto), *Smilax ornata* (sarsaparilla), *Tribulus terrestris* (tribulus), *Turnera diffusa* (damiana), *Withania somnifera* (ashwagandha), *Mucuna pruriens* (velvet bean) and *Eurycoma longifolia* (tongkat ali). Korean ginseng is especially indicated for men who require additional adaptogenic support or who are debilitated, and saw palmetto can provide support where lower urinary tract symptoms are also present. Tribulus is valuable to assist in increasing libido and damiana can provide additional mood support. Ashwagandha is of value where an adaptogen and an anxiolytic are required and both velvet bean and tongkat ali are of value for their aphrodisiac and androgenic properties.

NERVINES

Effective management of mood disorders is an essential strategy in ED patients where depression is present, as this is likely to have bearing on erectile function. The primary prescription to be considered here is *Crocus sativus* (saffron), due to its well-recognised historical use and modern evidence as an effective antidepressant agent, with erection-enhancing properties.[131,132] *Ptychopetalum olacoides* (muira puama), a nervine tonic with adaptogen, antioxidant and aphrodisiac qualities, also has a reputation for improving erectile function.[347] Other considerations are *Turnera diffusa* (damiana) due to its additional male tonic properties; *Leonurus cardiaca* (motherwort), particularly if anxiety is also present; and *Hypericum perforatum* (St John's wort).

APHRODISIACS

Changes in erectile function can accompany reductions in libido, or vice versa. Therefore, the inclusion of herbal medicines with a reputation for increasing sexual interest is an important consideration in ED. These herbs also typically have a reputation for improving erectile function. Herbs to consider include *Eurycoma longifolia* (tongkat ali), *Panax ginseng* (Korean ginseng), *Turnera diffusa* (damiana), *Crocus sativus* (saffron), *Tribulus terrestris* (tribulus), *Withania somnifera* (ashwagandha), *Mucuna pruriens* (velvet bean), *Lepidium meyenii* (maca) and *Ptychopetalum olacoides* (muira puama).

CIRCULATORY STIMULANTS

Because of the role of vascular health in erectile function, the role of supporting optimal circulation in ED cannot be understated. The efficacy of such herbal medicines that support healthy circulation is supported by concurrent lifestyle changes and optimal hydration. Important examples of circulatory stimulants are *Capsicum* spp. (chilli or cayenne), *Ginkgo biloba* (ginkgo), *Panax ginseng* (Korean ginseng), *Rosmarinus officinalis* (rosemary), *Zanthoxylum clava-herculis* (prickly ash bark), *Zingiber officinalis* (ginger) and *Cinnamomum zeylanicum* (cinnamon). The heat of the chosen circulatory stimulant should be assessed based on the patient's presentation. Prickly ash bark and rosemary are cooler options, while chilli, cinnamon and ginger are hotter alternatives.

HORMONE MODULATORS (TESTOSTEROGENIC)

Herbal medicines with a reputation for modulating testosterone production should be considered in ED, especially where low testosterone is demonstrated to be a contributing factor. Those that have some evidence demonstrating potential phytoandrogenic properties include *Eurycoma longifolia* (tongkat ali),[348] *Tribulus terrestris* (tribulus),[349] *Withania somnifera* (withania)[350] and *Mucuna pruriens* (velvet bean).[351] Traditionally *Panax ginseng* (Korean ginseng), *Smilax ornata* (sarsaparilla), *Turnera diffusa* (damiana) and *Avena sativa* seed (oat seed) would also be considered for this purpose.

CARDIAC TONICS/CARDIO-PROTECTIVES

These herbal medicines are indicated for inclusion in holistic herbal formulas for older men with ED due to compromised cardiovascular function. Important examples include *Crataegus* spp. (hawthorn leaves and berries), *Leonurus cardiaca* (motherwort), *Panax ginseng* (Korean ginseng), *Panax notoginseng* (tienchi ginseng), *Astragalus membranaceus* (astragalus), *Coleus forskholii* (coleus), *Salvia miltiorrhiza* (dan shen) and *Terminalia arjuna* (arjuna).

VASCULAR TONICS

Vascular tonics are indicated to support vascular integrity. Important herbal medicines of this type include *Pinus pinaster* (maritime pine), *Aesculus hippocastanum* (horse chestnut), *Ginkgo biloba* (ginkgo), *Vitis vinifera* (grape seed extract) and *Centella asiatica*. Ginkgo, grape seed extract and maritime pine also provide antioxidant support, which may contribute to reducing oxidative stress implicated in ED pathogenesis.

PERIPHERAL VASODILATORS

These herbal medicines have been observed to improve blood supply to peripheral tissues, especially to the extremities, which therefore could make them indicated in ED. Generally these herbal medicines also are indicated in cardiovascular disease, and appear useful in normalising blood pressure. They include *Achillea millefolium* (yarrow), *Crataegus* spp. (hawthorn leaves and berries), *Ginkgo biloba* (ginkgo), *Tilia* spp. (lime flowers, or linden), *Viburnum opulus* (cramp bark) and *Viscum album* (mistletoe). *Hibiscus sabdariffa* (roselle) could also be included here, due to its value in normalising blood pressure.

Specific herbal medicines

SAFFRON (*CROCUS SATIVUS*)

Saffron has a diverse range of traditional applications, including use in cardiovascular disease, as an antidepressant, aphrodisiac and erection-enhancing agent.[132] Its traditional application in improving erectile function has been explored in three relatively recent studies.[131,352,353]

An open label study demonstrated significant improvements in the total IIEF-15 from a baseline of 22.15 to 39.2 after 10 days treatment with 200 mg dried saffron stigma daily.[131] All domains of the IIEF-15 were shown to significantly improve, including erectile function, sexual desire and orgasmic function; the erectile function domain score increasing from a baseline of 11.75 to 17.15 at the end of the study.[131] Nocturnal penile tumescence testing also demonstrated improvements in tip rigidity and tumescence, base rigidity and tumescence, and the number of nocturnal erectile episodes.[131]

A much larger open label, randomised, fixed-dose crossover study compared the efficacy of 30 mg saffron stigma twice daily with on-demand sildenafil treatment.[352] No significant improvement was seen in regards to erectile function with 12 weeks treatment as assessed with the IIEF-15, sexual encounter profile (SEP) questions, Erectile Dysfunction Inventory of Treatment Satisfaction (EDITS) questionnaire or Global Efficacy Question (GEQ).[352] It is worth noting the lower dose used in this study (60 mg daily),[352] compared to the higher dose (200 mg daily) used previously that demonstrated efficacy.[131]

Saffron may be indicated in the management of SSRI-induced sexual dysfunction. Four-week treatment with 15 mg twice daily saffron stigma in men with sexual impairment taking fluoxetine treatment for major depressive disorder resulted in significant improvements in total IIEF score (mean increase 8.2), erectile function (mean increase 4.5) and satisfaction with intercourse (mean increase 2.1) scores.[353]

PANAX GINSENG (KOREAN GINSENG)

Numerous studies have investigated the role of *Panax ginseng* for the treatment of ED, a systematic review finding that there is good evidence to support the use of red *Panax ginseng* root to treat this condition.[354] However, as the studies were described as being of variable methodological quality, more rigorous evidence is required. The studies undertaken involved the use of red ginseng (steamed *Panax ginseng*) and doses of extracts varied from approximately 1800 mg to 3000 mg.[354] More recent evidence into the efficacy of Korean ginseng is however limited to research on the berry extract, which demonstrated small clinically insignificant increases in erectile function domain scores on the IIEF-15 (from 17.17 to 18.59).[355]

The mechanism by which ginseng exerts its effects is unknown, although animal and in-vitro studies would suggest that ginsenosides present in the root and berry extract exhibit nitric oxide upregulating activity.[355] The traditional application of *Panax ginseng* as an adaptogen may also be implicated in its therapeutic role in ED.

SERENOA REPENS (SAW PALMETTO)

In typical modern day practice of naturopathic medicine, *S. repens* is not a first-line treatment for ED. However, it was prized by the Eclectic physicians, particularly for cases where dysfunction was associated with excessive sexual intercourse and thus fatigue:

> *It will overcome the excitability from exhaustion and increase sexual power in those newly married who, having been anxious concerning their sexual strength or ability, have become suddenly almost entirely impotent after marriage. If the patient is instructed to abstain, for from*

> *four to six weeks, and to have confidence in his ultimate recovery, this agent in doses of from twenty to thirty drops three or four times daily, combined with a direct nerve tonic, such as avena sativa in doses of fifteen drops, or the one one-hundredth of a grain of phosphorus, will establish a cure.*
>
> ***Ellingwood (1919)***

Modern evidence for a role of *S. repens* in treating ED is limited to an animal study that suggested the extract exerted an increased inducible nitric oxide synthase (iNOS) messenger RNA (mRNA) expression in corpus cavernosum smooth muscles, and inhibits phosphodiesterase-5 activity.[356]

Although there have been no studies examining the effect of *S. repens* in men with ED, traditional application and limited animal research suggests a potential therapeutic application in the management of ED.

TRIBULUS TERRESTRIS (TRIBULUS)

T. terrestris has a reputation as improving sexual function and physical performance in men, and is a commonly recommended herbal strategy for improving erectile function. While its use as a libido-enhancing agent is well supported by the literature,[349] studies on its effects on improving erectile function have been conflicting. The effects of tribulus on sexual function are thought to relate to an endothelial and nitric oxide dependent mechanism which have been demonstrated in animal studies.[357]

A recent uncontrolled pilot study evaluating the effect of tribulus on erectile function in men with androgen deficiency found that 3-month daily treatment with 750 mg *Tribulus terrestris* extract significantly increased IIEF-5 scores from a baseline of 12.48 to 15.96.[358] Total and free testosterone were also demonstrated to significantly improve, although within normal limits for total testosterone, and below normal for free testosterone.[358] An earlier placebo-controlled randomised double-blind study evaluating the effect of 800 mg *Tribulus terrestris* daily for 30 days did not demonstrate any difference between placebo and tribulus treatment on IIEF-5 and total testosterone.[359]

A multi-herb ingredient product delivering *Tribulus terrestris* (900 mg), *Ecklonia bicyclis* (600 mg) and glucosamine oligosaccharide (500 mg) daily was demonstrated to improve total IIEF-15 by 11.54 after 3 months of treatment in men with mild to moderate erectile dysfunction.[360] Intercourse satisfaction, orgasmic function, sexual desire and overall satisfaction sub scores of the IIEF-15 were improved; however, changes in the erectile function sub-score were seen only in men with identified moderate arterial dysfunction (defined as a peak systolic velocity of 25 to 35) and in these men it was only modestly increased by 1.82.[360]

TONGKAT ALI (*EURYCOMA LONGIFOLIA*)

Tongkat ali is native to forests of Malaysia, Indonesia and Thailand, with a traditional reputation as an aphrodisiac and sexual performance enhancing plant medicine. Clinical trial evidence suggests that it can exert testosterone-modulating activity, and appears to have demonstrated clinical value in men with sexual dysfunction related to late-onset hypogonadism.[348] The mechanism of action is unknown but suggested to be mediated by phenolic compounds, polypetides, diterpenoids, alkaloids and quassinoids present in the water extract.[361]

A systematic review identified two randomised controlled trials that evaluated the effect of *Eurycoma longifolia* on erectile function. A significant increase in IIEF-5 score was demonstrated; however, it was limited to men with lower baseline IIEF-5 scores, with an increased mean score of 2.15.[361] While significant, the increase in IIEF-5 was modest, and not considered to be clinically important.[361]

LIFESTYLE RECOMMENDATIONS

Aerobic exercise

The role of exercise in managing ED appears obvious, given the intimate links between cardiovascular disease, metabolic syndrome and insulin resistance with ED, and the benefits that physical activity has on these conditions. Measures of exercise tolerance have been found to be correlated to erection quality[362] and, more importantly, clinical trials have consistently demonstrated the beneficial effect of exercise in improving erectile function.[363,364]

A meta-analysis of five randomised controlled trials found that aerobic exercise training as a single treatment modality significantly improved erectile function, increasing the mean IIEF from 13.91 to 16.74.[363] Exercise has also been shown to improve the efficacy of pharmacological treatment of ED; a 2-month exercise program consisting of tri-weekly 30-minute aerobic exercise sessions in combination with tadalafil resulted in much greater improvements in erectile function compared with tadalafil alone.[364] In this study, an increase in the IIEF from a baseline of 11.2 to 14.24 was seen in the men treated only with tadalafil, compared to an increase from 10.8 to 20.1 in the group who combined it with exercise training.[364]

Thus, given the diverse health benefits of physical activity, exercise therapy is an essential modality to incorporate into any ED management plan and is likely to improve treatment efficacy.

Pelvic floor exercises

Pelvic floor musculature, especially the ischiocavernosus and bulbospongiosus muscles, are involved in erectile function and ejaculation.[365] Stimulation of the glans penis and distension of the corpus cavernosum lead to reflex contractions of the pelvic musculature. Contraction of the ischiocavernosus muscle contributes rigidity to the penis during the muscular phase of an erection, and compresses the root of the corpus cavernosum, reducing venous outflow and thereby increasing intracavernosus pressure.[366,367] Any reduced tone in these muscles could therefore plausibly contribute to reduced erectile function, and thus exercises that aim to improve pelvic muscular strength could be used to treat ED.

The efficacy of pelvic floor exercises in the management of ED is supported by clinical trial evidence. Men with ED who practised pelvic floor strengthening exercises twice daily for 6 months demonstrated significant improvements in erectile function, the majority of improvement being seen to occur in the first 3 months of treatment.[365] After 6 months 40% of men regained normal erectile function, 35.5% saw some improvement and 24.5% saw no improvement.[365]

Surgical treatment for prostate cancer frequently results in erectile dysfunction. In men who developed sexual dysfunction following radical prostatectomy, twice daily pelvic floor exercises improved recovery of sexual function in 34.3% of the men by 12 months, compared to 7.4% in the control group.[368] The degree of erectile function recovered was also greater in men who undertook pelvic floor exercises than in the control group.[368]

A pelvic floor exercise routine that can be recommended to men with ED, consistent with those used in trials discussed here, is outlined in Box 19.8.

Weight loss

Maintaining a healthy body weight and abdominal circumference should be included in any erectile dysfunction treatment plan, due to the relationship between erectile dysfunction, reduced sexual desire and reduced enjoyment in sexual activity with obesity.[369] The role of obesity in erectile dysfunction is thought to relate to the effect of chronic inflammation and insulin resistance on endothelial function[125] and via hormonal mechanisms such as testosterone deficiency.[370]

Weight loss in obese men has been demonstrated to improve erectile function. Obese men with or without type 2 diabetes mellitus who followed a low-kilojoule diet for 8 weeks experienced improvements in erectile function and sexual desire.[369] An average weight loss of approximately 10% was associated with increases in IIEF-5 of 2.2 in non-diabetic men, and 2.1 in diabetic men.[369] These improvements in erectile function were associated with the degree of weight loss, with greater weight loss resulting in better erectile function.[369]

Smoking cessation

Smoking is a recognised risk factor for the development of ED[280] and smoking cessation has been demonstrated to improve erectile function.[371,372]

Six months after smoking cessation, 53.8% of men experienced improvements in erectile function, compared to 28.1% of men who did not quit.[371] Benefits to sexual function may be seen relatively soon after smoking cessation. Four weeks following an 8-week smoking cessation program, significant improvements in erectile

BOX 19.8 Pelvic floor exercises for men

In lying position

Lie on your back with your knees bent and your feet and knees slightly apart.

Tighten your pelvic floor as if you are trying to stop wind escaping and urine leaking. You should feel the base of your penis move towards your body and your testicles rise. Hold the pelvic floor muscle contraction as strongly as you can. Try to avoid holding your breath or tensing your buttocks.

Perform a maximum of three contractions while lying down in the morning holding for up to 10 seconds, each followed by a 10-second rest. Repeat in the afternoon.

In sitting position

Sit on a chair with your knees slightly apart and tighten your pelvic floor muscles as if you were trying to stop wind escaping and urine leaking. You should feel the base of your penis move towards your body and your testicles rise. Hold the pelvic floor muscle contraction as strongly as you can. Try to avoid holding your breath or tensing your buttocks.

Perform a maximum of three contractions sitting down in the morning holding for up to 10 seconds, each followed by a 10-second rest. Repeat in the afternoon.

In standing position

Stand with your feet apart and tighten your pelvic floor muscles. If you look in a mirror you should be able to see the base of your penis move nearer to your body and your testicles gradually rise. Hold the pelvic floor muscle contraction as strong as you can. Try to avoid holding your breath or tensing your buttocks.

Perform a maximum of three contractions standing up in the morning holding for up to 10 seconds, each followed by a 10-second rest. Repeat in the afternoon.

Fast contractions

Some of these pelvic floor muscle contractions can start quickly with a fast contraction and some can begin slowly with a slow build-up of strength.

While walking

Try lifting your pelvic floor up slightly when walking in order to use the muscles during activity. This should become a habit.

After urinating

After you have urinated while standing, try tightening your pelvic floor muscles up strongly to eliminate the urine left in the u-shaped portion of the urethra and avoid the embarrassing after-dribble of urine.

After passing a motion

After passing a motion tighten your anal sphincter before wiping your bottom.

This helps to return any faeces not voided back up the anal canal to the rectum and makes it easier to wipe your bottom.

'The knack'

Tighten your pelvic floor muscles quickly just before and during any activities that increase your abdominal pressure, such as coughing, sneezing, lifting, shouting, bending and getting out of a chair.

Source: Dorey G. Pelvic dysfunction in men. Diagnosis and treatment of male urinary incontinence and erectile dysfunction; a textbook for physiotherapists, nurses and doctors, 2006.

tumescence responses and a quicker onset to reach maximum subjective sexual arousal were demonstrated in men who were successful quitters.[372] Interestingly, the improvements in objective erectile measures were not seen during the 8-week intervention period, when men were receiving nicotine patches,[372] suggesting that nicotine is specifically implicated in the deleterious impacts of smoking on erectile function. This is consistent with a previous study that demonstrated that administration of nicotine replacement gum acutely reduced physiological sexual arousal by 23% in non-smokers.[373]

CASE STUDY

OVERVIEW

Harry is a 36-year-old male who presents with a 6-month history of difficulty attaining and maintaining an erection. He reports that erections have been especially difficult for the past 4 months. He has been in his current relationship for the past 6 months, which is monogamous. Prior to this he had not been in a sexual relationship for 12 months following the breakup with his wife of 10 years. Intercourse frequency during the latter part of the relationship was infrequent, and generally he reported it as unsatisfying, although during this time he felt he did not experience erectile difficulties.

IIEF-5 total score was 16, indicating mild to moderate erectile dysfunction. Harry reports that since having the erectile difficulties, he rarely wakes with erections. Libido is generally low, although he is attracted to his current partner and other than the difficulties experienced with erections, he feels that his current relationship is healthy and has no real concerns.

Harry reports that due to his low libido, he rarely masturbates (at the moment once a week at the most) although when he does, erections, while taking a little longer to develop, are satisfactory.

Currently Harry reports high levels of stress regarding custody disputes over his two children, aged 9 and 6. Interactions with his previous partner are always difficult, and have worsened considerably since he started seeing his current partner. Harry works for an insurance firm and finds the workload demanding, particularly in light of his personal life stresses.

Sleep is disrupted. Harry reports that he typically goes to bed at around 10 pm; however he wakes usually around 2 am, typically taking around an hour or so to get back to sleep. Any sleep he gets from this point is restless, generally waking again at 5 am, at which time he feels unrefreshed. As a consequence, Harry says he needs at least 4 coffees during the morning to function. He does however avoid drinking coffee in the afternoon.

Harry has been a smoker for the past 12 years, typically smoking 5 cigarettes a day. For the past 12 months he says he has been smoking closer to 10 cigarettes daily which he puts down to his current personal life stresses.

Harry consumes a glass of red wine most nights after dinner and binges with his mates once or twice a fortnight during which he can consume 6–10 beers.

CASE STUDY CONTINUED

Current exercise is infrequent, although Harry says he used to be quite fit, previously being a member of a gym, and doing weights and aerobic exercise at least 3 times a week. For the past 2–3 years he has been relatively sedentary in his office work, and has noticed he has put on a bit of weight, especially around his abdomen.

Harry says he generally enjoys cooking, but found previously that on his own he was eating mostly take-away and easy-to-prepare frozen meals. More recently, with the encouragement of his current partner (whom he affectionately refers to as a 'health nut') he has adopted a more plant-based, wholefood diet. Fish is consumed 1 or 2 times a week, kangaroo or lean beef twice weekly, and on other days meals are based around beans or tofu. Nuts are however infrequently consumed.

Systems review is otherwise unremarkable, with Harry not reporting any other health problems, and he does not take any prescribed medications. He is currently taking an unspecified men's multivitamin, and 1000 IU daily vitamin D.

Physical examination findings were as follows:

- The patient looks well
- Pulse: 72 bpm regular
- Respiratory rate: 12 respirations/minute
- Temperature: 37.1°C
- Blood pressure: 140/90 mmHg
- Weight: 81 kg
- Height: 1.72 cm
- Body mass index (BMI): 27 kg/m^2
- Conjunctiva: pink
- Nails: nicotine staining right index and middle fingers
- Capillary refill: 2 seconds
- Random blood glucose: 5.6 mmol/L.

A thorough genital examination was previously performed by a general practitioner in relation to the erectile dysfunction, the findings of which were unremarkable. Investigations were also performed in relation to the presentation: the relevant findings were:

- Total testosterone: 15 nmol/L
- Total cholesterol: 5.1 mmol/L
- HDL cholesterol: 1.2 mmol/L
- LDL cholesterol: 3.3 mmol/L
- Triglycerides: 1.3 mmol/L.

INITIAL TREATMENT

The initial treatment was aimed at improving erectile function and libido, with particular emphasis on addressing contributing factors that were likely to bring about the most rapid improvement, namely the contribution of nicotine, stress and physical inactivity. The patient was counselled about both the acute and long-term impacts of smoking on sexual function and the important role smoking cessation is likely to play on improving erections. The patient was also counselled about the role of other cardiovascular risk factors (hypertension, hyperlipidaemia, overweight) both in the short term in regards to his erectile function, but also long-term cardiovascular health.

HERBAL MEDICINE

- Herbal complex: 200 mL
  Withania somnifera 1:2: 80 mL
  Crocus sativus 1:20: 40 mL

CASE STUDY CONTINUED

Pinus pinaster 1:2: 20 mL
Turnera diffusa 1:2: 60 mL
Dose: 5 mL three times daily

NUTRITIONAL MEDICINE (DIETARY)

- Incorporate regular consumption of nuts and seeds, especially unsalted pistachios, almonds and Brazil nuts. Aim for at least a big handful daily
- Incorporate cholesterol-modifying dietary components. Include oats daily as either breakfast or in smoothies. Include 1–2 tablespoons ground flaxseeds daily. Try to incorporate soy protein most days, in particular tempeh as a rich source of dietary isoflavones.

NUTRITIONAL MEDICINE (SUPPLEMENTAL)

- Magnesium (as magnesium citrate) 135 mg: 1 capsule twice daily
- Increase vitamin D to 2000 IU daily, or get serum tested and dose accordingly.

LIFESTYLE EDUCATION

- Quit smoking. Harry expressed that his current levels of stress made him reluctant to quit at this stage, although he was open to in the future
- Incorporate regular exercise at least 3–4 times a week. Find ways of increasing incidental exercise, such as walking or cycling to work
- Referral to a counsellor/psychologist who also teaches mindfulness meditation for learning effective stress management techniques
- Have non-sex focused intimacy with partner, such as exchanging regular massage
- Have at least 2 alcohol-free days a week and avoid binge drinking.

FOLLOW-UP CONSULTATION 3 WEEKS LATER

Harry reported mild improvement in both his interest in sex and sexual function. He and his partner were enjoying exchanging massage, which occasionally had led to sex during which most recently he felt his capacity to maintain an erection had improved somewhat. Harry was sleeping better; in the past week he had only woken in the early hours twice, and both times he was able to go back to sleep more easily.

Harry reported that he had joined a gym and was taking a longer lunch break during which he was incorporating 30–40 minutes of a mix of treadmill/exercise bike and weights. At this stage he could do this 3 lunchtimes a week, but was looking at ways of increasing it to 5 times.

Overall, Harry reported that his management of stress had improved significantly, putting it down to the increase in exercise. He also felt that his energy levels were better.

Harry discussed that he was booked in to see a psychologist specifically to address stress management strategies, and to assist directly with smoking cessation strategies as he felt he was now ready for this.

ADDITIONAL RECOMMENDATIONS

Advice was to continue with previous dietary and lifestyle suggestions. The herbal complex was modified to incorporate the acute anxiolytic properties of *Leonurus cardiaca* as it was anticipated that irritability and agitation were likely to increase with smoking cessation. A herbal tea was also formulated to continue to support libido and to address hypertension.

- Herbal complex: 200 mL
  Withania somnifera 1:2: 70 mL
  Crocus sativus 1:20: 30 mL
  Pinus pinaster 1:2: 20 mL
  Leonurus cardiaca 1:2: 80 mL
  Dose: 5 mL three times daily. Take up to 6 times daily as needed for anxiety and irritability
- Herbal tea: 100 g
  Turnera diffusa: 30 g
  Hibiscus sabdariffa: 60 g
  Zingiber officinalis: 5 g
  Rosmarinus officinalis: 5 g
  Dose: 3 rounded tablespoons into a large teapot of hot water. Drink throughout the day.

THIRD CONSULTATION (6 WEEKS LATER)

Harry had maintained all recommendations including dietary, lifestyle, herbal and nutritional medicines. With the help of his psychologist he had successfully ceased smoking 'cold-turkey' 5 weeks previously. During that time he used increased exercise (going for a run or bicycle ride), or having a cup of his herbal tea as a distraction whenever he felt a craving for a cigarette. He also increased the dose of his herbal complex to 6 times daily when he felt irritable. Harry reported that he was feeling fitter and healthier than he had 'in ages'. His interest in sex had increased substantially over the past month. He was also feeling a lot more confident about his ability to both attain and maintain an erection and noticed that he was having morning erections, particularly after a good night's sleep.

LATE-ONSET HYPOGONADISM

Epidemiology

The true incidence and prevalence of late-onset hypogonadism (LOH) is difficult to ascertain due to varying definitions of the syndrome used, ages and comorbidities of study participants and laboratory methods used in epidemiological research.[309] The European Male Aging Study (EMAS) estimated prevalence of late-onset hypogonadism to be 2.1% overall in 40–79-year-old men, combining symptomatology and the presence of a total testosterone level of less than 11 nmol/L and free testosterone level of less than 220 pmol/L.[374] This is in contrast to findings of the Baltimore Area Longitudinal Study on Aging (BALSA) that found a prevalence of from 12% of men in their 50s to 49% of men over 80, based on a criteria of total testosterone levels of less than 11.3 nmol/L. The results were higher when based on the free testosterone index of less than 0.153 nmol/L, finding that 9% of men in their 50s and 91% of men over 80 were androgen deficient.[375] (See Fig. 19.5.)

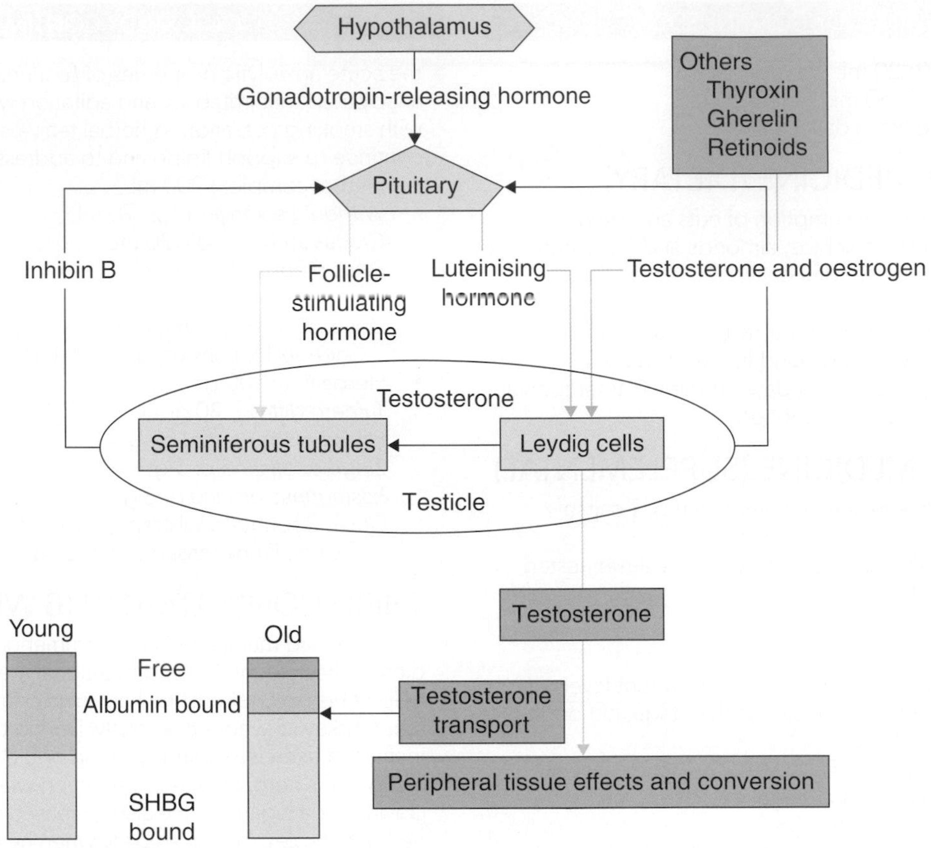

FIGURE 19.5 The effect of ageing on the production, transport and metabolism of testosterone. Testosterone production is regulated by LH, which is reduced together with GRH by the ageing process affecting the hypothalamus and pituitary gland. SHBG increases with ageing and binds to total testosterone, making it unavailable to tissues. The same occurs with albumin levels. Bioavailable testosterone can be converted to other hormones (dihydrotestosterone, dehydroepiandrosterone, oestradiol).

Source: Wein AJ, Kavoussi LR, Novick AC et al (editors). Campbell-Walsh urology. 9th edn. Saunders; 2007.

Classification

While low testosterone is found commonly in men worldwide, there is debate about whether or not LOH is in itself a clinical entity related to a physiological adaptation to ageing, pathology or rather the result of accumulating comorbidities in the ageing male.

LOH can be described as both a clinical and biochemical syndrome associated with age and comorbidity, with a characteristic decline of testosterone and relevant symptomatology. The function of multiple organ systems may be impacted upon, with a resulting detrimental effect on quality of life including changes in sexual function.[267] Results from the EMAS support a definition of late-onset hypogonadism (LOH) as the combination of three sexual symptoms (reduced sexual interest, reduced morning erections and erectile dysfunction) with a total testosterone (T) below 11 nmol/L and free testosterone below 220 pmol/L. This combination, rather than low T irrespective of sexual symptoms, was found to confer greater specificity on the presence of the end organ features attributed to LOH; reductions in muscle mass and bone mineral density, and mild anaemia.[376]

Other names that have been used to describe LOH include 'the andropause', 'male menopause', 'androgen deficiency in ageing men', 'partial androgen decline in ageing males', 'male climacteria' and 'viropause'.[335]

Aetiology

The cause of testosterone decline in ageing men is still poorly understood. While a number of risks have been proposed for LOH, other than age,[377] the most consistent evidence for a cause and effect relationship exists for obesity,[370,377], metabolic syndrome[377,378] and poor general health.[378] Vitamin D status[379] and sleep disruption[380] also appear to be contributing factors for some men.

AGE

Advancing age has been identified as a risk factor for the development of testosterone deficiency in a number of longitudinal studies, with decreases in testosterone per year of increased age ranging from 0.05 to 0.110 nmol/L.[377]

OBESITY

An age-independent inverse relationship of body mass index (BMI) with testosterone levels has been demonstrated consistently in a number of longitudinal population or community-based studies.[376] A three-fold increased incidence of LOH (as defined by the EMAS) is associated with a BMI ≥30 kg/m^2, or waist circumference >102 cm.[370]

METABOLIC SYNDROME

Metabolic syndrome has been demonstrated in longitudinal studies to be predictive for the development of hypogonadism.[377] Men with metabolic syndrome at baseline were found to be 2.2 times more likely to develop testosterone deficiency, with the presence of dyslipidaemia and diabetes also conferring increased risk.[378]

GENERAL HEALTH, COMORBIDITIES AND MEDICATIONS

The relationship between androgen deficiency and systemic disease has been extensively documented. Traumatic injury, chronic liver disease, chronic renal failure, rheumatoid arthritis, chronic obstructive pulmonary disease[381] and obstructive sleep apnoea[382] have all been associated with declines in testosterone levels. It is therefore unsurprising that longitudinal population studies exploring the characteristics of LOH have identified that the number of comorbid conditions and prescribed medications (more than 6) at baseline predicted later development of lower testosterone and higher incidence of testosterone deficiency.[378] Similarly, men enrolled in the Massachusetts Male Aging Study (MMAS) who had a higher medication usage, physician diagnosis of comorbidity or self-perceived assessment of health as 'less than excellent', had an increased probability of later symptomatic androgen deficiency.[383]

VITAMIN D STATUS

The EMAS identified an increased incidence of biochemical primary and secondary hypogonadism in men who were vitamin D deficient.[379] This result was supported by a Korean cross-sectional study that associated vitamin D deficiency with biochemical total testosterone deficiency (<7.98 nmol/L) and biochemical free testosterone deficiency (<22.5 pmol/L).[384]

The role of vitamin D in male hypogonadism is currently unclear, although its effects appear to be on multiple levels of the hypothalamic pituitary testicular axis. This is indicated by the presence of vitamin D receptors and vitamin D metabolising enzyme expression in Leydig cells,[385] the anterior pituitary and the hypothalamus.[386]

SLEEP DEPRIVATION

Insomnia as measured by the Insomnia Severity Index (ISI) was found to be a predictor of ageing male symptoms (AMS) in a cross-sectional hospital-based study of ageing men.[387] A cause and effect relationship is supported by studies that restrict sleep in healthy men, indicating a reduction in testosterone levels of 10–15% with restricting sleep to 5 hours per night (sleep between 12.30 am and 5.30 am) compared to 10 hours sleep (10 pm to 8 am) for 8 nights.[380]

Sleep timing may modulate the effect of sleep deprivation on testosterone levels. Total sleep deprivation and 4.5 hours sleep restricted to the first half of the night (sleep between 10.30 pm and 3.30 am) resulted in reduced morning testosterone and prolactin levels when compared to 8 hours regular sleep (sleep between 10.45 pm and 7.00 am). However, when sleep was restricted to 4 hours in the later part of the night (2.45 am to 7.00 am), no effect was seen on testosterone, prolactin or LH levels.[388] This implies that early morning waking or wakefulness in the later part of the night has the biggest impact of sleep deprivation on morning testosterone.

Overview

Testosterone levels decline progressively from 30 years onwards at a rate of 0.4–2%.[389] Conversely, the concentration of SHBG progressively increases with age and thus due to the high binding capacity of SHBG, there is a more pronounced decrease in free and bioavailable testosterone than in total testosterone.[390]

The hormone decline in men differs greatly from what women experience during the menopause, during which female hormones almost always decline rapidly over just a few years, with the rate of testosterone decline varying greatly between men.

Signs and symptoms attributed to declining testosterone levels in men are nonspecific and vary in severity and onset. The combination of severely reduced morning erections and sexual desire has the highest value in predicting low total testosterone and low free testosterone, with severe erectile dysfunction only slightly improving the accuracy of predicting low testosterone.[262]

Pathogenesis

Androgens are produced in the testes and the adrenal glands, and regulate the primary and secondary sex characteristics in men. The age-associated decline in testosterone levels appears to be multifactorial.

PRIMARY HYPOGONADISM

Primary hypogonadism is characterised by low testosterone and elevated follicle-stimulating hormone (FSH) and luteinising hormone (LH).[389] This reflects a primary testicular failure eventuating in reduced production of testosterone by Leydig cells, and reduced inhibin from Sertoli cells. Results from the EMAS suggest that a primary testicular failure cause for LOH is most associated with ageing and obesity (BMI ≥30 kg/m^2), with 0.1% of men aged 40–49 and 5.4% of men at 70–79 demonstrating primary hypogonadism.[389]

There appears to be a relationship with age and reduced Leydig and Sertoli cell numbers in men, as demonstrated in autopsy studies performed in the 1980s.[391,392] More recent ultrasonography studies have supported these earlier findings, with a reduced testicular volume shown to be associated with increasing age.[393,394] A 31% smaller testicular volume in men over 75 years old compared to men 18–45 years old was associated with higher serum LH and FSH, and lower serum bioavailable testosterone and inhibin B.[394]

In addition to reduced androgen production by declining endocrine tissue, reduced Leydig cell responsiveness to LH is another way in which testosterone production may be reduced in the ageing man. This possible mechanism was demonstrated in a study that found elevations in free and bioavailable testosterone concentrations in older men were half that produced in younger men, after overnight suppression of LH with a GnRH antagonist, followed by infusions of biosynthetic LH to provoke a testosterone response.[395]

SECONDARY MALE HYPOGONADISM (HYPOTHALAMIC PITUITARY FAILURE)

Secondary male hypogonadism is characterised by low testosterone and low or normal LH and FSH, reflecting normal testicular function with inadequate stimulation by gonadotrophins.[369]

An increase in frequency and reduction in amplitude of LH pulses has been observed in older men compared to young men. GnRH responsiveness by the pituitary appears to be preserved, suggesting that the smaller pulses of LH are a result of reduced GnRH secretion to the pituitary gland.[395] Reduced production of gonadotrophins may be a consequence of altered testosterone mediated negative feedback regulation, animal studies demonstrating reduced androgen-receptor expression in the brain and pituitary of ageing male rats, plausibly resulting in a reduced efficacy of the testosterone feedback mechanism.[395]

Results from the EMAS demonstrated a much higher prevalence of secondary hypogonadism than primary hypogonadism, finding that 10.9% of men aged 40–59 and 10.4% of men 70–79 demonstrated this hormonal profile.[389] The prevalence of secondary hypogonadism was not associated with ageing, but instead BMI was found to be a strong predictor. Men with a BMI ≥30 kg/m^2 were 8.74 times more likely to have secondary hypogonadism than men with a BMI ≤25 kg/m^2.[389]

How obesity induces hypogonadism is an area of current debate, with downregulation of GnRH release as a consequence of hypothalamic inflammation and glucose-sensitive downregulation of the hypothalamic pituitary neuronal network likely to be implicated.[370] Additionally, increases in oestrogens due to a high expression of P450 aromatase in adipose tissue may result in reduced LH production as a result of negative feedback inhibition by oestrogen on the hypothalamus and pituitary.[396]

Adrenal androgen production

Adrenal secretion of dehydroepiandrosterone (DHEA) and its sulfated form (DHEA-S) contribute to 30% of total androgens in men, being converted to androgens and oestrogens in non-reproductive tissues in the periphery.[397] The secretion of DHEA and DHEA-S has a clear relationship to age, with the highest circulating levels occurring between 20 and 30 years of age, steadily declining to 10–20% of the levels of a young adult by the age of 70–80.[397]

This decline in adrenal androgen production may have bearing on symptoms associated with LOH. Reduced DHEA/DHEA-S levels have been associated with increased erectile dysfunction,[398] increased partial androgen deficiency of the ageing male (PADAM) symptoms (especially sexual symptoms),[399] reduced physical performance[400] and reduced bone mineral density.[401]

Oestrogens

Oestradiol and oestrone also play a vital role in the health and wellbeing of men; however, their roles as determinants of health consequences are at this stage complex and unclear.

In men, around 80% of circulating oestradiol (E2) is a result of peripheral conversion of testosterone via aromatase, with the remaining 20% being produced predominantly by Leydig cells.[37] Androstenedione produced by the adrenal gland is also a source of oestrone (E1), a small amount of which also gets converted to E2.[37] Of the oestrogens, E2 is the most biologically active, having the highest affinity for oestrogen receptors.[37]

It is unclear how oestrogen levels in men vary with age, with some studies suggesting a decline, and others an increase or no change.[37] More recently, the Concord Health and Aging in Men Project Study (CHAMPS) found that while E1 declined with ageing significantly, E2 was found to increase.[402] The MMAS demonstrated a 3.6% yearly decline in E1 over a 7–10 year period.[403]

It has been well demonstrated that oestrogens play an important part in bone health in men. In vivo both testosterone and oestrogen inhibit osteoclast activity and proliferation and stimulate osteoclast apoptosis, thus reducing bone resorption. A deficiency in oestrogen leads to increased osteoblast apoptosis, reducing bone formation. In vivo, oestrogen in men is responsible for more than two-thirds of the antiresorptive effects of sex hormones on bone.[404] Longitudinal studies have demonstrated that E2 levels below 74 pmol/L increase the risk of low bone density. Men who had low baseline total serum oestradiol levels were 3 times more likely to have a hip fracture in the following 18 years compared to men who were in the high E2 group (≥126 pmol/L). When this was combined with low testosterone, the risk increased to 6.5 times, compared to men who had both hormones in the middle to high ranges.[405] More recently, low E1, but not low E2, was found to be predictive of increased bone loss in men.[402]

Progressive decline of serum E2, but not E1, was associated with a greater risk of all-cause, cancer-specific and cardiovascular-specific mortality.[402] Low baseline E1 was however found to predict the development of self-rated poor health in older men (OR 1.84).[406]

There may however be risks associated with elevated oestrogens in men. The upper limit for E2 has been suggested to be 160 pmol/L. Higher levels of E2 may be related to obesity due to a high level of aromatase expression in subcutaneous and gluteal fat, resulting in bioconversion of testosterone to E2. Genetic differences in aromatase activity can also account for E2 difference in men.[37]

The Framingham Heart Study found that higher E1 levels was predictive of an increased risk of diabetes development in older men,[407] while a lower E2/T ratio was found to be protective against metabolic syndrome in the EMAS.[408]

Elevated oestrogens have been suggested to be responsible for T deficiency in some men, with oestrogen signalling having an inhibitory effect on the hypothalamus, decreasing GnRH pulse frequency and gonadotrophin secretion from the pituitary gland.[37]

Signs and symptoms

Signs and symptoms attributed to LOH are often subtle and nonspecific, the majority of which have an unclear

> **BOX 19.9 Signs and symptoms associated with late-onset hypogonadism**
>
> - *Sexual:* Decreased libido; erectile dysfunction; decreased frequency of morning erections; decreased sexual performance; decreased testicular size; delayed ejaculation
> - *Somatic:* Increased visceral body fat/obesity; decreased lean muscle mass; decreased strength; fatigue/loss of energy; decreased physical activity/vitality; low bone mineral density; anaemia; hot flushes; loss of facial, axillary and pubic hair/slow beard growth; decline in general feeling of wellbeing
> - *Psychological:* Depression/depressed mood; mood changes; irritability; inability to concentrate; insomnia/sleep disturbances
>
> Sources: Buvat J, Maggi M, Guay A et al. Testosterone deficiency in men: systematic review and standard operating procedures for diagnosis and treatment. J Sex Med 2013 Jan;10(1):245–84; Morales A, Bebb RA, Manjoo P et al. Diagnosis and management of testosterone deficiency syndrome in men: clinical practice guideline. Can Med Assoc J 2015 Dec 8;187(18):1369–77.

relationship to reduced testosterone levels. Additionally, the presentation is complicated by the influence of ageing, comorbid illness, medications and environmental factors.[309]

The symptoms found to have a true syndromic relationship to declines in testosterone levels are the three sexual symptoms of reduced sexual interest, reduced morning erections and erectile dysfunction.[374] It has been suggested that the presence of these three symptoms in combination with identified low total (<11 nmol/L) and free testosterone (<220 pmol/L) is necessary for a diagnosis of androgen deficiency.[374] A recent study however found that a dual combination of either of the three sexual symptoms (especially severely reduced sexual desire and morning erections) was able to accurately detect low androgen levels in men presenting with sexual dysfunction.[261] An inability to perform vigorous activity, depression and fatigue have also been found to have independent associations with reduced testosterone levels.[389]

Other symptoms and signs attributed to late-onset hypogonadism are summarised in Box 19.9.

Systemic consequences

Of particular concern to the clinician are the systemic consequences on target organs of low levels of testosterone. A growing body of evidence supports the role of LOH in increasing the risk of metabolic syndrome, cardiovascular disease, osteoporosis and all-cause mortality.

Metabolic syndrome

Several longitudinal studies have demonstrated a potential causal link between testosterone deficiency and the risk of developing metabolic syndrome (MetS). The EMAS demonstrated that men who had a lower baseline testosterone level had a 40–70% increased risk of developing MetS at follow-up compared to eugonadal men.[408] These results support earlier findings from the Baltimore Longitudinal Study of Aging,[409] the Kuopio Ischemic Heart Disease Risk Factor Study[410] and the MMAS,[411] that also demonstrated this association. These studies also found that lower sex hormone binding globulin (SHBG) is predictive of metabolic syndrome development.[409–411]

Osteoporosis

Low bone mineral density is a physical sign associated with androgen decline. The role of testosterone in bone health is thought to be mostly due to its role as a precursor to E2; however there is evidence that an independent association between testosterone levels and markers of bone health also exists.

Total testosterone and E2 deficiency increased the incidence of osteoporosis and the risk of rapid hip bone loss, testosterone deficient men having twice the incidence of osteoporosis compared to men with normal testosterone (12.3% vs 6.0%).[412] Declines in E2 and testosterone, with a concomitant increase in SHBG, were associated with an increase in risk of incident fractures,[413] and low free testosterone at baseline predicted bone loss at the femoral neck within 3 years, but not at 7 or 10 years.[414]

Cardiovascular disease

In addition to its role as associated with metabolic syndrome, an increased risk of cardiovascular disease (CVD) has been associated with hypogonadism in a number of observational studies. A meta-analysis performed by Corona et al identified low testerosterone and elevated E2 as associated with overall cardiovascular disease and coronary heart disease risk in men.[415] Longitudinal studies found that low testosterone was predictive of overall and cardiovascular mortality.[415] Risk of abdominal aortic atherosclerosis, degree of angiographic coronary disease and carotid intimal thickness, atherosclerotic plaques and endothelial dysfunction have all been found to be increased with lower levels of testosterone in men.[416]

All-cause mortality

A significant association between low testosterone and an increased risk of all-cause mortality has been demonstrated in most studies identified in a systematic review by Zaratosky et al. Over a 4–16 year period, increased risk of all-cause mortality in men with low testosterone generally ranged from 24% to 124%.[377] A recent longitudinal study also found that progressive declines in testosterone, dihydrotestosterone (DHT), calculated free testosterone (cFT) as well as E2 were predictive of increased all-cause mortality.[402]

Mortality has been seen to be increased in CVD, respiratory disease and cancer in association with low testosterone.[377]

Differential diagnosis

Given the nonspecific symptoms attributed to LOH, and the contribution of comorbidities to testosterone deficiency, the differential diagnosis can be quite complicated.

Pathologies that can impact upon testosterone and the HPA axis must be considered, as should chronic conditions that can give rise to the syndrome. These include but are not limited to:

- Chronic liver disease
- Chronic kidney failure
- Hypothyroidism
- Haemochromatosis
- Anaemia (iron deficiency, B_{12} deficiency)
- Pituitary tumour
- Cushing's syndrome
- Obstructive sleep apnoea
- Cardiovascular disease
- Metabolic syndrome.

Naturopathic diagnosis

In the naturopathic diagnosis, clinical assessment, thorough history taking and the use of screening questionnaires are useful to help arrive at a proper diagnosis. History taking should include specific questions about sexual function, especially regarding the presence and severity of erectile dysfunction, low libido and absence of morning erections. The most used and easily available screening questionnaires are the Androgen Deficiency in the Aging Male (ADAM), the Aging Male Study (AMS) and the Massachusetts Male Aging Study (MMAS) questionnaires. These can be useful to guide history taking; however, as they demonstrate high sensitivity but low specificity in detecting low testosterone, they cannot be relied upon solely for the diagnosis of androgen deficiency.[309] For men presenting with sexual dysfunction, ANDROTEST may have greater clinical utility in detecting low total testosterone (Box 19.10). The naturopath interprets a patient's presentation holistically, and may formulate a provisional diagnosis prior to allopathic confirmation, which waits for significant decline. A review of all investigations, both general and functional, provides supportive evidence to formulate a conclusion and begin treatment.

BOX 19.10 ANDROTEST structured interview

ANDROTEST© is a structured interview for the screening of hypogonadism (total testosterone <10.4 nmol/L or 300 ng/dL in patients with sexual dysfunction). The test is applicable only to patients reporting at least one incidence of sexual intercourse during the past 3 months.

The interview is composed of 12 key items. The interviewer should ask the questions written in bold, using the exact words proposed. The further questions written in normal characters can be used to clarify the patient's answers if needed. The patient should be permitted to answer freely, using his own words.

The patient's answers are codified on a 0–3 scale by the interviewer, following detailed instructions reported after each item. For some of the items, the answers have a yes/no format.

The order in which the questions are presented should be observed, as alterations in this sequence could theoretically modify the patient's answers.

Interpretation

A total score of more than 8 has a sensitivity of 76% and specificity of 66% in identifying low total testosterone (<10.4 nmol/L)

1. **How old are you?**
   After asking the patient how old he is, rank a progressive score as a function of patient's age at the time of the visit.
   0 <40 years
   1 40–49 years
   2 50–59 years
   3 >59 years
2. **When did you undergo your sexual development (puberty)?**
   At what age did you undergo your sexual development? Did you experience puberty at the same time as your schoolmates? Did you notice that pubic hairs and the development of genitalia happened to you as well as to your schoolmates?
   Rank 0 if patient reports sexual development at the same time or before that of his schoolmates; 3 if patient reports delayed puberty.
   0 9–14 years (normal)
   3 >14 years (delayed)
3. **Have you ever had a pituitary disease?**
   Have you ever undergone surgery for pituitary disease? Have you ever been treated with medical therapy for pituitary disease?
   The score will be 0 if patient does not report a pituitary disease, and 3 for an affirmative response.
   0 No
   3 Yes
4. **Have you ever had a diagnosis of undescended testes (cryptorchidism)?**
   Have you ever undergone surgery for cryptorchidism? Have you ever been treated with medical therapy for cryptorchidism?
   The score will be 0 if patient does not report a history of cryptorchidism (even monolateral), and 3 for an affirmative response.
   0 No
   3 Yes
5. **Describe what happens during sexual intercourse: how often do you have lack of an erection?**
   The description of the problem refers to the last 3 months. Sometimes = <25%, quite often = 25–49%, often = 50–74%, and always = >75% of cases.
   0 Sometimes
   1 Quite often
   2 Often
   3 Always

BOX 19.10 ANDROTEST structured interview—cont'd

6. **Do you ever wake up with an erection?**
   How often has it happened in the last 3 months?
   Rank 0 if patient reports spontaneous nocturnal/morning erection with the same frequency previously observed: 1 if nocturnal/morning erections are present, but their frequency during the last 3 months is somewhat lower than that observed previously; 2 if the frequency of nocturnal/morning erections of the last 3 months is reduced by at least 50%; 3 if nocturnal/morning erections are not present.
   - 0 Yes, regularly
   - 1 Less frequently than in the past
   - 2 Only occasionally
   - 3 Never
7. **How often have you practised autoerotism (masturbation) in the last 3 months?**
   0 >8 times/month
   1 3–7 times/month
   2 1–2 times/month
   3 Never
   If the patient does not practise autoerotism (answer 3), the following question (#8) is not applicable. In this case rank 1 to question 8 and continue to question #9.
8. **How do you feel during autoerotism?**
   After asking the question above, rank with the following score:
   0 Well
   1 With a little sense of guilt
   2 With a big sense of guilt
   3 With a very big sense of guilt
9. **Have you had more or less desire to make love in the last 3 months?**
   Has your desire increased or reduced in comparison to the past?
   Rank 0 when the patient's desire is unmodified or increased; 1 if desire is reduced.
   0 Unmodified or increased desire
   1 Reduced desire
10. **Have you noticed a reduction in the quantity of ejaculate?**
    Rank 0 if the patient does not notice any modification of the volume of ejaculate; 1 if the patient has the feeling that the volume of ejaculate could be slightly reduced; 2 if the volume of ejaculate is markedly reduced; 3 if no ejaculation occurs.
    0 No modification
    1 Slightly reduced
    2 Markedly reduced
    3 Ejaculation absent
11. **In the last 3 months has it been difficult to ejaculate (or to achieve climax) during sexual intercourse?**
    Are you able to ejaculate during sexual intercourse with penetration or only with manual or oral stimulation by your partner?
    Rank 0 if patient does not report difficulties in ejaculating or, as in some rare cases, if ejaculation and climax could be obtained but only with autoerotism conducted in the absence of the partner or if it could not be obtained at all;1 if ejaculation and climax are still possible, but only with great effort and after prolonged intercourse, or if they are possible only with autoerotism, although in the presence of the partner, but not during coitus.
    0 No
    1 Yes
12. **How much do you weigh and how tall are you?**
    After asking the patient his weight and height the interviewer should rank a progressive score as a function of the calculation (body mass index = weight [kg]/height [m²]).
    0 <25 kg/m²
    1 25–29.9 kg/m²
    2 30–34.9 kg/m²
    3 >34.9 kg/m²

Source: Corona G, Mannucci E, Petrone L et al. A structured interview for the screening of hypogonadism in patients with sexual dysfunction. J Sex Med 2006;3(4):706–15.

Investigations

The diagnosis of androgen deficiency should be based on a combination of clinical findings that include a thorough patient history, physical examination and laboratory testing. Diagnosing androgen deficiency is complicated, as testosterone declines over several years and does not give rise to well-defined signs and symptoms. As previously mentioned, the clinical features of androgen deficiency are similar to those that occur in some diseases of ageing, and thus it can be misdiagnosed by clinicians or go unrecognised by patients. Therefore, androgen deficiency is diagnosed by exclusion, and it is recommended that pathological causes of androgen deficiency in the ageing male should be explored before assuming it is age-related.[417]

Like the history, lack of specificity limits the diagnostic accuracy of the physical examination in identifying androgen deficiency; however, collectively with a comprehensive history the examination can help make a strong provisional diagnosis. The physical examination is usually focused on secondary characteristics. Findings such as a decrease in facial, pubic and axillary hair and small testicular size are suggestive of hypogonadism.[309] Prostate examination is performed, especially if testosterone replacement therapy is to be considered.[418] Height, weight, BMI and abdominal circumference are relevant, as obesity is a significant contributor to androgen deficiency.[419] Gynaecomastia may be present due to increased oestrogen levels.[420]

TABLE 19.7 Biochemical definition of hypogonadism proposed by various international societies

Societies	Total testosterone concentration (nmol/L)
EAA, ISA, ISSAM	Mild <12
EAU, ASA, ISSM	Severe <8
ES	<10.4
AACE	<7

AACE, American Association of Clinical Endocrinologists; ASA, American Society of Andrology; EAA, European Academy of Andrology; EAU, European Association of Urology; ES, Endocrine Society; ISA, International Society of Andrology; ISSAM, International Society for the Study of the Aging Male; ISSM, International Society of Sexual Medicine

LABORATORY TESTS

Testosterone

A diagnosis of late-onset hypogonadism requires measurement of serum testosterone; however, the biochemical threshold at which symptoms of androgen deficiency and adverse outcomes occur is at this stage still unclear, resulting in the different suggested biochemical definitions of hypogonadism proposed by the relevant international societies (see Table 19.7).

Serum total testosterone, obtained with more than one morning sampling, is the screening test recommended for hypogonadism by the Endocrine Society.[303] Serum total testosterone is a measure of both bioavailable testosterone (free and loosely bound to albumin) and testosterone that is relatively unavailable to tissues being tightly bound to SHBG.[421] Because of this, a measure of total serum testosterone may not be a true indicator of tissue exposure to testosterone, as changes to SHBG levels (either increased or decreased levels) will alter testosterone bioavailability.[309] Conditions that are known to increase SHBG and therefore reduce testosterone bioavailability include ageing, liver disease, hyperthyroidism and some medications such as anticonvulsants.[303] Reductions in SHBG occur in obesity, hypothyroidism and acromegaly.[303]

For this reason, direct testing of free testosterone (FT) by equilibrium dialysis or centrifugal ultrafiltration is theoretically the best measure of tissue exposure to testosterone in men.[303] However, limited availability and cost limitations at this stage make it impractical for use in most clinical situations.[309]

An alternative to direct testing of FT is calculated free testosterone (cFT), an estimate of FT (using the Vermuelen equation) based on measures of total serum testosterone, SHBG and albumin.[303] While not a direct measure of FT, it is considered a suitable alternative due to its wide availability and low cost, and its validation by comparison to equilibrium dialysis methods.[303]

A free androgen index (FAI), calculated as a simple ratio of total testosterone/SHBG, while useful in estimating FT in women and children (where concentrations of SHBG are much higher), correlates poorly to FT in men and is therefore not recommended.[309]

Other hormones

If testosterone levels are low, additional pathology tests are usually performed to identify whether the hypogonadism is primary or secondary, or a combination of both, and to identify other pathologies that may account for abnormal levels. An elevation in FSH and LH suggests a primary hypogonadism (testicular), whereas normal to low FSH and LH suggest a secondary cause (pituitary hypothalamic).[389] In LOH the presentation is often a mixture of primary and secondary causes, resulting in variable gonadotrophin levels depending on the predominant cause.[418] Measurement of prolactin is essential, the presence of hyperprolactinaemia prompting further investigation.[309,418] In this case, diagnostic imaging (e.g. magnetic resonance imaging, computed tomography) is recommended to rule out a pituitary adenoma.

Other investigations relate to the systemic illness and comorbidities that can contribute to androgen deficiency. Considering the contribution of metabolic syndrome, glucose studies (HbA1c, fasting blood glucose, glucose tolerance) and blood lipids (total cholesterol, LDL cholesterol, HDL cholesterol, triglycerides) should be performed as part of a thorough work-up. Assessment of serum circulating 25(OH)D would also be appropriate for those at risk of vitamin D deficiency.

Thorough screening investigations should also include LFT, kidney function and thyroid function to detect any chronic disease (liver disease, chronic kidney disease, hypothyroidism) that could account for the hypogonadism or explain the symptoms. Assessment of 24-hour urinary cortisol may be indicated if Cushing's syndrome is suspected.

Iron studies (serum iron, ferritin, iron, transferrin saturation) in combination with a full blood count should be performed to screen for haemochromatosis and anaemia.

An assessment of bone mineral density (BMD) would also be appropriate, given the role of LOH in the development of osteoporosis.[412]

Assessment of DHEA-S and oestradiol may also be considered given their possible role in hypogonadism symptoms.

SPECIFIC NATUROPATHIC INVESTIGATIONS

Diagnostic tools available to naturopaths include the patient's clinical history, appropriate physical examination (within the realms of appropriate practice) and a symptom review incorporating at least one of the available screening questionnaires assessing androgen deficiency (ADAM, ANDROTEST).

Salivary hormone analysis

While the current recommended investigation for the diagnosis of testosterone deficiency is total serum testosterone,[303] assessment of salivary steroid hormones is popularly used by naturopathic clinicians and may offer a potential tool for screening, assessing overall steroid hormone balance and monitoring treatment efficacy. Commonly assessed hormones in men relevant to LOH are testosterone, oestradiol (E2), oestrone (E1) and DHEA. Dihydrotestosterone (DHT), androstenedione, cortisol and melatonin may also be of interest.

Advantages of salivary hormone analysis are the ease of use and the non-invasive nature of collection. It is also understood that saliva levels better measure tissue exposure to hormones as they reflect unbound, active concentrations.[422]

While salivary hormone measurements are used extensively in research, with the exception of salivary cortisol, the clinical application of most salivary hormone analysis is at this stage questioned due to limited research correlating salivary hormone levels to serum.[423] A limited number of studies in men have demonstrated a high correlation of salivary testosterone with total testosterone and calculated free testosterone;[424,425] however, a more recent study demonstrated poor correlation.[426] Fiers et al found that that while salivary testosterone correlated fairly well to serum free testosterone in men, variability did occur, potentially due to the effect of salivary protein binding of hormones.[427]

Similarly, the value of measuring other salivary hormones of interest (E2, DHEA and melatonin) is limited by scarce research correlating serum measures with salivary measures, although the research conducted thus far does suggest that salivary measures of these hormones do correlate well to serum levels in some but not all populations studied.[423,428–430]

Other issues that challenge clinical utility of salivary hormone analysis are the effects of different salivary collection methods, blood contamination of samples and bacterial contamination on salivary hormone concentrations.[431–433] A recent study also demonstrated high levels of inter-laboratory variation of results from testing the same saliva samples for melatonin, cortisol and testosterone.[422]

With this in mind, it is suggested that the naturopathic clinician, if using salivary investigations in assessment, interprets results cautiously and not at the expense of a thorough clinical history. It is also suggested that diagnosis of LOH follow the current criteria as determined by the combination of characteristic symptoms and a measure of serum testosterone levels.

Therapeutic considerations

CLINICAL DECISION MAKING AND RATIONALE

Following a thorough assessment, it is imperative to assess the patient and any compounding factors holistically. Important considerations include:

- Hormone status
- Cardiovascular function
- Renal and liver function
- Risk factors for metabolic syndrome
- Quality of life (ADAM questionnaire)
- Sexual function (ANDROTEST)
- Height, weight, BMI, hip/waist ratio and percentage body fat
- Sleep quality, duration and timing
- Diet and lifestyle
- Mood
- General health.

When sufficient information has been obtained, clinical decisions should be made considering all the aetiological and pathogenic factors that may contribute to the presentation. All aspects should be appropriately addressed for optimal holistic management of the patient.

Therapeutic application

HISTORICAL PERSPECTIVE

As the diagnosis of late-onset hypogonadism is a relatively modern concept, we would not expect to find much documentation regarding its treatment by the Eclectic physicians. That said, as ever ahead of their time, they appear to have had some inkling about the condition, documenting the use of *Delphinium staphisagria* for impotence.[2]

The 'impotence' they mention appears to be androgen deficiency, of which ED was merely a symptom. The Eclectics administered concurrent treatment with nervine herbs such as *Avena sativa*, which is likely to have a rebuilding and restorative effect, and male tonics such as *Serenoa repens*, which also functions to protect the health of the prostate. This is very much in line with modern botanical treatment today.

ALLOPATHIC TREATMENT

Testosterone replacement therapy (TRT) may take the form of bioidentical hormone replacement therapy or standard pharmaceutical preparations. Testosterone preparations are available in many forms including oral tablets, intramuscular injections, subcutaneous implants, transdermal patches, skin gels or topical solutions and troches.[317] Bioidentical prescriptions are formulated by a pharmacist who bases the prescription upon a patient's blood (and saliva) levels of hormones, and calculates the amounts of hormones to be included in the prescription.

Benefits and risks are associated with TRT, although the availability of high-quality data is limited, and intense debate is evident with contradictory findings in the literature. Currently no consensus exists for the benefits of TRT on osteoporosis, sexual function, type 2 diabetes mellitus, metabolic syndrome and obesity.[317] Benefits are suggested in men with type 2 diabetes with better survival, improved sexual function, improved glycaemic control, cholesterol concentration and body composition; and improved quality of life.[314–316]

The potential risks of TRT include gynaecomastia, acne or oily skin, erythrocytosis, sleep apnoea, aggravation of subclinical prostate cancer, growth of breast cancer and male pattern balding.[317] Impairments of male fertility often occur with TRT, via suppression of intratesticular testosterone production and thus spermatogenesis, sometimes to the extent of azoospermia.[434] Cardiovascular risks associated with TRT are at this stage unclear. Some reports suggest a cardiovascular risk, especially to those with preexisting cardiovascular disease,[435,436] with others suggesting no cardiovascular risk[437] or even a cardiovascular benefit.[438] The balance between risks and benefits must be evaluated for each individual patient.

Absolute contraindications to TRT are prostate and/or breast cancer, severe lower urinary tract symptoms associated with an enlarged prostate, unevaluated prostatic nodule or induration, a PSA >4 ng/mL, poorly controlled congestive heart failure, and a haematocrit greater than 50%.[317] Thus, before starting TRT, the haematocrit level (especially in patients with chronic respiratory disease) and a thorough assessment of prostate health (including assessment of PSA) should be performed.

NATUROPATHIC PERSPECTIVE

TRT (both allopathic and naturopathic) may result in an improvement in the quality of life for the ageing male. However, it takes time and experience to treat men with hypogonadal symptoms, and hormone therapy needs to be individualised to each patient.[439] Therefore, treatment is focused on addressing underlying comorbidities to testosterone deficiency, and hormone modulation and stabilisation. Concurrent treatment should also aim to achieve the following:

- Restore sexual function, libido and wellbeing
- Increase bone mineral density
- Increase energy levels
- Improve muscle mass, strength and stamina
- Decrease total body fat, especially central adiposity
- Modify cardiovascular risk factors
- Support optimal glycaemic control
- Support optimal sleep hygiene
- Support an optimal stress response.

Among the other factors that need to be holistically assessed and addressed is the patient's emotional history, which may have led to adrenal exhaustion and affected steroid hormone synthesis or other steroid hormone pathways, such as cholesterol metabolism, cortisol production (excessive) or circadian rhythm (dysregulation).

NUTRITIONAL MEDICINE (DIETARY)

Therapeutic objectives

1. Encourage general wholefood diet with a focus on antioxidant-rich fruits and vegetables
2. Ensure appropriate protein intake to avoid muscle wasting
3. Support optimal glycaemic control
4. Prevent associated comorbidities such as metabolic syndrome, cardiovascular disease and osteoporosis
5. Avoid potentially aggravating substances such alcohol.

Dietary inclusions

The diet should be predominantly based on whole, fresh foods, with ample variety, vegetables and adequate fresh fruit. A diet based on these principles will ensure maximum nutrition and thus optimal health benefits. Good-quality protein should be included with each meal for growth and healing, as well as to ensure stable blood sugar, as the prevalence of diabetes increases with age, and is associated with declines in testosterone. Essential fatty acids such as those found in fish, seeds and nuts should also be included. Optimal intake of calcium is required to ensure bone health, as bone loss may increase in the presence of androgen deficiency.

PROTEIN

Androgen deficiency is characterised by loss of muscle strength and a reduction in physical function.[309] Protein is required for structural, transport, storage, immune and hormonal roles. As the body is constantly using protein, adequate intake is necessary to ensure that the body has a steady supply for all body functions, including muscle mass and growth and development. It is essential that protein requirements are calculated based on the patient's weight and energy expenditure.

Dietary exclusions

ALCOHOL

In the presence of androgen deficiency, limited available human evidence suggests that alcohol consumption is best avoided. It is clear that alcoholism and its impacts on liver disease are associated with disruption of testosterone synthesis.[440] Earlier reports indicate that intoxication with alcohol (1.5 g alcohol per kilogram of body weight) reduces plasma testosterone by as much as 25% approximately 10–16 hours after consumption.[441] A small study found that moderate alcohol consumption (40 g/day) for 3 weeks resulted in plasma testosterone reductions by 6.8%; however, this was also accompanied by elevations of DHEA-S by 16.5%.[442]

NUTRITIONAL MEDICINE (SUPPLEMENTAL)

Therapeutic objectives

1. Support optimal hormonal status, using supplements demonstrated to improve testosterone levels
2. Prevent and treat associated comorbidities such as metabolic syndrome, diabetes, cardiovascular disease, osteoporosis and muscle wasting
3. Treat sexual dysfunction, specifically erectile dysfunction (refer to the relevant section in this chapter).

Specific nutrients required

Very little research has been conducted on the role of nutritional supplementation in augmenting sex hormones in men with late-onset hypogonadism. Those that have some rationale for specific treatment of LOH, especially for altering the decline in testosterone, are discussed below. Given the strong relationship between comorbidities and declines in testosterone, especially the role of metabolic syndrome, and the associated consequences of cardiovascular disease, low bone density and sexual dysfunction, the naturopathic clinician would be well

SAMPLE DAILY DIET

BREAKFAST	
Poached eggs with rocket and avocado and stone-ground toast	Eggs provide an optimal source of both protein and fats. Fats are essential for the production of testosterone while the protein reduces the risk of sarcopenia/decreased muscle strength and mass associated with ageing and andropause. Gastric acid is reported to decline with ageing, thus the addition of bitter greens such as rocket functions to stimulate digestive secretions so that absorption of nutrients is adequate.
LUNCH	
Roast chicken with Greek salad (cucumbers, onion, olives, tomato, oregano and fetta) and vitamin D enriched mushrooms	Chicken provides a source of zinc which is essential for the manufacture of testosterone, as is vitamin D. Insulin resistance is implicated in the pathogenesis of andropause, thus this meal provides a balance of protein and carbohydrates to ensure adequate blood sugar regulation.
DINNER	
Grilled salmon with lemon, sweet potato and cruciferous vegetables	Andropause is closely tied in with cardiovascular disease, thus nutritional recommendations should address this. The Mediterranean style of diet may be useful for its cardioprotective effects as well as its anti-inflammatory and weight loss benefits.
SNACK	
Brazil nuts and a fresh vegetable and fruit juice	Brazil nuts are a rich source of selenium which is required for testosterone production. Decline in testosterone levels can result in loss of energy and mood, thus the inclusion of nutrient-dense food sources such as a juice is suggested to provide adequate carbohydrates for energy.

advised to develop therapeutic strategies that incorporate management of these factors. This is likely to have an influence not only on improving health outcomes, but hormonal status also. Suggested supplements for underlying comorbidities are summarised here, although the reader is advised to refer to relevant chapters in this text for comprehensive coverage. The reader is also directed to the section of this chapter for treatments specific to erectile dysfunction.

VITAMIN D

Given the association of vitamin D status with testosterone levels, and its contribution to comorbidities associated with hypogonadism such as cardiovascular disease,[443] low bone mineral density and sarcopenia,[444] correcting vitamin D deficiency and subclinical deficiency is an important consideration in LOH management. In vitamin D deficient, overweight, non-diabetic men, 12-month daily supplementation of vitamin D (3332 IU) resulted in an increase in total testosterone (10.7 nmol/L to 13.4 nmol/L), bioactive testosterone (5.21 nmol/L to 6.25 nmol/L) and free testosterone (5.21 nmol/L to 6.25 nmol/L).[445]

ZINC

Zinc is a biologically essential trace element involved in over 300 enzyme functions within the body.[446] A number of these functions, such as testosterone synthesis, relate directly to the male reproductive system, and would seemingly be compromised in men with complaints related to low androgen levels. Interestingly, many of the symptoms attributed to LOH are synonymous with zinc deficiency, yet in spite of this there have been limited clinical studies investigating the action of zinc in androgen-deficient men. A study exploring the effect of zinc supplementation in men on haemodialysis with end-stage renal disease demonstrated significant increases in testosterone (from 1.55 nm/dL to 2.94 nm/dL) and LH (from 4.85 mg/dL to 15.77 mg/dL), with no significant changes in prolactin or FSH as a result of daily supplementation of 250 mg zinc sulfate for 6 weeks.[447]

Zinc supplementation may also help treat underlying comorbidities associated with LOH. Zinc supplementation has been shown to modify blood sugar regulation by improving insulin receptor function, insulin signalling and structural integrity of insulin.[448] In patients identified as prediabetic, supplementation has been observed to improve fasting blood glucose, triglyceride levels, HDL and LDL cholesterol, and C-reactive protein.[449]

MAGNESIUM

Few investigations have been performed in relation to the role of magnesium in LOH; however, cross-sectional studies in older men demonstrating a positive correlation between serum magnesium levels and testosterone levels[450,451] and measures of muscle performance[451] suggest a possible clinical application in this group.

A small study exploring the effect of 4 weeks supplementation of magnesium (magnesium sulfate 10 mg/kg body weight) in healthy young males (18–22 years) found that magnesium supplementation increased free and total testosterone levels at rest and following exhaustive exercise in both sedentary and exercising men. The effect was more pronounced when combined with regular exercise.[452] While this study was in young men, it is plausible that supplementing in an older age group may have similar favourable impacts on androgen levels, especially when combined with an exercise program.

Magnesium supplementation may also have a role in addressing underlying comorbidities in LOH. Benefits in insulin sensitivity, triglycerides, and diastolic and systolic blood pressure have been demonstrated by supplementing hypertensive type 2 diabetic patients with 300 mg magnesium daily.[453]

L-CARNITINE

There is a small amount of evidence that suggests carnitine status and supplementation have a role in LOH. In men with end-stage renal disease on haemodialysis, total carnitine and free carnitine were found to have a positive correlation with the Aging Male Symptoms and the Self Rating Depression scale,[454] and low serum carnitine was found to predict low free testosterone.[455]

Supplementation of carnitine has been demonstrated to improve measures of sexual function in men with LOH associated with renal disease. Treatment with 2 g propionyl-L-carnitine and 2 g acetyl-L-carnitine, compared to testosterone replacement therapy or placebo for 6 months demonstrated significant improvements in erectile function (as measured by vascular studies, nocturnal penile tumescence and IIEF-15), other aspects of sexual function (libido, general sexual wellbeing, sexual intercourse satisfaction and orgasm) and mood and fatigue levels.[456] No noted impact on total or free testosterone levels occurred, however. Effects on nocturnal penile tumescence and International Index of Erectile Function (IIEF-15) scores were greater for carnitine supplementation than for testosterone replacement therapy.[457] (See also Table 19.8.)

Dosage requirements

The doses listed below are based on adult doses reported in the literature:

- Zinc: 20–60 mg/day.
- Vitamin D: the Endocrine Society recommends supplementing 6000 IU daily in adults who are vitamin D deficient for 8 weeks to achieve a 25(OH)D blood level of above 75 nmol/L. 1500–2000 IU daily is then suggested to maintain blood levels[123]
- Magnesium:100 mg–500 mg/day
- Carnitine: 4 g daily as 2 g propionyl-L-carnitine and 2 g acetyl-L-carnitine
- Chromium: 200 micrograms to 600 micrograms daily
- Selenium: 50 micrograms to 200 micrograms daily. Care should be taken not to exceed this dose, as cardiovascular benefits of selenium have demonstrated a narrow therapeutic range[122]
- Co-enzyme Q10: 100–300 mg daily
- Essential fatty acids (fish oil): 1100 mg to 5600 mg EPA/DHA daily
- Calcium: Up to 1500 mg/daily in combination with vitamin D. An emphasis on dietary sources is suggested due to concerns about the cardiovascular risk of high-dose supplementation[456]
- Protein: initially this should be modified through the diet; however, if supplementation is required the dose should be calculated according to the patient's weight and energy expenditure (in general, prescription is 0.8–1.2 g protein per kilogram of body weight).

HERBAL MEDICINE

Therapeutic objectives

1. Address hormone modulation and regulation of testosterone production and release
2. Address underlying comorbidities such as metabolic syndrome and cardiovascular disease
3. Improve energy and wellbeing, with an emphasis on using male tonics and general tonics
4. Improve sexual function with an emphasis on libido and erectile function.

Herbal medicine classes

MALE TONICS

Male tonics are used to provide hormonal support and increase vitality and energy in the male patient. They have been used for centuries to support ageing men. Examples include *Panax ginseng* (Korean ginseng), *Smilax ornata* (sarsaparilla), *Turnera diffusa* (damiana), *Tribulus terrestris* (tribulus), *Serenoa repens* (saw palmetto), *Eurycoma longifolia* (tongkat ali), *Withania somnifera* (ashwagandha) and *Mucuna pruriens* (velvet bean). *Avena sativa* (oats) has a traditional use as a tonic appropriate for ageing men, and should also be considered here.

TABLE 19.8 Nutritional supplementation for associated comorbidities in late-onset hypogonadism

Nutrient	Supportive evidence
Chromium	Numerous human studies demonstrate beneficial effects of chromium supplementation, particularly in the form of chromium picolinate, on glycaemic control and blood lipids in patients with type 2 diabetes. Negative effects on insulin sensitivity have however been seen in non-obese, non-diabetic patients, suggesting that chromium supplementation is best avoided in this group.
Selenium	Selenium supplementation has been demonstrated to have beneficial effects on cardiovascular disease risk and blood glucose control.
Coenzyme Q10	CoQ10 demonstrates improvements in cardiovascular function, improving vascular endothelial function, blood pressure, blood lipids, antioxidant status and blood glucose control.
Essential fatty acids (EPA/DHA)	EPA and DHA supplementation may improve insulin resistance, blood lipids and hypertension. Protection against vascular disease and vascular death has been reported.
Calcium	In combination with vitamin D supplementation, calcium has been shown to modestly reduce hip and total fracture risk.

Sources: [122, 343–346, 489–491, 493–499, 501, 506]

APHRODISIACS

Reduced sexual interest is a defining symptom of LOH, therefore the inclusion of herbal medicines with a reputation for improving libido is of importance when indicated. Those to consider include *Eurycoma longifolia* (tongkat ali), *Panax ginseng* (Korean ginseng), *Turnera diffusa* (damiana), *Crocus sativus* (saffron), *Tribulus terrestris* (tribulus), *Withania somnifera* (ashwagandha), *Mucuna pruriens* (velvet bean), *Lepidium meyenii* (maca) and *Ptychopetalum olacoides* (muira puama). All have a traditional reputation in improving erectile function, with *Eurycoma longifolia*,[361] *Panax ginseng*,[354] *Crocus sativus*[131] and *Tribulus terrestris*[358] also having some modern evidence to support this use.

ANTIOXIDANTS

Because of the potential impact of free radicals on the ageing process, antioxidant herbal medicines are worthy of consideration. Important herbs in this class include *Allium sativum* (garlic), *Astragalus membranaceus* (astragalus), *Camellia sinensis* (green tea), *Crataegus* spp. (hawthorn leaves and berries), *Curcuma longa* (turmeric), *Ginkgo biloba* (ginkgo), *Olea europaea* (olive leaves), *Polygonum multiflorum* (polygonum), *Rosmarinus officinalis* (rosemary), *Silybum marianum* (St Mary's thistle), *Vaccinium myrtillus* (bilberry), *Vitis vinifera* (grape seed extract) and *Pinus pinaster* (French maritime pine bark).

Specific herbal medicines

TONGKAT ALI (*EURYCOMA LONGIFOLIA*)

Tongkat ali is a herb from the South-East Asian traditions of herbal medicine. It is traditionally reputed to have male reproductive tonic properties, being used to enhance libido and improve erectile function, stamina and endurance.[458]

Studies have supported the traditional use of *Eurycoma longifolia* as a male reproductive tonic, suggesting its value in treating men diagnosed with LOH.

In an open label study, 1-month treatment with 200 mg of a proprietary *Eurycoma longifolia* freeze-dried water extract (Physta®) decreased mean ageing male symptoms (AMS) scores from 38.05 to 23.67 and increased mean testosterone concentrations from 5.66 nmol/L to 8.31 nmol/L.[348] The rise in testosterone represented an increase of 46.8% on average in the study participants. Before treatment with the extract, 35.5% of men had serum testosterone concentrations considered normal, but after treatment this increased to 90.8% of men with normal testosterone levels.[348]

Another study using 300 mg of the same proprietary extract found that 12-week treatment in healthy men aged 30–50 resulted in significant improvements in physical functioning, role physical and vitality domains of the Quality of Life SF-36 scale.[459] Erectile function, sexual libido and sexual satisfaction scores as evaluated by the IIEF-15 scale also increased significantly.[459] The overall scores of these scales did not, however, show significant change. Hormonal profile (testosterone, SHBG, DHEA-S) also failed to be altered in this study.[459]

PANAX GINSENG (KOREAN GINSENG)

P. ginseng has long been thought of as a rejuvenating male tonic, and has been used in traditional Chinese medicine for lowered vitality and where physical performance and sexual function require enhancement. To date there have been no studies on the specific action of *P. ginseng* in men diagnosed with LOH. However its traditional use as a male tonic along with animal and human studies of *P. ginseng* under other circumstances suggest a supportive role for symptoms associated with LOH. These actions include improvements in erectile function,[460] and adaptogenic,[461] antioxidant, immune-modulating and glucose modification.[462]

TRIBULUS TERRESTRIS (TRIBULUS)

T. terrestris is a popular botanical suggested for men because of its purported energising and revitalising effects on male physiology and sexual function. A recent review of *Tribulus terrestris* supported its use as a treatment for sexual desire problems in both men and women;[349] however, evidence in men specifically affected by LOH is lacking.

T. terrestris has been purported to influence testosterone and other hormones of the pituitary-gonadal axis but evidence from human studies and animal studies is conflicting, suggesting other mechanisms for its action.[349] The most likely means by which tribulus improves sexual function is via an endothelial and nitric oxide (NO) dependent mechanism which has been demonstrated in animal studies.[357] Another hypothesis is of a possible androgen receptor modulating activity that does not alter endogenous testosterone levels.[349] Regardless of this, the efficacy of tribulus in improving the symptom of low sexual desire in men makes it worthy of consideration as part of a herbal strategy for androgen-deficient men with these symptoms.

SERENOA REPENS (SAW PALMETTO)

Although no studies have directly assessed the efficacy of *S. repens* in LOH, tradition provides a rationale for its therapeutic use. The Eclectic physicians used it for 'wasting away of the testicles' and 'to strengthen the sexual appetite particularly in the aged',[463] descriptions that mirror the modern-day diagnosis of LOH. The Eclectics used *S. repens* in many ways, describing it as a male tonic, an aphrodisiac and much more.

A small open label study comparing two doses (800 mg/day vs 2000 mg/day) of a proprietary combination of *Serenoa repens* berry and astaxanthin in healthy men (aged 37 to 70) for 14 days demonstrated significant increases in total testosterone and decreases in dihydrotestosterone at both dosages, and significant decreases in oestradiol in those who received the higher dose.[464] While modern clinical studies have typically focused on its role in lower urinary tract symptoms, broadening the research to assess the mode of action of *S. repens* in androgen deficiency and other male conditions described by the Eclectics is likely to benefit many and further increase the modern-day application of this herb.

ASHWAGANDHA (*WITHANIA SOMNIFERA*)

Traditionally indicated as an aphrodisiac and male rejuvenative tonic, ashwagandha finds particular value in the herbal management of men with hypogonadism. No studies are available assessing its role in late-onset hypogonadism, although extrapolations from available human research exploring its role in male fertility and resistance training, in combination with its noted traditional use, indicate its worthy consideration in the herbal treatment of LOH.

Amounts of 5 g daily of *Withania somnifera* powder given to 'stressed', normozoospermic infertile men for 3 months improved various male fertility measures with accompanying significant alterations in sex hormone status. Testosterone levels increased by up to 22% and LH by up to 22%. Men in the study were found to have raised FSH and PRL at baseline, which was reduced by withania treatment.[350]

Treeatments of 600 mg daily of concentrated ashwagandha extract (5% withanolides) were given to men 18–50 years old for 8 weeks. Combined with resistance training, significantly greater muscle mass, strength and testosterone levels were demonstrated compared to placebo treatment.[465] The increase in testosterone seen over the 8-week intervention period with ashwagandha treatment was 3.335 nmol/L, compared to 0.624 nmol/L for placebo.[465]

VELVET BEAN (*MUCUNA PRURIENS*)

The traditional indications for velvet bean as a restoring and invigorating male reproductive tonic, aphrodisiac and fertility-enhancing agent suggest its indication as part of the management of LOH. Again, no studies yet exist exploring this specific indication; however, combining extrapolation from its modern evidence in male infertility and traditional indications we can see a potential role for its use here.

In infertile men, 5 g daily of *Mucuna pruriens* seed powder for 3 months improved male fertility parameters with accompanying alterations in sex hormones. Testosterone was significantly increased by 17% and LH was increased by 23%. Elevated FSH and PRL was significantly reduced as well.[351] These results are supported by a more recent study using the same dosage regime that also reported increases in testosterone and LH, and reductions in FSH and PRL.[466]

TURNERA DIFFUSA (DAMIANA)

LOH is associated with depression and sexual dysfunction. Therefore, the use of *T. diffusa*, a male tonic indicated for its mild antidepressant and nervine effects, is likely to be of value. The administration of *T. diffusa* has been shown to increase sexual behaviour in castrated male rats[467] and to recover copulation in sexually exhausted rats.[468] These effects appear to be mediated via a central nitric oxide (NO) pathway, possibly by the action of flavonoids present within *T. diffusa*.[469] While the research is limited, coupled with traditional evidence and clinical experience, *T. diffusa* may be useful in managing loss of desire and low sex drive in men presenting with LOH.

AVENA SATIVA SEED (OAT SEED)

The immature seed of *A. sativa* was used traditionally for its mild tonic and stimulant actions, and was indicated specifically for male complaints associated with nervous debility, exhaustion and convalescence.[2] Because of its gentle restorative action, *A. sativa* may be considered as an adjuvant and supportive botanical therapy in the management of symptoms associated with low androgen levels, such as low mood and loss of energy.

LIFESTYLE RECOMMENDATIONS

Weight management and exercise

Achieving and maintaining a healthy body weight and waist circumference are essential in the effective management of hypogonadism. Numerous studies identified by Corona et al assessing the effect of weight loss on sex hormone levels found that significant increases in plasma total testosterone (both bound and unbound) were associated with weight loss whether by kilojoule-restricted diets or bariatric surgery.[396] Greater increases in androgens were associated with higher degrees of weight loss.[396] FSH and LH were also shown to increase and E2 was shown to decrease.[396]

An exercise program will form an important component in any weight loss strategy, and will be essential to manage the metabolic risk factors often associated with androgen deficiency. The advice of an exercise physiologist may be required to assess what the patient can accommodate based on their preexisting health concerns and physical ailments. Increasing upper body strength is especially beneficial for cardiac function and hormone stimulation, weight-bearing exercise is important for improving bone density and muscle mass, while aerobic exercise improves circulation and reduces cardiac risk.

CASE STUDY

OVERVIEW

Peter is a 70-year-old male who presents with fatigue and low mood that has been progressively worsening over the past 2–3 years. His partner Gerald says that he is often irritable and has low motivation, which Peter agrees with, stating that it often takes him quite some time to pluck up the energy to do anything. Afternoons are particularly worse for his energy levels, when he typically needs a nap after lunch, otherwise finding it 'impossible' to function.

Peter also thinks his muscle strength has reduced, although he does not report any muscle pain. He and Gerald live on a large suburban block that backs onto bushland and needs regular maintenance, which Peter says he is having difficulty with. As a result the bulk of the work is falling to Gerald. Peter's work as an academic is sedentary and he works mostly from home, which he enjoys the flexibility of. Other than yard work and the occasional bit of gardening (which he is finding difficult at the moment) he does not engage in any other physical activity.

CASE STUDY CONTINUED

Peter says he has very little interest in sex, which according to Gerald is putting significant strain upon their relationship. When they do make love, Peter experiences some difficulty attaining and maintaining an erection, although he puts it down to a low level of arousal. He also finds it can take him a while to reach climax. Similarly, Peter says he masturbates infrequently, generally no more often than once a month, and that even then reaching climax feels prolonged. His ejaculate volume he has noticed is also of a smaller volume. Peter says he very infrequently wakes with a morning erection. While Peter says he is not overly bothered by his changes in sexual function, Gerald makes it clear that he is finding it particularly difficult.

Peter has steadily gained weight over the last 8–9 years or so, which he is concerned about.

Peter says his diet is based heavily on easy-to-prepare foods, because 'I just don't have the energy'. Gerald is a vegetarian, which Peter says is not 'really his cup of tea', so as a consequence he often prepares his own meals, which he says regularly come out of a packet, or will consist of a cheese and ham toasted sandwich. Peter finds he likes to nibble on something sweet while he is working. This may be honey or jam on sourdough wholemeal toast, but is often a sweet biscuit or a bit of milk chocolate. Most evenings, Peter and Gerald share a bottle of wine; however, Gerald is quick to point out that he typically only has one small glass, whereas Peter finishes off the rest. On Friday nights, Peter admits that he may sometimes drink more than a bottle of wine.

Two years ago Peter was diagnosed with type 2 diabetes mellitus and is taking metformin hydrochloride 500 mg twice daily. He is also taking Coveram (perindopril arginine/amlodipine) 10 mg/10 mg once daily to manage high blood pressure. Peter also has hypercholesterolaemia, which is currently being treated with Crestor (rosuvastatin) 5 mg once daily. Peter reports that his most recent blood tests indicated that his blood sugar control was not ideal, and that his doctor wanted him to increase his metformin dose; however, he is reluctant to do. Peter is also taking a standard concentration fish oil supplement one capsule daily.

Systems review is otherwise unremarkable, except that Peter passes a bowel motion once every 2–3 days and he usually has to strain.

PHYSICAL EXAMINATION

- The patient looks tired
- Weight: 80 kg
- Height: 164 cm
- BMI: 29.7 kg/m^2 (overweight)
- Abdominal circumference: 101 cm
- Liver size: within normal limits
- Blood pressure: 140/85 mmHg
- Pulse: 85 bpm regular
- Respiratory rate: 16 breaths per minute
- Conjunctiva: pink
- Nails: mild spooning left ring and middle finger, right index and middle finger. Longitudinal ridging. Some nails peeling
- Capillary refill: 3 seconds
- Urinalysis: NAD (no protein, no blood, no ketones, no glucose)

CASE STUDY CONTINUED

- Random blood glucose: 9.2 mmol/L (breakfast was eaten 1 hour previously consisting of a bowl of commercial breakfast cereal with milk and a cup of coffee).

RELEVANT INVESTIGATION FINDINGS

- Serum total testosterone: 8.4 nmol/L (low)
- Calculated free testosterone: 198 pmol/L (low)
- Follicle-stimulating hormone: 1.2 U/L (normal)
- Luteinising hormone: 1.9 U/L (normal)
- 25-OH vitamin D: 26 nmol/L (moderate deficiency)
- HbA1c: 7.8% (high)
- Full blood count: NAD
- Thyroid: NAD
- Kidney function: eGFR 65 (low), otherwise NAD
- Liver function gamma GT: 81 (high), otherwise NAD
- Iron studies: NAD
- B_{12} studies: NAD
- Dual-energy x-ray absorptiometry (DXA) scanning T-score: 1.9 (osteopenia).

INITIAL TREATMENT

The initial treatment aims were to increase energy and motivation, and to implement dietary and lifestyle changes targeted towards sustained weight loss and improving blood sugar management. Discussions were had with Peter regarding the potential role testosterone replacement therapy may have in the interim in improving his blood sugar control and quality of life; however, he wanted to explore options other than hormone replacement at this stage.

HERBAL MEDICINE

- Herbal complex 100 mL
  Panax ginseng 1:2: 40 mL
  Crocus sativus 1:20: 40 mL
  Pinus pinaster 1:2: 20 mL
  Dose: 5 mL in water or juice in the morning and at lunchtime
- *Withania somnifera* powder: 1 teaspoon in milk or milk alternative twice daily
- *Hibiscus sabdariffa* tea: 1 rounded tablespoon (10 g) infused in 2 cups of hot water. Drink daily.

NUTRITIONAL MEDICINE (DIETARY)

- Eliminate processed breakfast cereal for breakfast. Replace with oats either as porridge or soaked overnight in calcium fortified soy milk and/or yoghurt. Top with blueberries/raspberries and 1 tablespoon of ground flaxseeds (as both a bulk laxative and source of lignans)
- Have a salad a day for lunch. Mixed dark greens, raw vegetables, sprouts topped with a healthy protein (tuna/salmon/sardines, mixed beans, couple of eggs or strips of lean beef/kangaroo)
- Share evening meals with Gerald. Have a piece of lean beef or fish as a side with the vegetarian meals prepared together, although try having vegetarian at least 2–3 times a week, using legumes or tofu/tempeh as a protein source
- Keep a container of mixed nuts for snacking (e.g. almonds, Brazil nuts, macadamias). Aim to eat at least 3 Brazil nuts daily for selenium

CASE STUDY CONTINUED

- Other than nuts, preference fruit as a snack when something sweet is desired.

NUTRITIONAL MEDICINE (SUPPLEMENTAL)

- Vitamin D_3: 6000 IU daily for at least 8 weeks or until deficiency is corrected
- Chromium picolinate: 800 micrograms once daily
- Increase fish oil supplementation to at least 4 capsules daily
- Combination supplement containing calcium (250 mg), magnesium (125 mg), zinc (6 mg) and boron (500 micrograms). Take 1 capsule 3 times daily.

LIFESTYLE EDUCATION

- Minimum 30 minutes exercise daily. Start with a brisk walk in the mornings
- Limit alcohol consumption to 1 standard drink a day, with at least 2 alcohol-free days a week. An emphasis was placed on the energy intake contribution made by alcohol, and that eliminating it is an easy way of restricting kilojoule intake.

FOLLOW-UP CONSULTATION 2 WEEKS LATER

Peter had noticed some improvement in his energy levels, more so in the last week or so. He had cut back his alcohol consumption typically to 1, sometimes 2 glasses of wine most nights, and had not binged since our last appointment. He found that since cutting back his alcohol he was waking with a bit more energy. As a consequence he had started walking in the mornings, although had only managed to go 3 times since our last appointment. He was finding that the dietary changes suggested were positively affecting his appetite and dietary choices. He found that he was really enjoying oats in the morning, as he was feeling fuller and found that his inclination to snack on sweets was lower. He was still enjoying the odd bit of chocolate; however, he was favouring an organic dark chocolate that Gerald had recently discovered. Since our last appointment, Peter and Gerald had decided to consult with a relationship counsellor, particularly in regards to their challenges with desire discrepancy and other dissatisfactions in their relationship. As a consequence, Peter felt that improvement in his libido was more of a priority for him now.

ADDITIONAL RECOMMENDATIONS

Tribulus terrestris tablets (equivalent to 9 g dried herb, standardised to furostanol saponins 110 mg): 1 tablet twice daily.

THIRD CONSULTATION (4 WEEKS LATER)

Peter reported that he was implementing all dietary suggestions made and was enjoying sharing meals with Gerald again. Peter was having a brisk walk most mornings, and had found a substantial hill nearby that he had begun challenging himself with. Although he felt he still had a way to go, Peter felt that his energy was continuing to improve and as such he was feeling happier and more motivated. He had cut back further on his alcohol consumption, which he felt

CASE STUDY CONTINUED

was also making a significant difference to his energy. Peter was also happy to report that he had lost around 2 kg since our last appointment, and was feeling fitter than he had in ages. Peter also was happy to report that he had noticed improvements in his libido and he and Gerald had made love 3 times in the last 4 weeks, the most recent time initiated by himself. He had also noticed that sexual function was gradually improving, which he was also happy about.

REFERENCES

[1] Tortora G, Grabowski S. Principles of anatomy and physiology. 9th ed. New York: Biological Sciences Textbooks/Wiley; 2000.

[2] Ellingwood F. The American materia medica, therapeutics and pharmacognosy. Evanston, Illinois: Ellingwoods Therapeutist; 1919.

[3] Jones EG. Definite medication. Boston: The Therapeutic Publishing Company; 1911.

[4] Andrology Australia Prostate Cancer Advisory Group. The early detection of prostate cancer: Review and summary of current professional guidelines & position statements. Andrology Australia; 2015. Available from: www.andrologyaustralia.org/wp-content/uploads/review-early-detection-of-prostate-cancer.pdf.

[5] Bolla M, van Casteren NJ, Cornford P, et al. Guidelines on prostate cancer. European Association of Urology 2015.

[6] Hayes JH, Barry MJ. Screening for prostate cancer with the prostate-specific antigen test: a review of current evidence. JAMA 2014;311(11):1143.

[7] Arthur R. Zinc. Herbs and natural supplements: an evidence-based guide. 4th ed. Sydney: Elsevier; 2015. p. 1197–223.

[8] Gratzke C, Bachmann A, Descazeaud A, et al. EAU guidelines on the assessment of non-neurogenic male lower urinary tract symptoms including benign prostatic obstruction. Eur Urol 2015;67(6):1099–2109.

[9] Roehrborn CG. Male lower urinary tract symptoms (LUTS) and benign prostatic hyperplasia (BPH). Med Clin North Am 2011 Jan;95(1):87–100.

[10] Madersbacher S, Pycha A, Klingler CH, et al. The International Prostate Symptom Score in both sexes: a urodynamics-based comparison. Neurourol Urodyn 1999;18:173–82.

[11] Vignozzi L, Gacci M, Maggi M. Lower urinary tract symptoms, benign prostatic hyperplasia and metabolic syndrome. Nat Rev Urol 2016;13(2):108–19.

[12] Roosen A, Chapple CR, Dmochowski RR, et al. A refocus on the bladder as the originator of storage lower urinary tract symptoms: a systematic review of the latest literature. Eur Urol 2009;56(5):810–20.

[13] Osman NI, Chapple CR, Abrams P, et al. Detrusor underactivity and the underactive bladder: a new clinical entity? A review of current terminology, definitions, epidemiology, aetiology, and diagnosis. Eur Urol 2014;65(2):389–98.

[14] Thiruchelvam N. Benign prostatic hyperplasia. Surg Oxf 2014;32(6):314–22.

[15] Roehrborn C. Benign prostatic hyperplasia: etiology, pathophysiology, epidemiology, and natural history. In: Wein W, Kavoussi L, Partin A, editors. Campbell-Walsh urology. 11th ed. Philadelphia: Elsevier; 2016. p. 2425–62.

[16] Wang C-C, Liao C-H, Kuo H-C. Clinical guidelines for male lower urinary tract symptoms associated with non-neurogenic overactive bladder. Urol Sci 2015;26(1):7–16.

[17] Griebling TL. Overactive bladder in elderly men: epidemiology, evaluation, clinical effects, and management. Curr Urol Rep 2013 Oct;14(5):418–25.

[18] Smith PP, Birder LA, Abrams P, et al. Detrusor underactivity and the underactive bladder: Symptoms, function, cause — what do we mean? ICI-RS Think Tank 2014. Neurourol Urodyn 2016;35(2):312–17.

[19] Gammie A, Kaper M, Dorrepaal C, et al. Signs and symptoms of detrusor underactivity: an analysis of clinical presentation and urodynamic tests from a large group of patients undergoing pressure flow studies. Eur Urol 2016;69(2):361–9.

[20] Weiss JP, Ruud Bosch JLH, Drake M, et al. Nocturia think tank: Focus on nocturnal polyuria: ICI-RS 2011. Neurourol Urodyn 2012;31(3):330–9.
[21] Homma Y, Kawabe K, Tsukamoto T, et al. Epidemiologic survey of lower urinary tract symptoms in Asia and Australia using the international prostate symptom score. Int J Urol 1997;4(1):40–6.
[22] Yamaguchi O, Aikawa K, Shishido K, et al. Place of overactive bladder in male lower urinary tract symptoms. World J Urol 2009 Dec;27(6):723–8.
[23] Wein AJ. Neuromuscular dysfunction of the lower urinary tract. In: Wein W, Kavoussi L, Partin A, editors. Campbell-Walsh urology. 11th ed. Philadelphia: Elsevier; 2016. p. 1761–95.
[24] Lepor H. Alpha-blockers for the treatment of benign prostatic hyperplasia. Urol Clin North Am 2016;43(3):311–23.
[25] Nicholson TM, Ricke WA. Androgens and estrogens in benign prostatic hyperplasia: past, present and future. Differentiation 2011;82(4–5):184–99.
[26] Mazur DJ, Helfand BT, McVary KT. Influences of neuroregulatory factors on the development of lower urinary tract symptoms/benign prostatic hyperplasia and erectile dysfunction in aging men. Urol Clin North Am 2012;39(1):77–88.
[27] Gacci M, Andersson K-E, Chapple C, et al. Latest evidence on the use of phosphodiesterase type 5 inhibitors for the treatment of lower urinary tract symptoms secondary to benign prostatic hyperplasia. Eur Urol 2016;70(1):124–33.
[28] Shimizu S, Tsounapi P, Shimizu T, et al. Lower urinary tract symptoms, benign prostatic hyperplasia/benign prostatic enlargement and erectile dysfunction: are these conditions related to vascular dysfunction? LUTS, BPH/BPE, ED and pelvic blood flow. Int J Urol 2014;21(9):856–64.
[29] Matsumoto S, Kakizaki H. Causative significance of bladder blood flow in lower urinary tract symptoms: LUTS and bladder blood flow. Int J Urol 2012;19(1):20–5.
[30] Thurmond P, Yang J-H, Azadzoi KM. LUTS in pelvic ischemia: a new concept in voiding dysfunction. Am J Physiol Renal Physiol 2016;310(8):F738–43.
[31] Yoshida M, Yamaguchi O. Detrusor underactivity: the current concept of the pathophysiology. LUTS Low Urin Tract Symptoms 2014;6(3):131–7.
[32] La Vignera S, Condorelli RA, Russo GI, et al. Endocrine control of benign prostatic hyperplasia. Andrology 2016;4(3):404–11.
[33] Bardan R, Dumache R, Dema A, et al. The role of prostatic inflammation biomarkers in the diagnosis of prostate diseases. Clin Biochem 2014;47(10–11):909–15.
[34] Izumi K, Mizokami A, Lin W-J, et al. Androgen receptor roles in the development of benign prostate hyperplasia. Am J Pathol 2013;182(6):1942–9.
[35] Jarvis TR, Chughtai B, Kaplan SA, et al. Testosterone and benign prostatic hyperplasia. Asian J Androl 2015;17(2):212.
[36] van der Sluis TM, Vis AN, van Moorselaar RJA, et al. Intraprostatic testosterone and dihydrotestosterone. Part I: concentrations and methods of determination in men with benign prostatic hyperplasia and prostate cancer: intraprostatic androgen assessment in untreated BPH and prostate cancer. BJU Int 2012;109(2):176–82.
[37] Kacker R, Traish AM, Morgentaler A. Estrogens in men: clinical implications for sexual function and the treatment of testosterone deficiency. J Sex Med 2012;9(6):1681–96.
[38] Roberts RO, Jacobson DJ, Rhodes T, et al. Serum sex hormones and measures of benign prostatic hyperplasia. Prostate 2004;61(2):124–31.
[39] Timms BG, Hofkamp LE. Prostate development and growth in benign prostatic hyperplasia. Differentiation 2011;82(4–5):173–83.
[40] Kim S, Chung J, Park H, et al. Association between polymorphisms of estrogen receptor 2 and benign prostatic hyperplasia. Exp Ther Med 2015;10(5):1990–4.
[41] Nickel JC. Role of prostatic inflammation in the clinical presentation of benign prostatic hyperplasia. Eur Urol Suppl 2015;14(9):e1459–63.
[42] Bartoletti R. Chronic inflammatory infiltrate and benign prostatic hyperplasia: what do we know? Eur Urol Suppl 2013;12(5):99–102.
[43] Camoes J, Coelho A, Castro-Diaz D, et al. Lower urinary tract symptoms and aging: the impact of chronic bladder ischemia on overactive bladder syndrome. Urol Int 2015;95(4):373–9.
[44] Liao C-H, Chung S-D, Kuo H-C, et al. Reactive protein levels are associated with residual urgency symptoms in patients with benign prostatic hyperplasia after medical treatment. Urology 2011;78(6):1373–8.
[45] Berger AP, Horninger W, Bektic J, et al. Vascular resistance in the prostate evaluated by colour Doppler ultrasonography: is benign prostatic hyperplasia a vascular disease? BJU Int 2006 Sep;98(3):587–90.
[46] Pinggera G-M, Mitterberger M, Steiner E, et al. Association of lower urinary tract symptoms and chronic ischaemia of the lower urinary tract in elderly women and men: assessment using colour Doppler ultrasonography. BJU Int 2008;102(4):470–4.
[47] Pinggera G-M, Mitterberger M, Pallwein L, et al. α-blockers improve chronic ischaemia of the lower urinary tract in patients with lower urinary tract symptoms. BJU Int 2008;101(3):319–24.
[48] Gacci M, Corona G, Vignozzi L, et al. Metabolic syndrome and benign prostatic enlargement: a systematic review and meta-analysis: metabolic syndrome and BPE. BJU Int 2015;115(1):24–31.
[49] Zou C, Gong D, Fang N, et al. Meta-analysis of metabolic syndrome and benign prostatic hyperplasia in Chinese patients. World J Urol 2016;34(2):281–9.
[50] Russo GI, Castelli T, Urzì D, et al. Emerging links between non-neurogenic lower urinary tract symptoms secondary to benign prostatic obstruction, metabolic syndrome and its components: a systematic review. Int J Urol 2015;22(11):982–90.
[51] Uzun H, Zorba OÜ. Metabolic syndrome in female patients with overactive bladder. Urology 2012;79(1):72–5.
[52] Parsons JK, Sarma AV, McVary K, et al. Obesity and benign prostatic hyperplasia: clinical connections, emerging etiological paradigms and future directions. J Urol 2013;189(1):S102–6.
[53] Mondul AM, Giovannucci E, Platz EA. A prospective study of obesity, and the incidence and progression of lower urinary tract symptoms. J Urol 2014;191(3):715–21.
[54] Gacci M, Sebastianelli A, Salvi M, et al. Central obesity is predictive of persistent storage lower urinary tract symptoms (LUTS) after surgery for benign prostatic enlargement: results of a multicentre prospective study. BJU Int 2015;116(2):271–7.
[55] Russo GI, Castelli T, Privitera S, et al. Increase of Framingham cardiovascular disease risk score is associated with severity of lower urinary tract symptoms. BJU Int 2015;116(5):791–6.
[56] Bouwman II, Blanker MH, Schouten BWV, et al. Are lower urinary tract symptoms associated with cardiovascular disease in the Dutch general population? Results from the Krimpen study. World J Urol 2015;33(5):669–76.
[57] Uzun H, Çiçek Y, Kocaman SA, et al. Increased pulse-wave velocity and carotid intima-media thickness in patients with lower urinary tract symptoms. Scand J Urol 2013;47(5):393–8.
[58] Takahashi N, Shishido K, Sato Y, et al. The association between severity of atherosclerosis and lower urinary tract function in male patients with lower urinary tract symptoms. LUTS: Low Urin Tract Symptoms 2012;4(1):9–13.
[59] Hwang EC, Kim S-O, Nam D-H, et al. Men with hypertension are more likely to have severe lower urinary tract symptoms and large prostate volume: hypertension and LUTS. LUTS: Low Urin Tract Symptoms 2015;7(1):32–6.
[60] Ito H, Yoshiyasu T, Yamaguchi O, et al. Male lower urinary tract symptoms: hypertension as a risk factor for storage symptoms, but not voiding symptoms. LUTS: Low Urin Tract Symptoms 2012;4(2):68–72.
[61] Barbosa JABA, Muracca E, Nakano É, et al. Interactions between lower urinary tract symptoms and cardiovascular risk factors determine distinct patterns of erectile dysfunction: a latent class analysis. J Urol 2013;190(6):2177–82.
[62] Kirby M, Chapple C, Jackson G, et al. Erectile dysfunction and lower urinary tract symptoms: a consensus on the importance of co-diagnosis. Int J Clin Pract 2013;67(7):606–18.
[63] Gravas S, Bach T, Bachmann A, et al. Guidelines on the management of non-neurogenic male lower urinary tract symptoms (LUTS), incl. benign prostatic obstruction (BPO). European Association of Urology 2015. Available from: http://uroweb.org/wp-content/uploads/EAU-Guidelines-Non-Neurogenic-Male-LUTS_LR.pdf.

[64] Liu Z-M, Wong C, Chan D, et al. Association of circulating 25(OH)D and lower urinary tract symptoms: a four-year prospective study among elderly Chinese men. Nutrients 2016;8(5):273.
[65] McNicholas TA, Speakman MJ, Kirby RS. Evaluation and nonsurgical management of benign prostatic hyperplasia. In: Wein W, Kavoussi L, Partin A, editors. Campbell-Walsh urology. 11th ed. Philadelphia: Elsevier; 2016.
[66] Kristal AR, Arnold KB, Schenk JM, et al. Dietary patterns, supplement use, and the risk of symptomatic benign prostatic hyperplasia: results from the Prostate Cancer Prevention Trial. Am J Epidemiol 2008;167(8):925–34.
[67] Liu Z, Wong CKM, Chan D, et al. Fruit and vegetable intake in relation to lower urinary tract symptoms and erectile dysfunction among southern Chinese elderly men: a 4-year prospective study of Mr OS Hong Kong. Medicine (Baltimore) 2016;95(4):e2557.
[68] Bravi F, Bosetti C, Dal Maso L, et al. Food groups and risk of benign prostatic hyperplasia. Urology 2006;67(1):73–9.
[69] USDA Food Composition Databases. 12 Nov 2016. Available from: https://ndb.nal.usda.gov/ndb/nutrients/index.
[70] Ambrosini GL, de Klerk NH, Mackerras D, et al. Dietary patterns and surgically treated benign prostatic hyperplasia: a case control study in Western Australia. BJU Int 2008;101(7):853–60.
[71] Espinosa G. Nutrition and benign prostatic hyperplasia. Curr Opin Urol 2013;23(1):38–41.
[72] Salas-Salvado J, Guasch-Ferre M, Lee C-H, et al. Protective effects of the Mediterranean diet on type 2 diabetes and metabolic syndrome. J Nutr 2016;146(4):920S–927S.
[73] Chiva-Blanch G, Badimon L, Estruch R. Latest evidence of the effects of the Mediterranean diet in prevention of cardiovascular disease. Curr Atheroscler Rep 2014;16(10):446.
[74] Esposito K, Ciotola M, Giugliano F, et al. Mediterranean diet improves erectile function in subjects with the metabolic syndrome. Int J Impot Res 2006;18(4):405–10.
[75] Parsons JK, Im R. Alcohol consumption is associated with a decreased risk of benign prostatic hyperplasia. J Urol 2009 Oct;182(4):1463–8.
[76] Wong SYS, Lau WWY, Leung PC, et al. The association between isoflavone and lower urinary tract symptoms in elderly men. Br J Nutr 2007;98:1237–42.
[77] Tavani A, Longoni E, Bosetti C, et al. Intake of selected micronutrients and the risk of surgically treated benign prostatic hyperplasia: a case-control study from Italy. Eur Urol 2006 Sep;50(3):549–54.
[78] Rohrmann S, Smit E, Giovannucci E, et al. Association between serum concentrations of micronutrients and lower urinary tract symptoms in older men in the Third National Health and Nutrition Examination Survey. Urology 2004;64(3):504–9.
[79] Holton KF, Marshall LM, Shannon J, et al. Dietary antioxidants and longitudinal changes in lower urinary tract symptoms in elderly men: the Osteoporotic Fractures in Men Study. Eur Urol Focus 2016;2(3):310–18.
[80] Bravi F, Bosetti C, Dal Maso L, et al. Macronutrients, fatty acids, cholesterol, and risk of benign prostatic hyperplasia. Urology 2006;67(6):1205–11.
[81] Lagiou P, Wuu J, Trichopoulou A, et al. Diet and benign prostatic hyperplasia: a study in Greece. Urology 1999;54(2):284–90.
[82] Erickson BA, Vaughan-Sarrazin M, Liu X, et al. Lower urinary tract symptoms and diet quality: findings from the 2000–2001 National Health and Nutrition Examination Survey. Urology 2012;79(6):1262–7.
[83] Demark-Wahnefried W, Robertson CN, Walther PJ, et al. Pilot study to explore effects of low-fat, flaxseed-supplemented diet on proliferation of benign prostatic epithelium and prostate-specific antigen. Urology 2004;63(5):900–4.
[84] Simons R, Sonawane N, Verbruggen M, et al. Efficacy and safety of a flaxseed hull extract in the symptomatic management of benign prostatic hyperplasia: a parallel, randomized, double-blind, placebo-controlled, pilot study. J Med Food 2015;18(2):233–40.
[85] Zhang W, Wang X, Liu Y, et al. Effects of dietary flaxseed lignan extract on symptoms of benign prostatic hyperplasia. J Med Food 2008;11(2):207–14.
[86] Demark-Wahnefried W, Polascik TJ, George SL, et al. Flaxseed supplementation (not dietary fat restriction) reduces prostate cancer proliferation rates in men presurgery. Cancer Epidemiol Biomarkers Prev 2008;17(12):3577–87.
[87] Wilt TJ, Macdonald R, Ishani A. β-sitosterol for the treatment of benign prostatic hyperplasia: a systematic review. BJU Int 1999;83:976–83.
[88] Vahlensieck W, Theurer C, Pfitzer E, et al. Effects of pumpkin seed in men with lower urinary tract symptoms due to benign prostatic hyperplasia in the one-year, randomized, placebo-controlled GRANU Study. Urol Int 2014;94(3):286–95.
[89] Allkanjari O, Vitalone A. What do we know about phytotherapy of benign prostatic hyperplasia? Life Sci 2015;126:42–56.
[90] Shirvan MK, Mahboob MRD, Masuminia M, et al. Pumpkin seed oil (Prostafit) or Prazosin? Which one is better in the treatment of symptomatic benign prostatic hyperplasia. J Pak Med Assoc 2014;64:683–5.
[91] Hong H, Kim C-S, Maeng S. Effects of pumpkin seed oil and saw palmetto oil in Korean men with symptomatic benign prostatic hyperplasia. Nutr Res Pract 2009;3(4):323.
[92] USDA-Iowa State University database on the isoflavone content of foods. Beltsville, MD: U.S. Dept of Agriculture, Agricultural Research Service, Beltsville Human Nutrition Research Center, Nutrient Data Laboratory; 2007. Available from: www.ars.usda.gov/ARSUserFiles/80400525/Data/isoflav/isoflav1-4.pdf.
[93] Xu M-L, Liu J, Zhu C, et al. Interactions between soy isoflavones and other bioactive compounds: a review of their potentially beneficial health effects. Phytochem Rev 2015 Jun;14(3):459–67.
[94] Hong SJ, Kim SI, Kwon SM, et al. Comparative study of concentration of isoflavones and lignans in plasma and prostatic tissues of normal control and benign prostatic hyperplasia. Yonsei Med J 2002;43(2):236–41.
[95] Brössner C, Petritsch K, Fink K, et al. Phytoestrogen tissue levels in benign prostatic hyperplasia and prostate cancer and their association with prostatic diseases. Urology 2004 Oct;64(4):707–11.
[96] Wong WCW, Wong ELY, Li H, et al. Isoflavones in treating watchful waiting benign prostate hyperplasia: a double-blinded, randomized controlled trial. J Altern Complement Med 2012 Jan;18(1):54–60.
[97] Bae WJ, Park HJ, Koo HC, et al. The effect of seoritae extract in men with mild to moderate lower urinary tract symptoms suggestive of benign prostatic hyperplasia. Evid Based Complement Alternat Med 2016;2016:1–6.
[98] Jang H, Bae W-J, Yuk S-M, et al. Seoritae extract reduces prostate weight and suppresses prostate cell proliferation in a rat model of benign prostate hyperplasia. Evid Based Complement Alternat Med 2014;2014:1–7.
[99] Isanga J, Zhang G-N. Soybean bioactive components and their implications to health — a review. Food Rev Int 2008;24(2):252–76.
[100] van Die MD, Bone KM, Williams SG, et al. Soy and soy isoflavones in prostate cancer: a systematic review and meta-analysis of randomized controlled trials. BJU Int 2014;113(5b):E119–30.
[101] Suh B, Shin DW, Hwang S, et al. Alcohol is longitudinally associated with lower urinary tract symptoms partially via high-density lipoprotein. Alcohol Clin Exp Res 2014;38(11):2878–83.
[102] Choo MS, Han JH, Shin TY, et al. Alcohol, smoking, physical activity, protein, and lower urinary tract symptoms: prospective longitudinal cohort. Int Neurourol J 2015;19(3):197–206.
[103] Roerecke M, Rehm J. Alcohol consumption, drinking patterns, and ischemic heart disease: a narrative review of meta-analyses and a systematic review and meta-analysis of the impact of heavy drinking occasions on risk for moderate drinkers. BMC Med 2014;12(1):1.
[104] Maserejian NN, Wager CG, Giovannucci EL, et al. Intake of caffeinated, carbonated, or citrus beverage types and development of lower urinary tract symptoms in men and women. Am J Epidemiol 2013;177(12):1399–410.
[105] Lohsiriwat S, Hirunsai M, Chaiyaprasithi B. Effect of caffeine on bladder function in patients with overactive bladder symptoms. Urol Ann 2011;3(1):14.
[106] Zhao J, Wu Q, Hu X, et al. Comparative study of serum zinc concentrations in benign and malignant prostate disease: a systematic review and meta-analysis. Sci Rep 2016;6:25778.

[107] Goel T, Sankhwar SN. Comparative study of zinc levels in benign and malignant lesions of the prostate. Scand J Urol Nephrol 2006;40(2):108–12.

[108] Eichholzer M, Steinbrecher A, Kaaks R, et al. Effects of selenium status, dietary glucosinolate intake and serum glutathione *S*-transferase α activity on the risk of benign prostatic hyperplasia: modifiable factors in the aetiology of BPH. BJU Int 2012;110(11c):E879–85.

[109] Minciullo PL, Inferrera A, Navarra M, et al. Oxidative stress in benign prostatic hyperplasia: a systematic review. Urol Int 2014;94(3):249–54.

[110] Bonvissuto G, Minutoli L, Morgia G, et al. Effect of *Serenoa repens*, lycopene, and selenium on proinflammatory phenotype activation: an in vitro and in vivo comparison study. Urology 2011;77(1):248.e9–e248.

[111] Minutoli L, Bitto A, Squadrito F, et al. *Serenoa repens*, lycopene and selenium: a triple therapeutic approach to manage benign prostatic hyperplasia. Curr Med Chem 2013;20(10):1306–12.

[112] Schwarz S, Obermüller-Jevic UC, Hellmis E, et al. Lycopene inhibits disease progression in patients with benign prostate hyperplasia. J Nutr 2008;138(1):49–53.

[113] Muti P, Awad AB, Schünemann H, et al. A plant food–based diet modifies the serum β-sitosterol concentration in hyperandrogenic postmenopausal women. J Nutr 2003;133(12):4252–5.

[114] Stanislavov R, Nikolova V. Treatment of erectile dysfunction with pycnogenol and L-arginine. J Sex Marital Ther 2003 Jan;29(3):207–13.

[115] Stanislavov R, Nikolova V, Rohdewald P. Improvement of erectile function with Prelox: a randomized, double-blind, placebo-controlled, crossover trial. Int J Impot Res 2008;20(2):173–80.

[116] Aoki H, Nagao J, Ueda T, et al. Clinical assessment of a supplement of Pycnogenol® and L-arginine in Japanese patients with mild to moderate erectile dysfunction: Pycnogenol® and L-arginine supplement for erectile dysfunction. Phytother Res 2012 Feb;26(2):204–7.

[117] Yagi H, Sato R, Nishio K, et al. Effects of a supplement combining Pycnogenol® and L-arginine aspartate on lower urinary dysfunction compared with saw palmetto extract. J Tradit Complement Med 2017;7(1):117–20.

[118] Shoskes DA, Zeitlin SI, Shahed A, et al. Quercetin in men with category III chronic prostatitis: a preliminary prospective, double-blind, placebo-controlled trial. Urology 1999;54(6):960–3.

[119] Ghorbanibirgani A. Efficacy of quercetin in treatment of benign prostatic hyperplasia in a double-blind randomized clinical trial in Iran — 2011. Contraception 2012;85(3):321.

[120] Zhang W, Zheng X, Wang Y, et al. Vitamin D deficiency as a potential marker of benign prostatic hyperplasia. Urology 2016 Nov;97:212–18.

[121] Colli E, Rigatti P, Montorsi F, et al. BXL628, a novel vitamin D_3 analog arrests prostate growth in patients with benign prostatic hyperplasia: a randomized clinical trial. Eur Urol 2006 Jan;49(1):82–6.

[122] Zhang X, Liu C, Guo J, et al. Selenium status and cardiovascular diseases: meta-analysis of prospective observational studies and randomized controlled trials. Eur J Clin Nutr 2016;70(2):162–9.

[123] Holick MF, Binkley NC, Bischoff-Ferrari HA, et al. Evaluation, treatment, and prevention of vitamin D deficiency: an Endocrine Society Clinical Practice Guideline. J Clin Endocrinol Metab 2011;96(7):1911–30.

[124] Scaglione F. How to choose the right *Serenoa repens* extract. Eur Urol Suppl 2015;14(9):e1464–9.

[125] Chrubasik JE, Roufogalis BD, Wagner H, et al. A comprehensive review on the stinging nettle effect and efficacy profiles. Part II: *Urticae radix*. Phytomedicine 2007;14(7–8):568–79.

[126] Edgar AD, Levin R, Constantinou CE, et al. A critical review of the pharmacology of the plant extract of *Pygeum africanum* in the treatment of LUTS. Neurourol Urodyn 2007;26(4):458–63.

[127] Cunningham AB, Tientcheu MLA, Anoncho VF, et al. Power, profits and policy: a reality check on the *Prunus africana* bark trade. CIFOR Working Paper no 2014;153.

[128] MacDonald R, Ishani A, Rutks I, et al. A systematic review of Cernilton for the treatment of benign prostatic hyperplasia. BJU Int 2000;85(7):836–41.

[129] Atawia RT, Tadros MG, Khalifa AE, et al. Role of the phytoestrogenic, pro-apoptotic and antioxidative properties of silymarin in inhibiting experimental benign prostatic hyperplasia in rats. Toxicol Lett 2013;219(2):160–9.

[130] Granica S, Piwowarski JP, Czerwińska ME, et al. Phytochemistry, pharmacology and traditional uses of different Epilobium species (Onagraceae): a review. J Ethnopharmacol 2014;156:316–46.

[131] Shamsa A, Hosseinzadeh H, Molaei M, et al. Evaluation of *Crocus sativus* L. (saffron) on male erectile dysfunction: a pilot study. Phytomedicine 2009;16(8):690–3.

[132] Hosseinzadeh H, Nassiri-Asl M. Avicenna's (Ibn Sina) the canon of medicine and saffron (*Crocus sativus*): a review. Phytother Res 2013;27(4):475–83.

[133] Kim SK, Seok H, Park HJ, et al. Inhibitory effect of curcumin on testosterone induced benign prostatic hyperplasia rat model. BMC Complement Altern Med 2015;15:380.

[134] Chen J, Song H. Protective potential of epigallocatechin-3-gallate against benign prostatic hyperplasia in metabolic syndrome rats. Environ Toxicol Pharmacol 2016;45:315–20.

[135] Li Y-F, Tang L-P, He R-R, et al. Anthocyanins extract from bilberry enhances the therapeutic effect of pollen of *Brassica napus* L. on stress-provoked benign prostatic hyperplasia in restrained mice. J Funct Foods 2013;5(3):1357–65.

[136] Lei Y, Liu D, Ren X, et al. Potential of grape seed-derived polyphenols extract for protection against testosterone-induced benign prostatic hyperplasia in castrated rats. RSC Adv 2014;4(108):62996–3004.

[137] Boyle P, Robertson C, Lowe F, et al. Updated meta-analysis of clinical trials of *Serenoa repens* extract in the treatment of symptomatic benign prostatic hyperplasia. BJU Int 2004;93(6):751–6.

[138] Tacklind J, MacDonald R, Rutks I, et al. *Serenoa repens* for benign prostatic hyperplasia. Cochrane Database Syst Rev 2009;(2):CD001423.

[139] Bent S, Kane C, Shinohara K, et al. Saw palmetto for benign prostatic hyperplasia. N Engl J Med 2006;354(6):557–66.

[140] Barry MJ, Meleth S, Lee JY, et al. Effect of increasing doses of saw palmetto extract on lower urinary tract symptoms. JAMA 2011;306(12):1344–51.

[141] Novara G, Giannarini G, Alcaraz A, et al. Efficacy and safety of hexanic lipidosterolic extract of *Serenoa repens* (Permixon) in the treatment of lower urinary tract symptoms due to benign prostatic hyperplasia: systematic review and meta-analysis of randomized controlled trials. Eur Urol Focus 2016;2(5): 553–61.

[142] Morgia G, Russo GI, Voce S, et al. *Serenoa repens*, lycopene and selenium versus tamsulosin for the treatment of LUTS/BPH. An Italian multicenter double-blinded randomized study between single or combination therapy (PROCOMB trial). Prostate 2014;74(15):1471–80.

[143] Morgia G, Cimino S, Favilla V, et al. Effects of *Serenoa repens*, selenium and lycopene (Profluss®) on chronic inflammation associated with benign prostatic hyperplasia: results of "FLOG" (flogosis and Profluss in prostatic and genital disease), a multicenter Italian study. Int Braz J Urol 2013;39(2):214–21.

[144] Morgia G, Mucciardi G, Galì A, et al. Treatment of chronic prostatitis/chronic pelvic pain syndrome category IIIA with *Serenoa repens* plus selenium and lycopene (Profluss®) versus *S. repens* alone: an Italian randomized multicenter-controlled study. Urol Int 2010;84(4):400–6.

[145] Wagenlehner FME, Bschleipfer T, Pilatz A, et al. Pollen extract for chronic prostatitis — chronic pelvic pain syndrome. Urol Clin North Am 2011;38(3):285–92.

[146] Qian X, Kong X, Qian Y, et al. Therapeutic efficacy of Cernilton in benign prostatic hyperplasia patients with histological prostatitis after transurethral resection of the prostate. Int J Clin Exp Med 2015;8(7):11268–75.

[147] Murakami M, Tsukada O, Okihara K, et al. Beneficial effect of honeybee-collected pollen lump extract on benign prostatic hyperplasia (BPH): a double-blind, placebo-controlled clinical trial. Food Sci Technol Res 2008;14(3):306–10.

[148] Safarinejad MR. *Urtica dioica* for treatment of benign prostatic hyperplasia: a prospective, randomized, double-blind, placebo-controlled, crossover study. J Herb Pharmacother 2005;5(4):1–11.

[149] Vostalova J, Vidlar A, Ulrichova J, et al. Use of selenium–silymarin mix reduces lower urinary tract symptoms and prostate specific antigen in men. Phytomedicine 2013;21(1):75–81.
[150] Atawia RT, Mosli HH, Tadros MG, et al. Modulatory effect of silymarin on inflammatory mediators in experimentally induced benign prostatic hyperplasia: emphasis on PTEN, HIF-1α, and NF-κB. Naunyn Schmiedebergs Arch Pharmacol 2014;387(12):1131–40.
[151] Vidlar A, Vostalova J, Ulrichova J, et al. The effectiveness of dried cranberries (*Vaccinium macrocarpon*) in men with lower urinary tract symptoms. Br J Nutr 2010;104(8):1181–9.
[152] Papaioannou M, Schleich S, Roell D, et al. NBBS isolated from *Pygeum africanum* bark exhibits androgen antagonistic activity, inhibits AR nuclear translocation and prostate cancer cell growth. Invest New Drugs 2010;28(6):729–43.
[153] Wilt TJ, Ishani A. *Pygeum africanum* for benign prostatic hyperplasia. Cochrane Database Syst Reviews 2002;(1):CD001044.
[154] Ingram VJ, van Loo J, Vinceti B, et al Ensuring the future of the pygeum tree (*Prunus africana*). Factsheet. LEI Wageningen UR; 2015. Available from: http://library.wur.nl/WebQuery/wurpubs/fulltext/342604.
[155] Maximillian JR, O'Laughlin J. Toward sustainable harvesting of Africa's largest medicinal plant export (*Prunus africana*): a case study in Tanzania. South For J For Sci 2009;71(4):303–9.
[156] Fowke JH, Phillips S, Koyama T, et al. Association between physical activity, lower urinary tract symptoms (LUTS) and prostate volume. BJU Int 2013;111(1):122–8.
[157] Wolin KY, Grubb RL, Pakpahan R, et al. Physical activity and benign prostatic hyperplasia-related outcomes and nocturia. Med Sci Sports Exerc 2015;47(3):581–92.
[158] Hou C-P, Chen T-Y, Chang C-C, et al. Use of the SF-36 quality of life scale to assess the effect of pelvic floor muscle exercise on aging males who received transurethral prostate surgery. Clin Interv Aging 2013;8:667–83.
[159] Burgio KL, Goode PS, Johnson TM, et al. Behavioral versus drug treatment for overactive bladder in men: the Male Overactive Bladder Treatment in Veterans (MOTIVE) Trial. J Am Geriatr Soc 2011;59(12):2209–16.
[160] Dorey G. Pelvic floor exercises after radical prostatectomy. Br J Nurs 2013;22(9):S4–9.
[161] Luzzi G. Prostatitis and male chronic pelvic pain. Medicine (Baltimore) 2010;38(6):314–17.
[162] Nickel C. Inflammatory and pain conditions of the male genitourinary tract: prostatitis and related pain conditions, orchitis, and epididymitis. In: Wein W, Kavoussi L, Partin A, editors. Campbell-Walsh urology. 11th ed. Philadelphia: Elsevier; 2016.
[163] Krieger JN, Nyberg L, Nickel JC. NIH consensus definition and classification of prostatitis. JAMA 1999;281(3):236–7.
[164] Yoon BI, Kim S, Han D-S, et al. Acute bacterial prostatitis: how to prevent and manage chronic infection? J Infect Chemother 2012;18(4):444–50.
[165] Wagenlehner FME, Weidner W, Pilatz A, et al. Urinary tract infections and bacterial prostatitis in men. Curr Opin Infect Dis 2014;27(1):97–101.
[166] Gill BC, Shoskes DA. Bacterial prostatitis. Curr Opin Infect Dis 2016;29(1):86–91.
[167] Deem S, Piesman M, Costabile R. Acute bacterial prostatitis: background, pathophysiology, etiology. Medscape 2015. Available from: http://emedicine.medscape.com/article/2002872-overview #showall.
[168] Wagenlehner FME, Pilatz A, Bschleipfer T, et al. Bacterial prostatitis. World J Urol 2013;31(4):711–16.
[169] Ahuja S, Mobley J. Chronic bacterial prostatitis. Medscape 2016. Available from: http://emedicine.medscape.com/article/458391-overview#showall.
[170] Polackwich A, Shoskes D. Chronic prostatitis/chronic pelvic pain syndrome: a review of evaluation and therapy. Prostate Cancer Prostate Dis 2016;19:132–8.
[171] True LD, Berger RE, Rothman I, et al. Prostate histopathology and the chronic prostatitis/chronic pelvic pain syndrome: a prospective biopsy study. J Urol 1999;162(6):2014–18.
[172] Schaeffer AJ, Knauss JS, Landis JR, et al. Leukocyte and bacterial counts do not correlate with severity of symptoms in men with chronic prostatitis: the National Institutes of Health Chronic Prostatitis Cohort Study. J Urol 2002;168(3):1048–53.
[173] Pontari MA, Ruggieri MR. Mechanisms in prostatitis/chronic pelvic pain syndrome. J Urol 2004;172(3):839–45.
[174] Pontari MA. Etiology of chronic prostatitis/chronic pelvic pain syndrome: psychoimmunoneurendocrine dysfunction (PINE syndrome) or just a really bad infection? World J Urol 2013;31(4):725–32.
[175] Penna G, Fibbi B, Maggi M, et al. Prostate autoimmunity: from experimental models to clinical counterparts. Expert Rev Clin Immunol 2009;5(5):577–86.
[176] Badalyan RR, Fanarjyan SV, Aghajanyan IG. Chlamydial and ureaplasmal infections in patients with nonbacterial chronic prostatitis. Andrologia 2003;35(5):263–5.
[177] Perletti G, Marras E, Wagenlehner FM, et al. Antimicrobial therapy for chronic bacterial prostatitis. Cochrane Database Syst Reviews 2013;(8):CD009071.
[178] Liu L, Yang J, Lu F. Urethral dysbacteriosis as an underlying, primary cause of chronic prostatitis: Potential implications for probiotic therapy. Med Hypotheses 2009;73(5):741–3.
[179] Mändar R. Microbiota of male genital tract: Impact on the health of man and his partner. Pharmacol Res 2013;69(1):32–41.
[180] Shoskes DA, Altemus J, Polackwich AS, et al. The urinary microbiome differs significantly between patients with chronic prostatitis/chronic pelvic pain syndrome and controls as well as between patients with different clinical phenotypes. Urology 2016;92:26–32.
[181] Ivanov IB, Kuzmin MD, Gritsenko VA. Microflora of the seminal fluid of healthy men and men suffering from chronic prostatitis syndrome. Int J Androl 2009;32(5):462–7.
[182] Ivanov IB, Gritsenko VA, Kuzmin MD, et al. Phenotypic differences between coryneform bacteria isolated from seminal fluid of healthy men and men with chronic prostatitis syndrome. Asian J Androl 2009;11(4):517–20.
[183] Shoskes DA, Wang H, Polackwich AS, et al. Analysis of gut microbiome reveals significant differences between men with chronic prostatitis/chronic pelvic pain syndrome and controls. J Urol 2016;196(2):435–41.
[184] Woolf CJ. Central sensitization: Implications for the diagnosis and treatment of pain. Pain 2011;152(Suppl.):S2–15.
[185] Davis SNP, Maykut CA, Binik YM, et al. Tenderness as measured by pressure pain thresholds extends beyond the pelvis in chronic pelvic pain syndrome in men. J Sex Med 2011;8(1):232–9.
[186] Hetrick DC, Ciol MA, Rothman I, et al. Musculoskeletal dysfunction in men with chronic pelvic pain syndrome type III: a case-control study. J Urol 2003;170(3):828–31.
[187] Zermann D-H, Ishigooka M, Doggweiler R, et al. Neurourological insights into the etiology of genitourinary pain in men. J Urol 1999;161(3):903–8.
[188] Khorasani B, Arab AM, Sedighi Gilani MA, et al. Transabdominal ultrasound measurement of pelvic floor muscle mobility in men with and without chronic prostatitis/chronic pelvic pain syndrome. Urology 2012;80(3):673–7.
[189] Anderson RU, Sawyer T, Wise D, et al. Painful myofascial trigger points and pain sites in men with chronic prostatitis/chronic pelvic pain syndrome. J Urol 2009;182(6):2753–8.
[190] Shoskes DA, Lee C-T, Murphy D, et al. Incidence and significance of prostatic stones in men with chronic prostatitis/chronic pelvic pain syndrome. Urology 2007;70(2):235–8.
[191] Riegel B, Bruenahl CA, Ahyai S, et al. Assessing psychological factors, social aspects and psychiatric co-morbidity associated with chronic prostatitis/chronic pelvic pain syndrome (CP/CPPS) in men — a systematic review. J Psychosom Res 2014;77(5):333–50.
[192] Samplaski MK, Li J, Shoskes DA. Clustering of UPOINT domains and subdomains in men with chronic prostatitis/chronic pelvic pain syndrome and contribution to symptom severity. J Urol 2012;188(5):1788–93.
[193] Clemens JQ, Brown SO, Calhoun EA. Mental health diagnoses in patients with interstitial cystitis/painful bladder syndrome and chronic prostatitis/chronic pelvic pain syndrome: a case/control study. J Urol 2008;180(4):1378–82.
[194] Chung S-D, Lin H-C. Association between chronic prostatitis/chronic pelvic pain syndrome and anxiety disorder: a population-based study. PLoS ONE 2013;8(5):e64630.

[195] Clemens JQ, Brown SO, Kozloff L, et al. Predictors of symptom severity in patients with chronic prostatitis and interstitial cystitis. J Urol 2006;175(3):963–7.
[196] Tripp DA, Curtis Nickel J, Landis JR, et al. Predictors of quality of life and pain in chronic prostatitis/chronic pelvic pain syndrome: findings from the National Institutes of Health Chronic Prostatitis Cohort Study. BJU Int 2004;94(9):1279–82.
[197] Ginting JV, Tripp DA, Nickel JC. Self-reported spousal support modifies the negative impact of pain on disability in men with chronic prostatitis/chronic pelvic pain syndrome. Urology 2011;78(5):1136–41.
[198] Liao C-H, Lin H-C, Huang C-Y. Chronic prostatitis/chronic pelvic pain syndrome is associated with irritable bowel syndrome: a population-based study. Sci Rep 2016;6:26939.
[199] Rodríguez MÁB, Afari N, Buchwald DS. Evidence for overlap between urological and nonurological unexplained clinical conditions. J Urol 2009;182(5):2123–31.
[200] Alshahrani S, McGill J, Agarwal A. Prostatitis and male infertility. J Reprod Immunol 2013;100(1):30–6.
[201] Jiang J, Li J, Yunxia Z, et al. The role of prostatitis in prostate cancer: meta-analysis. PLoS ONE 2013;8(12):e85179.
[202] Vaarala M, Mehik A, Ohtonen P, et al. Prostate cancer incidence in men with self-reported prostatitis after 15 years of follow-up. Oncol Lett 2016;12(2):1149–53.
[203] Pontari MA, McNaughton-Collins M, O'Leary MP, et al. A case-control study of risk factors in men with chronic pelvic pain syndrome. BJU Int 2005;96(4):559–65.
[204] Chen H-M, Lin C-C, Kang C-S, et al. Bladder pain syndrome/interstitial cystitis increase the risk of coronary heart disease: interstitial cystitis and cardiovascular disease. Neurourol Urodyn 2014;33(5):511–15.
[205] Shoskes DA, Prots D, Karns J, et al. Greater endothelial dysfunction and arterial stiffness in men with chronic prostatitis/chronic pelvic pain syndrome — a possible link to cardiovascular disease. J Urol 2011;186(3):907–10.
[206] Wagenlehner FME, van Till JWO, Magri V, et al. National Institutes of Health Chronic Prostatitis Symptom Index (NIH-CPSI) symptom evaluation in multinational cohorts of patients with chronic prostatitis/chronic pelvic pain syndrome. Eur Urol 2013;63(5):953–9.
[207] Pavone-Macaluso M. Chronic prostatitis syndrome: a common, but poorly understood condition. Part I. EAU-EBU Update Ser 2007;5(1):1–15.
[208] Mykletun A, Dahl AA, O'Leary MP, et al. Assessment of male sexual function by the Brief Sexual Function Inventory. BJU Int 2006;97(2):316–23.
[209] Magistro G, Wagenlehner FME, Grabe M, et al. Contemporary management of chronic prostatitis/chronic pelvic pain syndrome. Eur Urol 2016;69(2):286–97.
[210] Watson RA. Chronic pelvic pain in men differential diagnoses. Medscape 2016. Available from: http://emedicine.medscape.com/article/437745-differential.
[211] Nickel JC, Shoskes DA, Wagenlehner FME. Management of chronic prostatitis/chronic pelvic pain syndrome (CP/CPPS): the studies, the evidence, and the impact. World J Urol 2013;31(4):747–53.
[212] Nickel JC, Xiang J. Clinical significance of nontraditional bacterial uropathogens in the management of chronic prostatitis. J Urol 2008;179(4):1391–5.
[213] Szajewska H, Kołodziej M. Systematic review with meta-analysis: *Lactobacillus rhamnosus* GG in the prevention of antibiotic-associated diarrhoea in children and adults. Aliment Pharmacol Ther 2015;42(10):1149–57.
[214] Cai T, Mazzoli S, Bechi A, et al. *Serenoa repens* associated with *Urtica dioica* (ProstaMEV®) and curcumin and quercitin (FlogMEV®) extracts are able to improve the efficacy of prulifloxacin in bacterial prostatitis patients: results from a prospective randomised study. Int J Antimicrob Agents 2009;33(6):549–53.
[215] Busetto GM, Giovannone R, Ferro M, et al. Chronic bacterial prostatitis: efficacy of short-lasting antibiotic therapy with prulifloxacin (Unidrox®) in association with saw palmetto extract, *Lactobacillus sporogenes* and arbutin (Lactorepens®). BMC Urol 2014;14(1):1.
[216] Sohn DW, Han CH, Jung YS, et al. Anti-inflammatory and antimicrobial effects of garlic and synergistic effect between garlic and ciprofloxacin in a chronic bacterial prostatitis rat model. Int J Antimicrob Agents 2009;34(3):215–19.
[217] Shoskes DA, Nickel JC, Kattan MW. Phenotypically directed multimodal therapy for chronic prostatitis/chronic pelvic pain syndrome: a prospective study using UPOINT. Urology 2010;75(6):1249–53.
[218] Shoskes DA, Nickel JC. Classification and treatment of men with chronic prostatitis/chronic pelvic pain syndrome using the UPOINT system. World J Urol 2013;31(4):755–60.
[219] Magri V, Wagenlehner F, Perletti G, et al. Use of the UPOINT chronic prostatitis/chronic pelvic pain syndrome classification in European patient cohorts: sexual function domain improves correlations. J Urol 2010;184(6):2339–45.
[220] Samplaski MK, Li J, Shoskes DA. Inclusion of erectile domain to UPOINT phenotype does not improve correlation with symptom severity in men with chronic prostatitis/chronic pelvic pain syndrome. Urology 2011;78(3):653–8.
[221] Gallo L. Effectiveness of diet, sexual habits and lifestyle modifications on treatment of chronic pelvic pain syndrome. Prostate Cancer Prostatic Dis 2014;17(3):238–45.
[222] Tuohy KM, Conterno L, Gasperotti M, et al. Up-regulating the human intestinal microbiome using whole plant foods, polyphenols, and/or fiber. J Agric Food Chem 2012;60(36):8776–82.
[223] Cui D, Han G, Shang Y, et al. The effect of chronic prostatitis on zinc concentration of prostatic fluid and seminal plasma: a systematic review and meta-analysis. Curr Med Res Opin 2015;31(9):1763–9.
[224] Deng C, Zheng B, She S. Clinical study of zinc for the treatment of chronic bacterial prostatitis. Zhonghua Nan Ke Xue 2004;10(5):368–70.
[225] Goodarzi D, Cyrus A. Baghinia MR. The efficacy of zinc for treatment of chronic prostatitis. Acta Med Indones 2013;45(4):259–64.
[226] Lee LK, Foo KY. An appraisal of the therapeutic value of lycopene for the chemoprevention of prostate cancer: A nutrigenomic approach. Food Res Int 2013;54(1):1217–28.
[227] Han CH, Yang CH, Sohn DW, et al. Synergistic effect between lycopene and ciprofloxacin on a chronic bacterial prostatitis rat model. Int J Antimicrob Agents 2008;31:102–7.
[228] Herati AS, Shorter B, Srinivasan AK, et al. Effects of foods and beverages on the symptoms of chronic prostatitis/chronic pelvic pain syndrome. Urology 2013;82(6):1376–80.
[229] Shoskes DA, Nickel JC. Quercetin for chronic prostatitis/chronic pelvic pain syndrome. Urol Clin North Am 2011;38(3):279–84.
[230] Kullisaar T, Türk S, Punab M, et al. Oxidative stress in leucocytospermic prostatitis patients: preliminary results. Andrologia 2008;40(3):161–72.
[231] Arisan ED, Arisan S, Kiremit MC, et al. Manganase superoxide dismutase polymorphism in chronic pelvic pain syndrome patients. Prostate Cancer Prostatic Dis 2006;9(4):426–31.
[232] Zhou J-F, Xiao W-Q, Zheng Y-C, et al. Increased oxidative stress and oxidative damage associated with chronic bacterial prostatitis. Asian J Androl 2006;8(3):317–23.
[233] Lombardo F, Fiducia M, Lunghi R, et al. Effects of a dietary supplement on chronic pelvic pain syndrome (Category IIIA), leucocytospermia and semen parameters: dietary supplement and CPPS. Andrologia 2012;44:672–8.
[234] Wagenlehner FME, Schneider H, Ludwig M, et al. A pollen extract (Cernilton) in patients with inflammatory chronic prostatitis–chronic pelvic pain syndrome: a multicentre, randomised, prospective, double-blind, placebo-controlled phase 3 study. Eur Urol 2009;56(3):544–51.
[235] Kim HW, Ha U-S, Woo JC, et al. Preventive effect of selenium on chronic bacterial prostatitis. J Infect Chemother 2012;18(1):30–4.
[236] Williamson E. Major herbs of Ayurveda. Edinburgh: Churchill Livingston; 2002. p. 190–5, 321–5.
[237] Shukla KK, Mahdi AA, Ahmad MK, et al. *Mucuna pruriens* reduces stress and improves the quality of semen in infertile men. Evid Based Complement Alternat Med 2010;7(1):137–44.
[238] Robert GY. Comparison of the effects of hexanic extract of *Serenoa repens* (Permixon) and tamsulosin on inflammatory biomarkers in

the treatment of benign prostatic hyperplasia-related lower urinary tract symptoms. Eur Urol Suppl 2015;14(9):e1470–4.
[239] Reissigl A, Pointner J, Marberger J, et al. Safety and efficacy of phytotherapy in the treatment of chronic prostatitis/chronic pelvic pain syndrome: results of the prospective placebo-controlled multicentre Austrian trial. Eur Urol Suppl 2004;3(2):89.
[240] Kaplan SA, Volpe MA, Te AE. A prospective, 1-year trial using saw palmetto versus finasteride in the treatment of category III prostatitis/chronic pelvic pain syndrome. J Urol 2004;171(1):284–8.
[241] Elist J. Effects of pollen extract preparation Prostat/Poltit on lower urinary tract symptoms in patients with chronic nonbacterial prostatitis/chronic pelvic pain syndrome: a randomized, double-blind, placebo-controlled study. Urology 2006;67(1):60–3.
[242] Cai T, Wagenlehner F, Luciani L, et al. Pollen extract in association with vitamins provides early pain relief in patients affected by chronic prostatitis/chronic pelvic pain syndrome. Exp Ther Med 2014;8(4):1032–8.
[243] Cai T, Luciani LG, Caola I, et al. Effects of pollen extract in association with vitamins (DEPROX 500®) for pain relief in patients affected by chronic prostatitis/chronic pelvic pain syndrome: results from a pilot study. Riv Urol 2013;80(Suppl. 22):5–10.
[244] Zhang R, Chomistek AK, Dimitrakoff JD, et al. Physical activity and chronic prostatitis/chronic pelvic pain syndrome. Med Sci Sports Exerc 2015;47(4):757–64.
[245] Giubilei G, Mondaini N, Minervini A, et al. Physical activity of men with chronic prostatitis/chronic pelvic pain syndrome not satisfied with conventional treatments — could it represent a valid option? The Physical Activity and Male Pelvic Pain Trial: a double-blind, randomized study. J Urol 2007;177(1):159–65.
[246] Cornel EB, van Haarst EP, Schaarsberg RWMB-G, et al. The effect of biofeedback physical therapy in men with chronic pelvic pain syndrome type III. Eur Urol 2005;47(5):607–11.
[247] FitzGerald MP, Anderson RU, Potts J, et al. Randomized multicenter feasibility trial of myofascial physical therapy for the treatment of urological chronic pelvic pain syndromes. J Urol 2009;182(2):570–80.
[248] Anderson RU, Wise D, Sawyer T, et al. 6-day intensive treatment protocol for refractory chronic prostatitis/chronic pelvic pain syndrome using myofascial release and paradoxical relaxation training. J Urol 2011;185(4):1294–9.
[249] Anderson RU, Wise D, Sawyer T, et al. Sexual dysfunction in men with chronic prostatitis/chronic pelvic pain syndrome: improvement after trigger point release and paradoxical relaxation training. J Urol 2006;176(4):1534–9.
[250] Bella AJ, Lee JC, Carrier S, et al. 2015 CUA practice guidelines for erectile dysfunction. Can Urol Assoc J 2015;9(1–2):23–9.
[251] DeRogatis LR, Burnett AL. The epidemiology of sexual dysfunctions. J Sex Med 2008;5(2):289–300.
[252] Lewis RW, Fugl-Meyer KS, Corona G, et al. Definitions/epidemiology/risk factors for sexual dysfunction. J Sex Med 2010;7(4):1598–607.
[253] Aytac IA, McKinlay JB, Krane RJ, et al. The likely worldwide increase in erectile dysfunction between 1995 and 2025 and some possible policy consequences. BJU Int 1999;84:50–6.
[254] Lue TF. Physiology of penile erection and pathophysiology of erectile dysfunction. In: Wein W, Kavoussi L, Partin A, editors. Campbell-Walsh urology. 11th ed. Philadelphia: Elsevier; 2016. p. 612–42.
[255] Lizza E, Rosen R. Definition and classification of erectile dysfunction: Report of the Nomenclature Committee of the International Society of Impotence Research. Int J Impot Res 1999;11:141–3.
[256] Huang S-S, Lin C-H, Chan C-H, et al. Newly diagnosed major depressive disorder and the risk of erectile dysfunction: a population-based cohort study in Taiwan. Psychiatry Res 2013 Dec;210(2):601–6.
[257] Mills JN, Dall'Era JE, Carlsen SN, et al. Gene therapy for erectile dysfunction. Pharmacogenomics 2007;8(8):979–84.
[258] Gandaglia G, Briganti A, Jackson G, et al. A systematic review of the association between erectile dysfunction and cardiovascular disease. Eur Urol 2014;65(5):968–78.
[259] Linsenmeyer TA. Treatment of erectile dysfunction following spinal cord injury. Curr Urol Rep 2009;10(6):478–84.
[260] Defeudis G, Gianfrilli D, Di Emidio C, et al. Erectile dysfunction and its management in patients with diabetes mellitus. Rev Endocr Metab Disord 2015;16(3):213–31.
[261] Rastrelli G, Corona G, Tarocchi M, et al. How to define hypogonadism? Results from a population of men consulting for sexual dysfunction. J Endocrinol Invest 2016;39(4):473–84.
[262] Shiri R, Koskimäki J, Tammela TLJ, et al. Bidirectional relationship between depression and erectile dysfunction. J Urol 2007;177(2):669–73.
[263] Chou P, Chou W, Chen M, et al. Newly diagnosed erectile dysfunction and risk of depression: a population-based 5-year follow-up study in Taiwan. J Sex Med 2015;12(3):804–12.
[264] Corona G, Lee DM, Forti G, et al. Age-related changes in general and sexual health in middle-aged and older men: results from the European Male Ageing Study (EMAS). J Sex Med 2010;7(4):1362–80.
[265] Albersen M, Orabi H, Lue TF. Evaluation and treatment of erectile dysfunction in the aging male: a mini-review. Gerontology 2012;58(1):3–14.
[266] Wespes E. Erectile dysfunction in the ageing male. Curr Opin Urol 2000;10(6):625–8.
[267] Buvat J, Maggi M, Guay A, et al. Testosterone deficiency in men: systematic review and standard operating procedures for diagnosis and treatment. J Sex Med 2013;10(1):245–84.
[268] Johannes CB, Araujo AB, Feldman HA, et al. Incidence of erectile dysfunction in men 40 to 69 years old: longitudinal results from the Massachusetts male aging study. J Urol 2000;163(2):460–3.
[269] Skeldon SC, Detsky AS, Goldenberg SL, et al. Erectile dysfunction and undiagnosed diabetes, hypertension, and hypercholesterolemia. Ann Fam Med 2015;13(4):331–5.
[270] Kalter-Leibovici O, Wainstein J, Ziv A, et al. Clinical, socioeconomic, and lifestyle parameters associated with erectile dysfunction among diabetic men. Diabetes Care 2005;28(7):1739–44.
[271] Garimella PS, Paudel ML, Ensrud KE, et al. Association between body size and composition and erectile dysfunction in older men: Osteoporotic Fractures in Men Study. J Am Geriatr Soc 2013;61(1):46–54.
[272] Vlachopoulos CV, Terentes-Printzios DG, Ioakeimidis NK, et al. Prediction of cardiovascular events and all-cause mortality with erectile dysfunction a systematic review and meta-analysis of cohort studies. Circ Cardiovasc Qual Outcomes 2013;6(1):99–109.
[273] Montorsi P, Ravagnani PM, Galli S, et al. Association between erectile dysfunction and coronary artery disease. Role of coronary clinical presentation and extent of coronary vessels involvement: the COBRA trial. Eur Heart J 2006;27(22):2632–9.
[274] Besiroglu H, Otunctemur A, Ozbek E. The relationship between metabolic syndrome, its components, and erectile dysfunction: a systematic review and a meta-analysis of observational studies. J Sex Med 2015;12(6):1309–18.
[275] Fung MM, Bettencourt R, Barrett-Connor E. Heart disease risk factors predict erectile dysfunction 25 years later. J Am Coll Cardiol 2004;43(8):1405–11.
[276] Corona G, Bianchini S, Sforza A, et al. Hypogonadism as a possible link between metabolic diseases and erectile dysfunction in aging men. Horm Athens Greece 2015;14(4):569–78.
[277] Zohdy W, Kamal EE, Ibrahim Y. Androgen deficiency and abnormal penile duplex parameters in obese men with erectile dysfunction. J Sex Med 2011;4(3):797–808.
[278] Corona G, Rastrelli G, Filippi S, et al. Erectile dysfunction and central obesity: an Italian perspective. Asian J Androl 2014;16(4):581.
[279] Kaya E, Sikka SC, Gur S. A comprehensive review of metabolic syndrome affecting erectile dysfunction. J Sex Med 2015;12(4):856–75.
[280] Cao S, Yin X, Wang Y, et al. Smoking and risk of erectile dysfunction: systematic review of observational studies with meta-analysis. PLoS ONE 2013;8(4):e60443.
[281] Cao S, Gan Y, Dong X, et al. Association of quantity and duration of smoking with erectile dysfunction: a dose–response meta-analysis. J Sex Med 2014;11(10):2376–84.
[282] Kovac JR, Labbate C, Ramasamy R, et al. Effects of cigarette smoking on erectile dysfunction. Andrologia 2015;47(10):1087–92.

[283] Salonia A, Castagna G, Capogrosso P, et al. Prevention and management of post prostatectomy erectile dysfunction. Transl Androl Urol 2015;4(4):421–37.
[284] Koehler N, Holze S, Gansera L, et al. Erectile dysfunction after radical prostatectomy: the impact of nerve-sparing status and surgical approach. Int J Impot Res 2012;24(4):155–60.
[285] Incrocci L, Jensen PT. Pelvic radiotherapy and sexual function in men and women. J Sex Med 2013;10:53–64.
[286] Del Campo ER, Thomas K, Weinberg V, et al. Erectile dysfunction after radiotherapy for prostate cancer: a model assessing the conflicting literature on dose–volume effects. Int J Impot Res 2013;25(5):161–5.
[287] Wang Y, Liu T, Rossi PJ, et al. Influence of vascular comorbidities and race on erectile dysfunction after prostate cancer radiotherapy. J Sex Med 2013;10(8):2108–14.
[288] Cornu J-N, Ahyai S, Bachmann A, et al. A systematic review and meta-analysis of functional outcomes and complications following transurethral procedures for lower urinary tract symptoms resulting from benign prostatic obstruction: an update. Eur Urol 2015;67(6):1066–96.
[289] Sommer F, Goldstein I, Korda JB. Bicycle riding and erectile dysfunction: a review. J Sex Med 2010;7(7):2346–58.
[290] Michiels M, Van der Aa F. Bicycle riding and the bedroom: can riding a bicycle cause erectile dysfunction? Urology 2015;85(4):725–30.
[291] Chung E, De Young L, Brock GB. Penile duplex ultrasonography in men with Peyronie's disease: is it veno-occlusive dysfunction or poor cavernosal arterial inflow that contributes to erectile dysfunction? J Sex Med 2011;8(12):3446–51.
[292] Miner MM, Seftel AD. Peyronie's disease: epidemiology, diagnosis, and management. Curr Med Res Opin 2014;30(1):113–20.
[293] Nehra A, Alterowitz R, Culkin DJ, et al. Peyronie's disease: AUA guideline. J Urol 2015;194(3):745–53.
[294] Langston JP, Carson CC. Peyronie's disease: review and recent advances. Maturitas 2014;78(4):341–3.
[295] Ventimiglia E, Capogrosso P, Colicchia M, et al. Peyronie's disease and autoimmunity — a real-life clinical study and comprehensive review. J Sex Med 2015;12(4):1062–9.
[296] Al-Qudah HS, Parraga-Marquez M. Priapism: Practice essentials, background, pathophysiology. Medscape 2016. Available from: http://emedicine.medscape.com/article/437237-overview.
[297] Cirino G, Fusco F, Imbimbo C, et al. Pharmacology of erectile dysfunction in man. Pharmacol Ther 2006;111(2): 400–23.
[298] Burnett AL II. Evaluation and management of erectile dysfunction. In: Wein W, Kavoussi L, Partin A, editors. Campbell-Walsh urology. 11th ed. Elsevier; 2016. p. 643–68.
[299] McCabe MP, Connaughton C. Psychosocial factors associated with male sexual difficulties. J Sex Res 2014;51(1):31–42.
[300] Kim ED, Brosman SA Erectile dysfunction differential diagnoses Medscape 2016. Available from: http://emedicine.medscape.com/article/444220-differential.
[301] Karadag F, Ozcan H, Karul AB, et al. Correlates of erectile dysfunction in moderate-to-severe chronic obstructive pulmonary disease patients. Respirology 2007;12(2):248–53.
[302] Taken K, Ekin S, Arısoy A, et al. Erectile dysfunction is a marker for obstructive sleep apnea. Aging Male 2016;19(2):102–5.
[303] Corona G, Rastrelli G, Maggi M. Diagnosis and treatment of late-onset hypogonadism: systematic review and meta-analysis of TRT outcomes. Best Pract Res Clin Endocrinol Metab 2013;27(4):557–79.
[304] Tiefer L, Schuetz-Mueller D. Psychological issues in diagnosis and treatment of erectile disorders. Urol Clin North Am 1995;22(4):267–73.
[305] Cohen SD. The challenge of erectile dysfunction management in the young man. Curr Urol Rep 2015;16(12):84.
[306] Wespes E, Amar E, Hatzichristou D, et al. EAU Guidelines on erectile dysfunction: an update. Eur Urol 2006;49(5):806–15.
[307] Dorey G. Restoring pelvic floor function in men: review of RCTs. Br J Nurs 2005;14(19):1014–18, 1020–1021.
[308] Burnett AL. Erectile dysfunction. J Urol 2006;175(3):S25–31.
[309] Morales A, Bebb RA, Manjoo P, et al. Diagnosis and management of testosterone deficiency syndrome in men: clinical practice guideline. Can Med Assoc J 2015;187(18):1369–77.
[310] Lennartsson A-K, Kushnir MM, Bergquist J, et al. DHEA and DHEA-S response to acute psychosocial stress in healthy men and women. Biol Psychol 2012;90(2):143–9.
[311] An K, Salyer J, Brown RE, et al. Salivary biomarkers of chronic psychosocial stress and CVD risks: a systematic review. Biol Res Nurs 2016;18(3):241–63.
[312] Kramer H, Sprenger J Malleus Maleficarum. 1487. Translated by Summer M, p. 86. Available from: www.malleusmaleficarum.org.
[313] Madani AH, Asadolahzade A, Mokhtari G, et al. Assessment of the efficacy of combination therapy with folic acid and tadalafil for the management of erectile dysfunction in men with type 2 diabetes mellitus. J Sex Med 2013;10(4):1146–50.
[314] Hackett G, Cole N, Bhartia M, et al. Testosterone replacement therapy with long-acting testosterone undecanoate improves sexual function and quality-of-life parameters vs. placebo in a population of men with type 2 diabetes. J Sex Med 2013;10(6):1612–27.
[315] Jones TH, Arver S, Behre HM, et al. Testosterone replacement in hypogonadal men with type 2 diabetes and/or metabolic syndrome (the TIMES2 study). Diabetes Care 2011;34(4):828–37.
[316] Muraleedharan V, Marsh H, Kapoor D, et al. Testosterone deficiency is associated with increased risk of mortality and testosterone replacement improves survival in men with type 2 diabetes. Eur J Endocrinol 2013;169(6):725–33.
[317] Dimopoulou C, Ceausu I, Depypere H, et al. EMAS position statement: testosterone replacement therapy in the aging male. Maturitas 2016;84:94–9.
[318] Hatzimouratidis K, Amar E, Eardley I, et al. Guidelines on male sexual dysfunction: erectile dysfunction and premature ejaculation. Eur Urol 2010;57(5):804–14.
[319] Meldrum DR, Gambone JC, Morris MA, et al. The link between erectile and cardiovascular health: the canary in the coal mine. Am J Cardiol 2011;108(4):599–606.
[320] Esposito K, Giugliano F, De Sio M, et al. Dietary factors in erectile dysfunction. Int J Impot Res 2006;18(4):370–4.
[321] Esposito K, Ciotola M, Giugliano F, et al. Effects of intensive lifestyle changes on erectile dysfunction in men. J Sex Med 2009;6(1):243–50.
[322] Wang Q, Xia W, Zhao Z, et al. Effects comparison between low glycemic index diets and high glycemic index diets on HbA1c and fructosamine for patients with diabetes: a systematic review and meta-analysis. Prim Care Diabetes 2015;9(5):362–9.
[323] Juanola-Falgarona M, Salas-Salvado J, Ibarrola-Jurado N, et al. Effect of the glycemic index of the diet on weight loss, modulation of satiety, inflammation, and other metabolic risk factors: a randomized controlled trial. Am J Clin Nutr 2014;100(1): 27–35.
[324] Grosso G, Yang J, Marventano S, et al. Nut consumption on all-cause, cardiovascular, and cancer mortality risk: a systematic review and meta-analysis of epidemiologic studies. Am J Clin Nutr 2015;101(4):783–93.
[325] Aldemir M, Okulu E, Neselioglu S, et al. Pistachio diet improves erectile function parameters and serum lipid profiles in patients with erectile dysfunction. Int J Impot Res 2011;23:32–8.
[326] Cheng JYW, Ng EML, Chen RYL, et al. Alcohol consumption and erectile dysfunction: meta-analysis of population-based studies. Int J Impot Res 2007;19(4):343–52.
[327] Lee A, Ho L, Yip A, et al. The effect of alcohol drinking on erectile dysfunction in Chinese men. Int J Impot Res 2010;22:272–8.
[328] Mak R, De Backer G, Kornitzer M, et al. Prevalence and correlates of erectile dysfunction in a population-based study in Belgium. Eur Urol 2002;41(2):132–8.
[329] Chen J, Wollman Y, Chernichovsky T, et al. Effect of oral administration of high-dose nitric oxide donor L-arginine in men with organic erectile dysfunction: results of a double-blind, randomized, placebo-controlled study. BJU Int 1999;83:269–73.
[330] Klotz T, Mathers M, Braun M, et al. Effectiveness of oral L-arginine in first-line treatment of erectile dysfunction in a controlled crossover study. Urol Int 1999;63(4):220–3.
[331] Young L, Yu D, Bateman RM, et al. Oxidative stress and antioxidant therapy: their impact in diabetes-associated erectile dysfunction. J Androl 2004;25(5):830–6.
[332] Ushiyama M, Kuramochi T, Yagi S, et al. Antioxidant treatment with alpha-tocopherol improves erectile function in hypertensive rats. Hypertens Res 2008;31(5):1007–13.

[333] Helmy MM, Senbel AM. Evaluation of vitamin E in the treatment of erectile dysfunction in aged rats. Life Sci 2012 Apr;90(13–14):489–94.
[334] Kondoh N, Higuchi Y, Maruyama T, et al. Salvage therapy trial for erectile dysfunction using phosphodiesterase type 5 inhibitors and vitamin E: Preliminary report. Aging Male 2008;11(4):167–70.
[335] Lombardo F, Tsamatropoulos P, Piroli E, et al. Treatment of erectile dysfunction due to C677T mutation of the MTHFR gene with vitamin B_6 and folic acid in patients non responders to PDE5i. J Sex Med 2010;7(1):216–23.
[336] Agostini R, Rossi F, Pajalich R. Myoinositol/folic acid combination for the treatment of erectile dysfunction in type 2 diabetes men: a double-blind, randomized, placebo-controlled study. Eur Rev Med Pharmacol Sci 2006;10(5):247.
[337] Ng C, Lee C, Ho AL, et al. Effect of niacin on erectile function in men suffering erectile dysfunction and dyslipidemia. J Sex Med 2011;8(10):2883–93.
[338] Gentile V, Antonini G, Antonella Bertozzi M, et al. Effect of propionyl-L-carnitine, L-arginine and nicotinic acid on the efficacy of vardenafil in the treatment of erectile dysfunction in diabetes. Curr Med Res Opin 2009;25(9):2223–8.
[339] Gianfrilli D, Lauretta R, Di Dato C, et al. Propionyl-L-carnitine, L-arginine and niacin in sexual medicine: a nutraceutical approach to erectile dysfunction. Andrologia 2012;44:600–4.
[340] Vicari E, La Vignera S, Condorelli R, et al. Endothelial antioxidant administration ameliorates the erectile response to PDE5 regardless of the extension of the atherosclerotic process. J Sex Med 2010;7(3):1247–53.
[341] Miles C, Candy B, Jones L, et al. Interventions for sexual dysfunction following treatments for cancer. Cochrane Database Syst Rev 2007;(4):CD005540.
[342] Safarinejad M. Safety and efficacy of coenzyme Q10 supplementation in early chronic Peyronie's disease: a double-blind, placebo-controlled randomized study. Int J Impot Res 2010;22:298–309.
[343] Gao L, Mao Q, Cao J, et al. Effects of coenzyme Q10 on vascular endothelial function in humans: a meta-analysis of randomized controlled trials. Atherosclerosis 2012;221(2):311–16.
[344] Rosen RC, Cappelleri JC, Smith MD, et al. Development and evaluation of an abridged, 5-item version of the International Index of Erectile Function (IIEF-5) as a diagnostic tool for erectile dysfunction. Int J Impot Res 2000;11(6):319–26.
[345] Abdollahzad H, Alipour B, Aghdashi MA, et al. Coenzyme Q10 supplementation in patients with rheumatoid arthritis: are there any effects on cardiovascular risk factors? Eur J Integr Med 2015;7(5):534–9.
[346] Kolahdouz MR, Hosseinzadeh-Attar M, Eshraghian M, et al. The effect of coenzyme Q10 supplementation on metabolic status of type 2 diabetic patients. Minerva Gastroenterol Dietol 2013;59(2):231–6.
[347] Melnyk JP, Marcone MF. Aphrodisiacs from plant and animal sources — a review of current scientific literature. Food Res Int 2011;44(4):840–50.
[348] Tambi MIBM, Imran MK, Henkel RR. Standardised water-soluble extract of *Eurycoma longifolia*, tongkat ali, as testosterone booster for managing men with late-onset hypogonadism: treatment of hypogonadism with tongkat ali. Andrologia 2012;44:226–30.
[349] Neychev V, Mitev V. Pro-sexual and androgen enhancing effects of *Tribulus terrestris* L.: fact or fiction. J Ethnopharmacol 2016;179:345–55.
[350] Mahdi AA, Shukla KK, Ahmad MK, et al. *Withania somnifera* improves semen quality in stress-related male fertility. Evid Based Complement Alternat Med 2011;2011:1–9.
[351] Shukla KK, Mahdi AA, Ahmad MK, et al. *Mucuna pruriens* improves male fertility by its action on the hypothalamus–pituitary–gonadal axis. Fertil Steril 2009;92(6):1934–40.
[352] Safarinejad MR, Shafiei N, Safarinejad S. An open label, randomized, fixed-dose, crossover study comparing efficacy and safety of sildenafil citrate and saffron (*Crocus sativus* Linn.) for treating erectile dysfunction in men naïve to treatment. Int J Impot Res 2010;22(4):240–50.
[353] Modabbernia A, Sohrabi H, Nasehi A-A, et al. Effect of saffron on fluoxetine-induced sexual impairment in men: randomized double-blind placebo-controlled trial. Psychopharmacology (Berl) 2012;223(4):381–8.
[354] Jang D-J, Lee MS, Shin B-C, et al. Red ginseng for treating erectile dysfunction: a systematic review. Br J Clin Pharmacol 2008;66(4):444–50.
[355] Choi YD, Park CW, Jang J, et al. Effects of Korean ginseng berry extract on sexual function in men with erectile dysfunction: a multicenter, placebo-controlled, double-blind clinical study. Int J Impot Res 2013;25(2):45–50.
[356] Yang S, Chen C, Li Y, et al. Saw palmetto extract enhances erectile responses by inhibition of phosphodiesterase 5 activity and increase in inducible nitric oxide synthase messenger ribonucleic acid expression in rat and rabbit corpus cavernosum. Urology 2013;81(6):1380.e7–e13.
[357] Kam SC, Do JM, Choi JH, et al. In vivo and in vitro animal investigation of the effect of a mixture of herbal extracts from *Tribulus terrestris* and *Cornus officinalis* on penile erection. J Sex Med 2012;9(10):2544–51.
[358] Roaiah MF, El Khayat YI, Gamal El Din SF, et al. Pilot study on the effect of botanical medicine (*Tribulus terrestris*) on serum testosterone level and erectile function in aging males with partial androgen deficiency (PADAM). J Sex Marital Ther 2016;42(4):297–301.
[359] Santos CA, Reis LO, Destro-Saade R, et al. *Tribulus terrestris* versus placebo in the treatment of erectile dysfunction: a prospective, randomized, double-blind study. Actas Urol Esp Engl Ed 2014;38(4):244–8.
[360] Sansalone S, Leonardi R, Antonini G, et al. Alga *Ecklonia bicyclis*, *Tribulus terrestris*, and glucosamine oligosaccharide improve erectile function, sexual quality of life, and ejaculation function in patients with moderate mild-moderate erectile dysfunction: a prospective, randomized, placebo-controlled, single-blinded study. Biomed Res Int 2014;2014:1–7.
[361] Kotirum S, Ismail SB, Chaiyakunapruk N. Efficacy of tongkat ali (*Eurycoma longifolia*) on erectile function improvement: systematic review and meta-analysis of randomized controlled trials. Complement Ther Med 2015;23(5):693–8.
[362] Kałka D, Domagała Z, Dworak J, et al. Association between physical exercise and quality of erection in men with ischaemic heart disease and erectile dysfunction subjected to physical training. Kardiol Pol 2013;71(6):573–80.
[363] Sikiru L, Agbanusi EC, Nwacha CR. Effects of aerobic exercise in the management of erectile dysfunction: a meta-analysis study on randomized controlled trials. Ethiop J Health Sci 2011;21(3). Available from: www.ajol.info/index.php/ejhs/article/view/73760.
[364] Maresca L, D'Agostino M, Castaldo L, et al. Exercise training improves erectile dysfunction (ED) in patients with metabolic syndrome on phosphodiesterase-5 (PDE-5) inhibitors. Monaldi Arch Chest Dis 2013;80:177–83.
[365] Dorey G, Speakman MJ, Feneley RCL, et al. Pelvic floor exercises for erectile dysfunction. BJU Int 2005;96(4):595–7.
[366] Lavoisier P, Roy P, Dantony E, et al. Pelvic-floor muscle rehabilitation in erectile dysfunction and premature ejaculation. Phys Ther 2014;94(12):1731–43.
[367] Meldrum DR, Burnett AL, Dorey G, et al. Erectile hydraulics: maximizing inflow while minimizing outflow. J Sex Med 2014;11(5):1208–20.
[368] Lin Y-H, Yu T-J, Lin VC-H, et al. Effects of early pelvic-floor muscle exercise for sexual dysfunction in radical prostatectomy recipients. Cancer Nurs 2012;35(2):106–14.
[369] Khoo J, Piantadosi C, Worthley S, et al. Effects of a low-energy diet on sexual function and lower urinary tract symptoms in obese men. Int J Obes 2010;34(9):1396–403.
[370] Corona G, Vignozzi L, Sforza A, et al. Obesity and late-onset hypogonadism. Mol Cell Endocrinol 2015;418:120–33.
[371] Chan SSC, Leung DYP, Abdullah ASM, et al. Smoking cessation and adherence intervention among Chinese patients with erectile dysfunction. Am J Prev Med 2010;39(3):251–8.
[372] Harte CB, Meston CM. Association between smoking cessation and sexual health in men. BJU Int 2012;109(6):888–96.

[373] Harte CB, Meston CM. Acute effects of nicotine on physiological and subjective sexual arousal in nonsmoking men: a randomized, double-blind, placebo-controlled trial. J Sex Med 2008;5(1):110–21.
[374] Wu FC, Tajar A, Beynon JM, et al. Identification of late-onset hypogonadism in middle-aged and elderly men. N Engl J Med 2010;363(2):123–35.
[375] Harman SM, Metter EJ, Tobin JD, et al. Longitudinal effects of aging on serum total and free testosterone levels in healthy men. J Clin Endocrinol Metab 2001;86(2):724–31.
[376] Tajar A, Huhtaniemi IT, O'Neill TW, et al. Characteristics of androgen deficiency in late-onset hypogonadism: results from the European Male Aging Study (EMAS). J Clin Endocrinol Metab 2012;97(5):1508–16.
[377] Zarotsky V, Huang M-Y, Carman W, et al. Systematic literature review of the risk factors, comorbidities, and consequences of hypogonadism in men. Andrology 2014;2(6):819–34.
[378] Haring R, Ittermann T, Völzke H, et al. Prevalence, incidence and risk factors of testosterone deficiency in a population-based cohort of men: results from the study of health in Pomerania. Aging Male 2010;13(4):247–57.
[379] Lee DM, Tajar A, Pye SR, et al. Association of hypogonadism with vitamin D status: the European Male Ageing Study. Eur J Endocrinol 2012;166(1):77–85.
[380] Leproult R, Cauter EV. Effect of 1 week of sleep restriction on testosterone levels in young healthy men. JAMA 2011;305(21):2173–4.
[381] Kalyani RR, Gavini S, Dobs AS. Male hypogonadism in systemic disease. Endocrinol Metab Clin North Am 2007;36(2):333–48.
[382] Burschtin O, Wang J. Testosterone deficiency and sleep apnea. Urol Clin North Am 2016;43(2):233–7.
[383] Travison TG, Shackelton R, Araujo AB, et al. The natural history of symptomatic androgen deficiency in men: onset, progression, and spontaneous remission deficiency. J Am Geriatr Soc 2008;56(5):831–9.
[384] Tak YJ, Lee JG, Kim YJ, et al. Serum 25-hydroxyvitamin D levels and testosterone deficiency in middle-aged Korean men: a cross-sectional study. Asian J Androl 2014;17(2):324–8.
[385] Blomberg Jensen M, Nielsen JE, Jorgensen A, et al. Vitamin D receptor and vitamin D metabolizing enzymes are expressed in the human male reproductive tract. Hum Reprod 2010;25(5):1303–11.
[386] Eyles DW, Smith S, Kinobe R, et al. Distribution of the vitamin D receptor and 1α-hydroxylase in human brain. J Chem Neuroanat 2005;29(1):21–30.
[387] Chiu Y-W, Chu C-L, Chen Y, et al. Complaint of insomnia as a predictor of aging symptoms in males at a men's health clinic. Aging Male 2012;15(1):7–13.
[388] Schmid SM, Hallschmid M, Jauch-Chara K, et al. Sleep timing may modulate the effect of sleep loss on testosterone. Clin Endocrinol (Oxf) 2012;77(5):749–54.
[389] Tajar A, Forti G, O'Neill TW, et al. Characteristics of secondary, primary, and compensated hypogonadism in aging men: evidence from the European Male Ageing Study. J Clin Endocrinol Metab 2010;95(4):1810–18.
[390] Taylor SR, Meadowcraft LM, Williamson B. Prevalence, pathophysiology, and management of androgen deficiency in men with metabolic syndrome, type 2 diabetes mellitus, or both. Pharmacother J Hum Pharmacol Drug Ther 2015;35(8):780–92.
[391] Neaves WB, Johnson L, Porter JC, et al. Leydig cell numbers, daily sperm production, and serum gonadotropin levels in aging men. J Clin Endocrinol Metab 1984;59(4):756–63.
[392] Johnson L, Zane R, Petty C, et al. Quantification of the human Sertoli cell population: its distribution, relation to germ cell numbers, and age-related decline. Biol Reprod 1984;31:785–95.
[393] Well D, Yang H, Houseni M, et al. Age-related structural and metabolic changes in the pelvic reproductive end organs. Semin Nucl Med 2007;37(3):173–84.
[394] Mahmoud AM, Goemaere S, El-Garem Y, et al. Testicular volume in relation to hormonal indices of gonadal function in community-dwelling elderly men. J Clin Endocrinol Metab 2003;88(1):179–84.
[395] Veldhuis JD, Keenan DM, Liu PY, et al. The aging male hypothalamic–pituitary–gonadal axis: Pulsatility and feedback. Mol Cell Endocrinol 2009;299(1):14–22.
[396] Corona G, Rastrelli G, Monami M, et al. Body weight loss reverts obesity-associated hypogonadotropic hypogonadism: a systematic review and meta-analysis. Eur J Endocrinol 2013;168(6):829–43.
[397] Rutkowski K, Sowa P, Rutkowska-Talipska J, et al. Dehydroepiandrosterone (DHEA): hypes and hopes. Drugs 2014;74(11):1195–207.
[398] Reiter WJ, Pycha A, Schatzl G, et al. Serum dehydroepiandrosterone sulfate concentrations in men with erectile dysfunction. Urology 2000;55(5):755–8.
[399] Ponholzer A, Plas E, Schatzl G, et al. Association of DHEA-S and estradiol serum levels to symptoms of aging men. Aging Male 2002;5(4):233–8.
[400] O'Donnell AB, Travison TG, Harris SS, et al. Testosterone, dehydroepiandrosterone, and physical performance in older men: results from the Massachusetts Male Aging Study. J Clin Endocrinol Metab 2006;91(2):425–31.
[401] Lee D, Kim H, Ahn SH, et al. The association between serum dehydroepiandrosterone sulphate (DHEA-S) level and bone mineral density in Korean men. Clin Endocrinol (Oxf) 2015;83(2):173–9.
[402] Hsu B, Cumming RG, Naganathan V, et al. Temporal changes in androgens and estrogens are associated with all-cause and cause-specific mortality in older men. J Clin Endocrinol Metab 2016;101(5):2201–10.
[403] Feldman HA, Longcope C, Derby CA, et al. Age trends in the level of serum testosterone and other hormones in middle-aged men: longitudinal results from the Massachusetts male aging study. J Clin Endocrinol Metab 2002;87(2):589–98.
[404] Mosekilde L, Vestergaard P, Rejnmark L. The pathogenesis, treatment and prevention of osteoporosis in men. Drugs 2013;73(1):15–29.
[405] Amin S, Zhang Y, Felson DT, et al. Estradiol, testosterone, and the risk for hip fractures in elderly men from the Framingham Study. Am J Med 2006;119(5):426–33.
[406] Hsu B, Cumming RG, Blyth FM, et al. Longitudinal and cross-sectional relationships of circulating reproductive hormone levels to self-rated health and health-related quality of life in community-dwelling older men. J Clin Endocrinol Metab 2014;99(5):1638–47.
[407] Jasuja GK, Travison TG, Davda M, et al. Circulating estrone levels are associated prospectively with diabetes risk in men of the Framingham Heart Study. Diabetes Care 2013;36(9):2591–6.
[408] Antonio L, Wu FCW, O'Neill TW, et al. Associations between sex steroids and the development of metabolic syndrome: a longitudinal study in European Men. J Clin Endocrinol Metab 2015;100(4):1396–404.
[409] Rodriguez A, Muller DC, Metter EJ, et al. Aging, androgens, and the metabolic syndrome in a longitudinal study of aging. J Clin Endocrinol Metab 2007;92(9):3568–72.
[410] Laaksonen DE, Niskanen L, Punnonen K, et al. Testosterone and sex hormone–binding globulin predict the metabolic syndrome and diabetes in middle-aged men. Diabetes Care 2004;27(5):1036–41.
[411] Kupelian V, Page ST, Araujo AB, et al. Low sex hormone-binding globulin, total testosterone, and symptomatic androgen deficiency are associated with development of the metabolic syndrome in nonobese men. J Clin Endocrinol Metab 2006;91(3):843–50.
[412] Fink HA, Ewing SK, Ensrud KE, et al. Association of testosterone and estradiol deficiency with osteoporosis and rapid bone loss in older men. J Clin Endocrinol Metab 2006;91(10):3908–15.
[413] Woo J, Kwok T, Leung JCS, et al. Sex steroids and bone health in older Chinese men. Osteoporos Int 2012;23(5):1553–62.
[414] Yoshimura N, Muraki S, Oka H, et al. Capacity of endogenous sex steroids to predict bone loss in Japanese men: 10-year follow-up of the Taiji Cohort Study. J Bone Miner Metab 2011;29(1):96–102.
[415] Corona G, Rastrelli G, Monami M, et al. Hypogonadism as a risk factor for cardiovascular mortality in men: a meta-analytic study. Eur J Endocrinol 2011;165(5):687–701.
[416] Kloner RA, Carson C, Dobs A, et al. Testosterone and cardiovascular disease. J Am Coll Cardiol 2016;67(5):545–57.
[417] Harvey J, Berry JA. Andropause in the aging male. J Nurse Pract 2009;5(3):207–12.
[418] Chan I, Tang Fui MN, Zajac JD, et al. Assessment and management of male androgen disorders: an update. Aust Fam Physician 2014;43(5):277.

[419] Corona G, Maseroli E, Rastrelli G, et al. Characteristics of compensated hypogonadism in patients with sexual dysfunction. J Sex Med 2014;11(7):1823–34.
[420] Holcomb SS. Andropause in the aging male patient. Nurse Pract 2007;32(12):5–7.
[421] Wang C, Swerdloff RS. Measuring and interpreting serum testosterone levels in men. Medscape 2009. Available from: www.medscape.org/viewarticle/709653_3.
[422] Jensen MA, Mortier L, Koh E, et al. An interlaboratory comparison between similar methods for determination of melatonin, cortisol and testosterone in saliva. Scand J Clin Lab Invest 2014;74(5):454–61.
[423] Wood P. Salivary steroid assays — research or routine? Ann Clin Biochem 2009;46(3):183–96.
[424] Morley JE, Perry HM, Patrick P, et al. Validation of salivary testosterone as a screening test for male hypogonadism. Aging Male 2006;9(3):165–9.
[425] Cardoso EML, Contreras LN, Tumilasci EG, et al. Salivary testosterone for the diagnosis of androgen deficiency in end-stage renal disease. Nephrol Dial Transplant 2011;26(2):677–83.
[426] González-Sánchez V, Moreno-Pérez O, García de Guadiana L, et al. Reference ranges for serum and salivary testosterone in young men of Mediterranean region. Endocrinol Nutr 2015;62(1):4–10.
[427] Fiers T, Delanghe J, T'Sjoen G, et al. A critical evaluation of salivary testosterone as a method for the assessment of serum testosterone. Steroids 2014;86:5–9.
[428] Bagci S, Mueller A, Reinsberg J, et al. Saliva as a valid alternative in monitoring melatonin concentrations in newborn infants. Early Hum Dev 2009;85(9):595–8.
[429] Hampson E, Phillips S-D, Soares CN, et al. Steroid concentrations in antepartum and postpartum saliva: normative values in women and correlations with serum. Biol Sex Differ 2013;4(1):1.
[430] Tivis LJ, Richardson MD, Peddi E, et al. Saliva versus serum estradiol: implications for research studies using postmenopausal women. Prog Neuropsychopharmacol Biol Psychiatry 2005;29(5):727–32.
[431] Celec P, Ostatníková D. Saliva collection devices affect sex steroid concentrations. Clin Chim Acta 2012;413(19–20):1625–8.
[432] Durdiaková J, Fábryová H, Koborová I, et al. The effects of saliva collection, handling and storage on salivary testosterone measurement. Steroids 2013;78(14):1325–31.
[433] Whembolua G-LS, Granger DA, Singer S, et al. Bacteria in the oral mucosa and its effects on the measurement of cortisol, dehydroepiandrosterone, and testosterone in saliva. Horm Behav 2006;49(4):478–83.
[434] Kim ED, Crosnoe L, Bar-Chama N, et al. The treatment of hypogonadism in men of reproductive age. Fertil Steril 2013;99(3):718–24.
[435] Finkle WD, Greenland S, Ridgeway GK, et al. Increased risk of non-fatal myocardial infarction following testosterone therapy prescription in men. PLoS ONE 2014;9(1):e85805.
[436] Vigen R. Association of testosterone therapy with mortality, myocardial infarction, and stroke in men with low testosterone levels. JAMA 2013;310(17):1829.
[437] Shores MM, Smith NL, Forsberg CW, et al. Testosterone treatment and mortality in men with low testosterone levels. J Clin Endocrinol Metab 2012;97(6):2050–8.
[438] Haider KS, Yassin A, Doros G, et al. Men with testosterone deficiency and a history of cardiovascular diseases benefit from long-term testosterone therapy: observational, real-life data from a registry study. Vasc Health Risk Manag 2016;251.
[439] Salazar J, Tan RS. Therapeutic dilemmas for androgen deficiency in aging males. Aging Health 2005;1(1):157–66.
[440] Muthusami K, Chinnaswamy P. Effect of chronic alcoholism on male fertility hormones and semen quality. Fertil Steril 2005;84(4):919–24.
[441] Vermeulen A. Environment, human reproduction, menopause, and andropause. Environ Health Perspect 1993;101(Suppl. 2):91.
[442] Sierksma A, Sarkola T, Eriksson CJP, et al. Effect of moderate alcohol consumption on plasma dehydroepiandrosterone sulfate, testosterone, and estradiol levels in middle-aged men and postmenopausal women: a diet-controlled intervention study. Alcohol Clin Exp Res 2004;28(5):780–5.
[443] Schnatz PF, Manson JE, Vitamin D. and cardiovascular disease: an appraisal of the evidence. Clin Chem 2014;60(4):600–9.
[444] Binkley N. Vitamin D. and osteoporosis-related fracture. Arch Biochem Biophys 2012;523(1):115–22.
[445] Pilz S, Frisch S, Koertke H, et al. Effect of vitamin D supplementation on testosterone levels in men. Horm Metab Res 2011;43(3):223–5.
[446] Meunier N, O'Connor JM, Maiani G, et al. Importance of zinc in the elderly: the ZENITH study. Eur J Clin Nutr 2005;59:S1–4.
[447] Jalali GR, Roozbeh J, Mohammadzadeh A, et al. Impact of oral zinc therapy on the level of sex hormones in male patients on hemodialysis. Ren Fail 2010;32(4):417–19.
[448] Capdor J, Foster M, Petocz P, et al. Zinc and glycemic control: a meta-analysis of randomised placebo controlled supplementation trials in humans. J Trace Elem Med Biol 2013;27(2):137–42.
[449] Islam MR, Attia J, Ali L, et al. Zinc supplementation for improving glucose handling in pre-diabetes: a double blind randomized placebo controlled pilot study. Diabetes Res Clin Pract 2016;115:39–46.
[450] Rotter I, Kosik-Bogacka DI, Dołęgowska B, et al. Analysis of the relationship between the blood concentration of several metals, macro- and micronutrients and endocrine disorders associated with male aging. Environ Geochem Health 2016;38(3):749–61.
[451] Maggio M, Ceda GP, Lauretani F, et al. Magnesium and anabolic hormones in older men: magnesium and anabolic status in older men. Int J Androl 2011;34(6pt2):e594–600.
[452] Cinar V, Polat Y, Baltaci AK, et al. Effects of magnesium supplementation on testosterone levels of athletes and sedentary subjects at rest and after exhaustion. Biol Trace Elem Res 2011;140(1):18–23.
[453] Yokota K, Kato M, Lister F, et al. Clinical efficacy of magnesium supplementation in patients with type 2 diabetes. J Am Coll Nutr 2004;23(5):506S–509S.
[454] Fukami K, Yamagishi S, Sakai K, et al. Carnitine deficiency is associated with late-onset hypogonadism and depression in uremic men with hemodialysis. Aging Male 2014;17(4):238–42.
[455] Sakai K, Fukami K, Yamagishi S, et al. Evidence for a positive association between serum carnitine and free testosterone levels in uremic men with hemodialysis. Rejuvenation Res 2013;16(3):200–5.
[456] Cavallini G, Caracciolo S, Vitali G, et al. Carnitine versus androgen administration in the treatment of sexual dysfunction, depressed mood, and fatigue associated with male aging. Urology 2004;63(4):641–6.
[457] Reid IR, Bristow SM, Bolland MJ. Cardiovascular complications of calcium supplements: heart safety of calcium supplements. J Cell Biochem 2015;116(4):494–501.
[458] George A, Henkel R. Phytoandrogenic properties of *Eurycoma longifolia* as natural alternative to testosterone replacement therapy. Andrologia 2014;46(7):708–21.
[459] Ismail SB, Wan Mohammad WMZ, George A, et al. Randomized clinical trial on the use of physta freeze-dried water extract of *Eurycoma longifolia* for the improvement of quality of life and sexual well-being in men. Evid Based Complement Alternat Med 2012;2012:1–10.
[460] Kim T-H, Jeon SH, Hahn E-J, et al. Effects of tissue-cultured mountain ginseng (*Panax ginseng* CA Meyer) extract on male patients with erectile dysfunction. Asian J Androl 2009;11(3):356–61.
[461] Chan S-W. *Panax ginseng*, *Rhodiola rosea* and *Schisandra chinensis*. Int J Food Sci Nutr 2012;63(sup1):75–81.
[462] Shergis JL, Zhang AL, Zhou W, et al. *Panax ginseng* in randomised controlled trials: a systematic review. Phytother Res 2013;27(7):949–65.
[463] Felter HW, Lloyd JU. Kings American dispensatory. 11th ed. Cincinnati: The Ohio Valley Company; 1898.
[464] Angwafor F, Anderson ML. An open label, dose response study to determine the effect of a dietary supplement on dihydrotestosterone, testosterone and estradiol levels in healthy males. J Int Soc Sports Nutr 2008;5(1):12.
[465] Wankhede S, Langade D, Joshi K, et al. Examining the effect of *Withania somnifera* supplementation on muscle strength and recovery: a randomized controlled trial. J Int Soc Sports Nutr 2015;12:43.

[466] Gupta A, Mahdi AA, Ahmad MK, et al. A proton NMR study of the effect of *Mucuna pruriens* on seminal plasma metabolites of infertile males. J Pharm Biomed Anal 2011;55(5):1060–6.
[467] Gauthaman K, Adaikan PG, Prasad RNV. Aphrodisiac properties of *Tribulus terrestris* extract (Protodioscin) in normal and castrated rats. Life Sci 2002;71(12):1385–96.
[468] Estrada-Reyes R, Ortiz-López P, Gutiérrez-Ortíz J, et al. *Turnera diffusa* wild (Turneraceae) recovers sexual behavior in sexually exhausted males. J Ethnopharmacol 2009;123(3):423–9.
[469] Estrada-Reyes R, Carro-Juárez M, Martínez-Mota L. Pro-sexual effects of *Turnera diffusa* Wild (Turneraceae) in male rats involves the nitric oxide pathway. J Ethnopharmacol 2013;146(1):164–72.
[470] Li Y-Y, Feng J, Zhang X-L, et al. Pine bark extracts: nutraceutical, pharmacological, and toxicological evaluation. J Pharmacol Exp Ther 2015;353(1):9–16.
[471] de Souza KZD, Vale FBC, Geber S. Efficacy of *Tribulus terrestris* for the treatment of hypoactive sexual desire disorder in postmenopausal women: a randomized, double-blinded, placebo-controlled trial. Menopause 2016;23(11):1252–6.
[472] Colagar AH, Marzony ET, Chaichi MJ. Zinc levels in seminal plasma are associated with sperm quality in fertile and infertile men. Nutr Res 2009;29(2):82–8.
[473] Prasad AS. Discovery of human zinc deficiency: its impact on human health and disease. Adv Nutr Int Rev J 2013;4(2): 176–90.
[474] Mahajan S, Abbasi A, Prasad A, et al. Effect of oral zinc therapy on gonadal function in hemodialysis patients. A double-blind study. Ann Intern Med 1982;97(3):357–61.
[475] Fairweather-Tait SJ, Bao Y, Broadley MR, et al. Selenium in human health and disease. Antioxid Redox Signal 2011;14(7):1337–83.
[476] Sudar-Milovanovic E, Obradovic M, Jovanovic A, et al. Benefits of L-arginine on cardiovascular system. Mini Rev Med Chem 2016;16(2):94–103.
[477] Erlund I. Review of the flavonoids quercetin, hesperetin, and naringenin. Dietary sources, bioactivities, bioavailability, and epidemiology. Nutr Res 2004;24(10):851–74.
[478] Nishimuro H, Ohnishi H, Sato M, et al. Estimated daily intake and seasonal food sources of quercetin in Japan. Nutrients 2015;7(4):2345–58.
[479] Barassi A, Pezzilli R, Colpi GM, et al. Vitamin D and erectile dysfunction. J Sex Med 2014;11(11):2792–800.
[480] Levett K. Vitamin D. In: Braun L, Cohen M, editors. Herbs and natural supplements: an evidence-based guide. 4th ed. Sydney: Elsevier; 2015. p. 1125–49.
[481] Mitchell-Paterson T. Magnesium. In: Braun L, Cohen M, editors. Herbs and natural supplements: an evidence-based guide. 4th ed. Sydney: Elsevier; 2015. p. 677–92.
[482] Baines SK. Carnitine. In: Braun L, Cohen M, editors. Herbs and natural supplements: an evidence-based guide. 4th ed. Sydney: Elsevier; 2015. p. 142–56.
[483] Mitchell-Paterson T, Vitamin E. Braun L, Cohen M, editors. Herbs and natural supplements: an evidence-based guide. 4th ed. Sydney: Elsevier; 2015. p. 1149–76.
[484] Noventa M, Vitagliano A, Quaranta M, et al. Preventive and therapeutic role of dietary inositol supplementation in periconceptional period and during pregnancy: a summary of evidences and future applications. Reprod Sci 2016;23(3):278–88.
[485] Bradely E. Coenzyme Q10. In: Braun L, Cohen M, editors. Coenzyme Q10, Herbs and natural supplements: an evidence-based guide. 4th ed. Sydney: Elsevier; 2015. p. 214–36.
[486] Myles M. Vitamin B6. In: Braun L, Cohen M, editors. Herbs and natural supplements: an evidence-based guide. 4th ed. Sydney: Elsevier; 2015. p. 1078–91.
[487] Braun L, Cohen M. Folate. In: Braun L, Cohen M, editors. Herbs and natural supplements: an evidence-based guide. 4th ed. Sydney: Elsevier; 2015. p. 364–80.
[488] Ranasinghe P, Wathurapatha W, Ishara M, et al. Effects of zinc supplementation on serum lipids: a systematic review and meta-analysis. Nutr Metab (Lond) 2015;12:26.
[489] Lorente-Cebrián S, Costa AGV, Navas-Carretero S, et al. Role of omega-3 fatty acids in obesity, metabolic syndrome, and cardiovascular diseases: a review of the evidence. J Physiol Biochem 2013;69(3):633–51.
[490] Miller PE, Van Elswyk M, Alexander DD. Long-chain omega-3 fatty acids eicosapentaenoic acid and docosahexaenoic acid and blood pressure: a meta-analysis of randomized controlled trials. Am J Hypertens 2014;27(7):885–96.
[491] Kotwal S, Jun M, Sullivan D, et al. Omega-3 fatty acids and cardiovascular outcomes systematic review and meta-analysis. Circ Cardiovasc Qual Outcomes 2012;5(6):808–18.
[492] Wang Q, Liang X, Wang L, et al. Effect of omega-3 fatty acids supplementation on endothelial function: a meta-analysis of randomized controlled trials. Atherosclerosis 2012;221(2):536–43.
[493] Albarracin CA, Fuqua BC, Evans JL. Chromium picolinate and biotin combination improves glucose metabolism in treated, uncontrolled overweight to obese patients with type 2 diabetes. Diabetes Metab Res Rev 2008;24(1):41–51.
[494] Chen Y-L, Lin J-D, Hsia T-L, et al. The effect of chromium on inflammatory markers, 1st and 2nd phase insulin secretion in type 2 diabetes. Eur J Nutr 2014;53(1):127–33.
[495] Kleefstra N, Houweling ST, Jansman FG, et al. Chromium treatment has no effect in patients with poorly controlled, insulin-treated type 2 diabetes in an obese Western population a randomized, double-blind, placebo-controlled trial. Diabetes Care 2006;29(3):521–5.
[496] Martin J, Wang ZQ, Zhang XH, et al. Chromium picolinate supplementation attenuates body weight gain and increases insulin sensitivity in subjects with type 2 diabetes. Diabetes Care 2006;29(8):1826–32.
[497] Paiva AN, de Lima JG, de Medeiros ACQ, et al. Beneficial effects of oral chromium picolinate supplementation on glycemic control in patients with type 2 diabetes: a randomized clinical study. J Trace Elem Med Biol 2015;32:66–72.
[498] Masharani U, Gjerde C, McCoy S, et al. Chromium supplementation in non-obese non-diabetic subjects is associated with a decline in insulin sensitivity. BMC Endocr Disord 2012;12(1):1.
[499] Lee B-J, Huang Y-C, Chen S-J, et al. Coenzyme Q10 supplementation reduces oxidative stress and increases antioxidant enzyme activity in patients with coronary artery disease. Nutrition 2012;28(3):250–5.
[500] Lai J, Moxey A, Nowak G, et al. The efficacy of zinc supplementation in depression: systematic review of randomised controlled trials. J Affect Disord 2012;136(1–2):e31–9.
[501] Bahmani F, Kia M, Soleimani A, et al. Effect of selenium supplementation on glycemic control and lipid profiles in patients with diabetic nephropathy. Biol Trace Elem Res 2016;172(2):282–9.
[502] Asatiani M, Georgian T. Successful results of treatment of male patient with vitamin D deficiency associated with erectile dysfunction (ED). J Sex Med 2016;13(5 Suppl. 2):S175.
[503] Papandreou D, Hamid Z-T-N. The role of vitamin D in diabetes and cardiovascular disease: an updated review of the literature. Dis Markers 2015;2015:1–15.
[504] Tiemeier H, Van Tuijl HR, Hofman A, et al. Vitamin B_{12}, folate, and homocysteine in depression: the Rotterdam Study. Am J Psychiatry 2002;159(12):2099–101.
[505] Almeida OP, Ford AH, Flicker L. Systematic review and meta-analysis of randomized placebo-controlled trials of folate and vitamin B_{12} for depression. Int Psychogeriatr 2015;27(5):727–37.
[506] The DIPART (Vitamin D Individual Patient Analysis of Randomized Trials) group. Patient level pooled analysis of 68 500 patients from seven major vitamin D fracture trials in US and Europe. BMJ 2010;340(1):b5463.

20 The cardiovascular system

Leah Hechtman, Ian Breakspear

SECTION A

OVERVIEW OF THE CARDIOVASCULAR SYSTEM

The cardiovascular system (Fig. 20.1) is the body's main transport system and encompasses three essential components: the heart, the blood and the blood vessels (consisting of the arteries, capillaries and veins). Its primary function is to ensure that blood is circulated to and from the body's tissues as well as to carry waste products away from the body's cells.

The heart

The heart is a cone-shaped organ located between the two lungs close to the left-hand side of the body. In the average adult female the heart weighs approximately 200 g, while in the average adult male it weighs 300 g.[1] The heart rests on the diaphragm in the mediastinum, the middle section of the chest cavity. Interestingly, despite the mammoth role the heart plays within our body, it is surprisingly small and is actually only the size of a small closed human fist.

The pericardium is a thin, fluid-filled sac. It functions to surround and protect the heart, to keep the heart resting within the mediastinum while still allowing the heart enough space to contract as blood volume increases.

The wall of the heart is rich in blood vessels and comprises three layers:

- The epicardium: The outer layer of the heart that functions to protect the other layers
- The myocardium: The middle layer of the heart that is responsible for the vigorous pumping action of the heart. It is composed of involuntary striated cardiac muscle tissue
- The endocardium: The inner layer of the heart that controls myocardial function and provides a lining of the heart chambers and a cover for the heart valves.

FUNCTIONS OF THE HEART

The heart contracts continuously, functioning to pump out blood to the rest of the body. It is estimated that the heart circulates the blood through approximately 100 000 km of blood vessels — all without once ever resting; astounding! This pumping action is caused by a flow of electricity through the heart that repeats itself in a cycle.

The heart is divided into four chambers: two at the top (the atria) and two at the bottom (the ventricles). Each chamber has a very specific and important function and the walls of the chambers vary in thickness depending on the difficulty of its function.

The right side of the heart functions to collect de-oxygenated blood and is involved with the pulmonary circulation. The right atrium receives blood from three veins: the superior and inferior vena cava and the coronary sinus. This blood then exits through the tricuspid valve into the right ventricle.

The right ventricle receives blood from the right atrium and pumps blood to the lungs via the pulmonary semilunar valve and pulmonary trunk so that carbon dioxide can be dropped off and oxygen picked up.

The left side of the heart receives oxygenated blood from the lungs and is the pump for the systemic circulation. It pumps blood into the left atrium via four pulmonary veins. The left atrium forms the base of the heart.

The left ventricle forms the apex of the heart and has the biggest workload, hence has the thickest wall. It pumps out the oxygenated blood into the circulation via the aorta and aortic semilunar valve which eventually passes through smaller systemic arteries which carry blood throughout the body.

CARDIAC CYCLE

The cardiac cycle consists of all the events that take place in one heart beat:

- Electrical signals of the conduction system (can be measured by an electrocardiogram (ECG))
- Mechanical events including changes in both pressure and volume of the blood in the four chambers of the heart. Atria and ventricles alternately contract and relax. The phase of contraction is called systole and the phase of relaxation is called diastole
- Heart sounds which are the sound of turbulence caused by the closing of the heart valves. The closure of the atrioventricular (AV) valves cause the loud first sound (S1) and the closure of the semilunar valves causes the softer second sound (S2).

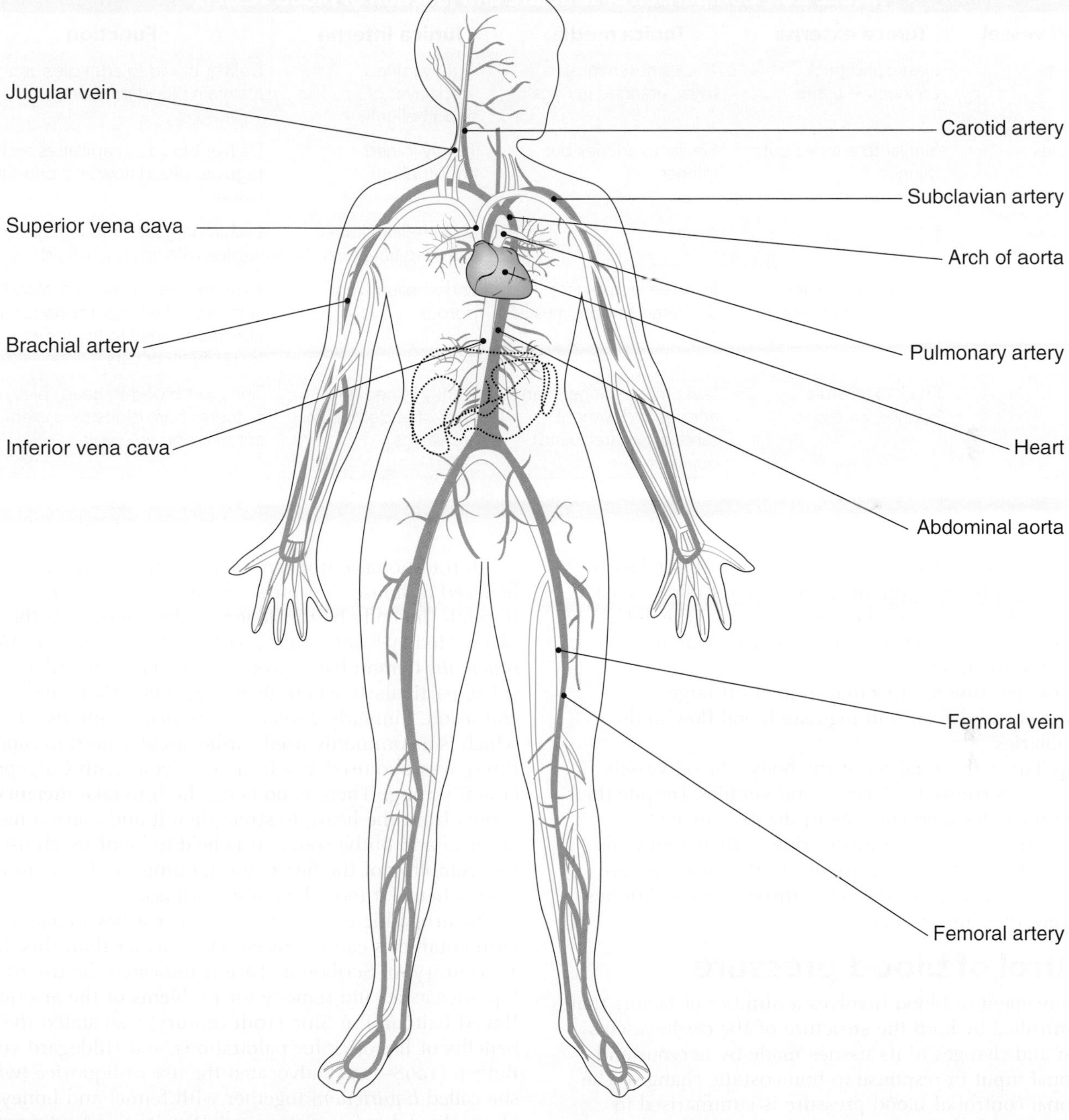

FIGURE 20.1 The cardiovascular system.
Source: Standring S, Ellis H, Wigley C. Gray's anatomy. 39th edn. New York: Elsevier Churchill Livingstone; 2005.

The blood

Blood is a type of connective tissue and is made from the endothelium (the thin layer of cells that line the interior surface of the blood vessels). Blood makes up approximately 8% of total body weight in adults and its volume comprises 4–6 L.[1]

Blood assists in regulating the temperature, pH and water content of the cells. It acts as a transporter, assisting the movement of gases such as oxygen (bound to haemoglobin) and carbon dioxide around the body as well as nutrients (e.g. glucose), wastes (e.g. lactic acid and urea), regulatory substance (e.g. hormones and enzymes) and proteins (e.g. albumins, interferon).

Blood also exerts protective mechanisms such as coagulation (which is life-saving after an injury) as well as immunological functions such as circulation of white blood cells.

The blood vessels

The blood vessels are a group of tubes responsible for circulating blood around the body (Table 20.1).

TABLE 20.1 Comparison of structure and function of blood vessels

Blood vessel	Tunica externa	Tunica media	Tunica interna	Function
Arteries	Elastic and thick connective tissue	Thick smooth muscle Layer arranged in rings	Tightly joined Thick layer of endothelium	Deliver blood to arterioles and maintain blood pressure
Arterioles	Similar to arteries but thinner	Similar to arteries but thinner	Tightly joined endothelium	Deliver blood to capillaries and regulate blood flow and pressure to tissues
Capillaries	None	None	Endothelium joined with gap junctions	Exchange gases, nutrients and wastes with interstitial fluid
Venules	Increased thickness similar to arterioles	Increase in thickness Scattered smooth muscle cells	Endothelium very porous	Transport deoxygenated blood to veins and allow macrophages and fibroblasts entry to tissues when tissue injury occurs
Veins	Thick extensible connective tissue	Layer much thinner than arteries and without same elastic (rebound) qualities	Tightly joined thin layer of endothelium has valves	Transport blood to heart, pick up nutrients from digestive system and act as blood reservoir

- Arteries: large blood vessels made up of three layers: the tunica interna (the inner coat), the tunica media (the middle coat) and the tunica externa (the outer coat). Arteries function to carry blood away from the heart to the tissues
- Arterioles: tiny arteries that branch off large arteries and deliver and regulate blood flow to the capillaries
- Capillaries: the smallest of the body's blood vessels, capillaries connect arterioles and venules. Despite their size they play a crucial role in the exchange of nutrients, oxygen and wastes due to their thin walls
- Veins: carry blood from tissues to the heart and are structurally made of the same three layers as arteries except they are thinner.

Control of blood pressure

The movement of blood involves a number of factors that are controlled by both the structure of the cardiovascular system and changes to its tissues made by nervous and hormonal input in response to homeostatic changes. The hormonal control of blood pressure is summarised in Table 20.2.

ROLE OF THE NATUROPATH

Traditional interpretation

Traditional naturopathic practitioners viewed the heart as an organ of great importance, even implying that it was the governing organ in the body. Nicholas Culpeper stated: 'Regard the heart, keep that upon the wheels, because the sun is the foundation of life, and therefore those universal remedies Aurum Potabile cure all diseases by fortifying the heart'.[2] This implies that the heart was considered central to any treatment procedure and that by nurturing the heart, resolution of the disease condition would surely come about.

In traditional European medicine the heart was believed to house the spirit, which was thought to move through the body by the action of the arteries via the blood. Hedley[3] notes that 'heart' medicines such as *Melissa officinalis* (lemon balm) were usually taken to enhance the spirit, particularly where there was melancholy and confusion. Similarly, *Leonurus cardiaca* (motherwort), which is a commonly used cardiovascular herb in modern times, was also used as a heart medicine, with Culpeper (1693) stating: 'There is no better herb to take melancholy vapors from the heart, to strengthen it and make a merry, cheerful and blithe soul ... It is held to be of much use for the trembling of the heart, and faintings and swoonings; from whence it took the name Cardiaca'.[2]

Naturopathic management of the cardiovascular system with botanicals can be traced back further than this. In the 1st century AD Scribonius Largus indicated the use of liquorice as a valid remedy for problems of the arteries. Ibn Al Baithar, Ibn Sina (10th century) also stated the benefits of liquorice for palpitations, and Hildegard von Bingen (1098–1179) advocated the use of liquorice (which she called *liquiricium*) together with fennel and honey for 'de cordis dolore', angina pain.[4] Despite this traditional use, in modern times liquorice is not a first-line treatment for management of cardiovascular disorders, particularly where there is hypertension present.

It was discovered that the heart contained valves around the 4th century BC, but not with the same understanding as we have now. The ancient anatomists believed that the arteries of the heart were filled with air (rather than blood) and thought they functioned to transport air. It was in the 2nd century AD that the Greek physician Galen realised that blood vessels carried blood rather than air and noted the differences visually and functionally between venous (dark red) and arterial (brighter and thinner) blood. However, Galen thought that the arterial and venous systems were separate entities, a concept we know today to be untrue.

TABLE 20.2 Hormonal control of blood pressure

Control mechanism	Description
Blood flow (velocity)	
Branching structure of blood vessels	Arterial increased branching which slows flow. Decreasing branching in venous system maintains flow
Cardiovascular centre in medulla oblongata	Changes blood vessel diameter via the sympathetic division of autonomic nervous system to increase or decrease flow
Hormonal control	Angiotensin II (a hormone controlled by sensors in the kidneys), adrenaline and antidiuretic hormone all constrict blood vessels
Blood pressure	
Branching structure of blood vessels	The same decreasing and increasing effects are achieved for blood pressure
Cardiovascular centre in medulla oblongata	Increases or decreases contractility of ventricles by autonomic nervous system stimulation in response to sensory input (e.g. proprioceptors measuring increased or decreased frequency of joint movement)
Hormonal control	Concentrations of adrenaline and noradrenaline in the blood alter the force of contraction of the heart
Blood vessel length	The longer the vessel, the greater the accumulated friction, the greater the blood pressure. The larger number of blood vessels in the adipose tissue of an obese person increases overall blood pressure (hypertension)
Blood vessel diameter	Smaller diameter means greater resistance so greater blood pressure. Clogging of arteries or atherosclerosis causes an increase in pressure in that vessel
Blood viscosity (thickness)	The change in water content due to dehydration or an increase in formed elements increase the thickness of blood, increasing resistance and blood pressure
Venous return	Muscle activity increases pressure in the venous system through mechanical action of contraction and relaxation pumping the vessel walls Respiratory activity — when the diaphragm moves in breathing it puts more or less pressure on veins in the thoracic or abdominal cavity

Central to naturopathic philosophy was the importance of addressing the causative factor of the diseased state of the heart. The Eclectic physicians emphasised this:[5] 'The first consideration in the treatment is the removal of the cause. In fact, but little can be done in regulating the action of the heart unless the cause is removed.' This idea of treating the cause is still close to the heart of modern naturopathic philosophy today.

Modern interpretation

With the powerful and highly technical pharmacological and surgical interventions available to cardiologists, it is even more important to accurately define the role of the modern naturopath in the context of cardiovascular disease. Modern naturopathic medicine provides a unique, multifaceted approach, incorporating: herbal medicines; nutritional modifications and prescriptions (dietary and supplemental); lifestyle modifications including stress management, exercise and sufficient sleep; and functional and biochemical testing to thoroughly and accurately assess the patient. Key to this approach is the core naturopathic principle of individualised patient-centred care.

The situation of a patient post-myocardial infarction is a good example. Clinical research indicates that even after successful coronary bypass and angioplasty, patient recovery in the fullest sense can be impeded by problems such as depression,[6] and lack of education around their situation.[7] It is in this context that the treatment approach — and not just the treatment modalities — of naturopathic medicine may offer significant benefit.

Modern naturopaths believe the pathogenesis of cardiovascular disease is a cumulative effect of many causative factors rather than just the emotions. These factors include:

- Widespread oxidative stress
- Inflammation
- Impaired cellular respiration
- Toxicity
- Excesses of stress
- Deficiency of nutrients and minerals
- Lifestyle factors such as lack of exercise.

A cornerstone of modern cardiovascular therapy is the reduction of oxidative stress and inflammation while simultaneously restoring circulatory equilibrium throughout the whole system, particularly in the context of atherosclerosis and its resultant problems. Focus is placed on the peripheral circulation and the balance between the blood vessels. The modern naturopath can also call on physical examination and clinical signs that may help to identify cardiovascular risk including both allopathic and naturopathic interpretations of signs and symptoms. Individual and family history, genetic factors and diagnostic laboratory markers give the modern naturopath the advantage that they can assess risk factors of cardiovascular disease in their patients.

The modern naturopath also has access to a wide range of cardiovascular supportive prescriptions. Their understanding of these nutrients is far greater than the knowledge available to their ancestors. Modern naturopaths, for example, are aware that all forms of magnesium are not equal in the management of cardiovascular disorders, and can choose magnesium orotate, a form of magnesium with an affinity for cardiac muscles.

Despite the benefits of technology and scientific breakthroughs, modern naturopaths still retain many of the lessons from their traditional forebearers. *Crataegus monogyna* (hawthorn), a cardio-tonic widely used by the Eclectics for 'very feeble and irregular heart action particularly for its sedative action in cross, irritable patients with cardiac symptoms'[8] is still one of the primary herbs used for cardiovascular disease today. Using such foundation knowledge the modern naturopath can successfully support their patients in a holistic manner (see Table 20.3).

NUTRITIONAL MEDICINES

The nutritional medicines available to treat the cardiovascular system are listed in Table 20.4.

TABLE 20.3 Stages of naturopathic intervention in cardiovascular disease

Intervention	Description	Key goals	Examples
Primary prevention	Prevention of disease through risk reduction	Individual or population-level reduction of disease incidence	Education leading to lifestyle and dietary modifications such as increased exercise, reduction of processed foods
Secondary prevention	Early detection of pre-clinical changes associated with subsequent disease progression	Stabilisation or reversal of early pathophysiological changes and pathological markers Prolongation of the pre-clinical stage (i.e. where major disease is not yet present)	Lowering of C-reactive protein Normalisation of blood glucose and triglycerides Normalisation of blood pressure
Tertiary prevention	Reducing the impact of existing disease on the patient as a whole	Improved quality of life in both reversible and irreversible conditions Prolonged survival and reduced symptom severity/frequency	Reduction of frequency and severity of dyspnoea and chest pain angina Improved patient-rating of quality of life in Class III heart failure

TABLE 20.4 Nutritional medicine

Requirement	Justification	Therapeutic dose	Food sources
Magnesium (orotate)	Essential for the normal rhythm of the heart and a healthy cardiovascular system. Protects cardiac cells from free radical damage and is a vasodilator. Plays a crucial role in the biosynthetic pathway of glycogen and improves the energy status of the heart cells and recovery from cardioplegic arrest	300–1000 mg/day	Eggs, cocoa, almonds, brewer's yeasts, cashews, kelp, wheat bran, wheatgerm, buckwheat
Calcium	Essential for healthy function of the cardiac muscle and its contraction including heart beat. Also required for regulation of blood pressure and blood clotting. Deficiency is associated with hypertension	1000–2000 mg/day	Tinned sardines and salmon (with the bones), almonds, dairy products (milk, yoghurt, cheese), tahini, sesame seeds, leafy green vegetables (spinach, broccoli, bok choy), dried figs
Potassium	Essential mineral needed for maintaining a healthy cardiovascular system particularly with regards to blood pressure. Enhances normal muscle contraction	2800–3800 mg/day up to 4700 mg/day (including food) (only provide under medical supervision)	All vegetables, avocado, apricots, bananas, almonds, cashews, pecans, sunflower seeds, potatoes
Vitamin B complex	The B vitamins provide energy and support during physically demanding periods. As the cardiovascular system has an affinity for a number of key B vitamins, it is imperative to prescribed a B complex to maintain B vitamin balance	Comprehensive complex containing all individual B vitamins	Legumes, wholegrains, nuts, beans, brewer's yeast, leafy green vegetables
Vitamin B_3	Involved in regulation of cholesterol and reducing the risk of cardiovascular disease. Promotes peripheral vasodilation	100–1000 mg/day niacinamide with upper dose to 3000 mg/day under close medical supervision and monitoring of LFTs	Almonds, chicken, eggs, legumes, salmon, sardines, sunflower seeds

TABLE 20.4 Nutritional medicine—cont'd

Requirement	Justification	Therapeutic dose	Food sources
Vitamin B_6	Work together to regulate homocysteine in the blood. Elevated levels of homocysteine are an independent risk factor for cardiovascular disease including atherosclerosis, stroke and coronary heart disease. Low intake of these vitamins increases homocysteine in the blood. Specific doses are to reduce homocysteine levels and may be warranted for the cardiovascular patient	Vitamin B_6: 20–60 mg	Brewer's yeast, cereal, chicken, egg yolk, oatmeal, salmon
Vitamin B_9		Folic acid: 400 micrograms–5 mg/day	Beans, eggs, green leafy vegetables, lentils, yeast
Vitamin B_{12}		Vitamin B_{12}: 400–800 micrograms/day	Egg yolk, milk, oysters, salmon, sardines, meat
Vitamin C	Functions as an antioxidant to enhance the synthesis or prevent the breakdown of nitric oxide and protect against fat oxidation by free radicals. Reduces the risk of platelet aggregation and may help to lower blood cholesterol	250–5000 mg/day in divided doses	Kiwi fruit, guava, papaya, mangoes, strawberries, acerola cherries, broccoli
Vitamin E	Antioxidant which supports normal healthy heart function and the maintenance of normal cardiovascular health by lowering LDL cholesterol and reducing the risk of platelet aggregation. Vitamin E may aid healthy blood circulation and helps to maintain cell integrity. Vitamin E protects polyunsaturated fatty acids from oxidation and helps maintain healthy arteries and capillaries	100–1000 IU/day	Almonds, wheat germ, safflower, egg yolks, corn
Lipoic acid	Oxidative stress and endothelial dysfunction play an important role in the aetiology of cardiovascular disease. Lipoic acid regenerates other antioxidants such as coenzyme Q10, glutathione, vitamin C and E, strengthening the antioxidant network and improving endothelial function	200–1800 mg/day	Typical dietary sources of lipoic acid are muscle meats, heart, kidney and liver, and to a lesser degree, fruits and vegetables, spinach, broccoli, tomatos, garden peas, Brussels sprouts and rice bran
Acetyl L-carnitine	The heart possesses 5000 mitochondria per cell and is one of the most susceptible organs to free radical damage Acetyl L-carnitine is a source of carnitine, a naturally occurring amino acid. The addition of an acetyl group gives acetyl L-carnitine a wide range of therapeutic applications in the body as the acetyl form is able to cross the blood–brain barrier. Carnitine plays a central role in the oxidation of fatty acids for energy and is particularly important in the myocardium. Carnitine is the 'shuttle' that carries fatty acids into the mitochondria so that they can be utilised for energy. This is important in the heart muscle when energy needs are high	600–2500 mg/day Higher doses can be given intravenously such as 15 g/day pre-open heart surgery	Avocado, beef, chicken, fish, milk, liver
Fish oil (DHA and EPA)	Fish oil is a natural source of the essential omega-3 triglycerides, eicosapentaenoic acid (EPA) and docosahexaenoic acid (DHA). Omega-3 fats (DHA and EPA) are precursors to prostaglandins that lower blood pressure and reduce platelet aggregation thus helping to protect against atherosclerosis and heart disease. Humans require a dietary source of omega-3 fatty acids as they cannot be synthesised	250 mg/day–882 mg/day EPA and DHA in the average ratio of EPA/DHA 1 : 2	Pilchards, salmon, trout, herring, salmon, mackerel

Continued

TABLE 20.4 Nutritional medicine—cont'd

Requirement	Justification	Therapeutic dose	Food sources
Coenzyme Q10	Coenzyme Q10 is a lipid-soluble substance that is found in all cells of the body, particularly in high concentrations in the heart. It helps to support and protect the heart and is essential for heart muscle contraction Coenzyme Q10 may assist in the maintenance of normal healthy blood pressure. As a lipid-soluble antioxidant it can inhibit the oxidation of lipids, including LDL cholesterol, and restores oxidised vitamin E back into its antioxidant form	30–300 mg/day with doses increasing to up to 800 mg/day under medical supervision of a cardiologist	Almonds, broccoli, chestnuts, hazelnuts, mackerel, rice bran, salmon, sardines, sesame seeds, soy beans
L-arginine	L-arginine is an amino acid and a precursor to nitric oxide. It has multiple functions, including vasodilation, improving endothelial function, regulating blood and intracellular pH and the effect on the depolarisation of endothelial cell membranes, antihypertensive and antioxidant properties, as well as influencing blood viscosity and the coagulation system	400–6000 mg/day	Almonds, cashews, garlic, peanuts, peas, pecans
Taurine	Taurine is essential for proper bile acid function and absorption of lipids	250–2000 mg/day	Animal protein
Choline	Choline is an essential component of the phospholipids and promotes the export of fats from the body	1000–3500 mg/day	Beans, egg yolks, lecithin, wholegrains
Inositol	Inositol promotes the export of fat from the liver and is involved in the control of blood cholesterol	750–6000 mg/day	Beans, cantaloupe, citrus fruits, corn, grains, seeds

Sources: Braun L, Cohen M. Herbs and natural supplements an evidence-based guide. 2nd edn. Edinburgh: Churchill Livingstone Elsevier; 2007, p. 653. Frishman WH, Beravol P, Carosella C et al. Alternative and complementary medicine for preventing and treating cardiovascular disease. Disease-a-Month 2009; 55(3):121–192. GISSI-Prevenzione Investigators (Gruppo Italiano per lo Studio della Sopravvivenza nell'Infarto miocardico). Dietary supplementation with omega-3 polyunsaturated fatty acids and vitamin E after myocardial infarction: results of the GISSi-prevenzione trial. Lancet 1999; 354:447–455. Hadj A, Pepe S, Marasco S, Rosenfeldt F et al. The principles of metabolic therapy in heart disease. Heart Lung Circ 2003; 12; (Supplement). Mozaffarian D. Fish and n-3 fatty acids for the prevention of fatal coronary heart disease and sudden cardiac death. Am J Clin Nutr 2008; 87(6):1991S–1996S. Pastoris O, Dossena M, Foppa P et al. Effect of L-carnitine on myocardial metabolism: results of a balanced, placebo-controlled, double-blind study in patients undergoing open heart surgery. Pharmacol Res 1998; 37(2):115–122. Tousoulis D, Antoniades C, Tentolouris C et al. L-arginine in cardiovascular disease: dream or reality? Vasc Med 2002; 7(3):203–211. Wollin SD, Jones PJ. Alpha-lipoic acid and cardiovascular disease. J Nutr 2003; 133(11):3327–3330. Zimmermann M. Burgenstein's handbook of nutrition, micronutrients in the prevention and therapy of diseases. New York: Thieme; 2001.

HERBAL MEDICINES

The herbal medicines available to treat the cardiovascular system are listed in Table 20.5.

INVESTIGATIONS

The goals of testing for heart disease are to distinguish between symptoms that are heart related and those that are caused by another condition. Testing is ordered to help determine which heart disease is present, to determine whether the disorder is acute or chronic, to monitor a cardiac event that is in progress — such as a heart attack — and to determine the severity and extent of the disease.

When a patient presents to the emergency room with acute coronary syndrome — a group of symptoms that suggest heart injury due to lack of blood flow — they are evaluated with a variety of laboratory blood tests and other tests. These are used to determine the cause of the pain and the severity of the condition. Since some treatments for a heart attack must be given within a short period of time to minimise heart damage, an accurate diagnosis must be confirmed quickly.

Testing patients for existing heart disease is not the same as cardiac risk testing (which actually mostly determines risk of coronary heart disease). Cardiac risk testing is performed to screen asymptomatic people and to help determine their risk of developing coronary heart disease.

Cardiac biomarkers (post heart attack)

Tests for cardiac biomarkers, proteins that are released when muscle cells are damaged, are frequently ordered when patients have symptoms of acute coronary syndrome, such as chest pain, pain in the jaw, neck, abdomen, back or that radiates to the shoulder or arms, nausea, dyspnoea and lightheadedness.

Such tests include:

- Troponin — the most commonly ordered and cardiac-specific of the markers; will be elevated within

TABLE 20.5 Herbal medicine for the cardiovascular system

Class	Example	Justification
Anti-arrhythmic	*Crataegus monogyna* (hawthorn)	Anti-arrhythmic herbal medicines are those that normalise the rhythm of the heart. Hawthorn is one of the oldest known medicinal plants used in European medicine and its cardiovascular benefits are well supported by both traditional and modern-day research. The German Commission E indicates the use of hawthorn flower for cases of mild bradyarrhythmia, paroxysmal tachycardia and for decreasing cardiac output. The flavonoids (active constituents within hawthorn) appear to be responsible for the majority of hawthorn's cardiovascular benefits
Antioxidant	*Vitis vinifera* (grapeseed)	Antioxidants protect against free radical damage and oxidation. Grape seed extract is a good source of oligomeric proanthocyanidins (OPCs). These are a type of bioflavonoid and are powerful antioxidants that are many times more potent than vitamins E and C in their antioxidant effect. OCPs help strengthen and protect cell membranes from oxidative damage and may assist in maintaining healthy blood vessels and capillaries
Antiplatelet	*Allium sativum* (garlic)	Increased platelet aggregation plays a significant role in the aetiology of cardiovascular disease and is complex, involving multiple mechanisms. Garlic belongs to the family Liliaceae and is one of the most ancient medicinal plants known to man. Animal studies suggest that odourless garlic not only activates fibrinolytic activity by accelerating t-PA-mediated plasminogen activation, but also suppresses the coagulation system by downregulating thrombin formation. This antiplatelet action suggests a beneficial role in preventing pathological thrombus formation
Cardioprotective	*Salvia miltiorrhiza* (dan shen)	Cardioprotective herbal medicines are those that protect the heart muscle and decrease the risk of heart damage from toxicity or ischaemia. Dan shen is a traditional Chinese medicine widely used in the treatment of acute ischaemic stroke, and myocardial infarction in China. Tanshinone, isotanshinone and hydroxytanshinone have been identified as some of the active constituents of importance. Pharmacological studies indicate that dan shen can be used for protecting against ischaemic reperfusion injury, improving circulation, dilating the cardio-cerebral vessels, suppressing the aggregation of platelets, removing blood stasis, enhancing the tolerance of ischaemic tissue to hypoxia and hence contributing to its protective action on the heart
Cardio-tonic	*Leonurus cardiaca* (motherwort)	Cardio-tonics are herbal medicines that protect the cardiac tissue from oxygen deficiency and improve the tone, vigour and strength of the cardiac muscle. *Leonurus* has traditionally been used as cardio-tonic. Ellingwood states it to be: 'a simple heart tonic, promoting normal action, probably very mild in its influence.' *Leonurus* is said to strengthen heart function and has hypotensive and anti-arrhythmic actions, supporting its use as a cardio-tonic. It is supported by the German Commission E for nervous cardiac disorders
Circulatory stimulant	*Ginkgo biloba* (ginkgo)	Circulatory stimulants improve blood flow to the body's tissues. In patients with coronary artery disease, coronary blood flow is usually impaired due to imbalanced vasoactive substances such as nitric oxide (NO) and endothelin-1 (ET-1). *Ginkgo biloba* can improve coronary blood flow and circulation in healthy adults as well as those with coronary heart disease
Fibrinolytic	*Centella asiatica* (gotu kola)	Fibrinolytic herbal medicines are those which help to prevent and break down insoluble fibrin clots. *Centella asiatica* has long been used in Ayurvedic medicine to treat a wide array of conditions. 3, 5-di-*O*-caffeoylquinic acid, a constituent of gotu kola, has been found to display an antithrombotic and inhibitory effect on dynamic coagulation. The results of this are significant when one considers fibrin clots play a pivotal role in cardiovascular conditions such as stroke
Hypertensive	*Glycyrrhiza glabra* (liquorice)	Hypertensive herbal medicines are those which increase blood pressure. *Glycyrrhiza glabra* exerts a hypertensive action and as a result mineralocorticoid activity is brought about by the glycoside glycyrrhizin, a major triterpenoid constituent of liquorice root. Glycyrrhizin inhibits hepatic and renal 11beta-OHSD and 5a-reductase, thereby blocking the inactivation of mineralocorticoids and increasing blood pressure
Hypocholesterolaemic	*Cynara scolymus* (globe artichoke)	Hypocholesterolaemic herbal medicines are those that reduce cholesterol in the body. Globe artichoke leaf has been used traditionally to increase bile flow and to act as a protective agent against various toxins. Data from various studies reveal that artichoke leaf and cynarin (the active constituent within artichoke leaf) have lipid-lowering effects

Continued

TABLE 20.5 Herbal medicine for the cardiovascular system—cont'd		
Class	**Example**	**Justification**
Hypolipidaemic	*Curcuma longa* (turmeric)	Hypolipidaemic medicines are those that reduce the concentrations of blood lipids (cholesterol and triglycerides). Curcumin, the principal ingredient of turmeric, is a potential cholesterol-lowering agent as indicated by clinical studies which reveal decreased levels of total cholesterol and non-HDL cholesterol in the plasma, following supplementation
Hypotensive	*Coleus forskohlii* (coleus)	Hypotensive herbs are those that lower blood pressure. *Coleus forskohlii* is a traditional Ayurvedic herb that has been a part of Indian medicine for centuries. In the 1970s researchers isolated a chemically active extract from the herb and called it forskolin. Clinical studies have demonstrated that forskolin significantly lowers blood pressure via relaxation of vascular smooth muscle. Another constituent of *Coleus*, known as coleonol, also reduces blood pressure, though to date this has only been seen in animals
Peripheral vasodilator	*Achillea millefolium* (yarrow)	Peripheral vasodilators widen blood vessels by relaxing the smooth muscle in the walls and decrease blood pressure. *Achillea millefolium* lowers high blood pressure and improves venous circulation by dilating the peripheral vessels. It is considered to be a specific in thrombotic conditions associated with high blood pressure
Vasoconstrictor	*Hydrastis canadensis* (goldenseal)	Vasoconstrictors cause narrowing of the blood vessels resulting from contraction of the muscular wall of the vessels so that flow of blood is restricted or decreased. Hydrastine, the active constituent of *Hydrastis canadensis*, may theoretically induce vasoconstriction, possibly resulting in hypertension
Vasoprotective	*Vaccinium myrtillus* (bilberry)	Bilberry helps to protect and maintain the capillaries. The dark-blue, sometimes velvet-black, berries of *V. myrtillus* contain anthocyanidins which are considered to be responsible for the main pharmacological effects of bilberry due to their antioxidative and free radical-scavenging properties
Venotonic	*Aesculus hippocastanum* (horse chestnut)	Venotonics help to maintain the structure and integrity of the veins. Horse chestnut has been used extensively in traditional European herbal medicine since the 16th century for conditions of venous congestion, particularly with dull, aching pain and fullness. In venous congestion, lysosomal enzymes break down the glycocalyx (mucopolysaccharides) in the capillary walls and as a result low-molecular proteins, electrolytes and water are filtered into the interstitium, leading to increased vascular permeability. Horse chestnut has been shown to prevent this from happening

Sources: Blumenthal M, Goldberg A, Brinckmann J. Herbal medicine: the expanded Commission E monographs. Newton, MA: Integrative Medicine Communications; 2000. Chevallier A. Encyclopedia of medicinal plants. London: Dorling Kindersley; 1996. Dubey MP, Srimal RC, Nityanand S et al. Pharmacological studies on coleonol, a hypotensive diterpene from *Coleus forskohlii*. J Ethnopharmacol 1981; 3(1):1–13. Ellingwood F. The American materia medica, therapeutics and pharmacognosy. Portland, OR: Eclectic Medical Publications; 1919. Felter HW. *Aesculus hippocastanum* — horsechestnut. In: The Eclectic materia medica, pharmacology and therapeutics. Portland, OR: Eclectic Materia Medica Publications; 1922. Fukao H, Yoshida H, Tazawa Y et al. Antithrombotic effects of odourless garlic powder both in vitro and in vivo. Biosci Biotechnol Biochem 2007; 71(1):84–90. Natural Standard Research Collaboration. Natural Standard Monographs (*Hydrastis canedensis*). Online. Available from: www.naturalstandard.com. Satake T, Kamiya K, An Y et al. The anti-thrombotic active constituents from *Centella asiatica*. Biol Pharm Bull 2007; 30(5):935–940. Wu B, Liu M, Zhang S. Dan shen agents for acute ischaemic stroke. Cochrane Database Syst Rev 2007(2); CD004295. Wu Y, Li S, Cui W et al. *Ginkgo biloba* extract improves coronary blood flow in healthy elderly adults: role of endothelium-dependent vasodilatation. Phytomedicine 2008; 15(3):164–169. Mancia G, Bombelli M, Fachetti R, et al. Long-term risk of sustained hypertension in white-coat or masked hypertension. Hypertension 2009;54(2):226–32.

a few hours of heart damage and remain elevated for up to 2 weeks

- CK-MB — one particular form of the enzyme creatine kinase that is found mostly in heart muscle and rises when there is damage to the heart muscle cells
- Myoglobin — a protein released into the blood when heart or other skeletal muscle is injured
- BNP or NT-proBNP — released by the body as a natural response to heart failure. Increased levels of BNP, while not diagnostic for a heart attack, indicate an increased risk of cardiac problems in patients with acute coronary syndrome. Because BNP is also released by the heart when it is stretched, it is also measured in those who have swelling of the legs or abdomen, or shortness of breath, to see if heart failure is present.

Cardiac risk assessment

This is a group of tests that are used to assess one's risk of having a heart attack.

COMPONENTS

- Personal health history — age, family history of heart disease, weight, smoking and exercise history, blood pressure, and diabetes
- Lipid profile — HDL, LDL, VLDL, triglycerides, total cholesterol
- Folate (B_9) and B_{12}.

HOMOCYSTEINE

Recent studies have suggested that people who have raised homocysteine levels have a much greater risk of heart attack or stroke than those with average levels. Blockage of a coronary artery, an event that can lead to a heart attack, occurs with more than double the average frequency in people with homocysteine levels in the highest 25% as compared with those in the lowest 25%. This evidence suggests that measurement of homocysteine may be an even better indicator of who is at risk of having a heart attack or stroke than other tests, such as cholesterol or lipid profile.

APOLIPOPROTEINS

ApoA-I and apoB may be measured as an alternative to HDL and LDL cholesterol respectively in the assessment of atherosclerosis risk factors, and may offer better prediction of risk. ApoB together with LDL cholesterol can be used to define hyperapobetalipoproteinaemia, a condition associated with small dense LDL and increased risk of atherosclerosis.

The apoA-I/apoB-100 ratio can be used as a coronary artery disease risk indicator. An increase of apoA-I is usually not a problem, but decreased levels are associated with low levels of HDL and decreased clearance of excess cholesterol from the body. Decreased levels of apoA-I coupled with increased concentrations of apoB-100 are associated with an increased risk of coronary artery disease.

Certain genetic disorders lead to deficiencies in apoA-I (and therefore to low levels of HDL). People with these disorders tend to have hyperlipidaemia and higher levels of LDL cholesterol. Frequently, they have accelerated rates of atherosclerosis.

ApoA-I may be decreased with:

- Chronic renal failure
- Drugs such as: androgens, beta blockers, diuretics and progestins (synthetic progesterone)
- Familial hypoalphalipoproteinaemia — a rare genetic disorder
- Smoking
- Uncontrolled diabetes.

ApoA-I may be increased with:

- Drugs such as carbamazepine, oestrogens, ethanol, niacin, oral contraceptives and phenobarbital (phenobarbitone)
- Familial hyperalphalipoproteinaemia (a rare genetic disorder)
- Physical exercise
- Pregnancy
- Weight reduction
- Use of statins such as pravastatin and simvastatin.

Lipoprotein a

Lipoprotein a (Lp(a)) is an independent risk factor for atherosclerosis and may be indicated in the assessment of a patient with premature coronary or cerebral arterial disease, especially if there is a suggestive family history.

Lp(a) levels are genetically determined and remain relatively constant over an individual's lifetime. They are not affected by lifestyle changes or by most drugs.

High Lp(a) levels may increase a person's risk for developing coronary artery disease and cerebral vascular disease and can occur in patients with a normal lipid profile. Elevated levels of Lp(a) are thought to work independently, to add to any underlying heart or vascular disease processes.

Other conditions that may cause elevated levels of Lp(a) include:

- Chronic renal failure
- Oestrogen depletion
- Familial hypercholesterolaemia
- Severe hypothyroidism
- Uncontrolled diabetes
- Nephrotic syndrome.

Low levels of Lp(a) do not appear to cause problems.

HIGH-SENSITIVITY C-REACTIVE PROTEIN

If a person's high-sensitivity C-reactive protein (hsCRP) level is on the high end of the normal range, it may be a sign that they are at risk for cardiovascular (heart and blood vessel) disease and other heart conditions. People who seem to be healthy but who have hsCRP results in the highest quartile have 2–4 times the risk of developing blocked arteries, compared with those in the lowest quartile.

The CRP molecule itself is not a harmful molecule in the body. The higher level of CRP is simply a sign of higher than normal inflammation. Because half of heart attacks and strokes happen in patients who do not have high levels of fat in their blood, measurement of hsCRP may help doctors identify patients who are at risk and in need of medical treatment.

Unfortunately, there is no agreement about exactly when the test should be used, and who should have it and there is currently no consensus about its value. Nevertheless, the test is being promoted by some as a test to help cardiologists assess risk of acute coronary syndrome (clogged blood vessels around the heart).

The results are generally interpreted on a relative scale. People with the highest values have the highest risk of heart disease and those with the lowest values have the lowest risk. This is often expressed in quintiles (five divisions) with those in the top fifth (the highest 20%) having risk of heart disease about twice that of those in the bottom fifth (lowest 20%).

General health assessment

More general blood tests that may be ordered include:

- Blood gases — performed to evaluate oxygen, carbon dioxide and pH levels
- Electrolytes, kidney and liver function tests (E/LFTs) — a group of tests that evaluate organ function
- Full blood count (FBC) — looks at the body's cells, checks for anaemia.

Other evaluations

A range of other evaluations and tests are used to assess chest pain and other symptoms. These include:

- A medical history, including an evaluation of risk factors such as age, CAD, diabetes, and smoking
- A physical examination, including blood pressure and others
- An electrocardiogram (ECG) — a test that looks at the heart's electrical activity and rhythm

- Echocardiography — ultrasound imaging of the heart.

Based on the findings of these tests, other procedures may be necessary, including:

- Stress testing
- Chest x-ray (CXR)
- CT (computed tomography) scan
- Continuous ECG monitoring (sometimes also called Holter monitoring) — the patient wears a monitor that evaluates heart rhythm over a period of time
- MRI (magnetic resonance imaging)
- PET (positron emission tomography)
- Radionuclide imaging
- Coronary angiography — x-rays of arteries using a radio-opaque dye to help diagnose CAD; this procedure is performed during coronary catheterisation
- Cardiac catheterisation — a thin flexible tube is inserted into an artery in the leg and threaded up to the coronary arteries to evaluate blood flow and pressure in the heart and the status of the arteries in the heart
- Tilt table test — to evaluate syncope.

Investigations

Investigations used for the cardiovascular system are listed in Table 20.6.

TABLE 20.6 Investigations

Assessment	Normal result	Clinical significance
Myoglobin	<70 micrograms/L	Increased levels are found in any condition causing muscle cell damage including myocardial infarction Myoglobin levels rise rapidly following myocardial infarction, peaking by about 90 min, but the protein is cleared rapidly by the kidneys This test is nonspecific and, if myocardial infarction is suspected, any raised value should be followed by a troponin assay
Erythrocyte sedimentation rate (ESR)	Child: 2–15 mm in 1 h Adult female 17–50 years: 3–19 mm in 1 h; 51–70 years: <20 mm in 1 h; >70 years: <35 mm in 1 h Adult male 17–50 years: 1–10 mm in 1 h; 51–70 years: <14 mm in 1 h; >70 years: <30 mm in 1 h	The ESR reflects an increase in the plasma concentration of acute-phase proteins, especially fibrinogen. This test shows the presence of inflammation in the body. A rising ESR can mean an increase in inflammation
C-reactive protein (CRP) test	<5.0 mg/L	CRP is an acute-phase protein that plays a major role in the regulation of the inflammatory response. The level of CRP rises when there is inflammation throughout the body. Inflammation plays a central role in the process of heart disease, particularly atherosclerosis Marginally raised CRP, and values within the normal range, have been demonstrated to be an independent risk factor for coronary artery disease. However, the applicability of measuring serum CRP for screening in asymptomatic populations for coronary artery disease risk remains unclear Note: hsCRP is considered more accurate with varying levels of accepted results from various pathology laboratories. Elevated hsCRP is believed to be a strong predictor of cardiovascular risk and recurrent events in patients with known coronary heart disease
Fibrinogen	1.5–4.0 g/L. Some variation with method	Fibrinogen is produced by the liver and is a protein in the blood to help blood clot. Excess amounts can increase the risk of clotting, leading to stroke or a heart attack. Excess fibrinogen can also signify inflammation associated with atherosclerosis Low levels indicate reduced production (liver disease, inherited deficiency) or increased consumption (DIC, fibrinolysis). Levels are elevated in an acute phase response
Apolipoproteins — serum	apoA-I: 1.0–1.8 g/L apoB: Optimally <0.9 g/L Lp(a): Optimally <200 mg/L — depends on method	Decreased apoA-I and increased apoB or apo(a) are associated with an increased risk of atherosclerosis Raised Lp(a) is associated with increased vascular risk. Homozygous apoE2 may result in type III hyperlipidaemia
Total cholesterol	For minimal risk of coronary artery disease, the Australian Heart Foundation recommends a treatment target of <4.0 mmol/L	Assessment of lipid status, particularly as a risk factor for coronary artery disease To assess atherosclerotic risk, cholesterol should be performed with triglyceride and HDL assays, as part of a global risk assessment

TABLE 20.6 Investigations—cont'd

Assessment	Normal result	Clinical significance
HDL cholesterol	Female — population reference range: 1.0–2.2 mmol/L; therapeutic targets: >1.0 mmol/L Male — population reference range: 0.9–2.0 mmol/L; therapeutic targets: >1.0 mmol/L	The optimal level is <4.0 mmol/L and higher levels are associated with an increased risk of coronary artery disease in all age groups. The cause may be primary (familial hypercholesterolaemia and other genetic disorders) or secondary (e.g. associated with biliary obstruction, hypothyroidism, nephrotic syndrome)
LDL cholesterol	LDL — population reference range: 2.0–3.4 mmol/L; therapeutic targets: <2.5 mmol/L LDL cholesterol is usually calculated rather than measured directly although this is unreliable if levels of triglyceride are >4.5 mmol/L The usual calculation using mmol/L for LDL cholesterol (Friedewald formula) is: LDL cholesterol = total cholesterol – HDL cholesterol – triglyceride/2.2	Low levels of HDL and high levels of LDL cholesterol are associated with an increased risk of atherosclerotic vascular disease Levels are reduced for up to 8 weeks with acute illness (e.g. myocardial infarction, acute infection) and assessment should not be attempted during this time Values increase in hyperlipidaemia, hypercholesterolaemia, atherosclerosis and hypertension
Triglycerides	<1.7 mmol/L (fasting)	Assessment of lipid status, especially in patients at high risk of developing hyperlipidaemia, e.g. diabetes mellitus, hypothyroidism Used in the calculation of LDL cholesterol by the Friedewald formula Lipoprotein electrophoresis should only be performed in patients with triglyceride levels of >4 mmol/L Increased levels seen in primary hypertriglyceridaemic states, and secondary to nephrotic syndrome, hypothyroidism, pancreatitis, diabetes mellitus, alcoholism, oral contraceptive use or corticosteroid medication Now generally accepted as an independent risk factor for coronary artery disease
Lipoprotein electrophoresis	Qualitative assessment	Investigation of patients with fasting triglyceride levels >4.0 mmol/L, to determine whether they have a type I, IIb, III, IV or V pattern. The test is not needed under other circumstances (e.g. isolated hypercholesterolaemia) to assess a lipoprotein abnormality. The main importance of the test is the diagnosis of patients with a type III pattern (dysbetalipoproteinaemia) who are at marked risk of premature vascular disease and xanthomata. This diagnosis should be confirmed by apoE genotyping or phenotyping
Troponin (serum)	Detected/undetected	Troponin is a protein released by dying heart cells and is a specific marker of myocardial injury and diagnoses previous myocardial infarction. The assays are specific for a cardiac isoform that occurs only in myocardium The test is very specific and sensitive for myocardial damage In myocardial infarction, elevation occurs from 4–12 h after the onset of pain and lasts for about 7 days. Some research indicates that it can remain elevated for up to 2 weeks post infarction In 'unstable angina' even a minor increase in troponin I should be regarded as defining the episode as a myocardial infarction
Red cell or serum folate	Red cell: 360–1400 nmol/L Serum: 7–45 nmol/L	Values are reduced in hyperhomocysteinaemia
Serum vitamin B_{12}	Serum B_{12}: Generally 120–680 pmol/L	Values are reduced in hyperhomocysteinaemia
Magnesium (plasma or serum)	Neonate: 0.6–0.9 mmol/L; adult: 0.8–1.0 mmol/L	Reliance on readings is controversial; however, detection of hypomagnesaemia as the cause of unexplained cardiac arrhythmias, neuromuscular disorders, refractory hypocalcaemia Patients with clinical features suggesting hypocalcaemia and a normal plasma calcium, or with refractory hypocalcaemia/hypokalaemia, should have plasma magnesium measured

Continued

TABLE 20.6 Investigations—cont'd

Assessment	Normal result	Clinical significance
Methylenetetrahydrafolate reductase mutation	Detected/undetected	MTHFR irreversibly reduces 5,10-methylenetetrahydrofolate (substrate) to 5-methyltetrahydrofolate (product) C677 — The MTHFR nucleotide at position 677 in the gene has 2 possibilities: C (cytosine) or T (thymine). 677C is the normal allele. 677T encodes a thermolabile enzyme with reduced activity. Individuals who are homozygous normal 677CC have both normal alleles, while individuals with 677TT are homozygous for the MTHFR deficiency. Individuals who code for 677CT are considered heterozygous for the mutation Low folate intake affects individuals with the 677TT genotype to a greater extent than those with the 677CC/CT genotypes. 677TT (but not 677CC/CT) individuals with lower plasma folate levels are at risk for elevated plasma homocysteine levels A1298 — Additionally, the nucleotide 1298 can have additional outcomes. At nucleotide 1298 of the MTHFR, there are two possibilities: A or C. 1298A (leading to a Glu at amino acid 429) is the most common while 1298C (leading to an Ala substitution at amino acid 429) is less common. 1298AA is the 'normal' homozygous, 1298AC the heterozygous, and 1298CC the homozygous for the 'variant'. In studies of human recombinant MTHFR, the protein encoded by 1298C cannot be distinguished from 1298A in terms of activity, thermolability, FAD release, or the protective effect of 5-methyl-THF. The C mutation does not appear to affect the MTHFR protein. It does not result in thermolabile MTHFR and does not appear to affect homocysteine levels
Homocysteine	5–15 μmol/L. If there is established vascular disease it is desirable that the fasting concentration is <10 μmol/L	Mild hyperhomocysteinaemia is an established risk factor for atherosclerosis and vascular disease Elevated homocysteine levels may result from low levels of folic acid, vitamin B_6, or vitamin B_{12}, some drugs and renal impairment, as well as a number of inherited defects

SECTION B

CARDIOVASCULAR RISK MANAGEMENT

It is widely recognised that a number of cardiovascular conditions are the result of the cumulative effect of multiple risk factors.[9] Management of these risk factors can be beneficial not just in secondary prevention, but also in the context of tertiary prevention, where addressing these factors may reduce the severity and progression of an existing condition.

Thus a whole system view is essential in the naturopathic understanding of cardiovascular risk factors. The contribution of individual factors versus combinations of factors is difficult to quantify, nevertheless a number of examples exist where certain combinations are well known as contributing to proportionally higher risk.[9] While the importance of dietary and lifestyle risk factors and their effect on population-level primary prevention should not be underestimated, it is largely beyond the scope of this chapter. Henceforth the focus will be on naturopathically modifiable risk factors in the context of secondary and tertiary prevention. These include:

- hypertension
- oxidative stress
- dyslipidaemia
- inflammation
- psychological stress and mood disorders
- atherosclerosis (itself seen as a pathological change resulting from many of the above risk factors).

HYPERTENSION

Epidemiology

Hypertension is an increasingly common problem. It affects approximately 1 billion people worldwide[10] and is the most common condition managed by Australian general practitioners.[11] Hypertension and associated cardiovascular conditions are the most expensive diseases in terms of health expenditure, absorbing up to 11% of allocated health funds.[12] There is evidence to suggest that the gradual increase in public health education has reduced the risk factors for hypertension,[13] reducing cardiovascular death rates and increasing life expectancy.[14] However, statistics still show that one in three Australians over the age of 24 has reported high blood pressure.[15]

Classification

Hypertension is classified according to the amount by which the blood pressure is elevated, the causative factors (if known) and concurrent pathology (Table 20.7).

TABLE 20.7 Classification of hypertension

Classification	Systolic pressure		Diastolic pressure
Normal	<120 mmHg	and	<80 mmHg
Prehypertension (high–normal)	120–139 mmHg	or	80–89 mmHg
Stage 1 hypertension	140–159 mmHg	or	and/or 90–99 mmHg
Stage 2 hypertension	>159 mmHg	or	and/or >99 mmHg

Source: Adapted from Chobhain A, Bakris G, Black H, et al. The Seventh Report of the Joint National Committee On Prevention, Detection, Evaluation, and Treatment of High Blood Pressure. US Department of Health and Human Services, 2004.

THERAPEUTIC CLASSIFICATION

The level of arterial pressure in hypertension will impact upon the diagnosis, intervention and treatment of the condition.[16]

Essential hypertension

When a direct cause cannot be established, the condition is known as essential hypertension. It is estimated that the majority of cases, 90–95% of hypertensive patients, have essential hypertension.[17] Of these cases, many have identifiable behaviours that contribute to the condition, including lifestyle factors such as high intake of kilojoules, salt and alcohol.

Secondary hypertension

Only 5–10% of hypertensive patients have the condition as the result of an identifiable cause. Secondary causes are more common in those under the age of 20 and over the age of 50 at the time of onset, with no other risk factors.[18]

White coat hypertension

Whie coat hypertension occurs when blood pressure is persistently elevated in an office or clinical setting. Often considered an 'innocent' phenomenon, the condition requires monitoring to ensure sustained hypertension does not develop. Longitudinal studies have shown that individuals who present with white coat hypertension are more at risk than their normotensive counterparts for developing hypertension and/or cardiovascular complications later in life.[19]

Aetiology

The pathogenesis of hypertension is not fully understood. It is generally acknowledged as a multifactorial condition, resulting in the disruption of arterial pressure and fluid volume. Hypertension rarely occurs in isolation. Persistently elevated blood pressure will often manifest clinically in major organs such as the heart, brain and kidneys.[20]

GENETICS

The rate of hypertension is greater within family groups than in unrelated individuals.[21] One longitudinal study investigating African-American and Caucasian hypertensive siblings over a period of 5 years demonstrated that certain factors, such as left ventricular mass, appear to be genetically predisposed, implying greater risk of disease progression in related individuals.[22,23]

ETHNICITY

Hypertension is more common in certain ethnic groups. The African-American population has a much higher prevalence of hypertension than the rest of the American population, concurrent with a tendency to develop the condition earlier in life.[24] People of African descent living in the United Kingdom have also historically had higher blood pressure in comparison to the rest of the population.[25] However, interestingly, hypertension is far less common among Africans living in Africa, suggesting greater significance of environmental and socioeconomic factors. In addition, European studies have shown more cases of hypertension in the non-African population of some countries (Finland, Germany and Spain) than in African-Americans.[24]

SOCIOECONOMIC STATUS

Unfortunately, individuals from lower socioeconomic backgrounds and those with poor access to education are at increased risk of developing hypertension.[13] Those in regional, or non-urban, communities also have poor general health and a higher incidence than their urban equivalents of hypertension and cardiovascular disease.[26] The Australian Indigenous population has a much lower overall health projection, with many individuals living in non-urban communities and low socioeconomic environments, concomitant with significantly higher rates of illness and mortality than the rest of the Australian population.[27] Indigenous Australians have much higher rates of cardiovascular disease, with an increased frequency of risk factors including smoking, alcohol consumption, excess body weight, poor nutrition and diabetes. There is a significant trend towards the development of hypertension from a younger age, affecting approximately 7% of the Indigenous population — 1.6 times higher than that in the rest of Australia.[28]

AGE

Hypertension is a problem inherent in an ageing population. Systemic blood pressure naturally rises with age and with it the incidence of hypertension and cardiovascular disease.[17] Hypertension occurs in over two-thirds of individuals over the age of 65,[29] which is also the population group with the lowest rate of adequate blood pressure control.[30] With an increment of 20 mmHg in systolic blood pressure or 10 mmHg in diastolic blood pressure, individuals between 40 and 70 years of age have a dramatically increased risk of cardiovascular disease.[31] The Framingham Heart Study showed that even those who are normotensive up to 55 years of age have a 90% chance of developing hypertension later in life.[32]

SEX

By and large, young to early middle-age women have a much lower prevalence of hypertension than their male counterparts, which is commonly attributed to the protective effects of oestrogen.[33] However, following menopause the incidence of cardiovascular disease among women increases significantly, and with it hypertension.[34]

OBESITY

Australian statistics show that more than one-third of the adult population are overweight, with over half of this group classified as obese. More alarming is that these numbers are on the rise.[35] Individuals who are overweight or obese carry a much greater risk of hypertension and dyslipidaemia.[36] In obese people, insulin resistance and hyperinsulinaemia have also been linked to the development of hypertension.[37]

DIET

One of the most important determinants of essential hypertension is diet.[21] A nutrient-poor diet, low in fresh produce and high in saturated fats, is both predisposing and sustaining for high blood pressure.[38] High salt consumption is also correlated with hypertension and its associated comorbidities.[39] Regular alcohol consumption can also influence the progression of hypertension if large amounts (>2 drinks per day) are involved. The pattern of consumption is important, as studies have shown that daily alcohol consumption as well as alcohol consumed predominantly outside of mealtimes significantly increases the risk of hypertension.[40]

STRESS

Stress can cause blood pressure elevation. Acutely, this occurs through sympathetic hyperactivity: resulting in increased production of catecholamines, stimulated renin production, constriction of arterioles and veins and, ultimately, increased cardiac output.[41] Chronic stress has, obviously, a more enduring effect on the body, including an increased likelihood of developing hypertension.[42]

SMOKING

Smoking has numerous deleterious health effects. It is independently and significantly associated with the onset of hypertension.[43] Smoking also increases arterial stiffness — a precursor to hypertension and other cardiovascular conditions.[44]

HEAVY METAL EXPOSURE

Exposure to heavy metals such as lead, mercury, cadmium and arsenic may also be a significant factor in some patients. The kidneys are end-organ targets of heavy metals. Although the link between blood lead levels and hypertension is still in debate, one study comparing male hypertensive (222 patients), normotensive (322 patients), and prehypertensive patients (432 patients) showed that hypertensive patients had higher blood lead levels.[45]

HYPERHOMOCYSTEINAEMIA

In 1969 McCully discovered severe atherosclerotic disease in the autopsy of two children with congenital homocysteine disorder. He postulated that the atherosclerotic change was directly linked to elevated blood levels of homocysteine (hyperhomocysteinaemia) (Fig. 20.2).

Homocysteine has been shown to be an independent risk factor of similar importance to cholesterol. Mild hyperhomocysteinaemia is asymptomatic, but evidence strongly suggests that it causes vascular damage via a number of mechanisms:

- Decreasing available NO (nitric oxide)
- Contributing to oxidation
- Damaging the vascular matrix.

Overview

Hypertension is a condition characterised by persistently elevated blood pressure. Comorbid conditions include cardiovascular disease events, diabetes and kidney disease.

Pathogenesis

Hypertension may result from any number of factors — vascular, hormonal, renal and neurological aspects are all involved in maintenance of blood pressure and disruption in any one will invariably upset the balance of regulatory mechanisms.[21] Essentially, blood pressure increases as a response to systemic and intrarenal vasoconstriction — it can be an acute or chronic reaction. Over time, this will cause tissue degradation and microvascular damage, involving immune and inflammatory processes.[46]

SIGNS AND SYMPTOMS

Hypertension is often asymptomatic; the most common presentations include headaches, dizziness, tinnitus and fainting, although these occur just as commonly in the normotensive population. As a result, hypertension is often referred to as the silent killer, because it can cause damage to blood vessels, heart, brain and kidneys if undetected and untreated long term.[41]

COMPLICATIONS

Cardiovascular disease

Hypertensive patients have a much higher risk of developing cardiovascular disease compared with normotensive individuals. This rate rises significantly for those whose condition is not treated.[47] Ischaemic heart disease is the most common form of organ damage associated with hypertension.[29] Heart failure — systolic or diastolic ventricular dysfunction — results primarily from systolic hypertension and ischaemic heart disease.[48]

Diabetes

Hypertension is very common in diabetic patients, playing a major role in both macro- and microvascular complications of the condition.[49] While apparent in type 1

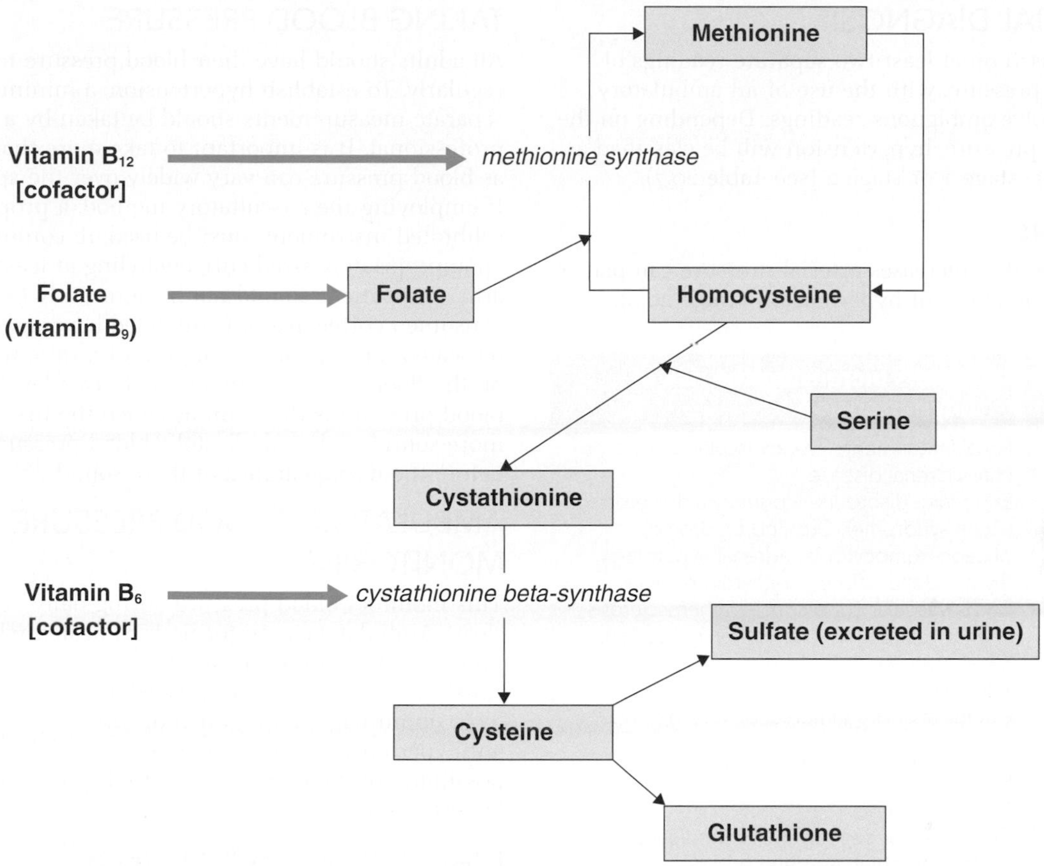

FIGURE 20.2 Homocysteine metabolism.

diabetes, in the absence of renal impairment hypertension is similar to that in the non-diabetic population. However, it is far more common in type 2 diabetes, with over 70% of patients reporting elevated blood pressure.[50] Hypertension in cases of type 1 diabetes can indicate nephropathy — a leading cause of renal disease, associated with significant cardiovascular mortality.[51] Diabetic hypertension can be difficult to control, often fluctuating dramatically; and combination therapy of two or more drugs is often prescribed by physicians.[52]

Renal disease

Chronic renal disease commonly presents with hypertension and treatment is usually aimed at slowing the deterioration of kidney function, in conjunction with preventing further deterioration of cardiovascular symptoms.[53] Renovascular disease is another condition linked to hypertension, and involves progressive narrowing of the renal arteries or veins. Although relatively uncommon, it is a frequent (curable) cause of hypertension. Factors indicating the presence of this condition include: hypertension before the age of 30; sudden onset of hypertension in middle age; resistant hypertension (to multiple combination therapy); idiopathic renal impairment; peripheral vascular disease; recurrent pulmonary oedema or heart failure with no known cause.[54]

Cerebrovascular disease

Cerebrovascular disease is associated with hypertension, and lowering blood pressure, particularly during acute treatment, reduces recurrent stroke rate.[55]

Autonomic nervous system

Elderly hypertensive patients have been shown to present more regularly with dementia and cognitive impairment than those with normal blood pressure.[56] Longitudinal studies have shown beneficial results in managing hypertension and its effect on dementia and cognitive decline.[57]

Pregnancy

Hypertension is one of the most common medical complications of pregnancy, affecting up to 10% of expectant mothers.[58] It may be a relatively benign event, or a harbinger of a more serious condition, such as the development of pre-eclampsia. The level of hypertension, involvement of other systems (e.g. kidneys), stage of pregnancy, health of mother and fetus will all dictate treatment and intervention recommendations. At all times, the aim should be to reduce blood pressure consistently and safely in order to prevent maternal and neonatal complications.[59]

DIFFERENTIAL DIAGNOSIS

Diagnosis is based on at least two separate readings of elevated blood pressure, with the use of an ambulatory measure to resolve ambiguous readings. Depending on the patient's blood pressure, hypertension will be classified as prehypertensive, stage 1 or stage 2 (see Table 20.7).

Other factors

Any mechanism that increases arterial pressure can play a part in the development of hypertension (Table 20.8).

TABLE 20.8 Factors increasing the risk of hypertension

Identifiable causes of hypertension	Renal impairment — renovascular disease, chronic renal disease Endocrine disorders — primary aldosteronism (Conn syndrome), Cushing syndrome, phaeochromocytoma, adrenal hyperplasia, thyroid dysfunction, parathyroid disease Cardiovascular conditions — atherosclerosis, arterial obstruction, coarctation of the aorta Sleep apnoea Pregnancy Chemical or drug interaction (see below)
Medications that may increase blood pressure	Immunosuppressive agents NSAIDs COX-2 inhibitors Oestrogen or oestrogen-like medication Certain weight-loss agents Stimulants Mineralocorticoids Antiparkinsonian drugs MAO inhibitors Anabolic steroids Sympathomimetics, such as pseudoephedrine

Sources: Adapted from Gray H, Dawkins K, Morgan J, et al. Cardiology. 5th ed. Oxford: Blackwell Publishing; 2008. Taylor G. Primary care cardiology. 2nd ed. Oxford: Blackwell Publishing; 2005.

NATUROPATHIC DIAGNOSIS

Diagnosis of hypertension largely relies on allopathic determinants. Assessment of predisposing risk factors is also important, and can be evaluated via a thorough case history. Nutritional intake, exercise factor, digestive and metabolic function, hormonal status, mental health, environment and comorbidities all play a role in the incidence of hypertension and should be considered in any treatment strategy.

Investigations

FAMILY/PERSONAL HISTORY

It is important to establish whether the patient has a strong family history of hypertension and heart disease, as this may predispose them to developing the condition during their own lifetime. A full case history, including diagnosed conditions and present medication is necessary in order to rule out any potentiating factors or possible causes.

TAKING BLOOD PRESSURE

All adults should have their blood pressure measured regularly. To establish hypertension, a minimum of two separate measurements should be taken by a health professional. It is important to take more than one reading, as blood pressure can vary widely over the space of 24 h. If employing the auscultatory method, a properly calibrated instrument must be used, in conjunction with an appropriately sized cuff, encircling at least 80% of the arm. The patient should not have recently (within 1 h) consumed coffee, tea or caffeinated beverages. They should be seated quietly for a minimum of 5 min, with the feet on the floor and arm supported at heart level. Systolic blood pressure is the point at which the first of two or more sounds is heard; diastolic blood pressure is the point before the disappearance of these sounds.[10]

AMBULATORY BLOOD PRESSURE MONITORING

This monitors blood pressure during daily activities and sleep. Ambulatory monitoring is indicated when blood pressure shows unusual variability; in hypertension resistant to drug therapy (defined as blood pressure >150/90 mmHg on a regimen of three or more antihypertensive drugs); when symptoms suggest the possibility of hypotension; and to diagnose white coat hypertension.[60]

DIAGNOSTIC PROCEDURES[61]

Routine investigations for hypertension are usually limited and used in order to rule out more insidious pathology (Table 20.9).

NATUROPATHIC INVESTIGATIONS

A full case history in conjunction with conventional investigations should inform any treatment strategy for a hypertensive patient. The condition is often enmeshed with lifestyle factors such as dietary intake, exercise, weight, ethnic background, socioeconomic status and environment, so it is important to discuss these points with the patient in order to identify areas for improvement and change. There are also several functional medicine tests that can be used for additional clarification.

Out of the relationship formed in a naturopathic consultation, the clinician can assist with the proper diagnosis and monitoring of a patient by considering the following factors:

- White coat syndrome — ensure that the patient has settled and is emotionally comfortable prior to assessment
- Home monitoring — home assessments are notoriously inaccurate. It is a good idea to get the patient to bring in their home unit and compare readings with in-clinic readings
- Take care to avoid over-monitoring — this can increase anxiety for the patient.

In addition, significant importance should be placed on technique:

- Assess positioning of the sphygmomanometer and ensure it is not overdue for calibration

TABLE 20.9 Routine investigations for hypertension

Investigation	Finding
Urinalysis	Urinary glucose is a crude screen for diabetes Albuminuria is a sign of kidney disease, even if serum creatinine is normal. It is linked to the development of diabetes, hypertension and kidney inflammation Haematuria can also indicate kidney disease. In isolation it may be idiopathic, or indicative of a localised infection and inflammation
Serum — electrolytes	Potassium plays an important role in cardiovascular function and hormone regulation. Hypokalaemia may indicate hyperaldosteronism (Conn's syndrome), one of the most common causes of secondary hypertension. Certain medications, namely diuretics, can also deplete potassium and should therefore be monitored Sodium can be low in patients with more developed cardiovascular conditions, such as congestive heart failure, and indicates the need for immediate intervention Calcium and phosphate levels are markers for hyperparathyroidism, which can cause hypertension
Serum — metabolites	Creatinine is elevated in cases of renal dysfunction Urea is elevated in cases of renal dysfunction Glucose (fasting) is an effective screen for possible diabetes. Hyperglycaemia is also associated with secondary causes of hypertension, including Cushing's syndrome and primary aldosteronism
Serum — lipid analysis	Elevated triglycerides, elevated LDL cholesterol and/or low HDL cholesterol are risk factors for cardiovascular disease and features of a constellation of symptoms known as metabolic syndrome
Serum — full blood count	This will identify underlying inflammation or infection Haematocrit will indicate whether anaemia is a marker for the condition polycythaemia, with can result in hypertension
Serum — vitamin D	Vitamin D deficiency can contribute to hypertension and cardiovascular disease[76]
Electrocardiogram (ECG)	This will identify arrhythmias and screen for left-ventricular hypertrophy, indicative of hypertensive heart disease
Homocysteine	Assess associated risk factors for hypertension

- Check that cuff size is appropriate for the patient
- Ensure that the stethoscope is tested.

Essential fatty acids

Various tests can be used to measure essential fatty acids in the body, which can be deficient or imbalanced in hypertension and cardiovascular disease.

Functional liver detoxification profile

Poor liver function can compromise essential fatty acid status. It can also indicate insufficient detoxification, subsequently increasing the load on the heart, liver and kidneys.

Total antioxidant status

Poor, or low, antioxidant status can reflect high free-radical load, which is often apparent in hypertensive patients.[62] It may also indicate compromised liver function.

Toxic nutrient screen

It may also be appropriate to investigate heavy metal toxicity if exposure to heavy metals like lead, mercury, cadmium and arsenic is relevant to the patient's case. The kidneys are end-organ targets of heavy metals and toxicity is implicated in hypertension.[63]

Therapeutic considerations

CLINICAL DECISION MAKING AND RATIONALE

It is imperative to differentiate between the types of hypertension when developing treatment protocols.

Primary hypertension (2–5% of cases)

- Renal or adrenal disease.

Essential hypertension (95–98% of cases)

- Obesity
- Smoking
- High alcohol intake
- High salt intake
- Excessive sympathetic nervous dominance
- Increased vascular resistance.

With this information, the clinician can then reflect on a number of key contributing factors. Without acknowledgement of these areas, it is unlikely that treatment will be successful. These include:

- Ethnicity and genetics: While no change can be made to a person's genes, it is important to acknowledge associated risk factors and support potential triggers for hypertensive development.
- Socioeconomic status: In the development of a treatment plan, it is essential to prioritise treatment recommendations so as not to aggravate any underlying financial stressors. Strong focus on dietary and lifestyle practices can provide much improvement long term; however, in the short term other treatments are required additionally.
- Age and sex: Considering the patient's age is beneficial to assess potential progression of the disease over time. Assessing a woman's menopausal status can elucidate potential future developments.
- Obesity: If a patient is overweight, a major component of the success of treatment will depend on if they can lose weight and reach a healthy weight level.
- Diet: Patients must adhere to dietary changes for successful intervention. For example if sodium intake is

not reduced, hyperstimulation of blood pressure (electrolyte imbalance) will perpetuate levels.

- Stress: While stress reduction is likely to take time throughout treatment, it is essential to provide stress-reducing strategies and treatments to support hypotensive effects.
- Smoking and other lifestyle factors: If a patient is not committed to compliance and cessation of smoking and other lifestyle practices, it is unlikely that treatment will be successful and judicious referral is advised.
- Heavy metal exposure: It is essential to properly assess patients first through case taking and then by referral for additional assessment as required. If heavy metal toxicity is not addressed, treatment potential will be significantly hindered due to competition of nutrient site.

Therapeutic application

ALLOPATHIC PERSPECTIVE

The treatment of hypertension (Fig. 20.3) will depend on whether it is associated with another treatable condition, as well as the level of hypertension. The ultimate goal lies in reducing latent hypertension and comorbid risk factors (Table 20.10).

TABLE 20.10 Allopathic medication regimen

BP classification	Hypertension without other risk factors	Hypertension with risk factors (e.g. diabetes)
Prehypertension	No antihypertensive medication is indicated	Medication specific to risk factor
Stage 1 hypertension	Thiazide-type diuretics for most; may consider ACE inhibitor, ARB, beta-blocker, CCB or combination	Medication specific to risk factor. Other antihypertensive drugs (diuretics, ACE inhibitor, ARB, beta-blocker, CCB) as needed
Stage 2 hypertension	Combination therapy for most (usually thiazide-type diuretic and ACE inhibitor or ARB or beta-blocker or CCB)	Medication specific to risk factor. Other antihypertensive drugs (diuretics, ACE inhibitor, ARB, beta-blocker, CCB) as needed

Abbreviations: angiotensin receptor blockers (ARB); calcium channel blockers (CCB); angiotensin-converting enzyme (ACE).
Source: Adapted from Chobhain A, Bakris G, Black H, et al. The Seventh Report of the Joint National Committee On Prevention, Detection, Evaluation, and Treatment of High Blood Pressure. US Department of Health and Human Services, 2004.

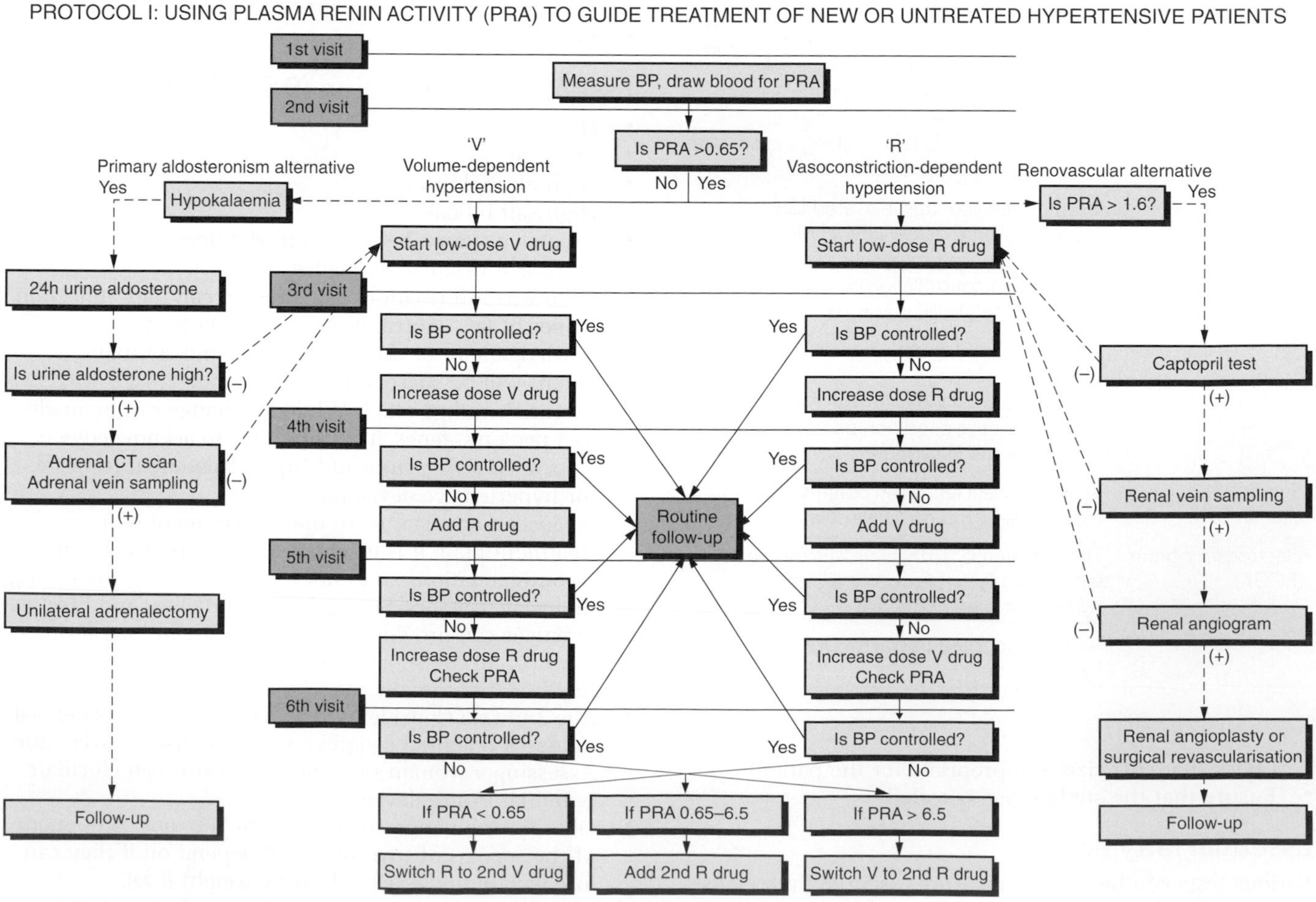

FIGURE 20.3 Hypertension.

Source: Brenner BM: Brenner and Rector's the kidney. 8th edn. Philadelphia: Saunders; 2007.

Non-pharmacological treatment is the primary intervention, and even when drug therapy is employed, dietary and lifestyle therapy is recommended for hypertensive and borderline hypertensive patients:[64]

- Weight reduction/maintenance of healthy weight (BMI 19–25)
- Dietary modification — increasing fruits and vegetables, reducing saturated and total fat
- Restrict dietary sodium — reduce intake to 2.4 g sodium (6 g sodium chloride) daily
- Physical exercise — maintain regular aerobic activity, ideally 30 min per day
- Limit alcohol consumption — no more than 2 standard drinks per day for men and 1 standard drink per day for women.

Allopathic medicine commonly employs antihypertensive medication in order to reduce blood pressure. Many hypertensive patients require two or more antihypertensive drugs to reach a healthy goal blood pressure.[65] Controlling systolic (as opposed to diastolic) blood pressure is the most important cardiovascular risk factor in patients younger than 50 years, although it can pose a considerable challenge.[66]

HISTORICAL PERSPECTIVE

Hypertension was first identified in the early 1800s and the famous cuff sphygmomanometer was in use by the early 20th century.[46] Although there is little description of hypertension in the pages of the Eclectic texts, gelsenium is described for its use in 'softening the blood pressure, slowly reducing the pulse'. Nervines such as *Scutellaria lateriflora* are likely to have been used; the latter was advocated for 'functional heart disorders of a purely nervous character, with intermittent pulse whether accompanied or not by hysterical excitement'. *Viscum album* and *Crataegus* were suggested for valvular insufficiency, as was cactus which was said to be useful for all cardiac irregularities.

NATUROPATHIC PERSPECTIVE

The naturopathic perspective addresses all key aspects of the patient's health. It takes a similar strong approach to weight, dietary influences and lifestyle practices and uses key nutritional supplements and herbal medicine prescriptions to lower blood pressure. As over 80% of patients with hypertension are in the borderline-to-moderate range, most cases of hypertension are generally able to be brought under control through changes in diet and lifestyle modifications.

For all patients, treatment aims to reduce blood pressure to <140/90 mmHg; for those with a kidney disorder or diabetes, the goal is <130/80 mmHg or as near this level as can be tolerated. Even the elderly and frail elderly can tolerate a diastolic blood pressure as low as 60–65 mmHg well and without an increase in cardiovascular events.[67] Ideally, patients or family members should measure blood pressure at home, provided they have been trained to do so, they are closely monitored, and the sphygmomanometer is regularly calibrated.

In stage 1 (mild) hypertension with no signs of target-organ damage, lifestyle changes may make drugs unnecessary. Patients with uncomplicated hypertension do not need to restrict their activities as long as blood pressure is controlled. Dietary modifications can also help control diabetes, obesity and dyslipidaemia. Patients with prehypertension are encouraged to follow these lifestyle recommendations.

If systolic blood pressure remains higher than 140 mmHg or diastolic blood pressure remains over 90 mmHg after 6 months of lifestyle modifications, antihypertensive drugs are required. Unless hypertension is severe, drugs are usually started at low doses. Drugs are initiated simultaneously with lifestyle changes for all patients with prehypertension or hypertension plus diabetes, a kidney disorder, target-organ damage or cardiovascular risk factors and for those with an initial blood pressure of >160/100 mmHg. Signs of hypertensive emergencies require immediate blood pressure reduction with parenteral antihypertensives.

The general recommendation is that medications are required if blood pressure is initially high (>160/100 mmHg) or unresponsive to lifestyle modifications. If a patient presents with elevated readings as listed above, it is imperative to work closely with their GP and ensure that they are regularly monitored and assessed.

NUTRITIONAL MEDICINE (DIETARY)

Dietary therapeutic objectives

- Aim to reduce all dietary sources of sodium and assess processed food intake for 'hidden' sources
- Increase fresh (preferably organic) fruit and vegetables
  - Fruit 2–3 servings per day
  - Vegetables 5–7 servings per day
  - Celery and its juice and bananas for potassium
  - Green leafy vegetables for increased calcium and magnesium sources
  - Garlic and onions for hypolipidaemic effects
- Increase non-mercury rich sources of fish (2–3 times per week minimum). Important sources include mackerel, non-farmed salmon and sardines
- Increase essential fatty acids from vegetarian sources including fresh (unroasted, unsalted) raw nuts and seeds or their oils for EFA content
- Increase fibre from wholegrains and legumes
- Reduce or avoid alcohol
- Reduce and avoid caffeine stimulants from coffee, black tea, cola and other soft drinks especially. Green tea and chocolate appear to be less stimulating; however, reduction is beneficial.

Specific dietary treatments

DIETARY INCLUSIONS

Vegetarian diet

Diet plays a major role in the development of hypertension, so it can also be used therapeutically to protect against the disorder. The benefits of a vegetarian diet in patients with hypertension have been observed in a number of studies in which vegetarians have been shown to have lower blood pressure then their meat-eating counterparts. The key point here is that a hypotensive vegetarian diet refers to one that is plant based; a vegetarian diet based upon copious amounts of cheese (high in salt) and processed foods is unlikely to confer the same benefits. A review of observational studies suggests that patients who switch to a plant-based vegetarian diet can expect a significant decrease in their blood pressure, with systolic and diastolic blood pressure of vegetarians observed to be 3–14/5–6 mmHg lower, respectively, than that of non-vegetarians.[68]

Fresh fruits and vegetables

A diet rich in fruit and vegetables is associated with reduced blood pressure. This is not surprising when one considers the vast and varied nutrient content (such as potassium, magnesium and fibre) available in these foods, all of which are likely to contribute to this hypotensive action. Trials[69] assessing the effects of diets rich in fruit and vegetables as well as the DASH diet (Box 20.1) which is also high in fruit and vegetables, have demonstrated significant reductions in blood pressure in individuals with hypertension after only 2 months of consuming more fruit and vegetables.

Potassium

Increasing potassium has been shown to promote urinary sodium excretion,[70] which is why numerous studies have demonstrated that higher intake of potassium is associated with lower blood pressure.[71–73] In the DASH Trial a potassium-rich diet (containing 4100 mg/day potassium and on average 8 pieces of fruit/vegetables) was found to lower blood pressure by an average of 7.2/2.8 mmHg in hypertensive individuals[71] compared with the controls who were on a diet which contained only 1700 mg/day potassium and 3 pieces of fruit/vegetables. This further emphasises the argument for fruit and vegetables in hypertensive patients, particularly those that are potassium rich, such as leafy green vegetables, zucchini, bananas, beans, cucumbers and pumpkin.[70] As potassium is readily absorbed from a diet rich in fresh fruits and vegetables, supplementation is typically not required.

BOX 20.1 The Dietary Approaches to Stop Hypertension (DASH) diet

The Dietary Approaches to Stop Hypertension (DASH) diet emphasises foods that are rich in fruit, vegetables, low-fat milk and milk products, wholegrains, fish, poultry, beans, seeds and nuts. It also contains less salt and sodium; sweets, added sugars and sugar-containing beverages; fats; and red meats than the typical Australian diet. The diet is also lower in saturated fat, trans fat and cholesterol and rich in nutrients such as magnesium, potassium, calcium, protein and fibre, all of which are associated with reduced blood pressure. The positive antihypertensive effects of the DASH diet are well published hence the recommendation to follow its basic principles in patients with hypertension.

Sources: Appel LJ, Moore TJ, Obarzanek E et al. A clinical trial of the effects of dietary patterns on blood pressure. DASH Collaborative Research Group. N Engl J Med 1997; 336(16):1117–1124. Harsha DW, Lin PH, Obarzanek E et al. Dietary Approaches to Stop Hypertension: a summary of study results. DASH Collaborative Research Group. J Am Diet Assoc 1999; 99(Suppl. 8):S35–S39. National Heart, Lung, and Blood Institute. Your guide to lowering your blood pressure with DASH. Available from: www.nhlbi.nih.gov/health/public/heart/hbp/dash/dash_brief.pdf. Sacks FM, Svetkey LP, Vollmer WM et al. DASH-Sodium Collaborative Research Group. Effects on blood pressure of reduced dietary sodium and the Dietary Approaches to Stop Hypertension (DASH) diet. DASH-Sodium Collaborative Research Group. N Engl J Med 2001; 344(1):3–10.

Garlic and onions

Both garlic and onion are rich in thiosulfinates and sulfur compounds and have been demonstrated to play a positive role in the management of hypertension. A meta-analysis by Reid et al[74] demonstrated garlic preparations to be useful in hypertension. The majority of studies used garlic powder dosages of 600–900 mg/day, providing potentially 3.6–5.4 mg of allicin; comparatively fresh garlic cloves each contain 5–9 mg allicin and are thus likely to be a better option. Garlic may be consumed in the form of pestos or baked with roast vegetables for those who find raw garlic unpalatable.

There has been little in the way of human clinical studies assessing the effects of onion on hypertension, but a study by Kalus et al[75] observed that supplementation with an onion/olive oil maceration capsule resulted in a decrease in arterial blood pressure. Animal studies reveal the ability of onion to inhibit production of angiotensin II, scavenge free radicals and save nitric oxide, all of which are suggested to contribute to its hypotensive action.[76]

DIETARY EXCLUSIONS

Sodium

The majority of diets in the West contain an excess of sodium, as well as an excess of sodium relative to potassium.[77] At least two meta-analyses have provided a link between excessive sodium intake and elevated blood pressure.[78,79]

Food Standards Australia and New Zealand (FSANZ) has estimated current sodium intakes from salt for the Australian population. These results show that Australians aged 2 years and older consume an average of 2150 mg of sodium per day from an average of 5500 mg of salt (5.5 g). About 80% of this is from processed foods and 20% from salt used at the table or in home cooking. This estimate does not include the smaller amounts of sodium coming from naturally occurring sodium or sodium-containing food additives. Some Australians (34%) are estimated to consume sodium at levels above that recommended from salt alone.[80]

The recommended daily intake of sodium in Australia is 8–9 times the amount required. The National Health and Medical Research Council (NHMRC) recommends that adults should aim to consume no more than 4 g/day of salt (equivalent to 1600 mg sodium). The Heart Foundation suggests that adults should reduce their salt intake to <6 g/day (approximately 2300 mg sodium/day).

Guidelines for hypertensive patients indicate that they should maintain their sodium intake below <2.4 g/day (equivalent to <6 g NaCl/day) to significantly improve their

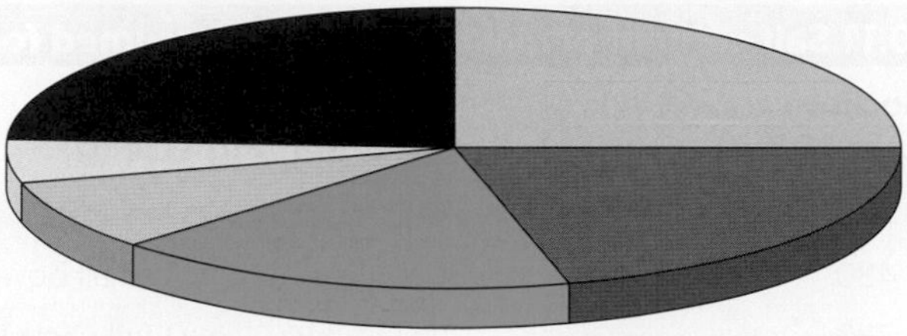

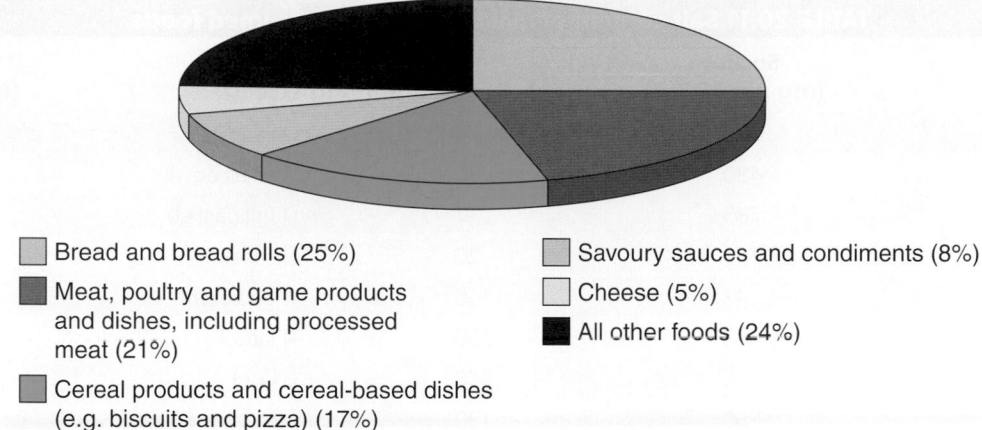

FIGURE 20.4 Processed foods that contribute to sodium intake from salt in Australia.

Source: Food Standards Australia. Available from: www.foodstandards.gov.au/scienceandeducation/factsheets/factsheets2009/howmuchsodiumandsalt4340.cfm

BOX 20.2 Sodium in food

Many foods — wholegrains, meat and dairy products — naturally contain traces of sodium, while processed foods tend to contain high quantities of salt. Some foods contain higher amounts of salt than expected:

- A jam sandwich has only 30% less salt than a Vegemite sandwich because most of the salt comes from the bread
- Sea salt, onion, celery and garlic salts are not low-sodium substitutes
- A bowl of cornflakes has approximately the same amount of salt as a small packet of plain potato chips
- Some sweet biscuits contain as much or more salt than savoury biscuits
- Ricotta, cottage, mozzarella and Swiss cheeses are lower in salt than most other cheeses.

blood pressure readings and cardiovascular health. The majority of diets in the West exceed this, containing an excess of sodium relative to potassium.[77]

Contrary to what many patients may think, the majority of sodium is not consumed in the form of table salt but rather in the form of the vast quantities of processed food many people consume (Fig. 20.4, Box 20.2). NHMRC guidelines suggest than more than 75% of dietary salt intake is from processed foods. Cereals, canned soups, bread, tinned fish, tomato sauce, frozen dinners and processed meats all contain added sodium. When making recommendations to hypertensive patients, emphasis should be placed on fresh wholefoods as close to their natural state as possible. An important strategy is to educate patients how to read nutritional panels on products so that they can make informed choices. Fresh herbs and spices should be encouraged as a replacement to salt in cooking.

Reducing salt in the diet

Some suggestions for reducing the amount of salt in the diet include:

- Avoid adding salt to cooking and at the table
- Choose reduced salt bread and breakfast cereals — bread is a major source of sodium in the diet
- Avoid high-salt foods
- Cut back on processed foods
- Cut back on takeaway and fast foods
- Buy fresh vegetables rather than canned
- Buy 'low salt' (contains less than 120 mg/100 g) or 'salt free' versions of commonly used foods, such as commercial sauces
- Use herbs and spices such as garlic, oregano and lemon juice to add flavour to meals
- Both sea salt and table salt are composed of sodium chloride
- Avoid processed foods.

High salt-containing foods that should be eaten sparingly include:

- Most fast foods, such as pizza
- Most snack foods, such as potato chips
- Processed meats, such as sausages, salami, hotdogs and luncheon meats
- Canned vegetables
- Dehydrated or packet foods, such as instant pasta or soups
- Pre-packaged sauces and condiments, such as tomato sauce and soy sauce, and processed tomato products in general
- White bread and bread rolls.

The salt content of some common foodstuffs is listed in Table 20.11.

Saturated fats

A diet high in saturated fat is associated with increased risk of cardiovascular mortality[81,82] and may impact hypertension by altering blood viscosity,[68] thus saturated fat should be kept to a minimum and replaced with good fats such as the omega-3 fatty acids which have known benefits in cardiovascular disease, including hypertension.

Caffeine

Acute intake of caffeine has been observed to exert a hypertensive effect[83] by increasing peripheral vascular

TABLE 20.11 Salt content of most commonly consumed foods

Food	Sodium (mg per 100 g)	Serving size (g)		Sodium (mg per serve)
Beef sausage*	790	70	(1 sausage)	553
Breakfast cereal	480	30	(1 small bowl)	144
Butter	780	7	(1 foil packet)	55
Cheddar cheese	730	20	(1 slice)	146
Chicken breast*	43	160	(1 cooked)	69
Hamburger*	440	200	(1 large)	880
Milk (full fat)	36	258	(1 cup)	93
Pizza*	550	130	(1/4 large pizza)	715
Potato chips (salt and vinegar flavour)	1180	45	(small packet)	531
Potato chips (other flavour)	580	45	(small packet)	261
White bread	450	30	(1 slice)	135
Yeast spread	3000	6	(1 tsp)	180

*Cooked.
Source: Food Standards Australia. Available from: www.foodstandards.gov.au/scienceandeducation/factsheets/factsheets2009/howmuchsodiumandsalt4340.cfm.

resistance. Habitual coffee consumption has also been shown to worsen BP control in patients 63 years or over, with the risk of uncontrolled blood pressure proportionally increasing with increased coffee consumption.[84] Additionally, a correlation between coffee consumption and cardiovascular events (defined as myocardial, aortic or lower limb revascularisation procedures, myocardial infarction, heart failure requiring hospitalisation, stroke, or renal events) was shown in an Italian long-term follow-up study, with participants showing high consumption (≥4 cups daily) being at even greater risk.[85] Thus patients presenting with hypertension should be questioned on all sources of caffeine, including coffee, tea (including green tea), energy drinks, soft drinks and dark chocolate. However, it is important to remember that not all dietary sources of caffeine are equivalent in terms of their potential hypertensive effect or effect on cardiovascular event frequency. For example, a small RCT of 37 hypertensive men and women showed a flavonoid and polyphenol enriched diet (dark chocolate plus green tea plus red apple) combined with antihypertensive medication improved blood pressure control and triglyceride levels.[86] Additionally a Cochrane review examining 20 studies showed that flavonol-rich cocoa and chocolate products appear to have a small but statistically significant positive effect on lowering blood pressure.[87]

Alcohol

Alcohol consumption should be reduced or avoided. Recommendations indicate that alcohol consumption of ≤30 mL/day in men and ≤15 mL/day in women is advisable, but if patients can be influenced to cease consumption, health improvements are markedly increased.

NUTRITIONAL MEDICINE (SUPPLEMENTAL)

Nutritional medicine therapeutic objectives

- Reduce hypertension through nutritional modulation of blood pressure
- Regulate transmembrane transport of calcium, potassium and sodium
- Reduce markers of oxidation: downregulate reactive oxygen species in the vascular wall, upregulate endothelial nitric oxide synthase (reduce nitric oxide)
- Increase mitochondrial energy production
- Reduce plasma homocysteine levels
- Lower blood viscosity
- Improve diastolic function
- Induce vasodilation.

Specific nutrients required

B COMPLEX

With any B vitamin prescription it is commonly accepted that all B vitamins should be prescribed in combination due to their synergy and the supportive interrelationship between each B vitamin. As such, when considering the following B vitamins, it is essential to prescribe a B complex to synergistically enhance the therapeutic outcome.

B_6, B_9 AND B_{12}

Increased plasma homocysteine levels have been recognised as an important risk factor for cardiovascular

SAMPLE DAILY DIET

BREAKFAST	
Beetroot juice (150–500 mL/d) Oats with 2–3 tbsp of LSA and 2 pieces of seasonal potassium-rich fruit	Consumption of beetroot juice has the ability to reduce hypertension attributed due to its nitrate content. A small study observed consumption of oats was associated with a reduced incidence of hypertension. Oats are also a source of fibre, the latter of which is associated with a reduction in hypertension. Consumption of approx. 30–50 g of flaxseed is associated with a small but significant decrease in blood pressure. 4–5 pieces of fruit per day is suggested to reduce hypertension.
LUNCH	
Large salad with leafy greens including baby spinach, celery and roasted vegetables. Served with legumes and a garlic/olive oil/vinegar dressing	Leafy greens are a source of potassium and magnesium both of which play a key role in management of hypertension. Fresh herbs can be used to replace some dietary sodium intake in order to enhance flavour and manipulate dietary sodium/potassium balance. Similarly to beetroot detailed above, spinach is also a source of dietary nitrates which may help reduce hypertension. The addition of fresh garlic in the dressing serves to further reduce hypertension.
DINNER	
Trout served with salad made from watercress, chives, new potato, snowpeas and Spanish onion. Drizzle with lemon and olive oil	Oily fish consumption plays an important role in the modulation of BP in hypertensive and normotensive adults and can be consumed at least 3 times per week. At least 5 serves of vegetables are suggested to reduce hypertension. Virgin olive oil is proposed to have anti-hypertensive effects and should be used as the oil of choice to protect against cardiovascular disease.
SNACKS	
Green tea Nuts (especially pistachios) and fresh fruit Dark chocolate (polyphenol rich)	The antioxidant ability of green tea appears to assist reductions in blood pressure. Pistachios seemed to have the strongest effect on reducing SBP and DBP. Consumption of polyphenol-rich dark chocolate improves endothelial function.

Chan Q, Stamler J, Griep LM, et al. An update on nutrients and blood pressure. J Atheroscler Thromb 2016;23(3):276–89. Colussi G, Catena C, Dialti V, et al. Fish meal supplementation and ambulatory blood pressure in patients with hypertension: relevance of baseline membrane fatty acid composition. Am J Hypertens 2014;27:471–481. Del Brutto OH, Mera RM, Gillman J, et al. Dietary oily fish intake and blood pressure levels: a population-based study. J Clin Hypertens 2016;18(4):337–41. Lopez S, Bermudez B, Montserrat-de la Paz S, et al. Virgin olive oil and hypertension. Curr Vasc Pharmacol 2016;14(4):323–9. Nogueira Lde P, Knibel MP, Torres MR, et al. Consumption of high-polyphenol dark chocolate improves endothelial function in individuals with stage 1 hypertension and excess body weight. Int J Hypertens 2012;2012:147321. Oza R, Garcellano M. Nonpharmacologic management of hypertension: what works? Am Fam Physician 2015;91(11):772–6. Siervo M, Lara J, Ogbonmwan I, et al. Inorganic nitrate and beetroot juice supplementation reduces blood pressure in adults: a systematic review and meta-analysis. J Nutr 2013;143(6):818–26.

disease. Supplementation with folic acid and other B vitamins, a relatively inexpensive way of reducing plasma homocysteine levels, might be a way to lower cardiovascular disease risk. All three B vitamins have a strong evidence base to lower plasma homocysteine levels.

Several studies have shown that folic acid in combination with B_{12} lowers homocysteine levels, but what has not been quantified is the contribution of vitamin B_{12} alone to the lowering of homocysteine levels.

One study[88] demonstrated that a supplement consisting of 5 mg folic acid and 250 micrograms vitamin B_{12} lowered fasting plasma homocysteine levels by 32% after 12 weeks in patients with coronary artery disease. In another study[89] of healthy men and women ranging in age from 70 to 93 years, daily supplementation for 4 months with 500 micrograms vitamin B_{12}, 0.8 mg folic acid and 3 mg vitamin B_6 significantly reduced plasma homocysteine levels ($p < 0.001$). The authors of the study suggested that suboptimal vitamin status is an important cause of elevated homocysteine even among the healthy elderly.

MAGNESIUM

Magnesium plays a key role in the regulation of healthy blood pressure via regulating transmembrane transport of calcium, sodium and potassium. Changes in intracellular and extracellular magnesium affect cardiac and vascular tone and reactivity, hence it should come as no surprise that deficiency of magnesium is linked to hypertension. Magnesium supplementation may also enhance the effect of antihypertensive medications in stage 1 hypertensive patients.[90]

ESSENTIAL FATTY ACIDS (EFAs)

The use of omega-3 fatty acids in the prevention of cardiovascular disease is supported by data from epidemiological studies in which the intake of even small amounts of fish seems to be protective and have beneficial effects on risk factors for coronary heart disease.

There is strong evidence to support the use of omega-3 fatty acids in hypertension with a meta-analysis of 17 trials by Appel et al showing a reduction of approximately −5.5/−3.5 mmHg in untreated hypertensive patients given omega-3 fish oils.[91] Beneficial results were also observed in a meta-analysis by Morris et al.[92] Omega-3 fatty acids in fish oil are believed to exert their hypotensive properties through stimulation of the prostaglandins that control sodium and water excretion, as well as their ability to cause vasodilation and inhibition of the vasoconstrictor thromboxane, regulate renin release and decrease response to vasopressor hormones.

DHA or EPA?

Until recently, it was unclear whether eicosapentaenoic acid (EPA) and docosahexaenoic acid (DHA) were equally important in relation to cardiovascular protection. A limiting factor was the lack of sufficient quantities of purified EPA or DHA. Data now demonstrate that DHA, like EPA, has important haemodynamic and anti-atherogenic properties. Mori et al[93] showed that DHA, but not EPA, significantly reduced 24-h (−5.8/−3.3 mmHg) and daytime (awake; −3.5/−2.0 mmHg) blood pressure relative to placebo in overweight, mildly hypercholesterolaemic individuals. Patients were given 4 g daily of highly purified EPA, DHA or olive oil (placebo) capsules while continuing their usual diets for 6 weeks. The blood pressure-lowering effects were accompanied by significant improvements in endothelial and smooth muscle function, as well as reduced vasoconstrictor responses, in forearm microcirculation with DHA but not EPA.[94] The study also demonstrated that DHA, but not EPA, significantly reduced 24-h, awake and asleep heart rate by −3.5, −3.7 and −2.8 bpm, respectively.[93]

The favourable effects of DHA on vasoreactivity are most likely attributable to direct and indirect effects of DHA on the arterial wall and may include DHA incorporation into endothelial membranes, increasing membrane fluidity, calcium influx and endogenous synthesis and release of NO.[95] DHA could also have direct effects on receptor-stimulated NO release, enhanced release of vasodilator prostanoids and/or endothelial-derived hyperpolarising factor, consistent with experimental evidence.[96]

Data suggest that EPA and DHA have differing haemodynamic and anti-atherogenic properties. DHA may be more favourable in lowering blood pressure and heart rate and improving vascular function. However, further studies are required to elucidate the independent effects of EPA and DHA on other clinical and biochemical measures. It is also likely that, to some extent, the effects of EPA and DHA may differ depending on the target population.[95]

VITAMINS C AND E

Oxidative stress has been implicated in the pathogenesis of hypertension due to an imbalance between antioxidant mechanisms and reactive oxygen species, thus vitamins C and E are often employed to target oxidative stress. Both vitamins C and E have been found to exert a range of mechanisms that help to reduce blood pressure including:

- Antioxidant activity
- Downregulation of NADPH oxidase, a major source of ROS in the vascular wall
- Upregulation of endothelial nitric oxide synthase.

A randomised double-blind placebo-controlled trial involving 110 men with grade 1 essential hypertension aged between 35 and 60 years of age investigated the effects of supplementation with the antioxidants vitamin C as ascorbic acid (1 g/day) and vitamin E (400 IU/day) and its effects on blood pressure over an 8-week period.[97] The participants were all non-smokers, with a healthy BMI range and were negative for dyslipidaemia and diabetes mellitus. They were also not undergoing vigorous physical exercise, did not use any medications and were not consuming a diet rich in fruit and vegetables.

Following the period of supplementation, individuals in the antioxidant groups had a significantly lower systolic, diastolic and mean arterial blood pressure and higher erythrocyte and serum antioxidant capacity compared with their original scores at baseline as well as with the placebo group. This result supports the use of antioxidant therapy with vitamins C and E to enhance blood antioxidant status resulting in a decrease in blood pressure in patients with mild to moderate essential hypertension.

COENZYME Q10

Coenzyme Q10 is an efficacious antioxidant and endogenous cofactor in mitochondrial energy production. A deficiency of coenzyme Q10 has been observed in 39% of hypertensive patients, in sharp contrast to 6% of healthy controls.[98] A number of different actions have been proposed for coenzyme Q10's hypotensive action, including its ability to lower blood viscosity, improve diastolic function, induce vasodilation, scavenge free radicals that deactivate endothelium-derived relaxing factor and/or fibrosis of arteriolar smooth muscle as well as to reduce aldosterone secretion. Interestingly, individuals with chronic hypertension have been noted to have a deficiency in the enzyme succinate dehydrogenase-CoQ10 reductase, leading to a decrease in levels of coenzyme Q10 in the body.[99] If levels of succinate dehydrogenase CoQ10 reductase in the body are increased, coenzyme Q10 levels increase and systolic and diastolic blood pressure decrease.

A number of clinical trials have shown that coenzyme Q10 has the ability to lower blood pressure. A systematic review involving 12 studies and a total of 362 individuals with hypertension observed that coenzyme Q10 (in combination with allopathic antihypertensive medications) reduced systolic blood pressure by as much as 17 mmHg and diastolic blood pressure by up to 10 mmHg over a 2–3 month period.[98] A Cochrane review of three trials totalling 96 individuals with hypertension observed that coenzyme Q10 taken over 8–12 weeks reduced systolic blood pressure by approximately 11 mmHg and diastolic blood pressure by 7 mmHg compared with placebo.[100] While these results are promising, the authors noted that there were several questionable issues with regards to methodology, suggesting that before a definite recommendation can be made further studies of sound quality need to be undertaken.

TAURINE

Taurine is an amino acid that has been shown to reduce blood pressure in both experimental and human studies, the majority of which have been undertaken in Japanese populations. In their review, Milatante and Lombardini[101] detail two small studies in which taurine at doses of 6 g/day reduced blood pressure in between 1 and 6 weeks. Taurine did not appear to lower blood pressure in those whose blood pressure was normal.

ARGININE

The amino acid arginine is an important contributor to nitric oxide (NO) formation and determines the tone of blood vessels (relaxing effect) and renal function. Through these roles it achieves the following key functions:

- Improves blood flow
- Improves renal plasma flow
- Improves glomerular filtration rate.

Although the body generally manufactures enough arginine, supplementation is warranted in some situations. Arginine is not an essential amino acid but is classified as 'conditionally essential' for adults. It is required in large amounts during growth, and although children can manufacture it, they are unable to do so in high enough quantities. Food sources include legumes, wholegrains, nuts and chocolate, but dietary intake may not be sufficient for all people.

In the hypertensive patient, even in mild cases, there appears to be a derangement of endothelial nitric oxide production. Arginine supplementation has been shown to improve blood flow, as described above, reducing the risk of blood clot formation.

Because loss of NO bioactivity is a central feature of endothelial dysfunction in hypertension, providing supplemental substrate to bolster NO production has been suggested as a rational treatment approach. Administration of L-arginine has been shown to improve endothelium-dependent vasodilation in a number of human clinical studies of hypercholesterolaemia and atherosclerosis.[102,103]

Potential mechanisms of L-arginine action in hypertension include:[104]

- Improved endothelial vasomotor function
- Enhanced vascular NO synthesis
- Reduced endothelin-1 and angiotensin II activity
- Favourable alteration of asymmetrical dimethylarginine (ADMA):L-arginine ratio
- Modulation of renal haemodynamics
- Reduced oxidative stress
- Improved insulin sensitivity.

Dosage requirements

The dosage requirements listed below are based on adult doses that have been reported in the literature.

- B complex (all B vitamins) high-dose combination, preferably activated forms
  - Thiamine 20–40 mg/day
  - Riboflavin 20–40 mg/day
  - Nicotinic acid 50–100 mg/day
  - Pantothenic acid 150–300 mg/day
  - Pyridoxine 20–60 mg/day
  - Folinic acid 500–1000 micrograms/day
  - Hydroxocobalamin 500–1000 micrograms/day
  - Choline 50–100 mg/day
  - Inositol 50–100 mg/day
  - Biotin 250–500 micrograms/day
- Additional B vitamin support:
  - Vitamin B_3 (nicotinic acid): extra B_3 (100 mg+) is indicated with elevated cholesterol levels
  - Vitamin B_6 (pyridoxine): extra B_6 (75–100 mg) is indicated with elevated homocysteine levels
  - Vitamin B_9 (folate): extra B_9 (500–5000 micrograms/day, i.e. UL = 5 mg/day) is indicated with elevated homocysteine levels
  - Vitamin B_{12} (hydroxocobalamin): extra B_{12} (500–1000 micrograms/day) is indicated with elevated homocysteine levels
- Magnesium: 460 mg/day,[90] however, the general recommendation is to prescribe between 600 and 1000 mg in divided doses throughout the day
- Essential fatty acids: 3–4 g/day total omega-3 fatty acids (50% DHA and 50% EPA)
- Coenzyme Q10 150–600 mg/day
- Vitamin C 500–1000 mg t.d.s.
- Vitamin E 400–500 IU b.i.d.
- Arginine 0.5 g/10 kg body weight for BP >140–180/105–114 mmHg (moderate classification)
- Taurine 2–3 g/day.

HERBAL MEDICINE

Herbal medicine therapeutic objectives

- Reduce hypertension through hypotensive herbal medicines
- Reduce markers of oxidation including downregulation of ROS in the vascular wall, upregulation of endothelial nitric oxide synthase (reduce NO)
- Provide cardiac tonification through the prescription of cardio-tonics
- Reduce peripheral vascular resistance: lower blood viscosity, induce vasodilation
- Reduce sympathetic dominance if a contributing or aggravating factor.

Herbal medicine classes

The herbal medicine classes used in hypertension are summarised in Table 20.12.

TABLE 20.12 Herbal medicine classes used for hypertension

Class	Action
Cardioprotective	Protective to the myocardium and decrease the risk of heart damage due to toxins, ischaemia or the oxidative effects of hypertension
Cardio-tonic	Increase the force of contraction of the heart (i.e. positively inotropic), and restore tone and vigour to the heart muscle (i.e. myocardium)
Hypotensive	Lower blood pressure levels by supporting cardiac integrity
Peripheral vasodilator	Reduce peripheral vascular resistance, dilate/widen peripheral blood vessels and thereby improve circulation to peripheral tissues to assist in reducing blood pressure
Nervines, adaptogens	Reduce sympathetic dominance
Other	Sedatives, nervines, anxiolytics, antidepressants, spasmolytics as required

Specific herbal medicines

CRATAEGUS SPP. (HAWTHORN)

Crataegus monogyna/oxycantha is considered a central cardiac medicine in Western herbal medicine, with a number of positive benefits on cardiac contractility, coronary blood flow, and blood pressure.[105,106] While the use of *Crataegus* as a hypotensive agent is not classically described in traditional herbal medicine, it is important to also realise that hypertension was not a recognised complaint in traditional herbal medicine, having only been understood as an important clinical entity in the first half of the 20th century.[107] Nevertheless hawthorn became a primary choice hypotensive medicine for Western herbalists during the second half of the 20th century, especially with the publication of the British Herbal Pharmacopoeia of 1983 (BHP1983), which listed hypertension among its indications, and listed 'Hypertension with myocardial weakness' as a specific indication.[108] A small pilot study assessing the effects of 500 mg/day *Crataegus* extract in mildly hypertensive patients observed a reduction ($p = 0.081$) in the resting diastolic blood pressure at 2.5 months in participants assigned the *Crataegus* spp. compared with the other groups.[109] A secondary observation was the trend towards less anxiety ($p = 0.094$), also experienced in the *Crataegus* group.

Despite widespread usage as a hypotensive, controversy remains, with most of the research focusing on extracts prepared from the leaves and flowers, and their application in heart failure.[106] Weiss explicitly states '*Crataegus* does not have hypotensive properties'; however, it may normalise blood pressure due to its effect on generally improving cardiac function. It is important to remember though that Weiss was discussing the use of preparations made from the leaves and flowers.[110] Some practitioners find berries more effective at reducing hypertension than a combination of berries and leaves, which is consistent with the BHP1983 description which only mentions berries.[108] For marked hypertension, the recommendation is to prescribe 2 mL t.d.s. (1 : 2) of a fluid extract of hawthorn berries, and usually in combination with other valuable hypotensives.

TILIA PLATYPHYLLOS, T. CORDATA, OR ACHILLEA MILLEFOLIUM (LIME FLOWERS, AND YARROW)

Increased peripheral vascular resistance has been implicated as a contributing factor in primary hypertension,[111] and classical peripheral vasodilators such as yarrow and lime flowers (lime blossoms) have been recommended as a component of therapy for many years.[108] While clinical usage suggests that these medicines are not sufficient alone in most cases of primary hypertension, when used in combination with core medicines such as *Crataegus*, additional benefit can be obtained.

VALERIANA OFFICINALIS (VALERIAN)

While the attention of very little modern clinical research, the hypotensive action of European valerian should not be ignored.[108,112] As nervous excitability can play a role in hypertension in many individuals, herbal sedatives are worthy of consideration, especially when patients present with a clear pattern of stress-related blood pressure variability. Valerian is a well-indicated medicine in many of these cases, and especially in combination with specific medicines such as hawthorn. A classic German tea preparation containing equal parts of mistletoe, hawthorn flowers, chamomile and valerian is a good example of such a formulation.[110]

SALVIA MILTIORRHIZA (DAN SHEN)

Dan shen has been traditionally used for treatment of hypertension in China, Korea and Japan.[113] Its hypotensive effect is mediated through the inhibition of an angiotensin-converting enzyme, an essential regulatory enzyme of the renin–angiotensin system.[113–116] The two components of dan shen responsible for its antihypertensive effect are lithospermic acid B[113] and salvianolic acid B.[115] One study concluded that lithospermic acid B and salvianolic acid B are actually the same compound, with identical chemical structures except for their stereochemistry.[117]

INULA RACEMOSA (INULA)

Inula racemosa is an Ayurvedic botanical that has been identified as containing a number of active constituents including beta sitosterols, daucosterol, inunolide, alantolactone, isoalantolactone, dihydroalantolactone and dihydroisoalantolactone.[118] The dried roots have been found to display hypotensive and anti-angina activity.[119] *Inula racemosa* administered to individuals with angina was found to decrease diastolic blood pressure over a 12-week treatment period.[119] In addition, plasma cortisol and catecholamine levels also decreased. This is interesting given the relationship between elevated cortisol and subsequent risk of hypertension in Cushing's syndrome.[120,121]

ALLIUM SATIVUM (GARLIC)

Allium sativum, commonly known as garlic, is a species of the Alliaceae family and has been shown to exert hypotensive properties, making it useful in hypertension. A meta-analysis involving 10 trials that examined the effects of *Allium sativum* supplementation in people with elevated systolic blood pressure as well as in those without elevated systolic blood pressure[122] produced promising results. In this meta-analysis the use of *Allium sativum* appeared to significantly reduce systolic and diastolic blood pressure by 16 and 9 mmHg, respectively, in patients with a mean systolic blood pressure greater than 140 mmHg at baseline. Of these trials, however, only three studies were found to evaluate patients with a baseline mean systolic blood pressure greater than 140 mmHg; the other seven involved patients with lower systolic blood pressures.

Despite these positive results the true effects of *Allium sativum* cannot be clearly ascertained due to inadequate study designs and with too little information about blood pressure measurements. Furthermore, in the meta-analysis discussed above all studies except one were funded by different manufacturers of garlic products, hence potential bias may come into play. Further unbiased studies are thus required.

OLEA EUROPAEA (OLIVE LEAF)

Olea europaea has been used medicinally in Europe for management of hypertension for centuries.

Its leaves contain a number of compounds that have been identified as important in hypertension; these include the secoiridoid compounds oleacein and oleuropein.[123] A small open, controlled, parallel-group co-twin study involving borderline hypertensive monozygotic twins investigated the effects of either:

- 500 mg/day of *Olea europaea* extract versus a control group who received lifestyle advice or
- 500 mg/day of *Olea europaea* extract versus 1000 mg/day of *Olea europaea* extract.

Following completion of the 8-week study it was noted that the 500 mg/day dose did not result in any significant change of mean blood pressure levels from baseline, but the 1000 mg/day dose resulted in a decrease of up to 19/10 mmHg and a continuous reduction of 11/5 mmHg of mean levels over the 8 weeks, highlighting the efficacy of *Olea europaea* at this dose.

VISCUM ALBUM (MISTLETOE)

Viscum album was traditionally used for cardiac hypertrophy and valvular insufficiency.[124] In modern times in Germany it is widely used for its hypotensive properties. *Viscum album* contains constituents known as viscotoxins; in animal studies these have been found to produce significant cardiovascular effects, including reflex bradycardia, negative inotropic effects and vasoconstriction in the cardiac muscle. Phenylpropanoids from mistletoe are thought to play a role by inhibiting cAMP phosphodiesterase, although data are currently inconclusive.

LIFESTYLE RECOMMENDATIONS

Weight management

Maintaining a healthy weight is always important, particularly to help prevent against hypertension. Weight loss to achieve a body mass index of 18.5–24.9 is generally advised. In one study participants involved in an 18-month weight loss intervention program who were followed up after 7 years had a 77% reduction in the incidence of hypertension.[125]

Stress

Increased stress is associated with a rise in blood pressure, hence the importance of implementing stress-reduction techniques such as meditation and regular massage.

Exercise

Regular exercise and a reduction in sedentary habits are recommended in patients with hypertension. The importance of exercise in reducing blood pressure and cardiovascular risk is profound. Introduction can be difficult due to patient compliance and safety concerns with existing cardiovascular history. It is beneficial to recommend a staggered approach to the introduction to exercise, starting with walking and increasing on a weekly basis. Assistance from a personal trainer is advisable where possible.

The general recommendation is to encourage regular aerobic physical activity of at least 30 minutes per day most days of the week.

Exercise and Sports Science Australia (ESSA)[126] suggests that exercise for individuals with hypertension should consist of a mixture of moderate-to-vigorous aerobic exercise, such as jogging (up to 5 days/week) as well as resistance exercise, such as weights, on 2 or more non-consecutive days per week. Aerobic exercise even at low intensity (50% VO_{2max}) has been demonstrated to reduce blood pressure in hypertensive patients, and these results may last several hours. Individuals with hypertension who undertake aerobic exercise consistently should expect a reduction in systolic and diastolic blood pressure of approximately 7/6 mmHg.

EXERCISE RECOMMENDATIONS

Patients with clinically stable and moderate severity of their cardiovascular disease should aim for 30 minutes per day of moderate intensity exercise, 5–7 days per week. Moderate intensity is individual: noticeable increase in rate and depth of breathing, while still allowing the person to comfortably talk. Examples include walking, cycling, cleaning the house, swimming.

In addition, light-to-moderate resistance exercise is recommended (under professional guidance) for all hypertensive patients.

EXERCISE CONTRAINDICATIONS

- Unstable angina
- Uncontrolled heart failure
- Severe aortic stenosis

- Uncontrolled or severe hypertension (e.g. blood pressure ≥180 mmHg (systolic) or ≥110 mmHg (diastolic))
- Symptomatic hypotension <90/60 mmHg
- Acute infection or fever
- Resting tachycardia or arrhythmias
- Poorly controlled diabetes.

SIGNS TO TERMINATE EXERCISE

- Ischaemic chest pain
- Dizziness, lightheadedness or feeling faint
- Dyspnoea
- Nausea or uncharacteristic excessive sweating
- Palpitations associated with feeling unwell
- Undue fatigue
- Leg ache that curtails function
- Physical inability to continue
- Diabetics: shakiness, tingling lips, hunger, weakness.

Smoking

A longitudinal study[127] reported on the link between smoking and increased risk of hypertension, but the results assessing the effects of smoking on hypertension were inconsistent. Given the other detrimental effects of smoking on the body, including its reputation as a risk factor for cardiovascular disease, smoking should be excluded in patients with hypertension.

CASE STUDY

OVERVIEW

LF was a 56-year-old female presenting with treatment-resistant hypertension. Hypertension was diagnosed at around age 50, and for the first year remained untreated, but in the past 5 years treatment has consisted of first an ACE-inhibitor, then a combination of ACE-inhibitor and calcium channel blocker.

The patient monitored her blood pressure twice weekly using home-monitoring equipment (which had been checked as accurate by her general practitioner). Systolic readings over the previous 2 months were 140–180 mmHg and diastolic readings were 80–120 mmHg.

Current antihypertensive medication consisted of:

- Enalapril 30 mg once daily
- Nifedipine 20 mg morning and 10 mg in the evening.

LF's general practitioner wished to increase the dosage of both the enalapril and nifedipine due to poor control of her blood pressure; however, the patient was reluctant to continue with this pattern of continually elevating drug dosages, and was thus seeking alternative options.

OTHER MEDICAL HISTORY

LF was also a type 2 diabetic, diagnosed 10 years ago, and managed with dietary control combined with 500 mg metformin twice daily. Her last HbA_{1c} test was conducted 11

CASE STUDY CONTINUED

months prior with a result of 8.3%. Additionally LF was obese, with a height of 168 cm and weight of 98 kg (BMI 34.0). LF had tried various weight loss diets over the last 4 years, but in each case with minimal impact, and the stress seemed to cause a slight but noticeable increase in blood pressure readings.

DIET AND LIFESTYLE

LF had been carefully controlling her dietary intake of sodium, trying to choose low-salt foods, and not adding salt to cooking or during the meal. However her intake of refined carbohydrates was relatively high, with a minimum of 2–3 slices of seeded white bread per day, sugared muesli for breakfast each morning, and snacks during the day usually consisting of dried fruit and nuts, or savoury crackers with marmalade.

Red meat consumption was approximately 4 serves per week, fish one serve, and chicken 2 serves. Vegetable intake was moderate, however, consisting mostly of boiled mixed vegetables for dinner, with only occasional raw vegetable intake. Fruit consumption usually consisted of 1–2 apples or oranges per day.

The patient described moderate to high stress levels (self-rated as 7 out of 10 in severity), due to a combination of serious family trauma and financial concerns due to her husband's business being quite erratic.

Exercise levels were minimal, consisting of a 20–30 minute slow walk twice a week, and incidental walking from housework and shopping.

CLINICAL EXAMINATION AND PATHOLOGY

BP at this first consultation was 165/100 mmHg. Recent blood tests (1 month prior) also showed elevated total cholesterol (6.0 mmol/L) and elevated fasting triglycerides (2.7 mmol/L).

ASSESSMENT

The patient had treatment-resistant hypertension. While the blood pressure during the initial consultation was clearly high, this single reading during an initial consultation is often unreliable. However consistent home monitoring confirmed hypertension and, especially given her current drug regimen, these readings were far from favourable.

Complicating the situation was the presence of type 2 diabetes combined with obesity, which increases the risk of hypertension, and increases the risk of coronary and cerebrovascular disease. Her HbA1c levels were in the inadequate control range, indicating consistently elevated blood glucose.

THERAPEUTIC OBJECTIVES

The initial treatment objectives for this first consultation were:

- Reduce blood pressure
- Reduce impact of stress on cardiovascular function
- Reduce blood glucose levels
- Reduce long-term cardiovascular risk.

CASE STUDY CONTINUED

TREATMENT

HERBAL TREATMENT

Herbal medicine	DER	Quantity/ week	Rationale
Crataegus monogyna berries and leaves	1:2	40 mL	Hypotensive, cardiovascular tonic
Codonopsis pilosula	1:2	60 mL	Adaptogen, mild hypoglycaemic
Trigonella foenum-graecum	1:2	40 mL	Hypoglycaemic, hypolipidaemic
Valeriana officinalis	1:2	20 mL	Hypotensive, sedative

Dosage: 8 mL three times daily before food.

NUTRITIONAL TREATMENT

Initial nutritional treatment was conservative to avoid overloading the patient, and involved:

- Changing afternoon snack to small mixed leaf salad with olive oil and balsamic vinegar dressing, with a small handful of raw seeds and nuts (not peanuts)
- Removing one serving of red meat per week and replacing with a vegetarian meal or fish-based meal
- Fish oil 1000 mg three times daily

OUTCOMES (0–4 MONTHS)

Over the next 4 months LF found her blood pressure readings dropping to a systolic range of 140–160 mmHg, and a diastolic range of 80–100 mmHg. HbA_{1c} reading was 7.9% at the fourth month of treatment. She described a significant decrease in perceived stress levels. However body weight remained largely unchanged. The assessment was that there was a significant, albeit still inadequate, improvement in her blood pressure, and a modest improvement in glucose control. She had been largely compliant with the dietary advice, indicating that more aggressive weight loss measures were needed. After having observed improved blood pressure control in other patients from changing the hawthorn prescription from a mixture of berries and leaves to berries only, the decision was made to pursue the same change for LF to see if control improved.

FROM MONTH 4: HERBAL TREATMENT

Herbal medicine	DER	Quantity/ week	Rationale
Crataegus monogyna berries	1:2	40 mL	Hypotensive, cardiovascular tonic
Codonopsis pilosula	1:2	60 mL	Adaptogen, mild hypoglycaemic
Trigonella foenum-graecum	1:2	40 mL	Hypoglycaemic, hypolipidaemic
Valeriana officinalis	1:2	20 mL	Hypotensive, sedative

Dosage: 8 mL three times daily before food

CASE STUDY CONTINUED

NUTRITIONAL TREATMENT

Continue with previous advice, and additionally:

- Replace morning cereal with a fruit and protein powder smoothie, with no added sugar.

LIFESTYLE TREATMENT

Convert her existing walks into more rapid walking over a minimum of 30 minutes per week, and commence gentle weight and exercise bike training at a gym three times a week.

OUTCOMES (5–9 MONTHS)

Over the next few months blood pressure control continued to improve dropping to a systolic range of 130–150 mmHg, and a diastolic range of 75–90 mmHg. The HbA_{1c} reading was 7.7% at the eighth month of treatment. Body weight had reduced slightly (4 kg over 4 months), and while the patient had been walking more vigorously, she had not commenced the advised gym-based exercise. Fasting triglyceride levels had dropped to 2.1 mmol/L; total cholesterol remained unchanged.

The assessment at this stage was the change to hawthorn berries had further improved the patient's blood pressure, and that there was a continued improvement in blood glucose levels.

At this point the patient wanted to reduce her enalapril dosage to 20 mg per day as she believed she was getting the nocturnal non-productive cough which is a reasonably common adverse reaction with ACE inhibitors. While her GP advised against it, she decided to pursue this option herself.

OUTCOMES (>10 MONTHS)

Over the next 6 months, blood pressure levels remained consistent despite her lowered ACE inhibitor dosage. Continued counselling around body weight and exercise had not resulted in any significant change. However at about the 18-month mark since commencement of treatment, the patient purchased an exercise bike for home and some resistance bands and began using them regularly during the week. Subsequent to this, over the next few months the patient lost 17 kg due to a combination of exercise and strict kilojoule counting, blood pressure continued dropping, and HbA_{1c} reached a low of 7.4%. The patient was able to discontinue the enalapril and reduce her nifedipine dosage to 10 mg twice daily, and maintain a blood pressure range of 130–150 mmHg systolic, and 75–90 mmHg diastolic.

ATHEROSCLEROSIS AND DYSLIPIDAEMIA

Classification

ATHEROSCLEROSIS

Atherosclerosis is defined as a chronic inflammatory change within blood vessels, involving accumulation of lipid and fibrous tissue on, and within arterial walls (plaque).[33,128] Atherosclerosis is not a single disease, but a common response to numerous, varied assaults.[129]

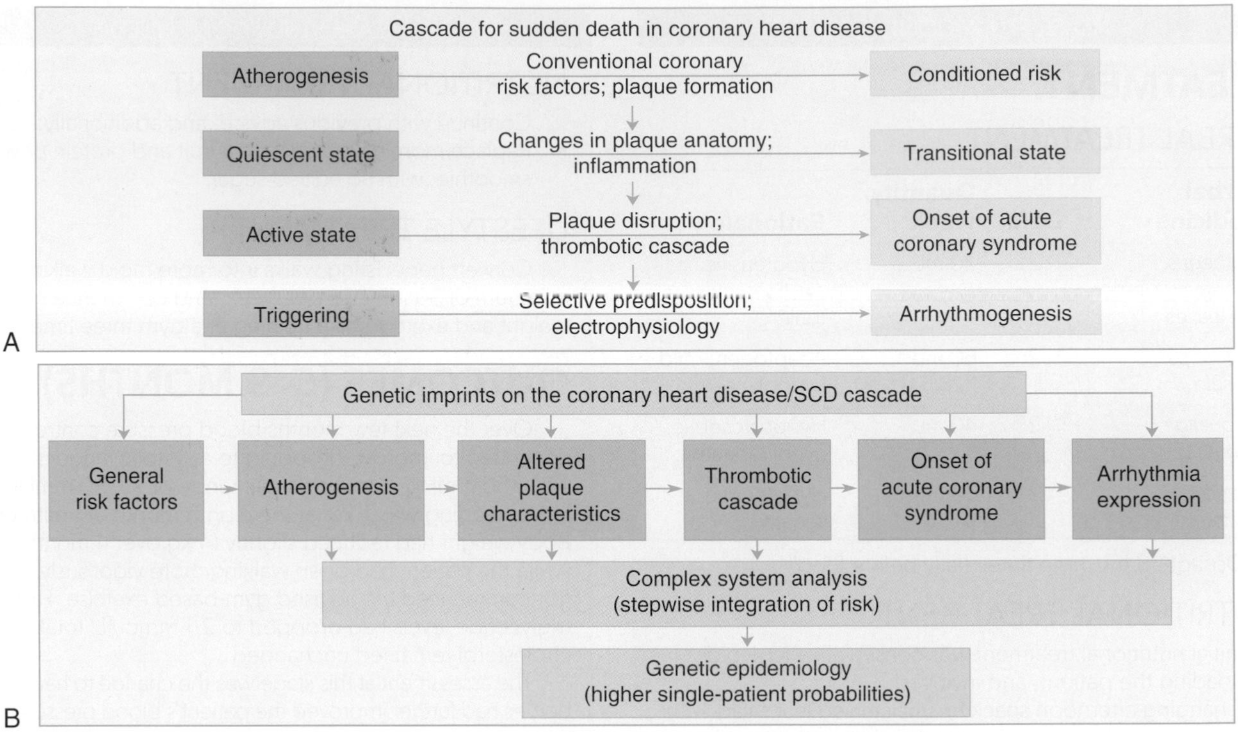

FIGURE 20.5 Coronary artery disease (atherosclerosis, dyslipidaemia).

Source: Libby P, Bonow R, Zipes D. Braunwald's heart disease: a textbook of cardiovascular medicine. 8th edn. Philadelphia: Saunders; 2007.

The condition progresses through several stages, affecting clinical presentation and health outcomes (Fig. 20.5, Table 20.13). It is typically clinically silent for a number of years, with symptoms eventually arising from erosion or fragmenting of plaque-triggering thrombus formation, which subsequently results in acute ischaemia of an end organ (such as with angina or myocardial infarction resulting from atherosclerotic changes in coronary arteries).[128]

TABLE 20.13 Stages of coronary artery disease

Phase 1	Small lesions, with a possibility of progression over time. Most commonly found in individuals <30 years
Phase 2	Vulnerable, or high-risk, plaques. Susceptible to disruption due to high lipid content, inflammation and thin, fibrous cap
Phases 3 and 4	Complicated lesions. May be obstructive or non-obstructive. Approximately two-thirds of acute coronary syndromes (e.g. myocardial infarction, angina) are related to phase 4, or occlusive thrombosis
Phase 5	Phase 3 or 4 plaques that evolve into fibrotic lesions. Can result in conditions such as angina
Phase 6	Complicated, occlusive thrombus of acute coronary syndromes. High risk

Source: Adapted from Therapeutic Guidelines Limited. Therapeutic guidelines, cardiovascular (version 5). 2008. Available from: http://online.tg.org.au/complete/

DYSLIPIDAEMIA

Lipids are a fundamental component of atherosclerotic plaque.[129] Assessment of an individual's lipid state involves the measurement of total cholesterol (TC), high-density lipoprotein (HDL) cholesterol, low-density lipoprotein (LDL) cholesterol and fasting triglyceride (TG). Elevated LDL cholesterol is positively associated with cardiovascular risk; as are elevated TG, along with comorbid counterparts diabetes and obesity.[130] Elevated TG, with high LDL cholesterol and high LDL:HDL cholesterol ratio, significantly increases the likelihood of coronary artery disease.[131] Plasma TG predicts coronary artery disease risk, independent of cholesterol, with even minor lipid elevation substantially increasing the risk of morbidity (Table 20.14).[132]

TABLE 20.14 Target lipid levels

Total cholesterol	<4.0 mmol/L
HDL cholesterol	>1.0 mmol/L
LDL cholesterol	<2.5 mmol/L (2.0 mmol/L for high-risk patients with existing cardiovascular disease)
Triglyceride	<1.5 mmol/L

Source: Adapted from Therapeutic Guidelines Limited. Therapeutic guidelines, cardiovascular (version 5). 2008. Available from: http://online.tg.org.au/complete/

Aetiology

While risk factors are useful predictors for those predisposed to developing coronary artery disease (CAD), they do not automatically prove causality. Nonetheless, addressing prominent risk factors has been shown to prevent disease development (primary prevention), and halt the progress of an established condition (secondary prevention).[133]

DYSLIPIDAEMIA

Dyslipidaemia is a common accompaniment to cardiovascular disease, and a significant risk factor for CAD and atherosclerotic conditions.[134] The process can begin in childhood with lipid-rich lesions, fatty streaks, appearing in the coronary arteries from around the age of 15 and increasing over time. More advanced lesions develop from the mid-20s, forming fibrous plaques that may protrude into the lumen of the artery, compromising vascular supply of the tissues involved.[129] Dyslipidaemia can be classed as primary or secondary. Primary dyslipidaemia may be caused by genetic, metabolic or environmental (e.g. diet) factors.[135] There are a number of secondary causes (Table 20.15) that may be considered in the evaluation and treatment of dyslipidaemia.

TABLE 20.15 Secondary causes of dyslipidaemia

Cause	Effect on lipid profile
Hypothyroidism Nephrotic syndrome Cholestasis Anorexia nervosa	Increased LDL cholesterol
Type 2 diabetes Obesity Renal impairment Smoking	Increased TG and/or decreased HDL cholesterol
Alcohol use Oestrogen use	Increased triglycerides; HDL cholesterol may increase; cardiovascular risk may not be increased

Source: Adapted from Anderson J, Carlquist J, Horne B, et al. Progress in unraveling the genetics of coronary artery disease and myocardial infarction. Curr Atheroscler Rep 2007;9(3):179–83.

HOMOCYSTEINE

Elevated homocysteine is one of the underlying causes of vascular disorders, through the stimulation of pro-inflammatory pathways in vascular cells.[136] Homocysteine is thought to induce atherosclerosis via oxidative stress and methylation modification.[137] One study showed that hyperhomocysteinaemia influences atherosclerosis by enhancing T-cell response, engaging an inappropriate immune reaction.[138] Dietary deficiency in B_6, folic acid and absorptive deficiency of B_{12} have all been implicated in elevated homocysteine and subsequent cardiovascular risk.[139]

C-REACTIVE PROTEIN

C-reactive protein is a sensitive, non-specific, marker of inflammation.[140] It is expressed in the liver, where production is stimulated by inflammatory cytokines,[141] and is also expressed in adipocytes, coronary artery smooth muscle and atherosclerotic plaque and may enhance local adhesions.[142] Observational studies demonstrate that a doubling of C-reactive protein levels increases the prevalence of CAD by 50%.[143]

HYPERTENSION

Hypertension is a common risk factor, present in three out of four patients with CAD.[144] Hypertensive patients have a much higher risk of developing cardiovascular disease, including sequelae of dyslipidaemia and atherosclerosis.[47]

DIABETES MELLITUS/INSULIN RESISTANCE/ METABOLIC SYNDROME

Individuals with CAD and abnormal glucose metabolism — as found in diabetes, insulin resistance and metabolic syndrome — have a much higher risk of subsequent cardiovascular events.[145] The increased risk is related to hyperglycaemia and hyperinsulinaemia, both of which are atherogenic.[146] Metabolic syndrome (Box 20.3) is associated with an inflammatory state, increased levels of coagulation factors, reduction in fibrinolysis, and endothelial dysfunction that significantly increases the risk of cardiovascular events.[147] Type 2 diabetes is independently associated with a significant increase in risk of CAD — sometimes considered a surrogate — much of which is attributed to hyperlipidaemia.[148] People with diabetes are 2–4 times more likely to develop CAD and coronary ischaemia than others.[149] The usual gender advantage conferred to premenopausal women does not apply to women with diabetes.[150]

BOX 20.3 Diagnostic criteria for metabolic syndrome (three or more indicates syndrome)

- Abdominal obesity: waist circumference >102 cm (men), or >88 cm (women)
- Plasma triglycerides ≥1.6 mmol/L
- HDL cholesterol <1.0 mmol/L (men) or 1.2 mmol/L (women)
- Blood pressure ≥130/85 mmHg
- Fasting glucose ≥6 mmol/L (or diabetes diagnosed)

Source: Adapted from Stampfer M, Hu F, Manson J et al. Primary prevention of coronary heart disease in women through diet and lifestyle. N Engl J Med 2000; 343(1):16–22.

GENETICS/ETHNICITY

Numerous studies have implicated ethnicity and genetics in the pathogenesis of atherosclerosis and CAD, however results are varied.[151] Studies in the United Kingdom have shown that otherwise healthy Indian Asians have greater insulin resistance and higher levels of the inflammatory marker C-reactive protein than the white population, an independent risk factor for CAD and cardiovascular events.[152,153] This population group has also been shown to have elevated homocysteine, concurrent with much lower B_{12} and folate.[154] In the United States, despite higher prevalence of risk factors in the African-American and Hispanic populations, it is the white population that has higher incidence of dyslipidaemia and atherosclerosis.[155] In Australia, there is a much higher prevalence of cardiovascular conditions and comorbidities among the Indigenous population, with many individuals living in non-urban communities and low socioeconomic environments, predisposing them to greater illness and mortality.[28]

OBESITY

The risk of developing heart disease is increased by 20% in overweight and 50% in obese individuals.[156] Excess body mass is associated with elevated free fatty acids, increased hepatic lipase, reduced HDL cholesterol and high triglycerides.[61] Increased circulation of free fatty acids mediates insulin resistance, which is in and of itself a risk factor for CAD.[157] Current evidence also shows that excess adipose tissue secretes inflammatory mediators, inducing systemic low-grade inflammation that can underlie metabolic and cardiovascular conditions.[158] In Australia, over half the adult population is classified as overweight or obese, and current trends suggest this number is increasing.[159]

DIET

Poor nutritional intake, high consumption of processed foods, saturated fats and low intake of fibre is associated with increased risk of atherosclerosis and cardiovascular conditions.[160] Conversely, modified fat intake (favouring mono- and polyunsaturated fats) and increased fibre consumption (and associated weight loss) have been shown to significantly lower C-reactive protein concentrations (25–54%).[160] Diets rich in wholegrains, fruit and low saturated fat intake have been linked to lower risk of atherosclerosis.[161] Certain nutritional deficiencies are implicated in pathogenesis of CAD, notably B_6, folic acid and B_{12} — all of which accord with elevated homocysteine.[139]

SMOKING

Tobacco smoking dramatically increases the risk of cardiovascular events, including atherosclerosis and CAD.[162] Smoking promotes atherogenesis, thrombogenesis and ischaemia, while reducing oxygen-carrying capacity of the blood.[41]

STRESS/MOOD

Psychological stress and depression may instigate or sustain the inflammatory processes involved in CAD.[163] There is strong and consistent evidence that stress, isolation and depression are independent risk factors for cardiovascular disease, with a three- to fivefold increase following major depressive episodes.[164]

Overview

Coronary artery disease is a syndrome typified by formation of atherosclerotic lesions, which obstruct the coronary arteries; these obstructions may be total, partial or mixed.[165]

Pathogenesis

The lesions of atherosclerosis form principally within the innermost layer of the artery wall, the intima. The condition initiates as an inflammatory response and is commonly associated with hyperlipidaemia, involving both intracellular and extracellular lipid accumulation.[129]

SIGNS AND SYMPTOMS

Atherosclerosis does not present with any one specific group of symptoms, and may be clinically silent for many years. However, due to its correlation with obesity, hypertension and metabolic disorders, any diagnosis of these should highlight the possibility of concurrent dyslipidaemia and atherosclerosis.[41] Clinical presentation will often involve one or more of the comorbidities discussed earlier, alerting patient and practitioner to the possibility of more insidious pathology. In such cases, a blood test exhibiting inappropriate cholesterol balance (see Table 20.14) should act as a red flag for dyslipidaemia and may indicate need for further investigation. Obstructive sleep apnoea is also linked with early-stage atherosclerosis — both conditions are associated with endothelial dysfunction, increased C-reactive protein, interleukin-6, fibrinogen and plasminogen activator inhibitor, with reduced fibrinolytic activity.[166]

COMPLICATIONS

Atherosclerosis may affect almost any artery, and thus the clinical sequelae are highly variable, depending upon which organ or tissue has been impacted by the reduced blood flow and subsequent ischaemia. It is important to remember that many manifestations of peripheral vascular disease are due to such atherosclerotic change; however, the conditions getting the most attention tend to be those resulting from ischaemia of the heart, lungs and brain.[128]

Angina

Angina is a common, pervasive, condition associated with CAD. This is due to myocardial ischaemia — when oxygen supply falls below myocardial oxygen demand — as a result of obstructed coronary blood flow.[167] The condition is typified by chest pain or discomfort and always requires further investigation.[61] Increased levels of C-reactive protein are also implicated in the inflammatory progression of CAD in patients with existing, stable angina.[168]

Myocardial infarction

The ultimate clinical manifestation of CAD is myocardial infarction. This occurs when an atherosclerotic plaque ruptures or erodes, inducing platelet activation, thrombus formation and subsequent occlusion of a blood vessel.[169] Inflammation of the endothelium, as occurs in atherosclerosis and CAD, and ongoing oxidative stress, inactivates nitric oxide, thereby impairing endothelium-dependent vasodilation, enhancing platelet susceptibility and adhesion.[170] In over 80% of fatal myocardial events, unstable plaque is implicated.[171]

Congestive heart failure

CAD is a predisposing factor for congestive heart failure, a serious condition in which the heart is unable to pump sufficient blood to meet the body's metabolic needs.[125]

Elevated homocysteine, associated atherosclerosis and CAD are also implicated in congestive heart failure.[172]

DIFFERENTIAL DIAGNOSIS

Atherosclerosis is multifactorial and differential diagnosis may depend on a number of presenting symptoms and comorbidities. A patient presenting with symptoms (e.g. chest pain) will usually have more advanced disease, and thus diagnosis of symptomatic patients will be discussed under the relevant conditions (such as angina, myocardial infarction and peripheral arterial disease).

However, an asymptomatic patient who is high risk (e.g. obese, poor nutritional intake, family history) should still be considered for:

- Atherosclerosis and/or dyslipidaemia
- Hypertension
- Insulin resistance/metabolic syndrome
- Peripheral vascular disease.

NATUROPATHIC DIAGNOSIS

Naturopathic diagnosis of atherosclerosis is largely dependent on allopathic determinants and consideration of concurrent conditions. However, naturopathic medicine also takes into consideration several other factors:

- Digestive capability and subsequent nutrient absorption
- Quality and quantity of nutritional intake
- Emotional health and stress levels, which may be impacting on hormonal balance and circulatory activity.

In many cases, understanding the interrelationship of conditions, combined with fundamental dietary and lifestyle modifications, can bring about significant change in a patient's condition.

Investigations

A full case history must be taken, assessing health history and current risk factors including diet, lifestyle, exercise, smoking, etc. Blood pressure must also be measured at each visit. When atherosclerosis with associated symptomatic pathology is suspected, more specific diagnostic procedures are involved (Table 20.16).

Naturopathic investigations

Naturopathic evaluation of atherosclerosis and dyslipidaemia will rely initially on thorough case taking, physical evaluation and standard pathology tests. There are also a number of functional investigations that will aid treatment and diagnosis.

ESSENTIAL FATTY ACIDS

Used to measure essential fatty acid status and identify deficiency, this is particularly relevant for the diagnosis and treatment of dyslipidaemia, as well as alleviating the inflammation associated with atherosclerosis.

TOTAL ANTIOXIDANT STATUS

This measures serum antioxidant status, important for the management of atherosclerosis, as much of the inflammation associated with the condition is a result of oxidative stress.

TABLE 20.16 Diagnostic procedures for coronary artery disease (CAD)

Electrocardiograph (ECG)	This will identify arrhythmias and/or left ventricular hypertrophy, although findings can be normal in up to 50% of patients with severe CAD. Nonetheless, left ventricular function is a significant predictor of long-term survival in patients with CAD
Exercise stress test	This is usually recommended, with an ECG, in patients with a moderate to high risk of CAD. It enables the physician to assess the activity of the heart under stress
Diagnostic imaging: Magnetic resonance imaging (MRI) Positron emission tomography (PET) Single-photon computed tomography (SPECT) Echocardiogram (ECHO)	These rely on the stress-inducible ischaemia, evidenced by perfusion abnormalities or systolic dysfunction, as a marker for CAD. They may be used with or without an accompanying stress test
Glucose tolerance test (GTT), fasting glucose, insulin and HbA_{1c}	This is recommended as abnormal glucose metabolism is highly correlated with CAD and subsequent cardiovascular disease events
Serum pathology — based on risk and/or comorbidity	Total cholesterol LDL cholesterol HDL cholesterol Triglycerides C-reactive protein Lipoprotein(a) Fibrinogen Homocysteine Ferritin (an iron-binding protein) Lipid peroxides

Sources: Bartnik M, Ryden L, Malmberg K et al. Oral glucose tolerance test is needed for appropriate classification of glucose regulation in patients with coronary artery disease: a report from the Euro Heart Survey on Diabetes and the Heart. Heart 2007; 93(1):72–77. Cassar A, Holmes D, Rihal C et al. Chronic coronary artery disease: diagnosis and management. Mayo Clinic Proc 2009; 84(12):1130–1146. Connolly D, Elveback L, Oxman H. Coronary heart disease in residents of Rochester, Minnesota: IV. Prognostic value of the resting electrocardiogram at the time of initial diagnosis of angina pectoris. Mayo Clin Proc 1984; 59(4):247–250. Emond M, Mock M, Davis K et al. Long-term survival of medically treated patients in the Coronary Artery Surgery Study (CASS) Registry. Circulation 1994; 90(6):2645–2657. Schuijf J, Poldermans D, Shaw L et al. Diagnostic and prognostic value of non-invasive imaging in known or suspected coronary artery disease. Eur J Nucl Med Mol Imaging 2006; 33(1):93–104.

Therapeutic considerations

CLINICAL DECISION MAKING AND RATIONALE

In assessing patients and deciding on a treatment approach for atherosclerosis, it is important to consider the context in terms of primary, secondary or tertiary prevention. Table 20.17 details an approach and rationale.

TABLE 20.17 Stages of naturopathic intervention in cardiovascular disease

Scenario	Broad treatment aim	Key goals	Treatment examples
Patient presents with no symptoms, no risk factors, wishing to prevent future disease	Primary prevention	Enable/encourage dietary and lifestyle changes known or suspected to prevent the development of atherosclerotic risk factors	Public health initiatives to reduce sodium and sugar intake, increase exercise, maintain appropriate body weight, increase fish consumption
Patient presents with no symptoms, but markers for increased risk (such as hypertension, dyslipidaemia, obesity, etc) or … Patient presents with clinical silent atherosclerosis discovered on routine testing	Secondary prevention	Reduction in severity of each individual risk factor and total cumulative risk	Same as primary prevention, plus … Interventions to specifically address risk factors (e.g. herbal medicines to lower blood pressure; herbal and nutritional medicines to alter lipid profile)
Patient presents with symptoms consistent with advanced atherosclerotic change resulting in some degree of tissue ischaemia	Tertiary prevention	Slowing, stopping or reversing progression of atherosclerotic change Managing the impact of ischaemia on affected tissues/organs	Same as primary and secondary prevention plus … Interventions to specifically manage the impact of ischaemia and prevent infarction in relevant tissues/organs (e.g. herbal and nutritional medicines to reduce coagulation, improve tissue oxygen utilisation efficiency)

Therapeutic application

ALLOPATHIC PERSPECTIVE

The allopathic treatment of atherosclerosis often begins if a patient presents with elevated risk factors associated with atherosclerosis, or becomes symptomatic with ischaemic conditions such as angina, myocardial infarction, or stroke. Treatment aims to achieve several aspects: reduce clinical symptoms (if present), reduce further progression of atherosclerosis and, ultimately, prevent an early death. This is managed through the control of risk factors, alongside medical and surgical intervention as appropriate (see Table 20.18 and Box 20.4).

HISTORICAL PERSPECTIVE

To ameliorate symptoms associated with what we now understand to be atherosclerosis, remedies that lowered blood tension and decreased the force of the heart such as the 'heart sedatives' were suggested, including *Crataegus*, which was thought to guard against arteriosclerosis.[173] The Eclectics advocated the use of diet and lifestyle habits, suggesting it was wise to change the patient's habits of life and to 'subject him to conditions which are unusual but in every way agreeable'.[174] The use of potassium or sodium iodide was believed to retard fatty deposits, restoring the normal condition of the arterial walls, while alcohol intake and stimulating condiments within the food was prohibited. The patient was advised to rest and keep away from active muscular effort, from anxiety, despondency or worry and from anger. Low altitude was also thought to help relieve atherosclerosis.

NATUROPATHIC PERSPECTIVE

The naturopathic perspective is similar in many ways to the allopathic interpretation for the atherosclerotic patient. Specific goals are to:

- Control risk factors (hypertension, dyslipidaemia, inflammation)
- Ensure appropriate weight, and regulate blood sugar levels
- Improve lifestyle and dietary practices, emotional and mental wellbeing
- Reduce and prevent ischaemia by improving blood supply to the affected organs
- Prevent an early death by working with a healthcare team that includes the patient's GP and cardiologist.

Other considerations the naturopath must review include:

- Thyroid function
- Antioxidant status
- 'Type A' personality.

When reviewing risk factors, it is additionally beneficial to also consider the compounding effect of multiple risk factors in lieu of simply one (Table 20.19).

NUTRITIONAL MEDICINE (DIETARY)

Dietary therapeutic objectives

- Prevent oxidative and free radical damage to cell membranes by consuming a high level of antioxidants and phytochemicals
- Improve the structure and composition of cell membranes by encouraging monounsaturated and

TABLE 20.18 Risk reduction/treatment for patients with CAD

Risk factor/ treatment	Recommendation
Physical activity	30–45 min activity/day (minimum 5 days/week) Cardiac rehabilitation for high-risk patients (e.g. recent myocardial infarction)
Weight management	BMI between 18.5 and 24.9 kg/m^2 Waist circumference <88 cm (women) and <102 cm (men)
Smoking cessation	Avoid exposure to tobacco smoke (passive or active)
Blood pressure control	Lifestyle modification (weight management, exercise, dietary improvement, reduced alcohol consumption) Target BP <140/90 mmHg or <130/80 mmHg for diabetic or renal patients Initial drug treatment with beta-blockers and/or ACE inhibitors, with addition of other medication as required to reach target BP
Lipid management	Diet low in saturated fat (<7% diet), trans fatty acids and cholesterol (<200 mg/day) Daily exercise and weight management Plant sterol (2 g/day), viscous fibre (>10 g/day) for LDL cholesterol reduction Omega-3 fatty acid (1 g/day) If LDL cholesterol ≥2.5 mmol/L then drug therapy (first choice: statins) to a goal of <2.0 mmol/L[134] If triglyceride >2.0 mmol/L then drug therapy with niacin or fibrates
Diabetes management	Normalise blood glucose and insulin with lifestyle and pharmacotherapy
Antiplatelet agents	Aspirin (75–162 mg/day) to be continued indefinitely, unless contraindicated Clopidogrel (75 mg/day) in the case that aspirin is contraindicated
Beta-blockers	Start and continue indefinitely with beta-blocker therapy in all patients with past myocardial infarction, acute coronary syndrome or left ventricular dysfunction Use as needed for angina, hypertension and arrhythmia
Renin–angiotensin–aldosterone system blockers	Start ACE inhibitors and continue indefinitely in all patients with left-ventricular dysfunction, hypertension, diabetes or chronic kidney disease, unless contraindicated Consider ACE inhibitors for all CAD patients, unless contraindicated Angiotensin II receptor blockers are used for those intolerant to ACE inhibitors
Nitrates	Sublingual glyceryl trinitrate or glyceryl trinitrate spray for immediate relief of angina, or for prophylaxis before exercising Long-acting nitrates for symptom relief if beta-blocker treatment is unsuccessful or contraindicated
Calcium antagonists	For symptom relief if beta-blocker treatment is unsuccessful or contraindicated Specific for coronary vasospasm
Influenza vaccine	Annual vaccine is often recommended for patients with CAD

Source: Adapted from Cassar A, Holmes D, Rihal C et al. Chronic coronary artery disease: diagnosis and management. Mayo Clinic Proc 2009; 84(12):1130–1146.

BOX 20.4 Statins, cholesterol and cardiovascular outcomes — a statistical deception?

A 2015 review provided an interesting insight into the ongoing controversial debate as to the role, efficacy, and risk versus benefit analysis of statin drugs. This review looked at the statistical analysis of the results of three major statin trials.

The first was the JUPITER trial of rosuvastatin compared to placebo in 17 802 healthy people with elevated C-reactive protein levels, and normal cholesterol levels. The primary outcome measure was the occurrence of a major cardiovascular event, with a median follow-up of 1.9 years. In this study 0.76% of people in the control group, and 0.35% of people in the statin group had a fatal or non-fatal heart attack. This was reported to the public and healthcare workers as a 54% reduction in heart attack in those people taking rosuvastatin, which appears clinically impressive. However, this is what is statistically known as relative risk reduction (RRR) — where risk is reported as a percentage difference between the two groups. This is quite different to absolute risk reduction (ARR), which is the actual difference in risk between the two groups. The ARR in this study is 0.41% (i.e. 0.76 minus 0.35), and the RRR is found by dividing the ARR by the risk in the control group (i.e. 0.41 divided by 0.76 = 54%). Therefore while the figures are correct, the way they are interpreted is questionable. When reporting a 54% reduction in the risk of heart attacks, people generally assume this means absolute risk reduction.

Additionally the study seemed to conceal the fact that while the ARR was a combination of non-fatal and fatal heart attacks, more people had fatal heart attacks in the statin group (*n* = 11) than in the placebo group (*n* = 6). Finally the JUPITER study also reported that in the rosuvastatin group

Continued

BOX 20.4 Statins, cholesterol and cardiovascular outcomes — a statistical deception?—cont'd

there were 270 new cases of diabetes, compared to 216 in the control group; unlike the beneficial effects that were amplified in appearance by reporting them as RRR, this difference in new-onset diabetes was reported using only ARR. The review authors suggest that the JUPITER trial finding should be reported to patients differently:

> *An objective assessment of the JUPITER findings should therefore be conveyed to potential patients in the following manner: 'Your chance to avoid a nonfatal heart attack during the next 2 years is about 97% without treatment, but you can increase it to about 98% by taking a Crestor every day. However, you will not prolong your life and there is a risk you may develop diabetes.'*

A similar issue is noticed with in-depth analysis of the ASCOT-LLA trial. This study compared atorvastatin with placebo in 10 305 patients with hypertension and at least three additional risk factors from the following list: peripheral arterial disease, previous stroke or transient ischaemic attack, type 2 diabetes, left ventricular hypertrophy and smoking. The primary outcome measure was occurrence of fatal and non-fatal coronary heart disease, with the trial planned for 5-years duration but terminated at 3.3 years due to an apparently impressive result reported as 36% reduction in fatal coronary heart disease and non-fatal myocardial infarction. Again, however, this 36% reduction is actually relative risk reduction, not absolute risk reduction (which in this case was 1.1%). The review authors again suggest the following:

> *If a patient with a risk profile of subjects in ASCOT asks a physician about the likelihood that he or she will not experience an MI or a fatal coronary event without treatment ... 97%, virtually all of the placebo-treated subjects, did not have a nonfatal MI or die of CHD.*

Finally the review analysed the British Heart Protection Study of 20 000 people comparing simvastatin and placebo, and discussed what appears to be systematic bias in minimising the reported frequency of adverse events from statins.

The review authors conclude that:

> *the presentation of statin trial findings can be characterized as a deceptive strategy in which negligible benefits of statin treatment have been amplified with the use of relative risk statistics, and that serious adverse effects are either ignored or explained away as a chance occurrences.*

Source: Diamond DM, Ravnskov U. How statistical deception created the appearance that statins are safe and effective in primary and secondary prevention of cardiovascular disease. Expert Rev Clin Pharmacol 2015; 8(2):201–210. Reprinted with permission of Taylor & Francis Ltd, http://www.tandfonline.com

TABLE 20.19 Association of risk factors with incidence of atherosclerosis

Major risk factors	Increase in incidence
Presence of one of the major risk factors	30%
High cholesterol and high blood pressure	300%
High cholesterol and a smoker	350%
High blood pressure and a smoker	350%
Smoker, high blood cholesterol and high blood pressure	720%

Source: Pizzorno J, Murray M. Textbook of natural medicine. 3rd ed. Oxford: Elsevier; 1999.

omega-3 fatty acids to provide the basic building blocks for structural components
- Discourage saturated, trans or hydrogenated fat sources
- Exclude caffeine, sodium and alcohol
- Encourage fibre-rich sources from a variety of wholegrains and pulses
- Encourage principles of the Mediterranean diet.

FOODS TO DECREASE BLOOD LIPIDS

Foods to decrease blood lipids include fermented soy foods, garlic and onions, foods high in soluble fibre (oats, barley, legumes, psyllium), omega-3 oils (fish oil, flaxseed, walnuts, hemp oil, canola oil), monounsaturated oils (olive oil), fresh fruits and vegetables (avocado, tomato, apples, pears, raspberries), nuts and seeds (walnuts, almonds, hazelnuts, flaxseed, sunflower seed), tea (contains antioxidant flavonoids including catechin) and yoghurt.

Specific dietary treatments

DIETARY INCLUSIONS

Dietary fibre

Intake of dietary fibre should be encouraged due to its cholesterol-lowering properties. An Australian study assessing the cholesterol-lowering effect of a ready-to-eat cereal containing soluble fibre in the form of psyllium (86%), oatmeal and barley (total soluble fibre 12 g) on the plasma lipids of otherwise healthy men with mild hypercholesterolaemia already eating a diet low in saturated fats, observed that total cholesterol and LDL cholesterol concentrations fell significantly in men eating the psyllium cereal when compared with those eating conventional wheat cereal containing 2 g soluble fibre.[175] This type of product is easy to implement into the daily routine of patients and is likely to assist with mild hypercholesterolaemia.

Garlic and onions

Garlic and onions have both been suggested to be useful for reducing hypercholesterolaemia and their intake should be encouraged in the diet.[176] For a full discussion, please see below in the section on herbal medicines. In general it is recommended to increase garlic in the diet; however, formalised prescriptions are recommended for some patients. Food dosage recommendations are 2–5 g/day of fresh garlic. Ensure it is bruised, crushed or chewed to obtain all active constituents.

MEDITERRANEAN DIET

The Mediterranean diet is associated with a protective effect on the cardiovascular system.[177,178] It is made up primarily of wholefoods that are plant based and high in fibre, such as fruit, vegetables, grains, breads, nuts and seeds, and is minimally processed and based upon fresh, in season foods (Box 20.5).[179] Olive oil and omega-3 fatty acids are used as the primary source of fat, and dairy, poultry and fish are consumed low to moderately, while red meat is consumed infrequently and in small portions. Fruit is consumed as dessert, while low to moderate amounts of wine (1–2 glasses for men and 1 glass per day for women) may be consumed in terms of alcohol. Given the protective effects of the Mediterranean diet on the cardiovascular system, particularly with regard to its cholesterol-lowering properties,[180] the basic principles that make up this diet are recommended for patients with coronary heart disease.

BOX 20.5 Principles of the Mediterranean diet

- Wholefood dietary principles prevail — food is fresh, unprocessed, seasonal and locally grown
- Abundance of (vegetarian) plant foods
- Fresh fruit and vegetables, pulses, bread, pasta, nuts and seeds
- Fresh fruit is the general source of sweets — sweets containing concentrated sugars or honey consumed a few times per week at the most
- Essential fatty acids are primarily obtained from olive oil
- Animal protein
- Dairy products are full fat and consumed daily in low to moderate amounts. Cheese and yoghurt are the richest sources
- Fresh fish is consumed regularly
- Poultry and eggs are consumed in moderate amounts (up to four times weekly) or not at all
- Red meat is consumed in low amounts
- Wine is consumed in low to moderate amounts, normally with meals
- Low GI/GL dietary principles

It is recommended that sugar and refined carbohydrates are reduced and a blood sugar-stabilising diet encouraged. For a full discussion, see the section on diabetes mellitus in Chapter 21.

DIETARY EXCLUSIONS

Trans fatty acids

There is strong evidence to support the relationship between trans fatty acids and heart disease. Trans fats have been linked to vascular inflammation and sudden cardiac death in animal studies[181] as well as endothelial dysfunction. Studies have shown that even an intake of small quantities (2% of total energy intake) is associated with increased risk of coronary heart disease.[182]

Caffeine

Caffeine has been found to increase homocysteine levels. This is significant since elevated homocysteine is associated with increased risk of coronary heart disease. Coffee, a source of caffeine, has long been linked to coronary heart disease, although, surprisingly, a recent meta-analysis could not support the hypothesis that coffee consumption increases the long-term risk of coronary heart disease.[183]

In spite of the latter result, it is important to note that coffee contains a diterpene known as cafestol which has been found to increase serum LDL cholesterol (cafestol is higher in unfiltered coffee). Coffee is also associated with increased blood pressure, aortic stiffness and endothelial dysfunction and should thus be omitted from the diet of patients with coronary heart disease.

Alcohol

Numerous studies have been undertaken examining the effects of alcohol in coronary artery disease. Some have observed a harmful[184] effect of alcohol in terms of coronary supply–demand relations, while others have observed a protective effect. Given the inconsistencies on this topic, along with the overall hazardous effects of alcohol as a whole, it would appear unethical to suggest that patients increase their alcohol intake on the premise of these studies.

Sodium

It is recommended to reduce sodium in the diet. For a full discussion, see the section on hypertension.

NUTRITIONAL MEDICINE (SUPPLEMENTAL)

Nutritional medicine therapeutic objectives

- Reduce atherosclerotic plaques, improve blood flow
- Reduce blood lipid levels (cholesterol and triglycerides)
- Improve hepatobiliary function to assist with balancing lipid profile
- Reduce existing oxidation and protect all sources of lipids from oxidation
- Improve cardiac function by controlling cardiac excitability, regular neuromuscular transmission, vasomotor tone and blood pressure
- Prevent ischaemic reperfusion damage
- Reduce reperfusion arrhythmias
- Lower total inotropic requirement and improve mediastinal drainage
- Balance blood sugar levels (as required)
- Support weight management.

Specific nutrients required

B COMPLEX

The importance of a B complex with potential additions of B_3, B_6, B_9 or B_{12} depending on patient presentation cannot be underestimated. Vitamin B_3 is composed of niacin (nicotinic acid) and its amide, niacinamide, and can be found in many foods, including yeast, meat, fish, milk, eggs, green vegetables and cereal grains. Dietary tryptophan, found in protein-containing foods such as red meat, poultry, eggs and dairy products, is also converted to niacin after ingestion. Vitamin B_3 is frequently found in combination with other

SAMPLE DAILY DIET

BREAKFAST	
Banana, oats, leafy greens and blueberry breakfast smoothie	Oats in part owe their cholesterol-lowering action to their beta-glucan content as well as their soluble fibre. Beta-glucans form a viscous mass in the small intestine, preventing reabsorption of bile salts and limiting intestinal absorption of dietary cholesterol, resulting in lower cholesterol levels. Leafy greens provide an optimal source of folate, which along with vitamins B_{12} and B_6 may assist with elevated levels of homocysteine, a common cause of inflammation in vascular disorders.
LUNCH	
Waldorf salad: witlof, celery, sliced red apple, thinly sliced red onion, poached chicken and raw walnuts. Drizzle with natural yoghurt and lemon juice	Consumption of nuts at least 2 × per week is associated with lower total cholesterol, LDL cholesterol. Since elevated levels of cholesterol are linked with inflammation ensuring the intake of large quantities of fruit and vegetables to downregulate inflammation is imperative. Fruit and vegetables are also fibre rich, ensuring removal of cholesterol from the body.
DINNER	
Grilled fish with peperonata (made with ample onions, red capsicum and garlic)	Intake of fatty fish is associated with an increase in HDL cholesterol. Grilling and steaming are healthier cooking methods than frying. Ample onions, red capsicum and garlic should be consumed in the diet due to their hypocholesterolaemic action. Onion and garlic enhance cholesterol conversion to bile acids through activation of hepatic cholesterol-7α-hydroxylase while capsaicin found in red capsicum has been shown to be hypotriglyceridaemic, preventing accumulation of fat in the liver by enhancing triglyceride transport out of the liver.
SNACKS	
1 cup of dhal soup containing a range of spices including fenugreek, turmeric 2 × kiwi fruit	Fenugreek and turmeric both display hypocholesterolaemic action. In men with high cholesterol levels consumption of two green kiwi fruit per day in combination with a healthy diet has been shown to improve HDL cholesterol and decrease total cholesterol compared to simply consuming a healthy diet alone.

B vitamins and so it is essential to combine the prescription with a comprehensive B vitamin complex.

Higher doses of vitamin B_3 have been shown to improve a number of parameters (Table 20.20).

Doses are usually started low and gradually increased to reduce the adverse effects of facial flushing. In addition, it is essential to remind patients to take the dose with a full meal containing adequate lipids and protein to slow absorption and prevent the flush response. Use of an antihistamine 15 minutes prior to a niacin dose may also suppress cutaneous flushing, but this is usually unnecessary. In most patients, the flushing response spontaneously diminishes after 1–2 weeks of therapy, especially when the dose is slowly increased over time.

A number of beneficial properties have been found:

- Decreased fibrinogen levels
- Reductions in LDL levels, with stronger effects generally occurring at higher doses than required for raising HDL levels (up to 3–4.5 g daily)
- Decreased hepatic synthesis of very low-density lipoprotein (VLDL) levels, the precursor of LDL
- Increase in LDL particle size and a shift from small LDL to the less atherogenic large LDL subclasses
- Conversion of LDL subclass patterns
- Decreased serum triglyceride levels by reducing the size of VLDL particles
- Increased large HDL particles without a net effect on small HDL particles
- Decreased smaller, denser LDL particles (L1 and L2) and increased larger, more buoyant L3 subclass
- Reductions in hepatic cholesterol synthesis have also been demonstrated in human studies.

VITAMIN E

Vitamin E protects polyunsaturated fatty acids from oxidation, decreases the deposition of atherogenic oxidised LDL in arterial walls and aids healthy blood circulation, helping to maintain cell integrity and health. The knowledge that free radical damage may be related to the pathogenesis of cardiovascular disease logically led many experts to suggest the use of vitamin E for coronary artery disease, particularly due to its purported ability to suppress oxidative stress-induced tissue factor expression in human coronary artery endothelial cells,[185] but results from clinical trials have been inconsistent, leading many to question the use of vitamin E in CAD.

TABLE 20.20 Evidence to support the prescription of vitamin B_3 with atherosclerosis or dyslipidaemia

Study design	Author, year	Number	Statistically significant	Quality of study 0–5	Magnitude of benefit	Comments
Hyperlipidaemia						
Meta-analysis	Goldberg, 2004	432	Yes	NA	Large	Five trials showed greater decreases in LDL and TG; effects were slightly better in women
Systematic review	Schectman, 1996	6 studies	NA	NA	Large	Three trials of niacin monotherapy demonstrated efficacy; three trials combining niacin with statins found additive effects
Randomised controlled trial	Elam, 2000	468	Yes	5	Large	3 g of niacin daily was associated with significant increase in HDL and decrease in LDL and triglyceride levels vs. placebo
Randomised controlled trial	Morgan, 1996 and 1998	122	Yes	4	Large	Niaspan® 1 g vs. 2 g vs. placebo. Niaspan® lowered LDL and increased HDL levels at both doses vs. placebo, with few adverse effects
Randomised controlled trial	Vacek, 1995	25	Yes	4	Large	Niacin plus was associated with superior lowering of total cholesterol and LDL than either agent alone
Randomised controlled trial	Davignon, 1994	158	Yes	4	Large	Niacin plus pravastatin was associated with superior HDL-raising and LDL-lowering effects than either therapy alone. Pravastatin monotherapy lowered LDL levels better than niacin
Randomised controlled trial	Keenan, 1991	201	Yes	4	Large	1.5 g of niacin daily was associated with significant increases in serum HDL vs. placebo. Greater effects in older patients (aged 50–70), but small subgroup sample sizes
Randomised controlled trial	Hunninghake, 2003	237	Yes	3	Medium	Combination of niacin and statin more effective than niacin monotherapy or statin monotherapy for improving LDL, HDL, and triglycerides
Randomised controlled trial	Goldberg, 2000	132	Yes	3	Large	Niaspan® (up to 3 g daily) for 25 weeks was associated with significant improvement in plasma lipids vs. placebo
Randomised controlled trial (plus dosing study)	Goldberg, 1998	131	Yes	3	Large	Dose escalation study of sustained-release niacin found HDL increases at 500 mg daily and LDL decreases at 1000 mg daily
Randomised controlled trial (crossover)	Aronov, 1996	89	Yes	3	Medium	Wax-matrix sustained-release niacin (1.5–2 g daily vs. placebo). Niacin was associated with significant decreases in total cholesterol and LDL
Randomised controlled trial (plus dosing)	Keenan, 1992	201	Yes	3	Medium	Older vs. younger subjects. More effective in older subjects

Continued

TABLE 20.20 Evidence to support the prescription of vitamin B_3 with atherosclerosis or dyslipidaemia—cont'd

Study design	Author, year	Number	Statistically significant	Quality of study 0–5	Magnitude of benefit	Comments
Hyperlipidaemia—cont'd						
Randomised controlled trial	Grundy, 2002	143	Yes	2	Small	Niacin significantly improved HDL and TG levels vs. placebo over 16 weeks
Randomised controlled and equivalence trial	Superko, 2004	180	Yes	1	Large	Niacin IR 3 g daily vs. niacin ER 1.5 g daily vs. placebo; niacin IR and niacin ER had differential effects on LDL subclass distribution in patients classified as LDL pattern A, B, or I
Randomised controlled trial (historical samples)	Morgan, 2003	60	Yes	3	Large	Post analysis of 60 samples showed influence of niacin on different lipoprotein blood classes
Randomised controlled trial (open-label, multicentre)	Capuzzi, 2003	270	Yes	3	Medium	Rosuvastatin alone superior to ER niacin for LDL reduction and better tolerated. Additive effect of niacin for HDL lowering
Randomised controlled trial (open-label, multicentre)	Capuzzi, 2004	270	No (cholesterol lowering above rosuvastatin); Yes (HDL cholesterol increase)	2	NA	Niacin ER combined therapy produced significantly greater rises in HDL-C and apoA-I than rosuvastatin monotherapy but had no additive effect on cholesterol lowering
Randomised controlled trial (open-label; crossover)	Lal, 1995	17	Yes	2	Large	Minimum of 1.5 g daily niacin for 16 weeks lowered TC, LDL, and TG
Equivalence trial (open-label)	McKenney, 2007	292	Yes (increased HDL above statin alone)	2	Large	Extended-release niacin increased HDL levels above statin alone
Equivalence trial (open-label)	Vega, 2003	47	Yes (less effective than statins)	2	Medium	Niacin decreased cholesterol levels in Alzheimer's patients
Equivalence trial (open-label)	McKenney, 2001	P	Yes	NA	Large	3000 mg of IR niacin vs. 10 mg of atorvastatin for 12 weeks lowered VLDL and small LDL
Open-label comparison	Superko,1992	26	Yes	NA	Large	Pattern A subjects vs. pattern B subjects
Open-label study	Dube, 2006	33	Yes	1	Large	Open-label study with ER niacin in HIV patients with dyslipidaemia
Before-and-after study	Gerber, 2004	14	Yes	1	Medium	Niacin ER significantly reduced TG, TC, and non-HDL-C in HIV-infected individuals
Atherosclerosis (as adjunct therapy; niacin)						
Randomised controlled trial	Taylor, 2004	167	No (carotid intima-media thickness)	4	Medium	Niacin only significantly reduced the rate of intima-media thickness progression in subjects without insulin resistance using statins
Follow-up open-label study	Taylor, 2006	130	Yes (carotid intima-media thickness)	NA	Medium	Niacin significantly reduced the rate of intima-media thickness progression in subjects in this 12–24 month follow-up

TABLE 20.20 Evidence to support the prescription of vitamin B_3 with atherosclerosis or dyslipidaemia—cont'd

Study design	Author, year	Number	Statistically significant	Quality of study 0–5	Magnitude of benefit	Comments
Cardiovascular disease (niacin)						
Meta-analysis	Birjmohun, 2005	4749	Yes	NA	Small	30 trials; limited data on cardiovascular event rate. 10 trials included Acipimox®
Systematic review	Studer, 2005	97 studies (only 2 niacin trials)	No (mortality)	NA	NA	Risk ratio for overall mortality (95% confidence interval (CI): 0.86–1.08), cardiac mortality and non-cardiovascular mortality indicated no benefit from niacin
Systematic review	Bucher, 1999	59 studies; 2 studies on niacin	No (mortality)	NA	NA	Review of mortality and all cholesterol-lowering treatments. Included two trials of niacin therapy. Pooled results showed a non-significant risk ratio of 0.95 for cardiac mortality, 0.96 for all-cause mortality, and 0.9 for non-cardiac mortality
Randomised controlled trial	Taylor, 2004	167	No (carotid intima-media thickness)	4	Medium	Niacin only significantly reduced the rate of intima-media thickness progression in subjects without insulin resistance using statins
Randomised controlled trial	Anonymous, 1975; Canner, 1996; Berge, 1991	8341; 1119 in niacin group	Yes	4	Medium	Coronary Drug Project: 1119 subjects randomised to 3 g of niacin daily. At 15 years, significant decrease in mortality seen with niacin
Randomised controlled trial (patients and data derived from the Coronary Drug Project)	Canner, 2005	8341	Yes	3	Small	Study conducted only in men; niacin found to have favourable effects on clinical outcome in patients including those with evidence of abnormal glucose metabolism or overt diabetes
Randomised controlled trial (patients and data derived from the Coronary Drug Project)	Canner, 2006	2787 + 1119	No	NA	NA	No statistical significance between individuals with or without metabolic syndrome
Randomised controlled trial	Kuvin, 2006	60	Yes	3	Large	Niacin in addition to existing medication reduced inflammatory and lipid parameters
Randomised controlled trial	Schoch, 1968	570	Yes	3	Large	4 g of niacin daily over 5 years associated with 20% decrease in total cholesterol and no significant effect on mortality
Randomised controlled trial	Chesney, 2000	80	Yes	2	Medium	1500 mg decreased fibrinogen by 14% and prothrombin by 60%
Before-and-after study	Lavie, 1992	36	Yes	NA	Large	Slo-Niacin® decreased TC, LDL, and TG

TC, total cholesterol; LDL, low-density lipoprotein; TG, triglycerides; ER, extended release; IR, immediate release.
Source: Adapted from Natural Standard, Vitamin B_3 monograph, 2010, www.naturalstandard.com

Results from the Cambridge Heart Antioxidant Study demonstrated positive results with regard to cardiovascular health, seeking to dispel some of the inconsistency. In this study, the effects of vitamin E (400 or 800 IU/day) were assessed in 2002 patients in the UK with angiographically proven CAD.[186] Patients received either a placebo or vitamin E and were assessed over a mean period of 1.4 years. At the end of the study it was observed that while there was no difference in overall mortality between the groups, the group consuming vitamin E had a significant decrease in the combined end point of cardiovascular death and non-fatal myocardial infarction, suggesting that vitamin E supplementation may decrease cardiac events in high-risk patients. Notably there were some methodological flaws with this study; for example, the groups were not equal at baseline with regard to gender or serum cholesterol level and some patients received 800 IU/day vitamin E while others received 400 IU/day. These results are promising nevertheless and warrant further investigation.

VITAMIN C

Vitamin C is the body's primary water-soluble antioxidant and is present in the blood, body fluids and all cells. Vitamin C helps protect against fat oxidation by free radicals and lowers the tendency for platelet aggregation. A meta-analysis comprising 15 RCTs demonstrated that supplementation with vitamin C 500–2000 mg/day for at least 1 month (though the longest study lasted 24 weeks) may help to decrease serum LDL cholesterol (−7.9 mg/dL) and triglyceride concentrations (−20.1 mg/dL).[187] While HDL cholesterol increased, the result was not found to be statistically significant.

ESSENTIAL FATTY ACIDS

Fish oil supplementation appears to be extremely beneficial for hyperlipidaemia with a 2009 systematic review and meta-analysis comprising 47 studies and involving 16 511 patients showing a clinically significant dose-dependent effect of fish oils. On average a dose of 3.25 g/day, comprising 1.9 g EPA/day and 1.35 g DHA/day was found to be effective in reducing triglycerides, though no changes in total cholesterol were observed.[188] The authors observed that beneficial effects could be expected in as little as 24 weeks for individuals with hypertriglyceridaemia. In one paper EPA and DHA both improved arterial compliance by 35% and 27%, respectively, in patients with dyslipidaemia.[189]

Fish oil is readily incorporated into atherosclerotic plaques. Plaques from patients given fish oil have been shown to be less heavily infiltrated with macrophages than those in controls; they are also less likely to be thin and rupture, signifying the protective effects of the fish oil.[190]

MAGNESIUM

Magnesium is an essential mineral in the body and has several important roles with regard to healthy cardiovascular function, including its role as a natural calcium channel blocker, the ability to control cardiac excitability and its roles in neuromuscular transmission, vasomotor tone and blood pressure. It is no wonder then that decreased quantities have been suggested to negatively affect myocardial cells, resulting in their death.[191] The Honolulu Heart Program, a longitudinal clinical trial assessing the relationship between dietary magnesium intake and future risk of chronic heart disease in male patients, observed a 1.7- to 2.1-fold increase in the risk of chronic heart disease in lowest versus highest quintiles of magnesium intake ($p < 0.001$), suggesting that intake of dietary magnesium is associated with a reduced risk of chronic heart disease.[192] Similar results were also seen following analysis of questionnaires from the Health Professionals Follow-up Study which involved 39 633 men and demonstrated that increased magnesium intake was associated with a modestly lower risk of heart disease among men.[193] Oral magnesium therapy (365 mg/day) has been observed to improve endothelial function and exercise tolerance in patients with coronary artery disease.[194]

COENZYME Q10

Coenzyme Q10 is an effective antioxidant that may help to prevent the oxidative modification of LDLs as well as reduce the risk of atherosclerosis. Following 1 year of supplementation with coenzyme Q10 120 mg/day in patients postacute myocardial infarction, total cardiac events including non-fatal infarction and cardiac deaths were significantly lower in the coenzyme Q10 group compared with the control.[195] Plasma levels of vitamin E and HDL cholesterol showed significant increases and oxidants showed significant reduction, respectively, in the coenzyme Q10 group compared with the control, suggesting that treatment with coenzyme Q10 may be beneficial in patients with recent myocardial infarction.

Coenzyme Q10 also shows great promise for patients undergoing coronary bypass graft surgery. Patients given coenzyme Q10 (150–180 mg/day) 7–10 days prior to the operation until the morning of surgery in an attempt to prevent ischaemic reperfusion damage show less reperfusion arrhythmias, lower total inotropic requirement, less mediastinal drainage, lower blood requirement and shorter hospitalisation compared with controls.[196]

OTHERS

In considering the holistic management of a patient, other nutrients as noted in the sections on hypertension (within this chapter) or diabetes mellitus (Chapter 21) may be indicated.

Dosage requirements

The dosage requirements listed below are based on adult doses that have been reported in the literature.

- B complex (all B vitamins) high-dose combination, preferably activated forms
  - Thiamine 20–40 mg/day
  - Riboflavin 20–40 mg
  - Niacinamide 50–100 mg/day
  - Pantothenic acid 150–300 mg/day
  - Pyridoxine 20–60 mg/day
  - Folinic acid or L-5MTHF 500–1000 micrograms/day
    - Selection based on methylation assessment
  - Hydroxocobalamin or methylcobalamin 500–1000 micrograms/day
    - Selection based on methylation assessment

  - Choline 50–100 mg/day
  - Inositol 50–100 mg/day
  - Biotin 250–500 microgram/day

  Additional B vitamin support:
  - Vitamin B_3 (niacinamide): extra B_3 (100 mg+) is indicated with elevated cholesterol levels
  - Vitamin B_6 (pyridoxine): extra B_6 (75–100 mg) is indicated with elevated homocysteine levels
  - Vitamin B_9 (folinic acid or L-5MTHF): extra B_9 (500 micrograms–5 mg) is indicated with elevated homocysteine levels
  - Vitamin B_{12} (hydroxocobalamin or methylcobalamin): extra B_{12} (500–1000 micrograms) is indicated with elevated homocysteine levels
- Magnesium 460 mg/day,[90] but general recommendation is to prescribe between 600 and 1000 mg in divided doses throughout the day
- Vitamin E 400 IU b.i.d.[186,197]
- Vitamin C 500–1000 mg t.d.s.
- Essential fatty acids: 3.25 g/day, comprising 1.9 g EPA/day and 1.35 g DHA/day
- Coenzyme Q10 30–200 mg/day.

HERBAL MEDICINE

Herbal medicine therapeutic objectives

- Reduce blood lipid profile
- Improve hepatobiliary function to normalise blood lipid profile
- Reduce oxidation
- Reduce blood pressure
- Protect and tonify the heart to regulate function
- Reduce peripheral resistance
- Reduce platelet aggregation.

Herbal medicine classes

The herbal medicine classes used for atherosclerosis are listed in Table 20.21.

TABLE 20.21 Herbal medicine classes used for atherosclerosis

Class	Action
Antioxidant	Protect against oxidation and free radical damage and improve circulation to tissues
Hypocholesterolaemic	Reduce cholesterol levels within the blood
Hypolipidaemic	Reduce the concentration of blood lipids, cholesterol and triglycerides, and also include phospholipids (chylomicrons, very low density lipoproteins (VLDL), intermediate-density lipoproteins (IDL), low-density lipoproteins (LDL) and high-density lipoproteins (HDL) and cholesterol esters
Cardioprotective	Protective to the myocardium especially when oxygen supply to the heart is reduced
Hypotensive	Lower blood pressure levels
Peripheral vasodilator	Reduce peripheral vascular resistance, dilate/widen peripheral blood vessels and thereby improve circulation to peripheral tissues to assist in reducing blood pressure
Platelet aggregation inhibitor	Reduce platelet aggregation and hence prolong bleeding time and prevent thrombus formation
Other	Sedatives, nervines, anxiolytics, antidepressants, spasmolytics, blood sugar regulators, thyroid stimulants as required

Specific herbal medicines

ALLIUM SATIVUM (GARLIC)

Garlic has been used as a food and medicine in many countries since antiquity. The German Commission E has approved its use as a support to dietary measures at elevated levels of lipids in the blood and as a preventive measure for age-dependent vascular changes.[198]

Garlic provides numerous benefits for the patient with atherosclerosis, including:

- Hypolipidaemic activity — meta-analysis of 13 clinical trials concluded that garlic was superior to placebo in reducing total cholesterol levels[199]
- Homocysteine-lowering activity — postulated to be due to its ability to inhibit CD36 expression and OxLDL uptake in the macrophages involved in the formation of atherosclerotic plaques[200]
- Antioxidant activity — capable of directly scavenging free radicals and indirectly enhancing endogenous antioxidant systems such as glutathione, superoxide dismutase, catalase and glutathione peroxidase[201]
- Protection against ischaemic perfusion injury — evident in in-vitro and animal models and showed marked improvement in protection against renal and hepatic ischaemia/reperfusion injury[202]
- Anti-inflammatory effects — although acknowledged, the mechanism of action is unresolved. Possible mechanisms include NF-κB activation, modification of COX expression, or suppression of iNOS and NO production[203,204]
- Inhibition of platelet aggregation — proposed mechanisms include inhibition of COX activity and thromboxane A2 production via suppression of intraplatelet Ca^{2+} mobilisation and by increasing cAMP and cGMP levels or through antioxidant pathways that increase platelet-derived NP and interaction with GPIIb/IIIa receptors to induce platelet ability to bind to fibrinogen[205–207]
- Antisclerotic activity — significantly decreases accumulation of aortic tissue cholesterol, fatty streak formation and the size of atherosclerotic plaque in vivo.[208]

Other important effects of garlic include hypotensive activity, hypoglycaemic activity and hepatoprotective effects.

CURCUMA LONGA (TURMERIC)

Curcumin, the active constituent within *Curcuma longa*, has been observed to have a beneficial effect on serum cholesterol and lipid peroxide levels. In one study, healthy volunteers administered 500 mg/day of curcumin daily for 7 days experienced a 33% reduction in serum lipid peroxides, a 12% reduction in total cholesterol and a 29% increase in serum HDL cholesterol. Ramirez Bosca et al[209] observed that 10 mg/day of curcumin administered twice daily for 2 weeks had an antifibrinolytic action. High levels of fibrinogen are associated with coronary heart disease.[209]

SALVIA MILTIORRHIZA (DAN SHEN)

Dan shen products have been widely reported to be useful for the treatment of cardiovascular diseases in China. Its effects of improving circulation and 'removing blood stasis' have been well documented in ancient traditional Chinese medicine writings. Because of its properties in improving microcirculation, causing coronary vasodilation, suppressing the formation of thromboxane, inhibiting platelet adhesion and aggregation, and protecting against myocardial ischaemia, it is widely used either alone or in combination with other herbal ingredients for patients with CAD and other cardiovascular diseases in both China and other countries.[210]

Various in-vitro and in-vivo studies suggested that dan shen could improve microcirculation, dilate the coronary arteries, increase blood flow and prevent myocardial ischaemia. In recent years, pharmacological studies have concentrated on dan shen components such as danshensu, salvianolic acid B and tanshinone IIA. Primary research has been conducted in China and with intravenous preparations, but extrapolation for internal prescriptions can be achieved in some instances.

The effect of dan shen products on cholesterol, triglyceride and LDL and HDL cholesterol levels has also been evaluated. In patients with angina pectoris, Xiang and Li[211] showed a greater reduction of cholesterol and triglyceride following Fufang danshen dripping pill (TCM product) treatment than with isosorbide dinitrate. At least four other studies have also shown that total cholesterol, triglyceride and LDL cholesterol levels are significantly reduced by 28.3%, 34.3%, and 29.9%, respectively, and HDL cholesterol was significantly raised by 33.2% by the Fufang danshen dripping pill.[212–215]

OLEA EUROPAEA (OLIVE LEAVES)

Olive leaves have been widely used in traditional remedies in European and Mediterranean countries such as Greece, Spain, Italy, France, Turkey, Israel, Morocco and Tunisia. They have been used in the human diet as an extract, a herbal tea and a powder, and they contain many potentially bioactive compounds that have antioxidant, antihypertensive, anti-atherogenic, anti-inflammatory, hypoglycaemic, cardioprotective and hypocholesterolaemic/hypolipidaemic properties. One of these potentially bioactive compounds is the secoiridoid oleuropein, which can constitute up to 6–9% of dry matter in the leaves. Other bioactive components found in olive leaves include related secoiridoids, flavonoids and triterpenes.

The phenolic compounds of olive leaves and olive oils in the Mediterranean diet have been associated with a reduced incidence of heart disease. It is thought that these antioxidant-rich diets might prevent the deleterious effects of oxidative metabolism by scavenging free radicals, thus inhibiting oxidation and delaying atherosclerosis. The process may involve phospholipase C activation and arachidonic acid metabolism, and is thought to reduce hydrogen peroxide.[216] The cardiovascular effects of olive leaf extracts are well studied and attributed to the main components of the leaves — oleuropein and oleacein.[217]

In a study by Pignatelli et al,[218] oleuropein and hydroxytyrosol inhibited the phorbol 12-myristate 13-acetate-induced respiratory burst of human neutrophils in a dose-dependent fashion. It was suggested that the effect was due to their capacity to scavenge hydrogen peroxide, which is produced during the arachidonic acid metabolism cascade and leads to platelet aggregation.

Singh et al[216] studied the effect of olive leaves on platelet function in 11 healthy male volunteers, 18–54 years of age. Food records of the volunteers were obtained using a food frequency questionnaire over a 7-day period. The results showed that polyphenols found in olive leaves were capable of in-vitro platelet activation in healthy, non-smoking males. There is a need to follow-up on this in-vivo study to validate its findings and to establish the bioavailability of these polyphenols.

The antioxidant effects of olive leaf extracts are summarised in Table 20.22.

TABLE 20.22 Antioxidant properties of olive leaf extract

Phenolic compound	TEAC (mmol/L)
Olive-leaf extract	1.58 ± 0.06
Rutin	2.75 ± 0.05
Catechin	2.28 ± 0.04
Luteolin	2.25 ± 0.11
Hydroxytyrosol	1.57 ± 0.12
Diosmetin	1.42 ± 0.07
Caffeic acid	1.37 ± 0.08
Verbascoside	1.02 ± 0.07
Oleuropein	0.88 ± 0.09
Luteolin-7-glucoside	0.71 ± 0.04
Vanillic acid	0.67 ± 0.09
Diosmetin-7-glucoside	0.64 ± 0.09
Apigenin-7-glucoside	0.42 ± 0.03
Tyrosol	0.35 ± 0.05
Vanillin	0.13 ± 0.01

Trolox equivalent antioxidant capacity (TEAC) measures the antioxidant capacity of a given substance, as compared to the standard, Trolox.
Source: Benavente-Garcia J, Castillo J, Lorente A et al. Antioxidant activity of phenolics extracted from *Olea europaea* L. leaves. Food Chem 2000; 68:457–462.

CYNARA SCOLYMUS (GLOBE ARTICHOKE)

Globe artichoke leaf has been used traditionally to increase bile flow and act as a protective agent against various toxins. Data from various studies reveal that artichoke leaf and cynarin (the active constituent within artichoke leaf) have lipid-lowering effects, highlighting the possibility of their role as an adjuvant in the management of high lipid levels. A randomised, double-blind, placebo-controlled clinical trial published in 2008[219] revealed that artichoke leaf extract reduced plasma cholesterol in otherwise healthy hypercholesterolaemic adults. Seventy-five healthy adults with mild to moderate hypercholesterolaemia consumed 1280 mg of a standardised artichoke leaf extract, or matched placebo, daily for 12 weeks. Plasma total cholesterol decreased in the treatment group by an average of 4.2% but increased in the control group by an average of 1.9%, the difference between groups being statistically significant ($p = 0.025$). General wellbeing improved significantly in both the treatment group (11%) and the control group (9%) with no significant differences between the groups. The authors concluded that consumption of artichoke leaf resulted in a modest but statistically significant difference in total cholesterol after 12 weeks.

COMMIPHORA MUKUL (GUGGUL)

The resin from *Commiphora mukul* has been demonstrated to have hypolipidaemic properties and is used in India as a cholesterol-lowering agent. The constituents known as guggulsterones appear to be responsible for the botanical's ability to lower cholesterol by antagonising two nuclear hormone receptors involved in cholesterol metabolism, resulting in a cholesterol-lowering action. A double-blind, randomised, placebo-controlled trial undertaken in the Norwegian population involving individuals with moderately increased cholesterol administered 2160 mg/day guggul or placebo for 12 weeks observed a reduction in mean levels of total cholesterol compared with placebo, although no corresponding changes were seen for LDL cholesterol and triglycerides. Furthermore the total cholesterol/HDL cholesterol ratio did not differ significantly between the two groups.[220] However, it is important to note that in Australia at this time, *Commiphora mukul* is not approved for use in therapeutic products, due to some concerns regarding lack of post-market safety surveillance for the specific extract Gugulipid® (an ethyl acetate extract of the oleo-resin) and some known safety issues involving thyroid stimulation, topical (skin) hypersensitivity and gastrointestinal distress.[221]

Lifestyle recommendations

WEIGHT MANAGEMENT

Maintaining a healthy weight is crucial for wellbeing, particularly with regard to overall cardiovascular health. A systematic review conducted by Poobalan et al[222] assessed the effects of weight loss in overweight or obese individuals and long-term lipid outcomes. Weight was lost using a variety of methods — some akin to naturopathy such as exercise and behaviour therapy, others less so such as surgical bypass. It was concluded that for every 10 kg of weight lost, a drop of 0.23 mmol/L in cholesterol may be expected for an obese or greatly overweight person. This highlights the possible benefits of weight loss on low-density lipoproteins and cholesterol.

EXERCISE

Regular exercise is known to be beneficial for cardiovascular health and lipid levels, but it appears that certain forms of exercise may be superior for specific subgroups. For example, the effects of an 8-month exercise program on lipid profiles in women aged 60–79 years was examined.[223] The women were separated into two groups, and took part in either:

- A multicomponent exercise program (consisting of aerobic exercise, muscular endurance exercises and activities targeted to improve balance and flexibility) or
- A resistance exercise program (e.g. leg extensions and curls, double chest raises, lateral raises, overhead press and abdominal exercise).

After 8 months, women in the multicomponent exercise program were found to have reduced triglycerides and increased high-density lipoproteins, while these changes were not observed in the resistance training group. This suggests that for this subgroup of people, multicomponent exercise had a better effect on lipid profiles than resistance. It would be interesting to observe in further studies if a combination of the two forms of exercise produced even better results than the one type in isolation, as well as whether results varied if frequency of exercise was increased.

SMOKING

Cigarette smoking and elevated total cholesterol levels are both associated with increased risk of mortality and cardiovascular disease. A number of studies have indicated that smoking may aggravate LDL cholesterol cardiovascular risk.[224] This view was confirmed using the large database of the Asia Pacific Cohort Studies Collaboration which assessed the effects of cigarette smoking, its effects on total cholesterol and HDL cholesterol as well as the subsequent risk of cardiovascular disease.[225] Researchers from this study observed that within the Asia-Pacific region cigarette smoking potentiates the harmful effects of total cholesterol and reduces the cardioprotective properties of high-density lipoproteins, subsequently increasing the risk of coronary heart disease.

Given the results from this large study it would appear that cessation of smoking is imperative, as is avoidance of exposure to secondhand smoke for patients at risk of coronary heart disease. Barriers to completing this goal should be discussed with patients. Naturopathy can offer some wonderful nutritional and herbal therapies to help support patients through their smoking cessation program. Concurrent counselling[226] is usually recommended.

CASE STUDY

OVERVIEW

JM was a 69-year-old woman who presented with hypercholesterolaemia. She was considerably overweight and did minimal exercise due to her physical symptoms. She experienced mild osteoarthritis in her knees and hands for which she self-prescribed glucosamine but felt no improvement.

Her diet was poor due to her history of disordered eating. She was preoccupied with her weight but was not making any changes to improve it. She drank at least half a bottle of wine per night (shared bottle with her husband), drank 2 cups of coffee per day and consumed high quantities of carbohydrates and sugar (especially processed biscuits). Essential fatty acids were excluded from the diet.

INVESTIGATION RESULTS

Recent pathology investigations provided the following results:

- Lipid profile:
  - Total cholesterol 6.3 mmol/L
  - Triglycerides 2.6 mmol/L
  - LDL 4.1 mmol/L
  - HDL 1.8 mmol/L
- Vitamin D (25-hydroxy) 19 nmol/L
- Fasting glucose 5.2 mmol/L
- HbA_{1c} 5.3%
- CRP 7.0 mg/L
- Rheumatoid factor: negative
- ANA: negative

CLINICAL EXAMINATION

- Height 165 cm
- Weight 104 kg
- BMI 38.2 (obese)
- BP 132/81 mmHg

TREATMENT PROTOCOL

HERBAL MEDICINE

Herbal medicine	Ratio	Quantity	Justification
Ginkgo biloba	STD ext	40 mL	Improve coronary blood flow
Salvia miltiorrhiza	1:2	50 mL	Improve microcirculation, hypotensive, platelet aggregating inhibitor, peripheral vasodilator
Olea europaea	1:2	50 mL	Hypolipidaemic, cardioprotective, hypoglycaemic
Cynara scolymus	1:2	80 mL	Hypolipidaemic, cholagogue

TOTAL: 220 mL. Dose: 11 mL b.i.d. (calculated based on weight, slowly increased).

CASE STUDY CONTINUED

NUTRITIONAL MEDICINE

Dietary

- Encourage dietary intake of *Curcuma longa*, preferably mixed into yoghurt to enable it to be eaten cold and not heated: 1 heaped teaspoon of organic turmeric mixed into yoghurt 2 times/day
- Encourage dietary sources of garlic (aim for 2 g/day, i.e. as much as possible)
- Prevent oxidative and free radical damage to cell membranes by consuming a high level of antioxidants and phytochemicals
- Improve the structure and composition of cell membranes by encouraging monounsaturated and omega-3 fatty acids to provide the basic building blocks for structural components
- Discourage saturated, trans or hydrogenated fat sources
- Exclude caffeine, sodium and alcohol
- Encourage fibre-rich sources from a variety of wholegrains and pulses
- Encourage principles of the Mediterranean diet
- Monitor and ensure hydration requirements are met.

Supplemental

Nutrient	Dosage	Justification
B complex (activated forms)	2 caps/day	High B_3 to reduce LDL, normalise lipid profile, improve hepatic cholesterol synthesis
Vitamin E	400 IU b.i.d.	Reduce oxidative stress, reduce atherogenic deposits
Vitamin C	500 mg b.i.d.	Reduce oxidative stress, decrease serum LDL
Concentrated fish oil supplementation	1 cap b.i.d. total:EPA: 650 mg, DHA: 450 mg, other omega-3s: 180 mg	Anti-inflammatory, hypolipidaemic, hypotensive, reduce inflammation and improve joint health
Vitamin D_3	4000 IU/day	To address deficiency and utilise positive blood sugar, mood and immune effects

LIFESTYLE/EDUCATION

- Weight loss was paramount — daily exercise as possible, slowly increasing over time. Encourage to partake in swimming to reduce impact on joints
- Cardiovascular self-assessment — blood pressure, pulse and associated symptom diary
- Avoidance of exposure to all passive smoke (patient was not an active smoker)
- Educate regarding principles of the Mediterranean diet and the importance of essential fatty acids.

CARDIOVASCULAR ISCHAEMIA (ANGINA)

Epidemiology

Angina pectoris is a condition characterised by chest pain due to ischaemia of the heart muscle. The condition is most commonly a sequelae of coronary artery disease, the leading cause of death in men with high cholesterol levels in Australia.[226] Angina comprises almost one-third of all Australian heart and vascular conditions, often found alongside more than one cardiovascular complication.[35] Each minute in the United States more than one person dies of a heart disease-related event.[227]

Classification

STABLE ANGINA

Stable angina pectoris is a chronic condition that produces symptoms at a predictable (reproducible) level of exertion, and can be relieved in a matter of minutes by rest or glyceryl trinitrate. To classify as stable angina, the symptoms must be consistent for a minimum of 2 months, with no change in either frequency or severity.[61]

UNSTABLE ANGINA

Unstable angina is considered in the presence of a crescendo pattern of chest pain, particularly one that has had recent onset (under 2 months), and it may be symptomatic at rest. This acute coronary state can be either troponin-positive or troponin-negative, determining the presence or absence of myocardial necrosis. The prognosis for troponin-negative patients is far better, with a lower incidence of subsequent myocardial infarction.[228]

Unstable angina is classified based on symptoms and severity (Table 20.23).

Aetiology

ATHEROSCLEROSIS

Atherosclerosis is the most common anatomical cause of angina. Ischaemia develops when fibrous plaques obstruct coronary blood flow. Angina is the most frequent clinical expression of myocardial ischaemia.[21] Atherosclerosis usually features with dyslipidaemia, as lipids are a fundamental component of atherosclerotic plaque.[129]

CHOLESTEROL

Elevated cholesterol, in particular the ratio of LDL to HDL cholesterol, is a well-known risk factor for ischaemic heart disease.[229] Lowering elevated cholesterol plays a significant role in decreasing mortality from ischaemic heart disease, and even just small reductions have been shown to be protective. The benefits of serum cholesterol reduction are also related to age. For example, a study published in the *British Medical Journal* observed that a 10% reduction in serum cholesterol concentration produced a reduction in ischaemic heart disease of 50% at age 40, 40% at age 50, 30% at age 60, and 20% at age 70.[230]

HYPERTENSION

Hypertension is becoming increasingly widespread, and a considerable risk factor for angina.[144] Hypertensive patients have a significantly higher risk of developing cardiovascular disease, particularly atherosclerotic sequelae such as angina.[47]

GENDER

Australian statistics show that men are almost twice as likely as women to develop angina and associated complications such as myocardial infarction.[226] This disparity is most commonly attributed to a protective effect of oestrogen. However, generalised over time and at different ages, women have a similar or slightly higher prevalence of angina than men across countries with widely differing myocardial infarction mortality rates.[231]

TABLE 20.23 Classification of unstable angina based on symptoms and severity, including troponin-positive and troponin-negative subgroups

Severity	Clinical circumstances		
	A — occurs as a result of extracardiac condition that increases myocardial ischaemia (secondary unstable angina)	B — occurs when an extracardiac condition (primary unstable angina) is absent	C — develops within 2 weeks of acute myocardial infarction
I — new onset of accelerated angina or severe angina with no pain while resting	IA	IB	IC
II — within the past month, onset of angina at rest, but without symptoms within previous 48 hours	IIA	IIB	IIC
III — acute symptoms of angina at rest within 48 hours	IIIA	IIIB-Tpos IIIB-Tneg	IIIC

Source: Adapted from Hamm C, Braunwald E. A classification of unstable angina revisited. Circulation 2000; 102(1):118–122.

AGE

Systemic blood pressure naturally rises with age and with it the incidence of hypertension and cardiovascular disease.[17] The elderly are also more likely to have silent ischaemia and to suffer silent myocardial infarct.[232]

GASTRO-OESOPHAGEAL REFLUX

The pain and discomfort of reflux can be mistaken for angina; and there appears to be an increased incidence of reflux among patients with unstable angina and established CAD.[233] A number of studies have shown that more than half of coronary patients complaining of recurrent retrosternal pain are experiencing symptoms of both reflux and angina.[234]

MYOCARDIAL INFARCTION OR PREVIOUS CORONARY EVENT

More than a quarter of patients treated for myocardial infarction are likely to develop angina; the incidence is higher in women, younger patients, smokers, those who have had previous coronary bypass and those who developed postinfarct angina while hospitalised.[235]

INFLAMMATION

Inflammatory markers, particularly interleukin-6 and C-reactive protein, play a significant role in the pathogenesis of coronary heart disease. They are also strong predictors of more serious coronary events in unstable angina.[236] C-reactive protein is a sensitive, nonspecific, marker of inflammation and an independent risk factor for atherosclerosis, a precursor to angina.[140]

SMOKING

Tobacco smoking dramatically increases the risk of developing atherosclerosis and subsequent angina.[237] Smoking reduces the oxygen-carrying capacity of blood and also increases arterial stiffness — a precursor to hypertension, atherosclerosis and angina.[44]

CARDIAC SYNDROME X

Syndrome X encompasses a heterogeneous group of patients who have angina-like chest symptoms but normal epicardial coronary arteries at angiography.[238] The syndrome is defined by exercise-induced, angina-like chest discomfort, normal coronary arteries, and ST-segment depression suggestive of ischaemia during spontaneous or provoked angina.[239]

Overview

Angina is a serious condition, characterised by severe chest pain. It may be chronic or acute.

Pathogenesis

Angina commonly occurs as a result of the hardening and damage of coronary arteries, associated with atherosclerosis and ischaemia.[240] Myocardial ischaemia occurs when myocardial oxygen supply falls below the oxygen demand. The typical causes of an increased oxygen demand, and subsequent angina, are hypertension, arrhythmias and coronary stenosis (caused by an atherosclerotic lesion) restricting the blood vessel by more than 70%.[61]

Myocardial ischaemia is associated with cellular sodium and calcium homeostasis. Ischaemia results in a rise of intracellular sodium concentration and thus sodium overload, which then activates the sodium calcium exchanger and leads to increased intracellular calcium. When this occurs there is electrical instability and mechanical dysfunction, which increases oxygen demand and decreases oxygen supply.[241]

SIGNS AND SYMPTOMS

Although angina presents with a number of individual variations, one of the earliest published observations of angina, by William Heberden in 1772, describes the essential manifestation of the condition:

> *There is a disorder of the breast, marked with strong and peculiar symptoms, considerable for the danger belonging to it. ... Those who are afflicted with it are seized, while they are walking, and more particularly when they walk soon after eating, with a painful and most disagreeable sensation in the breast ... the moment they stand still all this uneasiness vanishes ... After it has continued some months, it will not cease so instantaneous upon standing still ... (most) whom I have seen, who are at least twenty, were men, and almost all above 50 years old, and most of them with a short neck, and inclining to be fat ... But the natural tendency of this illness be to kill the patients suddenly ... The os sterni is usually pointed to as the seat of this malady ... and sometimes there is with it a pain about the middle of the left arm.*[242]

Chest pain

Angina is most often identified by chest pain that typically presents as tightness, squeezing or constriction, building rapidly within 30 seconds and disappearing in decrescendo within 5–15 minutes. The discomfort is commonly midsternal, radiating to the neck, left shoulder and left arm; with intensity of pain ranging from mild to severe discomfort.[21] Patients often have more than one type of chest pain, and musculoskeletal and gastro-oesophageal pains commonly coexist with angina, as well as forming part of the differential diagnosis.[240]

Exertion

Physical exertion is the most likely precipitant of angina symptoms. However, emotional tension, cold weather or a large meal may also aggravate the condition.[243]

Dyspnoea

For some patients, dyspnoea is the only sensation experienced during myocardial ischaemia, a so-called 'angina equivalent'. Often, dyspnoea occurs together with angina — many patients experience tightness across the chest both as a pain and as a sense of restriction in breathing.[244]

Levine's sign

A clenching of the fist over the sternum, while describing the pain, is a classic presentation of angina.[21]

COMPLICATIONS

Angina often acts as a harbinger of more serious cardiovascular disease events, requiring ongoing treatment and evaluation.[245] Patients presenting with angina-associated chest discomfort are more likely to experience acute myocardial infarction within a year.[246] Quality of life is another significant factor in the pervasive nature of angina, as recurrent symptoms, impaired activity and associated stress all impact upon general patient wellbeing.[247]

DIFFERENTIAL DIAGNOSIS

Differential diagnosis is largely focused on identifying causality for the most predominant symptom of chest pain, as there are a number of factors that may contribute (Table 20.24).

TABLE 20.24 Distinguishing differences in chest pain

Cardiac origin	Non-cardiac origin
Ischaemic pain	
Decreased oxygen supply Coronary atherosclerosis: significant atherosclerosis, coronary thrombosis Coronary, non-atherosclerotic causes: aortic or coronary dissection, coronary spasm, microvascular spasm, cocaine-induced vasoconstriction	Decreased oxygen supply Anaemia, sickle cell disease, hypoxaemia (e.g. sleep apnoea), carbon monoxide intoxication, hyperviscosity (e.g. polycythaemia)
Increased oxygen demand Hypertrophic cardiomyopathy, aortic stenosis, dilated cardiomyopathy, increased preloads (e.g. mitral valve regurgitation), tachycardia, myocardial bridging, congenital abnormality of the coronary circulation	Increased oxygen demand Hyperthyroidism, hyperthermia, high inotropic state (e.g. adrenergic stimulation)
Non-ischaemic pain	
Pericarditis Aortic dissection	Gastrointestinal: oesophageal (e.g. reflux), biliary (e.g. cholecystitis), gastric (e.g. peptic ulcer), pancreatitis Psychogenic: anxiety disorders (e.g. panic), affective disorders (e.g. depression), cardiac psychosis, somatisation Pulmonary: pulmonary embolism, pneumothorax, pleuritis, pneumonia, pulmonary hypertension Neuromuscular: costochondritis, fibrositis, Tietze's syndrome, rib fracture, herpes zoster, thoracic outlet syndrome, sternoclavicular arthritis

Source: Adapted from Goldman L, Ausiello D, editors. Cecil medicine. 23th ed. Philadelphia: Saunders, Elsevier; 2008.

NATUROPATHIC DIAGNOSIS

Angina is a serious, chronic condition and naturopathic diagnosis must assess a number of factors that impact upon cardiovascular function. As with all patients, it is essential to take a thorough case history, evaluating physical signs, clinical symptoms and allopathic diagnostic measures.

Other features that should form a naturopathic evaluation include:

- Hormonal status, with particular reference to thyroid and adrenal function
- Metabolism, specifically glucose metabolism
- Stress and anxiety levels, as the nervous system has significant impact upon cardiovascular health
- Digestive function, particularly of the upper digestive tract — including absorption and motility
- Dietary evaluation and assessment of the patient's nutritional intake, with particular focus on quality and quantity of dietary fat and antioxidant consumption.

Investigations

PHYSICAL EXAMINATION

Physical examination includes blood pressure monitoring, auscultation of chest and assessment for alternative diagnosis such as chest wall pain and other musculoskeletal pain.[240]

RESTING ECG

Electrocardiogram (ECG) is usually stable, but will identify any arrhythmias. A pathological Q wave almost always indicates myocardial infarction.[240]

TREADMILL ECG (AKA STRESS TEST)

Treadmill evaluation of a patient's endurance and cardiac activity while exercising establishes disease prognosis. The goal is to provoke ischaemia in a controlled setting so that both symptoms and ECG can be observed.[243] Angina (exercise-induced, chronic-stable) is indicated when coronary stenosis is tight enough to limit flow, reducing luminal diameter more than 70%.[61]

PERFUSION IMAGING

A perfusion imaging agent, such as thallium, is injected and two scans carried out, the first with stress (i.e. exertion/exercise). The injected agent perfuses muscle, with myocardial accumulation representing blood flow. In cases of ischaemia a 'cold spot' on the scan indicates diminished uptake and a stenosed or occluded coronary artery.[61]

CT AND MRI SCANNING

Imaging of the heart and greater vessels allows diagnosis of conditions inducing angina, including coronary artery disease, pericardial disease, neoplastic disease of the heart, myocardial thickness, chamber size and congenital defects.[243]

CORONARY ANGIOGRAPHY

An x-ray of the heart using a contrast dye to assess coronary blood flow is considered for patients with angina or suspected angina, particularly those at high risk of other coronary complications.[248]

PATHOLOGY TESTING

Pathology testing includes full blood count, to detect anaemia; thyroid function to detect over- or underactivity of the thyroid, which can result in angina or coronary disease; urea and electrolytes to assess renal and liver function.[240]

Troponin, which is more specific than creatine kinase MB isoenzyme — though both markers are often measured together — is used to assess risk of myocardial infarction following acute, unstable angina.[249]

Lipid profile, including HDL cholesterol, LDL cholesterol, triglycerides and glucose measurement, is also important to ascertain dyslipidaemia or impaired glucose tolerance.[240]

NATUROPATHIC INVESTIGATIONS

Naturopathic investigation aligns with the allopathic model insofar as determining the class of angina and risk of more insidious pathology. Some functional tests may also be appropriate in evaluating treatment and disease progression.

Essential fatty acids

Essential fatty acids are used to measure essential fatty acid status and identify deficiency. Insufficient essential fatty acids are pro-inflammatory and may exacerbate cardiovascular conditions. This test is also relevant for the diagnosis and treatment of dyslipidaemia and atherosclerosis, predisposing conditions of angina.

Functional liver detoxification profile

The functional liver detoxification profile identifies liver activity and detoxification capacity. Poor liver function can compromise essential fatty acid status and increase circulation of inflammatory mediators. It can also indicate insufficient detoxification, subsequently increasing the load on the heart, liver and kidneys.

Total antioxidant status

Total antioxidant status measures serum antioxidant status, important for the management of cardiovascular conditions such as angina, as much of the associated inflammation can result from oxidative stress.

IgG and IgE food profile

Because of the links between food allergens and angina (see below) it is prudent to investigate patients in whom dietary influences are concerning.

Therapeutic considerations

CLINICAL DECISION MAKING AND RATIONALE

At all times when examining a cardiovascular patient, it is essential to assess their risk for potential complications. It is also essential to communicate with the patient's GP (and cardiologist) to foster joint care and co-management.

Although ischaemic heart disease is prevalent within the Western world, many other cardiovascular diseases exist. Each of these diseases has its own pathophysiological and clinical features, which largely dictate the chosen treatment.

Patients with cardiovascular disease rarely understand the nature or patterns of their disease. Rehabilitation programs are often not maintained or completed. Patients routinely describe a feeling of 'lack of control' and continually reducing quality of life. The concept of patient-centred medicine encourages the clinician to shift their focus from only critical and drastic interventions to also consider quality of life of the patient. Holistic medicine can provide the patient with more personal care.

'Best care' in cardiology involves the patient seeking and acquiring rational and effective healthcare. 'Rational and effective healthcare' should include the strengths of both modern orthodox medicine and modern herbal medicine, used together, by experts in each field.

Naturopathic medicine is often said to be ineffective in the treatment of cardiovascular diseases. This is far from true — effectiveness hinges on understanding both the disease and the patient, the rational application of medicines and understanding limitations.

Therapeutic application

ALLOPATHIC PERSPECTIVE

Where aggravating factors have been identified (e.g. hypertension, strenuous activity, cold temperature, anxiety and emotional states) these are obviously avoided, reduced or controlled so as to prevent the recurrence of angina.

Some therapies used for the treatment of angina are listed in Table 20.25.

HISTORICAL PERSPECTIVE

The Eclectics make reference to angina as 'breast pang' and though amusing, this provides an accurate description of the nature of pain associated with angina as well as its location. The Eclectics give a detailed description of pain associated with angina, describing it as 'an acute paroxysmal pain in the heart that radiated through the shoulder and arm ... bringing with it agonising fear and severe prostration'.[5] Angina was believed to be caused by neuroses, suggesting a link between the physical and emotional realms, although the Eclectics also noted that it could be hereditary.[5] Prognosis if diagnosed with angina was said to be bleak, and it was rare for a patient to survive a third attack. Gelsemium and *Macrotys* (black cohosh) were used to prevent attacks, as were nervine sedatives. In those who were deemed 'feeble', stimulating sedatives such as ammonium valerianate were favoured.

NATUROPATHIC PERSPECTIVE

Naturopathic perspective for treatment focuses on dietary and lifestyle modifications as the primary objective for long-term health improvement. These include smoking cessation, weight reduction and exercise. If a patient is not compliant with these variables, treatment outcome can be

TABLE 20.25 Therapies used for treatment of angina

Glyceryl trinitrate	In acute management, sublingual glyceryl trinitrate is most commonly prescribed, providing relief from symptoms in 1–2 min. It may also be taken prophylactically, 5 min before an activity likely to precipitate angina
Long-acting nitrates	Depending on dose and application, taken 2–4 times daily The main limitation to long-term therapy is tolerance, which can be limited by establishing an 8–10 h period per day without nitrates. It may also be limited by headache, nausea, lightheadedness and hypotension
Beta-blockers	The most common first-line therapy in patients with chronic angina. The only anti-anginal agents shown to prolong life in patients with coronary disease. Contraindicated in severe bronchospastic disease, bradyarrhythmias, and decompensated heart failure
Calcium channel blockers	Considered third-line anti-ischaemic drug in post-infarction patients with angina. Some evidence to show they have increased ischaemia and mortality rates
Alternative and combination therapies	Patients may respond to one class of anti-anginal medication, but not another. Subsequently, alternative agents are often trialled before progressing to combinations Combinations may include a beta-blocker and long-acting nitrate, or beta-blocker and calcium channel blocker
Platelet-inhibiting agents	Unless contraindicated, aspirin is commonly prescribed for all patients with angina
Risk reduction	Dependent on the patient's condition, risk modification is recommended to prevent disease progression. This includes: statin treatment, antihypertensives, stopping smoking, weight reduction and exercise

Source: Adapted from Conti C. Re-thinking angina. Clin Cardiol 2007;30(Suppl. 1):I1–3.

unsuccessful. It is therefore imperative to assess a patient's compliance and willingness to be an active participant in their care.

As the progression to more serious conditions is possible (see Fig. 20.6), it is essential to thoroughly assess patients, and review all aspects of their health, diet, lifestyle, occupation, emotional and mental health. A number of key areas should be considered:

- Antioxidant status and general cardiovascular health
- Stress, stress management and adrenal health
- Level of activity and potential impairments to oxygenation of blood supply
- Thyroid, metabolism and weight management
- Blood glucose control and insulin sensitivity
- Digestive function and potential hindrances to nutrient absorption
- Hepatobiliary function and lipid profile
- Level of systemic inflammation and potential aggravating factors that contribute to inflammation (i.e. oxidation, lipid profile)
- Food allergens.

NUTRITIONAL MEDICINE (DIETARY)

Dietary therapeutic objectives

- Increase antioxidant status by ensuring diet is rich in fresh fruit and vegetables (especially leafy green types)
- Encourage liver-supportive foods, such as fibre and leafy green vegetables
- Encourage onions and garlic to protect against cardiovascular disease
- Encourage fibre to protect against ischaemia
- Encourage low-methylmercury fish sources for optimal protein and omega-3 fatty acid sources
- Avoid coffee and other caffeinated substances
- Avoid alcohol, saturated, trans and hydrogenated sources of fats and high animal protein consumption
- Avoid processed and refined carbohydrate sources and sugars.

Specific dietary treatments

DIETARY INCLUSIONS

Dietary fibre, especially the gel-forming or mucilaginous fibres (e.g. flaxseed, oat bran, pectin)

Dietary fibre has been found to protect against ischaemic heart disease in a number of studies[250,251] hence the benefits of increasing fibre in the diet. Soluble fibres such as *Plantago ovata* husk appear to work better than insoluble fibres such as plantago ovata seeds.[251] Other soluble fibres include flaxseed, oat bran and pectin.

Onions and garlic (both raw and cooked)

Diets rich in garlic and onions have been observed to have a protective effect against a range of cardiovascular diseases[252] so their intake should be increased in the diet of patients with or at risk of ischaemic heart disease. Both cooked and raw onion and garlic are likely to be therapeutically beneficial.

Vegetable consumption (especially leafy greens)

It has been suggested that just by increasing fruit and vegetable consumption up to 600 g per day the total worldwide burden of ischaemic heart disease could be lowered by 31%. Increased consumption of vegetables is known to be associated with a reduced incidence of ischaemic heart disease,[230] but in Australia many people do not get the recommended daily intake of fruits and vegetables. In fact in Australia low consumption of fruit and vegetables is associated with 2.8% of the burden of disease.[253] Given this fact and the protective effects fruit and vegetables have on the cardiovascular system, optimal amounts of fresh vegetables should be consumed; in particular leafy green vegetables are recommended due to their high magnesium content.

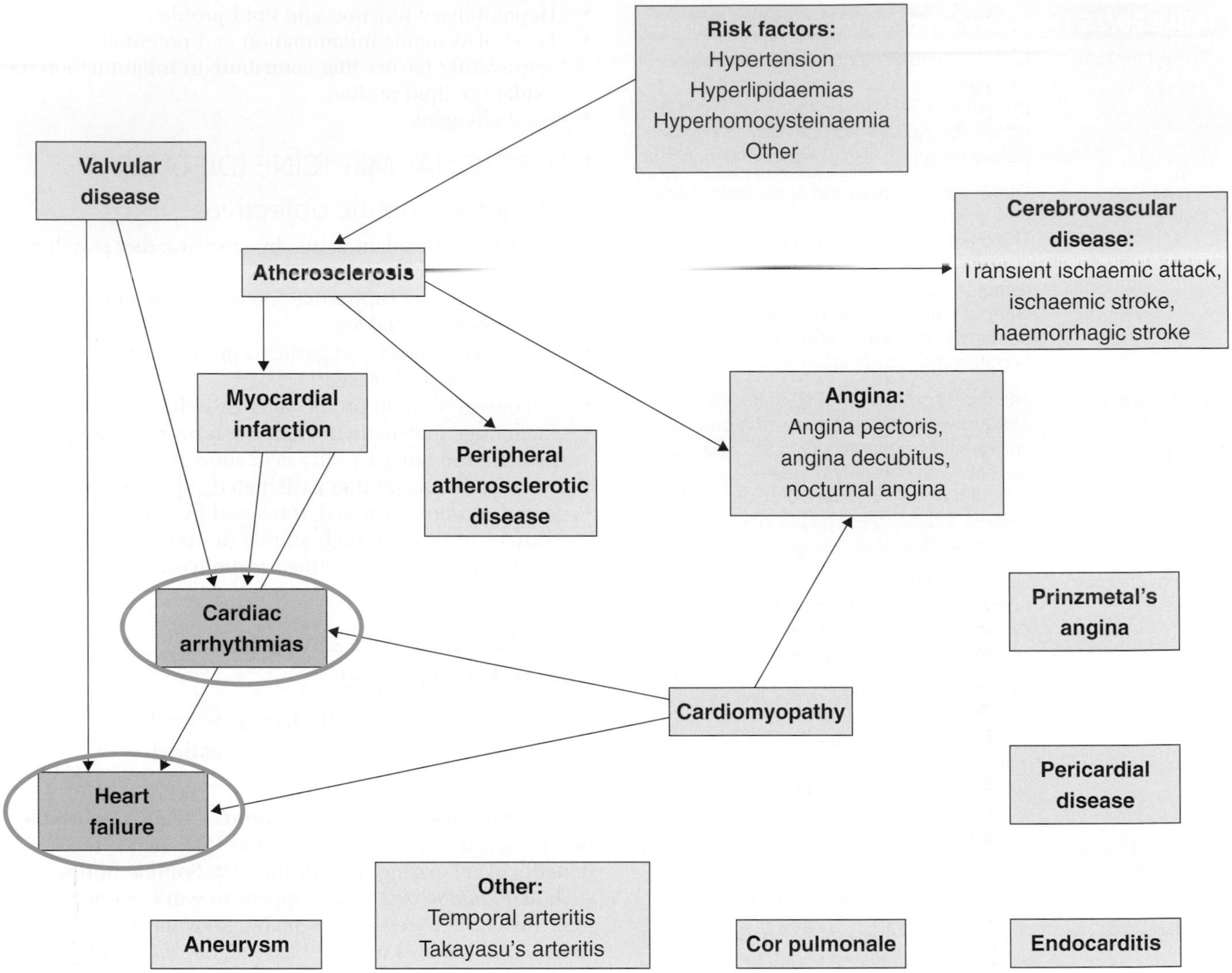

FIGURE 20.6 Risk factors and development for disease progression.

Breakspear I. Not just ischaemia. Sydney: WholMed; 2010.

Fish

Epidemiological research suggests that dietary intake of fish helps to protect against ischaemic heart disease.[254] Fish known to have low methylmercury contents should be chosen (see Box 20.6).

DIETARY EXCLUSIONS

Coffee and other caffeinated substances

Caffeine has been found to cause an acute increase in arterial wave reflection increasing the pulsatile load of the heart[255] and thus should be excluded in patients with angina. Boiled coffee has been demonstrated to increase cholesterol and LDL cholesterol dose dependently, further heightening the argument against coffee and caffeinated substances.[256] An Australian study[257] observed an increased risk of unstable angina and myocardial infarction among patients who consumed five or more cups of coffee daily. This type of dose is excessive and warrants further investigation as to why, or what individuals feel they are gaining from this quantity of coffee (e.g. 'I drink coffee for more energy' or 'It makes me feel alert' warrants further investigation of adrenal health).

Alcohol

A large number of studies have been published suggesting that alcohol may exert a protective effect in ischaemic heart disease. Naturopathic medicine emphasises the whole body, rather than just one system, and the benefits of alcohol in ischaemic heart disease are debatable when one considers the deleterious effects of alcohol to other parts of the body, particularly with regard to the liver and immune health. Alcohol increases the requirements of many of the body's nutrients such as the B vitamins, which are generally required in higher amounts in ischaemic heart disease. Overall, it can be seen that drinking alcohol is actually detrimental to the health of the whole body and should be omitted from the diet.

BOX 20.6 Mercury and fish

Mercury occurs naturally in the environment, and can be released into the air through industrial pollution and accumulate in streams and oceans where it is turned into methylmercury. Fish absorb the methylmercury as they feed in these waters and it accumulates, and then when we consume the fish we are exposed to the mercury. Nearly all fish and shellfish contain methylmercury. Fish that are more likely to have higher levels of mercury are larger, longer living or predatory species.

There are numerous nutritional benefits from regularly eating fish, but given the ongoing and unresolved concerns regarding mercury exposure, it is recommended that people should limit their consumption of some types of fish to 1–2 portions per 2 week period (150 g or 75 g for children under 6) and have no other fish for that 2 weeks.

High methylmercury-containing fish

High methylmercury-containing fish include: billfish (swordfish/broadbill and marlin), shark/flake, orange roughy (sea perch) and catfish (bassa). Other important species to limit include barramundi, gemfish, ling, bluefin tuna, other types of tuna — including canned white chunk or albacore, halibut, mahi mahi, pike, ray, seabass, tilefish, walleye and white croaker. Freshwater fish in geothermal lakes and rivers in New Zealand may also accumulate high levels of mercury.

The canned tuna debate is problematic. It is believed that smaller and younger species of tuna are used for canned varieties. Unfortunately, most canned tuna in Australia is from Thai waters where mercury control standards differ from Australian guidelines. As such, it is best to advise patients to limit consumption and replace with tinned salmon, sardines or mackerel.

Low methylmercury fish sources

Blue mackerel, herring, John Dory, ocean trout, salmon, sardines, silver trevally, silver warehou, anchovy, blue-eyed cod, bream, flathead, garfish, mullet, snapper, whiting and many others are all safer choices.

Saturated fats

Saturated fat promotes the deposit of cholesterol around the arteries of the cardiovascular system and should thus be minimised in the diet of any patient at risk of cardiovascular disease. Examples of foods high in saturated fat include butter, biscuits, pastries, hard cheeses, processed meats such as salami and cabanossi, deep-fried foods and some meat.

Sugar

Early studies in the 1960s proposed that an excess of sugar (sucrose) in the diet may be implicated in the pathogenesis of ischaemic heart disease.[258] The authors had observed that men with heart disease consumed much higher amounts of sugar than their healthy counterparts. The authors proposed that in order to prevent ischaemic heart disease, sugar intake should be reduced. Patients presenting with, or at risk of ischaemic heart disease should be questioned on sugar content in their diet. The majority of sugary foods and drinks (with the exception of fruit) generally offer little in the way of nutrients or vital force and are likely to aggravate inflammation in the body. Given that sugar is a highly addictive substance and is constantly overused in Western society its intake should be restricted.

Animal proteins

A large percentage of animal protein is high in cholesterol and saturated fat. Given the links between the latter and ischaemic heart disease, animal protein should be minimised. If animal protein is to be consumed lean sources of white meat (such as chicken or turkey) or fish are preferable.

Fried foods

Fried foods are high in trans fats, saturated fats and cholesterol. They also tend to offer little in the way of nutrition so they should be avoided and replaced with foods that have been cooked using healthier methods such as steaming or grilling.

Food allergens

Food and other allergens should be eliminated in patients with ischaemic heart disease due to a rare yet serious link found between food allergy and myocardial infarction. Gupta et al[259] reported a woman with no history of cardiovascular disease who presented with urticaria and concurrent chest pain. Electrocardiogram and enzymes revealed evidence of an acute myocardial infarction due to histamine release and subsequent spasm of the coronary vasculature leading to myocardial ischaemia and infarction. This isolated case highlights the importance of investigating all possibilities, particularly in patients with no previous history of cardiovascular disease.

NUTRITIONAL MEDICINE (SUPPLEMENTAL)

Nutritional medicine therapeutic objectives

- Address any deficiencies — commonly B vitamins and iron (assess prior to prescription)
- Increase antioxidant status to protect the cardiovascular system
- Improve endothelial function and fibrinolytic activity
- Protect the cardiac muscles from hypoxia, ischaemia and oxidative stress
- Reduce cardiac spasm with appropriate nutrient prescriptions.

Specific nutrients required

B COMPLEX

The importance of a B complex with potential additions of B_3, B_6, B_9 or B_{12} depending on patient presentation cannot be underestimated. For a full discussion, see other conditions throughout this chapter.

VITAMIN C

As a potent antioxidant, vitamin C supports patients with angina. It is especially indicated in those with high stress

SAMPLE DAILY DIET

While the sample diet below has been formulated based upon the fact that a wholefood plant-based diet can reduce the risk of ischaemic heart disease, it is important with prolonged dietary modification to ensure that the patient does not become anaemic. Patients with ischaemic heart disease and anaemia have been shown to have greater morbidity and mortality, and markers for anaemia such as low haemoglobin, iron concentration, total iron binding capacity and mean cell volume were all inversely correlated with disease severity.[260]

BREAKFAST	
Fresh fruit salad made from pineapple (including core), fig and berries served with home-made chia seed and raw nut mix	Ample fruit and vegetables in the diet have been hypothesised to result in favourable effects on CVD risk factors due to their protective effects via anti-inflammatory and antioxidant mechanisms. Pineapple core contains bromelain which has been shown to have fibrinolytic, antithrombotic and anti-inflammatory activities that might be especially useful in angina.
LUNCH	
Vegetarian chilli made with cooked tomato, beans, sweet potato and ample spices including onion, garlic, turmeric, chilli and fenugreek	Epidemiological research suggests lycopene found in cooked tomato products may have potential cardioprotective potential. Lycopene is highly antioxidant thus protecting against free radical damage and improving circulation in the tissues while also modulating HDL functionality towards an anti-atherogenic phenotype.
DINNER	
Mushroom, lentil and vegetable bolognese with wholemeal pasta Serve with a big raw salad	A low-fat, vegetarian wholefood plant-based diet, consisting primarily of vegetables, fruit, wholegrains, potatoes, beans, legumes and nuts has been shown to reverse angina, as well as reduce excess weight and elevated levels of cholesterol.
SNACKS	
Raw nuts and seeds	Nut consumption is associated with lower incidence of CVD. Nuts should be raw, unsalted and as fresh as possible.

levels due to compounding depletion of this vital nutrient. Vitamin C is required for collagen synthesis and thus structure of the blood vessels, including those of the cardiovascular system. It has also been found to improve vasodilation,[261] which may be altered in patients with ischaemic heart disease. Vitamin C has been observed in numerous studies to exert a protective effect on the cardiovascular system, and levels have been shown to be reduced in women with undiagnosed angina.[262] In clinical trials, vitamin C (via infusion) has been found to improve both endothelial function and insulin sensitivity in patients with coronary spastic angina.[263]

VITAMIN E

Vitamin E is a lipid-soluble antioxidant that has been shown to exert a protective effect on the cardiovascular system. Low levels of plasma vitamin E have been found in individuals with variant angina,[264] and supplementation is likely to be helpful, with oral administration of vitamin E (400 IU/day) shown to exert antioxidant effects while also improving fibrinolytic activity in patients with coronary spastic angina.[265]

COENZYME Q10

Coenzyme Q10 is a fat-soluble antioxidant. Levels decrease with age and have also been observed to be low in patients with cardiovascular diseases, muscular dystrophies, Parkinson's disease, cancers, diabetes and HIV/AIDS.[266]

Coenzyme Q10 is normally produced by the human body, although deficiency may occur in patients with impaired coenzyme Q10 biosynthesis due to severe metabolic or mitochondrial disorders, insufficient dietary intake or excessive use by the body. Symptoms of deficiency include angina and other cardiovascular anomalies. It is endogenously produced and serves as a cofactor in oxidative respiration for the Krebs cycle and the electron transport chain.

The biosynthesis of coenzyme Q10 is a 17-step process that requires riboflavin, niacinamide, panthothenic acid (B_5), pyridoxine, cobalamin (B_{12}), folic acid, vitamin C and other trace elements. Deficiencies of serum coenzyme Q10 may be caused by inadequate intake of these nutrients. Co-supplementation with these nutrients is beneficial to ensure appropriate absorption and utilisation.

One double-blind, placebo-controlled, randomised crossover trial observing the effects of coenzyme Q10 (150 mg/day in 3 daily doses) with regards to exercise tolerance in individuals with angina, found that coenzyme Q10 reduced the frequency of angina attacks as well as glyceryl trinitrate consumption when compared with placebo. It should be noted that the result, while clinically relevant, was not statistically significant and that the study

TABLE 20.26 Studies showing positive responses for coenzyme Q10

Study design	Author, year	Number	Statistically significant	Quality of study 0–5	Magnitude of benefit	Comments
Randomised, controlled, double-blind	Mazzola, 1987	20	Yes	3	Small	Patients had stable angina
Randomised, controlled, double-blind	Kamikawa, 1985	12	Yes	3	Small	Exercise-induced angina in patients with stable angina pectoris
Double-blind, placebo controlled crossover	Schardt, 1985	15	Yes	2	Small	Participants had exercise-induced angina

Source: Adapted from Natural Standard, CoEnzyme Q10 monograph, 2010, www.naturalstandard.com.

was conducted over a relatively short period of time (1 month, with only 2 weeks of supplementing with coenzyme Q10 due to crossover design) and involved only 12 participants.[267] Studies of longer duration, involving greater numbers are required to determine the true efficacy of coenzyme Q10 in angina.

Additional studies (Table 20.26) have shown positive responses.[266]

L-CARNITINE

L-carnitine is a naturally occurring amino acid that plays a key role in energy production by mobilising fatty acids into the mitochondria for the production of ATP. Supplementation with carnitine, an antioxidant, has been suggested to protect the cardiac muscles from hypoxia, ischaemia and oxidative stress. In their review, Pauly and Pepine[268] highlight the use of carnitine in stress-induced angina where it appears that carnitine increases lactate extraction and exerts a favourable action on myocardial free fatty acid levels. Iyer et al[269] conducted a study to examine the effects of oral L-carnitine in chronic stable angina. Forty-seven patients, a mix of men and women, each received L-carnitine (2 g/day for 12 weeks) or placebo. Patient parameters tested included exercise duration, time to onset of stress test changes, total stress test score at peak exercise, rate–pressure product at peak exercise and time needed for the stress test changes to recover to baseline as evaluated by a computerised stress test. Following the end of the study no changes were noted in the placebo group, but the L-carnitine group were noted to have a statistically significant improvement in exercise duration as well as time needed for the stress test changes to revert to baseline. This study suggests that L-carnitine improved the duration of exercise and time to recovery of stress test changes in patients with chronic stable angina.

MAGNESIUM

Magnesium deficiency has been associated with the development of variant angina[270] as well as coronary spasm, which has been implicated in the pathogenesis of various forms of angina including vasospastic angina. Satake et al[270] noted that severity of magnesium deficiency was directly related to the frequency of the attacks in both patient groups. To date, the majority of clinical trials utilising magnesium for treatment of angina have used an intravenous form, thus it is uncertain whether magnesium administered orally would produce the same beneficial results. Further clinical trials are required to determine this but, given the other effects of magnesium on the heart, supplementation is likely to be beneficial. Clinical experience suggests that oral forms are both effective and positive prescriptions.

ESSENTIAL FATTY ACIDS

The target EPA + DHA consumption should be at least 500 mg/day for individuals without underlying overt cardiovascular disease and at least 800 to 1000 mg/day for individuals with known coronary heart disease and heart failure. Further studies are needed to determine optimal dosing and the relative ratio of DHA and EPA omega-3 polyunsaturated fatty acids that provides maximal cardioprotection in those at risk of cardiovascular disease as well in the treatment of atherosclerotic, arrhythmic and primary myocardial disorders.

Potential EPA and DHA effects include:[271]

- Anti-arrhythmic effects
- Improvements in autonomic function
- Decreased platelet aggregation
- Vasodilation
- Decreased blood pressure
- Anti-inflammatory effects
- Improvements in endothelial function
- Plaque stabilisation
- Reduced atherosclerosis
- Reduced free fatty acids and triglycerides
- Upregulated adiponectin synthesis
- Reduced collagen deposition.

The major classes of fatty acids and their sources are listed in Table 20.27.

Dosage requirements

The dosage requirements listed below are based on adult doses that have been reported in the literature.

- B complex (all B vitamins) high-dose combination, preferably activated forms:
  - Thiamine 20–40 mg/day
  - Riboflavin 20–40 mg/day

TABLE 20.27 Major classes of fatty acids

Family*	Fatty acids	Formula†	Source
I omega-9	Oleic acid	c18:1	Most vegetable oils (canola, olive); animal fats
II omega-6	Linoleic acid Arachidonic acid	c18:2 c20:4	Many vegetable oils (corn, safflower, soybean) Poultry, meats
III omega-3	α-linolenic acid EPA DHA	c18:3 c20:5 c22:6	Selected vegetable oil (flaxseed, canola) Marine oils and fish Marine oils and fish
IV saturated fats	Palmitic acid Stearic acid	c16:0 c18:0	Animal and vegetable fats Butter, palm oil, kernel oil, coconut oil, and animal fats

DHA = docosahexaenoic acid; EPA = eicosapentaenoic acid.
*The omega number refers to the position of the first double bond from the methyl end of the molecule.
†The notation shows the total number of carbon atoms and total number of double bonds.
Source: Adapted with permission from Lavie Carl J, Milani Richard V, Mehra Mandeep R et al. Omega-3 polyunsaturated fatty acids and cardiovascular diseases. J Am Coll Cardiol 2009; 54(7):585–594.

  - Niacinamide/nicotinic acid 50–100 mg/day
  - Pantothenic acid 150–300 mg/day
  - Pyridoxine 20–60 mg/day
  - Folic acid 500–1000 micrograms/day
  - Cyanocobalamin 500–1000 micrograms/day
  - Choline 50–100 mg/day
  - Inositol 50–100 mg/day
  - Biotin 250–500 microgram/day
- Vitamin C: 500 mg–1 g t.d.s.
- Vitamin E: 400–800 IU/day
- Coenzyme Q10: 150–300 mg/day
- L-carnitine: 2 g/day
- Magnesium: 600–1000 mg/day
- Essential fatty acids: 3–4 g/day total omega-3 fatty acids (50% DHA and 50% EPA).

HERBAL MEDICINE

Herbal medicine therapeutic objectives

- Dilate coronary arteries
- Increase coronary blood flow
- Inhibit platelet aggregation and adhesion
- Protect against myocardial ischaemia (improve myocardial oxygen utilisation efficiency)
- Protect cardiac tissues against oxidation and free radical damage
- Provide negative chronotropic activity
- Reduce associated symptomatology, including stress, anxiety, systemic tension
- Reduce cardiac spasm and associated pain
- Reduce compounding factors, including hyperlipidaemia, obesity
- Restore tone and vigour to the heart muscle
- Scavenge free radicals
- Suppress formation of thromboxane.

Herbal medicine classes

Herbal medicine classes used in angina are listed in Table 20.28.

TABLE 20.28 Herbal medicine classes used in angina

Class	Action
Anti-arrhythmic	Prevent and/or alleviate palpitations and reduce heart rate (i.e. have a negatively chronotropic activity)
Antioxidant	Protect against oxidation and free radical damage and improve circulation to tissues
Cardioprotective	Protective to the myocardium and decrease the risk of heart damage due to toxins, ischaemia or the oxidative effects of hypertension
Cardio-tonic	Restore tone and vigour to the heart muscle
Peripheral vasodilator	Reduce peripheral vascular resistance, dilate/widen peripheral blood vessels and thereby improve circulation to peripheral tissues to assist in reducing blood pressure
Fibrinolytic	Prevent and reduce the development of insoluble fibrin clots
Hypolipidaemic	Reduce the concentration of blood lipids, cholesterol and triglycerides, and also include phospholipids (chylomicrons, very low-density lipoproteins (VLDL), intermediate-density lipoproteins (IDL), low-density lipoproteins (LDL) and high-density lipoproteins (HDL) and cholesterol esters
Spasmolytic	Relieve spasm symptomatically
Other	Nervine, sedative, analgesic, adaptogen as required

Specific herbal medicines

CRATAEGUS MONOGYNA (HAWTHORN LEAVES AND BERRIES)

Hawthorn has been discussed previously in regards to its antihypertensive action; however, it can be useful in a number of different cardiovascular conditions, including coronary ischaemia. While most human clinical research on hawthorn has focused on its efficacy and safety in heart failure, numerous in-vitro and in-vivo studies (in both animal and human tissue), as well as human clinical usage, have shown the value of hawthorn in reduced coronary blood flow. In relation to angina, two of its most important actions are in:

- improving coronary circulation[105,272,273]
- improving myocardial oxygen utilisation efficiency. It is thus a cardioprotective agent in oxygen states.[272,273]

Clinical usage reveals that hawthorn is a slow-acting medicine with long duration of activity (with activity persisting for some weeks after discontinuation), and thus the onset of measurable clinical response — in terms of reduction in symptom severity and frequency — often takes 6–8 weeks.[272] While this medicine clearly does improve coronary blood flow, it should not be considered as an alternative to conventional coronary vasodilators (such as nitrates) especially in the acute treatment of angina pain. Rather it should be used as the centrepiece of long-term management of coronary artery disease and angina.

TERMINALIA ARJUNA (ARJUN)

Terminalia arjuna is a traditional Ayurvedic herb that has undergone a substantial amount of research in its homeland in relation to management of cardiovascular disorders. The powdered tree bark has been used traditionally for cardiac ailments including 'hritshool' (angina) and has been found to contain a wide array of constituents including terpenoids, glycosides, flavonoids, tannins and minerals such as calcium and magnesium.[274] Several studies have shown *Terminalia arjuna* to be effective in reducing the frequency of angina attacks.[274] In one study *Terminalia arjuna* administered to 15 individuals with stable angina was found to reduce angina episodes by 50%, lower systolic blood pressure and slightly increase HDL cholesterol. The results were not so significant for patients with unstable angina, who also required conventional medication in addition to *Terminalia arjuna*.[275]

The majority of studies undertaken, although promising and supported by traditional evidence, have been small and of unsound methodological quality by Western standards. Double-blind randomised clinical trials in a wider population are required to confirm the effects of the studies reviewed.

AMMI VISNAGA (KHELLA)

Ammi visnaga is a botanical native to the Middle East containing a number of constituents, including khellin (0.3–1.2%), visnadine and visnagin,[276] which is thought to be of benefit to the cardiovascular system. At one time there was much interest in its anti-angina properties but this botanical appears to have faded into the background for several years, at least in the West. More recently it appears interest has been renewed with newer studies extracting active constituents from *Ammi visnaga*, such as visnadine and visnagin, and observing their mechanism of action. *Ammi visnaga* appears to be useful for management of angina due to its antispasmolytic action, whereby it relaxes the smooth muscles, as well as peripheral and coronary vasodilatory properties on the arteries.[277] The latter property leads to increased blood flow to the myocardium, providing relief from angina.[277] It is important to note that in Australia *Ammi visnaga* is a Schedule 4 medicine on the Standard for the Uniform Scheduling of Medicines and Poisons and thus unavailable for herbal and naturopathic dispensing.

GINKGO BILOBA (GINKGO)

Ginkgo biloba is well known for its circulatory effects but it may also be useful in angina for other reasons. A small group of patients with unstable angina pectoris taking conventional allopathic medication were divided into two groups: one was treated with conventional allopathic medication alone, and the other with conventional medication plus *Ginkgo biloba*.[278] Ginkgolide B with *Ginkgo biloba* was observed to suppress inflammation in these patients. The authors suggested this may be one way in which *Ginkgo biloba* assists patients with unstable angina pectoris. *Ginkgo biloba* extract (EGb761) has also been observed to provide protective effects in ischaemia and reperfusion in in-vivo studies. This is thought to be due to the antioxidant properties of terpenoid constituents within *Ginkgo biloba* and flavonoid metabolites produced after ginkgo administration.[278]

CORYDALIS AMBIGUA (CORYDALIS)

Corydalis ambigua is a traditional Chinese botanical that may be useful in angina. In TCM it is used for its ability to improve blood circulation and remove stasis.[279] Clinically, its application is primarily as an analgesic[280] and this property is well suited to the angina patient.

Unfortunately there is limited research in this area. Additional studies are needed to determine if corydalis is an effective treatment for this indication.

Corydalis has been shown to contain alkaloid constituents such as dehydrocavidine (YHL-I), coptisine (YHL-II), dehydroapocavidine (YHL-III) and tetradehydroscoulerine (YHL-IV).[281] The alkaloid L-tetrahydropalmatine (rotundium) has been identified in *Corydalis turtschanino*.[282] This substance has been shown in animal studies to have a positive anti-arrhythmic effect in blocking calcium channels.[282] The effective rate of rotundium on paroxysmal atrial fibrillation and sustained atrial fibrillation of 45 mm (left atrium diameter (LAD)) or more was 30%; LAD of less than 45 mm was 80% ($p <0.01$). The investigators believed that the anti-arrhythmic mechanism of rotundium might be related to its ability to prolong the effective refractory period of the atrial and atrioventricular nodes.

SALVIA MILTIORRHIZA (DAN SHEN)

Salvia miltiorrhiza is used extensively in China for treatment of cardiovascular disorders. It has been shown to:

- Protect against myocardial ischaemia
- Dilate coronary arteries
- Increase coronary blood flow
- Scavenge free radicals
- Suppress formation of thromboxane
- Inhibit platelet aggregation and adhesion.

These properties make it highly useful for the treatment of angina. In China, *Salvia miltiorrhiza* is most commonly used for angina or post-myocardial infarction support.[210] Its anti-angina effects have been confirmed by a meta-analysis[210] and a systematic review,[283] both of which found *Salvia miltiorrhiza* more effective at relieving angina and improving ECG readings than nitrate therapy — notably with fewer adverse reactions and better tolerance. In spite of these convincing results, it is recognised that the majority of studies undertaken have methodological flaws, thus further studies of better quality are required.

INULA RACEMOSA (PUSHKARMOOL, INULA)

Inula racemosa is another Ayurvedic botanical that has been found to exert benefits on the cardiovascular system, including where there is angina. A small study comparing the effects of *Inula racemosa* (3 g/day root powder) with glyceryl trinitrate for relief of angina in individuals with ischaemic heart disease observed favourable results.[118] The individuals were required to exert themselves and experienced chest pain and ECG ST-segment depression, a sign of myocardial ischaemia, but when treated with *Inula racemosa* 1.5 h before the test the individuals showed improved ST-segment depression on ECG.

VIBURNUM OPULUS (CRAMP BARK)

Modern herbalists have found much benefit when prescribing *Viburnum opulus* for a variety of spasmolytic conditions. The bark has been traditionally used for cramps, including menstrual cramps and cramping associated with arthritis. In angina *Viburnum opulus* is beneficial to reduce the generalised muscular tension commonly seen with angina patients and is specifically beneficial when prescribed in combination with *Corydalis ambigua* for symptomatic alleviation.

An in-vitro study found that viopudial isolated from *Viburnum opulus* had antispasmodic effects on smooth muscle,[284] but there is currently insufficient available evidence in humans to support the use of cramp bark specifically for angina.

LIFESTYLE RECOMMENDATIONS

Smoking

Patients who smoke need to be counselled on the link between smoking and attenuation of symptoms. The negative effect of smoking on ischaemic heart disease has been known for several years. This effect is apparent even with regard to passive smoke[285] and patients who do not smoke but are exposed to passive smoke are also at increased risk of ischaemic heart disease.

Stress

Stress, both emotional and physical, has been suggested to aggravate angina. Furthermore, symptoms such as anxiety and depression have been associated with more frequent angina,[286] hence the importance of the patient having appropriate stress management techniques. Patients need to be questioned on stressors personally relevant to them and what techniques (if any) they have to cope with these stressors. Education in stress management techniques such as meditation, cognitive behaviour therapy, deep breathing and the like is warranted in patients who exhibit high stress with concurrent angina.

Exercise

Although some patients may express concern, exercise is actually beneficial for patients with ischaemic heart disease and has been shown to improve cardiac function.[287,288] Exercise should be undertaken under the care and supervision of a suitably qualified healthcare professional such as an exercise physiologist.

CARDIAC REHABILITATION

According to the Australian Institute of Health and Welfare cardiac rehabilitation encompasses all measures used to help heart patients return to an active life. It aims to:

1. *Maximise physical, psychological and social functioning to enable patients to live productively and with confidence; and*
2. *Assist and encourage behaviours that are likely to reduce the risk of further heart, stroke and vascular events and conditions, such as identifying and modifying risk factors and encouraging adherence to recommended medical therapies.*[289]

While clearly the acute care of a patient who has suffered a myocardial infarction is not within the domain of naturopathic medicine, based upon the above aims it seems clear that individualised naturopathic care can have a useful place within long-term cardiac rehabilitation programs. Unfortunately evidence suggests that despite significant long-term benefits,[289,290] cardiac rehabilitation programs remain underutilised.[291] Therefore it seems prudent to consider the role that naturopaths can play in encouraging a multidisciplinary approach to cardiac rehabilitation, and encouraging greater levels of participation in these programs as well as cooperation and coordination between care providers.

CASE STUDY

OVERVIEW

JI is a 57-year-old retired male, presenting with angina. First diagnosed 6 years ago, the initial presentation was similar to episodes of heartburn with some shortness of breath, and his previous GP recognised the problem when the apparent heartburn was unresponsive to proton pump inhibitors. Stress ECG revealed some abnormalities, and angiography showed disease in two coronary arteries (although copies of the angiography report were unavailable to the patient, so details are lacking).

Over the last 3 years the patient's condition has worsened; however, the patient finds communication with the cardiologist and current GP difficult and has been provided little information about severity, prognosis and rationale for treatment.

CASE STUDY CONTINUED

A review of the patient's symptom pattern reveals that walking roughly 50–100 m up a very slight incline causes significant dyspnoea requiring a rest period, and sometimes also resulting in some chest pain (relieved quickly with sublingual nitrates). The patient has a supermarket less than 100 m from his flat but has stopped shopping there and instead orders online, because of the difficulty in carrying any shopping over that short distance. He lives alone on the 5th (top) floor of a block of flats, which has lifts for access. He recently experienced significant anxiety when a small fire in one of the flats caused an evacuation, and he found using the fire stairs to exit the building to be extremely difficult.

OTHER MEDICAL HISTORY

JI describes having been hypertensive since age 45, when a routine check-up revealed a blood pressure of 170/110 mmHg. A follow-up 2 weeks later showed 165/100 mmHg, and treatment was commenced immediately. He does not recall the details of the drug, but knows that over the last 10 years the drug has been changed once, and the dosage of the second drug has been increased over that time as well.

JI states that his mood has been quite low over the last 12 months or more, due mostly to the fact that his physical activity is impaired significantly. He does go for an hour-long walk 3 times a week, however finds these walks quite slow and very strenuous and fatiguing even though they are on relatively level ground and broken up by regular resting periods (estimated total walking time around 30 minutes or less). He has been considering purchasing an electric scooter to increase his mobility; however, he realises that he may end up relying on this too much thus further reducing his exercise.

The patient also describes noticeable muscle fatigue and some dull pain, which he has found to be more obvious in the last 6 months or so. The fatigue and pain seem to occur mainly in large muscle groups such as the thigh and upper arms, and in the thoracic and lumbar spine area. He initially assumed it was related to poor physical fitness but he does notice it at rest as well.

DIET AND LIFESTYLE

JI's diet is rich in refined carbohydrates. Breakfast usually consisting of wholegrain toast and jam or sweetened peanut butter, or sweetened muesli (roughly 30% sugar content according to the nutritional panel) with low-fat milk. Lunch is usually a wholegrain sandwich with low-fat cheese and salami in a hot sandwich press. Dinner 3 nights a week consists of home-delivery Thai or Vietnamese food, 2 nights a week a small portion of lean red meat and 3 boiled vegetables, and 2 nights a week a chicken stir fry with brown rice and multiple vegetables. Snacks between meals are mostly sweet biscuits (roughly 4 per day) or plain salted potato chips (roughly 100 g every 2 days). He eats one piece of fruit each day, and has recently replaced his after-dinner dessert (which previously consisted of low-fat ice-cream and chocolate fudge sauce) with either 4 squares of dark chocolate (Lindt 70%) or a low-fat flavoured and sweetened yoghurt.

Drinks are mostly water (roughly 1 litre per day), some packaged but unsweetened orange juice, and 3 cups of reduced-fat milk coffee per day, with 3 teaspoons of sugar per cup.

CASE STUDY CONTINUED

MEDICATIONS

- Aspirin 100 mg daily
- Nitrolingual pump spray (400 micrograms glyceryl trinitrate per dose) sublingually, 1 spray when walking and begins to get chest discomfort
- Lisinopril 20 mg daily
- Pravastatin 40 mg daily.

CLINICAL EXAMINATION AND PATHOLOGY

Copies of investigations were not available, except for his fasting blood lipids, full blood count, and fasting sugar:

- Total cholesterol 5.5 mmol/L
- Triglycerides 2.6 mmol/L
- HDL cholesterol 1.0 mmol/L
- LDL cholesterol 3.5 mmol/L
- Cholesterol/HDL cholesterol ratio 5.5
- Fasting glucose 5.2 mmol/L
- Normal full blood count.

The patient is noticeably obese and weighs 98 kg and is 173 cm tall, with a BMI of 32. Blood pressure during the first consultation was 155/95 mmHg.

ASSESSMENT

Based upon his symptoms and exercise tolerance, it can be estimated that the patient has stable Class III angina under the Canadian Cardiovascular Society Functional Classification. This is quite severe, and is obviously complicated by obesity and the fact that communication with his cardiologist was not possible. While he has low mood, it does not appear that he is suffering from clinical depression, although this is a possibility which must be considered and monitored long term. Additionally it seems likely that he is suffering from low-grade statin-induced myopathy.

THERAPEUTIC OBJECTIVES

The initial treatment objectives were:

- Reduce blood pressure
- Improve myocardial oxygen utilisation efficiency
- Reduce clotting risk
- Commence lowering patient's body weight.

TREATMENT

HERBAL TREATMENT

Herbal medicine	DER	Quantity/ week	Rationale
Crataegus monogyna berries	1:2	40 mL	Hypotensive, improves myocardial oxygen utilisation efficiency
Salvia miltiorrhiza	1:2	60 mL	Fibrinolytic, antiplatelet
Olea europea	1:2	40 mL	Hypotensive

Dosage: 10 mL twice daily before food

CASE STUDY CONTINUED

NUTRITIONAL TREATMENT

Initial nutritional treatment included:

- Omega capsules (1280 mg, with EPA 650 mg, DHA 450 mg). 1 capsule 3 times daily with food
- Vitamin E 500 IU daily
- CoQ10 150 mg, 2 capsules in the morning, 1 at lunch (total of 450 mg per day)
- Advice to cut coffee down to 1 cup per day, and to reduce sugar to 1.5 teaspoons per cup.

OUTCOMES (0–2 MONTHS)

The first follow-up consultation at 4 weeks showed some degree of blood pressure improvement, with a reading of 150/90 mmHg, although this change is minimum at this stage. JI described significantly improved exercise tolerance, with his 3 times weekly walk being of the same duration but punctuated by fewer rest periods and less severe dyspnoea. Recovery time after the walks was also reduced. Patient had reduced the coffee to 1 every 2 days in the last week, noticing that the CoQ10 had boosted his energy considerably, thus feeling less like he needed the coffee.

JI's mood had improved significantly, as he now felt like he was 'turning a corner and heading in the right direction'.

JI had been doing a lot of reading about angina and his medications, and in the last week had decided to stop his statin medication due to coming to the same conclusion (as his naturopath) that he was suffering statin-induced myopathy. This decision was discussed with the patient and he was encouraged to communicate this change to his cardiologist and GP; however, JI was disinclined to do so as he felt they were not offering effective care. He was also disinclined to seek a second medical opinion despite being encouraged to do so.

Having observed significant improvement in exercise tolerance, treatment objectives remained the same, with some additional dietary advice to focus more on weight loss.

FROM MONTH 2: HERBAL TREATMENT

Herbal medicine	DER	Quantity/ week	Rationale
Crataegus monogyna berries	1:2	40 mL	Hypotensive, improves myocardial oxygen utilisation efficiency
Salvia miltiorrhiza	1:2	60 mL	Fibrinolytic, antiplatelet
Olea europea	1:2	40 mL	Hypotensive

Dosage: 10 mL twice daily before food

NUTRITIONAL TREATMENT

Nutritional treatment included:

- Omega capsules (1280 mg, with EPA 650 mg, DHA 450 mg). 1 capsule 3 times daily with food
- Vitamin E 500 IU daily
- CoQ10 150 mg, 2 capsules in the morning, 1 at lunch (total of 450 mg per day)
- Advice to continue at 1 cup of coffee every 2 days, with 1 teaspoon of sugar per cup
- Replace breakfast regimen with a low-sugar muesli with added fresh fruit and 2 heaped teaspoons of psyllium hulls, or 1 boiled egg with avocado on wholemeal toast
- Replace lunch with a pre-washed packaged salad mix, with some nuts and seeds, and home-made balsamic vinegar and olive oil dressing
- Replace 2 nights of home delivery with grilled frozen packaged fish (with no coatings or additives) combined with salad or steamed mixed vegetables and brown rice
- Replace snacks with fresh fruit and/or mixed unsalted nuts and seeds.

OUTCOMES (2–9 MONTHS)

Over the next 7 months JI's blood pressure dropped to 140/90 mmHg. Exercise tolerance continued to improve with his walking distance being at least twice what it was on the first consultation, with fewer periods of rest and less exertional fatigue and dyspnoea. Additionally the patient added 2 days a week of gentle pool exercise for 30 minutes (walking and wading in the pool within his building).

Body weight had dropped to 89 kg by the end of the first 9 months. The patient was also now able to eat fresh fish, as he was able to take a short walk to purchase fresh fish from the nearby supermarket, and was able to carry it home with other light shopping.

Blood work at the end of 8 months showed the following (despite cessation of the statin more than 6 months previously):

- Total cholesterol 5.4 mmol/L
- Triglycerides 2.0 mmol/L
- HDL cholesterol 1.3 mmol/L
- LDL cholesterol 3.1 mmol/L
- Cholesterol/HDL cholesterol ratio 4.2
- Fasting glucose 4.8 mmol/L
- Normal full blood count.

Unfortunately the patient was reluctant to tell his GP that he was under herbal and naturopathic treatment; however, the GP was happy with his weight loss and improved blood pressure and blood results. (The patient did not tell the GP that he had discontinued the statin.)

Based on the patient's symptom picture it appears that the patient has reverted to Class II angina, which is a significant improvement. Treatment is ongoing with a target body weight of 80 kg. It is unfortunate that the patient felt uncomfortable with his other health professionals and thus unwilling to communicate that he was also under herbal and naturopathic care.

CEREBROVASCULAR ISCHAEMIA

Epidemiology

Cerebrovascular ischaemia (or ischaemic stroke) involves reduced blood flow to a section of the brain caused by a thrombus forming at the site of an atherosclerotic plaque, or an embolism arising from other areas of the body,[128] which in the case of a stroke (as opposed to a transient ischaemic attack) results in infarction within that part of the brain. Depending upon both the location and size of the infarct, various neurological and cognitive deficits can arise.[128]

Australian data indicate stroke prevalence increasing with age, with 8.1% of men and 5.3% of women aged 65–74 years having suffered either an ischaemic or a haemorrhagic stroke, increasing to 15.1% of men and 17.1% of women aged 85 years and over.[291]

Classification

Most strokes are ischaemic in nature, although roughly 15% of strokes are haemorrhagic in nature (and thus treated quite differently).[128] It is important to differentiate between an actual stroke (resulting in an infarct) and a transient ischaemic attack (TIA). Brain imaging after TIAs does not reveal permanent damage, and the symptoms of TIAs do not persist beyond a few hours. However patients who have had a TIA have a considerably elevated risk of having an actual stroke, often within hours or days of the TIA.[128]

Aetiology

Ischaemic strokes are caused by blockage of arterial blood flow to part of the brain. This may be caused by either a thrombus forming at the site of an atherosclerotic plaque, or an embolism arising from other areas of the body, most commonly from the heart (especially as a result of cardiac arrhythmias or valvular disease).[128]

Pathogenesis

The primary mechanism behind ischaemic stroke is obviously inadequate blood flow to areas of the brain. However, due to the vascular anatomy of the brain, inadequate blood supply in one artery can often be compensated for by a well-structured and efficient collateral blood flow system. Other existing arterial lesions, normal variations in collateral vessel diameter and in the circle of Willis, can increase the risk that single arterial occlusion can cause ischaemia.[292]

The extent of brain damage depends upon the severity of ischaemia. Mild and slowly developing (3–6 hours) neurological damage can occur even when tissue perfusion is 40% of normal. More rapid damage occurs when ischaemia is more severe; for example, when tissue perfusion drops below 5% for 5 minutes or more, then significant damage is likely.[292]

SIGNS AND SYMPTOMS

Signs and symptoms of ischaemic stroke are largely dependent upon the blood vessel occluded and thus the area of the brain affected, as can be clearly seen in Table 20.29. It is important to note that a number of other neurological disorders, such as migraine and seizure disorders, can exhibit symptoms and signs similar to TIAs and ischaemic strokes,[128] and thus differentiation is essential.

TABLE 20.29 Clinical manifestations of ischaemic stroke

Occluded blood vessel	Clinical manifestations
Internal carotid artery	Ipsilateral blindness (variable) Middle cerebral artery syndrome (see below)
Middle cerebral artery	Contralateral hemiparesis, sensory loss (worst in arm and face) Expressive aphasia or anosognosia and spatial disorientation Contralateral inferior quadrantanopsia
Anterior cerebral artery	Contralateral hemiparesis, sensory loss (worst in leg)
Posterior cerebral artery	Contralateral homonymous hemianopia or superior quadrantanopia Memory impairment
Basilar apex	Bilateral blindness Amnesia
Basilar artery	Contralateral hemiparesis, sensory loss Ipsilateral bulbar or cerebral signs
Vertebral artery or posterior inferior cerebellar artery	Ipsilateral loss of facial sensation, ataxia, contralateral hemiparesis, sensory loss
Superior cerebellar artery	Gait ataxia, nausea, dizziness, headache progressing to ipsilateral hemiataxia, dysathria, gaze paresis, contralateral hemiparesis, somnolence

Source: Adapted from Goldman L, Schafer AI, editors. Goldman's Cecil medicine. 24th ed. Philadelphia: Elsevier Saunders; 2012.

COMPLICATIONS

The complications of ischaemic stroke are many and varied. Provided the patient survives the initial ischaemic episode, the most obvious problems are neurological deficits related to the size and area of infarct. Common neurological issues include gait disturbances, dysphonia, dysphagia, fine motor coordination difficulties, sensory deficits, and cognitive deficits.[292]

Extraneurological complications are also an important consideration. Reduced motor function and subsequent mobility can result in issues such as pressure ulcers and peripheral thromboembolic complications. Urinary infections secondary to inadequate bladder control, aspiration pneumonia as a result of dysphagia, dehydration and malnutrition, and muscular deconditioning are additional issues to consider. Finally, mood and sleep disturbances (regardless of whether they are due to primary neurological damage or secondary to situational frustration) are important issues to be addressed.[293]

DIFFERENTIAL DIAGNOSIS

Differential diagnosis is largely focused on differentiating from other neurological complaints, and if it is clearly cerebrovascular in nature, then determining whether it constitutes a transient ischaemic attack (TIA) or whether it has been a true ischaemic or haemorrhagic stroke. Some key neurological conditions which can appear similar to a TIA or stroke include:[128]

- migraine
- brain tumour
- seizure disorders
- acute hypo- or hyperglycaemia
- acute cerebral anoxia of other causes (e.g. carbon monoxide poisoning).

NATUROPATHIC DIAGNOSIS

It is unlikely that naturopaths will be involved in initial diagnosis of an acutely ischaemic patient, as emergency medical care is required. Therefore the focus of naturopathic evaluation is predominantly concerned with establishing the severity and extent of complications and their impact on the patient's daily life and quality of life. In this context a detailed case history will be required but sometimes difficult to obtain, especially if the patient has lasting speech impediments and/or cognitive deficits. The involvement of relatives, friends or neighbours in the consultation may be valuable in obtaining the necessary information. The questioning should be broad, remembering that many neurological and extraneurological complications are possible. Physical examination is also valuable, especially evaluation of gait, fine motor coordination and muscular strength.

Investigations

GENERAL INVESTIGATIONS

Most investigations are initially focused on excluding other causes of neurological symptoms, and evaluating the extent of neurological damage. This is conducted primarily in the hospital setting and will involve a combination of initial history review as well as physical examination, followed by neuroimaging including computed tomography and magnetic resonance imaging. These studies are conducted to exclude other diagnoses such as intracerebral haemorrhage or subdural or epidural haematoma and to evaluate the location and severity of infarct.[292]

Later investigations to determine likely causes of ischaemic stroke, as well as risk of future stroke and other complications, are required. These may include cardiac rhythm evaluation (to exclude atrial fibrillation as a cause for example), vascular imaging to check for critical areas of stenosis, and blood coagulation tests.[292]

NATUROPATHIC INVESTIGATIONS

Apart from clinical evaluation (including history taking and physical examination — see 'Naturopathic diagnosis') there are no naturopathic-specific investigations of relevance in the context of long-term care of ischaemic stroke patients.

Therapeutic considerations

CLINICAL DECISION MAKING AND RATIONALE

In managing a patient who has been diagnosed as having had an ischaemic stroke, it is important to note that infarct size does not always correlate to level of functional impairment and the impact on individual quality of life can also be highly variable. Therefore a thorough case history, combined with physical and cognitive investigation is necessary. It is also often helpful to have family members or close friends present in some consultations to provide an additional perspective, provided the patient is comfortable with this. The involvement of other people with whom the patient regularly interacts can assist the clinician in understanding the level of long-term patient impairment, as well as assist in application and monitoring of therapeutic interventions (especially those involving lifestyle, exercise and diet).

Therapeutic application

ALLOPATHIC PERSPECTIVE

In managing a patient who has acute ischaemic stroke, the most immediate concern is life support, usually in the form of thrombolytic therapy and supportive measures such as acute blood pressure management, blood sugar regulation and other critical care measures.[128,292]

After discharge from hospital longer term care is generally initiated, which includes physical rehabilitation, counselling and management of risk factors (such as control of coagulation, reduction of blood pressure and better control of cardiac arrhythmias if relevant).[128]

HISTORICAL PERSPECTIVE

During the Middle Ages in Europe (1000–1450 AD), there was considerable debate about whether to treat patients with what was then known as 'apoplexy', with treatment being withheld from those deemed terminal. When treatment was administered, it often focused on bloodletting (to reduce an 'abundance of blood' believed to be causative), as well as vomiting and other purging treatments. While purging and vomiting continued to be the focus of treatment right through to the late 1800s, bloodletting began to be less commonly used. Other treatment and prevention guidelines such as avoiding emotional excitation and passion, avoiding excess food consumption and ensuring proper body and neck position, were also recommended from the late 1800s onwards. From the mid-1950s surgical intervention began to be employed to encourage reperfusion, and later pharmacological intervention with a similar goal began to be included in the treatment guidelines.[294]

NATUROPATHIC PERSPECTIVE

Naturopathic treatment of ischaemic stroke is primarily applicable after discharge and while similar to the allopathic approach (risk reduction, rehabilitation), it will usually focus more on additional methods to improve ongoing quality of life. Some key considerations include:

- Reducing clotting (with care as in most cases the patient is already on long-term platelet aggregation inhibiting drugs, or in some cases thrombolytic drugs)
- Managing blood pressure
- Lowering other atherosclerotic risk factors (such as improving blood lipid profile)
- Improving control of cardiac rhythm in patients whose stroke is secondary to atrial fibrillation
- Directly assisting with physical rehabilitation where that is within the scope of the clinician, or encouraging referral for effective physical rehabilitation (Note: the benefit of normal therapeutic massage as an addition to formal physiotherapy should not be discounted)[295]
- Improving mood and patient confidence
- Supporting neurological recovery.

NUTRITIONAL MEDICINE (DIETARY)

The dietary prevention of ischaemic stroke is somewhat controversial, but is considered to be largely the same as for any atherosclerotic disease. A US-based study published in 2011 involving 2568 participants (mean age 69 years, 64% female, 55% Hispanic, 24% black, 21% white) showed that while a higher adherence to a Mediterranean-style diet resulted in lower risk for the composite of ischaemic stroke, myocardial infarction or vascular causes of death, there was no decreased risk of ischaemic stroke alone.[296] However, a study of 32921 Swedish women published in 2015 showed high adherence to a Mediterranean diet was associated with a slight relative risk reduction in ischaemic stroke incidence versus low adherence to a Mediterranean diet.[297]

Another dietary study from 2017 demonstrated that factors such as high sodium intake, low nuts and seeds intake, low omega-3 fatty acid intake, high processed meat intake and low fruit and vegetable intake are associated with higher risk of mortality from cardiometabolic diseases in general (ischaemic heart disease, stroke and type 2 diabetes).[298] The same study demonstrated a lesser but still significant association between mortality from the same conditions and intake of sugar-sweetened beverages; however, another recent study of 2888 participants aged 45 years or older showed no association between stroke incidence and sugar-sweetened beverages, but interestingly showed an increased risk of stroke associated with intake of artificially sweetened beverages, even when risk was adjusted for age, gender, education, kilojoule intake, physical activity and smoking.[299]

Dietary management of patients post-ischaemic stroke is often complicated by dysphagia, with up to 15% still having difficulties swallowing more than 1 month after a stroke. This dysphagia can result in malnutrition, but also chest infections due to aspiration.[300] A macro- and micronutrient dense diet in an easily swallowed form (for example smoothies) may be beneficial in helping to avoid long-term malnutrition.

NUTRITIONAL MEDICINE (SUPPLEMENTAL)

As the mechanism of ischaemic cerebrovascular disease is similar to that of ischaemic heart disease, a similar supplementation plan may be hypothesised to be useful in prevention. However, more long-term rigorous studies with large sample sizes and well-defined supplementation regimens are needed to evaluate the true potential (if any) of nutritional supplementation in the prevention of ischaemic stroke, as some studies of supplementation of nutrients such as vitamin C, vitamin E and beta-carotene have shown no reduction in ischaemic stroke risk.[301,302]

Studies of B vitamins and some other supplements in humans show promise in terms of reduction in stroke recurrence. A meta-analysis of 12 studies consisting of a total of 7474 patients indicated that B vitamin supplementation in stroke patients reduced the risk of stroke recurrence, and the risk of other vascular events.[303] Of course, from a clinical standpoint, practical issues with administration of any tablet- or capsule-based treatment to patients with dysphagia must be considered.

HERBAL MEDICINE

Herbal medicine therapeutic objectives

Primary herbal objectives in treating patients who have had an ischaemic stroke include:

- Reduce clotting (with care, especially if the patient is on conventional antiplatelet or fibrinolytic drugs)
- Manage blood pressure (see earlier section on hypertension)
- Reduce total atherosclerotic risk (see earlier section on atherosclerosis)
- Improve neurological recovery
- Improve mood, vitality and patient confidence.

Herbal medicine classes

Classes of herbal medicines valuable in ischaemic stroke recovery are listed in Table 20.30. It is important to note that in the prevention of future cerebrovascular ischaemic events treatment should focus on total cardiovascular risk reduction, as well incorporate some of the elements of treatment employed in managing coronary ischaemia (such as reducing thrombolic and embolic risk and blood pressure).

TABLE 20.30 Specific herbal medicine classes used in ischaemic stroke recovery

Class	Action
Antioxidants	Reduce atherosclerotic deterioriation which may contribute to future ischaemic events
Cerebrovascular tonics	Improve function and structural integrity of cerebral blood vessels
Neuroprotectives and neurorestoratives	Improve neurological recovery
Adaptogens and nervines (including antidepressants, sedatives, and anxiolytics)	Normalise mood (where relevant) and improve vitality

Specific herbal medicines

GINKGO BILOBA (GINKGO)

Standardised extract of ginkgo is possibly the single most well-indicated herbal medicine in the context of ischaemic

SAMPLE DAILY DIET

BREAKFAST	
Smoothie: high-quality protein powder, blueberries, strawberries, kiwi fruit, cacao plus wheatgerm oil	Supplementation with a protein powder (20 g/d) has been shown to enhance recovery of neurological alterations in individuals who have experienced ischaemic stroke. Protein powder increases brain content of amino acids restoring protein synthesis and improving neuron energy formation. Protein powders also lead to provision of amino acids such as tyrosine which are needed for adrenergic neurotransmitters such as dopamine, adrenaline (epinephrine) and noradrenaline (norepinephrine) which influence activity-dependent plasticity and learning. A low-allergen, high-quality protein powder is suggested. Fruits such as berries and kiwi fruit are advocated for their antioxidant activity to neutralise damage by free radicals. Ischaemia results in production of free radicals via multiple pathways including inflammatory cells such as neutrophils, as well as glutamate and aspartate toxicity; the resultant effect is oxidative stress which damages cerebral cells. As well as providing antioxidant activity, blueberries are known to cross the blood–brain barrier. In animal studies examining the effects of diet in transient focal ischaemia, consumption of blueberries was shown to exert a neuroprotective action reducing the extension of cerebral infarction, thus it is hypothesised similar results may be observed in humans. Flavonoid-rich cacao may be used for its antioxidant, anti-hypertensive activity and ability to reduce platelet adhesion. Higher intake of dietary vitamin E is associated with lower risk of cerebral infarct, in part due to its antioxidant action as well as anticoagulant activity. Foods such as wheatgerm which contain high quantities of dietary vitamin E can be added to a smoothie.
LUNCH	
Fish chowder made with white fish, potato (to thicken), spinach, onion, sweetcorn, celery and chives (pureed)	Following stroke, self-feeding individuals have been recommended to consume a portion of protein (e.g. fish) per day to obtain 12–15 mg of zinc. Zinc plays a vital role in maintaining brain function and may contribute to cerebral repair due to its antioxidant action. Individuals with ischaemic stroke have been shown to have lower than recommended dietary intake of zinc and when their zinc is normalised may experience better recovery of neurological deficits. Ample antioxidant-rich vegetables such as onions, which contain quercetin, and spinach are recommended. Both have been shown in animal studies to reduce cell death in models of cerebral ischaemia. Observational studies suggest a protective effect of fruit and vegetable consumption against risk of ischaemic stroke, thus these foods should be promoted to protect against further strokes. At least 500 g/d of fruit and vegetables has been suggested to be beneficial.
DINNER	
Guacamole with refried beans, corn plus sweet potato	One-carbon metabolism plays an essential role in aiding recovery and increasing neuroplasticity after stroke, thus folate-containing foods such as avocado are essential. Refried beans provide a source of B vitamins. Supplementation of B group vitamins as well as antioxidants such as vitamins C and E has been demonstrated to reduce tissue levels of malondialdehyde and levels of C-reactive protein, a marker of tissue inflammation, thus foods that contain these nutrients should be promoted in the diet. These foods may be pureed to assist individuals with dysphagia. Ideally, dinner will be largely plant based, taking influence from the Mediterranean diet. Long-term adherence to this diet has been shown to decrease 5-year stroke risk by approximately 30%.
SNACKS	
Green tea Stewed, pureed fruit with natural yoghurt	Ingestion of green tea catechins is associated with reduced incidence of stroke. Green tea catechins possess potent antioxidative properties. In rodent studies green tea exerted a neuroprotective role, preventing recognition memory deficits and ameliorating hippocampal oxidative stress, indicating less cerebral ischaemic damage. Stroke may result in intestinal barrier breakdown and microbiota changes, with translocation of selective bacterial strains from the host gut microbiota to peripheral tissues such as the lungs; this may induce post-stroke infections. Natural yoghurt provides live cultures to optimise gut and immune health, while fruit provides prebiotics, vitamins and antioxidants to further enhance immunity.

stroke. Various applicable positive actions have been demonstrated in both animal and human research, including:

- Antioxidant[273]
- Antiplatelet (although there is debate about clinical significance of this action, especially in regards to safety, with some research indicating very little to no change in clotting)[273]
- Neuroprotective[273,304]
- Antidepressant (especially in the context of cerebrovascular insufficiency)[304]
- Nootropic[273,304]
- Mild anticholinergic activity.[273]

Research as well as clinical experience demonstrates that in most cases high doses of high-quality standardised extract are required. Much of the research has been conducted on a specific extract known as EGb 761, and some similar extracts, and these are concentrated extracts (usually around 50 : 1) with well-characterised levels of the flavone glycosides and terpenes which seem to be important in ginkgo's activity.[304] Dosages employed range from 100–360 mg of the extract daily, with some research demonstrating better effects at the higher end of the range.[304] Unfortunately there is a significant issue with adulteration of some ginkgo extracts with various flavonoid fractions to artificially boost total flavonoid levels.[304] Thus it is important to only use well-researched concentrated extracts, or galenical preparations which have been carefully characterised phytochemically.

BACOPA MONNIERA (BACOPA)

Bacopa has traditionally been seen as a tonic useful for improving memory and rehabilitation after any injury resulting in neurological deficit.[273] While human clinical studies on the relevance of bacopa in stroke recovery are lacking, animal research points to it having antioxidant, neuroprotective and antidepressant activity which may be beneficial.[273] However, many of these animal studies have focused on pre-treatment with bacopa or constituents from bacopa, prior to induction of an ischaemic brain event in rats, so the clinical benefit of post-ischaemic stroke administration is difficult to ascertain.[305,306]

CAMELLIA SINENSIS (GREEN TEA)

Green tea shows some promise in the prevention of ischaemic stroke. A systematic review from 2013 showed that green tea or green tea flavonoid consumption reduced both stroke incidence and mortality, with a dose-response relationship noted (with 3 cups per day or greater showing the best results).[307] An additional mouse study also indicated that green tea consumption exerted a preventive reduction of post-ischaemic stroke depressive symptoms, and improved endogenous oxidative defences.[308]

Lifestyle recommendations

Rehabilitation after ischaemic stroke is an essential part of treatment, and must be customised for the individual patient, depending upon motivation, social situation, learning ability, physical ability, and coping skills.[309] This will require attention from rehabilitation specialists such as physiotherapists and occupational therapists. The key aims of rehabilitation include:[309]

- Improving range of motion
- Improving muscle strength and function (including fine motor coordination)
- Normalising bowel and bladder function
- Improving cognitive abilities.

Addressing mood in the patient is no less important. While it may be possible in part to address depression using pharmacological methods, research indicates that collaborative goal setting, written information, screening for adverse sequelae, home visits, telephone contact and review of achievement towards goals results in reduced depressive symptoms compared to patients receiving a standard management program.[310]

In addition to exercise programs, and heat and cold therapy for muscle spasticity, assistive devices in the home, as well as mobility devices for use outside the home, can be extremely valuable.[309]

Acupuncture shows promise in a number of areas of stroke recovery, with studies demonstrating improvement in dysphagia (especially when combined with swallowing training),[311,312] neurological and cognitive impairment and lower limb function, but not upper limb function.[311]

CASE STUDY

OVERVIEW

DV was a 67-year-old female presenting with what appeared to be 3 transient ischaemic attacks (TIAs) over the previous 5 months. The attacks occurred during a particularly stressful period (her husband had recently died rather suddenly from metastatic prostate cancer), with the first occurring while she was with friends and being dismissed as just anxiety and fatigue. The second occurred roughly 2 months later and resulted in more obvious neurological deficits while babysitting her grandchildren, with the deficits lasting less than 1 hour.

This prompted her to see her GP who then referred her for further investigations, revealing no signs of vertebral or carotid artery occlusion, and no signs of cerebral infarct. Blood work showed normal blood sugar and lipid levels, and blood pressure was 140/80 mmHg unmedicated; however, the GP recommended commencing statins and 100 mg aspirin daily. The patient agreed with the aspirin but informed her doctor that she was disinclined to take the statins given her normal blood lipids and having read about the adverse effects. The GP also prescribed an antidepressant to help with her mood since her husband's death, which she also declined.

Her third TIA was just 2 days after commencing the aspirin and again resulted in overt neurological deficits lasting approximately 30 minutes, occurring in the evening while cooking dinner at home.

DV's sleep had been disturbed since her husband's death, with the patient waking regularly during the night feeling moderately anxious and she found returning to sleep difficult.

DIET AND LIFESTYLE

DV's diet was generally excellent with good fruit and vegetable intake, fish two to three times weekly, low sugar

CASE STUDY CONTINUED

intake, 1 cup of black tea with half a teaspoon of sugar daily, no coffee and an extremely occasional glass of white wine.

DV described low mood and significant fatigue during the day, resulting in less social activity than normal. Cognitive function however appeared normal, with no obvious signs of age-related cognitive decline. Previous to her husband's sudden diagnosis and death, she had been a relatively fit and active person, walking regularly, participating in a twice-weekly card game with her friends, and babysitting for her grandchildren at least twice weekly. Since these TIAs she had stopped babysitting as she was fearful of further TIAs while with the children and had reduced her card game to once every fortnight because of fatigue.

CLINICAL EXAMINATION AND PATHOLOGY

DV's body weight was normal, and blood pressure was 165/95 mmHg on presentation, which was higher than it had been at her previous doctor's visit.

ASSESSMENT

DV obviously had increased clotting risk, although her presentation was somewhat unusual with no history of hypertension, no history of cardiovascular disease and normal blood lipids. The situation was made worse by recent stressful trauma and subsequent decreasing confidence in her own health and capabilities.

THERAPEUTIC OBJECTIVES

The initial treatment objectives were:

- Reduce coagulation risk
- Reduce impact of stress on cardiovascular function
- Improve vitality and mood
- Improve cerebrovascular blood flow.

TREATMENT

HERBAL TREATMENT

Herbal medicine	DER	Quantity/ week	Rationale
Eleutherococcus senticosus	1:2	50 mL	Adaptogen
Crataegus monogyna berries	1:2	20 mL	Hypotensive, cardiovascular tonic

Dosage: 5 mL twice daily before food

Tebonin (EGb 761) *Ginkgo biloba* extract 12 mg, 1 tablet twice daily with food.

OUTCOMES (0–24 MONTHS)

Over the next 2 years of monitoring DV had no further TIA episodes. Mood, vitality and confidence improved rapidly and significantly after the first consultation, allowing her to resume her normal active life over the next few months. Aspirin at 100 mg daily was continued during this entire period. Blood pressure normalised with readings of 135–145/80–90 mmHg from the fourth month of treatment onwards.

CHRONIC HEART FAILURE

Epidemiology

Chronic heart failure is a major public health issue and one of the most significant causes of morbidity and mortality for older adults in Western countries.[313] It is estimated that about 30 000 new cases are diagnosed in Australia each year.[226] However, public awareness of the condition remains low,[312] and less than one in five eligible patients receives specialist heart failure management after hospitalisation for an acute episode.[314] Recent population studies suggest that diagnosed heart failure represents only the 'tip of the iceberg', with a much higher proportion of subclinical or preclinical stages of the disease.[315]

The prevalence of coronary heart failure in industrialised countries is rising and Australian estimates are 1.5–2% of the population.[316] The prevalence dramatically increases with age, doubling every decade,[317] and it is estimated that prevalence in Australians ≥65 years is at least 10%.[318] A sustained epidemic of chronic heart failure is predicted, with incidence increasing by 20–30% in the next 2 decades.[319]

Classification

CHRONIC HEART FAILURE

Congestive heart failure is a complex condition that usually occurs as a result of both heart failure and changes in peripheral circulation. It involves bouts of gradually worsening symptoms, often accompanied by activation of the sympathetic nervous system and renin–angiotensin system.[243] The condition is often complicated by periods of acute worsening.[313]

ACUTE HEART FAILURE

The term acute heart failure most often refers to acute dyspnoea characterised by signs of pulmonary congestion, including pulmonary oedema.[320] It can develop during acute ischaemia of the ventricle, following myocardial infarction, tachycardia or the rupture of a cardiac structure; there is usually a swift progression of severe symptoms and signs.[318]

SYSTOLIC VENTRICULAR FAILURE

Most heart failure is associated with evidence of left ventricular systolic dysfunction, characterised by ischaemic heart disease.[321] The resultant decrease in emptying capacity is associated with a compensatory increase in diastolic volume.[129]

DIASTOLIC VENTRICULAR DYSFUNCTION/FAILURE

Predominant diastolic dysfunction is relatively uncommon in younger patients, but highly prevalent in the elderly, in whom systolic hypertension and myocardial hypertrophy are contributors to cardiac dysfunction.[320] The condition impairs filling of one or both ventricles, with normal emptying capacity; leading to increased ventricular filling pressures and eventually pulmonary oedema.[129]

LEFT VS. RIGHT HEART FAILURE

Heart failure can be designated as either left or right, referring to the area of primary impairment of heart function, but since both sides of the heart form a circuit, degradation in one will invariably affect the other. In general, right-sided failure follows left-sided failure. Left-sided failure is used to refer to signs and symptoms of elevated pressure and congestion in the pulmonary veins and capillaries; right-sided failure refers to signs and symptoms of elevated pressure and congestion in the systemic veins and capillaries.[129]

Aetiology

Heart failure is one of the most complex cardiovascular conditions, encompassing several aetiologies and comorbidities. The condition results primarily from systolic hypertension and ischaemic heart disease.[48] It can be difficult to ascertain the primary cause of heart failure in a patient with multiple risk factors, such as hypertension and coronary artery disease. The condition usually arises as a consequence of an aberration in cardiac structure, function, rhythm or conduction. There are numerous factors that will influence this (see Box 20.7).[322]

HYPERTENSION

Hypertension, particularly systolic hypertension, is an independent risk factor for eventual development of congestive heart failure.[323] It is the most commonly occurring risk for heart failure, implicated in over 70% of cases.[318] Hypertension may predispose patients to heart failure through a number of pathological mechanisms — particularly left ventricular hypertrophy, associated with an increased risk of myocardial infarction.[324]

CORONARY ARTERY DISEASE

More than half of the cases of heart failure in patients under 75 years are a result of coronary artery disease.[325] Either alone or with hypertension, coronary artery disease appears to be the most common cause of heart failure in the West.[322]

KIDNEY DISEASE

Patients with chronic kidney disease are at significant risk of having or developing cardiovascular disease, including heart failure.[41]

METABOLIC DISORDERS

Disorders of glucose metabolism (i.e. insulin resistance, metabolic syndrome, diabetes) are independent risk factors for cardiovascular disease and heart failure. These conditions are associated with obesity and central adiposity, which has a significant and incremental relationship with the incidence of heart failure.[326] Longitudinal studies have shown that diabetes can increase the likelihood of progression to heart failure twofold in men and fivefold in women.[327]

BOX 20.7 The various causes in the progression of heart failure

- Coronary artery disease
- Myocardial infarction
- Ischaemia
- Hypertension
- Cardiomyopathy
- Dilated (congestive)
- Hypertrophic/obstructive
- Restrictive — for example, amyloidosis, sarcoidosis, haemochromatosis
- Obliterative
- Valvar and congenital heart disease
- Mitral valve disease
- Aortic valve disease
- Atrial septal defect, ventricular septal defect
- Arrhythmias
- Tachycardia
- Bradycardia (complete heart block, the sick sinus syndrome)
- Loss of atrial transport — for example, atrial fibrillation
- Alcohol and drugs
- Cardiac depressant drugs (beta-blockers, calcium antagonists)
- 'High output' failure
- Anaemia, thyrotoxicosis, arteriovenous fistulae, Paget's disease
- Pericardial disease
- Constrictive pericarditis
- Pericardial effusion
- Primary right heart failure
- Pulmonary hypertension — for example, pulmonary embolism, cor pulmonale
- Tricuspid incompetence

Source: Adapted from Lip G, Gibbs C, Beevers D. ABC of heart failure. BMJ 2000;320:104–7.

AGE

Individuals under 50 years are rarely found to have heart failure.[318] However, the prevalence increases with age and approximately 80% of patients with heart failure are over 65 years.[318] In Australia, over 90% of cases of heart failure resulting in death occur in patients over the age of 75.[226]

ANAEMIA

Anaemia is a common comorbidity in patients with heart failure and is associated with poor prognosis, though the mechanisms are poorly understood. Anaemic patients are likely to be older, with concomitant diabetes or chronic renal failure.[227] Anaemia and low haemoglobin are consistently associated with an increased risk of heart failure mortality, by up to 20–50%.[328]

Overview

Heart failure is a clinical event that arises when the heart is unable to pump sufficient blood to meet the metabolic needs of the body. It is defined as an impaired ventricular filling and/or ejection (unable to meet body's demands), especially during physical activity or stress.

- Systolic heart failure is characterised by weakened systolic contraction. It is the most common form.
- Diastolic dysfunction (heart failure with preserved systolic function) is characterised by impaired diastolic filling of the left ventricle.

Pathogenesis

When there is fundamental disturbance of myocardial contractility, or when excessive haemodynamic burden is placed on a normal ventricle, the heart will employ a number of adaptive mechanisms to maintain cardiac output and blood pressure.[41] These mechanisms are compensatory at first, but will become part of the pathological process over time, eventually worsening cardiac function. Neurohormonal changes, such as upregulated sympathetic nervous system function, will initially provide inotropic support to the failing heart — increasing stroke volume and peripheral vasoconstriction. This maintains mean arterial perfusion pressure but eventually accelerates disease progression, affecting survival.[329]

SIGNS AND SYMPTOMS

Breathlessness, ankle swelling and fatigue are characteristic symptoms of heart failure, but may be difficult to confirm in high-risk patients, particularly among the elderly, the obese and in women.[320] Heart failure is a clinical state defined by the physical presentation of symptoms and signs (Table 20.31).

TABLE 20.31 Symptoms and signs of heart failure

Symptoms	Signs
Dyspnoea (on exertion, nocturnal) Reduced exercise tolerance Fatigue, lethargy Orthopnoea Nocturnal cough Wheeze Anorexia Confusion/delirium (elderly)	Oedema, ascites Elevated jugular vein pressure Crepitations or wheeze Tachycardia Third heart sound, murmurs Hepatomegaly Displaced apex beat Cachexia and muscle wasting

Source: Mosterd A, Hoes A. Clinical epidemiology of heart failure. Heart 2007;93(9):1137–1146, with permission from BMJ Publishing Group Ltd.

Differentiation between left-sided and right-sided heart failure can be made with regard to the symptoms listed in Table 20.32.

COMPLICATIONS

The prognosis following heart failure is poor, with a 5-year survival rate of 25% for men and 38% for women.[330]

DIFFERENTIAL DIAGNOSIS

Heart failure may present, initially, as a symptom or complication of existing cardiovascular and/or metabolic conditions. While these may be comorbid, they must be considered in the differential diagnosis:

- Hypertension
- Coronary artery disease — atherosclerosis/dyslipidaemia/ischaemia
- Diabetes
- Insulin resistance
- Metabolic syndrome
- Anaemia.

The European Society of Cardiology definition of heart failure[320]

- Symptoms of heart failure (at rest or during exercise) and
- Objective evidence (preferably echocardiography) of cardiac dysfunction (systolic/diastolic) at rest and (in cases where diagnosis is in doubt)
- Response to treatment directed at heart failure.

TABLE 20.32 Differentiation between left-sided and right-sided heart failure

Left-sided heart failure	Right-sided heart failure
Reduced exercise capacity Dyspnoea (wheeze, orthopnoea, PND) Cough (haemoptysis) Lethargy and fatigue Reduced appetite Weight loss	Ankle swelling Dyspnoea (but not orthopnoea or PND) Reduced exercise capacity Chest pain
Cool skin Pulse normal or low volume (tachycardia, arrhythmias) Displaced apex Third sound, summation gallop Functional mitral regurgitation Pulmonary crepitations ± Pleural effusion	Pulse (tachycardia arrhythmias) Raised jugular venous pressure (JVP) Oedema Hepatomegaly and ascites Parasternal heave RV S3 or S4 Pleural effusion

PND, paroxysmal nocturnal dyspnoea.
Source: Adapted from Gray H, Dawkins K, Morgan J, et al. Cardiology. 5th ed. Oxford: Blackwell Publishing; 2008.

NATUROPATHIC DIAGNOSIS

Heart failure is a serious, potentially fatal, cardiac condition. If heart failure is suspected during consultation, the patient must be referred immediately to a hospital or emergency medicine physician for further investigation and treatment.

Naturopathic case taking should encompass current patient health, physical evaluation, clinical signs and all predisposing risk factors in an assessment of the patient's condition. Other features that should form a naturopathic evaluation include:

- Metabolism, specifically glucose metabolism and general muscle energetics (i.e. functional ability of muscle tissue, especially myocardial tissue)
- Stress and anxiety levels, as the nervous system has significant impact upon cardiovascular health

- Mood assessment, as depression is quite prevalent in patients with chronic heart failure, contributes to poor quality of life, and is an important risk factor for hospital readmission[304]
- Digestive function, particularly of the upper digestive tract — including absorption and motility
- Dietary evaluation and assessment of the patient's nutritional intake, with particular focus on hydration, plus quality and quantity of food.

Investigations

Clinical signs of heart failure should be assessed in a thorough examination including observation, palpation and auscultation. Where heart failure is suspected, further investigations will be carried out (Table 20.33).

TABLE 20.33 Investigations for heart failure

Test	Clinical implication
Full blood count	Anaemia
Iron studies	Haemochromatosis
Serum chemistry profile	Electrolyte disturbance Diabetes mellitus Renal insufficiency Hypoproteinaemia
Thyroid function	Hyper-/hypothyroidism
Urinalysis	Proteinuria (indicating nephrotic syndrome or glomerulonephritis, which can cause oedema)
Electrocardiogram (ECG)	Myocardial infarction Ventricular hypertrophy
Chest x-ray	Confirm congestion as cause of dyspnoea (important in cases of obstructive lung disease) Pulmonary infiltrates/fibrosis Presence of pleural effusion
Echocardiogram	Differentiate systolic vs diastolic function Document left-ventricular function and chamber size Wall motion abnormalities (with coronary artery disease aetiology) Valve abnormalities Pericardial effusion Intracardiac masses

Source: Adapted from Taylor G. Primary care cardiology. 2nd ed. Oxford: Blackwell Publishing; 2005.

NATUROPATHIC INVESTIGATIONS

The diagnosis of heart failure relies largely on clinical observations and allopathic investigations; however, there are several other investigations that can be useful when monitoring treatment and progression of this condition. In patients with a suspected cardiovascular condition, or history of heart failure, blood pressure should be taken at each visit.

25(OH)D — serum vitamin D

Vitamin D deficiency is increasingly, and surprisingly, prevalent; deficiency is implicated in myocardial dysfunction and poor prognosis for heart failure.[331]

Essential fatty acids

Essential fatty acids may be deficient or imbalanced in cardiovascular disease states.

Cardiovascular disability scales

Cardiovascular disability scales are important components for the naturopathic consultation. They are discussed in detail below.

Therapeutic considerations

CLINICAL DECISION MAKING AND RATIONALE

Assessing heart failure patients

It is imperative that a thorough history is taken, focusing on quantifiable functional assessment. It may be beneficial to include the use of cardiovascular disability scales to add depth and greater specificity to the assessment. The cardiovascular disability scales should be used to conduct an initial severity assessment and then throughout treatment to assess treatment effectiveness (or lack thereof).

When assessing the patient, it is important to also gain information about occupation, mood, stress, family life and so on. These can be important targets for lifestyle modification or adjuvant treatment and may also help provide further insight into situation/prognosis.

Cardiovascular disability scales

Cardiovascular disability scales are standardised scales for classifying the severity of disease process. Functional capability (i.e. physical activity) before the onset of symptoms is used as the measurement criteria. It is therefore essential that accurate information about exercise/activity tolerance is obtained. This is not always easy with some patients.

Three main scales are employed. All use a four-tier system, with class I being least severe and class IV being most severe:

- Canadian Cardiovascular Society Functional Classification — used for anginal syndrome
- Specific Activity Scale — for heart failure or anginal syndrome. Very specific with regard to metabolic strain of activity. Less commonly used
- New York Heart Association (NYHA) Functional Classification — for heart failure or anginal syndrome. Most commonly used.

USING THE NYHA CLASSIFICATION

'Ordinary physical activity' is open to individual interpretation: 10 kg of shopping up 8 steps, light jogging at 7 km/h for at least a few minutes. Increased respiratory rate and challenge at these levels is normal, but true dyspnoea, anginal pain and serious fatigue indicate pathology.

New York Heart Association (NYHA) functional classification

NYHA Class I	Patients with cardiac disease but without resulting limitations of physical activity. Ordinary physical activity does not cause undue fatigue, palpitation, dyspnoea or anginal pain
NYHA Class II	Patients with cardiac disease resulting in slight limitation of physical activity. They are comfortable at rest. Ordinary physical activity results in fatigue, palpitation, dyspnoea or anginal pain
NYHA Class III	Patients with cardiac disease resulting in marked limitation of physical activity. They are comfortable at rest. Less than ordinary activity causes fatigue, palpitation, dyspnoea or anginal pain
NYHA Class IV	Patients with cardiac disease resulting in inability to carry on any physical activity without discomfort. Symptoms of cardiac insufficiency or of anginal syndrome may be present even at rest. If any physical activity is undertaken, discomfort is increased

Detailed questioning about normal physical activities and occasional physical activities, along with accompanying symptoms, is essential:

- Gradient
- Distance
- Speed
- Weight (both carried and body weight)
- Actual symptoms
- Recovery time
- Use of nitrates (in angina).

Some male patients particularly may be inaccurate in their recall of nitrate use and this makes it difficult to assess severity. As such, a patient diary (for both sexes) is a useful tool. It may be beneficial to use one or more consistent activities as main monitor during successive consultations.

Educate the patient about what you are doing when you ask these detailed questions; better understanding means better awareness and cooperation.

Prognosis

Prognosis for patients is complicated and variable. It is imperative to realise that it is crucial to reduce severity indices. The use of ACE inhibitors in conventional medicine has been shown to increase survival rates. A few keys factors are listed below:

1 Severity
 All NYHA classes: 30% survival at 8 years
 NYHA class II and III: 34% mortality at 1 year
 NYHA class IV: 60% mortality at 1 year
 These figures are prior to use of ACE inhibitors
2 Duration
3 Type of therapy utilised.

Therapeutic application

ALLOPATHIC PERSPECTIVE

Allopathic treatment for heart failure will depend on the cause, severity and comorbid presentation. The aim, at all times, is to restore heart function, reduce symptomatology and prolong life. The measures used in allopathic management of heart failure are summarised in Table 20.34.

HISTORICAL PERSPECTIVE

The Eclectics used a wide range of botanicals to support the failing heart. Gentle restoratives such as *Avena sativa* were used for their enfeebled action of the heart[173] while more stimulating botanicals such as *Cactus grandiflora* and *Digitalis* were suggested for their impressive action upon the sympathetic nervous system, cactus being described as being especially active in its power over the cardiac plexus working upon the circular cardiac fibres. Dose was important as an excessive dose may instigate heart failure. *Crataegus* was also suggested for cardiac weakness, with valvular murmurs, sighing respiration or other difficult breathing and valvular insufficiency; cardiac pain and irregularity, and rapid and feeble heart action.

NATUROPATHIC PERSPECTIVE

- Watch patients at risk (those with chronic hypertension, ischaemic heart disease, chronic/recurrent anaemia). Instigate possible preventive treatment (e.g. *Crataegus*, co-enzyme Q10) early if risk is high, and ensure they are properly investigated intermittently to exclude heart failure or discover it when asymptomatic
- Ensure those who are diagnosed are getting adequate care
- GP care alone is not generally sufficient
- Even mildly symptomatic patients should have a cardiology consult at least once every year
- Adequate care is not just focused directly on the heart failure itself — psychological support and management of any psychological and/or physiological comorbidities are essential.

Improved control

To improve the health and control of the disease progression in patients a few key areas must be considered:

- All patients will be under conventional care. If they are not, ensure that you develop an integrated relationship with a GP and cardiologist and facilitate close monitoring and communication between all healthcare practitioners
- The addition of herbal or naturopathic medicines can result in better control of heart failure. There is some good clinical data for some interventions, and mentoring from experienced cardiovascular naturopaths is beneficial to support the care of patients through this condition.

Improved quality of life (QOL)

- Regardless of mortality rate, heart failure significantly affects quality of life.[332] An important role of the

TABLE 20.34 Allopathic management of heart failure

Stage	Clinical presentation	Therapy
Stage A High risk for heart failure Without structural heart disease or symptoms of heart failure	Hypertension Atherosclerosis Diabetes mellitus Obesity Metabolic syndrome OR patient using cardiotoxins, with family history of cardiomyopathy	**Goals** Treat hypertension Control risk factors, e.g. smoking, alcohol, drug use Treat lipid disorders Treat metabolic syndrome Encourage regular exercise **Medication** ACE inhibitors, in appropriate patients
	↓ Structural heart disease ↓	
Stage B Structural heart disease Without signs or symptoms of heart failure	Previous myocardial infarction Left ventricular remodelling, including LV hypertrophy and low ejection fraction Asymptomatic valvular disease	**Goals** All measures under stage A **Medication** ACE inhibitors or ARBs in appropriate patients Beta-blockers in appropriate patients **Devices** Implantable defibrillators
	↓ Development of symptoms of heart failure ↓	
Stage C Structural heart disease With prior or current symptoms of heart failure	Known structural heart disease Shortness of breath and fatigue Reduced exercise tolerance	**Goals** All measures under stages A and B Dietary salt restriction **Medications** Diuretics for fluid retention ACE inhibitors Beta-blockers — in selected patients Aldosterone antagonist ARBs Digoxin Hydralazine/nitrates **Devices** Biventricular pacing Implantable defibrillators
	↓ Refractory symptoms of heart failure at rest ↓	
Stage D Refractory heart failure requiring specialised interventions	Patients with marked symptoms at rest despite maximal medical therapy, e.g. those who are recurrently hospitalised or cannot be safely discharged from hospital without specialist intervention	**Goals** Appropriate measures under stages A, B and C Decisions regarding appropriate level of care **Decisions** Compassionate end-of-life care/hospice **Extraordinary measures** Heart transplantation Chronic inotropes Permanent medical support Experimental surgery or drug therapy

Source: Adapted from Centers for Disease Control and Prevention. Division for Heart Disease and Stroke Prevention. Heart disease fact sheet. 2017. Available from: www.cdc.gov/dhdsp/data_statistics/fact_sheets/ fs_heart_disease.htm.

naturopath is to improve quality of life in all situations.

- Direct interventions aimed at better control of congestive heart failure include herbal medicines, nutritional (dietary and supplemental), lifestyle and education support for patients.
- It is important to manage concurrent illnesses and always ensure that treatment focuses on individualised, patient-centred care.
- In managing heart failure it is essential to use reliable interventions only, so that an accurate assessment can be made of both the cost versus benefit of the treatment, as well as how the naturopathic and conventional treatment can integrate for better outcomes.

Chronic heart failure is a serious disease, with serious consequences. Some of these patients will be on the cardiac transplant waiting list. We have an ethical responsibility to:

- Manage the disease using reliable interventions only. Do not rely on product manufacturers or extrapolations without evidence as they can be dangerous (e.g. ginger, garlic, vitamin C, bioflavonoids). Above all, manage the individual, not just the disease.

Specific treatment objectives

PRIMARY TREATMENT OBJECTIVES

- Improved exercise tolerance (patient-reported change upon 'standardised exercise')
- Improved contractility (and relaxation) of ventricles
- Reduced fluid load (if relevant)
- Reduced pressure load
- Improved subjective quality of life and vitality.

SECONDARY TREATMENT OBJECTIVES

- Control hypertension
- Treat ischaemia if present
- Manage physiological stress, improve stress adaptation and mood
- Investigate psychological state of the patient and manage any depression
- Manage opportunistic, preexisting, complicating or unrelated illnesses
- Rule out anaemia as a comorbidity, and if present then manage the anaemia with urgency
- Watch for signs of infections, especially lung infections. Manage concurrent lung infections quickly and reliably, and consider referral for investigation to ensure cough and dyspnoea are not secondary to worsening pulmonary oedema
- Ensure B vitamin dietary intake is adequate, and if not then supplement
- In obese patients instigate a plan for long-term weight reduction
- Evaluate patient for hypothyroidism, especially if body weight is unresponsive to normal weight loss treatment, or if other signs indicate the possibility of hypothyroidism. Note that many of the symptoms of chronic heart failure and hypothyroidism are similar and therefore become a diagnostic challenge
- While not common, thyrotoxicosis can be life-threatening in patients with chronic heart failure, especially if it is secondary to coronary ischaemia.

NUTRITIONAL MEDICINE (DIETARY)

Dietary therapeutic objectives

Control hypertension
- Regulate sodium intake
- Increase fibre, fresh fruit and vegetables and essential fatty acids
- Reduce saturated and trans fats
- Avoid alcohol, smoking

Treat ischaemia if present
- Encourage adequate hydration
- Encourage fresh fruits and vegetables
- Avoid sodium excess

Manage physiological stress, improve stress adaptation and mood
- Balance blood sugar levels
- Encourage adequate protein (vegetarian and fish especially)

Manage opportunistic, preexisting, complicating or unrelated illnesses
- Anaemia — iron and vitamin B-rich foods, reduce carbohydrate intake (especially refined)
- Infections — vitamin C-rich foods, avoid sugar

Treat complicating factors
- B vitamin deficiencies — vitamin B-rich foods, reduce carbohydrate intake (especially refined)
- Liver disease — avoid alcohol and caffeine and encourage adequate fibre and leafy green vegetables
- Obesity — modify dietary intake to balance weight for healthy weight range.

Specific dietary treatments

DIETARY INCLUSIONS

Water

Given that many patients with heart failure will concurrently be taking diuretics, adequate intake of water is imperative to ensure proper hydration. Many physicians recommend restricting fluid intake to counteract fluid retention; however, adequate fluid intake for healthy bodily functioning is still important. In more advanced cases of heart failure, careful monitoring of fluid intake is essential and will be guided by the cardiologist. In this case it is important to ensure that whatever fluid volume the patient is consuming does not include potentially pathogenic influences (e.g. coffee, tea, sugar, phosphates) which may increase diuresis, worsen sympathetic compensation or lead to electrolyte disturbances.

Essential fatty acids

Essential fatty acids, in particular those found in fish, appear to be therapeutically beneficial in heart failure. Mozafarrian et al[333] observed that regular consumption of baked and boiled fish was linked to a lower incidence of heart failure. Similarly, a Japanese study noted that consumption of fish was associated with a reduced mortality from heart failure.[334] More recently, fatty fish consumed as little as 1–2 times per week was found to be associated with a lower rate of heart failure hospitalisation or death in Swedish middle-aged and older women.[335]

Fresh fruit and vegetables

Fresh fruit and vegetables are a natural source of vitamins, minerals and antioxidants, all of which are likely to be useful in promoting cardiovascular health. Intake of fruit and vegetables is associated with a reduction in the risk of heart failure in men,[336] hence the diet should include a variety of in-season fruit and vegetables, preferably with each meal.

DIETARY EXCLUSIONS

Sodium

In the West, many people consume excessive amounts of salt. This is detrimental at the best of times but never more so than in heart failure, when the excess of salt causes the body to retain water, resulting in fluid retention. Patients with heart failure are typically advised to reduce their sodium intake to <2.4 g/day (ideally <2 g/day). See the discussion in the section on hypertension for a full review of this dietary aspect.

Coffee and other caffeinated substances

Caffeine has been shown to have a detrimental effect on arterial stiffness in numerous studies[337] and is a risk factor for heart failure,[338], however some methyl xanthines (such as theobromine) may be beneficial. In fact theobromine (found in *Theobroma cacao*) and related xanthine derivatives were previously used in the management of heart failure,[339] especially in combination with digitalis.[340]

Alcohol

Heavy alcohol consumption plays a role in the development of heart failure[341] and will aggravate symptoms. Not only does alcohol rob the body of vital nutrients, it has also been suggested to depress myocardial contractibility.[342] Some studies have suggested that light drinking may exert a protective effect in heart failure, but given the other detrimental effects of alcohol in the body, intake is not recommended from a naturopathic perspective.

Saturated fats and fried foods

A diet that is high in saturated fat, in particular trans fats, is associated with increased monocyte production of pro-inflammatory cytokines such as tumour necrosis factor alpha and interleukin (IL)-1β and IL-6.[343] These cytokines have been linked to increased mortality from heart failure[344] hence a thorough analysis is required of the diet to check saturated fat content. Trans fats are non-essential in the body therefore they should be removed and replaced with good fats. Fried foods are generally high in saturated and trans fats and retain little if anything in the way of nutrition, thus these in particular must be removed from the diet.

Sugar

Animal studies have shown that a diet high in sugar results in cardiac dysfunction.[345] Intake of sugar affects insulin release and in the presence of hypertension stimulates cardiac signalling mechanisms leading to an increase in left ventricular hypertrophy, larger end-diastolic and end-systolic diameters, decreased ejection fraction and subsequent development of heart failure.[345,346] Patients should be advised on the link between sugar and heart failure and educated on the different terminology used to describe sugar (e.g. corn starch, maltodextrin).

NUTRITIONAL MEDICINE (SUPPLEMENTAL)

Nutritional medicine therapeutic objectives

- Improve myocardial contractility
- Control hypertension
- Treat ischaemia if present
- Improve myocardial energy metabolism: K^+/Mg^{2+}, coenzyme Q10, B complex
- Manage physiological stress, improve stress adaptation and mood
- Manage opportunistic, preexisting, complicating or unrelated illnesses: anaemia, infections
- Treat complicating factors: B vitamin deficiencies, liver disease, obesity, thyrotoxicosis.

Specific nutrients required

B COMPLEX

The B vitamins are highly important in heart failure due to their multiple functions in the body, including energy production, particularly that for the failing heart. Deficiencies are highly common and can complicate patient health and improvement. Hospitalised patients with heart failure have been found to be deficient in several B vitamins, including thiamine, riboflavin and pyridoxine.[347,348] This is astounding given the low recommended daily intake levels of B vitamins by conventional standards; realistically this intake should be easily met. Optimal thiamine status in particular is recognised as being crucial in patients with heart failure, as deficiency of thiamine results in altered cardiac function and may mimic the signs and symptoms of heart failure.[349] Stress increases requirements for B vitamins as does the use of certain medications such as the loop diuretics used extensively in patients with heart failure. The latter may cause hyperexcretion of B vitamins, increasing risk of deficiency and further highlighting the importance of maintaining good levels of B vitamins. Elevated levels of homocysteine have been linked to heart failure,[350,351] hence the importance of the B vitamins in particular vitamins B_6, B_9 and B_{12} as low levels of these vitamins are associated with hyperhomocysteinaemia.

MAGNESIUM

Magnesium is required for over 300 metabolic reactions within the body,[352] including transport of calcium and potassium ions across the cell membrane and ATP production. Individuals with heart failure have been found to be deficient in magnesium; this may be in part due to urinary loss of magnesium as a result of diuretic use or other medications such as digitalis (digoxin). The determination of serum magnesium is an unreliable method to estimate the magnesium status of a patient, because most magnesium is bound within cells and tissues. Thus the clinician must rely on careful case taking and symptomatic relief following prescription. Due to the non-toxic nature of the prescription, a starting dose of 500 mg is safe and realistic, with increases dependent on patient presentation and their response.

In a monocentric, controlled, double-blind study,[353] 79 patients with severe congestive heart failure (NYHA class IV) under optimal medical cardiovascular treatment were randomised to receive either magnesium orotate (6000 mg for 1 month, 3000 mg for about 11 months, $n = 40$) or placebo ($n = 39$). Both groups were comparable in demographic data, duration of heart failure and pre- and concomitant treatment.

After mean treatment duration of 1 year (magnesium orotate: 364.1 ± 14.7 days, placebo: 361.2 ± 12.7 days) the survival rate was 75.7% compared with 51.6% under placebo ($p < 0.05$). Clinical symptoms improved in 38.5% of patients under magnesium orotate, whereas they deteriorated in 56.3% of patients under placebo ($p < 0.001$). The results of this study support former epidemiological studies in which for 7–37% of patients with heart failure a magnesium deficit was found, caused

SAMPLE DAILY DIET

BREAKFAST	
Heart healthy smoothie: coconut water, soaked oats, cocoa, spinach, avocado plus banana	Cocoa and spinach are rich in antioxidants and electrolytes. They both contain magnesium to improve myocardial energy metabolism. Adequate nutrition is particularly important for individuals with heart failure as the risk for developing electrolyte imbalances and vitamin and micronutrient deficiencies increases with the use of diuretics, in particular vitamin B_1. Coconut water and fruit such as banana replenish electrolytes such as potassium while oats provide a source of thiamine.
LUNCH	
Ratatouille served on top of sweet potato mash	A low-fat and low-sodium, largely vegetarian diet is associated with better cardiovascular health. A low-sodium diet is also associated with better quality of life in individuals with heart failure. Ample herbs and spices can be used to ensure adequate flavour when replacing sodium. Lycopene found in cooked tomato products exhibits cardioprotective potential.
DINNER	
Warm brown rice salad made from organic brown rice, crushed garlic, cherry tomatoes, blanched asparagus and green beans, artichokes, lettuce and fresh turkey/chicken breast Dress with the juice of ½ lemon and a splash of olive oil Herb-crusted oily fish with green beans, broccoli, new potatoes drizzled with lemon juice and vinegar	This is based on a variety of nutrient-dense wholefoods and thus is low in salt. Brown rice is a good source of B vitamins which are required for energy production and a number of enzyme processes within the body. The addition of protein in the form of chicken/turkey helps to prevent cachexia, but ensure it is not smoked or salted. Asparagus provides a natural diuretic. This dinner is modelled from recommendations detailed on the DASH sodium-restricted diet which observed improved energy substrate utilisation in individuals with heart failure, following a diet that was low in sodium. Vegetables are potassium rich and can be dressed with herbs and lemon to flavour food.
SNACKS	
Raw nuts and seeds Chopped banana served with natural yoghurt and pumpkin seeds Carrot and celery sticks with home-made hummus	Nut consumption is associated with lower incidence of CVD. Choose raw, unsalted nuts that are as fresh as possible. Bananas are a rich source of potassium; yoghurt and pumpkin seeds provide protein and essential fatty acid requirements. Celery is a rich source of potassium and hummus provides protein and essential fatty acids.

for example by reduced absorption, neurohormonal disturbances and/or increased magnesium excretion.[353]

ESSENTIAL FATTY ACIDS

Omega-3 fatty acids show great potential in the therapeutic management of heart disease. Fatty acids have numerous functions in the body, including use as energy substrates within the heart as well as involvement in the regulation of gene-encoding proteins required for myocardial fatty acid uptake and metabolism.[271] In a small pilot study[354] lasting 4.5 months 14 patients with class III to IV heart failure received 5.1 g/day of EPA and DHA and were observed to have reductions in inflammatory mediators, highlighting the anti-inflammatory property of fish oil. In this same study, fish oil was also found to have a positive effect on body weight in patients with heart failure, seemingly reducing cachexia.

Leaf et al have shown that omega-3 fatty acids are incorporated into myocardial cells, altering electrophysiological function in a manner that reduces the vulnerability to ventricular fibrillation. It is thought the anti-arrhythmic effects of omega-3 fatty acids are related to their ability to inhibit the fast, voltage-dependent sodium current and the L-type calcium currents, although evidence of potassium channel modulation has also been suggested.[355]

VITAMIN E

Vitamin E is a fat-soluble antioxidant vitamin. Theoretically, because heart failure is associated with oxidative stress, increased free radical production and subsequent deterioration of the cardiovascular structures, the antioxidant activity of vitamin E would appear to be useful; however, studies have been inconsistent. In a small, uncontrolled study of patients with advanced heart failure given 400 mg/day, vitamin E was found to exert a protective role against a number of oxidants.[356] However, in another study although vitamin E improved antioxidant parameters, no improvements in prognostic or functional indices of heart failure were observed.[357] Further studies are required to elucidate the true efficacy of vitamin E in heart failure.

COENZYME Q10

Coenzyme Q10 may be valuable in congestive heart failure due to its antioxidant properties and role in ATP production and aerobic respiration. Coenzyme Q10 levels are typically decreased in patients with heart failure,[358] highlighting the necessity of supplementation to restore levels. Supplementation with coenzyme Q10 100 mg twice daily has been observed to improve left ventricular function in patients with heart failure,[359] but much higher doses may be used (450–900 mg/day) as patients with advanced heart failure have been observed to have impaired absorption of coenzyme Q10 due to intestinal oedema.[360] A 2014 Cochrane review on coenzyme Q10 in heart failure was inconclusive due to significant methodological heterogeneity in the seven included studies. Additionally it should be noted that the included studies mostly used low-dosage regimens of 100–200 mg daily, with the lowest dosage employed being 100 mg daily and the highest being 10 mg/kg body weight per day.[361] From clinical experience, the minimum effective dosage in heart failure is 150 mg twice daily, with 450–600 mg per day being commonly needed.

VITAMIN C

Vitamin C is a water-soluble vitamin and levels may be decreased in patients with heart failure. Vitamin C has many uses in heart failure including:

- Scavenging of free radicals that aggravate inflammation
- Improving myocardial efficiency[362]
- Improving endothelial function and cardiomyocyte apoptosis[363]
- Improving vagal sinus modulation.[364]

The majority of studies have used infusions as a means of administration but oral supplementation also appears to be beneficial at doses of >2 g.[365] These are best prescribed in divided doses for optimal outcome.

Dosage requirements

The dosage requirements listed below are based on adult doses that have been reported in the literature.

- B complex (all B vitamins) high-dose combination, preferably activated forms. Best to start on lower end of prescription and increase as investigations suggest
  - Thiamine 20–40 mg/day
  - Riboflavin 20–40 mg/day
  - Niacinamide 50–100 mg/day
  - Pantothenic acid 150–300 mg/day
  - Pyridoxine 20–60 mg/day
  - Folinic acid or L-5MTHF 500–1000 micrograms/day
    - > Selection based on methylation assessment
  - Hydroxocobalamin or methylcobalamin 500–1000 micrograms/day
    - > Selection based on methylation assessment
  - Choline 50–100 mg/day
  - Inositol 50–100 mg/day
  - Biotin 250–500 micrograms/day

  Additional B vitamin support:
  - Vitamin B_3 (niacinamide): extra B_3 (100 mg+) is indicated with elevated cholesterol levels
  - Vitamin B_6 (pyridoxine): extra B_6 (75–100 mg) is indicated with elevated homocysteine levels
  - Vitamin B_9 (folinic acid/L5MTHF): extra B_9 (500 micrograms–5 mg) is indicated with elevated homocysteine levels
  - Vitamin B_{12} (hydroxocobalamin or methylcobalamin): extra B_{12} (500–1000 micrograms) is indicated with elevated homocysteine levels
- Magnesium 500–1000 mg/day
- EFAs 5.1 g/day
- Vitamin E 400 IU b.i.d.
- Coenzyme Q10 200–600 mg/day with medical supervision
- Vitamin C >2 g/day in divided doses.

HERBAL MEDICINE

Herbal medicine therapeutic objectives

- Improve myocardial contractility: *Crataegus* spp., *Coleus forskohlii, Panax ginseng, Eleutherococcus senticosus, Terminalia arjuna, Astragalus membranaceus*
- Control hypertension: *Olea europaea, Crataegus* spp., *Coleus forskohlii*
- Avoid depressant sedatives, especially *Humulus lupulus*
- Provide diuretics as required: *Olea europaea*
- Treat ischaemia if present
- Manage physiological stress, improve stress adaptation: *Withania somnifera, Panax ginseng, Eleutherococcus senticosus*, relaxation
- Support mood and address depression if present: *Hypericum perforatum, Panax ginseng, Avena sativa* seed, *Verbena officinalis*
- Manage opportunistic, preexisting, complicating or unrelated illnesses: anaemia, infections
- Treat complicating factors: obesity, anaemia, thyroid disease.

Herbal medicine classes

The herbal medicine classes used for heart failure are summarised in Table 20.35.

TABLE 20.35 Herbal medicine classes used for heart failure

Class	Action
Antioxidant	Protect against oxidation and free radical damage and improve circulation to tissues
Cardioprotective	Protective to the myocardium and decrease the risk of heart damage due to toxins, ischaemia or the oxidative effects of hypertension
Cardio-tonic	Increase the force of contraction of the heart (i.e. positively inotropic), and restore tone and vigour to the heart muscle (i.e. myocardium)
Fibrinolytic	Prevent and reduce the development of insoluble fibrin clots
Other	Nervines, adaptogens, spasmolytics as required

Specific herbal medicines

CRATAEGUS SPP. (HAWTHORN) — BERRIES AND LEAF

Crataegus spp. is one of the most researched botanicals for the management of heart failure. Evidence suggests it has a slight positively inotropic effect, without increasing O_2 demand. While clinical research indicates best results in NYHA classes I–III[366] there is no reason it shouldn't be applied and expected to have some positive impact in class IV: research on *Crataegus spp.* in this more advanced state of heart failure is lacking. Its safety profile is excellent. Most research has been done in Europe and the United States on standardised extracts of leaf and flower.

Crataegus spp. contains a number of different constituents, including flavonoids such as rutin, oligomeric procyanidins, triterpene acids, organic acids and sterols, but the flavonoids and oligomeric procyanidins appear to be the most useful with regard to cardiovascular effects.[367] In Europe the leaves, flowers and berries or a combination have all been used therapeutically.[367] While the leaves and flowers of *Crataegus* have undergone much research, there is relatively little information on the berries apart from traditional evidence. A 2008 study demonstrated significant antioxidant and anti-inflammatory properties of the berries[367] likely to be of use in heart failure. *Crataegus* spp. as a whole exerts numerous functions useful in heart failure including:

- Positive inotropic effects (increases the strength of muscular contraction)
- Increased coronary blood flow
- Increased exercise tolerance
- Increased left ventricular ejection fraction (the fraction of blood pumped out of the left ventricle with each heartbeat).

The German Commission E approves the use of *Crataegus* leaf with flowers for decreasing cardiac output as described in functional NYHA class II.[198] A Cochrane meta-analysis[366] of 10 trials (using leaf and flower extract preparations only) confirms the efficacy of *Crataegus* spp., revealing it to increase the maximal workload in patients with chronic heart failure. Analysis of the data reveals that following supplementation with *Crataegus*, patients with heart failure report improvements in shortness of breath and fatigue when compared with placebo, as well as left ventricular ejection fraction and a subjective sense of wellbeing.

When taken in the dose recommended, *Crataegus* spp. is considered safe with mild side effects,[366] although self-medication in patients with heart failure is unwise. While there has been much speculation about potential drug interactions with hawthorn, with particular concern around the combined use of hawthorn and digitalis drugs, the theoretical concerns remain unsubstantiated in both the clinical research,[368] as well as routine clinical usage.

In Australia, and in Western herbal medicine in general, the berries of hawthorn are historically the favoured part of the plant; however, most of the existing research has been done on extracts of the leaf and flower. Though comparative research on these parts and their relative effectiveness is not yet available, from clinical experience the berries do exert significant positive effects in heart failure.

The authors of the 2008 Cochrane review conclude that:

> *The best evidence that is available suggests that hawthorn extract has significant benefits, compared with placebo, as an adjunctive treatment for patients with chronic heart failure. Reported adverse events were infrequent, mild, and transient.*[366]

Crataegus combined with low-dosage *Panax ginseng* (approximately 125–200 mg dry root twice daily) can be particularly effective in patients with class II or III heart failure with significant debility and/or depression.

WITHANIA SOMNIFERA (ASHWAGANDHA)

Withania somnifera is a rejuvenating tonic that may be useful in heart failure due to its ability to replenish the body and increase longevity, particularly where there is debility. As well as its adaptogen properties, animal studies have suggested that *Withania somnifera* may have cardio-tonic[369] and cardioprotective properties,[370] demonstrated through its ability to restore antioxidant status to the myocardium as well as preservation of left ventricular function.

ASTRAGALUS MEMBRANACEUS (ASTRAGALUS)

Astragalus membranaceus has been studied extensively in Chinese medicine for its effects on the cardiovascular system. It contains a number of constituents, including astragaloside IV, a saponin observed to have a protective effect on cardiac function via its antioxidant abilities. In-vivo studies reveal the ability of astragaloside IV to prevent biochemical and haemodynamic changes in the failing heart as well as depression in sarcoplasmic reticulum Ca^{2+} transport thus promoting cardiovascular health.[371] The majority of studies to date have been of poor quality and clinical research evidence to support prescription is lacking. There is some convincing laboratory and animal research. Clinical experience supports usage for positive inotropic (mild) and adaptogen (especially for debilitated patients) prescriptions.

LEONURUS CARDIACA (MOTHERWORT)

Leonurus cardiaca has been used traditionally since the 15th century for the treatment of cardiovascular disorders.[372] It has hypotensive and sedative properties, making it useful for cardiac debility.[215] The German Commission E approves the use of *Leonurus cardiaca* for nervous cardiac disorders[198] and also makes mention of its cardio-tonic action. While modern studies in humans are lacking, its clinical use should be considered, especially in tachyarrhythmias associated with heart failure.

OLEA EUROPAEA FOLIA (OLIVE LEAF)

Research has been carried out into the use of *Olea europaea* for the treatment and prevention of infections, but supportive evidence for heart failure is variable and generally unreliable. Olive leaf's primary cardiovascular actions have been defined as diuretic, and in-vitro and in-vivo animal research indicates calcium channel blockage-like activity.[373]

Clinically, olive leaf is an excellent choice to reduce fluid load in combination with hawthorn. From clinical experience, it is more beneficial than *Taraxacum officinale* folia for cardiovascular applications and can be coadministered with conventional diuretics if required. This can be beneficial if the fluid load is still high or if sufficient diuretic dose causes significant adverse reactions.

LIFESTYLE RECOMMENDATIONS

Counselling and education

- Educate patients as to what congestive heart failure is and how it works
- Encourage self-monitoring of symptoms, weight, etc. (diary useful)
- Counsel how quality of life can be improved and the things patients can still do in their lives
- Review work/home environment, encouraging purpose and usefulness in life
- Do not underestimate the incidence of depression. Support and refer accordingly
- While appropriate exercise regimens don't seem to impact all-cause mortality in the short term, they can improve quality of life outcomes and reduce hospitalisation risk in patients with heart failure.[374] Before exercise advice is given, expert guidance should be sought.

Smoking

Smoking is a risk factor for heart failure and is likely to further aggravate symptoms such as shortness of breath. In one study, smoking was associated with a 45% higher risk of heart failure in men and an 88% higher risk of heart failure in women, hence the benefits of quitting.[375]

Stress

Stress has been shown to impact cardiovascular function in numerous studies. One interesting example is the increased incidence of pulmonary embolism that has been noted to occur after earthquakes due to the stress![376] Similarly, Wittstein et al[377] observed patients who had undergone intensely stressful emotional experiences, such as death in the family, and subsequently presented with altered left ventricular function. Stress management techniques that are personally relevant for the patient should be discussed and implemented.

Exercise

A meta-analysis of randomised controlled trials published in the *British Medical Journal* found exercise training to significantly improve survival time in patients with chronic heart failure due to left ventricular systolic dysfunction.[378] The studies involved patients working within 50–80% of peak oxygen consumption and used a mixture of different exercise techniques including cycling and walking. Importantly, all exercise undertaken in these studies was supervised, thus the use of an exercise physiologist or the like is likely to be beneficial in terms of both skills and safety for patients with heart failure. It is essential to obtain approval and recommendation from the patient's cardiologist prior to prescription.

When the patient is stable, exercise should only be recommended within tolerance levels. If they are unstable, bed rest is required. Exercise objectives should be conservative and achievable but should encourage long-term increase in duration and intensity.

Weight

Congestive heart failure prognosis is negatively associated with obesity. As such, supporting patients to reach their optimal weight is beneficial. It is important to prevent any dietary extremes and encourage supervised exercise and regulated dietary measures to achieve this. It is also imperative that weight is assessed holistically and determination of fluid content vs fat content is achieved prior to assuming specific weight loss requirements.

Contraceptive options

As female patients with congestive heart failure (especially those in class III or IV) are at risk of maternal death from pregnancy/childbirth it is imperative that contraceptive options are discussed thoroughly. Barrier methods are the preferred option due to risk of thromboembolism with some hormonal preparations.

CASE STUDY

OVERVIEW

RJ was a 61-year-old man with NYHA class III, borderline class IV congestive heart failure. Walking on level ground slowly for more than 75 m caused dyspnoea and severe fatigue. Recovery time for such exertion was approximately 10 minutes. The origin of the patient's congestive heart failure was a viral cardiomyopathy contracted 26 years prior. He experienced occasional resting fatigue and dyspnoea and was overweight; however, examination revealed that the excessive weight was at least in part due to fluid retention. Resting blood pressure was 125/75 mmHg. He suffered from mild-to-moderate depression and was poorly educated regarding congestive heart failure and its effects on his health. His quality of life was low — he lived on a country property but was unable to maintain the upkeep (his wife managed most of it), which contributed to his depression.

Current treatment consisted of:

- Enalapril 30 mg daily, which was causing a mild bradykinin cough in the patient
- Furosemide (frusemide) 60 mg daily, with this high dose causing a feeling of 'dryness' and further reducing

CASE STUDY CONTINUED

quality of life due to regular urination. There was a distinct possibility that this diuretic was also bringing out latent mild benign prostatic hyperplasia manifesting with nocturia, further reducing the patient's quality of life
- Vitamin E: 500 IU daily
- Coenzyme Q10: 10 mg daily combined with a B complex supplement.

The patient believed these combined treatments provided mild improvement in heart failure and quality of life, but not significant improvement.

THERAPEUTIC OBJECTIVES

The initial treatment objectives were:
- Improve myocardial capability, thus increasing cardiac output
- Further reduce fluid load, without worsening adverse effects from furosemide (frusemide).

HERBAL TREATMENT

Herbal medicine	DER	Quantity per week	Rationale
Crataegus monogyna berries and leaves	1:2	50 mL	Mild cardio-tonic
Olea europaea	1:1	50 mL	Diuretic

Dose: 5 mL three times daily, or if more convenient 7.5 mL twice daily.

NUTRITIONAL TREATMENT

Initial nutritional treatment was conservative to avoid overloading the patient and involved:
- Increased dose of coenzyme Q10 to 150 mg daily.

OUTCOMES (WEEK 6)

RJ expressed a slight improvement in exercise tolerance — his 75 m level walk resulted in less severe dyspnoea and fatigue. Recovery time from this exertion was also reduced to about 5 minutes. The patient also mentioned that his resting fatigue had improved as well.

The assessment at this stage was that possible early improvement was being noted; however, more time was required for more significant improvement.

As a result the same treatment was continued.

OUTCOMES (WEEKS 7–12)

RJ's wife phoned during week 10 of treatment, stating that the patient had accidentally been taking 3 of the 150 mg coenzyme Q10 for 3 weeks. The cause of this accidental dosage increase was related to the geographical separation between the patient and the clinic. He ran out of the prescribed coenzyme Q10 supplement, and the only product readily available in the local area was a 50 mg capsule, so I advised him to purchase this and take 3 per day until I was able to send more of the previous capsules by post. Once

CASE STUDY CONTINUED

these arrived with the patient, he mistakenly continued taking 3 of the capsules per day, but they were now 150 mg, resulting in a total dose of 450 mg per day as opposed to the prescribed 150 mg. RJ's initial response to this increased dosage was massive fluid loss, and then significant improvement in exercise tolerance after 2 weeks. The cost versus benefit was discussed with the patient, and it was decided to continue same dose. Herbal prescription remained unchanged.

OUTCOMES (WEEK 21)

RJ had a recent cardiology consultation, during which his cardiologist apparently stated 'Unbelievable! Keep up whatever you are doing.' The patient had lost more than 8 kg of fluid. Exercise tolerance was also significantly improved with a 400 m walk on a 20–30 degree incline being sustainable, even with about 5 kg of weight carried. While RJ experienced moderate dyspnoea at the end of this exertion, combined with moderate fatigue, his recovery time was only 5 min. The patient's mood had also improved significantly.

This increased CoQ10 dosage resulted in very significant improvement. During the time this patient was under my care, CoQ10 was a very expensive supplement, and thus my prescribing was quite conservative in regards to dosage. This episode was a significant lesson in the need for substantive dosages of CoQ10 in heart failure.

CARDIAC ARRHYTHMIAS

Epidemiology

Cardiac arrhythmias (also known as dysrhythmias) are a group of conditions defined by abnormalities in the generation and/or conduction of myocardial electrical impulses, which result in rhythm disturbances of the heart. Almost any structural or functional abnormality of the heart can lead to cardiac rhythm disturbance, as can a number of systemic neurological, endocrine and haematological abnormalities.[378]

Classification

There are a number of ways cardiac arrhythmias may be classified, however one of the most common is based on whether episodic or continual rhythm tends to be slower than normal — bradyarrhythmias — or faster than normal — tachyarrhythmias. Episodes of bradycardia are defined as a resting heart rate of less than 60 beats per minute, and episodes of tachycardia as a resting heart rate of more than 100 beats per minute.[111] Of course this is contextual; some highly trained athletes can have extremely low resting heart rates, and normal individuals during intense exercise or under acute stress (e.g. fear) can have very fast heart rates.

The various tachy- and bradyarrhythmias can be subclassified based upon the nature and location of the conduction disturbance, and whether or not the rhythm disturbance primarily affects the atria or ventricles.

Aetiology

The causes of cardiac arrhythmias are many and diverse. Broadly they can be divided into intracardiac and extracardiac causes.

Intracardiac causes can include:[379]

- Congenital abnormalities of structure (such as accessory atrioventricular connection)
- Congenital abnormalities of function (such as hereditary ion channelopathies)
- Structural damage (such as occurs from myocardial infarction or cardiac hypertrophy).

Extracardiac causes can include:[379]

- Hypoxia
- Endocrine disorders (e.g. hypothyroidism or hyperthyroidism)
- Electrolyte imbalances
- Toxins (such as ethanol, caffeine and some drugs).

Overview

The most common presenting symptoms of cardiac arrhythmias include palpitations, dizziness and syncope,[128] but additional symptoms can include fatigue, dyspnoea, and chest pain. However all three of these symptoms can be due to a variety of different non-cardiac causes, and different cardiac arrhythmias present with different combinations and frequency of occurrence of these primary symptoms.

As palpitations are one of the most common symptoms, it is essential for both the clinician and the patient to understand the definition and nature of palpitations. Strictly speaking, palpitations are defined as an uncomfortable awareness of the heartbeat, and while they are a common symptom of cardiac arrhythmias, their presence in the patient does not always equate to a true arrhythmia. Conversely some cardiac arrhythmias can be entirely asymptomatic.[380]

Pathogenesis (general)

The primary mechanisms of tachycardia are:[111]

- An increase in automaticity (i.e. where there is repeated spontaneous ectopic depolarisation)
- Re-entry circuit (i.e. where two alternative conduction pathways exist resulting in different conduction and recovery speeds) which is the most common mechanism of tachyarrhythmias
- Secondary depolarisation from an incompletely repolarised membrane.

The primary mechanisms of bradycardia are:[111]

- A reduction in automaticity
- A blocked or slow conduction (e.g. atrioventricular block).

DIFFERENTIAL DIAGNOSIS

Due to the fact that the symptoms of arrhythmias can be highly variable and mimic many other cardiac and non-cardiac conditions, careful evaluation is essential. This will be a combination of clinical evaluation (patient history and physical examination) and electrophysiological studies of various forms (discussed at length under 'Investigations').

If a patient presents with palpitations, the first approach should be thorough questioning of the patient's medical history. Some key issues and questions to be considered are shown in the Table 20.36.

TABLE 20.36 Clinical questions and issues in the evaluation of palpitations

Nature of the palpitations	Duration of episodes? Frequency of episodes? Associated chest pain? Associated dyspnoea? Associated lightheadness? How and when does the episode commence? How and when does the episode stop?
Underlying heart disease	Angina or prior myocardial infarction? Valvular heart disease? Congenital heart disease? Cardiomyopathy? Coronary risk factors? Congestive heart failure? Prior antiarrhythmic treatment?
Precipitating factors	Psychological stress? Exercise? Caffeine, cocaine, amphetamine or other CNS/sympathetic nervous system stimulants? Alcohol? Thyroid disease? Anaemia or hypoxia?

Source: Adapted from Table 10.1 in Hlatky MA. Approach to the patient with palpitations. In: Goldman L, Braunwald E, editors. Primary cardiology. Philadelphia: WB Saunders Company; 1998.

Investigations (general)

GENERAL INVESTIGATIONS

Medical history and physical examination

A complete medical history will be the first investigation, which may then trigger further investigations. Physical examination is generally the next step, involving thorough chest auscultation. The first question is whether auscultation reveals signs of other cardiac disease (such as valvular disease, heart failure) which may explain the symptoms.[380] As this requires a highly trained and experienced ear, such examination is usually outside the scope of most naturopaths and is better conducted by a cardiologist. It is also important to remember that true arrhythmias are often episodic in nature, so physical examination between episodes may reveal no abnormalities.

Electrocardiography

A baseline electrocardiograph (ECG) is essential in the early evaluation of any patient with symptoms of possible cardiac arrhythmia. Interpretation of ECG traces requires significant expertise, and may be normal in patients with paroxysmal episodes, thus a normal baseline ECG does not necessarily rule out a cardiac arrhythmia. Ideally an ECG should be conducted during an episode, but obviously this may not be practical in the standard setting, hence ambulatory monitoring may be very useful.[381]

Ambulatory monitoring

There are three types of ambulatory monitoring used to monitor patients with paroxysmal episodes over an extended period in a normal daily environment, in an effort to capture one or more episodes. Holter monitors are wearable ECG monitors which can record for 24–48 hours. Event monitors record when an aberration of normal rhythm is detected (some can be activated by the patient when they feel symptomatic), and can be worn for days to weeks or even months if needed. Implantable loop recorders are similar to event monitors but more invasive as they require a minor surgical procedure to implant; however, they can offer greater accuracy in difficult to diagnose conditions.[381]

NATUROPATHIC INVESTIGATIONS

There are no specific naturopathic investigations for cardiac arrhythmias. If rhythm disorders are suspected to be secondary to electrolyte disturbances, blood potassium, magnesium and calcium evaluation may be valuable and guide treatment.

ATRIAL FIBRILLATION

Epidemiology

The most common sustained arrhythmia is atrial fibrillation (AF). The prevalence increases with age, with approximately 2–5% of 70-year-olds and 9% of those over 80 years of age being affected.[111]

Classification

Atrial fibrillation is a type of tachyarrhythmia involving fast and uncoordinated atrial beats. It may be classified into five different types based upon onset, frequency, and ability for return to normal sinus rhythm. The five classifications are:[382]

- Acute atrial fibrillation — new onset, lasting less than 48 hours
- Paroxysmal atrial fibrillation — recurrent episodes, lasting less than 48 hours, converting spontaneously to sinus rhythm without treatment
- Persistent atrial fibrillation — episodes lasting more than 1 week or requiring treatment to convert back to sinus rhythm
- Long-standing persistent atrial fibrillation — episodes lasting more than 1 year, still with the possibility of restoring sinus rhythm with appropriate treatment (usually electrical cardioversion)
- Permanent atrial fibrillation — spontaneous or treatment-induced conversion to sinus rhythm is not possible.

Aetiology

The primary causes of AF are:[111]

- Ischaemic heart disease
- Valvular heart disease
- Hypertension
- Sinoatrial disease
- Hyperthyroidism
- Alcohol
- Cardiomyopathy
- Congenital heart disease
- Chest infection
- Pulmonary embolism
- Pericardial disease
- Idiopathic (roughly 50% of all patients are diagnosed with paroxysmal AF, and 20% with persistent or permanent AF).

Pathogenesis

In AF there are multiple re-entry circuits interacting and looping around the atria. During an episode the atria beats very rapidly and in an uncoordinated manner, resulting in ineffective atrial contraction, with subsequent irregular activation of the ventricles.[111]

SIGNS AND SYMPTOMS

Atrial fibrillation can be asymptomatic and only discovered on routine examination or ECG. Most commonly though it presents with a combination of palpitations, breathlessness, general and vague chest discomfort, and fatigue and sometimes weakness and lightheadness.[111,382] These symptoms are more common in patients with a very rapid episodic ventricular rate of around 140–160 beats per minute.[382]

COMPLICATIONS

The primary complication in AF is thromboembolism, due to blood stasis in the left atrium, and can lead to ischaemic stroke or other ischaemic events systemically. There are many factors which can increase thromboembolic risk in AF patients, including previous ischaemic stroke or transient ischaemic attack, mitral valve disease, diabetes and hypertension, as well as an age over 65 years.[111]

DIFFERENTIAL DIAGNOSIS

One of the primary differential diagnostic considerations in AF is hyperthyroidism, with AF occurring in 15% of patients with hyperthyroidism, as opposed to 4% in the general population, and sub-clinical hyperthyroidism is associated with a three times increase in risk of AF.[383] Additionally it has been shown that treatment of hyperthyroidism can result in conversion to sinus rhythm in approximately two-thirds of patients,[384] therefore evaluation of thyroid function is essential in any patient presenting with the characteristic symptoms and electrophysiological pattern of AF.

NATUROPATHIC DIAGNOSIS

The naturopathic diagnosis of AF largely follows conventional diagnostic guidelines; however, it is more common with naturopathic assessment that close attention will be paid to other precipitating factors. For example, while caffeine is regarded as a rare cause of AF,[385] in naturopathic care it is considered a common precipitating factor, as is frequent consumption of large meals or binge consumption of alcoholic beverages. Therefore in the naturopathic assessment of a patient with AF, it is important to carefully consider the lifestyle and dietary factors which may lower the threshold for the triggering of an AF episode.

Investigations

GENERAL INVESTIGATIONS

Electrocardiography is the primary tool of diagnosis for AF. A classic presentation will involve the absence of P waves, presence of f (fibrillatory) waves between the QRS complexes, and irregularly irregular R-R intervals.[382]

Echocardiography is also important to determine whether structural defects (such as cardiomyopathies) may be present, which can both help in the understanding of causative factors as well as assist in determining the risk of complications.[382]

Finally thyroid function tests are essential as thyrotoxicosis is a well understood cause of AF, and if present should be specifically managed, thus making direct pharmacological or electrophysiological treatment of the AF potentially unnecessary.[382,385]

NATUROPATHIC INVESTIGATIONS

In naturopathic care, the main investigation of clinical relevance is a thorough medical and lifestyle history, in order to understand the impact of AF on the patient's daily life, and also understand more subtle contributing factors and triggers for AF episodes.

Therapeutic considerations

CLINICAL DECISION MAKING AND RATIONALE

A key issue in managing AF is to ensure accurate diagnosis and monitoring, which requires conventional cardiology care. Due to the complexity and enormous variety of possible rhythm disturbances, and the resultant variations in prognosis, such care is essential.

Therapeutic application

ALLOPATHIC PERSPECTIVE

Treatment of AF is dependant first on identifying whether the patient is in an acute state rapid heart rate or in a less immediately severe chronic state.[382] First-line treatment is generally pharmacological, with a range of options being available, the main types of which are illustrated in Table 20.37.

Electrical cardioversion, whereby the heart is totally depolarised by passing an appropriate strength of electrical current through it, is another option. The aim is to 'shock' the heart back into normal rhythm, by totally interrupting the arrhythmia for a brief period. This is conducted under general anaesthetic, and comes with some risk (such as systemic embolism in patients with prolonged atrial arrhythmias).[111] While in many cases cardioversion can be successful in normalising or reducing severity of the

TABLE 20.37 Pharmacological options in the management of cardiac arrhythmias

Type	General mechanism	Main uses	Specific examples
Class 1	Mostly reduction in electrical excitability and slowing of conduction in atrial or ventricular muscle	Prevention and/or treatment of either atrial or ventricular tachyarrhythmias. Some of these are intravenous use within an in-patient setting	Lidocaine, flecainide, propafenone
Class II	Beta-adrenoceptor antagonists (beta-blockers) which reduce the sympathetic nervous stimulation of heart rate	Treatment and prevention of SVT and AF	Atenolol, metaprolol
Class III	Prolong plateau phase of the action potential, resulting in a lengthening of refractory period	Treatment-resistant or serious atrial or ventricular tachyarrhythmias	Amiodarone
Class IV	Calcium channel antagonists — slowing impulse generation and conduction	Continued control of AF; treatment of SVT	Verapamil

Source: Boon NA, Colledge NR, Walker BR, editors. Davidson's principles & practice of medicine. 20th ed. Edinburgh: Churchill Livingstone; 2006.

arrhythmia for a prolonged period, in many cases the arrhythmia can reappear and subsequent cardioversions months or years later may be necessary. If subsequent cardioversion fails, other treatment options may be required.

Cardiac catheter ablation is a relatively new intervention and can be remarkably effective. A series of catheter electrodes are inserted into the heart and activity is monitored and sometimes altered to observe the focal location contributing to the arrhythmia. Then a steerable catheter is introduced into that area of the heart, and through application of heat, cold or radiofrequency, that area is partially ablated.[111] Ablation therapy can be far more successful in more intractable cases when combined with appropriate lifestyle and dietary treatment.

In addition to direct rhythm control, anticoagulant treatment is required, due to the increased risk of thromboembolic events (especially stroke). Guidelines vary as to the most appropriate medication; the most commonly employed is aspirin or warfarin. Warfarin appears superior in terms of stroke risk reduction, however issues such as an increase in bleeding risk and the need for constant monitoring need to be taken into consideration with warfarin prescription.[111]

HISTORICAL PERSPECTIVE

In the 1960s AF was primarily controlled with an early form of cardioversion using either quinidine or a direct current electrical shock, and digitalis was commonly recommended for rate control. Warfarin was only generally used prior to cardioversion, with the discovery of the benefit of persistent anticoagulation therapy in stroke prevention only occurring in the 1990s.[386]

NATUROPATHIC PERSPECTIVE

The naturopathic management of diagnosed AF is primarily supportive and complementary. While modern cardiology offers very specific and often very effective primary care for the patient with AF, there remain a number of therapeutic gaps which can be well managed through the addition of naturopathic care.

Identifying and addressing known/suspected triggers

Whether the patient has intermittent or constant arrhythmia, finding and minimising dietary, lifestyle and psychosocial triggers is important. This approach, combined with specific herbal treatment, can further reduce the frequency, severity and duration of episodes. However in persistent/constant arrhythmia, while still somewhat beneficial, this approach may be less effective and other treatment goals such as general wellbeing will be a more significant objective.

Reducing drug adverse reactions

Some of the commonly used medications can have significant impact on the patient's quality of life in other areas. For example beta-blockers can commonly induce fatigue and mild depression,[111] and amiodarone has a long list of common mild side effects (such as nausea, vomiting, constipation, long-term skin discolouration, photosensitivity, sleep disturbances) and less common but severe adverse reactions (such as liver damage, peripheral neuropathy and thyroid dysfunction).[387] Minimising the adverse impact of these drugs can improve the patient's quality of life, although care must be taken to avoid interfering in the efficacy of these medications by contributing to increased clearance and thus decreased blood/tissue levels.

NUTRITIONAL MEDICINE (DIETARY)

Alcohol and dietary stimulants such as caffeine are known triggers in many patients with existing episodic tachyarrhythmias.[111,388] Thus avoidance is important in these patients.

However the effect of caffeine in increasing AF risk in those without existing rhythm disturbances is controversial. A meta-analysis of 7 studies (6 cohort studies, and 1 case controlled study) with a total of 115 933 patients without existing AF, showed that dietary caffeine was not associated with an increased risk of developing AF and low dose may in fact be associated with a decreased risk.[389]

NUTRITIONAL MEDICINE (SUPPLEMENTAL)

Magnesium

The value of magnesium supplementation in various tachyarrhythmias should not be underestimated, although the most appropriate dosage and form of administration needs further investigation. Research indicates magnesium plays a number of roles in regulating cardiac rhythm, and some studies have shown improvement in patient outcomes when used in combination with antiarrhythmic drugs.[390] From clinical experience, supplemental magnesium in dosages of 300–450 mg (elemental) per day can improve the control of paroxysmal AF, alone or in combination with drug treatment.

Essential fatty acids

While the benefit of fish oil on cardiac rhythm remains controversial,[391] the clinical benefit in AF may lie in helping to reduce thromboembolic complications.[273]

HERBAL MEDICINE

Herbal medicine therapeutic objectives

The main herbal objectives in managing tachyarrhythmias are:

- Reduce known and suspected triggers in episodic tachyarrhythmias
- Assist in normalising sustained rhythm and reducing sensitivity to known/suspected triggers
- Improving quality of life factors (such as fatigue, depression) directly related to the arrhythmia, or as a result of drug therapy
- Reducing the risk of complications (such as stroke risk in AF patients)
- Managing any contributing diseases (such as thyroid disorders).

SAMPLE DAILY DIET

BREAKFAST	
Fruit salad with ground flaxseed plus rooibos tea	Seasonal fruit provides a range of vitamins and antioxidants. Those with atrial fibrillation with higher intakes of antioxidants were shown to have 80% greater odds of spontaneously reverting back to a normal heart rhythm. Fruits rich in lycopene such as guava, watermelon and pink grapefruit can be favoured, since lycopene has an affinity for the cardiovascular system. Flaxseed is used as a source of fibre and healthy fats. It may be used to assist with reducing hypertension, the latter of which may commonly coexist with AF and increase risk of an incident of AF.
LUNCH	
Gazpacho with crusty sourdough	In patients with atrial fibrillation, management of hypertension may reverse structural changes in the heart, reduce thromboembolic complications, and retard or prevent the occurrence of atrial fibrillation. Gazpacho is a Mediterranean vegetable-based cold soup rich in phytochemicals. Consumption is inversely associated with a reduction in prevalence of hypertension in individuals with high CVD risk. The association between gazpacho intake and reduction of BP is probably due to synergy among several bioactive compounds present in the vegetable ingredients used to make the recipe. A Mediterranean diet is associated with reduced incidence of vascular events in those with atrial fibrillation. This appears to be due to its ability to improve antioxidant levels as well as reducing thromboxane A2 production improving platelet function. This diet was shown to not effect anticoagulant medication and thus can be recommended for AF patients who are taking vitamin K analogues.
DINNER	
Salad: rocket, spinach, roast pumpkin, sesame, tempeh, nori, cucumber and ginger	Green leafy vegetables provide magnesium, folate and vitamin K. Magnesium functions as an atrial antiarrhythmic agent and low serum magnesium is moderately associated with the development of AF in individuals without cardiovascular disease. Elevated homocysteine is a risk factor for both AF and stroke, thus foods rich in folate (e.g. leafy greens) and vitamin B_{12} (nori) are recommended to lower homocysteine. Stroke risk can be modified in individuals with AF by using foods that exhibit natural anticoagulant with antiplatelet activity such as ginger, garlic and turmeric.

Herbal medicine classes

The primary classes of herbal medicines of benefit in AF include:

- Mild sedatives
- Adaptogens (most especially calming adaptogens such as *Withania somnifera*, with stimulating adaptogens such as *Panax ginseng* usually being contraindicated in tachyarrhythmias)
- Antiarrhythmics

Specific herbal medicines

LEONURUS CARDIACA (MOTHERWORT)

A number of the medicinal plants regarded as useful in arrhythmias — such as *Sarothamnus scoparius* and *Gelsemium sempervirens*[110] — are Scheduled medicines in Australia and thus not available to naturopaths or herbalists.

However *Leonurus cardiaca* (motherwort), while gentle, is of considerable value in tachyarrhythmias. While lacking in human clinical trials, *Leonurus* is listed in the British Herbal Pharmacopoeia of 1983 as a specific for 'cardiac symptoms associated with neurosis' and is said to be indicated for tachycardia.[108] Historically it was regarded as mild in action, with Cook stating that it was useful in 'hysterical forms of nervousness and palpitation' and 'as a tonic for nervousness, pains and palpitation of the heart',[392] and Ellingwood stating that it 'would work well combined with cactus or crataegus or both'.[5]

From clinical experience, motherwort is the single most effective anti-arrhythmic herbal medicine currently available for use in Australia, especially when it is combined with *Crataegus monogyna/laevigata* berries.

CRATAEGUS MONOGYNA (HAWTHORN)

While not a specific antiarrhythmic medicine, the overall tonic and normalising effect of hawthorn berries on the heart is highly valued, and traditional literature indicates that it is useful in paroxysmal tachycardia.[108] It should generally be used as a supportive medicine in conjunction with more specific medicines such as *Leonurus*.

SALVIA MILTIORRHIZA (DAN SHEN) OR *ALLIUM SATIVUM* (GARLIC)

With the increased risk of thromboembolic events in patients with atrial fibrillation, consideration should be given to reducing clotting risk. While the conventional use of warfarin and aspirin has already been discussed, there is a place (particularly when the patient is maintained on aspirin alone, or when they are unable to tolerate either medication) for herbal medicine in this role.

Both *Salvia miltiorrhiza* and *Allium sativum* are clinically relevant anticoagulants[273,393] and while it is generally accepted that *Salvia miltiorrhiza* should not be used in conjunction with warfarin,[393] a number of studies suggest garlic can be used safely with warfarin despite theoretical pharmacodynamic concerns.[273]

From clinical experience, if the patient is taking warfarin there is little if any need for additional herbal anticoagulants; however, if the patient is maintained on aspirin alone, then addition of one of these two herbal medicines, as well as fish oil, is a sensible intervention.

LIFESTYLE RECOMMENDATIONS

Atrial fibrillation can have a significant impact on the lifestyle of patients. Many patients become understandably nervous of involving themselves in activities which may trigger episodes, or activities where, if an episode was triggered, the patient would become at risk of accident or trauma (for example, swimming, rock climbing). Thus lifestyle counselling can be of benefit, and must be tailored to the nature and severity of the arrhythmia and the patient's particular needs and desires. In turn this can alter the focus of pharmacological or surgical treatment in some cases.[394]

SUPRAVENTRICULAR TACHYCARDIA

Epidemiology

Supraventricular tachycardias (SVTs or re-entrant supraventricular tachycardias) involve re-entrant electrical pathways resulting in sudden onset of palpitations with equally sudden resolution. The various types of SVTs occur in approximately 2 or 3 people out of 1000, more commonly in females (62%), with the average age of onset being 45 years.[395]

Classification

Supraventricular tachycardia (SVT) describes a range of tachycardic conditions with similar electrocardiograph appearance, caused either by a re-entry circuit in the right atrium and atrioventricular node, or an abnormal strip of conductive tissue connecting the atria and the ventricles (e.g. Wolff-Parkinson-White syndrome).[111,396]

Aetiology

Supraventricular tachycardias are regarded as idiopathic in nature; however, this type of rhythm disturbance is more common in patients with some types of existing cardiac dysfunction, such as cardiomyopathy.[396]

Pathogenesis

SIGNS AND SYMPTOMS

Commonly SVTs present from early adulthood to early middle age, and patients usually present with episodes of palpitations followed by dyspnoea, chest discomfort, lethargy and lightheadness, and heart rates usually between 160 and 240 beats per minute. These episodes are usually of rapid onset, and in many cases also cease very abruptly, and may last for a few minutes to a few hours, but rarely more than 12 hours.[396]

COMPLICATIONS

While major complications of SVTs do not generally occur, prolonged lethargy is a common occurrence, often lasting for a few hours after the episode of tachycardia has ceased (author's observation).

DIFFERENTIAL DIAGNOSIS

For naturopaths one of the most important clinical issues in the diagnosis of SVT is differentiation from acute anxiety attacks. As acute episodes of tachycardia can be triggered by stress and/or stimulant usage (such as caffeine),[395] and the presenting somatic signs and symptoms are extremely similar to acute panic attacks,[397] this differentiation can be difficult initially. While it is always wise to investigate panic attacks with significant chest/cardiac symptoms, a key differentiating factor is the heart rate. Palpitations and faster heart rate are normal in panic attacks; however, in SVTs the heart rate elevation is much more significant, commonly over 160 beats per minute.[396]

Additionally, while the clinical features of SVTs are quite specific, it is important to fully investigate the rhythm using ECG. Most SVTs have narrow QRS complex on ECG; however, some do present with a wide QRS complex, and in these cases must be carefully distinguished from ventricular tachycardia.[396]

NATUROPATHIC DIAGNOSIS

Patients presenting to naturopaths with SVTs usually have had the diagnosis confirmed through a cardiology consultation. Nevertheless there are some instances where patients may present with symptoms and signs consistent with the pattern of an SVT without having yet sought conventional medical care. Also patients with existing cardiomyopathy whose symptom picture changes may actually be developing a secondary SVT.[396] In all of these cases a cardiology referral for further diagnostic examination is essential.

Investigations

GENERAL INVESTIGATIONS

Once SVT is suspected through the patient's clinical history, ECG should be performed. Typically a narrow QRS complex is noted; however, occasionally a wide QRS complex is present, associated with a bundle branch block or an accessory pathway.[395] However due to the paroxysmal pattern of SVT, a 24–48 hour Holter monitor is often required; in some cases an event monitor may be more appropriate.[395]

NATUROPATHIC INVESTIGATIONS

There are no specific naturopathic investigations of relevance in SVTs. However thorough evaluation of the patient's clinical history, especially looking for dietary and lifestyle triggers, is key to the long-term naturopathic care of patients with SVT.

Therapeutic considerations

CLINICAL DECISION MAKING AND RATIONALE

While atrial fibrillation and supraventricular tachycardias are different in terms of their electrophysiological foundations, both AF and SVT are examples of fast rhythms and there are considerable similarities in the naturopathic treatment of both.

Therapeutic application

ALLOPATHIC PERSPECTIVE

The allopathic treatment of SVTs can essentially be divided into acute or long-term management. In acute management, the goal is to slow the heart rate and re-establish sinus rhythm, which can be achieved with either vagal manoeuvres, medications such as adenosine, amiodarone, calcium channel blockers or beta-blockers, or if necessary cardioversion.[395] Long-term management focuses more on prevention of acute episodes, using mostly sodium/calcium channel blockers or beta-blockers. If drug treatment is not satisfactory, catheter ablation may be employed provided an electrophysiological focus point can be located. Cryoablation or radiofrequency ablation techniques can in some cases be highly effective, with success rates in the high 90%.[395]

HISTORICAL PERSPECTIVE

In recent years the treatment of SVT has significantly changed with the introduction of catheter ablation techniques. Dr Melvin Scheinman conducted the first electrical cardiac catheter ablation in 1981 (in this case to treat AF) which, although pioneering, was eventually abandoned due to limited efficacy compared to later techniques employing radiofrequency energy or cryotherapy.[398]

NATUROPATHIC PERSPECTIVE

The naturopathic management of diagnosed SVTs is primarily supportive and complementary. While allopathic pharmacological treatment can be effective, in many cases adverse effects can result in less improvement in the patient's quality of life than might otherwise be expected. Combined care can assist in reducing adverse reactions as well as focusing directly on reducing the frequency and severity of acute episodes.

In managing patients with SVT, finding and minimising dietary, lifestyle and psychosocial triggers is extremely valuable. This will usually require an individualised care plan specific to the patient's particular circumstances and needs, in combination with herbal and/or nutritional pharmacological intervention.

NUTRITIONAL MEDICINE (DIETARY)

There is little research specifically on dietary influences on SVTs, however there are a specific items of interest.

Magnesium

The role of dietary magnesium is interesting. A small randomised double-blind crossover study of 29 postmenopausal women involved two groups, one receiving a magnesium-deficient standardised diet (mean dietary magnesium of 130 mg/day), and one receiving the same diet plus a magnesium supplement (mean dietary magnesium of 411 mg/day — to bring daily magnesium intake to a little above the recommended daily intake). Each phase of the study lasted 81 days, and a total of 22 women completed the full study. Holter monitor data showed that the participants maintained on a magnesium-deficient diet alone had more frequent supraventricular beats, and the sum of supraventricular and ventricular ectopic beats was also greater, compared with the participants maintained on the same diet with supplemental magnesium. The researchers conclude that it is not known whether a magnesium-deficient diet will cause SVT directly, but they do state that 'a diet low in magnesium will probably not benefit persons with valvular disease or cardiac hypertrophy or persons who consume toxins such as alcohol or caffeine, which predispose to this arrhythmia'.[399]

Caffeine

The role of caffeine in SVTs is very controversial. Numerous anecdotal reports exist for caffeine-containing beverages inducing paroxysmal episodes of SVT, and there is some biochemical and pharmacological basis to suspect that caffeine may adversely alter cardiac electrophysiology. However a review published in 2012 which looked at a number of controlled studies of caffeine and coffee use in patients with arrhythmias came to the conclusion that normal caffeine usage does not have a significant impact on cardiac electrophysiology and does not trigger increased frequency of episodes.[400] What is interesting in this review, however, is the narrow focus on the question of whether caffeine adversely alters cardiac electrophysiology and triggers paroxysmal arrhythmias or whether the patient's symptomatology and quality of life could be the cause of the arrhythmias. In fact, the review opens with a clinical scenario which in fact emphasises this issue:

> *"Every time I drink an espresso, my heart just races and races!" lamented our forty-year-old, otherwise healthy female patient ... Ironically, she was in sinus rhythm on the monitor while drinking coffee, although she noted "heart palpitations" on the record at that time.*
>
> *Should we restrict our patient's caffeine intake? Would cutting out coffee help eliminate any arrhythmias?*

Then in conclusion they state:

> *To summarize, caffeine does not appear to promote arrhythmias, at least for most patients who drink a moderate amount of caffeinated beverages daily. Although it is tempting to blame the double espresso for our patient's lone atrial fibrillation, it probably plays little role in its occurrence. We encouraged her to continue her espresso habit with moderation.*[400]

While this conclusion seems to be well supported, it ignores the patient experience that when she drinks coffee her heart races. It is well understood that while palpitations are a symptom of arrhythmia, they can still occur when the patient is in normal sinus rhythm. Regardless of whether or not the patient is in normal sinus rhythm, palpitations can be an uncomfortable and even distressing experience for the patient. Thus, the patient's perception that something is not right when she drinks coffee should not be ignored.

NUTRITIONAL MEDICINE (SUPPLEMENTAL)

Magnesium

As discussed in the section on atrial fibrillation, magnesium supplementation may be valuable in various tachyarrhythmias, although the most appropriate dosage and form of administration need further investigation.[390] From clinical experience, supplemental magnesium in dosages of 300–450 mg (elemental) per day can improve the control of SVT, alone or in combination with drug treatment.

HERBAL MEDICINE

Herbal medicine therapeutic objectives

The main herbal objectives in managing SVTs are:

- Reduce known and suspected triggers of episodic tachyarrhythmias
- Assist in maintaining normal sinus rhythm
- Improve quality of life factors (such as fatigue, depression) directly related to the arrhythmia, or as a result of drug therapy
- Manage any contributing conditions (such as thyroid disorders).

Herbal medicine classes

The primary classes of herbal medicines of benefit in SVT include:

- Mild sedatives
- Adaptogens (most especially calming adaptogens such as *Withania somnifera*, with stimulating adaptogens

SAMPLE DAILY DIET

BREAKFAST	
Fruit salad with walnut crumble	Consumption of fruits and vegetables is associated reduced risk of CVD. Eating 10 portions, or 800 g, of fruit and vegetables a day is associated with a 28% per decrease in CVD and 33% reduce risk of stroke. Though there are no specific foods that have been studied for management of supraventricular tachycardia, consumption of walnuts has been shown to decrease overall CVD risk and are thus a worthy inclusion in the diet. Walnuts improve endothelial function, decrease oxidative stress and inflammation, while decreasing cholesterol (9–16%) and blood pressure (diastolic blood pressure by ~2–3 mmHg).
LUNCH	
Greek salad (tomatoes, olives, oregano, feta, cucumber, drizzled with EVO)	Adherence to a Mediterranean dietary pattern is suggested because of its well-established protection against cardiovascular disease. This is largely due to the high concentration of bioactive compounds including polyphenols, phytosterols, vitamins and minerals, all of which exert antioxidant, anti-inflammatory and antithrombotic effects contributing to the delay of CVD initiation and progression.
DINNER	
Spinach and red lentil dhal with coriander, garlic, ginger and turmeric	Leafy greens and lentils are both excellent sources of magnesium. Low dietary magnesium significantly increases supraventricular plus ventricular beats when the dietary magnesium concentration is low. The large amount of vegetables in this meal can contribute to the 10 servings/d suggested to protect against CVD.
SNACKS	
Tomato juice	Tomato juice displays cardioprotective abilities, irrespective of its lycopene content. In-vivo studies demonstrate that tomato juice functions as an antioxidant and improves post-ischaemic ventricular function while reducing myocardial infarct size and cardiomyocyte apoptosis. Interestingly, these effects are not seen when lycopene is used alone.

such as *Panax ginseng* usually being contraindicated in tachyarrhythmias)
- Antiarrhythmics.

Specific herbal medicines

LEONURUS CARDIACA (MOTHERWORT)

Leonurus cardiaca (motherwort) is of great value in patients with SVT. While lacking in human clinical trials, *Leonurus* is listed in the British Herbal Pharmacopoeia of 1983 as a specific for 'cardiac symptoms associated with neurosis' and is said to be indicated for tachycardia.[108] Historically it was regarded as mild in action, with Cook stating that it was useful in 'hysterical forms of nervousness and palpitation' and 'as a tonic for nervousness, pains and palpitation of the heart',[392] and Ellingwood stating that it 'would work well combined with cactus or Crataegus or both'.[5]

From clinical experience, motherwort is the single most effective anti-arrhythmic herbal medicine currently available for use in Australia, especially when it is combined with *Crataegus monogyna/laevigata* berries.

CRATAEGUS MONOGYNA (HAWTHORN)

While not a specific antiarrhythmic medicine, the overall tonic and normalising effect of hawthorn berries on the heart is highly valued, and traditional literature indicates that it is useful in paroxysmal tachycardia.[108] It should generally be used as a supportive medicine in conjunction with more specific medicines such as *Leonurus*.

LIFESTYLE RECOMMENDATIONS

Vagal stimulation in supraventricular tachycardia

During acute episodes of supraventricular tachycardia (SVT), increasing vagal tone can terminate an episode in many cases. The two main techniques used are the valsalva manoeuvre (moderately forceful attempted exhalation while mouth is closed and nose pinched shut) and carotid sinus massage (gentle rhythmic circular pressure applied over the carotid sinus on one side of the neck for roughly 5–10 seconds).[111] The patient can be taught these techniques quite easily and they can provide actual benefit as well as additional peace of mind for the patient who knows that during an acute episode they have an option to try to control it. It is important to note however that if the patient is at risk or has known carotid artery disease, carotid sinus massage is contraindicated.[394]

CASE STUDIES

Because of the potential complexity and variability of cardiac rhythm disturbances, it is necessary to evaluate the risks and likelihood of complications on an individual basis. This allows the clinician to consciously address the seriousness of the presenting problem, in terms of the risk of

CASE STUDY CONTINUED

life-changing or life-ending complications. Relative 'levels of concern' are useful when reviewing a arrhythmic patient — a simple relative classification such as low, medium, high levels of concern can be adequate. It is important to recognise in arrhythmia that a high level of patient discomfort may not equate to a high level of concern (in terms of complications). In contrast a arrhythmia with a low level of concern may still present with very significant patient discomfort and a correspondingly very low quality of life for the patient.

OVERVIEW

DW is a 41-year-old journalist presenting with recently diagnosed dilated cardiomyopathy and atrial fibrillation.

HISTORY OF PRESENTING COMPLAINT

Approximately 5 years ago DW contracted an unidentified lower respiratory infection resulting in approximately 4 weeks of illness, including intermittent fever, severe fatigue, alternating productive and unproductive coughing and dyspnoea. Treatment at the time consistent of two courses of antibiotics, along with self-medication with an over-the-counter echinacea product, garlic and bed rest.

Recovery from the infection was very slow, with lasting fatigue and regular dyspnoea. Prior to this the patient was quite physically active, rowing and running for pleasure (including training and competing in an average of two marathons per year). Due to his persistent fatigue and dyspnoea he had to give up both activities, and instead purchased a bike for exercise which he rode an average of 30 minutes 3 times weekly, though he still found this considerably challenging, progressing to only 20 minutes of gentle cycling twice weekly.

Over the next 3 years DW gained weight (upon initial presentation he was 92 kg, but had previously peaked at 98 kg, with a height of 187 cm), and developed depression. Investigations during this period included spirometry and thyroid function tests, which were both normal. He was diagnosed with postviral fatigue/chronic fatigue syndrome. His depression resulted in considerable relationship strain and, combined with his fatigue, created difficulty in reaching deadlines at work. He commenced antidepressants 2.5 years ago, which did help with consistency with his writing and general social interaction, but the patient felt that his creative abilities were impaired. His general practitioner also prescribed counselling while the patient was on antidepressants and after a 9-month course of treatment the antidepressants were discontinued. The patient described his mood as currently stable (more than 1.5 years after discontinuing the antidepressant), however he did not feel 'really alive like I used to' and still suffered significantly with fatigue and shortness of breath.

About 8 months ago the patient started noticing episodes of palpitations and tachycardia (around 100–120 bpm) even when at rest. This was occasional at first, but became progressively more frequent over the next few months, averaging roughly one episode every 10 days now. Each episode lasted around 20 minutes, and was sometimes triggered by obviously stressful situations (arguments with his partner, deadlines), but sometimes seemed to occur with no obvious trigger. Most episodes would also result in

CASE STUDY CONTINUED

mild-to-moderate anxiety during the episode, and in even more severe fatigue for the next 12–24 hours.

Recent investigation of these palpitations (ECG, chest x-ray, event monitor and echocardiography) revealed that the patient had mild dilated cardiomyopathy and paroxysmal atrial fibrillation.

CURRENT TREATMENT

Upon diagnosis of the dilated cardiomyopathy and AF, ACE inhibitors were commenced; however, he had an adverse reaction (allergic response) so these were quickly discontinued. Beta-blockers were also commenced but after 3 months of treatment DW noticed an obvious return of depression, so the patient told the cardiologist he was stopping them and upon discontinuation his mood again improved. Warfarin was commenced 4 months ago, with a currently stable dosage and target INR range. This was currently the only pharmaceutical medicine the patient was taking.

DIETARY HISTORY

DW generally eats well, with a good balance of fruit and vegetables, wholegrains, and moderate meat intake (3–4 serves per week, 2–3 serves of fish per week, 1–2 serves of chicken per week). His sugar intake was a little high, with a daily sweet pastry for breakfast, and 2 teaspoons of sugar in his coffee (currently 1 cup per day, but prior to the recent diagnosis of AF had been an average of 3–4 cups per day), and a late afternoon sweet snack consisting of a dark chocolate and hazelnut spread on crusty white bread, or a piece of cake.

The patient had a history of high alcohol consumption between age 25–36, normally 1.5 glasses of wine or two shots of spirits per night when at home, and then at social events usually 3–5 glasses of wine or 3–5 shots of spirits (usually 3 times per week). DW dramatically reduced his alcohol intake after the infection 5 years ago as he became far more sensitive to it, and it seemed to really 'knock me about' the next day. He now averages 1 shot of spirits or 1 glass of wine per week.

PATIENT ASSESSMENT

Mild dilated cardiomyopathy (likely secondary to a viral infection years ago) with paroxysmal atrial fibrillation (likely secondary to the dilated cardiomyopathy). Blood pressure is normal at 130/75 mmHg.

In terms of risk of complications, there is a reasonably high level of concern, due to the fact that in both dilated cardiomyopathy and in atrial fibrillation the risk of thrombotic episodes is significantly elevated. This concern is somewhat mitigated by the recent commencement of warfarin.

There is a moderate to high level of patient discomfort. The patient has somewhat adapted to prolonged fatigue (likely as a result of the cardiomyopathy); however, it has adversely affected both his physical and psychological wellbeing. The relatively recent addition of paroxysmal AF has further complicated his physical wellbeing and is probably worsening his psychological wellbeing as well.

CASE STUDY CONTINUED

TREATMENT OBJECTIVES

- Improve cardiac output
- Reduce exposure, and sensitivity, to potential triggers of paroxysmal AF
- Note: mood and fatigue were judged as highly likely to respond to improvements in cardiac output.

HERBAL TREATMENT

Botanical name	DER	Amount per week	Rationale
Crataegus monogyna berries	1:2	50 mL	Positively inotropic; assists in normalising cardiac rhythm
Leonurus cardiaca	1:2	50 mL	Reduces both severity and frequency of tachycardia episodes
Panax ginseng	1:2	15 mL	Adaptogenic, seems to have a positively inotropic effect (author's clinical observation)
Withania somnifera	1:2	25 mL	Adaptogenic, with a calming effect (specifically to reduce sympathetic nervous system triggers for AF episodes)

Dose: 10 mL twice daily, morning and mid-afternoon (not evening due to risk of overstimulation in the evening from *Panax ginseng*)

NUTRITIONAL SUPPLEMENTATION

- Coenzyme Q10 150 mg, 1 capsule twice daily (morning and lunch, total of 300 mg per day). Rationale: improve cardiac output and general vitality. Note: a potential for interaction between warfarin and CoQ10 exists, so the patient was instructed to return to his GP and have more frequent INR monitoring until impact was understood
- Bioactivated magnesium tablets, 1 tablet three times daily (total of 275 mg of elemental magnesium per day, plus small doses of zinc, calcium, potassium and a range of B vitamins as well as taurine). Rationale: stabilise cardiac rhythm; improve myocardial function; support general vitality.

DIETARY RECOMMENDATIONS

- Ensure no more than 1 cup of coffee per day, and ideally reduce sugar to 1 teaspoon per cup.
- Eliminate afternoon cake or chocolate and hazelnut spread, and replace with 4–5 squares of 85% chocolate.

OUTCOMES (4 WEEKS)

DW described a significant improvement in vitality within less than 2 weeks of commencing treatment. He stated that both his physical stamina and dyspnoea seemed to improve, as well as his cognitive function (concentration and cognitive

CASE STUDY CONTINUED

stamina). While he was still fatigued, he estimated a 30% improvement since his first visit.

In the last 4 weeks he had two episodes of palpitations and tachycardia, with the second resulting in less severe and less prolonged fatigue.

The patient had been adhering to the dietary recommendations, and stated that the afternoon chocolate was both pleasurable and 'a fantastic pick-me-up'.

INR seemed unchanged.

TREATMENT OBJECTIVES

- Continue as previously, but increase emphasis on positively inotropic activity

HERBAL TREATMENT

- Continue as previously

NUTRITIONAL SUPPLEMENTATION

- Continue as previously, however increase CoQ10 dosage to 2 capsules twice daily (total of 600 mg per day)

OUTCOMES (38 WEEKS)

Over the next 34 weeks DW continued to improve. By week 38 of treatment, he estimated that his physical fatigue and dyspnoea had improved approximately 80%, and he had returned to gentle rowing once a week (not competitively, but in his own kayak), as well as cycling roughly 30 minutes at moderate intensity 3 times per week.

He reported that cognitive function and mood was excellent, and no longer an issue for him. He stated that his relationship with his wife had also improved considerably, due to his improved mood and also improved sexual activity frequency and quality.

The frequency and severity of palpitations and tachycardia also declined steadily over these 38 weeks, with the last noticeable episode being more than 40 days before the most recent consultation.

He had lost 4 kg of body weight in that period, which seemed to be a combination of fluid loss (likely due to improved cardiac output) as well as loss of some body fat.

DW did have a few weeks of disturbed sleep due to feeling more physically and mentally energetic in the evenings, so he was advised to stop his morning coffee and instead move his afternoon chocolate dosage to the morning. This seemed to reduce the evening overstimulation and his sleep went back to normal.

A follow-up cardiology consultation which included an echocardiogram seemed to indicate reduced cardiomegaly, and resting ECG was normal. The cardiologist was very happy with the patient's progress, and indicated that he should continue whatever he is doing. The warfarin prescription was maintained, and DW's INR remained within the target range.

The following case study is an example of a situation involving a low level of concern but high level of patient discomfort.

OVERVIEW

LN, a 33-year-old woman, presented with paroxysmal supraventricular tachycardia. She was diagnosed only

CASE STUDY CONTINUED

4 months ago, after at least 3 years of 'anxiety attacks'. She experiences severe anxiety, palpitations, facial flushing, mild chest discomfort and 'never feels well'. She is also mildly hypertensive (variable, averaging 155/85 mmHg).

Triggers for episodes of severe palpitations and tachycardia (occurring approximately 2–3 times per week) include:

- Relationship stress with brother
- Work stress (runs a fashion business)
- Too much coffee or chocolate (likes Lindt 70%, but can't have too much).

Her current treatment:

- 'Try to calm down'
- 'Wash your face in cold water'.

Her cardiologist has stated that the severity is not sufficient to warrant any further conventional treatment.

HEALTH REVIEW

Review of her health revealed that her stress was considerable. She worked long hours, had significant stress with her brother due to his poor relationships, and her work and other issues were always on her mind. She had a busy life and an overactive mind resulting in 6 h of broken sleep for the last 7–8 years.

She exercised for 2 × 10 min walking per day, and experienced persistent fatigue. Thyrotoxicosis was excluded, ECG was normal, patient was mildly overweight.

Her diet was generally good — moderate fat, moderate red meat, good intake of fruit and vegetables and water. Coffee — strong black once every 2 days. Chocolate once every 2–3 days (dark).

Emotionally she felt totally overwhelmed. 'On edge of collapse.' Irritable. Feels like diagnosis means that she now has no choice but to live like this for the rest of her life.

ASSESSMENT AND OBJECTIVES

- Risk of concern — risk of complications and sudden death minimal. High level of patient discomfort — patient is 'on edge of collapse'
- Objectives were to promote stress adaptation, promote effective sleep and normalise heart rhythm.

HERBAL MEDICINE

Herbal medicine	Ratio	Quantity per dose	Quantity per 200 mL
Crataegus spp. berries	1:2	1.5 mL	60 mL
Leonurus cardiaca	1:2	1 mL	40 mL
Verbena officinalis	1:2	1 mL	40 mL
Withania somnifera	1:2	1.5 mL	60 mL

Dose: 5 mL t.d.s. dispensed 1 × 200 mL bottles.

OTHER

Valeriana edulis 500 mg, 3 tabs once daily 30 min before sleep.

NUTRITIONAL SUPPLEMENTATION

B complex 50 mg b.i.d.

CASE STUDY CONTINUED

OUTCOMES (2 WEEKS LATER)

- Feeling only a little calmer
- Sleep more restful
- Arrhythmia: Same frequency, but might be a little less severe
- Fatigue same
- BP 155/90 mmHg.

OBJECTIVES

- Promote stress adaptation
- Promote effective sleep
- Normalise heart rhythm
- More emphasis on daytime sedation.

HERBAL MEDICINE

Herbal medicine	Ratio	Quantity per dose	Quantity per 200 mL
Crataegus spp. berries	1:2	2 mL	60 mL
Leonurus cardiaca	1:2	1 mL	30 mL
Zizyphus spinosa	1:2	2 mL	60 mL
Withania somnifera	1:2	2 mL	60 mL

Dose: 7 mL t.d.s. — dispensed 2 × 200 mL bottles.

OTHER

Valeriana edulis 500 mg, 3 tabs once daily 30 min before sleep.

NUTRITIONAL SUPPLEMENTATION

B complex 50 mg b.i.d.

OUTCOMES (3 WEEKS LATER)

- Feeling much calmer
- Sleeping 7 h per night, less broken
- Arrhythmia: Once in last week, severity reduced
- Fatigue 25% better
- BP 150/80 mmHg.

OBJECTIVES

- Continue previous
- Increase exercise to walking daily for 30 min if can
- Evaluate again in another 6 weeks.

HERBAL MEDICINE

Herbal medicine	Ratio	Quantity per dose	Quantity per 200 mL
Crataegus spp. berries	1:2	2 mL	60 mL
Leonurus cardiaca	1:2	1 mL	30 mL
Zizyphus spinosa	1:2	2 mL	60 mL
Withania somnifera	1:2	2 mL	60 mL

Dose: 7 mL t.d.s. — dispensed 2 × 600 mL bottle. Pick up repeat as required.

CASE STUDY CONTINUED

OTHER

Valeriana edulis 500 mg, 3 tabs once daily 30 min before sleep.

NUTRITIONAL SUPPLEMENTATION

B complex 50 mg b.i.d.

OUTCOMES (6 WEEKS LATER)

- 'New person!'
- Sleeping 7 h+ per night, less broken
- Arrhythmia: Once every 2 weeks, severity reduced
- Fatigue continuing to improve
- BP 135/75 mmHg
- Self-regulating *Valeriana* dose. Down to 2 tabs most nights
- Been exercising well. Wants to go to gym if can in another few weeks.

OBJECTIVES

- Continue previous.

PERIPHERAL ARTERIAL AND VENOUS DISORDERS

Epidemiology

Disorders of peripheral circulation can be divided into those affecting the arterial system and those affecting the venous system.

Peripheral arterial disorders are quite common, with the most common and specific disorder of peripheral atherosclerotic disease manifesting in approximately 12% of people in the United States, with males being more commonly affected.[401]

Peripheral venous disorders are also reasonably common, with chronic venous insufficiency affecting approximately 5% of people in the United States.[402]

Classification

Within the grouping of peripheral arterial disorders, there are a number of specific conditions.[403,404] The disorders which will be considered here include:

- Peripheral atherosclerotic disease (also known as peripheral arterial disease)
- Raynaud's syndrome
- Chilblains (also known as pernio)
- Thromboangiitis obliterans (also known as Buerger's disease).

Within the grouping of peripheral venous disorders, there are again a number of specific conditions.[405] The primary disorders of interest include:

- Deep venous thrombosis
- Chronic venous insufficiency and postphlebitic (also known as post-thrombotic) syndrome.

Aetiology

PERIPHERAL ATHEROSCLEROTIC DISEASE (PAD)

Peripheral atherosclerotic disease (PAD) occurs most commonly in older men, and while atherosclerosis is a systemic disorder, with 50–75% of those with PAD also having coronary artery disease, it is not uncommon for the coronary artery disease to be asymptomatic. This is in part likely due to patients with PAD being unable to exert themselves physically to the point of causing cardiac ischaemic symptoms, due to the ischaemic symptoms of PAD manifesting first.[401]

The risk factors for PAD are the same as for any atherosclerotic disease; however, cigarette smoking is even more important: in fact it is estimated that smokers are 2–3 times more likely to develop PAD than coronary artery disease.[403] Diabetes also dramatically increases risk, with an estimated 28% increase in risk with every 1% increase in glycosylated haemoglobin (HbA1c). Additionally diabetics with PAD are 7–15 times more likely to require major amputation than non-diabetic patients with PAD.[403]

RAYNAUD'S SYNDROME

Raynaud's syndrome is a vasospastic disorder predominantly affecting the fingers, which is marked by acute symptomatic episodes usually triggered by exposure to cold or acute stress.[404] It occurs in roughly 3–5% of the population, affects women more commonly than men, and younger people more than the elderly.[406] Primary Raynaud's syndrome has no known contributing factors and comprises roughly 80% of cases, whereas secondary Raynaud's syndrome occurs commonly as a component of an underlying chronic immune-mediated connective tissue disease (such as scleroderma — where roughly 90% of scleroderma patients suffer from Raynaud's — or lupus).[404,406]

CHILBLAINS

Chilblains is an old Anglo-Saxon term translating to 'cold sore'. The condition is also known by its Latin name, 'pernio' which translates to 'frostbite'. However it is important not to confuse chilblains (an abnormal response to non-freezing temperatures) with what is known in modern times as frostbite (a normal, but pathological, response to actual freezing of tissues).[404]

Chilblains most commonly occurs in women aged 15–30 years, but can also occur in older patients and even children, and is mostly seen in geographical areas prone to colder temperatures. It usually occurs on the toes 12–24 hours after exposure to low temperatures, and results in single or multiple oedematous blister-like lesions of a red to purple colour, which may turn yellow/brown in colour. The cause is vasospasm similar in basic nature to Raynaud's syndrome but more prolonged, resulting in localised inflammation.[404]

THROMBOANGIITIS OBLITERANS (BUERGER'S DISEASE)

Thromboangiitis obliterans, also known as Buerger's disease, is an inflammatory condition affecting small- and medium-sized arteries and veins primarily in the lower limbs, but sometimes the upper limbs. It almost exclusively occurs in tobacco users, mostly men aged between 20 and 40 years, and is more prevalent in the Middle East and Asia than in North America (in part likely due to decreasing tobacco use in North America).[404,407] The exact cause is unknown; however, the correlation with tobacco use is obviously important, and immune involvement is suspected due to it occurring more commonly in certain HLA genotypes (specifically HLA-A9 and HLA-B5).[407]

The inflammatory process results in ischaemia of the affected extremities as well as superficial thrombophlebitis. It is important to note that this is a non-atherosclerotic disease, and thus quite different in pathology to PAD.[407]

DEEP VENOUS THROMBOSIS

Deep venous thrombosis (DVT) is a clotting disorder occurring in a deep vein in the leg (usually the calf, but sometimes the thigh) which can subsequently lead to pulmonary embolism and thus is potentially fatal.[408]

The pathophysiological process leading to DVT usually involves a combination of two or more of the following:[405,408]

- Impaired venous return, such as may occur in pregnancy, or in patients who are immobilised for long periods (e.g. long aeroplane flights, or injury which limits mobility)
- Endothelial injury, often secondary to a bone fracture or surgery
- Hypercoagulation — either true hypercoagulation disorders (such as antiphospholipid syndrome, or factor V Leiden mutation, among others) or a suspected general tendency towards hypercoagulation.

The frequency and pattern of occurrence of DVT is hard to estimate, as it is suspected that in a great many cases it goes unrecognised as it may be asymptomatic.[405]

The combination of endothelial damage, venous stasis, and hypercoagulability (the so-called Virchow's triad) is regarded as essential in the development of DVT. In many cases a general tendency towards hypercoagulability (as opposed to true hypercoagulation disorders) is thought to contribute; however, this general tendency is harder to measure.[405]

Other factors known risk factors for DVT include:[408]

- Age of 60 years or older
- Cancer
- Cigarette smoking
- Oral contraceptives, oestrogen therapy, or oestrogen receptor modifying drugs
- Venous catheters
- Heart failure
- Obesity
- Pregnancy
- Sickle cell anaemia.

CHRONIC VENOUS INSUFFICIENCY AND POSTPHLEBITIC SYNDROME

Chronic venous insufficiency is defined as impaired venous return which often causes lower limb oedema and associated discomfort, and may cause skin changes. Postphlebitic syndrome is similar but it is always proceeded by the occurrence of deep venous thrombosis.[409]

It is estimated that chronic venous insufficiency affects approximately 5% of people in the United States,[409] and roughly 50% of patients with DVT go on to develop postphlebitic syndrome within 1–2 years.[405]

Risk factors for chronic venous insufficiency include venous obstruction, venous hypertension, inadequate lower limb muscle exercise, venous valvular incompetence/weakness, local tissue trauma, ageing and obesity.[409] As postphlebitic syndrome occurs after DVT, the primary risk factor is past DVT.[405]

Pathogenesis

SIGNS AND SYMPTOMS

Peripheral atherosclerotic disease

The primary symptom of PAD is intermittent claudication, where patients develop pain and/or cramping in the legs, typically the calves but sometimes the feet, thighs, hips, buttocks and, very rarely, the arms. This claudication is usually brought on by walking, and is improved with rest, with the distance patients can walk without discomfort decreasing as the severity of the PAD increases. As the disease becomes advanced, pain may occur when at rest and is usually worse at night due to leg elevation while lying down.[401]

In mild PAD there are often no obvious signs, however as it develops reduced peripheral pulses may be detected, and eventually changes of colour become obvious. Dependant rubor is characteristic — when the leg in below the heart the skin appears dusky red, and then when elevated it loses colour and ischaemic pain can develop, then when the limb is lowered again there is prolonged venous filling.[401]

Additionally atrophic skin changes may appear, with thinning or loss of hair on the lower limbs. The distal lower limb and feet may feel cool to the touch. In more advanced ischaemia skin ulcers may develop, typically with a border of black necrotic tissue, and are usually painful unless the patient has additional neurological impairment (as may be seen in diabetics and alcoholics) where the patient may not notice their presence. Infection of the ulcers can commonly develop and lead to rapidly progressing cellulitis.[401]

Raynaud's syndrome

Raynaud's presents with episodic vasospasm, most commonly in the fingers (especially the middle three fingers),[406] but can occur in the toes, and even more rarely the nose, ears or lips.[404] The patient notices sudden onset of coldness of the digits with pallor, which then often progresses to cyanosis with pain or numbness, followed often by reactive hyperaemia resulting in erythema and commonly swelling.[404] The vasospastic episodes usually last for a few minutes, but may occasionally last as long as 2 hours, are usually triggered by exposure to cold or acute stress and resolve quickly upon rewarming the affected hand.[406]

Chilblains

The lesions of chilblains are quite characteristic (erythematous blister-like lesions of a red/purple colour, progressing to yellow/brown), and are usually associated with intense localised burning pain or itching or both. Chronic chilblains occur when the patient has repeated exposure to cold conditions resulting in persistent lesions, and they can result in scarring and dermal atrophy, including ulceration of the lesions.[404]

Thromboangiitis obliterans

The onset of symptoms in thromboangiitis obliterans is slow and progressive, with early manifestations including Raynaud's phenomenon, numbness and tingling, coldness or burning in the extremities of the limbs, with intermittent claudication in the affected extremity (predominantly in the foot), and it can progress to pain on rest. Peripheral pulses are significantly reduced.[407]

As the condition worsens, the pain becomes persistent and severe, the affected limb feels cold and damp to the touch (due to excessive local perspiration) and it can become cyanotic.[407]

Deep venous thrombosis

It is suspected that many cases of DVT are asymptomatic, and are only discovered when the patient presents with pulmonary embolism, and a search for the cause results in discovery of a deep venous thrombosis still present (as in many cases only part of the thrombosis embolises).[405]

When it is symptomatic, the patient commonly experiences aching leg pain and swelling and tenderness over the area of the veins, sometimes with erythema or cynanosis.[405,408]

Chronic venous insufficiency and postphlebitic syndrome

Chronic venous insufficiency and postphlebitic syndrome exhibit almost the same clinical picture; however, chronic venous insufficiency may cause signs but be asymptomatic, whereas postphlebitic syndrome is always symptomatic.[409]

Primary symptoms and signs include:[409]

- Sensation of fullness and heaviness in the lower limb
- Lower limb oedema
- Lower limb aching, tiredness and sometimes cramping
- Lower limb pruritus
- Varicose veins.

The symptoms and the oedema are usually worse for walking or standing (especially if prolonged) and better for rest and elevation of the affected limbs.[409]

COMPLICATIONS

Peripheral atherosclerotic disease

The primary complications of PAD are as follows:[403]

- Acute limb ischaemia, which is a medical emergency and in some cases may require amputation of part (e.g. a toe) or the entire leg

- Atrophic skin changes including ulceration
- Acute infection of ulcers and subsequent acute cellulitis.

Raynaud's syndrome

Primary Raynaud's syndrome, while obviously uncomfortable for the patient, rarely leads to any trophic changes of the skin or other complications. However, secondary Raynaud's syndrome more commonly progresses to cause complications such as ulceration of the fingertips and in some cases gangrene.[406]

Chilblains

The primary complication of chilblains relates mostly to chronicity. Recurrent exposure to cold conditions results in recurrent and persistent lesions, and the recurrent prolonged vasospasm combined with healing and reappearance of lesions can create localised scarring and ulceration of the lesions. Infection of the ulcers is another possible complication.[404]

Thromboangiitis obliterans

The primary complications of thromboangiitis obliterans are ischaemic ulcers on one or more affected digits, which can progress to gangrene.[407]

Deep venous thrombosis

The most important and critical complication of DVT is pulmonary embolism, which may be fatal. In cases where embolism doesn't occur, chronic venous insufficiency and postphlebitic syndrome can result.[408]

Chronic venous insufficiency and postphlebitic syndrome

The primary complications of chronic venous insufficiency and postphlebitic syndrome are skin changes collectively referred to as venous stasis dermatitis. This is a reddish/brown discolouration and hardening (induration) of the skin over the affected area of the lower limb, with venous ectasia, and it may progress to include venous stasis ulcers. The ulcers develop after mild skin injury (such as scratching) or can even develop spontaneously, and mostly occur around the inside of the ankle, although they can occur higher up the lower half of the leg. They are shallow rather than deep, but their diameter can be highly variable, and they generally appear moist and, if not cleaned and dressed regularly, they can have an objectionable odour.[409] Some patients complain of significant pain from the ulcers; however, this is not always the case (especially in diabetic patients who may also have peripheral neuropathy).

DIFFERENTIAL DIAGNOSIS

Peripheral atherosclerotic disease

In many cases the early symptoms of PAD may go unrecognised, as they can be intermittent, variable, and in some cases the patient may not even report them to the clinician. Common conditions which may cause diagnostic confusion include:[401,403]

- Lower limb arthritis (evaluate joint mobility and pain)
- Venous disorders (more likely to have lower limb oedema)
- Spinal degeneration leading to stenosis (likely to have history of lower back discomfort and often have lower limb neurological symptoms)
- Compartment syndrome (more likely after a history of excessive exercise and relieved slowly through leg elevation).

Raynaud's syndrome

The diagnosis of Raynaud's is relatively easy and primarily based on the patient's description of the episodes,[404] and is even easier if the clinician is able to observe an active episode (or if the patient provides photographs of their hands during an episode). Diagnostic confusion is unlikely; however, the primary issue is determining whether the complaint is primary, or secondary to an existing or as yet undiagnosed immune-mediated connective tissue inflammatory disease, as the prognosis is obviously quite different.[406]

Chilblains

Conditions which may cause diagnostic confusion with chilblains include:[404]

- Nodular vasculitis or erythema nodosum (more likely to have systemic infectious or inflammatory symptoms such as fever, malaise, arthralgia)
- Peripheral atherosclerotic disease (more likely to have calf pain on walking, regardless of the temperature).

Thromboangiitis obliterans

The most obvious conditions to differentiate from thromboangiitis obliterans are primary or secondary Raynaud's syndrome (more likely episodic in nature and triggered by exposure to cold), and peripheral atherosclerotic disease (not as easily to clinically differentiate, but can be clearly differentiated with angiography).[404]

Due to its inflammatory nature, other conditions which may cause diagnostic confusion with thromboangiitis obliterans are:[404]

- Scleroderma
- Systemic lupus erythematosus
- Antiphospholipid syndrome
- Rheumatoid vasculitis
- Any other immune-mediated connective tissue inflammatory disease
- Chronic cocaine abuse.

Deep venous thrombosis

The diagnosis of DVT commences usually with the patient complaining of the characteristic lower limb symptoms,[408] or as a result of the investigation of acute pulmonary embolism.[405]

Conditions which can mimic the symptoms of DVT include:[405]

- Muscle strain or tearing
- General venous stasis and chronic venous insufficiency without thrombus development
- Lymphatic obstruction
- Cellulitis.

Chronic venous insufficiency and postphlebitic syndrome

The first diagnostic priority in patients with suspected chronic venous insufficiency or postphlebitic syndrome is to rule out the presence of deep venous thrombosis.[409]

Lower limb oedema of other causes may appear similar to early-stage chronic venous insufficiency (before commencement of venous stasis dermatitis), so the following causes must be ruled out:[409]

- Right heart failure
- Acute inflammation from trauma or infection
- Renal impairment.

NATUROPATHIC DIAGNOSIS

Naturopathic diagnosis of peripheral arterial or venous disorders commences with a combination of medical history and physical examination. In suspected PAD a simple evaluation and comparison of peripheral pulses in both lower limbs can be easily performed (remembering that in early disease peripheral pulses may appear normal). If symptoms or signs point to possible disorders, particularly in the presence of various risk factors in the history of the patient, then immediate referral is required for medical investigation. In many cases patients will present to naturopaths and herbalists with existing diagnosed disease, in which case the diagnostic role of the clinician is focused firstly on monitoring severity over time (to evaluate progression or regression with treatment), and watching for the occurrence of complications so that they may be rapidly addressed.

Investigations

GENERAL INVESTIGATIONS

For suspected PAD, a simple investigation involves determining the ankle-brachial index (ABI). This is a ratio of ankle to brachial systolic pressures calculated by first measuring the systolic brachial pressures in both arms and both legs (the highest reading for the dorsalis pedis and posterior tibial arteries are used) then dividing the ankle pressure by the arm pressure for each side. A ratio of 0.9 or above is regarded as normal, 0.71–0.8 is designated as mild obstruction, 0.41–0.7 as moderate obstruction, and 0.00–0.4 as severe obstruction. It is important to note that this assessment may not be possible with simple cuff-based sphygmomanometers especially in the ankles if there is existing disease, and handheld Doppler instruments may be required.[403]

Doppler ultrasonography is a non-invasive imaging method useful in determining peripheral arterial blood flow, and diagnosing stenosis or vascular obstructions. It is often a first-line investigation for confirming the presence of PAD and estimating severity.[401,403] It is also valuable in some venous disorders, such as deep venous thrombosis.[408]

Computed tomography angiography (CTA), magnetic resonance angiography (MRA) and invasive digital angiography are imaging methods employed in suspected arterial disease. Digital subtraction angiography (DSA) is still regarded as the gold standard despite a number of limitations (including the two-dimensional nature of the resultant imagery, and the greater level of exposure to ionising radiation), but all three investigations do have some degree of associated risk. However, the information gained from these investigations can be essential especially if surgical revascularisation is required.[403]

D-dimer testing is used in the evaluation of DVT (both diagnosis and prediction of future recurrence). D-dimer is a plasma protein produced in the process of fibrinolysis and elevated levels indicate the possible presence and lysis of thrombi. Thus it is a valuable blood test in suspected DVT and/or pulmonary embolism as it is quite sensitive and almost always elevated in DVT or pulmonary embolism. However, it does not have a high specificity, with a number of non-thrombotic conditions also causing elevated D-dimer levels, including heart failure, renal failure, liver disease, recent surgery, pregnancy and sepsis. Therefore it is most valuable as a test for excluding DVT if the levels are not elevated.[405]

NATUROPATHIC INVESTIGATIONS

Naturopathic investigation is similar to conventional investigation in terms of physical examination; however, in most cases referral for more technical investigations is required.

Therapeutic considerations

CLINICAL DECISION MAKING AND RATIONALE

Peripheral atherosclerotic disease

Ideally PAD is a preventable disease, with prevention involving the same lifestyle and dietary interventions as for any atherosclerotic disease.[401] However, in most cases the patient who presents to the naturopath will have existing or suspected PAD, in which case the focus is on reducing the progression of the disease, preventing and managing complications and, especially in cases of mild-to-moderate obstruction, attempting to reverse the arterial degeneration and re-establish normal or close to normal peripheral arterial blood flow. Additionally it is important to consider the systemic atherosclerotic change and focus on reducing contributing risk factors and preventing other ischaemic diseases (such as ischaemic stroke or myocardial ischaemia).

Raynaud's syndrome

The first objective in a patient who presents with Raynaud's is to determine if it is primary or secondary in nature. The management of secondary Raynaud's syndrome is obviously far more complex, due to the need to focus on the underlying immune dysregulation and connective tissue inflammation and damage.

Chilblains

Most patients presenting for naturopathic care for chilblains are suffering from chronic chilblains. Therefore while eliminating exposure to the precipitating cold temperatures might be ideal, it may not be entirely possible. Therefore maximising peripheral circulation is essential.

Thromboangiitis obliterans

Once other potential causes of arterial and venous inflammation have been ruled out, the next objective in the management of thromboangiitis obliterans is to avoid serious ischaemic change which may result in the need for digital amputation.[404]

Deep venous thrombosis

As DVT has a high risk of causing pulmonary embolism, which can be fatal, suspected DVT requires immediate medical evaluation and management. As a result there is very little that naturopathic medicine can offer in this acute stage. However, naturopathic medicine does lend itself to the long-term care of patients who have had a DVT, as lifestyle and risk modifications are essential in preventing future occurrences. Additionally, naturopathic treatment soon after the initial medical treatment may have a role to play in reducing the risk of the long-term complication of postphlebitic syndrome.

Chronic venous insufficiency and postphlebitic syndrome

Once DVT has been ruled out in patients with chronic venous insufficiency or postphlebitic syndrome, the focus should be on improving patient comfort and managing the skin changes, especially if ulceration is present.

Therapeutic application

ALLOPATHIC PERSPECTIVE

Peripheral atherosclerotic disease

The conventional treatment of PAD focuses on first sparing the limb from amputation, then improving walking distance and reducing the risk of complications (including complications of the systemic atherosclerotic changes such as coronary artery disease).

Pharmacologically pentoxifylline or cilostazol can be employed to reduce blood viscosity;[403] however, some studies indicate that pentoxifylline does not improve pain-free treadmill walking distance.[401] Aspirin and ACE inhibitors are also commonly prescribed for general risk reduction.[401]

Exercise is an extremely important — if underused — intervention and regarded as the preferred initial treatment (along with elimination of classic risk factors such as smoking).[403] Specifically a program of treadmill or track walking of more than 30 minutes duration (ideally 35–50 minutes) 3–4 times per week has been shown in various studies to be extremely beneficial.[401,403] Ideally a supervised program is initiated, whereby the patient is advised that while pain will occur it is not harmful, and they are encouraged to continue walking until pain is near maximal tolerance. Generally benefits are noticed within 1–2 months and increase over the next several months.[403]

Surgical revascularisation including percutaneous transluminal angioplasty is indicated if exercise and drug treatment combined have failed to result in improvement.[403]

Raynaud's syndrome

Physical measures such as cold avoidance, wearing gloves when appropriate, and using gentle heating devices (such as chemical or electrical hand warmers) are the first consideration for prevention of acute episodes.[404] During an acute episode, warming the hands is essential; however, this should be conducted carefully. If the fingers are numb, the patient may not be aware of excessive heat exposure (such as immersion of the fingers in very hot water) and thus worsen the hyperaemia and potentially cause local scalding.

Pharmacologically the main agents used are calcium channel blockers, which can be used daily or, in the case of short-acting versions, may be taken prophylactically when exposure to cold is unavoidable.[404]

Chilblains

Avoidance of exposure to cold temperatures and ensuring adequate protection for the feet is the primary treatment consideration; however, in some cases of chronic chilblains pharmacological therapy involving calcium channel blockers may be used. Additionally local antipruritic creams may be used in the management of the itching and pain of existing lesions.[404]

Thromboangiitis obliterans

The most immediate intervention in patients with thromboangiitis obliterans should be rapid and complete cessation of consumption of tobacco products of any kind (cigarettes, cigars, pipes, chewing tobacco, and even nicotine patches). Almost all patients who immediately stop using tobacco products avoid the need for amputations, whereas of those who continue, roughly 40% eventually require one or multiple amputations.[404]

Pharmacologically, intravenous iloprost (a synthetic PGI_2 analogue) can be used, but other drugs such as calcium channel blockers, while commonly used, are not well studied in terms of their effectiveness in thromboangiitis obliterans.[407]

Deep venous thrombosis

The specific treatment for DVT is immediate anticoagulant therapy, with heparin (for inpatient care) or low molecular weight heparin (for outpatient care). This is preferred due to the immediacy of its action, and is usually administered for approximately 1 week in total. Additionally oral warfarin dosage is usually commenced 24–48 hours after the commencement of the heparin or derivatives, allowing time for the warfarin to act prior to cessation of the heparin or derivatives. The target International Normalised Ratio (INR) is 2.0–3.0, and warfarin dosage is adjusted individually to achieve this target. Higher targets of 3.0–4.0 appear to have no better efficacy; however, they do increase the risk of bleeding complications.[405]

Oral warfarin dosing is generally sustained for approximately 3 months, although this may be individualised, depending on a number of factors.[405]

Chronic venous insufficiency and postphlebitic syndrome

Allopathic treatment of chronic venous insufficiency and of postphlebitic syndrome is identical, and focuses first on reducing venous stasis/congestion, and second on managing any skin complications.[409]

Reducing venous stasis is mostly accomplished through physical therapy such as regular leg elevation. The ideal process is to raise the leg above the level of the right atrium for minimum of 30 minutes, three times daily.[409] However, this may be impractical for many patients, therefore any level of elevation frequently during the day is recommended.[405] Additionally the frequent use of compression stockings is commonly recommended; however, many patients find them cumbersome and undesirable from an appearance viewpoint, and especially in summer they can be very hot and uncomfortable.[405]

Management of venous stasis ulcers is through appropriate wound care involving regular cleansing and dressing of the wound. The Unna boot is the preferred dressing, which is a type of bandage impregnated with zinc oxide paste, which in turn should be covered by compression bandages and changed weekly.[409]

While it is common for aspirin to be given to patients with chronic venous insufficiency and for topical steroids and oral or topical antibiotics to be used in treatment of venous stasis ulcers, none of these approaches tend to be effective in most cases.[409]

NATUROPATHIC PERSPECTIVE

Peripheral atherosclerotic disease

The objectives of naturopathic treatment of PAD align with allopathic treatment; however, there is a broader range of pharmacological options available, especially in herbal medicine.

Raynaud's syndrome

Primary Raynaud's syndrome can be considered a neurovascular dysfunction from a naturopathic perspective. The focus is on assessing whether the patient is generally susceptible to exposure to cold and has a relatively cold constitution, or whether the patient's digital susceptibility to cold stands alone. In the case of the former, generally warming agents such as consumption of spicy foods and circulatory stimulant herbal medicines are beneficial; however, in the latter the focus is on reducing stress triggers for vasospasm and normalising vascular motility.

In secondary Raynaud's syndrome the primary focus will be on the underlying connective tissue disease, with secondary focus on the Raynaud's itself as a manifestation of the underlying disease.

In either case, avoidance of vasoconstricting agents is essential, such as pseudoephedrine and nicotine.

Chilblains

Ideally chilblains should be prevented by reducing exposure to precipitating cold temperatures; however, it is important to note that not everybody exposed to the same cold conditions develops chilblains. Thus in the naturopathic approach, assessment of peripheral microcirculation is regarded as important especially in chronic chilblains, and subsequently treatment will focus not solely on the lesions themselves, but on prevention through improvement of peripheral circulation.

Thromboangiitis obliterans

As tobacco use is strongly associated with thromboangiitis obliterans, and cessation is correlated with significant reduction in severity and risk of amputation, this should be the first therapeutic target. As tobacco products can be remarkably addictive in some patients, general support measures such as counselling, stress management and herbal support for the nervous system may be helpful. It is important to realise and educate the patient that while withdrawal symptoms may be uncomfortable, it is critical that tobacco use is discontinued immediately.

As thromboangiitis obliterans is not an atherosclerotic disease, but instead the result of an inflammatory process, the naturopathic management will involve reduction of inflammation and inflammatory triggers, and oxidative change in the vascular system. Avoidance of other vasoconstricting agents (such as ephedrine and pseudoephedrine) is also essential.

Deep venous thrombosis

As previously stated, the primary naturopathic objective in the management of DVT is to reduce the risk of long-term complications such as postphlebitic syndrome and future recurrence of DVT. Management of dietary and lifestyle risk factors which may contribute to hypercoagulability is essential, and herbal treatment focusing on this as well as venous function and endothelial protection can be of benefit. Care needs to be taken while the patient is still being administered heparin derivatives or warfarin to ensure that naturopathic treatment does not interfere with the efficacy of the anticoagulant therapy or increase the risk of bleeding.

Chronic venous insufficiency and postphlebitic syndrome

Chronic venous insufficiency and postphlebitic syndrome are seen in naturopathic medicine as a failure of peripheral venous tone and competence thus focusing on improving these issues is core to management. This longer term objective complements the allopathic treatment involving rest, elevation and, where possible compression, as well as the wound care for venous stasis ulcers. Additionally, where ulceration exists, focusing on measures which speed tissue healing is of benefit to the patient.

NUTRITIONAL MEDICINE (DIETARY)

Nuts

While nut consumption has been associated with a lower risk of coronary heart disease, a study from 2015 has suggested that it may also be important in the prevention of peripheral arterial disease (PAD). Dietary information from self-referred participants at more than 20000 sites in the US, totalling 3312403 individuals was gathered, and in total 219 527 individuals were diagnosed with PAD through the use of ankle brachial indices. It was found that even after multivariable adjustment, daily nut consumption compared to consumption of nuts less than once a month was associated with 21% lower odds of PAD.[410]

Fruit and vegetables

Another study published by many of the same authors, and using a slightly expanded sample size from the same source, showed that consumption of three or more servings of fruit and vegetables per day, as compared to less than monthly consumption, showed 18% lower odds of PAD. Interestingly, this association was only present among current or former smokers, indicating that fruit and vegetable consumption may reduce some of the negative impacts of tobacco smoking.[411]

The Mediterranean diet

The Mediterranean diet has long been suspected of being beneficial in the prevention and treatment of peripheral arterial disease, with this suspicion being confirmed through a large randomised and blinded dietary intervention study in Spain. A total of 7477 individuals were initially included in the study, with 12 being subsequently excluded due to intermittent claudication symptoms at baseline. The participants were men aged 55–80 years, and women aged 60–80 years, all without PAD or baseline cardiovascular disease, but with at least three cardiovascular risk factors or type 2 diabetes. The participants were divided into three groups: a Mediterranean diet supplemented with extra-virgin olive oil; a Mediterranean diet supplemented with nuts; and counselling on a low-fat diet (control group). Compared to the control group, the Mediterranean diet plus extra-virgin olive oil group showed a hazard ratio of 0.34 (95% CI, 0.20–0.58) when adjusted for classic atherosclerotic risk factors. The Mediterranean diet plus nuts group also showed an improvement in the hazard ratio (0.5, 95% CI, 0.30–0.81).[412]

Beetroot juice and peripheral arterial disease

Beetroot juice is rich in inorganic nitrates, which can be converted to nitric oxide after ingestion, with nitric oxide being important in regulating vascular function.[413] In a small randomised crossover study of beetroot juice (500 mL) compared to an orange juice control, beetroot juice increased plasma nitrite concentration after 3 hours (a marker of nitric oxide activity), and lowered diastolic blood pressure at rest and after cardiopulmonary exercise, and most importantly improved walking duration before onset of claudication pain by 18% and also increased peak walking time by 17%.[413]

NUTRITIONAL MEDICINE (SUPPLEMENTAL)

Omega-3 fatty acids and peripheral arterial disease

The question as to the efficacy of fish oil and omega-3 fatty acids in peripheral arterial disease was considered by a Cochrane review published in 2013. The review considered all randomised controlled trials involving omega-3 fatty acids compared to either placebo or other medications (such as statins) in patients with intermittent claudication of greater than 6 months duration who had not had vascular surgery or angioplasty within the previous 3 months. The findings were summarised by the authors as follows:

> *Omega-3 fatty acids appear to have little haematological benefit in people with intermittent claudication and there is no evidence of consistently improved clinical outcomes (quality of life, walking distance, ankle brachial pressure index or angiographic findings). Supplementation may also cause adverse effects such as nausea, diarrhoea and flatulence. Further research is needed to evaluate fully short- and long-term effects of omega-3 fatty acids on the most clinically relevant outcomes in people with intermittent claudication before they can be recommended for routine use.*[414]

This disappointing finding may however be a product of the highly variable nature of the included studies (a total of 9 studies). The omega-3 interventions varied considerably in both form and dosage (from a dairy drink enriched with EPA and DHA as well as vitamins and other oils, to fish oil capsules with different total dosages and varying EPA and DHA content). Additionally the duration of treatment in the studies varied from 7 weeks to 2 years.[414] Another factor not considered is quality of the supplement. Various studies have suggested that issues such as whether or not the lipids are emulsified,[415] the presence of saturated fats in the supplements (in some cases up to 36% of total fatty acid content),[416] and oxidation status of the lipids[416,417] may alter rheological effects and clinical outcomes.

Flavonoids and chronic venous insufficiency or postphlebitic syndrome

While supplemental flavonoid preparations have been shown to have many interesting pharmacological actions of potential relevance to the prevention and treatment of chronic venous insufficiency (such as improving venous tone, reducing capillary leakage and reducing inflammation),[418] systematic reviews examining the benefit of flavonoid preparations on patient symptoms have concluded that while there may be some benefit, it appears slight and that there is a distinct need for higher quality studies.[419,420] The effects may be different with herbal preparations rich in flavonoids compared to isolated flavonoid preparations, due to the more complicated chemistry of herbal preparation. This is indicated by trends towards greater efficacy from preparations which are a combination of different constituents found commonly in herbal phlebotonics, such as a combination of coumarins and flavonoids, and use of compression stockings which had an oedema-protective effect greater than compression stockings and placebo.[421]

HERBAL MEDICINE

Herbal medicine therapeutic objectives

PERIPHERAL ATHEROSCLEROTIC DISEASE

The primary objectives in managing peripheral atherosclerotic disease are:

- Manage all known risk factors for atherosclerosis, including hypertension, oxidative risk, clotting risk, dyslipidaemia and obesity
- Increase peripheral vasodilation
- Improve arterial endothelial function
- Improve peripheral vascular integrity.

RAYNAUD'S SYNDROME

The primary objectives in managing Raynaud's syndrome are:

- If it is secondary to chronic inflammatory connective tissue disease, then directly address the inflammatory and autoimmune aspects contributing to the connective tissue dysfunction
- Stabilise peripheral vascular motility
- Increase peripheral vasodilation.

CHILBLAINS

The primary objectives in managing chilblains are:

- Increase peripheral circulation and vasodilation
- Reduce localised inflammation and pruritus.

THROMBOANGIITIS OBLITERANS

The primary objectives in managing thromboangiitis obliterans are:

- Reduce vascular inflammation
- Reduce vascular oxidation
- Stabilise peripheral vascular motility
- Reduce clotting risk
- Improve peripheral vascular integrity.

DEEP VENOUS THROMBOSIS

It is important to remember that acute DVT is most appropriately managed with conventional medical care. However in patients at risk of DVT, the following objectives are relevant:

- Reduce clotting risk
- Reduce other risk factors, especially immobility and hypertension
- Improve venous return
- Improve peripheral vascular integrity.

CHRONIC VENOUS INSUFFICIENCY AND POSTPHLEBITIC SYNDROME

The primary objectives in managing chronic venous insufficiency and/or postphlebitic syndrome are:

- Improve venous return
- Reduce clotting risk
- Improve peripheral vascular integrity
- Reduce peripheral oedema
- Encourage healing if skin lesions are present.

HERBAL MEDICINE CLASSES

A range of herbal medicine classes are directly relevant in peripheral arterial and venous disorders, as well as many which are indirectly relevant (such as antihypertensives). The primary classes of use are listed below:

- Anticoagulants
- Circulatory stimulants (specifically the types traditionally regarded as heating in nature)
- Peripheral vasodilators (often also classified as diaphoretics when applied in the context of fevers)
- Antioxidants
- Anti-inflammatories
- Connective tissue tonics
- Lymphatics (to improve peripheral oedema, especially in chronic venous insufficiency)
- Peripheral vascular tonics (as opposed to the circulatory stimulants, these are not heating in traditional nomenclature)
- Vulneraries (for wound healing).

Specific herbal medicines

VITIS VINIFERA SEED (GRAPE SEED), *PINUS PINASTA* (MARITIME PINE BARK) AND PYCNOGENOL

Flavonoids and their derivatives are a large and diverse group of plant constituents, found in a range of foods and medicinal plants. Often collectively referred to as polyphenolic constituents, these compounds can occur as simple monomers, glycosylated monomers (i.e. bound naturally to one or more sugar units), or as dimers, oligomers and polymers, and in some cases bound to other plant metabolites (such as gallate in the range of tea-based polyphenols including epigallocatechin gallate). They have a complex and diverse nomenclature, and names such as catechins, anthocyanidins, anthocyanins (which are simply glycosides of anthocyanidins), proanthocyanidins, and procyanidins are used to describe various groups and subgroups of these plant constituents.[422,423] Their effect on vascular function has been known since Rusznyák and Szent-Györgyi reported their early experiments in the journal *Nature* in 1936,[424] and remain a continued topic of clinical and experimental interest.

While there has yet to be extensive and repeated human clinical research on the various indications, a proprietary extract of *Pinus pinasta* known as Pycnogenol with a high concentration of proanthocyanidins has extensive in-vitro evidence and some human clinical trials supporting its anti-inflammatory, antioxidant, wound healing, vasodilatory and platelet aggregation inhibitory actions.[425] In terms of vascular indications, this specific extract has been shown to be of benefit (in small-scale human studies) in hypertension, chronic venous insufficiency and retinopathy.[425]

Grape seed extract (GSE) and the extracts of the bark of the maritime bark (*Pinus pinasta*) have similar chemistry, both having a high concentration of proanthocyanidins.[426] In-vitro, in-vivo and limited human clinical studies show the actions and indications of GSE and Pycnogenol to be very similar, especially in terms of cardiovascular applications.[273]

The dosages utilised in research are highly variable; however, the limited positive human studies on the vascular effects of Pycnogenol have utilised dosages of 100–360 mg of extract (standardised to 70% ± 5% procyanidins).[425]

For GSE the dosages are even less clear due to the multiple types and specifications of extracts available (such as the proprietary Leucoselect with specifications of ≥95% total proanthocyanidins with 13–19% catechin and epicatechin,[427] as well as a range of more generic extracts) and also the differences in how these specifications can be declared on products based on the regulatory requirements of individual countries. A general Australian guideline of extract equivalent to 24 000–36 000 mg of dried seed per day has been published;[273] however, many products and their dosage recommendations are far lower than this, therefore it is important for the clinician to ensure the patient is given an adequate dosage. In most cases this may be between 36 000 and 48 000 mg of dried seed equivalent per day for use in existing peripheral arterial and venous disorders — especially in more acute and severe scenarios such as thromboangiitis obliterans where it can be particularly valuable — with clear benefit being observed in 2–4 weeks in most cases, with venous conditions usually taking 4–8 weeks for observable change (see Box 20.8).

BOX 20.8 Is your grape seed extract actually peanut skin?

A study published in 2015 has illustrated the various concerns around lack of effective standardisation in relation to grape seed extract (GSE). In this study 21 different commercially available extracts of grape seed were chemically evaluated, and compared to three authenticated extracts of grape seed, an authenticated extract of peanut skin, and an authenticated extract of pine bark. Additionally antioxidant capacity of each was evaluated and compared using the Trolox equivalent antioxidant capacity test.

The first issue identified in this study was the enormous variation in the comparative chemical profile of the commercial GSEs to the authenticated GSEs, which raised questions as to clinical reliability when different products are utilised in practice and research.

Even more troubling was the discovery that 9 of the 21 samples of grape seed extract were found to be adulterated with peanut skin, with the researchers strongly suspecting that 6 of these 9 samples were solely peanut skin extract (with no GSE content) based upon comparison of their profiles. This raises the additional issue of patient safety, given the relatively widespread (and often serious nature) of peanut allergy in the community.

The researchers have proposed a relatively simple and inexpensive quality screening method involving thin layer chromatography which can be used to test samples for peanut skin adulteration.

The clinical end point is that herbalists and naturopaths should be raising questions with product suppliers (regardless of whether they are practitioner-only or over-the-counter products) as to their source of GSE, and if and how it has been authenticated.

Source: Villani TS, Reichert W, Ferruzzi MG et al. Chemical investigation of commercial grape seed derived products to assess quality and detect adulteration. Food Chem 2015; 170:271–280.

GINKGO BILOBA (GINKGO)

Ginkgo biloba is a specific for peripheral vascular disease of all types, arterial or venous. In-vitro and in-vivo research has demonstrated that ginkgo extract possesses a number of highly relevant actions:[273]

- Antioxidant
- Peripheral and coronary vasodilator
- Antiplatelet (although limited human studies as well as clinical use raise the question of whether this effect is significant or relevant in humans at normal dosages)
- Anti-oedematous
- Anti-inflammatory.

Human clinical trial evidence to support the benefit of ginkgo in peripheral vascular disease is often inconclusive however,[273] in part due to inadequate sample sizes, the possible risk of study bias and the variable dosages employed.[428] While a 2005 review examining complementary therapies for the management of peripheral arterial disease concluded that ginkgo was the only complementary treatment clearly effective for intermittent claudication when compared to placebo,[429] a 2013 Cochrane review came to the conclusion that it was no more effective than placebo.[428]

The conundrum for the clinician is whether to ignore the favourable in-vitro and in-vivo evidence in the face of a lack of high-quality and conflicting human research, or to also consider the wealth of clinical experience supporting the efficacy of ginkgo. In finding an answer to this conundrum consideration should be given to published guidelines such those of the German health authority and the World Health Organization both of which list intermittent claudication (from peripheral arterial disease) as an approved indication for ginkgo.[430] Additionally, the principles of evidence-based practice must come into play, the definition of which is 'the integration of the best research evidence with our clinical expertise and our patient's unique values and circumstances'.[431] In the face of inconclusive research evidence due consideration must be given to clinical experience which generally supports the safe and efficacious use of medicines such as ginkgo in peripheral arterial disease.

A full discussion of the complexity of *Ginkgo biloba* is beyond the scope of this text; however, comprehensive reviews such as found in the American Herbal Pharmacopoeia[430] are valuable in this regard, documenting its potential value in PAD and in Raynaud's syndrome. It is important to note that there are a number of issues around dosage and extract equivalency which are likely to affect clinical outcomes. For example, while a considerable amount of research has been conducted on one specific extract (EGb761) at a daily dosage of 120 mg of extract (which has an approximate drug extract ratio of 50:1), more recent research is often demonstrating better outcomes at higher dosages of 240 mg of extract daily.[430] This, in addition to the known issues around variation of extract type and quality, and adulteration of some extracts with isolated flavonoids[430] means that clinicians should expend considerable effort in determining the source and quality of the extract, as well as the dosage they employ in practice.

ALLIUM SATIVUM (GARLIC)

While human studies on garlic in peripheral arterial disease are conflicting,[273] the various positive benefits on components of atherosclerotic risk (such as hypertension, hyperlipidaemia, platelet and fibrin clotting) make it worthy of consideration.[273] A double-blind randomised control trial published in 2013 examined the effect of 2 years dosing of a specific extract of garlic on carotid intima-media thickness (as a marker for atherosclerosis progression) in a total of 196 men. Compared to placebo the garlic group had a statistically significant decrease in carotid intima-media thickness.[432] While this is not specific to PAD, given that PAD is associated with systemic atherosclerotic change, it follows that long-term use of garlic may be of benefit in reducing the atherosclerotic progression of PAD.

CURCUMA LONGA (TURMERIC)

While there appears to be no published human research on turmeric in thromboangiitis obliterans, the combination of well-researched anti-inflammatory and antioxidant activities[273] make it an obvious choice for the management of this condition.

From clinical experience, it is quite valuable even in the acute phases of thromboangiitis obliterans, provided high dosages are used. The primary preparation form which has been used by the author for this purpose is the proprietary curcumin C3 complex (standardised for 95% curcumin) at a dosage of 1052 mg of the extract two to three times daily in the early stages. Once significant clinical improvement is noticed, maintain this dosage for another 2 weeks, then reduce to 526 mg of extract 3 times daily. While other turmeric extracts may or may not be as effective, the author has limited clinical experience with these other extracts.

ZANTHOXYLUM CLAVA-HERCULIS, Z. AMERICANUM (PRICKLY ASH)

Prickly ash has traditionally been regarded as a diffusive circulatory stimulant, which can improve peripheral arterial and capillary circulation.[433] It is indicated in intermittent claudication and Raynaud's syndrome[108] and valuable in debilitated patients.[433] From clinical experience, its benefit in PAD and Raynaud's syndrome is significant, but takes around 3–4 weeks to be observed when employed at normal dosages.

ACHILLEA MILLEFOLIUM (YARROW)

The flowers and leaves of yarrow contain high levels of flavonoids and their derivatives, as well as some volatile oil components, which have demonstrated anti-inflammatory effects in in-vitro and in-vivo animal models.[106,434] Traditionally it has been known as a diaphoretic, hypotensive and peripheral vasodilator, indicated for thrombotic conditions.[108] While human research is lacking, the author has found it valuable as a component of treatment for peripheral venous disorders such as chronic venous insufficiency and postphlebitic syndrome.

CENTELLA ASIATICA (GOTU KOLA)

Gotu kola, also known as Indian pennywort, has traditionally been employed orally as an antirheumatic, and topically for wounds and ulcers.[108] In-vitro and animal research has demonstrated that the triterpenoid constituents are anti-inflammatory and encourage wound healing. While human research data are limited, it has been applied for chronic venous insufficiency, and a 2013 systematic review of 8 studies published noted that while there were considerable methodological and reporting issues in some of the included studies, *Centella* seemed to improve parameters of microcirculation (such as transcutaneous partial O_2 and CO_2 pressures, ankle swelling and venoarteriolar response) as well as symptoms and signs such as leg oedema, leg heaviness and pain.[435]

AESCULUS HIPPOCASTANUM (HORSECHESTNUT)

Horsechestnut extract is a well-researched herbal medicine specifically valuable for chronic venous insufficiency and postphlebitic syndrome, and varicose veins.[106,273] Its interesting chemistry including triterpenoid saponins, coumarins, flavonoids and allantoin, combine to exhibit vasoprotective effects, reducing vascular permeability, inflammation and oedema associated with chronic venous insufficiency.[273] A Cochrane review published in 2012, which considered 17 randomised controlled trials all employing extracts standardised for escin compared to either placebo or other reference medication, concluded that horsechestnut extract is a safe and efficacious treatment for chronic venous insufficiency.[436] According to both the research evidence and clinical application by the author, it is important to ensure preparations standardised for escin are employed, with a dosage of approximately 50–100 mg of escin twice daily, and if significant improvement is noticed after 8 weeks the dosage may be reduced to 50 mg escin once daily.[273] Mild gastrointestinal adverse reactions (including nausea) have been reported in studies (likely due to its saponin content), and thus extracts should be taken with food to minimise the risk.[273]

LIFESTYLE RECOMMENDATIONS

Weight loss and peripheral arterial disease

A meta-analysis involving a total of 4231 patients which examined the impact of weight loss by energy restriction (mean weight loss across participants was 11% of initial body weight) on measures of peripheral arterial function including cardio-ankle vascular index, beta-stiffness index, arterial compliance, pulse pressure and pulse wave analysis, showed that weight loss improvement most measures.[437]

Exercise and peripheral arterial disease

A Cochrane review of exercise programs in a total of 1816 patients with intermittent claudication showed improvements in maximal walking time, walking distance, as well as quality of life markers (as assessed by the SF-36 — used in only 2 of the included 30 studies).[438]

Thus dietary advice and exercise programs for patients who are medically able should be a component of therapy for peripheral arterial disease. However, despite the significant evidence as to the importance of diet and lifestyle in reducing progression of peripheral arterial disease, according to a study which reviewed 1982 outpatient visits for people with peripheral arterial disease (obtained from the United States National Ambulatory Medical Care Survey and National Hospital Ambulatory Medical Care Survey) exercise or dietary counselling was only provided to 22% of patients.[439]

Elastic compression stockings and postthrombotic syndrome

A Cochrane review of the effect of elastic compression stockings (ECS) on prevention of postthrombotic (also known as postphlebitic) syndrome in patients with a history of deep venous thrombosis, showed that ECS significantly reduced the incidence of postthrombotic syndrome, and improved pain and swelling. The authors concluded that ECS should be added to the therapy of patients who have been affected by deep venous thrombosis.[440] However, in the experience of this author, patient compliance with the usage recommendations of ECS is poor, with many patients discontinuing early, or only using them intermittently. Thus it is advised that patients be counselled directly on both the short- and long-term benefit of ECS.

CASE STUDY

OVERVIEW

TA was a 41-year-old male presenting with thromboangiitis obliterans mostly affecting his left leg, but also affecting his right to a lesser degree. The disease became an overt problem for the patient 8 weeks prior, with severe claudication pain at rest appearing in his left foot, combined with cyanosis of the lower areas of the limb. However, prior to this the patient recalls approximately 9 months of progressive numbness and tingling sensations in his left leg and foot, progressively frequent and severe episodes of intermittent claudication, and some swelling and redness of the lower areas of the left limb. Three poorly healing wounds (which from the patient's description appeared ulcerative) had occurred on this left leg over the course of the last 6 months, with the only treatment being non-adherent gauze covered by bandages.

Initial treatment involved hospitalisation where the patient was placed on an intravenous solution (likely iloprost), and later discharged with nifedipine 20 mg twice daily.

Upon presentation TA was still suffering with frequent claudication pain in the left leg and foot, including some

CASE STUDY CONTINUED

episodes at rest, as well as some episodes of claudication in the right leg as well (only on walking). Due to this pain the patient was not very mobile. One ulcerative lesion was visible on the left upper tibial surface, approximately 5 mm in diameter. While there appeared to be some erythema surrounding the lesion, it was difficult to judge due to diffuse redness of the entire lower limb. The patient described that the skin temperature of his lower left leg sometimes felt very hot to touch and sometimes very cold. At the time of presentation it was warmer than his upper limb, and somewhat oedematous.

The patient had been a cigarette smoker since his early 20s; however, based on recommendations from his doctor he had stopped smoking 7 weeks ago. He is still finding the cravings difficult but has not used nicotine replacement therapy as he was advised against this by his doctor.

DIET AND LIFESTYLE

Previously an active man, participating in coaching football as a hobby, and working as a bricklayer, TA also had a long history of poor diet. On average he would have 2 servings of vegetables per day, red meat often twice a day, eggs almost every day, white bread only and usually 2–4 slices per day, sweet biscuits or chocolate bars as snacks every day, ice-cream every second day, and 3 cups of sweetened white coffee per day on work days. His alcohol consumption was usually 1–2 beers per day during the working week, and usually once every second weekend he would consume roughly 6–8 beers and 2–4 shots of spirits at social events.

The recent increase in severity of his peripheral vascular issues has resulted in TA's work and social activities being considerably restricted.

CLINICAL EXAMINATION AND PATHOLOGY

The patient's weight was 84 kg, with a height of 178 cm (BMI of 26). His blood pressure on presentation was 130/80 mmHg; however, he said he had 4 years previously been diagnosed as hypertensive and had not bothered to take the prescribed medications 'because I didn't feel sick'. Clearly the nifedipine was now reducing his blood pressure.

No copies of blood test results were available but the patient said that the doctor had been pleased with his cholesterol levels. Additionally the doctor did tell him to 'knock out the alcohol because your liver is struggling'.

ASSESSMENT

TA has obvious thromboangiitis obliterans, with the possibility of some degree of peripheral vascular disease also being present. The recent cessation of smoking has been a good change though the patient understands little about his condition or issues such as healthy eating.

THERAPEUTIC OBJECTIVES

The initial treatment objectives for this first consultation were:

- Reduce vascular inflammation
- Reduce vascular oxidation

CASE STUDY CONTINUED

- Reduce peripheral clotting
- Normalise peripheral vascular motility.

TREATMENT

HERBAL TREATMENT

Herbal medicine	DER	Quantity/ week	Rationale
Ginkgo biloba	3:2	45 mL	Antioxidant, normalises peripheral vascular motility, antiplatelet
Salvia miltiorrhiza	1:2	55 mL	Antifibrin and antiplatelet

Dosage: 7 mL twice daily with breakfast and dinner.

Antioxidant tablets (breakdown of each tablet is below), 2 tablets 3 times daily with food.

- *Vitis vinifera* extract equivalent to dry seed 6000 mg, standardised to procyanidins 42.5 mg
- *Camellia sinensis* extract equivalent to dry leaf 4170 mg, standardised to catechins 83.35 mg
- *Curcuma longa* extract equivalent to dry rhizome 2000 mg, standardised to curcuminoids 76 mg
- *Rosmarinus officinalis* extract equivalent to dry leaf 1000 mg.

NUTRITIONAL TREATMENT

Initial nutritional treatment was conservative to avoid overloading the patient:

- For lunch 5 days a week change to a mixed leaf salad with olive oil and balsamic vinegar dressing, with a small handful of brown rice and a small handful of pre-cooked chicken breast or thigh
- Reduce red meat to once daily
- Eliminate ice-cream and replace with a piece of fresh fruit
- Omega capsules (1280 mg, with EPA 650 mg, DHA 450 mg). 1 capsule twice daily with food
- Vitamin E 500 IU per day.

PATIENT OUTCOMES

At the first follow-up 4 weeks later TA stated that his claudication pain had reduced in severity and frequency by 'about 30%'. Examination of his left leg revealed that the ulcerative lesion was healing and now was roughly 2 mm in diameter, with less erythema. Generalised lower limb erythema had reduced significantly and the lower limb was only slightly colder than the upper limb.

The patient had continued avoiding cigarette smoking and had enacted the requested dietary changes.

At this point the patient was told of the importance of reducing his alcohol intake given the previous comments from his doctor.

Treatment was continued the same, with the addition of (MZ80) silymarin capsules at a dosage of 1 capsule 3 times daily to address the probability that his liver function tests were not ideal.

At the next follow-up (12 weeks since the initial visit), further symptomatic improvement in the thromboangiitis obliterans was expressed by TA, with claudication pain

CASE STUDY CONTINUED

occurring only once every few days, and only on exercise. TA had returned to work and was starting to help with coaching football again, although without a lot of running at this stage. Examination of his lower limbs revealed almost no oedema, much less erythema and almost normalised skin temperature. No ulcerative lesions were present. The patient presented copies of recent blood tests showing normalisation of liver function enzymes from their previously elevated state. TA's alcohol consumption had significantly reduced to 4 beers per week. Treatment was continued unchanged.

REFERENCES

[1] Tortora JG, Grabowski SR. Principles of anatomy and physiology. 9th ed. New York: John Wiley; 2000.

[2] Culpeper N. A complete herbal. 1693. Available from: www.bibliomania.com/2/1/66/113/frameset.html.

[3] Hedley C as cited in Bergner. Medical herbalism: a journal for the clinical practitioner. 2001. Available from: http://medherb.com/Therapeutics/Cardiovascular_system_Case_Studies.htm.

[4] Fiore C. A history of the therapeutic use of liquorice in Europe. J Ethnopharmacol 2005;99(3):317–24.

[5] Ellingwood F. The American materia medica, therapeutics and pharmacognosy. Portland, OR: Eclectic Medical Publications; 1919.

[6] Shiozaki M, Iso H, Ohira T, et al. Longitudinal risk of cardiovascular events in relation to depression symptoms after discharge among survivors of myocardial infarction. Osaka Acute Coronary Insufficiency Study. Circ J 2011;75(12):2878–84.

[7] Uysal H, Özcan Ş. The effect of individual training and counselling programme for patients with myocardial infarction over patients' quality of life. Int J Nurs Pract 2012;18(5):445–53.

[8] Boericke W. Boericke's materia medica excerpt: the tinctures. 1901. Available from: http://www.henriettesherbal.com/eclectic/boericke/crataegus.html.

[9] Levy RI. Prevalence and epidemiology of cardiovascular disease. In: Wyngaarden JB, Smith LH, editors. Cecil textbook of medicine. 17th ed. Philadelphia: WB Saunders Company; 1985.

[10] Chobhain A, Bakris G, Black H, et al. The Seventh Report of the Joint National Committee On Prevention, Detection, Evaluation, and Treatment of High Blood Pressure. JAMA 2003;289(19):2560–71.

[11] Britt H, Miller GC, Charles J, et al. General practice activity in Australia 2006–07. Cat. no. GEP 21. General Practice Series no. 21. Canberra: AIHW; 2008.

[12] Australian Institute of Health and Welfare. Health care expenditure on cardiovascular diseases 2004–05. CVD43. Canberra: AIHW; 2008.

[13] Bennet S. Cardiovascular risk factors in Australia: trends in socioeconomic inequalities. J Epidemiol Community Health 1995;49(4):363–72.

[14] Broadbent A. Impact of falling cardiovascular disease death rates: deaths delayed and years of life extended, AUS113. Canberra: AIHW; 2009.

[15] International Diabetes Institute. Tracking the accelerating epidemic: its causes and outcomes, The Australian Diabetes, Obesity and Lifestyle Study (AusDiab). Melbourne: International Diabetes Institute; 2006.

[16] Vasan R, Larson M, Leip E, et al. Assessment of frequency of progression to hypertension in nonhypertensive participants in The Framingham Heart Study. Lancet 2001;358:1682–6.

[17] Boon N, Colledge N, Walker B, et al, editors. Davidson's principles and practice of medicine. 20th ed. Edinburgh: Elsevier, Churchill Livingstone; 2006.

[18] Holler T. Cardiology essentials. Sudbury: Jones & Bartlett Publishers; 2008.

[19] Mancia G, Bombelli M, Fachetti R, et al. Long-term risk of sustained hypertension in white-coat or masked hypertension. Hypertension 2009;54(2):226–32.

[20] Fuster V, Topol E, Nabel E, editors. Atherothrombosis and coronary artery disease. 2nd ed. Philadelphia: Lippincott Williams & Wilkins; 2005.
[21] Goldman L, Ausiello D, editors. Cecil medicine. 23th ed. Philadelphia: Saunders, Elsevier; 2008.
[22] Williams R, Rao D, Ellison R, et al. NHLBI family blood pressure program: methodology and recruitment in the HyperGEN network. Hypertension genetic epidemiology network. Ann Epidemiol 2000;10(6):389–400.
[23] Arnett D, Hong Y, Bella J, et al. Sibling correlation of left ventricular mass and geometry in hypertensive African Americans and whites: the HyperGEN study. Hypertension Genetic Epidemiology Network. Am J Hypertens 2001;14(12):1226–30.
[24] Cooper R, Wolf-Maier K, Luke A, et al. An international comparative study of blood pressure in populations of European vs. African descent. BMC Med 2005;3(2):1–8.
[25] Agyemang C, Bhopal R. Is the blood pressure of people from African origin adults in the UK higher or lower than that in European origin white people? A review of cross-sectional data. J Hum Hypertens 2003;17(8):523–34.
[26] Australian Institute of Health and Welfare. Cardiovascular medicines and primary health care: a regional analysis, CVD48. Canberra: AIHW; 2010.
[27] Brown A. Bridging the survival gap between Indigenous and non-Indigenous Australians: priorities for the road ahead. Heart Lung Circ 2009;18(2):29–100.
[28] Penm E. Cardiovascular disease and its associated risk factors in Aboriginal and Torres Strait Islander peoples 2004–05, CVD41. Canberra: AIHW; 2008.
[29] Joint National Committee on Prevention Detection. Evaluation, and Treatment of High Blood Pressure. The sixth report of the Joint National Committee on Prevention, Detection, Evaluation, and Treatment of High Blood Pressure. Arch Intern Med 1997;157(21):2413–46.
[30] Hyman D, Pavlik V. Characteristics of patients with uncontrolled hypertension in the United States. New Engl J Med 2001;345(7):479–86.
[31] Lewington S, Clarke R, Qizilbash N, et al. Age-specific relevance of usual blood pressure to vascular mortality: a meta-analysis of individual data for one million adults in 61 prospective studies. Lancet 2002;360(9349):1903–13.
[32] Vasan R, Beiser A, Seshadri S, et al. Residual lifetime risk for developing hypertension in middle-aged women and men: The Framingham Heart Study. JAMA 2002;287:1003–10.
[33] Durstine J, Moore G, LaMonte M, et al. Pollock's textbook of cardiovascular disease and rehabilitation. Champaign, IL: Human Kinetics; 2008.
[34] Azizi F, Ainy E. Coronary heart disease risk factors and menopause: a study in 1980 Tehranian women, the Tehran Lipid and Glucose Study. Climacteric 2003;6(4):330–6.
[35] Australian Bureau of Statistics. National Health Survey: summary of results, Australia, 2004–05. Cat. no. 4364.0. Canberra: ABS; 2006.
[36] Brown C, Higgins M, Donato K, et al. Body mass index and the prevalence of hypertension and dyslipidemia. Obes Res 2000;8(9):605–19.
[37] McGill J, Haffner S, Rees T, et al. Progress and controversies: treating obesity and insulin resistance in the context of hypertension. J Clin Hypertens (Greenwich) 2009;11(1):36–41.
[38] Lin P, Aickin M, Champagne C, et al. Food group sources of nutrients in the dietary patterns of the DASH-Sodium trial. J Am Diet Assoc 2003;103(4):488–96.
[39] He F, MacGregor G. A comprehensive review on salt and health and current experience of worldwide salt reduction programmes. J Hum Hypertens 2009;23(6):363–84.
[40] Stranges S, Wu T, Dorn J, et al. Relationship of alcohol drinking pattern to risk of hypertension: a population-based study. Hypertension 2004;44(6):813–19.
[41] Gray H, Dawkins K, Morgan J, et al. Cardiology. 5th ed. Oxford: Blackwell Publishing; 2008.
[42] Sparrenberger F, Cichelero F, Ascoli A, et al. Does psychosocial stress cause hypertension? A systematic review of observational studies. J Hum Hypertens 2009;23(1):12–19.
[43] Dochi M, Sakata K, Oishi M, et al. Smoking as an independent risk factor for hypertension: a 14-year longitudinal study in male Japanese workers. Tohoku J Exp Med 2009;217:37–43.
[44] Rhee M, Na S, Kim Y, et al. Acute effects of cigarette smoking on arterial stiffness and blood pressure in male smokers with hypertension. Am J Hypertens 2007;20(6):637–41.
[45] Sirivarasai J, Kaojarern S, Chanprasertyothin S, et al. Environmental lead exposure, catalase gene, and markers of antioxidant and oxidative stress relation to hypertension: an analysis based on the EGAT study. Biomed Res Int 2015;2015:856319.
[46] Johnson R, Feig D, Nakagawa T, et al. Pathogenesis of essential hypertension: historical paradigms and modern insights. J Hypertens 2008;26(3):381–91.
[47] Wang W, Lee E, Fabsitz R, et al. A longitudinal study of hypertension risk factors and their relation to cardiovascular disease: the Strong Heart Study. Hypertension 2006;47(3): 403–9.
[48] Hunt SA, et al. American College of Cardiology; American Heart Association Task Force on Practice Guidelines (Writing Committee to Update the 2001 Guidelines for the Evaluation and Management of Heart Failure). J Am Coll Cardiol 2005;46(6):e1–82.
[49] United Kingdom Prospective Diabetes Study Group. Tight blood pressure control and risk of macrovascular and microvascular complications in type 2 diabetes: UKPDS 38. BMJ 1998;317(7160):703–13.
[50] Colhoun H, Dong W, Barakat M, et al. The scope for cardiovascular disease risk factor intervention among people with diabetes mellitus in England: a population-based analysis from the Health Surveys for England 1991–94. Diabet Med 1999;16(1):35–40.
[51] Zelmanovitz T, Gerchman F, Balthazar A, et al. Diabetic nephropathy. Diabetol Metab Syndr 2009;1(1):10.
[52] American Diabetes Association. Hypertension management in adults with diabetes. Diabetes Care 2000;(Suppl. 1):S65–7.
[53] Bakris G, Williams M, Dworkin L, et al. Preserving renal function in adults with hypertension and diabetes: a consensus approach. National Kidney Foundation Hypertension and Diabetes Executive Committees Working Group. Am J Kidney Dis 2000;36(3):646–61.
[54] Ramsay L, Williams B, Johnston G, et al. Guidelines for management of hypertension: report of the third working party of the British Hypertension Society. J Hum Hypertens 1999;13(9):569–92.
[55] PROGRESS Collaborative Group. Randomised trial of a perindopril-based blood-pressure-lowering regimen among 6105 individuals with previous stroke or transient ischaemic attack. Lancet 2001;358(9287):1033–41.
[56] Peters R, Beckett N, Forette F, et al. Incidence of dementia and blood pressure lowering in the Hypertension in the Very Elderly Trial cognitive function assessment (HYVET-COG): a double-blind, placebo controlled trial. Lancet Neurol 2008;7(8):683–9.
[57] Duron E, Hanon O. Hypertension, cognitive decline and dementia. Arch Cardiovasc Dis 2008;101(3):181–9.
[58] Broughton Pipkin F. The hypertensive disorders of pregnancy. BMJ 1995;311(7005):609–13.
[59] Leeman L, Fontaine P. Hypertensive disorders of pregnancy. Am Fam Physician 2008;78(1):93–100.
[60] Myers M. Ambulatory blood pressure monitoring: guidelines for use in clinical practice. Can J Cardiol 1996;12(12):1271–5.
[61] Taylor G. Primary care cardiology. 2nd ed. Oxford: Blackwell Publishing; 2005.
[62] Pettit A, Wong R, Lee V, et al. Increased free radical production in hypertension due to increased expression of the NADPH oxidase subunit p22(phox) in lymphoblast cell lines. J Hypertens 2002;20(4):677–83.
[63] Pizzorno J, Murray M. Textbook of natural medicine. 3rd ed. Oxford: Elsevier; 1999.
[64] Kahn N, Hemmelgarn B, Herman R, et al. The 2008 Canadian Hypertension Education Program recommendations for the management of hypertension: part 2 — therapy. Can J Cardiol 2008;24(6):465–75.
[65] Cushman W, Ford C, Cutler J, et al. Success and predictors of blood pressure control in diverse North American settings: the antihypertensive and lipid-lowering treatment to prevent heart attack trial (ALLHAT). J Clin Hypertens (Greenwich) 2002;4(6):393–404.
[66] Izzo J, Levy D, Black H. Clinical Advisory Statement. Importance of systolic blood pressure in older Americans. Hypertension 2000;35:1021–4.

[67] Porter RS, Kaplan JL. The Merck manual online. Merck Sharp & Dohme Corp; 2010.

[68] Berkow S, Barnard N. Blood pressure regulation and vegetarian diets. Nutr Rev 2008;63(1):1–8.

[69] Sacks FM, Appel LJ, Moore TJ, et al. A dietary approach to prevent hypertension: a review of the Dietary Approaches to Stop Hypertension (DASH) Study. Clin Cardiol 1999;22(Suppl. 7):III6–II10.

[70] Australian National Health and Medical Research Council. The nutrient reference values. Available from: http://www.nrv.gov.au/nutrients/sodium.htm.

[71] Appel LJ, Moore TJ, Obarzanek E, et al. A clinical trial of the effects of dietary patterns on blood pressure. DASH Collaborative Research Group. N Engl J Med 1997;336(16):1117–24.

[72] Whelton PK, He J, Cutler JA, et al. Effects of oral potassium on blood pressure. Meta-analysis of randomized controlled clinical trials. JAMA 1997;277(20):1624–32.

[73] Barri YM, Wingo CS. The effects of potassium depletion and supplementation on blood pressure: a clinical review. Am J Med Sci 1997;314(1):37–40.

[74] Reid K, Frank OR, Stocks NP, et al. Effect of garlic on blood pressure: a systematic review and meta-analysis. BMC Cardiovasc Disord 2008;8:13.

[75] Chen ZY, Peng C, Jiao R, et al. Anti-hypertensive nutraceuticals and functional foods. J Agric Food Chem 2009;57(11):4485–99.

[76] Chen YJ, Peng C, Jiao R, et al. Anti-hypertensive nutraceuticals and functional foods. J Agric Food Chem 2009;57(11):4485–99.

[77] Karppanen H, Mervaala E. Sodium intake and hypertension. Prog Cardiovasc Dis 2006;49(2):59–75.

[78] Graudal NA, Galloe AM, Garred P. Effects of sodium restriction on blood pressure, renin, aldosterone, catecholamines, cholesterols and triglyceride: a meta-analysis. JAMA 1998;279:1383–91.

[79] Cutler JA, Follmann D, Allender PS. Randomised trials of sodium reduction: an overview. Am J Clin Nutr 1997;65:643S–651S.

[80] Food Standards Australia. Available from: www.foodstandards.gov.au/scienceandeducation/factsheets/factsheets2009/howmuchsodiumandsalt4340.cfm.

[81] Warensjö E, Sundström J, Vessby B, et al. Markers of dietary fat quality and fatty acid desaturation as predictors of total and cardiovascular mortality: a population-based prospective study. Am J Clin Nutr 2008;88(1):203–9.

[82] Erkkilä A, de Mello VD, Risérus U, et al. Dietary fatty acids and cardiovascular disease: an epidemiological approach. Prog Lipid Res 2008;47(3):172–87.

[83] Shirlow MJ, Berry G, Stokes G. Caffeine consumption and blood pressure: an epidemiological study. Int J Epidemiol 1988;17:90–7.

[84] Lopez-Garcia E, Orozco-Arbeláez E, Leon-Muñoz LM, et al. Habitual coffee consumption and 24-h blood pressure control in older adults with hypertension. Clin Nutr 2016;35(6):1457–63.

[85] Palatini P, Fania C, Mos L, et al. Coffee consumption and risk of cardiovascular events in hypertensive patients. Results from the HARVEST. Int J Cardiol 2016;212:131–7.

[86] Orozco-Arbeáez E, Guallar-Castillón P, Graciani A, et al. Habitual chocolate consumption and 24-hour blood pressure control in older adults with hypertension (letter to the editor). J Am Geriatr Soc 2015;63(12):2637–9.

[87] Ried K, Sullivan TR, Fakler P, et al. Effect of cocoa on blood pressure. Cochrane Database Syst Rev 2012;(8):CD008893.

[88] Lee BJ, Huang MC, Chung LJ, et al. Folic acid and vitamin B_{12} are more effective than vitamin B_6 in lowering fasting plasma homocysteine concentration in patients with coronary artery disease. Eur J Clin Nutr 2004;58:481–7.

[89] Lewerin C, Nilsson-Ehle H, Matousek M, et al. Reduction of plasma homocysteine and serum methymalonate concentrations in apparently healthy elderly subjects after treatment with folic acid, vitamin B_{12} and vitamin B_6: a randomized trial. Eur J Clin Nutr 2003;57:1426–36.

[90] Rosanoff A. Magnesium supplements may enhance the effect of antihypertensive medications in stage 1 hypertensive subjects. Magnesium Res 2010;23(1):27–40.

[91] Appel LJ, Miller ER 3rd, Seidler AJ, et al. Does supplementation of diet with 'fish oil' reduce blood pressure? A meta-analysis of controlled clinical trials. Arch Intern Med 1993;153(12):1429–38.

[92] Morris MC, Sacks F, Rosner B. Does fish oil lower blood pressure? A meta-analysis of controlled trials. Circulation 1993;88(2):523–33.

[93] Mori TA, Bao DQ, Burke V, et al. Docosahexaenoic acid but not eicosapentaenoic acid lowers ambulatory blood pressure and heart rate in humans. Hypertension 1999;34:253–60.

[94] Mori TA, Watts GF, Burke V, et al. Differential effects of eicosapentaenoic acid and docosahexaenoic acid on forearm vascular reactivity of the microcirculation in hyperlipidaemic, overweight men. Circulation 2000;102:1264–9.

[95] Mori TA. Omega-3 fatty acids and hypertension in humans. Clin Exp Pharmacol Physiol 2006;33:842–6.

[96] Yin K, Chu ZM, Beilin LJ. Study of mechanisms of glucocorticoid hypertension in rats: endothelial related changes and their amelioration by dietary fish oils. Br J Pharmacol 1992;106:435–42.

[97] Rodrigo R, Prat H, Passalacqua W, et al. Decrease in oxidative stress through supplementation of vitamins C and E is associated with a reduction in blood pressure in patients with essential hypertension. Clin Sci 2008;114(10):625–34.

[98] Kumar A, Kaur H, Devi P, et al. Role of coenzyme Q10 (CoQ10) in cardiac disease, hypertension and Menière-like syndrome. Pharmacol Ther 2009;124(3):259–68.

[99] Yamagami T, Iwamoto Y, Folkers K. Deficiency of activity of succinate dehydrogenase-coenzyme Q10 reductase in leucocytes from patients with essential hypertension. Int J Vitam Nutr Res 1974;44:404–14.

[100] Ho MJ, Bellusci A, Wright JM. Blood pressure lowering efficacy of coenzyme Q10 for primary hypertension. Cochrane Database Syst Rev 2009;(4):CD007435.

[101] Militante JD, Lombardini JB. Treatment of hypertension with oral taurine: experimental and clinical studies. Amino Acids 2002;23(4):381–93.

[102] Quyyumi AA, Dakak N, Diodati JG, et al. Effect of L-arginine on human coronary endothelium dependent and physiologic vasodilation. J Am Coll Cardiol 1997;30:1220–7.

[103] Lerman A, Burnett JCJ, Higano ST, et al. Long-term L-arginine supplementation improves small-vessel coronary endothelial function in humans. Circulation 1998;97:2123–8.

[104] Gokce N. L-Arginine and hypertension. J Nutr 2004;134:2807S–2811S.

[105] Schulz V, Hänsel R, Tyler VE. Rational phytotherapy: a physician's guide to herbal medicine. 4th ed. New York: Springer; 2001.

[106] Barnes J, Anderson LA, Phillipson JD. Herbal medicines. 3rd ed. London: Pharmaceutical Press; 2007.

[107] Korner PI. Essential hypertension and its causes: neuronal and non-neuronal mechanisms. New York: Oxford University Press; 2007.

[108] British Herbal Medicine Association. British herbal pharmacopoeia 1983. Bournemouth: British Herbal Medicine Association; 1991 (reprint).

[109] Walker AF, Marakis G, Morris AP, et al. Promising hypotensive effect of hawthorn extract: a randomized double-blind pilot study of mild, essential hypertension. Phytother Res 2001;16(1):48–54.

[110] Weiss RF. Herbal medicine classic edition. New York: Thieme; 2001 (reprint of 1985 English translation of German 6th edition of Lehrbuch der Phytotherapie).

[111] Boon NA, Colledge NR, Walker BR, editors. Davidson's principles & practice of medicine. 20th ed. Edinburgh: Churchill Livingstone; 2006.

[112] Circosta C, De Pasquale R, Samperi S, et al. Biological and analytical characterization of two extracts from *Valeriana officinalis*. J Ethnopharmacol 2007;112:361–7.

[113] Kang DG, Oh H, Chung HT, et al. Inhibition of angiotensin converting enzyme by lithospermic acid B isolated from Radix *Salviae miltiorrhiza* Bunge. Phytother Res 2003;17:917–20.

[114] Kang DG, Yun YG, Ryoo JH, et al. Anti-hypertensive effect of water extract of Danshen on renovascular hypertension through inhibition of the renin angiotensin system. Am J Chin Med 2002;30:87–93.

[115] Gao XP, Xu DY, Deng YL, et al. Screening of angiotensin converting enzyme inhibitors from *Salvia miltiorrhizae*. Zhongguo Zhong Yao Za Zhi 2004;29:359–62.

[116] Jiang RW, Lau KM, Hon PM, et al. Chemistry and biological activities of caffeic acid derivatives from *Salvia miltiorrhiza*. Curr Med Chem 2005;12:237–46.

[117] Watzke A, O'Malley SJ, Bergman RG, et al. Reassignment of the configuration of salvianolic acid B and establishment of its identity with lithospermic acid B. J Nat Prod 2006;69:1231–3.

[118] Miller AL. Botanical influences on cardiovascular disease. Altern Med Rev 1998;3(6):422–31.
[119] Dwivedi P, Somani K, Udupa N. Role of *Inula racemosa* and *Saussurea lappa* in management of angina pectoris. Pharmac Biol 1989;27(4):217–22.
[120] Hammer F, Stewart PM. Cortisol metabolism in hypertension. Best Pract Res Clin Endocrinol Metab 2006;20(3):337–53.
[121] Quinkler M, Stewart PM. Hypertension and the cortisol-cortisone shuttle. J Clin Endocrinol Metab 2003;88(6):2384–92.
[122] Reinhart KM, Coleman CI, Teevan C, et al. Effects of garlic on blood pressure in patients with and without systolic hypertension: a meta-analysis. Ann Pharmacother 2008;42(12):1766–71.
[123] El SN, Karakaya S. Olive tree (*Olea europaea*) leaves: potential beneficial effects on human health. Nutr Rev 2009;67(11): 632–8.
[124] Felter HW, Lloyd JR. King's American dispensatory. 18th ed. Rev. 3. Portland, OR: Eclectic Materia Medica Publications; 1905, reprinted 1983.
[125] He J, Whelton PK, Appel LJ, et al. Long-term effects of weight loss and dietary sodium reduction on incidence of hypertension. Hypertension 2000;35(2):544–9.
[126] Sharman JE, Stowasser M. Australian Association for Exercise and Sports Science position statement on exercise and hypertension. J Sci Med Sport 2009;12(2):252–7.
[127] Onat A, Uğur M, Hergenç G, et al. Lifestyle and metabolic determinants of incident hypertension, with special reference to cigarette smoking: a longitudinal population-based study. Am J Hypertens 2009;22(2):156–62.
[128] Goldman L, Schafer AI, editors. Goldman's Cecil medicine. 24th ed. Philadelphia: Elsevier Saunders; 2012.
[129] Alexander R, Schlant R, Fuster V, editors. Hurst's the heart: arteries and veins. New York: McGraw-Hill; 1998.
[130] Rizzo M, Kotur-Stevujevic J, Berneis K, et al. Atherogenic dyslipidemia and oxidative stress: a new look. Transl Res 2009;153(5):217–23.
[131] Cullen P. Evidence that triglycerides are an independent coronary heart disease risk factor. Am J Cardiol 2000;86(9):943–9.
[132] Hopkins P, Wu L, Hunt S, et al. Plasma triglycerides and type III hyperlipidaemia are independently associated with premature familial coronary artery disease. J Am Coll Cardiol 2005;45(7):1003–12.
[133] Bonow R. Primary prevention of cardiovascular disease: a call to action. Circulation 2002;106(25):3140–1.
[134] Arora S, Nicholls S. Atherosclerotic plaque reduction: blood pressure, dyslipidemia, atherothrombosis. Drugs Today (Barc) 2008;44(9):711–18.
[135] Smit J, Diamant M. Genetically defined hyperlipidaemia. Pharmacogenomics 2004;5(3):295–304.
[136] Papatheodorou L, Weiss N. Vascular oxidant stress and inflammation in hyperhomocysteinemia. Antioxid Redox Signal 2007;9(11):1941–58.
[137] Su J, Wang S, Hunang Y, et al. A comparative study on pathogenic effects of homocysteine and cysteine on atherosclerosis. Wei Sheng Yan Jiu 2009;38(1):43–6.
[138] Gokkusa C, Tulubas F, Unlucerci Y, et al. Homocysteine and pro-inflammatory cytokine concentrations in acute heart disease. Cytokine 2010;50:15–18.
[139] McCully K. Homocysteine, vitamins, and vascular disease prevention. Am J Clin Nutr 2007;86(5):1563S–1568S.
[140] Gotto A. Role of C-reactive protein in coronary risk reduction: focus on primary prevention. Am J Cardiol 2007;99(5):718–25.
[141] Calabro P, Willerson J, Yeh E. Inflammatory cytokines stimulated C-reactive protein production by human coronary artery smooth muscle cells. Circulation 2003;108(16):1930–2.
[142] Liapis C, Avgerinos E, Kadoglou N, et al. What a vascular surgeon should know and do about atherosclerotic risk factors. J Vasc Surg 2009;49(5):1348–54.
[143] Link N, Tanner M. Coronary artery disease: part 1. Epidemiology and diagnosis. West J Med 2001;174(4):257–61.
[144] Vongpatanasin W. Management of hypertension in patients with coronary artery disease. Curr Hypertens Rep 2008;10(5):349–54.
[145] Bartnik M, Ryden L, Malmberg K, et al. Oral glucose tolerance test is needed for appropriate classification of glucose regulation in patients with coronary artery disease: a report from the Euro Heart Survey on Diabetes and the Heart. Heart 2007;93(1):72–7.
[146] Carnethon M, Fortmann S, Palaniappan L, et al. Risk factors for progression to incident hyperinsulinemia: the Atherosclerosis Risk in Communities Study, 1987–1998. Am J Epidemiol 2003;158(11):1058–67.
[147] Dentali F, Squizzato A, Ageno W. The metabolic syndrome as a risk factor for venous and arterial thrombosis. Semin Thromb Hemost 2009;35(5):451–7.
[148] Haffner S. Diabetes, hyperlipidaemia, and coronary artery disease. Am J Cardiol 1999;83(9B):17F–21F.
[149] Celik T, Iyisoy A, Kardesoglu E, et al. The clinical significance of microvascular impairment in patients with pure uncomplicated diabetes mellitus. Int J Cardiol 2008;131(1):123–4.
[150] Booth G, Kapral M, Fung K, et al. Relation between age and cardiovascular disease in men and women with diabetes compared with non diabetic people: a population-based retrospective cohort study. Lancet 2006;368(9529):29–36.
[151] Roy H, Bhardwaj S, Yla-Herttuala S. Molecular genetics of atherosclerosis. Hum Genet 2009;125:467–91.
[152] Chambers J, Eda S, Basset P, et al. C-reactive protein, insulin resistance, central obesity, and coronary heart disease risk in Indian Asians from the United Kingdom compared with European whites. Circulation 2001;104(2):145–50.
[153] Chandalia M, Cabo-Chan A, Devaraj S, et al. Elevated plasma high-sensitivity C-reactive protein concentrations in Asian Indians living in the United States. J Clin Endocrinol Metab 2003;88(8):3773–6.
[154] Chambers J, Obeid O, Refsum H, et al. Plasma homocysteine concentrations and risk of coronary heart disease in UK Indian Asian and European men. Lancet 2000;355(9203):523–7.
[155] Budoff M, Nasir K, Mao S, et al. Ethnic differences of the presence and severity of coronary atherosclerosis. Atherosclerosis 2006;187(2):343–50.
[156] Lenz M, Richter T, Muhlhauser I. The morbidity and mortality associated with overweight and obesity in adulthood. Dtsch Arztebl Int 2009;106(40):641–8.
[157] Guilherme A, Virbasius J, Puri V, et al. Adipocyte dysfunctions linking obesity to insulin resistance and type 2 diabetes. Nat Rev Mol Cell Biol 2008;9(5):367–77.
[158] Ikeoka D, Mader J, Pieber T. Adipose tissue, inflammation and cardiovascular disease. Rev Assoc Med Bras 2010;56(1):116–21.
[159] Australian Bureau of Statistics (ABS). Australian social trends 2007: overweight and obesity. Cat. no. 4102.0. Canberra: ABS; 2007.
[160] North C, Venter C, Jerling J. The effects of dietary fibre on C-reactive protein, an inflammation marker predicting cardiovascular disease. Eur J Clin Nutr 2009;63(8):921–33.
[161] Nettleton J, Steffen L, Palmas W, et al. Associations between microalbuminuria and animal foods, plant foods, and dietary patterns in the Multiethnic Study of Atherosclerosis. Am J Clin Nutr 2009;87(6):1825–36.
[162] Chouraki V, Wagner A, Ferriers J, et al. Smoking habits, waist circumference and coronary artery disease risk relationship: the PRIME study. Eur J Cardiovasc Prev Rehabil 2008;15(6): 625–30.
[163] Ware W. Psychological stress, insulin resistance, inflammation and the assessment of heart disease risk. Time for a paradigm shift? Med Hypotheses 2008;71(1):45–52.
[164] Bunker S, Colquhoun D, Esler M, et al. 'Stress' and coronary heart disease: psychosocial risk factors. Med J Aust 2003;178(6):272–6.
[165] Thomas G. Classification and nomenclature for coronary artery disease. Int J Cardiol 2003;88(2–3):315–16.
[166] Parish J, Somers V. Obstructive sleep apnea and cardiovascular disease. Mayo Clin Proc 2004;79(8):1036–48.
[167] Bhatt A, Stone P. Current strategies for the prevention of angina in patients with stable coronary artery disease. Curr Opin Cardiol 2006;21(5):492–502.
[168] Zouridakis E, Avanzas P, Arroyo-Espliguero R, et al. Markers of inflammation and rapid coronary artery disease progression in patients with stable angina pectoris. Circulation 2004;110(13):1747–53.
[169] Anderson J, Carlquist J, Horne B, et al. Progress in unraveling the genetics of coronary artery disease and myocardial infarction. Curr Atheroscler Rep 2007;9(3):179–83.
[170] Schafer A, Bauersachs J. Endothelial dysfunction, impaired endogenous platelet inhibition and platelet activation in diabetes and atherosclerosis. Curr Vasc Pharmacol 2008;6(1):52–60.

[171] Virmani R, Burke A, Farb A, et al. Pathology of the unstable plaque. Prog Cardiovasc Dis 2002;44(5):349–56.
[172] May H, Alharethi R, Anderson J, et al. Homocysteine levels are associated with increased risk of congestive heart failure in patients with and without coronary artery disease. Cardiology 2007;107(3):178–84.
[173] Felter HW. The Eclectic materia medica, pharmacology and therapeutics. Portland, OR: Eclectic Materia Medica Publications; 1922.
[174] Ellingwood F. The Eclectic practice of medicine with especial reference to the treatment of disease. Portland, OR: Eclectic Materia Medica Publications; 1910.
[175] Roberts DC, Truswell AS, Bencke A, et al. The cholesterol-lowering effect of a breakfast cereal containing psyllium fibre. Med J Aust 1994;161(11–12):660–4.
[176] Lanzotti V. The analysis of onion and garlic. J Chromatogr A 2006;1112(1–2):3–22.
[177] de Lorgeril M, Salen P, Martin JL, et al. Mediterranean diet, traditional risk factors, and the rate of cardiovascular complications after myocardial infarction: final report of the Lyon Diet Heart Study. Circulation 1999;99:779–85.
[178] Bautista MC, Engler MM. The Mediterranean diet: is it cardioprotective? Prog Cardiovasc Nurs 2005;20(2):70–6.
[179] Katcher HI, Hill AM, Lanford JLG, et al. Lifestyle approaches and dietary strategies to lower LDL-cholesterol and triglycerides and raise HDL-cholesterol. Endocrinol Metab Clin North Am 2009;38(1):45–78.
[180] Singh RB, Dubnov G, Niaz MA, et al. Effect of an Indo-Mediterranean diet on progression of coronary artery disease in high risk patients (The Indo-Mediterranean Diet Heart Study): a randomised single blind trial. Lancet 2002;360:1455–61.
[181] Siddiqui RA, Harvey KA, Ruzmetov N, et al. n-3 fatty acids prevent whereas trans-fatty acids induce vascular inflammation and sudden cardiac death. Br J Nutr 2009;102(12):1811–19.
[182] Micha R, Mozaffarian D. Trans fatty acids: effects on cardiometabolic health and implications for policy. Prostag Leukotr Essent Fatty Acids 2008;79(3–5):147–52.
[183] Wu JN, Ho SC, Zhou C, et al. Coffee consumption and risk of coronary heart diseases: a meta-analysis of 21 prospective cohort studies. Int J Cardiol 2009;137(3):216–25.
[184] Ahlawat SK, Siwach SB. Alcohol and coronary artery disease. Int J Cardiol 1994;44:157–62.
[185] De Rosa S, Cirillo P, Paglia A, et al. Reactive oxygen species and antioxidants in the pathophysiology of cardiovascular disease: does the actual knowledge justify a clinical approach? Curr Vasc Pharmacol 2010;8(2):259–75.
[186] Stephens NG, Parsons A, Schofield PM, et al. Randomised controlled trial of vitamin E in-patients with coronary disease: Cambridge Heart Antioxidant Study. Lancet 1996;347:781–6.
[187] McRae MP. Vitamin C supplementation lowers serum low-density lipoprotein cholesterol and triglycerides: a meta-analysis of 13 randomized controlled trials. J Chiropr Med 2008;7(2):48–58.
[188] Eslick GD, Howe PR, Smith C, et al. Benefits of fish oil supplementation in hyperlipidaemia: a systematic review and meta-analysis. Int J Cardiol 2009;136(1):4–16.
[189] Nestel P, Shige H, Pomeroy S, et al. The n-3 fatty acids eicosapentaenoic acid and docosahexaenoic acid increase systemic arterial compliance in humans. Am J Clin Nutr 2002;76:326–30.
[190] Thies F, Garry J, Yaqoob P, et al. Association of n-3 polyunsaturated fatty acids with stability of atherosclerotic plaques: a randomised controlled trial. Lancet 2003;361:477–85.
[191] Pokan R, Hofmann P, von Duvillard SP, et al. Oral magnesium therapy, exercise heart rate, exercise tolerance, and myocardial function in coronary artery disease patients. Br J Sports Med 2006;40(9):773–8.
[192] Abbott RD, Ando F, Masaki KH, et al. Dietary magnesium intake and the future risk of coronary heart disease (The Honolulu Heart Program). Am J Cardiol 2003;92(6):665–9.
[193] Al-Delaimy WK, Rimm EB, Willett WC, et al. Magnesium intake and risk of coronary heart disease among men. J Am Coll Nutr 2004;23(1):63–70.
[194] Shechter M, Sharir M, Paul-Labrador M, et al. Oral magnesium therapy improves endothelial function in patients with coronary artery disease. Circulation 2000;102:2353–8.
[195] Singh RB, Neki NS, Kartikey K, et al. Effect of coenzyme Q10 on risk of atherosclerosis in patients with recent myocardial infarction. Mol Cell Biochem 2003;246(1–2):75–82.
[196] Makhija N, Sendasgupta C, Kiran U, et al. The role of oral coenzyme Q_{10} in patients undergoing coronary artery bypass graft surgery. J Cardiothorac Vasc Anesth 2008;22:832–9.
[197] Spencer AP, Carson DS, Crouch MA. Vitamin E and coronary artery disease. Arch Intern Med 1999;159(12):1313–20.
[198] Blumenthal M. The complete German Commission E monographs. Austin, TX: American Botanical Council; 1998.
[199] Stevinson C, Pittler MH, Ernst E. Garlic for treating hypercholesterolaemia. A meta-analysis of randomised clinical trials. Ann Intern Med 2000;133(6):420–9.
[200] Ide N, Keller C, Weiss N. Aged garlic extract inhibits homocysteine–induced CD36 expression and foam cell formation in human macrophages. J Nutr 2006;136(Suppl. 3):755S–758S.
[201] Arhan M, Oztürk HS, Turhan N, et al. Hepatic oxidant/antioxidant status in cholesterol fed rabbits: effects of garlic extract. Hepatol Res 2009;39(1):70–7.
[202] Kabaskal L, Sehirli O, Cetinel S, et al. Protective effects of aqueous garlic extract against renal ischaemia/reperfusion in rats. J Med Food 2005;8(3):319–26.
[203] Youn HS, Lim HJ, Lee HJ, et al. Garlic (*Allium sativum*) extract inhibits lipopolysaccharide-induced Toll-like receptor 4 dimerization. Biosci Biotechnol Biochem 2008;72(2):234–42.
[204] Thomson M, Al-Qattan KK, Bordia T, et al. Including garlic in the diet may help lower blood glucose, cholesterol, triglycerides. J Nutr 2006;136(Suppl. 3):800S–802S.
[205] Allison GL, Lowe GM, Rahman K. Aged garlic extract and its constituents inhibit platelet aggregation through multiple mechanisms. Am Soc Nutr J Nutr 2006;136:782S–788S.
[206] Chen C, Pung D, Leong V, et al. Induction of detoxifying enzymes by garlic organosulfur compounds through transcription factor Nrf2: effect of chemical structure and stress signals. Free Radic Biol Med 2004;37(10):1578–90.
[207] Rahman K. Effects of garlic on platelet biochemistry and physiology. Mol Nutr Food Res 2007;51(11):1335–44.
[208] Campbell JH, Efendy JL, Smith NJ, et al. Molecular basis by which garlic suppresses atherosclerosis. J Nutr 2001;131:1006S–1009S.
[209] Ramirez Bosca A, Soler A, Carrion-Gutierrez MA, et al. An hydroalcoholic extract of *Curcuma longa* lowers the abnormally high values of human-plasma fibrinogen. Mech Ageing Dev 2000;114(3):207–10.
[210] Cheng TO. Cardiovascular effects of Danshen. Int J Cardio 2007;121(1):9–22.
[211] Xiang NZ, Li XY. A observation on the effect of Guttae *S. miltiorrhiza* to alleviate angina in patients with CHD. Zhongguo Linchuang Baojian Zazhi 2004;7:110–11.
[212] Ma JY. Clinical observation of the treatment of hyperlipidemia with Danshen composite. Tianjin Zhongyi 1998;15:24.
[213] Wu XY, Guo XL. Clinical observation of the treatment of 60 hyperlipaemia with Fufang Danshen Dripping Pill. Hebei Zhongyi 2000;22:671.
[214] Ma WY, Yang JS, Gong CC, et al. Effect of Danshen composite on hyperlipaemia and blood rheology. Jiefangjun Yaoxue Xuebao 2001;17:47–8.
[215] Cui SK, Li GH. Clinical effect of Fufang Danshen Dripping Pill on hyperlipemia. Xiandai Zhongxiyi Jiehe Zazhi 2003;11:1029–30.
[216] Singh I, Mok M, Christensen AM, et al. The effects of polyphenols in olive leaves on platelet function. Nutr Metab Cardiovasc Dis 2008;18:127–32.
[217] Lasserre B, Kaiser R, Chanh PH. Effects on rats of aqueous extracts of plants used in folk medicine as antihypertensive agents. Naturwissenschaften 1983;70:95–6.
[218] Pignatelli P, Pulcinelli FM, Lenti L, et al. Hydrogen peroxide is involved in collagen-induced platelet activation. Blood 1998;91:484–90.
[219] Bundy R, Walker AF, Middleton RW, et al. Artichoke leaf extract (*Cynara scolymus*) reduces plasma cholesterol in otherwise healthy hypercholesterolemic adults: a randomized, double blind placebo controlled trial. Phytomedicine 2008;15(9):668–75.
[220] Nohr LA, Rasmussen LB, Straand J. Resin from the mukul myrrh tree, guggul, can it be used for treating hypercholesterolemia? A randomized, controlled study. Complement Ther Med 2009;17(1):16–22.

[221] Complementary Medicines Evaluation Committee. CMEC 43 Extracted Ratified Minutes Forty-third Meeting. 28 November 2013. Available from www.tga.gov.au/sites/default/files/cmec-minutes-43.pdf.
[222] Poobalan A, Aucott L, Smith WC, et al. Effects of weight loss in overweight/obese individuals and long-term lipid outcomes — a systematic review. Obes Rev 2004;5(1):43–50.
[223] Marques E, Carvalho J, Soares JM, et al. Effects of resistance and multicomponent exercise on lipid profiles of older women. Maturitas 2009;63(1):84–8.
[224] Jee SH, Suh I, Kim IS, et al. Smoking and atherosclerotic cardiovascular disease in men with low levels of serum cholesterol: the Korea Medical Insurance Corporation Study. JAMA 1999;282:2149–55.
[225] Nakamura K, Barzi F, Huxley R, et al. Asia Pacific Cohort Studies Collaboration. Does cigarette smoking exacerbate the effect of total cholesterol and high-density lipoprotein cholesterol on the risk of cardiovascular diseases? Heart 2009;95(11):909–16.
[226] Australian Institute of Health and Welfare (AIHW). Australia's Health 2008: the eleventh biennial health report of the Australian Institute of Health and Welfare. Cat. no. AUS 99. Canberra: AIHW; 2008.
[227] Centers for Disease Control and Prevention. Division for Heart Disease and Stroke Prevention. Heart disease fact sheet. 2017. Available from: www.cdc.gov/dhdsp/data_statistics/fact_sheets/fs_heart_disease.htm.
[228] Conti C. Re-thinking angina. Clin Cardiol 2007;30(Suppl. 1): I1–3.
[229] Marshall T. Exploring a fiscal food policy: the case of diet and ischaemic heart disease. BMJ 2000;320:301–5.
[230] Law MR, Wald NJ, Thompson SG. By how much and how quickly does reduction in serum cholesterol concentration lower risk of ischaemic heart disease? BMJ 1994;308:367–72.
[231] Hemingway H, Langenberg C, Damant J, et al. Prevalence of angina in women versus men: a systematic review and meta-analysis of international variations across 31 countries. Circulation 2008;117(12):1526–36.
[232] Sheifer S, Gersh B, Yanez N, et al. Prevalence, predisposing factors, and prognosis of clinically unrecognized myocardial infarction in the elderly. J Am Coll Cardiol 2000;35(1):119–26.
[233] Schultz T, Mannheimer C, Dellborg M, et al. High prevalence of gastroesophageal reflux in patients with clinical unstable angina and known coronary artery disease. Acute Card Care 2008;10(1):37–42.
[234] Liuzzo J, Ambrose J. Chest pain from gastroesophageal reflux disease in patients with coronary artery disease. Cardiol Rev 2005;13(4):167–73.
[235] Spertus J, Dawson J, Masoudi F, et al. Prevalence and predictors of angina pectoris one month after myocardial infarction. Am J Cardiol 2006;98(3):282–8.
[236] Koukkunen H, Penttil A, Kemppainen A, et al. C-reactive protein, fibrinogen, interleukin-6 and tumour necrosis factor-alpha in the prognostic classification of unstable angina pectoris. Ann Med 2001;33(1):37–47.
[237] Chouraki V, Wagner A, Ferriers J, et al. Smoking habits, waist circumference and coronary artery disease risk relationship: the PRIME study. Eur J Cardiovasc Prev Rehabil 2008;15(6): 625–30.
[238] Melikian N, DeBruyne B, Fearon W, et al. The pathophysiology and clinical course of the normal coronary angina syndrome (cardiac syndrome X). Prog Cardiovasc Dis 2008;50(4):294–310.
[239] Kaski J. Overview of gender aspects of cardiac syndrome X. Cardiovasc Res 2002;53(3):620–6.
[240] Davies S. Clinical presentation and diagnosis of coronary artery disease: stable angina. Br Med Bull 2001;59:17–27.
[241] Conti C. Inhibition of sodium-dependent calcium overload to treat myocardial ischemia. Clin Cardiol 2006;29(4):141–3.
[242] Heberden W. Some account of a disorder of the breast. Med Trans R Coll Physicians (Lond) 1772;2:59–67.
[243] McPhee S, Papadakis M, editors. Current medical diagnosis and treatment. 48th ed. New York: McGraw-Hill; 2009.
[244] Cheng O. Acute dyspnea on exertion is an angina equivalent. Int J Cardiol 2007;115(1):116.
[245] Peterson E. The burden of angina pectoris and its complications. Clin Cardiol 2007;30(2 Suppl. 1):I10–15.
[246] Hemingway H, McCallum A, Shipley M, et al. Incidence and prognostic implications of stable angina pectoris among women and men. JAMA 2006;295(12):1404–11.
[247] Gandjour A, Lauterbach K. Review of quality-of-life evaluations in patients with angina pectoris. Pharmacoeconomics 1999;16(2):141–52.
[248] Hemingway H, Chen R, Junghans C, et al. Appropriateness criteria for coronary angiography in angina: reliability and validity. Ann Intern Med 2008;149(4):221–31.
[249] McErlean E, VanLente C, Nissen S. Using troponin T to diagnose acute coronary syndromes. Cleve Clin J Med 2000;67(11):843–9.
[250] Trowell H. Dietary fibre, ischaemic heart disease and diabetes mellitus. Proc Nutr Soc 1973;32(3):151–7.
[251] Solà R, Godàs G, Ribalta J, et al. Effects of soluble fiber (*Plantago ovata* husk) on plasma lipids, lipoproteins, and apolipoproteins in men with ischemic heart disease. Am J Clin Nutr 2007;85(4):1157–63.
[252] Galeone C, Tavani A, Pelucchi C, et al. Allium vegetable intake and risk of acute myocardial infarction in Italy. Eur J Nutr 2009;48(2):120–3.
[253] Mathers C, Vos T, Stevenson C. The burden of disease and injury in Australia. Canberra: AIHW; 1999.
[254] Kristensen SD, De Caterina R, Schmidt EB, et al. Fish oil and ischaemic heart disease. Br Heart J 1993;70(3):212–14.
[255] Kachopoulos C, O'Rourke M. Caffeine alters arterial wave reflection: a new insight into its cardiovascular effects. Circulation 2000;102(Suppl. 2):519. (Abstract).
[256] Urgert R, Katan MB. The cholesterol-raising factor from coffee beans. J R Soc Med 1996;89:618–23.
[257] Tofler O, Foy S, Ng K, et al. Coffee and coronary heart disease. Heart Lung Circ 2001;10(3):116–20.
[258] Yudkin J. Dietary fat and dietary sugar in relation to ischaemic heart disease and diabetes. Lancet 1964;2(7349):4–5.
[259] Gupta MK, Gupta P, Rezai F. Histamine — can it cause an acute coronary event? Clin Cardiol 2001;24(3):258–9.
[260] Zeidman A, Fradin Z, Blecher A, et al. Anemia as a risk factor for ischemic heart disease. Isr Med Assoc J 2004;6(1):16–18.
[261] Gokce N, Keaney JF Jr, Frei B, et al. Long-term ascorbic acid administration reverses endothelial vasomotor dysfunction in patients with coronary artery disease. Circulation 1999;99(25):3234–40.
[262] Ness AR, Khaw KT, Bingham S, et al. Vitamin C status and undiagnosed angina. J Cardiovasc Risk 1996;3(4):373–7.
[263] Hirashima O, Kawano H, Motoyama T, et al. Improvement of endothelial function and insulin sensitivity with vitamin C in patients with coronary spastic angina: possible role of reactive oxygen species. J Am Coll Cardiol 2000;35(7):1860–6.
[264] Miwa K, Miyagi Y, Igawa A, et al. Vitamin E deficiency in variant angina. Circulation 1996;94(1):14–18.
[265] Miyamoto S, Kawano H, Takazoe K, et al. Vitamin E improves fibrinolytic activity in patients with coronary spastic angina. Thromb Res 2004;113(6):345–51.
[266] Natural Medicine. CoEnzyme Q10 monograph. 2010. Available from: www.naturalstandard.com.
[267] Kamikawa T, Kobayashi A, Yamashita T, et al. Effects of coenzyme Q10 on exercise tolerance in chronic stable angina pectoris. Am J Cardiol 1985;56(4):247–51.
[268] Pauly DF, Pepine CJ. The role of carnitine in myocardial dysfunction. Am J Kidney Dis 2003;41(4).
[269] Iyer RN, Khan AA, Gupta A, et al. L-carnitine moderately improves the exercise tolerance in chronic stable angina. J Assoc Physicians India 2000;48(11):1050–2.
[270] Satake K, Lee J-D, Shimizu H, et al. Relation between severity of magnesium deficiency and frequency of anginal attacks in men with variant angina. J Am Coll Cardiol 1996;28(4):897–902.
[271] Lavie CJ, Milani RV, Mehra MR, et al. Omega-3 polyunsaturated fatty acids and cardiovascular diseases. J Am Coll Cardiol 2009;54(7):585–94.
[272] Weiss RF, Fintelmann V. Herbal medicine. 2nd ed. New York: Thieme; 2000. (English translation of the German 9th edition of Lehrbuch der Phytotherapie).
[273] Braun L, Cohen M, editors. Herbs and natural supplements. An evidence-based guide. 3rd ed. Sydney: Churchill Livingstone Elsevier; 2010.

[274] Dwivedi S. *Terminalia arjuna* Wight, Arn. — a useful drug for cardiovascular disorders. J Ethnopharmacol 2007;114(2):114–29.

[275] Dwivedi S, Agarwal MP. Antianginal and cardioprotective effects of *Terminalia arjuna*, an indigenous drug, in coronary artery disease (Abstract only). J Assoc Physicians India 1994;42(4):287–9.

[276] Natural Medicine. Ammi visnaga monograph. 2010. Available from: www.naturalstandard.com.

[277] Duarte J, Pérez-Vizcaíno F, Torres AI, et al. Vasodilator effects of visnagin in isolated rat vascular smooth muscle. Eur J Pharmacol 1995;286(2):115–22.

[278] Li DZ, Sharma R, Zeng QT. Effects of ginkgo leaf extract on function of dendritic cells and Th1/Th2 cytokines in patients with unstable angina pectoris (Abstract only). Chin J Integr Med 2005;11(4):260–3.

[279] Hermann Hempen C, Fische N. Herbs that regulate the blood. In: A materia medica for Chinese medicine: plants, minerals, and animal products. 1st ed. Edinburgh: Churchill Livingstone; 2009. p. 514–617.

[280] Yuan CS, Mehendale SR, Wang CZ, et al. Effects of *Corydalis yanhusuo* and *Angelicae dahuricae* on cold pressor-induced pain in humans: a controlled trial. J Clin Pharmacol 2004; 44(11):1323–7.

[281] Li HL, Zhang WD, Liu RH, et al. Simultaneous determination of four active alkaloids from a traditional Chinese medicine *Corydalis saxicola* Bunting (Yanhuanglian) in plasma and urine samples by LC-MS-MS. J Chromatogr B Analyt Technol Biomed Life Sci 2006;831(1–2):140–6.

[282] Wang DJ, Mao HY, Lei M. [Rotundium in the treatment of atrial fibrillation]. Zhongguo Zhong Xi Yi Jie He Za Zhi 1993;13(8):455–7, 451.

[283] Wang L, Xiong ZY, Wang G. [Systematic assessment on randomized controlled trials for treatment of stable angina pectoris by compound salvia pellet]. Zhongguo Zhong Xi Yi Jie He Za Zhi 2004;24(6):500–4.

[284] Nicholson JA, Darby TD, Jarboe CH. Viopudial, a hypotensive and smooth muscle antispasmodic from *Viburnum opulus.* Proc Soc Exp Biol Med 1972;140(2):457–61.

[285] Gan Q, Smith KR, Hammond SK, et al. Disease burden of adult lung cancer and ischaemic heart disease from passive tobacco smoking in. China Tob Control 2007;16(6):417–22.

[286] Arnold SV, Spertus JA, Ciechanowski PS, et al. Psychosocial modulators of angina response to myocardial ischemia. Circulation 2009;120(2):126–33.

[287] Brehm M, Picard F, Ebner P, et al. Effects of exercise training on mobilization and functional activity of blood-derived progenitor cells in patients with acute myocardial infarction. Eur J Med Res 2009;14(9):393–405.

[288] Blumenthal JA, Sherwood A, Babyak MA, et al. Effects of exercise and stress management training on markers of cardiovascular risk in patients with ischemic heart disease: a randomized controlled trial. JAMA 2005;293(13):1626–34.

[289] AIHW. Heart, stroke and vascular diseases. Australian facts 2004. Available from: www.aihw.gov.au/WorkArea/DownloadAsset.aspx?id=6442454948.

[290] Ades PA. Cardiac rehabilitation and secondary prevention of coronary heart disease. N Engl J Med 2001;345:892–902.

[291] AIHW. Cardiovascular disease. Australian facts 2011. Available from: www.aihw.gov.au/WorkArea/DownloadAsset.aspx?id=10737418530.

[292] Giraldo EA. Ischemic stroke. In: Merck manual professional edition online. 2017. Available from www.merckmanuals.com/professional/neurologic-disorders/stroke/ischemic-stroke.

[293] Giraldo EA. Overview of stroke. In: Merck manual professional edition online. 2017. Available from: www.merckmanuals.com/professional/neurologic-disorders/stroke/overview-of-stroke.

[294] Nilsen ML. A historical account of stroke and the evolution of nursing care for stroke patients. J Neurosci Nurs 2010;42(1):19–27.

[295] Mok E, Woo CP. The effects of slow-stroke back massage on anxiety and shoulder pain in elderly stroke patients. Complement Ther Nurs Midwifery 2004;10:209–16.

[296] Gardener H, Wright CB, Gu Y, et al. Mediterranean-style diet and risk of ischemic stroke, myocardial infarction, and vascular death: the Northern Manhattan Study. Am J Clin Nutr 2011;94(6):1458–64.

[297] Tektonidis TG, Åkesson A, Gigante B, et al. A Mediterranean diet and risk of myocardial infarction, heart failure and stroke: a population-based cohort study. Atherosclerosis 2015;243(1):93–8.

[298] Micha R, Peñalvo JL, Cudhea F, et al. Association between dietary factors and mortality from heart disease, stroke, and type 2 diabetes in the United States. JAMA 2017;317(9):912–24.

[299] Pase MP, Himali JJ, Beiser AS, et al. Sugar- and artificially sweetened beverages and the risks of incident stroke and dementia: a prospective cohort study. Stroke 2017;48(5):1139–46.

[300] Geeganage C, Beavan J, Ellender S, et al. Interventions for dysphagia and nutritional support in acute and subacute stroke. Cochrane Database Syst Rev 2012;(10):CD000323.

[301] Sesso HD, Buring JE, Christen WG, et al. Vitamins E and C in the prevention of cardiovascular disease in men; the Physicians' Health Study II randomized controlled trial. JAMA 2008;300(18):2123–33.

[302] Cook NR, Albert CM, Gaziano JM, et al. A randomized factorial trial of vitamins C and E and beta carotene in the secondary prevention of cardiovascular events in women: results from the Women's Antioxidant Cardiovascular Study. Arch Intern Med 2007;167(15):1610–18.

[303] Wang L, Cui W, Nan G, et al. Meta-analysis reveals protective effects of vitamin B on stroke patients. Transl Neurosci 2015;6(1):150–6.

[304] Upton R, editor. Ginkgo leaf, ginkgo lead dry extract. In: American herbal pharmacopoeia and therapeutic compendium. Scotts Valley: American Herbal Pharmacopoeia; 2003.

[305] Saraf MK, Prabhakar S, Anand A. Neuroprotective effect of *Bacopa monniera* on ischemia induced brain injury. Pharmacol Biochem Behav 2010;97(2):192–7.

[306] Liu X, Yue R, Zhang J, et al. Neuroprotective effects of bacopaside I in ischemic brain injury. Restor Neurol Neurosci 2013;31(2):109–23.

[307] Arab L, Khan F, Lam H. Tea consumption and cardiovascular disease risk. Am J Clin Nutr 2013;98(6 Suppl.):1651S–1659S.

[308] Di Lorenzo A, Nabavi SF, Sureda A, et al. Antidepressive-like effects and antioxidant activity of green tea and GABA green tea in a mouse model of post-stroke depression. Mol Nutr Food Res 2016;60(3):566–79.

[309] Moroz A. Stroke rehabilitation. In: Merck manual professional edition online. 2017. Available from: www.merckmanuals.com/professional/special-subjects/rehabilitation/stroke-rehabilitation.

[310] Graven C, Brock K, Hill KD, et al. First year after stroke: an integrated approach focusing on participation goals aiming to reduce depressive symptoms. Stroke 2016;47(11):2820–7.

[311] Xia W, Zheng C, Zhu S, et al. Does the addition of specific acupuncture to standard swallowing training improve outcomes in patients with dysphagia after stroke? A randomized controlled trial. Clin Rehab 2016;30(3):237–46.

[312] Chen L, Fang J, Ma R, et al. Additional effects of acupuncture on early comprehensive rehabilitation in patients with mild to moderate acute ischemic stroke: a multicenter randomized controlled trial. BMC Comp Altern Med 2016;16:226.

[313] Nieminen M, Harjola V. Definition and epidemiology of acute heart failure syndromes. Am J Cardiol 2005;96(6):5–10.

[314] Driscoll A, Worrall-Carter L, McLennan S, et al. Heterogeneity of heart failure management programmes in Australia. Eur J Cardiovasc Nurs 2006;5(1):71–82.

[315] Abhayaratna W, Smith W, Becks N, et al. Prevalence of heart failure and systolic ventricular dysfunction in older Australians: the Canberra Heart Study. Med J Aust 2006;184(4):151–4.

[316] National Heart Foundation of Australia & the Cardiac Society of Australia & New Zealand (Chronic Heart Failure Guidelines Expert Writing Panel). Guidelines for the prevention, detection and management of chronic heart failure in Australia; 2006.

[317] Davis RC, Hobbs FDR, Lip GYH, et al. ABC of heart failure — history and epidemiology. BMJ 2000;320:39–42.

[318] Mosterd A, Hoes A. Clinical epidemiology of heart failure. Heart 2007;93(9):1137–46.

[319] Stewart S, MacIntyre K, Capewell S, et al. An ageing population and heart failure: an increasing burden in the 21st century? Heart 2003;89(1):49–53.

[320] Remme W, Swedeberg K. Guidelines for the diagnosis and treatment of chronic heart failure: Task Force Report. Eur Heart J 2001;22:1527–60.

[321] Remme W, McMurray J, Rauch B, et al. Public awareness of heart failure in Europe: first results from SHAPE. Eur Heart J 2005;26:2413–21.

[322] McMurray J, Stewart S. Heart failure: epidemiology, aetiology, and prognosis of heart failure. Heart 2000;83:596–602.

[323] Haider A, Larson M, Franklin S, et al. Systolic blood pressure, diastolic blood pressure, and pulse pressure as predictors of risk for congestive heart failure in the Framingham Heart Study. Ann Intern Med 2003;138(1):10–16.

[324] Lip G, Gibbs C, Beevers D. ABC of heart failure. BMJ 2000;320:104–7.

[325] Fox K, Cowie M, Wood D, et al. Coronary artery disease as the cause of incident heart failure in the population. Eur Heart J 2001;22(3):228–36.

[326] Horwich T, Fonarow G. Glucose, obesity, metabolic syndrome, and diabetes. J Am Coll Cardiol 2010;55(4):283–93.

[327] Kannel W, Hjortland M, Castelli W. Role of diabetes in congestive heart failure: the Framingham Study. Am J Cardiol 1974;34(1):29–34.

[328] Anand I. Heart failure and anemia: mechanisms and pathophysiology. Heart Fail Rev 2008;13(4):379–86.

[329] Tripodskiadis F, Karayannis G, Giamouzis G, et al. The sympathetic nervous system in heart failure physiology, pathophysiology, and clinical implications. J Am Coll Cardiol 2009;54(19):1747–62.

[330] Sharpe N, Doughty R. Epidemiology of heart failure and ventricular dysfunction. Lancet 1998;352(Suppl. 1):S13–17.

[331] Pilz S, Marz W, Wellnitz B, et al. Association of vitamin D deficiency with heart failure and sudden cardiac death in a large cross-sectional study of patients referred for coronary angiography. J Clin Endocrinol Metab 2008;93(10):3927–35.

[332] Ghosh RK, Ball S, Prasad V, et al. Depression in heart failure: intricate relationship, pathophysiology and most updated evidence of interventions from recent clinical studies. Int J Cardiol 2016;224:170–7.

[333] Mozaffarian D, Bryson CL, Lemaitre RN, et al. Fish intake and risk of incident heart failure. J Am Coll Cardiol 2005;45:2015–21.

[334] Yamagishi K, Iso H, Date C, et al. Fish, omega-3 polyunsaturated fatty acids, and mortality from cardiovascular diseases in a nationwide community-based cohort of Japanese men and women the JACC (Japan Collaborative Cohort Study for Evaluation of Cancer Risk) Study. J Am Coll Cardiol 2008;52: 988–96.

[335] Levitan EB, Wolk A, Mittleman MA. Fatty fish, marine omega-3 fatty acids and incidence of heart failure. Eur J Clin Nutr 2010;64(6):587–94.

[336] Djoussé L, Driver JA, Gaziano JM. Relation between modifiable lifestyle factors and lifetime risk of heart failure. JAMA 2009;302(4):394–400.

[337] Vlachopoulos C, Panagiotakos D, Ioakeimidis N, et al. Chronic coffee consumption has a detrimental effect on aortic stiffness and wave reflections. Am J Clin Nutr 2005;81(6):1307–12.

[338] Wilhelmsen L, Rosengren A, Eriksson H, et al. Heart failure in the general population of men — morbidity, risk factors and prognosis. J Intern Med 2001;249:253–61.

[339] Marvin HM. The value of xanthine diuretics in congestive heart failure. JAMA 1926;87(25):2043–6.

[340] Marvin HM. Digitalis and diuretics in heart failure with regular rhythm, with especial reference to the importance of etiologic classification of heart disease. J Clin Invest 1927;3(3):521–39.

[341] Djoussé L, Gaziano JM. Alcohol consumption and heart failure: a systematic review. Curr Atheroscler Rep 2008;10(2):117–20.

[342] Piano MR. Alcohol and heart failure. J Card Fail 2002;8:239–46.

[343] Han SN, Leka LS, Lichtenstein AH, et al. Effect of hydrogenated and saturated, relative to polyunsaturated, fat on immune and inflammatory responses of adults with moderate hypercholesterolemia. J Lipid Res 2002;43:445–52.

[344] Rauchhaus M, Doehner W, Francis DP, et al. Plasma cytokine parameters and mortality in patients with chronic heart failure. Circulation 2000;102:3060–7.

[345] Sharma N, Okere IC, Barrows BR, et al. High-sugar diets increase cardiac dysfunction and mortality in hypertension compared to low-carbohydrate or high-starch diets. J Hypertens 2008;26(7):1402–10.

[346] Chess DJ, Lei B, Hoit BD, et al. Deleterious effects of sugar and protective effects of starch on cardiac remodeling, contractile dysfunction, and mortality in response to pressure overload. Am J Physiol Heart Circ Physiol 2007;293(3):H1853–60.

[347] Hanninen SA, Darling PB, Sole MJ, et al. The prevalence of thiamin deficiency in hospitalized patients with congestive heart failure. J Am Coll Cardiol 2006;47(2):354–61.

[348] Keith ME, Walsh NA, Darling PB, et al. B-vitamin deficiency in hospitalized patients with heart failure. J Am Diet Assoc 2009;109(8):1406–10.

[349] Wooley JA. Characteristics of thiamin and its relevance to the management of heart failure. Nutr Clin Pract 2008;23(5):487–93.

[350] Vasan RS, Beiser A, D'Agostino RB, et al. Plasma homocysteine and risk for congestive heart failure in adults without prior myocardial infarction. JAMA 2003;289(10):1251–7.

[351] Sundström J, Vasan RS. Homocysteine and heart failure: a review of investigations from the Framingham Heart Study. Clin Chem Lab Med 2005;43(10):987–92.

[352] Higdon J. An evidence based approach to vitamins and minerals. New York: Thieme; 2003.

[353] Stepura OB, Martynow AI. Magnesium orotate in severe congestive heart failure (MACH). Int J Cardiol 2009;134(1):145–7.

[354] Mehra MR, Lavie CJ, Ventura HO, et al. Fish oils produce anti-inflammatory effects and improved body weight in severe heart failure. J Heart Lung Transplant 2006;25:834–8.

[355] Leaf A, Kang JX, Xiao YF, et al. Clinical prevention of sudden cardiac death by n-3 polyunsaturated fatty acids and mechanism of prevention of arrhythmias by n-3 fish oils. Circulation 2003;107:2646–52.

[356] Ghatak A, Brar MJ, Agarwal A, et al. Oxy free radical system in heart failure and therapeutic role of oral vitamin E. Int J Cardiol 1996;57(2):119–27.

[357] Keith ME, Jeejeebhoy KN, Langer A, et al. A controlled clinical trial of vitamin E supplementation in patients with congestive heart failure. Am J Clin Nutr 2001;73(2):219–24.

[358] Weant KA, Smith KM. The role of coenzyme Q10 in heart failure. Ann Pharmacother 2005;39(9):1522–6.

[359] Munkholm H, Hansen HH, Rasmussen K. Coenzyme Q10 treatment in serious heart failure. Biofactors 1999;9(2–4):285–9.

[360] Langsjoen PH, Langsjoen AM. Supplemental ubiquinol in patients with advanced congestive heart failure. Biofactors 2008;32(1–4):119–28.

[361] Madmani ME, Yusuf Solaiman A, Tamr Agha K, et al. Coenzyme Q10 for heart failure. Cochrane Database Syst Rev 2014;(6):CD008684.

[362] Shinke T, Shite J, Takaoka H, et al. Vitamin C restores the contractile response to dobutamine and improves myocardial efficiency in patients with heart failure after anterior myocardial infarction. Am Heart J 2007;154(4):645, e1–e8.

[363] Rössig L, Hoffmann J, Hugel B, et al. Vitamin C inhibits endothelial cell apoptosis in congestive heart failure. Circulation 2001;104(18):2182–7.

[364] Piccirillo G, Nocco M, Moise A, et al. Influence of vitamin C on baroreflex sensitivity in chronic heart failure. Hypertension 2003;41:1240–5.

[365] Witte KK, Clark AL. Micronutrients and their supplementation in chronic cardiac failure. An update beyond theoretical perspectives. Heart Fail Rev 2006;11(1):65–74.

[366] Guo R, Pittler MH, Ernst E. Hawthorn extract for treating chronic heart failure. Cochrane Database Syst Rev 2008;(1):CD005312.

[367] Tadić VM, Dobrić S, Marković GM, et al. Anti-inflammatory, gastroprotective, free-radical-scavenging, and antimicrobial activities of hawthorn berries ethanol extract. J Agric Food Chem 2008;56(17):7700–9.

[368] Tassell MC, Kingston R, Gilroy D, et al. Hawthorn (*Crataegus* spp.) in the treatment of cardiovascular disease. Pharmacogn Rev 2010;4(7):32–41.

[369] Mishra LC, Singh BB, Dagenais S. Scientific basis for the therapeutic use of *Withania somnifera* (ashwagandha) a review. Altern Med Rev 2000;5:334–46.

[370] Mohanty I, Arya DS, Dinda A, et al. Mechanisms of cardioprotective effect of *Withania somnifera* in experimentally induced myocardial infarction. Basic Clin Pharmacol Toxicol 2004;94:184–90.

[371] Xu XL, Ji H, Gu SY, et al. Modification of alterations in cardiac function and sarcoplasmic reticulum by astragaloside IV in myocardial injury in vivo. Eur J Pharmacol 2007;568(1–3):203–12.

[372] Mikowska-Leyck K, Filipek B, Strzelecka H. Pharmacological effects of lavandulifolioside from *Leonurus cardiaca*. J Ethnopharmacol 2002;80(1):85–90.
[373] Gilani AH, Khan AU, Shah AJ, et al. Blood pressure lowering effect of olive is mediated through calcium channel blockade. Int J Food Sci Nutr 2005;56(8):613–20.
[374] Taylor RS, Sagar VA, Davies EJ, et al. Exercise-based rehabilitation for heart failure. Cochrane Database Syst Rev 2014;(4):CD003331.
[375] He J, Ogden LG, Bazzano LA, et al. Risk factors for congestive heart failure in US men and women: NHANES I epidemiologic follow-up study. Arch Intern Med 2001;161:996–1002.
[376] Dimsdale JE. Psychological stress and cardiovascular disease. J Am Coll Cardiol 2008;51(13):1237–46.
[377] Wittstein I, Thiemann D, Lima J, et al. Neurohumoral features of myocardial stunning due to sudden emotional stress. N Engl J Med 2005;352:539–48.
[378] Piepoli MF, Davos C, Francis DP, et al. ExTraMATCH Collaborative. Exercise training meta-analysis of trials in patients with chronic heart failure (ExTraMATCH). BMJ 2004;328(7433):189.
[379] Mitchell LB. Overview of arrythmias. In: Merck manual professional edition online. 2016. Available from: www.merckmanuals.com/professional/cardiovascular-disorders/arrhythmias-and-conduction-disorders/overview-of-arrhythmias.
[380] Hlatky MA. Approach to the patient with palpitations. In: Goldman L, Braunwald E, editors. Primary cardiology. Philadelphia: WB Saunders Company; 1998.
[381] Olgin JE. Approach to the patient with suspected arrythmia. In: Goldman L, Schafer AI, editors. Goldman's Cecil medicine. 24th ed. Philadelphia: Elsevier Saunders; 2012.
[382] Mitchel LB. Atrial fibrillation. In: Merck manual professional edition online. 2017. Available from: www.merckmanuals.com/professional/cardiovascular-disorders/arrhythmias-and-conductio n-disorders/atrial-fibrillation.
[383] Bielecka-Dabrowa A, Mikhailidis DP, Rysz J, et al. The mechanisms of atrial fibrillation in hyperthyroidism. Thyroid Res 2009;2(1):4.
[384] Jayaprasad N, Johnson F. Atrial fibrillation and hyperthyroidism. Indian Pacing Electrophysiol J 2005;5(4):305–11.
[385] Zimetbaum P. Cardiac arrhythmias with supraventricular origin. In: Goldman L, Schafer AI, editors. Goldman's Cecil medicine. 24th ed. Philadelphia: Elsevier Saunders; 2012.
[386] Prystowsky EN. The history of atrial fibrillation: the last 100 years. J Cardiovasc Electrophysiol 2008;19(6):575–82.
[387] Campbell TJ. Amiodarone. Australian Prescriber 2005;28(6):150–4.
[388] Lee SH, Park SJ, Byeon K, et al. Risk factors between patients with lone and non-lone atrial fibrillation. J Korean Med Sci 2013;28(8):1174–80.
[389] Caldeira D, Martins C, Alves LB, et al. Caffeine does not increase the risk of atrial fibrillation: a systematic review and meta-analysis of observational studies. Heart 2013;99(19):1383–9.
[390] Baker WL. Treating arrhythmias with adjunctive magnesium: identifying future research directions. Eur Heart J Cardiovasc Pharmacother 2017;3(2):108–17.
[391] Christou GA, Christou KA, Korantzopoulos P, et al. The current role of omega-3 fatty acids in the management of atrial fibrillation. Int J Mol Sci 2015;16(9):22870–87.
[392] Cook WMH. The physio-medical dispensatory: a treatise on therapeutics, materia medica, and pharmacy in accordance with the principles of physiological medication. Cincinnati: WMH Cook; 1869.
[393] Chan TY. Interaction between warfarin and danshen (*Salvia miltiorrhiza*). Ann Pharmacother 2001;35(4):501–4.
[394] Medi C, Kalman JM, Freedman SB. Supraventricular tachycardia. Med J Aust 2009;190(5):255–60.
[395] Helton MR. Diagnosis and management of common types of supraventricular tachycardia. Am Fam Physician 2015;92(9):793–802.
[396] Mitchell LB. Reentrant supraventricular tachycardias. In: Merck manual professional edition online. 2016. Available from: www.merckmanuals.com/professional/cardiovascular-disorders/arrhythmias-and-conduction-disorders/reentrant-supraventricula r-tachycardias.
[397] Greist JH. Panic attacks and panic disorder. In: Merck manual professional edition online. 2017. Available from: www.merckmanuals.com/professional/psychiatric-disorders/anxiety-and-stressor-related-disorders/panic-attacks-and-panic-disorder.
[398] Yang Y, Keung EC, Scheinman MM. History of supraventricular tachycardia. In: Yan GX, Kowey PR, editors. Management of cardiac arrhythmias. 2nd ed. New York: Springer Press; 2011.
[399] Klevay LM, Milne DB. Low dietary magnesium increases supraventricular ectopy. Am J Clin Nutr 2002;75(3):550–4.
[400] Glatter KA, Myers R, Chiamvimonvat N. Recommendations regarding dietary intake and caffeine and alcohol consumption in patients with cardiac arrhythmias: what do you tell your patients to do or not to do? Curr Treat Options Cardiovasc Med 2012;14(5):529–35.
[401] Hallett JW. Peripheral arterial disease. In: Merck manual professional edition online. 2016. Available from: www.merckmanuals.com/professional/cardiovascular-disorders/peripheral-arterial-disorders/peripheral-arterial-disease.
[402] Douketis JD. Chronic venous insufficiency and postphlebitic syndrome. In: Merck manual professional edition online. 2016. Available from: www.merckmanuals.com/professional/cardiovascular-disorders/peripheral-venous-disorders/chronic-venou s-insufficiency-and-postphlebitic-syndrome.
[403] White CJ. Atherosclerotic peripheral arterial disease. In: Goldman L, Schafer AI, editors. Goldman's Cecil medicine. 24th ed. Philadelphia: Elsevier Saunders; 2012.
[404] Olin JW. Other peripheral arterial disease. In: Goldman L, Schafer AI, editors. Goldman's Cecil medicine. 24th ed. Philadelphia: Elsevier Saunders; 2012.
[405] Ginsberg J. Peripheral venous disease. In: Goldman L, Schafer AI, editors. Goldman's Cecil medicine. 24th ed. Philadelphia: Elsevier Saunders; 2012.
[406] Hallett JW. Raynaud syndrome. In: Merck manual professional edition online. 2016. Available from: www.merckmanuals.com/professional/cardiovascular-disorders/peripheral-arterial-disorders/raynaud-syndrome.
[407] Hallett JW. Thromboangiitis obliterans. In: Merck manual professional edition online. 2016. Available from: www.merckmanuals.com/professional/cardiovascular-disorders/peripheral-arterial-disorders/thromboangiitis-obliterans.
[408] Douketis JD. Deep venous thrombosis. In: Merck manual professional edition online. 2016. Available from: www.merckmanuals.com/professional/cardiovascular-disorders/peripheral-venous-disorders/deep-venous-thrombosis-dvt.
[409] Douketis JD. Chronic venous insufficiency and postphlebitic syndrome. In: Merck manual professional edition online. 2016. Available from: www.merckmanuals.com/professional/cardiovascular-disorders/peripheral-venous-disorders/chronic-venous-insufficiency-and-postphlebitic-syndrome.
[410] Heffron SP, Rockman CB, Gianos E, et al. Greater frequency of nut consumption is associated with lower prevalence of peripheral arterial disease. Prev Med 2015;72:15–18.
[411] Heffron SP, Rockman CB, Adelman MA, et al. Greater frequency of fruit and vegetable consumption is associated with lower prevalence of peripheral artery disease. Arterioscl Thromb Vasc Biol 2017;37(6):1234–40.
[412] Ruiz-Canela M, Estruch R, Corella D, et al. Association of Mediterranean diet with peripheral artery disease: the PREDIMED randomized trial. JAMA 2014;311(4):415–17.
[413] Kenjale AA, Ham KL, Stabler T, et al. Dietary nitrate supplementation enhances exercise performance in peripheral arterial disease. J Appl Physiol 2011;110(6):1582–91.
[414] Campbell A, Price J, Hiatt WR. Omega-3 fatty acids for intermittent claudication. Cochrane Database Syst Rev 2013;(7):CD003833.
[415] Ottestad I, Nordvi B, Vogt G, et al. Bioavailability of n-3 fatty acids from n-3-enriched foods and fish oil with different oxidative quality in healthy human subjects: a randomised single-meal cross-over study. J Nutr Sci 2016;5:e43.
[416] Mason RP, Sherratt SC. Omega-3 fatty acid fish oil dietary supplements contain saturated fats and oxidized lipids that may interfere with their intended biological benefits. Biochem Biophys Res Commun 2017;483(1):425–9.
[417] Rundblad A, Holven KB, Ottestad I, et al. High-quality fish oil has a more favourable effect than oxidised fish oil on intermediate-density lipoprotein and LDL subclasses: a randomised controlled trial. Br J Nutr 2017;117(9):1291–8.
[418] Perrin M, Ramelet AA. Pharmacological treatment of primary chronic venous disease: rationale, results and unanswered questions. Eur J Vasc Endovasc Surg 2011;41(1):117–25.

[419] Aziz Z, Tang WL, Chong NJ, et al. A systematic review of the efficacy and tolerability of hydroxyethylrutosides for improvement of the signs and symptoms of chronic venous insufficiency. J Clin Pharm Ther 2015;40(2):177–85.
[420] Morling JR, Yeoh SE, Kolbach DN. Rutosides for treatment of post-thrombotic syndrome. Cochrane Database Syst Rev 2015;(9):CD005625.
[421] Vanscheidt W, Rabe E, Naser-Hijazi B, et al. The efficacy and safety of a coumarin-/troxerutin-combination (SB-LOT) in patients with chronic venous insufficiency: a double blind placebo-controlled randomised study. Vasa 2002;31(3):185–90.
[422] Kumar S, Pandey AK. Chemistry and biological activities of flavonoids: an overview. ScientificWorldJournal 2013;2013: 162750.
[423] de Pascual-Teresa S, Moreno DA, García-Viguera C. Flavonols and anthocyanins in cardiovascular health: a review of current evidence. Int J Mol Sci 2010;11(4):1679–703.
[424] Rusznyák ST, Szent-Györgyi A. Vitamin P: flavonols as vitamins. Nature 1936;138:27.
[425] Oliff H. Proprietary botanical ingredient scientific and clinical monograph: Pycnogenol®. American Botanical Council; 2010. Available from:: http://abc.herbalgram.org/site/DocServer/Pycnog_FullMono120809_LOW.pdf?docID=1741.
[426] Fine AM. Oligomeric proanthocyanidin complexes: history, structure, and phytopharmaceutical applications. Altern Med Rev 2000;5(2):144–51.
[427] Leucoselect product page. Indena. 2016. Available from: www.indena.com/products/leucoselect.
[428] Nicolaï SPA, Kruidenier LM, Bendermacher BLW, et al. *Ginkgo biloba* for intermittent claudication. Cochrane Database Syst Rev 2013;(6):CD006888.
[429] Pittler MH, Ernst E. Complementary therapies for peripheral arterial disease: systematic review. Atherosclerosis 2005;181(1):1–7.
[430] Upton R, editor. Ginkgo leaf, ginkgo leaf dry extract. American herbal pharmacopoeia and therapeutic compendium. Scotts Valley: American Herbal Pharmacopoeia; 2003.
[431] Straus SE, Richardson WS, Glasziou P, et al. Evidence-based medicine. How to practice and teach EBM. 3rd ed. Edinburgh: Elsevier Churchill Livingstone; 2005.
[432] Orekhov AN, Sobenin IA, Korneev NV, et al. Anti-atherosclerotic therapy based on botanicals. Recent Pat Cardiovasc Drug Discov 2013;8(1):56–66.
[433] Priest AW, Priest LR. Herbal medication. A clinical and dispensary handbook. London: LN Fowler & Co; 1983.
[434] Dall'Acqua S, Bolego C, Cignarella A, et al. Vasoprotective activity of standardized *Achillea millefolium* extract. Phytomedicine 2011;18(12):1031–6.
[435] Chong NJ, Aziz Z. A systematic review of the efficacy of *Centella asiatica* for improvement of the signs and symptoms of chronic venous insufficiency. Evid Based Complement Alternat Med 2013;627182.
[436] Pittler MH, Ernst E. Horse chestnut seed extract for chronic venous insufficiency. Cochrane Database Syst Rev 2012;(11):CD003230.
[437] Petersen KS, Clifton PM, Lister N, et al. Effect of weight loss induced by energy restriction on measures of arterial compliance: a systematic review and meta-analysis. Atherosclerosis 2016;247:7–20.
[438] Lane R, Ellis B, Watson L, et al. Exercise for intermittent claudication. Cochrane Database Syst Rev 2014;(7):CD000990.
[439] Berger JS, Ladapo JA. Underuse of prevention and lifestyle counseling in patients with peripheral artery disease. J Am Coll Cardiol 2017;69(18):2293–300.
[440] Kolbach DN, Sandbrink MWC, Hamulyak K, et al. Non-pharmaceutical measures for prevention of post-thrombotic syndrome. Cochrane Database Syst Rev 2003;(3):CD004174.

SAMPLE DAILY DIET REFERENCES

Atherosclerosis and dyslipidaemia

Gammon CS, Kruger R, Minihane AM, et al. Kiwifruit consumption favourably affects plasma lipids in a randomised controlled trial in hypercholesterolaemic men. Br J Nutr 2013;109(12): 2208–18.
Hagen IV, Helland A, Bratlie M, et al. High intake of fatty fish, but not of lean fish, affects serum concentrations of TAG and HDL-cholesterol in healthy, normal-weight adults: a randomised trial. Br J Nutr 2016;116(4):648–57.
Nwachukwu ID, Devassy JG, Aluko RE, et al. Cholesterol-lowering properties of oat β-glucan and the promotion of cardiovascular health: did Health Canada make the right call? Appl Physiol Nutr Metab 2015;40(6):535–42.
Srinivasan K. Dietary spices as beneficial modulators of lipid profile in conditions of metabolic disorders and diseases. Food Funct 2013;4(4):503–21.

Cardiovascular ischaemia (angina)

Aune D, Keum N, Giovannucci E, et al. Nut consumption and risk of cardiovascular disease, total cancer, all-cause and cause-specific mortality: a systematic review and dose-response meta-analysis of prospective studies. BMC Med 2016;14(1):207.
Hartley L, Igbinedion E, Holmes J, et al. Increased consumption of fruit and vegetables for the primary prevention of cardiovascular diseases. Cochrane Database Syst Rev 2013;(6):CD009874.
Massera D, Graf L, Barba S, et al. Angina rapidly improved with a plant-based diet and returned after resuming a Western diet. J Geriatr Cardiol 2016;13(4):364–6.
Massera D, Zaman T, Farren GE, et al. A whole-food plant-based diet reversed angina without medications or procedures. Case Rep Cardiol 2015;2015:978906.
Müller L, Caris-Veyrat C, Lowe G, et al. Lycopene and its antioxidant role in the prevention of cardiovascular diseases — a critical review. Crit Rev Food Sci Nutr 2016;56(11):1868–79.

Cerebrovascular ischaemia

Altermann CDC, Souza MA, Schimidt HL, et al. Short-term green tea supplementation prevents recognition memory deficits and ameliorates hippocampal oxidative stress induced by different stroke models in rats. Brain Res Bull 2017;131:78–84.
Aquilani R, Baiardi P, Scocchi M, et al. Normalization of zinc intake enhances neurological retrieval of patients suffering from ischemic strokes. Nutr Neurosci 2009;12(5):219–25.
Aquilani R, Scocchi M, Iadarola P, et al. Spontaneous neurocognitive retrieval of patients with sub-acute ischemic stroke is associated with dietary protein. Nutr Neurosci 2010;13(3):129–34.
Aquilani R, Sessarego P, Iadarola P, et al. Nutrition for brain recovery after ischemic stroke: an added value to rehabilitation. Nutr Clin Pract 2011;26(3):339–45.
Cherubini A, Ruggiero C, Morand C, et al. Dietary antioxidants as potential pharmacological agents for ischemic stroke. Curr Med Chem 2008;15(12):1236–48.
Estruch R, Ros E, Martínez-González MA. Mediterranean diet for primary prevention of cardiovascular disease. N Engl J Med 2013;369(7):676–7.
Fraser ML, Mok GS, Lee AH. Green tea and stroke prevention: emerging evidence. Complement Ther Med 2007;15(1):46–53.
Jadavji NM, Emmerson JT, MacFarlane AJ, et al. B-vitamin and choline supplementation increases neuroplasticity and recovery after stroke. Neurobiol Dis 2017;103:89–100.
Leppälä JM, Virtamo J, Fogelholm R, et al. Different risk factors for different stroke subtypes: association of blood pressure, cholesterol, and antioxidants. Stroke 1999;30(12):2535–40.
Sato Y, Nakatsuka H, Watanabe T, et al. Possible contribution of green tea drinking habits to the prevention of stroke. Tohoku J Exp Med 1989;157(4):337–43.
Wang Y, Chang CF, Chou J, et al. Dietary supplementation with blueberries, spinach, or spirulina reduces ischemic brain damage. Exp Neurol 2005;193(1):75–84.
Wen SW, Wong CHY. An unexplored brain-gut microbiota axis in stroke. Gut Microbes 2017;22:1–6.

Chronic heart failure

Aune D, Keum N, Giovannucci E, et al. Nut consumption and risk of cardiovascular disease, total cancer, all-cause and cause-specific mortality: a systematic review and dose-response meta-analysis of prospective studies. BMC Med 2016;14(1):207.
Colin-Ramirez E, McAlister FA, Zheng Y, et al. The long-term effects of dietary sodium restriction on clinical outcomes in patients with heart

failure. The SODIUM-HF (Study of Dietary Intervention Under 100 mmol in Heart Failure): a pilot study. Am Heart J 2015;169(2):274 81, e1.
Mathew AV, Seymour EM, Byun J, et al. Altered metabolic profile with sodium-restricted dietary approaches to stop hypertension diet in hypertensive heart failure with preserved ejection fraction. J Card Fail 2015;21(12):963–7.

Atrial fibrillation

Ganga HV, Noyes A, White CM, et al. Magnesium adjunctive therapy in atrial arrhythmias. Pacing Clin Electrophysiol 2013;36(10):1308–18.
Healey JS, Connolly SJ. Atrial fibrillation: hypertension as a causative agent, risk factor for complications, and potential therapeutic target. Am J Cardiol 2003;91(10A):9G–14G.
Khan AM, Lubitz SA, Sullivan LM, et al. Low serum magnesium and the development of atrial fibrillation in the community: the Framingham Heart Study. Circulation 2013;127(1):33–8.
Lip GY. Atrial fibrillation in patients with hypertension: trajectories of risk factors in yet another manifestation of hypertensive target organ damage. Hypertension 2016;68(3):544–5.
Mattioli AV, Miloro C, Pennella S, et al. Adherence to Mediterranean diet and intake of antioxidants influence spontaneous conversion of atrial fibrillation. Nutr Metab Cardiovasc Dis 2013;23(2):115–21.
Medina-Remón A, Vallverdú-Queralt A, Arranz S, et al. Gazpacho consumption is associated with lower blood pressure and reduced hypertension in a high cardiovascular risk cohort. Cross-sectional study of the PREDIMED trial. Nutr Metab Cardiovasc Dis 2013;23(10):944–52.
Pastori D, Carnevale R, Menichelli D, et al. Is there an interplay between adherence to Mediterranean diet, antioxidant status, and vascular disease in atrial fibrillation patients? Antioxid Redox Signal 2016;25(14):751–5.
Pignatelli P, Pastori D, Farcomeni A, et al. Mediterranean diet reduces thromboxane A2 production in atrial fibrillation patients. Clin Nutr 2015;34(5):899–903.
Pignatelli P, Pastori D, Vicario T, et al. Relationship between Mediterranean diet and time in therapeutic range in atrial fibrillation patients taking vitamin K antagonists. Europace 2015;17(8):1223–8.

Supraventricular tachycardia

Aune D, Giovannucci E, et al. Fruit and vegetable intake and the risk of cardiovascular disease, total cancer and all-cause mortality — a systematic review and dose-response meta-analysis of prospective studies. Int J Epidemiol 2017;46(3):1029–56.
Das S, Otani H, Maulik N, et al. Lycopene, tomatoes, and coronary heart disease. Free Radic Res 2005;39(4):449–55.
Klevay LM, Milne DB. Low dietary magnesium increases supraventricular ectopy. Am J Clin Nutr 2002;75(3):550–4.
Kris-Etherton PM. Walnuts decrease risk of cardiovascular disease: a summary of efficacy and biologic mechanisms. J Nutr 2014;144 (4 Suppl.):547S–554S.

21

The endocrine system

Leah Hechtman

SECTION A

OVERVIEW OF THE ENDOCRINE SYSTEM

See Fig. 21.1 for an overview of the endocrine system.[1]

The endocrine system is a complex system of glands and their secretions, known as hormones (a term first used by Starling in 1905).[2] The functions of these hormones have far-reaching implications for our health and wellbeing, as they play a vital role in multiple essential life functions. This includes our ability to reproduce, metabolise food, fight infection, grow and develop. The endocrine system comprises both the endocrine glands (pituitary, thyroid, parathyroid, adrenal and pineal) and their associated hormone-secreting tissues and organs (which have the ability to secrete hormones) including adipose tissue, the hypothalamus, ovaries, testes, pancreas, thymus, kidneys, stomach, liver, small intestine, skin, heart and placenta.[3]

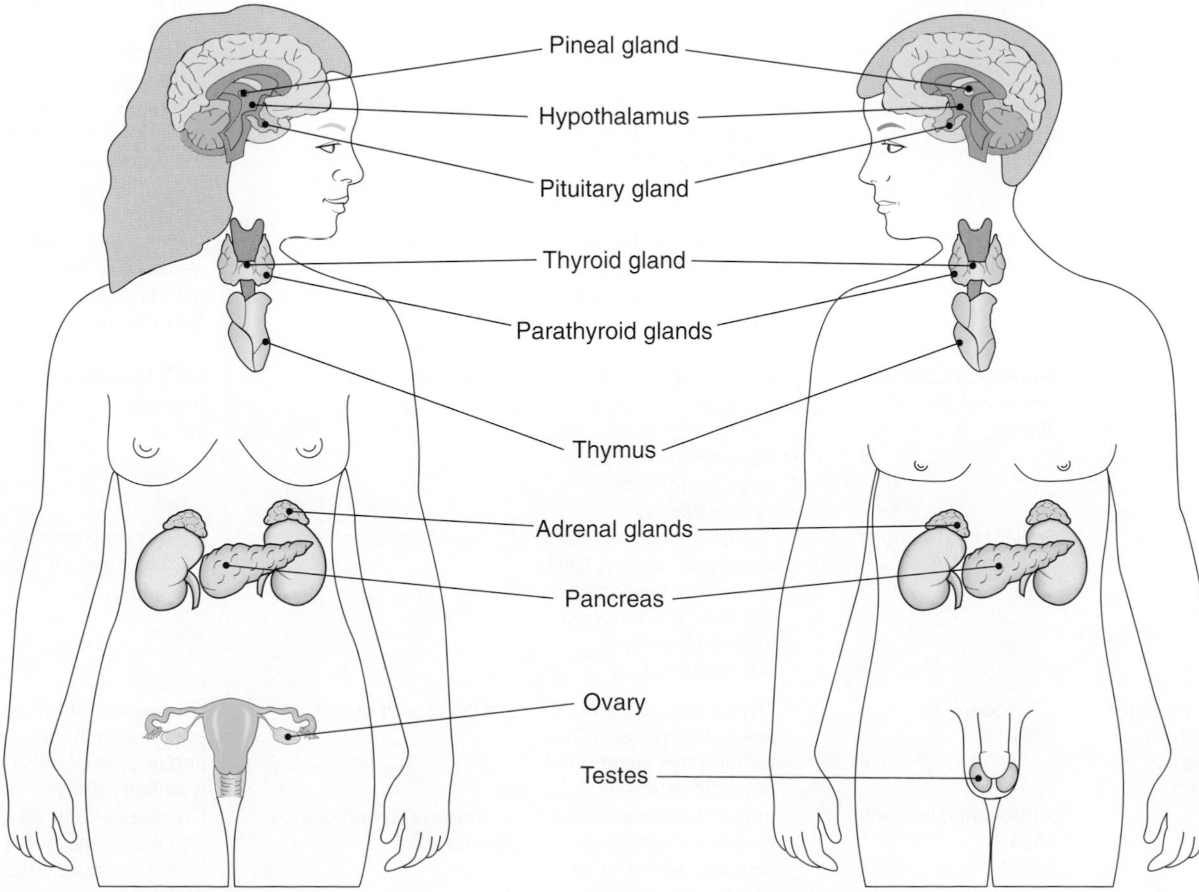

FIGURE 21.1 The endocrine system.

Talley N, O'Connor S. Clinical examination. 6th edn. Sydney: Churchill Livingstone; 2009.

GLANDS AND HORMONES OF THE ENDOCRINE SYSTEM

See Table 21.1 for a summary of the glands and the associated hormones.

Glands

PITUITARY GLAND

The pituitary gland is a 1–1.5 cm pea-shaped structure that has two anatomically separated lobes, known as the anterior

TABLE 21.1 Summary of hormone function

Gland	Hormone	Control condition	Target	Effect of secretion
Anterior pituitary	Human growth hormone (hGH) or somatotropin (WS)*	Hypothalamus monitors low blood sugar then secretes growth hormone-releasing hormone (GHRH). A rise in blood sugar causes the secretion of growth hormone-inhibiting hormone (GHIH)	Liver, muscle and connective tissues	Stimulates tissues to synthesise and release insulin-like growth factors (IGFs). These cause a rise in blood glucose and build proteins
	Thyroid-stimulating hormone (TSH) or thyrotrophin (WS)*	Hypothalamus monitors low blood levels of thyroid hormone and secretes TSH. A rise causes the secretion of GHIH	Thyroid gland	Stimulates the thyroid gland to secrete T_3 and T_4. The secretion of TSH may also be due to lowering of blood temperature or blood sugar
	Follicle-stimulating hormone (FSH) (WS)*	Hypothalamus matures at puberty and begins to secrete gonadotrophin-releasing hormone (GnRH)	Ovaries and testes	In females causes the development of egg cells and the ovarian secretion of oestrogen. In males the production of sperm is increased
	Luteinising hormone (LH) (WS)*	Hypothalamus matures at puberty and begins to secrete GnRH	Ovaries and testes	In females causes the ovulation and stimulates the secretion of progesterone. In males the secretion of testosterone
	Prolactin (PRL) (WS)*	Fall in sex hormones before menstruation inhibits. Pregnancy and suckling increase secretion	Mammary glands	Initiates and maintains milk secretion in the mammary glands together with oxytocin and sex hormones
	Adrenocorticotropic hormone (ACTH) (WS)*	Hypothalamus monitors stress and secretes corticotropin-releasing hormone (CRH). A negative feedback system inhibits	Adrenal cortex	ACTH causes secretion of glucocorticoids, e.g. cortisol
	Melanocyte-stimulating hormone (MSH) (WS)*	Hypothalamus monitors stress and releases CRH secretion of melanocyte-stimulating hormones (MSH). Dopamine inhibits secretion	Melanocytes in skin	Causes melanocytes to secrete pigment called melanin
Posterior pituitary (secreted by hypothalamus and stored)	Oxytocin (OT) (WS)*	Hypothalamus controls levels after puberty. In birthing the secretion of oxytocin increases	Uterus and breast	Causes smooth muscle contraction in the uterus and release of milk from mammary ducts
	Antidiuretic hormone (ADH) (WS)*	In hypothalamus, osmo (water)-receptors stimulate secretion of ADH in response to high blood concentration	Kidneys, sweat glands, arterioles	Decreases volumes of urine and perspiration. Raises blood pressure. The overall effect is to increase movement of nutrients from capillaries

TABLE 21.1 Summary of hormone function—cont'd

Gland	Hormone	Control condition	Target	Effect of secretion
Thyroid	Triiodothyronine (T_3), thyroxine (T_4) (LS)**	Hypothalamus monitors body temperature and metabolic rate. If either falls TSH is released	All cells of body	Increases oxygen use in cells, cellular metabolism and growth
	Calcitonin (CT) (WS)*	High levels of blood calcium increase and low blood calcium decreases calcitonin	Osteoclasts and osteoblasts	Decreases the activity of osteoclasts and increases uptake of calcium and phosphate into the bone matrix
Parathyroid	Parathyroid hormone (PTH) (WS)*	High levels of blood calcium decrease and low blood calcium increases secretion of PTH	Osteoclasts	Increases the activity of osteoclasts, and absorption of calcium from foods. In the presence of vitamin D
Adrenal cortex	Mineralocorticoids, aldosterone (LS)**	Formation of angiotensin or increased blood potassium (K+)	Nephron in kidneys, blood filtration tissues	Increases the reabsorption of Na+ from the kidneys and loss of potassium in the urine. Regulating blood ion concentration
	Glucocorticoids, cortisol (LS)**	Homeostasis disrupted, hypothalamus secretes CRH, this along with low levels of blood glucocorticoid stimulate anterior pituitary to secrete ACTH	Muscles, liver, adipose tissue, blood vessels and immune cells	Increases protein breakdown (muscles) and formation of glucose from amino acids and lactate. Increases fat breakdown and use of fatty acids for energy. Depresses inflammatory and immune responses. Overall aim to increase energy availability
	Androgens, other and sex hormones (LS)**	Hypothalamus matures and stimulates secretion of androgens	All body cells	Promotes growth particularly, secondary sexual characteristics. Continues to produce oestrogens after menopause in women
Adrenal medulla	Adrenaline (epinephrine), noradrenaline (norepinephrine) (LS)**	Receive direct stimulation from sympathetic division of autonomic nervous system (ANS) to cause secretion when homeostasis disrupted	Heart, circulatory system and lungs	Increase heart output of blood, blood flow to liver/muscles and airway size in lungs. Suppress blood flow to skin and digestive system. Actions of the fight or flight response as neurotransmitters
Pancreatic alpha cells	Glucagon (WS)*	Low blood glucose level causes secretion of glucagon from alpha cells in pancreas	Liver	Increase blood glucose level by formation of glucose from glycogen (glycogenolysis), lactic acid and amino acids (gluconeogenesis)
Pancreatic beta cells	Insulin (WS)*	High blood glucose levels stimulate secretion of insulin from beta cells in the pancreas	Liver, muscle and adipose tissue	Decreases blood glucose level by increasing permeability of glucose to cells. Increases formation of glycogen, proteins and lipids
Pancreatic delta cells	Somatostatin (WS)*	High levels of free glucagon and insulin stimulate secretion. Also suppresses secretion of hGH	Alpha and beta cells. Small intestine	Stabilises levels of glucose, amino acids and lipids in blood. Reduces cell metabolic processes that promote growth

Continued

TABLE 21.1 Summary of hormone function—cont'd				
Gland	**Hormone**	**Control condition**	**Target**	**Effect of secretion**
Pancreatic F-cells	Pancreatic polypeptide (WS)*	Pancreatic polypeptide is secreted by intake of high protein meal and exercise	Delta cells, pancreatic digestive enzymes and gall bladder	Increases ability of digestive system to absorb proteins (as amino acids) and fats. Increases availability of nutrients for cell growth
Ovaries	Oestrogens and progesterone (LS)**	FSH stimulates the production of oestrogens and progesterone	Female reproductive system, mammary glands	Regulate female reproductive cycle and promote development of feminine secondary sexual characteristics
	Relaxin (WS)*	Secreted in later stages of pregnancy	Connective tissues (esp. cartilage)	Increases elastic qualities of pubic symphysis and cervix to facilitate movement of child through the birth canal
	Inhibin (WS)*	Stimulated by increased secretion of oestrogens and progesterone	Anterior pituitary	Inhibits secretion of FSH
Testes	Testosterone (LS)**	FSH stimulates the production of testosterone	Male reproductive system	Regulates production of sperm cells and promotes development of masculine secondary sexual characteristics
	Inhibin (WS)*	Stimulated by increased secretion of testosterone	Anterior pituitary	Inhibits secretion of FSH
Pineal	Melatonin (WS)*	Released in darkened environment	Hypothalamus, possibly reproductive organs	Contributes to setting of body clock and sleeping rhythms. Inhibits activity of reproduction in animals
Thymus	Thymosin, thymopoeitin (WS)*	Production begins in utero and thymus shrinks after puberty	T-cell maturation	These hormones control development of T-cells into functioning immune cells

*WS, water soluble, target receptor on cell membrane.
**LS, lipid soluble, target receptor in nucleus.

and posterior pituitary. Of these two lobes the anterior pituitary is the larger and it secretes more hormones. However, both are regulated by the hypothalamus region of the brain, with the hypothalamic hormones being transported through the hypophyseal portal system. These hormones act on the anterior pituitary to produce numerous hormones, but are released directly from the posterior pituitary (which acts as a storage and releasing conduit rather than a synthesiser of hormones). This direct link between the hypothalamus and pituitary ensures immediate communication between the two, without the hormones being diluted into the general circulatory system. This gland is a key link between the nervous and endocrine systems, as emotional, painful and stressful experiences all affect the secretion of pituitary hormones due to its vital connection with the hypothalamus.

THYROID GLAND

The thyroid is a highly vascularised butterfly-shaped gland that weighs approximately 30 g and receives 80–120 mL of blood per minute. It is located below the larynx and straddles the trachea. The thyroid is influenced by the anterior pituitary hormone thyroid-stimulating hormone (TSH) and produces thyroxine (T_4), triiodothyronine (T_3) and calcitonin. It is the only endocrine gland that stores its hormones in large quantities, with a normally functioning thyroid storing approximately a 100-day supply of hormones. The control of thyroid hormone secretion is via a negative feedback system, although the level of iodine also contributes to this by influencing the amount of viable thyroid hormones.

PARATHYROID GLANDS

The parathyroid glands are located behind the 'wings' of the thyroid, and normally consist of four small round glands (two on each lateral lobe of the thyroid, with one superior and one inferior). Parathyroid hormone (PTH) regulates the concentrations of calcium, magnesium and phosphate ions in the blood. The level of calcitonin (from the thyroid) and PTH is directly linked to the blood calcium level via a negative feedback system. PTH has the following functions: it promotes the activity of osteoclasts, it acts on the kidneys to release calcitriol (in order to increase the amount of calcium that is absorbed from foods in the presence of vitamin D), slows the loss of both calcium and magnesium through urine and increases the loss of phosphate through the urine.

ADRENAL GLANDS

The adrenal (also called suprarenal) glands are two highly vascularised pyramid-shaped glands lying superior to each kidney. Both weigh approximately 3.5–5 g with a height of 3–5 cm, width of 2–3 cm and thickness of approximately 1 cm, and they double in size from birth. Each gland comprises an adrenal cortex (which accounts for 80–90% of its size) and a centrally located adrenal medulla. The adrenal cortex is subdivided into three zones: the zona glomerulosa (producing the mineralocorticoid aldosterone), the zona fasciculata (producing glucocorticoids cortisol, corticosterone and cortisone) and the zona reticularis (producing androgens). The production of aldosterone is related to increased blood levels of potassium and angiotensin II, while the production of both the glucocorticoids and androgens is linked with the release of adrenocorticotropic hormone (ACTH). The adrenal medulla is a part of the autonomic nervous system (ANS). Instead of having nerve ganglions and neurotransmitters, the adrenal medulla releases the hormones adrenaline (epinephrine) and noradrenaline (norepinephrine) from chromaffin cells. Eighty per cent of the adrenal medulla cells produce adrenaline, with only 20% producing noradrenaline. It is cortisol from the adrenal cortex that induces the production of an enzyme to convert noradrenaline to adrenaline. The secretion of adrenaline and noradrenaline is induced when a person is in a stressful situation. Impulses from the hypothalamus stimulate the preganglionic neurons, which then stimulate the chromaffin cells to produce adrenaline and noradrenaline. These hormones then add to the fight-or-flight response by acting on the autonomic nervous system.

PINEAL GLAND

The pineal gland is located on the midline roof of the third ventricle of the brain, and has a mass of only 0.1–0.2 g. It consists of both neuroglia and pinealocytes, which secrete melatonin. Melatonin is a water-soluble hormone that is derived from serotonin, and is released in higher quantities when a person is away from sunlight (for instance, at night-time). It plays a role in the setting of the 'body clock', in the setting of sleeping rhythms, and has been found to inhibit reproductive activity in some animals during non-reproductive seasons.

Pancreas

The pancreas is located in the curve of the duodenum. It is not only an endocrine gland but also an exocrine gland, due to the release of pancreatic enzymes via the pancreatic and accessory ducts. In this section we are concerned

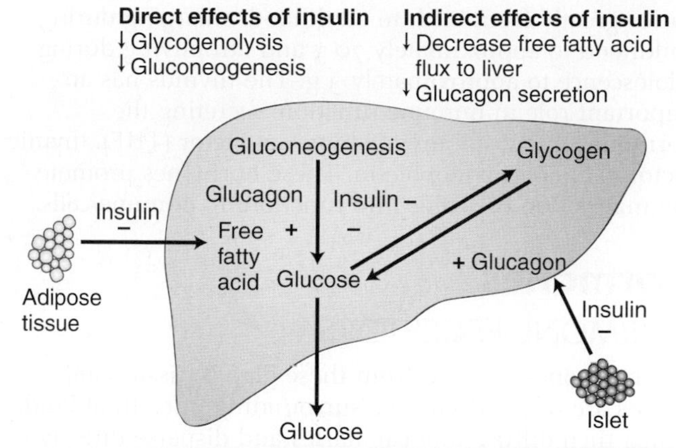

FIGURE 21.2 Flow diagram of negative feedback between glucagon and insulin.

Source: Kronenberg H. Williams textbook of endocrinology. 11th edn. Philadelphia: Saunders; 2007.

about the function of the endocrine alpha (secrete glucagon), beta (secrete insulin), delta (secrete somatostatin) and F (secrete pancreatic polypeptide) cells of the pancreas. These occur in tiny clusters throughout the pancreas, called pancreatic islets or islets of Langerhans (after Paul Langerhans who discovered these cells in 1869). To date the interactions between these hormones is not fully understood. See Fig. 21.2 for more detailed information on the negative feedback between glucagon and insulin.

Ovaries and testes

The ovaries and testes are the vital endocrine glands responsible for sexual maturation and reproduction. They are also referred to as the gonads due to their production of gametes (sperm in males and oocytes in females).

The ovaries are the two female gonads. They are the size and shape of two unshelled almonds and are located on either side of the uterus. They produce two steroid hormones (oestradiol and oestrone, which are both oestrogens), as well as inhibin (a hormone that inhibits the secretion of follicle-stimulating hormone (FSH)) and relaxin (a hormone that increases flexibility and dilates the cervix during the later stages of pregnancy).

The testes are two oval glands measuring approximately 5 cm in length and 2.5 cm in diameter, each weighing approximately 10–15 g. Developing near the kidneys, they descend via the inguinal canals during the seventh month of fetal development, and eventually sit in the scrotum. The testes produce both testosterone and inhibin, which regulate the production of sperm and masculine secondary sexual characteristics via a negative feedback system.

Thymus

The thymus consists of two lobes, located posterior to the sternum and anterior to the aorta. The size of the lobes varies greatly from birth to adulthood, enlarging during childhood to approximately 70 g and atrophying during adolescence to approximately 3 g. The thymus has an important role in immune function, secreting the hormones thymosin, thymic humoral factor (THF), thymic factor (TF) and thymopoietin. These hormones promote the maturation of T-cells into functioning immune cells.

Hormones

HORMONE RECEPTORS

The hormones secreted from these glands, tissues and organs are released into the surrounding interstitial fluid, which then diffuse into capillaries and disperse directly into the bloodstream. This distinguishing feature differentiates them from exocrine glands (such as oil and sweat glands), which utilise ducts to transport their secretions. These hormones act as signals to their target tissues, and to the system as a whole. While exocrine gland secretions are delivered to their targets via ducts, endocrine hormones circulate freely in the bloodstream. They are only able to promote a response in tissues by 'fitting' to the target tissue's glycoprotein receptors, just as a lock and key fit together to open a door. If a cell does not contain any receptors for that type of hormone, it will not be able to produce an effect on that cell. For example, thyroid cells do not have any receptors for oxytocin, thus oxytocin does not affect the function of the thyroid. This is despite its general presence in the bloodstream.

Hormone receptors are constantly being produced and broken down according to their perceived requirement. The perceived requirement is altered if there is too much or too little of a hormone present, with a target cell having anywhere from 2000 to 100 000 receptors. For example, if a patient has a consistently high level of blood insulin the number of insulin receptors in target tissues will reduce.

The location of hormone receptors differs according to the type of hormone that binds to it. For lipid-soluble hormones (e.g. steroid and thyroid hormones) the receptors are inside the target cells, and for water-soluble hormones (e.g. thyroid-stimulating hormone (TSH), oxytocin and antidiuretic hormone) they are part of the plasma membrane surrounding cells. A target cell will have a greater response to a hormone depending upon the level of hormone in the bloodstream, the number of receptors and the influence of other hormones. For example, the presence of both FSH and oestrogen has a greater effect on the production of oocytes in the ovaries than either hormone acting alone. In contrast some hormones act antagonistically with one another, for example glucagon and insulin.

HORMONE SECRETION

The secretion of hormones is dependent upon the stimulation of the gland. This is regulated by chemical changes in the blood, the presence of other hormones and signals from the nervous system. Regulatory systems within the endocrine system primarily operate via a negative feedback system. This means that if a level of the hormone is low, more is secreted, and when this level is high again the secretion is inhibited. For example, low blood levels of T_3 and T_4 stimulate the release of thyrotrophin-releasing hormone (TRH) in the hypothalamus, which then causes the anterior pituitary gland to secrete TSH. This then leads the thyroid to release more T_3 and T_4, but when the hypothalamus and anterior pituitary detect elevated T_3 levels, TRH and TSH release is inhibited. Most hormones are released into the bloodstream in short bursts, stopping and starting due to this negative feedback mechanism (Fig. 21.3). In contrast, the release of a hormone in a positive feedback system then stimulates more to be released, with no direct stopping mechanism. An example of a positive feedback system is the production of oxytocin during childbirth. The presence of oxytocin continues to rise with each contraction of the smooth muscle of the uterus, and this rising level leads to more contractions, and so the cycle continues until the delivery of the child. This feedback system has been used traditionally to ensure the prompt delivery of the placenta after the birth of a child, as the stimulation caused by breastfeeding immediately after birth further enhances the release of oxytocin, thus aiding the contraction of the uterus.

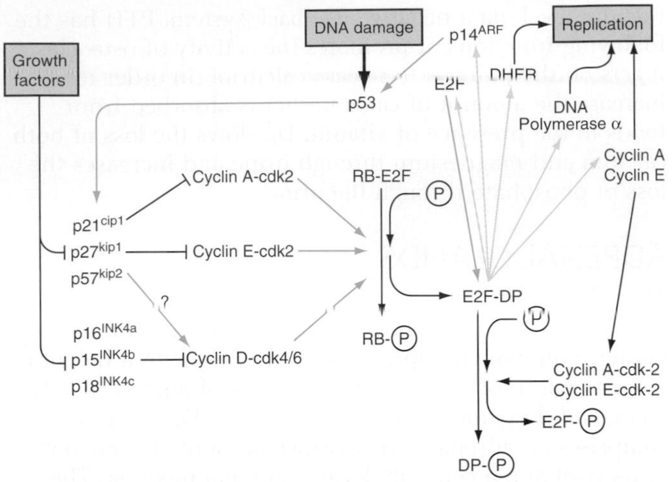

FIGURE 21.3 Flow diagram of negative and positive feedback systems.

Source: Wein AJ. Campbell-Walsh urology. 9th edn. Philadelphia: Saunders; 2007.

ROLE OF THE NATUROPATH

Traditional interpretation

The traditional understanding of the endocrine glands was largely reliant upon symptomatic evidence, as there was no deeper knowledge of the functions of the endocrine system until the mid-19th century. More comprehensive theories were developed in the mid- to late 20th century, but many questions still remain to be answered today.

The developmental changes caused by the castration of calves and humans (as evident in eunuchs) caught the attention of many enquiring minds in ancient Egypt and China, and led philosophers of those times to wonder at the mechanism of action of the testes. Similarly goitres were first recognised in China in 2700 BC,[4] and repeatedly noted in numerous cultures since. Avicenna (Abou Ali Sina, 980–1037), in his medicinal and philosophical masterpiece *al-Qanun* ('The Canon of Medicine'), outlined the physical symptoms of both insulin-dependent and non-insulin-dependent diabetes.[5] However, it was many centuries later, in 1869, before the pancreatic insula were discovered by Langerhans.

The anatomical discoveries of each of the endocrine glands greatly predated the understanding of their functions. The thymus gland was known to the Alexandrians in the 3rd century BC, and the thyroid, pineal and pituitary glands were anatomically described by Galen.[6] The adrenal glands were not discovered until the 16th century and the pancreatic and parathyroid glands in the latter 19th century. Predating each of these discoveries was the anatomical observation by the earliest physicians of both the gonads and the liver.[6]

Although the functions of individual endocrine 'hormones' were unknown, symptomatic treatment of endocrine diseases was widespread. For example, goat's rue (*Galega officinalis*) was used in medieval Europe for the treatment of diabetes and became the basis of the modern drug metformin. Goat's rue continues to be used by modern herbalists for its blood sugar regulating actions. Similarly fenugreek (*Trigonella foenum-graecum*) was used by Avicenna in the treatment of diabetes, and also continues to be used for this condition in modern naturopathic treatment.[7] The treatment of the endocrine system initially centred on the humoral beliefs of Galen. The pituitary was thought to be a sump for phlegm (waste products) from the brain which were then expelled via the nasal passage.[8] Similarly, goitres were thought to be caused from excess phlegm; however, they were treated with empirical treatments of marine sponge and seaweed.[4] These humoral theories were largely believed until 1855, when a number of scientists and physicians disproved them, although they had been anatomically disproved some 200 years previously by anatomists such as Conrad Victor Schneider and Richard Lower.[2]

Modern interpretation

The modern interpretation of the endocrine system is based on both the traditional use of herbs (for both symptomatic relief and treating the cause) and the scientific understanding of the connection between the nervous and endocrine systems. The scientific experimentation of the mid-19th century saw a radical shift and deeper understanding of the endocrine system, as experiments such as those carried out by AA Berthold (in 1849) were able to show that the action of the endocrine glands was not local, but systemic.[9] Berthold castrated four out of six young male chickens. Two of these four had their testes transplanted to the abdominal cavity, while the remaining two had their testes removed completely. The growth of the two uncastrated chickens was normal, and they developed into roosters with fully developed cones, wattles and plumage. The two fully castrated chickens failed to develop any male rooster characteristics, displaying only atrophied combs and wattles. Surprisingly for the scientists of the time, the two chickens with the transplanted testes grew to become fully developed roosters, displaying the same male characteristics as the control roosters. This was among the first evidence that hormones existed, that they were transported throughout the body in the bloodstream, and that they had a decisive role in sexual growth and maturation. Further experiments and observations conducted around this time helped to prove this theory, such as the observations of Thomas Addison (also in 1849) on patients with what he termed 'melasma suprarenale' (adrenal disease), a disorder which is now called Addison's disease in his honour.[6]

The understanding of the endocrine system progressed rapidly from this point, as these 'internal secretions' were eventually shown to be chemical structures called 'hormones'.[6] The discovery of each individual hormone quickly ensued at the turn of the 20th century. Following this the role of the hormones on the overall process of metabolism (a term first used by Michael Foster in 1876) and regulation was discovered via the work of Harvey Cushing and Langdon-Brown.[6] Until the mid-20th century the symptomatic approach to treatment remained, with varying results. This is evident in the quote below from Ellingwood (1910)[10] discussing the treatment and prognosis of diabetes mellitus:

> *Treatment: — As yet no specifics have been discovered, either for this disease as a whole, or for any of its attendant conditions. Various measures have been devised but these have usually been ultimately abandoned. While dietary measures are by far the most important.*
>
> *Prognosis: — The prognosis as to cure is always unfavourable.*

The most recent development in the understanding and subsequent treatment approach to the endocrine system has developed since the 1920s due to the knowledge of the interconnected nature of both the endocrine and nervous systems.[11] Specifically, it is the vast amount of research conducted in the latter part of the 20th century regarding the hypothalamic–pituitary–adrenal (HPA) axis and psychoneuroimmunology (PNI) that has most significantly altered the understanding of the endocrine system.[12] This innate link between the brain, the body and health has given a greater scientific basis to the holistic nature of the naturopathic treatment approach. For example, studies conducted in Russia on Siberian ginseng (*Eleutherococcus senticosus*) during the great 'space race' have helped to establish that the use of single herbs can alter immune function, physical stamina and aid stress adaptation, all via the endocrine system.[13] This holistic treatment of the endocrine system is often a key factor in treatment due to the role stress plays in many patients' lives. However, the power of what Bellamy and Pfister (1992)[14] term 'the largest endocrine gland' (the brain) is yet to be fully realised. They quote Albert Schweitzer's musings to better explain their point:

The witch doctor succeeds for the same reason all the rest of us succeed. Each patient carries his own doctor inside him. They come to us not knowing that cure. We are at our best when we give the doctor who resides within each patient a chance to go to work. (p. 259)

This concept of the patient's innate healing ability is central to the naturopathic approach to treatment, and is rapidly being given a scientific basis of evidence via the function of the endocrine system.

INVESTIGATIONS

Investigations used in endocrine disorders are summarised in Table 21.2

Testosterone and sex hormone-binding globulin (SHBG)

Normal values of testosterone and sex hormone-binding globulin are shown in Table 21.3

TABLE 21.2 Investigations

Test category	Normal result	Clinical significance
Growth hormone	Plasma/serum: dependent on age and assay method Stimulation test: peak growth hormone ≥20 mU/L (10 micrograms/L) Suppression test: suppression to <4 mU/L (<2 micrograms/L) in at least one specimen	**Decreased levels** that are unable to be stimulated indicate pituitary dwarfism **Increased levels** that are unable to be suppressed indicate gigantism or acromegaly
Insulin-like growth factor-1 (IGF-1)	Adult: 13–50 nmol/L NOTE: varies with age, gender and pubertal status	**Increased levels**: indicate acromegaly or gigantism; this test should be followed by GH suppression test for more conclusive results **Decreased levels**: used to diagnose Laron dwarfism
Follicle-stimulating hormone (FSH)	Female: 1.0–8.0 U/L ADD luteal/follicular/midcycle levels Post-menopausal female: >18.0 U/L Adult male: 1.0–5.0 U/L (age related) NOTE: method-dependent and related to menstrual cycle in females	**Increased levels**: indicate primary gonadal hypofunction, post-menopausal state, castration or pituitary gonadotroph tumours **Decreased levels**: pituitary or hypothalamic disease causing ovarian or testicular failure
Luteinising hormone (LH)	Adult male: 2–10 U/L Adult female: 2–15 U/L ADD luteal/follicular/midcycle levels Post-menopausal: 15–100 U/L NOTE: LH secretion is pulsatile and single results may be misleading	**Increased levels**: primary gonadal failure, indication of ovulation (peak occurs just prior to ovulation). An increased LH:FSH ratio can help diagnose polycystic ovary syndrome. High levels are found in primary gonadal failure **Decreased levels**: indication of hypothalamic failure (this responds to gonadotrophin-releasing hormone) or pituitary failure (no response to gonadotrophin-releasing hormone)
Prolactin (PRL)	Female: <750 mU/L Male: 150–500 mU/L	**Increased levels**: indication of prolactinomas, hypothalamic disorders (these may be associated with amenorrhoea-galactorrhoea syndrome). NOTE: some drugs cause increased levels (e.g. phenothiazines, metoclopramide and oestrogens). It is normal for levels to increase during pregnancy and lactation. Stress, nipple stimulation and strenuous exercise prior to testing can produce misleading results **Decreased levels**: general hypopituitarism. NOTE: low levels may also be caused by drugs such as dopamine, levodopa and ergot alkaloid derivatives
Adrenocorticotrophic hormone (ACTH)	<50 ng/L (dependent on time of collection)	**Increased levels**: can indicate corticosteroid excess (when caused by ectopic or pituitary source) or corticosteroid deficiency (due to primary adrenal insufficiency) **Decreased levels**: can indicate corticosteroid excess (due to adrenal tumour) or corticosteroid deficiency (due to pituitary deficiency)
Antidiuretic hormone (ADH)	Depends on plasma osmolality and intravascular volume	**Increased levels**: can indicate diabetes insipidus related to nephrogenic causes (when ADH level increases as plasma osmolality also increases) **Decreased levels**: central diabetes insipidus is linked with decreased ADH levels irrespective of plasma osmolality

TABLE 21.2 Investigations—cont'd

Test category	Normal result	Clinical significance
Thyroid-stimulating hormone (TSH)	0.4–5.0 mIU/L (depends on method)	**Increased levels**: high levels are found in primary hypothyroidism **Decreased levels**: may indicate hyperthyroidism, pituitary overproduction of TSH, concurrent treatment of thyroid cancer or hypopituitarism
Free T_3 (fT3)	4.0–8.0 pmol/L	**Increased levels**: indication of Graves' disease (hyperthyroidism). Able to give early warning of this as fT3 can become abnormal earlier than fT4 **Decreased levels**: indication of Hashimoto's disease (hypothyroidism)
Free T_4 (fT4)	10–25 pmol/L Values up to 35 pmol/L may be acceptable for patients on full replacement therapy with thyroxine	**Increased levels**: indication of Graves' disease (hyperthyroidism) **Decreased levels**: indication of Hashimoto's disease (hypothyroidism)
Antithyroid peroxidase activity (anti-TPO)	Negative	**Positive**: detects presence of antibodies against protein in thyroid cells. Positive result is highly associated with Hashimoto's disease (often also a positive in Graves' disease)
TSH receptor antibodies (TRAbs)	Negative	**Positive**: this test shows the presence of antibodies against proteins in the TSH receptors. A positive result is associated with Graves' disease
Thyroglobulin	<38 micrograms/L Thyroglobulin should be undetectable in a patient who has had a total thyroidectomy	**Increased levels**: associated with thyroiditis or thyrotoxicosis **Decreased levels**: associated with thyrotoxicosis due to self-medication with thyroid hormone
Calcitonin	<15 pmol/L	**Increased levels**: indication of C-cell hyperplasia or medullary thyroid cancer (MTC). Further testing is required to confirm the diagnosis (e.g. biopsy, scan, and ultrasound)
Parathyroid hormone (PTH)	Serum: 1.0–7.0 pmol/L (method dependent)	**Increased levels**: hyperparathyroidism (with concurrent hypercalcaemia) **Decreased levels**: if concurrent with hypercalcaemia and elevated parathyroid hormone-related protein (PTHrP), can indicate PTH malignancy NOTE: interpretation is dependent upon corrected calcium or ionised calcium, and the timing of the blood specimen
Parathyroid hormone related protein (PTHrP)	Plasma: <5 pmol/L (method dependent)	**Increased levels**: elevated levels with concurrent hypercalcaemia are indicative of malignancy, specifically of squamous carcinoma. Increasing levels suggest progression of the tumour
Aldosterone	Dependent on sodium intake, posture, drugs including ACE inhibitors and diuretics	**Increased levels**: high ratio of aldosterone to renin is indicative of a mineralocorticoid abnormality. Elevated aldosterone and renin is indicative of renal disease **Decreased levels**: indicates adrenal insufficiency (Addison's disease) with concurrently high renin levels NOTE: interpretation is dependent on aldosterone:renin ratio
Renin	Related to patient preparation, posture and drug therapy (e.g. levels increased by diuretics and ACE inhibitors)	**Increased levels**: high renin and aldosterone is indicative of renal disease. Increased levels also indicate secondary hyperaldosteronism or adrenal insufficiency (Addison's disease) **Decreased levels**: primary hyperaldosteronism (Conn's syndrome) or Cushing's syndrome NOTE: interpretation is dependent on aldosterone:renin ratio
Cortisol serum/ plasma	200–650 nmol/L (morning peak) NOTE: higher levels may be seen in stressed patients and in those on oral contraceptives Trough level (2000 h) should be <50% of the morning peak	**Increased levels**: indicative of Cushing's syndrome **Decreased levels**: indicates adrenal insufficiency (Addison's syndrome)

Continued

TABLE 21.2 Investigations—cont'd		
Test category	**Normal result**	**Clinical significance**
Cortisol (free) urinary	100–300 nmol/24 hours	**Increased levels**: primary or secondary adrenocortical hyperfunction, also seen in obesity, stress, depression and alcoholism
C-peptide	Fasting: 0.8–1.9 micrograms/L	**Increased levels**: indication of insulinomas, hypokalaemia, pregnancy, Cushing's syndrome and kidney disease. Also common in a newly diagnosed type 2 diabetic patient **Decreased levels**: can be seen in a newly diagnosed type 1 diabetic patient or a chronic long-term type 2 diabetic. Diuretics and alcohol can also cause low levels
Insulin	<5 mU/L during hypoglycaemia 4–10 mU/L after 8-hour fast, and with a normal plasma glucose	**Increased levels**: suggestive of non-insulin-dependent diabetes mellitus (early stages), insulin resistance (metabolic syndrome), fructose/galactose intolerance, Cushing's syndrome, acromegaly, and if concurrent with increased insulin:glucose ratio it can indicate pancreatic islet beta cell hyperplasia or insulinomas **Decreased levels**: diabetes, hypopituitarism NOTE: insulin levels must be compared with glucose results for a more complete diagnosis
Glucose	Venous plasma or serum Fasting: 3.0–5.4 mmol/L ≥2 hour post-prandial 'Random': 3.0–7.7 mmol/L	**Increased levels**: fasting glucose >7.0 mmol/L, or plasma glucose >11.1 mmol/L (2 h after a meal) on two occasions, is diagnostic of diabetes mellitus. Patients with fasting plasma level 5.5–6.9 mmol/L or random plasma glucose levels 7.8–11.0 mmol/L indicate further testing with a GTT. Increased glucose levels can also indicate acromegaly, acute stress, chronic kidney disease, Cushing's syndrome, hyperthyroidism, pancreatic cancer, pancreatitis NOTE: certain drugs can increase glucose levels (e.g. corticosteroids, tricyclic antidepressants, diuretics, adrenaline, oestrogens, lithium and asprin) **Decreased levels**: associated with Addison's disease, alcohol consumption, paracetamol and anabolic steroid use, extensive liver disease, hypopituitarism, hypothyroidism, insulinomas and starvation
Glucose tolerance test (GTT)	Fasting <5.5 mmol/L 2 hour <7.8 mmol/L	**Increased levels**: **Impaired glucose tolerance:** fasting <5.5 mmol/L; 2 h 7.8–11.0 mmol/L **Impaired fasting glycaemia**: fasting 5.5–6.9 mmol/L; 2 h <7.8 mmol/L **Diabetes mellitus:** fasting ≥7.0 mmol/L; 2 h ≥11.1 mmol/L
Glycated haemoglobin (HbA_{1c})	HbA_{1c}: 3.5–6.0% HbA_{1}: 4.5–7.0%	**Increased levels**: this is a reflection of the patient's average glucose concentration over the previous 3 months. If it is elevated >7%, this indicates suboptimal glucose control, and an increase in associated health risks **Decreased levels**: low levels can indicate the presence of a reticulocytosis
Diabetes-related auto-antibodies (ICA), (IAA), (GADA), (IA-2A)	Negative	**Positive:** if one or more antibodies are detected in a symptomatic diabetes type 1 patient, diagnosis is considered confirmed. A non-diabetic individual who is positive for antibodies has an increased risk of developing type 1 diabetes
Oestradiol [oestradiol-17 beta] (E2)	Female (serum) Early follicular phase: 100–200 pmol/L Preovulatory phase: 500–1700 pmol/L Luteal phase: 500–900 pmol/L Postmenopausal: 70–200 pmol/L	**Increased levels**: an endogenous or exogenous source of increased oestradiol **Decreased levels**: cycle time dependent. If lowered levels detected, failing ovulatory reserve can be considered and further investigations are warranted (anti-Müllerian hormone, FSH)

TABLE 21.2 Investigations—cont'd

Test category	Normal result	Clinical significance
Oestriol (E3)	Depends on gestational age and whether total (free and conjugated) or free oestriol is measured Normally tested in high-risk pregnancies from 26 weeks of gestation Unconjugated oestriol forms part of the antenatal 'triple test' for Down syndrome	**Decreased levels**: associated with placental insufficiency and/or fetal problems, anencephaly, congenital adrenal hyperplasia, adrenal hypoplasia and steroid therapy NOTE: impaired maternal liver function increases oestriol levels, making interpretation of results difficult
Progesterone	Method dependent, typically: Follicular phase: 2.0–4.5 nmol/L Luteal phase: 7.0–70.0 nmol/L	**Increased levels**: higher levels indicate pregnancy (with corresponding positive hCG test). Progesterone levels increase in multiple pregnancies (e.g. twins and triplets). In a non-pregnant state this can indicate luteal ovarian cysts, molar pregnancies or ovarian cancer **Decreased levels**: in luteal phase, this indicates an anovulatory cycle or corpus luteum inadequacy. In early pregnancy this can indicate an ectopic pregnancy. In late pregnancy this is associated with pre-eclampsia and toxaemia
Testosterone	See Table 21.3	**Increased levels**: in women this can be associated with hirsutism or virilisation **Decreased levels**: in males this is associated with testicular failure (either primary or secondary to hypopituitarism)
Androstenedione	Serum: Adult female: 3.5–9.0 nmol/L	**Increased levels**: can indicate polycystic ovary syndrome (PCOS), congenital adrenal hyperplasia or virilising tumours
Sex hormone-binding globulin (SHBG)	See Table 21.3	**Increased levels**: commonly seen in children of both sexes. After puberty levels should decrease. Increased levels may be seen in males with infertility. Increased levels are also associated with hyperthyroidism, liver disease, anorexia and oestrogen use (e.g. oral contraceptive pill). **Decreased levels**: associated with PCOS in females, hypothyroidism, obesity, androgen use and Cushing's disease
Free androgen index	Use individual pathology laboratory reference ranges	**Increased levels**: associated with PCOS and hirsutism in women **Decreased levels**: associated with testosterone deficiency in males, the following symptoms are common: erectile dysfunction, fatigue, weight gain and loss of secondary sex characteristics
Melatonin	Fluctuations occur during a 24 h cycle. The peak levels are seen between 2 and 4 am. These levels should drop between 6 and 8 am	**Increased levels**: associated with high levels of fatigue; higher levels have been found in patients with chronic fatigue syndrome (CFS) in the early part of the sleep cycle. It is normal for children and adolescents to have higher levels than adults **Decreased:** associated with autism spectrum disorder, insomnia, poor sleep quality, seasonal affective disorder (SAD) and mood disorders. It is normal for levels to decrease with age

Source: Reference ranges taken from the Royal College of Pathologists of Australasia Manual (v5). www.rcpamanual.edu.au

TABLE 21.3 Normal testosterone and SHBG values according to age and gender

	Male		Female	
	Prepubescent	Adult (age related)	Prepubescent	Adult (age related)
Free testosterone (pmol/L)		170–510		<4.0
Total testosterone (nmol/L)	<0.5	8–35	<0.5	<4.0
SHBG (nmol/L)	55–100	10–50	55–100	30–90 (250–500 in third trimester)
Dihydro-testosterone (nmol/L)		1–2.5		

SHBG, sex hormone-binding globulin.

Human chorionic gonadotrophin (hCG) test (urine pregnancy test)

This test is used to diagnose pregnancy, monitor 'high-risk' pregnancy, and as a tumour marker for certain tumours (Table 21.4). hCG hormone is normally secreted by the placental tissue after the ovum is fertilised (i.e. from the earliest stages of development). hCG will appear in the blood of pregnant women as early as 10 days after conception.

Urinary hormone assessment

An assessment of the urinary levels of oestrogen metabolites 2-hydroxyoestrone (2-OHE1) and 16α-hydroxyoestrone (16α-OHE1) provides information about the way in which oestrogen is being metabolised by the patient. A result showing a low ratio (a reduced 2-hydroxyoestrone) indicates that there is a state of oestrogen excess within the patient. Alternatively a high ratio (increased 2-hydroxyoestrone) indicates an oestrogen-deficient state. This test is suitable for males and females and is conducted using the first morning urine sample (the patient must fast from 10 pm the evening before). Females taking the test are advised to take it between days 18 and 25 of their menstrual cycle.

Urinary iodine

Excess iodine is excreted via the kidneys, thus providing an accurate measurement of recent iodine usage/requirement (Table 21.5). First morning urine samples provide the most accurate results; 24-hour urine samples are not required for this test. A study conducted in Indonesian children found urinary iodine excretion to be the best method for detecting iodine deficiency when compared with TSH, goitre palpation, ultrasonography, intellectual performance and anthropometric indices.[15]

TABLE 21.4 Clinical significance of hCG test

Test category	Normal result	Clinical significance
Positive	Pregnant state	Abnormal positive result can indicate: Ectopic pregnancy Hydatidiform mole of uterus Choriocarcinoma of the uterus Germ cell tumours of the testes or ovaries Other tumours
Negative	Non-pregnant state	Clinical significance of this result can include: Threatened abortion Incomplete abortion Fetal death

THERAPEUTIC APPLICATION

Nutritional medicine treatment of endocrine disorders is described in Table 21.6. Some useful herbal medicines are listed in Table 21.7

TABLE 21.5 Urinary iodine results

Median value (micrograms/L)	Severity of deficiency
<20	Severe deficiency
20–49	Moderate deficiency
50–99	Mild deficiency
>100	No deficiency

TABLE 21.6 Nutritional medicine

Requirement	Justification	RDI	Therapeutic dose	Food sources
A high-strength, sustained release multivitamin/mineral preparation	The excess production of thyroid hormones that occurs in hyperthyroidism leads to a higher metabolic rate and subsequently nutrients are depleted at a higher rate. Additionally, in hyperthyroidism there is malabsorption. Due to these factors a greater number of nutrients are required by the body. Similarly where there is adrenal exhaustion the body has higher requirements to meet increased demands	–	–	N/A
Vitamin B complex	The B vitamins provide energy and support during physically demanding periods. They are involved in maintaining the health of the hormone-producing glands	Comprehensive complex containing individual B vitamins as per below	–	Legumes, wholegrains, nuts, beans, brewer's yeast, leafy green vegetables

TABLE 21.6 Nutritional medicine—cont'd

Requirement	Justification	RDI	Therapeutic dose	Food sources
Thiamin (vitamin B_1)	Vitamin B_1 is involved with other B vitamins in energy metabolism and the normal functioning of nerves. Vitamin B_1 may be needed during periods of increased physical and mental stress and has been clinically proven to protect the adrenal gland from functional exhaustion	Men: 19–30 years 1.2 mg/day 31–50 years 1.2 mg/day 51–70 years 1.2 mg/day >70 years 1.0–1.2 mg/day Women: 19–30 years 1.1 mg/day 31–50 years 1.1 mg/day 51–70 years 1.1 mg/day >70 years 1.1 mg/d	5–100 mg/day	Legumes, liver, nuts, wholegrains, wheatgerm
Riboflavin (vitamin B_2)	Vitamin B_2 is crucial in the production of energy and may be needed in periods of heightened stress. Along with vitamins B_5, B_{12}, folic acid, potassium and sodium it stabilises the activity of the adrenal glands	Men: 19–30 years 1.3 mg/day 31–50 years 1.3 mg/day 51–70 years 1.3 mg/day >70 years 1.6 mg/day Women: 19–30 years 1.1 mg/day 31–50 years 1.1 mg/day 51–70 years 1.1 mg/day >70 years 1.3 mg/day	10–100 mg/day	Avocados, beans, currants, eggs, milk and dairy products, sprouts, wholegrains
Niacin (vitamin B_3)	Niacinamide is converted into the active forms of niacin in the body. Niacin is required for the function of more than 200 enzymes throughout the body and is a component of the glucose tolerance factor, which helps to control blood glucose, delaying or preventing the need for insulin by interfering with immune-mediated beta cell destruction. Vitamin B_3 has also been found to help slow down the development of nephropathy in diabetes	(As niacin equivalents) Men: 19–30 years 16 mg/day 31–50 years 16 mg/day 51–70 years 16 mg/day >70 years 16 mg/day Women: 19–30 years 14 mg/day 31–50 years 14 mg/day 51–70 years 14 mg/day >70 years 14 mg/day	10–1000 mg/day	Almonds, eggs, chicken, mackerel, meat, peanuts, salmon, sardines, sunflower seeds
Pantothenic acid (vitamin B_5)	Vitamin B_5 enhances adrenal cortex function. Deficiency leads to a compromised adrenal cortex function. Vitamin B_5 down-regulates hypersecretion of cortisol secondary to high-stress situations	Men: 19–30 years 6 mg/day 31–50 years 6 mg/day 51–70 years 6 mg/day >70 years 6 mg/day Women: 19–30 years 4 mg/day 31–50 years 4 mg/day 51–70 years 4 mg/day >70 years 4 mg/day	20–500 mg/day	Avocados, beans, egg yolks, green vegetables, milk, mushrooms, oranges, royal jelly, sweet potato, wholegrain cereals
Pyridoxine (vitamin B_6)	Along with the other B vitamins, vitamin B_6 is important during periods of stress, providing support to the nervous system and adrenal glands. Vitamin B_6 deficiency has been shown to cause symptoms of hypoglycaemia, increased insulin sensitivity and degeneration of beta cells	Men: 19–50 years 1.3 mg/day 51–70 years 1.7 mg/day Women: 19–50 years 1.3 mg/day 51–70 years 1.5 mg/day	10–150 mg/day	Brewer's yeast, chicken, egg yolk, legumes, mackerel, oatmeal, salmon, tuna, walnuts
Folate (vitamin B_9)	Along with vitamins B_2, B_5, B_{12}, potassium and sodium, vitamin B_9 stabilises the activity of the adrenal glands	Men: 19–70 years 400 micrograms/day Women: 19–70 years 400 micrograms/day	500–1000 micrograms/day	Beans, eggs, green leafy vegetables, lentils, yeast

Continued

TABLE 21.6 Nutritional medicine—cont'd				
Requirement	**Justification**	**RDI**	**Therapeutic dose**	**Food sources**
Cyanocobalamin (vitamin B_{12})	Along with vitamins B_2, B_5, folic acid, potassium and sodium, vitamin B_{12} stabilises the activity of the adrenal glands	Men: 19–70 years 2.4 micrograms/day Women: 19–70 years 2.4 micrograms/day	300–2000 micrograms/day	Clams, egg yolk, herring, milk, meat, oysters, salmon, sardines
Biotin	Supplementation with biotin has been found to help maintain healthy blood sugar levels in individuals with diabetes as the generation of glucose is dependent on a biotin-containing enzyme	Men: 19–70 years: 30 micrograms/day Women: 19–70 years: 25 micrograms/day	500–1500 micrograms/day	Bean sprouts, egg yolk, milk, peanuts, soy beans, wholegrain cereals
Vitamin C	Vitamin C is a water-soluble antioxidant that protects against oxidative stress associated with thyroid diseases. The adrenal gland is among the organs with the highest concentration of vitamin C in the body. Interestingly, both the adrenal cortex and the medulla accumulate such high levels of ascorbate. Vitamin C is a co-factor required both in catecholamine biosynthesis and adrenal steroidogenesis. Production of adrenaline (epinephrine) and noradrenaline (norepinephrine) are dependent on vitamin C Vitamin C can also help to regulate blood glucose	Men: 19–70 years 45 mg/day Women: 19–70 years 45 mg/day	250–5000 mg/day in divided doses	Blackcurrant, broccoli, citrus fruits, kiwi fruit, strawberries, rosehips, guava, mangoes, pineapple
Vitamin D	Glucose intolerance and insulin secretion have been observed during vitamin D deficiency, resulting in type 2 diabetes. It is theorised that this is due to vitamin D receptors in several tissues and cells, including the pancreatic beta-cells	Men: 19–50 years 5.0 micrograms/day 51–70 years 10.0 micrograms/day >70 years 15.0 micrograms/day Women: 19–50 years 5.0 micrograms/day 51–70 years 10.0 micrograms/day >70 years 15.0 micrograms/day	1000–2000 IU/day	Fish liver oils–cod, halibut, herring, tuna, egg yolk, milk, sprouted seeds
Vitamin E	Hypothyroidism is accompanied with increased oxidative stress and fat-soluble antioxidant vitamin E supplementation exerts beneficial effects on this situation. Vitamin E can enhance insulin sensitivity thus reducing the need for insulin and other hypoglycaemics	There is no Australian RDI but the AI for men of all ages is 10 mg/day and for women it is 7 mg/day	100–800 IU/day	Almonds, beef, corn, egg yolks, nuts, safflower, sunflower, wheatgerm

TABLE 21.6 Nutritional medicine—cont'd

Requirement	Justification	RDI	Therapeutic dose	Food sources
L-tyrosine	L-tyrosine is an essential precursor for the synthesis of the catecholamines adrenaline (epinephrine), noradrenaline (norepinephrine), and dopamine and the thyroid hormone thyroxine. Supplementation with tyrosine aids adrenal function helping during periods of prolonged stress, to support the body and improve stress adaptation	500–1000 mg/day	1120 mg/day	Almonds, beef, cheese, chicken, eggs, fish, soy beans, wild game
Zinc	Zinc is required for healthy thyroid function and the synthesis and metabolism of thyroid hormones. Deficiency of zinc-dependent enzymes may result in decreased thyroid hormone levels and resting metabolic rate (RMR). Changes in zinc metabolism are commonly observed in diabetic patients	Men of all ages: 12 mg/day Women: 6.5 mg/day	10–75 mg/day	Beef, baked beans, cashews, egg yolks, ginger, herrings, liver, milk, lamb, oysters, sunflower and pumpkin seeds, wholegrains
Selenium	Selenium is essential for the biosynthesis and function of the iodothyronine deiodinase enzymes that are essential for the conversion of T_4 to T_3. Selenium-dependent glutathione peroxidases protect against oxidative damage to the thyroid gland. Deficiency leads to decreased conversion of T_4 to T_3, and oxidative stress on the thyroid gland as a result of reduced glutathione peroxidise activity. The thyroid gland contains more selenium per gram than any other tissue in the body. Selenium is also important for healthy blood sugar regulation. Deficiency may reduce insulin secretion	Men: 19–70 years 70 micrograms/day Women: 19–70 years 60 micrograms/day	200–400 micrograms/day	Alfalfa, brazil nuts, cashews, crab, eggs, fish, garlic, kidney, liver, mackerel, oysters, peanuts, tuna, wholegrain cereals, broccoli, onions
Magnesium	Magnesium assists in the maintenance of normal healthy blood glucose metabolism. Hypomagnesaemia is frequently present in diabetic patients hence magnesium is often suggested in patients with diabetes mellitus who have proven hypomagnesaemia and the presence of its complications	Men: 19–30 years 400 mg/day 31–70 years 420 mg/day Women: 19–30 years 310 mg/day 31–70 years 320 mg/day	300–750 mg/day	Eggs, cocoa, almonds, brewer's yeast, cashews, kelp, wheatbran, wheatgerm, buckwheat
Manganese	Manganese plays a crucial role as part of its role in the glucose tolerance factor and is required for metabolism of carbohydrates as the synthesis of new glucose from puyruvate is necessary on manganese-containing enzymes as well as for normal insulin secretion. Deficiency may contribute to blood sugar abnormalities and reduced pancreatic cell function Manganese is required for thyroid hormone function	Men: 19–70 years 5.5 mg/day Women: 19–70 years 5 mg/day	2–11 mg/day	Almonds, beans, coconuts, corn, kelp, sunflower seeds, legumes, walnuts, wholegrains

Continued

TABLE 21.6 Nutritional medicine—cont'd				
Requirement	**Justification**	**RDI**	**Therapeutic dose**	**Food sources**
R-alpha lipoic acid	R-alpha lipoic acid, also known as thioctic acid, is an antioxidant and decreases the risk of cell damage attributed to free radicals. R-alpha lipoic acid is unique in that it is soluble in water as well as fat and is therefore able to scavenge both fat- and water soluble free radicals. It also has the ability to recycle or regenerate endogenous antioxidants including vitamins C and E, CoQ10 and glutathione. R-alpha lipoic acid plays a role in glucose metabolism and is involved in the transport of blood glucose into cells. It may therefore help maintain healthy blood sugar levels and has been used in diabetics to assist with the conversion of sugar to energy and is thought to be beneficial in reducing the effects of oxidative stress which are associated with this condition, as well as decreasing symptoms associated with diabetes such as diabetic polyneuropathy	50–600 mg/day	600 mg/day	Typical dietary sources of lipoic acid are muscle meats, heart, kidney, and liver, and to a lesser degree, fruits and vegetables; potatoes
Chromium	Chromium is an essential micronutrient for humans. It plays a role as a co-factor in all insulin-regulated activities including carbohydrate, lipid and protein metabolism and is an essential component of glucose tolerance factor, a compound that helps to regulate blood sugar. Chromium is particularly important for normal carbohydrate metabolism and assists in maintaining healthy blood glucose levels, by aiding the transport of glucose from the blood into the cells Chromium may be used where diets are high in simple sugars and refined carbohydrates, which may have increased chromium requirements	There is no Australian RDI but the AI for men of all ages is 35 micrograms/day and for women it is 25 micrograms/day	100–400 micrograms/day	Asparagus, beer, cheese, egg yolk, molasses, nuts, oysters, peanuts, prunes, raisins
Iodine	Iodine is an essential component of the thyroid hormones thyroxine (T_4) and triiodothyronine (T_3), and deficiency impairs synthesis of these hormones. Approximately 60 micrograms of iodine is absorbed each day by the thyroid gland; however, it is estimated that 150 micrograms is required each day for optimum functioning of the thyroid gland	Men: 19–70 years 150 micrograms/day Women: 19–70 years 150 micrograms/day	100–400 micrograms/day Ensure closely monitored	Seaweed (e.g. wakame), cod, iodised salt, lima beans, mushrooms, oysters

Sources: Anderson RA, Cheng N, Bryden NA et al. Elevated intakes of supplemental chromium improve glucose and insulin variables in individuals with type 2 diabetes. Diabetes 1997; 46(11):1786–1791. Borcea V, Nourooz-Zadeh J, Wolff SP et al. Alpha-lipoic acid decreases oxidative stress even in diabetic patients with poor glycemic control and albuminuria. Free Radic Biol Med 2005; 26(11–12):1495–1500. Institute of Medicine (IOM), Academy of Sciences, USA, Dietary reference intakes for vitamin A, vitamin K, arsenic, boron, chromium, copper, iodine, iron, manganese, molybdenum, nickel, silicon, vanadium and zinc. National Academy Press, Washington, DC. As cited in Zimmermann, MD. Iodine: it's important in patients that require parenteral nutrition. Gastroenterology 2001; 137(5):536–546. Jacob S, Ruus P, Hermann R et al. Oral administration of RA-α-lipoic acid modulates insulin sensitivity in patients with type-2 diabetes mellitus: a placebo controlled pilot trial. Free Radic Biol Med 1999; 27(3–4):309–314. National Health and Medical Research Council. Nutrient reference values for Australia and New Zealand. www.nrv.gov.au/nutrients/index.htm. Osiecki H. The nutrient bible. Eagle Farm, Queensland: Bioconcepts; 2003. Reavley N. The encyclopaedia of vitamins, minerals, supplements and herbs. Bookman Press, Victoria; 1998. Rheault S, Olmstead M, Ralston J et al. Iodine and iodide: functions and benefits beyond the thyroid. Townsend Letter for Doctors and Patients 2008 Dec; 99–101. Ziegler D, Nowak H, Kempler P et al. Effects of treatment with the antioxidant alpha-lipoic acid improves symptomatic diabetic polyneuropathy: the SYDNEY 2 trial. Diabetes Care 2006; 29:2365–2370. Zimmermann MD. Burgerstein's handbook of nutrition, micronutrients in the prevention and therapy of disease. New York: Thieme; 2001.

TABLE 21.7 Herbal medicine

Class	Example	Justification
Adaptogen	*Eleuthrococcus senticosus* (Siberian ginseng)	Adaptogens improve nonspecific responses to stress by increasing the resistance of the recipient to a variety of physical, chemical, or biological stressors while also promoting recovery and acting as a general regulator in the body. Siberian ginseng has traditionally been used as a prophylactic to build resistance, reduce susceptibility to illness, and promote health and longevity. Its activity appears to be based on whole body effects rather than particular organs or systems, which lends support to the traditional view that ginseng is a tonic that can revitalise the functioning of the organism as a whole. Siberian ginseng increases levels of noradrenaline (norepinephrine), serotonin, adrenaline (epinephrine) and cortisol (improving positive and negative responses to stress)
Adrenal restorative	*Rehmannia glutinosa* (rehmannia)	Rehmannia is an adrenal tonic that has been used in Traditional Chinese Medicine to nourish qi (vital energy). Rehmannia works by supporting the adrenal cortex and pituitary gland during prolonged stress and regulates cortisol levels. In trials done on rabbits, rehmannia reversed morphological changes to the pituitary and adrenal cortex, antagonising the suppressive effect of glucocorticoids on the hypothalamus–pituitary–adrenal axis
Tonic	*Withania glutinosa* (ashwagandha)	*Withania glutinosa* is a gentle tonic that is considered to be the pre-eminent adaptogen from the Ayurvedic medical system. *Withania* improves responses to stress, possibly via an action on the adrenal glands, and also has anti-inflammatory and sedative effects. It is used to treat nervous exhaustion, convalescence and debility associated with chronic inflammatory conditions
Aldose reductase inhibitor	*Glycyrrhiza glabra* (liquorice)	Aldose reductase is an enzyme in carbohydrate metabolism that converts glucose to sorbitol. Its activity increases as the glucose concentration rises in diabetes, particularly in the lens of the eyes, the peripheral nerves and glomerulus, leading to retinopathy and neuropathy. Liquorice in its role as an aldose reductase inhibitor helps to prevent eye and nerve damage in people with diabetes
Antiobesity	*Coleus forskohlii* (coleus)	The exact mechanism of *Coleus forskohlii* in weight loss is unknown; however, based on in-vitro data it is hypothesised that *Coleus forskohlii* may cause an increase in cyclic adenosine phosphate (cAMP) which in turn leads to an activation of protein kinase which activates lipase (an enzyme involved in the breakdown of triglycerides, fatty substances in the blood and components of LDL cholesterol). This results in thermogenesis, loss of body fat and the maintenance of lean body mass. *Coleus forskohlii* may have a thyroid stimulating action, thus possibly increasing metabolic rate and thermogenesis and may regulate insulin secretion thus positively affecting fat and protein metabolism
Appetite inhibiting	*Gymnema sylvestre* (gymnema)	Gymnema is an Ayurvedic herb with the ability to inhibit the taste of sweetness, hence its nickname 'sugar destroyer'. Gymnema reduces desire for food, particularly foods that are sweet in taste, leading to its action as an appetite inhibitor. This action also means it is a useful addition to any weight-loss program
Hypoglycaemic	*Galega officinalis* (goat's rue)	Galegine in goat's rue has been associated with marked reductions in blood sugar levels. Studies in the 1970s demonstrated that the alkaloid galegine within goat's rue is responsible for reducing blood sugar levels. The British Herbal Pharmacopeia confirms the action of *Galega* as a hypoglycaemic agent with anti-diabetic activity and indicates its use for diabetes
Hepatic, hepatoprotective, hepatotrophorestorative	*Bupleurum falcatum* (bupleurum)	The liver plays an important role in the effective metabolism of the thyroid hormones as well as the regulation of their systemic endocrine effects. Suboptimal liver function can affect thyroid hormone metabolism hence the application of hepatics in the management of thyroid conditions. *Bupleurum falcatum* is a Traditional Chinese Medicine which displays hepatoprotective activity. It is highly indicated where there is poor liver function

Continued

TABLE 21.7 Herbal medicine—cont'd		
Class	**Example**	**Justification**
Pancreatic trophorestorative (endocrine functions)	*Gymnema sylvestre* (gymnema)	The exact mode of action by which gymnema exerts its pancreatic trophorestorative action is unknown. It appears that gymnema helps to support healthy pancreatic function via a wide array of actions rather than just one; these include the inhibition of intestinal absorption of glucose and promotion of glucose homeostasis, and also increasing the number of cells in the pancreas responsible for insulin production
Thyroid stimulant	*Fucus vesiculosus* (bladderwrack)	*Fucus vesiculosus* is a valuable source of iodine, a trace element necessary for regulating the body's metabolism and normal production of thyroid hormones. Organic iodine, such as that found in bladderwrack, is likely to be better utilised by the body in terms of bioavailability and less likely to be excreted than potassium iodide
Thyroid suppressant/ regulator	*Lycopus* spp. (bugleweed)	*Lycopus* is a perennial herb containing phenolic acids. In the 19th century *Lycopus* was given to calm the nerves. Today *Lycopus* is primarily used to help manage hyperthyroid conditions as well as the associated cardiac symptoms. High doses of *Lycopus* cause a reduction of thyroid stimulating hormone in animal experiments; conversely in hyperthyroid patients treated with low doses of *Lycopus* improvement of cardiac symptoms was reported

Sources: British Herbal Medicine Association's Scientific Committee. British Herbal Pharmacopoeia. Bournemouth: BHMA; 1983. Chevallier A. Encyclopedia of medicinal plants. New York: DK Publishing; 1996. Kirschmann G, Kirschmann. Nutrition almanac. 4th edn. New York: McGraw-Hill; 1996. Morgan M. *Coleus forskohlii* root: the benefits of forskolin. A Phytotherapists Perspective 2006; 9:92. Vonhoff C, Baumgartner A, Hegger M et al. Extract of *Lycopus europaeus* L. reduces cardiac signs of hyperthyroidism in rats. Life Sciences 2006; 78(10):1063–1070. Zha LL. Experimental effect of *Rehmannia glutinosa* on the pituitary and adrenal cortex in a glucocorticoid inhibition model using rabbits. Zhong Xi Yi Jie He Za Zhi 1998; 8(2):70;95–97.

SECTION B: THYROID DISORDERS

Fig. 21.4 illustrates the thyroid gland.

HYPOTHYROIDISM

Epidemiology

Hypothyroidism is the most common pathological hormone deficiency.[16] Hypothyroidism and subclinical hypothyroidism are considered more common than their counterpart, hyperthyroidism.[17,18] According to a 1995 report from the Australian Bureau of Statistics (ABS), 5.3/1000 males and 27.3/1000 females experience thyroid dysfunction in Australia.[19] This figure is higher in the elderly, postmenopausal women and various groups presenting with psychological dysfunction.[17,20,21]

In the United States hypothyroidism is the second most common endocrine disorder and it has been estimated that 18/1000 people display decreased thyroid hormone levels.[17] It is present in 4.6% of the population (clinical, 0.3%; and subclinical, 4.3%).[22,23] In the UK, 15 in 1000 women and 1 in 1000 men are affected annually.[24]

It is important to note that most estimates on the rate of hypothyroidism are based on the levels of thyroid hormones in the blood. This may result in a large number of people with mild hypothyroidism going undetected. Thyroid hormones fluctuate consistently throughout the day and false negatives can occur for subclinical hypothyroid patients.

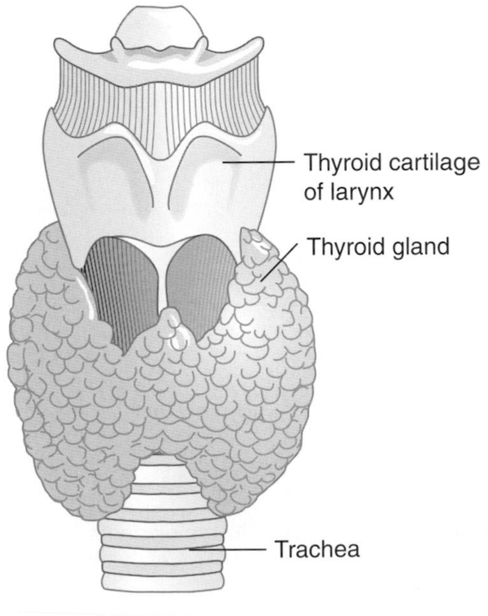

FIGURE 21.4 Thyroid gland.

The rate of hypothyroidism increases steadily with advancing age.[25] When considering multiple factors such as medical history, physical examination, and basal body temperatures along with the blood thyroid levels as the diagnostic criteria, the rate of hypothyroidism in the general adult population has been considered as high as 25% and is significantly higher in the elderly.[26]

TABLE 21.8 Definitions of hypothyroidism

	Thyroid-stimulating hormone	Thyroxine	Symptoms
Subclinical hypothyroidism	Raised	Normal	Usually absent; some authorities require the absence of symptoms as a criterion and use the term mild hypothyroidism for subclinical hypothyroidism plus symptoms
Grade 1	Above upper limit of reference range (10 mIU/L)	Normal	Symptoms are increasingly likely with higher thyroid stimulating hormone concentrations
Grade 2	10.1–20 mIU/L	Normal	
Grade 3	>20 mIU/L	Normal	
Clinical or overt hypothyroidism	Raised	Low	Usually present; symptoms are not considered a criterion by some authorities

A systematic international review indicated that the reported incidence of autoimmune hypothyroidism varied between 2.2/100 000/year (males) and 498.4/100 000/year (females). Higher incidence rates were found in women compared with men for all types of autoimmune thyroid disease.[25,27]

Classification

The subclassification of hypothyroidism reflects TSH readings primarily and considers additional thyroid hormone status (Table 21.8). The pituitary gland regulates thyroid activity through the secretion of thyroid-stimulating hormone (TSH).

PRIMARY HYPOTHYROIDISM

Primary hypothyroidism is characterised by the combination of low thyroid hormone and elevated TSH blood levels. This typically indicates defective thyroid hormone synthesis.

SECONDARY HYPOTHYROIDISM

Secondary hypothyroidism is characterised by low TSH and low thyroid hormone levels which indicates an issue with the pituitary gland.

CELLULAR HYPOTHYROIDISM

Cellular hypothyroidism is characterised by normal blood thyroid hormone and TSH blood levels combined with low functional thyroid activity (as defined by a low basal metabolic rate).

Aetiology

Primary hypothyroidism is caused by two variations:

1. Dysgenesis — abnormal formation of the thyroid gland
2. Dyshormogenesis — abnormal formation of thyroid hormone.

See Table 21.9 for further information on the aetiology of hypothyroidism.

TABLE 21.9 Aetiology of hypothyroidism

Autoimmune	Hashimoto's thyroiditis, Reidel's disease, previous Graves' disease, de Quervain's thyroiditis, postpartum thyroiditis, Down syndrome, family history of autoimmune disease or associated disorders (vitiligo, adrenal insufficiency, diabetes mellitus type 1, Sjögren's, coeliac disease), Turner's syndrome, multiple sclerosis, primary pulmonary hypertension
Nutritional	Iodine deficiency, excess intake of goitrogens, excessive iodine intake
Environmental	Radiation exposure, exposure to polybrominated and polychlorinated biphenyls and resorcinol
Iatrogenic	Radioactive iodine therapy, medical radiation exposure, total or subtotal thyroidectomy, drugs impairing thyroid function (amiodarone, thalidomide, betaroxine, lithium carbonate, stavudine, aminoglutethimide)
Hypothalamic	Hypothalamic or suprasellar mass, history of hypothalamic radiotherapy or surgery, disorders causing hypothalamic dysfunction (e.g. sarcoidosis, haemochromatosis)
Pituitary	Known pituitary tumour, other elements of hypopituitarism, manifestations of sellar mass, history of pituitary surgery or radiotherapy, history of head trauma
Other	Postpartum status

Source: Brown BT, Bonello R, Pollard H. The biopsychosocial model and hypothyroidism. Chiropractic and Osteopathic 2005; 13:5. © Brown et al; licensee BioMed Central Ltd, 2005.

FLUORIDE

A cross-sectional observational study in the UK concluded that regions with fluoridated drinking water were more likely to have a high prevalence of known hypothyroidism. The mechanism of action is unknown. It is unknown whether lower iodine and selenium levels play a role in increased incidence of hypothyroidism in these populations.[28]

Overview

A deficiency of thyroid hormones can affect virtually all bodily functions as thyroid gland hormones regulate metabolism in every cell of the body. The degree of severity of symptoms ranges from subclinical hypothyroidism to severe deficiency states which can be life threatening (myxoedema).

Pathogenesis

COMMON CAUSES OF DEFICIENCY OF T_3

- Lack of stimulation by the pituitary gland
- Defective hormone synthesis
- Impaired cellular conversion of T_4 to T_3.

SIGNS AND SYMPTOMS (Table 21.10)

Endocrine

Due to the dynamic interrelationship of all glands within the endocrine system, concurrent abnormalities in other glands are common both in initial stages and as the disease develops.

Loss of libido in both males and females is especially common. Women also frequently experience menstrual irregularities, as the impact of hypothyroidism on the menstrual cycle has been known since 1950.[29] It is important to note that the menstrual abnormality may precede clinical symptoms and signs of hypothyroidism. Symptoms include:

- Amenorrhoea or prolonged and heavy menstrual bleeding with a shorter cycle
- Menorrhagia (+/– menometrorrhagia) and associated Fe deficiency
- Shorter menstrual cycle
- Polycystic ovary syndrome (PCOS) tendencies.

Thyroid dysfunction adversely affects fertility. Many studies imply a role for immunology, including thyroid autoimmunity, in conception failure. Infertility can also be a problem for women. Lack of conception is common; however, if the woman does conceive, miscarriages, premature deliveries and stillbirths are common. It is unlikely for a woman to follow through to a successful pregnancy and labour/delivery if she is overtly hypothyroid (and untreated).

In women of fertile age, autoimmune thyroid disease (AITD) is undoubtedly the most common cause of hypothyroidism and in most patients thyroid peroxidase antibodies are found.[23,30] Other, though rarer, causes of hypothyroidism include post-iodine prescription, post-thyroiditis and drug-induced hypothyroidism. Hypothyroidism is associated with a broad spectrum of reproductive disorders ranging from abnormal sexual development to menstrual irregularities and infertility.

A number of hypotheses for these occurrences include the following:

- Subclinical hypothyroidism can be seen to alter the dynamics of prolactin release, with unknown consequences for gonadal function and fertility.[31]
- Hyperprolactinaemia resulting from increased production of TRH has been implicated in ovulatory dysfunction and in 1–3% of cases, with galactorrhoea.[32]
- Diminished synthesis and secretion of dopamine in the hypothalamus could account for loss of dopaminergic inhibitory influences on prolactin, TSH and luteinising hormone (LH).[33]
- Hypothyroidism interferes with normal physiological pulsatile gonadotrophin-releasing hormone (GnRH) secretion, a prerequisite for normal follicular development and ovulation. A delay in LH response may lead to inadequate corpus luteum progesterone

TABLE 21.10 Signs and symptoms of hypothyroidism

System	Symptoms
Central nervous system	Depression, fatigue (despite adequate sleep), lethargy, forgetfulness, decreased concentration, memory deficit, slow thinking, cold intolerance, nerve entrapment syndromes, decreased sweating, ataxia, headaches
Musculoskeletal	Muscular weakness, cramps, myalgia, arthralgia, and delayed relaxation phase of reflexes
Cardiovascular	Bradycardia, diastolic hypertension, hyperlipidaemia +/– hypercholesterolaemia (raised LDL), ascites, hyperhomocysteinaemia, poor circulation (cold extremities)
Haematological	Iron deficiency anaemia
Respiratory	Shortness of breath
Gastrointestinal	Anorexia or reduced appetite; constipation and sluggish bowel transit time – associated digestive symptoms are common including flatulence, bloating
Ear, nose and throat	Puffy eyes, enlarged tongue, hearing impairment, goitre, hoarseness of voice, dysphagia, sore throat
Immune	Lowered or poor immune response; recurrent infections
Genitourinary	Impaired kidney function
Female reproductive	Low libido, infertility, menstrual irregularities, menorrhagia, galactorrhoea, hyperprolactinaemia, fibrocystic breast disease (if related to iodine deficiency)
Male reproductive	Low libido, infertility, impotence, hyperprolactinaemia
Integumentary	Dry skin and mucous membranes (mouth, vagina, anus), skin can be covered with superficial scales; coarse skin, brittle and coarse hair, hair loss, thin and brittle nails (can present with transverse grooves)
Radiological	Pericardial and pleural effusions, pituitary gland enlargement
General	Weight gain or difficulty in losing weight, oedema causing facial features to swell and look puffy

secretion. Disturbances in normal pulsatile release of LH and hyperprolactinaemia can result in menstrual dysfunction, ranging from anovulatory cycles with menorrhagia, oligomenorrhoea or amenorrhoea.

Thyroid hormone receptors are expressed in human oocytes, cumulus cells and granulosa cells.[34]

Testing for thyroid disease is warranted in all women and men with unexplained infertility.[35]

Neuropsychiatric

Initial symptoms of thyroid dysfunction include lowered mood (progressing towards depression), fatigue, poor concentration and poor memory. It is prudent to consider the neuropsychiatric effects of lowered thyroid hormones.

Subclinical hypothyroidism is common in those suffering from affective disorders. Unfortunately more research is required to accurately assess this link as such observations have been uncontrolled or the effects of thyroxine replacement have not been assessed.[36,37]

Postpartum symptoms of depression are more common in women who have thyroid antibodies than in those without, irrespective of biochemical thyroid dysfunction.[38] Also, in patients with rapid cycles of a bipolar affective disorder the most significantly associated thyroid disorder was thyroid antibody positivity and not raised thyroid-stimulating hormone concentration.[39] Autoimmune considerations and referral for thyroid antibody status are essential as some mood disturbances in subclinical hypothyroidism appear to have an immunological rather than an endocrinological basis.

Musculoskeletal

Generalised muscle weakness and joint stiffness is a common observable symptom for hypothyroid patients. Asymptomatic polyneuropathy can be identified in subclinical hypothyroidism.[40] Slow reflexes (diagnostic is Achilles reflex time).

Cardiovascular

Both overt and subclinical hypothyroidism are associated with an increase in cholesterol and triglyceride levels, homocysteine and C-reactive protein. They are believed to predispose the person to atherosclerosis. One study found an association of subclinical hypothyroidism not only with raised low-density lipoprotein cholesterol and low high-density lipoprotein cholesterol concentrations but also with raised lipoprotein(a).[41] The effects of thyroxine replacement on cholesterol lowering alone are modest. A re-analysis of intervention studies between 1976 and 1995 led to the following conclusions:[42]

- Subclinical hypothyroidism is two to three times more common than expected in people with increased total plasma cholesterol concentrations
- Total cholesterol is only slightly raised (0–30% above normal) in subclinical hypothyroidism.

Hypothyroidism can also cause hypertension, reduce the function of the heart, and reduce heart rate. Minor alterations in heart muscle contractility, determined by systolic time intervals, occur in around half of patients, although not all studies agree.[43] Only a subgroup with the most serious abnormalities improves with thyroxine replacement suggesting other factors require treatment consideration.[44]

CAUSES OF HYPOTHYROIDISM

Primary hypothyroidism

A major cause of primary hypothyroidism is iodine deficiency. As iodine status among Australians reduces, incidences of primary hypothyroidism are expected to increase. The only function of iodine in the body is as part of the structure of thyroid hormones. The average healthy human adult contains 20–50 mg of iodine. Between 70% and 80% of this is converted in the thyroid gland with almost all in the form of thyroglobulin (storage form of thyroid hormone). The remainder is found in the ovaries, anterior pituitary, eye, bile, salivary glands, and distributed throughout the rest of the body. Only 1 mg is found in blood (as thyroid hormones).

Iodine is an essential component of the thyroid hormones T_3 and T_4 and is required for human growth and development throughout the body. The thyroid gland adds iodine to the amino acid tyrosine to create the thyroid hormones. The thyroid concentrates iodine in a process known as iodination in order not only to form the thyroid hormones but also to produce enough of its daily iodine requirements. The concentration of iodine in the thyroid is carefully regulated but is usually in the range 8–10 mg.[45]

Goitre development

Iodine deficiency leads to hypothyroidism or the development of an enlarged thyroid gland (i.e. a goitre), or both. Goitres are estimated to affect more than 200 million people worldwide — most being related to an iodine deficiency. Deficiency may be caused by low amounts of iodine in soil and there are large areas of soil around the world which are low in iodine (known as the 'goitre belts') — middle USA, the Midlands and south-west England, Tasmania, areas of China, South America, New Guinea, Africa, New Zealand, Russia. Deficiency is induced by an intake of less than 50 micrograms/day.

GOITROGENIC FOODS

Some foods contain goitrogenic substances that prevent the utilisation of iodine. These compounds are primarily isothiocyanates that are similar in action and structure to propylthiouracil (thionamide drug taken in hyperthyroidism). They are found in a number of foods including those from the *Brassica* family (broccoli, Brussels sprouts, kale, cauliflower, turnips, cabbage, rutabagas, mustard greens, radishes, horseradishes), cassava root, soybeans, peanuts, pine nuts, and millet.

In order to achieve clinical results (i.e. in hyperthyroid patients), large amounts of these foods must be consumed in their raw state, and iodine intake must be restricted. The highest levels of isothiocyanates are found in raw soymilk (0.46 to 2.5 mg/dL). In the *Brassica* family swedes, cabbage, and turnips usually contain the highest levels. However, the quantity varies considerably according to climatic and soil factors. Cooking typically deactivates

Iodine in Australia

Iodine deficiency is not a new phenomenon in Australia or New Zealand. Efforts to address iodine deficiency in both countries were implemented during the early and mid-1900s.[46] During the latter part of the 20th century, additional, though unplanned, protection from iodine deficiency was provided from residues in milk resulting from the widespread use of iodine-containing sanitising agents in the dairy industry in Australia and New Zealand.

Iodine was believed to not be deficient in Australians as recently as 1998.[47] Between 1999 and 2001, various research papers documented a re-emergence of the condition[48] and current statistics suggest that iodine deficiency affects a number of Australians. In 2011–12 the Australian Health Survey was conducted across the country (Table 21.11).[49,50] Urinary iodine concentration was determined from 31 837 people (30 329 aged 5 years and over; 27 636 aged 12 years and over). In all states across Australia the median urinary iodine concentration (MUIC) levels fell within the optimal range of 100–199 micrograms/L; Tasmania had the lowest status of 108 micrograms/L and Western Australia had the highest at 157.4 micrograms/L. Iodine status is considered optimal if population MUIC falls between 100 and 200 micrograms/L and is not considered excessive until MUIC exceeds 300 micrograms/L. Mild iodine deficiency is defined as MUIC between 50 and 100 micrograms/L.[51]

The recommended daily intake (RDI) of iodine is 150 micrograms daily for the general population and 150–200 micrograms daily for women who are pregnant or breastfeeding[52–55] (iodine demand increases during pregnancy because of increased renal clearance and fetal iodine transfer).

TABLE 21.11 Iodine status in Australia from the Australian Health Survey 2011–12

State/ territory	MUIC (micrograms/L)	Population iodine status
New South Wales	120.0	optimal
Victoria	112.5	optimal
South Australia	136.0	optimal
Western Australia	157.4	optimal
Queensland	132.0	optimal
Australian Capital Territory	113.0	optimal
Northern Territory	144.0	optimal
Tasmania	108.0	borderline optimal
Total: Australia	124.0	optimal

MUIC, median urinary iodine concentration. Mild deficiency = MUIC 50–100 micrograms/L; optimal = MUIC 100–200 micrograms/L
Source: Australian Population Health Development Principal Committee (APHDPC). The prevalence and severity of iodine deficiency in Australia — Report, 2007. Department of Health and Human Services, Tasmania with input from NSW Health, Ministry of Health NZ, Vic Health, Queensland Health and the Department of Health and Ageing.

(breaks down) dietary goitrogens enabling consumption by most patients.

IODINE EXCRETION

- Excess is excreted via urine
- 90–97% is excreted via the kidneys — approximately 175 micrograms/day
- 3–10% via bile (reabsorbed) and faeces (lost) — 20 micrograms/day
- Small amount is lost via sweat, saliva and gastric juices (6 micrograms/day)
- Total excretion is approximately 200 micrograms/day.

SOME FACTS

- In the past, an increased incidence of goitre and iodine deficiency was documented in certain parts of Australia.[56–58]
- Prevention of iodine deficiency in industrialised countries most commonly relies on iodised salt, iodine in milk, or iodine-supplemented bread.[44,53,54,59]
- The upper limit of the recommended daily intake of salt (NaCl) is 6 g (a heaped teaspoon); 100 mmol of iodised salt per day would provide 175–240 micrograms of iodine. However, most salt is incorporated into foods before purchase and most major Australian manufacturers of processed food use non-iodised salt only.
- Milk products, which used to contain significant concentrations of iodine (up to 300 micrograms/ 100 mL) by virtue of iodine-containing solutions used to clean the milk vats, now contain low levels of iodine because volatile cleaning solutions are used (chlorine is the standard cleaning agent).
- In addition, the re-emergence of iodine deficiency appears to be due to the increased consumption of commercially-prepared foods (manufactured mostly with non-iodised salt) and less salt being used in home prepared foods as a response to the health messages to reduce salt intake.
- While the incidence of iodine deficiency and goitre was decreased by legislation requiring iodine supplementation of bread in 1966,[56] this is no longer a requirement (because of concerns about an increased incidence of thyrotoxicosis).
- Food Standards Australia New Zealand (FSANZ) developed a mandatory iodine fortification regulation to help address the re-emergence of iodine deficiency across most of the population. This regulation requires the replacement of non-iodised salt with iodised salt in all bread, except organic bread. Since October 2009, most bread in Australia and New Zealand has contained added iodine.
- Marine fish, shellfish, seaweed and kelp contain high amounts of iodine[50,59] and such ocean seafood, as well

TABLE 21.12 Iodine content of various foods

Food	Micrograms of iodine per 100 g
Oysters	160
Sushi (containing seaweed)	92
Canned salmon	60
Bread (with added iodised salt)	46
Steamed snapper	40
Cheddar cheese	23
Eggs	22
Ice-cream	21
Chocolate milk	20
Flavoured yoghurt	16
Regular milk	13
Canned tuna	10
Bread	13
Beef, pork, lamb	<1.5
Apple, oranges, grapes, bananas	<0.5

Source: Food Standards Australia and New Zealand (FSANZ). Iodine in food and iodine requirements, 2016. © Food Standards Australia and New Zealand.

as added iodised salt, provide most of the iodine in the Australian diet. However, many people may consume these products rarely, if at all.

The iodine content of various foods is shown in Table 21.12.

Primary congenital hypothyroidism

Primary congenital hypothyroidism occurs when a patient with an increased plasma TSH has radiological evidence of either ectopic thyroid tissue, hemithyroid, athyreosis or dyshormonogenesis, *or* when a patient with documented persistent increase of TSH and inadequate fT4 is being treated with thyroxine. This definition does not exclude transient hypothyroidism, which usually requires monitoring of thyroid function following a withdrawal of treatment at age 2–3 years.

NEWBORN SCREENING

Congenital hypothyroidism is the most common disorder identified by routine screening. It has been assessed through newborn screening (heel prick tests) since 1977 in Australia. In NSW/ACT, it has an incidence of 1:3500.[60] Most (85%) is due to abnormal thyroid gland formation (thyroid dysgenesis) which is usually not familial and presents sporadically and 10%–15% is due to abnormal thyroid hormone biosynthesis (dyshormonogenesis type) which is usually autosomal recessive.[61] There is a higher incidence of congenital hypothyroidism reported in females than males (ratio of 2:1) however at the milder end of the spectrum, the sex ratio is equal.[62] As a result of newborn screening, thyroid hormone medication (thyroxine) can be given early which enables normal development and prevents mental and growth retardation.

Hashimoto's disease

In Australia, the most common cause of hypothyroidism is autoimmune chronic lymphocytic thyroiditis. It is more common in women than men (ratio, 9:1)[63] and is most common during the third to fifth decades, when the prevalence of antithyroid antibodies in women is 10%.[64]

Hashimoto's disease is an inflammatory autoimmune disease in which cells within the thyroid are gradually destroyed by autoantibodies. The antibodies bind to the thyroid (specifically against the thyroid peroxidase enzyme, thyroglobulin, and TSH receptors) and prevent the manufacture of sufficient levels of thyroid hormone. In addition to binding to thyroid tissue, these antibodies may also bind to the adrenal glands, pancreas, and acid-producing cells of the stomach (parietal cells). This reduces the capacity for thyroxine production and causes hypothyroidism.

Postpartum thyroiditis

Postpartum hypothyroidism is a transient form of hypothyroidism and is believed to affect 5–10% of women in the Western world. Women with insulin-dependent diabetes mellitus are three times more likely to develop postpartum thyroid dysfunction than non-diabetic controls and may have unsuspected thyroid disease in pregnancy.[65] Ideally, all diabetic women should have thyroid antibody measurements in the first trimester, with careful follow-up of those with positive results. Also, any woman who develops postpartum thyroiditis should be offered annual follow-up, as about a quarter of these women will develop overt hypothyroidism within the next 5 years.[66]

Other

Thyroid surgery and ablation.

Subclinical hypothyroidism

Subclinical hypothyroidism is characterised by elevations in TSH but with normal thyroid hormones. In this condition, the body compensates for decreased thyroid function by increasing TSH pituitary output. It is graded based on severity of TSH levels (Table 21.13).

TABLE 21.13 Subclinical hypothyroidism grading system

Grade	TSH levels	Thyroxine (T_4) levels
1	Above normal limits of reference range	Normal
2	10.1–20 mIU/L	Normal
3	>20 mIU/L	Normal

Source: Brown BT, Bonello R, Pollard H. The biopsychosocial model and hypothyroidism. Chiropathic and Osteopathic 2005; 13:5. © Brown et al; licensee BioMed Central Ltd, 2005.

Basal metabolic rate

Heat is released whenever the body breaks down carbohydrate, fat or protein for energy and again when that energy is used to do work. The work itself generates heat as well. The body's generation of heat is known as thermogenesis and is measured to determine the amount of energy expended. There are three main categories of thermogenesis:

1 Basal thermogenesis (basal metabolism)
2 Exercise-induced thermogenesis (physical activity)
3 Diet-induced thermogenesis (thermic effect of food).

People spend energy when they are physically active; however, they also spend energy when they are resting quietly. Interestingly 'quiet' metabolic activities account for a large proportion of most people's energy expenditures.

Basal metabolism constitutes approximately 60–80% of the energy the average person spends in a day to support the body's metabolism. Basal metabolism supports the basic processes of life; for example, body temperature, heart rate and kidney filtration and can be described as the 'quiet' metabolic activities.

Technically basal metabolism is defined as: 'The energy needed to maintain life when a body is at complete digestive, physical and emotional rest'.

BASAL METABOLIC RATE

The basal metabolic rate (BMR) is the rate at which the body spends energy for these maintenance activities. The rate may vary dramatically from person to person and may vary in the same individual with a change in circumstances or physical condition.

It is technically determined as: 'The rate of energy use for metabolism under specified conditions: after 12 hours of restful sleep, without any physical activity or emotional excitement and in a comfortable setting'. It is usually expressed as kcal/kg by weight/hour.

FACTORS THAT AFFECT BMR

There are many factors that raise or lower the BMR including:[68]

Factor	Effect on BMR
Age	Lean body mass diminishes with age, slowing BMR
Height	BMR is higher in tall, thin people
Growth	BMR is higher in children and pregnant women
Body composition	The more lean tissue, the higher the BMR The more fat tissue, the lower the BMR (this is why men usually have a higher BMR than women)
Fever	Fever raises BMR
Stresses	Stresses (including many diseases and certain drugs) raise BMR
Environmental temperature	Raises BMR
Fasting/starvation	Lowers BMR
Malnutrition	Lowers BMR
Hormones	Thyroxine speeds up BMR
Smoking	Increases energy expenditure
Caffeine	Increases energy expenditure
Sleep	BMR is lowest when sleeping

BMR is basically highest in people who are growing (children and pregnant women) and those with considerable lean body mass (physically fit people and males).

Source: Weetman AP. Fortnightly review: hypothyroidism: screening and subclinical disease — clinical review. BMJ 1997; 314:1175

Causes include:

- Mild autoimmune thyroid destruction
- Medication/iatrogenic
- Surgical intervention.

Functional hypothyroidism

Functional hypothyroidism is considered to be more prevalent than current laboratory assessments predict. It assesses thyroid function based on clinical assessment, reverse T_3 status and a person's resting metabolic rate — assessed via temperature measurements (basal body temperature).

Broda Otto Barnes, an American physician, was an expert in endocrine physiology. He studied thyroid disorders at length (in particular hypothyroidism) and proposed that hypothyroidism was more prevalent than standard measurements were predicting.[67] He believed that standard assays of thyroid function were inadequate, and that undiagnosed thyroid dysfunction was responsible for a wide range of health problems. Barnes found that measuring basal body temperature was a good way of assessing basal metabolic rate and thus the body's response to thyroid hormones, regardless of their blood level. If this test is clinically applied, it is essential that a number of key parameters are adopted:

- Digital thermometer to two decimal places with battery power checked regularly
- A minimum of 6 hours solid, unbroken, restful sleep
- Temperature taken at the same time each morning before any activity or movement
- Time has to be adhered to and any unusual variations documented
- Illness, impending illness, emotional upset, nightmares/difficult dreams, alcohol or excessive caffeine consumption on previous day must be documented
- Nocturia will understandably affect readings.

Functional assessments display a far greater incidence of low thyroid than blood tests for several reasons:

- Typical blood tests measure thyroxine (T_4), which accounts for 90% of the hormone secretion by the thyroid. However, the form that affects the cells the most is T_3 (triiodothyronine), which cells make from T_4.

- If the cells cannot convert T_4 to the four times more active T_3, a person can have normal levels of thyroid hormone in the blood yet be thyroid deficient. This condition is characterised as Wilson's syndrome — deficient peripheral conversion of T_4 to T_3.
- A high reverse T_3 reading is the most effective diagnostic of Wilson's syndrome.

Detecting fluctuations in basal metabolic rate

Low basal metabolic rate (<36.4°C may indicate hypothyroidism, and high rate >36.8°C may indicate hyperthyroidism). According to Barnes, the normal basal body temperature is 36.4°C–36.8°C (37.0°C is accepted; or 97.6°F–98.2°F). Please note that Barnes' approach can elicit an error, as a low basal metabolic rate could also indicate, for instance, nutritional deficiencies or inadequate physical activity while fever from an infection or other disease can result in an inaccurately high body temperature.

Underlying triggers (all types)

- Leaky gut — food allergies/sensitivities, alcohol, NSAIDs, corticosteroids
- Microflora imbalance in GIT
- Poor digestion and elimination
- Chemical overload
- Food additives, agricultural chemical run-off (organochloride exposure especially), environmental pollutants, chemical exposure, household cleaners and sprays, herbicides and pesticides, hair dyes
- Stress, depression, inadequate rest and relaxation
- Low-grade chronic acute infections.

Investigations

In order to distinguish between autoimmune Hashimoto's thyroiditis and other non-autoimmune subclinical and functional conditions, laboratory TSH, antithyroid peroxidase, and antithyroglobulin antibody tests should be performed. Wilson's syndrome may be suspected via observing low basal body temperature and a high reverse T_3 level (Table 21.14).

CLINICAL INTERPRETATION

When a thyroid disorder or possible thyroid involvement in a health problem is suspected, the first laboratory test that a GP will order is thyroid-stimulating hormone (TSH). The reference range is usually 0.3–5 mU/L. However, stimulating hormones should be on the low end of normal when the system is running smoothly and efficiently. In clinical experience, TSH values >2 or 2.5 mU/L constitute a 'labouring' thyroid and require support. In that case, T_3 and T_4 should also be measured, together with antibodies to rule out any autoimmune involvement. The actual hormones (in this case T_3 and T_4) should ideally be in the upper half of the range. Tendencies for TSH to rise over time or T_3/T_4 to fall would indicate impending hypothyroid. At this stage overt symptoms may not yet have manifested. In addition, it is typical for endocrinologists to refer for antibody testing when TSH is higher than 2–2.5 mU/L.

It may be advisable to measure iodine, selenium, iron and zinc, as they are involved in proper thyroid function (see below). In the case of thyroid antibodies, the ideal range is as low as possible (simply because they should not be there at all). In that case, further testing is indicated to establish the source of the autoimmunity. A functional thyroid assessment (see below) will also help to establish a correct diagnosis. It is advisable to start herbal and nutritional intervention at this point, before the development of a full-blown disease picture.

TSH (thyrotrophin)

It is now recognised that the thyroid-stimulating hormone (thyrotrophin, TSH) measurement is a more sensitive test than free T_4 (fT4) for detecting both hypo- and hyperthyroidism. As a result, some countries (Australia included) now promote a TSH-first strategy for diagnosing thyroid dysfunction (provided that the TSH method has a functional sensitivity ≤0.02 mIU/L). The diagnostic accuracy of thyroid dysfunction is mainly affected by the validity of reference intervals of TSH. The International Federation of Clinical Chemistry (IFCC) and the Clinical & Laboratory Standards Institute (CLSI) have recommended that each laboratory define its own reference intervals, and the AACC Academy (formerly National Academy of Clinical Biochemistry) recently proposed a protocol for establishing reference intervals of TSH.[69] Clinicians are advised to select laboratories for investigations carefully and consistently use the same reference values. The upper level of TSH is routinely criticised and specialists make a general

TABLE 21.14 Thyroid function tests in hypothyroidism

Physiological state	Serum TSH	Serum T_4	Serum T_3	THBR (T_3 resin uptake)	24-h radioiodine uptake (thyroid)
Hypothyroidism, untreated	High	Low	Low	Low	Low/normal
Euthyroid, on iodine	Normal	Normal	Normal	Normal	Low
Euthyroid, on exogenous thyroid hormone	Normal or low	High/normal T_4, low T_3	High T_3, normal T_4	Normal	Low
Euthyroid, on oestrogen	Normal	High	High	Low	Normal
Euthyroid, on phenytoin	Normal	Low/normal	Low/normal	High/normal	Normal
Euthyroid sick syndrome	Normal/low/high	Normal/low	Low	Normal/high	Normal

recommendation that patients with TSH readings higher than 2.0 mIU/L (potential Hashimoto's thyroiditis) be referred for antibody screening.

Thyroid antibodies

Thyroid autoantibodies are proteins manufactured by the immune system that are directed against proteins in the thyroid. Although nearly all patients with chronic autoimmune thyroid disease have high concentrations of circulating thyroid autoantibodies, for the most part the disorder appears to be the consequence of tissue damage initiated by T lymphocytes. Measurement of autoantibodies against thyroid peroxidase (TPO-Ab) and thyroglobulin (Tg-Ab) has for many years been a major tool in the diagnosis of autoimmune thyroid diseases such as Hashimoto's thyroiditis, primary myxoedema and postpartum thyroiditis.[70] Nearly all patients with chronic autoimmune thyroid disease have high concentrations of thyroglobulin antibodies (Tg-Ab) and thyroperoxidase antibodies (TPO-Ab) in serum.

Among the many environmental factors that have been suggested to take part in the development of thyroid autoimmunity, iodine intake may be the most important.[71]

THYROPEROXIDASE ANTIBODIES (TPO-Ab)

Thyroid peroxidase (TPO) is a 100 kDa poorly glycosylated membrane-bound enzyme containing a haem prosthetic group. The enzyme is expressed on the apical membrane of thyrocytes, facing the colloid, where it is responsible for catalysing iodine oxidation, iodination of tyrosine residues and coupling of iodotyrosines to generate thyroid hormones. TPO is identical with the previously defined thyroid microsomal antigen, and measurement of TPO-Ab has replaced measurements of antibodies against the microsomal antigen (Mic-Ab).[70]

Certain factors may lead to increased TPO levels including:

- Excess oestrogen conditions including pregnancy and oral oestrogen supplementation regimens from the oral contraceptive pill and hormone replacement therapy
- Tamoxifen therapy for breast cancer
- Liver diseases.

High TPO levels can hinder the availability of free thyroid hormone for use in the peripheral tissues, thus contributing to a hypothyroid symptomatology. It is elevated in both Hashimoto's thyroiditis and Graves' disease.

THYROGLOBULIN ANTIBODIES (Tg-Ab)

Thyroglobulin (Tg) is a large 660 kDa dimeric glycoprotein composed of two identical polypeptide chains, and is unique in its content of iodinated amino acids. Most iodinated amino acids in Tg are iodotyrosines, which serve as precursors of the biologically active thyroid hormones, thyroxine and triiodothyronine. Tg is produced by the thyroid follicular cells and secreted into the follicular lumen, where it is stored as colloid. Small amounts of Tg are present in the circulation, which is primarily of clinical importance in diagnosing the persistence or recurrence of thyroid cancer after ablative therapy. However, Tg in serum is increased in almost all kinds of thyroid disease, including goitre and subacute thyroiditis, the concentrations overlapping with those in healthy individuals.[70]

Tg influences the function and growth of the gland. It is typically elevated in thyroid cancer or Hashimoto's thyroiditis. The heterogeneous nature of Tg is well accepted. Besides their long-known thyroid-stimulating activity, Tg-Ab can act as blocking antibodies or growth-promoting antibodies and, thus, cause hypothyroidism (primary myxoedema) or endemic and sporadic goitres, respectively.

Urinary iodine

The measurement of urinary iodine (UI) provides an approximation of dietary iodine intake. Approximately 90% of iodine is excreted in the urine,[72] and measuring urinary iodine concentration usually assesses iodine status. The accepted minimum adequate level of urinary iodine is 100 micrograms/L, and levels above this are considered normal.[73,74] Urinary iodine concentrations below 25 micrograms/L are classified as severe deficiency, and are associated with an increased risk of cretinism; 26–50 micrograms/L is classified as moderate deficiency; and 51–100 micrograms/L is regarded as mild iodine deficiency.[74]

The World Health Organization (WHO) recommends that the median urinary iodine concentration for populations as a whole should be more than 100 micrograms/L, that less than 20% of the population should have a urinary iodine concentration below 50 micrograms/L, and that no cretinism occurs.[74] In constructing a reasonable health-based standard using the precautionary approach, it is clear that urinary iodine levels below 100 micrograms/L, which are in the mild iodine deficiency range, warrant intervention.[51]

As iodine's main action is involved in thyroid function and the numerous actions carried out by the thyroid, the implications of iodine deficiency are vast. The major hormone secreted by the thyroid is thyroxine (also called T_4 because it contains four iodine atoms). To exert its effects, T_4 is converted to T_3 by the removal of one iodine atom. This occurs mainly in the liver and other tissues where T_3 acts, such as the brain. When conducting the assessment, for optimal results it is essential that urinary iodine levels are measured from the first morning urine.

Alternatives include 24-hour urinary iodine and spot urinary assessment.

REVERSE T_3

Triiodothyronine (T_3) is the most active of the thyroid hormones. Approximately 85% of circulating T_3 is produced by monodeiodination of thyroxine (T_4) in tissues such as liver, muscle and kidney. Reverse T_3 (rT3) is an inactive form of T_3 that is produced in the body particularly during periods of stress. rT3 differs from T_3 in that the missing deiodinated iodine is from the inner ring of the thyroxine molecule compared with outer ring on T_3. Under normal conditions T_4 will convert to both T_3 and rT3 continually and the body eliminates rT3 quickly. Under certain conditions, more rT3 is produced and the desirable conversion of T_4 to T_3 decreases. This occurs during fasting, starvation, illness such as liver disease and during times of increased stress. This becomes a vicious cycle as rT3 competes with T_3 as a substrate for the 5-deiodinase enzyme. This inhibits the conversion of T_4 to T_3, with more T_4 being converted to more rT3. An increased production of rT3 is often seen in patients with disorders such as fibromyalgia, chronic fatigue syndrome (CFS), Wilson's thyroid syndrome and stress. Measurement of rT3 is also valuable in identifying sick euthyroid syndrome where active T_3 is within normal range and rT3 is elevated.

Coeliac profile and genetic screen

It is advisable that in the instance of suspected autoimmune thyroid conditions concurrent investigation into suspected coeliac disease is organised. It is prudent to include coeliac genetic screening in addition to standard assays (transglutimase and endomysial antibodies) due to fluctuations from dietary intake. Please see Chapter 12 for a comprehensive discussion of this assessment.

Other

Basal metabolic rate assessment via temperature measure and reflex assessment (Achilles).

Indications for screening hypothyroidism

ESTABLISHED

- Congenital hypothyroidism
- Treatment of hyperthyroidism
- Neck irradiation
- Pituitary surgery or irradiation
- Patients taking amiodarone or lithium.

ESSENTIAL CONSIDERATION

- Type 1 diabetes antepartum
- Previous episode of postpartum thyroiditis
- Unexplained infertility
- Women over 40 with nonspecific complaints
- Refractory depression; bipolar affective disorder with rapid cycling
- Turner's syndrome; Down syndrome
- Autoimmune Addison's disease.

UNCERTAIN

- Breast cancer
- Dementia
- Patients with a family history of autoimmune thyroid disease
- Pregnancy, looking for postpartum thyroiditis (check thyroid antibodies; screen positive patients postpartum using thyroid-stimulating hormone)
- Obesity
- Idiopathic oedema.

NOT INDICATED

- Acutely ill patients with no clinical reason to suspect thyroid disease.

Source: Weetman AP. Fortnightly review: hypothyroidism: screening and subclinical disease — clinical review. BMJ 1997; 314:1175

Therapeutic considerations

CLINICAL DECISION MAKING AND RATIONALE

- Sufficient investigations are required to accurately assess and establish the form of hypothyroidism detected. Treatment is adjusted accordingly
- Holistic consideration of current stressors — nutritional, environmental, emotional, physical, mental, and others are essential
- Assessment of hindrances to metabolic and endocrinological function
- Support and assessment of other endocrinological glands and associated symptoms as required.

Therapeutic application

HISTORICAL PERSPECTIVE

The treatment of hypothyroid conditions by the Eclectics differed greatly to the way in which modern naturopaths treat today; however, the knowledge that goitre may occur as a result of nutritional deficiency was still apparent to the Eclectics. Ellingwood[10] discusses the frequency of goitre seen in pregnancy (which today we know increases bodily requirements for iodine) as well as in women who worked hard, lived in drudgery and ate poor, coarse food; from a modern point of view these women were obviously nutritionally deficient. Ellingwood also suggests the use of iron in the treatment of goitre which we now know to play an important role in the manufacture of the thyroid hormones. Not in line with modern prescribing, Ellingwood suggests iron in conjunction with *Phytolacca americana,* a herb not commonly recommended in modern day naturopathy for goitre. There is little else mentioned in the eclectic texts regarding hypothyroidism bar the discussions Ellingwood and Thomas[75] both have on the treatment of myxoedema (as a result of hypothyroidism). Both suggest the use of animal-derived thymus gland. The lack of information available on the traditional treatment of hypothyroidism reveals the substantial growth in modern naturopathic understanding of the endocrine system.

ALLOPATHIC PERSPECTIVE

Replacement therapy with thyroxine is the cornerstone of therapy (1.6 micrograms/kg lean body weight daily, taken on an empty stomach); combination therapy with thyroxine and liothyronine (T_3) is promoted, but there is little evidence of its clinical benefit.[64]

NATUROPATHIC PERSPECTIVE

Treatment is aimed at normalising thyroid function. This is achieved when TSH is in the low-normal range, T_3 and T_4 is in the high-normal range and there are no antibodies present. On a day-to-day basis thyroid function can also be monitored through basal temperature readings. The symptoms, if any had developed before treatment had begun, should also normalise or at least show a trend towards normal.

As stated above, hypothyroidism can present on its own or as part of an autoimmune disease (Hashimoto's thyroiditis). Testing for TSH, T_3, T_4, thyroxine-binding globulins, thyroid antibodies and thyroid receptor antibodies will ascertain the kind of hypothyroid the patient is presenting with.[76–78]

Firstly, it needs to be established if antibodies are present. If they are, the source of the autoimmunity needs to be found (e.g. allergies, food intolerances, intestinal dysbiosis and permeability) and addressed. Anti-inflammatory herbs (e.g. turmeric) and nutrients (e.g. flavonoids and antioxidants) will be indicated. An elimination diet (avoidance of commonly reactive food items such as dairy and gluten) and low intake of sugar and chemicals is highly advisable. Dysbiosis should be tested for and treated, otherwise even the best supplementation is not going to produce lasting effects.

Iodine is generally the first nutrient thought of in hypothyroid conditions. It is commonly low in Australia and New Zealand.[79–84] In order to find out if it is indeed iodine that is needed iodine can be measured in urine, either in a spot sample (relative to creatinine) or better still in a 24-hour sample. Values <100 micrograms/L indicate deficiency.[77,85] Supplementation can be achieved through potassium iodide or iodate (often added to table salt), Lugol's solution or iodised vegetable oil. Any forms of seaweed are also rich sources of iodine. A daily amount of 150 micrograms per day is usually recommended.[77,86] Pregnancy and lactation require higher amounts, closer to 300 micrograms per day.[85] If the patient is already on thyroid medication such as thyroxine (T_4) iodine is generally contraindicated as it can lead to hyperthyroidism.

Supplements for the thyroid itself include not only iodine but also tyrosine, the amino acid needed for thyroid hormone (T_3, T_4) production. Situations that can lead to low levels of tyrosine include low protein intake, anorexia, infections, stress (adrenaline is derived from tyrosine and may compete with the thyroid for this amino acid) or any other condition that leaves the body protein deficit.

Geographically, most hypothyroid problems occur in areas where both iodine and selenium are deficient in the soil. Both minerals are vitally important in thyroid hormone production and should both be considered when hypothyroidism is diagnosed.[87] The conversion of T_4 to T_3 (the active form of the hormone), which mainly occurs in the liver but also in other tissues, is dependent on selenium. To activate T_4, one iodine atom needs to be removed from the tyrosine backbone of thyroxine. The enzymes involved in this reaction, iodothyronine deiodinases, are selenium dependent.[86,88] The most common way to ascertain selenium status is serum/plasma or whole blood.[85] However, selenium supplementation should only be advocated after iodine deficiency has been ruled out or iodine supplementation has been instituted (whichever applies). People on thyroxine treatment may also benefit from selenium supplementation, not only to ensure the conversion to T_3 but also to maximise thyroid hormone feedback to the pituitary gland in order to reduce TSH secretion.[89]

If selenium is not available in sufficient amounts a T_3 analogue, reverse T_3 (rT_3), is produced. rT3 has a hindering action on thyroid hormone activity as less T_3 is available, and therefore can produce hypothyroid symptoms and clinical presentation.[77] It is rT3 which is thought to be responsible for the brain damage in cretinism observed in iodine-deficient children.[90] In workers exposed to mercury vapours an inverse correlation between urinary iodine excretion and rT3 was found, indicating a detrimental effect of mercury on the iodothyronine deiodinases.[91] rT3 can be measured by laboratories (and will be an out-of-pocket expense to the patient).

Another mineral that plays an important role in thyroid metabolism, especially in the production of T_3, is zinc.[92,93] Zinc (in zinc fingers) is required to bind thyroxine to affect gene expression. Cadmium can replace zinc in zinc fingers, thus interfering with their proper functioning.[94]

Other nutrients that are required for optimal thyroid function include vitamin A and iron.[94]

Inflammation is part of the autoimmune picture and therefore involved in Hashimoto's thyroiditis. Anti-inflammatory nutrients (see hyperthyroidism) as well as fatty acids are indicated. The latter are of particular importance as hypothyroidism (with or without autoimmunity) causes alterations in fatty acid composition in plasma, erythrocytes, neutrophils and mitochondrial membranes, due to an inhibition of delta 5 and 6 desaturases and therefore altered eicosanoid synthesis. Supplementing with omega-3 fatty acids can ameliorate this problem.[95,96]

SPECIFIC TREATMENT APPROACHES

Natural treatment strategies for normalising thyroid function vary depending on the type of hypothyroid abnormality. Additional specifics are listed below.

Autoimmune hypothyroidism (Hashimoto's disease)

As per other autoimmune conditions, food elimination, detoxification, stress management and digestive healing options may be useful treatments aimed at ameliorating a possible root factor of antigenic autoimmune activity. Autoimmune support focusing on immune modulation through nutritional and botanical treatments is advisable. Avoid gluten-containing foods if indicated.

Non-autoimmune or subclinical hypothyroid disorder

Treatment of hypothyroidism of a non-autoimmune overt or subclinical nature should begin with optimisation of the nutrients needed not only for thyroid hormone production, but also for the critical cellular conversion of T_4 to T_3. If, after a few months, the patient does not respond, then thyroid hormone replacement is indicated. Obviously referral to a patient's GP and endocrinologist to appropriately diagnose and manage care is essential.

NUTRITIONAL MEDICINE (DIETARY)

Dietary therapeutic objectives

The diet should be low in goitrogens and high in foods rich in the trace minerals needed for thyroid hormone production and activation. A small study found that in children with subclinical hypothyroidism, consuming a nutrient-dense diet (nutrients required for thyroid function) for 3 months resulted in normalisation of TSH levels. Foods in the diet included green vegetables (boiled spinach, broccoli, cauliflower and chicory), beef, full-fat milk, and butter.[97] Due to sluggish digestive function, it is advisable to encourage small frequent meals to maintain metabolic rate, reduce carbohydrate (refined) consumption and optimise dietary intake as per nutritional needs to assist with weight reduction (if present).

DIETARY INCLUSIONS

- Good sources of iodine include seafoods (especially haddock, mackerel and cod), sea vegetables (kelp, dulse, arame, hijiki, nori, wakame, kombu), iodised salt, vegetables (including spinach, garlic, watercress and artichokes), egg yolks, pineapple and citrus fruits.
- Good sources of zinc include seafood (especially oysters), beef, oatmeal, chicken, liver, spinach, nuts and seeds.
- Copper is found in liver and other organ meats, eggs, yeast, beans, nuts, and seeds.
- Best sources of the B vitamins are yeast, wholegrains, and liver.
- The best source of selenium is Brazil nuts, especially those that are unshelled.
- Organically grown foods should be recommended due to their higher levels of trace minerals.

DIETARY EXCLUSIONS

Goitrogens to be limited include *Brassica* family foods (turnips, cabbage, broccoli, swedes, mustard greens, radishes, horseradishes), cassava root, soybeans, peanuts, pine nuts, and millet. If eaten, these foods should be cooked to break down their goitrogenic constituents. Consumption of soy products was associated with elevated TSH levels in women, but no association was found in men. Soy contains the isoflavones genenstein and daidzein, and may be associated with iodine deficiency and hypothyroidism.[98]

Patients who are on thyroid replacement therapy should avoid taking their medication in conjunction with fibre, soy products and coffee, as these may potentially negatively affect L-T_4 absorption.[99]

NUTRITIONAL MEDICINE (SUPPLEMENTAL)

Nutritional medicine therapeutic objectives

- Address underlying deficiencies present due to increased requirements, poor nutritional assimilation and absorption and poor dietary intake
- Address specific deficiencies to improve thyroid hormone synthesis and relieve symptom presentation.

Specific nutrients required

R-ALPHA LIPOIC ACID

R-alpha lipoic acid is a potent antioxidant that significantly influences the way in which the thyroid hormones work. Clinical experiments administrating lipoic acid together with thyroxine (T_4) for 9 days found that it suppressed the T_4 induced increase of T_3 generation by 56%.[100] It appears lipoic acid interferes with the production of T_3 from T_4 when it is co-administered with T_4. Elevated levels of T_3, after T_4 administration, may be reduced by treatment with lipoic acid.

B VITAMINS

The B vitamins function as coenzymes within the body where they are required for energy production, particularly in the mitochondria. Patients with hypothyroidism often present with fatigue and lethargy hence the application of the B vitamins is important to help with energy reserves. Vitamin B_1 is part of enzyme system known as thiamin pyrophosphate and is required for almost every cellular reaction in the body. Similarly vitamin B_2 forms part of two enzyme systems known as flavin adenine dinucleotide (FAD) and flavin mononucleotide (FMN) and is required to generate energy. Vitamin B_{12} is required for energy release from food and is involved in the production of genetic material. Studies show that approximately 40% of patients with hypothyroidism were also deficient in vitamin B_{12}.[101–103] The B vitamins (in particular vitamins B_6, B_{12} and folic acid) are also required if there is coexisting homocystinaemia which often presents in the hypothyroid patient.

L-CARNITINE

Endocrine disorders such as hypothyroidism are characterised by mitochondrial dysfunction and are often characterised by reduced cellular energy. Carnitine is an amino acid that mobilises fatty acids into the mitochondria for ATP energy production. Deficiency is associated with elevated cholesterol and triglycerides[104] (seen in hypothyroidism), hence supplementation may be warranted. Studies show that physical and mental fatigue was improved in hypothyroid patients, particularly those under 50 years of age and in those whose hypothyroidism developed after thyroidectomy.[105–107]

COENZYME Q10

Coenzyme Q10 is found in virtually every cell in the body and plays a vital role in all energy-dependent processes. The thyroid hormones have an important role in modulating coenzyme Q10 and its metabolism and alterations of coenzyme Q10 have been seen in patients with secondary hypothyroidism.[108] Coenzyme Q10 plays an essential physiological role in oxidative phosphorylation and also helps to inhibit oxidation of LDL cholesterol. This is significant considering the prevalence of dyslipidaemia that presents in patients with hypothyroidism. Care needs to be taken when using coenzyme Q10 in patients who are on thyroid medication.[109] It is worth noting that coenzyme Q10 is usually elevated in patients with hypothyroidism[110] (it is important to measure this before supplementing).

ESSENTIAL FATTY ACIDS

Omega-3 fatty acids play an important role in protecting against disease; however, it is well accepted that the majority of individuals living in Western countries generally have a low intake of the omega-3 fatty acids

SAMPLE DAILY DIET

BREAKFAST	
Green smoothie: Spinach, Brazil nuts, banana, 2 dates, water, natural yoghurt and LSA Dandelion tea	A smoothie provides an easy to assimilate nutrient-dense meal. Banana and dates provide fibre and carbohydrates. Adequate wholefood carbohydrates are essential in hypothyroid not only for energy production but due to the fact that low-carbohydrate diets and skipping meals have been shown to be capable of initiating thyroid dysfunction. Brazil nuts provide a source of selenium which is essential for thyroid hormone synthesis and function as well as to reduce thyroid antibodies. Leafy greens and dates provide a source of vitamins and minerals. This includes calcium and magnesium, an important consideration since osteoporosis risk is increased in hypothyroid individuals. Natural yoghurt if tolerated can be used to promote microbiome health since SIBO is commonly observed in individuals with hypothyroid. Dandelion tea may be used to gently stimulate the gallbladder and liver, reducing the chance of constipation, hypercholesterolaemia, gallstones and other common hepatic dysfunction manifestations of hypothyroid. The bitter nature of dandelion may also be useful since a high percentage of hypothyroid individuals produce antibodies against the parietal cells in the stomach which compromise digestion.
LUNCH	
Home-made nori rolls with avocado, carrot, ginger, tuna/salmon/chicken/tofu and lettuce served with tamari Miso soup containing sea vegetables such as wakame	Nori provides a source of iodine and vitamin B_{12}. Iodine is essential for thyroid hormone synthesis and function. Adequate vitamin B_{12} is imperative since Hashimoto's disease is associated with pernicious anaemia and atrophic gastritis. Tamari provides a gluten-free alternative to soya sauce. Lean protein is required as a source of tyrosine; however, it should be marinated to ensure proteins are broken down since protein digestion may be impaired due to compromised parietal cell function.
DINNER	
Lightly spiced vegetable and lentil shepherd's potato-topped pie	Vegetables and lentils provide fibre to facilitate bowel frequency and act as a prebiotic. Fibre also stabilises blood sugar levels, an important consideration since insulin resistance is associated with increased incidence of thyroid nodules. Note use of spices such as turmeric that are associated with reduced incidence of goitre due to their antioxidant and immune-regulating properties.
SNACK	
Trail mix comprising of pumpkin and sunflower seeds, Brazil nuts and goji berries Ginger tea	Nuts and seeds provide zinc which is also required for optimal thyroid function. Ginger can be used to energetically warm the client as hypothyroid is associated with cold sensitivity.

eicosapentaenoic acid (EPA) and docosahexaenoic acid (DHA). Omega-3 fatty acids have been found to influence cell membranes and membrane protein-mediated responses, cell signalling and gene expression throughout the body and thus play a key role through their influence on the cells.[111] In addition, they help maintain healthy cardiovascular function. Dyslipidaemia, particularly hypercholesterolaemia, commonly manifests in hypothyroidism and may be managed with the application of omega-3 fatty acids.

IODINE

Iodine is an essential component of the thyroid hormones T_3 and T_4 and is required for human growth and development throughout the body.[112] The thyroid concentrates iodine in a process known as iodination in order not only to form the thyroid hormones but also to produce enough of its daily iodine requirements. The body of a healthy adult contains 10–20 mg of iodine.[113] The concentration of iodine in the thyroid is carefully regulated but is usually in the range 8–10 mg.[45,113] Deficiency of iodine prevents the formation and production of thyroid hormones leading to suboptimal thyroid function and complaints such as low basal temperature.

IRON

Iron is an essential element in the body and plays a wide variety of physiological and biochemical roles particularly with regards to healthy thyroid function. Iron deficiency affects the thyroid-stimulating hormone axis. The first two steps of thyroid hormone synthesis are catalysed by thyroid peroxidase and require the presence of iron.[114,115] Any deficiency of iron will prevent this from happening, the result being thyroid dysfunction. Hypothyroidism may lead to low iron levels due to decreased GIT absorption, decreased digestive enzymes, or associated autoimmune diseases such as coeliac disease.[116] Monitoring of serum ferritin levels before and after treatment might be useful in tracking disease progression.[115] Iron deficiency in primary hypothyroidism affects a significant proportion of patients (up to 34%).[117] Monitoring of iron levels while treating hypothyroidism is advised.[118]

MAGNESIUM

Magnesium functions as a co-factor in 300+ enzyme systems within the body. Defects in magnesium metabolism and transport mechanisms have been noted in hypothyroid patients. In two studies, patients with hypothyroidism were found to have elevated plasma and faecal magnesium while urinary and total cellular magnesium was decreased.[119,120] Neuromuscular symptoms such as muscle and joint pain are also a common complaint in hypothyroidism and further highlight the necessity for extra magnesium via supplementation or through diet.

N-ACETYLCYSTEINE (NAC)

Keeping reactive oxygen species at a minimum is imperative in thyroid disorders to help maintain healthy thyrocyte function. Studies have shown that when reactive oxygen species drop below a basal threshold, the expression of proteins involved in thyroid cell function becomes disrupted. The antioxidant activity of *N*-acetylcysteine when incubated in vivo[121] inside thyrocytes has been found to block the production of intracellular reactive oxygen species while also decreasing dual oxidases, thyroperoxidase, pendrin and thyroglobulin protein and/or gene expression. This implies *N*-acetylcysteine exerts a protective mechanism and safeguards the function of thyroid cells; it also provides a good reason for its application in hypothyroidism, a condition in which reactive oxygen species have been implicated.

QUERCETIN AND BIOFLAVONOIDS

Quercetin is a source of flavonoids and has been shown to inhibit the growth of the thyroid, a useful action in the treatment of hypothyroidism. The mechanism by which quercetin does this remains undetermined but seems at least to be in some part due to inhibition of insulin-modulated phosphatidylinositol 3-kinase-Akt kinase activity.[122,123] Furthermore, quercetin decreases TSH-modulated RNA levels of the thyroid-restricted gene sodium/iodide symporter (NIS).

SELENIUM

Selenium is a trace mineral required for healthy function of the thyroid gland. Insufficient amounts of selenium have been linked with a number of disease manifestations, especially those affecting the thyroid hormone axis.[124] The endocrine glands, in particular the thyroid, contain some of the highest amounts of selenium among the human tissues.[125–127] Selenoproteins play an important role in antioxidant defence systems, such as the action of glutathione peroxidase (GPx), that occur within the cells. These defence mechanisms help to protect the thyroid gland from free radicals such as reactive oxygen species (ROS) that are produced by the follicles for biosynthesis of thyroid hormones.[126]

The conversion of T_3 to T_4 is also dependent on the presence of selenium and involves the work of selenoproteins. The majority of active T_3 is found within the body's cells and involves three important enzymes (which are also selenoproteins) known as the iodothyronine deiodinases (DIO1, 2, 3). The iodothyronine deiodinases instigate the removal of one iodine atom from T_4 (the non-active thyroid hormone). Through their actions on T_3, T_4 and other thyroid hormone metabolites the iodothyronine deiodinases are involved in activating and inactivating the thyroid hormones.[86] The role of the iodothyronine deiodinases in thyroid hormone regulation is very important and would not be possible without selenium.

Selenium was found to reduce serum thyroid antibody levels in autoimmune thyroiditis; however, further research is needed to determine the clinical relevance of these results and the impact for selenium supplementation.[128–130] A review found that selenium supplementation during pregnancy had a favourable impact on postpartum thyroid function, resulting in a decreased incidence of moderate to advanced postpartum thyroiditis.[131]

TYROSINE

Tyrosine is an amino acid with an affinity for the thyroid gland. Tyrosine is a precursor of the thyroid hormones T_3 and T_4; deficiency of tyrosine is seen regularly in the plasma of patients with hypothyroidism.

VITAMIN A

Vitamin A deficiency has been associated as one of the factors contributing to iodine deficiency and increasing intake is associated with improved iodine status and thyroid function. Vitamin A is involved in multiple roles with regards to the healthy function of the thyroid including the uptake of iodine by the thyroid, the modulation of thyroid hormone metabolism, peripheral metabolism of the thyroid hormones and the production of TSH by the pituitary to name but a few.[132] Deficiency of vitamin A has been found to exert multiple effects on the pituitary–thyroid axis. Supplementation with vitamin A (concurrently with iodine) in iodine-deficient children in Africa has been found to decrease thyrotrophin stimulation of the thyroid and reduce the rate of goitre, highlighting the efficacy of vitamin A supplementation for hypothyroid conditions.[133]

In addition, a study in Iran found that vitamin A supplementation reduces the risk of subclinical hypothyroidism in premenopausal women.[134]

VITAMIN C

Vitamin C is an antioxidant compound capable of scavenging superoxide anions at high concentrations.

Subclinical hypothyroidism is associated with low-grade inflammation and the production of free radicals of which vitamin C may help to scavenge, lessening oxidative damage to the thyroid gland. In hypothyroid patients with gastrointestinal pathology undergoing L-T_4 replacement therapy, vitamin C was found to improve the abnormalities in serum free T_4, T_3, and TSH concentrations.[135]

VITAMIN D

Vitamin D displays significant benefits as an immune modulator. While human clinical studies examining the link between vitamin D and autoimmune hypothyroid disorders such as Hashimoto's thyroiditis are under investigation, we know that deficiency of vitamin D has been associated with a predisposition towards autoimmune disorders. Due to these immune-modulating effects, its role in the management of thyroid autoimmune conditions such as Hashimoto's thyroiditis is justified. Appropriate investigations prior to prescription are essential for optimal and safe outcome.

Low vitamin D concentrations, certain vitamin D receptor (VDR) gene polymorphisms and pathologies of vitamin D-binding proteins and their genes may favour the development of Hashimoto's thyroiditis.[136,137]

Studies have found that serum vitamin D levels were significantly lower in premenopausal women with autoimmune thyroid disease,[138] and in elderly patients with autoimmune thyroiditis,[139] while another study found that early stages of thyroid autoimmunity are not associated with low vitamin D levels.[140]

Patients with hypothyroidism do seem to suffer from low vitamin D levels;[141] however, more research is needed in order to consolidate the existing research, to determine whether an association exists and the benefits of supplementation.[142,143]

VITAMIN E

Vitamin E is also a powerful free radical scavenger. Free radical-mediated oxidative stress has frequently been implicated in the pathogenesis of thyroid disorders. Studies[144] of patients with a range of thyroid disorders including hypothyroidism due to Hashimoto's thyroiditis have found increased generation of reactive oxygen species and impairment of the antioxidant system *particularly* in those patients with hypothyroidism. This indicates the thyroid hormones have a strong impact on oxidative stress and the antioxidant system, hence supplementation with antioxidants such as vitamin E in the management of hypothyroidism is a necessity. Data from animal studies support the use of vitamin E supplementation in hypothyroidism. Supplementing with vitamin E while undergoing L-T_4 replacement therapy might prevent oxidative stress and apoptosis of the hippocampus.[145,146] It was also found that vitamin E and curcumin regulate hepatic antioxidant gene expression in hypothyroid rats.[147]

ZINC

Normal thyroid function is dependent on the presence of many trace minerals, one of which is zinc, known to be involved in many biochemical reactions occurring within the thyroid. The direct effect of dietary zinc deficiency on thyroid hormone metabolism is unclear; however, epidemiological studies suggest an association between goitre and zinc deficiency, not a surprise when one considers zinc is required for the functioning of 1,50-deiodinase, the enzyme required to convert thyroxine to T_3. Researchers in a study undertaken in Pakistan observing the effect of zinc supplementation on zinc level in serum and urine and their relation to thyroid hormone profile in male and female goitrous patients concluded that pathogenesis of goitre disease is associated with changes in the balance of zinc in biological samples (serum and urine) of goitrous patients. They noted that even after 6 months of treatment, hypothyroid patients still had a lower level of zinc as compared with control participants.[148]

A small study showed that zinc supplementation (either on its own (30 mg) or in combination with selenium (200 micrograms)) positively affected thyroid function in overweight or obese female hypothyroid patients.[149]

Dosage requirements

The dosage requirements listed below are based on adult doses that have been reported in the literature:

- R-alpha lipoic acid: 50–400 mg/day
- B complex (all B vitamins) high-dose combination, preferably activated forms:
  - Thiamin: 20–40 mg/day
  - Riboflavin: 20–40 mg/day
  - Niacinamide: 50–100 mg/day
  - Pantothenic acid: 150–300 mg/day
  - Pyridoxine: 20–60 mg/day
  - Folinic acid (or L-5MTHF): 500–1000 micrograms/day
  - Hydroxocobalamin (or methylcobalamin): 500–1000 micrograms/day
  - Choline: 50–100 mg/day
  - Inositol: 50–100 mg/day
  - Biotin: 250–500 micrograms/day
- L-carnitine: 500–2000 mg/day[105,106]
- Coenzyme Q10: 100–300 mg/day
- Essential fatty acids: 3 g b.i.d.
- Iodine: 150[150,151]–400 micrograms/day[152]
- Iron: 5–80 mg/day:
  - If indicated on pathology
  - Literature: 60 mg/day (as sulfate — given to children, not adults, who were anaemic),[153] 300 mg/day (as ferrous sulfate — given to adolescent girls with iron deficiency, 5/7[154])
- Magnesium: 300–600 mg/day
- *N*-acetylcysteine: 200–1000 mg/day
- Probiotics — 25–50 × 10^{12}:
  - If digestive symptoms are present or if poor absorption concerns are evident
- Quercetin and bioflavonoids: 50–500 mg/day
- Selenium: 200–250 micrograms/day[155]
- Tyrosine: 400–6000 mg/day[104]
- Vitamin A: 5000–10 000 IU/day
- Vitamin C: 500–3000 mg/day in divided doses
  - In autoimmune presentation, dose will be increased

- Vitamin D: 1000 IU/day minimum (based on deficiency presentation)
- Vitamin: E 400–600 IU/day
- Zinc: 25–50 mg/day.

HERBAL MEDICINE

Herbal medicine therapeutic objectives

- To increase thyroxine production and output from the thyroid gland and subsequent reduction in TSH hyperstimulation
- To reduce the inflammatory process and the increased free radicals that result from inflammation
- To treat symptoms such as fatigue, cognitive deficits and weight gain
- To reduce the production of thyroid antibodies by regulating immune function (if autoimmune present).

Herbal medicine classes

ADAPTOGEN

Due to the direct interrelationship between stress and its impact on endocrinological function, it is important to consider the potential effects of stress, poor stress response and the fatigued presentation. Herbal adaptogens offer restorative capabilities that enable significant improvements when considered in the holistic paradigm of cause and effect for disease manifestation. Useful herbal medicines within this class include *Bacopa monnieri* (bacopa) for significant mental and cognitive support; *Codonopsis pilosula* (codonopsis) to support associated weight gain and potential blood sugar relationship; *Eleutherococcus senticosus* (Siberian ginseng), *Panax ginseng* (Korean ginseng) or *Rhodiola rosea* (rhodiola) to increase energy and vitality; and *Withania somnifera* (ashwagandha) for the depleted and weak patient.

ADRENAL RESTORATIVE

Glycyrrhiza glabra (liquorice) or *Rehmannia glutinosa* (rehmannia) is useful for additional adrenal restorative support. In addition, rehmannia can be chosen for support for autoimmune presentations, and liquorice for additional blood sugar regulating and mild laxative properties.

THYROID STIMULANT

Thyroid stimulant herbal medicines are an obvious essential inclusion in prescriptions. Those that have shown the most effect include *Coleus forskohlii* (coleus) as a weight loss stimulant and *Fucus vesiculosus* (bladderwrack) for iodine supplementation and to stimulate the function of the thyroid gland.

ANTIOBESITY

Both *Coleus forskohlii* (coleus) and *Fucus vesiculosus* (bladderwrack) can be used to assist in stimulating the metabolic rate of the patient and assisting with weight loss due to poor thyroid function.

PANCREATIC RESTORATIVE

Gymnema sylvestre (gymnema) is indicated to assist with reducing sugar cravings and inhibiting high carbohydrate consumption due to its effects on taste buds and restorative properties to endocrinological pancreatic functions.

NERVINE TONIC

If depression is evident, *Hypericum perforatum* (St John's wort), *Rhodiola rosea* (rhodiola) or *Turnera diffusa* (damiana) is indicated. If exhaustion has been preceded by overwork and mental worry *Bacopa monnieri* (bacopa) can assist in improving cognitive function and mental repair. Systemic depletion is best suited to general nervine tonics including *Passiflora incarnata* (passion flower), *Avena sativa* (oats) or *Scutellaria lateriflora* (skullcap).

TONIC (GENERAL)

Due to the depleted presentation, general tonic herbal medicines are indicated to rebuild and stimulate the system. Indicated herbal medicines include the ginsengs (*Eleutherococcus senticosus* (Siberian ginseng), *Panax ginseng* (Korean ginseng)) and mushrooms (*Ganoderma lucidum* (reishi), *Grifola frondosa* (maitake) and *Lentinus edodes* (shiitake)). Care must be taken when prescribing ginsengs to depleted patients. Ensure that the prescription is appropriate for the presentation and temperament. The herbal medicine par excellence is arguably *Withania somnifera* (ashwagandha) with its strengthening and restorative qualities typically required with these presentations. Clinically it rebuilds and enables the patient to be gently stimulated back towards health.

IMMUNE SUPPORT

Immune support and modulation are indicated primarily as hypothyroid patients can often present with poor immune function. In these presentations *Andrographis paniculata* (andrographis) can be prescribed for immune support especially when post stress; *Astragalus membranaceus* (astragalus) when chronic low immune history dominates; or *Echinacea* spp. (echinacea) for general immune stimulation and recovery.

In an autoimmune presentation, immune modulation should be encouraged. Herbal medicines required include *Echinacea* spp. (echinacea), *Rehmannia glutinosa* (rehmannia), *Hemidesmus indicus* (hemidesmus), *Calendula officinalis* (calendula) and other similar herbal medicines. *Handroanthus* spp. (pau d'arco) and *Uncaria tomentosa* (cat's claw) are indicated if a marked infective trigger or history has perpetuated the autoimmune process.

ADDITIONAL CLASSES

Hepatoprotectives and other liver restorative herbal medicines are indicated due to the role of the liver in regulating endocrinological function and hormonal cascade. Antioxidants are especially beneficial to reduce free radical synthesis and damage commonly experienced in this condition and associated development in an autoimmune context.

Specific herbal medicines

BACOPA MONNIERI (BACOPA)

Bacopa monnieri exhibits many actions that are desirable for therapeutic application in the hypothyroid patient including cognition enhancing, nervine tonifying and possible adaptogenic activity. In mice models *B. monnieri* was found to exhibit thyroid-stimulating abilities through an increase of T_4 serum concentrations without any increase in T_3. The authors conclude that since only T_4, and not T_3, was enhanced by *B. monnieri*, it appears that the plant extract might be stimulating the synthesis and/or release of T_4 directly at the glandular level but not through the peripheral conversion of T_4 to T_3.[156] Currently there are no human studies evaluating the efficacy of *B. monnieri* in hypothyroid patients.

WITHANIA SOMNIFERA (ASHWAGANDHA)

Data from animal studies suggest that *Withania somnifera* is able to increase serum concentrations of thyroid hormones, thereby stimulating thyroid function. In female rats daily administration of *Withania somnifera* root extract (1.4 g/kg body weight) for 20 days enhanced serum concentrations of T_4; however, it produced no significant changes to T_3.[157] The same study found that *Withania somnifera* also increased hepatic activity of glucose-6-phosphatase (Glc-6-Pase), an enzyme involved in energy production influenced by thyroid activity. A randomised controlled study on the use of *Withania somnifera* in patients with bipolar disorder found, as a secondary outcome to the study, that supplementation with *Withania somnifera* elevated T4 levels.[158] While these results are promising, further studies are required with a larger sample size in a non-bipolar population.

Withania is also a gentle adaptogen and tonic indicated to enhance immune function, making it useful for the treatment of hypothyroidism. It is traditionally used in Ayurveda for promoting growth in children, improving general debility, aiding recovery from illness, assisting in loss of muscular energy and promoting learning and memory retrieval. It is also said to 'provide fresh energy and vigour in a system worn out by any constitutional disease'.

FUCUS VESICULOSUS (BLADDERWRACK)

Fucus vesiculosis is a type of seaweed and is known as a thyroid stimulant due to its ability to stimulate production of thyroxine and increase basal metabolism. *Fucus vesiculosis* was used to treat goitre after it was identified to contain high amounts of iodine. The British Herbal Pharmacopoeia advocates the use of *Fucus vesiculosis* for underactive thyroid glands (hypothyroidism) and goitre.[159] Organic iodine, such as that found in bladderwrack, is better utilised by the body in terms of bioavailability and less likely to be excreted than potassium iodide.

COLEUS FORSKOHLII (COLEUS)

Forskolin, the active constituent derived from the roots of *Coleus forskohlii*, is known to assist in the maintenance of a healthy metabolism due to its beneficial effect on cyclic adenosine monophosphate (cAMP) levels in many systems of the body including endocrine tissues such as the thyroid gland.[160] Forskolin has been found to increase thyroid hormone production and may have many similar effects on the thyroid gland to TSH leading to its reputation as a thyroid stimulant. Recommended dosage is 50–100 mg two to three times per day; [161] however, dosages of up to 250 mg two times a day have been shown to be well tolerated with no apparent adverse effects.[162]

GENTIANA LUTEA (GENTIAN)

In hypothyroidism the healthy function of the gastrointestinal system is seemingly compromised. Sluggish intestinal motility, constipation and abdominal distension are all gastrointestinal symptoms that have been observed; in fact in one study 50% of patients with hypothyroidism were shown to have delayed gastric emptying.[163] *Gentiana lutea* is a bitter herb that may be well utilised in hypothyroidism due to its traditional application[164] for ailments of the gastrointestinal system. *Gentiana lutea* has the ability to stimulate digestive function. The principles responsible for its bitter property have been identified as secoiridoid compounds and include amarogentin, gentiopicroside and swertiamarine; these act as digestive/appetite stimulants[165] and thus increase the absorption and assimilation of nutrients.

VITEX AGNUS-CASTUS (CHASTE TREE)

Regulation of thyroid hormone synthesis is complex and involves the thyroid, pituitary, brain and peripheral tissues. *Vitex agnus-castus* contains constituents that act on the pituitary gland, the body's master gland that produces hormones and from its location at the base of the brain directs the other endocrine glands to produce hormones. Since hypothyroidism is a disorder of the hypothalamic–pituitary tract this provides a basis for its prescription in the treatment of suboptimal thyroid function.

Thyroid autoimmunity may be increased among infertile women (particularly those with endometriosis or ovarian dysfunction).[166] Hypothyroidism has the ability to influence a woman's fertility through its effects on ovarian function where it may reduce levels of sex hormone-binding globulin while increasing secretion of prolactin.[166] Corpus luteum insufficiency is a manifestation of ovarian dysfunction and is characterised by abnormally low progesterone levels. Abnormalities of other hormones have also been associated with corpus luteum insufficiency including an amplified response to the thyroid-releasing hormone (TRH) test associated with hypothyroidism.[167] Clinical studies reveal the efficacy of *Vitex agnus-castus* in the regulation of the reproductive hormones involved in ovulation, cycle balance and menstrual regularity.[168–170] *Vitex agnus-castus* appears to exert its effects via a hormonal cascade within the body termed the hypothalamic–pituitary–ovarian axis.[171] This secretes hormones or triggers other areas of the body to release hormones. *Vitex agnus-castus* inhibits prolactin release from the anterior pituitary and has been shown to increase levels of luteinising hormone while suppressing the secretion of follicle-stimulating hormone.

NIGELLA SATIVA (BLACK CUMIN)

The seeds of *Nigella sativa* and their oil have been widely used for centuries in the treatment of various ailments throughout the world. And it is an important drug in the Indian traditional systems of medicine like Unani and

Ayurveda. Among people of Islamic background, it is considered one of the greatest forms of healing medicine available because it was mentioned that black seed is the remedy for all diseases except death in one of the Prophetic hadith. It is also recommended for use on a regular basis in *Tibb-e-Nabawi* (Prophetic medicine). It has been extensively studied and exhibits many pharmacological actions including antidiabetic, anticancer, immunomodulator, analgesic, antimicrobial, anti-inflammatory, spasmolytic, bronchodilator, hepatoprotective, renal protective, gastroprotective, and antioxidant.

Supplementation (1 g of black powder) b.i.d. over a period of 8 weeks in conjunction with L-T_4 therapy in patients with Hashimoto's thyroiditis, resulted in a significant decrease in TSH, IL-23 and anti-TPO levels, and an increase in free T_3 and free T_4 levels.[172] The major component of *N. sativa* is thymoquinone, which has cytoprotective and antioxidant actions, as well as anti-inflammatory.[173]

LIFESTYLE RECOMMENDATIONS

Exercise is particularly important in the treatment of hypothyroidism. Exercise stimulates thyroid gland secretion and increases tissue sensitivity to thyroid hormone. Many of the health benefits of exercise may be a result of improved thyroid function.

The health benefits of exercise are especially important in overweight hypothyroid individuals who are dieting. A consistent effect of dieting is a decrease in the metabolic rate as the body strives to conserve fuel. Exercise has been shown to prevent the decline in metabolic rate in response to dieting.

Invigorating activity such as water sports, avoidance of overheated environments, and cold hydrotherapy can stimulate thyroid function.

Interaction between thyroxine, iodine, iodine-rich food sources and bladderwrack

It is imperative to work closely with the patient's endocrinologist (or GP) if concurrent iodine or bladderwrack (*Fucus vesiculosis*) prescriptions are considered. Bladderwrack preparations contain a maximum daily dosage of 150 micrograms of iodine. Doses higher than 150 micrograms of iodine per day increase the risk of inducing hyperthyroidism. In rare cases allergic reactions involving serious overall effects may occur. This risk is similar to a prescription of iodine as a supplement or food at the same dose.

Thyroxine prescriptions contain iodine and will free additional iodine when it is converted to T_3. Any concurrent iodine source — either from iodine-rich foods, iodine supplementation or the herbal prescription of bladderwrack increases the risk of overload.

CASE STUDY

OVERVIEW

DD was a 32-year-old female presenting with fatigue, weight gain and depression. Subsequent questioning elicited constipation, dry skin and mucous membranes and a past history of two miscarriages (and two live births).

TREATMENT PROTOCOL

INITIAL APPOINTMENT

Initial assessment referred her for investigations, which produced the following results:

- TSH — 5.84 mU/L, fT_4 9.6 pmol/L, fT_3 3.0 pmol/L
- Ferritin — 10 micrograms/L, iron 12 umol/L, transferrin 2.3 g/L, TIBC (calc) 52 umol/L, saturation 10%
- Urinary iodine — 42 micrograms/L
- TPO Ab — 473 IU/mL
- Tg Ab — <20 IU/mL
- Vitamin D — 95 nmol/L.

On receipt of these results, the patient was advised to obtain a referral to an endocrinologist and a thyroid ultrasound was requested through her GP.

SECOND APPOINTMENT

The ultrasound was negative for any abnormalities, and the endocrinologist was comfortable to monitor progress and allow naturopathic treatment, with review in 6 weeks to ascertain if thyroxine prescription would be required following patient's request to focus solely on naturopathic treatment. The endocrinologist was aware of concurrent treatment at all times.

Naturopathic treatment began consisting of dietary and lifestyle changes, nutritional and herbal medicine prescriptions and counselling.

HERBAL MEDICINE

Herbal medicine	Ratio	Quantity	Rationale
Hypericum perforatum	STD	30 mL	Antidepressant, nervine tonic
Coleus forskohlii	1:1	70 mL	Thyroid stimulant, anti-obesity, digestive tonic, stimulates cAMP which acts as a second messenger for TSH
Hemidesmus indicus	1:2	60 mL	Immune modulating (suppressant)
Rehmannia glutinosa	1:2	60 mL	Anti-inflammatory, immune modulating, adaptogen, adrenal restorative
TOTAL: 220 mL			
Dose: 7.5 mL b.i.d.			

CASE STUDY CONTINUED

NUTRITIONAL MEDICINE

DIETARY

- Organic wholefood diet
- Avoidance of all goitrogen containing foods
- Encourage iodine rich food
- Daily intake of organic sea vegetables (arame, kombu, wakame, hijiki)
- Avoidance of sugar, caffeine, refined foods, preservatives, colourings, additives
- Increase dietary sources of essential fatty acids

SUPPLEMENTAL

Nutrient	Dosage	Rationale
Iodine	400 micrograms (initial dose, then reduced)	Address deficiency, formation of thyroid hormones
Selenium	200 micrograms/day	Antioxidant defence, synthesis of thyroid hormones, regulation of autoimmune process
Zinc	60 mg/day	Conversion of thyroxine to T_3, production of thyroid hormones, stabilisation of thyroid function and regulation of autoimmune process
Vitamin C	500–1000 mg b.i.d.	Immune modulation, antioxidant and reduction in free radical damage to thyroid gland
Vitamin B complex	1 cap b.i.d. (activated forms)	Address deficiencies, energy production and assistance in weight stabilisation
Iron	24 mg b.i.d. with protein-rich meal	Address deficiency, improve thyroid function
Tyrosine	1000 mg/d with review	Production of thyroid hormones and stabilisation of thyroid function

LIFESTYLE/EDUCATION

- Counselling and discussion surrounding previous miscarriages
- Stress management and relaxation
- Adequate sleep including afternoon naps
- Daily exercise of at least 30 minutes per day — starting with walking and increasing as energy increases

See the box on the interaction between thyroxine, iodine, iodine-rich food sources and bladderwrack for a full discussion. With this particular patient, the patient's endocrinologist was completely informed and involved in the patient's treatment

CASE STUDY CONTINUED

and closely monitored her thyroid function and iodine status to prevent any reaction. As soon as iodine status was replete and thyroid hormone levels stabilised, the prescription of thyroxine was no longer considered. The patient continued to maintain a dose-regulated iodine prescription with concurrent iodine and thyroid hormone level assessments.

HYPERTHYROIDISM

Fig. 21.5 illustrates the symptoms of hyperthyroidism.

Epidemiology

Australian statistics pertaining specifically to hyperthyroidism are lacking. According to the 2007–8 National Health Survey[174] from the Australian Bureau of Statistics, 64700 males and 421 700 females experience thyroid dysfunction in Australia; however, because these results do not differentiate between types of thyroid disorders it is impossible to know what percentage of these relate to a diagnosis of hyperthyroidism. We do know, however, that the most common cause of hyperthyroidism in Australia is Graves' disease.[175]

In the United States hyperthyroidism is present in 1.3% of the population (clinical, 0.5%; subclinical, 0.7%),[22] while in the UK a long-term study found that the incidence of hyperthyroidism was 0.8 per 1000 women annually.[176] Canadian statistics reveal a significantly higher incidence in women (2%) as compared with men (0.2%).[177]

A recent systematic international review indicated that the reported incidence of autoimmune hyperthyroidism ranged from 0.70/100 000/year (Black males) to

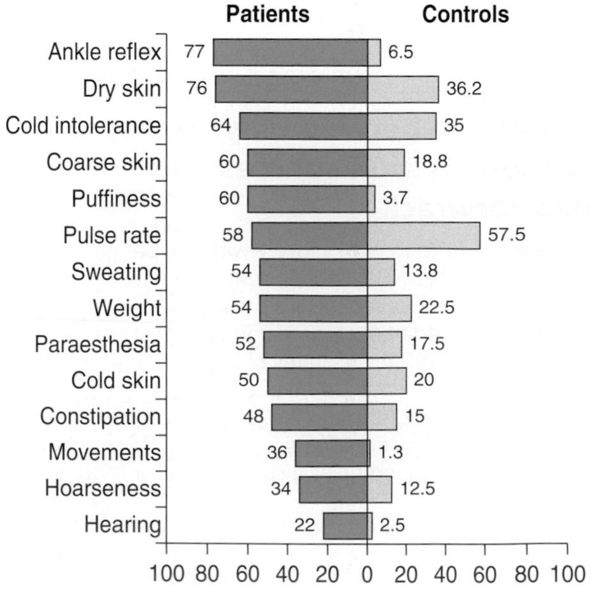

FIGURE 21.5 Symptoms of hyperthyroidism.

Source: Ferri F et al. Ferri's clinical advisor. St Louis: Mosby; 2011.

99/100 000/year (Caucasian females). Higher incidence rates were found in women compared with men for all types of autoimmune thyroid disease.[178]

Subclinical hyperthyroidism prevalence is estimated at 1–10% depending on the population studied. Prevalence increases with age.[179]

Classification

Hyperthyroidism is classified as a general or autoimmune type (Graves' disease). Due to the high prevalence of Graves' disease with any presentation (up to 85%), consideration of autoimmune factors will be discussed throughout.

Aetiology

Hyperthyroidism, also known as thyrotoxicosis, denotes a group of clinical disorders characterised by increased levels of free thyroxine, also known as tetraiodothyronine (T_4) and triiodothyronine (T_3).

Graves' disease, named after Dr Robert J Graves[180] (1830), is an autoimmune disease characterised by hyperthyroidism due to circulating autoantibodies. Thyrotrophin (TSH) receptor antibodies (TRAbs) bind to and activate thyrotrophin receptors, causing the thyroid gland to grow and the thyroid follicles to increase synthesis of thyroid hormone. It is a chronic inflammatory autoimmune disease of the thyroid resulting in excessive production of thyroxine and hyperthyroidism.

GENDER

The most obvious pattern is that of gender. Practically all the original cases described by Parry, von Basedow and Graves were women. As with most autoimmune diseases, susceptibility is increased in females. Hyperthyroidism due to Graves' disease has a female-to-male ratio of 7–8 : 1. The female-to-male ratio for pretibial myxoedema is 3.5 : 1. Only 7% of patients with localised myxoedema have thyroid acropachy. Unlike the other manifestations of Graves' disease, the female-to-male ratio for thyroid acropachy is 1 : 1 and the ratio of those with ophthalmic complications is about 1 : 1.

AGE

Typically, Graves' disease is a disease of young women, but it may occur in persons of any age. The typical age range is 20–40 years. Most affected women are aged 30–60 years.

STRESS

Stress can be a factor for thyroid autoimmunity. Recent stress has long been recognised as a precipitating factor for the development of Graves' disease. Studies now support the long-held observation that the onset of Graves' disease often follows some kind of emotional shock, in particular some sort of loss, such as divorce, death or difficult separations.

Acute stress-induced immunosuppression may be followed by immune system hyperactivity, which could precipitate autoimmune thyroid disease:

- This may occur during the postpartum period, in which Graves' disease may occur 3–9 months after delivery.
- Oestrogen may influence the immune system, particularly the B-cell repertoire.
- Both T- and B-cell function are diminished during pregnancy, and the rebound from this immunosuppression is thought to contribute to the development of postpartum thyroid syndrome.
- Experimental evidence suggests that androgens protect against, and oestrogens enhance, thyroiditis. The experimental results provide evidence for a major influence of sex steroids on the development of Graves' disease.
- Depression, inadequate rest and relaxation are all linked with increased stress levels and subsequent aggravation and development of the disease.

SMOKING

Cigarette smoking is a well-recognised risk factor of hyperthyroidism[181] and, particularly, Graves' ophthalmopathy. The effect of smoking is dose dependent and is more pronounced in women than in men.[182] Hence, germline polymorphisms of detoxification genes and genes belonging to the major DNA repair–apoptosis pathways might have an important role in disease susceptibility. In addition, as some of these genes are regulated by thyroid hormones, they may affect patient outcomes.

A recent prospective case-controlled study[183] identified an intriguing polymorphism linkage with smoking-related Graves' disease susceptibility. GSTP1, CYP1A1 and TP53 germline polymorphisms were found to be associated with smoking-related Graves' disease susceptibility and configure a risk profile for the disease. Of importance, these polymorphisms do not influence the patient's response to treatment.

GENETICS

Several autoimmune thyroid disease susceptibility genes have been identified: CD40, CTLA-4, thyroglobulin, TSH receptor, PTPN22 and FCRL3.[184] Some of these susceptibility genes are specific to either Graves' disease or Hashimoto's thyroiditis, while others confer susceptibility to both conditions. *HLA-DRB1* and *HLA-DQB1* also appear to be associated with Graves' disease susceptibility. Genetic factors contribute approximately 20–30% of overall disease susceptibility. Other identified polymorphisms associated with the development of Graves' disease include ESR2, PTPN22 and CTLA4 CT60 loci (OR ~ 1·7).[185] This research is in the developmental stage and thus is likely to evolve in the next few years when a conclusive diagnostic investigation may be determined.

Genetic regulation is a particularly important determinant of TSH and the fT4 × TSH product, and is a less important determinant of fT4 and fT3 concentrations determined in one fascinating twin study.[186] Data from a large well-characterised cohort suggest that while there is a strong heritable contribution to serum TSH, variation in fT4 and fT3 concentrations may be less explained by genetic factors and more driven by environmental effects than previously thought. The tight control of TSH has a strong heritable influence suggesting that the genetic predeterminance of developing either hyper- (or hypo-) thyroidism warrants regular and routine investigation of TSH in genetically susceptible individuals.

INFECTIVE ORGANISMS

Graves' disease has been associated with a variety of infectious agents such as *Yersinia enterocolitica* and *Borrelia burgdorferi*. Homologies have been shown between proteins of these organisms and thyroid autoantigens.[187,188] *Helicobacter pylori* is also associated with the onset and/or maintenance of Graves' disease.[189] In addition, it is important to consider the presence of low-grade chronic acute infections.

IATROGENIC

In older patients with hyperthyroidism, a toxic reaction to prescription drugs must be considered. The most common cause of hyperthyroidism in the elderly is a low intake of iodine and higher use of amiodarone (antiarrhythmic). In addition, symptoms of hyperthyroidism vary somewhat in older adults, with apathy, tachycardia and weight loss being more common.

DIGESTIVE FUNCTION

- Leaky GIT — food allergies/sensitivities, alcohol, NSAIDs, corticosteroids
- Microflora imbalance in GIT
- Poor digestion and elimination.

ENVIRONMENTAL TOXINS

- Chemical overload — food additives, agricultural chemical run-off, environmental pollutants, chemical exposure, household cleaners and sprays, herbicides and pesticides, hair dyes
  - Especially mercury and cadmium exposure
- Moderate alcohol consumption was found to be associated with reduced risk of Graves' disease with hyperthyroidism (irrespective of age and gender). The specific mechanism of action in Graves' hyperthyroidism is not known, but alcohol consumption appears to have a protective role in the development or autoimmune conditions in general.[190]

OTHER IMPORTANT FACTORS

- Left-handedness
- Excessive iodine supplementation
- Prevalence of hyperthyroidism was found to be higher in patients with major depressive disorder, particularly in females. Underlying aetiology is not known, but may be due to an autoimmune response.[191]

Overview

A hyperstimulated system and excessive levels of thyroid hormones will affect all bodily functions as thyroid gland hormones regulate metabolism in every cell of the body. The degree of severity of symptoms will vary. Autoimmune presentation will compound the manifestation of the disease progression. Consideration of autoimmune triggers and subsequent impact is essential.

Pathogenesis

In Graves' disease, B and T lymphocyte-mediated autoimmunity is known to be directed at four well-known thyroid antigens: thyroglobulin, thyroid peroxidase, sodium-iodide symporter and the thyrotrophin receptor. However, the thyrotrophin receptor is the primary autoantigen of Graves' disease and is responsible for the manifestation of hyperthyroidism. In this disease, the antibody and cell-mediated thyroid antigen-specific immune responses are well defined. Direct proof of an autoimmune disorder that is mediated by autoantibodies is the development of hyperthyroidism in healthy people by transferring thyrotrophin receptor antibodies in serum from patients with Graves' disease and the passive transfer of thyrotrophin receptor antibodies to the fetus in pregnant women.

The thyroid gland is under continuous stimulation by circulating autoantibodies against the thyrotrophin receptor, and pituitary thyrotrophin secretion is suppressed because of the increased production of thyroid hormones. The stimulating activity of thyrotrophin receptor antibodies is found mostly in the immunoglobulin G1 subclass. These thyroid-stimulating antibodies cause release of thyroid hormone and thyroglobulin that is mediated by 3′,5′-cyclic adenosine monophosphate (cyclic AMP), and they also stimulate iodine uptake, protein synthesis and thyroid gland growth.

SIGNS AND SYMPTOMS

See Table 21.15 for an outline of the major signs and symptoms of hyperthyroidism.

Clinical presentation

The typical clinical presentation of hyperthyroidism is a young adult female complaining of the following:

- Fatigue
- Frequent, loose stools (diarrhoea)
- Heat intolerance
- Insomnia
- Irritability
- Nervousness
- Palpitations and tachycardia
- Stare
- Sweating
- Tremor
- Weakness
- Weight loss despite a good appetite.

NOTE:

- Not all patients present with such classic features. A subset of patients with euthyroid Graves' disease can occur.
- In elderly individuals, fewer symptoms are apparent to the patient. Clues may include unexplained weight loss, hyperhidrosis or rapid heart beat.

TABLE 21.15 Signs and symptoms of hyperthyroidism

General	Fatigue, general weakness
Dermatological	Warm, moist, fine skin; sweating; fine hair; onycholysis; vitiligo; alopecia; pretibial myxoedema
Neuromuscular	Tremors, proximal muscle weakness, easy fatigability, periodic paralysis in persons of susceptible ethnic groups
Skeletal	Back pain, loss of stamina, history of fractures
Cardiovascular	Palpitations, dyspnoea on exertion, chest pain, oedema
Respiratory	Dyspnoea
Gastrointestinal	Increased bowel motility, hyperdefecation with or without diarrhoea
Ophthalmological	Tearing, gritty sensation in the eye, photophobia, eye pain, protruding eye, diplopia, visual loss
Renal	Polyuria, polydipsia
Haematological	Easy bruising
Metabolic	Heat intolerance, weight loss despite increased or similar appetite, worsening diabetes control
Endocrine/reproductive	Irregular menstrual periods, decreased menstrual volume, gynaecomastia, impotence
Psychiatric	Restlessness, anxiety, irritability, insomnia

Physical examination

See Table 21.16.

Other associated symptoms

Glucose intolerance, dyspnoea, polyuria and polydipsia, myopathy, paralysis, parkinsonian or choreoathetoid affect, diabetes mellitus, lung diseases[192] and others. Graves' disease, if left untreated, results in increased morbidity and mortality, primarily due to cardiovascular (atrial fibrillation, pulmonary hypertension, stroke and heart failure) and skeletal (osteoporosis) complications.[193] Subclinical hyperthyroidism is also associated with increased risk of coronary heart disease.[194] Hyperthyroidism is associated with accelerated bone turnover (two-fold) and a net loss of bone. Bone contains receptors for thyroid hormones and TSH and these hormones may act directly on osteoclasts and osteoblasts.[195]

Hyperthyroidism in adults is associated with mood symptoms and an increased risk of being hospitalised with psychiatric diagnoses.[196] High thyroid hormone levels can exert oestrogen-like effects, promoting breast cancer cell proliferation. Previous studies investigating the association of thyroid dysfunction and breast cancer have been inconclusive; however, a 2016 population-based cohort study in Denmark found an increased risk of breast cancer in women with a prior diagnosis of hyperthyroidism.[197]

TABLE 21.16 Physical examination in hyperthyroidism

General	Increased basal metabolic rate, weight loss despite increased or similar appetite, increased perspiration as a response to increased body temperature and heat intolerance
Skin	Warm, moist, finely textured skin; increased sweating; fine hair; vitiligo or pigment changes (especially to knuckes or skin creases); alopecia or thinning hair; pretibial myxoedema
Head, eyes, ears, nose, and throat	Chemosis, widening of the palpebral fissures, proptosis, impairment of extraocular motion, visual loss in severe optic nerve involvement, periorbital oedema, ophthalmopathy, mild proptosis, lid retraction, lid lag, conjunctival irritation
Neck	Upon examination, the thyroid gland generally is diffusely enlarged and smooth; a well-delineated pyramidal lobe may be appreciated upon palpation; thyroid bruits and, rarely, thrills may be appreciated; thyroid nodules may be palpable
Cardiovascular	Gynaecomastia, tachypnoea, tachycardia (especially after exercise), loud heart sounds (often a systolic murmur), hyperdynamic praecordium, S3/S4 heart sounds, ectopic beats, irregular heart rate and rhythm
Abdomen	Hyperactive bowel sound
Extremities	Localised, non-pitting oedema typically occurs along the shins (myxoedema) but may occur elsewhere, generally on the extensor surfaces, and is often pruritic and red, acropahy, onycholysis
Neurological	Hand tremor (fine and usually bilateral), hyperactive deep tendon reflexes
Musculoskeletal	Kyphosis, lordosis, loss of height, proximal muscle weakness, hypokalaemic periodic paralysis in persons of susceptible ethnic groups
Psychiatric	Restlessness, anxiety, irritability, insomnia, depression

Infertility

Menstrual disturbances in hyperthyroidism were described by Von Basedow in 1840 and have been confirmed by other groups over time.[198] One study found menstrual irregularities in 64.7% of hyperthyroid women compared with 17.2% of healthy controls.[199] More recently, Krassas et al observed irregular cycles in 46 of 214 hyperthyroid women (21.5%): 24 had hypomenorrhoea, 15 polymenorrhoea, 5 oligomenorrhoea, 2 hypermenorrhoea and none had amenorrhoea. The prevalence of menstrual abnormalities was two-and-a-half times higher than in the control population (8.4%).[200] Usually, treatment corrects cycle changes observed with hyperthyroidism and the exact impact of hyperthyroidism on fertility remains ill-defined.[201]

Most studies on the prevalence of hyperthyroidism in infertility are derived from uncontrolled, retrospective cohort studies. One study showed that out of 53 hyperthyroid patients, 5.8% had primary or secondary infertility.[199]

Autoimmune thyroid disease (AITD) is the most common autoimmune disorder in the female population, affecting 5–10% of women of childbearing age and it is the most frequent cause of thyroid failure (subclinical and overt hyperthyroidism).[202,203A] AITD can be present without thyroid dysfunction and may thus be undiagnosed. There are numerous studies that examine the prevalence of AITD in patients with infertility. A difficulty arising from the interpretation of the available data is that studies are often of heterogeneous groups with infertility problems, of retrospective design and often no control data are available. Some variability between studies can further be explained by differences in sample size (small series), by differences of the assays used to detect AITD and different geographical locations of the studies. Overall the studies favour an increased prevalence of AITD in infertility clinics.

Due to the impact of thyroid antibodies on implantation and potential risk of miscarriage, all patients with autoimmune subtype should be appropriately assessed and managed to protect against any subsequent negative outcomes.

DIFFERENTIAL DIAGNOSIS (Table 21.17)

Graves' disease is the most common diagnosis of hyperthyroidism, but several other conditions present with a similar symptom picture.

Several types of thyroiditis cause hyperthyroidism including:

- Hashimoto's thyroiditis (early stage)
- Subacute thyroiditis
- Painless thyroiditis
- Radiation thyroiditis.

Hyperthyroidism can also result from exogenous causes including:

- Iatrogenic hyperthyroidism
- Factitious hyperthyroidism (often seen in dieters who are taking thyroxine for weight loss, iodinated contrast, amiodarone)
- Iodine-induced hyperthyroidism (Jod–Basdow disease)
- Drug-induced thyroiditis (e.g. amiodarone, interferon-alfa)
- Radiation-induced thyroiditis.

Toxic nodular goitres are another source of hyperthyroidism including:

- Toxic adenoma
- Multinodular goitre.

Other rare causes of hyperthyroidism include:

- Thyroid carcinoma
- Ectopic hyperthyroidism
- Trophoblastic tumours (hydatidiform mole, choriocarcinoma, embryonic carcinoma of the testes)
- Excessive thyroid-stimulating hormone (pituitary adenoma, non-neoplastic pituitary secretion of TSH)
- Struma ovarii
- Exogenous thyroid hormone (intentional or unintentional)
- Silent thyroiditis
- Postpartum thyroiditis
- Pituitary resistance to thyroid hormone
- Abnormal thyroid-binding protein (e.g. thyroxine autoantibodies, abnormal concentration or binding of thyroxine-binding globulin or transthyretin).

TABLE 21.17 Comparative table in hyperthyroidism

Graves' disease	Special features include a diffusely enlarged thyroid gland, thyroid bruits, ophthalmopathy, pretibial myxoedema, and the presence of thyroid-stimulating immunoglobulins (TSIs)
Subacute thyroiditis	Special features include a history of antecedent respiratory tract infection, neck tenderness, elevated sedimentation rate, low or absent radioactive iodine uptake, and a self-limited course
Silent thyroiditis	Special features include painless thyroiditis, which may be seen in postpartum women (postpartum thyroiditis); a self-limited course; and low radioiodine uptake
Multinodular toxic goitre	Special features include a propensity to occur in elderly individuals and multiple nodules palpated or observed after thyroid scanning
Toxic adenoma	Special features include a solitary palpable nodule and a hot nodule observed after thyroid scanning
Factitious thyrotoxicosis	Special features include no goitre, a low thyroglobulin level, and low radioiodine uptake
Iatrogenic thyrotoxicosis	The special feature is a history of thyroid hormone intake
Iodide-induced thyrotoxicosis	The special feature is a propensity to occur in patients with a history of nodular thyroid disease who have been exposed to iodine-containing contrast agents or drugs such as amiodarone
Thyrotrophin-secreting pituitary adenoma	Special features include inappropriately elevated or normal thyrotrophin levels in the setting of elevated free thyroxine (T_4) and free triiodothyronine (T_3) levels, evidence of other pituitary hormone deficiencies, elevated alpha subunit level, and compressive symptoms
Beta-human choriogonadotrophin-induced thyrotoxicosis	Special features include a positive pregnancy test result, a history of hydatidiform mole, choriocarcinoma, and embryonal carcinoma of the testis. Also, rarely, it may be observed in normal gestation

TABLE 21.18 Thyroid function tests in hyperthyroidism

Physiological state	Serum TSH	Serum T_4	Serum T_3	Free T_4	THBR (T_3 resin uptake)	24-h radioiodine uptake (thyroid)
Hyperthyroidism, untreated	Low	High	High	High	High	High
Hyperthyroidism, T_3 toxicosis	Low	Normal	High	High	Normal	Normal

NATUROPATHIC DIAGNOSIS

Because Graves' disease is an autoimmune disorder that also affects other organ systems, taking a careful patient history is essential to establish the diagnosis. In some cases, the history might suggest a triggering factor such as trauma to the thyroid (including surgery of the thyroid gland), percutaneous injection of ethanol and infarction of a thyroid adenoma. Other factors might include interferon (e.g. interferon beta-1b) or interleukin (IL-4) therapy.

Investigations

Although many tests are available, for the vast majority of cases a few simple tests will confirm the diagnosis (Table 21.18):

- Serum T_3, T_4, thyroid resin uptake, and free thyroxine (T_4) and free T_4 index are usually all elevated
- A reliable, sensitive TSH assay will show low levels, except in rare cases
- Thyroglobulin antibodies (Tg-Ab) or thyrotrophin (TSH) receptor antibodies (TRAbs) are present in 80% of cases of hyperthyroidism suggesting a high prevalence of Graves' disease.

Due to the frequency of Graves' disease, it is advisable to conduct laboratory TSH, T_3, T_4 and thyroid antibody assessments for all suspected presentations.

TSH (THYROTROPHIN)

As indicated in hypothyroidism, it is now recognised that the thyroid-stimulating hormone (thyrotrophin, TSH) measurement is a more sensitive test than free T_4 (fT4) for detecting both hypo- and hyperthyroidism. As a result, some countries (Australia included) now promote a TSH-first strategy for diagnosing thyroid dysfunction (provided that the TSH method has a functional sensitivity ≤0.02 mIU/l).[69] Clinicians are advised to select laboratories for investigations carefully and consistently use the same reference values. Specialists make a general recommendation that patients with TSH readings lower than 0.75 mIU/L (potential Graves' disease) be referred for antibody screening.

THYROID ANTIBODIES

As indicated in hypothyroidism, thyroid autoantibodies are proteins manufactured by the immune system that are directed against proteins in the thyroid.

Thyroglobulin antibodies (Tg-Ab)

Thyroglobulin (Tg) in serum is increased in almost all kinds of thyroid disease, including goitre and subacute thyroiditis, the concentrations overlapping with those in healthy individuals.[70] Tg influences the function and growth of the gland and plays a major role in the pathogenesis of hyperthyroidism. Please see earlier in 'Hypothyroidism' for a more detailed discussion.

Thyroperoxidase antibodies (TPO-Ab)

Thyroperoxidase (TPO) antibodies are typically elevated in Hashimoto's or Graves' disease.

Thyrotrophin (TSH) receptor antibodies (TRAbs)

Thyrotrophin receptor antibodies (TRAbs) are antibodies directed against TSH receptor protein — a protein found on thyroid cells. These antibodies include two main groups: thyroid-stimulating immunoglobulins (TSI) which are characteristic of Graves' disease; and thyrotrophin binding inhibitory immunoglobins (TBII) which compete with thyrotrophin (TSH) for binding to the receptor without necessarily leading to its stimulation. Elevations in TRAbs are a direct indicator of Graves' disease.

URINARY IODINE

The measurement of urinary iodine (UI) provides an approximation of dietary iodine intake. Approximately 90% of iodine is excreted in the urine,[72] and measuring urinary iodine concentration usually assesses iodine status. Due to iodine's involvement in T_3 and T_4 synthesis and its effect on hyperthyroid symptoms and presentation it is essential to assess levels and amend dietary (and supplemental) intake as necessary.

IMAGING STUDIES

Radioactive iodine scanning and measurements of iodine uptake are useful in differentiating the causes of hyperthyroidism. In Graves' disease, the radioactive iodine uptake is increased and the uptake is diffusely distributed over the entire gland.

Ultrasounds with colour Doppler evaluation have been found to be cost-effective and should be performed as a first step in all hyperthyroid patients; scintigraphic examination should be limited to the uncommon cases in which the physician's observation, laboratory assays and/or ultrasounds are not diagnostic.

Computed tomography scanning or magnetic resonance imaging (of the orbits) may be necessary in the evaluation of proptosis. If routinely performed, most patients have evidence of orbitopathy, such as an increased volume of extraocular muscles and/or retrobulbar connective tissue. These techniques are useful to monitor changes over time or to ascertain the effects of treatment.

SPECIFIC NATUROPATHIC INVESTIGATIONS

Stress profile and cortisol levels

As stress is a major contributor to the development of Graves' disease, a stress profile and cortisol assessment is warranted. 24-hour urinary cortisol or adrenal hormonal profile (salivary) is the best initial assessment.

Antioxidant status

Due to the increased production of oxidation, assessment and determination of antioxidant nutrients is applicable to accurately determine dosages for prescriptions. Appropriate investigations are fat-soluble vitamin profile (serum), nutrient and toxic element assessment (erythrocyte and whole blood or hair) or Organix profiles (urine).

Environmental toxicities

Due to the potential impact of environmental toxins and heavy metal exposure and subsequent development of both hyperthyroid presentation and autoimmune subtype, it is essential to accurately determine the toxin load of the patient and to ensure appropriate nutritional chelation is conducted for efficacious outcome. Assessments may include a porphyrin profile (urine), chlorinated pesticides (blood), volatile solvents (blood), PCBs (serum) or nutrient levels — toxic and nutritional (hair). Individual heavy metal screening via urine or blood is dependent on active chelation — active excretion phase (urine) and current exposure (blood). A urinary chelation challenge test may be more appropriate.

Therapeutic considerations

CLINICAL DECISION MAKING AND RATIONALE

- Prime objective is to integrate treatment with allopathic interventions. Complementary approach may be primary strategy due to necessity for medication for some patients
- Reduction and alleviation of presenting symptoms
- Support for and re-establishment of normal thyroid status and function
- Reduction in free radical damage and appropriate antioxidant support
- Restoration of depletion due to overfunctioning systems.

Therapeutic application

HISTORICAL PERSPECTIVE

Though the endocrine system as we know it today had not yet been discovered, the Eclectics recognised 'exophthalmic goitre' (said to be synonymous with Graves' disease) as a condition in its own right. Ellingwood (1910) places the condition in his materia medica within the chapter 'Diseases of the blood, lymphatic system and ductless glands'. Ever insightful, he recognised the concurrent involvement of the nervous and gastrointestinal systems though he realised that these were distinct from the pathogenesis of goitre. Furthermore he acknowledged the role of stress in the pathogenesis of hyperthyroidism, writing:

> *It occurs in young women who are very sensitive and inclined to be slightly neurotic, who have much responsibility, anxiety and worry, and at the same time whose labor requires severe mental action or mental concentration.*[10]

Thomas (1907) also implicates stress and the involvement of the nervous system, writing:

> *Of the exciting causes no specific factor has been found, though nearly all writers agree that wrongs either of the cerebro-spinal or sympathetic system of nerves lie at the foundation of the disease. Thus great and prolonged worry, excessive grief, anger, or fright, excessive mental or physical exertion, and severe shock precede the disease.*[75]

These traditional observations and recognition of the involvement of the nervous system highlight the importance today of the application of botanicals and nutritionals that work on the nervous system in the prevention of thyroid dysfunction.

In a manner similar to today's naturopaths who prescribe relaxants, the Eclectics employed 'heart sedatives' such as *Lycopus* and *Veratrum* to ease symptoms. They also advocated the use of mistletoe for its effects on the heart (which today is scheduled). Lymphatic herbs such as echinacea and *Phytolacca* were also employed to regulate metabolism, a seemingly different use from those we have today. Interestingly the Eclectics also suggest the use of *Fucus vesiculosus* as they believed it to directly affect several of the existing conditions. Today *Fucus vesiculosus* is not a first-line treatment for Graves' disease; however, it does have many merits in the treatment of goitre. Lastly, and most definitely contraindicated today, the Eclectics advocated the use of electricity for the treatment of 'exophthalmic goitre' ... but cautioned that its stimulating influence must be guarded against!

NATUROPATHIC PERSPECTIVE

Due to the complex hyperstimulation of the patient's systems, comprehensive holistic treatment is required. Support for all effective systems by rebuilding and restoring them and restrengthening the patient, is important. Ascertaining triggers and causative agents and modifying treatment is understandably the prime objective.

As autoimmune Graves' disease is especially prevalent, as per other autoimmune conditions food elimination, detoxification, stress management and digestive healing options may be useful treatments aimed at ameliorating a possible root factor of antigenic autoimmune activity. Autoimmune support focusing on immune modulation through nutritional and botanical treatments is advisable, as well as avoidance of gluten-containing foods if indicated. Thorough investigations to ascertain if environmental toxins are causative triggers are also indicated.

NUTRITIONAL MEDICINE (DIETARY)

Dietary inclusions

- Due to increased metabolic rate and elimination, the diet should be nutritionally dense, high protein and have high kilojoule content.
- Patients should be asked to eat small frequent meals throughout the day.

Specific dietary treatments

PROTEIN

If the patient is significantly deficient protein requirements should be assessed on a kilojoule basis and supplemented if dietary intake is inadequate or too challenging to restore. Due to high energy output, normal requirements of 0.8–1.0 g/kg should be increased to at least 1.2 g/kg and up to 1.4 or 1.6 g/kg depending on the presentation.

DIETARY GOITROGENS

As previously discussed in the section on hypothyroidism, there are some foods (isothiocyanate foods) which contain goitrogenic substances that prevent the utilisation of iodine. These substances have been shown to be similar in action and structure to propylthiouracil (thionamide drug used to treat hyperthyroidism). The quantity required to provide a strong therapeutic effect is marked and due to the low goitrogen content, unreliable in lieu of medication. Foods need to be consumed in their raw state (goitrogenic substances inactivated by cooking). Of prime importance is to establish iodine status as naturally occurring goitrogens rely on this interaction. Iodine-rich foods need to be discouraged. A typical prescription is to encourage the *Brassica* family (especially raw cabbage) and raw soy milk (watch for kombu and iodine content). Homemade soy milk is preferred to store-bought soy milk.

Dietary exclusions

All stimulants, including caffeine, sugar, alcohol and other damaging foods should be avoided at all times.

A recent study found an association between vegetarian and vegan diets and decreased prevalence of hyperthyroidism. Results were more pronounced in a vegan diet (half the risk of an omnivore diet), and a vegetarian diet was found to have a moderate effect on hyperthyroidism risk. Semi-vegetarian diets did not offer any reduced risk. Possible explanations for this association are the lower BMI found in plant-based diets, and the increased antioxidant intake, a protective factor against autoimmune disease.[202]

NUTRITIONAL MEDICINE (SUPPLEMENTAL)

Nutritional medicine therapeutic objectives

With the increased metabolic activity in hyperthyroidism, the best nutritional approach, apart from recommending goitrogens such as coleslaw in the diet, is to support the overactive metabolism. The higher metabolic rate increases oxidative stress, and antioxidants would be well advised.[203A] Both endogenous (such as superoxide dismutase, glutathione peroxidise, catalase and nitric oxide synthase) and exogenous (such as vitamins A, C, E, selenium, zinc, R-alpha lipoic acid, *N*-acetylcysteine, coenzyme Q10) antioxidant systems are drawn upon with increased inflammation.[203A] For instance, oxidative damage has been found in hyperthyroid patients, and vitamin C, supplemented at 1000 mg per day, has shown an improved antioxidant capacity.[203B]

The autoimmunity encountered in Graves' disease (see also the section on hypothyroidism and autoimmune conditions) requires treatment with anti-inflammatory compounds, such as flavonoids and antioxidants.[203A] One feature of autoimmune diseases is enhanced angiogenesis, and flavonoids have proved to be of use in controlling this.[204] In the mouse model, conflicting evidence was obtained. One study found beneficial effects from quercetin treatment in Th1-mediated autoimmunity,[205] whereas another study showed delayed recovery in autoimmunity after flavonoid therapy.[206] However, Ma et al provide convincing evidence that antioxidants and flavonoids (such as quercetin) are of help in any inflammatory condition, including autoimmunity.[203A]

With the increased metabolic rate encountered in hyperthyroidism, energy production is upregulated. One explanation for this is the discovery that hyperthyroid patients have significant (three-fold) increased brown adipose tissue glucose uptake as well as a 90% increase in skeletal glucose uptake. Brown adipose tissue is metabolically active and involved in the regulation of energy expenditure. It was also found that hyperthyroid patients have a significantly higher lipid oxidation rate, and use more lipids for energy production in preference to carbohydrates.[207] To keep up with the additional demands it would be prudent to provide nutritional support for the Krebs cycle and oxidative phosphorylation (electron transport chain). Nutrients involved in these pathways include the B vitamins, magnesium, coenzyme Q10 and carnitine.[77,208] Other nutrients may also be affected, and regular testing is advisable. Thyroid function is associated with dyslipidaemia and altered mineral metabolism. One study found that total cholesterol levels are reduced in hyperthyroidism, as well as potassium and magnesium levels. Serum calcium and phosphate were increased. It would be prudent to check mineral profiles in patients with hyperthyroidism and try to normalise them through diet and/or supplementation.[209]

Specific nutrients required

VITAMIN A

Vitamin A is vital for healthy thyroid function. Deficiency is common in thyroid disorders. From 190 goitrous patients (106 euthyroid, 53 hyperthyroid, 31 hypothyroid) serum levels of vitamin A were obtained. The serum levels of vitamin A were significantly decreased in both hyperthyroidism and hypothyroidism.[210]

VITAMIN C

The application of vitamin C in patients with hyperthyroidism is likely to provide much needed antioxidant support. As free radicals and oxidative stress

SAMPLE DAILY DIET

BREAKFAST	
Green smoothie: kale, rocket, Brazil nuts, hemp protein powder, 2 ripe bananas, 4 dates, tahini, ½ an avocado	The smoothie provides nutritive fats, protein and carbohydrates to sustain the increased nutritional requirements needed by the body due to hypermetabolism. Nuts, dates, avocado and tahini can be added to increase kilojoule content to reduce weight loss. It is estimated that energy requirements may need to increase by up to 10–30% in mild cases and up to 60% in severe cases. Brazil nuts provide a source of selenium which is essential for thyroid hormone synthesis and function. Selenium has been shown to downregulate thyroid antibodies in Graves' disease.
LUNCH	
Stir-fried vegetables: bok choy, choy sum, broccoli, carrots, snow peas with marinated tempeh. Serve with basmati rice	Overall and throughout the day the diet contains a large variety of cruciferous vegetables including kale, rocket, Asian greens, broccoli, cabbage and Brussels sprouts. Small quantities of cruciferous vegetables in isolation are unlikely to suppress thyroid function; however, when consumed in large quantities over the day, they are likely to contain sufficient goitrin to potentially decrease iodine uptake by the thyroid, assisting in reducing thyroid function. The addition of basmati rice provides a low GI source of carbohydrates to support energy levels.
DINNER	
Home-made slaw: red and green cabbage, shaved Brussels sprouts dressed in tahini, served with marinated tofu, quinoa and guacamole	Soybean-related foods such as tempeh and tofu contain goitrogens, which interfere with thyroid hormone production or utilisation, thus may be useful to slow down thyroid function. Due to the widespread inflammation that exists with hyperthyroidism a variety of vegetables are included to maximise intake of phytochemicals with anti-inflammatory and antioxidant properties. These also support immunity should an infection be involved in the development of autoimmunity due to molecular mimicry. Wholegrains such as quinoa are a source of B vitamins to support adaption stress. Psychological stress, both acute and chronic, may precipitate Graves' disease by suppressing the immune system.
SNACK	
Blueberries plus carrot juice	Though no studies exist, blueberries and carrots contain constituents that have an affinity for the eye thus it is hypothesised that these may be useful to minimise damage as a result of Graves' ophthalmopathy.

have been implicated as playing a role in hypothyroidism, the same is true for hyperthyroidism, hence the application of antioxidant vitamin C. Animal studies examining the effects of vitamin C on plasma lipid peroxidation and the susceptibility of apolipoprotein B-containing lipoproteins to oxidation in experimental hyperthyroidism found an increased susceptibility of apo B-containing lipoproteins to oxidation in hyperthyroidism; however, vitamin C supplementation protected these lipoproteins from copper-induced oxidation.[211]

VITAMIN E

As with vitamin C above, vitamin E is employed in hyperthyroidism in an attempt to decrease oxidative stress due to its antioxidant activity.[212] The application of antioxidants such as vitamin E is imperative as normal antioxidant mechanisms appear to be defective or unable to cope with the amount of free radicals being generated. Elevated circulating levels of thyroid hormones are associated with tissue oxidative injury, and a review of available evidence found that vitamin E supplementation is able to reduce this oxidative stress and its consequences.[213]

SELENIUM

Patients with newly diagnosed Graves' disease had lower serum selenium levels than in controls, supporting a hypothetical link between selenium deficiency and Graves' disease.[214] Deficiency of selenium has been theorised to influence the generation of free radicals, the conversion of thyroxine (T_4) to T_3 and a thyroidal autoimmune process.[215] A small clinical trial concluded that high serum selenium levels (>120 micrograms/L) may influence the outcome of Graves' disease, supporting the idea of a positive effect of selenium on thyroidal autoimmune processes.[216] Clinical evidence supports the view that selenium prescriptions regulate thyroid antibodies. A small randomised clinical trial found that supplementation with selenium in conjunction with methimazole treatment did not confer any additional benefits in the short-term control of Graves' disease; however, selenium supplementation is still beneficial in patients who are selenium deficient and it may have a role to play in long-term antithyroid treatment.[217] A randomised double-blind placebo-controlled study of 159 patients with mild Graves' orbitopathy showed that supplementation with sodium selenium (100 micrograms b.i.d) for 6 months significantly improved quality of life, slowed the progression of the disease and reduced the ocular symptoms.[218] A study in Australia of 198 patients with Graves' disease (101 of whom had Graves' orbitopathy) found that patients with orbitopathy had lower serum selenium levels than those with Graves' disease without orbitopathy.[219] These results are in contradiction to another study of 84 Graves' orbitopathy (or ophthalmopathy) patients in which no association was found between disease severity or activity and selenium levels.[220]

ZINC

Marked alterations of zinc homeostasis have been observed in patients with hyperthyroidism. Researchers assessing hyperthyroid patients to evaluate their ability to metabolise zinc found plasma zinc concentration to be normal; however, red blood cell zinc content was significantly lower in hyperthyroid patients and was inversely related to plasma thyroxine concentration. The hyperthyroid patients also excreted significantly greater amounts of zinc than controls, indicative of a catabolic process.[221]

VITAMIN D

Low serum vitamin D status is associated with the development of autoimmune diseases, particularly hyperthyroidism and new-onset Graves' disease.[222,223] Vitamin D status is not changed by the treatment of Graves' disease; therefore it is likely that low vitamin D status favours the onset of the disease.[224] Furthermore, it was found that patients with higher vitamin D status had increased rates of remission.[225] Both of these observations are based on small studies and further research is required before definitive clinical implications can be determined.[226]

In people with malabsorption conditions, including those suffering from hyperthyroidism (due to increased metabolic rate and systemic functioning), vitamin D supplementation is recommended to maintain bone mineral density and to normalise circulating vitamin D concentrations. Adequate vitamin D is required to upregulate calcium absorption during these times of increased demand. Vitamin D also has other roles within the body, specifically immune function support and immune modulation in instances of autoimmunity. Data from supplementation studies indicate that vitamin D intakes of at least 800–1000 IU/day are required by adults living in temperate latitudes to achieve serum 25(OH)D levels of at least 80 nmol/L. It is prudent to assess vitamin D status in hyperthyroid patients prior to increasing prescription; however, it can be expected that doses of greater than 4000 IU may be required.

COENZYME Q10

Coenzyme Q10 (CoQ_{10}) has multiple applications for the management of hyperthyroidism. In its role as an antioxidant it helps to prevent oxidative stress to the thyroid gland. In its involvement in electron transport in the respiratory chain it is involved in production of energy to the mitochondria of the cells. And it may be used to reduce cardiovascular risk common in hyperthyroid patients.

Low serum levels of CoQ_{10} have been found in thyrotoxic patients and as a result congestive heart failure is a risk. Mancini et al report that CoQ_{10} levels in hyperthyroid patients were the lowest reported in different human diseases. This could be due to increased utilisation (due to increased metabolic demand), increased degradation, or decreased carriers in the serum (VLDL release from the liver is decreased in hyperthyroidism).[227] A dose of 120 mg of CoQ_{10} administered daily for 1 week to 12 hyperthyroid patients was found to produce a positive change in cardiac performance. The authors concluded that CoQ_{10} has a therapeutic value for congestive heart failure induced by severe thyrotoxicosis.[228]

MAGNESIUM

Magnesium is fundamental for healthy nerve conduction and muscular contraction and relaxation, while being intricately involved in normal healthy heart rhythm, important factors in the hyperthyroid patient. Magnesium is also required for cellular metabolism where it is involved in energy production for the body. Patients with hyperthyroidism are at increased risk of magnesium deficiency[229] and disturbances in magnesium metabolism are common in most hyperthyroid patients.[230] Supplementation is likely to aid hyperthyroid symptoms such as tremors and muscular aches which are also magnesium deficiency symptoms.

B COMPLEX (ALL B VITAMINS)

B vitamins may assist in supporting the body during times of physical and mental stress; they also play an important role in relieving and preventing nervous tension and mild anxiety. Deficiencies of B vitamins have been linked to nervous and psychological disorders such as anxiety and mild depression, both of which present in hyperthyroidism. The B vitamins are required for the metabolism and production of energy from food, which in turn contributes to the overall energy levels of an individual. Exhaustion and feeling tired quickly (fickle energy) are a common complaint of the hyperthyroid patient, even after they go into remission, with 53% of patients reporting a lack of energy.[231] Logic tells us that in hyperthyroidism due to increased demands on the body and concurrent malabsorption, requirements for the B vitamins are likely to be increased.

QUERCETIN AND BIOFLAVONOIDS

Plasma total antioxidant capacity in patients with Graves' disease has been found to be significantly lower than that in healthy persons while DNA damage has been found to be higher. After treatment with melatonin, quercetin or *N*-acetylcysteine for 4 h in vitro, DNA damage in lymphocytes in Graves' disease patients declined significantly. While these results were undertaken in vitro they provide a rationale for the use of antioxidants such as quercetin and *N*-acetylcysteine in Graves' disease patients.[232]

ESSENTIAL FATTY ACIDS

Alterations in thyroid function are associated with low-grade inflammation.[233] Omega-3 fatty acids display anti-inflammatory activity and therefore may be indicated to reduce inflammation in hypothyroidism. Furthermore omega-3 fatty acids are also cardioprotective and thus may be beneficial for the cardiovascular abnormalities that present in hyperthyroidism.

L-CARNITINE

L-carnitine may be effective in both reversing and preventing symptoms of hyperthyroidism. Studies suggest that L-carnitine may prevent thyroid hormone entry into certain areas of the body including the nucleus of hepatocytes, neurons, and fibroblasts.[234] Since hyperthyroidism depletes the body's regular stores of many nutrients, including L-carnitine, supplementation appears warranted (dose 1–2 g/day.)

R-ALPHA LIPOIC ACID

R-alpha lipoic acid is an antioxidant that has been found to decrease the risk of cell damage attributed to free radicals. R-alpha lipoic acid may be beneficial in conditions that are associated with oxidative stress; however, it also raises mitochondrial energy-producing capabilities of a cell by reversing the age-associated decline in mitochondrial enzyme activities and thereby protects mitochondria from ageing.

IODINE

Iodine is a highly controversial nutrient for hyperthyroidism. There are countless conflicting studies both supporting and refuting iodine's efficacy — primarily for the treatment of autoimmune Graves' disease. Therefore, prior to any prescriptions, it is essential that urinary iodine measurements be conducted and dietary review for iodine content established.

Caution

The effects of iodine in patients with hyperthyroidism can follow three distinct and unpredictable paths. Prescription of iodine in these instances is refuted and debatable and thorough investigations are essential.

1. Wolff–Chaikoff effect: in large doses, iodine temporarily reduces symptoms by stopping hormone synthesis.
2. Variation from Wolff–Chaikoff: the thyroid can remain suppressed or can eventually resume hormone synthesis at a reduced, former or even increased rate.
3. Jod–Basedow disease or normalisation to euthyroidic state: excess iodine can trigger hyperthyroidism in a euthyroid person or can trigger an overactive thyroid to return to normal.

Positive prescription?

A number of studies on the epidemiology of thyroid autoantibodies have been performed as descriptive studies in iodine-deficient areas (Table 21.19). Results from some population-based studies from both iodine-deficient and iodine-sufficient areas are shown in the table. The results are ambiguous. A number of studies suggest that the presence of a goitre is a cardinal diagnostic for the prescription.

Dosage requirements

The dosage requirements listed below are based on adult doses that have been reported in the literature:

- Vitamin A: 10000–20000 IU/day or beta-carotene — 6 mg/day[235]
- Vitamin C: 1000 mg/t.d.s.:[235]
  - Watch bowel tolerance and consider reducing to 500 mg t.d.s. and increasing slowly
- Vitamin E: 400–800 IU/day[235]
- Selenium: 60–200 micrograms/day[236,237]
- Zinc: 20–60 mg/day (increase for autoimmune presentation)
- Vitamin D: 1000–4000 IU/day (dependent on investigations and may require higher dose)
- Coenzyme Q10: 120–200 mg/day[228]
- Magnesium: 200–600 mg/day
- B complex (all B vitamins): high-dose combination, preferably activated forms:
  - Thiamine: 20–40 mg/day
  - Riboflavin: 20–40 mg/day
  - Niacinamide: 50–100 mg/day
  - Pantothenic acid: 150–300 mg/day
  - Pyridoxine: 20–60 mg/day
  - Folinic acid (or L5MTHF as indicated): 500–1000 micrograms/day
  - Hydroxocobalamin (or methylcobalamin as indicated): 500–1000 micrograms/day
  - Choline: 50–100 mg/day
  - Inositol: 50–100 mg/day
  - Biotin: 250–500 micrograms/day
- Quercetin and bioflavonoids: 500 mg b.i.d.
- Essential fatty acids: 2–4 g b.i.d.
- L-carnitine: 2–4 g/day[234]
- R-alpha lipoic acid: 50–400 mg/day.

Important note

Ensure that nutritional supplements are properly scrutinised for iodine content. Many multivitamin–mineral preparations (especially pregnancy formulations) contain supplemental iodine.

HERBAL MEDICINE

Herbal medicine therapeutic objectives

- To reduce thyroxine output from the thyroid gland
- To reduce the inflammatory process and the increased free radicals that result from inflammation
- To treat symptoms such as palpitations and restlessness
- To reduce the production of thyroid antibodies by regulating immune function (if autoimmune present).

TABLE 21.19 Thyroid autoantibodies in population studies from areas with different iodine intake

Author [country]	Iodine status	Antibody assays	Cutoff	Age (years)	Prevalence of antibody (%)
Laurberg et al. (1998) [Denmark]	Moderate ID	Tg-Ab: radioimmunoprecipitation	Detection limits	68	Tg-Ab: 31
		TPO-Ab: enzyme-linked immunosorbent assay			TPO-Ab: 29
Pedersen et al. (2003) [Denmark]	Moderate and mild ID	Tg-Ab: radioimmunoassay	Detection limits	18–65	Tg-Ab: 13.0
		TPO-Ab: radioimmunoassay			TPO-Ab: 13.1
Hintze et al. (1991) [Germany]	Mild ID	Tg-Ab: radioimmunoassay	Detection limits	60+	Tg-Ab: 10.1
		Mic-Ab: radioimmunoassay			Mic-Ab: 23.2
Knudsen et al. (1999) [Denmark]	Mild ID	TPO-Ab: enzyme linked immunosorbent assay	100 U/mL; detection limits not given	41 and 71 years	TPO-Ab: 22.8
Aghini-Lombardi et al. (1999) [Italy]	Mild ID	Tg-Ab: agglutination	≥1 : 100; detection limits not given	1+	Tg-Ab and/or TPO-Ab: 12.6
		TPO-Ab: agglutination			
Teng et al. (2006) [Panshan, China]	Mild ID	Tg-Ab: chemiluminescence	Detection limits	36±13(SD)	Tg-Ab: 9.0
		TPO-Ab: chemiluminescence			TPO-Ab: 9.2
Fenzi et al. (1986) [Italy]	Mild ID	Tg-Ab: agglutination	≥1 : 100; detection limits not given	Young adults	Tg-Ab and/or Mic-Ab: 14.4
		Mic-Ab: agglutination			
Hollowell et al. (1998) [United States]	Iodine sufficient	Tg-Ab: radioimmunoassay	Detection limits	12+	Tg-Ab: 11.5
		TPO-Ab: radioimmunoassay			TPO-Ab: 13.0
Bjøro et al. (2000) [Norway]	Iodine sufficient	TPO-Ab: luminoimmunoassay	200 U/mL; detection limits not given	40+	TPO-Ab: 9.7
Tunbridge et al. (1977) [UK]	Iodine sufficient	Tg-Ab: tanned red cell technique	Tg-Ab: ≥1 : 20	18+	Tg-Ab and/or Mic-Ab: 7.3
		Mic-Ab: microhaemagglutination	Mic-Ab: ≥1 : 100		
Bryhni et al. (1996) [Norway]	Iodine sufficient	Tg-Ab: agglutination	1 : 10 and 1 : 100; detection limits not given	34±8.4 (SD)	Tg-Ab: 2.8
		Mic-Ab: agglutination			Mic-Ab: 6.1
Laurberg et al. (1998) [Iceland]	Iodine sufficient	Tg-Ab: radioimmunoprecipitation	Detection limits	66–70	Tg-Ab: 13
		TPO-Ab: enzyme-linked immunosorbent			TPO-Ab: 18
Teng et al. (2006) [Zhangwu,China]	More than adequate	Tg-Ab: chemiluminescence	Detection limits	36±13 (SD)	Tg-Ab: 9.0
		TPO-Ab: chemiluminescence			TPO-Ab: 9.8

NOTE: Prevalence rates of TPO-Ab and/or Tg-Ab in populations with different iodine intake. All studies included both females and males. ID, iodine deficiency.

Adapted from Pedersen IB, Laurberg P. Comprehensive handbook of of iodine: nutritional biochemical, pathological and therapeutic aspects. Burlington: Elsevier; 2009, pp. 575–585.

Herbal medicine classes

ADAPTOGEN

Similarly to hypothyroidism, the importance of the impact of stress cannot be overestimated nor should it be ignored. The holistic practitioner is aware of the impact and potential damage stress can cause to a person. In addition, due to the typical preceding stressful trigger that initiates Graves' disease, a strong 'switch effect' for developing the autoimmune subtype is suggested.

The class of adaptogens offers much therapeutic merit. As the hypothyroid patient is already hyperstimulated, care needs to be taken to appropriately select the best herbal medicines. Generally avoidance of all stimulant adaptogens is recommended, including *Eleutherococcus senticosus* (Siberian ginseng), *Panax notoginseng* (Tienchi ginseng), *Panax quinquefolius* (American ginseng) or *Panax ginseng* (Korean ginseng). More appropriate prescriptions include *Withania somnifera* (ashwagandha) for the highly strung and overactive patient, *Ganoderma lucidum* (reishi) as a systemic tonic adaptogen or *Rhodiola rosea* (rhodiola) to regulate mood and modulate energy.

While not a clinically strong adaptogen, *Centella asiatica* (gotu kola) can offer systemic tonic and restorative functions specific to the musculoskeletal system and connective tissue. Because of the increased metabolic processing and lax ligament tension, this herbal medicine is appropriate for this condition.

ADRENAL RESTORATIVE

Rehmannia glutinosa (rehmannia) provides additional adrenal restorative support as well as autoimmune modulation, anti-inflammatory properties and is a general tonic. It is advisable to avoid *Glycyrrhiza glabra* (liquorice) due to its potential laxative and hypertensive effects.

THYROID SUPRESSANT/REGULATOR

The primary herbal medicine that provides this important function is *Lycopus* spp. (bugleweed). Traditional, scientific and clinical research supports this classification. The antithyroid activity of *Leonurus cardiaca* (motherwort) is less well supported in terms of research; however the German Commission E supports its prescription for hyperthyroidism. Traditional application focuses on support for the cardiovascular symptoms produced by hyperthyroidism such as tachycardia and palpitations. Strong clinical efficacy supports this prescription. *Melissa officinalis* (lemon balm) provides clinical support for anxiety, restlessness and associated digestive hyperactivity. The combination of three herbal medicines produces marked clinical outcome and is advisable as a primary component of any herbal medicine prescription.

TONIC (GENERAL)

Due to the depleted presentation, general tonic herbal medicines are indicated to rebuild and restore the system. Indicated herbal medicines include the mushrooms (*Ganoderma lucidum* (reishi), *Grifola frondosa* (maitake) and *Lentinus edodes* (shiitake)), *Avena sativa* (oats) and *Withania somnifera* (ashwagandha).

NERVINE TONIC

Tonification for the nervous system is especially important as the patient typically presents with insomnia, energy fluctuations and overstimulation. Systemic depletion is best treated with general nervine tonics including *Passiflora incarnata* (passion flower), *Avena sativa* (oats) or *Scutellaria lateriflora* (skullcap). If depression or preceding emotional trauma is present, *Hypericum perforatum* (St John's wort) or *Turnera diffusa* (damiana) is indicated. If insomnia and restlessness are strong, sedative hypnotics are warranted and effective. Clinically it is typical to find that strong sedatives are required to effectively 'slow' the patient.

IMMUNE SUPPORT

If the patient presents with frequent infections and lowered immune function, generally due to hyperstimulation, immune tonics are indicated and include *Andrographis paniculata* (andrographis), *Astragalus membranaceus* (astragalus) or *Echinacea* spp. (echinacea). It is advisable to avoid astragalus in cases of acute infection; however, Traditional Chinese Medicine does not adhere to this caution. Clinical expertise and assessment should enable accurate prescription.

If immune modulation is required (Graves' disease), herbal medicines including *Echinacea* spp. (echinacea), *Rehmannia glutinosa* (rehmannia), *Hemidesmus indicus* (hemidesmus), *Calendula officinalis* (calendula) and other similar herbal medicines are indicated.

ANTIOXIDANT

Due to the increased burden of free radical damage — both in the autoimmune type and general hyperthyroid patient — antioxidant herbal medicines should be encouraged to reduce the burden in the body. Important herbal medicines include *Crataegus* spp. (hawthorn leaves and berries), *Curcuma longa* (turmeric), *Ginkgo biloba* (ginkgo) or *Silybum marianum* (St Mary's thistle). St Mary's thistle has the added benefit of hepatotrophorestorative functions that assist with the hepatic clearance of increased hormonal production and free radical damage.

ANTI-INFLAMMATORY

Systemic inflammation is paramount to the presentation. Effective prescriptions include those that offer dual actions such as *Curcuma longa* — both a potent antioxidant and an anti-inflammatory; *Matricaria chamomilla* which provides both mild sedative, nervine tonic and anti-inflammatory properties; or if a female patient presents, *Dioscorea villosa* (wild yam) for hormonal support to regulate menstrual cycle or postmenopausal symptoms in addition to steroidal anti-inflammatory properties.

SYMPTOMATIC SUPPORT

Crataegus monogyna (hawthorn) and *Leonurus cardiaca* (motherwort) are specifically indicated to reduce palpitations and blood pressure and restore optimal cardiovascular function. As an antiarrhythmic, motherwort produces marked clinical outcome in a short period of time with patients experiencing calmness, centring and relief from internal anxiety. Additional anxiolytics may be warranted for extreme presentations. Efficacious prescriptions include *Piper methysticum* (kava), *Piscidia piscipula* (Jamaican dogwood) or *Scutellaria lateriflora* (skullcap).

Specific herbal medicines

AVENA SATIVA (OATS)

The excess of thyroid hormones in hyperthyroidism results in a hypermetabolic state and one in which the sympathetic nervous system goes into overdrive. This places stress upon the body and results in great fatigue and weakness for the person. *Avena sativa* has traditionally been used as a tonic for exhaustion and debility. The Eclectics considered it to be a mild stimulant and nerve tonic for use in nervous debility, and for affections bordering closely upon nervous prostration, saying 'It seemingly acts well ... where there is much nervous involvement and enfeebled action of the heart'.[238] Given the prevalence of these symptoms in hyperthyroid patients, the use of tonics such *Avena sativa* is recommended.

CRATAEGUS MONOGYNA (HAWTHORN)

Hyperthyroidism is characterised by widespread cardiovascular dysfunction manifesting as hyperdynamic circulation with increased cardiac output, increased heart rate, decreased peripheral resistance and increased oxidative stress.[239] Hawthorn is one of the oldest known medicinal plants used in European medicine and its cardiovascular benefits are well supported by both traditional and modern research. Hawthorn displays positive inotropic activity, improves coronary blood flow, increases the integrity of the blood vessel walls and improves the utilisation of energy[240] as well as having antioxidant and anti-inflammatory actions specific to the cardiovascular system. These actions make it the herb of choice for cardiovascular symptoms associated with hyperthyroid conditions.

CURCUMA LONGA (TURMERIC)

Curcumin (the primary active principle in turmeric, *Curcuma longa*) is an antioxidant and anti-inflammatory agent with phytonutrient and bioprotective properties that may be well used in the management of hyperthyroidism. Though no specific studies have been undertaken investigating the use of *Curcuma longa* in hyperthyroidism, this condition is characterised by widespread oxidative damage that results in damage to the thyroid gland and inflammation. Thus the application of *Curcuma longa* for its anti-inflammatory and antioxidant action is highly warranted.

IRIS VERSICOLOR (BLUE FLAG)

During the time of the Eclectic physicians, *Iris versicolor* was considered a specific herb to be employed for the treatment of goitre, particularly that which had recently presented. Ellingwood (1919) revealed his appreciation saying:

> *It is a favorite remedy in the treatment of enlargement of the thyroid and other glandular affections. In recent cases of goitre, iris is used to good advantage. With many, if used in the form of a recent preparation, it is believed to be specific ... They push it to a mild cathartic effect so that it will keep the bowels free.*[241]

This traditional application of *Iris versicolor* provides a novel way in which to prescribe as in modern naturopathy it is first and foremost prescribed for its depurative action.

LEONURUS CARDIACA (MOTHERWORT)

Leonurus cardiaca was traditionally employed by the Eclectics for nervous debility with irritation and unrest.[238] As the name suggests, *Leonurus cardiaca* exerts an effect on the heart, and is particularly efficacious where there are palpitations, such as in hyperthyroidism. The German Commission E approves the use of *Leonurus cardiaca* as an adjuvant therapy in the management of thyroid hyperfunction, a true sign of its efficacy.[242]

LITHOSPERMUM OFFICINALE (GROMWELL)

Lithospermum officinale is a botanical that has been found to exhibit antithyrotropic activity in animal studies. A study undertaken on rats given *Lithospermum officinale* cold-water freeze-dried extracts found that *Lithospermum officinale* significantly lowered thyroid hormone content in the serum.[243] Taken with the same authors' report of a goitre suppression test, in which the chronic administration of *Lithospermum officinale* freeze-dried extracts was found to suppress TSH levels resulting in reduced goitre weight, these findings suggest a possible role for the use of *Lithospermum officinale* in hyperthyroidism.

LYCOPUS SPP. (BUGLEWEED)

Lycopus spp. is a specific for hyperthyroidism. It has been shown to attach to the TSH receptor in the thyroid (inhibiting its effect), thereby reducing receptor binding of TSH receptor-stimulating IgE antibodies. This in turn reduces the output of thyroxine, reduces the conversion of T_4 to T_3 and inhibits peripheral T_3 formation.

Lycopus spp. has been used traditionally for cardiac palpitations. The Eclectics used it for thyroid conditions, stating: 'It has favorably influenced exophthalmic goiter'.[244] A prospective two-armed open study examining the effect of *Lycopus europaeus* on thyroid function and associated symptoms during a 3-month follow-up phase on a population of patients with a basal TSH <1.0 mU/L and hyperthyroidism-associated symptoms found that *Lycopus europaeus* increased urinary T_4 excretion.[245] Symptoms specific to the thyroid gland were diminished, for example increased heart rate in the morning. The authors concluded their findings confirm the positive effects of *Lycopus europaeus* in slight forms of hyperthyroidism. The German Commission E approves the use of *Lycopus* for mild thyroid dysfunction.

MELISSA OFFICINALIS (LEMON BALM)

In-vitro studies[246] reveal *Melissa officinalis* to be a thyroid-stimulating antagonist; however, little has been undertaken in the way of human clinical studies. *Melissa officinalis* may be utilised as a herbal remedy in the treatment of anxiety[247] and for mild depression. A high prevalence of mood disorders such as anxiety has been reported in hyperthyroid women[248] and symptoms of depression are also high and are estimated to occur in 40% of hyperthyroid patients.[249] This dual action of *Melissa officinalis* as a TSH antagonist and nervine tonic makes it highly indicated for the treatment of hyperthyroidism.

SCUTELLARIA LATERIFLORA (SKULLCAP)

Scutellaria lateriflora was used traditionally for disorders affecting the nervous system and in modern herbal medicine it has been investigated for this same purpose. A double-blind placebo-controlled crossover study of healthy adults ($n = 19$) revealed that skullcap dose-dependently reduced symptoms of anxiety and tension after acute administration compared with control.[250] This appears due to *Scutellaria*'s anxiolytic action. *Scutellaria* is therefore a useful addition to the herbalist's formula.

SILYBUM MARIANUM (ST MARY'S THISTLE)

The liver is frequently affected in hyperthyroid patients and relative hypoxia has been suggested as precipitating factor.[251] Liver function tests in hyperthyroid patients frequently present with abnormalities; in fact in one study as many as 46.9% of patients had at least one liver function abnormality detected.[251] *Silybum marianum* is a botanical that has been applied extensively in traditional and contemporary herbalism for disorders affecting the liver. The ability of *Silybum marianum* to enhance the antioxidant ability of the hepatocytes, to counteract oxidative stress and contribute to blocking liver disease provides good reasoning for its application in hyperthyroid patients who show signs of liver dysfunction.

VALERIANA OFFICINALIS (VALERIAN)

Hyperthyroidism causes a wide array of actions that negatively affect the nervous system; as a result symptoms associated with the nervous system such as anxiety and alterations in normal sleep patterns commonly afflict the hyperthyroid patient.[252] It is also interesting to note that a percentage of patients still continue to have sleep disturbances and neuropsychological deficits after they are diagnosed as euthyroid.[231] In these instances, the application of *Valeriana officinalis*, a mild sedative, relaxant and anxiolytic, may be useful. *Valeriana officinalis* has been used traditionally to calm the body and mind, with the Eclectics stating it to be: 'One of the best of calmatives for that collective condition termed "nervousness"'.

LIFESTYLE RECOMMENDATIONS

Stress reduction

The most important recommendation is for patients to avoid all forms of stress and triggers for agitation. This may involve changing choices of music, movies, books, television and social engagements. Stress management, meditation and counselling are advisable to help retrain patients and promote a calm, relaxed state. Patients will need to be reminded that their lifestyle and outlook require radical modification for optimal outcome. Avoidance of all stimulants including nicotine and recreational drugs is understandably indicated. Regulation of circadian rhythm and ensuring patients get adequate rest and sleep is essential. Afternoon naps and at least 8 hours of sound sleep per night should be encouraged.

Hydrotherapy

The strong traditional approach is to use hydrotherapy, such as a cold compress to the throat 15 minutes a day, to improve symptoms. Research is scarce to support this prescription; however, an animal trial highlighting a number of considerations showed positive effects. Rats were exposed to acute cold (4°C for 2 h), chronic cold (4°C) continuously, and chronic–intermittent cold (4°C for 2 h daily) and the control group was maintained at 25°C. In each animal, the plasma concentration of thyrotrophin (TSH), triiodothyronine (T_3), and thyroxine (T_4) was determined by radioimmunoassay. The results indicate that exposure to chronic–intermittent cold produces an inhibition in the secretion of TSH and thyroid hormones.[253]

CASE STUDY

OVERVIEW

CD was a 37-year-old speech pathologist who specialised in children with learning difficulties and disabilities. She presented with insomnia, diarrhoea (4–6 bowel movements per day), difficulty swallowing (sore throat), recent weight loss (5 kg in past month), increased appetite (unsatiated), increased thirst, anxiety and hair loss.

CLINICAL EXAMINATION

Alert, cooperative, thin, anxious. BP — 127/80 mmHg, BMI — 21 kg/m^2, fine motor tremor and mild hyperreflexia. No visible or palpable goitre, mild exophthalmos and warm, moist skin.

Investigation results confirmed hyperthyroidism due to:

- TSH — 0.3 mU/L
- T_4 — 26 pmol/L
- T_3 — WNR (within normal range)
- Stool analysis — NAD.

TREATMENT PROTOCOL

INITIAL APPOINTMENT

Due to the early diagnosis and mild laboratory readings, the patient chose to pursue naturopathic treatments in lieu of medication. The patient's GP was consulted and informed of progress throughout treatment.

CASE STUDY CONTINUED

HERBAL MEDICINE

Herbal medicine	Ratio	Quantity	Rationale
Avena sativa (green)	1:2	60 mL	Nervine tonic
Melissa officinalis	1:2	60 mL	Reduces the conversion of T_4 to T_3 and also has mild sedative activity
Leonurus cardiaca	1:2	40 mL	Reduces palpitations and is a specific for palpitations associated with hyperthyroidism
Lycopus spp.	1:2	60 mL	Attaches to the TSH receptor in the thyroid, thereby reducing receptor binding of TSH receptor-stimulating antibodies. This in turn reduces the output of thyroxine. *Lycopus* spp. are also thought to reduce the conversion of T_4 to T_3
TOTAL: 220 mL			
DOSE: 7.5 mL b.i.d.			

NUTRITIONAL MEDICINE

Dietary

- Encourage goitrogen-rich foods in the diet
- Avoid iodine-rich foods
- Ensure protein requirements are replete for both current and ideal body weight in easily digestible forms
- Encourage wholefood, organic diet
- Avoid all stimulants including caffeine, sugar, alcohol and others
- Increase hydration focusing on herbal teas (lemon balm, chamomile) and spring water.

Supplemental

Nutrient	Dosage	Rationale
Concentrated omega-3 fatty acids	325 mg EPA and 225 mg DHA b.i.d.	Anti-inflammatory, cardioprotective and restorative
High-potency antioxidant formulation consisting of selenium, zinc, vitamins A, E and C and phytochemical antioxidants	2 tabs b.i.d.	Antioxidants are essential for reducing free radical damage and oxidative stress and assisting with normalising thyroid hormonal cascades. In addition, they help to prevent complications

CASE STUDY CONTINUED

Nutrient	Dosage	Rationale
Vitamin B complex	1 cap b.i.d. (activated forms)	Address deficiencies, energy production and assistance in weight stabilisation
Magnesium	600 mg	Healthy nerve conduction, muscular contraction and relaxation, cardiac function and energy production

LIFESTYLE/EDUCATION

- Stress reduction, relaxation
- Adequate sleep — including resting in the afternoon
- Reduction of stimulus — electromagnetics and radiation, loud music, violent TV or movies, others
- Reduction of exercise for weight loss — exercise for relaxation only.

SECTION C: PANCREATIC DISORDERS

DIABETES MELLITUS

Epidemiology

Diabetes represents a major health and cost burden to the people of Australia. According to statistics from the Australian Diabetes, Obesity and Lifestyle follow-up study (AusDiab) 2012, approximately 12% of adults in Australia have diabetes.[254,255]

ABS figures for the 2014–15 period estimated that 5.1% of the Australian population had diabetes.[256,257] This includes people over the age of 2, of whom 0.7% had type 1 diabetes, 4.4% had type 2 diabetes. These figures exclude gestational diabetes. The prevalence of diabetes appears to increase with age, with the age bracket 55–64 years being the most likely age of diagnosis for men, and 65–74 years the most likely age of diagnosis for women. The prevalence of diabetes in people aged over 75 years is 18.4%.[257] With regards to type 2 diabetes, men are more likely to be afflicted than women. By 2025 it is estimated that up to 3 million Australians over the age of 25 will have diabetes.[258]

Classification (Table 21.20)

TYPE 1 DIABETES MELLITUS

Otherwise known as juvenile-onset diabetes or insulin-dependent diabetes mellitus (IDDM), type 1

TABLE 21.20 Comparison of type 1 and type 2 diabetes		
	Type 1 diabetes	**Type 2 diabetes**
Phenotype	Onset primarily in childhood and adolescence	Onset predominantly after 40 years of age but can occur earlier
	Often thin or normal weight	Often obese
	Prone to ketoacidosis	No ketoacidosis
	Insulin administration required for survival	Insulin administration not required for survival
	Pancreas is damaged by an autoimmune attack	Pancreas is not damaged by an autoimmune attack
	Absolute insulin deficiency	Relative insulin deficiency and/or insulin resistance
	Treatment: insulin injections	Treatment: (1) healthy diet and increased exercise; (2) hypoglycaemic tablets; (3) insulin injections
Genotype	Increased prevalence in relatives	Increased prevalence in relatives
	Identical twin studies: <50% concordance	Identical twin studies: usually above 70% concordance
	HLA association: yes (HLA-DR3 or HLA-DR4)	HLA association: no

diabetes is the result of injury to the insulin-producing beta cells coupled with some defect in tissue regeneration capacity. Most commonly it is an autoimmune disorder in which the body attacks its pancreatic beta cells, but it may also have no known aetiology (*idiopathic diabetes*).[259] The onset of type 1 diabetes is attributed to both an inherited risk and external triggers, such as diet or an infection.

Individuals will require lifelong insulin for the control of blood glucose levels. Individuals must learn how to manage blood glucose levels on a day-by-day basis, modifying insulin types and dosages as necessary, according to the results of regular blood glucose testing.

Genetics

Approximately 40 loci of the genome have been linked with influencing type 1 diabetes risk. The most well studied is IDDM1, which contains the human leucocyte antigen (HLA) genes that encode immune response proteins. Variations in HLA genes are an important genetic risk factor, accounting for up to half of the genetic susceptibility that leads to risk of type 1diabetes, but they alone do not account for the disease and other genes are involved. Of the remaining non-HLA genes, only those for the insulin VNTR, PTPN22, CTLA4, and IL2RA are associated with increased odds ratios. Most of the loci associated with risk of type 1 diabetes are thought to involve immune processes.[260]

TYPE 2 DIABETES MELLITUS

Type 2 diabetes has been loosely defined as 'adult onset' diabetes, although as diabetes becomes more common throughout the world, cases of type 2 diabetes are being observed in younger people. It is increasingly common in children.

Insulin levels are typically elevated, indicating a loss of sensitivity to insulin by the cells of the body. Later, as type 2 diabetes progresses, insulin levels can drop and insulin deficiency can magnify further the effects of insulin resistance. In determining the risk of developing diabetes, environmental factors such as food intake and exercise play an important role. The majority of individuals with type 2 diabetes are either overweight or obese. Achieving ideal body weight in these patients is associated with restoration of normal blood glucose levels in many cases. Inherited factors are also important, but the genes involved remain poorly defined. Recent statistics suggest an alarming increase in children and adolescents. Furthermore, it is generally thought that up to 90% of all diabetics are type 2, with misdiagnosis of approximately 15% of type 2 adults as they actually have type 1.

Genetics

In rare forms of diabetes, mutations of one gene can result in disease. However, in type 2 diabetes many genes are thought to be involved. 'Diabetes genes' may show only a subtle variation in the gene sequence, and these variations may be extremely common. The difficulty lies in linking such common gene variations, known as single nucleotide polymorphisms (SNPs), with an increased risk of developing diabetes. Genome-wide association scans (GWAS) have identified the strongest effect for type 2 diabetes is the rs7903146 SNP in the *TCF7L2* gene.[261]

One method of finding the diabetes susceptibility genes is by whole-genome linkage studies. The entire genome of affected family members is scanned, and the families are followed over several generations and/or large numbers of affected sibling pairs are studied. Associations between parts of the genome and the risk of developing diabetes are looked for. To date only two genes, calpain 10 (CAPN10) and hepatocyte nuclear factor 4 alpha (HNF4A), have been identified by this method.

SUBTYPE 2 DIABETES MELLITUS: LATENT AUTOIMMUNE DIABETES IN ADULTS (LADA)

Attempts to distinguish adult-onset type 1 diabetes cases from type 2 diabetes resulted in the proposal of new disease classifications, including latent autoimmune diabetes in adults (LADA) and ketosis-prone diabetes; however, the lack of firm diagnostic criteria for LADA has resulted in it not being officially adopted as a new category for diabetes.[260] There are, however, cases of this intermediate type of diabetes seen in practice (up to 9% of diabetes cases in Europe, and exceeding the number of cases of type 1 diabetes in some parts of the world),[262,263] and research is emerging showing that the condition includes genetic risks that overlap both type 1 and typ2 diabetes.[264] Recent research in Sweden has identified that coffee consumption (while reducing the risk of type 2 diabetes) might increase the risk of LADA[265]; and another Swedish study has shown high intake of sweetened beverages was associated with increased risk of LADA, similar to the relationship observed in type 2 diabetes, suggesting common pathways involving insulin resistance.[266] The consumption of omega-3 fatty acids is associated with a decreased risk of LADA and type 1 diabetes in children, but not type 2 diabetes.[267] Moderate alcohol consumption is associated with reduced risk for type 2 diabetes; however, similar results were observed in LADA only for those with low GADA levels (no beneficial effects on diabetes-related autoimmunity).[268]

While no firm diagnostic criteria exist for LADA, three criteria have often been used, although each of these has drawbacks. The criteria are:

- positivity for GADA
- older than 35 years at diagnosis
- no insulin therapy in the first 6–12 months after diagnosis[263]

Other types of diabetes — secondary development

Other types of diabetes include a form of diabetes that is secondary to certain conditions and syndromes:[259]

- Pancreatic disease including pancreatitis, trauma, neoplasia, cystic fibrosis, haemochromatosis
- Hormone disturbances (e.g. acromegaly, Cushing's syndrome, hyperthyroidism, aldosteronoma)
- Medication/recreational drug usage
- Gestational diabetes (pregnancy related)
- Genetic defects of β-cell function
- Genetic defects in insulin action
- Infections.

TYPE 3 DIABETES MELLITUS

Emerging evidence supports the notion that Alzheimer's disease (AD) is a metabolic disease resulting from impaired insulin responsiveness, glucose utilisation and energy metabolism in the brain. The fundamental abnormalities in AD represent insulin resistance and insulin deficiency in the brain, leading some researchers to classify it as a type of diabetes. The molecular and biochemical consequences of AD overlap with type 1and type 2 diabetes. Insulin and IGF signalling pathways in the central nervous system perform critical roles in cognitive function. The highest levels of insulin, IGF-1 and IGF-2 polypeptides and receptor genes are in structures that are heavily affected by neurodegeneration, particularly in AD. The pathological indicators of AD include amyloid-β-peptide (Aβ) (forming plaques) and hyperphosphorylated tau-based neurofibrillary tangles and synapse loss. It has been hypothesised that insulin resistance in the brain leads to increased oxidative stress, which is one mechanism responsible for the neurodegeneration seen in AD. There is a strong association between type 2 diabetes and AD risk, and AD as a complication of diabetes mellitus might explain its increasing incidence worldwide. Common mechanisms shared between diabetes and AD include inflammation, insulin resistance and mitochondrial dysfunction.[269–272] This is an emerging area of research and further studies are required to determine causality and therapeutic implications of AD as a type of diabetes.

Metabolic syndrome

IMPAIRED GLUCOSE TOLERANCE, PRE-DIABETES, SYNDROME X AND INSULIN RESISTANCE

All of the above-mentioned conditions can be viewed as different facets of the same disease with similar aetiological factors such as dietary, lifestyle and genetic influences. The modern diet and modern lifestyle practices are not conducive to the optimal functioning of the human body. The conditions under discussion occur when a person's blood glucose levels are higher than normal but not high enough for a diagnosis of type 2 diabetes. These conditions are believed to be precursors to the development of full-blown type 2 diabetes. Management is imperative as most cases are typically reversible, and development of diabetes can be avoided.

They are typically accompanied by the following abnormalities:

- Cholesterol abnormalities
- Elevations of blood pressure
- Inflammation
- Blood clotting irregularities and subsequent risk of development of cardiovascular disease, stroke and other health problems.

METABOLIC SYNDROME

Metabolic syndrome is a broad term typically used to describe numerous abnormalities that are triggered by a high intake of refined carbohydrates/sugars in individuals who are genetically predisposed to blood sugar irregularities. The underlying metabolic factor in metabolic syndrome is elevated insulin levels, which result from high intake of refined carbohydrates coupled with insulin resistance (cells that respond poorly to the effects of insulin).

Specific parameters include:

- Central obesity (increased waist to hip ratio due to excessive fat tissue in and around the abdomen)
- Raised blood pressure (130/85 mmHg or higher)
- Dyslipidaemia (mainly high triglycerides, high LDL and low HDL)
- Insulin resistance (hyperinsulinaemia) or elevated insulin levels
- Proinflammatory state (elevated plasma AA/EPA ratio), abnormal blood clotting
- Impaired glucose tolerance
- Fatty liver (note: fatty liver in metabolic syndrome has been found to predict type 2 diabetes, independently of age and obesity).[273]

Secondary features

- May suffer hypoglycaemic symptoms
- May have polycystic ovary syndrome (PCOS)
- Often exhausted, depressed
- Family history of diabetes and hypertension.

Aetiology

Diabetes is a disorder of metabolism — how we process carbohydrates, lipids and protein is inextricably linked to our blood glucose control, manufacture and energy production. After digestion, glucose passes into the bloodstream, where it is used by cells for growth and energy. For glucose entry into cells, we require insulin. Diabetes can occur when the pancreas does not secrete enough insulin or if the cells of the body become resistant to insulin; hence the blood glucose cannot get into the cells, which then leads to serious complications. Diabetes is characterised by poor glucose control (or elevated fasting blood glucose readings) and an increased risk of cardiovascular disease, renal disease and other health complications.

Patients typically present with polyuria, polydipsia, and polyphagia in type 1 diabetes mellitus (DM). These symptoms can occur with type 2 diabetes; however, as the symptoms are generally milder, they can go unnoticed until complications eventuate. Progression of the disease prompts the development of additional symptoms including fatigue, blurred vision, poor wound healing, periodontal disease, and frequent infections.

Pathogenesis

TYPE 1 — RISK FACTORS

It is well documented that type 1 diabetes is a truly multifactorial disease that creates immune deregulation and eventual destruction of the pancreatic insulin-producing cells. While popular opinion confers a genetic predisposition, there are many other risk factors that trigger the immune sensitivity such as dietary and environmental factors. The genetic predisposition simply sets the stage for the environmental or dietary factor to initiate the destructive process. The very term predisposition clearly indicates that something else needs to occur: less than 10% of those with increased genetic susceptibility for type 1 diabetes actually develop the disease.

The following risk factors require consideration.

Autoimmune triggers

Typical autoimmune triggers must be considered:

- Chemical or free radical damage
- Viral infection
- Food allergy
- Environmental:
  - Been shown to develop more often in winter than summer and is more common in colder climates
- Dietary risk factors
- Poor gastrointestinal health/integrity
- Nutritional deficiencies
- Nitrate/nitrosamines.

Poor gastrointestinal health/integrity

Several important factors contribute to developing tolerance to foods that might otherwise lead to autoimmune reactions: the type of gut microflora[274], the protection offered by breastfeeding, infections of the gastrointestinal tract and nutritional status. Bekkering et al have proposed that the composition of the gut microbiota contributes to the development of all types of diabetes, via increased intestinal permeability (due to microbiota changes in combination with specific diets) leading to a state of chronic low-grade inflammation and the development of insulin resistance.[275]

The intestinal immune system serves a vital role in processing the many food and microbial antigens to protect the body from infection or allergy. What appears to happen in the development of some cases of type 1 diabetes is the development of antibodies by the gastrointestinal immune system that ultimately attack the beta cells. It is interesting to consider that an underlying factor that may contribute to type 1 diabetes is poor protein digestion.

Numerous studies have shown that diets containing partially digested proteins produce a lower rate of autoimmune diabetes than diets containing whole proteins. Whole proteins are more likely to result in the formation of antibodies against them. Next, some of these proteins cross-react with antigens on or within the beta cells of the pancreas. In humans, two proteins that have had the highest degree of incrimination are those found in milk (bovine serum albumin, as well as bovine insulin) and wheat (gluten).

Strong evidence implicates dietary factors like cow's milk and gluten as important triggers of the autoimmune process that leads to type 1diabetes. In contrast, breastfeeding has been identified as an important factor in establishing proper intestinal immune function and reducing type 1 diabetes risk. It is well known that breastfeeding confers a reduction in the risk of food allergies, as well as better protection against both bacterial and viral intestinal infections. Sensitivity to gluten within other grains such as wheat, rye and barley has been shown to be the main culprit. Fruit and berry juices have also been shown to be associated with increased risk for advanced β cell autoimmunity.[276]

Cow's milk

The early introduction of cow's milk in infancy holds a strong case for the subsequent development of type 1 DM. This is supported by several lines of evidence: ecological data,[276,278] the observation of antibodies to bovine serum albumin (BSA) and beta-casein in type 1 DM,[279] a lymphocyte-mediated immune response to beta-casein in recently diagnosed type 1 DM patients,[280] enhanced levels of cow's milk antibodies in infancy in children who later develop type 1 DM,[281] and pilot data demonstrating that casein hydrolysate reduces the cumulative incidence of auto-antibodies in infants at increased risk for type 1 DM compared with a conventional cow's milk formula.[282] These data have led to speculation that the cow's milk responses might be cross-reactive with self-antigens and thus induce autoimmunity.[279,280]

Results from the Diabetes Autoimmunity Study in the Young (DAISY) indicate that cow's milk intake is associated with increased risk for islet autoimmunity and progression to type 1 diabetes, but only in children with a low-moderate risk HLA-DR genotype.[283] Other research found that polymorphisms in the PTPN22 gene are associated with type 1 diabetes in children exposed to cow's milk before 6 months, but not after.[284] These genetic influences on environmental factors such as cow's milk intake could account for the inconclusive results in previous studies. More research is needed in this complex interplay of factors.

While convincing, it is difficult to determine whether the data implicating early cow's milk consumption in type 1 DM are due to the removal of the protection offered by breastfeeding (for example, antibodies in breast milk protect from enteroviral infections,[285] a known type 1 DM trigger[277]), or the introduction of a diabetogenic factor in cow's milk per se,[278] or even the increased calorific content of cow's milk (the accelerator hypothesis).[277] It is essential to encourage breastfeeding where possible in conjunction with prevention of cow's milk exposure.

A number of studies link formula feeding and introduction of solids with the development of type 1 DM at later ages. Babies that are breastfed and eat solids at later ages have been shown to be less likely to develop type 1 DM than those that are fed formula (especially cow's milk formula) or those that are introduced solids too early or certain foods prematurely. This association is strongest in infants with a strong genetic risk profile, and inconclusive in those with lower risk.[286]

Enteroviruses and type 1 diabetes

Due to lack of concordance in identical twins, an environmental trigger is believed to be involved with the development of type 1 DM. This trigger has been suggested to be a virus and several lines of epidemiological evidence suggest that a viral infection might cause or trigger type 1 DM. Viruses have long been suspected to contribute to the development of human type 1 diabetes, largely by temporal and geographic association between the disease and viral infection, serological evidence of infection in patients recently diagnosed with type 1 diabetes, and isolation of viruses from the pancreas of diabetic patients in a few cases. In addition, some viruses have been reported to be associated with the development of type 1 diabetes in animals. Viruses can induce type 1 diabetes either by direct infection and cytolytic killing of beta cells or by triggering beta cell autoimmunity with or without direct infection of the beta cells.[287] Viruses may also initiate type 1 diabetes through molecular mimicry once autoimmunity has been initiated.[288]

There are instances where the diagnosis of type 1 DM in one member of a family has been rapidly followed by its appearance in other members of the same family.[289] One paper published a case report where an enterovirus was isolated from a mother and from her son diagnosed with type 1 DM the same day.[290] Such clustering of type 1 DM cases in time within a family is a strong indication of an infectious agent as a trigger or cause of the disease.[291] Evidence for enterovirus (EV) involvement has been presented in several studies, EV-IgM antibodies have been reported in type 1 DM patients, EV-RNA has been found in the blood from type 1 DM patients at onset, and EV has been isolated from newly diagnosed type 1 DM.[292] A meta-analysis of 26 studies showed that the likelihood of enterovirus is 10-fold higher in type 1 diabetic patients than non-diabetic controls, and four times higher in individuals with diabetes-related immunity[293] Evidence is emerging suggesting that enteroviral infections during pregnancy might result in islet autoimmunity in the mother as well as the offspring.[294] (See also Fig. 21.6.)

Common causative viral infections include:

- Enteroviruses (polioviruses, Coxsackie viruses, echoviruses)
- Rotavirus (common cause of diarrhoea in children)
- Epstein–Barr virus
- Herpes virus
- Mumps
- Rubella
- Cytomegalovirus.[288,295]

Specific deficiencies

Interesting research supports the links between the development of type 1 diabetes with the following deficiencies during pregnancy and/or in childhood:

- Vitamin D
- Omega-3 fatty acids (sources cod liver oil and fish oils).

In humans, serum vitamin D levels are lowered in recently diagnosed type 1 DM patients,[296–300] and dietary vitamin D supplementation to young children reduces the risk of type 1 DM. (Meta-analysis of four observational studies totalling 1429 cases and 5026 controls, which had assessed the effect of childhood vitamin D supplementation on type 1 DM risk, showed a protective effect of odds ratio = 0.71 (95% confidence interval 0.60–0.84)).[301] And studies report that increased vitamin D intake during pregnancy reduces evidence of pancreatic autoimmunity.[302–305] Association with genes involved in vitamin D metabolism and action also provides direct evidence for an involvement of vitamin D metabolism in the causation of type 1 DM.[306,307] Studies to date have produced conflicting results, and support the need for randomised clinical trials to evaluate the effect of vitamin D supplementation in pregnancy and infancy on type 1 DM.[307–309] Maternal vitamin D receptor (VDR) genetic variants have been found to be associated with the infant's risk of type 1 diabetes, regardless of the infant's genetic risk profile.[310] The risk is greater in the presence of maternal vitamin D deficiency.

Omega-3 fatty acid intake in childhood was found to be associated with a reduced risk of islet autoimmunity in children with an increased genetic risk for type 1 diabetes,[311] whereas no conclusive association was found between maternal fatty acid intake during pregnancy and incidence of type 1 diabetes in the offspring.[312] Further research is required in this area.

Polychlorinated biphenyls

In a small study of pregnant women, serum levels of PCBs were 30% higher among those with diabetes (primarily type 1) than among those without.[313] While the data are few, it is prudent to recommend that all women of

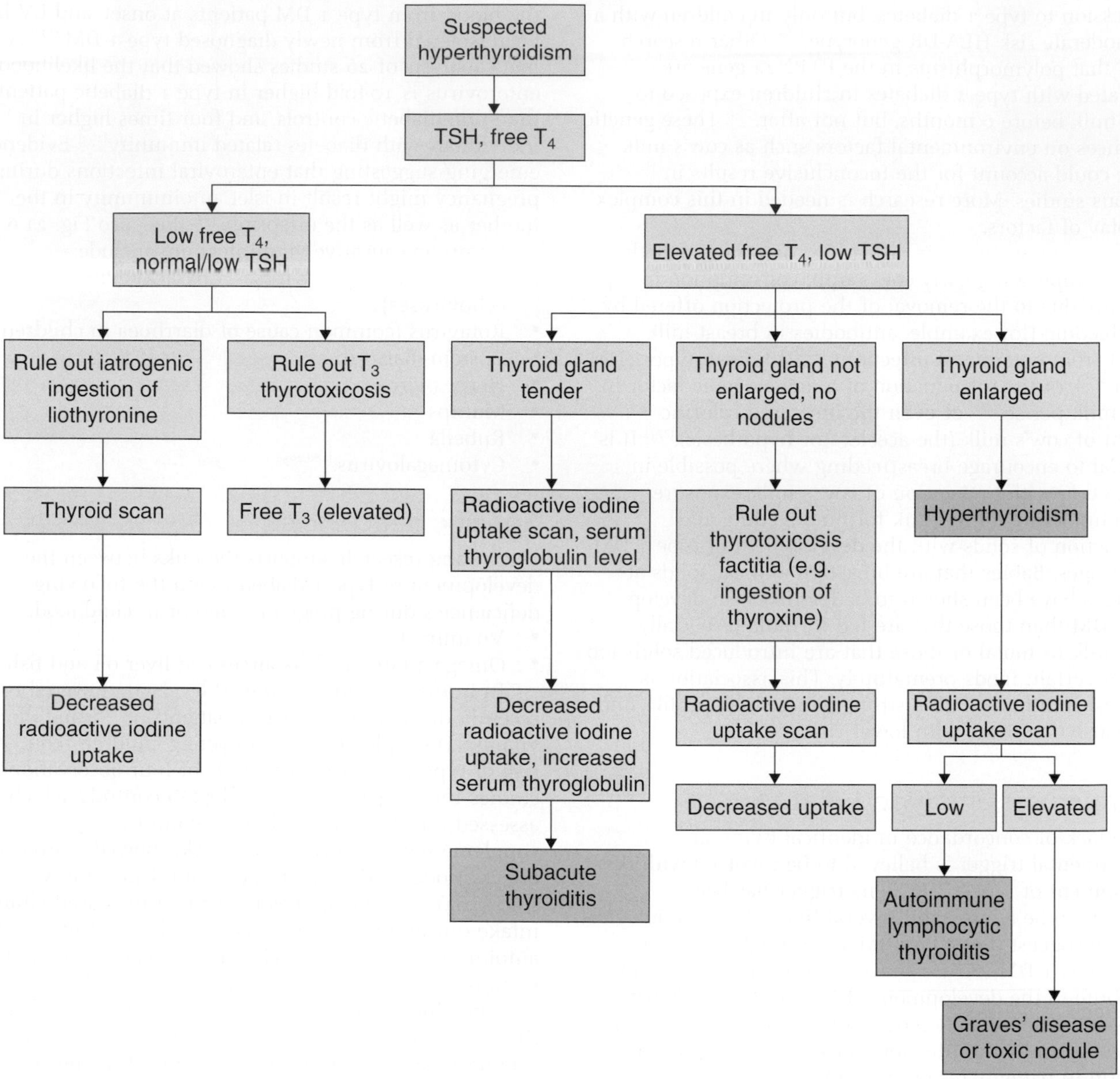

FIGURE 21.6 **Environmental triggers and protective factors for islet autoimmunity and promoters of progression to type 1 diabetes for which an association has been suggested.**

reproductive age and those who are considering becoming or are pregnant avoid exposure.

N-nitroso compounds (nitrates, nitrites and nitrosamines)

In 1981 Helgason and Jonasson[314] first drew attention to the possibility that *N*-nitroso compounds may cause type 1 diabetes in humans. Consumption early in pregnancy of cured mutton, a source of *N*-nitroso compounds, was followed by a high incidence of type 1 diabetes in male offspring. The authors proposed that dietary nitrosamine activity was inhibited by oestrogen and promoted by testosterone, as with streptozotocin, thus accounting for the male specificity. Helgason et al[315] subsequently induced diabetes in the progeny of mice fed *N*-nitroso-laden mutton, and males were preferentially affected. Subsequent in-vitro work revealed that selected *N*-nitroso compounds were especially toxic to pancreatic β cells.[316]

In the gastrointestinal tract, nitrates can be converted to nitrites, and nitrites can react with amines to form *N*-nitroso compounds. Nitrates are produced by agricultural run-off from fertilisers and are in cured or smoked foods including cold cuts, hot dogs, smoked fish (salmon), smoked cheese, jerky and other foods to keep the food from spoiling. Nitrates react within the body to form compounds known as nitrosamines. Case-controlled studies have not produced conclusive evidence of the effects of these compounds on development of type 1 diabetes, and additional studies are required to consolidate the results of previous studies.[288]

TYPE 2 — RISK FACTORS[317,318]

Early identification is crucial. If patients present with any of the following and are <30 years of age, they are considered to be at high risk:

- Age — risk increases above 45 years of age
- Cardiovascular disease (or family history of cardiovascular disease)
- Elevated triglycerides, low HDL or both
- Family history of diabetes (parent or sibling with type 1 or 2 diabetes or hypoglycaemia)
- Spousal diabetes — a meta-analysis found that a spousal history of diabetes is associated with a 26% increased risk[319]
- History of gestational diabetes or delivery of baby weighing more than 4.1 kg (9 lb)
- Hypertension (BP >140/90 mmHg)
- Increased waist-to-hip ratio
- Low adiponectin levels, elevated fasting insulin levels
- Obesity
- Overweight
- Polycystic ovary syndrome
- Previously identified impaired fasting glucose or impaired glucose tolerance
- Previously identified impaired glucose tolerance or impaired fasting glucose
- Race — African American, Hispanic American, Native American/Canadian, Indigenous Australian or New Zealander, Asian American, Asian, Pacific Islander. In the US the increased risk among racial/ethnic minorities has been found to be associated with socioeconomic factors[320]
- Sedentary lifestyle[321]; a systematic review and meta-analysis showed that all subtypes (vigorous, low intensity and leisure time activity) of physical activity (5–7 hours per week) reduce the risk of type 2 diabetes[322]
- Consumption of sugar-sweetened beverages[323–325]
- Low intake of dietary fibre[326]
- Psychosocial stress in adulthood and low stress resilience[327]
- Long working hours in low socioeconomic groups is associated with an increased risk[328]
- Short and long sleep duration (outside of 7–8 hours per night): 1 hour less per night was associated with a 9% increased risk, and 1 hour more per night a 14% increased risk[329,330]
- Results of the Adventist Health Study-2 showed that participants who followed vegetarian diets (including vegan, semi-vegetarian and lacto-ovo vegetarians) had a substantial and independent reduction in diabetes incidence and improved glycaemic control in type 2 diabetes.[331,332] These results are supported by an analysis of the EPIC-InterAct Study (240 234 adults from eight European countries) that found a positive association between meat consumption (particularly red meat) and the incidence of type 2 diabetes[333,334]
- Higher haem iron intake and increased iron body stores (measured by ferritin, soluble transferrin receptor (sTfR) and the sTfR:ferritin ratio) were significantly associated with type 2 diabetes risk in a 2012 systematic review and meta-analysis. No association was found with total dietary iron, non-haem iron or supplementation iron intakes[335–337]
- Eating patterns — irregular breakfast consumption (skipping breakfast one or more times per week) was associated with higher risk for type 2 diabetes in women (result from the Nurses' Health Study).[338] Similar results were found in the Health Professional Follow-Up Study in men who skipped breakfast (resulting in a 21% increased risk of type 2 diabetes) and in men who ate 1–2 meals per day compared to 3[339]
- Non-alcoholic fatty liver disease (NAFLD) — excess hepatic lipid causes hepatic insulin resistance and type 2 diabetes.[340]

Toxin exposure

The alarming increase in global incidence of diabetes has led researchers to investigate the link between increased environmental toxin exposure and rates of diabetes. Toxins that interfere with blood sugar control have been termed 'diabetogens'. Toxins which have the potential to cause or increase the risk of diabetes include toxic metals, dichlorodiphenyldichloroethylene, phthalates, bisphenol A (BPA), tributyltin, persistent organic pollutants (POPs), air pollution and pesticides.[341–344] A preliminary study found that a genetic risk for type 2 diabetes may modify susceptibility to air pollution through alterations in insulin sensitivity.[345] Nickel exposure is highlighted as a metal of concern requiring further research.[346] Association is inferred from epidemiological studies, however causality is difficult to establish.

Arsenic exposure

A strong theory for the development of type 2 DM is the proposed link between arsenic exposure and increased incidence. Epidemiological data for populations with high exposure to arsenic, including selected industrial groups, are generally consistent with an increased risk of type 2 diabetes (Table 21.21).

Arsenic is metabolised in vivo to trivalent arsenic. A trivalent arsenical, phenylarsine oxide, has adverse effects on the insulin receptor and glucose transport in in-vitro experiments.[347] The available epidemiological data on arsenic and diabetes are suggestive but inconclusive because of the limited number of studies, their small size and the possibility of publication bias.

If arsenic exposure via drinking water does increase risk of type 2 diabetes, this may occur only among those consuming water with an arsenic concentration of more than 0.1 mg/L. This is potentially an extremely serious problem in certain countries such as Bangladesh, where up to 30 million people may be drinking arsenic-contaminated water.[348] In several studies of other populations with high arsenic exposure, investigators have not specifically reported results for diabetes, raising the

TABLE 21.21 Risk of type 2 diabetes in groups exposed to arsenic relative to less exposed groups by type of exposure

First author, year	Place or type	Number of exposed cases	Mean exposure level[a,b]	*RR*[a]	Study design
Exposure via drinking water					
Tseng, 2000	Taiwan	41	0.8 mg/L water	4*	Ecological
Tsai, 1999	Taiwan	188	0.8 mg/L water	1.4*	Ecological[c]
Rahman, 1998	Bangladesh	21	0.5 mg/L water	6*	Cross-sectional
Occupational exposure					
Rahman, 1995	Copper smelter	10	0.5 mg/m^3 air	4	Nested case–control
Rahman, 1996	Glass workers	31	Unknown	1.4	Nested case–control
Bartoli, 1998	Glass workers	3	Unknown	0.34	Occupational cohort

[a]Approximate.
[b]Among the exposed group.
[c]The participants in the Tseng et al. study (39) and Tsai et al. study (40) overlapped somewhat (Putai Township). Value shown is reported SMR/100.
*$p < 0.05$.
Source: LongneckerMP, Daniels JL. Environmental contaminants as etiological factors for diabetes. Enviro health Perspect 2001; 109((Suppl 6):871–876.

possibility that no notable associations were present. It is essential to assess patients thoroughly; however, a direct correlation cannot be assumed. More recent studies have found associations between arsenic levels in drinking water, but still no causative effect has been established.[349–352] An interesting hypothesis put forward by Bell[353] proposing that the worldwide increase in type 2 diabetes risk is associated with higher consumption of white rice, may be not only due to rice's high glycaemic index value, but also partially attributed to its high inorganic arsenic content. This is of a particular concern in populations where white rice is a staple of the diet.

2,3,7,8-TETRACHLORODIBENZO-P-DIOXIN (TCDD)

Overall, the data on TCDD exposure in relation to diabetes and hyperglycaemia is mixed. Work by Enan et al[354] has shown that TCDD decreases cellular glucose update, thus a diabetogenic effect of TCDD is biologically plausible. One study elicited positive findings[355] of an association of TCDD level with hyperinsulinaemia on glucose tolerance test (GTT). While studies have reported positive associations, a causal effect has not been established and more research is needed before a conclusion can be reached.[356,357] Henley et al[358] conducted a systematic review and concluded that the risk of developing type 2 diabetes significantly increased with recurring exposure to TCDD in conjunction with other persistent chlorinated pesticides, but not with accidental isolated exposure.

From the naturopathic framework, avoidance of all environmental toxins is encouraged regardless of specific outcome; however, it is advisable that all type 2 DM patients avoid exposure to these substances.

Diet, exercise, lifestyle

Weight loss and maintenance of weight loss result in a decrease in the insulin resistance that is the hallmark of most patients with type 2 diabetes. Put simply, a negative kilojoule balance can decrease insulin resistance. The endpoint does not have to be weight loss. In the process of attaining a decrease in weight, blood glucose levels will improve. By monitoring the blood glucose levels and the kilojoule intake and output, the patient can understand the effect of a negative kilojoule balance on the blood glucose. These measurements and observations will help promote adherence. Patients do not have to achieve ideal body weight to improve control of blood glucose, control of hypertension and lipid levels. Loss of as little as 4.5–9 kg will be helpful, but the weight loss must then be maintained and exercise programs must be continued.

Numerous reports of individuals suffering with type 2 diabetes confirm that it is a disease of diet and lifestyle. Important considerations include:

- Dietary intake high in refined carbohydrates
- Dietary intake high in GI (glycaemic index) and GL (glycaemic load) foods
- Insufficient dietary fibre to modify glycaemic index/glycaemic load
- High dietary intake of saturated and trans fatty acids
- Low intake of antioxidant nutrients
- Excessive free radicals and pro-oxidants (increased production of reactive oxygen species (ROS) and reactive nitrogen species (RNS)).

Traditional communities

The diagnosis of type 2 DM is typically (but not always) made after the age of 50 years in Caucasians, but it is seen at much younger age in these high prevalence populations, which also include Pacific Islanders, Native Americans and migrant Asian Indians and Chinese. There is enormous variation in type 2 DM prevalence between populations, and exceptionally high rates have been documented in populations who have changed from a traditional to a modern lifestyle; for example, American Pima Indians, Micronesians and other Pacific Islanders, Indigenous Australians, migrant Asian Indians, and Mexican-Americans.

Research conducted on the Pima Indians for the past 30 years has helped scientists prove that obesity is a major risk factor in the development of diabetes. One-half of adult Pima Indians have diabetes and 95% of those with diabetes are overweight. These studies, carried out with the help of the Pima Indians, have shown that in overweight people, prior to them gaining weight they have a slower metabolic rate compared with people of the same weight. This slower metabolic rate, combined with a high-fat diet and a genetic tendency to retain fat may cause the epidemic overweight seen in the Pima Indians.

Along with genetic make-up, diet is a key factor to a healthy lifestyle. The influence of traditional desert crops on the metabolism of the Pima Indians is being studied to determine how to prevent the onset of diabetes and obesity. Researchers use the 'thrifty gene' theory proposed in 1962 by geneticist James Neel to help explain why many Pima Indians are overweight.[359] Neel's theory is based on the fact that for thousands of years populations which relied on farming, hunting and fishing for food, such as the Pima Indians, experienced alternating periods of feast and famine. Neel said that to adapt to these extreme changes in kilojoule needs, these people developed a thrifty gene that allowed them to store fat during times of plenty so that they would not starve during times of famine.

The thrifty gene

The first and most famous articulation of the genetic theory of diabetes was by University of Michigan geneticist James V Neel. In 1962, before the scope of the Pima health crisis was discovered, Neel published a paper entitled 'Diabetes mellitus: a "thrifty" genotype rendered detrimental by "progress"?' Calling diabetes an 'enigma', Neel wondered why it should be so common and heritable when it was so destructive. (His essay merged the juvenile 'early onset' type with the 'late onset' type.) Perhaps the individuals who had acquired the so-called thrifty gene were 'exceptionally efficient in the intake and/or utilisation of food', Neel wrote. 'It must be remembered that during the first 99 percent or more of man's life on Earth, while he existed as a hunter-gatherer, it was often feast or famine. Periods of gorging alternated with periods of greatly reduced food intake.' In short, a gene variant that may have been helpful in times of hunger would be harmful in times of unrelenting plenty.

Between 1983 and 1993, the National Institute of Diabetes and Digestive and Kidney Diseases (NIDDK) studied the genetic codes of almost 300 non-diabetic Pima Indians in great detail. In 1993, it identified a gene called *FABP2* that may contribute to insulin resistance. This gene makes an intestinal fatty acid binding protein using one of two amino acids. When the gene makes the protein with threonine, one of those amino acids, the body seems to absorb more fatty acids from the fat in meals. Scientists think that could lead to a higher level of certain fats and fatty acids in the blood, which could contribute to insulin resistance. This is obviously further evidence that diet and lifestyle appear to be able to overcome even the strongest genetic predispositions.

Lifestyle vs medication

Several well-designed, large trials have shown that lifestyle and dietary modifications can be used to effectively prevent type 2 diabetes. Clinical experience indicates that if patients can be encouraged to exercise frequently they can avoid most medications and reverse their blood sugar fluctuations.

In one study the risk of diabetes was reduced by 58% (p <0.001) in the intervention group.[360] The reduction in the incidence of diabetes was directly associated with changes in lifestyle enabling the authors to conclude that type 2 diabetes can be prevented by changes in the lifestyles of high-risk patients. Several studies have subsequently shown the success of lifestyle intervention programs at preventing or delaying the onset of diabetes in high-risk individuals.[361,362]

Complications

Repeated elevations in blood glucose levels and the loss of insulin sensitivity prevent systemic homeostasis. Complications can and will eventuate if proper maintenance is not maintained.

ACUTE COMPLICATIONS

The acute complications of diabetes represent a medical emergency and possible life or death situation. Any diabetic experiencing any symptom even remotely suggestive of an acute complication of diabetes should consult medical care immediately:

- Hypoglycaemia — this is a serious complication of diabetes. Please see the section on hypoglycaemia for more details
- Diabetic ketoacidosis
- Non-ketotic hyperosmolar hyperglycaemia.

CHRONIC COMPLICATIONS

Table 21.22 summarises some of the chronic complications encountered in diabetes.

CONTRIBUTING FACTORS TO LONG-TERM COMPLICATIONS

The major contributors to the long-term complications of diabetes include:

- Elevated homocysteine levels
- Endothelial cell dysfunction
- Glycosylation of proteins — binding of glucose to proteins causing inactivation of enzymes, inhibition of regulatory molecule binding, and the formation of abnormal protein structures
- Increased blood pressure
- Increased oxidative damage
- Intracellular accumulation of sorbitol
- Nutrient deficiency
- Poor glucose control.

TABLE 21.22 Chronic complications in diabetes

System	Effect
Endocrine	Due to the complexity and synchronistic nature of the endocrine system, it can be expected that subsequent irregularities within this system will eventuate. Common expectations can include subsequent negative effects to the reproductive system (male and female); cortisol fluctuations or poor stress coping abilities; emotional fluctuations; circadian rhythm disturbances; metabolic/thyroid fluctuations; and immune responses
Circulatory	Amputation, poor wound healing, foot ulcers
Cardiovascular	Atherosclerosis, hyperlipidaemia, cardiovascular disease, hypertension
Immune	Increased incidence of autoimmune conditions, immune system dysfunction, thyroid disease
Neurological	Depression, cognitive deficits, neuropathy, chronic pain
Hepatobiliary	Elevations in LFTs, hypercholesterolaemia
Renal	Nephropathy, renal disease
Ocular	Retinopathy, cataracts
Oral	Periodontal disease
Cancer	Increased risk of incidence and overall mortality for a number of site-specific cancers: Type 2: strongest relationship observed for liver and pancreatic cancer; followed by endometrial, post-menopausal breast cancer, colorectal, bladder, non-Hodgkin's lymphoma and kidney cancer Type 1: evidence is limited and inconclusive

DIFFERENTIAL DIAGNOSIS

- Diabetes insipidus
- Fructosuria
- L-xylulosuria
- Pancreatitis (acute and chronic)
- Glucagonoma
- Haemochromatosis
- Hypothyroidism
- Multiple sclerosis
- Cushing's syndrome
- Phaeochromocytoma
- PCOS
- Reye's syndrome.

NATUROPATHIC DIAGNOSIS

In addition to previous considerations, naturopathic diagnosis also carefully considers a patient's lifestyle, diet and family history in full detail. Additional assessments may be required determined on an individual basis.

Regulation of blood glucose concentrations

Every cell in the body relies to some extent on the availability of glucose to meet its energy needs. The glucose needed by the cells is obtained from glucose in the bloodstream. Therefore blood glucose levels must be maintained within strict limits to ensure that adequate (but not excessive) glucose is available. If glucose levels fall below normal an individual may feel weak and dizzy, while elevations of blood glucose can also cause problems, as is seen in diabetes.

Blood glucose homeostasis is maintained via the interaction of hormones. The two main hormones involved are insulin (which causes blood glucose to fall) and glucagon (which causes blood glucose to rise). Other hormones including adrenaline (epinephrine) may also influence blood glucose. The effects of these hormones and their roles in the regulation of blood glucose are outlined below.

INSULIN

Insulin is secreted by specialised cells in the pancreas (called beta cells) in response to increases in blood glucose levels (as may occur just *after* a meal). Insulin then travels in the bloodstream and instructs the body's cells to take glucose from the blood and into the cells — thus lowering blood glucose concentrations. Insulin also encourages the production of glycogen and fat from excess glucose. Again, these actions cause blood glucose levels to fall until they are within the normal range.

Insulin is said to be a hormone of the absorptive state — that is immediately after we have eaten and absorbed a meal. The actions of this hormone are therefore all about the use or storage of the nutrients and energy obtained from food.

GLUCAGON

Glucagon is also secreted by specialised cells in the pancreas (this time called alpha cells) in response to falls in blood glucose concentrations (as may occur *between* meals). Glucagon instructs the liver to break down glycogen and release glucose into the blood, and also stimulates gluconeogenesis — the production of glucose from non-carbohydrate sources. This causes blood glucose levels to rise until they are within the normal range.

Glucagon is said to be a hormone of the post-absorptive state — that is the time between meals and after absorption is complete. The actions of this hormone are therefore all about releasing nutrients and energy from storage.

ADRENALINE (EPINEPHRINE)

This hormone is an important part of the body's stress response and ensures that adequate energy is available for 'fight-or-flight' during danger and emergencies by instructing the liver to release glucose from glycogen storage.

Investigations

The standard method for diagnosing diabetes involves the measurement of blood glucose levels (Table 21.23).

Fasting plasma glucose

The initial measurement is generally a fasting blood glucose level taken after avoiding food for at least 10 hours but not more than 16 hours.

CLASSIFICATION

Fasting (overnight): venous plasma glucose concentration greater than or equal to 7 mmol/L (126 mg/dL) on at least two separate occasions.

Oral glucose tolerance test

A glucose tolerance test (GTT) is the administration of glucose to determine how quickly it is cleared from the blood and homeostasis is maintained (Table 21.24). The test is usually used to assess for diabetes, insulin resistance and reactive hypoglycaemia. The patient is instructed to increase carbohydrate intake in the days before the test. A full adult dose should not be given to a person weighing less than 43 kg (94 lb), or exaggerated glucoses may produce a false positive result.

The oral glucose tolerance test is considered a standard diagnostic test; however, it is not the most accurate or convenient test. It is fairly invasive and traumatic for the patient, and is mainly used because of its longstanding usage. In fact, according to some studies the GTT is significantly less reliable than fasting blood glucose, especially if combined with a glycosylated haemoglobin level ($HgbA_{1c}$).

CLASSIFICATION

Following ingestion of 75 g of glucose: venous plasma glucose concentration greater than or equal to 11 mmol/L (200 mg/dL) at 2 hours post-ingestion and at least one other sample during the 2-hour test.

Random blood glucose

CLASSIFICATION

A random blood glucose level of 11 mmol/L (200 mg/dL) or more, plus the presence of suggestive symptoms including polyuria, polydipsia, and polyphagia or fatigue, blurred vision, poor wound healing, periodontal disease and frequent infections are often presenting symptoms as well in type 2 diabetes.

TABLE 21.23 WHO diagnostic criteria for measuring blood glucose levels in diabetes (2006)

	1965	1980	1985	1999
Normal Fasting glucose 2-h glucose	Not specified <6 1 mmol/1	Not defined	Not defined	<6.1 mmol/1 Not specified but <7.8 mmol/1
Diabetes Fasting glucose 2-h glucose	Not specified ≥7.2 mmol/1	≥0.0 mmol/1 and/or ≥11.0 mmol/1	≥7.8 mmol/1 or ≥11.1 mmol/1	≥7.0 mmol/1 or ≥11.1 mmol/1
IGT Fasting glucose 2-h glucose	Referred to as borderline state 1 7.1 mmol/1	<8.0 mmol/1 and ≥8.0 and <11.0 mmol/1	<7.8 mmol/1 and ≥7.8 and <11.1 mmol/1	<7.0 mmol/1 and ≥7.8 and <11.1 mmol/1
IFG Fasting glucose 2-h glucose	Not defined	Not defined	Not defined	≥6.1 and <7.0 mmol/1 and <7.8 mmol/1 (if measured)

Values represent venous plasma glucose

	WHO 1999	ADA 2003
Diabetes Fasting glucose 2-h glucose*	≥7.0 mmol/1 or ≥11.1 mmol/1	≥7.0 mmol/1 or ≥11.1 mmol/1
IGT Fasting glucose 2-h glucose	<7.0 mmol/1 (if measured) and ≥7.8 and <11.1 mmol/1	Not required ≥7.8 and <11.1 mmol/1
IFG Fasting glucose 2-h glucose	6.1 to 6.9 mmol/1 (if measured) (measurement recommended)	5.6 to 6.9 mmol/1 measurement not recommended (but if measured should be <11.1 mmol/1)

*Venous plasma glucose 2 h after ingestion of 75 g oral glucose load
Source: World Health Organization (WHO). Definition and diagnosis of diabetes mellitus and intermediate hyperglycaemia: a report of a WHO/IDF consultation. Geneva: WHO; 2006.

TABLE 21.24 Glucose tolerance test response criteria

Response	Criteria
Normal	No elevation >9 mmol/L (160 mg) <8.3 mmol/L (150 mg) at the end of first hour <6.6 mmol/L (120 mg) at the end of second hour Never <1.1 mmol/L (20 mg) below fasting
Flat	No variation more than ± 1.1 mmol/L (20 mg) from fasting value
Pre-diabetic	Blood glucose levels of 7.8 mmol/L (140 mg/dl) to 10 mmol/L (180 mg/dL) at the end of second hour
Diabetic	>10 mmol/L (180 mg/dL) during first hour ≥11.1 mmol/L (200 mg) at the end of first hour ≥8.3 mmol/L (150 mg) at the end of second hour
Reactive hypoglycaemia	A normal 2- or 3-hour response curve followed by a decrease of ≥1.1 mmol/L (20 mg) from the fasting level during the final hours
Probable reactive hypoglycaemia	A normal 2- or 3-hour response curve followed by a decrease of 0.5–1.1 mmol/L (10–20 mg) from the fasting level during the final hours
Flat hypoglycaemia	An elevation of ≤1.1 mmol/L (20 mg), followed by a decrease of ≥1.1 mmol/L (20 mg) below the fasting level
Pre-diabetic hypoglycaemia	A 2-hour response identical to the pre-diabetic but showing a hypoglycaemic response during the final 3 hours
Hyperinsulinism	A marked hypoglycaemic response, with a value of <50 mg during the third, fourth, or fifth hour

Source: Adapted from Murray M, Pizzorno J. Textbook of natural medicine. 3rd edn. St Louis: Elsevier; 2004.

Important consideration when assessing blood glucose

It is important to acknowledge the effects of stress on the interpretation of blood sugar readings. Acute stress (even from blood draw) or vigorous exercise can affect readings.

Glycosylated haemoglobin (HbA_{1c})

HbA_{1c} measures a patient's average blood glucose control for the past 2–4 months. It determines the relative glucose load on the system by measuring the percentage of glycated (glycosylated) haemoglobin in the blood (Table 21.25). It is a prime reflection of the patient's (and the clinician's) management of blood glucose and patient compliance and enables assessment of current treatment.

TABLE 21.25 HbA_{1c} interpretation

HbA_{1c}	eAG (estimated average glucose)	
(%)	(mmol/L)	(mg/dL)
5	5.4 (4.2–6.7)	97 (76–120)
6	7.0 (5.5–8.5)	126 (100–152)
7	8.6 (6.8–10.3)	154 (123–185)
8	10.2 (8.1–12.1)	183 (147–217)
9	11.8 (9.4–13.9)	212 (170–249)
10	13.4 (10.7–15.7)	240 (193–282)
11	14.9 (12.0–17.5)	269 (217–314)
12	16.5 (13.3–19.3)	298 (240–347)

In the normal 120-day lifespan of the red blood cell, glucose molecules react with haemoglobin, forming glycated haemoglobin. In individuals with poorly controlled diabetes, the quantities of these glycated haemoglobins are much higher than in healthy people. Once a haemoglobin molecule is glycated, it remains that way. A build-up of glycated haemoglobin within the red cell therefore reflects the average level of glucose to which the cell has been exposed during its life cycle. HbA_{1c} can be used to diagnose diabetes (with a fasting blood glucose level); however, it is beneficial to confirm diagnosis with a 2-hour postprandial glucose level. It is recommended to check HbA_{1c} every 3 months once diagnosis is confirmed. It does not replace daily self-testing of blood glucose.

CLASSIFICATION

- Optimal: <6–7% (optimal)
- Mild: 7–8%
- Moderate: 8–9%
- Severe: >9%
- Diagnosis of DM: ≥6.5%

C-peptide

Also known as insulin C-peptide, connecting peptide, C-peptide is a peptide that is made when proinsulin is split into insulin and C-peptide. Insulin and peptide split before proinsulin is released from endocytic vesicles within the pancreas — one C-peptide for each insulin molecule. Measurement of C-peptide determines the level of damage to the pancreas and if the pancreas is still producing insulin. At the start, the pancreas manufactures a large protein called proinsulin. A piece of this protein (C-peptide) is then snipped off by enzymes, and both C-peptide and the remaining insulin are released into the bloodstream. Injected insulin has no C-peptide. Therefore even in diabetics already on insulin, a measurement of C-peptide can help to determine the degree of remaining pancreatic function.

C-peptide assessment can confirm treatment direction for newly diagnosed type 1 DM patients specifically if remaining pancreatic function can be conserved and

TABLE 21.26 C-peptide interpretation

C-peptide results	Interpretation
Normal	Normal insulin production
Low levels	Low levels are associated with low levels of insulin production. This can occur when insufficient insulin is being produced by the beta cells (newly diagnosed type 1 diabetic or chronic, long-term type 2 diabetic) or when production is suppressed by exogenous insulin or with suppression tests that involve substances such as somatostatin
High levels	Indicate high levels of endogenous insulin production such as in newly diagnosed type 2 diabetes, insulin resistance or similar. Can also indicate insulinomas (insulin-producing tumours) and may be seen with hypokalaemia, pregnancy, Cushing's syndrome, and renal failure
Undetectable	Chronic type 1 diabetic

encouraged. In type 2 DM patients, high or normal C-peptide levels confirm that their pancreas is making insulin, and should therefore motivate patients to comply with treatment to reduce insulin resistance and improve insulin sensitivity. If C-peptide levels indicate poor or declining pancreatic function, other treatment strategies can be implemented to encourage preservation of pancreatic function and stimulate insulin production (concurrent with obvious blood sugar regulation support) (Table 21.26).

Other

C-peptide testing is not widely used and may not be available in every laboratory. Repeated assessments should be conducted in the same laboratory for accuracy of interpretation. Even though they are produced at the same rate, C-peptide and insulin leave the body by different routes. Insulin is processed and eliminated mostly by the liver, while C-peptide is removed by the kidneys. Since the half-life of C-peptide is about 30 minutes to insulin's 5 minutes, normally there will be about 5–6 times as much C-peptide in the bloodstream as insulin.

MONITORING DIABETES

For optimal long-term health, it is essential that both type 1 and type 2 DM patients monitor their blood sugar levels regularly. Essential monitoring can be achieved through the use of the following assessments:

- Urine glucose monitoring
- Urine ketone testing
- Self-monitoring of blood glucose.

NATUROPATHIC INVESTIGATIONS

Naturopathic diagnosis considers dietary and lifestyle history to be paramount to the correct assessment of patients. In addition, a number of functional assessments have proven beneficial including those shown in Table 21.27.

TABLE 21.27 Naturopathic investigations

Homocysteine	To assess cardiovascular risk and associated complications
Metabolic syndrome profile	Assesses underlying factors of nitric oxide and eicosanoid cell response regulators including ADMA (asymmetric dimethylarginine), arachidonic acid (AA), eicosapentaenoic acid (EPA) and AA/EPA ratio
Nutrient elements	Assesses nutrient levels for appropriate therapeutic prescriptions
Toxic elements	Assesses presence of toxic elements to enable correct treatment and chelation as necessary
Hormone profile	As necessary to assess endocrine risk and associated effects. May include cortisol and DHEA assessment (saliva) to determine impact of stress hormones on presentation and development of condition
Functional liver detoxification profile	To assess liver function and ability to assist with glucose regulation
Gastrointestinal stool profile	To determine if underlying gastrointestinal pathogen is present and treat accordingly
Coeliac profile and genetic screen	It is prudent to include coeliac genetic screening in addition to standard assays (transglutaminase and endomysial antibodies) due to fluctuations from dietary intake
Food allergy profile (IgE, IgG)	Assess for instance of food allergy/ intolerance

Therapeutic considerations

CLINICAL DECISION MAKING AND RATIONALE

In type 1 DM, autoimmune factors play a major role. If there is a family history of type 1 DM or allergies/ intolerances, avoidance of food known to be reactive, such as gluten or dairy, may avert this disease.

In type 2 DM, insulin resistance (IR) and metabolic syndrome, Western diet and lifestyle have been linked to their development. Diets high in saturated fats and processed, refined carbohydrates and low in fibre and lean protein play a major role in the aetiology of insulin resistance, made worse by a sedentary lifestyle, high alcohol consumption and smoking.[363–365] Certain prescription medications influence carbohydrate metabolism and may thus contribute to glucose intolerance and IR.[11] Foundations for IR seem to be laid even before birth, correlating to suboptimal nutritional status, toxin exposure and elevated cortisol levels in the mother.[366]

Carbohydrates require insulin for their utilisation by the cells. Therefore, reducing carbohydrates may seem a logical step to take. However, concerns have been raised about the higher fat content of these diets which may increase total kilojoules and therefore promote further

Homocysteine

Homocysteine creates oxidative stress by blocking nitric oxide synthase (NOS).[374–376] It is a byproduct of methylation where methionine (as *S*-adenosyl methionine or SAM) donates methyl groups to any metabolic reaction in the body requiring them (such as purine and neurotransmitter formation). Thus, methionine converts to homocysteine and needs to be remethylated. This reaction requires folate and vitamin B_{12} as co-factors.[208] Alternatively, homocysteine can be degraded via the trans sulfuration pathway to cysteine, requiring vitamin B_6.[208] A range of supplements are available containing the three vitamins involved in homocysteine metabolism.

In polycystic ovary syndrome (PCOS) higher insulin levels have been found, indicative of IR. Further, homocysteine has also been found to be elevated, and treatment to reduce both these factors may improve outcome not only in PCOS but also in cardiovascular disease.[377–379] The latter is often linked to non-insulin-dependent diabetes mellitus (NIDDM) as part of the metabolic syndrome.

Suggested tests to ascertain homocysteine status are serum homocysteine, holotranscobalamin II ('active B_{12}') and red cell folate. The latter two tests make a differentiation possible as to which vitamin is likely to contribute to a high homocysteine. Ideal values for homocysteine are between 5 and 10 μmol/L. If the value is too low there may not be enough substrate for remethylation. Values higher than 10 μmol/L have been associated with higher morbidity. These tests are unreliable in persons with kidney impairment.

Inflammation and oxidative damage are part of the diabetic picture. The insulin secreting beta cells of the pancreas are particularly sensitive to oxidative damage which may be prevented by antioxidant supplementation.[363] Haemoglobin becomes glycosylated, the redox potential of the cells shift, levels of lipid peroxides increase and transition metals become decompartmentalised. Proteins and DNA become damaged.[380] It is therefore prudent to guard against such damage by prescribing antioxidants. However, single antioxidant nutrients are likely to produce mixed results as they become oxidised themselves in the process. It is therefore advisable to take them in combination as they do recycle each other.[208]

weight gain. Particular attention needs to be paid to the elements of the diet that are introduced/increased to replace the reduced carbohydrate intake, particularly the types of fats. Trials comparing diets of varying fat and carbohydrate content found significantly more weight loss for people following a low-carbohydrate (LC) diet than following a low-fat (LF) diet, yet this advantage was mostly lost after one year.[367] This begs the question of how many people were actually still strictly following their assigned diet after that time? When comparing cardiovascular profiles, people on a LF diet had better LDL values, whereas the LC dieters had better triglyceride and HDL values. In addition, people on an LC diet had lost more fat weight than those on a LF diet, thus showing an improved metabolic profile. Glucose control also seems to be enhanced on an LC diet.[367,368] Compliance with either of these diets is also linked to palatability of the food. For this reason olestra, a carbohydrate with smooth texture like fat, has been used to replace the fat in many LF food items. However, this can lead dieters to believe they are eating a healthy low-fat food and therefore they may be inclined to eat more. Olestra, being a carbohydrate, obviously contains kilojoules. These factors may be contributing to obesity in the first place.[369] It has also been shown that olestra reduces the absorption of fat-soluble vitamins.[370]

Other helpful food items in the diet include walnuts[371,372] and fish for essential fatty acids as well as sources of protein. Fibre is important to induce a feeling of satiety and to bind fats for elimination.[373]

Therapeutic application

TYPE 1 DIABETES MELLITUS

The flow diagram in Fig. 21.7, in the order shown, should be considered for treatment.

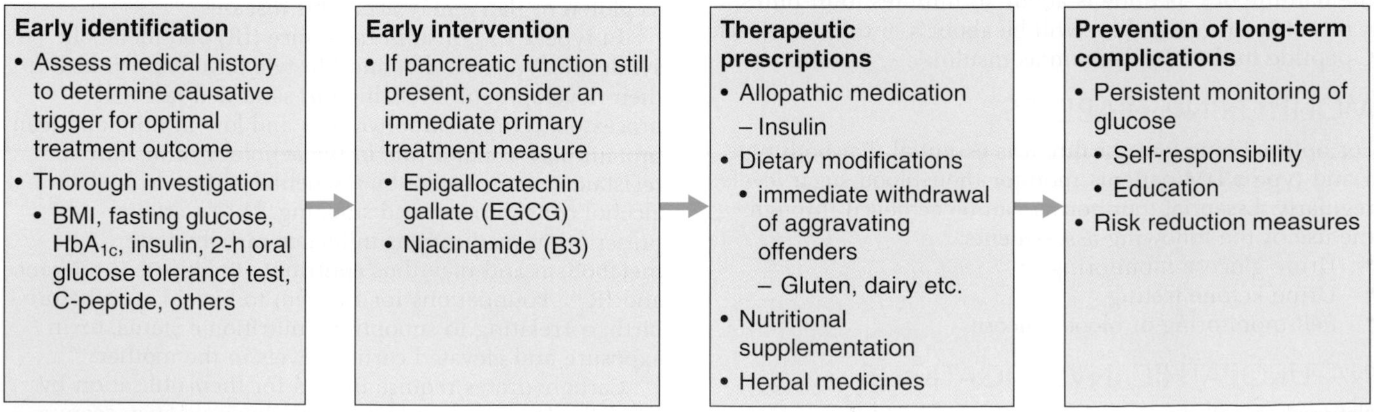

Early identification
• Assess medical history to determine causative trigger for optimal treatment outcome
• Thorough investigation
• BMI, fasting glucose, HbA1c, insulin, 2-h oral glucose tolerance test, C-peptide, others
Early intervention
• If pancreatic function still present, consider an immediate primary treatment measure
• Epigallocatechin gallate (EGCG)
• Niacinamide (B3)
Therapeutic prescriptions
• Allopathic medication
– Insulin
• Dietary modifications
• immediate withdrawal of aggravating offenders
– Gluten, dairy etc.
• Nutritional supplementation
• Herbal medicines
Prevention of long-term complications
• Persistent monitoring of glucose
• Self-responsibility
• Education
• Risk reduction measures

FIGURE 21.7 Type 1 diabetes mellitus.

Source: Adapted from Davidson JA, Blonde L, Jelliger PS et al. 2006. ACE/AACE Diabetes Road Map Task Force, ACE/AACE Diabetes Recommendations Implementation Conference.

TYPE 2 DIABETES MELLITUS

The flow diagram in Fig. 21.8, in the order shown, should be considered for treatment.

Patient and practitioner responsibilities in intensive diabetes self-management are shown in Table 21.28.

ALLOPATHIC PERSPECTIVE

See Table 21.29.

NATUROPATHIC PERSPECTIVE

An overview of naturopathic treatment for diabetes is shown in Fig. 21.9.

Type 1 DM

In type 1 DM, which is an autoimmune disease, there is progressive destruction of the pancreatic beta cells that produce insulin. Usually by the time of diagnosis there is little or no beta cell function. Therefore the majority of treatments will focus on:

- Blood sugar control
- Reducing the long-term complications that affect eyes, kidneys, nerves and blood vessels.

However, in some cases, particularly in early diagnosis, it may be possible to regenerate some of the beta cells.

Type 2 DM

In the treatment of type 2 DM, treatment should focus on:

- Enhancing blood sugar metabolism
- Reducing blood sugar levels
- Improving sensitivity to insulin
- Reducing long-term complications
- Achieving weight loss (if indicated) and lifestyle modifications as there can be beta cell defects resulting in inadequate secretion of insulin, and insulin resistance.

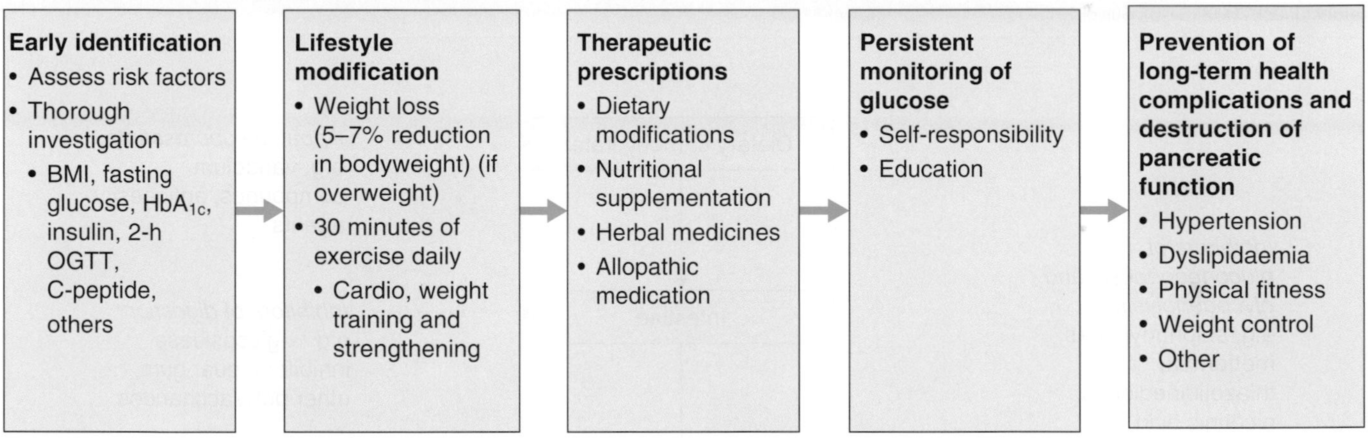

FIGURE 21.8 Type 2 diabetes mellitus.

Source: Adapted from Davidson JA, Blonde L, Jelliger PS et al. 2006. ACE/AACE Diabetes Road Map Task Force, ACE/AACE Diabetes Recommendations Implementation Conference.

TABLE 21.28 Patient and practitioner responsibilities in intensive diabetes self-management system

Patient responsibilities	Practitioner responsibilities
Monitoring of blood glucose	Adherence to the system of intensive self-management
Exercise program of diabetes	Measurement of outcomes
Adherence to dietary guidelines	Determination of patient satisfaction
Blood pressure monitoring	Maintenance of communication with team
Smoking cessation	Development of evaluation programs; include safety in taking medication and identification of patient misconceptions
Consistent use of prescriptions	Listening to patient concerns
Overcoming psychological and other barriers	Establishing and maintaining follow-up schedule
Healthy expression of feelings	Patient diabetes education – integrated approach with other members of healthcare team
Foot and eye care	Documentation of patient care

Continued

TABLE 21.28 Patient and practitioner responsibilities in intensive diabetes self-management system—cont'd

Patient responsibilities	Practitioner responsibilities
Understanding 'targets' for control of blood glucose and blood pressure	Encouragement of patient in use of preventive measures and risk reduction
Communication with physician and diabetes care team	Supervision of proper foot care procedures
Keeping appointments	Regular review of laboratory markers to assess progress and health status of patient
Record keeping	Regular communication with healthcare team of patient to ensure cohesive patient care and education
Adherence to medication regimen	Support, motivation and encouragement for ongoing healthcare
Evaluation of physician and diabetes care team	
Treating and modifying 'targets' in collaboration with physician	
Knowledge of personal glycosylated haemoglobin value and its meaning	

Adapted from American Association of Clinical Endocrinologists and the American College of Endocrinology. The American Association of Clinical Endocrinologists medical guidelines for the management of diabetes mellitus: The AACE system of intensive diabetes self-management — 2002 update. Endocr Pract 2002; 57(8): Suppl 1.

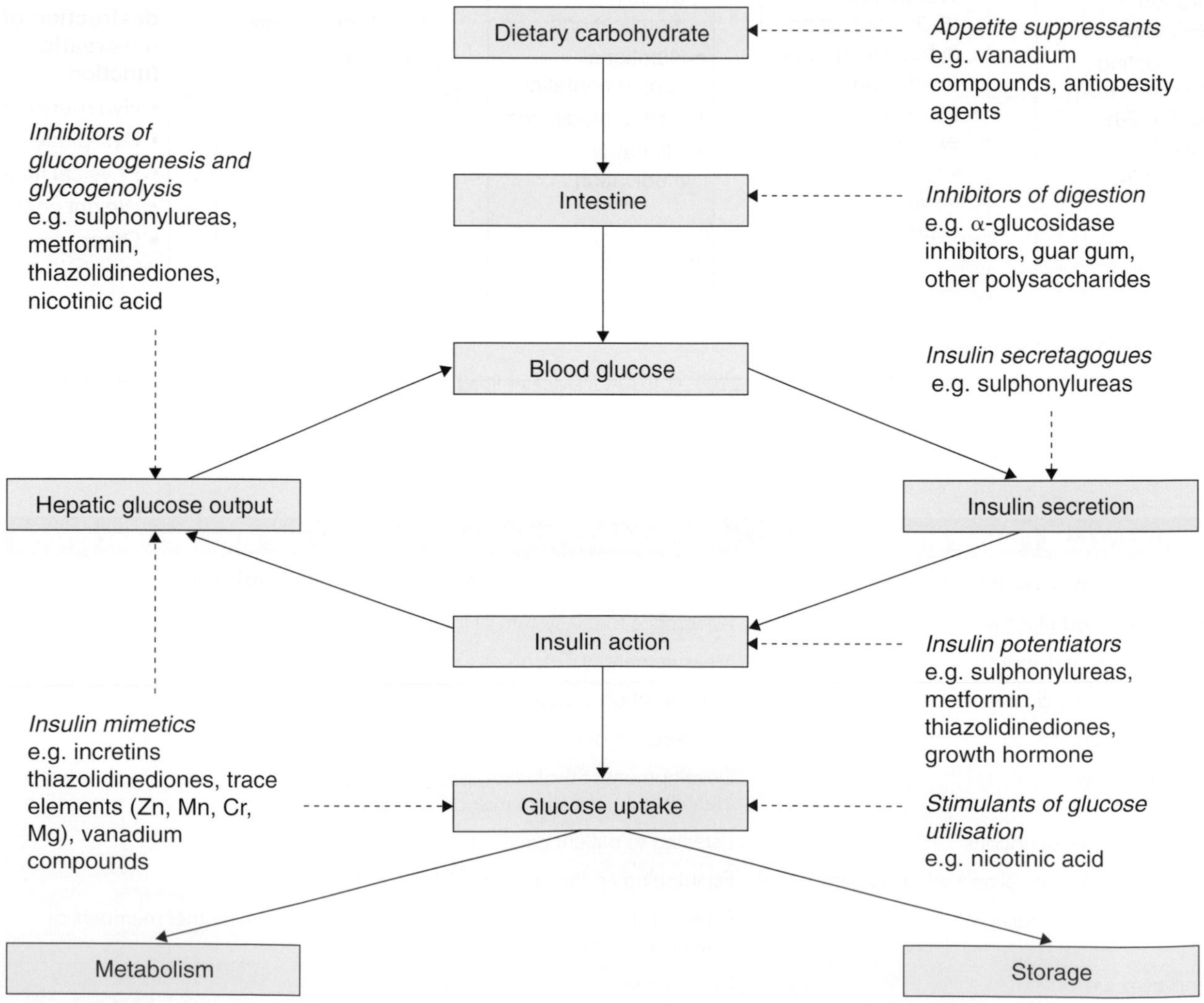

FIGURE 21.9 Overview of treatment for diabetes.

Source: Gray AM, Flatt PR. Nature's own pharmacy: the diabetes perspective. Proceedings of the Nutrition Society, 1997(56):507–517.

TABLE 21.29 Diabetes: medications and actions taken, persons — counts — estimates (National Health Survey: summary of results, 2007–8)

Persons – counts – estimates	Age group (years)						Totals		
Persons with diabetes	0–34	35–44	45–54	55–64	65–74	75 and over	Males	Females	Persons
Persons – counts – estimates									
Type of action taken									
Discussed self-management with GP or specialist ('000)	27.7	52.9	102.2	192.1	146.9	107.7	360.4	269.0	629.4
Had days away from work, school or study ('000)	5.3	9.9	5.5	4.3			15.3	10.6	25.9
Consulted an 'other' health professional ('000)	23.8	42.4	59.3	96.5	74.0	58.7	193.8	160.8	354.6
Type of action taken									
Followed changed eating pattern/diet ('000)	20.6	51.4	101.6	183.6	158.6	93.5	361.0	248.3	609.3
Losing weight ('000)	5.1	23.4	24.6	50.4	24.0	9.6	76.7	60.4	137.1
Exercised most days ('000)	10.8	20.3	46.5	65.6	52.3	23.4	137.3	81.6	218.9
Other actions taken ('000)			4.6	9.2			12.8	6.2	18.9
No action taken ('000)			2.9	5.0	9.9	12.0	17.9	17.3	35.2
Blood glucose checked									
At least once a day ('000)	19.3	35.2	61.0	103.5	84.5	68.5	207.2	164.7	371.9
At least once a week ('000)	4.6	14.1	28.0	53.0	53.7	28.5	113.7	68.2	181.9
At least once a month ('000)	3.3	5.3	9.8	31.4	14.1	17.5	40.6	40.9	81.4
Every 2 to less than 3 months ('000)			11.2	13.1	18.7	8.2	35.5	17.1	52.6
Every 3 to less than 6 months ('000)			8.3	21.3	14.2	10.4	36.6	22.9	59.5
Every 6 months ('000)				4.0	13.9	8.7	13.2	21.0	34.2
Every 7 to 12 months ('000)	0.0			2.6	5.6	3.6	6.5	11.2	17.7
Not at all in the past 12 months ('000)	0.0	3.4	0.8	4.3	1.9	5.7	9.8	6.3	16.1
Feet checked									
At least once a day ('000)			19.4	25.0	20.5	12.2	42.1	43.7	85.7
At least once a week ('000)	5.7	5.9	16.2	22.8	22.7	3.3	49.8	27.0	76.7
At least once a month('000)			16.4	28.7	17.3	13.8	44.9	38.3	83.2
Every 2 to less than 3 months ('000)			11.3	18.9	28.5	48.5	61.0	51.3	112.2
Every 3 to less than 6 months ('000)			7.5	13.0	16.8	10.9	30.3	21.5	51.8
Every 6 months ('000)	0.0	8.1	9.4	23.2	9.9	11.2	31.6	30.2	61.8
Every 7 to 12 months ('000)	7.2	15.2	12.8	17.9	33.6	24.7	68.9	42.6	111.5
Not at all in the past 12 months ('000)	5.5	21.8	36.0	79.4	56.7	25.7	130.9	94.1	225.0
Type of medication used									
Insulin ('000)	18.6	20.6	28.4	41.3	27.6	32.3	83.2	85.4	168.7
Gliclazide ('000)	0.0	5.3	21.7	47.9	43.9	40.1	89.6	69.3	159.0
Metformin ('000)	2.0	29.8	84.7	137.6	117.7	74.4	254.7	191.4	446.1
Other oral blood glucose lowering drugs ('000)			8.5	25.1	23.2	18.0	48.3	29.9	78.2
Other diabetes medication ('000)	11.6	22.0	29.8	31.8	39.2	29.8	90.4	73.6	164.1
Total pharmaceutical medication ('000)	21.5	52.2	105.7	168.5	147.8	120.6	348.8	267.5	616.3
Vitamins, minerals and herbal or natural treatments ('000)		5.0	20.7	8.8		4.7	21.2	25.7	46.9
Total ('000)	21.5	52.2	114.9	171.9	148.5	122.5	354.1	277.3	631.5
Total persons with diabetes ('000)	29.0	65.9	129.6	233.2	206.7	153.7	463.8	354.4	818.2

Source: Australian Bureau of Statistics (ABS). National Health Survey summary of results, 2007–2008. Long-term conditions (Reissue). Cat. no. 4340. Canberra: ABS; 2009.

NUTRITIONAL MEDICINE (DIETARY)

Dietary therapeutic objectives

The optimal diet for the treatment of diabetes is an even stricter avoidance of foods with a high GL. What determines how strict the diet needs to be with the intake of carbohydrates is based on the ability to get blood glucose measurements and A_{1c} levels under control and achieve/maintain ideal body weight. Obviously, the poorer the control, the more the carbohydrate intake must be restricted. Initially, some people with diabetes — especially those who have poorly controlled blood glucose levels — may need to avoid meals with a total GL of more than 20 and space these meals at least 3 hours apart. Higher GL meals can be consumed if one of the special natural products designed to slow gastric emptying and blunt after-meal blood glucose levels is used (these compounds are discussed later).

A number of diets have been studied with regards to the management of diabetes, yet there is still uncertainty over which diet is optimal for diabetics. The quality of dietary fats and carbohydrates consumed is more important than the quantity. Diets that are low in refined grains, red meat, processed meats and sugary beverages, and high in wholegrains,[381,382] fruits, vegetables, legumes, nuts and moderate alcohol consumption have been shown to reduce diabetes risk and improve glycaemic control and blood lipids in diabetic patients.[383] A systematic review and meta-analysis of 20 RCTs (3460 individuals) found that low-carbohydrate, low-GI, Mediterranean and high-protein diets are effective in improving glycaemic control in diabetics, with the greatest effect seen with the Mediterranean diet. The low-carbohydrate and Mediterranean diets both led to the greatest weight loss.[384] Higher adherence to a Mediterranean diet is associated with a 20–23% reduced risk of developing type 2 diabetes. The Mediterranean diet reduces glycosylated haemoglobin levels by 0.30–0.47 %, and is also associated with a 28–30% reduced risk for cardiovascular events in individuals with type 2 diabetes. These benefits are for the most part due to the anti-inflammatory and antioxidative stress effects of the diet.[385]

Dietary carbohydrate restriction in diabetes has been shown to reliably reduce high blood glucose levels (irrespective of weight loss, although carbohydrate restriction is sure to result in weight loss) and can lead to the reduction or elimination of the need for medication.[386–389] A randomised trial of 93 participants over 24 weeks showed that a low-carbohydrate diet (14% CHO, 28% protein, 58% fat (<10% saturated fat)) had a greater improvement on reducing glycaemic variability and reducing medication than an energy-matched high-carbohydrate diet (53% CHO, 17% protein, 30% fat (<10% saturated fat)).[390] A 2015 review of the data indicated that carbohydrate restriction appears to be safe and effective in the short term, but longer term results are not sustained and inconclusive.[391] The evidence so far is compelling, and further research is required.

A 2016 meta-analysis investigating different types of fats in the diet concluded that diets high in monounsaturated fatty acids improves metabolic risk factors in patients with type 2 diabetes, compared to high polyunsaturated fatty acids and high carbohydrate diets. High MUFA-diets when compared to both high-PUFA diets and high-carbohydrate diets resulted in significant reductions in fasting plasma glucose.[392]

The glycaemic index

The glycaemic index (or GI) is a way of ranking carbohydrate-containing foods according to their effect on blood glucose. Foods are given a number between 0 and 100 according to how fast their carbohydrate is converted to glucose and enters the bloodstream — the lower the number, the slower the rise in glucose.

Carbohydrates that break down quickly during digestion have high GIs, and cause a large, rapid increase in blood glucose that is not sustained over time. Carbohydrates that break down slowly during digestion have low GIs, and produce gradual, sustained increases in blood glucose — this is most desirable and is being demonstrated to be beneficial for our health.

The glycaemic index allows us to compare the effects of different carbohydrate-containing foods on the levels of glucose in the blood. In most cases pure glucose is used as the standard and is given a score of 100. All other foods are compared with the standard and given a rating. Some GIs are now using white bread as a standard as this is thought to be more typical of the type of foods we eat.

Fig. 21.10 visually represents the effects of high and low GI foods on blood glucose over a period of time.

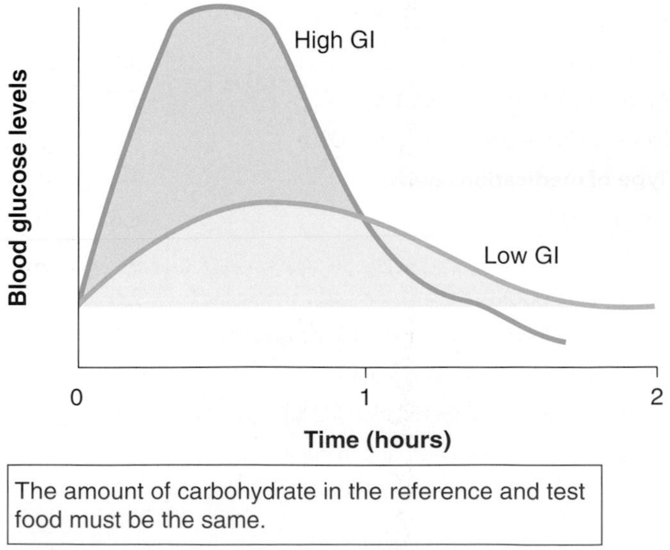

FIGURE 21.10 Glycaemic response in healthy adults.

COMPARING THE GI OF FOODS

Foods can be divided into three main groups to provide a quick indication of a food's effect on blood glucose:
- Foods with a GI of 55 or less are *low* GI foods
- Foods with a GI of between 56 and 69 are *moderate* GI foods
- Foods with a GI of 70 or over are *high* GI foods.

Note that a food's GI is *not* determined by whether the food contains simple or complex carbohydrates. Some simple carbohydrates like table sugar have a medium GI, while potatoes, which are starchy vegetables rich in complex carbohydrates, generally have a very high GI. So, often the GI of a food may not be what you would expect; as another example of this, brown rice has a higher GI than table sugar.

Examples

Low GI	Moderate GI	High GI
Most fruits and vegetables	Sucrose (table sugar)	White and wholemeal bread
Wholegrain and mixed grain breads	Basmati rice	White rice
Beans, legumes, lentils	Ice-cream	Weet-Bix
Soy products	Chocolate bars	Brown rice
Nuts	Buckwheat	Boiled potatoes
Pasta	Couscous	Cooked carrots
Porridge	Beetroot	Parsnip
Milk	Mango (just ripe)	Pumpkin
	Paw paw (just ripe)	Watermelon
	Sultanas (just ripe)	Dates
	Bananas (just ripe)	Rockmelon
		Cornflakes
		Rice bubbles
		Doughnuts
		Popcorn
		Rice pasta

FACTORS THAT AFFECT GI

Foods have different effects on blood glucose due to a number of factors, such as how rapidly they are digested and absorbed, and due to the presence of other nutrients or non-nutrients in the food. Importantly, the glycaemic effect of a food changes depending upon whether it is eaten alone, or with other foods as part of a meal. The factors that influence a food's GI are outlined below.

The degree of processing, cooking or chewing

As a general rule the more processed and refined a food is, the higher we would expect its GI to be. On the other hand, foods which are more textured, chewy, crunchy and fibrous tend to take longer to digest, and would therefore have a lower GI than foods that are soft, refined or pre-cooked. For example, whole rolled oats have a lower GI than processed 'quick cooking' oats, and regular white rice has a lower GI than quick cooking brown rice. As another example, wholegrain breads have a lower GI than wholemeal breads.

Traditional methods of raising bread dough (such as sourdough fermentation) are slower and produce breads with a lower GI than breads made with rapid-rise dough.

Whether the food is found in large pieces or broken down into fine particles also affects the GI. As a result, food that has not been chewed properly has a lower GI because it will be in larger pieces and harder to digest. However, this does *not* mean that you should not chew your food as a way of lowering the GI of your diet. Chewing is important for adequate digestion and nutrient absorption, and inadequate chewing can lead to indigestion.

Pasta has a low GI because the method of producing this food traps the starch in a sponge-like matrix of protein molecules within the pasta dough — and it takes longer to digest.

The type of fibre in the food

Soluble fibre slows the digestion of starches and the absorption of glucose into the bloodstream. Soluble fibre is found in oats, barley, fruits high in pectin (apples, stone fruits, pears, oranges), legumes (beans, lentils), and psyllium (a type of fibre used as a supplement and found in products like Metamucil). As a result, porridge has a lower GI than wheat-based cereals like Weet-Bix, and apples have a lower GI than watermelon.

The type of starch in the food

Resistant starch is a type of starch that is digested more slowly, and therefore releases glucose to the bloodstream more slowly. Starch in foods may be found either as amylose (a linear polymer of glucose that is a long chain of sugars joined together) or as amylopectin (a branched polymer of glucose). Amylose is digested more slowly than amylopectin, and as a consequence foods that are rich in amylose have a low GI. Remember also that starchy foods like potatoes and pasta contain more resistant fibre when they are eaten cold after cooking.

Cold cooked potato has a lower GI than freshly cooked white potato, new potatoes have a lower GI than Desiree potatoes, and long grain rice has a lower GI than short grain rice — these differences are due to the amount of amylose and resistant fibre present in these foods. Most types of rice have a high GI, but basmati rice has a medium GI due to its higher amylose content.

The degree of ripeness of the food

Generally, the riper the food, the higher the GI of the food would be. For example, ripe or very ripe bananas have a higher GI than unripe bananas.

The acidity and saltiness of the food

Acidic foods slow down the digestion of starches by slowing stomach emptying and so reduce the GI of a meal. This includes foods such as vinegar, lemon juice, acidic fruit, vinaigrette and pickled foods like gherkins.

Salt and salty foods or condiments increase the rate of starch digestion and glucose absorption, and so increase the GI of a meal.

The type of sugar in the food

Of the different sugars glucose has the most pronounced effect on blood glucose, therefore foods high in glucose have a higher GI. Foods that contain glucose syrup, including some sports drinks, have a high GI.

Fructose, a sugar found in fruits, honey, and as one of the sugars in sucrose (or table sugar), is absorbed as fructose and so does not immediately influence blood glucose — as a consequence high-fructose foods have a lower GI. Fructose is also found in some vegetables including sweet corn and sweet potato, and in corn syrup.

Lactose (the disaccharide found in milk) and sucrose (table sugar) both have an intermediate effect on blood glucose. This means that a food with a lot of refined sugar in it, such as a chocolate bar, could have a medium GI. Obviously this does not mean that these foods are good choices — they are high in refined sugars, kilojoules and saturated fat and low in other nutrients.

The amount of fat in a food

High-fat foods generally have a lower GI because fat slows down the rate of stomach emptying, and so slows the digestion and absorption of carbohydrates. This is why many foods that are obviously not the healthiest of choices (such as chocolate bars, ice-cream, chocolate milk powders and chocolate sandwich spreads) state that they have a low GI! Food with a low GI is not necessarily a healthy food or a good food choice. Evaluation of other aspects of the food's nutritional makeup is essential when making a decision about what to eat. If a food has a low GI, but is high in saturated fats and/or is a processed food, it may not be a good food choice.

The combination of foods eaten together

Generally foods are not eaten by themselves but as part of a meal with other foods. While we can establish the GI of individual foods, it may not accurately reflect the effect on blood glucose of eating that food once it is consumed with other foods as part of a meal. Eating foods that are high in protein, fat or fibre as part of a meal lowers the overall GI of the meal, as these nutrients slow stomach emptying. For example, eating pasta with a meat-based sauce has a lower GI (due to the fat and protein in the meat) than eating pasta with a tomato sauce.

A LOW GI DIET

It is generally recommended that foods with a low or moderate GI are consumed more often than those with a high GI, as this results in more desirable and controlled fluctuations in blood glucose. Although the beneficial effects of a low GI diet are controversial and still being researched, there is some evidence that low GI diets can be useful in helping to control blood glucose levels in those with diabetes — diabetics have blood glucose levels that are much higher than normal, so low GI foods can help to control this. An analysis of the EPIC cohort (across eight European countries) did not find any association between dietary GI, GL or digestible carbohydrates. Current evidence regarding the association of GI and GL with diabetes is still mixed, but does tend towards an increased risk of diabetes with higher GI/GL food intake. Mixed results might be explained by discrepancies in GI values assigned to foods across studies/study populations,[393] or because studies often investigated a combination of high-fibre and low-GI foods and the benefits of one component over the other can't be easily distinguished.[383]

Other possible benefits of a low GI diet include:

- May delay hunger and control appetite, and assist with weight loss
- May improve lipid metabolism and control blood lipid levels (because when blood glucose is high the pancreas releases insulin, and one of the actions of this hormone is to instruct the liver to manufacture lipids)
- May improve cellular sensitivity to insulin (the cells of some individuals, including those with diabetes, do not respond normally to insulin and so blood glucose stays high even when insulin has been released)
- May reduce the risk of obesity, diabetes and heart disease
- May improve endurance in athletes.

HIGH GI FOODS

High GI foods produce rapid increases in blood glucose and can be useful for athletes after heavy exercise to provide energy and to replace glycogen stores. High GI foods are also important in the treatment of hypoglycaemic episodes in diabetics — a situation where blood glucose levels become too low, which can be very dangerous and even fatal.

However, high GI foods may increase the risk of heart disease, diabetes and obesity, and in some individuals may cause a surge in blood glucose that is followed by a plunge below the normal range, resulting in hypoglycaemia. This would cause symptoms such as dizziness, blurred vision, nausea, sweating, and even fainting.

Table 21.30 shows the average GI of 62 common foods.

THE GLYCAEMIC LOAD

Some foods may have a high GI but do not actually contain very much carbohydrate, and so the actual effect on blood glucose may be minimal. For example, carrots, pumpkin and parsnips have a high GI (because the carbohydrate they contain is readily digested and absorbed) but they do not actually contain very much carbohydrate. Again this means that we cannot rely solely on the GI of a food to determine whether it is a good choice or not.

When calculating the GI researchers give volunteers enough of the food they are testing to provide 50 g of carbohydrate. This is what would be found in two slices of bread, 500 mL of soft drink, or 1 kg of carrots. But you are not going to eat 1 kg of carrots! So even though carrots have a high GI, the amount of carbohydrate present is small as is the real effect on blood glucose.

The GI can be regarded as a measure of the quality of carbohydrate in a food and of how easily it is digested and absorbed — not of how much is there. For this reason there is another way of ranking foods according to the amount of carbohydrate they contain — this is called the glycaemic load.

The glycaemic load is a measure of how much carbohydrate is present in a typical serving of a particular food, which is a more accurate representation of what we are really eating. The GL is calculated by multiplying the GI value of the food by the amount of carbohydrate in a serve, and then by dividing by 100. For example, a slice of white bread contains 15 g of carbohydrate and has a GI of 70, so the GL is $(70 \times 15) \div 100 = 10.5$.

TABLE 21.30 Average GI of some common foods

Fruit and fruit products		High-carbohydrate foods		Vegetables		Breakfast cereals	
Apple juice	41 ± 2	Barley	28 ± 2	Carrots, boiled	39 ± 4	Cornflakes	81 ± 6
Apple, raw†	36 ± 2	Brown rice, boiled	68 ± 4	Plantain/green banana	55 ± 6	Instant oat porridge	79 ± 3
Banana, raw†	51 ± 3	Chapatti	52 ± 4	Potato, boiled	78 ± 4	Millet porridge	67 ± 5
Dates, raw	42 ± 4	Corn tortilla	46 ± 4	Potato, French fries	63 ± 5	Muesli	57 ± 2
Mango, raw†	51 ± 5	Couscous†	65 ± 4	Potato, instant mash	87 ± 3	Porridge, rolled oats	55 ± 2
Orange juice	50 ± 2	Rice noodles†	53 ± 7	Pumpkin, boiled	64 ± 7	Rice porridge/ congee	78 ± 9
Orange, raw†	43 ± 3	Spaghetti, white	49 ± 2	Sweet potato, boiled	63 ± 6	Wheat flake biscuits	69 ± 2
Peaches, canned†	43 ± 5	Spaghetti, wholemeal	48 ± 5	Taro, boiled	53 ± 2		
Pineapple, raw	59 ± 8	Specialty grain bread	53 ± 2	Vegetable soup	48 ± 5		
Strawberry jam/jelly	49 ± 3	Sweet corn	52 ± 5				
Watermelon, raw	76 ± 4	Udon noodles	55 ± 7				
		Unleavened wheat bread	70 ± 5				
		Wheat roti	62 ± 3				
		White rice, boiled*	73 ± 4				
		White wheat bread*	74 ± 2				
		Wholewheat/wholemeal bread	74 ± 2				
Snack products		**Dairy products and alternatives**		**Sugars**		**Legumes**	
Chocolate	40 ± 3	Ice-cream	51 ± 3	Fructose	15 ± 4	Chickpeas	28 ± 9
Popcorn	65 ± 5	Milk, full fat	39 ± 3	Glucose	103 ± 3	Kidney beans	24 ± 4
Potato crisps	56 ± 3	Milk, skim	37 ± 4	Honey	61 ± 3	Lentils	32 ± 5
Rice crackers/crisps	87 ± 2	Rice milk	86 ± 7	Sucrose	65 ± 4	Soy beans	16 ± 1
Soft drink/soda	59 ± 3	Soy milk	34 ± 4				
		Yoghurt, fruit	41 ± 2				

Data are means ± SEM.
*Low-GI varieties were also identified.
†Average of all variable data.
Source: Adapted from Atkinson FS, Foster-Powell K, Brand-Miller J. International tables of glycemic index and glycemic load values. Diabetes Care 2008; 31(12):2281–2283.

Foods can be divided into three main groups to provide a quick indication of a food's carbohydrate content:

- Foods with a GL of 10 or less are *low* GL foods
- Foods with a GL of between 11 and 19 are *moderate* GL foods
- Foods with a GL of 20 or over are *high* GL foods.

When evaluating foods it is important to consider both its GI and the GL. A food with a high GI *and* high GL is probably not the best choice; however, a food with a high GI but a low GL may still be a good choice (for example, carrots) especially when other nutritional considerations (such as fat and kilojoule content, and the presence of vitamins, minerals and phytochemicals) is taken into account. So, while GI is a measure of quality, GL is a measure of quantity. Food tables that tell you the GI of a food now usually also state the GL. A 2013 meta-analysis of 24 prospective cohort studies found that low-GL diets are associated with a significantly lower risk of type 2 diabetes.[394] This is further supported by a 2014 systematic review of observational studies which found a protective effect of low dietary GI and GL,[395] as well as a meta-analysis from three large US cohorts.[396]

Food insulin index (FII)

The newest index is the food insulin index (FII) which directly quantifies the postprandial insulin response to an isoenergetic portion of a test food in comparison to a reference food. It allows testing of foods with little or no carbohydrate content and is able to predict the relative insulin demand evoked by mixed meals.[397,398]

It measures blood insulin response to a food compared to a reference food glucose (FII = 100). It measures incremental insulin area under the curve (AUC) over two hours in response to consumption of a 1000 kJ portion of the test food divided by the AUC after ingestion of a 1000 kJ portion of the reference food.

See Table 21.31 for a comparison of FII vs GI when assessing impact of food on blood glucose levels.

TABLE 21.31 Comparison of food insulin index (FII) with glycaemic index (GI)

Food insulin index	Glycaemic index
Measures postprandial increase in **insulin** secretion of a whole **food**	Measures effect of **carbohydrate-**containing foods on postprandial increase in **blood-glucose** levels
Dependent on carbohydrate, quantity and quality of protein and fat and their interactions	GI is not always proportional to the insulin response

COMMON FOODS ON USING FII

Highest analysed:

- Jelly beans (120)
- Pancakes (112)
- Honeydew melon (95)
- Potatoes (90)
- Breakfast cereals (70–113).

Lowest analysed:

- Most vegetables are negligible
- Olive oil (3)
- Avocado (5)
- Walnuts (6)
- Tuna (16)
- Chicken (20).

FII variability within some food groups complicated interpretation — for example dairy foods can range from cream cheese (18) to fruit yoghurt (86). Consideration of this is important when interpreting and applying this information to dietary recommendations for patients.

Other considerations

As FII is a measure of a food's relative insulin demand compared with other foods, it is a fixed value that doesn't change as the food portion size changes.

Conversely, food insulin demand (FID) combines a food's FII with the kilojoules in the portion size; that is, the FID changes as the food portion size changes and can therefore be used to determine the mealtime insulin dose (if required).

$$\text{FID} = \text{energy (kJ)} \times \text{food insulin index (FII)}$$

DIETARY INCLUSIONS

- Consumption of organic fresh fruits and vegetables should be encouraged (low GI/GL types). Blueberries, grapes and apples have been significantly associated with a lower risk of type 2 diabetes.[399]
- Complex carbohydrates should be chosen for carbohydrate requirements.
- Lean protein should be consumed at each meal from both animal and vegetarian sources. Vegetarian proteins should be balanced for complete intake. A randomised control study of 140 participants with type 2 diabetes, found that a high egg diet (2 eggs/day for 6 weeks) did not have an adverse effect on lipid profile (previous results have been inconclusive). Eggs can be included in the diet as they provide satiety.[400]

DIETARY EXCLUSIONS

- All high GI/GL foods; high FII foods
- Alcohol, refined foods, caffeine, sugar in any form (including artificial sources), soft drinks (especially diet types), and fruit juices[399]
- High consumption of white rice is associated with a significantly increased risk of type 2 diabetes (particularly in Asian populations)[401]
- Trans-fats, deep-fried foods and oxidised fats (stale nuts and seeds, rancid oils, smoked oils)
- All smoked and cured foods (nitrosamine content).

OTHER DIETARY CONSIDERATIONS

All simple, processed, concentrated carbohydrates must be avoided. Complex carbohydrate, high-fibre foods should be encouraged[402], and fats should be kept to a minimum. Legumes, onions and garlic are particularly useful and should be encouraged.[403] A crossover randomised clinical trial with 31 overweight type 2 diabetes participants found that substituting red meat intake with legumes improved lipid profiles and glycaemic control, independent of BMI changes.[404]

See Tables 21.32 and 21.33 for bioactive compounds and functional properties of some preferred fruits and vegetables and other foods.

NUTRITIONAL MEDICINE (SUPPLEMENTAL)

Nutritional medicine therapeutic objectives

There is evidence for a number of micronutrients beneficial in the treatment of diabetes and IR.[363,373,405] The major nutrients will be discussed below. In addition, vitamin A, biotin, *N*-acetylcysteine and fructo-oligo saccharides (FOS) have all shown favourable effects in diabetes.[405]

Specific nutrients required

CHROMIUM

Chromium (Cr), in its trivalent state Cr3+, is required for the uptake of insulin into the cells. The proposed

TABLE 21.32 Bioactive compounds and functional properties of some preferred fruits and vegetables

Fruits and vegetables	Nutrients	Bioactive components	Functional properties
Grapefruit	–	Lycopene, pectin, naringin, hesperidin	Regulates appetite Reduces triglyceride levels Antioxidant defence stimulator
Watermelon	–	Carotenoids, lycopene, cytrolin	Reduces blood pressure, insulin resistance and adipocyte size Improves endothelial function and nitric oxide biosynthesis
Grapes and grape byproducts	–	Anthocyanidins, resveratrol	Reduces blood pressure, renin-angiotensin activity, oxidative damage, cardiovascular disease, platelet aggregation and hyperactivity Increases nitric oxide production, bone marrow-derived endothelial progenitor cells
Cherries	Beta-carotene	Xanthine, lutein, gallic acid, phenolic acids, melatonin, carotenoids, quercetin, anthocyanidins, hydrocinnamic acid	Reduces diabetic neuropathy, cytokine production, oxidative stress, microalbuminuria, abdominal fat, HbA_{1c}, hyperglycaemia Anti-inflammatory — inhibits cyclooxygenase Improves metabolic syndrome and fatty liver features
Garlic and onions	–	Quercetin, flavonoids, dihydroflavonols, anthocyanidins (red onions), allyl sulfurs	Reduces platelet aggregation and hyperactivity, lipid peroxidation, blood pressure, hyperglycaemia Increases insulin sensitivity Regulates glycolysis, gluconeogenesis and carbohydrate pathways

TABLE 21.33 Bioactive compounds and functional properties of some preferred functional foods for diabetes mellitus

Functional foods	Nutrients	Bioactive components	Functional properties
Fish and seafood	Taurine Selenium Omega-3 fatty acids — docohexaenoic, eicosapentaenoic Antioxidant compounds	Bioactive peptides	Reduces triglycerides Reduces blood pressure Improves cardiovascular function Improves metabolic syndrome features
Dairy products	Conjugated linoleic acids Calcium B vitamins	Bioactive proteins: casein, whey Bioactive peptides: alpha and beta lactophines, lactoferrin, lactoferricin, alpha-lactalbumin, beta-lactoglobulin, growth factors Bacteria: lactic acid bacteria, bifidobacteria	Modulates digestive bacteria Improves metabolic syndrome features Regulates satiety and food intake
Cinnamon	–	Cinnamaldehyde, cinnamic acid, coumarin, catechins, epicatechin, procyanidins	Improves insulin sensitivity and peripheral uptake of glucose Increases glycolysis and gluconuogenesis
Olive oil	–	Flavonoids, oleic acid, omega-3 fatty acids, cinnamic acid, cumaric acid, ferulic acid, benzoic acid, lignans, carotenoids, oleuropein, oleocanthal	Reduces pro-inflammatory cyctokines Reduces atherosclerotic plaque, LDL oxidation Regulates cholesterol metabolism Protects against atherogenesis
Green tea	–	Catechins, epigallocatechin-3-gallat Pectin Plant sterols Chlorophyll Polyphenols, phenolic acids	Improves insulin sensitivity, glycaemic control, glycogen content, thermogenesis Reduces gluconeogenesis, glycation of collagen and fibrosis, proliferation and differentiation of adipocytes, proinflammatory cytokines

SAMPLE DAILY DIET

BREAKFAST	
Blueberry smoothie: blueberries, oats, cinnamon, chia seeds, almond milk	A gluten-free diet (GFD) has been found to protect against type 1 diabetes and has been shown to improve glycaemic control as measured by lower HBA_{1c} in individuals with type 1 diabetes following a GF diet compared to those not following a GF diet. Oats provide a low GI, complex carbohydrate which when combined with chia, a source of healthy fats, maintains blood sugar control. Blueberries and cinnamon both exhibit gluco-regulatory mechanisms and have been shown to improve insulin sensitivity.
LUNCH	
Corn, potato and zucchini fritters served with sauerkraut and salad dressed with miso	A diet rich in nutrient-rich starchy foods (such as potato and corn) is suggested. A diet rich in starch has been shown to be fermented by bacteria and results in production of the SCFAs acetate and butyrate, both of which have been shown to protect mice against type 1 diabetes by inhibiting the expansion of the autoimmune effector T-cells and improving gut barrier function. Considerable shifts in the bacterial communities found in the gut have been linked to increased autoimmune diseases thus use of prebiotic- and probiotic-rich foods (e.g. miso and sauerkraut) may provide a medium for improving microbial balance in the intestinal tract, promoting a return to normal microbial community.
DINNER	
Sweet potato wedges dusted with cinnamon served with turmeric and coconut crusted fish. Serve with salad dressed with vinegar	Sweet potato is rich in fibre and may help to regulate insulin metabolism. Antioxidant spices such as turmeric are used to downregulate inflammation associated with autoimmune disease. Consumption of vinegar has been shown to reduce gastric emptying times decreasing postprandial hyperglycaemia in individuals with type 1 diabetes.
SNACK	
Fruit with nuts plus green tea Coconut yoghurt with fruit, cinnamon, cacao and macadamias	Green tea contains polyphenols which have been shown to reduce the release of pro-inflammatory mediators in people at risk of chronic inflammation. Cacao may reduce inflammation. Fruit is antioxidant rich and anti-inflammatory.

mechanism of action is that transferrin-bound Cr is taken up by cells in response to elevated blood insulin levels. Inside the cell, Cr is released from transferrin and subsequently binds to apo-chromodulin, an oligopeptide consisting of the amino acids glycine, cysteine, aspartate and glutamate. The Cr-chromodulin complex (also called holo-chromodulin or simply chromodulin) carries four Cr ions and binds to insulin receptors on the cell wall. It also stimulates a number of enzymes involved in insulin signalling, thus potentiating the action of insulin.[208]

Dietary sources of Cr include wholegrains, fruit and vegetables, cheese, red and white meat (especially organ meat), fish and Cr-rich yeast. Absorption requires an acidic environment, and acid-lowering treatment has been linked to lower the uptake of the mineral. Phytates also reduce Cr absorption.[208]

Although Cr has been shown to be useful in impaired glucose tolerance only if levels are suboptimal,[86,208] the body has higher requirements under certain circumstances, such as in type 2 DM, being under stress, performing strenuous exercise or consuming a diet high in sugar, where higher urinary losses have been reported.[86,405] Studies in type 2 DM showed reduced insulin levels and glycated haemoglobin, and improved blood glucose and lipid profiles with supplemental Cr.[86] Claims on improved body composition and weight/fat loss have to date not been substantiated.[85,86] In stressed animals Cr supplementation has lowered cortisol levels,[85] and considering that increased cortisol is a factor in insulin resistance (IR),[406] there may be a role for Cr in preventing stress-induced elevations in blood glucose and IR.

To date, there is no gold standard for measuring Cr status in the body. Serum, red blood cell Cr, and urinary Cr excretion are commonly employed. Best approximations of body stores may be achieved by combining two or more methods. Chromium serum concentrations were significantly reduced in type 2 diabetes patients, but urinary levels were higher than in the healthy controls.[407]

Supplements in the range 200–1000 micrograms Cr per day have been considered safe, with increased benefits from higher dosages. Absorption of Cr is poor. Picolinate, showing higher solubility, has been preferred to other forms (such as chlorides). However, some doubt as to its safety have arisen which are not entirely conclusive regarding human consumption, leading to restrictions regarding the amount of Cr picolinate in supplements.

Organically bound Cr has superior uptake to inorganic salts, and the nicotinate forms (Cr bound to niacin) have been available under the name of 'glucose tolerance factor'. It was first discovered in Cr-rich yeast.[208]

VANADIUM

Vanadium (V) has similar action to Cr and works well in combination with this mineral. Amounts between 20 and 100 micrograms per day have been recommended.[408] Higher doses may be harmful to humans and caution is advised. In patients with type 2 diabetes, vanadium supplementation increased insulin sensitivity, glucose oxidation and glycogen synthesis.[407]

MAGNESIUM

Magnesium (Mg) deficiency, often associated with a Western diet,[6] has been found to be related to poor glycaemic control and impairment of insulin secretion and function due to reduced absorption and increased urinary losses.[208] IR in return can interfere with cellular Mg uptake, thus creating a vicious circle.[363] A meta-analysis of 13 prospective cohort studies found that magnesium intake is significantly associated with an inverse risk of type 2 diabetes (in a dose response manner).[409]

Food sources of magnesium include green leafy vegetables (magnesium is an essential part of chlorophyll), wholegrains and nuts.[86] High dietary intake as well as supplementation have improved the metabolic function in diabetes and metabolic syndrome. Improvements in IR and lipids and reductions in inflammation and oxidative stress have been shown, in addition to magnesium's beneficial effects in cardiovascular disease.[410,411] However, not all studies have shown a positive effect.[208]

Magnesium's actions include energy production, post-receptor insulin signalling, fatty acid synthesis and glucose utilisation.[411] The mechanism is thought to be linked to magnesium's role in stabilising ATP.[208]

Assessing magnesium status can be done through serum and red cell magnesium, and 24-hour urinary output. Serum reflects recent dietary intake, whereas red cells reflect longer term storage of magnesium. Urine is more reflective of surplus.

Supplementation of 400 mg elemental magnesium has been shown to improve glucose tolerance in those individuals testing low for the mineral.[86] Inorganic salts can have a laxative effect; therefore chelated forms of the mineral are preferable.[86]

VITAMIN C

Vitamin C, which most animals produce in response to stress, is made from glucose. Humans lack the enzyme for the final conversion and therefore rely on nutritional sources.[208] This similarity in structure may be the reason for competitive cellular uptake of glucose and vitamin C. The vitamin is also involved in releasing insulin in response to glucose and in restoring nitric oxide levels.[363] Hypercholesterolaemia in diabetic patients was reduced by the administration of vitamin C. The proposed mechanism of action includes the saturation of tissue levels, thus enhancing the liver's ability to increase cholesterol excretion through upregulated bile salts production.[412] A low to moderate dose (around 500 mg/day) has been shown to be most effective.[363,412]

VITAMIN E

Vitamin E, another antioxidant, not only reduces oxidative stress, it is also involved in the regeneration of other antioxidants. Vitamin E also reduces risk factors of IR and diabetic complications, such as LDL. Amounts between 100 and 900 IU have been used.[363]

SELENIUM

Selenium, alone or even more so in combination with vitamin E, reduces oxidative stress in obese diabetic rats. Both vitamins are involved in glutathione synthesis.[363]

VITAMIN D

Vitamin D deficiency has been shown to be correlated not only to IR and diabetes (both type 1 and type 2 DM)[405,413,414] but also to comorbidities such as cardiovascular disease.[415,416] Considering that vitamin D deficiency is high in Australia despite its high sunshine hours (due to fear of skin cancer and the 'slip, slop, slap' approach), these findings are not surprising. Vitamin D status correlates with insulin and glucose levels, and supplementation with the vitamin has improved not only glucose and insulin control but also hypertension, regardless of vitamin D status.[417] This vitamin plays a crucial role in immunomodulation as well as in the production and secretion of insulin. Deficiency has been linked to increased risk of type 1 DM, type 2 DM and metabolic syndrome.[417] Supplementation has improved both IR and glucose levels.[418]

Vitamin D can be measured as 25-hydroxy vitamin D and also as its activated form of 1,25-dihydroxy vitamin D. In general, 1000 IU vitamin D per day is needed if sun exposure is inadequate.[418]

ESSENTIAL FATTY ACIDS

Essential fatty acids (EFAs), notably the omega-3 series, are needed for energy and glucose regulation. They positively influence fat burning and negatively influence fat storage by increasing beta oxidation and glycogen synthesis.[419] EFAs reduce elevated triglycerides. Rat models have shown a protective effect regarding IR.[363] Apart from their beneficial effect on blood lipids and inflammation, they prevent organ damage in diabetes.[420] High fish intake in diabetic patients has delayed the onset of cardiovascular symptoms. As delta-6 desaturase, the enzyme converting linoleic acid to EPA and DHA is impaired in diabetes, supplemental fish oils are of higher therapeutic value than plant sources.[405] Dosage recommendations are 3 g twice a day.[373] Results of a systematic review and meta-analysis of sixteen studies (527 441 participants, 24082 diabetes cases) showed geographical variations in the association with fish consumption and EFAs with risk for type 2 diabetes. No association was found in European studies, a direct association in US studies, and an inverse association in Asian and Australian studies.[421] It is possible that contaminants in the fish, such as mercury, may modify the effects on diabetes risk.[422] A long-term lower risk of type 2 diabetes was associated with increased levels of fish consumption in Finnish men.[422] Further investigations are required.

CONJUGATED LINOLEIC ACID

Conjugated linoleic acid (CLA), found in ruminant fat (beef, lamb, dairy), has been associated with a protective role in type 2 DM and metabolic syndrome.[423,424] It has been estimated that people consume less than half the amount of dairy fat needed to benefit from its protective properties.[425] This is obviously a factor worth considering when recommending a low-fat diet. Low-fat fermented dairy products (largely yoghurt) have been associated with a decreased risk of type 2 diabetes. High-fat dairy, milk, cheese and high fat fermented dairy product intake was not associated with increased incidence of type 2 diabetes, indicating the protective role of these products.[426–428]

R-ALPHA LIPOIC ACID

R-alpha lipoic acid (r-ALA), a water- as well as fat-soluble antioxidant, protects against the development of diabetes and its comorbidities.[363] r-ALA has been shown to guard against diabetic complications such as damage to eyes, blood vessels and kidneys. These beneficial effects have been attributed to r-ALA's ability to enhance glucose uptake via the GLUT4 transport system, similarly to the uptake of glucose that is initiated by insulin.[380] A 2012 systematic review and meta-analysis on omega-3 fatty acids and type 2 diabetes incidence found that estimated dietary r-ALA and circulating r-ALA were both associated with a non-significant trend towards lower risk of type 2 diabetes.[429]

COENZYME Q10

Coenzyme Q10 (CoQ10) is known for its cardiovascular action and may therefore contribute to the protection against metabolic syndrome.[363] Cellular energy production depends on oxidative phosphorylation, where CoQ10 is an important co-factor. Various tissues, such as the nervous system, kidneys and pancreatic beta cells, are particularly dependent on this kind of energy production.[430] Statin drugs, commonly prescribed for elevated cholesterol which is part of the metabolic syndrome pathology, competitively inhibit HMG-CoA reductase. This enzyme is involved in cholesterol as well as CoQ10 synthesis.[431] Although there is some difference in the effect of various statins on CoQ10, even short-term administration of atorvastatin has led to marked decreases in CoQ10. It is hypothesised that the side effects commonly encountered with statin treatment, notably reduced exercise tolerance, myalgia and myoglobinuria, may well be due to this effect.[432] A daily dose of 30–100 mg has been recommended. A meta-analysis on CoQ10 supplementation in diabetes showed that there is no beneficial effect on glycaemic control, lipid profile, or blood pressure; however, it may reduce triglycerides.[433] Another review found that CoQ10 supplementation is beneficial in diabetes management through its effect on alleviating oxidative stress and preserving mitochondrial function.[434] The effect on oxidative stress in type 2 diabetes is supported by a randomised placebo-controlled study of 52 patients. Again, in this study there was no effect on glycaemic control with 100 mg/day CoQ10 supplementation.[435] It is noted that CoQ10 deficiency is often seen in patients with type 2 diabetes.

ACETYL-L-CARNITINE

Acetyl-L-carnitine is made from lysine which has been methylated, where the methyl groups have been donated by *S*-adenosyl methionine (SAM — see box on 'Homocysteine'). It facilitates the transport of fatty acids (especially long chain fatty acids) across the mitochondrial membrane for beta-oxidation. For this reason weight-loss claims have been made about acetyl-L-carnitine which do not stand up to scrutiny. However, acetyl-L-carnitine is essential for increased mitochondrial energy production.[illegible] It is generally decreased in type 1 DM. Doses of 3 g/day have been used in some trials.[405]

B COMPLEX (ALL B VITAMINS)

The B vitamins as a whole are responsible for numerous functions within the body, one of the most important in terms of diabetes being the metabolism of carbohydrates. Each B vitamin has its own individual role in the prevention of diabetes, for example thiamine (vitamin B_1) is an essential coenzyme for the enzymes transketolase, pyruvate dehydrogenase and alpha-ketoglutarate dehydrogenase, complexes that are all involved in intracellular glucose metabolism. Numerous clinical studies have investigated the importance of thiamine in the management of diabetes not least because of the increased requirements of thiamine by the body due to increased glucose metabolism[436] but also because thiamine deficiency involves impaired glucose tolerance. Of similar importance though less researched is riboflavin (vitamin B_2), which is part of flavin adenine dinucleotide, a coenzyme required for metabolism of carbohydrates. The merits of niacinamide (vitamin B_3) are discussed below. The B vitamins may also be used to help manage diabetic complications such as diabetic nephropathy.[437] A study of 174 type 2 diabetes patients showed that type 2 diabetes is associated with decreased plasma levels of thiamine and pyridoxal 5′-phosphate, and alterations in vitamin B_6 metabolism.[438]

ZINC

Diabetic patients commonly exhibit a disruption in their metabolism of zinc, evidenced by increased loss of zinc particularly via the urine.[439] It has been suggested that supplementation with zinc for diabetic patients would be advantageous as diabetic patients are commonly deficient in this important mineral.[440] Zinc has been proposed to mimic insulin by assisting in the signal transduction of insulin while also reducing beta cell insulin secretion and decreasing cytokine production;[441] however, the benefits of zinc are not limited to diabetes itself but also relate to diabetic complications such as diabetic retinopathy where zinc may exert a beneficial effect through its action as an antioxidant.

A study undertaken in Saudi Arabia investigating the effects of zinc supplementation in type 2 diabetic patients receiving 30 mg of elemental zinc for 3 months produced favourable results. Researchers discovered that the diabetic patients had significantly lower mean serum zinc levels when compared with healthy controls and at the end of the study zinc supplementation type-2 diabetics showed beneficial effects in elevating their serum zinc level, and in improving their glycaemic control shown by a decreased their HbA1c% concentration.[440] A systematic review and meta-analysis of 25 studies on zinc supplementation in diabetic patients (3 studies on type 1 diabetes, and 22 on type 2 diabetes) showed that zinc supplementation resulted in reductions in fasting blood glucose levels, 2 hour post-prandial blood sugar levels and HbA1c. There was also a reduction in cholesterol levels and systolic and diastolic blood pressure. Different zinc formulations were used across the studies and dosages ranged from 10–30 mg/day (elemental zinc) and 30–660 mg/day (as a zinc formula). Duration of supplementation ranged from 3 weeks to 5 years. Zinc supplementation has been shown to have potential beneficial antioxidant effects in type 2 diabetes.[442] A more recent meta-analysis of randomised placebo controlled trials found that zinc supplementation resulted in significant but modest glucose concentrations and a tendency for a decrease in HbA1c. In trials using zinc as the sole supplement, the median dose was 50 mg/day, and in trials supplementing with zinc in combination with other supplements, the median dose of zinc was 20 mg/day.[443]

MANGANESE

Manganese is a co-factor involved in many enzyme systems within the body including the synthesis and secretion of insulin as well as normal carbohydrate metabolism.[444] Patients with diabetes have been shown to have lower levels of manganese than normal healthy people.[445]

POLYPHENOLS

Several studies, mostly in-vitro and animal models, and some human studies, indicate that dietary plant polyphenols and polyphenol-rich products modulate carbohydrate and lipid metabolism, reduce hyperglycaemia, dyslipidaemia and insulin resistance and improve adipose tissue metabolism. Their role in alleviating oxidative stress and inflammatory processes is well known. Polyphenols can prevent long-term complication in diabetes including CVD, neuropathy, nephropathy and retinopathy.

Polyphenols are natural compounds found in plant-based foods (e.g. fruits, vegetables, wholegrains, cereals, legumes, tea, coffee, wine and cocoa). Flavonoids are the most abundant polyphenols in the human diet.[446,447] See Fig. 21.11 for a useful summary of effects of

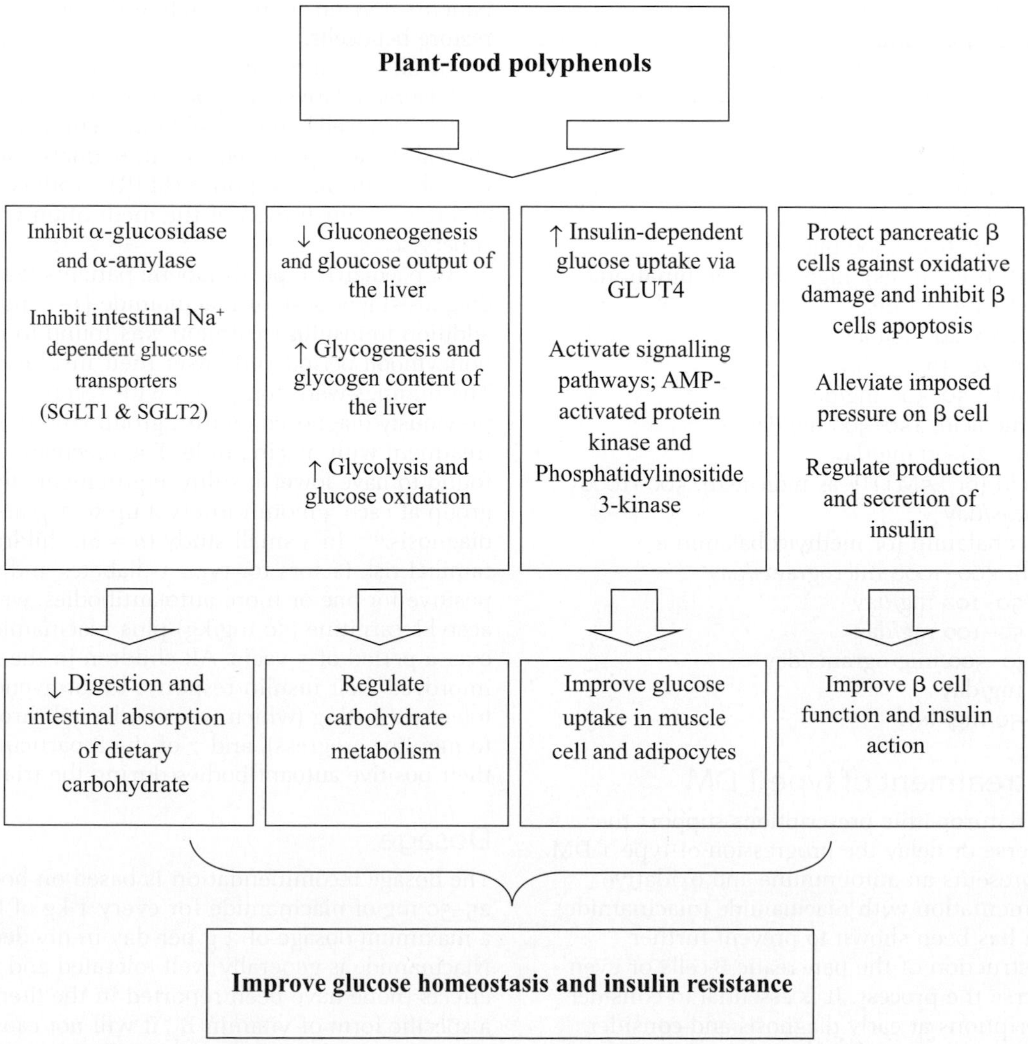

FIGURE 21.11 Beneficial effects of polyphenols on management of blood glucose in diabetes.

Bahadoran Z, Mirmiran P, Azizi F. Dietary polyphenols as potential nutraceuticals in management of diabetes: a review. J Diab Metab Disord 2013; 12(1):1.

polyphenols on the management of blood glucose levels in diabetes.

A large prospective case-cohort study across eight European countries showed that individual flavonoid subclasses (flavan-3-ol monomers, proanthocyanidins of low polymerisation degree, and the flavonol myricetin) were more beneficial in lowering type 2 diabetes risk than others.[448] Results from the Nurses' Health Study found that higher consumption of anthocyanins and anthocyanin rich fruit was associated with a lower risk of type 2 diabetes.[449] Further studies are needed to determine dosages required for supplementation in diabetes management as well as actions of specific polyphenol subclasses. It is prudent to include high polyphenol foods in the diet for management and prevention of diabetes.

Dosage requirements

The dosage requirements listed below are based on adult doses that have been reported in the literature:

- Chromium: 200–1000 micrograms/day(best to calculate on weight)
- Vanadium: 20–100 micrograms/day
- Magnesium: 400–800 mg/day
- Vitamin C: 500–1000 mg/day
- Vitamin E: 100–900 IU/day
- Selenium: 100–200 micrograms/day
- Vitamin D: 1000 IU/day (or greater if pathology results indicate)
- Essential fatty acids: 3 g b.i.d.
- R-alpha lipoic acid: 100–500 mg/day
- Coenzyme Q10: 30–150 mg/day
- Acetyl-L-carnitine: 600–2500 mg/day
- B complex (all B vitamins): high-dose combination, preferably activated forms:
  - Thiamine: 20–40 mg/day
  - Riboflavin: 20–40 mg/day
  - Niacinamide: 50–500 mg/day
  - Pantothenic acid: 150–300 mg/day
  - Pyridoxine: 20–60 mg/day
  - Folinic acid (or L5MTHF as indicated): 500–1000 micrograms/day
  - Hydroxocobalamin (or methylcobalamin as indicated): 500–1000 micrograms/day
  - Choline: 50–100 mg/day
  - Inositol: 50–100 mg/day
  - Biotin: 250–500 micrograms/day
- Zinc: 30–50 mg/day
- Manganese: 50 mg/day.

Preliminary treatment of type 1 DM

Two important naturopathic prescriptions support the potential to reverse or delay the progression of type 1 DM. As type 1 DM presents an autoimmune and oxidative process, supplementation with niacinamide (niacinamide) and epicatechin has been shown to prevent further damage and destruction of the pancreatic B-cells or even completely reverse the process. It is essential to consider these two prescriptions at early diagnosis and consider their prescription concurrent with consideration of C-peptide levels.

NIACINAMIDE

Niacinamide, the amide form of vitamin B_3 (niacin), is changed to its mononucleotide compound with the enzyme nicotinic acid/niacinamide adenylyl-transferase, and participates in the cellular energy metabolism that directly impacts normal physiology. It also influences oxidative stress and modulates multiple pathways tied to both cellular survival and death. During disorders that include immune system dysfunction such as in type 1 DM, niacinamide is a robust cytoprotectant that blocks cellular inflammatory cell activation, early apoptotic phosphatidylserine exposure, and late nuclear DNA degradation. It relies upon unique cellular pathways that involve forkhead transcription factors, sirtuins, protein kinase B (Akt), Bad, caspases and poly (ADP-ribose) polymerase that may offer a fine line with determining cellular longevity, cell survival and unwanted cancer progression.[450]

Specifically in DM, niacinamide has been shown to prevent some of the immune-mediated destruction of the pancreatic beta cells and may actually help to reverse the process. A few studies have suggested that it can prevent type 1 diabetes from progressing in some patients if given soon enough at the onset by helping restore beta cells.

In Chile, oral niacinamide used in ICA-positive first-degree relatives of type-1 diabetics was found to protect beta cells and possibly prevent some cases of clinical disease, provided the individuals had a baseline first-phase insulin response (FPIR) >10th centile for age and the administration of the medication was supervised.[451]

In paediatric type 1 diabetic patients (24 h within diagnosis) low dose of niacinamide (1–2 mg/kg) in addition to insulin treatment was found to prolong the honeymoon period and lower their insulin requirements. The findings were compared with records from a previously diagnosed control group who did not receive treatment with niacinamide. The niacinamide group was found to have lower insulin requirements than control group at each 3-month interval up to 2 years after diagnosis.[452] In a small study ($n = 8$), children with familial risk factors for type 1 diabetes and who were positive for one or more auto-antibodies, were treated with acetyl-L-carnitine (50 mg/kg) plus niacinamide (25 mg/kg) over a period of 5 years. All children in the study improved their insulin response to intravenous glucose tolerance testing (which was conducted through the study to monitor progress), and 7 of the 8 participants reversed their positive autoantibodies during the trial.[453]

Dosage

The dosage recommendation is based on body weight, 25–50 mg of niacinamide for every 1 kg of body weight or a maximum dosage of 3 g per day in divided dosages.[26] Niacinamide is generally well tolerated and without side effects (none have been reported in the literature). As it is a specific form of vitamin B_3, it will not cause the commonly associated flushing reaction as experienced with niacin (or specifically nicotinic acid). As the prescription is at a higher level, it is essential that patients be co-managed with their GP and monitored closely. Regular liver function tests (LFTs) are advised due to potential effects on the liver if dose is incorrectly prescribed or maintained.

EPIGALLOCATECHIN GALLATE (EGCG)

Epigallocatechin gallate (EGCG), also known as epigallocatechin 3-gallate, is the ester of epigallocatechin and gallic acid and a type of catechin. It is the most abundant catechin in green tea (*Camellia sinensis*) and is found in a number of other plants. It is unavailable in black tea as ECGC is converted into thearubigins during the fermentation process. It is a potent antioxidant. Primary research has been conducted on the bark from the Malabar kino tree (*Pterocarpus marsupium*) due to its epicatechin content; however, green tea (*Camellia sinensis*) extract is a superior choice due to higher levels of epicatechin and polyphenols.

A small study of healthy Japanese volunteers (18–24 years old) were fasted 12 h before the starting point of experiments and then administered with either a suspension of green tea powder (1.5 g) containing 84 mg EGCG or hot water. Ten minutes after the administration the volunteers were administered with 75 g glucose and blood glucose levels were measured before and 30, 60, and 120 min after the administration of glucose. Researchers observed that green tea improved oral glucose tolerance in humans, suggesting that green tea consumption at moderate doses may be associated with a reduced risk of type 2 diabetes in apparently healthy individuals by controlling postprandial hyperglycaemia.[454] In a more recent study investigating the effects of green tea extract powder (containing 544 mg polyphenols, 456 mg catechins) in borderline diabetic patients, researchers observed that supplementation with green tea improved glucose abnormality and resulted in a significant reduction in haemoglobin A1c levels.[455] Similarly beneficial results have been seen in other studies.[456]

HERBAL MEDICINE

Besides providing active raw materials, plants can offer molecules that serve as templates for the development of new drugs. Goat's rue *(Galega officinalis),* used in Europe as a treatment for diabetes since medieval times, yields a hypoglycaemic principle rich in guanidine.[457] Further derivatives of this principle have given rise to biguanides and the present antidiabetic agent, metformin.[458] A balanced approach to traditional plant treatments for diabetes is required which allows for proper scientific and medical evaluation together with cautious optimism in the face of sometimes conflicting scientific evidence.

Herbal medicine therapeutic objectives

- To rejuvenate and aid the functioning of pancreatic beta cells
- To reduce insulin resistance
- To regulate and lower blood sugar levels
- To aid in the prevention and treatment of long-term complications.

Herbal medicine classes

ADAPTOGEN

Adaptogens are ideally prescribed to support the patient's cortisol release and reduce blood sugar destabilising effects of high cortisol secretion. Additionally, as it is known that stress compounds the presentation and development of negative health effects, prescription of adaptogens is highly beneficial. Important medicines include the traditional TCM herbal medicine *Codonopsis pilosula* (codonopsis) due to its adaptogen and blood sugar regulating effects; the herb of five flavours, *Schisandra chinensis* (schisandra), due to its additional hepatotrophorestorative effects and medication support; *Panax ginseng* (Korean ginseng) for its joint adaptogen and hypoglycaemic properties; and *Glycyrrhiza glabra* (liquorice) due to its additional adrenal restorative properties and blood sugar regulating effects. It is important to note that liquorice can negatively affect blood sugar regulation so close monitoring of patients is encouraged.

TONIC (GENERAL)

Tonic herbal medicines are indicated to support and nourish the body. In particular it is beneficial to prescribe a tonic specific to pancreatic function — *Gymnema sylvestre* (gymnema).

PANCREATIC TROPHORESTORATIVE (ENDOCRINE FUNCTIONS)

Gymnema sylvestre (gymnema) is the primary herbal medicine of this class and is prescribed due to its multifaceted role in the treatment of diabetes. Its trophorestorative effects have been shown to clinically improve patients' responses to insulin thereby reducing dosages for type 1 patients. Close monitoring of the patient's blood sugar levels is essential. In type 2 patients, it improves pancreatic function and endocrine role thus improving blood sugar control and insulin sensitivity.

ALDOSE REDUCTASE INHIBITOR

Aldose reductase is an enzyme in carbohydrate metabolism that converts glucose to sorbitol. Its activity increases as the glucose concentration rises in diabetes, particularly in the lens of the eyes, the peripheral nerves and glomerulus leading to retinopathy and neuropathy. Both *Glycyrrhiza glabra* (liquorice) and *Scutellaria baicalensis* (Baikal skullcap) have been shown to help prevent eye and nerve damage in people with diabetes. Baikal skullcap would be selected in instances requiring greater antioxidant potential, while *Glycyrrhiza glabra* would be selected for additional adaptogenic and adrenal restorative functions.

ANTIOBESITY

Patients suffering from type 2 DM will require weight management assistance. A number of herbal medicines have shown promise as antiobesity agents through various functions. *Coleus forskohlii* (coleus) assists by increasing cyclic adenosine phosphate (cAMP), which in turn leads to an activation of protein kinase, which activates lipase (an enzyme involved in the breakdown of triglycerides, fatty substances in the blood and components of LDL cholesterol). This results in thermogenesis, loss of body fat and the maintenance of lean body mass. It also has a thyroid-stimulating action, thus possibly increasing metabolic rate and thermogenesis, and may regulate insulin secretion, thus positively affecting fat and protein metabolism. *Fucus vesiculosus* (bladderwrack) stimulates thryoid function and can be prescribed for those with iodine deficiency and concurrent hypothyroid presentation.

HYPOGLYCAEMIC

The effectiveness of blood sugar regulating herbal medicines should not be underestimated. It is therefore imperative that patients who are currently taking medications (either insulin or other) be properly assessed and monitored as interactions are possible. The most efficacious herbal medicines within this category include *Galega officinalis* (goat's rue), *Gymnema sylvestre* (gymnema), *Panax ginseng* (Korean ginseng), *Phyllanthus amarus* (phyllanthus), *Stevia rebaudiana* (stevia) and *Trigonella foenum-graecum* (fenugreek).

LIVER SUPPORT — INCLUDING ANTIOXIDANTS, HEPATICS, HEPATOTROPHORESTORATIVES, HEPATOPROTECTIVES

Additional liver support is essential when treating patients with DM. Medications, the increased burden of irregular blood sugar levels and the highly oxidised system support these prescriptions. Important herbal medicines within these classes include those with strong antioxidant properties. These include: *Camellia sinensis* (green tea), *Crataegus* spp. (hawthorn), *Curcuma longa* (turmeric), *Ginkgo biloba* (ginkgo), *Larrea Mexicana/tridentate* (chaparral), *Olea europaea* (olive leaves), *Polygonum multiflorum* (polygonum), *Rosmarinus officinalis* (rosemary), *Scutellaria baicalensis* (Baikal skullcap), *Silybum marianum* (St Mary's thistle), *Uncaria tomentosa* (cat's claw), *Vaccinium myrtillus* (bilberry) and *Vitis vinifera* (grape seed extract). These herbal medicines should form a part of every herbal medicine prescription both for current and preventive health management.

Specific herbal medicines

GYMNEMA SYLVESTRE (GYMNEMA)

Gymnema sylvestre is the key herb in the treatment of both type 1 and type 2 diabetes, and in the treatment of dysglycaemia. It is also known as the sugar destroyer and has been used in traditional Ayurvedic medicine for centuries to treat diabetes. A number of different theories have been proposed for the mechanism of action of *Gymnema sylvestre* including its ability to reduce intestinal absorption of glucose and inhibit active glucose transport in the small intestine as well as its ability to increase the number of cells in the pancreas responsible for insulin production.[459] This is believed to be achieved by the active constituent gymnemic acid, a mixture of many different saponins;[460] however, a number of other constituents have also been identified including the gymnemasaponins, gurmarin, gymnamine and gymnemasins B, C, and D to enable these blood sugar lowering effects.[459]

Gymnema has much to offer in the treatment of diabetes including the ability to regenerate beta cells and hence improve insulin secretion.[461] Several clinical trials demonstrate the effectiveness of gymnema in both type 1 and type 2 DM. Outcomes include a reduction in blood sugar levels; reduction of insulin or hypoglycaemic medications; reduction in glycosylated haemoglobin and glycosylated plasma protein levels; and reduction in serum cholesterol, triglycerides and free fatty acids. Gymnema also appears to increase the activity of enzymes which facilitate the use of glucose by insulin-dependent pathways.

Clinical trials reveal the efficacy of traditional knowledge. In a small open trial investigating the antidiabetic effect of a leaf extract (200 mg/day) from *Gymnema sylvestre* in non-insulin-dependent diabetes mellitus patients given either *Gymnema sylvestre* or their normal medication for 18–20 months, researchers observed improvements in fasting blood glucose and HbA1c levels ($p < 0.001$ for both).[462]

In a clinical context, it is important to acknowledge that the effects of gymnema are not immediate. Patients need to continue treatment for at least 120 days (life cycle of red blood cell) for optimal benefit to be seen and then maintained on a lower dose. Benefits will then be able to be measured by HbA1c levels improving over time.

With respect to type 1 patients, it is essential that they closely monitor their insulin prescription, as dosages may have to be decreased to avoid hypoglycaemia. This may be due to research suggesting that use by insulin-dependent diabetics may result in an increase in C-peptides indicating that pancreatic function has improved or stabilised. This is obviously most likely in patients whose C-peptide levels suggest some pancreatic function remained prior to treatment.

Liquid extract

Some practitioners consider the liquid extract to be more therapeutically effective due to additional desensitisation of tastebuds and thus an appetite lowering effect advantage. Researchers have found that appetite can be suppressed for up to 90 minutes after taking gymnema in liquid form. The mechanism is unclear but seems to be associated with the numbing of the sweet taste buds, hence the need to take it in liquid form for this purpose. Thus, for greater weight reduction liquid extracts may prove beneficial if sugar cravings are otherwise uncontrollable. If food cravings suggest other foods, it may help to reduce quantity consumed in its effect to reduce all taste sensation and 'ruin one's meal'.

Dosage

The dosage for gymnema extract (standardised to contain 24% gymnemic acid) is 200 mg twice a day.

TRIGONELLA FOENUM-GRAECUM (FENUGREEK)

Trigonella foenum-graecum has also been used to treat diabetes in Ayurvedic medicine. Though the hypoglycaemic effect was once thought to be due to an alkaloid known as trigonelline, many now believe that the fibre and gum within *Trigonella foenium-graecum* may be responsible by delaying gastric emptying by direct interference with glucose absorption.[463]

The mechanism behind the hypoglycaemic activity of *Trigonella foenum-graecum* and the components responsible are not certain. The following results have been obtained:

- 4-hydroxyisoleucine, a free amino acid from *Trigonella foenum-graecum*, stimulated glucose-induced insulin secretion from pancreatic islet cells and has demonstrated hypoglycaemic activity in vivo
- Trigonelline displayed hypoglycaemic activity in early research.

Fenugreek improves peripheral glucose utilisation and may exert antidiabetic activity at the insulin receptor as well as at the gastrointestinal level.

A small randomised clinical trial investigating the hypoglycaemic effects of fenugreek in 15 non-insulin-dependent diabetic patients receiving 100 g of defatted seed powder for 10 days observed improvements in fasting blood glucose values.[464] Unfortunately because of the short time period, HbA1c levels were not investigated.

In a recent study, 24 type 2 diabetic patients were given an 8-week prescription of 10 g/day of powdered fenugreek seeds either mixed with yoghurt or soaked in hot water. Six cases were excluded and the results of the remaining 18 patients (11 consumed fenugreek in hot water and 7 in yoghurt) were studied. Fasting blood sugar decreased by approximately 25% in those taking fenugreek seeds soaked in hot water whereas there were no significant changes in lab parameters in those who consumed fenugreek mixed with yoghurt.[465]

A 2016 meta-analysis of 12 RCTs, with a total sample size of 1173, evaluated the overall effects of fenugreek on hyperglycaemia and hyperlipidaemia in diabetic and prediabetic patients. Across the studies fenugreek supplementation was shown to significantly decrease the levels of fasting blood glucose, postprandial 2-hour blood glucose, HbA1c and total cholesterol. The median treatment dose used across the trials was 6.3 g, dispensed in the form of capsules or powder.[466]

CINNAMOMUM ZEYLANICUM (CINNAMON)

Cinnamomum zeylanicum is an aromatic spice with moderate clinical evidence to support its ability to lower blood glucose levels and associated cardiovascular effects present in the type 2 diabetic patient. A double-blind trial involving 60 people with poorly controlled diabetes administered 1, 3 or 6 g of cinnamon for 40 days found that all three levels of cinnamon reduced the mean fasting serum glucose (18–29%), triglyceride (23–30%), LDL cholesterol (7–27%), and total cholesterol (12–26%) levels with no significant changes noted in the placebo groups.[467] In a 2012 double blind, randomised, placebo controlled trial, participants with type 2 diabetes were randomly assigned to take either a 3 g/day *C. zeylanicum* supplement or a placebo for 8 weeks. In the treatment group, significant decreases were seen in the levels of fasting blood glucose, HbA1c, triglycerides and body fat mass compared to baseline.[468] Therefore, the inclusion of cinnamon in the diet of people with type 2 diabetes is likely to reduce risk factors associated with diabetes and cardiovascular diseases.

GALEGA OFFICINALIS (GOAT'S RUE)

The aerial parts of *Galega officinalis* are well used in Western herbal medicine for their hypoglycaemic and antidiabetic actions. The *British Herbal Pharmacopoeia* approves the use of *Galega officinalis* for use in diabetes.[469] In 1927, it was found that an active constituent, the alkaloid galegine, possessed hypoglycaemic properties. This led to the development of the related biguanide drugs (oral hypoglycaemics) such as metformin that have been shown to increase the activity of insulin and improve insulin resistance. *Galega officinalis* is currently the only example of a botanical that has been used to make an approved antidiabetic drug. Laboratory and early clinical research support the hypoglycaemic activity of goat's rue.

MOMORDICA CHARANTIA (BITTER MELON)

Momordica charantia also known as bitter melon, bitter gourd and karela, has long been used in Ayurvedic medicine for the treatment of diabetes and eaten as a vegetable in Asia. The blood glucose-lowering action of the fresh juice or extract of the unripe fruit has been clearly established in modern scientific studies in both type 1 and type 2 diabetes. The active constituents responsible for its hypoglycaemic action include charantin, insulin-like peptide (plant (p)-insulin), cucurbutanoids, momordicin, and oleanolic acids.[470] Charantin, extracted by alcohol, is a hypoglycaemic agent composed of mixed steroids that is more potent than the oral hypoglycaemic drug tolbutamide. Bitter melon also contains an insulin-like polypeptide, polypeptide-P, which lowers blood glucose levels when injected like insulin into type 1 diabetics. Because it appears to have fewer side effects than insulin, it has been suggested as a replacement for some patients, although the likelihood of this application ever being developed is extremely remote. Fortunately, taking as little as 60 mL of the juice has shown good results in clinical trials.

A 2015 study examined 95 diabetic participants randomised into 3 groups (groups 1 and 2 received freeze-dried *Mormodica charantia* powder (2 g/day or 4 g/day) and group 3 received glibenclamide (5 mg/day) for 10 weeks). Both groups receiving *Mormodica charantia* showed significant reduction in HbA1c and fasting plasma glucose. While *Mormodica charantia* had weaker hypoglycaemic activity compared with the medication glibenclamide, it imparted additional cardiovascular benefits by improving blood lipids, atherogenic index, body weight and systolic blood pressure — all parameters which had deteriorated in patients receiving glibenclamide.[471] Unfortunately the majority of the trials undertaken on *Mormodica charantia* are small and uncontrolled, therefore more rigorous clinical trials of better quality that also examine HbA1c levels are required.

In a clinical context, drinking the fresh extract is both unpalatable and challenging for compliance. The extract has thankfully been incorporated into a number of blood-glucose-regulating products. Further studies are needed to assess the quality of the various *Momordica charantia* preparations.[472]

PANAX QUINQUEFOLIUM (AMERICAN GINSENG) AND *PANAX GINSENG* (KOREAN GINSENG)

Panax quinquefolium is the cousin of *Panax ginseng*.[473] However, it is much less stimulating in nature. The root of *Panax quinquefolium* has been found to exert a mild hypoglycaemic action by affecting pancreatic beta cells and increasing insulin production.[474]

The use of *Panax ginseng* for the treatment of blood sugar irregularities can be traced back thousands of years to the *Compendium of Materia Medica* (Ben Cao Gang Mu) written by Dr Li (Li, ShiZhen), during the Ming dynasty (1368–1644) in China. This text is a favoured botanical textbook that detailed the symptom 'Xiao Ke' which can be translated as overindulging in food and drink and then losing energy and weight, synonymous with diabetic symptoms in modern day medicine.[475]

A 2016 meta-analysis of seven RCTs, totalling 195 cases and 195 controls, evaluated ginseng-induced improvement in glucose control and insulin sensitivity in patients with type 2 diabetes or impaired glucose tolerance. Both Asian (*Panax ginseng*) and American (*Panax quinquefolius*) ginseng species were assessed in this systematic review. Across the studies ginseng supplementation was shown to significantly improve fasting glucose, postprandial insulin and insulin resistance levels compared with controls. No significant difference in HbA1c levels were seen.[476]

ALLIUM CEPA (ONION) AND *ALLIUM SATIVUM* (GARLIC)

Allium cepa and *Allium sativum* are two of the oldest botanicals and are both documented in animal and human trials to be blood-glucose lowering. This activity is related to volatile sulfur compound constituents known as thiosulfinates — allyl propyl disulfide (APDS) and diallyl disulfide oxide (allicin),[477] although other constituents such as flavonoids may play a role as well. Although garlic generally has more potent effects, onions can be given at higher dosages and the active compounds appear to be more stable than allicin.

A clinical trial investigating the effect of graded doses of 25, 50, 100 and 200 g of an aqueous onion extract on healthy volunteers found no effect on fasting blood sugar levels; however, a dose-dependent reduction in blood glucose levels was observed when extracts were administered with glucose in glucose tolerance tests. The authors suggest that onion is an antihyperglycaemic rather than a hypoglycaemic agent.[478] Effects were similar in both raw and boiled onion extracts, indicating that the active components are probably stable.

A 2015 meta-analysis of RCTs of garlic or garlic extracts on markers of glycaemic control concluded that garlic intake results in a statistically significant lowering in fasting blood glucose. Garlic powder was the most commonly prescribed preparation of the seven RCTs assessed, with doses ranging from 600 to 900 mg/day. Other forms included garlic oil, garlic extract and spray dried garlic.[479]

CODONOPSIS PILOSULA (CODONOPSIS)

Codonopsis pilosula is a Chinese herb that has traditionally been used in Chinese medicine for the treatment of diabetes. As well as displaying hypoglycaemic activity, *Codonopsis pilosula* is also an antioxidant with an affinity for the pancreatic beta cells. In diabetes, increased levels of sugars in the blood increase the production of reactive oxygen species which damage the body, including the pancreatic beta cells. A preparation of *Codonopsis*, *Astragalus* and *Lycii* administered to diabetic mice was found to not only decrease high blood sugar levels but also protect the pancreatic beta cells via antioxidant activity.[480,481]

GLYCYRRHIZA GLABRA (LIQUORICE)

Glycyrrhiza glabra contains glycyrrhizic acid, a constituent reported to be 50 times sweeter than sugar![473] Several studies undertaken in vitro and in vivo have reported on the antidiabetic insulin effects of components within *Glycyrrhiza glabra* radix which appear to improve disordered glucose tolerance, possibly by enhancing the sensitivity of insulin.[482] Further studies need to be undertaken in humans to confirm the hypoglycaemic activity of *Glycyrrhiza glabra*.

COLEUS FORSKOHLII (COLEUS)

Coleus forskholli contains the active constituent colenol, a diterpenoid that has been found in studies undertaken on rats to stimulate the release of insulin and glucagon from the islets both in vitro and in vivo via stimulation of pancreatic alpha cells.[483] A 2015 clinical trial assessed the effects of supplementation with *C. forskohlii* extract on key markers of obesity and metabolic parameters in overweight and obese individuals. Participants were randomly assigned to receive either 250 mg of *C. forskohlii* extract or a placebo twice daily for 12 weeks. Both groups were instructed to follow a hypocaloric diet (deficit of approximately 500 kcal/day of estimated energy requirements). Those that supplemented with *C. forskohlii* extract were shown to have significant reduction in insulin concentration compared with the control group.[484] As with *Glycyrrhiza glabra*, further studies in humans are required to consolidate clinical efficacy.

OLEA EUROPAEA (OLIVE LEAF)

Olive leaf tea and chewing olive leaves are traditional folk remedies for diabetes. The biologically active component, oleuropein, has been associated with improved glucose metabolism. A randomised controlled clinical trial of

79 adults with type 2 diabetes, with administration of 500 mg/day olive leaf extract tablets over a period of 14 weeks, showed significantly lower HbA1c levels than the placebo group.[485] The oleuropein in olive leaves accelerates the cellular uptake of glucose and may also improve glucose-induced insulin release. Olive leaf extract also inhibits pancreatin amylase activity which is another mechanism by which it might reduce hyperglycaemic effects.

LIFESTYLE RECOMMENDATIONS

Psychological support in diabetes

Helping people with diabetes deal with their diagnosis, develop a sense of empowerment and make important lifestyle changes is an extremely important aspect of proper medical care. Counselling from various models (cognitive behavioural, psychodynamic, narrative, Gestalt and others) has proven especially effective in helping adolescents with type 1 diabetes deal with their disease, leading to improvements in both mood and blood glucose control.

GROUP-BASED COUNSELLING FOR BOTH TYPE 1 AND TYPE 2 DM

Karlsen et al designed a study to determine whether participation in a group-based counselling program would result in reduced diabetes-related stress, improved coping and psychological wellbeing as well as achieving glycaemic control closer to an acceptable level. Effects of the program were evaluated implementing an experimental design with a sample comprising 63 Norwegian adults with both types of diabetes aged between 25 and 70. At the 6-month follow-up, results indicated that the group-based counselling program tested in the study has the potential to reduce diabetes-related stress and self-blame as well as to improve coping in adults with diabetes. The results suggest too that the program can help participants to achieve more acceptable HbA1c levels as well. The authors concluded that the group-based counselling program is feasible in the sense of suggesting that cognitive restructuring and problem-solving approaches in groups may be useful in helping people adjust to diabetes.[486]

TYPE 2 DM

An interesting study was conducted that explored the beliefs of patients with type 2 diabetes, in the framework of the cognitive orientation model which assumes that cognitions could promote disease. The major hypotheses are that there is a cluster of beliefs characteristic for type 2 diabetes and that it does not differ with disease duration. The participants of the study were 112 individuals with type 2 diabetes and 103 matched healthy controls. They filled out a questionnaire about beliefs on goals, self, rules and norms, and other general relevant themes. The results showed that the questionnaire scores identified correctly patients and controls in 85%. The themes supported by the patients focus on maintaining the status quo, formal relations, authority, following rules and relying on powerful others. A major conclusion by Kreitler et al is that there is a unique cluster of beliefs characteristic for patients with type 2 diabetes. The findings can aid these patients to apply self-care procedures and cope with particular stresses.[487]

Dealing with stress

Increases in cortisol and adrenalin (epinephrine) have an immediate reaction to increase blood glucose levels and to blunt the response of insulin. In addition, these hormones cause immune suppression and aggravate autoimmune mechanisms in the body. Higher stress levels are associated with higher blood glucose levels in both type 1 and type 2 DM. Thus it is imperative that patients with either type 1 or type 2 DM be instructed on optimal stress-management techniques including relaxation, meditation, yoga, counselling and exercise.

EXERCISE AND DIABETES

Regular exercise is an important part of diabetes management. It directly improves insulin sensitivity and blood glucose control from a combination of increased lean muscle mass and an improvement in muscle cell metabolism. It regulates weight to a healthy balance, lowers blood pressure and reduces risk of cardiovascular disease. This occurs directly (improved cardiac output) and indirectly by improvements in blood lipids (especially in HDL levels). In addition, it helps patients manage stress, which has numerous health benefits. Exercise improves physical fitness, insulin resistance, lipids and macrovascular risk in people with type 1 diabetes, but studies on effects of glycaemic control are conflicting. In contrast, different forms of exercise (aerobic and resistance) have been shown to be beneficial in glycaemic control in type 2 diabetes.[488] Note: It is important to avoid exercise in type 1 patients if fasting BGL is >14 mmol/L and urinary ketones are present until normal levels have resumed. Exercise in these circumstances can actually elevate blood glucose and increase ketone production.

At least 30 minutes of exercise daily is advised with a focus on aerobic exercises, weight training and strengthening and stretching exercises. Reduction of abdominal adiposity (in type 2 DM patients) is a prime objective.

IDEAL BODY WEIGHT

Weight loss of >5% reduction in body weight (if overweight) is essential for type 2 DM patients especially in order to improve glucose, lipids and blood pressure control.[489] Often type 1 patients are underweight, but if weight issues are present maintaining ideal body weight will further contribute to improved health outcomes. Weight reduction will improve insulin sensitivity and function. There are numerous cases of type 2 DM patients whose weight has stabilised, enabling subsequent ceasing of medication.

OTHER

Avoidance of smoking, recreational drugs and alcohol is recommended, for obvious reasons.

CASE STUDY

OVERVIEW

RS was a 42-year-old man presenting with obesity, type 2 DM and depression. He had been prescribed metformin (1500 mg at night); however, his blood sugar control was poor and frequently produced high readings (13 mmol/L and above). He weighed 121 kg with significant abdominal adiposity. He had a strong family history of obesity, type 2 DM and depression. He did not partake in any formal exercise and diet was predictably poor consisting of high consumption of refined and processed carbohydrates, caffeine, sugar and artificial sweeteners (diet drinks, chewing gum, sweets).

INVESTIGATIONS

The patient was referred for a number of additional assessments including: HbA_{1c}, C-peptide, insulin, fasting glucose, vitamin D, urinary iodine, TSH and thyroid antibodies, homocysteine, cholesterol profile, LFT, FBC, hormone profile, red cell zinc and copper, MSU and ANA.

CLINICAL EXAMINATION

Review of previous investigations indicated LFT abnormalities concurrent with metformin prescription (marked GTT elevations), hypercholesterolaemia and low protein. Urinalysis showed no presence of infection; however, RS had experienced two UTIs in the past 3 months. BP was 140/95 mmHg with marked white coat hypertension.

Important results included: HbA_{1c}, 7.2%; C-peptide — normal; insulin — 19; fasting glucose — 7.2 mmol/L; vitamin D — 23 IU; homocysteine — 8.1.

TREATMENT PROTOCOL

INITIAL APPOINTMENT

Initial treatment focused on immediate blood sugar support due to concerning readings. Dietary, lifestyle and nutritional education was stressed and a structured program was developed with the patient's consent and involvement.

HERBAL MEDICINE

Due to elevations in GTT, liquid herbal medicines were avoided until repeat LFT was conducted. Initial blood sugar prescription relied on nutritional supplementation as optimal herbal medicine formulation in tablet preparation was unavailable. Patient was prescribed St John's wort tablet (Ze117) 1 tab t.d.s. for psychological support.

NUTRITIONAL MEDICINE

Dietary

- Avoid all stimulants including caffeine, sugar, alcohol and others
- High protein, low carbohydrate diet — ensure protein requirements are sufficient for both current and ideal body weight and in easily digestible forms
- Encourage consumption of low GI/GL foods

CASE STUDY CONTINUED

- Increase hydration, focusing on herbal teas and spring water
- Encourage consumption of wholefood, organic diet
- Encourage consumption of garlic, onion, cinnamon and fenugreek in meals where possible.

Supplemental

Note: Due to the weight of this patient, all doses were calculated using Clark's rule to enable optimal results. Standard adult doses are listed below.

Nutrient	Dosage	Rationale
Chromium	600 micrograms/day	Improved insulin sensitivity, weight loss and blood sugar regulation
R-alpha lipoic acid	400 mg/day	Blood sugar regulation, protection against diabetic complications, antioxidant
B complex (activated forms)	1 cap b.i.d.	Metabolism of carbohydrates, glucose metabolism, management and prevention of complications
Magnesium	800 mg/day	Improved insulin signalling and blood sugar regulation, energy production, lipid lowering
Antioxidant formulation consisting of vitamins A, C, E, selenium and zinc	2 tabs b.i.d.	To reduce oxidation and use each of the nutrients for blood sugar regulation and prevention of complications (especially cardiac)
Coenzyme Q10	200 mg/day	Cardiac support, energy production, antioxidant
Vitamin D_3	5000 IU/day	To address deficiency and utilise positive blood sugar, mood and immune effects
Essential fatty acids	3 g b.i.d.	Energy and glucose regulation, cholesterol lowering

LIFESTYLE/EDUCATION

- Daily exercise starting at 20 mins twice a day (morning and night) of walking and slowly increased by duration and intensity over 2 weeks
- Referral to a counsellor for emotional issues and grief from father's death
- Stress reduction, relaxation, adequate sleep.

HYPOGLYCAEMIA

Classification

Hypoglycaemia (low blood glucose) provokes characteristic symptoms of cognitive dysfunction and counter-regulatory hormonal secretion that occur at different glycaemic thresholds. Sympathoadrenal activation provokes physiological responses and neuroglycopenia affects cerebral function. Hypoglycaemia can promote untoward physiological changes in the body. Insulin-induced hypoglycaemia is known to increase the levels of C-reactive protein, a known cardiac risk factor. Because glucose is the primary fuel for the brain, low levels affect the brain first. Hypoglycaemia is divided into two main categories: reactive hypoglycaemia and fasting hypoglycaemia.

REACTIVE HYPOGLYCAEMIA

Reactive hypoglycaemia, the most common, is characterised by the development of symptoms of hypoglycaemia 3–5 hours after a meal and may herald the onset of early type 2 diabetes. Gastric surgeries may induce this condition, and anorexia nervosa has been a reported cause in the literature. Reactive hypoglycaemia may also result from the use of oral hypoglycaemic drugs.

FASTING HYPOGLYCAEMIA

Also called postabsorptive hypoglycaemia, fasting hypoglycaemia is often related to an underlying disease. Fasting hypoglycaemia is rare, as it usually appears only in severe disease states such as pancreatic tumours, extensive liver damage, prolonged starvation, autoantibodies against insulin or its receptor, various cancers, or as a result of excessive exogenous insulin in diabetics. Pregnant diabetic women using insulin or oral glycaemic medications also have a high incidence of asymptomatic hypoglycaemic events.

Aetiology

Medicine defines 'true' reactive hypoglycaemia as a manifestation of the dumping syndrome, for example in those who have had previous gastric surgery or who have a gastrointestinal motility disorder. However, healthcare professionals have commonly observed patients with symptoms related to low blood sugar occurring in the mid to late mornings and afternoons which are relieved by eating.

Both low and high blood glucose levels can cause significant physiological dysfunction. Normally, the body maintains blood sugar levels within a narrow range through the coordinated effort of several glands and their hormones. If these control mechanisms are disrupted, hypoglycaemia (low blood sugar) or diabetes (high blood sugar) may result.

People overstress these control mechanisms through improper diet and lifestyle. As a result, diabetes and hypoglycaemia are common diseases. Hypoglycaemia is, without question, a valid clinical entity. A substantial amount of information indicates that hypoglycaemia is caused by an excessive intake of refined carbohydrates.

Overview

Hypoglycaemia is a biochemical abnormality that can be arbitrarily defined by a low blood glucose concentration:

- In a person with type 1, blood glucose below 3.5 mmol/L (61 mg/dL) is considered to represent hypoglycaemia[490]
- In a non-diabetic person, blood glucose below 2.2 mmol/L (38 mg/dL) is almost always pathological.[490]

Diagnosis is made with the following readings:

- Blood glucose level at or below 2.2–3.1 mmol/L (40–50 mg/dL) (non-diabetic)
- A normal response curve during the first 2–3 hours of a glucose tolerance test (GTT) followed by a decrease of 20 mg or more below the fasting glucose level during the final hours of the test, with symptoms developing during the decrease.

Pathogenesis

The human brain requires a continuous supply of glucose as its principal source of energy and malfunctions rapidly if deprived of this substrate. To protect the brain and prevent a dangerous fall in blood glucose, multiple counter-regulatory mechanisms have evolved to maintain glucose homeostasis. These include:

- Secretion of counter-regulatory hormones including glucagon, adrenaline (epinephrine), cortisol and growth hormone
- Centrally activated release of various neurotransmitters
- Simultaneous inhibition of endogenous insulin secretion
- Hepatic autoregulation can release glucose during profound hypoglycaemia.

The secretion of pancreatic glucagon occurs independently of the activation of counter-regulatory mechanisms within the brain. In contrast, adrenaline is secreted secondary to the stimulation of the sympathetic division of the autonomic nervous system following the activation of autonomic centres within the hypothalamus. The other counter-regulatory hormones are released through the activation of the hypothalamic–pituitary–adrenal axis. These hormones promote the breakdown of glycogen to glucose within the liver (hepatic glycogenolysis) and the production of three carbon precursors from proteolysis and glycogenolysis in the skeletal muscle that are used for glucose formation (gluconeogenesis) within the liver and kidney. The oxidation of free fatty acids, produced by lipolysis, provides energy for gluconeogenesis.[490]

SIGNS AND SYMPTOMS (Fig. 21.12)

Hypoglycaemia generates symptoms as a direct consequence of glucose deprivation of neurons in the brain (neuroglycopenia) and secondary to acute autonomic stimulation. Symptoms are idiosyncratic and age specific, varying considerably among individuals, both in nature

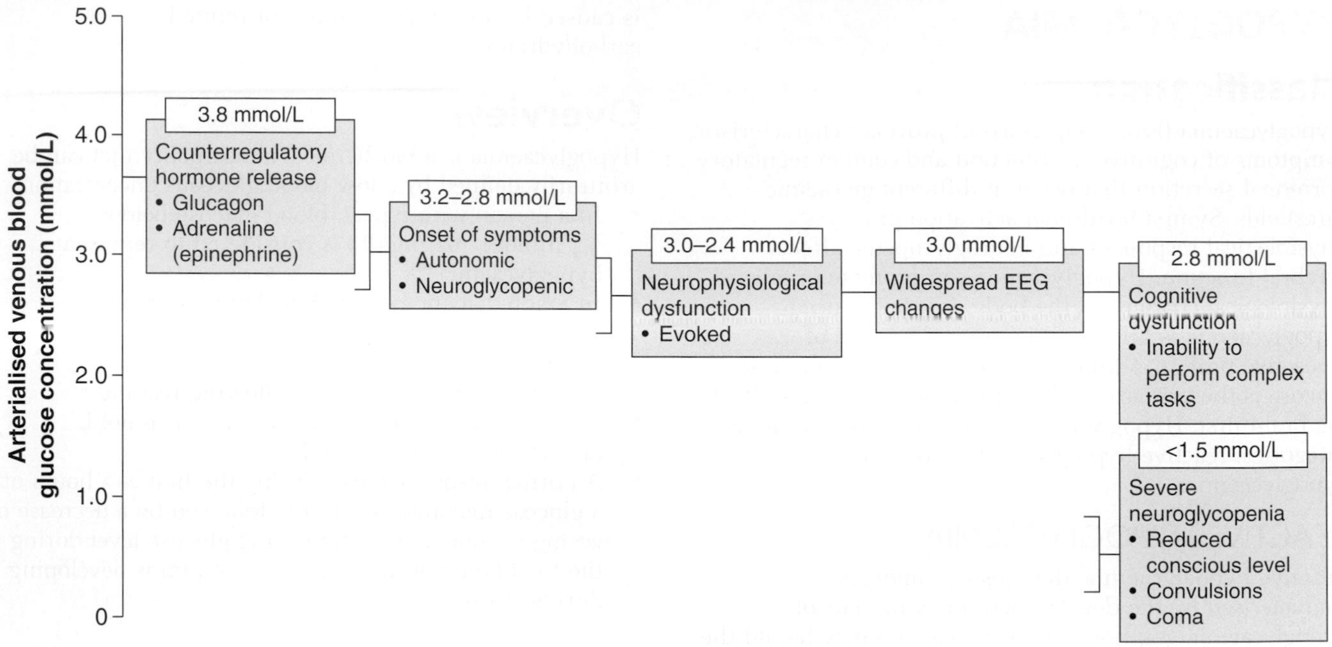

FIGURE 21.12 Glycaemic thresholds for the secretion of counter-regulatory hormones and the onset of physiological, symptomatic and cognitive changes in response to acute hypoglycaemia in non-diabetic adults. Glycaemic thresholds are shown in relation to glucose values in arterialised venous blood.

Source: Republished with permission of John Wiley & Sons, from Frier BM, Fisher BM, eds. Hypoglycaemia and clinical diabetes, Chichester, UK: John Wiley; 1999. Permission covered through Copyright Clearance Center, Inc.

and intensity. Symptoms can range from mild to severe and are similar to diabetes-related hypoglycaemia.

Common autonomic symptoms include sweating, trembling, pounding heart, hunger and anxiety. Neuroglycopenic symptoms include inability to concentrate, drowsiness, confusion, difficulty with speech and incoordination. Common nonspecific symptoms include nausea, tiredness, and headache.[490]

CONTRIBUTING FACTORS

The factors that contribute to reactive hypoglycaemia are:

- Individuals who suffer this disorder are likely to be more sensitive to drops in blood sugar (it may not be how far the blood sugar drops, but how sensitive they are to the drop)
- Caffeine intake
- Stress
- Low income and education levels are social risk factors in diabetic patients[491]
- Poor cerebral blood flow
- Diet (an extremely important factor): generally there is an excessive consumption of high glycaemic refined carbohydrates and low protein intake, especially at breakfast. Hypoglycaemia in diabetic patients is commonly (approximately 50% of the time) preceded by a food-related incident — either a missed or delayed meal, or one that had less carbohydrate composition than expected[492]
- The adrenal glands are probably weak from previous stress, resulting in inadequate counter-regulatory mechanisms in blood sugar control
- Old age: a risk factor for hypoglycaemia, possibly due to increased sensitivity to medication and compromised glucose counter-regulation. The elderly are also more likely to miss meals and/or suffer from malnutrition, due to problems preparing food, chewing food or swallowing[493]
- Some medications, such as ACE inhibitors and beta-blockers, may mask the symptoms of hypoglycaemia, causing a hypoglycaemic event to be aggravated[494]
- Alcohol intake
- Infection
- Renal dysfunction
- Cognitive impairment (note, this is a risk factor for hypoglycaemia, as well as a symptom).[495]

DIFFERENTIAL DIAGNOSIS

- Insulin-dependent diabetes mellitus
- Non-insulin-dependent diabetes mellitus
- Metabolic syndrome
- Disordered eating (anorexia nervosa)
- Stress related.

NATUROPATHIC DIAGNOSIS

Questions for the hypoglycaemic patient

The following questions should be asked of patients to determine the severity of symptoms and arrive at a diagnosis:

- Cravings for sweet foods
- Irritable if a meal is missed

- Feel tired or weak if a meal is missed
- Dizziness when standing suddenly
- Frequent headaches[494]
- Poor memory (forgetful) or concentration[494]
- Feel tired an hour or so after eating
- Heart palpitations and sweating[494]
- Feel shaky at times
- Afternoon fatigue
- Vision blurs on occasion[494]
- Slurred speech[494]
- Loss of balance due to impaired cognitive function; can lead to falls and accidents[496]
- Depression or mood swings
- Overweight or pronounced weight fluctuations
- Frequently anxious or nervous.

HEALTH IMPACT OF HYPOGLYCAEMIA

- Effects on brain function — dizziness, headache, clouding of vision, blunted mental acuity, emotional instability, confusion, abnormal behaviour and irritability.[494] Erratic and irrational behaviour, including aggression and criminal behaviour
- Cardiovascular effects including atherosclerosis, intermittent claudication, angina, cardiac arrhythmias and myocardial ischaemia[496]
- Metabolic syndrome
- Migraine headaches
- Premenstrual syndrome
- Oxidative stress through the generation of free radicals and inhibition of antioxidant enzymes[497]
- In older adults, recurrent exposure to hypoglycaemic events has a greater effect on the brain than in young and middle-aged patients, potentially promoting the development of dementia.[496]

OTHER CONSEQUENCES OF HYPOGLYCAEMIA

- Difficulty finding and/or keeping employment
- Weight gain
- Effect on social interactions (including sport and leisure activities)
- Low self-confidence
- Fear of hypoglycaemic episode, leading to reduced quality of life
- Sleep disturbances
- Difficulty obtaining and/or keeping a driver's licence.[494]

Investigations

Hypoglycaemia is characterised by a drop in blood glucose to a level where first it causes nervous system symptoms (sweating, palpitations, hunger, trembling and anxiety), then begins to affect the brain (causing confusion, hallucinations, blurred vision and sometimes even coma and death). An actual diagnosis of hypoglycaemia requires satisfying the following three criteria:

1. Documented low glucose levels (less than 2.2 mmol/L (40 mg/dL) often tested along with insulin levels and sometimes with C-peptide levels)
2. Symptoms of hypoglycaemia — central nervous system symptoms including confusion, aberrant behaviour, or coma
3. Reversal of the symptoms when blood glucose levels are returned to normal.

Therapeutic considerations

CLINICAL DECISION MAKING AND RATIONALE

The primary treatment of hypoglycaemia is the use of dietary therapy to stabilise blood sugar levels. Reactive hypoglycaemia is not a disease; it is simply a complex set of symptoms caused by faulty carbohydrate metabolism induced by an inappropriate diet.

Therapeutic application

NATUROPATHIC PERSPECTIVE

Of importance, dietary carbohydrate consumption is a primary cause and treatment for hypoglycaemia. It is essential to educate patients about the advantages of wholegrains, and the health effects of refined grains, excessive sugar and sugar-containing products.

During the milling of grain into flour and the refining of grains, the germ and bran are usually detached from the endosperm. Wholegrain flours will contain most of the germ, bran and endosperm, while white flour is just made from the endosperm. This means that the nutritional content of a processed grain will depend partly on which parts of the grain are present, although many cereal products will have been fortified with certain nutrients as outlined above. Whole, unprocessed foods are more slowly absorbed, as they are contained within cells and are associated with fibre and other food elements. In addition, methods that are used to refine grains and produce flours also generate significant amounts of heat, which can destroy some vitamins (especially water-soluble vitamins). It is important to remember that refined products not only increase the use of B vitamins for their digestion but also destroy any that are present.

When high-sugar foods are eaten alone, blood sugar levels rise quickly, producing a strain on blood sugar control. Patients should be instructed how to read food labels and be educated about sugar's many names, including brown or white sugar, castor sugar, icing sugar/mixture, glucose, dextrose, sucrose, fructose, polydextrose, maltose, galactose, mannose, lactose, syrup, modified carbohydrate, invert/raw/brown/cane/Demerara/Muscovado sugar, malt/malt extract, corn fructose/starch/sweetener/syrup, barley malt, beet sugar, blackstrap molasses, molasses, caramel, date sugar, dextrin, fruit fructose, grape sugar, grape sweetener, sucanat, turbinado, golden syrup, maple syrup, treacle and others.

In addition, patients should be instructed to ensure adequate intake of fibre, ensure dietary intakes of dietary sources of chromium are sufficient, and reduce high GI/GL food sources.

NUTRITIONAL MEDICINE (DIETARY)

Dietary therapeutic objectives

- Alcohol must be avoided as it can cause hypoglycaemia[498]
- All simple, processed, refined and concentrated carbohydrates, as well as food choices with a high GL, must be avoided
- Dietary sources of chromium should be encouraged including wholegrains, oysters, beef liver, beef, molasses, mushrooms and legumes
- Foods rich in soluble fibre such as legumes and low glycaemic vegetables should be consumed regularly
- Frequent, small meals may be more effective in stabilising blood sugar levels; skipped or inadequate meals are a likely factor causing hypoglycaemia[494,498]
- Intake of caffeine is best avoided
- Protein intake at each meal (protein stimulates gluconeogenesis which results in a consistent output of glucose from the liver).

NUTRITIONAL MEDICINE (SUPPLEMENTAL)

Specific nutrients required

The recommendations for the daily intake levels of vitamins and minerals were given previously and are critical to proper carbohydrate metabolism. Because of the nature of this condition, a potent multivitamin and mineral formulation with added chromium may be sufficient as a primary prescription. Chromium is critically important. It is essential that an appropriate dose is prescribed (minimum: 200–400 micrograms/day). It is essential to calculate this dose based on the patient's weight for optimal therapeutic outcome. The most important nutrient prescriptions are listed in Table 21.34.

TABLE 21.34 Dosage requirements of the most important nutrient prescriptions

Nutrient	Daily dosage	Rationale
Chromium	200–400 micrograms/day	Blood sugar regulation, improves insulin signalling and response
Magnesium	400–800 mg/day	Blood sugar control, regulate insulin secretion, post-receptor insulin signalling, fatty acid synthesis and glucose utilisation
Vitamin B complex	High-dose complex b.i.d.	Carbohydrate metabolism, to enhance the action of cortisol and improve adrenal function. In addition, blood sugar regulating properties are achieved from optimal doses of B_3

SAMPLE DAILY DIET

BREAKFAST	
1 piece of stone-ground toast topped with sardines, spinach, avocado, tomatoes Cinnamon tea	Adequate complex wholefood carbohydrates are required for management of hypoglycaemia and may prevent episodes occurring; most low glucose concentrations can be predicted in advance and the glucose levels can be raised back to the desired levels by consuming an appropriate amount of carbohydrate. This meal combines complex, wholefood carbohydrate in the form of bread with quality protein, fats and fibre to ensure stable blood sugar to prevent hypoglycaemia.
LUNCH	
Chicken salad: poached chicken, avocado, sweet potato, leafy greens, grated carrot, capers. Herb and vinegar dressing	Lunch combines protein (chicken) with low GI carbohydrates (sweet potato) to ensure stable blood sugar to prevent hypoglycaemia. Sweet potato is rich in fibre and can increase adiponectin, which helps to regulate insulin metabolism; consumption of sweet potato may improve HbA_{1c} when eaten over a 5-month period, highlighting its ability to improve glycaemic control. Vinegar reduces postprandial glucose and insulin levels resulting in better glycaemic control.
DINNER	
Tofu served with Thai herbs and a range of vegetables: carrots, broccoli, mushrooms, bok choy, ginger etc. Serve with a small quantity of basmati rice	Low GI grains, e.g. basmati rice should be chosen over refined high GI grains, e.g. jasmine rice, though portion control should be exercised. Combining with a protein such as tofu ensures glycaemic control. Adequate vegetables provide fibre, important for blood sugar control. Additionally, vegetables provide nutrients that support the liver, which plays a crucial role in regulating blood sugar.

As the nutrients listed in the table are suggestions only, recommendations for specific quantities of nutrients prescribed should be ascertained on an individual basis.

HERBAL MEDICINE

Herbal medicine therapeutic objectives

- Decrease sensitivity to a drop in blood sugar caused by caffeine intake, stress, poor cerebral blood flow
- Support adrenal gland function
- Improve the body's metabolism of simple sugars and response to insulin
- Support the role of the liver in regulating blood sugar.

Herbal medicine classes

- Adaptogen
- Adrenal restorative
- Bitter
- Circulatory stimulants (cerebral)
- Hypoglycaemic
- Pancreatic trophorestorative (endocrine).

Treatment protocol

See formula in Table 21.35.

TABLE 21.35 Herbal formula for hypoglycaemia

Herbal medicine	Ratio	Quantity	Rationale
Gentiana lutea	1:2	30 mL	Bitter, assists protein digestion
Ginkgo biloba	STD	40 mL	Circulatory stimulant (cerebral)
Gymnema sylvestre	1:1	70 mL	Pancreatic trophorestorative, hypoglycaemic, blood sugar regulator
Codonopsis pilosula	1:2	70 mL	Adaptogen, hypoglycaemic, blood sugar regulator, blood tonic
TOTAL: 210 mL			
DOSE: 5 mL t.d.s., before meals			

ADJUNCT FORMULA

Gymnema sylvestre 1 : 1 liquid extract: 10–20 drops p.r.n. for immediate relief from sugar cravings and to desensitise sugar tastebuds. Can also be used to reduce food intake due to taste effects.

LIFESTYLE RECOMMENDATIONS

The following lifestyle factors need to be considered and modified where appropriate:

- Alcohol must be avoided as it severely stresses blood sugar control
- Exercise must be encouraged and maintained regularly for optimal blood sugar control and weight management. However, unusual exertion, prolonged exercise duration or unaccustomed exercise intensity increases glucose utilisation and the risk of hypoglycaemia. Pre-exercise snacks should be eaten where falling glucose levels are indicated.[498] Hypoglycaemia is also common 7 to 11 hours post exercise, something to bear in mind when considering the risk of over-night hypoglycaemia, particularly in patients with type 1 diabetes.[499]

SECTION D: ADRENAL DISORDERS

STRESS

See Fig. 21.13.

Classification

The term 'stress' needs to be clarified as it is used rather loosely in our society. Stress is defined as any demand on the body to adjust; it is any arousal, be it negative (such as fear or injury) or positive (such as falling in love). However, what is generally meant by 'stress' is 'distress': a situation or event that challenges or exceeds the person's ability to cope or to adjust.

During stress a cascade of physiological reactions take place within the body, starting from the hypothalamus via the pituitary gland to the adrenals (and often other end-organs such as thyroid or ovaries). This is commonly known as HPA axis activation or stress response.[500] How individuals handle stress plays a major role in determining their level of health. Comprehensive stress management involves a truly holistic approach designed to counteract the everyday stresses of life. Most often stressors and the body's response to them are so mild they go entirely unnoticed and the body returns to normality or 'homeostasis'. Each time we experience a situation as stressful in such a way that the adaptation to a changed external and internal environment becomes necessary, the body cannot return to homeostasis. A new equilibrium is established termed 'allostasis'. This adaptation enhances the individual's survival chances.

However, when these stresses are perceived as overwhelming, threatening one's sense of control, the stress response can be severe. Too much stress and a resulting unhealthy lifestyle leads to wear and tear on the system, termed 'allostatic load', and can damage organs and body systems.[501,502] It is directly linked with all-cause mortality, and specific health outcomes (CVD, diabetes, osteoporosis, CKD and COPD). Allostatic load has also been linked to the general decline in physical and cognitive function associated with ageing, possibly due to an increase in oxidative stress, increase in innate immunity activation and constant low-grade inflammation associated with overload of allostatic mechanisms.[503] Another possible mechanism of action of allostatic load in ageing is the shortening of telomeres which occurs when cells are chronically exposed to oxidative stress.[504–506]

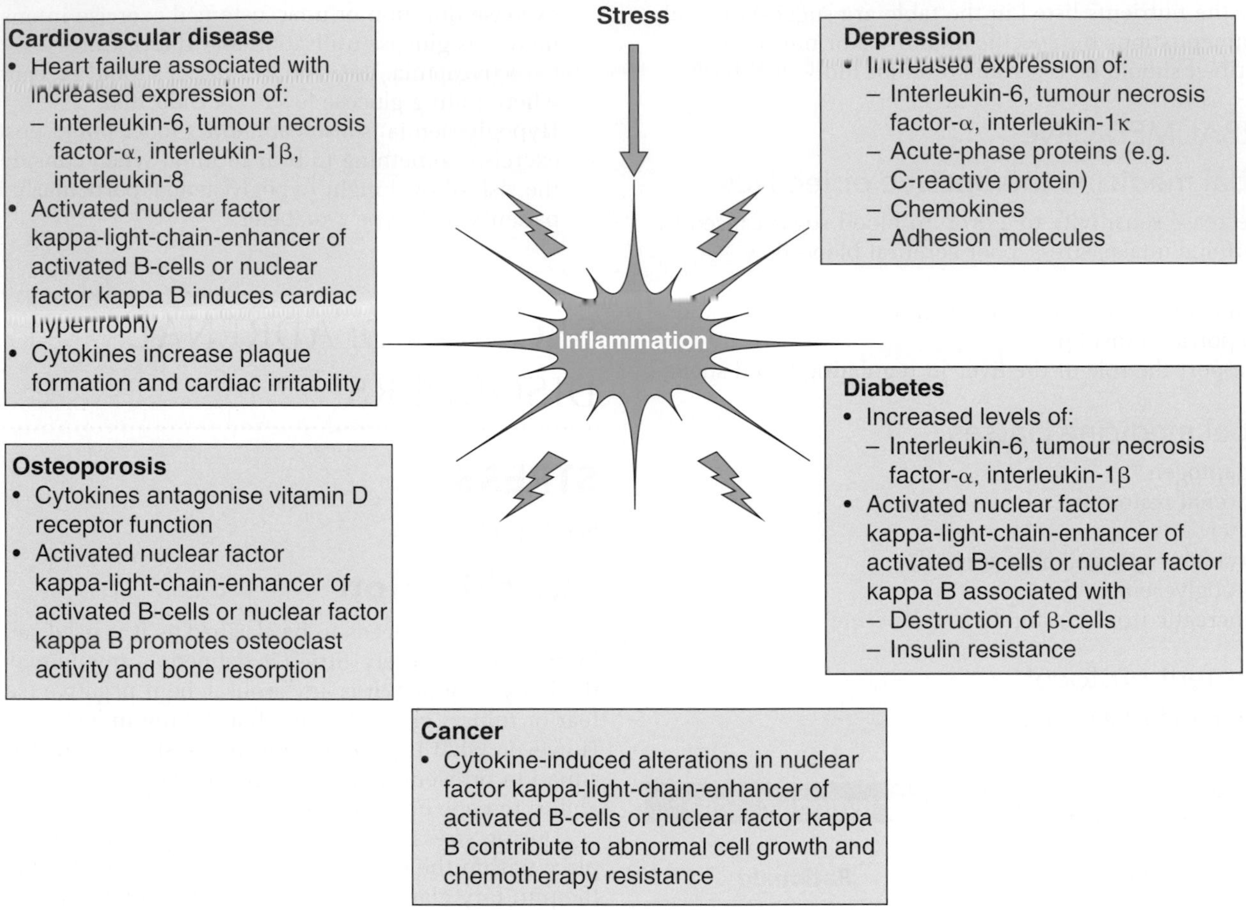

Stress
Inflammation
Cardiovascular disease
• Heart failure associated with increased expression of:
– interleukin-6, tumour necrosis factor-α, interleukin-1β, interleukin-8
• Activated nuclear factor kappa-light-chain-enhancer of activated B-cells or nuclear factor kappa B induces cardiac hypertrophy
• Cytokines increase plaque formation and cardiac irritability
Depression
• Increased expression of:
– Interleukin-6, tumour necrosis factor-α, interleukin-1κ
– Acute-phase proteins (e.g. C-reactive protein)
– Chemokines
– Adhesion molecules
Osteoporosis
• Cytokines antagonise vitamin D receptor function
• Activated nuclear factor kappa-light-chain-enhancer of activated B-cells or nuclear factor kappa B promotes osteoclast activity and bone resorption
Diabetes
• Increased levels of:
– Interleukin-6, tumour necrosis factor-α, interleukin-1β
• Activated nuclear factor kappa-light-chain-enhancer of activated B-cells or nuclear factor kappa B associated with
– Destruction of β-cells
– Insulin resistance
Cancer
• Cytokine-induced alterations in nuclear factor kappa-light-chain-enhancer of activated B-cells or nuclear factor kappa B contribute to abnormal cell growth and chemotherapy resistance

FIGURE 21.13 Stress and inflammation — triggering disease processes.
Source: Auerbach. Wilderness medicine. 5th edn. Mosby, 2007.

Ultimately, the success of any stress management program depends on its ability to improve an individual's immediate and long-term responses to stress; that is, to resource the individual physically and mentally to become more resilient.

Overview

One cannot discuss stress without mentioning the founder of the concept — Hans Selye. Selye, in 1935, was inspired to identify the general adaptation syndrome (GAS), a theory for stress, from various endocrinological experiments in which he injected mice with extracts of various organs. At first he believed he had discovered a new hormone, but multiple failed experiments and the observation that people with different diseases exhibited similar symptoms led to his description of the effects of 'noxious agents'. He then later coined the term 'stress' which has since been accepted into contemporary language.

According to Selye, stress in itself should not be viewed in a negative context. It is not the stressor that determines the effect; instead, it is the individual's internal reaction which then triggers the individualised response. What one person may experience as stress, the next person may view entirely differently:

> *Stress is both the soldier who sustains wounds in battle, the mother who worries about her soldier son, the gambler who watches the races — whether he wins or loses — the horse and the jockey he bet on: they are all under stress ... The mother who tries to keep her children out of trouble, the child who scalds himself — and especially the particular cells of the skin over which he spilled the coffee — they, too, are under stress ... What is the nature of stress?*[507]

Stress is all around us but it is the individual's interpretation of the stress that determines the potential health impact. A significant body of knowledge has now been accumulated, delineating methodologies for helping patients develop healthful, rather than disease-facilitating, responses to both short-term and long-term stress.

Pathogenesis

THE GENERAL ADAPTATION SYNDROME

The stress response is actually part of a larger response known as the general adaptation syndrome (GAS), a term coined by Selye.[508] To fully understand how the body reacts to stress, one must understand the GAS. The syndrome is composed of three phases: alarm, resistance and exhaustion.

Alarm phase (reaction)

The initial response to stress is the *alarm* reaction, which is often referred to as the fight-or-flight response. Fear is the strongest activator of the stress response.[509] Immediately, noradrenaline (norepinephrine) and adrenaline (epinephrine) are released by the adrenal medulla in response to stimulation of the sympathetic nervous system (SNS) by the hypothalamus (Fig. 21.14, right side). These hormones alert and mobilise the body's resources for immediate physical activity. As a result, the heart rate and its force of contraction increase to provide blood to areas necessary for response to the stressful situation. Blood is shunted away from the skin and internal organs, except the heart and lungs, while the amount of blood supplying required oxygen and glucose to the muscles and brain is increased. The rate of breathing rises to supply necessary oxygen to the heart, brain and exercising muscle. Blood sugar levels rise dramatically as the liver converts stored glycogen into glucose for release into the bloodstream. Adrenaline (epinephrine) also activates pro-inflammatory cytokines (notably interleukin-6)[510] (and vice versa),[511] leading to oxidative stress.[512] This response is at the expense of the parasympathetic nervous system (PNS) as activities such as digestion, relaxation and reproduction are deemed to be of minor importance in the face of a stressor.

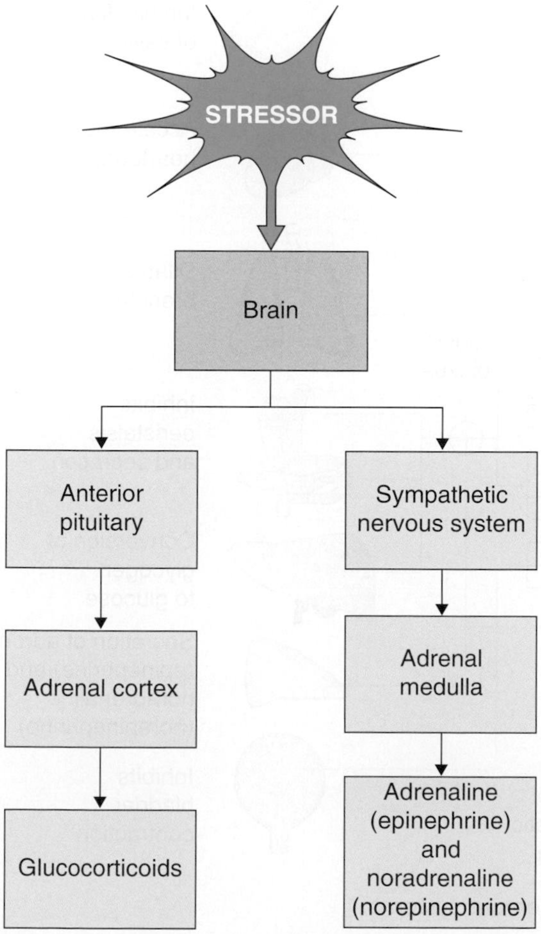

FIGURE 21.14 Effects of stressor on hormone release.

The hypothalamus also activates the anterior pituitary gland via corticotrophin-releasing hormone (CRP) to secrete adrenocorticotropic hormone (ACTH). ACTH triggers the release of glucocorticoids (cortisol) from the adrenal cortex (Fig. 21.14, left side). Cortisol's response is slower and more prolonged than that of adrenaline (epinephrine). Its role is to provide further glucose from protein and fat breakdown (gluconeogenesis), to dampen any inflammatory response (e.g. from any potential wounds sustained during fighting), and it elevates the pain threshold.

These changes are thought to be protective of the individual's survival.[513] As well as providing the necessary energy and circulatory changes required to deal effectively with stress, the alarm reaction provides the changes required to meet emotional crises, perform strenuous tasks and fight infection.

Resistance phase

When the stressor has passed, the above-mentioned physical reactions return to (near) normal (homeostasis), or the individual finds a new equilibrium (allostasis) after adjusting to a changed situation (e.g. a student leaving home to study in a different town). Humans go through these first two stages repeatedly in life as there will always be stressors. Without them, we would not evolve as human beings; in fact, we would not be alive.

However, if stress is prolonged or intense, the body may become overwhelmed and cannot resist the stressor any longer. It becomes incapable of returning to any kind of equilibrium, and exhaustion sets in.

Exhaustion phase

The effects of adrenal hormones are quite necessary when the body is faced with danger, but continued stress increases the risk of significant disease (including diabetes, high blood pressure and cancer)[514,515] and results in the final stage of the general adaptation syndrome, *exhaustion*. In severe or prolonged stress the system becomes overwhelmed and the body is unable to maintain the hormonal responses to stress. Cortisol and adrenaline (epinephrine) levels decline and physical illness sets in — the allostatic load takes its toll. For instance, adrenal glucocorticoid dysregulation diminishes glucose control, leading to reactive hypoglycaemia.[406,516]

Selye found that when rats were exposed to severe stress they all responded in the same manner, regardless of the stressor: their adrenals enlarged, their thymus gland and lymph nodes atrophied, and they developed gastric ulcers.[508] He then hypothesised that these responses are general; that is, they occurred as a response to any kind of prolonged stress, hence the notion of the GAS. In extreme cases death will ensue.

The three stages of the GAS are shown in Fig. 21.15.

To appreciate the effects of stress an understanding of the autonomic nervous system can give clues regarding the far-reaching effects on the whole system. The two divisions mentioned earlier, the sympathetic nervous system (SNS) and parasympathetic nervous system (PNS), each have vital functions within the body (Fig. 21.16). Stress is a

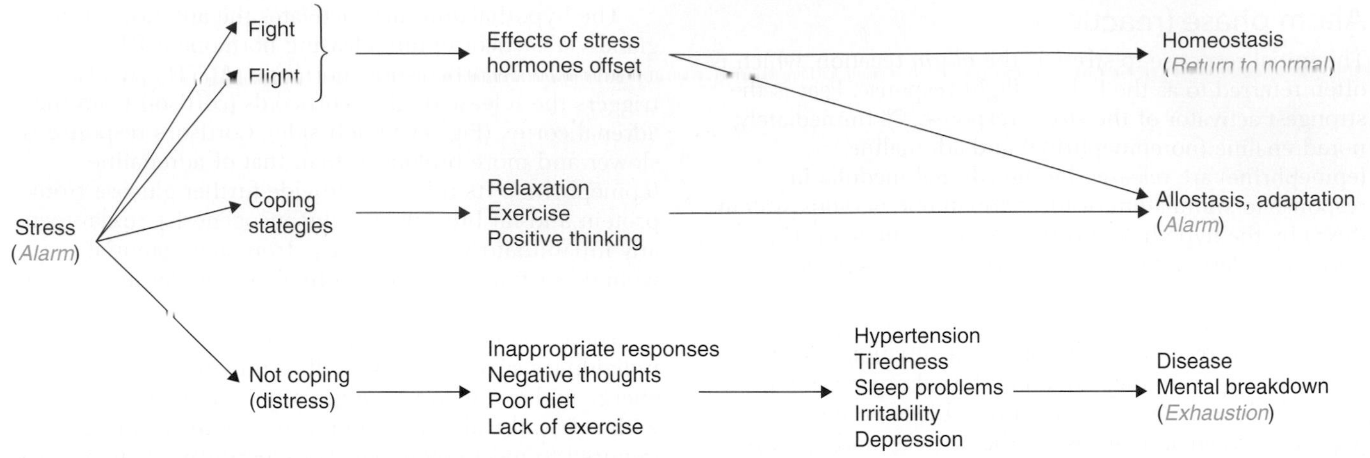

FIGURE 21.15 Effects of stress and the general adaptation syndrome.

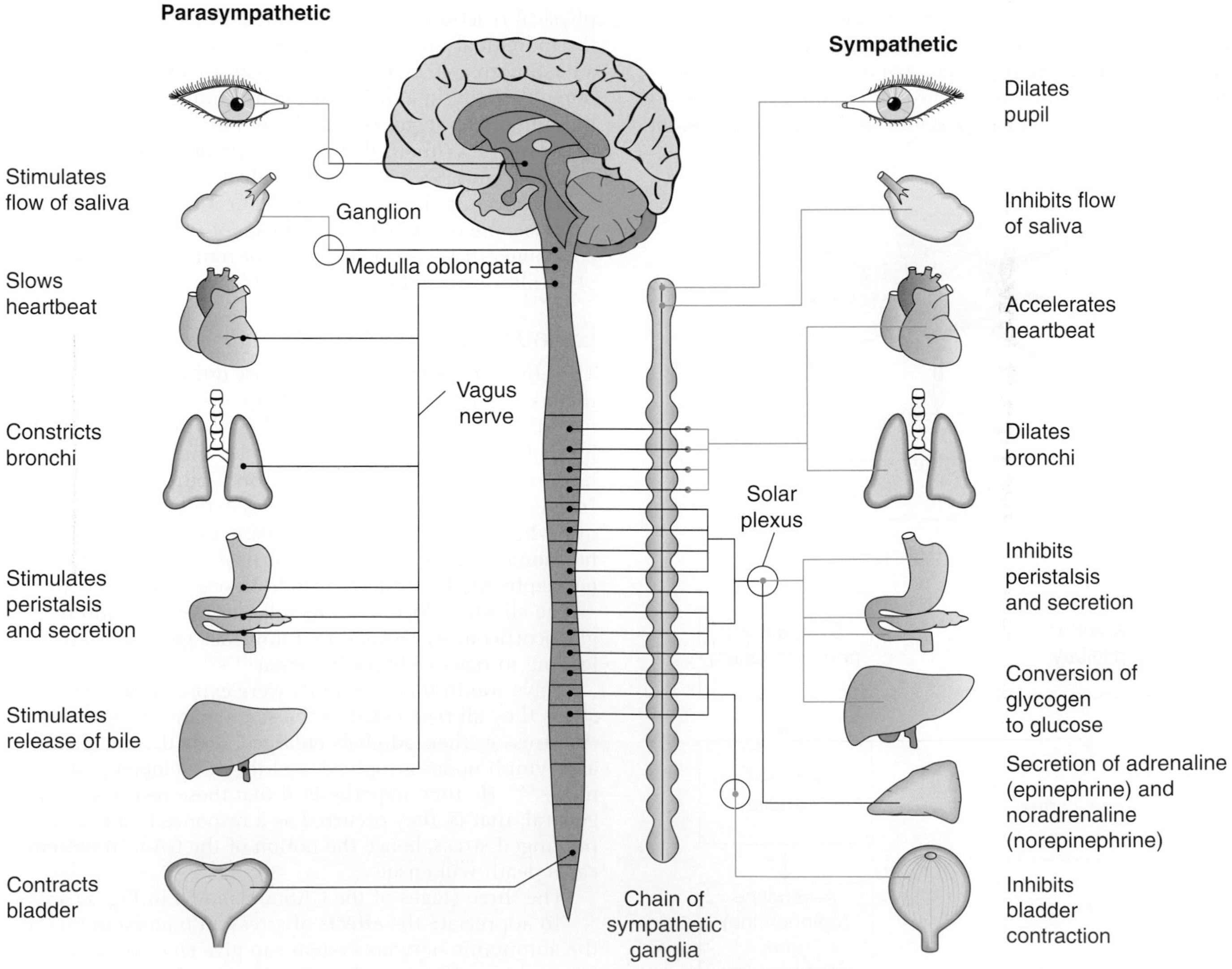

FIGURE 21.16 Functions of the sympathetic and parasympathetic nervous systems.

disruptor of these functions, and the secretions of adrenaline (epinephrine) and cortisol tend to have a suppressive effect on the inhibitory neurotransmitters of the PNS; that is, serotonin and gamma-aminobutyric acid (GABA). Prolonged stress places a tremendous load on many organ systems, especially the heart, blood vessels, adrenals and immune system, and is associated with many common diseases.

DIAGNOSTIC CONSIDERATIONS

Many people who are 'stressed out' may not be able to identify exactly what is causing them to feel stressed. Typical presenting symptoms include insomnia, depression, fatigue, headache, upset stomach, digestive disturbances and irritability.

To determine the role that stress may play, the Social Readjustment Rating Scale, developed by Holmes and Rahe,[517,518] may be used (Table 21.36). The scale was originally designed to predict the risk of a serious disease due to stress. Various life-changing events are numerically rated according to their potential to cause disease. Notice that even events commonly viewed as positive, such as an outstanding personal achievement, carry a measure of stress.

The standard interpretation of the Social Readjustment Rating Scale is that a total of 200 or more units in one year is considered to be predictive of a high likelihood of experiencing a serious disease. However, rather than using the scale solely to predict the chance of disease, the practitioner can use the scale to evaluate a patient's level of stressor exposure. This information, together with findings from case taking, determine an individual's risk of succumbing to stress, because everyone reacts differently to stressful events.

Diseases strongly linked to stress

- Angina
- Anorexia nervosa
- Asthma
- Autoimmune disease
- Cancer
- Cardiovascular disease
- Chronic fatigue syndrome
- Common cold
- Depression
- Diabetes (adult onset-type 2)
- Digestive disturbances
- Headaches
- Heart disease
- Hypertension
- Immune suppression
- Insulin resistance
- Irritable bowel syndrome
- Menstrual irregularities
- Premenstrual tension syndrome
- Rheumatoid arthritis
- Thyroid disorders
- Ulcerative colitis
- Ulcers

Sources: Benson H. The relaxation response. New York: William Morrow; 1975. Dantzer R. Somatization: a psychoneuroimmune perspective. Psychoneuroendocrinology 2005; 30(10):947–952. Hellhammer J, Schlotz W, Stone AA et al. Allostatic load, perceived stress, and health: a prospective study in two age groups. Ann New York Acad Sci 2004; 1032:8–13. Korte SM, Koolhaas JM, Wingfield JC et al. The Darwinian concept of stress: benefits of allostasis and costs of allostatic load and the trade-offs in health and disease. Neurosci Biobehav Rev 2005; 29(1):3–38. McCabe D, Colbeck M. The effectiveness of essential fatty acid, B vitamins, vitamin C, magnesium and zinc supplementation for managing stress in women: a systematic review protocol. JBI Database System Rev Implement Rep 2017; 15(2):402–453. McEwen BS. The end of stress as we know it. Washington DC: Dana Press (Joseph Henry Press); 2002. Miller DB, O'Callaghan JP. Neuroendocrine aspects of the response to stress. Metab Clin Exper 2002; 51(6 Suppl. 1):5–10. Tsigos C, Chrousos GP. Hypothalamic–pituitary–adrenal axis, neuroendocrine factors and stress. J Psychosom Res 2002; 53(4):865–871. Vitetta L, Anton B, Cortizo F et al. Mind–body medicine: stress and its impact on overall health and longevity. Ann New York Acad Sci 2005; 1057:492–505.

TABLE 21.36 The Social Readjustment Rating Scale

A: adults

Rank	Life event	Mean value	Rank	Life event	Mean value
1	Death of spouse	100	14	Gain of a new family member	39
2	Divorce	73	15	Business adjustment	39
3	Marital separation	65	16	Change in financial state	38
4	Imprisonment	63	17	Death of a close friend	37
5	Death of a close family member	63	18	Change to different line of work	36
6	Personal injury or illness	53	19	Change in frequency of arguments (with spouse)	35
7	Marriage	50	20	Large/major mortgage	31
8	Fired/dismissal from work	47	21	Foreclosure of mortgage or loan	30
9	Marital reconciliation	45	22	Change in responsibilities at work	29
10	Retirement	45	23	Son or daughter leaving home	29
11	Change in health of family member	44	24	Trouble with in-laws	29
12	Pregnancy	40	25	Outstanding personal achievement	28
13	Sexual difficulties	39	26	Spouse starts or stops work	26

Continued

TABLE 21.36 The Social Readjustment Rating Scale—cont'd

Rank	Life event	Mean value	Rank	Life event	Mean value
27	Beginning or end of school	26	36	Change in social activities	18
28	Change in living conditions	25	37	Minor mortgage or loan	17
29	Revision of personal habits	24	38	Change in sleeping habits	16
30	Trouble with boss	23	39	Change in number of family get-togethers	15
31	Change in work hours or conditions	20	40	Change in eating habits	15
32	Change in residence	20	41	Vacation	13
33	Change in schools	20	42	Christmas	12
34	Change in recreation	19	43	Minor violations of the law	11
35	Change in church activities	19			

Score of 200+: At risk of illness.
Score of 150–200+: Risk of illness is moderate (reduced by 30% from the above risk).
Score <150: Only have a slight risk of illness.
Sources: Holmes TH, Rahe RH. The Social Readjustment Rating Scale. J Psychosom Res 1967; 11(2):213–218.

B: children

A modified scale has also been developed for children. Similar to the adult scale, stress points for life events in the past year are added and compared with the rough estimate of how stress affects health.

Rank	Life event	Mean value	Rank	Life event	Mean value
1	Getting married	101	21	Jail sentence of parent for over 30 days	53
2	Unwed pregnancy	92	22	Breaking up with boyfriend or girlfriend	53
3	Death of parent	87	23	Beginning to date	51
4	Acquiring a visible deformity	81	24	Suspension from school	50
5	Divorce of parents	77	25	Birth of a brother or sister	50
6	Fathering an unwed pregnancy	77	26	Increase in arguments between parents	47
7	Becoming involved with drugs or alcohol	76	27	Loss of job by parent	46
8	Jail sentence of parent for over 1 year	75	28	Outstanding personal achievement	46
9	Marital separation of parents	69	29	Change in parent's financial status	45
10	Death of a brother or sister	68	30	Accepted at university/college of choice	43
11	Change in acceptance by peers	67	31	Being a senior in high school	42
12	Pregnancy of unwed sister	64	32	Hospitalisation of a sibling	41
13	Discovery of being an adopted child	63	33	Increased absence of parent from home	38
14	Marriage of parent to step-parent	63	34	Brother or sister leaving home	37
15	Death of a close friend	63	35	Addition of third adult to family	34
16	Having a visible congenital deformity	62	36	Becoming a fully-fledged member of a church	31
17	Serious illness requiring hospitalisation	58	37	Decrease in arguments between parents	27
18	Failure of a grade in school	56	38	Decrease in arguments with parents	26
19	Not making an extracurricular activity	55	39	Mother or father beginning work	26
20	Hospitalisation of a parent	55			

Score of 200+: At risk of illness.
Score of 150–200+: Risk of illness is moderate (reduced by 30% from the above risk).
Score <150: Slight risk of illness.

Investigations

If a person is under a great deal of immediate stress or has endured a fair amount of stress for some time, it is appropriate to assess adrenal dysfunction more accurately with in-clinic and laboratory methods. The tests in Table 21.37 have been recommended.

Therapeutic considerations

CLINICAL DECISION MAKING AND RATIONALE

Stress is part of everyday life and only becomes pathological when it is severe or prolonged. A stressful event initiates a hormone cascade, leading to increased levels of adrenaline and cortisol, which facilitates alertness and readiness for action. When these hormones do not return to normal (e.g. due to continual or severe stress) a myriad of health problems could result. The better resourced a patient is mentally and physically, the better the coping skills and the less impact any stressor will have.

The primary objectives of treatment include:

- To nourish and repair the nervous system
- To regulate and restore neurotransmitter release
- To regulate endocrinological function and hormonal release
- To enhance the body's capacity to recover and tolerate stress
- To enable the body to recover from primary and secondary health developments.

TABLE 21.37 Assessing stress

In-clinic assessment	
Waist circumference	High cortisol has been linked to visceral adiposity and insulin resistance. Waist circumference should be <102 cm for men and <88 cm for women
BMI	This is calculated from weight and height: BMI = weight (kg)/height $(m)^2$ The normal range is 18.5–25
Stress questionnaires	These include the Social Readjustment Rating Scale (see Table 21.36) and the Perceived Stress Scale
Blood pressure	One effect of adrenaline is to raise blood pressure to rapidly provide nutrients to sites of action (muscles)
Urinalysis	General MSU to exclude additional irregularities such as dehydration, elevated glucose or other abnormalities
Blood glucose	Adrenaline also increases blood glucose for the necessary energy to fight or flee. The link between high cortisol and hyperglycaemia glucose can stay elevated, predisposing the person to insulin resistance and type 2 diabetes
Pathology tests	
Cortisol	This is a diurnal hormone with highest levels in the morning and lowest around midnight. It is therefore best measured in blood early morning, and again in the late afternoon if required. Ideal values are in the upper half of the reference range A 24-hour urinary cortisol can give information on the overall amount produced
ACTH	As this hormone stimulates the release of cortisol (and should be silenced by high cortisol through negative feedback) information can be gained whether this cycle is still intact or whether these two hormones are becoming resistant to each other's actions
DHEA	Used to assess the hypothalamus-pituitary-adrenal axis. DHEA levels are high or normal during the acute stage of adrenal fatigue, and low during adaptation and depletion phases
Inflammatory markers (ESR, CRP)	High adrenaline (epinephrine) promotes inflammatory cytokines. These markers can give information regarding the extent of inflammation in the body. Under normal circumstances they should be as low as possible
Lipid studies	Stress, heart disease and insulin resistance are linked. The relationship of cholesterol to HDL will indicate the patient's risk of heart disease, and high triglycerides are linked to insulin resistance. Low HDL may be linked to inflammatory cytokines
HbA_{1c}	This is a measure of glycaemic control. It should be <4.8% in non-diabetic people. A value <6% in diabetic individuals indicates good control
Other	
Due to the interrelationship between all glands, clinical assessment of all endocrine function is advised	

ACTH, adrenocorticotropic hormone; BMI, body mass index; CRP, C-reactive protein; DHEA, dehydroepiandrosterone; ESR, erythrocyte sedimentation rate; MSU, mid-stream urine.

Sources: Anderson D. Assessment and nutraceutical management of stress-induced adrenal dysfunction. Integ Med 2008; 7(5):18–25. Cutshall SM, Bergstrom LR, Kalish DJ. Evaluation of a functional medicine approach to treating fatigue, stress, and digestive issues in women. Comp Ther Clin Pract 2016; 23:75–81. McEwen BS. The end of stress as we know it. Washington DC: Dana Press (Joseph Henry Press); 2002. Munroe S, Kelley J. Measurement of stress appraisal. In: Cohen S, Kessler RLG, eds. Measuring stress: a guide for health and social scientists. New York: Oxford University Press; 1995, pp. 122–147. Pagana KD, Pagana TJ. Mosby's manual of diagnostic and laboratory tests. 2nd edn. St Louis: Mosby; 2002. Schnorpfeil P, Noll A, Schulze R et al. Allostatic load and work conditions. Social Sci Med 2003; 57(4):647–656.

Therapeutic application

NATUROPATHIC PERSPECTIVE

Typically, the majority of individuals have little problem adjusting to life stressors when they appear, and once these stressors dissipate, these people display 'healthy' psychophysiological function in that the hormone levels achieved to deal with the stressor return to baseline levels.[519] However, when one is unable to continually adapt after prolonged periods of stress, adrenal dysfunction becomes clinically apparent.[520] Most often, these people are unable to maintain previous levels of energy in all realms of life and progressively deteriorate as times goes on. In fact, depression and substantial decreases in performance are considered hallmark symptoms of maladaptation to stress.[521,522]

Stress is undoubtedly going to factor into every treatment program a practitioner develops for patients — whether they present with stress or the effects of stress, or for something completely unrelated.

Patients have their own inbuilt coping strategies — some positive and some negative. They are often not able to determine the difference in the early stages. It is beneficial for the practitioner to assess the patient's lifestyle and habits in great detail and illuminate these patterns to the patient. Subsequent positive recommendations for a number of key areas are optimally beneficial.

The primary objective of the practitioner is neither to chastise the patient nor to highlight their deficiencies of character. The stress that the patient is feeling is very real to them and likely stems from emotional issues or trauma. A systematic, sequential and empathetic manner is the most effective. For example, if negative food behaviour is the primary coping strategy for the patient, presenting them with a perfect wholefood diet and expecting them to walk away and be cured is both unrealistic and insensitive. The objective should be to support, encourage and guide patients to their optimal health in a pace and manner that is gentle and comfortable for them.

Key areas for stress management include:

- Appropriate referral to address underlying emotional issues or direction to techniques to calm the mind and promote positive mental and emotional health
- Healthy lifestyle practices that encourage daily exercise, regular and restful sleep and positive social contact
- Nutritionally sound and easily digested dietary regimen
- Specific supplementation of nutrients to address deficiencies and regulate hormonal and neurotransmitter cascades
- Herbal medicines to re-educate and restore optimal neurological and psychological function
- Other treatments as necessary for secondary afflictions, for example digestive support for gastrointestinal ulcers.

NUTRITIONAL MEDICINE (DIETARY)

Dietary therapeutic objectives

Whether or not stress is harmful is based on how well the system is resourced. From a purely physiological perspective, it can be strongly argued that delivery of high-quality nutrition (nutrient-dense foods) to the cells of the body is the critical factor in determining the system's ability to withstand stress. An individual suffering from stress or anxiety must support the biochemistry of the body by following some important dietary guidelines. Poor eating habits and food choices create a burden on the stress response, as well as leaving the body without essential nutrients.[522]

Specific dietary treatments

DIETARY INCLUSIONS

- Consume high-quality protein (e.g. lean meat, fish, eggs, legumes, seeds and nuts) with every meal. Under stress people often crave carbohydrate-rich food (sweets and treats) at the expense of eating a balanced meal. Stress also induces protein breakdown from muscle tissue to sustain the fuel needed for the stress response. Sufficient protein is therefore essential.[522]
- Eat a diverse range of wholefoods. The greater the variety of foods, the higher the variety of essential nutrients.
- Eat regular planned meals in a relaxed environment. Skipping meals deprives the body of nutrients, and eating on the run does not allow for optimal digestive juices to be secreted.
- Increase the potassium-to-sodium ratio. This can be achieved by avoiding fruit (high potassium, low sodium) in the morning.[522]
- Encourage patients to chew food thoroughly, focus on optimal digestion and remind patients that stress relief can be encouraged with optimal digestion to enable adequate nutrient release and absorption.

DIETARY EXCLUSIONS

- Eliminate or restrict the intake of caffeine. Replace with herbal teas and filtered water.
- Eliminate or restrict the intake of alcohol. It has a detrimental effect on the brain, liver and glucose regulation.
- Eliminate refined carbohydrates from the diet. For better blood glucose regulation wholegrains, containing particularly B vitamins for energy production and fibre for slow glucose release, are much more beneficial.

Other dietary considerations

Control food allergies and intolerances. Many people react to food that is commonly over-consumed, such as wheat and dairy. Often symptoms are delayed, making it difficult to establish a link between a certain food and one's health problems. Eliminating a suspect food from one's diet for a couple of weeks and then reintroducing it is a good way of finding out one's reactivity. On the other hand, preexisting food reactivity contributes to the stress burden.[523]

SAMPLE DAILY DIET

BREAKFAST	
Oats with cinnamon, strawberries, cacao, dates and walnuts	Wholefood carbohydrates are required to ensure there is adequate glucose available to fuel the metabolic demands of stress responses. Oats are a complex carbohydrate which is also rich in B vitamins. The addition of strawberries provides vitamin C which is also critical for adaption to stress. Dates and cinnamon provide natural sweetness; research shows that the rewarding properties of sweet palatable foods confer stress relief. Intake of carbohydrate 'comfort' foods is associated with improved mood, decreased perceived stress and reduced plasma cortisol concentration in people who are sensitive to stress.
LUNCH	
Slow-cooked lamb with quinoa and root vegetables	Slow-cooked lamb with roasted vegetables provides an easy-to-digest, energetically grounding meal. The addition of quinoa provides additional protein and fibre for glycaemic control as well as B vitamins for energy.
DINNER	
Green vegetable, potato and brown lentil soup with GF toast spread with avocado and hummus	Meals should be nutritious but easy to prepare to conserve energy. Small frequent meals are suggested to ensure hypoglycaemia does not occur. Green vegetables provide magnesium which is required for adaption to stress. In-vivo studies reveal magnesium deficiency induces anxiety and HPA axis dysregulation.
SNACK	
Fresh juice: blueberry plus other seasonal fruits with nuts and seeds Liquorice tea	A fresh juice can be used to provide energy and reduce reliance on caffeine and less nutritive forms of sugar in the morning. In-vivo studies reveal plasma noradrenaline (norepinephrine) and dopamine concentrations were decreased by chronic stress resulting in cognitive impairment; however, these concentrations were improved when blueberry juice was consumed. Liquorice extends the half-life of cortisol in the body and thus may be useful for improving adaption to stress.

NUTRITIONAL MEDICINE (SUPPLEMENTAL)

Nutritional medicine treatment objectives

Nutritional support involves supporting the adrenal glands and the nervous system. Many of the B vitamins, as well as vitamin C, magnesium and zinc are used to regulate the stress response and synthesise the hormones necessary for increased physical activity, such as adrenaline (epinephrine) and cortisol. Conversely, the synthesis of the calming neurotransmitter serotonin also requires many of the same nutrients.[524] Hormones such as adrenaline (epinephrine) and cortisol are usually elevated in acute stress, leading to anxiety and hyperarousal.[509] They tend to decline in prolonged stress. Depletion of these hormones leads to chronic fatigue[525] and flat depression.[501,509]

Specific nutrients required

VITAMIN C

Vitamin C is a crucial vitamin in combating stress. Animals are able to produce vitamin C when under stress. Unfortunately, human beings cannot.[94] The adrenal glands need more vitamin C than any other organ or tissue.[522,524] Vitamin C is a co-factor in adrenalin (epinephrine) and neurotransmitter synthesis, as well as being an important antioxidant in the brain, which can help to affect cognitive functioning and the ability to cope with stress.[524] To reduce allopathic load, a dose of 1500 mg/day has been used to lower cortisol and adrenaline (epinephrine) in runners.[526]

B VITAMINS AND COENZYME Q10

B vitamins and coenzyme Q10 are co-factors in the Krebs cycle and hence indispensable for energy production.[94] They are particularly important in chronic health conditions[527] and energy-compromised states such as chronic fatigue.[528,529] Coenzyme Q10 tends to be low with low cortisol levels.[530]

The anti-stress vitamin, vitamin B_5 (pantothenic acid), gains its reputation in its role as CoA (coenzyme A). CoA is involved in adrenal cortex function, as it serves in increasing production of glucocorticoids and other adrenal hormones.[531] It has been shown to enhance adrenal cortical function in laboratory animals[532] and reduce the elevation of urinary cortisol metabolites that were expected to be produced as a byproduct of adrenal stimulation using ACTH, thus implying that B_5 can also potentially lower secretion of cortisol in periods of stress.[533]

MAGNESIUM

Magnesium is a co-factor in energy production neurotransmitter synthesis and glucose regulation.[illegible] In adrenergic stimulation such as in acute stress magnesium levels fell markedly.[534] Supplementation in high physical stress (triathlon) resulted in an improved response to stress without negatively affecting performance.[535]

ANTIOXIDANTS — VITAMINS A, C, E; ZINC, SELENIUM AND VARIOUS PHYTOCHEMICALS

Antioxidants are needed in situations of oxidative stress which tends to accompany the stress response, particularly in chronic stress.[536] Neurodegenerative diseases in particular have benefited from antioxidant supplementation.[537]

S-ADENOSYL METHIONINE (SAM OR SAM-E)

S-adenosyl methionine is derived from remethylating homocysteine with vitamin B_{12} and folate, or with betaine (trimethylglycine). SAM is the body's universal methyl donor, needed (among other functions) for neurotransmitter synthesis such as adrenaline (epinephrine) and serotonin. Where indicated, vitamin B_{12} and folate will also enhance methylation. These nutrients have all been shown to be helpful in depression.[538,539]

Supplementation of actual SAM is only indicated if the patient is not an over-methylator. If cautioned, high doses of methylation co-factors are a primary treatment prescription.

CO-FACTORS FOR NEUROTRANSMITTER SYNTHESIS

Include the amino acids tyrosine (substrate for adrenaline (epinephrine)), tryptophan (substrate for serotonin) and glutamine (substrate for GABA). Main co-factors for their metabolism include vitamin B_6 (in its activated form as pyridoxyl 5-phosphate), B_{12} and folate. Several other vitamins and minerals play a role in the conversion of these amino acids to neurotransmitters, vitamins B_2 and B_3, C, iron, copper, calcium and zinc, and need to be present in the body in adequate amounts.

DIGESTIVE SUPPORT

Digestive support may be needed as the aroused SNS has a negative impact on the ability to secrete hydrochloric acid and digestive enzymes.[540]

ESSENTIAL FATTY ACIDS

Omega-3 fatty acids are required for optimal functioning of the nervous system, in both neuronal membrane structure and neurotransmitter release. A deficiency of essential fatty acids may affect the ability to effectively cope with stress as a result of cognitive functioning deficits.[524] They have a beneficial effect on depression[538] and inflammation.[541]

MULTIVITAMIN/MULTIMINERAL

Given the wide array of nutrients required to support the complex mechanisms of the stress response, and the prevalence of chronic stress exposure in today's modern lifestyle, if a patient is not eating an optimal nutrient-dense diet, a good-quality multivitamin supplement might be beneficial while new dietary habits and stress management techniques are introduced.

Dosage requirements

The daily dosage requirements listed below are based on adult doses that have been reported in the literature:

- Calcium: 400–1000 mg/day
- Coenzyme Q10: 100–300 mg/day
- Copper: 2–4 mg/day:
  - Only prescribe if indicated on pathology, ensure zinc:copper ratio is maintained and prescribe for methylation support
- Iron: 5–80 mg/day:
  - If indicated on pathology
- Magnesium: 400–800 mg/day in divided doses
- Probiotics: 25–50 × 10^{12}:
  - If digestive symptoms are present or if poor absorption concerns are evident
- *S*-adenosyl methionine (SAM or SAM-e): 200–400 mg/day
  - Assess SAM:SAH ratio to confirm appropriateness prior to prescribing)
  - Can increase, depending on presentation and methylation status
  - Monitor closely and cease prescription after short term
- Selenium: 100–250 micrograms/day
- Vitamin A: 5000–15 000 IU/day
- Vitamin B complex: high-dose combination, preferably activated forms:
  - Thiamine: 40–80 mg/day
  - Riboflavin: 20–60 mg/day
  - Niacinamide 100–200 mg/day
  - Pantothenic acid: 150–300 mg/day
  - Pyridoxine: 20–100 mg/day
  - Folinic acid (or L5MTHF as indicated): 500–2000 micrograms/day
  - Hydroxocobalamin (or methylcobalamin as indicated): 500–2000 micrograms/day
  - Choline: 100–200 mg/day
  - Inositol: 100–200 mg/day
  - Biotin: 500–1000 micrograms/day
- Vitamin C: 1–2 g/day
- Vitamin E: 400–800 IU/day
- Zinc: 20–50 mg/day
- Essential fatty acids: minimum of 0.5–1 g of DHA in a combined essential fatty acid prescription.

HERBAL MEDICINE

Herbal medicine therapeutic objectives and relevant classes

1 Reduce stress (long term and short term)
   a Adaptogen
   b Adrenal restorative
   c Nervine tonic
   d Nervine trophorestorative
   e Sedative (if indicated)
   f Euphoric

2 Increase energy levels
Nervine stimulant (caution in some)
  a Nervine tonic
  b Nervine trophorestorative
  c Adaptogen
  d Adrenal restorative
3 Stabilise mood
  a Nervine trophorestorative
  b Adaptogen
  c Adrenal restorative
4 Reduce depression
  a Antidepressant
  b Thymoleptic
  c Euphoric
  d Serotonin agonist
5 Improve cognition
  a Cerebro-circulatory stimulants
  b Antioxidant
  c Cognitive enhancer
6 Restore nervous system function and integrity
  a Nervine tonic
  b Nervine trophorestorative
  c Sedative (if indicated)
7 Circadian rhythm stabilisation
  a Sedative
  b Nervine tonic
  c Nervine stimulant (caution with some)
  d Melatonin stimulation
    i Sunlight/moonlight
    ii Serotonin agonist
8 General body tonification
  a Tonic
  b Nutritive
9 Hormonal modulation
  a Serotonin agonist
  b HPA modulator
  c Melatonin stimulation (sunlight/moonlight)
  d Specific to sex of patient as needed (female and male).

Herbal medicine classes

NERVINE TONIC

Nervine tonics are indicated to repair neurological function. Their strong traditional application and marked clinical benefit highlight the importance of these prescriptions. Specific materia medica that are most appropriate for the recovery and treatment of stress include *Avena sativa* (oats, green and seed), *Bacopa monnieri* (bacopa), *Hypericum perforatum* (St John's wort), *Passiflora incarnata* (passion flower) and *Scutellaria lateriflora* (skullcap).

NERVINE TROPHORESTORATIVE

Nervine trophorestoratives are a subclass of herbal medicines within nervine tonics. These herbal medicines are specifically effective at restoring damaged neurological tissue. This can be especially evident in cases of stress or a stressful history when a person's reaction is stronger than intended or 'hyperreactive'. These three herbal medicines can provide much benefit, for example: *Avena sativa* (oats, green or seed) is known as a useful prescription both as a food and as a liquid extract (preferably both parts combined in equal portion) to settle and restore damaged neuronal communication. *Bacopa monnieri* (bacopa) is especially indicated for mentally overworked and overstressed patients who present with poor mental capacity and overactive mental processes with poor outcome. Its trophorestorative effects are best displayed in cognitive improvements and improvements from mental exertion/stress histories. *Hypericum perforatum* (St John's wort), often prescribed for depression, can be successfully prescribed to patients who require trophorestorative benefits specifically when depletion produces emotional fragility/lability, insomnia and generalised tension.

HYPNOTIC/SEDATIVE

Highly stressed patients will commonly experience poor-quality sleep and/or sleep difficulties. Hypnotic herbal medicines are classified as the deeper, more intoxicating prescriptions, while sedatives are seen to gently sedate patients and support deeper quality sleep. Sedatives as a general class can be applied to various organs/systems and will have varying effects. Examples include *Eschscholzia californica* (Californian poppy), *Humulus lupulus* (hops), *Lavandula angustifolia* (lavender), and *Piscidia piscipula* (Jamaican dogwood) within the hypnotic class. *Passiflora incarnata* (passion flower), *Piper methysticum* (kava), *Corydalis ambigua* (corydalis), *Valeriana officinalis* (valerian) and *Ziziphus jujuba* var. *spinosa* (zizyphus) within the sedative class. Above all, it is important to acknowledge that responses to herbal medicines are individual.

NERVINE RELAXANT

A subcategory within the sedative/hypnotic class is a gentler class known as nervine relaxants. Their prescription is generally made to relax the nervous system. They include a general group of herbal medicines including *Anemone pulsatilla* (pulsatilla), *Avena sativa* green (oats green), *Matricaria chamomilla* (chamomile), *Actaea racemosa* (black cohosh), *Corydalis ambigua* (corydalis), *Eschscholzia californica* (Californian poppy), *Humulus lupulus* (hops), *Hyssopus officinalis* (hyssop), *Lavandula angustifolia* (lavender), *Leonurus cardiaca* (motherwort), *Melissa officinalis* (lemon balm), *Nicotiana* spp. (tobacco), *Passiflora incarnata* (passion flower), *Piper methysticum* (kava), *Piscidia piscipula* (Jamaican dogwood), *Scutellaria lateriflora* (skullcap), *Tilia* spp. (lime flowers), *Valeriana officinalis* (valerian), *Verbena officinalis* (verbena), *Viburnum opulus* (cramp bark), *Viscum album* (mistletoe), *Withania somnifera* (withania) and *Ziziphus jujuba* var. *spinosa* (zizyphus).

ADAPTOGEN

The adaptogenic approach to adrenal fatigue is perhaps one of the most remarkable concepts in naturopathic medicine. To approach the patient from this perspective (bolstering their adaptive capabilities through modulation of hormone and neurotransmitter physiology) is a true approach to assisting the body in healing itself, rather than approaching symptoms directly. In fact, treatment of symptoms only in adrenal dysfunction is highly unlikely to produce any lasting benefit for the patient.[519]

Adaptogen herbal medicines are those that provide support and tonification to the whole body so that it can cope with current stressors. They are said to increase the body's resistance to stress on multiple levels. The following herbal medicines must be considered for any case of stress presentation. Practitioners will often prescribe multiple adaptogens within a formula in strong stress presentations. Important examples include: *Andrographis paniculata* (andrographis), *Asparagus racemosus* (shatavari), *Astragalus membranaceus* (astragalus), *Atractylodes macrocephala* (atractylodes), *Bacopa monnieri* (bacopa), *Codonopsis pilosula* (codonopsis), *Eleutherococcus senticosus* (Siberian ginseng), *Ganoderma lucidum* (reishi), *Glycyrrhiza glabra* (liquorice), *Grifola frondosa* (maitake), *Lentinus edodes* (shiitake), *Panax ginseng* (Korean ginseng), *Panax notoginseng* (Tienchi ginseng), *Panax quinquefolius* (American ginseng), *Rehmannia glutinosa* (rehmannia), *Rhodiola rosea* (rhodiola), *Schisandra chinensis* (schisandra) and *Withania somnifera* (ashwagandha).

ADRENAL RESTORATIVE

Adrenal restorative herbal medicines consist of two herbal medicines that have shown significant clinical benefit in assisting the adrenal glands to be restored to normal function. Their prescription is often made in instances of adrenal exhaustion, fatigue, emotional depletion and when a patient is worn out. Differentiating between *Glycyrrhiza glabra* (liquorice) and *Rehmannia glutinosa* (rehmannia) can be challenging clinically and practitioners may find benefit from the combined prescription in one formula. *Glycyrrhiza glabra* exhibits cautionary aspects and can increase blood pressure when prescribed long term. As adrenal restorative herbal medicines typically require extended prescription for best outcome, *Rehmannia glutinosa* may be a better prescription. Alternatively, alternating prescriptions can be considered.

TONIC

Tonic herbal medicines are best prescribed for stressful situations that affect a particular organ or organ system. They present with an affinity to a specific system. For example, a highly stressed patient may present with reflux and digestive ulceration. The herbal medicine *Filipendula ulmaria* (meadowsweet) would be an ideal prescription as a stomach tonic herbal medicine. A summary of some relevant herbal medicines is shown in Table 21.38. Please note that the list includes some of the main herbal medicines used in phytotherapy and is not complete.

Specific herbal medicines

PANAX GINSENG (KOREAN GINSENG)

The rejuvenating action of *Panax ginseng* has been known for thousands of years having been recorded in one of the most comprehensive materia medicas of traditional Chinese medicine, the *Shen Nong Ben Cao Jing*.[542] The Eclectic physicians also prized *Panax ginseng*, recommending its use as a tonic for mental exhaustion from overwork.[543] Clinical studies confirm traditional

TABLE 21.38 Tonic herbal medicines

Herbal medicines	Tonic properties
Astragalus membranaceus	Immune, renal and general tonic; qi tonic – repairs active spleen and lung energies
Avena sativa	Tonic for nervous and digestive systems (green is a tonic while seed is stimulating)
Berberis vulgaris	Liver tonic
Bupleurum falcatum	Liver, kidney, blood and general tonic
Codonopsis pillosula	Adrenal, liver and blood tonic; qi tonic – repairs active spleen and lung energies
Crataegus monogyna	Heart tonic
Crataeva nurvala	Bladder tonic
Filipendula ulmaria	Stomach tonic
Foeniculum vulgare	Digestive tonic
Glycyrrhiza glabra	General tonic that has an affinity for the GIT and lungs Qi tonic – repairs active spleen and lung energies
Gymnema sylvestre	Pancreatic tonic
Hydrastis canadensis	Tonic and stimulant for the GIT and entire system (all mucous membranes)
Hypericum perforatum	General tonic with specific emotional and mental support as well as gentle liver support
Medicago sativa	General nutritive and tonic
Paeonia lactiflora	Female tonic
Panax ginseng	Constitutional tonic; qi tonic – repairs active spleen and lung energies
Panax quinquefolius	Yin tonic – replaces bodily fluids and essence
Piper methysticum	Bladder tonic
Rehmannia glutinosa	Kidney tonic; xue tonic – repairs from pathology or substantial disturbance
Serenoa serrulata	Male tonic
Shatavari racemosa	Female tonic
Silybum marianum	Liver tonic
Trigonella foenum-graecum	General nutritive and tonic; yang tonic – repairs active kidney and heart energies
Turnera diffusa	Male tonic, general tonic, and tonic for menopausal women
Urtica dioica folia	Nutritive and general tonic
Verbascum thapsus	Lung tonic
Verbena officinalis	General tonic and nervous system tonic
Withania glutinosa	General tonic and nutritive, adrenal and nervous system tonic

knowledge on the adaptogenic properties of *Panax ginseng*, with it being shown to increase resistance to a number of stressors. A 2011 systematic review[544] indicates strong evidence of efficacy for the use of *P. ginseng* to support cognitive function and improve glucose metabolism (to aid patients with diminished glucose control due to adrenal glucocorticoid dysregulation). Additional actions include reduction in fatigue[545] and biological stress,[546] and improved antioxidant function.[546–548]

The active constituents within *Panax ginseng*, known as ginsenoside, which are saponin glycosides, have been suggested to produce a corticosteroid-like action and may supplement adrenal steroidogenesis through an indirect action on the pituitary gland.[549] The German Commission E and the World Health Organization both approve *Panax ginseng* for use during convalescence and for invigoration and fortification in times of fatigue and debility or declining capacity for work and concentration.[542]

ELEUTHEROCOCCUS SENTICOSUS (SIBERIAN GINSENG)

Though *Eleutherococcus senticosus* and *Panax ginseng* come from the same family, the chemical structure that makes them up is very different.[550] *Eleutherococcus senticosus* is considered to be much gentler and without the stimulating actions of *Panax ginseng*. A number of clinical trials have investigated the use of *Eleutherococcus senticosus* as an adaptogen and while there is evidence to support the use of *Eleutherococcus senticosus* for increasing endurance and mental performance in patients with mild fatigue and weakness[551] studies of a better quality are required. In their review, Panossian and Wagner (2005)[552] report of a study in which sailors undertaking night watch were given a single dose of *Eleutherococcus senticosus* extract (4 mL) which subsequently instigated a number of physiological changes within the body, including increasing the tonus of the parasympathetic part of the autonomic nervous system, intensifying excitation of the central nervous system and decreasing activity in the adrenal cortex. Other trials have reported similar benefits including the ability of *Eleutherococcus senticosus* to influence aerobic metabolism of tissues and increase oxygen consumption during maximal physical exercise (a form of stress on the body).[553] A 2013 multicentric, RCT compared three treatment schedules on participants suffering from stress-related low energy and reduced working capacity: (i) 2-day structured stress management training; (ii) oral treatment with *Eleutherococcus senticosus* root capsules (ES 120 mg dry extract WS 1070) 1 capsule daily for 8 weeks; (iii) combination of stress management training and ES capsules. Results revealed that the addition of ES capsules to stress management training did not show any additional benefit compared with stress management training alone in alleviating subjective and physiological stress parameters.[554]

RHODIOLA ROSEA (RHODIOLA)

There is strong scientific evidence to support the use of *Rhodiola rosea* as an adaptogen. A randomised, double-blind, placebo-controlled, parallel-group study investigating the standardised extract SHR-5 of the roots of *Rhodiola rosea* in the treatment of patients with stress-related fatigue found that repeated administration of *Rhodiola rosea* extract SHR-5 exerted an antifatigue effect that increased mental performance, particularly the ability to concentrate while also decreasing cortisol response to awakening stress in burnout patients with fatigue syndrome.[555] Similarly a double-blind crossover study investigating the antifatigue effect of *Rhodiola rosea* on the mental performance of healthy physicians during night duty found that supplementation with *Rhodiola rosea* reduced general fatigue under certain stressful conditions in just 2 weeks.[556]

HYPERICUM PERFORATUM (ST JOHN'S WORT)

It has been suggested that patients with depression have alterations in the hypothalamo-pituitary–adrenal (HPA) axis that may be normalised by certain antidepressants due to their ability to induce favourable modifications in the HPA axis reactivity to stress.[557] St John's wort is well known for its effects as a nervine tonic and as an antidepressant. A small study examining the effects of 600 mg of WS 5570 *Hypericum perforatum* extract in 12 physically and mentally healthy males found that between 30 and 90 minutes after taking the *Hypericum* extract a clear-cut cortisol stimulation was observed. The authors proposed that *Hypericum* extract WS 5570 is able to influence central neurotransmitters thus causing cortisol stimulation in a dose-dependent manner.[558] A second study examining the effect of subchronic treatment with Jarsin (extract of St John's wort, *Hypericum perforatum*) at two dose levels on evening salivary melatonin and cortisol concentrations in healthy male volunteers found that salivary cortisol was enhanced in the low-dose group only.[559]

SCUTELLARIA LATERIFLORA (SKULLCAP)

Scutellaria lateriflora has been used traditionally for its restorative effects on the nervous system where it was prescribed for disorders such as nervousness or insomnia stemming from mental and physical exhaustion.[560] A double-blind, placebo-controlled crossover study found that *Scutellaria lateriflora* administered daily to healthy adults reduced symptoms of anxiety and tension (common in stressful situations) after acute administration compared with control.[250] This anxiolytic activity of *Scutellaria* is likely to influence the body's adaption to stressors via its effects on the nervous system and provides a basis for its application in adrenal disorders, particularly those originating from nervous tension. A 2014 crossover RCT assessed the mood effects of *Scutellaria lateriflora* administered at a dose of 350 mg daily, over a 2-week period. Significant improvements in anxiety scores were observed in patients with higher mean Beck Anxiety Inventory (BAI) scores at baseline, but not in those with lower mean BAI scores at baseline.[561]

GLYCYRRHIZA GLABRA (LIQUORICE)

Glycyrrhiza glabra may be of benefit in patients experiencing chronic stress who are unable to mount their own natural healthy stress response. It contains glycyrrhetinic acid, a constituent that inhibits the enzyme

11-beta-hydroxysteroid dehydrogenase inhibiting cortisol metabolism. In a study involving 10 healthy young normotensive volunteers, glycyrrhetinic acid (500 mg/day), administered orally for 7 days resulted in elevated urinary excretion of free cortisol and virtually unchanged plasma cortisol levels. The authors concluded that this result provides direct clinical support for the hypothesis that glycyrrhetinic acid induces an inhibition of the activity of 11-beta-dehydrogenase, resulting in a blockade in the conversion of cortisol to cortisone.[562]

REHMANNIA GLUTINOSA (REHMANNIA)

Rehmannia glutinosa is a prime adrenal tonic[563] and adrenal restorative that has been used in Traditional Chinese Medicine to nourish the yin and invigorate the kidneys.[564] In-vitro studies show that uncured rehmannia supports the adrenal cortex and pituitary gland possibly by antagonising the suppressive effect of glucocorticoids on the HPA axis.[563]

Lifestyle recommendations

A patient's lifestyle is a major determinant of their stress levels.

The primary areas of concern are as follows:

- Negative coping patterns — recreational drugs, occupation, technology use, alcohol, caffeine, sugar and other stimulant substances
- Time management
- Exercise
- Quality and quantity of sleep — sleep deprivation and circadian disruption alter allostasis and elevate the allostatic load, predisposing a person to altered responses to stressors.[565] In particular, loss of sleep lowers the threshold at which a person experiences an event as stressful[566] and is associated with elevated resting cortisol release and an elevated HPA axis response to stressors[567]
- Dietary factors
- Relationships.

Mind and body therapies

Therapies that increase awareness of one's learned response to stress and which are able to modify future behaviour in a stressful situation include counselling and mindfulness,[568] cognitive behavioural therapy[569] and hypnosis.[570] If the problem is more of a spiritual nature pastoral advice may be appropriate.[571] Great works of art (painting, music) have been created out of an urge to express inner distress, and many people find these kinds of therapy help them deal with stressors in their lives.[572] It helps to find creative ways to problem solving through imagination and visualisation.[573] A person's mindset is an important factor in determining how they respond to stress and the extent of the resulting symptoms. Being aware of one's mindset and mindful of reaction style can be beneficial in implementing behavioural changes when dealing with stress.[574]

Various physical therapies, such as relaxation techniques, massage,[575] aromatherapy[576] and reiki[577] have been used successfully to invoke a relaxation response. The healing touch has been proved beneficial not only for muscular tension but also for anxiety and depression.[575]

Lifestyle factors

Patients often suffer from poor time management and feel overwhelmed and time restricted to accomplish everything. Time-saving gadgets often turn out to consume more time and energy than they allegedly save. The need to be instantly available (via mobile phone, for instance) does not allow undisturbed leisure activities. New knowledge and inventions tax, even overwhelm, our ability to absorb this ever growing information. To be able to say 'no' (without feeling guilty) to some of the demands on us and to be realistic of what can be achieved in a given time span is essential for finding balance between work, play and sleep.

With so much to think about and take in, with increasing pace of life, it is not surprising that sleep quality suffers. Yet a good night's sleep is the prerequisite for a productive day. Writing a journal or meditation before retiring may help some people to leave some of the stressors of the day behind them.

Feeling stressed and rushed for time can take its toll on those near and dear. Relationships can deteriorate and lead to estrangement of parents and children as communication and quality family time are suffering. Yet it is exactly the support from caring friends and family members that is so essential in coping with stress. Social isolation is one of the reasons for depression and perceived high allostatic load. People with a network of friends and peers tend to have less allostatic load and better coping skills than the ones without,[505,578,579] perhaps because they have an outlet to share their experiences. Sometimes a conscious effort is needed to create space in one's life for activities that enhance relationships. Buddy systems are another way to provide support and lower stress levels.

Exercise

When under stress ('fight or flight'), the body is geared for action. Since most stressful situations we encounter now do not require us to either fight or run, it is essential that stress hormones are brought back under control. Exercise is the best way to facilitate regulation of these hormonal irregularities.[573] It has been shown that regular physical activity is beneficial for most stress-related conditions and chronic diseases, including heart disease, diabetes, osteoporosis and mental functioning.[580] It needs to be done regularly several times a week and should be planned into one's schedule.

Supervised stress management program

A practitioner can help a patient learn new coping skills by setting small tasks or goals to be accomplished each week, such as introducing a regular exercise or changing to a healthier eating pattern. Under supervision patients are usually more inclined to adhere to the regimen, especially if there is regular follow-up and reporting. How much practitioner input each patient needs depends on the initial coping skills, willingness to change and the individual allostatic load. Guidance can gradually be withdrawn as patients manage to integrate better coping skills into their daily life.

CASE STUDY

OVERVIEW

JY was a 36-year-old male presenting with fatigue and exhaustion. He had previously overworked himself by working 16-hour days, sleeping 5–6 hours per night and relying on caffeine and stimulants to keep him going. This pattern of behaviour had been perpetuated for a number of years culminating in panic attacks and withdrawal from work due to exhaustion.

CLINICAL EXAMINATION

JY was thin, with dark circles under his eyes, marked stress history exhibited by numerous cramp rings in his iris, quickened pulse and white coat hypertension (normalised when he calmed down), marked reactions to noise and movement and excessive consumption of stimulants (6–8 cups of coffee per day).

INVESTIGATIONS

Patient was referred for some general assessments primarily as a routine health check as his clinical picture clearly supported adrenal exhaustion.

TREATMENT PROTOCOL

INITIAL APPOINTMENT

Initial treatment focused on adrenal restoration, nervine tonification, nutritional supplementation to replace lost nutrients and dietary modifications to repair his body and eliminate further stimulant exposure.

HERBAL MEDICINE

Herbal medicine	Ratio	Quantity	Rationale
Rehmannia glutinosa	1:2	80 mL	Anti-inflammatory, adaptogen, adrenal restorative
Hypericum perforatum	STD Ext	40 mL	Antidepressant, nervine tonic — due to planned caffeine withdrawal lowered mood was further expected
Scutellaria laterifolia	1:2	50 mL	Nervine tonic
Withania somnifera	1:1	50 mL	Adaptogen, nutritive, tonic
TOTAL: 220 mL			
DOSE: 7.5 mL b.i.d.			

NUTRITIONAL MEDICINE

Dietary

- Avoid all stimulants including caffeine, sugar, alcohol and others:

CASE STUDY CONTINUED

  – Withdrawal was planned for with a systematic reduction over a number of days. Patient was advised to increase water, herbal teas and vitamin C supplementation if withdrawal symptoms were problematic. Patient was allowed to consume green tea in the short term if headaches were severe, with plans to reduce following successful elimination of coffee
- Consume a high-protein, low-carbohydrate diet — ensure protein requirements are sufficient for both current and ideal body weight in easily digestible forms
- Increase hydration focusing on herbal teas and spring water
- Encourage consumption of a wholefood, organic diet.

Supplemental

Nutrient	Dosage	Rationale
Vitamin C	1 g t.d.s.–q.i.d.	Lower cortisol and adrenaline (epinephrine), nourish adrenal glands
B complex (activated forms)	1 cap b.i.d.	Co-factors in Krebs cycle for energy production
Pantothenic acid	300 mg b.i.d.	Adrenal support
Magnesium	200 mg t.d.s.	Co-factor in energy production and glucose regulation
Essential fatty acids	2 g b.i.d.	Required for optimal functioning of the nervous system
Coenzyme Q10	150 mg b.i.d.	Co-factor in Krebs cycle for energy production

LIFESTYLE/EDUCATION

- Daily exercise starting at 30 min/day of gentle walking and slowly increased by duration and intensity over 2 weeks. Yoga, breathing exercises and meditation throughout the day
- Referral to a counsellor for emotional issues and stress management strategies
- Adequate sleep including daytime naps as required
- Time off from work for a few weeks (as sick leave allowed)
- Avoidance of cigarette smoke (passive and active).

ADDISON'S DISEASE

Classification

Addison's disease is a condition characterised by hormone deficiency caused by damage to the outer layer of the adrenal gland (adrenal cortex).

The adrenal glands are small hormone-secreting organs located on top of each kidney. They consist of the outer portion (called the cortex) and the inner portion (called the medulla). The cortex produces three types of hormones: glucocorticoid hormones, mineralocorticoid hormones and sex hormones:

- The glucocorticoid hormones (such as cortisol) maintain glucose control, suppress immune response and help the body respond to stress
- The mineralocorticoid hormones (such as aldosterone) regulate sodium and potassium balance
- The sex hormones, androgens and oestrogens, affect sexual development and reproduction.

ALTERNATIVE NAMES

- Adrenocortical hypofunction
- Chronic adrenocortical insufficiency
- Primary adrenal insufficiency.

Aetiology

See Table 21.39.

Pathogenesis

Addison's disease results from damage to the adrenal cortex. The damage causes decreased production of the hormones produced by the cortex. This damage may be caused by the following:

- Autoimmune process
- Infections such as tuberculosis, HIV, or fungal infections[581]
- Haemorrhage, blood loss
- Tumours, most frequently pituitary[581]
- Trauma to the adrenals[582]
- Iatrogenic (e.g. surgery or medications such as glucocorticoids)[581,582]
- Use of blood-thinning drugs (anticoagulants).

Addison's disease, as a result of its low cortisol production, can also contribute to or cause autoimmune diseases, such as is seen in autoimmune thyroiditis. Autoimmune markers should therefore be tested for when the diagnosis of Addison's disease is made, and repeated at regular intervals.[582]

RISK FACTORS FOR AUTOIMMUNE TYPE

- Type 1 diabetes
- Hypoparathyroidism
- Hypopituitarism
- Pernicious anaemia
- Testicular dysfunction
- Graves' disease
- Chronic thyroiditis
- Dermatitis herpetiformis
- Vitiligo
- Myasthenia gravis
- Genetic defects
- Genetic predisposition.[581]

TRIGGERS/EXACERBATIONS

- Times of stress, infection, or injury
- Adrenal crisis is an extreme form of symptoms of adrenal insufficiency, brought on by physical stress. The most frequent causes are gastroenteritis and fever (60–70%), but other stresses include trauma, surgery, a dental procedure and major psychological distress.[581] Hydrocortisone must be injected immediately to sustain life. Supportive treatment for low blood pressure is usually necessary as well.

SIGNS AND SYMPTOMS

- Extreme weakness
- Fatigue (84–95% of patients)[581]
- Unintentional weight loss (66–76% of patients)[581]
- Nausea, vomiting and abdominal pain (49–62% of patients)[581]
- Chronic diarrhoea
- Loss of appetite/anorexia (53–67% of patients)[581]
- Hypoglycaemia

TABLE 21.39 Hormonal influences of addison's disease

Hormone	Control condition	Target	Effect of secretion
Adrenal cortex			
Mineralocorticoids, aldosterone	Formation of angiotensin or increased blood potassium (K^+)	Nephron in kidneys, blood filtration tissues	Increases the reabsorption of Na+ from the kidneys and loss of potassium in the urine. Regulating blood ion concentration
Glucocorticoids Cortisol	Homeostasis disrupted, hypothalamus secretes CRH; this, along with low levels of blood glucocorticoid, stimulates anterior pituitary to secrete ACTH. With low cortisol negative feedback and ACTH inhibition are lost	Muscles, liver, adipose tissue, blood vessels and immune cells	Increases protein breakdown (muscles) and formation of glucose from amino acids and lactate. Increases fat breakdown and use of fatty acids for energy. Depresses inflammatory and immune responses. Overall aim to increase energy availability
Androgens and other sex hormones	Hypothalamus matures and stimulates secretion of androgens	All body cells	Promote growth particularly secondary sexual characteristics. Continue to produce oestrogens after menopause in women

ACTH, adrenocortocotropic hormone; CRH, corticotropin-releasing hormone.

- Muscle and joint pain (36–40% of patients)[581]
- Pigmentation changes:
  - Darkening of the skin (41–74% of patients) — patchy skin colour, unnaturally dark colour in some locations particularly areas of skin subjected to increased friction, such as elbows, knees, knuckles, palmar creases, lips and buccal mucosa.[583] This is from enhanced activation of skin melanocortin 1 receptors by concentrations of high adrenocorticotropic hormone[581]
  - Paleness may also occur
- Mouth lesions on the buccal mucosa — pigmentation
- Slow, sluggish movement
- Changes in blood pressure or heart rate, including postural hypotension (55–68% of patients) [581]
- Salt cravings (38–64% of patients)[581]
- Women may lose pubic and axillary hair due to adrenal androgen insufficiency.[583,584]

See Table 21.40 for more signs and symptoms.

TABLE 21.40 Clinical manifestations and biochemical findings in adrenal insufficiency

	Pathophysiological mechanism	Prevalence (%)
Symptoms		
Fatigue, lack of energy or stamina, reduced strength	Glucocorticoid deficiency, adrenal androgen deficiency	100
Anorexia, weight loss (in children failure to thrive)	Glucocorticoid deficiency	100
Gastric pain, nausea, vomiting (most common in primary adrenal insufficiency)	Glucocorticoid deficiency, mineralocorticoid deficiency	92
Myalgia, joint pain	Glucocorticoid deficiency	6–13
Dizziness	Mineralocorticoid deficiency, glucocorticoid deficiency	12
Salt craving (primary adrenal insufficiency only)	Mineralocorticoid deficiency	16
Dry and itchy skin (in women)	Adrenal androgen deficiency	
Loss or impairment of libido (in women)	Adrenal androgen deficiency	
Signs		
Skin hyperpigmentation (primary adrenal insufficiency only)	Excess of pro-opiomelanocortin-derived peptides	94
Alabaster-coloured pale skin (secondary adrenal insufficiency only)	Deficiency of pro-opiomelanocortin-derived peptides	
Fever	Glucocorticoid deficiency	
Low blood pressure, postural hypotension, dehydration (pronounced in primary adrenal insufficiency)	Mineralocorticoid deficiency, glucocorticoid deficiency	88–94
Loss of axillary or pubic hair (in women), absence of adrenarche or pubarche in children	Adrenal androgen deficiency	
Biochemical findings		
Raised serum creatinine (primary adrenal insufficiency only)	Mineralocorticoid deficiency	
Hyponatraemia	Mineralocorticoid deficiency, glucocorticoid deficiency (leading to SIADH)	88
Hyperkalaemia (primary adrenal insufficiency only)	Mineralocorticoid deficiency	64
Anaemia, lymphocytosis, eosinophilia	Glucocorticoid deficiency	
Increased thyrotrophin (primary adrenal insufficiency only)	Glucocorticoid deficiency (or autoimmune thyroid failure)	
Hypercalcaemia (primary adrenal insufficiency only)	Glucocorticoid deficiency (mostly concurrent hyperthyroidism)	6
Hypoglycaemia	Glucocorticoid deficiency	

If prevalence is not given, data are not available. SIADH, syndrome of inappropriate antidiuretic hormone secretion.
Source: Charmandari E, Nicolaides NC, Chrousos GP. Adrenal insufficiency. The Lancet. 2014 Jun 27;383(9935):2152–67.

Investigations

- Low blood pressure
- Low serum cortisol
- Low serum sodium
- +/– increased potassium
- Abdominal x-ray — adrenal calcification
- Abdominal CT — adrenal calcification, enlargement or atrophy
- Androgens and oestrogens will probably remain normal, because these hormones are also made by the ovaries or testes (and in larger amounts). However, since they are steroid hormones and therefore linked to cortisol, measuring sex hormones may be prudent.

ADDITIONAL MARKERS

This disease may also alter the results of the following tests.

Blood

- Renin
- Potassium
- Aldosterone
- ACTH
- Eosinophil count.

Urine (24-hour)

- Cortisol
- Aldosterone excretion rate
- Potassium
- Sodium
- 17-ketosteroids
- 17-hydroxycorticosteroids.

Other

- Positive Cortrosyn (cosyntropin, also called synacthen) stimulation test (Cortrosyn is an artificial form of part of the ACTH hormone).

> **Cortisol**
>
> The amount of cortisol present in the blood undergoes diurnal variation, with the highest levels present in the early morning, and the lowest levels present around midnight, or 3–5 hours after the onset of sleep. Information about the light/dark cycle is transmitted from the retina to the paired suprachiasmatic nuclei in the hypothalamus. The pattern is not present at birth (estimates of when it starts vary from two weeks to 9 months). In normal release, cortisol (like other glucocorticoid agents) has widespread actions which help restore homeostasis after stress.

Therapeutic considerations

ALLOPATHIC TREATMENT

Treatment with replacement corticosteroids will control the symptoms of this disease. However, these drugs are usually continued for life.

Typically, people receive a combination of glucocorticoids (cortisone or hydrocortisone) and mineralocorticoids (fludrocortisone). Treatment regimens need to be carefully monitored and optimised. Under-replacement might lead to adrenal insufficiency with symptoms such as weight loss, loss of appetite, nausea and fatigue. Over-treatment can lead to symptoms of steroid excess including weight gain, hypertension, oedema and insomnia.[583]

It has been found that adding DHEA to the above prescriptions can lower total cholesterol, low-density lipoproteins (LDL) and fat mass significantly, thus improving body profile and cardiovascular risk factors.[585]

CLINICAL DECISION MAKING AND RATIONALE

- Elevation, balance and regulation of cortisol secretion
- Restoration of adrenal gland
- Nervous system repair and restoration
- Regulation of stress response
- Regulation of anterior pituitary function (if indicated)
- Restoration of electrolyte balance
- Alleviation of associated symptoms.

OTHER TREATMENT CONSIDERATIONS

- Immune modulation and general autoimmune principles (if indicated).

Therapeutic application

NUTRITIONAL MEDICINE (DIETARY)

Since both glucocorticoids and mineralocorticoids are affected by this disease, care needs to be taken to balance electrolytes. Salt intake should not be restricted unless there is convincing evidence to the contrary as low sodium and high potassium is common.[582] Hot weather often leads to increased perspiration and patients can report increased problems due to increased salt loss. Salt intake should be increased to compensate for this scenario.[586]

Careful consideration needs to be given to blood sugar regulation to avoid hypoglycaemia. Diets high in fast-release carbohydrates such as food containing sugar or fructose should be restricted and substituted with low glycaemic index food (see section on hypoglycaemia). If nocturnal hypoglycaemia is suspected, resulting in severe fatigue and/or headaches on waking in the morning, a low GI snack in the evening, including dietary fats might resolve the nocturnal hypoglycaemia.[587]

A small study found that symptoms such as fatigue, faintness, memory deficits and decreased concentration were alleviated somewhat by consumption of high-kilojoule 'comfort food', indicating that these symptoms may be linked to a deficit in cerebral energy supply (neuroglycopenia).[588] Introducing palatable, high-energy and nutrient-dense foods may be warranted, depending on the individual's glycaemic response and risk factors.

SAMPLE DAILY DIET

BREAKFAST	
Grapefruit juice Mixed berries, mango and kiwi fruit with quinoa porridge and LSA	Grapefruit juice has been shown to increase cortisone acetate (CA) available to the tissues, thus it can be used to prolong the effects of medication for Addison's disease in the body, allowing enhanced effects and possibly a reduction in medication dosage. Berries and other fruits rich in vitamin C such as mango and kiwi should be encouraged. High doses of vitamin C have been shown to accelerate cortisol recovery after response to acute psychological stress thus should be encouraged in the diet. The primary cause of adrenal insufficiency is of autoimmune origin; since individuals with Addison's disease experience a higher comorbidity with coeliac disease, implementation of a GF diet is essential. Quinoa is a gluten-free seed that is rich in both protein and minerals. Teamed with LSA, a source of healthy fats and fibre, this meal provides sustained energy to reduce hypoglycaemia, a common problem in Addison's disease.
LUNCH	
Sushi bento box: miso soup, edamame, brown rice, sushi/sashimi/tamari	Hyponatraemia is commonly seen in Addison's due to lack of cortisol and deficiency of mineralocorticoids. Sodium-rich foods that are of wholefood origin and exert medicinal action such as miso and tamari can be suggested to contribute to sodium levels to assist in restoring balance. Iodine-rich foods such as seaweed are also encouraged to ensure there is healthy thyroid function since autoimmune thyroid disease is a common comorbidity with Addison's disease.
DINNER	
Meat balls in a tomato-based sauce with brown lentils, onion, celery, carrots and baby spinach served on top of mashed potato	Dinner is fibre rich and comprises complex carbohydrates, protein and a small quantity of essential fats. It will assist in maintaining stable blood sugar levels, important since hypoglycaemia will lead to loss of cortisol. An emphasis is placed on foods that provide magnesium and B vitamins. Magnesium has been shown to be able to downregulate HPA activity thereby conserving cortisol levels while B vitamins are involved in metabolism and production of cortisol.
SNACKS	
Liquorice tea Fresh fruit/Brazil nuts with cacao and dried fruits	Liquorice has been shown to increase cortisone acetate (CA) available to the tissues, thus it can be used to prolong the effects of medication in the body, allowing enhanced effects and possibly a reduction in medication dosage. Liquorice provides glycyrrhizic acid and glycyrrhetinic acid, which act on the 11-beta hydroxysteroid dehydrogenase enzyme, extending the half-life of cortisol in the body. Small frequent meals are important to prevent hypoglycaemia and thus conserve cortisol in the body. Glucose-rich foods such as dried fruit may be promoted to reduce neuroglycopenic symptoms. Individuals with Addison's display deficits in cerebral energy supply which lead to neuroglycopenic symptoms such as fatigue, lack of concentration and poor memory. These symptoms can be partially alleviated with ingestion of glucose-rich foods.

NUTRITIONAL MEDICINE (SUPPLEMENTAL)

Specific nutrients required

Coenzyme Q10 has been found to be low in hypoadrenalism,[530] and its supplementation may therefore provide some health benefits.

Vitamin C, produced by most animals in the adrenal glands in response to increased stress (and therefore raised adrenaline (epinephrine) and cortisol levels — see section on stress),[94] may well be needed in this condition. In autoimmune conditions intravenous vitamin C has been shown to enhance the action of cortisol, thus dampening autoimmune and allergic responses.[589]

Neurotransmitter function may be compromised and support for their production warranted. Choice of nutrients include tyrosine, glutamate and aspartate as excitatory neurotransmitter precursors, together with their co-factors (which include vitamin B_6 and zinc). However, with compromised adrenal function adrenaline (epinephrine) may not be able to be produced, even with supplementation. Glucocorticoids act on glucocorticoid receptors which are found throughout the brain, and mineralocorticoids act on mineralocorticoid receptors, found predominantly in the hippocampus. This indicates a potential for decreased cognitive function in patients with Addison's disease. Small studies have found that decreased cognitive function is not very marked in Addison's patients, except in areas of verbal learning, concentration, depressive symptoms and episodic memory.[590,591]

There is a higher incidence of hypothyroidism in Addison's disease[77,592,593] so this should also be tested for. If proven that this is the case, tyrosine, an amino acid common to both adrenaline (epinephrine) and thyroid hormone pathways, may be indicated.

Dosage requirements

As the nutrients in Table 21.41 are suggestions only, recommendations for specific quantity of nutrients prescribed should be ascertained on an individual basis.

TABLE 21.41 Nutritional medicine

Nutrient	Daily dosage	Rationale
Coenzyme Q10	100–200 mg	Found to be low in hypoadrenalism
Vitamin C	1500–3000 mg	To enhance the action of cortisol
Vitamin B complex	High-dose complex b.i.d.	To enhance the action of cortisol, to improve adrenal function. NOTE: high doses of B_5 are not recommended
Tyrosine	500–1000 mg	To enhance thyroid function
Iodine and co-factors	150–300 micrograms/day	To enhance thyroid function

HERBAL MEDICINE

Herbal medicine classes

ADRENAL RESTORATIVES

This is the primary class of prescription and includes *Glycyrrhiza glabra* (liquorice) and *Rehmannia glutinosa* (rehmannia).

Specific herbal medicines

REHMANNIA GLUTINOSA (REHMANNIA)

Rehmannia is advised to be prescribed in large doses for extended periods of time with close monitoring.

GLYCYRRHIZA GLABRA (LIQUORICE)

Liquorice cannot be prescribed long term (especially in high-grade form) due to its effects on mineralocorticoids. It is also important to acknowledge its potential to potentiate the effects of prednisolone and other corticosteroid drugs.[583]

Other relevant classes

- Adaptogen
- Nervine tonic
- Additional classes (if indicated): sedative, hypnotic, antidepressant, anti-inflammatory, blood tonic, cardio-tonic, circulatory stimulant, renal tonic, tonic
- Other treatment considerations: immune modulation and general autoimmune principles (if indicated).

TREATMENT PROTOCOL

See suggested formula in Table 21.42.

TABLE 21.42 Herbal medicine

Herbal medicine	Ratio	Quantity	Rationale
Glycyrrhiza glabra	HG	40 mL	Adaptogen, adrenal restorative, anti-inflammatory, blood sugar regulator, inhibition of enzyme that catabolises cortisol
Rehmannia glutinosa	1:2	90 mL	Adaptogen, adrenal restorative, renal tonic, anti-inflammatory
Astragalus membranaceus	1:2	80 mL	Adaptogen, renal tonic, immune tonic
TOTAL: 210 mL			
DOSE: 5 mL t.d.s.			

LIFESTYLE MODIFICATIONS

To avoid further strain on the adrenals, stimulants such as tea, coffee and alcohol should be avoided. Stress levels need to be carefully monitored and excesses avoided. A low-stress job would be beneficial, as well as learning cognitive stress-management skills.[77]

CUSHING'S SYNDROME

Classification

Cushing's syndrome is caused by increased production of cortisol by the adrenal glands, or by excessive use of cortisol or other steroid hormones.

Epidemiology

Cushing's syndrome is a rare disorder with an annual estimated incidence of 0.2 to 3 per million people, and prevalence of 39–79 per million people in various populations.[594–596] The median age of onset is 41.4 years of age.[595]

ALTERNATIVE NAME

- Hypercortisolism.

Aetiology (Table 21.43)

CRH triggers ACTH which in turn triggers cortisol. High levels of cortisol, via negative feedback, inhibit ACTH secretion.

TABLE 21.43 Aetiology of Cushing's disease

Hormone	Control condition	Target	Effect of secretion
Anterior pituitary			
ACTH	Hypothalamus monitors stress and secretes CRH. A negative feedback system inhibits this process	Adrenal cortex	ACTH causes secretion of glucocorticoids, e.g. cortisol
Adrenal cortex			
Glucocorticoids Cortisol	Homeostasis disrupted, hypothalamus secretes CRH; this along with low levels of blood glucocorticoid stimulate anterior pituitary to secrete ACTH	Muscles, liver, adipose tissue, blood vessels and immune cells	Increases protein breakdown (muscles) and formation of glucose from amino acids and lactate. Increases fat breakdown and use of fatty acids for energy. Depresses inflammatory and immune responses. Overall aim to increase energy availability

ACTH, adrenocortocotropic hormone; CRH, corticotropin-releasing hormone.

Overview

CORTISOL

Production

Normally, the production of cortisol follows a precise chain of events:

1. Hypothalamus sends corticotrophin-releasing hormone (CRH) to the pituitary gland
2. CRH causes the pituitary gland to secrete ACTH, which stimulates the adrenal glands
3. When the adrenals receive the ACTH, they respond by releasing cortisol into the bloodstream.

Functions

Cortisol performs vital tasks in the body including:

- Maintaining blood pressure and cardiovascular function
- Reducing the immune system's inflammatory response
- Balancing the effects of insulin:
  - Cortisol counteracts insulin, contributing to hyperglycaemia by stimulus of hepatic gluconeogenesis and inhibition of the peripheral utilisation of glucose by decreasing the translocation of glucose transporters to the cell membrane, especially GLUT4. However, cortisol increases glycogen synthesis (glycogenesis) in the liver
- Regulating metabolism of protein, carbohydrate and lipids
- Supporting and regulating the body's stress response.

When the amount of cortisol in the blood is adequate, the hypothalamus and pituitary release less CRH and ACTH. This ensures that the amount of cortisol released by the adrenal glands is precisely balanced to meet the body's daily needs. However, if something goes wrong with the adrenals (or with their regulating switches in the pituitary gland or the hypothalamus) the level of cortisol produced may be more or less than what the body needs.

Pathogenesis

The most common cause of Cushing's syndrome is Cushing's disease, caused by excessive production of ACTH by the pituitary gland. ACTH stimulates the adrenal glands to produce cortisol.

TYPES AND ASSOCIATED RISK FACTORS

- Cushing's syndrome — adrenal or pituitary tumours
- Cushing's disease (pituitary Cushing's) — pituitary gland releases too much ACTH
- Cushing's syndrome (exogenous) — long-term therapy with corticosteroids
- Ectopic Cushing's syndrome — tumour somewhere other than the pituitary or adrenal glands
- Being female increases the risk of developing Cushing's syndrome:
  - The female-to-male incidence ratio is approximately 3 : 1[595] and 5 : 1 for Cushing's syndrome due to an adrenal or pituitary tumour
  - The female-to-male incidence ratio in ectopic ACTH production is 1 : 1.[595]

SIGNS AND SYMPTOMS

- Moon face (round, red, and full)
- Buffalo hump (a collection of fat between the shoulders)
- Central obesity with protruding abdomen and thin extremities
- Weight gain (unintentional)
- Weakness
- Backache
- Headache
- Acne or superficial skin infections
- Thin skin with easy bruising
- Thirst
- Increased urination
- Purple striations on the skin of the abdomen, thighs, and breasts
- Mental changes
- Impotence or cessation of menses
- Facial hair growth.

Additional symptoms

- Skin spots, red
- Skin blushing/flushing

- Muscle atrophy
- Fatigue
- Bone pain or tenderness
- High blood pressure.

Investigations

TESTS TO CONFIRM HIGH CORTISOL LEVEL

- Cortisol (urine), although late-night salivary cortisol might be more accurate[597]
- Dexamethasone suppression test:
  - Measures the response of the adrenal glands to ACTH. Dexamethasone is given and levels of cortisol are measured. Cortisol levels should decrease in response to the administration of dexamethasone
- Serial serum cortisol levels (blood).

TESTS TO DETERMINE THE CAUSE

- ACTH (blood)
- Cranial MRI or cranial CT scan may show pituitary tumour
- Abdominal CT may show adrenal mass.

GENERAL

- Glucose test is elevated
- Serum potassium may be low
- White blood cell count may be elevated.

DIFFERENTIAL DIAGNOSIS

See Table 21.44.

TABLE 21.44 Differential diagnosis

Disorder	Aldosterone	Cortisol	Renin
Primary hyperaldosteronism (Conn's syndrome)	High	Normal	Low
Secondary hyperaldosteronism	High	Normal	High
Cushing's syndrome	Low-normal	High	Low
Adrenal insufficiency (Addison's disease)	Low	Low	High

ALLOPATHIC TREATMENT

Treatment depends upon the cause of the disorder. In Cushing's syndrome caused by drug therapy with corticosteroids, the drug dose must be slowly decreased under medical supervision.

In Cushing's disease caused by a pituitary tumour, surgery to remove the tumour is recommended. Radiation is sometimes needed as well. Hydrocortisone (cortisol) replacement therapy is needed after surgery. In some cases, lifelong cortisol replacement therapy becomes necessary.

Cushing's syndrome caused by an adrenal tumour is usually treated by surgical removal of the tumour. If the tumour cannot be removed, certain medications can suppress the secretion of cortisol.

In Cushing's syndrome caused by a tumour secreting ACTH, removal of the tumour is the best way to treat the Cushing's syndrome. Cortisol replacement therapy is needed after surgery until cortisol production resumes. In some cases, lifelong therapy with cortisone drugs becomes necessary.

PROGNOSIS

Tumour removal may lead to full recovery, but there is a chance of recurrence. Survival for people with ectopic tumours depends upon the overall outcome associated with the particular tumour type. Untreated, Cushing's syndrome can lead to death.

Therapeutic considerations

CLINICAL DECISION MAKING AND RATIONALE

- Adrenal gland restoration
- Nervous system repair and restoration
- Regulation of stress response
- Regulation and balance of ACTH release
- Regulation of anterior pituitary function
- Alleviation of associated symptoms.

Therapeutic application

NUTRITIONAL MEDICINE (DIETARY)

High cortisol levels are also encountered in stress. One of the consequences is increased blood glucose due to gluconeogenesis from protein and fat. This gives rise to insulin resistance and metabolic syndrome which in turn favours fat gain. It would be prudent to address the diet accordingly to ensure that it contains low glycaemic load carbohydrates and higher amounts of protein to account for the loss due to gluconeogenesis. In short, the advice given in the section on stress would also be indicated here. Endogenous hypercortisolism is associated with an increased risk of cardiovascular disease through the features of visceral obesity, insulin resistance, impaired glucose tolerance and diabetes, hypertension and hyperlipidaemia.[598] These factors can be addressed as per CVD management protocols.

Patients with Cushing's disease are also at a high risk for metabolic complications, osteoporosis, kidney stones, autoimmune diseases, major depression, dyslipidemia and opportunistic infection susceptibility.[599] In particular, patients often experience severe fatigue, emotional instability, depression and cognitive impairment.[600]

Diabetes mellitus is one of the most frequent complications of Cushing's syndrome, with glucose tolerance defects occurring in as much as 70% of cases.[601] These comorbidities contribute to an impaired quality of life and the associated burden of the disease and practitioners should be aware of the role of dietary advice in decreasing their risk of comorbidities and treating comorbidity symptoms.

Insulin resistance and metabolic syndrome have been linked to an inflammatory condition,[602,603] fuelled by the pro-inflammatory central adiposity.[604] Reduction of unnatural and saturated fats would therefore be advisable, to be replaced with anti-inflammatory omega-3 oils from nuts and cold-water fish. Other natural anti-inflammatory substances include plant enzymes and bioflavonoids. These are high in pineapple (bromelain), papaya (papain), onions (quercetin) and coloured berries (proanthocyanidins). In general, a healthy diet is associated with decreased low-grade inflammation. Protective components of the diet include wholegrains, fibre, vegetables, fruit, fish, PUFAs, vitamin C, vitamin E and carotenoids. These are all components of the Mediterranean diet, which might be recommended for treating low-grade inflammation in Cushing's syndrome.[598]

NUTRITIONAL MEDICINE (SUPPLEMENTAL)

Inflammation causes oxidative damage through the creation of highly reactive species, and antioxidants have proven to be of benefit.[603,605] Due to their interactive nature it is advisable not to use single antioxidants but rather a combination to ensure reciprocal recycling. The above-mentioned enzymes and bioflavonoids are also available as supplements, either singly or in combination.

Other supplements need to be advised on an individual basis, such as magnesium and chromium because of their effect on insulin signalling (see section on diabetes), and curcumin for its effect on inflammation and for cardiovascular support.

A small study showed promising results in the use of retinoic acid supplementation in reducing urinary free cortisol levels in patients with Cushing's disease. The dosage used was 10 mg/day initially, increasing to 80 mg/day for 6–12 months.[606]

SAMPLE DAILY DIET

BREAKFAST	
Stone-ground toast with mashed sardines, avocado, leafy greens and a boiled egg plus chamomile tea	Skipping breakfast is associated with a disrupted HPA axis and elevated cortisol thus it is essential breakfast is consumed reasonably soon after waking. Phosphatidylserine reduces stress reactivity of the HPA axis blunting release of cortisol thus dietary sources are advocated. Eggs are a dietary source of phosphatidylserine and serine is found in protein-rich foods including sardines. The meal is protein rich to assist with glucose control, a common issue in Cushing's disease. Chamomile and other nervine teas may be used to support GABA pathways. GABA reduces secretion of corticoliberin and thus ultimately cortisol.
LUNCH	
GF wrap filled with black beans, onions, garlic, capsicum, leafy greens e.g. spinach, avocado and spicy yoghurt Passion flower tea	Lunch contains ample magnesium-rich foods (dark-green leafy vegetables, black beans and avocado). Magnesium inhibits NMDA (*N*-metil-d-aspartate) receptors, leading to reduction in adrenocorticotrophin secretion by the anterior pituitary and inhibition of cortisol synthesis at the stage of conversion of cholesterol to pregnenolone. Lunch is primarily plant based and thus rich in fibre and nutritive. Long-term high levels of cortisol contribute to the development of insulin resistance, dyslipidaemia and hypertension, thus foods with medicinal value to protect against these comorbidities are required.
DINNER	
Lamb and leafy green pie (made with mince, kale, spinach, chard, parsley, garlic and onion)	High levels of homocysteine are observed in individuals with Cushing's disease and may increase CVD risk, thus foods rich in folate (such as leafy greens) and vitamin B_{12} (red meat) are needed since these are known to reduce homocysteine and will decrease CVD risk. Adequate protein is required to prevent loss of muscle which occurs due to elevated cortisol. Leafy greens are beneficial as a calcium source to reduce bone loss associated with high cortisol levels. They also provide potassium to assist with reducing hypertension.
SNACKS	
Fresh fruit with nuts and seeds Salmon sushi roll with edamame 2 × rice cakes with avocado, tomato and goats cheese	Skipping meals disrupts normal HPA functioning resulting in cortisol and insulin spikes, thus snacks comprising wholefood carbohydrates teamed with proteins and/or healthy fats are essential to maintain glycaemic control and maintain a balanced HPA axis.

TABLE 21.45 Nutritional requirements			
Prescription	**Inclusions**	**Daily dosage**	**Rationale**
B vitamin complex	All B vitamins ensuring adequate doses of vitamin B_5 are met	Vitamin B complex — high-dose combination, preferably activated forms Thiamin 20–40 mg Riboflavin 20–40 mg Niacinamide 50–100 mg Pantothenic acid 150–300 mg Pyridoxine 20–60 mg Folinic acid or L5MTHF 500 –1000 micrograms Hydroxocobalamin or methylcobalamin 500–1000 micrograms Choline 50–100 mg Inositol 50–100 mg Biotin 250–500 micrograms	As indicated within the context of stress, vitamin B_5 has been shown to enhance adrenal cortical function in laboratory animals and reduces the elevation of urinary cortisol metabolites that were expected to be produced as a byproduct of adrenal stimulation using ACTH, thus implying that B_5 can also potentially lower secretion of cortisol in periods of stress
Antioxidant combination	Vitamin A Vitamin C Vitamin E Zinc Selenium Phytochemicals including lycopene, resveratrol and procyanidins	5000–10 000 IU 500–1500 mg 200–800 IU 20–40 mg 100–250 micrograms As available	Inflammation causes oxidative stress
Anti-inflammatory phytochemicals	Bioflavonoids Quercetin	50–200 mg 50–200 mg	To dampen inflammation caused by insulin resistance
Chromium		200–300 micrograms	To support insulin signalling
Magnesium		300–600 mg	To support insulin signalling

Dosage requirements

See Table 21.45.

HERBAL MEDICINE

Herbal medicine classes

- Adaptogen
- Adrenal restorative
- Nervine tonic
- Blood sugar regulator
- Antioxidant
- Anti-inflammatory
- Additional classes (if indicated): sedative, hypnotic, antidepressant, antioedematous, diuretic, circulatory stimulant, renal tonic, tonic.

Specific herbal medicines

Because of its restorative effects on the adrenal gland, *Rehmannia glutinosa* is especially indicated in this prescription. *Glycyrrhiza glabra* is contraindicated due to its potential to increase cortisol production.

Treatment protocol

See Table 21.46.

LIFESTYLE MODIFICATIONS

As with other adrenal disorders, stimulants such as tea, coffee and alcohol should be avoided. Stress levels need to be carefully monitored and excesses avoided. A low-stress job would be beneficial, as well as learning cognitive stress-management skills.[77]

TABLE 21.46 Herbal medicine			
Herbal medicine	**Ratio**	**Quantity**	**Rationale**
Curcuma longa	1:1	80 mL	Antioxidant, anti-inflammatory, hepatoprotective
Rehmannia glutinosa	1:2	80 mL	Adaptogen, adrenal restorative, renal tonic, anti-inflammatory
Codonopsis pillosula	1:2	60 mL	Adaptogen, anti-inflammatory, blood sugar regulating, blood tonic
TOTAL: 220 mL			
DOSE: 5 mL t.d.s.			

ACKNOWLEDGEMENT

This chapter was originally written by Dr Tini Gruner and Leah Hechtman. Dr Gruner spent her working life being tenaciously passionate about progressing naturopathic medicine. To this end, she knew the biggest impact could be made through focusing her efforts on improving the knowledge and skills, especially critical thinking and self-belief, of the next generation of practitioners. She was fearless in her passion and conviction regarding the power of nutrition and herbs. Like any good teacher, she inspired this in her students and others she taught or crossed paths with.

REFERENCES

[1] Talley NJ, O'Connor S. Clinical examination. 6th ed. Elsevier Australia; 2009.
[2] Everett John W. Pituitary and hypothalamus: perspectives and overview. In: Neil JD, editor. Knobil and Neill's physiology of reproduction. 3rd ed. St Louis: Elsevier; 2006. p. 1289–307.
[3] Tortora G, Grabowski SR. Principles of anatomy and physiology. 9th ed. New York: John Wiley and Sons; 2003.
[4] Werner SC, Ingbar SH, Braverman LE, et al. Werner & Ingbar's the thyroid: a fundamental and clinical text. 9th ed. Lippincott Williams & Wilkins; 2005.
[5] Nabipour I. Clinical endocrinology in the Islamic civilization in Iran. Int J Endocrinol Metab 2003;1:43–5. [44–5].
[6] Cawadias AP. The history of endocrinology: (Section of the history of medicine). Proc R Soc Med 1941;34(6):303–8.
[7] Medvei VC. The history of clinical endocrinology. Carnforth, Lancs: The Parthenon Publishing Group Ltd; 1993.
[8] Conn PM, Freeman ME. Neuroendocrinology in physiology and medicine. New Jersey: Human Press; 1999.
[9] Kochakian CD. Anabolic steroid abuse: history of anabolic-androgenic steroids. Rockville: US Department of Health and Human Services; 1996.
[10] Ellingwood F. The Eclectic practice of medicine with especial reference to the treatment of disease. Chicago: Ellingwood's Therapeutist Publishing Co; 1910.
[11] Pandit MK, Burke J, Gustafson AB, et al. Drug-induced disorders of glucose tolerance.[comment]. Ann Intern Med 1993;118(7): 529–39.
[12] Levine S. Stress: a historical perspective. In: Steckler T, Kalin NH, Reul JM, editors. Handbook of stress and the brain. Part 1: The neurobiology of stress, vol 15, part 1. Amsterdam: Elsevier Science Publication; 2005. p. 15.
[13] Brekhman II, Kirillov OI. Effect of *Eleutherococcus* on alarm-phase of stress. Life Sci 1969;8(3 Pt 2):113–21.
[14] Bellamy D, Pfister A. World medicine: plants, patients and people. Oxford: Blackwell; 1992.
[15] Pardede LV, Hardjowasito W, Gross R, et al. Urinary iodine excretion is the most appropriate outcome indicator for iodine deficiency at field conditions at district level. J Nut 1998;128(7):1122–6.
[16] Roberts CGP, Ladenson PW. Hypothyroidism. Lancet 2004;363(9411):793–831.
[17] Hueston WJ. Treatment of hypothyroidism. Am Fam Physician 2001;64(10):1717–24.
[18] Woeber KA. Update on the management of hyperthyroidism and hypothyroidism. Arch Fam Med 2000;9(8):743.
[19] Australian Bureau of Statistics (ABS). Prevalence of serious conditions. ABS; 1995.
[20] Simmons-Holcomb S. Detecting thyroid disease, part 1. Nursing 2003;33(8).
[21] Adlin V. Subclinical hypothyroidism: deciding when to treat. Am Fam Physician 1998;57(4):776–81.
[22] Hollowell JG, Staehling NW, Flanders WD, et al. Serum TSH, T4 and thyroid antibodies in the United States population (1988–1994): National Health and Nutrition Survey (NHANES III). J Clin Endocrinol Metab 2002;87(2):486–8.
[23] Vanderpump MP, Tunbridge WM, French JM, et al. The incidence of thyroid disorders in the community: a twenty-year follow-up of the Whickham Survey. Clin Endocrinol 1995;43: 55–68.
[24] NHS Choices [Internet]. United Kingdom: National Health Service (England). Underactive thyroid (hypothyroidism). 2015. Available from: http://www.nhs.uk/conditions/Thyroid-under-active/Pages/Introduction.aspx.
[25] McLeod DS, Cooper DS. The incidence and prevalence of thyroid autoimmunity. Endocrine 2012;42(2):252–65.
[26] Murray M, Pizzorno J. Textbook of natural medicine. 3rd ed. St Louis: Elsevier; 2004.
[27] McGrogan A, Seaman HE, Wright JW, et al. The incidence of autoimmune thyroid disease: a systematic review of the literature. Clin Endocrinol 2008;69:687–96.
[28] Pearce EN. Is fluoridated drinking water associated with increased hypothyroidism risk? Clin Thyroidol 2015;27(4):100–1.
[29] Benson RC, Dailey ME. The menstrual pattern in hyperthyroidism and subsequent posttherapy hypothyroidism. Surg Gynecol Obstet 1955;100:19–26.
[30] Hollowell JG, Staehling NW, Flanders WD, et al. T(4), and thyroid antibodies in the United States population (1988 to 1994): National Health and Nutrition Examination Survey (NHANES III). J Clin Endocrinol Metab 2002;87:489–99.
[31] Staub J-J, Althaus BU, Engler H, et al. Spectrum of subclinical and overt hypothyroidism: effect on thyrotropin, prolactin, and thyroid reserve, and metabolic impact on peripheral target tissues. Am J Med 1992;92:631–42.
[32] Longcope C, Abend S, Braverman LE, et al. Androstenedione and estrone dynamics in hypothyroid women. J Clin Endocrinol Metab 1990;70:903–7.
[33] Scanlon MF, Chan V, Heath M, et al. Dopaminergic control of thyrotropin, alpha-subunit, thyrotropin beta-subunit, and prolactin in euthyroidism and hypothyroidism: dissociated responses to dopamine receptor blockade with metoclopramide in hypothyroid subjects. J Clin Endocrinol Metab 1981;53:360–5.
[34] Wakim AN, Polizotto SL, Buffo MJ, et al. Thyroid hormones in human follicular fluid and thyroid hormone receptors in human granulosa cells. Fertil Steril 1993;59:1187–90.
[35] Mancini A, Silvestrini A, Di Segni C, et al. Hypothyroidism, oxidative stress and reproduction. INTECH Open Access Publisher; 2012.
[36] Haggerty JJ Jr, Stern RA, Mason GA, et al. Subclinical hypothyroidism: a modifiable risk factor for depression. Am J Psychiatry 1993;150:508–10.
[37] Joffe RT, Levitt AJ. Major depression and subclinical (grade 2) hypothyroidism. Psychoneuroendocrinology 1992;17:215–21.
[38] Harris B, Othman S, Davies JA, et al. Association between postpartum thyroid dysfunction and thyroid antibodies and depression. BMJ 1992;305:152–6.
[39] Oomen HAPC, Schipperijn AMJ, Drexhage HA. The prevalence of affective disorder and in particular of a rapid cycling of bipolar disorder in patients with abnormal thyroid function tests. Clin Endocrinol 1996;45:215–23.
[40] Misiunas A, Niepomniszcze H, Ravera B, et al. Peripheral neuropathy in subclinical hypothyroidism. Thyroid 1995;5:283–6.
[41] Kung AWC, Pang RWC, Janus ED. Elevated serum lipoprotein(a) in subclinical hypothyroidism. Clin Endocrinol 1995;43:445–9.
[42] Tanis BC, Westendorp RGJ, Smelt AHM. Effect of thyroid substitution on hypercholesterolaemia in patients with subclinical hypothyroidism: a re-analysis of intervention studies. Clin Endocrinol 1996;44:643–9.
[43] Surks MI, Ocampo E. Subclinical thyroid disease. Am J Med 1996;100:217–23.
[44] Cooper DS, Halpern R, Wood LC, et al. l-Thyroxine therapy in subclinical hypothyroidism. A double-blind, placebo-controlled trial. Ann Int Med 1984;101:18–24.
[45] Tran HA. Iodine, thyroid diseases and neuromuscular dysfunction. In: Preedy V, Burrow G, Watson R, editors. Comprehensive handbook of iodine. Burlington: Elsevier; 2009. p. 701–11.
[46] Gibson HB. Surveillance of iodine deficiency disorders in Tasmania 1949–1984. 2nd ed. Launceston: Myola House of Publishing; 2006.
[47] Mortimer RH. Thyroid disease and pregnancy. Aust N Z J Med 1998;28:647–53.
[48] Gunto JE, Hams G, Fiegert M, et al. Iodine deficiency in ambulatory participants at a Sydney teaching hospital: is Australia truly iodine replete? MJA 1999;171:467–70.
[49] Li M, Eastman CJ, Waite KV, et al. Are Australian children iodine deficient? Results of the Australian National Iodine Nutrition Study. Med J Aust 2006;184:165–9.
[50] Australian Health Survey: Biomedical results for nutrients, 2011–12. Feature article: Iodine. Canberra: ABS; c2013. Available from: http://www.abs.gov.au/ausstats/abs@.nsf/Lookup/4364.0.55.006Chapter1202011-12.
[51] Australian Population Health Development Principal Committee (APHDPC). The prevalence and severity of iodine deficiency in Australia — Report, 2007. Department of Health and Human Services, Tasmania with input from NSW Health, Ministry of Health NZ, Vic Health, Queensland Health and the Department of Health and Ageing.
[52] Boyages S. Iodine deficiency disorders. J Clin Endocrinol Metab 1993;77:587–91.

[53] Clugston GA, Hetzel BS. Iodine. In: Shils ME, Olson JA, Shike M, editors. Modern nutrition in health and disease, vol. 1. 18th ed. Philadelphia: Lea and Febiger; 1994. p. 252–63.
[54] Delange F. The disorders induced by iodine deficiency. Thyroid 1994;4:107–28.
[55] Smyth PPA, Hetherton AMT, Smith DF, et al. Maternal iodine status and thyroid volume during pregnancy: correlation with neonatal iodine intake. J Clin Endocrinol Metab 1997;82:2840–3.
[56] Tasmanian Thyroid Advisory Committee. Study in disease surveillance. 1950–1979. Med J Aust 1981;2:234–8.
[57] Clements FW. Goitre studies. 1. The incidence of endemic goitre in three areas in Australia. Med J Aust 1948;21:637–9.
[58] Hales I. Studies in diseases of the thyroid gland. Unpublished MD thesis. Sydney: University of Sydney; 1971.
[59] Hetzel BS. Iodine deficiency disorders. In: Garrow JS, James WPT, editors. Human nutrition and dietetics. Edinburgh: Churchill Livingstone; 1993. p. 534–55.
[60] The Sydney Children's Hospitals Network. Westmead NSW: NSW Ministry of Health; c2011. Disorders we test for: congenital hypothyroidism (CH); 2011. Available from: https://www.schn.health.nsw.gov.au/health-professionals/statewide-laboratory-services/nsw-newborn-screening-programme/disorders-we-test.
[61] Salim FA, Varma SK. Congenital hypothyroidism and the importance of universal newborn screening. Ind J Pediatr 2014;81(1):53–7.
[62] Lane LC, Cheetham T. Congenital hypothyroidism–what's new? Paediatr Child Health 2015;25(7):302–7.
[63] Pearce RN, Farwell AP, Braverman LE. Thyroiditis. N Engl J Med 2003;348:2646–55.
[64] Topliss DJ, Eastman CJ. Diagnosis and management of hyperthyroidism and hypothyroidism. Med J Aust 2004;180:186–93.
[65] Weetman AP. Postpartum thyroiditis and insulin-dependent diabetes mellitus: an important association. J Clin Endocrinol Metab 1994;79:7–9.
[66] Othman S, Philips DIW, Parkes AB, et al. A long-term follow-up of postpartum thyroiditis. Clin Endocrinol 1990;32:559–64.
[67] Broda O, Barnes MD Research Foundation Inc. http://www.brodabarnes.org.
[68] Whitney EN, Rolfes SR. Understanding nutrition. California: Wadsworth; 2002.
[69] Haixia G, Zhongyan S, Xiaochun T, et al. Influence of iodine on the reference interval of TSH and the optimal interval of TSH: results of a follow-up study in areas with different iodine intakes. Clin Endocrinol 2008;69:136–41.
[70] Pedersen IB, Laurberg P. Antibodies to thyroid peroxidase and thyroglobulin in iodine deficiencies. In: Preedy V, Burrow G, Watson R, editors. Comprehensive handbook of iodine. Burlington: Elsevier; 2009. p. 575–85.
[71] Prummel MF, Strieder T, Wiersinga WM. The environment and autoimmune thyroid diseases. Eur J Endocrinol 2004;150:605–18.
[72] Dunn JT. What's happening to our iodine? [editorial]. J Clin Endocrinol Metab 1998;83:3398–400.
[73] Hollowell JG, Staehling NW, Hannon WH, et al. Iodine nutrition in the United States. Trends and public health implications: iodine excretion data from the National Health and Nutrition Examination Surveys I and III (1971–1974 and 1988–1994). J Clin Endocrinol Metab 1998;83:3401–8.
[74] World Health Organization Nutrition Unit. Indicators for assessing iodine deficiency disorders and their control through salt iodization. Document No. WHO/NUT 94.6. Geneva: WHO; 1994. p. 36.
[75] Thomas R. The Eclectic practice of medicine. Cincinnati: Scudder Brothers: Eclectic Medical Publications; 1907.
[76] Pagana KD, Pagana TJ. Mosby's manual of diagnostic and laboratory tests. 2nd ed. St Louis: Mosby; 2002.
[77] Lord RS, Alexander BJ. Laboratory evaluations for integrative and functional medicine. 2nd ed. Duluth: Georgia: Metametrix Institute; 2008.
[78] Ochi Y, Kajita Y. [Determination of thyroid hormone]. Nippon Rinsho 1999;57(8):1794–9.
[79] Gunton JE, Hams G, Fiegert M, et al. Iodine deficiency in ambulatory participants at a Sydney teaching hospital: is Australia truly iodine replete? [see comment]. Med J Aust 1999;171(9):467–70.
[80] Li M, Ma G, Boyages SC, et al. Re-emergence of iodine deficiency in Australia. Asia Pac J Clin Nutr 2001;10(3):200–3.
[81] Guttikonda K, Burgess JR, Hynes K, et al. Recurrent iodine deficiency in Tasmania, Australia: a salutary lesson in sustainable iodine prophylaxis and its monitoring. J Clin Endocrinol Metab 2002;87(6):2809–15.
[82] Thomson CD. Selenium and iodine intakes and status in New Zealand and Australia. Br J Nutr 2004;91(5):661–72.
[83] Mann JI, Aitken E. The re-emergence of iodine deficiency in New Zealand? N Z Med J 2003;116(1170):U351.
[84] McDonnell CM, Harris M, Zacharin MR. Iodine deficiency and goitre in schoolchildren in Melbourne, 2001. Med J Aust 2003;178(4):159–62.
[85] Shils ME, Shike M, Ross AC, et al. Modern nutrition in health and disease. Philadelphia: Lippincott Williams & Wilkins; 2006.
[86] Higdon J. An evidence-based approach to vitamins and minerals. New York: Thieme; 2003.
[87] Utiger RD. Kashin–Beck disease — expanding the spectrum of iodine-deficiency disorders. New Engl J Med 1998;339(16):1156–8.
[88] Brown KM, Arthur JR. Selenium, selenoproteins and human health: a review. Public Health Nutr 2001;4(2B):593–9.
[89] Chanoine JP. Selenium and thyroid function in infants, children and adolescents. Biofactors 2003;19(3–4):137–43.
[90] Leonard JL. Non-genomic actions of thyroid hormone in brain development. Steroids 2008;73(9–10):1008–12.
[91] Ellingsen DG, Efskind J, Haug E, et al. Effects of low mercury vapour exposure on the thyroid function in chloralkali workers. J Applied Toxicol 2000;20(6):483–9.
[92] Ganapathy S, Volpe SL. Zinc, exercise, and thyroid hormone function. Crit Rev Food Sci Nutr Zinc 1999;39(4):369–90.
[93] Maxwell C, Volpe SL. Effect of zinc supplementation on thyroid hormone function. A case study of two college females. Ann Nutr Metab 2007;51(2):188–94.
[94] Gropper S, Smith J, Groff J. Advanced nutrition and human metabolism. 5th ed. Belmont, CA: Wadsworth/Cengage Learning; 2009.
[95] Pehowich DJ. Thyroid hormone status and membrane n-3 fatty acid content influence mitochondrial proton leak. Biochim Biophys Acta 1999;1411(1):192–200.
[96] van Doormaal JJ, Muskiet FA, Martini IA, et al. Changes in fatty acid profiles of plasma, erythrocytes and polymorphonuclear leucocytes in induced hypothyroidism in man: indirect evidence for altered delta 6 desaturase activity. Clin Chim Acta 1986;156(3):299–313.
[97] Kuiper MW, van der Gaag EJ. Subclinical hypothyroidism in children can normalize after changes in dietary intake. Food Nutr Sci 2012;3(3):411.
[98] Tonstad S, Jaceldo-Siegl K, Messina M, et al. The association between soya consumption and serum thyroid-stimulating hormone concentrations in the Adventist Health Study-2. Public Health Nutr 2016;19(08):1464–70.
[99] Jonklaas J, Bianco AC, Bauer AJ, et al. Guidelines for the treatment of hypothyroidism: prepared by the American Thyroid Association task force on thyroid hormone replacement. Thyroid 2014;24(12):1670–751.
[100] Segermann J, Hotze A, Ulrich H, et al. Effect of alpha-lipoic acid on the peripheral conversion of thyroxine to triiodothyronine and on serum lipid-, protein- and glucose levels. Arzneimittelforschung 1991;41(12):1294–8.
[101] Jabbar A, Yawar A, Waseem S, et al. Vitamin B_{12} deficiency common in primary hypothyroidism. J Pak Med Assoc 2008;58(5):258–61.
[102] Kumari SJ, Bantwal G, Devanath A, et al. Evaluation of serum vitamin B12 levels and its correlation with anti-thyroperoxidase antibody in patients with autoimmune thyroid disorders. Indi J Clin Biochem 2015;30(2):217–20.
[103] Wang YP, Lin HP, Chen HM, et al. Hemoglobin, iron, and vitamin B12 deficiencies and high blood homocysteine levels in patients with anti-thyroid autoantibodies. J Formos Med Assoc 2014;113(3):155–60.
[104] Osieki H. The nutrient bible. 6th ed. Australia: Bioconcepts Publishing; 2004.
[105] An JH, Kim YJ, Kim KJ, et al. L-carnitine supplementation for the management of fatigue in patients with hypothyroidism on

levothyroxine treatment: a randomized, double-blind, placebo-controlled trial. Endocr J 2016;63(10):885–95.
[106] An JH, Kim SG. L-carnitine supplementation in hypothyroidism [Letter to the editor]. Endocr J 2016;63(10):939–40.
[107] Benvenga S, Sindoni A. L-carnitine supplementation for the management of fatigue in patients with hypothyroidism on levothyroxine treatment [Letter to the editor]. Endocr J 2016;63(10):937–8.
[108] Giampietro A, Principi F, De Marinis L, et al. Coenzyme Q10 evaluation in pituitary–adrenal axis disease: preliminary data. Biofactors 2005;25(1–4):197–9.
[109] Coenzyme Q10: An evidence-based systematic review by the Natural Standard Research Collaboration. Alternative and Complementary Therapies 2014;20(5):279–84.
[110] Mancini A, Raimondo S, Di Segni C, et al. Thyroid hormones and antioxidant systems: focus on oxidative stress in cardiovascular and pulmonary diseases. Int J Mol Sci 2013;14(12):23893–909.
[111] Calder PC, Yaqoob P. Understanding omega-3 polyunsaturated fatty acids. Postgrad Med 2009;121(6):148–57.
[112] Zimmermann MB, Boelaert K. Iodine deficiency and thyroid disorders. Lancet Diab Endocrinol 2015;3(4):286–95.
[113] Zimmermann M, Trumbo PR. Iodine. Adv Nutr 2013;4(2):262–4.
[114] Gul Kazi T, Kandhro G, Afridi Hassan I, et al. Interaction of copper with iron, iodine, and thyroid hormone status in goitrous patients. Biolo Trace Elem Res 2010;134(3):265–79.
[115] Sachdeva A, Singh V, Malik I, et al. Association between serum ferritin and thyroid hormone profile in hypothyroidism. Int J Med Sci Public Health 2015;4(6):863–5.
[116] Dahiya K, Verma M, Dhankhar R, et al. Thyroid profile and iron metabolism: mutual relationship in hypothyroidism. Biomed Res 2016;27(4):1212–15.
[117] Banday TH, Bhat SB, Bhat SB, et al. To study prevalence of incipient iron deficiency in primary hypothyroidism. Int J Res Med Sci 2014;2(2):472–5.
[118] Khan MK, Mohiuddin MN. A prospective study on prevalence and characteristics of hematologic effects associated with subclinical hypothyroidism. Int J Res Med Sci 2016;4(9):3934–8.
[119] Jones JE, Desper PC, Shane SR, et al. Magnesium metabolism in hyperthyroidism and hypothyroidism. J Clin Invest 1966;45(6):891–900.
[120] Shrestha S, Bharti A, Rai R, et al. Assessment of serum minerals and electrolytes in thyroid patients. Int J Adv Sci Res 2015;1(6):259–63.
[121] Poncin S, Collin I, Gerard A. Minimal oxidative load: a prerequisite for thyroid cell function. J Endocrinol 2009;201:161–7.
[122] Giuliani C, Noguchi Y, Harii N, et al. The flavonoid quercetin regulates growth and gene expression in rat FRTL-5 thyroid cells. Endocrinology 2008;149(1):84–92.
[123] Giuliani C, Bucci I, Di Santo S, et al. The flavonoid quercetin inhibits thyroid-restricted genes expression and thyroid function. Food Chem Toxicol 2014;66:23–9.
[124] Wu Q, Rayman MP, Lv H, et al. Low population selenium status is associated with increased prevalence of thyroid disease. J Clin Endocrinol Metab 2015;100(11):4037–47.
[125] Köhrle J. Selenium and thyroid. Best Pract Res Clin Endocrinol Metab 2009;23(6):815–27, 6.
[126] Drutel A, Archambeaud F, Caron P. Selenium and the thyroid gland: more good news for clinicians. Clin Endocrinol 2013;78(2):155–64.
[127] Köhrle J. Selenium and the thyroid. Curr Opin Endocrinol Diab Obesity 2015;22(5):392–401.
[128] Wichman J, Winther KH, Bonnema SJ, et al. Selenium supplementation significantly reduces thyroid autoantibody levels in patients with chronic autoimmune thyroiditis: a systematic review and meta-analysis. Thyroid 2016;26(12):1681–92.
[129] Hegedüs L, Bonnema SJ, Winther KH. Selenium in the treatment of thyroid diseases: an element in search of the relevant indications. Eur Thyroid J 2016;5(3):149–51.
[130] van Zuuren EJ, Albusta AY, Fedorowicz Z, et al. Selenium supplementation for Hashimoto's thyroiditis. Cochrane Database Syst Rev 2013;(6):CD010223.
[131] Reid SM, Middleton P, Cossich MC, et al. Interventions for clinical and subclinical hypothyroidism pre-pregnancy and during pregnancy. Cochrane Database Syst Rev 2013;(5):CD007752.
[132] Zimmermann MB. Interactions of vitamin A and iodine deficiencies: effects on the pituitary–thyroid axis. Int J Vitam Nutr Res 2007;77(3):236–40.
[133] Zimmermann MB, Jooste PL, Mabapa NS, et al. Vitamin A supplementation in iodine-deficient African children decreases thyrotropin stimulation of the thyroid and reduces the goiter rate. Am J Clin Nutr 2007;86(4):1040–4.
[134] Farhangi MA, Keshavarz SA, Eshraghian M, et al. The effect of vitamin A supplementation on thyroid function in premenopausal women. J Am Coll Nutr 2012;31(4):268–74.
[135] Jubiz W, Ramirez M. Effect of vitamin C on the absorption of levothyroxine in patients with hypothyroidism and gastritis. J Clin Endocrinol Metab 2014;99(6):E1031–4.
[136] Feng M, Li H, Chen SF, et al. Polymorphisms in the vitamin D receptor gene and risk of autoimmune thyroid diseases: a meta-analysis. Endocrine 2013;43(2):318–26.
[137] Muscogiuri G, Tirabassi G, Bizzaro G, et al. Vitamin D and thyroid disease: to D or not to D? Eur J Clin Nutr 2015;69(3):291–6.
[138] Choi YM, Kim WG, Kim TY, et al. Low levels of serum vitamin D3 are associated with autoimmune thyroid disease in pre-menopausal women. Thyroid 2014;24(4):655–61.
[139] Muscogiuri G, Mari D, Prolo S, et al. 25 hydroxyvitamin D deficiency and its relationship to autoimmune thyroid disease in the elderly. Int J Environ Res Public Health 2016;13(9):850.
[140] Effraimidis G, Badenhoop K, Tijssen JG, et al. Vitamin D deficiency is not associated with early stages of thyroid autoimmunity. Eur J Endocrinol 2012;167(1):43–8.
[141] Mackawy AM, Al-Ayed BM, Al-Rashidi BM. Vitamin D deficiency and its association with thyroid disease. Int J Health Sci 2013;7(3):267.
[142] D'Aurizio F, Villalta D, Metus P, et al. Is vitamin D a player or not in the pathophysiology of autoimmune thyroid diseases? Autoimmun Rev 2015;14(5):363–9.
[143] Wang J, Lv S, Chen G, et al. Meta-analysis of the association between vitamin D and autoimmune thyroid disease. Nutrients 2015;7(4):2485–98.
[144] Erdamar H, Demirci H, Yaman H, et al. The effect of hypothyroidism, hyperthyroidism, and their treatment on parameters of oxidative stress and antioxidant status. Clin Chem Lab Med 2008;46(7):1004–10.
[145] Guo Y, Wan XY, Zhong X, et al. Levothyroxine replacement therapy with vitamin E supplementation prevents the oxidative stress and apoptosis in hippocampus of hypothyroid rats. Neuroendocrinology Letters 2014;35(8):684–90.
[146] Pan T, Zhong M, Zhong X, et al. Levothyroxine replacement therapy with vitamin E supplementation prevents oxidative stress and cognitive deficit in experimental hypothyroidism. Endocrine 2013;43(2):434–9.
[147] Subudhi U, Chainy GB. Curcumin and vitamin E modulate hepatic antioxidant gene expression in PTU-induced hypothyroid rats. Mol Biol Rep 2012;39(11):9849–61.
[148] Gul Kazi T, Afridi Hassan I, Naveed K, et al. Effect of zinc supplementation on the zinc level in serum and urine and their relation to thyroid hormone profile in male and female goitrous patients. Clin Nutr 2009;28:162–8.
[149] Mahmoodianfard S, Vafa M, Golgiri F, et al. Effects of zinc and selenium supplementation on thyroid function in overweight and obese hypothyroid female patients: a randomized double-blind controlled trial. J Am Coll Nutr 2015;34(5):391–9.
[150] Department of Health and Ageing, National Health and Medical Research Council, Ministry of Health. Nutrient reference values for Australia and New Zealand including recommended dietary intakes. 2005. Available from: http://www.nhmrc.gov.au/_files_nhmrc/file/publications/synopses/n35.pdf.
[151] Rheault S, Olmstead S, Ralston J, et al. Iodine and iodide: functions and benefits beyond the thyroid. Townsend Letter for Doctors and Patients 2008;99–101.
[152] Hintze G, Emrich D, Köbberling J. Therapy of endemic goitre: controlled study on the effect of iodine and thyroxine. Horm Metab Res 1985;17(7):362–5.
[153] Zimmermann MB, Köhrle J. The impact of iron and selenium deficiencies on iodine and thyroid metabolism: biochemistry and relevance to public health. Thyroid 2002;12(10):867–78.
[154] Eftekhari MH, Eshraghian MR, Mozaffari-Khosravi H, et al. Effect of iron repletion and correction of iron deficiency on thyroid

function in iron-deficient Iranian adolescent girls. Pak J Biol Sci 2007;10(2):255–60.
[155] Balázs C. [The effect of selenium therapy on autoimmune thyroiditis]. Orv Hetil 2008;149(26):1227–32.
[156] Kar A, Bhanda S, Bharti S. Relative efficacy of three medicinal plant extracts in the alteration of thyroid hormone concentrations in male mice. J Ethnopharmacol 2002;81(2):281–5.
[157] Panda S, Kar A. *Withania somnifera* and *Bauhinia purpurea* in the regulation of circulating thyroid hormone concentrations in female mice. J Ethnopharmacol 1999;67(2):233–9.
[158] Gannon JM, Forrest PE, Chengappa KR. Subtle changes in thyroid indices during a placebo-controlled study of an extract of *Withania somnifera* in persons with bipolar disorder. J Ayurveda Integr Med 2014;5(4):241.
[159] British Herbal Medicine Association Scientific Committee. British herbal pharmacopoeia. West Yorks, UK: British Herbal Medicine Association; 1983.
[160] Ealey PA, Kohn LD, Marshall NJ, et al. Forskolin stimulation of naphthylamidase in guinea pig thyroid sections detected with a cytochemical bioassay. Acta Endocrinol (Copenh) 1985;108(3):367–71.
[161] Onumah BM. Alternative and complementary treatment of thyroid disorders. In: Wartovsky L, Van Nostrand D, editors. Thyroid cancer. A comprehensive guide to clinical management. Springer New York: Springer; 2016. p. 759–65.
[162] Henderson S, Magu B, Rasmussen C, et al. Effects of *Coleus forskohlii* supplementation on body composition and hematological profiles in mildly overweight women. J Int Soc Sports Nutr 2005;2(2):1.
[163] Gunsar F, Yilmaz S, Bor S, et al. Effect of hypo- and hyperthyroidism on gastric myoelectrical activity. Digest Dis Sci 2003;48(4):706–12.
[164] Felter HW, Lloyd J. King's American dispensatory. Ohio Valley Co. in Cincinnati: Eclectic Medical Publications; 1898.
[165] Citová I, Ganzera M, Stuppner H, et al. Determination of gentisin, isogentisin, and amarogentin in *Gentiana lutea* L. by capillary electrophoresis. J Sep Sci 2008;31(1):195–200.
[166] Poppe K, Velkeniers B, Glinoer D. The role of thyroid autoimmunity in fertility and pregnancy. Nat Clin Pract Endocrinol Metab 2008;4(7):394–405.
[167] Brown, Donald J, ND. *Vitex agnus castus*. Clinical monograph. Townsend Letter for Doctors and Patients Oct 1995:139.
[168] He Z, Chen R, Zhou Y, et al. Treatment for premenstrual syndrome with *Vitex agnus castus*: a prospective, randomized, multi-center placebo controlled study in China. Maturitas 2009;63(1):99–103.
[169] Carmichael AR. Can *Vitex agnus castus* be used for the treatment of mastalgia? What is the current evidence? Evid Based Complement Alternat Med 2008;5(3):247–50.
[170] Milewicz A, Gejdel E, Sworen H, et al. [*Vitex agnus castus* extract in the treatment of luteal phase defects due to latent hyperprolactinemia. Results of a randomized placebo-controlled double-blind study]. Arzneimittelforschung 1993;43(7):752–6.
[171] Trickey R. Women, hormones and the menstrual cycle. 2nd ed. Crows Nest, NSW: Allen & Unwin; 1998.
[172] Tajmiri S, Farhangi MA, Dehghan P. *Nigella sativa* treatment and serum concentrations of thyroid hormones, transforming growth factor β (TGF-β) and interleukin 23 (IL-23) in patients with Hashimoto's thyroiditis. Eur J Integr Med 2016;8:576–80.
[173] Salem ML. Immunomodulatory and therapeutic properties of the *Nigella sativa* L. seed. Int Immunopharmacol 2005;5(13):1749–70.
[174] Australian Bureau of Statistics (ABS). National Health Survey summary of results, 2007–2008. Long-term conditions (Reissue). Cat. no. 4340. Camberra: ABS; 2009.
[175] Duncan JT, Creswell JE. Diagnosis and management of hyperthyroidism and hypothyroidism. Med J Aust 2004;180(4):186–93.
[176] Vanderpump MP, Tunbridge WM, French JM, et al. The incidence of thyroid disorders in the community: a twenty-year follow-up of the Whickham survey. Clin Endocrinol (Oxf) 1995;43:55–6.
[177] Thyroid Foundation of Canada Thyrobulletin. Summer 1998; 19(2). http://www.thyroid.org.au/Information/Conditions.html.
[178] McGrogan A, Seaman HE, Wright JW, et al. The incidence of autoimmune thyroid disease: a systematic review of the literature. Clin Endocrinol 2008;69:687–96.
[179] Mitchell AL, Pearce SH. Subclinical hyperthyroidism: first do no harm. Clin Endocrinol 2016;85(1):15–16.
[180] Ellis H. Robert Graves: 1796–1852. Br J Hosp Med (Lond) 2006;67(6):313.
[181] Andersen SL, Olsen J, Wu CS, et al. Smoking reduces the risk of hypothyroidism and increases the risk of hyperthyroidism: evidence from 450 842 mothers giving birth in Denmark. Clin Endocrinol 2014;80(2):307–14.
[182] Wiersinga WM. Smoking and thyroid. Clin Endocrinol 2013;79(2):145–51.
[183] Bufalo NE, Santos RB, Cury AN, et al. Genetic polymorphisms associated with cigarette smoking and the risk of Graves' disease. Clin Endocrinol 2008;68:982–7.
[184] Marinò M, Latrofa F, Menconi F, et al. Role of genetic and non-genetic factors in the etiology of Graves' disease. J Endocrinol Invest 2015;38(3):283–94.
[185] Kisiel B, Bednarczuk T, Kostrzewa G, et al. Polymorphism of the oestrogen receptor beta gene (ESR2) is associated with susceptibility to Graves' disease. Clin Endocrinol 2008;68:429–34.
[186] Panicker V, Wilson SG, Spector TD, et al. Heritability of serum TSH, free T4 and free T3 concentrations: a study of a large UK twin cohort. Clin Endocrinol 2008;68:652–9.
[187] Benvenga S, Guarneri F, Vaccaro M, et al. Homologies between proteins of *Borrelia burgdorferi* and thyroid autoantigens. Thyroid 2004;14:964–6.
[188] Gangi E, Kapatral V, El-Azami El-Idrissi M, et al. Characterization of a recombinant *Yersinia enterocolitica* lipoprotein: implications for its role in autoimmune response against thyrotropin receptor. Autoimmunity 2004;37(6–7):515–20.
[189] Bassi V, Santinelli C, Iengo A, et al. Identification of a correlation between *Helicobacter pylori* infection and Graves' disease. Helicobacter 2010;15(6):558–62.
[190] Carlé A, Bülow Pedersen I, Knudsen N, et al. Graves' hyperthyroidism and moderate alcohol consumption: evidence for disease prevention. Clin Endocrinol 2013;79(1):111–19.
[191] Wu EL, Chien IC, Lin CH, et al. Increased risk of hypothyroidism and hyperthyroidism in patients with major depressive disorder: a population-based study. J Psychosom Res 2013;74(3):233–7.
[192] Brandt F, Thvilum M, Almind D, et al. Morbidity before and after the diagnosis of hyperthyroidism: a nationwide register-based study. PLoS ONE 2013;8(6):e66711.
[193] Sundaresh V, Brito JP, Wang Z, et al. Comparative effectiveness of therapies for Graves' hyperthyroidism: a systematic review and network meta-analysis. J Clin Endocrinol Metab 2013;98(9):3671–7.
[194] Collet TH, Gussekloo J, Bauer DC, et al. Subclinical hyperthyroidism and the risk of coronary heart disease and mortality. Arch Intern Med 2012;172(10):799–809.
[195] Gorka J, Taylor-Gjevre RM, Arnason T. Metabolic and clinical consequences of hyperthyroidism on bone density. Int J Endocrinol 2013;3:638727.
[196] Brandt F, Thvilum M, Almind D, et al. Hyperthyroidism and psychiatric morbidity: evidence from a Danish nationwide register study. Eur J Endocrinol 2014;170(2):341–8.
[197] Pearce EN. Women with a history of hyperthyroidism may be at increased risk for breast cancer. Clin Thyroidol 2016;28(4):103–5.
[198] Goldsmith RE, Sturgis SH, Lerman J, et al. The menstrual pattern in thyroid disease. J Clin Endocrinol Metab 1952;12:846–55.
[199] Joshi JV, Bhandarkar SD, Chadha M, et al. Menstrual irregularities and lactation failure may precede thyroid dysfunction or goitre. J Postgrad Med 1993;39:137–41.
[200] Krassas GE, Pontikides N, Kaltsas T, et al. Menstrual disturbances in thyrotoxicosis. Clin Endocrinol 1994;40:641–4.
[201] Poppe K, Velkeniers B. Female infertility and the thyroid. Best Pract and Res Clin Endocrinol Metab 2004;18(2):153–65.
[202] Tonstad S, Nathan E, Oda K, et al. Prevalence of hyperthyroidism according to type of vegetarian diet. Public Health Nutr 2015;18(08):1482–7.
[203A] Ma A, Qi S, Chen H. Antioxidant therapy for prevention of inflammation, ischemic reperfusion injuries and allograft rejection. Cardiovasc Hematol Agents Med Chem 2008;6(1):20–43.
[203B] Abboud L, Carrns A. Even a diet of fat-free foods can pose a weighty problem. New York, NY: Wall Street Journal; 2002. Sect. D4.
[204] Mojzis J, Varinska L, Mojzisova G, et al. Antiangiogenic effects of flavonoids and chalcones. Pharmacol Res 2008;57(4):259–65.

[205] Muthian G, Bright JJ. Quercetin, a flavonoid phytoestrogen, ameliorates experimental allergic encephalomyelitis by blocking IL-12 signaling through JAK-STAT pathway in T lymphocyte. J Clin Immunol 2004;24(5):542–52.
[206] Verbeek R, van Tol EA, van Noort JM. Oral flavonoids delay recovery from experimental autoimmune encephalomyelitis in SJL mice. Biochem Pharmacol 2005;70(2):220–8.
[207] Lahesmaa M, Orava J, Schalin-Jäntti C, et al. Hyperthyroidism increases brown fat metabolism in humans. J Clin Endocrinol Metab 2013;99(1):E28–35.
[208] Gropper S, Smith J, Groff J. Advanced nutrition and human metabolism. 5th ed. Australia: Wadsworth/Cengage Learning; 2009.
[209] Abdel-Gayoum AA. Dyslipidemia and serum mineral profiles in patients with thyroid disorders. Saudi Med J 2014;35(12):1469.
[210] Smolle J, Wawschinek O, Hayn H, et al. Vitamin A and carotene in thyroid diseases. Acta Med Austriaca 1983;10(2–3):71–3.
[211] Dirican M, Taş S. Effects of vitamin E and vitamin C supplementation on plasma lipid peroxidation and on oxidation of apolipoprotein B-containing lipoproteins in experimental hyperthyroidism. J Med Invest 1999;46(1–2):29–33.
[212] Subudhi U, Das K, Paital B, et al. Alleviation of enhanced oxidative stress and oxygen consumption of l-thyroxine induced hyperthyroid rat liver mitochondria by vitamin E and curcumin. Chem Biol Interact 2008;173(2):105–14.
[213] Venditti P, Di Stefano L, Di Meo S. Vitamin E management of oxidative damage-linked dysfunctions of hyperthyroid tissues. Cell Mol Life Sci 2013;70(17):3125–44.
[214] Bülow Pedersen I, Knudsen N, Carlé A, et al. Serum selenium is low in newly diagnosed Graves' disease: a population-based study. Clin Endocrinol 2013;79(4):584–90.
[215] Bjoro T, Holmen J, Kruger O, et al. Prevalence of thyroid disease, thyroid dysfunction and thyroid peroxidase antibodies in a large, unselected population. Health Study of Nord-Trondelag (HUNT). Eur J Endocrinol 2000;143:639–47.
[216] Wertenbruch T, Willenberg HS, Sagert C, et al. Serum selenium levels in patients with remission and relapse of Graves' disease. Med Chem 2007;3(3):281–4.
[217] Leo M, Bartalena L, Dottore GR, et al. Effects of selenium on short-term control of hyperthyroidism due to Graves' disease treated with methimazole: results of a randomized clinical trial. J Endocrinol Invest 2016;40(3):281–7.
[218] Marcocci C, Kahaly GJ, Krassas GE, et al. Selenium and the course of mild Graves' orbitopathy. New Engl J Med 2011;364(20):1920–31.
[219] Khong JJ, Goldstein RF, Sanders KM, et al. Serum selenium status in Graves' disease with and without orbitopathy: a case–control study. Clin Endocrinol 2014;80(6):905–10.
[220] Dehina N, Hofmann PJ, Behrends T, et al. Lack of association between selenium status and disease severity and activity in patients with Graves' ophthalmopathy. Eur Thyroid J 2016;5(1):57–64.
[221] Dolev E, Deuster PA, Solomon B, et al. Alterations in magnesium and zinc metabolism in thyroid disease. Metabolism 1988;37(1):61–7.
[222] Skaaby T, Husemoen LL, Thuesen BH, et al. Prospective population-based study of the association between vitamin D status and incidence of autoimmune disease. Endocrine 2015;50(1):231–8.
[223] Wang J, Lv S, Chen G, et al. Meta-analysis of the association between vitamin D and autoimmune thyroid disease. Nutrients 2015;7(4):2485–98.
[224] Yasuda T, Okamoto Y, Hamada N, et al. Serum vitamin D levels are decreased and associated with thyroid volume in female patients with newly onset Graves' disease. Endocrine 2012;42(3):739–41.
[225] Yasuda T, Okamoto Y, Hamada N, et al. Serum vitamin D levels are decreased in patients without remission of Graves' disease. Endocrine 2013;43:230–2.
[226] Rotondi M, Chiovato L. Vitamin D deficiency in patients with Graves' disease: probably something more than a casual association. Endocrine 2013;43(1):3–5.
[227] Mancini A, Festa R, Raimondo S, et al. Hormonal influence on coenzyme Q10 levels in blood plasma. Int J Mol Sci 2011;12(12):9216–625.
[228] Suzuki H, Naitoh T, Kuniyoshi S, et al. Cardiac performance and coenzyme Q10 in thyroid disorders. Endocrinol Jpn 1984;31(6):755–61.
[229] Longmore JM, Wilkinson I, Turmezei T, et al. Oxford handbook of clinical medicine. 7th ed. New York: Oxford University Press; 2008.
[230] Ford H, Crooke M, Murphy C. Disturbances of calcium and magnesiumm metabolism occur in most hyperthyroid patients. Clin Biochem 1989;22(5):373–6.
[231] Fahrenfort J, Wilterdink A, Van der Veen E. Long-term residual complaints and psychosocial sequelae after remission of hyperthyroidism. Psychoneuroendocrinology 2000;25(2):201–11.
[232] Tang XL, Liu XJ, Sun WM, et al. Oxidative stress in Graves' disease patients and antioxidant protection against lymphocytes DNA damage in vitro. Pharmazie 2005;60(9):696–700.
[233] Ozkaya M, Sahin M, Cakal E, et al. Visfatin plasma concentrations in patients with hyperthyroidism and hypothyroidism before and after control of thyroid function. J Endocrinol Invest 2009;32(5):435–9.
[234] Benvenga S, Ruggeri R, Russo A, et al. Usefulness of L-carnitine, a naturally occurring peripheral antagonist of thyroid hormone action, in iatrogenic hyperthyroidism: a randomized, double-blind, placebo-controlled clinical trial. J Clin Endocrinol Metab 2001;86(8):3579–94.
[235] Guerra LN, Moiguer S, Karner M, et al. Antioxidants in the treatment of Graves' disease. IUBMB Life 2001;51(2):105–9.
[236] Duntas LH, Mantzou E, Koutras DA. Effects of a six month treatment with selenomethionine in patients with autoimmune thyroiditis. Eur J Endocrinol 2003;148:389–93.
[237] Mazopakis EE, Papadakis JA, Papadomanolakimg MG, et al. Effects of 12 months treatment with L-selenomethionine on serum anti-TPO levels in patients with Hashimoto's thyroiditis. Thyroid 2007;17:609–12.
[238] Felter HW. The Eclectic materia medica. Pharmacol Ther 1922.
[239] Oztay F, Ergin B, Ustunova S, et al. Effects of coenzyme Q10 on the heart ultrastructure and nitric oxide synthase during hyperthyroidism. Chin J Physiol 2007;50(5):217–24.
[240] Rigelsky JM, Sweet BV. Hawthorn: pharmacology and therapeutic uses. Am J Health Syst Pharm 2002;59(5):417–22.
[241] Ellingwood F. American materia medica. 2nd ed. Evanston, Ill; 1919.
[242] Blumenthal M, Goldberg A, Gruenwald J, et al. The complete German Commission E monographs: therapeutic guide to herbal medicines. Austin: American Botanical Council; 1998.
[243] Sourgens H, Winterhoff H, Gumbinger HG, et al. Effects of *Lithospermum officinale* and related plants on hypophyseal and thyroid hormones in the rat. Pharm Biol 1986;24(2):53–63.
[244] Felter HW, Lloyd JU. Kings American dispensatory. Eclectic Medical Publications; 1903. reprinted 1983.
[245] Beer AM, Wiebelitz KR, Schmidt-Gayk H. *Lycopus europaeus* (gypsy wort): effects on the thyroidal parameters and symptoms associated with thyroid function. Phytomedicine 2008;15(1–2):16–22.
[246] Bone K. A clinical guide to blending liquid herbs. St Louis: Churchill Livingstone; 2003.
[247] Awad R, Levac D, Cybulska P, et al. Effects of traditionally used anxiolytic botanicals on enzymes of the gamma-aminobutyric acid (GABA) system. Can J Physiol Pharmacol 2007;85(9):933–42.
[248] Bunevicius R, Velickiene D, Prange AJ Jr. Mood and anxiety disorders in women with treated hyperthyroidism and ophthalmopathy caused by Graves' disease. Gen Hosp Psychiatry 2005;27(2):133–9.
[249] Suwalska A, Lacka K, Lojko D, et al. Quality of life, depressive symptoms and anxiety in hyperthyroid patients. Rocz Akad Med Bialymst 2005;50(Suppl. 1):61–3.
[250] Wolfson P, Hoffmann DL. An investigation into the efficacy of *Scutellaria lateriflora* in healthy volunteers. Altern Ther Health Med 2003;9(2):74–8.
[251] Aydemir S, Bayraktaroglu T, Demircan N, et al. Effect of hyperthyroidism and propylthiouracil treatment on liver biochemical tests. Int J Clin Pract 2005;59(11):1304–8.
[252] Lu CL, Lee YC, Tsai SJ, et al. Psychiatric disturbances associated with hyperthyroidism: an analysis report of 30 cases. Zhonghua Yi Xue Za Zhi (Taipei) 1995;56(6):393–8.
[253] Quintanar-Stephano JL, Quintanar-Stephano A, Castillo-Hernandez L. Effect of the exposure to chronic-intermittent cold on the thyrotropin and thyroid hormones in the rat. Cryobiology 1991;28(4):400–3.
[254] Barr ELM, Magliano DJ, Zimmet PZ, et al. AusDiab 2005 Australian diabetes, obesity and lifestyle study 2005. Melbourne: International Diabetes Institute; 2006. Available from: www.baker.edu.au/Assets/Files/AUSDIAB_Report_2005.pdf.

[255] Tanamas SK, Magliano DJ, Lynch B, et al. AusDiab 2012 Australian diabetes, obesity and lifestyle study 2012. Melbourne: Baker IDI Heart and Diabetes Institute; 2013. Available from: www.bakeridi.edu.au/Assets/Files/Baker%20IDI%20Ausdiab%20Report_interactive_FINAL.pdf.

[256] Australian Bureau of Statistics (ABS). Diabetes in Australia: a snapshot 2004–05. Cat. no. 4820.0.55.001. Canberra: ABS; 2006.

[257] Australian Bureau of Statistics (ABS). Australian health survey: first results, 2014–2015. Cat. no. 4364.0.55.001. Canberra: ABS; 2015.

[258] Shaw J, Tanamas SK. Diabetes: the silent pandemic and its impact on Australia. Melbourne: Baker IDI Heart and Diabetes Institute; 2012.

[259] American Diabetes Association. Diagnosis and classification of diabetes mellitus. Diabetes Care 2014;37:S81–90.

[260] Atkinson MA, Eisenbarth GS, Michels AW. Type 1 diabetes. Lancet 2014;383(9911):69–82.

[261] Norris JM, Rich SS. Genetics of glucose homeostasis implications for insulin resistance and metabolic syndrome. Arterioscler Thromb Vasc Biol 2012;32(9):2091–6.

[262] Hawa MI, Kolb H, Schloot N, et al. Adult-onset autoimmune diabetes in Europe is prevalent with a broad clinical phenotype action LADA 7. Diabetes Care 2013;36(4):908–13.

[263] Tuomi T, Santoro N, Caprio S, et al. The many faces of diabetes: a disease with increasing heterogeneity. Lancet 2014;383(9922):1084–94.

[264] Basile KJ, Guy VC, Schwartz S, et al. Overlap of genetic susceptibility to type 1 diabetes, type 2 diabetes, and latent autoimmune diabetes in adults. Curr Diab Rep 2014;14(11):1–7.

[265] Löfvenborg JE, Andersson T, Carlsson PO, et al. Coffee consumption and the risk of latent autoimmune diabetes in adults — results from a Swedish case-control study. Diab Med 2014;31(7):799–805.

[266] Löfvenborg JE, Andersson T, Carlsson PO, et al. Sweetened beverage intake and risk of latent autoimmune diabetes in adults (LADA) and type 2 diabetes. Eur J Endocrinol 2016;175(6):605–14.

[267] Löfvenborg JE, Andersson T, Carlsson PO, et al. Fatty fish consumption and risk of latent autoimmune diabetes in adults. Nutr Diab 2014;4(10):e139.

[268] Rasouli B, Andersson T, Carlsson PO, et al. Alcohol and the risk for latent autoimmune diabetes in adults: results based on Swedish ESTRID study. Eur J Endocrinol 2014;171(5):535–43.

[269] de la Monte SM. Type 3 diabetes is sporadic Alzheimer's disease: mini-review. Eur Neuropsychopharmacol 2014;24(12):1954–60.

[270] Butterfield DA, Di Domenico F, Barone E. Elevated risk of type 2 diabetes for development of Alzheimer disease: a key role for oxidative stress in brain. Biochim Biophys Acta 2014;1842(9):1693–706.

[271] Kandimalla R, Thirumala V, Reddy PH. Is Alzheimer's disease a type 3 diabetes? A critical appraisal. Biochim Biophys Acta 2017;863(5):1078–89.

[272] De Felice FG, Ferreira ST. Inflammation, defective insulin signaling, and mitochondrial dysfunction as common molecular denominators connecting type 2 diabetes to Alzheimer disease. Diabetes 2014;63(7):2262–72.

[273] Lallukka S, Yki-Järvinen H. Non-alcoholic fatty liver disease and risk of type 2 diabetes. Best Pract Res Clin Endocrinol Metab 2016;30(3):385–95.

[274] Kostic AD, Gevers D, Siljander H, et al. The dynamics of the human infant gut microbiome in development and in progression toward type 1 diabetes. Cell Host Microbe 2015;17(2):260–73.

[275] Bekkering P, Jafri I, Van Overveld FJ, et al. The intricate association between gut microbiota and development of type 1, type 2 and type 3 diabetes. Exp Rev Clin Immunol 2013;9(11):1031–41.

[276] Virtanen SM, Nevalainen J, Kronberg-Kippilä C, et al. Food consumption and advanced β cell autoimmunity in young children with HLA-conferred susceptibility to type 1 diabetes: a nested case-control design. Am J Clin Nutr 2012;95(2):471–8.

[277] Peng H, Hagopian W. Environmental factors in the development of type 1 diabetes. Rev Endocr Metab Disord 2006;7:149–62.

[278] Rosenbauer J, Herzig P, Giani G. Early infant feeding and risk of type 1 diabetes mellitus — a nationwide population-based case-control study in pre-school children. Diabetes Metab Res Rev 2007;24:211–22.

[279] Monetini L, Cavallo MG, Manfrini S, et al. IMDIAB Group. Antibodies to bovine beta-casein in diabetes and other autoimmune diseases. Horm Metab Res 2002;34:455–9.

[280] Monetini L, Barone F, Stefanini L, et al. Establishment of T cell lines to bovine beta-casein and beta-casein-derived epitopes in patients with type 1 diabetes. J Endocrinol 2003;176:143–50.

[281] Luopajärvi K, Savilahti E, Virtanen SM, et al. Enhanced levels of cows' milk antibodies in infancy in children who develop type 1 diabetes later in childhood. Pediatr Diabetes 2008;9:434–41.

[282] Åkerblom HK, Virtanen SM, et al. Dietary manipulation of beta cell autoimmunity in infants at increased risk of type 1 diabetes: a pilot study. Diabetologia 2005;48:829–37.

[283] Lamb MM, Miller M, Seifert JA, et al. The effect of childhood cow's milk intake and HLA-DR genotype on risk of islet autoimmunity and type 1 diabetes: the Diabetes Autoimmunity Study in the Young. Pediatr Diabetes 2015;16(1):31–8.

[284] Lempainen J, Vaarala O, Mäkelä M, et al. Interplay between PTPN22 C1858T polymorphism and cow's milk formula exposure in type 1 diabetes. J Autoimmun 2009;33(2):155–64.

[285] Sadeharju K, Knip M, Virtanen SM, et al. Finnish TRIGR Study Group. Maternal antibodies in breast milk protect the child from enterovirus infections. Pediatrics 2007;119:941–6.

[286] Nucci AM, Virtanen SM, Becker DJ. Infant feeding and timing of complementary foods in the development of type 1 diabetes. Curr Diab Rep 2015;15(9):1–6.

[287] Jun HS, Yoon JW. A new look at viruses in type 1 diabetes. Diabetes Metab Res Rev 2003;19:8–31.

[288] Butalia S, Kaplan GG, Khokhar B, et al. Environmental risk factors and type 1 diabetes: past, present, and future. Can J Diabetes 2016;40(6):586–93.

[289] Phillips WR, Pauli R. Simultaneous onset of insulin dependent diabetes mellitus in siblings. Lancet 1981;2:807.

[290] Hindersson M, Elshebani A, Orn A, et al. Simultaneous type 1 diabetes onset in mother and son coincident with an enteroviral infection. J Clin Virol 2005;33:158–67.

[291] Craig ME, Nair S, Stein H, et al. Viruses and type 1 diabetes: a new look at an old story. Pediatr Diabetes 2013;14(3):149–58.

[292] Elshebania A, Olssonb A, Westmanc J, et al. Effects on isolated human pancreatic islet cells after infection with strains of enterovirus isolated at clinical presentation of type 1 diabetes. Virus Res 2007;124(1–2):193–203.

[293] Yeung WC, Rawlinson WD, Craig ME. Enterovirus infection and type 1 diabetes mellitus: systematic review and meta-analysis of observational molecular studies. BMJ 2011;342:d35.

[294] Rewers M, Ludvigsson J. Environmental risk factors for type 1 diabetes. Lancet 2016;387(10035):2340–8.

[295] Richardson SJ, Horwitz MS. Is type 1 diabetes "going viral"? Diabetes 2014;63(7):2203–5.

[296] Baumgartl HJ, Standl E, Schmidt-Gayk H, et al. Changes of vitamin D3 serum concentrations at the onset of immune-mediated type 1 (insulin-dependent) diabetes mellitus. Diabetes Res 1991;16:145–8.

[297] Greer RM, Rogers MA, Bowling FG, et al. Australian children and adolescents with type 1 diabetes have low vitamin D levels. Med J Aust 2007;187:59–60.

[298] Littorin B, Blom P, Schölin A, et al. Lower levels of plasma 25-hydroxyvitamin D among young adults at diagnosis of autoimmune type 1 diabetes compared with control subjects: results from the nationwide Diabetes Incidence Study in Sweden (DISS). Diabetologia 2006;49:2847–52.

[299] Raab J, Giannopoulou EZ, Schneider S, et al. Prevalence of vitamin D deficiency in pre-type 1 diabetes and its association with disease progression. Diabetologia 2014;57(5):902–8.

[300] Greer RM, Portelli SL, Hung BS, et al. Serum vitamin D levels are lower in Australian children and adolescents with type 1 diabetes than in children without diabetes. Pediatr Diabetes 2013;14(1):31–41.

[301] Zipitis CS, Akobeng AK. Vitamin D supplementation in early childhood and risk of type 1 diabetes: a systematic review and meta-analysis. Arch Dis Child 2008;93:512–17.

[302] Brekke HK, Ludvigsson J. Vitamin D supplementation and diabetes-related autoimmunity in the ABIS study. Pediatr Diabetes 2007;8:11–14.

[303] The EURODIAB Substudy 2 Study Group. Vitamin D supplement in early childhood and risk for type 1 (insulin-dependent) diabetes mellitus. Diabetologia 1999;42:51–4.

[304] Hypponen E, Laara E, Reunanen A, et al. Intake of vitamin D and risk of type 1 diabetes: a birth-cohort study. Lancet 2001;358:1500–3.
[305] Sørensen IM, Joner G, Jenum PA, et al. Maternal serum levels of 25-hydroxy-vitamin D during pregnancy and risk of type 1 diabetes in the offspring. Diabetes 2012;61(1):175–8.
[306] Bailey R, Cooper JD, Zeitels L, et al. Association of the vitamin D metabolism gene CYP27B1 with type 1 diabetes. Diabetes 2007;56:2616–21.
[307] Ponsonby AL, Pezic A, Ellis J, et al. Variation in associations between allelic variants of the vitamin D receptor gene and onset of type 1 diabetes mellitus by ambient winter ultraviolet radiation levels: a metaregression analysis. Am J Epidemiol 2008;168(4):358–65.
[308] Takiishi T, Van Belle T, Gysemans C, et al. Effects of vitamin D on antigen-specific and non-antigen-specific immune modulation: relevance for type 1 diabetes. Pediatr Diabetes 2013;14(2):81–9.
[309] Dong JY, Zhang W, Chen JJ, et al. Vitamin D intake and risk of type 1 diabetes: a meta-analysis of observational studies. Nutrients 2013;5(9):3551–62.
[310] Miettinen ME, Smart MC, Kinnunen L, et al. Maternal VDR variants rather than 25-hydroxyvitamin D concentration during early pregnancy are associated with type 1 diabetes in the offspring. Diabetologia 2015;58(10):2278–22783.
[311] Norris JM, Yin X, Lamb MM, et al. Omega-3 polyunsaturated fatty acid intake and islet autoimmunity in children at increased risk for type 1 diabetes. JAMA 2007;298(12):1420–8.
[312] Niinistö S, Takkinen HM, Uusitalo L, et al. Maternal dietary fatty acid intake during pregnancy and the risk of preclinical and clinical type 1 diabetes in the offspring. Br J Nutr 2014;111(05):895–903.
[313] Longnecker MP, Klebanoff MA, Brock JW, et al. Polychlorinated biphenyl serum levels in pregnant subjects with diabetes. Diabetes Care 2001;24:1099–101.
[314] Helgason T, Jonasson MR. Evidence for a food additive as a cause of ketosis-prone diabetes. Lancet 1981;2:716–20.
[315] Helgason T, Ewen SWB, Ross IS, et al. Diabetes produced in mice by smoked/cured mutton. Lancet 1982;2:1017–22.
[316] Wilson GL, Mossman BT, Craighead JE. Use of pancreatic beta cells in culture to identify diabetogenic N-nitroso compounds. In Vitro 1983;19:25–30.
[317] Davidson JA, Blonde L, Jelliger PS, et al ACE/AACE Diabetes Road Map Task Force, ACE/AACE Diabetes Recommendations Implementation Conference; 2006.
[318] Ding D, Chong S, Jalaludin B, et al. Risk factors of incident type 2-diabetes mellitus over a 3-year follow-up: Results from a large Australian sample. Diab Res Clin Pract 2015;108(2):306–15.
[319] Leong A, Rahme E, Dasgupta K. Spousal diabetes as a diabetes risk factor: a systematic review and meta-analysis. BMC Med 2014;12(1):1.
[320] Piccolo RS, Subramanian SV, Pearce N, et al. Relative contributions of socioeconomic, local environmental, psychosocial, lifestyle/behavioral, biophysiological, and ancestral factors to racial/ethnic disparities in type 2 diabetes. Diabetes Care 2016;39(7):1208–17.
[321] InterAct Consortium. Physical activity reduces the risk of incident type 2 diabetes in general and in abdominally lean and obese men and women: the EPIC–InterAct Study. Diabetologia 2012;55(7):1944–52.
[322] Aune D, Norat T, Leitzmann M, et al. Physical activity and the risk of type 2 diabetes: a systematic review and dose-response meta-analysis. Eur J Epidemiol 2015;30(7):529–42.
[323] Imamura F, O'Connor L, Ye Z, et al. Consumption of sugar sweetened beverages, artificially sweetened beverages, and fruit juice and incidence of type 2 diabetes: systematic review, meta-analysis, and estimation of population attributable fraction. BMJ 2015;351:h3576.
[324] Malik VS, Hu FB. Sweeteners and risk of obesity and type 2 diabetes: the role of sugar-sweetened beverages. Curr Diab Rep 2012;12(2):195–203.
[325] Basu S, McKee M, Galea G, et al. Relationship of soft drink consumption to global overweight, obesity, and diabetes: a cross-national analysis of 75 countries. Am J Public Health 2013;103(11):2071–7.
[326] InterAct Consortium. Dietary fibre and incidence of type 2 diabetes in eight European countries: the EPIC-InterAct Study and a meta-analysis of prospective studies. Diabetologia 2015;58(7):1394–408.
[327] Crump C, Sundquist J, Winkleby MA, et al. Stress resilience and subsequent risk of type 2 diabetes in 1.5 million young men. Diabetologia 2016;59(4):728–33.
[328] Kivimäki M, Virtanen M, Kawachi I, et al. Long working hours, socioeconomic status, and the risk of incident type 2 diabetes: a meta-analysis of published and unpublished data from 222 120 individuals. Lancet Diab Endocrinol 2015;3(1):27–34.
[329] Shan Z, Ma H, Xie M, et al. Sleep duration and risk of type 2 diabetes: a meta-analysis of prospective studies. Diabetes Care 2015;38(3):529–37.
[330] Anothaisintawee T, Reutrakul S, Van Cauter E, et al. Sleep disturbances compared to traditional risk factors for diabetes development: systematic review and meta-analysis. Sleep Med Rev 2016;30:11–24.
[331] Tonstad S, Stewart K, Oda K, et al. Vegetarian diets and incidence of diabetes in the Adventist Health Study-2. Nutr Metab Cardiovasc Dis 2013;23(4):292–9.
[332] Yokoyama Y, Barnard ND, Levin SM, et al. Vegetarian diets and glycemic control in diabetes: a systematic review and meta-analysis. Cardiovasc Diag Ther 2014;4(5):373–82.
[333] InterAct Consortium. Association between dietary meat consumption and incident type 2 diabetes: the EPIC-InterAct study. Diabetologia 2013;56(1):47–59.
[334] Pan A, Sun Q, Bernstein AM, et al. Changes in red meat consumption and subsequent risk of type 2 diabetes mellitus: three cohorts of US men and women. JAMA Intern Med 2013;173(14):1328–35.
[335] Bao W, Rong Y, Rong S, et al. Dietary iron intake, body iron stores, and the risk of type 2 diabetes: a systematic review and meta-analysis. BMC Med 2012;10(1):1.
[336] Simcox JA, McClain DA. Iron and diabetes risk. Cell Metab 2013;17(3):329–41.
[337] Zhao Z, Li S, Liu G, et al. Body iron stores and heme-iron intake in relation to risk of type 2 diabetes: a systematic review and meta-analysis. PLoS ONE 2012;7(7):e41641.
[338] Mekary RA, Giovannucci E, Cahill L, et al. Eating patterns and type 2 diabetes risk in older women: breakfast consumption and eating frequency. Am J Clin Nutr 2013;98(2):436–43.
[339] Mekary RA, Giovannucci E, Willett WC, et al. Eating patterns and type 2 diabetes risk in men: breakfast omission, eating frequency, and snacking. Am J Clin Nutr 2012;95(5):1182–9.
[340] Perry RJ, Samuel VT, Petersen KF, et al. The role of hepatic lipids in hepatic insulin resistance and type 2 diabetes. Nature 2014;510(7503):84.
[341] Legler J, Fletcher T, Govarts E, et al. Obesity, diabetes, and associated costs of exposure to endocrine-disrupting chemicals in the European Union. J Clin Endocrinol Metab 2015;100(4):1278–88.
[342] Gore AC. Endocrine-disrupting chemicals. JAMA Intern Med 2016;176(11):1705–6.
[343] Rajagopalan S, Brook RD. Air pollution and type 2 diabetes mechanistic insights. Diabetes 2012;61(12):3037–45.
[344] Esposito K, Petrizzo M, Maiorino MI, et al. Particulate matter pollutants and risk of type 2 diabetes: a time for concern? Endocrine 2016;51(1):32–7.
[345] Eze IC, Imboden M, Kumar A, et al. Air pollution and diabetes association: modification by type 2 diabetes genetic risk score. Environ Int 2016;94:263–71.
[346] Kuo CC, Navas-Acien A. Commentary: environmental chemicals and diabetes: which ones are we missing? Int J Epidemiol 2015;44(1):248.
[347] Douen AG, Jones MN. Phenylarsine oxide and the mechanism of insulin-stimulated sugar transport. Biofactors 1990;2:153–61.
[348] Hoque BA, Mahmood AA, Quadiruzzaman M, et al. Recommendations for water supply in arsenic mitigation: a case study from Bangladesh. Public Health 2000;114:488–94.
[349] Bräuner EV, Nordsborg RB, Andersen ZJ, et al. Long-term exposure to low-level arsenic in drinking water and diabetes incidence: a prospective study of the diet, cancer and health cohort. Environ Health Pers 2014;122(10).
[350] Gribble MO, Howard BV, Umans JG, et al. Arsenic exposure, diabetes prevalence, and diabetes control in the Strong Heart Study. Am J Epidemiol 2012;176(10):865–74.

[351] Kuo CC, Howard BV, Umans JG, et al. Arsenic exposure, arsenic metabolism, and incident diabetes in the strong heart study. Diabetes Care 2015;38(4):620–7.

[352] Kuo CC, Moon K, Thayer KA, et al. Environmental chemicals and type 2 diabetes: an updated systematic review of the epidemiologic evidence. Curr Diab Rep 2013;13(6):831–49.

[353] Bell DS. Riceabetes: is the association of type 2 diabetes with rice intake due to a high carbohydrate intake or due to exposure to excess inorganic arsenic? Postgrad Med 2015;127(8):781–2.

[354] Enan E, Lasley B, Stewart D, et al. 2,3,7,8-tetrachlor odibenzo-p-dioxin (TCDD) modulates function of human luteinizing granulosa cells via cAMP signaling and early reduction of glucose transporting activity. Reprod Toxicol 1996;10:191–8.

[355] Cranmer M, Louie S, Kennedy RH, et al. Exposure to 2,3,7,8-tetrac hlorodibenzo-p-dioxin (TCDD) is associated with hyperinsulinemia and insulin resistance. Toxicol Sci 2000;56:431–6.

[356] Starling AP, Hoppin JA. Environmental chemical risk factors for Type 2 diabetes: an update. Diab Manage 2015;5(4):285–99.

[357] Tuomisto J, Airaksinen R, Kiviranta H, et al. A pharmacokinetic analysis and dietary information are necessary to confirm or reject the hypothesis on persistent organic pollutants causing type 2 diabetes. Toxicol Letters 2016;261:41–8.

[358] Henley P, Hill J, Moretti ME, et al. Relationships between exposure to polyhalogenated aromatic hydrocarbons and organochlorine pesticides and the risk for developing type 2 diabetes: a systematic review and a meta-analysis of exposures to 2, 3, 7, 8-tetrachlorodibenzo-p-dioxin (TCDD). Toxicol Environ Chem 2012;94(5):814–45.

[359] Neel JV. Diabetes mellitus: A "thrifty" genotype rendered detrimental by "progress"? Am J Hum Genet 1962;14(4): 353–62.

[360] Tuomilehto J, Lindström J, Eriksson JG, et al. Prevention of type 2 diabetes mellitus by changes in lifestyle among subjects with impaired glucose tolerance. N Engl J Med 2001;344:1343–50.

[361] Aguiar EJ, Morgan PJ, Collins CE, et al. Efficacy of the type 2 diabetes Prevention Using Lifestyle Education Program RCT. Am J Prev Med 2016;50(3):353–64.

[362] Albright AL, Gregg EW. Preventing type 2 diabetes in communities across the US: the National Diabetes Prevention Program. Am J Prev Med 2013;44(4):S346–51.

[363] Roberts K, Dunn K, Jean SK, et al. Syndrome X: medical nutrition therapy. Nutr Rev 2000;58(5):154–60.

[364] Kelly GS. Insulin resistance: lifestyle and nutritional interventions. Altern Med Rev 2000;5(2):109–32.

[365] León-Latre M, Moreno-Franco B, Andrés-Esteban EM, et al. Sedentary lifestyle and its relation to cardiovascular risk factors, insulin resistance and inflammatory profile. Revista Española de Cardiología (English edition) 2014;67(6):449–55.

[366] Mota M, Pănuş C, Mota E, et al. The metabolic syndrome — a multifaceted disease. Rom J Intern Med 2004;42(2):247–55.

[367] Brehm BJ, D'Alessio DA. Weight loss and metabolic benefits with diets of varying fat and carbohydrate content: separating the wheat from the chaff. Nat Clin Pract Endocrinol Metab 2008;4(3):140–6.

[368] Pelkman CL, Fishell VK, Maddox DH, et al. Effects of moderate-fat (from monounsaturated fat) and low-fat weight-loss diets on the serum lipid profile in overweight and obese men and women. Am J Clin Nutr 2004;79(2):204–12.

[369] Carroll J. Attack on the food pyramid. New York, NY: Wall Street Journal; 2002. Sect. B1.

[370] Abboud L, Carrns A. Even a diet of fat-free foods can pose a weighty problem. New York, NY: Wall Street Journal; 2002. Sect. D4.

[371] Tapsell LC, Gillen LJ, Patch CS, et al. Including walnuts in a low-fat/modified-fat diet improves HDL cholesterol-to-total cholesterol ratios in patients with type 2 diabetes. Diabetes Care 2004;27(12):2777–83.

[372] Pan A, Sun Q, Manson JE, et al. Walnut consumption is associated with lower risk of type 2 diabetes in women. J Nutr 2013;143(4):512–18.

[373] Neff LM. Evidence-based dietary recommendations for patients with type 2 diabetes mellitus. Nutr Clin Care 2003;6(2):51–61.

[374] Weiss N. Mechanisms of increased vascular oxidant stress in hyperhomocysteinemia and its impact on endothelial function. Curr Drug Metab 2005;6(1):27–36.

[375] Tyagi SC, Hayden MR. Role of nitric oxide in matrix remodeling in diabetes and heart failure. Heart Fail Rev 2003;8(1):23–8.

[376] Hayden MR, Tyagi SC. Homocysteine and reactive oxygen species in metabolic syndrome, type 2 diabetes mellitus, and atheroscleropathy: the pleiotropic effects of folate supplementation. Nutr J 2004;3:4.

[377] Badawy A, State O, El Gawad SSA, et al. Plasma homocysteine and polycystic ovary syndrome: the missed link. Eur J Obstet Gynecol Reprod Biol 2007;131(1):68–72.

[378] Yilmaz N, Pektas M, Tonguc E, et al. The correlation of plasma homocysteine with insulin resistance in polycystic ovary syndrome. J Obstet Gynaecol Res 2008;34(3):384–91.

[379] Gupta MM, Chari S, Chandankhede M, et al. Insulin resistance and homocysteine levels in patients with polycystic ovarian syndrome. J South Asian Fed Obstet Gynaecol 2013;5(2):49–51.

[380] Packer L, Kraemer K, Rimbach G. Molecular aspects of lipoic acid in the prevention of diabetes complications. Nutrition 2001;17(10):888–95.

[381] Ye EQ, Chacko SA, Chou EL, et al. Greater whole-grain intake is associated with lower risk of type 2 diabetes, cardiovascular disease, and weight gain. J Nutr 2012;142(7):1304–13.

[382] Aune D, Norat T, Romundstad P, et al. Whole grain and refined grain consumption and the risk of type 2 diabetes: a systematic review and dose-response meta-analysis of cohort studies. Eur J Epidemiol 2013;28(11):845–58.

[383] Ley SH, Hamdy O, Mohan V, et al. Prevention and management of type 2 diabetes: dietary components and nutritional strategies. Lancet 2014;383(9933):1999–2007.

[384] Ajala O, English P, Pinkney J. Systematic review and meta-analysis of different dietary approaches to the management of type 2 diabetes. Am J Clin Nutr 2013;97(3):505–16.

[385] Esposito K, Maiorino MI, Bellastella G, et al. Mediterranean diet for type 2 diabetes: cardiometabolic benefits. Endocrine 2017;56(1):27–32.

[386] Feinman RD, Pogozelski WK, Astrup A, et al. Dietary carbohydrate restriction as the first approach in diabetes management: critical review and evidence base. Nutrition 2015;31(1):1–3.

[387] Saslow LR, Kim S, Daubenmier JJ, et al. A randomized pilot trial of a moderate carbohydrate diet compared to a very low carbohydrate diet in overweight or obese individuals with type 2 diabetes mellitus or prediabetes. PLoS ONE 2014;9(4):e91027.

[388] Hussain TA, Mathew TC, Dashti AA, et al. Effect of low-calorie versus low-carbohydrate ketogenic diet in type 2 diabetes. Nutrition 2012;28(10):1016–21.

[389] Schofield G, Henderson G, Thornley S, et al. Very low-carbohydrate diets in the management of diabetes revisited. N Z Med J 2016;129:1432.

[390] Tay J, Luscombe-Marsh ND, Thompson CH, et al. A very low-carbohydrate, low–saturated fat diet for type 2 diabetes management: a randomized trial. Diabetes Care 2014;37(11):2909–18.

[391] Dyson P. Low carbohydrate diets and type 2 diabetes: what is the latest evidence? Diab Ther 2015;6(4):411–24.

[392] Qian F, Korat AA, Malik V, et al. Metabolic effects of monounsaturated fatty acid-enriched diets compared with carbohydrate or polyunsaturated fatty acid-enriched diets in patients with type 2 diabetes: a systematic review and meta-analysis of randomized controlled trials. Diabetes Care 2016;39(8):1448–57.

[393] Sluijs I, Beulens JW, van der Schouw YT, et al. Dietary glycemic index, glycemic load, and digestible carbohydrate intake are not associated with risk of type 2 diabetes in eight European countries. J Nutr 2013;143(1):93–9.

[394] Livesey G, Taylor R, Livesey H, et al. Is there a dose-response relation of dietary glycemic load to risk of type 2 diabetes? Meta-analysis of prospective cohort studies. Am J Clin Nutr 2013;97(3):584–96.

[395] Greenwood DC, Threapleton DE, Evans CE, et al. Glycemic index, glycemic load, carbohydrates, and type 2 diabetes: systematic review and dose-response meta-analysis of prospective studies. Diabetes Care 2013;36(12):4166–471.

[396] Bhupathiraju SN, Tobias DK, Malik VS, et al. Glycemic index, glycemic load, and risk of type 2 diabetes: results from 3 large US cohorts and an updated meta-analysis. Am J Clin Nutr 2014;100(1):218–32.

[397] Bao J, de Jong V, Atkinson F, et al. Food insulin index: physiologic basis for predicting insulin demand evoked by composite meals. Am J Clin Nutr 2009;90:986–92.
[398] Holt SH, Miller JC, Petocz P. An insulin index of foods: the insulin demand generated by 1000-kJ portions of common foods. Am J Clin Nutr 1997;66:1264–7.
[399] Muraki I, Imamura F, Manson JE, et al. Fruit consumption and risk of type 2 diabetes: results from three prospective longitudinal cohort studies. BMJ 2013;347:f5001.
[400] Fuller NR, Caterson ID, Sainsbury A, et al. The effect of a high-egg diet on cardiovascular risk factors in people with type 2 diabetes: the Diabetes and Egg (DIABEGG) study—a 3-mo randomized controlled trial. Am J Clin Nutr 2015;101(4):705–13.
[401] Hu EA, Pan A, Malik V, et al. White rice consumption and risk of type 2 diabetes: meta-analysis and systematic review. BMJ 2012;344:e1454.
[402] Post RE, Mainous AG, King DE, et al. Dietary fiber for the treatment of type 2 diabetes mellitus: a meta-analysis. J Am Board Fam Med 2012;25(1):16–23.
[403] Jenkins DJ, Kendall CW, Augustin LS, et al. Effect of legumes as part of a low glycemic index diet on glycemic control and cardiovascular risk factors in type 2 diabetes mellitus: a randomized controlled trial. Arch Intern Med 2012;172(21):1653–60.
[404] Hosseinpour-Niazi S, Mirmiran P, Hedayati M, et al. Substitution of red meat with legumes in the therapeutic lifestyle change diet based on dietary advice improves cardiometabolic risk factors in overweight type 2 diabetes patients: a cross-over randomized clinical trial. Eur J Clin Nutr 2015;69(5):592–7.
[405] Triggiani V, Resta F, Guastamacchia E, et al. Role of antioxidants, essential fatty acids, carnitine, vitamins, phytochemicals and trace elements in the treatment of diabetes mellitus and its chronic complications. Endocr Metab Immune Disord Drug Targets 2006;6(1):77–93.
[406] Mechanick JI. Metabolic mechanisms of stress hyperglycemia. J Parenter Enteral Nutr 2006;30(2):157–63.
[407] Siddiqui K, Bawazeer N, Scaria Joy S. Variation in macro and trace elements in progression of type 2 diabetes. Sci World J 2014;2014:article ID 46159.
[408] Anderson JW, et al. Diabetes mellitus: medical nutrition therapy. In: Shils ME, Shike M, Ross AC, editors. Modern nutrition in health and disease. Philadelphia: Lippincott Williams & Wilkins; 2006. p. 1043–66.
[409] Dong JY, Xun P, He K, et al. Magnesium intake and risk of type 2 diabetes meta-analysis of prospective cohort studies. Diabetes Care 2011;34(9):2116–22.
[410] Belin RJ, He K. Magnesium physiology and pathogenic mechanisms that contribute to the development of the metabolic syndrome. Magnes Res 2007;20(2):107–29.
[411] Bo S, Pisu E. Role of dietary magnesium in cardiovascular disease prevention, insulin sensitivity and diabetes. Curr Opin Lipidol 2008;19(1):50–6.
[412] Ginter E, Zdichynec B, Holzerová O, et al. Hypocholesterolemic effect of ascorbic acid in maturity-onset diabetes mellitus. Int J Vitam Nutr Res 1978;48(4):368–73.
[413] Chakhtoura M, Azar ST. The role of vitamin D deficiency in the incidence, progression, and complications of type 1 diabetes mellitus. Int J Endocrinol 2013;2013:148673.
[414] Song Y, Wang L, Pittas AG, et al. Blood 25-hydroxy vitamin D levels and incident type 2 diabetes: a meta-analysis of prospective studies. Diabetes Care 2013;36(5):1422–8.
[415] Coyne DW. Vitamin D and the diabetic patient. Medscape Nephrology 2008;Available from:: http://cme.medscape.com/viewarticle/573383.
[416] Boucher BJ. Inadequate vitamin D status: does it contribute to the disorders comprising syndrome 'X'? Br J Nutr 1998;79(4):315–27.
[417] Khan H, Kunutsor S, Franco OH, et al. Vitamin D, type 2 diabetes and other metabolic outcomes: a systematic review and meta-analysis of prospective studies. Proc Nutr Soc 2013;72(01):89–97.
[418] Holick MF. Diabetes and the vitamin D connection. Curr Diab Rep 2008;8(5):393–8.
[419] Clarke SD. Polyunsaturated fatty acid regulation of gene transcription: a mechanism to improve energy balance and insulin resistance. Br J Nutr 2000;83(Suppl. 1):S59–66.
[420] Das UN. Essential fatty acids in health and disease. J Assoc Physicians India 1999;47(9):906–11.
[421] Wallin A, Di Giuseppe D, Orsini N, et al. Fish consumption, dietary long-chain n-3 fatty acids, and risk of type 2 diabetes. Diabetes Care 2012;35(4):918–29.
[422] Van Woudenbergh GJ, van Ballegooijen AJ, Kuijsten A, et al. Eating fish and risk of type 2 diabetes: a population-based, prospective follow-up study. Diabetes Care 2009;32(11):2021–6.
[423] Belury MA, Mahon A, Banni S. The conjugated linoleic acid (CLA) isomer, t10c12-CLA, is inversely associated with changes in body weight and serum leptin in subjects with type 2 diabetes mellitus. J Nutr 2003;133(1):257S–260S.
[424] Choi JS, Song J. Conjugated linoleic acid, obesity, and insulin resistance: waiting for the day of liberation from chronic disease. Nutrition 2005;21(11–12):1170–2.
[425] Dhiman TR, Nam S-H, Ure AL. Factors affecting conjugated linoleic acid content in milk and meat. Crit Rev Food Sci Nutr 2005;45(6):463–82.
[426] Aune D, Norat T, Romundstad P, et al. Dairy products and the risk of type 2 diabetes: a systematic review and dose-response meta-analysis of cohort studies. Am J Clin Nutr 2013;98(4):1066–83.
[427] Chen M, Sun Q, Giovannucci E, et al. Dairy consumption and risk of type 2 diabetes: 3 cohorts of US adults and an updated meta-analysis. BMC Med 2014;12(1):1.
[428] O'Connor LM, Lentjes MA, Luben RN, et al. Dietary dairy product intake and incident type 2 diabetes: a prospective study using dietary data from a 7-day food diary. Diabetologia 2014;57(5):909–17.
[429] Wu JH, Micha R, Imamura F, et al. Omega-3 fatty acids and incident type 2 diabetes: a systematic review and meta-analysis. Br J Nutr 2012;107(S2):S214–27.
[430] Fosslien E. Mitochondrial medicine — molecular pathology of defective oxidative phosphorylation. Ann Clin Lab Sci 2001;31(1):25–67.
[431] Hargreaves IP, Duncan AJ, Heales SJR, et al. The effect of HMG-CoA reductase inhibitors on coenzyme Q10: possible biochemical/clinical implications. Drug Saf 2005;28(8):659–76.
[432] Rundek T, Naini A, Sacco R, et al. Atorvastatin decreases the coenzyme Q10 level in the blood of patients at risk for cardiovascular disease and stroke. Arch Neurol 2004;61(6):889–92.
[433] Suksomboon N, Poolsup N, Juanak N. Effects of coenzyme Q10 supplementation on metabolic profile in diabetes: a systematic review and meta-analysis. J Clin Pharm Ther 2015;40(4):413–18.
[434] Shen Q, Pierce JD. Supplementation of coenzyme Q10 among patients with type 2 diabetes mellitus. Healthcare (Basel) 2015;3(2):296–309.
[435] Moazen M, Mazloom Z, Ahmadi A, et al. Effect of coenzyme Q10 on glycaemic control, oxidative stress and adiponectin in type 2 diabetes. J Pak Med Assoc 2015;65(4):404–8.
[436] Thornalley PJ. The potential role of thiamine (vitamin B_1) in diabetic complications. Curr Diabetes Rev 2005;1(3):287–98.
[437] Rabbani N, Alam SS, Riaz S, et al. High-dose thiamine therapy for patients with type 2 diabetes and microalbuminuria: a randomised, double-blind placebo-controlled pilot study. Diabetologia 2009;52(2):208–12.
[438] Nix WA, Zirwes R, Bangert V, et al. Vitamin B status in patients with type 2 diabetes mellitus with and without incipient nephropathy. Diabetes Res Clin Pract 2015;107(1):157–65.
[439] Kinlaw WB, Levine AS, Morley JE, et al. Abnormal zinc metabolism in type II diabetes mellitus. Am J Med 1983;75(2):273–7.
[440] Al-Maroof RA, Al-Sharbatti SS. Serum zinc levels in diabetic patients and effect of zinc supplementation on glycemic control of type 2 diabetics. Saudi Med J 2006;27(3):344–50.
[441] Jansen J, Karges W, Rink L. Zinc and diabetes clinical links and molecular mechanisms. J Nutr Biochem 2009;20(6):399–417.
[442] Jayawardena R, Ranasinghe P, Galappatthy P, et al. Effects of zinc supplementation on diabetes mellitus: a systematic review and meta-analysis. Diabetol Metab Syndr 2012;4(1):13.
[443] Capdor J, Foster M, Petocz P, et al. Zinc and glycemic control: a meta-analysis of randomised placebo controlled supplementation trials in humans. J Trace Elem Med Biol 2013;27(2):137–42.
[444] Zimmermann MD. Burgerstein's handbook of nutrition. Micronutrients in the prevention and therapy of disease. New York: Thieme; 2001.

[445] Ekmekcioglu C, Prohaska C, Pomazal K, et al. Concentrations of seven trace elements in different hematological matrices in patients with type 2 diabetes as compared with healthy controls. Biol Trace Elem Res 2001;79(3):205–19.
[446] Bahadoran Z, Mirmiran P, Azizi F. Dietary polyphenols as potential nutraceuticals in management of diabetes: a review. J Diab Metab Disord 2013;12(1):1.
[447] Liu YJ, Zhan J, Liu XL, et al. Dietary flavonoids intake and risk of type 2 diabetes: a meta-analysis of prospective cohort studies. Clin Nutr 2014;33(1):59–63.
[448] Zamora-Ros R, Forouhi NG, Sharp SJ, et al. Dietary intakes of individual flavonols and flavonols are inversely associated with incident type 2 diabetes in European populations. J Nutr 2014;144(3):335–43.
[449] Wedick NM, Pan A, Cassidy A, et al. Dietary flavonoid intakes and risk of type 2 diabetes in US men and women. Am J Clin Nutr 2012;95(4):925–33.
[450] Maiese K, Chong ZZ, Hou J, et al. The vitamin nicotinamide: translating nutrition into clinical care. Molecules 2009;14:3446–85.
[451] Olmos PR, Hodgson MI, Maiz A, et al. Nicotinamide protected first-phase insulin response (FPIR) and prevented clinical disease in first-degree relatives of type-1 diabetics. Diabetes Res Clin Pract 2006;71(3):320–33.
[452] Kamal M, Abbasy AJ, Muslemani AA, et al. Effect of nicotinamide on newly diagnosed type 1 diabetic children. Acta Pharmacol Sin 2006;27(6):724–7.
[453] Fernandez I, Tonietti M, del Carmen Camberos M, et al. Acetyl-L-carnitine and nicotinamide for prevention of type 1 diabetes. I — literature review which gave support to the treatment. II — case report, evaluation of five years treatment. Immunome Res 2015;11:094.
[454] Tsuneki H, Ishizuka M, Terasawa M, et al. Effect of green tea on blood glucose levels and serum proteomic patterns in diabetic (db/db) mice and on glucose metabolism in healthy humans. BMC Pharmacol 2004;4(1):18.
[455] Fukino Y, Ikeda A, Maruyama K, et al. Randomized controlled trial for an effect of green tea-extract powder supplementation on glucose abnormalities. Eur J Clin Nutr 2008;62:953–60.
[456] Nagao T, Meguro S, Hase T, et al. A catechin-rich beverage improves obesity and blood glucose control in patients with type 2 diabetes. Obesity (Silver Spring) 2009;17(2):310–17.
[457] Bailey CJ. The anti-hyperglycaemic action of metformin. In: Krans HMJ, editor. Diabetes, metformin, a research and clinical update. London: Royal Society of Medicine; 1985. p. 17–26.
[458] Sterne J. Pharmacology and mode of action of the hypoglycaemic guanidine derivatives. In: Campbell GD, editor. Oral hypoglycemic agents. New York: New York Academic Press; 1969. p. 193–245.
[459] Leach MJ. *Gymnema sylvestre* for diabetes mellitus: a systematic review. J Altern Complement Med 2007;13(9):977–83.
[460] Nahas R, Moher M. Complementary and alternative medicine for the treatment of type 2 diabetes. Can Fam Physician 2009;556:591–6.
[461] Porchezhian E, Dobriyal RM. An overview on the advances of *Gymnema sylvestre*: chemistry, pharmacology and patents. Pharmazie 2003;58:5–12.
[462] Baskaran K, Kizar Ahamath B, Radha Shanmugasundaram K, et al. Antidiabetic effect of a leaf extract from *Gymnema sylvestre* in non-insulin-dependent diabetes mellitus patients. J Ethnopharmacol 1990;30(3):295–305.
[463] Srinivasan K. Plant foods in the management of diabetes mellitus: spices as beneficial antidiabetic food adjuncts. Int J Food Sci Nutr 2005;56(6):399–414.
[464] Sharma RD, Raghuram TC. Hypoglycaemic effect of fenugreek seeds in non-insulin dependent diabetics subjects. Nutr Res 1990;10(7):731–9.
[465] Kassaian N, Azadbakht L, Forghani B, et al. Effect of fenugreek seeds on blood glucose and lipid profiles in type 2 diabetic patients. Int J Vitam Nutr Res 2009;79(1):34–9.
[466] Gong J, Fang K, Dong H, et al. Effect of fenugreek on hyperglycaemia and hyperlipidemia in diabetes and prediabetes: a meta-analysis. J Ethnopharmacol 2016;194:260–8.
[467] Khan A, Safdar M, Ali Khan MM, et al. Cinnamon improves glucose and lipids of people with type 2 diabetes. Diabetes Care 2003;26(12):3215–18.
[468] Vafa MR, Mohammadi F, Shidfar F, et al. Effects of cinnamon consumption on glycemic status, lipid profile and body composition in type 2 diabetes patients. Int J Prev Med 2012;3(8):531–6.
[469] British Herbal Medicine Association's Scientific Committee. British herbal pharmacopoeia. Bournemouth: BHMA; 1983.
[470] *Momordica charantia* (bitter melon). Monograph. Altern Med Rev 2007;12(4):360–3.
[471] Rahman IU, Khan RU, Rahman KU, et al. Lower hypoglycemic but higher antiatherogenic effects of bitter melon than glibenclamide in type 2 diabetic patients. Nutr J 2015;14(1):1.
[472] Ooi CP, Yassin Z, Hamid TA. *Momordica charantia* for type 2 diabetes mellitus. Cochrane Database Syst Rev 2012;(8):CD007845.
[473] Chevallier A. Encylopedia of medicinal plants. St Leonards: Dorling Kindersley; 2001.
[474] Luo JZ, Luo L. American ginseng stimulates insulin production and prevents apoptosis through regulation of uncoupling protein-2 in cultured beta cells. Evid Based Complement Alternat Med 2006;3:365–72.
[475] Luo J, Luo L. Ginseng on hyperglycemia: effects and mechanisms. Evid Based Complement Alternat Med 2009;6(4):423–7.
[476] Gui QF, Xu ZR, Xu KY, et al. The efficacy of ginseng-related therapies in type 2 diabetes mellitus: an updated systematic review and meta-analysis. Medicine (Baltimore) 2016;95(6):e2584.
[477] Lanzotti V. The analysis of onion and garlic. J Chromatog A 2006;1112(1–2):3–22.
[478] Sharma KK, Gupta RK, Gupta S, et al. as cited in Srinivasan K. Plant foods in the management of diabetes mellitus: spices as beneficial antidiabetic food adjuncts. Int J Food Sci Nutr 2005;56(6):399–414.
[479] Hou LQ, Liu YH, Zhang YY. Garlic intake lowers fasting blood glucose: meta-analysis of randomized controlled trials. Asia Pac J Clin Nutr 2015;24(4):575–82.
[480] Chan YJ, Lam FC, Leung PC, et al. Antihyperglycemic and antioxidative effects of a herbal formulation of *Radix astragali, Radix codonopsis* and *Cortex lycii* in a mouse model of type 2 diabetes mellitus. Phytother Res 2009;23:658–65.
[481] Chan JY, Leung PC, Che CT, et al. Protective effects of an herbal formulation of *Radix astragali, Radix codonopsis* and *Cortex lycii* on streptozotocin-induced apoptosis in pancreatic beta-cells: an implication for its treatment of diabetes mellitus. Phytother Res 2008;22(2):190–6.
[482] Ko BS, Jang JS, Hong SM, et al. Changes in components, glycyrrhizin and glycyrrhetinic acid in raw *Glycyrrhiza uralensis* Fisch modify insulin sensitizing and insulinotrophic actions. Biochem Biosci Biotechnol Biochem 2007;71(6):1452–61.
[483] Ahmad F, Khan MM, Rastogi AK, et al. Insulin and glucagon releasing activity of coleonol (forskolin) and its effect on blood glucose level in normal and alloxan diabetic rats. Acta Diabetol Lat 1991;28(1):71–7.
[484] Loftus HL, Astell KJ, Mathai ML, et al. *Coleus forskohlii* extract supplementation in conjunction with a hypocaloric diet reduces the risk factors of metabolic syndrome in overweight and obese subjects: a randomized controlled trial. Nutrients 2015;7(11):9508–22.
[485] Wainstein J, Ganz T, Boaz M, et al. Olive leaf extract as a hypoglycemic agent in both human diabetic subjects and in rats. J Med Food 2012;15(7):605–10.
[486] Karlsen B, Idsoe T, Dirdal I, et al. Effects of a group-based counseling program on diabetes-related stress, coping, psychological well-being and metabolic control in adults with type 1 or type 2 diabetes. Patient Educ Couns 2004;53:299–308.
[487] Kreitler S, Weissler K, Nurymberg K. The cognitive orientation of patients with type 2 diabetes in Israel. Patient Educ Couns 2004;53:257–67.
[488] Kennedy A, Nirantharakumar K, Chimen M, et al. Does exercise improve glycaemic control in type 1 diabetes? A systematic review and meta-analysis. PLoS ONE 2013;8(3):e58861.
[489] Franz MJ, Boucher JL, Rutten-Ramos S, et al. Lifestyle weight-loss intervention outcomes in overweight and obese adults with type 2 diabetes: a systematic review and meta-analysis of randomized clinical trials. J Acad Nutr Diet 2015;115(9):1447–63.
[490] Frier BM. Hypoglycemia. In: Fink G, editor. Encyclopedia of stress. 2nd ed. Elsevier; 2007. p. 408–13.
[491] Berkowitz SA, Karter AJ, Lyles CR, et al. Low socioeconomic status is associated with increased risk for hypoglycemia in diabetes

patients: the Diabetes Study of Northern California (DISTANCE). J Health Care Poor Underserved 2014;25(2):478–90.
[492] Bonds DE, Miller ME, Dudl J, et al. Severe hypoglycemia symptoms, antecedent behaviors, immediate consequences and association with glycemia medication usage: secondary analysis of the ACCORD clinical trial data. BMC Endocr Disord 2012;12(1):1.
[493] Ha WC, Oh SJ, Kim JH, et al. Severe hypoglycemia is a serious complication and becoming an economic burden in diabetes. Diabetes Metabol J 2012;36(4):280–4.
[494] Ahrén B. Avoiding hypoglycemia: a key to success for glucose-lowering therapy in type 2 diabetes. Vasc Health Risk Manage 2013;9:155–63.
[495] Moghissi E, Ismail-Beigi F, Devine R. Hypoglycemia: minimizing its impact in type 2 diabetes. Endocr Pract 2013;19(3):526–35.
[496] Frier BM. Hypoglycaemia in diabetes mellitus: epidemiology and clinical implications. Nat Rev Endocrinol 2014;10(12):711–22.
[497] Yousefzade G, Nakhaee A. Insulin-induced hypoglycemia and stress oxidative state in healthy people. Acta Diabetol 2012;49(1):81–5.
[498] Seaquist ER, Anderson J, Childs B, et al. Hypoglycemia and diabetes: a report of a workgroup of the American Diabetes Association and the Endocrine Society. Diabetes Care 2013;36(5):1384–95.
[499] McGill DE, Levitsky LL. Management of hypoglycemia in children and adolescents with type 1 diabetes mellitus. Curr Diab Rep 2016;16(9):88.
[500] Miller DB, O'Callaghan JP. Neuroendocrine aspects of the response to stress. Metab Clin Exper 2002;51(6 Suppl. 1):5–10.
[501] McEwen BS. Mood disorders and allostatic load. Biol Psychiatry 2003;54(3):200–7.
[502] McEwen BS. The brain on stress toward an integrative approach to brain, body, and behavior. Perspect Psychol Sci 2013;8(6):673–5.
[503] Shiels PG, Stenvinkel P, Kooman JP, et al. Circulating markers of ageing and allostatic load: a slow train coming. Pract Lab Med 2016;7:49–54.
[504] Tomiyama AJ, O'Donovan A, Lin J, et al. Does cellular aging relate to patterns of allostasis? An examination of basal and stress reactive HPA axis activity and telomere length. Physiol Behav 2012;106(1):40–5.
[505] McEwen BS. Interacting mediators of allostasis and allostatic load: towards an understanding of resilience in ageing. Metab Clin Exper 2003;52(10 Suppl. 2):10–16.
[506] McEwen BS. Sex, stress and the hippocampus: allostasis, allostatic load and the ageing process. Neurobiol Ageing 2002;23(5):921–39.
[507] Selye H. The stress of life. 2nd ed. New York: McGraw-Hill; 1978. p. 3.
[508] Selye H. Stress without distress. London: Hodder and Stoughton; 1974.
[509] McEwen BS. The end of stress as we know it. Washington DC: Dana Press (Joseph Henry Press); 2002.
[510] Bornstein SR, Rutkowski H. The adrenal hormone metabolism in the immune/inflammatory reaction. Endocr Res 2002;28(4):719–28.
[511] Path G, Scherbaum WA, Bornstein SR. The role of interleukin-6 in the human adrenal gland. Eur J Clin Invest 2000;30(Suppl. 3):91–5.
[512] Haddad JJ, Saade NE, Safieh-Garabedian B. Cytokines and neuro-immune-endocrine interactions: a role for the hypothalamic-pituitary-adrenal revolving axis. J Neuroimmunol 2002;133(1–2):1–19.
[513] Thibodeau G, Patton K. Anatomy and physiology. 5th ed. St Louis: Mosby; 2003.
[514] Abercrombie HC, Giese-Davis J, Sephton S, et al. Flattened cortisol rhythms in metastatic breast cancer patients. Psychoneuroendocrinology 2004;29(8):1082–92.
[515] McEwen B, Lasley EN. Allostatic load: when protection gives way to damage. Adv Mind Body Med 2003;19(1):28–33.
[516] Vanitallie TB. Stress: a risk factor for serious illness. Metab Clin Exper 2002;51(6 Suppl. 1):40–5.
[517] Holmes TH, Rahe RH. The Social Readjustment Rating Scale. J Psychosom Res 1967;11(2):213–18.
[518] Holmes TH, Rahe RH. Life Event Stress Scale. Adapted from Social Readjustment Rating Scale. J Psychosom Res 1967;11:213–18.
[519] Barker J, Meletis C Naturopathic perspectives — the naturopathic approach to adrenal dysfunction. Townsend Letter for Doctors and Patients Feb/Mar 2005.
[520] Morgan WP, Brown DR, Raglin JS, et al. Psychological monitoring of overtraining and staleness. Br J Sports Med 1987;21:408–14.
[521] Szabo S. Hans Selye and the development of the stress concept. Ann NY Acad Sci 1998;851:19–27.
[522] Wilson JL. Clinical perspective on stress, cortisol and adrenal fatigue. Adv Integr Med 2014;1(2):93–6.
[523] Teufel M, Biedermann T, Rapps N, et al. Psychological burden of food allergy. World J Gastroenterol 2007;13(25):3456–65.
[524] McCabe D, Colbeck M. The effectiveness of essential fatty acid, B vitamins, vitamin C, magnesium and zinc supplementation for managing stress in women: a systematic review protocol. JBI Database System Rev Implement Rep 2017;15(2):402–53.
[525] Maloney EM, Gurbaxani BM, Jones JF, et al. Chronic fatigue syndrome and high allostatic load. Pharmacogenomics 2006;7(3):467–73.
[526] Peters EM, Anderson R, Nieman DC, et al. Vitamin C supplementation attenuates the increases in circulating cortisol, adrenaline and anti-inflammatory polypeptides following ultramarathon running. Int J Sports Med 2001;22(7):537–43.
[527] Dhanasekaran M, Ren J. The emerging role of coenzyme Q-10 in ageing, neurodegeneration, cardiovascular disease, cancer and diabetes mellitus. Curr Neurovasc Res 2005;2(5):447–59.
[528] Werbach MR. Nutritional strategies for treating chronic fatigue syndrome.[see comment]. Altern Med Rev 2000;5(2):93–108.
[529] Regland B, Andersson M, Abrahamsson L, et al. Increased concentrations of homocysteine in the cerebrospinal fluid in patients with fibromyalgia and chronic fatigue syndrome. Scand J Rheumatol 1997;26(4):301–7.
[530] Mancini A, Bianchi A, Fusco A, et al. Coenzyme Q10 evaluation in pituitary–adrenal axis disease: preliminary data. Biofactors 2005;25(1–4):197–9.
[531] McKevoy GK, editor. AHFS drug information. Bethesda, MD: American Society of Health-System Pharmacists; 1998.
[532] Kosaka C, Okida M, Kaneyuki T, et al. Action of pantethine on the adrenal cortex of hypophysectomized rats. Horumon to Rinsho 1973;21:517–25.
[533] Onuki M, Suzawa A. Effect of pantethine on the function of the adrenal cortex: clinical experience using pantethine in cases under steroid hormone treatment. Horumon to Rinsho 1970;18:937–40.
[534] Whyte KF, Addis GJ, Whitesmith R, et al. Adrenergic control of plasma magnesium in man. Clin Sci 1987;72(1):135–8.
[535] Golf SW, Bender S, Gratten J. On the significance of magnesium in extreme physical stress. Cardiovasc Drugs Ther 1998;12(Suppl. 2):197–202.
[536] Aschbacher K, O'Donovan A, Wolkowitz OM, et al. Good stress, bad stress and oxidative stress: insights from anticipatory cortisol reactivity. Psychoneuroendocrinology 2013;38(9):1698–708.
[537] Rao AV, Balachandran B. Role of oxidative stress and antioxidants in neurodegenerative diseases. Nutr Neurosci 2002;5(5):291–309.
[538] Freeman MP, Helgason C, Hill RA. Selected integrative medicine treatments for depression: considerations for women. J Am Med Women's Assoc 2004;59(3):216–24.
[539] Coppen A, Bolander-Gouaille C. Treatment of depression: time to consider folic acid and vitamin B_{12}. J Psychopharmacol 2005;19(1):59–65.
[540] Lenz HJ. [Central regulation of gastrointestinal motility and secretion]. Zeitschrift Für Gastroenterologie 1991;29(Suppl. 3):5–9.
[541] Kidd P. Th1/Th2 balance: the hypothesis, its limitations, and implications for health and disease. Altern Med Rev 2003;8(3):223–46.
[542] Blumenthal M, Goldberg A, Gruenwald J, et al. The complete German Commission E monographs: therapeutic guide to herbal medicines. American Botanical Council, Integrative Medicine Communications; 1998.
[543] Felter HW, Lloyd JU. King's American dispensatory. 18th ed. Rev 3. Portland: Eclectic Medical Publications; 1905. [reprinted 1983].
[544] Lee NH, Son CG. Systematic review of randomized controlled trials evaluating the efficacy and safety of ginseng. J Acupunct Meridian Stud 2011;4(2):85–97.
[545] Kim HG, Cho JH, Yoo SR, et al. Antifatigue effects of *Panax ginseng* CA Meyer: a randomised, double-blind, placebo-controlled trial. PLoS ONE 2013;8(4):e61271.
[546] Kim JY, Park JY, Kang HJ, et al. Beneficial effects of Korean red ginseng on lymphocyte DNA damage, antioxidant enzyme activity, and LDL oxidation in healthy participants: a randomized, double-blind, placebo-controlled trial. Nutr J 2012;11(1):1.

[547] Shergis JL, Zhang AL, Zhou W, et al. *Panax ginseng* in randomised controlled trials: a systematic review. Phytother Res 2013;27(7):949–65.
[548] Kim HG, Yoo SR, Park HJ, et al. Antioxidant effects of *Panax ginseng* CA Meyer in healthy subjects: a randomized, placebo-controlled clinical trial. Food Chem Toxicol 2011;49(9):2229–35.
[549] Hiai S, Yokoyama H, Oura H, et al. Stimulation of pituitary-adrenocortical system by ginseng saponin. Endocrinol Jpn 1979;26:661–5.
[550] Davydov M, Krikorian AD. *Eleutherococcus senticosus* (Rupr. and Maxim.) Maxim. (Araliaceae) as an adaptogen: a closer look. J Ethnopharmacol 2000;72(3):345–93.
[551] Panossian A, Wikman G. Evidence-based efficacy of adaptogens in fatigue, and molecular mechanisms related to their stress-protective activity. Curr Clin Pharmacol 2009;4(3):198–219.
[552] Panossian A, Wikman G. Stimulating effect of adaptogens: an overview with particular reference to their efficacy following single dose administration. Phytother Res 2005;19(10):819–38.
[553] Szotomicki S, Samochowiec L, Wójcicki J, et al. The influence of active components of *Eleutherococcus senticosus* on cellular defence and physical fitness in man. Phytother Res 2000;14:30–5.
[554] Schaffler K, Wolf OT, Burkart M. No benefit adding *Eleutherococcus senticosus* to stress management training in stress-related fatigue/weakness, impaired work or concentration, a randomized controlled study. Pharmacopsychiatry 2013;46(05):181–90.
[555] Olsson EM, von Schéele B, Panossian AG. A randomised, double-blind, placebo-controlled, parallel-group study of the standardised extract SHR-5 of the roots of *Rhodiola rosea* in the treatment of subjects with stress-related fatigue. Planta Med 2009;75(2):105–12.
[556] Darbinyan V. *Rhodiola rosea* in stress- induced fatigue. A double blind cross-over study of standardised extract of SHR-5 with a repeated low-dose regimen on the mental performance of healthy physicians during night duty. Phytomedicine 2000;7(5):365–71.
[557] Viana A, Rates S, Naudin B, et al. Effects of acute or 3-day treatments of *Hypericum caprifoliatum* Cham. and Schltdt. (Guttiferae) extract or of two established antidepressants on basal and stress-induced increase in serum and brain corticosterone levels. Psychopharmacol 2008;22(6):681–90.
[558] Schüle C, Baghai T, Ferrera A, et al. Neuroendocrine effects of *Hypericum* extract WS 5570 in 12 healthy male volunteers. Pharmacopsychiatry 2001;34(Suppl. 1):S127–33.
[559] Franklin M, Hafizi S, Reed A, et al. Effect of sub-chronic treatment with Jarsin (extract of St John's wort, *Hypericum perforatum*) at two dose levels on evening salivary melatonin and cortisol concentrations in healthy male volunteers. Pharmacopsychiatry 2006;39(1):13–15.
[560] Felter HW. The Eclectic materia medica. Pharmacol Ther 1922.
[561] Brock C, Whitehouse J, Tewfik I, et al. American skullcap (*Scutellaria lateriflora*): a randomised, double-blind placebo-controlled crossover study of its effects on mood in healthy volunteers. Phytother Res 2014;28(5):692–8.
[562] MacKenzie MA, Hoefnagels WH, Jansen RW, et al. The influence of glycyrrhetinic acid on plasma cortisol and cortisone in healthy young volunteers. J Clin Endocrinol Metab 1990;70(6):1637–43.
[563] Bone KA. A clinical guide to blending liquid herbs. London: Churchill Livingstone; 2003.
[564] Zhang RX, Li XM, Jia PZ. *Rehmannia glutinosa*: review of botany, chemistry and pharmacology. J Ethnopharmacol 2008;117(2):199–214.
[565] McEwen BS, Karatsoreos IN. Sleep deprivation and circadian disruption: stress, allostasis, and allostatic load. Sleep Med Clin 2015;10(1):1–10.
[566] Minkel JD, Banks S, Htaik O, et al. Sleep deprivation and stressors: evidence for elevated negative affect in response to mild stressors when sleep deprived. Emotion 2012;12(5):1015.
[567] Minkel J, Moreta M, Muto J, et al. Sleep deprivation potentiates HPA axis stress reactivity in healthy adults. Health Psychol 2014;33(11):1430.
[568] Adelman EM. Mind–body intelligence: a new perspective integrating Eastern and Western healing traditions. Hol Nurs Pract 2006;20(3):147–51.
[569] Butler AC, Chapman JE, Forman EM, et al. The empirical status of cognitive-behavioral therapy: a review of meta-analyses. Clin Psychol Rev 2006;26(1):17–31.
[570] Richardson J, Smith JE, McCall G, et al. Hypnosis for procedure-related pain and distress in pediatric cancer patients: a systematic review of effectiveness and methodology related to hypnosis interventions. J Pain Symptom Manage 2006;31(1):70–84.
[571] Pronk K. Role of the doctor in relieving spiritual distress at the end of life. Am J Hosp Pall Care 2005;22(6):419–25.
[572] Pratt RR. Art, dance, and music therapy. Phys Med Rehab Clin North Am 2004;15(4):827–41.
[573] Eliopoulus C. Invitation to holistic health. Boston: Jones and Bartlett Publishers; 2004.
[574] Crum AJ, Salovey P, Achor S. Rethinking stress: The role of mindsets in determining the stress response. J Personal Social Psychol 2013;104(4):716.
[575] Robson T. An introduction to complementary medicine. Sydney: Allen & Unwin; 2003.
[576] Murakami S, Shirota T, Hayashi S, et al. Aromatherapy for outpatients with menopausal symptoms in obstetrics and gynecology. J Altern Comp Med 2005;11(3):491–4.
[577] Burden B, Herron-Marx S, Clifford C. The increasing use of reiki as a complementary therapy in specialist palliative care. Int J Pall Nurs 2005;11(5):248–53.
[578] Loucks EB, Berkman LF, Gruenewald TL, et al. Social integration is associated with fibrinogen concentration in elderly men. Psychosom Med 2005;67(3):353–8.
[579] Loucks EB, Berkman LF, Gruenewald TL, et al. Relation of social integration to inflammatory marker concentrations in men and women 70 to 79 years. Am J Cardiol 2006;97(7):1010–16.
[580] Stear S. Health and fitness series–1. The importance of physical activity for health. J Fam Health Care 2003;13(1):10–13.
[581] Bancos I, Hahner S, Tomlinson J, et al. Diagnosis and management of adrenal insufficiency. Lancet Diabetes Endocrinol 2015;3(3):216–26.
[582] Nelms M, Sucher K, Long S. Nutrition therapy and pathophysiology. Ch 12. Australia: Thomson Wadsworth; 2007.
[583] Napier C, Pearce SH. Autoimmune Addison's disease. Presse Med 2012;41(12 P 2):e626–35.
[584] Charmandari E, Nicolaides NC, Chrousos GP. Adrenal insufficiency. Lancet 2014;383(9935):2152–67.
[585] Libè R, Barbetta L, Dall'Asta C, et al. Effects of dehydroepiandrosterone (DHEA) supplementation on hormonal, metabolic and behavioral status in patients with hypoadrenalism. J Endocrinol Invest 2004;27(8):736–41.
[586] Quinkler M, Oelkers W, Remde H, et al. Mineralocorticoid substitution and monitoring in primary adrenal insufficiency. Best Pract Res Clin Endocrinol Metab 2015;29(1):17–24.
[587] Petersen KS, Rushworth RL, Clifton PM, et al. Recurrent nocturnal hypoglycaemia as a cause of morning fatigue in treated Addison's disease — favourable response to dietary management: a case report. BMC Endocr Disord 2015;15:61.
[588] Klement J, Hubold C, Cords H, et al. High-calorie glucose-rich food attenuates neuroglycopenic symptoms in patients with Addison's disease. J Clin Endocrinol Metab 2010;95(2):522–8.
[589] Kodama M, Kodama T, Murakami M, et al. Vitamin C infusion treatment enhances cortisol production of the adrenal via the pituitary ACTH route. In Vivo 1994;8(6):1079–85.
[590] Henry M, Thomas KG. Episodic memory impairment in Addison's disease: results from a telephonic cognitive assessment. Metab Brain Dis 2014;29(2):421–30.
[591] Schultebraucks K, Wingenfeld K, Qinkler M, et al. Cognitive function in patients with primary adrenal insufficiency (Addison's disease) and the role of mineralocorticoid receptors. Psychoneuroendocrinology 2015;61:45.
[592] Faber J, Cohn D, Kirkegaard C, et al. Subclinical hypothyroidism in Addison's disease. Acta Endocrinol (Copenh) 1979;91(4):674–9.
[593] Burrows AW. Reversible hypothyroidism after steroid replacement for Addison's disease. Postgrad Med J 1981;57(668):368–70.
[594] Bolland MJ, Holdaway IM, Berkeley JE, et al. Mortality and morbidity in Cushing's syndrome in New Zealand. Clin Endocrinol 2011;75(4):436–42.
[595] Steffensen C, Bak AM, Zøylner Rubeck K, et al. Epidemiology of Cushing's syndrome. Neuroendocrinology 2010;92(Suppl. 1): 1–5.

[596] Valassi E, Santos A, Yaneva M, et al. The European Registry on Cushing's syndrome: 2-year experience. Baseline demographic and clinical characteristics. Eur J Endocrinol 2011;165(3):383–92.
[597] Elias PC, Martinez EZ, Barone BF, et al. Late-night salivary cortisol has a better performance than urinary free cortisol in the diagnosis of Cushing's syndrome. J Clin Endocrinol Metab 2014;99(6):2045–51.
[598] Esposito K, Bellastella G, Maiorino MI, et al. Cushing syndrome, metabolic syndrome and inflammation: a suggested way out. Rev Endocrinol Metab 2013;1(1):41–5.
[599] Colao A, De Block C, Gaztambide MS, et al. Managing hyperglycemia in patients with Cushing's disease treated with pasireotide: medical expert recommendations. Pituitary 2014;17(2):180–6.
[600] Feelders RA, Pulgar SJ, Kempel A, et al. Management of endocrine disease: the burden of Cushing's disease: clinical and health-related quality of life aspects. Eur J Endocrinol 2012;167(3):311–26.
[601] Giordano C, Guarnotta V, Pivonello R, et al. Is diabetes in Cushing's syndrome only a consequence of hypercortisolism? Eur J Endocrinol 2014;170(2):311–19.
[602] Hristova M, Aloe L. Metabolic syndrome — neurotrophic hypothesis. Med Hypotheses 2006;66(3):545–9.
[603] Evans JL, Maddux BA, Goldfine ID. The molecular basis for oxidative stress-induced insulin resistances. Antioxid Redox Signal 2005;7(7–8):1040–52.
[604] Tsigos C, Chrousos GP. Hypothalamic–pituitary–adrenal axis, neuroendocrine factors and stress. J Psychosom Res 2002;53(4):865–71.
[605] Sebeková K, Boor P, Valachovicová M, et al. Association of metabolic syndrome risk factors with selected markers of oxidative status and microinflammation in healthy omnivores and vegetarians. Mol Nutr Food Res 2006;50(9):858–68.
[606] Pecori Giraldi F, Ambrogio AG, Andrioli M, et al. Potential role for retinoic acid in patients with Cushing's disease. J Clin Endocrinol Metab 2012;97(10):3577–37-83.

SAMPLE DAILY DIET REFERENCES

Hypothyroid

Acar B, Ozay AC, Ozay OE, et al. Evaluation of thyroid function status among postmenopausal women with and without osteoporosis. Int J Gynaecol Obstet 2016;134(1):53–7.
Chang JY, Chiang CP, Wang YP, et al. Antigastric parietal cell and antithyroid autoantibodies in patients with desquamative gingivitis. J Oral Pathol Med 2017;46(4):307–12.
Collins AB, Pawlak R. Prevalence of vitamin B-12 deficiency among patients with thyroid dysfunction. Asia Pac J Clin Nutr 2016;25(2):221–6.
Jawa A, Jawad A, Riaz SH, et al. Turmeric use is associated with reduced goitrogenesis: thyroid disorder prevalence in Pakistan. Ind J Endocrinol Metab 2016;20(1):147.
Kose E, Guzel O, Demir K, et al. Changes of thyroid hormonal status in patients receiving ketogenic diet due to intractable epilepsy. J Pediatr Endocrinol Metab 2017;30(4):411–16.
Lauritano EC, Bilotta AL, Gabrielli M, et al. Association between hypothyroidism and small intestinal bacterial overgrowth. J Clin Endocrinol Metab 2007;92:4180–4.

Hyperthyroidism

Cunningham E. Are there foods that support thyroid health? J Acad Nutr Diet 2012;112(4):588.
Felker P, Bunch R, Leung AM. Concentrations of thiocyanate and goitrin in human plasma, their precursor concentrations in Brassica vegetables, and associated potential risk for hypothyroidism. Nutr Rev 2016;74(4):248–58.

Type 1 diabetes

Coit P, Sawalha AH. The human microbiome in rheumatic autoimmune diseases: a comprehensive review. Clin Immunol 2016;170:70–9.
Ellinger S, Stehle P. Impact of cocoa consumption on inflammation processes — a critical review of randomized controlled trials. Nutrients 2016;8(6):321.
Mariño E, Richards JL, McLeod KH, et al. Gut microbial metabolites limit the frequency of autoimmune T cells and protect against type 1 diabetes. Nat Immunol 2017;18:552–62.
Medagama AB. The glycaemic outcomes of cinnamon, a review of the experimental evidence and clinical trials. Nutr J 2015;14:108.
Mitrou P, Raptis AE, Lambadiari V, et al. Vinegar decreases postprandial hyperglycemia in patients with type 1 diabetes. Diabetes Care 2010;33(2):e27.
Ooi CP, Loke SC. Sweet potato for type 2 diabetes mellitus. Cochrane Database Syst Rev 2013;(9):CD009128.

Hypoglycaemia

Lavernia F, Kushner P, Trence D, et al. Recognizing and minimizing hypoglycemia: the need for individualized care. Postgrad Med 2015;127(8):801–7.
Medagama AB. The glycaemic outcomes of cinnamon, a review of the experimental evidence and clinical trials. Nutr J 2015;14:108.
Ooi CP, Loke SC. Sweet potato for type 2 diabetes mellitus. Cochrane Database Syst Rev 2013;(9):CD009128.
Shishehbor F, Mansoori A, Shirani F. Vinegar consumption can attenuate postprandial glucose and insulin responses; a systematic review and meta-analysis of clinical trials. Diabetes Res Clin Pract 2017;127:1–9.
Turksoy K, Kilkus J, Hajizadeh I, et al. Hypoglycemia detection and carbohydrate suggestion in an artificial pancreas. J Diabetes Sci Technol 2016;10(6):1236–44.

Stress

Guo Q, Kim YN, Lee BH. Protective effects of blueberry drink on cognitive impairment induced by chronic mild stress in adult rats. Nutr Res Pract 2017;11(1):25–32.
Sartori SB, Whittle N, Hetzenauer A, et al. Magnesium deficiency induces anxiety and HPA axis dysregulation: modulation by therapeutic drug treatment. Neuropharmacology 2012;62(1):304–12.
Ulrich-Lai YM, Fulton S, Wilson M, et al. Stress exposure, food intake and emotional state. Stress 2015;18(4):381–99.

Addison's disease

Brody S, Preut R, Schommer K, et al. A randomized controlled trial of high dose ascorbic acid for reduction of blood pressure, cortisol and subjective responses to psychological stress. Psychopharmacology (Berl) 2002;159(3):319–423.
Dmitrašinović G, Pešić V, Stanić D, et al. ACTH, cortisol and IL-6 levels in athletes following magnesium supplementation. J Med Biochem 2016;35(4):375–84.
Klement J, Hubold C, Cords H, et al. High-calorie glucose-rich food attenuates neuroglycopenic symptoms in patients with Addison's disease. J Clin Endocrinol Metab 2010;95(2):522–8.
Methlie P, Husebye EE, Hustad S, et al. Grapefruit juice and licorice increase cortisol availability in patients with Addison's disease. Eur J Endocrinol 2011;165(5):761–9.
O'Leary C, Walsh CH, Wieneke P, et al. Coeliac disease and autoimmune Addison's disease: a clinical pitfall. QJM 2002;95(2):79–82.
Pihlanto A, Mattila P, Mäkinen S, et al. Bioactivities of alternative protein sources and their potential health benefits. Food Funct 2017;8(10):3443–58.

Cushing's syndrome

Faggiano A, Melis D, Alfieri R, et al. Sulfur amino acids in Cushing's disease: insight in homocysteine and taurine levels in patients with active and cured disease. J Clin Endocrinol Metab 2005;90(12):6616–22.
Monteleone P, Maj M, Beinat L, et al. Blunting by chronic phosphatidylserine administration of the stress-induced activation of the hypothalamo-pituitary-adrenal axis in healthy men. Eur J Clin Pharmacol 1992;42(4):385–8.
Stachowicz M, Lebiedzińska A. The effect of diet components on the level of cortisol. Eur Food Res Technol 2016;242(12):2001–9.

22 The neurological system

Leah Hechtman, Cheryl le Roux

SECTION A

PRINCIPLES OF THE NATUROPATHIC APPROACH TO THE NEUROLOGICAL SYSTEM

Overview of the neurological system

The neurological system (Fig. 22.1) is one of the most intricate systems within the human body and functions as our control centre where it gathers, conveys, processes and stores information. Experiencing a memory, being 'rational' and speaking coherently are all activities that occur as a result of the complex independent workings of the neurological system.

The nervous tissue of the neurological system contains cells known as neurons and neuroglia. Neurons are responsible for the specialised functions of the neurological system (for example, those that allow us to think) while neuroglia function to support and protect the neurons (very much like bodyguards). To understand the workings of the nervous system we can split it into structures:

- The brain and the spinal cord together make up the central nervous system (CNS) and function to process and respond to information communicated from the peripheral nervous system
- The cranial nerves (except cranial nerve II), the spinal nerves, the enteric plexuses and the sensory neurons together make up the peripheral nervous system (PNS) and function to oversee the nervous tissue outside the central nervous system.

THE CNS STRUCTURES

The brain

The brain sits within the cranium protected by the cranial bones and the meninges. Though we may think of it as being quite small, the brain is actually one of the largest organs in the body comprising approximately 100 billion neurons and even more neuroglia.[1]

THE SPINAL CORD

The spinal cord acts as a pathway to connect the brain to the peripheral nervous system so that sensory and motor information may be conveyed. The spinal cord is made up of grey and white matter and contains approximately 100 million neurons.[1]

THE PNS STRUCTURES

The 12 cranial nerves and their branches

The 12 cranial nerves are nerves that emerge from the brain. Each exerts a different function:

- Cranial nerve I, olfactory nerve, is responsible for the sense of smell
- Cranial nerve II, optic nerve, is responsible for visual fields and acuity. It is an exception to the rule as it belongs in the CNS category. The optic nerve is actually an out-pouching of the optic stalk during embryonic development thus making it part of the central nervous system
- Cranial nerves III, IV, VI, oculomotor, trochlear and abducens nerves, are responsible for eye movements
- Cranial nerve V, trigeminal nerve, is responsible for the sensory function of the face
- Cranial nerve VII, facial nerve, is responsible for the strength of facial muscle
- Cranial nerve XI, accessory nerve, is responsible for the strength of the girdle of shoulder muscle
- Cranial nerves VII, VIII, facial and vestibulocochlear nerves, are responsible for hearing
- Cranial nerves VII, IX, X, facial, glossopharyngeal, and vagus nerves, are responsible for taste
- Cranial nerve XI, glossopharyngeal nerve, is responsible for pharyngeal movement and reflex
- Cranial nerve X, vagus nerve, is also responsible for controlling the heart rate, breathing and digestive peristalsis
- Cranial nerve XII, hypoglossal nerve, is responsible for tongue movements.

The spinal nerves and their branches

There are 31 pairs of spinal nerves. These may be found passing out of the spinal cord and function to form a

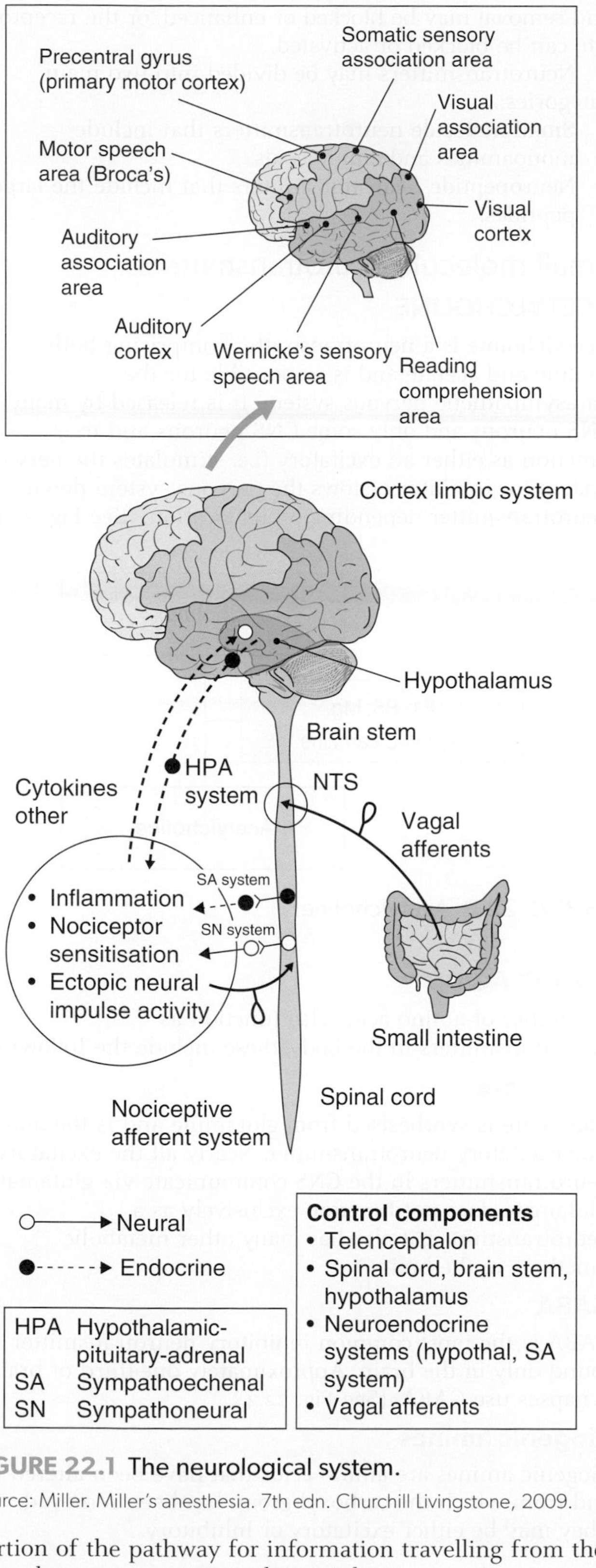

FIGURE 22.1 The neurological system.

Source: Miller. Miller's anesthesia. 7th edn. Churchill Livingstone, 2009.

portion of the pathway for information travelling from the central nervous system to the periphery.

Ganglia

The ganglia are nuclei found in the brain of vertebrates and have been found to play an important role in a wide number of neurological conditions.

Somatic, autonomic and enteric nervous systems

As discussed, the neurological system consists of the CNS and PNS. However, the PNS can be further divided into three subsystems: the somatic nervous system, the autonomic nervous system and the enteric nervous system.

The somatic nervous system (SNS) is made up of two types of neurons known as sensory and motor neurons. The sensory neurons of the SNS provide information from the somatic and special sensory receptors in the head, limbs and body wall to the CNS while the motor neurons function to conduct impulses from the CNS to the skeletal muscle. This system is involved in voluntary movement.

The autonomic nervous system (ANS) also contains sensory and motor neurons. However, they function differently from those above. The sensory neurons of the ANS system function to provide information from visceral autonomic sensory receptors to the CNS while the motor neurons of the CNS function to conduct impulses from the CNS to the smooth and cardiac muscle, the glands and adipose tissue. This system is involved in involuntary movement. The motor portion of the ANS can be further divided into the sympathetic nervous system and the parasympathetic nervous system.

The enteric nervous system is also known as the intrinsic nervous system. It directly controls the gastrointestinal system by its weave and extensions of mesh-like neurons throughout the structures of gastrointestinal system. It consists of the Auerbach's (myenteric) and Meissner's (submucosal) ganglia plexuses.

FUNCTIONS OF THE NEUROLOGICAL SYSTEM

The neurological system works closely with the other systems of the body to maintain homeostasis. Three primary functions (known as sensory, integrative, and motor functions) allow the neurological system to clearly convey and process information so that this can successfully occur.

Sensory function involves sensory receptors of the nervous system sensing internal and external changes occurring in and to the body. An example of this is the burning sensation of your hand when touching a hot surface such as a hotplate.

Integrative function involves the nervous system assimilating sensory information (the changes occurring in the body) and deciding what to do with this information. An example of this is the neurological system processing the information that your hand is burning on the hotplate and weighing up the pros and cons of leaving it there to burn or removing it.

Motor function involves the nervous system responding and reacting to the change occurring. An example of this is moving your hand off the burning surface as your neurological system has conveyed the dangers to the rest of your body.

NEUROTRANSMITTERS AND THE NEUROLOGICAL SYSTEM

Neurotransmitters are endogenous chemicals stored in the nerve cells. As their name suggests, neurotransmitters 'transmit' signals/information between neurons and other cells of the body allowing them to effectively communicate with each other. In this way, the neurotransmitters influence numerous bodily processes including mood and pain. Disruptions in their function occur when the neurotransmitters are unable to transmit the electrical signal (discussed below) from one neuron to another. This scenario is implicated in numerous neurological disorders. The main neurotransmitters are summarised in Table 22.1.

How neurotransmitters work in the body

Action potentials can be likened to electrical signals and allow neurons to communicate with each other. As action potentials depolarise, they cause Ca^{2+} ion channels to open and Ca^{2+} flows inwards allowing the release of thousands of neurotransmitters. These then flow into the synaptic cleft binding to neurotransmitter receptors. When enough neurotransmitters have bound to ligand-gated receptors, polarisation or hyperpolarisation occurs and an action potential pulsates down the cell causing release of its neurotransmitters. Action potentials move in one direction only, hence information is only transferred one way. It is important to note that neurotransmitter effects may be modified. Synthesis can be stimulated or inhibited, release and removal may be blocked or enhanced, or the receptor site can be blocked or activated.

Neurotransmitters may be divided into two main categories:

1. Small molecule neurotransmitters that include monoamines and amino acids
2. Neuropeptide neurotransmitters that include the larger peptides.

Small molecule neurotransmitters

ACETYLCHOLINE

Acetylcholine is a neurotransmitter comprising both choline and acetate and is responsible for the parasympathetic nervous system. It is released by many PNS neurons and only some CNS neurons and may function as either an excitatory (i.e. stimulates the nervous system) or inhibitory (slows the nervous system down) neurotransmitter depending on its location. (See Fig. 22.2.)

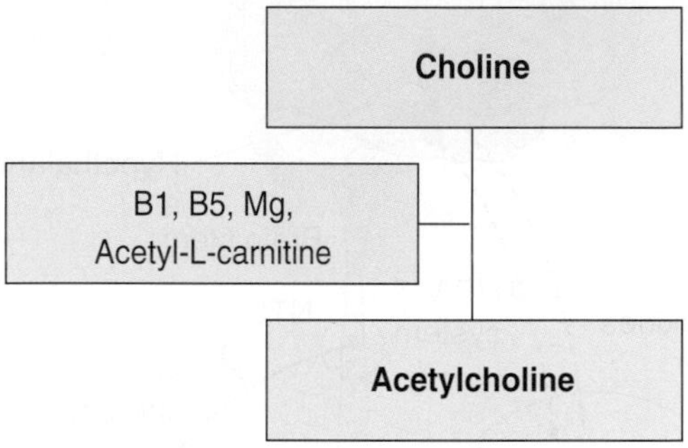

FIGURE 22.2 Acetylcholine.

TABLE 22.1 Main neurotransmitters

Type	Neurotransmitter	Postsynaptic effect
Amino acids	Gamma aminobutyric acid (GABA)	Inhibitory
	Glycine	Inhibitory
	Glutamate	Excitatory
	Aspartate	Excitatory
Biogenic amines	Dopamine	Excitatory
	Noradrenaline (norepinephrine)	Excitatory
	Serotonin	Excitatory
	Histamine	Excitatory
Other	Acetylcholine	Excitatory
	Endogenous opioids (encephalins, endorphins, dynorphin)	Excitatory
Main neuropeptide neurotransmitters		
Neuropeptide neurotransmitter		
Corticotrophin-releasing hormone		
Corticotrophin (ACTH)		
Beta-endorphin		
Substance P		
Neurotensin		
Somatostatin		
Bradykinin		
Vasopressin angiotensin II		

AMINO ACIDS

A number of amino acids also function as neurotransmitters in the body, these include the following.

Glutamate

Glutamate is synthesised from glutamine and is the only true excitatory neurotransmitter. Nearly all the excitatory neurotransmitters in the CNS communicate via glutamate. Glutamate does not function exclusively as a neurotransmitter: it also has many other metabolic functions in the brain.[2]

GABA

GABA is the most common inhibitory neurotransmitter found only in the brain. Approximately one-third of brain synapses use GABA. (See Fig. 22.3.)

Biogenic amines

Biogenic amines are amino acids that have been altered and from which the carboxyl group has been removed. They may be either excitatory or inhibitory.

Noradrenaline

Noradrenaline (norepinephrine) is a stimulating neurotransmitter[3] released by the adrenal medulla. As well as serving as a neurotransmitter, it also functions as a hormone and helps to maintain arousal as well as regulate mood and dreaming. (See Fig. 22.4.)

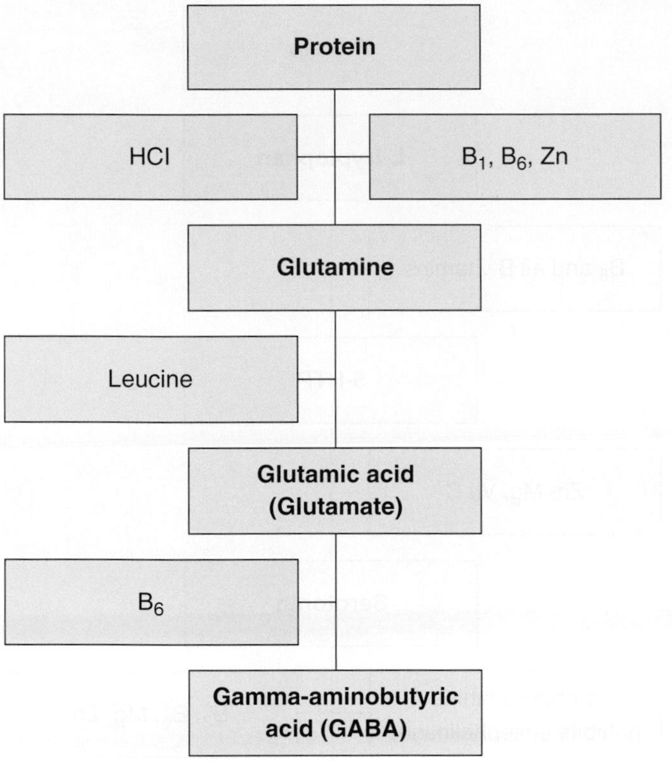

FIGURE 22.3 GABA.

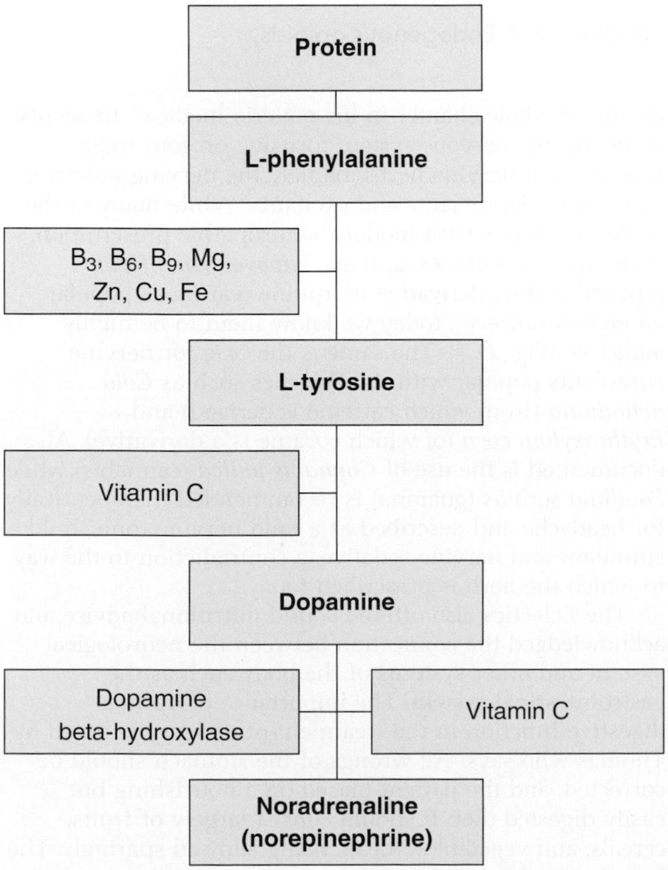

FIGURE 22.4 Noradrenaline cofactors.

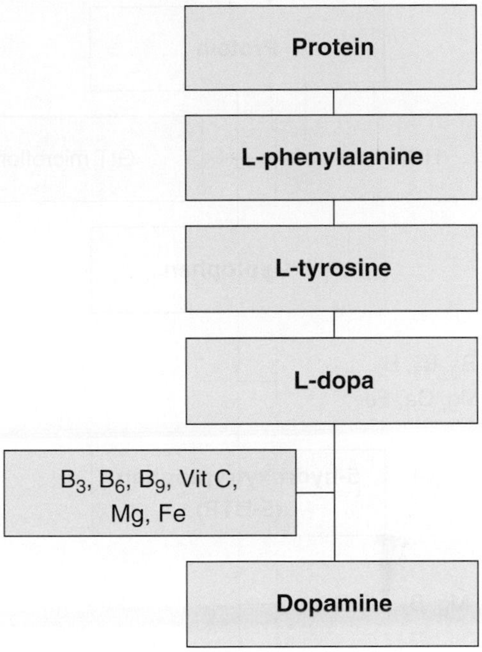

FIGURE 22.5 Dopamine cofactors.

Dopamine

Dopamine is involved in emotional responses as well as movement.[1] Deficiency of dopamine is associated with neurological disorders such as Parkinson's disease. (See Fig. 22.5.)

Serotonin

Serotonin is an inhibitory neurotransmitter that assists with regulation of temperature, mood and sleep.[1] (See Fig. 22.6.)

Neuropeptides

Neuropeptides are neurotransmitters (though they may also function as hormones) composed of 3–40 amino acids linked by peptide bonds. They can be found in both the CNS and PNS and are both excitatory and inhibitory.

Substance P is a neuropeptide found in sensory neurons, the spinal cord and the brain. Substance P enhances perception of pain.

Encephalins are neuropeptides that suppress release of substance P, producing pain-relieving effects.

Endorphins are neuropeptides also linked to pain-relieving effects and pleasure by blocking substance P.

Other neuropeptides include hypothalamic releasing and inhibiting hormones, angiotensin II and cholecystokinin (CKK).

ROLE OF THE NATUROPATH — NEUROLOGICAL SYSTEM

Traditional interpretation

Treatment of the neurological system with botanicals can be traced back to 6000 BC to the ancient practice of Ayurveda, which documents the use of *Withania somnifera*

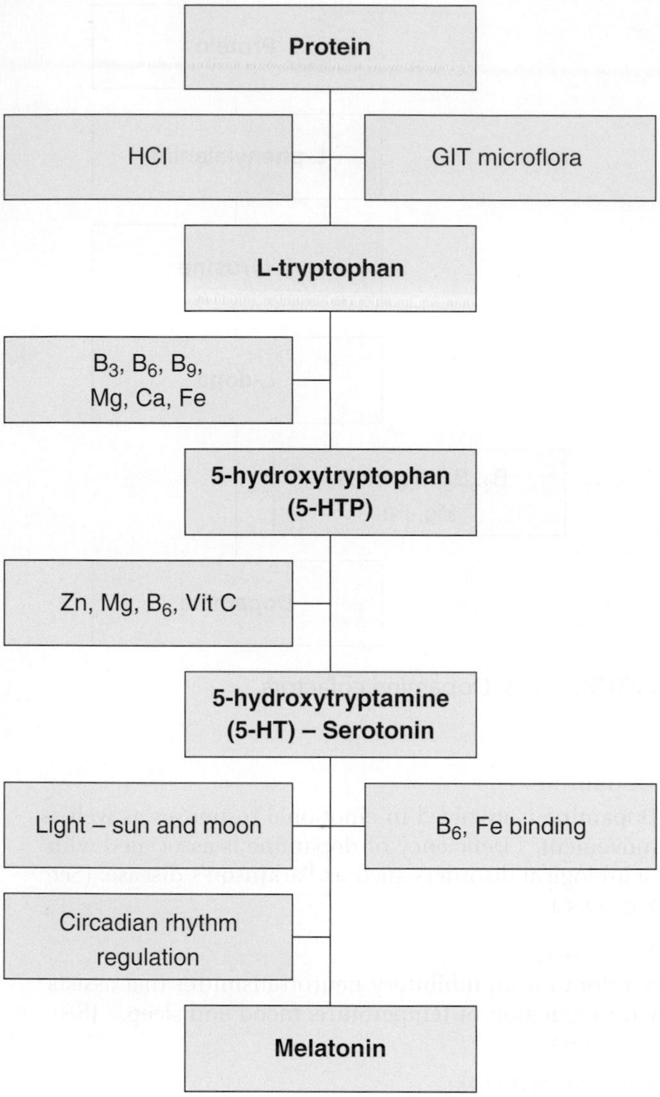

FIGURE 22.6 Serotonin cofactors.

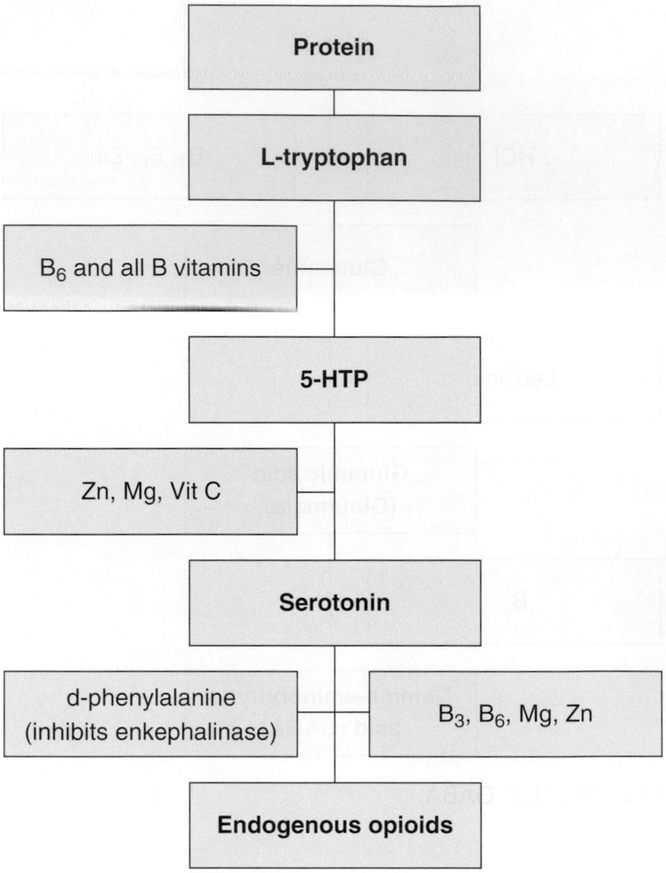

FIGURE 22.7 Endogenous opioids.

and the brahmi species for the management of seizures and convulsions.[4]

Despite these early applications, the structure and function of the neurological system appears to have been a source of much confusion to the early philosophers. Aristotle believed that the nerves stemmed from the heart as the heart was thought to be the controlling organ of the body; however, this view was soon challenged. Galen was advanced for his time and categorised the nerves into two distinct types, 'hard' nerves and 'soft', believing them to have two separate functions: first to convey sensation and second to convey motion, both to the extremities of the body. Galen challenged Aristotle's view that the nerves stemmed from the heart, saying 'I have shown in my book *On the Teachings of Hippocrates and Plato* that the source of the nerves, of all sensation, and of voluntary motion is the encephalon [the brain] and that the source of the arteries and of the innate heat is the heart'.[5]

The Eclectic physicians' management of the neurological system centred upon the use of homeopathics and the herbal class known as nervines. Ellingwood devotes a whole chapter in his materia medica[6] to agents acting on the nervous system focusing on four main categories of nervine herbs, namely the nervine sedatives, stimulants, depressants and excitants. While many of the herbs are in line with modern naturopathic prescription, there are also some exceptions. *Papaver somniferum* (opium) and its derivative morphine feature as popular anodynes, however, today we know them to be highly addictive (Fig. 22.7). The same is the case for nervine stimulants popular with the Eclectics such as *Cola acuminata* (from which caffeine is derived) and *Erythroxylum coca* (of which cocaine is a derivative). Also documented is the use of *Cannabis indica* (cannabis) while *Paullinia sorbilis* (guarana) is recommended therapeutically for headache and described as a mild nervine tonic, mild stimulant and nervine sedative, a contradiction to the way in which the herb is prescribed today.

The Eclectics also offered sound nutritional advice and acknowledged the connection between the neurological system and other systems of the body such as the gastrointestinal system. The importance of optimal digestive function in the treatment of epilepsy is noted by Thomas who says: 'All wrongs of the stomach should be corrected, and the patient placed on a nourishing but easily digested diet: It should consist largely of fruits, cereals, and vegetables, meats being allowed sparingly. The bowels should receive careful attention, constipation being avoided'.[7] Goldenseal, a herb renowned for its gastrointestinal system effects, was also advocated as a nervine by the Eclectics.[6] This is a prime example of the insights traditional prescribing can offer modern naturopaths with regards to new therapeutic applications of herbs, which may not have been considered as first-line treatments for the nervous system.

Modern interpretation

One cannot deny that there has been a substantial increase in knowledge on the workings of the neurological system since the time of the Eclectics. In-depth research into the structure and function of the nervous system at a biochemical level has increased naturopathic knowledge and there is now a greater understanding of the structures that make up the neurological system. Galen with his belief that the organs of the neurological system were hollow could not have fathomed the presence of ganglia and the enteric plexuses. Nor could he know what we know today regarding the necessity of balanced nutrition and the important role individual amino acids and nutrients in their correct amounts play for the proper and healthy functioning of the peripheral and central nervous system.

Modern naturopathy has identified a range of possible causes or contributing factors for the pathogenesis of neurological disorders including:

- Nutrition (deficiencies/excesses)
- Hormonal balance
- Infection
- Inflammation
- Stress
- Toxicity (e.g. heavy metal)
- Poor detoxification
- Elevated homocysteine levels.

The modern naturopath works closely with other allied specialist healthcare professionals in the management of neurological conditions such as multiple sclerosis, Parkinson's disease and sleep disorders. Specific nutritional objectives are summarised in Table 22.2 and specific herbal medicine in Table 22.3.

TABLE 22.2 Specific nutritional objectives — neurological system

Nutrient	Justification	Therapeutic dosage	Dietary source
Adenosine	Inhibitory neurotransmitter that produces a calming effect in the brain. Adenosine receptors modulate neuronal and synaptic function	100–200 mg/day	Purine containing foods especially offal
L-arginine	Reduces neuropathic pain. Agmatine is an amine formed by the decarboxylation of L-arginine by the enzyme arginine decarboxylase that has been found to modulate morphine analgesia	400–6000 mg/day	Almonds, pecans, cashews, chocolate, whole wheat
Vitamin B complex	Required to help maintain the health of the nervous system. In high doses sufficient to elevate mitochondrial enzyme factors, the B vitamins function as antioxidants while improving mitochondrial function suggesting a role in preventing Parkinson's disease (and possibly other neurological disorders)	Required dosage is specific to individual B vitamin	Legumes, wholegrains, nuts, beans, brewer's yeast, leafy green vegetables
Vitamin B_1	Glucose is a primary energy source for the brain. Thiamine (with the other B vitamins) is required by the nervous tissue to produce this energy. Required for the production of certain neurotransmitters and also found in the cell membrane of the nerves where it is involved in the transmission of nerve cells to and from the CNS/PNS. Deficiency is common in neurological disorders	5–150 mg/day	Legumes, liver, nuts, wholegrains, wheatgerm
Vitamin B_2	Required for development and metabolism of neurotransmitters. Deficiency is common in neurological disorders. Possible role in the treatment of headache and migraine	10–40 mg/day (standard therapeutic dose), 100–200 mg/day in the treatment of migraines	Avocado, beans, currants, eggs, milk and dairy products, sprouts, wholegrains
Vitamin B_3	Required for healthy nervous system function including proper sleep and may have a role in the prevention of headache. A source of the coenzymes NAD+ and NADP+, which are required for many metabolic processes. May indirectly increase serotonin	50–3000 mg/day depending on form prescribed	Salmon, sardines, sunflower seeds, almonds, chicken, eggs

Continued

TABLE 22.2 Specific nutritional objectives — neurological system—cont'd			
Nutrient	**Justification**	**Therapeutic dosage**	**Dietary source**
Vitamin B_5	Pantothenic acid (from vitamin B_5) is used in the synthesis of coenzyme A, which is a cofactor in over 70 enzymatic pathways in the body including the synthesis and formation of the neurotransmitter acetylcholine. Deficiency of vitamin B_5 causes acetylcholine synthesis to become impaired, and hence neurological symptoms may appear	100 mg–500 mg/day	Avocado, beans, egg yolks, green vegetables, milk, mushrooms, oranges, royal jelly, sweet potato, wholegrain cereals
Vitamin B_6	Pyridoxal 5′-phosphate (P5P) is the active form of vitamin B_6 and plays an important role in the synthesis of several neurotransmitters including serotonin, noradrenaline, adrenaline and GABA. Deficiency is common in neurological disorders	20–200 mg/day	Brewer's yeast, chicken, yolk, legumes, mackerel, oatmeal, salmon, tuna, walnuts
Vitamin B_9	Deficiency of folic acid presents with neurological symptoms such as cognitive decline, unrest, irritability, sleep disturbances and the like, as well as specific neurological disorders such as epilepsy	1000–5000 micrograms/day (as folic acid) 400–6000 micrograms/day (as folinic acid)	Eggs, green leafy vegetables, lentils
Vitamin B_{12}	Vitamin B_{12} is essential for healthy brain function through its role as manufacturer of the myelin sheath. Vitamin B_{12} is also required for the production of neurotransmitters	300–2000 micrograms/day	Clams, egg yolk, herring, milk, meat, oysters, salmon, sardines
Vitamins B_6, B_9, B_{12}	Deficiency of this trio of vitamins as well as secondary changes in the concentrations of associated metabolites, such as homocysteine, may contribute to the onset and progression of neurological conditions such as Parkinson's disease	B_6: 20–100 mg/day B_{12}: 125–2000 micrograms/day folic acid: 20–2500 micrograms/day	See above
Vitamin A	Vitamin A is required for the growth and maintenance of neural tissue, in particular the myelin sheath	10 000–50 000 IU as retinol palmitate for a few days	Carrots, egg yolk, apricots, fish liver oils
Vitamin C	Vitamin C is crucial for the conversion of certain substances into neurotransmitters such as serotonin, dopamine, and noradrenaline. Nerve endings contain the highest amount of vitamin C in the human body (after the suprarenal glands)	250–10 000 mg/day (up to bowel tolerance)	Kiwi fruit, guava, papaya, mangoes, strawberries, acerola cherries, broccoli
Vitamin D	Vitamin D exerts numerous positive effects on both the immune and neural cells. Deficiency has been suggested to predispose to a range of neurological disorders including depression and Parkinson's disease	400–1600 IU/day (NB increase in dosage may be required in instances of significant deficiency. Pathology interpretation is essential)	Synthesised by the action of sunlight on fish liver oils such as cod, tuna; also found in egg yolks, sprouted seeds and milk
Vitamin E	Vitamin E is essential for the maintenance and structure of the neurological system. It maintains the integrity and stability of membranes and protects phospholipids from peroxidation. Interestingly, vitamin E concentrations vary according to neuroanatomical regions. In the brain, the cerebral cortex has the highest concentration of vitamin E while the cerebellum has the lowest. It appears that only alphatocopherol is involved in nervous membranes	100–450 IU/day	Almonds, wheatgerm, safflower, egg yolks, corn, beef, nuts

TABLE 22.2 Specific nutritional objectives — neurological system—cont'd

Nutrient	Justification	Therapeutic dosage	Dietary source
Calcium	Calcium ions (Ca^{2+}) play a role in several important functions in the central nervous system including the release of neurotransmitters, production of action potentials, nerve depolarisation of membranes and neuronal plasticity. Ca^{2+} mediated toxicity is associated in the pathogenesis of neurodegenerative diseases including Parkinson's and epilepsy. Taken with magnesium, the two exert a calming effect in the body	1000–2000 mg/day	Tinned sardines and salmon (with the bones), almonds, dairy products (milk, yoghurt, cheese), tahini, sesame seeds, leafy green vegetables (spinach, broccoli, bok choy), dried figs
Quercetin	Quercetin displays antioxidant activity against reactive oxygen species involved in inflammatory pain synonymous with many disorders of the nervous system as well as analgesic effects thought to be through inhibition of pronociceptive cytokine production	600–1500 mg/day	Fruits and vegetables particularly citrus fruits, apples, onions, parsley, tea, and red wine are the primary dietary sources of quercetin. Olive oil, grapes, dark cherries, and dark berries such as blueberries, blackberries and bilberries are also high in flavonoids, including quercetin
Bromelain	Bromelain has been theorised to possibly have some beneficial effects on the clinical course of neurological symptoms related to multiple sclerosis though studies are scarce and remain inconclusive. However, the efficacy of bromelain in the treatment of other inflammatory disorders provides a rationale for its application in neurological disorders where there is inflammation such as headache	150–1600 mg/day	Pineapple
Magnesium	Magnesium has multiple functions in the neurological system. It is involved in nerve depolarisation of membranes and can reduce central sensitisation that causes abnormal responses to pain by blocking NMDA receptors that bind to glutamate preventing neuronal excitement. Magnesium also functions as a muscle relaxant useful in stress, headaches and the like	300–800 mg/day	Green leafy vegetables, eggs, cocoa, almonds, brewer's yeast, cashews, kelp, wheat bran, wheatgerm, buck wheat
Manganese	Manganese is an essential trace element for the development and function of the central nervous system through its participation in various antioxidant enzymatic mechanisms. Manganese is found in the brain especially in the basal ganglia. Changes in the concentration of manganese in the body (either too much or too little) may result in increased susceptibility to convulsions; movement of manganese in the brain is associated with increased neuronal activity	2.5–7 mg/day	Almonds, beans, coconuts, corn, kelp, sunflower seeds, legumes, walnuts, wholegrains
Copper	Copper is required for the proper functioning of the central nervous system where it participates in enzymatic mechanisms that protect against free radical scavengers. Deficiencies and excesses have also been implicated in neurological disorders	2–5 mg/day	Almonds, dried legumes, mushrooms, oysters, prunes, sunflower seeds, wholegrain cereals

Continued

TABLE 22.2 Specific nutritional objectives — neurological system—cont'd			
Nutrient	**Justification**	**Therapeutic dosage**	**Dietary source**
Iron	Iron is required to ensure there is adequate oxygenation to the cerebral structures, for energy production in the parenchyma and for neurotransmitter and myelin production	15–100 mg/day	Apricots, pine nuts, sunflower and pumpkin seeds, red meat
Zinc	Zinc is an essential mineral with multiple functions in the central nervous system including the modulation of certain neurotransmitters and involvement in secretory signalling of certain neurons in the brain. Deficiency results in disorders of the central nervous system	10–60 mg/day	Pumpkin seeds, sunflower seeds, oysters, wholegrains, beef, baked beans, cashews, egg yolks, ginger, herring, liver (organic), milk, lamb
Alpha lipoic acid	Alpha lipoic acid exhibits significant neuroprotective properties. Deficiency is associated with changes in the course of brain development and disturbs the make-up of the brain cell membranes and their structures	600–1200 mg/day	Typical dietary sources of lipoic acid are muscle meats, heart, kidney, and liver, and to a lesser degree, fruits and vegetables
Omega-3 fatty acids	The omega-3 fatty acids are vital for healthy neurological function. This is due to them being a structural component of neuronal membranes and glial cells. Additionally, they act as a precursor for lipid derived messengers. Omega-3 fatty acids are also involved in the neuroplasticity of nerve membranes, remyelination, synaptogenesis, synaptic transmission and regulation of prostaglandins. As such, they are indicated as a therapeutic prescription for a number of neurological conditions.	1–6 g/day	Pilchards, salmon, trout, herring, mackerel
Coenzyme Q10	Reactive oxygen species are known to play a role in neuronal loss and dysfunction therefore the neuroprotective coenzyme Q10 in its role as an antioxidant may help to prevent the neurological system from damage free radicals. Coenzyme Q10 may also be well utilised in the management of neurological disorders characterised by altered mitochondrial function because of its role in energy production within the mitochondria	90–600 mg/day	Almonds, broccoli, salmon, sardines, sesame seeds, hazelnuts
Acetyl L-carnitine	Acetyl L-carnitine crosses the blood–brain barrier, providing direct benefit to the central nervous system while also supporting the synthesis of the neurotransmitter acetylcholine. Acetyl L-carnitine also mobilises fatty acids into the mitochondria for ATP energy production helping to improve fatigue associated with chronic fatigue and multiple sclerosis	500–2000 mg/day	Avocado, chicken, beef, milk, fish
L-histidine	L-histidine is a precursor for neuronal synthesis of histamine, a central nervous system neurotransmitter mediating wakefulness, reaction time and alertness	14 mg/kg/day with an upper limit of 2 g/day	First-class proteins: chicken, cottage cheese, fish, eggs, etc
dl-phenylalanine	dl-phenylalanine is an essential amino acid, which may be converted into tyrosine. Preliminary evidence suggests therapeutic functions as an antidepressant and analgesic for chronic pain where it appears to increase opioid levels	150–600 mg/day	First-class proteins, e.g. eggs and chicken as well as fish, lentils, cottage cheese

TABLE 22.2 Specific nutritional objectives — neurological system—cont'd

Nutrient	Justification	Therapeutic dosage	Dietary source
Glycine	Glycine is an inhibitory neurotransmitter found within the central nervous system where it is involved in numerous functions including the processing of motor and sensory information that allows movement, vision and audition. Glycine also modulates excitatory neurotransmission by enhancing the way in which glutamate functions at N-methyl-D-aspartate (NMDA) receptors	4–40 g/day	Gelatine and protein sources, e.g. eggs
Glutamine	Precursor for gamma-aminobutyric acid (GABA) is an inhibitory neurotransmitter found in the central nervous system and glutamate. GABA reduces neuronal firing resulting in increased calmness and relaxation	500–3000 mg/day	First-class protein, e.g. meat as well as cottage cheese, ricotta cheese, rolled oats
Tryptophan	Amino acid required for the production of several important substances within the body including vitamin B and serotonin, a precursor of melatonin	5 mg/kg/day up to 2 g/day	Fish, cottage cheese, sesame seeds, pumpkin seeds, peanuts, soybeans
Tyrosine	Amino acid and precursor to several important neurotransmitters including dopamine, noradrenaline and adrenaline	33 mg/kg/day up to 6 g/day	Almonds, beef, chicken, egg, fish
5-hydroxytryptophan	Derived from tryptophan, increases serotonin within the central nervous system	150 mg/day	Beef, cottage cheese, fish, pepitas, peanuts, sesame seeds
Phosphatidyl serine	Phospholipid that makes up part of the myelin sheath and is found as a component of cell membranes. Facilitates neurotransmitter and synaptic release. Improves memory, learning, mood and stress	100–400 mg/day	Soy lecithin, egg lecithin
Selenium	Selenium is a powerful antioxidant. Oxidative stress has been associated with neuronal loss and pathological conditions of the nervous system as the brain is considered to be highly sensitive to damage as a result of oxidation.	25–400 micrograms/day	Brazil nuts, fish, shellfish, lentils and pulses, kidney and liver (choose organic)

Source: see page 1358.

TABLE 22.3 Specific herbal medicine classes — neurological system

Class	Example	Justification
Analgesic and anodynes (anodynes are usually used externally)	*Piscidia erythrina* (Jamaican dogwood)	The analgesic and anodyne classes of herbs are primarily used to provide pain relief. The root of *Piscidia erythrina* is thought to be one of the most powerful painkillers. It has been proposed to exert its pain relieving effects via its action as a smooth muscle relaxant, sedative and anti-inflammatory action. As early as 1844 the analgesic property of the root bark of *Piscidia erythrina* was discovered, yet despite this early discovery there have been little in the way of clinical trials
Anti-headache/ anti-migraine	*Tanacetum parthenium* (feverfew)	This class of herbs works to prevent and alleviate headaches and migraines. Traditionally *Tanacetum parthenium* was used for female reproductive complaints. However in the 17th century England's John Parkinson noted that *Tanacetum parthenium* was 'very effectual for all paines in the head'. Clinical research confirms the knowledge of the 17th century revealing that *Tanacetum parthenium* reduces inflammation and inhibits vasoconstriction thus providing a biochemical basis for its migraine-relieving action
Circulatory stimulants (cerebral)	*Vinca minor* (lesser periwinkle)	The circulatory stimulant class of herbal medicines comprises those that improve circulation. *Vinca minor* is a shrub native to Europe that has a particular affinity for improving circulation and thus blood flow and oxygen to the cerebral structures. It contains vincamine, a constituent widely used in allopathic medicine and identified to have neuroprotective, antioxidant and vasodilatory actions. These actions provide a rationale for its cerebral circulatory stimulant action

Continued

TABLE 22.3 Specific herbal medicine classes — neurological system—cont'd

Class	Example	Justification
Cognition enhancers	*Rosmarinus officinalis* (rosemary)	Herbs such as *Rosmarinus officinalis* enhance memory and cognition. While the antioxidants in *Rosmarinus officinalis* appear to play some part with regards to cognitive enhancement it is interesting to note that even the olfactory properties of *Rosmarinus officinalis* can influence cognition. In a clinical study, rosemary essential oil produced a significant enhancement on cognitive performance (in particular overall quality of memory and secondary memory factors) in people who smelt it and were then tested on different aspects of cognitive functioning
Hypnotic/sedative	*Valeriana officinalis* (valerian)	Herbs in the hypnotic/sedative class are vital in the management of those with sleep disorders where their prime function is to induce sleep. Valerian root is one of the most widely used botanicals for this purpose. Valerenic acid, one of the many constituents within valerian, influences the activity of neurons mediated by the GABAergic system, thought to be involved in sleep induction and sleep maintenance.
Musculoskeletal spasmolytic/ relaxant	*Viburnum opulus* (cramp bark)	Musculoskeletal spasmolytic/relaxants, such as the bark of *Viburnum opulus* help to reduce or relieve involuntary muscle contractions, common in neurological conditions such as Parkinson's disease. Greive suggests the benefit of *Viburnum opulus* in all nervous symptom conditions stating it 'has been used with success in cramps and spasms of all kinds'
Nervine trophorestorative	*Avena sativa* (oat seed)	Nervine trophorestoratives are those herbs that return the nervous system back to its natural balance. Oat seed is a gentle, rejuvenating herb with a restorative effect on the nervous system. It is specific as a supportive tonic for nervous exhaustion. The Eclectics considered oat seed tincture a primary nerve tonic stating, 'It ranks among the most important restoratives for conditions depending upon nervous prostration, and for the nervous exhaustion'
Nervine tonic	*Passiflora incarnata* (passionflower)	The botanical class of herbs known as nervine tonic improves the tone, vigour and function of the nervous system. *Passiflora incarnata* is a visually stunning purple flower indigenous to the Southern USA and Central and South America. Interestingly it contains constituents that are sedating (such as passiflorine) but also contains constituents that are stimulating (the harmala compounds). The aerial parts of passionflower are multifaceted and include mild sedative, anxiolytic, spasmolytic and hypnotic actions upon the neurological system making it the ideal nervine tonic.
Nervine relaxant	*Eschscholzia californica* (Californian poppy)	Nervine relaxants such as *Eschscholzia californica* calm and relax the nervous system thereby defusing nervous tension. *Eschscholzia californica* is a member of the Papaveraceae family yet differs from its family member the opium poppy in that it has a normalising effect on the nervous system rather than a narcotic effect. It is specifically indicated for anxiety and conditions or situations in which anxiety plays a role, such as fear of public speaking. In vivo *Eschscholzia californica* prevents the synthesis of adrenaline and also activates benzodiazepine receptors, leading to less anxiety and has a sedative effect thus providing a possible explanation for its relaxant properties
Nervine stimulant	*Theobroma cacao* (cocoa)	Nervine stimulants stimulate the nervous system and increase energy levels. *Theobroma cacao* contains compounds known as methylxanthines, two of which, caffeine and theobromine (a metabolite of caffeine), appear to be the most likely for the stimulant effects of *Theobroma cacao*. Caffeine increases feelings of alertness and mental energy while also providing improvement in feelings of wellbeing at lower doses

Source: see page 1359.

ROLE OF THE NATUROPATH — PSYCHOLOGICAL SYSTEM

Traditional interpretation

The in-depth coverage pertaining to disorders of the psychological system in the Eclectics' scripts suggests their occurrence was common. While there was certainly no understanding of the effects of neurotransmitters, amino acids and the like, the involvement of other body systems (such as the reproductive system) in the pathogenesis of psychological disorders was well established. Similarly to modern naturopathic practice, the Eclectics largely prescribed nervine herbs for treatment of psychological dysfunction, favouring botanicals such as pulsatilla, passiflora, viburnum, gossypium, gelsemium, ammoniated tincture of valerian, scutellaria and cypripedium.[8] While Ellingwood makes mention of *Hypericum perforatum*, one of the most well-used botanicals in modern practice, there is no discussion of its therapeutic application for melancholy; rather, he singles out its use as a sedative herb useful for diseases afflicting women.[6] Felter[9] also questions *Hypericum perforatum* stating: 'It has, without question, a value in nervous disorders and should be more fully studied and tested, but miraculous powers should not be hoped for from it'. Little could the Eclectics know that *Hypericum perforatum* would gain such epic popularity in the treatment of psychological disorders.

As for the treatment of patients with psychological disorders there are hints that they may have been treated with some indifference. Thomas stresses that 'they (the patients) should not be allowed to observe annoyance or disgust or disinterestedness on the part of the medical adviser…' a hint perhaps that patients were not viewed by practitioners with the same seriousness and care as they are today. However, the Eclectics did not rely solely on the prescription of botanicals in their therapy of the psychological system. External factors such as a change of environment were also recognised as being therapeutic, particularly a move away from the excitements of the city to the country where there was fresh air, plenty of sunshine, a nourishing diet and regular hours — the cornerstones of naturopathic therapy.[8] While there is no discussion of psychologists and the like, the Eclectics document that the 'patient's mind must be gotten away from self'[8] an acknowledgement that mental status was most definitely taken into consideration.

Modern interpretation

The understanding of the structures that make up the psychological system and subsequent naturopathic treatment of it has increased substantially over time. Modern naturopathy acknowledges that there is no one causative factor in the pathogenesis of psychological disease applicable to the general population, instead it is recognised that a range of factors that include stress, dietary, and lifestyle habits such as substance abuse or nutritional deficiency, genetics and/or hormonal status may all influence an individual's risk of psychological illness. The modern naturopath draws upon specific botanical classes such as the antidepressants and adaptogens (discussed below) to regulate the workings of the psychological system. Simultaneously they assist with better assimilation and absorption of nutrients and the use of food as medicine or work on other symptoms of the body such as the reproductive system if applicable. Where necessary they may prescribe the use of vitamin, mineral, and amino acid supplements to further enhance the workings on the psychological system.

Specific herbal medicine classes

There are a number of herbal medicines for the modern naturopath to choose from when treating dysfunctions of the psychological system. However, it is imperative that these botanicals be prescribed in the correct context as well as checked against interactions with any allopathic medicines the patient may already be taking. (See the interactions tables at the end of the book.)

The *adaptogens* are particularly useful in the treatment of depression and anxiety where they assist the patient in adapting to stressful situations. Equally useful for the same situations are the *adrenal trophorestoratives* which function to support and restore the proper functioning of the adrenal glands. Tonics are indicated in most diseased states, however, none more so than when the psychological system is not functioning optimally.

Antidepressants are the first line of treatment in patients presenting with depression as these function to alleviate depression. *Thymoleptics* are equally important and work to elevate the mood. *Anxiolytics* are a first-line treatment for patients presenting with anxiety. Depending on the severity of symptoms *antiarrhythmics*, that help to regulate the heartbeat, may also be prescribed in conjunction. Modern clinical research has also provided a number of herbs that work directly to alter neurotransmitter status. These include *dopaminergic and serotonin agonists* and may be useful in a number of conditions affecting the nervous system. Herbs that alter neurotransmitter status are summarised in Table 22.3.

INVESTIGATIONS

Allopathic testing

The recommended approach with suspected neurological or psychological conditions is to organise a general health screen with follow-up testing specific for a condition. A general summary is included in Table 22.4.

TABLE 22.4 Investigations

Assessment	Reference range	Interpretation
Full blood count	Various	Elucidates any underlying pathology. Refer to Ch 12 for a full discussion
Liver function test	Various	Elucidates any underlying pathology. Refer to Ch 11 for a full discussion
C-reactive protein test (CRP)	<5.0 mg/L	C-reactive protein (CRP) is an acute phase protein that plays a major role in the regulation of the inflammatory response. The level of CRP rises when there is inflammation throughout the body. Inflammation plays a central role in the process of heart disease particularly atherosclerosis
Vitamin B_{12} (serum)	120–680 pmol/L	Levels may be reduced in folate deficiency or megaloblastic anaemia due to vitamin B_{12} deficiency
Folate (red cell and serum)	Red cell: 360–1400 nmol/L Serum: 7–45 nmol/L	Levels may be reduced in megaloblastic anaemia
Vitamin D (25-hydroxy)	General consensus is that readings should be >100 nmol/L, however many labs use the range 51–160 Mild deficiency: 25–50 nmol/L Moderate deficiency: 12.5–25 nmol/L Severe deficiency: <12.5 nmol/L	Essential to assess for deficiency, however assesses post-liver hydroxylation only

Continued

TABLE 22.4 Investigations—cont'd

Assessment	Reference range	Interpretation
Vitamin D (1,25-dihydroxy)	35–120 pmol/L	Assesses useable vitamin D levels in the body post liver and kidney hydroxylation
Iron studies	Ferritin:15–200 micrograms/L Iron:10–30 μmol/L Iron binding capacity: 45–80 μmol/L Transferrin saturation: 0.15–0.45 (15–45%) Transferrin: 1.7–3.0 g/L	Assesses anaemia and associated neurological and/or psychological manifestations. Also assesses for overload or acute iron poisoning
Magnesium (plasma or serum)	Neonate: 0.6–0.9 mmol/L Adult: 0.8–1.0 mmol/L	Reliance on readings is controversial; however, detection of hypomagnesaemia may be the cause of unexplained cardiac arrhythmias, neuromuscular disorders, refractory hypocalcaemia Patients with clinical features suggesting hypocalcaemia and a normal plasma calcium, or with refractory hypocalcaemia/hypokalaemia, should have plasma magnesium measured
Calcium (serum or plasma)	Total calcium: 2.10–2.60 mmol/L Corrected calcium: 2.15–2.60 mmol/L Ionised calcium: 1.16–1.30 mmol/L	(i) Diagnosis of hypercalcaemia. Investigation of patients with clinical features of hypercalcaemia or other features of hyperparathyroidism; malignancy, especially lung, multiple myeloma, kidney, bony metastases; sarcoidosis; vitamin D or vitamin A toxicity (ii) Diagnosis of hypocalcaemia. Investigation of patients with clinical features of hypocalcaemia or other features of hypoparathyroidism, renal failure, osteomalacia or rickets. Evaluation of patients after thyroid or parathyroid surgery, or during massive blood transfusion
Homocysteine	5–15 μmol/L If there is established vascular disease it is desirable that the fasting concentration is <10 μmol/L	Mild hyperhomocysteinaemia is an established risk factor for atherosclerosis and vascular disease Elevated homocysteine levels may result from low levels of folic acid, vitamin B_6, or vitamin B_{12}, some drugs and renal impairment, as well as a number of inherited defects
Urea and electrolytes	Various	Abnormalities in electrolytes or urea can cause marked effects on neurological and psychological function (see Ch 17 for full description)
Creatinine	Child (<12 years): 0.04–0.08 mmol/L Adult female: 0.05–0.11 mmol/L Adult male: 0.06–0.12 mmol/L	Indicates impaired renal filtration which can affect neurological and psychological function
Glucose	Venous plasma or serum fasting: 3.0–5.4 mmol/L ≥2 hour post-prandial 'Random': 3.0–7.7 mmol/L	Assesses blood sugar levels. Full discussion in Ch 21
Thyroid function (TSH, T3, T4), thyroid antibodies, urinary iodine	TSH: 0.4–5.0m IU/L (depends on method) fT3: 4.0–8.0 pmol/L fT4: 10–25 pmol/L. Values up to 35 pmol/L may be acceptable for patients on full replacement therapy with thyroxine Urinary iodine: >100 micrograms/L	Assesses thyroid function. Dysfunctional thyroid function is associated with alterations in the neurological and psychological systems. Full discussion in Ch 21
Cortisol (free) — urinary	100–300 nmol/24 hours	**Increased levels**: primary or secondary adrenocortical hyperfunction, also seen in obesity, stress, depression and alcoholism
Melatonin	Fluctuations occur during a 24 hr cycle. The peak levels are seen between 2 and 4 am. These levels should drop between 6 and 8 am	**Increased levels**: associated with high levels of fatigue, higher levels have been found in patients with systemic exertion intolerance disease (SEID) in the early part of the sleep cycle. It is normal for children and adolescents to have higher levels than adults **Decreased levels:** associated with autism spectrum disorder, insomnia, poor sleep quality, seasonal affective disorder (SAD) and mood disorders. It is normal for levels to decrease with age

Other evaluations

A range of other evaluations and tests are used to assess neurological and psychological function, including:

- A **medical history**, including an evaluation of risk factors such as age, CAD, diabetes and smoking
- A **mental status examination:**
  - Intellect
  - Orientation
  - Attention span
  - Recent memory
  - Remote memory
  - New learning
  - Judgement
  - Perception
- Cranial nerve assessment
- Reflex testing
  - Biceps
  - Triceps
  - Brachioradialis
  - Patellar
  - Achilles
- Motor system assessment
  - Strength assessment
  - Muscle strength
  - Coordination and balance assessment
- Sensory system assessment
- General physical examination
  - Including blood pressure, temperature, auscultation, palpation and others
  - An electroencephalograph (EEG) — the recording of electrical activity along the scalp produced by the firing of neurons within the brain

Based on the findings of these tests, other procedures may be necessary, including:

- CT (computed tomography) scan
- MRI (magnetic resonance imaging)
- Tilt table test — ordered to evaluate syncope.

Naturopathic investigations

Naturopathic investigations are summarised in Table 22.5.

TABLE 22.5 Naturopathic investigations

Assessment	Justification
Essential fatty acid profile	Essential fatty acids play a significant role in healthy neurological function. The essential fatty acid profile provides an indication of essential fatty acid status in the body
Amino acid profile	A definitive link between amino acid imbalance and disorders of the neurological and psychological systems exists. The amino acid profile measures the status of various amino acids providing information on metabolic and nutritional imbalances
Urinary organic acids — metabolic analysis profile and cellular energy profile	Organic acids play a role in critical areas of metabolism including cellular energy production and neurotransmitter processing. This profile provides an overall assessment of the patient's health with regards to cellular health and metabolic analysis
Environmental screen	Assesses environmental toxin exposure including chlorinated pesticides, PCBs, volatile solvents, porphyrins, phthalates and parabens
Toxic metal/mineral screen	Useful tools for screening nutrient and metal status within the body. Heavy metal toxicity is known to cause neurotoxicity and is implicated in a number of neurological disorders
Functional liver detoxification profile	Impaired detoxification has been suggested in several neurological disorders and is considered to be impaired in various psychological states. Additionally, medications often impair the hepatobiliary pathways thus impeding various pathways. The functional liver detoxification profile identifies an individual's detoxification capacity and assists in the direction of treatment
Baseline hormone profile	The baseline hormone profile provides information on an individual's hormonal status and the potential impact this may have on the neurological system, e.g. disturbed sleep pattern
Adrenal hormone profile	Monitors the levels of the stress hormones cortisol and DHEA-S
Melatonin profile	Useful tool when dealing with sleep disorders. Decreased levels of melatonin may result in sleep disturbance and mood disorders
IgG/IgE/IgA food sensitivity profile	Food sensitivities are indicated in the pathogenesis of certain neurological disorders and can interfere with neurotransmitter synthesis and release
Neuroendocrine metabolites	Interprets levels of neuroendocrine metabolites such as dopamine, noradrenaline, adrenaline and serotonin within the body
Histamine	Histamine is a central nervous system neurotransmitter High levels are associated with over-methylation (>75) histadelia Low levels are associated with under-methylation (<28) histapenia
Kryptopyroles	High kryptopyroles are associated with low vitamin B_6, zinc and fatty acids

Sources: Osiecki H, Meeke F, Smith J. The encyclopaedia of clinical nutrition — the nervous system. Eagle Farm, QLD: Bioconcepts Publishing; 2004. p. 269. Buchwald D, Umali P, Umali J, et al. Chronic fatigue and the chronic fatigue syndrome: prevalence in a Pacific Northwest healthcare system. Ann Intern Med 1995; 123:81–88.

SECTION B

NEUROLOGICAL SYSTEM

Systemic exertion intolerance disease (SEID)

Throughout this chapter we will refer to this condition as SEID; however, it is also known as chronic fatigue syndrome (CFS) and myalgic encephalopathy (encephalomyelitis) (see Fig. 22.8).

Epidemiology

Variations in sampling methods, surgery instruments and diagnostic criteria are responsible for large variations in the reported prevalence estimates of SEID. The true prevalence of SEID can be determined only in large-scale community studies with adequate case detection and characterisation techniques. In the US and UK, four studies have provided a more realistic estimate of 0.2–0.7% (i.e. 200–700 cases per 100 000 population). In primary care, preliminary estimate of incidence of SEID is about 0.4%.[10,11] The prevalence of fatigue states is summarised in Table 22.6.

SEID is estimated to affect about 17 million people worldwide. It commonly affects young adults, with a peak age of onset between 20 and 40 years. The illness also appears to be more common in women (in a ratio of 2–3 : 1). Individuals from upper socioeconomic groups are not widely affected by SEID.[12] Rather, some studies suggest that fatigue syndromes may be more common in people from more socially disadvantaged groups.[11] One study has suggested that nurses and similar healthcare professionals have a high rate of SEID, indicating that specific occupations may be at risk.[13]

SEID is less common in children than adults, affecting between 0.2% and 2.3% of children and adolescents, and is more common in adolescents than younger children.[14] Reporting of somatic symptoms, including fatigue, increases during adolescence and early adulthood. Most children with SEID have impaired school attendance or

TABLE 22.6 Prevalence of fatigue states

	Prolonged fatigue	Chronic fatigue	SEID
Community studies	5–20%	1–10%	0.2–0.7%
Primary care	10–25%	5–15%	0.5–2.5%
Tertiary referrals for fatigue	70%	40%	10–15%

Prolonged fatigue = prolonged and disabling fatigue lasting for at least 1 month; chronic fatigue = prolonged and disabling fatigue lasting for at least 6 months; SEID = prolonged and disabling fatigue lasting for at least 6 months, unexplained by other medical or psychological conditions. *Source:* Lawrie SM, Manders DN, Geddes JR et al. A population-based incidence study of chronic fatigue. Psychol Med 1997; 27:343–353.

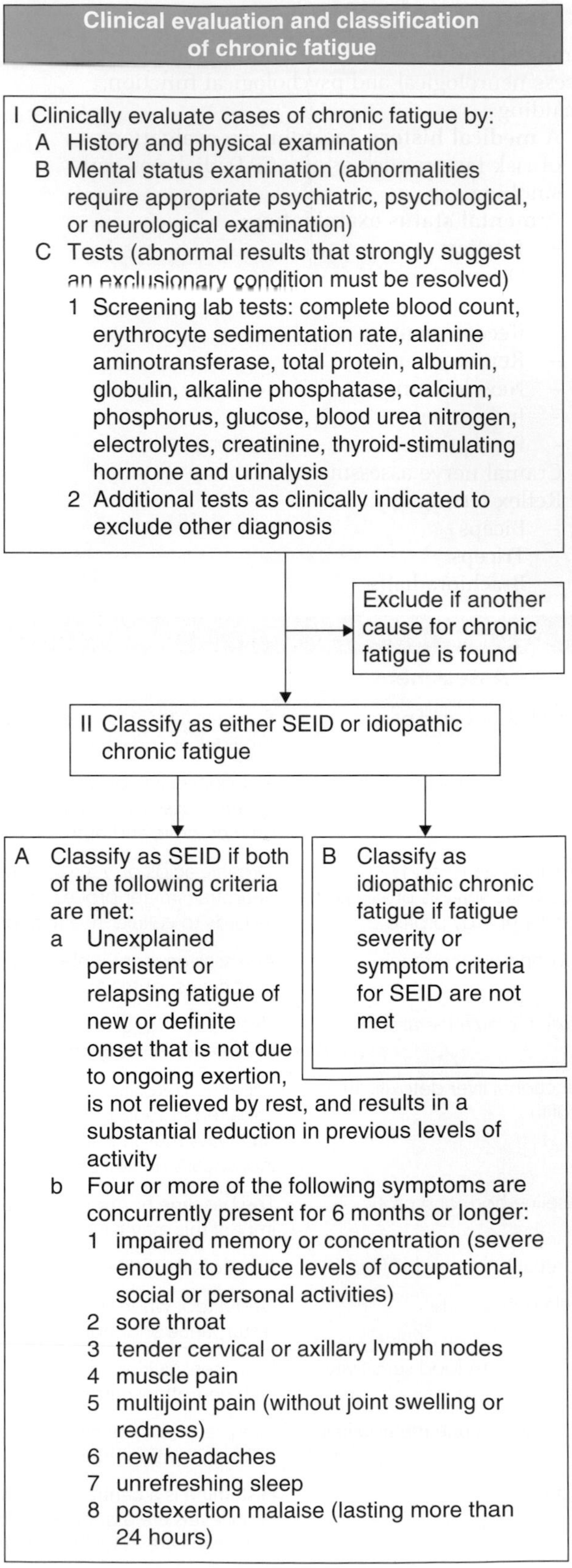

Clinical evaluation and classification of chronic fatigue
I Clinically evaluate cases of chronic fatigue by:
A History and physical examination
B Mental status examination (abnormalities require appropriate psychiatric, psychological, or neurological examination)
C Tests (abnormal results that strongly suggest an exclusionary condition must be resolved)
1 Screening lab tests: complete blood count, erythrocyte sedimentation rate, alanine aminotransferase, total protein, albumin, globulin, alkaline phosphatase, calcium, phosphorus, glucose, blood urea nitrogen, electrolytes, creatinine, thyroid-stimulating hormone and urinalysis
2 Additional tests as clinically indicated to exclude other diagnosis
Exclude if another cause for chronic fatigue is found
II Classify as either SEID or idiopathic chronic fatigue
A Classify as SEID if both of the following criteria are met:
a Unexplained persistent or relapsing fatigue of new or definite onset that is not due to ongoing exertion, is not relieved by rest, and results in a substantial reduction in previous levels of activity
b Four or more of the following symptoms are concurrently present for 6 months or longer:
1 impaired memory or concentration (severe enough to reduce levels of occupational, social or personal activities)
2 sore throat
3 tender cervical or axillary lymph nodes
4 muscle pain
5 multijoint pain (without joint swelling or redness)
6 new headaches
7 unrefreshing sleep
8 postexertion malaise (lasting more than 24 hours)
B Classify as idiopathic chronic fatigue if fatigue severity or symptom criteria for SEID are not met

FIGURE 22.8 Chronic fatigue and SEID.
Source: Kliegman. Nelson textbook of pediatrics. 18th edn. Saunders, 2007.

performance and a decrease in social activities and it is thought to be the commonest current cause of long-term absence from school. Studies of adolescents have found a point prevalence of 0.4–1.1% for chronic fatigue and 0.1–0.5% for SEID using the adult diagnostic criteria.[15]

Classification

While it is unlikely that SEID is a single illness, defining different subgroups by symptom profile or aetiological factors has been difficult. One suggestion is to classify on the basis of onset of symptoms — from those with an abrupt onset to those with more insidious origins. Patients with an abrupt onset seem to have a favourable prognosis. There is one more difference that has been observed: a minority of cases have long-term illness with severe disability, multiple symptoms, and overlapping with other functional somatic disorders; most cases have short-term illness with less disability and fewer symptoms.[16]

Aetiology

Clinically, SEID has the characteristics of a neuropsychiatric disorder. Its major symptoms (disturbed perception of fatigue and pain, sleep disturbance, neurocognitive difficulties and mood disturbances) suggest a non-localised disturbance of central nervous system function. However, its pathophysiological basis remains obscure. There is no established single cause for SEID. A diverse array of aetiologies has been proposed (including immunological, infective, metabolic, central nervous system dysfunction, neuroendocrine and psychiatric hypotheses, genetic polymorphisms, neuroinflammation, nutritional deficiencies, autoimmunity), but no simple explanatory model has been supported by well-controlled studies. Indeed, the heterogeneity within patient groups labelled as having SEID makes it likely that aetiology and pathogenesis are multifactorial.[17–20]

INFECTION

The infective triggers are a strong argument for the development of SEID. According to most research, viral and/or fungal infections are deemed the most common causes with a significant amount of supportive research including:

- Numerous geographical clusters of SEID-like illnesses have been reported suggesting an infectious component to those possible 'epidemics'
- Many patients with SEID report that the illness began with a flu-like illness, particularly in children and adolescents[18]
- Sore throat, myalgias and lymphadenopathy (some of SEID minor criteria) resemble symptoms of an acute viral infection
- Viral and infections provoke the immune system to increase production of cytokines and alteration of HPA axis. This can induce variable fatigue and alter sleep pattern.

Various viruses and virus groups have been implicated in SEID at some time; these include Epstein-Barr virus (EBV), cytomegalovirus, parvovirus B_{19}, Brucellae, *Toxoplasma gondii, Chlamydia burnetii, Chlamydia pneumoniae*, human herpes virus-6 (HHV-6), group B coxsackieviruses (CVB), human T-cell leukaemia virus II-like virus, spumavirus, hepatitis C virus, human lentiviruses, mycoplasma, *Rickettsia rickettsii, Borrelia burgdorferi*, herpes virus-7, candida, *Giardia*[21] and others. Organisms associated with SEID are listed in Table 22.7. It seems likely that an initial infection or stress leads to a state of decreased immunological resistance and immune memory dysfunction, which promotes reactivation of previously acquired infections, thereby maintaining SEID symptoms.[22]

TABLE 22.7 Organisms associated with SEID

Organism	Evidence
Epstein-Barr virus (EBV)	Infectious mononucleosis (glandular fever) can trigger SEID. Studies have shown evidence for active EBV infection in patients with persistent, unexplained chronic illnesses including chronic fatigue Higher antibody titres in patients with symptoms compatible with SEID
Human herpes virus (HHV-6)	Active infection with HHV-6 may trigger and perpetuate some cases of SEID, because HHV-6 infection is also associated with encephalitis, multiple sclerosis and seizure disorders, each of which has clinical features that overlap with SEID Active infection with HHV-6 is present in a substantial fraction of patients with SEID. In some patients with SEID and multiple sclerosis, increased levels of HHV-6 antibody and HHV-6 DNA were detected
Non-viral infections: Q fever, Lyme disease (*Borrelia burgdorferi*), *Mycoplasma*	In one study, the percentage of *M. genus* infection was found to be 52% in SEID patients and only 15% in healthy individuals. *Mycoplasma fermentans*, *M. hominis* and *M. penetrans* were detected in 32%, 9% and 6% of the SEID patients while they were detected in 8%, 3% and 2% of the healthy control subjects respectively

Sources: Abashi DV, Eastman HB, Owen CB et al. Frequent HHV-6 reactivation in multiple sclerosis (MS) and chronic fatigue syndrome (CFS) patients. J ClinVirol 2000; 16(3):179–191. Choppa PC, Vojdani A, Tagle C et al. Multiplex PCR for the detection of *Mycoplasma fermentans*, *M. hominis* and *M. penetrans* in cell cultures and blood samples of patients with chronic fatigue syndrome. Mol Cell Probes 1998; 12:301–308. Homes GP, Kaplan JE, Stewart JA et al. A cluster of patients with a chronic mononucleosis-like syndrome. Is Epstein- Barr virus the cause? JAMA 1987; 257(17):2297–2302. Jones JF, Nisenbaum R, Soloman L et al. Chronic fatigue syndrome and other fatiguing illnesses in adolescents: a population-based study. J Adolesc Health 2004; 35:34–40. Komaroff AL. Is human herpesvirus-6 a trigger for chronic fatigue syndrome? J Clin Virol 2006; 37(1):839–846. Straus SE, Tosato G, Armstrong G et al. Persisting illness and fatigue in adults with evidence of Epstein-Barr virus infection. Ann Intern Med 1985; 102(1):7–16.

A 2013 study found the presence of mycotoxins in the urine of 104 out of 112 (93%) SEID patients. An environmental history found that 90% of the patients had current or past exposure to water-damaged buildings, therefore the finding is not surprising. Prior testing on a healthy control population with no history of exposure to water-damaged buildings or other mouldy environments found no trace of mycotoxins in the urine. What this study indicates is that exposure to mouldy environments likely leads to the presence of mycotoxins in the urine, regardless of SEID state. What is interesting is that patients with mycotoxin exposure in water-damaged buildings often present with clinical features that resemble SEID. This is an area that warrants further investigation. The three mycotoxins which were tested for and found to be present were aflatoxins, ochratoxin A and macrocyclic trichothecenes.[23]

IMMUNOLOGICAL

Immune dysfunction is recognised as part of the SEID pathogenesis but has received less attention than other theories such as neurological or endocrine dysfunction. Substantial evidence suggests that many SEID patients have one or more immunological abnormalities:[18,24,25]

- As discussed earlier, SEID might be related to virus reactivation, e.g. Epstein-Barr and human herpes-virus 6
- Fungal infections and mycotoxins can influence the immune system
- Increased production of some cytokines has been reported, especially interleukins (IL-1, IL-2, IL-6) and other cytokines, which can explain the symptom of fatigue
- Many studies have shown dysfunction of natural killer (NK) cells. Some people with SEID have a reduced number and responsiveness of natural killer cells; others have shown an increased number (along with increased B lymphocytes). A study found that SEID patients tend to have lower circulating levels of IL-16 and IL-7. IL-7 is required for T-cell, B-cell and NK-cell proliferation and survival, and might explain the reduced level of NK cells noted in SEID[26]
- A reduced CD8 suppressor cell population and increased activation markers on CD8 cells were found in patients with major SEID symptoms
- Recent research results suggest that early life immune insults (ELII) including developmental immunotoxicity (DIT), which is induced by xenobiotics, may offer an important clue to the origin(s) of SEID. The developing immune system is a sensitive and novel target for environmental insult (xenobiotic, infectious agents, stress) with major ramifications for postnatal health risks[27]
- EBV viraemia is associated with cell-mediated immune activation and increased tryptophan (a precursor of the neurotransmitter 5-hydroxytryptamine or serotonin), degradation, which may partly account for the symptoms (such as mood disturbances) found in this disorder. It has been shown that ongoing EBV replication increases levels of interferon-gamma (IFN-γ), which triggers several antiviral mechanisms in target cells including the induction of indoleamine-2,3-dioxygenase (IDO), which degrades the essential amino acid tryptophan[28]
- A systematic review of 23 case control studies found that patients with SEID had a different immune response to exercise compared to controls. This included a more pronounced response to oxidative stress and immune cell gene expression profile alteration[29]
- An analysis of responses to a mild stressor found that in patients with SEID, a distinct plasma immune signature occurred in the first 3 years of the illness which is not present in patients who have had SEID for longer than 3 years. Cytokine levels remain high until the 3-year mark after which the immune system shows signs of exhaustion and cytokine levels drop.[30]

Collectively these results point to chronic low-level immune system activation, but their relationship to the symptoms of SEID remains unclear. Some findings suggest that the degree of cellular immune activation could be associated with the severity of the physical symptoms, cognitive complaints, and perceived impairment associated with SEID.

DISTURBANCE OF CNS FUNCTION

Several symptoms reported by SEID patients — fatigue; impaired concentration, attention and memory; and headache — suggest that the central nervous system may be involved in the pathophysiology of the syndrome. Several lines of evidence support this theory.

Neuroendocrine and neurochemical dysfunction

Several studies have demonstrated abnormal function of the hypothalamic-pituitary-adrenocortical (HPA) axis. Reduced basal cortisol output has been found in serial samples of blood or saliva or 24-h urinary output (reverse of that seen in major depression). About one-third of patients with SEID have been shown to exhibit hypocortisolism. There is evidence for heightened negative feedback and glucocorticoid receptor function and for impaired ACTH and cortisol responses to a variety of challenges. No evidence indicates a specific or uniform dysfunction of the HPA axis. On the contrary, the dysfunction seems to be heterogeneous and of multifactorial origin as many factors such as inactivity, sleep disturbance, associated psychiatric disorders, medication, and ongoing stress can impinge on the HPA axis.[31] One thing that is unclear is at what stage of the disease these changes occur, as most studies were largely undertaken on samples of patients who had been ill for several years. Changes occurring in the HPA axis at a later stage of the illness do appear to be of clinical importance, since their reversal using supplementation with a low dose of hydrocortisone can improve fatigue in some patients.

In addition, studies have demonstrated abnormalities of CNS serotonin (5-HT) physiology in patients with SEID. Studies suggest an increased turnover or an up-regulation of 5-HT in the CNS. In contrast, patients with clinical depression demonstrate an opposite pattern of hypercortisolism and have a reduced serotonergic function. 5-HT is known to be important in the physiological control of sleep, appetite and mood.

Abnormalities in the hypothalamic-pituitary-adrenal (HPA) axis and serotonin pathways in SEID patients, suggest an altered physiological response to stress.[32]

Other studies have looked at dehydroepiandrostenedione (DHEA) and its sulfate (DHEA-s) in SEID patients. The role of DHEA and DHEA-s, though unclear, could be related to mood, sleep and energy. Some results reported DHEA and DHEA-s levels significantly lower in SEID patients as compared with healthy subjects. However, there were conflicting results with other studies.[33]

Neuroimaging studies

Magnetic resonance imaging (MRI) and single photon emission computed tomography (SPECT) studies are generally consistent in demonstrating some abnormalities, such as abnormalities in the subcortical white matter and reduced blood flow to many areas of the brain, most notably the brain stem in SEID patients. However, the significance and clinical application of these findings remain uncertain.

Autonomic nervous system

Several symptoms of SEID patients evoke features of an altered autonomic nervous system: hypotension with bradycardia or orthostatic tachycardia, hypothermia, episodes of sweating, profound pallor, syncope and palpitations.[34]

A number of studies have found an increased rate of neural mediated hypotension, while other studies have shown evidence of increased sympathetic activity and/or parasympathetic underactivity.

Neuropsychological factors

Cognitive problems are some of the most disruptive and disabling symptoms of SEID, as many as 85% of patients complain of impairments in attention, concentration, and memory abilities.[35] As a recent review of neuropsychological studies in SEID confirmed, the weight of the evidence suggests a modest but significant deficit in information processing, impaired working memory, and poor learning of information.[36] Coexisting psychological distress or psychiatric disorder also may contribute to neurocognitive deficits.

Psychiatric disorders

Some researchers have postulated that SEID is primarily a psychiatric disorder because of absence of a consistent biological marker. Several researchers believe that SEID and related disorders are manifestations of a psychiatric condition such as somatisation disorder, hypochondriasis, major depression or atypical depression.

Indeed, persons with SEID have an increased prevalence of current and lifetime mood disorders, primarily major depression, compared with other chronically ill subjects or healthy comparison subjects.

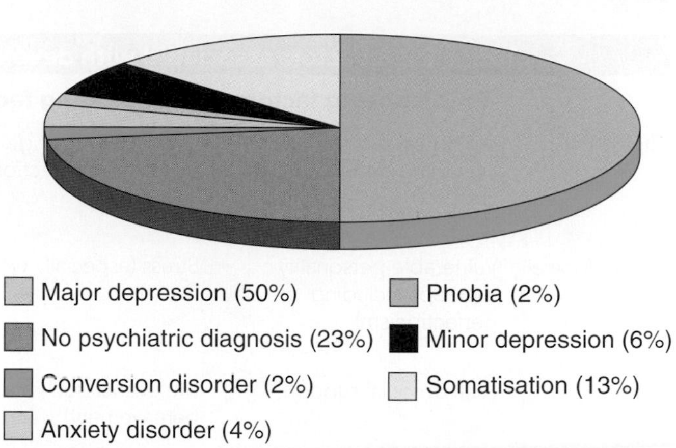

FIGURE 22.9 Psychiatric conditions associated with SEID.
Source: Browne T, Chalder T. Chronic fatigue syndrome. Psychiatry 2009; 8(5):153–157.

Generalised anxiety disorder and somatoform disorder also occur at a higher rate in SEID subjects than in the general population.[37]

In most, but not all cases, the mood or anxiety disorder precedes the onset of SEID as illustrated in Fig. 22.9.

Genetic factors

The family and twin data suggest that prolonged fatigue and SEID–like illness may be familial and that genetic effects could be important. Studies suggest that there is a genetic propensity to suffer from chronic fatigue, with the concordance between monozygotic twins more than twice that of dizygotic twins.[38]

Food and environmental intolerances

Some patients with SEID have reported various food intolerances that can exacerbate symptoms. It has been suggested that intolerances to multiple foods is probably not a cause or the effect of chronic fatigue, but can be one of the manifestations of the somatisation trait expressed in these patients.[39] A 2-year prospective study of 55 adolescents and young adults with SEID found that cow's milk protein intolerance is a common problem and contributor to SEID symptoms.[40] There is also evidence linking SEID to sick building syndrome (SBS). The study also showed that the fatigue related to SBS including SEID is significantly more likely to improve than fatigue identified in sporadic cases of SEID.[41] Overlapping of symptoms also occurs between SEID and Gulf War syndrome[42] and multiple chemical sensitivity syndrome (MCS).[43] Heavy metals may play a role and cadmium has been hypothesised to be a causative agent.[44]

Oxidative stress

Overlapping that occurs between SEID and MCS is not with regard to symptoms only, but possibly in aetiology as well. It has been suggested that in both of these conditions stress can lead to a chronic pathology by inducing a self-perpetuating vicious cycle based on elevated levels of

TABLE 22.8 Factors associated with development systemic exertion intolerance disease

	Predisposing factors	Precipitating factors	Perpetuating factors
Biological	Biological vulnerability (including genetic factors)	Acute disease (e.g. Epstein-Barr infection)	Pathophysiology (mainly neuroendocrine) Excessive inactivity (or oscillation between activity and inactivity 0 Sleep disorder
Psychological	Vulnerable personality (perhaps including perfectionism)	Stress (especially work stress)	Depression and anxiety Unhelpful beliefs (such as 'activity is harmful') Avoidance of activity Heightened perception of fatigue and other symptoms
Social	Lack of social support	Life events (such as bereavement)	Reinforcement of unhelpful beliefs (e.g. by misleading information) Chronic social or work stress

Source: Sharpe M. Chronic fatigue syndrome. Psychiatric Aspects of General Medicine 2008; 36(9):452–453.

nitric oxide and its potent oxidant product, peroxynitrite.[44] ML Pall[45] has proposed a theory explaining the aetiology of SEID based on these biochemical mechanisms. This theory starts with the observation that about 70% of cases of SEID are preceded by an infectious episode and viral, bacterial or other infections are known to induce elevated levels of inflammatory cytokines, including TNF-α, IL-6 and IFN-γ. These cytokines in turn induce elevated levels of inducible nitric oxide synthetase (iNOS) which then synthesises increased amounts of nitric oxide. Nitric oxide reacts rapidly with superoxide to form the potent oxidant peroxynitrite. Six different positive feedback loops are proposed such that elevated peroxynitrite can act to increase levels of both nitric oxide and superoxide, thus generating more peroxynitrite. The elevated levels of peroxynitrite and nitric oxide affect the tissues involved, producing symptoms of SEID. This can be summarised as follows:

Six positive feedback loops, each increasing nitric oxide or superoxide:

1. Inactivation of the mitochondrial Mn-superoxide dismutase (SOD)
2. Activation of iNOS transcription via NF-κB
3. Activation of TNF-α, IL-1β, IL-6 and IFN-γ transcription via NF-κB
4. Activation of constitutive NOS activities via increase in cytoplasmic calcium ion
5. Increased superoxide generation via xanthine oxide activation
6. Increased superoxide generation by nitric oxide and peroxynitrite via the mitochondrial electron transport chain.

Neuromuscular disorder

Although muscle pain and complaints of muscle fatigability are common, there is little objective evidence that symptoms have a primary neuromuscular origin. Given the importance of mental fatigue and fatigability, central rather than peripheral explanations are more likely. There is increasing evidence suggesting that muscular biochemical abnormalities may play a role in SEID associated fatigue. There appears to be profound intramuscular dysfunction regarding acid generation and clearance, tending towards an overutilisation of the lactate dehydrogenase pathway following relatively low-level activity. The precise mechanism underlying the dysfunction is still not known.[46]

Poisoning

Exposure to industrial solvents, insecticides or pesticides might induce a syndrome resembling SEID. Long-term, low-dose exposure to pentachlorophenol (PCP), hexachlorocyclohexanes (HCH), polychlorinated biphenyls (PCBs), and hexachlorobenzene (HCB) is suspected to cause clinical symptoms, such as chronic infections of the upper respiratory tract, general fatigue and neurotoxicity. Some patients with SEID showed elevated HCB serum levels. The incidence of HCB contamination (>2.0 ppb) was 45% in a SEID group compared with 21% in a non-SEID control group.[47]

Others

Other aetiological factors including anaemia, hypoglycaemia, thyroid function, genetics and epigenetic factors, blatant nutritional deficiencies, peripheral tissue issues and other considerations should be reviewed for the SEID patient. Thorough assessment, questioning and investigations should elucidate the cause — see Table 22.8.

Overview

SEID is a condition characterised by persistent, medically unexplained fatigue, lasting for at least 6 months and accompanied by several other unexplained physical, constitutional and neuropsychological symptoms and severe functional disability.[48]

DEFINITION

As there were no proper diagnostic features and definitions, early studies of SEID were limited. In 1994, a consensus was reached on a case definition from the US Centers for Disease Control and Prevention (CDC) based upon symptoms and the exclusion of other illnesses.[48] Many questions have been raised about these symptom criteria, such as a lack of specificity with regard to the symptom severity.[49] Heterogeneity has also been found within samples of patients with chronic fatigue.[50]

SEID was first proposed as a diagnostic label in 1988 to classify a condition characterised by severe fatigue and exhaustion after minimal physical and mental effort accompanied by other unexplained somatic symptoms. It was first introduced partly as an acceptable clinical alternative to the term myalgic encephalomyelitis, which described a similar presentation and had been coined in 1956 to describe an illness that affected the medical staff of the Royal Free Hospital. The most widely supported scientific case definition is the 1994 definition from the CDC, which was considered the standard. However, in 2015, the Institute of Medicine redefined the diagnostic criteria for SEID/CFS while requesting its name be changed from CFS to SEID.[51] These diagnostic criteria focus on the most specific clinical features of the disease. While these criteria are intentionally restrictive to aid in research identification of symptoms, they may not always be an appropriate tool in a clinical setting with a patient.

SEID is a symptom-based diagnosis without distinguishing physical examination findings. Regardless of the pathogenesis, those with SEID have substantially impaired functional status resulting in significant personal and economic morbidity.

SEID is best regarded as an 'illness' (a subjective state that can only be defined by reference to the sick individual) rather than a 'disease'. 'Disability' arises when illness interferes with the individual's ability to function normally. People with SEID are clearly ill, and are often significantly disabled, even though an underlying disease process has not yet been identified.[52]

Many theories (immunological, infective, metabolic, central nervous system dysfunction, neuroendocrine and psychiatric) have been put forward to explain the cause of SEID. Many pathogens have been proposed as aetiological agents in SEID. However, to date there is no consistent evidence that a single infectious agent causes SEID. Despite almost two decades of intensive study the condition remains without diagnostic laboratory findings or an established pathophysiology. This lack of aetiological clarity contributes to the stigmatisation of patients and represents a primary impediment towards progress in understanding and treating the condition. The immune system and interrelated central nervous system stress outflow pathways such as the autonomic nervous system (ANS) and hypothalamic-pituitary-adrenal (HPA) axis have remained active areas of investigation.

1994 case definition for CFS [SEID] from Centers for Disease Control and Prevention (CDC)

Characterised by persistent or relapsing unexplained chronic fatigue:

- Fatigue lasts for at least 6 months
- Fatigue is of new or definite onset
- Fatigue is not the result of organic disease or of continuing exertion
- Fatigue is not alleviated by rest
- Fatigue results in a substantial reduction in previous occupational, educational, social and personal activities

Four or more of the following symptoms concurrently present for 6 months:

- Impaired memory or concentration
- Sore throat
- Tender cervical or axillary lymph nodes
- Muscle pain
- Pain in several joints
- New headaches
- Unrefreshing sleep
- Malaise after exertion.

Exclusion criteria:

- Medical condition explaining fatigue
- Major depressive disorder (psychotic features) or bipolar disorder
- Schizophrenia, dementia, or delusional disorder
- Anorexia nervosa, bulimia nervosa
- Alcohol or substance abuse
- Severe obesity.

Source: Prins J B, van der Meer JWM, Bleijenberg G. Chronic fatigue syndrome: a review. Lancet 2006; 367:346–355.

Oxford Criteria

The 1995 Oxford consensus meeting agreed to establish a set of diagnostic criteria for CFS [SEID] now known as Oxford Criteria, which include:

- Fatigue of at least 6 months' duration
- Definite onset
- Impaired function (in activities of daily living and/or social engagement)
- Physical and mental fatigability
- Myalgia
- Mood and sleep disturbance.

Exclusion criteria:

- Extensive list of physical causes
- Psychosis
- Bipolar disorder
- Substance abuse.

Source: Everett T, Stewart A. Chronic fatigue syndrome. In Donaghy M, Nicol M, eds. Cognitive-behavioural interventions in physiotherapy and occupational therapy. Elsevier; 2008, pp.147–164.

Definition for SEID from Institute of Medicine (IOM)

- Symptoms should be present for 6 months or more
- Symptoms should have moderate, substantial, or severe intensity at least one half of the time
- Postexertional malaise
- Sleep problems
- Cognitive impairment
- Orthostatic related symptoms.

Source: Beyond myalgic encephalomyelitis/chronic fatigue syndrome: redefining an illness. Committee on the Diagnostic Criteria for Myalgic Encephalomyelitis/Chronic Fatigue Syndrome; Board on the Health of Select Populations; Institute of Medicine. Washington (DC): National Academies Press (US); 2015 Feb 10.

OTHER NAMES

Systemic exertion intolerance disease (SEID, as of 2015) and chronic fatigue syndrome (CFS) are the current names accepted by most research groups for a disease that has been known by various other names in the past. Other names for SEID include: vapours, yuppie flu, neurasthenia, effort syndrome, chronic brucellosis, epidemic neuromyasthenia, chronic mononucleosis-like syndrome or chronic EBV syndrome, postviral fatigue syndrome, Iceland disease, chronic candidiasis, multichemical sensitivity syndrome, chronic fatigue and immune dysfunction syndrome (CFIDS), Royal Free Hospital disease, myalgic encephalomyelitis (ME), and others.[53,54] Currently, some of the above terms are still in use in various parts of the world. In the UK the earlier term myalgic encephalomyelitis (ME) is still in use and in the USA, the term chronic fatigue and immune dysfunction syndrome is still popular though systemic exertion intolerance disease is slowly gaining popularity.

The term myalgic encephalomyelitis was first introduced into medical publications by a *Lancet* editorial in 1956 for an epidemic of neurological symptoms among staff at the Royal Free Hospital in London, UK. Similar clusters of outbreaks were reported in other parts of the world, which then led the researchers to think a possibility of infection as an underlying cause. The term ME is pathologically incorrect for this condition (even though some research has shown the role of inflammation) as this is a heterogeneous disorder involving various factors that both precipitate and perpetuate the symptoms and disability.[55]

The scientists agreed on naming the condition chronic fatigue syndrome in the early 1990s, whereas patients preferred the terms ME or CFIDS. Patients' preference for those terms was based on the fact that in the WHO 1992 classification, neuraesthenia, which was associated with CFS was linked to psychiatry, and postviral fatigue syndrome or benign myalgic encephalitis was linked to neurology, even though the description of both disorders was identical. Currently many patients' organisations have adopted the name CFS/ME;[56] however, political lobbying suggested a possible modification of the name by terming the condition myalgic encephalopathy (encephalomyelitis). A 2016 study compared 131 people who were previously diagnosed with CFS and found that the SEID criteria categorised a similar percentage of people as the previous criteria did and noted that SEID may have an advantage in that it is easier to use.[57]

Pathogenesis

Although many aetiological factors (as discussed earlier) have been suggested, the exact pathogenesis of SEID is not completely understood. It seems obvious that the illness is the result of interactions between host and environmental factors. The following figure includes some of the suggested pathways of these interactions (Fig. 22.10).[16]

As the name indicates, fatigue is the hallmark of SEID. Patients often report excellent pre-illness physical fitness and energy and an abrupt onset of fatigue, typically with a flu-like illness, such as fever, sore throat, cough, myalgias and fatigue. After illness onset, patients indicate that physical exertion tends to exacerbate the fatigue. Many patients with SEID also often experience anorexia, nausea, drenching night sweats, dizziness and intolerance to alcohol and pharmaceuticals that affect the central nervous system (see Fig. 22.11 for specific CNS pathways). The illness then tends to proceed to a chronic state of fatigue

Risk factors or predisposing factors
Genetic
Female gender
Past psychological illness
Somatic in close family members
Childhood experiences
History of fatigue
History of other medically unexplained symptoms

Triggering or precipitating factors
Serious infective illness (EBV, Q fever, viral meningitis, viral hepatitis)
Life events
Operative stress
Overstraining
Depression/anxiety
Cancer
Physical trauma?
Head injury?

ACUTE OR SUBACUTE FATIGUE

Maintaining or perpetuating factors
Response to fatigue: prolonged bed rest or time off work; fixed somatic attribution of cause; demoralisation; depression; anxiety
Effects of inactivity: fatigue; physical deconditioning
Response of doctor: imprecise diagnosis
Behavioural factors: use of avoidance as coping strategy
Cognitive factors: loss of control; belief that exercise will cause damage or worsen fatigue
Biological factors: reduced cortisol levels; hypothalamic disturbance; disruption of circadian rhythm; altered central 5-HT receptor sensitivity; autonomic disturbances
Sleep: insomnia; hypersomnia; or poor sleep efficiency
Social factors: reinforcement by others; work-related problems; lack of social support

FIGURE 22.10 Interaction of predisposing, precipitating and perpetuating factors of SEID.

Source: Cleare AJ, Wesseley S. Chronic fatigue syndrome. In: Encyclopedia of stress. 2nd edn. Oxford: Elsevier; 2007; pp. 484–493.

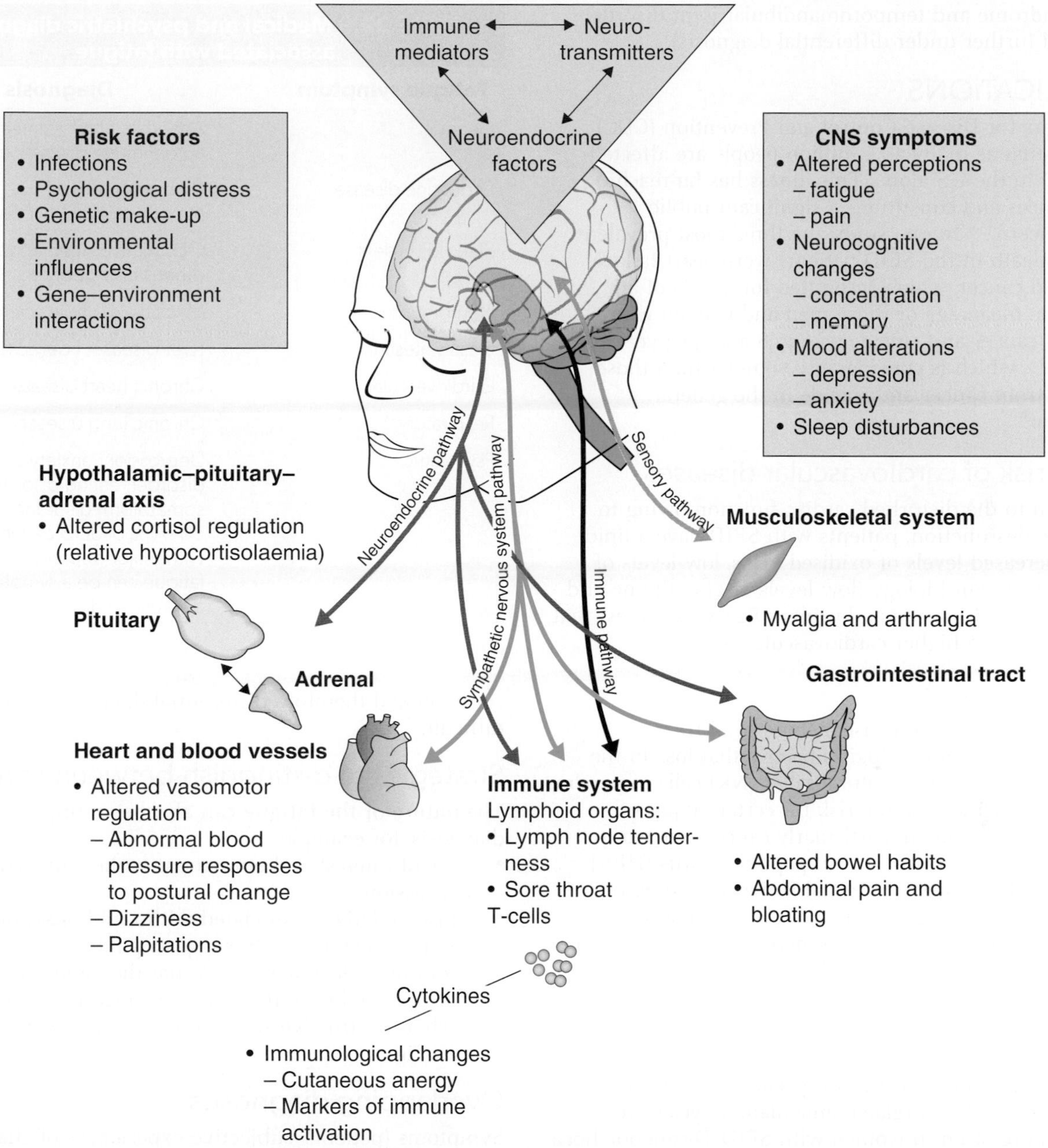

FIGURE 22.11 Potential central nervous system pathways to SEID.

Source: Toulkidis V and produced by a working group convened under the auspices of the Royal Australasian College of Physicians. Chronic fatigue syndrome. Clinical practice guidelines — 2002. Med J Aust 2002; 176(Suppl 6): S17–S55. © Copyright 2002 The Medical Journal of Australia. Reproduced with permission.

with other symptoms and signs such as headaches, myalgias, cognitive difficulties, sleep disturbances, sore throat, muscle weakness, prolonged postexertional fatigue and affective symptoms as well as low-grade fever and cervical adenopathy. These symptoms usually become quite debilitating.

Nearly all patients with SEID note a decrease in social relationships in addition to other unwanted consequences of illness; about one-third are unable to work, and another one-third can only work part-time. It has been found that the reaction and beliefs of people with whom the patient has close interpersonal relationships can affect the patient outcome and there may be a role for intervention/education of significant others to help to improve outcome chances.[58] Recent findings from community-based studies suggest that women, members of minority ethnic groups, and non-working individuals with SEID may experience greater functional disability and symptom severity than men, whites, and working individuals, respectively. Fortunately, the diagnosis of SEID is not associated with increased mortality.[59]

The symptoms of chronic fatigue, as well as SEID itself, often co-occur with other so-called functional illnesses such as fibromyalgia, multiple chemical sensitivities, irritable bowel syndrome and temporomandibular joint disorder (discussed further under differential diagnosis).

COMPLICATIONS

The Centers for Disease Control and Prevention (CDC) estimates that as many as 4 million people are affected with SEID in the US alone. This illness has far-reaching consequences and constitutes a significant public health concern.[60] In one study, the three most prevalent causes of death in the SEID patients were heart failure, suicide and cancer, which accounted for 59.6% of all deaths. The mean age of those men and women who died from cancer and suicide was 47.8 and 39.3 years, respectively, which is considerably younger than those who died from cancer and suicide in the general population.[61]

Higher risk of cardiovascular diseases

In addition to the disturbed cardiac function owing to autonomic dysfunction, patients with SEID have a lipid profile (increased levels of oxidised LDLs, low levels of HDLs) and oxidant biology (low levels of glutathione and elevated levels of plasma and urinary F2-isoprostanes) that is consistent with higher cardiovascular risk.

SEID and cancer

Although the long-term consequences of SEID are unknown, many immunologists believe that loss in the function and number of natural killer (NK) cells in persons with SEID may increase the risk for certain types of malignancies in women, particularly cancers related to viral reactivation such as human papillomavirus (HPV)-induced cervical cancer. A DePaul University study of causes of death among persons with SEID showed that women with SEID may have an increased incidence and younger onset of cancer from abnormalities in immune function.[61]

SEID and pregnancy

SEID may adversely affect fertility. Polycystic ovary syndrome (PCOS) and related anovulatory cycles are reported more often in women with SEID. Dysmenorrhoea is almost universal in women with SEID. Endometriosis, where dysmenorrhoea is a common symptom, may also be more common in women with SEID.[62] Rate of first trimester spontaneous miscarriage was four times higher than normal in women with SEID. Developmental delays were also reported more often in offspring of women who became pregnant after as opposed to before the onset of SEID. Low maternal cortisol levels (hypocortisolism) may be responsible for the delays in the fetal growth and development.

DIFFERENTIAL DIAGNOSIS

Medical conditions associated with fatigue

The following are some important medical and psychiatric diagnoses associated with fatigue — see Table 22.9. It is important to look for evidence of underlying medical conditions. The complaints relating to fatigue appear quite common and therefore differential diagnosis remains difficult.

TABLE 22.9 Medical and psychiatric diagnoses associated with fatigue

Fatigue symptom	Diagnosis
General	Anaemia, chronic infection, autoimmune disease, cancer
Endocrine disease	Diabetes mellitus, hypothyroidism, hypoadrenalism
Sleep disorders	Obstructive sleep apnoea and other sleep disorders
Neuromuscular	Myositis, multiple sclerosis
Gastrointestinal	Liver disease, coeliac disease
Cardiovascular	Chronic heart disease
Respiratory	Chronic lung disease
Psychiatric	Depression, anxiety and panic disorder, eating disorders, somatoform disorders 30–70% of SEID patients present with major depression, while fatigue can be a symptom in depressive disorders

Strategies to distinguish between conditions

The **nature of the fatigue** can also be an important clue to diagnosis, for example:

- Loss of interest and enjoyment (anhedonia) suggests depression
- Episodic fatigue associated with rapid onset of multiple symptoms and anxiety suggests panic
- Prominent sleepiness, such that the patient repeatedly falls asleep during the day, can suggest a sleep disorder such as obstructive sleep apnoea or, rarely, narcolepsy (see Fig. 22.12).

Overlapping diagnoses

Symptoms (patients' subjective experiences of changes occurring in the body) are the reasons for seeking medical help. Doctors diagnose diseases to explain these symptoms. Sometimes doctors experience difficulties in providing explanation for some of those symptoms as they cannot find any objective reason. These symptoms are then referred to as 'medically unexplained' or 'functional'. Various names are given to medically unexplained symptoms, such as somatisation, somatoform disorders, and functional somatic symptoms. These symptoms are common, frequently consistent and associated with significant distress and disability. Many such different functional syndromes have been described — see Table 22.10.

Some of the findings suggestive of overlap between these syndromes are:

- There is substantial overlap in the case definitions of specific functional somatic symptoms. Therefore, patients with one functional syndrome frequently meet

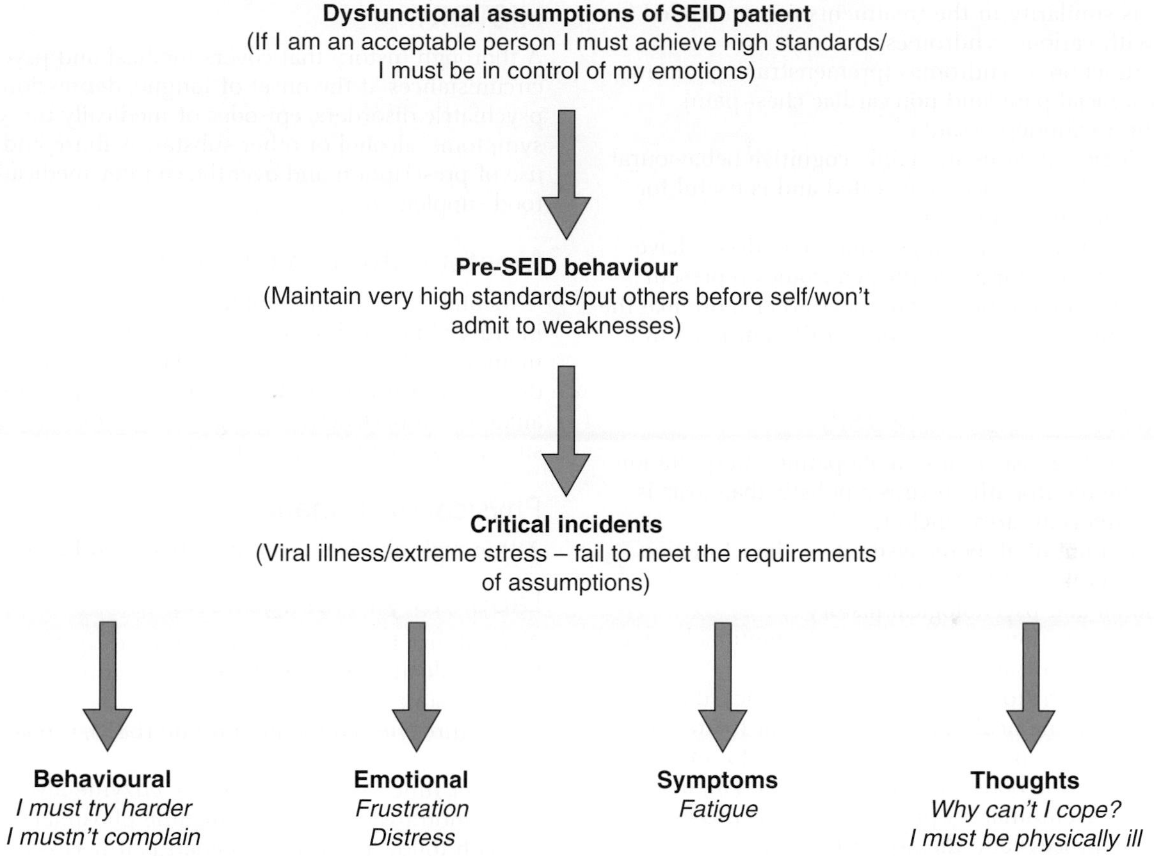

FIGURE 22.12 Theoretical cognitive model of the aetiology of SEID.

Source: Browne T, Chalder T. Chronic fatigue syndrome. Psychiatry 2009; 8(5):153–157.

TABLE 22.10 Examples of functional somatic syndromes by specialty

Speciality	Functional somatic syndrome
Gastroenterology	Irritable bowel syndrome, non-ulcer dyspepsia
Gynaecology	Premenstrual syndrome, chronic pelvic pain
Rheumatology	Fibromyalgia
Cardiology	Atypical or non-cardiac chest pain
Respiratory medicine	Hyperventilation syndrome
Infectious diseases	Chronic (postviral) syndrome
Dentistry	Temporomandibular joint dysfunction, atypical facial pain
Ear, nose and throat	Globus syndrome
Allergy	Multiple chemical sensitivity

Sources: Maquet D, Demoulin C, Crielaard JM. Chronic fatigue syndrome: a systematic review. Annales de Réadaptation et de Médecine Physique 2006; 49(6):418–427. Wessely S, Nimnuan C, Sharpe M. Functional somatic syndromes: one or many? Lancet 1999; 354:936–939.

diagnostic criteria of other syndromes, e.g. symptoms of SEID overlap with fibromyalgia (FM), tension headache, multiple chemical sensitivity, food allergy, premenstrual syndrome (PMS) and irritable bowel syndrome (IBS). Irritable bowel syndrome has similarities to SEID with several complaints (nausea, diarrhoea) overlapping. Fibromyalgia can be confused with SEID, as approximately 70% of SEID patients report FM features, whereas 42% of patients with FM were found to have SEID symptoms and 37% of SEID patients were found to meet FM criteria.

- Some other common characteristics are:
  - Almost all functional somatic symptoms are more common in women than in men
  - There is strong association between many functional somatic syndromes and emotional distress such as anxiety and depression
  - There are no clear pathophysiological mechanisms to explain them
  - History of childhood trauma or abuse has been reported by patients with many of the syndromes, e.g. functional pelvic pain, irritable bowel syndrome, premenstrual syndrome, tension headache, fibromyalgia and SEID.

There is similarity in the treatments recommended for patients with various syndromes:

- Some functional syndromes (premenstrual syndrome, atypical facial pain, and non-cardiac chest pain) respond to antidepressants
- Psychological treatment, mainly cognitive behavioural therapy (CBT), has been advocated and is useful for many of these syndromes.

Based on the above findings, some scientists[63] have raised a question, asking, 'Do the syndromes represent specific diagnostic entities or are they rather more like the elephant to the blind man — simply different parts of a larger animal?'

NATUROPATHIC DIAGNOSIS

Naturopathic diagnosis relies on allopathic interpretation. However, the naturopath ensures a holistic diagnosis is achieved. Important areas include:

- Consideration of all body systems — their function both currently and historically
- Emotional and psychological history
- Stress — nutritional, environmental, emotional, mental, occupational, social, toxin exposure
- Full infective history — recovery, frequency, duration, current immune health, past and current treatment
- Immune function — particular attention to immune processes in the body, i.e. lymphatic function, blood parameters, eliminatory processes, mucus presentation
- Digestive process and dietary correlation
- Dietary intake — past and present with a focus on cravings, alcohol, stimulant (sugar and caffeine) intake
- Medication and recreational drug use (past and present)
- Occupation (past and present)
- Hobbies (past and present)
- Home environment — mould, chemical and toxin exposure
- Sleep, exercise and energy assessment
- The patient's own prenatal experience
- Birth and childhood health
- Family and genetics — infective history, adrenal exhaustion, and transgeneration epigenetics.

Investigations

The clinical diagnosis of SEID is based on specific criteria (as described above) associated with the absence of any organic or psychiatric affliction that could explain fatigue. Results of medical examination appear normal, and a validated diagnostic test for SEID is lacking.

Investigations are needed to exclude other explanations of fatigue, such as infectious disease (human immunodeficiency virus (HIV), hepatitis, Lyme's disease), autoimmune disorders (systemic lupus erythematosus, rheumatoid arthritis), neuromuscular disease (myasthenia), neurological disease (multiple sclerosis), cardiorespiratory disease, metabolic disease (hypocalcaemia, hypercalcaemia), psychiatric disease (major depression, anxiety, somatisation), sleep disorders (apnoea, insomnia), or haematological (anaemia) or side effects related to medication.

HISTORY

A thorough history that covers medical and psychological circumstances at the onset of fatigue, depression or other psychiatric disorders, episodes of medically unexplained symptoms, alcohol or other substance abuse and current use of prescription and over-the-counter medications and food supplements.

Mental status examination

A mental status examination should be carried out to identify abnormalities in mood, intellectual function, memory and personality. Particular attention should be directed towards current symptoms of depression or anxiety, self-destructive thoughts, and observable signs such as psychomotor retardation.

Physical examination

A thorough physical examination should be performed.

Laboratory investigations

A minimum battery of laboratory investigations including:

- Full blood count (FBC) with differential white blood cell count
- Erythrocyte sedimentation rate (ESR), C-reactive protein (CRP)
- Liver function tests, especially enzyme levels: alanine aminotransferase (ALT), alkaline phosphatase (ALP), with follow-up tests for hepatitis if necessary
- Blood proteins: total, albumin, globulin
- Blood glucose
- Blood urea nitrogen and serum creatinine
- Serum electrolytes
- Calcium, phosphorus
- Thyroid function tests
- Iron studies
- Vitamin D
- DHEA-S
- Red cell folate and B_{12}.

Additional specific tests should be directed towards confirming or excluding other causes. Some specific tests that do not confirm or exclude the diagnosis of SEID are: serological tests for Epstein-Barr virus, retroviruses, human herpesvirus 6, enteroviruses, and *Candida albicans*; tests of immunological function including cell population and function studies and imaging studies, including magnetic resonance imaging scans and radionuclide scans of the head. If mould is suspected, blood, urine and stool tests can be obtained to identify the culprit.

Naturopathic investigations

See Table 22.11.

Therapeutic considerations

CLINICAL DECISION MAKING AND RATIONALE

When presented with a SEID patient it is essential to focus on supporting a sense of possibility. Often patients have experienced significant fatigue for extended periods of

TABLE 22.11 Specific naturopathic investigations

Assessment	Justification
Coeliac serology and genetic screen	Common trigger, essential to eliminate
Full thyroid profile including urinary iodine, reverse T3 and thyroid antibodies	Restrictions with assessment allowances for GPs often cause limitation for assessment of thyroid function. TSH can be misleading and full assessment should be encouraged
Red cell zinc and copper (assess ratio)	Determine effectiveness of zinc status
Infective trigger assessment (various)	From assessing and questioning the patient, it is often easier to streamline the potential infective triggers. Pending this, referral to determine underlying infection is essential, i.e. mycoplasma PCR or serology, Lyme and co-infection testing
Environmental screen	Assess environmental toxin exposure including chlorinated pesticides, PCBs, volatile solvents, porphyrins, toxic metals, phthalates and parabens
Amino acid profile	Assess amino acid status for energy production and neurotransmitter synthesis. Assesses protein metabolism and utilisation
Urinary organic acids	Metabolism analysis. Assess cellular energy production and neurotransmitter processing
IgG/IgE food sensitivity profile	Assess for food intolerance/allergy contributing to or causing fatigue
Adrenal hormone profile	Assess adrenal exhaustion and adrenal hormone status
Candida antibodies	*Candida* screen to assess for residual infection
Comprehensive stool analysis	Assess for underlying GIT pathogen triggering presentation
Genetic testing (SNPs)	Predominantly to assess detoxification pathways but other variables may be applicable

time. Understandably, their mood often deteriorates consistent with their reduced energy levels. Hope is likely to be the most powerful stimulating treatment the clinician can provide.

Holistic interpretation and thought focusing on all key areas outlined in naturopathic diagnosis provides powerful considerations for SEID sufferers. Often they have been 'boxed' by their diagnosis and it is the naturopathic framework that considers all variables and pieces together a multitude of seemingly unrelated factors into a cohesive and consistent picture.

Do not underestimate the power of a current or previous infection. Often the patient may casually mention repeated chest infections or repeated thrush. This provides clues for the clinician to understand that the immune system has been deranged and requires a 're-set'. Infections can exist mildly or aggressively, often undetected by standard investigations. A careful review and comparison of percentages and levels of white blood cell readings can provide clues to the presence of immune irregularity. For example, neutrophils and lymphocytes are best kept within a close 2 : 1 ratio,; however, SEID sufferers often have a 1 : 1 or even a 1 : 2 ratio, suggesting viral activity.

Working in a team with psychological intervention, GPs, exercise physiologists and/or bodyworkers can enable a clear path towards recovery for most patients. However, patient motivation and compliance are paramount.

The concept of energy balance and regulation is crucial for the education and future positive outcome for patients. When on the road to recovery, patients often experience energy surges and may abuse their newfound vitality. It is essential to explain to them the concept of energy reserve — keeping some for the future. If the patient exhausts their energy reserve, recovery from this experience often sets them back, perpetuating the exhaustion. This can often continue in a cycle contributing to the long-standing fatigue.

PROGNOSIS

The nature of SEID is that it 'waxes and wanes', following a cyclical pattern of improvement alternating with unpredictable relapses of variable severity. The percentage of people who recover from SEID is unknown, although preliminary estimates are that at least partial recovery is possible in 40–60% of patients. Delays in SEID diagnosis and treatment may lead to a more complicated course of illness and poorer prognosis for recovery.[64] The prognosis of untreated SEID is poor: however, about two-thirds of patients improve with a comprehensive approach including CBT and graded-exercise therapy.[65]

Some of the risk factors for poor prognosis are:

- Sensation of severe fatigue
- Longer duration of illness
- Comorbid psychiatric disorder, such as depression and/or anxiety
- Holding an exclusively physical attribution for SEID
- Not receiving rehabilitation
- Older age.

Children and adolescents appear to recover more readily than adults. Specific therapies directed at underlying mechanisms may significantly improve outcome and should offer hope for SEID patients. Patients with higher levels of depressive symptoms require more intensive, longer treatment, or cognitive behavioural therapy in order to achieve a significant improvement in fatigue.[66]

Therapeutic application

ALLOPATHIC PERSPECTIVE

SEID should be recognised as a biopsychosocial model including biological, physical and psychological aspects. A variety of therapeutic approaches have been described as being beneficial to patients with SEID. The treatments should be tailored to the individual needs of the patient who should be encouraged to remain as active as possible. The immediate aim is the relief of symptoms, which will enable the patient to regain some level of preexisting function and wellbeing.

PHARMACOLOGICAL THERAPY

A range of antibiotics, antiviral, antifungal, immunoregulatory, antidepressant and metabolic drug regimens have been evaluated in double-blind, placebo-controlled trials in people with SEID. Although limited positive responses have been reported, no agent has consistently shown long-term efficacy in well-designed studies. Rintatolimod (Ampligen), a restricted toll-like receptor 3 agonist, is currently undergoing clinical trials and awaiting US FDA approval. Evidence to date indicates that it may be beneficial in 30–40% of SEID patients and appears to be generally well tolerated and safe.[67]

Antidepressants

Given the rate of depression-related symptoms (anxiety, poor concentration, sleep disturbances, fatigue and memory impairment) and the high prevalence of depression, antidepressant drugs are prescribed. Two placebo-controlled studies of fluoxetine (a selective serotonin reuptake inhibitor) in SEID have shown divergent results, one study indicating no benefit, even in depressed SEID patients, while the other showing mild benefit to both fatigue and depression. Two other studies of monoamine oxidase inhibitors (moclobemide and phenelzine) also have shown mild benefit, primarily on symptoms rather than disability. Low-dose tricyclic antidepressants can be helpful if pain or insomnia predominates.[31]

Corticosteroids

Because of the finding of reduced cortisol levels, some studies investigated a replacement strategy. Hydrocortisone (cortisol) in small doses (5–10 mg daily) produced large reduction in fatigue (in about 28% compared with 9% in the placebo group). Potential side effects of corticosteroids preclude their use as routine treatment. Other randomised controlled studies using the mineralocorticoid, fludrocortisone, alone or in combination with hydrocortisone, found no benefits.

Other drugs

Other agents, such as analgesics, antihistamines, antivirals, dehydroepiandrosterone (DHEA), magnesium sulfate (intramuscular), nutritional IV therapy, and immunotherapy have also been used.

NON-PHARMACOLOGICAL TREATMENT

Rehabilitation, behavioural and cognitive approaches link the principles of good clinical management with varying degrees of graded physical activity and psychological intervention. Such treatments are not designed to achieve rapid symptomatic relief. Rather, they are aimed at maximising functional capacity over longer periods. The initial treatment strategy is usually individualised according to the patient's level of disability and personal preferences, and subsequently modified according to the response, sometimes referred to as 'pacing'.

Graded aerobic exercises

Aerobic exercise therapy represents a key component in any treatment of SEID patients. Inactivity seems to perpetuate the symptoms of SEID, especially fatigue and sleep disturbances; graded exercise is an obvious treatment for SEID. A 2016 meta-analysis of 8 RCTs (n = 1518) found positive effects of aerobic exercise on sleep, physical function and self-perceived general health. No conclusions could be drawn for the effect on pain, quality of life, anxiety or depression. In none of the studies did aerobic exercise result in adverse effects.[68] However, one researcher does point out that outside of clinical trials, many patients report deterioration with graded exercise therapy and it is prudent to tailor the treatment program accordingly.[69] The benefits of exercise appear to be more behavioural than physiological. It may reflect increased confidence and decreased avoidance behaviour. Nevertheless, many patients are reluctant to engage in such programs, usually because of fears of possible adverse consequences. Graded aerobic exercise (30 min/day of cycling, walking or swimming) significantly increases the feeling of wellbeing. A study on Chinese *qigong* exercise showed significant improvements in sleep quality, anxiety and depression.[70]

Prolonged rest

No study observed harmful effects with prolonged rest in SEID patients. But it seems to perpetuate or increase fatigue.

Cognitive behavioural therapy (CBT)

CBT is a promising line of treatment. This is the only effective common therapy that has been shown to result in beneficial outcomes in patients with SEID. It encourages a collaborative approach to treatment, emphasises the importance of engagement and has lower dropout rates than those encountered in single exercise programs. Treatment depends upon challenging some of the unhelpful illness beliefs, overcoming behavioural avoidance by encouraging consistent, modest activity followed by graded increases, and looking at cognitive factors associated with predisposition and relapse. Good outcome is associated with altered beliefs about the relative merits of rest versus exercise.[31,71] CBT may also reverse some of the HPA axis changes seen in SEID.[72] A 2015 randomised controlled trial found that CBT delivered in group settings was as effective as individual treatment in SEID patients.[73]

Sleep management

Sleeping for long does not appear to improve physical or mental functioning in patients with SEID, and excessive periods of daytime sleep or frequent napping can further disrupt circadian rhythm. The aim is to establish a regular, normalised sleep–wake pattern:

- Avoid stimulants during the evening
- Avoid going to bed too early in the evening
- Try to avoid excessive night-time sleep periods
- Establish a routine morning wake up time (e.g. 7 am)
- Reduce (to less than 30 minutes) or abolish daytime naps
- Engage in daytime physical and mental activities (within the limits of the individual's functional capacity).

HISTORICAL PERSPECTIVE

SEID is not a new condition. As early as 1750 Sir Richard Manningham describes a condition strikingly similar known as 'febricula', characterised by fever, chilliness, listlessness, lassitude and weariness within the body.[74] Not long after, neurologist George Beard discovered another condition strikingly similar to the yet-to-be-defined chronic fatigue. This was termed 'neurasthenia', a reference to the weakness and debility experienced in chronic fatigue. Obviously because it had not yet been defined, there is no mention of SEID within the texts of the Eclectics; however, one can hypothesise that the Eclectics would have administered a range of restorative and immune-stimulating botanicals. These include botanicals such as *Avena sativa*, prized for its restorative effects, with the Eclectics saying, 'It is regarded by many as a remedy of some importance for nervous debility, and for affections bordering closely upon nervous prostration'. It seemingly acts well in the exhaustion following typhoid and other low fevers,[75] as well as herbs that influenced the immune system such as *Echinacea purpurea* and *Phytolacca decandra*. It is important to note that many of the botanicals prescribed today for SEID have been borrowed from other countries, e.g. *Astragalus membranaceous* and *Panax ginseng* from Traditional Chinese Medicine as well as *Withania somnifera* from Ayurvedic medicine; hence there is no mention of them in the traditional texts of the Eclectics.

NATUROPATHIC PERSPECTIVE

The naturopathic approach to treatment addresses a few key areas with a comprehensive treatment management plan:

- Identify and eradicate underlying infection (if present)
- Re-educate and rebuild the immune system
- Stabilise energy balance — educate requirement of energy reserves and prevent burn out when energy begins to increase
- Normalise circadian rhythm
- Repair adrenal exhaustion
- Full nutritional review — address deficiencies for optimal repletion and assess and correct dietary requirements.

NUTRITIONAL MEDICINE (DIETARY)

Dietary therapeutic objectives

- Avoid all dietary stimulants, such as caffeine, that will compound the presentation and delay recovery
- Avoid all substances that will hamper immune function. Provide sufficient protein (calculation is essential based on body weight) to ensure energy can be acquired from sustainable sources and immune recovery can be achieved
- Identify and eliminate any present food allergy or intolerance
- Consume small meals throughout the day to maintain ease of digestion, regularity of blood sugar levels and frequent supply of vital nutrients to sustain energy
- Focus dietary prescriptions on foods that provide energy and do not require energy for their metabolism, i.e. avoid all those that contain chemicals, preservatives, additives or substances that cause unnecessary pressure on the body to process and assimilate
- Can add digestive enzymes and probiotics to help enhance absorption and assimilate nutrients.

Specific dietary treatments

DIETARY INCLUSIONS

Protein

Adequate protein is imperative in SEID as protein is required to make up components of the immune system including interferons which protect uninfected host cells from viral infection as well as the complementary system which promotes phagocytosis.[1] Without adequate protein the body is unable to mount and facilitate a healthy immune defence. A variety of proteins (vegetable and animal — if appropriate) are encouraged, these should be well cooked and consumed in small quantities (for example in a stew or soup rather than a steak) so as not to place too much strain on the digestive system. Again, digestive aids can be helpful.

Essential fatty acids

The few clinical trials assessing supplementation with essential fatty acids in individuals with chronic fatigue have suggested a beneficial effect particularly with regards to cognitive function and relapse frequency (see 'Essential fatty acids' under supplements for more details). A wide variety of essential fatty acids should be consumed including oily fish, nuts and seeds. However, those foods which are rich in EPA are particularly encouraged as this constituent has thus far shown the most benefit.

Pre- and probiotics

SEID is associated with lowered diversity in the gut microbiome and changes in abundance of various bacterial species (for example lower levels of *Bifidobacterium* and *Faecalibacterium* have been found in SEID). There is greater translocation of gut bacteria into the blood in SEID than in healthy controls (leaky gut), leading to inflammation. Gut dysbiosis is a likely contributor to symptoms of SEID including, but not limited to, GIT disturbances.[76–78] Prebiotics and probiotics can be administered to aid in restoring the bacterial diversity of the gut microbiome and helping to resolve GIT issues. It is recommended that strain-specific probiotics are administered based on the results of a CDSA.

DIETARY EXCLUSIONS

Caffeine

Caffeine is a commonly abused dietary substance found in chocolate, colas, energy drinks, coffee and tea and is popular for its ability to temporarily counteract fatigue. Though tempting for the fatigued patient this stimulating action is unfortunately short lived and has a rebound effect causing greater fatigue and thus is discouraged in the patient with SEID. Caffeine overuse may further weaken the impaired immune system, place strain on the adrenal glands and cause depletion of important nutrients (such as B vitamins) needed to nourish the body in SEID.

Alcohol

Alcohol use in SEID is commonly associated with subjective worsening of symptoms.[79] Individuals may report feeling more tired, nauseous, with sleep interference, exacerbation of hangovers as well as more anxiety and/or depression after drinking alcohol and thus many seek of their own accord to eliminate alcohol from their diet.[79] Aside from the reasons cited above, alcohol like caffeine depletes the body of vital nutrients and impairs immunity, thus it is wise to avoid consumption in individuals with chronic fatigue.

Sugar and artificial sweeteners

Sugar is an immune-depressant and like caffeine produces a quick burst of energy that is quickly accompanied by a rebound effect, thus it needs to be avoided. Artificial sweeteners are found in many foods including diet soft drinks, chewing gums, shakes and even some vitamin supplements. Aspartame is one of the most researched sweeteners and there is a strong connection between dietary excitotoxin excess (such as aspartates) and neurological abnormalities. Aspartame contains methanol, which is converted to formaldehyde, a dangerous neurotoxin that may cause a range of (direct and indirect) cellular effects in sensitive individuals,[80] such as those with chronic fatigue, thus it should be avoided.

Food allergy

Manu et al[39] showed that 13.5% of individuals with SEID exhibited food intolerances and there are other reports of individuals improving on a wheat-free or coeliac diet.[81] Logically the removal of offending items from the diet places less stress on the immune system and body as a whole, thus individuals with allergies and intolerances to specific constituents/foods need to avoid the offending item/s.

OTHER DIETARY CONSIDERATIONS

Hypoglycaemia

Individuals who suffer from hypoglycaemia often state that symptoms such as fatigue are worsened, thus functional hypoglycaemia in the patient with SEID is likely to further aggravate symptoms. Care should be taken to prevent hypoglycaemia by consuming small, frequent balanced meals with a protein component.

NUTRITIONAL MEDICINE (SUPPLEMENTAL)

Nutritional medicine therapeutic objectives

- Provision of key nutrients for energy synthesis and regulation and production of ATP
- Nutrient repletion to restore immunological function and eradicate infection (if present)
- Restoration of neurological and psychological requirements and pathways
- Antioxidant support to reduce oxidation and inflammation
- Regulation of energy balance and circadian rhythm.

Specific nutrients required

B COMPLEX

Deficits of B vitamins have been observed in individuals with SEID.[82,83] Acknowledging that the B vitamins play an imperative role in mitochondrial cellular energy production one can assume that deficiency in any B vitamin is likely to induce an energy deficit and/or abnormality of the intramitochondria resulting in general fatigue and postexertional malaise in patients. While all the B vitamins are important, folate (in folinic acid form) in particular has shown great promise in SEID particularly with regards to B-cell immunodeficiency and chronic reactivated Epstein-Barr virus infection where supplementation has been found to reduce symptomatology.[84] Clinically, prescription of injectable or sublingual B_{12} and activated B complex can provide energy stimulation that can support and rectify energy pathways for the patient. A 2015 study found the frequent injections of methylcobalamin combined with a daily high dose of folic acid (oral supplementation) may be safe and effective for fatigue and other SEID symptoms. Response to treatment is generally seen within a few weeks.[85]

Additionally, it is important to consider the important role that B vitamins have in regulating mood and psychological status of the patient. Please review the discussion under 'Depression' in Chapter 23 of this text for more information.

VITAMIN C

SEID is characterised by alterations in normal immunology and similarly an infectious theory has also been proposed. Individuals with chronic fatigue often display impaired immune and infective signs such as sore throat, fever and tender lymph nodes[86] and subsequent clinical laboratory testing demonstrates decreased function of natural killer cells and macrophages[87] all of which vitamin C owing to its immune stimulant and anti-infective actions may remedy. Oxidative stress has also been implicated in SEID and here, vitamin C as an antioxidant may exert a protective role. In Japan mega-doses of vitamin C have been used as an infusion in combination with antibiotics as a prophylactic.[88] However, in spite of its potential use in SEID there is a scarcity of clinical trials assessing its role and large, well-designed clinical trials are yet to be seen.

SAMPLE DAILY DIET

BREAKFAST	
Smoothie: blueberries, banana, low allergen vegan protein powder, leafy greens, sesame seeds	Mitochondrial dysfunction is implicated in the pathogenesis of SEID. Dietary strategies that are protective of the mitochondria are advocated with foods rich in magnesium (leafy greens) as well as coenzyme Q10 (strawberries and sesame seed) suggested. A smoothie also provides a concentrated source of nutrients in an easy-to-assimilate form.
LUNCH	
Vegetable casserole with spices, okra and ¾ cup of lentils. Serve with sauerkraut	Altered intestinal microflora may contribute to the pathogenesis of SEID. Supplementation with probiotics has been shown to improve neurocognitive function thus fibre as a source of prebiotics and probiotic-rich foods such as miso and sauerkraut are suggested. Intestinal permeability is implicated in the pathogenesis of SEID. Lentils provide a source of zinc, important for gut barrier function. Spices like turmeric and ginger can be used to downregulate inflammation. In-vitro studies have identified that the seeds of okra contain anti-fatigue activity whereby they may reduce levels of blood lactic acid, enhance hepatic glycogen storage and promote antioxidant ability by lowering malondialdehyde (MDA) level and increasing superoxide dismutase (SOD) and glutathione peroxidase (GSH-PX) levels.
DINNER	
Brown rice congee made with vegetables, nori, ginger, miso and organic chicken	Energetically a congee is restorative and easy to digest. The brown rice contains B vitamins for energy while the chicken provides protein to balance blood sugar levels. It can be made in bulk to reduce exertion spent cooking. SEID has a distinct inflammatory component with evidence of cytokine abnormalities and pathogenic inflammation, therefore an anti-inflammatory diet is hypothesised to be likely to be useful. Meals that minimise pro-inflammatory constituents and promote foods with known anti-inflammatory activity such as ginger and immune-boosting herbs and vegetables are suggested.
SNACKS	
High-quality polyphenol-rich chocolate Fresh fruit/fruit juice Liquorice tea	High cocoa liquor/polyphenol-rich chocolate was shown to reduce fatigue and improve mood in individuals with SEID when compared to placebo. Oxidative stress may impair muscle repair increasing fatigue in SEID, thus antioxidant-rich foods are suggested. Adrenal fatigue is commonly seen in SEID with abnormalities of the HPA axis including low cortisol, enhanced cortisol negative feedback, and blunted HPA axis response. Liquorice root is used to increase the cortisol level by increasing the half-life of cortisol.

VITAMIN E

Vitamin E may be used in SEID owing to its antioxidant and immune roles. A clinical study undertaken by Miwa and Fujita[89] suggests that oxidative stress may be higher in patients with SEID compared with healthy controls as manifested by lower alpha-tocopherol levels in the serum. However, as yet there has been little in the way of clinical testing with vitamin E in individuals with SEID.

MAGNESIUM

Magnesium is beneficial in SEID, with Cox et al observing a decrease in myalgia and fatigue in 70% of individuals administered magnesium although this was via injection.[90] Many of the signs of magnesium deficiency such as muscular and neurological symptoms mimic that of SEID. However, measurements of magnesium levels within patients with chronic fatigue have been inconsistent, with decreased magnesium observed in some trials yet normal and even increased magnesium observed in other trials.[82] SEID is characterised by mitochondrial abnormalities and magnesium plays an important role in healthy cellular metabolism and mitochondrial function with ATP energy production dependent upon the presence of magnesium. Myalgia and muscle fatigue are commonly reported symptoms in chronic fatigue; however, magnesium supplementation may aid in the relief of muscular aches and cramps.

GLUTATHIONE (GSH)

Glutathione is termed as the mother of all antioxidants in the body. When there is excessive oxidative stress in the body, GSH can be added to the treatment program to reduce and quench oxidative stress. Note that while other supplements mentioned like magnesium, vitamin C and B-complex help recycle GSH in the body, adding GSH through IV, intramuscular injection, dermal or oral delivery (if product viable) can help reduce oxidative stress faster. While research is still inconclusive about the severity of GSH utilisation/depletion in a person with SEID, there is evidence that patients have reported better outcomes when their GSH levels increase.[91]

L-CARNITINE

L-carnitine is an amino acid that has a number of important functions with regards to the maintenance of mitochondrial health, hence acknowledging that impaired mitochondrial function has been implicated in the pathogenesis of SEID, L-carnitine has been proposed to be of use. L-carnitine is essential for the transport of long-chain fatty acids across the mitochondrial membrane and mitochondrial energy metabolism; serum levels obtained from individuals with SEID have been largely inconsistent, producing contradictory results with some individuals showing decreased levels[92–94] and other study groups revealing normal levels.[95] Improvements in mental fatigue and general fatigue have been seen following supplementation with acetyl-L-carnitine and L-carnitine respectively.[96]

ESSENTIAL FATTY ACIDS

Essential fatty acids exert anti-inflammatory, immune regulatory and antiviral functions and thus have been suggested to be of use in SEID.[97,98] There have been mixed results seen in double-blind placebo-controlled studies assessing the effects of omega-3 fatty acids in individuals with SEID. In one study, individuals with SEID of 1–3 years duration after an apparent viral infection were administered a combination that contained linoleic, gamma-linolenic, eicosapentaenoic and docosahexaenoic acids or placebo for 12 weeks.[99] After only 1 month of treatment 74% of patients consuming essential fatty acids assessed themselves as improved compared with 23% in the placebo group. Surprisingly, however, when Warren et al tried, the results were not significant and no real differences were seen between placebo and the control group.[100] Puri[101] details a series of case reports of individuals with SEID in which participants consumed on average 1116 mg/day eicosapentaenoic acid, 348 mg/day docosahexaenoic acid, 120 mg gamma-linolenic acid and 19.2 mg natural vitamin E (in the form of D alpha-tocopheryl acetate). The authors report an improvement in symptomatology within 2–3 months with testimonials such as 'The first thing is that the fogginess of the brain has gone completely' as well as reports of a reduction in frequency and severity of relapses.

ZINC

Lower zinc concentrations have been observed in the serum of individuals with chronic fatigue when compared with controls. Interestingly, a trend may be seen between the severity of illness and serum zinc.[102] Low zinc concentrations are associated with immune activation and inflammation both of which are observed in SEID, thus individuals with chronic fatigue are recommended to use zinc supplements in order to prevent defects associated with early T-cell activation.[103] Zinc via its role as an antioxidant is also likely to be of use in protecting against oxidative damage. Werbech[104] also highlights the use of zinc to decrease pain and fatigue and increase muscle strength and endurance in chronic fatigue.

5-HYDROXYTRYPTOPHAN (5-HTP)

Depression is common in individuals with chronic fatigue and a serious factor that needs to be investigated in all presenting patients. Results from one representative study reveal that 36% of respondents were depressed and 22% of respondents surveyed had seriously considered suicide in the past year.[105] 5-HTP is a serotonin precursor and has been used successfully to help manage depression. As yet no published clinical studies have been found assessing the efficacy of 5-HTP in patients with SEID.

SAMe

SAMe like 5-HTP may be useful in SEID due to its success in managing depression. An added benefit of SAMe is its musculoskeletal benefits, whereby it may also help to relieve musculoskeletal-related pain such as fibromyalgia.[106] In instances of under-methylation, short-term SAMe prescription can assist in optimising the methylation cycle which has been shown to produce significant positive clinical outcomes.

COENZYME Q10

Coenzyme Q10 is a mitochondrial nutrient that acts as an essential cofactor for the production of ATP in mitochondria and displays significant antioxidant activities, hence it is commonly used by patients with SEID. Individuals with SEID have been observed to have lower plasma levels of coenzyme Q10 than healthy controls, and thus it has been hypothesised that this deficiency may be one influencing factor in the aetiology of SEID as well as a reason for symptoms, such as fatigue, experienced by patients.[107] Despite the popularity of coenzyme Q10 there have been surprisingly few formalised clinical studies. A small randomised, double-blind placebo-controlled study ($n = 73$) administering CoQ10 (200 mg/day) with NADH (20 mg/day) to SEID patients over a period of 8 weeks showed a significant improvement in fatigue scores in the patients, as well as a significant improvement in their biochemical markers.[108] Further large-scale trials are warranted.

MULTIVITAMIN SUPPLEMENT

A prospective study of 38 women aged 18–50 with SEID found that after 2 months of supplementation with a multivitamin mineral, there was a significant decrease in fatigue, sleep disorders, ANS symptoms and headache intensity. There was also a significant improvement in antioxidant status. No positive effect on quality of life was found in this study.[109]

Dosage requirements

The dosage requirements listed below are based on adult doses that have been reported in the literature.

- B complex (all B vitamins) high-dose combination, preferably activated forms
  - Thiamine 20–40 mg/day
  - Riboflavin 20–40 mg/day
  - Niacinamide 50–100 mg/day
  - Pantothenic acid 150–300 mg/day
  - Pyridoxine 50–100 mg/day
  - Folate (as folinic acid or L-5MTHF as indicated) 500–1000 micrograms/day
    - Higher doses will be required in instances of anaemia
    - Doses as high as 1000–10 000 micrograms/day for 3 months may be required[104]
  - Hydroxocobalamin or methylcobalamin 500–1000 micrograms/day
  - Doses as high as 6–70 000 micrograms/day for 3 months may be required[104]
  - Choline 50–100 mg/day
  - Inositol 50–100 mg/day
  - Biotin 250–500 micrograms/day
- Vitamin C: up to 10 000–15 000 mg/day[104] intravenously OR 500–1000 mg t.d.s.-q.i.d. orally; doses this high are typically given intravenously. Oral doses are best limited to up to 5 g in divided doses
- Vitamin E: 400–800 IU/day
- Magnesium: 300 mg/day t.d.s.
- Glutathione: 400 mg dermal or oral, 1–4 g weekly infusion
- L-carnitine: 2 g/day OR 3–4 g/day in divided doses
- Essential fatty acids: minimum of 280 mg/day GLA and 135 mg/day EPA daily,[104] however, total active constituents (EPA and DHA) of fish oil should contain at least 1000 mg/day taken in divided doses
- Zinc: 80–135 mg/day[104]
- 5-HTP: 100 mg/day or higher[104]
- SAM-e: 400–1200 mg/day (divided doses)
- Coenzyme Q10: 100–400 mg/day.[104]

HERBAL MEDICINE

The therapeutic objectives and associated classes of herbal medicine are detailed in Table 22.12.

Specific herbal medicines

ELEUTHEROCOCCUS SENTICOSUS (SIBERIAN GINSENG)

SEID implies the presence of prolonged fatigue and debility hence botanicals that display adaptogen and anti-fatigue properties are likely to be of particular use. *Eleutherococcus senticosus* is one such herb and has shown promising results for the management of moderate SEID. Hartz et al[110] conducted a randomised, double-blind, controlled trial involving 96 patients with SEID administered eleutherococcus extract (200 mg/day containing 2.24 mg eleutherosides) or placebo for 2 months. At the end of the study, overall results were found to be statistically insignificant when compared with placebo; however, the authors hypothesised that not all patients respond the same way to an intervention (also, an individual's degree of fatigue may impact treatment outcome) and decided to divide patients into a subset of those with moderate fatigue. This group of individuals demonstrated a statistically significant improvement in Rand Vitality Index scores compared with placebo and when those in the placebo group with moderate fatigue were administered *Eleutherococcus senticosus* they too experienced a statistically significant improvement after 2 months. Interestingly, *Eleutherococcus senticosus* did not appear to continue to be effective in those who remained on the treatment for 4 months suggesting short periods of treatment may be best in this group of individuals.

GLYCYRRHIZA GLABRA (LIQUORICE) AND *REHMANNIA GLUTINOSA* (REHMANNIA)

Suboptimal function of the hypothalamic-pituitary-adrenal axis has been implicated in SEID and subsequently hypocortisolism has been observed.[111,112] In these instances, both *Glycyrrhiza glabra* and *Rehmannia glutinosa* may be of use due to their restorative effects on the adrenal glands and their ability to increase cortisol in the body; increases in cortisol are associated with reductions in fatigue[113] and thus may help to alleviate fatigue in patients with SEID.

HYPERICUM PERFORATUM (ST JOHN'S WORT)

Acknowledging the prevalence of depression in SEID, *Hypericum perforatum* should be considered for any patients exhibiting signs of despondency. *Hypericum perforatum* has proven itself to be a reliable and efficacious antidepressant herb in numerous clinical trials. *Hypericum perforatum* may also be of use if chronic fatigue is believed to be of viral infectious origin due to its antiviral action.

PANAX GINSENG (KOREAN GINSENG)

Panax ginseng is a perennial herb indigenous to Asia that has been used medicinally for centuries. The evidence reviewed suggests that *Panax ginseng* and its components, the ginsenosides, can help to regulate a wide array of physiological mechanisms within the body leading to the ability of *Panax ginseng* to enhance recovery from illness, help provide resistance against stress and fatigue via its adaptogen action, enhance cognitive performance, stimulate immune function as well as support overall health via its tonic effects; all of which may be of use for sufferers of SEID.

As yet there have been no human clinical trials assessing the effects of *Panax ginseng* in SEID. However, in-vitro studies of peripheral blood mononuclear cells treated with *Panax ginseng* reveal an immune-enhancing action evidenced by improved cellular immune function and increased antibody-dependent cellular cytotoxicity and NK-function.[114]

In addition, one study in 2013 found that a daily 2 g dose of *Panax ginseng* helped significantly reduce self-reported fatigue in patients ($n = 90$) with idiopathic chronic fatigue by increasing their glutathione concentrations and antioxidant activity.[115]

ASTRAGALUS MEMBRANACEUS (ASTRAGALUS)

Astragalus is an adaptogen that has a regulating effect on the immune system. In animal studies flavonoids from

TABLE 22.12 Herbal medicine therapeutic objectives and associated classes

Symptomatic support

Objective	Herbal medicine class
Increase energy levels	Nervine stimulant (caution in some) Nervine tonic Nervine trophorestorative Adaptogen Adrenal restorative
Stabilise mood	Nervine trophorestorative Adaptogen Adrenal restorative
Reduce depression	Antidepressant Thymoleptic Euphoric Serotonin agonist
Improve cognition	Cerebro-circulatory stimulants Antioxidant Cognitive enhancer
Restore nervous system function and integrity	Nervine tonic Nervine trophorestorative Sedative (if indicated)
Circadian rhythm stabilisation	Sedative Nervine tonic Nervine stimulant (caution with some) Melatonin stimulation — sunlight/ moonlight, serotonin agonist
General body tonification	Tonic Nutritive

Causative

Objective	Herbal medicine class
Eradicate infection	Antimicrobial Antiseptic Specific 'anti-' for infective organism, e.g. Antiviral (due to viral infection)
Reduce stress (long term and short term)	Adaptogen Adrenal restorative Nervine tonic Nervine trophorestorative Sedative (if indicated) Euphoric

Causative—cont'd

Objective	Herbal medicine class
Hormonal modulation	Serotonin agonist HPA modulator Melatonin stimulation (sunlight/ moonlight)
Female hormonal modulation	HPO modulator Menstrual cycle regulator Female tonics Other specific hormonal modification (e.g. progesterone stimulant
Male hormonal modulation	HPT modulator Male tonics Other specific hormonal modification (e.g. testosterone stimulant)
Allergies or intolerances	Anti-allergic Anti-inflammatory GIT restoration Improve liver detoxification
Eliminate heavy metal toxicity	Cerebro-circulatory stimulants Antioxidant Hepatoprotective Hepatotrophorestorative Hepatotonic Detoxicant

Long-term effects

Objective	Herbal medicine class
Improve liver function	Hepatoprotective Hepatotrophorestorative Hepatotonic Choleretic Cholagogue Detoxicant Antioxidant
Restore GIT integrity and function	Bitter Mucous membrane trophorestorative Astringent Vulnerary/demulcent Antacid

Astragalus membranaceus have been shown to ameliorate SEID by counteracting abnormal production of cytokines.[116] Highlighting the adaptogen properties of astragalus, rats with SEID that were administered astragalus have been found to display higher endurance capacity than those without. Acknowledging the severe fatigue and alterations in immunity that accompany SEID, *Astragalus membranaceus* appears to be an extremely useful botanical for use in SEID. A combination of *Astragalus membranaceus* and the roots from *Salvia miltiorrhiza* have been used in a combination known as Myelophil to treat chronic fatigue (but not SEID).[117] While an anti-fatigue effect was observed by participants no changes were observed in terms of cytokine expression.

RHODIOLA ROSEA (RHODIOLA)

Rhodiola rosea has recently emerged in Australia as a new botanical for use as an adaptogen. However, it has been used medicinally in Europe for this for centuries. The therapeutic potential of *Rhodiola rosea* and its components have been well documented in a range of in vitro, in vivo and human clinical studies. In randomised human clinical studies *Rhodiola rosea* has been found to be able to improve mental, physical and emotional fatigue and exhaustion[118-120] and salivary cortisol levels;[118] other human studies have also noted a reduction in insomnia and emotional lability[121] in individuals administered *Rhodiola rosea*. It must be noted that a specific extract of *Rhodiola rosea* known as '*Rhodiola rosea* SHR-5 extract' was used in all the aforementioned studies, thus results at this point can only be theorised to be obtained if using this specific extract. Other studies suggest that *Rhodiola rosea* may be useful in improving cognitive function,[122] immune function as well as inhibiting monamine oxidases A and B suggesting it to be of use as an antidepressant. An 8-week trial conducted on 100 patients with prolonged or chronic fatigue symptoms showed marked improvement over time in all eight outcome measures including fatigue, stress, overload and tension. The greatest change was measured after 1 week of treatment and symptoms continued to decline over the remainder of the trial. Treatment was a dry ethanolic *Rhodiola rosea* extract (WS® 1375) 200 mg, administered twice daily.[123] Given the numerous potential clinical applications of this herb for sufferers of SEID, it is clear that more research is warranted.

ECHINACEA SPP. (ECHINACEA)

SEID is associated with abnormal cellular immune function such as decreased natural killer (NK) cell function[124] and manifestations of flu-like symptoms and fever in a large number of patients;[125] interestingly many individuals also recall an infective episode preceded the onset of their symptoms, suggesting that an infective microbial agent may be involved. However, despite these findings, a 2003 systematic review, while acknowledging the role of immunological dysfunction in SEID, failed to observe any replicable immune abnormalities.[126]

Echinacea, a purple coneflower native to North America, is well known and widely used for its ability to strengthen the body's resistance to illness through its effects on the immune system. Interesting results have been observed in vitro[114] with regards to chronic fatigue in which increasing concentrations of *Echinacea purpurea* administered to peripheral blood mononuclear cells from patients with SEID resulted in enhancement of cellular immune function, and increases in both antibody-dependent cellular cytotoxicity and NK-function. As yet it appears that studies are yet to be re-created in well-designed clinical studies. However, this result indicates that use of the *Echinacea* spp. and possibly other botanicals that support immunity may be useful to improve cellular immunity in individuals with SEID.

WITHANIA SOMNIFERA (ASHWAGANDHA)

Withania somnifera, also known as ashwagandha, is a green shrub that has been used extensively in Ayurvedic medicine for centuries to promote physical and mental well-being.[127] As with most herbs *Withania somnifera* contains a range of constituents, however, the 'withanolides' have been identified as some of the major constituents of importance. In the practice of Ayurvedic medicine *Withania somnifera* is classified as a rasayana, that is, it has 'rejuvenating' qualities. This rejuvenating action is likely to be influenced by the nervine and adaptogen[128] properties also suggested of *Withania somnifera* whereby it helps to restore the body providing support from fatigue and debility.

Though *Withania somnifera* has been used for centuries in Ayurvedic medicine there is a scarcity of human clinical research assessing its use. However, in-vitro and in-vivo studies provide an indication and explanation of its usefulness in SEID. In vivo, mice with chronic fatigue administered antioxidants and *Withania somnifera* were shown to have greater endurance than controls, highlighting the adaptogen action of *Withania somnifera*.[129] Interestingly, the mice were found to have decreased antioxidant defence mechanisms after swimming which were able to be restored using *Withania* in conjunction with other antioxidants. The authors suggest oxidative stress may be implicated in the pathogenesis of chronic fatigue; however, this may be attenuated with use of *Withania somnifera* and other antioxidants. Aside from this antioxidant role, *Withania* has also been observed to exert antistress and immunological functions restoring stress-induced altered T-cell function,[130] as well as neuroprotective effects attributed to down-regulation of nNOS and neurochemical alterations of specific neurotransmitter systems.[131] *Withania somnifera* appears to be of great use for SEID, warranting further human trials.

LIFESTYLE RECOMMENDATIONS

Counselling

Coming to terms with a chronic illness particularly one characterised by chronic fatigue and no known aetiology is a difficult and challenging experience for many sufferers. Though there has not been a great deal of research undertaken with regards to psychological therapies and SEID, counselling is recommended for all individuals particularly when one considers the high incidence of depression and other mood deviations many sufferers experience. Counselling offers individuals the chance to learn coping strategies to deal with their condition as well as the change of pace in life many experience. Counselling may be individual but some have also suggested that group and supportive psychotherapy as well as marital and family therapy may be beneficial,[132] particularly as often family members and carers are also affected by the condition. Though not classically defined as counselling, cognitive behavioural therapy has been studied and appears to be helpful in reducing fatigue.[133]

Exercise

There is good evidence to suggest exercise is beneficial in SEID.[134,135] However, care must be taken to not over-exercise owing to exacerbation of chronic fatigue symptoms.[136] Following supervised exercise therapy a number of improvements in fatigue, functional capacity, and fitness may be observed. In a study by Fulcher et al[135] these benefits appeared to be higher in those following aerobic-style exercise rather than flexibility treatment. As always a supervised exercise program designed by an individual with specialised qualifications in designing programs for special needs (such as an exercise physiologist) is likely to be most beneficial.

Circadian rhythm regulation

The circadian rhythm helps to maintain normal sleep–wake cycle, feelings of alertness and tiredness as well as cognitive function.[137] It can be seen that abnormalities and alterations in normal circadian rhythm would be similar to many of the symptoms experienced in SEID. This leads and supports the hypothesis of a link between altered circadian rhythms and chronic fatigue.[138] To regulate circadian rhythm it is important to connect the SEID sufferer with normal daylight and moonlight exposure. Patients need to understand the importance of sunlight exposure to stimulate and activate the anterior pituitary gland and the importance of settling and allowing a reduction in stimulation for the nervous system at night-time. A few simple strategies include:

- Waking with the sun rising regardless of fatigue — resetting the sleep–wake cycle
- Going to bed at a reasonable hour that allows for sufficient sleep (at least 8 hours per night)
- Settling the nervous system prior to getting into bed — darkness, lack of electronic stimulation
- General sleep hygiene principles mentioned in sleep disorders.

Energy conservation

Fatigue is one of the defining symptoms associated with SEID and directly affects quality of life. Energy conservation is planned management of an individual's energy resources in an attempt to prevent depletion. This may involve such things as delegation of tasks to others, scheduled rest times and undertaking physical activity when energy levels are at their highest. Studies have been conducted using the energy conservation model in other conditions characterised by fatigue including multiple sclerosis,[139] rheumatoid arthritis[140] and cancer and have worked well, thus energy conservation is also expected to work similarly in SEID.

CASE STUDY

OVERVIEW

LY, a 17-year-old female, presented with SEID of 2 years duration. Diagnosis was confirmed after she was unable to attend school for more than 6 months owing to fatigue. Prior to her SEID diagnosis LY had two infections with Epstein-Barr virus. Both episodes lasted 4–6 weeks and caused considerable fatigue and immune compromise. Following both infections, her immune system continued to remain low and fatigue increased over time. On presentation her fatigue had perpetuated and energy levels were as low as 1–2/10. This reduction in energy reduced her appetite thus reducing her BMI to its low level.

CLINICAL EXAMINATION

- Neck: Cervical lymphadenopathy — small nodes in right and left
- Eyes: Darkened circles under eyes
- BMI: 17

CASE STUDY CONTINUED

TREATMENT PROTOCOL

Herbal medicine as listed here.

Herbal medicine	Ratio	Quantity	Rationale
Andrographis panniculata	1:2	70 mL	Immune stimulating, adaptogen
Echinacea spp. (blend)	1:2	60 mL	Immune stimulating
Withania somnifera	1:1	60 mL	Adaptogen, nervine, restorative
Hypericum perforatum	STD ext	30 mL	Thymoleptic, anxiolytic, antiviral
TOTAL: 220 mL			

Dose: 5 mL t.d.s.

NUTRITIONAL MEDICINE

Dietary

- Marked increase in protein to both increase weight but also to provide building blocks for neurotransmitters, energy stabilisation and immune function
- Dietary aperitifs (bitters) to stimulate appetite and improve digestion and assimilation of nutrients
- Avoidance of all stimulants — e.g. sugar, artificial sweeteners, caffeine, alcohol
- Significant dietary education and meal planning to balance energy levels and blood sugar levels
- Protein smoothie at least once per day consisting of protein powder, yoghurt, LSA or nut meal, hulled tahini, cinnamon and fruit to provide easily digestible protein in high levels.

Supplemental

- High-dose B complex (activated): one cap × b.i.d.
- Zinc: 250 mg t.d.s.
- Vitamin C: 1 g t.d.s.
- Magnesium: 250 mg t.d.s.
- Coenzyme Q10: 150 mg b.i.d.

LIFESTYLE/EDUCATION

- Education: Energy conservation
- Circadian rhythm regulation
- Introduction of gentle exercise to be increased over time.

SLEEP DISORDERS

Epidemiology

Sleep disorders (see Fig. 22.13) are a common problem in Australia with over 1.2 million (6%) Australians estimated to experience sleeping problems.[141] In 2016, the Report to the Sleep Health Foundation estimated that more and more Australians are experiencing some kind of sleep

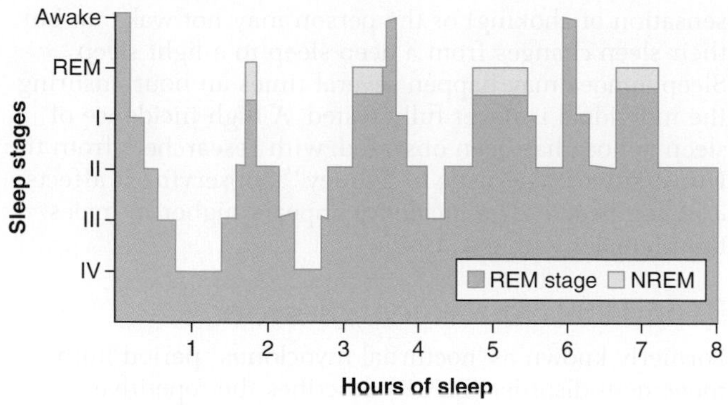

FIGURE 22.13 Sleep disorders.
Source: Ferri. Ferri's clinical advisor 2011. Mosby, 2010.

difficulty, with prevalence as high as 33–45% of adults. Insomnia, restless leg syndrome, and obstructive sleep apnoea appear to be the most common sleep problems affecting Australians. However, according to a 2004 report by Access Economics for Sleep Australia, over 70 other different sleep disorders have been diagnosed.[141] Results from the Australian Bureau of Statistics in 1999 indicated that 4% of the population had recently used sleeping medication; females were more likely to use these medications than males.[142] In 2011, 4.3% of the Australian population or 921 100 people used at least one prescription for anxiolytic/hypnotic and sedative medications to fall asleep. The highest ratio was in people aged 65–74.[143]

Classification

DIAGNOSTIC CRITERIA FOR INSOMNIA ACCORDING TO ICSD-3[144]

The International Classification of Sleep Disorders (ICSD) third edition was released in 2014. It is the key reference work for diagnosis of sleep disorders. Prior to this, insomnia was categorised into different subtypes based on duration and presumed pathophysiology, but the new edition consolidates all insomnia diagnoses into one: chronic insomnia disorder.

A Complaint of difficulty initiating sleep, difficulty maintaining sleep, or waking up too early, or sleep that is chronically non-restorative or poor in quality
B The above sleep difficulty occurs despite adequate opportunity and circumstances for sleep
C At least one of the following forms of daytime impairment related to the night-time sleep difficulty is reported by the patient:
  1 Fatigue or malaise
  2 Attention, concentration or memory impairment
  3 Social or vocational dysfunction or poor school performance
  4 Mood disturbances or irritability
  5 Daytime sleepiness
  6 Motivation, energy or initiative reduction
  7 Proneness for errors/accidents at work or while driving
  8 Tension, headaches, or gastrointestinal symptoms in response to sleep loss
  9 Concerns or worries about sleep.
D The problem persists for at least 3 months and occurs at least 3 times per week.

DSM-5 sleep–wake disorders are summarised in Table 22.13.

TABLE 22.13 DSM-5 sleep-wake disorders

Disorder	Sub-type
Insomnia disorder	None
Hypersomnolence disorder	None
Narcolepsy	None
Breathing-related sleep disorders	Obstructive sleep apnoea hypopnoea Central sleep apnoea Sleep-related hypoventilation
Circadian rhythm sleep–wake disorders	Delayed sleep type Advanced sleep phase type Irregular sleep–wake type Non-24-hour sleep–wake type Shift work type
Parasomnias	Non-rapid eye movement (NREM) sleep arousal disorders Nightmare disorder Rapid eye movement (REM) sleep behaviour disorder Restless legs syndrome Substance/medication-induced sleep disorder

Source: American Psychiatric Association. Diagnostic and statistical manual of mental disorders. 5th edn. Arlington: American Psychiatric Publishing. 2013.

Aetiology

SLEEP-ONSET INSOMNIA (DIFFICULTY FALLING ASLEEP)

Anxiety or tension

Psychiatric influences such as anxiety or tension are commonly associated with insomnia and thus questioning of the naturopathic patient should address whether there have been any recent worrying events that may be influencing the individual's current sleep complaints. Often the individual will only become aware of the link between a worrying event and their lack of sleep upon questioning. As well as being caused by anxiety or tension, insomnia is common in those with anxiety disorders. EEG sleep studies of individuals with generalised anxiety disorders show increased sleep latency and decreased sleep continuity in comparison to control participants.[145]

Environmental change

A change in an individual's usual environment may contribute to sleep-onset insomnia. These include factors such as a new place of sleep, such as sleeping at a hotel, as well as such things as a new bed partner or a new mattress.

Emotional arousal

Emotional arousal (strong feelings) such as anger or sadness may also affect an individual's ability to fall asleep. An example of this is having an argument with one's partner prior to bed time and then feeling so angry that one is not able to sleep.

Fear of insomnia

Often a few nights of troubled sleep can cause fear of insomnia which in itself may pre-empt sleep, causing anxiety that prevents onset of sleep. Cognitive behavioural therapy should be encouraged in these patients.

Disruptive environment

A disruptive environment can increase the risk of sleep-onset insomnia. Disruptions may include noise (loud music coming from the neighbours, a crying baby or a restless child), clutter, light or deviations in temperature.

Pain or discomfort

There is a strong link between sleep disorders and chronically painful conditions such as rheumatoid arthritis and fibromyalgia whereby the arousing effects of pain are believed to prevent sleep initiation. The presence of chronic pain is associated with worsening of insomnia, in particular a greater number of insomnia symptoms such as shorter sleep periods as well as anxiety, depression, irritability and mental and physical fatigue.[146,147] Pain clinics estimate that as many as 90% of individuals suffering from chronic pain also have a sleep disturbance.[148] It is important to note that sleep deprivation (even partially) has been found to increase pain sensitivity (hyperanalgesia) and is associated with pain complaints[149] hence the importance of ensuring good restorative sleep not only for healing and repair but also to reduce pain.

SLEEP-MAINTENANCE INSOMNIA

Environmental change

As with sleep-onset insomnia discussed above, a change in an individual's usual environment may also contribute to sleep-maintenance insomnia; for example, moving to a new house, sleeping at a hotel, sleeping next to a new bed partner.

Sleep apnoea (cessation of airflow)

A high prevalence of insomnia has been observed in patients with obstructive sleep apnoea, a sleep-related breathing disorder characterised by a cessation of breathing and subsequent hypoxia during sleep due to partial or complete obstruction of the airway by pharyngeal structures.[150,151] Cessation of airflow can cause the individual to wake with a shock (due to the sensation of choking) or the person may not wake up but their sleep changes from a deep sleep to a light sleep. Sleep apnoea may happen several times an hour ensuring the individual is never fully rested. A high incidence of sleep apnoea has been observed, with researchers from the University of Newcastle in Sydney[152] observing it affects 4 in 100 people. The incidence appears higher in males than females with a 4 : 1 ratio.

Period limb movement disorder

Formerly known as 'nocturnal myoclonus', period limb movement disorder (PLMD) describes the repetitive movements of the lower limbs such as in restless leg syndrome and is a common cause of disturbed sleep having been frequently observed on polysomnography.[153] Prevalence in Australia is unknown, however, an epidemiological study undertaken in Europe observed an incidence of 3.9% in 18 980 people surveyed.[154] PLMD is associated with female gender, caffeine intake, stress and the presence of mental disorders.

Parasomnias

Parasomnias are a common cause of sleep disturbance and describe a set of undesirable physical or behavioural phenomena that take place while asleep. Disorders of arousal are the most common parasomnias and include such things as sleepwalking, night terrors, dressing, driving, and eating (all while asleep, usually with no recollection in the morning). Other parasomnias include rapid eye movement sleep behaviour disorder (acting out dream content), nocturnal seizures, hypnagogic hallucinations (visual or auditory sensations while drifting off to sleep), sleep-onset paralysis, bruxism (tooth grinding) as well as rhythmic-movement disorder (rhythmic moving such as body rocking and head banging while asleep).[155] As well as the disturbance in sleep that parasomnias may cause, they may also put the individual or others at risk (e.g. driving while asleep) and thus need to be investigated thoroughly.

Pain or discomfort

As with sleep-onset insomnia discussed above, pain and discomfort may also impair sleep-maintenance insomnia whereby pain prevents the continuation of sleep. Individuals suffering from chronic pain have been shown to have increased difficulty resuming sleep once awake, others may also experience the inability to resume sleep altogether. According to Ukponmwan,[156] the pain-relieving action of endogenous and exogenous opioids requires undisturbed sleep architecture. Clearly when there is disrupted sleep, deprivation of REM sleep prevents the pain-relieving effects of opioids and may explain increased pain sensitivity.

Drugs

Several drugs have been identified as hindering normal sleep (see Table 22.14). These include commonly used over-the-counter prescription medications as well as recreational drugs such as marijuana, amphetamines and

TABLE 22.14 Common contributing medications and substances

Category	Examples
Antidepressants	SSRIs (fluoxetine, paroxetine, sertraline, citalopram, escitalopram, fluvoxamine), venlafaxine, duloxetine, monoamine oxidase inhibitors
Stimulants	Caffeine, methylphenidate, amphetamine derivatives, ephedrine and derivatives, cocaine
Decongestants	Pseudoephedrine, phenylephrine
Narcotic analgesics	Oxycodone, codeine, dextropropoxyphene
Cardiovascular	β-blockers, α-receptor agonists and antagonists, diuretics, lipid-lowering agents
Pulmonary alcohol	Theophylline, salbutamol

Source: Adapted from Schutte-Rodin S, Broch L, Buysse D et al. Clinical guideline for the evaluation and management of chronic insomnia in adults. J Clin Sleep Med 2008; 4(5):487–504.

ecstasy. These are discussed in more detail later in this chapter.

Overview

Periods of good quality sleep are recognised as necessary to maintain a good balance of health. The physiological changes that occur in the body during wakefulness, NREM sleep, and REM sleep are detailed in Table 22.15, and the behavioural and physiological criteria of wakefulness and sleep are summarised in Tables 22.15 and 22.16; see also Fig. 22.14. Life is filled with events that may cause occasional insomnia in an individual who usually sleeps well; however, for many people, this condition occurs repetitively (nightly, weekly) over a prolonged period that may last from some months to several years. Over the years, the concept of insomnia has changed to reflect the advancement of our understanding. Initially the concept of 'unsatisfactory sleep' was promoted by the American Institute of Medicine in 1979.[157] In 1990, it then progressed to the International Classification of Sleep Disorders of the almost nightly complaint of insufficient sleep or the feeling of being unrested after the habitual

TABLE 22.15 Physiological changes in the body during wakefulness, NREM sleep, and REM sleep

Physiology	Wakefulness	Non-rapid eye movement sleep (NREM)	Rapid eye movement sleep (REM)
Respiratory rate	Normal	Decreases variable	Apnoeas may occur
Upper airway resistance	++	+++	++++
Peripheral vascular resistance	Normal	Normal or decrease slightly	Decreases further
Heart rate	Normal sinus rhythm	Bradycardia	Bradytachyarrhythmia
Cardiac output	Normal	Decrease	Decreases further
Blood pressure	Normal	Decreases	Variable
Cerebral blood flow	++	Decreased	++++
Alveolar ventilation	Normal	Decreases	Decreases further
Upper airway muscle tone	++	+	Decreases or absent
Penile or clitoral tumescence	Normal	Normal	Markedly increased
Sympathetic activity	++	+	Decreases or variable (++)
Parasympathetic activity	++	+++	++++
Swallowing	Normal	Decreases	Decreases
Gastric motility	Normal	Decreases	Decreases
Salivary flow	Normal	Decrease	Decreases
Gastric acid secretion	Normal	Variable	Variable
Thermoregulation	++	+	–
Migrating motor complex	Normal	Slow velocity	Slow velocity
Hypoxic and hypercapnic ventilatory (a special type of intestinal motor activity	Normal	Decreases	Decreases further

Key: + mild, ++ moderate, +++ marked, ++++ very marked, – absent
Source: Adapted from Chokroverty S. Overview of sleep and sleep disorders. Indian J Med Res 2010;131:126–140.

TABLE 22.16 Behavioural and physiological criteria of wakefulness and sleep

Criteria	Awake	Non-rapid eye movement (NREM) sleep	Rapid eye movement (REM) sleep
Mobility	Normal	Postural shifts; immobile or reduced slightly	Immobile or reduced moderately with myoclonic jerks
Eye movements	Waking eye movements	Slow rolling eye movements	Rapid eye movements
Eyelids	Open	Closed	Closed
Level of alertness	Alert	Unconscious but reversible	Unconscious but reversible
Posture	Erect, sitting, or recumbent	Recumbent	Recumbent
Response to stimulation	Normal	Mildly to moderately reduced	Moderately reduced to no response
Electro-oculography	Waking eye movements	Slow rolling eye movements	Rapid eye movements
Electroencephalography	Alpha waves; desynchronised	Synchronised	Theta or saw tooth waves; desynchronised
Electroencephalography (muscle tone)	Normal	Mildly reduced	Moderately to severely reduced or absent

Source: Adapted from Chokroverty S. Overview of sleep and sleep disorders. Indian J Med Res 2010; 131:126–140.

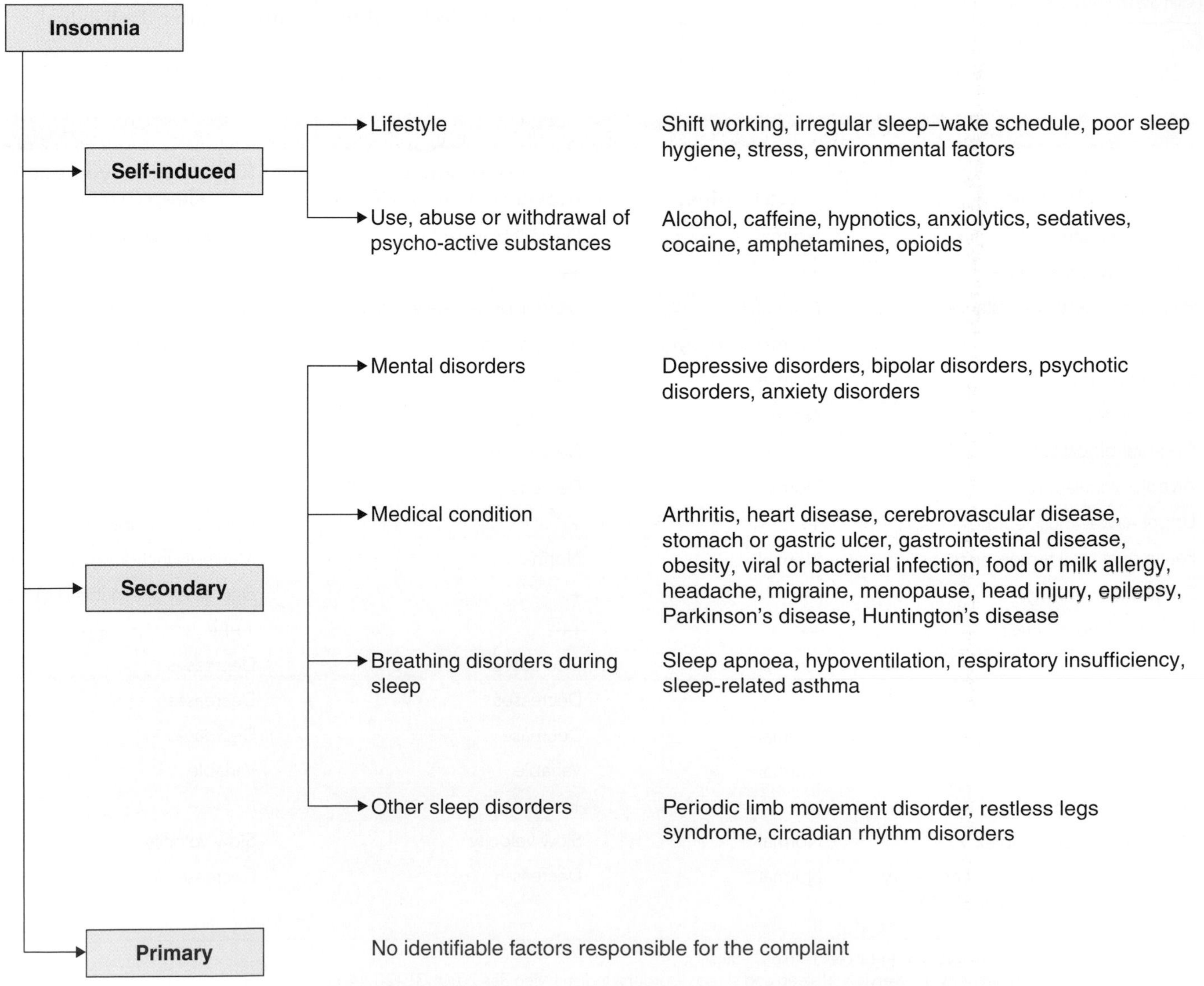

FIGURE 22.14 Factors associated with insomnia.

Source: Ohayon MM. Epidemiology of insomnia: what we know and what we still need to learn. Sleep Medicine Reviews 2002; 6(2): 97–111.

sleep period.[158] Most of the studies focus on three forms of insomnia symptoms:

- Difficulty in initiating sleep
- Disrupted sleep
- Early morning awakenings.

Non-restorative sleep, an insomnia symptom described in the DSM-IV and the International Classification of Sleep Disorders, is rarely studied. The daytime consequences of these symptoms are also often unexplored.

Pathogenesis

SIGNS AND SYMPTOMS

- Difficulty maintaining sleep
- Difficulty initiating sleep
- Early wakening
- Non-restorative sleep.

In addition to these night-time symptoms, individuals with insomnia may experience daytime symptoms such as fatigue, cognitive problems (difficulty concentrating, decreased efficiency), psychological disturbance (depression, anxiety, irritability), impaired psychomotor performance (e.g. driving a car) as well as nonspecific physical complaints such as headache and muscular aches and pains. (See also Fig. 22.15.)

COMPLICATIONS

Insomnia symptoms are present in the majority (over 80%) of people with a major depressive illness and persistent insomnia symptoms increase the likelihood of developing a major depressive illness within a one-year period with a risk factor of at least 4. Insomnia symptoms are associated with a mental disorder in more than one-third of cases.[154]

Common comorbid medical disorders, conditions and symptoms are summarised in Table 22.17.

DIFFERENTIAL DIAGNOSIS

Insomnia differential diagnosis and common comorbidities[159]

MEDICAL CONDITIONS

- Cardiovascular: congestive heart failure, arrhythmia, coronary artery disease
- Pulmonary: COPD, asthma
- Neurological: stroke, Parkinson's disease, neuropathy traumatic brain injury
- Gastrointestinal: gastro-oesophageal reflux
- Renal: chronic renal failure, nocturia
- Endocrine: diabetes, hyperthyroidism
- Rheumatological: rheumatoid arthritis, osteoarthritis, fibromyalgia, headaches.

SLEEP DISORDERS

- Restless legs syndrome
- Periodic limb movement disorder
- Sleep apnoea
- Circadian rhythm disorder
- Nightmares
- REM behaviour disorder.

PSYCHIATRIC CONDITIONS

- Depression
- Anxiety
- Panic disorder
- Posttraumatic stress disorder.

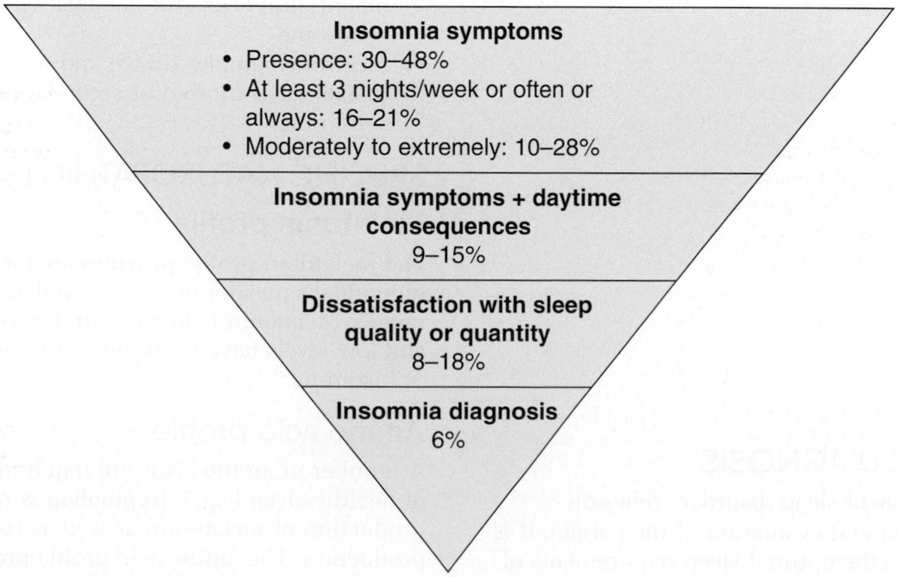

FIGURE 22.15 Average prevalence of insomnia symptoms and diagnoses.

Source: Ohayon MM. Epidemiology of insomnia: what we know and what we still need to learn. Sleep Medicine Reviews 2002; 6(2): 97–111.

TABLE 22.17 Common comorbid medical disorders, conditions and symptoms

System	Examples of disorders, conditions and symptoms
Musculoskeletal	Osteoarthritis, fibromyalgia, rheumatoid arthritis, kyphosis, Sjögren's syndrome
Pulmonary	COPD, emphysema, asthma, laryngospasm
Neurological	Chronic pain disorders, dementia, stroke, Parkinson's, traumatic brain injury, seizure disorders, headache disorders, neuromuscular disorders, peripheral neuropathy
Digestive	Irritable bowel syndrome, colitis, peptic ulcer disease, cholelithiasis, reflux
Cardiovascular	Angina, congestive heart failure, dyspnoea, arrhythmias
Endocrine	Hypothyroidism, hyperthyroidism, diabetes mellitus
Reproductive	Pregnancy, menopause, menstrual cycle variations
Genitourinary	Incontinence, benign prostatic hypertrophy, nocturia, enuresis, interstitial cystitis
Sleep disorders	Periodic limb movement disorder, circadian rhythm sleep disorders, parasomnias, central sleep apnoea, obstructive sleep apnoea, restless legs syndrome
Other	Allergies, rhinitis, sinusitis, bruxism, alcohol and other substance use/dependence/withdrawal

Source: Adapted from Schutte-Rodin S, Broch L, Buysse D et al. Clinical guideline for the evaluation and management of chronic insomnia in adults. J Clin Sleep Med 2008; 4(5):487–504.

MEDICATIONS

- Decongestants
- Antidepressants
- Corticosteroids
- Beta-agonists
- Stimulants
- Statins
- Diuretics.

SUBSTANCES

- Caffeine
- Alcohol
- Nicotine
- Cocaine.

NATUROPATHIC DIAGNOSIS

Naturopathic diagnosis of sleep disorders relies on discussion, assessment and evaluation of the patient. It is essential to determine the optimal sleep requirements of the patient and assess the severity of the disorder. The investigations outlined in 'Naturopathic investigations' should be considered with each patient. This enables an understanding of the effects of the presentation and determination of the cause.

Investigations

DIAGNOSTIC WORKUP FOR THE PRIMARY OR COMORBID CONDITION CAUSING SLEEP DISTURBANCE[160]

- Laboratory tests for the diagnosis and monitoring of sleep disorders
- Overnight polysomnography (PSG)
- Multiple sleep latency tests (MSLT)
- Maintenance of wakefulness test
- Actigraphy
- Video-PSG
- Standard electroencephalography (EEG) and video-EEG monitoring for suspected seizure disorders.

IMAGING STUDIES[160]

- Upper airway imaging for obstructive sleep apnoea syndrome
- Neuroimaging studies (e.g. computed tomography, magnetic resonance imaging) and cerebral angiography in cases of suspected neurological illness causing sleep disorder
- Positron emission tomography and single-photon emission computed tomography in special situations.

MISCELLANEOUS TESTS[161]

- Pulmonary function tests in cases of suspected bronchopulmonary and neuromuscular disorders causing sleep-disordered breathing
- Histocompatibility leucocyte antigen for suspected narcolepsy
- Cerebrospinal fluid hypocretin 1 levels in suspected narcolepsy
- Serum iron and ferritin levels as well as serum magnesium levels for patients with restless legs syndrome
- Electromyography (EMG) and nerve conduction studies to exclude comorbid or secondary restless legs syndrome.

SPECIFIC NATUROPATHIC INVESTIGATIONS

Melatonin profile

The melatonin profile provides an analysis of an individual's melatonin level as well as targeted reference ranges. Melatonin is involved in the regulation of sleep and low levels have been linked to sleep disturbances such as insomnia.

Amino acid profile

A number of amino acids are required for the maintenance of healthy sleep (e.g. L-tryptophan is required for production of melatonin) as well as for neurotransmitter production. The amino acid profile provides an analysis of amino acid status including essential and non-essential amino acids so that excess and deficiency can be observed. This may also be a useful test where comorbid conditions such as anxiety and depression coexist with impaired sleep.

Female or male hormone profile

The female hormone profile provides an assessment of the female's hormonal status. Hormonal imbalance (e.g. hot sweats during menopause) may interfere with normal sleep mechanisms hence the benefit of this test where indicated. Similarly, it is beneficial to review a male hormone profile to assess the impact of andropause or benign prostatic hyperplasia.

Essential fatty acids

Essential fatty acids play an essential role both structurally and functionally in sleep, thus analysis to ensure status is adequate is important. This is discussed in more detail in the section on nutrients for sleep.

Nutrient screen: vitamins, minerals and antioxidants

Nutritional deficiencies such as zinc and magnesium may impair neurological function thereby compromising sleep. Results from the vitamin, mineral and antioxidant analysis can be used to back up findings observed while case taking.

Thyroid hormone profile

Dysfunctional thyroid function may affect sleep hence females presenting with insomnia should be assessed for thyroid function where appropriate.

Cortisol/adrenal hormone profile

Consistently high cortisol levels throughout the day and into the night can make falling asleep and staying asleep difficult. High cortisol levels can be due to a stressful lifestyle, constant stress, or health-related issue. Cortisol levels can be tested easily by doing the Adrenal Stress Index (ADI) test. This test measures salivary cortisol levels at different times throughout the day and into the night. For a more in-depth approach, a 24-hour urinary free cortisol (UFC) can be collected and measured. In one study, a high 24-hour UFC was positively correlated with longer total wake time in insomniacs.[161]

QUESTIONING AND ASSESSMENT

Thorough assessment and case taking will typically elucidate a comprehensive overview. Appropriate questioning should include the following.[162]

Primary insomnia complaint

- Characterisation of complaint(s) — difficulty falling asleep, awakenings, poor or unrefreshing sleep
- Onset
- Duration
- Frequency
- Severity
- Course
- Perpetuating factors
- Past and current treatments and responses.

Pre-sleep conditions

- Pre-bedtime activities
- Bedroom environment
- Evening physical and mental status.

Sleep–wake schedule (average, variability)

- Bedtime — time to fall asleep, factors prolonging sleep onset, factors shortening sleep
- Awakenings — number, characterisation, duration; associated symptoms; associated behaviours
- Final awakening versus time out of bed
- Amount of sleep obtained.

Nocturnal symptoms

- Respiratory
- Motor
- Other medical
- Behavioural and psychological.

Daytime activities and function

- Identify sleepiness versus fatigue
- Napping
- Work
- Lifestyle
- Travel
- Daytime consequences — quality of life, mood disturbance, cognitive dysfunction, exacerbation of comorbid conditions.

Therapeutic considerations

CLINICAL DECISION MAKING AND RATIONALE

When considering the sleep-disordered patient, it is essential to determine compliance. If the patient expects to receive a natural sedative and take no responsibility to change their life, then treatment outcome will be minimal. Holistic naturopathy considers sleep to be a comprehensive reflection of the patient's emotional, mental, physical, and spiritual self. Sleep is seen as the time with which the body can relax, recharge and repair. Deficits in this process can erode the patient's equilibrium and can promote or initiate a variety of defects in health. At times one can be presented with a patient with, for example, digestive concerns whereby their perpetual sleep deficits have affected serotonin production and created anxiety-induced diarrhoea (morning diarrhoea) or similar.

When determining the course of treatment it is beneficial to thoroughly discuss the importance of a comprehensive and holistic treatment approach. The patient must be aware that they will need to adopt a variety of changes in all areas of their life for optimal outcome. Initial treatment must address the sedative requirement; however, it is beneficial to ascertain the trigger and make modifications as necessary for full recovery.

Therapeutic application

ALLOPATHIC PERSPECTIVE[163]

Non-pharmacological management

- Sleep hygiene strategies
- Stimulus control
- Sleep restriction
- Cognitive therapy
- Various relaxation therapies such as hypnosis, meditation, deep breathing and progressive muscle relaxation.

Pharmacological management

Pharmacological treatment may be indicated for short-term management of acute insomnia and for chronic insomnia when the non-pharmacological strategies described above are not effective.

Two types of hypnotic are available: benzodiazepines and the non-benzodiazepine drugs, zopiclone and zolpidem. Compared with benzodiazepines, zolpidem and zopiclone generally cause less morning sedation and have a less disruptive effect on normal sleep patterns.

Primary options include:

- Temazepam 10 mg orally
- Zolpidem 5–10 mg orally
- Zolpidem (controlled-release) 6.25–12.5 mg orally
- Zopiclone 3.75–7.5 mg orally.

Sedating antidepressants, such as the tricyclic antidepressants (TCAs) and mirtazapine, are sometimes used as hypnotics. A drug called Suvorexant has been approved for insomnia since 2015. It is a selective dual orexin receptor antagonist neuropeptide that blocks the brain's mechanism for generating wakefulness. It is available in 15 mg and 20 mg tablets.

HISTORICAL PERSPECTIVE

From the numerous botanicals recorded in the texts of the Eclectics it is clear that they had a wide array of sedative herbs at their disposal to induce sleep. The nervine tonic passiflora was observed to have hypnotic properties, as it produced a quality of sleep different from other sedatives. As written by Ellingwood: 'The patient goes to sleep naturally, can be awakened as usual at any time, to fall into a quiet, natural slumber. He awakens at the usual time rested and refreshed, with no disturbance of the cerebral functions, no languor, dullness or other disagreeable sensations'.[164]

Another nervine, *Scutellaria lateriflora*, was also employed particularly where insomnia was due to worry, nervous irritability or exhaustion, as was pulsatilla, the latter particularly for females and children. *Hyoscyamus niger* appears to have belonged to a stronger class of sedatives. It was indicated where there was mental excitement, as well as agitation and insomnia of exhaustion. Analgesic herb *Piscidia erythrina* was also prized in moderate dose for its sedative action. Not only did it lessen sensation (thus making it useful for sleep impairment due to pain) it also was useful for insomnia due to nervous, mental worry and anxiety where it produced a quiet and restful sleep.[164]

The Eclectic physicians also recommend the use of *Cannabis sativa* to enhance sleep, writing: 'Finally drowsiness overtakes him and he drops into a heavy sleep, which may last for hours, and from which he awakens with no other discomfort than a ravenous hunger',[9] highlighting the strong sedative action of this herb. The fact that we now know that this botanical does actually bring with it a lot of discomfort including alterations in normal sleeping patterns is an indication of the growth and development of herbal medicine today.

NATUROPATHIC PERSPECTIVE

The treatment goals for the sleep-disordered patient include:

- Improvement in sleep quality and/or time
- Improvement of insomnia-related daytime impairments such as improvement of energy, attention or memory difficulties, cognitive dysfunction, fatigue, or somatic symptoms
- Improvement in insomnia symptoms such as:
  - Formation of a positive and clear association between the bed and sleeping
  - Improvement in sleep-related psychological distress
  - Restoration of adrenal and nervine function.

NUTRITIONAL MEDICINE (DIETARY)

Dietary therapeutic objectives

- Meals must be regulated throughout the day to ensure blood sugar levels maintain equilibrium
- Protein requires repletion which is best delivered in larger doses at night-time in combination with essential fatty acids to enable sufficient relaxation to initiate and sustain sleep
- Ensure that night-time meals are light and easily digestible
- Avoid all stimulant foods entirely, particularly after midnight
- Assess and determine if any food allergy or intolerance is present that precipitates an adrenaline (epinephrine) reaction interfering with sleep initiation.

Specific dietary treatments

DIETARY INCLUSIONS

Protein

Protein is made up of amino acids in particular L-tryptophan, which plays an important role in the regulation of sleep due to its part in serotonin and melatonin synthesis. Adequate protein may also help to prevent nocturnal hypoglycaemia by stabilising blood sugar levels.

When presented with a patient suffering from insomnia it is essential to calculate their protein requirements based on their weight and energy expenditure. Of importance, reviewing their intake after 5 pm can elucidate clues that may contribute to mood and neurological fluctuations in the evening.

Essential fatty acids

Essential fatty acids have been shown to play an important part in sleep regulation where they are required structurally for neuronal membrane health as well as for production and regulation of prostaglandins that promote and suppress sleep.[165]

DIETARY EXCLUSIONS

Caffeine

Caffeine in all its forms (beverages, foods and medication) is discouraged owing to its stimulating nature. Caffeine has an antagonistic effect on adenosine receptors which are critically involved in sleep regulation and energy homeostasis. It has been found that the relationship between caffeine and adenosine is affected by genetic polymorphism ADA G22A.[166] Ageing also affects the adenosine receptors and adenosine formation, and a positive association has been found between caffeine-induced insomnia and age, for both men and women.[167] Ingestion of caffeine is associated with decreased sleep quality and an increased incidence of sleep complaints. A systematic review assessing the effectiveness of caffeine abstinence on quality of sleep observed that the removal of caffeine from the diet was associated with increased sleep duration and improved sleep quality.[168] It is important not to underestimate its effect. For example, a few squares of dark chocolate after dinner can be sufficient to prevent sleep initiation or to sustain sleep.

Alcohol

Sleep disturbance following alcohol ingestion is well documented. It is imperative to assess alcohol consumption in all patients who report alterations in normal sleep patterns. Although many individuals (particularly those with insomnia) may use alcohol to promote sleep, it is important to educate patients that while alcohol does contain sedative properties it is also a stimulant and will negatively affect the quality of their sleep. Alcohol ingestion in the evening is associated with greater incidence and loudness of snoring in males who already snore[169] as well as increased incidence of nocturnal respiratory events such as sleep apnoea.

Sugar and artificial sweeteners

Sugar is a stimulant and thus should be avoided throughout the day. It is essential to advise sleep-challenged patients to avoid the sugar addictive pattern throughout the day but especially close to sleep times.

Artificial sweeteners including aspartame have been associated with insomnia.[80] The consumption of aspartame can elevate levels of phenylalanine and aspartic acid in the brain, compounds which can change cerebral catecholamine metabolism and inhibit the synthesis and release of neurotransmitters, dopamine, noradrenaline (norepinephrine) and serotonin.[170] Aspartame and other artificial sweeteners should be avoided.

Food allergy

The concept of food allergy and its relationship with disordered sleep has been studied extensively in infants[171,172] many of whom experienced disordered sleep due to food allergy. Taking this into account it is also possible that in adults food allergy may play a part in aggravating sleep thus a thorough analysis should be undertaken of the diet.

NUTRITIONAL MEDICINE (SUPPLEMENTAL)

Nutritional medicine therapeutic objectives

- Optimise nutrient status for neurotransmitter regulation
- Provide key neurotransmitter energy by-products such as adenosine or other substances where possible to regulate sleep cycles
- Supply nutrients for serotonin regulation to support and improve melatonin pathways
- Provide nutritional cofactors for neuronal membrane structure and integrity.

Specific nutrients required

5-HYDROXYTRYPTOPHAN (5-HTP), TRYPTOPHAN

5-HTP and tryptophan are serotonin precursors and will thus be useful in promoting sleep due to the fact that serotonin is involved in the regulation of proper sleep. In his review Birdsall[173] reports on early studies undertaken in the early 1970s demonstrating the role of 5-HTP as a useful supplement for this purpose. In one study, supplementation with 5-HTP (600 mg) divided into two doses, one of 200 mg administered at 9.15 pm and a larger 400 mg dose at 11.15 pm resulted in an increase in REM sleep in a small study involving 8 individuals. A smaller dose 200 mg/day was also found to increase REM sleep (though to a lesser degree). However, the authors stipulate that this smaller dose is probably preferable as high doses of 5-HTP can paradoxically cause vivid dreams and nightmares. More recently 5-HTP was also found to be useful for sleep disturbances in children where it works to modulate arousal levels thus helping to alleviate 'night terrors'.[174] The availability of ingested tryptophan depends on the presence of other amino acids, macronutrient balance and adequate cofactors such as vitamin B_6 and EFAs for enzyme conversion.[175]

MELATONIN

Melatonin is a hormone secreted by the pineal gland in the brain that endogenously modulates sleep. It is controlled by the central circadian rhythm generator known as the suprachiasmatic nucleus of the anterior hypothalamus which adjusts melatonin levels in response to light cues. Melatonin production is inhibited during the day and enhanced at night.[176] Melatonin has been used to encourage sleep in people suffering from insomnia, jet lag and other dysfunctional circadian rhythm. It is believed to assist in the restorative value of sleep (perceived sleep quality).[177]

A 2017 systematic review of melatonin sleep studies included 1510 patients (aged 18–80) and found that melatonin had significant effects on treating primary insomnia, delayed sleep phase disorders and non-24-hour

SAMPLE DAILY DIET

BREAKFAST	
Turkey with smashed avocado and sliced tomato on stoneground bread Dandelion tea	Turkey is a source of tryptophan. Tryptophan stimulates serotonergic activity, promoting sleep. A tryptophan-rich breakfast in combination with exposure to daytime light increases night-time melatonin secretion and has been found to induce better onset of night sleep and higher quality of sleep in some individuals. Stimulants containing caffeine such as coffee and tea should be avoided and replaced with caffeine-free herbal alternatives particularly those with sedative properties such as chamomile.
LUNCH	
Beef, spinach and potato curry made with ground almonds and served with brown rice	Beef provides a source of vitamin B_{12}. Vitamin B_{12} is required for secretion of melatonin and may improve sleep–wake disorders. Leafy greens and almonds are sources of magnesium. Magnesium is a GABA agonist and plays a key role in sleep regulation. Brown rice is preferred to white rice as it retains GABA, calcium and magnesium.
DINNER	
Sweet potato chips with grilled salmon and a kiwi fruit, lime and pineapple salsa	Sweet potato provides high-quality carbohydrates. A carbohydrate-rich evening meal prior to bed may decrease time taken to fall asleep. Adequate protein is also important and appears to reduce waking episodes. Essential fatty acids are required for neuronal health. Consuming 2 kiwi fruits an hour before bedtime improves sleep onset, time taken to fall asleep, and increases total sleep time and sleep efficiency, both the total sleep time as well as sleep efficiency. Animal studies of kiwi fruit show it may exert its hypnotic action by modulating a GABAergic mechanism.
SNACK	
Tart cherry juice	Tart Montmorency cherries contain high levels of melatonin and may increase total sleep time and sleep efficiency. Fresh tart cherry juice, consumed twice daily, produced reductions in insomnia in 15 elderly people, and the time required to fall asleep was reduced by 17 minutes.

sleep–wake syndrome in blind individuals. Doses ranged from 0.1 mg to 10 mg over periods of 2 to 5 weeks.[178] A pilot study on 84 children with chronic sleep-onset insomnia showed that 3 mg of melatonin decreased sleep latency.[179] Melatonin has a low risk profile for physical dependence, and does not cause significant memory and cognitive impairment, psychomotor retardation or next-day hangover effect.[180] Melatonin is available in immediate and slow/controlled release formulas which might more accurately reflect natural melatonin cycles, but there is concern that extended durations of extended levels may be unsafe.[181]

Common doses range from 0.2 mg to 3 mg 1–2 hours before bed and away from food. Please note this is a Schedule 3 substance and is available by prescription only.

L-THEANINE

L-theanine is an amino acid commonly found in *Camellia sinensis* (a species commonly used for the production of green tea). Studies have shown that L-theanine (50 mg–200 mg) increases α-wave activity in areas of the cerebral cortex, leading to a relaxed state without drowsiness. Studies in animal models and human trials show that higher doses (250 mg–400 mg) have profound modulatory effects that result in improved sleep quality.[182,183] It's important to note that if green tea is to be used as a source of theanine in the diet to aid with sleep, then a lowered caffeine or decaf variety is needed. Studies have demonstrated that low-caffeine green tea can still be beneficial through its effect on lowering stress.[184,185]

B COMPLEX

The B vitamins play a pivotal role in the regulation of sleep mechanisms due to their multifaceted role within the body. One of the most important mechanisms with regards to sleep is the role of the B vitamins in the metabolism of serotonin: without adequate intake of B vitamins the body is unable to manufacture serotonin. Of the B vitamins both vitamin B_3 and B_6 are required for the synthesis of serotonin. Depletion of vitamin B_3 has also been linked to sleep-deprivation induced neuronal damage whereby Reimund[186] suggests that alterations in neuronal energy metabolism in sleep deprivation occur due to NADH and ATP depletion secondary to vitamin B_3. Lastly, acknowledging the stress as well as the fatigue that accompanies sleep disorders, a B complex will also be required to provide support to the body.

ZINC

Zinc functions as a cofactor in numerous essential bodily processes where it is required structurally and as a modulator for many proteins and enzymes for neurotransmission cell signalling[187] including that of the monoamine oxidases. Any disruption to this cell signalling and neurotransmission is likely to affect sleep. Zinc status should be screened in all patients presenting with insomnia.

A recent randomised controlled trial in healthy individuals (n = 120) showed that zinc enrichment led to improved sleep-onset latency and sleep efficiency.[188]

Clinical experience provides a rationale for this important recommendation. When prescribing zinc it is optimal to select a vitamin B_6-free prescription if taking this nutrient immediately prior to sleep. This prevents the common occurrence of nausea or dream interference initiated by vitamin B_6. Zinc citrate or picolinate appears to provide the strongest clinical outcome for this purpose.

ESSENTIAL FATTY ACIDS

The amount and type of particular fatty acids and the ratio between them have been hypothesised to play an important role in the regulation of sleep. Structurally fatty acids are required to make up the neuronal membrane and ensure its fluidity. Any impairment to these membranes due to inadequate supply of essential fatty acids results in changed sleep patterns as evidenced by Fagioli et al[189] who demonstrated decreased slow wave sleep in children with prolonged absence of essential fatty acids. Of particular importance is the ratio of omega-3 fatty acids to omega-6 acids. Two prostaglandins derived from the fatty acids have been identified as of particular importance. PGD2 functions to promote sleep while PGE2 functions to suppress sleep.[165] Without the presence of essential fatty acids production of PGD2 becomes impaired and hence alterations in normal sleep patterns ensue. Acknowledging the importance of fatty acids for sleep regulation, patients with sleep abnormalities should be screened for essential fatty acid intake.

ADENOSINE

The sedative and sleep-promoting effects of adenosine, an energy byproduct and inhibitory neurotransmitter, have been studied since the 1950s. Adenosine functions in the central nervous system to inhibit excitatory neurotransmitters as well as some inhibitory ones.[190] Extracellular levels of adenosine increase in the basal forebrain during periods of wakefulness: thus it has been revealed to be an important nutrient for sleep where it functions as a sleep–wakefulness modulator inhibiting wakefulness-promoting neurons.[191] Increases in duration and depth of sleep after wakefulness have been observed to be carefully modulated by increased concentrations of adenosine.[192] Interestingly, caffeine acts as an antagonist to adenosine affecting both the A1 and A2A receptors, the latter of which promote wakefulness. Ethanol increases extracellular adenosine thereby promoting sleepiness, however chronic exposure to alcohol reduces extracellular adenosine levels leading to a reduction in quality of sleep.[193] A polymorphism in the adenosine deaminase gene (ADA G22A) has been associated with deeper and more efficient sleep.[194]

MAGNESIUM

Magnesium is a cofactor for serotonin synthesis and thus deficiency will result in inadequate serotonin, a considerable problem since serotonin is involved in the regulation of sleep. Magnesium is a natural N-methyl-D-aspartic acid (NMDA) antagonist and GABA agonist, other factors which explain its role in sleep regulation. Magnesium, because of its relaxant action, may also be useful to help ease muscle tension and relieve nervous tension stress. Clinical efficacy warrants the prescription of magnesium for sleep disorders owing to its marked relaxing and muscular spasmolytic properties. A 2014 systematic review and meta-analysis found that magnesium does not appear to be an effective treatment for nocturnal leg cramps in the general population, but it may have a small effect in pregnant women.[195] A double-blind randomised clinical trial involving 46 elderly participants showed that administering magnesium oxide twice a day (total 500 mg elemental magnesium) over 8 weeks resulted in improvements in both objective and subjective sleep measures. There was a statistically significant increase in sleep time and sleep efficiency, and significant decrease in Insomnia Severity Score and sleep-onset latency in the supplemented group compared to placebo.[196] Combining magnesium with zinc is another treatment option. A trial conducted at a long-term care facility showed that in residents who suffered from insomnia, administering magnesium (225 mg) with melatonin (5 mg) and zinc (11.25 mg) daily for 2 months improved quality of sleep as well as quality of life.[197] The limited amount of formalised research warrants future research opportunities.

OTHER

Certain nutrients have been found to affect different aspects of sleep. For example, reduced selenium intake was found to be associated with difficulty falling asleep and lower vitamin C intake was associated with non-restorative sleep. Calcium intake was associated with both of these measures. Vitamin D was associated with less difficulty maintaining sleep. Lycopene was associated with less difficulty falling asleep.[198] Further detailed research is required on these specific nutrients.

Dosage requirements

The dosage requirements listed below are based on adult doses that have been reported in the literature.

- 5-HTP 2 mg/kg/day, typically given as 100–300 mg/day
- L-tryptophan: 1 g/day taken 20 minutes before bed. 0.25–0.5 g doses might also provide some benefit[177]
- L-theanine: 50 mg–400 mg taken 30-60 minutes before bed[175]
- Melatonin: 0.2–3 mg an hour before bed. Start at low doses and increase as necessary (up to 6 mg)[177]
- B complex (all B vitamins) high-dose combination, preferably activated forms
  - Thiamine 20–40 mg/day
  - Riboflavin 20–40 mg/day
  - Niacinamide 50–100 mg/day
  - Pantothenic acid 150–300 mg/day
  - Pyridoxine 50–250 mg/day

  - Folate as folinic acid or L5MTHF (as indicated) 500–2000 micrograms/day
  - Hydroxocobalamin or methylcobalamin 500–2000 micrograms/day
  - Choline 50–100 mg/day
  - Inositol 50–100 mg/day
  - Biotin 250–500 micrograms/day
- Zinc: 60 mg/day
- Essential fatty acids: total active constituents (EPA, GLA and DHA) should contain at least 1000 mg/day taken in divided doses in 3–6 g total fish oil/day
- Adenosine: 200 mg/day
- Magnesium: 250–750 mg/day in divided doses
- Protein: calculated based on patient's weight and energy expenditure, however, minimum dosage is ideally 0.8–1.4 g/kg body weight
- Tryptophan: 300–1000 mg/day
  - Or 5-HTP 50–150 mg/day (in some instances, doses as high as 400 mg/day may be required).

HERBAL MEDICINE

The therapeutic objectives and associated classes of herbal medicine are detailed in Table 22.18.

Specific herbal medicines

WITHANIA SOMNIFERA (ASHWAGANDHA)

Ashwagandha is an Ayurvedic herb long used for its adaptogenic effects. It has a balancing effect on the adrenal glands and immune system. It is believed to rejuvenate and promote longevity. In 2017, a group found that the active component of ashwagandha responsible for inducing sleep is triethylene glycol.[199] In addition, an animal study found that ashwagandha promoted anxiolytic effects and reduced acute stress. If stress is the main reason for insomnia, adding ashwagandha may help reduce stress and promote better sleep.[200]

HUMULUS LUPULUS (HOPS)

Humulus lupulus is a climbing perennial whose use as a herbal sedative for insomnia can be traced back to numerous traditional healing systems including that of Ayurvedic medicine, Chinese medicine and that of the Aboriginal Cherokees.[201] The German Commission E[201] approves the use of *Humulus lupulus* for sleep disturbances especially where there is anxiety and nervousness, while the British Herbal Compendium and ESCOP also highlight its use for sleep disorders. In-vivo studies reveal *Humulus lupulus* to have a central sedative effect increasing ketamine-induced sleeping time and reducing spontaneous locomotor activity.[202] However, despite the validation from well-regarded authorities on herbal medicine there have been relatively few human clinical studies undertaken using *Humulus lupulus* in isolation; rather, many of the studies assessed combine *Humulus lupulus* with *Valeriana officinalis*. A specific extract of *Humulus lupulus* in combination with *Valeriana officinalis* (known as extract Ze 91109) has been shown to decrease sleep latency in patients with non-organic sleep disorder compared with use of *Valeriana officinalis* in isolation.[203] In another double-blind, randomised, placebo-controlled sleep-EEG

TABLE 22.18 Herbal medicine therapeutic objectives and associated classes

Objective	Herbal medicine class
Symptomatic support	
Sedate patient	Sedative Hypnotic
Circadian rhythm stabilisation	Sedative Nervine tonic Nervine stimulant (caution with some) Melatonin stimulation Sunlight/moonlight, serotonin agonist
Restore nervous system function and integrity	Nervine tonic Nervine trophorestorative
Restore adrenal gland function and integrity	Nervine trophorestorative Adaptogen Adrenal restorative
Improve daytime cognition	Cerebro-circulatory stimulants Antioxidant Cognitive enhancer
General body tonification	Tonic Nutritive
Causative	
Reduce depression	Antidepressant Thymoleptic Euphoric Serotonin agonist
Reduce pain (if present)	Analgesic Anodyne
Alleviate anxiety	Anxiolytic Nervine tonic Sedative
Reduce addiction (narcotics, OTC)	Nervine tonic Nervine trophorestorative Antidepressant Thymoleptic Euphoric Serotonin agonist
Other	
Reduce stress (long and short term)	Adaptogen Adrenal restorative Nervine tonic Nervine trophorestorative Sedative (if indicated) Euphoric
Hormonal modulation	Serotonin agonist HPA modulator Melatonin stimulation (sunlight/moonlight)
Female or male hormonal modulation	As required: Female: HPO modulator, menstrual cycle regulator, female tonics, other specific hormonal modification (e.g. progesterone stimulant) Male: HPT modulator, male tonics, other specific hormonal modification (e.g. testosterone stimulant)

study using electrohypnograms, a single dose administration of a valerian/hops fluid extract was found to increase time spent in sleep when compared with placebo; time spent in deeper sleep was also statistically significant, suggesting better sleep quality.[204] In a 2010 trial of 101 adults with chronic primary insomnia, no improvement in quality of sleep or sleep duration was found with supplementation with 100 mg *Humulus lupulus* extract pills, taken nightly for 1 month, compared with placebo.[205]

A small trial ($n = 17$) found that drinking 333 mL non-alcoholic beer (containing around 1 g of hops) at dinner time, compared to no beer, reduced sleep latency and improved sleep quality in healthy nurses doing shift work.[206] The same researchers did another study with the same intervention on stressed university students ($n = 30$). Once again, there was a decrease in sleep latency, and improvement in subjective sleep quality.[207]

PASSIFLORA INCARNATA (PASSIONFLOWER)

The British Herbal Compendium[208] supports the use of *Passiflora incarnata* for sleep disorders as well as restlessness and nervous stress, the latter two indications useful since both may accompany sleep disorders. As with *Humulus lupulus* above, human clinical trials assessing the efficacy of *Passiflora incarnata* for sleep are lacking. However, a review of the *Passiflora* spp. suggests that *Passiflora incarnata* promotes REM sleep resulting in freshness on awakening.[209] The sedative properties of *Passiflora incarnata* have been confirmed in vivo, with a combination of *Passiflora incarnata* and *Piper methysticum* shown to significantly decrease amphetamine-induced hypermotility as well as prolong sleeping induced by subcutaneous injection of barbiturates. Interestingly, the combination of the two botanicals appeared to work better than when either extract was used alone.[210] In a randomised, double-blind trial, a combination of *Valeriana officinalis* (300 mg), *Humulus lupulus* (30 mg) and *Passiflora incarnata* (80 mg) was compared to zolpidem (10 mg) at bedtime in 78 patients with chronic insomnia. After 2 weeks the two treatments were equally effective at reducing sleep latency and improving sleep quality. Daytime drowsiness was not different between the groups and there were no serious adverse events.[211] Drinking one cup of *Passiflora incarnata* tea (2 g of dried leaves, stems, seeds, flowers) per night for just 1 week was shown to improve sleep quality in healthy adults with mild intermittent disturbed sleep in a small RCT.[212] *Passiflora incarnata* has been shown in vitro to affect GABA-A and GABA-B channels and to affect GABA uptake into neurons.[213]

PIPER METHYSTICUM (KAVA)

The roots of *Piper methysticum*, a Polynesian plant from the South Pacific Islands, function as a central nervous system depressant displaying sedative, muscle relaxant and anxiolytic actions, all of use in sleep disorders.[214] The kava lactones or pyrones (including kavain, methysticin, yangonin and dihydrokawain) have been shown to be responsible for these actions.[214]

In animal studies *Piper methysticum* has been shown to promote sedation, evidenced by a decrease in locomotor activity.[215] *Piper methysticum* may also enhance sleep quality seen by decreased sleep latency (time it takes to fall asleep) and increased delta activity during NREM sleep in sleep-deprived animals administered *Piper methysticum*.[216]

In human studies *Piper methysticum* has been shown to improve sleep disturbance associated with menopause,[217] as well as to decrease sleep latency, duration of wake phase and sleep stage 1.[218] *Piper methysticum* has also been shown to increase in sleep spindle density in a manner likened to that of tranquillisers and has also been shown to be effective for stress-induced insomnia.[219] The precise mechanism of *Piper methysticum* is unknown; however, the leading theory is that kavalactones interact with GABA receptors, acting as a positive allosteric modulator of the $GABA_A$ receptor. The binding site of kavain is unknown, but it is clearly different from the benzodiazepine site, as the action of kavain is not affected by a benzodiazepine antagonist, flumazenil.[220] *Piper methysticum* appears safe for use,[221] the usual recommended dose for insomnia is 210 mg of kavalactones, 1 hour before bedtime.[222] The German Commission E recommends 60–120 mg kavalactones.

PISCIDIA ERYTHRINA (JAMAICAN DOGWOOD)

The root bark of *Piscidia erythrina* has been traditionally documented for its use in sleep disorders. It was employed by the Eclectic physicians for its sedative and analgesic action and was said to be especially useful for prolonged insomnia particularly in the elderly and in those with a nervous temperament.[223]

SCUTELLARIA LATERIFLORA (SKULLCAP)

Scutellaria lateriflora is a gentle nervine sedative that was traditionally employed as a sedative due to its soothing action on the nervous system whereby it alleviated nervous excitability and irritability, promoting quiet and restful sleep.[164] *Scutellaria lateriflora* was also suggested for sleep disorders associated with the presence of pain. As yet clinical trials are lacking.

VALERIANA OFFICINALIS (VALERIAN)

Probably the most widely recognised herbal sedative and tranquilliser in Australia, *Valeriana officinalis* is a popular herb for the treatment of sleep disorders. Approved by the German Commission E for restlessness and sleeping disorders based on nervous conditions,[201] this odorous botanical contains a range of active constituents including valtrates, didrovaltrates and isovaltrates, monoterpenes and sesquiterpenes[201] — all of which are believed to work in synergy to produce its sedative effects.

Valeriana officinalis constituents are believed to inhibit sympathetic nervous system neurons activating gamma-aminobutyric acid (GABA) receptors involved in sleep promotion and regulation. However, *Valeriana officinalis* has also been shown to affect other receptors such as adenosine that are involved in the regulation of sleep.

A number of clinical trials have been undertaken assessing the efficacy of *Valeriana officinalis*. One such meta-analysis undertaken by Bent et al[224] suggested that *Valeriana officinalis* may improve quality of sleep. A more recent meta-analysis undertaken by Fernández-San-Martín et al[225] involved 18 randomised placebo-controlled trials which found a statistically significant improvement in the subjective variable of sleep quality but not in quantitative or objective measurements. In an early trial undertaken by Leathwood et al[226] *Valeriana officinalis* was found to decrease self-evaluated subjective sleep latency scores as well as to improve night-time quality, particularly among those who considered themselves poor or irregular sleepers and those who believed it took them a long time to fall asleep. A pilot study undertaken by Schultz et al[227] also observed positive results: *Valeriana officinalis* was shown to increase slow wave sleep in poor sleepers. However, no changes were observed on sleep-onset time or time waking after sleep. Though some studies have suggested that a single dose of *Valeriana officinalis* (when used in combination with *Humulus lupulus*) may be efficacious[204] the majority of the data reviewed suggest that *Valeriana officinalis* works better for long maintenance of sleep thus it would be better utilised for chronic insomnia then for acute insomnia (as in jet lag).[222] A randomised triple-blind controlled trial of 100 postmenopausal women found that 530 mg of concentrated *Valeriana officinalis* extract administered twice a day improved sleep quality.[228] A follow-up study by the same authors found that a combination of *Valeriana officinalis* (160 mg) and *Melissa officinalis* (80 mg) administered twice a day assisted in promoting sleep and improved sleep quality in menopausal women, compared to placebo.[229]

A 2017 randomised controlled trial using a combination of *Valeriana officinalis* (250 mg), *Humulus lupulus* (100 mg) and a Chinese medicine herb *Ziziphus jujube* (50 mg), administered twice daily for 20 days, showed improvement in sleep latency, total sleep time, and night wakenings in 120 people suffering from sleep disturbance symptoms.[230]

Not all studies have produced favourable results. A phase 2 randomised crossover trial both of 1-day and 2-week nightly treatment with *Valeriana officinalis* did not improve self-reports, polysomnography or actigraphic sleep outcomes in older women with insomnia; however, nocturnal wakefulness increased with *Valeriana officinalis*.[231] A 2015 systematic review and meta-analysis found that trials using high-dose *Valeriana officinalis* reported more favourable outcomes than those using lower doses.[232] Use of *Valeriana officinalis* is considered to be safe when taken in the doses recommended (300–900 mg standardised extract of 0.8%, or as a tea 1.5–3 g of root).[177] There is no evidence of any pharmacokinetic interactions between valerian and any drug.[233]

ZIZYPHUS SPINOSA (ZIZYPHUS)

Zizyphus spinosa has been widely used in Traditional Chinese Medicine to provide relief from sleep-related problems such as insomnia, anxiety and nervousness[234,235] because of its sedative and hypnotic effects. A number of constituents within *Zizyphus spinosa* have been identified as having sleep-promoting actions including alkaloids,[236] flavonoids and saponins,[237] in particular the saponin constituents known as the jujubosides.[235] Rats administered jujubosides during both the daytime and night-time were found to experience increases in total sleep time. During daytime (the equivalent of humans' night-time as rats are nocturnal) the jujubosides were found to increase REM sleep while during night-time (the equivalent of humans' daytime) the jujubosides significantly increased light sleep and showed no effect on REM sleep.

A significant amount of research[234] has focused on the use of *Zizyphus spinosa* in combination with *Magnolia officinalis*, a botanical with similar indications. The combination of the two herbs taken for 15 days consecutively has been shown to provide beneficial sedative properties in a number of unpublished studies. Further research is required to substantiate these findings. However, clinical evidence provides much efficacy for prescription.

A combination of *Zizyphus spinosa* and *Schisandra chinensis* was shown to have sedative-hypnotic effects that may be related to regulating amino acid neurotransmitter (GABA) in the hypothalamus of rats.[238]

MATRICARIA RECUTITA (CHAMOMILE)

A 28-day randomised, double-blind, placebo-controlled pilot trial in 34 patients with chronic primary insomnia, found that 270 mg (twice daily) of *M. recutita* did not find statistically significant improvements in sleep measures. Sleep measure results were mixed. A modest improvement in daytime functioning was reported.[239]

A trial of 80 Taiwanese postnatal women with poor sleep quality who were instructed to drink one cup of chamomile tea (2 g dried flowers) per day in addition to regular postpartum care, found significant improvements in sleep inefficiency and symptoms of depression compared to the control group who received regular postpartum care only. Effects were evident at 2 weeks follow up, however after stopping the treatment, the positive effects did not last long enough to be detectable at 4 weeks follow up.[240] A trial of chamomile (400 mg oral capsule administered twice daily, after lunch and dinner, for 4 weeks) to elderly patients in a nursing home showed that sleep quality was significantly improved after 4 weeks in the experimental group, compared to control. This shows promising results which can be applied in similar cases and nursing care.[241]

LIFESTYLE RECOMMENDATIONS

Sleep hygiene principles

Often individuals who present with problems sleeping will be helped simply from integrating good sleep hygiene principles into their usual routine. The concept of sleep hygiene has been around since the late 1970s and describes a set of principles and behaviours designed to enhance and promote sleep. The patient should seek to practise these principles on a daily basis. Examples of sleep hygiene principles include the following.[242,243]

SLEEP–WAKE ACTIVITY REGULATION

- Encourage regular time of arising, avoiding oversleeping
- Avoid lying in bed for long periods of time worrying about sleeping, instead set up a regular relaxing bedtime routing in a pleasant sleep environment
- Avoid napping (if necessary, limit to afternoon 'powernap' of 10–15 minutes)
- Encourage regular exercise well before bedtime.

The National Sleep Foundation shares similar sleep hygiene practices with the additions of avoiding stimulants like caffeine and nicotine close to bedtime, avoiding foods that disrupt sleep such as citrus and fatty foods that may cause gastro-oesophageal reflux and trigger indigestion, and ensuring adequate exposure to natural light during the day.

SLEEP SETTING AND INFLUENCES

- Avoid bright light exposure in late evening or night, particularly blue light from electronic device screens
- Encourage exposure to bright light after rising
- Avoid heavy meals or vigorous physical activity within 3 hours of bedtime
- Encourage a quiet, dark room for sleeping (remove television, stereo, laptop, internet access, mobile phone, etc.)
- Use a suitable mattress and pillow for comfort and support
- Reserve bedroom for sleep and intimacy
- Avoid alerting and stressful ruminations before bedtime. Allocate time earlier in the evening to go through worrying issues where possible
- If the individual cannot fall asleep after 15 minutes, suggest going to another room and returning to bed when tired
- Eliminate all stimulants such as caffeine, sugar, soft drinks and nicotine from the diet
- Reduce excessive alcohol intake
- Avoid illicit drugs
- Avoid having pets and highly illuminated digital clocks in the bedroom.

SLEEP-PROMOTING ADJUVANTS

- Encourage a light snack or a warm drink (preferably herbal tea)
- Encourage a warm bath before bed
- Ensure a comfortable temperature (19°C is optimal) and maximal darkness (can use blackout curtains)
- Encourage a 30–60 minute 'wind down' period before bed, setting aside some time to relax with a bedtime routine, such as warm bath, self-massage, breathing/ yoga nidra/relaxation CDs. Music may be effective for improving subjective sleep quality in insomnia.[244]

Warm bath

The humble hot bath should not be ignored. Horne et al[245] observed that a hot bath taken before bedtime resulted in passive body heating that increased the perception of sleepiness at bedtime, slow wave sleep and stage 4 sleep. REM sleep was reduced, particularly in the first REM sleep period. In contrast, a cold bath produced no effects.

Exercise

Regular exercise forms part of the sleep hygiene principles and is often promoted as encouraging sleep. A number of mechanisms have been suggested as to how exercise promotes better sleep including thermoregulation, energy conservation and body restoration,[246] all of which appear likely. The best effects appear to occur with aerobic endurance training and acute exercise of one hour or more. Overtraining, however, is a problem with exhaustive exercise of high intensity and long duration also suggested to inhibit sleep.[246]

RECREATIONAL DRUGS — MARIJUANA

Marijuana is commonly used to induce sleep.[247] However, a review of studies[248] suggests that chronic use of marijuana can result in increased tolerance to its sleep-inducing effects and subsequently more of the drug is required to get the desired effect. Marijuana use also interferes with normal sleep conduction; studies have generally been very small. However, decreased REM sleep has been consistently observed. Sleepiness may also be pronounced the following morning, particularly if there is poor clearance of D-9-tetrahydrocannabinol (THC), the constituent found within cannabis responsible for many of its psychotropic effects.[248] Withdrawal from marijuana is also associated with sleep abnormalities hence patients need to be supported appropriately.

STIMULANT SUBSTANCES

Where appropriate the prospect that sleep disturbances may be associated with use of illicit drugs must be considered. Use of stimulant substances such as cocaine, 3,4-methylenedioxymethamphetamine (ecstasy) and amphetamines are illicit substances that have a stimulating effect in the body and are associated with a range of sleep disturbances.[248] Polysomnography studies of individuals' sleep patterns following cocaine use reveal longer sleep latency, reduced total sleep time and suppression of REM sleep.[249,250] Meanwhile, ecstasy users may experience wakefulness, no REM sleep[251] and abnormal circadian rhythm patterns due to serotonergic dysfunction. Thorough education on the relationship of recreational habits and subsequent altered sleep patterns must ensue.

OTC MEDICATION REVIEW

Illicit substances are not the only drugs that need to be considered. Over-the-counter (OTC) medications may also cause sleep disturbance hence a case history should include questioning of all medications being used (in addition to OTC) as well as a thorough investigation of their side effects. A number of medications have been indicated as possible sleep disturbers including: anticholinergic agents, antidepressants (SSRIs, bupropion), MAOIs, antiepileptics (lamotrigine, phenytoin), antineoplastics, beta-blockers, bronchodilators (beta agonists), CNS stimulants (methylphenidate dexamphetamine, nicotine), interferon alfa, steroids, oral contraceptives, progesterone, thyroid hormones, and miscellaneous (diuretics, atorvastatin, levodopa).[252]

CASE STUDY

OVERVIEW

JP, a 42-year-old male presented with insomnia of extended duration. It had progressed from a period of significant stress 6 months prior. JP had not been able to break the cycle. He felt that the occupational stress had dissipated but that he continued poor habits that perpetuated the cycle. Upon discussion, it was clear that JP had an extended history of anxiety and had been medicated previously (Aropax) but he had discontinued it due to side effects of erectile dysfunction and poor sleep quality. His anxiety continued but was mildly managed through self-directed cognitive behavioural therapy (CBT) strategies and avoidance tactics including excessive television watching, and alcohol consumption (up to 2 bottles of wine at night).

He explained that he often fell asleep on the couch (at approximately 10 pm) while watching television and rose at 1–2 am, then showered and got into bed. From then on he tossed and turned throughout the night and eventually got out of bed and exercised at 4.30 am.

CLINICAL EXAMINATION

- Magnesium deficiency signs: bitten fingernails, eye twitches and leg cramping (especially at night)
- B vitamin deficiency signs: glossitis, cracks at the corner of mouth, mouth ulcers

TREATMENT PROTOCOL

HERBAL MEDICINE

Both a day and night formula were prescribed to sustain and nourish energy throughout the day and sedate, repair and restore during the night.

Day formula

Herbal medicine	Ratio	Quantity	Rationale
Scutellaria lateriflora	1:2	50 mL	Nervine tonic, mild sedative
Withania somnifera	1:1	60 mL	Nervine tonic, adaptogen, restorative
Bacopa moniera	1:2	70 mL	Cognitive enhancer, nervine tonic
Panax ginseng	STD Ext	40 mL	Adaptogen, tonic
TOTAL: 220 mL			

Dose: 7.5 mL twice a day

Night formula

Herbal medicine	Ratio	Quantity	Rationale
Zizyphus spinosa	1:2	80 mL	Sedative, anxiolytic
Piscidia erythrina	1:2	30 mL	Sedative, nervine
Lavandula angustifolia	1:2	30 mL	Sedative, hypnotic, mild antidepressant, anxiolytic
Humulus lupulus	1:2	20 mL	Hypnotic, sedative, anodyne, anxiolytic
Passiflora incarnata	1:2	60 mL	Hypnotic, nervine relaxant, sedative, anxiolytic
TOTAL: 220 mL			

CASE STUDY CONTINUED

Dose: 5 mL 1–3 times at night (one dose with dinner and another before bed as required)

NUTRITIONAL MEDICINE

Dietary

- Protein (especially consumed at dinner) calculated based on weight at 1.2 g/kg body weight
- Adequate essential fatty acids in the diet (primarily at dinner)
- Ensure that night-time meals are light and easily digestible
- Avoidance of all stimulants including caffeine, alcohol, sugar and preservatives (MSG especially).

Supplemental

- Magnesium: 400 mg twice a day
- B complex (activated and high dose): 1 capsule twice a day
- Zinc picolinate 60 mg before bed.

LIFESTYLE/EDUCATION

- Educate in and encourage full sleep hygiene:
  - Avoid all electromagnetic exposure at night (including lights) with use of candles only
  - Relax for 30 minutes (breathing or meditation) prior to showering or bathing before getting into bed
  - Avoid all stimulants (dietary, television, emotional, occupational, other) from 1 hour prior to anticipation of going to bed
  - Plan to go to bed at a time when the patient could calculate at least 8 hours of quality, solid sleep
- Observe circadian rhythm principles
- Continue daily exercise to assist with reducing anxiety and stress, and promoting energy levels.

HEADACHES AND MIGRAINES

Epidemiology

Headaches (Fig. 22.16) are among the most common neurological symptoms experienced, and are characteristic for the recurrent head pain that they cause. The worldwide prevalence of adults with an active headache disorder is estimated to be 47% for headache in general, 10% for migraine, 38% for tension-type headache, and 3% for

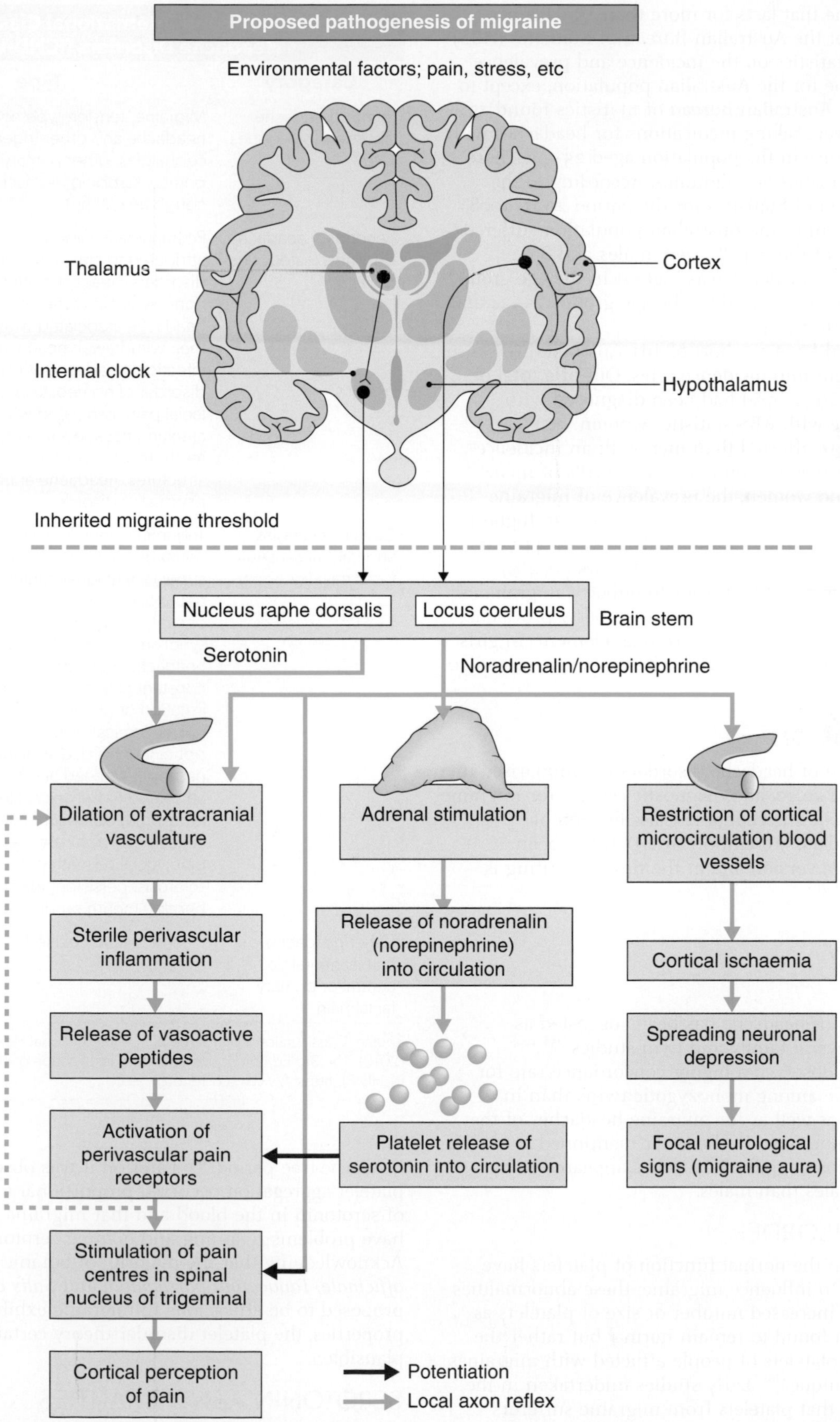

FIGURE 22.16 Headaches and migraines.

Source: Yanoff, Duker. Ophthalmology. 3rd edn. Mosby, 2008.

chronic headache that lasts for more than 15 days per month.[253] As yet the Australian Bureau of Statistics (ABS) does not hold statistics on the incidence and prevalence rates of headache for the Australian population, except to say in 1995, the Australian Bureau of Statistics found 15% of Australians were taking medications for headaches with a higher prevalence in the population aged 25–44. There are, however, statistics on migraines. According to the Australian Bureau of Statistics for the period 2007–2008, 5.7% (1.66 million) of the Australian population suffered from migraines, of these 3.3% were males and 8% females. Migraine incidence was highest in the age group 35–44 years (9.7%), followed by the age groups 25–34 and 45–54 years (both 7.4%).[254]

Data collected from a cohort of 191 Australian GPs also provide an insight into incidence rates. Out of a total of 5663 patients, 649 (11.5%) had been diagnosed with migraine. In line with ABS statistics women were significantly more affected than men with an incidence rate of 14.9% in women compared with 6.1% of men.[255] For both men and women, the prevalence of migraine appeared to rise throughout early adult life with highest incidence observed among individuals aged 25–44 years (17.6%), followed by those aged 45–64 years (15.4%). Interestingly, it is noted that prior to puberty, migraine is more common in males but following puberty prevalence increases in girls suggesting a hormonal element. In girls and women, the rate almost triples between age 10 and 30 years.[256]

Classification

The classification of headache disorders is summarised in Tables 22.19 and 22.20, and diagnostic criteria for migraine in Table 22.21. The International Classification of Headache Disorders, 3rd edition (ICHD-3) has been released as a beta version and at the time of writing is being finalised.[257]

TABLE 22.19 Second International Classification of Headache Disorders (ICHD-II)

Category	Type
Primary headache disorders (categories 1–4)	Migraine, tension-type headache, cluster headache and other trigeminal cephalgias, other primary headache (e.g. primary stabbing headache, primary cough headache)
Secondary headache disorders (categories 5–12)	Posttraumatic headache; headache attributed to cranial or cervical vascular disorders; headache attributed to nonvascular intracranial disorder; headache associated with substances or their withdrawal; headache attributed to infection; headache attributed to disorder of homeostasis; headache or facial pain associated with disorder of cranium, neck, eyes, ears, nose sinuses, teeth, mouth, or other facial or cranial structures; headache attributed to psychiatric disorder
Cranial neuralgias and central causes of facial pain (category 13)	Trigeminal neuralgia; glossopharyngeal neuralgia; nervus intermedius neuralgia; superior laryngeal neuralgia; nasociliary neuralgia; supraorbital neuralgia; occipital neuralgia; neck-tongue syndrome; external compression headache; cold stimulus headache; constant pain caused by compression, irritation or distortion of cranial nerves or upper cervical roots by structural lesions; optic neuritis; ocular diabetic neuropathy; head and facial pain attributed to herpes zoster; Tolosa-Hunt syndrome; ophthalmoplegic migraine; anaesthesia dolorosa; central poststroke pain; facial pain attributed to multiple sclerosis; persistent idiopathic facial pain; buming mouth syndrome
Other headache, cranial neuralgia, central or primary facial pain	Headache unspecified

Source: Classification Committee of The International Headache Society (2018). The 3rd Edition of International Classification of Headache Disorders (ICHD-3), https://www.ichd-3.org/

Aetiology

GENETICS

A genetic basis for headache has been suggested as evidenced by several family and twin studies.[258–260] Larsson et al[259] observed a higher concordance rate for lifetime migraine among monozygotic twins than in dizygotic twins as well as for migraine headaches of the recurrent disabling type. In the latter mentioned study the genetic effects for migraine headaches appeared to be stronger in females than males.

PLATELET DISORDER

Abnormalities in the normal function of platelets have been suggested to influence migraine; these abnormalities do not relate to increased number or size of platelets as those have been found to remain normal but rather the composition of platelets of people afflicted with migraines appears to be unique.[261] Early studies undertaken in the 1980s observed that platelets from migraine sufferers demonstrated higher spontaneous platelet aggregation and platelet adhesion than platelets from controls during a headache-free period.[262] Later on it was observed that platelet aggregation occurred proportional to the content of serotonin in the blood and that migraine platelets may have problems retaining and holding serotonin.[261] Acknowledging that the majority of botanicals (*Zingiber officinale*, *Tanacetum parthenium* and *Salix alba*) that are proposed to be efficacious in migraine exhibit antiplatelet properties, the platelet disorder theory certainly appears plausible.

SEROTONIN ABNORMALITIES

The relationship between serotonin and migraine is complex and the exact mechanism that links abnormal

TABLE 22.20 Classification of headaches		
Type	**Symptoms**	**Precipitating factors**
Hangover headache	Migraine-like symptoms of throbbing pain and nausea not localised to one side	Alcohol, which causes dilation and irritation of the blood vessels of the brain and surrounding tissue
Caffeine-withdrawal headache	Throbbing headache caused by rebound dilation of the blood vessels, occurring multiple days after consumption of large quantities of caffeine	Caffeine
Exertion headache	Generalised head pain of short duration (minutes to 1 hour) during or following physical exertion (running, jumping, or sexual intercourse) or passive exertion (sneezing, coughing, moving one's bowels, etc.)	10% caused by organic diseases (aneurysms, tumours, or blood-vessel malformation). 90% are related to migraine or cluster headaches
Posttraumatic headache	Localised or generalised pain, can mimic migraine or tension-type headache symptoms	Headaches usually occur on daily basis and are frequently resistant to treatment. Pain can occur after relatively minor traumas
Hunger headache	Pain strikes just before mealtime. Caused by muscle tension, low blood sugar and rebound dilation of the blood vessels, oversleeping or missing a meal	Strenuous dieting or skipping meals
Temporomandibular joint (TMJ) headache	A muscle-contraction type of pain, sometimes accompanied by a painful 'clicking' sound on opening the jaw. Infrequent cause of headache	Caused by malocclusion (poor bite), stress, and jaw clenching
Tic douloureux headaches	Short, jab like pain in trigger areas found in the face around the mouth or jaw. Frequency and longevity of pain vary	Relatively rare disease of the neural impulses; more common in women after age 55. Cause unknown. Pain from chewing, cold air, touching face. If under age 55, may result from neurological disease such as MS
Fever headache	Generalised head pain that develops with fever. Caused by swelling of the blood vessels of the head	Infection
Arthritis headache	Pain at the back of head or neck. Intensifies on movement. Caused by inflammation of the blood vessels of the head or bony changes in the structures of the neck	Unknown. Possible inflammatory cascade or mediation
Eyestrain headache	Headaches usually frontal, bilateral pain, directly related to eye strain	Muscle imbalance. Uncorrected vision, astigmatism
Temporal arteritis headache	Boring, burning, or jabbing pain caused by inflammation of the temporal arteries. Pain, often around ear, on chewing	Weight loss, eyesight problems. Rarely affects people under 50
Tumour headache	Pain progressively worsens, projectile vomiting, possible visual disturbances speech or personality changes; problems with equilibrium, gait or coordination; seizures. Extremely rare condition	Cause of tumour is usually unknown
Tension-type headache	Dull, non-throbbing pain, frequently bilateral, associated with tightness of scalp or neck. Degree of severity remains constant	Emotional stress. Hidden depression
Migraine without aura	Severe, one-sided throbbing pain, often accompanied by nausea, vomiting, cold hands, sensitivity to sound and light	Certain foods, the Pill or hormones, excessive hunger, changes in altitude, weather, lights, excessive smoking, and emotional stress. Hereditary component
Migraine with aura	Similar to migraine without aura, except warning symptoms develop. May include visual disturbances, numbness in arm or leg. Warning symptoms subside within one-half hour, followed by severe pain	Certain foods, the contraceptive pill or hormones, excessive hunger, changes in altitude, weather, lights, excessive smoking, and emotional stress. Hereditary component
Cluster headaches	Headaches of excruciating pain in vicinity of eye. Tearing of eye, nose congestion, flushing of face. Pain frequently develops during sleep and may last for several hours. Attacks occur every day for weeks/month, then disappear for up to a year. 90% of cluster patients are male, most ages 20–50	Alcoholic beverages, excessive smoking

Continued

TABLE 22.20 Classification of headaches—cont'd

Type	Symptoms	Precipitating factors
Menstrual-related headaches	Headaches–migraine-type pain that occurs shortly before, during, or immediately after menstruation or at mid-cycle (at time of ovulation)	Hormonal imbalance
Hypertension	Generalised or 'hairband' type pain, most severe in the morning. Diminishes throughout day	Severe hypertension: >200 mmHg systolic and >110 mmHg diastolic
Aneurysm	Symptoms may mimic frequent migraine or cluster headaches, caused by balloon-like weakness or bulge in blood-vessel wall. May rupture (stroke) or allow blood to leak slowly resulting in a sudden, unbearable headache, double vision, rigid neck. Individual rapidly becomes unconscious. Congenital tendency	Extreme hypertension
Sinus headaches	Gnawing pain over nasal area, often increasing in severity throughout day. Caused by acute infection, usually with fever, producing blockage of sinus ducts and preventing normal drainage. Sinus headaches are rare. Migraine and cluster headaches are often misdiagnosed as sinus in origin	Infection, nasal polyps, anatomical deformities, such as a deviated septum, that block the sinus ducts
Allergy headache	Generalised headache. Nasal congestion, watery eyes. Seasonal allergens, such as pollen, moulds	Allergy

Source: Adapted from National Headache Foundation. Headache topic sheets. Available from: https://headaches.org/resources/headache-topic-sheet/

TABLE 22.21 Diagnostic criteria for migraine

Migraine without aura	A At least five attacks fulfilling B–D B Headache attacks lasting 4–72 hrs (untreated or unsuccessfully treated) C Headache has at least two of the following characteristics: unilateral location, pulsating quality, moderate or severe pain intensity, aggravation by or causing avoidance of routine physical activity (e.g. walking or climbing stairs) D During headache at least one of the following: nausea and/or vomiting, photophobia and phonophobia E Not attributed to another disorder
Migraine with typical aura	A At least two attacks fulfilling B–C B Aura consisting of at least one of the following, but no motor weakness: fully reversible visual symptoms including positive features (e.g. flickering lights, spots, or lines) and/or negative features (i.e. loss of vision), fully reversible sensory symptoms including positive features (e.g. pins and needles) and/or negative features (i.e. numbness), fully reversible dysphasic speech disturbance C At least two of the following: headache fulfilling criteria B–D for migraine without aura; begins during the aura or follows aura within 60 min; headache that does not fulfil criteria B–D for migraine without aura; begins during the aura or follows aura within 60 min; headache does not occur during aura or follow aura within 60 min D Not attributed to another disorder

Source: Classification Committee of The International Headache Society (2018). The 3rd Edition of International Classification of Headache Disorders (ICHD-3), https://www.ichd-3.org/

serotonin neurotransmission to headaches is still unknown. It is clear that serotonin plays a large role in the pathogenesis of migraine as evidenced by the numerous studies available on the topic.[263] Consider that serotonin is involved in the regulation of pain, low concentrations of serotonin then can be seen to contribute to the considerable pain associated with migraine. Early studies showed that serotonin was released by platelets during migraine attack and it was initially proposed that hyposerotonergic status was a causative factor in migraine and tension headache. It now appears that low serotonin turnover and serotonin vascular hyperreactivity both contribute to the pathogenesis of migraine.[264] Serotonin vascular hyperreactivity has been shown to be more pronounced in females than males perhaps accounting for the high prevalence of migraine headache seen in women.

TABLE 22.22 Characteristics of headaches attributed to drugs and drug classes

Type of headache	Medication associated with headache
Migraine without aura	Cyclosporin, dipyridamole, nitric oxide donors, phosphodiesterase inhibitors, interferon-β, ondansetron, tacrolimus, sertraline
Migraine with aura	Nitric oxide donors, phosphodiesterase inhibitors, tacrolimus, fluoxetine
Typical aura w/out headache	Tadalafil
Cluster headache	Nitric oxide donors, phosphodiesterase inhibitors

Source: Ferrari A, Spaccapelo L, Gallesi D et al. Focus on headache as an adverse reaction to drugs. J Headache Pain 2009; 10(4):235–239.

VASOMOTOR INSTABILITY

Changes in blood vessels and cerebral vascular flow as a result of constriction or dilation of the blood vessels have been found to be involved in the pathogenesis of migraine.[265] Animal studies reveal that stimulation of the brainstem nuclei, locus coeruleus and raphe dorsalis alters both intracranial and extracranial blood flow. Blau[266] notes that in cluster headaches vasodilation provokes a headache while vasoconstriction stops attacks, thus promoting vasomotor stability may be one way in which to help relieve migraines of this origin.

NEURONAL DISORDER/SENSORY DEFECTS

Migraines have also been suggested to occur as a result of sensory defects in which the sensory system of the nervous system becomes hyperactive.[267] In this model, platelet composition abnormalities and subsequent release of serotonin and other components during an attack are considered to be secondary events to sensory defects and neuronal disorder.[268]

MEDICATION REACTION

Headache may be associated as an adverse drug reaction to medication due to vasodilation or increased intracranial pressure, an example of this may be seen with the use of the antihypertensive ACE inhibitors and calcium channel blockers which may cause headaches due to their vasodilator effects (see Table 22.22 for more examples).

MEDICATION-OVERUSE HEADACHE (MOH)

Overuse of headache medication paradoxically leads to 'medication-overuse headache' a headache induced by abuse of analgesics, triptans or other acute headache medications. Amazingly, this type of headache is estimated to be the third most common type of headache after tension-type headache and migraine and is estimated to affect approximately 1% of the world's population.[269] The current recommendation is to limit headache treatment to 10–15 days a month so as to minimise the risk of MOH. However, a recent discussion paper brought up many observational studies. The researchers concluded that perhaps we should consider frequent symptom-relieving headache medications as an indication of poorly controlled headaches and not as a cause until further research says otherwise.[270]

HORMONES/MENSTRUAL RELATED MIGRAINE HEADACHE

A large proportion of women who experience migraine report an association between menstruation and migraine[271] thus migraine has been hypothesised to be influenced by fluctuating hormonal levels[272] or possibly iron loss from menses. Consideration of the menstrual cycle and relevant questioning is required when conducting a history intake.

FOOD ALLERGY/INTOLERANCE

Migraine has been called an allergic disease[273] due to the proposed link between migraine and food allergies/intolerances/sensitivities. A high incidence of migraine and headache have been found in patients with coeliac disease compared with controls;[274] moreover, adherence to a strict gluten-free diet is associated with a significant reduction of headache. Similar results were seen in a study by Bushara et al in which individuals with coeliac disease observed a reduction in the incidence of migraine headaches.[275] Early proponents suggested testing for IgE-specific food allergy but a later review proposed that an IgE mediated immune reaction seemed to be unimportant in the process of food-induced migraine.[276] Nevertheless, as seen by the studies mentioned in Table 22.23, many individuals report favourable effect following removal of allergy/intolerance promoting items in their diet. With new laboratory advancements, other immunoglobulins that affect food intolerances such as IgA and IgG can be tested. Both these immunoglobulins are linked to food sensitivities and can further help clinicians assist patients with individualised elimination diets.

DIETARY AMINES

Diet appears able to trigger a migraine, with a number of different dietary components implicated in the pathogenesis of migraine, including MSG, tyramine, phenylethylamine, nitrites and nitrates, alcohol and caffeine. These are discussed in more detail further on in this chapter.

Overview

Headaches are neurological disorders affecting the head region owing to alterations in the pain sensitive structures of the brain. Subsequent discomfort and pain are experienced by the sufferer. Headaches may be interspersed by periods of remission.

PATHOGENESIS

Although headaches and migraines are common, clear pathogenesis remains unclear. Vascular and neuronal

TABLE 22.23 Foods that most commonly induce migraine headaches

Food	Egger et al(%)	Hughes et al(%)	Monro et al(%)
Cow's milk	67	57	65
Wheat	52	43	57
Chocolate	55	57	26
Egg	60	24	22
Orange	52	-	13
Benzoic acid	35	-	-
Cheese	32	-	-
Tomato	32	14	-
Tartrazine	30	-	-
Rye	30	-	-
Rice	-	-	30
Fish	22	29 (shell)	17
Grapes	12	33	-
Onion	-	24	-
Soy	17	24	-
Pork	22	-	17
Peanuts	12	29	-
Alcohol	-	29	9
Monosodium glutamate	-	19	-
Walnuts	-	19	-
Beef	20	14	-
Tea	17	-	17
Coffee	15	19	17
Nuts	12	19 (cashew)	17
Goats' milk	15	14	-
Corn	20	9	-
Oats	15	-	-
Cane sugar	7	19	-
Yeast	12	14	-
Apple	12	-	-
Peach	12	-	-
Potato	12	-	-
Chicken	7	14	-
Banana	7	-	-
Strawberry	7	-	-
Melon	7	-	-
Carrot	7	-	-

Sources: Egger J, Carter CM, Wilson J et al. Is migraine food allergy? A double-blind controlled trial of oligoantigenic diet treatment. Lancet 1983; 2:865–869. Hughes EC, Gott PS, Weinstein RC et al. Migraine: a diagnostic test for etiology of food sensitivity by a nutritionally supported fast and confirmed by long-term report. Ann Allergy 1985; 55:28–32. Monro J, Brostoff J, Carini C et al. Food allergy in migraine. Study of dietary exclusion and RAST. Lancet 1980; 2:1–4. Murray M, Pizzorno J. Textbook of natural medicine. Elsevier; 2006.

abnormalities have both been proposed as playing an important role in the pathogenesis of migraine as have muscular tension and mitochondrial dysfunction.

Signs and symptoms

Signs and symptoms of headache and migraine are highly variable and dependent upon the type of headache/migraine experienced. The most defining trait is the recurrent pain experienced in the head area. Over 100 different types of headache have been found, and typically while head pain is experienced in all, the location, duration and nature of the pain will usually provide a clue as to what type of headache is being experienced, hence the importance of taking a thorough history.

The classical description of migraine headache as defined by the International Headache Classification Society is quite specific and defines migraines as unilateral and throbbing in nature with photophobia and/or phonophobia. This definition has led to criticism owing to its narrowness, particularly as it has been noted that a third of migraine headaches are bilateral and not all throb or are accompanied by nausea and photophobia. Thus it is important to take into account that not all individuals will fit into the rigid guidelines set out in the classification criteria.

For a thorough discussion of signs and symptoms please refer to Table 22.20.

COMPLICATIONS

Headaches and migraine may be indicative of other health problems. Warning signs in the diagnosis of headache are summarised in Table 22.24.

Cardiovascular health

The link between impaired cardiovascular health and migraine has undergone much research and there appears to be a definite relationship thus cardiovascular risk as well as support is an area that also needs to be considered when the migraine patient presents. Migraine sufferers who also experience aura are at a twofold-increased risk of developing ischaemic stroke.[277] A population study[278] also demonstrated that migraines are associated with an increased risk of stroke, myocardial infarction and claudication. Though extremely rare, a recent case of migrainous infarction was published in Autopsy & Case Reports when a 16-year-old female was hospitalised for migraines and concurrently suffered a midbrain ischaemic stroke.[279]

Affective disorders

Affective disorders including anxiety, depression, bipolar and panic disorder have all been implicated as comorbid with migraine. Aside from the impaired quality of life and pain that may contribute to the sufferer's experience, abnormalities of serotonin implicated in the pathogenesis of migraine are also likely to influence mood. Statistics vary but suggest that 33–40%,[280,281] of individuals with migraine and 35%[281] of those with cluster headache may suffer from depression.

TABLE 22.24 Warning signs in the diagnosis of headache

Type of headache	Possible organic causes
Sudden onset, accompanied by drowsiness, vomiting and confusion; mild stroke-like symptoms may be present (diplopia, sixth nerve palsy, ataxia, mild hemiparesis, Horner's syndrome)	Cerebral venous thrombosis, intracranial or subarachnoid haemorrhage, vertebral or carotid artery dissection
Recent onset, accompanied by drowsiness, confusion or fever	Intracranial abscess, meningitis, severe hypertension, encephalitis
Recent onset, in young obese individual	Idiopathic (benign) intracranial hypertension (look for papilloedema)
Recent onset, in a patient over 50 years of age	Sinusitis, brain tumour, cervicogenic, medication overuse, subdural collection, herpes zoster, giant cell arteritis
Recent onset as a result of sexual activity, cough or exertion	Subarachnoid haemorrhage, brain tumour
After head injury, particularly with loss of consciousness, or if prolonged or severe	Intracranial haemorrhage

Source: Adapted from eTG complete. Headache, Therapeutic Guidelines. November 2009.

Epilepsy

A strong link between migraine and epilepsy has been demonstrated: not only do they share many of the same symptoms, there is also a high incidence of epilepsy in those with migraine. Bigal et al[282] refer to interesting statistics in which the incidence of epilepsy in individuals with migraine (median 5.9%) has been found to be substantially higher than that of the epilepsy population prevalence (0.5%). Taking this into account it is important that the practitioner be aware that an individual with migraine may also have an increased risk of epilepsy.

DIFFERENTIAL DIAGNOSIS

Chronic daily headache may be attributed to a variety of causes; the differential diagnosis is summarised in Table 22.25.

NATUROPATHIC DIAGNOSIS

A comprehensive assessment of the patient is essential. It is imperative to consider all compounding variables and bodily processes.

Questioning

- When did you start having headaches?
- How often do they occur? At what time of day? During the week or on weekends? How long do they last?
- Where is the pain?

TABLE 22.25 Differential diagnosis of chronic daily headache

Primary headaches	Secondary headaches
Duration of headache >4 hours (with or without medication overuse) New daily persistent headache Duration of headache <4 hours Cluster headache Headache from coughing Chronic tension headache Idiopathic stabbing headache Headache from sexual activity Exertional benign headache Chronic (transformed) migraine Trigeminal neuralgia Paroxysmal hemicrania Hemicrania continua Strictly unilateral, with prominent autonomic features Bilateral or unilateral with no autonomic features	Posttraumatic headache Vascular disorders headache Non-vascular intracranial disorders headache Sleep disorders headache Obstructive sleep apnoea Headache from infection Myofascial pain Idiopathic intracranial hypertension Subdural haematoma Disorders of the cervical spine Temporomandibular joint dysfunction Giant cell arteritis Arteriovenous malformation Carotid dissection Neoplasm Vasculitis

Source: Adapted from Maizels M. The patient with daily headaches. Am Fam Physician 2004; 70(12):2299–2306.

- Which word best describes it: throbbing, pounding, splitting, stabbing, blinding?
- How bad is the pain? (rate from 1–10)
- What makes them better?
- What makes them worse?
- Are your headaches associated with your menstrual cycle?
- What triggers your headache: certain foods, specific physical activities, bright light, strong odours, change in temperature, or altitude, noise, smoke, stress, oversleeping?
- What symptoms do you experience prior to the headache?
- Does anyone else in your family suffer from headaches?
- Do you notice visual disturbances before or after your headaches?
- Do you suffer from more than one type of headache?
- Does anything else hurt around the time that you have your headache?

Investigations

There is no specific laboratory diagnostic marker for headaches or migraine thus diagnosis is usually made on the patient's subjective complaints.

Imaging studies and blood work may be required when a more severe pathology such as encephalitis or meningitis is suspected.[283]

Subarachnoid haemorrhage may mimic a sudden onset headache; however, this is a medical emergency. It is typically associated with visual disturbance, nausea and vomiting, numbness on one side of the body and even seizures. Do not delay; send the patient to emergency where clinicians will further evaluate the patient.

SPECIFIC NATUROPATHIC INVESTIGATIONS

Functional liver detoxification profile and genetic testing

Assessing an individual's liver function can be useful to assess their detoxification profile. Inadequate detoxification mechanisms may result in hormones and toxins building up in the body, contributing to headaches/migraines. This may be especially important for individuals regularly exposed to chemicals (e.g. dental nurse, hairdresser, painter).

Amino acid profile

Amino acids are required for the synthesis of neurotransmitters including serotonin, which has been implicated in the pathogenesis of migraine. The amino acid profile provides an analysis of amino acid status including essential and non-essential amino acids.

Female hormone profile

The female hormone profile provides an assessment of the female's hormonal status. Many females with migraine/headache report accentuation of symptoms during the time of menstrual cycle; this is in part due to hormonal dysregulation and requires hormonal balance to be reinstated for resolution of symptoms. Similar symptoms may be experienced during perimenopause.

Food allergy/intolerance testing

As previously discussed, food allergy including such things as nitrites, amines and sulfites is frequently implicated in migraines, hence the benefit of identifying problematic foods. Once offending items have been identified and eliminated a decrease in migraine severity and frequency is expected.

Essential fatty acids

Essential fatty acids may reduce inflammation and prostaglandin activity in headache disorders, thus analysis to ensure status is adequate is important.

Environmental screen (especially toxic mineral profile and mould exposure)

Both heavy metal toxicity and mould exposure may cause neurological alterations including headache, thus individuals at risk should be screened.

Nutritional profile: vitamins, minerals and antioxidants

Nutritional deficiencies may increase the risk of migraine/headache. An example of this is magnesium, which has been demonstrated to be low in migraine sufferers during an attack.[284] Vitamin, mineral and antioxidant status (particularly coenzyme Q10 which plays an important role in the resolution of migraines) should be assessed in individuals presenting with depression.

Vitamin D status

A 2017 study of 2601 men in Finland (aged 42–60 years) found that low serum 25(OH)D concentration was associated with a markedly higher risk of frequent headache.[285]

Therapeutic considerations

CLINICAL DECISION MAKING AND RATIONALE

Headaches and migraines are individual and multifactorial. While naturopathy adheres to the philosophy of individualised treatment at all times, headaches and migraines present the clinician with a challenge to explore this philosophy to its utmost. One patient may be successfully treated by simply increasing their water intake and reducing their caffeine intake while another may require careful deliberation and a comprehensive treatment protocol that considers each and every variable that the person consumes, experiences or is exposed to. It is essential to treat each patient respectfully and uniquely. Treatment should consider all variables as listed below; however, consideration of the functioning of all other systems should be supported as well.

Therapeutic application

ALLOPATHIC PERSPECTIVE

Treatment is centred upon reducing attack frequency, severity and duration as well as improving function and reducing disability. Tricyclic antidepressants, analgesics and certain anticonvulsants may be administered, as may beta-blockers if there is a migraine component. Maizels[286] notes that often individuals with refractory headaches require multi-agent therapy; for example, antidepressant with anticonvulsant plus a beta-blocker.

PHARMACOLOGICAL MANAGEMENT[163]

Short-lived attacks

PAEDIATRIC

- Ibuprofen: 5–10 mg/kg orally, 6- to 8-hourly, up to 40 mg/kg/day (up to 2 g daily) (do not use in children under the age of 6 months) OR
- Paracetamol: 20 mg/kg orally, immediately, then 15 mg/kg 4- to 6-hourly, up to 90 mg/kg/day under medical supervision (up to 4 g daily).

ADULTS

- Aspirin: soluble 600 to 900 mg orally, repeat in 4 hours if required
- Diclofenac potassium: 12.5–25 mg orally, repeat in 6 hours if required
- Ibuprofen: 200–400 mg orally, repeat in 6 hours if required
- Naproxen sodium: 275–550 mg orally, repeat in 6 hours if required

- Paracetamol: soluble 1–1.5 g orally, 4-hourly, up to 4 g daily.

FREQUENT ATTACKS

For frequent or constant tension headache, or transformed migraine: Amitriptyline: initial doses of 10 mg can be given orally throughout the day with an average of 75 mg daily. It can be increased to 150 mg per day and the increases are preferable in the afternoon or bedtime as it can cause some sedative effects. The usual maintenance dose is 50–100 mg. Preventive medication should be continued for a minimum of 3–6 months and then tapered.

For patients with tension headache and sleep disturbance, depression should be considered. Counselling in conjunction with appropriate antidepressant therapy may be helpful.

For patients with tension headache and symptoms of anxiety, counselling should be first-line therapy. A short course of an anxiolytic (e.g. diazepam) may occasionally be of benefit.

Anticonvulsants (sodium valproate and gabapentin) and botulinum toxin have been advocated for treatment of frequent tension headache. In 2014, a study from the UK showed that patients suffering from chronic migraines had significantly reduced the number of headaches/migraines days with Botox injections.[287] Sodium valproate may cause thrombocytopenia and platelet dysfunction; it should be used cautiously with aspirin.

HISTORICAL PERSPECTIVE

The use of botanicals for the alleviation of migraines and headache can be traced back to the time of the Eclectic physicians. Though *Tanacetum parthenium* (feverfew) is probably the most well-recognised botanical used in migraine in modern times, there is no mention of its application in *King's American Dispensatory*, or in Felter's *Pharmacology and Therapeutics*, two of the most popular compendiums of the time. Instead, popular nervine tonic *Passiflora incarnata* (passionflower) in the form of an application of bruised leaves as a poultice to the head is proposed for relief from headache. *Passiflora incarnata* is also documented to have temporarily reduced pulse and arterial tension. This is thought to be due to an action upon the vasomotor centre of the medulla oblongata, this latter action probably assisted its reputation in headache.[164] Other botanicals for use include *Valeriana officinalis* (valerian) which was suggested for nervous headache, hemicrania and enfeebled circulation. Interestingly, it was noted that large doses of *Valeriana officinalis* may also cause headache.[223]

Piscidia erythrina (Jamaican dogwood) was prized for its analgesic action where Eclectic physician Ellingwood recommended it for spasmodic and neuralgic afflictions as well as cerebral excitation. *King's American Dispensatory* also suggests the use of *Piscidia erythrina* for use in migraine and to allay spasm.[223] Last but not least, a plaster of *Sinapis nigra* (mustard) was said to be useful when applied to the nape of the neck for the relief of congestive headache or headache with fullness of the cerebral vessels.[223] This is likely due to its counterirritant action.

Pulsatilla was considered a useful remedy in headache of various types where it was said to relieve frontal headache from nasal catarrh; nervous headache, particularly when due to gastric disturbances with greasy taste or debility as well as menstrual headache.[288] Macrotys (black cohosh) was suggested for headache, whether congestive or from cold, neuralgia, dysmenorrhoea, or from la grippe. The Eclectics also describe its use in detail for headache pertaining to eye strain, saying: 'In eye strain from over-use of the eyes, giving rise to headache associated with a sensation of stiffness in the ocular muscles, or a bruised feeling in the muscles of the frontal region, macrotys is one of the most successful of remedies'.[288]

NATUROPATHIC PERSPECTIVE

The naturopathic treatment of various types of headaches is summarised in Table 22.26.

NUTRITIONAL MEDICINE (DIETARY)

Dietary therapeutic objectives

- Calculate water requirements for each patient and ensure hydration needs are met
- Avoid all dehydrating fluids and stimulant substances
- Avoid all known dietary triggers or general unknown food triggers such as amines, preservatives, aspartame, nitrites and alcohol
- Regulate blood sugar levels with wholefood dietary principles and avoidance of processed foods
- Identify and avoid food allergies or intolerances and modify intake to meet nutritional requirements
- A low-fat diet may be beneficial in some patients. It has been shown to decrease number and severity of migraine attacks[289]
- Ensure that meals are eaten frequently. Hunger is the most frequently reported dietary trigger for migraine[290]
- Increase salt intake and reduce carbohydrate intake to prevent glucose induced electrolyte changes which have been shown to increase migraine frequency[291]
- A ketogenic diet may be beneficial in some patients. Evidence suggests that it may be an effective prophylactic treatment for episodic and chronic migraine.[292,293]

SPECIFIC DIETARY TREATMENTS

Dietary inclusions

HYDRATION

Dehydration is a trigger of migraine headache hence optimal hydration should be maintained. Martins and Gouveia[294] detail a number of case reports in which dehydrated individuals who increased their water intake experienced a reduction in migraine incidence. One particularly interesting case is documented in which a participant who installed a reminder on his computer monitor with the message *'it is time to drink water'*

TABLE 22.26 Naturopathic treatment of the various types of headaches

Type	Avoidance or modification of precipitating factors	Treatment and prevention
Hangover headache	Alcohol, which causes dilation and irritation of the blood vessels of the brain and surrounding tissue	Removal or reduction of alcohol. Ensure adequate hydration and detoxification mechanisms are functioning correctly. Support the body with adaptogens and botanicals that work on phase 1 and 2 detoxification
Caffeine-withdrawal headache	Caffeine (in all forms)	Removal or reduction of caffeine (in all its forms). Ensure adequate hydration and detoxification mechanisms are functioning correctly. Support the body with adaptogens and botanicals that work on phase 1 and 2 detoxification
Exertion headache	10% caused by organic diseases (aneurysms, tumours, or blood-vessel malformation). 90% are related to migraine or cluster headaches	Review of physical fitness and cardiovascular function. Assessment and prescription of adequate hydration and electrolyte repletion
Posttraumatic headache	Headaches usually occur on daily basis and are frequently resistant to treatment. Pain can occur after relatively minor traumas	Support the body with herbal anti-inflammatories, adaptogens and nervines. Counselling and biofeedback may be useful
Hunger headache	Strenuous dieting or skipping meals	Encourage regular, nourishing meals containing adequate protein and complex carbohydrates. Support with blood-sugar regulators such as chromium, magnesium and botanicals such as *Gymnema sylvestre*
Temporomandibular joint (TMJ) headache	Caused by malocclusion (poor bite), stress, and jaw clenching	Relaxation, biofeedback, use of bite plate. Support with muscle relaxants such as magnesium, herbal medicine nervines and relaxants such as *Piper methysticum* and *Viburnum opulus*
Tic douloureux headaches	Relatively rare disease of the neural impulses; more common in women after age 55. Cause unknown. Pain from chewing, cold air, touching face. If under age 55, may result from neurological disease such as MS	Support with botanical antioxidants, antispasmodics and relaxants
Fever headache	Infection	Provide immune support (see Ch 12)
Arthritis headache	Unknown. Possible inflammatory cascade or mediation	Support with herbal anti-inflammatories *Curcuma longa*. Antioxidants such as *Vitis vinifera* may also be of use
Eyestrain headache	Muscle imbalance. Uncorrected vision, astigmatism	Correction of vision — referral for eye assessment and possible prescription of glasses, etc. Skeletal alignment support adjustments (chiropractor, osteopath) Regular breaks from the computer Eye exercises Antioxidant nutrients to provide sufficient oxygen to the eye area, musculoskeletal spasmolytic herbal medicines to relieve muscle spasm around eye area
Temporal arteritis headache	Weight loss, eyesight problems. Rarely affects people under 50	Herbal medicines that support arterial health and reduce inflammation
Tumour headache	Cause of tumour is usually unknown	Refer to specialist
Tension-type headache	Emotional stress. Hidden depression	Rest. Stress support. Coping strategies. Learning to delegate. Counselling, relaxation. Support with herbal medicine adaptogens and nervines and nutritional prescriptions of B vitamins, magnesium and zinc
Migraine without aura	Certain foods, the Pill or hormones, excessive hunger, changes in altitude, weather, lights, excessive smoking, and emotional stress. Hereditary component	Support as listed in this chapter

TABLE 22.26 Naturopathic treatment of the various types of headaches—cont'd

Type	Avoidance or modification of precipitating factors	Treatment and prevention
Migraine with aura	Certain foods, the Pill or hormones, excessive hunger, changes in altitude, weather, lights, excessive smoking, and emotional stress. Hereditary component	Support as listed in this chapter
Cluster headaches	Alcoholic beverages, excessive smoking	Removal of precipitating factors. Use of herbal anti-inflammatories, liver support and hydration. Adherence to principles as set out in this chapter
Menstrual related headaches	Hormonal imbalance	Regulate and restore normal hormonal balance (see Ch 18)
Hypertension	Severe hypertension: over 200 mmHg systolic and 110 mmHg diastolic	To prevent, keep blood pressure under control using protocols set out in Ch 20
Aneurysm	Extreme hypertension	Keep blood pressure under control using protocols set out in Ch 20 and support with antioxidants and venotonics such as *Vitis vinifera* (grapeseed) and *Centella asiatica* (gotu kola)
Sinus headaches	Infection, nasal polyps, anatomical deformities, such as a deviated septum, that block the sinus ducts	Eliminate infective organism and support mucosal health. For protocols see Ch 14
Allergy headache	Allergy	Reduce allergic response and support the immune system. For protocols see Ch 14

Source: Adapted from National Headache Foundation. Headache topic sheets. Available from: https://headaches.org/resources/headache-topic-sheet/

resulted in the individual increasing his water intake by 150% and led to a significant decrease in the frequency of migraines. This example highlights just how powerful simple dietary changes can be in reducing the incidence of migraine, as well as how lifestyle changes may be implemented into the daily routine of patients with migraine.

FREQUENT PROTEIN-RICH MEALS

Skipping meals and subsequent hypoglycaemia has been identified as a headache trigger with more than 50% of participants in one study acknowledging 'not eating' as a trigger of acute migraine attack.[295] Acknowledging this, small, frequent meals with optimal quantities of both fibre and protein are suggested to prevent hypoglycaemia for patients with migraine.

Dietary exclusions

CAFFEINE

Caffeine abuse has been identified as a common trigger of migraines and has also been shown to cause headache in patients withdrawing from caffeine intake.[296] All caffeine sources (energy drinks, coffee, tea, chocolate) as well as their quantity in the diet need to be identified in the migraine patient. It is important to acknowledge that intake may need to be withdrawn slowly to prevent severe side effects.[297] Some migraine sufferers report aggravation from caffeine at doses as low as 10 mg/day; however, some find benefit from high doses owing to its effects on blood pressure and vasodilation of blood vessels. Metabolites of caffeine also contribute to caffeine's effects. Theobromine is a vasodilator that increases the amount of oxygen and nutrient flow to the brain and muscles. Theophylline acts as a smooth muscle relaxant that chiefly affects bronchioles and acts as a chronotrope and inotrope that increases heart rate and efficiency. Paraxanthine is responsible for an increase in the lipolysis process, which releases glycerol and fatty acids into the blood to be used as a source of fuel by the muscles. In these individuals, withdrawal is best achieved with concurrent activated vitamin B_3 and vitamin C prescriptions to ease the transition. These individuals may benefit from activated B_3 regularly for headache and migraine prevention. Table 22.27 summarises common sources of caffeine content.

ALCOHOL

Alcohol is also a common trigger of migraines. Of the alcohols, red wine is commonly identified as a major trigger (possibly because it contains higher amounts of histamine and phenolic flavonoids than white wine).[298] However, white wine and other alcoholic beverages such as champagne have also been implicated. Wine contains a number of substances that have been implicated in migraine, including histamine and tyramine, discussed below. Furthermore, alcohol intake contributes to magnesium deficiency[256] and dehydration.

ASPARTAME

There is significant research to suggest that prolonged use of the artificial sweetener aspartame may trigger headaches in individuals with migraine,[299] thus all foods and drinks containing artificial sweetener should be omitted from the diet.

NITRITES

Nitrites have been identified as a common trigger of migraines and thus need to be avoided.[298] Nitrites are used in food as preservatives to inhibit the growth of bacteria that cause botulism as well as to give food a smoked or cured flavour. Common foods that contain nitrites include tinned meats, delicatessen meats such as smoked ham, salami, certain sausages, hot dogs and bacon. When concerned, check the label.

TABLE 22.27 Common caffeine content

Beverage/Item	Container/ size	Typical caffeine content
Coffee		
Instant	150 mL cup	60–100 mg
Percolated/drip	150 mL cup	100–150 mg
Espresso	150 mL cup	90 mg
Decaffeinated	150 mL cup	2–4 mg
Tea	150 mL cup	30–100 mg
Cocoa	150 mL cup	30–60 mg
Cola soft drink	250 mL	35 mg
Energy drink	250 mL	80 mg
Chocolate bar	30 g bar	20–60 mg
Prescription/ over-the-counter medicines	Tablet	20–100 mg

DIETARY AMINE FOODS

Dietary consumption of amines such as tyramine and phenylethylamine has been identified as triggers of migraine in some individuals.[298] Tyramine is a biogenic amine that may cause migraines via its release of noradrenaline and subsequent agonist effect on alpha-adrenergic receptors. Phenylethylamine is a component within chocolate that has also been implicated in migraine. In a double-blind clinical study individuals with migraine were challenged with either chocolate (40 g bar) or a placebo.[300] Of those in the chocolate group 41% experienced a migraine headache compared with 0% in the placebo group, highlighting the extent to which chocolate may provoke migraines. Other common foods that contain amines include aged cheese, cured meats, smoked fish such as smoked salmon, beer, wine, fermented food and yeast extract;[256] thus these need to be avoided in patients who display sensitivity towards them (see Table 22.28).

HISTAMINE FOODS

High intake of histamine foods or histamine sensitivity may occur as a result of reduced diamine oxidase activity, an enzyme required for breakdown of histamine. This may induce headache via release of nitrate monoxide.[301]

Other dietary considerations

FOOD ALLERGY AND INTOLERANCE

Early studies undertaken in the 1980s suggested that food intolerances may be common triggers of migraine.[302] Interestingly, there appears to be multiple intolerances rather than an intolerance to just a single food. Egger et al[268] observed that 93% of 88 children with severe frequent migraine recovered on oligoantigenic diets; thus patients should be tested for food intolerances/ allergies and, if necessary, tried on an oligoantigenic diet.

TABLE 22.28 Low tyramine diet

Food group	Safe to use	Use with caution	Avoid using
Breads, cereals, pasta	Pancakes, coffee cakes, biscuits and any commercial product prepared with yeast and baking powder All pasta both cooked and dry: macaroni, spaghetti, ravioli, egg noodles	Homemade yeast leavened breads and coffee cakes Sourdough breads	Any with a restricted ingredient
Nuts and seeds			All nuts: peanuts, peanut butter, pumpkin seeds, sesame seeds, walnuts, pecans
Dairy	Milk: whole, 2% or skim Cheese: cottage, farmer, ricotta, cream cheese, low-fat processed	Yoghurt, buttermilk, sour cream: ½ cup per day Parmesan or Romano as a garnish (2 tsp) or minor ingredient	Aged cheeses: mozzarella, cheddar, Swiss, brie, blue cheese, Roquefort, stilton, provolone
Meat, fish, poultry, eggs	Freshly purchased and prepared meats, fish, and poultry, eggs, tuna fish, tuna salad (with allowed ingredients)	Sausage, hot dogs, corned beef, bacon, any luncheon meats with nitrates or nitrites such as ham and bologna Meats with tenderiser, caviar	Aged, dried, fermented, salted, smoked, or pickled products. Pepperoni, salami, and liverwurst. Non-fresh meat or liver, pickled herring

TABLE 22.28 Low tyramine diet—cont'd			
Food group	**Safe to use**	**Use with caution**	**Avoid using**
Fruits	Apple, applesauce, cherries, apricots, peaches, any not on restricted list	½ cup per day allowed of: banana, passionfruit, plums, avocado, raisins, dried fruit, papaya, lemon, lime, orange, tangerine, pineapple, grapefruit	
Vegetables	Broccoli, asparagus, spinach, pumpkin, zucchini, carrots, beetroot, string beans, onions, potatoes, peas, beans, soy beans	Raw onion	Snow peas, fava or broad beans, sauerkraut, pickles and olives Fermented soy products such as miso, soy sauce, and teriyaki sauce
Beverages	Decaffeinated coffee, fruit juices, club soda, caffeine-free carbonated beverages	No more than 2 servings per day of coffee, tea, carbonated beverages, hot cocoa and chocolate milk Limit alcohol to one serving of riesling wine, vodka or scotch per day	Alcoholic beverages: Chianti, sherry, burgundy, vermouth, ale, beer and non-alcoholic fermented beverages All others not specified in 'Use with caution' column
Desserts and sweets	Items made with allowed foods and ingredients: cakes, cookies, jam, lollies, sugar, jelly	Chocolate-based products: ice-cream (1 cup), pudding (1 cup), cookies (1 average size), cakes (10 cm cube), and chocolate lollies 15 g) (All count as one serving of caffeinated beverage)	Fruit mince pie
Soups	Soups made from allowed ingredients, homemade broths	Canned soups with autolysed or hydrolysed yeast, meat extracts, or monosodium glutamate (MSG)	
Fats, oils, and miscellaneous	Commercial salad dressings with allowed ingredients Spices not listed on the restricted ingredient list White vinegar All cooking oils and fats, such as olive oil and vegetable oil	Wine, apple, or other fermented vinegars	
Ingredients listed on food labels	Any not listed in the restricted section		MSG (in large amounts), nitrates and nitrites (found mainly in processed meats), yeast, yeast extracts, brewer's yeast, hydrolysed or autolysed yeast, meat extracts, meat tenderisers (papain, bromelin), seasoned salt (containing MSG), soy sauce, teriyaki sauce

Source: Adapted from National Headache Foundation. Available from: www.headaches.org/

Table 22.29 lists some dietary items that have been identified as containing chemical triggers of migraine.

GIT ISSUES

There is increasing evidence indicating an increased frequency of GI disorders in patients with migraine. These include *Helicobacter pylori* infection,[303] irritable bowel syndrome, gastroparesis, hepatobiliary disorders, coeliac disease, GORD and alterations in the microbiota. The gut-brain axis plays an important role in this association.[304,305] Migraine has been associated with increased gut permeability, and an improvement in the gut microbiota and reduction of inflammation can have positive effects on strengthening gut and brain function. Probiotics may have a beneficial effect on migraine frequency and severity.[306,307] A thorough assessment of the patients GIT functioning is required and treating of these underlying issues may well contribute to better quality of life or remission. A case report of a 23-year-old woman with severe GORD who developed migraines after changing her diet to accommodate the GORD, experienced complete remission from migraines after receiving dietary advice and supplements to treat her GORD.[308]

SAMPLE DAILY DIET

BREAKFAST	
Juice: celery, carrot, ginger, beetroot Brown rice porridge with figs, maple syrup and raw nuts and seeds	Dehydration can trigger headaches/migraines. Increasing water intake by 1 L per day is associated with an average reduction of headaches by 21 h in 2 weeks as well as a reduction in subjective headache intensity. The higher potassium content of the juice may also be useful in correcting Na/K balance since reduced sodium intake is associated with a significantly reduced risk of headaches, possibly through reducing hypertension. Ginger functions as an anti-inflammatory. Brown rice provides B vitamins which may assist in migraine reduction. Raw nuts and seeds provide a source of magnesium.
LUNCH	
Poached salmon salad with fennel, walnuts and pear	Salmon and walnuts are sources of essential fatty acids. Plentiful research exists highlighting the benefits of manipulating the diet to reduce pain and inflammation. Omega-3 and omega-6 fatty acids are precursors to lipid mediators with antinociceptive and pronociceptive properties. The typical Western diet has a high ratio of omega-6 PUFAs compared with omega-3 PUFAs; however, by altering the diet in favour of omega-3 fatty acids, it is possible to achieve a reduction in headache pain and improve quality of life.
DINNER	
Moroccan harira soup with garlic, leafy greens, chickpeas and lamb	Harira contains a range of spices including turmeric and ginger, both powerful anti-inflammatory spices. Garlic provides antiplatelet activity. Leafy greens provide magnesium. Prolonged stress can initiate vasospasm resulting in migraine. Magnesium assists with stress adaption but also with vaso-relaxation. This meal contains a range of nutrients including fibre, complex carbohydrates and proteins to ensure blood sugar levels remain stable, thus reducing hypoglycaemia.
SNACK	
Rice crackers with avocado and cherry tomatoes Fresh seasonal fruit	Small frequent snacks are suggested since hypoglycaemia is positively correlated with the development of migraines in some individuals. Focus should be placed on wholefood snacks to avoid exposure to common migraine triggers such as amines found in processed foods.

TABLE 22.29 Dietary items and chemical migraine triggers

Offending food item	Chemical trigger
Cheese	Tyramine
Chocolate	Phenylethylamine, theobromine
Citrus fruits	Phenolic amines, octopamine
Hot dogs, ham, cured meats	Nitrites, nitric oxide
Dairy products, yoghurt	Allergenic proteins (e.g. casein)
Fatty and fried foods	Linoleic and oleic fatty acids
Asian, frozen, snack foods	Monosodium glutamate
Coffee, tea, cola	Caffeine, caffeine withdrawal
Food dyes, additives	Tartrazine, sulfites
Artificial sweetener	Aspartame
Wine, beer	Histamine, tyramine, sulfites
Fasting	Stress hormone release, hypoglycaemia

Source: Millichap JG, Yee MM. The diet factor in pediatric and adolescent migraine. Pediatr Neurol 2003; 28(1):9–15.

NUTRITIONAL MEDICINE (SUPPLEMENTAL)

Nutritional medicine therapeutic objectives

- Support cellular energy metabolism
- Regulate mitochondrial function
- Provide peripheral vasodilation to relieve pain and tension
- Modulate hormonal cascades to prevent hormonally induced episodes
- Reduce inflammation
- Promote optimal blood pressure
- Prevent spasm and platelet aggregation
- Alter neurotransmitter release to stabilise cascades
- Stabilise serotonergic and adrenergic pathways.

Specific nutrients required

B COMPLEX

The B complex vitamins are required for numerous enzyme systems within the body particularly those involved in cellular energy metabolism. A number of individual B vitamins have been identified for use in treatment of migraine (such as vitamin B_2 and B_3 discussed below) owing to their role in regulating mitochondrial dysfunction, a factor which has been implicated in the aetiology of migraine. B vitamin requirements increase in the presence of stress; stress is a known trigger of migraines and migraines are also likely to produce stress, hence the argument for B vitamins. Vitamin B_6 (discussed below) may also be of use for menstrual-related migraines owing to its hormone regulating effects. The B vitamins are also required as a whole for activation and normal functioning of other nutrients required for the prevention of migraines such as magnesium. Acknowledging the synergistic action of the B vitamins and their multiple therapeutic roles for management of migraine, a B complex is recommended for all patients with migraine.

VITAMIN B_2

Vitamin B_2 plays a key role in cellular energy metabolism of the mitochondria via its role in the enzyme system flavin mononucleotide: because inadequate mitochondrial energy reserve has been suggested to be an influencing factor in migraine, use of vitamin B_2 has thus been suggested to correct this deficiency. In addition, B_2 ameliorates oxidative stress, neuroinflammation, and glutamate excitotoxicity, all of which play a part in the pathogenesis of migraine.[309]

A number of studies have demonstrated the efficacy of vitamin B_2 as a prophylactic to reduce the incidence of migraine; these studies include benefits in adults as well as adolescents and children.[310] An open pilot study involving 25 individuals with migraine observed on average a 68% improvement in migraine severity index when individuals were administered riboflavin (400 mg/day) as a prophylactic treatment for migraine.[311] Following the success of this open trial study, a randomised placebo-controlled trial study was conducted in which riboflavin (400 mg/day) was again administered to individuals with migraine in a trial of 3 months' duration.[312] In this study, riboflavin was found to be superior to placebo in reducing attack frequency and number of days with headache. A 2017 systematic review of 11 clinical trials showed mixed results from riboflavin treatment in migraine. Five trials showed positive results in adults with dosages of 400 mg/day. As a prophylactic agent, 400 mg/day was found to be comparable with 500 mg/day of sodium valproate, and 100 mg/day was comparable with 80 mg/day of propranolol. On the other hand, clinical trials in children and adolescents have mixed results. Trials using 20 mg–200 mg/day of riboflavin in 5–15-year-olds failed to produce any significant benefit. However, a trial using 400 mg/day in 12–19-year-olds demonstrated significant positive results in reducing migraine frequency and related disability.[313] Clearly, riboflavin appears to be a useful nutrient for management of migraine where impaired cellular metabolism appears to play a role.

VITAMIN B_3

While the majority of evidence is clinically based, it appears that vitamin B_3 may exert benefits for sufferers of migraine headaches, tension-type headaches and headaches of other aetiologies.[314] The mechanism that vitamin B_3 exerts is undetermined; however, due to its role as a peripheral vasodilator it is believed to assist in cerebral circulation and relieve tension and constriction evident in migraines and headaches.

Studies demonstrating niacin's effectiveness for the treatment of migraine headaches and headaches of other aetiologies are summarised in Table 22.30.

VITAMIN B_6

Migraines occur more frequently in women suggesting that hormonal imbalance may be in some way implicated. This is further emphasised with figures that estimate that up to 10% of migraines may be triggered by menstruation.[315] Vitamin B_6 plays a key role in hormonal regulation, thus it may be useful for hormone-related headaches and migraines, in particular those that are related to premenstrual syndrome.

FOLATE

A 2015 study found that folic acid may influence migraine frequency in females who suffer from migraine with aura. The study included 245 women. Total dietary folate intake was assessed through food diaries and correlated with serum folate levels, and genetic testing for the MTHFR C677T polymorphism. There is an interaction between the genotype for the polymorphism, folate intake and its effect on migraines. In women with the CC genotype, increased folic acid intake was related to decreased migraine frequency. Individuals who carry the T allele for the MTHFR C677T variant may require higher levels of folic acid in order to reduce migraine frequency, due to their genetically slower homocysteine metabolism rate.[316] A 2016 case-control study found that in general, migraine patients have lower dietary intake of folate compared with non-migraine patients.[317] A recent double-blind randomised placebo-controlled study in adult patients with migraine with aura found that folic acid plus pyridoxine resulted in significant decreases in migraine severity and frequency but not duration. Folic acid without pyridoxine did not lead to any significant benefits compared to placebo. Patients ($n = 95$) were given either folic acid (5 mg/day) plus pyridoxine (80 mg/day), or folic acid alone (5 mg/day) or placebo for 3 months.[318] Further rigorous trials are needed to confirm these promising results.

OMEGA-3 FATTY ACIDS

Theoretically omega-3 fatty acids appear to be a viable option for treatment of migraines given their anti-inflammatory and vaso-relaxant properties. Omega-3 fatty acids decrease production of inflammatory mediators such as prostaglandin E2 metabolites and leukotriene B4 while decreasing production of thromboxane A2, a platelet aggregator and vasoconstrictor.[319] They also increase the production of prostacyclin PGI3, a vasodilator and inhibitor of platelet aggregation. Early studies undertaken in the 1980s suggested benefit of omega-3 fatty acids for use in ameliorating severe migraine. However, more recently a double-blind, placebo-controlled study failed to find omega-3 fish oils more effective than placebo at preventing migraine.[320] A randomised controlled trial ($n = 67$) carried out over 12 weeks found that dietary

TABLE 22.30 Summary of articles demonstrating niacin's effectiveness for the treatment of migraine headaches and headaches of other aetiologies

Condition	*n*	Protocol	Outcome	Evidence grade
Migraine headaches	21	One initial intramuscular injection (IM) followed by a series of 6 or 8 intravenous (IV) treatments (maximum 50 mg), then regular IM injections (25–50 mg) combined with 50–150 mg of oral administration	17 of the 21 subjects had a positive response	C: case-series
Headaches of different aetiologic types	100	100 mg of IV sodium nicotinate or niacin	75 of the 100 subjects had complete relief	C: case-series
Migraine headaches	15	100 mg IV niacin, and an additional 50–200 mg if necessary to ensure a flushing response of more than 15 minutes	13 of the 45 subjects had a positive response. The headaches were relieved in 27 of the 31 times when niacin was administered by IV	C: case-series
Tension headaches	35	22 subjects received 100–200 mg of IV niacin for a total of 53 times	13 of the 22 subjects had a positive response. The headaches were relieved in 41 of the 53 times when niacin was administered by IV	C: case-series
Emotional or tension headaches	5	100 mg of IV niacin regularly for 12 weeks combined with a graded schedule of oral dosing, beginning at 300 mg daily, increasing to 900 mg daily, and tapering down to 300 mg daily	All 5 cases of emotional or tension headaches were very responsive to both IV and oral niacin	C: case-series
Tension headaches accompanied with depression	50	100 mg of IV niacin regularly for 23 weeks and then continued once every 2 months and as needed. This was combined with a graded schedule of oral dosing, beginning at 300 mg daily, increasing to 900 mg daily, and tapering down to 300 mg daily	In 44 of the 50 subjects the results with niacin therapy were very satisfactory or favourable	C: case-series
Migraine headaches	1	300–500 mg of niacin were chewed and allowed to slightly dissolve in the mouth	Resolution of migraine headaches	C: case-report
Migraine headaches	2	500 mg of oral niacin taken at the onset of acute symptoms	In two of the subjects, niacin aborted the acute migraine symptoms. In the first subject, niacin resolved the acute attacks in 4 of 4 occasions. In the other subject, niacin resolved the attack on one occasion	C: case-report
Migraine headaches	1	375 mg of oral sustained-release niacin twice daily for 1 month, and 375 mg once daily for 2 months	Migraine-free for the first month, and a marked reduction in migraine headaches over the next 2 months	C: case-report

n = number

Source: Atkinson M. Migraine headache: some clinical observations on the vascular mechanism and its control. Ann Intern Med 1944;21:990-7. Goldzieher JW, Popkin GL. Treatment of headaches with intravenous sodium nicotinate. JAMA 1946, 131:103-5. Grenfell RF. Treatment of migraine with nicotinic acid. Am Pract 1949;3:542-4. Grenfell RF. Treatment of tension headache. Am Pract Dig Treat 1951;2:933-6. Hall JA. Enhancing niacin's effect for migraine. Cortlandt Forum 1991:46. Morgan ZR. Nicotinic acid therapy in vasoconstriction type of headache. Md State Med J 1953;2:377-82. Morgan ZR. A newer method of nicotinic acid therapy in headache of the vasoconstrictive type. J Am Geriatr Soc 1955;3:545-51. Prousky J, Seely D. The treatment of migraines and tension-type headaches with intravenous and oral niacin (nicotinic acid): systematic review of the literature. Nut J 2005(4):3. Prousky J, Sykes E. Two case reports on the treatment of acute migraine with niacin. Its hypothetical mechanism of action upon calcitonin-gene related peptide and platelets. J Orthomol Med 2003;18:108-10. Velling DA, Dodick DW, Muir JJ. Sustained-release niacin for prevention of migraine headache. Mayo Clin Proc 2003;78:770-1.

intervention which increased omega-3 and decreased omega-6 fatty acids produced improvements in headache frequency and severity, compared to the control group which had decreased omega-6 fatty acids only.[321] A follow-up analysis by the researchers demonstrated that the beneficial effects of the intervention extended beyond pain reduction and had favourable impacts on quality of life and improvements on psychological distress. These were accompanied by improvements in physical and mental function.[322] It has been shown that low levels of both EPA and DHA fatty acids are associated with higher frequency of migraine attacks.[323]

A randomised trial ($n = 74$) on migraine patients found that a formulation of fish oil (2500 mg) with curcumin (using nanotechnology, 160 mg) significantly reduced the frequency of migraine attacks compared to either treatment on its own.[324]

ALPHA LIPOIC ACID

The trend of success with use of supplements that aid in the relief of migraine owing to their effects on energy metabolism in the mitochondria also implies that alpha lipoic acid may be of use. In a randomised double-blind placebo-controlled trial of alpha lipoic acid (600 mg/day) in migraine prophylaxis for 3 months (with a 1-month run-in period), monthly attack frequency, headache days and headache severity all declined in comparison to the placebo group,[325] and though results were not statistically significant, they were clinically significant. While the results from this study are heartening, the authors note that this study was underpowered, thus, before definite conclusions can be made, further studies involving a larger study group are required to confirm the efficacy of these results.

MAGNESIUM

Magnesium plays an important role in the pathogenesis of migraine headaches where it exerts numerous functions all likely to influence the resolution of migraine headache. Magnesium functions as a vasodilator and relaxant, preventing spasm and altering neurotransmitter release and hyper-aggregation of platelets. Magnesium also influences serotonin receptors and inflammatory mediators that may be involved in the pathogenesis of migraine.[326] Deficiency of magnesium is common in migraine headache;[327–329] however, despite its multifaceted action within the body and the widespread deficiency observed, there have been relatively few clinical trials examining its efficacy in migraine. In a prospective, multi-centre, placebo-controlled double-blind study oral magnesium was found to exert a prophylactic action in individuals with migraine.[330] Patients received magnesium 600 mg/day (as trimagnesium dicitrate) for 3 months or placebo. At weeks 9–12 the attack frequency was reduced by 41.6% in the magnesium group compared with only 15.8% in the placebo group. The number of days with migraine as well as use of analgesic medication also decreased significantly in those taking the magnesium, revealing magnesium to be effective in migraine prophylaxis. Magnesium citrate (600 mg/day) was also found to be useful as a prophylactic in migraine without aura whereby migraine attack frequency, severity and amplitude decreased after magnesium treatment with respect to pretreatment values.[331] Magnesium may also be useful for menstrual-related migraine. In a double-blind, placebo-controlled study 360 mg/day of magnesium or placebo started on the 15th day of the menstrual cycle and continued until the next menses for several months was found to exert beneficial effects.[332] After 2 months of supplementation, magnesium was found to reduce the number of days experienced with headache in the treatment group, as well as improve premenstrual complaints. A clinical trial with 133 patients with migraine found that 3 months treatment with magnesium oxide resulted in a significant reduction in all migraine indicators. Subjects were randomly assigned into one of 3 treatment groups: magnesium oxide (500 mg/day), L-carnitine (500 mg/day) or a combination of both. Both the magnesium groups had significant reductions in migraine frequency, severity and index. L-carnitine on its own resulted in decreased frequency and duration, but not severity.[333]

A comparison trial involving 70 migraine patients who had been referred to an emergency department, found that magnesium sulfate (1 g) was more effective and fast-acting than dexamethasone (8 mg)/metoclopramide (10 mg) for treatment of acute migraine.[334,335]

5-HYDROXYTRYPTOPHAN (5-HTP)

A defect in the serotonergic and adrenergic systems has been implicated in the pathogenesis of migraine with many individuals with migraines showing altered serotonin (5-HT) metabolism[336] and thus low levels of serotonin.[337] Low levels of serotonin enhance the effects of substance P resulting in vasodilation, inflammation and of course the sensation of pain. 5-hydroxytryptophan as a serotonin precursor seems the obvious choice here to help relieve symptoms of headache and migraine where migraine and headache are caused by altered serotonin metabolism, however as yet clinical trials while promising are not entirely convincing.[338]

COENZYME Q10

Mitochondrial dysfunction has been suggested to be involved in the pathogenesis of migraine, thus coenzyme Q10, which has been demonstrated to improve mitochondrial function, is an obvious choice when it comes to preventive solutions for the treatment of migraines. In an open-label trial study coenzyme Q10 (150 mg/day) was administered to individuals with a history of episodic migraine with or without aura.[339] Approximately 60% of patients experienced a reduction in number of migraines by at least 50% with the average number of days with migraine reducing from 7.34 to 2.95 after 3 months of therapy. These fantastic results were confirmed in a randomised, placebo-controlled double-blind trial using double the dose of coenzyme Q10 (100 mg 3 times daily) in migraine patients. Coenzyme Q10 was found to be superior to placebo for reducing frequency of attacks, days with headaches as well as days with nausea after 3 months of treatment.[340] More recently, another study confirmed that using one dose of 100 mg of coenzyme Q10 daily in addition to their regular prophylactic medication over 3 months, reduced the number of migraines and might also reduce the duration and severity in migraine sufferers.[341]

Dosage requirements

The dosage requirements listed below are based on adult doses that have been reported in the literature.

- B complex (all B vitamins) high-dose combination, preferably activated forms
  - Thiamine 20–40 mg/day
  - Riboflavin 20–40 mg/day

  - Riboflavin 5 phosphate as a single therapy in doses up to 500 mg/day
  - Niacinamide 50–100 mg/day
  - Niacinamide as a single therapy in doses up to 200 mg/day
  - Pantothenic acid 150–300 mg/day
  - Pyridoxine 50–100 mg/day
  - Folate as folinic acid or L5MTHF 500–1000 micrograms/day
    > In instances of MTHFR genetic mutations, higher requirements may be indicated
  - Hydroxocobalamin or methylcobalamin 500–1000 micrograms/day
    > In instances of methylation errors or dysfunction, higher does may be required
  - Choline 50–100 mg/day
  - Inositol 50–100 mg/day
  - Biotin 250–500 micrograms/day
- Omega-3 fatty acids: with a minimum of 600 mg/day EPA (in divided doses)[342]
- Alpha lipoic acid: 600 mg/day
- Magnesium: 400–1200 mg/day
- 5-HTP: 150 md b.i.d.
- Coenzyme Q10: 300 mg/day.

HERBAL MEDICINE

Herbal medicine therapeutic objectives

The therapeutic objectives and associated classes of herbal medicine are summarised in Tables 22.31 and 22.32.

TABLE 22.31 General herbal objectives and associated classes

Objective	Associated class
Improve liver function	Hepatoprotective Hepatotrophorestorative Hepatotonic Choleretic Cholagogue Detoxicant Antioxidant
Restore GIT integrity and function	Mucous membrane trophorestorative Astringent Bitter Vulnerary/demulcent
Modulate immune response, eradicate infection if present	Immune enhancer (be specific for infective organism) Immunomodulator Diaphoretic
Restore nervous system function and integrity	Nervine tonic Nervine trophorestorative
Restore natural stress response	Adaptogen Adrenal restorative Nervine tonic Nervine trophorestorative Sedative (if indicated)
Reduce oxidation, free radical damage and production	Antioxidant
Elliminate allergies (if present)	Anti-allergic Anti-inflammatory GIT restoration
General body tonification	Tonic (organ specific and general)
Hormonal modulation	Serotonin agonist HPA modulator HPO modulator Menstrual cycle regulator Male or female tonics Melatonin stimulation (sunlight/moonlight)

Specific herbal medicines

ESCHSCHOLZIA CALIFORNICA (CALIFORNIAN POPPY)

Eschscholzia californica belongs to the Papaveraceae family and displays hypnotic and analgesic properties that make it a valuable botanical for managing conditions characterised by pain such as migraine and headache. Studies show that *Eschscholzia californica* exerts a peripheral analgesic action in animals;[343] as yet no studies have been conducted in clinical trials assessing its effects in migraine and headache.

LAVANDULA ANGUSTIFOLIA (LAVENDER)

So powerful is the scent of *Lavandula angustifolia* that the Eclectic physicians suggested that it constituted as 'smelling salts' for the relief of headache and tendency to fainting.[344] In modern day herbal medicine *Lavandula angustifolia*, owing to its nervine and anti-anxiolytic actions, may be employed (particularly in the form of an essential oil on the pillow or the patient's temples) as an adjuvant for the relief of headaches and migraines, in teas, and oral capsule form. A study of 60 Iranian adults with migraine who received lavender therapy for 3 months found that the number and severity of migraines decreased significantly compared to the placebo group. The lavender therapy consisted of 10 drops of Spanish lavender extract dissolved in water, and drunk each evening.[345] An earlier placebo-controlled clinical trial of 47 patients with migraine showed that inhaling lavender essential oil for 15 minutes (2–3 drops rubbed onto the upper lip) reduced migraine severity.[346]

PISCIDIA ERYTHRINA (JAMAICAN DOGWOOD)

Based on its historical use as an analgesic for 'lessening sensation' *Piscidia erythrina* may be employed in migraine and headache to provide relief from pain. *Piscidia erythrina* also functions as a nervine sedative, inducing sleep, reducing distress and functioning as a mild antispasmodic.[164] Yarnell and Abascal[347] suggest a dose of *Piscidia erythrina* tincture at 1–2 mL every 2–3 hours for relief from strong migraine or cluster headache.

TANACETUM PARTHENIUM (FEVERFEW)

Tanacetum parthenium has a long history of use for the treatment of migraine and is probably the most

TABLE 22.32 Herbal medicine classes

Specific causes	Relevant herbal medicine class
Alcohol, dehydration	Hydrate Nutritive Hepatoprotective
Caffeine withdrawal	Analgesic General tonic Adaptogen Antioxidant Hepatotonic
Hypertension	NB: Requires urgent and aggressive treatment Antihypertensive Antioxidant Cardio-tonic
Eyestrain	Visual tonic Antioxidant Cerebral circulatory stimulant
Allergies or intolerances	Antiallergic Anti-inflammatory GIT restoration Improve liver detoxification
Sinusitis, ear infections, dental trauma/infection	Treat underlying condition Immune enhancement, eradicate underlying infection Upper respiratory support — e.g. antimicrobial, vulnerary, decongestant
Anxiety, depression	Anxiolytic Antidepressant, thymoleptic Adaptogen, adrenal restorative Nervine tonic, nervine trophorestorative Sedative
Muscular tension, malalignment	Musculoskeletal spasmolytic Anti-inflammatory Analgesic Sedative, relaxant
Migraine specific	Vascular tonic Analgesic Anti-inflammatory Liver support

well-known botanical for relief of migraines in modern day Western herbal medicine. The sesquiterpene lactone parthenolide has been identified as the main constituent to be of use for migraine. Clinical evidence reviewing the efficacy of *Tanacetum parthenium* has been mixed. In 2000 in a systematic review, Pittler et al[348] reviewed 4 trials that supported the use of *Tanacetum parthenium* as a migraine prophylactic. However, the largest trial which was also of the highest quality suggested no difference between placebo and *Tanacetum parthenium*. In a subsequent review in 2004 Pittler and Ernst[349] suggested there to be inconclusive evidence to suggest an effect of *Tanacetum parthenium* over placebo for preventing migraine because of the mixed results obtained in the studies reviewed.

Note that the majority of studies that produced positive results used *Tanacetum parthenium* in dried or freeze-dried form while in those studies that used alcoholic extract a negative outcome was observed; thus clearly the form of herb used is extremely important to efficacy and thus treatment outcomes. More recently the combination of *Tanacetum parthenium* and *Salix alba* (white willow bark) was found to be more effective than *Tanacetum parthenium* alone for prevention of migraine. In a small, prospective, open-label study involving 12 individuals diagnosed with migraine without aura individuals were administered 'Mig-RL', a combination of *Tanacetum parthenium* 300 mg plus *Salix alba* 300 mg twice daily.[350] Treatment period was approximately 3 months; at completion of the study there were 2 drop-outs (for reasons unrelated to the study). Reductions in frequency of attacks, attack intensity and attack duration were observed in sufferers of migraine. Interestingly, self-assessment of general health as well as anxiety was also improved. Given the small sample involved in this study, further studies of double-blind, randomised, placebo-controlled design involving a larger patient population are warranted.

Summary of results at 12 weeks of taking *T. parthenium* and *S. alba* combination 'Mig-RL':

- Attack frequency: reduced by 61.7% in 9 of 10 patients
- Attack intensity: reduced by 62.6% in 10 of 10 patients
- Attack duration: decreased by 76.2% in 10 of 10 patients.

A 2015 update[351] to the 2004 Cochrane review included one newer (2005), larger ($n = 218$), more rigorous study which adds positive evidence to the mixed and inconclusive findings of the previous report. This study reported that feverfew reduced migraine frequency compared to placebo.[352] Larger vigorous trials with stable feverfew extracts are required.

VERBENA OFFICINALIS (VERVAIN)

Verbena officinalis, also known as 'vervain', is a slender perennial from the Verbenaceae family from which a number of different constituents have been identified including iridoids, verbascosides, flavonoids, triterpenic acids and sterols.[353] *Verbena officinalis* displays nervine tonic and mild sedative properties that may be of use during migraine and headache to help relieve nervous tension associated with the situation. As yet the use of *Verbena officinalis* for migraine has not been researched. However, it is employed in Traditional Chinese Medicine for treatment of migraines associated with hormonal imbalance such as in menopause.[354]

VIBURNUM OPULUS (CRAMP BARK)

Vascular spasm and constriction are key components of migraine hence *Viburnum opulus*, with its antispasmodic and relaxant actions, may be of use. As yet, however, there are no well-designed human clinical studies detailing the effects of *Viburnum opulus* in migraine.

ZINGIBER OFFICINALE (GINGER)

Zingiber officinale exhibits anti-inflammatory and platelet aggregate inhibition roles, which indicates that it may be of use for migraines since inflammation and platelet aggregation have both been implicated in the pathogenesis of migraine. The use of *Zingiber officinale* for migraine has been hypothesised by Mustafa and Srivastava,[355] who describe a case study in which a patient with a history of migraine consumed 500–600 mg/day of *Zingiber officinale* as powder at the onset of aura. Remarkably, a decrease in the migraine was observed within 30 minutes of administration. A double-blind randomised clinical trial on 100 patients who had acute migraine without aura received either ginger powder (250 mg powder of ginger rhizome) or sumatriptan. Two hours after using either drug, headache severity decreased significantly. Adverse effects with the ginger treatment were less than the sumatriptan.[356] The use of *Zingiber officinale* requires more controlled trials; however, these results plus its demonstrated actions indicate that it would be useful. Anecdotal evidence suggests that it is a very powerful herb for use in migraine patients. Maghbooli et al[356] report on a 42-year-old woman with a 16-year history of migraines, who experienced significant relief after supplementing her diet with 1.5–2 g of dried ginger daily.

GINKGO BILOBA (GINKGO)

Ginkgolide B, a constituent extract from *Ginkgo biloba* tree leaves and root bark, is the most potent platelet-activating factor (PAF) antagonist and modulator of glutamate via pharmacological actions in NMDA receptors. Ginkgolide B has been clinically tested for efficacy in migraine. A study of a proprietary compound (Migrasoll), of which Ginkgolide B (60 mg) was the main component in addition to coenzyme Q10 (11 mg) and riboflavin (8.7 mg) on 50 patients suffering from migraine with aura who had the compound administered twice daily over a 4-month treatment period, found that the migraines with aura decreased significantly in frequency and duration.[357] In a smaller preliminary open trial ($n = 21$) the same compound was shown to be clinically effective at treating an acute attack of migraine aura. Taking the compound at the first symptoms of an aura reduced the aura duration. In four of the patients in the trial, the pain phase of the aura disappeared.[358] A similar study was carried out on 119 school-age children with migraine. The treatment compound consisted of Ginkgolide B (80 mg), coenzymeQ10 (20 mg) and riboflavin (1.6 mg) and magnesium (300 mg). It was administered prophylactically twice a day for 3 months. The study found that after 3 months of treatment the frequency of migraine was significantly reduced.[359]

LIFESTYLE RECOMMENDATIONS

Structural support

Underlying structural imbalances may contribute to migraine thus structural support in the form of modalities such as craniosacral, chiropractic, and osteopathy may be considered, particularly in individuals who exhibit symptoms such as neck pain and tenderness in the suboccipital areas.[360] As yet the majority of evidence involves case studies.

Circadian rhythm regulation

Disordered circadian rhythm has been observed in individuals with migraine. However, evidence suggests that migraine may improve with regulation of sleep, thus strategies to restore sleep are likely to be effective for resolution of migraine. Sleep hygiene principles discussed under the section 'Sleep disorders' earlier in this chapter should be recommended.

Psychological therapies

There is good evidence to support the use of psychological therapies for relief of symptoms associated with migraine and headache.[361,362] Therapies with the most evidence include cognitive behavioural therapy,[363] relaxation and biofeedback therapy which is especially useful for adolescents and children. Given the lack of invasiveness of psychological therapies and their lack of interaction with other therapies they should be considered for all patients with migraines.

Reduce environmental toxin exposure

The patient's exposure to possible occupational environmental toxins must be clearly discussed as exposure to such toxins has been implicated as a migraine trigger or precipitant. The World Health Organization has suggested that new or refurbished commercial offices may contribute to symptoms such as headache owing to the high levels of volatile organic compounds (from paints, lacquers, plastics and glues).[364] Other factors such as poor or excessive lighting and air conditioning may also influence headache. Clearly, occupation in the migraine headache patient is something that needs to be carefully considered, for example perfume[365] is a trigger of migraine thus should be avoided in those with migraine. Avoidance of environmental toxins is recommended: simple lifestyle measures may also replace old habits such as replacing highly chemical-derived cleaning products with strong odour such as bleach with natural products such as white vinegar and clove oil.

CASE STUDY

OVERVIEW

MD, a 34-year-old male, presented with headaches. He was a barrister specialising in taxation law. He had suffered from headaches for many years. However, they had recently worsened. MD explained that he often has disturbed vision before the onset of the headache accompanied with nausea, vomiting and photophobia. He had been experiencing these headaches every second week with one of the severe headaches every 3 weeks. In severe cases he had to stop working and sleep to ameliorate his symptoms. Paracetamol did not alleviate sufficiently. He was under significant stress with his company. He has recently acquired a new client that

CASE STUDY CONTINUED

requires a lot of research and attention. He has been working around the clock with limited relaxation time. He has been eating takeaway food for all meals and has been sleeping at the office on some nights. He drinks 14 cups of coffee per day and 6 glasses of water. System review showed that MD had an intolerance to alcohol while all other areas were unremarkable. MD performed 30 minutes of exercise daily on the treadmill at work.

CLINICAL EXAMINATION

Marked trigger points in musculoskeletal system focusing on upper back and neck regions. BMI 21.7 kg/m^2.

INVESTIGATIONS FROM GP

All unremarkable.

TREATMENT PROTOCOL

MD's headaches and migraines were interpreted as strong indicators of stress, dehydration, caffeine overload and general overwork and burnout. Significant discussion considered work–life balance and MD's happiness and enjoyment of life. He concluded that his headaches and migraines were warning signs that warranted changes in his life. MD became an active participant in the development of his treatment program with prioritised treatment objectives that were staggered for greater implementation and change motivation.

His treatment priorities included:

- Immediate reduction with goal of ceasing caffeine intake
- Caffeine withdrawal prescription (as listed below)
- Optimisation and encouragement of hydration as pure water (at a quantity calculated based on his weight)
- Encouragement to leave work early and reduce work hours and pressure
- Education regarding wholefood diet principles and discussion of simple recipes and menu ideas to reduce takeaway intake
- Encouragement to enjoy life, spend time outdoors, encourage hobbies and socialising, and live more happily
- Supplementation for daily health and headache and migraine prevention
  - B complex — activated (2 capsules/day) to assist with stress relief and provide migraine prevention through B_3's role in vasodilation. He was recommended to avoid taking the second capsule after 4 pm as it may affect sleeping and was encouraged to take one with breakfast and one with lunch
  - Magnesium 400 mg twice a day to reduce stress levels, muscular spasm and tension and prevent and treat headaches and migraines
- Referral for massage/body therapy to relieve muscular tension and spasm
- Discuss workload with human resources manager at work to assess options.

CAFFEINE WITHDRAWAL TREATMENT

- Reduce coffee intake by 1 cup each day over 14 days — can speed up the process if patient desires once intake reaches <5 cups per day
- Replace coffee with herbal teas (non-caffeinated)

CASE STUDY CONTINUED

- Encourage sufficient water (30 mL/kg body weight) + 250–300 mL per cup of coffee drunk
- Supplementation as listed above plus
- Vitamin C 500 mg q.i.d.
- Green tea as a coffee replacement if withdrawal significant
- *Hypericum perforatum* (St John's wort) 1.375 g (standardised to hypericin 500 micrograms): 1 tab 3 times a day.

MULTIPLE SCLEROSIS

Epidemiology

Multiple sclerosis (MS) (see Fig. 22.17), first described by the French neurologist, Charcot, in 1868, is a demyelinating immune-mediated disease of the CNS, and is the leading cause of disability in young and middle-aged people in the developed world. The total number of people living with MS worldwide is estimated to be 2–2.5 million.[366] The prevalence of MS in Australia is about 23 000 people.[367]

The most striking epidemiological characteristic is the apparent uneven distribution of the disease across the world. The incidence of MS has traditionally been extremely low in regions near the equator and the incidence rates rise to approximately one case per thousand in some areas at around 54° latitude north or south.[368] The traditional view, based on many early studies and reviews, is that MS is particularly prevalent where white people of Nordic origin live, in temperate zones, and in high-income countries. Conversely, MS is uncommon where non-whites live, in low-income countries, and in tropical zones.[369]

This traditional view (theory of a latitudinal gradient of incidence of MS) has been challenged by a new literature search and meta-regression analyses.[369] This study has observed a universal increase in prevalence and incidence of MS over time, more particularly a general increase in the incidence of MS in females. It was also observed that MS frequency varies substantially between the continents.

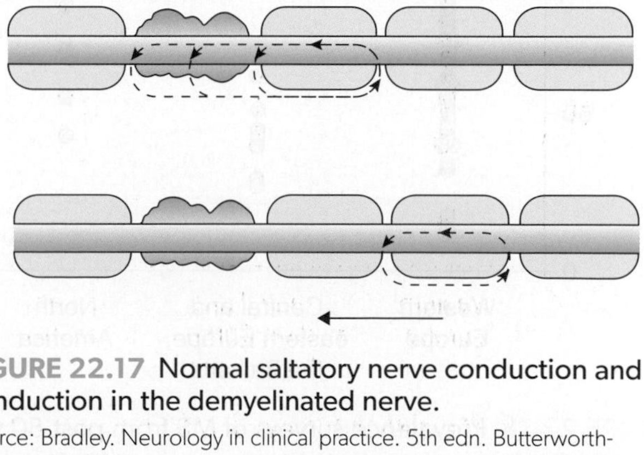

FIGURE 22.17 Normal saltatory nerve conduction and conduction in the demyelinated nerve.

Source: Bradley. Neurology in clinical practice. 5th edn. Butterworth-Heinemann, 2008.

MS is twice as common in females. It typically presents in young adults between 20 and 50 years of age, with a peak occurring at 30 years of age, although childhood or older age cases occasionally occur.[366] (See also Figs 22.18 and 22.19.)

Classification

There are four major types of MS, depending on how the disease acts on the body: relapsing-remitting MS (RRMS), secondary-progressive MS (SPMS), primary-progressive MS (PPMS), and progressive-relapsing MS (PRMS). Though controversial, some scientists believe there are an additional two types worth noting: benign MS and malignant MS (see Table 22.33).

Aetiology

Multiple sclerosis is a chronic inflammatory demyelinating disorder of the central nervous system.[366] Its aetiology still remains unclear. A cell-mediated autoimmune demyelination possibly precipitated by an unknown antigen or groups of antigens is thought to be the common underlying pathology.[366]

Two other theories proposed for development of MS are infective (viral such as Epstein-Barr virus and human herpes virus 6) and neurodegeneration.[366]

Two factors are in effect:

- Population genetics
- The interplay between genetic and environmental factors.

GENETIC FACTORS

Genetic factors can be helpful in explaining the geographic variation of MS. It is suggested that the geographic distribution can be explained in part by geographical clustering of northern Europeans and their descendants.[370]

Following is the evidence suggestive of genetic susceptibility to MS:

A There is a higher incidence of MS in some ethnic populations compared with others. Caucasians from Scandinavia and Scotland are extremely susceptible to the disease; while it is less frequent in African blacks, Aboriginal, Norwegian Lapps and Gypsies. MS is rare in the Mongolian race, Japanese,

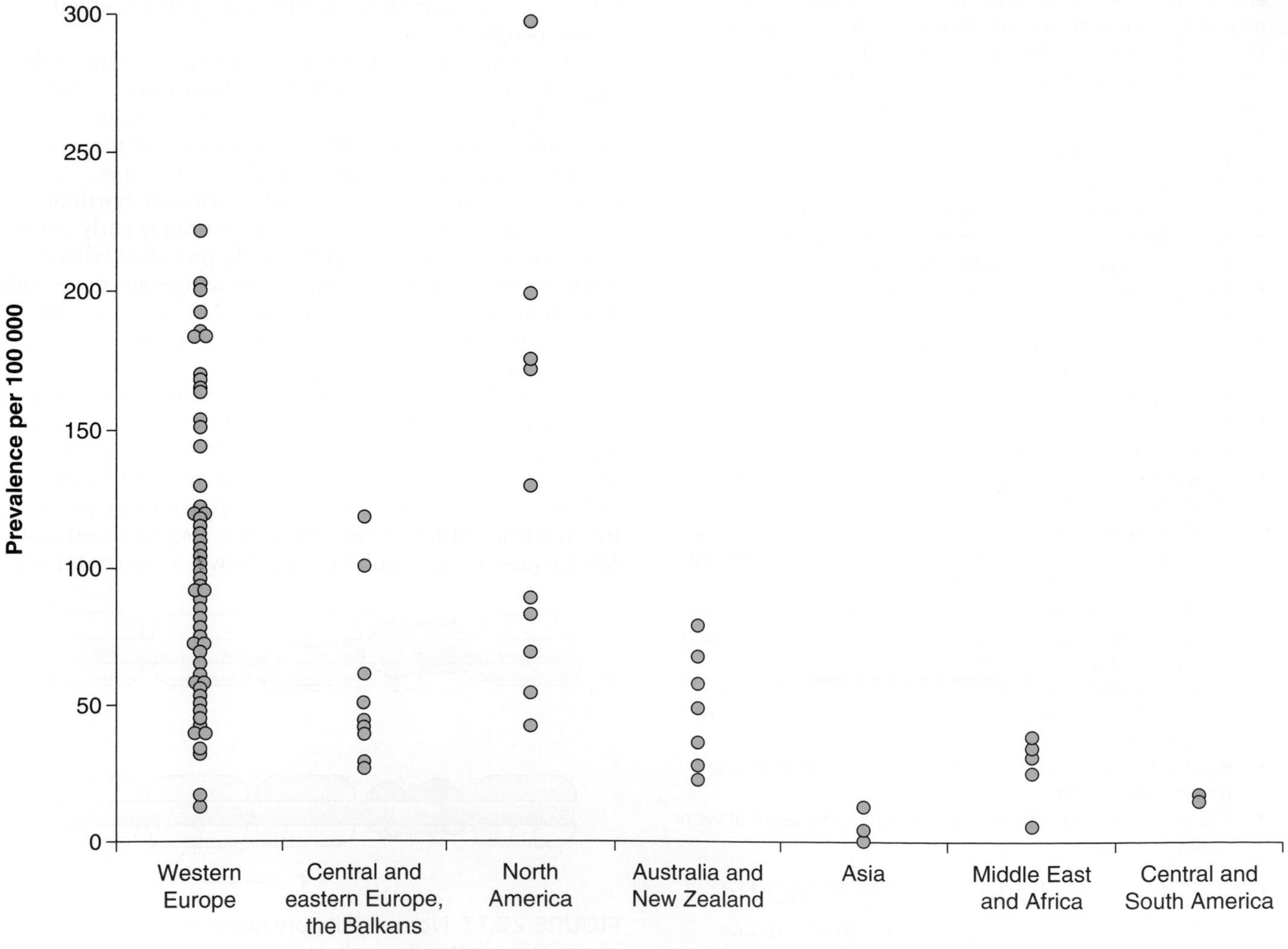

FIGURE 22.18 Prevalence surveys of MS from past 50 years.

Source: Koch-Henriksen N, Sorensen PS. The changing demographic pattern of multiple sclerosis epidemiology. Lancet Neurol 2010; 9(5):520–532.

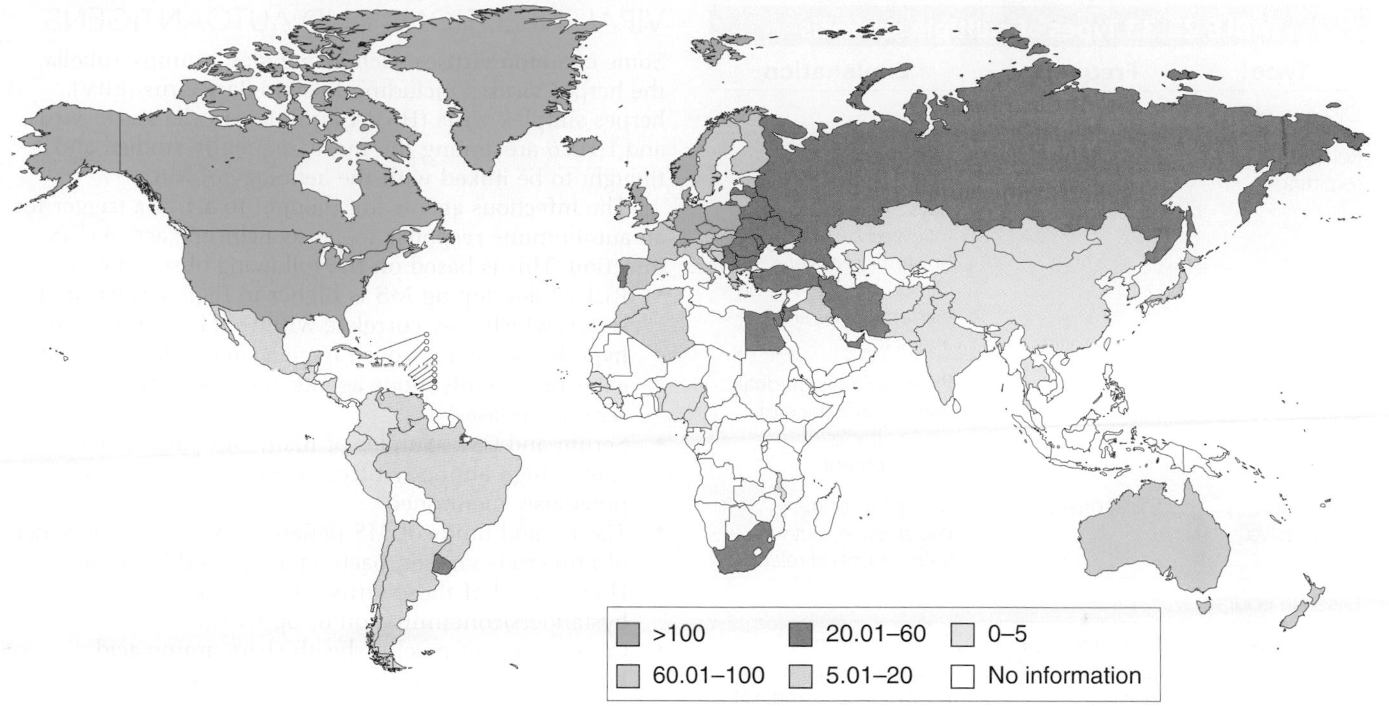

FIGURE 22.19 The geography of MS: prevalence per 100 000 population.

Source: *Atlas multiple sclerosis resources in the world* 2008, p. 15. © 2008, reproduced with permission from the World Health Organization.

Chinese, Native American Indians and New Zealand Māori.

B Twin studies also indicate genetic susceptibility with a concordance rate of 25–30% and in identical twins compared with 2–5% in non-identical twins.[366,370]

C About 20% of MS patients have at least one affected relative. Research in various countries has revealed that the risk for developing MS in first-degree relatives is increased.[366]

The genetic inheritance of MS is probably polygenic with the possibility of genetic heterogenicity (different susceptibility among individuals). Studies so far have revealed linkage mainly with the HLA allele DRB1*1501 (on chromosome 6p21), accounting for less than 50% of the total genetic basis of the disease. It is not yet clear how this *HLA-DRB1* gene influences genetic susceptibility, but it might be related to the physiological function of HLA molecules in immune responses such as antigen-binding and presentation and T-cell activation. Studies have recently identified new MS susceptibility loci within and outside the HLA region. *HLA-DRB1* is also associated with autoimmune diseases such as rheumatoid arthritis and type 1 diabetes.[371]

According to Duke University's Molecular Physiology Institute, there are other chromosomes to consider and investigate for MS. The ones of interest are chromosomes 3, 5 and 19. It is interesting to note that currently chromosome 3p21 is being investigated and patients with this deletion had an age of onset 3 years later than MS patients without this deletion.

The autoimmune and MS risk gene ZMIZ1 is underexpressed in blood in people with MS. Expression is partly heritable, relatively stable over time and levels of ZMIZ1 protein expression are reduced in MS. ZMIZ1 gene expression is affected by and interacts with environmental risk factors EBV and vitamin D. ZMIZ1 gene expression is increased in response to vitamin D_3.[372]

ENVIRONMENTAL FACTORS

A large number of environmental agents, which include viral, fungal and bacterial infections, nutritional and dietary factors, well-water consumption, exposure to animals, minerals, trauma due to accident or surgery, pollution, solar radiation, temperature, rainfall, humidity, chemical agents, heavy metals, organic solvents, various occupational hazards have been investigated.[370]

Sunlight and UV radiation

The intensity of sunlight and UV radiation was thought to be one of the strongest correlations of the latitudinal effect of MS incidence. A study done in Tasmania showed that higher exposure to sunlight (average 2–3 h or more per day during weekends and holidays) when aged 6–15 years was associated with a decreased risk of MS. Studies done on the populations of Israel do not support actinic exposure as a sole factor in MS risk.[366]

Vitamin D

A number of clinical observations were made in MS populations that support a role for vitamin D. These include associations with plasma 25(OH)D levels, the geographic distribution of MS prevalence, the low bone mass density found in MS patients, the seasonal

TABLE 22.33 Types of multiple sclerosis

Type	Frequency	Explanation
Disease onset		
Relapsing-remitting	85% at onset	Neurological dysfunction may last days to weeks and be followed by complete or partial recovery; clinical stability will be evident between attacks
Primary-progressive	10% at onset	Progression is gradual with no evidence of acute attacks or improvement
Relapsing-progressive	5% at onset	Similar to primary progressive, but with superimposed relapses
Disease course		
Secondary-progressive	50% of relapsing-remitting after 10 years	Changes from relapsing-remitting to progressive; some will have only relapses or progression
Benign	10–30% in different studies	Infrequent attacks with minimal or no disability after a period of 15 years; chances of recovery are excellent
Malignant	Rare	Rapid progression to severe attacks with poor recovery; death or profound disability within 2 years

Source: Adapted from eTG complete. Multiple sclerosis: introduction. Available from: http://online.tg.org.au/complete/

fluctuation of plasma 25(OH)D, MS disease parameters and MS births, the clinical remission of disease during pregnancy and the associations of various genetic polymorphisms of the VDR gene (associated with vitamin D receptor) with MS. The postulated mechanism of the beneficial effects of vitamin D involves inhibition of inflammatory cytokines by activated macrophages, as well as enhanced production of anti-inflammatory cytokines and reduction of IL-2 mRNA in the peripheral blood, enhancing immunological self-tolerance. Vitamin D is metabolised into calcitrol, which in turn regulates the haematopoietic system, including the immune system.[370] Vitamin D may also influence remyelination of nerves by inducing an increase in the expression of calcium-binding proteins like calretinin involving calcium homeostasis and mitochondrial activity.[373] In a recent study, vitamin D supplementation was found to reduce seasonal MS activity during late winter/early spring when the vitamin D levels are low due to low ultraviolet-B radiation.[374]

VIRAL INFECTIONS AND AUTOANTIGENS

Some common viruses such as measles, mumps, rubella, the herpes viruses including Epstein Barr virus (EBV), herpes simplex virus (HSV-1 and 2), varicella zoster virus, and HHV6 are among the most frequently studied and thought to be linked with the aetiology of MS.

The infectious agents are thought to act as a trigger for an autoimmune response to cause a chronic active CNS infection. This is based on the following observations:

- Risk of developing MS is higher in high socioeconomic status, which may correlate with well known hygiene hypothesis (i.e. improved hygiene and delayed initial exposures to infectious agents, increasing risk for more serious diseases)
- Serum and CSF samples of many MS patients have shown high antibody titres against many viruses previously mentioned
- Tissues and fluids of MS patients have shown presence of numerous viruses, bacteria, fungi and bacteria. However, all of these viruses may simply be bystanders/contamination or opportunistic
- Components of myelin sheath share amino acid homologies with proteins of measles, influenza, herpes, papilloma and other viruses ('molecular mimicry' theory of autoimmunity). This may activate myelin-specific T-cells to produce a misguided immune response.[370]

Epstein-Barr virus (EBV)

EBV (having a worldwide distribution) in particular seems to have the strongest evidence in this regard based on biological and epidemiological studies:

- Higher risk of infectious mononucleosis and higher antibody titres to the latency-associated antigen (EBNA1), associated with late EBV infection, are associated with MS
- Individual nerves infected by EBV are at low risk of developing MS.[370]

ROLE OF FREE RADICALS

Free radical damage and subsequent oxidative damage is emerging as an important factor contributing to the pathogenesis of multiple sclerosis.[375–377] Free radicals are produced from the mitochondria which under normal circumstances function as powerhouses of the body. Less known is the fact that the mitochondria are also a cellular source of reactive oxygen species (ROS) and reactive nitrogen species (RNS). When appropriate defence mechanisms are in place a fine balance is maintained between the two. However, when there is mitochondrial dysfunction and inadequate antioxidant defence mechanisms, ROS and RNS generate excessively. ROS and RNS have been suggested to contribute to inflammation and oxidative stress resulting in demyelination and the loss of the oligodendrocyte complex.[377] ROS have been identified as causes of dysfunction in the blood–brain barrier and contribute to the formation and persistence of multiple sclerosis lesions.[378] Antioxidant support would appear imperative to quench this oxidative stress.

HEAVY METALS AND MULTIPLE SCLEROSIS

Exposure to heavy metals is a potential risk factor for MS. Patients with MS are more likely to report lead and mercury exposures. The potential gene–environment interactions include the single nucleotide polymorphisms (SNPs) of TNF-alpha and TNF-beta. Both are pro-inflammatory cytokines that may potentially cause greater inflammation in a patient.[379] In addition, a study in 2016 found that repeat exposure to mercury accelerated the progression of MS by damaging the mitochondria enough to increase oxidative stress and finally cell death.[380] Not only does it seem that there are various ways heavy metals can cause damage and increase risk for MS, but continuous exposure to these metals seems to worsen the progression of MS. A case study of a patient with MS who had been unsuccessfully treated for many years, revealed how urinary testing for heavy metals found elevated levels of aluminium, lead and mercury. After undergoing chelation therapy, his MS symptoms improved to the extent that he was in remission.[381]

STRESS AND MULTIPLE SCLEROSIS

Stress has been demonstrated to influence the occurrence of new brain lesions in multiple sclerosis. In a prospective longitudinal study Mohr et al[382] observed that patients with relapsing multiple sclerosis who experienced increased conflict and disruption in their routine had an increased risk of developing new Gd+ brain lesions 8 weeks later evidenced by MRI. Interestingly, psychological stress or distress did not correlate with clinical exacerbation. However, a subsequent meta-analysis has suggested that stressful life events may cause exacerbation in multiple sclerosis.[383]

FOOD ALLERGY

Food allergy, in particular gluten (allergy or sensitivity/intolerance), has also been implicated in the pathogenesis of multiple sclerosis; refer to the section 'Dietary exclusions' for more information.

GUT MICROBIOME

Studies show that the gut microbiome composition differs between MS patients and healthy individuals. The microbiomes of 71 MS patients were compared with 71 healthy patients and it was found that *Akkermansia muciniphila* and *Acinetobacter calcoaceticus* were increased in MS patients, while *Parabacteroides distasonis* species was decreased. All of these species are significantly associated with MS. The researchers then conducted in-vivo and in-vitro experiments with these bacteria species and found that *A. muciniphila* and *A. calcoaceticus* induced pro-inflammatory responses, and *P. distasonis* stimulated anti-inflammatory IL-10 cells. All *Acinetobacter* species are rare in the healthy human gut microbiome. *A. calcoaceticus* has been shown to encode peptides that mimic the amino acid sequences of myelin basic protein and myelin oligodendrocyte glycoprotein, both of which are myelin components. This indicates that an immune response against *A. calcoaceticus* could trigger an autoimmune response against myelin.[384] A second study compared the gut microbial composition of 34 monozygotic twin pairs discordant for MS and found significantly higher rates of *Akkermansia* in untreated MS twins. When the microbiota from selected twin pairs were transplanted to germ-free mice that expressed a myelin autoantigen-specific T-cell receptor, the MS-twin derived microbiota induced a significantly higher incidence of autoimmunity than the healthy twin-derived microbiota.[385] This line of research is a new development showing promising potential for treatment options. Further clinical trials are needed in humans.

OBESITY

Strong evidence now supports obesity during adolescence as a factor which increases MS risk in females. Adolescent obesity interacts with human leucocyte antigen MS risk genes, with substantial risk increases in individuals who carry genes that predispose them to MS. The association is strongest for a BMI >27; however, being more modestly overweight is also associated with increased risk. Individuals with a high BMI who carry DRB1*15:01 and do not have the protective HLA–A*02 have a ~14–fold increased risk of MS. Obesity is also associated with increased risk of paediatric-onset MS.[386]

INFLAMMATORY BOWEL DISEASE

Inflammatory bowel diseases are a common cause of malabsorption in multiple sclerosis.[387–389] One large study involving 7988 Crohn's disease and 12 185 ulcerative colitis patients observed a greater incidence of demyelinating diseases in patients with irritable bowel disease than among non-irritable bowel disease patients.[388] It is prudent to thoroughly consider all malabsorptive processes including coeliac disease and fructose intolerance when holistically assessing the MS patient.

Overview

MS is the most common inflammatory disorder of the central nervous system and a leading cause of disability in young adults. Strong evidence suggests that MS is an autoimmune disease directed against CNS myelin or oligodendrocytes. Pathologically, it is characterised by perivascular infiltrates of mononuclear inflammatory cells, demyelination, axonal loss and gliosis mainly in the white matter, with the formation of multiple plaques in the brain and spinal cord. Epidemiology of MS follows a latitudinal gradient. Combined genetic and environmental factors determine the risk for developing MS. The leading environmental factors are some infectious agents, particularly EBV, heavy metals and vitamin D.[366]

Pathogenesis

There are two pathological processes responsible for the symptoms and signs of MS including inflammation and neurodegeneration. These two processes are explained in Fig. 22.20.

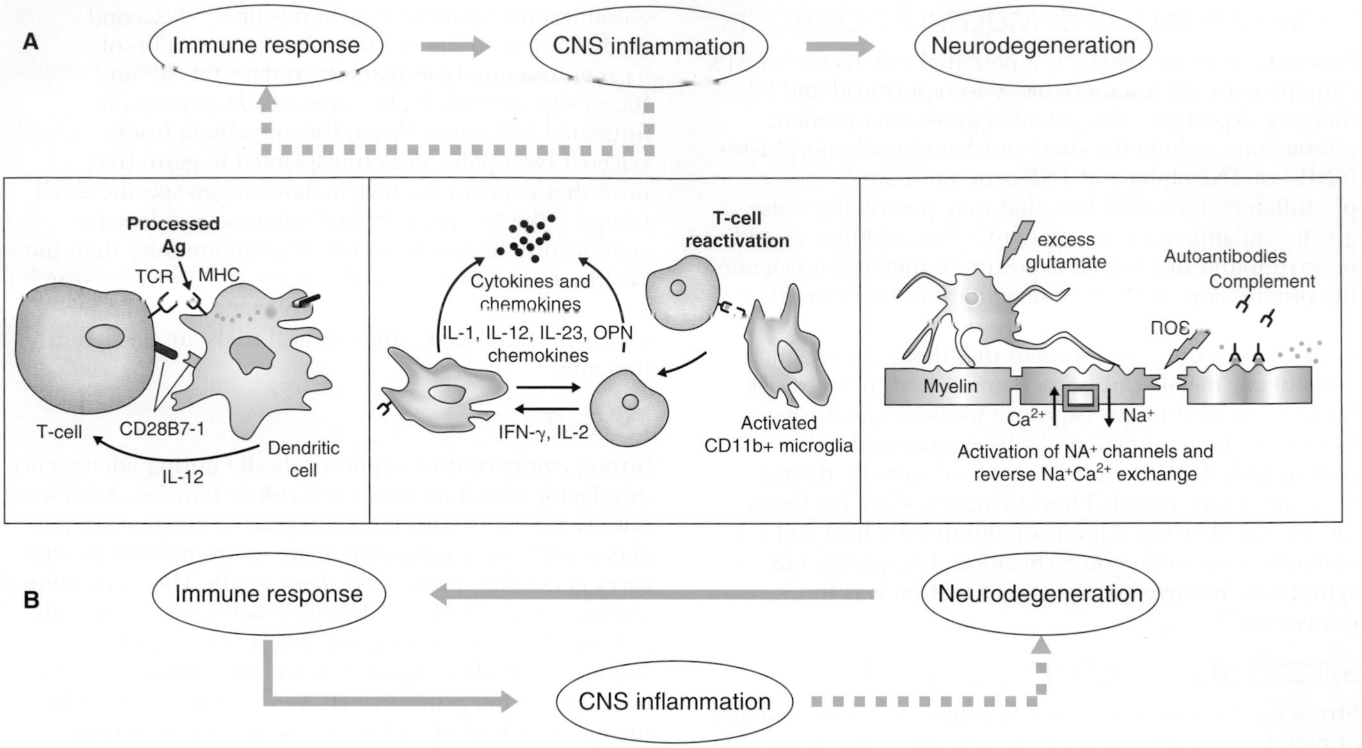

FIGURE 22.20 Models of disease pathogenesis in MS. (**A**) Highlights the traditional view of MS, which is an autoimmune response, causes inflammation, which in turn causes CNS injury/degeneration. (**B**) Proposes that activation of autoimmune cells occurs as a consequence of toxic damage to CNS cells; e.g. asymptomatic infections cause damage to the cells releasing neural antigens, which induce inflammatory response.

TCR, T-cell receptor; MHC, major histocompatibility complex; Ag, antigen; OPN, osteopontin; CD1, cluster of differentiation; ROS, reactive oxygen species; IL, interleukin.

Source: Hauser SL, Oksenberg JR. The neurobiology of multiple sclerosis: genes, inflammation, and neurodegeneration. Neuron 2006; 52:61–76.

AUTOIMMUNE RESPONSE

It is thought that in MS, there is a loss of immune homeostasis and uncontrolled immune responses against structural CNS components, mainly protein components of myelin sheath and the oligodendrocytes (see Fig. 22.21).

Additionally, B-cell activation and antibody responses appear to be necessary for the full development of demyelination.

NEURODEGENERATION

Popular thought has suggested that myelin loss has been the key event causing impaired propagation of impulses across the affected part of the axon, resulting in the neurological deficits. Studies with advanced MRI techniques and some pathological studies have shown that axonal damage/loss is responsible for the progressive and irreversible neurological dysfunction in patients with MS.[370]

SIGNS AND SYMPTOMS

Clinical features of MS are attributed to impaired impulse conduction and later to axonal damage due to demyelination of the tracts in the central nervous system (CNS). The peripheral nervous system (PNS) is not affected. Symptoms of MS are extremely varied and depend upon the location of lesions within the CNS.[370] The most common presenting symptoms of MS are given in Table 22.34 and other symptoms are in Table 22.35.

TABLE 22.34 Most common presenting symptoms of multiple sclerosis

Symptom	%
Weakness in one or more limbs	50
Numbness in one or more limbs	45
Optic neuritis	20
Unsteady gait	15
Diplopia	10
Vertigo or dizziness	5

Source: Rolak LA. The diagnosis of multiple sclerosis. Diagnostic Testing in Neurology 1996; (14):1.

Onset

Onset may be abrupt or insidious. Symptoms can be quite severe from the very beginning or can be so trivial that a patient may not seek medical attention for months or

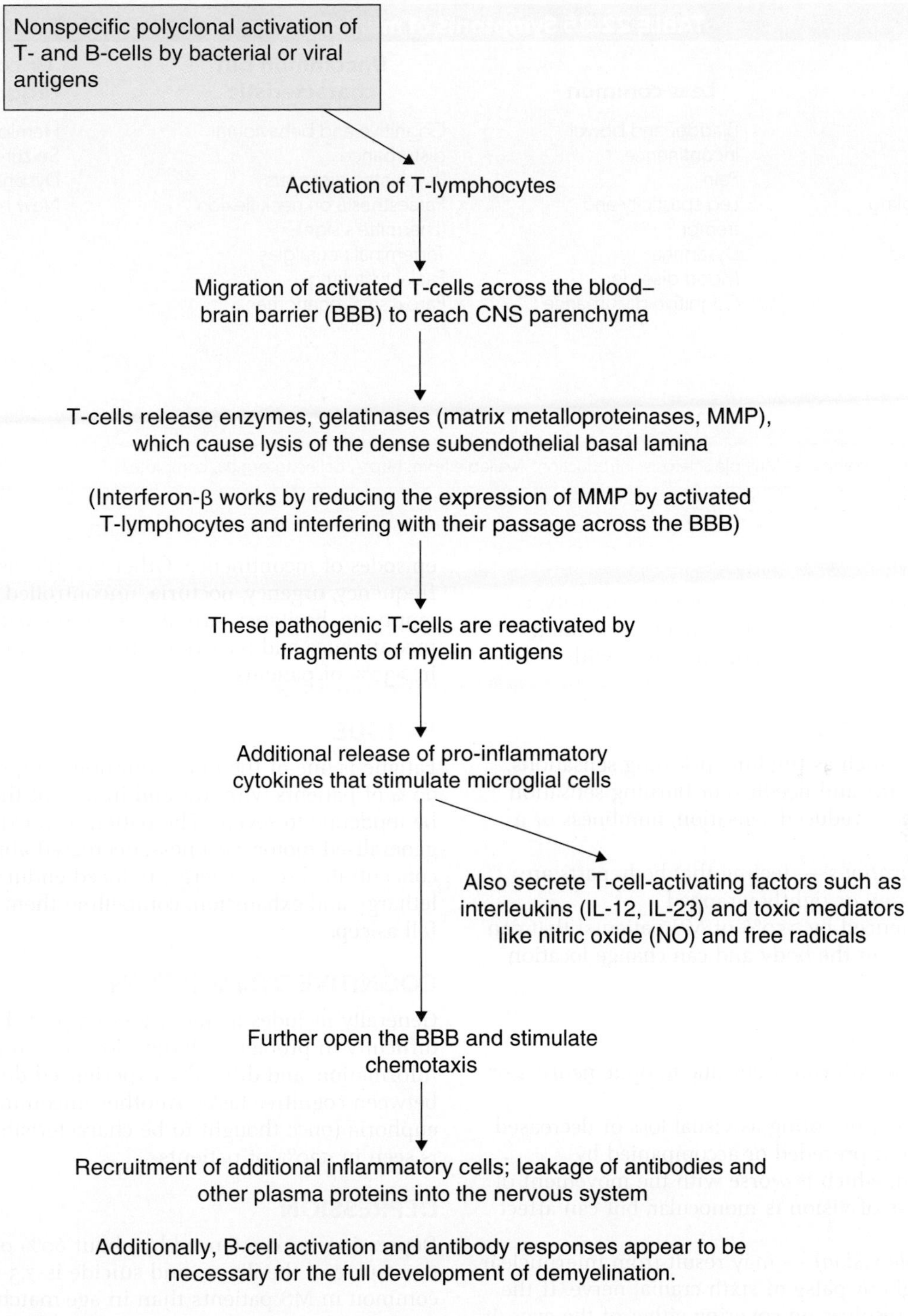

FIGURE 22.21 **Autoimmune theory — pathway of inflammation.**

years. Indeed, autopsy findings have confirmed MS in individuals who have remained asymptomatic during their life. In other instances, an MRI scan performed for other reasons has identified lesions of MS in asymptomatic individuals.[370,390]

Initial symptoms

Patients can present with one or more of the following.

WEAKNESS IN ONE OR MORE LIMBS

This can present as loss of strength or dexterity, disturbance of gait or fatigue. It can be accompanied by other pyramidal signs such as spasticity, hyperreflexia and Babinski's sign (upper motor neuron type weakness). Loss of tendon reflex can be observed in occasional cases due to the lesion affecting the afferent reflex fibres in the spinal cord.

TABLE 22.35 Symptoms of multiple sclerosis

Common	Less common	Uncommon but characteristic	Uncommon but requiring review
Incoordination Weakness of limbs Dizziness Numbness and tingling Diplopia Blurring of vision and visual loss Bladder urgency or constipation Depression and anxiety Sexual issues Heat sensitivity Fatigue	Bladder and bowel incontinence Pain Leg spasticity and tremor Dysarthria Mood disorders Cognitive disturbance	Cognitive and behavioural disturbances Psychiatric disorders Paraesthesia on neck flexion (Lhermitte's sign) Trigeminal neuralgias Facial twitching Paroxysmal phenomena	Hemiplegia Seizures Dysphasia New headaches

Source: Adapted from eTG complete. Multiple sclerosis: introduction. Available from: http://online.tg.org.au/complete/

SPASTICITY

Especially in the legs, of moderate to severe intensity, is observed in more than 30% of MS patients. It is often associated with painful spasms and interferes with patients' ambulation.

SENSORY DISTURBANCE

- *Paraesthesia* — such as tingling, prickling sensations, formications, 'pins and needles', or burning sensation
- *Hyperaesthesia* — reduced sensation, numbness or a 'dead' feeling
- *Unpleasant sensations* — feeling that body parts are swollen, tight, raw or tightly wrapped
- *Pain* — (experienced by >50% of MS patients) that can occur anywhere on the body and can change location over time.

VISUAL SYMPTOMS

Blurring of vision in MS can occur due to optic neuritis or diplopia:
- *Optic neuritis* — presenting as visual loss or decreased colour perception preceded or accompanied by periorbital pain, which is worse with the movement of the eyeball. Loss of vision is monocular, but can affect bilaterally
- *Diplopia (double vision)* — may result from internuclear ophthalmoplegia or palsy of sixth cranial nerve. If the blurred vision resolves on covering either of the eyes, it is due to diplopia.

ATAXIA

Ataxia presents as cerebellar tremors. It may also involve the head and trunk or the voice resulting in a characteristic cerebellar dysarthria (*slurring speech*).

Advanced symptoms

BLADDER AND BOWEL DYSFUNCTION

Symptoms of bladder dysfunction are seen in >90% of MS patients. In one-third of these patients, there are frequent episodes of incontinence. Other symptoms can be urinary frequency, urgency, nocturia, uncontrolled bladder emptying, hesitancy, urinary retention, overflow incontinence and recurrent infection. Constipation occurs in >30% of patients.

FATIGUE

Fatigue is one of the most common symptoms affecting 90% of patients with MS and in half of them it can be moderate to severe. The patient can experience generalised motor weakness, decreased ability to concentrate, loss of energy, reduced endurance, extreme lethargy and exhaustion, compelling them to take rest or fall asleep.

COGNITIVE DYSFUNCTION

Generally includes memory loss, impaired attention, difficulty in problem solving, slowness in processing information, and difficulty experienced during shifting between cognitive tasks. Another uncommon symptom is euphoria (once thought to be characteristic of MS), which is seen in <20% of patients.

DEPRESSION

Depression is experienced by about 60% of patients during the course of the illness and suicide is 7.5-fold more common in MS patients than in age-matched controls.

OTHER

Other symptoms can be sexual dysfunction, facial weakness and vertigo.

Ancillary symptoms

HEAT SENSITIVITY

Heat sensitivity refers to the production or aggravation of neurological symptoms as a result of elevation in body's core temperature (causes transient conduction block). For example, physical exercise or a hot shower can cause transient unilateral visual blurring or loss (known as

Uhthoff's symptom). Fever also causes transient worsening of the symptoms.

LHERMITTE'S SYMPTOM

Lhermitte's symptom is an electric shock-like sensation down the spine and into the limbs (more commonly lower limbs) produced by flexion of the neck. It is also present in other disorders of the cervical spine, such as cervical spondylosis.

PAROXYSMAL SYMPTOMS

These are characterised by their brief duration (30 sec to 2 min), high frequency (5–40 episodes per day) and generally lasting weeks to months (self-limited course). Included in these symptoms are: Lhermitte's symptom, tonic seizures, paroxysmal dysarthria/ataxia, paroxysmal sensory disturbances and some other less characteristic symptoms.

OTHER

Some uncommon symptoms include trigeminal neuralgia, hemifacial spasm and glossopharyngeal neuralgia when 5th, 7th and 9th cranial nerve roots are affected.

Complications

DISEASE PROGRESSION

Chronic progressive worsening usually manifests as progressive spastic weakness of the limbs leading to permanent disability. Fifteen years after diagnosis, fewer than 20% of patients have no functional limitation, 50 to 60% require assistance when ambulating, 70% are limited or unable to perform major activities of daily living and 75% are not employed. The NSW, Australia, MS Society surveyed 2618 people with MS (estimated to be 70% of the NSW MS population) in 2001. The mobility disability profile of the sample covered the entire spectrum with half reporting being able to walk without an aid and only 17% being confined to a wheelchair. The average age of patients confined to a wheelchair was 56 years.[391]

Other factors affecting prognosis include:[370]

- Gender — research indicates that females reach disability endpoints at an older age than males
- Age at onset — the younger the age of onset, the earlier the onset of disability.

SUICIDE

Due to the disease process, suicide rates are significantly higher among individuals with multiple sclerosis than with the population in general.[392] Thus it is important to monitor and screen patients thoroughly.

Differential diagnosis

For differential diagnosis of multiple sclerosis, see Table 22.36.

TABLE 22.36 Differential diagnosis of multiple sclerosis

Inflammatory/ autoimmune diseases	Dysmyelinating disorders
Systemic lupus erythematosus	Metachromatic leukodystrophy
Antiphospholipid antibody syndrome	Krabbe's leukoencephalopathy
Primary Sjögren's syndrome	Multiple sulfatase deficiency
Neurosar coidosis	Alexander disease
Neuro-Behcet's disease	Adrenoleukodystrophy
Primary angiitis of the CNS	Pelizacus-Merzbacher disease
Polyarteritis nodosa	Other demyelinating disorders
Wegener's granulomatosis	Neuromyelitis optica (Devic disease)
Susac syndrome	Acute disseminated encephalomyelitis
Infectious aetiologies	Concentric sclerosis
Neuroborreliosis	Schilder's disease
Progressive multifocal leukoencephalopathy	Optic neuritis
Tropical spastic paraparesis	CNS neoplasms
HIV-related disorders	CNS lymphoma
Genetic/hereditary disorders	
Migraine	
CADASIL	
Leber's hereditary optic atrophy	

Source: Fadil H, Kelley RE, Gonzalez-Toledo E. Differential diagnoses of multiple sclerosis. Int Rev Microb 2007; (79):393–422.

Naturopathic diagnosis

Due to the complexity of the disease, naturopathic diagnosis relies on conventional opinion. The naturopathic framework interprets the disease manifestation as a consequence of some stress and consideration of stress to be a vital part of formulating a diagnosis. Stress may be:

- Nutritional (deficiency or excess)
- Environmental
- Occupational
- Emotional or mental
- Infective (or immune derangement).

Investigations

MS remains a clinical diagnosis, as there is no single test that can diagnose MS. Diagnosis relies on a knowledgeable doctor taking a history, performing a neurological examination, conducting various tests, and then making a diagnosis on the basis of all of the data.

Diagnosis of multiple sclerosis is aided by magnetic resonance imaging (MRI), cerebrospinal fluid examination and visual tests. The traditional requirement for diagnosis includes lesions that are 'multiple in time and multiple in space'. However, for every clinical attack there are now known to be 6 to 10 asymptomatic brain lesions on MRI.

The MRI scan can allow earlier diagnosis, as a single scan can demonstrate dissemination in space, while repeat scans may demonstrate dissemination in time.

International criteria for diagnosis (the McDonald Criteria) incorporate the traditional clinical and new MRI methods of diagnosis.[393]

McDonald Criteria for the diagnosis of MS

McDonald Criteria are formulated by an international panel and enable the diagnosis of multiple sclerosis. Key issues are the occurrence of multiple attacks in multiple parts of the nervous system. These may be identified by clinical symptoms and signs, MRI-detected lesions (which may be subclinical), and oligoclonal bands in the CSF.

RELEVANT ASSESSMENTS

MRI of the brain and spinal cord

MRI scanning (Fig. 22.22) has significantly improved the ability to diagnose MS in its early stages, as it allows imaging of areas of demyelination in the brain and spinal cord. It also helps exclude the presence of other diseases that might explain the patient's symptoms.

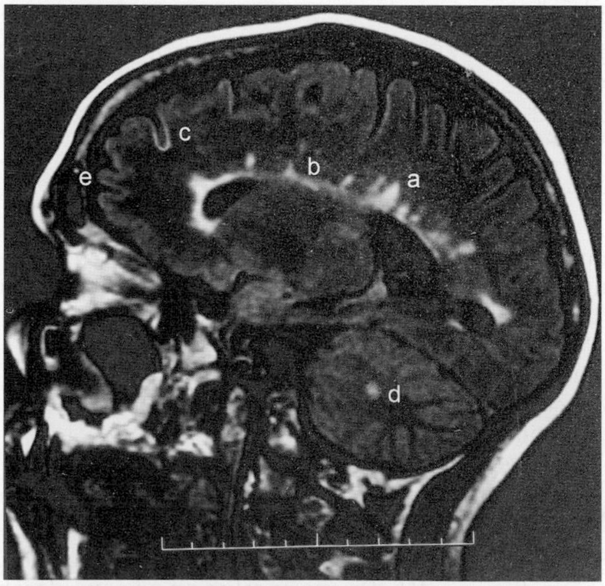

FIGURE 22.22 Sagittal MRI in a patient with MS. a, classical lesions perpendicular to ventricles and in corpus callosum — Dawson's fingers; b, lesions tend to be periventricular whereas in vasculitis they are more peripheral; c, subcortical U fibres, characteristic of MS; d, cerebellar (infratentorial) plaque; e, cortex may show atrophy.

Source: Waldman S et al. Pharmacology and therapeutics: principles to practice. Saunders, 2009.

Neurological examination

Demonstration of areas of demyelination through comprehensive neurological examination.

Electrophysiological tests

Tests to evoke neuronal electrical potentials that assess visual, auditory and somatosensory pathways.

CSF examination

Evaluated for the presence of plasma cells that are producing immunoglobulins (Igs) within the CNS by assessing for qualitative (oligoclonal bands) and quantitative (total IgG, IgG index and IgG synthesis rate) immunoglobulin changes.

Fundoscopic (ophthalmoscopic) examination

Examination of retina may be normal or may show optic disc swelling (papillitis), and pallor of the optic disc that indicates optic atrophy and commonly follows optic neuritis. Uveitis is very rare.

SPECIFIC NATUROPATHIC INVESTIGATIONS

Stool analysis

Malabsorption and inflammatory bowel disorders are common in individuals with multiple sclerosis hence the usefulness of a stool analysis which provides an insight into absorption, general gut function, and bacterial/fungal dysbiosis. If absorption and assimilation are impaired or if there is an imbalance in the gut flora, the patient may not be getting the desired nutrients required to ensure neurological health and may be releasing toxins through the digestive tract. This needs to be identified and corrected.

Oxidative stress markers

A strong relationship exists demonstrating the adverse effects of free radicals with regards to inflammation and axonal degeneration in multiple sclerosis. Analysis of antioxidant status as well as oxidative risk provides a rationale for use of antioxidants to improve patient symptomatology and outcomes.

Essential fatty acids

Essential fatty acid screening needs to be considered in individuals with multiple sclerosis as essential fatty acids promote the production of substances involved in myelinogenesis and possess immune regulatory actions.

Adrenal hormone profile

The adrenal hormone profile monitors the levels of stress hormones cortisol and DHEA-S over the course of a day; stress may cause reactivations of multiple sclerosis owing to its ability to influence the occurrence of new brain lesions. The adrenal hormone profile provides a useful tool to measure the stress response particularly in those individuals who may not be aware of the extent of their stress.

Food allergy/intolerance testing

Due to the links discussed between food allergy and multiple sclerosis, potential allergy and intolerances should be identified and removed from the diet. A number of allergens have been linked to impaired neurological function.

Therapeutic considerations

CLINICAL DECISION MAKING AND RATIONALE

When presented with an MS patient the naturopath should recognise that their role is multifaceted and understandably primarily supportive. Fundamentally MS is a degenerative nerve disease characterised by multiple areas of inflammation and demyelination in the brain and spinal cord. Specific approaches should consider a few key variables including:

1. Delay/halt disease progression
2. Encourage remission if disease treatment occurs in early stages and delay progressive stage for as long as possible
3. Assess and determine contributing cause of disease development to support objective #1
4. Address and treat relevant factors ascertained in #3 (as possible)
5. Modulate immune response and protect autoimmune aggravation
6. Treat medication reactions or side effects as evident
7. Provide symptomatic support for the whole person as required; this may require referral to other health practitioners
8. Address patient requirements and symptomatology as disease progresses.

Therapeutic application

ALLOPATHIC PERSPECTIVE

Neuroprotective therapeutic strategies for MS

There is currently no cure for MS; however, treatments are available to modify the disease course and treat exacerbations to manage symptoms. There are currently six disease-modifying drugs (DMT) that reduce the relapse rates in MS. These include interferon-beta preparations (IFN-β; IFN-β-1a; IFN-β-1b) as well as glatiramer acetate (GA), mitoxantrone and natalizumab. All of these agents have shown moderate to high efficacy in reducing relapse rates in large-scale, randomised, placebo-controlled phase III trials.[394]

Sodium-channel blockers

Sodium-channel blockers such as carbamazepine are used widely in MS for the symptomatic treatment of tonic spasms, neuropathic pain and trigeminal neuralgia. These drugs might prevent the axonal injury due to increased sodium permeability.[395]

Treatment of acute attack:

- Corticosteroids
- Intravenous immunoglobulins
- Plasma exchange.

HISTORICAL PERSPECTIVE

Jean-Martin Charcot is credited with first describing a condition strikingly similar to multiple sclerosis in 1868, where he details symptoms such as nystagmus, intention tremor and scanning speech.[396] There is no mention of multiple sclerosis in the texts of the Eclectics and this is, of course, because it was yet to be defined, thus we can only hypothesise what the Eclectic physicians may have used. Antidepressants and nervines such as *Hypericum perforatum* would likely have been useful for help to manage the depressive symptoms that occur with this condition. Adaptogens such as *Panax ginseng* and restoratives such as *Avena sativa* may have been useful to counteract fatigue and weakness. Analgesics such as *Piscidia erythrina* may have been used to help control and allay spasm[344] and tremor. Antispasmodics such as *Dioscorea villosa* were believed to be useful in neuralgic afflictions and in irritable conditions of the nervous system — especially when combined with pain.

NATUROPATHIC PERSPECTIVE

As MS treatment is primarily supportive, it requires a thorough assessment and overview to accurately ascertain the current health status of the patient. From this perspective, the clinician is able to then develop a comprehensive approach that includes support for all levels of health. The patient must take an active role in their healthcare management and is required to embrace health responsibility on all levels. This must include vigilance in the home and work environment with respect to potential exposure and lifestyle practices. As the disease progresses, treatment modification will be directed to more specific needs; for example, cognitive improvement, incontinence support and mobility relief.

NUTRITIONAL MEDICINE (DIETARY)

Dietary therapeutic objectives

- Follow basic principles of the Swank diet where possible with a focus on reducing saturated (animal) fats and aiming to avoid red meat where possible
- Avoid all sources of hydrogenated, rancid or poor quality oils
- Encourage cold-pressed, fresh and organic pure oils such as flaxseed, olive, sunflower, safflower and similar. All oils must adhere to the above criteria. Oils should be purchased in dark bottles and stored out of direct light (or refrigerated as indicated)
- Avoid caffeine, sugar, artificial sweeteners (all types)
- Follow naturopathic wholefood principles that encourage individualised dietary programs rich in organic vegetables, lean meats and wild caught or sustainably farmed fish that is guaranteed to be free of heavy metals, antibiotics and other concerning ingredients

- Avoid all smoked and cured meats due to nitrite/nitrophenol content which may induce autoantibodies against the myelin sheath
- Identify any food allergies/intolerances and avoid as indicated
- Encourage small, frequent meals to optimise and ease digestive processes
- Encourage dietary antioxidant sources such as organic fruits and vegetables — especially those that are brightly coloured for flavonoid content
- Control dietary salt intake.[397]

Specific dietary treatments

DIETARY INCLUSIONS

The Swank diet

Neurologist Roy Swank was one of the first to suggest a link between dietary factors and multiple sclerosis. His diet, the Swank diet, has become one of the most popular therapeutic diets for individuals suffering from this condition. Swank proposed that MS is caused in part by excessive consumption of saturated animal fat[398] and has conducted numerous studies over the years in individuals with multiple sclerosis following a low saturated fat diet. Swank proposes that saturated fat aggregates are larger than those of unsaturated and, when consumed in large amounts, due to their sheer size they may get lodged in the capillaries or very slowly pass through. Subsequently, tissues reliant on fats fail to receive adequate nourishment and are not able to optimally function causing lesions to appear in the central nervous system.[399] Results from the long-term studies Swank has conducted show beneficial effects with one 34-year study showing that those individuals who had adhered to the Swank diet (20 g/day or less of saturated fat daily) showed significantly less neurological deterioration, disability and death rates than those who consumed more fat than prescribed (greater than 20 g fat/day);[400] similar benefits were observed at 50 years.[401] In 2003 Swank recommended that saturated fat content should be even lower suggesting the diet should contain no more than 10–15 g/day of saturated fat. Note that some fat is important, so while Swank minimises saturated fat he highlights the importance of essential fatty acids and encourages the use of cod liver oil to prevent nutritional deficiencies. By following the principles of the Swank diet, it is suggested by Swank, individuals with multiple sclerosis can expect to survive and be ambulant and otherwise normal to an advanced age.

Basic principles of the Swank diet[402]

- Saturated fat should not exceed 15 g/day
- Unsaturated fat (oils) should be kept to 20–50 g/day
- No red meat for the first year, after the first year, 85 g of red meat is allowed once per week
- Dairy products must contain 1% or less butterfat
- No processed foods containing saturated fat
- Fats not allowed: margarine, hydrogenated peanut butter, coconut oil, palm oil
- Additional supplementation with cod liver oil, multi mineral and vitamin and vitamin C and E to prevent nutritional deficiency

While Swank's work has been published in *The Lancet*, a Cochrane review disputes its usefulness owing to the lack of double-blind testing involved in the studies.[403] Further research is required.

Other popular dietary programs include but are not limited to the Mediterranean diet, ketogenic diet, Paleolithic diet, and anti-inflammatory diet. Each patient requires a personalised diet in order to achieve the best adherence and overall healthier lifestyle. Interestingly, the Mediterranean diet showed the greatest patient adherence.[404] While much available research compares the different diets and their efficacies, no two people are alike when it comes to their dietary needs. Working with your patients to come up with the best diet (within a set of MS guidelines) for that particular person and their particular health needs exceeds the proposed benefits of a set universal dietary program. By being attentive, this is where you, the healthcare provider, can really help your patient.

DIETARY EXCLUSIONS

Caffeine

Spasticity results in a high incidence of bladder and bowel dysfunction in individuals with multiple sclerosis. As a result of hyperactivity of the bladder up to 75%[405] of individuals are estimated to suffer from symptoms such as frequency, urgency and incontinence. Similarly, though less studied, constipation and faecal incontinence may affect almost half of all individuals with multiple sclerosis.[406] Caffeine is a bladder and bowel irritant and thus it promotes urination and bowel movements — this is undesirable given that the organs of elimination are already hypersensitive. Paradoxically, because caffeine is a diuretic and many people do not follow it up with proper hydration, it may also cause constipation. Caffeine also places strain on the adrenal glands and contributes to fatigue, a complaint that already predominates in individuals with multiple sclerosis. For those patients who are able to tolerate caffeine, a pilot study of 63 MS patients has shown that participants who consumed two or more cups of caffeine daily outperformed those consuming less on scores of verbal memory. No differences were reported on processing speed or depressive symptoms.[407]

Sugar

Refined sugars offer no nutritional value and contribute to impaired immunity, gut dysbiosis and glucose metabolism. Because individuals with multiple sclerosis may also be at increased risk of bladder infection and gut dysbiosis, sugar intake should be excluded from the diet.

Artificial sweeteners

A number of reports exist associating use of artificial sweeteners, in particular the sweetener aspartame, with neurological and behavioural complications in humans including depression[408] and headaches.[299] Aspartame may be marketed as NutraSweet or Equal and is predominantly found in diet and sugar-free products such as soft drinks and low-joule jams and jellies. A number of papers have suggested that aspartame causes neurodegeneration.[80]

However, because studies have not as yet been conducted, evidence does not support links between aspartame and multiple sclerosis; this is not to say that a link does not exist. As noted by Briffa[409] 100% of the studies that conclude that aspartame is safe are industry funded either wholly or in part. Interestingly, 92% of independently funded studies have found that aspartame has the potential for adverse effects, including those that are neurological. While aspartame-induced neurological toxicity will not occur in all individuals, in those who are more susceptible to neurological damage, such as those with multiple sclerosis, risk would logically appear to be higher, hence exclusion from the diet should be mandatory.

OTHER DIETARY CONSIDERATIONS

Food allergy/intolerance

The role of allergy and food intolerance in the aetiology and pathogenesis of multiple sclerosis has been explored in numerous studies. Gluten sensitivity in particular is known to produce a range of abnormalities with regards to neurological function. Recently, Shor et al[410] observed an association between antibodies against gliadin and tissue transglutaminase in patients with multiple sclerosis confirming the work of Reichelt et al[411] who observed increased IgA and IgG antibodies against gliadin and gluten. Others have found no such association.[412] However, given this possible link between food intolerance and multiple sclerosis, diagnostic testing particularly for gluten and casein is highly warranted. The importance of this is further emphasised when one considers that many individuals with multiple sclerosis show signs of intestinal malabsorption,[413] further highlighting the importance of thoroughly investigating gut health in all patients.

NUTRITIONAL MEDICINE (SUPPLEMENTAL)

Nutritional medicine therapeutic objectives

- Address deficiency states and replete supportive or deficient nutrients
- Provide antioxidants to prevent free radical damage, reduce oxidation and protect neurons

SAMPLE DAILY DIET

BREAKFAST	
Papaya breakfast bowl: papaya filled with blueberries, banana, strawberries and a small quantity of chia seeds	A nutritional intervention that takes into account inflammatory and autoimmune processes involved in MS is likely to be most beneficial. MS may present as a neurological manifestation of coeliac disease and an increased prevalence of coeliac disease has been observed in individuals with MS and their first-degree relatives; therefore implementation of an anti-inflammatory, immune regulating GF diet is suggested. Papaya provides papain to assist with digestion while blueberries have an affinity for the neurological system, their constituents being found to cross the blood–brain barrier. Chia seeds provide omega-3 fatty acids to downregulate inflammation (see below).
LUNCH	
Walnut and flaxseed tacos (walnuts pulsed with coriander, lime, turmeric, cumin) served in iceberg lettuce cups with shredded red cabbage, carrot, avocado and tomato	Walnuts and flaxseeds are a source of PUFAs which include omega-3 PUFAs. PUFAs may reduce inflammation by inhibiting arachidonic acid, and reducing T-cell proliferation. As well as being anti-inflammatory, omega-3 fatty acids make up glial and neuronal membrane phospholipids and are involved in myelin protein expression. Ample vegetables (cabbage, carrot and lettuce) and fruits (avocado and tomato) provide antioxidants to reduce the impact of free radicals that cause peroxidation of myelin sheaths.
DINNER	
Pad Thai salad with rice or kelp noodles, tempeh, bean sprouts, carrots, tamari, snow peas, lemon, coriander and ginger	Alterations in gut microbiota have been implicated in the pathogenesis of MS, therefore a high-fibre diet which contains prebiotics and fermented foods may be useful. Dinner contains ample herbs and spices. Herbs and spices should be used to flavour food to reduce consumption of sodium since some studies suggests that a high-sodium diet (>5 g/day) may contribute to the development of MS through the induction of pathogenic Th17 cells and pro-inflammatory cytokines.
SNACKS	
Fruit salad with Brazil nuts	Fruit salad provides a high-fibre option to assist with removal of heavy metals. It also provides vitamin C to assist as an adjuvant with chelation therapy if heavy metal exposure is considered to be a causative factor. Brazil nuts contain selenium which may be useful in assisting the removal of mercury.

- Address neurotransmitter insufficiency and provide symptomatic relief as required for associated mood effects
- Support myelination and promote myelin repair with appropriate nutritional cofactors
- Decrease proinflammatory cytokines, matrix metalloproteinase levels
- Prevent neuronal injury and alleviate symptoms associated with injury that is existing
- Regulate immune response and reduce autoimmunity.

Specific nutrients required

5-HYDROXYTRYPTOPHAN (5-HTP)

Depression is estimated to occur in 50% of individuals with multiple sclerosis[414] and thus is an important factor that needs to be considered and acknowledged throughout the health management of the patient. 5-hydroxytryptophan is a useful antidepressant that functions by increasing levels of serotonin in the central nervous system. The results from two meta-analyses suggest positive results for the ability of 5-HTP to assist with depression. However, they also state that a definitive answer cannot be given with regards to efficacy due to the poor quality of trials conducted.[415,416] Additionally, 5-HTP may also help with cerebellar ataxia[417] which may manifest with multiple sclerosis.

B COMPLEX

The B vitamins are highly indicated in multiple sclerosis owing to their indispensable role within the body. One of their main roles in neurological health is to help prevent conditions associated with multiple sclerosis such as fatigue, cognitive function and depression. Structurally the B vitamins are essential for synthesis of the myelin sheath and maintaining the health of the neurons.[403,418] Inadequate B vitamins will therefore impair normal myelination.

A number of studies have proposed a link between vitamin B_{12} and multiple sclerosis,[419] particularly as deficiency symptoms are so similar. However, as yet the relationship remains undetermined though it is recognised that many individuals with multiple sclerosis are deficient in vitamin B_{12}.[420] A 2003 experimental study revealed vitamin B_{12} to exert a neurotrophic action[421] thus it would appear to be a much-needed vitamin in multiple sclerosis and its role warrants further study.

COENZYME Q10

Coenzyme Q10 is a powerful antioxidant and transporter within the mitochondria where it is required for ATP generation and cellular energy production as well as a free radical scavenger. This latter role has led to its recommendation for use in a number of neurodegenerative conditions including Parkinson's syndromes and Alzheimer's disease.[422] Mitochondrial abnormalities have been proposed to drive inflammation in multiple sclerosis[423] hence coenzyme Q10 with its antioxidant action and key role within the mitochondria is likely to be of use. Serum coenzyme Q10 levels of individuals with multiple sclerosis were measured in one small study but were observed to be not dissimilar to those of healthy subjects.[424]

A randomised placebo-controlled double-blind study (n = 24) of coenzyme Q10 supplementation (500 mg/d) over 12 weeks in patients with relapsing and remitting MS demonstrated a reduction in IL-6 and MMP-9 levels.[425] The results of another similar trial by the same group demonstrated a reduction in depression and fatigue.[426] Further studies are required to confirm these promising results.

ESSENTIAL FATTY ACIDS

Essential fatty acids have been shown to play a key role in the treatment of multiple sclerosis. Not only do they promote the production of substances involved in myelinogenesis[427,428] but they also exert significant anti-inflammatory and immuno-modulatory functions required in multiple sclerosis. The benefits of omega-3 fatty acids are not lost to those afflicted with multiple sclerosis in a South Australian study.[429] The researchers observed that fish oil was the most commonly used CAM medication with 62.5% of the participants surveyed found to use it.

DHA AND EPA

Gallai et al[430] observed a decrease in levels of interleukin-1β, TNF-α, IL-2 and IFN-γ produced from unstimulated and stimulated peripheral blood mononuclear cells in patients with multiple sclerosis after 12 weeks of omega-3 fatty acids supplementation (3 g/day of EPA and 1.8 g/day DHA), highlighting the ability of omega-3 fatty acids to decrease proinflammatory cytokine levels in multiple sclerosis.

Clinical trials also reveal the ability of the omega-3 fatty acids to decrease matrix metalloproteinase levels which may also promote inflammation and disease state in multiple sclerosis. In an open-label study involving 10 subjects with relapsing-remitting multiple sclerosis Shinto et al, administering omega-3 fatty acids (9.6 g of fish oil concentrate per day containing 2.9 g EPA and 1.9 g DHA), observed a significant decrease in matrix metalloproteinase-9 levels secreted from peripheral blood mononuclear cells after 3 months of supplementation.[431] A randomised double-blind placebo-controlled trial (n = 80, duration 30 months) showed that an intervention composed of omega-3 and omega-6 fatty acids (EPA 1650 mg, DHA 4650 mg, GLA 2000 mg, LA 3850 mg) with small amounts of vitamin A (0.6 mg) and E (22 mg) plus γ-tocopherol (760 mg) significantly reduced the annual relapse rate, and the risk of sustained disability progression, compared to placebo. The authors reported that the γ-tocopherol was a necessary component of this combination. One of the control groups in the study had the same combination without γ-tocopherol and did not get the same results. This was a small trial and had a high dropout rate.[432] Further research is required.

GLA

Animal studies reveal the ability of GLA to promote oligodendrocyte differentiation, thus promoting myelin repair evidenced by increased myelin sheath formation.[433] Small decreases in relapse rate and relapse severity in patients with multiple sclerosis have been observed when consuming omega-6 fatty acids. However, a Cochrane review observed studies were small and findings are limited because of methodological errors.[403]

MAGNESIUM

Magnesium is an essential mineral essential for healthy neurological function. Magnesium blocks NMDA channels and prevents influx of calcium that otherwise may result in neuronal injury and death. Low levels of magnesium lead to uncontrollable muscle contraction as magnesium inhibits the release of acetylcholine.[434] Thus inadequate magnesium has also been suggested to cause alterations in normal functioning of nerve cells contributing to multiple sclerosis.[435] Action tremor, cramps, spasticity, Babinski's sign and hyperreflexia are all signs associated with multiple sclerosis. Magnesium, via its action as a muscle relaxant, might help to ease these symptoms though clinical studies are lacking. A case-controlled study illustrates the use of magnesium for managing spasticity, in which magnesium (elemental) 125 mg/day administered in conjunction with dietary magnesium (estimated to contain approximately 300–350 mg/day of magnesium) significantly improved spasticity in a young woman with multiple sclerosis.[436]

SELENIUM

Free radicals and oxidative stress promote neurodegeneration in multiple sclerosis[376] contributing to neuronal demyelination and axonal injury. However, the brain contains decreased quantities of antioxidants when compared with other areas of the body and is thus at greater risk of damage from free radicals.[437] Individuals with multiple sclerosis show signs of increased oxidative stress and increased lipid peroxides. They have been hypothesised to be involved in multiple sclerosis[438] as well as in reduced glutathione peroxidase activity.[439] Thus, due to these factors, antioxidant supplementation with selenium, a powerful antioxidant, has been suggested.[440] Selenium status has been measured in individuals with multiple sclerosis but provides mixed results.[441] A more recent study of 101 relapsing-remitting MS patients found that their selenium concentrations were significantly lower when compared with healthy controls.[442] A definitive link between deficiency and multiple sclerosis cannot be made. However, selenium has been useful in a number of autoimmune conditions due to its immune regulating role. Since multiple sclerosis has been proposed to involve an autoimmune component, selenium may be of use from this perspective. Selenium via its detoxification capacities may also aid the removal of toxic metals from the body. Heavy metal toxicity such as mercury from dental work has also been implicated in multiple sclerosis but is as yet unproven.[443]

VITAMIN A

Vitamin A exerts immune regulatory and antioxidant functions that may be of use in multiple sclerosis. Low levels of vitamin A have been hypothesised to be involved in the development of multiple sclerosis. However, there has been little undertaken in the way of clinical trials. Vitamin A may also be of use to inhibit leukotriene synthesis,[444] which is implicated in retrobulbar neuritis, an eye disorder characterised by inflammation and destruction of the myelin sheath covering the optic nerve, commonly seen in multiple sclerosis. A placebo-controlled randomised trial of 101 relapse-remitting MS patients showed that administering 25 000 IU/d retinyl palmitate for 6 months, followed by 10 000 UI/d retinyl palmitate for a further 6 months improved cognitive ability and countered disability in the upper extremity of the trunk. It did not change the relapse rate or the EDSS score which measured neurological disability.[445] A randomised double-blind placebo-controlled phase III clinical trial showed that vitamin A (25 000 IU/d retinyl palmitate for 6 months) affects the gene expression of negative modulators of regulatory autoimmune T-cells, indicating that vitamin A may have a role to play in MS disease prevention and treatment.[446]

VITAMIN D

For many decades, the lower MS mortality and disability rates in the coastal regions compared with inland were hypothesised to be attributable to vitamin D levels.[447] Strong evidence that directly supports the hypothesis that vitamin D is able to modulate disease in MS is lacking. However, significant clinical observations have been made in MS populations that support a role for vitamin D in the treatment of MS. These include associations with plasma 25(OH)D levels, the geographic distribution of MS prevalence, the low bone mass density found in MS patients, the seasonal fluctuation of plasma 25(OH)D, MS disease parameters and MS births, the clinical remission of disease during pregnancy and the associations of various genetic polymorphisms of the vitamin D receptor with MS patients.

Most of the biological effects of 1,25(OH)2D are mediated by the vitamin D receptor (VDR). This receptor is a member of the steroid receptor super-family and it influences the rate of transcription of vitamin D responsive genes by a ligand-activated transcription factor that binds to the vitamin D response elements in those genes.[448] In the CNS, expression of VDR has been described in different cell types.[449] 1α-hydroxylase and 24-hydroxylase are also expressed in the CNS.[450,451] Therefore, the CNS may be a site of action, metabolism and catabolism of vitamin D.

In a large observational study in the United States, the use of supplemental vitamin D, mostly in the form of multivitamins, by healthy female nurses seemed to lower their risk of MS by 40%.[452] However, several methodological weaknesses in the study design made the results inconclusive.

VITAMIN E

Vitamin E is a powerful antioxidant and free radical scavenger that shows great potential for use in multiple sclerosis owing to its neuroprotective effects.[378] When administered to animals, vitamin E has been shown to increase endogenous remyelination in the rat's hippocampus[453], suggesting it may exert the same effects in humans. Decreased quantities of vitamin E have been observed in the plaques of demyelination of brains of those with multiple sclerosis[454] and in a study analysing blood lipids, homocysteine, stress factors and vitamins in clinically stable multiple sclerosis patients, decreased concentrations of vitamin E were found in individuals with multiple sclerosis.[455] These results signifying that reserves of vitamin E may have been used up to counterbalance the neurodegeneration associated with multiple sclerosis and supplementation may be of benefit.

ZINC

Zinc levels in subjects with multiple sclerosis have been conflicting, with some studies revealing low serum levels of zinc in individuals with multiple sclerosis compared with healthy subjects[456] while others show high levels or even no difference. A recent meta-analysis reports a significant reduction in overall serum or plasma zinc levels in patients with MS.[457] Mixed results from studies might be due to differences in age, gender, disease subtype and duration of the disease. Zinc plays a crucial role in numerous enzymatic reactions within the body. Matrix metalloproteinases are a group of proteases which are dependent on zinc for their proteolytic activity. They are involved in modifying cell–matrix interactions and remodelling of the extracellular matrix. Their proteolytic substrates include myelin basic protein, components of the blood–brain barrier, and neural/glial antigen 2, important for proper myelinisation in the CNS. This is a potentially important role in both the pathogenesis of MS, as well as in the development of new treatments.[457] Zinc's role in regulation of the immune system as well as its antioxidant activity (where it may help protect against lipid peroxidation) is also likely to be of use in patients with multiple sclerosis who present with inadequate zinc levels. A randomised controlled trial of zinc sulphate supplementation (220 mg containing 50 mg elemental zinc) in MS patients ($n = 43$) found that depression was reduced compared to placebo, but there was no improvement in neurological signs.[458]

Dosage requirements

The dosage requirements listed below are based on adult doses that have been reported in the literature.

- 5-HTP: 50–150 mg/day
- B complex (all B vitamins) high-dose combination, preferably activated forms
  - Thiamine 20–40 mg/day
  - Riboflavin 20–40 mg/day
  - Niacinamide 50–100 mg/day
  - Pantothenic acid 150–300 mg/day
  - Pyridoxine 50–100 mg/day
  - Folate as folinic acid or L5MTHF (as indicated) 500–1000 micrograms/day
    - > Higher doses may be applicable pending testing and genetic screening
  - Hydroxocobalamin or methylcobalamin 500–1000 micrograms/day
    - > Extra vitamin B_{12} is often warranted at doses greater than 2000 micrograms/day (deficiency assessment dependent)
  - Choline 50–100 mg/day
  - Inositol 50–100 mg/day
  - Biotin 250–500 micrograms/day
- Coenzyme Q10: 200–600 mg/day
- Essential fatty acids
  - DHA: 1.9 g/day
  - EPA: 3 g/day
- Magnesium: 400–1000 mg/day
- Selenium: 200–400 micrograms/day
- Vitamin A: 5000 IU/day or beta-carotene: 25 000 IU/day
- Vitamin C: 500–1000 mg 3 times a day
- Vitamin D_3: 1000–10 000 IU/day (pathology results dependent)
  - Higher doses require careful monitoring and are only indicated for short term or for those with genetic issues for vitamin D processing
- Vitamin E: 400–500 IU twice a day
- Zinc: 40–80 mg/day based on plasma levels

HERBAL MEDICINE

The therapeutic objectives and relevant classes of herbal medicine are outlined in Table 22.37.

TABLE 22.37 Herbal medicine therapeutic objectives and relevant classes

Objective	Herbal medicine class
Reduce degeneration	Nervine tonic Nervine trophorestorative
Modulate immune response, eradicate infection if present	Immune enhancer (infective organism specific) Immunomodulator
Restore nervous system function and integrity	Nervine tonic Nervine trophorestorative
Restore natural stress response	Adaptogen Adrenal restorative Nervine tonic Nervine trophorestorative Sedative (if indicated)
Reduce oxidation, free radical damage and production	Antioxidant
Restore GIT integrity and function	Mucous membrane trophorestorative Astringent Bitter Vulnerary/demulcent Antacid
Eliminate allergies (if present)	Anti-allergic GIT restoration
General body tonification	Tonic (organ specific and general)

Specific herbal medicines

GINKGO BILOBA (GINKGO)

Ginkgo biloba is one of the oldest living tree species in the world and has been used since antiquity. It contains a range of constituents including flavonoids, terpenoids and the terpene lactones, ginkgolides and bilobalide. The majority of research undertaken has used a specific *Ginkgo biloba* extract known as EGb 761, which is produced from the ground-up leaves and contains 24% w/w (weight of active compound/total weight of extract) flavone glycosides and 6% w/w terpenelactones.[459]

Ginkgo exerts a range of actions[460] which may be of use in multiple sclerosis including:

- Antioxidant activity
- Antiplatelet-activating factor properties
- Enhancement of blood flow including cerebral
- Potentiates neurotransmitter activity
- Modulation of cerebrovascular tone and glucose metabolism.

A double-blind, placebo-controlled parallel pilot study undertaken by Johnson et al[460] investigating the use of *Ginkgo biloba* extract (EGb 761) 240 mg/day for 1 month in individuals with multiple sclerosis observed an improvement in functional parameters (e.g. fatigue) when compared with placebo.

Owing to the small study group and short duration of the study, preliminary results, though promising, clearly indicate that further studies are warranted. Cognitive impairment is a commonly noted symptom. *Ginkgo biloba* has proved useful in a number of conditions related to cognitive impairment, hence it has also been examined with regards to its role in improving cognitive function in individuals with multiple sclerosis. Though overall statistical significance was not displayed in a randomised, double-blind, placebo-controlled trial by Lovera et al[461] which examined the effects of *Ginkgo biloba* 120 mg twice a day for 12 weeks in improving cognitive function in patients with multiple sclerosis, treatment effect was seen in one neurophysical test suggesting it may improve some aspects of mental flexibility.[461] For this particular study a longer treatment period may have been more efficacious. In a larger follow-up trial 5 years later ($n = 120$), 120 mg treatment twice a day for 12 weeks was found to have no benefit in improving cognitive performance in people with MS.[462] An 8-week open-label trial ($n = 30$) using *Ginkgo biloba* 240 mg/day (in 3 divided doses) showed that MS patients had significant improvement on the Weschler memory test after treatment.[463]

PANAX GINSENG (KOREAN GINSENG)

Experimental and in-vivo studies suggest that constituents within *Panax ginseng* known as the ginsenosides exert significant neuroprotective[464] and neurotrophic effects as well as the ability to indirectly promote neuroregeneration by stimulating endothelial growth and angiogenesis.[465] The ginsenosides have been found to prevent neuronal loss and axonal degeneration by protecting against factors such as free radicals, environmental toxins, excitotoxic action of glutamate[466] and rises in intracellular calcium, all of which may promote neuronal cell death.[464] Aside from its neuroprotective effects, *Panax ginseng* may also be used as a general tonic and adaptogen for adaption to stress and to assist with complaints of fatigue by patients with multiple sclerosis. A trial of 60 female patients with MS treated with *Panax ginseng* (250 mg tablets, twice daily) for 3 months showed a significant improvement in fatigue and quality of life.[467] Further larger scale trials are needed.

VITIS VINIFERA (GRAPESEED EXTRACT)

Much of the literature reviewed alludes to the fact that the excessive generation of reactive oxygen species and subsequent oxidative damage that ensues plays a key role in the neuropathology of multiple sclerosis.[375,468,469] Due to the pathogenic role of free radicals, antioxidants that help to prevent inflammation and damage to the neuronal structures are highly indicated to minimise disease progression. *Vitis vinifera*, also known as grapeseed extract, contains a range of pharmacological actions including widespread anti-inflammatory, antioxidant and neuroprotective[470] ability. Evidence for the effects of *Vitis vinifera* as a whole is extensive. However, there is a lack of information pertaining specifically to multiple sclerosis. Nevertheless, acknowledging the significant antioxidant and neuroprotective effects, from experimental models involving other neurological conditions such as stroke[471] and Parkinson's disease,[472] it is likely to be extremely beneficial. Further research in human clinical studies is recommended.

ROSMARINUS OFFICINALIS (ROSEMARY)

Rosmarinus officinalis is an aromatic shrub that has been used medicinally for centuries for its tonic effects. *Rosmarinus officinalis* contains a range of constituents including the neuroprotective agent carnosic acid. Carnosic acid may be of use in multiple sclerosis due to its antioxidant action[473] and subsequent ability to protect neurons against excitotoxicity and free radical mediated damage the latter of which is thought to contribute to the pathogenesis of multiple sclerosis. Carnosic acid has been found to protect dopaminergic neuronal cells by enhancing brain-derived neurotrophic factor and repressing apoptotic molecules.[474] Aside from this antioxidant action, *Rosmarinus officinalis* may also be of use for its mild antidepressant[475] action. Depression is commonly seen in multiple sclerosis, as is impaired cognitive function, with estimates that up to 65% of individuals with MS may experience alterations in such things as learning/memory, processing speed and working memory.[476]

CURCUMA LONGA (TURMERIC)

The pigment that gives curry powder its characteristic yellow colour may also be of use in helping to manage multiple sclerosis. Curcumin, the active constituent within Ayurvedic botanical *Curcuma longa*, has been shown to exhibit anti-inflammatory, antioxidant and anti-protein-aggregate properties leading to its reputation as a neuroprotective agent.[477] So powerful is this yellow spice that in-vivo studies reveal its ability to stimulate adult neurogenesis.[478] Multiple sclerosis is characterised by inflammation of the central nervous system; IL-17-producing T-cells have been identified as playing a dominant role in the pathogenesis of multiple sclerosis and more recently the Th17 cells have been implicated for their pro-inflammatory role in multiple sclerosis. However, *Curcuma longa* may play a role in correcting this. As yet the majority of published research is limited to animal studies but findings demonstrate that when curcumin is administered to experimental autoimmune encephalomyelitis (EAE, an animal mode of multiple sclerosis), it blocks IL-6 and IL-21 activated STAT3 signal pathway, inhibiting the proliferation and differentiation of Th17 cells in EAE, suggesting a beneficial role in multiple sclerosis.[479,480,481] Curcumin protects axons from NO-mediated degeneration. Local exposure of axons to inflammatory mediators causes axon degeneration, and curcumin protects axons from local inflammation, suggesting a potential therapeutic role for curcumin in axon protection in MS.[482] As yet research is in its early stages; whether these results can be replicated in human clinical studies remains to be seen but it is not unreasonable to think that an early blockade of inflammatory processes by *Curcuma longa* may subsequently delay disability progression.

POLYGALA TENUIFOLIA (YUAN ZHI)

Polygala tenuifolia is a Traditional Chinese Medicine that displays favourable effects upon the central nervous system. *Polygala tenuifolia* has shown neuroprotective effects against serum deficiency and glutamate in experimental studies while in-vivo studies reveal it to exert an antidepressant-like activity in chronically mildly stressed rats possibly due to modulation of the HPO axis.[483] If the same action can be reproduced in human clinical studies it shows potential for assisting with depression, a common symptom in patients with multiple sclerosis. Human studies reveal the ability of *Polygala tenuifolia* to enhance cognition in elderly subjects[484] as well as healthy adults[485] thus this botanical appears to have a wide range of actions that would appear to benefit the neurological system. As yet there have been no studies undertaken specifically in multiple sclerosis; however, it certainly appears to be a promising herb to monitor in the future.

CAMELLIA SINENSIS (GREEN TEA)

Concomitant use of immunomodulatory and neuroprotective agents has been suggested to reduce inflammation and neurodegeneration to target autoimmune demyelination[486] such as in multiple sclerosis; epigallocatechin-3-gallate, a constituent within *Camellia sinensis,* has been shown to do this. Extracts of *Camellia sinensis* have enjoyed a steady rise in popularity in the West due to their potential health benefits; however, *Camellia sinensis* has been used medicinally in China for centuries. In animal studies epigallocatechin-3-gallate reveals itself to be a neuroprotective and anti-inflammatory antioxidant suppressing experimental autoimmune encephalomyelitis (a condition similar to multiple sclerosis) and directly blocking the formation of neurotoxic reactive oxygen species in neurons.[487] As well as suppressing activity of experimental autoimmune encephalomyelitis, epigallocatechin-3-gallate also limits its severity, reducing inflammation and neuronal damage when given at initiation or after the onset of experimental autoimmune encephalomyelitis. Future studies are welcomed to see if these results can be transferred to humans. However, if so, constituents from within *Camellia sinensis* such as epigallocatechin-3-gallate certainly appear to be potential candidates to protect against neuronal injury and destruction of the myelin sheaths that surround the axons of the central nervous system.

LIFESTYLE RECOMMENDATIONS

Temperature control

Heat sensitivity is a commonly associated symptom experienced by those with multiple sclerosis[488] and causes sufferers much anguish:

> *[The humidity] kills me. It saps whatever energy is there to begin with. It makes my muscles feel heavier. It makes me feel sluggish, groggy... It is one of the few things that I can count on as creating some cognitive symptoms as well.*[489]

Adequate means must be taken to ensure the body's thermoregulatory centre is kept in balance. This may include wearing cooling garments, ensuring surroundings provide enough ventilation as well as using cool compresses, fans and the like. Care must be taken to avoid hot situations such as a day outside in the sun; even a hot bath though initially relaxing may cause fatigue in some individuals.

Meditation and relaxation

Many individuals with multiple sclerosis find meditation a useful means of self-care to help manage their symptoms.[490] Meditation not only provides a relaxing experience for many, participants also report that it may help relieve specific physical symptoms assisting with better sleep, muscle tension[490] and reducing fatigue.[491] Psychologically, meditation may also promote a better sense of wellbeing and help control the frustration associated with the disease. There is a wide range of literature available on meditation in local bookstores as well as libraries. Alternatively, guided meditation CDs can be recommended by the practitioner and many local community colleges run casual meditation classes.

Exercise

Exercise forms an important part of management of multiple sclerosis not only for symptomatic improvement but also for psychological wellbeing. Results from meta-analysis studies demonstrate improved walking mobility,[492] improved quality of life[493] and a range of other physical and mental benefits such as enhanced mood,[494] hence it is imperative that regular exercise be implemented. A 2015 Cochrane review investigating exercise for fatigue in MS concluded that exercise therapy can be prescribed in MS patients without harm. Exercise therapy, particularly endurance or mixed training, may reduce self-reported fatigue.[495]

Exercise programs should be undertaken with a trained healthcare professional with relevant qualifications in putting together specialised exercise programs, such as an exercise physiologist.

Stress management

Though controversial, there is a large body of evidence suggesting a link between high levels of stress and exacerbations of multiple sclerosis,[383,496] hence stress management is imperative. Patients may be questioned on whether they believe that stressful life events cause exacerbations of their illness, on their major sources of stress, how they deal with stress, what they do to relax and how often they actually implement stress management and relaxation strategies. Accordingly, a stress management plan needs to be set out so that patients can develop the necessary skills required to cope with stressful events. In saying this, it is acknowledged of course that not all exacerbations of illness will be caused by stress, hence patients should not feel guilty and personally responsible if they experience an exacerbation in disease.

Memory rehabilitation

Impairments in cognitive function, particularly memory, are common in MS patients and can potentially affect the patient's ability to complete functional activities. A 2016 Cochrane review concluded that there is some evidence to support the effectiveness of memory rehabilitation on memory function as well as quality of life.[497]

CASE STUDY

OVERVIEW

AP, a 25-year-old female, presented with a recent diagnosis of MS (confirmed by specialist). Her aunt and grandmother also suffered from the condition. On review, initiation of an appointment to ascertain diagnosis was due to recent episodes of diplopia, fatigue and muscle weakness in her left hand and arm. This had concerned her especially as she was a pianist in an orchestra and was finding it difficult to sustain her job. Following diagnosis, AP decided to cease performances and focus on music tuition. Her energy levels were still positive but she was concerned about increasing fatigue similar to her family members suffering from MS.

History revealed a previous Epstein-Barr infection when she was 13 years of age. She felt her recovery was poor and has never felt well since with frequent colds and flus most years. Her diet consisted of minimal protein, high intake of artificial sweeteners in the form of chewing gum and Diet Coke, 2–4 cups of coffee per day and frequent skipping of meals.

As her diagnosis was recent, she chose to wait to begin interferon-beta preparations to assess the impact of naturopathic treatment initially. While discussed in detail, the patient's personal choice was respected.

Blood testing revealed:

- Vitamin D: 19 nmol/L
- Vitamin B_{12}: 102 pmol/L
- Folate (red cell): 375 nmol/L
- FBC: Hb: 110 g/L,
- Iron studies: NAD
- Coeliac screen: negative.

CASE STUDY CONTINUED

PHYSICAL EXAMINATION

- Tone: Weakened tone in lower limbs
- Power: Reduced coordination of arms
- Sensation: Reduced vibratory sensation
- Reflexes: Absent abdominal reflex, hyperactive tendon reflex
- Neck: Positive Lhermitte's sign.

TREATMENT PROTOCOL

Treatment protocol focused on:

- Addressing historical infection and modulating immune response to halt disease progression
- Modifying dietary intake to improve nutritional status
- Addressing nutritional deficiencies
- Reducing MS symptomatology and improving tone, power, sensation and reflexes in musculoskeletal system.

HERBAL MEDICINE

Herbal medicine	Ratio	Quantity	Rationale
Ginkgo biloba	STD ext	50 mL	Antioxidant, antiplatelet activator, cerebral blood flow enhancement, circulatory stimulant
Rosemary officinalis	1:2	40 mL	Neuroprotective, antioxidant, mild antidepressant, cognitive support
Rehmannia glutinosa	1:2	60 mL	Adaptogen, immune modulation
Andrographis panniculata	1:2	70 mL	Adaptogen, immune modulating
TOTAL: 220 mL			

Dose: 7.5 mL twice a day

NUTRITIONAL MEDICINE

Dietary

- 1 tspn organic turmeric daily in yoghurt
- Avoidance of all artificial sweeteners and sugar
- Avoidance of all caffeine and other stimulants
- Encourage cold-pressed, fresh and organic pure oils such as flaxseed, olive, sunflower, safflower oil
- Avoid all sources of hydrogenated, rancid or poor-quality oils
- General Swank diet principles
- Follow naturopathic wholefood principles that encourage organic vegetarian (or pesco-vegetarian) principles
- Encourage dietary antioxidant sources such as organic fruits and vegetables.

CASE STUDY CONTINUED

Supplemental

- Vitamin D: 5000 IU/day
- Vitamin B_{12}: 1000 micrograms sublingually twice a day
- B complex (high potency, activated): 2 capsules/day
- Concentrated fish oil supplementation: 1 capsule twice a day (EPA: 650 mg, DHA: 450 mg, Other omega-3s: 180 mg)
- Selenium: 250 micrograms/day
- Coenzyme Q10: 300 mg/day
- Zinc: 60 mq/day
- Vitamin E: 500 IU twice a day.

LIFESTYLE/EDUCATION

- Meditation and relaxation
- Temperature control
- Daily exercise (gentle)
- Stress management.

REFERRAL

- Counselling due to diagnosis.

REFERENCES

[1] Tortora G, Grabowski S. Principles of anatomy and physiology. Biological sciences textbooks. 9th ed. New York: John Wiley; 2000.
[2] Ottersen OP, Mathisen JS. Handbook of clinical neuroanatomy-glutamate. New York: Elsevier; 2000.
[3] Osiecki H, Meeke F, Smith J. The encyclopaedia of clinical nutrition — the nervous system. Eagle Farm, QLD: Bioconcepts Publishing; 2004. p. 269.
[4] Schachter S. Botanicals and herb: a traditional approach to treating epilepsy. Neurother 2009;6(2):415–20.
[5] A history of the nervous system. Available from: www.stanford.edu/class/history13/earlysciencelab/body/nervespages/nerves.html.
[6] Ellingwood F. American materia medica, therapeutics and pharmacognosy. Portland, OR: Eclectic Medical Publications; 1983. (reprint of 1919 original).
[7 and 8] Thomas R. The eclectic practice of medicine. Portland OR: Eclectic Medical Publications; (reprint of 1907 original).
[9] Felter HW. The Eclectic materia medica, pharmacology and therapeutics. Eclectic Materia Medica Publications; 1922.
[10] Buchwald D, Umali P, Umali J, et al. Chronic fatigue and the chronic fatigue syndrome: prevalence in a Pacific Northwest health care system. Ann Intern Med 1995;123:81–8.
[11] Lawrie SM, Manders DN, Geddes JR, et al. A population-based incidence study of chronic fatigue. Psychol Med 1997;27:343–53.
[12] Lloyd AR, Hickie I, Boughton CR, et al. Prevalence of chronic fatigue syndrome in an Australian population. Med J Aust 1990;153:522–8.
[13] Jason LA, Wagner L, Rosenthal S, et al. Estimating the prevalence of chronic fatigue syndrome among nurses. Am J Med 1998;105:S91–3.
[14] Centers for Disease Control and Prevention. ME/CFS in children. Available from: www.cdc.gov/me-cfs/me-cfs-children/index.html.
[15] Jones TF, Ray CG, Minnich LL, et al. Evidence for active Epstein-Barr virus infection in patients with persistent, unexplained illnesses: elevated anti-early antigen antibodies. Ann Intern Med 1985;102(1):1–7.
[16] Cleare AJ, Wesseley S. Chronic fatigue syndrome. In: Encyclopedia of stress. 2nd ed. Oxford: Elsevier; 2007. p. 484–93.
[17] Hickie I, Lloyd A, Hadzi-Pavlovic D, et al. Can the chronic fatigue syndrome be defined by distinct clinical features? Psychol Med 1995;25:925–35.
[18] Horowitz S. Chronic fatigue syndrome: case definitions, possible causes, and therapies. Altern Complement Ther 2015;21(5):217–23.
[19] Glassford JA. The neuroinflammatory etiopathology of myalgic encephalomyelitis/chronic fatigue syndrome (ME/CFS). Front Physiol 2017;8:88.
[20] Morris G, Berk M, Galecki P, et al. The emerging role of autoimmunity in myalgic encephalomyelitis/chronic fatigue syndrome (ME/CFs). Mol Neurobiol 2014;49(2):741–56.
[21] Naess H, Nyland M, Hausken T, et al. Chronic fatigue syndrome after Giardia enteritis: clinical characteristics, disability and long-term sickness absence. BMC Gastroenterol 2012;12(1):13.
[22] Bansal AS, Bradley AS, Bishop KN, et al. Chronic fatigue syndrome, the immune system and viral infection. Brain Behav Immun 2012;26(1):24–31.
[23] Brewer JH, Thrasher JD, Straus DC, et al. Detection of mycotoxins in patients with chronic fatigue syndrome. Toxins (Basel) 2013;5(4):605–17.
[24] Broderick G, Fuite J, Kreitz A, et al. A formal analysis of cytokine networks in chronic fatigue syndrome. Brain Behav Immun 2010;24(7):1209–17.
[25] Maquet D, Demoulin C, Crielaard JM. Chronic fatigue syndrome: a systematic review. Ann Med Phys (Lille) 2006;49(6):418–27.
[26] Landi A, Broadhurst D, Vernon SD, et al. Reductions in circulating levels of IL-16, IL-7 and VEGF-A in myalgic encephalomyelitis/chronic fatigue syndrome. Cytokine 2016;78:27–36.
[27] Dietert RR, Dietert JM. Possible role for early life immune insult including developmental immunotoxicity in chronic fatigue syndrome (CFS) or myalgic encephalomyelitis (ME). Toxicology 2008;247(1):61–72.
[28] Bellmann-Weiler R, Schroecksnadel K, Larcher C, et al. IFN-gamma mediated pathways in patients with fatigue and chronic active Epstein-Barr virus-infection. J Affect Disord 2008;108(1–2):171–6.
[29] Nijs J, Nees A, Paul L, et al. Altered immune response to exercise in patients with chronic fatigue syndrome/myalgic encephalomyelitis: a systematic literature review. Exerc Immunol Rev 2014;20:94–116.
[30] Hornig M, Montoya JG, Klimas NG, et al. Distinct plasma immune signatures in ME/CFS are present early in the course of illness. Sci Adv 2015;1(1):e1400121.
[31] Cleare AJ. The neuroendocrinology of chronic fatigue syndrome. Endocr Rev 2003;2:236–52.
[32] Scott LV, Svec F, Dinan T. A preliminary study of dehydroepiandrosterone response to low-dose ACTH in chronic fatigue syndrome and in healthy subjects. Psychiatry Res 2000;97:21–8.
[33] Kuratsune H, Yamaguti K, Sawada M, et al. Dehydroepiandrosterone sulfate deficiency in chronic fatigue syndrome. Int J Mol Med 1998;1:143–6.
[34] Cauwenbergh D, Nijs J, Kos D, et al. Malfunctioning of the autonomic nervous system in patients with chronic fatigue syndrome: a systematic literature review. Eur J Clin Invest 2014;44(5):516–26.
[35] DeLuca J, Johnson SK, Beldowicz D, et al. Neuropsychological impairments in chronic fatigue syndrome, multiple sclerosis, and depression. J Neurol Neurosurg Psych 1995;58:38–43.
[36] Michiels V, Cluydts R. Neuropsychological functioning in chronic fatigue syndrome: a review. Acta Psychiatr Scand 2001;103:84–93.
[37] Wessely S, Chalder T, Hirsch S, et al. Psychological symptoms, somatic symptoms, and psychiatric disorder in chronic fatigue and chronic fatigue syndrome: a prospective study in the primary care setting. Am J Psychiatry 1996;153:1050–9.
[38] Buchwald D, Herrell R, Ashton S, et al. A twin study of chronic fatigue. Psychosom Med 2001;63:936–43.
[39] Manu P, Matthews DA, Lane TJ. Food intolerance in patients with chronic fatigue. Int J Eat Disord 1993;13(2):203–9.
[40] Rowe PC, Marden CL, Jasion SE, et al. Cow's milk protein intolerance in adolescents and young adults with chronic fatigue syndrome. Acta Paediatr 2016;105(9).
[41] Chester AC, Levine PH. The natural history of concurrent sick building syndrome and chronic fatigue syndrome. J Psychiatr Res 1997;31:51–7.
[42] Kilshaw S. Gulf War syndrome. Psychiatry 2004;3(8):17–20.
[43] Kilburn KH. Symptoms, syndrome, and semantics: multiple chemical sensitivity and chronic fatigue syndrome. Arch Environ Health 1993;48:368–9.

[44] Pacini S, Fiore MG, Magherini S, et al. Could cadmium be responsible for some of the neurological signs and symptoms of myalgic encephalomyelitis/chronic fatigue syndrome. Med Hypotheses 2012;79(3):403–37.
[45] Pall ML. Common aetiology of posttraumatic stress disorder, fibromyalgia, chronic fatigue syndrome and multiple chemical sensitivity syndrome via elevated nitric oxide/peroxynitrite. Med Hypotheses 2001;57(2):139–45.
[46] Rutherford G, Manning P, Newton JL. Understanding muscle dysfunction in chronic fatigue syndrome. J Aging Res 2016;2016:2497348.
[47] Daniel V, Huber W, Bauer K, et al. Associations of blood levels of PCB, HCHs, and HCB with numbers of lymphocyte subpopulations, in vitro lymphocyte response, plasma cytokine levels and immunoglobulin antibodies. Environ Health Perspec 2001; 109(2).
[48] Fukuda K, Straus SE, Hickie I, et al. The chronic fatigue syndrome: a comprehensive approach to its definition and study. International Chronic Fatigue Syndrome Study Group. Ann Intern Med 1994;121:953–9.
[49] Kennedy G, Abbot NC, Spence V, et al. The specificity of the CDC-1994 criteria for chronic fatigue syndrome: comparison of health status in three groups of patients who fulfil the criteria. Ann Epidemiol 2004;14:95–100.
[50] Wilson A, Hickie I, Hadzi-Pavlovic D, et al. What is chronic fatigue syndrome? Heterogeneity within an international multicentre study. Aust N Z J Psychiatry 2001;35:520–7.
[51] Beyond myalgic encephalomyelitis/chronic fatigue syndrome: redefining an illness. Committee on the Diagnostic Criteria for Myalgic Encephalomyelitis/Chronic Fatigue Syndrome; Board on the Health of Select Populations; Institute of Medicine. Washington (DC): National Academies Press (US); 2015.
[52] Lloyd AR, Hickie IB, Loblay RH. Illness or disease? The case of chronic fatigue syndrome. Med J Aust 2000;172:471–2.
[53] Kasper DL, Braunwald E, Fauci AS, et al, editors. Harrison's principles of internal medicine. 16th ed. Part XV Neurologic disorders; chronic fatigue syndrome. New York: McGraw-Hill; 2005. p. 2545–7.
[54] Pizzorno J, Murray M. Textbook of natural medicine. 3rd edn. Oxford: Elsevier, pp. 1579–1580.
[55] Shepherd C. Chronic fatigue syndrome. Lancet 1997;349(9044):57–8.
[56] David A, Wessely S. Chronic fatigue, ME and ICD-10. Lancet 1993;342:1247–8.
[57] Chu L, Norris JL, Valencia IJ, et al. Patients diagnosed with myalgic encephalomyelitis/chronic fatigue syndrome also fit systemic exertion intolerance disease criteria. Fatigue 2017;5(2):114–28.
[58] Band R, Wearden A, Barrowclough C. Patient outcomes in association with significant other responses to chronic fatigue syndrome: a systematic review of the literature. Clin Psychol: Sci Pract 2015;22(1):29–46.
[59] Roberts E, Wessely S, Chalder T, et al. Mortality of people with chronic fatigue syndrome: a retrospective cohort study in England and Wales from the South London and Maudsley NHS Foundation Trust Biomedical Research Centre (SLaM BRC) Clinical Record Interactive Search (CRIS) Register. Lancet 2016;387(10028):1638–43.
[60] Broderick G, Fuite J, Kreitz A, et al. A formal analysis of cytokine networks in chronic fatigue syndrome. Brain Behav Immun 2010;24(7):1209–17.
[61] Jason LA, Corradi K, Gress S, et al. Causes of death among patients with chronic fatigue syndrome. Health Care Women Int 2006;27:615–26.
[62] Harlow BL, Signorello LB. Reproductive correlates of chronic fatigue syndrome. Am J Med 1998;108:S94–9.
[63] Wessely S, Nimnuan C, Sharpe M. Functional somatic syndromes: one or many? Lancet 1999;354:936–9.
[64] Allen PR. Chronic fatigue syndrome: implications for women and their health care providers during the childbearing years. J Midwif Womens Health 2008;53(4):289–301.
[65] Cairns R, Hotopf M. A systematic review describing the prognosis of chronic fatigue syndrome. Occup Med (Lond) 2005;55:20–31.
[66] Wearden AJ, Dunn G, Dowrick C, et al. Depressive symptoms and pragmatic rehabilitation for chronic fatigue syndrome. Br J Psychiatry 2012;201(3):227–32.
[67] Mitchell WM. Efficacy of rintatolimod in the treatment of chronic fatigue syndrome/myalgic encephalomyelitis (CFS/ME). Expert Rev Clin Pharmacol 2016;9(6):755–70.
[68] Larun L, Brurberg KG, Odgaard-Jensen J, et al. Exercise therapy for chronic fatigue syndrome. Cochrane Database Syst Rev 2016;(2):CD003200.
[69] Kindlon T. Do graded activity therapies cause harm in chronic fatigue syndrome? J Health Psychol 2017;22(9):1146–54.
[70] Chan JS, Ho RT, Chung KF, et al. Qigong exercise alleviates fatigue, anxiety, and depressive symptoms, improves sleep quality, and shortens sleep latency in persons with chronic fatigue syndrome-like illness. Evid Based Complement Alternat Med 2014;2014:106048.
[71] Tanaka M, Watanabe Y. A new hypothesis of chronic fatigue syndrome: Co-conditioning theory. Med Hypotheses 2010;75(2):244–9.
[72] Roberts AD, Papadopoulos AS, Wessely S, et al. Salivary cortisol output before and after cognitive behavioural therapy for chronic fatigue syndrome. J Affect Disord 2009;115(1–2):280–6.
[73] Wiborg JF, van Bussel J, van Dijk A, et al. Randomised controlled trial of cognitive behaviour therapy delivered in groups of patients with chronic fatigue syndrome. Psychother Psychosom 2015;84(6):368–76.
[74] Straus S. History of chronic fatigue syndrome reviews of infectious diseases. Considerations in the design of studies of chronic fatigue syndrome 1991;13(Suppl. 1):S2–S7.
[75] Felter HW, Lloyd F. King's American dispensatory. Eclectic Materia Medica Publications; 1898.
[76] Giloteaux L, Goodrich JK, Walters WA, et al. Reduced diversity and altered composition of the gut microbiome in individuals with myalgic encephalomyelitis/chronic fatigue syndrome. Microbiome 2016;4(1):30.
[77] Giloteaux L, Hanson MR, Keller BA. A pair of identical twins discordant for myalgic encephalomyelitis/chronic fatigue syndrome differ in physiological parameters and gut microbiome composition. Am J Case Rep 2016;17:720.
[78] Maes M, Twisk FN, Kubera M, et al. Increased IgA responses to the LPS of commensal bacteria is associated with inflammation and activation of cell-mediated immunity in chronic fatigue syndrome. J Affect Disord 2012;136(3):909–17.
[79] Woolley J, Allen R, Wessely S. Alcohol use in chronic fatigue syndrome. J Psychosom Res 2004;56(2):203–6.
[80] Humphries P, Pretorius E, Naudé H. Direct and indirect cellular effects of aspartame on the brain. Eur J Clin Nutr 2008;62(4):451–62.
[81] Logan AC, Wong C. Chronic fatigue syndrome: oxidative stress and dietary modifications. Altern Med Rev 2001;6(5):450–9.
[82] Werbach MR. Nutritional strategies for treating chronic fatigue syndrome. Altern Med Rev 2000;5(2):93–108.
[83] Heap LC, Peters TJ, Wessely S. Vitamin B status in patients with chronic fatigue syndrome. J R Soc Med 1999;92(4):183–5.
[84] Lundell K, Qazi S, Eddy L, et al. Clinical activity of folinic acid in patients with chronic fatigue syndrome (Abstract only). Arzneimittelforschung 2006;56(6):399–404.
[85] Regland B, Forsmark S, Halaouate L, et al. Response to vitamin B12 and folic acid in myalgic encephalomyelitis and fibromyalgia. PLoS ONE 2015;10(4):e0124648.
[86] Avellaneda FA, Pérez MA, Izquierdo MM, et al. Chronic fatigue syndrome: aetiology, diagnosis and treatment BMC. Psychiatry 2009;(9 Suppl. 1):S1.
[87] Bates DW, Buchwald D, Lee J, et al. Clinical laboratory test findings in patients with chronic fatigue syndrome. Arch Intern Med 1995;155:97–103.
[88] Kodama M, Kodama T. Four problems with the clinical control of interstitial pneumonia, or chronic fatigue syndrome, using the megadose vitamin C infusion system with dehydroepiandrosterone-cortisol annex. Vivo 2006;20(2): 285–91.
[89] Miwa K, Fujita M. Increased oxidative stress suggested by low serum vitamin E concentrations in patients with chronic fatigue syndrome. Int J Cardiol 2009;136(2):238–9.
[90] Cox IM, Campbell MJ, Dowson D. Red blood cell magnesium and chronic fatigue syndrome. Lancet 1991;337:757–60.
[91] Morris G, Anderson G, Dean O, et al. The glutathione system: a new drug target in neuroimmune disorders. Mol Neurobiol 2014;50(3):1059–84.

[92] Kuratsune H, Yamaguti K, Takahashi M, et al. Acylcarnitine deficiency in chronic fatigue syndrome. Clin Infect Dis 1994;18(Suppl. 1):S62–7.
[93] Kuratsune H, Yamaguti K, Lindh G, et al. Low levels of serum acylcarnitine in chronic fatigue syndrome and chronic hepatitis type C, but not seen in other diseases (Abstract only). Int J Mol Med 1998;2(1):51–6.
[94] Plioplys AV, Plioplys S. Serum levels of carnitine in chronic fatigue syndrome: clinical correlates. Neuropsychobiology 1995;32(3):132–8.
[95] Soetekouw PM, Wevers RA, Vreken P, et al. Normal carnitine levels in patients with chronic fatigue syndrome. Neth J Med 2000;57(1):20–4.
[96] Vermeulen RC, Scholte HR. Exploratory open label, randomized study of acetyl- and propionylcarnitine in chronic fatigue syndrome. Psychosom Med 2004;66(2):276–82.
[97] Tamizi far B, Tamizi B. Treatment of chronic fatigue syndrome by dietary supplementation with omega-3 fatty acids — a good idea? Med Hypotheses 2002;58(3):249–50.
[98] Puri BK. Long-chain polyunsaturated fatty acids and the pathophysiology of myalgic encephalomyelitis (chronic fatigue syndrome). J Clin Pathol 2007;60(2):122–4.
[99] Behan PO, Behan WM, Horrobin D. Effect of high doses of essential fatty acids on the postviral fatigue syndrome. Acta Neurol Scand 1990;82(3):209–16.
[100] Warren G, McKendrick M, Peet M. The role of essential fatty acids in chronic fatigue syndrome. A case-controlled study of red-cell membrane essential fatty acids (EFA) and a placebo-controlled treatment study with high dose of EFA. Acta Neurol Scand 1999;99(2):112–16.
[101] Puri BK. The use of eicosapentaenoic acid in the treatment of chronic fatigue syndrome. Prostaglandins Leukot Essent Fatty Acids 2004;70(4):399–401.
[102 and 103] Maes M, Mihaylova I, De Ruyter M. Lower serum zinc in chronic fatigue syndrome (CFS): relationships to immune dysfunctions and relevance for the oxidative stress status in CFS. J Affect Disord 2006;90(2–3):141–147.
[104] Werbach M. Nutritional strategies for treating chronic fatigue syndrome. Altern Med Rev 2000;5(2):93–108.
[105] Fuller-Thomson E, Nimigoon J. Factors associated with depression among individuals with chronic fatigue syndrome: findings from a nationally representative survey. Fam Pract 2008;25(6):414–22.
[106] De Silva V, El-Metwally A, Ernst E, et al. Arthritis Research Campaign working group on complementary and alternative medicines. Evidence for the efficacy of complementary and alternative medicines in the management of fibromyalgia: a systematic review. Rheumatology (Oxford) 2010;49(6):1063–8.
[107] Maes M, Mihaylova I, Kubera M, et al. Coenzyme Q10 deficiency in myalgic encephalomyelitis/chronic fatigue syndrome (ME/CFS) is related to fatigue, autonomic and neurocognitive symptoms and is another risk factor explaining the early mortality in ME/CFS due to cardiovascular disorder. Neuro Endocrinol Lett 2009;30(4):470–6.
[108] Castro-Marrero J, Cordero MD, Segundo MJ, et al. Does oral coenzyme Q10 plus NADH supplementation improve fatigue and biochemical parameters in chronic fatigue syndrome? Antioxid Redox Signal 2015;22(8):679–85.
[109] Maric D, Brkic S, Mikic AN, et al. Multivitamin mineral supplementation in patients with chronic fatigue syndrome. Med Sci Monitor 2014;20:47.
[110] Hartz AJ, Bentler S, Noyes R, et al. Randomized controlled trial of Siberian ginseng for chronic fatigue. Psychol Med 2004;34:51–61.
[111] Van Den Eede F, Moorkens G, Van Houdenhove B, et al. Hypothalamic-pituitary-adrenal axis function in chronic fatigue syndrome. Neuropsychobiology 2007;55(2):112–20.
[112] Cleare AJ. The HPA axis and the genesis of chronic fatigue syndrome. Trends Endocrinol Metab 2004;15(2):55–9.
[113] Cleare AJ, Heap E, Malhi GS, et al. Low-dose hydrocortisone in chronic fatigue syndrome: a randomised crossover trial. Lancet 1999;353:455–8.
[114] See DM, Broumand N, Sahl L, et al. In vitro effects of echinacea and ginseng on natural killer and antibody-dependent cell cytotoxicity in healthy subjects and chronic fatigue syndrome or acquired immunodeficiency syndrome patients. Immunopharmacology 1997;35(3):229–35.
[115] Kim HG, Cho JH, Yoo SR, et al. Antifatigue effects of Panax ginseng CA Meyer: a randomised, double-blind, placebo-controlled trial. PLoS ONE 2013;8(4):e61271.
[116] Kuo YH, Tsai WJ, Loke SH, et al. Astragalus membranaceus flavonoids (AMF) ameliorate chronic fatigue syndrome induced by food intake restriction plus forced swimming. J Ethnopharmacol 2009;122(1):28–34.
[117] Cho JH, Cho CK, Shin JW, et al. Myelophil, an extract mix of *Astragali radix* and *Salviae radix*, ameliorates chronic fatigue: a randomised, double-blind, controlled pilot study. Comp Ther Med 2009;17(3):141–6.
[118] Olsson EMG, von Schéele B, Panossian AG. A randomized double-blind placebo controlled parallel group study of SHR-5 extract of *Rhodiola rosea* roots as treatment for patients with stress related fatigue. Planta Med 2009;75:105–12.
[119] Darbinyan V, Kteyan A, Panossian A, et al. *Rhodiola rosea* in stress induced fatigue — a double blind cross-over study of a standardized extract SHR-5 with a repeated low-dose regimen on the mental performance of healthy physicians during night duty. Phytomedicine 2000;7:365–71, 909–914.
[120] Spasov AA, Wikman GK, Mandrikov VB, et al. A double-blind, placebo-controlled pilot study of the stimulating and adaptogenic effect of *Rhodiola rosea* SHR-5 extract on the fatigue of students caused by stress during an examination period with a repeated low-dose regimen. Phytomedicine 2000;7:85–9.
[121] Darbinyan V, Aslanyan G, Amroyan E, et al. Clinical trial of *Rhodiola rosea* L. extract SHR-5 in the treatment of mild to moderate depression. Nord J Psychiatry 2007;61:2343–8.
[122] Fintelmann V, Gruenwald J. Efficacy and tolerability of a *Rhodiola rosea* extract in adults with physical and cognitive deficiencies. Adv Ther 2007;24:929–39.
[123] Lekomtseva Y, Zhukova I, Wacker A. *Rhodiola rosea* in subjects with prolonged or chronic fatigue symptoms: results of an open-label clinical trial. Complement Med Res 2017;24(1):46–52.
[124] Aoki T, Miyakoshi H, Usuda Y, et al. Low NK syndrome and its relationship to chronic fatigue syndrome. Clin Immunol Immunopathol 1993;69:253–65.
[125] Lorusso L, Mikhaylova SV, Capelli E, et al. Immunological aspects of chronic fatigue syndrome. Autoimmun Rev 2009;8(4):287–91.
[126] Lyall M, Peakman M, Wessely S. A systematic review and critical evaluation of the immunology of chronic fatigue syndrome. J Psychosom Res 2003;55:79–90.
[127] Kulkarni SK, Dhir A. *Withania somnifera*: an Indian ginseng. Prog Neuropsychopharmacol Biol Psychiatry 2008;32(5):1093–105.
[128] Singh RH, Narsimhamurthy K, Singh G. Neuronutrient impact of Ayurvedic Rasayana therapy in brain ageing. Biogerontology 2008;9(6):369–74.
[129] Singh A, Naidu PS, Gupta S, et al. Effect of natural and synthetic antioxidants in a mouse model of chronic fatigue syndrome. J Med Food 2002;5211–20.
[130] Kour K, Pandey A, Suri KA, et al. Restoration of stress-induced altered T cell function and corresponding cytokines patterns by withanolide. Int Immunopharmacol 2009;9(10):1137–44.
[131] Bhatnagar M, Sharma D, Salvi M. Neuroprotective effects of *Withania somnifera* dunal: a possible mechanism. Neurochem Res 2009;34(11):1975–83.
[132] Ax S, Gregg VH, Jones D. Coping and illness cognitions: chronic fatigue syndrome. Clin Psychol Rev 2001;21(2):161–82.
[133] Price JR, Mitchell E, Tidy E, et al. Cognitive behaviour therapy for chronic fatigue syndrome in adults. Cochrane Database Syst Rev 2008;(3):CD001027.
[134] Powell P, Bentall RP, Nye FJ, et al. Randomised controlled trial of patient education to encourage graded exercise in chronic fatigue syndrome. BMJ 2001;322:387–92.
[135] Fulcher KY, White PD. Randomised controlled trial of graded exercise in patients with the chronic fatigue syndrome. BMJ 1997;314:1647–52.
[136] Reid SF, Chalder T, Cleare A, et al. Chronic fatigue syndrome. BMJ Clin Evid 2011;2011:pii: 1101.
[137] Siemionow V, Fang Y, Calabrese L, et al. Altered central nervous signal during motor performance in chronic fatigue syndrome. Clin Neurophysiol 2004;115:2372–81.

[138] Tryon WW, Jason L, Frankenberry E, et al. Chronic fatigue syndrome impairs circadian rhythm of activity level. Physiol Behav 2004;82(5):849–53.
[139] Mathiowetz V, Matuska KM, Murphy ME. Efficacy of an energy conservation course for persons with multiple sclerosis. Arch Phys Med Rehabil 2001;82:449–56.
[140] Furst GP, Gerber LH, Smith CC, et al. A program for improving energy conservation behaviors in adults with rheumatoid arthritis. Am J Occup Ther 1987;41(2):102–11.
[141] Access Economics. Wake up Australia: the value of healthy sleep. Report to Sleep Health Australia, October 2004.
[142] Australian Bureau of Statistics (ABS). National health survey: use of medications. Canberra: ABS; 1999. Cat. no. 4377.0.
[143] Australian Bureau of Statistics (ABS). Patterns of use of mental health services and prescription medications, 2011. Canberra: ABS; 2016. Cat. no. 4329.0.00.003.
[144] Sateia MJ. International classification of sleep disorders — highlights and modifications. Chest J 2014;146(5):1387–94.
[145] Papadimitriou G, Kerkhofs M, Kempenaers C, et al. EEG sleep studies in patients with generalized anxiety disorder. Psychiatry Res 1988;26(2):183–90.
[146] Lautenbacher S, Kundermann B, Krieg JC. Sleep deprivation and pain perception. Sleep Med Rev 2006;10:357–69.
[147] Sutton DA, Moldofsky H, Badley EM. Insomnia and health problems in Canadians. Sleep 2001;24:665–70.
[148] McCracken LM, Iverson GL. Disrupted sleep patterns and daily functioning in patients with chronic pain. Pain Res Manage 2002;7:75–9.
[149] Kundermann B, Hemmeter-Spernal J, Huber MT, et al. Effects of total sleep deprivation in major depression: overnight improvement of mood is accompanied by increased pain sensitivity and augmented pain complaints. Psychosom Med 2008;70:92–101.
[150] Victor LD. Treatment of obstructive sleep apnea in primary care. Am Fam Physician 2004;69(3):561–8.
[151] Benetó A, Gomez-Siurana E, Rubio-Sanchez P. Comorbidity between sleep apnea and insomnia. Sleep Med Rev 2009;13(4):287–93.
[152] Punjabi NM. The epidemiology of adult obstructive sleep apnea. Proc Am Thorac Soc 2008;5(2):136–43.
[153] Hornyak M, Feige B, Riemann D, et al. Periodic leg movements in sleep and periodic limb movement disorder: prevalence, clinical significance and treatment. Sleep Med Rev 2006;10(3):169–77.
[154] Ohayon MM, Roth T. Prevalence of restless legs syndrome and periodic limb movement disorder in the general population. J Psychosom Res 2002;53:547–54.
[155] Wills L, Garcia J. Parasomnias: epidemiology and management. CNS Drugs 2002;16(12):803–10.
[156] Ukponmwan OE, Rupreht J, Dzoljic MR. REM sleep deprivation decreases the antinociceptive property of enkephalinase-inhibition, morphine and cold-water-swim. Gen Pharmacol 1984;15: 255–8.[157] Association of Sleep Disorders Centers. Diagnostic classification of sleep and arousal disorders. Sleep 1979;2:5–122.
[158] Diagnostic Classification Steering Committee, Thorpe JM. Chairman. International classification of sleep disorders: diagnostic and coding manual (ICSD). Rochester MN: American Sleep Disorders Association; 1990.
[159] Mai E, Buysse DJ. Insomnia: prevalence, impact, pathogenesis, differential diagnosis, and evaluation. Sleep Med Clin 2008;3(2):167–74.
[160] Chokroverty S. Overview of sleep and sleep disorders. Indian J Med Res 2010;131:126–40.
[161] Basta M, Chrousos GP, Vela-Bueno A, et al. Chronic insomnia and the stress system. Sleep Med Clin 2007;2(2):279–91.
[162] Schutte-Rodin S, Broch L, Buysse D, et al. Clinical guideline for the evaluation and management of chronic insomnia in adults. J Clin Sleep Med 2008;4:5.
[163] eTG complete Headache, Therapeutic Guidelines. November 2009.
[164] Ellingwood F. The American materia medica, therapeutics and pharmacognosy. Eclectic Materia Medica Publications; 1919.
[165] Yehuda S, Rabinovitz S, Mostovsky DI. Essential fatty acids and sleep: mini-review and hypothesis. Med Hypotheses 1998;50:139–45.
[166] Mazzotti DR, Guindalini C, Pellegrino R, et al. Effects of the adenosine deaminase polymorphism and caffeine intake on sleep parameters in a large population sample. Sleep 2011;34(3):399.
[167] Frozi J, de Carvalho HW, Ottoni GL, et al. Distinct sensitivity to caffeine-induced insomnia related to age. J Psychopharmacol 2018;32(1):89–95.
[168] Sin CW, Ho JS, Chung JW. Systematic review on the effectiveness of caffeine abstinence on the quality of sleep. J Clin Nurs 2009;18(1):13–21.
[169] Riemann R, Volk R, Müller A, et al. The influence of nocturnal alcohol ingestion on snoring. Eur Arch Otorhinolaryngol 2010;267(7):1147–56.
[170] Choudhary AK, Lee YY. Neurophysiological symptoms and aspartame: What is the connection? Nutr Neurosci 2017;1–11.
[171] Kahn A, Mozin MJ, Rebuffat E, et al. Milk intolerance in children with persistent sleeplessness: a prospective double-blind crossover evaluation. Pediatrics 1989;84(4):595–603.
[172] Kahn A, Mozin MJ, Casimir G, et al. Insomnia and cows' milk allergy in infants. Pediatrics 1985;76(6):880–4.
[173] Birdsall T. 5-Hydroxytryptophan: a clinically-effective serotonin precursor. Altern Med Rev 1998;3(4):271–80.
[174] Bruni O, Ferri R, Miano S, et al. L-5-Hydroxytryptophan treatment of sleep terrors in children. Eur J Pediatr 2004;163(7):402–7.
[175] Peuhkuri K, Sihvola N, Korpela R. Diet promotes sleep duration and quality. Nutr Res 2012;32(5):309–19.
[176] Ring M, Marchlewski A, Kaplan J. Dietary supplements for insomnia. Curr Sleep Med Rep 2017;3(4):306–15.
[177] Zisapel N. New perspectives on the role of melatonin in human sleep, circadian rhythms and their regulation. Br J Pharmacol 2018;doi:10.1111/bph.14116. [Epub ahead of print].
[178] Auld F, Maschauer EL, Morrison I, et al. Evidence for the efficacy of melatonin in the treatment of primary adult sleep disorders. Sleep Med Rev 2017;34:10–22.
[179] van Maanen A, Meijer AM, Smits MG, et al. Classical conditioning for preserving the effects of short melatonin treatment in children with delayed sleep: a pilot study. Nat Sci Sleep 2017;9:67–79.
[180] Wilson SJ, Nutt DJ, Alford C, et al. British Association for Psychopharmacology consensus statement on evidence-based treatment of insomnia, parasomnias and circadian rhythm disorders. J Psychopharmacol 2010;24(11):1577–601.
[181] Vural EM, Van Munster BC, De Rooij SE. Optimal dosages for melatonin supplementation therapy in older adults: a systematic review of current literature. Drugs Aging 2014;31(6):441–51.
[182] Williams J, Kellett J, Roach PD, et al. L-Theanine as a functional food additive: its role in disease prevention and health promotion. Beverages 2016;2(2):13.
[183] Rao TP, Ozeki M, Juneja LR. In search of a safe natural sleep aid. J Am Coll Nutr 2015;34(5):436–47.
[184] Unno K, Noda S, Kawasaki Y, et al. Ingestion of green tea with lowered caffeine improves sleep quality of the elderly via suppression of stress. J Clin Biochem Nutr 2017;61(3):210–16.
[185] Unno K, Noda S, Kawasaki Y, et al. Reduced stress and improved sleep quality caused by green tea are associated with a reduced caffeine content. Nutrients 2017;9(7):777.
[186] Reimund E. Sleep deprivation-induced neuronal damage may be due to nicotinic acid depletion. Med Hypotheses 1991;34(3): 275–7.
[187] Adamo AM, Oteiza PI. Zinc deficiency and neurodevelopment: the case of neurons. Biofactors 2010;36(2):117–24.
[188] Saito H, Cherasse Y, Suzuki R, et al. Zinc-rich oysters as well as zinc-yeast-and astaxanthin-enriched food improved sleep efficiency and sleep onset in a randomized controlled trial of healthy individuals. Mol Nutr Food Res 2017;61(5).
[189] Fagioli I, Baroncini P, Ricour C, et al. Decrease of slow wave sleep in children with prolonged absence of essential lipids intake. Sleep 1989;12:495–9.
[190] Porkka-Heiskanen T, Alanko L, Kalinchuk A, et al. Adenosine and sleep. Sleep Med Rev 2002;6(4):321–32.
[191] Basheer R, Strecker RE, Thakkar MM, et al. Adenosine and sleep–wake regulation. Prog Neurobiol 2004;73(6):379–96.
[192] Porkka-Heiskanen T, Strecker RE, Thakkar M, et al. Adenosine: a mediator of the sleep-inducing effects of prolonged wakefulness. Science 1997;276.

[193] Wiers CE. Adenosine sheds light on the relationship between alcohol and sleep. J Neurosci 2014;34(23):7733–4.
[194] Mazzotti DR, Guindalini C, de Souza AA, et al. Adenosine deaminase polymorphism affects sleep EEG spectral power in a large epidemiological sample. PLoS ONE 2012;7(8):e44154.
[195] Sebo P, Cerutti B, Haller DM. Effect of magnesium therapy on nocturnal leg cramps: a systematic review of randomized controlled trials with meta-analysis using simulations. Family Pract 2013;31(1):7–19.
[196] Abbasi B, Kimiagar M, Sadeghniiat K, et al. The effect of magnesium supplementation on primary insomnia in elderly: a double-blind placebo-controlled clinical trial. J Res Med Sci 2012;17(12):1161.
[197] Rondanelli M, Opizzi A, Monteferrario F, et al. The effect of melatonin, magnesium, and zinc on primary insomnia in long-term care facility residents in Italy: a double-blind, placebo-controlled clinical trial. J Am Geriatr Soc 2011;59(1):82–90.
[198] Grandner MA, Jackson N, Gerstner J, et al. Sleep symptoms associated with intake of specific dietary nutrients. J Sleep Res 2014;23(1):22–34.
[199] Kaushik MK, Kaul SC, Wadhwa R, et al. Triethylene glycol, an active component of ashwagandha (*Withania somnifera*) leaves, is responsible for sleep induction. PLoS ONE 2017;12(2):e0172508.
[200] Kaur T, Singh H, Mishra R, et al. *Withania somnifera* as a potential anxiolytic and immunomodulatory agent in acute sleep deprived female Wistar rats. Mol Cell Biochem 2017;427(1–2):91–101.
[201] Blumenthal M, Goldberg A, Brinckmann J. Herbal medicine: expanded commission E monographs. Newton, MA: Integrative Medicine Communication; 2000.
[202] Schiller H, Forster A, Vonhoff C, et al. Sedating effects of *Humulus lupulus* L. extracts. Phytomedicine 2006;13(8):535–41.
[203] Koetter U, Schrader E, Käufeler R, et al. A randomized, double blind, placebo-controlled, prospective clinical study to demonstrate clinical efficacy of a fixed valerian hops extract combination (Ze 91019) in patients suffering from non-organic sleep disorder. Phytother Res 2007;21(9):847–51.
[204] Dimpfel W, Suter A. Sleep improving effects of a single dose administration of a valerian/hops fluid extract - a double blind, randomized, placebo-controlled sleep-EEG study in a parallel design using electrohypnograms. Eur J Med Res 2008;13(5):200–4.
[205] Cornu C, Remontet L, Noel-Baron F, et al. A dietary supplement to improve the quality of sleep: a randomized placebo controlled trial. BMC Comp Alter Med 2010;10(1):29.
[206] Franco L, Sánchez C, Bravo R, et al. The sedative effect of non-alcoholic beer in healthy female nurses. PLoS ONE 2012;7(7):e37290.
[207] Franco L, Bravo R, Galán C, et al. Effect of non-alcoholic beer on subjective sleep quality in a university stressed population. Acta Physiol Hung 2014;101(3):353–61.
[208] Bradley PR, editor. British herbal compendium, vol. 1. Bournemouth: British Herbal Medicine Association; 1992.
[209] Dhawan K, Dhawan S, Sharma A. Passiflora: a review update. J Ethnopharmacol 2004;94(1):1–23.
[210] Capasso A, Sorrentino L. Pharmacological studies on the sedative and hypnotic effect of Kava kava and Passiflora extracts combination. Phytomedicine 2005;12(1–2):39–45.
[211] Maroo N, Hazra A, Das T. Efficacy and safety of a polyherbal sedative-hypnotic formulation NSF-3 in primary insomnia in comparison to zolpidem: a randomized controlled trial. Ind J Pharmacol 2013;45(1):34.
[212] Ngan A, Conduit R. A double-blind, placebo-controlled investigation of the effects of *Passiflora incarnata* (Passionflower) herbal tea on subjective sleep quality. Phytother Res 2011;25(8):1153–9.
[213] Appel K, Rose T, Fiebich B, et al. Modulation of the γ-aminobutyric acid (GABA) system by *Passiflora incarnata* L. Phytother Res 2011;25(6):838–43.
[214] Gyllenhaal C, Merritt S, Peterson SD, et al. Efficacy and safety of herbal stimulants and sedatives in sleep disorders. Sleep Med Rev 2000;4(3):229–51.
[215] Garrett KM, Basmadjian G, Khan IA, et al. Extracts of kava (*Piper methysticum*) induce acute anxiolytic-like behavioral changes in mice. Psychopharmacology (Berl) 2003;170(1):33–41.
[216] Shinomiya K, Inoue T, Utsu Y, et al. Effects of kava-kava extract on the sleep–wake cycle in sleep-disturbed rats. Psychopharmacology (Berl) 2005;180(3):564–9.
[217] Warnecke G. Psychosomatic disorders in the female climacterium, clinical efficacy and tolerance of kava extract WS 1490. As cited in: Gyllenhaal C, Merritt SL, Peterson SD et al, eds. Efficacy and safety of herbal stimulants and sedatives in sleep disorders. Sleep Med Rev 2000;4(3):229–51.
[218] Emser W, Bartylla K. Improvement of sleep quality As cited in: Gyllenhaal C, Merritt SL, Peterson SD et al, eds. Efficacy and safety of herbal stimulants and sedatives in sleep disorders. Sleep Med Rev 2000;4(3):229–51.
[219] Wheatley D. Kava and valerian in the treatment of stress-induced insomnia. Phytother Res 2001;15(6):549–51.
[220] Chua HC, Christensen ET, Hoestgaard-Jensen K, et al. Kavain, the major constituent of the anxiolytic kava extract, potentiates GABAA receptors: functional characteristics and molecular mechanism. PLoS ONE 2016;11(6):e0157700.
[221] Pittler MH, Ernst E. Kava extract for treating anxiety. Cochrane Database Syst Rev 2003;(1):CD003383.
[222] Wheatley D. Medicinal plants for insomnia: a review of their pharmacology, efficacy and tolerability. J Psychopharmacol 2005;19(4):414–21.
[223] Felter HW, Lloyd F. King's American dispensatory. Eclectic Matera Medica Publications; 1898.
[224] Bent S, Padula A, Moore D, et al. Valerian for sleep: a systematic review and meta-analysis. Am J Med 2006;119(12):1005–12.
[225] Fernández-San-Martín MA, Masa-Font R, Palacios-Soler L, et al. Effectiveness of Valerian on insomnia: a meta-analysis of randomized placebo-controlled trials. Sleep Med 2010;11(6): 505–11.
[226] Leathwood PD, Chauffard F, Heck E, et al. Aqueous extract of valerian root (*Valeriana officinalis* L.) improves sleep quality in man. Pharmacol Biochem Behav 1982;17(1):65–71.
[227] Schulz H, Stolz C, Müller J. The effect of valerian extract on sleep polygraphy in poor sleepers: a pilot study. Pharmacopsychiatry 1994;27(4):147–51.
[228] Taavoni S, Ekbatani N, Kashaniyan M, et al. Effect of valerian on sleep quality in postmenopausal women: a randomized placebo-controlled clinical trial. Menopause 2011;18(9):951–5.
[229] Taavoni S, Haghani H. Valerian/lemon balm use for sleep disorders during menopause. Comp Ther Clin Pract 2013;19(4):193–6.
[230] Palmieri G, Contaldi P, Fogliame G. Evaluation of effectiveness and safety of a herbal compound in primary insomnia symptoms and sleep disturbances not related to medical or psychiatric causes. Nature Sci Sleep 2017;9:163.
[231] Taibi DM, Vitiello MV, Barsness S, et al. A randomized clinical trial of valerian fails to improve self-reported, polysomnographic, and actigraphic sleep in older women with insomnia. Sleep Med 2009;10(3):319–28.
[232] Leach MJ, Page AT. Herbal medicine for insomnia: a systematic review and meta-analysis. Sleep Med Rev 2015;24:1–2.
[233] Kelber O, Nieber K, Kraft K. Valerian: no evidence for clinically relevant interactions. Evid Based Complement Alternat Med 2014;2014:Art–no. 879396.
[234] Koetter U, Barrett M, Lacher S, et al. Interactions of Magnolia and *Ziziphus* extracts with selected central nervous system receptors. J Ethnopharmacol 2009;124(3):421–5.
[235] Cao JX, Zhang QY, Cui SY, et al. Hypnotic effect of jujubosides from semen *Ziziphi spinosae*. J Ethnopharmacol 2010;130(1): 163–6.
[236] Ma Y, Han H, Nam SY, et al. Cyclopeptide alkaloid fraction from *Zizyphi spinosi* semen enhances pentobarbital-induced sleeping behaviors. J Ethnopharmacol 2008;117:318–24.
[237] Jiang JG, Huang XJ, Chen J, et al. Comparison of the sedative and hypnotic effects of flavonoids, saponins, and polysaccharides extracted from semen *Ziziphus* jujube. Nat Prod Res 2007;21(4):310–20.
[238] Gao JR, Ji WB, Jiang H, et al. Effects of extracts from *Ziziphi spinosae* semen and *schisandrae chinensis* fructus on amino acid neurotransmitter in rats with insomnia induced by PCPA. Zhong Yao Cai 2013;36(10):1635–9.
[239] Zick SM, Wright BD, Sen A, et al. Preliminary examination of the efficacy and safety of a standardized chamomile extract for chronic primary insomnia: a randomized placebo-controlled pilot study. BMC Comp Alter Med 2011;11(1):78.
[240] Chang SM, Chen CH. Effects of an intervention with drinking chamomile tea on sleep quality and depression in sleep disturbed

postnatal women: a randomized controlled trial. J Adv Nurs 2016;72(2):306–15.
[241] Abdullahzadeh M, Matourypour P, Naji SA. Investigation effect of oral chamomilla on sleep quality in elderly people in Isfahan: a randomized control trial. J Educ Health Promot 2017;6.
[242] American Academy of Family Physicians. Information from your family doctor. Help with chronic insomnia. Am Fam Physician 2009;79(2):131–2.
[243] Harsora P, Kessmann J. Nonpharmacologic management of chronic insomnia. Am Fam Physician 2009;79(2):125–30.
[244] Jespersen KV, Koenig J, Jennum P, et al. Music for insomnia in adults. Cochrane Database Syst Rev 2015;(8):CD010459.
[245] Horne JA, Reid AJ. Night-time sleep EEG changes following body heating in a warm bath (Abstract only). Electroencephalogr Clin Neurophysiol 1985;60:154–7.
[246] Driver HS, Taylor SR. Exercise and sleep. Sleep Med Rev 2000;4:387–402.
[247] Tringale R, Jensen C. Cannabis and insomnia. Depression 2011;4(12):0–68.
[248] Schierenbeck T, Riemann D, Berger M, et al. Effect of illicit recreational drugs upon sleep: cocaine, ecstasy and marijuana. Sleep Med Rev 2008;12(5):381–9.
[249] Johanson CE, Roehrs T, Schuh K, et al. The effects of cocaine on mood and sleep in cocaine-dependent males. Exp Clin Psychopharmacol 1999;7(4):E338–46.
[250] Watson R, Bakos L, Compton P, et al. Cocaine use and withdrawal: the effect on sleep and mood. Am J Drug Alcohol Abuse 1992;18(1):21–8.
[251] Gouzoulis E, Steiger A, Ensslin M, et al. Sleep EEG effects of 3,4-methylenedioxyethamphetamine (MDE; "eve") in healthy volunteers. Biol Psychiatry 1992;32(12):1108–17.
[252] Ramakrishnan K, Scheid DC. Treatment options for insomnia. Am Fam Physician 2007;76(4):517–26.
[253] Stovner L, Hagen K, Jensen R, et al. The global burden of headache: a documentation of headache prevalence and disability worldwide. Cephalalgia 2007;27:193–210.
[254] ABS. Australian health survey: users' guide, 2011–13. Canberra: ABS; 2013. Cat. no. 4363.0.55.001.
[255] Stark RJ, Valenti L, Miller GC. Management of migraine in Australian general practice. Med J Aust 2007;187(3):142–6.
[256] Sun-Edelstein C, Mauskop A. Foods and supplements in the management of migraine headaches. Clin J Pain 2009;25(5): 446–52.
[257] The International Classification of Headache Disorders. 3rd edn (Beta version). 2016 International Headache Society. Available from: www.ichd-3.org/.
[258] Russel MB, Iselius L, Olesen J. Migraine without and migraine with aura are inherited disorders. Cephalalgia 1997;16:305–9.
[259] Larsson B, Bille B, Pedersen NL. Genetic influence in headaches: a Swedish twin study. Headache 1995;35(9):513–19.
[260] Schürks M. Genetics of cluster headache. Curr Pain Headache Rep 2010;14(2):132–9.
[261] Hanington E. Migraine: the platelet hypothesis after 10 years. Biomed Pharmacother 1989;43(10):719–26.
[262] Hanington E, Jones RJ, Amess JA, et al. Migraine: a platelet disorder. Lancet 1981;2(8249):720–3.
[263] Hamel E. Serotonin and migraine: biology and clinical implications. Cephalalgia 2007;27(11):1293–300.
[264] Panconesi A. Serotonin and migraine: a reconsideration of the central theory. J Headache Pain 2008;9(5):267–76.
[265] Bartolini M, Baruffaldi R, Paolino I, et al. Cerebral blood flow changes in the different phases of migraine. Funct Neurol 2005;20(4):209–11.
[266] Blau JN. Feeling and seeing headaches. J Headache Pain 2005;6(1):10–19.
[267] Taylor F. Lifestyle changes, dietary restrictions, and nutraceuticals in migraine prevention. Tech Reg Anesth Pain Manag 2009;13(1):28–37.
[268] Welch KM, Ramadan NM. Mitochondria, magnesium and migraine. J Neurol Sci 1995;134(1–2):9–14.
[269] Obermann M, Katsarava Z. Management of medication-overuse headache. Expert Rev Neurother 2007;7(9):1145–55.
[270] Scher AI, Rizzoli PB, Loder EW. Medication overuse headache. An entrenched idea in need of scrutiny. Neurology 2017;89(12):1296–304.
[271] Vetvik KG, MacGregor EA, Lundqvist C, et al. Self-reported menstrual migraine in the general population. J Headache Pain 2010;11(2):87–92.
[272] Rothrock JF. Menstrual migraine. Headache 2009;49(9):1399–400.
[273] Monro J, Carini C, Brostoff J. Migraine is a food-allergic disease. Lancet 1984;2(8405):719–21.
[274] Cicarelli G, Della Rocca G, Amboni M, et al. Clinical and neurological abnormalities in adult celiac disease. Neurol Sci 2003;24:311–17.
[275] Bushara KO. Neurologic presentation of celiac disease. Gastroenterology 2005;128:S92–7.
[276] Pradalier A, Launay JM. Immunological aspects of migraine. Biomed Pharmacother 1996;50(2):64–70.
[277] Schürks M, Rist PM, Bigal ME, et al. Migraine and cardiovascular disease: systematic review and meta-analysis. BMJ 2009;339: b3914.
[278] Bigal ME, Kurth T, Santanello N, et al. Migraine and cardiovascular disease: a population-based study. Neurology 2010;74(8):628–35.
[279] Kreling GA, de Almeida NR, Neto PJ. Migrainous infarction: a rare and often overlooked diagnosis. Autops Case Rep 2017;7(2):61.
[280] Beghi E, Bussone G, D'Amico D, et al. Headache, anxiety and depressive disorders: the HADAS study. Headache Pain 2010;11(2):141–50.
[281] Breslau N, Lipton RB, Stewart WF, et al. Comorbidity of migraine and depression. Investigating potential etiology and prognosis. Neurology 2003;60:1308–12.
[282] Bigal ME, Lipton RB, Cohen J, et al. Epilepsy and migraine. Epilep Behav 2003;4(Suppl. 2):13–24.
[283] Stark R. How to treat severe headache. Australian Doctor 2005; 19.
[284] Ramadan NM, Halvorson H, Vande-Linde A. Low brain magnesium in migraine. Headache 1989;29:590–3.
[285] Virtanen JK, Giniatullin R, Mäntyselkä P, et al. Low serum 25-hydroxyvitamin D is associated with higher risk of frequent headache in middle-aged and older men. Sci Rep 2017;7:39697.
[286] Maizels M. The patient with daily headaches. Am Fam Physician 2004;70(12):2299–306.
[287] Khalil M, Zafar HW, Quarshie V, et al. Prospective analysis of the use of OnabotulinumtoxinA (BOTOX) in the treatment of chronic migraine; real-life data in 254 patients from Hull, UK. J Headache Pain 2014;15:54.
[288] Felter HW. The Eclectic materia medica, pharmacology and therapeutics. Eclectic Materia Medica Publications; 1922.
[289] Ferrara LA, Pacioni D, Di Fronzo V, et al. Low-lipid diet reduces frequency and severity of acute migraine attacks. Nutr Metab Cardiovasc Dis 2015;25(4):370–5.
[290] Özturan A, Şanlıer N, Coşkun Ö. The relationship between migraine and nutrition. Turk Noroloji Dergisi 2016;22(2).
[291] Stanton AA. Migraine cause and treatment. SSRN 2015;doi:10.2139/ssrn.2690927.
[292] Di Lorenzo C, Currà A, Sirianni G, et al. Diet transiently improves migraine in two twin sisters: possible role of ketogenesis? Funct Neurol 2013;28(4):305.
[293] Barbanti P, Fofi L, Aurilia C, et al. Ketogenic diet in migraine: rationale, findings and perspectives. Neurol Sci 2017;38(1): 111–15.
[294] Martins IP, Gouveia RG. More on water and migraine. Cephalalgia 2007;27:372–4.
[295] Kelman L. The triggers or precipitants of the acute migraine attack. Cephalalgia 2007;27:394–402, 43.
[296] Silverman K, Evans SM, Strain EC, et al. Withdrawal syndrome after the double-blind cessation of caffeine consumption. N Engl J Med 1992;327:1109–14.
[297] Kalladka D, Siddiqui A, Tyagi A, et al. Reversible cerebral vasoconstriction syndrome secondary to caffeine withdrawal. Scot Med J 2017;0036933017706892.
[298] Millichap JG, Yee MM. The diet factor in pediatric and adolescent migraine. Pediatr Neurol 2003;28(1):9–15.
[299] Van Den Eeden SK, Koepsell TD, Longstreth WT Jr, et al. Aspartame ingestion and headaches: a randomized, crossover trial. Neurology 1994;44:1787–93.
[300] Gibb CM, Davies PT, Glover V, et al. Chocolate is a migraine-provoking agent. Cephalalgia 1991;11:93–5.
[301] Maintz L, Novak N. Histamine and histamine intolerance. Am J Clin Nutr 2007;85(5):1185–96.

[302] Egger J, Carter CM, Wilson J, et al. Is migraine food allergy? A double-blind controlled trial of oligoantigenic diet treatment. Lancet 1983;2:865–9.
[303] Ansari B, Basiri K, Meamar R, et al. Association of *Helicobacter pylori* antibodies and severity of migraine attack. Iran J Neurol 2015;14(3):125.
[304] Cámara-Lemarroy CR, Rodriguez-Gutierrez R, Monreal-Robles R, et al. Gastrointestinal disorders associated with migraine: a comprehensive review. World J Gastroenterol 2016;22(36):8149.
[305] Hindiyeh N, Aurora SK. What the gut can teach us about migraine. Curr Pain Headache Rep 2015;19(7):33.
[306] Dai Yu-Jie, Wang Hai-Yan, Wang Xi-Jian, et al. Potential beneficial effects of probiotics on human migraine headache: a literature review. Pain Physician 2017;20:E251–5.
[307] De Roos NM, Giezenaar CG, Rovers JM, et al. The effects of the multispecies probiotic mixture Ecologic® Barrier on migraine: results of an open-label pilot study. Benef Microbes 2015;6(5):641–6.
[308] Martin BR, Seaman DR. Dietary and lifestyle changes in the treatment of a 23-year-old female patient with migraine. J Chiropr Med 2015;14(3):205–11.
[309] Marashly ET, Bohlega SA. Riboflavin has neuroprotective potential: focus on Parkinson's disease and migraine. Front Neurol 2017;8.
[310] Condò M, Posar A, Arbizzani A, et al. Riboflavin prophylaxis in pediatric and adolescent migraine. J Headache Pain 2009;10(5):361–5.
[311] Schoenen J, Lenaerts M, Bastings E. High-dose riboflavin as a prophylactic treatment of migraine: results of an open pilot study. Cephalalgia 1994;14:328–9.
[312] Schoenen J, Jacquy J, Lenaerts M. Effectiveness of high-dose riboflavin in migraine prophylaxis: a randomized controlled trial. Neurology 1998;50:466–70.
[313] Thompson DF, Saluja HS. Prophylaxis of migraine headaches with riboflavin: a systematic review. J Clin Pharm Ther 2017;42(4):394–403.
[314] Prousky J, Seely D. The treatment of migraines and tension-type headaches with intravenous and oral niacin (nicotinic acid): systematic review of the literature. Nutr J 2005;4:3.
[315] Elrington G. Migraine diagnosis and management. J Neurol Neurosurg Psychiatry 2002;72(Suppl. 2):ii10–15.
[316] Menon S, Lea RA, Ingle S, et al. Effects of dietary folate intake on migraine disability and frequency. Headache 2015;55(2):301–9.
[317] Sadeghi O, Maghsoudi Z, Khorvash F, et al. Assessment of pyridoxine and folate intake in migraine patients. Adv Biomed Res 2016;5.
[318] Askari G, Nasiri M, Mozaffari-Khosravi H, et al. The effects of folic acid and pyridoxine supplementation on characteristics of migraine attacks in migraine patients with aura: a double-blind, randomized placebo-controlled, clinical trial. Nutrition 2017;38:74–9.
[319] Simopoulos AP. Omega-3 fatty acids in inflammation and autoimmune diseases. J Am Coll Nutr 2002;21(6):495–505.
[320] Pradalier A, Bakouche P, Baudesson G, et al. Failure of omega-3 polyunsaturated fatty acids in prevention of migraine: a double-blind study versus placebo. Cephalalgia 2001;21(8):818–22.
[321] Ramsden CE, Faurot KR, Zamora D, et al. Targeted alteration of dietary n-3 and n-6 fatty acids for the treatment of chronic headaches: a randomized trial. Pain 2013;154(11):2441–51.
[322] Ramsden CE, Faurot KR, Zamora D, et al. Targeted alterations in dietary n-3 and n-6 fatty acids improve life functioning and reduce psychological distress among chronic headache patients: secondary analysis of a randomized trial. Pain 2015;156(4):587.
[323] Sadeghi O, Maghsoudi Z, Khorvash F, et al. The relationship between different fatty acids intake and frequency of migraine attacks. Iran J Nurs Midwifery Res 2015;20(3):334.
[324] Abdolahi M, Tafakhori A, Togha M, et al. The synergistic effects of ω-3 fatty acids and nano-curcumin supplementation on tumor necrosis factor (TNF)-α gene expression and serum level in migraine patients. Immunogenetics 2017;1–8.
[325] Magis D, Ambrosini A, Sándor P, et al. A randomized double-blind placebo-controlled trial of thioctic acid in migraine prophylaxis. Headache 2007;47(1):52–7.
[326] Bianchi A, Salomone S, Caraci F, et al. Role of magnesium, coenzyme Q10, riboflavin, and vitamin B_{12} in migraine prophylaxis. Vitam Horm 2004;69:297–312, 82.
[327] Mauskop A, Altura BT, Altura BM. Serum ionized magnesium levels and serum ionized calcium/ionized magnesium ratios in women with menstrual migraine. Headache 2002;42(4):242–8.
[328] Durlach J, Pagès N, Bac P, et al. Headache due to photosensitive magnesium depletion. Magnes Res 2005;18(2):109–22.
[329] Trauninger A, Pfund Z, Koszegi T, et al. Oral magnesium load test in patients with migraine. Headache 2002;42(2):114–19.
[330] Peikert A, Wilimzig C, Köhne-Volland R. Prophylaxis of migraine with oral magnesium: results from a prospective, multi-center, placebo-controlled and double-blind randomized study. Cephalalgia 1996;16(4):257–63.
[331] Köseoglu E, Talaslioglu A, Gönül AS, et al. The effects of magnesium prophylaxis in migraine without aura. Magnes Res 2008;21(2):101–8.
[332] Facchinetti F, Sances G, Borella P, et al. Magnesium prophylaxis of menstrual migraine: effects on intracellular magnesium. Headache 1991;31(5):298–301.
[333] Esfanjani AT, Mahdavi R, Mameghani ME, et al. The effects of magnesium, L-carnitine, and concurrent magnesium–L-carnitine supplementation in migraine prophylaxis. Biol Trace Elem Res 2012;150(1–3):42–8.
[334 and 335] Shahrami A, Assarzadegan F, Hatamabadi HR, et al. Comparison of therapeutic effects of magnesium sulfate vs. dexamethasone/metoclopramide on alleviating acute migraine headache. J Emerg Med 2015;48(1):69–76.
[336] Nagata E, Hamada J, Shimizu T, et al. Altered levels of serotonin in lymphoblasts derived from migraine patients. Neurosci Res 2007;57(2):179–83.
[337] Nagata E, Shibata M, Hamada J, et al. Plasma 5-hydroxytryptamine (5-HT) in migraine during an attack-free period. Headache 2006;46(4):592–6.
[338] Ribeiro CA. L-5-Hydroxytryptophan in the prophylaxis of chronic tension-type headache: a double-blind, randomized, placebo-controlled study for the Portuguese Head Society. Headache 2000;40(6):451–6.
[339] Rozen TD, Oshinsky ML, Gebeline CA, et al. Open label trial of coenzyme Q10 as a migraine preventive. Cephalalgia 2002;22:137–41.
[340] Sándor PS, Di Clemente L, Coppola G, et al. Efficacy of coenzyme Q10 in migraine prophylaxis: a randomized controlled trial. Neurology 2005;64(4):713–15.
[341] Shoeibi A, Olfati N, Sabi MS, et al. Effectiveness of coenzyme Q10 in prophylactic treatment of migraine headache: an open-label, add-on, controlled trial. Acta Neurol Belg 2017;117(1):103–9.
[342] Dupois S. A comprehensive approach to treatment of intractable headaches. Townsend Lett Doctors 1990;88:740–4.
[343] Rolland A, Fleurentin J, Lanhers MC, et al. Neurophysiological effects of an extract of *Eschscholzia californica* Cham. (Papaveraceae). Phytother Res 2001;15(5):377–81.
[344] Felter HW, Lloyd F. King's American dispensatory. Eclectic Matera Medica Publications; 1898.
[345] Rafie S, Namjoyan F, Golfakhrabadi F, et al. Effect of lavender essential oil as a prophylactic therapy for migraine: a randomized controlled clinical trial. J Herbal Med 2016;6(1):18–23.
[346] Sasannejad P, Saeedi M, Shoeibi A, et al. Lavender essential oil in the treatment of migraine headache: a placebo-controlled clinical trial. Eur Neurol 2012;67(5):288–91.
[347] Yarnell E, Abascal K. Botanical medicines for headache. Altern Complement Ther 2007;148–52.
[348] Pittler MH, Vogler BK, Ernst E. Feverfew for preventing migraine. Cochrane Database Syst Rev 2000;(3):CD002286.
[349] Pittler MH, Ernst E. Feverfew for preventing migraine. Cochrane Database Syst Rev 2004;(1):CD002286.
[350] Shrivastava R, Pechadre JC, John GW. *Tanacetum parthenium* and *Salix alba* (Mig-RL) combination in migraine prophylaxis: a prospective, open-label study. Clin Drug Investig 2006;26(5):287–96.
[351] Wider B, Pittler MH, Ernst E. Feverfew for preventing migraine. Cochrane Database Syst Rev 2015;(4):CD002286.
[352] Diener H, Pfaffenrath V, Schnitker J, et al. Efficacy and safety of 6.25 mg tid feverfew CO_2-extract (MIG-99) in migraine prevention–a randomized, double-blind, multicentre, placebo-controlled study. Cephalalgia 2005;25(11):1031–41.

[353] Calvo MI. Anti-inflammatory and analgesic activity of the topical preparation of *Verbena officinalis* L. J Ethnopharmacol 2006;107(3):380–2.
[354] Chevallier A. Encyclopedia of medicinal plants. London: Dorling Kindersley; 2001.
[355] Mustafa T, Srivastava KC. Ginger (*Zingiber officinale*) in migraine headache. J Ethnopharmacol 1990;29(3):267–73.
[356] Maghbooli M, Golipour F, Moghimi Esfandabadi A, et al. Comparison between the efficacy of ginger and sumatriptan in the ablative treatment of the common migraine. Phytother Res 2014;28(3):412–15.
[357] D'Andrea G, Bussone G, Allais G, et al. Efficacy of ginkgolide B in the prophylaxis of migraine with aura. Neurol Sci 2009;30(1):121–4.
[358] Allais G, D'Andrea G, Maggio M, et al. The efficacy of ginkgolide B in the acute treatment of migraine aura: an open preliminary trial. Neurol Sci 2013;34(1):161–3.
[359] Esposito M, Carotenuto M. Ginkgolide B complex efficacy for brief prophylaxis of migraine in school-aged children: an open-label study. Neurol Sci 2011;32(1):79–81.
[360] Tuchin PJ. A case of chronic migraine remission after chiropractic care. J Chiropr Med 2008;7(2):66–70.
[361] Trautmann E, Lackschewitz H, Kröner-Herwig B. Psychological treatment of recurrent headache in children and adolescents — a meta-analysis. Cephalalgia 2006;26:1411–26.
[362] Eccleston C, Yorke L, Morley S, et al. Psychological therapies for the management of chronic and recurrent pain in children and adolescents. Cochrane Database Syst Rev 2003;(1):CD003968.
[363] Holroyd KA, Penzien DB. Pharmacological versus non-pharmacological prophylaxis of recurrent migraine headache: a meta-analytic review of clinical trials. Pain 1990;42:1–13.
[364] Woolhouse M. Migraine and tension headache — a complementary and alternative medicine approach. Aust Fam Physician 2005;34(8).
[365] Kelman L. The triggers or precipitants of the acute migraine attack. Cephalalgia 2007;27(5):394–402.
[366] Milo R, Kathana E. Multiple sclerosis: geoepidemiology, genetics and the environment. Autoimmun Rev 2010;9(5):A387–94.
[367] MS Australia. Key facts and figures about MS. 2015. Available from: www.msaustralia.org.au.
[368] Moynihan J, Moore H. Endocrine system dynamics and MS epidemiology. Med Hypotheses 2010;74(5):814–17.
[369] Koch-Henriksen N, Sorensen PS. The changing demographic pattern of multiple sclerosis epidemiology. Lancet Neurol 2010;9(5):520–32.
[370] Hauser SL, Oksenberg JR. The neurobiology of multiple sclerosis: genes, inflammation, and neurodegeneration. Neuron 2006;52:61–76.
[371] Simmonds MJ, Gough SC. The HLA region and autoimmune disease: associations and mechanisms of action. Curr Genom 2007;8(7):453–65.
[372] Fewings NL, Gatt PN, McKay FC, et al. The autoimmune risk gene ZMIZ1 is a vitamin D responsive marker of a molecular phenotype of multiple sclerosis. J Autoimmun 2017;78:57–69.
[373] Oveland E, Nystad A, Berven F, et al. 1, 25-Dihydroxyvitamin-D3 induces brain proteomic changes in cuprizone mice during remyelination involving calcium proteins. Neurochem Inter 2017;112:267–77.
[374] Miclea A, Miclea M, Pistor M, et al. Vitamin D supplementation differentially affects seasonal multiple sclerosis disease activity. Brain Behav 2017;7(8).
[375] Gilgun-Sherki Y, Melamed E, Offen D. The role of oxidative stress in the pathogenesis of multiple sclerosis: the need for effective antioxidant therapy. J Neurol 2004;251(3):261–8.
[376] Gonsette RE. Neurodegeneration in multiple sclerosis: the role of oxidative stress and excitotoxicity. J Neurol Sci 2008;274(1–2):48–53.
[377] Ghafourifar P, Mousavizadeh K, Parihar MS, et al. Mitochondria in multiple sclerosis. Front Biosci 2008;13:3116–26.
[378] Mirshafiey A, Mohsenzadegan M. Antioxidant therapy in multiple sclerosis. Immunopharmacol Immunotoxicol 2009;31(1):13–29.
[379] Napier MD, Poole C, Satten GA, et al. Heavy metals, organic solvents, and multiple sclerosis: an exploratory look at gene-environment interactions. Arch Environ Occup Health 2016;71(1):26–34.
[380] Kahrizi F, Salimi A, Noorbakhsh F, et al. Repeated administration of mercury intensifies brain damage in multiple sclerosis through mitochondrial dysfunction. Iran J Pharmaceut Res 2016;15(4):834.
[381] Fulgenzi A, Zanella SG, Mariani MM, et al. A case of multiple sclerosis improvement following removal of heavy metal intoxication. Biometals 2012;25(3):569–76.
[382] Mohr DC, Goodkin DE, Bacchetti P, et al. Psychological stress and the subsequent appearance of new brain MRI lesions in MS. Neurology 2000;55(1):55–61.
[383] Mohr DC, Hart SL, Julian L, et al. Association between stressful life events and exacerbation in multiple sclerosis: a meta-analysis. BMJ 2004;328(7442):731.
[384] Cekanaviciute E, Yoo BB, Runia TF, et al. Gut bacteria from multiple sclerosis patients modulate human T cells and exacerbate symptoms in mouse models. Proc Nat Acad Sci 2017;114(40):10713–18.
[385] Berer K, Gerdes LA, Cekanaviciute E, et al. Gut microbiota from multiple sclerosis patients enables spontaneous autoimmune encephalomyelitis in mice. Proc Nat Acad Sci 2017;114(40):10719–24.
[386] Olsson T, Barcellos LF, Alfredsson L. Interactions between genetic, lifestyle and environmental risk factors for multiple sclerosis. Nat Rev Neurol 2017;13(1):25–36.
[387] Kimura K, Hunter SF, Thollander MS, et al. Concurrence of inflammatory bowel disease and multiple sclerosis. Mayo Clin Proc 2000;75(8):802–6, 85.
[388] Gupta G, Gelfand JM, Lewis JD. Increased risk for demyelinating diseases in patients with inflammatory bowel disease. Gastroenterology 2005;129(3):819–26.
[389] Rang EH, Brooke BN, Hermon-Taylor J. Association of ulcerative colitis with multiple sclerosis. Lancet 1982;2(8297):555.
[390] Kasper DL, Braunwald E, Fauci AS, et al, editors. Harrison's principles of internal medicine. 16th ed. Part XV — Neurologic disorders. New York: McGraw-Hill; 2005. p. 2461–71.
[391] Tribe KL, Longley WA, Fulcher G, et al. Living with multiple sclerosis in New South Wales, Australia, at the beginning of the 21st century: impact of mobility disability. Inter J MS Care 2006;8:19–30.
[392] Giannini MJ, Bergmark B, Kreshover S, et al. Understanding suicide and disability through three major disabling conditions: intellectual disability, spinal cord injury, and multiple sclerosis. Disab Health J 2010;3(2):74–8.
[393] Multiple sclerosis: Introduction, eTG complete. http://online.tg.org.au/complete/.
[394] Van der Walt A, Butzkueven H, Kolbe S, et al. Neuroprotection in multiple sclerosis: a therapeutic challenge for the next decade. Pharmacol Ther 2010;126(1):82–93.
[395] Trapp B, Stys P. Virtual hypoxia and chronic necrosis of demyelinated axons in multiple sclerosis. Lancet Neurol 2009;8(3):280–91.
[396] Poser CM, Brinar VV. Diagnostic criteria for multiple sclerosis: an historical review. Clin Neurol Neurosurg 2004;106(3):147–58.
[397] Riccio P, Rossano R. Nutrition facts in multiple sclerosis. ASN Neuro 2015;7(1):1759091414568185.
[398] Swank RL, Goodwin J. Review of MS patient survival on a Swank low saturated fat diet. Nutrition 2003;19(2):161–2.
[399] Swank RL, Goodwin JW. How saturated fats may be a causative factor in multiple sclerosis and other diseases. Nutrition 2003;19(5):478.
[400] Swank RL, Dugan BB. Effect of low saturated fat diet in early and late cases of multiple sclerosis. Lancet 1990;336(8706):37–9.
[401] Swank RL, Goodwin JW. Review of MS patient survival on a Swank low saturated fat diet. Nutrition 2003;19:161.
[402] Swank MS Foundation. http://swankmsdiet.charityfinders.org.
[403] Farinotti M, Simi S, Di Pietrantoni C, et al. Dietary interventions for multiple sclerosis. Cochrane Database Syst Rev 2007;(1):CD004192.
[404] Riemann-Lorenz K, Eilers M, von Geldern G, et al. Dietary interventions in multiple sclerosis: development and pilot-testing of an evidence based patient education program. PLoS ONE 2016;11(10):e0165246.
[405] Das Gupta R, Fowler CJ. Bladder, bowel and sexual dysfunction in multiple sclerosis: management strategies. Drugs 2003;63(2):153–66.

[406] Bakke A, Myhr KM, Grønning M, et al. Bladder, bowel and sexual dysfunction in patients with multiple sclerosis — a cohort study (Abstract only). Scand J Urol Nephrol Suppl 1996;179:61–6.

[407] Segala L, Forte M, Ortega MR, et al. Moderate caffeine intake and verbal memory in multiple sclerosis: a pilot study. J Caff Res 2016;6(3):134–8.

[408] Walton RG, Hudak R, Green-Waite RJ. Adverse reactions to aspartame: double-blind challenge in patients from a vulnerable population. Biol Psychiatry 1993;34(1–2):13–17.

[409] Briffa J. Aspartame and its effects on health: independently funded studies have found potential for adverse effects. BMJ 2005;330(7486):309–10, author reply 310.

[410] Shor DB, Barzilai O, Ram M, et al. Gluten sensitivity in multiple sclerosis: experimental myth or clinical truth? Ann N Y Acad Sci 2009;1173:343–9.

[411] Reichelt KL, Jensen D. IgA antibodies against gliadin and gluten in multiple sclerosis. Acta Neurol Scand 2004;110(4):239–41.

[412] Borhani Haghighi A, Ansari N, Mokhtari M, et al. Multiple sclerosis and gluten sensitivity. Clin Neurol Neurosurg 2007;109(8):651–3.

[413] Gupta JK, Ingegno AP, Cook AW, et al. Multiple sclerosis and malabsorption. Am J Gastroenterol 1977;68(6):560–5.

[414] Feinstein A, Feinstein K. Depression associated with multiple sclerosis. Looking beyond diagnosis to symptom expression. J Affect Disord 2001;66:193–8.

[415] Shaw K, Turner J, Del Mar C. Tryptophan and 5-hydroxytryptophan for depression. Cochrane Database Syst Rev 2002;(1):CD003198.

[416] Shaw K, Turner J, Del Mar C. Are tryptophan and 5-hydroxytryptophan effective treatments for depression? A meta-analysis. Aust N Z J Psychiatry 2002;36(4):488–91.

[417] Trouillas P. Regression of cerebellar syndrome with long-term administration of 5-HTP or the combination 5-HTP-benserazide (Abstract only). Ital J Neurol Sci 1984;5(3):253–66.

[418] Nakashima Y, Suzue R. Effect of nicotinic acid on myelin lipids in brain of developing rat (Abstract only). J Nutr Sci Vitaminol (Tokyo) 1982;28(5):491–500.

[419] Miller A, Korem M, Almog R, et al. Vitamin B_{12}, demyelination, remyelination and repair in multiple sclerosis. J Neurol Sci 2005;233(1–2):93–7.

[420] Reynolds EH, Bottiglieri T, Laundy M, et al. Vitamin B_{12} metabolism in multiple sclerosis. Arch Neurol 1992;49: 649–52.

[421] Scalabrino G, Buccellato F, Veber D, et al. New basis of the neurotrophic action of vitamin B_{12}. Clin Chem Lab Med 2003;41:1435–37.

[422] Spindler M, Beal MF, Henchcliffe C. Coenzyme Q10 effects in neurodegenerative disease. Neuropsychiatr Dis Treat 2009;5:597–610.

[423] Kidd PM. Neurodegeneration from mitochondrial insufficiency: nutrients, stem cells, growth factors, and prospects for brain rebuilding using integrative management. Altern Med Rev 2005;10(4):268–93.

[424] de Bustos F, Jiménez-Jiménez FJ, Molina JA, et al. Serum levels of coenzyme Q10 in patients with multiple sclerosis. Acta Neurol Scand 2000;101(3):209–11.

[425] Sanoobar M, Eghtesadi S, Azimi A, et al. Coenzyme Q10 supplementation ameliorates inflammatory markers in patients with multiple sclerosis: a double blind, placebo, controlled randomized clinical trial. Nutr Neurosci 2015;18(4):169–76.

[426] Sanoobar M, Dehghan P, Khalili M, et al. Coenzyme Q10 as a treatment for fatigue and depression in multiple sclerosis patients: a double blind randomized clinical trial. Nutr Neurosci 2016;19(3):138–43.

[427] Hon G, Hassan M, van Rensburg SJ, et al. Immune cell membrane fatty acids and inflammatory marker, C-reactive protein, in patients with multiple sclerosis. Br J Nutr 2009;102(9):1334–40.

[428] Salvati S, Natali F, Attorri L, et al. Eicosapentaenoic acid stimulates the expression of myelin proteins in rat brain. J Neurosci Res 2008;86:776–84.

[429] Leong EM, Semple SJ, Angley M, et al. Complementary and alternative medicines and dietary interventions in multiple sclerosis: what is being used in South Australia and why? Complement Ther Med 2009;17(4):216–23.

[430] Gallai V, Sarchielli P, Trequattrini A, et al. Cytokine secretion and eicosanoid production in the peripheral blood mononuclear cells of MS patients undergoing dietary supplementation with n-3 polyunsaturated fatty acids. J Neuroimmunol 1995;56(2): 143–53.

[431] Shinto L, Marracci G, Baldauf-Wagner S, et al. Omega-3 fatty acid supplementation decreases matrix metalloproteinase-9 production in relapsing-remitting multiple sclerosis. Prostaglandins Leukot Essent Fatty Acids 2009;80(2–3):131–6.

[432] Pantzaris MC, Loukaides GN, Ntzani EE, et al. A novel oral nutraceutical formula of omega-3 and omega-6 fatty acids with vitamins (PLP10) in relapsing remitting multiple sclerosis: a randomised, double-blind, placebo-controlled proof-of-concept clinical trial. BMJ Open 2013;3(4):e002170.

[433] van Meeteren ME, Baron W, Beermann C, et al. Polyunsaturated fatty acid supplementation stimulates differentiation of oligodendroglia cells. Dev Neurosci 2006;28(3):196–208.

[434] Johnson S. The multifaceted and widespread pathology of magnesium deficiency. Med Hypotheses 2001;56(2):163–70.

[435] Yasui M, Ota K. Experimental and clinical studies on dysregulation of magnesium metabolism and the aetiopathogenesis of multiple sclerosis. Magnes Res 1992;5(4):295–302.

[436] Rossier P, van Erven S, Wade DT. The effect of magnesium oral therapy on spasticity in a patient with multiple sclerosis. Eur J Neurol 2000;7(6):741–4.

[437] Syburra C, Passi S. Oxidative stress in patients with multiple sclerosis. Ukr Biokhim Zh 1999;71(3):112–15.

[438] Korpela H, Kinnunen E, Juntunen J, et al. Serum selenium concentration, glutathione peroxidase activity and lipid peroxides in a co-twin control study on multiple sclerosis. J Neurol Sci 1989;91(1–2):79–84.

[439] Mai J, Sørensen PS, Hansen JC. High dose antioxidant supplementation to MS patients. Effects on glutathione peroxidase, clinical safety, and absorption of selenium. Biol Trace Elem Res 1990;24(2):109–17.

[440] Clausen J, Jensen GE, Nielsen SA. Selenium in chronic neurologic diseases. Multiple sclerosis and Batten's disease. Biol Trace Elem Res 1988;15:179–203.

[441] Smith DK, Feldman EB, Feldman DS. Trace element status in multiple sclerosis. Am J Clin Nutr 1989;50(1):136–40.

[442] Socha K, Kochanowicz J, Karpińska E, et al. Dietary habits and selenium, glutathione peroxidase and total antioxidant status in the serum of patients with relapsing-remitting multiple sclerosis. Nutr J 2014;13(1):62.

[443] Aminzadeh KK, Etminan M. Dental amalgam and multiple sclerosis: a systematic review and meta-analysis. J Public Health Dent 2007;67(1):64–6.

[444] Hutter C. On the causes of multiple sclerosis. Med Hypotheses 1993;41(2):93–6.

[445] Sahraian MA, Nafissi S, Roostaei T, et al. Impact of vitamin A supplementation on disease progression in patients with multiple sclerosis. Archiv Iran Med 2015;18(7):435.

[446] Saboor-Yaraghi AA, Harirchian MH, Honarvar NM, et al. The effect of vitamin A supplementation on FoxP3 and TGF-β gene expression in avonex-treated multiple sclerosis patients. J Mol Neurosci 2015;56(3):608–12.

[447] Westlund K. Distribution and mortality time trend of multiple sclerosis and some other diseases in Norway. Acta Neurol Scand 1970;46:455–83.

[448] Carlberg C, Quack M, Herdick M, et al. Central role of VDR conformations for understanding selective actions of vitamin D(3) analogues. Steroids 2001;66:213–21.

[449] Garcion E, Wion-Barbot N, Montero-Menei CN, et al. New clues about vitamin D functions in the nervous system. Trends Endocrinol Metab 2002;13:100–5.

[450] Overbergh L, Decallonne B, Valckx D, et al. Identification and immune regulation of 25-hydroxyvitamin D-1-alphahydroxylase in murine macrophages. Clin Exp Immunol 2000;120:139–46.

[451] Zehnder D, Bland R, Williams MC, et al. Extrarenal expression of 25-hydroxyvitamin d(3)- 1 alpha-hydroxylase. J Clin Endocrinol Metab 2001;86:888–94.

[452] Munger KL, Zhang SM, O'Reilly E, et al. Vitamin D intake and incidence of multiple sclerosis. Neurology 2004;62:60–5.

[453] Goudarzvand M, Javan M, Mirnajafi-Zadeh J, et al. Vitamins E and D3 attenuate demyelination and potentiate remyelination processes of hippocampal formation of rats following local injection of ethidium bromide. Cell Mol Neurobiol 2010;30(2): 289–99.

[454] Jiménez-Jiménez FJ, de Bustos F, Molina JA, et al. Cerebrospinal fluid levels of alpha-tocopherol in patients with multiple sclerosis. Neurosci Lett 1998;249:65–7.
[455] Salemi G, Gueli MC, Vitale F, et al. Blood lipids, homocysteine, stress factors, and vitamins in clinically stable multiple sclerosis patients. Lipids Health Dis 2010;9:19.
[456] Palm R, Hallmans G. Zinc and copper in multiple sclerosis. J Neurol Neurosurg Psychiatry 1982;45(8):691–8.
[457] Bredholt M, Frederiksen JL. Zinc in multiple sclerosis: a systematic review and meta-analysis. ASN Neuro 2016;8(3):1759091416651511.
[458] Salari S, Khomand P, Arasteh M, et al. Zinc sulphate: a reasonable choice for depression management in patients with multiple sclerosis: a randomized, double-blind, placebo-controlled clinical trial. Pharmacol Rep 2015;67(3):606–9.
[459] Birks J, Grimley EV, Van Dongen M. *Ginkgo biloba* for cognitive impairment and dementia. Cochrane Database Syst Rev 2002;(4):CD003120.
[460] Johnson SK, Diamond BJ, Rausch S, et al. The effect of *Ginkgo biloba* on functional measures in multiple sclerosis: a pilot randomized controlled trial. Explore (NY) 2006;2:19–24.
[461] Lovera J, Bagert B, Smoot K, et al. *Ginkgo biloba* for the improvement of cognitive performance in multiple sclerosis: a randomized, placebo-controlled trial. Mult Scler 2007;13(3):376–85.
[462] Lovera JF, Kim E, Heriza E, et al. *Ginkgo biloba* does not improve cognitive function in MS: A randomized placebo-controlled trial. Neurology 2012;79(12):1278–84.
[463] Noroozian M, Mohebbi-Rasa S, Tasviechi AK, et al. *Ginkgo biloba* for improvement of memory and quality of life in multiple sclerosis: an open trial. J Med Plants 2011;3(39):33–42.
[464] Rausch WD, Liu S, Gille G, et al. Neuroprotective effects of ginsenosides. Neurobiol Exp (Wars) 2006;66(4):369–75.
[465] Huang YC, Chen CT, Chen SC, et al. A natural compound (ginsenoside Re) isolated from *Panax ginseng* as a novel angiogenic agent for tissue regeneration. Pharm Res 2005;22(4):636–46.
[466] Liao B, Newmark H, Zhou R. Neuroprotective effects of ginseng total saponin and ginsenosides Rb1 and Rg1 on spinal cord neurons in vitro. Exp Neurol 2002;173(2):224–34.
[467] Etemadifar M, Sayahi F, Abtahi SH, et al. Ginseng in the treatment of fatigue in multiple sclerosis: a randomized, placebo-controlled, double-blind pilot study. Inter J Neurosci 2013;123(7):480–6.
[468] Gonsette RE. Oxidative stress and excitotoxicity: a therapeutic issue in multiple sclerosis? Mult Scler 2008;14(1):22–34.
[469] Mossberg N, Movitz C, Hellstrand K, et al. Oxygen radical production in leucocytes and disease severity in multiple sclerosis. J Neuroimmunol 2009;213(1–2):131–4.
[470] Nassiri-Asl M, Hosseinzadeh H. Review of the pharmacological effects of *Vitis vinifera* (grape) and its bioactive compounds. Phytother Res 2009;23(9):1197–204.
[471] Chun HS, Kim JM, Choi EH, et al. Neuroprotective effects of several Korean medicinal plants traditionally used for stroke remedy. J Med Food 2008;11(2):246–51.
[472] Long J, Gao H, Sun L, et al. Grape extract protects mitochondria from oxidative damage and improves locomotor dysfunction and extends lifespan in a *Drosophila* Parkinson's disease model. Rejuvenation Res 2009;12(5):321–31.
[473] Satoh T, Kosaka K, Itoh K, et al. Carnosic acid, a catechol-type electrophilic compound, protects neurons both in vitro and in vivo through activation of the Keap1/Nrf2 pathway via S-alkylation of targeted cysteines on Keap1. J Neurochem 2008;104(4):1116–31.
[474] Park JA, Kim S, Lee SY, et al. Beneficial effects of carnosic acid on dieldrin-induced dopaminergic neuronal cell death. Neuroreport 2008;19(13):1301–4.
[475] Machado DG, Bettio LE, Cunha MP, et al. Antidepressant-like effect of the extract of *Rosmarinus officinalis* in mice: involvement of the monoaminergic system. Prog Neuropsychopharmacol Biol Psychiatry 2009;33(4):642–50.
[476] Genova HM, Sumowski JF, Chiaravalloti N, et al. Cognition in multiple sclerosis: a review of neuropsychological and fMRI research. Front Biosci 2009;14:1730–44.
[477] Cole GM, Teter B, Frautschy SA. Neuroprotective effects of curcumin. Adv Exp Med Biol 2007;595:197–212.
[478] Kang SK, Cha SH, Jeon HG. Curcumin-induced histone hypoacetylation enhances caspase-3-dependent glioma cell death and neurogenesis of neural progenitor cells. Stem Cells Dev 2006;15:165–74.
[479] Xie L, Li XK, Funeshima-Fuji N, et al. Amelioration of experimental autoimmune encephalomyelitis by curcumin treatment through inhibition of IL-17 production. Int Immunopharmacol 2009;9(5):575–81.
[480] Kocaadam B, Şanlier N. Curcumin, an active component of turmeric (*Curcuma longa*), and its effects on health. Crit Rev Food Sci Nutr 2017;57(13):2889–95.
[481] Tegenge MA, Rajbhandari L, Shrestha S, et al. Curcumin protects axons from degeneration in the setting of local neuroinflammation. Exp Neurol 2014;253:102–10.
[482] Xie L, Li XK, Takahara S. Curcumin has bright prospects for the treatment of multiple sclerosis. Inter Immunopharmacol 2011;11(3):323–30.
[483] Hu Y, Liao HB, Dai-Hong G, et al. Antidepressant-like effects of 3,6′-disinapoyl sucrose on hippocampal neuronal plasticity and neurotrophic signal pathway in chronically mild stressed rats. Neurochem Int 2010;56(3):461–5.
[484] Shin KY, Lee JY, Won BY, et al. BT-11 is effective for enhancing cognitive functions in the elderly humans. Neurosci Lett 2009;465(2):157–9.
[485] Lee JY, Kim KY, Shin KY, et al. Effects of BT-11 on memory in healthy humans. Neurosci Lett 2009;454(2):111–14.
[486] Aktas O, Waiczies S, Zipp F. Neurodegeneration in autoimmune demyelination: recent mechanistic insights reveal novel therapeutic targets. J Neuroimmunol 2007;184(1–2):17–26.
[487] Aktas O, Prozorovski T, Smorodchenko A, et al. Green tea epigallocatechin-3-gallate mediates T cellular NF-kappa B inhibition and exerts neuroprotection in autoimmune encephalomyelitis. J Immunol 2004;173(9):5794–800.
[488] Calebresi P. Diagnosis and management of multiple sclerosis. Am Fam Physician 2004;70(4).
[489] Stuifbergen AK, Rogers S. The experience of fatigue and strategies of self-care among persons with multiple sclerosis. Appl Nurs Res 1997;10(1):2–10.
[490] Esmonde L, Long AF. Complementary therapy use by persons with multiple sclerosis: benefits and research priorities. Complement Ther Clin Pract 2008;14(3):176–84.
[491] Freal JE, Kraft GH, Coryell JK. Symptomatic fatigue in multiple sclerosis. Arch Phys Med Rehabil 1984;65(3):135–8.
[492] Snook EM, Motl RW. Effect of exercise training on walking mobility in multiple sclerosis: a meta-analysis. Neurorehabil Neural Repair 2009;23(2):108–16.
[493] Motl RW, Gosney JL. Effect of exercise training on quality of life in multiple sclerosis: a meta-analysis. Mult Scler 2008;14(1):129–35.
[494] Rietberg MB, Brooks D, Uitdehaag BM, et al. Exercise therapy for multiple sclerosis. Cochrane Database Syst Rev 2005;(1):CD003980.
[495] Heine M, van der Port I, Rietberg MB, et al. Exercise therapy for fatigue in multiple sclerosis. Cochrane Database Syst Rev 2015;(9):CD009956.
[496] Mitsonis CI, Potagas C, Zervas I, et al. The effects of stressful life events on the course of multiple sclerosis: a review. Int J Neurosci 2009;119(3):315–35.
[497] das Nair R, Martin KJ, Lincoln NB. Memory rehabilitation for people with multiple sclerosis. Cochrane Database Syst Rev 2016;(3):CD008754.

SAMPLE DAILY DIETS: REFERENCES

SEID

Arick CT. Chiropractic management of a patient with chronic fatigue: a case report. J Chiropr Med. 2016;15(4):314–20.

Gerwyn M, Maes M. Mechanisms explaining muscle fatigue and muscle pain in patients with myalgic encephalomyelitis/chronic fatigue syndrome (ME/CFS): a review of recent findings. Curr Rheumatol Rep 2017;19(1):1.

Morris G, Berk M, Carvalho AF, et al. The role of microbiota and intestinal permeability in the pathophysiology of autoimmune and neuroimmune processes with an emphasis on inflammatory bowel disease type 1 diabetes and chronic fatigue syndrome. Curr Pharm Des 2016;22(40):6058–75.

Myhill S, Booth NE, McLaren-Howard J. Targeting mitochondrial dysfunction in the treatment of myalgic encephalomyelitis/chronic

fatigue syndrome (ME/CFS) — a clinical audit. Int J Clin Exp Med 2013;6(1):1–15.
Nijhof SL, Rutten JM, Uiterwaal CS, et al. The role of hypocortisolism in chronic fatigue syndrome. Psychoneuroendocrinology 2014;42:199–206.
Sathyapalan T, Beckett S, Rigby AS, et al. High cocoa polyphenol rich chocolate may reduce the burden of the symptoms in chronic fatigue syndrome. Nutr J 2010;9:55.
Sullivan A, Nord CE, Evengård B. Effect of supplement with lactic-acid producing bacteria on fatigue and physical activity in patients with chronic fatigue syndrome. Nutr J 2009;8:4.
Xia F, Zhong Y, Li M, et al. Antioxidant and anti-fatigue constituents of okra. Nutrients 2015;7(10):8846–58.

Sleep

Abbasi B, Kimiagar M, Sadeghniiat K, et al. The effect of magnesium supplementation on primary insomnia in elderly: a double-blind placebo-controlled clinical trial. J Res Med Sci 2012;17(12): 1161–9.
Fukushige H, Fukuda Y, Tanaka M, et al. Effects of tryptophan-rich breakfast and light exposure during the daytime on melatonin secretion at night. J Physiol Anthropol 2014;33:33.
Howatson G, Bell PG, Tallent J, et al. Effect of tart cherry juice (*Prunus cerasus*) on melatonin levels and enhanced sleep quality. Eur J Nutr 2012;51(8):909–16.
Lin HH, Tsai PS, Fang SC, et al. Effect of kiwifruit consumption on sleep quality in adults with sleep problems. Asia Pac J Clin Nutr 2011;20(2):169–74.
Lindseth G, Lindseth P, Thompson M. Nutritional effects on sleep. West J Nurs Res 2013;35(4):497–513.
Pigeon W, Carr M, Gorman C, et al. Effects of a tart cherry juice beverage on the sleep of older adults with insomnia: a pilot study. J Med Food 2010;13:579–83.
Wada K, Yata S, Akimitsu O, et al. A tryptophan-rich breakfast and exposure to light with low color temperature at night improve sleep and salivary melatonin level in Japanese students. J Circadian Rhythms 2013;11:4.
Yang H, Lee YC, Han KS, et al. Green and gold kiwifruit peel ethanol extracts potentiate pentobarbital-induced sleep in mice via a GABAergic mechanism. Food Chem 2013;136(1):160–3.
Zeng Y, Yang J, Du J, et al. Strategies of functional foods promote sleep in human being. Curr Signal Transduct Ther 2014;9(3):148–55.

Headache

Amer M, Woodward M, Appel LJ. Effects of dietary sodium and the DASH diet on the occurrence of headaches: results from randomised multicentre DASH-Sodium clinical trial. BMJ Open 2014;4:1–7.
Finocchi C, Sivori G. Food as trigger and aggravating factor of migraine. Neurol Sci 2012;10:10070–2.
Gröber U, Schmidt J, Kisters K. Magnesium in prevention and therapy. Nutrients 2015;7(9):8199–226.
Ramsden CE, Faurot KR, Zamora D, et al. Targeted alteration of dietary n-3 and n-6 fatty acids for the treatment of chronic headaches: a randomized trial. Pain 2013;154(11):2441–51.
Ramsden CE, Zamora D, Makriyannis A, et al. Diet-induced changes in n-3- and n-6-derived endocannabinoids and reductions in headache pain and psychological distress. J Pain 2015;16(8):707–16.
Spigt MG, Kuijper EC, Schayck CP, et al. Increasing the daily water intake for the prophylactic treatment of headache: a pilot trial. Eur J Neurol 2005;12:715–18.

Multiple sclerosis

Casella G, Bordo BM, Schalling R, et al. Neurological disorders and celiac disease. Minerva Gastroenterol Dietol 2016;62(2):197–206.
Finsterer J, Leutmezer F. Celiac disease with cerebral and peripheral nerve involvement mimicking multiple sclerosis. J Med Life 2014;7(3):440–4.
Newland PK, Heitkemper M, Zhou Y. The emerging role of the gut microbiome in adult patients with multiple sclerosis. J Neurosci Nurs 2016;48(6):358–64.
Hernández-Lahoz RL, Fuentes D, Alvarez N, et al. Prevalence of celiac disease in multiple sclerosis. BMC Neurol 2011;11:31.
Sears ME. Chelation: harnessing and enhancing heavy metal detoxification—a review. ScientificWorldJournal 2013;2013: 219840.
von Geldern G, Mowry EM. The influence of nutritional factors on the prognosis of multiple sclerosis. Nat Rev Neurol 2012;8(12):678–89.
Zostawa J, Adamczyk J, Sowa P, et al. The influence of sodium on pathophysiology of multiple sclerosis. Neurol Sci 2017;38(3): 389–98.

TABLE REFERENCES

Table 22.2

Anonymous. 5-hydroxytryptophan. Altern Med Rev 1998;3(3):224–6.
Baker SK, Tarnopolsky MA. Targeting cellular energy production in neurological disorders. Expert Opin Investig Drugs 2003;12(10):1655–79.
Bastianetto S, Quirion R. Natural antioxidants and neurodegenerative diseases. Front Biosci 2004;9:3447–52.
Baumhackl U, Kappos L, Radue EW, et al. A randomized, double blind, placebo controlled study of oral hydrolytic enzymes in relapsing multiple sclerosis. Mult Scler 2005;11(2):166–8.
Bourre JM. The role of nutritional factors on the structure and function of the brain: an update on dietary requirements (Abstract only). Rev Neurol (Paris) 2004;160(8–9):767–92.
Braun L, Cohen M. An evidence-based guide to herbs and natural supplements. Edinburgh: Elsevier, Churchill Livingstone; 2007.
de Abreu DA, Eyles D, Féron F, et al. A neuro-immunomodulator: implications for neurodegenerative and autoimmune diseases. Psychoneuroendocrinology 2009;34(Suppl. 1):S265–77.
Dyall SC, Michael-Titus AT. Neurological benefits of omega-3 fatty acids. Neuromolecular Med 2008;10(4):219–35.
Fitzhugh DJ, Shan S, Dewhirst MW, et al. Bromelain treatment decreases neutrophil migration to sites of inflammation. Clin Immunol 2008;128(1):66–74.
Jia H, Liu Z, Li X, et al. Synergistic anti-Parkinsonism activity of high doses of B vitamins in a chronic cellular model. Neurobiol Ageing 2010;31(4):636–46.
Jiménez-Jiménez FJ. Calcium, neuronal death and neurological disease (Abstract only). Rev Neurol 1996;24(134):1199–209.
Keck T, White JA. Glycinergic inhibition in the hippocampus. Rev Neurosci 2009;20(1):13–22.
Langohr HD, Petruch F, Schroth G. Vitamin B1, B2 and B6 deficiency in neurological disorders. J Neurol 1981;225(2):95–108.
Lieberman P. Histamine, antihistamines, and the central nervous system. Allergy Asthma Proc 2009;30(5):482–6.
López-Corcuera B, Geerlings A, Aragón C. Glycine neurotransmitter transporters: an update. Mol Membr Biol 2001;18(1):13–20.
Mazza M, Pomponi M, Janiri L, et al. Omega-3 fatty acids and antioxidants in neurological and psychiatric diseases: an overview. Prog Neuropsychopharmacol Biol Psychiatry 2007;31(1):12–26.
Moja EA, Lucini V, Benedetti F, et al. Decrease in plasma phenylalanine and tyrosine after phenylalanine-tyrosine free amino acid solutions in man. Life Sci 1996;58:2389–95.
Muller DP, Vitamin E: its role in neurological function. Postgrad Med J 1986;62(724):107–12.
Obeid R, McCaddon A, Herrmann W. The role of hyperhomocysteinemia and B-vitamin deficiency in neurological and psychiatric diseases. Clin Chem Lab Med 2007;45(12):1590–606.
Osiecki H, Meeke F, Smith J. The encyclopaedia of clinical nutrition — the nervous system. Eagle Farm, QLD: Bioconcepts Publishing; 2004. p. 269.
Osiecki H. The nutrient bible. 6th ed. Eagle Farm, QLD: Bioconcepts Publishing; 2004.
Ramaekers VT, Blau N. Cerebral folate deficiency. Dev Med Child Neurol 2004;46(12):843–51.
Reavley N. The new encyclopedia of vitamins, minerals, supplements and herbs. VIC: Bookman Press; 1998.
Regunathan S, Dozier D, Takkalapalli R, et al. Agmatine levels in the cerebrospinal fluid of normal human volunteers. J Pain Palliat Care Pharmacother 2009;23(1):35–9.
Reimund E. Sleep deprivation-induced neuronal damage may be due to nicotinic acid depletion. Med Hypotheses 1991;34(3):275.
Reynolds EH. Benefits and risks of folic acid to the nervous system. J Neurol Neurosurg Psychiatry 2002;72(5):567–71.
Rossi L, Arciello M, Capo C, et al. Copper imbalance and oxidative stress in neurodegeneration. Ital J Biochem 2006;55(3–4):212–21.

Russell AL, McCarty MF. DL-phenylalanine markedly potentiates opiate analgesia — an example of nutrient/pharmaceutical up-regulation of the endogenous analgesia system. Med Hypotheses 2000;55(4):283–8.
Schoenen J, Jacquy J, Lenaerts M. Effectiveness of high dose riboflavin in migraine prophylaxis. A randomised controlled trial. Neurology 1998;50(2):466–70.
Stone TW, Ceruti S, Abbracchio MP. Adenosine receptors and neurological disease: neuroprotection and neurodegeneration. Handb Exp Pharmacol 2009;193:535–87.
Storch A. Coenzyme Q10 in Parkinson's disease. Symptomatic or neuroprotective effects? Nervenarzt 2007;78(12):1378–82.
Taked A. Manganese action in brain function (review). Brain Res Rev 2003;41:79–87.
Tomassini V, Pozzilli C, Onesti E, et al. Comparison of the effects of acetyl L-carnitine and amantadine for the treatment of fatigue in multiple sclerosis: results of a pilot, randomised, double-blind, crossover trial. J Neurol Sci 2004;218(1–2):103–8.
Valerio D, Georgetti SR, Magro DA, et al. Quercetin reduces inflammatory pain: inhibition of oxidative stress and cytokine production. J Nat Prod 2009;72(11):1975–9.
Walsh NE, Ramamurthy S, Schoenfeld L, et al. Analgesic effectiveness of D-phenylalanine in chronic pain patients. Arch Phys Med Rehabil 1986;67(7):436–9.
Yasiu M, Verity A. Mineral and metal neurotoxicology. CRC Press; 1997. [Chapter 14].
Zimmermann MD. Burgerstein's handbook of nutrition: micronutrients in the prevention and therapy of disease. New York: Thieme; 2001.

Table 22.3

Anonymous. Vinpocetine monograph. Altern Med Rev 2002.
Barker J, Meletis C. Naturopathic pain management. Altern Complement Ther 2004;10(4):188–93.
Bone K. A clinician's guide to blending liquid herbs. Churchill-Livingstone Elsevier; 2003.
Castleman M. The new healing herbs. VIC: Hinkler Books Pty Ltd; 2001.
Felter HW, Lloyd F. King's American dispensatory. Eclectic Materia Medica Publications; 1898.
Greive M. A modern herbal 1931 Available at: www.botanical.com/botanical/mgmh/mgmh.html.
Moss M. Aromas of rosemary and lavender essential oils differentially affect cognition and mood in healthy adults. Inter J Neurosci 2003;113(1):15–38.
National Standards Research Collaboration. National Standards Monographs (*Tanacetum parthenium*). Available at: www.nationalstandards.com.
Smit HJ, Gaffan EA, Rogers PJ. Methylxanthines are the psycho-pharmacologically active constituents of chocolate. Psychopharmacology (Berl) 2004;176:412–19.

23 Psychological system

Kate Worsfold, Erica McIntyre, Rachel Arthur

SECTION A

OVERVIEW OF PSYCHOLOGY

Psychology as a science seeks to understand and explain the functioning of the mind. Psychology involves a complex interaction between multiple body systems. Biopsychology seeks to understand and explain interactions between the two primary systems involved in maintaining psychological health: the neurological system (Chapter 22), and the endocrine system (Chapter 21). The role of the gastrointestinal system (Chapter 10) and the immune system (Chapter 12) are increasingly being recognised as playing an important role in maintaining psychological health. Psychological disorders reflect a dysfunction in either one or a number of these body systems. Below is an overview of the aetiology of psychological disorders and the paradigms used to describe them.

Aetiology of psychological disorders

In order to discuss how psychological disorders develop it is important to appreciate the body systems outlined in other chapters of this text, in particular two of the body's 'internal communication systems' — the 'fast-acting first responder' neurological system and the 'slower second responder' endocrine system.[1] The neurological system, which encompasses a vast network of nerve cells facilitating electrochemical messages, can quickly increase your heart rate and breathing to prepare your body for a challenge.[1] The 'second-on-the-scene' endocrine system releases hormonal messages from major glands (pituitary, thyroid, adrenals, gonads). The hormones released may be a slower-acting type of message, but these help to sustain the neurological system's initial response.[1] The brain may be thought of as the body's 'conductor of the orchestra' and thankfully coordinates these two key systems to enable effective communication within the body. This concept is key to understanding, as these two communication systems 'are the biological bedrock for all our thoughts, emotions and behaviours'.[1] Given increasing research is also highlighting the importance of acknowledging the interrelationships between the brain and many other body systems, our review is holistic in perspective and includes emerging research about the brain's connections with these other body systems and associations with psychological disorders.

A PARADIGM SHIFT: MOVING FROM 'SPLITTING' TO 'LUMPING'

Prior research and the *Diagnostic and Statistical Manual of Mental Disorders*, 5th edition (DSM-5)[2] have engaged a 'splitting' approach and predominantly looked at specific disorders and treatment protocols, leading to an increasing number of discrete treatment approaches for the various emotional disorders, considered as ranging from the anxiety, trauma and depressive disorders to somatic, dissociative and to some degree eating disorders.[3] Apart from increasing difficulty for the student in learning about each disorder, keeping abreast of all current best practices as a clinician is also time consuming. However, a recent review by Payne et al highlights the large comorbidity and shared aetiology between such disorders and posits the rationale for a more parsimonious 'lumping' approach and a unified trans-diagnostic protocol (UP) to the understanding and treatment of such disorders given their commonalities.[3]

In this chapter we explain the aetiology of the two most common psychological disorders: major depressive disorder (MDD), and generalised anxiety disorder (GAD). Instead of providing separate aetiological explanations, we draw from this newer lumping approach and Barlow's aetiological model referred to as the 'triple vulnerability theory',[3–5] where emotional disorders (including both MDD and GAD) can all be explained as arising from same the *interaction* of three vulnerabilities (displayed in Fig. 23.1):

1. General biological vulnerability (heritable genetic vulnerability/neurobiology)
2. General psychological vulnerability (early learning that events are unpredictable/uncontrollable, with the person having low confidence in coping)
3. Specific psychological vulnerability (disorder-specific learning)

The following section describes each of these vulnerabilities in more detail and explains some of the relevant body systems that have been associated with psychological functioning.

GENERAL BIOLOGICAL VULNERABILITY

A large body of prior research has highlighted the importance of vulnerabilities such as temperament on the development of psychological disorders. Neuroticism is known as a dimension of temperament where the person has a tendency to react negatively to stressors, which can be external or internal events. The associated negative reactions involve negative emotions (e.g. irritability, anger, anxiety, fear, sadness), along with negative perceptions and beliefs (e.g. a 'pervasive perception that the world is a dangerous and threatening place, along with beliefs about one's inability to manage or cope with challenging events'.).[6] It is unsurprising that neuroticism and research around related constructs such as behavioural inhibition or trait anxiety have been linked with the development of mood disorders (see Box 23.1).

Individuals can have a biological/genetic vulnerability to neuroticism. Barlow et al's review of the research indicates 40–60% of neuroticism is inherited (nature), where particular genetic polymorphisms (e.g. in the 5HTTPR serotonin transporter gene) are associated with differences in neurobiology (e.g. having a tendency towards a hyperexcitable amygdala and reduced inhibitory input from the prefrontal cortex). While neuroticism has been viewed as a stable, genetically based trait, gene–environment interactions occur on an ongoing basis. Because of this continuing nature–nurture interaction (see Box 23.2), temperament or biology does not purely dictate destiny and can be shaped (for better or worse) by the environment and learning experiences. In the triple vulnerability model, the three vulnerabilities, while separate, serve to contribute to emotional disorder development through their interaction, as seen in Fig. 23.1.

BOX 23.1 Applied learning

Kagan's behavioural inhibition baby experiment — predicting shyness and sociability

Can we have a temperamental predisposition towards anxiety? What age can we start to determine this and what are the signs?

Jerome Kagan pioneered research into the influence of temperament on behaviour. In Kagan's baby experiment, he measured 4-month-old infants' reactivity to new things (e.g. a mobile) and how easily upset they became. Twenty percent of Kagan's infant participants were high reactives, a behavioural profile marked by vigorous motor activity and crying to unfamiliar experiences. Forty percent were low reactors as they showed the opposite behaviours. Both temperaments are modest predictors of future personalities, depending on how children responded to their environments. Thus, as evidenced by Kagan, behavioural inhibition, a specific temperamental trait, can be identified during infancy and is marked by a tendency to display fear or inhibition when faced with novelty/unfamiliarity.

'The high-reactive infants are biased to become children who are timid, shy, and cautious in unfamiliar situations. This is a personality trait known as inhibited', said Kagan. 'The low reactives are biased to develop into outgoing, spontaneous, fearless children — uninhibited.'

Barlow DH, Ellard KK, Sauer-Zavala S et al. The origins of neuroticism. Perspect Psychol Sci 2014; 9(5):481–496; Sweeney S. Often, we are what we were. Harvard Gazette; 2010. Available from: http://news.harvard.edu/gazette/story/2010/04/often-we-are-what-we-were/

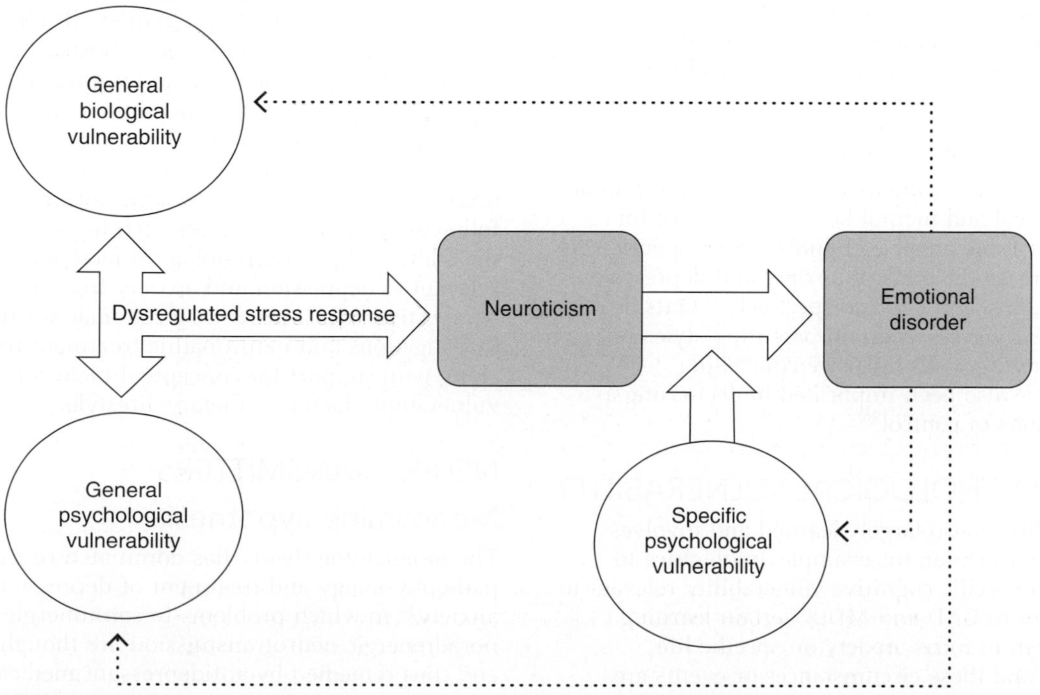

FIGURE 23.1 Triple vulnerability theory in the development of neuroticism and emotional disorders.

Source: Barlow DH, Ellard KK, Sauer-Zavala S et al. The origins of neuroticism. Perspect Psychol Sci 2014; 9(5):481–496.

BOX 23.2 What causes disorders — is it nature or nurture?

The nature vs nurture debate is clearly highlighted by research involving identical twins (who have identical genes), which reveals the concordance rate (the presence of the disorder in both) for schizophrenia is only 50%. Schizophrenia, as with all psychological disorders, requires an interaction between biological, cognitive, behavioural, sociocultural and environmental factors where, for example, the environment (e.g. chemical toxins or a healthy family environment) can switch on or off a biological predisposition.

Note: Despite what future biological research finds in terms of genetics or nutritional factors and mental health, we must also be aware that how we *think* and *behave* continually affects not only how we feel, but also the chemicals in our brain along with the activity and connectivity of particular brain areas. This is a key tenet of cognitive behavioural therapy (CBT), an evidence-based psychological treatment for depression and anxiety.

Source: Zimbardo PG, Johnson RL, McCann V. Psychology: core concepts. 7th edn. Boston: Pearson; 2012.

GENERAL PSYCHOLOGICAL VULNERABILITY

General psychological vulnerability relates to a person's perceived control over stress, events or emotional states. Early disruptive life experiences that promote development of beliefs that negative events are unpredictable or uncontrollable, and perceptions that they have an inability to cope may contribute to a generalised psychological vulnerability.[3] Poor levels of perceived control have featured across time in different research (e.g. Seligman's learned helplessness theory of depression),[3] with more recent research (e.g. Adverse Childhood Experiences studies) revealing the strong association between trauma and many physical and mental health conditions; for example, five or more adverse childhood experiences were revealed to increase the odds of anxiety and depressive symptoms by 420% and 810% respectively.[7] Outside of these adverse early events, certain parenting styles (e.g. 'helicopter' parenting with intrusive/controlling behaviours) have also been implicated in decreasing a child's perceptions of control.[6]

SPECIFIC PSYCHOLOGICAL VULNERABILITY

This vulnerability is also largely learned and involves disorder-specific learning; for example, intolerance to uncertainty is a specific cognitive vulnerability relevant to the development of GAD and MDD. Certain learning experiences seem to focus anxiety on specific life circumstances, and these circumstances or events are associated with a heightened sense of threat or danger. This vulnerability factor and learning can determine whether a person develops a particular type of anxiety disorder over another; for example, they may view somatic sensations (panic), intrusive thoughts (obsessive compulsive disorder), or social evaluation (social anxiety) as dangerous. Some individuals may have had early learning experiences or messages from their family members; for example, to be on their best behaviour or to look their best and to avoid being disapproved of by others, which is linked with social anxiety.[3] Intolerance to uncertainty involves an individual developing a set of negative beliefs about uncertainty (e.g. 'I can't relax if I don't know what is happening'; 'uncertainty is bad and/or makes me sad') which may lead to maladaptive coping behaviours such as excessive planning/organisation/preparation, rumination, worry, or avoidance of evaluation and particular activities/procrastination and so on. If the person has both generalised biological and psychological vulnerabilities towards being more marked in neuroticism, when combined with disorder-specific learning, development of an emotional disorder is more likely,[3] as displayed in Fig. 23.1.

A quadruple vulnerability theory?

Extending on from Barlow's triple vulnerability theory and in particular the biological vulnerability factor and the influence of genetics, psychological functioning is associated not only with the nervous system but also other body systems (the immune and gastrointestinal systems for example). Given the emerging evidence around dietary and lifestyle factors being associated with psychological disorders, we propose including an additional dietary–lifestyle vulnerability factor to the model, an approach which conceptually aligns with the Royal Australian and New Zealand College of Psychiatrists (RANZCP) clinical practice guidelines (CPGs) biopsychosocial and lifestyle (BPSL) model. Compared to earlier guidelines for other disorders (e.g. anxiety disorders) the current RANZCP model focuses on explaining how mood disorders are maintained by diet along with other lifestyle factors (exercise, sleep, smoking and substance misuse).[8] The following section reviews research highlighting some of the additional pathophysiological factors and body systems relevant to depression and anxiety from a biological perspective, which provides a rationale for future investigations and naturopathic treatment recommended, along with support for conceptual inclusion of the fourth vulnerability factor — dietary–lifestyle.

NEUROTRANSMITTERS

Monoamine hypothesis

The monoamine theory has dominated research into the pathophysiology and treatment of depression and anxiety,[9] in which problems in serotonergic and noradrenergic neurotransmission are thought to be key and thus remedied by antidepressant medication (e.g. selective serotonin reuptake inhibitors [SSRIs] or selective noradrenaline reuptake inhibitors (SNRIs)). While various studies associate amino acid depletion with mood disturbance, many problems exist in the monoamine hypothesis — for a review see Massart's work.[10] More recently, research has begun to focus on improving dopaminergic neurotransmission in depression as dopamine plays a role in symptoms such as anhedonia (the motivational/appetitive phase), with symptoms such as decreased motivation, drive or initiation of behaviour that could ultimately be reinforcing.[11] Subsequently, more studies involving dopaminergic medication (e.g. trials involving nomifensine, pramipexole or modafinil[12]) have been done, with buproprion recommended as a first-line medication for MDD in some countries.[8]

Role of other neurotransmitters

Dysregulation of endogenous opioids, GABA and glutamate have been associated with depression or anxiety disorders.[11–13] Recent trials using low-dose buprenorphine (an opioid modulator) have revealed improvements in treatment-resistant depression within 1 week and suggest that it may be useful as a rapid-acting antidepressant with other studies revealing anxiolytic effects and reductions in suicidality.[14] Such findings could be particularly important, given that the pervasively held belief that only dopamine is related to anhedonia is being abandoned in favour or dissecting anhedonia into the appetitive or drive component (dopamine dependent) and consummatory anhedonia, the latter of which is related to the experience of reward/enjoyment and dependent on opioid functioning.[11]

NEUROENDOCRINE CHANGES

Hypothalamic-pituitary-adrenal (HPA) axis dysregulation

Both hyperactivity and hypoactivity of the HPA axis have been linked with mood disorders.[10,15] HPA axis activity is directed by changes in neuropeptides such as corticotrophin-releasing hormone (CRH) and arginine-vasopressin (AVP) from the hypothalamus, which activate the release of adrenocorticotropic hormone (ACTH) from the pituitary and then corticoid secretion from the adrenals.[10] While the glucocorticoids should have a negative feedback loop on CRH and AVP in the brain, depressed patients have been found to have a deficit in this negative feedback loop.[10] Cortisol appears to have a U-shaped relationship with depression; for example, research by Maripuu and colleagues has shown an increased frequency of depression with both hypercortisolism and hypocortisolism.[15]

Various studies reveal AVP and oxytocin to be involved in modulating stress, learning and memory, where AVP has anxiogenic effects compared to oxytocin's anxiolytic actions.[9] From a dietary perspective, low fluid intake leads to increased AVP levels.[16]

Sex hormones and neurosteroids

The brain may be thought of as the 'third ovary' as it is capable of producing neurosteroids. Made from circulating steroid hormones (e.g. progesterone), neurosteroids such as allopregnanolone can bind to distinct sites on $GABA_A$ receptors and have been implicated in the experience of mood disorders and premenstrual syndrome.[17] Various psychotropic medications (e.g. SSRIs, antipsychotics) have been found to affect neurosteroid levels in the brain.[17] Other hormones such as melatonin affect not only brain function but also progesterone function and have been shown to improve luteal phase defects.[18] Similarly, receptors for progesterone and oestradiol have been found in the brain, with the concentration levels of such hormones in the brain found to be associated with peripheral levels.[17] The role of testosterone in mood for both men and women should also be considered. Polycystic ovary syndrome (PCOS) has been found in approximately 12% to 21% of Australian women of reproductive age.[19,20] A large number of women with PCOS (70%) remain undiagnosed[20] and PCOS has been associated with increased rates of psychological issues (e.g. depression, anxiety and eating disorders).[19,21]

Inflammation and oxidative stress

Increased cortisol production and inflammation/cytokine production can disrupt production of neurotransmitters like serotonin[10] as displayed in Fig. 23.2; for example, IDO catabolises the amino acid (tryptophan) into metabolites (kynurenine and quinolinic acid), which bind to NMDA receptors and lead to glutamate release. Quinolinic acid has been linked with a number of effects (oxidative stress, lipid peroxidation, decreased dopamine and cognitive function, exitoxicity of the brain, mood and neurodegenerative disorders).[22] It is unsurprising then to see increased rates of depression and anxiety among patients with conditions involving infections, allergies or other immune dysregulation/autoimmunity.[10] Other studies highlight the importance of poor mitochondrial function[23] and oxidative stress upon mood[24] along with, for example, the association between biomarkers such as uric acid and social anxiety.[25]

Neurogenesis and neuroplasticity

Elevated cortisol can also impair brain-derived neurotrophic factor (BDNF) and neurogenesis (birth of new neurons),[10] whereby prolonged cortisol elevation can act as a 'chemical blanket' to impede growth in the brain.[26] Neuroplasticity refers to the brain's ability to adapt and change in response to experience.[1] Changes in the brain's architecture have been found across psychiatric disorders and those highly trained in particular skills. For example, the left prefrontal cortex is up to 40% smaller in survivors of child trauma, and as left prefrontal cortex functioning is related to positive affect and approach behaviours, damage to this area has been found to result in depressive symptoms.[27,28] Similarly, other studies reveal increased right hemisphere hyperactivation in emotional disorders such as anxiety, insomnia and pain (where vigilance, rumination, withdrawal and avoidant coping behaviours predominate).[29] While it was previously thought that neurogenesis did not occur in adulthood, this notion has been shown to be false, with neurogenesis

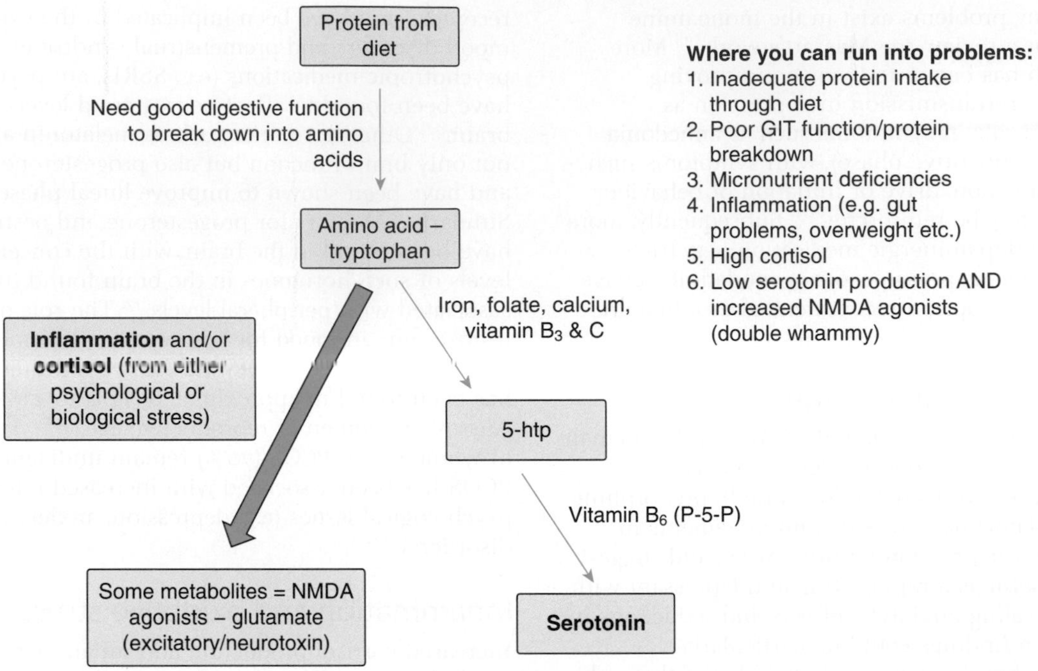

FIGURE 23.2 Inflammatory effects upon serotonin production.

possible even into older adulthood.[30] What stimulates neurogenesis? The brain requires the 'right conditions' for neurogenesis (e.g. enriched environments which include 'physical exercise, learning new things, sleep, reflection, complex problem solving and social interaction'.[26] The brain is a 'social organ' and thus ideally requires a safe but stimulating social environment or 'soil' to continue growing.

While the development of mood disorders is no longer thought of merely in terms of the monoamine hypothesis or a 'serotonin deficiency' syndrome, antidepressants (and other psychotropic medications) have wider effects apart from affecting neurotransmitters, and may improve BDNF/neurogenesis along with affecting neurosteroid levels and reducing neuroinflammation. While research trials have not been conducted with similar nutraceutical interventions, it would be interesting for future research to explore the potential for nutritional agents (historically used to upregulate neurotransmitter levels; for example, SAM-e, and 5-HTP) to affect these other factors such as neurogenesis and neurosteroid levels as well. Preliminary evidence of increased BDNF with some nutritional interventions has been an important first step.[31,32] See Box 23.3.

Gastrointestinal system: the microbiome and mood connection

Communication between the brain and the gastrointestinal tract (GIT) is not a one-way street, comprising a rich array of pathways including endocrine (hormonal), immune modulation (cytokines/immune cells) and neural (vagal nerve and the enteric nervous system),[33] as seen in Fig. 23.3. Similarly, while the influence of serotonin has been narrowly thought of in terms of brain and psychological functioning, in contrast most of the body's serotonin appears to be synthesised and stored in the GIT.[34] Various neurotransmitters and hormones are involved in gut functioning, with serotonin being a major player.[35]

Animal studies (along with more recent human trials) have established an emerging marriage between neuroscience and microbiology via the effect of gut microbes on the brain.[33] A continuous release of stress hormones can be deleterious to the gut microbiome, diminishing particular *Lactobacillus* and *Bifidobacterium* species, and is also associated with increased proliferation of pathogenic species.[33,36] Gut microbial changes have been linked with anxious and depressive behaviour;[37] for example, stress, appetite and eating disorders.[33] Interestingly, other recent research shows bacteria from various *Lactobacillus* and *Bifidobacterium* species can impact mood and vagal nerve activity and vice versa, with gut microbes dependent on the vagal nerve to impact the brain.[33,38] Because of the capabilities of our gut microflora, the microbiome is often referred to as the 'forgotten organ': our GIT can generate neural input to the brain; our flora has the ability to produce some vitamins and neurotransmitters — where, for example, *Lactobacillus* and *Bifidobacterium* species have been shown to produce GABA;[33,39] and where we are equally 'bacterial as human', given an approximately equal number of microbial to human cells.[40] Such is the growing awareness of the impact of gut microbes on the brain, that new research is using the terminology of psychobiotics.[38] Thus arises the potential for novel treatments targeting the gut and brain to help either gastrointestinal or mood conditions.[33]

BOX 23.3 Applied learning

Neuroplasticity — taxi drivers, POWs and sea gypsies

Does our environment have the potential to medicate or mould the brain? Can being a taxi driver literally change your brain? What does being a prisoner of war (POW) or a sea gypsy do to the brain?

London taxi drivers

Becoming a London taxi driver is no easy feat. All drivers must pass 'The Knowledge' test, renowned as one of the hardest to pass in the world, given it requires memorising a map of London's 25 000 streets. A famous experiment has shown that taxi drivers' hippocampi (the part of the brain that holds spatial memory) were larger than that of bus drivers who don't exercise that part of the brain as much, given they drive the same route daily. Learning may be more difficult than routine, but with such exercise, we unlock the potential for continued brain growth throughout life.

POWs and mathematical powers

Psychiatrist and neuroscientist Dr Dennis Charney reviewed research with POWs and how having only cognitive exercises changed their brain and their maths ability! Charney states, 'in general we do not make full use of the capacity of the brain'. POWs in solitary confinement, with *only* the ability to think, given they had no other activities, were found to develop unusual cognitive capacities that they did not have before. Through this type of cognitive exercise, one POW interviewed was able to correctly multiply 12-digit numbers by 12-digit numbers. Thus even in the impoverished conditions of solitary confinement, 'when you exercise the brain … you can find enormous capacities' states Charney.

Moken people of Myanmar (sea gypsies)

Humans usually have poor underwater vision. The Moken people have been hunter-gatherers for centuries. Living on the coasts of Myanmar and Thailand, they gather food from the sea and have developed underwater sea vision. The Moken brains' adaptation to the environment is such that they do not require masks or diving gear to collect small shellfish or other food from the ocean floor at depths of approximately 25 metres. Despite their vision being no different to European children's on land, the Moken children's underwater vision was found to be twice as sharp as their European participants.

Charney D. The resilient brain: big think. 2017. Available from: http://bcove.me/3gchixos; Gislen A, Dacke M, Kroger RHH et al. Superior underwater vision in a human population of sea gypsies. Current Biology 2003; (10):833–836; Handwerk B. Sea Gypsies of Asia boast 'incredible' underwater vision. National Geographic News,14 May, 2004. Available from: http://news.nationalgeographic.com/news/2004/05/0514_040514_seagypsies.html

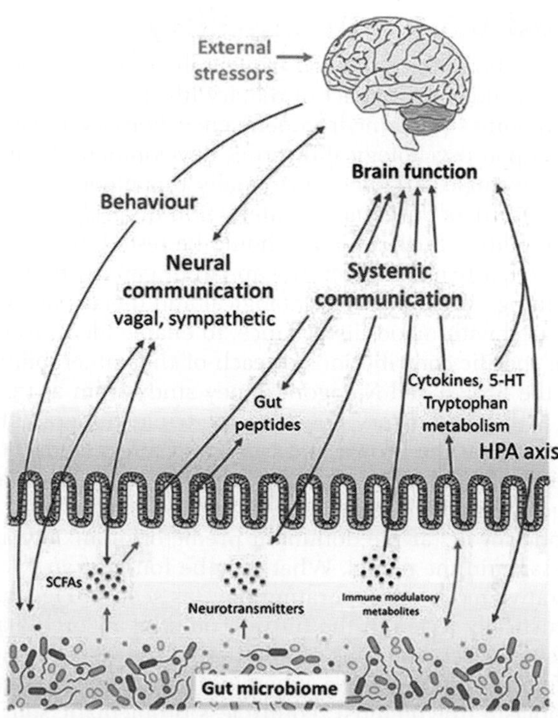

FIGURE 23.3 Communication pathways linking the gut microbiome with brain function.

Source: Rogers GB et al. From gut dysbiosis to altered brain function and mental illness: mechanisms and pathways. Mol Psychiatry 2016; 21(6):738–748. Reprinted by permission of Macmillan Publishers. https://www.nature.com/mp/journal/v21/n6/full/mp201650a.html

Lymphatic system

Until very recently we thought the brain did not have a lymphatic system. New research reveals this widely held belief to be incorrect, with the brain having what is termed a glymphatic system.[41] How does one of the most energy-hungry organs in the body clear itself of quickly rising waste? The glymphatic system — similar to the body's lymphatic system but in the brain — is a 'perivascular system of tunnels formed by astroglial cells' that are responsible for the transport and removal of nutrients and waste.[41] While the dysregulation of this system has not been directly associated with depression or anxiety to date, we know the operation of the glymphatic system is highly reliant upon sleep[41] and sleep disturbance is a symptom common in both MDD and GAD (see Box 23.4).

Genetic contributions

As indicated, genetic contributions have been associated with neuroticism and the development of depression and anxiety.[3,12] In terms of depression, a review of research reports the influence of genetics to be between 30% and 40%.[12] More recently research has shown that genetic polymorphisms (e.g. serotonin transporter gene 5HTTPR) are linked to differences in the structure and function of neural pathways (e.g. hyperexcitability of the amygdala and reduced inhibitory input from the prefrontal cortex).[6] It should be noted that apart from genetics, traumatic experiences (particularly during crucial developmental stages) can also lead to hyperexcitability of the amygdala.[6]

BOX 23.4 Applied learning

The 'garbage trucks' of the brain

The brain uses a quarter of the body's entire energy supply, yet only accounts for about 2% of the body's mass. So how does this unique organ receive and, perhaps more importantly, rid itself of vital nutrients? New research suggests it has to do with sleep. In his TED Talk 'One more reason to get a good night's sleep' neuroscientist Jeff Lliff discusses how the brain's waste clearance system is dependent on sleep. Jeff was part of a University of Rochester Medical Center team that discovered a brain cleansing system, which they dubbed the glymphatic system.

> *If sleep, then, is part of the brain's solution to the problem of waste clearance, then this may dramatically change how we think about the relationship between sleep, amyloid-beta, and Alzheimer's disease. A series of recent clinical studies suggest that among patients who haven't yet developed Alzheimer's disease, worsening sleep quality and sleep duration are associated with a greater amount of amyloid-beta building up in the brain, and while it's important to point out that these studies don't prove that lack of sleep or poor sleep cause Alzheimer's disease, they do suggest that the failure of the brain to keep its house clean by clearing away waste like amyloid-beta may contribute to the development of conditions like Alzheimer's.*

© Jeff Illif, TEDMED 2014. Lliff J. One more reason to get a good night's sleep. 2014. Available from: www.ted.com/talks/jeff_iliff_one_more_reason_to_get_a_good_night_s_sleep?language=en

A recent review suggests a pleiotropic effect, where neuroticism is polygenic and influenced by 'many genetic variants of small effect', and these variants also affect risk of depression along with other mental and physical health conditions.[42] While alterations in folate metabolism and MTHFR polymorphisms have been widely investigated, with some studies showing an association of certain polymorphisms and increased frequency of depression or relapse rates for those with a childhood trauma background,[43] it must be remembered this is but *one* potential genetic vulnerability and that mood disorders are polygenic in nature.

Diet and lifestyle

Various studies also implicate nutritional deficiencies (e.g. low-kilojoule dieting and associated increased cortisol output along with amino acid/tryptophan depletion, dysglycaemia, zinc, iron, and depletion of B vitamins that are associated with the homocysteine hypothesis) as potentially relevant pathophysiological factors in either depression or anxiety.[43–48] It should be noted that while many of these nutritional issues have been implicated as associated factors with psychological disorders, far less research has studied whether treatment trials aimed to correct such factors remediate the mood disorder and whether improvements in the nutritional parameters mediate symptom improvement.

A relevant example of this research disparity pertains to zinc. A growing evidence base of research highlights zinc deficiency to be associated with depression: a recent meta-analysis[49] reveals that while differences between the zinc levels of those who were depressed (median zinc level of 12 mmol/L) compared to healthy individuals (median of 14 mmol/L) were small (i.e. 2 mmol/L), this difference was clinically meaningful and, notably, the zinc level of the depressed participants was still within general laboratory reference range of 'normal'. In comparison, while some intervention studies show zinc as a stand-alone intervention or, in augmentation with antidepressants, to be effective in improving depression scores in people with depression symptoms, further well-designed randomised-control treatment trials are needed before firmer conclusions can be made.[50]

Intoxication/drug reactions

Illicit drugs, prescription medications, chemical toxins and heavy metals have been associated with mood disorders, and should be considered as a potential cause of mood disorders.[2,51] An interesting example is antibiomania, where an episode of mania or psychosis has been experienced following ingestion of particular antibiotics (e.g. triple therapy treatment for *Heliobacter pylori*).[51]

Quadruple vulnerability

Fig. 23.4 shows the extended triple vulnerability model which includes the impact of dietary/lifestyle vulnerabilities (e.g. zinc/iron deficiency, homocysteine levels) upon psychological disorder development. Rather than one single variable, conceptually this model suggests mood disorders arise via the interaction of all the vulnerabilities. Such a model should be tested in future research, particularly given the apparent gap in studies combining well-known psychological and dietary factors associated with mood disturbance, to enable identification of the specific contributions of each of the vulnerabilities, as in the Brown and Naragon-Gainey study from 2013.[5] Such is the explanatory power of the triple vulnerability model, that in the Brown and Naragon-Gainey study[5] this model explained 61% to 70% of variance in depression and generalised anxiety scores respectively, with neuroticism by far the dominant predictor of anxiety and depression in the model. What may be found if an integrative model incorporating diet (as seen in Fig. 23.4) is statistically tested in the future, could be an 'orchid and dandelion' effect in terms of emotional disorder development/performance, whereby those higher in neuroticism (the orchids) require less problematic soil (dietary/lifestyle factors) compared to hardier dandelions (low on neuroticism) who can survive in far worse soil. Essentially the orchids may wilt more easily in stressful or problematic environments, but can blossom when given the right soil compared to the dandelions who fare well wherever they are planted.

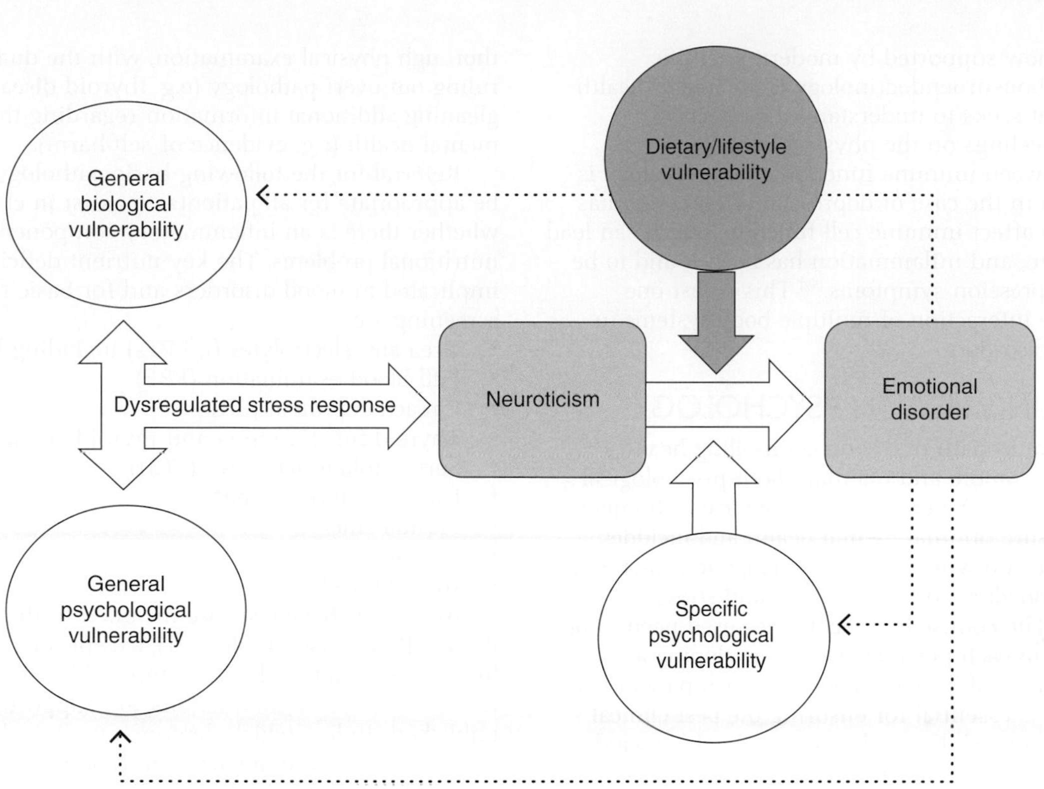

FIGURE 23.4 A quadruple theory explanation of emotional disorder development.

Source: Adapted from Barlow DH, Ellard KK, Sauer-Zavala S et al. The origins of neuroticism. Perspect Psychol Sci 2014; 9(5):481–496.

ROLE OF THE NATUROPATH

Traditional interpretation

Psychological disorders were frequently mentioned in texts of the Eclectic physicians; however, they were primarily referred to as disorders of the nervous system. The study of psychology as a discipline was in its infancy at the turn of the 20th century, and modern psychological terminology had yet to be adopted. The Eclectics largely prescribed nervine and tonic herbs to treat psychological dysfunction; including botanicals such as *Panax quinquefolium, Pulsatilla vulgaris, Passiflora incarnata, Viburnum opulus, Gossypium herbaceum, Gelsemium sempervirens, Valeriana officinalis, Scutellaria lateriflora, Matricaria recutita.*[52,53]

Hypericum perforatum is one of the most widely used nervine herbs in modern practice, and is commonly used to treat depression symptoms. The Eclectics did not consider melancholy (now known as depression) as a specific indication for the herb — it was instead more frequently described as being specifically indicated for neuralgic pain in the body and hysteria (which we now refer to as anxiety).[53] Interestingly, Felter questioned the value of *Hypericum perforatum* as a medicine, stating: 'It has, without question, a value in nervous disorders and should be more fully studied and tested, but miraculous powers should not be hoped for from it'.[53]

In the seminal naturopathic text *Nature Cure*, holistic beliefs about the connection between the mind and body were described by Lindlahr,[54] who believed that dysfunction in the body was influenced by biological, social and psychological processes. This hypothesis was later developed as the biopsychosocial model of health and illness,[55] which is now supported by a substantial amount of research evidence.

Modern interpretation

Modern naturopathy recognises the importance of both the body and mind, and considers psychological disorders within a holistic context where a person's psychology, biology, and environment interact in complex ways to cause dysfunction. The naturopathic approach also acknowledges the complex interaction between the different body systems that create homeostasis to ensure a healthy state of mind and body. Consequently, naturopaths use a range of therapeutic techniques from various modalities to support each person's unique psychological and physical needs. They are considered to be technical Eclectics.[56] In addition, naturopaths are teachers who enable people to remove obstacles to maintaining good psychological health, which includes dietary and lifestyle modification, the prescription of herbal, nutritional and homeopathic medicines, and counselling health psychology techniques that support the person and address behaviour change.

THE BIOPSYCHOSOCIAL MODEL

The biopsychosocial model of health and illness — initially proposed by Engel[55] — hypothesises that a number of factors interact to contribute to ill health including psychological (e.g. stress, beliefs, behaviour), biological (e.g. infections, nutritional deficiencies), and social (e.g. relationships, employment) factors. This model of illness aligns with the holistic naturopathic approach described above, and is now supported by modern scientific evidence. Psychoneuroendocrinology is an area of health psychology that seeks to understand the effects of thoughts and feelings on the physical body. This interaction between immune function and psychology is well illustrated in the case of depression. Depression has been shown to affect immune cell function, which can lead to inflammation, and inflammation has been found to be involved in depression symptoms.[57] This is just one example of the interaction of multiple body systems in psychological disorders.

COUNSELLING HEALTH PSYCHOLOGY

The modern naturopath draws on counselling health psychology to promote and maintain both psychological and physical health. A range of psychological techniques are used to ensure optimal mental health and include: assisting the person with behaviour change (e.g. diet and lifestyle), psychoeducation, counselling and stress management. The counselling techniques used need to be individualised to each person's needs. Developing a therapeutic relationship that aligns with each patient is a technique that is essential for ensuring the best clinical outcomes. Essential skills needed to achieve this include:

- Therapeutic alliance in individual psychotherapy
- Empathy
- Collecting patient feedback
- Goal consensus and collaboration
- Positive regard
- Congruence/genuineness
- Repairing alliance ruptures
- Managing countertransference.

INTEGRATIVE MENTAL HEALTHCARE

As psychological disorders are complex, naturopaths work with a range of mental health practitioners and services to get the best outcomes for people with psychological disorders. While naturopaths are not currently considered part of the mental healthcare system it is important that they are familiar with this system so they can refer to other specialist practitioners (e.g. psychologists, psychiatrists) and mental health service providers (e.g. hospitals, community outreach) to ensure their clients receive appropriate care.[58] Knowing when to refer is critical; therefore, naturopaths need to be able to identify more serious psychological disorders (e.g. bipolar disorder, schizophrenia), as people with these disorders commonly present with comorbid common mental health problems.[59] Naturopaths need to be aware of their skills and scope of practice related to treating psychological disorders in order to avoid acts of commission, which may cause harm to the person.[60]

INVESTIGATIONS

Biological

Given the long list of medical conditions that should be considered as differential diagnoses (see below), it is essential that all patients presenting with mental health issues be comprehensively investigated. This starts with a thorough physical examination, with the dual purpose of ruling out overt pathology (e.g. thyroid disease), and gleaning additional information regarding the patient's mental health (e.g. evidence of self-harm).

Referral for the following basic pathology tests would be appropriate for all patients, to assist in clarifying whether there is an inflammatory component or overt nutritional problems. The key nutrient deficiencies implicated in mood disorders and for basic thyroid disease screening are:

- Urea and electrolytes (E/LFTs) including bilirubin
- Full blood examination (FBE)
- C reactive protein (CRP)
- Thyroid function tests and thyroid autoantibodies
- Serum folate, active B_{12} (TCII)
- Fasting homocysteine*
- Plasma zinc*
- Serum copper*
- Iron studies*.

All of the above tests are included in the current RANZCP CPGs (see Table 23.1), except for those indicated by *. These additional parameters, while not included in the RANZCP recommendations, are supported by several published studies, which demonstrate links between imbalances of these nutrients and mental health presentations.[46,49,61]

A second tier of investigations might be considered where first round results have not revealed anything of significance. Some of these may, at the clinician's discretion, be included in first round investigations; however, as most of these are 'pay-out-of-pocket' tests, the clinician needs a strong rationale to justify requesting these. Some examples of second tier investigations and their rationale are included in Table 23.2.

Psychological

As part of a clinical psychological assessment, the following investigations are typically undertaken: file/record review, clinical interview, observations and psychometric testing.

CLINICAL INTERVIEW

Apart from gathering the required clinical information, a second key goal of the interview is to establish a therapeutic relationship with the patient. Experiencing any health condition, particularly one that is psychological in nature, can be distressing and difficult to make sense of. By virtue of a comprehensive clinical assessment, the clinician can help to formulate a clearer plan of the patient's presenting problems, predisposing vulnerability factors, precipitating triggers and perpetuating factors that may be maintaining the presenting problems, along with the patient's potentials or strengths (given that these can easily be forgotten if a disorder-centric assessment approach is taken). Such data can then inform diagnosis and individualised case formulation, which serves to directly inform individualised treatment planning. Formulation offers the patient a clearer understanding of why particular psychological issues may exist along with a way forward with individualised treatment, an approach

TABLE 23.1 Physical examination and biological investigations recommended by RANZCP CPGs

Examination	Rationale
Vital signs	Blood pressure may be altered by certain psychotropic medications and anxiety Bradycardia may occur in hypothyroid states Sinus tachycardia may reflect anxiety
Body mass index and waist circumference	To assess current general health status and gauge subsequent psychotropic associated weight gain
Signs of possible self-harm	Old scars (including tracheostomy scars)
Endocrine disorders	Goitre, hyper-/hypothyroid features, Cushingoid features
Respiratory disorders	Observed sleep apnoea/snoring, restless leg syndrome, COPD features, wheeze/asthma, lung malignancy
Neurological disorders	Parkinsonism, motor/sensory deficits, cerebrovascular disease features, motor tics
Organ insufficiency	Jaundice, AV fistula for dialysis, dyspnoea, peripheral oedema
Investigation	**Rationale**
Full blood examination (FBE)	Some psychotropics are associated with neutropenia and agranulocytosis Neutropenia has been particularly associated with clozapine and carbamazepine, and reported with olanzapine Macrocytosis is seen in heavy drinkers (20–30% in the community and in 50–70% of hospital patients)
Urea and electrolytes (U&Es) and liver function tests (LFTs)	Psychotropics may alter LFTs and U&Es Psychotropic pharmacokinetics may be influenced by otherwise clinically silent renal or hepatic impairments Possibility of hyponatraemia especially in elderly patients on multiple medications Isolated escalation of gamma-glutamyltransferase (GGT) suggests alcohol misuse GGT is elevated in 30–50% of heavy drinkers in the community and in 50–80% of hospital patients
Electrocardiogram (ECG)	Some psychotropics are associated with a prolonged QTc interval QTc prolongation has been particularly associated with TCAs, citalopram at high doses, ziprasidone, paliperidone, and lurasidone
Thyroid function tests (TFTs) and thyroid auto-antibodies	Thyroid dysfunction can cause changes in mood Thyroid dysfunction can be induced by treatments such as lithium
Inflammatory markers and microbial serology	Needs assessment on a case by case basis
Vitamin levels	There is an association between vitamin deficiencies and mood disorders Vitamin B_{12}, folate and vitamin D, studies are relevant in some cases
Sexually transmitted infection (STI) testing	If history suggests impulsive unprotected behaviour with sexual activity
Pregnancy testing (beta hCG)	If history suggests impulsive unprotected sexual activity Necessary prior to starting psychotropics in any woman who is potentially pregnant
Urine and blood drug screening	Screen for benzodiazepines, opioids, psychostimulants, cannabis, hallucinogens

Source: Malhi GS, Bassett D, Boyce P et al. Royal Australian and New Zealand College of Psychiatrists clinical practice guidelines for mood disorders. Aust N Z J Psychiatry 2015; 49(12):1087–1206.

that differs from diagnosis-based treatment (e.g. treating all depressed patients with St John's wort).

Key information gathered includes: biographical data; presenting problems, history of presenting problems, past psychiatric and medical history, family history, personal history (prenatal and perinatal, childhood to adulthood and any forensic history), in conjunction with ascertaining premorbid personality and functioning. Sources of information may also include third parties (e.g. family/partner or from other treating practitioners' observations and records).

MENTAL STATUS EXAMINATION (MSE)

While symptoms reported by the patient form one core source of data for the clinician, objective signs that can be directly observed by the clinician are an important secondary source of information. An MSE can be

TABLE 23.2 Potential second tier investigations

Test	Test explanation	Examples of indications for requesting
Whole blood histamine or SAM/SAH ratio	Based on the Pfeiffer model of under- and over-methylation	Prescreening using an informal methylation questionnaire suggests strong possibility of high or low histamine
Urinary pyrroles	Based on the Hoffer/Pfeiffer model of mental health and 'pyrroluria'	Prescreening using an informal pyrrole checklist indicates many characteristic features or primary relative has confirmed pyrroles
Hair heavy metal analysis and/or urinary provocation testing	Heavy metal toxicity has been implicated in mental health; for example, mercury and depression	History of or current significant exposure. Other features of heavy metal toxicity; for example, marked fatigue, mitochondrial or detoxification dysfunction
Red blood cell fatty acid levels	An imbalance of omega-3 and omega-6 fatty acids is involved in the pathogenesis of depression and correlates with presence and severity of bipolar disorder	Patient presents with marked pro-inflammatory picture
am blood cortisol, saliva or 24-hour urine cortisol	While 'typical' depression often correlates with HPA overactivity, only 50% of patients exhibit this feature and there is a sub-group of depressed patients, such as in the PTSD cohort, who can have HPA underactivity	History of adverse childhood experiences (high ACE scale core) or prescreening with the PTSD checklist that suggests possibility of significant trauma exposure
Sex hormone investigation	MDD should be differentiated from premenstrual dysphoric disorder (PMDD) (DSM-5). PCOS is found in up to 21% of Australian women of reproductive age and is associated with mental health disorders Several studies show correlation between free testosterone levels and depressive or dysthymic symptoms in men	In women mood symptoms are prominent in the premenstrual phase and tend to improve with the onset of menses (e.g. PMDD) In men, features suggestive of hypoandrogenism
Complete digestive stool analysis including PCR-based bacteriology, parasitology and inflammatory markers	There is increasing evidence of the role gut microbiome plays in mental health	Significant digestive symptoms or apparent risk for dysbiosis
Gene profile including MTHFR	Psychiatric genome-wide association study analyses implicate genetic differences in neuronal, immune and histone pathways. Several SNPs have also been independently implicated, e.g. MTHFR polymorphisms	Pervasive family history of any mental health issues

Sources: [19,20,62–73]

conducted at each session and entails the clinician's observations and impressions of the patient's appearance, behaviour, attitude, mood and affect, speech, perceptual disturbances, thought, cognition, impulse control, judgment/insight, and capacity to report reliably. Each of these factors can help to reveal underlying psychiatric disturbances and may serve to guide further testing (e.g. psychomotor agitation can be indicative of anxiety, mania or possible substance misuse).

PSYCHOMETRIC TESTING

Various psychometric assessments may be undertaken to screen for potential disorders, aid diagnosis (and assist in making appropriate referrals), gauge symptom severity, and to quantify therapeutic alliance and outcome progress across sessions to monitor treatment. Effective use of these psychometric assessments can reduce therapy failures. A range of psychological functions can be assessed if needed by psychometric tests, including, for example, personality, emotion, cognition, intelligence and executive functioning. Assessments can range from self-report instruments to performance-based tests. Psychometric tests have been used across large standardised samples so that a patient's score may be compared to the normative data of similar demographics (e.g. a young female patient's score can be compared to the average score of similarly aged girls aged 8–12 years). Many assessment tools are freely available, such as the Kessler Psychological Distress Scale (K–10) and the Depression Anxiety Stress Scale Short Version (DASS–21), which are often used by general medical practitioners, as they are brief tools that are relatively easy to score and interpret. More sophisticated instruments are restricted for use by trained mental health professionals only, such as psychologists. While psychometric assessments afford the clinician many benefits in practice, ethical administration of them requires the user to understand what the test actually measures, the test's limitations and what constitutes correct interpretation.

RISK ASSESSMENT AND REFERRAL

Risk assessment is a critical consideration when patients present with psychological symptoms. People who are actively psychotic, manic or who represent a danger to themselves or others should be referred for inpatient treatment and stabilisation with medication. Risk assessment should include assessing the risk of the person causing harm not only to themselves but also to others and risk for violent behaviour. Various factors shown to be associated with increased suicide risk, as outlined in the Mental Health First Aid Guidelines for Suicide,[74] are listed in Box 23.5.

> *Suicide can be prevented. Most suicidal people do not want to die. They simply do not want to live with the pain. Openly talking about suicidal thoughts and feelings can save a life. Do not underestimate your ability to help a suicidal person, even to save a life.*[74]

BOX 23.5 Factors associated with increased suicide risk

The various factors associated with increased risk of suicide include if individuals have:

- Mental illness
- Poor physical health and disabilities
- Attempted suicide or harmed themselves in the past
- Had bad things happen recently, particularly with relationships or their health
- Been physically or sexually abused as a child
- Been recently exposed to suicide by someone else.
- Been recently exposed to suicide by someone else.

Suicide is also more common across some groups — males, Indigenous people, unemployed, prisoners and gay, lesbian and bisexual people.

Source: Adapted from Mental Health First Aid Australia. Suicidal thoughts and behaviours: first aid guidelines (Revised 2014). Melbourne: Mental Health First Aid Australia; 2014.

Either as a community member or health clinician, if you are concerned someone may be at risk of suicide, direct questions about suicidal thoughts and feelings must be asked. Given the increased risk of suicide with psychiatric disorders, it is sound practice for a risk assessment to be undertaken by a mental health clinician formally trained in conducting suicide risk assessment and intervention planning. Risk assessment is a required competency for mental health professionals when working with suicidal clients, as outlined by the National Practice Standards for the Mental Health Workforce 2013.[75] As part of a risk assessment, key variables shown by evidence to increase risk (e.g. current suicide ideation, previous suicide attempts and resolved plans and preparations) are specifically assessed.[76] Box 23.6 lists a sample of typical suicide risk assessment questions.

BOX 23.6 Sample of suicide assessment questions

Current mood

- How are you feeling now? (Probe for severity)
- How do you feel when you think about the future? Are you hopeful you can do something about your problems?

Suicidal thoughts

- Have you been thinking about suicide recently?
- When you think about suicide, what kinds of thoughts do you have? How frequent? Duration?
- What are some of the reasons you would consider attempting suicide?

Plans and access

- Have you made any plans for attempting suicide? For example, have you obtained the means to complete suicide, like purchasing a gun or obtaining pills? Do you have access to rope/gun/pills etc?
- Do you have the confidence that you could attempt suicide?

History

- Have you ever attempted suicide previously? (Probe for lethality, detail, rehearsal, rescue)
- Have you ever deliberately harmed yourself? For example, cut yourself, swallowed pills or burned yourself?

Risk factors

- Do you use alcohol/drugs?
- Tell me about your support system. Do you feel isolated? Are you able to talk to friends and family about your problems?

Source: Cukrowicz KC, Wingate LR, Driscoll KA et al. A standard of care for the assessment of suicide risk and associated treatment: the Florida State University Psychology Clinic as an example. J Contemp Psychother 2004; 34(1):87–100. With permission of Springer.

Additional Australian resources relevant to suicidality include:*

- Mental Health First Aid Australia. Suicidal thoughts and behaviours: First aid guidelines. www.mhfa.com.au
- Government — local acute mental health/triage services. Australian practitioners and the public may seek further advice from their local acute mental health/triage service. Examples of 24-hour government triage services include: Queensland, 24-hour government-operated mental health services which can be reached on 1300MHCALL (1300 64 2255) and NSW, where 24-hour support is available on the Mental Health Access Line 1800 011 511. Other Australian states such as Victoria have separate triage numbers for their local public hospitals
- Suicide Callback Service: 1300 659 467 www.suicidecallbackservice.org.au

While the treating mental health clinician (e.g. psychologist) would typically formulate a coping plan with the patient, if you as the treating naturopathic practitioner were concerned about the risk level of a patient, provide them with the following 24-hour support services* as part of a coping plan while also liaising with the other treating professionals:

- Emergency services: 000
- Government acute care/triage number (e.g. QLD — 1300MHCALL (1300 64 22 55))
- Suicide Callback Service: 1300 659 467
- Lifeline: 13 11 14
- Domestic Violence Hotline (QLD): 1800 811 811
- Kids Helpline: 1800 551 800

*Note: these resources/contact details may be changed or updated over time. Please check the relevant organisation's website for the most current details.

MANDATORY REPORTING OF CHILD NEGLECT AND ABUSE

As part of assessing risk, the treating mental health clinician would also assess for 'vulnerability risk' (e.g. sexual assault risk, self-neglect) and for 'child protection risk'. However, naturopathic practitioners should be aware of the legislative requirement imposed on selected classes of people to report suspected cases of child abuse and neglect to government authorities. Legal requirements for reporting vary by state and the reader is strongly encouraged to visit the Australian Government's Australian Institute of Family Studies website, especially regarding mandatory reporting of child abuse and neglect.

- Main website: www.aifs.gov.au
- Reporting: https://aifs.gov.au/cfca/bibliography/mandatory-reporting

FUTURE TRAINING?

While discussion of assessing risk for violent behaviour is beyond the scope of this chapter, clinicians would do well to undertake further training in this area given that Andersen's review of studies showed the potential for aggressive and violent behaviour in mental health settings is up to four times greater than in general medical settings.[77] It is strongly recommended that naturopaths be trained in mental health first aid to ensure the best outcomes for their patients.

Therapeutic considerations

OBJECTIVES

To provide guidance for best practice and management of mood disorders based on scientific evidence and expert clinical consensus, the National Institute for Health and Care Excellence (NICE) in the United Kingdom and the Royal Australian and New Zealand College of Psychiatrists (RANZCP) provide clinical practice guidelines (CPGs) for the assessment and treatment of mental health disorders. The CPGs are intended for clinical use not only by medical doctors and psychologists, but for anyone involved in mental healthcare and the treatment of individuals with mood disorders, which includes naturopaths. If a clinician suspects a patient is experiencing depressive or other mental health symptoms and the clinician is 'not competent to perform a mental health assessment, they should refer the person to an appropriate professional. If this professional is not the person's GP, inform the GP of the referral'.[78] The evidence for informing these treatment guidelines is tied to diagnosis, thus it is imperative to have a correct diagnosis for the patient so the correct evidence-informed treatment can be commenced.
You will find NICE guidelines for depression at: www.nice.org.uk

Drawing from a biopsychosocial approach to understanding and treating psychological disorders Fig. 23.5, derived from the recently released 2015 RANZCP CPGs, has expanded on the BPSL model previously employed by mental health clinicians to specifically address lifestyle factors such as diet as a foundational strategy in treating mood disorders, as seen in 'Step 0'.[8] While achieving a healthful dietary pattern has been the historical naturopathic treatment for assisting depression/anxiety, achieving a healthy diet is now being formally recognised as an evidence-based treatment strategy, with the CPGs noting the 'exponential rise' in scientific evidence linking higher dietary quality with reduced risk for depression.[8] This treatment approach aligns with the CPG-recommended biological investigations, which make more reference to checking for nutritional deficiencies and inflammatory/microbial pathology tests where appropriate than earlier guidelines or those from NICE.[8]

Nutritional medicine

A NUTRITIONAL APPROACH TO PSYCHOLOGICAL DISORDERS

Therapeutic nutrition can take multiple forms, from correction of basic dietary choices and practices, right through to using nutrients as supplements in a more pharmacological manner. Each aspect of nutritional medicine should be considered in each patient for best outcomes.

NUTRITIONAL MEDICINE

Dietary correction

Many would argue that dietary correction typically constitutes the starting place for a nutritional approach and this remains pertinent in mental health. Educating and supporting patients with regard to the basic healthy eating tenets, such as regular food intake, balanced blood sugar, whole food choices, caffeine and alcohol minimisation, can have a powerful normalising or corrective effect on mood. These basic principles should always constitute the first nutritional treatment objectives. See Chapter 3 for a detailed discussion of naturopathic nutritional medicine philosophy.

There is a growing body of evidence to support the understanding that different diets can either reduce or increase vulnerability to depression and anxiety. Studies have confirmed this in adolescents, with a clear correlation between increasing unhealthy eating behaviours and higher incidence of symptomatic depression.[79,80] In

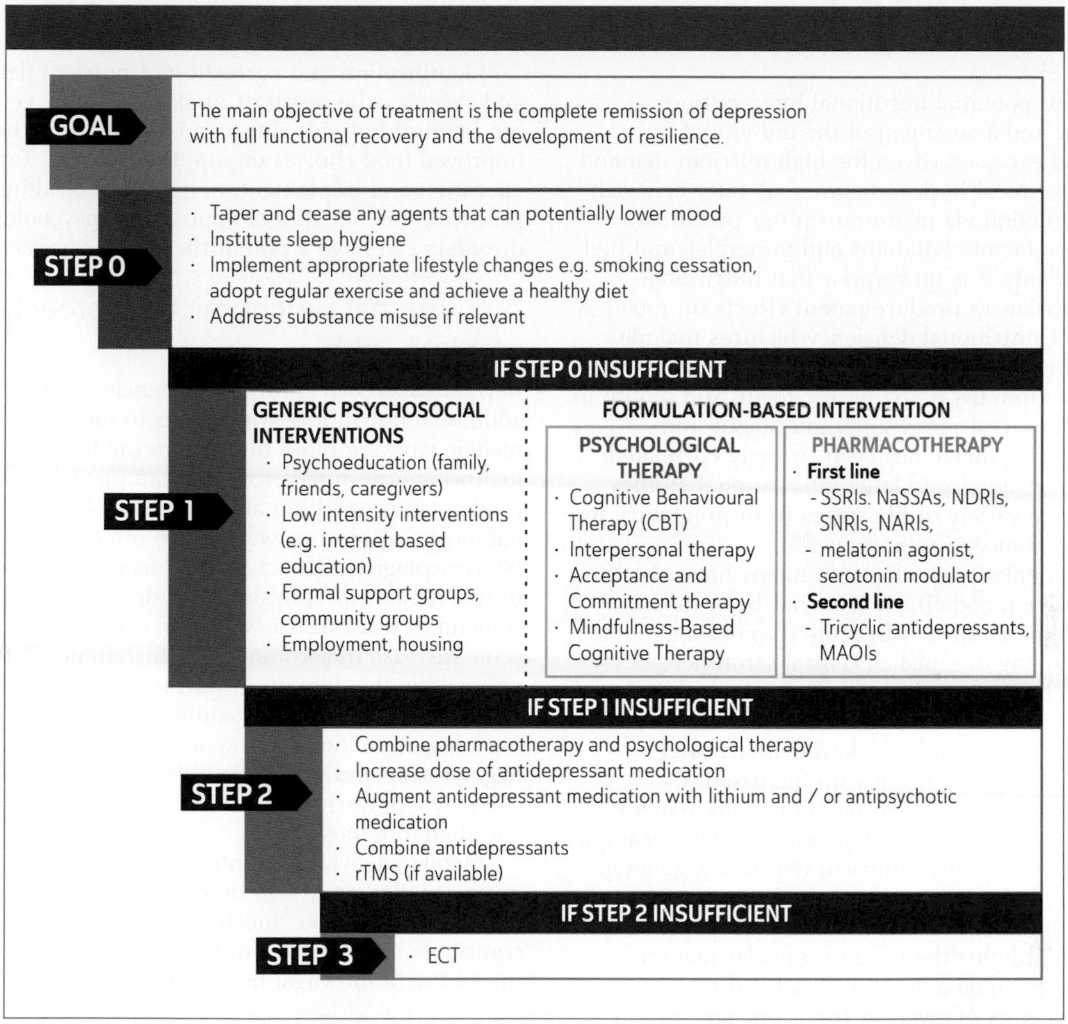

GOAL
The main objective of treatment is the complete remission of depression with full functional recovery and the development of resilience.
STEP 0
· Taper and cease any agents that can potentially lower mood
· Institute sleep hygiene
· Implement appropriate lifestyle changes e.g. smoking cessation, adopt regular exercise and achieve a healthy diet
· Address substance misuse if relevant
IF STEP 0 INSUFFICIENT
STEP 1
GENERIC PSYCHOSOCIAL INTERVENTIONS
· Psychoeducation (family, friends, caregivers)
· Low intensity interventions (e.g. internet based education)
· Formal support groups, community groups
· Employment, housing
FORMULATION-BASED INTERVENTION
PSYCHOLOGICAL THERAPY
· Cognitive Behavioural Therapy (CBT)
· Interpersonal therapy
· Acceptance and Commitment therapy
· Mindfulness-Based Cognitive Therapy
PHARMACOTHERAPY
· First line
- SSRIs. NaSSAs, NDRIs, SNRIs, NARIs,
- melatonin agonist, serotonin modulator
· Second line
- Tricyclic antidepressants, MAOIs
IF STEP 1 INSUFFICIENT
STEP 2
· Combine pharmacotherapy and psychological therapy
· Increase dose of antidepressant medication
· Augment antidepressant medication with lithium and / or antipsychotic medication
· Combine antidepressants
· rTMS (if available)
IF STEP 2 INSUFFICIENT
STEP 3
· ECT

Schematic illustration of step-wise management of major depressive disorder: In Step 1 a whole host of interventions and therapies need to be considered and choice of treatment should be based on individual formulation. Note the various steps are not necessarily sequential and in some instances treatment may commence with options from Step 2 and Step 3.

FIGURE 23.5 Management of major depressive disorder.

Source: Malhi GS, Bassett D, Boyce P et al. Royal Australian and New Zealand College of Psychiatrists clinical practice guidelines for mood disorders. Aust N Z J Psychiatry 2015; 49(12):1087–1206.

addition, females (but not males) aged 20 to 79 years consuming a 'healthy dietary pattern' (characterised by high intakes of wholegrains, vegetables, fruits, fish, nuts and seeds) recorded lower depression scores on the Patient Health Questionnaire-9 (PHQ-9).[81] In this latter study, based on data from over 8000 individuals from the National Health and Nutrition Examination Survey (NHANES), those women in the highest quintile for healthy eating patterns had an OR of 0.6 for depression (CI): 0.42–0.85, P <0.001, which translates to roughly a 40% reduced likelihood of being diagnosed with depression compared with women eating less healthy diets. Not all studies exploring this relationship, however, have found a statistically significant correlation between diet and depression symptoms independent of other factors[82] and the current consensus is that there is limited evidence and an urgent need for more research.

A counter-argument to the diet→mood association is one of reverse causality; for example, patients with mental health issues make poorer dietary choices as a result of impaired appetite and self-care;[83] however, a study which specifically explored this possibility found this was not likely to be the explanation.[84] Prospective studies of diet and subsequent depression incidence have focused on adherence to the Mediterranean diet (characterised by plant-dominated foods: vegetables, fruit, nuts and unprocessed cereals and relatively low intake of both meat and dairy).[85] One key study investigating the dietary patterns of over 8000 women aged 50 to 55 years found that higher consumption of a Mediterranean diet was associated with lower incidence of depression during the subsequent 3 years. The authors concluded that consumption of a Mediterranean-style dietary pattern by middle-aged women may have a protective influence against the onset of depression.[85]

Correction of nutritional deficiencies and excesses

The next level of potential nutritional intervention involves review and assessment of the individual for deficiencies and excesses. Given the high nutrient demand of the CNS in terms of basic structure (e.g. fatty acid rich membranes), function via neurotransmitter precursors (amino acids), co-factors (vitamins and minerals), and fuel (glucose dependent), it is no surprise that nutritional deficits and imbalances produce potent effects on mood. A large number of nutritional deficiency pictures include psychological impairment, such as the deficiencies associated with vitamins B_1, B_3, B_6, B_{12}, folate and biotin; in addition to the minerals, iron, zinc, and magnesium. Inadequate omega-3 intake has been strongly correlated with depression incidence in large international studies and across a wide variety of life stages from pregnancy to childhood, adolescence to senescence.[86]

Amino acid depletion studies in humans have also produced negative mood effects. This has been most convincingly demonstrated with acute tryptophan depletion, producing diminished central serotonergic transmission, which can induce or trigger a relapse of depression in vulnerable people, such as patients with chronic MDD in remission,[87] or detrimentally alter emotional processing consistent with increased vulnerability to a depressive episode in healthy patients with a strong family history of depression.[88] This example of the interaction between a nutrient deficiency, genotype and depression phenotype underscores the increasing complexity in the nutritional management of psychological disorders and highlights the need to consider factors beyond basic nutritional adequacy as defined by recommended dietary allowances (i.e. a 'one size fits all' approach). Therefore, individual genetic, biochemical and psychological factors need to be considered together.

While there are additional nutritional deficiencies that are found to occur at higher rates in depressed cohorts[89] (e.g. vitamin D), depression is not traditionally thought to be part of the deficiency picture of these nutrients, and follow-up intervention studies have failed to provide evidence of benefit in depressed individuals. Correction of these deficiencies is still important in the whole-care approach to these patients but is not likely to improve mood.

Due to high comorbidity between depression and substance use, the nutritional impact from recreational and illicit substances may play a major role in declining nutritional status of the depressed or anxious patient. A good example of this is the potent folate depletion seen with alcohol use. Several small studies of alcoholics found correction of this depletion via folate supplementation produced significant reductions in depression scores.[90] In addition to promoting increased intake of these negatively affected nutrients, reduced drug use is of course also important to address as the source of ongoing nutrient depletion.

The psychological impact from nutritional excesses is less well documented and understood; however, there is evidence to suggest copper excess[61] and manganese toxicity (most likely from occupational or environmental exposure)[91] can produce psychiatric presentations.

Identification and correction of nutrient deficiencies and excesses, the result of intake, exposure, genetic and biochemical individuality, can be achieved either via improved food choices or supplementation. Together with education and implementation of basic healthy dietary practices, this nutritional approach to psychological disorders can have a potent therapeutic impact.

A nutritional biochemical approach to mental health

Beyond basic correction of deficiencies and excesses, additional nutritional approaches to mental health may include working more directly on the hypothesised neurochemical imbalance; for example, increasing production or working at the receptor level, or other pathophysiological drivers. These often necessitate pharmacological-like actions but using nutrients in lieu of drugs. While supraphysiological doses of nutrients can sometimes work in this way (e.g. excess B_3 can produce an acute increase in serotonin and histamine),[92] this is particularly the domain of nutraceuticals, such as S-adenosyl methionine, theanine, phosphatidyl serine and high-dose individual amino acids or amino acid derivatives (e.g. tyrosine and 5HTP). In this form, nutritional medicine can play a powerful direct role in changing neurochemistry and therefore mood.[93,94]

Mood-beneficial probiotic supplements, recently termed 'psychobiotics', may also be regarded as having 'pharmacological-like' mechanisms, via their ability to both contribute to neurotransmitter production and directly interact with the vagal nerve.[95,96]

GENERAL DIETARY TREATMENTS

In line with Step 0 of the CPGs, the following section highlights the importance of adopting a healthful dietary pattern and addressing substance misuse (e.g. illicit drugs, nicotine, alcohol, caffeine) in relation to managing depression.

Dietary therapeutic objectives

- Encourage regular food intake to maintain stable blood sugar levels and varied nutrient consumption
- Focus on 'wholefood' choices such as vegetables, fruits, unrefined grains, unprocessed protein, nuts and seeds
- Include regular lean-quality red meat
- Increase dietary sources of omega-3 essential fatty acids
- Minimise caffeine and alcohol.

KEY DIETARY INCLUSIONS

Nutrient-dense wholefoods

Diets characterised by plant-dominated foods, or of a Mediterranean-style with varied vegetables, fruit, fish, nuts and seeds have been shown to have a protective effect against depression. A varied, nutrient-dense diet also promotes a diverse intake of vitamins and minerals, addressing potential deficiencies associated with psychological impairment.

SAMPLE DAILY DIET

BREAKFAST

Smoothie: avocado, spinach, banana, oats and chia seeds	Diet should be nutrient dense and wholefood in composition to provide resilience. Adults following a wholefood dietary pattern have a reduced risk of developing depression compared to those following a higher processed food dietary pattern. Diets characterised by low intakes of nutrient-dense foods and higher intakes of unhealthy foods are each independently associated with smaller left hippocampal volume. Altered hippocampal function and smaller hippocampus are seen in individuals with depression. Oats are a source of B vitamins which are required for proper neuronal function. Raw greens and avocado are both excellent sources of folate. Folate deficiency is associated with increased risk of depression as folate is needed in the brain for the synthesis of noradrenaline (norepinephrine) serotonin, and dopamine. As well as folate, leafy greens are also a source of magnesium. Magnesium plays a vital modulatory role in brain biochemistry, influencing several neurotransmission pathways associated with the development of depression. The addition of chia seeds provides fatty acids and fibre.

LUNCH

Sardines with salad greens, capers, sweet potato, avocado, sauerkraut and beetroot relish	High intake of fish is associated with reduced risk of depression; constituents in fish are thought to change membrane microstructure modifying serotonergic and dopaminergic neurotransmission. Potatoes are a source of carbohydrates. Adequate wholefood carbohydrates are required since carbohydrate intake increases the plasma ratio of tryptophan to other large neutral amino acids. The gut microbiota play a role in influencing behaviour and mood in humans and may interact bidirectionally with diet hence optimal fibre and intake of fermented foods, if tolerated, are advocated.

DINNER

Turkey san choy bow made with turkey mince, tamari, rice vermicelli, carrots, corn, coriander, shallots	Turkey is a source of tryptophan which is as a precursor for production of neurotransmitter serotonin. In-vivo research suggests that high inflammatory and oxidative states may deplete tryptophan; however, it is hypothesised that by combining tryptophan with antioxidants brain tryptophan levels may be more available for serotonin, hence the benefit of consuming turkey with ample vegetables and herbs. Turkey is also rich in zinc. Low dietary zinc is associated with depression.

SNACK

Walnuts Fresh fruit salad Dark chocolate	Walnuts are highly antioxidant, folate rich and contain ALA, a precursor of eicosapentaenoic acid (EPA) and docosahexaenoic acid (DHA). DHA assists with modulation of serotonin and dopamine concentrations which may influence mood. Walnut consumption over a period of 8 weeks has been shown to improve mood in healthy young adult males, but had no effect in females. Higher fruit and vegetable consumption is related to fewer internalising and externalising behaviours in adolescents. Chocolate is proposed to impact mood by increasing tryptophan and resultant synthesis of serotonin, leading to mood modulation. Chocolate must be low in protein (i.e. preferably dark chocolate) to exert this action.

Dipnall JF, Pasco JA, Meyer D et al. The association between dietary patterns, diabetes and depression. J Affect Disord 2015 Mar 15; 174:215–224; Eby GA, Eby KL. Rapid recovery from major depression using magnesium treatment. Med Hypotheses 2006; 67(2):362–370; Fava M, Mischoulon D. Folate in depression: efficacy, safety, differences in formulations, and clinical issues. J Clin Psychiatry 2009; 70 Suppl 5:12–17; Finkelmeyer A, Nilsson J, He J et al. Altered hippocampal function in major depression despite intact structure and resting perfusion. Psychol Med 2016 Jul; 46(10):2157–2168; Jacka FN, Cherbuin N, Anstey KJ et al. Western diet is associated with a smaller hippocampus: a longitudinal investigation. BMC Med 2015 Sep 8; 13:215; Jacka FN, Pasco JA, Mykletun A et al. Association of Western and traditional diets with depression and anxiety in women. Am J Psychiatry 2010; 167: 305–311; Li F, Liu X, Zhang D. Fish consumption and risk of depression: a meta-analysis. J Epidemiol Community Health 2016 Mar; 70(3):299–304; Li Z, Li B, Song X, Zhang D. Dietary zinc and iron intake and risk of depression: a meta-analysis. Psychiatry Res 2017 Feb 3; 251:41–47; Møller SE. Serotonin, carbohydrates, and atypical depression. Pharmacol Toxicol 1992; 71:61–71; Oddy WH, Robinson M, Ambrosini GL et al. The association between dietary patterns and mental health in early adolescence. Prev Med 2009; 49: 39–44; Opie RS, O'Neil A, Itsiopoulos C et al. The impact of whole-of-diet interventions on depression and anxiety: a systematic review of randomised controlled trials. Public Health Nutr 2015 Aug; 18(11):2074–2093; Pribis P. Effects of walnut consumption on mood in young adults—a randomized controlled trial. Nutrients 2016; 8(11):668; Serefko A, Szopa A, Poleszak E. Magnesium and depression. Magnes Res 2016 Mar 1; 29(3):112–119; Silva NR. Chocolate consumption and effects on serotonin synthesis. Arch Intern Med 2010 Sep 27; 170(17):1608; author reply 1608–1609; Strasser B, Gostner JM, Fuchs D. Mood, food, and cognition: role of tryptophan and serotonin. Curr Opin Clin Nutr Metab Care 2016 Jan; 19(1):55–61.

Essential fatty acids

Include omega-3 fatty fish in diet such as salmon, sardines, anchovies, herring, tuna, or mackerel. Increase other essential fatty acid containing foods such as walnuts, chia seeds, avocado, flaxseed oil, dark leafy greens.

Protein

Assess protein requirements of the individual and ensure adequate intake. Protein plays an important role in blood sugar regulation and also provides substrates for neurotransmitter synthesis.

SUBSTANCE MISUSE MANAGEMENT

Substance misuse can be a comorbid issue for individuals with mood or anxiety disorders. As such, implementing lifestyle changes to manage substance misuse (e.g. alcohol, illicit drugs, nicotine, caffeine) can have therapeutic effects upon mood.

Caffeine (found in energy drinks, soft drinks, coffee, regular tea and chocolate) is a stimulant that can negatively impact mood in high doses (500 mg), so management of caffeine misuse is recommended, particularly in patients with anxious features. Those prone to anxiety disorders may have a genetic vulnerability (e.g. adenosine SNPs) that may lead to increased sensitivity to the stimulating effects of caffeine.

Alcohol has anti-nutrient actions, depleting the body of many essential nutrients; therefore, alcohol misuse should be managed appropriately. While treatment of substance misuse is recommended to help mood, it should be remembered that with all substances, including caffeine, individuals can develop drug dependence, leading to withdrawal symptoms when levels are reduced and thus possible mood/sleep deterioration as part of the withdrawal process.

OTHER DIETARY CONSIDERATIONS

Reduce pro-inflammatory foods such as processed meats, alcohol, sugar and additives. Increase antioxidant intake by including a rainbow of wholefoods (fruits, vegetables, grains, legumes) in the diet. Include anti-inflammatory herbs and spices such as turmeric and ginger.

HERBAL MEDICINE

Specific herbal medicine classes for psychological disorders

Many herbal medicines are available to naturopaths for use in the management of psychological disorders. It needs to be noted that herbal medicines need to be used with due consideration of prescribed psychotropic medications because of the potential to interact. Limited evidence is available for the efficacy of herbal medicines in the treatment of more complex psychological disorders; therefore, practitioners are advised to consult with specialist mental health practitioners, such as psychiatrists and psychologists, when treating people with these conditions. Table 23.3 provides a summary of commonly prescribed herbal medicines for the treatment of common psychological disorders and their medicinal actions.

ADAPTOGENS

Adaptogenic substances assist the body to adapt to, or cope with, stressors (either psychological or physical). They are also considered tonics that revitalise and restore physiological function to the body. Herbal adaptogens include *Centella asiatica, Eleutherococcus senticosus, Schisandra chinensis, Rhodiola rosea* and *Withania somnifera.* Adaptogens with antidepressant action include *Panax ginseng* and *Rhodiola rosea.*

ADRENAL RESTORATIVES

Adrenal restoratives are substances that restore functioning of the adrenal glands. The two primary herbs used are *Glycyrrhiza glabra* and *Rhemannia glutinosa.*

ANTI-INFLAMMATORIES

Anti-inflammatory substances reduce inflammation in the body. The anti-inflammatory action occurs via a variety of mechanisms, such as decreasing cytokines. Anti-inflammatory herbs relevant to psychological disorders include *Centella asiatica, Curcumin longa, Echinacea* spp., *Matricaria recutita* and *Rhodiola rosea.*

ANTIDEPRESSANTS

Herbal antidepressants act in various ways, primarily in the nervous system, to reduce depression symptoms; for example, they may inhibit the reuptake of neurotransmitters such as serotonin, noradrenalin (norepinephrine) and dopamine, or act as neuro-endocrine modulators.[97] These herbs include *Crocus sativus, Curcumin longa, Echium amoenum, Hypericum perforatum, Lavendula angustifolia* and *Rhodiola rosea.*

ANXIOLYTICS

An anxyolitic substance has the effect of reducing anxiety symptoms. This effect has been found most commonly to act on the GABA system; however, it may also involve regulation of the stress response via the HPA axis.[98] These herbal medicines may also have a sedative effect at higher doses. Herbal medicines in this class are used to treat anxiety and related disorders, and include *Bacopa monnieri, Ginkgo biloba, Centella asiatica, Piper methysticum, Melisa officinalis, Matricaria recutita, Passiflora incarnata, Rhodiola rosea, Salvia* spp., *Scutellaria lateriflora, Valeriana officinalis* and *Withania somnifera.*

COGNITION ENHANCERS

Cognition-enhancing substances improve various aspects of cognitive functioning, including problems with learning, memory, alertness and concentration that often occur as features of anxiety, depression and other mental health disorders. Herbs that have been shown to have cognitive-enhancing effects include *Bacopa monnieri, Camellia sinensis, Ginkgo biloba, Melissa officinalis, Rosmarinus officinalis* and *Salvia* spp.

NERVINE STIMULANTS

Herbal nervine stimulants increase energy by stimulating the nervous system; examples include *Camellia sinensis, Coffea arabica, Eleuthrococus senticosis, Panax ginseng* and *Rosemarinus officinalis.*

TABLE 23.3 Commonly prescribed herbal medicines for the treatment of psychological disorders and their medicinal actions

Herbal medicine	Adaptogen	Adrenal restorative	Anti-inflammatory	Antidepressant	Anxiolytic	Cognition enhancer	Nervine stimulant	Nervine tonic	Sedative/relaxant
Bacopa monnieri			X		X	X		X	X
Centella asiatica	X		X		X			X	X
Curcuma longa			X	X					
Eleuthorococcus senticosis	X					X	X	X	
Ginkgo biloba			X		X	X			
Hypericum perforatum				X				X	
Lavandula angustifolia				X					X
Matricaria recutita			X		X			X	X
Melisa officinalis				X		X			
Panax ginseng	X						X		
Passiflora incarnata					X			X	X
Piper methysticum					X			X	X
Rehmannia somnifera		X	X						
Rhodiola rosea	X		X	X	X	X	X		
Rosmarinus officinalis				X		X	X	X	
Salvia spp.						X			
Valeriana officinalis					X			X	X
Withania somnifera	X		X		X	X			X

NERVINE TONICS/TROPHORESTORATIVES

Nervine tonics help restore tone and assist to strengthen the nervous system; these include *Avena sativa, Centella asiatica, Hypericum perforatum, Schizandra chinensis, Scutellaria laterifolia, Turnera diffusa, Verbena officinalis* and *Withania somnifera.*

SEDATIVES (HYPNOTICS)/RELAXANTS

Herbal sedatives/hypnotics/relaxants often act via the same biochemical pathways as herbal anxiolytics. Many of the herbal anxiolytics mentioned above have sedative actions that are dose dependent (i.e. higher doses = sedation, lower doses = anxiolysis). Herbal sedatives and relaxants are particularly useful when sleep problems occur with anxiety, depression and other mental health problems. Herbal sedatives include *Eschscholzia californica, Piper methysticum, Matricaria recutita, Melissa officinalis, Passiflora incarnata, Scutellaria lateriflora, Valeriana officinalis* and *Zizyphus spinosa.*

Psychological therapies

Evidence-based practice (EBP) is a particular method for delivering healthcare and should strongly influence the chosen psychological treatment. Mental health conditions are posing an increasing social and economic burden on society and, with a multitude of treatments available, it is important to choose a treatment that has evidence for being effective for the particular condition and one which does not cause harm. For example, exposure-based therapies have been shown to be highly effective in treating different anxiety disorders.[99] Yet, despite these therapies being a first-line treatment for such disorders, an overview of research by Kaplin and Tolin[99] revealed that only a small proportion of patients typically receive exposure therapy that seeks to reduce anxiety via encouragement of the patient to systematically approach feared external or internal triggers. Insomnia can also be a comorbid issue with anxiety, and similarly new research reveals a specific form of cognitive behavioural therapy (CBT) for insomnia (known as CBT-i) has had remarkable success and superiority to sleep medications.[100] Yet again, Barlow notes how CBT-i, despite being acknowledged as a first-line treatment for insomnia by the American Academy of Sleep Medicine, is under-utilised by clinicians who are said to be still largely unaware of such treatments. A variety of evidence-based psychological therapies for MDD and GAD exist, including CBT, interpersonal therapy (IPT) and mindfulness-based cognitive therapy (MBCT).

SECTION B

DEPRESSION

Description and classification

The DSM-5 highlights a family of depressive disorders, including disruptive mood dysregulation disorder, major depressive disorder, persistent depressive disorder (dysthymia), premenstrual dysphoric disorder, substance/medication-induced depressive disorder, depressive disorder due to another medical condition, other specified depressive disorder, and unspecified depressive disorder.[2] A core feature in all disorders is the existence of a mood disturbance (either sad, empty or irritable mood), in addition to both cognitive and somatic changes that impair the person's functioning.[2] This chapter focuses on one of these disorders, namely major depressive disorder (MDD). Clinicians should note that if symptoms of clinical depression are suspected, referral to a health professional competent in undertaking a comprehensive mental health assessment to enable accurate diagnosis and risk assessment is imperative,[78] particularly given depressive symptoms can overlap with bipolar and psychotic symptoms along with increased risk for suicidality.

Differentiating between clinical depression, sadness and grief

Depression differs from typical mood fluctuations and reactions to daily life challenges, with depressive symptoms typically occurring 'most of the day, nearly every day' during at least a 2-week period. Clinical depression may be classified using the DSM-5 or the International Classification of Diseases (ICD-10). Criteria for Major Depressive Episode (MDE) taken directly from DSM-5 (p. 160),[2] are as follows:

A Five (or more) of the following symptoms have been present during the same 2-week period and represent a change from previous functioning; at least one of the symptoms is either (1) depressed mood or (2) loss of interest or pleasure.
Note: Do not include symptoms that are clearly due to a general medical condition, or mood-incongruent delusions or hallucinations.
1 Depressed mood most of the day, nearly every day, as indicated by either subjective report (e.g. feels sad or empty) or observation made by others (e.g. appears tearful). Note: In children and adolescents, can be irritable mood.
2 Markedly diminished interest or pleasure in all, or almost all, activities most of the day, nearly every day (as indicated by either subjective account or observation made by others).
3 Significant weight loss when not dieting, or weight gain (e.g. a change of more than 5% of body weight in a month), or decrease or increase in appetite nearly every day. Note: In children, consider failure to make expected weight gains.
4 Insomnia or hypersomnia nearly every day.
5 Psychomotor agitation or retardation nearly every day (observable by others, not merely subjective feelings of restlessness or being slowed down).
6 Fatigue or loss of energy nearly every day.
7 Feelings of worthlessness or excessive or inappropriate guilt (which may be delusional)

nearly every day (not merely self-reproach or guilt about being sick).

8 Diminished ability to think or concentrate, or indecisiveness, nearly every day (either by subjective account or as observed by others).

9 Recurrent thoughts of death (not just fear of dying), recurrent suicidal ideation without a specific plan, or a suicide attempt or a specific plan for committing suicide.

B The symptoms cause clinically significant distress or impairment in social, occupational, or other important areas of functioning.

C The episode is not attributable to the physiological effects of a substance or to another medical condition.

D The occurrence of the major depressive episode is not better explained by schizoaffective disorder, schizophrenia, schizophreniform disorder, delusional disorder, or other specified and unspecified schizophrenia spectrum and other psychotic disorders.

E There has never been a manic episode or a hypomanic episode.

Note: In distinguishing grief from an MDE, it is useful to consider that in grief the predominant affect is feelings of emptiness and loss, while in MDE it is persistent depressed mood and the inability to anticipate happiness or pleasure. The dysphoria in grief is likely to decrease in intensity over days to weeks and occurs in waves, the so-called pangs of grief. These waves tend to be associated with thoughts or reminders of the deceased. Table 23.4 shows these MDE symptoms in an easy-to-assess mnemonic to aid your recall of symptoms.

TABLE 23.4 Major depressive episode symptoms using the mnemonic DIGS-E-CAPS

2-week duration of 5 or more of the following symptoms, 1 of which includes either depressed mood or loss of interest/pleasure:	
1	**D**epressed mood (sad or irritable)
2	**I**nterest/pleasure loss (can lead to social/activity withdrawal, lack of sexual desire)
3	**G**uilt or worthlessness
4	**S**leep disturbance (insomnia or hypersomnia)
5	**E**nergy loss/fatigue
6	**C**ognitive symptoms (decreased concentration ability or indecisiveness)
7	**A**ppetite change or weight loss/gain
8	**P**sychomotor agitation or retardation (e.g. agitation — pacing, inability to sit still, rubbing of skin/clothing, or retardation — slowed speech, thinking, body movements)
9	**S**uicidality

Source: Barlow DH, Ellard KK, Sauer-Zavala S et al. The origins of neuroticism. Perspect Psychol Sci 2014; 9(5):481–496.

Epidemiology

A review of research in relation to depression reveals the following:

- Depression is one of the most common psychiatric disorders and is estimated to affect approximately 350 million people worldwide.[101] Lifetime prevalence estimates reveal a significant proportion (30%) of the United States population will experience a major depressive episode at some during their life.[102] Almost half (45%) of Australians are estimated to experience a psychiatric disorder of some kind during their lifetime,[103] with antidepressant medication taken by more than 1 in 10 Americans aged 12 and over[104] and with Australia also having one of the highest rates of antidepressant use in the world.[105] Twelve-month prevalence rates for major depressive disorder are estimated at 9% for the United States[102] and 6% in Australia.[103]
- Onset of depression can occur at any age, but incidence significantly increases with puberty.[2] Age-of-onset is most common in adults aged early to mid-twenties.[106] In contrast to ageist myths, rates of depression decline into older adulthood, with 12-month prevalence rates for Australians peaking at 8% in middle adulthood (35 to 45 years) and only 4% for those 66 years and over.[103]
- Depression is the leading cause of disability, with the burden estimated to be 50% higher for females than males.[107] Internationally for women depression is: twice as high as in men, it is their most common mental health problem and is possibly more chronic in course.[108] In women there is a higher risk of suicide attempts compared to males who have higher rates of suicide completion.[2]
- Depression has a high comorbidity with other psychiatric disorders (e.g. anxiety disorders, substance misuse, eating disorders and borderline personality disorder) and co-occurs commonly with health conditions (e.g. cardiovascular disease, diabetes, cancer, osteoporosis, obesity). It should be differentiated from premenstrual dysphoric disorder or a mood disorder induced by a medication/substance or a medical condition.[2,109,110] Clinicians should also note that bipolar spectrum disorders often begin with a major depressive episode,[2] and that antidepressant use has been linked to increased risk for mania.[111,112] While recovery from depression commonly starts within 3 months of onset for approximately 40% of individuals and within 1 year for 80%, chronic depressive symptoms considerably increase the probability of an underlying personality disorder, anxiety or substance misuse disorder.[2]
- Recurrence of depression is not uncommon, with various studies showing relapse rates of 50% to 80%.[113] While various psychotherapy options exist (e.g. emotional freedom technique and so on), given the worldwide social and economic costs associated with depression, it is imperative that naturopaths consider options for which there is current evidence that they prevent relapse of depression. An important finding in depression treatment, described by Young and colleagues, is how patients treated with cognitive therapy only or in

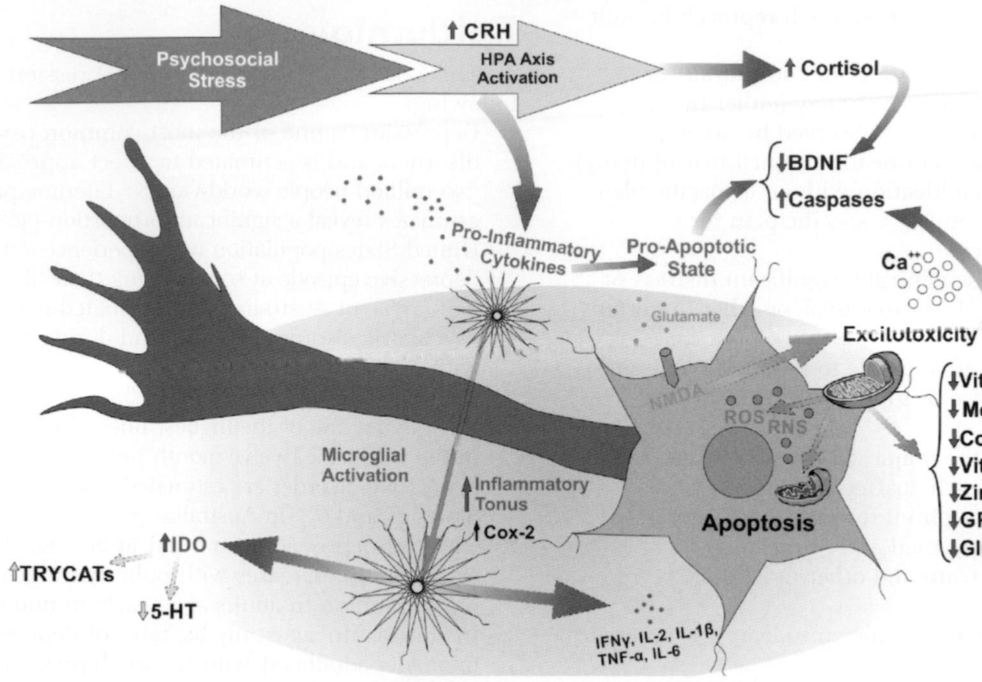

FIGURE 23.6 Pathways implicated in the progressive cognitive decline of MDD.

Source: Carvalho AF, Miskowiak KK, Hyphantis TN et al. Cognitive dysfunction in depression — pathophysiology and novel targets. CNS Neurol Disord Drug Targets (formerly Curr Drug Targets) 2014; 13(10):1819–1835. Permission conveyed through Copyright Clearance Center, Inc.

combination with medication have lower relapse rates than do patients using medication only; numerous studies reveal far lower relapse rates for cognitive therapy than for antidepressants (e.g. 12% vs 66%).[114]

- The potential side effects of a treatment are also an important consideration; for example, antidepressants commonly have unwanted side effects such as lowered sexual functioning or have been associated with increased suicide risk.[114] Currently there is an increasing recognition in research of dietary/lifestyle factors correlating with MDD (Fig. 23.6) but further evidence and intervention trials are needed to quantify the efficacy of such factors as treatments, a viewed shared by Berk and colleagues.[115]

Note: Pathways include: an overactive HPA axis; a decrease in BDNF and neurotrophic support; excitotoxicity through over-stimulation of glutamate NMDA receptors which leads to an increase in intracellular Ca2+ and activation of pro-apoptotic caspases (e.g. caspase 3); an increase in the generation of ROS and RNS along with decreased levels of antioxidants and/or decreased activities of antioxidant enzymes (e.g. GPX, glutathione) leading to oxidative and nitrosative stress; increased production of pro-inflammatory cytokines (e.g. IFNγ and IL-1β) by the activated microglia; inflammatory cytokines stimulate the enzyme IDO which metabolises tryptophan resulting in a decrease in 5-HT and melatonin. Some TRYCATs are neurotoxic and depressogenic; cyclooxygenase-2 (cox-2) is increased in MDD.

Signs and symptoms

The DSM-5 highlights how sleep disturbance and loss of energy are common presenting symptoms in people with depression, and that failure to probe for any associated depressive symptomology may lead to under-diagnosis of an MDE. Psychomotor changes are less common, but are indicative of increased symptom severity. While depressed mood is a core feature of an MDE, in children and adolescents the presentation may be more of irritable mood rather than a sad mood.[2] Men may also present with more irritable rather than sad mood, with many possibly going undetected due to diagnostic biases, for example:

> *Doctors are more likely to diagnose depression in women compared with men, even when they have similar scores on standardized measures of depression or present with identical symptoms.*[108]

Given the growing ageing population in Australia, increased consideration of older adult mental health is warranted. While mood disorder prevalence declines over the life span, Beattie et al (2010) warn that when depression is experienced in older adults, the duration is generally chronic with lower remission rates[116] — attributable to increased comorbidity of medical conditions, dementia, and more limited tangible social support.[117] Older adults often present with more somatic complaints particularly when the depression is comorbid with anxiety. When such comorbidity is present in older adults, overall psychopathology is more severe with increased suicide ideation and attempts.[116] One study showed that for 60% of older adults with MDD alone, recovery time was on average just under 1 year (300 days).[118] For those with comorbid MDD and GAD, recovery time was extended by some 300 days, with 60% taking approximately 600 days to remit.[118]

Differential diagnosis and comorbidities

The DSM-5[2] encourages consideration of the following differential diagnoses:

- Manic episodes with irritable or mixed episodes
- Mood disorder due to another medical condition
- Substance/medication-induced depressive or bipolar disorder
- Attention-deficit/hyperactivity disorder
- Adjustment disorder with depressed mood
- Sadness.

Many medical conditions can also mimic depression:

- Endocrine (e.g. hypo- or hyperthyroidism; Cushing's/Addison's disease)
- Neurological (e.g. Parkinson's disease, dementia)
- Immunological (e.g. viral conditions/pneumonia, 'sickness behaviour')
- Cardiovascular (e.g. stroke, heart disease)
- Substance/medication induced (e.g. withdrawal symptoms from cocaine, medications that can cause depression. Includes antibiotics, antimicrobials, antifungals, antivirals, cardiac and blood pressure medication and insomnia aids/sedatives among others).

Common comorbidities as indicated by the DSM-5:

- Substance-related disorders
- Anxiety disorders (e.g. panic disorder, obsessive-compulsive disorder)
- Anorexia nervosa, bulimia nervosa and borderline personality disorder.

See Box 23.7 for preexisting conditions associated with depression.

BOX 23.7 Preexisting conditions associated with depression

Acquired immunodeficiency syndrome (AIDS)
Addison's disease
Angina
Cancer (particularly of the pancreas)
Cerebral arteriosclerosis, cerebral infarction
Cushing's disease
Diabetes
Electrolyte abnormalities (e.g. hypernatraemia, hypercalcaemia, hypokalaemia, hyperkalaemia)
Folate and thiamine deficiencies
Hepatitis
Hypoglycaemia
Hypothyroidism, hyperthyroidism, hyperparathyroidism
Influenza
Intracranial tumours (malignant or benign)
Myocardial infarction
Parkinson's disease
Pernicious anaemia
Porphyria
Renal disease
Rheumatoid arthritis
Senile dementia
Syphilis
Systemic lupus erythematosus
Temporal arteritis
Temporal lobe epilepsy
Viral pneumonia

Source: Birrer RB, Vemuri SP. Depression in later life: a diagnostic and therapeutic challenge. Am Fam Physician 2004 May 15; 69(10):2375–2382.

Investigations: psychometric

The following denotes some of the self-report psychometric tools freely available to assess depressive symptoms in adults.

DASS-21

The Depression, Anxiety and Stress Scale — Short Version (DASS-21) is a tool with good psychometric properties that can be used for screening and discriminating between three emotional states and also symptom severity.[119] This scale was originally developed using a sample of individuals aged from 17 to 69 years and the scale was used previously with adolescents down to 14 years of age. Exercise caution when using the scale with adolescents, bearing in mind the individual's literacy skills and that there is limited validity data for younger samples. A more specific version is currently being constructed and tested for this youth population. Higher DASS-21 scores reflect greater severity (which can be compared against established cut-offs of severity). However, it must be acknowledged that the DASS-21 is not diagnostic, with 'no direct implications for the allocation of patients to discrete diagnostic categories' such as those in the DSM-5.[120]

The DASS may be administered and scored by non-psychologists, but decisions based on particular score profiles should be made only by experienced clinicians who have carried out an appropriate clinical examination. It should be noted also that none of the DASS items refers to suicidal tendencies because items relating to such tendencies were found not to load on any scale. The experienced clinician will recognise the need to determine the risk of suicide in seriously disturbed persons.[120]

More details and current research regarding the DASS-21 and its use can be found at: www2.psy.unsw.edu.au/dass/

PATIENT HEALTH QUESTIONNAIRE-9 (PHQ-9)

The PHQ-9 is a brief scale of nine items that is suitable for screening and monitoring of depression, with item content reflecting DSM-5 criteria for an MDE. The scale has good psychometrics (e.g. sensitivity and specificity of 88% each for depression with a cut-off of ≥10) along with cut-offs for severity levels. A 2010 study looked at using the PHQ-9 among 13–17-year-olds found a cut-off score ≥11 had a sensitivity of 90% and a specificity of 78% for detecting youth with clinical depression.[121] A modified version of the PHQ-9 for adolescents is also available online with wording adapted for this population.

GERIATRIC DEPRESSION SCALE — SHORT FORM (GDS-S)

The GDS-S is a unique depression-screening tool designed specifically for use with older adults aged 60 years and over.[122] The GDS-S is an easy-to-use scale comprised of 15 self-report items and a dichotomous (yes/no) response format. The GDS-S has demonstrated adequate psychometric statistics (Cronbach's $\alpha = 0.75$; and a sensitivity of 81% and specificity of 75% with a cut-off score of 6 for differentiating depressed from non-depressed older adults).[122,123] The original longer version 30-item GDS has very good psychometrics and provides additional cut-off scores for different severity levels.[122]

SCOFF

Given the highlighted comorbidity between depression and various eating disorders, and with many individuals with eating disorders instead seeking treatment for the factors known to perpetuate their eating disorder (e.g. weight loss and dieting), it is imperative that clinicians, particularly if providing dietary advice, screen for the presence of an eating disorder.[124] Recent research revealed poor detection rates with 'almost 4 in 10 psychologists, 7 in 10 natural therapists and 8 in 10 fitness instructors failing to detect a general eating disorder in a case scenario depicting bulimia, with the latter two groups more likely to believe the problem was a self-esteem issue'.[124] Use of standardised eating disorder screeners such as the SCOFF was remarkably low, with only 5% of practitioners using any standardised assessment tools.[124] Results revealed a strong need to increase practitioner literacy and, as a minimum, encourage the implementation of standardised and simple screening measures[124] such as the SCOFF[125] in front-line health practices. This is particularly important given the increased mortality and morbidity rates associated with eating disorders.[124] The SCOFF has good psychometric properties and within a primary care setting the SCOFF has been found to have a sensitivity of 85% and specificity of 90%.[126] A positive screen on the SCOFF is considered to be a score of 2 or more.

Note. Unlike the more sophisticated and restricted psychometric instruments, it must be remembered that these scales *do not* include impression management scales (to detect whether an individual may be 'faking good' and giving socially desirable answers, or 'faking bad' which could occur where a gain is to be had; e.g. monetary gain/insurance). Any psychometric scale data should also be triangulated or cross-verified with other clinical data (e.g. with clinical interview information and with objective observable signs/MSE information). Clinicians should also consider that while an individual can be of a certain age to complete the scale, results may be rendered invalid due to the individual's literacy level, cultural background and any medication or drugs taken.

Therapeutic application

OBJECTIVES

As naturopathy is based on the premise of biochemical individuality, the therapeutic objectives when treating depressed patients will depend on the sum effect of the combination of each patient's presenting features, pathophysiological drivers, psychosocial components, genetics, diet, lifestyle and health-related behaviours. This holistic approach requires extensive investigation that will take time; however that is often not possible in real-world practice. In the context of patients presenting with psychological disorders which can be severe, symptomatic treatment is often necessary and relief of depressive symptoms should remain the primary objective, whether CAM interventions are adjunctive or stand-alone.

As a result of the significant biopsychosocial contributors to depression, patients typically require a team approach; for example, naturopath, psychologist and GP. Therefore, another key objective for CAM practitioners in the management of depressed patients is to actively communicate with and contribute to the patient's healthcare team in a way that ensures best patient outcomes. See 'The healthcare team' below.

In the treatment of depressed patients the objectives of any CAM intervention are:

- Reducing depressive symptoms and stabilising mood
- Actively participating in and facilitating a healthcare team approach
- Determining and treating the underlying pathophysiological factors contributing to depression symptoms (e.g. stress, inflammation, methylation, pyrroles)
- Supporting healthy diet, exercise and lifestyle behaviours
- Managing associated symptoms (e.g. low energy, cognitive dysfunction and sleep disturbance)
- Addressing any secondary nutritional issues that may have arisen due to altered appetite and impaired self-care
- Addressing secondary physical symptoms that may be comorbid with depression (e.g. gut function).

Nutritional medicine

The therapeutic objective when using nutritional medicine to treat depression symptoms will depend on each person's unique presentation, dietary and nutritional context and pathology markers; therefore, a holistic approach is essential. It is important to note that the underlying psychosocial factors contributing to depression need to be addressed, in addition to any prescribed treatment. When choosing appropriate nutritional interventions, therapeutic objectives include:

- Reducing depression symptoms and stabilising mood
- Determining and treating the underlying pathophysiological factors contributing to depression symptoms (e.g. inflammation, methylation, pyrroles)
- Supporting improved food choices and good dietary practices in the face of altered appetite and impaired self-care
- Addressing secondary nutritional issues that may have arisen as a consequence of depression (e.g. vitamin D deficiency secondary to reduced time outdoors).

NUTRITIONAL MEDICINE (SUPPLEMENTAL)

Following are some of the most commonly used nutrients and nutraceuticals for treating depression, with supportive scientific evidence.

Folate

Given folate's central role in neurotransmitter synthesis and maintenance of healthy homocysteine levels, it is not surprising that it has been a key nutrient of interest in depression research, as both a stand-alone and adjunctive treatment.

EVIDENCE OF EFFICACY

Although earlier trials reported some positive results using the synthetic form, folic acid, a recent systematic review and meta-analysis challenges these findings and suggests folate's efficacy in depression is restricted to the active forms, in particular methylfolate at a dose of 15 mg/day, when used in combination with pharmaceutical antidepressants.[94]

However, there may be more to this story. The findings of one review of 10 studies of various forms of folate (with or without B_{12} and B_6) investigated as either a stand-alone or adjunctive treatment in depressed cohorts, concluded that while short-term studies failed to demonstrate efficacy, long-term supplementation, for example for ≥1 year, improved response to treatment, particularly in those individuals with elevated homocysteine at baseline.[127]

The other related consideration is that earlier folate intervention studies principally used patients with confirmed folate deficiency. Many clinical trials since, however, have administered folate as a treatment independent of patients' baseline folate status. There is strong evidence that blood folate levels tend to be lower in depressed populations which may be explained by the documented over-representation of folate polymorphisms (genetic variants that result in impaired utilisation of folate) in depressed populations.[128] However, very few studies investigating the efficacy of supplemented folate for depression have taken patients' genetics or even baseline folate status into account. One exception to this is an observational study in which pregnant women were given folic acid or placebo and followed up over 21 months postpartum to assess if supplementation reduced the risk of developing postpartum depression (PPD).[129] While the researchers found folic acid supplementation was not associated with depression scores generally across the sample, there was a particularly strong protective effect against subsequent development of PPD for those women with the most severe folate polymorphism: C677T homozygotes.

The primary safety concern regarding folate supplementation is in individuals with cancer, because of the theoretical risk of increasing cell proliferation.[94] Although meta-analyses have failed to reveal a definite relationship, caution should be encouraged.

S-adenosyl-methionine (SAMe)

SAMe is a naturally occurring amino acid derivative that is produced via the methylation cycle in the presence of adequate folate and B_{12} and constitutes the key 'methyl donor' in humans. This means that SAMe is central to the production of catecholamines, clearance of serotonin and histamine and enhances activity of both dopamine and noradrenaline (norepinephrine).[62]

EVIDENCE OF EFFICACY

There is a general consensus in the scientific literature that SAMe has demonstrated efficacy in the treatment of depression, as either a stand-alone treatment or as an adjunct to pharmaceutical antidepressants.[62] In particular SAMe, at doses between 800–1600 mg/day, has produced antidepressant effects comparable to those of both citalopram (an SSRI) and a range of tricyclic antidepressants,[62] with fewer side effects.[130] SAMe supplementation has also been found to be superior to placebo as an adjunct to standard antidepressants[130] for partial and non-responders to SSRIs and SNRIs.[131,132]

While both a recent Cochrane review[130] and a meta-analysis[94] have been critical of the quality of studies investigating SAMe in the treatment of depression, when many of the earlier Italian studies are excluded, SAMe is still regarded as having significant potential as an antidepressant. Researchers agree that larger studies of better design are now needed and more detailed information needs to be collected on the safety and side-effect profile of this nutraceutical, particularly given its capacity to induce mania in bipolar patients when administered intravenously or intramuscularly.[94] This makes it an unsuitable antidepressant choice for bipolar patients.

Given naturopathy's emphasis on biochemical individuality, Sarris and colleagues' ongoing research to elucidate which sub-groups of depressed individuals are most likely to benefit from SAMe are pertinent.[94,133] Initial findings suggest that depressed males may be more likely than females to positively respond to SAMe.[133]

Long-chain omega-3 fatty acids (LCPUFA-n3) — EPA

In spite of widespread epidemiological data documenting poor omega-3 status with a range of depressive disorders, including major depression, postpartum depression and seasonal affective disorder, and extensive evidence of the role of inflammation in depression,[134] there are surprisingly few interventional studies using fish oils in depressed patients. Those studies that have been done differ markedly in their forms, doses and other key study characteristics, making comparisons and conclusions difficult.[94,135] In spite of this there is a general consensus that improved LCPUFA-n3 levels has the potential to both prevent and treat depression.

ACTIONS

Fatty acids are major components of the brain and are found in high concentrations in two structural components: the neuronal membrane and the myelin sheath. About 50% of the neuronal membrane is composed of fatty acids (one-third from LCPUFA-n3), while in the myelin sheath lipids constitute about 70%.[136] The lipid component has a relatively high turnover, in contrast to the protein component, which is fundamentally stable.

LCPUFA-n3 play an active role in neuronal membrane function, fluidity and control of neuronal growth factors. They also potentially influence each step in biogenic amine function, including neurotransmitter synthesis, degradation, release, reuptake and binding.[137] Studies indicate that omega-3 fats may influence noradrenergic and serotonergic neurotransmission and receptor function in the nervous system and thus have a direct effect on function, mood and behaviour.

Recent reviews have focused on eliminating the confounding issue of variable omega-3 forms and dose used across the studies.[138–140] These reviews appear to have reached a consensus regarding the superiority of EPA over DHA for depression.[138] In particular, the research postulates that interventions providing >60% EPA and a minimum of 200–2200 mg EPA in excess of DHA were more effective. Although DHA is the more prevalent LCPUFA-n3 in the brain and possesses actions that would make it likely to be helpful in depression, several theories are proposed about why this does not translate into clinical effectiveness. Oral DHA supplementation has not been shown conclusively to increase brain DHA levels. In addition, it is EPA that directly competes with arachidonic acid for conversion to eicosanoids and therefore EPA may have the most relevant anti-inflammatory action.

EVIDENCE OF EFFICACY

Several placebo-controlled trials and open-label studies have investigated omega-3 supplementation in MDD and in depression associated with bipolar disorder, typically as an adjunct to psychiatric medication. In spite of substantial differences in the form and doses used as well as study design, recent reviews and a meta-analysis conclude that LCPUFA-n3 supplementation is superior to placebo for reducing depression severity and they concur with the finding of Sublette et al that greatest benefit is seen in those patients treated with supplements containing a higher EPA:DHA.[32,94]

The dosage range of EPA has varied between 930 mg and 4.4 g; however, the most common regimen used in both research and practice is 1–2 g/day.[94] If using a combination EPA and DHA supplement, then ensuring >60% EPA and a minimum of 200–2200 mg EPA in excess of DHA will produce best results.[138] All studies report good tolerance and, importantly, it is safe in children, pregnant women and patients at risk of mania.[141]

N-acetylcysteine (NAC)

N-acetylcysteine (NAC) is an acetylated form of the amino acid cysteine. This small modification translates to better stability, bioavailability and therapeutic potential beyond that of its amino acid precursor.[142,143] NAC has attracted particular interest in relation to its antioxidant and anti-inflammatory properties, making it a key nutraceutical for investigation, given the current inflammatory theory of depression.

ACTIONS

The chemistry of NAC means that it may modulate key pathophysiological processes that have been implicated in a wide range of psychological disorders, including depression. These actions include:[142]

- Antioxidant via increased glutathione levels
- Anti-inflammatory — ↓ TNFα, IL-1β, IL-6, IL-10 and suppressed microglial activation
- Glutaminergic modulation — suppressing excessive levels of glutamate release in the brain
- NMDA receptor modulation
- Regulation of dopamine-induced neurotoxicity
- Enhanced activity and protection of mitochondria
- Modulation of intracellular calcium
- Inhibition of neuronal apoptosis and promotion of neurogenesis.

EVIDENCE OF EFFICACY

Studies employing NAC for psychological disorders have spread over a wide range of diagnoses from addiction to autism. As a result, there isn't a concentration of NAC studies in major depressive disorder specifically. However, from the limited studies conducted in MDD, together with evidence of efficacy for NAC in bipolar-related depression, researchers generally regard NAC as a 'promising treatment'.[144] NAC has been administered at 2 g/day (in divided doses) as an adjunct to standard pharmaceutical treatment. When compared with placebo in the largest study to date, the addition of NAC produced statistically significant improvement in multiple outcomes; however, depression scores, response and remission rates did not become statistically significant until 16 weeks.[13]

Generally, oral NAC across clinical trials in a range of areas, not just depression, has proven to be well tolerated, with a low side-effect profile. Adverse effects reported as part of clinical trials have most commonly been mild gastrointestinal symptoms including abdominal pain, flatulence, heartburn, nausea and vomiting. Overall, however, rates of adverse effects appear to be comparable with placebo in most studies and very few studies have reported cases where discontinuation has been necessary.[144]

Zinc

Several studies have documented a correlation between low zinc levels and depression incidence generally[43,50] and, according to one study, in treatment-resistant depressed patients specifically.[145] Animal studies of induced zinc deficiency reliably producing depression-like behaviour resolved with zinc repletion add to this association, and we are now seeing the results of some human clinical trials using zinc as the intervention for depressed patients.[43,50] Currently there are only a small number of these studies and findings are preliminary; however, there is a strong rationale for its therapeutic potential in this area and some promising indications emerging from these trials.

ACTIONS

The brain possesses the highest zinc content of any organ in the body and it is particularly concentrated in the hippocampus, amygdala, cerebral cortex and olfactory bulbs.[146,147] Zinc has diverse critical roles within the brain, acting both as a co-factor to multiple enzymes and directly in regulatory roles. Its actions relevant to depression include:[31,146,148,149]

- Anti-inflammatory actions by reducing nuclear factor-kappaB (NF-κB), TNF-alpha and interleukin-beta[150–152]
- Modulation of neuronal excitability by inhibition of both GABA and glutamate receptors
- Increasing brain-derived neurotrophic factor (BDNF)
- Dopamine reuptake inhibition
- Roles in neurogenesis and synaptic plasticity
- Normalisation of the hypothalamic pituitary adrenal (HPA) axis — deficiency leads to activation.

EVIDENCE OF EFFICACY

Although several studies have been conducted using zinc as an intervention for depression, current conclusions are principally based on three small higher quality studies which all administered 25 mg of elemental zinc per day adjunctive to antidepressants over 12 weeks.[50,94] These studies produced largely positive results with statistically significant reductions in depression scores over placebo. An interesting study not included in these reviews administered 50 mg elemental zinc over 12 weeks to multiple sclerosis patients concurrently experiencing moderate to severe MDD.[148] The results of this study found that there was a statistically significant reduction in depression scores for those taking zinc. Other focus areas of research in zinc and depression have been in postpartum depression[153–155] and in the elderly;[156] again there is epidemiological evidence of a correlation between poor zinc status and incidence in these populations but no well-designed intervention studies to confirm efficacy as yet.

In terms of safety and tolerance, oral zinc at doses of 50–150 mg/day commonly produces mild gastrointestinal distress. Although acute toxicity would necessitate doses in the range of 4–8 g/d, single doses of 225–450 mg of zinc have been reported to induce vomiting and long-term excessive intake may induce a copper deficiency.[157]

L-tryptophan (L-Trp) and 5-hydroxytryptophan (5HTP)

The amino acid tryptophan is the precursor to serotonin via its intermediate metabolite, 5HTP. In numerous studies L-Trp deficiency has been demonstrated to correlate with depression development in susceptible individuals[87,88] and recently data from almost 30 000 individuals as part of the National Health and Nutrition Examination Survey (NHANES) 2001–2012 found a correlation between low L-Trp intake and self-reported depression and sleep duration.[158]

Given the dominance of the monoamine model of depression since the 1950s, interventions that increase serotonin such as SSRIs have attracted a strong rationale and L-Trp and 5HTP fall under this category. Consequently, much of the research into these two nutrients took place in the 1960s and 1970s, with the majority demonstrating efficacy for L-Trp or 5HTP as adjuncts to tricyclic antidepressants.[94]

In the current climate of reduced emphasis on the monoamine theory and the emergence of other models such as the 'inflamed brain', these serotonergic precursors continue to maintain some relevance. Specifically, this is because CNS inflammation leads to reciprocal changes in tryptophan metabolism, favouring production of the excitotoxic kynurenine and quinolinic acid at the expense of serotonin.[159]

From a supplement perspective, 5HTP has several advantages over L-Trp related to increased bioavailability, bioactivity and no concerns regarding contamination.[160]

ACTIONS

Both Trp and 5HTP are precursors to serotonin and therefore may promote increased serotonin production.[160]

EVIDENCE OF EFFICACY

Over 30 studies have investigated the use of 5HTP as either a stand-alone or adjunctive treatment. Several of these compared the efficacy of 5HTP as a monotherapy against a pharmaceutical antidepressant, with two demonstrating equal efficacy and another two studies suggesting 5HTP was less effective than a monoamine oxidase inhibitor (MAOI). The highest quality of 5HTP's evidence of efficacy comes from augmentation studies.[160]

A recent review of the evidence for L-Trp and 5HTP specifically as adjunctive treatments in depression included eight studies of variable quality.[94] Doses of L-Trp varied between 3–6 g/day and 5HTP was administered at 300 mg/day over 4–12 weeks. Four out of seven tryptophan studies found positive effects (note four of the seven studies used a DL-form which is less potent due to only 50% bioactivity) and one study of 5HTP also produced a superior antidepressant effect when compared with placebo.

For best results, 5HTP should be administered in divided doses, with some reviewers suggesting t.d.s. dosing as the ideal regimen, which also helps to reduce any associated nausea with the supplement.[160] Adverse effects associated with 5HTP are most commonly gastrointestinal (nausea, vomiting, diarrhoea) as a result of conversion into serotonin in the gut. Headaches, insomnia and palpitations have also been reported, which more likely signal an increase in CNS serotonin.[160]

Historically, there were safety concerns about both L-Trp and 5HTP borne out of a spate of deaths caused by supplemental L-Trp which led to eosinophilia myalgia syndrome (EMS). This event precipitated the banning of L-Trp as a supplement in many countries; however, subsequent research into the cause of these deaths has strongly suggested that they were the result of batch contamination but this is still debated.[160,161] Importantly, no new cases of EMS have been reported since 1998 and retrospectively authors have pointed out that 5HTP has never been implicated as the cause.[160]

The primary current safety concern regarding supplemental L-Trp or 5HTP, particularly when used in combination with other serotonergic agents (e.g. SSRIs), is the risk of serotonin syndrome. Animal studies suggest 5HTP doses of 100–200 mg/kg bodyweight are necessary to produce serotonin syndrome when administered alone and while there remains a theoretical risk for humans when combined with powerful serotonergic medications, as previously reported, 5HTP has frequently been employed in studies as an adjunct to antidepressants and no reports of this occurring have been made.[160]

Herbal medicine

The therapeutic objective when choosing herbal medicines to treat depression symptoms will depend on each person's unique presentation; therefore, a holistic approach is essential. It is important to note that the underlying psychosocial factors contributing to depression need to be addressed in addition to any prescribed herbal treatment. When choosing appropriate herbal medicines therapeutic objectives include:

- Reducing depression symptoms and stabilising mood
- Determining and treating the underlying factors contributing to depression symptoms (e.g. stress and inflammation)
- Managing associated symptoms (e.g. low energy, cognitive dysfunction and sleep disturbance)
- If chronic stress is involved, enhancing immune function and reducing oxidative stress
- Restoring nervous system function
- Addressing secondary physical symptoms that may be comorbid with depression (e.g. gut function).

Following are some of the most commonly used herbs for treating depression with both evidence of traditional use and scientific evidence. Note that the herbal medicines *Hypericum perforatum, Rhodiola rosea,* and *Lavendula angustifolia* covered in this section also have anxiolytic actions and are suitable for treating anxiety symptoms.

Hypericum perforatum (St John's wort)

Hypericum perforatum is a perennial with characteristic bright-yellow flowering tops, belonging to the *Guttiferae* family. This herb has a long history of traditional use for nervous system conditions, and is the most widely studied herb for the treatment of depression.

More than 150 different constituents have been identified in *Hypericum perforatum.* These include naphthodianthrons (hypericin, pseudohypericin), phloroglucinols (hyperforin, adhyperforin), amino acids (GABA), xanthons (norathyriol), phenylpropanes (caffeic acid, chlorogenic acid), flavonoids (quercetin, hyperoside, rutin), bioflavonoids (biapigenin), procyanidins and essential oils.[162] Of these constituents hypericin and hyperforin have been studied extensively for their antidepressant action, though other constituents have been identified as having antidepressant potential, suggesting that there is not one single constituent that is responsible for the antidepressant effects.

A number of different explanations have been proposed to explain *Hypericum perforatum*'s mechanism of action. These include:

- Monoamine oxidase (MAO) inhibition by both hypericin and flavonoids[162]
- Nonspecific inhibition of reuptake of serotonin, noradrenaline (norepinephrine), dopamine, GABA by hyperforin (in vitro)[162]
- Suppression of interleukin 6 (modulator of cortisol release)[162]
- Inhibition of catechol-O-methyltransferase (catalyses degradation of catecholamine neurotransmitters; e.g. dopamine, adrenaline (epinephrine) and noradrenaline (norepinephrine)).[162]

EVIDENCE OF EFFICACY

There is good evidence of the efficacy of *Hypericum* in the treatment of mild-to-moderate depression. While there is some evidence for *Hypericum*'s efficacy in severe depression, overall the research is inconclusive; therefore, use of *Hypericum* as a stand-alone treatment for severe depression is not recommended. A recent systematic review including 35 studies evaluated the efficacy and safety of *Hypericum* in MDD.[163] *Hypericum* was found to significantly improve depression symptoms compared to placebo and demonstrated equal efficacy to antidepressant pharmacotherapies; however, there was no difference between treatments in remission on follow-up (4 to 6 weeks post treatment), or relapse of depression (only assessed in one study). Another meta-analysis comparing pharmacological treatments for depressive disorders in primary care found that *Hypericum* extracts were equally as effective as conventional pharmacotherapies, with fewer adverse events.[164] While the pharmacokinetic properties of *Hypericum* are considered to be poor compared to antidepressant pharmacotherapies, there is a similar onset of action (4 to 6 weeks) and fewer side effects.[162]

There is good evidence for the efficacy of *Hypericum* in the short-term treatment of mild-to-moderate depression; however, more research is needed to establish the safety and efficacy of longer term treatment in more chronic forms of depression. The use of *Hypericum* for the treatment of major depression should only be considered in consultation with specialist mental health practitioners, such as psychiatrists. Dosage of *Hypericum* is dependent on standardisation, and ranges between 900 and 1800 mg per day (standardised to 0.3 % of hypericin and/or 1–5 % of hyperforin).

Rhodiola rosea

Rhodiola rosea has a long history of traditional use in Europe that is reputed to date back to the Vikings.[165] The traditional uses reported in Swedish materia medica from the 1700s included 'enhancing intellect', being a 'tonic against infirmity', and used to 'restore weak nerves'.[165] *Rhodiola* has now been widely studied for its effects on the nervous system and the stress response.

Numerous biologically active constituents have been identified in *Rhodiola* including rosavin, rhodioloside and salidroside. The following is a summary of *Rhodiola*'s pharmacological effects as identified in a review of the research literature:[165]

- Adaptogenic and stress-protective (neuro-cardio and hepato-protective)
- Cardioprotective
- Antioxidant
- Stimulation of the central nervous system including effects on cognitive functions such as attention, memory and learning
- Anti-fatigue
- Antidepressive and anxiolytic
- Endocrine activity normalising
- Life-span increasing.

EVIDENCE OF EFFICACY

A systematic review of randomised controlled trials (RCTs) on the efficacy of *Rhodiola* found evidence for the herb's effectiveness in reducing depression symptoms in patients with mild-to-moderate depression, and improved stress-related fatigue.[166] In a more recent study,[167] *Rhodiola* treatment reduced depression symptoms in patients with MDD to a lesser extent than the conventional pharmacotherapy (sertraline). This reduction was not statistically significant for either treatment; however, *Rhodiola* was better tolerated with significantly fewer adverse events. The results from this study may be related to the dosage regimen used. Another study on adults with mild-to-moderate depression demonstrated *Rhodiola* extract SHR-5 at two doses (340 mg/day and 680 mg/day) over 6 weeks significantly reduced depression symptoms compared to placebo, in addition to significant improvement in the depression-related symptoms of insomnia and somatisation.[168]

Rhodiola is indicated for mild-to-moderate depression, especially when stress-related symptoms are also involved. The most frequently studied extract is SHR-5 capsules standardised to rosavin 3.07%/rhodioloside 1.95%. The recommended dose is 300 to 680 mg per day (4 : 1 herb/extract ratio, 70% ethanol).

Lavandula angustifolia (lavender)

Lavandula angustifolia is a perennial evergreen indigenous to the Mediterranean and its use as a herbal medicine dates back to ancient times.[169] Lavender is best known for its use as an essential oil in aromatherapy; however, it is also used as a whole plant medicine with sedative, anxiolytic, antidepressant, carminative and antibacterial actions. Clinical trials have demonstrated *Lavandula* spp. to be effective in reducing depression symptoms in patients with mild-to-moderate depression. One clinical trial found that although *Lavandula angustifolia* significantly reduced depression symptoms, it was not as effective as imipramine (tricyclic antidepressant); however, when the treatments were combined they were more effective than either treatment alone.[170] The volatile oil linalool appears to be responsible for the antidepressant effect, which occurs via GABA modulation.[97]

Lavandula angustifolia is indicated for mild-to-moderate depression especially when there is also sleep disturbance. It may also be used as an adjunctive treatment with imipramine in consultation with the prescribing health practitioner. The recommended dose based on traditional use is 2–4.5 mL daily (1 : 2 liquid extract), or as a tea 1.5 g flowers or leaves steeped in 150 mL of boiling water. The dose used in the previously mentioned study was 60 drops daily (1 : 5, 50% alcohol).

Crocus sativus (saffron)

Crocus sativus, otherwise known as saffron, has not been widely used in Western herbal medicine; however, it has a history of traditional use in Western Asia and Iran as an anxiolytic, hypnotic, antidepressant, aphrodisiac, stimulant and adaptogen.[171,172] In recent years there has been an increasing body of evidence for the efficacy of *Crocus sativus* in the treatment of depression.

A systematic review found six studies evaluated the efficacy of *Crocus sativus* on depression symptoms in adults with MDD.[173] All RCTs reviewed used a dose of 15 mg twice daily; however various preparations, standardisation, and plant parts (stigma or petal) were used, for between 6 and 8 weeks. Treatment with *Crocus sativus* significantly improved mild-to-moderate depression symptoms compared to placebo, and had similar efficacy to antidepressant pharmacotherapy. Significant improvements in depression symptoms were seen following 1 week of treatment with progressive improvement over the 6 to 8 weeks.

Crocus sativus is an effective herb for the treatment of mild-to-moderate depression in MDD; however, its safety has only been evaluated in short-term treatment (8 weeks). When considering the secondary actions *Crocus* would be indicated in depression with associated sleep disturbance and fatigue. The effective dose for reducing depression symptoms is 30 mg/day.

Psychological

As outlined previously, the NICE and RANZCP guidelines for treating depression include a stepped care approach, in which, depending on the severity of the individual's depression, different treatment approaches are used:

- Risk assessment and monitoring
- Addressing diet/lifestyle factors
- Low-intensity psychosocial interventions (e.g. self-guided CBT, online CBT such as MoodGYM, structured group physical activity/support programs)
- Intensive psychological approaches (e.g. higher frequency individual CBT, IPT, short-term psychodynamic therapy or behavioural couples therapy) or combining the prior interventions with medication
- Brain stimulation methods indicated for severe or treatment-resistant patients.[78]

Given high relapse rates, CBT or mindfulness-based cognitive therapy is recommended in terms of relapse prevention.[78,114] Box 23.8 outlines some of these approaches as in the RANZCP CPGs.[8]

BOX 23.8 RANZCP CPGs: common psychological therapies for treating MDD

CBT Cognitive-behavioural therapy (CBT) aims to modify dysfunctional cognitions and related behaviours that are presumed to maintain depression. Among evidence-based psychological therapies, CBT is the most widely researched treatment for depression, and it is recommended by all international guidelines.

IPT Interpersonal psychotherapy (IPT) is a brief structured approach that addresses interpersonal issues and role transitions. It has Level I evidence for the treatment of major depression. IPT has Level I evidence for both acute depression and depression maintenance/relapse.

MBCT and **ACT** Recently developed structured therapies, such as mindfulness-based cognitive therapy (MBCT) and acceptance and commitment therapy (ACT) have not been evaluated as thoroughly as CBT and IPT, but appear to be effective in reducing depressive symptoms and in preventing relapse of depression (specificity for subtype and/or severity of depression remains unclear). MBCT may be better for patients prone to worry and ACT may be best for patients needing to accept and adjust to persisting problems.

Source: Malhi GS, Bassett D, Boyce P et al. Royal Australian and New Zealand College of Psychiatrists clinical practice guidelines for mood disorders. Aust N Z J Psychiatry 2015; 49(12):1087–1206.

Lifestyle recommendations

There are several environmental factors that contribute to the onset and maintenance of MDD and GAD symptoms. Some of these are social- or lifestyle-related factors that are modifiable. The RANZCP BPSL model denotes various social factors that may require management or treatment which can include: family psychoeducation; engaging with/or developing a supportive social network; addressing employment, finances and housing factors. It is the role of the naturopath to support their patients to adopt lifestyle changes to assist in managing depression symptoms and prevent relapse once in recovery. The lifestyle recommendations applied in MDD are also relevant to GAD, and other common mental health problems. Lifestyle treatments can comprise: exercise, diet, smoking/alcohol/drug cessation, managing substance misuse, and sleep.

EXERCISE

Physical activity is critical for maintaining both physical and mental health. Studies have demonstrated the benefits of exercise in reducing depression and anxiety symptoms and associated oxidative and nitrogen stress. One critical review concluded that exercise is preventive of some mental disorders, and there are positive effects of exercise on depression and anxiety symptoms.[174] A more recent review of 37 meta-analyses on the effects of exercise on anxiety and depression found that while exercise was beneficial for reducing both anxiety and depression symptoms, there was a greater benefit for depression.[175] The review also found that exercise was more beneficial for patients compared with symptom-free individuals. Large effect sizes were found for prescribed exercise programs lasting between 10 and 26 weeks. There is currently no clear evidence for the type, frequency and duration of exercise that provides the most benefit for each type of mental health condition; however, it is clear that some exercise is better than none.

There are inherent difficulties in getting patients with anxiety and depression to change health behaviours which relate to the nature of the mood disorders (involving sleep, appetite and energy issues for example) and the individual characteristics of the patient (e.g. personality, and social environment). Empowering a patient to enable behaviour change requires a unique set of skills that draw on psychological principles described above.

The healthcare team

There are several immutable reasons for electing, wherever possible, to work as part of a team of practitioners when treating patients with depression. The first relates to the patient who presents without a diagnosis, as a consequence of the long list of differential diagnoses that require consideration. See 'Differential diagnoses' above. The exclusion of differentials and confirmation of an MDD diagnosis requires the knowledge and skills of other health professionals (e.g. psychologists, psychiatrists, general practitioners). In the instance that a patient presents with an established diagnosis of MDD or GAD, the need for accurate ongoing monitoring of the severity of the illness arises. While naturopaths can and should administer validated depression and anxiety rating scales as part of their patient management, this remains rudimentary if practitioners have not undergone additional training in psychology. In addition, the insights of the psychologist or psychiatrist who cares for the same patient are critical.

Beyond identification, assessment and monitoring, working as part of a healthcare team with depressed patients is also fundamental to best treatment outcomes. Consistent with our recognition of the BPSL model of depression, all of these contributing elements require equal addressing. Naturopaths and GPs principally treat within the biological realm and many patients with psychological disorders present already taking medications. Therefore, communication and collaboration between the naturopath and the prescribing physician regarding a dual biological approach is important. Psychologists, psychiatrists and social workers are, for example, better placed to offer evidence-based psychological and social support and skills development.

The success of any healthcare team is overwhelmingly dependent on open reciprocal communication between the various practitioners, once the patient has granted permission for this to occur. Even in those instances where other team members may not be communicating optimally, naturopaths should continue to advise them of any important changes to either the intervention or the patient's presentation.

CASE STUDY

OVERVIEW

AB is a 63-year-old male presenting with low mood, depression, difficulty concentrating and insulin resistance (borderline type 2 diabetes mellitus). AB reports a long history of depression, with suicidal ideation in his 30s, and heavy self-medication with alcohol and smoking. He has been consulting with a psychologist long term, which he reports to have been helpful. AB has not had any pharmaceutical, herbal or nutritional intervention to date. AB recalls always being overweight and this is increasingly problematic as he laments the he is almost at his heaviest weight and 'at the edge of no return with diabetes'. He notes that 'good food' is his weakness and his current diet reflects a high-carbohydrate, low-nutrient intake.

CLINICAL EXAMINATION

IMPORTANT OBSERVATIONS

- Obese with central adiposity: BMI 32.8 kg/m^2, WC 120 cm
- Poor focus and low mood
- Hypertensive (worse for white coat syndrome)
- DASS — moderate depression, low anxiety, and low stress scores. SCOFF — below cut-off.

INVESTIGATION RESULTS

- Anion gap 15.5 mmol/L with HCO_3 levels at 26 mmol/L
- Urinary pH 5
- Blood histamine 0.3 μmol/L
- Homocysteine 10.4 μmol/L
- Serum B_{12} 300 pmol/L
- Serum folate 29 nmol/L
- Pyrroles 57.2 micrograms/dL
- Serum Zn 12.0 μmol/L (≈ 10 μmol/L)
- Plasma Cu 12.9 μmol/L
- FBGL 6.8 mmol/L and HbA_{1c} 6.1%

TREATMENT PROTOCOL

DIETARY

- Encourage protein, essential fatty acids and wholefood principles
- Encourage small frequent meals to stabilise blood sugar levels
- Reduce carbohydrate intake (including minimal fruit consumption).

SUPPLEMENTAL

Nutrition supplementation addressing methylation, pyroluria, blood glucose dysregulation and inflammation.

Formula providing per day:

- Folic acid 1800 micrograms
- Hydroxycobalamin 1500 micrograms
- Zinc 75 mg
- B_6 300 mg as pyridoxine and 150 mg as P5P
- Manganese 9 mg (as gluconate)

CASE STUDY CONTINUED

- Chromium 600 micrograms/day
- NAC 1 g/day
- Citrate-based mineral (calcium, magnesium, potassium) preparation for alkalising 1 scoop/day initially → increased to 2 scoops/day

LIFESTYLE

- Go for a walk after meals when possible
- Practise mindful eating (e.g. no eating in front of TV) and be aware of satiety
- Continue treatment with psychologist.

AFTER 6 MONTHS OF TREATMENT

- DASS — borderline mild depression, normal anxiety and normal stress scores
- AB appears more vibrant and reports experiencing 'incredible clarity, improved mood and productivity'.

ANXIETY DISORDERS

Description and classification

Anxiety disorders are a dysfunctional response to a threat or stressor that involves interacting physical, cognitive, and emotional factors. The symptoms of excessive fear and consequent behaviours are common features of anxiety disorders. An anxiety disorder diagnosis is dependent on how these symptoms manifest in each person and the classification system used for diagnosis. There are two primary classification systems used in the English-speaking world that define anxiety disorders: the DSM and the International Classification of Diseases (ICD); both vary in the way anxiety disorders are described and categorised, and in diagnostic criteria; however, both are continually revised as new research comes to light.

The anxiety disorders currently described in the DSM-5 or ICD-10 include social phobia (social anxiety disorder), panic disorder, specific phobia, selective mutism, agoraphobia and generalised anxiety disorder (GAD), substance/medication-induced anxiety disorder, mixed anxiety and depressive disorder, separation anxiety disorder, posttraumatic stress disorder (PTSD), and obsessive compulsive disorder (OCD).[2,176] Note that PTSD and OCD are no longer categorised as anxiety disorders in the DSM-5; however, anxiety symptoms are also a feature of these disorders.

Core anxiety symptoms occur on a continuum from normal to severe and include both somatic (sweating, palpitations, nervousness, trembling, muscular tension) and cognitive (intrusive thoughts, irrational fears, and worry) symptoms. People who do not meet the criteria for an anxiety disorder may still need treatment for anxiety symptoms; in order to prevent more serious disorders developing it is important to identify those with moderate 'sub-threshold' levels of anxiety.[177,178] This chapter focuses on GAD as it is currently the most prevalent anxiety disorder.

FEATURES OF GENERALISED ANXIETY DISORDER

Criteria for GAD, taken from the DSM-5[2] are:

A Excessive anxiety and worry (apprehensive expectation), occurring more days than not for at least 6 months, about a number of events or activities (such as work or school performance).

B The individual finds it difficult to control the worry.

C The anxiety and worry are associated with three (or more) of the following six symptoms (with at least some symptoms having been present for more days than not for the past 6 months):

Note: Only one item is required in children.

1. Restlessness or feeling keyed up or on edge
2. Being easily fatigued
3. Difficulty concentrating or mind going blank
4. Irritability
5. Muscle tension
6. Sleep disturbance (difficulty falling or staying asleep, or restless, unsatisfying sleep).

D The anxiety, worry, or physical symptoms cause clinically significant distress or impairment in social, occupational, or other important areas of functioning.

E The disturbance is not attributable to the physiological effects of a substance (e.g. a drug of abuse, a medication) or another medical condition (e.g. hyperthyroidism).

F The disturbance is not better explained by another mental disorder (e.g. anxiety or worry about having panic attacks in panic disorder, negative evaluation in social anxiety disorder (social phobia), contamination or other obsessions in obsessive-compulsive disorder, separation from attachment figures in separation anxiety disorder, reminders of traumatic events in posttraumatic stress disorder, gaining weight in anorexia nervosa, physical complaints in somatic symptom disorder, perceived appearance flaws in body dysmorphic disorder, having a serious illness in illness anxiety disorder, or the content of delusional beliefs in schizophrenia or delusional disorder).

It is important to note that there is a high comorbidity of GAD with other mental health and physical disorders.

Epidemiology

In relation to GAD, epidemiological research reveals the following:

- Anxiety disorders are among the most common of mental health disorders in Australia, with 12-month prevalence rates indicating that 14% or one in seven Australians are affected by some sort of anxiety disorder, with GAD specifically experienced by almost 3%.[103] Similarly 12-month prevalence rates reveal 2% of adults in the United States have GAD.[103]
- High comorbidity rates with over 90% of individuals with GAD also meeting criteria for another mental health disorder, with GAD also indicated as being a risk factor for the development of depression.[179] GAD is the most frequent anxiety disorder seen in general practice, with GAD patients having a higher frequency of medical visits than other patients. GAD is linked with a range of physical complaints (e.g. gastrointestinal, pain, cardiovascular) and patients are more likely to seek medical care as opposed to psychological care for their symptoms, leading to over-use and expenditure on medical care and under-use of psychological care.[179] Both anxiety and depression are often associated with substance misuse.[180]

Signs and symptoms

Excessive worry and anxiety ('apprehensive expectation') about a number of topics is the core feature of GAD.[2] Typical topics of worry include: work/performance at work, finance, health, family members or more trivial matters (e.g. being late). Children who have GAD often have worries about competence or performance as their core concerns. While all people worry, individuals with GAD typically have:

- Marked trouble controlling their worries, which are also disproportionate to the event of concern or the actual likelihood of the event happening. This leads to the anxiety impairing their functioning in some way
- Anxiety/worry is distressing and often longer in duration
- Physical symptoms in addition to the worry (keyed up, muscle tension, fatigue).[2]

Differential diagnosis and comorbidities

As there is frequently symptom overlap in common mental health problems it is important to consider the following differential diagnoses.[2]

Anxiety disorder due to another medical condition

This diagnosis should be made if the individual's anxiety and worry are a physiological effect of a medical condition such as phaeochromocytoma or hyperthyroidism.

Psychiatric disorders

Substance/medication-induced anxiety disorder, social anxiety disorder, obsessive-compulsive disorder, posttraumatic stress disorder and adjustment disorders, depressive, bipolar and psychotic disorders.

Comorbid psychiatric disorders

People with a GAD diagnosis are likely to have met the criteria for other anxiety and unipolar depressive disorders. Less common comorbidities include substance use, neurodevelopmental, neurocognitive, and psychotic disorders.

Investigations: psychometric

DASS-21

As already indicated, the DASS-21 can be used to assess anxiety levels. A review of sub-scale item content and research by Brown and colleagues reveals that high scores on the 'anxiety' scale may be reflective of panic disorder symptoms compared to high scores on the stress scale which are more reflective of GAD.[181]

THE GENERALISED ANXIETY DISORDER-7 (GAD-7)

The GAD-7 is a very brief tool consisting of seven Likert-scaled items designed to screen for and assess symptom severity of GAD.[182] The scale uses a threshold score of 10 and has been found to have a sensitivity of 89% and a specificity of 82% for detecting GAD. It is also a reasonable screening tool for three other common disorders that feature anxiety: panic disorder (sensitivity 74%, specificity 81%), social anxiety disorder (sensitivity 72%, specificity 80%), and posttraumatic stress disorder (sensitivity 66%, specificity 81%).[183] Given the overlap across anxiety disorders, a positive result would indicate further clinical assessment for other potential anxiety disorders. Note: Some clinicians prefer to use both the PHQ-9 (screener for depression) and the GAD-7, while others prefer to use the DASS-21. Alternatives for children include the freely available Spence Children's Anxiety Scale (SCAS), which may be obtained via www.scaswebsite.com

GERIATRIC ANXIETY INVENTORY (GAI)

The GAI is a 20-item self-report or clinician-administered scale assessing dimensional anxiety in the older adult. A cut-off score of 10 may be used (given research reflecting those with a DSM-5 diagnosis of GAD had a mean score of 10.64).[184] The scale is quick to administer with a dichotomous response format (agree/disagree). It has sound psychometric properties (internal reliability $\alpha = 0.93$ and good inter-rater and test–retest reliability; good concurrent validity; and adequate sensitivity and specificity at 75% and 84% respectively).[184] To obtain the GAI and for more information see: http://gai.net.au/

Therapeutic considerations

OBJECTIVES

The treatment objectives for GAD are similar to the principles applied to MMD. Refer to the previous section on MDD objectives for these.

NUTRITIONAL MEDICINE (DIETARY)

When treating any mental health problem the therapeutic objective when using nutritional medicine is dependent on each person's unique presentation, dietary and nutritional context and pathology markers; therefore, a holistic approach is needed. When treating anxiety it is essential to address the underlying psychosocial factors contributing to anxiety in addition to any nutritional prescription. Biological treatments need to be combined with appropriate psychological therapies that address dysfunctional cognitions (e.g. worry) and consequent behaviours, which are a key feature of GAD. When choosing appropriate nutritional interventions for treating generalised anxiety symptoms, therapeutic objectives are the same as those listed for treating MDD and include:

- Reducing anxiety symptoms and stabilising mood
- Determining and treating the underlying factors contributing to anxiety symptoms (e.g. inflammation, methylation, pyrroles)
- Supporting improved food choices and good dietary practices, with particular emphasis on regularity of food intake and low glycaemic index choices[185]
- Addressing secondary nutritional issues that may have arisen as a consequence of anxiety (e.g. depleted nervous system nutrients)
- Addressing secondary physical symptoms that may be comorbid with anxiety (e.g. gut function).

NUTRITIONAL MEDICINE (SUPPLEMENTAL)

Following are some of the most commonly used nutrients and nutraceuticals for treating anxiety symptoms.

Magnesium

Magnesium has a long tradition of being considered a nervous system nutrient by naturopaths, and is especially indicated for stress and anxiety. Preclinical data support the bidirectional relationships between magnesium and anxiety, with animal models confirming that magnesium deficiency induces HPA activation and anxiety-like behaviours,[186,187] while the acute experiences of stress and anxiety have been confirmed to produce increased losses of magnesium via urine.[188] Surprisingly, however, very few studies have been published using magnesium as an intervention for anxiety and the two key papers used magnesium in combination with other agents. One small study investigated magnesium (200 mg elemental) either alone or in combination with 50 mg B_6/day administered over one menstrual cycle to women suffering anxiety-related premenstrual symptoms. It reported a modest reduction in anxiety-related symptoms (nervous tension, mood swings, irritability or anxiety) for only those women taking the combination.[189] Another larger study administered magnesium (75 mg elemental) with *Crataegus oxycantha* extract (75 mg) and *Eschscholzia californica* extract (20 mg) to patients with mild-moderate anxiety over 3 months. Compared with placebo, the herbal magnesium combination lowered anxiety scores more; however, the difference was small.[190] It is important to note that both of these studies used magnesium oxide which is a form with documented poor bioavailability and also combined magnesium with other active ingredients. Therefore better designed studies that can elucidate the true efficacy of magnesium are needed.

Vitamin C

Recognition of the increased synthesis of vitamin C in other mammals under stress posits the notion that for humans incapable of vitamin C synthesis, exposed to chronic stressors, such as those experiencing anxiety, higher intakes may be warranted to meet this extra demand.[191] In addition to this, oxidative stress has been implicated as part of the pathophysiology of anxiety, which would therefore necessitate higher antioxidant defence.[192–194] Preliminary studies of antioxidant levels in patients diagnosed with GAD report significantly lower levels of vitamins C, A and E.[192]

ACTIONS

- Antioxidant and antioxidant recycler[193]
- Stimulates 3H-GABA binding to decrease arterial pressure and heart rate[191]
- NMDA receptor antagonism[191]
- Modulation of catecholamine release.[191]

EVIDENCE OF EFFICACY

Several small key studies have investigated vitamin C as a potential anxiolytic either on its own[191,195] or in conjunction with other antioxidants and antidepressant medications.[192] The shared design feature of these studies is using 'high' doses of vitamin C, 500 mg–2000 mg administered daily for a minimum of 14 days. Only one study sample included patients with confirmed GAD,[192] while the other two employed healthy people who were subjected to experimental stressors.[191,195] The results of these studies all found in favour of a demonstrable anxiety lowering effect of vitamin C, in terms of both subjective and objective measures. In particular, both studies that assessed stress-induced cardiovascular changes found either reduced blood pressure, faster blood pressure normalisation post-stressor, or lower heart rate in those people taking vitamin C.[191,195] The study by Brody et al also reported faster salivary cortisol recovery following stress exposure.[195] Interestingly, another study of type 2 diabetic patients administered either vitamin C 1 g/day or vitamin E 400 IU or placebo over 6 weeks, found only those taking the vitamin C showed significantly reduced anxiety scores after 6 weeks of treatment.[193] This would suggest that the efficacy of vitamin C is not limited to its antioxidant role.

The primary adverse effect associated with vitamin C is diarrhoea and loose stools; however, in one study where a sustained-release preparation was used, this effect appears to have been mitigated.[195]

N-acetylcysteine

N-acetylcysteine (NAC) is an acetylated form of the amino acid cysteine. This small modification translates to better stability, bioavailability and therapeutic potential beyond that of its amino acid precursor.[142,143] NAC has attracted particular interest in relation to its antioxidant and anti-inflammatory properties and has demonstrated some efficacy in a range of psychiatric disorders which have core features of anxiety; for example, obsessive compulsive disorder and nail biting, making it a nutraceutical of interest in anxiety disorders.[143]

ACTIONS

The chemistry of NAC means that it may modulate key pathophysiological processes that have been implicated in a wide range of psychological disorders, including anxiety. These actions include:[142,194]

- Antioxidant via increased glutathione levels
- Anti-inflammatory — ↓ TNFα, IL-1β, IL-6, IL-10 and suppressed microglial activation
- Glutaminergic modulation — suppressing excessive levels of glutamate release in the brain
- NMDA receptor modulation
- Regulation of dopamine-induced neurotoxicity
- Enhanced activity and protection of mitochondria
- Modulation of intracellular calcium
- Neuroprotective.

EVIDENCE OF EFFICACY

A recent animal study confirms the anxiolytic effects of IV NAC, without sedation, using five different anxiety models that translate well to human anxiety states. Of particular note, the researchers reported that daily dosing enabled a lowering of the dose without reduced efficacy when compared with acute pre-stress acute dosing.[194] One case report of a 17-year-old male with partially treatment-resistant GAD and social phobia administered an initial dose of NAC at 600 mg b.i.d. for 4 weeks, followed with 1200 mg b.i.d. for another 4 weeks, found that the addition of NAC, in particular, at this higher dose of 2.4 g/day, correlated with significant improvements in mental health scores, social functioning and anxiety-related insomnia.[196]

Evidence from other human studies is limited to clinical trials, which have investigated NAC in psychological disorders that have marked anxiety components, such as nail biting, trichotillomania, skin picking. These studies are a mixture of case series and open-label studies; not regarded as strong evidence and a small number of controlled trials. While their results have been mixed, these preliminary findings appear promising in specific areas such as skin picking and nail biting.[144] The typical doses used have been 1–2 g/day over 6–24 weeks.

Generally, oral NAC across clinical trials in a range of areas has proven to be well tolerated, with a low side-effect profile. Adverse effects reported as part of clinical trials have most commonly been mild gastrointestinal symptoms including abdominal pain, flatulence, heartburn, nausea and vomiting. Overall, however, rates of adverse effects appear to be comparable with placebo in most studies and very few studies have reported cases where discontinuation has been necessary.[144]

L-theanine

L-theanine (γ-glutamylethylamide) is a unique amino acid present almost exclusively in the tea plant (*Camellia sinensis*), where it constitutes only 1–2% of the dry weight.[197] Originally discovered by Japanese researchers in 1949, it has had limited investigation in the treatment of anxiety in spite of a long history of use as a relaxing agent and preliminary animal evidence of anxiolytic effects.[198,199]

ACTIONS

- Inhibits glutamate reuptake as a natural glutamate analogue[198–200]
- Increases GABA concentrations[200]
- Increases dopamine release via NMDA stimulation[200]
- Decreases CNS serotonin levels overall; however, increases serotonin levels specifically in the striatum, hippocampus and hypothalamus of rats[200]

- Exhibits neuroprotective effects via blocking NDMA receptors[200]
- Inhibits the excitatory effects of caffeine at high doses; for example, 0.781 mg/kg IV, augmentation at low oral (250 mg) and IV (0.174–0.348 mg/kg) doses.[198,201]

EVIDENCE OF EFFICACY

In spite of a range of preclinical and animal studies that document interesting cognitive and mood effects of theanine, with a net anxiolytic effect proposed,[200,202] there are limited human trials to confirm this. Most human studies have employed one-off doses of theanine between 200–250 mg administered 30 minutes prior to a mental task or other event designed to promote stress and anxiety in subjects. In these scenarios, the results have been mixed. Some studies have demonstrated theanine's ability to induce a more relaxed state and increase alpha brainwave activity at rest (prior to the stressor),[198,199,203] to attenuate both state anxiety and perceived stress following the stressor,[202] and to reduce physical responses to stress such as rises in systolic blood pressure, heart rate and salivary IgA.[202,204] Other similar study designs have failed to demonstrate a significant anxiety reduction following a stressor in those treated with theanine.[198,199]

Our limited understanding of theanine pharmacokinetics suggests that peak plasma levels occur within 30 minutes of taking which coincides with theanine reaching the brain so acute repeat dosing would appear to make sense in anxious patients. There are no reported side effects in either animal or human studies investigating theanine[200] although headache was reported more frequently 90 minutes post-dose in one study.[198]

HERBAL MEDICINE

When treating mental health problems, the therapeutic objective when choosing herbal medicines is dependent on the unique presentation of each person. When treating anxiety, it is essential to address the underlying psychosocial factors contributing to anxiety in addition to any prescribed herbal treatment. Biological treatments such as herbal medicines need to be combined with appropriate psychological therapies that address dysfunctional cognitions (e.g. worry) and consequent behaviours, which are a key feature of GAD. The safety of long-term use of herbal anxiolytics has yet to be established — this is an important consideration when treating GAD as it is a more chronic form of anxiety. When choosing appropriate herbal medicines for treating generalised anxiety symptoms, therapeutic objectives include:

- Reducing anxiety symptoms
- Determining and treating the underlying factors contributing to anxiety symptoms (e.g. stress, trauma, and inflammation)
- Managing associated symptoms (e.g. cognitive dysfunction, sleep disturbance, fatigue and muscular tension)
- Enhancing immune function and reducing oxidative and nitrogen stress
- Supporting and restoring nervous system and adrenal function
- Addressing secondary physical symptoms that may be comorbid with anxiety (e.g. gut function).

Following are some of the most commonly used herbs with evidence of efficacy for treating anxiety symptoms. Each of the herbs covered has an anxiolytic action. Secondary actions also need to be considered when developing a treatment plan, such as cognition enhancing, adaptogenic, sedative, antidepressant, anti-inflammatory and antioxidant. For further reading on herbal anxiolytics refer to the text *Evidence-Based Herbal and Nutritional Treatments for Anxiety in Psychiatric Disorders.*[205]

Piper methysticum (kava kava)

Piper methysticum is the most widely studied herbal medicine for treating generalised anxiety symptoms. A number of additional pharmacological actions have been identified including being analgesic, anti-stress, sedative, muscle relaxant, antithrombotic, neuroprotective, mild anaesthetic, hypnotic and anticonvulsant. The primary constituents reputed to be responsible for the anxiolytic effects of kava are kavalactones. The roots of the plant have the highest concentration of kavalactones, and are the plant part used in herbal preparations. In-vivo and in-vitro studies suggest possible mechanisms for kava's effects:[205]

- Blockage of voltage-gated sodium ion channels
- Reduced excitatory neurotransmitter release due to blockage of calcium ion channels
- Enhanced ligand binding to GABA type A receptors
- Reversible inhibition of monoamine oxidase B
- Reduced neuronal reuptake of noradrenaline (norepinephrine) and dopamine.

EVIDENCE OF EFFICACY

There is good evidence of the efficacy of *Piper methysticum* in the treatment of generalised anxiety symptoms, demonstrated in numerous clinical trials. For a recent comprehensive review see Camfield et al, 2017.[205] Two meta-analyses of RCTs have been conducted on the anxiolytic effects of various types of kava extracts.[206, 207] Both found that anxiety symptoms (assessed using the Hamilton Anxiety Scale) were significantly reduced in all studies reviewed. Types of anxiety included in these studies were GAD, state and trait anxiety, climacteric anxiety, acute preoperative anxiety, and nonpsychotic anxiety disorders.

In 2007 the World Health Organization (WHO) made safety recommendations for the use of water-based preparations following concerns over the safety of acetone and ethanol extracts.[208] Studies following this recommendation have used aqueous extracts to evaluate kava's efficacy in treating anxiety. In two studies kava significantly reduced anxiety symptoms in adults with generalised anxiety symptoms,[209] and in adults with a GAD diagnosis.[210] In the aforementioned study, there was also a significant reduction in depression symptoms. The aqueous extracts used in these studies were found to be well tolerated with no serious adverse effects reported.

Kava has also been found to have similar efficacy to the pharmaceuticals buspirone and opipramol in the treatment of GAD.[211] In contrast, a more recent study found kava did not reduce state anxiety, which was significantly reduced by oxazepam in moderately anxious adults.[212] A possible explanation for this result was that genetic analyses indicated that noradrenaline (SLC6A2) transporter polymorphisms may affect the treatment response to kava. The effects of kava vary depending on type of cultivar used, method of preparation, dose and individual genetics and biochemistry.

Kava is specifically indicated for generalised anxiety symptoms and GAD. This herb may also be useful for treating social anxiety and anxiety with sleep disturbance (due to its sedative effect at higher doses), and may be indicated for comorbid depression. Kava has also demonstrated acute anxiolytic effects without cognitive impairment; theoretically it may be helpful when acute anxiolysis is needed, such as panic attacks and exam anxiety, although more research is needed.

Use of traditional water-based extracts of the rhizome is recommended. Dosage of *Piper methysticum* for an anxiolytic effect is dependent on standardisation, and a total dose ranges between 50 mg and 250 mg of kavalactones per day (approx. 50–60 mg of kavalactones per tablet). Note that there is a potential for liver toxicity; however, this is considered to be very rare. Clinical advice is to avoid high doses, monitor patients, and use intermittently. Liver function tests and hepatobiliary clinical examination are recommended if there is a potential liver dysfunction, or if longer term use is needed. Avoid concurrent use with depressants such as benzodiazepines and alcohol.

Matricaria recutita (chamomile)

The flowering tops of *Matricaria recutita* (syn. *Matricaria chamomilla, Chamomilla recutita*) are well known for their calming effects, which have a long history of traditional use. Its actions have been described as being indicated for 'nervous irritability, with peevishness, fretfulness, discontent, and impatience'.[53] The anxiolytic effects of chamomile have been shown to involve the GABA system,[213,214] with the flavone apigenin being responsible for this action.[215,216] However, it is suggested that the anxiolytic effects may also involve other mechanisms.

EVIDENCE OF EFFICACY

Two RCTs have shown *Matricaria recutita* to be efficacious in the treatment of GAD symptoms. The first was a dose-escalation study (ranging from 220 to 1100 mg) over 8 weeks[217] and the second was a two-phase study (open-label for 12 weeks, then randomised to three groups for 24 weeks) over a total of 38 weeks.[218] The first study also found a significant reduction in depression symptoms. During the follow-up phase of the second study chamomile was found to reduce relapse of GAD symptoms at a dose of 3 capsules daily (500 mg of dry extract *Matricaria recutita*, equivalent to 2.0 g flowers, 6 mg of apigenin-7-glycosides). While this effect was not significantly different to placebo, the researchers considered it to be a clinically meaningful effect, and consistent with relapse response seen in pharmaceutical treatments. In addition, they found a number of significant differences compared to the placebo group in a range of biological measures including lower weight, lower mean arterial blood pressure, and lower systolic pressure, with a trend towards lower diastolic pressure (nonsignificant), but no difference in pulse.

Based on its traditional use and RCT evidence, *Matricaria recutita* is indicated for treatment of generalised anxiety disorder symptoms, and is suitable for long-term treatment (up to 36 weeks). The recommended dose for anxiolytic effect is dried herb 6 g per day standardised to apigenin.

Passiflora incarnata (passionflower)

Passiflora incarnata has long been used for stress, sleep and anxiety symptoms,[219,220] with a Spanish researcher in Peru reported to have first described its medical use in 1569.[221] Its traditional indication for 'worry' and 'mental overwork', as described in *King's American Dispensatory*,[53] is well suited to those with GAD.

EVIDENCE OF EFFICACY

While a number of passionflower species are used as medicines, *Passiflora incarnata* has shown the strongest anxiolytic action. The aerial parts of the plant are used for their medicinal effects with the leaves showing the strongest anxiolytic activity. The constituents responsible for the anxiolytic action are unconfirmed; however, the benzoflavone chrysin is considered the main constituent responsible for this action. Passionflower extracts are typically standardised to between 1.01 mg/500 mg[222] and 2.8 mg/5 mL.[223]

Only one double-blind RCT has investigated the chronic effects of *Passiflora incarnata* on anxiety symptoms in outpatients with GAD.[219] This study found that passionflower (45 drops daily) significantly reduced anxiety symptoms following 4 weeks of treatment that was similar to oxazepam (comparison treatment). The passionflower treatment was slower to act, taking 7 days, compared to 4 days for oxazepam, to achieve a significant reduction in anxiety symptoms. Acute effects of passionflower have been found in preoperative anxiety[226,223] and dental anxiety[224] using varying preparations and doses. Each of these studies found a significant reduction in anxiety symptoms compared to placebo. Reduction of anxiety symptoms peaked at 30 minutes in both the preoperative studies.

Passiflora incarnata is suitable for both chronic and acute forms of anxiety. More research is needed to determine its efficacy in specific anxiety disorders; however, its traditional indication for worry and restlessness, RCT evidence and safety profile suggests it is well suited to GAD. The recommended chronic dose is dried herb 1–3 g per day standardised to benzoflavones, and acute dose 500–700 mg standardised to benzoflavones.

Withania somnifera (ashwagandha)

Withania somnifera has been used for centuries as an Ayurvedic herb and is classified as a rejuvenative ('rasayana') medicine that improves mental and physical health and prolongs life.[225] The rhizome is the plant part used for its medical effects. *Withania* has antioxidant, anxiolytic, adaptogenic and anti-inflammatory actions. Many bioactive compounds have been identified; however, withaferin A and withanolide D are believed to be responsible for the adaptogenic effects.[226]

EVIDENCE OF EFFICACY

A number of clinical trials have demonstrated the efficacy of *Withania* in reducing anxiety- and stress-related symptoms; however these studies were not consistent in the dose or preparation type used, the type of anxiety treated or the length of treatment.[226] A systematic review of five clinical trials published in 2014 concluded that although all studies reviewed showed significant reductions in anxiety and stress symptoms, the evidence needed to be interpreted with caution as there was a risk of potential bias related to poor study design.[227] More well-designed clinical trials are needed to clarify *Withania*'s efficacy in generalised anxiety and obsessive-compulsive disorder and the most effective preparation and acute and chronic doses needed.

Of note, one RCT investigated the anxiolytic effects of *Withania* as part of naturopathic care compared to standardised CBT plus placebo over 12 weeks in adults (N = 75) with moderate-to-severe anxiety of at least 6 weeks duration.[228] A significant reduction in anxiety scores was found for both groups; however, the reduction in the *Withania* group was significantly greater than in the CBT group. The RCT also found significant differences between each treatment in other symptoms including mental health, concentration, fatigue, social functioning, vitality and quality of life — in addition to no adverse reactions for each group.

Withania somnifera is indicated in generalised anxiety that is more chronic in nature when there are fatigue and/or cognitive problems. It also has the potential be used for obsessive-compulsive disorder as an adjunct treatment to SSRIs.[229] The recommended dose is 500–1000 mg per day of dried extract standardised to withanolides or 4–6 g/day root powder.

PSYCHOLOGICAL

Again NICE guidelines recommend a stepped care approach and CBT. More recent research trials show third-wave psychological therapies such as an acceptance-based behavioural therapy approach for GAD to have high rates of success.[179] As outlined by Payne, growing evidence for a singular UP (unified transdiagnostic protocol) approach to treating all emotional disorders is increasing.[3]

LIFESTYLE RECOMMENDATIONS

There are several environmental factors that contribute to the onset and maintenance of GAD symptoms. Some of these are lifestyle related and modifiable. It is the role of the naturopath to support their patients to adopt lifestyle changes to assist in managing anxiety symptoms and prevent relapse once in recovery. The lifestyle recommendations applied in MDD are also relevant to GAD, and are described in the previous section.

THE HEALTHCARE TEAM

As with all mental health problems it is essential that patients with GAD are treated as part of a mental healthcare team to ensure the best outcome for their situation. The same approach applies to GAD as MDD described in the previous section.

CASE STUDY

OVERVIEW

Sarah is a 42-year-old married mother of two who self-referred to the clinic after being diagnosed by her psychologist with GAD and some obsessive-compulsive personality traits. She is continuing to see her psychologist who she is finding helpful. Sarah reported having difficulty relaxing, ongoing muscle tension, irritability and sleep disturbance where she awakens at night and ruminates on her perceived mistakes of the day. Sarah also self-castigates because she can't 'control' her thoughts very well, leading to feelings of shame. She also describes a tendency to just keep pushing until exhaustion, and feeling keyed up constantly. She reports being worried about her relationship with her daughter and that her perfectionist tendencies ('being controlling') are affecting her behaviour. Sarah describes her work as a nurse in ICU as being a 'high adrenaline' environment.

Sarah referred to herself as having a type A personality. In terms of the triple vulnerability model, possible predisposing factors to Sarah's presenting anxiety included: an anxious/inhibited temperament and earlier learning experiences/psychological vulnerabilities such as coming from a family that valued achievement highly, and an early environment where social inclusion and popularity were seen as an efficient route to gain power and success. Sarah described an intolerance to uncertainty (highly associated with GAD) in which she developed a set of negative beliefs about uncertainty (e.g. 'I can't relax if I don't know what is happening', 'I must not leave anything to chance'). This led to maladaptive coping behaviours such as excessive planning/organisation/preparation, rumination, worry, sensitivity to being evaluated at work (leading to avoidance of such situations) and procrastination (to avoid failing or not doing something perfectly). While these behaviours offered Sarah short-term relief, in the long term this cognitive-behavioural cycle was starting to wear Sarah down, leading to increased irritability towards her children, further strengthening her worries about not being a good enough mother.

CLINICAL EXAMINATION

Sarah's symptoms are chronic and typical of GAD, with long-term stress contributing to them. Physically she may have been conditioned to living in a state characterised by high sympathetic nervous system activity due to chronic stress related to perfectionism, her work environment and the difficult relationship with her daughter. Sarah is committed to the psychological treatments she is having with her psychologist, which she believes are helping her to better manage her worries, more accurately identify her own internal experiences/emotions and have a better relationship with her daughter.

CASE STUDY CONTINUED

Clinical observations included:
- Self-reported lifelong worries
- DASS Stress Scale: extremely severe (consistent with GAD)
- Previous 'mood and fatigue issues' (5 years ago). GP diagnosed depression and prescribed an SSRI (citalopram: 20 mg daily for 6 months) with minimal change in mood and unwanted side effects
- Sleep assessment (5 years ago) revealing sleep apnoea treated with a CPAP machine resulting in reduced fatigue
- BMI = 28 (overweight)
- Blood pressure 120/75 mmHg (normal)
- Currently not exercising.

TREATMENT PROTOCOL

Sarah is receiving an evidence-based psychological treatment for GAD (acceptance-based behavioural therapy) and was encouraged to continue this. The treatment following the initial consult was focused on supporting her to cope with the chronic stress and anxiety she is experiencing. This involved reducing anxiety symptoms (e.g. fatigue, sleep disturbance, muscle tension), supporting and normalising nervous system and adrenal function, regulating HPA-axis activity, and providing lifestyle strategies to assist with stress management. Weight management and diet were not addressed in the initial consult, as it was not a treatment priority for Sarah. In addition, too many behavioural interventions would likely be overwhelming, possibly increasing Sarah's stress and anxiety, and noncompliance at this stage. These would be addressed in follow-up consultations. Sarah was referred for basic pathology testing to identify any nutritional problems and other possible medical causes of her symptoms, to be reviewed at a follow-up consultation.

HERBAL MEDICINE

Piper methysticum (standardised 50 mg kavalactones) 2 tablets twice daily.

Herbal medicine	Ratio	mL/ bottle	Rationale
Passiflora incarnata	1:2	40	Anxiolytic, sedative, antispasmodic, traditional indication for 'worry'
Glycyrrhiza glabra	1:1	20	Adrenal tonic, anti-inflammatory
Centella asiatica (20 mg/mL triterpenes)	1:1	60	Adaptogen, anxiolytic, anti-inflammatory
Withania somnifera (4.0 mg/mL of withanolides)	2:1	40	Adaptogen, anxiolytic, antioxidant, anti-inflammatory
Scutellaria lateriflora	1:2	40	Anxiolytic, antispasmodic, anti-inflammatory, nervous system tonic

Total liquid: 200 mL
Dose: 7.5 mL twice daily

CASE STUDY CONTINUED

NUTRITIONAL MEDICINE

Tablet formula:
- Magnesium amino acid chelate 750 mg, equivalent to 150 mg elemental magnesium
- Pyridoxal-5-phosphate 50 mg, equivalent to 34.23 mg pyridoxine (B_6)
1 tablet twice daily.

LIFESTYLE

- Start walking and aim for at least 30 minutes 3 times a week
- Use massage to assist with muscle relaxation and stress management
- Follow the information provided on sleep hygiene to ensure environmental factors do not contribute to sleep problems.

COMPLEX PSYCHIATRIC DISORDERS

It is outside the scope of this text to cover more complex mental health conditions in detail. However, complex psychiatric disorders can be comorbid with MDD and GAD, and may present in a clinical situation. It is essential that naturopaths are familiar with how to manage a patient if they suspect the patient has a more complex mental health problem. This section provides enough information to naturopaths to have a general awareness of these mental health conditions. It is not recommended that naturopaths treat patients presenting with these disorders, unless appropriately trained to do so in consultation with their primary mental health practitioner. Complex psychiatric disorders are typically diagnosed by specialised mental health practitioners such as psychiatrists and psychologists. Following is a brief description of more complex psychiatric disorders that are more likely to present in naturopathic practice. If a naturopath suspects a patient is presenting with a serious psychiatric disorder they should refer to a GP for assessment and referral to specialist mental health care. For further reading on these disorders it is recommended that naturopaths refer to the DSM-5.

Bipolar and related disorders

The features of these disorders overlap between depressive disorders and psychotic disorders. Following are the bipolar and related disorders according to the DSM-5:[2]
- Bipolar I disorder (manic-depressive disorder): manic episode (at least 1 week duration) may be either preceded by or followed by hypomanic or depressive episodes
- Bipolar II disorder: current or past hypomanic episode and a current or past major depressive episode
- Cyclothymic disorder: hypomanic symptoms that have been present periodically for at least 2 years, and present for at least half that time

- Substance/medication-induced bipolar and related disorder
- Bipolar and related disorder due to another medical condition
- Other specified bipolar and related disorder, and unspecified bipolar and related disorder.

Trauma and stressor-related disorders

Trauma- and stressor-related disorders are characterised by exposure to a traumatic or stressful event. These disorders may present with anxiety and/or depression symptoms. It is important to note that trauma or stress as an underlying cause of anxiety and depression symptoms may not always be obvious, as patients may not disclose their exposure to trauma. Domestic violence is one example of trauma often occurring with chronic stress that can be difficult to identify. It is important that victims of domestic violence are adequately supported, and suspected cases need to be assessed for vulnerability risk and child protection risk. Refer to the previous risk assessment section on mandatory reporting of child neglect and abuse. Trauma- and stressor-related disorders include:

- Reactive attachment disorder
- Disinhibited social engagement disorder
- Posttraumatic stress disorder (PTSD)
- Acute stress disorder
- Adjustment disorders.

Obsessive-compulsive and related disorders

Obsessive-compulsive and related disorders often present with significant distress and anxiety symptoms. Key features of these disorders relate to the presence of obsessions ('recurrent and persistent thoughts, urges, or images that are experienced as intrusive and unwanted'), and compulsions ('repetitive behaviours or mental acts that an individual feels driven to perform in response to an obsession').[2] These disorders include:

- Obsessive-compulsive disorder (OCD)
- Body dysmorphic disorder
- Hoarding disorder
- Trichotillomania (hair-pulling disorder) and excoriation (skin-picking) disorder
- Substance/medication-induced obsessive-compulsive and related disorder, obsessive-compulsive and related disorder due to another medical condition, and other specified obsessive-compulsive and related disorder and unspecified obsessive-compulsive and related disorder (e.g. body-focused repetitive behaviour disorder, obsessional jealousy).

Substance-related and addictive disorders

The DSM-5 includes 10 classes of drugs in the category of substance-related disorders: 'alcohol; caffeine; cannabis; hallucinogens (with separate categories for phencyclidine [or similarly acting arylcyclohexylamines] and other hallucinogens); inhalants; opioids; sedatives, hypnotics, and anxiolytics; stimulants (amphetamine-type substances, cocaine, and other stimulants); tobacco; and other (or unknown) substances'.[2] Gambling disorder is the only behavioural disorder described in the DSM-5, as it has shown strong evidence of activation of reward centres similar to drugs of addiction; however, other behavioural addictions can cause significant distress and social dysfunction such as sex addiction, internet gaming addiction, exercise addiction and shopping addiction. People with substance-related and addictive disorders often have comorbid anxiety and depression symptoms. In the case of substance-related disorders anxiety and depression symptoms may be directly related to the substance being abused.

Psychotic disorders

The DSM-5[2] describes the key features of psychotic disorders as hallucinations (perception-like experiences occurring without an external stimulus), delusions (fixed beliefs that are unlikely to change despite conflicting evidence), disorganised thinking (usually identified in speech), negative symptoms (reduced emotional expression or motivation, alogia, anhedonia, asociality), and disorganised or abnormal motor behaviour. Psychotic disorders include:

- Schizotypical (personality) disorder
- Delusional disorder
- Brief psychotic disorder
- Schizophreniform disorder
- Schizophrenia
- Schizoaffective disorder
- Substance/medication-induced psychotic disorder
- Psychotic disorder due to another medical condition
- Catatonic disorders.

Neurodevelopmental disorders

There are a number of neurodevelopmental disorders, each of which has unique developmental deficits and varies considerably for each person. This section draws your attention to the two most likely to present in a naturopathic setting: autism spectrum disorder (ASD) and attention-deficit/hyperactivity disorder (ADHD). In both of these disorders the symptoms change throughout the life span.

The prevalence of ASD is estimated at 1% of the US population[2] and is characterised by problems with social functioning in a range of contexts and the presence of repetitive, restrictive behaviour, activities or interests.

The prevalence of ADHD is approximately 5% in children and 2.5% in adults in most cultures. ADHD is characterised by inattention and/or hyperactivity-impulsivity that is persistent and interferes with functioning or development. ADHD is often misdiagnosed as an anxiety disorder, particularly in adults, as it can share similar symptoms related to inattention; however, the inattention in ADHD is related to attraction to things (e.g. external stimuli) as opposed to worry and rumination seen in anxiety disorder populations.[2]

Personality disorders

The DSM-5 characterises personality disorders as an 'enduring pattern of inner experience and behaviour that deviates markedly from the expectations of the individual's culture, is pervasive and inflexible, has an onset in adolescence or early adulthood, is stable over time, and leads to distress or impairment'.[2] The enduring nature of personality disorders is their defining feature and the characteristics of each disorder occur before early adulthood. People with personality disorders can often present with anxiety and depressive disorder symptoms, which can be difficult to differentiate. Following are personality disorders as defined by the DSM-5.[7]

Cluster A: characterised as odd and eccentric
- Paranoid personality disorder is a pattern of distrust and suspiciousness such that others' motives are interpreted as malevolent
- Schizoid personality disorder is a pattern of detachment from social relationships and a restricted range of emotional expression
- Schizotypal personality disorder is a pattern of acute discomfort in close relationships, cognitive or perceptual distortions, and eccentricities of behaviour.

Cluster B: characterised as dramatic, emotional, or erratic
- Antisocial personality disorder is a pattern of disregard for, and violation of, the rights of others
- Borderline personality disorder is a pattern of instability in interpersonal relationships, self-image, and affects, and marked impulsivity
- Histrionic personality disorder is a pattern of excessive emotionality and attention seeking
- Narcissistic personality disorder is a pattern of grandiosity, need for admiration, and lack of empathy.

Cluster C: characterised as anxious or fearful
- Avoidant personality disorder is a pattern of social inhibition, feelings of inadequacy, and hypersensitivity to negative evaluation
- Dependent personality disorder is a pattern of submissive and clinging behaviour related to an excessive need to be taken care of
- Obsessive-compulsive personality disorder is a pattern of preoccupation with orderliness, perfectionism, and control.

Other:
- Personality change due to another medical condition is a persistent personality disturbance that is judged to be due to the direct physiological effects of a medical condition (e.g. frontal lobe lesion)
- Other specified personality disorder and unspecified personality disorder.

REFERENCES

[1] Zimbardo PG, Johnson RL, McCann V. Psychology: core concepts. 7th ed. Boston: Pearson; 2012.

[2] American Psychiatric Association. Diagnostic and statistical manual of mental disorders. 5th ed. Arlington, VA: American Psychiatric Publishing; 2013.

[3] Payne LA, Ellard KK, Farchione TJ, et al. Emotional disorders: a unified transdiagnostic protocol. In: Barlow DH, editor. Clinical handbook of psychological disorders: a step-by-step treatment manual. 5th ed. New York: Guilford Press; 2014.

[4] Farchione TJ, Fairholme CP, Ellard KK, et al. Unified protocol for transdiagnostic treatment of emotional disorders: a randomized controlled trial. Behav Ther 2012;43(3):666–78.

[5] Brown TA, Naragon-Gainey K. Evaluation of the unique and specific contributions of dimensions of the triple vulnerability model to the prediction of DSM-IV anxiety and mood disorder constructs. Behav Ther 2013;44(2):277–92.

[6] Barlow DH, Ellard KK, Sauer-Zavala S, et al. The origins of neuroticism. Perspect Psychol Sci 2014;9(5):481–96.

[7] Mersky JP, Topitzes J, Reynolds AJ. Impacts of adverse childhood experiences on health, mental health, and substance use in early adulthood: a cohort study of an urban, minority sample in the US. Child Abuse Negl 2013;37(11):917–25.

[8] Malhi GS, Bassett D, Boyce P, et al. Royal Australian and New Zealand College of Psychiatrists clinical practice guidelines for mood disorders. Aust N Z J Psychiatry 2015;49(12):1087–206.

[9] den Boer JA. Looking beyond the monoamine hypothesis. Eur Neurol Rev 2006;6(1):87–92.

[10] Massart R, Mongeau R, Lanfumey L. Beyond the monoaminergic hypothesis: neuroplasticity and epigenetic changes in a transgenic mouse model of depression. Philos Trans R Soc Lond B Biol Sci 2012;367(1601):2485–94.

[11] Soskin DP, Holt DJ, Sacco GR, et al. Incentive salience: novel treatment strategies for major depression. CNS Spectr 2013;18(6):307–14.

[12] Hasler G. Pathophysiology of depression: do we have any solid evidence of interest to clinicians? World Psychiatry 2010;9:155–61.

[13] Berk M, Dean OM, Cotton SM, et al. The efficacy of adjunctive N-acetylcysteine in major depressive disorder: a double-blind, randomized, placebo-controlled trial. J Clin Psychiatry 2014;75(6):628–36.

[14] Sher L. Buprenorphine and the treatment of depression, anxiety, non-suicidal self-injury, and suicidality. Acta Psychiatr Scand 2016;134(1):84–5.

[15] Maripuu M, Wikgren M, Karling P, et al. Relative hypo- and hypercortisolism are both associated with depression and lower quality of life in bipolar disorder: a cross-sectional study. PLoS ONE 2014;9(6):e98682.

[16] Cheuvront SN, Kenefick RW. Am I drinking enough? Yes, no, and maybe. J Am Coll Nutr 2016;35(2):185–92.

[17] Carta MG, Bhat KM, Preti A. GABAergic neuroactive steroids: a new frontier in bipolar disorders? Behav Brain Funct 2012;8:61.

[18] Taketani T, Tamura H, Takasaki A, et al. Protective role of melatonin in progesterone production by human luteal cells. J Pineal Res 2011;51:207–13.

[19] Hailes J. Evidence-based guidelines for the assessment and management of polycystic ovary syndrome. Melbourne: PCOS Australian Alliance; 2015.

[20] March WA, Moore VM, Willson KJ, et al. The prevalence of polycystic ovary syndrome in a community sample assessed under contrasting diagnostic criteria. Hum Reprod 2010;25(2):544–51.

[21] Boyle J, Teede HJ. Polycystic ovary syndrome. Aust Fam Phys 2012;41(10).

[22] Haroon E, Raison CL, Miller AH. Psychoneuroimmunology meets neuropsychopharmacology: translational implications of the impact of inflammation on behavior. Neuropsychopharmacology 2012;37(1):137–62.

[23] Morris G, Berk M. The many roads to mitochondrial dysfunction in neuroimmune and neuropsychiatric disorders. BMC Med 2015;13:68.

[24] Maes M, Berk M, Goehler L, et al. Depression and sickness behavior are Janus-faced responses to shared inflammatory pathways. BMC Med 2012;10:66.

[25] Lyngdoh T, Bochud M, Glaus J, et al. Associations of serum uric acid and SLC2A9 variant with depressive and anxiety disorders: a population-based study. PLoS ONE 2013;8(10):e76336.

[26] Neurogenesis, leadership and rewiring your own brain [press release]. 2016. http://www.abc.net.au/radionational/programs/ockhamsrazor/rewiring-your-own-brain/635841.

[27] Davidson RJ. Anxiety and affective style: role of prefrontal cortex and amygdala. Biol Psychiatry 2002;51:68–80.

[28] Berkman ET, Lieberman D. Approaching the bad and avoiding the good: lateral prefrontal cortical asymmetry distinguishes between action and valence. J Cogn Neurosci 2010;22(9):1970–9.
[29] Hect D. Depression and the hyperactive right-hemisphere. Neurosci Res 2010;68:77–87.
[30] Galvan V, Jin K. Neurogenesis in the aging brain. Clin Interv Aging 2007;2(4):605–10.
[31] Szewczyk B, Poleszak E, Sowa-Kucma M, et al. Antidepressant activity of zinc and magnesium in view of the current hypotheses of antidepressant action. Pharmacol Rep 2008;60(5):588–9.
[32] McNamara RK. Role of omega-3 fatty acids in the etiology, treatment, and prevention of depression: current status and future directions. J Nutr Intermed Metab 2016;5:96–106.
[33] Cryan JF, Dinan TG. Mind-altering microorganisms: the impact of the gut microbiota on brain and behaviour. Nat Rev Neurosci 2012;13(10):701–12.
[34] Bornstein JC. Serotonin in the gut: what does it do? Front Neurosci 2012;6:16.
[35] Chang L. Pathophysiology of chronic constipation and irritable bowel syndrome. Adv Stud Med 2006;6(4A):S232–6.
[36] Hawrelak J, Myers S. The causes of intestinal dysbiosis: a review. Altern Med Rev 2004;9(2):180–97.
[37] Naseribafrouei A, Hestad K, Avershina E, et al. Correlation between the human fecal microbiota and depression. Neurogastroenterol Motil 2014;26(8):1155–62.
[38] Dinan TG, Stanton C, Cryan JF. Psychobiotics: a novel class of psychotropic. Biol Psychiatry 2013;74(10):720–6.
[39] O'Hara AM, Shanahan F. The gut flora as a forgotten organ. EMBO Rep 2006;7(7):688–93.
[40] Sender R, Fuchs S, Milo R. Revised estimates for the number of human and bacteria cells in the body. PLoS Biol 2016;14(8):e1002533.
[41] Jessen NA, Munk AS, Lundgaard I, et al. The glymphatic system: a beginner's guide. Neurochem Res 2015;40(12):2583–99.
[42] Gale C, Hagenaars SP, Davies G, et al. Pleiotropy between neuroticism and physical and mental health: findings from 108 038 men and women in UK Biobank. Transl Psychiatry 2015.
[43] Lok A, Bockting CLH, Koeter MWJ, et al. Interaction between the MTHFR C677T polymorphism and traumatic childhood events predicts depression. Transl Psychiatry 2013;3(7):e288.
[44] Gronli O, Kvamme M, Friborg O, et al. Zinc deficiency is common in several psychiatric disorders. PLoS ONE 2013;8(12):e82793.
[45] Rao TS, Asha MR, Ramesh BN, et al. Understanding nutrition, depression and mental illnesses. Indian J Psychiatry 2008;50(2):77–82.
[46] Beard J, Hendricks MK, Perez EM, et al. Maternal iron deficiency anemia affects postpartum emotions and cognition. Nutr Epidemiol 2005;135:267–72.
[47] Gariballa S. Testing homocysteine-induced neurotransmitter deficiency, and depression of mood hypothesis in clinical practice. Age Ageing 2011;40(6):702–5.
[48] Tomiyama AJ, Mann T, Vinas D, et al. Low calorie dieting increases cortisol. Psychosom Med 2010;72(4):357–64.
[49] Swardfager W, Herrmann N, Mazereeuw G, et al. Zinc in depression: a meta-analysis. Biol Psychiatry 2013;74(12):872–8.
[50] Lai J, Moxey A, Nowak G, et al. The efficacy of zinc supplementation in depression: systematic review of randomised controlled trials. J Affect Disord 2012;136(1–2):e31–9.
[51] Shah M, Subhani M, Rizvon K, et al. Transient psychotic episode induced by *Helicobacter pylori* triple therapy treatment. Case Rep Gastroenterol 2012;6(2):381–6.
[52] Ellingwood F. Ellingwood's theraputics. Ellingwood's Theraputics; 1908.
[53] Felter HW, Lloyd JU. King's American dispensatory. 18th ed. Portland, OR: Eclectic Medical Publications; 1905. Reprinted 1983.
[54] Lindlahr H. Nature cure: philosophy & practice based on the unity of disease & cure. Chicago: The Nature Cure Publishing Company; 1922. Available from: www.soilandhealth.org/02/0201hyglibcat/020123lindlahr/020123toc.html.
[55] Engel GL. The need for a new medical model: a challenge for biomedicine. Science 1977;196(4286):129–36.
[56] Norcross J, Karpiak C, Lister K. What's an integrationist? A study of self-identified integrative and (occasionally) eclectic psychologists. J Clin Psychol 2005;61(12):1587–94.
[57] Miller AH, Maletic V, Raison CL. Inflammation and its discontents: the role of cytokines in the pathophysiology of major depression. Biol Psychiatry 2009;65(9):732–41.
[58] McIntyre E. Management of mental health in Australia: a critical role for herbalists and naturopaths. Aust J Herb Med 2016;28(3):69–72.
[59] Serrano-Blanco A, Palao DJ, Luciano JV, et al. Prevalence of mental disorders in primary care: results from the diagnosis and treatment of mental disorders in primary care study (DASMAP). Soc Psychiatry Psychiatr Epidemiol 2010;45(2):201–10.
[60] Wardle J, Adams J. Indirect and non-health risks associated with complementary and alternative medicine use: an integrative review. Eur J Int Med 2014;6:doi:10.1016/j.eujim.2014.01.001.
[61] Mlyniec K, Ostachowicz B, Krakowska A, et al. Chronic but not acute antidepresant treatment alters serum zinc/copper ratio under pathological/zinc-deficient conditions in mice. J Physiol Pharmacol 2014;65(5):673–8.
[62] Sarris J, Papakostas GI, Vitolo O, et al. S-adenosyl methionine (SAMe) versus escitalopram and placebo in major depression RCT: efficacy and effects of histamine and carnitine as moderators of response. J Affect Disord 2014;164:76–81.
[63] Mikirova N. Clinical test of pyrroles: usefulness and association with other biochemical markers. Clin Med Rev Case Rep 2015;2(2).
[64] Kern JK, Geier DA, Bjorklund G, et al. Evidence supporting a link between dental amalgams and chronic illness, fatigue, depression, anxiety, and suicide. Neuro Endocrinol Lett 2014;35(7):537–52.
[65] Pusceddu MM, Kelly P, Stanton C, et al. N-3 Polyunsaturated fatty acids through the lifespan: implication for psychopathology. Int J Neuropsychopharmacol 2016;19(12).
[66] Saunders EF, Ramsden CE, Sherazy MS, et al. Omega-3 and omega-6 polyunsaturated fatty acids in bipolar disorder: a review of biomarker and treatment studies. J Clin Psychiatry 2016;77(10):e1301–8.
[67] Palazidou E. The neurobiology of depression. Br Med Bull 2012;101:127–45.
[68] Morris MC, Compas BE, Garber J. Relations among posttraumatic stress disorder, comorbid major depression, and HPA function: a systematic review and meta-analysis. Clin Psychol Rev 2012;32(4):301–15.
[69] Amore M, Innamorati M, Costi S, et al. Partial androgen deficiency, depression, and testosterone supplementation in aging men. Int J Endocrinol 2012;2012:280724.
[70] Slyepchenko A, Maes M, Jacka FN, et al. Gut microbiota, bacterial translocation, and interactions with diet: pathophysiological links between major depressive disorder and non-communicable medical comorbidities. Psychother Psychosom 2017;86(1):31–46.
[71] Sherwin E, Sandhu KV, Dinan TG, et al. May the force be with you: the light and dark sides of the microbiota-gut-brain axis in neuropsychiatry. CNS Drugs 2016;30(11):1019–41.
[72] Consortium NaPASoPG. Psychiatric genome-wide association study analyses implicate neuronal, immune and histone pathways. Nat Neurosci 2015;18(2):199–209.
[73] Peerbooms OL, van Os J, Drukker M, et al. Meta-analysis of MTHFR gene variants in schizophrenia, bipolar disorder and unipolar depressive disorder: evidence for a common genetic vulnerability? Brain Behav Immun 2011;25(8):1530–43.
[74] Mental Health First Aid Australia. Suicidal thoughts and behaviours: first aid guidelines (revised 2014). Melbourne: Mental Health First Aid Australia; 2014. Available from: www.mhfa.com.au.
[75] Victorian Government Department of Health. National practice standards for the mental health workforce 2013.
[76] Cukrowicz KC, Wingate LR, Driscoll KA, et al. A standard of care for the assessment of suicide risk and associated treatment: the Florida State University Psychology Clinic as an example. J Contemp Psychother 2004;34(1):87–100.
[77] Anderson A, West SG. Violence against mental health professionals: when the treater becomes the victim. Innov Clin Neurosci 2011;8(3):34–9.
[78] NICE. Depression in adults: recognition and management. 2009, updated 2016. Available from: www.nice.org.uk/guidance/cg90.
[79] Jacka FN, Kremer PJ, Leslie ER, et al. Associations between diet quality and depressed mood in adolescents: results from the Australian Healthy Neighbourhoods Study. Aust N Z J Psychiatry 2010;44(5):435–42.

[80] Jacka FN, Rothon C, Taylor S, et al. Diet quality and mental health problems in adolescents from East London: a prospective study. Soc Psychiatry Psychiatr Epidemiol 2013;48(8):1297–306.
[81] Kim WK, Shin D, Song WO. Are dietary patterns associated with depression in US adults? J Med Food 2016;19(11):10741084.
[82] Lai JS, Oldmeadow C, Hure AJ, et al. Longitudinal diet quality is not associated with depressive symptoms in a cohort of middle-aged Australian women. Br J Nutr 2016;115(5):842–50.
[83] Andreasson A, Arborelius L, Erlanson-Albertsson C, et al. A putative role for cytokines in the impaired appetite in depression. Brain Behav Immun 2007;21(2):147–52.
[84] Jacka FN, Cherbuin N, Anstey KJ, et al. Does reverse causality explain the relationship between diet and depression? J Affect Disord 2015;175:248–50.
[85] Rienks J, Dobson AJ, Mishra GD. Mediterranean dietary pattern and prevalence and incidence of depressive symptoms in mid-aged women: results from a large community-based prospective study. Eur J Clin Nutr 2013;67(1):75–82.
[86] Messamore E, McNamara RK. Detection and treatment of omega-3 fatty acid deficiency in psychiatric practice: rationale and implementation. Lipids Health Dis 2016;15:25.
[87] Neumeister A. Tryptophan depletion, serotonin, and depression: where do we stand? Psychopharmacol Bull 2003;37(4):99–115.
[88] Feder A, Skipper J, Blair JR, et al. Tryptophan depletion and emotional processing in healthy volunteers at high risk for depression. Biol Psychiatry 2011;69(8):804–7.
[89] Roca M, Kohls E, Gili M, et al. Prevention of depression through nutritional strategies in high-risk persons: rationale and design of the MooDFOOD prevention trial. BMC Psychiatry 2016;16:192.
[90] Fava M, Mischoulon D. Folate in depression: efficacy, safety, differences in formulations, and clinical issues. J Clin Psychiatry 2009;70(Suppl. 5):12–17.
[91] Guilarte TR, Chen MK. Manganese inhibits NMDA receptor channel function: implications to psychiatric and cognitive effects. Neurotoxicology 2007;28(6):1147–52.
[92] Tian YJ, Li D, Ma Q, et al. Excess nicotinamide increases plasma serotonin and histamine levels. Sheng Li Xue Bao 2013;65(1):33–8.
[93] Sarris J, Mischoulon D, Schweitzer I. Adjunctive nutraceuticals with standard pharmacotherapies in bipolar disorder: a systematic review of clinical trials. Bipolar Disord 2011;13(5–6):454–65.
[94] Sarris J, Murphy J, Mischoulon D, et al. Adjunctive nutraceuticals for depression: a systematic review and meta-analyses. Am J Psychiatry 2016;173(6):575–87.
[95] Messaoudi M, Violle N, Bisson JF, et al. Beneficial psychological effects of a probiotic formulation (*Lactobacillus helveticus* R0052 and *Bifidobacterium longum* R0175) in healthy human volunteers. Gut Microbes 2011;2(4):256–61.
[96] McKean J, Naug H, Nikbakht E, et al. Probiotics and subclinical psychological symptoms in healthy participants: a systematic review and meta-analysis. J Altern Complement Med 2017;23(4):249–58.
[97] Sarris J, Panossian A, Schweitzer I, et al. Herbal medicine for depression, anxiety and insomnia: a review of psychopharmacology and clinical evidence. Eur Neuropsychopharmacol 2011;21(12):841–60.
[98] Sarris J, McIntyre E, Camfield DA. Plant-based medicines for anxiety disorders, part 2: a review of clinical studies with supporting preclinical evidence. CNS Drugs 2013;27:301–19.
[99] Kaplan JS, Tolin DF. Exposure therapy for anxiety disorders. Psychiatric Times 2011.
[100] Barlow DH. Preface. In: Barlow DH, editor. Clinical handbook of psychological disorders: a step-by-step treatment manual. 5th ed. New York: Guilford Press; 2014.
[101] World Health Organization. Depression 2016. Available from: http://apps.who.int/classifications/icd10/browse/2010/en.
[102] Kessler RC, Petukhova M, Sampson NA, et al. Twelve-month and lifetime prevalence and lifetime morbid risk of anxiety and mood disorders in the United States. Int J Methods Psychiatr Res 2012;21(3):169–84.
[103] Australian Bureau of Statistics. National survey of mental health and wellbeing: summary of results, Australia, 2007. ABS cat. no. 4326.0. Canberra: ABS; 2008.
[104] Pratt LA, Brody DJ, Gu Q. Antidepressant use in persons aged 12 and over: United States, 2005–2008. NCHS Data Brief 2011;76:1–8.
[105] OECD. Health at a glance 2015: how does Australia compare? 2015.
[106] Kessler RC, Bromet EJ. The epidemiology of depression across cultures. Annu Rev Public Health 2013;34:119–38.
[107] WHO Department of Mental Health and Substance Abuse, Marcus M, Yasamy MT, et al Depression: a global public health concern. 2012.
[108] World Health Organization. Gender and women's mental health 2016. Available from: www.who.int/mental_health/prevention/genderwomen/en/.
[109] Clarke DM, Currie KC. Depression, anxiety and their relationship with chronic diseases: a review of the epidemiology, risk and treatment evidence. Med J Aust 2009;190:S54–60.
[110] Stranges S, Samaraweera PC, Taggart F, et al. Major health-related behaviours and mental well-being in the general population: the Health Survey for England. BMJ Open 2014;4(9):e005878.
[111] Patel R, Reiss P, Shetty H, et al. Do antidepressants increase the risk of mania and bipolar disorder in people with depression? A retrospective electronic case register cohort study. BMJ Open 2015;5(12):e008341.
[112] Tondo L, Vázquez G, Baldessarini RJ. Mania associated with antidepressant treatment: comprehensive meta-analytic review. Acta Psychiatr Scand 2009;121(6):404–14.
[113] Williams JM, Crane C, Barnhofer T, et al. Mindfulness-based cognitive therapy for preventing relapse in recurrent depression: a randomized dismantling trial. J Consult Clin Psychol 2014;82(2):275–86.
[114] Young JE, Rygh J, Weinberger AD, et al. Cognitive therapy for depression. In: Barlow DH, editor. Clinical handbook of psychological disorders: a step-by-step treatment manual. 5th ed. New York: Guilford Press; 2014.
[115] Berk M, Jacka F. Preventive strategies in depression: gathering evidence for risk factors and potential interventions. Br J Psychiatry 2012;201(5):339–41.
[116] Beattie E, Pachana NA, Franklin SJ. Double jeopardy: comorbid anxiety and depression in late life. Res Gerontol Nurs 2010;3(3):209–20.
[117] Blazer DG. Depression in late life: review and commentary. J Gerontol A Biol Sci Med Sci 2002;58:249–65.
[118] Steffens DC, McQuoid DR. Impact of symptoms of generalized anxiety disorder on the course of late-life depression. Am J Geriatr Psychiatry 2005;13(1):40–7.
[119] Lovibond PF, Lovibond SH. The structure of negative emotional states: comparison of scales (DASS) with the Beck Depression and Anxiety Inventories. Behav Res Ther 1995;33(3):335–43.
[120] Lovibond PF Overview of the DASS and its uses. 2014. Available from: www2.psy.unsw.edu.au/dass/over.htm.
[121] Richardson LP, McCauley E, Grossman DC, et al. Evaluation of the Patient Health Questionnaire-9 Item for detecting major depression among adolescents. Pediatrics 2010;126(6):1117–23.
[122] Yesavage JA, Brink TL, Rose TL, et al. Development and validation of a geriatric depression screening scale: a preliminary report. J Psychiatr Res 1983;17:37–49.
[123] Friedman B, Heisel MJ, Delavan RL. Psychometric properties of the 15-item geriatric depression scale in functionally impaired, cognitively intact, community-dwelling elderly primary care patients. J Am Geriatr Soc 2005;53(9):1570–6.
[124] Worsfold K. Eating disorder mental health literacy: what do we know as health practitioners? A comparative study of psychologists, naturopaths and fitness instructors. [Master of Clinical Psychology]. Brisbane, Australia: University of Queensland; 2016.
[125] Morgan JF, Reid F, Lacey JH. The SCOFF questionnaire: assessment of a new screening tool for eating disorders. BMJ 1999;319:1467–78.
[126] Hill LS, Reid F, Morgan JF, et al. SCOFF, the development of an eating disorder screening questionnaire. Int J Eat Disord 2010;43(4):344–51.
[127] Almeida OP, Ford AH, Flicker L. Systematic review and meta-analysis of randomized placebo-controlled trials of folate and vitamin B12 for depression. Int Psychogeriatr 2015;27(5):727–37.
[128] Mischoulon D, Lamon-Fava S, Selhub J, et al. Prevalence of MTHFR C677T and MS A2756G polymorphisms in major depressive disorder, and their impact on response to fluoxetine treatment. CNS Spectr 2012;17(2):76–86.
[129] Lewis SJ, Araya R, Leary S, et al. Folic acid supplementation during pregnancy may protect against depression 21 months after

pregnancy, an effect modified by MTHFR C677T genotype. Eur J Clin Nutr 2012;66(1):97–103.
[130] Galizia I, Oldani L, Macritchie K, et al. S-adenosyl methionine (SAMe) for depression in adults. Cochrane Database Syst Rev 2016;(10):CD011286.
[131] Alpert JE, Papakostas G, Mischoulon D, et al. S-adenosyl-L-methionine (SAMe) as an adjunct for resistant major depressive disorder: an open trial following partial or nonresponse to selective serotonin reuptake inhibitors or venlafaxine. J Clin Psychopharmacol 2004;24(6):661–4.
[132] Papakostas GI, Mischoulon D, Shyu I, et al. S-adenosyl methionine (SAMe) augmentation of serotonin reuptake inhibitors for antidepressant nonresponders with major depressive disorder: a double-blind, randomized clinical trial. Am J Psychiatry 2010;167(8):942–8.
[133] Sarris J, Price LH, Carpenter LL, et al. Is S-adenosyl methionine (SAMe) for depression only effective in males? A re-analysis of data from a randomized clinical trial. Pharmacopsychiatry 2015;48(4–5):141–4.
[134] Kendall-Tackett K. Long-chain omega-3 fatty acids and women's mental health in the perinatal period and beyond. J Midwifery Womens Health 2010;55(6):561–7.
[135] Grenyer BF, Crowe T, Meyer B, et al. Fish oil supplementation in the treatment of major depression: a randomised double-blind placebo-controlled trial. Prog Neuropsychopharmacol Biol Psychiatry 2007;31(7):1393–6.
[136] Yehuda S, Rabinovitz S, Mostofsky DI. Essential fatty acids and the brain: from infancy to aging. Neurobiol Aging 2005;26(Suppl. 1):98–102.
[137] Bruinsma KA, Taren DL. Dieting, essential fatty acid intake, and depression. Nutr Rev 2000;58(4):98–108.
[138] Sublette ME, Ellis SP, Geant AL, et al. Meta-analysis of the effects of eicosapentaenoic acid (EPA) in clinical trials in depression. J Clin Psychiatry 2011;72(12):1577–84.
[139] Martins JG. EPA but not DHA appears to be responsible for the efficacy of omega-3 long chain polyunsaturated fatty acid supplementation in depression: evidence from a meta-analysis of randomized controlled trials. J Am Coll Nutr 2009;28(5):525–42.
[140] Ross BM, Seguin J, Sieswerda LE. Omega-3 fatty acids as treatments for mental illness: which disorder and which fatty acid? Lipids Health Dis 2007;6:21.
[141] Husted KS, Bouzinova EV. The importance of n-6/n-3 fatty acids ration in the major depressive disorder. Medicina (Kaunas) 2016;52(3):139–47.
[142] Samuni Y, Goldstein S, Dean OM, et al. The chemistry and biological activities of N-acetylcysteine. Biochim Biophys Acta 2013;1830(8):4117–29.
[143] Rushworth GF, Megson IL. Existing and potential therapeutic uses for N-acetylcysteine: the need for conversion to intracellular glutathione for antioxidant benefits. Pharmacol Ther 2014;141(2):150–9.
[144] Deepmala, Slattery J, Kumar N, et al. Clinical trials of N-acetylcysteine in psychiatry and neurology: a systematic review. Neurosci Biobehav Rev 2015;55:294–321.
[145] Maes M, Vandoolaeghe E, Neels H, et al. Lower serum zinc in major depression is a sensitive marker of treatment resistance and of the immune/inflammatory response in that illness. Biol Psychiatry 1997;42(5):349–58.
[146] Jurowski K, Szewczyk B, Nowak G, et al. Biological consequences of zinc deficiency in the pathomechanisms of selected diseases. J Biol Inorg Chem 2014;19(7):1069–79.
[147] Styczen K, Sowa-Kucma M, Siwek M, et al. The serum zinc concentration as a potential biological marker in patients with major depressive disorder. Metab Brain Dis 2017;32(1):97–103.
[148] Salari S, Khomand P, Arasteh M, et al. Zinc sulphate: a reasonable choice for depression management in patients with multiple sclerosis. A randomized, double-blind, placebo-controlled clinical trial. Pharmacol Rep 2015;67(3):606–9.
[149] Stockner T, Montgomery TR, Kudlacek O, et al. Mutational analysis of the high-affinity zinc binding site validates a refined human dopamine transporter homology model. PLoS Comput Biol 2013;9(2):e1002909.
[150] Feitosa MC, Lima VB, Moita Neto JM, et al. Plasma concentration of IL-6 and TNF-alpha and its relationship with zincemia in obese women. Rev Assoc Med Bras 2013;59(5):429–34.
[151] Prasad AS. Zinc: role in immunity, oxidative stress and chronic inflammation. Curr Opin Clin Nutr Metab Care 2009;12(6):646–52.
[152] Prasad AS. Discovery of human zinc deficiency: its impact on human health and disease. Adv Nutr 2013;4(2):176–90.
[153] Ellsworth-Bowers ER, Corwin EJ. Nutrition and the psychoneuroimmunology of postpartum depression. Nutr Res Rev 2012;25(1):180–92.
[154] Roomruangwong C, Kanchanatawan B, Sirivichayakul S, et al. Lower serum zinc and higher CRP strongly predict prenatal depression and physio-somatic symptoms, which all together predict postnatal depressive symptoms. Mol Neurobiol 2016;54(2):1500–12.
[155] Wojcik J, Dudek D, Schlegel-Zawadzka M, et al. Antepartum/postpartum depressive symptoms and serum zinc and magnesium levels. Pharmacol Rep 2006;58(4):571–6.
[156] Marcellini F, Giuli C, Papa R, et al. Zinc status, psychological and nutritional assessment in old people recruited in five European countries: Zincage study. Biogerontology 2006;7(5–6):339–45.
[157] International Zinc Nutrition Consultative Group (IZiNCG). Assessment of the risk of zinc deficiency in populations and options for its control. Food Nutr Bull 2004;25(1):suppl 2.
[158] Lieberman HR, Agarwal S, Fulgoni VL 3rd. Tryptophan intake in the US adult population is not related to liver or kidney function but is associated with depression and sleep outcomes. J Nutr 2016;146(12):2609s–2615s.
[159] Anderson GM, Maes M. How immune-inflammatory processes link CNS and psychiatric disorders: classification and treatment implications. CNS Neurol Disord Drug Targets 2017;16(1).
[160] Turner EH, Loftis JM, Blackwell AD. Serotonin a la carte: supplementation with the serotonin precursor 5-hydroxytryptophan. Pharmacol Ther 2006;109(3):325–38.
[161] Garlick PJ. Assessment of the safety of glutamine and other amino acids. J Nutr 2001;131(9 Suppl.):2556s–2561s.
[162] Russo E, Scicchitano F, Whalley BJ, et al. Hypericum perforatum: pharmacokinetic, mechanism of action, tolerability, and clinical drug–drug interactions. Phytother Res 2014;28(5):643–55.
[163] Apaydin EA, Maher AR, Shanman R, et al. A systematic review of St John's wort for major depressive disorder. Syst Rev 2016;5(1):148.
[164] Linde K, Kriston L, Rücker G, et al. Efficacy and acceptability of pharmacological treatments for depressive disorders in primary care: systematic review and network meta-analysis. Ann Fam Med 2015;13(1):69–79.
[165] Panossian A, Wikman G, Sarris J. Rosenroot (*Rhodiola rosea*): traditional use, chemical composition, pharmacology and clinical efficacy. Phytomedicine 2010;17(7):481–93.
[166] Hung SK, Perry R, Ernst E. The effectiveness and efficacy of *Rhodiola rosea* L.: A systematic review of randomized clinical trials. Phytomedicine 2011;18(4):235–44.
[167] Mao JJ, Xie SX, Zee J, et al. *Rhodiola rosea* versus sertraline for major depressive disorder: a randomized placebo-controlled trial. Phytomedicine 2015;22(3):394–9.
[168] Ross SM. *Rhodiola rosea* (SHR-5), part 2: a standardized extract of *Rhodiola rosea* is shown to be effective in the treatment of mild to moderate depression. Holist Nurs Pract 2014;28(3):217–21.
[169] Prusinowska R, Śmigielski Krzysztof B. Composition, biological properties and therapeutic effects of lavender (*Lavandula angustifolia* L). A review. Herba Polonica 2014;60(2):56–66.
[170] Akhondzadeh S, Kashani L, Fotouhi A, et al. Comparison of *Lavandula angustifolia* Mill. tincture and imipramine in the treatment of mild to moderate depression: a double-blind, randomized trial. Prog Neuropsychopharmacol Biol Psychiatry 2003;27(1):123–7.
[171] Rabbani M, Vaseghi G, Sajjadi SE, et al. Persian herbal medicines with anxiolytic properties. J Med Plants 2011;10(39):7–11.
[172] Schmidt M, Betti G, Hensel A. Saffron in phytotherapy: pharmacology and clinical uses. Wien Med Wochenschr 2007;157(13):315.
[173] Lopresti AL, Drummond PD. Saffron (*Crocus sativus*) for depression: a systematic review of clinical studies and examination of underlying antidepressant mechanisms of action. Hum Psychopharmacol 2014;29(6):517–27.
[174] Ströhle A. Physical activity, exercise, depression and anxiety disorders. J Neural Transm 2008;116(6):777.

[175] Wegner M, Helmich I, Machado S, et al. Effects of exercise on anxiety and depression disorders: review of meta-analyses and neurobiological mechanisms. CNS Neurol Disord Drug Targets 2014;13(6):1002–14.
[176] World Health Organization (WHO). The ICD-10 classification of mental and behavioural disorders: Clinical descriptions and diagnostic guidelines. Geneva: WHO; 2003.
[177] Kanuri N, Taylor CB, Cohen JM, et al. Classification models for subthreshold generalized anxiety disorder in a college population: implications for prevention. J Anxiety Dis 2015;34:43–52.
[178] Kessler RC, Wittchen H-U. Patterns and correlates of generalized anxiety disorder in community samples. J Clin Psychiatry 2002;63:4–10.
[179] Roemer L, Orsillo SM. An acceptance-based behavioural therapy for generalised anxiety. In: Barlow DH, editor. Clinical handbook of psychological disorders: a step-by-step treatment manual. 5th ed. New York: Guilford Press; 2014.
[180] Tiller JWG. Depression and anxiety. Med J Aust 2012;1(4):28–31.
[181] Brown TA, Chorpita BF, Korotitsch W, et al. Psychometric properties of the Depression Anxiety Stress Scales (DASS) in clinical samples. Behav Res Ther 1997;35:1.
[182] Spitzer RL, Kroenke K, Williams JBW, et al. A brief measure for assessing generalized anxiety disorder: the GAD-7. Arch Intern Med 2006;166(10):1092–7.
[183] Kroenke K, Spitzer RL, Williams JB, et al. Anxiety disorders in primary care: prevalence, impairment, comorbidity, and detection. Ann Intern Med 2007;146(5):317–25.
[184] Pachana NA, Byrne GJ, Siddle H, et al. Development and validation of the Geriatric Anxiety Inventory. Int Psychogeriatr 2007;19(1):103–14.
[185] Aucoin M, Bhardwaj S. Generalized anxiety disorder and hypoglycemia symptoms improved with diet modification. Case Rep Psychiatr 2016;2016:7165425.
[186] Sartori SB, Whittle N, Hetzenauer A, et al. Magnesium deficiency induces anxiety and HPA axis dysregulation: modulation by therapeutic drug treatment. Neuropharmacology 2012;62(1):304–12.
[187] Singewald N, Sinner C, Hetzenauer A, et al. Magnesium-deficient diet alters depression- and anxiety-related behavior in mice — influence of desipramine and *Hypericum perforatum* extract. Neuropharmacology 2004;47(8):1189–97.
[188] Grases G, Perez-Castello JA, Sanchis P, et al. Anxiety and stress among science students. Study of calcium and magnesium alterations. Magnes Res 2006;19(2):102–6.
[189] De Souza MC, Walker AF, Robinson PA, et al. A synergistic effect of a daily supplement for 1 month of 200 mg magnesium plus 50 mg vitamin B6 for the relief of anxiety-related premenstrual symptoms: a randomized, double-blind, crossover study. J Womens Health Gend Based Med 2000;9(2):131–9.
[190] Hanus M, Lafon J, Mathieu M. Double-blind, randomised, placebo-controlled study to evaluate the efficacy and safety of a fixed combination containing two plant extracts (*Crataegus oxyacantha* and *Eschscholtzia californica*) and magnesium in mild-to-moderate anxiety disorders. Curr Med Res Opin 2004;20(1):63–71.
[191] de Oliveira IJ, de Souza VV, Motta V, et al. Effects of oral vitamin C supplementation on anxiety in students: a double-blind, randomized, placebo-controlled trial. Pak J Biol Sci 2015;18(1):11–18.
[192] Gautam M, Agrawal M, Gautam M, et al. Role of antioxidants in generalised anxiety disorder and depression. Indian J Psychiatry 2012;54(3):244–7.
[193] Mazloom Z, Ekramzadeh M, Hejazi N. Efficacy of supplementary vitamins C and E on anxiety, depression and stress in type 2 diabetic patients: a randomized, single-blind, placebo-controlled trial. Pak J Biol Sci 2013;16(22):1597–600.
[194] Santos P, Herrmann AP, Benvenutti R, et al. Anxiolytic properties of N-acetylcysteine in mice. Behav Brain Res 2017;317:461–9.
[195] Brody S, Preut R, Schommer K, et al. A randomized controlled trial of high dose ascorbic acid for reduction of blood pressure, cortisol, and subjective responses to psychological stress. Psychopharmacology (Berl) 2002;159(3):319–24.
[196] Strawn JR, Saldana SN. Treatment with adjunctive N-acetylcysteine in an adolescent with selective serotonin reuptake inhibitor-resistant anxiety. J Child Adolesc Psychopharmacol 2012;22(6):472–3.
[197] L-theanine. Monograph. Altern Med Rev 2005;10(2):136–8.
[198] Haskell CF, Kennedy DO, Milne AL, et al. The effects of L-theanine, caffeine and their combination on cognition and mood. Biol Psychiatry 2008;77(2):113–22.
[199] Lu K, Gray MA, Oliver C, et al. The acute effects of L-theanine in comparison with alprazolam on anticipatory anxiety in humans. Hum Psychopharmacol 2004;19(7):457–65.
[200] Nathan PJ, Lu K, Gray M, et al. The neuropharmacology of L-theanine(N-ethyl-L-glutamine): a possible neuroprotective and cognitive enhancing agent. J Herb Pharmacother 2006;6(2):21–30.
[201] Kakuda T, Nozawa A, Unno T, et al. Inhibiting effects of theanine on caffeine stimulation evaluated by EEG in the rat. Biosci Biotechnol Biochem 2000;64(2):287–93.
[202] Kimura K, Ozeki M, Juneja LR, et al. L-theanine reduces psychological and physiological stress responses. Biol Psychiatry 2007;74(1):39–45.
[203] Kobayashi K, Nagato Y, Aoi N, et al. Effects of L-theanine on the release of alpha-brain waves in human volunteers. Nippon Nogeikagaku Kaishi 1998;72(2):153–7.
[204] Yoto A, Motoki M, Murao S, et al. Effects of L-theanine or caffeine intake on changes in blood pressure under physical and psychological stresses. J Physiolog Anthropol 2012;31:28.
[205] Camfield D, McIntyre E, Sarris J, editors. Evidence-based herbal and nutritional treatments for anxiety in psychiatric disorders. Switzerland: Springer International Publishing; 2017.
[206] Pittler MH, Ernst E. Efficacy of kava extract for treating anxiety: systematic review and meta-analysis. J Clin Psychopharmacol 2000;20(1):84–9.
[207] Witte S, Loew D, Gaus W. Meta-analysis of the efficacy of the acetonic kava-kava extract WS1490 in patients with non-psychotic anxiety disorders. Phytother Res 2005;19(3):183–8.
[208] Coulter D. Assessment of the risk of hepatotoxicity with kava products. WHO appointed committee. Geneva: WHO; 2007.
[209] Sarris J, Kavanagh D, Byrne G, et al. The Kava Anxiety Depression Spectrum Study (KADSS): a randomized, placebo-controlled, cross-over trial using an aqueous extract of *Piper methysticum.* Psychopharmacology (Berl) 2009;205(3):399–407.
[210] Sarris J, Stough C, Bousman CA, et al. Kava in the treatment of generalized anxiety disorder: a double-blind, randomized, placebo-controlled study. J Clin Psychopharmacol 2013;33(5): 643–8.
[211] Boerner RJ, Sommer H, Berger W, et al. Kava-kava extract LI 150 is as effective as opipramol and buspirone in generalised anxiety disorder — an 8-week randomized, double-blind multi-centre clinical trial in 129 out-patients. Phytomedicine 2003;10(Suppl. 4):38–49.
[212] Sarris J, Scholey A, Schweitzer I, et al. The acute effects of kava and oxazepam on anxiety, mood, neurocognition; and genetic correlates: a randomized, placebo-controlled, double-blind study. Hum Psychopharmacol 2012;27(3):262–9.
[213] Awad R, Levac D, Cybulska P, et al. Effects of traditionally used anxiolytic botanicals on enzymes of the γ-aminobutyric acid (GABA) system. Can J Physiol Pharmacol 2007;85(9):933–42.
[214] Avallone R, Zanoli P, Puia G, et al. Pharmacological profile of apigenin, a flavonoid isolated from *Matricaria chamomilla.* Biochem Pharmacol 2000;59(11):1387–94.
[215] Viola H, Wasowski C, Levi de Stein M, et al. Apigenin, a component of *Matricaria recutita* flowers, is a central benzodiazepine receptors-ligand with anxiolytic effects. Planta Med 1995;61(3):213–16.
[216] Salgueiro JB, Ardenghi P, Dias M, et al. Anxiolytic natural and synthetic flavonoid ligands of the central benzodiazepine receptor have no effect on memory tasks in rats. Pharmacol Biochem Behav 1997;58(4):887–91.
[217] Amsterdam JD, Li Y, Soeller I, et al. A randomized, double-blind, placebo-controlled trial of oral *Matricaria recutita* (chamomile) extract therapy for generalized anxiety disorder. J Clin Psychopharmacol 2009;29(4):378–82.
[218] Mao JJ, Xie SX, Keefe JR, et al. Long-term chamomile (*Matricaria chamomilla* L.) treatment for generalized anxiety disorder: a randomized clinical trial. Phytomedicine 2016;23(14):1735–42.
[219] Akhondzadeh S, Naghavi HR, Vazirian M, et al. Passionflower in the treatment of generalized anxiety: a pilot double-blind randomized controlled trial with oxazepam. J Clin Pharmac Ther 2001;26(5):363–7.

[220] Dhawan K, Kumar S, Sharma A. Anxiolytic activity of aerial and underground parts of *Passiflora incarnata*. J Ethnopharmacol 2001;72(8):922–6.
[221] Dhawan K, Dhawan S, Sharma A. *Passiflora*: a review update. J Ethnopharmacol 2004;94(1):1–23.
[222] Movafegh A, Alizadeh R, Hajimohamadi F, et al. Preoperative oral *Passiflora incarnata* reduces anxiety in ambulatory surgery patients: a double-blind, placebo-controlled study. Anesth Analg 2008;106(6):1728–32.
[223] Aslanargun P, Cuvas O, Dikmen B, et al. *Passiflora incarnata* Linneaus as an anxiolytic before spinal anesthesia. J Anesthes 2012;26(1):39–44.
[224] Kaviani N, Tavakoli M, Tabanmehr MR, et al. The efficacy of *Passiflora incarnata* Linnaeus in reducing dental anxiety in patients undergoing periodontal treatment. J Dent (Shiraz) 2013;14(2):68–72.
[225] Kulkarni SK, Dhir A. *Withania somnifera*: an Indian ginseng. Prog Neuropsychopharmacol Biol Psychiatry 2008;32(5):1093–105.
[226] Perry NL, Camfield DA. Adaptogens. In: Camfield D, McIntyre E, Sarris J, editors. Evidence-based herbal and nutritional treatments for anxiety in psychiatric disorders. Switzerland: Springer International Publishing; 2017.
[227] Pratte MA, Nanavati KB, Young V, et al. An alternative treatment for anxiety: a systematic review of human trial results reported for the ayurvedic herb ashwagandha (*Withania somnifera*). J Altern Complement Med 2014;20(12):901–8.
[228] Cooley K, Szczurko O, Perri D, et al. Naturopathic care for anxiety: a randomized controlled trial ISRCTN78958974. PLoS ONE 2009;4(8):e6628.
[229] Jahanbakhsh SP, Manteghi AA, Emami SA, et al. Evaluation of the efficacy of *Withania somnifera* (Ashwagandha) root extract in patients with obsessive-compulsive disorder: a randomized double-blind placebo-controlled trial. Complement Ther Med 2016;27:25–9.

CHAPTER APPENDICES

APPENDIX 12.1

Seven cluster events that trigger carcinogenesis and that can be targeted for strategies for treatment

Induction of cancer	Strategies to inhibit cancer
Genetic instability — all cancer cells have genetic instability which increases their chances of mutation — oxidative stress	Reduce genetic instability by increasing antioxidants such as SAMe, methylation factors and *Camellia sinensis* (green tea). This reduces mutations.
Abnormal gene expression — some genes produce proteins that increase cancer progression, some produce proteins that inhibit progression	Inhibit abnormal gene expression by modifying transcription factors (cytokines, growth factors, etc.) with melatonin, vitamins C and E and lipoic acid and *N*-acetylcysteine, curcumin, quercetin, selenium, etc.
Abnormal signal transduction — the signal comes from outside the cell into the nucleus where it can stimulate proliferation (e.g. growth factors) or otherwise. Cell to cell communication is regulated by portals between adjacent cells through gap junctions and cell adhesion molecules (proteins). Can produce growth factor and free radicals making growth factor more responsive to stimulation	Inhibit abnormal signal transduction with compounds that inhibit protein tyrosine kinases — such as curcumin, flavonoids, parthenolide, hypericin, omega-3 fatty acids, selenium and vitamins D and E and silymarin.
Abnormal cell to cell communication — cancer cells decrease contact with normal cells — acting more independently	Re-establish normal cell to cell communication with compounds such as genistein, EGCG (green tea), melatonin, resveratrol, selenium and vitamin D.
Angiogenesis is the growth of new blood vessels to feed the growing tumour. Solid tumours particularly require new blood vessels to provide the extra oxygen and nutrients. Angiogenesis also allows for metastases. Malignant cells also synthesise excess PGE2 (increasing inflammation)	Inhibit tumour angiogenesis with anthrocyanidins, *Centella asiatica*, flavonoids, garlic, omega-3 fatty acids, resveratrol, boswellic acids, curcumin, etc. These also inhibit inflammation.
Invasion and metastases — tumours can spread locally via invasion of adjacent tissues and distantly via metastases through blood and lymph	Inhibit invasion and metastases — inhibiting the enzymes that digest local tissue and invasion with apigenin, boswellic acids, *Centella asiatica*, vitamin C, resveratrol, EGCG, anthrocyanidins, EPA, PSK and polysaccharides, curcumin, vitamins A and C, flavonoids, *Panax ginseng*, *Astragalus membranaceus*, etc.
Immune evasion — cancer cells have the ability to shield themselves from immune attack by camouflaging techniques or by producing immunosuppressive compounds	Stimulation of the immune system with *Astragalus membranaceus*, *Eleutherococcus senticosus*, *Ganoderma lucidium*, *Panax ginseng*, mushroom polysaccharides, glutamine, selenium, vitamins C and E, melatonin, antioxidants generally, etc.

Source: Adapted from Boik J. Natural compounds in cancer therapy — promising non-toxic antitumour agents from plants and other natural sources. Minnesota: Oregon Medical Press; 2001.

APPENDIX 12.2

Tamoxifen and indoles (1)

Tested compound	Inhibition of tyrosine kinase (growth factor)	Inhibition of orthinine decarboxylase (growth factor)	Induction of glutathione (antioxidant)	Inhibition of free radicals (antioxidant)	Inhibition of PADPR (indicator of DNA damage)	Inhibition of DNA binding (prevents induced DNA damage)
Indoles (I3C)	+++	+	++	+++	+++	+++
Tamoxifen	+++	+++	+++	+++	+++	–

Source: Adapted from Life Extension Collectors Edition 1999; 26–32. I3C: The tamoxifen substitute. Cancer prevention for thinking people. http://www.lef.org/magazine/mag99/oct9

APPENDIX 12.3

Tamoxifen and indoles (2)

Activity	Tamoxifen	Indole-3-carbinole (I3C)
Works in oestrogen receptor negative breast cancer	√	√√√
Inhibits oestrogen-induced growth of cancer cells	√	√
Interrupts the cell cycle and triggers apoptosis	√	√
Inhibits protein kinase C (growth factors)	√	Maybe
Metabolises toxic forms of oestrogen to 'safe' forms in liver		√
Inhibits chemically activated cancer (dioxin receptor)		√
Restores tumour-suppressor gene p21		√
Antioxidant	√	√
Causes mutations in tumour-suppressor gene p53	√	

Source: Adapted from Life Extension Collectors Edition 1999; 26–32. I3C: The tamoxifen substitute. Cancer prevention for thinking people. http://www.lef.org/magazine/mag99/oct9

APPENDIX 15.1

The Fibromyalgia Impact Questionnaire (FIQ)

The Fibromyalgia Impact Questionnaire is a useful tool to evaluate the overall symptomatology of fibromyalgia.

PART 1

Directions: For questions 1 to 3, please circle the number that best describes how you were overall for the past week.

Question 1. Were you able to:

	Always (0)	Mostly (1)	Occasionally (2)	Never (3)
1. Do shoppinq?				
2. Do laundry with washer and dryer?				
3. Prepare meals?				
4. Wash dishes/cooking utensils by hand?				
5. Vaccum a rug?				
6. Makes beds?				
7. Walk several blocks?				
8. Visit friends/relatives?				
9. Do yard work?				
10. Drive a car?				
11. Climb stairs?				

Question 2: Of the 7 days in the past week, how many days did you feel good?

0 1 2 3 4 5 6 7

Question 3: How many days last week did you miss work, including housework, because of fibromyalgia?

0 1 2 3 4 5 6 7

PART 2

Directions: For the remaining items, mark the point on the line that best indicates how you felt overall for the past week.

1. Question 4: When you worked, how much did pain or other symptoms of your fibromyalgia interfere with your ability to do your work, including housework?

• ________ ☐ ________ ☐ ________ ☐ ________ ☐ ________ ☐ ________ ☐ ________ ☐ ________ ☐ ________ ☐ ________•.

No problem Great difficulty with work

2. Question 5: How bad has your pain been?

• ________ ☐ ________ ☐ ________ ☐ ________ ☐ ________ ☐ ________ ☐ ________ ☐ ________ ☐ ________ ☐ ________•.

No pain Very severe pain

3. Question 6.How tired have you been?

• ________ ☐ ________ ☐ ________ ☐ ________ ☐ ________ ☐ ________ ☐ ________ ☐ ________ ☐ ________ ☐ ________•.

No tiredness Very tired

4. Question 7: How have you felt when you get up in the morning?

• ________ ☐ ________ ☐ ________ ☐ ________ ☐ ________ ☐ ________ ☐ ________ ☐ ________ ☐ ________ ☐ ________•.

Awoke well Awoke rested Very tired

5. Question 8: How bad has your stiffness been?

• ________ ☐ ________ ☐ ________ ☐ ________ ☐ ________ ☐ ________ ☐ ________ ☐ ________ ☐ ________ ☐ ________•.

No stiffness Very stiff

6. Question 9. How nervous or anxious have you felt?

• ________ ☐ ________ ☐ ________ ☐ ________ ☐ ________ ☐ ________ ☐ ________ ☐ ________ ☐ ________ ☐ ________•.

Not anxious Very anxious

7. Question 10. How depressed or blue have you felt?

• ________ ☐ ________ ☐ ________ ☐ ________ ☐ ________ ☐ ________ ☐ ________ ☐ ________ ☐ ________ ☐ ________•.

Not depressed Very depressed

Reproduced from: Bennet R. The Fibromyalgia Impact Questionnaire (FIQ): a review of its development, current version, operating characteristics and uses. Clin Exp Rheumatol 2005; 23(Suppl. 39):S154–S162. www.myalgia.com/FIQ/FIQ_D.pdf

APPENDIX 15.2

DAS 28 assessment table

DAS 28 Assessment table

Date of assessment: ....

Patient name: ....

	Right swollen	Right tender	Left swollen	Left tender
Shoulder	☐	☐	☐	☐
Elbow	☐	☐	☐	☐
Wrist	☐	☐	☐	☐
MCP 1	☐	☐	☐	☐
MCP 2	☐	☐	☐	☐
MCP 3	☐	☐	☐	☐
MCP 4	☐	☐	☐	☐
MCP 5	☐	☐	☐	☐
PIP 1	☐	☐	☐	☐
PIP 2	☐	☐	☐	☐
PIP 3	☐	☐	☐	☐
PIP 4	☐	☐	☐	☐
PIP 5	☐	☐	☐	☐
Knee	☐	☐	☐	☐
Subtotal	....	....	....	....
	Total swollen:	....	**Total tender:**	....

Disease activity VAS (mark the degree of activity on the scale below by placing a vertical line)

|————————————————————————————————|

No disease activity — High disease activity

To calculate the DAS 28 access the online calculator at http://www.das-score.nl/das28/DAScalculators/dasculators.html *and enter the total number of tender joints, the total number of swollen joints, the ESR CRP and the VAS. The calculated DAS is a number between 0 and 10, indicating how active the patient's rheumatoid arthritis is at the moment. A number greater than 5.1 implies active disease, less than 3.2 low disease activity and less than 2.6 remission.*

Calculated DAS 28

APPENDIX 15.3

Health Assessment Questionnaire (HAQ-DI)©

HEALTH ASSESSMENT QUESTIONNAIRE (HAQ-DI)©

Name: ______________________________ Date: ______________

Please place an 'x' in the box which best describes your abilities OVER THE PAST WEEK:

	Without any difficulty	With some difficulty	With much difficulty	Unable to do
DRESSING & GROOMING				
Are you able to:				
Dress yourself, including shoelaces and buttons?	☐	☐	☐	☐
Shampoo your hair?	☐	☐	☐	☐
ARISING				
Are you able to:				
Stand up from a straight chair?	☐	☐	☐	☐
Get in and out of bed?	☐	☐	☐	☐
EATING				
Are you able to:				
Cut your own meat?	☐	☐	☐	☐
Lift a full cup or glass to your mouth?	☐	☐	☐	☐
Open a new milk carton?	☐	☐	☐	☐
WALKING				
Are you able to:				
Walk outdoors on flat ground?	☐	☐	☐	☐
Climb up five steps?	☐	☐	☐	☐

Please check any AIDS or DEVICES that you usually use for any of the above activities:

- ☐ Devices used for dressing (button hook, zipper pull, etc.)
- ☐ Special or built up chair
- ☐ Built up or special utensils
- ☐ Cane
- ☐ Walker
- ☐ Crutches
- ☐ Wheelchair

Please check any categories for which you usually need HELP FROM ANOTHER PERSON:

☐ Dressing and grooming ☐ Arising ☐ Eating ☐ Walking

	Without any difficulty	With some difficulty	With much difficulty	Unable to do
HYGIENE				
Are you able to:				
Wash and dry your body?	☐	☐	☐	☐
Take a tub bath?	☐	☐	☐	☐
Get on and off the toilet?	☐	☐	☐	☐

Please place an 'x' in the box which best describes your abilities OVER THE PAST WEEK:

	Without any difficulty	With some difficulty	With much difficulty	Unable to do
REACH				
Are you able to:				
Reach and get down a 5 pound object (such as a bag of sugar) from above your head?	☐	☐	☐	☐
Bend down to pick up clothing from the floor?	☐	☐	☐	☐
GRIP				
Are you able to:				
Open car doors?	☐	☐	☐	☐
Open previously opened jars?	☐	☐	☐	☐
Turn faucets on and off?	☐	☐	☐	☐
ACTIVITIES				
Are you able to:				
Run errands and shop?	☐	☐	☐	☐
Get in and out of a car?	☐	☐	☐	☐
Do chores such as vacuuming or yard work?	☐	☐	☐	☐

Please check any AIDS or DEVICES that you usually use for any of the above activities:

☐ Raised toilet set ☐ Bathtub bar ☐ Long handled appliances for reach

☐ Bathtub seat ☐ Long-handled appliances in bathroom ☐ Jar opener (for jars previously opened)

Please check any categories for which you usually need HELP FROM ANOTHER PERSON:

☐ Hygiene ☐ Reach ☐ Gripping and opening things ☐ Errands and chores

Your ACTIVITIES: To what extent are you able to carry out your everyday physical activities such as walking, climbing stairs carrying groceries, or moving a chair?

Completely	Mostly	Moderately	A little	Not at all
☐	☐	☐	☐	☐

Your PAIN: How much pain have you had IN THE PAST WEEK?

On a scale of 0 to 100 (where 0 represents 'no pain' and 100 represents 'severe pain'), please record the number below.

☐☐☐

Your HEALTH: Please rate how well you are doing on a scale of 0 to 100 (0 represents 'very well' and 100 represents 'very poor' health). Please record the number below.

☐☐☐

Source: Stanford University School of Medicine, Division of Immunology & Rheumatology. The Health Assessment Questionnaire 1995: status and review. Philadelphia: Lippincott-Raven, 1996. Fries JF, Spitz P, Kraines G, Holman H. Measurement of patient outcome in arthritis. Arthritis and Rheumatism 1980, 23:137–145.

APPENDIX 15.4

Functional assessment of chronic illness therapy — fatigue

FACIT-F (Version 4)

Below is a list of statements that other people with your illness have said are important. **Please circle or mark one number per line to indicate your response as it applies to the past 7 days.**

	PHYSICAL WELL-BEING	Not at all	A little bit	Some-what	Quite a bit	Very much
GP1	I have a lack of energy	0	1	2	3	4
GP2	I have nausea	0	1	2	3	4
GP3	Because of my physical condition, I have trouble meeting the needs of my family	0	1	2	3	4
GP4	I have pain	0	1	2	3	4
GP5	I am bothered by side effects of treatment	0	1	2	3	4
GP6	I feel ill	0	1	2	3	4
GP7	I am forced to spend time in bed	0	1	2	3	4

	SOCIAL/FAMILY WELL-BEING	Not at all	A little bit	Some-what	Quite a bit	Very much
GS1	I feel close to my friends	0	1	2	3	4
GS2	I get emotional support from my family	0	1	2	3	4
GS3	I get support from my friends	0	1	2	3	4
GS4	My family has accepted my illness	0	1	2	3	4
GS5	I am satisfied with family communication about my illness	0	1	2	3	4
GS6	I feel close to my partner (or the person who is my main support)	0	1	2	3	4
Q1	*Regardless of your current level of sexual activity, please answer the following question. If you prefer not to answer it, please mark this box* ☐ *and go to the next section.*					
GS7	I am satisfied with my sex life	0	1	2	3	4

FACIT-F (Version 4) cont'd

Please circle or mark one number per line to indicate your response as it applies to the past 7 days.

	EMOTIONAL WELL-BEING	Not at all	A little bit	Some-what	Quite a bit	Very much
GE1	I feel sad	0	1	2	3	4
GE2	I am satisfied with how I am coping with my illness	0	1	2	3	4
GE3	I am losing hope in the fight against my illness	0	1	2	3	4
GE4	I feel nervous	0	1	2	3	4
GE5	I worry about dying	0	1	2	3	4
GE6	I worry that my condition will get worse	0	1	2	3	4

	FUNCTIONAL WELL-BEING	Not at all	A little bit	Some-what	Quite a bit	Very much
GF1	I am able to work (include work at home)	0	1	2	3	4
GF2	My work (include work at home) is fulfilling	0	1	2	3	4
GF3	I am able to enjoy life	0	1	2	3	4
GF4	I have accepted my illness	0	1	2	3	4
GF5	I am sleeping well	0	1	2	3	4
GF6	I am enjoying the things I usually do for fun	0	1	2	3	4
GF7	I am content with the quality of my life right now	0	1	2	3	4

Continued

FACIT-F (Version 4) cont'd

Please circle or mark one number per line to indicate your response as it applies to the past 7 days.

	ADDITIONAL CONCERNS	Not at all	A little bit	Some-what	Quite a bit	Very much
HI7	I feel fatigued	0	1	2	3	4
HI12	I feel weak all over	0	1	2	3	4
An1	I feel listless ("washed out")	0	1	2	3	4
An2	I feel tired	0	1	2	3	4
An3	I have trouble starting things because I am tired	0	1	2	3	4
An4	I have trouble finishing things because I am tired	0	1	2	3	4
An5	I have energy	0	1	2	3	4
An7	I am able to do my usual activities	0	1	2	3	4
An8	I need to sleep during the day	0	1	2	3	4
An12	I am too tired to eat	0	1	2	3	4
An14	I need help doing my usual activities	0	1	2	3	4
An15	I am frustrated by being too tired to do the things I want to do	0	1	2	3	4
An16	I have to limit my social activity because I am tired	0	1	2	3	4

APPENDIX 18.1

Menstrual symptom diary

Symptom grading
1 mild
2 moderate
3 severe
4 debilitating

Menstrual flow grading
1 spotting
2 light
3 medium
4 heavy
5 extremely heavy

Cycle day	1	2	3	4	5	6	7	8	9	10	11	12	13	14	15	16	17	18	19	20	21	22	23	24	25	26	27	28
Date																												
Spotting																												
Menstruation																												
Menstruation description (flow, colour, consistency)																												
Menstrual clots																												
Menstrual pain																												
Fertile quality cervical fluid																												
Ovulation symptoms																												
Positive dietary habits																												
Negative dietary habits																												
Food cravings																												
Exercise																												
Depression																												
Anxiety																												
Obsessive thoughts																												
Crying, sad																												
Anger																												
Grief																												
Frustration																												
Irritation																												
Isolation, loneliness																												
Breast self-exam																												

Continued

Cycle day	1	2	3	4	5	6	7	8	9	10	11	12	13	14	15	16	17	18	19	20	21	22	23	24	25	26	27	28
Breast symptoms (nipple sensitivity)																												
Breast symptoms (tender)																												
Breast symptoms (fullness)																												
Fluid retention																												
Lowered energy/ fatigue																												
Headache or migraine																												
Increased libido																												
Decreased libido																												
Painful intercourse																												
Insomnia																												
Poor quality sleep																												
Acne																												
Increased oil production (hair, skin)																												
Increased facial hair or hirsutism																												
Hot flushes																												
Thrush																												
Urinary symptoms																												

APPENDIX 18.2

Endometriosis pain journal

Please use the keys under each category to fill out the chart. The first two lines are example entries.

Date	Day of cycle	Ovulation or menses	During or after sexual activity	Pain location	Intensity of pain (see key)	Quality of pain (see key)	Treatment, management	Associated symptoms
2 April 2019	14	Ovulation	NA	Abdomen (right side)	6	5 + 3	Ceased exercise, rest	Diarrhoea and nausea
27 April 2019	1	Day 1 menses	NA	Abdomen (central)	8	1 + 8 + 10	Complete bed rest	Heavy menstrual flow, large clots, diarrhoea

Scale	Pain intensity	Interference to activities
1	Minimal	Minor interference to daily life
2	Minimal	Mild exercise, full life activities
3	Mild	Mild exercise, all activities except for those with intense pressure to abdomen
4	Mild	No exercise, some interference to activities
5	Moderate	No exercise, able to work but fatigued
6	Moderate	Unable to exercise or perform significant activity, significant fatigue
7	Severe	Unable to exercise or perform significant activity, frequent resting
8	Severe	Minor activities only — showering, food preparation
9	Extreme	Unable to exercise or work, resting only
10	Unbearable	Unable to complete any activity, complete bedrest

Pain quality descriptors and associated keys for chart	
1	Flickering, quivering, pulsing, throbbing, beating, pounding
2	Jumping, flushing, shooting
3	Sharp, cutting, lacerating
4	Pinching, pressing, gnawing, cramping, crushing
5	Tugging, pulling, wrenching, dragging
6	Hot, burning, scalding, searing
7	Tingling, itchy, smarting, stinging
8	Dull, sore, hurting, aching, heavy
9	Tender, taut, rasping, splitting
10	Tiring, exhausting
11	Sickening, suffocating
12	Fearful, frightful, terrifying
13	Punishing, gruelling, cruel, vicious
14	Wretched, blinding
15	Annoying, troublesome, miserable, intense, unbearable
16	Spreading, radiating, penetrating, piercing
17	Tight, numb, drawing, squeezing, tearing
18	Cool, cold, freezing
19	Nagging, nauseating, agonising, dreadful, torturing

APPENDIX 18.3

Menopausal symptom diary

Although the listed symptoms can be related to other health problems individually, as a group they often appear around menopause. These symptoms are frequently due to a reduction in oestrogen and are related to other hormone levels such as DHEA, testosterone and progesterone. Rate each symptom: 0 (none), 1 (mild), 2 (moderate) or 3 (severe).

Hormone deficiency symptoms	Before treatment	2 months after starting	4 months after starting	6 months after starting
Hot flushes				
Lightheaded/dizzy				
Headache				
Migraine				
Depression				
Grief				
Irritability				
Anger				
Frustration				
Loneliness				
Anxiety				
Tearful, sadness				
Mood changes				
Creativity				
Unsociable, introspective				
Insomnia/difficulty sleeping				
Nightmares/disturbing dreams				
Excessive fatigue				
Backache				
Joint pains				
Muscle pains				
Weight gain				
Weight loss				
New facial hair				
Sore breasts				
Dry skin				
Dry anus, vagina, mouth				
Crawling feelings under skin				
Constipation				
Diarrhoea				
Reduced libido				
Uncomfortable intercourse				
Urinary frequency				
Urinary incontinence				
Forgetful, memory loss				
Reduced concentration/clarity				
Total				

APPENDIX 22.1

Sleep diary

	First day	Second day	Third day	Fourth day
COMPLETE IN MORNING				
Bedtime (dose/time)	11:00 pm (25/7)			
Rise time (date/time)	6:30 am (26/07)			
Estimated time to fall asleep	40 minutes			
Estimated number of awakenings and total time awake	6 times 2.5 hours			
Estimated amount of sleep obtained	4 hours			
COMPLETE AT BEDTIME				
Naps (number, time, and duration)	1 at 2:30 pm 1 hour			
Alcoholic drinks (number and time)	1 drink at 8:30 pm 1 drink at 9:00 pm 1 drink at 10:30 pm			
List stresses of the day	Work deadline Argued with partner			
Rate how you felt today 1 = Very tired/sleepy 2 = Somewhat tired/sleepy 3 = Fairly alert 4 = Wide awake	2			
Irritability level 1 = None 2 = Some 3 = Moderate 4 = Fairly high 5 = High	5			
Medications				

Sample sleep diary for use in patients with insomnia. The diary provides a night-to-night account of the patient's sleep schedule and perception of sleep.
Source: Adapted from Harsora P, Kessmann J. Nonpharmacological management of chronic insomnia, Am Fam Phys, 2009; 79(2):125–130.

APPENDIX 22.2

MIDAS (Migraine Disability Assessment) questionnaire

The MIDAS (Migraine Disability Assessment) questionnaire was put together to help patients measure the impact that their headaches have on their life. The information in this questionnaire is also helpful to determine the level of pain and disability caused by a patient's headaches and to find the best treatment for them.

INSTRUCTIONS

Please answer the following questions about ALL of the headaches you have had over the last 3 months. Mark your answer in the box next to each question. Select zero if you did not have the activity in the last 3 months. Please take the completed form to your healthcare professional.

Headache frequency

Question	Amount
On how many days in the last 3 months did you miss work or school because of your headaches?	
On how many days in the last 3 months was your productivity at work or school reduced by half or more because of your headaches? (Do not include days you counted in question 1 where you missed work or school.)	
On how many days in the last 3 months did you not do household work (such as housework, home repairs and maintenance, shopping, caring for children and relatives) because of your headaches?	
On how many days in the last 3 months was your productivity in household work reduced by half or more because of your headaches? (Do not include days you counted in question 3 where you did not do household work.)	
On how many days in the last 3 months did you miss family, social or leisure activities because of your headaches?	
Total	

Interpretation

Scores >6 require review and assessment

MIDAS grade	Definition	MIDAS score
I	Little or no disability	0–5
II	Mild disability	6–10
III	Moderate disability	11–20
IV	Severe disability	21+

Headache intensity

Question	Amount
On how many days in the last 3 months did you have a headache? (If a headache lasted more than 1 day, count each day.)	
On a scale of 0–10, on average how painful were these headaches? (0 = no pain at all, and 10 = pain as bad as it can be.)	
Total	

Interpretation

General questioning useful for interpretation for the clinician.

APPENDIX 22.3

Headache diary

Date	Time (start)	Time (finish)	Intensity (0–10)	Preceding symptoms	Triggers	Treatment	Relief

TREATMENT

Please provide details of type of treatment, dose taken and other specifics.

RELIEF

Please provide details if relief was moderate, mild, complete or none.

Index

A

Page numbers followed by '*f*' indicate figures, '*t*' indicate tables, and '*b*' indicate boxes.

D

E

G

I

J

M

P

W

X

Y

Z

HERB/NUTRIENT–DRUG INTERACTIONS TABLES

Compiled by Liesl Blott

Potential herb–drug and nutrient–drug interactions are described in the following tables. These tables have been formulated to include information on interactions between herbal medicines, nutrients/nutritional medicines and drugs. They include a summary of the potential outcome, a graded recommendation and a comments section that explains the nature of each interaction in more detail.

The recommendations are broadly divided into four categories: avoid, caution, monitor and beneficial. Factors that were taken into account when determining these interaction categories include currently available evidence and safety data; potential severity and clinical consequences; the likelihood of an interaction; whether the interaction is based on clinical studies or extrapolated from case studies, laboratory or animal studies; and commonly applied integrative prescribing principles. However, new safety data and evidence are constantly emerging, and best practice regarding some of these interactions may change with time.

The tables do not include information on possible contraindications, for example use in pregnancy, nor do they include herb–herb, herb–nutrient or nutrient–nutrient interactions.

Practitioners are encouraged to use the interactions tables as a guide, but to apply professional judgment on the appropriateness of use of a combination of herb–drug or nutrient–drug for each individual patient. It is imperative that health practitioners investigate whether there are any known safety concerns or interactions when prescribing herbal or nutritional medicines for patients already taking pharmaceutical medicines.

Health practitioners of all disciplines are encouraged to make use of available resources to allow for informed decisions, so as to optimise patient wellbeing without compromising patient safety. When recommending complementary medicines in combination with pharmaceutical medicines, both anticipated benefits and potential risks should be taken into consideration.

TABLE I.1 Herbal interactions

Herbal medicine	Drug/drug class	Potential outcome	Recommendations	Comments
Achillea millefolium	Acid reducing drugs (antacids, H_2 antagonists, proton pump inhibitors)	Theoretical decreased drug effect	Monitor — may not be clinically significant	Yarrow may increase gastric acidity. Use may theoretically antagonise drug action, resulting in decreased drug effect.
	Anticoagulant/ antiplatelet drugs	Theoretical increased risk of bleeding	Caution with use of this combination	Yarrow may have antiplatelet properties. Combined use with anticoagulant and antiplatelet drugs will theoretically increase the risk of bleeding and bruising.
	Barbiturates, e.g. phenobarbital (phenobarbitone)	Theoretical increased sedation	Caution with use of this combination	Yarrow may theoretically prolong barbiturate-induced sleep time.
	Lithium	Theoretical increased risk of drug toxicity	Caution with use of this combination	Yarrow may have diuretic properties. Combined use may theoretically precipitate lithium toxicity.
Actaea racemosa	Androgen blockade chemotherapies	Theoretical decreased drug adverse effects	May be beneficial — medical supervision recommended	Androgen deprivation in prostate cancer patients can result in hot flushes and decreased libido. Black cohosh may theoretically reduce vasomotor symptoms in patients taking drugs that reduce androgen levels. Benefits are speculative and more data are required.
	Cisplatin	Possible reduced drug effects	Avoid combination	Preliminary evidence suggests that black cohosh may decrease the cytotoxic effects of cisplatin on breast cells. Avoid combination until further data become available.

LEGEND

- Combination okay to use
- Use of combination should be monitored
- Use combination with caution
- Avoid combination

Continued

TABLE I.1 Herbal interactions—cont'd

Herbal medicine	Drug/drug class	Potential outcome	Recommendations	Comments
Actaea racemosa cont'd	Chemotherapy drugs	Variable effects possible	Avoid combination	Variable effects have been reported with concomitant use of black cohosh and chemotherapeutic agents. Some studies have shown a decreased effect and others an increased drug action and risk of toxicity, depending on the agent. Concomitant use should be avoided unless under strict medical supervision.
	CYP2D6 substrates	Theoretical increased drug levels	Caution with use of this combination	Limited evidence suggests black cohosh may modestly inhibit CYP2D6. Theoretically this can result in increased drug levels and risk of toxicity of drugs metabolised by this enzyme.
	Hepatotoxic drugs	Possible increased risk of liver toxicity	Caution with use of this combination	The risk of liver damage may be increased with concomitant use of black cohosh and hepatotoxic drugs.
	HMGCoA reductase inhibitors (statins)	Possible increased risk of liver toxicity	Caution with use of this combination	A case report describes a patient who was taking atorvastatin and developed significantly raised liver enzymes after commencement of black cohosh. It is unclear if this was due to the drug, the herb or the combination.
	Hormone replacement therapy (HRT)	Possible additive effects	Combination may be beneficial	Black cohosh may theoretically provide additive benefits for the reduction of menopause symptoms such as hot flushes and night sweats when used with HRT. Theoretically concomitant use may allow for lower HRT doses. Direct research investigating the safety and efficacy of combined use is lacking.
	Tamoxifen	Possible reduction of hot flushes	Caution with use of this combination	Some studies suggest that black cohosh may help to treat hot flushes in women with a history of breast cancer and taking tamoxifen. Appropriateness of use is however the subject of debate as the oestrogenic effects of black cohosh may also have potentially negative consequences. Medical supervision is recommended.
Aesculus hippocastanum	Anticoagulant/ antiplatelet drugs	Theoretical increased risk of bleeding	Caution with use of this combination	Horse chestnut may have antiplatelet properties. Concomitant use with anticoagulant or antiplatelet drugs will theoretically increase the risk of bleeding.
	Antidiabetic drugs	Possible additive effects possible	Caution with use of this combination	Horse chestnut may lower blood glucose levels. Additive effects are theoretically possible, increasing the risk of hypoglycaemia. Caution is advised until more data become available.
	Lithium	Increased risk of drug toxicity	Caution with use of this combination	Horse chestnut may have diuretic properties. Combined use may theoretically precipitate lithium toxicity. The combination should be used with caution or avoided.

TABLE I.1 Herbal interactions—cont'd				
Herbal medicine	**Drug/drug class**	**Potential outcome**	**Recommendations**	**Comments**
Agaricus blazei	Antidiabetic drugs	Possible additive effects	Caution with use of this combination	Clinical research suggests *Agaricus* mushrooms may lower blood glucose levels by decreasing insulin resistance in type 2 diabetics. Additive effects are theoretically possible, which increase the risk of hypoglycaemia.
Agrimonia eupatoria	Antidiabetic drugs	Theoretical additive effects	Caution with use of this combination	Agrimony may theoretically lower blood glucose levels; based on one animal study. Findings are inconclusive.
Albizia lebbeck	Antidepressant drugs (SSRIs, SNRIs)	Theoretical risk of serotonin syndrome	Monitor — may not be clinically significant	Animal studies show *Albizia* may theoretically increase serotonin levels. Patients should be monitored but this effect has not yet been demonstrated in humans.
	Antihistamines	Theoretical additive effects	Combination may be beneficial — monitor	Additive beneficial effects are theoretically possible as *Albizia* inhibits early processes of allergy sensitisation and may reduce allergic response.
	CNS depressant drugs including barbiturates	Theoretical increased risk of sedation	Monitor — may not be clinically significant	*Albizia* may theoretically enhance drug sedative adverse effects. Animal studies suggest that *Albizia* may potentiate phenobarbital (phenobarbitone)-induced sleep time.
Alchemilla vulgaris	Oral drugs	Theoretical decreased drug absorption	Monitor — may not be clinically significant	The high tannin content of lady's mantle may theoretically impair absorption of some drugs due to precipitation interactions. Significance is unknown, but dosage separation is advised.
Aletris farinosa	Acid reducing drugs (antacids, H_2 antagonists, proton pump inhibitors)	Theoretical decreased drug effect	Monitor — may not be clinically significant	True unicorn root may increase gastric acidity. Use may theoretically counteract drug action, resulting in decreased drug effect.
	Oestrogens	Theoretical altered drug effect	Monitor — may not be clinically significant	True unicorn root may have oestrogenic activity and so may theoretically interfere with the effects of hormone replacement therapy (HRT) or oral contraceptives due to competition for oestrogen receptors. Evidence of this interaction is lacking. Women with hormone-sensitive conditions should avoid this herb.
Allium cepa	Anticoagulant/ antiplatelet drugs	Theoretical increased risk of bleeding	Caution with use of this combination	Limited data suggest onion may have antiplatelet activity at high doses. There is a theoretical interaction with anticoagulant and antiplatelet drugs, increasing the risk of bleeding.
	Antidiabetic drugs	Possible additive effects possible	Caution with use of this combination	Onion may lower blood glucose levels. Additive effects are theoretically possible, increasing the risk of hypoglycaemia. Caution is advised until more data become available.
	CYP450 substrates (CYP2E1)	Theoretical risk of increased drug levels	Monitor — may not be clinically significant	Animal research suggests that onion powder may inhibit CYP2E1. This may theoretically increase drug levels of agents metabolised by this enzyme; however, this has not yet been demonstrated in humans.

Continued

TABLE I.1 Herbal interactions—cont'd				
Herbal medicine	**Drug/drug class**	**Potential outcome**	**Recommendations**	**Comments**
Allium cepa cont'd	Lithium	Increased risk of drug toxicity	Caution with use of this combination	Onion may have diuretic properties. Combined use may theoretically precipitate lithium toxicity. The combination should be used with caution.
Allium sativum	Anticoagulant/ antiplatelet drugs	Theoretical increased risk of bleeding	Caution with use of this combination	Garlic has antiplatelet activity and may theoretically interact with anticoagulant and antiplatelet drugs. Clinical studies have not reported changes to the pharmacokinetics or pharmacodynamics of warfarin, nor an increased incidence of adverse effects. Caution is urged however with doses >7 g/day of garlic. Normal therapeutic doses appear safe.
	Antihypertensive drugs	Theoretical additive effects	Combination may be beneficial — monitor	Garlic may have a small effect in lowering blood pressure, so additive effects are theoretically possible. The interaction may be beneficial but patients should be monitored for hypotension.
	Anti-retroviral drugs — protease inhibitors, e.g. saquinavir	Possible decreased drug effect	Avoid combination	Garlic extract has been shown to significantly reduce blood concentrations of saquinavir, potentially reducing drug effectiveness in the management of HIV. High-dose garlic supplements should be avoided with saquinavir. A study with ritonavir showed only a small non-statistically significant change in drug concentration, but caution is advised with use of supplemental garlic and all drugs in this class until more data become available. The effect of dietary garlic is unknown.
	CYP450 substrates (CYP2E1)	Theoretical increased risk of drug toxicity	Caution with use of this combination	Preliminary evidence suggests garlic oil may inhibit the activity of CYP2E1 by 39%. Theoretically this may increase the risk of toxicity of drugs metabolised by this enzyme.
	CYP450 substrates (CYP3A4)	Theoretical decreased drug effectiveness	Caution with use of this combination	Preliminary evidence suggests garlic may induce the activity of CYP3A4, although results from different studies have been mixed. Caution is advised due to a theoretical risk of decreased drug effectiveness with concurrent use of garlic and drugs metabolised by this enzyme.
	Isoniazid	Theoretical decreased drug effect	Avoid combination	Animal studies report that garlic can significantly reduce isoniazid plasma concentrations. The combination should be avoided until further data become available.
	Lipid-lowering agents, e.g. statins	Theoretical additive effects	Combination may be beneficial — monitor	Garlic is reported to lower cholesterol and a study suggests it may potentiate the effects of lipid-lowering drugs. The combination appears well tolerated and may be beneficial.

TABLE I.1 Herbal interactions—cont'd

Herbal medicine	Drug/drug class	Potential outcome	Recommendations	Comments
Aloe barbadencis	Antidiabetic drugs	Theoretically additive effects	Caution with use of this combination	Some clinical research has reported that oral aloe vera may lower blood glucose levels in patients with type 2 diabetes, although other studies have reported no effect. Concomitant use may theoretically be additive and beneficial, but caution is advised due to a risk of hypoglycaemia.
	Cancer therapy (chemotherapy or radiotherapy)	Possible improved response; possible reduced drug adverse effects	May be beneficial — medical supervision recommended	Results of a clinical study suggest that the addition of aloe vera to chemotherapy in patients with advanced cancer may lead to improved survival and reduced tumour progression, compared to placebo. More research is needed, but the combination may be beneficial under medical supervision. Topical aloe vera may also reduce inflammation of the oral mucosa caused by chemotherapeutic agents or radiation therapy.
	Corticosteroids — topical	Theoretical improved drug effect	Combination may be beneficial	An animal study conducted on rodent paws reported that the addition of topical aloe vera to topical hydrocortisone was more effective in reducing inflammation and oedema than topical hydrocortisone alone. Theoretically, combined use may be beneficial; however, the effect has not been demonstrated in clinical trials.
	Digoxin	Theoretical increased risk of adverse effects	Avoid combination	Long-term excessive use of oral aloe vera may theoretically lead to loss of potassium, which potentially increases the risk of drug toxicity.
	Diuretics	Theoretical increased risk of adverse effects	Caution with use of this combination	Oral aloe vera has a laxative effect. Excessive use may lead to loss of potassium, which increases the risk of hypokalaemia when used with potassium-depleting diuretics such as thiazide and loop diuretics.
	Laxatives	Additive effects with increased risk of adverse effects	Caution with use of this combination	The combination of oral aloe vera and stimulant laxatives may increase the risk of fluid and electrolyte loss.
	Sevoflurane	Theoretical increased risk of bleeding	Caution with use of this combination	A case report describes excessive intraoperative blood loss in a patient who was administered sevoflurane for anaesthesia and had taken high-dose oral aloe vera prior to surgery. While it was proposed that aloe vera may have enhanced drug antiplatelet effects, evidence is inconclusive.
Althaea officinalis	Antidiabetic drugs	Theoretical additive effects	Caution with use of this combination	Marshmallow may theoretically have hypoglycaemic effects. Concomitant use may theoretically be additive and beneficial, but caution is advised due to a risk of hypoglycaemia.
	Lithium	Theoretical increased risk of drug toxicity	Caution with use of this combination	Marshmallow may have diuretic properties. Theoretically, combined use may reduce lithium excretion and increase the risk of lithium toxicity.

Continued

TABLE I.1 Herbal interactions—cont'd

Herbal medicine	Drug/drug class	Potential outcome	Recommendations	Comments
Althaea officinalis cont'd	Oral drugs	Theoretical impaired drug absorption	Caution with use of this combination	The mucilage in marshmallow may theoretically impair absorption of some drugs.
Ammi visnaga	Digoxin	Theoretical decreased drug effect	Caution with use of this combination	In-vivo and in-vitro evidence suggests that a constituent of this herb, visnadin, may have negative inotropic effects. This may theoretically oppose drug action. Significance is unknown, but caution is advised.
	Hepatotoxic drugs	Theoretical additive effects	Monitor — may not be clinically significant	A constituent of this herb may increase liver transaminases. Theoretically, concomitant use with hepatotoxic drugs will increase the risk of the liver damage.
	Photosensitising drugs	Theoretical increased risk of photosensitivity	Monitor — may not be clinically significant	This herb may cause photosensitivity. Additive adverse effects are theoretically possible.
Andrographis paniculata	5-aminosalicylates, e.g. mesalazine, sulfasalzine	Possible additive effects possible	Combination may be beneficial — medical supervision recommended	The combination may lead to improved clinical response and mucosal healing, based on limited research in patients with ulcerative colitis. Caution is advised until more long-term safety data become available.
	Anticoagulant/ antiplatelet drugs	Theoretical increased risk of bleeding	Caution with use of this combination	Andrographis has antiplatelet activity. Concomitant use with anticoagulant or antiplatelet drugs will theoretically increase the risk of bleeding and bruising.
	Anti-rheumatoid arthritis agents, e.g. prednisone, methotrexate	Possible additive effects	May be beneficial — medical supervision recommended	In a small study andrographis was shown to reduce pain, swelling and inflammation associated with rheumatoid arthritis. The combination may be additive and beneficial, but caution is advised until more safety data become available.
	Immunosuppressant drugs	Theoretical risk of decreased drug effect	Caution with use of this combination	Andrographis has immunomodulatory activity which may theoretically counteract drug immunosuppressant effects.
Anethum graveolens	Antidiabetic drugs	Possible additive effects	Caution with use of this combination	Animal studies show that dill may theoretically lower blood glucose levels. Concomitant use may theoretically be additive and beneficial, but caution is advised due to a risk of hypoglycaemia.
	Lithium	Increased risk of drug toxicity	Caution with use of this combination	Dill may have diuretic properties. Theoretically, combined use may reduce lithium excretion and increase the risk of lithium toxicity.
Angelica sinensis	Anticoagulant/ antiplatelet drugs	Theoretical increased risk of bleeding	Caution with use of this combination	Dong quai may have antiplatelet activity based on limited data. Concomitant use with anticoagulant and antiplatelet drugs will theoretically increase the risk of bleeding and bruising. One case report describes a woman who was taking warfarin and experienced fluctuations in INR when she started taking dong quai.

TABLE I.1 Herbal interactions—cont'd

Herbal medicine	Drug/drug class	Potential outcome	Recommendations	Comments
Angelica sinensis cont'd	Oestrogens	Theoretical altered drug effect	Caution with use of this combination	Dong quai may have oestrogenic activity. Theoretically this herb may interfere with the effects of hormone replacement therapy (HRT) due to competition for oestrogen receptors. Evidence of this interaction is lacking.
Apium graveolens	Antidepressant drugs, e.g. venlafaxine	Theoretical increased risk of adverse effects	Avoid combination	A case report describes an interaction between celery root extract, St John's wort and venlafaxine, which led to mania and hallucinations.
	Anticoagulant/ antiplatelet drugs	Theoretical increased risk of bleeding	Caution with use of this combination	In-vitro research has reported that two of the constituents found in celery have antiplatelet activity. Concomitant use with anticoagulant and antiplatelet drugs theoretically increases the risk of bleeding and bruising.
	Antihypertensive drugs	Additive effects theoretically possible	Caution with use of this combination	Anecdotal evidence suggests that celery may lower blood pressure. Concomitant use may be additive, with a theoretical risk of hypotension. Clinical significance is unclear.
	CYP450 substrates (CYP1A2)	Theoretical increased drug effect	Caution with use of this combination	In-vitro and animal research suggests celery may inhibit CYP1A2. Theoretically, concomitant use with drugs that are CYP1A2 substrates may result in increased drug effects and risk of adverse effect.
	L-thyroxine (Levothyroxine)	Theoretical decrease in drug effect	Caution with use of this combination	Case reports suggest that celery seed tablets may interact with thyroxine, leading to reduced drug effect. Caution is advised until more data become available.
	Lithium	Increased risk of drug toxicity	Caution with use of this combination	Celery may have diuretic properties. Theoretically, combined use may reduce lithium excretion and increase the risk of lithium toxicity.
	Paracetamol	Theoretical increased drug effect	Monitor — may not be clinically significant	Animal research suggests celery juice may prolong the effects of paracetamol. It has been proposed that this is due to inhibition of CYP450 enzyme activity.
	PUVA therapy	Increased risk of phototoxicity	Caution with use of this combination	According to limited data celery may increase the risk of phototoxicity when used with PUVA therapy.
Arctium lappa	Anticoagulant/ antiplatelet drugs	Theoretical increased risk of bleeding	Caution with use of this combination	Burdock may have antiplatelet properties. Concomitant use with anticoagulant and antiplatelet drugs will theoretically increase the risk of bleeding and bruising.
	Antidiabetic drugs	Theoretical additive effects	Caution with use of this combination	Burdock may theoretically lower blood glucose levels, based on animal studies. Findings are inconclusive, but caution is advised due to a risk of hypoglycaemia.

Continued

TABLE I.1 Herbal interactions—cont'd

Herbal medicine	Drug/drug class	Potential outcome	Recommendations	Comments
Arctostaphylos uva-ursi	Lithium	Increased risk of drug toxicity	Caution with use of this combination	This herb may have diuretic properties. Theoretically, combined use may reduce lithium excretion and increase the risk of lithium toxicity. A case report describes an interaction between lithium and a herbal combination that included bearberry, which led to drug toxicity.
Armoracia rustica	L-thyroxine (Levothyroxine)	Theoretical decreased drug effect	Monitor — may not be clinically significant	Theoretically horseradish may exacerbate hypothyroidism or interfere with drug action. Clinical significance is unknown, but patients should be monitored.
Artemesia annua	CYP450 substrates (CYP2B6, CYP3A4)	Theoretical decreased drug effects	Monitor — clinical significance unknown	In-vitro evidence suggests this herb may induce CYP2B6 and CYP3A4 activity. Theoretically this may result in increased metabolism and decreased therapeutic effects of drugs that are CYP2B6 or CYP3A4 substrates.
Artemisia herba-alba	Antidiabetic drugs	Theoretical additive effects	Caution with use of this combination	Animal studies show that *Artemisia* may theoretically lower blood glucose levels. Findings are inconclusive, but caution is advised due to a theoretical risk of hypoglycaemia.
Asparagus racemosus	Lithium	Increased risk of drug toxicity	Caution with use of this combination	Shatavari may have diuretic properties. Theoretically, combined use may reduce lithium excretion and increase the risk of lithium toxicity.
	Metoclopramide	Possible additive effects	Caution with use of this combination	Limited evidence suggests that shatavari may help to promote lactation. Additive effects are theoretically possible when used concomitantly with metoclopramide, a drug sometimes prescribed to promote lactation. There are currently insufficient clear data on the effectiveness or safety of this combination and caution is advised.
Astragalus membranaceus	Chemotherapeutic agents, e.g. cyclophosphamide, cisplatin	Interaction may be beneficial — herb may improve patient quality of life measures	May be beneficial — medical supervision recommended	Limited research suggests that astragalus may improve quality of life and patient wellbeing while reducing drug-related adverse effects such as fatigue, nausea and vomiting, pain and loss of appetite. Further study is needed to confirm results but adjunctive use of astragalus may be beneficial.
	Immunosuppressant drugs	Theoretical decreased drug effect	Caution with use of this combination	Astragalus has immunostimulant activity which may theoretically counteract drug immunosuppressant effects. Clinical significance is unclear, but caution is advised.
	Interferon alpha (IFN-α)	Theoretical additive or synergistic effect	May be beneficial — medical supervision recommended	Limited data show that astragalus may increase endogenous interferon production by leucocytes. Theoretically, concomitant use with therapeutic interferon-alpha may have additive beneficial effects. Data are limited and medical supervision is strongly recommended.

TABLE I.1 Herbal interactions—cont'd

Herbal medicine	Drug/drug class	Potential outcome	Recommendations	Comments
Astragalus membranaceus cont'd	Lithium	Increased risk of drug toxicity	Caution with use of this combination	Astragalus may have diuretic properties. Theoretically, combined use may reduce lithium excretion and increase the risk of lithium toxicity.
Avena sativa	Antihypertensive drugs	Additive effects possible	Combination may be beneficial	Beta-glucan, found in oats, has been shown to reduce blood pressure, particularly in obese individuals with hypertension. Concurrent use may be additive and potentially beneficial, but monitor for hypotension.
	Immunosuppressant drugs	Theoretical risk of decreased drug effect	Caution with use of this combination	Beta-glucan, found in oats, may have immunostimulant effects. Theoretically this may counteract drug immunosuppressant action; however, clinical significance is unclear.
	Lipid-lowering drugs	Additive effects possible	Combination may be beneficial	Beta-glucan, found in oats, has been shown to significantly reduce cholesterol. Additive beneficial effects may be seen with concurrent use.
Azadirachta indica	Antidiabetic drugs	Theoretical additive effects	Caution with use of this combination	Limited data show that neem may theoretically lower blood glucose levels. Concomitant use may theoretically be additive and beneficial, but caution is advised due to a risk of hypoglycaemia.
	Immunosuppressant drugs	Theoretical decreased drug effect	Caution with use of this combination	According to animal studies neem may have immunostimulant activity. Theoretically this may counteract drug immunosuppressant effects. Clinical significance is unclear, but caution is advised.
	Lithium	Increased risk of drug toxicity	Caution with use of this combination	Neem may have diuretic properties. Theoretically, combined use may reduce lithium excretion and increase the risk of lithium toxicity.
Bacopa monniera	Acetylcholinesterase inhibitors	Possible increased drug effects and adverse effects	Caution with use of this combination	*Bacopa* appears to inhibit acetylcholinesterase, which can increase acetylcholine levels. Concomitant use of *Bacopa* and acetylcholinesterase (AChE) inhibitors, such as donepezil, used for Alzheimer's disease, may theoretically have additive beneficial effects. Caution is advised as there is an increased risk of cholinergic side effects.
	Anticholinergic drugs	Theoretical decreased drug effect	Caution with use of this combination	*Bacopa* appears to increase acetylcholine levels and may theoretically oppose the action of drugs with an anticholinergic action. Significance is unclear, but caution is advised.
	Cholinergic drugs	Theoretical additive drug effect	Caution with use of this combination	*Bacopa* appears to increase acetylcholine levels and may theoretically have additive effects when used in combination with drugs with cholinergic actions. Significance is unclear.
Barosma betulina	Anticoagulant/ antiplatelet drugs	Theoretical increased risk of bleeding	Caution with use of this combination	Buchu may have antiplatelet properties. Concomitant use with anticoagulant and antiplatelet drugs will theoretically increase the risk of bleeding and bruising.

Continued

TABLE I.1 Herbal interactions—cont'd

Herbal medicine	Drug/drug class	Potential outcome	Recommendations	Comments
Barosma betulina cont'd	Lithium	Increased risk of drug toxicity	Caution with use of this combination	Buchu may have diuretic properties. Theoretically, combined use may reduce lithium excretion and increase the risk of lithium toxicity.
Berberine extract/ berberine-containing herbs	Anticoagulant/ antiplatelet drugs	Theoretical increased risk of bleeding	Caution with use of this combination	In-vitro and animal studies suggest that berberine may inhibit platelet aggregation. There is a theoretical increased risk of bleeding, although this has not been demonstrated in human studies. Caution is advised.
	Antidiabetic drugs	Theoretical additive effects	Caution with use of this combination	Berberine may lower blood glucose levels and have additive effects when used concomitantly with antidiabetic drugs. Caution is advised due to an increased risk of hypoglycaemia.
	Antihypertensive drugs	Theoretical additive effects	Monitor — may not be clinically significant	Berberine may have hypotensive effects. Additive effects are theoretically possible if used in combination with antihypertensive drugs. Monitor for hypotension.
	Ciclosporin	Increased risk of drug toxicity	Avoid this combination	A clinical study reported that berberine significantly increased drug serum levels in renal-transplant patients. This may have been due to inhibition of CYP3A4. Theoretically, concomitant use will increase the risk of drug toxicity.
	CNS depressant drugs	Increased risk of sedative effects	Caution with use of this combination	Animal research suggests that berberine may have sedative effects. There is a theoretical risk of excessive drowsiness when used with CNS depressant drugs.
	CYP450 substrates (CYP2C9, CYP2D6, CYP3A4)	Theoretical increased risk of drug toxicity	Caution with use of this combination	Preliminary evidence suggests berberine may inhibit activity of CYP2C9, CYP2D6, CYP3A4. Theoretically, herbal medicines containing berberine may increase drug levels as they can increase the risk of toxicity if used concomitantly with substrates of these enzymes.
Berberis aquifolium	Ciclosporin	Theoretical increased risk of drug toxicity	Caution with use of this combination	A clinical study reported that berberine, which is a constituent of Oregon grape, significantly increased drug serum levels in renal-transplant patients. This may have been due to inhibition of CYP3A4. Theoretically, concomitant use will increase the risk of drug toxicity.
	CYP3A4 substrates	Theoretical increased drug levels	Caution with use of this combination	According to limited data Oregon grape may inhibit CYP3A4 activity. Theoretically this may lead to increased drug levels and risk of toxicity of drugs metabolised by this enzyme. More data are needed to determine significance of this interaction.
Berberis vulgaris	Anticholinergic drugs	Theoretical increased risk of adverse effects	Monitor — clinical significance unknown	In-vitro evidence has shown that barberry may have anticholinergic properties. Theoretically, concomitant use with anticholinergic drugs such as antihistamines and tricyclic antidepressants may result in additive effects and adverse effects.

TABLE I.1 Herbal interactions—cont'd

Herbal medicine	Drug/drug class	Potential outcome	Recommendations	Comments
Berberis vulgaris cont'd	Anticoagulant/antiplatelet drugs	Theoretical increased risk of bleeding	Caution with use of this combination	In-vitro and animal studies suggest that berberine, a constituent of barberry, may inhibit platelet aggregation. There is a theoretical increased risk of bleeding, although this has not been demonstrated in human studies.
	Antidiabetic drugs	Theoretical additive effects	Caution with use of this combination	Berberine, a constituent of barberry, may lower blood glucose levels and have additive effects. Caution is advised due to an increased risk of hypoglycaemia.
	Antihypertensive drugs	Theoretical additive effects	Monitor — may not be clinically significant	Berberine, a constituent of barberry, may have hypotensive effects. Additive effects are theoretically possible if used in combination with antihypertensive drugs. Monitor for hypotension.
	Cholinergic drugs	Theoretical decreased drug effect	Monitor — clinical significance unknown	In-vitro evidence has shown that barberry may have anticholinergic properties. Theoretically, concurrent use may decrease the effects of cholinergic drugs, e.g. donepezil, tacrine.
	Ciclosporin	Increased risk of drug toxicity	Avoid this combination	A clinical study reported that berberine, which is a constituent of barberry, significantly increased drug serum levels in renal transplant patients. This may have been due to inhibition of CYP3A4. Theoretically, concomitant use will increase the risk of drug toxicity.
	CNS depressant drugs	Increased risk of sedative effects	Caution with use of this combination	Animal research suggests that berberine, a constituent of barberry, may have sedative effects. There is a theoretical risk of excessive drowsiness when used with CNS depressant drugs.
	CYP450 substrates (CYP3A4)	Theoretical increased risk of drug toxicity	Caution with use of this combination	Preliminary evidence suggests berberine may inhibit activity of CYP3A4. Theoretically this may lead to increased drug levels and risk of toxicity of drugs metabolised by this enzyme. More data are needed to determine significance of this interaction.
Boswellia serrata	Antidiabetic drugs	Theoretical additive effects	May be beneficial — medical supervision recommended	One study reported that boswellia extract improved glucose levels and cholesterol levels compared to placebo when used in combination with conventional antidiabetic medication. More study is needed to confirm findings.
	Anti-inflammatory drugs	Theoretical additive effects	Combination may be beneficial	Boswellia has anti-inflammatory properties and may provide an additive effect when used with anti-inflammatory drugs for conditions such as arthritis.
	CYP450 substrates (CYP1A2, CYP2C9, CYP2C19, CYP2D6, CYP3A4)	Theoretical increased risk of drug toxicity	Caution with use of this combination	In-vitro studies suggest boswellia may inhibit activity of CYP1A2, CYP2C9, CYP2C19, CYP2D6 and CYP3A4. Concurrent use of boswellia may theoretically increase drugs levels of drugs metabolised by these enzymes and increase the risk of toxicity.

Continued

TABLE I.1 Herbal interactions—cont'd				
Herbal medicine	**Drug/drug class**	**Potential outcome**	**Recommendations**	**Comments**
Boswellia serrata cont'd	Immunosuppressant drugs	Theoretical decreased drug effectiveness	Caution with use of this combination	According to in-vitro studies boswellia may have immunostimulant activity. This may theoretically counteract drug immunosuppressant effects, although evidence is limited.
	Sulfasalazine	Additive effects possible	May be beneficial — medical supervision recommended	Clinical research suggests boswellia may improve symptoms of ulcerative colitis. Additive effects are theoretically possible with concomitant use, but medical supervision is recommended.
Brassica oleracea	CYP450 substrates (CYP1A2, CYP2A6)	Theoretical decreased drug effects	Monitor — clinical significance unknown	In-vitro evidence suggests broccoli may induce CYP1A2 and CYP2A6 activity. Theoretically this may result in increased metabolism and decreased therapeutic effects of drugs that are substrates for these enzymes.
Bupleurum falcatum	Anticoagulant/antiplatelet drugs	Theoretical increased risk of bleeding	Caution with use of this combination	Bupleurum may have antiplatelet properties. Concomitant use with anticoagulant and antiplatelet drugs will theoretically increase the risk of bleeding and bruising.
	Antidiabetic drugs	Theoretical compromised disease management	Caution with use of this combination	Animal research suggests that saikosaponins, constituents of bupleurum, can increase blood glucose. Concomitant use with antidiabetic drugs may theoretically interfere with blood glucose control and management of diabetes.
	Immunosuppressant drugs	Theoretical decrease in drug effectiveness	Caution with use of this combination	According to animal studies bupleurum may have immunostimulant activity. This may theoretically counteract drug immunosuppressant effects although evidence is limited.
Calendula officinalis	CNS depressant drugs	Theoretical increased risk of sedative effects	Monitor. Unlikely to be clinically significant	Animal studies suggest oral calendula may have sedative effects. Concomitant use with CNS depressant drugs may theoretically increase sedation.
	Radiation therapy	Possible decreased adverse effects	May be beneficial — medical supervision recommended	Preliminary evidence suggests that topical application of calendula may help to ameliorate dermatitis in patients receiving radiation therapy for breast cancer.
Camellia sinensis	Alcohol	Theoretical increased risk of adverse effects	Monitor. Unlikely to be clinically significant	Alcohol reduces caffeine metabolism. Theoretically, concomitant intake will increase the risk of caffeine-related adverse effects.
	Amphetamines	Theoretical increased risk of CNS effects	Caution with use of this combination	Caffeine in green tea may have additive CNS stimulant effects if taken concomitantly with amphetamines.
	Anticoagulant/antiplatelet drugs	Theoretical increased risk of bleeding	Caution with use of this combination	Catechins in green tea are reported to have antiplatelet activity. The interaction has not been reported in human studies; however, people taking warfarin should avoid excessive consumption of green tea.

TABLE I.1 Herbal interactions—cont'd

Herbal medicine	Drug/drug class	Potential outcome	Recommendations	Comments
Camellia sinensis cont'd	Antidiabetic drugs	Theoretical altered drug effects	Monitor. Unlikely to be clinically significant	Caffeine in green tea may affect blood glucose levels according to some sources, but data are conflicting. Patients should be monitored but, based on current data, it seems unlikely that the interactions will be clinically relevant.
	Antifungal agents	Theoretical increased caffeine effects	Monitor. Unlikely to be clinically significant	Preliminary evidence suggests that caffeine metabolism may be decreased by some antifungal agents such as fluconazole and terbinafine. Theoretically this may result in increased caffeine-related adverse effects. Evidence is inconclusive.
	Bortezomib	Theoretical decreased drug effect	Avoid combination	Green tea polyphenols such as EGCG were reported to block this drug's antineoplastic effects in animal studies. Avoid use of green tea in patients taking boronic acid-based proteasome inhibitors such as bortezomib until further data become available.
	Cimetidine	Theoretical increased caffeine effects	Monitor. Unlikely to be clinically significant	Cimetidine may reduce clearance of caffeine in green tea, which theoretically increases the risk of caffeine-related adverse effects.
	Clozapine	Theoretical decreased drug effects	Caution with use of this combination	Animal studies suggest green tea may reduce drug concentrations, although the clinical significance of these findings is unclear. Caffeine has also been shown to exacerbate psychotic symptoms. Caution is advised as this drug has a narrow therapeutic index.
	CNS depressants	Theoretical decreased CNS effects	Monitor — may not be clinically significant	Caffeine in green tea may theoretically oppose the action of CNS depressant drugs and reduce drug effects.
	CNS stimulants	Theoretical increased CNS effects	Monitor — may not be clinically significant	Caffeine in green tea may have additive CNS stimulant effects if taken concomitantly with CNS stimulant drugs.
	Disulfiram	Theoretical increased caffeine effects	Monitor — may not be clinically significant	Disulfiram may reduce clearance of caffeine in green tea, which theoretically increases the risk of caffeine-related adverse effects.
	Doxorubicin	Theoretical decreased adverse effects and increased drug effect	May theoretically be beneficial — medical supervision recommended	Preliminary evidence suggests green tea polyphenols may reduce doxorubicin-induced cardiotoxicity. In addition, experimental in-vitro data suggest that EGCG and theanine may enhance drug activity. While human studies are required to confirm these effects, there is a theoretical beneficial interaction.
	Ephedrine	Increased risk of stimulatory effects	Avoid combination	Use of ephedrine with caffeine-containing products may increase the risk of excessive stimulatory effects.
	Fluvoxamine	Theoretical increased caffeine levels	Monitor — may not be clinically significant	Fluvoxamine may reduce caffeine metabolism, theoretically increasing the risk of caffeine-related adverse effects.

Continued

TABLE I.1 Herbal interactions—cont'd

Herbal medicine	Drug/drug class	Potential outcome	Recommendations	Comments
Camellia sinensis cont'd	Hepatotoxic drugs	Increased risk of hepatotoxicity	Caution with use of this combination	Green tea extract supplements have been linked to several cases of hepatotoxicity. Concurrent use with hepatotoxic drugs will have additive effects.
	Iron	Theoretical decreased mineral absorption	Monitor — may not be clinically significant	Tea polyphenols may form chelates with non-haem iron and reduce absorption. This interaction may not be significant, but dose administration should be separated.
	Lithium	Increased risk of drug toxicity	Caution with use of this combination	Abrupt withdrawal of caffeine can increase serum lithium levels and increase risk of adverse effects and drug toxicity.
	Monoamine oxidase inhibitors (MAOIs)	Theoretical risk of hypertensive crisis	Caution with use of this combination	Theoretically, high intake of caffeine, which is found in green tea, may precipitate a hypertensive crisis in patients taking MAOIs.
	Nadolol	Possible decreased drug effect	Avoid combination	Clinical trial evidence suggests that green tea catechins may inhibit organic anion transporting polypeptides (OATP), resulting in decreased drug levels and antihypertensive effect.
	Oral contraceptives	Theoretical increased caffeine effects	Monitor — may not be clinically significant	Oral contraceptives may reduce clearance of caffeine in green tea, which theoretically increases the risk of caffeine-related adverse effects.
	Phenylpropanolamine	Theoretical increased risk of hypertension	Caution with use of this combination	Phenylpropanolamine and caffeine in green tea may have additive effects on raising blood pressure. Caution is advised with this combination.
	Quinolone antibiotics	Theoretical increased caffeine effects	Monitor — may not be clinically significant	Quinolone antibiotics may reduce clearance of caffeine in green tea, which theoretically increases the risk of caffeine-related adverse effects.
	Theophylline	Theoretical increased risk of adverse effects	Caution with use of this combination	Caffeine in green tea may theoretically increase drug effects and adverse effects. Caution is advised but the interaction may not be clinically significant.
	Verapamil	Theoretical increased caffeine effects	Caution with use of this combination	According to some research verapamil may increase plasma caffeine concentration by 25%. Concomitant use may theoretically increase the risk of caffeine-related adverse effects.
Cannabis spp.	CNS depressant drugs	Additive effects and adverse effects	Caution with use of this combination	Preliminary evidence suggests cannabidiol has sedative and hypnotic effects. Excessive sedation is theoretically possible when used in combination with CNS depressant drugs.
	CYP450 substrates (CYP1A1, CYP1A2, CYP1B1, CYP2B6, CYP2C9, CYP2C19, CYP2D6, CYP3A4, CYP3A5)	Theoretical increased risk of drug toxicity	Caution with use of this combination	In-vitro and animal research shows that cannabidiol, in cannabis, may inhibit CYP1A1, CYP1A2, CYP1B1, CYP2B6, CYP2C9, CYP2C19, CYP2D6, CYP3A4 and CYP3A5. Theoretically, concomitant use may increase the risk of drug toxicity of drugs metabolised by these enzymes. Caution is advised until more data become available.

TABLE I.1 Herbal interactions—cont'd

Herbal medicine	Drug/drug class	Potential outcome	Recommendations	Comments
Cantharanthus rosea	Antidiabetic drugs	Theoretical additive effects	Caution with use of this combination	Madagascar periwinkle may lower blood glucose levels. Additive effects are theoretically possible, increasing the risk of hypoglycaemia.
	Lithium	Increased risk of drug toxicity	Caution with use of this combination	Madagascar periwinkle may have diuretic properties. Theoretically, combined use may reduce lithium excretion and increase the risk of lithium toxicity.
Capsella bursa-pastoris	CNS depressant drugs	Theoretical additive effects	Monitor — may not be clinically significant	Limited data have shown that shepherd's purse may theoretically have additive sedative effects.
	Thyroid hormone	Theoretical altered drug effect	Monitor — may not be clinically significant	Limited data have shown that concomitant use may theoretically interfere with drug therapy. Significance is unknown.
Capsicum spp.	ACE-inhibitors (ACE-I)	Theoretical increased risk of drug-induced cough	Monitor — may not be clinically significant	A case report describes a woman, who was previously stabilised on an ACE-I, experiencing a cough when she applied topical capsaicin cream. This may be due to an increase in bradykinin levels. The interaction is unlikely to be of significance in most individuals.
	Acid-reducing medication	Worsening or improved outcomes — conflicting data	Monitor — unlikely to be beneficial	Data are conflicting. Preliminary observational evidence suggested that regular intake of dietary chilli may be associated with a lower incidence of peptic ulcers. Some sources have suggested that cayenne may have gastroprotective effects. Other sources have however stated that cayenne is gastro-irritant and may worsen gastric conditions. A small preliminary clinical study reported that 2.5 g/day of red pepper may improve symptoms of dyspepsia, possibly by desensitising gastric nociceptive C-fibres. Results of a clinical trial however showed no improvement in duodenal ulcers compared to placebo when patients consumed chilli peppers. No benefits were reported in a study investigating the use of capsicum or cayenne in IBS. On balance, any suggested benefit seems to be speculative.
	Analgesics and NSAIDs	Additive effects possible	Combination may be beneficial	Topical use of capsaicin may have additive effects for reduction of pain.
	Anticoagulant/antiplatelet drugs	Theoretical increased risk of bleeding	Caution with use of this combination	Capsicum (capsaicin) may have antiplatelet properties. Combined oral use with anticoagulant and antiplatelet drugs will theoretically increase the risk of bleeding and bruising. An observational study suggested that capsicum may increase the risk of bleeding when used with warfarin.
	Antidiabetic drugs	Theoretical additive effects	Caution with use of this combination	Limited data have shown that oral use of high-dose capsicum may increase the risk of hypoglycaemia.

Continued

TABLE I.1 Herbal interactions—cont'd				
Herbal medicine	**Drug/drug class**	**Potential outcome**	**Recommendations**	**Comments**
Capsicum spp. cont'd	Theophylline	Theoretical increased drug absorption and risk of adverse effects	Caution with use of this combination	Animal research has shown that oral capsaicin may enhance theophylline absorption.
Carica papaya	Anticoagulant/ antiplatelet drugs	Theoretical increased risk of bleeding	Caution with use of this combination	Papaya may have antiplatelet properties. Concomitant use with anticoagulant and antiplatelet drugs may theoretically increase the risk of bleeding and bruising. Significance is unknown.
	Antidiabetic drugs	Additive effects possible	Caution with use of this combination	Limited study has shown that fermented papaya may lower blood glucose levels. Additive, potentially beneficial effects are possible. Caution is advised until more data become available.
Carum carvi	Antidiabetic drugs	Theoretical additive effects	Monitor — may not be clinically significant	Animal data have shown that caraway may theoretically lower blood glucose levels. Additive effects are theoretically possible, increasing the risk of hypoglycaemia.
	CNS depressant drugs	Theoretical additive effects	Monitor — may not be clinically significant	According to animal studies caraway may theoretically have sedative effects, due to the constituent carvone. Significance in humans is unknown.
	L-thyroxine (Levothyroxine)	Theoretical increased risk of hypothyroidism	Avoid combination	A case report describes a significant increase in thyroid-stimulating hormone (TSH) in a patient who took caraway with thyroxine. TSH returned to normal once caraway was stopped. Caution is advised until further safety data become available.
	Lithium	Increased risk of drug toxicity	Caution with use of this combination	Caraway may have diuretic properties, which could theoretically precipitate lithium toxicity. The combination should be used with caution or avoided.
Centella asiatica	CNS depressant drugs	Theoretical additive effects	Caution with use of this combination	Gotu kola may have sedative effects, leading to a theoretical increased risk of sedation if used concomitantly with CNS depressant drugs.
	Hepatotoxic drugs	Theoretical increased risk of hepatotoxicity	Caution with use of this combination	Based on case reports, some concerns have been raised that concomitant use of gotu kola with hepatoxic drugs may theoretically increase the risk of liver damage.
Cetraria islandica	Oral drugs	Theoretical impaired drug absorption	Monitor — may not be clinically significant	The mucilage content of Iceland moss may theoretically interfere with drug absorption, although clinical significance has not been established.
Chamaelirium luteum	Lithium	Increased risk of drug toxicity	Caution with use of this combination	False unicorn may have diuretic properties, which could theoretically precipitate lithium toxicity. The combination should be used with caution.
Chelidonium majus	Hepatotoxic drugs	Theoretical increased risk of hepatotoxicity	Caution with use of this combination	Greater celandine has been linked to several cases of hepatotoxicity. Concerns have been raised that concomitant use of this herb with hepatoxic drugs may increase the risk of liver damage.

TABLE I.1 Herbal interactions—cont'd

Herbal medicine	Drug/drug class	Potential outcome	Recommendations	Comments
Chelidonium majus cont'd	Immunosuppressant drugs	Theoretical decreased drugs effects	Caution with use of this combination	According to preliminary evidence, a semi-synthetic derivative of chelidonine, a constituent of greater celandine, may stimulate the immune response in cancer patients. Theoretically this may decrease the effects of immunosuppressant drugs. Caution is advised until more data become available.
Cinnamomum zeylanicum	Antidiabetic drugs	Theoretical additive effects	Caution with use of this combination	Cinnamon may lower blood glucose levels and additive effects are theoretically possible. The combination may be beneficial, but caution is advised due to a risk of hypoglycaemia.
Citrus paradisi	Aliskiren	Decreased drug concentration	Caution with use of this combination	Studies have reported a significant decrease in drug concentration with this combination, which may lead to reduced drug effect. The proposed mechanism for this interaction is due to inhibition of the organic anion transporting polypeptide 2B1 (OATP2B1). Separate dose administration by at least 4 hours if concurrent use is deemed necessary.
	Amiodarone	Increased drug plasma concentration and risk of adverse effects	Avoid combination	Grapefruit juice has been shown to significantly inhibit CYP3A4 enzyme activity. Studies have reported a significant increase in drug concentration with this combination, which increases the risk of adverse effects and drug toxicity.
	Artemether	Increased drug plasma concentration and risk of adverse effects	Avoid combination	Grapefruit juice has been shown to significantly inhibit CYP450 enzyme activity. Studies have reported a significant increase in drug concentration with this combination, which increases the risk of adverse effects and drug toxicity.
	Benzodiazepines, e.g. midazolam, diazepam	Increased drug plasma concentration and risk of adverse effects	Avoid combination	Grapefruit juice has been shown to significantly inhibit CYP3A4 enzyme activity. Studies have reported a significant increase in drug concentration with this combination, which increases the risk of adverse effects and drug toxicity. This interaction has been reported especially with diazepam and midazolam. It does not appear to occur with alprazolam.
	Budesonide	Increased drug plasma concentration and risk of adverse effects	Caution with use of this combination	Grapefruit juice has been shown to significantly inhibit CYP3A4 enzyme activity. Studies have reported an increase in drug concentration with this combination, which increases the risk of adverse effects and drug toxicity.
	Buspirone	Increased drug plasma concentration and risk of adverse effects	Avoid combination	Studies have reported a significant increase in drug concentration with this combination, which increases the risk of adverse effects and drug toxicity.

Continued

TABLE I.1 Herbal interactions—cont'd				
Herbal medicine	**Drug/drug class**	**Potential outcome**	**Recommendations**	**Comments**
Citrus paradisi cont'd	Caffeine	Increased risk of caffeine-related adverse effects	Caution with use of this combination	Studies have reported an increase in caffeine concentration with this combination, which increases the risk of adverse effects.
	Calcium channel blockers, e.g. verapamil, amlodipine, nifedipine	Increased drug plasma concentration and risk of adverse effects	Avoid combination	Studies have reported a significant increase in drug concentration with this combination, which increases the risk of adverse effects and drug toxicity. It has been proposed that this is due to inhibition of CYP3A4 activity, but some sources suggest other mechanisms may also be involved.
	Carbamazepine	Increased drug plasma concentration	Avoid combination	Increased drug absorption and plasma concentrations have been reported.
	Carvedilol	Increased drug plasma concentration	Avoid combination	Grapefruit juice is reported to increase drug bioavailability.
	Celiprolol	Decreased drug concentration	Avoid combination	Grapefruit juice is reported to decrease drug bioavailability. The proposed mechanism for this interaction is due to inhibition of the organic anion transporting polypeptide (OATP).
	Ciclosporin	Increased drug bioavailability	Avoid combination	Evidence suggests an increase in drug bioavailability with use of this combination.
	Cisapride	Increased drug plasma concentration and risk of adverse effects	Avoid combination	Increased plasma concentrations have been reported.
	Clomipramine	Increased drug plasma concentration and risk of adverse effects	Caution with use of this combination	Increased plasma concentrations have been described in two case reports.
	Clopidogrel	Decreased drug concentration	Avoid combination	Grapefruit juice has been reported to significantly decrease drug concentrations, which could reduce effectiveness as an antiplatelet drug.
	Colchicine	Increased drug plasma concentration and risk of adverse effects	Caution with use of this combination	In-vitro evidence has reported that grapefruit juice increases drug absorption by inhibiting P-gp.
	CYP450 substrates (CYP1A2, CYP2C19, CYP2C9)	Risk of increased drug plasma concentration and adverse effects	Caution with use of this combination	Preliminary evidence suggests grapefruit juice may inhibit CYP1A2, CYP2C19, CYP2C9. Interactions have not been reported in human studies to date and significance is unclear.
	CYP450 substrates (CYP3A4)	Risk of increased drug plasma concentration and adverse effects	Avoid combination	Grapefruit juice has been shown to significantly inhibit CYP3A4 enzyme activity. When taken orally, effects of grapefruit juice on CYP3A4 appear to last at least 48 hours.
	Dextromethorphan	Increased drug concentration and risk of adverse effects	Caution with use of this combination	A pharmacokinetic study reported increased concentration of dextromethorphan when taken in combination with grapefruit juice. It has been proposed that the interaction is due to inhibition of CYP3A4.
	Docetaxel	Increased drug plasma concentration and risk of adverse effects	Avoid combination	A case report describes an interaction with use of this combination, leading to increased drug concentrations and a reduction in white blood cell count.

TABLE I.1 Herbal interactions—cont'd

Herbal medicine	Drug/drug class	Potential outcome	Recommendations	Comments
Citrus paradisi cont'd	Erythromycin	Increased drug plasma concentration and risk of adverse effects	Caution with use of this combination	A study reported increased absorption of erythromycin when taken in combination with grapefruit juice.
	Etoposide	Decreased drug concentration and effect	Avoid combination	Studies have reported a significant decrease in drug concentration with this combination, which may lead to reduced drug effect. The proposed mechanism for this interaction is inhibition of the organic anion transporting polypeptide (OATP).
	Fexofenadine	Decreased drug concentration and effect	Caution with use of this combination	Studies have reported a significant decrease in drug concentration with this combination, which may lead to reduced drug effect. The proposed mechanism for this interaction is inhibition of the organic anion transporting polypeptide (OATP).
	Fluvoxamine	Increased drug plasma concentration	Caution with use of this combination	Increased drug plasma concentrations have been reported.
	Halofantrine	Increased drug plasma concentration and risk of adverse effects	Avoid combination	Increased drug plasma concentrations have been reported in a small clinical study. This may lead to an increased risk of prolonged QT interval.
	HMGCoA reductase inhibitors (statins), e.g. atorvastatin, simvastatin	Increased drug plasma concentration and risk of adverse effects	Avoid combination	Grapefruit juice has been shown to significantly inhibit CYP3A4 enzyme activity. Studies have reported a significant increase in drug concentration with this combination, which increases the risk of adverse effects and drug toxicity.
	Itraconazole	Altered drug levels possible	Caution with use of this combination	Data on effect of grapefruit juice on this drug are conflicting and significance is unclear. Caution with use until further data become available.
	L-thyroxine (Levothyroxine)	Possible decreased drug effect	Caution with use of this combination	A modest decrease in drug effect has been reported. The proposed mechanism for this interaction is due to inhibition of the organic anion transporting polypeptide (OATP).
	Losartan	Possible decreased drug concentration	Caution with use of this combination	A study in healthy volunteers reported decreased drug concentrations with use of this combination. Clinical significance is unclear.
	Methadone	Increased drug plasma concentration	Caution with use of this combination	An increased drug concentration has been reported with this combination. Clinical significance is unclear.
	Methylprednisolone	Increased drug plasma concentration	Avoid combination	Studies have reported an increase in drug concentration with this combination, which increases the risk of adverse effects and drug toxicity.
	Nadolol	Theoretical decreased drug effect	Caution with use of this combination	Grapefruit juice may theoretically decrease drug bioavailability due to inhibition of the organic anion transporting polypeptide (OATP1A2). It is not known if this interaction is clinically significant.

Continued

TABLE I.1 Herbal interactions—cont'd

Herbal medicine	Drug/drug class	Potential outcome	Recommendations	Comments
Citrus paradisi cont'd	Nilotinib	Increased drug plasma concentration	Caution with use of this combination	Increased drug concentration and drug absorption have been reported with this combination.
	Oestrogens	Increased drug plasma concentration	Caution with use of this combination	Increased plasma concentrations have been reported. It has been proposed that this is due to inhibition of CYP3A4.
	Organic anion-transporting polypeptide (OATP) substrates	Possible decreased drug absorption and drug effect	Avoid combination	In-vitro and clinical evidence show that grapefruit juice inhibits organic anion-transporting polypeptides (OATP). This reduces bioavailability of oral drugs that are OATP substrates. Separation of dose administration by at least 4 hours may help to avoid this interaction as the effect appears to last only a short time.
	Oxycodone	Increased drug concentration and risk of adverse effects	Avoid combination	An increase in drug concentration has been reported with this combination. Oxycodone is metabolised by CYP3A4.
	Praziquantel	Increased drug concentration and risk of adverse effects	Avoid combination	Studies have reported a significant increase in drug concentration with this combination, which increases the risk of adverse effects and drug toxicity.
	Primaquine	Possible increased drug bioavailability	Caution with use of this combination	An increase in drug bioavailability has been reported. Clinical significance is unclear.
	Quinidine	Altered drug effect	Caution with use of this combination	Grapefruit juice has been reported to decrease drug absorption, clearance and metabolism, and to prolong drug half-life. Clinical significance is unclear.
	Regorafenib	Theoretical increased drug concentrations and risk of toxicity	Avoid combination	Grapefruit juice has been shown to significantly inhibit CYP3A4 enzyme activity. While no direct interaction has been reported, this drug is a CYP3A4 substrate.
	Repaglinide	Small increase in serum drug concentration	Caution with use of this combination	A small but significant increase in drug concentration has been reported with use of this combination.
	Saquinavir	Increased drug absorption	Caution with use of this combination	Increased drug absorption has been reported with use of this combination. This interaction does not appear to occur with indinavir, another protease-inhibitor.
	Scopolamine	Increased drug concentration and risk of adverse effects	Avoid combination	An increased drug concentration has been reported with this combination. Scopolamine is metabolised by CYP3A4.
	Sertraline	Increased drug plasma concentration and risk of adverse effects	Caution with use of this combination	Two studies have reported a significant increase in drug concentration with this combination, which increases the risk of adverse effects and drug toxicity.
	Sildenafil	Increased drug concentration and risk of adverse effects	Caution with use of this combination	An increased drug concentration has been reported with this combination. Sildenafil is metabolised by CYP3A4.
	Sunitinib	Possible increase in drug plasma concentration	Caution with use of this combination	A modest increase in drug levels has been reported with use of this combination. This interaction may not be clinically significant, but caution is advised.

TABLE I.1 Herbal interactions—cont'd				
Herbal medicine	**Drug/drug class**	**Potential outcome**	**Recommendations**	**Comments**
Citrus paradisi cont'd	Tacrolimus	Increased drug bioavailability and risk of adverse effects	Avoid combination unless under strict medical supervision	Studies have reported a significant increase in drug bioavailability with this combination. It has been proposed that this may enhance drug action, but strict medical supervision is required due to a lack of reliable safety and efficacy data.
	Talinolol	Possible increased drug bioavailability	Caution with use of this combination	An increase in drug bioavailability may occur with this combination. The clinical significance is unclear.
	Terfenadine	Possible increased drug concentrations	Avoid combination	An increase in drug absorption and plasma concentration has been reported with this combination. Clinical significance is unclear.
	Theophylline	Possible decreased drug concentrations	Caution with use of this combination	A modest decrease in drug levels has been reported. The mechanism of this interaction is unknown.
	Ticagrelor	Increased drug plasma concentration and risk of bleeding	Avoid combination	Grapefruit juice has been shown to significantly inhibit CYP3A4 enzyme activity. Studies have reported a significant increase in drug concentration with this combination, which increases the risk of adverse effects and drug toxicity.
	Tolvaptan	Increased drug plasma concentration and risk of adverse effects	Caution with use of this combination	Studies have reported an increase in drug concentration with this combination. This may lead to an increased extent and duration of diuretic effect, and an increased risk of adverse effects and drug toxicity.
	Toremifene	Theoretical increased drug plasma concentration and risk of adverse effects	Avoid combination	Grapefruit juice has been shown to significantly inhibit CYP3A4 enzyme activity. While an interaction between grapefruit juice and this drug has not been demonstrated directly, the drug is a CYP3A4 substrate. There is a theoretical risk of prolonged QT interval.
	Warfarin	Theoretical increased risk of bleeding	Caution with use of this combination	A case report describes an increase in INR in a patient taking large doses of grapefruit juice while on warfarin. A small clinical study, however, reported that daily consumption of grapefruit juice did not affect INR in a group of men taking warfarin. Caution is recommended until more safety data become available.
Cnicus benedictus	Acid reducing drugs, e.g. antacids, H_2 antagonists, proton pump inhibitors	Theoretical decreased drug effect	Monitor — may not be clinically significant	Blessed thistle may increase gastric acidity. Use may theoretically counteract drug acid-reducing action, resulting in decreased drug effect.
Codonopsis pilosula	Anticoagulant/ antiplatelet drugs	Theoretical increased risk of bleeding	Caution with use of this combination	Preliminary clinical research suggests codonopsis has antiplatelet activity. Concomitant use with anticoagulant and antiplatelet drugs may theoretically increase the risk of bleeding and bruising.

Continued

TABLE I.1 Herbal interactions—cont'd

Herbal medicine	Drug/drug class	Potential outcome	Recommendations	Comments
Coffea arabica	Alcohol	Theoretical increased caffeine effects	Monitor — may not be clinically significant	Alcohol reduces caffeine metabolism. Theoretically, concomitant intake will increase the risk of caffeine-related adverse effects.
	Alendronate	Reduced drug bioavailability	Caution with use of this combination — separate doses	Coffee significantly reduces drug bioavailability. Doses should be separated by at least 2 hours
	Anticoagulant/ antiplatelet drugs	Theoretical increased risk of bleeding	Monitor — may not be clinically significant	Caffeine is reported to have antiplatelet activity; however, interactions between coffee and anticoagulant/antiplatelet drugs have not been reported in humans.
	Clozapine	Theoretical disease exacerbation	Caution with use of this combination	The caffeine content of coffee may exacerbate psychotic symptoms and increase drug effects and toxicity at high doses (400–1000 mg daily of caffeine).
	CNS stimulant drugs	Enhanced stimulatory effects	Caution with use of this combination	Concomitant use of caffeine in coffee and CNS stimulant drugs will increase the risk of adverse effects due to additive stimulatory actions.
	Disulfiram	Theoretical increased caffeine effects	Monitor — may not be clinically significant	Disulfiram may reduce clearance of caffeine, which theoretically increases the risk of caffeine-related adverse effects.
	Ephedrine	Enhanced stimulatory effects	Avoid combination	Ephedrine may enhance the stimulatory effects of caffeine. The combination has been associated with an increased risk of life-threatening or debilitating adverse effects such as hypertension, myocardial infarction, stroke, seizures and death.
	L-thyroxine (Levothyroxine)	Possible decreased drug absorption	Caution with use of this combination	It has been proposed that coffee may form insoluble complexes with L-thyroxine in some patients. Dose administration should be separated.
	Monoamine oxidase inhibitors	Theoretical risk of hypertensive crisis	Caution with use of this combination	Theoretically high intake of caffeine in coffee may precipitate a hypertensive crisis in patients taking MAOIs.
	Phenylpropanolamine	Theoretical increased risk of hypertension	Caution with use of this combination	Phenylpropanolamine and caffeine may have additive effects on raising blood pressure. Caution is advised with this combination.
	Quinolone antibiotics	Theoretical increased caffeine effects	Monitor — may not be clinically significant	Quinolones reduce caffeine metabolism. Theoretically, there is an increased risk of caffeine-related adverse effects.
	Theophylline	Theoretical increased risk of drug toxicity	Caution with use of this combination	Caffeine in coffee may inhibit drug metabolism and increase the risk of adverse effects.
Coleus forskohlii	Anticoagulant/ antiplatelet drugs	Unpredictable effect	Caution with use of this combination	According to animal studies coleus may increase the rate of warfarin metabolism, leading to a reduced anticoagulant action. There is, however, evidence that forskolin, a constituent of coleus, may inhibit platelet aggregation and adhesion, which potentially increases the risk of bleeding and bruising.

TABLE I.1 Herbal interactions—cont'd

Herbal medicine	Drug/drug class	Potential outcome	Recommendations	Comments
Coleus forskohlii cont'd	Antihypertensive drugs	Theoretical additive effects	Caution with use of this combination	Coleus may lower blood pressure, based on limited studies. Additive effects are possible, increasing the risk of hypotension.
	CYP450 substrates (CYP2C9, CYP3A4)	Theoretical decrease in drug effects	Caution with use of this combination	Laboratory and animal studies suggest that coleus may induce CYP2C9 and CYP3A4. Theoretically this may result in an increased rate of drug metabolism and decreased drug effect. Clinical significance is unclear, but caution is advised.
	Nitrates	Additive coronary vasodilatory effect	Avoid combination	Limited research suggests that additive vasodilatory effects are possible, due to the constituent forskolin. The combination should be avoided unless under medical supervision.
	Vasodilatory drugs including calcium channel blockers	Additive vasodilatory effects	Caution with use of this combination	Limited research suggests that additive vasodilatory effects are possible, due to the constituent forskolin. Caution is advised.
Commiphora mukul	Anticoagulant/ antiplatelet drugs	Theoretical increased risk of bleeding	Caution with use of this combination	Guggul may have antiplatelet activity. Concomitant use may theoretically increase the risk of bleeding or bruising. Clinical significance is unclear.
	CYP450 substrates (CYP3A4)	Theoretical decreased drug effects	Monitor — clinical significance is unclear	In-vivo evidence suggests that guggul may induce CYP3A4 enzyme activity. Theoretically, this may result in increased rate of drug metabolism and decreased drug effects.
	Diltiazem	Possible decreased drug effects	Monitor — clinical significance is unclear	One small study reported that guggul may reduce drug bioavailability. Significance is unknown.
	L-thyroxine (Levothyroxine)	Theoretical altered drug effects	Monitor — clinical significance is unclear	High-dose intake of guggul may theoretically interfere with drug action.
	Propranolol	Possible decreased drug effects	Monitor — clinical significance is unclear	One small study reported that guggul may reduce drug bioavailability. Significance is unknown.
	Tamoxifen	Theoretical altered drug effects	Caution with use of this combination	High-dose intake of guggul may theoretically interfere with drug action through oestrogen-alpha receptor agonist activity.
Commiphora myrrha/mol mol	Anticoagulant/ antiplatelet drugs	Theoretical decreased drug effect	Caution with use of this combination	One case report and in-vitro studies suggest myrrh may decrease effectiveness of warfarin. Caution is advised, but clinically significance is unclear based on current data.
	Antidiabetic drugs	Theoretical additive effects	Caution with use of this combination	Myrrh may have hypoglycaemic effects. Additive effects are theoretically possible, increasing the risk of hypoglycaemia.

Continued

TABLE I.1 Herbal interactions—cont'd				
Herbal medicine	**Drug/drug class**	**Potential outcome**	**Recommendations**	**Comments**
Coptic chinensis	Ciclosporin	Theoretical increased risk of drug toxicity	Caution with use of this combination	Berberine, a constituent of this herb, may reduce rate of metabolism of ciclosporin and increase risk of drug toxicity.
	CYP3A4 substrates	Theoretical increased drug levels	Caution with use of this combination	This herb may inhibit CYP3A4 activity based on limited data. Theoretically, this may result in increased drug levels and risk of toxicity of drugs metabolised by this enzyme. More data are needed to determine significance of this interaction.
Cordyceps spp.	Anticoagulant/ antiplatelet drugs	Theoretical increased risk of bleeding	Caution with use of this combination	Animal research suggests cordyceps may have antiplatelet effects. There is a theoretical increased risk of bleeding with concomitant use, but this has not been reported in humans.
	Chemotherapy	Theoretical improved outcomes	Caution with use of this combination	Preliminary evidence suggests cordyceps may improve quality of life and cellular immunity in patients undergoing cancer chemotherapy. Concomitant use may be beneficial, but caution is advised until more data become available.
	Ciclosporin	Theoretical decreased drug effects	Avoid combination	A small clinical study reported that cordyceps reduced the immunosuppressive effects of ciclosporin in patients who had undergone renal transplantation. Other research has reported that cordyceps may help to ameliorate ciclosporin-induced nephrotoxicity. Avoid combination unless under strict medical supervision.
	Immunosuppressant drugs	Theoretical decreased drug effects; possible improved outcomes	Caution with use of this combination	Theoretically cordyceps may reduce drug immunosuppressive effects by stimulating the immune system. Preliminary evidence has suggested, however, that use of cordyceps in renal transplant patients may have beneficial effects. Research has suggested that adjunctive use of cordyceps with immunosuppressive therapy may result in reduced hepatotoxicity and nephrotoxicity, reduced number of infections and reduced drug requirements. Concomitant use may potentially be beneficial under strict medical supervision.
	Testosterone	Theoretical additive effects	Monitor — clinical significance is unclear	Animal research suggests cordyceps may increase testosterone levels. Clinical significance is unknown based on current data.
Crataegus spp.	Antihypertensive drugs	Possible additive effects	Caution with use of this combination	Hawthorn has been shown to lower blood pressure and may reduce heart rate. Additive, beneficial effects are possible with antihypertensive drugs, but caution is advised due to a risk of hypotension.

TABLE I.1 Herbal interactions—cont'd

Herbal medicine	Drug/drug class	Potential outcome	Recommendations	Comments
Crataegus spp. cont'd	Digoxin and cardiac glycosides	Theoretical additive effects	May be beneficial — medical supervision recommended	Hawthorn appears to improve cardiac output and combined use may theoretically potentiate drug effects. This interaction may be beneficial, but medical supervision is advised as there are currently insufficient data to determine risks and benefits of concomitant use.
	Diuretics	Theoretical additive effects in heart failure	May be beneficial — medical supervision recommended	Hawthorn may provide additional cardiovascular benefits in patients with congestive heart failure which could theoretically lead to improved outcomes. Limited data suggest a potential benefit with concurrent use. Caution is advised until more data become available.
	Doxorubicin	Theoretical decreased drug cardiotoxicity	May be beneficial — medical supervision recommended	It has been speculated that hawthorn may provide cardioprotective effects and help to reduce risk of cardiotoxicity in patients taking doxorubicin. Further research is needed to investigate the risks and benefits of this interaction.
	Lipid-lowering drugs	Theoretical additive effects	Combination may be beneficial	Hawthorn may theoretically reduce serum cholesterol and potentiate drug lipid-lowering effects.
	Nitrates	Theoretical additive effects	Avoid combination	Hawthorn may have additive vasodilatory effects when used with nitrates. The combination should be avoided unless under medical supervision.
	Phosphodiesterase-5 inhibitors	Theoretical additive effects	Avoid combination	Hawthorn may have additive vasodilatory effects when used with phosphodiesterase-5 inhibitors, such as sildenafil. The combination should be avoided unless under medical supervision.
Crocus sativus	Antihypertensive drugs	Theoretical additive effects	Monitor — clinical significance is unclear	Animal studies suggest saffron may have hypotensive properties. Additive effects are theoretically possible, with an increased risk of hypotension.
	Calcium channel blockers	Theoretical additive effects	Caution with use of this combination	Additive coronary vasodilatory effects are possible, which suggests saffron may have negative inotropic and chronotropic activity.
Curcuma longa	Alcohol	Possible reduced organ damage	May be beneficial — medical supervision recommended	Animal models suggest that curcumin may provide some protective effects against alcoholic liver and pancreatic disease. This may theoretically be a useful adjunct therapy in those with high alcohol ingestion.
	Anticoagulant/antiplatelet drugs	Theoretical increased risk of bleeding	Caution with use of this combination	Turmeric is reported to have antiplatelet activity in vitro. Theoretically, concurrent use with anticoagulant or antiplatelet drugs increases the risk of bleeding. Caution is advised until more data become available.

Continued

TABLE I.1 Herbal interactions—cont'd				
Herbal medicine	**Drug/drug class**	**Potential outcome**	**Recommendations**	**Comments**
Curcuma longa cont'd	Antidiabetic drugs	Theoretical additive effects	Caution with use of this combination	Turmeric may have hypoglycaemic effects. Clinical significance of this interaction is unclear, but additive effects are theoretically possible.
	CYP450 substrates (CYP1A1, CYP1A2, CYP3A4)	Theoretical increased drug effect	Monitor — may not be clinically significant	In-vitro and animal research suggests that curcumin may inhibit liver metabolising activity of CYP1A1, CYP1A2 and CYP3A4. This has not been demonstrated in humans, although a case report describes a possible interaction with tacrolimus, a CYP3A4 substrate.
	Dexamethasone	Theoretical increase in drug levels	Caution with use of this combination	Turmeric may increase drug blood levels, based on preliminary data. There is a theoretical increase in drug effects and adverse effects, although data are limited.
	Non-steroidal anti-inflammatory drugs (NSAIDs)	Theoretical additive effects	Combination may be beneficial	Additive effects are possible with concomitant use which may be beneficial for the management of conditions such as arthritis. No negative drug–herb interactions have been reported, but monitoring is suggested.
	Sulfasalazine	Theoretical increased drug levels	Caution with use of this combination	Preliminary evidence suggests turmeric may increase blood levels of drug. Combined use may theoretically increase drug effects and adverse effects.
	Tacrolimus	Theoretical increased drug levels	Caution with use of this combination	Animal studies and a case report suggest that turmeric may increase drug levels. Combined use may theoretically increase drug effects and adverse effects. Caution is advised until more safety data become available.
	Talinolol	Possible reduced drug bioavailability	Caution with use of this combination	Preliminary clinical evidence suggests curcumin may decrease drug bioavailability. Caution is advised until more data become available.
Cynara scolymus	Lipid-lowering drugs	Theoretical additive effects	Combination may be beneficial	Additive, beneficial effects are theoretically possible with high-dose intake of globe artichoke, although evidence is conflicting. No negative drug–herb interactions have been reported.
Dioscorea villosa	Oestrogens, e.g. HRT and oral contraceptives	Theoretical additive effects	Monitor — may not be clinically significant	In-vitro evidence suggests wild yam may have oestrogenic and anti-oestrogenic effects. Clinical evidence of an interaction is lacking, but monitoring is advised with concomitant use.
Echinacea spp.	Antineoplastic drugs, e.g. etoposide	Theoretical increased risk of drug toxicity	Avoid combination	A case report suggests that use of echinacea with etoposide resulted in increased drug toxicity. Avoid this combination until further data become available.

TABLE I.1 Herbal interactions—cont'd

Herbal medicine	Drug/drug class	Potential outcome	Recommendations	Comments
Echinacea spp. cont'd	Asthma or atopic medication	Herb may trigger allergic reactions and asthma	Avoid combination	There are several case reports that echinacea caused allergic reactions and exacerbated asthma in predisposed individuals, leading to effects including anaphylaxis, urticaria and bronchospasm. Although the incidence of reported interactions is rare, caution or avoidance of echinacea is recommended in patients requiring regular asthma or atopic medication.
	Cyclophosphamide	Theoretical decreased drug effect	Caution with use of this combination	Echinacea has immunostimulant activity which may theoretically counteract drug effect. The clinical significance is unknown, but caution is advised.
	CYP450 substrates (CYP1A2)	Theoretical increased drug levels	Caution with use of this combination	Limited study has shown that echinacea may inhibit CYP1A2. There is a theoretical risk of increased drug levels and toxicity.
	CYP450 substrates (CYP3A4)	Theoretical altered drug effect	Caution with use of this combination	Some literature suggests that echinacea may induce CYP3A4, while other sources suggest it may inhibit CYP3A4. It has been proposed that this herb may induce hepatic CYP3A4 and inhibit intestinal CYP3A4. The effects may theoretically balance each other out. The interaction may not be clinically relevant, but caution is advised until more data become available.
	Immunosuppressant drugs	Theoretical decreased drug effect	Caution with use of this combination	Echinacea has immunostimulant activity which may theoretically counteract drug immunosuppressant effects. Evidence of an interaction is limited, but caution is advised.
	Warfarin	Theoretical decreased drug	Monitor — may not be clinically significant	A study conducted in healthy male volunteers suggests that echinacea may increase drug clearance. This did not appear to have a clinically relevant effect on INR.
Echium amoenum	Antidepressant drugs (SSRIs)	Possible improved outcomes	Caution with use of this combination	Results of two small clinical trials suggest an additive beneficial effect with concomitant use of SSRIs and Iranian borage in the management of anxiety or depression. No differences in frequency of adverse effects have been reported so far. Patients should be monitored and caution is advised until more data become available.
	Benzodiazepines	Theoretical additive effects	Caution with use of this combination	According to animal studies and preliminary clinical research Iranian borage may have anxiolytic properties. Additive effects and an increased risk of adverse effects are theoretically possible. Patients should be monitored and caution is advised until more data become available.

Continued

TABLE I.1 Herbal interactions—cont'd				
Herbal medicine	**Drug/drug class**	**Potential outcome**	**Recommendations**	**Comments**
Eleutherococcus senticosus	Alcohol	Increased risk of sedation	Caution with use of this combination	Siberian ginseng may have additive sedative effects when used in combination with alcohol.
	Anticoagulant/ antiplatelet drugs	Theoretical increased risk of bleeding	Monitor — clinical significance is unclear	A constituent of Siberian ginseng is reported to have antiplatelet activity in vitro. There is a theoretical risk of increased bleeding, but significance is unclear.
	Antidiabetic drugs	Theoretical additive effects	Monitor — clinical significance is unclear	Siberian ginseng may have hypoglycaemic effects. Additive effects are theoretically possible, increasing the risk of hypoglycaemia. Caution is advised until more data become available.
	Chemotherapy	Possible reduced drug adverse effects	Combination may be beneficial — medical supervision recommended	Limited evidence suggests Siberian ginseng may reduce adverse effects associated with chemotherapy and enhance general stress resistance. Data are limited and medical supervision is recommended.
	CNS depressant drugs	Increased risk of sedation	Caution with use of this combination	Siberian ginseng may have additive sedative effects when used in combination with CNS depressant drugs.
	CYP450 substrates (CYP1A2, CYP2C9, CYP2D6, CYP3A4)	Theoretical increased risk of drugs effects and adverse effects	Caution with use of this combination	In-vitro and animal studies suggest that Siberian ginseng may inhibit activity of CYP1A2 and CYP2C9. Caution is advised until more data become available. Siberian ginseng has also been shown to inhibit CYP2D6 and CYP3A4 in in-vitro and animal models, but this effect does not appear to be relevant in human studies.
	Digoxin	Theoretical risk of increased drug levels	Caution with use of this combination	One case report associated Siberian ginseng with an elevation in serum digoxin levels. Drug toxicity was not reported, but caution is advised until further safety data become available.
	Immunosuppressant drugs	Theoretical decrease in drug effectiveness	Caution with use of this combination	Siberian ginseng may theoretically counteract drug immunosuppressant effects due to herb immunostimulating activity. Evidence of an interaction is limited, but caution is advised.
	Lithium	Theoretical increased risk of drug toxicity	Caution with use of this combination	Siberian ginseng may have diuretic properties. Theoretically, combined use may reduce lithium excretion and increase the risk of lithium toxicity.
	P-gp substrates	Theoretical increased risk of drug toxicity	Caution with use of this combination	Preliminary in-vitro evidence suggests that Siberian ginseng may inhibit P-gp. This could theoretically increase drug effects, although there is currently insufficient data to determine if the interactions would be clinically important.

TABLE I.1 Herbal interactions—cont'd

Herbal medicine	Drug/drug class	Potential outcome	Recommendations	Comments
Ephedra sineca	Anticonvulsants	Increased risk of seizures	Caution with use of this combination	Ephedra is associated with triggering seizure activity and may therefore interfere with drug effectiveness. Use would be inappropriate in people with epilepsy or a history of seizures.
	Antidiabetic drugs	Possible decreased drug effects	Caution with use of this combination	Limited research suggests ephedra may raise blood glucose and potentially interfere with drug effectiveness and impair disease management.
	B-agonists, e.g. salbutamol (Ventolin®)	Increased risk of adverse effects	Caution with use of this combination	Additive effects are possible, with an increased risk of adverse effects.
	Caffeine	Additive stimulant effects	Avoid combination	Evidence suggests that use of ephedra in combination with caffeine may increase the risk of potentially serious life-threatening or debilitating adverse effects.
	Cardiovascular drugs	Increased risk of cardiovascular events	Avoid combination	Ephedra has been reported to cause severe life-threatening or disabling adverse effects and there are case reports linking ephedra to hypertension, myocardial infarction and stroke. Those with preexisting cardiovascular conditions appear to be at greater risk.
	Dexamethasone	Theoretical decreased drug effects	Caution with use of this combination	The ephedrine in ephedra may theoretically increase the rate of dexamethasone clearance and reduce drug effectiveness.
	Ergot derivatives	Theoretical risk of hypertension	Caution with use of this combination	There is a theoretical risk of hypertension due to the ephedrine in ephedra.
	Monoamine oxidase inhibitors (MAOIs)	Theoretical increased risk of adverse effects	Avoid combination	There is a theoretical increased risk of drug adverse effects based on drug and herb mechanisms of action and limited case reports.
	Pseudoephedrine	Theoretical risk of hypertension	Caution with use of this combination	There is a theoretical risk of hypertension due to the ephedrine in ephedra.
	QT-interval prolonging drugs, e.g. amiodarone	Increased risk of arrhythmias	Avoid combination	A small study reported that use of a combination product containing ephedra and caffeine increased the QT-interval in healthy volunteers. Additive effects are theoretically possible with a combination of ephedra and drugs that prolong the QT-interval, and may increase the risk arrhythmias.
	Stimulant drugs	Increased risk of adverse effects	Avoid combination	There is a theoretical increased risk of hypertension and adverse cardiovascular effects with use of ephedra and drugs with CNS stimulant properties including phenylpropanolamine and pseudoephedrine.
	Theophylline	Increased risk of adverse effects	Avoid combination	The combination of ephedra with methylxanthine drugs such as theophylline will have additive stimulant actions and risk of adverse effects.

Continued

TABLE I.1 Herbal interactions—cont'd				
Herbal medicine	Drug/drug class	Potential outcome	Recommendations	Comments
Equisetum arvense	Antidiabetic drugs	Theoretical additive effects	Monitor — clinical significance is unclear	Horsetail may lower blood glucose levels, based on limited data. Additive effects are theoretically possible, increasing the risk of hypoglycaemia. Caution is advised until more data become available.
	Diuretic drugs	Increased risk of potassium depletion	Caution with use of this combination	Horsetail may have diuretic properties. Concurrent use with potassium-depleting diuretics will increase the risk of hypokalaemia.
	Lithium	Theoretical increased risk of drug toxicity	Caution with use of this combination	Horsetail may have diuretic properties. Theoretically, combined use may reduce lithium excretion and increase the risk of lithium toxicity.
Eriodictyon crassifolium	Lithium	Theoretical increased risk of drug toxicity	Caution with use of this combination	This herb may have diuretic properties. Theoretically, combined use may reduce lithium excretion and increase the risk of lithium toxicity.
Eschscholzia californica	Benzodiazepines	Theoretical additive effects and adverse effects	Caution with use of this combination	Concurrent use of Californian poppy with benzodiazepines may theoretically lead to additive effects and an increased risk of adverse effects such as excessive drowsiness.
	CNS depressants	Theoretical additive effects and adverse effects	Caution with use of this combination	Concurrent use of Californian poppy with CNS depressant drugs may theoretically lead to additive effects and risk of adverse effects such as excessive drowsiness.
Eucalyptus globus	Antidiabetic drugs	Theoretical additive effects	Monitor — clinical significance is unclear	Animal research suggests that eucalyptus may have hypoglycaemic effects. Significance is unknown, but additive effects are theoretically possible, increasing the risk of hypoglycaemia.
	CYP450 substrates (CYP1A2, CYP2C19, CYP2C9, CYP3A4)	Theoretical increased drug levels	Monitor — clinical significance is unclear	In-vitro evidence suggests eucalyptus oil may inhibit CYP450 enzyme activity. This has not been demonstrated in humans to date.
	Phenobarbital (phenobarbitone)	Theoretical decreased drug effect	Monitor — clinical significance is unclear	Preliminary animal research suggests that inhaling eucalyptus may reduce the amount of drug that reaches the brain. Clinical significance is not known.
Eugenia caryophyllata	Anticoagulant/ antiplatelet drugs	Theoretical increased risk of bleeding	Monitor — clinical significance is unclear	Laboratory studies suggest that eugenol, a constituent of clove, may have antiplatelet activity. This has not been demonstrated in humans, but monitoring is recommended.
Eupatorium perfoliatum	CYP450 substrates (CYP3A4)	Theoretical risk of decreased drug effect	Monitor — interaction is speculative	It has been proposed that boneset may theoretically induce CYP3A4, based on the fact that this herb belongs to the genus *Eupatorium*, and other plants of this genus have been shown to induce CYP3A4. There is no specific research investigating this effect with boneset.

TABLE I.1 Herbal interactions—cont'd

Herbal medicine	Drug/drug class	Potential outcome	Recommendations	Comments
Euphrasia spp.	Antidiabetic drugs	Theoretical additive effects	Monitor — clinical significance is unclear	Animal studies suggest that eyebright may have hypoglycaemic effects. Clinical significance has not been established, but additive effects are theoretically possible, increasing the risk of hypoglycaemia.
Eurycoma longifolia	Propranolol	Risk of decreased drug effects	Caution with use of this combination	Results of a small clinical trial found that concomitant use of this herb and propranolol led to reduced drug bioavailability. This appears to be due to decreased drug absorption.
Filipendula ulmaria	Anticoagulant/ antiplatelet drugs including aspirin	Theoretical additive effects	Caution with use of this combination	Meadowsweet contains plant salicylates which have been shown to have anticoagulant properties in vitro and in animal studies. There is a theoretical increased risk of bleeding, but this is speculative and clinical significance is unknown.
Foeniculum vulgare	Anticoagulant/ antiplatelet drugs	Theoretical increased risk of bleeding	Monitor — clinical significance is unclear	Animal research suggests fennel may have some antithrombotic and antiplatelet effects.
	Ciprofloxacin	Theoretical decreased drug effect	Caution with use of this combination	Preliminary evidence suggests fennel may reduce drug bioavailability by nearly 50%. Caution with combination and separate dose administration.
	CYP450 substrates (CYP3A4)	Theoretical increased risk of drugs effects and adverse effects	Caution with use of this combination	In-vitro evidence suggests fennel may inhibit activity of CYP3A4, which may theoretically increase the risk of drug effects and adverse effects.
	Oestrogens, e.g. oral contraceptives and HRT	Theoretical additive effects	Caution with use of this combination	Some constituents of fennel have oestrogenic activity. Theoretically large doses of fennel may affect drug action by competing for oestrogen receptor binding sites. Clinical significance is unclear.
	Tamoxifen	Theoretical decrease in drug effect	Caution with use of this combination	Some constituents of fennel have oestrogenic activity. Theoretically large doses of fennel may decrease drug effectiveness. Clinical significance is unclear, but caution is advised.
Fucus versiculosis	Anticoagulant/ antiplatelet drugs	Theoretical increased risk of bleeding	Monitor — may not be clinically significant	In-vitro evidence suggests a constituent of kelp may have anticoagulant properties. Clinical research, however, suggests that a clinically relevant interaction is unlikely due to poor absorption. Patients should be monitored.
	Lithium	Case report of hyperthyroidism	Caution with use of this combination	A case reports describes hyperthyroidism with concomitant use of lithium and kelp.

Continued

TABLE I.1 Herbal interactions—cont'd

Herbal medicine	Drug/drug class	Potential outcome	Recommendations	Comments
Fucus versiculosis cont'd	Thyroid medication	Additive effects	Caution with use of this combination	Kelp contains a significant amount of iodine. Evidence suggests concomitant use with thyroid medication may have additive effects and result in hypothyroidism. A case report describes iodine-induced thyrotoxicosis in a patient with an enlarged thyroid gland after ingestion of a kelp-containing tea.
Galega officinalis	Anticoagulant/ antiplatelet drugs	Theoretical increased risk of bleeding	Monitor — clinical significance is unclear	In-vitro studies suggest goat's rue may have antiplatelet properties. There is a theoretical increased risk of bleeding and bruising when used with anticoagulant or antiplatelet drugs.
	Antidiabetic drugs	Theoretical additive effects	Monitor — clinical significance is unclear	Goat's rue may theoretically potentiate the hypoglycaemic effects of antidiabetic drugs. Clinical significance has not been established, but caution is advised. Dosage adjustments may be required.
Ganoderma lucidum	Anti-cancer therapy	Theoretical improved outcomes	Combination may be beneficial — medical supervision recommended	Animal studies suggest reishi extracts may provide protective benefits against the adverse effects associated with some antineoplastic drugs, including myelosuppression, and may improve therapeutic outcomes. Several mechanisms have been proposed. Further clinical trial evidence is needed to establish the benefits and risks associated with concomitant use.
	Anticoagulant/ antiplatelet drugs	Theoretical increased risk of bleeding	Monitor — clinical significance is unclear	Limited evidence suggests that high-dose use (≥3 g daily) of reishi mushrooms may have antiplatelet properties. This effect has not been shown at doses of ≤1.5 g daily.
	Antidiabetic drugs	Theoretical additive effects	Monitor — clinical significance is unclear	Animal studies suggest that reishi mushrooms may have hypoglycaemic effects. Additive effects are theoretically possible, with an increased risk of hypoglycaemia.
	Antihypertensive drugs	Theoretical additive effects	Monitor — clinical significance is unclear	Animal studies suggest that reishi mushrooms may have hypotensive properties. Additive effects are theoretically possible, with an increased risk of hypotension.
	Antimicrobial therapy	Theoretical improved outcomes	Combination may be beneficial — medical supervision recommended	In-vitro research has demonstrated synergy between reishi mushrooms and several antibiotics. Reishi may have antibacterial properties and may enhance immune response.
	Antiviral therapy	Theoretical improved outcomes	Combination may be beneficial — medical supervision recommended	In-vitro research has demonstrated synergy between reishi mushrooms and aciclovir. Reishi may have antiviral effects against HSV1 and HSV2 and may enhance immune response. More research is needed to establish safety and efficacy of concomitant use.

TABLE I.1 Herbal interactions—cont'd

Herbal medicine	Drug/drug class	Potential outcome	Recommendations	Comments
Garcinia mangostana	Anticoagulant/ antiplatelet drugs	Theoretical increased risk of bleeding	Caution with use of this combination	In-vitro and animal research suggests mangosteen may have antiplatelet activity. There is a theoretical increased risk of bleeding, although data are limited.
Gentiana lutea	Antihypertensive drugs	Theoretical additive effects	Monitor — speculative	Traditional use suggests gentian may have hypotensive properties. Theoretically the combination may have additive effects, but the interaction is speculative.
Ginkgo biloba	Antibiotics — aminoglycosides, e.g. gentamycin	Theoretical decreased drug adverse effects	Monitor — unlikely to be of benefit	Animal research has reported that ginkgo may have protective effects against the ototoxicity and nephrotoxicity associated with use of gentamycin. Another study, however, reported that concomitant use of ginkgo increased the incidence of ototoxicity. Benefits in humans are considered unlikely. The doses used in animal studies were very high and do not translate to normal therapeutic doses of ginkgo. Theoretical benefits can also not be extrapolated to other antibiotics.
	Anticoagulants/ antiplatelet drugs	Possible increased risk of bleeding	Caution with use of this combination	Several studies suggest that ginkgo inhibits platelet aggregation, which appears to be due to the action of the constituent ginkgolide B. A number of case studies have described serious bleeding events in patients taking ginkgo. However, population-based studies and clinical trials have produced mixed results, with evidence suggesting that ginkgo may not exhibit significant effects on platelet aggregation with short-term use. Analysis of the records of a large medical database suggests that when warfarin and ginkgo are taken concurrently, there is a 38% increased risk of bleeding. This interaction has not been shown in studies with other anticoagulant or antiplatelet drugs. Caution is advised until further safety data become available, especially with longer-term use.
	Anticonvulsant drugs	Theoretical increased risk of seizures	Caution with use of this combination	Large amounts of ginkgotoxin, which is found in ginkgo seeds, have been shown to cause neurotoxicity and seizures. Only trace amounts of ginkgotoxin are found in ginkgo leaf and it has been proposed that toxicity and seizures are unlikely with use of ginkgo leaf extract. There are, however, anecdotal reports of seizures occurring in epileptic patients following use of ginkgo. Evidence is inconclusive, but caution is recommended.

Continued

TABLE I.1 Herbal interactions—cont'd

Herbal medicine	Drug/drug class	Potential outcome	Recommendations	Comments
Ginkgo biloba cont'd	Antidepressant drugs	Theoretical decreased drug effects	Caution with use of this combination	Animal and in-vitro studies suggest that ginkgo may increase serotonin reuptake, which could theoretically decrease drug efficacy. Significance is unclear.
	Antidiabetic drugs	Possible altered drug effects	Caution with use of this combination	Ginkgo may influence insulin secretion and metabolism in type 2 diabetics. Theoretically, ginkgo may alter response to antidiabetic drugs, with variable effects reported in different patients. The effect ginkgo has on insulin secretion may be patient specific, and also relate to which antidiabetic medications are being taken.
	Buspirone	Theoretical risk of adverse effects	Caution with use of this combination	A case report describes the development of hypomania in a patient after adding ginkgo and St John's wort to her existing regimen of fluoxetine and buspirone.
	CYP450 substrates (CYP1A2, CYP2C9, CYP2D6, CYP3A4)	Theoretical increased risk of toxicity	Caution with use of this combination	Preliminary evidence suggests that ginkgo may modestly inhibit CYP1A2, CYP2C9, and CYP2D6. There is conflicting evidence as to whether ginkgo inhibits or induces CYP3A4. Theoretically, inhibition of these enzymes can reduce the rate of drug metabolism and increase risk of toxicity. Caution is advised until further data become available.
	CYP450 substrates (CYP2C19, CYP3A4)	Theoretical decreased drug effect	Caution with use of this combination	Preliminary evidence suggests that ginkgo may modestly induce CYP2C19. There is conflicting evidence as to whether ginkgo inhibits or induces CYP3A4. Enzyme induction may theoretically increase the rate of drug metabolism and decrease drug effectiveness. Caution is advised until further data become available.
	Donepezil	Possible additive effects	May be beneficial — medical supervision recommended	Co-administration of ginkgo and donepezil in a group of patients with Alzheimer's disease did not have a major effect on drug pharmacokinetics and pharmacodynamics. Effects may therefore be additive and beneficial, but monitoring is recommended.
	Fluoxetine	Theoretical risk of adverse effects	Caution with use of this combination	A case report describes the development of hypomania in a patient after adding ginkgo and St John's wort to her existing regimen of fluoxetine and buspirone.
	Haloperidol	Possible enhanced drug effect	May be beneficial — medical supervision recommended	Research suggests that ginkgo may enhance drug effects and reduce drug adverse effects in schizophrenic patients. A small but well-designed study reported that ginkgo enhanced the effectiveness of haloperidol in schizophrenic patients.

TABLE I.1 Herbal interactions—cont'd

Herbal medicine	Drug/drug class	Potential outcome	Recommendations	Comments
Ginkgo biloba cont'd	HIV-drugs — non-nucleoside reverse transcriptase inhibitors (NNRTIs), e.g. efavirenz, raltegravir	Possible altered drug effect	Caution with use of this combination	Ginkgo may influence activity of drugs in this class, but results have been conflicting. Two case reports describe a reduction in concentration of efavirenz with use of ginkgo. A pharmacokinetic study showed a small effect on raltegravir, but clinical significance was unclear. It is possible that variations in response may relate to the different drugs in this class being metabolised by different CYP450 enzymes.
	HMGCoA reductase inhibitors (statins), e.g. atorvastatin and simvastatin	Theoretical decreased drug effects	Caution with use of this combination	Ginkgo has been shown to significantly increase the clearance of atorvastatin and simvastatin, which may theoretically reduce drug efficacy.
	Omeprazole	Possible decreased drug levels	Caution with use of this combination	Ginkgo has been shown to decrease plasma concentrations of omeprazole in a study conducted in healthy volunteers. It has been proposed that this was due to induction of CYP2C19.
	Selective serotonin-reuptake inhibitors (SSRIs)	Possible decreased drug-induced sexual dysfunction	May be beneficial — medical supervision recommended	Ginkgo may theoretically help to ameliorate symptoms of sexual dysfunction associated with use of SSRIs, based on limited and conflicting data. Preliminary data suggested a benefit, but subsequent data have not been as positive. Response may vary significantly between individuals.
Glycine max	Antibiotics	Theoretical decreased herbal action	Monitor — clinical significance is unclear	Theoretically, antibiotics may decrease the action of soy isoflavones by disturbing gastrointestinal bacteria. This may theoretically impair conversion of isoflavones to the active form. The interaction is speculative and only likely to be relevant with long-term antibiotic use.
	Antidiabetic drugs	Additive effects theoretically possible	Caution with use of this combination	Clinical research suggests that soy-based diets may reduce fasting blood glucose levels. Theoretically, concomitant use may have additive effects, which could be beneficial for the management of diabetes. Caution is advised due to the theoretical risk of hypoglycaemia.
	Antihypertensive drugs	Additive effects theoretically possible	Monitor — clinical significance is unclear	Clinical evidence suggests that soy protein may modestly lower blood pressure in individuals with hypertension. Effects may be additive, but patients should be monitored for hypotension.
	Chemotherapeutic drugs, e.g. vincristine, vinblastine, cisplatin, daunorubicin	Theoretical beneficial interaction	Caution with use of this combination	In-vitro evidence suggests soy isoflavones may potentially enhance drug antitumour effects with certain chemotherapeutic agents. Clinical significance is unknown and safety of this combination has not been established. Medical supervision is warranted.

Continued

TABLE I.1 Herbal interactions—cont'd				
Herbal medicine	**Drug/drug class**	**Potential outcome**	**Recommendations**	**Comments**
Glycine max cont'd	L-thyroxine (Levothyroxine)	Possible decreased drug effects	Caution with use of this combination	Preliminary evidence suggests that soy-based formulas may decrease thyroxine levels in infants with congenital hypothyroidism. It is unclear if this interaction occurs in other patient populations. Soy may theoretically affect thyroid function although, based on current evidence, this effect does not appear to be clinically significant.
	Monoamine oxidase inhibitors (MAOIs)	Theoretical increased risk of drug adverse effects	Avoid combination	Fermented soy products such as tofu and soy sauce contain tyramine, which may theoretically interact with MAOIs and increase the risk of a hypertensive crisis. The amount of tyramine in fermented soy products is usually relatively small, but concentrations can vary.
	Oestrogens, e.g. HRT	Theoretical altered drug action	May be beneficial — medical supervision recommended	Data are conflicting on the interaction between soy and oestrogenic drugs. Some sources suggest that soy isoflavones theoretically inhibit the effects of HRT due to competition for oestrogen-binding receptors, while others suggest soy may have additive beneficial effects. Caution is advised until more data become available.
	Progesterone	Possible increased bone loss	Monitor — clinical significance is unclear	Results of a small clinical study suggest that while both soy milk and progesterone patches had bone-sparing effects when used alone, when used in combination it resulted in bone loss. Further data are required to establish clinical significance.
	Tamoxifen	May antagonise drug effect	Avoid combination	Soy may interfere with drug action due to the oestrogenic effects of soy isoflavones. Preliminary evidence suggests that the soy isoflavones genistein and diadzen may antagonise drug antitumour effect. Results from studies have been conflicting, which may be due to dose variations. Caution is advised until more data become available.
	Warfarin	Theoretical decreased drug effect	Caution with use of this combination	A case report describes a possible interaction between soy milk and warfarin. The data are inconclusive.
Glycyrrhiza glabra	Antihypertensive drugs	Theoretical decreased drug effect and increased hypertension	Caution with use of this combination	Liquorice can significantly raise blood pressure with regular high-dose intake. This adverse effect appears to occur to a greater extent in patients with high blood pressure, than in those with normal blood pressure.
	Ciclosporin	Theoretical decreased drug effects	Caution with use of this combination	Liquorice has been reported to reduce drug therapeutic effects in animal models. Clinical significance is unclear, but caution is advised due to the risk of serious consequences.

TABLE I.1 Herbal interactions—cont'd

Herbal medicine	Drug/drug class	Potential outcome	Recommendations	Comments
Glycyrrhiza glabra cont'd	Cisplatin	Theoretical decreased drug effects	Caution with use of this combination	In animal models liquorice has been reported to reduce drug therapeutic effect. Clinical significance is unclear.
	Corticosteroids	Theoretical increased drug adverse effects	Caution with use of this combination	High-dose intake of liquorice may potentiate drug duration and activity and decrease drug excretion. This could theoretically lead to an increased risk of drug adverse effects. The combination may also increase the risk of potassium loss and potassium depletion.
	CYP450 substrates (CYP2B6)	Theoretical increased risk of adverse effects	Monitor — clinical significance is unclear	In-vitro studies suggest that liquorice may inhibit activity of CYP2B6. These interactions have not been demonstrated in humans.
	CYP450 substrates (CYP2C9)	Theoretical altered drug effects	Monitor — clinical significance is unclear	Evidence about the effect of liquorice on CYP2C9 activity is conflicting. Some studies suggest liquorice induces enzyme activity, while others suggest enzyme inhibition. Caution is advised until more data become available.
	CYP450 substrates (CYP3A4)	Theoretical decreased drug effects	Caution with use of this combination	Liquorice appears to induce CYP3A4 metabolism, which may theoretically reduce drug effectiveness. Caution is advised until further data become available.
	Digoxin	Increased risk of drug adverse effects	Caution with use of this combination	There is an increased risk of potassium loss and drug adverse effects with regular consumption of large quantities of liquorice. Small occasional consumption is not expected to affect digoxin efficacy or toxicity. Caution is advised.
	Diuretic drugs (thiazide and loop)	Increased risk of potassium loss	Caution with use of this combination	There is an increased risk of hypokalaemia with overuse of liquorice in combination with potassium-depleting diuretics such as thiazides and loop diuretics.
	Laxatives including herbal laxatives	Increased risk of potassium loss	Caution with use of this combination	The overuse or misuse of liquorice in combination with stimulant laxatives increases the risk of potassium depletion, which may have health consequences.
	Non-steroidal anti-inflammatory drugs (NSAIDs)	Decreased drug gastric adverse effects	Combination may be beneficial	Liquorice and deglycyrrhizinated liquorice confer gastroprotective effects which may help to reduce the incidence of gastric irritation associated with NSAIDs and aspirin.
	Oestrogens, e.g. oral contraceptives and HRT	Theoretical increased drug adverse effects	Caution with use of this combination	Case reports suggest that liquorice may increase the risk of drug adverse effects. Use with caution at high doses for >2 weeks.

Continued

TABLE I.1 Herbal interactions—cont'd

Herbal medicine	Drug/drug class	Potential outcome	Recommendations	Comments
Glycyrrhiza glabra cont'd	Warfarin	Theoretical decreased drug effects	Caution with use of this combination	An animal study suggested that liquorice may increase drug metabolism and decrease drug effects. The interaction is however speculative and there is currently no evidence that constituents of liquorice have anticoagulant effects
Grifolia frondosa	Antidiabetic drugs	Possible additive effects	Caution with use of this combination	Preliminary clinical research suggests maitake mushrooms may lower blood glucose levels in type 2 diabetic patients. Concomitant use with antidiabetic drugs may result in additive effects and an increased risk of hypoglycaemia.
	Antihypertensive drugs	Theoretical additive effects	Caution with use of this combination	Animal research suggests maitake mushrooms may lower blood pressure. Theoretically, concomitant use with antihypertensive drugs may result in additive effects and an increased risk of hypotension.
	Warfarin	Theoretical increased risk of bleeding	Caution with use of this combination	A case report describes an increase in INR when a patient who was previously stabilised on warfarin commenced taking maitake mushrooms. It has been proposed that this may have been due to protein displacement of warfarin, resulting in increased anticoagulant effect. Caution is advised until more data become available.
Guaiacum officinale	Lithium	Increased risk of drug toxicity	Caution with use of this combination	This herb may have diuretic properties. Theoretically, combined use may reduce lithium excretion and increase the risk of lithium toxicity.
Gymnena sylvestre	Antidiabetic drugs	Possible additive effects	Caution with use of this combination	According to a number of clinical studies gymnema has clinically relevant hypoglycaemic effects in type 2 diabetics. The combination will be additive and potentially be beneficial. Caution is recommended as dosage adjustments may be needed to avoid hypoglycaemia.
	Insulin	Additive effects possible	Caution with use of this combination	Gymnema has clinically relevant hypoglycaemic effects in type 1 diabetics. The combination will be additive and potentially beneficial. Caution is recommended as dosage adjustment may be needed to avoid hypoglycaemia.
Harpagophytum procumbens	Acid-reducing drugs, e.g. H_2 antagonists and proton pump inhibitors	Theoretical decreased drug effect	Monitor — clinical significance is unclear	Devil's claw may increase gastric acidity. Use may theoretically counteract drug acid-reducing action, resulting in decreased drug effect. More data are needed to establish relevance.
	CYP450 substrates (CYP2C19, CYP2C9, CYP3A4)	Theoretical increased risk of drug toxicity	Monitor — clinical significance is unclear	Limited in-vitro studies suggest that devil's claw may inhibit CYP2C19, CYP2C9 and CYP3A4. This may theoretically lead to increased drug serum levels and risk of toxicity with drugs metabolised by these enzymes. These interactions are speculative and have not been demonstrated in humans.

TABLE I.1 Herbal interactions—cont'd

Herbal medicine	Drug/drug class	Potential outcome	Recommendations	Comments
Harpagophytum procumbens cont'd	Non-steroidal anti-inflammatory drugs (NSAIDs)	Possible additive effects	Combination may be beneficial	Additive anti-inflammatory effects may allow for a decrease in NSAID dose and this will reduce the risk of drug adverse effects. This beneficial interaction is supported by evidence.
	Warfarin	Theoretical increased risk of bleeding	Caution with use of this combination	A case report describes symptoms of purpurea in a patient who took devil's claw with warfarin. Findings were inconclusive, but caution is recommended.
Hericium erinaceus	Anticoagulant/ antiplatelet drugs	Theoretical increased risk of bleeding	Caution with use of this combination	In-vitro evidence suggests this herb has antiplatelet activity. Combined use with anticoagulant and antiplatelet drugs will theoretically increase the risk of bleeding and bruising.
	Antidiabetic drugs	Theoretical additive effects	Caution with use of this combination	Animal studies suggest this herb may lower blood glucose levels. Additive effects are theoretically possible, increasing the risk of hypoglycaemia. Caution is advised until more data become available.
Hibiscus sabdariffa	Antidiabetic drugs	Theoretical additive effects	Caution with use of this combination	Preliminary evidence suggests roselle may lower blood glucose levels. Effects may be additive, with a theoretical risk of hypoglycaemia.
	Antihypertensive drugs	Theoretical increased risk of hypotension	Monitor — clinical significance is unclear	Limited studies suggest that roselle may lower blood pressure. The interaction may be beneficial but patients should be monitored for hypotension.
	Chloroquine	Reduced drug effect	Avoid combination	Roselle has been shown to significantly reduce the bioavailability of chloroquine. Concomitant use may reduce drug efficacy and should be avoided.
Hippophea rhamnoides	Anticoagulant/ antiplatelet drugs	Theoretical increased risk of bleeding	Caution with use of this combination	Limited research suggests sea buckthorn has antiplatelet properties. Concomitant use with anticoagulant and antiplatelet drugs will theoretically increase the risk of bleeding and bruising.
	Antihypertensive drugs	Theoretical increased risk of hypotension	Monitor — clinical significance is unclear	Limited studies suggest that sea buckthorn may have hypotensive properties. Additive beneficial effects are theoretically possible, but monitor for hypotension.
Humulus lupulus	Alcohol	Increased risk of sedation	Caution with use of this combination	Hops may potentiate the sedative effects of alcohol.
	CNS depressant drugs	Increased risk of sedation	Caution with use of this combination	Hops may potentiate the sedative effects of CNS depressant drugs.
	CYP450 substrates (CYP1A1, CYP1A2, CYP1B1)	Theoretical increased risk of adverse effects	Monitor — may not be clinically significant	Hops may inhibit CYP1A1, CYP1A2 and CYP1B1 enzymes according to in-vitro studies. This may theoretically increase the risk of drug adverse effects, although this interaction has not been reported in humans.

Continued

TABLE I.1 Herbal interactions—cont'd

Herbal medicine	Drug/drug class	Potential outcome	Recommendations	Comments
Humulus lupulus cont'd	CYP450 substrates (CYP3A4)	Theoretical decreased drug effects	Monitor — may not be clinically significant	In-vitro studies suggest that hops may induce CYP3A4 enzyme. Theoretically, combined use may decrease drug effect. Caution is advised although this interaction has not been demonstrated in humans.
	Oestrogen, e.g. oral contraceptives and HRT or anti-oestrogenic drugs	Theoretical altered drug effect	Monitor — may not be clinically significant	In-vitro studies suggest that certain hops constituents can bind to oestrogen receptors and potentially alter drug efficacy. The interaction may not be clinically relevant, but patients can be monitored.
Hydrastis canadensis	Anticoagulant/ antiplatelet drugs	Theoretical increased risk of bleeding	Caution with use of this combination	In-vitro and animal studies suggest that berberine, a constituent of goldenseal, may inhibit platelet aggregation. There is a theoretical increased risk of bleeding, although this has not been demonstrated in human studies. Caution is advised.
	Antidiabetic drugs	Theoretical additive effects	Caution with use of this combination	Berberine in goldenseal may lower blood glucose levels, theoretically increasing the risk of hypoglycaemia.
	Antihypertensive drugs	Theoretical additive effects	Caution with use of this combination	Berberine in goldenseal may have hypotensive effects, theoretically having additive effects. The interaction may not be clinically significant, but monitor for hypotension.
	Antimicrobial agents	Theoretical additive effects	Combination may be beneficial	Constituents of goldenseal have antimicrobial effects against several organisms. Due to poor absorption of the alkaloids, it is unclear if the serum concentrations will be sufficiently high to make a clinical difference. There is, however, a theoretical additive effect.
	Ciclosporin	Risk of increased drug effects	Caution with use of this combination	A clinical study reported that berberine, which is a constituent of goldenseal, significantly increased drug serum levels in renal-transplant patients. Theoretically, concomitant use may increase the risk of drug toxicity.
	CNS depressant drugs	Theoretical additive effects	Caution with use of this combination	Berberine in goldenseal may have sedative effects. Theoretically this may result in additive effects and a risk of excessive sedation, although clinical significance of this interaction is unclear.
	CYP2D6 substrates	Theoretical risk of increased drug effects	Caution with use of this combination	Goldenseal has been shown to significantly inhibit CYP2D6 enzyme activity, theoretically leading to an increased risk of drug toxicity and adverse effects.
	CYP450 substrates (CYP2C9, CYP2E1, CYP3A4)	Theoretical risk of increased drug effects	Caution with use of this combination	Goldenseal may inhibit CYP2C9, CYP2E1 and CYP3A4 enzyme activity based on in vitro studies. This may theoretically lead to an increased risk of drug toxicity and adverse effects, although clinical significance is unclear.

TABLE I.1 Herbal interactions—cont'd

Herbal medicine	Drug/drug class	Potential outcome	Recommendations	Comments
Hydrastis canadensis cont'd	Digoxin	Risk of increased drug effects	Caution with use of this combination	A small increase in drug peak levels has been reported with use of this combination. Caution is advised until more data become available.
	Laxatives	Risk of decreased drug effects	Monitor — may not be clinically significant	Goldenseal may have an anti-diarrhoeal effect. This may theoretically reduce effectiveness of laxatives.
	Midazolam	Risk of increased drug effects	Caution with use of this combination	Goldenseal has been shown to increase midazolam blood concentrations in two clinical studies.
	P-gp substrates	Possible altered drug effects	Caution with use of this combination	There is conflicting data as to whether goldenseal affects P-gp or not, and if so, whether it inhibits or induces P-gp. Caution is advised until more data become available.
	Tacrolimus	Risk of increased drug effects	Caution with use of this combination	An increased incidence of drug adverse effects was reported in a case study where goldenseal and tacrolimus were used concurrently.
Hypericum perforatum	Antidepressant drugs (SSRIs, e.g. paroxetine or SNRIs, e.g. venlafaxine)	Increased risk of serotonin-related adverse effects	Avoid combination	Concomitant use of St John's wort and selective serotonin antagonists (SSRI antidepressants) may increase the risk of adverse effects and serotonin syndrome. The combination should be avoided.
	Antidepressants (tricyclics, e.g. amitriptyline, nortriptyline)	Decreased drug effect	Caution with use of this combination	St John's wort may reduce drug effect due to induction of the CYP3A4 enzyme and P-gp drug transporter.
	Antiepileptic drugs — barbiturates, e.g. phenytoin, phenobarbital (phenobarbitone)	Decreased drug effect	Avoid combination	St John's wort may increase the rate of drug metabolism, which can potentially result in decreased drug effect. The interaction is considered likely to be clinically significant, and may lead to an increased risk of seizures.
	Antineoplastic drugs	Decreased drug effect	Avoid combination	St John's wort may increase the rate of drug metabolism, which can potentially result in decreased drug effect. The interaction is considered likely to be clinically significant.
	Benzodiazepines, e.g. alprazolam, midazolam	Decreased drug effect	Avoid combination	St John's wort may increase the rate of drug metabolism, which can potentially result in decreased drug effect. The interaction is considered likely to be clinically significant.
	Buproprion	Decreased drug effect	Caution with use of this combination	St John's wort may increase the rate of drug metabolism, which can potentially result in decreased drug effect. The interaction is considered likely to be clinically significant.
	Ciclosporin	Decreased drug effect	Avoid combination	St John's wort may increase the rate of drug metabolism, which can potentially result in decreased drug effect. The interaction is considered likely to be clinically significant.

Continued

TABLE I.1 Herbal interactions—cont'd

Herbal medicine	Drug/drug class	Potential outcome	Recommendations	Comments
Hypericum perforatum cont'd	Clopidogrel	Theoretical increased risk of bleeding	Caution with use of this combination	Preliminary evidence suggests St John's wort may increase antiplatelet activity of clopidogrel, which could potentially increase the risk of bleeding. Evidence is inconclusive.
	Contraceptive drugs	Decreased drug effect	Avoid combination	St John's wort may increase the rate of drug metabolism, which can potentially result in decreased drug effect. The interaction is considered likely to be clinically significant and may increase the risk of breakthrough bleeding and unplanned pregnancy.
	CYP450 substrates (CYP3A4 and CYP2C19)	Decreased drug effects	Avoid combination	St John's wort significantly induces cytochrome P450 enzymes CYP2C19 and CYP3A4. This has been shown to increase the rate of clearance of drugs metabolised via these pathways, potentially leading to reduced drug concentration and drug effectiveness. A significant number of medicinal drugs are metabolised via these two pathways, especially CYP3A4.
	CYP450 substrates (CYP1A2, CYP2B6, CYP2C9)	Decreased drug effects	Caution with use of this combination	St John's wort may moderately induce activity of CYP1A2, CYP2B6 and CYP2C9. This may increase the rate of drug metabolism, leading to reduced drug effect. The extent of enzyme induction appears to be less pronounced than the effect on CYP3A4 and CYP2C19.
	Dextromethorphan	Increased risk of serotonin-related adverse effects	Caution with use of this combination	Concomitant use of St John's wort and dextromethorphan may increase the risk of adverse effects and serotonin syndrome.
	Digoxin	Decreased drug effect	Avoid combination	St John's wort may increase the rate of drug metabolism, which can potentially result in decreased drug effect. The interaction is considered likely to be clinically significant.
	Docetaxel	Decreased drug effect	Avoid combination	St John's wort may increase the rate of drug metabolism, which can potentially result in decreased drug effect. The interaction is considered likely to be clinically significant and may compromise cancer treatment.
	Fenfluramine	Increased risk of serotonin-related adverse effects	Avoid combination	Concomitant use of St John's wort and fenfluramine may increase the risk of adverse effects and serotonin syndrome.
	Gliclazide	Decreased drug effect	Caution with use of this combination	St John's wort may increase the rate of drug metabolism, which can potentially result in decreased drug effect.

TABLE I.1 Herbal interactions—cont'd

Herbal medicine	Drug/drug class	Potential outcome	Recommendations	Comments
Hypericum perforatum cont'd	HMGCoA reductase inhibitors (statins) e.g. simvastatin	Decreased drug effect	Caution with use of this combination	St John's wort may increase the rate of drug metabolism, which can potentially result in decreased drug effect. A study describes a 28% reduction in plasma concentrations of simvastatin.
	Imatinib	Decreased drug effect	Avoid combination	St John's wort may increase the rate of drug metabolism, which can potentially result in decreased drug effect. The interaction is likely to be clinically significant.
	Irinotecan	Decreased drug effect	Avoid combination	St John's wort may increase the rate of drug metabolism, which can potentially result in decreased drug effect. The interaction is likely to be clinically significant.
	Methadone	Decreased drug effect	Avoid combination	St John's wort may increase the rate of drug metabolism, which can potentially result in decreased drug effect. The interaction is likely to be clinically significant.
	Methylphenidate	Decreased drug effect	Monitor — may not be clinically significant	A case report describes a decrease in drug effectiveness in a man who had been stabilised on methylphenidate commenced use of St John's wort.
	Monoamine oxidase inhibitors	Increased risk of adverse effects	Caution with use of this combination	Concomitant use of St John's wort and drugs in this class may increase the risk of adverse effects and serotonin syndrome.
	Non-nucleoside reverse transcriptase inhibitors (NNRTIs)	Decreased drug effect	Avoid combination	St John's wort may increase the rate of drug metabolism, which can potentially result in decreased drug effect. The interaction is likely to be clinically significant and may result in treatment failure of HIV.
	Omeprazole	Decreased drug effect	Caution with use of this combination	St John's wort may increase the rate of drug metabolism, which can potentially result in decreased drug effect.
	Photosensitising drugs	Increased risk of photosensitivity	Caution with use of this combination	St John's wort may increase the risk of photosensitivity due to the hypericin content. Clinical significance is unclear, but caution is recommended.
	P-glycoprotein (P-gp) substrates	Decreased efficacy with drugs that are P-gp substrates	Avoid combination	St John's wort induces P-glycoprotein (P-gp), which may lead to decreased drug effect. P-gp is a transport protein that can actively pump drugs out of cells.
	Psoralen plus UVA therapy	Increased risk of photosensitivity	Caution with use of this combination	St John's wort may increase the risk of photosensitivity reactions due to the hypericin content.
	Protease inhibitors, e.g. indinavir	Decreased drug effect	Avoid combination	St John's wort may increase the rate of drug metabolism, which can potentially result in decreased drug effect. The interaction is likely to be clinically significant and may result in treatment failure of HIV.

Continued

TABLE I.1 Herbal interactions—cont'd

Herbal medicine	Drug/drug class	Potential outcome	Recommendations	Comments
Hypericum perforatum cont'd	Proton-pup inhibitors, e.g. omeprazole	Decreased drug effect	Caution with use of this combination	St John's wort may increase the rate of drug metabolism, which can potentially result in decreased drug effect.
	Tacrolimus	Decreased drug effect	Avoid combination	St John's wort may increase the rate of drug metabolism, which can potentially result in decreased drug effect. The interaction is likely to be clinically significant.
	Tramadol	Increased risk of serotonin-related adverse effects	Avoid combination	Concomitant use of St John's wort and tramadol may theoretically increase the risk of adverse effects and serotonin syndrome.
	Triptans, e.g. sumatriptan, zolmitriptan for migraines	Increased risk of serotonin-related adverse effects	Avoid combination	Concomitant use of St John's wort and selective serotonin agonists (triptans) may theoretically increase the risk of adverse effects and serotonin syndrome. Case reports describe interactions between St John's wort and 'triptan' drugs, used for migraines.
	Tyrosine kinase inhibitors, e.g. imatinib	Decreased drug effect	Avoid combination	St John's wort may increase the rate of drug metabolism, which can potentially result in decreased drug effect. The interaction is likely to be clinically significant.
	Warfarin	Decreased drug effect — risk of clotting	Avoid combination	St John's wort may increase the rate of drug metabolism, which can potentially result in decreased drug effect. This may increase the risk of clotting. The interaction is likely to be clinically significant.
	Zolpidem	Decreased drug effect	Avoid combination	A small study reported a reduction in zolpidem serum levels with concurrent use of St John's wort.
Inula helenium	CYP450 substrates (CYP2C19, CYP3A4)	Theoretical decreased drug effects	Caution with use of this combination	In-vitro and animal studies suggest that a constituent of elecampane, alantolactone, may induce CYP3A4 and CYP2C19 enzyme activity. This may theoretically result in an increased rate of drug metabolism and decreased efficacy. Clinical significance is unknown.
	CNS depressant drugs	Theoretical additive sedative effects	Caution with use of this combination	Sedative effects have been observed with use of elecampane in animal models. There is a risk of additive sedation with concomitant use. Clinical significance is unclear.
Iris versicolor	Digoxin	Theoretical increased risk of drug adverse effects	Avoid combination	Theoretically, the combination of blue flag with digoxin increases the risk of drug adverse effects. Clinical evidence of this interaction is lacking, but caution is advised due to potentially serious consequences.
	Diuretics	Theoretical increased risk of potassium loss	Caution with use of this combination	There is an increased risk of hypokalaemia with overuse of blue flag in combination with potassium-depleting diuretics such as thiazides and loop diuretics.

TABLE I.1 Herbal interactions—cont'd

Herbal medicine	Drug/drug class	Potential outcome	Recommendations	Comments
Iris versicolor cont'd	Warfarin	Theoretical increased risk of bleeding	Caution with use of this combination	Blue flag has stimulant laxative effects and may cause diarrhoea. This may theoretically elevate INR and increase the risk of bleeding with excessive intake of herb.
Juglans cinerea	Corticosteroids	Increased risk of potassium loss	Caution with use of this combination	Overuse of this herb may compound drug-induced potassium loss.
	Digoxin	Increased risk of drug adverse effects	Caution with use of this combination	Overuse of this herb may compound drug-induced potassium loss, leading to an increased risk of drug adverse effects and toxicity.
	Diuretics	Increased risk of potassium loss	Caution with use of this combination	Overuse of this herb in combination with potassium-depleting diuretics, such as thiazides and loop diuretics, increases the risk of potassium loss.
	Stimulant laxatives	Increased risk of diarrhoea and loss of electrolytes	Caution with use of this combination	Both herb and drug have laxative effects, and may lead to loss of electrolytes.
Juniperus communis	Antidiabetic drugs	Theoretical additive effects	Monitor — clinical significance is unclear	Animal studies suggest that juniper may have hypoglycaemic properties. Additive effects are theoretically possible, increasing the risk of hypoglycaemia. Caution is advised until more data become available.
	Diuretics	Possible additive effects	Monitor — clinical significance is unclear	Juniper has been shown to have diuretic properties. Additive effects are theoretically possible, but the clinical significance has not been established.
Lavendula officinalis	Antidepressant drugs, including imipramine	Potentially beneficial additive effects	May be beneficial — medical supervision recommended	Oral lavender may improve management of mild to moderate depression. Concomitant use may be beneficial, but caution is recommended until more data become available.
	Antihypertensive drugs	Theoretical additive effects	Monitor — may not be clinically significant	Lavender oil in combination with other essential oils as aromatherapy may slightly lower blood pressure. Additive effects are theoretically possible. The interaction may be beneficial, but patients should be monitored for hypotension.
	Barbiturates	Theoretical increased effects and sedation	Caution with use of this combination	Lavender may theoretically potentiate the effects of barbiturates and increase the risk of sedation.
	Benzodiazepines	Possible additive effects and increased risk of sedation	Caution with use of this combination	Lavender may theoretically potentiate the effects of benzodiazepines and increase the risk of sedation. Clinical studies have reported that oral lavender has beneficial anxiolytic effects.
	CNS depressant drugs	Theoretical increased effects and sedation	Caution with use of this combination	Lavender may theoretically potentiate the effects of CNS depressant drugs increase the risk of sedation.

Continued

TABLE I.1 Herbal interactions—cont'd				
Herbal medicine	**Drug/drug class**	**Potential outcome**	**Recommendations**	**Comments**
Lentinus edodes	Immunosuppressant drugs	Theoretical decreased drug effect	Caution with use of this combination	Laboratory studies suggest that shiitake mushrooms may have immunostimulant activity. Theoretically this could counteract drug immunosuppressant effects. Clinical significance is unclear, but caution is advised.
Leonurus cardiaca	CNS depressant drugs including benzodiazepines	Possible additive effects and adverse effects	Caution with use of this combination	Evidence suggests motherwort has additive effects when used with CNS depressant drugs such as benzodiazepines. The combination may lead to excessive drowsiness.
Lepidium meyenii	Antidepressant drugs (SSRIs, SNRIs)	Possible decreased drug adverse effects	Combination may be beneficial	Maca may help to alleviate sexual dysfunction caused by SSRIs/SNRIs. This is according to the findings of a small clinical trial conducted in postmenopausal women who were taking these drugs for depression.
Leptandra virginica	Digoxin	Altered drug effects	Caution with use of this combination	Theoretically, overuse or abuse of black root may increase the risk of adverse effects of cardiac glycosides such as digoxin. Some other sources suggest black root may reduce drug effectiveness by binding to the drug in the GI tract. Evidence is inconclusive, but caution is advised.
	Diuretics	Theoretical risk of hypokalaemia	Caution with use of this combination	Black root may lead to diuretic-induced potassium loss. There is a theoretical increased risk of hypokalaemia when used with potassium-depleting diuretics.
Leptospermum scoparium	Antibiotics for wound healing	Theoretical additive effect	Combination may be beneficial	Topical use of manuka honey may improve wound healing and have antimicrobial properties. Theoretically, honey dressings may provide an additive beneficial effect when used with antibiotics.
Linum usitatissimum	Anticoagulant/antiplatelet drugs	Theoretical increased risk of bleeding	Monitor — may not be clinically significant	Flaxseed may have antiplatelet properties. Concomitant use with anticoagulant and antiplatelet drugs will theoretically increase the risk of bleeding and bruising. The interaction is unlikely to be clinically significant at normal therapeutic doses.
	Antidiabetic drugs	Theoretical additive effects	Monitor — may not be clinically significant	Flaxseed may lower blood glucose levels. Additive effects are theoretically possible, increasing the risk of hypoglycaemia. Clinical significance at normal therapeutic doses is unclear.
	Antihypertensive drugs	Theoretical additive effects	Monitor — may not be clinically significant	Flaxseed may slightly lower diastolic pressure, leading to a theoretical additive effect. Clinical significance at normal therapeutic doses is unclear.
	Furosemide (frusemide)	Theoretical decreased drug absorption	Monitor — may not be clinically significant	Preliminary in-vitro research suggests flaxseed may decrease drug absorption. The clinical significance is unknown.
	Ketoprofen	Theoretical decreased drug absorption	Monitor — may not be clinically significant	Preliminary in-vitro research suggests flaxseed may decrease drug absorption. The clinical significance is unknown.

TABLE I.1 Herbal interactions—cont'd

Herbal medicine	Drug/drug class	Potential outcome	Recommendations	Comments
Linum usitatissimum cont'd	Oestrogens, e.g. HRT and oral contraceptives	Theoretical decreased drug effect	Monitor — may not be clinically significant	Flaxseed may theoretically have mild oestrogenic effects. Theoretically, the lignans in flaxseed may compete with oestrogens for binding sites and reduce drug effect. The interaction is speculative.
	Paracetamol	Theoretical decreased drug absorption	Monitor — may not be clinically significant	Preliminary in-vitro research suggests flaxseed may decrease drug absorption. The clinical significance is unknown.
Lobelia inflata	Lithium	Theoretical increased risk of drug toxicity	Caution with use of this combination	Lobelia may have diuretic properties. Theoretically this might decrease drug excretion and potentiate the risk of drug toxicity.
	Nicotine replacement therapy	Theoretical additive effects	May be beneficial — medical supervision recommended	Some studies suggest a possible benefit for lobelia as an aid to smoking cessation, although results have been conflicting. Theoretically combined use may be beneficial, under appropriate medical supervision.
Lycopus virginicus	L-thyroxine (Levothyroxine)	Possible reduced drug effect	Avoid combination	Bugleweed may reduce drug effect by blocking peripheral conversion of thyroxine to T3.
Magnolia spp.	Alcohol	Theoretical additive sedative effects	Caution with use of this combination	Magnolia may have sedative properties. Theoretically, concomitant use with alcohol may lead to excessive drowsiness and decreased motor function.
	Anticoagulant/ antiplatelet drugs	Additive effects theoretically possible	Monitor — may not be clinically significant	Magnolia may have some antiplatelet properties. The combination may theoretically increase the risk of bleeding, although this has not been demonstrated in humans.
	Barbiturates	Theoretical additive sedative effects	Caution with use of this combination	Magnolia may have sedative properties. Theoretically, concomitant use with barbiturates may lead to excessive drowsiness and decreased motor function.
	Benzodiazepines	Theoretical additive sedative effects	Caution with use of this combination	Magnolia may have sedative properties. Theoretically concomitant use with benzodiazepines may lead to excessive drowsiness and decreased motor function.
	CNS depressant drugs	Theoretical additive sedative effects	Caution with use of this combination	Magnolia may have sedative properties. Theoretically concomitant use with CNS depressant drugs may lead to excessive drowsiness and decreased motor function.
Marrubium vulgare	Antidiabetic drugs	Theoretical additive effects	Monitor — may not be clinically significant	White horehound may slightly lower blood glucose. Preliminary clinical research suggests this effect may not be clinically significant when used in combination with antidiabetic drugs.
	Antihypertensive drugs	Theoretical additive effects	Monitor — may not be clinically significant	White horehound may lower blood pressure according to animal research. Theoretically this may increase the risk of hypotension when used with antihypertensive drugs.

Continued

TABLE I.1 Herbal interactions—cont'd				
Herbal medicine	**Drug/drug class**	**Potential outcome**	**Recommendations**	**Comments**
Matricaria recutita	Anticoagulant/ antiplatelet drugs	Case report of increased bleeding	Monitor — may not be clinically significant	One case report describes internal bleeding and raised INR following ingestion of 4–5 cups of chamomile tea and use of a chamomile-based skin lotion in an elderly woman taking warfarin. Caution is recommended until more data become available.
	Antidiabetic drugs	Theoretical additive effects	Combination may be beneficial	Chamomile may have hypoglycaemic effects. The interaction may be beneficial and improve outcomes based on limited research, but patients should be monitored for hypoglycaemia.
	CNS depressant drugs including benzodiazepines	Theoretical additive sedative effects	Caution with use of this combination	Chamomile has sedative effects and may theoretically interact with CNS depressants drugs, including benzodiazepines, leading to additive effects and adverse effects.
	CYP450 substrates (CYP2C9, CYP2D6, CYP3A4)	Theoretical risk of increased adverse effects	Monitor — may not be clinically significant	Chamomile may inhibit activity of CYP2D6, CYP2C9 and CYP3A4 according to in-vitro studies. This may theoretically increase the risk of drug-related adverse effects, although this interaction has not been reported in humans.
	Oestrogen, e.g. HRT and oral contraceptives	Theoretical altered drug effects	Monitor — may not be clinically significant	Chamomile may have oestrogenic effects and may theoretically interact with oestrogenic drugs. The interaction may not be clinically significant, but patients should be monitored.
	Tamoxifen	Theoretical altered drug effects	Caution with use of this combination	Chamomile may have oestrogenic effects and theoretically interact with anti-oestrogen drugs (e.g. tamoxifen). Oral chamomile should be avoided in hormone-sensitive tumours until more safety data become available.
Medicago sativa	Antidiabetic drugs	Theoretical additive effects	Monitor — may not be clinically significant	Alfalfa may have hypoglycaemic properties based on animal research and one case report. Additive effects are theoretically possible, increasing the risk of hypoglycaemia. Caution is advised until more data become available.
	Immunosuppressant drugs	Theoretical decreased drug effects	Caution with use of this combination	Alfalfa may theoretically counteract drug immunosuppressant effects due to herb immunostimulating activity. Evidence of an interaction is limited, but caution is advised. Alfalfa has been shown to exacerbate symptoms of SLE and should be avoided in these patients.
	Oestrogen, e.g. HRT and oral contraceptives	Theoretical altered drug effects	Caution with use of this combination	Alfalfa contains isoflavonoids with oestrogenic properties. Theoretically, this may interfere with drug effects at high dose, although data are limited.
	Photosensitising drugs	Increased risk of photosensitivity	Caution with use of this combination	Excessive intake of alfalfa may potentiate drug-induced photosensitivity reactions.
	Warfarin	Decreased drug effect	Avoid combination	Alfalfa contains high amounts of vitamin K. Concurrent use can oppose drug action and increase the risk of clotting.

TABLE I.1 Herbal interactions—cont'd

Herbal medicine	Drug/drug class	Potential outcome	Recommendations	Comments
Melissa officinalis	Alcohol	Increased risk of sedation	Caution with use of this combination	Lemon balm may potentiate the sedative effects of alcohol.
	Antidiabetic drugs	Theoretical additive effects	Monitor — may not be clinically significant	One animal study suggests that lemon balm may have hypoglycaemic properties. Additive effects are theoretically possible, increasing the risk of hypoglycaemia. More study is needed to assess the clinical significance of this effect.
	Barbiturates	Increased risk of sedation	Caution with use of this combination	Lemon balm may potentiate the sedative effects of barbiturates.
	CNS depressant drugs	Increased risk of sedation	Caution with use of this combination	Lemon balm may potentiate the sedative effects of CNS depressant drugs.
	Thyroid hormones	Theoretical altered thyroid function	Monitor — may not be clinically significant	Animal and in-vitro studies suggest that theoretically lemon balm may alter thyroid function and reduce thyroid hormone levels. Evidence is weak.
Mentha x piperita	Acid-reducing drugs (antacids, H_2-antagonsist and proton pump inhibitors)	Increased herbal adverse effects; decreased management of condition	Caution with use of this combination	Drugs that decrease stomach acid and raise gastric pH may cause premature dissolution of enteric-coated peppermint oil. In addition, peppermint oil may relax the lower oesophageal sphincter in some individuals, leading to increased risk of heartburn, reflux and GORD and potentially counteracting drug effects.
	Ciclosporin	Increased risk of drug effects and adverse effects	Caution with use of this combination	Peppermint oil may inhibit drug metabolism by inhibition of CYP3A4. This may theoretically increase drug bioavailability and the risk of adverse effects. An interaction between ciclosporin and peppermint oil has not been reported in human studies, but caution is advised.
	CYP450 substrates (CYP1A2, CYP2C19, CYP2C9, CYP3A4)	Decreased drug metabolism with theoretical increased risk of adverse effects	Caution with use of this combination	Peppermint oil may inhibit activity of CYP1A2, CYP2C19, CYP2C9 and CYP3A4. This may theoretically increase blood levels of drugs metabolised via these enzyme pathways. The interactions appear to only occur at very high doses of peppermint oil, but caution is advised.
	Felodipine	Increased risk of drug effects and adverse effects	Caution with use of this combination	A small clinical study reported that peppermint oil increased drug bioavailability and theoretically increased the risk of adverse effect. Peppermint has been shown to inhibit CYP3A4 enzyme activity in animal and in-vitro studies. Patients taking felodipine with peppermint oil should be monitored for hypotension and other drug adverse effects.
	Simvastatin	Increased risk of drug effects and adverse effects	Monitor — may not be clinically significant	Preliminary animal research suggests peppermint oil may increase drug bioavailability and theoretically increase the risk of adverse effects. Clinical significance is unclear.

Continued

TABLE I.1 Herbal interactions—cont'd				
Herbal medicine	**Drug/drug class**	**Potential outcome**	**Recommendations**	**Comments**
Mentha x piperita cont'd	Iron	Decreased iron absorption	Monitor — may not be clinically significant	High intake of peppermint tea has been shown to inhibit iron absorption. Dose separation is advised.
Mentha spicata	CNS depressant drugs	Increased risk of sedation	Monitor — may not be clinically significant	Spearmint may have sedative effects, based on animal studies. Theoretically this may potentiate the sedative effects of CNS depressant drugs, although clinical significance is unknown.
	Hepatotoxic drugs	Theoretical increased risk of liver damage	Monitor — may not be clinically significant	Animal research suggests that high-dose spearmint tea may increase markers of liver damage (AST and ALT). Theoretically excessive intake may have additive detrimental effects on the liver when used with hepatotoxic drugs.
Menyanthes trifoliata	Anticoagulant/ antiplatelet drugs	Theoretical additive effects	Monitor — may not be clinically significant	Bogbean may theoretically have some antiplatelet properties although data are limited. Concomitant use with anticoagulant and antiplatelet drugs will theoretically increase the risk of bleeding and bruising.
Momordica charantia	Antidiabetic drugs	Possible additive effects possible	Caution with use of this combination	Bitter melon has hypoglycaemic properties and may have additive effects when used with antidiabetic drugs. This interaction may be beneficial, but supervision is required due to the risk of hypoglycaemia.
Moringa oleifera folia	Antidiabetic drugs	Theoretical additive effects	Caution with use of this combination	Animal research suggests moringa may lower blood glucose levels. Concomitant use with antidiabetic drugs may result in additive effects and an increased risk of hypoglycaemia.
	Antihypertensive drugs	Theoretical additive effects	Monitor — may not be clinically significant	Animal research suggests moringa pod may lower blood pressure. Theoretically, concomitant use with antihypertensive drugs may result in additive effects and an increased risk of hypotension. This effect may not apply to other plant parts.
	CYP450 substrates (CYP3A4)	Theoretical increased drug levels	Monitor — may not be clinically significant	In-vitro evidence suggests moringa may inhibit CYP3A4 activity. Theoretically this may result in raised drug plasma levels and an increased risk of adverse effects and toxicity if taken with drugs that are CYP3A4 substrates.
	L-thyroxine (Levothyroxine)	Theoretical decreased drug effects	Monitor — may not be clinically significant	Theoretically, moringa may reduce effectiveness of L-thyroxine. Preliminary animal research suggests moringa may inhibit peripheral conversion of T4 to T3.
Morus alba	Antidiabetic drugs	Possible additive effects	Caution with use of this combination	Limited studies show that white mulberry has hypoglycaemic properties. Additive effects are theoretically possible, increasing the risk of hypoglycaemia. Caution is advised until more data become available.

TABLE I.1 Herbal interactions—cont'd				
Herbal medicine	**Drug/drug class**	**Potential outcome**	**Recommendations**	**Comments**
Mucuna pruriens	Anaesthesia	Possible increased risk of cardiac arrhythmias	Caution with use of this combination	Theoretically this herb may increase the risk of cardiac arrhythmias with certain anaesthetics (cyclopropane and halogenated hydrocarbons), due to the L-dopa constituent. Patients should be advised to withdraw herbal therapy 2 weeks prior to surgery.
	Antidiabetic drugs	Theoretical risk of hypoglycaemia	Caution with use of this combination	Limited data suggest this herb may have hypoglycaemic effects. Additive effects are theoretically possible, increasing the risk of hypoglycaemia. Caution is advised until more data become available.
	Anti-Parkinson's disease drugs	Possible additive effects	May be beneficial — medical supervision recommended	This herb contains L-dopa. Preliminary evidence suggests this herb may help to improve symptoms of Parkinson's disease when used in combination with conventional drug for Parkinson's disease.
	Antipsychotic drugs	Possible decreased drug effects	Caution with use of this combination	This herb appears to have dopaminergic effects and so may theoretically decrease the antidopaminergic effects of some antipsychotic medications. Caution is advised.
	Levodopa	Possible additive effects	May be beneficial — medical supervision recommended	This herb contains L-dopa. Preliminary evidence suggests this herb may lead to quicker onset of action, duration of action and higher drug levels when used with levodopa. While theoretically this may be beneficial, medical supervision is required due to a risk of toxicity.
	Methyldopa	Increased risk of adverse effects	Avoid combination	Additive hypotensive effects are possible when used with methyldopa. Methyldopa may also inhibit peripheral decarboxylation of the herb constituent, L-dopa, which increases the risk of L-dopa toxicity.
	Monoamine oxidase inhibitors (MAOIs)	Increased risk of adverse effects	Avoid combination	An increased risk of hypertensive crisis has been proposed with this combination, due to the L-dopa constituent. The risk appears greatest with non-selective MAOIs.
	Tricyclic antidepressants	Increased risk of adverse effects	Caution with use of this combination	Rare reports suggest concomitant use may lead to hypertension and dyskinesia. Caution is advised until further data become available.
Myrtilli fructus	Anticoagulant/ antiplatelet drugs	Additive effects theoretically possible	Caution with use of this combination	Preliminary evidence suggests that bilberry may inhibit platelet aggregation at high dose, due to the anthocyanidin content. Combined use may increase the risk of bleeding and bruising.
	Antidiabetic drugs	Additive effects theoretically possible	Caution with use of this combination	Bilberry may have hypoglycaemic properties according to limited animal and human research findings. Additive effects are theoretically possible, increasing the risk of hypoglycaemia.

Continued

TABLE I.1 Herbal interactions—cont'd				
Herbal medicine	**Drug/drug class**	**Potential outcome**	**Recommendations**	**Comments**
Nepeta cataria	CNS depressant drugs	Increased risk of sedation	Monitor — may not be clinically significant	Limited research suggests that catnip may have sedative effects. Theoretically this may potentiate the sedative effects of CNS depressant drugs, although clinical significance is unknown.
	Lithium	Increased risk of drug toxicity	Caution with use of this combination	Catnip may have diuretic properties. Theoretically, combined use may reduce lithium excretion and increase the risk of lithium toxicity.
Nigella sativa	Analgesics	Theoretical additive effects	Monitor — may not be clinically significant	Animal studies suggest that nigella may have analgesic effects at high doses.
	Anticoagulant/ antiplatelet drugs	Theoretical additive effects	Caution with use of this combination	Preliminary evidence suggests that nigella may inhibit platelet aggregation. Combined use with anticoagulants may theoretically may increase the risk of bleeding.
	Anticonvulsants	Theoretical additive effects	Monitor — may not be clinically significant	A small clinical study reported that nigella had anticonvulsant effects. Clinical significance is unknown, but caution is advised.
	Antidiabetic drugs	Theoretical additive effects	Monitor — may not be clinically significant	Limited animal and human research findings suggest that nigella may have hypoglycaemic properties. Additive effects are theoretically possible, increasing the risk of hypoglycaemia. Caution is advised until more data become available.
	Antihypertensive drugs	Possible additive effects	Monitor — may not be clinically significant	Nigella may have mild hypotensive effects, and so theoretically enhance the effects of drugs that lower blood pressure. Significance is unclear.
	Antineoplastic drugs	Additive beneficial effects theoretically possible	Combination may be beneficial — medical supervision recommended	Preliminary evidence suggests that constituents of nigella may have antineoplastic activity. Nigella may potentiate the drug effects of some antineoplastic drugs, according to some animal studies. There may theoretically be potential for beneficial interactions, but further research is required to determine significance.
	Cisplatin	Theoretical decreased drug adverse effects	Combination may be beneficial	Animal models suggest that the constituent thymoquinone may be protective against cisplatin-induced nephrotoxicity. More data are required.
	CNS depressant drugs	Theoretical increased risk of sedation	Monitor — may not be clinically significant	Animal studies suggest that nigella may have sedative effects. Theoretically this may potentiate the sedative effects of CNS depressant drugs.
	Doxorubicin	Theoretical decreased drug adverse effects	Combination may be beneficial	Animal studies suggest that the constituent thymoquinone may be protective against doxorubicin-induced cardiotoxicity. More data are required.

TABLE I.1 Herbal interactions—cont'd				
Herbal medicine	**Drug/drug class**	**Potential outcome**	**Recommendations**	**Comments**
Nigella sativa cont'd	Immunosuppressant drugs	Theoretical decreased drug effect	Caution with use of this combination	Animal and in-vitro research suggests that nigella may have immunostimulant properties, which could theoretically antagonise the effects of immunosuppressant drugs. Some animal studies have, however, suggested nigella may suppress immune function. Caution is advised until more data become available.
Nigra alba	Antidiabetic drugs	Additive effects theoretically possible	Monitor — may not be clinically significant	According to limited studies black mulberry may have hypoglycaemic properties. Additive effects are theoretically possible when used with antidiabetic drugs, but significance is unclear. Monitor for hypoglycaemia.
Ocimum tenuiflorum	Anticoagulant/ antiplatelet drugs	Theoretical additive effects	Monitor — may not be clinically significant	According to animal research holy basil may have antiplatelet properties. Concomitant use with anticoagulant and antiplatelet drugs will theoretically increase the risk of bleeding and bruising.
	Phenobarbital (phenobarbitone)	Theoretical increased risk of sedation	Monitor — may not be clinically significant	Results of an animal study suggest that holy basil may increase phenobarbital (phenobarbitone)-induced sleeping time. Clinical significance is unclear. It is unknown whether this interaction would apply to other barbiturates or CNS depressant drugs, but patients should be monitored.
Olea europea	Anticoagulant/ antiplatelet drugs	Theoretical additive effects	Monitor — may not be clinically significant	According to limited research olive leaf extract may have antiplatelet properties. Concomitant use with anticoagulant and antiplatelet drugs will theoretically increase the risk of bleeding and bruising.
	Antidiabetic drugs	Theoretical additive effects	Monitor — may not be clinically significant	In a small study olive leaf extract was found to lower blood glucose concentrations and improve glucose regulation. Additive effects are therefore theoretically possible. Patients should be monitored for hypoglycaemia with concomitant use.
	Antihypertensive drugs	Theoretical additive effects	Monitor — may not be clinically significant	Olive leaf extract may have hypotensive properties and additive effects are theoretically possible. The interaction may be beneficial but patients should be monitored for hypotension.
Origanum vulgare	Anticoagulant/ antiplatelet drugs	Theoretical additive effects	Monitor — may not be clinically significant	According to limited research oregano may have antiplatelet/anticoagulant properties. Concomitant use with anticoagulant and antiplatelet drugs will theoretically increase the risk of bleeding and bruising.
	Antidiabetic drugs	Theoretical additive effects	Monitor — may not be clinically significant	According to animal and in-vitro studies oregano may lower blood glucose concentrations. Additive effects are theoretically possible, increasing the risk of hypoglycaemia.

Continued

TABLE I.1 Herbal interactions—cont'd				
Herbal medicine	**Drug/drug class**	**Potential outcome**	**Recommendations**	**Comments**
Paeonia lactiflora	Anticoagulant/ antiplatelet drugs	Theoretical additive effects	Monitor — may not be clinically significant	White peony may have antiplatelet / anticoagulant properties according to limited research. Concomitant use with anticoagulant and antiplatelet drugs will theoretically increase the risk of bleeding and bruising.
	Phenytoin	Theoretical decreased drug effect	Caution with use of this combination	Limited research suggests white peony root may reduce phenytoin plasma levels, which could theoretically decrease drug effectiveness.
Panax ginseng	Anticoagulant/ antiplatelet drugs	Theoretical increased risk of bleeding	Caution with use of this combination	In-vitro studies suggest that *Panax ginseng* may inhibit platelet aggregation, however research conducted in humans has not shown a clinically relevant effect. Caution is advised until more data become available.
	Antidiabetic drugs	Possible additive effects	Caution with use of this combination	Evidence suggests that *Panax ginseng* may have hypoglycaemic properties. Additive effects are possible, with an increased risk of hypoglycaemia.
	Caffeine	Additive stimulant effects	Caution with use of this combination	Theoretically caffeine may exacerbate the stimulant effects of *Panax ginseng*.
	Cancer therapy (chemotherapy and radiotherapy)	Possible improved quality of life and outcomes	May be beneficial — medical supervision recommended	Preliminary research suggests *Panax ginseng* may improve quality of life, psychological and social wellbeing and reduce mortality in breast cancer patients. Medical supervision is recommended.
	CYP450 substrates (CYP2D6, CYP3A4)	Theoretical increased risk of drug toxicity	Caution with use of this combination	Limited evidence suggests that *Panax ginseng* may inhibit CYP2D6 and CYP3A4. However, findings of one study with midazolam suggested that *Panax ginseng* may induce CYP3A4. Caution is advised until further data become available about the nature and extent of effect on CYP450 enzymes.
	Digoxin	Theoretical increased risk of drug toxicity	Caution with use of this combination	*Panax ginseng* may lead to an increase in serum digoxin levels according to limited data. This would theoretically increase the risk of drug adverse effects and toxicity.
	Imatinib	Theoretical increased risk of hepatotoxicity	Caution with use of this combination	A case report describes drug-induced hepatotoxicity when *Panax ginseng* was added to an established regimen of imatinib.
	Immunosuppressant drugs	Theoretical decreased drug effectiveness	Caution with use of this combination	The immunostimulant properties of *Panax ginseng* may theoretically counteract the action of immunosuppressant drugs.
	Insulin	Possible additive effects	Caution with use of this combination	Evidence suggests that *Panax ginseng* may have hypoglycaemic properties. Additive effects are possible, with an increased risk of hypoglycaemia.

TABLE I.1 Herbal interactions—cont'd

Herbal medicine	Drug/drug class	Potential outcome	Recommendations	Comments
Panax ginseng cont'd	Midazolam	Possible decreased drugs effect	Caution with use of this combination	Clinical research suggests that *Panax ginseng* may reduce drug plasma concentration, theoretically decreasing drug effect. It has been proposed that this interaction was due to CYP3A4 induction.
	Monoamine oxidase inhibitors (MAOIs)	Possible increased risk of adverse effects	Caution with use of this combination	According to some case reports concomitant use of *Panax ginseng* and phenelzine may result in symptoms of mania, insomnia, headache and tremors. Caution is advised until more data become available.
	Nifedipine	Theoretical altered drug effects	Caution with use of this combination	One study reported that *Panax ginseng* may inhibit drug metabolism, which would theoretically increase the risk of adverse effects. This interaction has not been reported in other studies.
	Oestrogens	Theoretical altered drug effects	Caution with use of this combination	*Panax ginseng* appears to have oestrogenic effects due to ginsenosides. Theoretically, large doses may compete with hormone replacement therapy for oestrogen receptors and alter drug activity. Clinical significance is unclear.
	Raltegravir	Increased risk of liver toxicity	Caution with use of this combination	A case report suggests that concomitant use of *Panax ginseng* with raltegravir resulted in elevated liver enzymes.
	Stimulant drugs	Additive stimulant effects	Caution with use of this combination	Theoretically, *Panax ginseng* may exacerbate the effects of stimulant drugs. Caution is advised.
Panax notoginseng	Oestrogenic and anti-oestrogenic drugs	Speculative effects	Monitor — speculative interaction	In-vitro studies suggest that *Panax notoginseng* may have oestrogenic effects. Theoretically this herb may interact with oestrogens and anti-oestrogenic drugs; however, this interaction is speculative.
Panax quinquefolius	Antidiabetic drugs	Possible additive effects	Caution with use of this combination	Clinical evidence suggests that American ginseng has hypoglycaemic properties. Additive effects are theoretically possible, increasing the risk of hypoglycaemia. Caution is advised until more data become available.
	Antineoplastic drugs (breast cancer)	Improved quality of life	May be beneficial — medical supervision recommended	Clinical evidence suggests that use of American ginseng may improve quality of life in patients with breast cancer while undergoing treatment.
	Immunosuppressant drugs	Theoretical decrease in drug effectiveness	Caution with use of this combination	The immunostimulant properties of American ginseng may theoretically counteract the action of immunosuppressant drugs. Caution is advised.
	Monoamine oxidase inhibitors (MAOIs)	Increased risk of adverse effects	Caution with use of this combination	One case report describes how concomitant use of phenelzine and an unspecified ginseng resulted in insomnia, headache and tremors. Another case report suggests this combination may result in hypomania. Caution is advised.

Continued

TABLE I.1 Herbal interactions—cont'd

Herbal medicine	Drug/drug class	Potential outcome	Recommendations	Comments
Panax quinquefolius cont'd	Warfarin	Decreased drug effectiveness	Avoid combination	Evidence from a randomised controlled trial (RCT) reported that America ginseng significantly reduced INR, warfarin plasma concentrations and drug effectiveness. Concomitant use should be avoided.
Passiflora incarnata	Barbiturates	Increased risk of sedation	Caution with use of this combination	Passionflower may potentiate the sedative effects of barbiturates.
	Benzodiazepines	Increased risk of sedation	Caution with use of this combination	A case report describes a suspected interaction between lorazepam and a combination of passionflower and valerian. Concomitant use led to symptoms including excessive drowsiness, dizziness, shaking and palpitations.
	CNS depressant drugs	Increased risk of sedation	Caution with use of this combination	Passionflower may potentiate the sedative effects of CNS depressant drugs.
Pelargonium sidoides	Anticoagulant/antiplatelet drugs	Additive effects theoretically possible	Monitor — may not be clinically significant	According to limited research pelargonium (Umckaloabo) may have antiplatelet properties. The combination may theoretically increase the risk of bleeding and bruising, although this has not been shown in studies.
	Immunosuppressant drugs	Theoretical decrease in drug effect	Caution with use of this combination	Pelargonium may have immunostimulant properties which could theoretically antagonise the effects of immunosuppressant drugs.
Peumus boldo	Anticoagulant/antiplatelet drugs	Theoretical increased risk of bleeding	Caution with use of this combination	Boldo may have antiplatelet properties according to limited evidence and an isolated case report. Concomitant use may theoretically increase the risk of bleeding and bruising.
	Hepatotoxic drugs	Theoretical increased risk of liver damage	Caution with use of this combination	Boldo may cause hepatotoxicity. Theoretically, the risk of liver damage is increased if boldo is used concomitantly with hepatotoxic drugs.
	Lithium	Increased risk of drug toxicity	Caution with use of this combination	Boldo may have diuretic properties. Theoretically, combined use may reduce lithium excretion and increase the risk of lithium toxicity.
	Tacrolimus	Possible decreased drug effectiveness	Avoid combination	A case report describes sub-therapeutic drug levels of tacrolimus following co-administration of boldo. Avoid this combination until further data become available.
Picrorhiza kurroa	Antidiabetic drugs	Possible additive effects	Monitor — may not be clinically significant	According to limited animal studies picrorhiza may have hypoglycaemic properties. Additive effects are theoretically possible, increasing the risk of hypoglycaemia. Caution is advised until more data become available.

TABLE I.1 Herbal interactions—cont'd

Herbal medicine	Drug/drug class	Potential outcome	Recommendations	Comments
Picrorhiza kurroa cont'd	Immunosuppressant drugs	Theoretical decreased drug effects	Caution with use of this combination	Picrorhiza appears to have immunostimulant properties. This could theoretically antagonise the effects of immunosuppressant drugs. Caution is advised until further data become available.
Pimpinella anisum	Oestrogens, e.g. oral contraceptives and HRT	Theoretical altered drug effects	Monitor — may not be clinically significant	In-vitro studies have reported both oestrogenic and anti-oestrogenic effects with anise. This appears to be due to mechanisms relating to oestrogen-receptors modulation. The significance in humans is not known, but caution is advised.
	Tamoxifen	Theoretical altered drug effects	Caution with use of this combination	In-vitro studies have reported both oestrogenic and anti-oestrogenic effects with anise. This appears to be due to mechanisms relating to oestrogen-receptors modulation. The significance in humans is not known, but caution is advised.
Pinus pinaster	Anticoagulant/antiplatelet drugs	Theoretical increased risk of bleeding	Caution with use of this combination	According to clinical research pycnogenol may have antiplatelet properties. Concomitant use may theoretically increase the risk of bleeding and bruising.
	Antidiabetic drugs	Possible additive effects	Caution with use of this combination	Pycnogenol appears to have hypoglycaemic properties according to human studies. Additive effects are theoretically possible, increasing the risk of hypoglycaemia. Caution is advised until more data become available.
	Antihypertensive drugs, e.g. ramipril	Possible protective effects on renal function in patients at risk	May be beneficial — medical supervision recommended	A small study reported that pycnogenol conferred protective effects on renal function in a group of patients taking ramipril who had advanced hypertension and a history of cardiovascular events.
	Cardiovascular drugs	Possible improved disease management	May be beneficial — medical supervision recommended	Pycnogenol appears to have antioxidant, antiplatelet and anti-inflammatory effects. A small study reported that pycnogenol was effective in improving endothelial function and reducing oxidative stress in patients with stable coronary artery disease.
	Immunosuppressant drugs	Theoretical decreased drug effects	Caution with use of this combination	Pycnogenol may have immunostimulant properties which could theoretically antagonise the effects of immunosuppressant drugs. Significance is unclear, but caution is advised until further data become available.
Piper longum	Propranolol	Theoretical increased drug bioavailability	Monitor — may not be clinically significant	Piperine, a constituent of Indian long pepper, may increase drug bioavailability based on a small preliminary study.
	Theophylline	Theoretical increased drug bioavailability	Monitor — may not be clinically significant	Piperine, a constituent of Indian long pepper, may increase drug bioavailability based on a small preliminary study.

Continued

TABLE I.1 Herbal interactions—cont'd				
Herbal medicine	**Drug/drug class**	**Potential outcome**	**Recommendations**	**Comments**
Piper methysticum	Alcohol	Increased risk of sedation and liver damage	Avoid combination	Kava may potentiate the sedative effects of alcohol. There is also concern that concomitant use may increase the risk of hepatotoxicity.
	Benzodiazepines	Increased risk of sedation; may help with drug withdrawal	Avoid combination unless under medical supervision	Kava may potentiate the sedative effects of benzodiazepines. Kava may, however, also assist in benzodiazepine withdrawal. The combination should be avoided unless under close medical supervision.
	CNS depressant drugs	Increased risk of sedation	Avoid combination	Kava may potentiate the sedative effects of CNS depressant drugs.
	CYP450 substrates (CYP1A2, CYP2C19, CYP2C9, CYP2E1)	Increased risk of drug effects and adverse effects	Caution with use of this combination	Preliminary evidence suggests kava may significantly inhibit CYP2E1. This would theoretically decrease the rate of drug metabolism, which may result in an increased risk of adverse effects. According to current research it appears unlikely that kava will affect drugs metabolised by CYP1A2, CYP2C19, CYP2C9 or CYP2E1, but caution is advised.
	Haloperidol	Theoretical increased risk of adverse effects	Caution with use of this combination	A case report describes symptoms of atrial flutter and hypoxia following co-administration of oral kava and intramuscular haloperidol and lorazepam.
	Hepatotoxic drugs	Increased risk of hepatotoxicity	Caution with use of this combination	Concomitant use of kava with hepatotoxic drugs may increase the risk of liver damage. This may include high-dose paracetamol.
	Levodopa	Symptoms of Parkinson's disease may worsen based on a case reports	Avoid combination	Several case reports describe how the combination of kava with levodopa has led to a significant increase in the number and duration of severe Parkinson's symptoms.
	Paracetamol	Increased risk of hepatoxicity at high drug dose	Caution with use of this combination	Kava may theoretically increase the risk of paracetamol-induced liver damage. This is unlikely to be a concern with normal therapeutic doses, but caution is advised.
	P-glycoprotein substrates	Theoretical increased drug effect	Caution with use of this combination	Kava may inhibit P-gp, based on limited data. Theoretically this may increase drug effects of P-gp substrates, although this has not been demonstrated in human studies.
Piscidia erythrina	CNS depressant drugs	Theoretical increased risk of sedation	Caution with use of this combination	Jamaican dogwood may theoretically potentiate sedative adverse effects when used concomitantly with CNS depressant drugs.
Plantago ovata	Anticoagulants	Possible reduced drug absorption	Caution with use of this combination	Ispaghula may reduce drug absorption and theoretically reduce drug effect. No clinically significant interactions with warfarin have been reported.
	Antidiabetic drugs	Theoretical additive effects	May be beneficial — medical supervision recommended	Ispaghula may reduce blood glucose levels in patients with type 2 diabetes and potentially have additive effects. Close monitoring is recommended.

TABLE I.1 Herbal interactions—cont'd

Herbal medicine	Drug/drug class	Potential outcome	Recommendations	Comments
Plantago ovata cont'd	Antihypertensive drugs	Theoretical additive effects	May be beneficial — medical supervision recommended	Ispaghula may reduce blood pressure. Additive beneficial effects are theoretically possible when used concomitantly with antihypertensive drugs. Monitor for hypotension.
	Carbamazepine	Reduced drug absorption possible	Caution with use of this combination	Ispaghula may reduce drug absorption and may theoretically interfere with drug effect.
	Lithium	Reduced drug absorption possible	Caution with use of this combination	Ispaghula may reduce drug absorption and theoretically reduce drug effect. An interaction between ispaghula and lithium salts has been described in one case report.
Polygonum multiflorum	Antidiabetic drugs	Theoretical additive effects	Caution with use of this combination	This herb may have hypoglycaemic properties. Additive effects are theoretically possible when used with antidiabetic drugs. Significance is unclear based on current evidence, but caution is advised due to a risk of hypoglycaemia.
	CYP450 substrates (CYP1A2, CYP2C19, CYP2C9, CYP3A4)	Theoretical risk of increased drug levels	Caution with use of this combination	In-vitro evidence suggests this herb may inhibit activity of CYP1A2, CYP2C19, CYP2C9 and CYP3A4. There is a theoretical risk of increased drug levels and adverse effects with drugs metabolised by these enzymes. Clinical significance in humans is unknown based on current evidence.
	Digoxin	Theoretical increased risk of drug toxicity	Caution with use of this combination	Overuse of anthraquinone laxative herbs may theoretically increase the risk of hypokalaemia, which increases the risk of digoxin cardiotoxicity.
	Diuretics	Theoretical increased risk of hypokalaemia	Caution with use of this combination	This herb may result in potassium loss. Theoretically, there is an increased risk of hypokalaemia when used in combination with potassium-depleting diuretic drugs such as loop and thiazide diuretics.
	Hepatotoxic drugs	Increased risk of liver damage	Caution with use of this combination	Case reports suggest this herb may be hepatotoxic. There is a theoretical increased risk of liver damage when used concomitantly with hepatotoxic drugs.
	Oestrogens	Theoretical altered drug effect	Monitor — may not be clinically significant	This herb may have oestrogenic activity based on in-vitro studies. Theoretically high-dose use may interfere with HRT and oral contraceptive drugs due to competitive binding at oestrogen receptors.
	Stimulant laxatives	Theoretical additive effects	Caution with use of this combination	This herb has stimulant laxative properties. Theoretically, concomitant use with stimulant laxative drugs will increase the risk of fluid and electrolyte depletion.

Continued

TABLE I.1 Herbal interactions—cont'd				
Herbal medicine	**Drug/drug class**	**Potential outcome**	**Recommendations**	**Comments**
Polygonum multiflorum cont'd	Warfarin		Caution with use of this combination	A case report describes acute hepatitis and an elevated INR when a patient, previously stabilised on warfarin, commenced intake of this herb. It has been proposed that this may have been due to diarrhoea caused by the herb's laxative effect.
Punica grantum	ACE-inhibitors (ACE-I)	Theoretical additive effects	Caution with use of this combination	Pomegranate may have an action similar to ACE-inhibitors, leading to additive effects and an increased risk of hypotension. Monitor for hypotension and for signs of potassium depletion.
	Antihypertensive drugs	Theoretical additive effects	Caution with use of this combination	Pomegranate may modestly lower blood pressure. Additive effects are theoretically possible, with an increased risk of hypotension.
	Carbamazepine	Theoretical increased drug levels	Caution with use of this combination	Animal models suggest pomegranate juice may decrease the rate of carbamazepine metabolism and increase the serum levels.
	CYP450 substrates (CYP2C9, CYP2D6)	Theoretical increased drug levels	Caution with use of this combination	Animal models suggest pomegranate may inhibit activity of CYP2C9 and CYP2D6, which may theoretically lead to increased drug levels and adverse effects. Clinical significance in humans is currently unknown.
	CYP450 substrates (CYP3A4)	Theoretical altered drug levels	Caution with use of this combination	Evidence about the effect of pomegranate on CYP3A4 is contradictory. Some research has reported enzyme inhibition, while other studies have reported enzyme induction, and some have reported no effect. Caution is advised at high doses until more data become available.
	Rosuvastatin	Theoretical increased drug adverse effects	Caution with use of this combination	A case report describes a patient on rosuvastatin who developed rhabdomyolysis 3 weeks after commencing pomegranate juice, 200 mL taken twice weekly. It is possible the patient was predisposed to this adverse effect as there was a history of elevated levels of creatine kinase.
	Tacrolimus	Theoretical increased drug levels	Avoid combination	A case report describes elevated drug levels while consuming concentrated pomegranate popsicles. More data are required to determine significance.
	Warfarin	Theoretical increased risk of bleeding	Caution with use of this combination	Based on two case reports high intake of pomegranate juice may increase bleeding time in patients taking warfarin. Warfarin is a CYP2C9 substrate and animal models have reported that pomegranate juice may inhibit this metabolising enzyme, potentially leading to increased drug levels.

TABLE I.1 Herbal interactions—cont'd

Herbal medicine	Drug/drug class	Potential outcome	Recommendations	Comments
Rehmannia glutinosa	Antidiabetic drugs	Theoretical additive effects	Caution with use of this combination	Rehmannia may have hypoglycaemic properties. Additive effects are theoretically possible, increasing the risk of hypoglycaemia. Caution is advised until more data become available.
	Irbesartan	Improved disease management in chronic renal disease	May be beneficial — medical supervision recommended	The results of one study of 480 patients with chronic renal disease suggest that the combination of rehmannia with irbesartan is more effective in reducing proteinuria than irbesartan alone.
Rhamnus purshiana	Corticosteroids	Theoretical increased risk of potassium loss	Caution with use of this combination	Overuse of cascara may compound drug-induced potassium loss. The interaction is speculative, but caution is advised.
	Digoxin	Theoretical risk of increased drug adverse effects	Caution with use of this combination	Overuse of cascara may compound drug-induced potassium loss, which may theoretically increase the risk of drug toxicity. The interaction is speculative, but caution is advised.
	Diuretics	Increased risk of potassium loss	Caution with use of this combination	Overuse of cascara in combination with potassium-depleting diuretics, such as thiazide and loop diuretics, may increase the risk of hypokalaemia.
	Stimulant laxatives	Increased risk of diarrhoea and electrolyte loss	Caution with use of this combination	Additive stimulant laxative effects may occur with concomitant use of this drug class and cascara. This may result in diarrhoea and loss of electrolytes.
Rheum palmatum	Corticosteroids	Increased risk of potassium loss	Caution with use of this combination	Overuse of rhubarb may compound drug-induced potassium loss. The interaction is speculative, but caution is advised.
	Digoxin	Increased risk of drug toxicity	Caution with use of this combination	Overuse of rhubarb may compound drug-induced potassium loss, which theoretically increases the risk of drug toxicity. The interaction is speculative, but caution is advised.
	Diuretics	Increased risk of potassium loss	Caution with use of this combination	Overuse of rhubarb in combination with potassium-depleting diuretics, such as thiazide and loop diuretics, may increase the risk of hypokalaemia. The interaction is speculative, but caution is advised.
	Nephrotoxic drugs	Increased risk of renal failure	Caution with use of this combination	A case report described renal failure linked to a rhubarb-containing supplement, possibly due to the anthraquinone constituent. The patient was also taking diclofenac (NSAID). It is unclear how much effect was due to rhubarb alone.
	Stimulant laxatives	Increased risk of diarrhoea and loss of electrolytes	Caution with use of this combination	Additive stimulant laxative effects may occur with concomitant use of this drug class and rhubarb. This may result in diarrhoea and loss of electrolytes.

Continued

TABLE I.1 Herbal interactions—cont'd

Herbal medicine	Drug/drug class	Potential outcome	Recommendations	Comments
Rhodiola rosea	Adriamycin	Theoretical decreased drug adverse effects	Combination may be beneficial	Preliminary evidence suggests rhodiola may reduce severity of drug-induced liver dysfunction. More data are needed to determine significance and likelihood of benefit.
	Antidepressant drugs, e.g. paroxetine, escitalopram	Theoretical increased risk of adverse effects	Caution with use of this combination	A case report describes an interaction which appears to have been due to the addition of rhodiola to paroxetine in a patient with depression. The patient experienced restlessness, trembling and a disordered state of consciousness. Another case report describes significant tachycardia occurring in a patient who took rhodiola in combination with escitalopram. Caution is advised.
	Antidiabetic drugs	Theoretical additive effects	Caution with use of this combination	Animal and in-vitro studies suggest rhodiola may have hypoglycaemic properties due to alpha-glucosidase activity. Additive effects are theoretically possible, increasing the risk of hypoglycaemia. Caution is advised until more data become available.
	Antihypertensive drugs especially ACE-inhibitors	Possible additive effects	Monitor — may not be clinically significant	Animal and in-vitro studies suggest rhodiola may lower blood pressure due to inhibition of angiotensin-converting enzyme (ACE). Additive effects are theoretically possible, with an increased risk of hypotension.
	CYP3A4 substrates	Theoretical increased risk of adverse effects	Monitor — may not be clinically significant	In-vitro research suggests that rhodiola may inhibit CYP3A4. Theoretically this may increase drug levels and the risk of adverse effects, although significance in humans has not been established.
	Immunosuppressant drugs	Theoretical decreased drug effects	Caution with use of this combination	Rhodiola may have immunostimulant properties which could theoretically antagonise the effects of immunosuppressant drugs. Significance is unclear, but caution is advised until further data become available.
	Monoamine oxidase inhibitors (MAOIs)	Theoretical altered drug effects	Caution with use of this combination	In-vitro studies suggest that rhodiola may inhibit MAO-A receptors. There is a theoretical interaction with MAOI antidepressants, although effect and significance are unknown.
	P-glyocoprotein (P-gp) substrates	Theoretical increased drug effects	Caution with use of this combination	Limited data suggest that rhodiola may inhibit P-gp. This may theoretically increase drug effects, although this has not been demonstrated in human studies.
Ricinus communis	Diuretics	Increased risk of hypokalaemia	Caution with use of this combination	Overuse of castor oil may exacerbate potassium loss due to diuretics
Rosmarinus officinalis	Anticoagulant/ antiplatelet drugs	Theoretical increased risk of bleeding	Caution with use of this combination	In-vitro and animal research suggests that rosemary may have antithrombotic and antiplatelet effects. Concomitant use with anticoagulant and antiplatelet drugs will theoretically increase the risk of bleeding and bruising.

TABLE I.1 Herbal interactions—cont'd				
Herbal medicine	**Drug/drug class**	**Potential outcome**	**Recommendations**	**Comments**
Rosmarinus officinalis cont'd	Iron supplements	Reduced iron absorption	Caution with use of this combination	Rosemary has been shown to reduce absorption of dietary iron and may theoretically decrease absorption of iron supplements. Dosage separation is recommended.
	P-glyocoprotein (P-gp) substrates	Theoretical increased drug effect	Caution with use of this combination	Limited data suggest that rhodiola may inhibit P-gp. This may theoretically increase drug effects, although this has not been demonstrated in human studies.
Rumex acetosa	Mineral supplements (calcium, iron and zinc)	Possible reduced mineral absorption	Monitor — may not be clinically significant	Sorrel contains oxalates which may theoretically bind to minerals and reduce absorption. Clinical significance is unclear, but dosage separation is advised.
Rumex crispus	Digoxin	Theoretical increased risk of drug toxicity	Avoid this combination	Long-term use of yellow dock may result in potassium loss, which increases the risk of drug toxicity.
	Diuretics	Theoretical increased risk of potassium loss	Caution with use of this combination	Overuse of yellow dock in combination with potassium-depleting diuretics, such as thiazide and loop diuretics, will increase the risk of hypokalaemia.
Salix alba	Anticoagulant/antiplatelet drugs	Theoretical increased risk of bleeding	Avoid this combination	Willow bark has been shown to have antithrombotic and antiplatelet activity. Concomitant use with anticoagulant and antiplatelet drugs will theoretically increase the risk of bleeding and bruising. Caution is also recommended with use of willow bark in combination with other salicylate-containing herbs, or herbs with anticoagulant properties.
	NSAIDs and opioid analgesics	Theoretical additive effects	Combination may be beneficial — monitor	Willow bark extract has been shown to provide additive pain-relieving effects when used in combination with NSAIDs or opioid drugs for rheumatic pain. There was no direct evidence of an interaction in this study, but patients should be monitored.
Salvia miltiorrhiza	Anticoagulant/antiplatelet drugs	Possible increased risk of bleeding	Avoid this combination	Dan shen appears to have anticoagulant effects. A series of case reports suggest that dan shen may affect the pharmacokinetics of warfarin, leading to an increased INR and risk of bleeding. Avoid use with warfarin.
	Antihypertensive drugs	Possible additive effects	Caution with use of this combination	Dan shen may lower blood pressure therefore there is a theoretical increased risk of hypotension when used with antihypertensive drugs. An in-vitro study reported that dan shen may potentiate effects of captopril.
	CYP450 substrates (CYP3A4)	Theoretical decreased drug effects	Caution with use of this combination	Preliminary evidence suggests dan shen may induce CYP3A4 enzyme activity. This could theoretically lead to an increased rate of metabolism and decreased drug effect in drugs that are CYP3A4 substrates.

Continued

TABLE I.1 Herbal interactions—cont'd				
Herbal medicine	**Drug/drug class**	**Potential outcome**	**Recommendations**	**Comments**
Salvia miltiorrhiza cont'd	Digoxin	Theoretical increased risk of drug toxicity	Avoid this combination	Dan shen has structural and pharmacological similarities to cardiac glycosides. Concomitant use could theoretically have additive effect and increase the risk of arrhythmias and drug toxicity.
	Midazolam	Theoretical decreased drug effect	Caution with use of this combination	A small study reported that dan shen significantly increased the rate of drug clearance, leading to decreased drug effect.
Salvia officinalis	Acetylcholinesterase inhibitors	Theoretical increase in drug effects and adverse effects	Caution with use of this combination	In-vitro research suggests sage may inhibit acetylcholinesterase. Additive effects are theoretically possible with concomitant use of sage and acetylcholinesterase (AChE) inhibitors, such as donepezil, used for Alzheimer's disease. The interaction may potentially be beneficial, but there is an increased risk of cholinergic adverse effects.
	Anticholinergic drugs	Theoretical decreased drug effect	Monitor — may not be clinically significant	In-vitro research suggests sage may increase acetylcholine levels. This may theoretically oppose the action of drugs with an anticholinergic action. Significance has not been established.
	Antidiabetic drugs	Theoretical additive effects	Caution with use of this combination	Preliminary research suggests that sage may have hypoglycaemic properties. Additive effects are theoretically possible, increasing the risk of hypoglycaemia. Caution is advised until more data become available.
	Cholinergic drugs	Theoretical additive drug effect	Monitor — may not be clinically significant	In-vitro research suggests sage may increase acetylcholine levels. Theoretically there may be additive effects when used in combination with drugs with cholinergic actions. Significance is unclear.
	CNS depressant drugs	Theoretical increased sedative effects	Monitor — may not be clinically significant	Some constituents of sage may have sedative effects. There is a theoretical risk of additive effects and adverse effects.
	CYP450 substrates (CYP2C19, CYP2C9, CYP2D6, CYP3A4)	Theoretical increased risk of adverse effects	Monitor — may not be clinically significant	Preliminary evidence suggests that sage may inhibit activity of CYP2C19, CYP2C9, CYP2D6 and CYP3A4 enzymes. This may theoretically increase drug concentrations and the risk of adverse effects. These interactions have not been demonstrated in human studies.
Sambucus nigra	Antidiabetic drugs	Theoretical additive effects	Caution with use of this combination	Elderflower may have hypoglycaemic properties according to in-vitro studies. Additive effects are theoretically possible, increasing the risk of hypoglycaemia. Caution is advised until more data become available.
	Immunosuppressant drugs	Theoretical decreased drug effect	Caution with use of this combination	Elderberry may have immunostimulant properties which could theoretically antagonise the effects of immunosuppressant drugs. Caution is advised.

TABLE I.1 Herbal interactions—cont'd

Herbal medicine	Drug/drug class	Potential outcome	Recommendations	Comments
Sceletium tortuosum	CNS depressant drugs	Theoretical increased risk of sedation	Monitor — may not be clinically significant	Sceletium may have sedative effects, based on in-vitro studies. Theoretically this may potentiate the sedative effects of CNS depressant drugs.
Schisandra chinensis	Benzodiazepines, e.g. midazolam	Risk of increased drug levels and adverse effects	Caution with use of this combination	A small study reported an interaction between schisandra and midazolam, leading to an increased drug concentration and theoretical increased risk of adverse effects. It is unclear if this is a drug class affect, but caution is advised with all benzodiazepines.
	CYP2C9 substrates	Theoretical decreased drug effects	Monitor — may not be clinically significant	Animal models suggest that schisandra may induce activity of CYP2C9. This may theoretically lead to reduced drug effect of drugs metabolised by this enzyme pathway.
	CYP3A4 substrates	Theoretical altered drug effects	Monitor — may not be clinically significant	Schisandra has been shown to inhibit CYP3A4 enzyme activity in some animal studies, with other animal studies reporting that this herb induced CYP3A4 activity. Caution is advised until more data become available.
	Phenobarbital (phenobarbitone)	Increased risk of sedation	Caution with use of this combination	Schisandra may potentiate the sedative effects of phenobarbital (phenobarbitone) based on animal studies.
	Sirolimus and tacrolimus	Risk of increased drug levels and adverse effects	Avoid this combination	Schisandra has been shown to significantly increase concentration of both sirolimus and tacrolimus (immunosuppressants) in separate small studies conducted in healthy volunteers. Avoid this combination until further safety data become available.
	Warfarin	Theoretical decreased drug effects	Caution with use of this combination	Animal models suggest that schisandra may decrease warfarin levels, theoretically leading to decreased drug effect.
Scutellaria baicalensis	Alcohol	Increased risk of sedation	Caution with use of this combination	Baikal skullcap may theoretically potentiate the sedative effects of alcohol. Clinical significance is unclear, but caution is advised.
	Anticoagulant/ antiplatelet drugs	Theoretical increased risk of bleeding	Caution with use of this combination	Baikal skullcap may have antiplatelet activity. Concomitant use with anticoagulant and antiplatelet drugs will theoretically increase the risk of bleeding and bruising.
	Antidiabetic drugs	Theoretical additive effects	Caution with use of this combination	Animal research suggests that baikal skullcap may enhance the antidiabetic effect of metformin. Additive effects are theoretically possible, increasing the risk of hypoglycaemia. Caution is advised until more data become available.
	Antihypertensive drugs	Theoretical additive effects	Monitor — may not be clinically significant	Baikal skullcap may lower blood pressure. Additive effects are theoretically possible, with an increased risk of hypotension.

Continued

TABLE I.1 Herbal interactions—cont'd

Herbal medicine	Drug/drug class	Potential outcome	Recommendations	Comments
Scutellaria baicalensis cont'd	Benzodiazepines	Theoretical additive effects	Caution with use of this combination	Baikal skullcap may potentiate the therapeutic and sedative effects of benzodiazepines.
	Ciclosporin	Theoretical decreased drug effects	Avoid this combination	An animal study reported a significant decrease in drug plasma levels with use of this combination. Avoid until further data become available.
	CNS depressant drugs	Theoretical additive effects	Caution with use of this combination	Baikal skullcap may potentiate the therapeutic and sedative effects of CNS depressant drugs.
	CYP450 substrates (CYP1A2, CYP2C19)	Theoretical increased risk of adverse effects	Monitor — may not be clinically significant	In-vitro evidence suggests that baikal skullcap may inhibit CYP1A2 and CYP2C19 enzyme activity. Theoretically this may increase drug concentrations and risk of adverse effects.
	Oestrogens	Theoretical altered drug effects	Monitor — may not be clinically significant	In-vitro evidence suggests that baikal skullcap may have oestrogenic activity. Concomitant use of high doses may theoretically interfere with the action of oral contraceptives and HRT.
	Lithium	Theoretical increased risk of drug toxicity	Caution with use of this combination	Baikal skullcap may have diuretic properties. Theoretically, combined use may reduce lithium excretion and increase the risk of lithium toxicity.
	Rosuvastatin	Possible reduced drug effects	Avoid this combination	Baicalin, a constituent of baikal skullcap, was reported to reduce the serum concentration of rosuvastatin in one small study. It has been proposed that this may relate only to specific genotypes, but caution is advised until more data become available.
Scutellaria lateriflora	CNS depressant drugs	Theoretical additive effects	Caution with use of this combination	Skullcap may potentiate the therapeutic and sedative effects of CNS depressant drugs.
Serenoa repens	Androgenic drugs, e.g. testosterone	Theoretical decreased drug effects	Monitor — clinical significance is unclear	Saw palmetto may reduce the effectiveness of androgenic drugs such as testosterone. Monitor for signs of decreased drug effect.
	Anticoagulant/antiplatelet drugs	Theoretical increased risk of bleeding	Caution with use of this combination	Saw palmetto may have antiplatelet activity. Concomitant use with anticoagulant and antiplatelet drugs will theoretically increase the risk of bleeding and bruising.
	Finasteride and other drugs used for BPH	Possible additive effects	Combination may be beneficial	Additive effects are theoretically possible, which may improve disease management. There does not appear to be any evidence of negative interactions, but patients should be monitored.
	Oestrogen (HRT and oral contraceptives)	Theoretical altered drug effects	Caution with use of this combination	Saw palmetto may have anti-oestrogenic effects. Concomitant use with oestrogenic drugs such as HRT and oral contraceptives may theoretically interfere with drug action.

TABLE I.1 Herbal interactions—cont'd

Herbal medicine	Drug/drug class	Potential outcome	Recommendations	Comments
Silybum marianum	Antidiabetic drugs	Possible additive effects	May be beneficial — medical supervision recommended	Clinical research suggests that St Mary's thistle may lower blood glucose levels, HBA_{1c} and insulin resistance in type 2 diabetics. Additive, potentially beneficial effects are possible, but caution is advised due to an increased risk of hypoglycaemia.
	CYP450 substrates (CYP2C9, CYP2D6)	Theoretical increased drug concentrations and risk of adverse effects	Monitor — may not be clinically significant	Preliminary evidence suggests that St Mary's thistle may inhibit CYP2C9 and CYP2D6 enzymes, theoretically increasing drug concentrations and risk of adverse effects.
	CYP450 substrates (CYP2C9, CYP2D6, CYP3A4)	Theoretical altered drug effects	Monitor — may not be clinically significant	There is contradictory evidence as to whether St Mary's thistle has an effect on CYP3A4 and, if so, whether it inhibits or induces enzyme activity. Patients should be monitored.
	Doxorubicin and cisplatin	May increase drug effect	Combination may be beneficial — medical supervision recommended	Limited evidence suggests St Mary's thistle may increase tumour sensitivity to the chemotherapeutic action of these drugs, while also reducing drug toxicity. Clinical significance is unclear and medical supervision is recommended.
	Hepatotoxic substances	Theoretical protect effects	Combination may be beneficial — medical supervision recommended	St Mary's thistle is reported to have hepatoprotective effects and may be beneficial in combination with hepatotoxic drugs.
	Metronidazole	Risk of decreased drug concentrations	Monitor — may not be clinically significant	A constituent of St Mary's thistle, silymarin, was reported to reduce drug concentrations in a small study. The interaction may not be clinically significant, but patients should be monitored.
	Risperidone	Theoretical increased drug bioavailability	Caution with use of this combination	A pharmacokinetic study in rats reported that regular use of St Mary's thistle increased drug bioavailability, possibly due to inhibition of P-gp. Clinical significance has not been established.
	Sirolimus	Theoretical increase in drug concentration	Caution with use of this combination	Pharmacokinetic research suggests the constituent silymarin may decrease the clearance of sirolimus in hepatically impaired renal transplant patients. Caution is advised.
	Tamoxifen	Theoretical increase in drug concentration	Caution with use of this combination	Preliminary animal research suggests the constituent silibinin may increase drug plasma concentration. Clinical significance in humans is unknown, but caution is advised.
Smilax ornata	Digoxin	Theoretical increased drug effect and adverse effect	Caution with use of this combination	Sarsaparilla may theoretically increase drug absorption, which could theoretically lead to increased drug levels and risk of toxicity.
	Lithium	Theoretical increased risk of drug toxicity	Caution with use of this combination	Sarsaparilla may have diuretic properties. Theoretically concomitant use may reduce lithium excretion and increase the risk of lithium toxicity.

Continued

TABLE I.1 Herbal interactions—cont'd

Herbal medicine	Drug/drug class	Potential outcome	Recommendations	Comments
Solidago spp.	Diuretics	Theoretical additive effects	Monitor — may not be clinically significant	Goldenrod may have diuretic properties. Additive effects are theoretically possible. Monitor for hypotension and loss of fluid and electrolytes.
Syzygium aromaticum	Anticoagulant/ antiplatelet drugs	Theoretical increased risk of bleeding	Monitor — may not be clinically significant	In-vitro studies have reported that a constituent of clove, eugenol, appears to have antiplatelet activity. No interactions have been reported in humans, but patients should be monitored.
Tabebuia avellanedae	Anticoagulant/ antiplatelet drugs	Theoretical increased risk of bleeding	Caution with use of this combination	Limited evidence suggests that pau d'arco may have anticoagulant properties at high doses. Concomitant use with anticoagulant and antiplatelet drugs will theoretically increase the risk of bleeding and bruising.
Tanacetum parthenium	Anticoagulant/ antiplatelet drugs	Theoretical increased risk of bleeding	Caution with use of this combination	In-vitro studies suggest that feverfew may inhibit platelet aggregation. Concomitant use with anticoagulant and antiplatelet drugs will theoretically increase the risk of bleeding and bruising. This interaction has not been demonstrated in human studies.
	CYP450 substrates (CYP1A2, CYP2C19, CYP2C8, CYP2C9, CYP2D6, CYP3A4)	Theoretical increased risk of drug toxicity	Monitor — may not be clinically significant	Preliminary evidence suggests feverfew may inhibit several CYP450 enzymes (CYP1A2, CYP2C19, CYP2C8, CYP2C9, CYP2D6, CYP3A4). Theoretically this may reduce the rate of drug metabolism and increase the risk of toxicity. Interactions have not been demonstrated in human studies.
Taraxacum officinale	Anticoagulant/ antiplatelet drugs	Theoretical increased risk of bleeding	Caution with use of this combination	Dandelion root may inhibit platelet aggregation. Concomitant use with anticoagulant and antiplatelet drugs will theoretically increase the risk of bleeding and bruising. Significance is unclear, but caution is advised.
	Antidiabetic drugs	Theoretical additive effects	Caution with use of this combination	Dandelion extract may have hypoglycaemic properties. Additive effects are theoretically possible, increasing the risk of hypoglycaemia. Caution is advised until more data become available.
	CYP450 substrates (CYP1A2)	Theoretical increased risk of drug toxicity	Monitor — may not be clinically significant	Preliminary evidence suggests dandelion may inhibit CYP1A2. This interaction has not been demonstrated in human studies.
	Lithium	Theoretical increased risk of drug toxicity	Caution with use of this combination	Dandelion may have diuretic properties. Theoretically, concomitant use may reduce lithium excretion and increase the risk of lithium toxicity.
	Potassium-sparing diuretics, e.g. spironolactone	Increased risk of hyperkalaemia; possible additive diuretic actions	Monitor — may not be clinically significant	Dandelion leaf contains significant amounts of potassium. Theoretically, concomitant use of dandelion and potassium-sparing diuretics will have additive effects and an increased risk of hyperkalaemia. Additive diuretic actions are also possible with use of dandelion leaf in combination with diuretic drugs.

TABLE I.1 Herbal interactions—cont'd

Herbal medicine	Drug/drug class	Potential outcome	Recommendations	Comments
Taraxacum officinale cont'd	Quinolone antibiotics	Theoretical decreased drug bioavailability	Monitor and separate doses	The high mineral content of dandelion may theoretically form insoluble complexes with drugs in this class and reduce absorption and bioavailability. Doses should be separated.
Terminalia arjuna	Antidiabetic drugs	Theoretical additive effects	Caution with use of this combination	Animal research suggests that this herb may have hypoglycaemic properties. Theoretically, concomitant use with antidiabetic drugs may result in additive effects and a risk of hypoglycaemia.
Thuja occidentalis	Anticonvulsant drugs	Increased risk of seizures	Caution with use of this combination	Thuja may lower seizure threshold due to the constituent thujone, which has neurotoxic properties. This may theoretically increase the risk of seizures and reduce drug effectiveness.
	Immunosuppressant drugs	Theoretical decrease in drug effect	Caution with use of this combination	Thuja may have immunostimulant properties which could theoretically antagonise the effects of immunosuppressant drugs.
Thymus vulgaris	Anticoagulant/ antiplatelet drugs	Theoretical increased risk of bleeding	Caution with use of this combination	Thyme may have antiplatelet properties. Concomitant use with anticoagulant and antiplatelet drugs will theoretically increase the risk of bleeding and bruising.
Tilia spp.	Lithium	Theoretical increased risk of drug toxicity	Caution with use of this combination	Linden may have diuretic properties. Theoretically, concomitant use may reduce lithium excretion and increase the risk of lithium toxicity.
Tinospora cordifolia	Antidiabetic drugs	Theoretical additive effects	Caution with use of this combination	This herb may have hypoglycaemic properties, leading to theoretical additive effects. Clinical significance is unclear.
	Immunosuppressant drugs	Theoretical decrease in drug effect	Caution with use of this combination	This herb may have immunostimulant properties which could theoretically antagonise the effects of immunosuppressant drugs.
Tribulus terrestris	Antidiabetic drugs	Theoretical additive effects	Caution with use of this combination	Tribulus may have hypoglycaemic properties. Additive effects are theoretically possible, increasing the risk of hypoglycaemia. Caution is advised until more data become available.
	Antihypertensive drugs, e.g. ACE-inhibitors	Theoretical additive effects	Monitor — may not be clinically significant	Animal studies suggest that tribulus may lower blood pressure due to inhibition of angiotensin-converting enzyme (ACE). Additive effects are theoretically possible, with an increased risk of hypotension.
	Androgenic drugs	Theoretical additive effects	Caution with use of this combination	Theoretically the combination may have additive effects. There does not appear to be evidence of a negative interaction, but caution is advised.
	Erectile dysfunction drugs	Theoretical additive effects	Caution with use of this combination	Theoretically, concomitant use may have additive beneficial effects. There does not appear to be evidence of a negative interaction, but caution is advised.

Continued

TABLE I.1 Herbal interactions—cont'd

Herbal medicine	Drug/drug class	Potential outcome	Recommendations	Comments
Tribulus terrestris cont'd	Lithium	Theoretical increased risk of drug toxicity	Caution with use of this combination	Tribulus may have diuretic properties. Theoretically, concomitant use may reduce lithium excretion and increase the risk of lithium toxicity.
	Testosterone	Theoretical additive effects	Caution with use of this combination	Concomitant use may have additive effects. There does not appear to be evidence of a negative interaction, but caution is advised.
Trifolium pratense	Anticoagulant/antiplatelet drugs	Theoretical increased risk of bleeding	Caution with use of this combination	Red clover may inhibit platelet aggregation. Concomitant use with anticoagulant and antiplatelet drugs will theoretically increase the risk of bleeding and bruising. No effects on coagulation or prothrombin time were seen in a 12-month study using red clover 378 mg daily. Clinical significance is thus unclear, but caution is advised.
	Contraceptive drugs	Possible altered drug effect	Caution with use of this combination	Theoretically high-dose red clover may compete with contraceptive drugs for oestrogen receptor binding sites. Significance is unclear.
	CYP450 substrates (CYP1A2, CYP2C19, CYP2C9, CYP3A4)	Theoretical risk of increased drug adverse effects	Monitor — may not be clinically significant	Preliminary evidence suggests red clover may inhibit the activity of CYP1A2, CYP2C19, CYP2C9 and CYP3A4 enzymes. This may theoretically increase drug levels and risk of adverse effects when used concomitantly with drugs that are substrates for these enzymes. So far, interactions have not been reported in humans.
	Hormone replacement therapy (HRT)	Possible altered drug effects	Caution with use of this combination	Theoretically high-dose red clover may compete with HRT for oestrogen receptor binding sites. Significance is unclear.
	Lipid-lowering drugs	Possible additive effects	Combination may be beneficial — monitor	Red clover may have favourable effects on serum lipids, especially in postmenopausal women. It does not appear to have negative interactions with lipid-lowering drugs based on current evidence.
	Methotrexate	Theoretical increased risk of drug toxicity	Caution with use of this combination	A case study describes adverse effects consistent with drug toxicity including severe vomiting and epigastric pain when red clover was added to an existing regimen of methotrexate in a woman with psoriasis.
	Tamoxifen	Theoretical antagonistic action	Caution with use of this combination	It has been proposed that red clover may antagonise drug effects due to the herb's oestrogenic actions. Caution is advised until more data become available.
Trigonella-foenum graecum	Anticoagulant/antiplatelet drugs	Theoretical increased risk of bleeding	Caution with use of this combination	Fenugreek may inhibit platelet aggregation. Concomitant use with anticoagulant and antiplatelet drugs will theoretically increase the risk of bleeding and bruising.

TABLE I.1 Herbal interactions—cont'd

Herbal medicine	Drug/drug class	Potential outcome	Recommendations	Comments
Trigonella-foenum graecum cont'd	Antidiabetic drugs	Possible additive effects	Caution with use of this combination	Fenugreek has been shown to reduce blood glucose concentrations in patients with type 2 diabetes. Additive, beneficial effects are possible. Caution is advised as there is a risk of hypoglycaemia.
	Theophylline	Theoretical decreased drug effects	Monitor — may not be clinically significant	Limited animal research suggests fenugreek may reduce drug effects. Clinical significance is unknown, but patients should be monitored.
Turnera diffusa	Antidiabetic drugs	Theoretical additive effects	Caution with use of this combination	Animal research suggests that damiana may have hypoglycaemic properties. Additive effects are theoretically possible, increasing the risk of hypoglycaemia. Caution is advised until more data become available.
Ulmus rubra	Oral drugs	Possible decreased drug absorption	Monitor and separate dose — may not be clinically significant	The mucilage content of slippery elm may theoretically slow the absorption and reduce serum levels of some oral drugs. Clinical significance is unclear, but separation of dose administration is recommended. Caution is advised in particular with drugs with a narrow therapeutic index.
Uncaria tomentosa	Anticoagulants/ antiplatelet drugs	Theoretical increased risk of bleeding	Caution with use of this combination	Constituents in cat's claw may inhibit platelet aggregation. The combination will theoretically increase the risk of bleeding, although clinical significance is unclear.
	Antihypertensive drugs	Additive effects theoretically possible	Monitor — may not be clinically significant	Cat's claw may lower blood pressure. Additive effects are theoretically possible if used concomitantly with antihypertensive drugs. Monitor for hypotension.
	CYP3A4 substrates	Theoretical increased risk of drug adverse effects	Monitor — may not be clinically significant	Preliminary evidence suggests cat's claw may inhibit the activity of CYP3A4. This may theoretically increase drug levels and risk of adverse effects when used concomitantly with drugs that are CYP3A4 substrates.
	Immunosuppressant drugs	Theoretical decrease in drug effect	Caution with use of this combination	Cat's claw may have immunostimulant properties which could theoretically antagonise the effects of immunosuppressant drugs.
	Protease inhibitors, e.g. atazanavir, ritonavir, saquinavir	Theoretical increased risk of drug adverse effects	Caution with use of this combination	A case study describes a possible interaction between atazanavir and cat's claw leading to increased drug levels and risk of toxicity.
Urtica dioica	Antidiabetic drugs	Theoretical additive effects	Monitor — a clinically significant interaction appears unlikely	According to animal studies and limited clinical research stinging nettle may have hypoglycaemic properties. Additive effects are theoretically possible, increasing the risk of hypoglycaemia.

Continued

TABLE I.1 Herbal interactions—cont'd

Herbal medicine	Drug/drug class	Potential outcome	Recommendations	Comments
Urtica dioica cont'd	Antihypertensive drugs	Theoretically additive effects	Monitor — a clinically significant interaction appears unlikely	Stinging nettle may lower blood pressure according to animal studies. Additive effects are theoretically possible if used concomitantly with antihypertensive drugs. Monitor for hypotension.
	Lithium	Theoretical increased risk of drug toxicity	Caution with use of this combination	Stinging nettle may have diuretic properties. Theoretically, concomitant use may reduce lithium excretion and increase the risk of lithium toxicity.
	Warfarin	Theoretical decreased drug effect	Caution with use of this combination	Stinging nettle contains significant amounts of vitamin K. Concomitant use of stinging nettle with warfarin may antagonise drug effects.
Vaccinium macrocarpon	Atorvastatin	Theoretical increased risk of drug adverse effects	Caution with use of this combination	A case report describes upper back pain, rhabdomyolysis and abnormal liver function after high intake of cranberry juice in a patient taking atorvastatin. It has been proposed that this was due to inhibition of CYP3A4 activity, leading to increased drug concentration.
	CYP450 substrates (CYP2CP, CYP3A4)	Theoretical increased risk of drug adverse effects	Caution with use of this combination	Cranberry may inhibit activity of CYP2C9 and CYP3A4, although data have been conflicting. Current evidence suggests the effect on CYP2C9 may not be clinically relevant, but that some cranberry products may affect CYP3A4 activity. Variations in effect may relate to differences in the concentration of triterpenes in various cranberry products. Patients should be monitored and cranberry should be used with caution with drugs with a narrow therapeutic index.
	Non-steroidal anti-inflammatory drugs (NSAIDs)	Theoretical increased drug effect	Monitor — may not be clinically significant	In-vitro evidence suggests cranberry may inhibit metabolism of some NSAIDs due to an effect on CYP2C9. This has not been shown in human studies. Clinical research reported no significant changes to drug plasma levels when cranberry was used in combination with diclofenac, nor when used in combination with flurbiprofen.
	Warfarin	Possible increased INR, but data are conflicting	Caution with use of this combination	Evidence is conflicting. A small number of case reports have suggested that cranberry may interact with warfarin leading to increased INR. A possible interaction was also reported in two small studies. However, no clinically relevant interactions have been found between cranberry and warfarin in clinical pharmacokinetic studies. Other studies investigating this interaction have also failed to report changes to warfarin plasma levels or INR.

TABLE I.1 Herbal interactions—cont'd

Herbal medicine	Drug/drug class	Potential outcome	Recommendations	Comments
Vaccinium myrtillus	Anticoagulants/ antiplatelet drugs	Theoretical increased risk of bleeding	Caution with use of this combination	Anthocyanidin extracts from bilberry can inhibit platelet aggregation. Concomitant use with anticoagulant and antiplatelet drugs will theoretically increase the risk of bleeding and bruising. Clinical significance is unclear.
	Antidiabetic drugs	Possible additive effects	Caution with use of this combination	Bilberry may have hypoglycaemic properties. The combination could be additive and beneficial, but monitor for hypoglycaemia.
Valeriana officinalis	Alcohol	Increased risk of sedation	Caution with use of this combination	Valerian may potentiate the sedative effects of alcohol. Caution is advised.
	Benzodiazepines	Increased effects and risk of sedation	Caution with use of this combination	Valerian may have additive effects and potentiate the sedative effects of benzodiazepines.
	CNS depressant drugs including barbiturates	Increased effects and risk of sedation	Caution with use of this combination	Valerian may have additive effects and potentiate the sedative effects of CNS depressant drugs.
	CYP450 substrates (CYP3A4)	Theoretical altered drug effect	Monitor — interaction may not be clinically significant	Results from in-vitro studies have been conflicting. Some findings suggest valerian may inhibit CYP3A4 and other findings suggest it may induce CYP3A4. It has been proposed that a modest interaction may occur at doses of 1000 mg daily of valerian, but is unlikely at low doses. Caution is advised until further data become available.
Verbena officinalis	CYP450 substrates (CYP2B1)	Theoretical risk of increased adverse effects	Monitor — may not be clinically significant	In-vitro research suggests verbena can significantly inhibit CYP2B1 enzyme activity. Theoretically this may increase levels of drugs metabolised by this enzyme, however this interaction has not been reported in humans.
Viscum album	Antihypertensive drugs	Theoretical additive effects	Monitor — interaction may not be clinically significant	Preliminary research suggests European mistletoe may have hypotensive properties. Theoretically this may result in additive effects and a risk of hypotension. Clinical significance is unknown.
	Hepatotoxic drugs	Theoretical increased risk of liver damage	Monitor — may not be clinically significant	Case studies suggest European mistletoe may adversely affect liver function in some individuals. There is a theoretical increased risk of liver damage when used concomitantly with hepatotoxic drugs, but significance is unknown.
	Immunosuppressant drugs	Theoretical decrease in drug effect	Caution with use of this combination	European mistletoe may have immunostimulant properties which could theoretically antagonise the effects of immunosuppressant drugs.

Continued

TABLE I.1 Herbal interactions—cont'd

Herbal medicine	Drug/drug class	Potential outcome	Recommendations	Comments
Vitex agnus-castus	Dopamine receptor antagonists — including antipsychotic drugs	Theoretical decreased drug effects	Monitor — may not be clinically significant	Chaste tree may have dopaminergic activity. Concurrent use with dopamine antagonists may theoretically result in decreased drug effects. Caution is advised, although there are no clinical studies in humans to confirm this interaction.
	Dopamine agonists	Theoretical additive effects	Monitor — may not be clinically significant	Chaste tree may have dopaminergic effects and so may theoretically potentiate drug effects.
	Metoclopramide	Theoretical decreased drug effects	Monitor — may not be clinically significant	Chaste tree may interfere with drug action due to the dopaminergic effects of this drug.
	Oestrogenic drugs, e.g. contraceptive drugs and HRT	Theoretical decreased drug effects	Monitor — may not be clinically significant	Chaste tree appears to have weak hormone modulating activity and may theoretically interfere with drug action. This interaction is hypothetical and has not been supported by evidence.
Vitis vinifera	Anticoagulants/ antiplatelet drugs	Theoretical increased risk of bleeding	Caution with use of this combination	Grape may inhibit platelet aggregation. Concomitant use with anticoagulant and antiplatelet drugs will theoretically increase the risk of bleeding and bruising. Clinical significance is unclear.
	CYP450 substrates (CYP2C9, CYP3A4)	Theoretical increased risk of adverse effects	Monitor — may not be clinically significant	Preliminary in-vitro evidence suggests that grape may inhibit activity of CYP2C9 and CYP3A4. This interaction has not been reported in humans and significance is unknown.
Withania somnifera	Antidiabetic drugs	Additive effects theoretically possible	Caution with use of this combination	Preliminary evidence suggests that ashwagandha may have hypoglycaemic properties. Additive effects are theoretically possible, increasing the risk of hypoglycaemia. Caution is advised until more data become available.
	Antihypertensive drugs	Additive effects theoretically possible	Monitor — may not be clinically significant	According to animal studies ashwagandha may lower blood pressure. Additive effects are theoretically possible, with an increased risk of hypotension.
	Antipsychotic drugs, e.g. haloperidol	Theoretical decreased drug effects	May be beneficial — medical supervision recommended	Animal studies suggest ashwagandha may reduce drug-induced adverse effects such as dyskinesia. Clinical relevance is unclear, but may theoretically be beneficial.
	Benzodiazepines	Increased risk of sedation	Caution with use of this combination	Preliminary evidence suggests that ashwagandha may potentiate the effects of benzodiazepines. Caution is advised.
	Chemotherapeutic agents	Improved patient wellbeing	May be beneficial — medical supervision recommended	Ashwagandha has been found to significantly improve quality of life and reduce fatigue in breast cancer patients undergoing chemotherapy. Medical supervision is recommended.

TABLE I.1 Herbal interactions—cont'd

Herbal medicine	Drug/drug class	Potential outcome	Recommendations	Comments
Withania somnifera cont'd	Clomipramine	Improved management of obsessive compulsive disorder	May be beneficial — medical supervision recommended	A small study describes improved outcomes in patients with obsessive compulsive disorder when ashwagandha was added to existing drug therapy.
	CNS depressant drugs	Increased risk of sedation	Caution with use of this combination	Theoretically, concomitant use may have additive effects and an increased risk of excessive sedation.
	Immunosuppressant drugs	Theoretical decrease in drug effect	Caution with use of this combination	Ashwagandha may have immunostimulant properties which could theoretically antagonise the effects of immunosuppressant drugs.
Zanthoxylum spp.	Acid-reducing drugs (antacids, H_2 antagonists, proton pump inhibitors)	Theoretical decreased drug effect	Monitor — may not be clinically significant	Prickly ash may increase gastric acidity. Use may theoretically antagonise drug action, resulting in decreased drug effect.
Zanthoxylum simulans	Anticoagulants/ antiplatelet drugs	Theoretical increased risk of bleeding	Caution with use of this combination	In-vitro research suggests that Chinese prickly ash may inhibit platelet aggregation. Concomitant use with anticoagulant or antiplatelet drugs may theoretically increase the risk of bleeding.
Zea mays	Antidiabetic drugs	Theoretical additive effects	Caution with use of this combination	Corn silk may have hypoglycaemic properties according to animal research. Additive effects are theoretically possible, increasing the risk of hypoglycaemia. Caution is advised until more data become available.
	Antihypertensive drugs	Theoretical additive effects	Monitor — may not be clinically significant	Corn silk may theoretically lower blood pressure due to the herb's diuretic properties. Additive effects are theoretically possible, with an increased risk of hypotension. Clinical significance is unclear.
	Diuretics — potassium depleting, e.g. loop and thiazides	Theoretical increased risk of hypokalaemia	Monitor — may not be clinically significant	Diuretic effects with increased potassium loss have been reported in animal studies. Theoretically, concomitant use of corn silk with potassium depleting diuretics increases the risk of hypokalaemia. Monitor for signs of potassium depletion.
	Warfarin	Theoretical decreased drug anticoagulant effect	Caution with use of this combination	Corn silk contains vitamin K. Theoretically, high-dose intake of corn silk will increase vitamin K levels and could antagonise the activity of anticoagulants such as warfarin and reduce drug anticoagulant effect.

Continued

TABLE I.1 Herbal interactions—cont'd				
Herbal medicine	**Drug/drug class**	**Potential outcome**	**Recommendations**	**Comments**
Zingiber officinale	Anaesthetics	Possible decreased drug-induced nausea	May be beneficial — medical supervision recommended	Limited research suggests ginger may reduce severity of anaesthetic-induced postoperative nausea and vomiting if taken pre-treatment.
	Anticoagulant/ antiplatelet drugs	Theoretical increased risk of bleeding	Caution with use of this combination	Ginger appears to inhibit thromboxane synthetase and decrease platelet aggregation. Excessive intake of ginger may theoretically increase the risk of bleeding when used with anticoagulant/ antiplatelet drugs.
	Antidiabetic drugs	Additive effects theoretically possible	Monitor — may not be clinically significant	Preliminary evidence suggests that ginger may have hypoglycaemic properties, although data have been inconclusive. Additive effects are theoretically possible, increasing the risk of hypoglycaemia.
	Anti-emetic drugs	Additive effects theoretically possible	Combination may be beneficial	Ginger has anti-emetic properties and may have additive beneficial effects when used concomitantly with anti-emetic drugs. Theoretically, this may allow for a lower drug dose.
	Chemotherapy, e.g. cisplatin	Possible decreased drug-induced nausea	May be beneficial — medical supervision recommended	Limited research suggests ginger may reduce severity of nausea associated with certain chemotherapeutic agents.
	Nifedipine	Additive effects theoretically possible	Avoid combination	A synergistic effect on platelet aggregation was observed between ginger 1 g and nifedipine 10 mg in a small study of hypertensive patients. The combination should be avoided.
	Tacrolimus	Theoretical increased risk of drug toxicity	Avoid combination	An animal study reported increased drug levels when ginger was given concomitantly with tacrolimus. The combination should be avoided due to an increased risk of drug toxicity.
Zizyphus jujube/ spinosa	Antidiabetic drugs	Theoretical additive effects	Caution with use of this combination	Animal research suggests that zizyphus may have hypoglycaemic properties. Additive effects are theoretically possible, increasing the risk of hypoglycaemia. Clinical significance is unclear, but caution is advised until more data become available.
	CNS depressant drugs	Theoretical increased risk of sedation	Caution with use of this combination	Zizyphus may theoretically potentiate sedative adverse effects when used with CNS depressant drugs, based on animal studies.

TABLE I.2 Nutrient and nutritional supplement interactions

Nutrient/ supplement	Drug/drug class	Potential outcome	Recommendations	Comments
3,3′-diindolylmethane (DIM)	CYP450 substrates (CYP1A2)	Theoretical decreased drug effect	Monitor — may not be clinically significant	In-vitro evidence suggests that diindolylmethane may induce CYP1A2, which could theoretically increase the rate of drug metabolism and reduce drug efficacy. This has not been demonstrated in humans.
	Diuretics	Theoretical increased risk of hyponatraemia	Monitor — may not be clinically significant	A small study conducted in men with prostate cancer reported that high-dose intake of diindolylmethane resulted in asymptomatic hyponatraemia. Theoretically the risk of hyponatraemia is increased when used with diuretics.
	Oestrogens, e.g. HRT and oral contraceptives	Theoretical altered drug effect	Monitor — may not be clinically significant	Diindolylmethane may have mild oestrogenic and anti-oestrogenic effects. Theoretically high-dose intake may interfere with drug action.
5-hydroxytryptophan (5-HTP)	Antidepressant drugs (SSRIs and SNRIs)	Increased risk of serotonin-related adverse effects	Avoid combination	Concomitant use of 5-HTP and SSRIs or SNRIs may increase the risk of adverse effects and serotonin syndrome. The combination should be avoided as the consequences are potentially serious.
	Carbidopa	Increased risk of serotonin-related adverse effects	Caution with use of this combination	Concomitant use of 5-HTP and carbidopa may increase the risk of serotonergic adverse effects. Limited research suggests the combination may enhance drug therapy, but there are insufficient data to be clear on the benefits vs the risks.
	CNS depressants	Increased risk of drowsiness	Caution with use of this combination	Additive sedative effects are possible and may lead to excessive drowsiness.
	Dextromethorphan	Increased risk of serotonin-related adverse effects	Caution with use of this combination	Concomitant use of 5-HTP and dextromethorphan may increase the risk of adverse effects and serotonin syndrome.
	Monoamine oxidase inhibitors (MAOIs)	Increased risk of serotonin-related adverse effects	Avoid combination	Concomitant use of 5-HTP and MAOIs may increase the risk of adverse effects and serotonin syndrome.
	Tramadol	Increased risk of serotonin-related adverse effects	Caution with use of this combination	Concomitant use of 5-HTP and tramadol may increase the risk of adverse effects and serotonin syndrome.
Acetyl L-carnitine	Anticoagulants/ antiplatelet drugs	Theoretical increased risk of bleeding	Caution with use of this combination	Acetyl L-carnitine may theoretically potentiate drug effects and increase the risk of bleeding.
Activated charcoal	Oral medications	Theoretical decreased drug absorption	Caution with use of this combination	Activated charcoal may theoretically bind to, and reduce, absorption of several drugs and supplements. Dosages should be separated by a minimum of 2 hours.

LEGEND

- Combination okay to use
- Use of combination should be monitored
- Use combination with caution
- Avoid combination

Continued

TABLE I.2 Nutrient and nutritional supplement interactions—cont'd

Nutrient/ supplement	Drug/drug class	Potential outcome	Recommendations	Comments
Adenosine	Antigout drugs	Theoretical decreased drug effectiveness	Monitor — may not be clinically significant	Adenosine triphosphate can cause hyperuricaemia and uricosuria. This may theoretically reduce drug effectiveness.
	Dipyridamole	Risk of nutrient toxicity	Avoid combination	Dipyridamole decreases metabolism of adenosine and may increase risk of toxicity.
	Methylxanthines	Theoretical decreased nutrient effect	Monitor — may not be clinically significant	Aminophylline, caffeine and theophylline may theoretically block adenosine effects due to a competitive antagonist action.
Agaricus mushrooms	Antidiabetic drugs	Theoretical additive effects	Caution with use of this combination	Some evidence suggests that agaricus mushrooms may lower blood glucose levels by decreasing insulin resistance in type 2 diabetics. Additive effects are possible, with an increased risk of hypoglycaemia.
Alpha-casozepine milk protein (casein peptides)	Antihypertensive drugs	Theoretical additive effects	Monitor — may not be clinically significant	According to limited research alpha-casozepine may lower blood pressure slightly. Concomitant use will theoretically have additive effects. This may potentially be beneficial, but monitor for hypotension.
	Anxiolytic drugs, e.g. benzodiazepines	Theoretical additive effects	Monitor — may not be clinically significant	Alpha-casozepine may have anxiolytic properties. Concomitant use will theoretically have additive effects, which may be beneficial. Patients should be monitored due to insufficient research data on the effects of combined use.
Alpha-lipoic acid	Antidiabetic drugs	Theoretical additive effects	Caution with use of this combination	Alpha-lipoic acid may have hypoglycaemic effects. The combination could be additive and beneficial, but drug dosage adjustments may be required.
	Cisplatin	Possible decreased drug-induced adverse effects	May be beneficial — medical supervision recommended	Preliminary research suggests alpha-lipoic acid may have some protective effects against drug-induced ototoxicity, peripheral sensory neuropathy and oxidative stress.
	L-thryroxine (Levothyroxine)	Theoretical decreased drug effects	Caution with use of this combination	Animal research suggests that alpha-lipoic acid may reduce conversion of thyroxine to the active T3 form. Significance is unclear.
Apple cider vinegar	Antidiabetic drugs	Theoretical additive effects	Caution with use of this combination	Apple cider vinegar may have additive effects when used with antidiabetic drugs. It has been shown to reduce postprandial blood glucose levels and decrease gastric emptying time in people with diabetes. While this could potentially be beneficial, caution is recommended.

TABLE I.2 Nutrient and nutritional supplement interactions—cont'd				
Nutrient/ supplement	**Drug/drug class**	**Potential outcome**	**Recommendations**	**Comments**
Apple cider vinegar cont'd	Digoxin	Theoretical increased risk of drug toxicity	Caution with use of this combination	Overuse of apple cider vinegar may theoretically decrease potassium levels and increase the risk of drug toxicity.
	Diuretics	Theoretical increased risk of hypokalaemia	Caution with use of this combination	Overuse of apple cider vinegar may theoretically decrease potassium levels and increase the risk of hypokalaemia.
Arginine (L-arginine)	ACE-inhibitors (ACE-I)	Risk of hypotension and hyperkalaemia	Caution with use of this combination	Additive vasodilatory and blood pressure-lowering effects have been reported, which increases the risk of hypotension. Theoretically, combined use may also increase the risk of hyperkalaemia as both drug and nutrient can raise potassium levels. The combination may theoretically be beneficial, but careful monitoring is recommended.
	Angiotensin receptor blockers (ARBs)	Risk of hypotension and hyperkalaemia	Caution with use of this combination	Additive vasodilatory and blood pressure-lowering effects have been reported, which increases the risk of hypotension. Theoretically, combined use may also increase the risk of hyperkalaemia as both drug and nutrient can raise potassium levels. The combination may theoretically be beneficial, but careful monitoring is recommended.
	Anticoagulant/ antiplatelet drugs	Theoretical increased risk of bleeding	Caution with use of this combination	Preliminary evidence suggests arginine may decrease platelet aggregation. Concurrent use may theoretically increase the risk of bleeding.
	Antidiabetic drugs	Theoretical increased risk of hypoglycaemia	Caution with use of this combination	Preliminary evidence suggests arginine may decrease blood glucose levels in patients with type 2 diabetes. Concurrent use may theoretically be beneficial; however, there is an increased risk of hypoglycaemia.
	Antihypertensive drugs	Additive effect possible	Caution with use of this combination	Arginine increases nitric oxide levels which results in vasodilation. Additive blood pressure-lowering effects have been reported when used in combination with antihypertensive drugs. Concurrent use may theoretically be beneficial; however, there is an increased risk of hypotension.
	Diuretics	Increased risk of hyperkalaemia	Caution with use of this combination	Arginine intake may result in raised potassium levels. This is a theoretical increased risk of hyperkalaemia when used with potassium-sparing diuretics.

Continued

TABLE I.2 Nutrient and nutritional supplement interactions—cont'd

Nutrient/ supplement	Drug/drug class	Potential outcome	Recommendations	Comments
Arginine (L-arginine) cont'd	Herpes treatments including antiviral drugs and lysine	Possible decreased disease management	Caution with use of this combination	Arginine may oppose the therapeutic action of agents used for the management of herpes simplex. High levels of arginine may stimulate viral replication of herpes simplex virus.
	Nitrates	Additive vasodilatory effects possible	Caution with use of this combination	Caution is advised due to a risk of additive vasodilatory and hypotensive effects.
	Sildenafil and other phosphodiesterase-5 inhibitors	Additive effects possible	May be beneficial — medical supervision recommended	Arginine can lead to increased nitric oxide production, which may theoretically enhance drug effect in the management of erectile dysfunction. The combination may theoretically be beneficial; however, caution is advised due to an increased risk of vasodilation and hypotension.
Beta-carotene	Anthelmintic drugs	Possible improved response	Combination may be beneficial	Vitamin A deficiency is associated with an increased risk of parasitic worm infections. In addition, worm infections, especially roundworm, can interfere with vitamin A absorption. Concurrent use of beta-carotene or vitamin A may assist with management of this condition, as well as supporting immunity and epithelial integrity.
	Cholestyramine	Reduced nutrient absorption	May be beneficial to address nutrient depletion	Cholestyramine may reduce nutrient absorption. Supplements may be required in some individuals. Separate dose administration.
	Colchicine	Reduced nutrient absorption	May be beneficial to address nutrient depletion	Colchicine reduces absorption of fat-soluble vitamins including beta-carotene. Supplements may be required to address nutrient depletion.
	Mineral oil	Risk of vitamin depletion	May be beneficial to address nutrient depletion	A moderate risk of nutrient depletion has been reported and supplements may be required in some individuals.
	Neomycin	Risk of nutrient depletion	May be beneficial to address nutrient depletion	Neomycin may damage the structure and affect function of the digestive tract lining. Long-term use may reduce absorption and increase excretion of beta-carotene.
	Orlistat	Reduced nutrient absorption	May be beneficial to address nutrient depletion	Orlistat reduces absorption of fat-soluble vitamins including beta-carotene. Supplements may be required to address nutrient depletion.
	Proton pump inhibitors	Risk of nutrient depletion	Combination may be beneficial to address nutrient depletion	Proton pump inhibitors may theoretically reduce absorption of beta-carotene. Increased intake of dietary carotenoid-rich foods may be beneficial. Individuals taking proton pump inhibitors should be monitored for signs of nutrient deficiencies.

TABLE I.2 Nutrient and nutritional supplement interactions—cont'd

Nutrient/ supplement	Drug/drug class	Potential outcome	Recommendations	Comments
Beta-glucan	Antihypertensive drugs	Additive effects possible	Combination may be beneficial	Beta-glucan has been shown to reduce blood pressure, particularly in obese individuals with hypertension. Concurrent use may be additive and potentially beneficial, but monitor for hypotension.
	Immunosuppressant drugs	Theoretical risk of decreased drug effect	Caution with use of this combination	Beta-glucans may have immunostimulant effects. Theoretically this may counteract drug immunosuppressant action, however clinical significance is unclear.
	Lipid-lowering drugs	Additive effects possible	Combination may be beneficial	Beta-glucans have been shown to significantly reduce cholesterol. Additive beneficial effects may be seen with concurrent use.
Beta-sitosterol	Ezetimibe	Decreased β-sitosterol absorption	Caution with use of this combination	Ezetimibe has been shown to inhibit absorption of β-sitosterol and may reduce levels by up to 41%.
	Pravastatin	Theoretical decreased β-sitosterol levels	Monitor — may not be clinically significant	Limited data suggest that pravastatin may lower β-sitosterol levels.
Betaine HCl	Acid-reducing drugs (antacids, H_2-antagonists, proton pump inhibitors)	Theoretical decreased drug effect	Monitor — may not be clinically significant	Betaine may increase gastric acidity and concurrent use may theoretically counteract drug action.
Biotin	Anticonvulsant drugs	Nutrient depletion possible	May be beneficial to address nutrient depletion	Reduced plasma biotin levels have been observed in patients taking carbamazepine, phenobarbital (phenobarbitone) and phenytoin. Clinical significance is unclear.
Blackcurrant oil	Anticoagulant/ antiplatelet drugs	Theoretical increased risk of bleeding	Caution with use of this combination	Gamma-linolenic acid (GLA), which is found in blackcurrant oil, may have antiplatelet properties. Concurrent use may theoretically increase the risk of bleeding.
	Anticonvulsant drugs	Theoretical increased risk of seizures	Caution with use of this combination	Theoretically, products containing gamma-linolenic acid (GLA), including blackcurrant oil, may lower seizure threshold and increase the risk of seizures. This interaction is based on anecdotal evidence and significance is unclear.
	Antihypertensive drugs	Theoretical risk of hypotension	Monitor — may not be clinically significant	Blackcurrant oil may decrease systolic blood pressure, based on limited data. There is a theoretical increased risked of hypotension when used concurrently with antihypertensive drugs.
	Phenothiazines	Theoretical increased risk of seizures	Caution with use of this combination	Theoretically, products containing gamma-linolenic acid (GLA), including blackcurrant oil, may increase the risk of seizures in people taking phenothiazines. This interaction is based on anecdotal evidence and significance is unclear.

Continued

TABLE I.2 Nutrient and nutritional supplement interactions—cont'd

Nutrient/ supplement	Drug/drug class	Potential outcome	Recommendations	Comments
Blueberry	Antidiabetic drugs	Possible additive effects	May be beneficial — monitor	Evidence suggests that blueberries and blueberry extract may lower blood glucose and improve glycaemic status. Additive, beneficial effects are theoretically possible, but monitor for hypoglycaemia.
Branched chain amino acids (BCAAs)	Antidiabetic drugs	Possible additive hypoglycaemic effects	Caution with use of this combination	Some evidence suggests that BCAAs may stimulate release of insulin. Additive effects are theoretically possible, but may increase the risk of hypoglycaemia.
	Levodopa	Theoretical decreased drug effects	Caution with use of this combination	Theoretically, BCAAs may compete with levodopa for transport systems. This may result in decreased drug effectiveness, although clinical significance is unclear.
Bromelain	Anticoagulant/ antiplatelet drugs	Theoretical increased risk of bleeding	Caution with use of this combination	Bromelain may have antiplatelet properties, leading to a theoretical increased risk of bleeding.
Caffeine	Alcohol	Theoretical increased caffeine levels	Monitor — may not be clinically significant	Alcohol reduces caffeine metabolism, therefore there is a theoretical increased risk of caffeine-related adverse effects.
	Alendronate	Reduced drug bioavailability	Caution with use of this combination — separate doses	Caffeine significantly reduces drug bioavailability. Doses should be separated by at least 2 hours.
	Anticoagulant/ antiplatelet drugs	Theoretical increased risk of bleeding	Monitor — may not be clinically significant	Caffeine is reported to have antiplatelet activity, however an interaction between coffee and drugs in this class has not been reported in humans.
	Anticonvulsant drugs, e.g. carbamazepine, phenytoin, ethosuximide, valproate	Theoretical decreased drugs effects	Caution with use of this combination	Animal models suggest that high-dose intake of caffeine may reduce drug anticonvulsant effects. The mechanism of this interaction and clinical significance is unclear.
	Cimetidine	Theoretical increased caffeine levels	Caution with use of this combination	Cimetidine may reduce caffeine metabolism, theoretically increasing the risk of caffeine-related adverse effects.
	Clozapine	Theoretical disease exacerbation	Caution with use of this combination	Caffeine may exacerbate psychotic symptoms and increase drug effects and toxicity at high doses (400–1000 mg daily of caffeine).
	CNS stimulant drugs	Enhanced stimulatory effects	Caution with use of this combination	Concomitant use of caffeine and CNS stimulant drugs will increase the risk of adverse effects due to additive stimulatory actions.
	Disulfiram	Theoretical increased caffeine levels	Monitor — may not be clinically significant	Disulfiram may reduce caffeine metabolism, theoretically increasing the risk of caffeine-related adverse effects.

TABLE I.2 Nutrient and nutritional supplement interactions—cont'd

Nutrient/ supplement	Drug/drug class	Potential outcome	Recommendations	Comments
Caffeine cont'd	Diuretics	Theoretical increased risk of hypokalaemia	Caution with use of this combination	Excessive intake of caffeine may reduce potassium levels due to stimulation of the sodium-potassium pump. There is a theoretical increased risk of hypokalaemia when taken with potassium-depleting diuretics.
	Ephedrine	Enhanced stimulatory effects	Avoid combination	Ephedrine may enhance the stimulatory effects of caffeine. The combination has been associated with an increased risk of life-threatening or debilitating adverse effects such as hypertension, myocardial infarction, stroke, seizures and death.
	Fluvoxamine	Theoretical increased caffeine levels	Monitor — may not be clinically significant	Fluvoxamine may reduce caffeine metabolism, theoretically increasing the risk of caffeine-related adverse effects.
	L-thyroxine (Levothyroxine)	Possible reduced drug absorption	Caution with use of this combination	It has been proposed that coffee may form insoluble complexes with thyroxine in some patients. Dosage separation is advised.
	Lithium	Theoretical increased risk of drug toxicity	Caution with use of this combination	Case reports suggest that abrupt withdrawal from caffeine may increase serum lithium levels.
	Monoamine oxidase inhibitors (MAOIs)	Theoretical risk of hypertensive crisis	Caution with use of this combination	Theoretically, high intake of caffeine may precipitate a hypertensive crisis in patients taking MAOIs.
	Phenylpropanolamine	Theoretical increased risk of hypertension	Caution with use of this combination	Concomitant use may have additive effects in raising blood pressure. Phenylpropanolamine may also raise serum caffeine levels according to limited data.
	Quinolone antibiotics	Theoretical increased caffeine levels	Monitor — may not be clinically significant	Quinolones reduce caffeine metabolism, therefore there is a theoretical increased risk of caffeine-related adverse effects.
	Theophylline	Theoretical increased risk of drug toxicity	Caution with use of this combination	Caffeine may inhibit drug metabolism and increase the risk of adverse effects
	Verapamil	Theoretical increased caffeine levels	Caution with use of this combination	Verapamil may increase plasma caffeine concentration by 25% according to some research. Concomitant use may theoretically increase the risk of caffeine-related adverse effects.
Calcium	Acid-reducing drugs (H_2-antagonists and proton pump inhibitors (PPIs))	Risk of nutrient depletion	May be beneficial to address nutrient depletion	Some calcium salts, especially calcium carbonate, require adequate stomach acid to dissolve and allow for absorption. Drugs that raise gastric pH may theoretically reduce calcium absorption. Monitor for calcium depletion with long-term use of acid-reducing drugs.

Continued

TABLE I.2 Nutrient and nutritional supplement interactions—cont'd

Nutrient/ supplement	Drug/drug class	Potential outcome	Recommendations	Comments
Calcium cont'd	Aluminium salts, e.g. antacids	Increased risk of aluminium absorption	Caution with use of this combination	Calcium citrate may increase the absorption of aluminium as aluminium hydroxide. Aluminium may be toxic, especially in those with renal disease. This interaction appears to be specific to the citrate salt.
	Antibiotics (quinolones and tetracyclines)	Reduced drug effect	Monitor — separate doses	Calcium supplements form complexes with these drugs and may reduce drug effectiveness. Separate doses by at least 2 hours.
	Anticonvulsant drugs (carbamazepine, phenobarbital (phenobarbitone), phenytoin, fosphenytoin)	Risk of nutrient depletion with long-term use	May be beneficial to address nutrient depletion	Use of some anticonvulsant drugs may result in a major calcium depletion. This is due to increased vitamin D metabolism resulting in decreased calcium absorption. Hypocalcaemia and osteomalacia have occurred, especially with prolonged therapy or concurrent use of more than one anticonvulsant drug. Most patients will need calcium and vitamin D supplements.
	Bisphosphonates, e.g. alendronate, risedronate, ibrandronic acid	Reduced drug absorption	Beneficial interaction, but dosage separation is essential	Calcium significantly reduces absorption of oral bisphosphonates and may reduce drug effectiveness. Bisphosphonates should be taken at least 30 minutes before calcium supplements. It should be noted that use of bisphosphonates is contraindicated in individuals with hypocalcaemia, therefore adequate intake of calcium and vitamin D is important for both drug safety and efficacy and to enhance disease management.
	Caffeine	Risk of nutrient depletion with long-term use	May be beneficial to address nutrient depletion	High caffeine intake may increase urinary excretion of calcium and has been associated with increased bone loss and risk of fractures in the elderly. Calcium supplements may be required with regular high intake.
	Calcipotriene	Increased risk of hypercalcaemia	Caution with use of this combination	Rare cases of hypercalcaemia have been reported with use of calcipotriene. Calcium supplements should be used with caution or avoided due to an increased risk of hypercalcaemia.
	Calcium channel blockers	Theoretical antagonistic effect	Monitor — may not be clinically significant	Calcium supplements may antagonise the effects of intravenous calcium channel blockers. There is no evidence that dietary or supplemental calcium interacts with oral calcium channel blockers.

TABLE I.2 Nutrient and nutritional supplement interactions—cont'd				
Nutrient/ supplement	**Drug/drug class**	**Potential outcome**	**Recommendations**	**Comments**
Calcium cont'd	Ceftriaxone	Risk of deposition of a drug-nutrient complex	Avoid combination	Case reports describe an interaction in neonates where the combination of IV calcium with IV ceftriaxone has led to the precipitation of a drug-nutrient salt in the lungs and kidneys, which has led to death. While this interaction has not been reported in adults, caution and dosage separation are advised, especially with IV forms of calcium and ceftriaxone.
	Cholestyramine	Risk of nutrient depletion with long-term use	May be beneficial to address nutrient depletion	Cholestyramine may reduce vitamin D absorption which can then affect calcium absorption. Current evidence suggests this depletion is not significant in most patients, but monitoring is advised.
	Corticosteroids	Risk of mineral depletion with long-term use	May be beneficial to address nutrient depletion	Long-term intake of oral corticosteroids (equivalent to ≥7.5 mg prednisone daily) causes significant bone loss and increases the risk of osteoporosis and fractures. A major depletion is possible and supplements may be required.
	Digoxin	Increased risk of drug toxicity	Caution with use of this combination	Hypercalcaemia may potentiate digoxin toxicity. Caution is recommended with high-dose intake of supplemental calcium.
	Diuretics — loop	Risk of nutrient depletion	May be beneficial to address nutrient depletion	Loop diuretics *increase* urinary excretion of calcium. Moderate risk of depletion.
	Diuretics — thiazides	Increased risk of hypercalcaemia	Caution with use of this combination	Thiazide diuretics *decrease* urinary excretion of calcium, theoretically increasing the risk of hypercalcaemia with high calcium intake.
	Integrase inhibitors, e.g. dolutegravir, elvitegravir, raltegravir	Theoretical decreased drug effect	Avoid combination	Pharmacokinetic studies suggest calcium supplements decrease drug serum levels of integrase inhibitors, possibly due to a chelation interaction. These combinations should be avoided until more data become available as it may theoretically compromise HIV therapy.
	L-thyroxine (Levothyroxine)	Possible decreased drug absorption	Caution with use of this combination — separate doses	Calcium may theoretically reduce drug absorption by forming insoluble complexes. Separate doses by at least 4 hours.
	Lithium	Theoretical increased risk of hypercalcaemia	Caution with use of this combination	Evidence suggests that long-term use of lithium may result in hypercalcaemia. Combined use of calcium supplements with lithium will theoretically increase this risk.

Continued

TABLE I.2 Nutrient and nutritional supplement interactions—cont'd

Nutrient/ supplement	Drug/drug class	Potential outcome	Recommendations	Comments
Calcium cont'd	Minerals (iron, magnesium)	Reduced mineral absorption	Monitor — separate doses	Calcium supplements may interfere with absorption of dietary and supplemental iron and magnesium. The interaction may not be clinically relevant unless there is a deficiency, but separation of dose administration is generally advised.
	Mineral oil	Risk of nutrient depletion with long-term use	May be beneficial to address nutrient depletion	Mineral oil may interfere with absorption of vitamin D and calcium. Some patients will need supplements with long-term use.
	Sotalol	Possible decreased drug absorption	Caution with use of this combination — separate doses	Calcium appears to reduce drug absorption, possibly by forming insoluble complexes. Dose administration should be separated.
	Stimulant laxatives	Risk of nutrient depletion with long-term use	May be beneficial to address nutrient depletion	Stimulant laxatives can moderately reduce calcium and vitamin D absorption. Advise patients not to use stimulant laxatives long term, and monitor for signs of nutrient depletion.
Calcium D-glucarate	Alcohol	Theoretical decreased calcium D-glucarate activity	Caution with use of this combination	Clinical research suggests alcohol may increase urinary excretion of calcium D-glucarate and decrease nutrient activity.
	Glucuronidated drugs	Theoretical increased drug clearance	Monitor — clinical significance is unknown	Theoretically, calcium D-glucarate may increase clearance of drugs that undergo Phase II glucuronidation metabolism. Examples of drugs metabolised via this pathway include atorvastatin, diazepam, digoxin, lamotrigine, lorazepam, paracetamol, morphine, oxazepam.
Carnitine (L-carnitine)	Anticoagulants/ antiplatelet drugs	Theoretical increased risk of bleeding	Caution with use of this combination	L-carnitine may theoretically potentiate drug effects and increase the risk of bleeding.
	L-thyroxine (Levothyroxine)	Theoretical decreased drug effect	Caution with use of this combination	Theoretically L-carnitine may decrease effectiveness of L-thyroxine. L-carnitine appears to act as a peripheral thyroid hormone antagonist.
Choline	Atropine	Theoretical decreased drug effects	Monitor — may not be clinically significant	Animal research suggests that concomitant administration of choline and atropine may result in decreased effects of atropine.
Chondroitin sulfate	Anticoagulant/ antiplatelet drugs	Theoretical increased risk of bleeding	Caution with use of this combination	Evidence suggests that a combination of chondroitin with glucosamine may potentiate the effects of warfarin, leading to an increased risk of bleeding. It is unclear whether the interaction is due to chondroitin, glucosamine or both.
	Non-steroidal anti-inflammatory drugs (NSAIDs)	Increased disease management in OA	Combination may be beneficial	The combination may lead to improved outcomes in patients with osteoarthritis and may result in reduced NSAID requirements.

TABLE I.2 Nutrient and nutritional supplement interactions—cont'd

Nutrient/ supplement	Drug/drug class	Potential outcome	Recommendations	Comments
Chromium	Antidiabetic drugs	Possible additive effects	Caution with use of this combination	Chromium may lower blood glucose levels. Additive effects are possible when used with antidiabetic drugs, which may be beneficial, but caution is advised due to a risk of hypoglycaemia.
	Corticosteroids	Risk of nutrient depletion	May be beneficial to address nutrient depletion	Corticosteroids may increase urinary excretion of chromium. A moderate risk of chromium deficiency has been reported with long-term use.
	Insulin	Possible additive effects	Caution with use of this combination	Chromium has been shown to increase insulin sensitivity. Additive effects are possible and may be beneficial, but caution is advised due to a risk of hypoglycaemia.
	L-thyroxine (Levothyroxine)	Possible decreased drug bioavailability	Caution with use of this combination	Clinical research suggests that chromium may bind to thyroxine and decrease drug absorption. Intake should be separated.
	Lipid-lowering drugs	May improve disease management	Combination may be beneficial	Chromium may have lipid-lowering properties and could have additive benefits in disease management.
Coenzyme Q10 (ubiquinol, ubidecarenone)	Antidiabetic drugs	Possible improved disease management; possible nutrient depletion	Combination may be beneficial	Research reports that people with type 2 diabetes tend to have lower CoQ10 levels and that CoQ10 supplements may help to improve glycaemic control. CoQ10 has also been shown to improve nerve conduction and reduce neuropathic pain in diabetic patients. Observational studies have proposed that some oral antidiabetic drugs may deplete CoQ10 levels, although further research is needed to investigate significance. The combination maybe beneficial, but monitoring is advised.
	Antihypertensive drugs	Possible additive effects	Combination may be beneficial	CoQ10 can lower blood pressure according to research, with this effect being clinically relevant. Additive, beneficial effects are theoretically possible, but monitor for hypotension.
	β-blockers	Possible nutrient depletion	May be beneficial to address nutrient depletion	In-vitro studies suggest that β-blockers may lead to a reduction in CoQ10 levels, with secondary sources proposing that this may contribute to drug adverse effects such as fatigue. Concurrent use may theoretically be beneficial and could potentially support cardiovascular health in general.

Continued

TABLE I.2 Nutrient and nutritional supplement interactions—cont'd				
Nutrient/ supplement	**Drug/drug class**	**Potential outcome**	**Recommendations**	**Comments**
Coenzyme Q10 (ubiquinol, ubidecarenone) cont'd	Doxorubicin	Possible decreased risk of drug toxicity	May be beneficial — medical supervision recommended	Preliminary evidence suggests that doxorubicin may decrease CoQ10 synthesis and that this may contribute to drug cardiotoxicity. CoQ10 has not been shown to affect drug pharmacokinetics, therefore may be useful as an adjunct therapy, under medical supervision.
	HMGCoA reductase inhibitors (statins)	Possible decreased risk of drug adverse effects	May be beneficial to address nutrient depletion	Statins block endogenous synthesis of CoQ10, which may lead to reduced serum levels. This dose-dependent interaction is considered a contributing factor for statin-induced adverse effects such as myalgia, fatigue and headache. Concerns have also been raised about the potential negative impact of reduced CoQ10 levels on cardiovascular function, particularly in those at risk. While there is a lack of consensus as to whether CoQ10 should be recommended routinely with statins, there are no known risks to use of this combination and it is potentially beneficial.
	Warfarin	Theoretical decreased drug effect	Caution with use of this combination	Data on this interaction are conflicting. CoQ10 is structurally similar to menaquinone and may theoretically have a vitamin K-like effect. Case reports suggest use of CoQ10 may reduce drug anticoagulant effect. Results of a small RCT trial, however, reported no significant change to warfarin pharmacokinetics with concurrent use of warfarin and CoQ10. Caution is advised until more data become available.
Cod liver oil	Anticoagulant/ antiplatelet drugs	Theoretical increased risk of bleeding	Caution with use of this combination	Cod liver oil may have antiplatelet properties at high doses, leading to a theoretical increased risk of bleeding.
	Antihypertensive drugs	Possible additive effects	Caution with use of this combination	Cod liver oil may lower blood pressure. This may lead to additive beneficial effects, but monitor for hypotension.
Colloidal silver	Antibiotics (quinolones and tetracyclines)	Theoretical decreased drug absorption	Caution with use of this combination	Colloidal silver may theoretically reduce drug absorption.
	Hepatotoxic drugs	Increased risk of liver damage	Caution with use of this combination	According to preliminary animal studies colloidal silver may be hepatotoxic. Concurrent use with hepatotoxic drugs theoretically increases the risk of liver damage.
	L-thyroxine (Levothyroxine)	Theoretical decreased drug absorption	Caution with use of this combination	Colloidal silver may theoretically reduce drug absorption.
	Penicillamine	Theoretical decreased drug absorption	Caution with use of this combination	Colloidal silver may theoretically reduce drug absorption.

TABLE I.2 Nutrient and nutritional supplement interactions—cont'd

Nutrient/ supplement	Drug/drug class	Potential outcome	Recommendations	Comments
Conjugated linoleic acid (CLA)	Anticoagulant/ antiplatelet drugs	Theoretical increased risk of bleeding	Caution with use of this combination	CLA may have antiplatelet properties. There is a theoretical increased risk of bleeding with concurrent use.
	Antihypertensive drugs, e.g. ramipril	Additive effects	Caution with use of this combination	CLA may reduce blood pressure and enhance drug effects. One study reported that CLA enhanced ramipril's blood pressure-lowering effects in obese hypertensive patients. The combination of CLA with antihypertensive drugs may be beneficial, but monitor for hypotension.
Copper	Contraceptive drugs	Increased copper levels	Monitor — may not be clinically significant	Contraceptive drugs may increase copper levels above reference levels according to some studies. Intake of supplemental copper while taking the contraceptive pill may theoretically lead to excessive copper levels.
	Penicillamine	Decreased drug effects	Caution with use of this combination	Copper chelates penicillamine and decreases drug absorption. Separate dose administration by at least 2 hours.
Creatine	Nephrotoxic drugs	Theoretical increased risk of kidney damage	Caution with use of this combination	Some cases of renal impairment after intake of creatine supplements have been reported, although most research suggests no adverse effect on kidney function. Theoretically, creatine may increase the risk of kidney damage when used with nephrotoxic drugs, although this effect has not been reported in humans.
Ellagic acid — see *Punica grantum*				
Epigallocatechin-3-gallate — see *Camellia sinensis*				
Evening primrose oil	Anticoagulant/ antiplatelet drugs	Theoretical increased risk of bleeding	Caution with use of this combination	Gamma-linolenic acid (GLA), found in evening primrose oil, may have antiplatelet properties, leading to a theoretical increased risk of bleeding.
	Anticonvulsant drugs	Theoretical increased risk of seizures	Caution with use of this combination	Theoretically, products containing gamma-linolenic acid (GLA), including evening primrose oil, may lower seizure threshold and increase the risk of seizures. This interaction is based on anecdotal evidence and significance is unclear.
	Phenothiazines	Theoretical increased risk of seizures	Caution with use of this combination	Theoretically, products containing gamma-linolenic acid (GLA), including evening primrose oil, may increase the risk of seizures in people taking phenothiazines. This interaction is based on anecdotal evidence and significance is unclear.

Continued

TABLE I.2 Nutrient and nutritional supplement interactions—cont'd				
Nutrient/ supplement	**Drug/drug class**	**Potential outcome**	**Recommendations**	**Comments**
Evening primrose oil cont'd	Protease inhibitors, e.g. lopinavir	Possible increased drug levels	Caution with use of this combination	A case report describes a possible interaction between evening primrose oil and lopinavir in an HIV patient, which led to increased drug concentration.
	Tamoxifen	Possible improved outcomes	May be beneficial — medical supervision recommended	Preliminary evidence suggests that gamma-linolenic acid (GLA), found in evening primrose oil, may improve outcomes in patients with breast cancer who are taking tamoxifen. Data are limited and medical supervision is recommended.
Fermented wheatgerm extract	Immunosuppressant drugs	Theoretical risk of decreased drug effect	Caution with use of this combination	Fermented wheatgerm extract appears to stimulate immune function. This may theoretically oppose drug immunosuppressant effects.
Fibre	Oral medications	Theoretical decrease in drug effect possible	Monitor — separate doses	High-fibre intake may theoretically affect absorption of some drugs. Clinical significance is unclear and will be variable. Dosage separation is suggested.
Fish oil — see Omega-3 essential fatty acids				
Flaxseed	Anticoagulant/ antiplatelet drugs	Theoretical increased risk of bleeding	Monitor — may not be clinically significant	Flaxseed may have antiplatelet properties. There is a theoretical risk of additive effects, with an increased risk of bleeding. The interaction is unlikely to be clinically significant at normal therapeutic doses.
	Antidiabetic drugs	Theoretical additive effects	Monitor — may not be clinically significant	Flaxseed may have hypoglycaemic properties and additive effects are theoretically possible. Clinical significance at normal therapeutic doses is unclear.
	Antihypertensive drugs	Theoretical additive effects	Monitor — may not be clinically significant	Flaxseed may slightly lower diastolic pressure and additive effects are theoretically possible. Clinical significance at normal therapeutic doses is unclear.
	Furosemide (frusemide)	Theoretical decreased drug absorption	Monitor — may not be clinically significant	Preliminary in-vitro research suggests flaxseed may decrease drug absorption. Clinical significance is unknown.
	Ketoprofen	Theoretical decreased drug absorption	Monitor — may not be clinically significant	Preliminary in-vitro research suggests flaxseed may decrease drug absorption. Clinical significance is unknown.
	Oestrogens, e.g. HRT and oral contraceptives	Theoretical decreased drug effect	Monitor — may not be clinically significant	Flaxseed may theoretically have mild oestrogenic effects. Theoretically the lignans in flaxseed may compete with oestrogens for binding sites and reduce drug effect. The interaction is speculative.

TABLE I.2 Nutrient and nutritional supplement interactions—cont'd

Nutrient/ supplement	Drug/drug class	Potential outcome	Recommendations	Comments
Flaxseed cont'd	Paracetamol	Theoretical decreased drug absorption	Monitor — may not be clinically significant	Preliminary in-vitro research suggests flaxseed may decrease drug absorption. Clinical significance is unknown.
Gamma-aminobutyric acid (GABA)	Antihypertensive drugs	Theoretical additive effects	Caution with use of this combination	Some evidence suggests that GABA may lower blood pressure. Additive beneficial effects are theoretically possible, but caution is advised due to a risk of hypotension.
Gamma-linolenic acid (GLA)	Anticoagulant/ antiplatelet drugs	Theoretical increased risk of bleeding	Caution with use of this combination	Gamma-linolenic acid (GLA) may have antiplatelet properties, leading to a theoretical increased risk of bleeding.
	Anticonvulsant drugs	Theoretical increased risk of seizures	Caution with use of this combination	Theoretically gamma-linolenic acid (GLA) may lower seizure threshold and increase the risk of seizures. This interaction is based on anecdotal evidence and significance is unclear.
	Phenothiazines	Theoretical increased risk of seizures	Caution with use of this combination	Theoretically, gamma-linolenic acid (GLA) may increase the risk of seizures in people taking phenothiazines. This interaction is based on anecdotal evidence and significance is unclear.
Genistein — see Soy protein and soy isoflavones				
Germinated barley foodstuff	Antidiabetic drugs	Additive effects possible	Monitor — may not be clinically significant	Barley may theoretically enhance drug blood glucose lowering effects. Clinical significance is not clear.
Glucosamine sulfate	Anticoagulant/ antiplatelet drugs	Increased risk of bleeding	Avoid combination	Case reports suggest that the combination of warfarin and glucosamine, both with and without chondroitin, may increase INR and risk of bleeding and bruising. The combination should be avoided until more safety data become available.
	Antidiabetic drugs	Theoretical decreased disease management, although interaction appears unlikely	Monitor — may not be clinically significant	Preliminary research suggested that glucosamine may increase insulin resistance or decrease insulin production. Concerns were raised that use of glucosamine may decrease drug effectiveness and worsen disease management. Based on current clinical research, however, glucosamine does not appear to adversely affect blood glucose control or HbA_{1C}. Patients should still be monitored.
	Non-steroidal anti-inflammatory drugs (NSAIDs)	Possible improved disease management; reduced need for drug therapy	Combination may be beneficial	Glucosamine sulfate can help to improve cartilage synthesis and repair, reduce disease progression and reduce symptoms of osteoarthritis. According to clinical research glucosamine sulfate may reduce requirements for NSAID therapy in patients with knee osteoarthritis.

Continued

TABLE I.2 Nutrient and nutritional supplement interactions—cont'd				
Nutrient/ supplement	**Drug/drug class**	**Potential outcome**	**Recommendations**	**Comments**
Glucosamine sulfate cont'd	Paracetamol	Theoretical decreased pain management	Monitor — unlikely to be clinically relevant	Two case reports in a survey suggested that concomitant use of glucosamine sulfate and paracetamol may lead to decreased pain control in patients with osteoarthritis. This interaction is considered speculative and unlikely to be clinically relevant. The combination is frequently used in practice.
Glutamine (L-glutamine)	Anticonvulsant drugs	Theoretical antagonistic effect	Caution with use of this combination	Glutamine may be metabolised to the excitatory neurotransmitter glutamate which could theoretically antagonise the anticonvulsants effects. Clinical significance is unclear, but caution is advised.
	Antidiabetic drugs	Reduced cardiovascular risk	Combination may be beneficial	One study reported that glutamine supplementation was effective in improving cardiovascular risk factors in patients with type 2 diabetes.
	Antiretroviral therapy	Possible decreased drug adverse effect	May be beneficial — medical supervision recommended	Preliminary clinical research reported that glutamine reduced severity of diarrhoea in HIV patients taking nelfinavir. More research is needed to investigate this possible beneficial interaction.
	Chemotherapy	Possible improved disease management	May be beneficial — medical supervision recommended	Data are inconclusive, but glutamine may potentially have some benefits as an adjunct therapy in patients undergoing chemotherapy. Research suggests oral glutamine may decrease the incidence, severity and duration of mouth pain and oral mucositis in some patients undergoing cancer chemotherapy or bone marrow transplant. Research has suggested that glutamine may also help reduce drug-induced myalgia and arthralgia in patients taking paclitaxel. Other studies have suggested that glutamine may help to reduce chemotherapy-induced diarrhoea and chemotherapy-induced lymphocytopenia. More research is needed but current evidence is promising.
	Human growth hormone	Possible improved disease management	May be beneficial — medical supervision recommended	Glutamine in combination with human growth hormone may decrease dependence on parenteral nutrition in some patients with short bowel syndrome. Research findings have, however, been inconsistent.
	Lactulose	Theoretical decreased drug effects	Monitor — may not be clinically significant	Glutamine may theoretically reduce the drug effects due to an antagonistic action.

TABLE I.2 Nutrient and nutritional supplement interactions—cont'd

Nutrient/ supplement	Drug/drug class	Potential outcome	Recommendations	Comments
Glutathione	Alcohol	Risk of nutrient depletion	May be beneficial to address nutrient depletion	Alcohol may deplete glutathione levels and may theoretically reduce efficacy of glutathione supplements. Supplementation may be beneficial with regular excessive intake of alcohol.
	Chemotherapeutic agents	Reduced risk of drug toxicity	May be beneficial — medical supervision recommended	Evidence suggests that IV glutathione may help to prevent against toxicity induced by several chemotherapeutic agents. It is unclear if oral glutathione will have the same effect. More data are required to investigate clinical significance.
	Paracetamol	Risk of nutrient depletion	May be beneficial to address nutrient depletion	Paracetamol may deplete glutathione levels and may theoretically reduce efficacy of glutathione supplements. Supplementation may be beneficial with chronic or high-dose intake of paracetamol.
Glycine	Clozapine	Theoretical decrease in disease management	Caution with use of this combination	High-dose glycine was shown to interfere with drug antipsychotic activity in a small study of patients with schizophrenia.
Grapefruit	Aliskiren	Decreased drug concentration	Caution with use of this combination	Studies have reported a significant decrease in drug concentration with this combination, which may lead to reduced drug effect. The proposed mechanism for this interaction is due to inhibition of the organic anion transporting polypeptide 2B1 (OATP2B1). Separate dose administration by at least 4 hours if concurrent use is deemed necessary.
	Amiodarone	Increased drug plasma concentration and risk of adverse effects	Avoid combination	Grapefruit juice has been shown to significantly inhibit CYP3A4 enzyme activity. Studies have reported a significant increase in drug concentration with this combination, which increases the risk of adverse effects and drug toxicity.
	Artemether	Increased drug plasma concentration and risk of adverse effects	Avoid combination	Grapefruit juice has been shown to significantly inhibit CYP450 enzyme activity. Studies have reported a significant increase in drug concentration with this combination, which increases the risk of adverse effects and drug toxicity.
	Benzodiazepines, e.g. midazolam, diazepam	Increased drug plasma concentration and risk of adverse effects	Avoid combination	Grapefruit juice has been shown to significantly inhibit CYP3A4 enzyme activity. Studies have reported a significant increase in drug concentration with this combination, which increases the risk of adverse effects and drug toxicity. This interaction has been reported especially with diazepam and midazolam. It does not appear to occur with alprazolam.

Continued

TABLE I.2 Nutrient and nutritional supplement interactions—cont'd				
Nutrient/ supplement	**Drug/drug class**	**Potential outcome**	**Recommendations**	**Comments**
Grapefruit cont'd	Budesonide	Increased drug plasma concentration and risk of adverse effects	Caution with use of this combination	Grapefruit juice has been shown to significantly inhibit CYP3A4 enzyme activity. Studies have reported an increase in drug concentration with this combination, which increases the risk of adverse effects and drug toxicity.
	Buspirone	Increased drug plasma concentration and risk of adverse effects	Avoid combination	Studies have reported a significant increase in drug concentration with this combination, which increases the risk of adverse effects and drug toxicity.
	Caffeine	Increased risk of caffeine-related adverse effects	Caution with use of this combination	Studies have reported an increase in caffeine concentration with this combination, which increases the risk of adverse effects.
	Calcium channel blockers, e.g. verapamil, amlodipine, nifedipine	Increased drug plasma concentration and risk of adverse effects	Avoid combination	Studies have reported a significant increase in drug concentration with this combination, which increases the risk of adverse effects and drug toxicity. It has been proposed that this is due to inhibition of CYP3A4 activity, but some sources suggest other mechanisms may also be involved.
	Carbamazepine	Increased drug plasma concentration and risk of adverse effects	Avoid combination	Increased drug absorption and plasma concentrations have been reported.
	Carvedilol	Increased drug plasma concentration and risk of adverse effects	Avoid combination	Grapefruit juice is reported to increase drug bioavailability.
	Celiprolol	Decreased drug concentration	Avoid combination	Grapefruit juice is reported to decrease drug bioavailability. The proposed mechanism for this interaction is due to inhibition of the organic anion transporting polypeptide (OATP).
	Ciclosporin	Increased drug bioavailability	Avoid combination	Evidence suggests an increase in drug bioavailability with use of this combination.
	Cisapride	Increased drug plasma concentration and risk of adverse effects	Avoid combination	Increased plasma concentrations have been reported.
	Clomipramine	Increased drug plasma concentration and risk of adverse effects	Caution with use of this combination	Increased plasma concentrations have been described in two case reports.
	Clopidogrel	Decreased drug concentration	Avoid combination	Grapefruit juice has been reported to significantly decrease drug concentrations, which could reduce effectiveness as an antiplatelet drug.
	Colchicine	Increased drug plasma concentration and risk of adverse effects	Caution with use of this combination	In-vitro evidence has reported that grapefruit juice increases drug absorption by inhibiting P-gp.

TABLE I.2 Nutrient and nutritional supplement interactions—cont'd

Nutrient/ supplement	Drug/drug class	Potential outcome	Recommendations	Comments
Grapefruit cont'd	CYP450 substrates (CYP1A2, CYP2C19, CYP2C9)	Risk of increased drug plasma concentration and adverse effects	Caution with use of this combination	Preliminary evidence suggests grapefruit juice may inhibit CYP1A2, CYP2C19, CYP2C9. Interactions have not been reported in human studies to date and significance is unclear.
	CYP450 substrates (CYP3A4)	Risk of increased drug plasma concentration and adverse effects	Avoid combination	Grapefruit juice has been shown to significantly inhibit CYP34A enzyme activity. When taken orally, effects of grapefruit juice on CYP3A4 appear to last at least 48 hours.
	Dextromethorphan	Increased drug concentration and risk of adverse effects	Caution with use of this combination	A pharmacokinetic study reported increased concentration of dextromethorphan when taken in combination with grapefruit juice. It has been proposed that the interaction is due to inhibition of CYP3A4.
	Docetaxel	Increased drug plasma concentration and risk of adverse effects	Avoid combination	A case report describes an interaction with use of this combination, leading to increased drug concentrations and a reduction in white blood cell count.
	Erythromycin	Increased drug plasma concentration and risk of adverse effects	Caution with use of this combination	A study reported increased absorption of erythromycin when taken in combination with grapefruit juice.
	Etoposide	Decreased drug concentration and effect	Avoid combination	Studies have reported a significant decrease in drug concentration with this combination, which may lead to reduced drug effect. The proposed mechanism for this interaction is inhibition of the organic anion transporting polypeptide (OATP).
	Fexofenadine	Decreased drug concentration and effect	Caution with use of this combination	Studies have reported a significant decrease in drug concentration with this combination, which may lead to reduced drug effect. The proposed mechanism for this interaction is inhibition of the organic anion transporting polypeptide (OATP).
	Fluvoxamine	Increased drug plasma concentration and risk of adverse effects	Caution with use of this combination	Increased drug plasma concentrations have been reported.
	Halofantrine	Increased drug plasma concentration and risk of adverse effects	Avoid combination	Increased drug plasma concentrations have been reported in a small clinical study. This may lead to an increased risk of prolonged QT interval.
	HMGCoA reductase inhibitors (statins), e.g. atorvastatin, simvastatin	Increased drug plasma concentration and risk of adverse effects	Avoid combination	Grapefruit juice has been shown to significantly inhibit CYP3A4 enzyme activity. Studies have reported a significant increase in drug concentration with this combination, which increases the risk of adverse effects and drug toxicity.

Continued

TABLE I.2 Nutrient and nutritional supplement interactions—cont'd

Nutrient/ supplement	Drug/drug class	Potential outcome	Recommendations	Comments
Grapefruit cont'd	Itraconazole	Altered drug levels possible	Caution with use of this combination	Data on effect of grapefruit juice on this drug are conflicting and significance is unclear. Caution with use until further data become available.
	L-thyroxine (Levothyroxine)	Possible decreased drug effect	Caution with use of this combination	A modest decrease in drug effect has been reported. The proposed mechanism for this interaction is due to inhibition of the organic anion transporting polypeptide (OATP).
	Losartan	Possible decreased drug concentration	Caution with use of this combination	A study in healthy volunteers reported decreased drug concentrations with use of this combination. Clinical significance is unclear.
	Methadone	Increased drug plasma concentration and risk of adverse effects	Caution with use of this combination	An increased drug concentration has been reported with this combination. Clinical significance is unclear.
	Methylprednisolone	Increased drug plasma concentration and risk of adverse effects	Avoid combination	Studies have reported an increase in drug concentration with this combination, which increases the risk of adverse effects and drug toxicity.
	Nadolol	Theoretical decreased drug effect	Caution with use of this combination	Grapefruit juice may theoretically decrease drug bioavailability due to inhibition of the organic anion transporting polypeptide (OATP1A2). It is not known if this interaction is clinically significant.
	Nilotinib	Increased drug plasma concentration and increased absorption	Caution with use of this combination	Increased drug concentration and drug absorption have been reported with this combination.
	Oestrogens	Increased drug plasma concentration and risk of adverse effects	Caution with use of this combination	Increased plasma concentrations have been reported. It has been proposed that this is due to inhibition of CYP3A4.
	Organic anion-transporting polypeptide (OATP) substrates	Possible decreased drug absorption and drug effect	Avoid combination	In-vitro and clinical evidence show that grapefruit juice inhibits organic anion transporting polypeptides (OATP). This reduces bioavailability of oral drugs that are OATP substrates. Separation of dose administration by at least 4 hours may help to avoid this interaction as the effect appears to only last for a short time.
	Oxycodone	Increased drug concentration and risk of adverse effects	Avoid combination	An increase in drug concentration has been reported with this combination. Oxycodone is metabolised by CYP3A4.
	Praziquantel	Increased drug concentration and risk of adverse effects	Avoid combination	Studies have reported a significant increase in drug concentration with this combination, which increases the risk of adverse effects and drug toxicity.
	Primaquine	Possible increased drug bioavailability	Caution with use of this combination	An increase in drug bioavailability has been reported. Clinical significance is unclear.

TABLE I.2 Nutrient and nutritional supplement interactions—cont'd

Nutrient/ supplement	Drug/drug class	Potential outcome	Recommendations	Comments
Grapefruit cont'd	Quinidine	Altered drug effect	Caution with use of this combination	Grapefruit juice has been reported to decrease drug absorption, clearance and metabolism, and to prolong drug half-life. Clinical significance is unclear.
	Regorafenib	Theoretical increased drug concentrations and risk of toxicity	Avoid combination	Grapefruit juice has been shown to significantly inhibit CYP3A4 enzyme activity. While no direct interaction has been reported, this drug is a CYP3A4 substrate.
	Repaglinide	Small increase in serum drug concentration	Caution with use of this combination	A small but significant increase in drug concentration has been reported with use of this combination.
	Saquinavir	Increased drug absorption	Caution with use of this combination	Increased drug absorption has been reported with use of this combination. This interaction does not appear to occur with indinavir, another protease-inhibitor.
	Scopolamine	Increased drug concentration and risk of adverse effects	Avoid combination	An increased drug concentration has been reported with this combination. Scopolamine is metabolised by CYP3A4.
	Sertraline	Increased drug plasma concentration and risk of adverse effects	Caution with use of this combination	Two studies have reported a significant increase in drug concentration with this combination, which increases the risk of adverse effects and drug toxicity.
	Sildenafil	Increased drug concentration and risk of adverse effects	Caution with use of this combination	An increased drug concentration has been reported with this combination. Sildenafil is metabolised by CYP3A4.
	Sunitinib	Possible increase in drug plasma concentration	Caution with use of this combination	A modest increase in drug levels has been reported with use of this combination. This interaction may not be clinically significant, but caution is advised.
	Tacrolimus	Increased drug bioavailability and risk of adverse effects	Avoid combination unless under strict medical supervision	Studies have reported a significant increase in drug bioavailability with this combination. It has been proposed that this may enhance drug action, but strict medical supervision is required due to a lack of reliable safety and efficacy data.
	Talinolol	Possible increased drug bioavailability	Caution with use of this combination	An increase in drug bioavailability may occur with this combination. The clinical significance is unclear.
	Terfenadine	Possible increased drug concentrations	Avoid combination	An increase in drug absorption and plasma concentration have been reported with this combination. Clinical significance is unclear.
	Theophylline	Possible decreased drug concentrations	Caution with use of this combination	A modest decrease in drug levels has been reported. The mechanism of this interaction is unknown.

Continued

TABLE I.2 Nutrient and nutritional supplement interactions—cont'd				
Nutrient/ supplement	**Drug/drug class**	**Potential outcome**	**Recommendations**	**Comments**
Grapefruit cont'd	Ticagrelor	Increased drug plasma concentration and risk of bleeding	Avoid combination	Grapefruit juice has been shown to significantly inhibit CYP3A4 enzyme activity. Studies have reported a significant increase in drug concentration with this combination, which increases the risk of adverse effects and drug toxicity.
	Tolvaptan	Increased drug plasma concentration and risk of adverse effects	Caution with use of this combination	Studies have reported an increase in drug concentration with this combination. This may lead to an increased extent and duration of diuretic effect, and an increased risk of adverse effects and drug toxicity.
	Toremifene	Theoretical increased drug plasma concentration and risk of adverse effects	Avoid combination	Grapefruit juice has been shown to significantly inhibit CYP3A4 enzyme activity. While an interaction between grapefruit juice and this drug have not been demonstrated directly, the drug is a CYP3A4 substrate. There is a theoretical risk of prolonged QT interval.
	Warfarin	Theoretical increased risk of bleeding	Caution with use of this combination	A case report describes an increase in INR is a patient taking large doses of grapefruit juice while on warfarin. A small clinical study reported, however, that daily consumption of grapefruit juice did not affect INR in a group of men taking warfarin. Caution is recommended until more safety data become available.
Green-lipped mussel	NSAIDs	Possible additive effects	Combination may be beneficial	Additive, beneficial effects are theoretically possible due to the anti-inflammatory effects of green-lipped mussel. No negative interaction has been reported with this combination.
Guar gum	Antidiabetic drugs	Theoretical additive effects	Monitor — may not be clinically significant	Guar gum may decrease blood glucose levels. Additive effects are possible, which may be beneficial, but caution is advised to reduce risk of hypoglycaemia.
	Antihypertensive drugs	Theoretical additive effects	Monitor — may not be clinically significant	Some evidence suggests that guar gum may lower blood pressure. Additive effects are theoretically possible, but caution is advised to reduce risk of hypotension.
	Digoxin	Theoretical decreased drug absorption	Caution with use of this combination	Guar gum may reduce drug absorption and theoretically decrease drug effect. Significance has not been established, but caution is advised.
	Metformin	Theoretical decreased drug absorption	Monitor — may not be clinically significant	Guar gum may reduce drug absorption and theoretically decrease drug effect. Significance has not been established.

TABLE I.2 Nutrient and nutritional supplement interactions—cont'd

Nutrient/ supplement	Drug/drug class	Potential outcome	Recommendations	Comments
Guar gum cont'd	Oestrogens	Theoretical decreased drug absorption	Monitor — may not be clinically significant	Guar gum may reduce drug absorption and theoretically decrease drug effect. Significance has not been established.
	Penicillin	Theoretical decreased drug absorption	Monitor — may not be clinically significant	Guar gum may reduce drug absorption and theoretically decrease drug effect. Significance has not been established.
Hesperidin	Anticoagulant/ antiplatelet drugs	Theoretical increased risk of bleeding	Monitor — may not be clinically significant	Hesperidin may have antiplatelet activity. There is a theoretical increased risk of bleeding, but clinical significance has not been established.
	Antihypertensive drugs	Theoretical additive effects	Monitor — may not be clinically significant	Some evidence suggests that hesperidin may lower blood pressure. Additive beneficial effects are theoretically possible but caution is advised to reduce the risk of hypotension.
	CNS depressant drugs including benzodiazepines	Theoretical increased risk of sedation	Monitor — may not be clinically significant	Animal studies suggest hesperidin may have sedative effects due to opioid receptor activity. There is a theoretical increased risk of sedation when used with CNS depressant drugs.
	P-glycoprotein substrates	Theoretical increased drug effect	Monitor — may not be clinically significant	In-vitro studies suggest hesperidin may inhibit p-glycoprotein. Theoretically this could increase drug levels of p-glycoprotein substrates.
Indole-3-carbinol	CYP450 substrates (CYP1A2)	Theoretical increased drug levels	Monitor — clinical significance unclear	In-vitro and in-vivo evidence suggest indole-3-carbinol may inhibit CYP1A2. This could theoretically result in increased drug concentration and risk of drug toxicity, although clinical significance is not known.
Inositol	Anticonvulsant drugs, carbamazepine, valproic acid	Theoretical decrease in inositol levels in the brain.	Monitor — may not be clinically significant	Carbamazepine and valproic acid have been shown to reduce inositol levels in the brain. This is possibly due to these drugs inhibiting an enzyme involved in inositol synthesis. The clinical significance of this is unknown but caution is advised with use of inositol supplements in patients taking these drugs.
	Lithium	Possible reduced drug effect	Caution with use of this combination	Lithium reduces inositol levels in the brain by inhibition of an enzyme involved in synthesis of inositol. Preliminary data also suggest that inositol supplements may reduce the therapeutic effects of lithium, and that dietary restriction of inositol may enhance effects of lithium. Caution is advised until more data become available.

Continued

TABLE I.2 Nutrient and nutritional supplement interactions—cont'd

Nutrient/ supplement	Drug/drug class	Potential outcome	Recommendations	Comments
Iodine	Amiodarone	Risk of excessive iodine	Caution with use of this combination	Amiodarone contains nearly 40% iodine and can increase iodine levels. Concomitant use with iodine supplements may result in excessive iodine levels and may adversely affect thyroid function.
	Anti-thyroid medication, e.g. carbimazole, propylthiouracil	Increased risk of hypothyroidism	Avoid combination	Concomitant use may result in additive hypothyroid activity and may lead to hypothyroidism. The combination should be avoided.
	Lithium	Theoretical increased risk of hypothyroidism	Caution with use of this combination	Lithium may inhibit thyroid function. Combined use may have additive hypothyroid effects.
	Metronidazole	Risk of mineral depletion	May be beneficial to address nutrient depletion	There is a moderate risk of iodine depletion. Patients should be monitored as supplements may be required in some individuals.
Iron	ACE-inhibitors	Possible improvement of drug-induced cough	Combination may be beneficial	Oral iron supplementation may inhibit coughs induced by ACE-I, according to a study that used ferrous sulfate 200 mg. This appears to be due to an effect on nitric oxide generation.
	Acid-reducing agents, e.g. antacids, H_2-antagonists, proton pump inhibitors	Decreased iron absorption	Monitor — separate doses	Adequate gastric acid is important for iron absorption. Drugs that raise gastric pH may theoretically reduce iron absorption. Doses should be separated.
	Antibiotics (quinolones and tetracyclines)	Reduced drug effect	Caution with use of this combination	Iron supplements form complexes with these drugs and may reduce drug effectiveness. Separate doses by at least 2 hours.
	Bisphosphonates	Reduced drug absorption	Caution with use of this combination	Iron can reduce absorption of oral bisphosphonates and reduce drug efficacy. Separate doses by at least 2 hours.
	Chloramphenicol	Theoretical decreased response to mineral	Monitor — may not be clinically significant	Chloramphenicol interferes with maturation of erythrocytes and may reduce response to iron supplements in iron-deficiency anaemia. The interaction is unlikely to be clinically significant as the antibiotic is generally used only short term.
	Integrase inhibitors, e.g. dolutegravir	Reduced drug effect	Caution with use of this combination	Iron supplements may form complexes with drugs in this class and reduce drug effectiveness. Separate doses by at least 2 hours.
	L-thyroxine (Levothyroxine)	Reduced drug effect	Caution with use of this combination	Iron supplements may form complexes with L-thyroxine and reduce drug effectiveness. Separate doses by at least 2 hours.

TABLE I.2 Nutrient and nutritional supplement interactions—cont'd				
Nutrient/ supplement	**Drug/drug class**	**Potential outcome**	**Recommendations**	**Comments**
Iron cont'd	Levodopa	Reduced drug effect	Caution with use of this combination	Iron supplements may form complexes with levodopa and reduce drug effectiveness. Separate doses by at least 2 hours.
	Methyldopa	Reduced drug effect	Caution with use of this combination	Iron supplements are known to form complexes with methyldopa and reduce drug effectiveness. Separate doses by at least 2 hours or avoid combination.
	Minerals (calcium, zinc)	Reduced mineral absorption	Monitor — separate doses	Calcium may inhibit the absorption of haem and non-haem iron. This may not be clinically significant unless there is iron deficiency. Doses should be separated. Iron and zinc supplements can interfere with each other's absorption, especially if taken on an empty stomach due to competition for nonspecific carriers. The interaction does not appear to be significant if the supplements are taken with food as the ions complex with food components. Take supplements with food or separate intake.
	Mycophenolate mofetil	Theoretical decreased drug absorption	Caution with use of this combination	It has been proposed that iron may form an insoluble chelate with this drug and decrease absorption. This has not been demonstrated in clinical studies, but caution is advised and dose administration should be separated.
	Penicillamine	Reduced drug effect	Caution with use of this combination	Iron supplements may form complexes with penicillamine and reduce drug effectiveness. Separate doses by at least 2 hours.
	Vitamin C	Increased vitamin absorption	Combination may be beneficial	Vitamin C (dietary and supplemental) improves absorption of iron if ingested at the same time.
Krill oil — see Omega-3 essential fatty acids				
L-arginine — see Arginine				
L-carnitine — see Carnitine				
L-glutamine — see Glutamine				
L-tryptophan — see Tryptophan				
Lutein	Orlistat	Theoretical risk of nutrient depletion	May be beneficial to address nutrient depletion	Theoretically, long-term use of orlistat may result in lutein depletion due to reduced gastrointestinal absorption. Patients should be monitored. Supplements may be required in some individuals.
Lycopene	Anticoagulant/ antiplatelet drugs	Theoretical increased risk of bleeding	Caution with use of this combination	Lycopene may have antiplatelet effects based on in-vitro studies. There is a theoretical increased risk of bleeding.

Continued

TABLE I.2 Nutrient and nutritional supplement interactions—cont'd

Nutrient/ supplement	Drug/drug class	Potential outcome	Recommendations	Comments
Lysine	Antiviral therapy, e.g. aciclovir, famciclovir	Improved disease management	Combination may be beneficial	Lysine has been shown to be beneficial in reducing the recurrence of herpes simplex infections, and may reduce severity and healing times of herpes simplex infections. No negative interactions have been reported in the literature with use of lysine concurrently with antiviral therapy for herpes infection.
Magnesium	Alcohol	Risk of mineral depletion	May be beneficial to address nutrient depletion	High ingestion of alcohol may result in magnesium depletion. Alcohol impairs the kidney's ability to conserve magnesium and so may result in increased urinary excretion. Supplements may be indicated in some individuals.
	Anticoagulant/ antiplatelet drugs	Theoretical increased risk of bleeding	Monitor — clinical significance unclear	In-vitro evidence suggests magnesium sulfate may inhibit platelet aggregation. Some preliminary clinical research suggests that IV magnesium may increase bleeding time and reduce platelet activity, but results from research have been inconsistent and conflicting.
	Antibiotics (aminogylcosides)	Theoretical increased risk of neuromuscular adverse effects; theoretical risk of mineral depletion	Caution with use of this combination	An animal study reported that concurrent use of IV magnesium and aminoglycoside antibiotics led to neuromuscular weakness and possible paralysis. A case report describes respiratory failure in an infant with high blood magnesium levels after administration of gentamycin. Magnesium and aminoglycoside antibiotics both reduce presynaptic release of acetylcholine, which can affect neuromuscular function. Aminoglycosides have also been associated with nephrotoxicity which may increase urinary loss of magnesium.
	Antibiotics (tetracyclines and quinolones)	Reduced drug effect possible	Caution with use of this combination	Magnesium supplements form complexes with these drugs and may reduce drug effectiveness. Use with caution and separate doses by at least 2 hours.
	Antidiabetic drugs (sulfonylureas), e.g. glibenclamide, glipizide	Theoretical increased drug absorption	Monitor — clinical significance unclear	Antacids containing magnesium hydroxide raise gastric pH, which is reported to increase absorption of glibenclamide and glipizide. This may theoretically increase the risk of hypoglycaemia.
	Amphotericin-B	Major risk of mineral depletion	May be beneficial to address nutrient depletion	There is a major risk of magnesium depletion associated with use of this antifungal agent (not marketed in Australia). Supplements may be required with long-term use.

TABLE I.2 Nutrient and nutritional supplement interactions—cont'd				
Nutrient/ supplement	**Drug/drug class**	**Potential outcome**	**Recommendations**	**Comments**
Magnesium cont'd	Bisphosphonates	Risk of decreased drug absorption	Caution with use of this combination — separate doses	Magnesium may reduce drug absorption and bioavailability by forming drug-mineral complexes. Separate dose administration by 2 hours.
	Calcium channel blockers	Additive effect possible	Combination may be beneficial — monitor	Magnesium may theoretically have an additive effect when used with calcium channel blockers at high doses. The interaction is likely to be beneficial at normal therapeutic doses, although there is a theoretical risk of hypotension. Caution is advised as some research has reported severe hypotension and neuromuscular blockade with concurrent use of IV magnesium and nifedipine.
	Ciclosporin	Risk of mineral depletion	May be beneficial to address nutrient depletion	Moderate risk of depletion. Patients should be monitored and supplements may be required in some individuals.
	Corticosteroids (chronic use)	Risk of mineral depletion	May be beneficial to address nutrient depletion	Moderate risk of depletion. Patients should be monitored and supplements may be required in some individuals.
	Digoxin	Risk of decreased drug effect; risk of mineral depletion	Caution with use of this combination	Clinical evidence suggests that oral magnesium hydroxide or magnesium trisilicate may reduce digoxin absorption, which could lead to decreased therapeutic effects. Digoxin may also result in increased urinary excretion of magnesium, resulting in a moderate risk of depletion. Patients should be monitored and supplements may be required in some individuals. Depletion increases the risk of arrhythmias and may have serious consequences. The likelihood of depletion is increased if the patient is also taking diuretics, e.g. in heart failure.
	Diuretics (loop and thiazide)	Risk of mineral depletion	May be beneficial to address nutrient depletion	Moderate risk of depletion. Patients should be monitored and supplements may be required in some individuals.
	Diuretics (potassium-sparing)	Possible risk of excessive magnesium	Monitor — may not be clinically significant	Potassium-sparing diuretics may also spare magnesium. Theoretically concomitant use of magnesium supplements with potassium-sparing diuretics may result in raised magnesium levels; however, significance is not clear.

Continued

TABLE I.2 Nutrient and nutritional supplement interactions—cont'd

Nutrient/ supplement	Drug/drug class	Potential outcome	Recommendations	Comments
Magnesium cont'd	Foscarnet	Risk of mineral depletion	May be beneficial to address nutrient depletion	Foscarnet may result in symptomatic hypomagnesaemia, possibly due to magnesium chelation and increased elimination. Magnesium levels should be monitored and supplements may be required in some patients.
	Minerals (calcium, zinc)	Reduced mineral absorption	Monitor — separate doses	Calcium may decrease absorption of magnesium. Magnesium does not appear to affect calcium absorption. High-dose zinc supplements may decrease magnesium absorption and increase magnesium excretion. These interactions may not be clinically relevant unless there is a deficiency, but dosage separation is generally advised.
	Oestrogens, e.g. oral contraceptives, HRT	Risk of mineral depletion	May be beneficial to address nutrient depletion	There is a moderate risk of depletion with long-term use of oestrogens. Oestrogens enhance uptake of magnesium into soft tissue and bones which may lower serum levels. Patients should be monitored and supplements may be required in some individuals.
	Panitumumab	Risk of mineral depletion	May be beneficial to address nutrient depletion	Hypomagnesaemia has occurred with use of this drug, with decreased magnesium levels being reported in almost 40% of patients according to secondary sources. Monitor for signs of magnesium depletion.
	Penicillamine	Possible decreased drug absorption	Caution with use of this combination	Magnesium may reduce drug bioavailability by forming insoluble drug-mineral complexes. Dose administration should be separated and patients should be monitored for magnesium depletion with long-term drug use.
	Pentamidine	Major risk of mineral depletion	May be beneficial to address nutrient depletion	Symptomatic hypomagnesaemia has occurred with use of this drug, especially when given intravenously. Patients should be monitored and supplements will be needed in most patients with long-term use.
	Proguanil	Possible decreased drug absorption	Caution with use of this combination	A small study reported that concomitant use of magnesium trisilicate and the antimalarial drug proguanil resulted in a significant decrease in drug absorption. Separate dose administration by at least 3 hours.

TABLE I.2 Nutrient and nutritional supplement interactions—cont'd

Nutrient/ supplement	Drug/drug class	Potential outcome	Recommendations	Comments
Magnesium cont'd	Proton pump inhibitors (PPIs)	Major risk of mineral depletion	May be beneficial to address nutrient depletion	PPIs inhibit the active transport of magnesium and long-term use may lead to severe hypomagnesaemia with side effects including muscle spasm, tetany, hypokalaemia, hypoparathyroidism, hypocalcaemia, and seizures. A magnesium supplement will be required by most individuals who take PPIs long term.
	Tacrolimus	Major risk of mineral depletion	May be beneficial to address nutrient depletion	Tacrolimus reduces renal tubular reabsorption of magnesium. Hypomagnesaemia is reported in a significant proportion of people treated with tacrolimus. Supplements will be required in most individuals.
Manganese	Antibiotics, e.g. tetracyclines and quinolones	Reduced drug effect possible	Monitor — separate doses	Manganese supplements form complexes with these drugs, which may theoretically reduce drug effectiveness. Separate doses by at least 2 hours.
Melatonin	Anticoagulant/ antiplatelet drugs	Possible increased risk of bleeding	Caution with use of this combination	Isolated case reports describe bleeding with use of warfarin and melatonin which suggests a possible interaction. More data are needed to confirm interaction.
	Anticonvulsant drugs	Possible increased risk of seizures	Caution with use of this combination	Some clinical evidence suggests that melatonin may increase the risk of seizures in certain patients, especially in neurologically disabled children. Melatonin may inhibit drug effects in these patients.
	Antidiabetic drugs	Possible altered disease management	Caution with use of this combination	Some evidence suggests that melatonin may impair glucose utilisation and increase insulin resistance. Other studies have reported improved glycaemic control, while still others have reported that melatonin has no effect on glucose levels. Caution is advised until more data become available.
	Antihypertensive drugs, e.g. verapamil, nifedipine	Possible altered disease management	Caution with use of this combination	Melatonin may decrease blood pressure according to some studies. Other studies however report that melatonin may worsen blood pressure in patients taking antihypertensive drugs. Caution is advised until more data become available.
	Benzodiazepines	Possible reduced endogenous melatonin. Risk of excessive sedative effects with combined use.	Caution with use of this combination	Theoretically, chronic intake of benzodiazepines may decrease endogenous melatonin levels. Additive effects are possible with combined use which may lead to excessive drowsiness and sedation.

Continued

TABLE I.2 Nutrient and nutritional supplement interactions—cont'd				
Nutrient/ supplement	**Drug/drug class**	**Potential outcome**	**Recommendations**	**Comments**
Melatonin cont'd	CNS depressant drugs	Risk of excessive sedative effects	Caution with use of this combination	Additive effects are possible which may lead to excessive drowsiness and sedation.
	Fluvoxamine	Risk of increased melatonin levels	Caution with use of this combination	Fluvoxamine can significantly increase melatonin levels and may lead to excessive drowsiness.
	Hypnotic drugs including zolpidem	Risk of excessive sedative effects	Caution with use of this combination	Additive effects are possible which may lead to excessive drowsiness and sedation.
	Immunosuppressant drugs	Possible decreased drug effect	Caution with use of this combination	Melatonin may have immunostimulant activity. This may theoretically interfere with immunosuppressive drug action.
	Methamphetamine	Theoretical increased drug adverse effects	Caution with use of this combination	Animal research suggests melatonin may exacerbate adverse effects of methamphetamine.
	Nifedipine	Possible decreased drug effect	Caution with use of this combination	Preliminary evidence suggests that melatonin may impair antihypertensive activity of nifedipine. Caution is advised until further data become available.
	Oestrogens	Risk of excessive sedative effects	Caution with use of this combination	Oestrogens may inhibit metabolism of melatonin, which may result in increased drowsiness and sedation.
	Propofol	Possible decreased drug requirement for anaesthesia	Caution with use of this combination	A study reported that the combination resulted in a decreased dose requirement of propofol to induce anaesthesia.
	Psoralen medication, e.g. 5-methoxypsoralen	Risk of excessive sedative effects	Caution with use of this combination	Drugs in this class may inhibit metabolism of melatonin, which may result in increased drowsiness and sedation.
	Seizure threshold lowering drugs	Possible increased risk of seizures	Caution with use of this combination	Some clinical evidence suggests a risk of increased frequency of seizures with this combination, especially in neurologically disabled children.
N-acetyl cysteine (NAC)	ACE-inhibitors (ACE-I)	Theoretical additive effects	Caution with use of this combination	According to animal research NAC may potentiate the blood pressure-lowering effects of ACE-I. The interaction may potentially be beneficial, but caution is advised due to a risk of hypotension.
	Activated charcoal	Possible decreased effect of activated charcoal	Caution with use of this combination	According to some studies NAC may possibly reduce the ability of activated charcoal to adsorb paracetamol and aspirin. Activated charcoal does not appear to affect effectiveness of NAC.
	Anticoagulant/ antiplatelet drugs	Increased risk of bleeding	Caution with use of this combination	NAC may decrease platelet aggregation and prothrombin time, prolong coagulation time and increase blood loss in surgical patients.

TABLE I.2 Nutrient and nutritional supplement interactions—cont'd				
Nutrient/ supplement	**Drug/drug class**	**Potential outcome**	**Recommendations**	**Comments**
N-acetyl cysteine (NAC) cont'd	Antihypertensive drugs	Theoretical additive effects	Caution with use of this combination	According to animal research NAC may potentiate the blood pressure-lowering effects of ACE-I. This effect may theoretically also be seen with other antihypertensive drugs. The interaction may potentially be beneficial, but caution is advised due to a risk of hypotension.
	Chloroquine	Theoretical decreased drug effect	Caution with use of this combination	Animal research suggests NAC may reduce drug antimalarial effect by increasing cellular levels of glutathione.
	Clomiphene	Possible improved outcomes	May be beneficial — medical supervision recommended	NAC was shown to be a safe and effective adjuvant to clomiphene in improving induction of ovulation in patients with PCOS.
	Nitroglycerine (glyceryl trinitrate)	Increased risk of hypotension and severe headache	Avoid combination	Concurrent use of NAC and IV nitroglycerine may cause severe hypotension and intolerable headaches according to limited clinical research.
Nattokinase	Anticoagulant/ antiplatelet drugs	Theoretical increased risk of bleeding	Caution with use of this combination	In-vitro and animal studies suggest that nattokinase may have antiplatelet effects. There is a theoretical increased risk of bleeding.
	Antihypertensive drugs	Possible additive effects	Combination may be beneficial	Nattokinase has been shown to reduce blood pressure in clinical trials. Concurrent use may be additive and potentially beneficial, but monitor for hypotension.
Omega-3 essential fatty acids (EPA and DHA)	Anticoagulant/ antiplatelet drugs	Possible additive effects, with theoretical increased risk of bleeding	Monitor, but unlikely to be clinically significant	There has long been concern that use of fish or krill oil supplements may increase the risk of bleeding with anticoagulant/antiplatelet drugs, due to the antiplatelet activity of EPA. A recent large retrospective analysis, however, found no reports of an interaction between warfarin and fish or krill oil. This supports findings of other studies that found no evidence of an interaction between warfarin and fish oil. Monitoring is advised at very high-dose intake (equivalent to ≥12 g fish oil daily).
	Antihypertensive drugs	Possible additive effects	Combination may be beneficial	Omega-3 fatty acids as fish oils have been shown to have a small, but consistent blood pressure lowering effect. Additive beneficial effects may be seen when used concomitantly with antihypertensive drugs.
	Chemotherapy	Possible improved outcomes	Combination may be beneficial	Omega-3 fatty acids may provide nutritional, anti-inflammatory and cardiovascular support and enhance overall patient management. There does not appear to be evidence of a negative interaction.

Continued

TABLE I.2 Nutrient and nutritional supplement interactions—cont'd

Nutrient/ supplement	Drug/drug class	Potential outcome	Recommendations	Comments
Omega-3 essential fatty acids (EPA and DHA) cont'd	Ciclosporin	Possible reduced drug adverse effects	Combination may be beneficial	Some research evidence suggests omega-3 fatty acids may help to reduce blood pressure and preserve renal function in patients following organ transplantation. Results have been inconsistent.
	Corticosteroids	Possible improved outcomes	Combination may be beneficial	Omega-3 supplements may improve management of inflammatory conditions, including RA and IBD. Theoretically the combination may allow for lower dose requirements of corticosteroids. There does not appear to be evidence of a negative interaction.
	Lipid-lowering drugs — hypertriglyceridaemia	Possible additive effects	Combination may be beneficial	Omega-3 essential fatty acids as fish oils have been shown to significantly reduce triglyceride levels and may be beneficial as an adjunct therapy with drugs used to treat hypertriglyceridaemia.
	Non-steroidal anti-inflammatory drugs (NSAIDs)	Possible additive effects	Combination may be beneficial	Fish or krill oil can reduce inflammation, pain and swelling due to the EPA content. The combination will have an additive, beneficial effect especially in the management of conditions such as arthritis.
	Sulfasalazine	Possible improved outcomes	Combination may be beneficial	Omega-3 fatty acid supplements may improve management of inflammatory conditions, including RA and IBD. Theoretically the combination may allow for lower drug dose requirements. There does not appear to be evidence of a negative interaction.
Papain	Anticoagulants/ antiplatelet drugs	Theoretical increased risk of bleeding	Caution with use of this combination	Combined use may theoretically potentiate the effects of warfarin. Clinical significance is unclear.
Phosphatidylcholine	Acetylcholinesterase (AChE) inhibitors, e.g. donepezil, rivastigmine	Theoretical increased risk of cholinergic adverse effects	Caution with use of this combination	Phosphatidylcholine may theoretically increase acetylcholine levels. The combination could theoretically increase the risk of cholinergic adverse effects.
	Anticholinergic drugs	Theoretical decreased drug effect	Caution with use of this combination	Phosphatidylcholine may theoretically increase acetylcholine levels. The combination could theoretically decrease effectiveness of anticholinergic drugs.
	Cholinergic drugs	Theoretical increased risk of cholinergic adverse effects	Caution with use of this combination	Phosphatidylcholine may theoretically increase acetylcholine levels. The combination could theoretically increase the risk of cholinergic adverse effects.
Phosphatidylserine	Acetylcholinesterase (AChE) inhibitors, e.g. donepezil, rivastigmine	Theoretical increased risk of cholinergic adverse effects	Caution with use of this combination	Phosphatidylserine may theoretically increase acetylcholine levels. The combination could theoretically increase the risk of cholinergic adverse effects.

TABLE I.2 Nutrient and nutritional supplement interactions—cont'd

Nutrient/ supplement	Drug/drug class	Potential outcome	Recommendations	Comments
Phosphatidylserine cont'd	Anticholinergic drugs	Theoretical decreased drug effect	Caution with use of this combination	Phosphatidylserine may theoretically increase acetylcholine levels. The combination could theoretically decrease effectiveness of anticholinergic drugs.
	Cholinergic drugs	Theoretical increased risk of cholinergic adverse effects	Caution with use of this combination	Phosphatidylserine may theoretically increase acetylcholine levels. The combination could theoretically increase the risk of cholinergic adverse effects.
Pomegranate	ACE-inhibitors (ACE-I)	Theoretical additive effects	Caution with use of this combination	Pomegranate may have an action similar to ACE-inhibitors, leading to a theoretical increased risk of hypotension and potassium depletion.
	Antihypertensive drugs	Theoretical additive effects	Caution with use of this combination	Pomegranate may moderately lower blood pressure. There is a theoretical increased risk of hypotension.
	Carbamazepine	Theoretical risk of increased drug levels	Caution with use of this combination	Animal models suggest pomegranate juice may decrease the rate of drug metabolism and increase drug serum levels. Limited clinical research suggests this effect may not occur in humans. Caution is advised until more data become available.
	CYP450 substrates (CYP2C9, CYP2D6, CYP3A4)	Theoretical risk of increased drug levels	Caution with use of this combination	Animal models suggest pomegranate may inhibit activity of CYP2C9 and CYP2D6. There is a theoretical risk of increased drug levels and adverse effects, but clinical significance in humans is currently unknown. There is contradictory evidence as to the effect of pomegranate on CYP3A4, with some reports suggesting enzyme inhibition, others suggesting enzyme induction and still others showing no effect.
	Rosuvastatin	Theoretical increased risk of drug adverse effects	Caution with use of this combination	A case report describes a patient on rosuvastatin who developed rhabdomyolysis 3 weeks after commencing pomegranate juice, 200 mL taken twice weekly. It is possible the patient was predisposed to this adverse effect as there was a history of elevated creatine kinase levels.
	Tacrolimus	Theoretical increased drug levels	Avoid combination	A case report describes elevated drug levels while consuming concentrated pomegranate popsicles. More data are required to determine significance.

Continued

TABLE I.2 Nutrient and nutritional supplement interactions—cont'd

Nutrient/ supplement	Drug/drug class	Potential outcome	Recommendations	Comments
Pomegranate cont'd	Warfarin	Theoretical increased risk of bleeding	Caution with use of this combination	Two case reports suggest high intake of pomegranate juice may increase bleeding time in patients taking warfarin. Until more safety data become available, patients taking warfarin should neither significantly increase, nor decrease, intake of pomegranate juice without medical supervision.
Potassium	ACE-inhibitors (ACE-I)	Increased risk of hyperkalaemia	Caution with use of this combination	ACE-I have a potassium-sparing action. Concomitant use may theoretically increase the risk of hyperkalaemia. In practice, ACE-I are often prescribed with potassium-depleting diuretics, so this interaction may not be clinically relevant.
	Aminoglycosides	Risk of mineral depletion	Combination may be beneficial	Aminoglycosides may cause nephrotoxicity, which can lead to increased urinary loss of potassium. Patients should be monitored.
	Amphotericin-B	Major risk of mineral depletion	May be beneficial to address nutrient depletion	There is a major risk of potassium depletion associated with use of this anti-fungal agent (not marketed in Australia). Supplements may be required with long-term use.
	Angiotensin receptor blockers (ARBs)	Increased risk of hyperkalaemia	Caution with use of this combination	ARBs have a potassium-sparing action. Concomitant use may theoretically increase the risk of hyperkalaemia. In practice, ARBs are often prescribed with potassium-depleting diuretics, so this interaction may not be clinically relevant.
	Cisplatin	Risk of mineral depletion	May be beneficial to address nutrient depletion	Cisplatin can cause renal tubular damage which may result in increased loss of electrolytes, including potassium.
	Corticosteroids	Risk of mineral depletion	May be beneficial to address nutrient depletion	Corticosteroids can cause sodium retention, resulting in a compensatory renal loss of potassium. Risk of hypokalaemia has been associated with drugs such as hydrocortisone, cortisone, fludrocortisone, prednisone and prednisolone.
	Diuretics — potassium depleting e.g. loop and thiazides	Major risk of mineral depletion	May be beneficial to address nutrient depletion	There is a major risk of potassium depletion associated with use of potassium depleting diuretics. Supplements may be required with long-term use.
	Diuretics — potassium sparing	Increased risk of hyperkalaemia	Caution with use of this combination	Concomitant use of potassium supplements with potassium-sparing diuretics may increase the risk of hyperkalaemia.
	Methylxanthines	Possible risk of mineral depletion	May be beneficial to address nutrient depletion	Theophylline and related drugs have been shown to reduce serum potassium levels. Patients should be monitored for signs of hypokalaemia.

TABLE I.2 Nutrient and nutritional supplement interactions—cont'd

Nutrient/ supplement	Drug/drug class	Potential outcome	Recommendations	Comments
Potassium cont'd	Penicillins	Possible risk of mineral depletion	May be beneficial to address nutrient depletion	Penicillins may theoretically promote potassium excretion. This is unlikely to be a concern with short-term antibiotic use, but monitor for signs of hypokalaemia with long-term use. Supplements may be required in some individuals.
	Stimulant laxatives	Possible risk of mineral depletion	May be beneficial to address nutrient depletion	Hypokalaemia has been reported with long-term use of stimulant laxatives, or acute use of high doses. Monitor for signs of depletion.
	Succinylcholine	Theoretical increased risk of hyperkalaemia	Caution with use of this combination	A case report describes the occurrence of hyperkalaemia following administration of succinylcholine. Theoretically, concurrent use of this drug and potassium supplements may increase the risk of hyperkalaemia; however, clinical significance is unclear.
Probiotics	Antibiotics	Reduced drugs adverse effects	Combination may be beneficial	Probiotics can reduce the risk of adverse effects of antibiotics such as gastrointestinal disturbances including diarrhoea, and urogenital disturbances such as thrush/*Candida*. Dosage separation is recommended.
Propolis	Anticoagulant/ antiplatelet drugs	Theoretical increased risk of bleeding	Monitor — may not be clinically significant	In-vitro evidence suggests that a constituent of propolis may inhibit platelet aggregation. The interaction is speculative.
Proteolytic enzymes — see Bromelain, Papain				
Pumpkin seeds	Lithium	Theoretical increased risk of drug toxicity	Caution with use of this combination	Pumpkin may have diuretic properties. This may theoretically reduce drug excretion and increase the risk of drug toxicity. Significance is unclear.
Pycnogenol	Anticoagulant/ antiplatelet drugs	Theoretical increased risk of bleeding	Caution with use of this combination	According to clinical research pycnogenol may have antiplatelet properties. Concomitant use may theoretically increase the risk of bleeding and bruising.
	Antidiabetic drugs	Possible additive effects	Caution with use of this combination	Pycnogenol appears to have hypoglycaemic properties according to human studies. Additive effects are theoretically possible, increasing the risk of hypoglycaemia. Caution is advised until more data become available.
	Antihypertensive drugs, e.g. ramipril	Possible protective effects on renal function in patients at risk	May be beneficial — medical supervision recommended	A small study reported that pycnogenol conferred protective effects on renal function in a group of patients taking ramipril, who had advanced hypertension and a history of cardiovascular events.

Continued

TABLE I.2 Nutrient and nutritional supplement interactions—cont'd				
Nutrient/ supplement	**Drug/drug class**	**Potential outcome**	**Recommendations**	**Comments**
Pycnogenol cont'd	Cardiovascular drugs	Possible improved disease management	May be beneficial — medical supervision recommended	Pycnogenol appears to have antioxidant, antiplatelet and anti-inflammatory effects. A small study reported that pycnogenol was effective in improving endothelial function and reducing oxidative stress in patients with stable coronary artery disease.
	Immunosuppressant drugs	Theoretical decreased drug effects	Caution with use of this combination	Pycnogenol may have immunostimulant properties which could theoretically antagonise the effects of immunosuppressant drugs. Significance is unclear, but caution is advised until further data become available.
Quercetin	Adriamycin	Theoretical decreased risk of drug-induced cardiotoxicity	May be beneficial — medical supervision recommended	Animal studies suggest quercetin may have a protective effect against drug-induced cardiotoxicity.
	Antihypertensive drugs	Possible additive effects	May be beneficial — medical supervision recommended	Quercetin can modestly lower blood pressure in people with mild hypertension. The combination may be beneficial, but monitor for signs of hypotension.
	Ciclosporin	Possible increased drug effects	Caution with use of this combination	A small study in healthy volunteers found that pre-treatment with quercetin led to increased drug plasma levels and prolonged half-life. Caution is advised until more data become available.
	Cisplatin	Theoretical increased drug effect	May be beneficial — medical supervision recommended	In-vitro evidence suggests pre-treatment with quercetin may sensitise cervical cancer cells to drug-induced apoptosis. Clinical significance is not known.
	CYP450 substrates (CYP2C8, CYP2C9, CYP2D6, CYP3A4)	Theoretical increased drug levels	Monitor — may not be clinically significant	Preliminary evidence suggests quercetin may inhibit activity of CYP2C8, CYP2C9, CYP2D6 and CYP3A4. Theoretically, this may lead to increased drug levels and risk of adverse effects.
	Digoxin	Theoretical increased drug bioavailability	Caution with use of this combination	Quercetin may result in increased drug bioavailability according to the findings of an in-vivo study. Caution is advised until more data become available, especially as this drug has a narrow therapeutic index.
	Diltiazem	Theoretical increased drug bioavailability	Caution with use of this combination	Quercetin may result in increased drug bioavailability according to the findings of an animal study. The interaction may not be clinically significant, but caution is advised until more data become available.
	Doxorubicin	Theoretical increased drug effect	May be beneficial — medical supervision recommended	In-vitro studies suggest quercetin may potentiate drug antitumour effect. Further research is needed to investigate the relevance of this interaction.

TABLE I.2 Nutrient and nutritional supplement interactions—cont'd

Nutrient/ supplement	Drug/drug class	Potential outcome	Recommendations	Comments
Quercetin cont'd	Haloperidol	Possible increased drug effects	May be beneficial — medical supervision recommended	Results from animal studies suggest that quercetin may reduce haloperidol-induced tardive dyskinesia. A positive interaction is theoretically possible, although this effect has not yet been described in human studies.
	Iron	Possible decreased iron absorption	Monitor and separate dose administration	Quercetin chelates iron and may reduce bioavailability. Intake of quercetin and iron supplements should be separated by 2 hours.
	Paclitaxel	Theoretical increased drug effects	Caution with use of this combination	Quercetin may result in increased drug bioavailability according to the findings of an animal study. This drug is used in the treatment of cancer and the interaction could theoretically be beneficial under medical supervision, but drug dose adjustments may be required. Caution is advised until more data become available.
	P-glycoprotein substrates	Theoretical increased drug bioavailability	Caution with use of this combination	Preliminary evidence suggests quercetin may inhibit the gastrointestinal p-glycoprotein (P-gp) efflux pump. This may theoretically increase drug bioavailability of P-gp substrates. Significance is unclear based on current evidence, but caution is advised with use of high-dose quercetin in combination with P-gp substrates.
	Pioglitazone	Theoretical increased drug bioavailability	Caution with use of this combination	In-vitro evidence suggests quercetin may increase drug bioavailability. While human data are not yet available, there is a theoretical increased risk of adverse effects and drug toxicity. The antidiabetic drug has been associated with rare incidences of hepatic damage, heart failure and pulmonary oedema.
	Quinolone antibiotics	Theoretical decreased drug effect	Caution with use of this combination	Limited evidence suggests that quercetin may theoretically reduce drug action by competitive inhibition at the DNA gyrase binding site.
	Warfarin	Theoretical increased risk of bleeding	Caution with use of this combination	In-vitro evidence suggests quercetin may increase warfarin levels by displacement at the human serum albumin (HSA) binding site. Significance is unknown.
Resveratrol	Anticoagulant/ antiplatelet drugs	Theoretical increased risk of bleeding	Monitor — may not be clinically significant	Resveratrol may have antiplatelet effects. There is a theoretical increased risk of bleeding. Monitor patients taking this combination, but clinical significance is unclear.

Continued

TABLE I.2 Nutrient and nutritional supplement interactions—cont'd

Nutrient/ supplement	Drug/drug class	Potential outcome	Recommendations	Comments
Resveratrol cont'd	CYP450 substrates (CYP1A1, CYP1A2, CYP1B1, CYP2C19, CYP2E1, CYP3A4)	Theoretical increased drug levels	Monitor — may not be clinically significant	In-vitro evidence suggests resveratrol may inhibit activity of CYP1A1, CYP1A2, CYP1B1, CYP2C19, CYP2E1 and CYP3A4. Theoretically, this may lead to increased drug levels; however, these interactions have not been reported in humans.
Saccharomyces boulardii	Antifungal drugs	Theoretical decreased drug effectiveness	Monitor — clinical significance is unclear	Theoretically *Saccharomyces boulardii* may reduce antifungal action as it is a yeast, however this interaction is speculative.
SAMe (S-adenosyl-L-methionine)	Antidepressant drugs (SSRIs, SNRIs, TCAs)	Possible improved disease management. Increased risk of serotonin syndrome	Avoid combination unless under medical supervision	Some evidence suggests that concomitant use may be beneficial in patients who are not responding adequately to conventional antidepressant drugs. Strict medical supervision would be required with use of this combination as there is an increased risk of serotonergic effects and serotonin syndrome.
	Dextromethorphan	Theoretical increased risk of serotonin syndrome	Caution with use of this combination	Theoretically, concurrent use may have additive serotonergic effects at high doses, which increases the risk of serotonin syndrome.
	Levodopa	Theoretical decreased drug effects	Caution with use of this combination	SAMe methylates levodopa, which may reduce drug effectiveness and theoretically worsen symptoms of Parkinson's disease.
	Monoamine oxidase inhibitors (MAOIs)	Increased risk of serotonin syndrome	Avoid combination	Concurrent use may have additive serotonergic effects, which increases the risk of serotonin syndrome. SAMe should be avoided in patients taking MAOIs and for 2 weeks after discontinuation of MAOIs.
	Oral contraceptives	May be beneficial in women at risk of hepatobiliary dysfunction	Combination may be beneficial	Co-administration may be beneficial in patients at risk of hepatobiliary dysfunction, according to secondary sources. SAMe supports liver detoxification process, including production of glutathione.
	Tramadol	Theoretical increased risk of serotonin syndrome	Caution with use of this combination	Theoretically, concurrent use may have additive serotonergic effects at high doses, which increases the risk of serotonin syndrome.
Selenium	Antiplatelet/ anticoagulant drugs	Theoretical increased risk of bleeding	Caution with use of this combination	There is a theoretical increased risk of bleeding with this combination. Preliminary evidence suggests that selenium may reduce platelet aggregation. Animal studies suggest selenium may increase warfarin activity.
	Barbiturates	Theoretical prolonged sedative effects	Caution with use of this combination	Preliminary evidence suggests selenium may inhibit hepatic metabolism of barbiturates and prolong the sedative effects. This has not been demonstrated in humans but caution is advised.

TABLE I.2 Nutrient and nutritional supplement interactions—cont'd

Nutrient/ supplement	Drug/drug class	Potential outcome	Recommendations	Comments
Selenium cont'd	Cisplatin	Theoretical decrease in drug adverse effects	May be beneficial — more data are required	Preliminary evidence suggests cisplatin may lower selenium levels in humans. Furthermore, in-vitro and animal studies suggest that selenium may help to reduce drug-induced nephrotoxicity, myeloid suppression and weight loss. There is insufficient evidence to know if selenium supplements would be beneficial.
	Clozapine	Theoretical nutrient depletion	May be beneficial — more data are required	Low plasma selenium levels have been observed in some patients taking clozapine. It has been speculated that this may contribute to drug-induced adverse effects; however, there are insufficient data to routinely recommend selenium supplements for patients taking clozapine.
	Corticosteroids	Possible nutrient depletion	Combination may be beneficial	Some evidence suggests that high-dose corticosteroids may increase urinary excretion of selenium and reduce plasma levels. Data are, however, conflicting. Some inflammatory conditions have also been associated with low selenium status. Selenium supplementation may theoretically be beneficial and could also support immunity.
	Doxorubicin	Theoretical decrease in drug adverse effects	May be beneficial — medical supervision recommended	Animal research suggests selenium may help to reduce risk of drug-induced cardiotoxicity without affecting drug efficacy.
	Heavy metals, e.g. mercury, lead, arsenic, silver, cadmium	Theoretical decreased risk of heavy metal toxicity	Combination may be beneficial	Selenium may theoretically reduce risk of heavy metal toxicity by forming inert complexes with these metals.
	HMGCoA reductase inhibitors (statins)	Theoretical risk of decreased drug effect	Monitor — clinical significance is unclear	Reduced drug effectiveness was reported in a clinical study investigating the concomitant use of statins plus niacin, with an antioxidant combination of selenium, beta-carotene, vitamin C and vitamin E. It is not possible to determine how much of this can be attributed to selenium, or the clinical relevance of this interaction.
	Immunosuppressants	Theoretical risk of decreased drug effect	Monitor — clinical significance is unclear	Selenium may stimulate the immune system. There is a theoretical risk that this may interfere with immunosuppressant therapy, but appears unlikely at normal therapeutic doses.
Serrapeptase	Anticoagulant/ antiplatelet drugs	Theoretical increased risk of bleeding	Caution with use of this combination	Serrapeptase may have fibrinolytic activity. Combined use may theoretically increase the risk of bleeding.

Continued

TABLE I.2 Nutrient and nutritional supplement interactions—cont'd

Nutrient/ supplement	Drug/drug class	Potential outcome	Recommendations	Comments
Shark cartilage	Immunosuppressant drugs	Theoretical decreased drug effectiveness	Caution with use of this combination	Shark cartilage may stimulate immune response based on in-vitro evidence. Theoretically this could interfere with immunosuppressive therapy.
Sodium	Antihypertensive drugs	Reduced drug effect/ increased drug requirements	Caution with use of this combination	High dietary intake of sodium can raise blood pressure and may lead to increased drug requirements. Patients on antihypertensive medication should avoid high sodium intake.
	Didanosine (NRTI)	Possible excessive sodium intake	Caution with use of this combination	Didanosine formulations contain a significant amount of sodium. The combination may lead to excessive sodium levels.
	Glucocorticoids, e.g. hydrocortisone	Theoretical increased risk of hypernatraemia	Caution with use of this combination	Glucocorticoids may cause sodium retention. The magnitude of effect relates to drug dose and specific drug characteristics. Not all glucocorticoids result in clinically relevant sodium retention, but caution is advised with intake of sodium-containing foods and supplements.
	Lithium	Altered drug effect	Caution with use of this combination	High sodium intake can decrease drug concentrations by increasing lithium excretion. Conversely, a significant decrease in sodium intake can result in drug toxicity. Patients taking lithium should avoid significant alterations to sodium intake without medical supervision.
	Mineralocorticoids	Theoretical increased risk of hypernatraemia	Caution with use of this combination	Mineralocorticoids may cause sodium retention. The magnitude of effect relates to drug dose and drug mineralocorticoid potency.
	Tolvaptan	Theoretical increased risk of hypernatraemia	Caution with use of this combination	Concomitant use may increase the risk of sodium retention and hypernatraemia.
Sodium bicarbonate	Aminoglycosides	Theoretical increased risk of hypokalaemia	Caution with use of this combination	The combination theoretically increases the risk of hypokalaemia. Excessive intake of sodium bicarbonate has been associated with hypokalaemia. Aminoglycosides may cause nephrotoxicity, resulting in further loss of potassium.
	Amphotericin-B	Theoretical increased risk of hypokalaemia	Caution with use of this combination	The combination increases the risk of hypokalaemia, and potassium supplements may be required. Excessive intake of sodium bicarbonate has been associated with hypokalaemia This drug increases urinary loss of potassium.
	Aspirin	Possible reduced drug effects	Caution with use of this combination	Sodium bicarbonate may increase elimination of salicylates such as aspirin. It is proposed that this is due to increased urinary pH.

TABLE I.2 Nutrient and nutritional supplement interactions—cont'd

Nutrient/ supplement	Drug/drug class	Potential outcome	Recommendations	Comments
Sodium bicarbonate cont'd	B_2-agonists, e.g. salbutamol	Theoretical increased risk of hypokalaemia	Caution with use of this combination	Excessive intake of sodium bicarbonate has been associated with hypokalaemia. The combination theoretically increases the risk of hypokalaemia.
	Cefpodoxime proxetil	Decreased drug concentrations	Caution with use of this combination	High-dose sodium bicarbonate may increase gastric pH and inhibit conversion of drug to the active form. A clinical study reported a significant decrease in drug plasma concentration when taken concomitantly with 12.6 g oral sodium bicarbonate.
	Chlorpropamide	Possible reduced drug effect	Caution with use of this combination	High-dose sodium bicarbonate may alter urinary pH. A preliminary clinical study reported a significant increase in drug urinary excretion with this combination.
	Cisplatin	Theoretical increased risk of hypokalaemia	Caution with use of this combination	The combination theoretically increases the risk of hypokalaemia. Excessive intake of sodium bicarbonate has been associated with hypokalaemia. Cisplatin may affect renal function, resulting in further loss of potassium.
	Corticosteroids	Theoretical increased risk of hypokalaemia	Caution with use of this combination	The combination theoretically increases the risk of hypokalaemia. Excessive intake of sodium bicarbonate has been associated with hypokalaemia. Corticosteroids may cause hypokalaemia as a consequence of sodium retention and resulting compensatory renal excretion of potassium.
	Diuretics — loop and thiazide	Theoretical increased risk of hypokalaemia	Caution with use of this combination	Excessive intake of sodium bicarbonate has been associated with hypokalaemia. The combination theoretically increases the risk of hypokalaemia.
	Methylxanthines	Theoretical increased risk of hypokalaemia	Caution with use of this combination	Excessive intake of sodium bicarbonate has been associated with hypokalaemia. The combination theoretically increases the risk of hypokalaemia as theophylline and related compounds may reduce serum potassium levels.
	Penicillins	Theoretical increased risk of hypokalaemia	Caution with use of this combination	Excessive intake of sodium bicarbonate has been associated with hypokalaemia. Some penicillins are formulated as sodium salts, which may theoretically promote urinary excretion of potassium. The combination may theoretically increase the risk of hypokalaemia.

Continued

TABLE I.2 Nutrient and nutritional supplement interactions—cont'd

Nutrient/ supplement	Drug/drug class	Potential outcome	Recommendations	Comments
Sodium bicarbonate cont'd	Pseudoephedrine	Theoretical increased risk of drug toxicity	Caution with use of this combination	High intake of sodium bicarbonate may increase urinary pH. A case study describes a patient with persistent alkaline urine who experienced hallucinations and personality changes while taking pseudoephedrine. Theoretically the combination may reduce drug clearance and increase the risk of drug toxicity.
	Stimulant laxatives	Theoretical increased risk of hypokalaemia	Caution with use of this combination	Excessive use of stimulant laxatives may increase urinary excretion of potassium. Excessive intake of sodium bicarbonate has also been associated with hypokalaemia. The combination theoretically increases this risk.
Soy protein and soy isoflavones, e.g. genistein and daidzein	Antibiotics	Theoretical decreased effect of soy isoflavones	Monitor — clinical significance is unclear	Theoretically antibiotics may decrease the action of soy isoflavones by disturbing gastrointestinal bacteria, which may then impair conversion of isoflavones to the active form. The interaction is speculative and only likely to be relevant with long-term antibiotic use.
	Antidiabetic drugs	Possible additive effects	Caution with use of this combination	Clinical research suggests that soy-based diets may reduce fasting blood glucose levels. Theoretically concurrent use may have additive effects, which could be beneficial for the management of diabetes. Caution is advised due to the risk of hypoglycaemia.
	Antihypertensive drugs	Possible additive effects	Monitor — clinical significance is unclear	Clinical evidence suggests that soy protein may modestly lower blood pressure in individuals with hypertension. Effects may be additive, but there is a theoretical risk of hypotension.
	Chemotherapeutic drugs, e.g. vincristine, vinblastine, cisplatin, daunorubicin	Theoretical beneficial interaction	Caution with use of this combination	In-vitro evidence suggests soy isoflavones may potentially enhance drug antitumour effects with certain chemotherapeutic agents. Clinical significance is unknown and safety of this combination has not been established. Medical supervision is warranted.
	L-thyroxine (Levothyroxine)	Possible decreased drug effects	Caution with use of this combination	Preliminary evidence suggests that soy-based formulas may decrease thyroxine levels in infants with congenital hypothyroidism. It is unclear if this interaction occurs in other patient populations. Soy may theoretically affect thyroid function, although this effect does not appear to be clinically significant based on current evidence.

TABLE I.2 Nutrient and nutritional supplement interactions—cont'd

Nutrient/ supplement	Drug/drug class	Potential outcome	Recommendations	Comments
Soy protein and soy isoflavones, e.g. genistein and daidzein cont'd	Monoamine oxidase inhibitors (MAOIs)	Theoretical increased risk of drug adverse effects	Avoid combination	Fermented soy products such as tofu and soy sauce contain tyramine, which may theoretically interact with MAOIs and increase the risk of a hypertensive crisis. The amount of tyramine in fermented soy products is usually relatively small, but concentrations can vary.
	Oestrogens, e.g. HRT	Theoretical altered drug action	May be beneficial — medical supervision recommended	Data are conflicting on the interaction between soy and oestrogenic drugs. Some sources suggest that soy isoflavones may have additive beneficial effects when used with HRT, while others suggest soy theoretically inhibits the effects of HRT due to competition for oestrogen bind receptors. Caution is advised until more data become available.
	Progesterone	Possible increased bone loss	Monitor — clinical significance is unclear	Both soy milk and progesterone patches have bone sparing effects when used alone; however, results of a small clinical study suggest that use of this combination resulted in bone loss. Further data are required to establish clinical significance of this interaction.
	Tamoxifen	May antagonise drug effect	Avoid combination	Preliminary evidence suggests that the soy isoflavones genistein and diadzen may antagonise drug antitumour effect. Soy may interfere with drug action due to the oestrogenic effects of soy isoflavones. Results from studies have, however, been conflicting, which may be due to dose variations. Caution is advised until more data become available.
	Warfarin	Theoretical decreased drug effect	Caution with use of this combination	A case report describes a possible interaction between soy milk and warfarin. The data are inconclusive but caution is advised.
Spirulina (blue-green algae)	Anticoagulant/ antiplatelet drugs	Theoretical increased risk of bleeding	Caution with use of this combination	Spirulina may have antiplatelet properties. Concomitant use with anticoagulant and antiplatelet drugs will theoretically increase the risk of bleeding and bruising.
	Immunosuppressant drugs	Theoretical risk of decreased drug effect	Caution with use of this combination	Spirulina may have immunomodulatory activity which could theoretically oppose drug immunosuppressant effects.
Taurine	Antihypertensive drugs	Possible additive effects	Combination may be beneficial — monitor	Clinical evidence suggests taurine may lower blood pressure. Additive, beneficial effects may be seen with use of this combination, but monitor to reduce the risk of hypotension.

Continued

TABLE I.2 Nutrient and nutritional supplement interactions—cont'd

Nutrient/ supplement	Drug/drug class	Potential outcome	Recommendations	Comments
Taurine cont'd	Lithium	Theoretical increased risk of drug toxicity	Caution with use of this combination	Taurine may have diuretic properties, which can theoretically reduce drug excretion and increase the risk of toxicity.
Theanine (L-theanine)	Antihypertensive drugs	Theoretical additive effects	Combination may be beneficial — monitor	Animal studies suggest theanine may lower blood pressure. Additive, beneficial effects may theoretically be seen with use of this combination, but monitor to reduce the risk of hypotension.
	Stimulant drugs	Theoretical decreased drug effects	Caution with use of this combination	Animal studies suggest that theanine may decrease drug effects. Significance is unclear.
Theobroma cacao (also refer to interactions listed under caffeine)	ACE-inhibitors (ACE-I)	Additive effects possible	May be beneficial — medical supervision recommended	Cocoa may inhibit angiotensin-converting enzyme activity according to limited research. Additive blood pressure-lowering effects are theoretically possible, but monitor for hypotension.
	Anticoagulant/ antiplatelet drugs	Theoretical increased risk of bleeding	Caution with use of this combination	Cocoa may have antiplatelet properties according to limited research. There is a theoretical increased risk of bleeding with this combination.
	Antidiabetic drugs	Theoretical altered drug affects	Caution with use of this combination	Cocoa may affect blood glucose regulation, with some reports suggesting an increased level of blood sugar and other reports suggesting a decreased level. Clinical significance of this interaction is unclear and caution is advised.
	Antihypertensive drugs	Additive effects possible	May be beneficial — medical supervision recommended	Cocoa may lower blood pressure. The combination may theoretically be beneficial, but caution is advised due to a risk of hypotension.
	Cardiovascular drugs	Possible improved disease management	May be beneficial — medical supervision recommended	A preliminary study reported that increased intake of high-flavonol cocoa helped to improve endothelial function and blood pressure in patients with coronary artery disease who were taking a combination of statins, aspirin, beta-blockers and ACE-I/ARB.
	Clozapine	Theoretical disease exacerbation	Caution with use of this combination	Caffeine, found in cocoa, may exacerbate psychotic symptoms and increase drug effects and toxicity at high doses.
	Lipid-lowering drugs (statins)	Possible improved disease management	May be beneficial — medical supervision recommended	A preliminary study reported that increased intake of high-flavonol cocoa helped to improve endothelial function and blood pressure in patients with coronary artery disease who were taking a combination of statin, aspirin, beta-blocker and ACE-I/ARB.

TABLE I.2 Nutrient and nutritional supplement interactions—cont'd

Nutrient/ supplement	Drug/drug class	Potential outcome	Recommendations	Comments
Tocopherols and tocotrienols — see Vitamin E				
Tryptophan (L-tryptophan)	Antidepressant drugs (SSRIs and SNRIs)	Theoretical risk of serotonin syndrome	Caution with use of this combination	Tryptophan is an endogenous precursor for the production of serotonin. Theoretically, the combination may increase the risk of serotonin syndrome.
	Antidepressant drugs (tricyclic antidepressants)	Possible synergistic effects	Caution with use of this combination	Synergistic beneficial effects are theoretically possible, but medical supervision is required.
	Benzodiazepines	Theoretical increased risk of adverse effects	Caution with use of this combination	Secondary sources suggest that concomitant use may increase the risk of adverse effects such as sexual disinhibition, reversible dyskinesia and reversible Parkinson's-like rigidity. There are insufficient data to comment on clinical relevance of this interaction.
	CNS depressant drugs	Increased risk of sedation	Avoid combination	Concomitant use may have additive effects and increase the risk of excessive sedation.
	Dextromethorphan	Theoretical risk of serotonin syndrome	Caution with use of this combination	Tryptophan is an endogenous precursor for the production of serotonin. Theoretically, the combination may increase the risk of serotonin syndrome.
	Monoamine oxidase inhibitors (MAOIs)	Theoretical risk of serotonin syndrome	Avoid combination	Tryptophan is an endogenous precursor for the production of serotonin. Theoretically, the combination may increase the risk of serotonin syndrome. Case reports describe adverse reactions with this combination including myoclonus, hyperreflexia, diaphoresis, confusion, hypomania, ocular oscillation and ataxia.
	Phenothiazines	Theoretical increased risk of adverse effects	Caution with use of this combination	Secondary sources suggest that concomitant use may increase the risk of adverse effects such as sexual disinhibition, reversible dyskinesia and reversible Parkinson's-like rigidity. There are insufficient available data to comment on clinical relevance of this interaction.
	Tramadol	Theoretical risk of serotonin syndrome	Caution with use of this combination	Tryptophan is an endogenous precursor for the production of serotonin. Theoretically, the combination may increase the risk of serotonin syndrome.
Tyrosine	L-thyroxine (Levothyroxine)	Theoretical additive effects	Caution with use of this combination	Tyrosine is a precursor to thyroid hormone. There is some concern that concomitant use may have additive effects. Dose adjustments may be required.

Continued

TABLE I.2 Nutrient and nutritional supplement interactions—cont'd

Nutrient/ supplement	Drug/drug class	Potential outcome	Recommendations	Comments
Tyrosine cont'd	Levodopa	Theoretical decreased drug effect	Caution with use of this combination	Tyrosine and levodopa compete for absorption by the same transport system. Theoretically, concomitant use may lead to decreased drug effectiveness.
Ubiquinol/ubidecarenone — see Coenzyme Q10				
Vitamin A	Anthelmintic drugs	Possible improved response	Combination may be beneficial	Vitamin A deficiency is associated with an increased risk of parasitic worm infections. Concurrent use of beta-carotene or vitamin A may assist with management of condition, as well as supporting immunity and epithelial integrity.
	Bile acid sequestrants	Risk of vitamin depletion	May be beneficial to address nutrient depletion	Nutrient depletion has been reported, but may not be clinically significant unless there is long-term use of cholestyramine.
	Chemotherapeutic agents	Possible improved drug response	Caution with use of this combination	Epidemiological evidence suggests an association between higher dietary intake of vitamin A and a reduced risk of breast cancer and possibly some other forms of cancer although data are inconclusive. According to some preliminary data adjunctive use of vitamin A with chemotherapeutic agents may improve outcomes, although evidence is conflicting and inconclusive.
	Hepatotoxic drugs	Increased risk of hepatotoxicity	Caution with use of this combination	Theoretically high-dose vitamin A may increase the risk of liver damage when used in combination with hepatotoxic drugs.
	HMGCoA reductase inhibitors (statins)	Possible increased vitamin A levels	Caution with use of this combination	Preliminary research suggests statins may increase serum retinol levels. The clinical significance is not known. Caution is advised with high-dose vitamin A supplements, especially in those with compromised liver function, until more data become available.
	Mineral oil	Risk of vitamin depletion	May be beneficial to address nutrient depletion	A moderate risk of vitamin A depletion has been reported with long-term or regular use of mineral oil. Supplements may be required in some individuals.
	Neomycin	Risk of vitamin depletion	May be beneficial to address nutrient depletion	Neomycin may damage the structure and affect the function of the digestive tract lining. Long-term use may reduce absorption of vitamin A.
	Orlistat	Risk of vitamin depletion	May be beneficial to address nutrient depletion	A moderate risk of vitamin A depletion has been reported with long-term use of orlistat. Supplements may be required in some individuals.

TABLE I.2 Nutrient and nutritional supplement interactions—cont'd

Nutrient/ supplement	Drug/drug class	Potential outcome	Recommendations	Comments
Vitamin A cont'd	Retinoids, e.g. isotretinoin	Risk of drug toxicity	Avoid combination	There is a major risk of additive toxic effects with concomitant use of vitamin A and retinoid drugs such as isotretinoin. The interaction is well established and the combination should be avoided.
	Tetracycline antibiotics	Increased risk of adverse effects	Caution with use of this combination	Long-term tetracyclines in combination with vitamin A increases the risk of benign intercranial hypertension. This interaction has been described in case reports.
	Warfarin	Theoretical increased risk of bleeding	Caution with use of this combination	Theoretically high-dose vitamin A may increase the risk of bleeding if taken with warfarin. Vitamin A toxicity is associated with haemorrhage, possibly due to vitamin K antagonism.
Vitamin B_1 (thiamine)	Alcohol	Risk of vitamin depletion	May be beneficial to address nutrient depletion	It has been reported that 30–80% of alcoholics have clinical or biochemical signs of vitamin B_1 deficiency. Vitamin B_1 deficiency may lead to the development of Wernicke-Korsakoff syndrome and alcoholic neuropathy.
	Diuretic drugs	Risk of vitamin depletion	May be beneficial to address nutrient depletion	A moderate depletion of vitamin B_1 has been reported with long-term use of diuretics due to increased excretion. The risk of depletion appears greatest in those taking loop diuretics and if over 60 years, especially where dietary intake is inadequate. There is a concern that vitamin B_1 deficiency may worsen heart failure.
	Oestrogens, e.g. oral contraceptives	Risk of vitamin depletion	May be beneficial to address nutrient depletion	A small reduction in vitamin B_1 levels has been noted in women taking oral contraceptives long term. The depletion may not be clinically significant, but monitor for signs of deficiency.
Vitamin B_2 (riboflavin, riboflavin-5-phosphate)	Antibiotics	Risk of vitamin depletion	May be beneficial to address nutrient depletion	Long-term use of antibiotics may interfere with bacterial synthesis of vitamin B_2. This interaction may not be clinically relevant, but monitor for signs of depletion with long-term antibiotic use.
	Oestrogens, e.g. oral contraceptives	Risk of vitamin depletion	May be beneficial to address nutrient depletion	A small reduction in vitamin B_2 activity has been noted in women taking oral contraceptives long term. The depletion may not be clinically significant, but monitor for signs of deficiency.
	Tricyclic antidepressants (TCAs)	Risk of vitamin depletion	May be beneficial to address nutrient depletion	Tricyclic antidepressants may interfere with conversion of vitamin B_2 to the active form flavin adenine dinucleotide (FAD). The interaction does not appear to be important clinically, but monitor for signs of deficiency.

Continued

TABLE I.2 Nutrient and nutritional supplement interactions—cont'd				
Nutrient/ supplement	**Drug/drug class**	**Potential outcome**	**Recommendations**	**Comments**
Vitamin B_3 (niacin and nicotinamide)				
Niacin	Alcohol	Increased risk of adverse effects	Caution with use of this combination	Alcohol may exacerbate flushing and pruritic associated with high-dose niacin supplementation.
	Anticoagulant/ antiplatelet drugs	Theoretical increased risk of bleeding	Caution with use of this combination	High-dose sustained-release niacin may theoretically increase the risk of bleeding in patients taking anticoagulants and antiplatelet drugs.
	Antidiabetic drugs	Risk that condition may be exacerbated	Caution with use of this combination	High-dose niacin may impair glycaemic control, possibly aggravating insulin intolerance and increasing glucose production by the liver. About 10–35% of diabetic patients may need drug dose adjustments with high-dose niacin therapy.
	Antiepileptic drugs	Risk of vitamin depletion	May be beneficial to address nutrient depletion	A moderate risk of nutrient depletion has been reported with use of phenytoin and valproic acid.
	Antihypertensive drugs	Possible additive effects	Caution with use of this combination	Some evidence suggests that high-dose niacin may lower blood pressure in hypertensive individuals. This may potentially be beneficial, but monitor as there is an increased risk of hypotension.
	Antigout drugs	Possible decreased disease management	Caution with use of this combination	High-dose niacin may reduce urinary excretion of uric acid, potentially leading to hyperuricaemia. Drug dosage adjustment may be required for patients who commence treatment with high-dose niacin.
	Azathioprine	Risk of vitamin depletion	May be beneficial to address nutrient depletion	A moderate depletion of niacin has been reported with use of this drug. Supplements may be required in some individuals.
	Bile acid sequestrants	Possible decreased nutrient absorption and increased risk of myopathy	Caution with use of this combination	Bile acid sequestrants can bind niacin and decrease absorption. Doses should be separated. Some evidence suggests an increased risk of myopathy associated with concomitant use of high-dose niacin and bile acid sequestrants.
	Cycloserine	Risk of vitamin depletion	May be beneficial to address nutrient depletion	A moderate depletion of niacin has been reported with use of this drug. Supplements may be required in some individuals.
	Fluorouracil	Risk of vitamin depletion	May be beneficial to address nutrient depletion	A moderate depletion of niacin has been reported with use of this drug. Supplements may be required in some individuals.

TABLE I.2 Nutrient and nutritional supplement interactions—cont'd				
Nutrient/ supplement	**Drug/drug class**	**Potential outcome**	**Recommendations**	**Comments**
Niacin cont'd	HMGCoA reductase inhibitors (statins)	Possible additive lipid lowering effects	Combination may be beneficial	High-dose niacin may enhance drug lipid-lowering effects and the combination may be beneficial and result in improved outcomes. Case reports have however suggested an increased risk of muscle myopathy with this combination. Evidence of this interaction is limited and significance is unclear.
	Isoniazid	Risk of vitamin depletion	May be beneficial to address nutrient depletion	A moderate depletion of niacin has been reported with use of this drug. Supplements may be required in some individuals.
	Levodopa/ carbidopa	Risk of vitamin depletion	May be beneficial to address nutrient depletion	A moderate depletion of niacin has been reported with use of this drug. Supplements may be required in some individuals.
Nicotinamide	Anticoagulant/ antiplatelet drugs	Theoretical increased risk of bleeding	Caution with use of this combination	Case reports suggest that concomitant use of high-dose nicotinamide with anticoagulant/ antiplatelet drugs may increase the risk of bleeding. Caution is advised until further safety data become available.
	Carbamazepine	Theoretical increased drug levels	Caution with use of this combination	Two case reports suggest that high-dose nicotinamide may increase drug levels. There is currently insufficient data to determine significance.
	Ethionamide	Risk of nutrient depletion	May be beneficial to address nutrient depletion	This drug has structural similarities to nicotinamide and may interfere with nutrient activity. There is a moderate risk of nutrient depletion. Supplements may be required in some individuals.
	Hepatoxic drugs	Theoretical increased risk of hepatoxicity	Caution with use of this combination	Nicotinamide has been associated with increased liver enzymes and liver damage at high doses. Theoretically, concomitant use may result in an increased risk of liver damage.
	Primidone	Theoretical increased drug levels	Caution with use of this combination	Limited case reports suggest that high-dose nicotinamide may reduce drug metabolism and increase drug levels. There is currently insufficient data to determine significance.
	Pyrazinamide	Risk of nutrient depletion	May be beneficial to address nutrient depletion	This drug has structural similarities to nicotinamide and may interfere with nutrient activity. There is a moderate risk of nutrient depletion. Supplements may be required in some individuals.
Vitamin B_6 (pyridoxine, pyridoxyl-5-phosphate (PLP)	Amiodarone	Possible increased risk of photosensitivity	Caution with use of this combination	Preliminary evidence suggests that vitamin B_6 may exacerbate drug-induced photosensitivity. Data are conflicting and inconclusive, with some sources suggesting vitamin B_6 provides a protective effect.

Continued

TABLE I.2 Nutrient and nutritional supplement interactions—cont'd

Nutrient/ supplement	Drug/drug class	Potential outcome	Recommendations	Comments
Vitamin B_6 (pyridoxine, pyridoxyl-5-phosphate (PLP) cont'd	Anticonvulsant drugs, e.g. phenobarbital (phenobarbitone), phenytoin	Risk of decreased drug levels with high vitamin intake	Caution with use of this combination	Preliminary evidence suggests that high-dose vitamin B_6 (200 mg daily) can reduce plasma levels of phenobarbital (phenobarbitone) and phenytoin, possibly due to increased drug metabolism. Concerns have also been raised about the potential for interactions between high-dose vitamin B_6 and other anticonvulsant drugs.
	Antihypertensive drugs	Additive effects possible	Combination may be beneficial	Vitamin B_6 may lower blood pressure in hypertensive patients. Additive, beneficial effects are possible, but monitor for hypotension.
	Cycloserine	Major risk of vitamin depletion	May be beneficial to address nutrient depletion	A major risk of depletion of vitamin B_6 has been reported with use of cycloserine. It has been proposed that this depletion contributes to drug-induced neurotoxicity and seizures. Most patients will require supplementation with long-term use.
	Diuretics (loop)	Risk of vitamin depletion	May be beneficial to address nutrient depletion	Loop diuretics may theoretically increase urinary excretion of vitamin B_6. Monitor for signs of deficiency; however, based on current data, this depletion does not appear to be clinically significant.
	Hydralazine	Risk of vitamin depletion	May be beneficial to address nutrient depletion	This drug may lead to a moderate depletion of vitamin B_6 with long-term use. Patients should be monitored for depletion and supplements may be required in some individuals, especially in those presenting with paraesthesia, numbness and tingling.
	Isoniazid	Risk of vitamin depletion	May be beneficial to address nutrient depletion	This drug may lead to a moderate depletion of vitamin B_6 with long-term use, which could lead to a peripheral neuritis. Patients should be monitored for depletion and supplements may be required in some individuals.
	Levodopa (without carbidopa)	Theoretical decreased drug effect	Combination may be beneficial	Vitamin B_6 enhances levodopa peripheral metabolism and may reduce anti-Parkinson's disease effect. In practice, this interaction is unlikely as levodopa is usually co-prescribed with carbidopa, and this negates this effect.
	Methotrexate	Possible reduced vitamin levels	May be beneficial — medical supervision recommended	Some sources suggest that chronic inflammatory diseases such as rheumatoid arthritis may be associated with a lower vitamin B_6 status. Use of methotrexate has also been associated with raised homocysteine levels due to an interference in vitamin B_6 and folic acid-dependent reactions. Monitor for signs of deficiency, although based on current data, significance is unclear.

TABLE I.2 Nutrient and nutritional supplement interactions—cont'd

Nutrient/ supplement	Drug/drug class	Potential outcome	Recommendations	Comments
Vitamin B_6 (pyridoxine, pyridoxyl-5-phosphate (PLP) cont'd	Penicillamine	Major risk of vitamin depletion	May be beneficial to address nutrient depletion	A major risk of vitamin B_6 depletion has been associated with this drug. Penicillamine inhibits the activity of vitamin B_6 by forming an inactive complex with pyridoxal phosphate. Most patients will require supplementation with long-term use.
	Oestrogens (oral contraceptives and HRT)	Risk of vitamin depletion	May be beneficial to address nutrient depletion	Oestrogens can interfere with vitamin B_6 metabolism and may theoretically reduce levels, or increase nutrient requirements. Evidence from one recent study suggests that vitamin B_6 supplementation may help to reduce the incidence of drug-related adverse effects such as nausea, headache and depression. Monitor for signs of deficiency, but the risk of depletion is not considered to be clinically significant in most individuals.
	Theophylline	Risk of vitamin depletion	May be beneficial to address nutrient depletion	Theophylline intake may theoretically result in a moderate vitamin B_6 deficiency and it has been proposed that this may contribute to drug adverse effects. Theophylline inhibits pyridoxal kinase, which catalyses phosphorylation of vitamin B_6 to the active form pyridoxal-5-phosphate. Monitor for signs of deficiency. Supplements may be required in some individuals.
Vitamin B_9 (folic acid)				
Folic acid (folate, folinic acid, 5-methyltetrahydrofolate (L-5MTHF))	5-fluorouracil	Theoretical increased risk of drug toxicity	Caution with use of this combination	Theoretically, high-dose folic acid may increase drug toxicity. Increased gastrointestinal adverse effects including stomatitis and diarrhoea have been described in clinical studies.
	Anticonvulsants, e.g. phenytoin	Risk of vitamin depletion; risk of decreased seizure control	Caution with use of this combination — combination may be beneficial to address nutrient depletion, but medical supervision is recommended	Anticonvulsants such as phenytoin may lead to a moderate nutrient depletion, especially with low dietary intake. Patients should be monitored and supplements may be required in some individuals. Conversely, some studies have reported that high-dose folic acid may cause a reduction in phenytoin blood levels and lead to an increased risk of seizures. High-dose intake of folic acid should be avoided unless under medical supervision.

Continued

TABLE I.2 Nutrient and nutritional supplement interactions—cont'd

Nutrient/ supplement	Drug/drug class	Potential outcome	Recommendations	Comments
Folic acid (folate, folinic acid, 5-methyltetrahydrofolate (L-5MTHF)) cont'd	Carbamazepine	Risk of vitamin depletion; risk of decreased seizure control	Combination may be beneficial to address nutrient depletion, but medical supervision is recommended	Carbamazepine may reduce serum folate levels, which may theoretically contribute to drug-induced mild reductions in nerve conduction and mental changes. Megaloblastic anaemia has not been reported. Caution is advised, however, as folic acid supplements have been shown to reduce seizure control in some patients with epilepsy.
	Capecitabine	Theoretical increased risk of drug toxicity	Caution with use of this combination	Theoretically, high-dose folic acid may increase drug toxicity. A case report suggests that folic acid 15 mg daily contributed to drug toxicity symptoms including severe diarrhoea, vomiting, oedema, hand–foot syndrome and eventual death in a patient taking capecitabine. It is unclear if this interaction would occur at normal therapeutic doses.
	Cholestyramine	Risk of vitamin depletion	May be beneficial to address nutrient depletion	This drug is associated with a moderate risk of folic acid depletion. Patients should be monitored and doses should be separated. Supplements may be required in some individuals.
	Metformin	Risk of vitamin depletion	May be beneficial to address nutrient depletion	Metformin may reduce folic acid absorption according to some sources. Symptomatic folic acid deficiency seems unlikely, based on current evidence, but patients should be monitored. Long-term use of metformin is associated with an increased risk of raised homocysteine levels, although data on severity and clinical significance are conflicting.
	Methotrexate	Risk of vitamin depletion; risk of decreased drug efficacy in cancer	Caution with use of this combination	Methotrexate is a folic acid antagonist and can lead to a major folic acid depletion. Supplementation with folic acid is usually required in patients prescribed methotrexate for conditions such as rheumatoid arthritis or psoriasis. Use may help to reduce drug toxicity and side effects. Folic acid supplements may, however, oppose drug mechanism of action if methotrexate is prescribed for the management of cancer and could reduce drug efficacy. Medical supervision is required.
	Oral contraceptives	Risk of vitamin depletion	May be beneficial to address nutrient depletion	Folate levels may be reduced with long-term use of oral contraceptives. Supplements may be required in some individuals.

TABLE I.2 Nutrient and nutritional supplement interactions—cont'd

Nutrient/ supplement	Drug/drug class	Potential outcome	Recommendations	Comments
Folic acid (folate, folinic acid, 5-methyltetrahydrofolate (L-5MTHF)) cont'd	Pyrimethamine	Risk of vitamin depletion; risk of decreased drug efficacy	Caution with use of this combination	This drug is a folic acid antagonist and can reduce serum folate levels. Folic acid supplements may antagonise drug action and reduce drug efficacy, depending on indication. Medical supervision is recommended.
	Retinoids	Risk of vitamin depletion	May be beneficial to address nutrient depletion	Isotretinoin has been shown to reduce serum folic acid in patients with acne. Good dietary intake should be maintained. Supplements may be required in some individuals, due to a moderate risk of depletion.
	Sulfasalazine	Risk of vitamin depletion	May be beneficial to address nutrient depletion	Moderate risk of depletion as drug reduces folic acid absorption. Patients should be monitored and supplements may be required in some individuals.
Vitamin B_{12} (cyanocobalamin, methylcobalamin, hydroxycobalamin)	Acid-reducing drugs, e.g. H_2-antagonists and proton pump inhibitors (PPIs)	Risk of vitamin depletion	May be beneficial to address nutrient depletion	Absorption of dietary vitamin B_{12} may be compromised with regular intake of acid-reducing drugs. Stomach acid is required to release vitamin B_{12} from protein so that it can be absorbed. Monitor for vitamin B_{12} depletion with long-term use (>2 years) of acid-reducing drugs.
	Aminosalicylic acid	Risk of vitamin depletion	May be beneficial to address nutrient depletion	Aminosalicylic acid may significantly reduce absorption of vitamin B_{12}. Megaloblastic anaemia has been reported with long-term use of this drug. Monitor for signs of deficiency.
	Anticonvulsant drugs, e.g. phenytoin	Risk of vitamin depletion	May be beneficial to address nutrient depletion	A moderate vitamin B_{12} depletion has been reported with use of anticonvulsant drugs, especially phenytoin, phenobarbital (phenobarbitone) and primidone. Patients should be monitored and supplements may be required in some individuals.
	Aspirin	Risk of vitamin depletion	May be beneficial to address nutrient depletion	There is a moderate risk of depletion with long-term use of aspirin. Patients should be monitored and supplements may be required in some individuals.
	Chloramphenicol	Risk of delayed response to vitamin supplementation	Monitor — may not be clinically significant	Limited case reports suggest that chloramphenicol can delay response to vitamin B_{12} supplementation. Monitor if the combination is required.
	Colchicine	Risk of vitamin depletion	May be beneficial to address nutrient depletion	There is a moderate risk of vitamin B_{12} depletion with use of colchicine. Colchicine disrupts normal intestinal mucosal function, which may lead to malabsorption of some nutrients. Patients should be monitored and supplements may be required in some individuals.

Continued

TABLE I.2 Nutrient and nutritional supplement interactions—cont'd

Nutrient/ supplement	Drug/drug class	Potential outcome	Recommendations	Comments
Vitamin B_{12} (cyanocobalamin, methylcobalamin, hydroxycobalamin) cont'd	Metformin	Risk of vitamin depletion	May be beneficial to address nutrient depletion	Metformin can deplete vitamin B_{12} and folic acid with long-term use. This can lead to raised homocysteine levels and an increased risk of cardiovascular disease and other conditions related to hyperhomocysteinaemia. Megaloblastic anaemia has also been reported with long-term use of metformin. Patients should be monitored and supplements may be required in some individuals.
	Zidovudine	Possible increased risk of drug-related adverse effects	May be beneficial — medical supervision recommended	Some research suggests that low vitamin B_{12} levels may increase the risk of drug-related adverse effects. A higher incidence of comprised vitamin B_{12} status has also been reported in individuals with HIV infection. While data are inconclusive, vitamin B_{12} status should be monitored in HIV-positive patients.
Vitamin C (ascorbic acid)	Aluminium, e.g. in antacids	Risk of increased aluminium absorption and toxicity	Monitor and separate doses	Vitamin C may increase aluminium absorption which is potentially toxic. The interaction may not be clinically significant, unless renally impaired, but dosage separation is recommended.
	Chemotherapy	Possible enhanced disease management	May be beneficial with medical supervision	Use of high-dose IV vitamin C in the management of cancer is controversial. Vitamin C may enhance therapeutic effects of some drugs. There is, however, concern that the antioxidant action may also interfere with drug efficacy for certain chemotherapeutic agents. Medical supervision is required to determine appropriateness of use for the individual.
	Corticosteroids	Theoretical vitamin depletion	May be beneficial to address nutrient depletion	Vitamin C requirements may be increased in patients taking corticosteroids based on in-vitro and animal studies.
	Indinavir	Possible decreased drug absorption	Caution with use of this combination	Concomitant use of 1 g vitamin C with indinavir resulted in a small reduction in drug absorption in a preliminary pharmacokinetic study. Clinical significance is unclear but caution is advised.
	Iron	Enhanced iron absorption	Combination may be beneficial	Vitamin C enhances the absorption of iron. The combination is often used to manage iron deficiency.
	Oestrogens	Theoretical increase in plasma oestrogen levels	Monitor — interaction may not be clinically significant	Limited evidence suggests that vitamin C supplements may increase plasma oestrogen levels in women who are vitamin C deficient. Vitamin C supplements do not appear to have an effect on oestrogen in the absence of deficiency and a clinically relevant interaction appears unlikely.

TABLE I.2 Nutrient and nutritional supplement interactions—cont'd				
Nutrient/ supplement	**Drug/drug class**	**Potential outcome**	**Recommendations**	**Comments**
Vitamin C (ascorbic acid) cont'd	Propranolol	Theoretical decreased drug absorption	Monitor — interaction may not be clinically significant	Preliminary data suggest that pre-treatment with vitamin C 2 g may reduce propranolol absorption and metabolism. Patients should be monitored with use of this combination, but the interaction may not be clinically relevant.
	Warfarin	Theoretical decreased drug effect — conflicting data	Caution with use of this combination	Data on the interaction between warfarin and vitamin C are conflicting. A small study concluded that vitamin C does not affect warfarin's anticoagulant effects. However, several case reports describe a possible interaction between warfarin and high-dose vitamin C, leading to reduced drug effect. Caution is advised until more data become available.
Vitamin D	Aluminium, e.g. in antacids	Risk of increased aluminium absorption and toxicity	Monitor — separate doses	Vitamin D increases aluminium absorption which is potentially toxic. The interaction may not be clinically significant, but dosage separation is recommended.
	Anticonvulsant drugs, e.g. carbamazepine, phenobarbital (phenobarbitone), phenytoin	Risk of nutrient depletion	May be beneficial to address nutrient depletion	Anticonvulsant drugs may lead to a moderate vitamin D depletion by increasing liver metabolism of vitamin D to inactive compounds. Hypocalcaemia and osteomalacia have been reported with long-term use, especially where other risk factors for vitamin D deficiency are present. Patients taking anticonvulsant drugs should be monitored. Supplements may be required in some individuals.
	Atorvastatin	Possible decreased drug bioavailability	Caution with use of this combination	Limited evidence suggests that vitamin D supplements may decrease atorvastatin bioavailability. Caution is advised until more data become available.
	Calcipotriene	Theoretical increased risk of hypocalcaemia	Caution with use of this combination	Calcipotriene is a vitamin D analogue used in the management of psoriasis. Theoretically, concomitant use of vitamin D supplements with this drug may increase the risk of hypercalcaemia.
	Calcium channel blockers, e.g. diltiazem, verapamil	Theoretical risk of reduced drug effect	Caution with use of this combination	High-dose intake of vitamin D (in the absence of deficiency) may increase the risk of hypercalcaemia and theoretically reduce drug effectiveness. Clinical significance is unclear.
	Cholestyramine	Risk of nutrient depletion	May be beneficial to address nutrient depletion	There is a moderate risk of vitamin D depletion with use of cholestyramine. Patients should be monitored and supplements may be required in some individuals.

Continued

TABLE I.2 Nutrient and nutritional supplement interactions—cont'd

Nutrient/ supplement	Drug/drug class	Potential outcome	Recommendations	Comments
Vitamin D cont'd	Corticosteroids (chronic use)	Risk of nutrient depletion	May be beneficial to address nutrient depletion	Long-term intake of oral corticosteroids (equivalent to ≥7.5 mg prednisone daily) causes significant bone loss and increases the risk of osteoporosis and fractures. This is mainly due to disturbances in calcium metabolism; however, vitamin D supplements may be required to improve calcium absorption.
	Digoxin	Increased risk of hypercalcaemia	Avoid combination	High-dose intake of vitamin D, in the absence of a deficiency, can increase the risk of hypercalcaemia and risk of fatal cardiac arrhythmias in patients taking digoxin.
	Orlistat	Risk of major nutrient depletion	May be beneficial to address nutrient depletion	There is a significant risk of vitamin D depletion with use of orlistat. Patients should be monitored for vitamin D depletion and a supplement will be needed in most individuals. Doses should be separated by at least 2 hours.
	Rifampicin/rifampin	Risk of nutrient depletion	May be beneficial to address nutrient depletion	Rifampicin may increase vitamin D metabolism and may result in an increased risk of osteomalacia with long-term use. Patients should be monitored and supplements may be required in some individuals.
	Stimulant laxatives (chronic use)	Risk of nutrient depletion	May be beneficial to address nutrient depletion	Moderate risk of depletion. Patients should be monitored and supplements may be required in some individuals.
Vitamin E (tocopherols, tocotrienols)	Anticoagulant/ antiplatelet drugs	Theoretical increased risk of bleeding	Caution with use of this combination	There is an increased risk of bleeding with the combined use of warfarin and vitamin E, especially at higher doses. Vitamin E inhibits platelet aggregation and reduces vitamin K-dependent clotting factors. People with low levels of vitamin K appear to be at a greater risk of an interaction.
	Anticonvulsant drugs, e.g. phenytoin, phenobarbital (phenobarbitone)	Risk of nutrient depletion	May be beneficial to address nutrient depletion	A moderate risk of nutrient depletion has been reported with use of anticonvulsant drugs. Supplements may be required in some individuals.
	Beta-carotene	Reduced nutrient absorption	Monitor — may not be clinically significant	High-dose vitamin E (≥800 IU) may reduce absorption of beta-carotene. Clinical significance is unclear.
	Chemotherapeutic agents	Possible reduced drug effects — controversial	Caution with use of this combination	The use of antioxidants including vitamin E in patients on chemotherapy is controversial. It has been proposed that vitamin E may protect tumour cells from chemotherapeutic drugs that work by inducing oxidative stress and so theoretically reduce drug effectiveness. Avoid high-dose supplements unless under medical supervision.

TABLE I.2 Nutrient and nutritional supplement interactions—cont'd

Nutrient/ supplement	Drug/drug class	Potential outcome	Recommendations	Comments
Vitamin E (tocopherols, tocotrienols) cont'd	Cholestyramine	Risk of nutrient depletion	May be beneficial to address nutrient depletion	Vitamin E depletion has been reported with use of cholestyramine. This interaction may not be clinically significant unless there is long-term use. Patients on this drug should be monitored for signs of depletion.
	Ciclosporin	Theoretical increased risk of drug toxicity	Caution with use of this combination	Some evidence suggests that certain forms of vitamin E may increase ciclosporin absorption, which could theoretically lead to drug toxicity. The combination should be used with caution until further data become available.
	HMGCoA reductase inhibitors (statins)	Risk of nutrient depletion	May be beneficial to address nutrient depletion	Some current reports suggest that statins may lower vitamin E levels, however clinical significance is unclear.
	Nitrates	Decreased risk of drug adverse effects	May be beneficial to address nutrient depletion	Oral vitamin E (300–600 mg/day) may help to prevent development of nitrate tolerance to transdermal patches.
	Orlistat	Risk of nutrient depletion	May be beneficial to address nutrient depletion	Orlistat may result in a moderate vitamin E depletion. Supplements may be required in some individuals, but dose administration should be separated.
Vitamin K	Antibiotics (long term)	Risk of nutrient depletion	Monitor — may not be clinically significant	Long-term antibiotic use may alter synthesis of vitamin K_2 by disturbing normal gut flora. The clinical significance of this interaction is unclear.
	Anticoagulant/ antiplatelet drugs	Risk of decreased drug effect and clotting	Avoid combination	High intake of vitamin K antagonises the activity of anticoagulants such as warfarin and will reduce drug anticoagulant effect, leading to an increased risk of clotting. Anticoagulants will also affect the activity of vitamin K. Significant dietary changes that alter vitamin K intake may also potentially lead to an interaction. The combination should be avoided, or only used under medical supervision.
	Antidiabetic drugs	Theoretical risk of hypoglycaemia	Caution with use of this combination	High intake of vitamin K_1 has been reported to increase insulin sensitivity and reduce postprandial glucose levels. Clinical significance is unclear.
	Cholestyramine	Risk of nutrient depletion	May be beneficial to address nutrient depletion	Vitamin K depletion has been reported with use of cholestyramine. This interaction may not be clinically significant unless there is long-term use. Patients on this drug should be monitored for signs of depletion.
	Orlistat	Risk of nutrient depletion	May be beneficial to address nutrient depletion	Orlistat may result in a moderate vitamin K depletion. Supplements may be required in some individuals, but dose administration should be separated.

Continued

TABLE I.2 Nutrient and nutritional supplement interactions—cont'd

Nutrient/ supplement	Drug/drug class	Potential outcome	Recommendations	Comments
Vitamin K cont'd	Rifampicin	Risk of nutrient depletion	May be beneficial to address nutrient depletion	A moderate risk of nutrient depletion has been reported with long-term use of rifampicin. Supplements may be required in some individuals.
Whey protein	Albendazole	Theoretical risk of decreased drug effect	Monitor — separate doses	Animal research suggests high intake of whey protein prior to intake of oral albendazole may delay or hinder drug effects. Significance is unknown, but separation of dose administration is recommended.
	Antibiotics (quinolones and tetracyclines)	Possible decreased drug absorption	Monitor — separate doses	Secondary sources suggest intake of whey protein may decrease drug absorption. Significance is unknown, but separation of dose administration is recommended.
	Levodopa	Possible decreased drug absorption	Caution with use of this combination	Secondary sources suggest intake of whey protein may decrease drug absorption. Significance is unknown, but separation of dose administration is recommended.
Zinc	ACE-inhibitors	Risk of nutrient depletion	May be beneficial to address nutrient depletion	There is a moderate risk of zinc depletion with this class of antihypertensive drugs. Patients should be monitored and supplements may be required in some individuals.
	Androgens	Possible synergistic effects	Combination may be beneficial	Zinc helps to support male sexual function and to maintain male sexual health. Concurrent use may provide a synergistic benefit.
	Antibiotics (quinolones and tetracyclines)	Reduced drug effect	Monitor — separate doses	Zinc supplements form complexes with these drugs and may reduce drug effectiveness. Separate doses by at least 2 hours.
	Antibiotic — cefalexin	Reduced drug effect	Monitor — separate doses	Zinc supplements may reduce drug concentration and effectiveness. Separate doses by at least 3 hours.
	Antidepressant drugs	Possible improved outcomes	Combination may be beneficial	Zinc supplements may improve drug efficacy and the management of depression.
	Antiretroviral therapy, e.g. zidovudine	Possible improved outcomes	May be beneficial — medical supervision recommended	Preliminary evidence suggests that use of zinc supplements in combination with zidovudine (AZT) may reduce the risk of opportunistic infections in patients with HIV. Zinc supports immune function, but a higher incidence of zinc deficiency has been reported in patients with HIV. Drugs used for the management of HIV such as zidovudine and other NRTIs may theoretically deplete zinc due to their mechanism of action. Some concerns have been raised, however, that elevating zinc levels may not be appropriate, especially in later stages of disease. Supplements may be beneficial but medical supervision is recommended as data are inconsistent.

TABLE I.2 Nutrient and nutritional supplement interactions—cont'd

Nutrient/ supplement	Drug/drug class	Potential outcome	Recommendations	Comments
Zinc cont'd	Corticosteroids	Theoretical risk of nutrient depletion	May be beneficial to address nutrient depletion	Ongoing use of corticosteroids may theoretically lead to a reduction in zinc levels. Based on current evidence, the risk of depletion appears to be low and supplementation will not be needed in most patients.
	Diuretics	Risk of nutrient depletion	May be beneficial to address nutrient depletion	Diuretics may increase urinary extraction of zinc. Long-term use of diuretics will increase the risk of depletion. Many patients take diuretics in combination with ACE-I, which further increases the risk of zinc depletion.
	Methylphenidate	Increased drug effect possible	Combination may be beneficial	Drug efficacy has been shown to improve with supplementation of 15 mg elemental zinc/day for ≥6 weeks. Assess appropriateness of high-dose zinc for younger patients.
	Minerals (calcium, iron, magnesium)	Reduced nutrient absorption	Monitor — separate doses	Calcium supplements may decrease dietary zinc absorption. High-dose zinc supplements may decrease magnesium absorption and increase magnesium excretion. These interactions may not be clinically relevant unless there is a deficiency, but dosage separation is generally advised. Iron and zinc supplements can interfere with each other's absorption, especially if taken on an empty stomach due to competition for nonspecific carriers. The interaction does not appear to be significant if the supplements are taken with food as the ions complex with food components.
	Oestrogens (HRT and oral contraceptives)	Theoretical risk of nutrient depletion	May be beneficial to address nutrient depletion	Ongoing intake of oestrogens may lead to a reduction in zinc levels; however, data are conflicting. Based on current evidence, the risk of depletion appears to be low and supplementation will not be needed in most patients. Monitor.

SOURCES FOR INTERACTIONS TABLES

Al-Jenoobi FI, Al-Thukair AA, Alam MA, et al. Effect of *Curcuma longa* on CYP2D6- and CYP3A4-mediated metabolism of dextromethorphan in human liver microsomes and healthy human subjects. Eur J Drug Metab Pharmacokinet 2015;40(1):61–6.

Azadmehr A, Ziaee A, Ghanei L, et al. A randomized clinical trial study: anti-oxidant, anti-hyperglycemic and anti-hyperlipidemic effects of olibanum gum in type 2 diabetic patients. Iran J Pharm Res 2014;13(3):1003–9.

Baskaran K, Ahamath BK, Shanmugasundaram KR, et al. Antidiabetic effect of a leaf extract from *Gymnema sylvestre* in non-insulin dependent diabetes mellitus patients. J Ethnopharmacol 1990;30:295–305.

Biswal BM, Sulaiman SA, Ismail HC, et al. Effect of *Withania somnifera* (ashwagandha) on the development of chemotherapy-induced fatigue and quality of life in breast cancer patients. Integr Cancer Ther 2013;12(4):312–22.

Blonk M, Colbers A, Poirters A, et al. Effect of *ginkgo biloba* on the pharmacokinetics of raltegravir in healthy volunteers. Antimicrob Agents Chemother 2012;56(10):5070–5.

Bodinet C, Freundenstein J. Influence of *Cimicifuga racemosa* on the proliferation of estrogen receptor-positive human breast cancer cells. Breast Cancer Res 2002;76:1–10.

Bonetto N, Santelli L, Battistin L, et al. Serotonin syndrome and rhabdomyolysis induced by concomitant use of triptans, fluoxetine and hypericum. Cephalalgia 2007;27(12):1421–3.

Bossaer JB, Odle BL. Probable etoposide interaction with *Echinacea*. J Diet Suppl 2012;9(2):90–5.

Braun L, Cohen M. Herbs and natural supplements: an evidence-based guide. 4th ed. Elsevier Churchill Livingstone; 2015.

Brown BG, Zhao XQ, Chait A, et al. Simvastatin and niacin, antioxidant vitamins, or the combination for the prevention of coronary disease. N Engl J Med 2001;345:1583–93.

Burgos RA, Hancke JL, Bertoglio JC, et al. Efficacy of an *Andrographis paniculata* composition for the relief of rheumatoid arthritis symptoms: a prospective randomized placebo-controlled trial. Clin Rheumatol 2009;28(8):931–46.

Campbell NR, Kara M, Hasinoff BB, et al. Norfloxacin interaction with antacids and minerals. Br J Clin Pharmacol 1992;33(1):115–16.

Campbell N, Paddock V, Sundaram R. Alteration of methyldopa absorption, metabolism, and blood pressure control caused by ferrous sulfate and ferrous gluconate. Clin Pharmacol Ther 1988;43(4):381–6.

Chan TY. Drug interactions as a cause of overanticoagulation and bleedings in Chinese patients receiving warfarin. Int J Clin Pharmacol Ther 1998;36(7):403–5.

Chedraui P, San Miguel G, Hildago L, et al. Effect of *Trifolium pratense*-derived isoflavones on the lipid profile of postmenopausal women with increased body mass index. Gynecol Endocrinol 2008;24(11):620–4.

Chen HW, Lin IH, Chen YJ, et al. A novel infusible botanically-derived drug, PG2, for cancer-related fatigue: a phase II double-blind, randomized placebo-controlled study. Clin Invest Med 2012;35(1):E1–11.

Chen MF, Shimada F, Kato H, et al. Effect of oral administration of glycyrrhizin on the pharmacokinetics of prednisolone. Endocrinol Jpn 1991;38(2):167–74.

Chen MF, Shimanda F, Kato H, et al. Effect of oral administration of glycyrrhizin on the pharmacokinetics of prednisolone. Endocrinol Jpn 1991;38:167–75.

Cui Y, Shu X-O, Gao Y-T, et al. Association of ginseng use with survival and quality of life among breast cancer patients. Am J Epidemiol 2006;163:64553.

Day E, Bentham P, Callaghan R, et al. Thiamine for prevention and treatment of Wernicke-Korsakoff syndrome in people who abuse alcohol. Cochrane Database Syst Rev 2013;CD004033.

de Maat M, Hoetelmans MR, Mathot RMW, et al. Drug interaction between St John's wort and nevirapine. AIDS 2001;15(3):420–1.

Dhamija P, Malhotra S, Pandhi P. Effect of oral administration of crude aqueous extract of garlic on pharmacokinetic parameters of isoniazid and rifampicin in rabbits. Pharmacology 2006;77:100–4.

Ding Y, Jia Y, Li F, et al. The effect of staggered administration of zinc sulfate on the pharmacokinetics of oral cephalexin. Br J Clin Pharmacol 2012;73(3):422–7.

Enseleit F, Sudano I, Périat D, et al. Effects of pycnogenol on endothelial function in patients with stable coronary artery disease: a double-blind, randomized, placebo-controlled, cross-over study. Eur Heart J 2012;33(13):1589–97.

Fan L, Zhang W, Guo D, et al. The effect of herbal medicine baicalin on pharmacokinetics of rosuvastatin, substrate of organic anion-transporting polypeptide 1B1. Clin Pharmacol Ther 2008;83(3):471–6.

Golden EB, Lam PY, Kardosh A, et al. Green tea polyphenols block the anticancer effects of bortezomib and other boronic acid-based proteasome inhibitors. Blood 2009;113(23):5927–37.

Guo L, Bai SP, Zhao L, et al. Astragalus polysaccharide injection integrated with vinorelbine and cisplatin for patients with advanced non-small cell lung cancer: effects on quality of life and survival. Med Oncol 2012;29(3):1656–62.

Gupta I, Parihar A, Malhotra P, et al. Effects of gum resin of *Boswellia serrata* in patients with chronic colitis. Planta Med 2001;67(5):391–5.

Gupta A, Gupta R, Lal B. Effect of *Trigonella foenum-graecum* (fenugreek) seeds on glycaemic control and insulin resistance in type 2 diabetes mellitus: a double blind placebo controlled study. J Assoc Physicians India 2001;49:1057–61.

Harada T, Ohtaki E, Misu K, et al. Congestive heart failure caused by digitalis toxicity in an elderly man taking a liquorice-containing Chinese herbal laxative. Cardiology 2002;98(4):218.

Harkness R, Bratman S. Mosby's handbook of drug–herb and drug–supplement interactions. Mosby; 2003.

Heiss C, Jahn S, Taylor M, et al. Improvement of endothelial function with dietary flavanols is associated with mobilization of circulating angiogenic cells in patients with coronary artery disease. J Am Coll Cardiol 2010;56(3):218–24.

Hernandez-Munoz G, Pluchino S. *Cimicifuga racemosa* for the treatment of hot flushes in women surviving breast cancer. Maturitas 2003;44(Suppl. 1):S59–65.

Hurrel RF, Reddy M, Cook JD. Inhibition of non-haem iron absorption in man by polyphenolic-containing beverages. Br J Nutr 1999;81(4):289–95.

Jacobson JS, Troxel AB, Evans J, et al. Randomized trial of black cohosh for the treatment of hot flashes among women with a history of breast cancer. Am Soc Clin Oncol 2001;19(10):2739–45.

Jiang X, Williams K, Liauw WS, et al. Effect of ginkgo and ginger on the pharmacokinetics and pharmacodynamics of warfarin in healthy subjects. Br J Clin Pharmacol 2005;59(4):425–32.

Isso AA, Ernst E. Interactions between herbal medicines and prescribed drugs: an updated systematic review. Drugs 2009;69(13):1777–98.

Khalid Z, Osuagwu FC, Shah B, et al. Celery root extract as an inducer of mania induction in a patient on venlafaxine and St John's wort. Postgrad Med 2016;128(7):682–3.

Kassi E, Papoutsi Z, Fokialakis N, et al. Greek plant extracts exhibit selective estrogen receptor modulator (SERM)-like properties. J Agric Food Chem 2004;52(23):6956–61.

Kenny FS, Pinder SE, Ellis IO, et al. Gamma linolenic acid with tamoxifen as primary therapy in breast cancer. Int J Cancer 2000;85:643–8.

Krivoy N, Pavlotzky E, Chrubasik S, et al. Effect of *Salicis cortex* extract on human platelet aggregation. Planta Med 2001;67:209–12.

Kurnik D, Loebstein R, Rabinovitz H, et al. Over-the-counter vitamin K1-containing multivitamin supplements disrupt warfarin anticoagulation in vitamin K1-depleted patients. A prospective, controlled trial. Thromb Haemost 2004;92(5):1018–24.

Lau WC, Carville DG, Guyer KE, et al. St John's wort enhances the platelet inhibitory effect of clopidogrel in clopidogrel "resistant" healthy volunteers. J Am Coll Cardiol 2005;45:382A.

Lau WC, Welch TD, Shields T, et al. The effect of St John's wort on the pharmacodynamic response of clopidogrel in hyporesponsive volunteers and patients: increased platelet inhibition by enhancement of CYP3A4 metabolic activity. J Cardiovasc Pharmacol 2011;57(1):86–93.

Li R, Guo W, Fu Z, et al. A study about drug combination therapy of *Schisandra sphenanthera* extract and rapamycin in healthy subjects. Can J Physiol Pharmacol 2012;90(7):941–5.

Li Y, Xue WJ, Tian PX, et al. Clinical application of *Cordyceps sinensis* on immunosuppressive therapy in renal transplantation. Transplant Proc 2009;41(5):1565–9.

Lissoni P, Rovelli F, Brivio F, et al. A randomized study of chemotherapy versus biochemotherapy with chemotherapy plus *Aloe arborescens* in patients with metastatic cancer. In Vivo 2009;23(1):171–5.

Lydeking-Olsen E, Beck-Jensen JE, Setchell KD, et al. Soymilk or progesterone for prevention of bone loss — a 2 year randomized, placebo-controlled trial. Eur J Nutr 2004;43(4):246–57.

Maged AM, Elsawah H, Abdelhafez A, et al. The adjuvant effect of metformin and N-acetylcysteine to clomiphene citrate in induction of ovulation in patients with polycystic ovary syndrome. Gynecol Endocrinol 2015;31(8):635–8.

Malsch U, Kieser M. Efficacy of kava-kava in the treatment of non-psychotic anxiety, following pretreatment with benzodiazepines. Psychopharmacology (Berl) 2001;157:277–83.

Mansour A, Mohajeri-Tehrani MR, Qorbani M, et al. Effect of glutamine supplementation on cardiovascular risk factors in patients with type 2 diabetes. Nutrition 2015;31(1):119–26.

Mathijssen RHJ, Loos WJ, Sparreboom A, et al. Effects of St. John's wort on irinotecan metabolism. J Natl Cancer Inst 2002;94(16):1247–9.

McBride BF, Karapanos AK, Krudysz A, et al. Electrocardiographic and hemodynamic effects of a multicomponent dietary supplement containing ephedra and caffeine: a randomized controlled trial. JAMA 2004;291(2):216–21.

Mills S, Bone K. The essential guide to herbal safety. London: Churchill Livingstone; 2005.

Moltó J, Valle M, Miranda C, et al. Effect of milk thistle on the pharmacokinetics of darunavir-ritonavir in HIV-infected patients. Antimicrob Agents Chemother 2012;56(6):2837–41.

Neuvonen PJ. Interactions with the absorption of tetracyclines. Drugs 1976;11(1):45–54.

Persky VW, Turky ME, Wang L, et al. Effect of soy protein on endogenous hormones in postmenopausal women. Am J Clin Nutr 2002;75:145–53.

Piscitelli SC, Burstein AH, Welden N, et al. The effect of garlic supplements on the pharmacokinetics of saquinavir. Clin Infect Dis 2002;34:234–8.

Pryce R, Bernaitis N, Davey AK, et al. The use of fish oil with warfarin does not significantly affect either the international normalised ratio or incidence of adverse events in patients with atrial fibrillation and deep vein thrombosis: a retrospective study. Nutrients 2016;8(9):578.

Pyevich D, Bogenschutz MP. Herbal diuretics and lithium toxicity. Am J Psychiatry 2001;8(8):1329.

Qiu H, Fu P, Fan W, et al. Treatment of primary chronic glomerulonephritis with *Rehmannia glutinosa acteosides* in combination with the angiotensin receptor blocker irbesartan: a randomized controlled trial. Phytother Res 2014;28(1):132–6.

Rahimi R, Nikfar S, Abdollahi M. Induction of clinical response and remission of inflammatory bowel disease by use of herbal medicines: a meta-analysis. World J Gastroenterol 2013;34:5738–49.

Rajnarayana K, Reddy MS, Vidyasagar J, et al. Study on the influence of silymarin pretreatment on metabolism and disposition of metronidazole. Arzneimittelforschung 2004;54(2):109–13.

Raskin HN, Fishman RA. Pyridoxine-deficiency neuropathy due to hydralazine. N Engl J Med 1965;273:1182–5.

Rockwell S, Liu Y, Higgins SA. Alteration of the effects of cancer therapy agents on breast cancer cells by the herbal medicine black cohosh. Breast Cancer Res Treat 2005;90:233–9.

Samman S, Sandström B, Toft MB, et al. Green tea or rosemary extract added to foods reduces nonheme-iron absorption. Am J Clin Nutr 2001;73(3):607–12.

Sandborn WJ, Targan SR, Byers VS, et al. *Andrographis paniculata* extract (HMPL-004) for active ulcerative colitis. Am J Gastroenterol 2013;108(1):90–8.

Scambia G, De Vincenzo R, Ranelletti FO, et al. Antiproliferative effect of silybin on gynaelogical malignancies: synergism with cisplatin and doxorubicin. Eur J Cancer 1996;32:877–82.

Schelosky L, Raffauf C, Jendroska K, et al. Kava and dopamine antagonism. J Neurol Neurosurg Psychiatry 1995;58(5):639–40.

Segal R, Pilote L. Warfarin interaction with *Matricaria chamomilla*. CMAJ 2006;174(9):1281–2.

Sharma RD, Sarkar A, Hazra DK, et al. Use of fenugreek seed powder in the management of non-insulin dependent diabetes mellitus. Nutr Res 1996;16(8):1331–9.

Shi S, Klotz U. Drug interactions with herbal medicines. Clin Pharmacokinet 2012;51(2):77–104.

Sigurjónsdóttir HA, Franzson L, Manhem K, et al. Liquorice-induced rise in blood pressure: a linear dose-response relationship. J Hum Hypertens 2001;15(8):549–52.

Sigurjonsdottir HA, Manhem K, Axelson M, et al. Subjects with essential hypertension are more sensitive to the inhibition of 11 beta-HSD by liquorice. J Hum Hypertens 2003;17(2):125–31.

Shanmugasundaram ERB, Rafeswari G, Baskaran K, et al. Use of *Gymnema sylvestre* leaf extract in the control of blood glucose in insulin-dependent diabetes mellitus. J Ethnopharmacol 1990;30:281–94.

Stargrove MB, Treasure J, McKee DL. Herb, nutrient and drug interactions. Clinical implications and therapeutic strategies. Mosby; 2008.

Stoddard GJ, Archer M, Shane-McWhorter L, et al. Ginkgo and warfarin interaction in a large Veterans Administration population. AMIA Annu Symp Proc 2015;2015:1174–83.

Terzic MM, Dotlic J, Maricic S, et al. Influence of red clover-derived isoflavones on serum lipid profile in postmenopausal women. J Obstet Gynaecol Res 2009;35(6):1091–5.

Therapeutic Research Faculty. Natural medicines database; 2017. Available from: http://naturaldatabase.therapeuticresearch.com.

Turkistani A, Abdullah KM, Al-Shaer AA, et al. Melatonin premedication and the induction dose of propofol. Eur J Anaesthesiol 2007;24(5):399–402.

Uehleke B, Müller J, Stange R, et al. Willow bark extract STW 33-I in the long-term treatment of outpatients with rheumatic pain mainly osteoarthritis or back pain. Phytomedicine 2013;20(11):980–4.

Ulbricht CE, Basch EM. Natural standard herb and supplement reference. Evidence-based clinical reviews. Mosby; 2005.

Var C, Keller S, Tung R, et al. Supplementation with vitamin B_6 reduces side effects in Cambodian women using oral contraception. Nutrients 2014;6(9):3353–62.

Wainstein J, Ganz T, Boaz M, et al. Olive leaf extract as a hypoglycemic agent in both human diabetic subjects and in rats. J Med Food 2012;15(7):605–10.

Walker AF, Marakis G, Morris AP, et al. Promising hypotensive effect of hawthorn extract: a randomized double-blind pilot study of mild, essential hypertension. Phytother Res 2002;16(1):48–54.

Xin HW, Wu XC, Li Q, et al. Effects of *Schisandra sphenanthera* extract on the pharmacokinetics of midazolam in healthy volunteers. Br J Clin Pharmacol 2009;67(5):541–6.

Xin HW, Wu XC, Li Q, et al. Effects of *Schisandra sphenanthera* extract on the pharmacokinetics of tacrolimus in healthy volunteers. Br J Clin Pharmacol 2007;64(4):469–75.

Yamamoto T, Hatanaka M, Matsuda J, et al. Clinical characteristics of five elderly patients with severe hypokalemia induced by glycyrrhizin derivatives. Nippon Jinzo Gakkai Shi 2010;52(1):80–5.

Yuan CS, Wei G, Dey L. American ginseng reduces warfarin's effect in healthy patients. A randomized, controlled trial. Ann Intern Med 2004;141(1):123–6.

Zemestani M, Rafraf M, Asghari-Jafarabadi M. Chamomile tea improves glycemic indices and antioxidants status in patients with type 2 diabetes mellitus. Nutrition 2016;32(1):66–72.